DRUG INFORMATION HANDBOOK for NURSING

Including
Assessment, Administration, Monitoring
Guidelines and Patient Education

6th Edition

Lexicomp®

NOTICE

This data is intended to serve the user as a handy reference and not as a complete drug information resource. It does not include information on every therapeutic agent available. The publication covers over 1000 commonly used drugs and is specifically designed to present important aspects of drug data in a more concise format than is typically found in medical literature or product material supplied by manufacturers.

The nature of drug information is that it is constantly evolving because of ongoing research and clinical experience and is often subject to interpretation. While great care has been taken to ensure the accuracy of the information and recommendations presented, the reader is advised that the authors, editors, reviewers, contributors, and publishers cannot be responsible for the continued currency of the information or for any errors, omissions, or the application of this information, or for any consequences arising therefrom. Therefore, the author(s) and/or the publisher shall have no liability to any person or entity with regard to claims, loss, or damage caused, or alleged to be caused, directly or indirectly, by the use of information contained herein. Because of the dynamic nature of drug information, readers are advised that decisions regarding drug therapy must be based on the independent judgment of the clinician, changing information about a drug (eg, as reflected in the literature and manufacturer's most current product information), and changing medical practices. Therefore, this data is designed to be used in conjunction with other necessary information and is not designed to be solely relied upon by any user. The user of this data hereby and forever releases the authors and publishers of this data from any and all liability of any kind that might arise out of the use of this data. The editors are not responsible for any inaccuracy of quotation or for any false or misleading implication that may arise due to the text or formulas as used or due to the quotation of revisions no longer official.

Certain of the authors, editors, and contributors have written this book in their private capacities. No official support or endorsement by any federal or state agency or pharmaceutical company is intended or inferred.

The publishers have made every effort to trace any third party copyright holders, if any, for borrowed material. If they have inadvertently overlooked any, they will be pleased to make the necessary arrangements at the first opportunity.

If you have any suggestions or questions regarding any information presented in this data, please contact our drug information pharmacists at (330) 650-6506. Book revisions are available at our website at http://www.lexi.com/home/revisions/.

This manual was produced using Lexi-Comp's Information Management System™ (LIMS) — A complete publishing service of Lexi-Comp, Inc.

Lexicomp®

1100 Terex Road • Hudson, Ohio • 44236
(330) 650-6506

ISBN 978-1-59195-333-3

TABLE OF CONTENTS

NURSING EDITORIAL ADVISORY PANEL

EDITORIAL ADVISORY PANEL

Jason C. Gallagher, PharmD, BCPS
Clinical Pharmacy Specialist, Infectious Diseases
and *Clinical Associate Professor*
Temple University Hospital

Joyce Generali, RPh, MS, FASHP
Director, Synthesized Referential Content
Wolters Kluwer Health

Meredith D. Girard, MD, FACP
Medical Staff
Department of Internal Medicine
Summa Health Systems
Assistant Professor Internal Medicine
Northeast Ohio Medical University (NEOMED)

Morton P. Goldman, RPh, PharmD, BCPS, FCCP
Health Care Consultant
American Pharmacotherapy, Inc

Julie A. Golembiewski, PharmD
Clinical Associate Professor and
Clinical Pharmacist, Anesthesia/Pain
Colleges of Pharmacy and Medicine
University of Illinois

Jeffrey P. Gonzales, PharmD, BCPS
Critical Care Clinical Pharmacy Specialist
University of Maryland Medical Center

John Grabenstein, RPh, PhD, FAPhA
Pharmacotherapy Contributor
Wolters Kluwer Health

Roland Grad, MDCM, MSc, CCFP, FCFP
Associate Professor
Department of Family Medicine
McGill University

Larry D. Gray, PhD, ABMM
Director, Clinical Microbiology
TriHealth Laboratories
Bethesda and Good Samaritan Hospitals

Tracy Hagemann, PharmD
Associate Professor
College of Pharmacy
The University of Oklahoma

JoEllen L. Hanigosky, PharmD
Clinical Coordinator
Department of Hematology/Oncology/Bone
Marrow Transplant
Children's Hospital of Akron

Martin D. Higbee, PharmD
Associate Professor
Department of Pharmacy Practice and Science
The University of Arizona

Jane Hurlburt Hodding, PharmD
Executive Director, Inpatient Pharmacy Services
and *Clinical Nutrition Services*
Long Beach Memorial Medical Center and
Miller Children's Hospital

Mark T. Holdsworth, PharmD
Associate Professor of Pharmacy & Pediatrics
and *Pharmacy Practice Area Head*
College of Pharmacy
The University of New Mexico

Edward Horn, PharmD, BCPS
Clinical Specialist, Transplant Surgery
Allegheny General Hospital

Collin A. Hovinga, PharmD
Director of Research and *Associate Professor*
Dell Children's Medical Center
UT Austin School of Pharmacy

Darrell T. Hulisz, PharmD
Associate Professor
Department of Family Medicine
Case Western Reserve University

Douglas L. Jennings, PharmD, BCPS
Clinical Pharmacy Specialist, Cardiovascular Surgery
Jackson Memorial Hospital

Sallie Johnson, PharmD, BCPS, AQ Cardiology
Clinical Pharmacy Specialist, Cardiology
Penn State Milton S. Hershey Medical Center

Michael A. Kahn, DDS
Professor and Chairman
Department of Oral and Maxillofacial Pathology
Tufts University School of Dental Medicine

Jeannette Kaiser, MT, MBA
Medical Technologist
Akron General Medical Center

Julie J. Kelsey, PharmD
Clinical Specialist
Women's Health and Family Medicine
Department of Pharmacy Services
University of Virginia Health System

Patrick J. Kiel, PharmD, BCPS, BCOP
Clinical Pharmacy Specialist
Hematology and Stem Cell Transplant
Indiana University Simon Cancer Center

Polly E. Kintzel, PharmD, BCPS, BCOP
Clinical Pharmacy Specialist-Oncology
Spectrum Health

Michael Klepser, PharmD, FCCP
Professor of Pharmacy
Department of Pharmacy Practice
Ferris State University

Daren Knoell, PharmD
Associate Professor of Pharmacy Practice and
Internal Medicine
Davis Heart and Lung Research Institute
The Ohio State University

David Knoppert, MScPhm, FCCP, MSc, FCSHP
Clinical Leader - Paediatrics
Pharmacy Services
London Health Sciences Centre
Children's Health Research Institute

Stephanie S. Minich, PharmD, BCOP
Pharmacotherapy Specialist
Wolters Kluwer Health

Kim Moeller, MSN, RN, ACNS-BC, AOCNS
Unit Manager, Outpatient Infusion
Cooper Cancer Center
Advanced Practice Nurse
Summit Oncology Associates
Summa Health System

Kara M. Morris, DDS, MS
Pediatric Dentist
Olentangy Pediatric Dentistry

Kevin M. Mulieri, BS, PharmD
Pediatric Hematology/Oncology Clinical Specialist
Penn State Milton S. Hershey Medical Center
Instructor of Pharmacology
Penn State College of Medicine

Lynne Nakashima, PharmD
Professional Practice Leader, Clinical Professor
B.C. Cancer Agency, Vancouver Centre,
University of BC

Elizabeth A. Neuner, PharmD, BCPS
Infectious Diseases Clinical Specialist
Cleveland Clinic

Carlene N. Oliverio, PharmD, BCPS
Clinical Content Specialist
Wolters Kluwer Health

Tom Palma, MS, RPh
Medical Science Pharmacist
Wolters Kluwer Health

Susie H. Park, PharmD, BCPP
Assistant Professor of Clinical Pharmacy
University of Southern California

Nicole Passerrello, PharmD, BCPS
Pharmacotherapy Specialist
Wolters Kluwer Health

Alpa Patel, PharmD
Antimicrobial Clinical Pharmacist
University of Louisville Hospital

Gayle Pearson, BSPharm, MSA
Drug Information Pharmacist
Peter Lougheed Centre
Alberta Health Services

Jennifer L. Placencia, PharmD
Neonatal Clinical Pharmacy Specialist
Texas Children's Hospital

James A. Ponto, MS, RPh, BCNP
Chief Nuclear Pharmacist
Department of Radiology
University of Iowa, Hospitals and Clinics
Professor of Clinical Pharmacy
Department of Pharmacy Practice and Science
University of Iowa College of Pharmacy

Amy L. Potts, PharmD, BCPS
Assistant Director
Department of Pharmacy
PGY1 & PGY2 Residency Program Director
Monroe Carell Jr. Children's Hospital at Vanderbilt

Sally Rafie, PharmD, BCPS
Medical Safety Pharmacist
UC San Diego Health System

Esta Razavi, PharmD
Clinical Editor
Wolters Kluwer Health

James Reissig, PharmD
Assistant Director, Clinical Services
Akron General Medical Center

A.J. (Fred) Remillard, PharmD
Assistant Dean, Research and Graduate Affairs
College of Pharmacy and Nutrition
University of Saskatchewan

Elizabeth Rich, RN, BSN, BA
Registered Nurse, Critical Care
Hillcrest Hospital

Curtis M. Rimmermann, MD, MBA, FACC
Gus P. Karos Chair
Clinical Cardiovascular Medicine
Cleveland Clinic

Renee Rivard, PharmD
Consultant, Independent Medical Writer
Wolters Kluwer Health

P. David Rogers, PharmD, PhD, FCCP
Director, Clinical and Translational Therapeutics
University of Tennessee College of Pharmacy

James L. Rutkowski, DMD, PhD
Editor-in-Chief
Journal of Oral Implantology

Amy Rybarczyk, PharmD, BCPS
Pharmacotherapy Specialist, Internal Medicine
Akron General Medical Center

Jennifer K. Sekeres, PharmD, BCPS
Infectious Diseases Clinical Specialist
Cleveland Clinic

Todd P. Semla, MS, PharmD, BCPS, FCCP, AGSF
National PBM Clinical Program Manager – Mental Health & Geriatrics
Department of Veterans Affairs
Pharmacy Benefits Management Services
Associate Professor, Clinical
Department of Medicine, Psychiatry and
Behavioral Health
Feinberg School of Medicine
Northwestern University

Wende Wood, RPh, BSPharm, BCPP
Pharmacotherapy Contributor
Wolters Kluwer Health

Richard L. Wynn, BSPharm, PhD
Professor of Pharmacology
Baltimore College of Dental Surgery
University of Maryland

Jessica Zatroch, DDS
Private Practice Dentist
Willoughby Hills, OH

Jennifer Zimmer-Young, PharmD, CCRP
Educator, Clinical Pharmacist
ThedaCare

DESCRIPTION OF SECTIONS AND FIELDS IN THIS HANDBOOK

Introduction

This and other documents in this section provide guidelines for the use of the handbook including a brief overview of General Nursing Issues (Assessment, Administration, Monitoring, and Patient Education); Patient Factors That Influence Drug Therapy; and Therapeutic Nursing Management of Side Effects.

Individual Drug Monographs

Medications are arranged alphabetically by generic name. Abbreviated monographs contain unique information, commonly for combination formulations.

Monograph Fields

Generic Name	U.S. adopted name
Pronunciation	Phonetic pronunciation guide
Brand Names: U.S.	Trade names (manufacturer-specific) found in the United States. The symbol [DSC] appears after trade names that have been recently discontinued.
Index Terms	Other names or accepted abbreviations of the generic drug. May also include common brand names no longer available; this field is used to create cross-references to monographs.
Pharmacologic Category	Unique systematic classification of medications
Medication Safety Issues	In an effort to promote the safe use of medications, this field is intended to highlight possible sources of medication errors such as sound-alike/look-alike drugs or highly concentrated formulations which require vigilance on the part of healthcare professionals. In addition, medications which have been associated with severe consequences in the event of a medication error are also identified in this field.
Medication Guide Available	Identifies drugs that have an FDA-approved Medication Guide
Pregnancy Risk Factor	Five categories established by the FDA to indicate the potential of a systemically absorbed drug for causing risk to fetus
Lactation	Indicates if the drug listed in the monograph is present in breast milk and the manufacturer's recommendation for use while breast-feeding
Breast-Feeding Considerations	Information pertinent to or associated with the human use of the drug as it relates to clinical effects on the nursing infant or postpartum woman.
Use	Information pertaining to FDA- or Canadian-approved indications for the drug
Unlabeled Use	Information pertaining to non-FDA-approved indications of the drug
Mechanism of Action/Effect	How the drug works in the body to elicit a response
Contraindications	Information pertaining to inappropriate use of the drug as dictated by approved labeling
Warnings/Precautions	Precautionary considerations, hazardous conditions related to use of the drug, and disease states or patient populations in which the drug should be cautiously used. Boxed warnings, when present, are clearly identified and are adapted from the FDA-approved labeling. Consult the product labeling for the black box warning through the manufacturer's or the FDA website.
Drug Interactions	Agents that, when combined with the drug, may affect therapy; may include the following:
Avoid Concomitant Use	Designates drug combinations which should not be used concomitantly, due to an unacceptable risk:benefit assessment. Frequently, the concurrent use of the agents is explicitly prohibited or contraindicated by the product labeling.
Decreased Effect	Drug combinations that result in a decreased therapeutic effect between the drug listed in the monograph and other drugs or drug classes
Increased Effect/Toxicity	Drug combinations that result in an increased or toxic therapeutic effect between the drug listed in the monograph and other drugs or drug classes
Nutritional/Ethanol Interactions	Presents a description of the interaction between the drug listed in the monograph and ethanol, food, or herb/nutraceuticals
Adverse Reactions	Only side effects >1% are included and are grouped by percentage of incidence (if known)

Pharmacodynamics/Kinetics

May include the following:

Onset of Action

The time after drug administration when therapeutic effect is observed; may also include time for peak therapeutic effect

Duration of Action

Length of therapeutic effect

Product Availability

Provides availability information on products that have been approved by the FDA, but not yet available for use. Estimates for when a product may be available are included, when this information is known. May also provide any unique or critical drug availability issues.

Controlled Substance

The controlled substance classification from the Drug Enforcement Agency (DEA). U.S. schedules are I-V. Schedules vary by country and sometimes state (eg, Massachusetts uses I-VI).

Dosage Forms Considerations

More specific information regarding product concentrations, ingredients, package sizes, amount of doses per container, and other important details pertaining to various formulations of medications

Available Dosage Forms

Information with regard to form, strength, and availability of the drug in the United States. Please consult product labeling for further information.

General Dosage Range

The range of dosing typically used during therapy in children and adults based upon route of administration. The information included is useful for confirming the dose is within the range but should not be used for prescribing purposes. Medications with a variety of indication-specific doses that cannot be encompassed by a range will not have a dose.

Usual Infusion Concentrations

Information describing the usual concentrations of drugs for continuous infusion administration in the pediatric and adult populations as appropriate. Concentrations are derived from the literature, manufacturer's recommendation, or organizational recommendations (eg, the Institute for Safe Medication Practices [ISMP]) and are universally established. Institution-specific standard concentrations may differ from those listed.

Administration

I.M.
I.V.
Injectable Detail
Oral
Topical
Subcutaneous
Inhalation
Other
Endotracheal
Intra-arterial
Intracavernous
Intradermal
Intraosseous
Intrathecal
Intravaginal
Intravitreal
Ophthalmic
Otic
Rectal

The administration field contains subfields by route regarding issues relative to appropriately giving a medication; includes suggestions on final drug concentrations and/or rates of infusion for parenteral medications and comments regarding the timing of drug administration relative to meals.

Preparation for Administration

Provides information regarding the preparation of drug products prior to administration, including dilution, reconstitution, etc.

Storage/Stability

Information regarding storage and stability of commercially available products and products that have been reconstituted, diluted, or otherwise prepared. Provides the time and conditions for which a solution or mixture will maintain potency.

Nursing Actions

Physical Assessment   Monitoring guidelines

Patient Education   Some information that may be helpful regarding medications, including the reason the patient is prescribed the medication and common side effects associated with its use. Focus is directed towards the HCAHPS (Hospital Consumer Assessment of Healthcare Providers and Systems) survey as some of the questions patients are asked on that survey relate to medication education.

Intended Use and Disclaimer: Should not be printed and given to patients. This information is intended to serve as a concise initial reference for healthcare professionals to use when discussing medications with a patient. You must ultimately rely on your own discretion, experience, and judgment in diagnosing, treating, and advising patients. This information:

- Is not a complete reference source

- Does not contain all information that you may need to know about this medication, including possible interactions, contraindications, side effects, warnings, precautions, allergic reactions, adverse reactions, approved or off-label indications, dosing regimens, or duration of therapy

- Is generalized and does not contain all information that may be relevant to use by a particular patient

- Is not intended to endorse any medication as safe or effective for treating any particular patient or health condition

- Is developed from publicly available information, including manufacturer package inserts, and is not based upon any independent review, testing, or study of any medication by the publisher

Additional information about this medication is available in the full monograph for this medication.

Dietary Considerations   Specific dietary modifications and/or restrictions (eg, information about sodium content)

Related Information   Cross-reference to other pertinent drug information in this handbook

Appendix

The extensive appendix is filled with useful tables and text including conversions, laboratory information, and administration and therapy guidelines.

Alphabetical Index

This is an alphabetical index which provides a quick reference to the monograph section by using the generic names, index terms, and U.S. brand names.

PREGNANCY CATEGORIES

Pregnancy Categories (sometimes referred to as pregnancy risk factors) are a letter system currently required under the *Teratogenic Effects* subsection of the product labeling. The system was initiated in 1979. The categories are required to be part of the package insert for prescription drugs that are systemically absorbed.

The categories are defined as follows:

A   Adequate and well-controlled studies in pregnant women have not shown that the drug increases the risk of fetal abnormalities.

B   Animal reproduction studies show no evidence of impaired fertility or harm to the fetus; however, no adequate and well-controlled studies have been conducted in pregnant women.
or
Animal reproduction studies have shown adverse events; however, studies in pregnant women have not shown that the drug increases the risk of abnormalities.

C   Animal reproduction studies have shown an adverse effect on the fetus. There are no adequate and well-controlled studies in humans and the benefits from the use of the drug in pregnant women may be acceptable, despite its potential risks.
or
Animal reproduction studies have not been conducted.

D   Based on human data, the drug can cause fetal harm when administered to pregnant women, but the potential benefits from the use of the drug may be acceptable, despite its potential risks.

X   Studies in animals or humans have demonstrated fetal abnormalities (or there is positive evidence of fetal risk based on reports and/or marketing experience) and the risk of using the drug in pregnant women clearly outweighs any possible benefit (for example, safer drugs or other forms of therapy are available).

The categories do not take into consideration nonteratogenic effects (that information is currently presented separately). In 2008, the Food and Drug Administration (FDA) proposed new labeling requirements which would eliminate the use of the pregnancy category system and replace it with scientific data and other information specific to the use of the drug in pregnant women. These proposed changes were suggested because the current category system may be misleading. For instance, some practitioners may believe that risk increases from category A to B to C to D to X, which is not the intent. In addition, practitioners may not be aware that some medications are categorized based on animal data, while others are based on human data. When the new labeling requirements are approved, product labeling will contain pregnancy and lactation subsections, each describing a risk summary, clinical considerations, and section for specific data.

For full descriptions of the current and proposed labeling requirements, refer to the following websites:

Labeling Requirements for Prescription Drugs and/or Insulin (Code of Federal Regulations, Title 21, Volume 4, Revised April 1, 2010). http://www.accessdata.fda.gov/scripts/cdrh/cfdocs/cfCFR/CFRSearch.cfm?fr=201.57

Content and Format of Labeling for Human Prescription Drug and Biological Products; Requirements for Pregnancy and Lactation Labeling (Federal Register, May 29, 2008). https://www.federalregister.gov/articles/2008/05/29/E8-11806/content-and-format-of-labeling-for-human-prescription-drug-and-biological-products-requirements-for

GENERAL NURSING ISSUES

ASSESSMENT

Assessment is the *primary* action in the nursing process and it is also a vital part of optimal drug therapy. Assessment activities must precede administering any medication. Appropriate assessment includes not only details of the chief complaint, but also must include the patient's insight to his/her condition (eg, etiology and prognosis of complaint, impact of lifestyle habits). Information gathered in a primary assessment should serve as a guide to patient education and to identify specific areas that need close monitoring. Generally, assessment starts with a thorough patient history that can include:

- Current complaint: History, observation, laboratory results, other treatments, etc.
- Other concurrent conditions: Chronic illnesses
- Past health problems and treatments: Resolved, chronic, treatments effective/noneffective
- Current drugs: Prescription, OTC, home remedies, herbs and herbal medicines
- Past drugs: Reason for taking, effectiveness, adverse effects
- Allergies or adverse effects: Drugs, household products, food products, environmental factors
- Health habits: Caffeine, alcohol, nicotine, street drugs, sleep, activity, nutrition, hydration, sexual activity, pregnant, lactating, use of contraceptives (barrier or oral)
- Physical: Vital signs, weight, height; may include details (as necessary) about any body system: Pulmonary, cardiac, circulatory, hepatic, renal, gastrointestinal, genitourinary, integumentary, or musculoskeletal systems
- Psychosocial support: Financial, religious, personal, community

SAFE ADMINISTRATION

Safe administration is grounded in the five "Right" principles: *Right Drug, Right Dose, Right Patient, Right Route, Right Time.*

Right drug: Involves checking drug dispensed with the written prescription. Many drugs have similar-sounding names (terbutaline/tolbutamide, calciferol/calcitriol); caution must be used to determine the exact drug prescribed. In addition, a nurse must understand the indication for any medication being prescribed.

Right dose: Requires checking the prescribed dosage, being aware of the standard or "usual" dosage for that drug, and identifying any assessment findings which may rationalize an uncommon dosage. Determining the right dose for some medications means titrating the dose to monitored physiological parameters determined by hemodynamic or cardiac telemetry monitoring, according to kidney or liver function, or calculating the dose according to body weight or body surface area.

Right patient: Means identifying each individual patient. Patients in healthcare institutions generally wear identifying namebands that can be checked prior to administration. If patients are able to communicate, the nurse still asks for name and birthdate verification to check against the nameband and Medication Administration Record (MAR). When patients are not wearing namebands (eg, at home, in rehabilitation, in outpatient settings), asking patients to identify themselves will reduce medication misadventures.

Right route: Includes consideration of traditional routes (P.O., I.V., I.M., or SubQ, etc). Right route should also include knowledge about whether the dispensed oral drug form can safely be altered by crushing, chewing, dissolving, and being administered via a nasogastric or any other type of feeding tube? Extended release formulations should never be crushed, chewed, or dissolved (see Oral Medications That Should Not Be Crushed or Altered on page 1712 in the Appendix). Some intravenous drugs should be administered via a central line because the possibility of peripheral extravasation presents a serious risk for the patient. Extra care is needed when administering intravenous drugs that are vesicants and have extravasation risk. Some intravenous drugs (eg, etoposide, idarubicin, ifosfamide, irinotecan, mannitol, mechlorethamine, mitomycin, nafcillin, norepinephrine, phenobarbital, phenylephrine, phenytoin, potassium chloride, vasopressin) are extremely irritating to peripheral veins; this requires their administration via a central line or as dilute solutions at a slow rate given peripherally or with specific administration instructions. Consult with the administration field of the monograph for proper administration.

Right time: Necessitates knowledge of a drug's bioavailability; knowing whether the drug should be given at around-the-clock intervals, or whether doses need to be timed in a specific manner. Are there specific dietary considerations? Food will slow the absorption time of many drugs; however, their overall effect will not be affected. Administering medications with food will often reduce the nausea or vomiting that occurs when medications are given on an empty stomach. The drug monographs clearly identify the drugs that must be administered on an empty stomach or with food. Some monographs include the recommendation for administering the drug in the morning hours to reduce night-time sleep interruptions (eg, diuretics).

MONITORING

Nursing actions are found in each monograph and address a wide variety of assessment and monitoring activities. Advanced nurse practitioners may be responsible for both prescribing and monitoring. However, the nurse responsible for administering the medication or teaching the patient about administration is also responsible for monitoring effectiveness and adverse effects and communicating these details to the prescriber. Some common monitoring responsibilities are described in the following paragraphs.

Assessing patient knowledge/teaching. Educating the patient about the use and common side effects for his/her drug regimen is important. Educating the patient and/or caregiver about the proper use and administration of the medications is also critical, as well as using a teach-back method to assess the patient's understanding of that information. Linking the medication to its use in the disease process may help the patient to further his/her understanding of the disease and the medications used to treat it. If the patient's knowledge is incomplete or incorrect, then it is vital to teach the patient (or caregiver) the necessary information (eg, correct procedure for using inhalators, instilling ophthalmic medications, inserting a suppository, administering injectable medications, disposing of needles). Is the patient's knowledge about identifying signs and symptoms of opportunistic infections accurate? Is the patient aware of the precautions necessary with antihypertensives (eg, postural hypotension precautions)? Does the patient understand the rationale for contraception and the difference between oral and barrier forms of contraception? Sometimes patients need to be referred to other professionals for advanced education pertaining to their disease and the prescribed drugs (eg, drug monographs for medications used to treat diabetes suggest referring the patient to a diabetic educator).

Monitoring vital signs means more than just identifying a deviation from the norm. It also means communicating any adverse signs or symptoms to the prescriber. When the patient is in danger, it may be necessary to discontinue a medication and notify the prescriber. In other instances, it will mean contacting the prescriber for further instructions. Some monitoring is continuous, as with emergency drugs; and some is intermittent, as with patient-administered medications. Awareness of the need for monitoring, the rationale behind monitoring instructions, and the type of monitoring required is a nursing responsibility.

Monitoring for adverse/toxic response. Known adverse reactions are categorized according to body systems in the Adverse Reactions field. The Physical Assessment field also includes reminders about the necessity for monitoring the most threatening or severe of those possible side effects.

Monitoring laboratory test results includes knowing what tests are necessary to monitor drug response and ensuring that ordered tests are completed at appropriate times. Communicating laboratory test results to the appropriate prescriber is frequently a nursing responsibility.

Some laboratory tests must be completed prior to administering the first dose of a drug (eg, culture and sensitivity tests; tests that indicate premedication status of liver, kidney, or other systems' functions). Standard peak and trough serum concentration recommendations are available from most laboratories. Since these may change somewhat among laboratories, it is always best to check with the laboratory that will be completing peak and trough assays to identify their exact timing regulations.

Patient education sections provide some information that may be helpful regarding medications, including the reason the patient is prescribed the medication and common side effects associated with its use. Focus is directed towards the HCAHPS (Hospital Consumer Assessment of Healthcare Providers and Systems) survey as some of the questions patients are asked on that survey relate to medication education. **Intended Use and Disclaimer:** Should not be printed and given to patients. This information is intended to serve as a concise initial reference for healthcare professionals to use when discussing medications with a patient. You must ultimately rely on your own discretion, experience and judgment in diagnosing, treating and advising patients. This information:

- Is not a complete reference source

- Does not contain all information that you may need to know about this medication, including possible interactions, contraindications, side effects, warnings, precautions, allergic reactions, adverse reactions, approved or off-label indications, dosing regimens, or duration of therapy

- Is generalized and does not contain all information that may be relevant to use by a particular patient

- Is not intended to endorse any medication as safe or effective for treating any particular patient or health condition

- Is developed from publicly available information, including manufacturer package inserts, and is not based upon any independent review, testing, or study of any medication by the publisher

Additional information about this medication is available in the full monograph for this medication.

Geriatric considerations include information pertinent for that drug in relation to therapy for older patients. In addition to these precautions or information, it is necessary to remember the general effects of aging on drug response, especially the effects that impaired circulation or renal function may have on pharmacokinetics.

PATIENT FACTORS THAT INFLUENCE DRUG THERAPY

Many factors related to an individual patient, or a group of similar patients, can impact the pharmacokinetics of drugs and relate to adverse reactions.

PREGNANCY/LACTATION

The changes that occur during pregnancy may necessitate dosage changes for some drugs. Decreased gastric motility, increased blood volume, decreased protein binding sites, and increased glomerular filtration rates may alter the degree of anticipated pharmacotherapeutic response.

The primary concern about drugs during pregnancy is the effect the drug has on the fetus, either teratogenic (causing birth defects) or systemic (causing addiction). Although many drugs cross the placenta, the type of drug, the concentration of the drug, and the gestational age at time of exposure are primary determinants of fetal reaction. When prescribing or administering drugs to any female of childbearing age, it is vital to ask when her last menstrual period was and, if necessary, to wait for the results of a pregnancy test before starting any drug therapy. Of course, it is best to avoid all drugs during pregnancy. However, in some cases, the physiological context (eg, cardiac output, renal blood flow) may be altered enough by the pregnancy alone to require the use of drugs that are not needed by the same woman when she is not pregnant.

Most systematically absorbed drugs have been assigned a pregnancy risk factor based on the drug's potential to cause birth defects. This permits a necessary evaluation of the risk:benefit ratio when prescribing or administering drugs. Drugs in the risk factor class "A" are generally considered safe for use during pregnancy; class "X" drugs are never safe and are known to be positively teratogenic. See Pregnancy Categories on page 13.

Contraception note: Many drugs will interact with and decrease the effectiveness of oral contraceptives (eg, barbiturates, protease inhibitors, rifampin, carbamazepine). When a drug will decrease the effectiveness of oral contraceptives, the patient needs to be educated about the necessity for using an additional "barrier" (non-hormonal) form of contraception. Barrier contraception (alone or in combination with some form of oral contraception) is often recommended for the patient who must take selected drugs with pregnancy risk factors "D" (idarubicin) or class "X" (isotretinoin).

Because many drugs and substances used by a mother appear in breast milk, care must be taken to evaluate the drug effects on the lactating woman and the infant. Some drugs are identified as being clearly contra-indicated during lactation, others may cross into breast milk but adverse side effects on the fetus have not been identified, and for some drugs the administration times should be distanced from nursing time. Nurses should advise lactating women about the effects that drugs may have on the infant.

AGE

Pharmacokinetics (absorption, distribution, metabolism, and excretion) differ between infants, young adults, and elderly patients. Elderly patients may exhibit mildly decreased or severely decreased blood flow to all organs, slowed gastric motility, reduced kidney function, decreased nutrition, and sedentary lifestyles, which are all capable of impacting a drug's response and effectiveness. Slower gastric motility slows the rate of absorption of a drug, resulting in a delayed clinical response. Decreased blood flow means that distribution of the drug is altered, resulting in decreased response or longer response time. Excretion of the drug may be altered with decreased glomerular filtration rates or slower gastric emptying which can result in increased levels of the drug accumulating in the system.

The ratio between total body water and total body fat also changes with age; older persons have decreased amounts of total body water and higher body fat. This aspect of aging also influences the blood concentration of some drugs. In a person with increased body fat, fat-soluble drugs are distributed to tissues more than to plasma, resulting in a longer response time as the drug must then be redistributed from tissue to plasma. The idiosyncratic response incidence also increases with an aging population. Responses to drugs may be both more exaggerated or diminished with the standard dosage of some drugs.

In addition, and of major concern with elderly patients, is the incidence of poly-pharmacy. Poly-pharmacy is the use of multiple medications by a patient. Older patients may have several chronic conditions for which they are taking medication. In addition, they may be seeing a different prescriber for each of these conditions. Often, it is a nurse who identifies and coordinates the care of these elderly patients, and the nurse must be aware of the possibility for increased incidence of adverse effects. Enhanced medication reconciliation may be critical to improving readmission rates. Indeed, a growing body of research suggests that lack of attention to this area is a contributing factor to the revolving door effect of patients discharging and re-entering hospitals. A review of previously taken medications against a list of current discharge medications needs to occur, including use of over-the-counter and natural products. Duplicate therapies, new dosages, and new medications need to be identified. The medications no longer in use or with old doses or instructions should be appropriately discarded.

BODY WEIGHT/BUILD

Most recommended dosages of drugs are based on the average-sized, young or middle-aged adult (usually males). Extremely obese or extremely thin patients may be prone to adverse effects as a result of "non-individualized" prescribing. Creatinine is a breakdown product of skeletal muscle and its levels in the serum are used to estimate renal function. Decreased muscle mass can result in reduced creatinine from muscle breakdown, leading to an artificially low or normal serum creatinine. When dosing is based on estimated creatinine clearance (which is calculated based on the serum creatinine) rather than "actual" creatinine clearance, normal doses may be administered to patients with a diminished capacity for excretion, potentially leading to accumulation and toxicity. This is a particular problem in elderly and/or debilitated patients.

SMOKING, ALCOHOL, NUTRITION, AND HYDRATION

Smoking has a direct impact on liver enzyme activity, blood flow, and the central nervous system. Excessive alcohol intake impacts liver enzymes, renal function, and has an additive effect with most antipsychotic, sedative, or anxiolytic medications, as well as altering responses to many other medications. Nutrition and hydration also play an important part in drug responses and possible adverse reactions. Poor hydration may result in reduced blood flow and excretion. Decreased gastric motility can result in delayed excretion and/or prolonged absorption. Poor or inadequate nutrition may result in decreased protein available for binding.

It is vital that a patient's current habits are considered when prescribing, administering, or monitoring drug therapy. Patients must also be aware of the need to inform their professional care provider if they have changed their smoking, alcohol, or dietary patterns. For example, the dosage of theophylline is titrated in accordance with how much a patient smokes, so if the patient quits smoking, the dosage must be adjusted to prevent an overdose. Another example is seen with vitamin K during warfarin therapy. Drastic increases in the amount of vitamin K intake through green leafy vegetables can dramatically alter the effect of warfarin.

OTHER PATIENT FACTORS THAT INFLUENCE DRUG RESPONSE

- Genetic variations
- Differences in circadian patterns
- Disease states
- Psychological temperament

Genetic differences in enzymes may influence the effectiveness of therapy or the incidence of adverse effects (fast acetylators or slow acetylators). The emerging science of pharmacogenomics is devoted to the investigation of these genetic differences in drug response and offers the hope of truly individualized therapy. Circadian rhythms differ among individuals and have an impact on absorption patterns, hormone secretion, and urinary excretion patterns. Disease states can and do change all aspects of pharmacokinetics. Cirrhosis can impair liver enzyme metabolism rate. Kidney disease will reduce excretion rates for many drugs. Abnormal thyroid function can influence drug metabolism. Diseases which affect blood circulation (eg, hypertension, CHF, Raynaud's phenomena, malignancies) can have an impact on absorption, distribution, and excretion. Diabetes impacts the response to many drugs. Malnutrition, commonly associated with disease, can drastically reduce albumin levels.

See Therapeutic Nursing Management of Side Effects on page 19

THERAPEUTIC NURSING MANAGEMENT OF SIDE EFFECTS

MANAGEMENT OF DRUG-RELATED PROBLEMS

Patients may experience some type of side effect or adverse drug reaction as a result of their drug therapy. The type of effect, the severity, and the frequency of occurrence is dependent on the medication and dose being used, as well as the individual's response to therapy. The following information is presented as helpful tips to assist the patient through these drug-related problems. Pharmacological support may also be required for their management. May use the Lexicomp patient education leaflets on these topics to help the patient understand how to manage the drug-related problem he/she has.

Alopecia

- Your hair loss is temporary. Hair usually will begin to grow within 3-6 months of completing drug therapy.
- Your hair may come back with a different texture, color, or thickness.
- Avoid excessive shampooing and hair combing or harsh hair care products.
- Avoid excessive drying of hair.
- Avoid use of permanents, dyes, or hair sprays.
- Always cover head in cold weather or sunshine.

Anemia

- Observe all bleeding precautions (see Thrombocytopenia).
- Get adequate sleep and rest.
- Be alert for potential for dizziness, fainting, or extreme fatigue.
- Maintain adequate nutrition and hydration. Eat iron-rich foods such as dark leafy greens, beans, meat, nuts, and dried fruit; incorporate foods that increase iron absorption in the body (eg, vitamin C) and avoid the ones that inhibit absorption (eg, milk).
- Have laboratory tests done as recommended.
- If unusual bleeding occurs, notify prescriber.

Anorexia

- Small, frequent meals containing favorite foods may tempt appetite. The goal is to gradually increase the intake of food since the body is not used to normal meal sizes. Electrolyte abnormalities (hypophosphatemia, hypokalemia) may occur when refeeding starts.
- Eat simple foods such as toast, rice, bananas, mashed potatoes, and scrambled eggs.
- Eat in a pleasant environment conducive to eating.
- When possible, eat with others.
- Avoid noxious odors when eating.
- Use nutritional supplements high in protein and calories.
- Freezing nutritional supplements sometimes makes them more palatable.
- A small glass of wine (if not contraindicated) may stimulate appetite.
- Mild exercise or short walks may stimulate appetite.
- Request antiemetic medication to reduce nausea or vomiting.

Diarrhea

- Include fiber, high-protein foods, and fruits in dietary intake.
- Eat small, frequent, meals throughout the day (six meals/day). See http://www.guideline.gov/content.aspx?id=12679&search=diarrhea#Section420
- Drink plenty of liquids.
- Buttermilk, yogurt, or boiled milk may be helpful.

- Antidiarrheal agents may be needed. Consult your prescriber.
- Include regular rest periods in your activities.
- Institute skin care regimen to prevent breakdown and promote comfort.
- Maintain strict handwashing at all times.

Fluid Retention/Edema

- Elevate legs 3-4 times a day to improve circulation. See http://www.nhs.uk/conditions/oedema/pages/introduction.aspx.
- Avoid standing for long periods of time.
- Wear support hose.
- Increase physical exercise.
- Maintain adequate hydration; avoiding fluids will not reduce edema.
- Weigh yourself regularly.
- If your prescriber has advised you to limit your salt intake, avoid foods such as ham, bacon, processed meats, and canned foods. Many of these foods are high in salt content. Read all labels carefully.
- Report to prescriber if any of the following occur: Sudden weight gain, decrease in urination, swelling of hands or feet, increase in waist size, wet cough, or difficulty breathing.

Headache

- Lie down.
- Use cool cloth on forehead; massage temples and neck.
- Practice deep-breathing techniques.
- Take warm showers.
- Avoid caffeine.
- Use mild analgesics. Consult prescriber.
- Keep the same sleep routine and get enough sleep.
- Eat regular meals.
- Exercise often. Drink lots of fluids, especially in hot weather.
- Do not drink beer, wine, and mixed drinks (alcohol).
- Practice ways to control your stress. Learn and practice coping skills.
- Avoid foods that might cause your headaches.
- Stop smoking if you smoke.
- Keep a diary of your headaches (eg, when they happen, what causes them, what helps them).

Leukopenia/Neutropenia

- Monitor for signs of infections: Persistent sore throat, change in cough or new cough, shortness of breath, fever, chills, fatigue, headache, flu-like symptoms, vaginal discharge, burning or pain with urination, or foul-smelling stools. The CDC defines a neutropenic fever as a fever that is ≥38°C (100.4°F) for >1 hour or a one-time temperature of ≥38.3°C (101°F).
- Prevent infection. Maintain strict handwashing at all times. Avoid crowds when possible. Avoid exposure to infected persons.
- Do not share food, cups, utensils, or other personal items, such as toothbrushes.
- Avoid exposure to temperature changes.
- Maintain adequate nutrition and hydration. Cook meat and eggs all the way through to kill germs and carefully wash raw fruits and vegetables.
- Maintain good personal hygiene. Use a mouthwash to help with bad breath or mouth sores. Use this every day after meals or at least 3 times a day
- Wear gloves when handling waste from dogs, cats, or other pets. Then wash your hands afterward.

- Avoid injury or skin breaks.
- Avoid live vaccinations (unless recommended by healthcare provider). The seasonal flu shot may be helpful.
- Avoid sunburn.

Nausea and Vomiting

- Eat food served cold or at room temperature. Ice chips are sometimes helpful.
- Drink clear liquids in severe cases of nausea. Avoid carbonated beverages.
- Sip liquids slowly and often.
- Avoid spicy food. Bland foods are easier to digest.
- Rinse mouth with lemon water. Practice good oral hygiene.
- Avoid sweet, fatty, and salty foods and foods with strong odors.
- Eat small, frequent meals rather than heavy meals.
- Use relaxation techniques and guided imagery.
- Use distractions such as meals, television, reading, games, etc.
- Sleep during intense periods of nausea.
- Chew gum or suck on hard candy or lozenges.
- Eat in an upright (sitting) position, rather than a semirecumbent position.
- Avoid tight, constrictive clothing at meal time.
- Use some mild exercise following light meals rather than lying down.
- Request antiemetic medication to reduce nausea or vomiting.

Postural Hypotension

- Use care and rise slowly from sitting or lying position to standing, especially when awaking in the morning.
- Use care when climbing stairs.
- Initiate ambulation slowly. Get your bearings before you start walking.
- Do not bend over; always squat slowly if you must pick up something from the floor.
- Elevated environmental temperatures, a hot bath or shower, and sauna should be avoided.
- Elastic stockings and abdominal compression bands may be effective.

Stomatitis

- Perform good oral hygiene frequently, especially before and after meals.
- Avoid use of strong or alcoholic commercial mouthwashes.
- Keep lips well-lubricated.
- Avoid tobacco or other products that are irritating to the oral mucosa.
- Avoid hot, spicy, and excessively salty foods.
- Eat soft foods and drink adequate fluids.
- Request topical or systemic analgesics for painful ulcerations.
- Be alert for and report signs of oral fungal infections.

Thrombocytopenia

- Avoid aspirin and aspirin-containing products.
- Use electric or safety razor and blunt scissors.
- Use soft toothbrush or cotton swabs for oral care. Avoid the use of dental floss.
- Avoid the use of enemas, cathartics, and suppositories unless approved by prescriber.
- Avoid valsalva maneuvers such as straining at stool.

- Use stool softeners if necessary to prevent constipation. Consult prescriber.
- Avoid blowing nose forcefully.
- Never go barefoot; wear protective foot covering.
- Use care when trimming nails (if necessary).
- Maintain a safe environment; arrange furniture to provide safe passageway.
- Maintain adequate lighting in darkened areas to avoid bumping into objects.
- Avoid handling sharp tools or instruments.
- Avoid contact sports or activities that might result in bruising or bleeding.
- Promptly report signs of bleeding; abdominal pain; blood in stool, urine, or vomitus; unusual fatigue; easy bruising; bleeding around gums; or nosebleeds.
- If injection or bloodsticks are necessary, inform healthcare provider that you may have excess bleeding.
- If you've had your spleen removed, monitor for fever or other signs of infection.

Vertigo

- Observe postural hypotension precautions.
- Sleep with your head slightly raised on two or more pillows.
- Use caution when driving or using any machinery.
- Avoid sudden position shifts; do not "rush".
- Be careful while going down steps or escalators or in places with poor lighting to avoid falls.
- Utilize appropriate supports (eg, cane, walker) to prevent injury.
- Make your living environment safe by removing anything that may cause a fall risk. Get rid of loose electrical cords, clutter, and slippery rugs. Also, make sure that you wear sturdy, nonslip shoes and that your walkways are clear and well-lit.

ALPHABETICAL LISTING OF DRUGS

Abacavir (a BAK a veer)

Brand Names: U.S. Ziagen
Index Terms Abacavir Sulfate; ABC
Pharmacologic Category Antiretroviral, Reverse Transcriptase Inhibitor, Nucleoside (Anti-HIV)
Medication Guide Available Yes
Pregnancy Risk Factor C
Lactation Excretion in breast milk unknown/contraindicated
Breast-Feeding Considerations Maternal or infant antiretroviral therapy does not completely eliminate the risk of postnatal HIV transmission. In addition, multiclass-resistant virus has been detected in breast-feeding infants despite maternal therapy. Therefore, in the United States, where formula is accessible, affordable, safe, and sustainable, and the risk of infant mortality due to diarrhea and respiratory infections is low, complete avoidance of breast-feeding by HIV-infected women is recommended to decrease potential transmission of HIV (DHHS [perinatal], 2012).
Use Treatment of HIV infections in combination with other antiretroviral agents
Mechanism of Action/Effect Nucleoside reverse transcriptase inhibitor which interferes with HIV viral RNA-dependent DNA polymerase resulting in inhibition of viral replication
Contraindications Hypersensitivity to abacavir or any component of the formulation (do not rechallenge patients who have experienced hypersensitivity to abacavir regardless of *HLA-B*5701* status); moderate-to-severe hepatic impairment
Warnings/Precautions Abacavir should always be used as a component of a multidrug regimen. **[U.S. Boxed Warning]: Serious and sometimes fatal hypersensitivity reactions have occurred.** Patients testing positive for the presence of the *HLA-B*5701* allele are at an increased risk for hypersensitivity reactions. Screening for *HLA-B*5701* allele status is recommended prior to initiating therapy or reinitiating therapy in patients of unknown status, including patients who previously tolerated therapy. Therapy is **not** recommended in patients testing positive for the *HLA-B*5701* allele. An allergy to abacavir should be reported in the patient's medical record (DHHS, 2013a). Reactions usually occur within 9 days of starting abacavir; ~90% occur within 6 weeks. Patients exhibiting symptoms from two or more of the following: Fever, skin rash, constitutional symptoms (malaise, fatigue, aches), respiratory symptoms (eg, pharyngitis, dyspnea, cough), and GI symptoms (eg, abdominal pain, diarrhea, nausea, vomiting) should discontinue therapy immediately and call for medical attention. Abacavir should be permanently discontinued if hypersensitivity cannot be ruled out, even when other diagnoses are possible and regardless of *HLA-B*5701* status. Abacavir SHOULD NOT be restarted because more severe symptoms may occur within hours, including LIFE-THREATENING HYPOTENSION AND DEATH. Fatal hypersensitivity reactions have occurred following the reintroduction of abacavir in patients whose therapy was interrupted (ie, interruption in drug supply, temporary discontinuation while treating other conditions). In some cases, signs of hypersensitivity may have been previously present, but attributed to other medical conditions (eg, acute onset respiratory diseases, gastroenteritis, reactions to other medications). If abacavir is restarted following an interruption in therapy, evaluate the patient for previously unsuspected symptoms of hypersensitivity. A higher incidence of severe hypersensitivity reactions may be associated with a 600 mg once daily dosing regimen.

[U.S. Boxed Warning]: Lactic acidosis and severe hepatomegaly with steatosis (sometimes fatal) have occurred with antiretroviral nucleoside analogues. Female gender, prior liver disease, obesity, and prolonged treatment may increase the risk of hepatotoxicity. May be associated with fat redistribution. Immune reconstitution syndrome may develop, resulting in the occurrence of an inflammatory response to an indolent or residual opportunistic infection during initial HIV treatment or activation of autoimmune disorders (eg, Graves' disease, polymyositis, Guillain-Barré syndrome) later in therapy; further evaluation and treatment may be required.

Use has been associated with an increased risk of myocardial infarction (MI) in observational studies; however, based on a meta-analysis of 26 randomized trials, the FDA has concluded there is not an increased risk. Consider using with caution in patients with risks for coronary heart disease and minimizing modifiable risk factors (eg, hypertension, hyperlipidemia, diabetes mellitus, and smoking) prior to use. Products may contain propylene glycol. Safety and efficacy in children <3 months of age have not been established.

Drug Interactions
  Avoid Concomitant Use There are no known interactions where it is recommended to avoid concomitant use.
  Decreased Effect
    The levels/effects of Abacavir may be decreased by: Protease Inhibitors
  Increased Effect/Toxicity
    The levels/effects of Abacavir may be increased by: Ganciclovir-Valganciclovir; Ribavirin
  Nutritional/Ethanol Interactions Ethanol: Ethanol may increase the risk of toxicity.
  Adverse Reactions Hypersensitivity reactions (which may be fatal) occur in ~5% of patients. Symptoms may include anaphylaxis, fever, rash (including erythema multiforme), fatigue, diarrhea, abdominal pain; respiratory symptoms (eg, pharyngitis, dyspnea, cough, adult respiratory distress syndrome, or respiratory failure); headache,

malaise, lethargy, myalgia, myolysis, arthralgia, edema, paresthesia, nausea and vomiting, mouth ulcerations, conjunctivitis, lymphadenopathy, hepatic failure, and renal failure.

Note: Rates of adverse reactions were defined during combination therapy with other antiretrovirals (lamivudine and efavirenz **or** lamivudine and zidovudine). Only reactions which occurred at a higher frequency in adults (except where noted) than in the comparator group are noted. Adverse reaction rates attributable to abacavir alone are not available.

>10%:
  Central nervous system: Headache (7% to 13%)
  Gastrointestinal: Nausea (7% to 19%, children 9%)
1% to 10%:
  Central nervous system: Depression (6%), fever/chills (6%, children 9%), anxiety (5%)
  Dermatologic: Rash (5% to 6%, children 7%)
  Endocrine & metabolic: Triglycerides increased (2% to 6%)
  Gastrointestinal: Diarrhea (7%), vomiting (children 9%), amylase increased (2%)
  Hematologic: Thrombocytopenia (1%)
  Hepatic: AST increased (6%)
  Neuromuscular & skeletal: Musculoskeletal pain (5% to 6%)
  Miscellaneous: Hypersensitivity reactions (2% to 9%; may include reactions to other components of antiretroviral regimen), infection (ENT 5%)

Available Dosage Forms
Solution, Oral:
  Ziagen: 20 mg/mL (240 mL)
Tablet, Oral:
  Ziagen: 300 mg
  Generic: 300 mg
General Dosage Range Dosage adjustment recommended in patients with hepatic impairment
Oral:
  Infants and Children ≥3 months to <16 years: 8 mg/kg twice daily (maximum: 300 mg twice daily)
  Adolescents ≥16 years and Adults: 600 mg/day in 1-2 divided doses (maximum: 600 mg/day)
Administration
Oral May be administered with or without food.
Storage/Stability Store oral solution and tablets at controlled room temperature of 20°C to 25°C (68°F to 77°F). Oral solution may be refrigerated; do not freeze.
Nursing Actions
Physical Assessment Previous exposure/allergy to abacavir and risk factors for heart disease should be assessed prior to beginning treatment. A medication guide and a warning card (summarizing symptoms of hypersensitivity) are available in each bottle and patients should be provided with this information. Monitor patient closely for any sign of hypersensitivity reaction;

can occur within hours or at any time and may be fatal (can also occur at reintroduction with patients who have no history of previous reaction). Assess decrease in infections. Teach patient proper timing of multiple medications and importance of immediately reporting any sign of hypersensitivity or myocardial infarction.

Patient Education
• Discuss specific use of drug and side effects with patient as it relates to treatment. (HCAHPS: During this hospital stay, were you given any medicine that you had not taken before? Before giving you any new medicine, how often did hospital staff tell you what the medicine was for? How often did hospital staff describe possible side effects in a way you could understand?)
• Patient may experience headache, nausea, diarrhea, lack of appetite, lipodystrophy, insomnia, or nightmares. Have patient report immediately to prescriber signs of lactic acidosis, signs of hepatic impairment, signs of depression (ie, suicidal ideation, anxiety, emotional instability, illogical thinking), angina, severe dizziness, syncope, stomatitis, enlarged lymph nodes, or signs of infection (HCAHPS).
• Educate patient about signs of a significant reaction (eg, wheezing; chest tightness; fever; itching; bad cough; blue skin color; seizures; or swelling of face, lips, tongue, or throat). **Note:** This is not a comprehensive list of all side effects. Patient should consult prescriber for additional questions.

Intended Use and Disclaimer: Should not be printed and given to patients. This information is intended to serve as a concise initial reference for healthcare professionals to use when discussing medications with a patient. You must ultimately rely on your own discretion, experience and judgment in diagnosing, treating and advising patients.

Dietary Considerations May be taken with or without food.

Abacavir and Lamivudine
(a BAK a veer & la MI vyoo deen)

Brand Names: U.S. Epzicom®
Index Terms Abacavir Sulfate and Lamivudine; Lamivudine and Abacavir
Pharmacologic Category Antiretroviral, Reverse Transcriptase Inhibitor, Nucleoside (Anti-HIV)
Medication Guide Available Yes
Pregnancy Risk Factor C
Lactation See individual agents.
Use Treatment of HIV infections in combination with other antiretroviral agents
Available Dosage Forms
Tablet:
  Epzicom®: Abacavir 600 mg and lamivudine 300 mg

General Dosage Range Oral: *Adults:* One tablet (abacavir 600 mg and lamivudine 300 mg) once daily

Administration

Oral May be administered with or without food.

Nursing Actions

Physical Assessment See individual agents.

Patient Education
- Discuss specific use of drug and side effects with patient as it relates to treatment. (HCAHPS: During this hospital stay, were you given any medicine that you had not taken before? Before giving you any new medicine, how often did hospital staff tell you what the medicine was for? How often did hospital staff describe possible side effects in a way you could understand?)
- Patient may experience headache, lack of appetite, lipodystrophy, insomnia, or nightmares. Have patient report immediately to prescriber signs of hepatic impairment, signs of lactic acidosis, signs of pancreatitis, severe dizziness, syncope, angina, urinary retention, oliguria, depression, stomatitis, myalgia, asthenia, paresthesia, dyspnea, hyperhidrosis, edema, or signs of infection (HCAHPS).
- Educate patient about signs of a significant reaction (eg, wheezing; chest tightness; fever; itching; bad cough; blue skin color; seizures; or swelling of face, lips, tongue, or throat). **Note:** This is not a comprehensive list of all side effects. Patient should consult prescriber for additional questions.

Intended Use and Disclaimer: Should not be printed and given to patients. This information is intended to serve as a concise initial reference for healthcare professionals to use when discussing medications with a patient. You must ultimately rely on your own discretion, experience and judgment in diagnosing, treating and advising patients.

Related Information
Abacavir *on page 24*
LamiVUDine *on page 900*

Abacavir, Lamivudine, and Zidovudine
(a BAK a veer, la MI vyoo deen, & zye DOE vyoo deen)

Brand Names: U.S. Trizivir®

Index Terms 3TC, Abacavir, and Zidovudine; Azidothymidine, Abacavir, and Lamivudine; AZT, Abacavir, and Lamivudine; Compound S, Abacavir, and Lamivudine; Lamivudine, Abacavir, and Zidovudine; ZDV, Abacavir, and Lamivudine; Zidovudine, Abacavir, and Lamivudine

Pharmacologic Category Antiretroviral, Reverse Transcriptase Inhibitor, Nucleoside (Anti-HIV)

Medication Guide Available Yes

Pregnancy Risk Factor C

Lactation See individual agents.

Use Treatment of HIV infection (either alone or in combination with other antiretroviral agents) in patients whose regimen would otherwise contain the components of Trizivir®

Available Dosage Forms

Tablet, oral:

Trizivir®: Abacavir 300 mg, lamivudine 150 mg, and zidovudine 300 mg

Generic: Abacavir sulfate 300 mg, lamivudine 150 mg, and zidovudine 300 mg

General Dosage Range Oral: *Adolescents ≥40 kg and Adults:* One tablet twice daily

Administration

Oral Administer without regard to food.

Nursing Actions

Physical Assessment See individual agents.

Patient Education
- Discuss specific use of drug and side effects with patient as it relates to treatment. (HCAHPS: During this hospital stay, were you given any medicine that you had not taken before? Before giving you any new medicine, how often did hospital staff tell you what the medicine was for? How often did hospital staff describe possible side effects in a way you could understand?)
- Patient may experience headache, arthralgia, anxiety, lack of appetite, or lipodystrophy. Have patient report immediately to prescriber signs of hepatic impairment, signs of lactic acidosis, signs of pancreatitis, severe asthenia, angina, urinary retention, oliguria, depression, severe dizziness, syncope, stomatitis, myalgia, muscle cramps, paresthesia, dyspnea, hyperhidrosis, edema, ecchymosis, hemorrhaging, or signs of infection (HCAHPS).
- Educate patient about signs of a significant reaction (eg, wheezing; chest tightness; fever; itching; bad cough; blue skin color; seizures; or swelling of face, lips, tongue, or throat). **Note:** This is not a comprehensive list of all side effects. Patient should consult prescriber for additional questions.

Intended Use and Disclaimer: Should not be printed and given to patients. This information is intended to serve as a concise initial reference for healthcare professionals to use when discussing medications with a patient. You must ultimately rely on your own discretion, experience and judgment in diagnosing, treating and advising patients.

Related Information
Abacavir *on page 24*
LamiVUDine *on page 900*
Zidovudine *on page 1630*

Abatacept (ab a TA sept)

Brand Names: U.S. Orencia

Index Terms BMS-188667; CTLA-4Ig

Pharmacologic Category Antirheumatic, Disease Modifying; Selective T-Cell Costimulation Blocker
Medication Safety Issues
  Sound-alike/look-alike issues:
    Orencia may be confused with Oracea
Pregnancy Risk Factor C
Lactation Excretion in breast milk unknown/not recommended
Breast-Feeding Considerations It is not known if abatacept is excreted into human milk. Due to the potential for serious adverse reactions in the nursing infant, a decision should be made to discontinue nursing or to discontinue the drug, taking into account the importance of treatment to the mother.
Use
  Rheumatoid arthritis: Treatment of moderately to severely active adult rheumatoid arthritis (RA); may be used as monotherapy or in combination with other DMARDs
  Juvenile idiopathic arthritis: Treatment of moderately to severely active polyarticular juvenile idiopathic arthritis (JIA); may be used as monotherapy or in combination with methotrexate
  Note: Abatacept should **not** be used in combination with anakinra or TNF-blocking agents
Mechanism of Action/Effect Prevents activation of T cells
Contraindications There are no contraindications listed within the manufacturer's U.S. labeling.

Canadian labeling: Hypersensitivity to abatacept or any component of the formulation; patients with, or at risk of sepsis syndrome (eg, immunocompromised, HIV positive)
Warnings/Precautions Serious and potentially fatal infections (including tuberculosis and sepsis) have been reported, particularly in patients receiving concomitant immunosuppressive therapy. RA patients receiving a concomitant TNF antagonist experienced an even higher rate of serious infection. Caution should be exercised when considering the use of abatacept in any patient with a history of recurrent infections, with conditions that predispose them to infections, or with chronic, latent, or localized infections. Patients who develop a new infection while undergoing treatment should be monitored closely. If a patient develops a serious infection, abatacept should be discontinued. Screen patients for latent tuberculosis infection prior to initiating abatacept; safety in tuberculosis-positive patients has not been established. Treat patients testing positive according to standard therapy prior to initiating abatacept. Adult patients receiving abatacept in combination with TNF-blocking agents had higher rates of infections (including serious infections) than patients on TNF-blocking agents alone. Potentially significant drug-drug interactions may exist, requiring dose or frequency adjustment, additional monitoring, and/or selection of alternative therapy. The manufacturer does not recommend concurrent use with anakinra or TNF-blocking agents. Monitor for signs and symptoms of infection when transitioning from TNF-blocking agents to abatacept. Due to the effect of T-cell inhibition on host defenses, abatacept may affect immune responses against infections and malignancies; impact on the development and course of malignancies is not fully defined.

Use caution with chronic obstructive pulmonary disease (COPD), higher incidences of adverse effects (COPD exacerbation, cough, rhonchi, dyspnea) have been observed; monitor closely. Rare cases of hypersensitivity, anaphylaxis, or anaphylactoid reactions have been reported with intravenous administration; may occur with first infusion. Some reactions (hypotension, urticaria, dyspnea) occurred within 24 hours of infusion. Discontinue treatment if anaphylaxis or other serious allergic reaction occurs; medications for the treatment of hypersensitivity reactions should be available for immediate use. Patients should be screened for viral hepatitis prior to use; antirheumatic therapy may cause reactivation of hepatitis B. Patients should be brought up to date with all immunizations before initiating therapy. Live vaccines should not be given concurrently or within 3 months of discontinuation of therapy; there is no data available concerning secondary transmission of live vaccines in patients receiving therapy. Powder for injection may contain maltose, which may result in falsely-elevated serum glucose readings on the day of infusion. Higher incidences of infection and malignancy were observed in the elderly; use with caution.
Drug Interactions
  Avoid Concomitant Use
    Avoid concomitant use of Abatacept with any of the following: Anakinra; Anti-TNF Agents; BCG; Belimumab; Natalizumab; Pimecrolimus; RiTUXimab; Tacrolimus (Topical); Tocilizumab; Tofacitinib; Vaccines (Live)
  Decreased Effect
    Abatacept may decrease the levels/effects of: BCG; Coccidioidin Skin Test; Sipuleucel-T; Vaccines (Inactivated); Vaccines (Live)

    The levels/effects of Abatacept may be decreased by: Echinacea
  Increased Effect/Toxicity
    Abatacept may increase the levels/effects of: Belimumab; Leflunomide; Natalizumab; Tofacitinib; Vaccines (Live)

    The levels/effects of Abatacept may be increased by: Anakinra; Anti-TNF Agents; Denosumab; Pimecrolimus; RiTUXimab; Roflumilast; Tacrolimus (Topical); Tocilizumab; Trastuzumab
  Nutritional/Ethanol Interactions Herb/Nutraceutical: Avoid echinacea (has immunostimulant properties; consider therapy modifications).

Adverse Reactions Note: Percentages not always reported; COPD patients experienced a higher frequency of COPD-related adverse reactions (COPD exacerbation, cough, dyspnea, pneumonia, rhonchi)

>10%:
Central nervous system: Headache (≤18%)
Gastrointestinal: Nausea
Respiratory: Nasopharyngitis (12%), upper respiratory tract infection
Miscellaneous: Infection (adults 54%; children 36%), antibody development (2% to 41%)
1% to 10%:
Cardiovascular: Hypertension (7%)
Central nervous system: Dizziness (9%)
Dermatologic: Skin rash (4%)
Gastrointestinal: Dyspepsia (6%), abdominal pain, diarrhea
Genitourinary: Urinary tract infection (6%)
Immunologic: Immunogenicity (1% to 2%)
Infection: Herpes simplex infection, influenza
Local: Injection site reaction (3%)
Neuromuscular & skeletal: Back pain (7%), limb pain (3%)
Respiratory: Cough (8%), bronchitis, pneumonia, rhinitis, sinusitis
Miscellaneous: Infusion-related reaction (≤9%), fever

Available Dosage Forms

Solution, Subcutaneous [preservative free]:
Orencia: 125 mg/mL (1 mL)
Solution Reconstituted, Intravenous [preservative free]:
Orencia: 250 mg (1 ea)

General Dosage Range

I.V.: Repeat dose at 2 weeks and 4 weeks, then every 4 weeks thereafter
Children ≥6 years and <75 kg: 10 mg/kg/dose
Children ≥6 years and 75-100 kg: 750 mg/dose
Children ≥6 years and >100 kg: 1000 mg/dose
Adults <60 kg: 500 mg/dose
Adults 60-100 kg: 750 mg/dose
Adults >100 kg: 1000 mg/dose
SubQ: *Adults:* 125 mg/dose once weekly

Administration

I.V. Infuse over 30 minutes. Administer through a 0.2-1.2 micron low protein-binding filter

Injectable Detail pH: 7-8

Subcutaneous SubQ: Allow prefilled syringe to warm to room temperature (for 30-60 minutes) prior to administration. Inject into the front of the thigh (preferred), abdomen (except for 2-inch area around the navel), or the outer area of the upper arms (if administered by a caregiver). Rotate injection sites (≥1 inch apart); do not administer into tender, bruised, red, or hard skin.

Preparation for Administration

I.V.: Reconstitute each vial with 10 mL SWFI using the provided silicone-free disposable syringe (discard solutions accidentally reconstituted with siliconized syringe as they may develop translucent particles). Inject SWFI down the side of the vial to avoid foaming. The reconstituted solution contains 25 mg/mL abatacept. Further dilute (using a silicone-free syringe) in 100 mL NS to a final concentration of ≤10 mg/mL. Prior to adding abatacept to the 100 mL bag, the manufacturer recommends withdrawing a volume of NS equal to the abatacept volume required, resulting in a final volume of 100 mL. Mix gently; do not shake.

SubQ: Allow prefilled syringe to reach room temperature prior to administration by removing from refrigerator 30-60 minutes prior to administration.

Storage/Stability

Prefilled syringe: Store at 2°C to 8°C (36°F to 46°F); do not freeze. Protect from light.

Powder for injection: Prior to reconstitution, store at 2°C to 8°C (36°F to 46°F); do not freeze. Protect from light. After dilution, may be stored for up to 24 hours at room temperature or refrigerated at 2°C to 8°C (36°F to 46°F). Must be used within 24 hours of reconstitution.

Nursing Actions

Physical Assessment Perform testing for tuberculosis prior to initiating therapy. Assess for infection prior to initiating infusion.

Patient Education

- Discuss specific use of drug and side effects with patient as it relates to treatment. (HCAHPS: During this hospital stay, were you given any medicine that you had not taken before? Before giving you any new medicine, how often did hospital staff tell you what the medicine was for? How often did hospital staff describe possible side effects in a way you could understand?)

- Patient may experience pharyngitis, injection site pain or irritation, dyspepsia, hypertension, or back pain. Have patient report immediately to prescriber signs of infection, severe dizziness, considerable headache, dyspnea, wheezing, skin growth, weight loss, night sweats, intolerable nausea, or significant diarrhea (HCAHPS).

- Educate patient about signs of a significant reaction (eg, wheezing; chest tightness; fever; itching; bad cough; blue skin color; seizures; or swelling of face, lips, tongue, or throat). **Note:** This is not a comprehensive list of all side effects. Patient should consult prescriber for additional questions.

Intended Use and Disclaimer: Should not be printed and given to patients. This information is intended to serve as a concise initial reference for healthcare professionals to use when discussing medications with a patient. You must ultimately rely on your own discretion, experience and judgment in diagnosing, treating and advising patients.

Abiraterone Acetate (a bir A ter one AS e tate)

Brand Names: U.S. Zytiga
Index Terms Abiraterone; CB7630
Pharmacologic Category Antiandrogen; Antineoplastic Agent, Antiandrogen
Medication Safety Issues
Sound-alike/look-alike issues:
Zytiga may be confused with Jevtana, Xgeva, Xofigo, Xtandi, Zometa
Pregnancy Risk Factor X
Lactation Excretion in breast milk unknown/not recommended
Use Prostate cancer: Treatment of metastatic, castration-resistant prostate cancer (in combination with prednisone)
Available Dosage Forms
Tablet, Oral:
Zytiga: 250 mg
General Dosage Range Dosage adjustment recommended in patients with hepatic impairment, on concomitant therapy, or who develop toxicity.
Oral: *Adults:* 1000 mg once daily
Administration
Oral Administer on an empty stomach, at least 1 hour before and 2 hours after food. Swallow tablets whole with water. Do not crush or chew.

Hazardous agent; use appropriate precautions for handling and disposal (meets NIOSH, 2012 criteria). Women who are or may become pregnant should wear gloves if handling the tablets.
Nursing Actions
Physical Assessment Monitor for vital signs, liver function tests, electrolyte panel. May cause hypertension, multiple metabolic changes (glucose, sodium, potassium, phosphate, triglycerides), fluid retention, and signs and symptoms of adrenocorticoid insufficiency.
Patient Education
• Discuss specific use of drug and side effects with patient as it relates to treatment. (HCAHPS: During this hospital stay, were you given any medicine that you had not taken before? Before giving you any new medicine, how often did hospital staff tell you what the medicine was for? How often did hospital staff describe possible side effects in a way you could understand?)
• Patient may experience flushing, myalgia, arthralgia, pyrosis, or emesis. Have patient report immediately to prescriber signs of infection, signs of hypokalemia, signs of hepatic impairment, severe dizziness, syncope, angina, tachycardia, bradycardia, illogical thinking, dyspnea, excessive weight gain, edema of extremities, considerable headache, significant asthenia, ecchymosis, hemorrhaging, urinary retention, oliguria, dysuria, intolerable diarrhea, or osteodynia (HCAHPS).

• Educate patient about signs of a significant reaction (eg, wheezing; chest tightness; fever; itching; bad cough; blue skin color; seizures; or swelling of face, lips, tongue, or throat). **Note:** This is not a comprehensive list of all side effects. Patient should consult prescriber for additional questions.

Intended Use and Disclaimer: Should not be printed and given to patients. This information is intended to serve as a concise initial reference for healthcare professionals to use when discussing medications with a patient. You must ultimately rely on your own discretion, experience and judgment in diagnosing, treating and advising patients.
Related Information
Oral Medications That Should Not Be Crushed or Altered *on page 1712*

Acamprosate (a kam PROE sate)

Brand Names: U.S. Campral
Index Terms Acamprosate Calcium; Calcium Acetylhomotaurinate
Pharmacologic Category GABA Agonist/Glutamate Antagonist
Pregnancy Risk Factor C
Lactation Excretion in breast milk unknown/use caution
Use Maintenance of alcohol abstinence
Available Dosage Forms
Tablet Delayed Release, Oral:
Campral: 333 mg
Generic: 333 mg
General Dosage Range Dosage adjustment recommended in patients with renal impairment.
Oral: *Adults:* 666 mg 3 times/day (maximum: 1998 mg/day)
Administration
Oral May be administered without regard to meals (administered with meals during clinical trials to possibly increase compliance). Tablet should be swallowed whole; do not crush or chew.
Nursing Actions
Physical Assessment Can cause depression. Monitor for suicide ideation.
Patient Education
• Discuss specific use of drug and side effects with patient as it relates to treatment. (HCAHPS: During this hospital stay, were you given any medicine that you had not taken before? Before giving you any new medicine, how often did hospital staff tell you what the medicine was for? How often did hospital staff describe possible side effects in a way you could understand?)
• Patient may experience dyspepsia, diarrhea, asthenia, lack of appetite, flatulence, dizziness, xerostomia, insomnia, or hyperhidrosis. Have patient report immediately to prescriber paresthesia, behavioral changes, or depression (ie,

suicidal ideation, anxiety, emotional instability, illogical thinking) (HCAHPS).

- Educate patient about signs of a significant reaction (eg, wheezing; chest tightness; fever; itching; bad cough; blue skin color; seizures; or swelling of face, lips, tongue, or throat). **Note:** This is not a comprehensive list of all side effects. Patient should consult prescriber for additional questions.

Intended Use and Disclaimer: Should not be printed and given to patients. This information is intended to serve as a concise initial reference for healthcare professionals to use when discussing medications with a patient. You must ultimately rely on your own discretion, experience and judgment in diagnosing, treating and advising patients.

Related Information

Oral Medications That Should Not Be Crushed or Altered *on page 1712*

Acarbose (AY car bose)

Brand Names: U.S. Precose

Pharmacologic Category Antidiabetic Agent, Alpha-Glucosidase Inhibitor

Medication Safety Issues

Sound-alike/look-alike issues:

Precose® may be confused with PreCare®

High alert medication:

The Institute for Safe Medication Practices (ISMP) includes this medication among its list of drug classes which have a heightened risk of causing significant patient harm when used in error.

International issues:

Precose® [U.S., Malaysia] may be confused with Precosa brand name for *Saccharomyces boulardii* [Finland, Sweden]

Pregnancy Risk Factor B

Lactation Excretion in breast milk unknown/not recommended

Breast-Feeding Considerations It is not known if acarbose is found in breast milk; however, low amounts of acarbose are absorbed systemically in adults, which may limit the amount that could distribute into breast milk. Although breast-feeding is encouraged for all women, including those with diabetes, the safety of acarbose during breast-feeding has not yet been established (Metzger, 2007). Breast-feeding is not recommended by the manufacturer.

Use Adjunct to diet and exercise to lower blood glucose in patients with type 2 diabetes mellitus (noninsulin dependent, NIDDM)

Mechanism of Action/Effect Delays glucose absorption and lowers postprandial hyperglycemia.

Contraindications Hypersensitivity to acarbose or any component of the formulation; patients with diabetic ketoacidosis or cirrhosis; patients with inflammatory bowel disease, colonic ulceration, partial intestinal obstruction, or in patients predisposed to intestinal obstruction; patients who have chronic intestinal diseases associated with marked disorders of digestion or absorption, and in patients who have conditions that may deteriorate as a result of increased gas formation in the intestine

Warnings/Precautions Acarbose given in combination with a sulfonylurea or insulin will cause a further lowering of blood glucose and may increase the hypoglycemic potential of the sulfonylurea or insulin. Treatment-emergent elevations of serum transaminases (AST and/or ALT) occurred in up to 14% of acarbose-treated patients in long-term studies. These serum transaminase elevations appear to be dose related and were asymptomatic, reversible, more common in females, and, in general, were not associated with other evidence of liver dysfunction. Fulminant hepatitis has been reported rarely. It may be necessary to discontinue acarbose and administer insulin if the patient is exposed to stress (ie, fever, trauma, infection, surgery). Use not recommended in patients with significant impairment (S_{cr} >2 mg/dL); use with caution in other patients with renal impairment.

Drug Interactions

Avoid Concomitant Use There are no known interactions where it is recommended to avoid concomitant use.

Decreased Effect

Acarbose may decrease the levels/effects of: Digoxin

The levels/effects of Acarbose may be decreased by: Corticosteroids (Orally Inhaled); Corticosteroids (Systemic); Loop Diuretics; Luteinizing Hormone-Releasing Hormone Analogs; Somatropin; Thiazide Diuretics

Increased Effect/Toxicity

Acarbose may increase the levels/effects of: Hypoglycemic Agents

The levels/effects of Acarbose may be increased by: Herbs (Hypoglycemic Properties); MAO Inhibitors; Neomycin; Pegvisomant; Salicylates; Selective Serotonin Reuptake Inhibitors

Nutritional/Ethanol Interactions Ethanol: Limit ethanol.

Adverse Reactions >10%:

Gastrointestinal: Diarrhea (31%) and abdominal pain (19%) tend to return to pretreatment levels over time; frequency and intensity of flatulence (74%) tend to abate with time

Hepatic: Transaminases increased (≤4%)

Available Dosage Forms

Tablet, Oral:

Precose: 25 mg, 50 mg, 100 mg

Generic: 25 mg, 50 mg, 100 mg

General Dosage Range Dosage adjustment recommended in patients on concomitant therapy

Oral: *Adults:* Initial: 25 mg 1-3 times/day; Maintenance: 75-300 mg/day in 3 divided doses (maximum: ≤60 kg: 150 mg/day; >60 kg: 300 mg/day)

Administration

Oral Should be **administered with the first bite of each main meal.**

Storage/Stability Store at <25°C (77°F). Protect from moisture.

Nursing Actions

Physical Assessment Teach patient importance of diabetic control.

Patient Education

- Discuss specific use of drug and side effects with patient as it relates to treatment. (HCAHPS: During this hospital stay, were you given any medicine that you had not taken before? Before giving you any new medicine, how often did hospital staff tell you what the medicine was for? How often did hospital staff describe possible side effects in a way you could understand?)
- Patient may experience flatulence or bloating. Have patient report immediately to prescriber signs of hepatic impairment, severe diarrhea, significant dyspepsia, or signs of hypoglycemia (HCAHPS).
- Educate patient about signs of a significant reaction (eg, wheezing; chest tightness; fever; itching; bad cough; blue skin color; seizures; or swelling of face, lips, tongue, or throat). **Note:** This is not a comprehensive list of all side effects. Patient should consult prescriber for additional questions.

Intended Use and Disclaimer: Should not be printed and given to patients. This information is intended to serve as a concise initial reference for healthcare professionals to use when discussing medications with a patient. You must ultimately rely on your own discretion, experience and judgment in diagnosing, treating and advising patients.

Dietary Considerations Take with food (first bite of meal).

Acetaminophen (a seet a MIN oh fen)

Brand Names: U.S. Acephen [OTC]; APAP 500 [OTC]; Aspirin Free Anacin Extra Strength [OTC]; Cetafen Extra [OTC]; Cetafen [OTC]; Excedrin Tension Headache [OTC]; Feverall [OTC]; Little Fevers [OTC]; Mapap Arthritis Pain [OTC]; Mapap Children's [OTC]; Mapap Extra Strength [OTC]; Mapap Infant's [OTC]; Mapap Junior Rapid Tabs [OTC]; Mapap [OTC]; Non-Aspirin Pain Reliever [OTC]; Nortemp Children's [OTC]; Ofirmev; Pain & Fever Children's [OTC]; Pain Eze [OTC]; Q-Pap Children's [OTC]; Q-Pap Extra Strength [OTC]; Q-Pap Infant's [OTC]; Q-Pap [OTC]; RapiMed Children's [OTC]; RapiMed Junior [OTC]; Silapap Children's [OTC]; Silapap Infant's [OTC]; Triaminic Children's Fever Reducer Pain Reliever [OTC]; Tylenol 8 Hour [OTC]; Tylenol Arthritis Pain Extended Relief [OTC]; Tylenol Children's Meltaways [OTC]; Tylenol Children's [OTC]; Tylenol Extra Strength [OTC]; Tylenol Infant's Concentrated [OTC] [DSC]; Tylenol Jr. Meltaways [OTC]; Tylenol [OTC]; Valorin Extra [OTC]; Valorin [OTC]

Index Terms APAP (abbreviation is not recommended); N-Acetyl-P-Aminophenol; Paracetamol

Pharmacologic Category Analgesic, Miscellaneous

Medication Safety Issues

Sound-alike/look-alike issues:

Acephen may be confused with AcipHex

FeverALL may be confused with Fiberall

Triaminic Children's Fever Reducer Pain Reliever may be confused with Triaminic cough and cold products

Tylenol may be confused with atenolol, timolol, Tylenol PM, Tylox

Other safety concerns:

Duplicate therapy issues: This product contains acetaminophen, which may be a component of combination products. Do not exceed the maximum recommended daily dose of acetaminophen.

Infant concentration change: All children's and infant acetaminophen products are available as 160 mg/5mL. Some remaining infant concentrated solutions of 80 mg/0.8mL and 100 mg/mL may still be available on pharmacy shelves or in patient homes. Check concentrations closely prior to administering or dispensing and verify concentration available to patients prior to recommending a dose (November 2011).

Injection: Reports of 10-fold overdose errors using the parenteral product have occurred in the U.S. and Europe; calculation of doses in "mg" and subsequent administration of the dose in "mL" using the commercially available concentration of 10 mg/mL contributed to these errors. Expressing doses as mg **and** mL, as well as pharmacy preparation of doses, may decrease error potential (Dart, 2012; ISMP, 2012).

International issues:

Depon [Greece] may be confused with Depen brand name for penicillamine [U.S.]; Depin brand name for nifedipine [India]; Dipen brand name for diltiazem [Greece]

Duorol [Spain] may be confused with Diuril brand name for chlorothiazide [U.S., Canada]

Paralen [Czech Republic] may be confused with Aralen brand name for chloroquine [U.S., Mexico]

Pregnancy Risk Factor C (intravenous)

Lactation Enters breast milk/use caution

Breast-Feeding Considerations Low concentrations of acetaminophen are excreted into breast milk and can be detected in the urine of nursing infants. Adverse reactions have generally not been observed; however, a rash caused by acetaminophen exposure was reported in one breast-feeding infant.

Use Treatment of mild-to-moderate pain and fever (analgesic/antipyretic)

I.V.: Additional indication: Management of moderate-to-severe pain when combined with opioid analgesia

Mechanism of Action/Effect Reduces fever by acting on the hypothalamus to cause vasodilatation and sweating

Contraindications Hypersensitivity to acetaminophen or any component of the formulation; severe hepatic impairment or severe active liver disease (Ofirmev™)

Warnings/Precautions [U.S. Boxed Warning]: Acetaminophen injection formulation has been associated with acute liver failure, at times resulting in liver transplant and death. Take care to avoid dosing errors; ensure that the dose in mg is not confused with mL, dosing in patients <50 kg is based on body weight, infusion pumps are properly programmed, and total daily dose of acetaminophen from all sources does not exceed the maximum daily limits.

Limit acetaminophen dose from all sources (prescription, OTC, combination products) and all routes of administration (I.V., oral, rectal) to <4 g/day (adults). In addition, chronic daily dosing may result in liver damage in some patients; hepatotoxicity is usually associated with excessive acetaminophen intake (>4 g/day in adults). Use with caution in patients with alcoholic liver disease; consuming ≥3 alcoholic drinks/day may increase the risk of liver damage. Use caution in patients with hepatic impairment or active liver disease. Use of I.V. formulation is contraindicated in patients with severe hepatic impairment or severe active liver disease. Use caution in patients with known G6PD deficiency; rare reports of hemolysis have occurred. Use caution in patients with chronic malnutrition and hypovolemia (I.V. formulation). Use caution in patients with severe renal impairment; consider dosing adjustments. Hypersensitivity and anaphylactic reactions have been reported; discontinue immediately if symptoms of allergic or hypersensitivity reactions occur. Rarely, acetaminophen may cause serious and potentially fatal skin reactions such as acute generalized exanthematous pustulosis, Stevens-Johnson syndrome (SJS), and toxic epidermal necrolysis (TEN). Discontinue treatment if severe skin reactions develop.

OTC labeling: When used for self-medication, patients should be instructed to contact healthcare provider if used for fever lasting >3 days or for pain lasting >10 days in adults or >5 days in children. OTC labeling limits the maximum daily dose to ≤3250 mg (dosage form specific).

Drug Interactions

Avoid Concomitant Use

Avoid concomitant use of Acetaminophen with any of the following: Pimozide

Decreased Effect

The levels/effects of Acetaminophen may be decreased by: Anticonvulsants (Hydantoin); Barbiturates; CarBAMazepine; Cholestyramine Resin; Peginterferon Alfa-2b

Increased Effect/Toxicity

Acetaminophen may increase the levels/effects of: ARIPiprazole; Busulfan; Dasatinib; Dofetilide; Imatinib; Lomitapide; Mipomersen; Pimozide; Prilocaine; Sodium Nitrite; SORAfenib; Vitamin K Antagonists

The levels/effects of Acetaminophen may be increased by: Dasatinib; Isoniazid; Metyrapone; Nitric Oxide; Probenecid; SORAfenib

Nutritional/Ethanol Interactions

Ethanol: Excessive intake of ethanol may increase the risk of acetaminophen-induced hepatotoxicity. Avoid ethanol or limit to <3 drinks/day.

Food: Rate of absorption may be decreased when given with food.

Herb/Nutraceutical: St John's wort may decrease acetaminophen levels.

Adverse Reactions Oral, Rectal: Frequency not defined:

Dermatologic: Skin rash

Endocrine & metabolic: Decreased serum bicarbonate, decreased serum calcium, decreased serum sodium, hyperchloremia, hyperuricemia, increased serum glucose

Genitourinary: Nephrotoxicity (with chronic overdose)

Hematologic & oncologic: Anemia, leukopenia, neutropenia, pancytopenia

Hepatic: Increased serum alkaline phosphatase, increased serum bilirubin

Hypersensitivity: Hypersensitivity reaction (rare)

Renal: Hyperammonemia, renal disease (analgesic)

I.V.:

>10%: Gastrointestinal: Nausea (adults 34%; children ≥5%), vomiting (adults 15%; children ≥5%)

1% to 10%:

Cardiovascular: Hypertension, hypotension, peripheral edema, tachycardia

Central nervous system: Headache (adults 10%; children ≥1%), insomnia (adults 7%; children ≥1%), agitation (children ≥5%), anxiety, fatigue, trismus

Dermatologic: Pruritus (children ≥5%), skin rash

Endocrine & metabolic: Hypervolemia, hypoalbuminemia, hypokalemia, hypomagnesemia, hypophosphatemia

Gastrointestinal: Constipation (children ≥5%), abdominal pain, diarrhea

Genitourinary: Oliguria (children ≥1%)

Hematologic & oncologic: Anemia

Hepatic: Increased serum transaminases

Local: Infusion site reaction (pain)

Neuromuscular & skeletal: Limb pain, muscle spasm

Ophthalmic: Periorbital edema

Respiratory: Atelectasis (children ≥5%), abnormal breath sounds, dyspnea, hypoxia, pleural effusion, pulmonary edema, stridor, wheezing

Miscellaneous: Fever (children ≥1%)

Pharmacodynamics/Kinetics

Onset of Action

Oral: <1 hour

I.V.: Analgesia: 5-10 minutes; Antipyretic: Within 30 minutes

Peak effect: I.V.: Analgesic: 1 hour

Duration of Action

I.V., Oral: Analgesia: 4-6 hours

I.V.: Antipyretic: ≥6 hours

Available Dosage Forms

Caplet, oral: 500 mg

Cetafen® Extra [OTC]: 500 mg

Mapap® Extra Strength [OTC]: 500 mg

Pain Eze [OTC]: 650 mg

Tylenol® [OTC]: 325 mg

Tylenol® Extra Strength [OTC]: 500 mg

Caplet, extended release, oral:

Mapap® Arthritis Pain [OTC]: 650 mg

Tylenol® 8 Hour [OTC]: 650 mg

Tylenol® Arthritis Pain Extended Relief [OTC]: 650 mg

Capsule, oral:

Mapap® Extra Strength [OTC]: 500 mg

Captab, oral: 500 mg

Elixir, oral:

Mapap® Children's [OTC]: 160 mg/5 mL (118 mL, 480 mL)

Gelcap, oral: 500 mg

Mapap® [OTC]: 500 mg

Gelcap, rapid release, oral: 500 mg

Tylenol® Extra Strength [OTC]: 500 mg

Geltab, oral: 500 mg

Excedrin® Tension Headache [OTC]: 500 mg

Injection, solution [preservative free]:

Ofirmev™: 10 mg/mL (100 mL)

Liquid, oral: 160 mg/5 mL (120 mL, 473 mL); 500 mg/5 mL (240 mL)

APAP 500 [OTC]: 500 mg/5 mL (237 mL)

Mapap® Extra Strength [OTC]: 500 mg/5 mL (237 mL)

Q-Pap Children's [OTC]: 160 mg/5 mL (118 mL, 473 mL)

Silapap Children's [OTC]: 160 mg/5 mL (118 mL, 237 mL, 473 mL)

Tylenol® Extra Strength [OTC]: 500 mg/15 mL (240 mL)

Solution, oral: 160 mg/5 mL (5 mL, 10 mL, 20 mL, 118 mL, 473 mL)

Little Fevers™ [OTC]: 80 mg/mL (30 mL)

Pain & Fever Children's [OTC]: 160 mg/5 mL (118 mL, 473 mL)

Q-Pap Infant's [OTC]: 80 mg/0.8 mL (15 mL)

Silapap Infant's [OTC]: 80 mg/0.8 mL (15 mL, 30 mL)

Suppository, rectal: 120 mg (12s, 50s, 100s); 325 mg (12s); 650 mg (12s, 50s, 100s)

Acephen™ [OTC]: 120 mg (12s, 50s, 100s); 325 mg (6s, 12s, 50s, 100s); 650 mg (12s, 50s, 100s)

Feverall® [OTC]: 80 mg (6s, 50s); 120 mg (6s, 50s); 325 mg (6s, 50s); 650 mg (50s)

Suspension, oral: 160 mg/5 mL (5 mL, 10 mL, 10.15 mL, 20 mL, 20.3 mL)

Mapap® Children's [OTC]: 160 mg/5 mL (118 mL)

Mapap® Infant's [OTC]: 160 mg/5 mL (59 mL)

Nortemp Children's [OTC]: 160 mg/5 mL (118 mL)

Pain & Fever Children's [OTC]: 160 mg/5 mL (60 mL)

Q-Pap Children's [OTC]: 160 mg/5 mL (118 mL)

Tylenol® Children's [OTC]: 160 mg/5 mL (60 mL, 120 mL)

Syrup, oral:

Triaminic™ Children's Fever Reducer Pain Reliever [OTC]: 160 mg/5 mL (118 mL)

Tablet, oral: 325 mg, 500 mg

Aspirin Free Anacin® Extra Strength [OTC]: 500 mg

Cetafen® [OTC]: 325 mg

Mapap® [OTC]: 325 mg

Non-Aspirin Pain Reliever [OTC]: 325 mg

Q-Pap [OTC]: 325 mg

Q-Pap Extra Strength [OTC]: 500 mg

Tylenol® [OTC]: 325 mg

Tylenol® Extra Strength [OTC]: 500 mg

Valorin [OTC]: 325 mg

Valorin Extra [OTC]: 500 mg

Tablet, chewable, oral: 80 mg

Mapap® Children's [OTC]: 80 mg

Tablet, orally disintegrating, oral: 80 mg, 160 mg

Mapap® Children's [OTC]: 80 mg

Mapap® Junior Rapid Tabs [OTC]: 160 mg

RapiMed® Children's [OTC]: 80 mg

RapiMed® Junior [OTC]: 160 mg

Tylenol® Children's Meltaways [OTC]: 80 mg

Tylenol® Jr. Meltaways [OTC]: 160 mg

General Dosage Range Dosage adjustment recommended in patients with renal impairment

Oral, rectal:

Children 0-3 months: 10-15 mg/kg/dose **or** 40 mg/dose every 4-6 hours as needed (maximum: 2.6 g daily)

Children 4-11 months: 10-15 mg/kg/dose **or** 80 mg/dose every 4-6 hours as needed (maximum: 2.6 g daily)

Children 1-2 years: 10-15 mg/kg/dose **or** 120 mg/dose every 4-6 hours as needed (maximum: 2.6 g daily)

Children 2-3 years: 10-15 mg/kg/dose **or** 160 mg/dose every 4-6 hours as needed (maximum: 2.6 g daily)

Children 4-5 years: 10-15 mg/kg/dose **or** 240 mg/dose every 4-6 hours as needed (maximum: 2.6 g daily)

Children 6-8 years: 10-15 mg/kg/dose **or** 320 mg/dose every 4-6 hours as needed (maximum: 2.6 g daily)

Children 9-10 years: 10-15 mg/kg/dose **or** 400 mg/dose every 4-6 hours as needed (maximum: 2.6 g daily)

Children 11 years: 10-15 mg/kg/dose **or** 480 mg/dose every 4-6 hours as needed (maximum: 2.6 g daily)

Children ≥12 years, Adolescents, and Adults: Regular release: 325-650 mg every 4-6 hours as needed **or** 1000 mg 3-4 times daily as needed (maximum: 4 g daily); Extended release: 1300 mg every 8 hours (maximum: 3.9 g daily)

I.V.:

Children 2-12 years: 15 mg/kg every 6 hours **or** 12.5 mg/kg every 4 hours; maximum single dose: 15 mg/kg/dose (≤750 mg/dose); maximum daily dose: 75 mg/kg/day (≤3.75 g daily)

Adolescents and Adults <50 kg: 15 mg/kg every 6 hours **or** 12.5 mg/kg every 4 hours; maximum single dose: 15 mg/kg/dose (750 mg/dose); maximum daily dose: 75 mg/kg/day (≤3.75 g daily)

Adolescents and Adults ≥50 kg: 650 mg every 4 hours **or** 1000 mg every 6 hours; maximum single dose: 1000 mg; maximum daily dose: 4 g daily

Administration

I.V. For I.V. infusion only. May administer undiluted over 15 minutes.

Injectable Detail pH: 5.5

Oral Shake suspension well before pouring dose.

Preparation for Administration Injectable solution may be administered directly from the vial without further dilution.

Doses <1000 mg (<50 kg): Withdraw appropriate dose from vial and transfer to a separate sterile container (eg, glass bottle, plastic I.V. container, syringe) for administration. Small volume pediatric doses (up to 600 mg [60 mL]) may be placed in a syringe and infused over 15 minutes via syringe pump.

Doses of 1000 mg (≥50 kg): Insert vented I.V. set through vial stopper.

Storage/Stability

Injection: Store intact vials at 20°C to 25°C (68°F to 77°F); do not refrigerate or freeze. Use within 6 hours of opening vial or transferring to another container. Discard any unused portion; single use vials only.

Oral formulations: Store at controlled room temperature.

Suppositories: Store at <27°C (80°F); do not freeze.

Nursing Actions

Physical Assessment Assess patient for history of liver disease or ethanol abuse (acetaminophen and any ethanol may have adverse liver effects). Ensure adult patients keep daily dose to ≤4 g/day.

Patient Education

- Discuss specific use of drug and side effects with patient as it relates to treatment. (HCAHPS: During this hospital stay, were you given any medicine that you had not taken before? Before giving you any new medicine, how often did hospital staff tell you what the medicine was for? How often did hospital staff describe possible side effects in a way you could understand?)

- Have patient report immediately to prescriber signs of hepatic impairment, urinary retention, oliguria, illogical thinking, signs of Stevens-Johnson syndrome/toxic epidermal necrolysis, or injection site pain or irritation (HCAHPS).

- Educate patient about signs of a significant reaction (eg, wheezing; chest tightness; fever; itching; bad cough; blue skin color; seizures; or swelling of face, lips, tongue, or throat). **Note:** This is not a comprehensive list of all side effects. Patient should consult prescriber for additional questions.

Intended Use and Disclaimer: Should not be printed and given to patients. This information is intended to serve as a concise initial reference for healthcare professionals to use when discussing medications with a patient. You must ultimately rely on your own discretion, experience and judgment in diagnosing, treating and advising patients.

Dietary Considerations Some products may contain phenylalanine and/or sodium.

Related Information

Oral Medications That Should Not Be Crushed or Altered *on page 1712*

Acetaminophen and Codeine
(a seet a MIN oh fen & KOE deen)

Brand Names: U.S. Capital® and Codeine; Tylenol® with Codeine No. 3; Tylenol® with Codeine No. 4

Index Terms Codeine and Acetaminophen; Emtec; Tylenol #2; Tylenol #3; Tylenol Codeine

Pharmacologic Category Analgesic Combination (Opioid)

Medication Safety Issues

Sound-alike/look-alike issues:

Tylenol® may be confused with atenolol, timolol, Tylox®

High alert medication:

The Institute for Safe Medication Practices (ISMP) includes this medication among its list of drug classes which have a heightened risk of causing significant patient harm when used in error.

Other safety concerns:

Duplicate therapy issues: This product contains acetaminophen, which may be a component of other combination products. Do not exceed the maximum recommended daily dose of acetaminophen.

T3 is an error-prone abbreviation (mistaken as liothyronine)

International issues:

Codex: Brand name for acetaminophen/codeine [Brazil], but also the brand name for *saccharomyces boulardii* [Italy]

Codex [Brazil] may be confused with Cedax brand name for ceftibuten [U.S. and multiple international markets]

Pregnancy Risk Factor C

Lactation Enters breast milk/use caution

Use Relief of mild-to-moderate pain

Controlled Substance C-III; C-V

Available Dosage Forms

Solution, oral [C-V]: Acetaminophen 120 mg and codeine 12 mg per 5 mL

Suspension, oral [C-V]:

Capital® and Codeine [C-V]: Acetaminophen 120 mg and codeine 12 mg per 5 mL

Tablet, oral [C-III]: Acetaminophen 300 mg and codeine 15 mg; acetaminophen 300 mg and codeine 30 mg; acetaminophen 300 mg and codeine 60 mg

Tylenol® with Codeine No. 3: Acetaminophen 300 mg and codeine 30 mg

Tylenol® with Codeine No. 4: Acetaminophen 300 mg and codeine 60 mg

General Dosage Range Dosage adjustment recommended in patients with renal impairment

Oral:

Acetaminophen:

Children ≤12 years: 10-15 mg/kg/dose every 4-6 hours as needed (maximum: 2.6 g/day)

Children >12 years and Adults: 325-650 mg every 4-6 hours as needed (maximum: 4 g/day)

Codeine:

Children: 0.5-1 mg/kg/dose every 4-6 hours (maximum: 60 mg/dose)

Adults: 15-60 mg/dose every 4-6 hours (maximum: 360 mg/day)

Administration

Oral May be administered with food.

Nursing Actions

Physical Assessment See individual agents.

Patient Education

- Discuss specific use of drug and side effects with patient as it relates to treatment. (HCAHPS: During this hospital stay, were you given any medicine that you had not taken before? Before giving you any new medicine, how often did hospital staff tell you what the medicine was for? How often did hospital staff describe possible side effects in a way you could understand?)
- Patient may experience fatigue, dyspepsia, or nausea. Have patient report immediately to prescriber signs of hepatic impairment, severe dizziness, syncope, illogical thinking, considerable constipation, significant asthenia, urinary retention, oliguria, chills, pharyngitis, mood changes, intolerable headache, dyspnea, ecchymosis, hemorrhaging, vision changes, or signs of Stevens-Johnson syndrome/toxic epidermal necrolysis (HCAHPS).
- Educate patient about signs of a significant reaction (eg, wheezing; chest tightness; fever; itching; bad cough; blue skin color; seizures; or swelling of face, lips, tongue, or throat). **Note:** This is not a comprehensive list of all side effects. Patient should consult prescriber for additional questions.

Intended Use and Disclaimer: Should not be printed and given to patients. This information is intended to serve as a concise initial reference for healthcare professionals to use when discussing medications with a patient. You must ultimately rely on your own discretion, experience and judgment in diagnosing, treating and advising patients.

Related Information

Acetaminophen *on page 31*

Codeine *on page 363*

AcetaZOLAMIDE (a set a ZOLE a mide)

Brand Names: U.S. Diamox Sequels

Pharmacologic Category Anticonvulsant, Miscellaneous; Carbonic Anhydrase Inhibitor; Diuretic, Carbonic Anhydrase Inhibitor; Ophthalmic Agent, Antiglaucoma

Medication Safety Issues

International issues:

Diamox [Canada and multiple international markets] may be confused with Diabinese brand name for chlorpropamide [Multiple international markets]; Dobutrex brand name for dobutamine [Multiple international markets]; Trimox brand name for amoxicillin [Brazil]; Zimox brand name for amoxicillin [Italy] and carbidopa/levodopa [Greece]

Pregnancy Risk Factor C

Lactation Enters breast milk/not recommended

Use Treatment of glaucoma (chronic simple openangle, secondary glaucoma, preoperatively in acute angle-closure); drug-induced edema or edema due to congestive heart failure (adjunctive therapy; I.V. and immediate release dosage forms); centrencephalic epilepsies (I.V. and immediate release dosage forms); prevention or amelioration of symptoms associated with acute mountain sickness (immediate and extended release dosage forms)

Unlabeled Use Metabolic alkalosis; respiratory stimulant in stable hypercapnic COPD

Available Dosage Forms
Capsule Extended Release 12 Hour, Oral:
Diamox Sequels: 500 mg
Generic: 500 mg
Solution Reconstituted, Injection [preservative free]:
Generic: 500 mg (1 ea)
Tablet, Oral:
Generic: 125 mg, 250 mg
General Dosage Range Dosage adjustment recommended in patients with renal impairment
I.V.: Adults: 250-1000 mg/day
Oral:
Immediate release:
Children: 8-30 mg/kg/day divided in 1-4 doses (maximum: 30 mg/kg/day or 1 g/day)
Adults: 250-1000 mg/day **or** 8-30 mg/kg/day in 1-4 divided doses (maximum: 30 mg/kg/day or 1 g/day) **or** 125-250 mg every 4 hours
Elderly: Initial: 250-500 mg/day
Extended release:
Adults: 500-1000 mg/day

Administration
I.M. I.M. administration is painful because of the alkaline pH of the drug; use by this route is not recommended.
I.V. I.V.: Direct I.V. injection is the preferred parenteral route of administration. Specific I.V. push rates are not provided in the manufacturer's labeling. However, an I.V. push rate of up to 500 mg over 3 minutes has been reported in a clinical trial (Mazur, 1999). Additionally, a study to assess cerebrovascular reserve used a rapid I.V. push of up to 1 g over ≤1 minute (Piepgras, 1990).
Injectable Detail pH: 9.2
Oral May be administered with food. May cause an alteration in taste, especially carbonated beverages. Short-acting tablets may be crushed and suspended in cherry or chocolate syrup to disguise the bitter taste of the drug; do not use fruit juices. Alternatively, submerge tablet in 10 mL of hot water and add 10 mL honey or syrup.

Nursing Actions
Physical Assessment Assess allergy history prior to beginning therapy. Monitor for signs of excessive fatigue, malaise, and myalgia. Monitor growth in pediatric patients. Monitor blood glucose levels closely if patients have diabetes.
Patient Education
• Discuss specific use of drug and side effects with patient as it relates to treatment. (HCAHPS: During this hospital stay, were you given any medicine that you had not taken before? Before giving you any new medicine, how often did hospital staff tell you what the medicine was for? How often did hospital staff describe possible side effects in a way you could understand?)
• Patient may experience nausea, dysgeusia, diarrhea, lack of appetite, blurred vision, or fatigue. Have patient report immediately to prescriber signs of hepatic impairment, vision

changes, hearing impairment, tinnitus, ecchymosis, hemorrhaging, paresthesia, hematuria, tachypnea, chills, pharyngitis, or injection site pain or irritation (HCAHPS).
• Educate patient about signs of a significant reaction (eg, wheezing; chest tightness; fever; itching; bad cough; blue skin color; seizures; or swelling of face, lips, tongue, or throat). **Note:** This is not a comprehensive list of all side effects. Patient should consult prescriber for additional questions.

Intended Use and Disclaimer: Should not be printed and given to patients. This information is intended to serve as a concise initial reference for healthcare professionals to use when discussing medications with a patient. You must ultimately rely on your own discretion, experience and judgment in diagnosing, treating and advising patients.

Related Information
Oral Medications That Should Not Be Crushed or Altered *on page 1712*

Acetic Acid, Propylene Glycol Diacetate, and Hydrocortisone
(a SEE tik AS id, PRO pa leen GLY kole dye AS e tate, & hye droe KOR ti sone)

Brand Names: U.S. Acetasol® HC; VoSol® HC
Index Terms Acetic Acid, Hydrocortisone, and Propylene Glycol Diacetate; Hydrocortisone, Acetic Acid, and Propylene Glycol Diacetate; Propylene Glycol Diacetate, Acetic Acid, and Hydrocortisone
Pharmacologic Category Otic Agent, Anti-infective
Medication Safety Issues
Sound-alike/look-alike issues:
VoSol® may be confused with Vexol®
Use Treatment of superficial infections of the external auditory canal caused by organisms susceptible to the action of the antimicrobial, complicated by swelling
Available Dosage Forms
Solution, otic [drops]: Acetic acid 2%, propylene glycol diacetate 3%, and hydrocortisone 1% (10 mL)
Acetasol® HC, VoSol® HC: Acetic acid 2%, propylene glycol diacetate 3%, and hydrocortisone 1% (10 mL)
General Dosage Range Otic: *Children ≥3 years and Adults:* Instill 3-5 drops in ear(s) every 4-6 hours
Administration
Other After removing cerumen and debris, solution may be applied by inserting a cotton wick into the ear canal and saturating with the solution. Wick may remain in place for 24 hours and then removed; however, drops should continue to be instilled into ear canal as long as indicated.

Nursing Actions

Physical Assessment See individual agents.

Patient Education

- Discuss specific use of drug and side effects with patient as it relates to treatment. (HCAHPS: During this hospital stay, were you given any medicine that you had not taken before? Before giving you any new medicine, how often did hospital staff tell you what the medicine was for? How often did hospital staff describe possible side effects in a way you could understand?)
- Patient may experience ear discomfort. Have patient report immediately to prescriber severe otalgia or significant skin irritation (HCAHPS).
- Educate patient about signs of a significant reaction (eg, wheezing; chest tightness; fever; itching; bad cough; blue skin color; seizures; or swelling of face, lips, tongue, or throat). **Note:** This is not a comprehensive list of all side effects. Patient should consult prescriber for additional questions.

Intended Use and Disclaimer: Should not be printed and given to patients. This information is intended to serve as a concise initial reference for healthcare professionals to use when discussing medications with a patient. You must ultimately rely on your own discretion, experience and judgment in diagnosing, treating and advising patients.

Aclidinium (a kli DIN ee um)

Brand Names: U.S. Tudorza Pressair
Index Terms 14115700; Aclidinium Bromide; LAS-34273; LAS-34273 Micronized; LAS-W-330
Pharmacologic Category Anticholinergic Agent; Anticholinergic Agent, Long-Acting
Medication Safety Issues
Sound-alike/look-alike issues:
Aclidinium may be confused with clidinium
Tudorza™ may be confused with Jolessa™, Lodosyn®, Taclonex®, Tekturna HCT®, Tekturna®, Tikosyn®, Tobrex®, Toradol®, Truvada®, Tubersol®, Zaditor®
Pressair™ may be confused with Provera®, Precose®, Primacor®
Pregnancy Risk Factor C
Lactation Excretion in breast milk/unknown/use caution
Breast-Feeding Considerations Excretion of aclidinium into human milk is probable. The manufacturer recommends caution should be exercised when administering to nursing women.
Use Long-term maintenance treatment of bronchospasm associated with COPD (including bronchitis and emphysema)
Mechanism of Action/Effect Blocks the action of acetylcholine at parasympathetic sites in bronchial smooth muscle causing bronchodilation

Contraindications There are no contraindications listed in the manufacturer's labeling.

Warnings/Precautions Rarely, paradoxical bronchospasm may occur with use of inhaled bronchodilating agents; discontinue use and consider other therapy if bronchospasm occurs. Not indicated for the initial (rescue) treatment of acute episodes of bronchospasm. Use with caution in patients with myasthenia gravis, narrow-angle glaucoma, prostatic hyperplasia, bladder neck obstruction, or history of hypersensitivity to atropine. Immediate hypersensitivity reactions may occur; discontinue immediately if signs/symptoms occur. The Tudorza™ Pressair™ powder for inhalation contains lactose; use with caution in patients with severe milk protein allergy.

Drug Interactions

Avoid Concomitant Use
Avoid concomitant use of Aclidinium with any of the following: Anticholinergics; Ipratropium (Oral Inhalation); Potassium Chloride; Tiotropium; Umeclidinium

Decreased Effect
Aclidinium may decrease the levels/effects of: Acetylcholinesterase Inhibitors (Central); Secretin

The levels/effects of Aclidinium may be decreased by: Acetylcholinesterase Inhibitors (Central); Peginterferon Alfa-2b

Increased Effect/Toxicity
Aclidinium may increase the levels/effects of: AbobotulinumtoxinA; Analgesics (Opioid); Anticholinergics; Cannabinoids; Mirabegron; OnabotulinumtoxinA; Potassium Chloride; RimabotulinumtoxinB; Thiazide Diuretics; Tiotropium; Topiramate

The levels/effects of Aclidinium may be increased by: Ipratropium (Oral Inhalation); Pramlintide; Umeclidinium

Adverse Reactions 1% to 10%:
Central nervous system: Headache (7%)
Gastrointestinal: Diarrhea (3%), vomiting (1%)
Neuromuscular & skeletal: Fall (1%)
Respiratory: Nasopharyngitis (6%), cough (3%), rhinitis (2%), sinusitis (2%)
Miscellaneous: Toothache (1%)

Available Dosage Forms
Aerosol Powder Breath Activated, Inhalation:
Tudorza Pressair: 400 mcg/actuation (1 ea)
General Dosage Range Inhalation, oral: *Adults:* 400 mcg twice daily

Administration

Inhalation Administer via oral inhalation. Prior to first use, remove from sealed pouch immediately before use. Prior to each use, remove protective cap from Tudorza™ Pressair™ inhaler and prepare inhaler by pressing and releasing the green button (while keeping the green button straight up and avoiding tilting the inhaler). After this step, ensure that the inhaler is ready for use by the colored control window which should have changed from red to green. The green control window indicates the inhaler is ready for use. If the control window is red, retry activating the inhaler again by pressing and releasing the green button. Prior to inhaling the dose, exhale fully (do not exhale into the inhaler), then close lips tightly around the inhaler mouthpiece and inhale (rapidly, steadily, and deeply); do not hold the green button down while inhaling. Keep breathing in until a "click" is heard to ensure that the full dose has been given. Hold breath as long as possible, then breathe out slowly through nose. Ensure the dose was delivered correctly by observing the control window which should have changed from green to red. If the control window is still green, repeat inhalation steps. When control window has been verified as red, replace the protective cap for next use.

Storage/Stability Store at 25°C (77°F); excursions permitted between 15°C to 30°C (59°F to 86°F). Protect from moisture. Product should be stored inside sealed pouch and only removed immediately before use. Discard product 45 days after opening pouch, when device locks out, or when dose indicator displays "0", whichever comes first.

Nursing Actions

Patient Education

• Discuss specific use of drug and side effects with patient as it relates to treatment. (HCAHPS: During this hospital stay, were you given any medicine that you had not taken before? Before giving you any new medicine, how often did hospital staff tell you what the medicine was for? How often did hospital staff describe possible side effects in a way you could understand?)

• Patient may experience headache, pharyngitis, or rhinitis. Have patient report immediately to prescriber vision changes, ophthalmalgia, severe eye irritation, urinary retention, difficult urination, polyuria, dyspnea, or wheezing (HCAHPS).

• Educate patient about signs of a significant reaction (eg, wheezing; chest tightness; fever; itching; bad cough; blue skin color; seizures; or swelling of face, lips, tongue, or throat). **Note:** This is not a comprehensive list of all side effects. Patient should consult prescriber for additional questions.

Intended Use and Disclaimer: Should not be printed and given to patients. This information is intended to serve as a concise initial reference for healthcare professionals to use when discussing medications with a patient. You must ultimately rely on your own discretion, experience and judgment in diagnosing, treating and advising patients.

Acyclovir (Systemic) (ay SYE kloe veer)

Brand Names: U.S. Zovirax

Index Terms Aciclovir; ACV; Acycloguanosine

Pharmacologic Category Antiviral Agent

Medication Safety Issues

Sound-alike/look-alike issues:

Acyclovir may be confused with ganciclovir, Retrovir, valacyclovir

Zovirax may be confused with Doribax, Valtrex, Zithromax, Zostrix, Zyloprim, Zyvox

Pregnancy Risk Factor B

Lactation Enters breast milk/use with caution

Breast-Feeding Considerations Acyclovir is excreted in breast milk. The manufacturer recommends that caution be exercised when administering acyclovir to nursing women. Limited data suggest exposure to the nursing infant of ~0.3 mg/kg/day following oral administration of acyclovir to the mother. Nursing mothers with herpetic lesions near or on the breast should avoid breast-feeding (Gartner, 2005).

Use Treatment of genital herpes simplex virus (HSV) and HSV encephalitis

Unlabeled Use Prevention of HSV reactivation in HIV-positive patients; prevention of HSV reactivation in hematopoietic stem cell transplant (HSCT); prevention of HSV reactivation during periods of neutropenia in patients with cancer; prevention of varicella zoster virus (VZV) reactivation in allogenic HSCT; prevention of CMV reactivation in low-risk allogeneic HSCT; treatment of disseminated HSV or VZV in immunocompromised patients with cancer; empiric treatment of suspected encephalitis in immunocompromised patients with cancer; treatment of initial and prophylaxis of recurrent mucosal and cutaneous herpes simplex (HSV-1 and HSV-2) infections in immunocompromised patients

Mechanism of Action/Effect Inhibits DNA synthesis and viral replication

Contraindications Hypersensitivity to acyclovir, valacyclovir, or any component of the formulation

Warnings/Precautions Use with caution in immunocompromised patients; thrombocytopenic purpura/hemolytic uremic syndrome (TTP/HUS) has been reported. Use caution in the elderly, preexisting renal disease (may require dosage modification), or in those receiving other nephrotoxic drugs. Renal failure (sometimes fatal) has been reported. Maintain adequate hydration during oral or intravenous therapy. Use I.V. preparation with caution in patients with underlying neurologic abnormalities, serious hepatic or electrolyte abnormalities, or substantial hypoxia.

Varicella-zoster: Treatment should begin within 24 hours of appearance of rash; oral route not recommended for routine use in otherwise healthy children with varicella, but may be effective in patients at increased risk of moderate-to-severe infection (>12 years of age, chronic cutaneous or pulmonary disorders, long-term salicylate therapy, corticosteroid therapy).

Drug Interactions

Avoid Concomitant Use

Avoid concomitant use of Acyclovir (Systemic) with any of the following: Zoster Vaccine

Decreased Effect

Acyclovir (Systemic) may decrease the levels/effects of: Zoster Vaccine

Increased Effect/Toxicity

Acyclovir (Systemic) may increase the levels/effects of: Mycophenolate; Tenofovir; Zidovudine

The levels/effects of Acyclovir (Systemic) may be increased by: Mycophenolate

Nutritional/Ethanol Interactions Food: Does not affect absorption of oral acyclovir.

Adverse Reactions

Oral:

>10%: Central nervous system: Malaise (≤12%)

1% to 10%:

Central nervous system: Headache (≤2%)

Gastrointestinal: Nausea (2% to 5%), vomiting (≤3%), diarrhea (2% to 3%)

Parenteral:

1% to 10%:

Dermatologic: Hives (2%), itching (2%), rash (2%)

Gastrointestinal: Nausea/vomiting (7%)

Hepatic: Liver function tests increased (1% to 2%)

Local: Inflammation at injection site or phlebitis (9%)

Renal: BUN increased (5% to 10%), creatinine increased (5% to 10%), acute renal failure

Available Dosage Forms

Capsule, Oral:

Zovirax: 200 mg

Generic: 200 mg

Solution, Intravenous:

Generic: 50 mg/mL (10 mL, 20 mL)

Solution Reconstituted, Intravenous:

Generic: 500 mg (1 ea); 1000 mg (1 ea)

Suspension, Oral:

Zovirax: 200 mg/5 mL (473 mL)

Generic: 200 mg/5 mL (473 mL)

Tablet, Oral:

Zovirax: 400 mg, 800 mg

Generic: 400 mg, 800 mg

General Dosage Range Dosage adjustment recommended in patients with renal impairment

I.V.:

Children <12 years: 10-20 mg/kg/dose every 8 hours (maximum: 60 mg/kg/day)

Children ≥12 years and Adults: 5-10 mg/kg/dose or 500 mg/m^2/dose every 8 hours (maximum: 45 mg/kg/day)

Oral:

Children ≥2 years and ≤40 kg: 20 mg/kg/dose 4 times daily (maximum: 800 mg per dose)

Children ≥2 years and >40 kg: 800 mg 4 times daily

Adults: 200-800 mg/dose 3-5 times daily

Administration

I.V. For I.V. infusion only. Avoid rapid infusion. Infuse over 1 hour to prevent renal damage. Maintain adequate hydration of patient. Check for phlebitis and rotate infusion sites. Avoid I.M. or SubQ administration.

Injectable Detail pH: 10.5-11.6 (reconstituted solution)

Oral May be administered with or without food.

Preparation for Administration Powder for injection: Reconstitute acyclovir 500 mg powder with SWFI 10 mL; do not use bacteriostatic water containing benzyl alcohol or parabens. For intravenous infusion, dilute in D$_5$W, D$_5$NS, D$_5$1/4NS, D$_5$1/2NS, LR, or NS to a final concentration ≤7 mg/mL. Concentrations >10 mg/mL increase the risk of phlebitis.

Storage/Stability

Capsule, tablet: Store at controlled room temperature of 15°C to 25°C (59°F to 77°F); protect from moisture.

Injection: Store powder at controlled room temperature of 15°C to 25°C (59°F to 77°F). Reconstituted solutions remain stable for 12 hours at room temperature. Do not refrigerate reconstituted solutions or solutions diluted for infusion as they may precipitate. Once diluted for infusion, use within 24 hours.

Nursing Actions

Physical Assessment Patient should be adequately hydrated during I.V. therapy and monitored closely during intravenous administration.

Patient Education

• Discuss specific use of drug and side effects with patient as it relates to treatment. (HCAHPS: During this hospital stay, were you given any medicine that you had not taken before? Before giving you any new medicine, how often did hospital staff tell you what the medicine was for? How often did hospital staff describe possible side effects in a way you could understand?)

• Patient may experience headache, nausea, diarrhea, asthenia, or injection site irritation. Have patient report immediately to prescriber signs of hepatic impairment, behavioral changes, mood changes, hallucinations, tremors, chills, pharyngitis, severe renal impairment, or signs of thrombotic thrombocytopenic purpura/hemolytic uremic syndrome (TTP/HUS) (HCAHPS).

• Educate patient about signs of a significant reaction (eg, wheezing; chest tightness; fever; itching; bad cough; blue skin color; seizures; or swelling of face, lips, tongue, or throat). **Note:** This is not a comprehensive list of all side effects. Patient should consult prescriber for additional questions.

Intended Use and Disclaimer: Should not be printed and given to patients. This information is intended to serve as a concise initial reference for

healthcare professionals to use when discussing medications with a patient. You must ultimately rely on your own discretion, experience and judgment in diagnosing, treating and advising patients.

Dietary Considerations May be taken with or without food. Some products may contain sodium.

Related Information

Management of Drug Extravasations *on page 1700*

Acyclovir (Topical) (ay SYE kloe veer)

Brand Names: U.S. Zovirax

Index Terms Aciclovir; ACV; Acycloguanosine; Sitavig®

Pharmacologic Category Antiviral Agent, Topical

Medication Safety Issues

Sound-alike/look-alike issues:

Acyclovir may be confused with ganciclovir, Retrovir®, valacyclovir

Zovirax® may be confused with Doribax®, Valtrex®, Zithromax®, Zostrix®, Zyloprim®, Zyvox®

International issues:

Opthavir [Mexico] may be confused with Optivar brand name for azelastine [U.S.]

Pregnancy Risk Factor B

Use Treatment of herpes labialis (cold sores), mucocutaneous HSV in immunocompromised patients

Product Availability

Sitavig®: FDA approved April 2013; anticipated availability is currently unknown

Sitavig® buccal tablets are indicated for the treatment of recurrent herpes labialis (cold sores) in immunocompetent adults.

Available Dosage Forms

Cream, External:

Zovirax: 5% (5 g)

Ointment, External:

Zovirax: 5% (30 g)

Generic: 5% (5 g, 15 g, 30 g)

General Dosage Range Topical:

Children ≥12 years: Cream: Apply 5 times/day

Adults: Cream: Apply 5 times/day; Ointment: 1/2" ribbon for a 4" square surface area 6 times/day

Administration

Topical Not for use in the eye. Apply using a finger cot or rubber glove to avoid transmission to other parts of the body or to other persons.

Nursing Actions

Patient Education

• Discuss specific use of drug and side effects with patient as it relates to treatment. (HCAHPS: During this hospital stay, were you given any medicine that you had not taken before? Before giving you any new medicine, how often did hospital staff tell you what the medicine was

for? How often did hospital staff describe possible side effects in a way you could understand?)

• Patient may experience xeroderma. Have patient report immediately to prescriber severe application site irritation (HCAHPS).

• Educate patient about signs of a significant reaction (eg, wheezing; chest tightness; fever; itching; bad cough; blue skin color; seizures; or swelling of face, lips, tongue, or throat). **Note:** This is not a comprehensive list of all side effects. Patient should consult prescriber for additional questions.

Intended Use and Disclaimer: Should not be printed and given to patients. This information is intended to serve as a concise initial reference for healthcare professionals to use when discussing medications with a patient. You must ultimately rely on your own discretion, experience and judgment in diagnosing, treating and advising patients.

Acyclovir and Hydrocortisone
(ay SYE kloe veer & hye droe KOR ti sone)

Brand Names: U.S. Xerese™

Index Terms Hydrocortisone and Acyclovir; ME-609; Xerclear

Pharmacologic Category Antiviral Agent, Topical; Corticosteroid, Topical

Pregnancy Risk Factor B

Lactation Excretion in breast milk unknown/use caution

Use Treatment of recurrent herpes labialis (cold sores)

Available Dosage Forms

Cream, topical:

Xerese®: Acyclovir 5% and hydrocortisone 1% (5 g)

General Dosage Range Topical: *Children ≥12 years and Adults:* Apply 5 times/day

Administration

Topical For external use only; not for use in the eye, inside the mouth or nose, or on the genitals. Apply to clean, dry area using a finger cot or rubber glove to avoid transmission to other parts of the body or to other persons. Use sufficient amount to cover the affected area(s), including the outer margin of cold sore; do not rub affected area. Initiate therapy early (ie, during the prodrome or when lesions appear).

Nursing Actions

Physical Assessment See individual agents.

Patient Education

• Discuss specific use of drug and side effects with patient as it relates to treatment. (HCAHPS: During this hospital stay, were you given any medicine that you had not taken before? Before giving you any new medicine, how often did hospital staff tell you what the medicine was

for? How often did hospital staff describe possible side effects in a way you could understand?)
• Patient may experience parageusia or xeroderma. Have patient report immediately to prescriber severe skin irritation (HCAHPS).
• Educate patient about signs of a significant reaction (eg, wheezing; chest tightness; fever; itching; bad cough; blue skin color; seizures; or swelling of face, lips, tongue, or throat). **Note:** This is not a comprehensive list of all side effects. Patient should consult prescriber for additional questions.

Intended Use and Disclaimer: Should not be printed and given to patients. This information is intended to serve as a concise initial reference for healthcare professionals to use when discussing medications with a patient. You must ultimately rely on your own discretion, experience and judgment in diagnosing, treating and advising patients.

Adalimumab (a da LIM yoo mab)

Brand Names: U.S. Humira; Humira Pen; Humira Pen-Crohns Starter; Humira Pen-Psoriasis Starter
Index Terms Antitumor Necrosis Factor Alpha (Human); D2E7; Human Antitumor Necrosis Factor Alpha
Pharmacologic Category Antirheumatic, Disease Modifying; Gastrointestinal Agent, Miscellaneous; Monoclonal Antibody; Tumor Necrosis Factor (TNF) Blocking Agent
Medication Safety Issues
Sound-alike/look-alike issues:
Humira may be confused with Humulin, Humalog
Humira Pen may be confused with HumaPen Memoir
Medication Guide Available Yes
Pregnancy Risk Factor B
Lactation Enters breast milk/use caution
Breast-Feeding Considerations Low concentrations of adalimumab may be detected in breast milk but are unlikely to be absorbed by a nursing infant. The manufacturer recommends caution be used if administered to a nursing woman.
Use
Ankylosing spondylitis: Treatment of ankylosing spondylitis (may be used in combination with methotrexate or other nonbiologic disease-modifying antirheumatic drugs (DMARDS)
Crohn's disease: Treatment of active Crohn's disease (moderate-to-severe) in patients with inadequate response to conventional treatment, or patients who have lost response to or are intolerant of infliximab
Juvenile idiopathic arthritis: Treatment of active juvenile idiopathic arthritis (moderate-to-severe); may be used alone or in combination with methotrexate

Plaque psoriasis: Treatment of chronic plaque psoriasis (moderate-to-severe) when systemic therapy is required and other agents are less appropriate
Psoriatic arthritis: Treatment of active psoriatic arthritis; may be used alone or in combination with methotrexate or other DMARDs
Rheumatoid arthritis: Treatment of active rheumatoid arthritis (moderate-to-severe); may be used alone or in combination with methotrexate or other DMARDs
Ulcerative colitis: Treatment of active ulcerative colitis (moderate-to-severe) in patients unresponsive to immunosuppressants (**Note:** Efficacy in patients that are intolerant to or no longer responsive to other TNF blockers has not been established.)

Canadian labeling: Additional use (not in U.S. labeling): Crohn's disease, pediatric: Treatment of adolescents with active Crohn's disease (moderate-to-severe) who have had an inadequate response to conventional treatment and/or other TNF blockers
Mechanism of Action/Effect Adalimumab decreases signs and symptoms of psoriatic arthritis, rheumatoid arthritis, Crohn's disease, ulcerative colitis, and ankylosing spondylitis; inhibits progression of structural damage in rheumatoid and psoriatic arthritis
Contraindications There are no contraindications listed within the FDA-approved labeling.

Canadian labeling: Hypersensitivity to adalimumab or any component of the formulation; severe infection (eg, sepsis, tuberculosis, opportunistic infection); moderate-to-severe heart failure (NYHA class III/IV)
Warnings/Precautions [U.S. Boxed Warnings]: Patients should be evaluated for latent tuberculosis infection with a tuberculin skin test prior to therapy. Treatment of latent tuberculosis should be initiated before adalimumab is used. Tuberculosis (disseminated or extrapulmonary) has been reactivated while on adalimumab. Most cases have been reported within the first 8 months of treatment. **Patients with initial negative tuberculin skin tests should receive continued monitoring for tuberculosis throughout treatment; active tuberculosis has developed in this population during treatment.** Rare reactivation of hepatitis B virus (HBV) has occurred in chronic virus carriers; use with caution; evaluate prior to initiation and during treatment.

[U.S. Boxed Warning]: Patients receiving adalimumab are at increased risk for serious infections which may result in hospitalization and/or fatality; infections usually developed in patients receiving concomitant immunosuppressive agents (eg, methotrexate or corticosteroids) and may present as disseminated (rather than local) disease. Active tuberculosis ▶

(or reactivation of latent tuberculosis), invasive fungal (including aspergillosis, blastomycosis, candidiasis, coccidioidomycosis, histoplasmosis, and pneumocystosis) and bacterial, viral or other opportunistic infections (including legionellosis and listeriosis) have been reported in patients receiving TNF-blocking agents, including adalimumab. Monitor closely for signs/symptoms of infection. Discontinue for serious infection or sepsis. Consider risks versus benefits prior to use in patients with a history of chronic or recurrent infection. Consider empiric antifungal therapy in patients who are at risk for invasive fungal infection and develop severe systemic illness. Caution should be exercised when considering use in the elderly or in patients with conditions that predispose them to infections (eg, diabetes) or residence/travel from areas of endemic mycoses (blastomycosis, coccidioidomycosis, histoplasmosis), or with latent or localized infections. Do not initiate adalimumab therapy with clinically important active infection. Patients who develop a new infection while undergoing treatment should be monitored closely. There is limited experience with patients undergoing surgical procedures while on therapy; consider long half-life with planned procedures and monitor closely for infection.

[U.S. Boxed Warning]: Lymphoma and other malignancies (some fatal) have been reported in children and adolescent patients receiving TNF-blocking agents, including adalimumab. Half the cases are lymphomas (Hodgkin and non-Hodgkin) and the other cases are varied, but include malignancies not typically observed in this population. Most patients were receiving concomitant immunosuppressants. **[U.S. Boxed Warning]: Hepatosplenic T-cell lymphoma (HSTCL), a rare T-cell lymphoma, has also been reported primarily in patients with Crohn's disease or ulcerative colitis treated with adalimumab and who received concomitant azathioprine or mercaptopurine; reports occurred predominantly in adolescent and young adult males.** Rare cases of lymphoma have also been reported in association with adalimumab. A higher incidence of nonmelanoma skin cancers was noted in adalimumab treated patients, when compared to the control group. Impact on the development and course of malignancies is not fully defined. May exacerbate pre-existing or recent-onset central or peripheral nervous system demyelinating disorders. Consider discontinuing use in patients who develop peripheral or central nervous system demyelinating disorders during treatment.

May exacerbate pre-existing or recent-onset demyelinating CNS disorders. Worsening and new-onset heart failure (HF) has been reported; use caution in patients with decreased left ventricular function. Use caution in patients with HF (Canadian labeling contraindicates use in NYHA III/IV). Patients should be brought up to date with all immunizations before initiating therapy. No data are available concerning the effects of adalimumab on vaccination. Live vaccines should not be given concurrently. No data are available concerning secondary transmission of live vaccines in patients receiving adalimumab. Rare cases of pancytopenia (including aplastic anemia) have been reported with TNF-blocking agents; with significant hematologic abnormalities, consider discontinuing therapy. Positive antinuclear antibody titers have been detected in patients (with negative baselines) treated with adalimumab. Rare cases of autoimmune disorder, including lupus-like syndrome, have been reported; monitor and discontinue adalimumab if symptoms develop. May cause hypersensitivity reactions, including anaphylaxis; monitor. Infection and malignancy has been reported at a higher incidence in elderly patients compared to younger adults; use caution in elderly patients. Potentially significant drug-drug interactions may exist, requiring dose or frequency adjustment, additional monitoring, and/or selection of alternative therapy. The packaging (needle cover of prefilled syringe) may contain latex. Product may contain polysorbate 80. According to the Centers for Disease Control and Prevention (CDC), pen-shaped injection devices should never be used for more than one person (even when the needle is changed) because of the risk of infection. The injection device should be clearly labeled with individual patient information to ensure that the correct pen is used (CDC, 2012).

Drug Interactions

Avoid Concomitant Use

Avoid concomitant use of Adalimumab with any of the following: Abatacept; Anakinra; BCG; Belimumab; Canakinumab; Certolizumab Pegol; InFLIXimab; Natalizumab; Pimecrolimus; Rilonacept; Tacrolimus (Topical); Tocilizumab; Tofacitinib; Vaccines (Live)

Decreased Effect

Adalimumab may decrease the levels/effects of: BCG; Coccidioidin Skin Test; CycloSPORINE (Systemic); Sipuleucel-T; Theophylline Derivatives; Vaccines (Inactivated); Vaccines (Live); Warfarin

The levels/effects of Adalimumab may be decreased by: Echinacea

Increased Effect/Toxicity

Adalimumab may increase the levels/effects of: Abatacept; Anakinra; Belimumab; Canakinumab; Certolizumab Pegol; InFLIXimab; Leflunomide; Natalizumab; Rilonacept; Tofacitinib; Vaccines (Live)

The levels/effects of Adalimumab may be increased by: Abciximab; Denosumab; Pimecrolimus; Roflumilast; Tacrolimus (Topical); Tocilizumab; Trastuzumab

Nutritional/Ethanol Interactions Herb/nutraceutical: Echinacea may decrease the therapeutic effects of adalimumab; avoid concurrent use.

Adverse Reactions

>10%:

Central nervous system: Headache (12%)

Dermatologic: Skin rash (6% to 12%)

Hematologic & oncologic: Positive ANA titer (12%)

Immunologic: Antibody development (3% to 26%; significance unknown)

Infection: Serious infection (adults 1.4-6.7 events/ 100 person years; children 2 events/100 person years [Burmester, 2012])

Local: Injection site reaction (12% to 20%; includes erythema, itching, hemorrhage, pain, swelling)

Neuromuscular & skeletal: Increased creatine phosphokinase (15%)

Respiratory: Upper respiratory tract infection (17%), sinusitis (11%)

5% to 10%:

Cardiovascular: Hypertension (5%)

Endocrine & metabolic: Hyperlipidemia (7%), hypercholesterolemia (6%)

Gastrointestinal: Nausea (9%), abdominal pain (7%)

Genitourinary: Urinary tract infection (8%), hematuria (5%)

Hepatic: Increased serum alkaline phosphatase (5%)

Hypersensitivity: Hypersensitivity reaction (children 6%; adults 1%)

Local: Injection site reaction (8%; other than erythema, itching, hemorrhage, pain, swelling)

Neuromuscular & skeletal: Back pain (6%)

Respiratory: Flu-like symptoms (7%)

Miscellaneous: Accidental injury (10%)

1% to 5%:

Cardiovascular: Atrial fibrillation, cardiac arrest, cardiac arrhythmia, cardiac failure, chest pain, coronary artery disease, deep vein thrombosis, hypertensive encephalopathy, myocardial infarction, palpitations, pericardial effusion, pericarditis, peripheral edema, subdural hematoma, syncope, tachycardia, vascular disease

Central nervous system: Confusion, myasthenia, paresthesia

Dermatologic: Alopecia, cellulitis, erysipelas

Endocrine & metabolic: Dehydration, ketosis, menstrual disease, parathyroid disease

Gastrointestinal: Cholecystitis, cholelithiasis, diverticulitis, esophagitis, gastroenteritis, gastrointestinal hemorrhage, vomiting

Genitourinary: Cystitis, pelvic pain

Hematologic & oncologic: Adenoma, agranulocytosis, carcinoma (including breast, gastrointestinal, skin, urogenital), granulocytopenia, leukopenia, malignant lymphoma, malignant melanoma, pancytopenia, paraproteinemia, polycythemia

Hepatic: Hepatic necrosis

Infection: Herpes zoster, sepsis

Neuromuscular & skeletal: Arthralgia, arthritis, arthropathy, bone fracture, limb pain, multiple sclerosis, muscle cramps, myasthenia, osteonecrosis, septic arthritis, synovitis, systemic lupus erythematosus, tendon disease, tremor

Ophthalmic: Cataract

Renal: Nephrolithiasis, pyelonephritis

Respiratory: Asthma, bronchospasm, dyspnea, pleural effusion, pneumonia, respiratory depression, tuberculosis (including reactivation of latent infection; disseminated, miliary, lymphatic, peritoneal, and pulmonary)

Miscellaneous: Abnormal healing, fever, postoperative complication (infection)

Available Dosage Forms

Kit, Subcutaneous [preservative free]:

Humira: 20 mg/0.4 mL, 40 mg/0.8 mL

Humira Pen: 40 mg/0.8 mL

Humira Pen-Crohns Starter: 40 mg/0.8 mL

Humira Pen-Psoriasis Starter: 40 mg/0.8 mL

General Dosage Range SubQ:

Children ≥4 years: 15 kg to <30 kg: 20 mg every other week; ≥30 kg: 40 mg every other week

Adults: Initial: 40-160 mg; Maintenance: 40 mg every other week (maximum: 40 mg every week)

Administration

Subcutaneous For SubQ injection (into thigh or lower abdomen, avoiding areas within 2 inches of navel); rotate injection sites. Do not use if solution is discolored or contains particulate matter. Do not administer to skin which is red, tender, bruised, or hard. Needle cap of the prefilled syringe may contain latex. Prefilled pens and syringes are available for use by patients (self-administration); the vial is intended for institutional use only. Vials do not contain a preservative; discard unused portion.

Storage/Stability Store under refrigeration at 2°C to 8°C (36°F to 46°F); do not freeze. Protect from light.

Nursing Actions

Physical Assessment Monitor for signs and symptoms of tuberculosis, other infections, enlarged lymph nodes, or skin lesions/eruptions. Assess for liver dysfunction (unusual fatigue, easy bruising or bleeding, jaundice). Monitor PDD at regular intervals during treatment. Teach patient proper injection technique and syringe/ needle disposal. Latex-sensitive patients: Needle cap of prefilled syringe contains latex.

Patient Education

• Discuss specific use of drug and side effects with patient as it relates to treatment. (HCAHPS: During this hospital stay, were you given any medicine that you had not taken before? Before giving you any new medicine, how often did hospital staff tell you what the medicine was for? How often did hospital staff describe possible side effects in a way you could understand?)

• Patient may experience rhinitis, rhinorrhea, dyspepsia, back pain, or injection site irritation. Have patient report immediately to prescriber signs of infection, signs of lupus, dyspnea, excessive weight gain, edema of extremities, angina, severe headache, significant asthenia, paresthesia, considerable dizziness, syncope, ecchymosis, hemorrhaging, night sweats, mole changes, skin growth, hematuria, pallor, severe skin irritation, or signs of hepatic impairment (HCAHPS).

• Educate patient about signs of a significant reaction (eg, wheezing; chest tightness; fever; itching; bad cough; blue skin color; seizures; or swelling of face, lips, tongue, or throat). **Note:** This is not a comprehensive list of all side effects. Patient should consult prescriber for additional questions.

Intended Use and Disclaimer: Should not be printed and given to patients. This information is intended to serve as a concise initial reference for healthcare professionals to use when discussing medications with a patient. You must ultimately rely on your own discretion, experience and judgment in diagnosing, treating and advising patients.

Adapalene (a DAP a leen)

Brand Names: U.S. Differin
Pharmacologic Category Acne Products; Topical Skin Product, Acne
Pregnancy Risk Factor C
Lactation Excretion in breast milk unknown/use caution
Use Treatment of acne vulgaris
Available Dosage Forms
Cream, External:
Differin: 0.1% (45 g)
Generic: 0.1% (45 g)
Gel, External:
Differin: 0.1% (45 g); 0.3% (45 g)
Generic: 0.1% (45 g)
Lotion, External:
Differin: 0.1% (59 mL)
General Dosage Range Topical: *Children >12 years and Adults:* Apply once daily at bedtime
Administration
Topical For external use only. Apply a thin film at night to clean/dry skin; avoid contact with abraded, eczematous, or sunburned skin, mucous membranes, eyes, mouth and angles of the nose. Moisturizers may be used if necessary; avoid alpha hydroxy or glycolic acid-containing products.
Nursing Actions
Patient Education
• Discuss specific use of drug and side effects with patient as it relates to treatment. (HCAHPS: During this hospital stay, were you given any

medicine that you had not taken before? Before giving you any new medicine, how often did hospital staff tell you what the medicine was for? How often did hospital staff describe possible side effects in a way you could understand?)

• Patient may experience warmth sensation or xeroderma. Have patient report immediately to prescriber severe skin irritation or application site edema or peeling (HCAHPS).

• Educate patient about signs of a significant reaction (eg, wheezing; chest tightness; fever; itching; bad cough; blue skin color; seizures; or swelling of face, lips, tongue, or throat). **Note:** This is not a comprehensive list of all side effects. Patient should consult prescriber for additional questions.

Intended Use and Disclaimer: Should not be printed and given to patients. This information is intended to serve as a concise initial reference for healthcare professionals to use when discussing medications with a patient. You must ultimately rely on your own discretion, experience and judgment in diagnosing, treating and advising patients.

Adapalene and Benzoyl Peroxide
(a DAP a leen & BEN zoe il peer OKS ide)

Brand Names: U.S. Epiduo®
Index Terms Benzoyl Peroxide and Adapalene
Pharmacologic Category Acne Products; Topical Skin Product; Topical Skin Product, Acne
Pregnancy Risk Factor C
Lactation Excretion in breast milk unknown/use caution
Use Topical treatment of acne vulgaris
Available Dosage Forms
Gel, topical:
Epiduo®: Adapalene 0.1% and benzoyl peroxide 2.5% (45 g)
General Dosage Range Topical: *Children ≥9 years, Adolescents, and Adults:* Apply once daily
Administration
Topical Apply a pea-sized amount for each area of the face (eg, forehead, chin, each cheek). Skin should be clean and dry before applying. For external use only; avoid applying to eyes and mucous membranes.
Nursing Actions
Patient Education
• Discuss specific use of drug and side effects with patient as it relates to treatment. (HCAHPS: During this hospital stay, were you given any medicine that you had not taken before? Before giving you any new medicine, how often did hospital staff tell you what the medicine was for? How often did hospital staff describe possible side effects in a way you could understand?)
• Patient may experience warmth sensation, xeroderma, or application site scaling or burning.

Have patient report immediately to prescriber severe skin irritation or application site edema or peeling (HCAHPS).
• Educate patient about signs of a significant reaction (eg, wheezing; chest tightness; fever; itching; bad cough; blue skin color; seizures; or swelling of face, lips, tongue, or throat). **Note:** This is not a comprehensive list of all side effects. Patient should consult prescriber for additional questions.

Intended Use and Disclaimer: Should not be printed and given to patients. This information is intended to serve as a concise initial reference for healthcare professionals to use when discussing medications with a patient. You must ultimately rely on your own discretion, experience and judgment in diagnosing, treating and advising patients.

Adefovir (a DEF o veer)

Brand Names: U.S. Hepsera
Index Terms Adefovir Dipivoxil; Bis-POM PMEA
Pharmacologic Category Antihepadnaviral, Reverse Transcriptase Inhibitor, Nucleotide (Anti-HBV)
Pregnancy Risk Factor C
Lactation Excretion in breast milk unknown/not recommended
Breast-Feeding Considerations It is not known if adefovir is excreted in breast milk. Due to the potential for serious adverse reactions in the nursing infant, a decision should be made whether to discontinue nursing or to discontinue the drug, taking into account the importance of treatment to the mother.
Use Treatment of chronic hepatitis B with evidence of active viral replication (based on persistent elevation of ALT/AST or histologic evidence), including patients with lamivudine-resistant hepatitis B
Mechanism of Action/Effect Acyclic nucleotide reverse transcriptase inhibitor (adenosine analog) which interferes with HBV viral DNA polymerase resulting in inhibition of viral replication
Contraindications Hypersensitivity to adefovir or any component of the formulation
Warnings/Precautions [U.S. Boxed Warning]: Use with caution in patients with renal dysfunction or in patients at risk of renal toxicity (including concurrent nephrotoxic agents or NSAIDs). Chronic administration may result in nephrotoxicity. Dosage adjustment is required in adult patients with renal dysfunction or in patients who develop renal dysfunction during therapy; no data available for use in children ≥12 years or adolescents with renal impairment. Not recommended as first line therapy of chronic HBV due to weak antiviral activity and high rate of resistance after first year. May be more appropriate as second-line agent in treatment-naïve patients.

Combination therapy with lamivudine in nucleoside-naïve patients has not been shown to provide synergistic antiviral effects. In patients with lamivudine-resistant HBV, switching to adefovir monotherapy was associated with a higher risk of adefovir resistance compared to adding adefovir to lamivudine therapy (Lok, 2009).

Calculate creatinine clearance before initiation of therapy. Consider alternative therapy in patients who do not respond to adefovir monotherapy treatment. **[U.S. Boxed Warning]: May cause the development of HIV resistance in patients with unrecognized or untreated HIV infection.** Determine HIV status prior to initiating treatment with adefovir. **[U.S. Boxed Warning]: Fatal cases of lactic acidosis and severe hepatomegaly with steatosis have been reported with the use of nucleoside analogues alone or in combination with other antiretrovirals.** Female gender, obesity, and prolonged treatment may increase the risk of hepatotoxicity. Treatment should be discontinued in patients with lactic acidosis or signs/symptoms of hepatotoxicity (which may occur without marked transaminase elevations). **[U.S. Boxed Warning]: Acute exacerbations of hepatitis may occur (in up to 25% of patients) when antihepatitis therapy is discontinued.** Exacerbations typically occur within 12 weeks and may be self-limited or resolve upon resuming treatment; risk may be increased with advanced liver disease or cirrhosis. Monitor patients following discontinuation of therapy. Safety and efficacy in children <12 years of age have not been established. Do not use concurrently with tenofovir (Viread®) or any product containing tenofovir (eg, Truvada®, Atripla®, Complera®).

Drug Interactions
Avoid Concomitant Use
   Avoid concomitant use of Adefovir with any of the following: Tenofovir
Decreased Effect
   Adefovir may decrease the levels/effects of: Tenofovir
Increased Effect/Toxicity
   Adefovir may increase the levels/effects of: Tenofovir

   The levels/effects of Adefovir may be increased by: Ganciclovir-Valganciclovir; Ribavirin; Tenofovir
Nutritional/Ethanol Interactions
   Ethanol: Should be avoided in hepatitis B infection due to potential hepatic toxicity.
   Food: Does not have a significant effect on adefovir absorption.
Adverse Reactions
   >10%:
      Central nervous system: Headache (24% to 25%)
      Gastrointestinal: Abdominal pain (15%), diarrhea (up to 13%)

▶

Hepatic: Hepatitis exacerbation (up to 25% within 12 weeks of adefovir discontinuation)

Neuromuscular & skeletal: Weakness (up to 25%)

Renal: Hematuria (grade ≥3: 11%)

1% to 10%:

Dermatologic: Rash, pruritus

Endocrine & metabolic: Hypophosphatemia (<2 mg/dL: 1% and 3% in pre-/post-liver transplant patients, respectively)

Gastrointestinal: Flatulence (up to 8%), dyspepsia (5% to 9%), nausea, vomiting

Neuromuscular & skeletal: Back pain (up to 10%)

Renal: Serum creatinine increased (≥0.5 mg/dL: 2% to 3% in compensated liver disease; incidence may be higher in patients with decompensated cirrhosis or in liver transplant recipients), renal failure

Note: In liver transplant patients with baseline renal dysfunction, frequency of increased serum creatinine has been observed to be as high as 32% to 51% at 48 and 96 weeks post-transplantation, respectively; considering the concomitant use of other potentially nephrotoxic medications, baseline renal insufficiency, and predisposing comorbidities, the role of adefovir in these changes could not be established.

Respiratory: Cough (6% to 8%), rhinitis (up to 5%)

Available Dosage Forms

Tablet, Oral:

Hepsera: 10 mg

Generic: 10 mg

General Dosage Range Dosage adjustment recommended in patients with renal impairment

Oral: *Children ≥12 years and Adults:* 10 mg once daily

Administration

Oral May be administered without regard to food.

Storage/Stability Store controlled room temperature of 25°C (77°F).

Nursing Actions

Physical Assessment Assess adherence to regimen. Monitor for lactic acidosis and altered hepatic status on a regular basis throughout therapy.

Patient Education

• Discuss specific use of drug and side effects with patient as it relates to treatment. (HCAHPS: During this hospital stay, were you given any medicine that you had not taken before? Before giving you any new medicine, how often did hospital staff tell you what the medicine was for? How often did hospital staff describe possible side effects in a way you could understand?)

• Patient may experience headache, diarrhea, flatulence, dyspepsia, nausea, or asthenia. Have patient report immediately to prescriber signs of hepatic impairment, signs of lactic acidosis, signs of pancreatitis, osteodynia, urinary retention, or oliguria (HCAHPS).

• Educate patient about signs of a significant reaction (eg, wheezing; chest tightness; fever; itching; bad cough; blue skin color; seizures; or swelling of face, lips, tongue, or throat). **Note:** This is not a comprehensive list of all side effects. Patient should consult prescriber for additional questions.

Intended Use and Disclaimer: Should not be printed and given to patients. This information is intended to serve as a concise initial reference for healthcare professionals to use when discussing medications with a patient. You must ultimately rely on your own discretion, experience and judgment in diagnosing, treating and advising patients.

Dietary Considerations May be taken without regard to food.

Adenosine (a DEN oh seen)

Brand Names: U.S. Adenocard; Adenoscan

Index Terms 9-Beta-D-Ribofuranosyladenine

Pharmacologic Category Antiarrhythmic Agent, Miscellaneous; Diagnostic Agent

Medication Safety Issues

High alert medication:

This medication is in a class the Institute for Safe Medication Practices (ISMP) includes among its list of drug classes that have a heightened risk of causing significant patient harm when used in error.

Pregnancy Risk Factor C

Lactation Excretion in breast milk unknown

Use

Adenocard: Treatment of paroxysmal supraventricular tachycardia (PSVT) including that associated with accessory bypass tracts (Wolff-Parkinson-White syndrome); when clinically advisable, appropriate vagal maneuvers should be attempted prior to adenosine administration; **not effective for conversion of atrial fibrillation, atrial flutter, or ventricular tachycardia**

Adenoscan: Pharmacologic stress agent used in myocardial perfusion thallium-201 scintigraphy

Unlabeled Use

ACLS/PALS Guidelines (2010): Stable, narrow-complex regular tachycardias; unstable narrow-complex regular tachycardias while preparations are made for synchronized direct-current cardioversion; stable regular monomorphic, wide-complex tachycardia as a therapeutic (if SVT) and diagnostic maneuver

Adenoscan: Acute vasodilator testing in pulmonary artery hypertension

Available Dosage Forms

Solution, Intravenous:

Adenocard: 6 mg/2 mL (2 mL); 12 mg/4 mL (4 mL)

Adenoscan: 3 mg/mL (20 mL, 30 mL)

Generic: 6 mg/2 mL (2 mL); 12 mg/4 mL (4 mL)

Solution, Intravenous [preservative free]: Generic: 3 mg/mL (20 mL, 30 mL); 6 mg/2 mL (2 mL); 12 mg/4 mL (4 mL)

General Dosage Range I.V.:

Children <50 kg: Initial: 0.05-0.1 mg/kg/dose (maximum initial dose: 6 mg); repeat: 0.05-0.3 mg/kg/dose (maximum: 0.3 mg/kg/dose or 12 mg/dose)

Children ≥50 kg and Adults: Initial: 6 mg; if not effective, 12 mg may be given; may repeat 12 mg if needed (maximum: 12 mg/dose)

Administration

I.V.

Adenocard: For rapid bolus I.V. use only; administer I.V. push over 1-2 seconds at a peripheral I.V. site as proximal as possible to trunk (not in lower arm, hand, lower leg, or foot); follow each bolus with a rapid normal saline flush (infants and children ≥5 mL; adults 20 mL). Use of 2 syringes (one with adenosine dose and the other with NS flush) connected to a T-connector or stopcock is recommended. If administered via **central line** in adults, reduce initial dose (ACLS, 2010).

Adenoscan: For I.V. infusion only via peripheral line

Injectable Detail Do not mix with any other drug in syringe or solution.

Nursing Actions

Physical Assessment Requires use of infusion pump and continuous cardiac and hemodynamic monitoring during infusion. Emergency resuscitation equipment should be immediately available. Monitor for adverse reactions. Adenosine could produce bronchoconstriction in patients with asthma.

Patient Education

• Discuss specific use of drug and side effects with patient as it relates to treatment. (HCAHPS: During this hospital stay, were you given any medicine that you had not taken before? Before giving you any new medicine, how often did hospital staff tell you what the medicine was for? How often did hospital staff describe possible side effects in a way you could understand?)

• Patient may experience flushing, headache, injection site irritation, dyspepsia, or paresthesia. Have patient report immediately to prescriber angina, dyspnea, severe dizziness, syncope, tachycardia, bradycardia, or arrhythmia (HCAHPS).

• Educate patient about signs of a significant reaction (eg, wheezing; chest tightness; fever; itching; bad cough; blue skin color; seizures; or swelling of face, lips, tongue, or throat). **Note:** This is not a comprehensive list of all side effects. Patient should consult prescriber for additional questions.

Intended Use and Disclaimer: Should not be printed and given to patients. This information is intended to serve as a concise initial reference for healthcare professionals to use when discussing medications with a patient. You must ultimately rely on your own discretion, experience and judgment in diagnosing, treating and advising patients.

Adenovirus (Types 4, 7) Vaccine
(ad e noh VYE rus typs for SEV en vak SEEN)

Index Terms Adenovirus Type 4 and Type 7 Vaccine; Adenovirus Vaccine; Adenovirus Vaccine (Types 4 and 7); Type 4 and Type 7 Adenovirus Vaccine

Pharmacologic Category Vaccine, Live (Viral)

Lactation Excretion in breast milk unknown/use caution

Use Prevention of acute febrile respiratory disease caused by adenovirus types 4 and 7 (approved for use in military populations)

Available Dosage Forms

Tablet, enteric coated, oral [combination package]:

Adenovirus type 4 ≥4.5 log_{10} $TCID_{50}$ [contains albumin (human); 100 white tablets]

Adenovirus type 7 ≥4.5 log_{10} $TCID_{50}$ [contains albumin (human); 100 white tablets]

General Dosage Range Oral: *Adolescents ≥17 years and Adults ≤50 years:* One tablet each of type 4 and type 7 as a single vaccine dose

Administration

Oral Swallow tablets whole, do not chew, crush, or split. Both tablets (type 4 and type 7) are to be taken together as a single dose.

Nursing Actions

Patient Education

• Discuss specific use of vaccine and side effects with patient as it relates to treatment. (HCAHPS: During this hospital stay, were you given any medicine that you had not taken before? Before giving you any new medicine, how often did hospital staff tell you what the medicine was for? How often did hospital staff describe possible side effects in a way you could understand?)

• Patient may experience headache, nausea, diarrhea, or rhinitis. Have patient report immediately to prescriber severe asthenia (HCAHPS).

• Educate patient about signs of a significant reaction (eg, wheezing; chest tightness; fever; itching; bad cough; blue skin color; seizures; or swelling of face, lips, tongue, or throat). **Note:** This is not a comprehensive list of all side effects. Patient should consult prescriber for additional questions.

Intended Use and Disclaimer: Should not be printed and given to patients. This information is intended to serve as a concise initial reference for healthcare professionals to use when discussing medications with a patient. You must ultimately rely on your own discretion, experience and judgment in diagnosing, treating and advising patients.

Related Information
Immunization Administration Recommendations *on page 1675*
Oral Medications That Should Not Be Crushed or Altered *on page 1712*

Ado-Trastuzumab Emtansine
(a do tras TU zoo mab em TAN seen)

Brand Names: U.S. Kadcyla
Index Terms T-DM1; Trastuzumab Emtansine; Trastuzumab-DM1; Trastuzumab-MCC-DM1
Pharmacologic Category Antineoplastic Agent, Anti-HER2; Antineoplastic Agent, Antibody Drug Conjugate; Antineoplastic Agent, Antimicrotubular; Antineoplastic Agent, Monoclonal Antibody
Medication Safety Issues
Sound-alike/look-alike issues:
Ado-trastuzumab emtansine may be confused with pertuzumab, trastuzumab
Other safety concerns:
In the U.S., ado-trastuzumab emtansine (Kadcyla) may be confused with conventional trastuzumab (Herceptin); products are **not** interchangeable.
In Canada, trastuzumab emtansine (Kadcyla) may be confused with conventional trastuzumab (Herceptin); products are **not** interchangeable.
Pregnancy Risk Factor D
Lactation Excretion in breast milk unknown/not recommended
Use Treatment of HER2-positive, metastatic breast cancer in patients who previously received trastuzumab and a taxane, separately or in combination, and have either received prior therapy for metastatic disease or developed disease recurrence during or within 6 months of completing adjuvant therapy.
Available Dosage Forms
Solution Reconstituted, Intravenous [preservative free]:
Kadcyla: 100 mg (1 ea); 160 mg (1 ea)
General Dosage Range Dosage reduction recommended in patients who develop toxicities.
I.V.: *Adults:* 3.6 mg/kg every 3 weeks; maximum dose: 3.6 mg/kg
Administration
I.V. Check label to ensure appropriate product is being administered (ado-trastuzumab emtansine [U.S.] or trastuzumab emtansine [Canada] and conventional trastuzumab are different products and are **NOT** interchangeable).

Infuse over 90 minutes (first infusion) or over 30 minutes (subsequent infusions if prior infusions were well tolerated) through a 0.22 micron inline nonprotein adsorptive polyethersulfone filter. Do not administer I.V. push or bolus. Do not administer with other medications.

Closely monitor infusion site during administration. Monitor patient during infusion for signs of infusion-related reactions (eg, fever, chills); monitor for at least 90 minutes following initial infusion and (if tolerated) for at least 30 minutes following subsequent infusions.

Hazardous agent; use appropriate precautions for handling and disposal (meets NIOSH, 2012 criteria).

Injectable Detail pH: 5 (reconstituted solution)
Nursing Actions
Physical Assessment Monitor GI tolerance, fatigue, headache, and fever. Potential for hepatic toxicity necessitates monitoring of liver function tests. Check for results. Assess patient for signs and symptoms of heart failure or lung toxicity (dyspnea, cough, fatigue). Risk of local reaction, evaluate infusion site for redness or pain. Can cause thrombocytopenia; more common in patients of Asian descent; monitor for bleeding and check CBC results.
Patient Education
- Discuss specific use of drug and side effects with patient as it relates to treatment. (HCAHPS) During this hospital stay, were you given any medicine that you had not taken before? Before giving you any new medicine, how often did hospital staff tell you what the medicine was for? How often did hospital staff describe possible side effects in a way you could understand?
- Patient may experience xerostomia, stomatitis, dyspepsia, nausea, diarrhea, constipation, asthenia, myalgia, arthralgia, headache, epistaxis, insomnia, rash, or dizziness. Have patient report immediately to prescriber signs of infection, dyspnea, angina, tachycardia, excessive weight gain, edema of extremities, signs of hepatic impairment, paresthesia, ecchymosis, or hemorrhaging (HCAHPS).
- Educate patient about signs of a significant reaction (eg, wheezing; chest tightness; fever; itching; bad cough; blue skin color; seizures; or swelling of face, lips, tongue, or throat). **Note** This is not a comprehensive list of all side effects. Patient should consult prescriber for additional questions.

Intended Use and Disclaimer: Should not be printed and given to patients. This information is intended to serve as a concise initial reference for healthcare professionals to use when discussing medications with a patient. You must ultimately rely on your own discretion, experience and judgment in diagnosing, treating and advising patients.

Aflibercept (Ophthalmic) (a FLIB er sept)

Brand Names: U.S. Eylea
Index Terms AVE 0005; AVE 005; AVE-0005; VEGF Trap; VEGF Trap-Eye

Pharmacologic Category Ophthalmic Agent; Vascular Endothelial Growth Factor (VEGF) Inhibitor

Medication Safety Issues

Sound-alike/look-alike issues:

Aflibercept may be confused with Ziv-aflibercept

Pregnancy Risk Factor C

Lactation Excretion in breast milk unknown/not recommended

Use Treatment of neovascular (wet) age-related macular degeneration (AMD); treatment of macular edema following central retinal vein occlusion (CRVO)

Available Dosage Forms

Solution, Intraocular [preservative free]:

Eylea: 2 mg/0.05 mL (0.05 mL)

General Dosage Range Intravitreal: *Adults:* 2 mg (0.05 mL) every 4-8 weeks

Administration

Intravitreal Ophthalmic: For intravitreal injection only. Remove contents from vial using a 5 micron, 19-gauge 1½ inch filter needle (supplied) attached to a 1 mL syringe (supplied). Discard filter needle and replace with a sterile 30 gauge ½ inch needle (supplied) for intravitreal injection procedure (do not use filter needle for intravitreal injection). Depress plunger to expel excess air and medication (plunger tip should align with the 0.05 mL marking on syringe). Adequate anesthesia and a topical broad-spectrum antimicrobial agent should be administered prior to the procedure.

Nursing Actions

Physical Assessment

Assess allergy history before beginning therapy. Assess visual acuity and intraocular pressure prior to beginning treatment and periodically during treatment. Adequate anesthesia and broad spectrum antibiotic should be administered prior to intravitreous injection. Rare hypersensitivity reactions, including anaphylaxis, can occur within several hours of use; patient should be monitored closely following injection and appropriate emergency equipment should be immediately available. Teach patient/caregiver to report any signs of infection, intraocular discomfort, or visual disturbances.

Patient Education

• Discuss specific use of drug and side effects with patient as it relates to treatment. (HCAHPS: During this hospital stay, were you given any medicine that you had not taken before? Before giving you any new medicine, how often did hospital staff tell you what the medicine was for? How often did hospital staff describe possible side effects in a way you could understand?)

• Patient may experience eye floaters. Have patient report immediately to prescriber strength differences from one side to another, difficulty speaking or thinking, change in balance, blurred vision, angina, severe dizziness, syncope, significant nausea, dyspnea, hyperhidrosis, vision changes, ophthalmalgia, eye irritation, eyelid edema, or sensitivity to light (HCAHPS).

• Educate patient about signs of a significant reaction (eg, wheezing; chest tightness; fever; itching; bad cough; blue skin color; seizures; or swelling of face, lips, tongue, or throat). **Note:** This is not a comprehensive list of all side effects. Patient should consult prescriber for additional questions.

Intended Use and Disclaimer: Should not be printed and given to patients. This information is intended to serve as a concise initial reference for healthcare professionals to use when discussing medications with a patient. You must ultimately rely on your own discretion, experience and judgment in diagnosing, treating and advising patients.

Albendazole (al BEN da zole)

Brand Names: U.S. Albenza

Pharmacologic Category Anthelmintic

Medication Safety Issues

Sound-alike/look-alike issues:

Albenza® may be confused with Aplenzin™, Relenza®

International issues:

Albenza [U.S.] may be confused with Avanza brand name for mirtazapine [Australia]

Pregnancy Risk Factor C

Lactation Excreted in breast milk/use caution

Use Treatment of parenchymal neurocysticercosis caused by *Taenia solium* and cystic hydatid disease of the liver, lung, and peritoneum caused by *Echinococcus granulosus*

Unlabeled Use Albendazole has activity against *Ascaris lumbricoides* (roundworm); *Ancylostoma caninum*; *Ancylostoma duodenale* and *Necator americanus* (hookworms); cutaneous larva migrans; *Enterobius vermicularis* (pinworm); *Giardia duodenalis* (giardiasis); *Gnathostoma spinigerum*; *Gongylonema* sp; *Mansonella perstans* (filariasis); *Oesophagostomum bifurcum*; *Opisthorchis sinensis* (liver fluke); *Trichinella spiralis* (Trichinellosis); visceral larva migrans (toxocariasis); activity has also been shown against the liver fluke *Clonorchis sinensis*, *Giardia lamblia*, *Cysticercus cellulosae*, and *Echinococcus multilocularis*. Albendazole has also been used for the treatment of intestinal microsporidiosis (*Encephalitozoon intestinalis*), disseminated microsporidiosis (*E. hellem*, *E. cuniculi*, *E. intestinalis*, *Pleistophora* sp, *Trachipleistophora* sp, *Brachiola vesicularum*), and ocular microsporidiosis (*E. hellem*, *E. cuniculi*, *Vittaforma corneae*).

Available Dosage Forms

Tablet, Oral:

Albenza: 200 mg

General Dosage Range Oral:
Children and Adults <60 kg: 15 mg/kg/day in 2 divided doses (maximum: 800 mg/day)
Children and Adults ≥60 kg: 800 mg/day in 2 divided doses (maximum: 800 mg/day)

Administration
Oral Should be administered with a high-fat meal. Administer anticonvulsant and corticosteroid therapy during first week of neurocysticercosis therapy. If patients have difficulty swallowing, tablets may be crushed or chewed, then swallowed with a drink of water.

Nursing Actions
Physical Assessment Monitor laboratory tests for reduction or elimination of ova and parasites. Monitor for elevated LFTs.

Patient Education
• Discuss specific use of drug and side effects with patient as it relates to treatment. (HCAHPS: During this hospital stay, were you given any medicine that you had not taken before? Before giving you any new medicine, how often did hospital staff tell you what the medicine was for? How often did hospital staff describe possible side effects in a way you could understand?)
• Patient may experience dyspepsia or nausea. Have patient report immediately to prescriber signs of infection, signs of hepatic impairment, severe asthenia, considerable headache, vision changes, ecchymosis, hemorrhaging, urinary retention, or oliguria (HCAHPS).
• Educate patient about signs of a significant reaction (eg, wheezing; chest tightness; fever; itching; bad cough; blue skin color; seizures; or swelling of face, lips, tongue, or throat). **Note:** This is not a comprehensive list of all side effects. Patient should consult prescriber for additional questions.

Intended Use and Disclaimer: Should not be printed and given to patients. This information is intended to serve as a concise initial reference for healthcare professionals to use when discussing medications with a patient. You must ultimately rely on your own discretion, experience and judgment in diagnosing, treating and advising patients.

Albumin (al BYOO min)

Brand Names: U.S. Albuked 25; Albuked 5; Albumin-ZLB; Albuminar-25; Albuminar-5; AlbuRx; Albutein; Buminate; Flexbumin; Human Albumin Grifols; Kedbumin; Plasbumin-25; Plasbumin-5

Index Terms Albumin (Human); Normal Human Serum Albumin; Normal Serum Albumin (Human); Salt Poor Albumin; SPA

Pharmacologic Category Blood Product Derivative; Plasma Volume Expander, Colloid

Medication Safety Issues
Sound-alike/look-alike issues:
Albutein® may be confused with albuterol
Buminate® may be confused with bumetanide

Pregnancy Risk Factor C

Use Plasma volume expansion and maintenance of cardiac output in the treatment of certain types of shock or impending shock; may be useful for burn patients, ARDS, and cardiopulmonary bypass; other uses considered by some investigators (but not proven) are retroperitoneal surgery, peritonitis, and ascites; unless the condition responsible for hypoproteinemia can be corrected, albumin can provide only symptomatic relief or supportive treatment

Note: Nutritional supplementation is not an appropriate indication.

Unlabeled Use In patients with cirrhosis, administered with diuretics to help facilitate diuresis; large volume paracentesis; volume expansion in dehydrated, mildly hypotensive patients with cirrhosis; to prevent renal impairment and reduce mortality associated with spontaneous bacterial peritonitis (SBP) in patients with cirrhosis

Available Dosage Forms
Solution, Intravenous:
Albumin-ZLB: 5% (250 mL, 500 mL); 25% (50 mL, 100 mL)
Albuminar-5: 5% (250 mL, 500 mL)
Albuminar-25: 25% (50 mL, 100 mL)
AlbuRx: 5% (250 mL, 500 mL)
Albutein: 25% (50 mL, 100 mL)
Buminate: 5% (250 mL, 500 mL); 25% (20 mL)
Human Albumin Grifols: 25% (50 mL, 100 mL)
Plasbumin-5: 5% (50 mL, 250 mL)
Plasbumin-25: 25% (20 mL, 50 mL, 100 mL)
Generic: 5% (50 mL); 25% (50 mL, 100 mL)
Solution, Intravenous [preservative free]:
Albuked 5: 5% (250 mL)
Albuked 25: 25% (50 mL, 100 mL)
Albutein: 5% (250 mL, 500 mL); 25% (50 mL, 100 mL)
Flexbumin: 25% (50 mL, 100 mL)
Kedbumin: 25% (50 mL, 100 mL)
Plasbumin-5: 5% (50 mL, 250 mL)
Plasbumin-25: 25% (20 mL, 50 mL, 100 mL)
Generic: 5% (100 mL, 250 mL, 500 mL); 25% (50 mL, 100 mL)

General Dosage Range I.V.:
Children: 0.5-1 g/kg/dose (10-20 mL/kg/dose) as needed
Adults: 0.5-1 g/kg/dose as needed **or** 25 g/dose may repeat in 15-30 minutes if response inadequate (maximum: 250 g/48 hours)

Administration

I.V. For I.V. administration only. Use within 4 hours after opening vial; discard unused portion. In emergencies, may administer as rapidly as necessary to improve clinical condition. After initial volume replacement:

5%: Do not exceed 2-4 mL/minute in patients with normal plasma volume; 5-10 mL/minute in patients with hypoproteinemia

25%: Do not exceed 1 mL/minute in patients with normal plasma volume; 2-3 mL/minute in patients with hypoproteinemia

Injectable Detail Rapid infusion may cause vascular overload. Albumin 25% may be given undiluted or diluted in normal saline. May give in combination or through the same administration set as saline or carbohydrates. Do not use with ethanol or protein hydrolysates, precipitation may form.

pH: 6.4-7.4

Nursing Actions

Physical Assessment Monitor patient closely for pulmonary edema and cardiac failure (assess vital signs and central venous pressure) during administration. Monitor frequently for hypovolemia or fluid overload. If fever, tachycardia, hypotension, or dyspnea occurs, stop infusion and notify prescriber.

Patient Education

• Discuss specific use of drug and side effects with patient as it relates to treatment. (HCAHPS: During this hospital stay, were you given any medicine that you had not taken before? Before giving you any new medicine, how often did hospital staff tell you what the medicine was for? How often did hospital staff describe possible side effects in a way you could understand?)

• Patient may experience flushing. Have patient report immediately to prescriber chills, tachycardia, severe dizziness, syncope, or considerable nausea (HCAHPS).

• Educate patient about signs of a significant reaction (eg, wheezing; chest tightness; fever; itching; bad cough; blue skin color; seizures; or swelling of face, lips, tongue, or throat). **Note:** This is not a comprehensive list of all side effects. Patient should consult prescriber for additional questions.

Intended Use and Disclaimer: Should not be printed and given to patients. This information is intended to serve as a concise initial reference for healthcare professionals to use when discussing medications with a patient. You must ultimately rely on your own discretion, experience and judgment in diagnosing, treating and advising patients.

Related Information

Reference Values for Adults *on page 1665*

Albuterol (al BYOO ter ole)

Brand Names: U.S. AccuNeb; ProAir HFA; Proventil HFA; Ventolin HFA; VoSpire ER

Index Terms Albuterol Sulfate; Salbutamol; Salbutamol Sulphate

Pharmacologic Category Beta$_2$ Agonist

Medication Safety Issues

Sound-alike/look-alike issues:

Albuterol may be confused with Albutein®, atenolol

Proventil® may be confused with Bentyl®, PriLOSEC®, Prinivil®

Salbutamol may be confused with salmeterol

Ventolin® may be confused with phentolamine, Benylin®, Vantin

Pregnancy Risk Factor C

Lactation Excretion in breast milk unknown/not recommended

Breast-Feeding Considerations It is not known if albuterol is excreted into breast milk. The amount of albuterol available systemically following inhalation is significantly less in comparison to oral doses. According to the manufacturer, the decision to continue or discontinue breast-feeding during therapy should take into account the risk of exposure to the infant and the benefits of treatment to the mother. The use of beta-2-receptor agonists are not considered a contraindication to breast feeding (NAEPP, 2005).

Use Treatment or prevention of bronchospasm in patients with reversible obstructive airway disease; prevention of exercise-induced bronchospasm

Mechanism of Action/Effect Relaxes bronchial smooth muscle by action on beta$_2$-receptors with little effect on heart rate

Contraindications Hypersensitivity to albuterol or any component of the formulation

Injection formulation (Canadian labeling; product not available in U.S.): Hypersensitivity to albuterol or any component of the formulation; tachyarrhythmias; risk of abortion during first or second trimester

Warnings/Precautions Optimize anti-inflammatory treatment before initiating maintenance treatment with albuterol. Do not use as a component of chronic therapy without an anti-inflammatory agent. Only the mildest forms of asthma (Step 1 and/or exercise-induced) would not require concurrent use based upon asthma guidelines. Patient must be instructed to seek medical attention in cases where acute symptoms are not relieved or a previous level of response is diminished. The need to increase frequency of use may indicate deterioration of asthma, and treatment must not be delayed.

Use caution in patients with cardiovascular disease (arrhythmia or hypertension or HF), convulsive disorders, diabetes, glaucoma, hyperthyroidism, or hypokalemia. Beta-agonists may cause elevation in blood pressure, heart rate, and result in CNS stimulation/excitation. Beta$_2$-agonists may increase risk of arrhythmia, increase serum glucose, or decrease serum potassium.

Immediate hypersensitivity reactions (urticaria, angioedema, rash, bronchospasm) have been reported. Do not exceed recommended dose; serious adverse events, including fatalities, have been associated with excessive use of inhaled sympathomimetics. Rarely, paradoxical bronchospasm may occur with use of inhaled bronchodilating agents; this should be distinguished from inadequate response. All patients should utilize a spacer device or valved holding chamber when using a metered-dose inhaler; in addition, face masks should be used in children <4 years of age.

Drug Interactions
Avoid Concomitant Use
Avoid concomitant use of Albuterol with any of the following: Beta-Blockers (Nonselective); Iobenguane I 123
Decreased Effect
Albuterol may decrease the levels/effects of: Iobenguane I 123

The levels/effects of Albuterol may be decreased by: Beta-Blockers (Beta1 Selective); Beta-Blockers (Nonselective); Betahistine
Increased Effect/Toxicity
Albuterol may increase the levels/effects of: Atosiban; Loop Diuretics; Sympathomimetics; Thiazide Diuretics

The levels/effects of Albuterol may be increased by: AtoMOXetine; Cannabinoids; MAO Inhibitors; Tricyclic Antidepressants
Nutritional/Ethanol Interactions
Food: Avoid or limit caffeine (may cause CNS stimulation).
Herb/Nutraceutical: Avoid ephedra, yohimbe (may cause CNS stimulation). Avoid St John's wort (may decrease the levels/effects of albuterol).

Adverse Reactions Incidence of adverse effects is dependent upon age of patient, dose, and route of administration.

Cardiovascular: Angina pectoris, atrial fibrillation, cardiac arrhythmia, chest discomfort, chest pain, extrasystoles, flushing, hypertension, hypotension, palpitations, supraventricular tachycardia, tachycardia

Central nervous system: Central nervous system stimulation, dizziness, drowsiness, headache, insomnia, irritability, migraine, nervousness, nightmares, restlessness, seizure, vertigo

Dermatologic: Diaphoresis, skin rash, urticaria

Endocrine & metabolic: Hyperglycemia, hypokalemia, lactic acidosis

Gastrointestinal: Diarrhea, dysgeusia, dyspepsia, gastroenteritis, nausea, vomiting, xerostomia

Genitourinary: Difficulty in micturition

Hematologic & oncologic: Lymphadenopathy

Hypersensitivity: Anaphylaxis, angioedema, hypersensitivity reaction

Local: Pain at injection site

Neuromuscular & skeletal: Muscle cramps, musculoskeletal pain, tremor, weakness

Otic: Otitis media

Respiratory: Bronchospasm, cough, epistaxis, exacerbation of asthma, laryngitis, oropharyngeal edema, oropharyngeal irritation, pharyngitis, rhinitis, upper respiratory tract inflammation, viral upper respiratory tract infection

Pharmacodynamics/Kinetics
Onset of Action Peak effect:
Nebulization/oral inhalation: 0.5-2 hours
  CFC-propelled albuterol: 10 minutes
  Ventolin® HFA: 25 minutes
Oral: 2-3 hours

Duration of Action Nebulization/oral inhalation: 3-4 hours; Oral: 4-6 hours

Dosage Forms Considerations
ProAir HFA 8.5 g canisters and Proventil HFA 6.7 g canisters contain 200 inhalations.
Ventolin HFA 18 g canisters contain 200 inhalations and the 8 g canisters contain 60 inhalations.

Available Dosage Forms
Aerosol Solution, Inhalation:
ProAir HFA: 108 (90 Base) mcg/acutation (8.5 g)
Proventil HFA: 108 (90 Base) mcg/acutation (6.7 g)
Ventolin HFA: 108 (90 Base) mcg/acutation (8 g, 18 g)
Nebulization Solution, Inhalation:
Generic: 0.63 mg/3 mL (3 mL); (2.5 mg/3 mL) 0.083% (3 mL); (5 mg/mL) 0.5% (20 mL)
Nebulization Solution, Inhalation [preservative free]:
AccuNeb: 0.63 mg/3 mL (3 mL); 1.25 mg/3 mL (3 mL)
Generic: 0.63 mg/3 mL (3 mL); 1.25 mg/3 mL (3 mL); (2.5 mg/3 mL) 0.083% (3 mL); (5 mg/mL) 0.5% (1 ea); 0.083% (3 mL)
Syrup, Oral:
Generic: 2 mg/5 mL (473 mL)
Tablet, Oral:
Generic: 2 mg, 4 mg
Tablet Extended Release 12 Hour, Oral:
VoSpire ER: 4 mg, 8 mg
Generic: 4 mg, 8 mg
General Dosage Range
Inhalation via metered-dose inhaler (90 mcg/puff): *Children and Adults:* 2 puffs every 4-6 hours **or** 4-8 puffs every 1-4 hours [acute symptoms] **or** 1-2 puffs prior to exercise
Nebulization:
Children <12 years: 0.15-0.3 mg/kg (maximum: 10 mg) every 1-4 hours **or** 0.63-1.25 mg 3-4 times daily **or** 0.5 mg/kg/hour by continuous nebulization

Children ≥12 years: 2.5-10 mg every 1-4 hours **or** 10-15 mg/hour by continuous nebulization
Adults: 2.5-10 mg every 1-4 hours **or** 10-15 mg/hour by continuous nebulization

Oral:
Regular release:
Children 2-6 years: 0.1-0.2 mg/kg/dose 3 times daily (maximum: 12 mg daily)
Children 6-12 years: 2 mg/dose 3-4 times daily (maximum: 24 mg daily)
Children >12 years and Adults: 2-4 mg/dose 3-4 times daily (maximum: 32 mg daily)
Extended release:
Children 6-12 years: 4 mg every 12 hours (maximum: 24 mg daily)
Children >12 years and Adults: 8 mg every 12 hours (maximum: 32 mg daily)

Administration

I.V. Infusion solution (Canadian labeling; product not available in U.S.): Do not inject undiluted. Reduce concentration by at least 50% before infusing. Administer as a continuous infusion via infusion pump.

Oral Do not crush or chew extended release tablets.

Inhalation

Metered-dose inhaler: Shake well before use; prime prior to first use, and whenever inhaler has not been used for >2 weeks or when it has been dropped, by releasing 3-4 test sprays into the air (away from face). Airomir™ Canadian product labeling recommends releasing a minimum of 4 test sprays when priming. HFA inhalers should be cleaned with warm water at least once per week; allow to air dry completely prior to use. A spacer device or valved holding chamber is recommended for use with metered-dose inhalers.

Nebulization solution: Concentrated solution should be diluted prior to use. Blow-by administration is not recommended, use a mask device if patient unable to hold mouthpiece in mouth for administration.

Preparation for Administration Solution for nebulization: To prepare a 2.5 mg dose, dilute 0.5 mL of solution to a total of 3 mL with normal saline; also compatible with cromolyn or ipratropium nebulizer solutions.

Storage/Stability

HFA aerosols: Store at 15°C to 25°C (59°F to 77°F).
Ventolin® HFA: Discard when counter reads 000 or 12 months after removal from protective pouch, whichever comes first. Store with mouthpiece down.
Infusion solution (Canadian labeling; product not available in U.S.): Ventolin® I.V.: Store at 15°C to 30°C (59°F to 86°F). Protect from light. After dilution, discard unused portion after 24 hours.
Solution for nebulization (0.5%): Store at 2°C to 25°C (36°F to 77°F).

AccuNeb®: Store at 2°C to 25°C (36°F to 77°F). Do not use if solution changes color or becomes cloudy. Use within 1 week of opening foil pouch.
Syrup: Store at 20°C to 25°C (68°F to 77°F).
Tablet: Store at 20°C to 25°C (68°F to 77°F).
Tablet, extended release: Store at 20°C to 25°C (68°F to 77°F)

Nursing Actions

Physical Assessment Evaluate effectiveness of therapy (relief of airway obstruction). For inpatient care, monitor vital signs and lung sounds prior to and periodically during therapy.

Patient Education
• Discuss specific use of drug and side effects with patient as it relates to treatment. (HCAHPS: During this hospital stay, were you given any medicine that you had not taken before? Before giving you any new medicine, how often did hospital staff tell you what the medicine was for? How often did hospital staff describe possible side effects in a way you could understand?)
• Patient may experience dyspepsia, tremors, pharyngitis, rhinorrhea, or xerostomia. Have patient report immediately to prescriber hypokalemia, uncontrolled breathing attack, angina, tachycardia, considerable anxiety, significant headache, intolerable dizziness, syncope, low peak flow measurement, severe dyspnea, wheezing, or signs of Stevens-Johnson syndrome/toxic epidermal necrolysis (HCAHPS).
• Educate patient about signs of a significant reaction (eg, wheezing; chest tightness; fever; itching; bad cough; blue skin color; seizures; or swelling of face, lips, tongue, or throat). **Note:** This is not a comprehensive list of all side effects. Patient should consult prescriber for additional questions.

Intended Use and Disclaimer: Should not be printed and given to patients. This information is intended to serve as a concise initial reference for healthcare professionals to use when discussing medications with a patient. You must ultimately rely on your own discretion, experience and judgment in diagnosing, treating and advising patients.

Related Information

Oral Medications That Should Not Be Crushed or Altered on page 1712

Alcaftadine (al KAF ta deen)

Brand Names: U.S. Lastacaft
Pharmacologic Category Histamine H_1 Antagonist; Histamine H_1 Antagonist, Second Generation; Mast Cell Stabilizer
Pregnancy Risk Factor B
Lactation Excretion in breast milk unknown/use caution
Use Prevention of itching associated with allergic conjunctivitis

Available Dosage Forms

Solution, Ophthalmic:

Lastacaft: 0.25% (3 mL)

General Dosage Range Ophthalmic: *Children ≥2 years and Adults:* Instill 1 drop into each eye once daily

Administration

Other For topical ophthalmic use only. Contact lenses should be removed prior to application, and may be reinserted 10 minutes after administration. Do not insert contacts if eyes are red. Avoid contaminating the applicator tip with affected eye(s).

Nursing Actions

Patient Education

• Discuss specific use of drug and side effects with patient as it relates to treatment. (HCAHPS: During this hospital stay, were you given any medicine that you had not taken before? Before giving you any new medicine, how often did hospital staff tell you what the medicine was for? How often did hospital staff describe possible side effects in a way you could understand?)

• Patient may experience headache, rhinitis, or pharyngitis. Have patient report immediately to prescriber vision changes, ophthalmalgia, or severe eye irritation (HCAHPS).

• Educate patient about signs of a significant reaction (eg, wheezing; chest tightness; fever; itching; bad cough; blue skin color; seizures; or swelling of face, lips, tongue, or throat). **Note:** This is not a comprehensive list of all side effects. Patient should consult prescriber for additional questions.

Intended Use and Disclaimer: Should not be printed and given to patients. This information is intended to serve as a concise initial reference for healthcare professionals to use when discussing medications with a patient. You must ultimately rely on your own discretion, experience and judgment in diagnosing, treating and advising patients.

Aldesleukin (al des LOO kin)

Brand Names: U.S. Proleukin

Index Terms IL-2; Interleukin 2; Interleukin-2; Lymphocyte Mitogenic Factor; Recombinant Human Interleukin-2; T-Cell Growth Factor; TCGF; Thymocyte Stimulating Factor

Pharmacologic Category Antineoplastic Agent, Biological Response Modulator; Antineoplastic Agent, Miscellaneous

Medication Safety Issues

Sound-alike/look-alike issues:

Aldesleukin may be confused with oprelvekin

Proleukin® may be confused with oprelvekin

High alert medication:

The Institute for Safe Medication Practices (ISMP) includes this medication among its list of drug classes which have a heightened risk of causing significant patient harm when used in error.

Pregnancy Risk Factor C

Lactation Excretion in breast milk unknown/not recommended

Use Treatment of metastatic renal cell cancer, metastatic melanoma

Unlabeled Use Treatment of acute myeloid leukemia (AML)

Available Dosage Forms

Solution Reconstituted, Intravenous [preservative free]:

Proleukin: 22,000,000 units (1 ea)

General Dosage Range Dosage adjustment recommended in patients who develop toxicities

I.V.: *Adults:* 600,000 units/kg every 8 hours (maximum: 14 doses); may repeat after 9 days for a total of 28 doses/course

Administration

I.V. Infuse over 15 minutes. Allow solution to reach room temperature prior to administration. Do not administer with an inline filter. Flush before and after with D_5W, particularly if maintenance I.V. line contains sodium chloride.

Hazardous agent; use appropriate precautions for handling and disposal (NIOSH, 2012).

Other May be administered by SubQ injection (unlabeled route).

Hazardous agent; use appropriate precautions for handling and disposal (NIOSH, 2012).

Nursing Actions

Physical Assessment Monitor vital signs; cardiac, respiratory, and CNS status; fluid balance; signs of systemic sepsis; changes in mental status; and laboratory tests daily prior to beginning infusion and for 2 hours following infusion. Closely monitor infusion site for extravasation.

Patient Education

• Discuss specific use of drug and side effects with patient as it relates to treatment. (HCAHPS: During this hospital stay, were you given any medicine that you had not taken before? Before giving you any new medicine, how often did hospital staff tell you what the medicine was for? How often did hospital staff describe possible side effects in a way you could understand?)

• Patient may experience nausea, anxiety, lack of appetite, diarrhea, rhinorrhea, or fatigue. Have patient report immediately to prescriber signs of infection, signs of renal impairment, signs of hepatic impairment, signs of depression (ie, suicidal ideation, anxiety, emotional instability, illogical thinking), signs of hyperglycemia, arrhythmia, angina, tachycardia, severe dizziness, syncope, dyspnea, excessive weight gain, edema of extremities, hematemesis, melena, abdominal edema, stomatitis, considerable dyspepsia, hallucinations, difficulty speaking, abnormal gait, change in balance, blindness,

ecchymosis, hemorrhaging, significant asthenia, or signs of Stevens-Johnson syndrome/toxic epidermal necrolysis (HCAHPS).
• Educate patient about signs of a significant reaction (eg, wheezing; chest tightness; fever; itching; bad cough; blue skin color; seizures; or swelling of face, lips, tongue, or throat). **Note:** This is not a comprehensive list of all side effects. Patient should consult prescriber for additional questions.

Intended Use and Disclaimer: Should not be printed and given to patients. This information is intended to serve as a concise initial reference for healthcare professionals to use when discussing medications with a patient. You must ultimately rely on your own discretion, experience and judgment in diagnosing, treating and advising patients.

Alendronate (a LEN droe nate)

Brand Names: U.S. Binosto; Fosamax
Index Terms Alendronate Sodium; Alendronic Acid Monosodium Salt Trihydrate; MK-217
Pharmacologic Category Bisphosphonate Derivative
Medication Safety Issues
Sound-alike/look-alike issues:
Alendronate may be confused with risedronate
Fosamax® may be confused with Flomax®, Fosamax Plus D®, fosinopril, Zithromax®
International issues:
Fosamax [U.S., Canada, and multiple international markets] may be confused with Fisamox brand name for amoxicillin [Australia]
Medication Guide Available Yes
Pregnancy Risk Factor C
Lactation Excretion in breast milk unknown/use caution
Breast-Feeding Considerations It is not known if alendronate is excreted into breast milk. The manufacturer recommends that caution be exercised when administering alendronate to nursing women.
Use Treatment of osteoporosis in postmenopausal females (Fosamax®, Binosto®); prevention of osteoporosis in postmenopausal females (Fosamax®); treatment of osteoporosis in males (Fosamax®, Binosto®); treatment of Paget's disease of the bone in patients who are symptomatic, at risk for future complications, or with alkaline phosphatase ≥2 times the upper limit of normal (Fosamax®); treatment of glucocorticoid-induced osteoporosis in males and females with low bone mineral density who are receiving a daily dosage ≥7.5 mg of prednisone (or equivalent) (Fosamax®)
Mechanism of Action/Effect A bisphosphonate which inhibits bone resorption via actions on osteoclasts or on osteoclast precursors; decreases the rate of bone resorption, leading to an indirect increase in bone mineral density. In Paget's

disease, characterized by disordered resorption and formation of bone, inhibition of resorption leads to an indirect decrease in bone formation; but the newly-formed bone has a more normal architecture.
Contraindications Hypersensitivity to alendronate, other bisphosphonates, or any component of the formulation; hypocalcemia; abnormalities of the esophagus (eg, stricture, achalasia) which delay esophageal emptying; inability to stand or sit upright for at least 30 minutes; increased risk of aspiration (effervescent tablets; oral solution)
Warnings/Precautions Use caution in patients with renal impairment (not recommended for use in patients with CrCl <35 mL/minute); hypocalcemia must be corrected before therapy initiation; ensure adequate calcium and vitamin D intake. May cause irritation to upper gastrointestinal mucosa. Esophagitis, dysphagia, esophageal ulcers, esophageal erosions, and esophageal stricture (rare) have been reported; risk increases in patients unable to comply with dosing instructions. Use with caution in patients with dysphagia, esophageal disease, gastritis, duodenitis, or ulcers (may worsen underlying condition). Discontinue use if new or worsening symptoms develop.

Osteonecrosis of the jaw (ONJ) has been reported in patients receiving bisphosphonates. Risk factors include invasive dental procedures (eg, tooth extraction, dental implants, boney surgery); a diagnosis of cancer, with concomitant chemotherapy or corticosteroids; poor oral hygiene, ill-fitting dentures; and comorbid disorders (anemia, coagulopathy, infection, pre-existing dental disease); risk may increase with duration of bisphosphonate use. Most reported cases occurred after I.V. bisphosphonate therapy; however, cases have been reported following oral therapy. A dental exam and preventative dentistry should be performed prior to placing patients with risk factors on chronic bisphosphonate therapy. The manufacturer's labeling states that discontinuing bisphosphonates in patients requiring invasive dental procedures may reduce the risk of ONJ. However, other experts suggest that there is no evidence that discontinuing therapy reduces the risk of developing ONJ (Assael, 2009). The benefit/risk must be assessed by the treating physician and/or dentist/surgeon prior to any invasive dental procedure. Patients developing ONJ while on bisphosphonates should receive care by an oral surgeon.

Atypical femur fractures have been reported in patients receiving bisphosphonates for treatment/prevention of osteoporosis. The fractures include subtrochanteric femur (bone just below the hip joint) and diaphyseal femur (long segment of the thigh bone). Some patients experience prodromal pain weeks or months before the fracture occurs. It is unclear if bisphosphonate therapy is the cause for these fractures, although the majority of cases have been reported in patients taking bisphospho-nates. Patients receiving long-term (>3-5 years) therapy may be at an increased risk. Discontinue bisphosphonate therapy in patients who develop a femoral shaft fracture.

Severe (and occasionally debilitating) bone, joint, and/or muscle pain have been reported during bisphosphonate treatment. The onset of pain ranged from a single day to several months. Consider discontinuing therapy in patients who experience severe symptoms; symptoms usually resolve upon discontinuation. Some patients experienced recurrence when rechallenged with same drug or another bisphosphonate; avoid use in patients with a history of these symptoms in association with bisphosphonate therapy. In the management of osteoporosis, re-evaluate the need for continued therapy periodically; the optimal duration of treatment has not yet been determined. Consider discontinuing after 3-5 years of use in patients at low-risk for fracture; following discontinuation, re-evaluate fracture risk periodically.

Potentially significant drug-drug interactions may exist, requiring dose or frequency adjustment, additional monitoring, and/or selection of alternative therapy. Consult drug interactions database for more detailed information. Each effervescent tablet contains 650 mg of sodium (NaCl 1650 mg); use with caution in patients following a sodium-restricted diet.

Drug Interactions

Avoid Concomitant Use There are no known interactions where it is recommended to avoid concomitant use.

Decreased Effect
The levels/effects of Alendronate may be decreased by: Antacids; Calcium Salts; Iron Salts; Magnesium Salts; Multivitamins/Minerals (with ADEK, Folate, Iron); Multivitamins/Minerals (with AE, No Iron); Proton Pump Inhibitors; Sucroferric Oxyhydroxide

Increased Effect/Toxicity
Alendronate may increase the levels/effects of: Deferasirox; Phosphate Supplements

The levels/effects of Alendronate may be increased by: Aminoglycosides; Aspirin; Nonsteroidal Anti-Inflammatory Agents; Systemic Angiogenesis Inhibitors

Nutritional/Ethanol Interactions

Ethanol: May increase risk of osteoporosis and gastric irritation. Management: Avoid ethanol.

Food: All food and beverages interfere with absorption. Coadministration with caffeine may reduce alendronate efficacy. Coadministration with dairy products may decrease alendronate absorption. Beverages (especially orange juice, coffee, and mineral water) and food may reduce the absorption of alendronate as much as 60%. Management: Alendronate must be taken first thing in the morning and ≥30 minutes before the first food, beverage (except plain water), or other medication of the day.

Adverse Reactions Note: Incidence of adverse effects (mostly GI) increases significantly in patients treated for Paget's disease at 40 mg/day.

>10%: Endocrine & metabolic: Hypocalcemia (18%; transient, mild)
1% to 10%:
Central nervous system: Headache (≤3%)
Endocrine & metabolic: Hypophosphatemia (10%; transient, mild)
Gastrointestinal: Abdominal pain (1% to 7%), acid regurgitation (1% to 4%), dyspepsia (1% to 4%), nausea (1% to 4%), flatulence (≤4%), diarrhea (1% to 3%), gastroesophageal reflux disease (1% to 3%), constipation (≤3%), esophageal ulcer (≤2%), abdominal distension (≤1%), gastritis (≤1%), vomiting (≤1%), dysphagia (≤1%), gastric ulcer (1%), melena (1%)
Neuromuscular & skeletal: Musculoskeletal pain (≤6%), muscle cramps (≤1%)

Available Dosage Forms

Solution, Oral:
Generic: 70 mg/75 mL (75 mL)
Tablet, Oral:
Fosamax: 70 mg
Generic: 5 mg, 10 mg, 35 mg, 40 mg, 70 mg
Tablet Effervescent, Oral:
Binosto: 70 mg

General Dosage Range Oral: *Adults:* 5-10 mg daily **or** 35-70 mg once weekly (maximum: 70 mg weekly) **or** 40 mg once daily [Paget's disease]

Administration

Oral Administer first thing in the morning and ≥30 minutes before the first food, beverage (except plain water), or other medication(s) of the day. Do not take with mineral water or with other beverages. Patients should be instructed to stay upright (not to lie down) for at least 30 minutes and until after first food of the day (to reduce esophageal irritation).

Oral solution: Administer oral solution, followed with at least 2 oz of plain water.

Tablet (Fosamax®): Must be taken with 6-8 oz of plain water.

Tablet, effervescent (Binosto®): Dissolve one tablet in 4 oz of room temperature plain water only; once effervescence stops, wait ≥5 minutes and stir the solution for ~10 seconds and then drink

Preparation for Administration Tablet, effervescent (Binosto®): Dissolve effervescent tablet in 120 mL of room temperature plain water (not mineral water or flavored water); wait ≥5 minutes after effervescence stops, then stir for 10 seconds and administer.

Storage/Stability

Oral solution: Store at 25°C (77°F), excursions permitted to 15°C to 30°C (59°F to 86°F). Do not freeze.

Tablet (Fosamax®): Store at room temperature of 15°C to 30°C (59°F to 86°F). Keep in well-closed container.

Tablet, effervescent (Binosto®): Store at 20°C to 25°C (68°F to 77°F), excursions permitted to 15°C to 30°C (59°F to 86°F). Protect from moisture. Store in original blister package until use.

Nursing Actions

Physical Assessment Monitor for unusual or acute musculoskeletal pain. Monitor blood pressure at the beginning of therapy and periodically during use. Stress importance of proper administration and other preventative measures to prevent risk of osteoporosis. Educate patient about need for good oral hygiene and regular dental exams.

Patient Education
- Discuss specific use of drug and side effects with patient as it relates to treatment. (HCAHPS: During this hospital stay, were you given any medicine that you had not taken before? Before giving you any new medicine, how often did hospital staff tell you what the medicine was for? How often did hospital staff describe possible side effects in a way you could understand?)
- Patient may experience dizziness, bloating, flatulence, headache, dysgeusia, flu-like syndrome, constipation, diarrhea, or back pain. Have patient report immediately to prescriber signs of hypocalcemia; melena; angina; hemoptysis; severe dyspepsia; pyrosis; dysphagia; pharyngitis; significant nausea; hematemesis; intolerable osteodynia; considerable arthralgia or myalgia; groin, hip, or thigh pain; stomatitis; edema of extremities; or jaw edema or pain (HCAHPS).
- Educate patient about signs of a significant reaction (eg, wheezing; chest tightness; fever; itching; bad cough; blue skin color; seizures; or swelling of face, lips, tongue, or throat). **Note:** This is not a comprehensive list of all side effects. Patient should consult prescriber for additional questions.

Intended Use and Disclaimer: Should not be printed and given to patients. This information is intended to serve as a concise initial reference for healthcare professionals to use when discussing medications with a patient. You must ultimately rely on your own discretion, experience and judgment in diagnosing, treating and advising patients.

Dietary Considerations Ensure adequate calcium and vitamin D intake; if dietary intake is inadequate, dietary supplementation is recommended. Women and men should consume:
Calcium: 1000 mg/day (men: 50-70 years) **or** 1200 mg/day (women ≥51 years and men ≥71 years) (IOM, 2011; NOF, 2013)
Vitamin D: 800-1000 IU/day (men and women ≥50 years) (NOF, 2013). Recommended Dietary Allowance (RDA): 600 IU/day (men and women ≤70 years) **or** 800 IU/day (men and women ≥71 years) (IOM, 2011).

Related Information
Oral Medications That Should Not Be Crushed or Altered *on page 1712*

Alfuzosin (al FYOO zoe sin)

Brand Names: U.S. Uroxatral
Index Terms Alfuzosin Hydrochloride
Pharmacologic Category Alpha$_1$ Blocker
Pregnancy Risk Factor B
Use Treatment of the functional symptoms of benign prostatic hyperplasia (BPH)
Unlabeled Use Facilitation of expulsion of ureteral stones
Mechanism of Action/Effect An antagonist of alpha$_1$-adrenoreceptors in the lower urinary tract. Blockade of these adrenoreceptors can cause smooth muscles in the bladder neck and prostate to relax, resulting in an improvement in urine flow rate and a reduction in BPH symptoms.
Contraindications Hypersensitivity to alfuzosin or any component of the formulation; moderate or severe hepatic insufficiency (Child-Pugh class B and C); concurrent use with potent CYP3A4 inhibitors (eg, itraconazole, ketoconazole, ritonavir) or other alpha$_1$-blocking agents
Warnings/Precautions Not intended for use as an antihypertensive drug. May cause significant orthostatic hypotension and syncope, especially with first dose; anticipate a similar effect if therapy is interrupted for a few days, if dosage is rapidly increased, or used with antihypertensives (particularly vasodilators), PDE-5 inhibitors, nitrates or other medications which may result in hypotension. Discontinue if symptoms of angina occur or worsen. Alfuzosin has been shown to prolong the QT interval alone (minimal) and with other drugs with comparable effects on the QT interval (additive); use with caution in patients with known QT prolongation (congenital or acquired). Patients should be cautioned about performing hazardous tasks when starting new therapy or adjusting dosage upward. Discontinue if symptoms of angina occur or worsen. Rule out prostatic carcinoma before beginning therapy. Use caution with severe renal or mild hepatic impairment; contraindicated in moderate-to-severe hepatic impairment. Intraoperative floppy iris syndrome has been observed in cataract surgery patients who were on or were previously treated with alpha$_1$-blockers. Causality has not been established and there appears to be no benefit in discontinuing alpha-blocker therapy prior to surgery. May cause priapism. Contraindicated in patients taking strong CYP3A4 inhibitors or other alpha$_1$-blockers.

▶

Drug Interactions

Avoid Concomitant Use
Avoid concomitant use of Alfuzosin with any of the following: Alpha1-Blockers; CYP3A4 Inhibitors (Strong); Fusidic Acid (Systemic); Highest Risk QTc-Prolonging Agents; Ivabradine; Mifepristone; Protease Inhibitors; Telaprevir

Decreased Effect
Alfuzosin may decrease the levels/effects of: Alpha-/Beta-Agonists; Alpha1-Agonists

The levels/effects of Alfuzosin may be decreased by: Bosentan; CYP3A4 Inducers (Strong); Dabrafenib; Deferasirox; Herbs (CYP3A4 Inducers); Mitotane; Tocilizumab

Increased Effect/Toxicity
Alfuzosin may increase the levels/effects of: Alpha1-Blockers; Antihypertensives; Calcium Channel Blockers; Highest Risk QTc-Prolonging Agents; Moderate Risk QTc-Prolonging Agents; Nitroglycerin

The levels/effects of Alfuzosin may be increased by: Beta-Blockers; CYP3A4 Inhibitors (Moderate); CYP3A4 Inhibitors (Strong); Dasatinib; Fusidic Acid (Systemic); Ivabradine; Ivacaftor; Luliconazole; MAO Inhibitors; Mifepristone; Phosphodiesterase 5 Inhibitors; Protease Inhibitors; QTc-Prolonging Agents (Indeterminate Risk and Risk Modifying); Simeprevir; Telaprevir

Nutritional/Ethanol Interactions
Food: Food increases the extent of absorption. Management: Administer immediately following a meal at the same time each day.

Herb/Nutraceutical: St John's wort may decrease alfuzosin levels. Management: Avoid St John's wort.

Adverse Reactions 1% to 10%:
Central nervous system: Dizziness (6%), fatigue (3%), headache (3%), pain (1% to 2%)

Gastrointestinal: Abdominal pain (1% to 2%), constipation (1% to 2%), dyspepsia (1% to 2%), nausea (1% to 2%)

Genitourinary: Impotence (1% to 2%)

Respiratory: Upper respiratory tract infection (3%), bronchitis (1% to 2%), pharyngitis (1% to 2%), sinusitis (1% to 2%)

Available Dosage Forms
Tablet Extended Release 24 Hour, Oral:
Uroxatral: 10 mg
Generic: 10 mg

General Dosage Range Oral: *Adults:* 10 mg once daily

Administration
Oral Tablet should be swallowed whole; do not crush or chew. Administer once daily (immediately following a meal); should be taken at the same time each day.

Storage/Stability
Store at room temperature of 25°C (77°F); excursions permitted to 15°C to 30°C (59°F to 86°F). Protect from light and moisture.

Nursing Actions

Physical Assessment
Assess blood pressure and monitor for hypotension, dizziness, somnolence, and impotence at beginning of therapy and on a regular basis.

Patient Education
- Discuss specific use of drug and side effects with patient as it relates to treatment. (HCAHPS: During this hospital stay, were you given any medicine that you had not taken before? Before giving you any new medicine, how often did hospital staff tell you what the medicine was for? How often did hospital staff describe possible side effects in a way you could understand?)
- Patient may experience headache. Have patient report immediately to prescriber signs of hepatic impairment, severe dizziness, syncope, angina, back pain, sexual dysfunction, tachycardia, arrhythmia, chills, pharyngitis, arthralgia, considerable asthenia, or priapism (HCAHPS).
- Educate patient about signs of a significant reaction (eg, wheezing; chest tightness; fever; itching; bad cough; blue skin color; seizures; or swelling of face, lips, tongue, or throat). **Note:** This is not a comprehensive list of all side effects. Patient should consult prescriber for additional questions.

Intended Use and Disclaimer: Should not be printed and given to patients. This information is intended to serve as a concise initial reference for healthcare professionals to use when discussing medications with a patient. You must ultimately rely on your own discretion, experience and judgment in diagnosing, treating and advising patients.

Dietary Considerations Take immediately following a meal at the same time each day.

Related Information
Oral Medications That Should Not Be Crushed or Altered *on page 1712*

Aliskiren (a lis KYE ren)

Brand Names: U.S. Tekturna
Index Terms Aliskiren Hemifumarate; SPP100
Pharmacologic Category Renin Inhibitor
Medication Safety Issues
Sound-alike/look-alike issues:
Tekturna may be confused with Valturna
Pregnancy Risk Factor D
Lactation Excretion in breast milk unknown/not recommended
Breast-Feeding Considerations It is not known if aliskiren is excreted in breast milk. Due to the potential for serious adverse reactions in the nursing infant, a decision should be made whether to discontinue nursing or to discontinue the drug, taking into account the importance of treatment to the mother.

Use Hypertension: Treatment of hypertension, alone or in combination with other antihypertensive agents

Mechanism of Action/Effect Aliskiren is a direct renin inhibitor, resulting in blockade of the conversion of angiotensinogen to angiotensin I. Angiotensin I suppression decreases the formation of angiotensin II (Ang II), resulting in blood pressure reduction.

Contraindications

U.S. labeling: Concomitant use with an ACE inhibitor or ARB in patients with diabetes mellitus

Canada labeling: Additional contraindications (not in U.S. labeling): Hypersensitivity to aliskiren or any component of the formulation; history of angioedema with aliskiren, ACE inhibitors, or ARBs; hereditary or idiopathic angioedema; concomitant use with ACE inhibitors or ARBs in patients with GFR <60 mL/minute/1.73 m^2

Warnings/Precautions [U.S. Boxed Warning]: Drugs that act on the renin-angiotensin system can cause injury and death to the developing fetus. Discontinue as soon as possible once pregnancy is detected. Hypersensitivity reactions, including anaphylaxis and angioedema have been reported; since the effect of aliskiren on bradykinin levels is unknown, the risk of kinin-mediated etiologies of angioedema occurring is also unknown. Use with caution in any patient with a history of angioedema (of any etiology) as angioedema, some cases necessitating hospitalization and intubation, has been observed (rarely) with aliskiren use. Discontinue immediately following the occurrence of anaphylaxis or angioedema; do not readminister. Prolonged frequent monitoring may be required especially if tongue, glottis, or larynx are involved as they are associated with airway obstruction. Patients with a history of airway surgery may have a higher risk of airway obstruction. Early, aggressive, and appropriate management is critical. Hyperkalemia may occur (rarely) during monotherapy; risk may increase in patients with predisposing factors (eg, renal dysfunction, diabetes mellitus or concomitant use with ACE inhibitors, potassium-sparing diuretics, potassium supplements, and/or potassium-containing salts). Symptomatic hypotension may occur (rarely) during the initiation of therapy, particularly in volume or salt-depleted patients or with concomitant use of other agents acting on the renin-angiotensin-aldosterone system. If hypotension does occur, this is not a contraindication for further use; once blood pressure has been stabilized, aliskiren usually can be continued without difficulty. Use with caution or avoid in patients with deteriorating renal function or low renal blood flow (eg, renal artery stenosis, severe heart failure); may increase risk of developing acute renal failure and hyperkalemia. Concomitant use with an ACE inhibitor or ARB may increase risk of developing acute renal failure and

should be avoided in patient with GFR <60 mL/minute. Use (monotherapy or combined with ACE inhibitors or ARBs) in patients with type 2 diabetes mellitus has demonstrated an increased incidence of renal impairment, hypotension, and hyperkalemia; use is contraindicated in patients with diabetes mellitus who are taking an ACE inhibitor or ARB. Potentially significant drug-drug interactions may exist, requiring dose or frequency adjustment, additional monitoring, and/or selection of alternative therapy.

Drug Interactions

Avoid Concomitant Use

Avoid concomitant use of Aliskiren with any of the following: CycloSPORINE (Systemic); Itraconazole

Decreased Effect

Aliskiren may decrease the levels/effects of: Furosemide

The levels/effects of Aliskiren may be decreased by: Grapefruit Juice; Herbs (Hypertensive Properties); Methylphenidate; Nonsteroidal Anti-Inflammatory Agents; P-glycoprotein/ABCB1 Inducers; Yohimbine

Increased Effect/Toxicity

Aliskiren may increase the levels/effects of: ACE Inhibitors; Amifostine; Angiotensin II Receptor Blockers; Antihypertensives; DULoxetine; Hypotensive Agents; Obinutuzumab; RiTUXimab

The levels/effects of Aliskiren may be increased by: Alfuzosin; AtorvaSTATin; Brimonidine (Topical); Canagliflozin; CycloSPORINE (Systemic); Diazoxide; Heparin; Heparin (Low Molecular Weight); Herbs (Hypotensive Properties); Itraconazole; Ketoconazole (Systemic); MAO Inhibitors; Nonsteroidal Anti-Inflammatory Agents; Pentoxifylline; P-glycoprotein/ABCB1 Inhibitors; Phosphodiesterase 5 Inhibitors; Prostacyclin Analogues; Verapamil

Nutritional/Ethanol Interactions

Food: High-fat meals decrease absorption. Grapefruit juice may decrease the serum concentration of aliskiren. Management: Administer at the same time each day; may take with or without a meal, but consistent administration with regards to meals is recommended. Avoid concomitant use of aliskiren and grapefruit juice.

Herb/Nutraceutical: Some herbal medications may worsen hypertension (eg, licorice); others may increase the antihypertensive effect of aliskiren (eg, shepherd's purse). Management: Avoid bayberry, blue cohosh, cayenne, ephedra, ginger, ginseng (American), kola, licorice, and yohimbe. Avoid black cohosh, California poppy, coleus, golden seal, hawthorn, mistletoe, periwinkle, quinine, and shepherd's purse.

▶

Adverse Reactions
1% to 10%:
Dermatologic: Skin rash (1%)
Endocrine & metabolic: Hyperkalemia (monotherapy ≤1%; may be increased with concurrent ACE inhibitor or ARB)
Gastrointestinal: Diarrhea (2%)
Neuromuscular & skeletal: Increased creatine kinase (>300% increase: 1%)
Renal: Increased blood urea nitrogen (≤7%), increased serum creatinine (≤7%)
Respiratory: Cough (1%)

Pharmacodynamics/Kinetics
Onset of Action Maximum antihypertensive effect: Within 2 weeks

Available Dosage Forms
Tablet, Oral:
Tekturna: 150 mg, 300 mg

General Dosage Range Oral: *Adults:* 150-300 mg once daily (maximum: 300 mg daily)

Administration
Oral Administer at the same time daily; may take with or without a meal, but consistent administration with regards to meals is recommended.

Storage/Stability Store at 25°C (77°F); excursions permitted to 15°C to 30°C (59°F to 86°F). Protect from moisture.

Nursing Actions
Physical Assessment Monitor for angioedema and hypotension at beginning of therapy, when changing dose, and on a regular basis throughout.

Patient Education
• Discuss specific use of drug and side effects with patient as it relates to treatment. (HCAHPS: During this hospital stay, were you given any medicine that you had not taken before? Before giving you any new medicine, how often did hospital staff tell you what the medicine was for? How often did hospital staff describe possible side effects in a way you could understand?)
• Patient may experience diarrhea, back pain, or flu-like syndrome. Have patient report immediately to prescriber severe dizziness, syncope, urinary retention, oliguria, arrhythmia, dyspepsia, or emesis (HCAHPS).
• Educate patient about signs of a significant reaction (eg, wheezing; chest tightness; fever; itching; bad cough; blue skin color; seizures; or swelling of face, lips, tongue, or throat). **Note:** This is not a comprehensive list of all side effects. Patient should consult prescriber for additional questions.

Intended Use and Disclaimer: Should not be printed and given to patients. This information is intended to serve as a concise initial reference for healthcare professionals to use when discussing medications with a patient. You must ultimately rely on your own discretion, experience and judgment in diagnosing, treating and advising patients.

Dietary Considerations May be taken with or without food; however, a high-fat meal reduces absorption. Consistent administration with regards to meals is recommended.

Aliskiren, Amlodipine, and Hydrochlorothiazide
(a lis KYE ren, am LOE di peen, & hye droe klor oh THYE a zide)

Brand Names: U.S. Amturnide™

Index Terms Aliskiren, Hydrochlorothiazide, and Amlodipine; Amlodipine Besylate, Aliskiren Hemifumarate, and Hydrochlorothiazide; Amlodipine, Aliskiren, and Hydrochlorothiazide; Amlodipine, Hydrochlorothiazide, and Aliskiren; Hydrochlorothiazide, Aliskiren, and Amlodipine; Hydrochlorothiazide, Amlodipine, and Aliskiren

Pharmacologic Category Antianginal Agent; Antihypertensive; Calcium Channel Blocker; Calcium Channel Blocker, Dihydropyridine; Diuretic, Thiazide; Renin Inhibitor

Medication Safety Issues
Sound-alike/look-alike issues:
Amturnide™ may be confused with AMILoride

Pregnancy Risk Factor D

Use Treatment of hypertension (not for initial therapy)

Available Dosage Forms
Tablet, oral:
Amturnide: Aliskiren 150 mg, amlodipine 5 mg, and hydrochlorothiazide 12.5 mg; Aliskiren 300 mg, amlodipine 5 mg, and hydrochlorothiazide 12.5 mg; Aliskiren 300 mg, amlodipine 5 mg, and hydrochlorothiazide 25 mg; Aliskiren 300 mg, amlodipine 10 mg, and hydrochlorothiazide 12.5 mg; Aliskiren 300 mg, amlodipine 10 mg, and hydrochlorothiazide 25 mg

General Dosage Range Oral: *Adults:* Aliskiren 150-300 mg and Amlodipine 5-10 mg and Hydrochlorothiazide 12.5-25 mg once daily (maximum recommended daily dose: Aliskiren 300 mg; amlodipine 10 mg; hydrochlorothiazide 25 mg)

Administration
Oral Administer at the same time daily. May take with or without a meal, but consistent administration with regard to meals is recommended.

Nursing Actions
Physical Assessment See individual agents.
Patient Education
• Discuss specific use of drug and side effects with patient as it relates to treatment. (HCAHPS: During this hospital stay, were you given any medicine that you had not taken before? Before giving you any new medicine, how often did hospital staff tell you what the medicine was for? How often did hospital staff describe possible side effects in a way you could understand?)

- Patient may experience dizziness, diarrhea, headache, pharyngitis, rhinitis, rhinorrhea, or asthenia. Have patient report immediately to prescriber signs of infection, signs of hyperglycemia, signs of fluid and electrolyte imbalance, urine discoloration, jaundice, angina, bradycardia, dyspnea, excessive weight gain, edema of extremities, dyspepsia, ecchymosis, hemorrhaging, hyperhidrosis, vision changes, or ophthalmalgia (HCAHPS).
- Educate patient about signs of a significant reaction (eg, wheezing; chest tightness; fever; itching; bad cough; blue skin color; seizures; or swelling of face, lips, tongue, or throat). **Note:** This is not a comprehensive list of all side effects. Patient should consult prescriber for additional questions.

Intended Use and Disclaimer: Should not be printed and given to patients. This information is intended to serve as a concise initial reference for healthcare professionals to use when discussing medications with a patient. You must ultimately rely on your own discretion, experience and judgment in diagnosing, treating and advising patients.

Related Information
Aliskiren *on page 58*
AmLODIPine *on page 87*
Hydrochlorothiazide *on page 775*

Aliskiren and Amlodipine
(a lis KYE ren & am LOE di peen)

Brand Names: U.S. Tekamlo
Index Terms Aliskiren Hemifumarate and Amlodipine Besylate; Amlodipine and Aliskiren
Pharmacologic Category Antianginal Agent; Antihypertensive; Calcium Channel Blocker; Calcium Channel Blocker, Dihydropyridine; Renin Inhibitor
Pregnancy Risk Factor D
Use Treatment of hypertension, alone or in combination with other antihypertensive agents
Available Dosage Forms
Tablet, oral:
Tekamlo: 150/5: Aliskiren 150 mg and amlodipine 5 mg, 300/5: Aliskiren 300 mg and amlodipine 5 mg, 150/10: Aliskiren 150 mg and amlodipine 10 mg, 300/10: Aliskiren 300 mg and amlodipine 10 mg
General Dosage Range Oral: *Adults:* Aliskiren 150-300 mg and amlodipine 5-10 mg once daily (maximum: 300 mg daily [aliskiren]; 10 mg daily [amlodipine])
Administration
Oral Administer at the same time daily. May take with or without a meal, but consistent administration with regards to meals is recommended.

Nursing Actions
Physical Assessment See individual agents.
Patient Education
- Discuss specific use of drug and side effects with patient as it relates to treatment. (HCAHPS: During this hospital stay, were you given any medicine that you had not taken before? Before giving you any new medicine, how often did hospital staff tell you what the medicine was for? How often did hospital staff describe possible side effects in a way you could understand?)
- Patient may experience diarrhea or flu-like syndrome. Have patient report immediately to prescriber severe dizziness, syncope, urinary retention, oliguria, angina, urine discoloration, jaundice, tachycardia, bradycardia, arrhythmia, myalgia, dyspnea, excessive weight gain, edema of extremities, dyspepsia, significant nausea, hyperhidrosis, or considerable asthenia (HCAHPS).
- Educate patient about signs of a significant reaction (eg, wheezing; chest tightness; fever; itching; bad cough; blue skin color; seizures; or swelling of face, lips, tongue, or throat). **Note:** This is not a comprehensive list of all side effects. Patient should consult prescriber for additional questions.

Intended Use and Disclaimer: Should not be printed and given to patients. This information is intended to serve as a concise initial reference for healthcare professionals to use when discussing medications with a patient. You must ultimately rely on your own discretion, experience and judgment in diagnosing, treating and advising patients.
Related Information
Aliskiren *on page 58*
AmLODIPine *on page 87*

Aliskiren and Hydrochlorothiazide
(a lis KYE ren & hye droe klor oh THYE a zide)

Brand Names: U.S. Tekturna HCT
Index Terms Aliskiren Hemifumarate and Hydrochlorothiazide; Hydrochlorothiazide and Aliskiren
Pharmacologic Category Antihypertensive; Diuretic, Thiazide; Renin Inhibitor
Pregnancy Risk Factor D
Use
Hypertension: Treatment of hypertension, including use as initial therapy in patients likely to need multiple antihypertensives for adequate control
Canadian labeling: Treatment of hypertension when combination therapy is appropriate; not indicated for initial therapy.

Available Dosage Forms
Tablet, Oral:
Tekturna HCT: 150/12.5: Aliskiren 150 mg and hydrochlorothiazide 12.5 mg; 150/25: Aliskiren 150 mg and hydrochlorothiazide 25 mg; 300/12.5: Aliskiren 300 mg and hydrochlorothiazide 12.5 mg; 300/25: Aliskiren 300 mg and hydrochlorothiazide 25 mg

General Dosage Range Oral: *Adults:* Aliskiren 150-300 mg and hydrochlorothiazide 12.5-25 mg once daily (maximum: 300 mg daily [aliskiren]; 25 mg daily [hydrochlorothiazide])

Administration
Oral Administer at the same time daily; may take with or without a meal, but consistent administration with regards to meals is recommended.

Nursing Actions
Physical Assessment See individual agents.

Patient Education
- Discuss specific use of drug and side effects with patient as it relates to treatment. (HCAHPS: During this hospital stay, were you given any medicine that you had not taken before? Before giving you any new medicine, how often did hospital staff tell you what the medicine was for? How often did hospital staff describe possible side effects in a way you could understand?)
- Patient may experience dizziness, asthenia, diarrhea, or flu-like symptoms. Have patient report immediately to prescriber signs of hepatic impairment, signs of hyperglycemia, signs of fluid and electrolyte imbalance, dysphagia, dyspnea, significant weight gain, edema of extremities, vision changes, or signs of Stevens-Johnson syndrome/toxic epidermal necrolysis (HCAHPS).
- Educate patient about signs of a significant reaction (eg, wheezing; chest tightness; fever; itching; bad cough; blue skin color; seizures; or swelling of face, lips, tongue, or throat). **Note:** This is not a comprehensive list of all side effects. Patient should consult prescriber for additional questions.

Intended Use and Disclaimer: Should not be printed and given to patients. This information is intended to serve as a concise initial reference for healthcare professionals to use when discussing medications with a patient. You must ultimately rely on your own discretion, experience and judgment in diagnosing, treating and advising patients.

Related Information
Aliskiren *on page 58*
Hydrochlorothiazide *on page 775*

Alitretinoin (Systemic)

Index Terms 9-*cis*-Retinoic Acid; 9-*cis*-Tretinoin

Pharmacologic Category Anti-inflammatory Agent; Immunomodulator, Systemic; Retinoic Acid Derivative

Medication Safety Issues
Sound-alike/look-alike issues:
Alitretinoin may be confused with isotretinoin
Alitretinoin may be confused with tretinoin
High alert medication:
The Institute for Safe Medication Practices (ISMP) includes this medication among its list of drugs which have a heightened risk of causing significant patient harm when used in error.
International issues:
Panretin is a topical preparation of alitretinoin available in the U.S.
Other safety concerns:
ALERT: Canadian Boxed Warning: Health Canada-approved labeling includes a boxed warning. For verbatim wording of the boxed warning, consult the product labeling.

Lactation Excretion in breast milk unknown/contraindicated

Use Treatment of severe chronic hand eczema refractory to topical corticosteroids

Product Availability Not available in the U.S.

General Dosage Range Oral: *Adults:* 10-30 mg once daily

Administration
Oral Administer once daily with a meal. Missed doses should be taken as soon as possible; 2 doses should not be taken on the same day. Hazardous agent; use appropriate precautions for handling and disposal (NIOSH, 2012).

Nursing Actions
Patient Education
- Discuss specific use of drug and side effects with patient as it relates to treatment. (HCAHPS: During this hospital stay, were you given any medicine that you had not taken before? Before giving you any new medicine, how often did hospital staff tell you what the medicine was for? How often did hospital staff describe possible side effects in a way you could understand?)
- Patient may experience headache, flushing, xerophthalmia, contact lens discomfort, cheilitis, or xerostomia. Have patient report immediately to prescriber signs of depression (ie, suicidal ideation, anxiety, emotional instability, illogical thinking), signs of pancreatitis, signs of hepatic impairment, signs of hyperglycemia, asthenia, myalgia, severe arthralgia, significant osteodynia, ophthalmalgia, eye irritation, ecchymosis, hemorrhaging, decreased night vision, or signs of inflammatory bowel disease (HCAHPS).
- Educate patient about signs of a significant reaction (eg, wheezing; chest tightness; fever; itching; bad cough; blue skin color; seizures; or swelling of face, lips, tongue, or throat). **Note:** This is not a comprehensive list of all side effects. Patient should consult prescriber for additional questions.

Intended Use and Disclaimer: Should not be printed and given to patients. This information is intended to serve as a concise initial reference for healthcare professionals to use when discussing medications with a patient. You must ultimately rely on your own discretion, experience and judgment in diagnosing, treating and advising patients.

Alitretinoin (Topical) (a li TRET i noyn)

Brand Names: U.S. Panretin
Pharmacologic Category Antineoplastic Agent, Retinoic Acid Derivative
Medication Safety Issues
  Sound-alike/look-alike issues:
  Panretin® may be confused with pancreatin
  High alert medication:
  The Institute for Safe Medication Practices (ISMP) includes this medication among its list of drugs which have a heightened risk of causing significant patient harm when used in error.
Pregnancy Risk Factor D
Lactation Excretion in breast milk unknown/not recommended
Use Topical treatment of cutaneous lesions in AIDS-related Kaposi's sarcoma. Not indicated when systemic therapy is necessary (eg, >10 new lesions in previous month, symptomatic visceral involvement, symptomatic pulmonary Kaposi's sarcoma, symptomatic lymphedema)
Available Dosage Forms
  Gel, External:
  Panretin: 0.1% (60 g)
General Dosage Range Dosage adjustment may be necessary for application site toxicity.
  Topical: *Adults:* Initial: Apply twice daily; Range: Apply 2-4 times daily
Administration
  Topical Apply sufficient gel to cover lesion(s) with a generous coating; allow gel to dry 3-5 minutes after application before covering with clothing. Do not use occlusive dressings. Avoid applying gel to normal skin surrounding lesions. Do not apply to any lesions on or near mucosal surfaces.

  Hazardous agent; use appropriate precautions for handling and disposal (NIOSH, 2012).
Nursing Actions
  Patient Education
  • Discuss specific use of drug and side effects with patient as it relates to treatment. (HCAHPS: During this hospital stay, were you given any medicine that you had not taken before? Before giving you any new medicine, how often did hospital staff tell you what the medicine was for? How often did hospital staff describe possible side effects in a way you could understand?)
  • Have patient report immediately to prescriber paresthesia or severe application site irritation (HCAHPS).

• Educate patient about signs of a significant reaction (eg, wheezing; chest tightness; fever; itching; bad cough; blue skin color; seizures; or swelling of face, lips, tongue, or throat). **Note:** This is not a comprehensive list of all side effects. Patient should consult prescriber for additional questions.

Intended Use and Disclaimer: Should not be printed and given to patients. This information is intended to serve as a concise initial reference for healthcare professionals to use when discussing medications with a patient. You must ultimately rely on your own discretion, experience and judgment in diagnosing, treating and advising patients.

Allopurinol (al oh PURE i nole)

Brand Names: U.S. Aloprim; Zyloprim
Index Terms Allopurinol Sodium
Pharmacologic Category Antigout Agent; Xanthine Oxidase Inhibitor
Medication Safety Issues
  Sound-alike/look-alike issues:
  Allopurinol may be confused with Apresoline
  Zyloprim® may be confused with ZORprin®, Zovirax®
Pregnancy Risk Factor C
Lactation Enters breast milk/use caution
Breast-Feeding Considerations Allopurinol and its metabolite are excreted into breast milk; the metabolite was also detected in the serum of the nursing infant (Kamilli, 1993). The manufacturer recommends caution be used when administering allopurinol to nursing women.
Use
  Oral: Management of primary or secondary gout (acute attack, tophi, joint destruction, uric acid lithiasis, and/or nephropathy); management of hyperuricemia associated with cancer treatment for leukemia, lymphoma, or solid tumor malignancies; management of recurrent calcium oxalate calculi (with uric acid excretion >800 mg/day in men and >750 mg/day in women)
  I.V.: Management of hyperuricemia associated with cancer treatment for leukemia, lymphoma, or solid tumor malignancies
Mechanism of Action/Effect Allopurinol inhibits xanthine oxidase, the enzyme responsible for the conversion of hypoxanthine to xanthine to uric acid. Allopurinol is metabolized to oxypurinol which is also an inhibitor of xanthine oxidase; allopurinol acts on purine catabolism, reducing the production of uric acid without disrupting the biosynthesis of vital purines.
Contraindications Hypersensitivity to allopurinol or any component of the formulation
Warnings/Precautions Do not use to treat asymptomatic hyperuricemia. Has been associated with a number of hypersensitivity reactions,

including severe reactions (vasculitis and Stevens-Johnson syndrome); discontinue at first sign of rash. Reversible hepatotoxicity has been reported; use with caution in patients with pre-existing hepatic impairment. Bone marrow suppression has been reported; use caution with other drugs causing myelosuppression. Caution in renal impairment, dosage adjustments needed. Use with caution in patients taking diuretics concurrently. Risk of skin rash may be increased in patients receiving amoxicillin or ampicillin. The risk of hypersensitivity may be increased in patients receiving thiazides, and possibly ACE inhibitors. Use caution with mercaptopurine or azathioprine; dosage adjustment necessary. Full effect on serum uric acid levels in chronic gout may take several weeks to become evident; gradual titration is recommended.

Drug Interactions
Avoid Concomitant Use
Avoid concomitant use of Allopurinol with any of the following: Didanosine; Pegloticase; Tegafur
Decreased Effect
Allopurinol may decrease the levels/effects of: Tegafur

The levels/effects of Allopurinol may be decreased by: Antacids
Increased Effect/Toxicity
Allopurinol may increase the levels/effects of: Amoxicillin; Ampicillin; Anticonvulsants (Hydantoin); AzaTHIOprine; Bendamustine; CarBAMazepine; ChlorproPAMIDE; Cyclophosphamide; Didanosine; Mercaptopurine; Pegloticase; Theophylline Derivatives; Vitamin K Antagonists

The levels/effects of Allopurinol may be increased by: ACE Inhibitors; Loop Diuretics; Thiazide Diuretics
Nutritional/Ethanol Interactions
Ethanol: May decrease effectiveness.
Iron supplements: Hepatic iron uptake may be increased.
Vitamin C: Large amounts of vitamin C may acidify urine and increase kidney stone formation.

Adverse Reactions
Most commonly reported:
Dermatologic: Skin rash
Endocrine & metabolic: Gout (acute)
Gastrointestinal: Diarrhea, nausea
Hepatic: Increased liver enzymes, increased serum alkaline phosphatase

Pharmacodynamics/Kinetics
Onset of Action Peak effect: 1-2 weeks
Available Dosage Forms
Solution Reconstituted, Intravenous [preservative free]:
Aloprim: 500 mg (1 ea)
Generic: 500 mg (1 ea)
Tablet, Oral:
Zyloprim: 100 mg, 300 mg
Generic: 100 mg, 300 mg

General Dosage Range Dosage adjustment recommended in patients with renal impairment
I.V.:
Children: Initial: 200 mg/m^2/day as a single infusion or in equally divided doses at 6-, 8-, or 12-hour intervals
Adults: 200-400 mg/m^2/day as a single infusion or in equally divided doses at 6-, 8-, or 12-hour intervals (maximum: 600 mg/day)
Oral:
Children <6 years: 150 mg/day
Children 6-10 years: 10 mg/kg/day
Children >10 years and Adults: 100-800 mg/day in 1-3 divided doses (maximum: 800 mg/day)
Administration
I.V. The rate of infusion depends on the volume of the infusion; infuse maximum single daily doses (600 mg/day) over ≥30 minutes. Whenever possible, therapy should be initiated at 24-48 hours before the start of chemotherapy known to cause tumor lysis (including adrenocorticosteroids). I.V. daily dose can be administered as a single infusion or in equally divided doses at 6-, 8-, or 12-hour interval.

Oral Do not initiate or discontinue allopurinol during an acute gout attack. Should be administered after meals with plenty of fluid.
Preparation for Administration Reconstitute powder for injection with SWFI. Further dilution with NS or D$_5$W (50-100 mL) to ≤6 mg/mL is recommended.
Storage/Stability
Powder for injection: Store at controlled room temperature of 20°C to 25°C (68°F to 77°F). Following preparation, intravenous solutions should be stored at 20°C to 25°C (68°F to 77°F). Do not refrigerate reconstituted and/or diluted product. Must be administered within 10 hours of solution preparation.
Tablet: Store at controlled room temperature of 20°C to 25°C (68°F to 77°F). Protect from moisture and light.
Nursing Actions
Physical Assessment Monitor frequency and severity of gouty attacks.
Patient Education
• Discuss specific use of drug and side effects with patient as it relates to treatment. (HCAHPS: During this hospital stay, were you given any medicine that you had not taken before? Before giving you any new medicine, how often did hospital staff tell you what the medicine was for? How often did hospital staff describe possible side effects in a way you could understand?)
• Patient may experience diarrhea, dyspepsia, or injection site irritation. Have patient report immediately to prescriber signs of hepatic impairment, dysuria, hematuria, paresthesia, urinary retention, oliguria, chills, pharyngitis, eye irritation, severe arthralgia, ecchymosis, hemorrhaging, myalgia, significant asthenia, or signs of

Stevens-Johnson syndrome/toxic epidermal necrolysis (HCAHPS).

- Educate patient about signs of a significant reaction (eg, wheezing; chest tightness; fever; itching; bad cough; blue skin color; seizures; or swelling of face, lips, tongue, or throat). **Note:** This is not a comprehensive list of all side effects. Patient should consult prescriber for additional questions.

Intended Use and Disclaimer: Should not be printed and given to patients. This information is intended to serve as a concise initial reference for healthcare professionals to use when discussing medications with a patient. You must ultimately rely on your own discretion, experience and judgment in diagnosing, treating and advising patients.

Dietary Considerations Should take oral forms after meals with plenty of fluid. Fluid intake should be administered to yield neutral or slightly alkaline urine and an output of ~2 L (in adults).

Almotriptan (al moh TRIP tan)

Brand Names: U.S. Axert

Index Terms Almotriptan Malate

Pharmacologic Category Antimigraine Agent; Serotonin 5-HT$_{1B, 1D}$ Receptor Agonist

Medication Safety Issues

Sound-alike/look-alike issues:

Axert may be confused with Antivert

Pregnancy Risk Factor C

Lactation Excretion in breast milk unknown/use caution

Breast-Feeding Considerations It is not known if almotriptan is excreted in breast milk. The manufacturer recommends that caution be exercised when administering almotriptan to nursing women.

Use Acute treatment of migraine with or without aura in adults (with a history of migraine) and adolescents (with a history of migraine lasting ≥4 hours when left untreated)

Mechanism of Action/Effect Selective agonist for serotonin receptor in cranial arteries; causes vasoconstriction and relief of migraine.

Contraindications Hypersensitivity to almotriptan or any component of the formulation; hemiplegic or basilar migraine; known or suspected ischemic heart disease (eg, angina pectoris, MI, documented silent ischemia, coronary artery vasospasm, Prinzmetal's variant angina); cerebrovascular syndromes (eg, stroke, transient ischemic attacks); peripheral vascular disease (eg, ischemic bowel disease); uncontrolled hypertension; use within 24 hours of another 5-HT$_1$ agonist; use within 24 hours of ergotamine derivatives and/or ergotamine-containing medications (eg, dihydroergotamine, ergotamine)

Warnings/Precautions Almotriptan is only indicated for the treatment of acute migraine headache; not indicated for migraine prophylaxis, or the treatment of cluster headaches, hemiplegic migraine, or basilar migraine. If a patient does not respond to the first dose, the diagnosis of acute migraine should be reconsidered.

Almotriptan should not be given to patients with documented ischemic or vasospastic CAD. Patients with risk factors for CAD (eg, hypertension, hypercholesterolemia, smoker, obesity, diabetes, strong family history of CAD, menopause, male >40 years of age) should undergo adequate cardiac evaluation prior to administration; if the cardiac evaluation is "satisfactory," the first dose of almotriptan should be given in the healthcare provider's office (consider ECG monitoring). All patients should undergo periodic evaluation of cardiovascular status during treatment. Cardiac events (coronary artery vasospasm, transient ischemia, myocardial infarction, ventricular tachycardia/fibrillation, cardiac arrest, and death), cerebral/subarachnoid hemorrhage, stroke, peripheral vascular ischemia, and colonic ischemia have been reported with 5-HT$_1$ agonist administration. Patients who experience sensations of chest pain/pressure/tightness or symptoms suggestive of angina following dosing should be evaluated for coronary artery disease or Prinzmetal's angina before receiving additional doses; if dosing is resumed and similar symptoms recur, monitor with ECG. Significant elevation in blood pressure, including hypertensive crisis, has also been reported on rare occasions following 5-HT$_1$ agonist administration in patients with and without a history of hypertension.

Transient and permanent blindness and partial vision loss have been reported (rare) with 5-HT$_1$ agonist administration. Almotriptan contains a sulfonyl group which is structurally different from a sulfonamide. Cross-reactivity in patients with sulfonamide allergy has not been evaluated; however, the manufacturer recommends that caution be exercised in this patient population. Use with caution in liver or renal dysfunction. Symptoms of agitation, confusion, hallucinations, hyper-reflexia, myoclonus, shivering, and tachycardia (serotonin syndrome) may occur with concomitant proserotonergic drugs (ie, SSRIs/SNRIs or triptans) or agents which reduce almotriptan's metabolism. Concurrent use of serotonin precursors (eg, tryptophan) is not recommended. If concomitant administration with SSRIs is warranted, monitor closely, especially at initiation and with dose increases. Efficacy has not been demonstrated in improvement of migraine-associated symptoms (eg, phonophobia, nausea, photophobia) in patients aged 12-17 years (Linder, 2008).

Drug Interactions

Avoid Concomitant Use

Avoid concomitant use of Almotriptan with any of the following: Ergot Derivatives; MAO Inhibitors

Decreased Effect
The levels/effects of Almotriptan may be decreased by: Peginterferon Alfa-2b

Increased Effect/Toxicity
Almotriptan may increase the levels/effects of: Antipsychotics; Droxidopa; Ergot Derivatives; Metoclopramide; Serotonin Modulators

The levels/effects of Almotriptan may be increased by: Antipsychotics; CYP3A4 Inhibitors (Strong); Ergot Derivatives; MAO Inhibitors

Adverse Reactions 1% to 10%:
Central nervous system: Somnolence (≤5%), dizziness (≤4%), headache (≤2%)
Gastrointestinal: Nausea (1% to 3%), vomiting (≤2%), xerostomia (1%)
Neuromuscular & skeletal: Paresthesia (≤1%)

Available Dosage Forms
Tablet, Oral:
Axert: 6.25 mg, 12.5 mg

General Dosage Range Dosage adjustment recommended in patients with hepatic or renal impairment and/or on concomitant therapy
Oral: *Children ≥12 years and Adults:* 6.25-12.5 mg in a single dose; may repeat after 2 hours (maximum daily dose: 25 mg)

Administration
Oral Administer without regard to meals.

Storage/Stability Store at 25°C (77°F); excursions permitted to 15°C to 30°C (59°F to 86°F).

Nursing Actions
Physical Assessment Clear diagnosis of migraines and cardiac status should be determined before beginning treatment. Assess risk for coronary artery disease, liver or renal dysfunction, and sulfonamide allergy. Monitor for hypertension and cardiac events. Teach patient proper use (treatment of acute migraine; not prevention of migraine).

Patient Education
• Discuss specific use of drug and side effects with patient as it relates to treatment. (HCAHPS: During this hospital stay, were you given any medicine that you had not taken before? Before giving you any new medicine, how often did hospital staff tell you what the medicine was for? How often did hospital staff describe possible side effects in a way you could understand?)
• Patient may experience fatigue or xerostomia. Have patient report immediately to prescriber constipation, significant dyspepsia, melena, paresthesia, weight loss, leg cramps, leg pain, sensation of cold, burning or aching pain in feet or toes, dyspnea, vision changes, blindness, serotonin syndrome (ie, dizziness, severe headache, agitation, hallucinations, tachycardia, arrhythmia, flushing, tremors, hyperhidrosis, change in balance, illogical thinking, severe nausea, significant diarrhea), signs of severe cardiac abnormalities, strength differences from one side to another, or difficulty speaking or thinking (HCAHPS).
• Educate patient about signs of a significant reaction (eg, wheezing; chest tightness; fever; itching; bad cough; blue skin color; seizures; or swelling of face, lips, tongue, or throat). **Note:** This is not a comprehensive list of all side effects. Patient should consult prescriber for additional questions.

Intended Use and Disclaimer: Should not be printed and given to patients. This information is intended to serve as a concise initial reference for healthcare professionals to use when discussing medications with a patient. You must ultimately rely on your own discretion, experience and judgment in diagnosing, treating and advising patients.

Dietary Considerations May be taken without regard to meals.

Alogliptin (al oh GLIP tin)

Brand Names: U.S. Nesina
Index Terms Alogliptin Benzoate
Pharmacologic Category Antidiabetic Agent, Dipeptidyl Peptidase IV (DPP-IV) Inhibitor; Hypoglycemic Agent, Oral

Medication Safety Issues
High alert medication:
The Institute for Safe Medication Practices (ISMP) includes this medication among its list of drug classes which have a heightened risk of causing significant patient harm when used in error.

Medication Guide Available Yes
Pregnancy Risk Factor B
Lactation Excretion in breast milk unknown/use caution

Breast-Feeding Considerations It is not known if alogliptin is excreted in breast milk. The manufacturer recommends that caution be exercised when administering alogliptin to nursing women.

Use Management of type 2 diabetes mellitus (non-insulin dependent, NIDDM) as an adjunct to diet and exercise as monotherapy or in combination with other antidiabetic agents

Mechanism of Action/Effect Alogliptin inhibits dipeptidyl peptidase IV (DPP-IV) enzyme resulting in increased insulin synthesis and release and decreased hepatic glucose production.

Contraindications Serious hypersensitivity (eg, anaphylaxis, angioedema, severe dermatologic reactions) to products that contain alogliptin

Warnings/Precautions Cases of fatal and nonfatal hepatic failure have been reported in postmarketing surveillance. Baseline liver function tests (serum transaminases) are recommended to rule out underlying liver diseases. Use with caution in patients with abnormal serum transaminases. Monitor and promptly evaluate serum transaminase levels in patients with symptoms of hepatic injury (eg, fatigue, anorexia, jaundice, dark urine, and/or abdominal pain). In patients with clinically significant transaminase elevations and/or persistent or worsening elevations, alogliptin therapy should be interrupted. Therapy should only be resumed with caution in patients where an alternative cause of transaminase elevations has been determined.

Rare hypersensitivity reactions, including anaphylaxis, angioedema, and/or severe dermatologic reactions such as Stevens-Johnson syndrome, have been reported in postmarketing surveillance; discontinue if signs/symptoms of hypersensitivity reactions occur. Use with caution if patient has experienced angioedema with other DPP-IV inhibitor use. Cases of acute pancreatitis have been reported with use. Monitor for signs/symptoms of pancreatitis; discontinue use immediately if pancreatitis is suspected and initiate appropriate management. Use with caution in patients with a history of pancreatitis as it is not known if this population is at greater risk.

Not indicated for use in patients with type 1 diabetes mellitus (insulin dependent, IDDM) due to lack of efficacy in this population. Not indicated for use in patients with DKA due to lack of efficacy in this patient population. Safety and efficacy have not been established in severe hepatic dysfunction. Dosage adjustments are not required in mild or moderate hepatic dysfunction. Use with caution in patients with liver disease. Use with caution in patients with moderate-to-severe renal dysfunction and end-stage renal disease (ESRD) requiring hemodialysis; dosing adjustment required. Concomitant use of insulin may increase the risk of hypoglycemia. Monitor blood glucose closely; dosage reduction of insulin may be required. Concomitant use of an insulin secretagogue (eg, sulfonylurea) may increase the risk of hypoglycemia. Monitor blood glucose closely; dosage reduction of secretagogues may be required. Diabetes self-management education (DSME) is essential to maximize the effectiveness of therapy.

Drug Interactions

Avoid Concomitant Use There are no known interactions where it is recommended to avoid concomitant use.

Decreased Effect

The levels/effects of Alogliptin may be decreased by: Corticosteroids (Orally Inhaled); Corticosteroids (Systemic); Loop Diuretics; Luteinizing Hormone-Releasing Hormone Analogs; Peginterferon Alfa-2b; Somatropin; Thiazide Diuretics

Increased Effect/Toxicity

Alogliptin may increase the levels/effects of: ACE Inhibitors; Hypoglycemic Agents

The levels/effects of Alogliptin may be increased by: Herbs (Hypoglycemic Properties); MAO Inhibitors; Pegvisomant; Salicylates; Selective Serotonin Reuptake Inhibitors

Adverse Reactions

1% to 10%:

Central nervous system: Headache (4%)

Hepatic: Increased serum ALT (>3 times ULN: 1%)

Respiratory: Nasopharyngitis (4%), upper respiratory tract infection (4%)

Available Dosage Forms

Tablet, Oral:

Nesina: 6.25 mg, 12.5 mg, 25 mg

General Dosage Range Dosage adjustment recommended in patients with renal impairment.

Oral: *Adults:* 25 mg once daily

Administration

Oral May be taken with or without food.

Storage/Stability Store at 25°C (77°F); excursions permitted between 15°C to 30°C (59°F to 86°F).

Nursing Actions

Patient Education

- Discuss specific use of drug and side effects with patient as it relates to treatment. (HCAHPS: During this hospital stay, were you given any medicine that you had not taken before? Before giving you any new medicine, how often did hospital staff tell you what the medicine was for? How often did hospital staff describe possible side effects in a way you could understand?)
- Patient may experience pharyngitis, rhinitis, rhinorrhea, or headache. Have patient report immediately to prescriber signs of hypoglycemia, signs of pancreatitis, or signs of hepatic impairment (HCAHPS).
- Educate patient about signs of a significant reaction (eg, wheezing; chest tightness; fever; itching; bad cough; blue skin color; seizures; or swelling of face, lips, tongue, or throat). **Note:** This is not a comprehensive list of all side effects. Patient should consult prescriber for additional questions.

Intended Use and Disclaimer: Should not be printed and given to patients. This information is intended to serve as a concise initial reference for healthcare professionals to use when discussing medications with a patient. You must ultimately rely on your own discretion, experience and judgment in diagnosing, treating and advising patients.

Dietary Considerations May be taken with or without food. Individualized medical nutrition therapy (MNT) based on ADA recommendations is an integral part of therapy.

Alogliptin and Metformin
(al oh GLIP tin & met FOR min)

Brand Names: U.S. Kazano

Index Terms Alogliptin and Metformin Hydrochloride; Metformin and Alogliptin; Metformin Hydrochloride and Alogliptin

Pharmacologic Category Antidiabetic Agent, Biguanide; Antidiabetic Agent, Dipeptidyl Peptidase IV (DPP-IV) Inhibitor; Hypoglycemic Agent, Oral

Medication Safety Issues

Sound-alike/look-alike issues:

Alogliptin and Metformin may be confused with Linagliptin and Metformin, Saxagliptin and Metformin, Sitagliptin and Metformin

High alert medication:

The Institute for Safe Medication Practices (ISMP) includes this medication among its list of drug classes which have a heightened risk of causing significant patient harm when used in error.

Medication Guide Available Yes

Pregnancy Risk Factor B

Use Management of type 2 diabetes mellitus (non-insulin dependent, NIDDM) as an adjunct to diet and exercise in patients not adequately controlled on alogliptin or metformin monotherapy

Available Dosage Forms

Tablet, Oral:

Kazano: Alogliptin 12.5 mg and metformin hydrochloride 500 mg, Alogliptin 12.5 mg and metformin hydrochloride 1000 mg

General Dosage Range

Oral: *Adults:* Alogliptin 12.5 mg and metformin 500-1000 mg twice daily (maximum: 25 mg daily [alogliptin], 2000 mg per day [metformin])

Administration

Oral Administer twice daily with meals. Swallow tablets whole; do not split or divide.

Nursing Actions

Patient Education

• Discuss specific use of drug and side effects with patient as it relates to treatment. (HCAHPS: During this hospital stay, were you given any medicine that you had not taken before? Before giving you any new medicine, how often did hospital staff tell you what the medicine was for? How often did hospital staff describe possible side effects in a way you could understand?)

• Patient may experience pharyngitis, rhinitis, diarrhea, back pain, rhinorrhea, or headache. Have patient report immediately to prescriber angina, chills, dysuria, difficult urination, foul-smelling urine, signs of hypoglycemia, signs of pancreatitis, signs of hepatic impairment, or signs of lactic acidosis (HCAHPS).

• Educate patient about signs of a significant reaction (eg, wheezing; chest tightness; fever; itching; bad cough; blue skin color; seizures; or swelling of face, lips, tongue, or throat). **Note:** This is not a comprehensive list of all side effects. Patient should consult prescriber for additional questions.

Intended Use and Disclaimer: Should not be printed and given to patients. This information is intended to serve as a concise initial reference for healthcare professionals to use when discussing medications with a patient. You must ultimately rely on your own discretion, experience and judgment in diagnosing, treating and advising patients.

Related Information

Alogliptin *on page 66*

MetFORMIN *on page 1014*

Alogliptin and Pioglitazone
(al oh GLIP tin & pye oh GLI ta zone)

Brand Names: U.S. Oseni

Index Terms Pioglitazone and Alogliptin

Pharmacologic Category Antidiabetic Agent; Dipeptidyl Peptidase IV (DPP-IV) Inhibitor; Antidiabetic Agent, Thiazolidinedione; Hypoglycemic Agent, Oral

Medication Safety Issues

High alert medication:

The Institute for Safe Medication Practices (ISMP) includes this medication among its list of drug classes which have a heightened risk of causing significant patient harm when used in error.

Medication Guide Available Yes

Pregnancy Risk Factor C

Use Management of type 2 diabetes mellitus (non-insulin dependent, NIDDM) as an adjunct to diet and exercise in patients not adequately controlled on alogliptin or pioglitazone monotherapy

Available Dosage Forms

Tablet, Oral:

Oseni: Alogliptin 25 mg and pioglitazone 15 mg, Alogliptin 25 mg and pioglitazone 30 mg, Alogliptin 25 mg and pioglitazone 45 mg, Alogliptin 12.5 mg and pioglitazone 15 mg, Alogliptin 12.5 mg and pioglitazone 30 mg, Alogliptin 12.5 mg and pioglitazone 45 mg

General Dosage Range Dosage adjustment recommended in patients with renal impairment or concomitant drug therapy.

Oral: *Adults:* Alogliptin 25 mg and pioglitazone 15-45 mg once daily (Maximum: Alogliptin 25 mg/pioglitazone 45 mg once daily)

Administration

Oral May be taken with or without food. Swallow tablets whole; do not split or divide.

Nursing Actions

Patient Education

• Discuss specific use of drug and side effects with patient as it relates to treatment. (HCAHPS: During this hospital stay, were you given any medicine that you had not taken before? Before giving you any new medicine, how often did hospital staff tell you what the medicine was for? How often did hospital staff describe possible side effects in a way you could understand?

• Patient may experience headache, rhinitis, rhinorrhea, pharyngitis, or back pain. Have patient report immediately to prescriber strength differences from one side to another, difficulty speaking or thinking, change in balance, blurred vision, dysuria, hematuria, polyuria, osteodynia, severe asthenia, angina, vision changes, signs of hypoglycemia, signs of pancreatitis, or signs of hepatic impairment (HCAHPS).

• Educate patient about signs of a significant reaction (eg, wheezing; chest tightness; fever; itching; bad cough; blue skin color; seizures; or swelling of face, lips, tongue, or throat). **Note:** This is not a comprehensive list of all side effects. Patient should consult prescriber for additional questions.

Intended Use and Disclaimer: Should not be printed and given to patients. This information is intended to serve as a concise initial reference for healthcare professionals to use when discussing medications with a patient. You must ultimately rely on your own discretion, experience and judgment in diagnosing, treating and advising patients.

Related Information
Alogliptin on page 66
Pioglitazone on page 1250

ALPRAZolam (al PRAY zoe lam)

Brand Names: U.S. ALPRAZolam Intensol; ALPRAZolam XR; Niravam; Xanax; Xanax XR
Pharmacologic Category Benzodiazepine
Medication Safety Issues
 Sound-alike/look-alike issues:
  ALPRAZolam may be confused with alprostadil, LORazepam, triazolam
  Xanax® may be confused with Fanapt®, Lanoxin®, Tenex®, Tylox®, Xopenex®, Zantac®, ZyrTEC®
 BEERS Criteria medication:
  This drug may be potentially inappropriate for use in geriatric patients (Quality of evidence - high; Strength of recommendation - strong).

Pregnancy Risk Factor D
Lactation Enters breast milk/not recommended
Breast-Feeding Considerations Benzodiazepines are excreted into breast milk. In a study of eight postpartum women, peak concentrations of alprazolam were found in breast milk ~1 hour after the maternal dose and the half-life was ~14 hours. Samples were obtained over 36 hours following a single oral dose of alprazolam 0.5 mg. Metabolites were not detected in breast milk. In this study, the estimated exposure to the breast-feeding infant was ~3% of the weight-adjusted maternal dose (Oo, 1995). Drowsiness, lethargy, or weight loss in nursing infants have been observed in case reports following maternal use of some benzodiazepines (Iqbal, 2002). Breast-feeding is not recommended by the manufacturer.

Use Treatment of anxiety disorder (GAD); short-term relief of symptoms of anxiety; panic disorder, with or without agoraphobia; anxiety associated with depression
Unlabeled Use Anxiety in children
Mechanism of Action/Effect Binds to stereospecific benzodiazepine receptors on the postsynaptic GABA neuron at several sites within the central nervous system, including the limbic system, reticular formation. Enhancement of the inhibitory effect of GABA on neuronal excitability results by increased neuronal membrane permeability to chloride ions. This shift in chloride ions results in hyperpolarization (a less excitable state) and stabilization.
Contraindications Hypersensitivity to alprazolam or any component of the formulation (cross-sensitivity with other benzodiazepines may exist); narrow-angle glaucoma; concurrent use with ketoconazole or itraconazole
Warnings/Precautions Rebound or withdrawal symptoms, including seizures, may occur following abrupt discontinuation or large decreases in dose (more common in patients receiving >4 mg/day or prolonged treatment); the risk of seizures appears to be greatest 24-72 hours following discontinuation of therapy. Breakthrough anxiety may occur at the end of dosing interval. Use with caution in patients receiving concurrent CYP3A4 inhibitors, moderate or strong CYP3A4 inducers, and major CYP3A4 substrates; consider alternative agents that avoid or lessen the potential for CYP-mediated interactions. Use with caution in renal impairment or predisposition to urate nephropathy; has weak uricosuric properties. In older adults, benzodiazepines increase the risk of impaired cognition, delirium, falls, fractures, and motor vehicle accidents. Due to increased sensitivity in this age group, avoid use for treatment of insomnia, agitation, or delirium (Beers Criteria). Use with caution in or debilitated patients, patients with hepatic disease (including alcoholics) or respiratory disease, or obese patients.

Causes CNS depression (dose related) which may impair physical and mental capabilities. Patients must be cautioned about performing tasks that require mental alertness (eg, operating machinery or driving). Effects with other sedative drugs or ethanol may be potentiated. Benzodiazepines have been associated with falls and traumatic injury and should be used with extreme caution in patients who are at risk of these events.

Use caution in patients with depression, particularly if suicidal risk may be present. Episodes of mania or hypomania have occurred in depressed patients treated with alprazolam. May cause physical or psychological dependence. Acute ▶

withdrawal may be precipitated in patients after administration of flumazenil.

Benzodiazepines have been associated with anterograde amnesia. Paradoxical reactions have been reported with benzodiazepines, particularly in adolescent/pediatric or psychiatric patients. Does not have analgesic, antidepressant, or antipsychotic properties.

Drug Interactions

Avoid Concomitant Use
Avoid concomitant use of ALPRAZolam with any of the following: Azelastine (Nasal); Conivaptan; Fusidic Acid (Systemic); Indinavir; Itraconazole; Ketoconazole (Systemic); OLANZapine; Paraldehyde; Sodium Oxybate; Thalidomide

Decreased Effect
The levels/effects of ALPRAZolam may be decreased by: Bosentan; CarBAMazepine; CYP3A4 Inducers (Strong); Dabrafenib; Deferasirox; Herbs (CYP3A4 Inducers); Mitotane; Rifamycin Derivatives; Theophylline Derivatives; Tocilizumab; Yohimbine

Increased Effect/Toxicity
ALPRAZolam may increase the levels/effects of: Alcohol (Ethyl); Azelastine (Nasal); Buprenorphine; CloZAPine; CNS Depressants; Hydrocodone; Methotrimeprazine; Metyrosine; Mirtazapine; Paraldehyde; Pramipexole; ROPINIRole; Rotigotine; Selective Serotonin Reuptake Inhibitors; Sodium Oxybate; Thalidomide; Zolpidem

The levels/effects of ALPRAZolam may be increased by: Antifungal Agents (Azole Derivatives, Systemic); Aprepitant; Boceprevir; Brimonidine (Topical); Calcium Channel Blockers (Nondihydropyridine); Cimetidine; Conivaptan; Contraceptives (Estrogens); Contraceptives (Progestins); CYP3A4 Inhibitors (Moderate); CYP3A4 Inhibitors (Strong); Dasatinib; Doxylamine; Droperidol; Fosaprepitant; Fusidic Acid (Systemic); Grapefruit Juice; HydrOXYzine; Indinavir; Isoniazid; Itraconazole; Ivacaftor; Ketoconazole (Systemic); Luliconazole; Macrolide Antibiotics; Magnesium Sulfate; Methotrimeprazine; Mifepristone; OLANZapine; Perampanel; Protease Inhibitors; Proton Pump Inhibitors; Selective Serotonin Reuptake Inhibitors; Simeprevir; Stiripentol; Tapentadol; Telaprevir

Nutritional/Ethanol Interactions
Cigarette: Smoking may decrease alprazolam concentrations up to 50%.

Ethanol: Ethanol may increase CNS depression. Management: Avoid ethanol.

Food: Alprazolam serum concentration is unlikely to be increased by grapefruit juice because of alprazolam's high oral bioavailability. The C_{max} of the extended release formulation is increased by 25% when a high-fat meal is given 2 hours before dosing. T_{max} is decreased 33% when food is given immediately prior to dose and increased by 33% when food is given ≥1 hour after dose.

Herb/Nutraceutical: St John's wort may decrease alprazolam levels. Valerian, kava kava, and gotu kola may increase CNS depression. Management: Avoid St John's wort. Avoid valerian, kava kava, and gotu kola.

Adverse Reactions
>10%:
Central nervous system: Ataxia, cognitive dysfunction, depression, dizziness, drowsiness, dysarthria, fatigue, irritability, memory impairment, sedation
Endocrine & metabolic: Decreased libido, weight gain, weight loss
Gastrointestinal: Change in appetite, constipation, xerostomia
Genitourinary: Difficulty in micturition
Respiratory: Nasal congestion
1% to 10%:
Cardiovascular: Chest pain, hypotension, palpitations, sinus tachycardia, syncope
Central nervous system: Abnormal dreams, agitation, akathisia, altered mental status, confusion, depersonalization, derealization, disinhibition, disorientation, disturbance in attention, dystonia, fear, hallucination, headache, hypersomnia, hypoesthesia, insomnia, lethargy, malaise, nervousness, nightmares, paresthesia, restlessness, seizure, talkativeness, vertigo
Dermatologic: Dermatitis, diaphoresis, skin rash
Endocrine & metabolic: Increased libido, menstrual disease
Gastrointestinal: Abdominal pain, anorexia, diarrhea, dyspepsia, nausea, sialorrhea, vomiting
Genitourinary: Dysmenorrhea, sexual disorder, urinary incontinence
Hepatic: Increased liver enzymes, increased serum bilirubin, jaundice
Neuromuscular & skeletal: Arthralgia, back pain, dyskinesia, muscle cramps, muscle twitching, myalgia, tremor, weakness
Ophthalmic: Blurred vision
Respiratory: Allergic rhinitis, dyspnea, hyperventilation, upper respiratory tract infection

Pharmacodynamics/Kinetics
Onset of Action Immediate release and extended release formulations: 1 hour
Duration of Action Immediate release: 5.1 ± 1.7 hours; Extended release: 11.3 ± 4.2 hours
Controlled Substance C-IV
Available Dosage Forms
Concentrate, Oral:
ALPRAZolam Intensol: 1 mg/mL (30 mL)
Tablet, Oral:
Xanax: 0.25 mg, 0.5 mg, 1 mg, 2 mg
Generic: 0.25 mg, 0.5 mg, 1 mg, 2 mg
Tablet Dispersible, Oral:
Niravam: 0.25 mg, 0.5 mg, 1 mg, 2 mg
Generic: 0.25 mg, 0.5 mg, 1 mg, 2 mg

Tablet Extended Release 24 Hour, Oral:
ALPRAZolam XR: 0.5 mg, 1 mg, 2 mg, 3 mg
Xanax XR: 0.5 mg, 1 mg, 2 mg, 3 mg
Generic: 0.5 mg, 1 mg, 2 mg, 3 mg

General Dosage Range Dosage adjustment recommended in patients with hepatic impairment

Oral:
Immediate release:
Adults: Initial: 0.25-0.5 mg 3 times/day; titrate as needed and tolerated (maximum: 10 mg/day)
Elderly: Initial: 0.25 mg 2-3 times/day; titrate gradually if needed and tolerated
Extended release:
Adults: Initial: 0.5-1 mg once daily; Maintenance: 3-6 mg/day (maximum: 6 mg/day)
Elderly: Initial: 0.5 mg/day; titrate gradually if needed and tolerated

Administration

Oral
Immediate release preparations: Can be administered sublingually if oral administration is not possible; absorption and onset of effect are comparable to oral administration (Scavone,1987; Scavone, 1992)
Extended release tablet: Should be taken once daily in the morning; do not crush, break, or chew.
Orally-disintegrating tablets: Using dry hands, place tablet on top of tongue and allow to disintegrate. If using one-half of tablet, immediately discard remaining half (may not remain stable). Administration with water is not necessary.

Storage/Stability
Immediate release tablets: Store at 20°C to 25°C (68°F to 77°F).
Extended release tablets: Store at 25°C (77°F); excursions permitted to 15°C to 30°C (59°F to 86°F).
Orally-disintegrating tablet: Store at room temperature of 20°C to 25°C (68°F to 77°F). Protect from moisture. Seal bottle tightly and discard any cotton packaged inside bottle.

Nursing Actions

Physical Assessment Assess for signs of CNS depression (sedation, dizziness, confusion, or ataxia). Assess for history of addiction; long-term use can result in dependence, abuse, or tolerance; periodically evaluate need for continued use. For inpatient use, institute safety measures to prevent falls. Taper dosage slowly when discontinuing.

Patient Education
• Discuss specific use of drug and side effects with patient as it relates to treatment. (HCAHPS: During this hospital stay, were you given any medicine that you had not taken before? Before giving you any new medicine, how often did hospital staff tell you what the medicine was for? How often did hospital staff describe possible side effects in a way you could understand?)

• Patient may experience presyncope, fatigue, blurred vision, xerostomia, polyphagia, lack of appetite, dyspepsia, constipation, sexual dysfunction, or weight change. Have patient report immediately to prescriber dyspnea, paresthesia, angina, tachycardia, arrhythmia, severe dizziness, syncope, significant change in balance, signs of depression (ie, suicidal ideation, anxiety, emotional instability, illogical thinking), hallucinations, memory loss, difficulty speaking, considerable asthenia, fasciculations, tremors, urine discoloration, jaundice, or difficult urination (HCAHPS).
• Educate patient about signs of a significant reaction (eg, wheezing; chest tightness; fever; itching; bad cough; blue skin color; seizures; or swelling of face, lips, tongue, or throat). **Note:** This is not a comprehensive list of all side effects. Patient should consult prescriber for additional questions.

Intended Use and Disclaimer: Should not be printed and given to patients. This information is intended to serve as a concise initial reference for healthcare professionals to use when discussing medications with a patient. You must ultimately rely on your own discretion, experience and judgment in diagnosing, treating and advising patients.

Dietary Considerations Extended release tablet should be taken once daily in the morning.

Related Information
Oral Medications That Should Not Be Crushed or Altered on page 1712

Alprostadil (al PROS ta dill)

Brand Names: U.S. Caverject; Caverject Impulse; Edex; Muse; Prostin VR
Index Terms PGE$_1$; Prostaglandin E$_1$
Pharmacologic Category Prostaglandin; Vasodilator
Medication Safety Issues
Sound-alike/look-alike issues:
Alprostadil may be confused with alPRAZolam
Pregnancy Risk Factor X/C (Muse®)
Lactation Not indicated for use in women
Use
Prostin VR Pediatric®: Temporary maintenance of patency of ductus arteriosus in neonates with ductal-dependent congenital heart disease until surgery can be performed. These defects include cyanotic (eg, pulmonary atresia, pulmonary stenosis, tricuspid atresia, Fallot's tetralogy, transposition of the great vessels) and acyanotic (eg, interruption of aortic arch, coarctation of aorta, hypoplastic left ventricle) heart disease.
Caverject®: Treatment of erectile dysfunction of vasculogenic, psychogenic, or neurogenic etiology; adjunct in the diagnosis of erectile dysfunction

Edex®, Muse®: Treatment of erectile dysfunction of vasculogenic, psychogenic, or neurogenic etiology

Unlabeled Use Treatment of pulmonary hypertension in infants and children with congenital heart defects with left-to-right shunts

Available Dosage Forms
Kit, Intracavernosal:
Caverject Impulse: 10 mcg, 20 mcg
Edex: 10 mcg, 20 mcg, 40 mcg
Pellet, Urethral:
Muse: 125 mcg (1 ea, 6 ea); 250 mcg (1 ea, 6 ea); 500 mcg (1 ea, 6 ea); 1000 mcg (1 ea, 6 ea)
Solution, Injection:
Prostin VR: 500 mcg/mL (1 mL)
Generic: 500 mcg/mL (1 mL)
Solution Reconstituted, Intracavernosal:
Caverject: 20 mcg (1 ea); 40 mcg (1 ea)
General Dosage Range
I.V.: *Neonates:* Initial: 0.05-0.1 mcg/kg/minute; Maintenance: 0.01-0.4 mcg/kg/minute
Intracavernous: *Adults:* Initial: 1.25-2.5 mcg; Maintenance: Increase to effective dose no more than 3 times/week with at least 24 hours between doses (maximum: 40 mcg/dose [Edex®]; 60 mcg/dose [Caverject®])
Intraurethral: *Adults:* Initial: 125-250 mcg; Maintenance: As needed (maximum: 2 doses/day)
Usual Infusion Concentrations: Pediatric I.V. infusion: 10 mcg/mL **or** 20 mcg/mL
Administration
I.V. Patent ductus arteriosus (Prostin VR Pediatric®): I.V. continuous infusion into a large vein or alternatively through an umbilical artery catheter placed at the ductal opening; manufacturer recommended maximum concentration for I.V. infusion: 20 mcg/mL
Other Erectile dysfunction: Use a 1/2 inch, 27- to 30-gauge needle. Inject into the dorsolateral aspect of the proximal third of the penis, avoiding visible veins; alternate side of the penis for injections.
Nursing Actions
Physical Assessment Neonate: Monitor closely; apnea has occurred during first hour after administration. **Erectile dysfunction:** After individual dose titration is determined by prescriber, the medication is self-administered. Teach patient appropriate injection technique and syringe/needle disposal.
Patient Education
• Discuss specific use of drug and side effects with patient as it relates to treatment. (HCAHPS: During this hospital stay, were you given any medicine that you had not taken before? Before giving you any new medicine, how often did hospital staff tell you what the medicine was for? How often did hospital staff describe possible side effects in a way you could understand?)
• Have patient report immediately to prescriber severe penile pain, injection site irritation,

angina, tachycardia, significant dizziness, syncope, considerable headache, dyspnea, ecchymosis, hemorrhaging, or priapism (HCAHPS).
• Educate patient about signs of a significant reaction (eg, wheezing; chest tightness; fever; itching; bad cough; blue skin color; seizures; or swelling of face, lips, tongue, or throat). **Note:** This is not a comprehensive list of all side effects. Patient should consult prescriber for additional questions.

Intended Use and Disclaimer: Should not be printed and given to patients. This information is intended to serve as a concise initial reference for healthcare professionals to use when discussing medications with a patient. You must ultimately rely on your own discretion, experience and judgment in diagnosing, treating and advising patients.

Alteplase (AL te plase)

Brand Names: U.S. Activase; Cathflo Activase
Index Terms Alteplase, Recombinant; Alteplase, Tissue Plasminogen Activator, Recombinant; tPA
Pharmacologic Category Thrombolytic Agent
Medication Safety Issues
Sound-alike/look-alike issues:
Activase may be confused with Cathflo Activase, TNKase
Alteplase may be confused with Altace
"tPA" abbreviation should not be used when writing orders for this medication; has been misread as TNKase (tenecteplase)
High alert medication:
The Institute for Safe Medication Practices (ISMP) includes this medication (I.V.) among its list of drugs which have a heightened risk of causing significant patient harm when used in error.
Pregnancy Risk Factor C
Lactation Excretion in breast milk unknown/use caution
Breast-Feeding Considerations It is not known if alteplase is excreted in breast milk. The manufacturer recommends that caution be exercised when administering alteplase to nursing women.
Use Management of ST-elevation myocardial infarction (STEMI) for the lysis of thrombi in coronary arteries; management of acute ischemic stroke (AIS); management of acute pulmonary embolism (PE)
Recommended criteria for treatment:
STEMI (ACCF/AHA; O'Gara, 2013): Ischemic symptoms within 12 hours of treatment or evidence of ongoing ischemia 12-24 hours after symptom onset with a large area of myocardium at risk or hemodynamic instability.

STEMI ECG definition: New ST-segment elevation at the J point in at least 2 contiguous leads of ≥2 mm (0.2 mV) in men or ≥1.5 mm (0.15 mV) in women in leads V_2-V_3 and/or of ≥1 mm (0.1 mV) in other contiguous precordial leads or limb leads. New or presumably new left bundle branch block (LBBB) may interfere with ST-elevation analysis and should not be considered diagnostic in isolation.

At non-PCI-capable hospitals, the ACCF/AHA recommends thrombolytic therapy administration when the anticipated first medical contact (FMC)-to-device time at a PCI-capable hospital is >120 minutes due to unavoidable delays.

AIS: Onset of stroke symptoms within 3 hours of treatment

Acute pulmonary embolism: Age ≤75 years: Documented massive PE (defined as acute PE with sustained hypotension [SBP <90 mm Hg for ≤15 minutes or requiring inotropic support], persistent profound bradycardia [HR <40 bpm with signs or symptoms of shock], or pulselessness); alteplase may be considered for submassive PE with clinical evidence of adverse prognosis (eg, new hemodynamic instability, worsening respiratory insufficiency, severe RV dysfunction, or major myocardial necrosis) and low risk of bleeding complications. **Note:** Not recommended for patients with low-risk PE (eg, normotensive, no RV dysfunction, normal biomarkers) or submassive acute PE with minor RV dysfunction, minor myocardial necrosis, and no clinical worsening (Jaff, 2011).

Cathflo® Activase®: Restoration of central venous catheter function

Unlabeled Use Acute ischemic stroke presenting 3-4.5 hours after symptom onset; acute peripheral arterial occlusion; infected parapneumonic effusion (with [adult] or without [pediatric] dornase alfa); prosthetic valve thrombosis; intra-arterial administration for patients who have contraindications to I.V. use (**Note:** Intra-arterial administration requires patient to be at an experienced stroke center with rapid access to cerebral angiography and qualified interventionalists)

Mechanism of Action/Effect Dissolves thrombus (clot)

Contraindications Hypersensitivity to alteplase or any component of the formulation

Treatment of STEMI or PE: Active internal bleeding; history of CVA; ischemic stroke within 3 months except when within 4.5 hours (Jaff, 2011; O'Gara, 2013); recent intracranial or intraspinal surgery or trauma; intracranial neoplasm; prior intracranial hemorrhage (Jaff, 2011; O'Gara, 2013); arteriovenous malformation or aneurysm; active bleeding (excluding menses) (O'Gara, 2013); known bleeding diathesis; severe uncontrolled hypertension; suspected aortic dissection (Jaff, 2011; O'Gara, 2013); significant closed head or facial trauma (Jaff, 2011; O'Gara, 2013) within 3 months with radiographic evidence of bony fracture or brain injury (Jaff, 2011)

Treatment of acute ischemic stroke: Evidence/history of intracranial hemorrhage or suspicion of subarachnoid hemorrhage on pretreatment evaluation; recent intracranial or intraspinal surgery; stroke or serious head injury within 3 months; uncontrolled hypertension at time of treatment (eg, >185 mm Hg systolic or >110 mm Hg diastolic); seizure at the onset of stroke; active internal bleeding; intracranial neoplasm; arteriovenous malformation or aneurysm; multilobar cerebral infarction (hypodensity >1/3 cerebral hemisphere); known bleeding diathesis including but not limited to current use of oral anticoagulants with an INR >1.7 (or PT >15 seconds), current use of direct thrombin inhibitors or direct factor Xa inhibitors with elevated sensitive laboratory tests (eg, aPTT, INR, platelet count, and ECT, TT, or appropriate factor Xa activity assays) (See **"Note"**; Jauch, 2013), administration of heparin within 48 hours preceding the onset of stroke with an elevated aPTT at presentation, or platelet count <100,000/mm³.

Note: The AHA/ASA guidelines do allow the use of direct thrombin inhibitors (eg, dabigatran) or direct factor Xa inhibitors (eg, rivaroxaban) when sensitive laboratory tests (eg, aPTT, INR, platelet count, ECT, TT, or appropriate direct factor Xa activity assays) are normal or the patient has not received a dose of these agents for >2 days (assuming normal renal function).

Additional exclusion criteria within clinical trials:
Presentation <3 hours after initial symptoms (NINDS, 1995): Time of symptom onset unknown, rapidly improving or minor symptoms, major surgery within 2 weeks, GI or urinary tract hemorrhage within 3 weeks, aggressive treatment required to lower blood pressure, glucose level <50 or >400 mg/dL, and arterial puncture at a noncompressible site or lumbar puncture within 1 week.

Presentation 3-4.5 hours after initial symptoms (ECASS-III; Hacke, 2008; Jauch, 2013): Age >80 years, time of symptom onset unknown, rapidly improving or minor symptoms, current use of oral anticoagulants regardless of INR, glucose level <50 or >400 mg/dL, aggressive intravenous treatment required to lower blood pressure, major surgery or severe trauma within 3 months, baseline National Institutes of Health Stroke Scale (NIHSS) score >25 [ie, severe stroke], and history of both stroke and diabetes.

Warnings/Precautions The total dose should not exceed 90 mg for acute ischemic stroke or 100 mg for acute myocardial infarction or pulmonary embolism. Doses ≥150 mg associated with significantly increased risk of intracranial hemorrhage compared to doses ≤100 mg. Concurrent heparin anticoagulation may contribute to bleeding. In the ▶

treatment of acute ischemic stroke, concurrent use of anticoagulants was not permitted during the initial 24 hours of the <3 hour window trial (NINDS, 1995). The AHA/ASA does not recommend initiation of anticoagulant therapy within 24 hours of treatment with alteplase (Jauch, 2013). Initiation of SubQ heparin (≤10,000 units) or equivalent doses of low molecular weight heparin for prevention of DVT during the first 24 hours of the 3-4.5 hour window trial was permitted and did not increase the incidence of intracerebral hemorrhage (Hacke, 2008). For acute PE, withhold heparin during the 2-hour infusion period. Monitor all potential bleeding sites. Intramuscular injections and nonessential handling of the patient should be avoided. Venipunctures should be performed carefully and only when necessary. If arterial puncture is necessary, use an upper extremity vessel that can be manually compressed. If serious bleeding occurs, the infusion of alteplase and heparin should be stopped. Avoid aspirin for 24 hours following administration of alteplase; administration within 24 hours increases the risk of hemorrhagic transformation.

For the following conditions, the risk of bleeding is higher with use of thrombolytics and should be weighed against the benefits of therapy: Recent major surgery (eg, CABG, obstetrical delivery, organ biopsy, pregnancy, previous puncture of noncompressible vessels), prolonged CPR with evidence of thoracic trauma, lumbar puncture within 1 week, cerebrovascular disease, recent gastrointestinal or genitourinary bleeding, recent trauma, hypertension (systolic BP >175 mm Hg and/or diastolic BP >110 mm Hg), high likelihood of left heart thrombus (eg, mitral stenosis with atrial fibrillation), acute pericarditis, subacute bacterial endocarditis, hemostatic defects including ones caused by severe renal or hepatic dysfunction, significant hepatic dysfunction, pregnancy, diabetic hemorrhagic retinopathy or other hemorrhagic ophthalmic conditions, septic thrombophlebitis or occluded AV cannula at seriously infected site, advanced age (eg, >75 years), any other condition in which bleeding constitutes a significant hazard or would be particularly difficult to manage because of location. When treating acute MI or pulmonary embolism, use with caution in patients receiving oral anticoagulants. In the treatment of acute ischemic stroke (AIS) within 3 hours of symptom onset, the current use of oral anticoagulants is a contraindication per the manufacturer. According to the AHA/ASA, the current use of oral anticoagulants producing an INR >1.7, direct thrombin inhibitors, or direct factor Xa inhibitors with elevated sensitive laboratory tests are contraindications. However, alteplase may be administered to patients with AIS having received direct thrombin inhibitors (eg, dabigatran) or direct factor Xa inhibitors (eg, rivaroxaban) when sensitive laboratory tests (eg, aPTT, INR, platelet count, ECT, TT, or appropriate direct

factor Xa activity assays) are normal or the patient has not received a dose of these agents for >2 days (assuming normal renal function). When treating AIS 3-4.5 hours after symptom onset, the use of alteplase should be avoided with current use of any oral anticoagulant regardless of INR (Jauch, 2013). In the treatment of STEMI, adjunctive use of parenteral anticoagulants (eg, enoxaparin, heparin, or fondaparinux) is recommended to improve vessel patency and prevent reocclusion and may also contribute to bleeding; monitor for bleeding (ACCF/AHA; O'Gara, 2013).

Coronary thrombolysis may result in reperfusion arrhythmias. Patients who present **within 3 hours** of stroke symptom onset should be treated with alteplase unless contraindications exist. A longer time window (**3-4.5 hours** after symptom onset) has been shown to be safe and efficacious for select individuals (Hacke, 2008; Jauch, 2013). Treatment of patients with minor neurological deficit or with rapidly improving symptoms is not recommended. Follow standard management for STEMI while infusing alteplase.

Cathflo® Activase®: When used to restore catheter function, use Cathflo® cautiously in those patients with known or suspected catheter infections. Evaluate catheter for other causes of dysfunction before use. Avoid excessive pressure when instilling into catheter.

Drug Interactions
Avoid Concomitant Use There are no known interactions where it is recommended to avoid concomitant use.

Decreased Effect
The levels/effects of Alteplase may be decreased by: Aprotinin; Nitroglycerin

Increased Effect/Toxicity
Alteplase may increase the levels/effects of: Anticoagulants; Dabigatran Etexilate

The levels/effects of Alteplase may be increased by: Agents with Antiplatelet Properties; Herbs (Anticoagulant/Antiplatelet Properties); Salicylates

Nutritional/Ethanol Interactions Herb/Nutraceutical: Avoid cat's claw, dong quai, evening primrose, feverfew, red clover, horse chestnut, garlic, green tea, ginseng, ginkgo (all have additional antiplatelet activity).

Adverse Reactions As with all drugs which may affect hemostasis, bleeding is the major adverse effect associated with alteplase. Hemorrhage may occur at virtually any site. Risk is dependent on multiple variables, including the dosage administered, concurrent use of multiple agents which alter hemostasis, and patient predisposition. Rapid lysis of coronary artery thrombi by thrombolytic agents may be associated with reperfusion-related atrial and/or ventricular arrhythmia. **Note:** Lowest rate of bleeding complications expected with dose used to restore catheter function.

1% to 10%:

Cardiovascular: Hypotension

Central nervous system: Fever

Dermatologic: Bruising (1%)

Gastrointestinal: GI hemorrhage (5%), nausea, vomiting

Genitourinary: GU hemorrhage (4%)

Hematologic: Bleeding (0.5% major, 7% minor: GUSTO trial)

Local: Bleeding at catheter puncture site (15.3%, accelerated administration)

Additional cardiovascular events associated **with use in STEMI:** AV block, cardiogenic shock, heart failure, cardiac arrest, recurrent ischemia/infarction, myocardial rupture, electromechanical dissociation, pericardial effusion, pericarditis, mitral regurgitation, cardiac tamponade, thromboembolism, pulmonary edema, asystole, ventricular tachycardia, bradycardia, ruptured intracranial AV malformation, seizure, hemorrhagic bursitis, cholesterol crystal embolization

Additional events associated **with use in pulmonary embolism:** Pulmonary re-embolization, pulmonary edema, pleural effusion, thromboembolism

Additional events associated **with use in stroke:** Cerebral edema, cerebral herniation, seizure, new ischemic stroke

Pharmacodynamics/Kinetics

Duration of Action >50% present in plasma cleared ~5 minutes after infusion terminated, ~80% cleared within 10 minutes; fibrinolytic activity persists for up to 1 hour after infusion terminated (Semba, 2000)

Available Dosage Forms

Solution Reconstituted, Injection:

Cathflo Activase: 2 mg (1 ea)

Solution Reconstituted, Intravenous:

Activase: 50 mg (1 ea); 100 mg (1 ea)

General Dosage Range

Intracatheter:

Children <30 kg: 110% of the internal lumen volume of the catheter; retain in catheter for 0.5-2 hours; may repeat once (maximum: 2 mg/2 mL/dose)

Children ≥30 kg and Adults: 2 mg (2 mL) retain in catheter for 0.5-2 hours; may repeat once

I.V. infusion: *Adults:* Dosage varies greatly depending on indication

Usual Infusion Concentrations: Pediatric I.V. infusion: 0.5 mg/mL **or** 1 mg/mL

Usual Infusion Concentrations: Adult I.V. infusion: 1 mg/mL

Note: Concentrations for some indications (eg, peripheral arterial occlusion) may require further dilution (eg, 0.1-0.2 mg/mL [Chan, 2001; Semba, 2000]) and a usual concentration may not be established.

Administration

I.V.

Activase®: ST-elevation MI or acute ischemic stroke: Administer bolus dose (prepared by one of three methods) over 1 minute followed by infusion.

Infusion: Remaining dose for STEMI, AIS, or total dose for acute pulmonary embolism may be administered as follows: Any quantity of drug not to be administered to the patient must be removed from vial(s) prior to administration of remaining dose.

50 mg vial: Either PVC bag or glass vial and infusion set

100 mg vial: Insert spike end of the infusion set through the same puncture site created by transfer device and infuse from vial

If further dilution is desired, may be diluted in equal volume of 0.9% sodium chloride or D₅W to yield a final concentration of 0.5 mg/mL.

Injectable Detail Reconstituted solution should be clear or pale yellow and transparent. Avoid agitation during dilution.

pH: 5-7.3

Other

Cathflo® Activase®: Intracatheter: Instill dose into occluded catheter. Do not force solution into catheter. After a 30-minute dwell time, assess catheter function by attempting to aspirate blood. If catheter is functional, aspirate 4-5 mL of blood in patients ≥10 kg or 3 mL in patients <10 kg to remove Cathflo® Activase® and residual clots. Gently irrigate the catheter with NS. If catheter remains nonfunctional, let Cathflo® Activase® dwell for another 90 minutes (total dwell time: 120 minutes) and reassess function. If catheter function is not restored, a second dose may be instilled.

Parapneumonic effusion (unlabeled use): Intrapleural: Instill dose into chest tube and clamp drain. Although the optimum dwell time has not been determined, clinical trials more often have used either a 45 minute (Hawkins, 2004) or 1 hour (Rahman, 2011; St. Peter, 2009) dwell time; after dwell period, release clamp and connect chest tube to continuous suction.

Preparation for Administration

Activase®:

50 mg vial: Use accompanying diluent; mix by gentle swirling or slow inversion; do not shake. Vacuum is present in 50 mg vial. Final concentration: 1 mg/mL.

100 mg vial: Use transfer set with accompanying diluent (100 mL vial of sterile water for injection). No vacuum is present in 100 mg vial. Final concentration: 1 mg/mL.

Activase®: ST-elevation MI: Accelerated infusion: Bolus dose may be prepared by one of three methods:

1) Removal of 15 mL reconstituted (1 mg/mL) solution from vial
2) Removal of 15 mL from a port on the infusion line after priming
3) Programming an infusion pump to deliver a 15 mL bolus at the initiation of infusion

Activase®: Acute ischemic stroke: Bolus dose (10% of total dose) may be prepared by one of three methods:

1) Removal of the appropriate volume from reconstituted solution (1 mg/mL)
2) Removal of the appropriate volume from a port on the infusion line after priming
3) Programming an infusion pump to deliver the appropriate volume at the initiation of infusion

Cathflo® Activase®: Add 2.2 mL SWFI to vial; do not shake. Final concentration: 1 mg/mL.

Storage/Stability

Activase®: The lyophilized product may be stored at room temperature (not to exceed 30°C/86°F), or under refrigeration. Once reconstituted, it should be used within 8 hours.

Cathflo® Activase®: Store lyophilized product under refrigeration. Once reconstituted, it should be used within 8 hours.

Nursing Actions

Physical Assessment Monitor vital signs and ECG prior to, during, and after therapy. Report abnormalities to prescriber immediately. Arrhythmias may occur; treatment should be available. Assess infusion site and monitor for hemorrhage during therapy and for 1 hour following therapy. Maintain strict bedrest and monitor regularly for excess bleeding. Use bleeding precautions.

Patient Education

• Discuss specific use of drug and side effects with patient as it relates to treatment. (HCAHPS: During this hospital stay, were you given any medicine that you had not taken before? Before giving you any new medicine, how often did hospital staff tell you what the medicine was for? How often did hospital staff describe possible side effects in a way you could understand?)

• Have patient report immediately to prescriber angina, ecchymosis, hemorrhaging, hematemesis, hematuria, melena, hemoptysis, strength differences from one side to another, difficulty speaking or thinking, change in balance, blurred vision, painful extremities, dyspnea, tachycardia, bradycardia, arrhythmia, chills, paresthesia, illogical thinking, severe headache, significant back pain, considerable myalgia, intolerable asthenia, severe dyspepsia, skin or nail discoloration, injection site irritation, catheter site irritation, or signs of renal impairment (HCAHPS).

• Educate about signs of a significant reaction (eg, wheezing; chest tightness; fever; itching; bad cough; blue skin color; seizures; or

swelling of face, lips, tongue, or throat). **Note** This is not a comprehensive list of all side effects. Patient should consult prescriber for additional questions.

Intended Use and Disclaimer: Should not be printed and given to patients. This information is intended to serve as a concise initial reference for healthcare professionals to use when discussing medications with a patient. You must ultimately rely on your own discretion, experience and judgment in diagnosing, treating and advising patients.

Alvimopan (al VI moe pan)

Brand Names: U.S. Entereg

Index Terms ADL-2698; LY246736

Pharmacologic Category Gastrointestinal Agent, Miscellaneous; Opioid Antagonist, Peripherally-Acting

Medication Safety Issues

Sound-alike/look-alike issues:

Alvimopan may be confused with almotriptan

Pregnancy Risk Factor B

Lactation Excretion in breast milk unknown/use caution

Breast-Feeding Considerations It is not known if alvimopan is excreted in breast milk. The manufacturer recommends that caution be exercised when administering alvimopan to nursing women.

Use Postoperative ileus: To accelerate the time to upper and lower GI recovery following surgeries including partial bowel resection with primary anastomosis

Mechanism of Action/Effect An opioid receptor antagonist which blocks opioid binding at the mu receptor; alvimopan has restricted ability to cross the blood-brain barrier at therapeutic doses. It selectively and competitively binds to the GI tract mu opioid receptors and antagonizes the peripheral effects of opioids on gastrointestinal motility and secretion. Does not affect opioid analgesic effects or induce opioid withdrawal symptoms.

Contraindications Patients who have taken therapeutic doses of opioids for more than 7 consecutive days immediately prior to alvimopan

Warnings/Precautions [U.S. Boxed Warning]: For short-term (≤15 doses) hospital use only. Only hospitals that have registered through the ENTEREG Access Support and Education (E.A.S.E.™) Program and met all requirements may use. It will not be dispensed to patients who have been discharged from the hospital. Use not recommended in patients with complete bowel obstruction or in patients having gastric or pancreatic anastomosis. Use with caution in patients with hepatic or renal impairment; use not recommended in patients with severe hepatic impairment or ESRD. Use with caution is patients recently exposed to opioids; may be more sensitive to gastrointestinal adverse effects (eg, abdominal pain, diarrhea, nausea and vomiting). Contraindicated in patients who have received therapeutic opioids for >7 consecutive days immediately prior to use. **[U.S. Boxed Warning]: A trend towards an increased incidence of MI was observed in alvimopan (low dose) treated patients compared to placebo in a 12-month study in patients treated with opioids for chronic pain. Other short-term studies have not observed this trend and a causal relationship has not been found.** MI was generally observed more frequently in the initial 1-4 months of treatment. Patients of Japanese descent should be monitored closely for gastrointestinal side effects (eg, abdominal pain, cramping, diarrhea) due to possibility of greater drug exposure; discontinue use if side effects occur.

Drug Interactions

Avoid Concomitant Use There are no known interactions where it is recommended to avoid concomitant use.

Decreased Effect There are no known significant interactions involving a decrease in effect.

Increased Effect/Toxicity
The levels/effects of Alvimopan may be increased by: Analgesics (Opioid)

Nutritional/Ethanol Interactions Food: When administered with a high-fat meal, extent and rate of absorption may be reduced (C_{max} and AUC decreased by ~38% and 21%, respectively).

Adverse Reactions Note: Incidence reported limited to bowel resection patients only.
1% to 10%:
Endocrine & metabolic: Hypokalemia (10%)
Gastrointestinal: Dyspepsia (2% to 7%)
Genitourinary: Urinary retention (3%)
Hematologic and oncologic: Anemia (5%)
Neuromuscular & skeletal: Back pain (3%)
Frequency not defined:
Cardiovascular: Myocardial infarction

Available Dosage Forms
Capsule, Oral:
Entereg: 12 mg

General Dosage Range Oral: *Adults:* Initial: 12 mg prior to surgery; Maintenance: 12 mg twice daily (maximum: 15 doses)

Administration

Oral Patient must be hospitalized. Initial dose should be administered 30 minutes to 5 hours prior to surgery. May be administered with or without food.

Storage/Stability Store at 25°C (77°F); excursions permitted to 15°C to 30°C (59°F to 86°F).

Nursing Actions

Physical Assessment For restricted in-hospital use only to improve bowel function.

Patient Education
• Discuss specific use of drug and side effects with patient as it relates to treatment. (HCAHPS: During this hospital stay, were you given any

medicine that you had not taken before? Before giving you any new medicine, how often did hospital staff tell you what the medicine was for? How often did hospital staff describe possible side effects in a way you could understand?)
• Patient may experience flatulence. Have patient report immediately to prescriber signs of hypokalemia, severe constipation, considerable asthenia, angina, tachycardia, significant dizziness, syncope, intolerable headache, severe nausea, bradycardia, significant dyspepsia, abdominal cramps, urinary retention, or oliguria (HCAHPS).
• Educate patient about signs of a significant reaction (eg, wheezing; chest tightness; fever; itching; bad cough; blue skin color; seizures; or swelling of face, lips, tongue, or throat). **Note:** This is not a comprehensive list of all side effects. Patient should consult prescriber for additional questions.

Intended Use and Disclaimer: Should not be printed and given to patients. This information is intended to serve as a concise initial reference for healthcare professionals to use when discussing medications with a patient. You must ultimately rely on your own discretion, experience and judgment in diagnosing, treating and advising patients.

Dietary Considerations Take with or without food; high-fat meals may decrease the rate and extent of absorption

---

Amantadine (a MAN ta deen)

Index Terms Adamantanamine Hydrochloride; Amantadine Hydrochloride; Symmetrel

Pharmacologic Category Anti-Parkinson's Agent, Dopamine Agonist; Antiviral Agent; Antiviral Agent, Adamantane

Medication Safety Issues
Sound-alike/look-alike issues:
Amantadine may be confused with ranitidine, rimantadine
Symmetrel may be confused with Synthroid®

Pregnancy Risk Factor C

Lactation Enters breast milk/not recommended

Use Prophylaxis and treatment of influenza A viral infection (per manufacturer's labeling; also refer to current ACIP guidelines for recommendations during current flu season); treatment of parkinsonism; treatment of drug-induced extrapyramidal symptoms

Available Dosage Forms
Capsule, Oral:
Generic: 100 mg
Syrup, Oral:
Generic: 50 mg/5 mL (10 mL, 473 mL)
Tablet, Oral:
Generic: 100 mg

General Dosage Range Dosage adjustment recommended in patients with renal impairment

Oral:

Children 1-9 years: 4.4-8.8 mg/kg/day in 2 divided doses (maximum: 150 mg/day)

Children ≥10 years and <40 kg: 5 mg/kg/day in 2 divided doses

Children ≥10 years and ≥40 kg: 100 mg twice daily (maximum: 200 mg/day)

Adults: 200-400 mg/day in 2 divided doses (maximum: 400 mg/day)

Elderly: 100-400 mg/day in 2 divided doses (maximum: 400 mg/day)

Nursing Actions

Physical Assessment Recommendations for antiviral susceptibility and effectiveness have changed; amantadine is not recommended for use for the 2011 flu season. Monitor renal function at beginning of therapy and periodically throughout. Assess blood pressure; monitor for signs of fluid retention. When treating Parkinson's disease, taper slowly when discontinuing.

Patient Education

• Discuss specific use of drug and side effects with patient as it relates to treatment. (HCAHPS: During this hospital stay, were you given any medicine that you had not taken before? Before giving you any new medicine, how often did hospital staff tell you what the medicine was for? How often did hospital staff describe possible side effects in a way you could understand?)

• Patient may experience nausea, insomnia, lack of appetite, blurred vision, constipation, diarrhea, fatigue, xerostomia, headache, nightmares, or asthenia. Have patient report immediately to prescriber signs of depression (ie, suicidal ideation, anxiety, emotional instability, illogical thinking), mood changes, behavioral changes, severe dizziness, syncope, hallucinations, memory loss, dyspnea, pharyngitis, edema of extremities, urinary retention, vision changes, difficulty with motor activity, fasciculations, or signs of neuroleptic malignant syndrome (NMS) (HCAHPS).

• Educate patient about signs of a significant reaction (eg, wheezing; chest tightness; fever; itching; bad cough; blue skin color; seizures; or swelling of face, lips, tongue, or throat). **Note:** This is not a comprehensive list of all side effects. Patient should consult prescriber for additional questions.

Intended Use and Disclaimer: Should not be printed and given to patients. This information is intended to serve as a concise initial reference for healthcare professionals to use when discussing medications with a patient. You must ultimately rely on your own discretion, experience and judgment in diagnosing, treating and advising patients.

Ambrisentan (am bri SEN tan)

Brand Names: U.S. Letairis

Index Terms BSF208075

Pharmacologic Category Endothelin Receptor Antagonist; Vasodilator

Medication Safety Issues

International issues:

Letaris, a formerly marketed Dutch brand name product for letrozole, may be confused with Letairis, a U.S. brand name for ambrisentan.

Medication Guide Available Yes

Pregnancy Risk Factor X

Lactation Excretion in breast milk unknown/not recommended

Breast-Feeding Considerations It is not known if ambrisentan is excreted in breast milk. Due to the potential for serious adverse reactions in the nursing infant, the manufacturer recommends a decision be made whether to discontinue nursing or to discontinue the drug, taking into account the importance of treatment to the mother.

Use Pulmonary arterial hypertension: Treatment of pulmonary artery hypertension (PAH) World Health Organization (WHO) Group I to improve exercise ability and delay clinical worsening

Mechanism of Action/Effect Decreases symptoms of pulmonary arterial hypertension and slows progression of the disease by causing vasodilation of the pulmonary arteries.

Contraindications Pregnancy; idiopathic pulmonary fibrosis, including idiopathic pulmonary fibrosis with pulmonary hypertension (WHO Group 3)

Canadian labeling: Additional contraindications (not in U.S. labeling): Hypersensitivity to ambrisentan or any component of the formulation

Warnings/Precautions Hazardous agent - use appropriate precautions for handling and disposal (NIOSH, 2012). **[U.S. Boxed Warning]: May cause birth defects; use in pregnancy is contraindicated. Exclude pregnancy prior to initiation of therapy and obtain pregnancy tests monthly during treatment and for 1 month after therapy is complete. Reliable contraception must be used during therapy and for 1 month after stopping treatment.** Two reliable methods of contraception (eg, hormone method with a barrier method or 2 barrier methods) must be used throughout treatment and for 1 month after stopping treatment. Patients who have undergone a tubal ligation or the insertion of a contraceptive implant or intrauterine device (Copper T 380A or LNg 20) do not require additional contraceptive measures. A missed menses or suspected pregnancy should be reported to a healthcare provider and prompt immediate pregnancy testing. Women should also be educated on the appropriate use of emergency contraception if failure of contraceptive is known or suspected or in the event of unprotected sex.

[U.S. Boxed Warning]: Because of the high likelihood of teratogenic effects, ambrisentan is only available through the Letairis REMS restricted distribution program. Patients, prescribers, and pharmacies must be registered with and meet conditions of the program. Call 1-866-664-5327 or visit www.letairisrems.com for more information.

Use caution in patients with low hemoglobin levels. May cause decreases in hemoglobin and hematocrit (monitoring of hemoglobin is recommended. Use not recommended in patients with clinically significant anemia. Development of peripheral edema due to treatment and/or disease state (pulmonary arterial hypertension) may occur; a higher incidence is seen in elderly patients. Sperm count may be reduced in men during treatment (as observed with bosentan). No changes in sperm function or hormone levels have been noted. Fertility issues may require discussion with patient. Increases in serum liver aminotransferases have been reported during postmarketing use; however, in the majority of the cases, alternative causes of hepatotoxicity could be identified. Perform liver enzyme testing only when clinically indicated. Discontinue therapy if signs/symptoms of hepatic injury appear, if serum liver aminotransferases >5 times ULN are observed, or if aminotransferases are increased in the presence of bilirubin >2 times ULN. Hepatotoxicity has been reported with other endothelin receptor antagonists (eg, bosentan); however, ambrisentan may be tried in patients that have experienced asymptomatic increases in liver enzymes caused by another endothelin receptor antagonist after the liver enzymes have returned to normal. Use caution in patients with mild hepatic impairment; use not recommended in patients with moderate-to-severe impairment. There have also been postmarketing reports of fluid retention requiring treatment (eg, diuretics, fluid management, hospitalization). Further evaluation may be necessary to determine cause and appropriate treatment or discontinuation of therapy. Discontinue in any patient with pulmonary edema suggestive of pulmonary veno-occlusive disease (PVOD).

Drug Interactions

Avoid Concomitant Use There are no known interactions where it is recommended to avoid concomitant use.

Decreased Effect There are no known significant interactions involving a decrease in effect.

Increased Effect/Toxicity

The levels/effects of Ambrisentan may be increased by: CycloSPORINE (Systemic)

Nutritional/Ethanol Interactions

Food: Grapefruit/grapefruit juice may increase levels/effects of ambrisentan.

Herb/Nutraceutical: Avoid St John's wort (concurrent use may decrease levels/effects of ambrisentan).

Adverse Reactions

>10%:
Cardiovascular: Peripheral edema (17%)
Central nervous system: Headache (15%)
1% to 10%:
Cardiovascular: Palpitation (5%), flushing (4%)
Gastrointestinal: Constipation (4%), abdominal pain (3%)
Hematologic: Hemoglobin decreased (7% to 10%)
Respiratory: Nasal congestion (6%), dyspnea (4%), nasopharyngitis (3%), sinusitis (3%)

Available Dosage Forms

Tablet, Oral:
Letairis: 5 mg, 10 mg

General Dosage Range Dosage adjustment recommended in patients on concomitant therapy.

Oral: *Adults:* Initial: 5 mg once daily (maximum: 10 mg/day)

Administration

Oral Swallow tablet whole. Do not split, crush, or chew tablets. May be administered with or without food.

Hazardous agent; use appropriate precautions for handling and disposal (NIOSH, 2012).

Storage/Stability Store at 25°C (77°F); excursions are permitted between 15°C and 30°C (59°F and 86°F). Store in original packaging.

Nursing Actions

Physical Assessment Assess for symptoms of hepatic problems and fluid retention.

Patient Education

• Discuss specific use of drug and side effects with patient as it relates to treatment. (HCAHPS: During this hospital stay, were you given any medicine that you had not taken before? Before giving you any new medicine, how often did hospital staff tell you what the medicine was for? How often did hospital staff describe possible side effects in a way you could understand?)

• Patient may experience headache, flushing, rhinitis, pharyngitis, or rhinorrhea. Have patient report immediately to prescriber signs of hepatic impairment, dyspnea, excessive weight gain, edema of extremities, or severe asthenia (HCAHPS).

• Educate patient about signs of a significant reaction (eg, wheezing; chest tightness; fever; itching; bad cough; blue skin color; seizures; or swelling of face, lips, tongue, or throat). **Note:** This is not a comprehensive list of all side effects. Patient should consult prescriber for additional questions.

Intended Use and Disclaimer: Should not be printed and given to patients. This information is intended to serve as a concise initial reference for healthcare professionals to use when discussing medications with a patient. You must ultimately rely on your own discretion, experience and

judgment in diagnosing, treating and advising patients.

Dietary Considerations Avoid grapefruit and grapefruit juice.

Related Information
Oral Medications That Should Not Be Crushed or Altered *on page 1712*

Amikacin (am i KAY sin)

Index Terms Amikacin Sulfate

Pharmacologic Category Antibiotic, Aminoglycoside

Medication Safety Issues
Sound-alike/look-alike issues:
Amikacin may be confused with Amicar, anakinra
Amikin may be confused with Amicar, Kineret

Pregnancy Risk Factor D

Lactation Enters breast milk/not recommended

Use Treatment of serious infections (bone infections, respiratory tract infections, endocarditis, and septicemia) due to organisms resistant to gentamicin and tobramycin, including *Pseudomonas*, *Proteus*, *Serratia*, and other gram-negative bacilli; documented infection of mycobacterial organisms susceptible to amikacin

Unlabeled Use Bacterial endophthalmitis; *Mycobacterium avium* complex (MAC; fibrocavitary or severe nodular/bronchiectatic disease)

Available Dosage Forms
Solution, Injection:
Generic: 500 mg/2 mL (2 mL); 1 g/4 mL (4 mL)
Solution, Injection [preservative free]:
Generic: 500 mg/2 mL (2 mL); 1 g/4 mL (4 mL)

General Dosage Range Dosage adjustment recommended in patients with renal impairment
I.M.: *Infants, Children, and Adults:* 5-7.5 mg/kg/dose every 8 hours (maximum: 20 mg/kg/day)
I.V.:
Infants and Children: 5-7.5 mg/kg/dose every 8 hours (maximum: 20 mg/kg/day)
Adults: 5-7.5 mg/kg/dose every 8 hours **or** 15-20 mg/kg as a single daily dose (maximum: 20 mg/kg/day)

Administration
I.M. Administer I.M. injection in large muscle mass. Administer around-the-clock to promote less variation in peak and trough serum levels. Do not mix with other drugs, administer separately.
I.V. Infuse over 30-60 minutes; in infants, infusion over 1-2 hours is recommended by the manufacturer.
Some penicillins (eg, carbenicillin, ticarcillin, and piperacillin) have been shown to inactivate *in vitro*. This has been observed to a greater extent with tobramycin and gentamicin, while amikacin has shown greater stability against inactivation. Concurrent use of these agents may pose a risk of reduced antibacterial efficacy *in vivo*, particularly in the setting of profound renal impairment. However, definitive clinical evidence is lacking. If combination penicillin/aminoglycoside therapy is desired in a patient with renal dysfunction, separation of doses (if feasible), and routine monitoring of aminoglycoside levels, CBC, and clinical response should be considered.

Injectable Detail Administer around-the-clock to promote less variation in peak and trough serum levels. Do not mix with other drugs, administer separately.
pH: 3.5-5.5

Other Intrathecal/Intraventricular (unlabeled route): Reserved solely for meningitis due to susceptible gram-negative organisms. Available formulation contains sodium metabisulfite. If possible, consider alternative therapy with gentamicin or tobramycin as both of these agents are available as preservative-free formulations.

Nursing Actions

Physical Assessment Assess allergy history prior to beginning therapy. Monitor for ototoxicity, nephrotoxicity, and neurotoxicity. Hearing and renal status should be assessed before, during, and after therapy.

Patient Education
• Discuss specific use of drug and side effects with patient as it relates to treatment. (HCAHPS: During this hospital stay, were you given any medicine that you had not taken before? Before giving you any new medicine, how often did hospital staff tell you what the medicine was for? How often did hospital staff describe possible side effects in a way you could understand?)
• Have patient report immediately to prescriber significant change in balance, severe dizziness, urinary retention, oliguria, hearing impairment, asthenia, paresthesia, tinnitus, vaginal yeast infection, or signs of pseudomembranous colitis (HCAHPS).
• Educate patient about signs of a significant reaction (eg, wheezing; chest tightness; fever; itching; bad cough; blue skin color; seizures; or swelling of face, lips, tongue, or throat). **Note:** This is not a comprehensive list of all side effects. Patient should consult prescriber for additional questions.

Intended Use and Disclaimer: Should not be printed and given to patients. This information is intended to serve as a concise initial reference for healthcare professionals to use when discussing medications with a patient. You must ultimately rely on your own discretion, experience and judgment in diagnosing, treating and advising patients.

Related Information
Peak and Trough Guidelines *on page 1710*

AMILoride (a MIL oh ride)

Index Terms Amiloride Hydrochloride
Pharmacologic Category Antihypertensive; Diuretic, Potassium-Sparing
Medication Safety Issues
Sound-alike/look-alike issues:
AMILoride may be confused with amiodarone, amLODIPine, inamrinone
Pregnancy Risk Factor B
Lactation Excretion in breast milk unknown/not recommended
Breast-Feeding Considerations It is not known if amiloride is excreted in breast milk. Due to the potential for serious adverse reactions in the nursing infant, a decision should be made whether to discontinue nursing or to discontinue the drug, taking into account the importance of treatment to the mother.
Use Counteracts potassium loss induced by other diuretics in the treatment of hypertension or edematous conditions including CHF, hepatic cirrhosis, and hypoaldosteronism; usually used in conjunction with more potent diuretics such as thiazides or loop diuretics
Unlabeled Use Cystic fibrosis; reduction of lithium-induced polyuria; pediatric hypertension
Mechanism of Action/Effect Inhibits sodium reabsorption in the distal tubule, cortical collecting tubule, and collecting duct subsequently reducing both potassium and hydrogen excretion resulting in weak natriuretic, diuretic, and antihypertensive activity; increases sodium loss; increases potassium retention; decreases calcium excretion; decreases magnesium loss
Contraindications Hypersensitivity to amiloride or any component of the formulation; presence of elevated serum potassium levels (>5.5 mEq/L); if patient is receiving other potassium-conserving agents (eg, spironolactone, triamterene) or potassium supplementation (medicine, potassium-containing salt substitutes, potassium-rich diet); anuria; acute or chronic renal insufficiency; evidence of diabetic nephropathy. Patients with evidence of renal impairment or diabetes mellitus should not receive this medicine without close, frequent monitoring of serum electrolytes and renal function.
Warnings/Precautions [U.S. Boxed Warning]: Hyperkalemia can occur; patients at risk include those with renal impairment, diabetes, the elderly, and the severely ill. Serum potassium levels must be monitored at frequent intervals especially when dosages are changed or with any illness that may cause renal dysfunction. Excess amounts can lead to profound diuresis with fluid and electrolyte loss; close

medical supervision and dose evaluation are required. Watch for and correct electrolyte disturbances; adjust dose to avoid dehydration. In cirrhosis, avoid electrolyte and acid/base imbalances that might lead to hepatic encephalopathy. Use with extreme caution in patients with diabetes mellitus; monitor closely. Discontinue amiloride 3 days prior to glucose tolerance testing. Use with caution in patients who are at risk for metabolic or respiratory acidosis (eg, cardiopulmonary disease, uncontrolled diabetes). Safety and efficacy have not been established in children.
Drug Interactions
Avoid Concomitant Use
Avoid concomitant use of AMILoride with any of the following: CycloSPORINE (Systemic); Spironolactone; Tacrolimus (Systemic)
Decreased Effect
AMILoride may decrease the levels/effects of: Cardiac Glycosides; QuiNIDine

The levels/effects of AMILoride may be decreased by: Herbs (Hypertensive Properties); Methylphenidate; Nonsteroidal Anti-Inflammatory Agents; Yohimbine
Increased Effect/Toxicity
AMILoride may increase the levels/effects of: ACE Inhibitors; Amifostine; Ammonium Chloride; Antihypertensives; Cardiac Glycosides; CycloSPORINE (Systemic); Dofetilide; DULoxetine; Hypotensive Agents; Obinutuzumab; RiTUXimab; Sodium Phosphates; Spironolactone; Tacrolimus (Systemic)

The levels/effects of AMILoride may be increased by: Alfuzosin; Analgesics (Opioid); Angiotensin II Receptor Blockers; Brimonidine (Topical); Canagliflozin; Diazoxide; Drospirenone; Eplerenone; Heparin; Heparin (Low Molecular Weight); Herbs (Hypotensive Properties); MAO Inhibitors; Nonsteroidal Anti-Inflammatory Agents; Pentoxifylline; Phosphodiesterase 5 Inhibitors; Potassium Salts; Prostacyclin Analogues; Tolvaptan
Nutritional/Ethanol Interactions Food: Hyperkalemia may result if amiloride is taken with potassium-containing foods.
Adverse Reactions
1% to 10%:
Central nervous system: Dizziness, fatigue, headache
Endocrine & metabolic: Hyperkalemia (up to 10%; risk reduced in patients receiving kaliuretic diuretics), dehydration, gynecomastia, hyperchloremic metabolic acidosis, hyponatremia
Gastrointestinal: Abdominal pain, change in appetite, constipation, diarrhea, gas pain, nausea, vomiting
Genitourinary: Impotence
Neuromuscular & skeletal: Muscle cramps, weakness
Respiratory: Cough, dyspnea

◀ **Pharmacodynamics/Kinetics**
  Onset of Action 2 hours
  Duration of Action 24 hours
Available Dosage Forms
  Tablet, Oral:
    Generic: 5 mg
General Dosage Range Dosage adjustment recommended in patients with renal impairment
  Oral:
    Adults: 5-10 mg/day in 1-2 divided doses (maximum: 20 mg/day)
    Elderly: Initial: 5 mg once daily or every other day
Administration
  Oral Administer with food or meals to avoid GI upset.
Nursing Actions
  Physical Assessment Monitor electrolytes and fluid status (I & O, weight, blood pressure). Monitor for hyperkalemia.
  Patient Education
    • Discuss specific use of drug and side effects with patient as it relates to treatment. (HCAHPS: During this hospital stay, were you given any medicine that you had not taken before? Before giving you any new medicine, how often did hospital staff tell you what the medicine was for? How often did hospital staff describe possible side effects in a way you could understand?)
    • Patient may experience diarrhea, headache, or lack of appetite. Have patient report immediately to prescriber severe dizziness, syncope, significant asthenia, considerable nausea, xerostomia, polydipsia, bradycardia, arrhythmia, or myalgia (HCAHPS).
    • Educate patient about signs of a significant reaction (eg, wheezing; chest tightness; fever; itching; bad cough; blue skin color; seizures; or swelling of face, lips, tongue, or throat). **Note:** This is not a comprehensive list of all side effects. Patient should consult prescriber for additional questions.

    Intended Use and Disclaimer: Should not be printed and given to patients. This information is intended to serve as a concise initial reference for healthcare professionals to use when discussing medications with a patient. You must ultimately rely on your own discretion, experience and judgment in diagnosing, treating and advising patients.
  Dietary Considerations Take with food or meals to avoid GI upset. Do not use salt substitutes or low salt milk without checking with healthcare provider.

Amiloride and Hydrochlorothiazide
(a MIL oh ride & hye droe klor oh THYE a zide)

Index Terms Hydrochlorothiazide and Amiloride
Pharmacologic Category Antihypertensive; Diuretic, Combination
Pregnancy Risk Factor B

Lactation Enters breast milk/contraindicated
Use Potassium-sparing diuretic; antihypertensive
Available Dosage Forms
  Tablet: 5/50: Amiloride 5 mg and hydrochlorothiazide 50 mg
General Dosage Range Dosage adjustment recommended in patients with renal impairment
  Oral:
    Adults: 1-2 tablets (amiloride 5 mg/HCTZ 50 mg per tablet) once daily (maximum: 2 tablets/day)
    Elderly: Initial: 1/2 to 1 tablet/day (maximum: 2 tablets/day)
Administration
  Oral May administer with food.
Nursing Actions
  Physical Assessment See individual agents.
  Patient Education
    • Discuss specific use of drug and side effects with patient as it relates to treatment. (HCAHPS: During this hospital stay, were you given any medicine that you had not taken before? Before giving you any new medicine, how often did hospital staff tell you what the medicine was for? How often did hospital staff describe possible side effects in a way you could understand?)
    • Patient may experience dizziness, headache, lack of appetite, dyspepsia, or asthenia. Have patient report immediately to prescriber signs of hyperglycemia, signs of fluid and electrolyte imbalance, severe dizziness, syncope, vision changes, or ophthalmalgia (HCAHPS).
    • Educate patient about signs of a significant reaction (eg, wheezing; chest tightness; fever; itching; bad cough; blue skin color; seizures; or swelling of face, lips, tongue, or throat). **Note:** This is not a comprehensive list of all side effects. Patient should consult prescriber for additional questions.

    Intended Use and Disclaimer: Should not be printed and given to patients. This information is intended to serve as a concise initial reference for healthcare professionals to use when discussing medications with a patient. You must ultimately rely on your own discretion, experience and judgment in diagnosing, treating and advising patients.
  Related Information
    AMILoride *on page 81*
    Hydrochlorothiazide *on page 775*

Amiodarone (a MEE oh da rone)

Brand Names: U.S. Cordarone; Nexterone; Pacerone
Index Terms Amiodarone Hydrochloride
Pharmacologic Category Antiarrhythmic Agent, Class III

Medication Safety Issues

Sound-alike/look-alike issues:
Amiodarone may be confused with aMILoride, inamrinone
Cordarone may be confused with Cardura, Cordran

High alert medication:
The Institute for Safe Medication Practices (ISMP) includes this medication among its list of drugs which have a heightened risk of causing significant patient harm when used in error.

BEERS Criteria medication:
This drug may be potentially inappropriate for use in geriatric patients (Quality of evidence - high; Strength of recommendation - strong).

Medication Guide Available Yes

Pregnancy Risk Factor D

Lactation Enters breast milk/not recommended

Breast-Feeding Considerations Amiodarone and its active metabolite are excreted into human milk. Breast-feeding may lead to significant infant exposure and potential toxicity. Due to the long half-life, amiodarone may be present in breast milk for several days following discontinuation of maternal therapy (Hall, 2003). The manufacturer recommends that breast-feeding be discontinued if treatment is needed.

Use Management of life-threatening recurrent ventricular fibrillation (VF) or hemodynamically-unstable ventricular tachycardia (VT) refractory to other antiarrhythmic agents or in patients intolerant of other agents used for these conditions

Unlabeled Use
Atrial fibrillation (AF): Pharmacologic conversion of AF to and maintenance of normal sinus rhythm; treatment of AF in patients with heart failure [no accessory pathway] who require heart rate control (ACC/AHA/ESC Practice Guidelines) or in patients with hypertrophic cardiomyopathy (ACCF/AHA Practice Guidelines); prevention of postoperative AF associated with cardiothoracic surgery
Paroxysmal supraventricular tachycardia (SVT) (not initial drug of choice)
Ventricular tachyarrhythmias (ACLS/PALS guidelines): Cardiac arrest with persistent VT or VF if defibrillation, CPR, and vasopressor administration have failed; control of hemodynamically-stable monomorphic VT, polymorphic VT with a normal baseline QT interval, or wide-complex tachycardia of uncertain origin; control of rapid ventricular rate due to accessory pathway conduction in pre-excited atrial arrhythmias (ACLS guidelines) or stable narrow-complex tachycardia (ACLS guidelines)
Adjunct to ICD therapy to suppress symptomatic ventricular tachyarrhythmias in otherwise optimally-treated patients with heart failure (ACC/AHA/ESC Practice Guidelines)

Mechanism of Action/Effect Class III antiarrhythmic agent which inhibits adrenergic stimulation, prolongs the action potential and refractory period in myocardial tissue; decreases AV conduction and sinus node function. Amiodarone shows beta-blocker-like and calcium channel blocker-like effects on SA and AV nodes.

Contraindications Hypersensitivity to amiodarone, iodine, or any component of the formulation; severe sinus-node dysfunction; second- and third-degree heart block (except in patients with a functioning artificial pacemaker); bradycardia causing syncope (except in patients with a functioning artificial pacemaker); cardiogenic shock

Warnings/Precautions [U.S. Boxed Warning]: Only indicated for patients with life-threatening arrhythmias because of risk of toxicity. Alternative therapies should be tried first before using amiodarone. Patients should be hospitalized when amiodarone is initiated. Currently, the 2005 ACLS guidelines recommend I.V. amiodarone as the preferred antiarrhythmic for the treatment of pulseless VT/VF, both life-threatening arrhythmias. In patients with non-life-threatening arrhythmias (eg, atrial fibrillation), amiodarone should be used only if the use of other antiarrhythmics has proven ineffective or are contraindicated.

[U.S. Boxed Warning]: Lung damage (abnormal diffusion capacity) may occur without symptoms. Monitor for pulmonary toxicity. Evaluate new respiratory symptoms; pre-existing pulmonary disease does not increase risk of developing pulmonary toxicity, but if pulmonary toxicity develops then the prognosis is worse. The lowest effective dose should be used as appropriate for the acuity/severity of the arrhythmia being treated. **[U.S. Boxed Warning]: Liver toxicity is common, but usually mild with evidence of increased liver enzymes. Severe liver toxicity can occur and has been fatal in a few cases.**

[U.S. Boxed Warning]: Amiodarone can exacerbate arrhythmias, by making them more difficult to tolerate or reverse; other types of arrhythmias have occurred, including significant heart block, sinus bradycardia new ventricular fibrillation, incessant ventricular tachycardia, increased resistance to cardioversion, and polymorphic ventricular tachycardia associated with QT_c prolongation (torsade de pointes [TdP]). Risk may be increased with concomitant use of other antiarrhythmic agents or drugs that prolong the QT_c interval. Proarrhythmic effects may be prolonged.

Monitor pacing or defibrillation thresholds in patients with implantable cardiac devices (eg, pacemakers, defibrillators). Use very cautiously and with close monitoring in patients with thyroid or liver disease. May cause hyper- or hypothyroidism. Hyperthyroidism may result in thyrotoxicosis and may aggravate or cause breakthrough arrhythmias. If any new signs of arrhythmia appear, hyperthyroidism should be considered. Thyroid function should be monitored prior to treatment and periodically thereafter.

May cause optic neuropathy and/or optic neuritis, usually resulting in visual impairment. Corneal microdeposits occur in a majority of patients, and may cause visual disturbances in some patients (blurred vision, halos); these are not generally considered a reason to discontinue treatment. Corneal refractive laser surgery is generally contraindicated in amiodarone users. Avoid excessive exposure to sunlight; may cause photosensitivity.

Amiodarone is a potent inhibitor of CYP enzymes and transport proteins (including p-glycoprotein), which may lead to increased serum concentrations/toxicity of a number of medications. Particular caution must be used when a drug with QT_c-prolonging potential relies on metabolism via these enzymes, since the effect of elevated concentrations may be additive with the effect of amiodarone. Carefully assess risk:benefit of coadministration of other drugs which may prolong QT_c interval. Patients may still be at risk for amiodarone–related drug interactions after the drug has been discontinued. The pharmacokinetics are complex (due to prolonged duration of action and half-life) and difficult to predict. Correct electrolyte disturbances, especially hypokalemia or hypomagnesemia, prior to use and throughout therapy. Use caution when initiating amiodarone in patients on warfarin. Cases of increased INR with or without bleeding have occurred in patients treated with warfarin; monitor INR closely after initiating amiodarone in these patients.

In the treatment of atrial fibrillation in older adults, avoid antiarrhythmics as first-line treatment. In older adults, data suggests rate control may provide more benefits than risks compared to rhythm control for most patients (Beers Criteria).

May cause hypotension and bradycardia (infusion-rate related). Hypotension with rapid administration has been attributed to the emulsifier polysorbate 80. Commercially-prepared premixed solutions do not contain polysorbate 80 and may have a lower incidence of hypotension. Caution in surgical patients; may enhance hemodynamic effect of anesthetics; associated with increased risk of adult respiratory distress syndrome (ARDS) postoperatively. Vials for injection contain benzyl alcohol, which has been associated with "gasping syndrome" in neonates. Commercially-prepared premixed solutions do not contain benzyl alcohol. Commercially-prepared premixed infusion contains the excipient cyclodextrin (sulfobutyl ether beta-cyclodextrin), which may accumulate in patients with renal insufficiency.

Drug Interactions
Avoid Concomitant Use
Avoid concomitant use of Amiodarone with any of the following: Agalsidase Alfa; Agalsidase Beta; Antiarrhythmic Agents (Class Ia); Azithromycin (Systemic); Bosutinib; Conivaptan; Fingolimod; Fusidic Acid (Systemic); Grapefruit Juice; Highest Risk QTc-Prolonging Agents; Ivabradine; Mifepristone; Moderate Risk QTc-Prolonging Agents; Pomalidomide; Propafenone; Protease Inhibitors; Silodosin; Tegafur; Thioridazine; Topotecan; VinCRIStine (Liposomal)

Decreased Effect
Amiodarone may decrease the levels/effects of: Agalsidase Alfa; Agalsidase Beta; Clopidogrel; Codeine; Sodium Iodide I131; Tamoxifen; Tegafur; TraMADol

The levels/effects of Amiodarone may be decreased by: Bile Acid Sequestrants; Bosentan; CYP2C8 Inducers (Strong); CYP3A4 Inducers (Strong); Dabrafenib; Deferasirox; Etravirine; Fosphenytoin; Grapefruit Juice; Herbs (CYP3A4 Inducers); Mitotane; Orlistat; Peginterferon Alfa-2b; P-glycoprotein/ABCB1 Inducers; Phenytoin; Rifampin; Tocilizumab

Increased Effect/Toxicity
Amiodarone may increase the levels/effects of: Afatinib; Antiarrhythmic Agents (Class Ia); ARIPiprazole; Beta-Blockers; Bosentan; Bosutinib; Cardiac Glycosides; Colchicine; CycloSPORINE (Systemic); CYP2A6 Substrates; CYP2C9 Substrates; CYP2D6 Substrates; Dabigatran Etexilate; DOXOrubicin (Conventional); Everolimus; Fesoterodine; Flecainide; Fosphenytoin; Highest Risk QTc-Prolonging Agents; HMG-CoA Reductase Inhibitors; Lidocaine (Systemic); Lidocaine (Topical); Loratadine; Metoprolol; Mipomersen; P-glycoprotein/ABCB1 Substrates; Phenytoin; Pomalidomide; Porfimer; Propafenone; Prucalopride; Rivaroxaban; Silodosin; Thioridazine; Topotecan; VinCRIStine (Liposomal); Vitamin K Antagonists

The levels/effects of Amiodarone may be increased by: Azithromycin (Systemic); Boceprevir; Calcium Channel Blockers (Nondihydropyridine); Cimetidine; Conivaptan; CYP2C8 Inhibitors (Moderate); CYP2C8 Inhibitors (Strong); CYP3A4 Inhibitors (Moderate); CYP3A4 Inhibitors (Strong); Dasatinib; Deferasirox; Fingolimod; Fosphenytoin; Fusidic Acid (Systemic); Grapefruit Juice; Ivabradine; Ivacaftor; Lidocaine (Topical); Luliconazole; Mifepristone; Moderate Risk QTc-Prolonging Agents; P-glycoprotein/ABCB1 Inhibitors; Protease Inhibitors; QTc-Prolonging Agents (Indeterminate Risk and Risk Modifying); Simeprevir; Stiripentol; Telaprevir

Nutritional/Ethanol Interactions
Food: Increases the rate and extent of absorption of amiodarone. Grapefruit juice increases bioavailability of oral amiodarone by 50% and decreases the conversion of amiodarone to N-DEA (active metabolite); altered effects are possible. Management: Take consistently with regard

to meals; grapefruit juice should be avoided during therapy.

Herb/Nutraceutical: St John's wort may decrease amiodarone levels or enhance photosensitization. Ephedra may worsen arrythmia. Management: Avoid St John's wort, ephedra and dong quai.

Adverse Reactions In a recent meta-analysis, adult patients taking lower doses of amiodarone (152-330 mg daily for at least 12 months) were more likely to develop thyroid, neurologic, skin, ocular, and bradycardic abnormalities than those taking placebo (Vorperian, 1997). Pulmonary toxicity was similar in both the low-dose amiodarone group and in the placebo group, but there was a trend towards increased toxicity in the amiodarone group. Gastrointestinal and hepatic events were seen to a similar extent in both the low-dose amiodarone group and placebo group. As the frequency of adverse events varies considerably across studies as a function of route and dose, a consolidation of adverse event rates is provided by Goldschlager, 2000.

>10%:

Cardiovascular: Hypotension (I.V. 16%, refractory in rare cases)

Central nervous system (3% to 40%): Abnormal gait/ataxia, dizziness, fatigue, headache, malaise, impaired memory, involuntary movement, insomnia, poor coordination, peripheral neuropathy, sleep disturbances, tremor

Dermatologic: Photosensitivity (10% to 75%)

Endocrine & Metabolic: Hypothyroidism (1% to 22%)

Gastrointestinal: Nausea, vomiting, anorexia, and constipation (10% to 33%)

Hepatic: AST or ALT level >2x normal (15% to 50%)

Ocular: Corneal microdeposits (>90%; causes visual disturbance in <10%)

1% to 10%:

Cardiovascular: CHF (3%), bradycardia (3% to 5%), AV block (5%), conduction abnormalities, SA node dysfunction (1% to 3%), cardiac arrhythmia, flushing, edema. Additional effects associated with I.V. administration include asystole, atrial fibrillation, cardiac arrest, electromechanical dissociation, pulseless electrical activity (PEA), ventricular tachycardia, and cardiogenic shock.

Dermatologic: Slate blue skin discoloration (<10%)

Endocrine & metabolic: Hyperthyroidism (3% to 10%; more common in iodine-deficient regions of the world), libido decreased

Gastrointestinal: Abdominal pain, abnormal salivation, abnormal taste (oral), diarrhea, nausea (I.V.)

Hematologic: Coagulation abnormalities

Hepatic: Hepatitis and cirrhosis (<3%)

Local: Phlebitis (I.V., with concentrations >3 mg/mL)

Ocular: Visual disturbances (2% to 9%), halo vision (<5% occurring especially at night), optic neuritis (1%)

Respiratory: Pulmonary toxicity has been estimated to occur at a frequency between 2% and 7% of patients (some reports indicate a frequency as high as 17%). Toxicity may present as hypersensitivity pneumonitis; pulmonary fibrosis (cough, fever, malaise); pulmonary inflammation; interstitial pneumonitis; or alveolar pneumonitis. ARDS has been reported in up to 2% of patients receiving amiodarone, and postoperatively in patients receiving oral amiodarone.

Miscellaneous: Abnormal smell (oral)

Pharmacodynamics/Kinetics

Onset of Action Oral: 2 days to 3 weeks; I.V.: May be more rapid; Peak effect: 1 week to 5 months

Duration of Action After discontinuing therapy: 7-50 days

Note: Mean onset of effect and duration after discontinuation may be shorter in children than adults

Available Dosage Forms

Solution, Intravenous:

Nexterone: 150 mg/100 mL (100 mL); 360 mg/200 mL (200 mL)

Generic: 150 mg/3 mL (3 mL); 450 mg/9 mL (9 mL); 900 mg/18 mL (18 mL)

Tablet, Oral:

Cordarone: 200 mg

Pacerone: 100 mg, 200 mg, 400 mg

Generic: 100 mg, 200 mg, 400 mg

General Dosage Range

I.O.: *Children (PALS dosing):* 5 mg/kg (maximum: 300 mg per dose); may repeat twice up to maximum dose of 15 mg/kg/day

I.V.:

Children (PALS dosing): 5 mg/kg (maximum: 300 mg per dose); may repeat twice up to maximum dose of 15 mg/kg/day

Adults: Initial: 150-300 mg bolus **or** 5-7 mg/kg; Maintenance: 1200-1800 mg daily continuous infusion until 10 g total **or** 1 mg/minute infusion for 6 hours, then 0.5 mg/minute infusion for 18 hours (maximum: 2.1 g daily)

Oral: *Adults:* Initial: 600-1600 mg daily until 10 g total; Maintenance: 100-400 mg daily

Usual Infusion Concentrations: Pediatric

Note: Premixed solutions available.

I.V. infusion: 1.8 mg/mL

Usual Infusion Concentrations: Adult Note:

Premixed solutions available.

I.V. infusion: 450 mg in 250 mL (concentration: 1.8 mg/mL) of D_5W or NS

Administration

I.V. For infusions >1 hour, use concentrations ≤2 mg/mL unless a central venous catheter is used; commercially-prepared premixed solutions in concentrations of 1.5 mg/mL and 1.8 mg/mL ▶

are available. Use only volumetric infusion pump; use of drop counting may lead to underdosage. Administer through an I.V. line located as centrally as possible. For continuous infusions, an in-line filter has been recommended during administration to reduce the incidence of phlebitis. During pulseless VT/VF, administering **undiluted** is preferred (Dager, 2006; Skrifvars, 2004). *The Handbook of Emergency Cardiovascular Care* (Hazinski, 2010) and the 2010 ACLS guidelines do not make any specific recommendations regarding dilution of amiodarone in this setting.

Adjust administration rate to urgency (give more slowly when perfusing arrhythmia present). Slow the infusion rate if hypotension or bradycardia develops. Infusions >2 hours must be administered in a non-PVC container (eg, glass or polyolefin). PVC tubing is recommended for administration regardless of infusion duration. **Incompatible** with heparin; flush with saline prior to and following infusion. **Note:** I.V. administration at lower flow rates (potentially associated with use in pediatrics) and higher concentrations than recommended may result in leaching of plasticizers (DEHP) from intravenous tubing. DEHP may adversely affect male reproductive tract development. Alternative means of dosing and administration (1 mg/kg aliquots) may need to be considered.

Injectable Detail pH: 4.08

Oral Administer consistently with regard to meals. Take in divided doses with meals if GI upset occurs or if taking large daily dose. If GI intolerance occurs with single-dose therapy, use twice daily dosing.

Storage/Stability

Tablets: Store at 20°C to 25°C (68°F to 77°F); excursions are permitted between 15°C and 30°C (59°F and 86°F); protect from light.

Injection: Store undiluted vials and premixed solutions (Nexterone) at 20°C to 25°C (68°F to 77°F); excursions are permitted between 15°C and 30°C (59°F and 86°F). Protect from light during storage; protect from excessive heat. There is no need to protect solutions from light during administration. When vial contents are admixed in D$_5$W to a final concentration of 1-6 mg/mL, amiodarone is stable for 24 hours in glass or polyolefin bottles and for 2 hours in polyvinyl chloride (PVC) bags; do not use evacuated glass containers as buffer may cause precipitation. Nexterone is available as premixed solutions. Although amiodarone adsorbs to PVC tubing, all clinical studies used PVC tubing and the recommended doses account for adsorption; in adults, PVC tubing is recommended.

Nursing Actions

Physical Assessment Eye examinations should be performed periodically. Monitor cardiac status closely and assess for CNS changes (ie,

abnormal gait/ataxia, dizziness, impaired memory, involuntary movement, poor coordination, peripheral neuropathy, tremor). Monitor for signs of pulmonary toxicity (eg, nonproductive cough, dyspnea, pleuritic pain, weight loss, fever, malaise). **I.V.:** Requires continuous cardiac/hemodynamic monitoring during infusion. Be alert for adverse reactions. **Oral:** Monitor cardiac status prior to treatment and throughout.

Patient Education

• Discuss specific use of drug and side effects with patient as it relates to treatment. (HCAHPS: During this hospital stay, were you given any medicine that you had not taken before? Before giving you any new medicine, how often did hospital staff tell you what the medicine was for? How often did hospital staff describe possible side effects in a way you could understand?)

• Patient may experience constipation, headache, or insomnia. Have patient report immediately to prescriber signs of depression (ie, suicidal ideation, anxiety, emotional instability, illogical thinking), signs of hepatic impairment, mood changes, severe nausea, change in balance, temperature sensitivity, tremors, bradykinesia, rigidity, excessive weight gain or loss, alopecia, edema of neck, significant asthenia, skin discoloration, hemoptysis, chills, pharyngitis, angina, paresthesia, tachycardia, bradycardia, arrhythmia, vision loss, urinary retention, oliguria, severe dizziness, syncope, ophthalmalgia, difficulty with motor activity, arthralgia, myalgia, dyspnea, edema of extremities, ecchymosis, hemorrhaging, vision changes, hyperhydrosis, dehydration, or severe diarrhea (HCAHPS).

• Educate patient about signs of a significant reaction (eg, wheezing; chest tightness; fever; itching; bad cough; blue skin color; seizures; or swelling of face, lips, tongue, or throat). **Note:** This is not a comprehensive list of all side effects. Patient should consult prescriber for additional questions.

Intended Use and Disclaimer: Should not be printed and given to patients. This information is intended to serve as a concise initial reference for healthcare professionals to use when discussing medications with a patient. You must ultimately rely on your own discretion, experience and judgment in diagnosing, treating and advising patients.

Dietary Considerations Take consistently with regard to meals. Amiodarone is a potential source of large amounts of inorganic iodine; ~3 mg of inorganic iodine per 100 mg of amiodarone is released into the systemic circulation. Recommended daily allowance for iodine in adults is 150 mcg.

Grapefruit juice is not recommended.

Amitriptyline (a mee TRIP ti leen)

Index Terms Amitriptyline Hydrochloride; Elavil
Pharmacologic Category Antidepressant, Tricyclic (Tertiary Amine)
Medication Safety Issues
Sound-alike/look-alike issues:
Amitriptyline may be confused with aminophylline, imipramine, nortriptyline
Elavil may be confused with Aldoril, Eldepryl, enalapril, Equanil, Plavix
BEERS Criteria medication:
This drug may be potentially inappropriate for use in geriatric patients (Quality of evidence - high [moderate for SIADH]; Strength of recommendation - strong).
Medication Guide Available Yes
Pregnancy Risk Factor C
Lactation Enters breast milk/not recommended
Use Depression: Treatment of depression
Unlabeled Use Analgesic for certain chronic and neuropathic pain (including diabetic neuropathy); prophylaxis against migraine headaches; post-traumatic stress disorder (PTSD)
Available Dosage Forms
Tablet, Oral:
Generic: 10 mg, 25 mg, 50 mg, 75 mg, 100 mg, 150 mg
General Dosage Range Oral:
Adolescents: 10 mg 3 times daily and 20 mg at bedtime (recommended by the manufacturer).
Adults: 25-300 mg daily as a single dose at bedtime or in divided doses
*Elderly:*10 mg 3 times daily and 20 mg at bedtime (recommended by the manufacturer).
Administration
Oral Administer higher doses preferably at late afternoon or as bedtime doses to minimize daytime sedation.
Nursing Actions
Physical Assessment Assess for suicidal tendencies or unusual changes in behavior before beginning therapy and periodically thereafter. Caution patients with diabetes; may increase or decrease serum glucose levels. Taper dosage slowly when discontinuing.
Patient Education
- Discuss specific use of drug and side effects with patient as it relates to treatment. (HCAHPS: During this hospital stay, were you given any medicine that you had not taken before? Before giving you any new medicine, how often did hospital staff tell you what the medicine was for? How often did hospital staff describe possible side effects in a way you could understand?)
- Patient may experience fatigue, xerostomia, nausea, lack of appetite, or diarrhea. Have patient report immediately to prescriber signs of hepatic impairment, suicidal ideation, strength differences from one side to another, difficulty

speaking or thinking, change in balance, blurred vision, tachycardia, arrhythmia, severe dizziness, syncope, considerable headache, illogical thinking, urinary retention, significant asthenia, ecchymosis, hemorrhaging, edema of extremities, tremors, hallucinations, paresthesia, angina, sexual dysfunction, vision changes, chills, pharyngitis, intolerable dyspepsia, severe constipation, anhidrosis, or signs of tardive dyskinesia (HCAHPS).
- Educate patient about signs of a significant reaction (eg, wheezing; chest tightness; fever; itching; bad cough; blue skin color; seizures; or swelling of face, lips, tongue, or throat). **Note:** This is not a comprehensive list of all side effects. Patient should consult prescriber for additional questions.

Intended Use and Disclaimer: Should not be printed and given to patients. This information is intended to serve as a concise initial reference for healthcare professionals to use when discussing medications with a patient. You must ultimately rely on your own discretion, experience and judgment in diagnosing, treating and advising patients.
Related Information
Peak and Trough Guidelines on page 1710

AmLODIPine (am LOE di peen)

Brand Names: U.S. Norvasc
Index Terms Amlodipine Besylate
Pharmacologic Category Antianginal Agent; Antihypertensive; Calcium Channel Blocker; Calcium Channel Blocker, Dihydropyridine
Medication Safety Issues
Sound-alike/look-alike issues:
AmLODIPine may be confused with aMILoride
Norvasc may be confused with Navane, Norvir, Vascor
International issues:
Norvasc [U.S., Canada, and multiple international markets] may be confused with Vascor brand name for imidapril [Philippines] and simvastatin [Malaysia, Singapore, and Thailand]
Pregnancy Risk Factor C
Lactation Excretion in breast milk unknown/not recommended
Breast-Feeding Considerations It is not known if amlodipine is excreted into breast milk. The manufacturer recommends nursing be discontinued during treatment. Breast-fed infants of mothers taking medications for hypertension should be monitored for adverse effects (Chobanian, 2003).
Use Treatment of hypertension; treatment of symptomatic chronic stable angina, vasospastic (Prinzmetal's) angina (confirmed or suspected); prevention of hospitalization due to angina with documented CAD (limited to patients without heart failure or ejection fraction <40%)

The ACCF/AHA 2013 guidelines for management of heart failure state that, with the exception of amlodipine, calcium channel blockers should be avoided and withdrawn whenever possible in patients with heart failure with reduced ejection fraction (HFrEF). While amlodipine, like other calcium channel blockers, has no benefit on functioning or survival, it may be used for the treatment of hypertension or ischemic heart disease in patients with HFrEF (ACCF/AHA [Yancy, 2013]).

Mechanism of Action/Effect Inhibits calcium ion from entering the "slow channels" or select voltage-sensitive areas of vascular smooth muscle and myocardium during depolarization; a peripheral arterial vasodilator that causes a reduction in blood pressure

Contraindications Hypersensitivity to amlodipine or any component of the formulation

Warnings/Precautions Increased angina and/or MI has occurred with initiation or dosage titration of calcium channel blockers. Symptomatic hypotension with or without syncope can rarely occur; blood pressure must be lowered at a rate appropriate for the patient's clinical condition. Use caution in severe aortic stenosis and/or hypertrophic cardiomyopathy with outflow tract obstruction. Use caution in patients with hepatic impairment; may require lower starting dose; titrate slowly with severe hepatic impairment. The most common side effect is peripheral edema; occurs within 2-3 weeks of starting therapy. Reflex tachycardia may occur with use. Peak antihypertensive effect is delayed; dosage titration should occur after 7-14 days on a given dose. Initiate at a lower dose in the elderly.

Drug Interactions

Avoid Concomitant Use

Avoid concomitant use of AmLODIPine with any of the following: Conivaptan; Fusidic Acid (Systemic); Pimozide

Decreased Effect

AmLODIPine may decrease the levels/effects of: Clopidogrel; QuiNIDine

The levels/effects of AmLODIPine may be decreased by: Barbiturates; Bosentan; Calcium Salts; CarBAMazepine; CYP3A4 Inducers (Strong); Dabrafenib; Deferasirox; Herbs (CYP3A4 Inducers); Herbs (Hypertensive Properties); Melatonin; Methylphenidate; Mitotane; Nafcillin; Rifamycin Derivatives; Tocilizumab; Yohimbine

Increased Effect/Toxicity

AmLODIPine may increase the levels/effects of: Amifostine; Antihypertensives; ARIPiprazole; Atosiban; Beta-Blockers; Calcium Channel Blockers (Nondihydropyridine); Dofetilide; DULoxetine; Fosphenytoin; Hypotensive Agents; Lomitapide; Magnesium Salts; Neuromuscular-Blocking Agents (Nondepolarizing); Nitroprusside; Obinutuzumab; Phenytoin; Pimozide; QuiNIDine; RiTUXimab; Simvastatin; Tacrolimus (Systemic)

The levels/effects of AmLODIPine may be increased by: Alpha1-Blockers; Antifungal Agents (Azole Derivatives, Systemic); Brimonidine (Topical); Calcium Channel Blockers (Nondihydropyridine); Conivaptan; CycloSPORINE (Systemic); CYP3A4 Inhibitors (Moderate); CYP3A4 Inhibitors (Strong); Dasatinib; Diazoxide; Fluconazole; Fusidic Acid (Systemic); Grapefruit Juice; Herbs (Hypotensive Properties); Ivacaftor; Luliconazole; Macrolide Antibiotics; Magnesium Salts; MAO Inhibitors; Mifepristone; Pentoxifylline; Phosphodiesterase 5 Inhibitors; Prostacyclin Analogues; Protease Inhibitors; QuiNIDine; Simeprevir; Stiripentol

Nutritional/Ethanol Interactions

Food: Grapefruit juice may modestly increase amlodipine levels.

Herb/Nutraceutical: St John's wort may decrease amlodipine levels. Avoid herbs with *hypertensive* properties (bayberry, blue cohosh, cayenne, ephedra, ginger, ginseng [American], kola, licorice). Avoid herbs with *hypotensive* properties (black cohosh, California poppy, coleus, garlic, goldenseal, hawthorn, mistletoe, periwinkle, quinine, shepherd's purse).

Adverse Reactions

>10%:

Cardiovascular: Peripheral edema (2% to 11% dose related; female 15%; male 6%; HF patients 27% to 28% [Packer, 1996; Packer, 2013])

Respiratory: Pulmonary edema (HF patients 7% to 15% [Packer, 1996; Packer, 2013])

1% to 10%:

Cardiovascular: Palpitations (1% to 5% dose related), flushing (1% to 3% dose related, more frequent in females)

Central nervous system: Fatigue (5%), dizziness (1% to 3% dose related), male sexual disorder (1% to 2%), drowsiness (1%)

Dermatologic: Pruritus (1% to 2%), skin rash (1% to 2%)

Gastrointestinal: Nausea (3%), abdominal pain (2%)

Neuromuscular & skeletal: Muscle cramps (1% to 2%), weakness (1% to 2%)

Respiratory: Dyspnea (1% to 2%)

Pharmacodynamics/Kinetics

Duration of Action Antihypertensive effect: 24 hours

Available Dosage Forms

Tablet, Oral:

Norvasc: 2.5 mg, 5 mg, 10 mg

Generic: 2.5 mg, 5 mg, 10 mg

General Dosage Range Dosage adjustment recommended in patients with hepatic impairment

Oral:

Children 6-17 years: 2.5-5 mg once daily

Adults: Initial: 5 mg once daily; Maintenance: 2.5-10 mg once daily (maximum: 10 mg/day)

Elderly: 2.5-5 mg once daily

Administration

Oral May be administered without regard to meals.

Storage/Stability Store at room temperature of 15°C to 30°C (59°F to 86°F).

Nursing Actions

Physical Assessment Monitor blood pressure, pulse, frequency and intensity of angina, weight, and peripheral edema.

Patient Education

- Discuss specific use of drug and side effects with patient as it relates to treatment. (HCAHPS: During this hospital stay, were you given any medicine that you had not taken before? Before giving you any new medicine, how often did hospital staff tell you what the medicine was for? How often did hospital staff describe possible side effects in a way you could understand?)
- Patient may experience fatigue, asthenia, flushing, or dyspepsia. Have patient report immediately to prescriber severe dizziness, syncope, significant headache, angina, tachycardia, bradycardia, arrhythmia, dyspnea, excessive weight gain, edema of extremities, urine discoloration, jaundice, or changes to teeth or gums (HCAHPS).
- Educate patient about signs of a significant reaction (eg, wheezing; chest tightness; fever; itching; bad cough; blue skin color; seizures; or swelling of face, lips, tongue, or throat). **Note:** This is not a comprehensive list of all side effects. Patient should consult prescriber for additional questions.

Intended Use and Disclaimer: Should not be printed and given to patients. This information is intended to serve as a concise initial reference for healthcare professionals to use when discussing medications with a patient. You must ultimately rely on your own discretion, experience and judgment in diagnosing, treating and advising patients.

Dietary Considerations May be taken without regard to meals.

Amlodipine and Atorvastatin
(am LOW di peen & a TORE va sta tin)

Brand Names: U.S. Caduet®

Index Terms Atorvastatin and Amlodipine; Atorvastatin Calcium and Amlodipine Besylate

Pharmacologic Category Antianginal Agent; Antihypertensive; Antilipemic Agent, HMG-CoA Reductase Inhibitor; Calcium Channel Blocker; Calcium Channel Blocker, Dihydropyridine

Pregnancy Risk Factor X

Use For use when treatment with both amlodipine and atorvastatin is appropriate:

Amlodipine: Treatment of hypertension; treatment of chronic stable angina, vasospastic (Prinzmetal's) angina (confirmed or suspected); prevention of hospitalization or to decrease coronary revascularization procedure due to angina with documented CAD (limited to patients without heart failure or ejection fraction <40%)

Atorvastatin: Treatment of dyslipidemias or primary prevention of cardiovascular disease (atherosclerotic) as detailed here:

Primary prevention of cardiovascular disease (high-risk for CVD): To reduce the risk of MI or stroke in patients without evidence of coronary heart disease who have multiple CVD risk factors or type 2 diabetes; also reduces the risk for angina or revascularization procedures in patients with multiple CVD risk factors without evidence of coronary heart disease

Secondary prevention of cardiovascular disease: To reduce the risk of MI, stroke, revascularization procedures, angina, and hospitalization for heart failure

Treatment of dyslipidemias: To reduce elevations in total cholesterol, LDL-C, apolipoprotein B, and triglycerides in patients with elevations of one or more components, and/or to increase low HDL-C as present in heterozygous familial/nonfamilial hypercholesterolemia and mixed dyslipidemia (Fredrickson type IIa and IIb hyperlipidemias); treatment of primary dysbetalipoproteinemia (Fredrickson type III), elevated serum TG levels (Fredrickson type IV), and homozygous familial hypercholesterolemia

Treatment of heterozygous familial hypercholesterolemia (HeFH) in adolescent patients (10-17 years of age, females >1 year postmenarche) having LDL-C ≥190 mg/dL or LDL-C ≥160 mg/dL with positive family history of premature cardiovascular disease (CVD) or with two or more CVD risk factors.

Available Dosage Forms

Tablet, oral: Amlodipine 2.5 mg and atorvastatin 10 mg; Amlodipine 2.5 mg and atorvastatin 20 mg; Amlodipine 2.5 mg and atorvastatin 40 mg; Amlodipine 5 mg and atorvastatin 10 mg; Amlodipine 5 mg and atorvastatin 20 mg; Amlodipine 5 mg and atorvastatin 40 mg; Amlodipine 5 mg and atorvastatin 80 mg; Amlodipine 10 mg and atorvastatin 10 mg; Amlodipine 10 mg and atorvastatin 20 mg; Amlodipine 10 mg and atorvastatin 40 mg; Amlodipine 10 mg and atorvastatin 80 mg

Caduet®:

2.5/10: Amlodipine 2.5 mg and atorvastatin 10 mg; 2.5/20: Amlodipine 2.5 mg and atorvastatin 20 mg; 2.5/40: Amlodipine 2.5 mg and atorvastatin 40 mg

5/10: Amlodipine 5 mg and atorvastatin 10 mg; 5/20: Amlodipine 5 mg and atorvastatin 20 mg; 5/40: Amlodipine 5 mg and atorvastatin 40 mg; 5/80: Amlodipine 5 mg and atorvastatin 80 mg

10/10: Amlodipine 10 mg and atorvastatin 10 mg; 10/20: Amlodipine 10 mg and atorvastatin 20 mg; 10/40: Amlodipine 10 mg and atorvastatin 40 mg; 10/80: Amlodipine 10 mg and atorvastatin 80 mg

◄ **General Dosage Range** Dosage adjustment recommended in patients on concomitant therapy
Oral:
Children 10-17 years (females >1 year postmenarche): 2.5-5 mg (amlodipine) and 10-20 mg (atorvastatin) once daily (maximum: amlodipine 5 mg/day; atorvastatin 20 mg/day)
Adults: 2.5-10 mg (amlodipine) and 10-80 mg (atorvastatin) once daily (maximum: amlodipine 10 mg/day; atorvastatin 80 mg/day)
Administration
Oral May be administered without regard to meals.
Nursing Actions
Physical Assessment See individual agents.
Patient Education
- Discuss specific use of drug and side effects with patient as it relates to treatment. (HCAHPS: During this hospital stay, were you given any medicine that you had not taken before? Before giving you any new medicine, how often did hospital staff tell you what the medicine was for? How often did hospital staff describe possible side effects in a way you could understand?)
- Patient may experience diarrhea, dyspepsia, rhinorrhea, pharyngitis, or insomnia. Have patient report immediately to prescriber severe dizziness, syncope, dyspnea, excessive weight gain, edema of extremities, angina, tachycardia, bradycardia, arrhythmia, memory loss, considerable arthralgia, significant myalgia, intolerable asthenia, urinary retention, oliguria, signs of hepatic impairment, strength differences from one side to another, difficulty speaking or thinking, change in balance, or vision changes (HCAHPS).
- Educate patient about signs of a significant reaction (eg, wheezing; chest tightness; fever; itching; bad cough; blue skin color; seizures; or swelling of face, lips, tongue, or throat). **Note:** This is not a comprehensive list of all side effects. Patient should consult prescriber for additional questions.

Intended Use and Disclaimer: Should not be printed and given to patients. This information is intended to serve as a concise initial reference for healthcare professionals to use when discussing medications with a patient. You must ultimately rely on your own discretion, experience and judgment in diagnosing, treating and advising patients.

Related Information
AmLODIPine *on page* 87
AtorvaSTATin *on page* 139

Amlodipine and Benazepril
(am LOE di peen & ben AY ze pril)

Brand Names: U.S. Lotrel®
Index Terms Benazepril Hydrochloride and Amlodipine Besylate

Pharmacologic Category Angiotensin-Converting Enzyme (ACE) Inhibitor; Antianginal Agent; Antihypertensive; Calcium Channel Blocker; Calcium Channel Blocker, Dihydropyridine
Pregnancy Risk Factor D
Use Treatment of hypertension
Available Dosage Forms
Capsule, oral: 2.5/10: Amlodipine 2.5 mg and benazepril 10 mg; 5/10: Amlodipine 5 mg and benazepril 10 mg; 5/20: Amlodipine 5 mg and benazepril 20 mg; 5/40: Amlodipine 5 mg and benazepril hydrochloride 40 mg; 10/20: Amlodipine 10 mg and benazepril 20 mg; 10/40: Amlodipine 10 mg and benazepril hydrochloride 40 mg
Lotrel®: 2.5/10: Amlodipine 2.5 and benazepril 10 mg; 5/10: Amlodipine 5 mg and benazepril 10 mg; 5/20: Amlodipine 5 mg and benazepril 20 mg; 5/40: Amlodipine 5 mg and benazepril 40 mg; 10/20: Amlodipine 10 mg and benazepril 20 mg; 10/40: Amlodipine 10 mg and benazepril 40 mg
General Dosage Range Dosage adjustment recommended in patients with hepatic impairment
Oral:
Adults: 2.5-10 mg (amlodipine) and 10-40 mg (benazepril) once daily (maximum: Amlodipine 10 mg/day; benazepril 80 mg/day)
Elderly: Initial: 2.5 mg/day (based on amlodipine component)
Nursing Actions
Physical Assessment See individual agents.
Patient Education
- Discuss specific use of drug and side effects with patient as it relates to treatment. (HCAHPS: During this hospital stay, were you given any medicine that you had not taken before? Before giving you any new medicine, how often did hospital staff tell you what the medicine was for? How often did hospital staff describe possible side effects in a way you could understand?)
- Patient may experience headache. Have patient report immediately to prescriber signs of infection, signs of hepatic impairment, severe dizziness, syncope, angina, urinary retention, oliguria, tachycardia, bradycardia, arrhythmia, myalgia, dyspnea, excessive weight gain, edema of extremities, changes to teeth or gums, ecchymosis, hemorrhaging, hyperhidrosis, or significant asthenia (HCAHPS).
- Educate patient about signs of a significant reaction (eg, wheezing; chest tightness; fever; itching; bad cough; blue skin color; seizures; or swelling of face, lips, tongue, or throat). **Note:** This is not a comprehensive list of all side effects. Patient should consult prescriber for additional questions.

Intended Use and Disclaimer: Should not be printed and given to patients. This information is intended to serve as a concise initial reference for healthcare professionals to use when discussing

medications with a patient. You must ultimately rely on your own discretion, experience and judgment in diagnosing, treating and advising patients.

Related Information
AmLODIPine *on page* 87
Benazepril *on page* 168

Amlodipine and Olmesartan
(am LOE di peen & olme SAR tan)

Brand Names: U.S. Azor™
Index Terms Amlodipine Besylate and Olmesartan Medoxomil; Olmesartan and Amlodipine
Pharmacologic Category Angiotensin II Receptor Blocker; Antianginal Agent; Antihypertensive; Calcium Channel Blocker; Calcium Channel Blocker, Dihydropyridine
Pregnancy Risk Factor D
Use Treatment of hypertension, including initial treatment in patients who will require multiple antihypertensives for adequate control
Available Dosage Forms
Tablet:
Azor™: 5/20: Amlodipine 5 mg and olmesartan medoxomil 20 mg; 5/40: Amlodipine 5 mg and olmesartan medoxomil 40 mg; 10/20: Amlodipine 10 mg and olmesartan medoxomil 20 mg; 10/40: Amlodipine 10 mg and olmesartan medoxomil 40 mg
General Dosage Range Oral: *Adults:* Amlodipine 5-10 mg and olmesartan 20-40 mg once daily (maximum: 10 mg/day [amlodipine]; 40 mg/day [olmesartan])
Administration
Oral Administer with or without food.
Nursing Actions
Physical Assessment See individual agents.
Patient Education
• Discuss specific use of drug and side effects with patient as it relates to treatment. (HCAHPS: During this hospital stay, were you given any medicine that you had not taken before? Before giving you any new medicine, how often did hospital staff tell you what the medicine was for? How often did hospital staff describe possible side effects in a way you could understand?)
• Patient may experience flushing. Have patient report immediately to prescriber severe dizziness, syncope, significant headache, urinary retention, oliguria, angina, tachycardia, arrhythmia, myalgia, asthenia, dyspnea, excessive weight gain or loss, edema of extremities, vision changes, considerable diarrhea, jaundice, or changes to teeth or gums (HCAHPS).
• Educate patient about signs of a significant reaction (eg, wheezing; chest tightness; fever; itching; bad cough; blue skin color; seizures; or swelling of face, lips, tongue, or throat). **Note:** This is not a comprehensive list of all side effects. Patient should consult prescriber for additional questions.

Intended Use and Disclaimer: Should not be printed and given to patients. This information is intended to serve as a concise initial reference for healthcare professionals to use when discussing medications with a patient. You must ultimately rely on your own discretion, experience and judgment in diagnosing, treating and advising patients.

Related Information
AmLODIPine *on page* 87
Olmesartan *on page* 1150

Amlodipine and Valsartan
(am LOE di peen & val SAR tan)

Brand Names: U.S. Exforge®
Index Terms Amlodipine Besylate and Valsartan; Valsartan and Amlodipine
Pharmacologic Category Angiotensin II Receptor Blocker; Antianginal Agent; Antihypertensive; Calcium Channel Blocker; Calcium Channel Blocker, Dihydropyridine
Pregnancy Risk Factor D
Use Treatment of hypertension
Available Dosage Forms
Tablet:
Exforge®: 5/160: Amlodipine 5 mg and valsartan 160 mg; 5/320: Amlodipine 5 mg and valsartan 320 mg; 10/160: Amlodipine 10 mg and valsartan 160 mg; 10/320: Amlodipine 10 mg and valsartan 320 mg
General Dosage Range Oral: *Adults:* Amlodipine 5-10 mg and valsartan 160-320 mg once daily (maximum: 10 mg daily [amlodipine]; 320 mg daily [valsartan])
Administration
Oral Administer with or without food.
Nursing Actions
Physical Assessment See individual agents.
Patient Education
• Discuss specific use of drug and side effects with patient as it relates to treatment. (HCAHPS: During this hospital stay, were you given any medicine that you had not taken before? Before giving you any new medicine, how often did hospital staff tell you what the medicine was for? How often did hospital staff describe possible side effects in a way you could understand?)
• Patient may experience rhinitis. Have patient report immediately to prescriber signs of infection, signs of hepatic impairment, severe dizziness, syncope, paresthesia, urinary retention, oliguria, angina, tachycardia, bradycardia, arrhythmia, myalgia, dyspnea, excessive weight gain, edema of extremities, significant nausea, hyperhidrosis, or considerable asthenia (HCAHPS).

- Educate patient about signs of a significant reaction (eg, wheezing; chest tightness; fever; itching; bad cough; blue skin color; seizures; or swelling of face, lips, tongue, or throat). **Note:** This is not a comprehensive list of all side effects. Patient should consult prescriber for additional questions.

Intended Use and Disclaimer: Should not be printed and given to patients. This information is intended to serve as a concise initial reference for healthcare professionals to use when discussing medications with a patient. You must ultimately rely on your own discretion, experience and judgment in diagnosing, treating and advising patients.

Related Information
AmLODIPine *on page 87*
Valsartan *on page 1581*

Amlodipine, Valsartan, and Hydrochlorothiazide
(am LOE di peen, val SAR tan, & hye droe klor oh THYE a zide)

Brand Names: U.S. Exforge HCT®
Index Terms Amlodipine Besylate, Valsartan, and Hydrochlorothiazide; Amlodipine, Hydrochlorothiazide, and Valsartan; Hydrochlorothiazide, Amlodipine, and Valsartan; Valsartan, Hydrochlorothiazide, and Amlodipine
Pharmacologic Category Angiotensin II Receptor Blocker; Antianginal Agent; Antihypertensive; Calcium Channel Blocker; Calcium Channel Blocker, Dihydropyridine; Diuretic, Thiazide
Pregnancy Risk Factor D
Use Treatment of hypertension (not for initial therapy)
Available Dosage Forms
Tablet, oral:
Exforge HCT®: Amlodipine 5 mg, valsartan 160 mg, and hydrochlorothiazide 12.5 mg; Amlodipine 5 mg, valsartan 160 mg, and hydrochlorothiazide 25 mg; Amlodipine 10 mg, valsartan 160 mg, and hydrochlorothiazide 12.5 mg; Amlodipine 10 mg, valsartan 160 mg, and hydrochlorothiazide 25 mg; Amlodipine 10 mg, valsartan 320 mg, and hydrochlorothiazide 25 mg
General Dosage Range Oral: *Adults:* Amlodipine 5-10 mg and valsartan 160-320 mg and hydrochlorothiazide 12.5-25 mg once daily (maximum: 10 mg daily [amlodipine]; 25 mg daily [hydrochlorothiazide]; 320 mg daily [valsartan])
Administration
Oral Administer with or without food.
Nursing Actions
Physical Assessment See individual agents.
Patient Education
- Discuss specific use of drug and side effects with patient as it relates to treatment. (HCAHPS: During this hospital stay, were you given any

medicine that you had not taken before? Before giving you any new medicine, how often did hospital staff tell you what the medicine was for? How often did hospital staff describe possible side effects in a way you could understand?)
- Patient may experience dizziness, headache, rhinitis, or asthenia. Have patient report immediately to prescriber signs of infection, signs of hyperglycemia, signs of fluid and electrolyte imbalance, signs of hepatic impairment, signs of pancreatitis, paresthesia, angina, bradycardia, arthralgia, joint edema, akathisia, severe dyspepsia, considerable back pain, dyspnea, excessive weight gain, edema of extremities, ecchymosis, hemorrhaging, hyperhidrosis, ophthalmalgia, or vision changes (HCAHPS).
- Educate patient about signs of a significant reaction (eg, wheezing; chest tightness; fever; itching; bad cough; blue skin color; seizures; or swelling of face, lips, tongue, or throat). **Note:** This is not a comprehensive list of all side effects. Patient should consult prescriber for additional questions.

Intended Use and Disclaimer: Should not be printed and given to patients. This information is intended to serve as a concise initial reference for healthcare professionals to use when discussing medications with a patient. You must ultimately rely on your own discretion, experience and judgment in diagnosing, treating and advising patients.
Related Information
AmLODIPine *on page 87*
Hydrochlorothiazide *on page 775*
Valsartan *on page 1581*

Amoxicillin (a moks i SIL in)

Brand Names: U.S. Moxatag
Index Terms *p*-Hydroxyampicillin; Amoxicillin Trihydrate; Amoxil; Amoxycillin
Pharmacologic Category Antibiotic, Penicillin
Medication Safety Issues
Sound-alike/look-alike issues:
Amoxicillin may be confused with amoxapine, Augmentin®
Amoxil may be confused with amoxapine
International issues:
Fisamox [Australia] may be confused with Fosamax brand name for alendronate [U.S., Canada, and multiple international markets] and Vigamox brand name for moxifloxacin [U.S., Canada, and multiple international markets]
Limoxin [Mexico] may be confused with Lanoxin brand name for digoxin [U.S., Canada, and multiple international markets]; Lincocin brand name for lincomycin [U.S., Canada, and multiple international markets]

Zimox: Brand name for amoxicillin [Italy], but also the brand name for carbidopa/levodopa [Greece]

Zimox [Italy] may be confused with Diamox which is the brand name for acetazolamide [Canada and multiple international markets]

Pregnancy Risk Factor B

Lactation Enters breast milk/use caution

Breast-Feeding Considerations Very small amounts of amoxicillin are excreted in breast milk. The manufacturer recommends that caution be exercised when administering amoxicillin to nursing women. Nondose-related effects could include modification of bowel flora and allergic sensitization of the infant.

Use Treatment of otitis media, sinusitis, and infections caused by susceptible organisms involving the upper and lower respiratory tract, skin, and urinary tract; prophylaxis of infective endocarditis in patients undergoing surgical or dental procedures; as part of a multidrug regimen for *H. pylori* eradication; periodontitis

Unlabeled Use Postexposure prophylaxis for anthrax exposure with documented susceptible organisms; chronic oral antimicrobial suppression of prosthetic joint infection

Mechanism of Action/Effect Interferes with bacterial cell wall synthesis during active multiplication, causing cell wall death and resultant bactericidal activity against susceptible bacteria

Contraindications Hypersensitivity to amoxicillin, penicillin, other beta-lactams, or any component of the formulation

Warnings/Precautions In patients with renal impairment, doses and/or frequency of administration should be modified in response to the degree of renal impairment; in addition, use of certain dosage forms (eg, extended release 775 mg tablet and immediate release 875 mg tablet) should be avoided in patients with CrCl <30 mL/minute or patients requiring hemodialysis. A high percentage of patients with infectious mononucleosis have developed rash during therapy with amoxicillin; ampicillin-class antibiotics not recommended in these patients. Serious and occasionally severe or fatal hypersensitivity (anaphylactoid) reactions have been reported in patients on penicillin therapy, especially with a history of beta-lactam hypersensitivity, history of sensitivity to multiple allergens, or previous IgE-mediated reactions (eg, anaphylaxis, angioedema, urticaria). Use with caution in asthmatic patients. Prolonged use may result in fungal or bacterial superinfection, including *C. difficile*-associated diarrhea (CDAD) and pseudomembranous colitis; CDAD has been observed >2 months postantibiotic treatment. Chewable tablets contain phenylalanine.

Drug Interactions

Avoid Concomitant Use

Avoid concomitant use of Amoxicillin with any of the following: BCG

Decreased Effect

Amoxicillin may decrease the levels/effects of: BCG; Mycophenolate; Sodium Picosulfate; Typhoid Vaccine

The levels/effects of Amoxicillin may be decreased by: Tetracycline Derivatives

Increased Effect/Toxicity

Amoxicillin may increase the levels/effects of: Methotrexate; Vitamin K Antagonists

The levels/effects of Amoxicillin may be increased by: Allopurinol; Probenecid

Adverse Reactions Frequency not defined.

Cardiovascular: Hypersensitivity angiitis

Central nervous system: Agitation, anxiety, behavioral changes, confusion, dizziness, headache, hyperactivity (reversible), insomnia, seizure

Dermatologic: Acute generalized exanthematous pustulosis, erythematous maculopapular rash, erythema multiforme, exfoliative dermatitis, Stevens-Johnson syndrome, toxic epidermal necrolysis, urticaria

Gastrointestinal: Dental discoloration (brown, yellow, or gray; rare), diarrhea, hemorrhagic colitis, melanoglossia, mucocutaneous candidiasis, nausea, pseudomembranous colitis, vomiting

Genitourinary: Crystalluria

Hematologic & oncologic: Agranulocytosis, anemia, eosinophilia, hemolytic anemia, leukopenia, thrombocytopenia, thrombocytopenia purpura

Hepatic: Cholestatic hepatitis, cholestatic jaundice, hepatitis (acute cytolytic), increased serum ALT, increased serum AST

Hypersensitivity: Anaphylaxis

Immunologic: Serum sickness-like reaction

Available Dosage Forms

Capsule, Oral:

Generic: 250 mg, 500 mg

Suspension Reconstituted, Oral:

Generic: 125 mg/5 mL (80 mL, 100 mL, 150 mL); 200 mg/5 mL (50 mL, 75 mL, 100 mL); 250 mg/5 mL (80 mL, 100 mL, 150 mL); 400 mg/5 mL (50 mL, 75 mL, 100 mL)

Tablet, Oral:

Generic: 500 mg, 875 mg

Tablet Chewable, Oral:

Generic: 125 mg, 250 mg

Tablet Extended Release 24 Hour, Oral:

Moxatag: 775 mg

General Dosage Range Dosage adjustment recommended in patients with renal impairment

Oral:

Immediate release:

Infants ≤3 months: 20-30 mg/kg/day divided every 12 hours

Children >3 months and <40 kg: 20-100 mg/kg/day divided every 8-12 hours

Adults: 250-500 mg every 8 hours **or** 500-875 mg twice daily (maximum: 875 mg/dose)

Extended release: *Children ≥12 years and Adults:* 775 mg once daily

Administration

Oral Administer around-the-clock to promote less variation in peak and trough serum levels. The appropriate amount of suspension may be mixed with formula, milk, fruit juice, water, ginger ale, or cold drinks; administer dose immediately after mixing.

Moxatag™ extended release tablet: Administer within 1 hour of finishing a meal.

Some penicillins (eg, carbenicillin, ticarcillin, and piperacillin) have been shown to inactivate aminoglycosides *in vitro*. This has been observed to a greater extent with tobramycin and gentamicin, while amikacin has shown greater stability against inactivation. Concurrent use of these agents may pose a risk of reduced antibacterial efficacy *in vivo*, particularly in the setting of profound renal impairment. However, definitive clinical evidence is lacking. If combination penicillin/aminoglycoside therapy is desired in a patient with renal dysfunction, separation of doses (if feasible), and routine monitoring of aminoglycoside levels, CBC, and clinical response should be considered.

Storage/Stability

Amoxil®: Oral suspension remains stable for 14 days at room temperature or if refrigerated (refrigeration preferred). Unit-dose antibiotic oral syringes are stable at room temperature for at least 72 hours (Tu, 1988).

Moxatag™: Store at 25°C (77°F); excursions permitted to 15°C to 30°C (59°F to 86°F).

Nursing Actions

Physical Assessment Culture and sensitivity report and patient's allergies should be assessed prior to starting therapy. Monitor for opportunistic infection.

Patient Education

- Discuss specific use of drug and side effects with patient as it relates to treatment. (HCAHPS: During this hospital stay, were you given any medicine that you had not taken before? Before giving you any new medicine, how often did hospital staff tell you what the medicine was for? How often did hospital staff describe possible side effects in a way you could understand?)
- Patient may experience diarrhea or dizziness. Have patient report immediately to prescriber severe nausea, vaginal yeast infection, ecchymosis, hemorrhaging, stomatitis, considerable asthenia, chills, illogical thinking, tooth discoloration, signs of hepatic impairment, or signs of pseudomembranous colitis (HCAHPS).
- Educate patient about signs of a significant reaction (eg, wheezing; chest tightness; fever; itching; bad cough; blue skin color; seizures; or swelling of face, lips, tongue, or throat). **Note:** This is not a comprehensive list of all side effects. Patient should consult prescriber for additional questions.

Intended Use and Disclaimer: Should not be printed and given to patients. This information is intended to serve as a concise initial reference for healthcare professionals to use when discussing medications with a patient. You must ultimately rely on your own discretion, experience and judgment in diagnosing, treating and advising patients.

Dietary Considerations May be taken with food. Some products may contain phenylalanine. Moxatag™: Take within 1 hour of finishing a meal.

Related Information

Oral Medications That Should Not Be Crushed or Altered *on page 1712*

Amoxicillin and Clavulanate
(a moks i SIL in & klav yoo LAN ate)

Brand Names: U.S. Amoclan; Augmentin; Augmentin ES-600; Augmentin XR

Index Terms Amoxicillin and Clavulanate Potassium; Amoxicillin and Clavulanic Acid; Clavulanic Acid and Amoxicillin

Pharmacologic Category Antibiotic, Penicillin

Medication Safety Issues

Sound-alike/look-alike issues:

Augmentin® may be confused with amoxicillin, Azulfidine

Pregnancy Risk Factor B

Lactation Enters breast milk/use caution

Use Treatment of otitis media, sinusitis, and infections caused by susceptible organisms involving the lower respiratory tract, skin and skin structure, and urinary tract; spectrum same as amoxicillin with additional coverage of beta-lactamase producing *B. catarrhalis*, *H. influenzae*, *N. gonorrhoeae*, and *S. aureus* (not MRSA). The expanded coverage of this combination makes it a useful alternative when amoxicillin resistance is present and patients cannot tolerate alternative treatments.

Unlabeled Use Chronic antimicrobial suppression of prosthetic joint infection

Available Dosage Forms

Powder for suspension, oral:

Generic: 200: Amoxicillin 200 mg and clavulanate potassium 28.5 mg per 5 mL; 250: Amoxicillin 250 mg and clavulanate potassium 62.5 mg per 5 mL; 400: Amoxicillin 400 mg and clavulanate potassium 57 mg per 5 mL; 600: Amoxicillin 600 mg and clavulanate potassium 42.9 mg per 5 mL

Amoclan:

200: Amoxicillin 200 mg and clavulanate potassium 28.5 mg per 5 mL

400: Amoxicillin 400 mg and clavulanate potassium 57 mg per 5 mL

600: Amoxicillin 600 mg and clavulanate potassium 42.9 mg per 5 mL

Augmentin:

125: Amoxicillin 125 mg and clavulanate potassium 31.25 mg per 5 mL

250: Amoxicillin 250 mg and clavulanate potassium 62.5 mg per 5 mL

Augmentin ES-600:

600: Amoxicillin 600 mg and clavulanate potassium 42.9 mg per 5 mL (75 mL, 125 mL, 200 mL) [contains phenylalanine 7 mg/5 mL, potassium 0.23 mEq/5 mL; strawberry cream flavor]

Tablet, oral:

Generic: 250: Amoxicillin 250 mg and clavulanate potassium 125 mg; 500: Amoxicillin 500 mg and clavulanate potassium 125 mg; 875: Amoxicillin 875 mg and clavulanate potassium 125 mg

Augmentin:

500: Amoxicillin 500 mg and clavulanate potassium 125 mg

875: Amoxicillin 875 mg and clavulanate potassium 125 mg

Tablet, chewable, oral: Generic: 200: Amoxicillin 200 mg and clavulanate potassium 28.5 mg; 400: Amoxicillin 400 mg and clavulanate potassium 57 mg

Tablet, extended release, oral:

Generic: Amoxicillin 1000 mg and clavulanate acid 62.5 mg

Augmentin XR: 1000: Amoxicillin 1000 mg and clavulanate acid 62.5 mg

General Dosage Range Dosage adjustment recommended in patients with renal impairment

Oral:

Immediate release:

Infants <3 months: 30 mg/kg/day divided every 12 hours

Children ≥3 months and <40 kg: 25-90 mg/kg/day divided every 12 hours **or** 20-40 mg/kg/day divided every 8 hours

Children >40 kg and Adults: 250-500 mg every 8 hours **or** 875 mg every 12 hours

Extended release: *Children ≥16 years and Adults:* 2000 mg every 12 hours (maximum: 2000 mg/dose)

Administration

Oral Administer around-the-clock to promote less variation in peak and trough serum levels. Administer with food to increase absorption and decrease stomach upset; shake suspension well before use. Extended release tablets should be administered with food.

Some penicillins (eg, carbenicillin, ticarcillin, and piperacillin) have been shown to inactivate aminoglycosides *in vitro*. This has been observed to a greater extent with tobramycin and gentamicin, while amikacin has shown greater stability against inactivation. Concurrent use of these agents may pose a risk of reduced antibacterial efficacy *in vivo*, particularly in the setting of profound renal impairment. However, definitive clinical evidence is lacking. If combination penicillin/aminoglycoside therapy is desired in a patient with renal dysfunction, separation of doses (if feasible), and routine monitoring of aminoglycoside levels, CBC, and clinical response should be considered.

Nursing Actions

Physical Assessment See individual agents.

Patient Education

• Discuss specific use of drug and side effects with patient as it relates to treatment. (HCAHPS: During this hospital stay, were you given any medicine that you had not taken before? Before giving you any new medicine, how often did hospital staff tell you what the medicine was for? How often did hospital staff describe possible side effects in a way you could understand?)

• Patient may experience diarrhea or dizziness. Have patient report immediately to prescriber severe nausea, vaginal yeast infection, ecchymosis, hemorrhaging, stomatitis, considerable asthenia, chills, illogical thinking, tooth discoloration, signs of hepatic impairment, or signs of pseudomembranous colitis (HCAHPS).

• Educate patient about signs of a significant reaction (eg, wheezing; chest tightness; fever; itching; bad cough; blue skin color; seizures; or swelling of face, lips, tongue, or throat). **Note:** This is not a comprehensive list of all side effects. Patient should consult prescriber for additional questions.

Intended Use and Disclaimer: Should not be printed and given to patients. This information is intended to serve as a concise initial reference for healthcare professionals to use when discussing medications with a patient. You must ultimately rely on your own discretion, experience and judgment in diagnosing, treating and advising patients.

Related Information

Amoxicillin *on page 92*

Oral Medications That Should Not Be Crushed or Altered *on page 1712*

Amphotericin B Cholesteryl Sulfate Complex

(am foe TER i sin bee kole LES te ril SUL fate KOM plecks)

Brand Names: U.S. Amphotec

Index Terms ABCD; Amphotericin B Colloidal Dispersion

Pharmacologic Category Antifungal Agent, Parenteral

Medication Safety Issues

High alert medication:

The Institute for Safe Medication Practices (ISMP) includes this medication among its list ▶

of drugs which have a heightened risk of causing significant patient harm when used in error.

Other safety concerns:

Lipid-based amphotericin formulations (Amphotec®) may be confused with conventional formulations (Amphocin®, Fungizone®)

Large overdoses have occurred when conventional formulations were dispensed inadvertently for lipid-based products. Single daily doses of conventional amphotericin formulation never exceed 1.5 mg/kg.

Pregnancy Risk Factor B

Lactation Excretion in breast milk unknown/not recommended

Breast-Feeding Considerations It is not known if amphotericin is excreted into breast milk. Due to its poor oral absorption, systemic exposure to the nursing infant is expected to be decreased; however, because of the potential for toxicity, breast-feeding is not recommended (Mactal-Haaf, 2001).

Use Treatment of invasive aspergillosis in patients who have failed amphotericin B deoxycholate treatment, or who have renal impairment or experience unacceptable toxicity which precludes treatment with amphotericin B deoxycholate in effective doses.

Unlabeled Use Effective in patients with serious *Candida* species infections

Mechanism of Action/Effect Binds to ergosterol altering cell membrane permeability in susceptible fungi and causing leakage of cell components with subsequent cell death

Contraindications Hypersensitivity to amphotericin B or any component of the formulation (unless the benefits outweigh the possible risk to the patient)

Warnings/Precautions Anaphylaxis has been reported with amphotericin B-containing drugs. If severe respiratory distress occurs, the infusion should be immediately discontinued; the patient should not receive further infusions. During the initial dosing, the drug should be administered under close clinical observation. Acute infusion reactions, sometimes severe, may occur 1-3 hours after starting infusion. These reactions are usually more common with the first few doses and generally diminish with subsequent doses. Pretreatment with antihistamines/corticosteroids and/or decreasing the rate of infusion can be used to manage reactions. Avoid rapid infusion.

Drug Interactions

Avoid Concomitant Use

Avoid concomitant use of Amphotericin B Cholesteryl Sulfate Complex with any of the following: Gallium Nitrate

Decreased Effect

Amphotericin B Cholesteryl Sulfate Complex may decrease the levels/effects of: Saccharomyces boulardii

The levels/effects of Amphotericin B Cholesteryl Sulfate Complex may be decreased by: Antifungal Agents (Azole Derivatives, Systemic)

Increased Effect/Toxicity

Amphotericin B Cholesteryl Sulfate Complex may increase the levels/effects of: Aminoglycosides; Colistimethate; CycloSPORINE (Systemic); Flucytosine; Gallium Nitrate

The levels/effects of Amphotericin B Cholesteryl Sulfate Complex may be increased by: Corticosteroids (Orally Inhaled); Corticosteroids (Systemic)

Adverse Reactions

>10%:

Cardiovascular: Hypotension, tachycardia

Central nervous system: Chills, fever

Endocrine & metabolic: Hypokalemia

Gastrointestinal: Vomiting

Hepatic: Hyperbilirubinemia

Renal: Creatinine increased

5% to 10%:

Cardiovascular: Chest pain, facial edema, hypertension

Central nervous system: Abnormal thinking, headache, insomnia, somnolence, tremor

Dermatologic: Pruritus, rash, sweating

Endocrine & metabolic: Hyperglycemia, hypocalcemia, hypomagnesemia, hypophosphatemia

Gastrointestinal: Abdominal enlargement, abdominal pain, diarrhea, dry mouth, hematemesis, jaundice, nausea, stomatitis

Hematologic: Anemia, hemorrhage, thrombocytopenia

Hepatic: Alkaline phosphatase increased, liver function test abnormal

Neuromuscular & skeletal: Back pain, rigor

Respiratory: Cough increased, dyspnea, epistaxis, hypoxia, rhinitis

Note: Amphotericin B colloidal dispersion has an improved therapeutic index compared to conventional amphotericin B, and has been used safely in patients with amphotericin B-related nephrotoxicity; however, continued decline of renal function has occurred in some patients.

Available Dosage Forms

Suspension Reconstituted, Intravenous:

Amphotec: 50 mg (1 ea); 100 mg (1 ea)

General Dosage Range I.V.: *Children and Adults:* 3-4 mg/kg/day

Administration

I.V. Initially infuse at 1 mg/kg/hour. Rate of infusion may be increased with subsequent doses as patient tolerance allows (minimum infusion time: 2 hours). For a patient who experiences chills, fever, hypotension, nausea, or other nonanaphylactic infusion-related reactions, premedicate with the following drugs 30-60 minutes prior to drug administration: A nonsteroidal with or without diphenhydramine **or** acetaminophen with diphenhydramine **or** hydrocortisone 50-100 mg with or without a nonsteroidal and diphenhydramine (Paterson, 2008). If the patient experiences rigors during the infusion, meperidine may be administered. If severe respiratory distress occurs, the infusion should be immediately discontinued.

Preparation for Administration Reconstitute 50 mg and 100 mg vials with 10 mL and 20 mL of SWI, respectively. The reconstituted vials contain 5 mg/mL of amphotericin B. Shake the vial gently by hand until all solid particles have dissolved. Further dilute amphotericin B colloidal dispersion with D_5W.

Storage/Stability Store intact vials at 15°C to 30°C (59°F to 86°F). After reconstitution, the solution should be refrigerated at 2°C to 8°C (36°F to 46°F) and used within 24 hours. Concentrations of 0.1-2 mg/mL in D_5W are stable for 24 hours at 2°C to 8°C (36°F to 46°F).

Nursing Actions

Physical Assessment Culture and sensitivity and patient history of exposure to amphotericin B should be assessed prior to beginning treatment. Premedication may be ordered to reduce incidence/severity of infusion reaction. Monitor patient closely for infusion related reactions (eg, anaphylaxis, chills, fever, nausea, vomiting, rigors, hypotension, acute respiratory distress); facilities for cardiopulmonary resuscitation should be available.

Patient Education
- Discuss specific use of drug and side effects with patient as it relates to treatment. (HCAHPS: During this hospital stay, were you given any medicine that you had not taken before? Before giving you any new medicine, how often did hospital staff tell you what the medicine was for? How often did hospital staff describe possible side effects in a way you could understand?)
- Patient may experience flu-like syndrome, chills, nausea, lack of appetite, weight loss, arthralgia, or dyspepsia. Have patient report immediately to prescriber angina, melena, tachypnea, hearing impairment, urinary retention, oliguria, urine discoloration, jaundice, severe diarrhea, considerable asthenia, arrhythmia, significant myalgia, or injection site irritation (HCAHPS).
- Educate patient about signs of a significant reaction (eg, wheezing; chest tightness; fever; itching; bad cough; blue skin color; seizures; or swelling of face, lips, tongue, or throat). **Note:** This is not a comprehensive list of all side effects. Patient should consult prescriber for additional questions.

Intended Use and Disclaimer: Should not be printed and given to patients. This information is intended to serve as a concise initial reference for healthcare professionals to use when discussing medications with a patient. You must ultimately rely on your own discretion, experience and judgment in diagnosing, treating and advising patients.

Amphotericin B (Conventional)
(am foe TER i sin bee con VEN sha nal)

Index Terms Amphotericin B Deoxycholate; Amphotericin B Desoxycholate; Conventional Amphotericin B

Pharmacologic Category Antifungal Agent, Parenteral

Medication Safety Issues

High alert medication:

The Institute for Safe Medication Practices (ISMP) includes this medication (intrathecal administration) among its list of drugs which have a heightened risk of causing significant patient harm when used in error.

Other safety concerns:

Conventional amphotericin formulations (Amphocin, Fungizone) may be confused with lipid-based formulations (AmBisome, Abelcet, Amphotec).

Large overdoses have occurred when conventional formulations were dispensed inadvertently for lipid-based products. Single daily doses of conventional amphotericin formulation never exceed 1.5 mg/kg.

Pregnancy Risk Factor B

Lactation Excretion in breast milk unknown/not recommended

Use Treatment of severe systemic and central nervous system infections caused by susceptible fungi such as *Candida* species, *Histoplasma capsulatum*, *Cryptococcus neoformans*, *Aspergillus* species, *Blastomyces dermatitidis*, *Torulopsis glabrata*, and *Coccidioides immitis*; fungal peritonitis; irrigant for bladder fungal infections; used in fungal infection in patients with bone marrow transplantation, amebic meningoencephalitis, ocular aspergillosis (intraocular injection), candidal cystitis (bladder irrigation), chemoprophylaxis (low-dose I.V.), immunocompromised patients at risk of aspergillosis (intranasal/nebulized), refractory meningitis (intrathecal), coccidioidal arthritis (intraarticular/I.M.).

Low-dose amphotericin B has been administered after bone marrow transplantation to reduce the risk of invasive fungal disease.

Unlabeled Use Treatment of fungal endophthalmitis

Available Dosage Forms

Solution Reconstituted, Injection:

Generic: 50 mg (1 ea)

General Dosage Range Dosage adjustment recommended in patients who develop toxicities

I.V.:

Infants and Children: Test dose: 0.1 mg/kg/dose (maximum: 1 mg); Maintenance: 0.25-1 mg/kg/day given once daily; 1-1.5 mg/kg every other day may be given once therapy is established (maximum: 1.5-4 g cumulative dose)

Adults: Test dose: 1 mg infused; Maintenance: 0.3-1.5 mg/kg/day given once daily; 1-1.5 mg/kg every other day may be given once therapy is established (maximum: 1.5 mg/kg/day)

Administration

I.V. May be infused over 4-6 hours. For a patient who experiences chills, fever, hypotension, nausea, or other nonanaphylactic infusion-related reactions, premedicate with the following drugs 30-60 minutes prior to drug administration: A non-steroidal (eg, ibuprofen, choline magnesium trisalicylate) ± diphenhydramine **or** acetaminophen with diphenhydramine **or** hydrocortisone. If the patient experiences rigors during the infusion, meperidine may be administered. Bolus infusion of normal saline immediately preceding, or immediately preceding and following amphotericin B may reduce drug-induced nephrotoxicity. Risk of nephrotoxicity increases with amphotericin B doses >1 mg/kg/day. Infusion of admixtures more concentrated than 0.25 mg/mL should be limited to patients absolutely requiring volume contraction.

Injectable Detail Precipitate may form in ionic dialysate solutions.

pH: 5.7 (100 mg/L in D_5W)

Intravitreal Unlabeled use/route: Administer amphotericin intravitreally with a final concentration of 5 mcg/0.1 mL NS (John, 2007)

Nursing Actions

Physical Assessment Culture and sensitivity and patient history of exposure to amphotericin B should be assessed prior to beginning treatment. Premedication may be ordered to reduce incidence/severity of infusion reaction. Monitor patient closely for infusion-related reactions (eg, anaphylaxis, chills, fever, nausea, vomiting, rigors, hypotension, acute respiratory distress); facilities for cardiopulmonary resuscitation should be available. If acute respiratory distress occurs, stop infusion and notify prescriber.

Patient Education

• Discuss specific use of drug and side effects with patient as it relates to treatment. (HCAHPS: During this hospital stay, were you given any medicine that you had not taken before? Before giving you any new medicine, how often did hospital staff tell you what the medicine was for? How often did hospital staff describe possible side effects in a way you could understand?)

• Patient may experience flu-like syndrome, chills, pyrosis, nausea, lack of appetite, or arthralgia. Have patient report immediately to prescriber melena, urinary retention, oliguria, tachypnea, hearing impairment, urine discoloration, jaundice, severe diarrhea, considerable asthenia, significant myalgia, arrhythmia, or injection site irritation (HCAHPS).

• Educate patient about signs of a significant reaction (eg, wheezing; chest tightness; fever; itching; bad cough; blue skin color; seizures; or swelling of face, lips, tongue, or throat). **Note:** This is not a comprehensive list of all side effects. Patient should consult prescriber for additional questions.

Intended Use and Disclaimer: Should not be printed and given to patients. This information is intended to serve as a concise initial reference for healthcare professionals to use when discussing medications with a patient. You must ultimately rely on your own discretion, experience and judgment in diagnosing, treating and advising patients.

Amphotericin B (Lipid Complex)
(am foe TER i sin bee LIP id KOM pleks)

Brand Names: U.S. Abelcet

Index Terms ABLC

Pharmacologic Category Antifungal Agent, Parenteral

Medication Safety Issues

High alert medication:

The Institute for Safe Medication Practices (ISMP) includes this medication among its list of drugs which have a heightened risk of causing significant patient harm when used in error.

Other safety concerns:

Lipid-based amphotericin formulations (Abelcet®) may be confused with conventional formulations (Fungizone®) or with other lipid-based amphotericin formulations (amphotericin B liposomal [AmBisome®]; amphotericin B cholesteryl sulfate complex [Amphotec®])

Large overdoses have occurred when conventional formulations were dispensed inadvertently for lipid-based products. Single daily doses of conventional amphotericin formulation never exceed 1.5 mg/kg.

Pregnancy Risk Factor B

Lactation Enters breast milk/not recommended

Breast-Feeding Considerations It is not known if amphotericin is excreted into breast milk. Due to its poor oral absorption, systemic exposure to the nursing infant is expected to be decreased; however, because of the potential for toxicity, breast-feeding is not recommended (Mactal-Haaf, 2001).

Use Treatment of invasive fungal infection in patients who are refractory to or intolerant of conventional amphotericin B (amphotericin B deoxycholate) therapy

Mechanism of Action/Effect Mechanism is like amphotericin - includes binding to ergosterol altering cell membrane permeability in susceptible fungi and causing leakage of cell components with subsequent cell death.

Contraindications Hypersensitivity to amphotericin or any component of the formulation

Warnings/Precautions Anaphylaxis has been reported with amphotericin B-containing drugs. If severe respiratory distress occurs, the infusion should be immediately discontinued. During the initial dosing, the drug should be administered under close clinical observation. Acute reactions (including fever and chills) may occur 1-2 hours after starting an intravenous infusion. These reactions are usually more common with the first few doses and generally diminish with subsequent doses. Infusion has been rarely associated with hypotension, bronchospasm, arrhythmias, and shock. Acute pulmonary toxicity has been reported in patients receiving leukocyte transfusions and amphotericin B; amphotericin B lipid complex and concurrent leukocyte transfusions are not recommended. Concurrent use with antineoplastic agents may enhance the potential for renal toxicity, bronchospasm or hypotension; use with caution. Concurrent use of amphotericin B with other nephrotoxic drugs may enhance the potential for drug-induced renal toxicity.

Drug Interactions

Avoid Concomitant Use

Avoid concomitant use of Amphotericin B (Lipid Complex) with any of the following: Gallium Nitrate

Decreased Effect

Amphotericin B (Lipid Complex) may decrease the levels/effects of: Saccharomyces boulardii

The levels/effects of Amphotericin B (Lipid Complex) may be decreased by: Antifungal Agents (Azole Derivatives, Systemic)

Increased Effect/Toxicity

Amphotericin B (Lipid Complex) may increase the levels/effects of: Aminoglycosides; Colistimethate; CycloSPORINE (Systemic); Flucytosine; Gallium Nitrate

The levels/effects of Amphotericin B (Lipid Complex) may be increased by: Corticosteroids (Orally Inhaled); Corticosteroids (Systemic)

Adverse Reactions Nephrotoxicity and infusion-related hyperpyrexia, rigor, and chilling are reduced relative to amphotericin deoxycholate.

>10%:
  Central nervous system: Chills (18%), fever (14%)
  Renal: Serum creatinine increased (11%)
  Miscellaneous: Multiple organ failure (11%)

1% to 10%:
  Cardiovascular: Hypotension (8%), cardiac arrest (6%), hypertension (5%), chest pain (3%)
  Central nervous system: Headache (6%), pain (5%)
  Dermatologic: Rash (4%)
  Endocrine & metabolic: Hypokalemia (5%), bilirubinemia (4%)
  Gastrointestinal: Nausea (9%), vomiting (8%), diarrhea (6%), gastrointestinal hemorrhage (4%), abdominal pain (4%)

  Hematologic: Thrombocytopenia (5%), anemia (4%), leukopenia (4%)
  Renal: Renal failure (5%)
  Respiratory: Respiratory failure (8%), dyspnea (6%), respiratory disorder (4%)
  Miscellaneous: Sepsis (7%), infection (5%)

Available Dosage Forms

Suspension, Intravenous:
  Abelcet: 5 mg/mL (20 mL)

General Dosage Range I.V.: *Children and Adults:* 5 mg/kg once daily

Administration

I.V. For patients who experience nonanaphylactic infusion-related reactions, premedicate 30-60 minutes prior to drug administration with a nonsteroidal anti-inflammatory agent ± diphenhydramine **or** acetaminophen with diphenhydramine **or** hydrocortisone. If the patient experiences rigors during the infusion, meperidine may be administered.

Administer at an infusion rate of 2.5 mg/kg/hour (eg, over 2 hours for 5 mg/kg). Invert infusion container several times prior to administration and every 2 hours during infusion if it exceeds 2 hours. **Do not use an in-line filter during administration.** Flush line with dextrose; normal saline may cause precipitate.

Preparation for Administration Shake the vial gently until there is no evidence of any yellow sediment at the bottom. Withdraw the appropriate dose from the vial using an 18-gauge needle. Remove the 18-gauge needle and attach the provided 5-micron filter needle to filter, and dilute the dose with D_5W to a final concentration of 1 mg/mL. Limited data suggests $D_{10}W$ and $D_{15}W$ may also be used for dilution (data on file [Sigma-Tau Pharmaceuticals, 2014]). Each filter needle may be used to filter up to four 100 mg vials. A final concentration of 2 mg/mL may be used for pediatric patients and patients with cardiovascular disease.

Do not dilute with saline solutions or mix with other drugs or electrolytes - compatibility has not been established

Storage/Stability Intact vials should be stored at 2°C to 8°C (35°F to 46°F); do not freeze. Protect intact vials from exposure to light. Solutions for infusion are stable for 48 hours under refrigeration and for an additional 6 hours at room temperature.

Nursing Actions

Physical Assessment Patient history of previous exposure to amphotericin B should be assessed before beginning treatment. Premedication may be ordered to reduce incidence/severity of infusion reaction. Monitor patient closely for infusion related reactions (eg, anaphylaxis, chills, fever, nausea, vomiting, rigors, hypotension, acute respiratory distress); facilities for cardiopulmonary resuscitation should be available. If acute respiratory distress occurs, stop infusion and notify prescriber.

Patient Education

• Discuss specific use of drug and side effects with patient as it relates to treatment. (HCAHPS: During this hospital stay, were you given any medicine that you had not taken before? Before giving you any new medicine, how often did hospital staff tell you what the medicine was for? How often did hospital staff describe possible side effects in a way you could understand?)

• Patient may experience flu-like syndrome, chills, nausea, lack of appetite, weight loss, arthralgia, or dyspepsia. Have patient report immediately to prescriber hematuria, angina, melena, tachypnea, hearing impairment, urinary retention, oliguria, urine discoloration, jaundice, severe diarrhea, considerable asthenia, arrhythmia, significant myalgia, or injection site irritation (HCAHPS).

• Educate patient about signs of a significant reaction (eg, wheezing; chest tightness; fever; itching; bad cough; blue skin color; seizures; or swelling of face, lips, tongue, or throat). **Note:** This is not a comprehensive list of all side effects. Patient should consult prescriber for additional questions.

Intended Use and Disclaimer: Should not be printed and given to patients. This information is intended to serve as a concise initial reference for healthcare professionals to use when discussing medications with a patient. You must ultimately rely on your own discretion, experience and judgment in diagnosing, treating and advising patients.

Dietary Considerations If on parenteral nutrition, may need to adjust the amount of lipid infused. The lipid portion of amphotericin B (lipid complex) formulation contains 0.045 kcal per 5 mg (Sacks, 1997).

Amphotericin B (Liposomal)
(am foe TER i sin bee lye po SO mal)

Brand Names: U.S. AmBisome
Index Terms Amphotericin B Liposome; L-AmB
Pharmacologic Category Antifungal Agent, Parenteral
Medication Safety Issues
High alert medication:
The Institute for Safe Medication Practices (ISMP) includes this medication among its list of drugs which have a heightened risk of causing significant patient harm when used in error.

Other safety concerns:
Lipid-based amphotericin formulations (AmBisome®) may be confused with conventional formulations (Amphocin®, Fungizone®) or with other lipid-based amphotericin formulations (Abelcet®, Amphotec®)

Large overdoses have occurred when conventional formulations were dispensed inadvertently for lipid-based products. Single daily doses of conventional amphotericin formulation never exceed 1.5 mg/kg.

Pregnancy Risk Factor B

Lactation Excretion in breast milk unknown/not recommended

Breast-Feeding Considerations It is not known if amphotericin is excreted into breast milk. Due to its poor oral absorption, systemic exposure to the nursing infant is expected to be decreased; however, because of the potential for toxicity, breast-feeding is not recommended (Mactal-Haaf, 2001).

Use Empirical therapy for presumed fungal infection in febrile, neutropenic patients; treatment of patients with *Aspergillus* species, *Candida* species, and/or *Cryptococcus* species infections refractory to amphotericin B desoxycholate (conventional amphotericin), or in patients where renal impairment or unacceptable toxicity precludes the use of amphotericin B desoxycholate; treatment of cryptococcal meningitis in HIV-infected patients; treatment of visceral leishmaniasis

Unlabeled Use Treatment of systemic *Histoplasmosis* infection; empiric treatment of fungal meningitis or osteoarticular infections

Mechanism of Action/Effect Amphotericin B, the active ingredient, binds to the sterol component of a cell membrane leading to alterations in cell permeability and cell death. While amphotericin B has a higher affinity for the ergosterol component of the fungal cell membrane, it can also bind to the cholesterol component of the mammalian cell leading to cytotoxicity. AmBisome®, the liposomal preparation of amphotericin B, has been shown to penetrate the cell wall of both extracellular and intracellular forms of susceptible fungi.

Contraindications Hypersensitivity to amphotericin B deoxycholate or any component of the formulation

Warnings/Precautions Patients should be under close clinical observation during initial dosing. As with other amphotericin B-containing products, anaphylaxis has been reported. Facilities for cardiopulmonary resuscitation should be available during administration. Acute infusion reactions (including fever and chills) may occur 1-2 hours after starting infusions; reactions are more common with the first few doses and generally diminish with subsequent doses. Immediately discontinue infusion if severe respiratory distress occurs; the patient should not receive further infusions. Concurrent use of amphotericin B with other nephrotoxic drugs may enhance the potential for drug-induced renal toxicity. Concurrent use with antineoplastic agents may enhance the potential for renal toxicity, bronchospasm or hypotension. Acute pulmonary toxicity has been reported in patients receiving simultaneous leukocyte transfusions and amphotericin B. Safety and efficacy have not been established in patients <1 month of age.

Drug Interactions

Avoid Concomitant Use

Avoid concomitant use of Amphotericin B (Liposomal) with any of the following: Gallium Nitrate

Decreased Effect

Amphotericin B (Liposomal) may decrease the levels/effects of: Saccharomyces boulardii

The levels/effects of Amphotericin B (Liposomal) may be decreased by: Antifungal Agents (Azole Derivatives, Systemic)

Increased Effect/Toxicity

Amphotericin B (Liposomal) may increase the levels/effects of: Aminoglycosides; Colistimethate; CycloSPORINE (Systemic); Flucytosine; Gallium Nitrate

The levels/effects of Amphotericin B (Liposomal) may be increased by: Corticosteroids (Orally Inhaled); Corticosteroids (Systemic)

Adverse Reactions Percentage of adverse reactions is dependent upon population studied and may vary with respect to premedications and underlying illness. Incidence of decreased renal function and infusion-related events are lower than rates observed with amphotericin B deoxycholate.

>10%:

Cardiovascular: Peripheral edema (15%), edema (12% to 14%), tachycardia (9% to 19%), hypotension (7% to 14%), hypertension (8% to 20%), chest pain (8% to 12%), hypervolemia (8% to 12%)

Central nervous system: Chills (29% to 48%), insomnia (17% to 22%), headache (9% to 20%), anxiety (7% to 14%), pain (14%), confusion (9% to 13%)

Dermatologic: Rash (5% to 25%), pruritus (11%)

Endocrine & metabolic: Hypokalemia (31% to 51%), hypomagnesemia (15% to 50%), hyperglycemia (8% to 23%), hypocalcemia (5% to 18%), hyponatremia (9% to 12%)

Gastrointestinal: Nausea (16% to 40%), vomiting (11% to 32%), diarrhea (11% to 30%), abdominal pain (7% to 20%), constipation (15%), anorexia (10% to 14%)

Hematologic: Anemia (27% to 48%), blood transfusion reaction (9% to 18%), leukopenia (15% to 17%), thrombocytopenia (6% to 13%)

Hepatic: Alkaline phosphatase increased (7% to 22%), bilirubinemia (≤18%), ALT increased (15%), AST increased (13%), liver function tests abnormal (not specified) (4% to 13%)

Local: Phlebitis (9% to 11%)

Neuromuscular & skeletal: Weakness (6% to 13%), back pain (12%)

Renal: Nephrotoxicity (14% to 47%), creatinine increased (18% to 40%), BUN increased (7% to 21%), hematuria (14%)

Respiratory: Dyspnea (18% to 23%), lung disorder (14% to 18%), cough (2% to 18%), epistaxis (9% to 15%), pleural effusion (13%), rhinitis (11%)

Miscellaneous: Infusion reactions (4% to 21%), sepsis (7% to 14%), infection (11% to 13%)

2% to 10%:

Cardiovascular: Arrhythmia, atrial fibrillation, bradycardia, cardiac arrest, cardiomegaly, facial swelling, flushing, orthostatic hypotension, valvular heart disease, vascular disorder, vasodilation

Central nervous system: Agitation, abnormal thinking, coma, depression, dysesthesia, dizziness (7% to 9%), hallucinations, malaise, nervousness, seizure, somnolence

Dermatologic: Alopecia, bruising, cellulitis, dry skin, maculopapular rash, petechia, purpura, skin discoloration, skin disorder, skin ulcer, urticaria, vesiculobullous rash

Endocrine & metabolic: Acidosis, fluid overload, hypernatremia (4%), hyperchloremia, hyperkalemia, hypermagnesemia, hyperphosphatemia, hypophosphatemia, hypoproteinemia, lactate dehydrogenase increased, nonprotein nitrogen increased

Gastrointestinal: Abdomen enlarged, amylase increased, dyspepsia, dysphagia, eructation, fecal incontinence, flatulence, gastrointestinal hemorrhage (10%), hematemesis, hemorrhoids, gum/oral hemorrhage, ileus, mucositis, rectal disorder, stomatitis, ulcerative stomatitis, xerostomia

Genitourinary: Vaginal hemorrhage

Hematologic: Coagulation disorder, hemorrhage, prothrombin decreased

Hepatic: Hepatocellular damage, hepatomegaly, veno-occlusive liver disease

Local: Injection site inflammation

Neuromuscular & skeletal: Arthralgia, bone pain, dystonia, myalgia, neck pain, paresthesia, rigors, tremor

Ocular: Conjunctivitis, dry eyes, eye hemorrhage

Renal: Abnormal renal function, acute renal failure, dysuria, renal failure, toxic nephropathy, urinary incontinence

Respiratory: Asthma, atelectasis, dry nose, hemoptysis, hyperventilation, pharyngitis, pneumonia, pulmonary edema, respiratory alkalosis, respiratory insufficiency, respiratory failure, sinusitis, hypoxia (6% to 8%)

Miscellaneous: Allergic reaction, cell-mediated immunological reaction, flu-like syndrome, graft-versus-host disease, herpes simplex, hiccup, procedural complication (8% to 10%), diaphoresis (7%)

Available Dosage Forms

Suspension Reconstituted, Intravenous:

AmBisome: 50 mg (1 ea)

General Dosage Range I.V.: *Children and Adults:* 3-6 mg/kg/day as a single daily dose (maximum: 6 mg/kg/day)

Administration

I.V. Intravenous infusion, over a period of approximately 2 hours. Infusion time may be reduced to approximately 1 hour in patients in whom the treatment is well-tolerated. If the patient experiences discomfort during infusion, the duration of infusion may be increased. Discontinue if severe respiratory distress occurs.

For a patient who experiences chills, fever, hypotension, nausea, or other nonanaphylactic infusion-related reactions, premedicate with the following drugs, 30-60 minutes prior to drug administration: A nonsteroidal (eg, ibuprofen, choline magnesium trisalicylate) ± diphenhydramine **or** acetaminophen with diphenhydramine **or** hydrocortisone. If the patient experiences rigors during the infusion, meperidine may be administered.

Injectable Detail Existing intravenous line should be flushed with D₅W prior to infusion (if not feasible, administer through a separate line). An in-line membrane filter (not less than 1 micron) may be used.

Preparation for Administration Reconstitute with 12 mL SWFI to a concentration of 4 mg/mL. The use of any solution other than those recommended, or the presence of a bacteriostatic agent in the solution, may cause precipitation. **Shake the vial vigorously** for 30 seconds, until dispersed into a translucent yellow suspension.

Filtration and dilution: The 5-micron filter should be on the syringe used to remove the reconstituted AmBisome®. Dilute to a final concentration of 1-2 mg/mL (0.2-0.5 mg/mL for infants and small children).

Storage/Stability Store intact vials at ≤25°C (≤77°F). Reconstituted vials are stable refrigerated at 2°C to 8°C (36°F to 46°F) for 24 hours. Do not freeze. Manufacturer's labeling states infusion should begin within 6 hours of dilution with D₅W; data on file with Astellas Pharma shows extended formulation stability when admixed in D₅W at 0.2-2 mg/mL (in polyolefin or PVC bags) for up to 11 days when stored refrigerated at 2°C to 8°C (36°F to 46°F).

Nursing Actions

Physical Assessment Culture and sensitivity report and patient's previous exposure to Amphotericin B should be assessed before beginning treatment. Premedication may be ordered to reduce incidence/severity of infusion reaction. Monitor patient closely for infusion-related reactions (eg, anaphylaxis, chills, fever, nausea, vomiting, rigors, hypotension, acute respiratory distress); facilities for cardiopulmonary resuscitation should be available. If acute respiratory distress occurs, stop infusion and notify prescriber.

Patient Education

• Discuss specific use of drug and side effects with patient as it relates to treatment. (HCAHPS: During this hospital stay, were you given any medicine that you had not taken before? Before giving you any new medicine, how often did hospital staff tell you what the medicine was for? How often did hospital staff describe possible side effects in a way you could understand?)

• Patient may experience flu-like syndrome, chills, injection site irritation, nausea, lack of appetite, insomnia, back pain, or dyspepsia. Have patient report immediately to prescriber hematuria, angina, melena, excessive weight gain, significant edema, urine discoloration, jaundice, urinary retention, oliguria, considerable diarrhea, severe dizziness, intolerable headache, tachypnea, hearing loss, significant asthenia, ecchymosis, hemorrhaging, arrhythmia, or considerable myalgia (HCAHPS).

• Educate patient about signs of a significant reaction (eg, wheezing; chest tightness; fever; itching; bad cough; blue skin color; seizures; or swelling of face, lips, tongue, or throat). **Note:** This is not a comprehensive list of all side effects. Patient should consult prescriber for additional questions.

Intended Use and Disclaimer: Should not be printed and given to patients. This information is intended to serve as a concise initial reference for healthcare professionals to use when discussing medications with a patient. You must ultimately rely on your own discretion, experience and judgment in diagnosing, treating and advising patients.

Dietary Considerations If on parenteral nutrition, may need to adjust the amount of lipid infused. The lipid portion of amphotericin B (liposomal) formulation contains 0.27 kcal per 5 mg (Sacks, 1997).

Ampicillin (am pi SIL in)

Index Terms Aminobenzylpenicillin; Ampicillin Sodium; Ampicillin Trihydrate

Pharmacologic Category Antibiotic, Penicillin

Medication Safety Issues

Sound-alike/look-alike issues:

Ampicillin may be confused with aminophylline

Pregnancy Risk Factor B

Lactation Enters breast milk/use caution

Breast-Feeding Considerations Ampicillin is excreted in breast milk. The manufacturer recommends that caution be exercised when administering ampicillin to nursing women. Due to the low concentrations in human milk, minimal toxicity would be expected in the nursing infant. Non-dose-related effects could include modification of bowel flora and allergic sensitization.

Use Treatment of susceptible bacterial infections (nonbeta-lactamase-producing organisms); treatment or prophylaxis of infective endocarditis; susceptible bacterial infections caused by streptococci, pneumococci, nonpenicillinase-producing staphylococci, *Listeria*, meningococci; some strains of *H. influenzae, Salmonella, Shigella, E. coli, Enterobacter,* and *Klebsiella*

Unlabeled Use Surgical (perioperative) prophylaxis in patients undergoing liver transplantation (Bratzler, 2013)

Mechanism of Action/Effect Interferes with bacterial cell wall synthesis during active multiplication, causing cell wall death and resultant bactericidal activity against susceptible bacteria

Contraindications Hypersensitivity to ampicillin, any component of the formulation, or other penicillins

Warnings/Precautions Dosage adjustment may be necessary in patients with renal impairment. Serious and occasionally severe or fatal hypersensitivity (anaphylactoid) reactions have been reported in patients on penicillin therapy, especially with a history of beta-lactam hypersensitivity, history of sensitivity to multiple allergens, or previous IgE-mediated reactions (eg, anaphylaxis, angioedema, urticaria). Use with caution in asthmatic patients. High percentage of patients with infectious mononucleosis have developed rash during therapy with ampicillin; ampicillin-class antibiotics not recommended in these patients. Appearance of a rash should be carefully evaluated to differentiate a nonallergic ampicillin rash from a hypersensitivity reaction. Ampicillin rash occurs in 5% to 10% of children receiving ampicillin and is a generalized dull red, maculopapular rash, generally appearing 3-14 days after the start of therapy. It normally begins on the trunk and spreads over most of the body. It may be most intense at pressure areas, elbows, and knees. Prolonged use may result in fungal or bacterial superinfection, including *C. difficile*-associated diarrhea (CDAD) and pseudomembranous colitis; CDAD has been observed >2 months postantibiotic treatment.

Drug Interactions

Avoid Concomitant Use
Avoid concomitant use of Ampicillin with any of the following: BCG

Decreased Effect
Ampicillin may decrease the levels/effects of: Atenolol; BCG; Mycophenolate; Sodium Picosulfate; Typhoid Vaccine

The levels/effects of Ampicillin may be decreased by: Chloroquine; Lanthanum; Tetracycline Derivatives

Increased Effect/Toxicity
Ampicillin may increase the levels/effects of: Methotrexate; Vitamin K Antagonists

The levels/effects of Ampicillin may be increased by: Allopurinol; Probenecid

Nutritional/Ethanol Interactions Food: Food decreases ampicillin absorption rate; may decrease ampicillin serum concentration. Management: Take at equal intervals around-the-clock, preferably on an empty stomach (1 hour before or 2 hours after meals). Maintain adequate hydration, unless instructed to restrict fluid intake.

Adverse Reactions Frequency not defined.

Central nervous system: Fever, penicillin encephalopathy, seizure

Dermatologic: Erythema multiforme, exfoliative dermatitis, rash, urticaria

Note: Appearance of a rash should be carefully evaluated to differentiate (if possible) nonallergic ampicillin rash from hypersensitivity reaction. Incidence is higher in patients with viral infection, *Salmonella* infection, lymphocytic leukemia, or patients that have hyperuricemia.

Gastrointestinal: Black hairy tongue, diarrhea, enterocolitis, glossitis, nausea, oral candidiasis, pseudomembranous colitis, sore mouth or tongue, stomatitis, vomiting

Hematologic: Agranulocytosis, anemia, hemolytic anemia, eosinophilia, leukopenia, thrombocytopenia purpura

Hepatic: AST increased

Renal: Interstitial nephritis (rare)

Respiratory: Laryngeal stridor

Miscellaneous: Anaphylaxis, serum sickness-like reaction

Available Dosage Forms

Capsule, Oral:
Generic: 250 mg, 500 mg

Solution Reconstituted, Injection:
Generic: 125 mg (1 ea); 250 mg (1 ea); 500 mg (1 ea); 1 g (1 ea); 2 g (1 ea); 10 g (1 ea)

Solution Reconstituted, Injection [preservative free]:
Generic: 250 mg (1 ea); 500 mg (1 ea)

Solution Reconstituted, Intravenous:
Generic: 1 g (1 ea); 2 g (1 ea); 10 g (1 ea)

Solution Reconstituted, Intravenous [preservative free]:
Generic: 10 g (1 ea)

Suspension Reconstituted, Oral:
Generic: 125 mg/5 mL (100 mL, 200 mL); 250 mg/5 mL (100 mL, 200 mL)

General Dosage Range Dosage adjustment recommended in patients with renal impairment

I.M., I.V.:
Infants and Children: 100-400 mg/kg/day divided every 6 hours (maximum: 12 g/day)
Adults: 1-2 g every 4-6 hours or 50-250 mg/kg/day in divided doses (maximum: 12 g/day)

Oral:
Infants and Children: 50-100 mg/kg/day divided every 6 hours (maximum: 2-4 g/day)
Adults: 250-500 mg every 6 hours

◄ **Administration**

I.V. Administer around-the-clock to promote less variation in peak and trough serum levels. Administer over 3-5 minutes (125-500 mg) or over 10-15 minutes (1-2 g). More rapid infusion may cause seizures. Ampicillin and gentamicin should not be mixed in the same I.V. tubing.

Some penicillins (eg, carbenicillin, ticarcillin, and piperacillin) have been shown to inactivate aminoglycosides *in vitro*. This has been observed to a greater extent with tobramycin and gentamicin, while amikacin has shown greater stability against inactivation. Concurrent use of these agents may pose a risk of reduced antibacterial efficacy *in vivo*, particularly in the setting of profound renal impairment. However, definitive clinical evidence is lacking. If combination penicillin/aminoglycoside therapy is desired in a patient with renal dysfunction, separation of doses (if feasible), and routine monitoring of aminoglycoside levels, CBC, and clinical response should be considered.

Injectable Detail pH: 8-10 (reconstituted solution)

Oral Administer around-the-clock to promote less variation in peak and trough serum levels. Administer on an empty stomach (ie, 1 hour prior to, or 2 hours after meals) to increase total absorption.

Preparation for Administration I.V.: Minimum volume: Concentration should not exceed 30 mg/mL due to concentration-dependent stability restrictions. Standard diluent: 500 mg/50 mL NS; 1 g/50 mL NS; 2 g/100 mL NS.

Storage/Stability

Oral: Oral suspension is stable for 7 days at room temperature or for 14 days under refrigeration.

I.V.:

Solutions for I.M. or direct I.V. should be used within 1 hour. Solutions for I.V. infusion will be inactivated by dextrose at room temperature. If dextrose-containing solutions are to be used, the resultant solution will only be stable for 2 hours versus 8 hours in the 0.9% sodium chloride injection. D_5W has limited stability.

Stability of parenteral admixture in NS at room temperature (25°C) is 8 hours.

Stability of parenteral admixture in NS at refrigeration temperature (4°C) is 2 days.

Nursing Actions

Physical Assessment Allergy history should be assessed prior to starting therapy. Monitor for opportunistic infection (fever, chills, unhealed sores, white plaques in mouth or vagina, purulent vaginal discharge).

Patient Education

• Discuss specific use of drug and side effects with patient as it relates to treatment. (HCAHPS: During this hospital stay, were you given any medicine that you had not taken before? Before giving you any new medicine, how often did hospital staff tell you what the medicine was

for? How often did hospital staff describe possible side effects in a way you could understand?

• Patient may experience diarrhea. Have patient report immediately to prescriber severe nausea vaginal yeast infection, ecchymosis, hemorrhaging, stomatitis, significant asthenia, chills, or signs of pseudomembranous colitis (HCAHPS).

• Educate patient about signs of a significant reaction (eg, wheezing; chest tightness; fever itching; bad cough; blue skin color; seizures; or swelling of face, lips, tongue, or throat). **Note:** This is not a comprehensive list of all side effects. Patient should consult prescriber for additional questions.

Intended Use and Disclaimer: Should not be printed and given to patients. This information is intended to serve as a concise initial reference for healthcare professionals to use when discussing medications with a patient. You must ultimately rely on your own discretion, experience and judgment in diagnosing, treating and advising patients.

Dietary Considerations Take on an empty stomach 1 hour before or 2 hours after meals. Some products may contain sodium.

Ampicillin and Sulbactam
(am pi SIL in & SUL bak tam)

Brand Names: U.S. Unasyn®

Index Terms Sulbactam and Ampicillin

Pharmacologic Category Antibiotic, Penicillin

Pregnancy Risk Factor B

Lactation Enters breast milk/use caution

Use Treatment of susceptible bacterial infections involved with skin and skin structure, intra-abdominal infections, gynecological infections; spectrum is that of ampicillin plus organisms producing beta-lactamases such as *S. aureus*, *H. influenzae*, *E. coli*, *Klebsiella*, *Acinetobacter*, *Enterobacter*, and anaerobes

Unlabeled Use Treatment of acute bacterial rhinosinusitis (ABRS); endocarditis; intravascular catheter-associated bloodstream infection caused by susceptible bacteria; community-acquired pneumonia; early-onset hospital-acquired pneumonia; surgical (perioperative) prophylaxis

Available Dosage Forms

Injection, powder for reconstitution: 1.5 g [ampicillin 1 g and sulbactam 0.5 g]; 3 g [ampicillin 2 g and sulbactam 1 g]; 15 g [ampicillin 10 g and sulbactam 5 g]

Unasyn®: 1.5 g [ampicillin 1 g and sulbactam 0.5 g]; 3 g [ampicillin 2 g and sulbactam 1 g]; 15 g [ampicillin 10 g and sulbactam 5 g]; 15 g [ampicillin 10 g and sulbactam 5 g

General Dosage Range Dosage adjustment recommended in patients with renal impairment

I.M.: *Adults:* 1000-2000 mg (1500-3000 mg Unasyn®) ampicillin every 6 hours (maximum: 8 g ampicillin daily)

I.V.:

Children ≥1 year: 100-400 mg ampicillin/kg/day divided every 6 hours (maximum: 8 g ampicillin daily)

Adults: 1000-2000 mg (1500-3000 mg Unasyn®) ampicillin every 6 hours (maximum: 8 g ampicillin daily)

Administration

I.V. Administer around-the-clock to promote less variation in peak and trough serum levels. Administer by slow injection over 10-15 minutes or I.V. over 15-30 minutes. Ampicillin and gentamicin should not be mixed in the same I.V. tubing.

Some penicillins (eg, ampicillin, carbenicillin, ticarcillin, and piperacillin) have been shown to inactivate aminoglycosides *in vitro*. This has been observed to a greater extent with tobramycin and gentamicin, while amikacin has shown greater stability against inactivation. Concurrent Y-site administration should be avoided.

Injectable Detail pH: 8-10

Nursing Actions

Physical Assessment Monitor for signs of hypersensitivity reactions, kidney function tests, and urine output. Monitor for fluid and electrolyte imbalance in patients with diarrhea, nausea, and vomiting; may worsen condition.

Patient Education

• Discuss specific use of drug and side effects with patient as it relates to treatment. (HCAHPS: During this hospital stay, were you given any medicine that you had not taken before? Before giving you any new medicine, how often did hospital staff tell you what the medicine was for? How often did hospital staff describe possible side effects in a way you could understand?)

• Patient may experience diarrhea or injection site irritation. Have patient report immediately to prescriber severe nausea, vaginal yeast infection, ecchymosis, hemorrhaging, stomatitis, significant asthenia, chills, angina, or signs of pseudomembranous colitis (HCAHPS).

• Educate patient about signs of a significant reaction (eg, wheezing; chest tightness; fever; itching; bad cough; blue skin color; seizures; or swelling of face, lips, tongue, or throat). **Note:** This is not a comprehensive list of all side effects. Patient should consult prescriber for additional questions.

Intended Use and Disclaimer: Should not be printed and given to patients. This information is intended to serve as a concise initial reference for healthcare professionals to use when discussing medications with a patient. You must ultimately rely on your own discretion, experience and judgment in diagnosing, treating and advising patients.

Related Information

Ampicillin *on page 102*

Anastrozole (an AS troe zole)

Brand Names: U.S. Arimidex

Index Terms ICI-D1033; ZD1033

Pharmacologic Category Antineoplastic Agent, Aromatase Inhibitor

Medication Safety Issues

Sound-alike/look-alike issues:

Anastrozole may be confused with anagrelide, letrozole

Arimidex may be confused with Aromasin

Pregnancy Risk Factor X

Lactation Excretion in breast milk unknown/not recommended

Breast-Feeding Considerations It is not known if anastrozole is excreted in breast milk. Due to the potential for serious adverse reactions in the nursing infant, a decision should be made whether to discontinue nursing or to discontinue the drug, taking into account the importance of treatment to the mother. The Canadian labeling contraindicates use in lactating women.

Use Breast cancer:

First-line treatment of locally-advanced or metastatic breast cancer (hormone receptor-positive or unknown) in postmenopausal women

Adjuvant treatment of early hormone receptor-positive breast cancer in postmenopausal women

Treatment of advanced breast cancer in postmenopausal women with disease progression following tamoxifen therapy

Unlabeled Use Treatment of recurrent or metastatic endometrial or uterine cancers, treatment of recurrent ovarian cancer

Mechanism of Action/Effect Potent and selective nonsteroidal aromatase inhibitor. By inhibiting aromatase, the conversion of androstenedione to estrone, and testosterone to estradiol, is prevented, thereby decreasing tumor mass or delaying progression in patients with tumors responsive to hormones. Anastrozole causes an 85% decrease in estrone sulfate levels.

Contraindications Hypersensitivity to anastrozole or any component of the formulation; use in women who are or may become pregnant

Canadian labeling: Additional contraindications (not in U.S. labeling): Lactating women

Warnings/Precautions Hazardous agent - use appropriate precautions for handling and disposal (NIOSH, 2012). Use is contraindicated in women who are or may become pregnant. Anastrozole offers no clinical benefit in premenopausal women with breast cancer. Patients with pre-existing ischemic cardiac disease have an increased risk for ischemic cardiovascular events.

Due to decreased circulating estrogen levels, anastrozole is associated with a reduction in bone ▶

mineral density (BMD); decreases (from baseline) in total hip and lumbar spine BMD have been reported. Patients with pre-existing osteopenia are at higher risk for developing osteoporosis (Eastell, 2008). When initiating anastrozole treatment, follow available guidelines for bone mineral density management in postmenopausal women with similar fracture risk; concurrent use of bisphosphonates may be useful in patients at risk for fractures.

Elevated total cholesterol levels (contributed to by LDL cholesterol increases) have been reported in patients receiving anastrozole; use with caution in patients with hyperlipidemias; cholesterol levels should be monitored/managed in accordance with current guidelines for patients with LDL elevations. Plasma concentrations in patients with stable hepatic cirrhosis were within the range of concentrations seen in normal subjects across all clinical trials; use has not been studied in patients with severe hepatic impairment. Safety and efficacy in children have not been established.

Drug Interactions

Avoid Concomitant Use

Avoid concomitant use of Anastrozole with any of the following: Estrogen Derivatives; Pimozide

Decreased Effect

Anastrozole may decrease the levels/effects of: Cardiac Glycosides; Vitamin K Antagonists

The levels/effects of Anastrozole may be decreased by: Estrogen Derivatives; Tamoxifen

Increased Effect/Toxicity

Anastrozole may increase the levels/effects of: ARIPiprazole; Dofetilide; Lomitapide; Methadone; Pimozide; Vitamin K Antagonists

Adverse Reactions

>10%:

Cardiovascular: Vasodilatation (25% to 36%), ischemic heart disease (4%; 17% in patients with pre-existing ischemic heart disease), hypertension (2% to 13%), angina pectoris (2%; 12% in patients with pre-existing ischemic heart disease), edema (7% to 11%)

Central nervous system: Fatigue (19%), mood disorder (19%), headache (9% to 18%), pain (11% to 17%), depression (2% to 13%)

Dermatologic: Skin rash (6% to 11%)

Endocrine & metabolic: Hot flash (12% to 36%)

Gastrointestinal: Gastrointestinal distress (29% to 34%), nausea (11% to 20%), vomiting (8% to 13%)

Neuromuscular & skeletal: Weakness (13% to 19%), arthritis (17%), arthralgia (2% to 15%), back pain (10% to 12%), ostealgia (6% to 12%), osteoporosis (11%)

Respiratory: Pharyngitis (6% to 14%), dyspnea (8% to 11%), increased cough (7% to 11%)

1% to 10%:

Cardiovascular: Peripheral edema (5% to 10%), chest pain (5% to 7%), venous thrombosis (2%

to 4%; including pulmonary embolism, thrombophlebitis, retinal vein thrombosis), myocardial infarction (1%)

Central nervous system: Insomnia (2% to 10%), dizziness (5% to 8%), paresthesia (5% to 7%), anxiety (2% to 6%), confusion (2% to 5%), drowsiness (2% to 5%), malaise (2% to 5%), nervousness (2% to 5%), carpal tunnel syndrome (3%), hypertonia (3%), cerebrovascular insufficiency (2%), lethargy (1%)

Dermatologic: Alopecia (2% to 5%), pruritus (2% to 5%), diaphoresis (1% to 5%)

Endocrine & metabolic: Hypercholesterolemia (9%), increased serum cholesterol (9%), weight gain (2% to 9%), increased gamma-glutamyl transferase (2% to 5%), weight loss (2% to 5%)

Gastrointestinal: Constipation (7% to 9%), diarrhea (7% to 9%), abdominal pain (6% to 9%), anorexia (5% to 8%), dyspepsia (7%), gastrointestinal disease (7%), xerostomia (4% to 6%)

Genitourinary: Mastalgia (2% to 8%), urinary tract infection (2% to 8%), pelvic pain (5% to 7%), vulvovaginitis (6%), vaginal dryness (1% to 5%), vaginal hemorrhage (1% to 5%), vaginal discharge (4%), vaginitis (4%), leukorrhea (2% to 3%)

Hematologic & oncologic: Lymphedema (10%), breast neoplasm (5%), neoplasm (5%), anemia (2% to 5%), leukopenia (2% to 5%), tumor flare (3%)

Hepatic: Increased serum alkaline phosphatase (2% to 5%), increased serum ALT (2% to 5%), increased serum AST (2% to 5%)

Infection: Infection (2% to 9%)

Neuromuscular & skeletal: Bone fracture (1% to 10%), arthrosis (7%), myalgia (2% to 6%), neck pain (2% to 5%), pathological fracture (2% to 5%)

Ophthalmic: Cataract (6%)

Respiratory: Flu-like symptoms (2% to 7%), sinusitis (2% to 6%), bronchitis (2% to 5%), rhinitis (2% to 5%)

Miscellaneous: Accidental injury (2% to 10%), cyst (5%), fever (2% to 5%)

Pharmacodynamics/Kinetics

Onset of Action Onset of estradiol reduction: 70% reduction after 24 hours; 80% after 2 weeks therapy

Duration of Action Duration of estradiol reduction: 6 days

Available Dosage Forms

Tablet, Oral:

Arimidex: 1 mg

Generic: 1 mg

General Dosage Range Oral: *Adults:* 1 mg once daily

Administration

Oral May be administered with or without food.

Hazardous agent; use appropriate precautions for handling and disposal (NIOSH, 2012).

Storage/Stability Store at 20°C to 25°C (68°F to 77°F).

Nursing Actions

Physical Assessment Monitor bone mineral density and cholesterol levels. Monitor for hyperlipidemia, hypotension, CNS changes, thrombophlebitis, and bone pain or fracture at regular intervals during therapy.

Patient Education

- Discuss specific use of drug and side effects with patient as it relates to treatment. (HCAHPS: During this hospital stay, were you given any medicine that you had not taken before? Before giving you any new medicine, how often did hospital staff tell you what the medicine was for? How often did hospital staff describe possible side effects in a way you could understand?)
- Patient may experience flushing, nausea, arthralgia, insomnia, pharyngitis, or back pain. Have patient report immediately to prescriber signs of depression (ie, suicidal ideation, anxiety, emotional instability, illogical thinking), signs of hepatic impairment, signs of hypercalcemia, excessive weight gain, edema of extremities, strength differences from one side to another, difficulty speaking or thinking, change in balance, blurred vision, severe headache, paresthesia, arrhythmia, mood changes, significant dizziness, syncope, polyuria, difficult urination, considerable asthenia, enlarged lymph nodes, vaginal hemorrhaging, vaginitis, severe angina, or significant dyspnea (HCAHPS).
- Educate patient about signs of a significant reaction (eg, wheezing; chest tightness; fever; itching; bad cough; blue skin color; seizures; or swelling of face, lips, tongue, or throat). **Note:** This is not a comprehensive list of all side effects. Patient should consult prescriber for additional questions.

Intended Use and Disclaimer: Should not be printed and given to patients. This information is intended to serve as a concise initial reference for healthcare professionals to use when discussing medications with a patient. You must ultimately rely on your own discretion, experience and judgment in diagnosing, treating and advising patients.

Dietary Considerations May be taken with or without food.

Anidulafungin (ay nid yoo la FUN jin)

Brand Names: U.S. Eraxis
Index Terms LY303366
Pharmacologic Category Antifungal Agent, Parenteral; Echinocandin
Pregnancy Risk Factor B
Lactation Excretion in breast milk unknown/use caution

Breast-Feeding Considerations It is not known if anidulafungin is excreted in breast milk. The manufacturer recommends that caution be exercised when administering anidulafungin to nursing women.

Use Treatment of candidemia and other forms of *Candida* infections (including those of intra-abdominal, peritoneal, and esophageal locus)

Mechanism of Action/Effect Noncompetitive inhibitor of 1,3-beta-D-glucan synthase resulting in reduced formation of 1,3-beta-D-glucan, an essential polysaccharide comprising 30% to 60% of *Candida* cell walls (absent in mammalian cells); decreased glucan content leads to osmotic instability and cellular lysis

Contraindications Hypersensitivity to anidulafungin, other echinocandins, or any component of the formulation

Warnings/Precautions Severe hypersensitivity reactions, including anaphylactic reactions and anaphylactic shock have been reported; immediate treatment for hypersensitivity reactions should be available. Discontinue treatment immediately if reactions occur. Infusion reactions (eg, bronchospasm, dyspnea, flushing, hypotension, pruritus, rash, urticaria) may occur; do not exceed rate of infusion. Elevated liver function tests, hepatitis, and hepatic failure have been reported. Monitor for progressive hepatic impairment if increased transaminase enzymes noted. Safety and efficacy have not been established in other *Candida* infections (eg, endocarditis, osteomyelitis, meningitis).

Drug Interactions

Avoid Concomitant Use There are no known interactions where it is recommended to avoid concomitant use.

Decreased Effect
Anidulafungin may decrease the levels/effects of: Saccharomyces boulardii

Increased Effect/Toxicity There are no known significant interactions involving an increase in effect.

Adverse Reactions
>10%:
Cardiovascular: Hypotension (15%), hypertension (12%), peripheral edema (11%)
Central nervous system: Fever (9% to 18%), insomnia (15%)
Endocrine & metabolic: Hypokalemia (≤25%), hypomagnesemia (12%)
Gastrointestinal: Nausea (7% to 24%), diarrhea (9% to 18%), vomiting (7% to 18%)
Genitourinary: Urinary tract infection (15%)
Hepatic: Alkaline phosphatase increased (12%)
Respiratory: Dyspnea (12%)
Miscellaneous: Bacteremia (18%)
2% to 10%:
Cardiovascular: Deep vein thrombosis (10%), chest pain (5%)
Central nervous system: Confusion (8%), headache (8%), depression (6%)

◀ Dermatologic: Decubitus ulcer (5%)
Endocrine & metabolic: Hypoglycemia (7%), dehydration (6%), hyperglycemia (6%), hyperkalemia (6%)
Gastrointestinal: Constipation (8%), dyspepsia (7%), abdominal pain (6%), oral candidiasis (5%)
Hematologic: Anemia (8% to 9%), thrombocythemia (6%), leukocytosis (5% to 8%)
Hepatic: Transaminases increased (≤5%)
Neuromuscular & skeletal: Back pain (5%)
Renal: Creatinine increased (5%)
Respiratory: Pleural effusion (10%), cough (7%), pneumonia (6%), respiratory distress (6%)
Miscellaneous: Sepsis (7%)

Available Dosage Forms
Solution Reconstituted, Intravenous [preservative free]:
Eraxis: 50 mg (1 ea); 100 mg (1 ea)
General Dosage Range I.V.: *Adults:* Initial dose: 100-200 mg as a single dose; Subsequent dosing: 50-100 mg daily

Administration
I.V. For intravenous use only; infusion rate should not exceed 1.1 mg/minute (1.4 mL/minute or 84 mL/hour).
Preparation for Administration Aseptically add 15 mL (50 mg vial) or 30 mL (100 mg vial) of sterile water for injection to each vial. Further dilute 50 mg or 100 mg vials in 50 mL or 100 mL, respectively, of D$_5$W or NS.
Storage/Stability Store vials at 2°C to 8°C (36°F to 46°F); excursions at 25°C (77°F) are permitted for 96 hours and the vial may be returned to storage at 2°C to 8°C (36°F to 46°F). Do not freeze. The reconstituted solution can be stored for up to 24 hours at temperatures up to 25°C (77°F) prior to dilution into the infusion solution. The infusion solution may be stored for up to 48 hours at temperatures up to 25°C (77°F) or stored in the freezer for ≥72 hours prior to administration.

Nursing Actions
Patient Education
• Discuss specific use of drug and side effects with patient as it relates to treatment. (HCAHPS: During this hospital stay, were you given any medicine that you had not taken before? Before giving you any new medicine, how often did hospital staff tell you what the medicine was for? How often did hospital staff describe possible side effects in a way you could understand?)
• Patient may experience nausea, diarrhea, or insomnia. Have patient report immediately to prescriber signs of hepatic impairment, signs of hypokalemia, angina, illogical thinking, depression, difficult urination, dysuria, severe dizziness, syncope, chills, pharyngitis, flushing, edema of extremities, injection site pain or irritation, significant headache, dyspnea, ecchymosis, hemorrhaging, or vision changes (HCAHPS).

• Educate patient about signs of a significant reaction (eg, wheezing; chest tightness; fever; itching; bad cough; blue skin color; seizures; or swelling of face, lips, tongue, or throat). **Note:** This is not a comprehensive list of all side effects. Patient should consult prescriber for additional questions.

Intended Use and Disclaimer: Should not be printed and given to patients. This information is intended to serve as a concise initial reference for healthcare professionals to use when discussing medications with a patient. You must ultimately rely on your own discretion, experience and judgment in diagnosing, treating and advising patients.

Antihemophilic Factor (Human)
(an tee hee moe FIL ik FAK tor HYU man)

Brand Names: U.S. Hemofil M; Koāte®-DVI; Monoclate-P®
Index Terms AHF (Human); Factor VIII (Human); Kaote DVI
Pharmacologic Category Antihemophilic Agent; Blood Product Derivative
Medication Safety Issues
Sound-alike/look-alike issues:
Factor VIII may be confused with Factor XIII
Other safety concerns:
Confusion may occur due to the omitting of "Factor VIII" from some product labeling. Review product contents carefully prior to dispensing any antihemophilic factor.
Pregnancy Risk Factor C
Lactation Use caution
Use Prevention and treatment of hemorrhagic episodes in patients with hemophilia A (classic hemophilia); perioperative management of hemophilia A; can be of significant therapeutic value in patients with acquired factor VIII inhibitors not exceeding 10 Bethesda units/mL
Available Dosage Forms
Injection, powder for reconstitution:
Hemofil M: ~250 units, ~500 units, ~1000 units, ~1700 units
Koāte®-DVI: ~250 units, ~500 units, ~1000 units
Monoclate-P®: ~250 units, ~500 units, ~1000 units, ~1500 units
General Dosage Range I.V.: *Children and Adults:* Dosage varies greatly depending on indication
Administration
I.V. Over 5-10 minutes (maximum: 10 mL/minute). Infuse Monoclate-P® at 2 mL/minute.
Nursing Actions
Physical Assessment Monitor patient closely during and after infusion for any change in vital signs, cardiac and CNS status, or hypersensitivity reactions (eg, chills, fever, chest pain, respiratory difficulty). Assess results of hematocrit and

coagulation studies. Monitor bleeding and coagulation status. Monitor for anemia.

Patient Education
- Discuss specific use of drug and side effects with patient as it relates to treatment. (HCAHPS: During this hospital stay, were you given any medicine that you had not taken before? Before giving you any new medicine, how often did hospital staff tell you what the medicine was for? How often did hospital staff describe possible side effects in a way you could understand?)
- Have patient report immediately to prescriber signs of infection, dyspnea, severe dizziness, syncope, significant nausea, flushing, considerable asthenia, tachycardia, mouth discoloration, angina, strength differences from one side to another, difficulty speaking or thinking, change in balance, blurred vision, hemoptysis, or edema of extremities (HCAHPS).
- Educate patient about signs of a significant reaction (eg, wheezing; chest tightness; fever; itching; bad cough; blue skin color; seizures; or swelling of face, lips, tongue, or throat). **Note:** This is not a comprehensive list of all side effects. Patient should consult prescriber for additional questions.

Intended Use and Disclaimer: Should not be printed and given to patients. This information is intended to serve as a concise initial reference for healthcare professionals to use when discussing medications with a patient. You must ultimately rely on your own discretion, experience and judgment in diagnosing, treating and advising patients.

Antihemophilic Factor (Recombinant)
(an tee hee moe FIL ik FAK tor ree KOM be nant)

Brand Names: U.S. Advate; Helixate FS; Kogenate FS; Kogenate FS Bio-Set; Recombinate; Xyntha; Xyntha Solofuse

Index Terms AHF (Recombinant); Factor VIII (Recombinant); Novoeight; rAHF

Pharmacologic Category Antihemophilic Agent

Medication Safety Issues
Sound-alike/look-alike issues:
Factor VIII may be confused with Factor XIII
Other safety concerns:
Confusion may occur due to the omitting of "Factor VIII" from some product labeling. Review product contents carefully prior to dispensing any antihemophilic factor.

Pregnancy Risk Factor C

Lactation Excretion in breast milk unknown/use caution

Use Prevention and treatment of hemorrhagic episodes in patients with hemophilia A (classic hemophilia or congenital factor VIII deficiency); perioperative management of hemophilia A; routine prophylaxis in patients with hemophilia A to prevent bleeding episodes (Advate, Helixate® FS, Kogenate® FS)

Note: Helixate® FS and Kogenate® FS are also approved in children with hemophilia A with no pre-existing joint damage to reduce risk of joint damage. In addition, Recombinate can be of therapeutic value in patients with acquired factor VIII inhibitors ≤10 Bethesda units/mL.

Product Availability
Novoeight: FDA approved October 2013; availability anticipated in the second quarter of 2015.

Novoeight is indicated for use in children and adults with hemophilia A (congenital factor VIII deficiency or classic hemophilia) for control and prevention of bleeding episodes, perioperative management, and routine prophylaxis to prevent or reduce the frequency of bleeding episodes.

Available Dosage Forms
Kit, Intravenous:
Kogenate FS: 250 units, 500 units, 1000 units
Kit, Intravenous [preservative free]:
Helixate FS: 250 units, 500 units, 1000 units, 2000 units, 3000 units
Kogenate FS: 2000 units, 3000 units
Kogenate FS Bio-Set: 250 units, 500 units, 1000 units, 2000 units, 3000 units
Xyntha: 250 units, 500 units, 1000 units, 2000 units
Xyntha Solofuse: 250 units, 500 units, 1000 units, 2000 units, 3000 units
Solution Reconstituted, Intravenous:
Advate: 250 units (1 ea); 500 units (1 ea); 1000 units (1 ea); 1500 units (1 ea); 2000 units (1 ea); 3000 units (1 ea)
Solution Reconstituted, Intravenous [preservative free]:
Advate: 250 units (1 ea); 500 units (1 ea); 1000 units (1 ea); 1500 units (1 ea); 2000 units (1 ea); 3000 units (1 ea); 4000 units (1 ea)
Recombinate: 220-400 UNIT (1 ea); 401-800 UNIT (1 ea); 801-1240 UNIT (1 ea); 1241-1800 UNIT (1 ea); 1801-2400 UNIT (1 ea)

General Dosage Range I.V.: *Children and Adults:* Dosage varies greatly depending on indication

Administration
I.V. Use administration sets/tubing provided by manufacturer (if provided).
Advate: Infuse over ≤5 minutes (maximum: 10 mL/minute)
Helixate® FS, Kogenate® FS: Infuse over 1-15 minutes; based on patient tolerability
Recombinate reconstituted with 5 mL of SWFI: Infuse at a rate of ≤5 mL/minute (maximum: 5 mL/minute)
Recombinate reconstituted with 10 mL of SWFI: Infuse at a rate of ≤10 mL/minute (maximum: 10 mL/minute)
Xyntha®, Xyntha® Solofuse™: Infuse over several minutes; adjust based on patient comfort. ▶

Do not admix or administer in same tubing as other medications.

Nursing Actions

Physical Assessment Monitor patient closely during and after infusion for any change in vital signs, cardiac and CNS status, or hypersensitivity reactions (eg, chills, fever, chest pain, respiratory difficulty). Assess results of hematocrit and coagulation studies. Monitor bleeding and coagulation status. Monitor for anemia.

Patient Education
- Discuss specific use of drug and side effects with patient as it relates to treatment. (HCAHPS: During this hospital stay, were you given any medicine that you had not taken before? Before giving you any new medicine, how often did hospital staff tell you what the medicine was for? How often did hospital staff describe possible side effects in a way you could understand?)
- Patient may experience headache, rhinitis, pharyngitis, arthralgia, diarrhea, or injection site irritation. Have patient report immediately to prescriber severe dizziness, syncope, dyspnea, considerable nausea, flushing, significant asthenia, tachycardia, mouth discoloration, angina, paresthesia, strength differences from one side to another, difficulty speaking or thinking, change in balance, blurred vision, hemoptysis, or edema of extremities (HCAHPS).
- Educate patient about signs of a significant reaction (eg, wheezing; chest tightness; fever; itching; bad cough; blue skin color; seizures; or swelling of face, lips, tongue, or throat). **Note:** This is not a comprehensive list of all side effects. Patient should consult prescriber for additional questions.

Intended Use and Disclaimer: Should not be printed and given to patients. This information is intended to serve as a concise initial reference for healthcare professionals to use when discussing medications with a patient. You must ultimately rely on your own discretion, experience and judgment in diagnosing, treating and advising patients.

Antihemophilic Factor/von Willebrand Factor Complex (Human)
(an tee hee moe FIL ik FAK tor von WILL le brand FAK tor KOM plex HYU man)

Brand Names: U.S. Alphanate®; Humate-P®; Wilate®

Index Terms AHF (Human); Factor VIII (Human); Factor VIII Concentrate; FVIII/vWF; von Willebrand Factor/Factor VIII Complex; VWF/FVIII Concentrate; VWF:RCo; vWF:RCof

Pharmacologic Category Antihemophilic Agent; Blood Product Derivative

Medication Safety Issues
Sound-alike/look-alike issues:
Factor VIII may be confused with Factor XIII

Pregnancy Risk Factor C
Lactation Excretion in breast milk unknown/use caution
Use
Factor VIII deficiency: Alphanate®, Humate-P®: Prevention and treatment of hemorrhagic episodes in patients with hemophilia A (classical hemophilia) or acquired factor VIII deficiency (Alphanate® only); **Note:** Wilate® is not approved for use in patients with hemophilia A or acquired factor VIII deficiency

von Willebrand disease (VWD):
Alphanate®: Prophylaxis with surgical and/or invasive procedures in patients with VWD when desmopressin is either ineffective or contraindicated; **Note:** Not indicated for patients with severe VWD undergoing major surgery
Humate-P®: Treatment of spontaneous or trauma-induced bleeding, as well as prevention of excessive bleeding during and after surgery in patients with severe VWD, including mild or moderate disease where use of desmopressin is known or suspected to be inadequate; **Note:** Not indicated for the prophylaxis of spontaneous bleeding episodes
Wilate®: Treatment of spontaneous and trauma-induced bleeding in patients with severe VWD, including mild or moderate disease where use of desmopressin is known or suspected to be inadequate or contraindicated; **Note:** Not indicated for prophylaxis of spontaneous bleeding or prevention of excessive bleeding during and after surgery)

Available Dosage Forms
Injection, powder for reconstitution [human derived]:
Alphanate®:
250 units [Factor VIII and VWF:RCo ratio varies by lot]
500 units [Factor VIII and VWF:RCo ratio varies by lot]
1000 units [Factor VIII and VWF:RCo ratio varies by lot]
1500 units [Factor VIII and VWF:RCo ratio varies by lot]
Humate-P®:
FVIII 250 units and VWF:RCo 600 units
FVIII 500 units and VWF:RCo 1200 units
FVIII 1000 units and VWF:RCo 2400 units
Wilate®:
FVIII 500 units and VWF:RCo 500 units
FVIII 1000 units and VWF:RCo 1000 units

General Dosage Range I.V.: *Children and Adults:* Dosage varies greatly depending on indication
Administration
I.V.
Alphanate®: Infuse slowly (maximum rate: 10 mL/minute)
Humate-P®: Infuse slowly (maximum rate: 4 mL/minute)
Wilate®: Infuse slowly at a rate of 2-4 mL/minute

Nursing Actions

Physical Assessment Monitor patient closely during and after infusion for any change in vital signs, cardiac and CNS status, or hypersensitivity reactions (eg, chills, fever, chest pain, respiratory difficulty). Assess results of hematocrit and coagulation studies. Monitor bleeding and coagulation status. Monitor for anemia.

Patient Education

- Discuss specific use of drug and side effects with patient as it relates to treatment. (HCAHPS: During this hospital stay, were you given any medicine that you had not taken before? Before giving you any new medicine, how often did hospital staff tell you what the medicine was for? How often did hospital staff describe possible side effects in a way you could understand?)
- Patient may experience dyspepsia. Have patient report immediately to prescriber signs of hemorrhaging, signs of infection, flushing, severe dizziness, syncope, significant headache, paresthesia, edema, considerable nausea, intolerable asthenia, akathisia, jaundice, angina, dyspnea, hemoptysis, edema of extremities, tachycardia, mouth discoloration, strength differences from one side to another, difficulty speaking or thinking, change in balance, or blurred vision (HCAHPS).
- Educate patient about signs of a significant reaction (eg, wheezing; chest tightness; fever; itching; bad cough; blue skin color; seizures; or swelling of face, lips, tongue, or throat). **Note:** This is not a comprehensive list of all side effects. Patient should consult prescriber for additional questions.

Intended Use and Disclaimer: Should not be printed and given to patients. This information is intended to serve as a concise initial reference for healthcare professionals to use when discussing medications with a patient. You must ultimately rely on your own discretion, experience and judgment in diagnosing, treating and advising patients.

Anti-inhibitor Coagulant Complex (Human)
(an TEE in HI bi tor coe AG yoo lant KOM pleks HYU man)

Brand Names: U.S. Feiba NF

Index Terms Activated PCC; AICC; aPCC; Coagulant Complex Inhibitor; Factor Eight Inhibitor Bypassing Activity; Factor VIII Inhibitor Bypassing Activity; FEIBA VH

Pharmacologic Category Activated Prothrombin Complex Concentrate (aPCC); Antihemophilic Agent; Blood Product Derivative

Pregnancy Risk Factor C

Lactation Excretion in breast milk unknown/use caution

Use

Hemorrhage in patients with hemophilia: For use in patients with hemophilia A and B with inhibitors for control and prevention of bleeding episodes.

Perioperative bleeding management in patients with hemophilia: For use in patients with hemophilia A and B with inhibitors for perioperative management.

Routine prophylaxis of bleeding events in patients with hemophilia: For use in patients with hemophilia A and B for routine prophylaxis to prevent or reduce the frequency of bleeding episodes.

Unlabeled Use Acquired hemophilia with factor VIII or factor IX inhibitor titers >5 Bethesda units (BU); treatment of life-threatening bleeding associated with dabigatran

Available Dosage Forms

Solution Reconstituted, Intravenous:
Feiba NF: (1 ea)

Solution Reconstituted, Intravenous [preservative free]:
Feiba NF: 500 units (1 ea); 1000 units (1 ea); 2500 units (1 ea)

General Dosage Range I.V.: *Children, Adolescents, and Adults:* 50-100 units/kg every 6-12 hours (maximum: 100 units/kg [single dose]; 200 units/kg/day [total daily dose])

Administration

I.V. For I.V. injection or drip infusion only; maximum infusion rate: 2 units/kg/minute. Following reconstitution, complete infusion within 3 hours.

Nursing Actions

Physical Assessment Monitor patient closely during and after infusion for any change in vital signs, cardiac and CNS status, or hypersensitivity reactions. If hypotension develops, the rate of infusion should be slowed and prescriber notified. Monitor for signs of excessive clotting. Monitor coagulation labs: Fibrinogen, platelets, FDP, thrombin time, PT, PTT, and INR and report abnormalities. Monitor for signs of infection. Record the batch number of the product with each administration. Instruct patients to call doctor with fever, drowsiness, chills, and runny nose, followed by a rash and joint pain 2 weeks after infusion, or dark urine, yellow skin, or eyes.

Patient Education

- Discuss specific use of drug and side effects with patient as it relates to treatment. (HCAHPS: During this hospital stay, were you given any medicine that you had not taken before? Before giving you any new medicine, how often did hospital staff tell you what the medicine was for? How often did hospital staff describe possible side effects in a way you could understand?)
- Patient may experience fatigue or dysgeusia. Have patient report immediately to prescriber signs of infection, dyspnea, severe dizziness, syncope, considerable nausea, significant

headache, chills, tachycardia, mouth discoloration, angina, hemoptysis, strength differences from one side to another, difficulty speaking or thinking, change in balance, blurred vision, or edema of extremities (HCAHPS).

- Educate patient about signs of a significant reaction (eg, wheezing; chest tightness; fever; itching; bad cough; blue skin color; seizures; or swelling of face, lips, tongue, or throat). **Note:** This is not a comprehensive list of all side effects. Patient should consult prescriber for additional questions.

Intended Use and Disclaimer: Should not be printed and given to patients. This information is intended to serve as a concise initial reference for healthcare professionals to use when discussing medications with a patient. You must ultimately rely on your own discretion, experience and judgment in diagnosing, treating and advising patients.

Antithymocyte Globulin (Equine)
(an te THY moe site GLOB yu lin, E kwine)

Brand Names: U.S. Atgam

Index Terms Antithymocyte Immunoglobulin; ATG; Horse Antihuman Thymocyte Gamma Globulin; Lymphocyte Immune Globulin

Pharmacologic Category Immune Globulin; Immunosuppressant Agent; Polyclonal Antibody

Medication Safety Issues

Sound-alike/look-alike issues:

Antithymocyte globulin equine (Atgam®) may be confused with antithymocyte globulin rabbit (Thymoglobulin®)

Atgam® may be confused with Ativan®

Pregnancy Risk Factor C

Lactation Excretion in breast milk unknown/use caution

Use Prevention and treatment of acute renal allograft rejection; treatment of moderate-to-severe aplastic anemia in patients not considered suitable candidates for bone marrow transplantation

Unlabeled Use Prevention and treatment of other solid organ allograft rejection; prevention or treatment of graft-versus-host disease (GVHD) following allogeneic stem cell transplantation; treatment of myelodysplastic syndrome (MDS)

Available Dosage Forms

Injectable, Intravenous:

Atgam: 50 mg/mL (5 mL)

General Dosage Range I.V.:

Children: Initial: 5-25 mg/kg/day administered daily for 8-14 days; may be followed by administration every other day (maximum: 21 doses in 28 days)

Adults: Initial: 10-20 mg/kg/day administered daily; may be followed by administration every other day (maximum: 21 doses in 28 days)

Administration

I.V. Infuse dose over at least 4 hours. Any severe systemic reaction to the skin test, such as generalized rash, tachycardia, dyspnea, hypotension or anaphylaxis, should preclude further therapy. Epinephrine and resuscitative equipment should be nearby. Patient may need to be pretreated with an antipyretic, antihistamine, and/or corticosteroid. Mild itching and erythema can be treated with antihistamines. May cause vein irritation (chemical phlebitis) if administered peripherally. Infuse into a vascular shunt, arterial venous fistula, or high-flow central vein through a 0.2-1 micron in-line filter.

First dose: Premedicate with diphenhydramine orally 30 minutes prior to and hydrocortisone I.V. 15 minutes prior to infusion and acetaminophen 2 hours after start of infusion.

Nursing Actions

Physical Assessment Intradermal skin testing and premedication are recommended with the first dose. Treatment for hypersensitivity should be available. Assess for history of previous allergic reactions. Monitor vital signs during infusion and observe for adverse or allergic reactions closely.

Patient Education

- Discuss specific use of drug and side effects with patient as it relates to treatment. (HCAHPS: During this hospital stay, were you given any medicine that you had not taken before? Before giving you any new medicine, how often did hospital staff tell you what the medicine was for? How often did hospital staff describe possible side effects in a way you could understand?)
- Patient may experience arthralgia. Have patient report immediately to prescriber signs of infection, angina, tachycardia, bradycardia, arrhythmia, dyspnea, severe dizziness, syncope, ecchymosis, hemorrhaging, significant back pain, considerable asthenia, illogical thinking, intolerable headache, paresthesia, severe skin irritation, or injection site irritation (HCAHPS).
- Educate patient about signs of a significant reaction (eg, wheezing; chest tightness; fever; itching; bad cough; blue skin color; seizures; or swelling of face, lips, tongue, or throat). **Note:** This is not a comprehensive list of all side effects. Patient should consult prescriber for additional questions.

Intended Use and Disclaimer: Should not be printed and given to patients. This information is intended to serve as a concise initial reference for healthcare professionals to use when discussing medications with a patient. You must ultimately rely on your own discretion, experience and judgment in diagnosing, treating and advising patients.

Apixaban (a PIX a ban)

Brand Names: U.S. Eliquis

Pharmacologic Category Anticoagulant; Anticoagulant, Factor Xa Inhibitor

Medication Safety Issues

High alert medication:

This medication is in a class the Institute for Safe Medication Practices (ISMP) includes among its list of drug classes which have a heightened risk of causing significant patient harm when used in error.

Medication Guide Available Yes

Pregnancy Risk Factor B

Lactation Excretion unknown/not recommended

Breast-Feeding Considerations It is not known if apixaban is excreted in breast milk. Apixaban is not recommended for use in breast-feeding women; use of alternative anticoagulants is preferred (Bates, 2012)

Use

Nonvalvular atrial fibrillation: To reduce the risk of stroke and systemic embolism in patients with nonvalvular atrial fibrillation

Canadian labeling: Additional use (not in U.S. labeling): Postoperative prophylaxis of venous thromboembolism (VTE) following elective knee or hip replacement surgery

Unlabeled Use Initial treatment of VTE; extended treatment of VTE to reduce the risk of recurrent DVT and/or PE (in patients completing 6-12 months of standard anticoagulation for venous thromboembolism)

Mechanism of Action/Effect Inhibits platelet activation and fibrin clot formation by inhibiting free and clot-bound factor Xa (FXa). FXa, as part of the prothrombinase complex catalyzes the conversion of prothrombin to thrombin. Thrombin both activates platelets and catalyzes the conversion of fibrinogen to fibrin.

Contraindications

U.S. labeling: Severe hypersensitivity reaction (ie, anaphylaxis) to apixaban or any component of the formulation; active pathological bleeding

Canadian labeling: Hypersensitivity to apixaban or any component of the formulation; clinically-significant active bleeding (including gastrointestinal bleeding); lesions or conditions at increased risk of clinically-significant bleeding (eg, cerebral infarct [ischemic or hemorrhagic], active peptic ulcer disease with recent bleeding; patients with spontaneous or acquired impairment of hemostasis); hepatic disease associated with coagulopathy and clinically-relevant bleeding risk; concomitant systemic treatment with agents that are strong inhibitors of both CYP3A4 and P-glycoprotein (P-gp); concomitant treatment with any other anticoagulant including unfractionated heparin (except at doses used to maintain patency of central venous or arterial catheter), low molecular weight heparins, heparin derivatives (eg, fondaparinux), and oral anticoagulants including warfarin, dabigatran, rivaroxaban except when transitioning to or from apixaban therapy

Warnings/Precautions [U.S. Boxed Warning]: When used to prevent stroke in patients with nonvalvular atrial fibrillation, an increased risk of stroke may occur upon apixaban discontinuation if patient is not adequately anticoagulated with an alternative anticoagulant. If apixaban must be discontinued for reasons other than bleeding, consider the use of another anticoagulant to prevent stroke from occurring.

May increase the risk of bleeding; serious, potentially fatal bleeding may occur. Concomitant use of drugs that affect hemostasis increases the risk of bleeding. Monitor for signs and symptoms of bleeding. Discontinue therapy with active pathological hemorrhage and promptly evaluate for bleeding source. No specific antidote exists for apixaban reversal; hemodialysis does not appear to have a substantial impact on apixaban exposure. Although not evaluated in clinical trials, in the event of apixaban-related hemorrhage, the use of prothrombin complex concentrate (PCC), activated prothrombin complex concentrate, or recombinant factor VIIa may be considered. The use of activated oral charcoal may be considered if ingestion occurred within 2-6 hours of presentation.

Spinal or epidural hematomas, including subsequent paralysis, may occur with neuraxial anesthesia (epidural or spinal anesthesia) or spinal puncture in patients who are anticoagulated; the risk is increased with concomitant administration of other drugs that affect hemostasis (eg, NSAIDs, platelet inhibitors, other anticoagulants), in patients with a history of traumatic or repeated epidural or spinal punctures, or a history of spinal deformity or surgery. In patients who receive both apixaban and neuraxial anesthesia, Canadian labeling recommends to avoid removal of epidural catheter for at least 24 hours following last apixaban dose; avoid apixaban administration for at least 5 hours following epidural or intrathecal catheter removal. Monitor for signs of neurologic impairment (eg, numbness/weakness of legs, bowel/bladder dysfunction); prompt diagnosis and treatment are necessary.

In a clinical trial of high-risk, post-acute coronary syndrome (ACS) patients (unlabeled use), use of apixaban in addition to standard antiplatelet therapy increased the incidence of major bleeding (including intracranial and fatal bleeding) without any significant clinical benefit (Alexander, 2011). In acutely ill patients (eg, heart failure, respiratory failure) at risk for venous thromboembolism (VTE) receiving apixaban for extended VTE prophylaxis (unlabeled use), an increased incidence of major bleeding without greater efficacy was observed with extended apixaban therapy (eg, 30 days) ▶

versus low molecular weight heparin (enoxaparin) therapy for 1-2 weeks (Goldhaber, 2011). Use in patients undergoing hip fracture surgery has not been studied; avoid use in these patients.

Use with caution in moderate impairment (Child-Pugh class B) as there is limited clinical experience in these patients; dosing recommendations cannot be provided. Use in severe hepatic impairment (Child-Pugh class C) is not recommended. Patients with ALT/AST >2 times ULN or total bilirubin ≥1.5 times ULN and undergoing major orthopedic surgery (approved use in Canada; not an approved use in U.S.) were excluded from clinical trials; use with caution in these patients. Systemic exposure increases with worsening renal function. Bleeding risk may be increased in severe renal impairment (CrCl <15-29 mL/minute); use with caution. Patients with ESRD with or without hemodialysis have not been studied. Dosage reduction is recommended for patients with nonvalvular atrial fibrillation with a serum creatinine ≥1.5 mg/dL and are either ≥80 years of age or weigh ≤60 kg. Safety and efficacy have not been established in patients with prosthetic heart valves or significant rheumatic heart disease (eg, mitral stenosis); use is not recommended. Non-valvular atrial fibrillation is defined as atrial fibrillation that occurs in the absence of rheumatic mitral valve disease, mitral valve repair, or prosthetic heart valve (Fuster, 2011).

Potentially significant drug-drug interactions may exist, requiring dose or frequency adjustment, additional monitoring, and/or selection of alternative therapy. Systemic exposure is increased ~32% in patients >65 years of age and may be increased by 20% to 30% in patients <50 kg and decreased by 20% to 30% in patients >120 kg; dosage reduction is recommended for patients with nonvalvular atrial fibrillation with any 2 of the following: ≥80 years of age, weight ≤60 kg, or serum creatinine ≥1.5 mg/dL.

Discontinue apixaban at least 24-48 hours prior to elective surgery or invasive procedures depending on risk or location of bleeding.

Drug Interactions

Avoid Concomitant Use

Avoid concomitant use of Apixaban with any of the following: Anticoagulants; CYP3A4 Inducers (Strong); CYP3A4 Inhibitors (Strong); Dabigatran Etexilate; Omacetaxine; Rivaroxaban; St Johns Wort; Urokinase

Decreased Effect

The levels/effects of Apixaban may be decreased by: Bosentan; CYP3A4 Inducers (Strong); Dabrafenib; Deferasirox; Estrogen Derivatives; P-glycoprotein/ABCB1 Inducers; Progestins; St Johns Wort; Tocilizumab

Increased Effect/Toxicity

Apixaban may increase the levels/effects of: Anticoagulants; Collagenase (Systemic); Deferasirox; Ibritumomab; Omacetaxine; Rivaroxaban; Tositumomab and Iodine I 131 Tositumomab

The levels/effects of Apixaban may be increased by: Agents with Antiplatelet Properties; CYP3A4 Inhibitors (Moderate); CYP3A4 Inhibitors (Strong); Dabigatran Etexilate; Dasatinib; Fusidic Acid (Systemic); Herbs (Anticoagulant/Antiplatelet Properties); Ibrutinib; Ivacaftor; Luliconazole; Mifepristone; Nonsteroidal Anti-Inflammatory Agents; Omega-3 Fatty Acids; Pentosan Polysulfate Sodium; P-glycoprotein/ABCB1 Inhibitors; Prostacyclin Analogues; Salicylates; Simeprevir; Sugammadex; Thrombolytic Agents; Tibolone; Tipranavir; Urokinase; Vitamin E

Nutritional/Ethanol Interactions

Food: Grapefruit juice may increase levels/effects of apixaban. Management: Advise patients who consume grapefruit juice during therapy to use caution; monitor for increased effects (eg, bleeding).

Herb/Nutraceutical: St John's wort may reduce apixaban systemic exposure. Management: Advise patients to use St. John's wort with caution or if possible, avoid concomitant use.

Adverse Reactions Note: Includes adverse reactions from nonvalvular atrial fibrillation and hip/knee replacement surgery clinical trials.

>10%: Hematologic: Bleeding (5% to 12%; major: ≤2%; clinically-relevant non-major bleeding: 2% to 4%)

1% to 10%:

Dermatologic: Bruising (1%)

Gastrointestinal: Nausea (3%)

Hematologic: Anemia (3%), postprocedural hemorrhage (1%)

Hepatic: GGT increased (1%), transaminases increased (1%)

Pharmacodynamics/Kinetics

Onset of Action 3-4 hours

Available Dosage Forms

Tablet, Oral:

Eliquis: 2.5 mg, 5 mg

General Dosage Range Dosage adjustment recommended in patients with multiple risk factors for bleeding including renal impairment or patients on concomitant therapy.

Oral: *Adults:* 2.5-5 mg twice daily

Administration

Oral Administer without regard to meals. After hip/knee replacement (Canadian labeling), initial dose should be administered 12-24 hours postoperatively.

Storage/Stability Store at 20°C to 25°C (68°F to 77°F); excursions permitted between 15°C to 30°C (59°F to 86°F).

Nursing Actions

Physical Assessment Monitor for signs and symptoms of bleeding. After neuraxial anesthesia, monitor for development of hematoma at site of catheter. Monitor for unusual bleeding and for neurological compromise (eg, numbness or weakness of legs, bowel or bladder dysfunction) in the setting of epidural or spinal hematoma. Educate patient about signs and symptoms of bleeding and who to contact in the event of bleeding. Advise patient to tell all doctors and dentists about use of an anticoagulant.

Patient Education

- Discuss specific use of drug and side effects with patient as it relates to treatment. (HCAHPS: During this hospital stay, were you given any medicine that you had not taken before? Before giving you any new medicine, how often did hospital staff tell you what the medicine was for? How often did hospital staff describe possible side effects in a way you could understand?)
- Have patient report immediately to prescriber severe dizziness, syncope, paresthesia, illogical thinking, ecchymosis, or hemorrhaging (HCAHPS).
- Educate patient about signs of a significant reaction (eg, wheezing; chest tightness; fever; itching; bad cough; blue skin color; seizures; or swelling of face, lips, tongue, or throat). **Note:** This is not a comprehensive list of all side effects. Patient should consult prescriber for additional questions.

Intended Use and Disclaimer: Should not be printed and given to patients. This information is intended to serve as a concise initial reference for healthcare professionals to use when discussing medications with a patient. You must ultimately rely on your own discretion, experience and judgment in diagnosing, treating and advising patients.

Apomorphine (a poe MOR feen)

Brand Names: U.S. Apokyn
Index Terms Apomorphine Hydrochloride; Apomorphine Hydrochloride Hemihydrate
Pharmacologic Category Anti-Parkinson's Agent, Dopamine Agonist
Pregnancy Risk Factor C
Lactation Excretion in breast milk unknown/not recommended
Use Treatment of hypomobility, "off" episodes with Parkinson's disease
Unlabeled Use Treatment of erectile dysfunction
Available Dosage Forms
  Solution, Subcutaneous:
  Apokyn: 10 mg/mL (3 mL)
General Dosage Range Dosage adjustment recommended in patients with renal impairment

SubQ: *Adults:* Initial test dose: 2 mg; Starting dose: 2-3 mg/dose at time of "off" episode; Maintenance dose: 2-6 mg/dose at time of "off" episode (maximum: 20 mg/day; 6 mg/dose; 5 doses/day)

Administration

I.V. Not for I.V. administration.
Other SubQ: Initiate antiemetic 3 days before test dose of apomorphine and continue for 2 months (if patient to be treated) before reassessment. Administer in abdomen, upper arm, or upper leg; change site with each injection. 3 mL cartridges are used with a manual, reusable, multidose injector pen. Injector pen can deliver doses up to 1 mL in 0.02 mL increments. Do not give intravenously; thrombus formation or pulmonary embolism may occur.

Nursing Actions

Physical Assessment Monitor patient closely for 90 minutes following each test dose. Premedication with antiemetic is required prior to each dose. Monitor for orthostatic hypotension, nausea, vomiting, dyskinesias, and excessive sedation or somnolence. Teach patient or caregiver proper injection technique and needle disposal.

Patient Education

- Discuss specific use of drug and side effects with patient as it relates to treatment. (HCAHPS: During this hospital stay, were you given any medicine that you had not taken before? Before giving you any new medicine, how often did hospital staff tell you what the medicine was for? How often did hospital staff describe possible side effects in a way you could understand?)
- Patient may experience rhinorrhea, oscitation, injection site irritation, fatigue, headache, flushing, or pallor. Have patient report immediately to prescriber strength differences from one side to another, difficulty speaking or thinking, change in balance, blurred vision, severe dizziness, syncope, illogical thinking, narcolepsy, considerable nausea, skin growths, mole changes, uncontrollable urges, mood changes, behavioral changes, difficulty with motor activity, hallucinations, hyperhidrosis, arrhythmia, significant headache, dyspnea, excessive weight gain, edema of extremities, angina, tachycardia, or priapism (HCAHPS).
- Educate patient about signs of a significant reaction (eg, wheezing; chest tightness; fever; itching; bad cough; blue skin color; seizures; or swelling of face, lips, tongue, or throat). **Note:** This is not a comprehensive list of all side effects. Patient should consult prescriber for additional questions.

Intended Use and Disclaimer: Should not be printed and given to patients. This information is intended to serve as a concise initial reference for healthcare professionals to use when discussing medications with a patient. You must ultimately

◄ rely on your own discretion, experience and judgment in diagnosing, treating and advising patients.

Apraclonidine (a pra KLOE ni deen)

Brand Names: U.S. Iopidine
Index Terms Aplonidine; Apraclonidine Hydrochloride; p-Aminoclonidine
Pharmacologic Category Alpha₂ Agonist, Ophthalmic
Medication Safety Issues
Sound-alike/look-alike issues:
Iopidine® may be confused with indapamide, iodine, Lodine®
Pregnancy Risk Factor C
Lactation Excretion in breast milk unknown/use caution
Use Prevention and treatment of postsurgical intraocular pressure (IOP) elevation; short-term, adjunctive therapy in patients who require additional reduction of IOP
Available Dosage Forms
Solution, Ophthalmic:
Iopidine: 0.5% (5 mL, 10 mL); 1% (1 ea)
Generic: 0.5% (5 mL, 10 mL)
General Dosage Range Ophthalmic: *Adults:* 0.5%: Instill 1-2 drops in the affected eye(s) 3 times/day; 1%: Instill 1 drop in operative eye 1 hour prior to and upon completion of surgery
Administration
Other Wait 5 minutes between instillation of other ophthalmic agents to avoid washout of previous dose. After topical instillation, finger pressure should be applied to lacrimal sac to decrease drainage into the nose and throat and minimize possible systemic absorption.
Nursing Actions
Patient Education
• Discuss specific use of drug and side effects with patient as it relates to treatment. (HCAHPS: During this hospital stay, were you given any medicine that you had not taken before? Before giving you any new medicine, how often did hospital staff tell your what the medicine was for? How often did hospital staff describe possible side effects in a way you could understand?)
• Patient may experience blurred vision, xerophthalmia, nasal dryness, xerostomia, or sensitivity to light. Have patient report immediately to prescriber vision changes, ophthalmalgia, severe eye irritation, eyelid edema, eye discharge, significant dizziness, syncope, arrhythmia, or dyspnea (HCAHPS).
• Educate patient about signs of a significant reaction (eg, wheezing; chest tightness; fever; itching; bad cough; blue skin color; seizures; or swelling of face, lips, tongue, or throat). **Note:** This is not a comprehensive list of all side effects. Patient should consult prescriber for additional questions.

Intended Use and Disclaimer: Should not be printed and given to patients. This information is intended to serve as a concise initial reference for healthcare professionals to use when discussing medications with a patient. You must ultimately rely on your own discretion, experience and judgment in diagnosing, treating and advising patients.

Aprepitant (ap RE pi tant)

Brand Names: U.S. Emend
Index Terms L 754030; MK 869
Pharmacologic Category Antiemetic; Substance P/Neurokinin 1 Receptor Antagonist
Medication Safety Issues
Sound-alike/look-alike issues:
Aprepitant may be confused with fosaprepitant
Emend® (aprepitant) oral capsule formulation may be confused with Emend® for injection (fosaprepitant)
Pregnancy Risk Factor B
Lactation Excretion in breast milk unknown/not recommended
Breast-Feeding Considerations It is not known if aprepitant is excreted in breast milk. Due to the potential for adverse reactions in the nursing infant, the decision to discontinue aprepitant or to discontinue breast-feeding should take into account the benefits of treatment to the mother.
Use Prevention of acute and delayed nausea and vomiting associated with moderately- and highly-emetogenic chemotherapy (in combination with other antiemetics); prevention of postoperative nausea and vomiting (PONV)
Mechanism of Action/Effect Prevents acute and delayed vomiting at the substance P/neurokinin 1 (NK₁) receptor; augments the antiemetic activity of 5-HT₃ receptor antagonists and corticosteroids to inhibit acute and delayed phases of chemotherapy-induced emesis.
Contraindications Hypersensitivity to aprepitant or any component of the formulation; concurrent use with cisapride or pimozide
Warnings/Precautions Potentially significant drug-drug interactions may exist, requiring dose or frequency adjustment, additional monitoring, and/or selection of alternative therapy. Use caution with severe hepatic impairment (Child-Pugh class C); has not been studied. Not studied for treatment of existing nausea and vomiting. Chronic continuous administration is not recommended.
Drug Interactions
Avoid Concomitant Use
Avoid concomitant use of Aprepitant with any of the following: Axitinib; Bosutinib; Cisapride; Conivaptan; Fusidic Acid (Systemic); Ibrutinib;

Ivabradine; Lomitapide; Pimozide; Rivaroxaban; Simeprevir; Tolvaptan; Ulipristal

Decreased Effect

Aprepitant may decrease the levels/effects of: ARIPiprazole; Axitinib; Contraceptives (Estrogens); Contraceptives (Progestins); CYP2C9 Substrates; Diclofenac (Systemic); Ibrutinib; Ifosfamide; PARoxetine; Saxagliptin; Simeprevir; TOLBUTamide; Warfarin

The levels/effects of Aprepitant may be decreased by: Bosentan; CYP3A4 Inducers (Strong); Dabrafenib; Deferasirox; Herbs (CYP3A4 Inducers); Mitotane; PARoxetine; Rifampin; Tocilizumab

Increased Effect/Toxicity

Aprepitant may increase the levels/effects of: ARIPiprazole; Avanafil; Benzodiazepines (metabolized by oxidation); Bosentan; Bosutinib; Budesonide (Systemic, Oral Inhalation); Cisapride; Colchicine; Corticosteroids (Systemic); CYP3A4 Substrates; Diltiazem; Dofetilide; DOXOrubicin (Conventional); Eplerenone; Everolimus; FentaNYL; Halofantrine; Ibrutinib; Imatinib; Ivabradine; Ivacaftor; Lomitapide; Lurasidone; OxyCODONE; Pimecrolimus; Pimozide; Propafenone; Ranolazine; Rivaroxaban; Salmeterol; Saxagliptin; Simeprevir; Tolvaptan; Ulipristal; Vilazodone; Zuclopenthixol

The levels/effects of Aprepitant may be increased by: Conivaptan; CYP3A4 Inhibitors (Moderate); CYP3A4 Inhibitors (Strong); Dasatinib; Diltiazem; Fusidic Acid (Systemic); Ivacaftor; Luliconazole; Mifepristone; Simeprevir; Stiripentol

Nutritional/Ethanol Interactions

Food: Aprepitant serum concentration may be increased when taken with grapefruit juice; avoid concurrent use.

Herb/Nutraceutical: Avoid St John's wort (may decrease aprepitant levels).

Adverse Reactions Note: Adverse reactions reported as part of a combination chemotherapy regimen or with general anesthesia.

>10%:
Central nervous system: Fatigue (≤18%)
Gastrointestinal: Nausea (6% to 13%), constipation (9% to 10%)
Neuromuscular & skeletal: Weakness (≤18%)
Miscellaneous: Hiccups (11%)
1% to 10%:
Cardiovascular: Hypotension (≤6%), bradycardia (≤4%)
Central nervous system: Dizziness (≤7%)
Endocrine & metabolic: Dehydration (≤6%)
Gastrointestinal: Diarrhea (≤10%), dyspepsia (≤6%), abdominal pain (≤5%), epigastric discomfort (4%), gastritis (4%), stomatitis (3%)
Hepatic: ALT increased (≤6%), AST increased (3%)
Renal: Proteinuria (7%), BUN increased (5%)

Available Dosage Forms

Capsule, Oral:
Emend: 40 mg, 80 mg, 125 mg, 80 mg (2s) and 125 mg (1s)

General Dosage Range Oral: *Adults:* 125 mg on day 1, followed by 80 mg on days 2 and 3 **or** 40 mg within 3 hours prior to induction with anesthesia

Administration

Oral

Chemotherapy-induced nausea/vomiting: Administer with or without food. First dose should be given 1 hour prior to antineoplastic therapy; subsequent doses should be given in the morning.

PONV: Administer within 3 hours prior to induction; follow healthcare providers instructions about food/drink restrictions prior to surgery.

Storage/Stability Store at room temperature of 20°C to 25°C (68°F to 77°F).

Nursing Actions

Physical Assessment Monitor for fatigue, weakness, constipation, low blood pressure, and dizziness. Monitor patient for increased level of sedation.

Patient Education

• Discuss specific use of drug and side effects with patient as it relates to treatment. (HCAHPS: During this hospital stay, were you given any medicine that you had not taken before? Before giving you any new medicine, how often did hospital staff tell you what the medicine was for? How often did hospital staff describe possible side effects in a way you could understand?)

• Patient may experience asthenia, diarrhea, lack of appetite, hiccups, constipation, alopecia, headache, pyrosis, or nausea. Have patient report immediately to prescriber signs of infection, severe dizziness, syncope, flushing, or signs of Stevens-Johnson syndrome/toxic epidermal necrolysis (HCAHPS).

• Educate patient about signs of a significant reaction (eg, wheezing; chest tightness; fever; itching; bad cough; blue skin color; seizures; or swelling of face, lips, tongue, or throat). **Note:** This is not a comprehensive list of all side effects. Patient should consult prescriber for additional questions.

Intended Use and Disclaimer: Should not be printed and given to patients. This information is intended to serve as a concise initial reference for healthcare professionals to use when discussing medications with a patient. You must ultimately rely on your own discretion, experience and judgment in diagnosing, treating and advising patients.

Dietary Considerations May be taken with or without food.

Arformoterol (ar for MOE ter ol)

Brand Names: U.S. Brovana

Index Terms (R,R)-Formoterol L-Tartrate; Arformoterol Tartrate

Pharmacologic Category Beta$_2$-Adrenergic Agonist; Beta$_2$-Adrenergic Agonist, Long-Acting

Medication Guide Available Yes

Pregnancy Risk Factor C

Lactation Excretion in breast milk unknown/use caution

Use Long-term maintenance treatment of bronchoconstriction in chronic obstructive pulmonary disease (COPD), including chronic bronchitis and emphysema

Available Dosage Forms

Nebulization Solution, Inhalation:
Brovana: 15 mcg/2 mL (2 mL)

General Dosage Range Nebulization: *Adults:* 5 mcg twice daily (maximum: 30 mcg/day)

Administration

Inhalation Nebulization: Remove each vial from individually sealed foil pouch immediately before use. Use with standard jet nebulizer connected to an air compressor, administer with mouthpiece or face mask. Administer vial undiluted and do not mix with other medications in nebulizer.

Nursing Actions

Physical Assessment Teach patient appropriate use and care of nebulizer.

Patient Education

- Discuss specific use of drug and side effects with patient as it relates to treatment. (HCAHPS: During this hospital stay, were you given any medicine that you had not taken before? Before giving you any new medicine, how often did hospital staff tell you what the medicine was for? How often did hospital staff describe possible side effects in a way you could understand?)
- Patient may experience back pain, diarrhea, rhinitis. Have patient report immediately to prescriber signs of hyperglycemia, signs of hypokalemia, angina, tachycardia, severe anxiety, considerable dizziness, syncope, chills, pharyngitis, edema of extremities, significant headache, intolerable nausea, difficulty speaking, severe dyspnea (HCAHPS).
- Educate patient about signs of a significant reaction (eg, wheezing; chest tightness; fever; itching; bad cough; blue skin color; seizures; or swelling of face, lips, tongue, or throat). **Note:** This is not a comprehensive list of all side effects. Patient should consult prescriber for additional questions.

Intended Use and Disclaimer: Should not be printed and given to patients. This information is intended to serve as a concise initial reference for healthcare professionals to use when discussing medications with a patient. You must ultimately rely on your own discretion, experience and judgment in diagnosing, treating and advising patients.

Argatroban (ar GA troh ban)

Pharmacologic Category Anticoagulant; Anticoagulant, Direct Thrombin Inhibitor

Medication Safety Issues

Sound-alike/look-alike issues:
Argatroban may be confused with Aggrastat®, Orgaran®

High alert medication:
The Institute for Safe Medication Practices (ISMP) includes this medication among its list of drugs which have a heightened risk of causing significant patient harm when used in error.

Pregnancy Risk Factor B

Lactation Excretion in breast milk unknown/not recommended

Use Prophylaxis or treatment of thrombosis in patients with heparin-induced thrombocytopenia (HIT); adjunct to percutaneous coronary intervention (PCI) in patients who have or are at risk of thrombosis associated with HIT

Unlabeled Use To maintain extracorporeal circuit patency (prefilter administration) of continuous renal replacement therapy (CRRT) in critically-ill patients with HIT

Available Dosage Forms

Solution, Intravenous:
Generic: 125 mg/125 mL (125 mL); 100 mg/mL (2.5 mL)

Solution, Intravenous [preservative free]:
Generic: 50 mg/50 mL (50 mL)

General Dosage Range Dosage adjustment recommended in patients with hepatic impairment

I.V.:

Children: Initial dose: 0.75 mcg/kg/minute; dosage may be adjusted in increments of 0.1-0.25 mcg/kg/minute

Adults: Bolus dose: 150-350 mcg/kg during procedure; Infusion: Initial: 2 mcg/kg/minute **or** 25 mcg/kg/minute during procedure; Maintenance: 0.5-10 mcg/kg/minute (maximum: 10 mcg/kg/minute) **or** 25-40 mcg/kg/minute during procedure

Adults (critically-ill): Initial: 0.2 mcg/kg/minute; Maintenance: 0.5-1.3 mcg/kg/minute

Usual Infusion Concentrations: Pediatric Note: Premixed solutions available.

I.V. infusion: 1000 mcg/mL

Usual Infusion Concentrations: Adult Note: Premixed solutions available.

I.V. infusion: 250 mg in 250 mL (concentration: 1000 mcg/mL) in D$_5$W or NS

Administration

I.V. The 2.5 mL (100 mg/mL) **concentrated** vial **must be diluted to 1 mg/mL** prior to administration. The premixed 50 mL or 125 mL (1 mg/mL) vial requires no further dilution. The premixed

1 mg/mL vial may be inverted for use with an infusion set.

Nursing Actions

Physical Assessment Monitor for abnormal bleeding, GI pain, epistaxis, hematuria, and irritation at infusion site. Observe bleeding precautions.

Patient Education

- Discuss specific use of drug and side effects with patient as it relates to treatment. (HCAHPS: During this hospital stay, were you given any medicine that you had not taken before? Before giving you any new medicine, how often did hospital staff tell you what the medicine was for? How often did hospital staff describe possible side effects in a way you could understand?)
- Patient may experience diarrhea. Have patient report immediately to prescriber severe dizziness, syncope, angina, arrhythmia, strength differences from one side to another, difficulty speaking or thinking, change in balance, blurred vision, illogical thinking, considerable headache, ecchymosis, hemorrhaging, significant nausea, hematemesis, hematuria, or melena (HCAHPS).
- Educate patient about signs of a significant reaction (eg, wheezing; chest tightness; fever; itching; bad cough; blue skin color; seizures; or swelling of face, lips, tongue, or throat). **Note:** This is not a comprehensive list of all side effects. Patient should consult prescriber for additional questions.

Intended Use and Disclaimer: Should not be printed and given to patients. This information is intended to serve as a concise initial reference for healthcare professionals to use when discussing medications with a patient. You must ultimately rely on your own discretion, experience and judgment in diagnosing, treating and advising patients.

Aripiprazole (ay ri PIP ray zole)

Brand Names: U.S. Abilify; Abilify Discmelt; Abilify Maintena

Index Terms BMS 337039; OPC-14597

Pharmacologic Category Antipsychotic Agent, Atypical

Medication Safety Issues

Sound-alike/look-alike issues:

Abilify may be confused with Ambien

ARIPiprazole may be confused with proton pump inhibitors (dexlansoprazole, esomeprazole, lansoprazole, omeprazole, pantoprazole, RABEprazole)

BEERS Criteria medication:

This drug may be potentially inappropriate for use in geriatric patients (Quality of evidence - moderate; Strength of recommendation - strong).

Other safety issues:

There are two formulations available for intramuscular administration: Abilify is an immediate release short-acting formulation and Abilify Maintena is an extended-release formulation. These products are **not** interchangeable.

Medication Guide Available Yes

Pregnancy Risk Factor C

Lactation Enters breast milk/not recommended

Breast-Feeding Considerations Aripiprazole is excreted in breast milk (Schlotterbeck, 2007; Watanabe, 2011). In one case report, milk concentrations were ~20% of the maternal plasma concentration (maternal dose: 15 mg/day; ~6 months postpartum) (Schlotterbeck, 2007); however, aripiprazole was not detected in the breast milk in a second case (limit of detection 10 ng/mL; maternal dose: 15 mg/day; ~1 month postpartum) (Lutz, 2010). Aripiprazole was also detected in the neonatal blood 6 days after delivery in a breast-fed infant also exposed during pregnancy. In this case report, the authors suggest in utero exposure could have contributed to the findings due to the long elimination half-life of aripiprazole (Watanabe, 2011). In one report, lactation was not able to be established, possibly due to changes in maternal prolactin potentially caused by aripiprazole (Mendhekar, 2006). The manufacturer recommends a decision be made whether to discontinue nursing or to discontinue the drug, taking into account the importance of treatment to the mother.

Use

Oral:

Bipolar I disorder: For the acute treatment of manic and mixed episodes associated with bipolar I disorder in pediatric patients 10 to 17 years of age as monotherapy; for the acute and maintenance treatment of manic and mixed episodes associated with bipolar I disorder in adults, both as monotherapy and as an adjunct to lithium or valproate.

Irritability associated with autistic disorder: For the treatment of irritability associated with autistic disorder in pediatric patients 6 to 17 years of age.

Major depressive disorder: For use as an adjunctive treatment to antidepressants for the treatment of major depressive disorder in adults.

Schizophrenia: For the acute treatment of schizophrenia in adolescents 13 to 17 years of age; for the acute and maintenance treatment of schizophrenia in adults.

Injection:

Agitation associated with schizophrenia or bipolar mania (immediate-release injection only): For the acute treatment of agitation associated with schizophrenia or bipolar mania, manic or mixed in adults.

Schizophrenia (extended-release injection only): For the treatment of schizophrenia in adults.

Unlabeled Use Depression with psychotic features; aggression (children); conduct disorder (children); Tourette syndrome (children); pervasive developmental disorder not otherwise specified (PDD-NOS) (children); Asperger's Disorder (children); psychosis/agitation related to Alzheimer's dementia

Mechanism of Action/Effect Aripiprazole (quinolinone antipsychotic) is a dopamine-serotonin system stabilizer with activity at dopamine and serotonin receptors.

Contraindications Known hypersensitivity (eg, anaphylaxis, pruritus, urticaria) to aripiprazole.

Warnings/Precautions [U.S. Boxed Warning]: Elderly patients with dementia-related psychosis treated with antipsychotics are at an increased risk of death compared to placebo. Most deaths appeared to be either cardiovascular (eg, heart failure, sudden death) or infectious (eg, pneumonia) in nature. In addition, an increased incidence of cerebrovascular effects (eg, transient ischemic attack, cerebrovascular accidents) has been reported in studies of placebo-controlled trials of aripiprazole in elderly patients with dementia-related psychosis. Aripiprazole is not approved for the treatment of dementia-related psychosis.

[U.S. Boxed Warning]: Antidepressants increase the risk of suicidal thinking and behavior in children, adolescents, and young adults (18-24 years of age) with major depressive disorder (MDD) and other psychiatric disorders; consider risk prior to prescribing. The possibility of a suicide attempt is inherent in major depression and may persist until remission occurs. Patients treated with antidepressants should be observed for clinical worsening and suicidality, especially during the initial few months of a course of drug therapy, or at times of dose changes, either increases or decreases. Prescriptions should be written for the smallest quantity consistent with good patient care. The patient's family or caregiver should be alerted to monitor patients for the emergence of suicidality and associated behaviors; patients should be instructed to notify their healthcare provider if any of these symptoms or worsening depression or psychosis occur.

Leukopenia, neutropenia, and agranulocytosis (sometimes fatal) have been reported in clinical trials and postmarketing reports with antipsychotic use; presence of risk factors (eg, pre-existing low WBC or history of drug-induced leuko-/neutropenia) should prompt periodic blood count assessment. Discontinue therapy at first signs of blood dyscrasias or if absolute neutrophil count <1000/mm^3.

A medication guide concerning the use of antidepressants should be dispensed with each prescription. **Aripiprazole is not FDA approved for adjunctive treatment of depression in children**

May cause extrapyramidal symptoms (EPS) including pseudoparkinsonism, acute dystonic reactions, akathisia, and tardive dyskinesia (risk of these reactions is very low relative to typical conventional antipsychotics, frequencies reported are similar to placebo). Risk of dystonia (and probably other EPS) may be greater with increased doses, use of conventional antipsychotics, males and younger patients. May be associated with neuroleptic malignant syndrome (NMS).

May be sedating, use with caution in disorders where CNS depression is a feature. May cause orthostatic hypotension (although reported rates are similar to placebo); use caution in patients at risk of this effect or those who would not tolerate transient hypotensive episodes (cerebrovascular disease, cardiovascular disease, or other medications which may predispose).

Use caution in patients with Parkinson's disease; predisposition to seizures; and severe cardiac disease. May alter cardiac conduction; life-threatening arrhythmias have occurred with therapeutic doses of antipsychotics. Esophageal dysmotility and aspiration have been associated with antipsychotic use; use caution in patients at risk of pneumonia (eg, Alzheimer's disease). May alter temperature regulation.

Atypical antipsychotics have been associated with metabolic changes including loss of glucose control, lipid changes, and weight gain (risk profile varies with product). Development of hyperglycemia in some cases, may be extreme and associated with ketoacidosis, hyperosmolar coma, or death. Reports of hyperglycemia with aripiprazole therapy have been few and specific risk associated with this agent is not known. Use caution in patients with diabetes or other disorders of glucose regulation; monitor for worsening of glucose control.

Use in elderly patients with dementia is associated with an increased risk of mortality and cerebrovascular accidents; avoid antipsychotic use for behavioral problems associated with dementia unless alternative nonpharmacologic therapies have failed and patient may harm self or others. In addition, use may cause or exacerbate syndrome of inappropriate antidiuretic hormone secretion or hyponatremia; monitor sodium closely with initiation or dosage adjustments in older adults (Beers Criteria).

Tablets contain lactose; avoid use in patients with galactose intolerance or glucose-galactose malabsorption.

Abilify Discmelt®: Use caution in phenylketonuria; contains phenylalanine.

There are two formulations available for intramuscular administration: Abilify® is an immediate release short-acting formulation and Abilify Maintena™ is an extended-release formulation. These products are **not** interchangeable.

Drug Interactions

Avoid Concomitant Use

Avoid concomitant use of ARIPiprazole with any of the following: Amisulpride; Azelastine (Nasal); Fusidic Acid (Systemic); Metoclopramide; Paraldehyde; Sulpiride; Thalidomide

Decreased Effect

ARIPiprazole may decrease the levels/effects of: Amphetamines; Anti-Parkinson's Agents (Dopamine Agonist); Haloperidol; Quinagolide

The levels/effects of ARIPiprazole may be decreased by: Bosentan; CYP3A4 Inducers; CYP3A4 Inducers (Strong); Dabrafenib; Deferasirox; Lithium formulations; Mitotane; Peginterferon Alfa-2b; Tocilizumab

Increased Effect/Toxicity

ARIPiprazole may increase the levels/effects of: Alcohol (Ethyl); Amisulpride; Azelastine (Nasal); Buprenorphine; CNS Depressants; DULoxetine; FLUoxetine; Haloperidol; Highest Risk QTc-Prolonging Agents; Hydrocodone; Methylphenidate; Moderate Risk QTc-Prolonging Agents; Paraldehyde; PARoxetine; Ritonavir; Serotonin Modulators; Sulpiride; Thalidomide; Zolpidem

The levels/effects of ARIPiprazole may be increased by: Abiraterone Acetate; Acetylcholinesterase Inhibitors (Central); Brimonidine (Topical); CYP2D6 Inhibitors (Moderate); CYP2D6 Inhibitors (Strong); CYP2D6 Inhibitors (Weak); CYP3A4 Inhibitors (Moderate); CYP3A4 Inhibitors (Strong); CYP3A4 Inhibitors (Weak); Dasatinib; Doxylamine; Droperidol; DULoxetine; FLUoxetine; Fusidic Acid (Systemic); Haloperidol; HydrOXYzine; Ivacaftor; Lithium formulations; Luliconazole; Magnesium Sulfate; Methylphenidate; Metoclopramide; Metyrosine; Mifepristone; PARoxetine; Perampanel; Ritonavir; Serotonin Modulators; Sertraline; Simeprevir; Sodium Oxybate; Tetrabenazine

Nutritional/Ethanol Interactions

Ethanol: May increase CNS depression; monitor for increased effects with coadministration. Caution patients about effects.

Food: Ingestion with a high-fat meal delays time to peak plasma level.

Herb/Nutraceutical: St John's wort may decrease aripiprazole levels. Avoid kava kava, gotu kola, valerian, St John's wort (may increase CNS depression).

Adverse Reactions Unless otherwise noted, frequency of adverse reactions is shown as reported for adult patients receiving oral administration. Spectrum and incidence of adverse effects similar in children; exceptions noted when incidence much higher in children.

>10%:

Central nervous system: Headache (adults 27%; children 13%; injection 12%), extrapyramidal reaction (dose-related; 8% to 26%), akathisia (dose-related; adults 2% to 25%; children 6% to 10%), cognitive dysfunction (children 24%; adults 11%; injection 9%), drowsiness (children 10% to 24%; adults 11%; injection 11%), sedation (dose-related; children 8% to 24%; adults 4% to 13%; injection 3% to 9%), fatigue (dose-related; children 4% to 22%; adults 6% to 8%; injection 2%), agitation (19%), insomnia (8% to 18%), anxiety (4% to 17%), restlessness (2% to 12%)

Gastrointestinal: Nausea (8% to 15%; injection 9%), vomiting (4% to 14%; injection 3%), constipation (adults 5% to 11%; children 3%)

1% to 10%:

Cardiovascular: Chest pain (1% to 10%), tachycardia (2%; injection <1%), hypertension (≥1%), orthostatic hypotension (including injection, ≤1%), peripheral edema (≥1%)

Central nervous system: Dizziness (3% to 10%; injection 8%), drooling (children 4% to 9%), lethargy (children 2% to 5%), nervousness (3%), pain (3%), ataxia (≥1%), dystonia (children 1%), hypersomnia (children 1%)

Dermatologic: Skin rash (children ≥1% to 2%)

Endocrine & metabolic: Weight gain (≥7% body weight; 2% to 8%), weight loss (>1%), increased thirst (children 1%)

Gastrointestinal: Dyspepsia (9%), sialorrhea (dose-related; 3% to 8%), decreased appetite (children 4% to 7%), increased appetite (children 3% to 7%), diarrhea (children 5%), xerostomia (adults 2% to 5%; children 1%), toothache (4%), abdominal distress (3%), gastric distress (3%), upper abdominal pain (children 3%)

Genitourinary: Dysmenorrhea (children 2%)

Local: Injection site reaction (injection >1%)

Neuromuscular & skeletal: Increased creatine phosphokinase (1% to 10%), tremor (dose-related; 5% to 10%), weakness (1% to 10%), arthralgia (adults 4%; children 1%), limb pain (4%), stiffness (adults 4%; children 1%), myalgia (2% to 3%), muscle cramps (2%), muscle spasm (2%), dyskinesia (children 1%)

Ophthalmic: Blurred vision (3% to 8%), accommodation disturbance (3%)

Respiratory: Aspiration pneumonia (1% to 10%), dyspnea (1% to 10%), nasal congestion (1% to 10%), upper respiratory tract infection (6%), nasopharyngitis (children 3% to 6%), cough (3%), pharyngolaryngeal pain (3%), rhinorrhea (children 2%)

Miscellaneous: Fever (children 5% to 9%)

Pharmacodynamics/Kinetics

Onset of Action Initial: 1-3 weeks

Available Dosage Forms

Solution, Intramuscular:

Abilify: 9.75 mg/1.3 mL (1.3 mL)

Solution, Oral:

Abilify: 1 mg/mL (150 mL)

Suspension Reconstituted, Intramuscular:

Abilify Maintena: 300 mg (1 ea); 400 mg (1 ea)

Tablet, Oral:

Abilify: 2 mg, 5 mg, 10 mg, 15 mg, 20 mg, 30 mg

Tablet Dispersible, Oral:

Abilify Discmelt: 10 mg, 15 mg

General Dosage Range Dosage adjustment recommended in patients on concomitant therapy or with CYP2D6 poor metabolizer status

Oral:

Children 6-9 years: 5-15 mg once daily (maximum: 15 mg daily)

Children ≥10 years: 5-30 mg once daily (maximum: 30 mg daily)

Adults: 10-30 mg once daily (maximum: 30 mg daily)

I.M.: *Adults:* Immediate release: 5.25-30 mg daily (maximum: 30 mg daily); Extended release: 400 mg once monthly

Administration

I.M. Injection: For I.M. use only; do not administer SubQ or I.V.; **Note:** Immediate release and extended release parenteral products are **not** interchangeable.

Immediate release (Abilify®): Inject slowly into deep muscle mass

Extended release (Abilify Maintena™): Inject slowly into gluteal muscle using the provided 1.5 inch (38 mm) needle for nonobese patients or the provided 2 inch (50 mm) needle for obese patients. Do not massage muscle after administration. Rotate injection sites between the two gluteal muscles. Administer monthly (doses should be separated by ≥26 days).

Oral May be administered with or without food. Tablet and oral solution may be interchanged on a mg-per-mg basis, up to 25 mg. Doses using 30 mg tablets should be exchanged for 25 mg oral solution. Orally disintegrating tablets (Abilify Discmelt®) are bioequivalent to the immediate release tablets (Abilify®).

Orally disintegrating tablet: Remove from foil blister by peeling back (do not push tablet through the foil). Place tablet in mouth immediately upon removal. Tablet dissolves rapidly in saliva and may be swallowed without liquid. If needed, can be taken with liquid. Do not split tablet.

Preparation for Administration

Injection, powder for reconstitution: Reconstitute using 1.5 mL sterile water for injection (SWFI) (provided) for the 300 mg vial or 1.9 mL SWFI (provided) for the 400 mg vial to a final concentration of 200 mg/mL; residual SWFI should be discarded after reconstitution. Shake vigorously for 30 seconds or until the suspension is uniform; the resulting suspension will be milky white and opaque. If the suspension is not administered immediately after reconstitution, shake vigorously for 60 seconds prior to administration.

Storage/Stability

Injection, powder for reconstitution: Store unused vials at 25°C (77°F); excursions permitted to 15°C to 30°C (59°F to 86°F). If the suspension is not administered immediately after reconstitution, store at room temperature in the vial (do not store in a syringe); shake vigorously for 60 seconds prior to administration.

Injection solution: Store at 25°C (77°F); excursions permitted to 15°C to 30°C (59°F to 86°F). Protect from light.

Oral solution: Store at 25°C (77°F); excursions permitted to 15°C to 30°C (59°F to 86°F). Use within 6 months after opening.

Tablet: Store at 25°C (77°F); excursions permitted to 15°C to 30°C (59°F to 86°F).

Nursing Actions

Physical Assessment Educate patient about and monitor for insomnia, anxiety, oversedation, GI tolerance, and weight gain. Assess for signs and symptoms of hyperglycemia.

Assess vital signs, blood pressure, mental status including thoughts of suicide, abnormal involuntary movements, and extrapyramidal symptoms. Obtain weight and waist circumference prior to treatment, at 4 weeks, 8 weeks, 12 weeks, and then at quarterly intervals. Monitor for extrapyramidal symptoms prior to and periodically during therapy, particularly akathisia (restlessness).

Patient Education

• Discuss specific use of drug and side effects with patient as it relates to treatment. (HCAHPS: During this hospital stay, were you given any medicine that you had not taken before? Before giving you any new medicine, how often did hospital staff tell you what the medicine was for? How often did hospital staff describe possible side effects in a way you could understand?)

• Patient may experience fatigue, asthenia, akathisia, anxiety, headache, nausea, weight gain, constipation, insomnia, polyphagia, lack of appetite, rhinitis, pharyngitis, xerostomia, tremors, or sialorrhea. Have patient report immediately to prescriber signs of infection, signs of hyperglycemia, difficulty with motor activity, fasciculations, change in balance, dysphagia,

difficulty speaking, suicidal ideation, severe dizziness, syncope, severe asthenia, blurred vision, signs of neuroleptic malignant syndrome (NMS), or signs of tardive dyskinesia (HCAHPS).
- Educate patient about signs of a significant reaction (eg, wheezing; chest tightness; fever; itching; bad cough; blue skin color; swelling of face, lips, tongue, or throat). **Note:** This is not a comprehensive list of all side effects. Patient should consult prescriber for additional questions.

Intended Use and Disclaimer: Should not be printed and given to patients. This information is intended to serve as a concise initial reference for healthcare professionals to use when discussing medications with a patient. You must ultimately rely on your own discretion, experience and judgment in diagnosing, treating and advising patients.

Dietary Considerations May be taken with or without food. Some products may contain phenylalanine.

Armodafinil (ar moe DAF i nil)

Brand Names: U.S. Nuvigil
Index Terms R-modafinil
Pharmacologic Category Central Nervous System Stimulant
Medication Guide Available Yes
Pregnancy Risk Factor C
Lactation Excretion in breast milk unknown/use caution
Breast-Feeding Considerations It is not known if armodafinil or its metabolite is excreted into breast milk. The manufacture recommends caution be used if administered to a nursing woman.
Use Improve wakefulness in patients with excessive daytime sleepiness associated with narcolepsy and shift work sleep disorder (SWSD); adjunctive therapy for obstructive sleep apnea/hypopnea syndrome (OSAHS)
Mechanism of Action/Effect Armodafinil is a stimulant with effects. The exact mechanism of action of armodafinil is unknown.
Contraindications Hypersensitivity to armodafinil, modafinil, or any component of the formulation
Warnings/Precautions For use following complete evaluation of sleepiness and in conjunction with other standard treatments (eg, CPAP). The degree of sleepiness should be reassessed frequently; some patients may not return to a normal level of wakefulness. Patients with excessive sleepiness should be advised to avoid driving or any other potentially dangerous activity. Use >12 weeks has not been studied; patient should be reevaluated to determine effectiveness if use exceeds 12 weeks. Use is not recommended in patients with a history of angina or myocardial infarction, left ventricular hypertrophy, or patients with mitral valve prolapse who have developed mitral valve prolapse syndrome with previous CNS stimulant use. Patients with these conditions may also experience chest pain, palpitations, dyspnea, and transient ischemic T-wave changes on ECG. Increased blood pressure monitoring may be required in patients taking armodafinil. New or additional antihypertensive therapy may be needed.

Serious and life-threatening rashes including Stevens-Johnson syndrome, toxic epidermal necrolysis, and drug rash with eosinophilia and systemic symptoms (DRESS) have been reported. In modafinil clinical trials, rashes were more likely to occur in children; serious, postmarketing reactions have occurred with modafinil in adults and children as well as with armodafinil in adults. Most cases have been reported within the first 5 weeks of initiating therapy; however, rare cases have occurred after prolonged therapy. No risk factors have been identified to predict occurrence or severity of these reactions. Patients should be advised to discontinue use at first sign of rash (unless the rash is clearly not drug-related). Rare cases of multiorgan hypersensitivity reactions (with modafinil) and cases of angioedema and anaphylactoid reactions (armodafinil) have been reported. Signs and symptoms of multiorgan hypersensitivity reactions are diverse. Patients typically present with fever and rash associated with other organ system involvement. Patients should be advised to discontinue therapy and promptly report any signs or symptoms related to these adverse effects.

Caution should be exercised when modafinil is given to patients with a history of psychosis, depression, or mania; use may worsen symptoms (eg, mania, hallucinations, suicidal thoughts) of these disease; discontinue therapy if psychiatric symptoms develop. Use may impair the ability to engage in potentially hazardous activities; patients must be cautioned about performing tasks which require mental alertness (eg, operating machinery or driving). Stimulants may unmask tics in individuals with coexisting Tourette's syndrome. Use caution with hepatic impairment; consider use of a reduced dosage in patients with hepatic impairment or elderly patients. Safety and efficacy have not been established in patients with severe renal impairment. Use with caution in patients with a history of drug abuse; potential for drug dependency exists.

Drug Interactions
Avoid Concomitant Use
Avoid concomitant use of Armodafinil with any of the following: Axitinib; Conivaptan; Fusidic Acid (Systemic); Iobenguane I 123; Simeprevir

Decreased Effect
Armodafinil may decrease the levels/effects of: ARIPiprazole; Axitinib; Clopidogrel; Contraceptives (Estrogens); CycloSPORINE (Systemic);

Ibrutinib; Iobenguane I 123; Saxagliptin; Simeprevir

The levels/effects of Armodafinil may be decreased by: Bosentan; CYP3A4 Inducers (Strong); Dabrafenib; Deferasirox; Herbs (CYP3A4 Inducers); Mitotane; Tocilizumab

Increased Effect/Toxicity

Armodafinil may increase the levels/effects of: Citalopram; CYP2C19 Substrates; Sympathomimetics

The levels/effects of Armodafinil may be increased by: AtoMOXetine; Cannabinoids; Conivaptan; CYP3A4 Inhibitors (Moderate); CYP3A4 Inhibitors (Strong); Dasatinib; Fusidic Acid (Systemic); Ivacaftor; Linezolid; Luliconazole; Mifepristone; Simeprevir; Stiripentol

Nutritional/Ethanol Interactions

Ethanol: Avoid or limit ethanol.

Food: Delays absorption, but minimal effects on bioavailability. Food may affect the onset and time course of armodafinil.

Adverse Reactions

>10%: Central nervous system: Headache (14% to 23%; dose-related)

1% to 10%:

Cardiovascular: Palpitation (2%), heart rate increased (1%)

Central nervous system: Dizziness (5%), insomnia (4% to 6%; dose related), anxiety (4%), depression (1% to 3%; dose related), fatigue (2%), agitation (1%), attention disturbance (1%), depressed mood (1%), migraine (1%), nervousness (1%), pain (1%), pyrexia (1%), tremor (1%)

Dermatologic: Rash (1% to 4%; dose related), contact dermatitis (1%), hyperhidrosis (1%)

Gastrointestinal: Nausea (6% to 9%; dose related), xerostomia (2% to 7%; dose related), diarrhea (4%), abdominal pain (2%), dyspepsia (2%), anorexia (1%), appetite decreased (1%), constipation (1%), loose stools (1%), vomiting (1%)

Genitourinary: Polyuria (1%)

Hepatic: GGT increased (1%)

Neuromuscular & skeletal: Paresthesia (1%)

Respiratory: Dyspnea (1%)

Miscellaneous: Flu-like syndrome (1%), seasonal allergy (1%), thirst (1%)

Controlled Substance C-IV

Available Dosage Forms

Tablet, Oral:

Nuvigil: 50 mg, 150 mg, 200 mg, 250 mg

General Dosage Range

Oral: *Adults:* 150-250 mg once daily

Administration

Oral May be administered without regard to food.

Storage/Stability Store at 20°C to 25°C (68°F to 77°F).

Nursing Actions

Physical Assessment Monitor blood pressure at the beginning of therapy and periodically throughout.

Patient Education

- Discuss specific use of drug and side effects with patient as it relates to treatment. (HCAHPS: During this hospital stay, were you given any medicine that you had not taken before? Before giving you any new medicine, how often did hospital staff tell you what the medicine was for? How often did hospital staff describe possible side effects in a way you could understand?)
- Patient may experience anxiety, akathisia, diarrhea, insomnia, back pain, dizziness, dyspepsia, or rhinitis. Have patient report immediately to prescriber signs of hepatic impairment, signs of depression (ie, suicidal ideation, anxiety, emotional instability, illogical thinking), hallucinations, angina, tachycardia, severe headache, arrhythmia, chills, pharyngitis, dyspnea, edema of extremities, ecchymosis, hemorrhaging, significant asthenia, or signs of Stevens-Johnson syndrome/toxic epidermal necrolysis (HCAHPS).
- Educate patient about signs of a significant reaction (eg, wheezing; chest tightness; fever; itching; bad cough; blue skin color; seizures; or swelling of face, lips, tongue, or throat). **Note:** This is not a comprehensive list of all side effects. Patient should consult prescriber for additional questions.

Intended Use and Disclaimer: Should not be printed and given to patients. This information is intended to serve as a concise initial reference for healthcare professionals to use when discussing medications with a patient. You must ultimately rely on your own discretion, experience and judgment in diagnosing, treating and advising patients.

Dietary Considerations Take with or without meals.

Arsenic Trioxide (AR se nik tri OKS id)

Brand Names: U.S. Trisenox

Index Terms As_2O_3

Pharmacologic Category Antineoplastic Agent, Miscellaneous

Medication Safety Issues

High alert medication:

This medication is in a class the Institute for Safe Medication Practices (ISMP) includes among its list of drugs which have a heightened risk of causing significant patient harm when used in error.

Pregnancy Risk Factor D

Lactation Enters breast milk/not recommended

Use Remission induction and consolidation in patients with relapsed or refractory acute promyelocytic leukemia (APL) characterized by t(15;17) translocation or PML/RAR-alpha gene expression

Unlabeled Use Initial treatment of APL, treatment of myelodysplastic syndrome (MDS)

Available Dosage Forms

Solution, Intravenous:

Trisenox: 10 mg/10 mL (10 mL)

General Dosage Range Dosage adjustment recommended for renal impairment.

I.V.: *Children ≥4 years and Adults:* Induction: 0.15 mg/kg/day (maximum: 60 doses); Consolidation: 0.15 mg/kg/day (maximum: 25 doses over a period of up to 5 weeks)

Administration

I.V. I.V. infusion over 1-2 hours. If acute vasomotor reactions occur, infuse over a maximum of 4 hours. Does not require administration via a central venous catheter.

Hazardous agent; use appropriate precautions for handling and disposal (NIOSH, 2012).

Injectable Detail pH: 7.5-8.5

Nursing Actions

Physical Assessment Monitor cardiac and electrolyte status at beginning of and periodically during therapy.

Patient Education

• Discuss specific use of drug and side effects with patient as it relates to treatment. (HCAHPS: During this hospital stay, were you given any medicine that you had not taken before? Before giving you any new medicine, how often did hospital staff tell you what the medicine was for? How often did hospital staff describe possible side effects in a way you could understand?)

• Patient may experience nausea, constipation, lack of appetite, weight gain, insomnia, osteodynia, arthralgia, myalgia, back pain, pharyngitis, hyperhidrosis, tremors, eye irritation, or blurred vision. Have patient report immediately to prescriber signs of infection, signs of hyperglycemia, signs of hypokalemia, dyspnea, tachypnea, angina, tachycardia, arrhythmia, edema, severe dizziness, syncope, considerable headache, significant asthenia, depression, illogical thinking, anxiety, intolerable diarrhea, ecchymosis, hemorrhaging, vaginal hemorrhaging, severe dyspepsia, melena, hematemesis, pallor, urinary retention, oliguria, paresthesia, considerable injection site irritation (HCAHPS).

• Educate patient about signs of a significant reaction (eg, wheezing; chest tightness; fever; itching; bad cough; blue skin color; seizures; or swelling of face, lips, tongue, or throat). **Note:** This is not a comprehensive list of all side effects. Patient should consult prescriber for additional questions.

Intended Use and Disclaimer: Should not be printed and given to patients. This information is intended to serve as a concise initial reference for healthcare professionals to use when discussing medications with a patient. You must ultimately rely on your own discretion, experience and judgment in diagnosing, treating and advising patients.

Related Information

Management of Drug Extravasations *on page 1700*

Asenapine (a SEN a peen)

Brand Names: U.S. Saphris

Pharmacologic Category Antimanic Agent; Antipsychotic Agent, Atypical

Medication Safety Issues

BEERS Criteria medication:

This drug may be potentially inappropriate for use in geriatric patients (Quality of evidence - moderate; Strength of recommendation - strong).

Pregnancy Risk Factor C

Lactation Excretion in breast milk unknown/not recommended

Breast-Feeding Considerations It is not known if asenapine is excreted into breast milk. Breast-feeding is not recommended by the manufacturer.

Use Acute and maintenance treatment of schizophrenia; treatment of acute mania or mixed episodes associated with bipolar I disorder (as monotherapy or in combination with lithium or valproate)

Mechanism of Action/Effect Atypical antipsychotic with high affinity for serotonin, dopamine, alpha$_1$- and alpha$_2$-adrenergic receptors, and histamine receptors; no affinity for muscarinic receptors. Results in improvement of psychotic symptoms and reduction of extrapyramidal and antimuscarinic side effects as compared to typical antipsychotics.

Contraindications Hypersensitivity to asenapine or any component of the formulation

Warnings/Precautions [U.S. Boxed Warning]: Elderly patients with dementia-related psychosis treated with atypical antipsychotics are at an increased risk of death compared to placebo. Most deaths appeared to be either cardiovascular (eg, heart failure, sudden death) or infectious (eg, pneumonia) in nature. In addition, an increased incidence of cerebrovascular effects (eg, transient ischemic attack, cerebrovascular accidents) has been reported in studies of antipsychotics in elderly patients with dementia-related psychosis. Asenapine is not approved for the treatment of dementia-related psychosis.

Use in elderly patients with dementia is associated with an increased risk of mortality and cerebrovascular accidents; avoid antipsychotic use for behavioral problems associated with dementia unless alternative nonpharmacologic therapies have failed and patient may harm self or others. In addition, use may cause or exacerbate syndrome of inappropriate antidiuretic hormone secretion or hyponatremia; monitor sodium closely with initiation or dosage adjustments in older adults (Beers Criteria). Pharmacokinetic studies showed a decrease in clearance in older adults (65-85 years of age) with psychosis compared to younger adults; increased risk of adverse effects and orthostasis may occur.

Leukopenia, neutropenia, and agranulocytosis (sometimes fatal) have been reported in clinical trials and postmarketing reports with antipsychotic use; presence of risk factors (eg, pre-existing low WBC or history of drug-induced leuko/neutropenia) should prompt periodic blood count assessment. Discontinue therapy at first signs of blood dyscrasias or if absolute neutrophil count <1000/mm^3.

May be sedating; use with caution in disorders where CNS depression is a feature. Use with caution in Parkinson's disease. Use with caution in patients at risk of seizures, including those with a history of seizures, head trauma, brain damage, alcoholism, or concurrent therapy with medications which may lower seizure threshold. Use is not recommended in severe hepatic impairment; increased drug concentrations may occur. Esophageal dysmotility and aspiration have been associated with antipsychotic use; use with caution in patients at risk of aspiration pneumonia (ie, Alzheimer's disease). Elevates prolactin levels; use with caution in breast cancer or other prolactin-dependent tumors. May alter temperature regulation.

Use with caution in patients with cardiovascular diseases (eg, heart failure, history of myocardial infarction or ischemia, cerebrovascular disease, conduction abnormalities). May cause orthostatic hypotension; use with caution in patients at risk of this effect (eg, concurrent medication use which may predispose to hypotension/bradycardia or presence of hypovolemia) or in those who would not tolerate transient hypotensive episodes. May result in QT$_c$ prolongation. Risk may be increased by conditions or concomitant medications which cause bradycardia, hypokalemia, and/or hypomagnesemia. Avoid use in combination with QT$_c$-prolonging drugs and in patients with congenital long QT syndrome or patients with history of cardiac arrhythmia.

May cause extrapyramidal symptoms (EPS), including pseudoparkinsonism, acute dystonic reactions, akathisia, and tardive dyskinesia. Risk of dystonia (and probably other EPS) may be greater with increased doses, use of conventional antipsychotics, males, and younger patients. Risk of neuroleptic malignant syndrome (NMS) may be increased in patients with Parkinson's disease or Lewy body dementia. May cause hyperglycemia; in some cases may be extreme and associated with ketoacidosis, hyperosmolar coma, or death. Use with caution in patients with diabetes or other disorders of glucose regulation; monitor for worsening of glucose control. Dyslipidemia has been reported with atypical antipsychotics; risk profile may differ between agents. In clinical trials, the incidence of hypertriglyceridemia observed with asenapine was greater than that observed with placebo, while total cholesterol elevations were similar. Significant weight gain has been observed with antipsychotic therapy; incidence varies with product. Monitor waist circumference and BMI. May cause anaphylaxis or hypersensitivity reactions.

The possibility of a suicide attempt is inherent in psychotic illness or bipolar disorder; use caution in high-risk patients during initiation of therapy. Prescriptions should be written for the smallest quantity consistent with good patient care.

Drug Interactions

Avoid Concomitant Use

Avoid concomitant use of Asenapine with any of the following: Amisulpride; Azelastine (Nasal); Highest Risk QTc-Prolonging Agents; Ivabradine; Metoclopramide; Mifepristone; Moderate Risk QTc-Prolonging Agents; Paraldehyde; Sulpiride; Thalidomide

Decreased Effect

Asenapine may decrease the levels/effects of: Amphetamines; Anti-Parkinson's Agents (Dopamine Agonist); Quinagolide

The levels/effects of Asenapine may be decreased by: CYP1A2 Inducers (Strong); Cyproterone; Lithium formulations; Peginterferon Alfa-2b

Increased Effect/Toxicity

Asenapine may increase the levels/effects of: Alcohol (Ethyl); Amisulpride; ARIPiprazole; Azelastine (Nasal); Buprenorphine; CNS Depressants; Highest Risk QTc-Prolonging Agents; Hydrocodone; Methotrimeprazine; Methylphenidate; Paraldehyde; PARoxetine; Serotonin Modulators; Sulpiride; Thalidomide; Zolpidem

The levels/effects of Asenapine may be increased by: Abiraterone Acetate; Acetylcholinesterase Inhibitors (Central); Brimonidine (Topical); CYP1A2 Inhibitors (Moderate); CYP1A2 Inhibitors (Strong); Deferasirox; Doxylamine; FluvoxaMINE; HydrOXYzine; Ivabradine; Lithium formulations; Magnesium Sulfate; MAO Inhibitors; Methotrimeprazine; Methylphenidate; Metoclopramide; Metyrosine; Mifepristone; Moderate Risk QTc-Prolonging Agents; PARoxetine; Perampanel; QTc-Prolonging Agents (Indeterminate Risk and Risk Modifying); Serotonin Modulators; Sodium Oxybate; Tetrabenazine

Nutritional/Ethanol Interactions Ethanol: May increase CNS depression; monitor for increased effects with coadministration. Caution patients about effects.

Adverse Reactions Actual frequency may be dependent upon dose and/or indication.

>10%:

Central nervous system: Drowsiness (13% to 24%), insomnia (6% to 16%), extrapyramidal reaction (6% to 12%), headache (12%), akathisia (4% to 11%; dose related), dizziness (3% to 11%)

Endocrine & metabolic: Hypertriglyceridemia (13% to 15%), weight gain (2% to 15%)

Neuromuscular and skeletal: Increased creatine kinase (6% to 11%)

1% to 10%:

Cardiovascular: Peripheral edema (3%), hypertension (2% to 3%)

Central nervous system: Hypoesthesia (4% to 7%), fatigue (3% to 4%), anxiety (4%), depression (2%), irritability (1% to 2%)

Endocrine & metabolic: Increased serum cholesterol (8% to 9%), increased serum glucose (5% to 7%), hyperprolactinemia (2% to 3%)

Gastrointestinal: Constipation (4% to 7%), vomiting (4% to 7%), dyspepsia (3% to 4%), increased appetite (≤4%), increased salivation (≤4%), dysgeusia (3%), toothache (3%), abdominal distress (≤3%), xerostomia (1% to 3%)

Hepatic: Increased serum transaminases (<1% to 3%)

Neuromuscular & skeletal: Arthralgia (3%), limb pain (2%)

Available Dosage Forms

Tablet Sublingual, Sublingual:

Saphris: 5 mg, 10 mg

General Dosage Range Oral: *Adults:* 5-10 mg twice daily

Administration

Oral Sublingual tablets should be placed under the tongue and allowed to disintegrate. Do not crush, chew, or swallow. Avoid eating or drinking for at least 10 minutes after administration.

Storage/Stability Store at 15°C to 30°C (59°F to 86°F).

Nursing Actions

Physical Assessment Monitor weight prior to treatment and periodically throughout. Be alert to the potential for orthostatic hypotension, especially during the titration phase. Initiate at lower doses and titrate to target dose. Taper dosage slowly when discontinuing.

Patient Education

• Discuss specific use of drug and side effects with patient as it relates to treatment. (HCAHPS: During this hospital stay, were you given any medicine that you had not taken before? Before giving you any new medicine, how often did hospital staff tell you what the medicine was for? How often did hospital staff describe possible side effects in a way you could understand?)

• Patient may experience fatigue, headache, akathisia, emesis, paresthesia of mouth, insomnia, or constipation. Have patient report immediately to prescriber signs of hyperglycemia, suicidal ideation, arrhythmia, bradycardia, tachycardia, dyspnea, severe dizziness, syncope, difficulty with motor activity, fasciculations, change in balance, dysphagia, difficulty speaking, menstrual irregularities, macromastia, nipple discharge, sexual dysfunction, stomatitis, signs of neuroleptic malignant syndrome (NMS), or signs of tardive dyskinesia (HCAHPS).

• Educate patient about signs of a significant reaction (eg, wheezing; chest tightness; fever; itching; bad cough; blue skin color; seizures; or swelling of face, lips, tongue, or throat). **Note:** This is not a comprehensive list of all side effects. Patient should consult prescriber for additional questions.

Intended Use and Disclaimer: Should not be printed and given to patients. This information is intended to serve as a concise initial reference for healthcare professionals to use when discussing medications with a patient. You must ultimately rely on your own discretion, experience and judgment in diagnosing, treating and advising patients.

Dietary Considerations Avoid eating or drinking for at least 10 minutes after administration.

Related Information

Oral Medications That Should Not Be Crushed or Altered *on page 1712*

Asparaginase *(E. coli)*

(a SPEAR a ji nase e ko lye)

Brand Names: U.S. Elspar [DSC]

Index Terms *E. coli* Asparaginase; ASNase; Asparaginase; L-ASP; L-asparaginase (*E. coli*)

Pharmacologic Category Antineoplastic Agent, Enzyme; Antineoplastic Agent, Miscellaneous

Medication Safety Issues

Sound-alike/look-alike issues:

Asparaginase (*E. coli*) may be confused with asparaginase (*Erwinia*), pegaspargase

Elspar may be confused with Elaprase, Erwinaze, Oncaspar

High alert medication:

This medication is in a class the Institute for Safe Medication Practices (ISMP) includes among its list of drug classes which have a heightened risk of causing significant patient harm when used in error.

Pregnancy Risk Factor C

Lactation Excretion in breast milk unknown/not recommended

Use Acute lymphoblastic leukemia (ALL): Treatment (in combination with other chemotherapy) of ALL

Unlabeled Use Treatment of lymphoblastic lymphoma

◀ **Product Availability** Elspar: Manufacturing of asparaginase *(E. coli)* was discontinued by Lundbeck at the end of 2012. Elspar was acquired by Recordati Rare Diseases; availability information is currently unavailable.

General Dosage Range I.M., I.V.: *Children, Adolescents, and Adults:* 6000 units/m^2/dose 3 times weekly

Administration

I.M. Observe patients for 1 hour after administration; have epinephrine, diphenhydramine, and hydrocortisone at the bedside. A physician should be readily accessible. Doses should be given as a deep intramuscular injection into a large muscle; volumes >2 mL should be divided and administered in 2 separate sites.

Hazardous agent; use appropriate precautions for handling and disposal (NIOSH, 2012).

I.V.

Observe patients for 1 hour after administration; have epinephrine, diphenhydramine, and hydrocortisone at the bedside. A physician should be readily accessible.

Infuse over at least 30 minutes through the side arm of a NS or D$_5$W infusion.

Gelatinous fiber-like particles may develop on standing. Filtration through a 5-micron filter during administration will remove the particles with no loss of potency.

Hazardous agent; use appropriate precautions for handling and disposal (NIOSH, 2012).

Subcutaneous

Has been administered SubQ (unlabeled route) in specific protocols (Larson, 1995). Observe patients for 1 hour after administration; have epinephrine, diphenhydramine, and hydrocortisone at the bedside. A physician should be readily accessible.

Hazardous agent; use appropriate precautions for handling and disposal (NIOSH, 2012).

Nursing Actions

Physical Assessment With each dose, monitor patient closely for CNS changes, acute hypersensitivity reaction (may occur in 10% to 35% of patients and may be fatal), hyperglycemia, nausea, or vomiting. In the event of hypersensitivity or hyperglycemia, stop infusion and notify prescriber immediately.

Patient Education

• Discuss specific use of drug and side effects with patient as it relates to treatment. (HCAHPS: During this hospital stay, were you given any medicine that you had not taken before? Before giving you any new medicine, how often did hospital staff tell you what the medicine was for? How often did hospital staff describe possible side effects in a way you could understand?)

• Have patient report immediately to prescriber signs of pancreatitis, signs of hyperglycemia, signs of hepatic impairment, strength differences from one side to another, difficulty speaking or thinking, change in balance, blurred eyesight, edema of extremities, angina, hemoptysis, dyspnea, severe headache, ecchymosis, hemorrhaging, hallucinations, vision changes, illogical thinking, urinary retention, oliguria, or signs of tumor lysis syndrome (TLS) (HCAHPS).

• Educate patient about signs of a significant reaction (eg, wheezing; chest tightness; fever; itching; bad cough; blue skin color; seizures; swelling of face, lips, tongue, or throat). **Note:** This is not a comprehensive list of all side effects. Patient should consult prescriber for additional questions.

Intended Use and Disclaimer: Should not be printed and given to patients. This information is intended to serve as a concise initial reference for healthcare professionals to use when discussing medications with a patient. You must ultimately rely on your own discretion, experience and judgment in diagnosing, treating and advising patients.

Asparaginase *(Erwinia)*
(a SPEAR a ji nase er WIN i ah)

Brand Names: U.S. Erwinaze

Index Terms *Erwinia chrysanthemi*; Asparaginase *Erwinia chrysanthemi*; L-asparaginase *(Erwinia)*

Pharmacologic Category Antineoplastic Agent, Enzyme; Antineoplastic Agent, Miscellaneous

Medication Safety Issues

Sound-alike/look-alike issues:

Asparaginase *(Erwinia)* may be confused with asparaginase *(E. coli)*, pegaspargase

Erwinaze™ may be confused with Elaprase®, Elspar®, Oncaspar®

High alert medication:

This medication is in a class the Institute for Safe Medication Practices (ISMP) includes among its list of drug classes which have a heightened risk of causing significant patient harm when used in error.

Pregnancy Risk Factor C

Lactation Excretion in breast milk unknown/not recommended

Use Treatment (in combination with other chemotherapy) of acute lymphoblastic leukemia (ALL) in patients with hypersensitivity to *E. coli*-derived asparaginase

Available Dosage Forms

Solution Reconstituted, Intramuscular:

Erwinaze: 10,000 units (1 ea)

General Dosage Range I.M.: *Children and Adults:* 25,000 units/m^2 3 times/week (Mon, Wed, Fri) for 6 doses for each planned pegaspargase dose **or** 25,000 units/m^2 for each planned asparaginase *(E. coli)* dose

Administration

I.M. Volume of each single injection site should be limited to 2 mL; use multiple injections for volumes >2 mL

Hazardous agent; use appropriate precautions for handling and disposal (NIOSH, 2012).

I.V. *Canadian labeling (additional administration routes not in the U.S. labeling):* May also be administered I.V., although I.M. and SubQ are preferred.

Hazardous agent; use appropriate precautions for handling and disposal (NIOSH, 2012).

Other *Canadian labeling (additional administration routes not in the U.S. labeling):* May also be administered SubQ, (I.M. and SubQ are the preferred routes).

Hazardous agent; use appropriate precautions for handling and disposal (NIOSH, 2012).

Nursing Actions

Physical Assessment With each dose, patient should be monitored closely for acute hypersensitivity reactions, hyperglycemia, pancreatitis, and thrombosis. In event of hypersensitivity or hyperglycemia, infusion should be stopped and prescriber notified immediately.

Patient Education

• Discuss specific use of drug and side effects with patient as it relates to treatment. (HCAHPS: During this hospital stay, were you given any medicine that you had not taken before? Before giving you any new medicine, how often did hospital staff tell you what the medicine was for? How often did hospital staff describe possible side effects in a way you could understand?)

• Have patient report immediately to prescriber signs of pancreatitis, signs of hyperglycemia, strength differences from one side to another, difficulty speaking or thinking, change in balance, blurred eyesight, angina, edema of extremities, hemoptysis, dyspnea, severe headache, ecchymosis, hemorrhaging, hallucinations, vision changes, illogical thinking, urinary retention, or oliguria (HCAHPS).

• Educate patient about signs of a significant reaction (eg, wheezing; chest tightness; fever; itching; bad cough; blue skin color; seizures; or swelling of face, lips, tongue or throat). **Note:** This is not a comprehensive list of all side effects. Patient should consult prescriber for additional questions.

Intended Use and Disclaimer: Should not be printed and given to patients. This information is intended to serve as a concise initial reference for healthcare professionals to use when discussing medications with a patient. You must ultimately rely on your own discretion, experience and judgment in diagnosing, treating and advising patients.

Aspirin (AS pir in)

Brand Names: U.S. Ascriptin Maximum Strength [OTC]; Ascriptin Regular Strength [OTC]; Aspercin [OTC]; Aspergum [OTC]; Aspir-low [OTC]; Aspirtab [OTC]; Bayer Aspirin Extra Strength [OTC]; Bayer Aspirin Regimen Adult Low Strength [OTC]; Bayer Aspirin Regimen Children's [OTC]; Bayer Aspirin Regimen Regular Strength [OTC]; Bayer Genuine Aspirin [OTC]; Bayer Plus Extra Strength [OTC]; Bayer Women's Low Dose Aspirin [OTC]; Buffasal [OTC]; Bufferin Extra Strength [OTC]; Bufferin [OTC]; Buffinol [OTC]; Ecotrin Arthritis Strength [OTC]; Ecotrin Low Strength [OTC]; Ecotrin [OTC]; Halfprin [OTC]; St Joseph Adult Aspirin [OTC]; Tri-Buffered Aspirin [OTC]

Index Terms Acetylsalicylic Acid; ASA; Baby Aspirin

Pharmacologic Category Antiplatelet Agent; Salicylate

Medication Safety Issues

Sound-alike/look-alike issues:

Aspirin may be confused with Afrin

Ascriptin may be confused with Aricept

Ecotrin may be confused with Edecrin, Epogen

Halfprin may be confused with Haltran

ZORprin may be confused with Zyloprim

International issues:

Cartia [multiple international markets] may be confused with Cartia XT brand name for diltiazem [U.S.]

BEERS Criteria medication:

This drug may be potentially inappropriate for use in geriatric patients (Quality of evidence - moderate; Strength of recommendation - strong).

Lactation Enters breast milk

Breast-Feeding Considerations Low amounts of aspirin can be found in breast milk. Milk/plasma ratios ranging from 0.03-0.3 have been reported. Peak levels in breast milk are reported to be at ~9 hours after a dose. Metabolic acidosis was reported in one infant following an aspirin dose of 3.9 g/day in the mother. The WHO considers occasional doses of aspirin to be compatible with breast-feeding, but to avoid long-term therapy and consider monitoring the infant for adverse effects (WHO, 2002). Other sources suggest avoiding aspirin while breast-feeding due to the theoretical risk of Reye's syndrome (Bar-Oz, 2003; Spigset, 2000). When used for vascular indications, breast-feeding may be continued during low-dose aspirin therapy (Guyatt, 2012).

Use Treatment of mild-to-moderate pain, inflammation, and fever; prevention and treatment of acute coronary syndromes (ST-elevation MI, non-ST-elevation MI, unstable angina), acute ischemic stroke, and transient ischemic episodes; management of rheumatoid arthritis, rheumatic fever, osteoarthritis; adjunctive therapy in revascularization procedures (coronary artery bypass graft [CABG], ▶

percutaneous transluminal coronary angioplasty [PTCA], carotid endarterectomy), stent implantation

Unlabeled Use Low doses have been used in the prevention of pre-eclampsia, complications associated with autoimmune disorders such as lupus or antiphospholipid syndrome; colorectal cancer; Kawasaki disease; alternative therapy for prevention of thromboembolism associated with atrial fibrillation in patients not candidates for warfarin; pericarditis including pericarditis associated with MI; thromboprophylaxis for aortic valve repair, Blalock-Taussig shunt placement, carotid artery stenosis, coronary artery disease, Fontan surgery, peripheral arterial occlusive disease, peripheral artery percutaneous transluminal angioplasty, peripheral artery bypass graft surgery, prosthetic valves, ventricular assist device (VAD) placement

Mechanism of Action/Effect Irreversibly inhibits cyclooxygenase-1 and 2 (COX-1 and 2) enzymes, which results in decreased formation of prostaglandin precursors; has antipyretic, analgesic, and anti-inflammatory properties

Contraindications Hypersensitivity to salicylates, other NSAIDs, or any component of the formulation; asthma; rhinitis; nasal polyps; inherited or acquired bleeding disorders (including factor VII and factor IX deficiency); do not use in children (<16 years of age) for viral infections (chickenpox or flu symptoms), with or without fever, due to a potential association with Reye's syndrome

Warnings/Precautions Use with caution in patients with platelet and bleeding disorders, renal dysfunction, dehydration, erosive gastritis, or peptic ulcer disease. Heavy ethanol use (>3 drinks/day) can increase bleeding risks. Avoid use in severe renal failure or in severe hepatic failure. Low-dose aspirin for cardioprotective effects is associated with a two- to fourfold increase in UGI events (eg, symptomatic or complicated ulcers); risks of these events increase with increasing aspirin dose; during the chronic phase of aspirin dosing, doses >81 mg are not recommended unless indicated (Bhatt, 2008). Use of safer agents for routine management of pain or headache throughout pregnancy should be considered. If possible, avoid use during the third trimester of pregnancy.

Discontinue use if tinnitus or impaired hearing occurs. Caution in mild-to-moderate renal failure (only at high dosages). Patients with sensitivity to tartrazine dyes, nasal polyps, and asthma may have an increased risk of salicylate sensitivity. In the treatment of acute ischemic stroke, avoid aspirin for 24 hours following administration of alteplase; administration within 24 hours increases the risk of hemorrhagic transformation (Jauch, 2013). Concurrent use of aspirin and clopidogrel is not recommended for secondary prevention of ischemic stroke or TIA in patients unable to take oral anticoagulants due to hemorrhagic risk (Furie, 2011). Surgical patients should avoid ASA if possible, for 1-2 weeks prior to surgery, to reduce the risk of excessive bleeding (except in patients with cardiac stents that have not completed their full course of dual antiplatelet therapy [aspirin, clopidogrel]; patient-specific situations need to be discussed with cardiologist; AHA/ACC/SCAI/ACS/ADA Science Advisory provides recommendations). When used concomitantly with ≤325 mg of aspirin, NSAIDs (including selective COX-2 inhibitors) substantially increase the risk of gastrointestinal complications (eg, ulcer); concomitant gastroprotective therapy (eg, proton pump inhibitors) is recommended (Bhatt, 2008).

Elderly: Avoid chronic use of doses >325 mg/day (unless alternative agents ineffective and patient can receive concomitant gastroprotective agent); nonselective oral NSAID use is associated with an increased risk of GI bleeding and peptic ulcer disease in older adults in high risk category (eg, >75 years or age or receiving concomitant oral/parenteral corticosteroids, anticoagulants, or antiplatelet agents) (Beers Criteria).

When used for self-medication (OTC labeling): Children and teenagers who have or are recovering from chickenpox or flu-like symptoms should not use this product. Changes in behavior (along with nausea and vomiting) may be an early sign of Reye's syndrome; patients should be instructed to contact their healthcare provider if these occur.

Drug Interactions

Avoid Concomitant Use

Avoid concomitant use of Aspirin with any of the following: Floctafenine; Influenza Virus Vaccine (Live/Attenuated); Ketorolac (Nasal); Ketorolac (Systemic); Omacetaxine

Decreased Effect

Aspirin may decrease the levels/effects of: ACE Inhibitors; Carisoprodol; Hyaluronidase; Loop Diuretics; Multivitamins/Fluoride (with ADE); Multivitamins/Minerals (with ADEK, Folate, Iron); Multivitamins/Minerals (with AE, No Iron); NSAID (Nonselective); Probenecid; Ticagrelor; Tiludronate

The levels/effects of Aspirin may be decreased by: Corticosteroids (Systemic); Floctafenine; Ketorolac (Nasal); Ketorolac (Systemic); NSAID (Nonselective)

Increased Effect/Toxicity

Aspirin may increase the levels/effects of: Alendronate; Anticoagulants; Carbonic Anhydrase Inhibitors; Carisoprodol; Collagenase (Systemic); Corticosteroids (Systemic); Dabigatran Etexilate; Heparin; Hypoglycemic Agents; Ibritumomab; Methotrexate; NSAID (COX-2 Inhibitor); Omacetaxine; PRALAtrexate; Rivaroxaban; Salicylates; Thrombolytic Agents; Ticagrelor; Tositumomab and Iodine I 131 Tositumomab; Valproic Acid and Derivatives; Varicella Virus-Containing Vaccines; Vitamin K Antagonists

The levels/effects of Aspirin may be increased by: Agents with Antiplatelet Properties; Ammonium Chloride; Antidepressants (Tricyclic, Tertiary Amine); Calcium Channel Blockers (Nondihydropyridine); Dasatinib; Floctafenine; Ginkgo Biloba; Glucosamine; Herbs (Anticoagulant/Antiplatelet Properties); Ibrutinib; Influenza Virus Vaccine (Live/Attenuated); Ketorolac (Nasal); Ketorolac (Systemic); Loop Diuretics; Multivitamins/Fluoride (with ADE); Multivitamins/Minerals (with ADEK, Folate, Iron); Multivitamins/Minerals (with AE, No Iron); NSAID (Nonselective); Omega-3 Fatty Acids; Pentosan Polysulfate Sodium; Pentoxifylline; Potassium Acid Phosphate; Prostacyclin Analogues; Selective Serotonin Reuptake Inhibitors; Serotonin/Norepinephrine Reuptake Inhibitors; Tipranavir; Treprostinil; Vitamin E

Nutritional/Ethanol Interactions

Ethanol: Avoid ethanol (may enhance gastric mucosal damage).

Food: Food may decrease the rate but not the extent of oral absorption.

Folic acid: Hyperexcretion of folate; folic acid deficiency may result, leading to macrocytic anemia.

Iron: With chronic aspirin use and at doses of 3-4 g/day, iron-deficiency anemia may result.

Sodium: Hypernatremia resulting from buffered aspirin solutions or sodium salicylate containing high sodium content. Avoid or use with caution in CHF or any condition where hypernatremia would be detrimental.

Benedictine liqueur, prunes, raisins, tea, and gherkins: Potential salicylate accumulation.

Fresh fruits containing vitamin C: Displace drug from binding sites, resulting in increased urinary excretion of aspirin.

Herb/Nutraceutical: Avoid cat's claw, dong quai, evening primrose, feverfew, garlic, ginger, ginkgo, red clover, horse chestnut, green tea, ginseng (all have additional antiplatelet activity). Limit curry powder, paprika, licorice; may cause salicylate accumulation. These foods contain 6 mg salicylate/100 g. An ordinary American diet contains 10-200 mg/day of salicylate.

Adverse Reactions As with all drugs which may affect hemostasis, bleeding is associated with aspirin. Hemorrhage may occur at virtually any site. Risk is dependent on multiple variables including dosage, concurrent use of multiple agents which alter hemostasis, and patient susceptibility. Many adverse effects of aspirin are dose related, and are rare at low dosages. Other serious reactions are idiosyncratic, related to allergy or individual sensitivity. Accurate estimation of frequencies is not possible. The reactions listed below have been reported for aspirin (frequency not defined).

Cardiovascular: Hypotension, tachycardia, dysrhythmias, edema

Central nervous system: Fatigue, insomnia, nervousness, agitation, confusion, dizziness, headache, lethargy, cerebral edema, hyperthermia, coma

Dermatologic: Rash, angioedema, urticaria

Endocrine & metabolic: Acidosis, hyperkalemia, dehydration, hypoglycemia (children), hyperglycemia, hypernatremia (buffered forms)

Gastrointestinal: Nausea, vomiting, dyspepsia, epigastric discomfort, heartburn, stomach pain, gastrointestinal ulceration (6% to 31%), gastric erosions, gastric erythema, duodenal ulcers

Hematologic: Anemia, disseminated intravascular coagulation (DIC), prothrombin times prolonged, coagulopathy, thrombocytopenia, hemolytic anemia, bleeding, iron deficiency anemia

Hepatic: Hepatotoxicity, transaminases increased, hepatitis (reversible)

Neuromuscular & skeletal: Rhabdomyolysis, weakness, acetabular bone destruction (OA)

Otic: Hearing loss, tinnitus

Renal: Interstitial nephritis, papillary necrosis, proteinuria, renal impairment, renal failure (including cases caused by rhabdomyolysis), BUN increased, serum creatinine increased

Respiratory: Asthma, bronchospasm, dyspnea, laryngeal edema, hyperpnea, tachypnea, respiratory alkalosis, noncardiogenic pulmonary edema

Miscellaneous: Anaphylaxis, prolonged pregnancy and labor, stillbirths, low birth weight, peripartum bleeding, Reye's syndrome

Pharmacodynamics/Kinetics

Duration of Action 4-6 hours

Available Dosage Forms

Caplet, oral: 500 mg

Ascriptin® Maximum Strength [OTC]: 500 mg

Bayer® Aspirin Extra Strength [OTC]: 500 mg

Bayer® Genuine Aspirin [OTC]: 325 mg

Bayer® Plus Extra Strength [OTC]: 500 mg

Bayer® Women's Low Dose Aspirin [OTC]: 81 mg

Caplet, enteric coated, oral:

Bayer® Aspirin Regimen Regular Strength [OTC]: 325 mg

Gum, chewing, oral:

Aspergum® [OTC]: 227 mg (12s)

Suppository, rectal: 300 mg (12s); 600 mg (12s)

Tablet, oral: 325 mg

Ascriptin® Regular Strength [OTC]: 325 mg

Aspercin [OTC]: 325 mg

Aspirtab [OTC]: 325 mg

Bayer® Genuine Aspirin [OTC]: 325 mg

Buffasal [OTC]: 325 mg

Bufferin® [OTC]: 325 mg

Bufferin® Extra Strength [OTC]: 500 mg

Buffinol [OTC]: 324 mg

Tri-Buffered Aspirin [OTC]: 325 mg

◄ **Tablet, chewable, oral**: 81 mg
Bayer® Aspirin Regimen Children's [OTC]: 81 mg
St Joseph® Adult Aspirin [OTC]: 81 mg
Tablet, enteric coated, oral: 81 mg, 325 mg, 650 mg
Aspir-low [OTC]: 81 mg
Bayer® Aspirin Regimen Adult Low Strength [OTC]: 81 mg
Ecotrin® [OTC]: 325 mg
Ecotrin® Arthritis Strength [OTC]: 500 mg
Ecotrin® Low Strength [OTC]: 81 mg
Halfprin® [OTC]: 81 mg, 162 mg
St Joseph® Adult Aspirin [OTC]: 81 mg

General Dosage Range
Oral:
Children: 10-15 mg/kg/dose every 4-6 hours (maximum: 4 g/day) **or** 60-100 mg/kg/day divided every 4-8 hours **or** 1-20 mg/kg/day as a single dose
Adults: 325-650 mg every 4-6 hours (maximum: 4 g/day) **or** 2.4-5.4 g/day in divided doses **or** 40-325 mg/day as a single dose
Rectal:
Children: 10-15 mg/kg/dose every 4-6 hours (maximum: 4 g/day)
Adults: 300-600 mg every 4-6 hours (maximum: 4 g/day)

Administration
Oral Do not crush enteric coated tablet. Administer with food or a full glass of water to minimize GI distress. For acute myocardial infarction, have patient chew tablet.

Storage/Stability Keep suppositories in refrigerator; do not freeze. Hydrolysis of aspirin occurs upon exposure to water or moist air, resulting in salicylate and acetate, which possess a vinegar-like odor. Do not use if a strong odor is present.

Nursing Actions
Physical Assessment Monitor for signs of bleeding and hypersensitivity reactions.
Patient Education
• Discuss specific use of drug and side effects with patient as it relates to treatment. (HCAHPS: During this hospital stay, were you given any medicine that you had not taken before? Before giving you any new medicine, how often did hospital staff tell you what the medicine was for? How often did hospital staff describe possible side effects in a way you could understand?)
• Patient may experience pyrosis or nausea. Have patient report immediately to prescriber severe dizziness, syncope, illogical thinking, significant headache, tinnitus, hearing impairment, considerable dyspepsia, melena, hematemesis, ecchymosis, hemorrhaging, intolerable rectal pain or irritation, or hematochezia (HCAHPS).
• Educate patient about signs of a significant reaction (eg, wheezing; chest tightness; fever; itching; bad cough; blue skin color; seizures; or swelling of face, lips, tongue, or throat). **Note:** This is not a comprehensive list of all side

effects. Patient should consult prescriber for additional questions.

Intended Use and Disclaimer: Should not be printed and given to patients. This information is intended to serve as a concise initial reference for healthcare professionals to use when discussing medications with a patient. You must ultimately rely on your own discretion, experience and judgment in diagnosing, treating and advising patients.

Dietary Considerations Take with food or large volume of water or milk to minimize GI upset.

Related Information
Oral Medications That Should Not Be Crushed or Altered *on page 1712*

Aspirin and Diphenhydramine
(AS pir in & dye fen HYE dra meen)

Brand Names: U.S. Bayer® PM [OTC]
Index Terms ASA and Diphenhydramine; Aspirin and Diphenhydramine Citrate; Diphenhydramine and ASA; Diphenhydramine and Aspirin; Diphenhydramine Citrate and Aspirin
Pharmacologic Category Analgesic, Miscellaneous
Lactation See individual agents.
Use Aid in the relief of insomnia accompanied by minor pain or headache
Available Dosage Forms
Caplet, oral:
Bayer® PM [OTC]: Aspirin 500 mg and diphenhydramine 38.3 mg
General Dosage Range Oral: *Children ≥12 years and Adults:* Two caplets (1000 mg aspirin/77 mg diphenhydramine citrate) at bedtime
Administration
Oral Administer each dose with a full glass of water.
Nursing Actions
Physical Assessment See individual agents.
Patient Education
• Discuss specific use of drug and side effects with patient as it relates to treatment. (HCAHPS: During this hospital stay, were you given any medicine that you had not taken before? Before giving you any new medicine, how often did hospital staff tell you what the medicine was for? How often did hospital staff describe possible side effects in a way you could understand?)
• Patient may experience presyncope, fatigue, blurred vision, constipation, xerostomia, dyspepsia, pyrosis, or nausea. Have patient report immediately to prescriber dyspnea, tinnitus, illogical thinking, melena, hematuria, ecchymosis, hemorrhaging, urinary retention, or severe asthenia (HCAHPS).
• Educate patient about signs of a significant reaction (eg, wheezing; chest tightness; fever; itching; bad cough; blue skin color; seizures; or

swelling of face, lips, tongue, or throat). **Note:** This is not a comprehensive list of all side effects. Patient should consult prescriber for additional questions.

Intended Use and Disclaimer: Should not be printed and given to patients. This information is intended to serve as a concise initial reference for healthcare professionals to use when discussing medications with a patient. You must ultimately rely on your own discretion, experience and judgment in diagnosing, treating and advising patients.

Related Information

Aspirin on page 129
DiphenhydrAMINE (Systemic) on page 462

Aspirin and Dipyridamole
(AS pir in & dye peer ID a mole)

Brand Names: U.S. Aggrenox®
Index Terms Aspirin and Extended-Release Dipyridamole; Dipyridamole and Aspirin
Pharmacologic Category Antiplatelet Agent
Medication Safety Issues
Sound-alike/look-alike issues:
Aggrenox® may be confused with Aggrastat®
Pregnancy Risk Factor D
Lactation Enters breast milk/use caution
Breast-Feeding Considerations Both aspirin and dipyridamole are excreted in breast milk.
Use Reduction in the risk of stroke in patients who have had transient ischemia of the brain or ischemic stroke due to thrombosis
Unlabeled Use Hemodialysis graft patency; symptomatic carotid artery stenosis (including recent carotid endarterectomy)
Mechanism of Action/Effect Antithrombotic action results from additive antiplatelet effects of aspirin and dipyridamole.
Contraindications Hypersensitivity to dipyridamole, aspirin, or any component of the formulation; allergy to NSAIDs; patients with the syndrome of asthma, rhinitis, and nasal polyps; children <16 years of age with viral infections; pregnancy (third trimester; aspirin)

Canadian labeling: Additional contraindications (not in U.S. labeling): Patients with hereditary fructose and/or galactose intolerance
Warnings/Precautions Patients who consume ≥3 alcoholic drinks per day may be at risk of bleeding. Use cautiously use in patients with inherited or acquired bleeding disorders, renal impairment, hypotension, unstable angina, recent MI or hepatic dysfunction. Avoid use in patients with a history of active peptic ulcer disease, severe hepatic failure, or severe renal impairment (CrCl <10 mL/minute). Monitor for signs and symptoms of GI ulcers and bleeding. Discontinue use if dizziness, tinnitus, or impaired hearing occurs. Discontinue use 24 hours prior to pharmacologic (I.V. dipyridamole) stress

testing. Discontinue 1-2 weeks before elective surgical procedures to reduce the risk of bleeding. Use caution in the elderly who are at high risk for adverse events. Dose of aspirin in this combination may not be adequate to prevent for cardiac indications (eg, MI prophylaxis). Avoid use in children due to risk of Reye's syndrome in certain viral illness associated with aspirin component. Formulation may contain lactose and/or sucrose. Use in patients with fructose and/or galactose intolerance is contraindicated in the Canadian labeling.

Drug Interactions
Avoid Concomitant Use
Avoid concomitant use of Aspirin and Dipyridamole with any of the following: Bosutinib; Floctafenine; Influenza Virus Vaccine (Live/Attenuated); Ketorolac (Nasal); Ketorolac (Systemic); Omacetaxine; PAZOPanib; Pomalidomide; Riociguat; Silodosin; VinCRIStine (Liposomal)

Decreased Effect
Aspirin and Dipyridamole may decrease the levels/effects of: ACE Inhibitors; Acetylcholinesterase Inhibitors; Carisoprodol; Hyaluronidase; Loop Diuretics; Multivitamins/Fluoride (with ADE); Multivitamins/Minerals (with ADEK, Folate, Iron); Multivitamins/Minerals (with AE, No Iron); NSAID (Nonselective); Probenecid; Ticagrelor; Tiludronate

The levels/effects of Aspirin and Dipyridamole may be decreased by: Corticosteroids (Systemic); Floctafenine; Ketorolac (Nasal); Ketorolac (Systemic); NSAID (Nonselective)

Increased Effect/Toxicity
Aspirin and Dipyridamole may increase the levels/effects of: Adenosine; Afatinib; Alendronate; Anticoagulants; Beta-Blockers; Bosutinib; Carbonic Anhydrase Inhibitors; Carisoprodol; Colchicine; Collagenase (Systemic); Corticosteroids (Systemic); Dabigatran Etexilate; DOXOrubicin (Conventional); Everolimus; Heparin; Hypoglycemic Agents; Hypotensive Agents; Ibritumomab; Methotrexate; NSAID (COX-2 Inhibitor); Omacetaxine; PAZOPanib; P-glycoprotein/ABCB1 Substrates; Pomalidomide; PRALAtrexate; Prucalopride; Regadenoson; Riociguat; Rivaroxaban; Salicylates; Silodosin; Thrombolytic Agents; Ticagrelor; Topotecan; Tositumomab and Iodine I 131 Tositumomab; Valproic Acid and Derivatives; Varicella Virus-Containing Vaccines; VinCRIStine (Liposomal); Vitamin K Antagonists

The levels/effects of Aspirin and Dipyridamole may be increased by: Agents with Antiplatelet Properties; Ammonium Chloride; Antidepressants (Tricyclic, Tertiary Amine); Calcium Channel Blockers (Nondihydropyridine); Dasatinib; Floctafenine; Ginkgo Biloba; Glucosamine; Herbs (Anticoagulant/Antiplatelet Properties); Ibrutinib; Influenza Virus Vaccine (Live/Attenuated); Ketorolac (Nasal); Ketorolac (Systemic); Loop

Diuretics; Multivitamins/Fluoride (with ADE); Multivitamins/Minerals (with ADEK, Folate, Iron); Multivitamins/Minerals (with AE, No Iron); NSAID (Nonselective); Omega-3 Fatty Acids; Pentosan Polysulfate Sodium; Pentoxifylline; Potassium Acid Phosphate; Prostacyclin Analogues; Selective Serotonin Reuptake Inhibitors; Serotonin/Norepinephrine Reuptake Inhibitors; Tipranavir; Treprostinil; Vitamin E

Nutritional/Ethanol Interactions Ethanol: Avoid ethanol (due to GI irritation).

Adverse Reactions

>10%:

Central nervous system: Headache (39%; tolerance usually develops)

Gastrointestinal: Abdominal pain (18%), dyspepsia (18%), nausea (16%), diarrhea (13%)

1% to 10%:

Cardiovascular: Cardiac failure (2%), syncope (1%)

Central nervous system: Fatigue (6%), pain (6%), amnesia (2%), malaise (2%), seizure (2%), confusion (1%), somnolence (1%)

Dermatologic: Purpura (1%)

Gastrointestinal: Vomiting (8%), GI bleeding (4%), melena (2%), rectal bleeding (2%), hemorrhoids (1%), GI hemorrhage (1%), anorexia (1%)

Hematologic: Hemorrhage (3%), anemia (2%)

Neuromuscular & skeletal: Arthralgia (6%), back pain (5%), weakness (2%), arthritis (2%), arthrosis (1%), myalgia (1%)

Respiratory: Cough (2%), epistaxis (2%), upper respiratory tract infection (1%)

Available Dosage Forms

Capsule:

Aggrenox®: Aspirin 25 mg [immediate release] and dipyridamole 200 mg [extended release]

General Dosage Range Oral: *Adults:* 1 capsule (200 mg dipyridamole, 25 mg aspirin) twice daily

Administration

Oral Capsule should be swallowed whole; do not crush or chew. May be administered with or without food.

Storage/Stability Store at 25°C (77°F); excursions permitted to 15°C to 30°C (59°F to 86°F). Protect from excessive moisture.

Nursing Actions

Physical Assessment See individual agents.

Patient Education

• Discuss specific use of drug and side effects with patient as it relates to treatment. (HCAHPS: During this hospital stay, were you given any medicine that you had not taken before? Before giving you any new medicine, how often did hospital staff tell you what the medicine was for? How often did hospital staff describe possible side effects in a way you could understand?)

• Patient may experience pyrosis. Have patient report immediately to prescriber signs of hepatic impairment, strength differences from one side to another, difficulty speaking or thinking, change in balance, blurred vision, angina, arrhythmia, severe asthenia, significant headache, considerable dizziness, syncope, intolerable diarrhea, severe nausea, considerable dyspepsia, ecchymosis, hemorrhaging, melena, hematuria, hematemesis, sudden vision changes, tinnitus, loss of hearing, memory loss, illogical thinking, dyspnea, urinary retention, or oliguria (HCAHPS).

• Educate patient about signs of a significant reaction (eg, wheezing; chest tightness; fever; itching; bad cough; blue skin color; seizures; or swelling of face, lips, tongue, or throat). **Note:** This is not a comprehensive list of all side effects. Patient should consult prescriber for additional questions.

Intended Use and Disclaimer: Should not be printed and given to patients. This information is intended to serve as a concise initial reference for healthcare professionals to use when discussing medications with a patient. You must ultimately rely on your own discretion, experience and judgment in diagnosing, treating and advising patients.

Dietary Considerations May be taken with or without food.

Related Information

Aspirin *on page 129*

Dipyridamole *on page 473*

Oral Medications That Should Not Be Crushed or Altered *on page 1712*

Atenolol (a TEN oh lole)

Brand Names: U.S. Tenormin

Pharmacologic Category Antianginal Agent; Antihypertensive; Beta-Blocker, Beta-1 Selective

Medication Safety Issues

Sound-alike/look-alike issues:

Atenolol may be confused with albuterol, Altenol®, timolol, Tylenol®

Tenormin® may be confused with Imuran®, Norpramin®, thiamine, Trovan®

Pregnancy Risk Factor D

Lactation Enters breast milk/use caution

Breast-Feeding Considerations Atenolol is excreted in breast milk and has been detected in the serum and urine of nursing infants. Peak concentrations in breast milk have been reported to occur between 2-8 hours after the maternal dose and in some cases are higher than the peak maternal serum concentration. Although most studies have not reported adverse events in nursing infants, avoiding maternal use while nursing infants with renal dysfunction or infants <44 weeks postconceptual age has been suggested. Beta-blockers with less distribution into breast milk may be preferred. The manufacturer recommends that caution be exercised when administering atenolol to nursing women.

Use Treatment of hypertension, alone or in combination with other agents; management of angina pectoris; secondary prevention postmyocardial infarction

Unlabeled Use Acute ethanol withdrawal (in combination with a benzodiazepine), supraventricular and ventricular arrhythmias, and migraine headache prophylaxis

Mechanism of Action/Effect Competitively blocks response to beta-adrenergic stimulation, selectively blocks beta$_1$-receptors with little or no effect on beta$_2$-receptors except at high doses

Contraindications Hypersensitivity to atenolol or any component of the formulation; sinus bradycardia; sinus node dysfunction; heart block greater than first-degree (except in patients with a functioning artificial pacemaker); cardiogenic shock; uncompensated cardiac failure; pulmonary edema; pregnancy

Warnings/Precautions Consider pre-existing conditions such as sick sinus syndrome before initiating. Administer cautiously in compensated heart failure and monitor for a worsening of the condition (efficacy of atenolol in heart failure has not been established). **[U.S. Boxed Warning]: Beta-blocker therapy should not be withdrawn abruptly (particularly in patients with CAD), but gradually tapered to avoid acute tachycardia, hypertension, and/or ischemia.** Chronic beta-blocker therapy should not be routinely withdrawn prior to major surgery. Beta-blockers should be avoided in patients with bronchospastic disease (asthma). Atenolol, with B$_1$ selectivity, has been used cautiously in bronchospastic disease with close monitoring. May precipitate or aggravate symptoms of arterial insufficiency in patients with PVD and Raynaud's disease; use with caution and monitor for progression of arterial obstruction. Use cautiously in patients with diabetes - may mask hypoglycemic symptoms. May mask signs of hyperthyroidism (eg, tachycardia); use caution if hyperthyroidism is suspected, abrupt withdrawal may precipitate thyroid storm. Alterations in thyroid function tests may be observed. Use cautiously in the renally impaired (dosage adjustment required). Caution in myasthenia gravis or psychiatric disease (may cause CNS depression). Bradycardia may be observed more frequently in elderly patients (>65 years of age); dosage reductions may be necessary. Adequate alpha-blockade is required prior to use of any beta-blocker for patients with untreated pheochromocytoma. May induce or exacerbate psoriasis. Use caution with history of severe anaphylaxis to allergens; patients taking beta-blockers may become more sensitive to repeated challenges. Treatment of anaphylaxis (eg, epinephrine) in patients taking beta-blockers may be ineffective or promote undesirable effects. Use with caution in patients on concurrent digoxin, verapamil, or diltiazem; bradycardia or heart block can occur. Use with caution in patients receiving inhaled anesthetic agents known to depress myocardial contractility.

Drug Interactions

Avoid Concomitant Use

Avoid concomitant use of Atenolol with any of the following: Floctafenine; Methacholine

Decreased Effect

Atenolol may decrease the levels/effects of: Beta2-Agonists; Theophylline Derivatives

The levels/effects of Atenolol may be decreased by: Ampicillin; Herbs (Hypertensive Properties); Methylphenidate; Nonsteroidal Anti-Inflammatory Agents; Yohimbine

Increased Effect/Toxicity

Atenolol may increase the levels/effects of: Alpha-/Beta-Agonists (Direct-Acting); Alpha1-Blockers; Alpha2-Agonists; Amifostine; Antihypertensives; Bupivacaine; Cardiac Glycosides; Cholinergic Agonists; DULoxetine; Ergot Derivatives; Fingolimod; Hypotensive Agents; Insulin; Lidocaine (Systemic); Lidocaine (Topical); Mepivacaine; Methacholine; Midodrine; Obinutuzumab; RiTUXimab; Sulfonylureas

The levels/effects of Atenolol may be increased by: Acetylcholinesterase Inhibitors; Alpha2-Agonists; Amiodarone; Anilidopiperidine Opioids; Brimonidine (Topical); Calcium Channel Blockers (Dihydropyridine); Calcium Channel Blockers (Nondihydropyridine); Diazoxide; Dipyridamole; Disopyramide; Dronedarone; Floctafenine; Glycopyrrolate; Herbs (Hypotensive Properties); MAO Inhibitors; Pentoxifylline; Phosphodiesterase 5 Inhibitors; Prostacyclin Analogues; Regorafenib; Reserpine

Nutritional/Ethanol Interactions

Food: Atenolol serum concentrations may be decreased if taken with food.

Herb/Nutraceutical: Dong quai has estrogenic activity. Ephedra, yohimbe, and ginseng may worsen hypertension. Garlic may have increased antihypertensive effect. Management: Avoid dong quai, ephedra, yohimbe, ginseng, and garlic.

Adverse Reactions 1% to 10%:

Cardiovascular: Persistent bradycardia, hypotension, chest pain, edema, heart failure, second- or third-degree AV block, Raynaud's phenomenon

Central nervous system: Dizziness, fatigue, insomnia, lethargy, confusion, mental impairment, depression, headache, nightmares

Gastrointestinal: Constipation, diarrhea, nausea

Genitourinary: Impotence

Miscellaneous: Cold extremities

Pharmacodynamics/Kinetics

Onset of Action Peak effect: Oral: 2-4 hours

Duration of Action Normal renal function: 12-24 hours

Available Dosage Forms

Tablet, Oral:

Tenormin: 25 mg, 50 mg, 100 mg

Generic: 25 mg, 50 mg, 100 mg

General Dosage Range Dosage adjustment recommended in patients with renal impairment

Oral:

Children: 0.5-1 mg/kg/dose given daily; range of 0.5-1.5 mg/kg/day (maximum dose: 2 mg/kg/day up to 100 mg/day)

Adults: 25-100 mg/day as a single daily dose (maximum dose: 100 mg/day)

Administration

Oral When administered acutely for cardiac treatment, monitor ECG and blood pressure. May be administered without regard to meals.

Storage/Stability Protect from light.

Nursing Actions

Physical Assessment Monitor blood pressure and heart rate prior to and following first dose and after any change in dosage. Monitor for CHF, edema, new cough, dyspnea, unintentional weight gain, or unresolved fatigue. Advise patients with diabetes to monitor glucose levels closely; beta-blockers may alter glucose tolerance. Taper dosage slowly when discontinuing. Teach patient hypotension precautions to report.

Patient Education

• Discuss specific use of drug and side effects with patient as it relates to treatment. (HCAHPS: During this hospital stay, were you given any medicine that you had not taken before? Before giving you any new medicine, how often did hospital staff tell you what the medicine was for? How often did hospital staff describe possible side effects in a way you could understand?)

• Patient may experience diarrhea, sensation of cold, fatigue, dyspepsia, or asthenia. Have patient report immediately to prescriber signs of depression (ie, suicidal ideation, anxiety, emotional instability, illogical thinking), severe dizziness, syncope, dyspnea, skin discoloration, sexual dysfunction, mood changes, dyspnea, excessive weight gain, edema of extremities, ecchymosis, hemorrhaging, or bradycardia (HCAHPS).

• Educate patient about signs of a significant reaction (eg, wheezing; chest tightness; fever; itching; bad cough; blue skin color; seizures; or swelling of face, lips, tongue, or throat). **Note:** This is not a comprehensive list of all side effects. Patient should consult prescriber for additional questions.

Intended Use and Disclaimer: Should not be printed and given to patients. This information is intended to serve as a concise initial reference for healthcare professionals to use when discussing medications with a patient. You must ultimately rely on your own discretion, experience and judgment in diagnosing, treating and advising patients.

Dietary Considerations May be taken without regard to meals.

Atenolol and Chlorthalidone

(a TEN oh lole & klor THAL i done)

Brand Names: U.S. Tenoretic®

Index Terms Chlorthalidone and Atenolol

Pharmacologic Category Antihypertensive, Beta-Blocker, Beta-1 Selective; Diuretic, Thiazide

Pregnancy Risk Factor D

Lactation Excretion in breast milk unknown/use caution

Use Treatment of hypertension with a cardioselective beta-blocker and a diuretic

Available Dosage Forms

Tablet, oral: Atenolol 50 mg and chlorthalidone 25 mg; atenolol 100 mg and chlorthalidone 25 mg

Tenoretic®: Atenolol 50 mg and chlorthalidone 25 mg; atenolol 100 mg and chlorthalidone 25 mg

General Dosage Range Dosage adjustment recommended in patients with renal impairment.

Oral: *Adults:* Initial: Atenolol 50 mg and chlorthalidone 25 mg once daily; Maintenance: Atenolol 50-100 mg and chlorthalidone 25 mg once daily (maximum dose: Atenolol 100 mg/day; chlorthalidone 25 mg/day)

Nursing Actions

Physical Assessment See individual agents.

Patient Education

• Discuss specific use of drug and side effects with patient as it relates to treatment. (HCAHPS: During this hospital stay, were you given any medicine that you had not taken before? Before giving you any new medicine, how often did hospital staff tell you what the medicine was for? How often did hospital staff describe possible side effects in a way you could understand?)

• Patient may experience diarrhea, sensation of cold, fatigue, headache, dyspepsia, or asthenia. Have patient report immediately to prescriber signs of fluid and electrolyte imbalance, signs of hyperglycemia, signs of hepatic impairment, skin discoloration, severe dizziness, syncope, dyspnea, bradycardia, akathisia, significant arthralgia, edema of extremities, ecchymosis, or hemorrhaging (HCAHPS).

• Educate patient about signs of a significant reaction (eg, wheezing; chest tightness; fever; itching; bad cough; blue skin color; seizures; or swelling of face, lips, tongue, or throat). **Note:** This is not a comprehensive list of all side effects. Patient should consult prescriber for additional questions.

Intended Use and Disclaimer: Should not be printed and given to patients. This information is intended to serve as a concise initial reference for healthcare professionals to use when discussing medications with a patient. You must ultimately rely on your own discretion, experience and

judgment in diagnosing, treating and advising patients.

Related Information

Atenolol *on page 134*
Chlorthalidone *on page 310*

AtoMOXetine (AT oh mox e teen)

Brand Names: U.S. Strattera
Index Terms Atomoxetine Hydrochloride; LY139603; Methylphenoxy-Benzene Propanamine; Tomoxetine
Pharmacologic Category Norepinephrine Reuptake Inhibitor, Selective
Medication Safety Issues
Sound-alike/look-alike issues:
  AtoMOXetine may be confused with atorvaSTATin
Medication Guide Available Yes
Pregnancy Risk Factor C
Lactation Excretion in breast milk unknown/use caution
Breast-Feeding Considerations It is not known if atomoxetine is excreted in breast milk. The manufacturer recommends that caution be exercised when administering atomoxetine to nursing women.
Use Attention deficit hyperactivity disorder: Treatment of attention deficit hyperactivity disorder (ADHD)
Mechanism of Action/Effect Selectively inhibits the reuptake of norepinephrine (Ki 4.5nM) with little to no activity at the other neuronal reuptake pumps or receptor sites.
Contraindications Hypersensitivity to atomoxetine or any component of the formulation; use with or within 14 days of MAO inhibitors; narrow-angle glaucoma; current or past history of pheochromocytoma; severe cardiac or vascular disorders in which the condition would be expected to deteriorate with clinically important increases in blood pressure (eg, 15 to 20 mm Hg) or heart rate (eg, 20 beats/minute).

Canadian labeling: Additional contraindications (not in U.S. labeling): Symptomatic cardiovascular diseases, moderate-to-severe hypertension; advanced arteriosclerosis; uncontrolled hyperthyroidism

Warnings/Precautions [U.S. Boxed Warning]: Use caution in pediatric patients; may be an increased risk of suicidal ideation. Closely monitor for clinical worsening, suicidality, or unusual changes in behavior; especially during the initial few months of a course of drug therapy, or at times of dose changes, either increases or decreases. The family or caregiver should be instructed to closely observe the patient and communicate condition with healthcare provider. New or worsening symptoms of hostility or aggressive behaviors have been associated with atomoxetine, particularly with

the initiation of therapy. Treatment-emergent psychotic or manic symptoms (eg, hallucinations, delusional thinking, mania) may occur in children and adolescents without a prior history of psychotic illness or mania; consider discontinuation of treatment if symptoms occur. Use caution in patients with comorbid bipolar disorder; therapy may induce mixed/manic episode. Atomoxetine is not approved for major depressive disorder. Patients presenting with depressive symptoms should be screened for bipolar disorder. Recommended to be used as part of a comprehensive treatment program for attention deficit disorders. Atomoxetine does not worsen anxiety in patients with existing anxiety disorders or tics related to Tourette's disorder.

Use caution with hepatic disease (dosage adjustments necessary in moderate and severe hepatic impairment). Use may be associated with rare but severe hepatotoxicity, including hepatic failure; discontinue and do not restart if signs or symptoms of hepatotoxic reaction (eg, jaundice, pruritus, flu-like symptoms, dark urine, right upper quadrant tenderness) or laboratory evidence of liver disease are noted. Use caution in patients who are poor metabolizers of CYP2D6 metabolized drugs ("poor metabolizers"), bioavailability increases; dosage adjustments are recommended in patients known to be CYP2D6 poor metabolizers.

Orthostasis can occur; use caution in patients predisposed to hypotension or those with abrupt changes in heart rate or blood pressure. Atomoxetine has been associated with serious cardiovascular events including sudden death in patients with pre-existing structural cardiac abnormalities or other serious heart problems (sudden death in children and adolescents; sudden death, stroke, and MI in adults). Atomoxetine should be avoided in patients with known serious structural cardiac abnormalities, cardiomyopathy, serious heart rhythm abnormalities, or other serious cardiac problems that could increase the risk of sudden death that these conditions alone carry. Patients should be carefully evaluated for cardiac disease prior to initiation of therapy. Perform a prompt cardiac evaluation in patients who develop symptoms of exertional chest pain, unexplained syncope, or other symptoms suggestive of cardiac disease during treatment. May cause increased heart rate or blood pressure; use caution with hypertension or other cardiovascular or cerebrovascular disease; CYP2D6 poor metabolizers may experience greater increases in blood pressure and heart rate effects. Use caution in patients with a history of urinary retention or bladder outlet obstruction; may cause urinary retention/hesitancy; use caution in patients with history of urinary retention or bladder outlet obstruction. Priapism has been associated with use (rarely). Allergic reactions (including anaphylactic reactions, angioneurotic edema, urticaria, and rash) may occur (rare).

Growth in pediatric patients should be monitored during treatment. Height and weight gain may be reduced during the first 9-12 months of treatment, but should recover by 3 years of therapy.

Drug Interactions

Avoid Concomitant Use

Avoid concomitant use of AtoMOXetine with any of the following: Iobenguane I 123; MAO Inhibitors; Pimozide

Decreased Effect

AtoMOXetine may decrease the levels/effects of: Iobenguane I 123

The levels/effects of AtoMOXetine may be decreased by: Peginterferon Alfa-2b

Increased Effect/Toxicity

AtoMOXetine may increase the levels/effects of: ARIPiprazole; Beta2-Agonists; Dofetilide; Lomitapide; Pimozide; Sympathomimetics

The levels/effects of AtoMOXetine may be increased by: Abiraterone Acetate; CYP2D6 Inhibitors (Moderate); CYP2D6 Inhibitors (Strong); Darunavir; MAO Inhibitors

Nutritional/Ethanol Interactions Ethanol: May increase CNS depression; monitor for increased effects with coadministration. Caution patients about effects.

Adverse Reactions Percentages as reported in children and adults; some adverse reactions may be increased in "poor metabolizers" (CYP2D6).

>10%:
  Central nervous system: Headache (2% to 19%), insomnia (2% to 15%), drowsiness (4% to 11%)
  Gastrointestinal: Nausea (7% to 26%), xerostomia (20%), abdominal pain (7% to 18%), decreased appetite (11% to 16%), vomiting (3% to 11%)
1% to 10%:
  Cardiovascular: Systolic hypertension (4% to 5%), increased diastolic blood pressure (≤4%), palpitations (3%), syncope (1% to 3%), flushing (≥2%), tachycardia (<1% to ≥2%), orthostatic hypotension (<2%)
  Central nervous system: Fatigue (6% to 10%), dizziness (5% to 8%), depression (4% to 7%), irritability (≤6%), abnormal dreams (4%), chills (3%), disturbed sleep (3%; adults; postmarketing observation in children), agitation (2%), anxiety (2%), restlessness (2%), emotional lability (1% to 2%)
  Dermatologic: Hyperhidrosis (4%), excoriation (2% to 4%), skin rash (2%)
  Endocrine & metabolic: Weight loss (2% to 7%), decreased libido (3% to 4%), hot flash (3%), increased thirst (2%), menstrual disease (2%)
  Gastrointestinal: Constipation (1% to 9%), dyspepsia (4%), anorexia (≤3%), diarrhea (2%), dysgeusia (2%), flatulence (2%)

Genitourinary: Erectile dysfunction (8%), urinary retention (6%), ejaculatory disorder (4%), dysmenorrhea (3%), dysuria (3%), orgasm abnormal (2%), pollakiuria (2%), prostatitis (2%), urinary frequency (2%)
  Neuromuscular & skeletal: Tremor (1% to 5%), back pain (2%), muscle spasm (2%), weakness (2%)
  Ophthalmic: Conjunctivitis (1% to 3%), mydriasis (≥2%)
  Respiratory: Sinus headache (3%), pharyngolaryngeal pain (≥2%), oropharyngeal pain (2%)
  Miscellaneous: Jitteriness (2%), therapeutic response unexpected (2%)

Available Dosage Forms

Capsule, Oral:
  Strattera: 10 mg, 18 mg, 25 mg, 40 mg, 60 mg, 80 mg, 100 mg

General Dosage Range Dosage adjustment recommended in patients with hepatic impairment or on concomitant therapy.

Oral:
  Children ≥6 years and ≤70 kg: Initial: 0.5 mg/kg/day in 1-2 divided doses; Maintenance: 0.5-1.4 mg/kg/day in 1-2 divided doses (maximum: 1.4 mg/kg/day **or** 100 mg/day, whichever is less)
  Children ≥6 years and >70 kg and Adults: Initial: 40 mg/day in 1-2 divided doses; Maintenance: 40-100 mg/day in 1-2 divided doses (maximum: 100 mg/day)

Administration

Oral Administer with or without food as a single daily dose in the morning or as two evenly divided doses in morning and late afternoon/early evening. Swallow capsules whole; do not open capsules. If opened accidentally, do not touch eyes; wash hands immediately (product is an ocular irritant).

Storage/Stability Store at 25°C (77°F); excursions are permitted between 15°C and 30°C (59°F and 86°F).

Nursing Actions

Physical Assessment Pediatric patients should be screened/monitored for cardiovascular conditions prior to treatment. Monitor growth (height and weight) regularly and for risk of suicide ideation.

Patient Education
• Discuss specific use of drug and side effects with patient as it relates to treatment. (HCAHPS: During this hospital stay, were you given any medicine that you had not taken before? Before giving you any new medicine, how often did hospital staff tell you what the medicine was for? How often did hospital staff describe possible side effects in a way you could understand?)
• Patient may experience dyspepsia, insomnia, nausea, lack of appetite, xerostomia, constipation, sexual dysfunction, asthenia, or fatigue. Have patient report immediately to prescriber

signs of depression (ie, suicidal ideation, anxiety, emotional instability, illogical thinking), signs of hepatic impairment, behavioral changes, irritability, tachycardia, arrhythmia, severe headache, difficult urination, paresthesia, priapism, or strength differences from one side to another, difficulty speaking or thinking, change in balance, vision changes, angina, dyspnea, significant dizziness, or syncope (HCAHPS).
- Educate patient about signs of a significant reaction (eg, wheezing; chest tightness; fever; itching; bad cough; blue skin color; seizures; or swelling of face, lips, tongue, or throat). **Note:** This is not a comprehensive list of all side effects. Patient should consult prescriber for additional questions.

Intended Use and Disclaimer: Should not be printed and given to patients. This information is intended to serve as a concise initial reference for healthcare professionals to use when discussing medications with a patient. You must ultimately rely on your own discretion, experience and judgment in diagnosing, treating and advising patients.

Related Information
Oral Medications That Should Not Be Crushed or Altered *on page 1712*

AtorvaSTATin (a TORE va sta tin)

Brand Names: U.S. Lipitor
Index Terms Atorvastatin Calcium
Pharmacologic Category Antilipemic Agent, HMG-CoA Reductase Inhibitor
Medication Safety Issues
  Sound-alike/look-alike issues:
    AtorvaSTATin may be confused with atoMOXetine, lovastatin, nystatin, pitavastatin, pravastatin, rosuvastatin, simvastatin
    Lipitor may be confused with labetalol, Levatol, lisinopril, Loniten, Lopid, Mevacor, Zocor, Zyr-TEC
Pregnancy Risk Factor X
Lactation Excretion in breast milk unknown/contraindicated
Breast-Feeding Considerations It is not known if atorvastatin is excreted into breast milk. Due to the potential for serious adverse reactions in a nursing infant, use while breast-feeding is contraindicated by the manufacturer.
Use Treatment of dyslipidemias or primary prevention of cardiovascular disease (atherosclerotic) as detailed below:
Prevention of cardiovascular disease:
  Primary prevention of cardiovascular disease (high-risk for CVD): To reduce the risk of MI or stroke in patients without evidence of heart disease who have multiple CVD risk factors or type 2 diabetes. Treatment reduces the risk for

angina or revascularization procedures in patients with multiple risk factors.
  Secondary prevention of cardiovascular disease: To reduce the risk of nonfatal MI, nonfatal stroke, revascularization procedures, hospitalization for heart failure, and angina in patients with evidence of coronary heart disease.
  Primary and secondary prevention of atherosclerotic cardiovascular disease (ASCVD) according to the American College of Cardiology/American Heart Association: To reduce the risk of ASCVD in patients with clinical ASCVD (eg, coronary heart disease, stroke/TIA, or peripheral arterial disease presumed to be of atherosclerotic origin) who are less than 75 years of age; in patients without clinical ASCVD if LDL-C is 190 mg/dL or greater; in patients without clinical ASCVD who have type 1 or type 2 diabetes and are between 40 and 75 years of age with an estimated 10-year ASCVD risk 7.5% or greater; in patients with an estimated 10-year ASCVD risk 7.5% or greater and who are between 40 and 75 years of age (Stone, 2013)
  Treatment of dyslipidemias: To reduce elevations in total cholesterol (C), LDL-C, apolipoprotein B, and triglycerides in patients with elevations of one or more components, and/or to increase low HDL-C as present in Fredrickson type IIa, IIb, III, and IV hyperlipidemias, heterozygous familial and non-familial hypercholesterolemia, and homozygous familial hypercholesterolemia
  Treatment of heterozygous familial hypercholesterolemia (HeFH) in adolescent patients (10-17 years of age, females >1 year postmenarche) having LDL-C ≥190 mg/dL or LDL-C ≥160 mg/dL with positive family history of premature cardiovascular disease (CVD) or with two or more CVD risk factors.
Unlabeled Use Secondary prevention in patients who have experienced a noncardioembolic stroke/TIA or following an ACS event regardless of baseline LDL-C using intensive lipid-lowering therapy
Mechanism of Action/Effect Inhibitor of 3-hydroxy-3-methylglutaryl coenzyme A (HMG-CoA) reductase, the rate-limiting enzyme in cholesterol synthesis (reduces the production of mevalonic acid from HMG-CoA); this then results in a compensatory increase in the expression of LDL receptors on hepatocyte membranes and a stimulation of LDL catabolism
Contraindications Hypersensitivity to atorvastatin or any component of the formulation; active liver disease; unexplained persistent elevations of serum transaminases; pregnancy (or those who may become pregnant); breast-feeding

Note: Telaprevir Canadian product monograph contraindicates use with atorvastatin.
Warnings/Precautions Secondary causes of hyperlipidemia should be ruled out prior to therapy. Atorvastatin has not been studied when the ▶

primary lipid abnormality is chylomicron elevation (Fredrickson types I and V). Liver function tests must be obtained prior to initiating therapy, repeat if clinically indicated thereafter. May cause hepatic dysfunction. Use with caution in patients who consume large amounts of ethanol or have a history of liver disease; monitoring is recommended. Use is contraindicated in patients with active liver disease or unexplained persistent elevations of serum transaminases; monitoring is recommended. Use high-dose atorvastatin with caution in patients with prior stroke or TIA; the risk of hemorrhagic stroke may be increased.

Rhabdomyolysis with acute renal failure has occurred. Risk is dose related and is increased with concurrent use of lipid-lowering agents which may cause rhabdomyolysis (fibric acid derivatives or niacin at doses ≥1 g/day) or during concurrent use with potent CYP3A4 inhibitors (including amiodarone, clarithromycin, erythromycin, itraconazole, ketoconazole, nefazodone, grapefruit juice in large quantities, verapamil, or protease inhibitors such as indinavir, nelfinavir, or ritonavir). Ensure patient is on the lowest effective atorvastatin dose. If concurrent use of clarithromycin or combination protease inhibitors (eg, lopinavir/ritonavir or ritonavir/saquinavir) is warranted consider dose adjustment of atorvastatin. Do not use with cyclosporine, gemfibrozil, tipranavir plus ritonavir, or telaprevir. Monitor closely if used with other drugs associated with myopathy. Weigh the risk versus benefit when combining any of these drugs with atorvastatin. Discontinue in any patient in which CPK levels are markedly elevated (>10 times ULN) or if myopathy is suspected/diagnosed. The manufacturer recommends temporary discontinuation for elective major surgery, acute medical or surgical conditions, or in any patient experiencing an acute or serious condition predisposing to renal failure (eg, sepsis, hypotension, trauma, uncontrolled seizures). However, based upon current evidence, HMG-CoA reductase inhibitor therapy should be continued in the perioperative period unless risk outweighs cardioprotective benefit. Use with caution in patients with advanced age, these patients are predisposed to myopathy. Immune-mediated necrotizing myopathy (IMNM), an autoimmune-mediated myopathy, has been reported (rarely) with HMG-CoA reductase inhibitor therapy. IMNM presents as proximal muscle weakness with elevated CPK levels, which persists despite discontinuation of HMG-CoA reductase inhibitor therapy; additionally, muscle biopsy may show necrotizing myopathy with limited inflammation; immunosuppressive therapy (eg, corticosteroids, azathioprine) may be used for treatment.

Drug Interactions

Avoid Concomitant Use

Avoid concomitant use of AtorvaSTATin with any of the following: Bosutinib; Conivaptan; CycloSPORINE (Systemic); Fusidic Acid (Systemic); Gemfibrozil; Pimozide; Pomalidomide; Posaconazole; Red Yeast Rice; Silodosin; Telaprevir; Tipranavir; Topotecan; VinCRIStine (Liposomal)

Decreased Effect

AtorvaSTATin may decrease the levels/effects of: Dabigatran Etexilate; Lanthanum

The levels/effects of AtorvaSTATin may be decreased by: Antacids; Bexarotene (Systemic); Bile Acid Sequestrants; Bosentan; CYP3A4 Inducers (Strong); Dabrafenib; Deferasirox; Efavirenz; Etravirine; Fosphenytoin; Mitotane; P-glycoprotein/ABCB1 Inducers; Phenytoin; Rifamycin Derivatives; St Johns Wort; Tocilizumab

Increased Effect/Toxicity

AtorvaSTATin may increase the levels/effects of: Afatinib; Aliskiren; ARIPiprazole; Bosutinib; Cimetidine; DAPTOmycin; Digoxin; Diltiazem; Dofetilide; DOXOrubicin (Conventional); Everolimus; Ketoconazole (Systemic); Lomitapide; Midazolam; PAZOPanib; P-glycoprotein/ABCB1 Substrates; Pimozide; Pomalidomide; Prucalopride; Rivaroxaban; Silodosin; Spironolactone; Topotecan; Trabectedin; Verapamil; VinCRIStine (Liposomal)

The levels/effects of AtorvaSTATin may be increased by: Amiodarone; Azithromycin (Systemic); Bezafibrate; Boceprevir; Clarithromycin; Cobicistat; Colchicine; Conivaptan; CycloSPORINE (Systemic); CYP3A4 Inhibitors (Moderate); CYP3A4 Inhibitors (Strong); Cyproterone; Danazol; Dasatinib; Diltiazem; Dronedarone; Eltrombopag; Erythromycin (Systemic); Fenofibrate and Derivatives; Fluconazole; Fusidic Acid (Systemic); Gemfibrozil; Grapefruit Juice; Itraconazole; Ivacaftor; Ketoconazole (Systemic); Luliconazole; Mifepristone; Niacin; Niacinamide; P-glycoprotein/ABCB1 Inhibitors; Posaconazole; Protease Inhibitors; QuiNINE; Raltegravir; Ranolazine; Red Yeast Rice; Sildenafil; Simeprevir; Stiripentol; Telaprevir; Telithromycin; Tipranavir; Verapamil; Voriconazole

Nutritional/Ethanol Interactions

Ethanol: Ethanol may enhance the potential of adverse hepatic effects. Management: Avoid excessive ethanol consumption.

Food: Atorvastatin serum concentrations may be increased by grapefruit juice. Management: Avoid concurrent intake of large quantities of grapefruit juice (>1 quart/day). Red yeast rice contains an estimated 2.4 mg lovastatin per 600 mg rice.

Herb/Nutraceutical: St John's wort may decrease atorvastatin levels.

Adverse Reactions

>10%:

Gastrointestinal: Diarrhea (5% to 14%)
Neuromuscular & skeletal: Arthralgia (4% to 12%)
Respiratory: Nasopharyngitis (4% to 13%)

2% to 10%:
  Central nervous system: Insomnia (1% to 5%)
  Gastrointestinal: Nausea (4% to 7%), dyspepsia (3% to 6%)
  Genitourinary: Urinary tract infection (4% to 8%)
  Hepatic: Transaminases increased (2% to 3% with 80 mg/day dosing)
  Neuromuscular & skeletal: Limb pain (3% to 9%), myalgia (3% to 8%), muscle spasms (2% to 5%), musculoskeletal pain (2% to 5%)
  Respiratory: Pharyngolaryngeal pain (1% to 4%)
Additional class-related events or case reports (not necessarily reported with atorvastatin therapy): Cataracts, cirrhosis, dermatomyositis, eosinophilia, erectile dysfunction, extraocular muscle movement impaired, fulminant hepatic necrosis, gynecomastia, hemolytic anemia, immune-mediated necrotizing myopathy (IMNM), interstitial lung disease, ophthalmoplegia, peripheral nerve palsy, polymyalgia rheumatica, positive ANA, renal failure (secondary to rhabdomyolysis), systemic lupus erythematosus-like syndrome, thyroid dysfunction, tremor, vasculitis, vertigo

Pharmacodynamics/Kinetics
  Onset of Action Initial changes: 3-5 days; Maximal reduction in plasma cholesterol and triglycerides: 2 weeks

Available Dosage Forms
  Tablet, Oral:
    Lipitor: 10 mg, 20 mg, 40 mg, 80 mg
    Generic: 10 mg, 20 mg, 40 mg, 80 mg

General Dosage Range
  Dosage adjustment recommended in patients on concomitant therapy
  Oral:
    Children 10-17 years (females >1 year postmenarche): 10-20 mg/day (maximum: 20 mg/day)
    Adults: Maintenance: 10-80 mg once daily (maximum: 80 mg/day)

Administration
  Oral May be administered with food if desired; may take without regard to time of day.

Storage/Stability Store at controlled room temperature of 20°C to 25°C (68°F to 77°F).

Nursing Actions
  Physical Assessment Monitor for signs and symptoms of myopathy (muscle pain, weakness, fatigue). Assess risk potential for interactions with other prescriptions or herbal products patient may be taking that may increase risk of rhabdomyolysis. Monitor CPK prior to initiation and recheck when symptoms are suggestive of myopathy. Assess liver function tests prior to initiation, repeat LFTs if indicated thereafter. Consider dietary assessment and plan for teaching.
  Patient Education
  • Discuss specific use of drug and side effects with patient as it relates to treatment. (HCAHPS: During this hospital stay, were you given any medicine that you had not taken before? Before giving you any new medicine, how often did hospital staff tell you what the medicine was for? How often did hospital staff describe possible side effects in a way you could understand?)
  • Patient may experience diarrhea, pharyngitis, rhinorrhea, dyspepsia, or rhinitis. Have patient report immediately to prescriber signs of hepatic impairment, signs of pancreatitis, asthenia, severe arthralgia, paresthesia, urinary retention, oliguria, dysuria, illogical thinking, memory loss, or depression (HCAHPS).
  • Educate patient about signs of a significant reaction (eg, wheezing; chest tightness; fever; itching; bad cough; blue skin color; seizures; or swelling of face, lips, tongue, or throat). **Note:** This is not a comprehensive list of all side effects. Patient should consult prescriber for additional questions.

Intended Use and Disclaimer: Should not be printed and given to patients. This information is intended to serve as a concise initial reference for healthcare professionals to use when discussing medications with a patient. You must ultimately rely on your own discretion, experience and judgment in diagnosing, treating and advising patients.

Dietary Considerations May take with food if desired; may take without regard to time of day. Before initiation of therapy, patients should be placed on a standard cholesterol-lowering diet for 3-6 months and the diet should be continued during drug therapy. Red yeast rice contains an estimated 2.4 mg lovastatin per 600 mg rice. Atorvastatin serum concentration may be increased when taken with grapefruit juice; avoid concurrent intake of large quantities (>1 quart/day).

Atovaquone (a TOE va kwone)

Brand Names: U.S. Mepron
Pharmacologic Category Antiprotozoal
Pregnancy Risk Factor C
Lactation Excretion in breast milk unknown/use caution
Use
  Pneumocystis jirovecii pneumonia (PCP) prophylaxis: Prevention of PCP in patients who are intolerant to trimethoprim-sulfamethoxazole (TMP-SMZ)
  Pneumocystis jirovecii pneumonia (PCP) treatment: Acute oral treatment of mild-to-moderate PCP in patients who are intolerant to TMP-SMZ
Unlabeled Use Treatment of babesiosis; treatment/chronic maintenance of *Toxoplasma gondii* encephalitis; primary prophylaxis of HIV-infected persons at high risk for developing *Toxoplasma gondii* encephalitis
Available Dosage Forms
  Suspension, Oral:
    Mepron: 750 mg/5 mL (5 mL, 210 mL)

General Dosage Range Oral: *Adolescents ≥13 years and Adults:* 1500 mg daily in 1-2 divided doses

Administration

Oral Must be taken administered meals. Shake suspension gently before use. Once opened, the foil pouch can be emptied on a dosing spoon, in a cup, or directly into the mouth.

Nursing Actions

Physical Assessment Ensure patient is taking the medication properly. Needs to be taken with food. Most common side effects are: Rash, nausea/vomiting, diarrhea, headache, and fever.

Patient Education

• Discuss specific use of drug and side effects with patient as it relates to treatment. (HCAHPS: During this hospital stay, were you given any medicine that you had not taken before? Before giving you any new medicine, how often did hospital staff tell you what the medicine was for? How often did hospital staff describe possible side effects in a way you could understand?)

• Patient may experience headache, nausea, dyspepsia, diarrhea, myalgia, insomnia, dizziness, hyperhidrosis, lack of appetite, rhinitis, or rhinorrhea. Have patient report immediately to prescriber depression, dyspnea, stomatitis, severe asthenia, flu-like syndrome, or signs of hepatic impairment (HCAHPS).

• Educate patient about signs of a significant reaction (eg, wheezing; chest tightness; fever; itching; bad cough; blue skin color; seizures; or swelling of face, lips, tongue, or throat). **Note:** This is not a comprehensive list of all side effects. Patient should consult prescriber for additional questions.

Intended Use and Disclaimer: Should not be printed and given to patients. This information is intended to serve as a concise initial reference for healthcare professionals to use when discussing medications with a patient. You must ultimately rely on your own discretion, experience and judgment in diagnosing, treating and advising patients.

Atracurium (a tra KYOO ree um)

Index Terms Atracurium Besylate
Pharmacologic Category Neuromuscular Blocker Agent, Nondepolarizing
Medication Safety Issues
High alert medication:
The Institute for Safe Medication Practices (ISMP) includes this medication among its list of drugs which have a heightened risk of causing significant patient harm when used in error.
Other safety concerns:
United States Pharmacopeia (USP) 2006: The Interdisciplinary Safe Medication Use Expert Committee of the USP has recommended the following:
- Hospitals, clinics, and other practice sites should institute special safeguards in the storage, labeling, and use of these agents and should include these safeguards in staff orientation and competency training.
- Healthcare professionals should be on **high alert** (especially vigilant) whenever a neuromuscular-blocking agent (NMBA) is stocked, ordered, prepared, or administered.

Pregnancy Risk Factor C
Lactation Excretion in breast milk unknown/use caution
Breast-Feeding Considerations It is not known if atracurium is excreted in breast milk. The manufacturer recommends that caution be exercised when administering atracurium to nursing women.
Use Adjunct to general anesthesia to facilitate endotracheal intubation and to relax skeletal muscles during surgery; to facilitate mechanical ventilation in ICU patients; does not relieve pain or produce sedation
Mechanism of Action/Effect Blocks neural transmission at the myoneural junction by binding with cholinergic receptor sites
Contraindications Hypersensitivity to atracurium besylate or any component of the formulation
Warnings/Precautions Reduce initial dosage and inject slowly (over 1-2 minutes) in patients in whom substantial histamine release would be potentially hazardous (eg, patients with clinically-important cardiovascular disease). Maintenance of an adequate airway and respiratory support is critical. Certain clinical conditions may result in potentiation or antagonism of neuromuscular blockade:
Potentiation: Electrolyte abnormalities, severe hyponatremia, severe hypocalcemia, severe hypokalemia, hypermagnesemia, neuromuscular diseases, acidosis, acute intermittent porphyria, renal failure, hepatic failure
Antagonism: Alkalosis, hypercalcemia, demyelinating lesions, peripheral neuropathies, diabetes mellitus

Increased sensitivity in patients with myasthenia gravis, Eaton-Lambert syndrome; resistance in burn patients (>30% of body) for period of 5-70 days postinjury; resistance in patients with muscle trauma, denervation, immobilization, infection, chronic treatment with atracurium. Cross-sensitivity with other neuromuscular-blocking agents may occur; use extreme caution in patients with previous anaphylactic reactions. Use caution in the elderly. Bradycardia may be more common with atracurium than with other neuromuscular-blocking agents since it has no clinically-significant effects on heart rate to counteract the bradycardia produced by anesthetics. Should be administered by adequately trained individuals familiar with its use. Some dosage forms may contain benzyl alcohol which has been associated with "gasping syndrome" in neonates.

Drug Interactions

Avoid Concomitant Use

Avoid concomitant use of Atracurium with any of the following: QuiNINE

Decreased Effect

The levels/effects of Atracurium may be decreased by: Acetylcholinesterase Inhibitors; Fosphenytoin-Phenytoin; Loop Diuretics

Increased Effect/Toxicity

Atracurium may increase the levels/effects of: Cardiac Glycosides; Corticosteroids (Systemic); OnabotulinumtoxinA; RimabotulinumtoxinB

The levels/effects of Atracurium may be increased by: AbobotulinumtoxinA; Aminoglycosides; Calcium Channel Blockers; Capreomycin; Colistimethate; CycloSPORINE (Systemic); Fosphenytoin-Phenytoin; Inhalational Anesthetics; Ketorolac (Nasal); Ketorolac (Systemic); Lincosamide Antibiotics; Lithium; Loop Diuretics; Magnesium Salts; Polymyxin B; Procainamide; QuiNIDine; QuiNINE; Spironolactone; Tetracycline Derivatives; Vancomycin

Adverse Reactions Mild, rare, and generally suggestive of histamine release

1% to 10%: Cardiovascular: Flushing

Causes of prolonged neuromuscular blockade: Excessive drug administration; cumulative drug effect, metabolism/excretion decreased (hepatic and/or renal impairment); accumulation of active metabolites; electrolyte imbalance (hypokalemia, hypocalcemia, hypermagnesemia, hypernatremia); hypothermia

Pharmacodynamics/Kinetics

Onset of Action Dose dependent: 2-3 minutes

Duration of Action Recovery begins in 20-35 minutes following initial dose of 0.4-0.5 mg/kg under balanced anesthesia; recovery to 95% of control takes 60-70 minutes

Available Dosage Forms

Solution, Intravenous:
Generic: 50 mg/5 mL (5 mL); 100 mg/10 mL (10 mL)

Solution, Intravenous [preservative free]:
Generic: 50 mg/5 mL (5 mL)

General Dosage Range I.V.:

Children 1 month to 2 years: Initial: 0.3-0.4 mg/kg; Maintenance: Doses as needed to maintain neuromuscular blockade.

Children >2 years and Adults: Initial: 0.4-0.5 mg/kg; Maintenance: 0.08-1 mg/kg at 15- to 25-minute intervals; Infusion: 5-15 **mcg/kg/minute**

Administration

I.M. Not for I.M. injection due to tissue irritation.

I.V. May be given undiluted as a bolus injection. Administration via infusion requires the use of an infusion pump. Use infusion solutions within 24 hours of preparation.

Injectable Detail pH: 3.25-3.65 (adjusted)

Preparation for Administration Atracurium should not be mixed with alkaline solutions.

Storage/Stability Refrigerate intact vials at 2°C to 8°C (36°F to 46°F); protect from freezing. Use vials within 14 days upon removal from the refrigerator to room temperature of 25°C (77°F). Dilutions of 0.2 mg/mL or 0.5 mg/mL in 0.9% sodium chloride, dextrose 5% in water, or 5% dextrose in sodium chloride 0.9% are stable for up to 24 hours at room temperature or under refrigeration.

Nursing Actions

Physical Assessment Ventilatory support must be instituted and maintained until adequate respiratory muscle function and/or airway protection are assured. Other drugs that affect neuromuscular activity may increase/decrease neuromuscular block induced by atracurium. This drug is not an anesthetic or analgesic; pain must be treated with other agents. Continuous monitoring of vital signs, cardiac status, respiratory status, and degree of neuromuscular block (objective assessment with peripheral external nerve stimulator) is mandatory during infusion and until full muscle tone has returned. Safety precautions must be maintained until full muscle tone has returned. It may take longer for return of muscle tone in obese or elderly patients or patients with renal or hepatic disease, myasthenia gravis, myopathy, other neuromuscular disease, dehydration, electrolyte imbalance, or severe acid/base imbalance.

Long-term use: Monitor level of neuromuscular blockade, skeletal muscle movement, and respiratory effort. Reposition patient and provide appropriate skin care, mouth care, and care of patient's eyes every 2-3 hours while sedated. Provide appropriate emotional and sensory support (auditory and environmental).

Patient Education
- Discuss specific use of drug and side effects with patient as it relates to treatment. (HCAHPS: During this hospital stay, were you given any medicine that you had not taken before? Before giving you any new medicine, how often did hospital staff tell you what the medicine was for? How often did hospital staff describe possible side effects in a way you could understand?)
- Patient may experience flushing or myalgia. Have patient report immediately to prescriber tachycardia, severe dizziness, or syncope (HCAHPS).
- Educate patient about signs of a significant reaction (eg, wheezing; chest tightness; fever; itching; bad cough; blue skin color; seizures; or

swelling of face, lips, tongue, or throat). **Note:** This is not a comprehensive list of all side effects. Patient should consult prescriber for additional questions.

Intended Use and Disclaimer: Should not be printed and given to patients. This information is intended to serve as a concise initial reference for healthcare professionals to use when discussing medications with a patient. You must ultimately rely on your own discretion, experience and judgment in diagnosing, treating and advising patients.

Atropine (A troe peen)

Brand Names: U.S. AtroPen; Atropine-Care; Isopto Atropine
Index Terms Atropine Sulfate
Pharmacologic Category Anticholinergic Agent; Anticholinergic Agent, Ophthalmic; Antidote; Antispasmodic Agent, Gastrointestinal; Ophthalmic Agent, Mydriatic
Medication Safety Issues
BEERS Criteria medication:
 This drug may be potentially inappropriate for use in geriatric patients (Quality of evidence - varies based on comorbidity; Strength of recommendation - varies based on comorbidity)
Pregnancy Risk Factor B/C (manufacturer specific)
Lactation Enters breast milk/use caution
Breast-Feeding Considerations Trace amounts of atropine are excreted into breast milk. Anticholinergic agents may suppress lactation.
Use
Injection: Preoperative medication to inhibit salivation and secretions; treatment of symptomatic sinus bradycardia, AV block (nodal level); antidote for anticholinesterase poisoning (carbamate insecticides, nerve agents, organophosphate insecticides); adjuvant use with anticholinesterases (eg, edrophonium, neostigmine) to decrease their side effects during reversal of neuromuscular blockade
Note: Use is no longer recommended in the management of asystole or pulseless electrical activity (PEA) (ACLS, 2010).
Ophthalmic: Produce mydriasis and cycloplegia for examination of the retina and optic disc and accurate measurement of refractive errors; produce papillary dilation in inflammatory conditions (eg, uveitis)
Mechanism of Action/Effect Blocks the action of acetylcholine at parasympathetic sites in smooth muscle, secretory glands, and the CNS; increases cardiac output, dries secretions. Atropine reverses the muscarinic effects of cholinergic poisoning due to agents with acetylcholinesterase inhibitor activity by acting as a competitive antagonist of acetylcholine at muscarinic receptors. The primary goal in

cholinergic poisonings is reversal of bronchorrhea and bronchoconstriction. Atropine has no effect on the nicotinic receptors responsible for muscle weakness, fasciculations, and paralysis.
Contraindications Hypersensitivity to atropine or any component of the formulation; narrow-angle glaucoma; adhesions between the iris and lens (ophthalmic product); pyloric stenosis; prostatic hypertrophy

Note: No contraindications exist in the treatment of life-threatening organophosphate or carbamate insecticide or nerve agent poisoning.
Warnings/Precautions Heat prostration may occur in the presence of high environmental temperatures. Psychosis may occur in sensitive individuals or following use of excessive doses. Avoid use if possible in patients with obstructive uropathy or in other conditions resulting in urinary retention; use is contraindicated in patients with prostatic hypertrophy. Avoid use in patients with paralytic ileus, intestinal atony of the elderly or debilitated patient, severe ulcerative colitis, and toxic megacolon complicating ulcerative colitis. Use with caution in patients with autonomic neuropathy, hyperthyroidism, renal or hepatic impairment, myocardial ischemia, HF, tachyarrhythmias (including sinus tachycardia), hypertension, and hiatal hernia associated with reflux esophagitis. Treatment-related blood pressure increases and tachycardia may lead to ischemia, precipitate an MI, or increase arrhythmogenic potential. In heart transplant recipients, atropine will likely be ineffective in treatment of bradycardia due to lack of vagal innervation of the transplanted heart; cholinergic reinnervation may occur over time (years), so atropine may be used cautiously; however, some may experience paradoxical slowing of the heart rate and high-degree AV block upon administration (ACLS, 2010; Bernheim, 2004).

Avoid relying on atropine for effective treatment of type II second-degree or third-degree AV block (with or without a new wide QRS complex). Asystole or bradycardic pulseless electrical activity (PEA): Although no evidence exists for significant detrimental effects, routine use is unlikely to have a therapeutic benefit and is no longer recommended (ACLS, 2010).

AtroPen®: There are no absolute contraindications for the use of atropine in severe organophosphate or carbamate insecticide or nerve agent poisonings; however, in mild poisonings, use caution in those patients where the use of atropine would be otherwise contraindicated. Formulation for use by trained personnel only. Clinical symptoms consistent with highly-suspected organophosphate or carbamate insecticides or nerve agent poisoning should be treated with antidote immediately; administration should not be delayed for confirmatory laboratory tests. Signs of atropinization include flushing, mydriasis, tachycardia, and dryness of the mouth or nose. Monitor effects closely when administering subsequent injections as necessary. The presence of these effects is not indicative of the success of therapy; inappropriate use of mydriasis as an indicator of successful treatment has resulted in atropine toxicity. Reversal of bronchial secretions is the preferred indicator of success. Adjunct treatment with a cholinesterase reactivator (eg, pralidoxime) may be required in patients with toxicity secondary to organophosphorus insecticides or nerve agents. Treatment should always include proper evacuation and decontamination procedures; medical personnel should protect themselves from inadvertent contamination. Antidotal administration is intended only for initial management; definitive and more extensive medical care is required following administration. Individuals should not rely solely on antidote for treatment, as other supportive measures (eg, artificial respiration) may still be required. Atropine reverses the muscarinic but not the nicotinic effects associated with anticholinesterase toxicity.

Children may be more sensitive to the anticholinergic effects of atropine; use with caution in children with spastic paralysis. May be inappropriate in older adults depending on comorbidities (eg, dementia, delirium) due to its potent anticholinergic effects (Beers Criteria).

Drug Interactions

Avoid Concomitant Use

Avoid concomitant use of Atropine with any of the following: Aclidinium; Ipratropium (Oral Inhalation); Potassium Chloride; Tiotropium; Umeclidinium

Decreased Effect

Atropine may decrease the levels/effects of: Acetylcholinesterase Inhibitors (Central); Secretin

The levels/effects of Atropine may be decreased by: Acetylcholinesterase Inhibitors (Central)

Increased Effect/Toxicity

Atropine may increase the levels/effects of: AbobotulinumtoxinA; Analgesics (Opioid); Anticholinergics; Cannabinoids; Mirabegron; OnabotulinumtoxinA; Potassium Chloride; RimabotulinumtoxinB; Thiazide Diuretics; Tiotropium; Topiramate

The levels/effects of Atropine may be increased by: Aclidinium; Ipratropium (Oral Inhalation); Pramlintide; Umeclidinium

Adverse Reactions
Severity and frequency of adverse reactions are dose related and vary greatly; listed reactions are limited to significant and/or life-threatening.

Cardiovascular: Cardiac arrhythmia, flushing, hypotension, palpitations, tachycardia

Central nervous system: Ataxia, coma, delirium, disorientation, dizziness, drowsiness, excitement, hallucination, headache, insomnia, nervousness

Dermatologic: Anhidrosis, scarlatiniform rash, skin rash, urticaria

Gastrointestinal: Ageusia, bloating, constipation, delayed gastric emptying, nausea, paralytic ileus, vomiting, xerostomia

Genitourinary: Urinary hesitancy, urinary retention

Hypersensitivity: Anaphylaxis

Neuromuscular & skeletal: Laryngospasm, weakness

Ocular: Angle-closure glaucoma, blurred vision, cycloplegia, dry eye syndrome, increased intraocular pressure, mydriasis

Respiratory: Dry nose, dry throat, dyspnea, pulmonary edema

Miscellaneous: Fever

Pharmacodynamics/Kinetics

Onset of Action I.M., I.V.: Rapid

Available Dosage Forms

Device, Intramuscular:
AtroPen: 0.25 mg/0.3 mL (0.3 mL); 0.5 mg/0.7 mL (0.7 mL); 1 mg/0.7 mL (0.7 mL); 2 mg/0.7 mL (0.7 mL)

Ointment, Ophthalmic:
Generic: 1% (3.5 g)

Solution, Injection:
Generic: 0.05 mg/mL (5 mL); 0.1 mg/mL (5 mL, 10 mL); 0.4 mg/mL (1 mL, 20 mL); 1 mg/mL (1 mL)

Solution, Injection [preservative free]:
Generic: 0.4 mg/mL (1 mL); 0.8 mg/mL (0.5 mL); 1 mg/mL (1 mL)

Solution, Ophthalmic:
Atropine-Care: 1% (2 mL, 5 mL, 15 mL)
Isopto Atropine: 1% (5 mL, 15 mL)
Generic: 1% (5 mL, 15 mL)

General Dosage Range

I.M.; SubQ:
Children ≤5 kg: 0.02 mg/kg/dose every 4-6 hours as needed
Children >5 kg: 0.01-0.02 mg/kg/dose every 4-6 hours as needed (maximum: 0.4 mg/dose; minimum: 0.1 mg/dose)
Adults: 0.4-0.6 mg every 4-6 hours as needed
AtroPen® (I.M.):
Children <6.8 kg: 0.25 mg/dose (maximum: 3 doses)
Children 6.8-18 kg: 0.5 mg/dose (maximum: 3 doses)
Children 18-41 kg: 1 mg/dose (maximum: 3 doses)
Children >41 kg and Adults: 2 mg/dose (maximum: 3 doses)

I.V.: *Children and Adults:* Dosage varies greatly depending on indication

Ophthalmic: *Adults:* Ointment: Apply a small amount in the conjunctival sac up to 3 times/day; Solution (1%): Instill 1-2 drops up to 4 times/day

◄ **Administration**
I.M. AtroPen®: Administer to the outer thigh. Firmly grasp the autoinjector with the green tip (0.5 mg, 1 mg, and 2 mg autoinjector) or black tip (0.25 mg autoinjector) pointed down; remove the yellow safety release (0.5 mg, 1 mg, and 2 mg autoinjector) or gray safety release (0.25 autoinjector). Jab the green tip at a 90° angle against the outer thigh; may be administered through clothing as long as pockets at the injection site are empty. In thin patients or patients <6.8 kg (15 lb), bunch up the thigh prior to injection. Hold the autoinjector in place for 10 seconds following the injection; remove the autoinjector and massage the injection site. After administration, the needle will be visible; if the needle is not visible, repeat the above steps. After use, bend the needle against a hard surface (needle does not retract) to avoid accidental injury.
I.V. Administer undiluted by rapid I.V. injection; slow injection may result in paradoxical bradycardia. In bradycardia, atropine administration should not delay treatment with external pacing.
Injectable Detail pH: 3-6.5; AtroPen®: pH: 4-5
Other Endotracheal: Dilute in NS or sterile water. Absorption may be greater with sterile water. Stop compressions (if using for cardiac arrest), spray the drug quickly down the tube. Follow immediately with several quick insufflations and continue chest compressions.

Preparation for Administration Preparation of bulk atropine solution for mass chemical terrorism: Add atropine sulfate powder to 100 mL NS in polyvinyl chloride bags to yield a final concentration of 1 mg/mL. Stable for 72 hours at 4°C to 8°C (39°F to 46°F); 20°C to 25°C (68°F to 77°F); 32°C to 36°C (90°F to 97°F) (Dix, 2003).

Storage/Stability Store injection at controlled room temperature of 15°C to 30°C (59°F to 86°F); avoid freezing. In addition, AtroPen® should be protected from light.

Nursing Actions
Physical Assessment Monitor for tachycardia and hypotension, especially if cardiac problems are present. Ensure patient safety (side rails up, call light within reach), have patient void prior to administration, and ensure adequate hydration. Be alert to the potential of heat prostration in the presence of high temperatures.

Patient Education
• Discuss specific use of drug and side effects with patient as it relates to treatment. (HCAHPS: During this hospital stay, were you given any medicine that you had not taken before? Before giving you any new medicine, how often did hospital staff tell you what the medicine was for? How often did hospital staff describe possible side effects in a way you could understand?)
• Patient may experience blurred vision, constipation, anhydrosis, insomnia, dizziness, fatigue, anxiety, headache, polydipsia, dysgeusia,

mydriasis, or eye irritation. Have patient report immediately to prescriber urinary retention, oliguria, tachycardia, arrhythmia, flushing, illogical thinking, change in balance, hallucinations, severe asthenia, akathisia, dysphagia, difficulty speaking, xerostomia, xeroderma, or ophthalmalgia (HCAHPS).
• Educate patient about signs of a significant reaction (eg, wheezing; chest tightness; fever; itching; bad cough; blue skin color; seizures; or swelling of face, lips, tongue, or throat). **Note:** This is not a comprehensive list of all side effects. Patient should consult prescriber for additional questions.

Intended Use and Disclaimer: Should not be printed and given to patients. This information is intended to serve as a concise initial reference for healthcare professionals to use when discussing medications with a patient. You must ultimately rely on your own discretion, experience and judgment in diagnosing, treating and advising patients.

Avanafil (a VAN a fil)

Brand Names: U.S. Stendra
Index Terms Stendra
Pharmacologic Category Phosphodiesterase-5 Enzyme Inhibitor
Medication Safety Issues
Sound-alike/look-alike issues:
Avanafil may be confused with sildenafil, tadalafil, vardenafil
Pregnancy Risk Factor C
Breast-Feeding Considerations This product is not indicated for use in women.
Use Treatment of erectile dysfunction (ED)
Mechanism of Action/Effect Avanafil enhances the effect of nitric oxide by inhibiting phosphodiesterase type 5 (PDE-5), resulting in smooth muscle relaxation and inflow of blood into the corpus cavernosum with sexual stimulation.
Contraindications Hypersensitivity to avanafil or any component of the formulation; concurrent (regular or intermittent) use of organic nitrates in any form (eg, nitroglycerin, isosorbide dinitrate)
Warnings/Precautions There is a degree of cardiac risk associated with sexual activity; therefore, physicians may wish to consider the patient's cardiovascular status prior to initiating any treatment for erectile dysfunction. Use caution in patients with anatomical deformation of the penis (angulation, cavernosal fibrosis, or Peyronie's disease) and in patients who have conditions which may predispose them to priapism (sickle cell anemia, multiple myeloma, leukemia). Instruct patients to seek immediate medical attention if erection persists >4 hours.

Use is not recommended in patients with hypotension (<90/50 mm Hg); uncontrolled hypertension

(>170/100 mm Hg); unstable angina or angina during intercourse; life-threatening arrhythmias, stroke, or MI within the last 6 months; cardiac failure or coronary artery disease causing unstable angina. Safety and efficacy have not been studied in these patients. Use caution in patients with left ventricular outflow obstruction (eg, aortic stenosis). Use caution with alpha-blockers; dosage adjustment is needed. Avoid or limit concurrent substantial alcohol consumption as this may increase the risk of symptomatic hypotension.

Rare cases of nonarteritic ischemic optic neuropathy (NAION) have been reported; risk may be increased with history of vision loss. Other risk factors for NAION include heart disease, diabetes, hypertension, smoking, age >50 years, or history of certain eye problems. Sudden decrease or loss of hearing has been reported rarely; hearing changes may be accompanied by tinnitus and dizziness.

Safety and efficacy have not been studied in patients with the following conditions, therefore, use in these patients is not recommended at this time: Severe hepatic impairment (Child-Pugh class C); severe renal impairment; end-stage renal disease requiring dialysis; retinitis pigmentosa or other degenerative retinal disorders. The safety and efficacy of avanafil with other treatments for erectile dysfunction have not been studied and are not recommended as combination therapy. Concomitant use with all forms of nitrates is contraindicated. If nitrate administration is medically necessary, at least 12 hours should elapse from time of last dose of avanafil to time of nitrate administration; administer only under close medical supervision with appropriate hemodynamic monitoring. Avoid use in patients taking strong CYP3A4 inhibitors (see Drug Interactions); dosage reduction recommended in patients taking moderate CYP3A4 inhibitors. Potential underlying causes of erectile dysfunction should be evaluated prior to treatment.

Drug Interactions

Avoid Concomitant Use

Avoid concomitant use of Avanafil with any of the following: Alprostadil; Amyl Nitrite; CYP3A4 Inhibitors (Strong); Fusidic Acid (Systemic); Itraconazole; Ketoconazole (Systemic); Phosphodiesterase 5 Inhibitors; Posaconazole; Riociguat; Vasodilators (Organic Nitrates); Voriconazole

Decreased Effect

The levels/effects of Avanafil may be decreased by: Bosentan; CYP3A4 Inducers (Strong); Dabrafenib; Deferasirox; Etravirine; Herbs (CYP3A4 Inducers); Mitotane; Tocilizumab

Increased Effect/Toxicity

Avanafil may increase the levels/effects of: Alpha1-Blockers; Alprostadil; Amyl Nitrite; Antihypertensives; Bosentan; Phosphodiesterase 5 Inhibitors; Riociguat; Vasodilators (Organic Nitrates)

The levels/effects of Avanafil may be increased by: Alcohol (Ethyl); CYP3A4 Inhibitors (Moderate); CYP3A4 Inhibitors (Strong); Dasatinib; Fluconazole; Fusidic Acid (Systemic); Itraconazole; Ivacaftor; Ketoconazole (Systemic); Lorcaserin; Luliconazole; Mifepristone; Posaconazole; Sapropterin; Simeprevir; Voriconazole

Nutritional/Ethanol Interactions Ethanol: Substantial consumption of ethanol may increase the risk of hypotension and orthostasis. Lower ethanol consumption has not been associated with significant changes in blood pressure or increase in orthostatic symptoms. Management: Avoid or limit ethanol consumption. Food: Avoid grapefruit juice.

Adverse Reactions

>10%: Central nervous system: Headache (5% to 12%)

2% to 10%:

Cardiovascular: Flushing (3% to 10%), ECG abnormal (1% to 3%)

Central nervous system: Dizziness (1% to 2%)

Neuromuscular & skeletal: Back pain (1% to 3%)

Respiratory: Nasopharyngitis (1% to 5%), nasal congestion (1% to 3%), upper respiratory infection (1% to 3%)

Available Dosage Forms

Tablet, Oral:

Stendra: 50 mg, 100 mg, 200 mg

General Dosage Range Dosage adjustment recommended in patients on concomitant therapy.

Oral: *Adults:* Initial: 100 mg 30 minutes prior to sexual activity; to be given as one single dose and not given more than once daily; dosing range: 50-200 mg once daily

Administration

Oral May be administered with or without food, 30 minutes prior to sexual activity.

Storage/Stability Store at 20°C to 25°C (68°F to 77°F); excursions permitted to 30°C (86°F). Protect from light.

Nursing Actions

Physical Assessment Monitor for efficacy, blood pressure, and heart rate.

Patient Education

• Discuss specific use of drug and side effects with patient as it relates to treatment. (HCAHPS: During this hospital stay, were you given any medicine that you had not taken before? Before giving you any new medicine, how often did hospital staff tell you what the medicine was for? How often did hospital staff describe possible side effects in a way you could understand?)

• Patient may experience flushing, pharyngitis, back pain, rhinitis, or rhinorrhea. Have patient report immediately to prescriber angina, tachycardia, arrhythmia, severe dizziness, syncope, intolerable headache, considerable nausea, strength differences from one side to another, difficulty speaking or thinking, change in balance, blurred vision, vision changes, ophthalmalgia, significant eye irritation, blindness, hearing impairment, tinnitus, or priapism (HCAHPS).

- Educate patient about signs of a significant reaction (eg, wheezing; chest tightness; fever; itching; bad cough; blue skin color; seizures; or swelling of face, lips, tongue, or throat). **Note:** This is not a comprehensive list of all side effects. Patient should consult prescriber for additional questions.

Intended Use and Disclaimer: Should not be printed and given to patients. This information is intended to serve as a concise initial reference for healthcare professionals to use when discussing medications with a patient. You must ultimately rely on your own discretion, experience and judgment in diagnosing, treating and advising patients.

Dietary Considerations May take with or without food. Avoid grapefruit juice.

Axitinib (ax I ti nib)

Brand Names: U.S. Inlyta

Index Terms AG-013736; Inlyta®

Pharmacologic Category Antineoplastic Agent, Tyrosine Kinase Inhibitor; Antineoplastic Agent, Vascular Endothelial Growth Factor (VEGF) Inhibitor

Medication Safety Issues

Sound-alike/look-alike issues:

Axitinib may be confused with afatinib, gefitinib, imatinib, PAZOPanib, PONATinib, SORAfenib, SUNItinib, vandetanib, vemurafenib

High alert medication:

This medication is in a class the Institute for Safe Medication Practices (ISMP) includes among its list of drug classes which have a heightened risk of causing significant patient harm when used in error.

Pregnancy Risk Factor D

Lactation Excretion in breast milk unknown/not recommended

Use Treatment of advanced renal cell cancer (RCC) after failure of one prior systemic treatment

Available Dosage Forms

Tablet, Oral:

Inlyta: 1 mg, 5 mg

General Dosage Range Dosage adjustment recommended in patients with hepatic impairment, on concomitant therapy, or who develop toxicities.

Oral: *Adults:* 5 mg every 12 hours; maximum: 10 mg every 12 hours

Administration

Oral Swallow tablet whole with a glass of water. May be taken with or without food. If a dose is missed or vomited, do not make up; resume dosing with the next scheduled dose.

Hazardous agent; use appropriate precautions for handling and disposal (meets NIOSH, 2012 criteria).

Nursing Actions

Physical Assessment Blood pressure needs to be monitored closely from start of therapy. Due to altered wound healing, instruct patient to discuss any surgery or procedures with surgeons and dentists. Monitor for bleeding, symptoms of hypothyroidism, hyperglycemia, diarrhea, severe abdominal pain, and proper wound healing. Instruct patient to report symptoms of vision problems, severe headache, confusion, numbness, stomach pain, or seizures. Monitor kidney, thyroid, and hepatic function.

Patient Education

- Discuss specific use of drug and side effects with patient as it relates to treatment. (HCAHPS: During this hospital stay, were you given any medicine that you had not taken before? Before giving you any new medicine, how often did hospital staff tell you what the medicine was for? How often did hospital staff describe possible side effects in a way you could understand?)
- Patient may experience dysgeusia, diarrhea, nausea, lack of appetite, stomatitis, constipation, arthralgia, or xeroderma. Have patient report immediately to prescriber signs of hemorrhaging, signs of hyperglycemia, illogical thinking, severe headache, intolerable dyspepsia, significant asthenia, temperature sensitivity, weight gain or loss, eczema of hands or feet, myalgia, muscle cramps, blindness, dysphonia, alopecia, or signs of blood clots (HCAHPS).
- Educate patient about signs of a significant reaction (eg, wheezing; chest tightness; fever; itching; bad cough; blue skin color; seizures; or swelling of face, lips, tongue, or throat). **Note:** This is not a comprehensive list of all side effects. Patient should consult prescriber for additional questions.

Intended Use and Disclaimer: Should not be printed and given to patients. This information is intended to serve as a concise initial reference for healthcare professionals to use when discussing medications with a patient. You must ultimately rely on your own discretion, experience and judgment in diagnosing, treating and advising patients.

Related Information

Oral Medications That Should Not Be Crushed or Altered *on page 1712*

AzaCITIDine (ay za SYE ti deen)

Brand Names: U.S. Vidaza

Index Terms 5-Azacytidine; 5-AZC; AZA-CR; Azacytidine; Ladakamycin

Pharmacologic Category Antineoplastic Agent, Antimetabolite; Antineoplastic Agent, DNA Methylation Inhibitor

Medication Safety Issues
Sound-alike/look-alike issues:
AzaCITIDine may be confused with azaTHIOprine

High alert medication:
This medication is in a class the Institute for Safe Medication Practices (ISMP) includes among its list of drug classes which have a heightened risk of causing significant patient harm when used in error.

Pregnancy Risk Factor D

Lactation Excretion in breast milk unknown/not recommended

Use Myelodysplastic syndromes: Treatment of myelodysplastic syndrome (MDS) in patients with the following subtypes: Refractory anemia or refractory anemia with ringed sideroblasts (if accompanied by neutropenia or thrombocytopenia or requiring transfusions), refractory anemia with excess blasts, refractory anemia with excess blasts in transformation, and chronic myelomonocytic leukemia

Unlabeled Use Treatment of acute myelogenous leukemia (AML) in patients requiring low-intensity therapy

Available Dosage Forms
Suspension Reconstituted, Injection [preservative free]:
Vidaza: 100 mg (1 ea)
Generic: 100 mg (1 ea)

General Dosage Range Dosage adjustment recommended in patients who develop toxicities
I.V., SubQ: *Adults:* 75-100 mg/m^2/day for 7 days every 4 weeks

Administration
I.V. Azacitidine is associated with a moderate emetic potential (Basch, 2011); premedication to prevent nausea and vomiting is recommended. Infuse over 10-40 minutes; infusion must be completed within 1 hour of (vial) reconstitution.

Hazardous agent; use appropriate precautions for handling and disposal (NIOSH, 2012). If azacitidine suspension comes in contact with the skin, immediately wash with soap and water; if it comes into contact with mucous membranes, flush thoroughly with water.

Subcutaneous Azacitidine is associated with a moderate emetic potential (Basch, 2011); premedication to prevent nausea and vomiting is recommended.
SubQ: The manufacturer recommends equally dividing volumes >4 mL into 2 syringes and injecting into 2 separate sites; however, policies for maximum SubQ administration volume may vary by institution; interpatient variations may also apply. Rotate sites for each injection (thigh, abdomen, or upper arm). Administer subsequent injections at least 1 inch from previous injection sites; do not inject into tender, bruised, red, or hard areas. Allow refrigerated suspensions to come to room temperature (up to 30 minutes) prior to administration. Resuspend by inverting the syringe 2-3 times and then rolling the syringe between the palms for 30 seconds.

Hazardous agent; use appropriate precautions for handling and disposal (NIOSH, 2012). If azacitidine suspension comes in contact with the skin, immediately wash with soap and water. If it comes into contact with mucous membranes, flush thoroughly with water.

Nursing Actions
Physical Assessment Pretreatment with antiemetic may be ordered to reduce nausea and vomiting. Note specific reconstitution, administration, and storage instructions (I.V. and SubQ stability differs). Monitor patient closely for edema, chest pain, hypotension, CNS changes, gastrointestinal disturbances, and hematologic and hepatic effects.

Patient Education
• Discuss specific use of drug and side effects with patient as it relates to treatment. (HCAHPS: During this hospital stay, were you given any medicine that you had not taken before? Before giving you any new medicine, how often did hospital staff tell you what the medicine was for? How often did hospital staff describe possible side effects in a way you could understand?)
• Patient may experience stomatitis, insomnia, constipation, lack of appetite, xeroderma, rhinitis, pharyngitis, arthralgia, myalgia, anxiety, or dyspepsia. Have patient report immediately to prescriber signs of infection, signs of hemorrhaging, signs of hepatic impairment, signs of renal impairment, signs of hypokalemia, strength differences from one side to another, difficulty speaking or thinking, change in balance, blurred vision, angina, dyspnea, excessive weight gain, edema of extremities, severe dizziness, syncope, intolerable headache, considerable nausea, severe diarrhea, significant injection site irritation, or intolerable asthenia (HCAHPS).
• Educate patient about signs of a significant reaction (eg, wheezing; chest tightness; fever; itching; bad cough; blue skin color; seizures; or swelling of face, lips, tongue, or throat). **Note:** This is not a comprehensive list of all side effects. Patient should consult prescriber for additional questions.

Intended Use and Disclaimer: Should not be printed and given to patients. This information is intended to serve as a concise initial reference for healthcare professionals to use when discussing medications with a patient. You must ultimately rely on your own discretion, experience and judgment in diagnosing, treating and advising patients.

AzaTHIOprine (ay za THYE oh preen)

Brand Names: U.S. Azasan; Imuran
Index Terms Azathioprine Sodium
Pharmacologic Category Immunosuppressant Agent
Medication Safety Issues
Sound-alike/look-alike issues:
AzaTHIOprine may be confused with azaCITI-Dine, azidothymidine, azithromycin, Azulfidine
Imuran may be confused with Elmiron, Enduron, Imdur, Inderal, Tenormin
Other safety concerns:
Azathioprine is metabolized to mercaptopurine; concurrent use of these commercially-available products has resulted in profound myelosuppression.

Pregnancy Risk Factor D
Lactation Enters breast milk/not recommended
Breast-Feeding Considerations Azathioprine is excreted in breast milk. Due to potential for serious adverse reactions in the nursing infant, breast-feeding is not recommended by the manufacturer.
Use
Renal transplantation: Adjunctive therapy in prevention of rejection of kidney transplants
Rheumatoid arthritis: Treatment of active rheumatoid arthritis (RA), to reduce signs and symptoms
Unlabeled Use Adjunct in prevention of rejection of solid organ (nonrenal) transplants; remission maintenance or reduction of steroid use in Crohn disease (CD) and in ulcerative colitis (UC); dermatomyositis/polymyositis; erythema multiforme; pemphigus vulgaris; lupus nephritis (maintenance), chronic refractory immune thrombocytopenia (ITP), relapsed/remitting multiple sclerosis
Mechanism of Action/Effect Azathioprine is a derivative of mercaptopurine; metabolites halt DNA replication and block the pathway for purine synthesis (Taylor, 2005). The 6-thioguanine nucleotide metabolites appear to mediate the majority of azathioprine's immunosuppressive and toxic effects.
Contraindications Hypersensitivity to azathioprine or any component of the formulation; pregnancy (in patients with rheumatoid arthritis); patients with rheumatoid arthritis and a history of treatment with alkylating agents (eg, cyclophosphamide, chlorambucil, melphalan) may have a prohibitive risk of malignancy with azathioprine treatment
Warnings/Precautions Hazardous agent - use appropriate precautions for handling and disposal (NIOSH, 2012).

[U.S. Boxed Warning]:Immunosuppressive agents, including azathioprine, increase the risk of development of malignancy; lymphoma (in post-transplant patients) and hepatosplenic T-cell lymphoma (HSTCL) (in patients with inflammatory bowel disease) have been reported. Patients should be informed of the risk for malignancy development. HSTCL is a rare white blood cell cancer that is usually fatal and has predominantly occurred in adolescents and young adults treated for Crohn disease or ulcerative colitis and receiving TNF blockers (eg, adalimumab, certolizumab pegol, etanercept, golimumab), azathioprine, and/or mercaptopurine. Most cases of HSTCL have occurred in patients treated with a combination of immunosuppressant agents, although there have been reports of HSTCL in patients receiving azathioprine or mercaptopurine monotherapy. Renal transplant patients are also at increased risk for malignancy (eg, skin cancer, lymphoma); limit sun and ultraviolet light exposure and use appropriate sun protection.

Dose-related hematologic toxicities (leukopenia, thrombocytopenia, and anemias, including macrocytic anemia, or pancytopenia) may occur; may be severe and/or delayed. Patients with intermediate thiopurine methyltransferase (TPMT) activity may be at increased risk for hematologic toxicity at conventional azathioprine doses; patients with low or absent TPMT activity are at risk for severe, life-threatening myelotoxicity. Myelosuppression may be more severe with renal transplants undergoing rejection. Monitor CBC with differential and platelets weekly during the first month, then twice a month for 2 months, then monthly (or more frequently if clinically indicated). May require treatment interruption or dose reduction.

Chronic immunosuppression increases the risk of serious, sometimes fatal, infections (bacterial, viral, fungal, protozoal, and opportunistic). Progressive multifocal leukoencephalopathy (PML), an opportunistic CNS infection caused by reactivation of the JC virus, has been reported in patients receiving immunosuppressive therapy, including azathioprine; promptly evaluate any patient presenting with neurological changes. Consider decreasing the degree of immunosuppression with consideration to the risk of organ rejection in transplant patients.

Use with caution in patients with liver disease or renal impairment; monitor hematologic function closely. Azathioprine is metabolized to mercaptopurine; concomitant use may result in profound myelosuppression and should be avoided. Patients with genetic deficiency of thiopurine methyltransferase (TPMT) or concurrent therapy with drugs which may inhibit TPMT are more sensitive to myelosuppressive effects. Patients with intermediate TPMT activity may be at risk for increased myelosuppression; those with low or absent TPMT activity are at risk for developing severe myelotoxicity. TPMT genotyping or phenotyping may assist in identifying patients at risk for developing toxicity.

Consider TPMT testing in patients with abnormally low CBC unresponsive to dose reduction. TPMT testing does not substitute for CBC monitoring. Potentially significant drug-drug interactions may exist, requiring dose or frequency adjustment, additional monitoring, and/or selection of alternative therapy. Xanthine oxidase inhibitors may increase risk for hematologic toxicity; reduce azathioprine dose when used concurrently with allopurinol; patients with low or absent TPMT activity may require further dose reductions or discontinuation.

Hepatotoxicity (transaminase, bilirubin, and alkaline phosphatase elevations) may occur, usually in renal transplant patients and generally within 6 months of transplant; normally reversible with discontinuation; monitor liver function periodically. Rarely, hepatic sinusoidal obstruction syndrome (SOS; formerly called veno-occlusive disease) has been reported; discontinue if hepatic SOS is suspected. Severe nausea, vomiting, diarrhea, rash, fever, malaise, myalgia, hypotension, and liver enzyme abnormalities may occur within the first several weeks of treatment and are generally reversible upon discontinuation. **[U.S. Boxed Warning]: Should be prescribed by physicians familiar with the risks, including hematologic toxicities and mutagenic potential.** Immune response to vaccines may be diminished.

Drug Interactions

Avoid Concomitant Use
Avoid concomitant use of AzaTHIOprine with any of the following: BCG; Febuxostat; Mercaptopurine; Natalizumab; Pimecrolimus; Tacrolimus (Topical); Tofacitinib

Decreased Effect
AzaTHIOprine may decrease the levels/effects of: BCG; Coccidioidin Skin Test; Sipuleucel-T; Vaccines (Inactivated); Vitamin K Antagonists

The levels/effects of AzaTHIOprine may be decreased by: Echinacea

Increased Effect/Toxicity
AzaTHIOprine may increase the levels/effects of: Leflunomide; Mercaptopurine; Natalizumab; Tofacitinib; Vaccines (Live)

The levels/effects of AzaTHIOprine may be increased by: 5-ASA Derivatives; ACE Inhibitors; Allopurinol; Denosumab; Febuxostat; Pimecrolimus; Ribavirin; Roflumilast; Sulfamethoxazole; Tacrolimus (Topical); Trastuzumab; Trimethoprim

Nutritional/Ethanol Interactions Herb/Nutraceutical: Avoid cat's claw, echinacea (have immunostimulant properties).

Adverse Reactions Frequency not always defined; dependent upon dose, duration, indication, and concomitant therapy.

Central nervous system: Fever, malaise
Gastrointestinal: Nausea/vomiting (RA 12%), diarrhea

Hematologic: Leukopenia (renal transplant >50%; RA 28%), thrombocytopenia
Hepatic: Alkaline phosphatase increased, bilirubin increased, hepatotoxicity, transaminases increased
Neuromuscular & skeletal: Myalgia
Miscellaneous: Infection (renal transplant 20%; RA <1%; includes bacterial, fungal, protozoal, viral), neoplasia (renal transplant 3% [other than lymphoma], 0.5% [lymphoma])

Available Dosage Forms
Solution Reconstituted, Injection [preservative free]:
Generic: 100 mg (1 ea)
Tablet, Oral:
Azasan: 75 mg, 100 mg
Imuran: 50 mg
Generic: 50 mg

General Dosage Range Dosage adjustment recommended in patients with renal impairment, on concomitant therapy, or who develop toxicities
I.V.: *Adults:* Transplant immunosuppression: Initial: 3-5 mg/kg/day as a single daily dose; Maintenance: 1-3 mg/kg/day as a single daily dose
Oral: *Adults:*
Transplant immunosuppression: Initial: 3-5 mg/kg/day in 1-2 divided doses; Maintenance: 1-3 mg/kg/day in 1-2 divided doses
Rheumatoid arthritis: Initial: 1 mg/kg/day (50-100 mg) in 1-2 divided doses; Maintenance: 0.5-2.5 mg/kg/day in 1-2 divided doses

Administration
I.V. Can be administered IVP over 5 minutes at a concentration not to exceed 10 mg/mL **or** diluted and given as an intermittent infusion usually over 30-60 minutes or as an extended infusion over up to 8 hours.

Hazardous agent; use appropriate precautions for handling and disposal (NIOSH, 2012).
Injectable Detail pH: 9.6
Oral Administering tablets after meals or in divided doses may decrease adverse GI events.

Hazardous agent; use appropriate precautions for handling and disposal (NIOSH, 2012).
Preparation for Administration Hazardous agent; use appropriate precautions for handling and disposal (NIOSH, 2012).
Powder for injection: Reconstitute each vial with 10 mL sterile water for injection; may further dilute for infusion (in D_5W, 1/2NS, or NS).

Storage/Stability
Tablet: Store at 15°C to 25°C (59°F to 77°F). Protect from light and moisture.
Powder for injection: Store intact vials at 20°C to 25°C (68°F to 77°F). Protect from light. Reconstituted solution should be used within 24 hours; solutions diluted in D_5W, 1/2NS, or NS for infusion are stable at room temperature or refrigerated for up to 16 days (Johnson, 1981); however, the ▶

manufacturer recommends use within 24 hours of reconstitution.

Nursing Actions

Physical Assessment Monitor for opportunistic infection (eg, fever, mouth and vaginal sores or plaques, unhealed wounds) and signs/symptoms of malignancy (eg, splenomegaly, hepatomegaly, abdominal pain, persistent fever, night sweats, weight loss).

Patient Education

• Discuss specific use of drug and side effects with patient as it relates to treatment. (HCAHPS: During this hospital stay, were you given any medicine that you had not taken before? Before giving you any new medicine, how often did hospital staff tell you what the medicine was for? How often did hospital staff describe possible side effects in a way you could understand?)

• Have patient report immediately to prescriber signs of infection, signs of hepatic impairment, signs of pancreatitis, angina, severe nausea, significant asthenia, ecchymosis, hemorrhaging, considerable dizziness, syncope, diarrhea, myalgia, night sweats, excessive weight loss, mole changes, skin growths, or signs of progressive multifocal leukoencephalopathy (confusion, memory impairment, depression, behavioral changes, strength differences from one side to another, difficulty speaking or thinking, change in balance, vision changes) (HCAHPS).

• Educate patient about signs of a significant reaction (eg, wheezing; chest tightness; fever; itching; bad cough; blue skin color; seizures; or swelling of face, lips, tongue, or throat). **Note:** This is not a comprehensive list of all side effects. Patient should consult prescriber for additional questions.

Intended Use and Disclaimer: Should not be printed and given to patients. This information is intended to serve as a concise initial reference for healthcare professionals to use when discussing medications with a patient. You must ultimately rely on your own discretion, experience and judgment in diagnosing, treating and advising patients.

Azelastine and Fluticasone
(a ZEL as teen & floo TIK a sone)

Brand Names: U.S. Dymista™

Index Terms Fluticasone Propionate and Azelastine Hydrochloride

Pharmacologic Category Corticosteroid, Nasal; Histamine H$_1$ Antagonist, Second Generation

Pregnancy Risk Factor C

Use Symptomatic relief of seasonal allergic rhinitis

Available Dosage Forms

Suspension, intranasal [spray]:

Dymista™: Azelastine hydrochloride 0.1% [137 mcg/spray] and fluticasone propionate 0.037% [50 mcg /spray] (23 g)

General Dosage Range Intranasal: *Children ≥12 years and Adults:* 1 spray (137 mcg azelastine/50 mcg fluticasone) per nostril twice daily

Administration

Inhalation For intranasal administration only. Prime pump (press 6 times until fine spray appears) prior to first use. If 14 or more days have elapsed since last use, then reprime pump with 1 spray or until a fine mist appears. Shake bottle gently before using. Blow nose to clear nostrils. Keep head tilted downward when spraying. Insert applicator tip 1/4 to 1/2 inch into nostril, keeping bottle upright, and close off the other nostril. Breathe in through nose. While inhaling, press pump to release spray. Alternate sprays between nostrils. After each use, wipe the spray tip with a clean tissue or cloth and replace cap. Avoid spraying directly into nasal septum, eyes or mouth. Discard after 120 medicated sprays have been used, even if bottle is not completely empty.

Nursing Actions

Physical Assessment Educate patients about proper use of short-acting inhaler for acute asthma attacks; monitor for oral pain or oral fungal infection. Monitor for growth in pediatric patients.

Patient Education

• Discuss specific use of drug and side effects with patient as it relates to treatment. (HCAHPS: During this hospital stay, were you given any medicine that you had not taken before? Before giving you any new medicine, how often did hospital staff tell you what the medicine was for? How often did hospital staff describe possible side effects in a way you could understand?)

• Patient may experience headache or dysgeusia. Have patient report immediately to prescriber signs of infection, severe dizziness, syncope, considerable nausea, significant asthenia, intolerable rhinitis, wheezing, vision changes, ophthalmalgia, eye irritation, severe epistaxis, or stomatitis (HCAHPS).

• Educate patient about signs of a significant reaction (eg, wheezing; chest tightness; fever; itching; bad cough; blue skin color; seizures; or swelling of face, lips, tongue, or throat). **Note:** This is not a comprehensive list of all side effects. Patient should consult prescriber for additional questions.

Intended Use and Disclaimer: Should not be printed and given to patients. This information is intended to serve as a concise initial reference for healthcare professionals to use when discussing medications with a patient. You must ultimately rely on your own discretion, experience and

judgment in diagnosing, treating and advising patients.

Azilsartan (ay zil SAR tan)

Brand Names: U.S. Edarbi

Index Terms Azilsartan Medoxomil; AZL-M

Pharmacologic Category Angiotensin II Receptor Blocker; Antihypertensive

Pregnancy Risk Factor D

Lactation Excretion in breast milk unknown/not recommended

Breast-Feeding Considerations It is not known if azilsartan is excreted into breast milk. Due to the potential for serious adverse reactions in the nursing infant, the manufacturer recommends a decision be made whether to discontinue nursing or to discontinue the drug, taking into account the importance of treatment to the mother. Breast-fed infants of mothers taking medications for hypertension should be monitored for adverse effects (Chobanian, 2003).

Use Treatment of hypertension; may be used alone or in combination with other antihypertensives

Mechanism of Action/Effect Azilsartan is an angiotensin receptor antagonist which selectively blocks the vasoconstriction and aldosterone-secreting effects of angiotensin II.

Contraindications

U.S. labeling: Concomitant use with aliskiren in patients with diabetes mellitus

Canadian labeling: Hypersensitivity to azilsartan medoxomil or any component of the formulation; concomitant use with aliskiren in patients with diabetes or moderate-to-severe renal impairment (GFR <60 mL/minute/1.73 m^2).

Warnings/Precautions [U.S. Boxed Warning]: Drugs that act on the renin-angiotensin system can cause injury and death to the developing fetus. Discontinue as soon as possible once pregnancy is detected. Angiotensin II receptor blockers may cause hyperkalemia; avoid potassium supplementation unless specifically required by healthcare provider. Avoid use or use a smaller dose in patients who are volume depleted; correct depletion first. May be associated with deterioration of renal function and/or increases in serum creatinine, particularly in patients with low renal blood flow (eg, renal artery stenosis, heart failure, volume depletion) whose glomerular filtration rate (GFR) is dependent on efferent arteriolar vasoconstriction by angiotensin II. Use with caution in unstented unilateral/bilateral renal artery stenosis. When unstented bilateral renal artery stenosis is present, use is generally avoided due to the elevated risk of deterioration in renal function unless possible benefits outweigh risks. Use with caution in pre-existing renal insufficiency; significant aortic/mitral stenosis. Potentially significant drug-drug interactions may exist, requiring dose or frequency

adjustment, additional monitoring, and/or selection of alternative therapy.

Angioedema has been reported rarely with some angiotensin II receptor antagonists (ARBs) and may occur at any time during treatment (especially following first dose). It may involve the head and neck (potentially compromising airway) or the intestine (presenting with abdominal pain). Patients with idiopathic or hereditary angioedema or previous angioedema associated with ACE-inhibitor therapy may be at an increased risk. Prolonged frequent monitoring may be required, especially if tongue, glottis, or larynx are involved, as they are associated with airway obstruction. Patients with a history of airway surgery may have a higher risk of airway obstruction. Discontinue therapy immediately if angioedema occurs. Aggressive early management is critical. Intramuscular (I.M.) administration of epinephrine may be necessary. Do not readminister to patients who have had angioedema with ARBs.

Drug Interactions

Avoid Concomitant Use There are no known interactions where it is recommended to avoid concomitant use.

Decreased Effect

The levels/effects of Azilsartan may be decreased by: Herbs (Hypertensive Properties); Methylphenidate; Nonsteroidal Anti-Inflammatory Agents; Rifamycin Derivatives; Yohimbine

Increased Effect/Toxicity

Azilsartan may increase the levels/effects of: ACE Inhibitors; Amifostine; Antihypertensives; CycloSPORINE (Systemic); DULoxetine; Hypotensive Agents; Lithium; Nonsteroidal Anti-Inflammatory Agents; Obinutuzumab; Potassium-Sparing Diuretics; RiTUXimab; Sodium Phosphates

The levels/effects of Azilsartan may be increased by: Alfuzosin; Aliskiren; Brimonidine (Topical); Canagliflozin; Diazoxide; Eplerenone; Heparin; Heparin (Low Molecular Weight); Herbs (Hypotensive Properties); MAO Inhibitors; Pentoxifylline; Phosphodiesterase 5 Inhibitors; Potassium Salts; Prostacyclin Analogues; Tolvaptan; Trimethoprim

Nutritional/Ethanol Interactions Herb/Nutraceutical: Avoid ephedra, yohimbe, ginseng (may worsen hypertension). Avoid garlic (may have increased antihypertensive effect).

Adverse Reactions

Cardiovascular: Hypotension, orthostatic hypotension

Central nervous system: Dizziness, fatigue

Gastrointestinal: Diarrhea (2%), nausea

Hematologic: Hemoglobin decreased, hematocrit decreased, leukopenia (rare), RBC decreased, thrombocytopenia (rare)

Neuromuscular & skeletal: Muscle spasm, weakness

Renal: Serum creatinine increased

Respiratory: Cough

Available Dosage Forms
Tablet, Oral:
Edarbi: 40 mg, 80 mg
General Dosage Range Oral: *Adults:* 40-80 mg once daily
Administration
Oral Administer without regard to food.
Storage/Stability Store at 25°C (77°F); excursions permitted to 15°C to 30°C (59°F to 86°F). Protect from moisture and light. Dispense and store in original container.
Nursing Actions
Patient Education
- Discuss specific use of drug and side effects with patient as it relates to treatment. (HCAHPS: During this hospital stay, were you given any medicine that you had not taken before? Before giving you any new medicine, how often did hospital staff tell you what the medicine was for? How often did hospital staff describe possible side effects in a way you could understand?)
- Patient may experience diarrhea. Have patient report immediately to prescriber severe dizziness, syncope, urinary retention, oliguria, angina, tachycardia, bradycardia, arrhythmia, myalgia, significant nausea, or considerable asthenia (HCAHPS).
- Educate patient about signs of a significant reaction (eg, wheezing; chest tightness; fever; itching; bad cough; blue skin color; seizures; or swelling of face, lips, tongue, or throat). **Note:** This is not a comprehensive list of all side effects. Patient should consult prescriber for additional questions.

Intended Use and Disclaimer: Should not be printed and given to patients. This information is intended to serve as a concise initial reference for healthcare professionals to use when discussing medications with a patient. You must ultimately rely on your own discretion, experience and judgment in diagnosing, treating and advising patients.
Dietary Considerations May be taken with or without food.

Azilsartan and Chlorthalidone
(ay zil SAR tan & klor THAL i done)

Brand Names: U.S. Edarbyclor
Index Terms Azilsartan Medoxomil and Chlorthalidone; Chlorthalidone and Azilsartan
Pharmacologic Category Angiotensin II Receptor Blocker; Antihypertensive; Diuretic, Thiazide
Pregnancy Risk Factor D
Use Treatment of hypertension

Available Dosage Forms
Tablet, Oral:
Edarbyclor: 40/25: Azilsartan medoxomil 40 mg and chlorthalidone 25 mg, 40/12.5: Azilsartan medoxomil 40 mg and chlorthalidone 12.5 mg
General Dosage Range Oral: *Adults:* 40 mg (azilsartan) and 12.5-25 mg (chlorthalidone) once daily; (maximum: Azilsartan 40 mg/day; chlorthalidone 25 mg/day)
Administration
Oral May be administered without regard to meals.
Nursing Actions
Physical Assessment See individual agents.
Patient Education
- Discuss specific use of drug and side effects with patient as it relates to treatment. (HCAHPS: During this hospital stay, were you given any medicine that you had not taken before? Before giving you any new medicine, how often did hospital staff tell you what the medicine was for? How often did hospital staff describe possible side effects in a way you could understand?)
- Patient may experience dizziness or asthenia. Have patient report immediately to prescriber signs of fluid and electrolyte imbalance, angina, severe constipation, or akathisia (HCAHPS).
- Educate patient about signs of a significant reaction (eg, wheezing; chest tightness; fever; itching; bad cough; blue skin color; seizures; or swelling of face, lips, tongue, or throat). **Note:** This is not a comprehensive list of all side effects. Patient should consult prescriber for additional questions.

Intended Use and Disclaimer: Should not be printed and given to patients. This information is intended to serve as a concise initial reference for healthcare professionals to use when discussing medications with a patient. You must ultimately rely on your own discretion, experience and judgment in diagnosing, treating and advising patients.
Related Information
Azilsartan *on page* 153
Chlorthalidone *on page* 310

Azithromycin (Systemic) (az ith roe MYE sin)

Brand Names: U.S. Zithromax; Zithromax Tri-Pak; Zithromax Z-Pak; Zmax
Index Terms Azithromycin Dihydrate; Azithromycin Monohydrate; Z-Pak; Zithromax TRI-PAK™; Zithromax Z-PAK®
Pharmacologic Category Antibiotic, Macrolide
Medication Safety Issues
Sound-alike/look-alike issues:
Azithromycin may be confused with azathioprine, erythromycin
Zithromax® may be confused with Fosamax®, Zinacef®, Zovirax®
Pregnancy Risk Factor B

Lactation Enters breast milk/use caution

Breast-Feeding Considerations Azithromycin is excreted in low amounts into breast milk (Kelsey, 1994). Decreased appetite, diarrhea, rash, and somnolence have been reported in nursing infants exposed to macrolide antibiotics (Goldstein, 2009). The manufacturer recommends that caution be exercised when administering azithromycin to breast-feeding women.

Use Oral, I.V.: Treatment of acute otitis media due to *H. influenzae, M. catarrhalis,* or *S. pneumoniae;* pharyngitis/tonsillitis due to *S. pyogenes,* community-acquired pneumonia due to *Chlamydia pneumonia, H. influenzae, M. pneumoniae,* or *S. pneumoniae;* pelvic inflammatory disease (PID) due to *C. trachomatis, N. gonorrhoeae,* or *M. hominis;* genital ulcer disease (in men) due to *H. ducreyi* (chancroid); acute bacterial exacerbations of chronic obstructive pulmonary disease (COPD) due to *H. influenzae, M. catarrhalis,* or *S. pneumoniae;* acute bacterial sinusitis due to *H. influenzae, M. catarrhalis,* or *S. pneumoniae;* prevention of *Mycobacterium avium* complex (MAC) (alone or in combination with rifabutin) in patients with advanced HIV infection; treatment of disseminated MAC (in combination with ethambutol) in patients with advanced HIV infection; skin and skin structure infections (uncomplicated) due to *S. aureus, S. pyogenes,* or *S. agalactiae;* urethritis and cervicitis due to *C. trachomatis* or *N. gonorrhoeae*

Unlabeled Use Treatment of babesiosis; cat scratch disease; gonococcal infections of the pharynx or rectum (combination therapy) and expedited partner therapy; granuloma inguinale (donovanosis); *Mycoplasma genitalium* infections; pertussis; prophylaxis of infective endocarditis in select patients who are allergic to penicillin and undergoing dental procedures; prevention of pulmonary exacerbations in patients with noncystic fibrosis bronchiectasis; treatment of *Shigella dysenteriae* type 1

Mechanism of Action/Effect Inhibits RNA-dependent protein synthesis at the chain elongation step; binds to the 50S ribosomal subunit resulting in blockage of transpeptidation

Contraindications Hypersensitivity to azithromycin, other macrolide (eg, azalide or ketolide) antibiotics, or any component of the formulation; history of cholestatic jaundice/hepatic dysfunction associated with prior azithromycin use

Note: The manufacturer does not list concurrent use of pimozide as a contraindication; however, azithromycin is listed as a contraindication in the manufacturer's labeling for pimozide.

Warnings/Precautions Use with caution in patients with pre-existing liver disease; hepatocellular and/or cholestatic hepatitis, with or without jaundice, hepatic necrosis, failure and death have occurred. Discontinue immediately if symptoms of hepatitis occur (malaise, nausea, vomiting, abdominal colic, fever). Allergic reactions have been reported (rare); reappearance of allergic reaction may occur shortly after discontinuation without further azithromycin exposure. May mask or delay symptoms of incubating gonorrhea or syphilis, so appropriate culture and susceptibility tests should be performed prior to initiating a treatment regimen. Prolonged use may result in fungal or bacterial superinfection, including *C. difficile*-associated diarrhea (CDAD); CDAD has been observed >2 months postantibiotic treatment. Use caution with renal dysfunction. Macrolides (especially erythromycin) have been associated with rare QTc prolongation and ventricular arrhythmias, including torsade de pointes; consider avoiding use in patients with prolonged QT interval, congenital long QT syndrome, history of torsade de pointes, bradyarrhythmias, uncorrected hypokalemia or hypomagnesemia, clinically significant bradycardia, uncompensated heart failure, or concurrent use of Class IA (eg, quinidine, procainamide) or Class III (eg, amiodarone, dofetilide, sotalol) antiarrhythmic agents or other drugs known to prolong the QT interval. Use with caution in patients with myasthenia gravis.

Oral suspensions (immediate release and extended release) are not interchangeable.

Drug Interactions

Avoid Concomitant Use

Avoid concomitant use of Azithromycin (Systemic) with any of the following: Amiodarone; BCG; Highest Risk QTc-Prolonging Agents; Ivabradine; Mifepristone; Pimozide; QuiNINE; Terfenadine

Decreased Effect

Azithromycin (Systemic) may decrease the levels/effects of: BCG; Sodium Picosulfate; Typhoid Vaccine

Increased Effect/Toxicity

Azithromycin (Systemic) may increase the levels/effects of: Amiodarone; AtorvaSTATin; Cardiac Glycosides; CycloSPORINE (Systemic); Highest Risk QTc-Prolonging Agents; Ivermectin (Systemic); Lovastatin; Moderate Risk QTc-Prolonging Agents; Pimozide; QuiNINE; Rilpivirine; Rivaroxaban; Simvastatin; Tacrolimus (Systemic); Tacrolimus (Topical); Terfenadine; Vitamin K Antagonists

The levels/effects of Azithromycin (Systemic) may be increased by: Ivabradine; Mifepristone; Nelfinavir; QTc-Prolonging Agents (Indeterminate Risk and Risk Modifying)

Nutritional/Ethanol Interactions Food: Rate and extent of GI absorption may be altered depending upon the formulation. Azithromycin suspension, not tablet form, has significantly increased absorption (46%) with food.

▶

Adverse Reactions
>10%: Gastrointestinal: Diarrhea (4% to 9%; high single-dose regimens 12% to 14%), nausea (≤7%; high single-dose regimens 18%)

2% to 10%:

Dermatologic: Pruritus, rash

Gastrointestinal: Abdominal pain, anorexia, cramping, vomiting (especially with high single-dose regimens)

Genitourinary: Vaginitis

Local: (with I.V. administration): Injection site pain, inflammation

Available Dosage Forms
Packet, Oral:

Zithromax: 1 g (3 ea, 10 ea)

Generic: 1 g (3 ea, 10 ea)

Solution Reconstituted, Intravenous:

Zithromax: 500 mg (1 ea)

Generic: 500 mg (1 ea); 2.5 g (1 ea)

Solution Reconstituted, Intravenous [preservative free]:

Generic: 500 mg (1 ea)

Suspension Reconstituted, Oral:

Zithromax: 100 mg/5 mL (15 mL); 200 mg/5 mL (15 mL, 22.5 mL, 30 mL)

Zmax: 2 g (1 ea)

Generic: 100 mg/5 mL (15 mL); 200 mg/5 mL (15 mL, 22.5 mL, 30 mL)

Tablet, Oral:

Zithromax: 250 mg, 500 mg, 600 mg

Zithromax Tri-Pak: 500 mg

Zithromax Z-Pak: 250 mg

Generic: 250 mg, 500 mg, 600 mg

General Dosage Range
I.V.: *Adults:* 500 mg as a single daily dose

Oral:

Immediate release:

Children ≥6 months to 2 years: 5-10 mg/kg as a single daily dose (maximum: 500 mg/dose) **or** 30 mg/kg as a single dose (maximum: 1500 mg/dose)

Children ≥2 years: 5-12 mg/kg as single daily dose (maximum: 500 mg/dose) **or** 30 mg/kg as a single dose (maximum: 1500 mg/dose)

Adults: 250-500 mg as a single daily dose **or** 1-2 g as a single dose

Extended release (suspension):

Children ≥6 months and <34 kg: 60 mg/kg as a single dose

Children ≥6 months and ≥34 kg and Adults: 2 g as a single dose

Administration
I.V. Other medications should not be infused simultaneously through the same I.V. line.

Injectable Detail Infusate concentration and rate of infusion for azithromycin for injection should be either 1 mg/mL over 3 hours or 2 mg/mL over 1 hour.

Oral Immediate release suspension and tablet may be taken without regard to food; extended release suspension should be taken on an empty stomach (at least 1 hour before or 2 hours following a meal), within 12 hours of reconstitution.

Preparation for Administration Injection (Zithromax®): Prepare initiation solution by adding 4.8 mL of sterile water for injection to the 500 mg vial (resulting concentration: 100 mg/mL). Use of a standard syringe is recommended due to the vacuum in the vial (which may draw additional solution through an automated syringe).

The initial solution should be further diluted to a concentration of 1 mg/mL (500 mL) to 2 mg/mL (250 mL) in 0.9% sodium chloride, 5% dextrose in water, or lactated Ringer's. The diluted solution is stable for 24 hours at or below room temperature (30°C or 86°F) and for 7 days if stored under refrigeration (5°C or 41°F).

Storage/Stability
Injection (Zithromax®): Store intact vials of injection at room temperature. Reconstituted solution is stable for 24 hours when stored below 30°C (86°F).

Suspension, immediate release (Zithromax®): Store dry powder below 30°C (86°F). Following reconstitution, store at 5°C to 30°C (41°F to 86°F).

Suspension, extended release (Zmax®): Store dry powder ≤30°C (86°F). Following reconstitution, store at 25°C (77°F); excursions permitted to 15°C to 30°C (59°F to 86°F); do not refrigerate or freeze. Should be consumed within 12 hours following reconstitution.

Tablet (Zithromax®): Store between 15°C to 30°C (59°F to 86°F).

Nursing Actions
Physical Assessment Results of culture and sensitivity tests and patient's allergy history should be assessed prior to beginning therapy. Monitor LFTs and CBC with diff. Instruct patients being treated for STDs about preventing transmission.

Patient Education
• Discuss specific use of drug and side effects with patient as it relates to treatment. (HCAHPS: During this hospital stay, were you given any medicine that you had not taken before? Before giving you any new medicine, how often did hospital staff tell you what the medicine was for? How often did hospital staff describe possible side effects in a way you could understand?)

• Patient may experience dyspepsia, diarrhea, headache, nausea, or lack of appetite. Have patient report immediately to prescriber tachycardia, arrhythmia, hearing impairment, angina, vision changes, myalgia, tinnitus, severe dizziness, syncope, dysphagia, difficulty speaking, vaginitis, signs of pseudomembranous colitis, signs of hepatic impairment, signs of Stevens-Johnson syndrome/toxic epidermal necrolysis, emesis, or injection site irritation (HCAHPS).

- Educate patient about signs of a significant reaction (eg, wheezing; chest tightness; fever; itching; bad cough; blue skin color; seizures; or swelling of face, lips, tongue, or throat). **Note:** This is not a comprehensive list of all side effects. Patient should consult prescriber for additional questions.

Intended Use and Disclaimer: Should not be printed and given to patients. This information is intended to serve as a concise initial reference for healthcare professionals to use when discussing medications with a patient. You must ultimately rely on your own discretion, experience and judgment in diagnosing, treating and advising patients.

Dietary Considerations
Some products may contain sodium and/or sucrose.
Oral suspension, immediate release, may be administered with or without food.
Oral suspension, extended release, should be taken on an empty stomach (at least 1 hour before or 2 hours following a meal).
Tablet may be administered with food to decrease GI effects.

Aztreonam (AZ tree oh nam)

Brand Names: U.S. Azactam; Azactam in Dextrose; Cayston
Index Terms Azthreonam
Pharmacologic Category Antibiotic, Miscellaneous
Medication Safety Issues
Sound-alike/look-alike issues:
Aztreonam may be confused with azidothymidine
Pregnancy Risk Factor B
Lactation Enters breast milk/not recommended
Breast-Feeding Considerations Very small amounts of aztreonam are excreted in breast milk. The poor oral absorption of aztreonam (<1%) may limit adverse effects to the infant. Nondose-related effects could include modification of bowel flora. Maternal use of aztreonam inhalation is not likely to pose a risk to breast-feeding infants.
Use
Injection: Treatment of patients with urinary tract infections, lower respiratory tract infections, septicemia, skin/skin structure infections, intra-abdominal infections, and gynecological infections caused by susceptible gram-negative bacilli
Inhalation: Improve respiratory symptoms in cystic fibrosis (CF) patients with *Pseudomonas aeruginosa*
Unlabeled Use Surgical (perioperative) prophylaxis
Mechanism of Action/Effect Monobactam which is active only against gram-negative bacilli; inhibits bacterial cell wall synthesis during active multiplication, causing cell wall destruction

Contraindications Hypersensitivity to aztreonam or any component of the formulation
Warnings/Precautions Rare cross-allergenicity to penicillins, cephalosporins, or carbapenems may occur; use with caution in patients with a history of hypersensitivity to beta-lactams. Use caution in renal impairment; dosing adjustment required for the injectable formulation. Prolonged use may result in fungal or bacterial superinfection, including *C. difficile*-associated diarrhea (CDAD) and pseudomembranous colitis; CDAD has been observed >2 months postantibiotic treatment. Use with caution in bone marrow transplant patients with multiple risk factors for toxic epidermal necrolysis (TEN) (eg, sepsis, radiation therapy, drugs known to cause TEN); rare cases of TEN in this population have been reported. Patients colonized with *Burkholderia cepacia* have not been studied. Potentially significant interactions may exist, requiring dose or frequency adjustment, additional monitoring, and/or selection of alternative therapy. Safety and efficacy has not been established in patients with FEV_1 <25% or >75% predicted. To reduce the development of resistant bacteria and maintain efficacy reserve use for CF patients with known *Pseudomonas aeruginosa*. Bronchospasm may occur occur following nebulization; administer a bronchodilator prior to treatment.
Drug Interactions
Avoid Concomitant Use
Avoid concomitant use of Aztreonam with any of the following: BCG
Decreased Effect
Aztreonam may decrease the levels/effects of: BCG; Sodium Picosulfate; Typhoid Vaccine
Increased Effect/Toxicity There are no known significant interactions involving an increase in effect.
Adverse Reactions
Inhalation:
>10%:
Respiratory: Cough (54%), nasal congestion (16%), wheezing (16%), sore throat (12%)
Miscellaneous: Fever (13%; more common in children)
1% to 10%:
Cardiovascular: Chest discomfort (8%)
Dermatologic: Skin rash (2%)
Gastrointestinal: Abdominal pain (7%), vomiting (6%)
Respiratory: Bronchospasm (3%)
<1%, postmarketing, and/or case reports: Arthralgia, facial edema, hypersensitivity reaction, joint swelling, tightness in chest and throat

Injection:
>10%:
Hematologic & oncologic: Neutropenia (children 3% to 11%; adults <1%)

Hepatic: Increased serum transaminases (ALT/ AST; children 4% to 6%; >3 times ULN: 15% to 20%, high dose)

Local: Pain at injection site (children 12%, adults 2%)

1% to 10%:

Dermatologic: Skin rash (children 4%, adults 1%)

Gastrointestinal: Diarrhea (1%), nausea (1%), vomiting (1%)

Hematologic & oncologic: Eosinophilia (children 6%, adults <1%), thrombocythemia (children 4%, adults <1%)

Local: Injection site reaction (1% to 3%) (erythema, induration; more common in children), inflammation at injection site (2%)

Renal: Increased serum creatinine (children 6%)

Miscellaneous: Fever (≤1%)

Available Dosage Forms

Solution, Intravenous:

Azactam in Dextrose: 1 g (50 mL); 2 g (50 mL)

Solution Reconstituted, Inhalation [preservative free]:

Cayston: 75 mg (84 mL)

Solution Reconstituted, Injection:

Azactam: 1 g (1 ea); 2 g (1 ea)

Generic: 1 g (1 ea); 2 g (1 ea)

General Dosage Range Dosage adjustment recommended in patients with renal impairment

I.M.: *Adults:* 500 mg to 1 g every 8-12 hours

I.V.:

Children >1 month: 30-50 mg/kg/dose every 6-8 hours (maximum: 8 g daily)

Adults: 1-2 g every 6-12 hours (maximum: 8 g daily)

Oral inhalation: *Children ≥7 years and Adults:* 75 mg 3 times daily

Administration

I.M. Administer by deep injection into large muscle mass, such as upper outer quadrant of gluteus maximus or the lateral part of the thigh. Doses >1 g should be administered I.V.

I.V. I.V. route is preferred for doses >1 g or in patients with severe life-threatening infections. Administer by slow I.V. push over 3-5 minutes or by intermittent infusion over 20-60 minutes.

Injectable Detail Monitor infusion/injection sites carefully. Administer around-the-clock to promote less variation in peak and trough serum levels.

pH: 4.5-7.5 (aqueous solution)

Inhalation Administer using only an Altera nebulizer system; **administer alone; do not mix with other nebulizer medications**. Administer a bronchodilator before administration of aztreonam (short-acting: 15 minutes to 4 hours before; long-acting: 30 minutes to 12 hours before). For patients on multiple inhaled therapies, administer bronchodilator first, then mucolytic, and lastly, aztreonam.

To administer Cayston, pour reconstituted solution into the handset of the nebulizer system, turn unit on. Place the mouthpiece in the patient's mouth and encourage to breath normally through the mouth. Administration time is usually 2-3 minutes. Administer doses ≥4 hours apart.

Preparation for Administration

Inhalation: Reconstitute immediately prior to use. Squeeze diluent into opened glass vial. Replace rubber stopper and gently swirl vial until contents have completely dissolved.

I.M.: Reconstitute vial with at least 3 mL SWFI, sterile bacteriostatic water for injection, NS, or bacteriostatic sodium chloride per gram of aztreonam; immediately shake vigorously.

I.V.:

Bolus injection: Reconstitute vial with 6-10 mL SWFI; immediately shake vigorously.

Infusion: Reconstitute vial with at least 3 mL SWFI per gram of aztreonam; immediately shake vigorously. Reconstituted solutions are colorless to light yellow straw and may turn pink upon standing without affecting potency. Further dilute in an appropriate solution for infusion to a final concentration ≤2% (ie, final concentration should not exceed 20 mg/mL).

Storage/Stability

Inhalation: Prior to reconstitution, store at 2°C to 8°C (36°F to 46°F). Once removed from refrigeration, aztreonam and the diluent may be stored at room temperature (up to 25°C [77°F]) for ≤28 days. Protect from light. Use immediately after reconstitution.

Vials: Prior to reconstitution, store at room temperature; avoid excessive heat. After reconstitution, solutions for infusion with a final concentration of ≤20 mg/mL should be used within 48 hours if stored at room temperature or within 7 days if refrigerated. Solutions for infusion with a final concentration of >20 mg/mL (if prepared with SWFI or NS **only**) should also be used within 48 hours if stored at room temperature or within 7 days if refrigerated; all other solutions for infusion with a final concentration >20 mg/mL must be used immediately after preparation (unless prepared with SWFI or NS).

Premixed frozen containers: Store unused container frozen at ≤ -20°C (-4°F). Frozen container can be thawed at room temperature of 25°C (77°F) or in a refrigerator, 2°C to 8°C (36°F to 46°F). Thawed solution should be used within 48 hours if stored at room temperature or within 14 days if stored under refrigeration. **Do not freeze.**

Nursing Actions

Physical Assessment Allergy history should be assessed prior to beginning treatment. I.V.: Infusion site should be monitored closely. Monitor patient closely during first dose for anaphylaxis. Bronchospasm may occur following inhalation administration; a bronchodilator may be ordered prior to treatment.

Patient Education
- Discuss specific use of drug and side effects with patient as it relates to treatment. (HCAHPS: During this hospital stay, were you given any medicine that you had not taken before? Before giving you any new medicine, how often did hospital staff tell you what the medicine was for? How often did hospital staff describe possible side effects in a way you could understand?)
- Patient may experience diarrhea or rhinitis. Have patient report immediately to prescriber angina, dyspnea, severe nausea, injection site pain or irritation, asthenia, myalgia, ecchymosis, hemorrhaging, vaginitis, signs of pseudomembranous colitis, considerable pharyngitis, significant dyspepsia, arthralgia, or signs of severe pulmonary disorder (HCAHPS).
- Educate patient about signs of a significant reaction (eg, wheezing; chest tightness; fever; itching; bad cough; blue skin color; seizures; or swelling of face, lips, tongue, or throat). **Note:** This is not a comprehensive list of all side effects. Patient should consult prescriber for additional questions.

Intended Use and Disclaimer: Should not be printed and given to patients. This information is intended to serve as a concise initial reference for healthcare professionals to use when discussing medications with a patient. You must ultimately rely on your own discretion, experience and judgment in diagnosing, treating and advising patients.

Baclofen (BAK loe fen)

Brand Names: U.S. Gablofen; Lioresal
Pharmacologic Category Skeletal Muscle Relaxant
Medication Safety Issues
Sound-alike/look-alike issues:
Baclofen may be confused with Bactroban®
Lioresal® may be confused with lisinopril, Lotensin®
High alert medication:
The Institute for Safe Medication Practices (ISMP) includes this medication (intrathecal administration) among its list of drugs which have a heightened risk of causing significant patient harm when used in error.
Pregnancy Risk Factor C
Lactation Enters breast milk/not recommended
Breast-Feeding Considerations Baclofen is excreted into breast milk. Very small amounts were found in the breast milk of a woman 14 days postpartum after oral use. Following a single oral dose of baclofen 20 mg, the total amount of baclofen excreted in breast milk within 26 hours was 22 mcg (Eriksson, 1981). Adverse events were not observed in a nursing infant following maternal use of intrathecal baclofen 200 mcg/day

throughout pregnancy and while nursing (Morton, 2009). Due to the potential for adverse events in the nursing infant, breast-feeding is not recommended by the manufacturer.
Use Treatment of reversible spasticity associated with multiple sclerosis or spinal cord lesions
Orphan drug: Intrathecal: Treatment of intractable spasticity caused by spinal cord injury, multiple sclerosis, and other spinal disease (spinal ischemia or tumor, transverse myelitis, cervical spondylosis, degenerative myelopathy)
Unlabeled Use Intractable hiccups, intractable pain relief, bladder spasticity, trigeminal neuralgia, cerebral palsy, short-term treatment of spasticity in children with cerebral palsy, Huntington's chorea
Mechanism of Action/Effect Inhibits the transmission of both monosynaptic and polysynaptic reflexes at the spinal cord level, possibly by hyperpolarization of primary afferent fiber terminals, with resultant relief of muscle spasticity
Contraindications Hypersensitivity to baclofen or any component of the formulation
Warnings/Precautions Use with caution in patients with seizure disorder or impaired renal function. **[U.S. Boxed Warning]: Avoid abrupt withdrawal of the drug; abrupt withdrawal of intrathecal baclofen has resulted in severe sequelae (hyperpyrexia, obtundation, rebound/ exaggerated spasticity, muscle rigidity, and rhabdomyolysis), leading to organ failure and some fatalities.** Risk may be higher in patients with injuries at T-6 or above, history of baclofen withdrawal, or limited ability to communicate. May cause CNS depression, which may impair physical or mental abilities; patients must be cautioned about performing tasks which require mental alertness (eg, operating machinery or driving). Elderly are more sensitive to the effects of baclofen and are more likely to experience adverse CNS effects at higher doses.

Cases (most from pharmacy compounded preparations) of intrathecal mass formation at the implanted catheter tip have been reported; may lead to loss of clinical response, pain or new/ worsening neurological effects. Neurosurgical evaluation and/or an appropriate imaging study should be considered if a mass is suspected.
Drug Interactions
Avoid Concomitant Use
Avoid concomitant use of Baclofen with any of the following: Azelastine (Nasal); Paraldehyde; Thalidomide
Decreased Effect There are no known significant interactions involving a decrease in effect.
Increased Effect/Toxicity
Baclofen may increase the levels/effects of: Alcohol (Ethyl); Azelastine (Nasal); Buprenorphine; CNS Depressants; Hydrocodone; Methotrimeprazine; Metyrosine; Mirtazapine; Paraldehyde; Pramipexole; ROPINIRole; Rotigotine; Selective

Serotonin Reuptake Inhibitors; Thalidomide; Zolpidem

The levels/effects of Baclofen may be increased by: Brimonidine (Topical); Doxylamine; Droperidol; HydrOXYzine; Magnesium Sulfate; Methotrimeprazine; Perampanel; Sodium Oxybate; Tapentadol

Nutritional/Ethanol Interactions

Ethanol: May increase CNS depression; monitor for increased effects with coadministration. Caution patients about effects.

Herb/Nutraceutical: Avoid valerian, St John's wort, kava kava, gotu kola.

Adverse Reactions

>10%:

Central nervous system: Drowsiness, vertigo, psychiatric disturbances, insomnia, slurred speech, ataxia, hypotonia

Neuromuscular & skeletal: Weakness

1% to 10%:

Cardiovascular: Hypotension

Central nervous system: Fatigue, confusion, headache

Dermatologic: Rash

Gastrointestinal: Nausea, constipation

Genitourinary: Polyuria

Pharmacodynamics/Kinetics

Onset of Action 3-4 days; Peak effect: 5-10 days

Available Dosage Forms

Solution, Intrathecal:

Gablofen: 50 mcg/mL (1 mL)

Lioresal: 0.05 mg/mL (1 mL); 10 mg/20 mL (20 mL)

Solution, Intrathecal [preservative free]:

Gablofen: 10,000 mcg/20 mL (20 mL); 20,000 mcg/20 mL (20 mL); 40,000 mcg/20 mL (20 mL)

Lioresal: 10 mg/5 mL (5 mL); 40 mg/20 mL (20 mL)

Tablet, Oral:

Generic: 10 mg, 20 mg

General Dosage Range

Intrathecal:

Children: Test dose: 25-100 mcg; Initial infusion: Infuse at a 24-hourly rate dosed at twice the test dose

Adults: Test dose: 50-100 mcg; Initial infusion: Infuse at a 24-hourly rate dosed at twice the test dose

Oral:

Adults: Initial: 5 mg 3 times/day; Maintenance: Up to 80 mg/day in 2-3 divided doses

Elderly: Initial: 5 mg 2-3 times/day, increasing gradually as needed

Administration

Injectable Detail pH: 5-7

Intrathecal Intrathecal: For screening dosages, administer as a bolus injection (50 mcg/mL concentration) into the subarachnoid space followed by maintenance infusion (500-2000 mcg/mL concentration).

Preparation for Administration Intrathecal: For screening dosages, dilute with preservative-free sodium chloride to a final concentration of 50 mcg/mL. For maintenance infusions, concentrations of 500-2000 mcg/mL may be used.

Nursing Actions

Physical Assessment Assess cardiovascular and CNS status at beginning of therapy and periodically throughout.

Patient Education

• Discuss specific use of drug and side effects with patient as it relates to treatment. (HCAHPS: During this hospital stay, were you given any medicine that you had not taken before? Before giving you any new medicine, how often did hospital staff tell you what the medicine was for? How often did hospital staff describe possible side effects in a way you could understand?)

• Patient may experience fatigue, nausea, headache, or constipation. Have patient report immediately to prescriber considerable asthenia, severe dizziness, syncope, illogical thinking, behavioral changes, vision changes, angina, myalgia, muscle rigidity, paresthesia, dyspnea, urinary retention, oliguria, hematuria, mood changes, hallucinations, difficulty with motor activity, fasciculations, change in balance, dysphagia, difficulty speaking, involuntary eye movements, or arrhythmia (HCAHPS).

• Educate patient about signs of a significant reaction (eg, wheezing; chest tightness; fever; itching; bad cough; blue skin color; seizures; or swelling of face, lips, tongue, or throat). **Note:** This is not a comprehensive list of all side effects. Patient should consult prescriber for additional questions.

Intended Use and Disclaimer: Should not be printed and given to patients. This information is intended to serve as a concise initial reference for healthcare professionals to use when discussing medications with a patient. You must ultimately rely on your own discretion, experience and judgment in diagnosing, treating and advising patients.

Basiliximab (ba si LIK si mab)

Brand Names: U.S. Simulect

Pharmacologic Category Immunosuppressant Agent; Monoclonal Antibody

Pregnancy Risk Factor B

Lactation Excretion in breast milk unknown/not recommended

Breast-Feeding Considerations It is not known whether basiliximab is excreted in human milk. Because many immunoglobulins are secreted in milk and the potential for serious adverse reactions exists, a decision should be made whether to discontinue nursing or discontinue the drug, taking into account the importance of the drug to the mother.

Use Prophylaxis of acute organ rejection in renal transplantation (in combination with cyclosporine and corticosteroids)

Unlabeled Use Treatment of refractory acute graft-versus-host disease (GVHD); prevention of liver or cardiac transplant rejection

Mechanism of Action/Effect Chimeric (murine/human) immunosuppressant monoclonal antibody which blocks the alpha-chain of the interleukin-2 (IL-2) receptor complex; this receptor is expressed on activated T lymphocytes and is a critical pathway for activating cell-mediated allograft rejection

Contraindications Hypersensitivity to basiliximab or any component of the formulation

Warnings/Precautions To be used as a component of an immunosuppressive regimen which includes cyclosporine and corticosteroids. The incidence of lymphoproliferative disorders and/or opportunistic infections may be increased by immunosuppressive therapy. Severe hypersensitivity reactions, occurring within 24 hours, have been reported. Reactions, including anaphylaxis, have occurred both with the initial exposure and/or following re-exposure after several months. Use caution during re-exposure to a subsequent course of therapy in a patient who has previously received basiliximab; patients in whom concomitant immunosuppression was prematurely discontinued due to abandoned transplantation or early graft loss are at increased risk for developing a severe hypersensitivity reaction upon re-exposure. Discontinue permanently if a severe reaction occurs. Medications for the treatment of hypersensitivity reactions should be available for immediate use. Treatment may result in the development of human antimurine antibodies (HAMA); however, limited evidence suggesting the use of muromonab-CD3 or other murine products is not precluded. **[U.S. Boxed Warning]: Should be administered under the supervision of a physician experienced in immunosuppression therapy and organ transplant management.** In renal transplant patients receiving basiliximab plus prednisone, cyclosporine, and mycophenolate, new-onset diabetes, glucose intolerance, and impaired fasting glucose were observed at rates significantly higher than observed in patients receiving prednisone, cyclosporine, and mycophenolate without basiliximab (Aasebo, 2010).

Drug Interactions

Avoid Concomitant Use

Avoid concomitant use of Basiliximab with any of the following: BCG; Belimumab; Natalizumab; Pimecrolimus; Tacrolimus (Topical); Tofacitinib; Vaccines (Live)

Decreased Effect

Basiliximab may decrease the levels/effects of: BCG; Coccidioidin Skin Test; Sipuleucel-T; Vaccines (Inactivated); Vaccines (Live)

The levels/effects of Basiliximab may be decreased by: Echinacea; Loop Diuretics

Increased Effect/Toxicity

Basiliximab may increase the levels/effects of: Belimumab; Hypoglycemic Agents; Leflunomide; Natalizumab; Tofacitinib; Vaccines (Live)

The levels/effects of Basiliximab may be increased by: Abciximab; Denosumab; Herbs (Hypoglycemic Properties); MAO Inhibitors; Pimecrolimus; Roflumilast; Salicylates; Selective Serotonin Reuptake Inhibitors; Tacrolimus (Topical); Trastuzumab

Nutritional/Ethanol Interactions Herb/Nutraceutical: Echinacea may diminish the therapeutic effect of basiliximab. Avoid hypoglycemic herbs, including alfalfa, bilberry, bitter melon, burdock, celery, damiana, fenugreek, garcinia, garlic, ginger, ginseng, gymnema, marshmallow, and stinging nettle (may enhance the hypoglycemic effect of basiliximab).

Adverse Reactions Administration of basiliximab did not appear to increase the incidence or severity of adverse effects in clinical trials. Adverse events were reported in 96% of both the placebo and basiliximab groups.

>10%:

Cardiovascular: Hypertension, peripheral edema

Central nervous system: Fever, headache, insomnia, pain

Dermatologic: Acne, wound complications

Endocrine & metabolic: Hypercholesterolemia, hyperglycemia, hyper-/hypokalemia, hyperuricemia, hypophosphatemia

Gastrointestinal: Abdominal pain, constipation, diarrhea, dyspepsia, nausea, vomiting

Genitourinary: Urinary tract infection

Hematologic: Anemia

Neuromuscular & skeletal: Tremor

Respiratory: Dyspnea, infection (upper respiratory)

Miscellaneous: Viral infection

3% to 10%:

Cardiovascular: Abnormal heart sounds, angina, arrhythmia, atrial fibrillation, chest pain, generalized edema, heart failure, hypotension, tachycardia

Central nervous system: Agitation, anxiety, depression, dizziness, fatigue, hypoesthesia, malaise

Dermatologic: Cyst, hypertrichosis, pruritus, rash, skin disorder, skin ulceration

Endocrine & metabolic: Acidosis, dehydration, diabetes mellitus, fluid overload, glucocorticoids increased, hyper-/hypocalcemia, hyperlipemia, hypertriglyceridemia, hypoglycemia, hypomagnesemia, hyponatremia, hypoproteinemia

Gastrointestinal: Abdomen enlarged, esophagitis, flatulence, gastroenteritis, GI hemorrhage, gingival hyperplasia, melena, moniliasis, stomatitis (including ulcerative), weight gain

Genitourinary: Bladder disorder, dysuria, genital edema (male), impotence, ureteral disorder, urinary frequency, urinary retention

Hematologic: Hematoma, hemorrhage, leukopenia, polycythemia, purpura, thrombocytopenia, thrombosis

Neuromuscular & skeletal: Arthralgia, arthropathy, back pain, cramps, fracture, hernia, leg pain, myalgia, neuropathy, paresthesia, rigors, weakness

Ocular: Abnormal vision, cataract, conjunctivitis

Renal: Albuminuria, hematuria, nonprotein nitrogen increased, oliguria, renal function abnormal, renal tubular necrosis

Respiratory: Bronchitis, bronchospasm, cough, pharyngitis, pneumonia, pulmonary edema, sinusitis, rhinitis

Miscellaneous: Accidental trauma, cytomegalovirus (CMV) infection, herpes infection (simplex and zoster), infection, sepsis

Pharmacodynamics/Kinetics
Duration of Action Mean: 36 days (determined by IL-2R alpha saturation)

Available Dosage Forms
Solution Reconstituted, Intravenous [preservative free]:
Simulect: 10 mg (1 ea); 20 mg (1 ea)

General Dosage Range I.V.:
Children <35 kg: 10 mg within 2 hours prior to transplant surgery, followed by a second 10 mg dose 4 days after transplantation

Children ≥35 kg and Adults: 20 mg within 2 hours prior to transplant surgery, followed by a second 20 mg dose 4 days after transplantation

Administration
I.V. For intravenous administration only. Infuse as a bolus or I.V. infusion over 20-30 minutes. (Bolus dosing is associated with nausea, vomiting, and local pain at the injection site.) Administer only after assurance that patient will receive renal graft and immunosuppression. For the treatment of acute GVHD (unlabeled use), the dose was diluted in 250 mL NS and administered over 30 minutes (Schmidt-Hieber, 2005).

Preparation for Administration Reconstitute with preservative-free sterile water for injection (reconstitute 10 mg vial with 2.5 mL, 20 mg vial with 5 mL). Shake gently to dissolve. May further dilute reconstituted solution with 25 mL (10 mg) or 50 mL (20 mg) 0.9% sodium chloride or dextrose 5% in water. When mixing the solution, gently invert the bag to avoid foaming. Do not shake solutions diluted for infusion.

Storage/Stability Store intact vials refrigerated at 2°C to 8°C (36°F to 46°F). Should be used immediately after reconstitution; however, if not used immediately, reconstituted solution may be stored at 2°C to 8°C for up to 24 hours or at room temperature for up to 4 hours. Discard the reconstituted solution if not used within 24 hours.

Nursing Actions
Physical Assessment Monitor infusion site and cardiovascular, respiratory, and renal function during infusion. Allergic reactions, including anaphylaxis, have occurred both with the initial exposure and/or following re-exposure after several months. Treatment of hypersensitivity reactions should be available for immediate use. Monitor closely for opportunistic infection (eg, chills, fever, sore throat, easy bruising or bleeding, mouth sores, unhealed sores).

Patient Education
• Discuss specific use of drug and side effects with patient as it relates to treatment. (HCAHPS: During this hospital stay, were you given any medicine that you had not taken before? Before giving you any new medicine, how often did hospital staff tell you what the medicine was for? How often did hospital staff describe possible side effects in a way you could understand?)
• Patient may experience insomnia, acne vulgaris, constipation, diarrhea, nausea, dyspepsia, or pyrosis. Have patient report immediately to prescriber signs of infection, signs of hyperglycemia, signs of hypokalemia, severe dizziness, syncope, angina, tachycardia, dyspnea, excessive weight gain, edema of extremities, sternutation, considerable headache, tremors, significant asthenia, paresthesia, urinary retention, ecchymosis, hemorrhaging, or vision changes (HCAHPS).
• Educate patient about signs of a significant reaction (eg, wheezing; chest tightness; fever; itching; bad cough; blue skin color; seizures; or swelling of face, lips, tongue, or throat). **Note:** This is not a comprehensive list of all side effects. Patient should consult prescriber for additional questions.

Intended Use and Disclaimer: Should not be printed and given to patients. This information is intended to serve as a concise initial reference for healthcare professionals to use when discussing medications with a patient. You must ultimately rely on your own discretion, experience and judgment in diagnosing, treating and advising patients.

Beclomethasone (Oral Inhalation)
(be kloe METH a sone)

Brand Names: U.S. Qvar
Index Terms Vanceril
Pharmacologic Category Corticosteroid, Inhalant (Oral)
Pregnancy Risk Factor C
Lactation Excretion in breast milk unknown/use caution
Breast-Feeding Considerations Other corticosteroids have been found in breast milk; however, information for beclomethasone is not available. Due to the potential for serious adverse reactions

in the nursing infant, the manufacturer recommends a decision be made whether to discontinue nursing or to discontinue the drug, taking into account the importance of treatment to the mother. Use of inhaled corticosteroids is not a contraindication to breast-feeding (NAEPP, 2005).

Use Oral inhalation: Maintenance and prophylactic treatment of asthma; includes those who require corticosteroids and those who may benefit from a dose reduction/elimination of systemically-administered corticosteroids. Not for relief of acute bronchospasm.

Mechanism of Action/Effect Acts at cellular level to prevent or control inflammation

Contraindications Hypersensitivity to beclomethasone or any component of the formulation; status asthmaticus, or other acute asthma episodes requiring intensive measures

Canadian labeling: Additional contraindications (not in U.S. labeling): Moderate-to-severe bronchiectasis requiring intensive measures; untreated fungal, bacterial, or tubercular infections of the respiratory tract

Warnings/Precautions May cause hypercorticism or suppression of hypothalamic-pituitary-adrenal (HPA) axis, particularly in younger children or in patients receiving high doses for prolonged periods. HPA axis suppression may lead to adrenal crisis. Withdrawal and discontinuation of a corticosteroid should be done slowly and carefully. Particular care is required when patients are transferred from systemic corticosteroids to inhaled products due to possible adrenal insufficiency or withdrawal from steroids, including an increase in allergic symptoms. Patients receiving >20 mg per day of prednisone (or equivalent) may be most susceptible. Fatalities have occurred due to adrenal insufficiency in asthmatic patients during and after transfer from systemic corticosteroids to aerosol steroids; aerosol steroids do **not** provide the systemic steroid needed to treat patients having trauma, surgery, or infections.

Bronchospasm may occur with wheezing after inhalation; if this occurs, stop steroid and treat with a fast-acting bronchodilator. Supplemental steroids (oral or parenteral) may be needed during stress or severe asthma attacks. Not to be used in status asthmaticus or for the relief of acute bronchospasm. Corticosteroid use may cause psychiatric disturbances, including depression, euphoria, insomnia, mood swings, and personality changes. Pre-existing psychiatric conditions may be exacerbated by corticosteroid use. Prolonged use of corticosteroids may also increase the incidence of secondary infection, mask acute infection (including fungal infections), prolong or exacerbate viral infections, or limit response to vaccines. Avoid use in patients with ocular herpes or untreated viral, fungal, parasitic or bacterial systemic infections (Canadian labeling contraindicates use with

untreated respiratory infections). Exposure to chickenpox should be avoided. Close observation is required in patients with latent tuberculosis and/or TB reactivity; restrict use in active TB (only in conjunction with antituberculosis treatment). Prolonged treatment with corticosteroids has been associated with the development of Kaposi's sarcoma (case reports); if noted, discontinuation of therapy should be considered.

Use with caution in patients with thyroid disease, hepatic impairment, renal impairment, cardiovascular disease, diabetes, glaucoma, cataracts, myasthenia gravis, patients at risk for osteoporosis, patients at risk for seizures, or GI diseases (diverticulitis, peptic ulcer, ulcerative colitis) due to perforation risk. Use caution following acute MI (corticosteroids have been associated with myocardial rupture). Because of the risk of adverse effects, systemic corticosteroids should be used cautiously in the elderly in the smallest possible effective dose for the shortest duration.

Orally-inhaled corticosteroids may cause a reduction in growth velocity in pediatric patients (~1 centimeter per year [range: 0.3-1.8 cm per year] and related to dose and duration of exposure). To minimize the systemic effects of orally-inhaled corticosteroids, each patient should be titrated to the lowest effective dose. Growth should be routinely monitored in pediatric patients. Safety and efficacy have not been established in children <5 years of age. There have been reports of systemic corticosteroid withdrawal symptoms (eg, joint/muscle pain, lassitude, depression) when withdrawing oral inhalation therapy.

Drug Interactions

Avoid Concomitant Use

Avoid concomitant use of Beclomethasone (Oral Inhalation) with any of the following: Aldesleukin; BCG; Natalizumab; Pimecrolimus; Tacrolimus (Topical); Tofacitinib

Decreased Effect

Beclomethasone (Oral Inhalation) may decrease the levels/effects of: Aldesleukin; Antidiabetic Agents; BCG; Coccidioidin Skin Test; Corticorelin; Hyaluronidase; Sipuleucel-T; Telaprevir; Vaccines (Inactivated)

The levels/effects of Beclomethasone (Oral Inhalation) may be decreased by: Echinacea

Increased Effect/Toxicity

Beclomethasone (Oral Inhalation) may increase the levels/effects of: Amphotericin B; Deferasirox; Leflunomide; Loop Diuretics; Natalizumab; Thiazide Diuretics; Tofacitinib

The levels/effects of Beclomethasone (Oral Inhalation) may be increased by: Denosumab; Pimecrolimus; Tacrolimus (Topical); Telaprevir; Trastuzumab

▶

◄ **Adverse Reactions**
>10%: Central nervous system: Headache (12%)
1% to 10%:
Central nervous system: Dysphonia (1% to 3%),
pain (2%)
Endocrine & metabolic: Dysmenorrhea (1%
to 3%)
Gastrointestinal: Nausea (1%)
Neuromuscular & skeletal: Back pain (1%)
Respiratory: Upper respiratory tract infection
(9%), pharyngitis (8%), rhinitis (6%), sinusitis
(3%), cough (1% to 3%)
Pharmacodynamics/Kinetics
Onset of Action Therapeutic effect: 1-4 weeks
Dosage Forms Considerations
QVAR 8.7 g canisters contain 120 inhalations.
Available Dosage Forms
Aerosol Solution, Inhalation:
Qvar: 40 mcg/actuation (8.7 g); 80 mcg/actuation (8.7 g)
General Dosage Range Inhalation:
Children 5-11 years: Initial: 40 mcg twice daily;
Maintenance: 80-160 mcg/day in 2 divided doses
Children ≥12 years and Adults: Initial: 40-160 mcg
twice daily; Maintenance: 80-640 mcg/day in 2
divided doses
Administration
Inhalation Canister does not need shaken prior to
use. Prime canister by spraying twice into the air
prior to initial use or if not in use for >10 days.
Avoid spraying in face or eyes. Exhale fully prior
to bringing inhaler to mouth. Place inhaler in
mouth, close lips around mouthpiece, and inhale
slowly and deeply. Remove inhaler and hold
breath for approximately 5-10 seconds. Rinse
mouth and throat after use to prevent *Candida*
infection. Do not wash or put inhaler in water;
mouth piece may be cleaned with a dry tissue
or cloth. Discard after the "discard by" date or
after labeled number of doses has been used,
even if container is not completely empty. Patients
using a spacer should inhale immediately due to
decreased amount of medication that is delivered
with a delayed inspiration.
Storage/Stability Do not store near heat or open
flame. Do not puncture canisters. Store at 25°C
(77°F); excursions permitted between 15°C to
30°C (59°F to 86°F). Rest QVAR® on concave
end of canister with actuator on top.
Nursing Actions
Physical Assessment When changing from systemic steroids to inhalational steroids, taper
reduction of systemic medication slowly.
Patient Education
• Discuss specific use of drug and side effects
with patient as it relates to treatment. (HCAHPS:
During this hospital stay, were you given any
medicine that you had not taken before? Before
giving you any new medicine, how often did
hospital staff tell you what the medicine was

for? How often did hospital staff describe possible side effects in a way you could understand?)
• Patient may experience headache, rhinitis, or
pharyngitis. Have patient report immediately to
prescriber signs of infection, severe asthenia,
irritability, tremors, tachycardia, confusion, dizziness, or diaphoresis (HCAHPS).
• Educate patient about signs of a significant
reaction (eg, wheezing; chest tightness; fever;
itching; bad cough; blue skin color; seizures; or
swelling of face, lips, tongue, or throat). **Note:**
This is not a comprehensive list of all side
effects. Patient should consult prescriber for
additional questions.

Intended Use and Disclaimer: Should not be
printed and given to patients. This information is
intended to serve as a concise initial reference for
healthcare professionals to use when discussing
medications with a patient. You must ultimately
rely on your own discretion, experience and judgment in diagnosing, treating and advising
patients.

Bedaquiline (bed AK wi leen)

Brand Names: U.S. Sirturo
Index Terms AIDS222089; R207910; TMC207
Pharmacologic Category Antitubercular Agent
Medication Guide Available Yes
Pregnancy Risk Factor B
Lactation Excretion in breast milk unknown/not
recommended
Use Multidrug-resistant tuberculosis: Treatment
of pulmonary multidrug-resistant tuberculosis
(MDR-TB) in combination therapy in adults (≥18
years of age) when other alternatives are not
available
Available Dosage Forms
Tablet, Oral:
Sirturo: 100 mg
General Dosage Range Oral: *Adults:*
Weeks 1-2: 400 mg once daily
Weeks 3-24: 200 mg 3 times weekly (total weekly
dose: 600 mg)
Administration
Oral Administer with food; swallow tablets whole.
During weeks 3-24 of therapy, space doses at
least 48 hours apart. Administer by directly
observed therapy (DOT).
Nursing Actions
Physical Assessment Monitor ECG, electrolyte
panel, and liver function tests. Instruct patients to
report nausea, anorexia, joint pain, or chest pain.
Patient Education
• Discuss specific use of drug and side effects
with patient as it relates to treatment. (HCAHPS:
During this hospital stay, were you given any
medicine that you had not taken before? Before
giving you any new medicine, how often did
hospital staff tell you what the medicine was

for? How often did hospital staff describe possible side effects in a way you could understand?)
- Patient may experience headache or arthralgia. Have patient report immediately to prescriber tachycardia, severe dizziness, syncope, significant asthenia, considerable nausea, intolerable dyspepsia, urine discoloration, jaundice, inability to eat, severe diarrhea, or hemoptysis (HCAHPS).
- Educate patient about signs of a significant reaction (eg, wheezing; chest tightness; fever; itching; bad cough; blue skin color; seizures; or swelling of face, lips, tongue, or throat). **Note:** This is not a comprehensive list of all side effects. Patient should consult prescriber for additional questions.

Intended Use and Disclaimer: Should not be printed and given to patients. This information is intended to serve as a concise initial reference for healthcare professionals to use when discussing medications with a patient. You must ultimately rely on your own discretion, experience and judgment in diagnosing, treating and advising patients.

Belatacept (bel AT a sept)

Brand Names: U.S. Nulojix
Index Terms BMS-224818; LEA29Y
Pharmacologic Category Selective T-Cell Costimulation Blocker
Medication Guide Available Yes
Pregnancy Risk Factor C
Lactation Excretion in breast milk unknown/not recommended
Breast-Feeding Considerations It is not known if belatacept is excreted in breast milk. Due to the potential for adverse reactions and possible effects on the developing immune system, breast-feeding is not recommended.
Use Prophylaxis of organ rejection concomitantly with basiliximab induction, mycophenolate, and corticosteroids in Epstein-Barr virus (EBV) seropositive kidney transplant recipients
Mechanism of Action/Effect Prevents activation of T cells, a mediator in immunologic rejection associated with kidney transplantation
Contraindications Transplant patients who are Epstein-Barr virus (EBV) seronegative or with unknown EBV status
Warnings/Precautions [U.S. Boxed Warning]: Risk of post-transplant lymphoproliferative disorder (PTLD) is increased, primarily involving the CNS, in patients receiving belatacept compared to patients receiving cyclosporine-based regimens. Degree of immunosuppression is a risk factor for PTLD developing; do not exceed recommended dosing. Patients who are Epstein-Barr virus seronegative (EBV) are at an even higher risk; use is contraindicated in patients without

evidence of immunity to EBV. Therapy is only appropriate in patients who are EBV seropositive via evidence of acquired immunity, such as presence of IgG antibodies to viral capsid antigen [VCA] and EBV nuclear antigen [EBNA]. Cytomegalovirus (CMV) infection also increases the risk for PTLD; CMV prophylaxis is recommended for a minimum of 3 months following transplantation. Although CMV disease is a risk for PTLD and CMV seronegative patients are at an increased risk for CMV disease, the clinical role, if any, of determining CMV serology to determine risk of PTLD development has not been determined.

[U.S. Boxed Warning]: Risk for infection is increased. Immunosuppressive therapy may lead to opportunistic infections, sepsis, and/or fatal infections. Tuberculosis (TB) is increased; test patients for latent TB prior to initiation, and treat latent TB infection prior to use. Patients receiving immunosuppressive therapy are at an increased risk of activation of latent viral infections, including John Cunningham virus (JCV) and BK virus infection. Activation of JCV may result in progressive multifocal leukoencephalopathy (PML), a rare and potentially fatal condition affecting the CNS. Symptoms of PML include apathy, ataxia, cognitive deficiencies, confusion, and hemiparesis. Polyoma virus-associated nephropathy (PVAN), primarily from activation of BK virus, may also occur and lead to the deterioration of renal function and/or renal graft loss. Risk factors for the development of PML and PVAN include immunosuppression and treatment with immunosuppressant therapy. The onset of PML or PVAN may warrant a reduction in immunosuppressive therapy; however, in transplant recipients, the risk of reduced immunosuppression and graft rejection should be considered.

[U.S. Boxed Warning]: Risk for malignancy is increased. Malignancy, including skin malignancy and post-transplant lymphoproliferative disease, is associated with the use of immunosuppressants, including belatacept; higher than recommended doses or more frequent dosing is not recommended; patients should be advised to limit their exposure to sunlight/UV light.

[U.S. Boxed Warning]: Therapy is not recommended in liver transplant patients due to increased risk of graft loss and death. [U.S. Boxed Warning]: Should be administered under the supervision of a physician experienced in immunosuppressive therapy. Patients should not be immunized with attenuated or live viral vaccines during or shortly after treatment; safety of immunization following therapy has not been studied. An increased risk of acute rejection and graft loss has been observed with belatacept when corticosteroids were minimized to 5 mg daily between day 3 and week 6 post-transplant; corticosteroid dosing should be consistent with clinical trial experience (ie, tapered to ~15 mg daily by the first 6 weeks

▶

post-transplant and remain at ~10 mg daily for the first 6 months post-transplant). Patients should not be immunized with attenuated or live viral vaccines during or shortly after treatment; safety of immunization following therapy has not been studied.

Drug Interactions

Avoid Concomitant Use

Avoid concomitant use of Belatacept with any of the following: BCG; Belimumab; Natalizumab; Pimecrolimus; Tacrolimus (Topical); Tofacitinib; Vaccines (Live)

Decreased Effect

Belatacept may decrease the levels/effects of: BCG; Coccidioidin Skin Test; Sipuleucel-T; Vaccines (Inactivated); Vaccines (Live)

The levels/effects of Belatacept may be decreased by: Echinacea

Increased Effect/Toxicity

Belatacept may increase the levels/effects of: Belimumab; Leflunomide; Mycophenolate; Natalizumab; Tofacitinib; Vaccines (Live)

The levels/effects of Belatacept may be increased by: Denosumab; Pimecrolimus; Roflumilast; Tacrolimus (Topical); Trastuzumab

Adverse Reactions Incidences reported occurred during clinical trials using belatacept compared to a cyclosporine control regimen. All patients also received basiliximab induction, mycophenolate mofetil, and corticosteroids, and were followed up to 3 years.

>10%:

Cardiovascular: Peripheral edema (34%), hypertension (32%), hypotension (18%)

Central nervous system: Fever (28%), headache (21%), insomnia (15%)

Endocrine & metabolic: Hypokalemia (21%), hyperkalemia (20%), hypophosphatemia (19%), lipid metabolism disorder (19%), hyperglycemia (16%), hypocalcemia (13%), hypercholesterolemia (11%)

Gastrointestinal: Diarrhea (39%), constipation (33%), nausea (24%), vomiting (22%), abdominal pain (19%)

Genitourinary: Urinary tract infection (37%), dysuria (11%)

Hematologic & oncologic: Anemia (45%), leukopenia (20%)

Infection: Increased susceptibility to infection (72% to 82%), serious infection 24% to 36%), herpes (7% to 14%), cytomegalovirus disease (11% to 13%), influenza (11%)

Neuromuscular & skeletal: Arthralgia (17%), back pain (13%)

Renal: Proteinuria (16%; up to 33% 2+ proteinuria at 1 month post-transplant), renal graft dysfunction (25%), hematuria (16%), increased serum creatinine (15%)

Respiratory: Cough (24%), upper respiratory tract infection (15%), nasopharyngitis (13%), dyspnea (12%)

1% to 10%:

Cardiovascular: Arteriovenous fistula site complication (thrombosis, <10%), atrial fibrillation (<10%)

Central nervous system: Anxiety (10%), Guillain-Barré syndrome (<10%), dizziness (9%)

Dermatologic: Alopecia (<10%), hyperhidrosis (<10%), acne vulgaris (8%)

Endocrine & metabolic: Diabetes mellitus (new onset, 5% to 8%), hypomagnesemia (7%), hyperuricemia (5%)

Gastrointestinal: Stomatitis (<10%), upper abdominal pain (9%)

Genitourinary: Urinary incontinence (<10%)

Hematologic & oncologic: Hematoma (<10%), lymphocele (<10%), neutropenia (<10%), malignant neoplasm (4%), malignant neoplasm of skin (nonmelanoma, 2%)

Immunologic: Antibody development (2%)

Infection: Polyoma virus (3% to 4%)

Neuromuscular & skeletal: Musculoskeletal pain (<10%), tremor (8%)

Renal: Acute renal failure (<10%), chronic allograft nephropathy (<10%), hydronephrosis (<10%), renal insufficiency (<10%), renal artery stenosis (<10%), renal tubular necrosis (9%), renal disease (BK virus-associated, 1%)

Respiratory: Bronchitis (10%), tuberculosis (1% to 2%)

Miscellaneous: Infusion related reaction (5%)

Available Dosage Forms

Solution Reconstituted, Intravenous:

Nulojix: 250 mg (1 ea)

General Dosage Range I.V.: *Adults:* Initial phase: 10 mg/kg on day 1 (day of transplantation, prior to transplant) and day 5 (post-transplant), and at the end of week 2, 4, 8, and 12 post-transplant; maintenance phase: 5 mg/kg every 4 weeks beginning at the end of week 16 post-transplant

Administration

I.V. Administer as an I.V. infusion over 30 minutes using an infusion set with a 0.2-1.2 micron low protein-binding filter. Prior to administration, inspect visually and do not use if solution is discolored or contains particulate matter.

Preparation for Administration Reconstitute each vial with 10.5 mL of diluent (SWFI, NS, or D_5W) using the provided silicone-free disposable syringe, and an 18- to 21-gauge needle. Reconstitute using **only** the silicone-free syringe provided (discard if powder is inadvertently mixed using a siliconized syringe, translucent particles may develop). Inject the diluent down the side of the vial to avoid foaming. Rotate the vial and invert with gentle swirling until completely dissolved; do **not** shake vial. The reconstituted solution should be clear to slightly opalescent and colorless to pale yellow. Immediately transfer the reconstituted solution using the same silicone-free syringe to an infusion bag or bottle with NS or D_5W (if NS or D_5W were used to reconstitute, the same fluid should be used to further dilute). The final concentration should range from 2 mg/mL and 10 mg/mL (typical infusion volume is 100 mL). Prior to adding belatacept to the infusion solution, the manufacturer recommends withdrawing a volume equal to the amount of belatacept to be added. Mix gently; do not shake.

Storage/Stability Prior to use, store refrigerated at 2°C to 8°C (36°F to 46°F). Protect from light. After dilution, the infusion solution (reconstituted solution must be further diluted immediately) may be stored refrigerated for up to 24 hours, with a maximum of 4 hours of the 24 hours at room temperature, 20°C to 25°C (68°F to 77°F), and room light. Infusion must be completed within 24 hours of reconstitution.

Nursing Actions

Physical Assessment Monitor vital signs as changes in blood pressure can occur. Assess for signs or symptoms of infection, transplant rejection, changes in electrolytes (potassium, phosphorus, calcium, glucose), and cholesterol. Monitor for most common reactions: Infection, blood pressure changes (hypertension, hypotension), diarrhea, anemia, peripheral edema, constipation, fever, cough, nausea, vomiting, headache, electrolyte changes, and leukopenia. Educate patient to limit exposure to ultraviolet light and sunlight, on regular doctor visits, and on infection prevention measures.

Patient Education

• Discuss specific use of drug and side effects with patient as it relates to treatment. (HCAHPS: During this hospital stay, were you given any medicine that you had not taken before? Before giving you any new medicine, how often did hospital staff tell you what the medicine was for? How often did hospital staff describe possible side effects in a way you could understand?)

• Patient may experience constipation, diarrhea, nausea, dyspepsia, arthralgia, back pain, or insomnia. Have patient report immediately to prescriber signs of infection, signs of hypokalemia, signs of hyperglycemia, confusion, anxiety, irritability, diaphoresis, tremors, shivering, rigidity, severe dizziness, syncope, significant headache, considerable asthenia, urinary retention, oliguria, dysuria, hematuria, dyspnea, edema of extremities, excessive weight loss, night sweats, enlarged lymph nodes, mole changes, skin growths, signs of progressive multifocal leukoencephalopathy (PML), or signs of renal impairment (HCAHPS).

• Educate patient about signs of a significant reaction (eg, wheezing; chest tightness; fever; itching; bad cough; blue skin color; seizures; or swelling of face, lips, tongue, or throat). **Note:** This is not a comprehensive list of all side effects. Patient should consult prescriber for additional questions.

Intended Use and Disclaimer: Should not be printed and given to patients. This information is intended to serve as a concise initial reference for healthcare professionals to use when discussing medications with a patient. You must ultimately rely on your own discretion, experience and judgment in diagnosing, treating and advising patients.

Dietary Considerations May contain sucrose.

Belimumab (be LIM yoo mab)

Brand Names: U.S. Benlysta
Pharmacologic Category Monoclonal Antibody
Medication Guide Available Yes
Pregnancy Risk Factor C
Lactation Excretion in breast milk unknown/not recommended

Use

Systemic lupus erythematosus: Treatment of adult patients with active, autoantibody-positive systemic lupus erythematosus (SLE) who are receiving standard therapy.

Limitations of use: Use is not recommended in patients with severe active lupus nephritis, severe active CNS lupus, or in combination with other biologics, including B-cell targeted therapies or intravenous (IV) cyclophosphamide.

Available Dosage Forms

Solution Reconstituted, Intravenous [preservative free]:

Benlysta: 120 mg (1 ea); 400 mg (1 ea)

General Dosage Range I.V.: *Adults:* 10 mg/kg every 2 weeks for 3 doses; Maintenance: 10 mg/kg every 4 weeks

Administration

I.V. Administer intravenously over 1 hour through a dedicated I.V. line. Do **NOT** administer as an I.V. push or bolus. Discontinue infusion for severe hypersensitivity reaction (eg, anaphylaxis, angioedema). The infusion may be slowed or temporarily interrupted for minor reactions. Consider premedicating with an antihistamine and antipyretic for prophylaxis against hypersensitivity or infusion reactions.

Nursing Actions

Patient Education

• Discuss specific use of drug and side effects with patient as it relates to treatment. (HCAHPS: During this hospital stay, were you given any medicine that you had not taken before? Before giving you any new medicine, how often did hospital staff tell you what the medicine was for? How often did hospital staff describe possible side effects in a way you could understand?)

• Patient may experience insomnia, headache, diarrhea, dyspepsia, rhinitis, rhinorrhea, or pharyngitis. Have patient report immediately to prescriber signs of infection, signs of depression (ie, suicidal ideation, anxiety, emotional instability, ▸

illogical thinking), angina, bradycardia, severe dizziness, syncope, dyspnea, diaphoresis, or significant nausea (HCAHPS).
• Educate patient about signs of a significant reaction (eg, wheezing; chest tightness; fever; itching; bad cough; blue skin color; seizures; or swelling of face, lips, tongue, or throat). **Note:** This is not a comprehensive list of all side effects. Patient should consult prescriber for additional questions.

Intended Use and Disclaimer: Should not be printed and given to patients. This information is intended to serve as a concise initial reference for healthcare professionals to use when discussing medications with a patient. You must ultimately rely on your own discretion, experience and judgment in diagnosing, treating and advising patients.

Belladonna and Opium
(bel a DON a & OH pee um)

Index Terms B&O; Opium and Belladonna
Pharmacologic Category Analgesic Combination (Opioid); Antispasmodic Agent, Urinary
Medication Safety Issues
Sound-alike/look-alike issues:
B&O may be confused with beano®
High alert medication:
The Institute for Safe Medication Practices (ISMP) includes this medication among its list of drug classes which have a heightened risk of causing significant patient harm when used in error.
BEERS Criteria medication:
This drug may be potentially inappropriate for use in geriatric patients (Quality of evidence - moderate; Strength of recommendation - strong).
Pregnancy Risk Factor C
Lactation Excretion in breast milk unknown/use caution
Use Relief of moderate-to-severe pain associated with ureteral spasms not responsive to nonopioid analgesics and to space intervals between injections of opioids
Controlled Substance C-II
Available Dosage Forms
Suppository: Belladonna extract 16.2 mg and opium 30 mg; belladonna extract 16.2 mg and opium 60 mg
General Dosage Range Rectal: *Children >12 years and Adults:* 1 suppository 1-2 times/day (maximum: 4 doses/day)
Administration
Other Prior to rectal insertion, the finger and suppository should be moistened. Assist with ambulation.
Nursing Actions
Physical Assessment Monitor blood pressure, CNS and respiratory status, and degree of

sedation at beginning of therapy and at regular intervals. May cause physical and/or psychological dependence. For inpatients, implement safety measures (eg, side rails up, call light within reach, instructions to call for assistance) to prevent falls.
Patient Education
• Discuss specific use of drug and side effects with patient as it relates to treatment. (HCAHPS: During this hospital stay, were you given any medicine that you had not taken before? Before giving you any new medicine, how often did hospital staff tell you what the medicine was for? How often did hospital staff describe possible side effects in a way you could understand?)
• Patient may experience fatigue, xerostomia, constipation, or nausea. Have patient report immediately to prescriber severe dizziness, syncope, illogical thinking, tachycardia, vision changes, urinary retention, oliguria, or light sensitivity (HCAHPS).
• Educate patient about signs of a significant reaction (eg, wheezing; chest tightness; fever; itching; bad cough; blue skin color; seizures; or swelling of face, lips, tongue, or throat). **Note:** This is not a comprehensive list of all side effects. Patient should consult prescriber for additional questions.

Intended Use and Disclaimer: Should not be printed and given to patients. This information is intended to serve as a concise initial reference for healthcare professionals to use when discussing medications with a patient. You must ultimately rely on your own discretion, experience and judgment in diagnosing, treating and advising patients.
Related Information
Opium Tincture *on page 1164*

Benazepril (ben AY ze pril)

Brand Names: U.S. Lotensin
Index Terms Benazepril Hydrochloride
Pharmacologic Category Angiotensin-Converting Enzyme (ACE) Inhibitor; Antihypertensive
Medication Safety Issues
Sound-alike/look-alike issues:
Benazepril may be confused with Benadryl
Lotensin may be confused with Lioresal, lorcaserin, lovastatin
Pregnancy Risk Factor D
Lactation Enters breast milk
Breast-Feeding Considerations Small amounts of benazepril and benazeprilat are found in breast milk.
Use Treatment of hypertension, either alone or in combination with other antihypertensive agents
Unlabeled Use Heart failure (HF): The ACCF/AHA 2013 heart failure guidelines recommend the use of ACE inhibitors, along with other guideline directed medical therapies, to prevent heart failure

in patients with a reduced ejection fraction who have a history of MI (Stage B HF), to prevent heart failure in any patient with a reduced ejection fraction (Stage B HF), or to treat those with heart failure and reduced ejection fraction (Stage C HFrEF) (ACCF/AHA [Yancy, 2013]).

Mechanism of Action/Effect Competitive inhibitor of angiotensin-converting enzyme (ACE); prevents conversion of angiotensin I to angiotensin II, a potent vasoconstrictor; results in lower levels of angiotensin II which causes an increase in plasma renin activity and a reduction in aldosterone secretion

Contraindications Hypersensitivity to benazepril or any component of the formulation; patients with a history of angioedema (with or without prior ACE inhibitor therapy); concomitant use with aliskiren in patients with diabetes mellitus

Canadian labeling: Additional contraindications (not in U.S. labeling): Concomitant use with aliskiren in patients with moderate to severe renal impairment (GFR <60 mL/minute/1.73 m^2); pregnancy; breast-feeding; rare hereditary problems of galactose intolerance (eg, galactosemia, Lapp Lactase deficiency or glucose-galactose malabsorption)

Warnings/Precautions Anaphylactic reactions may occur rarely with ACE inhibitors. At any time during treatment (especially following first dose) angioedema may occur rarely with ACE inhibitors. It may involve the head and neck (potentially compromising airway) or the intestine (presenting with abdominal pain). African-Americans and patients with idiopathic or hereditary angioedema may be at an increased risk. Prolonged frequent monitoring may be required especially if tongue, glottis, or larynx are involved as they are associated with airway obstruction. Patients with a history of airway surgery may have a higher risk of airway obstruction. Aggressive early and appropriate management is critical. Contraindicated in patients with history of angioedema with or without prior ACE inhibitor therapy. Hypersensitivity reactions may be seen during hemodialysis (eg, CVVHD) with high-flux dialysis membranes (eg, AN69), and rarely, during low density lipoprotein apheresis with dextran sulfate cellulose. Rare cases of anaphylactoid reactions have been reported in patients undergoing sensitization treatment with hymenoptera (bee, wasp) venom while receiving ACE inhibitors.

Symptomatic hypotension with or without syncope can occur with ACE inhibitors (usually with the first several doses); effects are most often observed in volume depleted patients; close monitoring of patient is required especially with initial dosing and dosing increases; blood pressure must be lowered at a rate appropriate for the patient's clinical condition. Initiation of therapy in patients with ischemic heart disease or cerebrovascular disease warrants close observation due to the potential consequences posed by falling blood pressure (eg, MI, stroke). **[U.S. Boxed Warning]: Drugs that act on the renin-angiotensin system can cause injury and death to the developing fetus. Discontinue as soon as possible once pregnancy is detected.** Use with caution in hypertrophic cardiomyopathy with outflow tract obstruction, severe aortic stenosis, or before, during, or immediately after major surgery.

Hyperkalemia may occur with ACE inhibitors; risk factors include renal dysfunction, diabetes mellitus, concomitant use of potassium-sparing diuretics, potassium supplements and/or potassium-containing salts. Use cautiously, if at all, with these agents and monitor potassium periodically. Cough may occur with ACE inhibitors. Other causes of cough should be considered (eg, pulmonary congestion in patients with heart failure) and excluded prior to discontinuation. Use with caution in patients with diabetes receiving insulin or oral antidiabetic agents; may be at increased risk for episodes of hypoglycemia.

May be associated with deterioration of renal function and/or increases in serum creatinine, particularly in patients with low renal blood flow (eg, renal artery stenosis, heart failure) whose glomerular filtration rate (GFR) is dependent on efferent arteriolar vasoconstriction by angiotensin II; deterioration may result in oliguria, acute renal failure, and progressive azotemia. Small increases in serum creatinine may occur following initiation; consider discontinuation only in patients with progressive and/or significant deterioration in renal function. Use with caution in patients with unstented unilateral/bilateral renal artery stenosis. When unstented bilateral renal artery stenosis is present, use is generally avoided due to the elevated risk of deterioration in renal function unless possible benefits outweigh risks. Potentially significant drug-drug interactions may exist, requiring dose or frequency adjustment, additional monitoring, and/or selection of alternative therapy.

Rare toxicities associated with ACE inhibitors include cholestatic jaundice (which may progress to fulminant hepatic necrosis), agranulocytosis, neutropenia, or leukopenia with myeloid hypoplasia. Patients with collagen vascular diseases (especially with concomitant renal impairment) or renal impairment alone may be at increased risk for hematologic toxicity; periodically monitor CBC with differential in these patients.

Drug Interactions

Avoid Concomitant Use There are no known interactions where it is recommended to avoid concomitant use.

Decreased Effect

Benazepril may decrease the levels/effects of: Hydrochlorothiazide

The levels/effects of Benazepril may be decreased by: Antacids; Aprotinin; Herbs (Hypertensive Properties); Icatibant; Lanthanum; Methylphenidate; Nonsteroidal Anti-Inflammatory Agents; Salicylates; Yohimbine

Increased Effect/Toxicity

Benazepril may increase the levels/effects of: Allopurinol; Amifostine; Antihypertensives; Aza-THIOprine; CycloSPORINE (Systemic); DULoxetine; Ferric Gluconate; Gold Sodium Thiomalate; Hypotensive Agents; Iron Dextran Complex; Lithium; Nonsteroidal Anti-Inflammatory Agents; Obinutuzumab; RiTUXimab; Sodium Phosphates

The levels/effects of Benazepril may be increased by: Alfuzosin; Aliskiren; Angiotensin II Receptor Blockers; Brimonidine (Topical); Canagliflozin; Diazoxide; DPP-IV Inhibitors; Eplerenone; Everolimus; Heparin; Heparin (Low Molecular Weight); Herbs (Hypotensive Properties); Hydrochlorothiazide; Loop Diuretics; MAO Inhibitors; Pentoxifylline; Phosphodiesterase 5 Inhibitors; Potassium Salts; Potassium-Sparing Diuretics; Prostacyclin Analogues; Sirolimus; Temsirolimus; Thiazide Diuretics; TiZANidine; Tolvaptan; Trimethoprim

Nutritional/Ethanol Interactions

Food: Potassium supplements and/or potassium-containing salts may cause or worsen hyperkalemia. Management: Consult prescriber before consuming a potassium-rich diet, potassium supplements, or salt substitutes.

Herb/Nutraceutical: Some herbal medications may worsen hypertension (eg, licorice); others may increase the antihypertensive effect of benazepril (eg, shepherd's purse). Management: Avoid bayberry, blue cohosh, cayenne, ephedra, ginger, ginseng (American), kola, licorice, and yohimbe. Avoid black cohosh, California poppy, coleus, golden seal, hawthorn, mistletoe, periwinkle, quinine, and shepherd's purse.

Adverse Reactions

1% to 10%:
Cardiovascular: Postural dizziness (2%)
Central nervous system: Headache (6%), dizziness (4%), somnolence (2%)
Renal: Serum creatinine increased (2%), worsening of renal function may occur in patients with bilateral renal artery stenosis or hypovolemia
Respiratory: Cough (1% to 10%)
Eosinophilic pneumonitis, anaphylaxis, neutropenia, agranulocytosis, renal insufficiency, and renal failure have been reported with other ACE inhibitors. In addition, a syndrome including fever, myalgia, arthralgia, interstitial nephritis, vasculitis, rash, eosinophilia, and elevated ESR has been reported to be associated with ACE inhibitors.

Pharmacodynamics/Kinetics

Onset of Action

Reduction in plasma angiotensin-converting enzyme (ACE) activity: Peak effect: 1-2 hours after 2-20 mg dose

Reduction in blood pressure: Peak effect: Single dose: 2-4 hours; Continuous therapy: 2 weeks

Duration of Action Reduction in plasma angiotensin-converting enzyme (ACE) activity: >90% inhibition for 24 hours after 5-20 mg dose

Available Dosage Forms

Tablet, Oral:
Lotensin: 10 mg, 20 mg, 40 mg
Generic: 5 mg, 10 mg, 20 mg, 40 mg

General Dosage Range Dosage adjustment recommended in patients with renal impairment

Oral:
Children ≥6 years: Initial: 0.2 mg/kg/day (up to 10 mg/day); Maintenance: 0.1-0.6 mg/kg/day (maximum: 40 mg/day)
Adults: Initial: 5-10 mg/day; Maintenance: 20-80 mg/day in 1-2 divided doses

Storage/Stability Store at ≤30°C (86°F). Protect from moisture.

Nursing Actions

Physical Assessment Blood pressure should be monitored after first doses and periodically throughout.

Patient Education

- Discuss specific use of drug and side effects with patient as it relates to treatment. (HCAHPS: During this hospital stay, were you given any medicine that you had not taken before? Before giving you any new medicine, how often did hospital staff tell you what the medicine was for? How often did hospital staff describe possible side effects in a way you could understand?)
- Patient may experience headache or parageusia. Have patient report immediately to prescriber signs of infection, severe dizziness, syncope, urine discoloration, jaundice, angina, urinary retention, oliguria, bradycardia, arrhythmia, dyspnea, excessive weight gain, edema of extremities, ecchymosis, hemorrhaging, or significant dyspepsia (HCAHPS).
- Educate patient about signs of a significant reaction (eg, wheezing; chest tightness; fever; itching; bad cough; blue skin color; seizures; or swelling of face, lips, tongue, or throat). **Note:** This is not a comprehensive list of all side effects. Patient should consult prescriber for additional questions.

Intended Use and Disclaimer: Should not be printed and given to patients. This information is intended to serve as a concise initial reference for healthcare professionals to use when discussing medications with a patient. You must ultimately rely on your own discretion, experience and judgment in diagnosing, treating and advising patients.

Benazepril and Hydrochlorothiazide
(ben AY ze pril & hye droe klor oh THYE a zide)

Brand Names: U.S. Lotensin HCT®

Index Terms Benazepril Hydrochloride and Hydrochlorothiazide; Hydrochlorothiazide and Benazepril

Pharmacologic Category Angiotensin-Converting Enzyme (ACE) Inhibitor; Antihypertensive; Diuretic, Thiazide

Pregnancy Risk Factor D

Use Treatment of hypertension

Available Dosage Forms

Tablet:

Generics:

5/6.25: Benazepril 5 mg and hydrochlorothiazide 6.25 mg

10/12.5: Benazepril 10 mg and hydrochlorothiazide 12.5 mg

20/12.5: Benazepril 20 mg and hydrochlorothiazide 12.5 mg

20/25: Benazepril 20 mg and hydrochlorothiazide 25 mg

Brands:

Lotensin HCT® 10/12.5: Benazepril 10 mg and hydrochlorothiazide 12.5 mg

Lotensin HCT® 20/12.5: Benazepril 20 mg and hydrochlorothiazide 12.5 mg

Lotensin HCT® 20/25: Benazepril 20 mg and hydrochlorothiazide 25 mg

General Dosage Range Oral: *Adults:* Benazepril 5-20 mg and hydrochlorothiazide 6.25-25 mg daily

Nursing Actions

Physical Assessment See individual agents.

Patient Education

• Discuss specific use of drug and side effects with patient as it relates to treatment. (HCAHPS: During this hospital stay, were you given any medicine that you had not taken before? Before giving you any new medicine, how often did hospital staff tell you what the medicine was for? How often did hospital staff describe possible side effects in a way you could understand?)

• Patient may experience dizziness, headache, diarrhea, asthenia, or nausea. Have patient report immediately to prescriber signs of infection, signs of hyperglycemia, signs of fluid and electrolyte imbalance, urine discoloration, jaundice, angina, sexual dysfunction, bradycardia, akathisia, dyspnea, dyspepsia, ecchymosis, hemorrhaging, vision changes, or ophthalmalgia (HCAHPS).

• Educate patient about signs of a significant reaction (eg, wheezing; chest tightness; fever; itching; bad cough; blue skin color; seizures; or swelling of face, lips, tongue, or throat). **Note:** This is not a comprehensive list of all side effects. Patient should consult prescriber for additional questions.

Intended Use and Disclaimer: Should not be printed and given to patients. This information is intended to serve as a concise initial reference for healthcare professionals to use when discussing medications with a patient. You must ultimately rely on your own discretion, experience and judgment in diagnosing, treating and advising patients.

Related Information

Benazepril *on page 168*

Hydrochlorothiazide *on page 775*

Bendamustine (ben da MUS teen)

Brand Names: U.S. Treanda

Index Terms Bendamustine Hydrochloride; Cytostasan; SDX-105

Pharmacologic Category Antineoplastic Agent, Alkylating Agent; Antineoplastic Agent, Alkylating Agent (Nitrogen Mustard)

Medication Safety Issues

Sound-alike/look-alike issues:

Bendamustine may be confused with brentuximab, carmustine, lomustine

High alert medication:

This medication is in a class the Institute for Safe Medication Practices (ISMP) includes among its list of drug classes which have a heightened risk of causing significant patient harm when used in error.

Pregnancy Risk Factor D

Lactation Excretion in breast milk unknown/not recommended

Use

Chronic lymphocytic leukemia: Treatment of chronic lymphocytic leukemia (CLL)

Non-Hodgkin lymphoma: Treatment of indolent B-cell non-Hodgkin lymphoma (NHL) which has progressed during or within 6 months of rituximab treatment or a rituximab-containing regimen

Unlabeled Use Treatment of relapsed or refractory Hodgkin lymphoma; treatment of mantle cell lymphoma; salvage therapy for relapsed multiple myeloma; first-line therapy for follicular lymphoma; treatment of Waldenström's macroglobulinemia

Available Dosage Forms

Solution Reconstituted, Intravenous:

Treanda: 25 mg (1 ea); 100 mg (1 ea)

General Dosage Range Dosage adjustment recommended in patients who develop toxicities

I.V.: *Adults:* 100 mg/m^2 on days 1 and 2 of a 28-day treatment cycle **or** 120 mg/m^2 on days 1 and 2 of a 21-day treatment cycle

Administration

I.V. Infuse over 30 minutes for the treatment of CLL and over 60 minutes for NHL; administration times for unlabeled uses/doses vary by protocol. Consider premedication with antihistamines, antipyretics, and corticosteroids for patients with a previous grade 1 or 2 infusion reaction to bendamustine. Bendamustine is associated with a moderate emetic potential (Basch, 2011); antiemetics are recommended to prevent nausea and vomiting.

Irritant with vesicant-like properties; ensure proper needle or catheter placement prior to and during infusion. Avoid extravasation; monitor I.V. site for redness, swelling, or pain.

Extravasation management: If extravasation occurs, stop infusion immediately and disconnect (leave cannula/needle in place); gently aspirate extravasated solution (do **NOT** flush the line); remove needle/cannula; elevate extremity. Apply dry cold compresses for 20 minutes 4 times daily (Perez Fildago, 2012). May be managed with sodium thiosulfate in the same manner as mechlorethamine extravasation (Schulmeister, 2011). *Sodium thiosulfate 1/6 M solution (instructions for mechlorethamine):* Inject subcutaneously into extravasation area using 2 mL for each mg of drug suspected to have extravasated (Perez Fidalgo, 2012; Polovich, 2009).

Hazardous agent; use appropriate precautions for handling and disposal (NIOSH, 2012).

Injectable Detail pH: 2.5-3.5 (reconstituted solution)

Nursing Actions

Physical Assessment Monitor infusion site closely to avoid extravasation. Monitor infusion reactions, including skin reactions; can occur with first or subsequent cycles and may require premedication or discontinuation.

Patient Education

• Discuss specific use of drug and side effects with patient as it relates to treatment. (HCAHPS: During this hospital stay, were you given any medicine that you had not taken before? Before giving you any new medicine, how often did hospital staff tell you what the medicine was for? How often did hospital staff describe possible side effects in a way you could understand?)

• Patient may experience diarrhea, dyspepsia, lack of appetite, back pain, constipation, fatigue, insomnia, or weight loss. Have patient report immediately to prescriber signs of infection, dyspnea, severe nausea, ecchymosis, hemorrhaging, significant skin irritation, paresthesia, angina, melena, urine discoloration, depression, dysuria, polyuria, myalgia, considerable dizziness, syncope, intolerable headache, severe asthenia, dyspnea, excessive weight gain, edema of extremities, stomatitis, significant injection site edema or irritation, or signs of tumor lysis syndrome (TLS) (HCAHPS).

• Educate patient about signs of a significant reaction (eg, wheezing; chest tightness; fever; itching; bad cough; blue skin color; seizures; or swelling of face, lips, tongue, or throat). **Note:** This is not a comprehensive list of all side effects. Patient should consult prescriber for additional questions.

Intended Use and Disclaimer: Should not be printed and given to patients. This information is intended to serve as a concise initial reference for healthcare professionals to use when discussing medications with a patient. You must ultimately rely on your own discretion, experience and judgment in diagnosing, treating and advising patients.

Related Information
Management of Drug Extravasations *on page 1700*

Benzonatate (ben ZOE na tate)

Brand Names: U.S. Tessalon Perles; Zonatuss
Index Terms Tessalon Perles
Pharmacologic Category Antitussive
Pregnancy Risk Factor C
Lactation Excretion in breast milk unknown/use caution
Use Symptomatic relief of nonproductive cough
Available Dosage Forms
Capsule, Oral:
Tessalon Perles: 100 mg
Zonatuss: 150 mg
Generic: 100 mg, 200 mg
General Dosage Range Oral: *Children >10 years and Adults:* 100-200 mg 3 times/day as needed (maximum: 600 mg/day)
Administration
Oral Swallow capsule whole (do not break. chew, dissolve, cut, or crush).
Nursing Actions
Physical Assessment Assess effectiveness of therapy (relief of cough, lung sounds, and respiratory pattern). Monitor for CNS changes at beginning of therapy and periodically throughout.
Patient Education
• Discuss specific use of drug and side effects with patient as it relates to treatment. (HCAHPS: During this hospital stay, were you given any medicine that you had not taken before? Before giving you any new medicine, how often did hospital staff tell you what the medicine was for? How often did hospital staff describe possible side effects in a way you could understand?)
• Patient may experience constipation, dizziness, fatigue, rhinitis, nausea, or headache. Have patient report immediately to prescriber behavioral changes, illogical thinking, hallucinations, or paresthesia of mouth, throat, and face (HCAHPS).
• Educate patient about signs of a significant reaction (eg, wheezing; chest tightness; fever; itching; bad cough; blue skin color; seizures; or swelling of face, lips, tongue, or throat). **Note:** This is not a comprehensive list of all side effects. Patient should consult prescriber for additional questions.

Intended Use and Disclaimer: Should not be printed and given to patients. This information is intended to serve as a concise initial reference for

healthcare professionals to use when discussing medications with a patient. You must ultimately rely on your own discretion, experience and judgment in diagnosing, treating and advising patients.

Related Information

Oral Medications That Should Not Be Crushed or Altered *on page 1712*

Benztropine (BENZ troe peen)

Brand Names: U.S. Cogentin

Index Terms Benztropine Mesylate

Pharmacologic Category Anti-Parkinson's Agent, Anticholinergic; Anticholinergic Agent

Medication Safety Issues

Sound-alike/look-alike issues:

Benztropine may be confused with bromocriptine

BEERS Criteria medication:

This drug may be potentially inappropriate for use in geriatric patients (Parkinson's disease: Quality of evidence - moderate; Strength of recommendation - strong).

Lactation Excretion in breast milk unknown/use caution

Breast-Feeding Considerations It is not known if benztropine is excreted in breast milk. Anticholinergic agents may suppress lactation.

Use Adjunctive treatment of Parkinson's disease; aid in the treatment of drug-induced extrapyramidal symptoms (except tardive dyskinesia)

Mechanism of Action/Effect Possesses both anticholinergic and antihistaminic effects. *In vitro* anticholinergic activity approximates that of atropine; *in vivo* it is only about half as active as atropine. Animal data suggest its antihistaminic activity and duration of action approach that of pyrilamine maleate. May also inhibit the reuptake and storage of dopamine, thereby prolonging the action of dopamine.

Contraindications Hypersensitivity to benztropine or any component of the formulation; children <3 years of age (due to atropine-like adverse effects)

Warnings/Precautions Use with caution in children >3 years of age due to its anticholinergic effects (dose has not been established). Use is contraindicated in children <3 years of age. Use with caution in hot weather or during exercise. May cause anhydrosis and hyperthermia, which may be severe. The risk is increased in hot environments, particularly in the elderly, alcoholics, patients with CNS disease, and those with prolonged outdoor exposure.

Use with caution in patients >65 years of age; response in elderly may be altered. Initiate at low doses in the elderly and increase as needed while monitoring for adverse events. Avoid use of oral benztropine in older adults for prevention of extrapyramidal symptoms with antipsychotics and alternative agents preferred in the treatment of

Parkinson's disease. May be inappropriate in older adults depending on comorbidities (eg, dementia, delirium) due to its potent anticholinergic effects (Beers Criteria). Avoid use in patients with myasthenia gravis, may precipitate myasthenic crisis. Avoid use in angle-closure glaucoma.

Use with caution in patients with tachycardia, cardiac arrhythmias, hypertension, hypotension, glaucoma, prostatic hyperplasia (especially in the elderly), any tendency toward urinary retention, liver or kidney disorders, and obstructive disease of the GI or GU tracts. When given in large doses or to susceptible patients, may cause weakness and inability to move particular muscle groups.

May be associated with confusion, visual hallucinations, or excitement (generally at higher dosages). Intensification of symptoms or toxic psychosis may occur in patients with mental disorders. May cause CNS depression, which may impair physical or mental abilities; patients must be cautioned about performing tasks which require mental alertness (eg, operating machinery or driving). Benztropine does not relieve symptoms of tardive dyskinesia and may potentially exacerbate symptoms.

Potentially significant drug-drug interactions may exist, requiring dose or frequency adjustment, additional monitoring, and/or selection of alternative therapy.

Drug Interactions

Avoid Concomitant Use

Avoid concomitant use of Benztropine with any of the following: Aclidinium; Ipratropium (Oral Inhalation); Potassium Chloride; Tiotropium; Umeclidinium

Decreased Effect

Benztropine may decrease the levels/effects of: Acetylcholinesterase Inhibitors (Central); Ioflupane I 123; Secretin

The levels/effects of Benztropine may be decreased by: Acetylcholinesterase Inhibitors (Central); Peginterferon Alfa-2b

Increased Effect/Toxicity

Benztropine may increase the levels/effects of: AbobotulinumtoxinA; Analgesics (Opioid); Anticholinergics; Cannabinoids; Mirabegron; OnabotulinumtoxinA; Potassium Chloride; RimabotulinumtoxinB; Thiazide Diuretics; Tiotropium; Topiramate

The levels/effects of Benztropine may be increased by: Aclidinium; Ipratropium (Oral Inhalation); Pramlintide; Umeclidinium

Nutritional/Ethanol Interactions Ethanol: Avoid ethanol (may increase CNS depression).

Adverse Reactions Frequency not defined.

Cardiovascular: Tachycardia

Central nervous system: Confusion, depression, disorientation, exacerbation of pre-existing psychotic symptoms, fever, listlessness, memory impairment, nervousness, toxic psychosis, visual hallucinations

Dermatologic: Rash

Endocrine & metabolic: Heat stroke, hyperthermia

Gastrointestinal: Constipation, nausea, paralytic ileus, vomiting, xerostomia

Genitourinary: Urinary retention, dysuria

Neuromuscular & skeletal: Numbness of fingers

Ocular: Blurred vision, mydriasis

Pharmacodynamics/Kinetics

Onset of Action I.M., I.V.: Within a few minutes

Available Dosage Forms

Solution, Injection:

Cogentin: 1 mg/mL (2 mL)

Generic: 1 mg/mL (2 mL)

Tablet, Oral:

Generic: 0.5 mg, 1 mg, 2 mg

General Dosage Range I.M., I.V., Oral: *Adults:* Range: 0.5-8 mg daily

Administration

I.M. May administer I.M. if oral route is unacceptable.

I.V. May administer I.V. if oral route is unacceptable. Manufacturer's labeling states there is no difference in onset of effect after I.V. or I.M. injection and therefore there is usually no need to use the I.V. route. No specific instructions on administering benztropine I.V. are provided in the labeling. The I.V. route has been reported in the literature (slow I.V. push when reported), although specific instructions are lacking (Duncan, 2001; Lydon, 1998; Sachdev, 1993; Schramm, 2002).

Injectable Detail pH: 5-8

Oral May be given with or without food.

Nursing Actions

Physical Assessment Monitor renal function and therapeutic response (eg, Parkinsonian symptoms). Monitor for anticholinergic syndrome (dry mouth and mucous membranes, constipation, epigastric distress, CNS disturbances, paralytic ileus).

Patient Education

• Discuss specific use of drug and side effects with patient as it relates to treatment. (HCAHPS: During this hospital stay, were you given any medicine that you had not taken before? Before giving you any new medicine, how often did hospital staff tell you what the medicine was for? How often did hospital staff describe possible side effects in a way you could understand?)

• Patient may experience constipation, headache, nausea, lack of appetite, insomnia, blurred vision, fatigue, xerostomia, or light sensitivity. Have patient report immediately to prescriber signs of depression (ie, suicidal ideation, anxiety, emotional instability, illogical thinking), hallucinations, severe dizziness, syncope, ophthalmalgia, dysphagia, emesis, difficult urination, dysuria, difficulty with motor activity,

angina, tachycardia, arrhythmia, mydriasis, memory loss, paresthesia, tremors, asthenia, or muscle rigidity (HCAHPS).

• Educate patient about signs of a significant reaction (eg, wheezing; chest tightness; fever; itching; bad cough; blue skin color; seizures; or swelling of face, lips, tongue, or throat). **Note:** This is not a comprehensive list of all side effects. Patient should consult prescriber for additional questions.

Intended Use and Disclaimer: Should not be printed and given to patients. This information is intended to serve as a concise initial reference for healthcare professionals to use when discussing medications with a patient. You must ultimately rely on your own discretion, experience and judgment in diagnosing, treating and advising patients.

Dietary Considerations Tablet may be taken with or without food.

Benzylpenicilloyl Polylysine
(BEN zil pen i SIL oyl pol i LIE seen)

Brand Names: U.S. Pre-Pen®

Index Terms Benzylpenicilloyl-polylysine; Penicilloyl-polylysine; PPL

Pharmacologic Category Diagnostic Agent

Pregnancy Risk Factor C

Use Adjunct in assessing the risk of administering penicillin (penicillin G or benzylpenicillin) in patients suspected of clinical penicillin hypersensitivity

Unlabeled Use Adjunct in assessment of hypersensitivity to other beta-lactam antibiotics (penicillins and cephalosporins) to determine the safety of penicillin administration in patients with a history of reaction to cephalosporins

Available Dosage Forms

Injection, solution:

Pre-Pen®: 6 x 10^{-5} M (0.25 mL)

General Dosage Range

Intradermal: *Children and Adults:* Inject a volume of skin test solution sufficient to raise a small intradermal bleb ~3 mm in diameter, in duplicate

Puncture test (first step): *Children and Adults:* Apply a small drop of solution to make a single shallow puncture of the epidermis

Administration

Other

Puncture test: Administer initially by puncture technique on the inner volar aspect of the forearm, followed by an intradermal injection only in patients with a negative reaction.

Intradermal: Do **not** administer intradermally to patients with a positive reaction (wheal of 5-15 mm or more in diameter). Administer the intradermal test on the upper, outer arm, below the deltoid muscle in the event a severe hypersensitivity reaction occurs and a tourniquet needs to be applied. During the skin test, immediate treatment with epinephrine should also be available.

Nursing Actions

Patient Education

- Discuss specific use of drug and side effects with patient as it relates to treatment. (HCAHPS: During this hospital stay, were you given any medicine that you had not taken before? Before giving you any new medicine, how often did hospital staff tell you what the medicine was for? How often did hospital staff describe possible side effects in a way you could understand?)
- Educate patient about signs of a significant reaction (eg, wheezing; chest tightness; fever; itching; bad cough; blue skin color; seizures; or swelling of face, lips, tongue, or throat). **Note:** This is not a comprehensive list of all side effects. Patient should consult prescriber for additional questions.

Intended Use and Disclaimer: Should not be printed and given to patients. This information is intended to serve as a concise initial reference for healthcare professionals to use when discussing medications with a patient. You must ultimately rely on your own discretion, experience and judgment in diagnosing, treating and advising patients.

Bepotastine (be poe TAS teen)

Brand Names: U.S. Bepreve
Index Terms Bepotastine Besilate
Pharmacologic Category Histamine H_1 Antagonist; Histamine H_1 Antagonist, Second Generation; Mast Cell Stabilizer
Pregnancy Risk Factor C
Lactation Excretion in breast milk unknown/use caution
Use Treatment of itching associated with allergic conjunctivitis
Available Dosage Forms
  Solution, Ophthalmic:
    Bepreve: 1.5% (5 mL, 10 mL)
General Dosage Range Ophthalmic: *Children ≥2 years and Adults:* Instill 1 drop into the affected eye(s) twice daily
Administration
  Other For topical ophthalmic use only. Contact lenses should be removed prior to application, may be inserted after 10 minutes. Do not insert contacts if eyes are red. Avoid contaminating the applicator tip.
Nursing Actions
  Patient Education
  - Discuss specific use of drug and side effects with patient as it relates to treatment. (HCAHPS: During this hospital stay, were you given any medicine that you had not taken before? Before giving you any new medicine, how often did hospital staff tell you what the medicine was

for? How often did hospital staff describe possible side effects in a way you could understand?)
- Patient may experience parageusia. Have patient report immediately to prescriber vision changes, ophthalmalgia, or severe eye irritation (HCAHPS).
- Educate patient about signs of a significant reaction (eg, wheezing; chest tightness; fever; itching; bad cough; blue skin color; seizures; or swelling of face, lips, tongue, or throat). **Note:** This is not a comprehensive list of all side effects. Patient should consult prescriber for additional questions.

Intended Use and Disclaimer: Should not be printed and given to patients. This information is intended to serve as a concise initial reference for healthcare professionals to use when discussing medications with a patient. You must ultimately rely on your own discretion, experience and judgment in diagnosing, treating and advising patients.

Besifloxacin (be si FLOX a sin)

Brand Names: U.S. Besivance
Index Terms Besifloxacin Hydrochloride; BOL-303224-A; SS734
Pharmacologic Category Antibiotic, Fluoroquinolone; Antibiotic, Ophthalmic
Pregnancy Risk Factor C
Lactation Excretion in breast milk unknown/use caution
Use Treatment of bacterial conjunctivitis
Available Dosage Forms
  Suspension, Ophthalmic:
    Besivance: 0.6% (5 mL)
General Dosage Range Ophthalmic: *Children ≥1 year and Adults:* 1 drop into affected eye(s) 3 times/day (4-12 hours apart)
Administration
  Other Ophthalmic: Wash hands before and after instillation. Shake bottle once prior to each administration. Avoid contaminating the applicator tip with affected eye(s).
Nursing Actions
  Patient Education
  - Discuss specific use of drug and side effects with patient as it relates to treatment. (HCAHPS: During this hospital stay, were you given any medicine that you had not taken before? Before giving you any new medicine, how often did hospital staff tell you what the medicine was for? How often did hospital staff describe possible side effects in a way you could understand?)
  - Patient may experience short-term pain. Have patient report immediately to prescriber sudden vision changes, ophthalmalgia, or eye irritation (HCAHPS).
  - Educate patient about signs of a significant reaction (eg, wheezing; chest tightness; fever;

itching; bad cough; blue skin color; seizures; or swelling of face, lips, tongue, or throat). **Note:** This is not a comprehensive list of all side effects. Patient should consult prescriber for additional questions.

Intended Use and Disclaimer: Should not be printed and given to patients. This information is intended to serve as a concise initial reference for healthcare professionals to use when discussing medications with a patient. You must ultimately rely on your own discretion, experience and judgment in diagnosing, treating and advising patients.

Betamethasone (bay ta METH a sone)

Brand Names: U.S. AlphaTrex; Celestone; Celestone Soluspan; Diprolene; Diprolene AF; Luxiq
Index Terms Betamethasone Dipropionate; Betamethasone Dipropionate, Augmented; Betamethasone Sodium Phosphate; Betamethasone Valerate; Flubenisolone
Pharmacologic Category Corticosteroid, Systemic; Corticosteroid, Topical
Medication Safety Issues
Sound-alike/look-alike issues:
Luxiq may be confused with Lasix
International issues:
Beta-Val [U.S.] may be confused with Betanol brand name for metipranolol [Monaco]
Pregnancy Risk Factor C
Lactation Excretion in breast milk unknown/use caution
Breast-Feeding Considerations Corticosteroids are excreted in human milk. The onset of milk secretion after birth may be delayed and the volume of milk produced may be decreased by antenatal betamethasone therapy; this affect was seen when delivery occurred 3-9 days after the betamethasone dose in women between 28 and 34 weeks gestation. Antenatal betamethasone therapy did not affect milk production when birth occurred <3 days or >10 days of treatment (Henderson, 2008). It is not known if systemic absorption following topical administration results in detectable quantities in human milk. Do not apply topical corticosteroids to nipples; hypertension was noted in a nursing infant exposed to a topical corticosteroid while nursing (Leachman, 2006).

The manufacturer notes that when used systemically, maternal use of corticosteroids have the potential to cause adverse events in a nursing infant (eg, growth suppression, interfere with endogenous corticosteroid production) and therefore recommends that caution be exercised when administering betamethasone to nursing women. If there is concern about exposure to the infant, some guidelines recommend waiting 4 hours after the maternal dose of an oral systemic corticosteroid before breast-feeding in order to decrease potential exposure to the infant (based on a study using prednisolone) (Bae, 2011; Leachman, 2006; Makol, 2011; Ost, 1985).

Use Inflammatory dermatoses such as seborrheic or atopic dermatitis, neurodermatitis, anogenital pruritus, psoriasis, inflammatory phase of xerosis
Unlabeled Use Accelerate fetal lung maturation in patients with preterm labor
Mechanism of Action/Effect Binds to corticosteroid receptors in cell and acts to prevent or control inflammation
Contraindications Hypersensitivity to betamethasone, other corticosteroids, or any component of the formulation; systemic fungal infections; I.M. administration contraindicated in idiopathic thrombocytopenia purpura
Warnings/Precautions Very high potency topical products are not for treatment of rosacea, perioral dermatitis; not for use on face, groin, or axillae; not for use in a diapered area. Avoid concurrent use of other corticosteroids.

May cause hypercorticism or suppression of hypothalamic-pituitary-adrenal (HPA) axis, particularly in younger children or in patients receiving high doses for prolonged periods. HPA axis suppression may lead to adrenal crisis. Withdrawal and discontinuation of a corticosteroid should be done slowly and carefully. Particular care is required when patients are transferred from systemic corticosteroids to inhaled products due to possible adrenal insufficiency or withdrawal from steroids, including an increase in allergic symptoms. Patients receiving >20 mg per day of prednisone (or equivalent) may be most susceptible. Fatalities have occurred due to adrenal insufficiency in asthmatic patients during and after transfer from systemic corticosteroids to aerosol steroids; aerosol steroids do not provide the systemic steroid needed to treat patients having trauma, surgery, or infections. In stressful situations, HPA axis-suppressed patients should receive adequate supplementation with natural glucocorticoids (hydrocortisone or cortisone) rather than betamethasone (due to lack of mineralocorticoid activity).

Topical corticosteroids may be absorbed percutaneously. Absorption of topical corticosteroids may cause manifestations of Cushing's syndrome, hyperglycemia, or glycosuria. Absorption is increased by the use of occlusive dressings, application to denuded skin, or application to large surface areas.

Acute myopathy has been reported with high dose corticosteroids, usually in patients with neuromuscular transmission disorders; may involve ocular and/or respiratory muscles; monitor creatine kinase; recovery may be delayed. Corticosteroid use may cause psychiatric disturbances, including depression, euphoria, insomnia, mood swings, and personality changes. Pre-existing psychiatric conditions may be exacerbated by corticosteroid use. Prolonged use of corticosteroids may also increase the incidence of secondary infection, mask acute infection (including fungal infections), prolong or exacerbate viral infections, or limit response to vaccines. Exposure to chickenpox should be avoided; corticosteroids should not be used to treat ocular herpes simplex. Corticosteroids should not be used for cerebral malaria or viral hepatitis. Close observation is required in patients with latent tuberculosis and/or TB reactivity; restrict use in active TB (only in conjunction with antituberculosis treatment). Prolonged treatment with corticosteroids has been associated with the development of Kaposi's sarcoma (case reports); if noted, discontinuation of therapy should be considered. High-dose corticosteroids should not be used to manage acute head injury.

Use with caution in patients with thyroid disease, hepatic impairment, renal impairment, cardiovascular disease, diabetes, glaucoma, cataracts, myasthenia gravis, patients at risk for osteoporosis, patients at risk for seizures, or GI diseases (diverticulitis, peptic ulcer, ulcerative colitis) due to perforation risk. Use caution following acute MI (corticosteroids have been associated with myocardial rupture). Because of the risk of adverse effects, systemic corticosteroids should be used cautiously in the elderly in the smallest possible effective dose for the shortest duration. Discontinue if skin irritation or contact dermatitis should occur; do not use in patients with decreased skin circulation. Withdraw therapy with gradual tapering of dose.

Topical use in patients ≤12 years of age is not recommended. Children may absorb proportionally larger amounts after topical application and may be more prone to systemic effects. HPA axis suppression, intracranial hypertension, and Cushing's syndrome have been reported in children receiving topical corticosteroids. Prolonged use may affect growth velocity; growth should be routinely monitored in pediatric patients.

Drug Interactions

Avoid Concomitant Use

Avoid concomitant use of Betamethasone with any of the following: Aldesleukin; BCG; Indium 111 Capromab Pendetide; Mifepristone; Natalizumab; Pimecrolimus; Tacrolimus (Topical); Tofacitinib

Decreased Effect

Betamethasone may decrease the levels/effects of: Aldesleukin; Antidiabetic Agents; BCG; Calcitriol; Coccidioidin Skin Test; Corticorelin; Hyaluronidase; Indium 111 Capromab Pendetide; Isoniazid; Salicylates; Sipuleucel-T; Telaprevir; Urea Cycle Disorder Agents; Vaccines (Inactivated)

The levels/effects of Betamethasone may be decreased by: Aminoglutethimide; Antacids; Barbiturates; Bile Acid Sequestrants; Echinacea; Mifepristone; Mitotane; Primidone; Rifamycin Derivatives

Increased Effect/Toxicity

Betamethasone may increase the levels/effects of: Acetylcholinesterase Inhibitors; Amphotericin B; Deferasirox; Leflunomide; Loop Diuretics; Natalizumab; NSAID (COX-2 Inhibitor); NSAID (Nonselective); Thiazide Diuretics; Tofacitinib; Vaccines (Live); Warfarin

The levels/effects of Betamethasone may be increased by: Antifungal Agents (Azole Derivatives, Systemic); Aprepitant; Calcium Channel Blockers (Nondihydropyridine); Denosumab; Estrogen Derivatives; Fluconazole; Fosaprepitant; Indacaterol; Macrolide Antibiotics; Mifepristone; Neuromuscular-Blocking Agents (Nondepolarizing); Pimecrolimus; Quinolone Antibiotics; Roflumilast; Salicylates; Tacrolimus (Topical); Telaprevir; Trastuzumab

Nutritional/Ethanol Interactions

Ethanol: Avoid ethanol (may enhance gastric mucosal irritation).

Food: Betamethasone interferes with calcium absorption.

Herb/Nutraceutical: Avoid cat's claw, echinacea (have immunostimulant properties).

Adverse Reactions

Systemic:

Cardiovascular: Congestive heart failure, edema, hyper-/hypotension

Central nervous system: Dizziness, headache, insomnia, intracranial pressure increased, light-headedness, nervousness, pseudotumor cerebri, seizure, vertigo

Dermatologic: Ecchymoses, facial erythema, fragile skin, hirsutism, hyper-/hypopigmentation, perioral dermatitis (oral), petechiae, striae, wound healing impaired

Endocrine & metabolic: Amenorrhea, Cushing's syndrome, diabetes mellitus, growth suppression, hyperglycemia, hypokalemia, menstrual irregularities, pituitary-adrenal axis suppression, protein catabolism, sodium retention, water retention

Local: Injection site reactions (intra-articular use), sterile abscess

Neuromuscular & skeletal: Arthralgia, muscle atrophy, fractures, muscle weakness, myopathy, osteoporosis, necrosis (femoral and humeral heads)

Ocular: Cataracts, glaucoma, intraocular pressure increased

Miscellaneous: Anaphylactoid reaction, diaphoresis, hypersensitivity, secondary infection

Topical:
Dermatologic: Acneiform eruptions, allergic dermatitis, burning, dry skin, erythema, folliculitis, hypertrichosis, irritation, miliaria, pruritus, skin atrophy, striae, vesiculation
Endocrine and metabolic effects have occasionally been reported with topical use.

Available Dosage Forms
Cream, External:
Diprolene AF: 0.05% (15 g, 50 g)
Generic: 0.05% (15 g, 45 g, 50 g); 0.1% (15 g, 45 g)
Foam, External:
Luxiq: 0.12% (50 g, 100 g)
Generic: 0.12% (50 g, 100 g)
Gel, External:
AlphaTrex: 0.05% (15 g, 50 g)
Generic: 0.05% (15 g, 50 g)
Lotion, External:
Diprolene: 0.05% (30 mL, 60 mL)
Generic: 0.05% (30 mL, 60 mL); 0.1% (60 mL)
Ointment, External:
Diprolene: 0.05% (15 g, 50 g)
Generic: 0.05% (15 g, 45 g, 50 g); 0.1% (15 g, 45 g)
Solution, Oral:
Celestone: 0.6 mg/5 mL (118 mL)
Suspension, Injection:
Celestone Soluspan: Betamethasone sodium phosphate 3 mg and betamethasone acetate 3 mg per 1 mL (5 mL)
Generic: Betamethasone sodium phosphate 3 mg and betamethasone acetate 3 mg per 1 mL (5 mL)

General Dosage Range
I.M.:
Children ≤12 years: 0.0175-0.125 mg base/kg/day or 0.5-7.5 mg base/m²/day divided every 6-12 hours
Children ≥13 years and Adults: 0.6-9 mg/day divided every 12-24 hours
Intrabursal, intra-articular, intradermal: Adults: 0.25-2 mL
Intralesional: Adults: Very large joints: 1-2 mL; Large joints: 1 mL; Medium joints: 0.5-1 mL; Small joints: 0.25-0.5 mL
Oral:
Children ≤12 years: 0.0175-0.25 mg/kg/day or 0.5-7.5 mg/m²/day divided every 6-8 hours
Children ≥13 years and Adults: 0.6-7.2 mg/day in 2-4 divided doses
Topical: Children ≥13 years and Adults: Apply once or twice daily (maximum: 45-50 g/week; 50 mL/week)

Administration
I.M. Do **not** give injectable sodium phosphate/acetate suspension I.V.
Oral Not for alternate day therapy; once daily doses should be given in the morning. May be administered with food to decrease GI distress.

Topical Apply topical sparingly to areas. Not for use on broken skin or in areas of infection. Do not apply to wet skin unless directed; do not cover with occlusive dressing. Do not apply very high potency agents to face, groin, axillae, or diaper area.

Foam: Invert can and dispense a small amount onto a saucer or other cool surface. Do not dispense directly into hands. Pick up small amounts of foam and gently massage into affected areas until foam disappears. Repeat until entire affected scalp area is treated.

Nursing Actions
Physical Assessment Growth should be routinely monitored in pediatric patients. With systemic administration, caution patients with diabetes to monitor glucose levels closely (corticosteroids may alter glucose levels).

Patient Education
• Discuss specific use of drug and side effects with patient as it relates to treatment. (HCAHPS: During this hospital stay, were you given any medicine that you had not taken before? Before giving you any new medicine, how often did hospital staff tell you what the medicine was for? How often did hospital staff describe possible side effects in a way you could understand?)
• Patient may experience nausea, akathisia, or xeroderma. Have patient report immediately to prescriber signs of hyperglycemia, skin changes, signs of infection, signs of hypokalemia, signs of pancreatitis, severe asthenia, irritability, tremors, tachycardia, confusion, hyperhydrosis, dizziness, dyspnea, excessive weight gain, edema of extremities, moon face, buffalo hump, significant headache, tachycardia, bradycardia, arrhythmia, angina, menstrual irregularities, arthralgia, osteodynia, mood changes, behavioral changes, depression, paresthesia, ecchymosis, hemorrhaging, vision changes, considerable dyspepsia, melena, hematemesis, or intolerable application site irritation (HCAHPS).
• Educate patient about signs of a significant reaction (eg, wheezing; chest tightness; fever; itching; bad cough; blue skin color; seizures; or swelling of face, lips, tongue, or throat). **Note:** This is not a comprehensive list of all side effects. Patient should consult prescriber for additional questions.

Intended Use and Disclaimer: Should not be printed and given to patients. This information is intended to serve as a concise initial reference for healthcare professionals to use when discussing medications with a patient. You must ultimately rely on your own discretion, experience and judgment in diagnosing, treating and advising patients.

Dietary Considerations May be taken with food to decrease GI distress.

Betamethasone and Clotrimazole
(bay ta METH a sone & kloe TRIM a zole)

Brand Names: U.S. Lotrisone®
Index Terms Clotrimazole and Betamethasone
Pharmacologic Category Antifungal Agent, Topical; Corticosteroid, Topical
Medication Safety Issues
Sound-alike/look-alike issues:
Clotrimazole may be confused with co-trimoxazole
Lotrisone® may be confused with Lotrimin®
Pregnancy Risk Factor C
Lactation Excretion in breast milk unknown/use caution
Use Topical treatment of various dermal fungal infections (including tinea pedis, cruris, and corpora in patients ≥17 years of age)
Available Dosage Forms
Cream: Betamethasone 0.05% and clotrimazole 1% (15 g, 45 g)
Lotrisone®: Betamethasone 0.05% and clotrimazole 1% (15 g, 45 g)
Lotion: Betamethasone 0.05% and clotrimazole 1% (30 mL)
Lotrisone®: Betamethasone 0.05% and clotrimazole 1% (30 mL)
General Dosage Range Topical: *Adults:* Apply to affected area twice daily (maximum: 45 g cream/week; 45 mL lotion/week)
Administration
Topical For external use only. Do not use on open wounds. Do not cover with occlusive dressings. Shake lotion well prior to use
Nursing Actions
Physical Assessment See individual agents.
Patient Education
- Discuss specific use of drug and side effects with patient as it relates to treatment. (HCAHPS: During this hospital stay, were you given any medicine that you had not taken before? Before giving you any new medicine, how often did hospital staff tell you what the medicine was for? How often did hospital staff describe possible side effects in a way you could understand?)
- Patient may experience xeroderma. Have patient report immediately to prescriber signs of hyperglycemia, skin changes, skin discoloration, or severe application site irritation (HCAHPS).
- Educate patient about signs of a significant reaction (eg, wheezing; chest tightness; fever; itching; bad cough; blue skin color; seizures; or swelling of face, lips, tongue, or throat). **Note:** This is not a comprehensive list of all side effects. Patient should consult prescriber for additional questions.

Intended Use and Disclaimer: Should not be printed and given to patients. This information is intended to serve as a concise initial reference for healthcare professionals to use when discussing medications with a patient. You must ultimately rely on your own discretion, experience and judgment in diagnosing, treating and advising patients.
Related Information
Betamethasone *on page 176*

Betaxolol (Systemic) (be TAKS oh lol)

Brand Names: U.S. Kerlone
Index Terms Betaxolol Hydrochloride
Pharmacologic Category Antihypertensive; Beta-Blocker, Beta-1 Selective
Medication Safety Issues
Sound-alike/look-alike issues:
Betaxolol may be confused with bethanechol, labetalol
Pregnancy Risk Factor C
Lactation Enters breast milk/use caution
Breast-Feeding Considerations Betaxolol is excreted into breast milk in amounts which may have a pharmacologic effect in the nursing infant. The manufacturer recommends that caution be exercised when administering betaxolol to nursing women.
Use Management of hypertension
Unlabeled Use Treatment of coronary artery disease
Mechanism of Action/Effect Competitively blocks beta$_1$-receptors, with little or no effect on beta$_2$-receptors
Contraindications Hypersensitivity to betaxolol or any component of the formulation; sinus bradycardia; heart block greater than first-degree (except in patients with a functioning artificial pacemaker); cardiogenic shock; uncompensated cardiac failure
Warnings/Precautions Consider pre-existing conditions (such as sick sinus syndrome) before initiating. Administer cautiously in compensated heart failure and monitor for a worsening of the condition; efficacy of betaxolol in HF has not been demonstrated. Beta-blocker therapy should not be withdrawn abruptly (particularly in patients with CAD), but gradually tapered to avoid acute tachycardia, hypertension, and/or ischemia. Chronic beta-blocker therapy should not be routinely withdrawn prior to major surgery. Use caution with concurrent use of digoxin, verapamil, or diltiazem; bradycardia or heart block can occur. Use with caution in patients receiving inhaled anesthetic agents known to depress myocardial contractility. Bradycardia may be observed more frequently in elderly patients (>65 years of age); dosage reductions may be necessary.

May precipitate or aggravate symptoms of arterial insufficiency in patients with peripheral vascular disease (PVD) and Raynaud's disease; use with caution; monitor for progression of arterial obstruction. In general, beta-blockers should be avoided in ▶

patients with bronchospastic disease. Betaxolol, with beta$_1$ selectivity, may be used cautiously in bronchospastic disease with the lowest possible dose (eg, 5-10 mg/day), availability of a broncho-dilator, and close monitoring; if dosage increase is indicated, administer in divided doses. Use cautiously in patients with diabetes because it may potentiate and/or mask prominent hypoglycemic symptoms. May mask signs of hyperthyroidism (eg, tachycardia); use caution if hyperthyroidism is suspected, abrupt withdrawal may precipitate thyroid storm. May induce or exacerbate psoriasis. Use with caution in patients with cerebrovascular insufficiency; hypotension and decreased heart rate may reduce cerebral blood flow. Dosage adjustment required in severe renal impairment and in patients on dialysis. Use with caution in patients with myasthenia gravis (may potentiate myasthenia-related muscle weakness, including diplopia and ptosis) or psychiatric disease (may cause CNS depression). Adequate alpha-blockade is required prior to use of any beta-blocker for patients with untreated pheochromocytoma. Use caution with history of severe anaphylaxis to allergens; patients taking beta-blockers may become more sensitive to repeated challenges. Treatment of anaphylaxis (eg, epinephrine) in patients taking beta-blockers may be ineffective or promote undesirable effects.

Drug Interactions

Avoid Concomitant Use

Avoid concomitant use of Betaxolol (Systemic) with any of the following: Floctafenine; Methacholine

Decreased Effect

Betaxolol (Systemic) may decrease the levels/effects of: Beta2-Agonists; Theophylline Derivatives

The levels/effects of Betaxolol (Systemic) may be decreased by: Barbiturates; CYP1A2 Inducers (Strong); Cyproterone; Herbs (Hypertensive Properties); Methylphenidate; Nonsteroidal Anti-Inflammatory Agents; Peginterferon Alfa-2b; Rifamycin Derivatives; Yohimbine

Increased Effect/Toxicity

Betaxolol (Systemic) may increase the levels/effects of: Alpha-/Beta-Agonists (Direct-Acting); Alpha1-Blockers; Alpha2-Agonists; Amifostine; Antihypertensives; Antipsychotic Agents (Phenothiazines); ARIPiprazole; Bupivacaine; Cardiac Glycosides; Cholinergic Agonists; DULoxetine; Ergot Derivatives; Fingolimod; Hypotensive Agents; Insulin; Lidocaine (Systemic); Lidocaine (Topical); Mepivacaine; Methacholine; Midodrine; Obinutuzumab; RiTUXimab; Sulfonylureas

The levels/effects of Betaxolol (Systemic) may be increased by: Abiraterone Acetate; Acetylcholinesterase Inhibitors; Alpha2-Agonists; Aminoquinolines (Antimalarial); Amiodarone; Anilidopiperidine Opioids; Antipsychotic Agents (Phenothiazines); Brimonidine (Topical); Calcium Channel Blockers (Dihydropyridine); Calcium Channel Blockers (Nondihydropyridine); CYP1A2 Inhibitors (Moderate); CYP1A2 Inhibitors (Strong); Deferasirox; Diazoxide; Dipyridamole; Disopyramide; Dronedarone; Floctafenine; Herbs (Hypotensive Properties); MAO Inhibitors; Pentoxifylline; Phosphodiesterase 5 Inhibitors; Propafenone; Prostacyclin Analogues; Regorafenib; Reserpine; Vemurafenib

Nutritional/Ethanol Interactions Herb/Nutraceutical: Avoid bayberry; blue cohosh, cayenne, ephedra, ginger, ginseng (American), gotu kola, and licorice (may worsen hypertension). Avoid black cohosh, California poppy, coleus, golden seal, hawthorn, mistletoe, periwinkle, quinine, shepherd's purse (may have increased antihypertensive effects).

Adverse Reactions 2% to 10%:
Cardiovascular: Bradycardia (6% to 8%; symptomatic bradycardia: <1% to 2%; dose-dependent), chest pain (2% to 7%), palpitation (2%), edema (≤2%; similar to placebo)
Central nervous system: Fatigue (3% to 10%), insomnia (1% to 5%), lethargy (3%)
Gastrointestinal: Nausea (2% to 6%), dyspepsia (4% to 5%), diarrhea (2%)
Neuromuscular & skeletal: Arthralgia (3% to 5%), paresthesia (2%)
Respiratory: Dyspnea (2%), pharyngitis (2%)
Miscellaneous: Antinuclear antibody positive (5%), cold extremities (2%)

Pharmacodynamics/Kinetics

Onset of Action 1-1.5 hours

Available Dosage Forms

Tablet, Oral:
Kerlone: 10 mg, 20 mg
Generic: 10 mg, 20 mg

General Dosage Range Dosage adjustment recommended in patients with renal impairment
Oral:
Adults: 5-20 mg/day
Elderly: Initial dose: 5 mg/day

Administration

Oral Absorption is not affected by food.
Storage/Stability Avoid freezing. Store tablets at room temperature of 15°C to 25°C (59°F to 77°F).

Nursing Actions

Physical Assessment Advise patients with diabetes to monitor glucose levels closely; beta-blockers may alter glucose tolerance. Taper dosage slowly when discontinuing.

Patient Education
• Discuss specific use of drug and side effects with patient as it relates to treatment. (HCAHPS: During this hospital stay, were you given any medicine that you had not taken before? Before giving you any new medicine, how often did hospital staff tell you what the medicine was

for? How often did hospital staff describe possible side effects in a way you could understand?)
- Patient may experience diarrhea, headache, pyrosis, arthralgia, asthenia, or insomnia. Have patient report immediately to prescriber signs of depression (ie, suicidal ideation, anxiety, emotional instability, illogical thinking), severe dizziness, syncope, dyspnea, significant asthenia, excessive weight gain, edema of extremities, skin discoloration, sensation of cold, angina, sexual dysfunction, chills, pharyngitis, mood changes, memory loss, considerable dyspepsia, bradycardia, arrhythmia, ecchymosis, or hemorrhaging (HCAHPS).
- Educate patient about signs of a significant reaction (eg, wheezing; chest tightness; fever; itching; bad cough; blue skin color; seizures; or swelling of face, lips, tongue, or throat). **Note:** This is not a comprehensive list of all side effects. Patient should consult prescriber for additional questions.

Intended Use and Disclaimer: Should not be printed and given to patients. This information is intended to serve as a concise initial reference for healthcare professionals to use when discussing medications with a patient. You must ultimately rely on your own discretion, experience and judgment in diagnosing, treating and advising patients.

Bethanechol (be THAN e kole)

Brand Names: U.S. Urecholine
Index Terms Bethanechol Chloride
Pharmacologic Category Cholinergic Agonist
Medication Safety Issues
  Sound-alike/look-alike issues:
    Bethanechol may be confused with betaxolol
Pregnancy Risk Factor C
Lactation Excretion in breast milk unknown/not recommended
Use Treatment of acute postoperative and postpartum nonobstructive (functional) urinary retention; treatment of neurogenic atony of the urinary bladder with retention
Unlabeled Use Gastroesophageal reflux
Available Dosage Forms
  Tablet, Oral:
    Urecholine: 5 mg, 10 mg, 25 mg, 50 mg
    Generic: 5 mg, 10 mg, 25 mg, 50 mg
General Dosage Range Oral: *Adults:* 10-100 mg 2-4 times/day
Administration
  Oral Should be administered 1 hour before meals or 2 hours after meals.
Nursing Actions
  Physical Assessment Assess bladder and sphincter adequacy prior to administering medication.

- Patient may experience headache, dyspepsia, pyrosis, polyuria, hyperhidrosis, or lacrimation. Have patient report immediately to prescriber severe dizziness, syncope, dyspnea, significant flushing, considerable nausea, or intolerable diarrhea (HCAHPS).
- Educate patient about signs of a significant reaction (eg, wheezing; chest tightness; fever; itching; bad cough; blue skin color; seizures; or swelling of face, lips, tongue, or throat). **Note:** This is not a comprehensive list of all side effects. Patient should consult prescriber for additional questions.

Intended Use and Disclaimer: Should not be printed and given to patients. This information is intended to serve as a concise initial reference for healthcare professionals to use when discussing medications with a patient. You must ultimately rely on your own discretion, experience and judgment in diagnosing, treating and advising patients.

Bevacizumab (be vuh SIZ uh mab)

Brand Names: U.S. Avastin
Index Terms Anti-VEGF Monoclonal Antibody; Anti-VEGF rhuMAb; rhuMAb-VEGF
Pharmacologic Category Antineoplastic Agent, Monoclonal Antibody; Antineoplastic Agent, Vascular Endothelial Growth Factor (VEGF) Inhibitor; Vascular Endothelial Growth Factor (VEGF) Inhibitor
Medication Safety Issues
  Sound-alike/look-alike issues:
    Avastin may be confused with Astelin
    Bevacizumab may be confused with brentuximab, cetuximab, ranibizumab, riTUXimab
  High alert medication:
    This medication is in a class the Institute for Safe Medication Practices (ISMP) includes among its list of drug classes which have a heightened risk of causing significant patient harm when used in error.
  International issues:
    Avastin [U.S., Canada, and multiple international markets] may be confused with Avaxim, a brand name for hepatitis A vaccine [Canada and multiple international markets]
Pregnancy Risk Factor C
Lactation Excretion in breast milk unknown/not recommended

Use

Colorectal cancer, metastatic: First-or second-line treatment of metastatic colorectal cancer (CRC) (in combination with fluorouracil-based chemotherapy); second-line treatment of metastatic CRC (in combination with fluoropyrimidine-irinotecan- or fluoropyrimidine-oxaliplatin-based chemotherapy) after progression on a first-line treatment containing bevacizumab. **Note:** Not indicated for the adjuvant treatment of CRC.

Glioblastoma: Treatment of progressive glioblastoma (as a single agent). Effectiveness is based on improvement in objective response rate.

Non-small cell lung cancer, non-squamous: First-line treatment of unresectable, locally advanced, recurrent or metastatic nonsquamous non-small cell lung cancer (NSCLC) (in combination with carboplatin and paclitaxel).

Renal cell carcinoma, metastatic: Treatment of metastatic renal cell carcinoma (RCC) (in combination with interferon alfa). **Note:** Not an approved use in Canada.

Unlabeled Use Treatment of metastatic breast cancer, recurrent/metastatic cervical cancer, recurrent endometrial cancer, recurrent advanced ovarian cancer (platinum-sensitive), soft tissue sarcomas (angiosarcoma or hemangiopericytoma/solitary fibrous tumor), age-related macular degeneration (AMD)

Available Dosage Forms

Solution, Intravenous [preservative free]:
Avastin: 100 mg/4 mL (4 mL); 400 mg/16 mL (16 mL)

General Dosage Range I.V.: *Adults:* 5 or 10 mg/kg every 2 weeks **or** 15 mg/kg every 3 weeks

Administration

I.V. Infuse the initial dose over 90 minutes. The second infusion may be shortened to 60 minutes if the initial infusion is well tolerated. The third and subsequent infusions may be shortened to 30 minutes if the 60-minute infusion is well tolerated. Monitor closely during the infusion for signs/symptoms of an infusion reaction. After tolerance at the 90-, 60-, and 30-minute infusion rates has been established, some institutions use an unlabeled 10-minute infusion rate (0.5 mg/kg/minute) for bevacizumab dosed at 5 mg/kg (Reidy, 2007). In a study evaluating the safety of the 0.5 mg/kg/minute infusion rate, proteinuria and hypertension incidences were not increased with the shorter infusion time (Shah, 2013). Do not administer I.V. push. Do not administer with dextrose solutions.

Injectable Detail pH: 6.2

Intravitreal Intravitreal injection (unlabeled use/route): Adequate local anesthesia and a topical broad-spectrum antimicrobial agent should be administered prior to the procedure.

Nursing Actions

Physical Assessment Hypertensive crisis may occur; monitor blood pressure closely, even after discontinuation of therapy. Monitor patient closely during infusion for reaction such as hypertension, chest pain, wheezing, or diaphoresis. Drug may be discontinued with severe reactions. Severe complications include gastrointestinal perforation. Educate patient about seeking immediate help if severe abdominal pain, constipation, vomiting, nausea, or fever develop. Serious side effects include heart failure, hypertensive crisis, serious bleeding, and nephrotic syndrome.

Patient Education

- Discuss specific use of drug and side effects with patient as it relates to treatment. (HCAHPS: During this hospital stay, were you given any medicine that you had not taken before? Before giving you any new medicine, how often did hospital staff tell you what the medicine was for? How often did hospital staff describe possible side effects in a way you could understand?)
- Patient may experience back pain, myalgia, diarrhea, asthenia, lack of appetite, stomatitis, alopecia, xeroderma, dysgeusia, xerostomia, or voice changes. Have patient report immediately to prescriber signs of hemorrhaging, signs of infection, strength differences from one side to another, difficulty speaking or thinking, change in balance, blurred vision, edema of extremities, angina, severe dizziness, syncope, dyspnea, excessive weight gain, edema of extremities, significant headache, illogical thinking, blindness, considerable nausea, intolerable constipation, severe dyspepsia, wound healing impairment, vision changes, urinary retention, oliguria, or hyperhidrosis (HCAHPS).
- Educate patient about signs of a significant reaction (eg, wheezing; chest tightness; fever; itching; bad cough; blue skin color; seizures; or swelling of face, lips, tongue, or throat). **Note:** This is not a comprehensive list of all side effects. Patient should consult prescriber for additional questions.

Intended Use and Disclaimer: Should not be printed and given to patients. This information is intended to serve as a concise initial reference for healthcare professionals to use when discussing medications with a patient. You must ultimately rely on your own discretion, experience and judgment in diagnosing, treating and advising patients.

Bexarotene (Systemic) (beks AIR oh teen)

Brand Names: U.S. Targretin
Pharmacologic Category Antineoplastic Agent, Retinoic Acid Derivative

Medication Safety Issues

High alert medication:

This medication is in a class the Institute for Safe Medication Practices (ISMP) includes among its list of drug classes which have a heightened risk of causing significant patient harm when used in error.

Pregnancy Risk Factor X

Lactation Excretion in breast milk unknown/not recommended

Breast-Feeding Considerations It is not known if bexarotene is excreted into breast milk. Due to the potential for serious adverse reactions in a nursing infant, the decision to continue or discontinue breast-feeding during therapy should take into account the risk of exposure to the infant and the benefits of treatment to the mother.

Use Treatment of cutaneous manifestations of cutaneous T-cell lymphoma in patients who are refractory to at least one prior systemic therapy

Mechanism of Action/Effect Binds to and activates retinoid X receptors (RXRs) which then control cellular differentiation and proliferation.

Contraindications Hypersensitivity to bexarotene or any component of the formulation; pregnancy

Warnings/Precautions Hazardous agent - use appropriate precautions for handling and disposal (NIOSH, 2012). **[U.S. Boxed Warning]: Bexarotene is a retinoid, a drug class associated with birth defects in humans; do not administer during pregnancy.** Pregnancy test needed within 1 week before initiation and every month thereafter. Effective contraception must be in place 1 month before initiation, during therapy, and for at least 1 month after discontinuation. Male patients with sexual partners who are pregnant, possibly pregnant, or who could become pregnant, must use condoms during sexual intercourse during treatment and for at least 1 month after last dose. Induces significant lipid abnormalities in a majority of patients (triglyceride, total cholesterol, and HDL); monitor lipid panel; may require dose reduction, treatment interruption, and/or concomitant antilipemic therapy; reversible on discontinuation. Pancreatitis secondary to hypertriglyceridemia has been reported. Patients with risk factors for pancreatitis (eg, prior pancreatitis, uncontrolled hyperlipidemia, excessive ethanol consumption, uncontrolled diabetes, biliary tract disease, concomitant medications causing hyperlipidemia) should generally not receive bexarotene (oral). Dose-related elevations in ALT, AST, and bilirubin have been reported; monitor for liver function test abnormalities and temporarily hold or discontinue drug if tests are >3 times the upper limit of normal (ULN) values for AST, ALT, or bilirubin. Bexarotene rapidly suppresses TSH levels by directly inhibiting TSH secretion and also affects thyroid hormone metabolism (Hamnvik, 2011). Hypothyroidism occurs in about one third to the majority of all patients; monitor free T_4 levels closely. Thyroid supplementation is usually required; in patients already receiving thyroid hormone therapy, may require increased thyroid hormone doses to achieve therapeutic levels (Hamnvik, 2011). Monitor for signs and symptoms of infection about 4-8 weeks after initiation (leukopenia may occur). Any new visual abnormalities experienced by the patient should be evaluated by an ophthalmologist (cataracts may form, or worsen, especially in the geriatric population). Retinoids are associated with photosensitivity; mild phototoxicity (sunburn, sunlight sensitivity) has occurred with bexarotene; advise patients to limit sunlight and artificial ultraviolet light during treatment. Use only with extreme caution in patients with hepatic impairment; undergoes extensive hepatic elimination. Limit additional vitamin A intake (in studies, additional vitamin A was limited to <15,000 units/day). Use caution with diabetic patients; may enhance the actions of insulin, sulfonylureas or thiazolidinediones, resulting in hypoglycemia in patients receiving these agents (hypoglycemia has not been observed with bexarotene monotherapy). Monitor blood glucose as necessary.

Drug Interactions

Avoid Concomitant Use

Avoid concomitant use of Bexarotene (Systemic) with any of the following: Axitinib; CloZAPine; Gemfibrozil; Multivitamins/Fluoride (with ADE); Multivitamins/Minerals (with ADEK, Folate, Iron); Multivitamins/Minerals (with AE, No Iron); Simeprevir; Tetracycline Derivatives; Vitamin A

Decreased Effect

Bexarotene (Systemic) may decrease the levels/ effects of: ARIPiprazole; AtorvaSTATin; Axitinib; Contraceptives (Estrogens); Contraceptives (Progestins); Ibrutinib; PACLitaxel; Saxagliptin; Simeprevir; Tamoxifen

Increased Effect/Toxicity

Bexarotene (Systemic) may increase the levels/ effects of: CloZAPine; Porfimer; Vitamin A

The levels/effects of Bexarotene (Systemic) may be increased by: CARBOplatin; Gemfibrozil; Multivitamins/Fluoride (with ADE); Multivitamins/Minerals (with ADEK, Folate, Iron); Multivitamins/Minerals (with AE, No Iron); PACLitaxel; Tetracycline Derivatives

Nutritional/Ethanol Interactions

Food: Bioavailability is increased when administered with a fat-containing meal. Serum levels may be increased by grapefruit juice. Management: Administer with food. Avoid grapefruit juice. Herb/Nutraceutical: Dong quai and St John's wort may cause photosensitization. St John's wort may decrease bexarotene levels. Additional vitamin A supplementation may lead to vitamin A toxicity (dry skin, irritation, arthralgias, myalgias, abdominal pain, hepatic changes). Management: Avoid St John's wort and dong quai. Limit the use of vitamin A supplements.

Adverse Reactions

>10%:

Cardiovascular: Peripheral edema (11% to 13%)

Central nervous system: Headache (30% to 42%), fever (5% to 17%), chills (10% to 13%), insomnia (5% to 11%)

Dermatologic: Rash (17% to 23%), exfoliative dermatitis (10% to 28%), dry skin (9% to 11%), alopecia (4% to 11%)

Endocrine & metabolic: Hyperlipidemia (79%), hypercholesteremia (32% to 62%), hypothyroidism (29% to 53%)

Gastrointestinal: Diarrhea (7% to 42%), anorexia (2% to 23%), nausea (8% to 16%), vomiting (4% to 13%), abdominal pain (4% to 11%)

Hematologic: Leukopenia (17% to 47%), anemia (6% to 25%), hypochromic anemia (4% to 13%)

Hepatic: LDH increased (7% to 13%)

Neuromuscular & skeletal: Weakness (20% to 45%), back pain (2% to 11%)

Miscellaneous: Infection (13% to 23%; bacterial: 1% to 13%), flu-like syndrome (4% to 13%)

<10%:

Cardiovascular: Angina pectoris, cerebrovascular accident, chest pain, heart failure (right), hypertension, syncope, tachycardia

Central nervous system: Agitation, ataxia, confusion, depression, dizziness, hyperesthesia, subdural hematoma

Dermatologic: Acne, cellulitis, cheilitis, maculopapular rash, photosensitivity, pustular rash, serous drainage, skin nodule, skin rash, skin sensitivity, sunburn, vesicular bullous rash

Endocrine & metabolic: Breast pain, hypoproteinemia, hyperglycemia

Gastrointestinal: Amylase increased, colitis, constipation, dyspepsia, flatulence, gastroenteritis, gingivitis, melena, pancreatitis, weight loss/gain, xerostomia

Genitourinary: Dysuria, hematuria, urinary incontinence, urinary tract infection, urinary urgency

Hematologic: Coagulopathy, eosinophilia, hemorrhage, lymphocytosis, thrombocythemia, thrombocytopenia

Hepatic: ALT increased, AST increased, bilirubin increased, hepatic failure

Neuromuscular & skeletal: Arthralgia, arthrosis, bone pain, myalgia, myasthenia, neuropathy

Ocular: Blepharitis, cataracts (new and worsening), conjunctivitis, corneal lesion, dry eyes, keratitis, visual field defects

Otic: Ear pain, otitis externa

Renal: Albuminuria, creatinine increased, renal function abnormal

Respiratory: Bronchitis, cough, dyspnea, hemoptysis, hypoxia, pharyngitis, pleural effusion, pneumonia, pulmonary edema, rhinitis

Miscellaneous: Monilia, sepsis

Available Dosage Forms

Capsule, Oral:

Targretin: 75 mg

General Dosage Range Dosage adjustment recommended in patients who develop toxicities.

Oral: *Adults:* 300-400 mg/m² once daily

Administration

Oral Administer with a meal. Swallow capsule whole; do not chew or dissolve (per the manufacturer).

Hazardous agent; use appropriate precautions for handling and disposal (NIOSH, 2012).

Storage/Stability Store at 2°C to 25°C (36°F to 77°F). Protect from light. Avoid humidity and high temperatures after opening bottle.

Nursing Actions

Physical Assessment Monitor for CNS or cardiovascular effects, opportunistic infection, visual abnormalities, and hypoglycemia. Instruct patients that effectiveness of hormonal birth control may be decreased while taking this medication. Patient should avoid getting pregnant while on this medication. Avoid alcohol intake as increase in drug toxicity may occur. Teach patient about photosensitivity potential; use sunscreen and appropriate clothing. Teach patient the importance of keeping scheduled lab appointments to monitor lipid panel, LFTs, thyroid functions, and CBC throughout treatment. Instruct patient to report symptoms of pancreatitis, including nausea, vomiting, or abdominal and back pain. Harmful if medication gets on skin; wash with soap and water immediately.

Patient Education

• Discuss specific use of drug and side effects with patient as it relates to treatment. (HCAHPS: During this hospital stay, were you given any medicine that you had not taken before? Before giving you any new medicine, how often did hospital staff tell you what the medicine was for? How often did hospital staff describe possible side effects in a way you could understand?)

• Patient may experience insomnia, lack of appetite, dyspepsia, nausea, diarrhea, alopecia, xeroderma, or back pain. Have patient report immediately to prescriber signs of infection, signs of pancreatitis, signs of hepatic impairment, strength differences from one side to another, difficulty speaking or thinking, change in balance, blurred vision, severe headache, ecchymosis, hemorrhaging, temperature sensitivity, vision changes, edema of extremities, significant asthenia, angina, tachycardia, depression, or paresthesia (HCAHPS).

• Educate patient about signs of a significant reaction (eg, wheezing; chest tightness; fever; itching; bad cough; blue skin color; seizures; or swelling of face, lips, tongue, or throat). **Note:** This is not a comprehensive list of all side effects. Patient should consult prescriber for additional questions.

Intended Use and Disclaimer: Should not be printed and given to patients. This information is

intended to serve as a concise initial reference for healthcare professionals to use when discussing medications with a patient. You must ultimately rely on your own discretion, experience and judgment in diagnosing, treating and advising patients.

Dietary Considerations Take with food. Avoid grapefruit juice.

Related Information

Oral Medications That Should Not Be Crushed or Altered *on page 1712*

Bexarotene (Topical) (beks AIR oh teen)

Brand Names: U.S. Targretin

Pharmacologic Category Antineoplastic Agent, Retinoic Acid Derivative

Medication Safety Issues

High alert medication:

The Institute for Safe Medication Practices (ISMP) includes this medication among its list of drugs which have a heightened risk of causing significant patient harm when used in error.

Pregnancy Risk Factor X

Lactation Excretion in breast milk unknown/not recommended

Use Treatment of cutaneous lesions in patients with refractory cutaneous T-cell lymphoma (stage 1A and 1B) or who have not tolerated other therapies

Available Dosage Forms

Gel, External:

Targretin: 1% (60 g)

General Dosage Range Topical: *Adults:* Initial: Apply once every other day for first week; Maintenance: Apply 1-4 times/day

Administration

Topical Allow gel to dry before covering with clothing. Avoid application to normal skin. Use of occlusive dressings is not recommended.

Hazardous agent; use appropriate precautions for handling and disposal (NIOSH, 2012).

Nursing Actions

Patient Education

- Discuss specific use of drug and side effects with patient as it relates to treatment. (HCAHPS: During this hospital stay, were you given any medicine that you had not taken before? Before giving you any new medicine, how often did hospital staff tell you what the medicine was for? How often did hospital staff describe possible side effects in a way you could understand?)
- Patient may experience headache. Have patient report immediately to prescriber signs of infection, paresthesia, edema of extremities, or severe application site irritation (HCAHPS).
- Educate patient about signs of a significant reaction (eg, wheezing; chest tightness; fever; itching; bad cough; blue skin color; seizures; or swelling of face, lips, tongue, or throat). **Note:** This is not a comprehensive list of all side

effects. Patient should consult prescriber for additional questions.

Intended Use and Disclaimer: Should not be printed and given to patients. This information is intended to serve as a concise initial reference for healthcare professionals to use when discussing medications with a patient. You must ultimately rely on your own discretion, experience and judgment in diagnosing, treating and advising patients.

Related Information

Oral Medications That Should Not Be Crushed or Altered *on page 1712*

Bicalutamide (bye ka LOO ta mide)

Brand Names: U.S. Casodex

Index Terms CDX; ICI-176334

Pharmacologic Category Antineoplastic Agent, Antiandrogen

Medication Safety Issues

Sound-alike/look-alike issues:

Casodex® may be confused with Kapidex [DSC]

International issues:

Casodex [U.S., Canada, and multiple international markets] may be confused with Capadex brand name for propoxyphene/acetaminophen [Australia, New Zealand]

Pregnancy Risk Factor X

Lactation Excretion in breast milk unknown/contra-indicated

Use Treatment of metastatic prostate cancer (in combination with an LHRH agonist)

Unlabeled Use Monotherapy for locally-advanced prostate cancer

Available Dosage Forms

Tablet, Oral:

Casodex: 50 mg

Generic: 50 mg

General Dosage Range Oral: *Adults:* 50 mg once daily

Administration

Oral Dose should be taken at the same time each day with or without food. Treatment for metastatic cancer should be started concomitantly with an LHRH analogue.

Hazardous agent; use appropriate precautions for handling and disposal (NIOSH, 2012).

Nursing Actions

Physical Assessment Monitor LFTs at baseline and regularly during therapy. Advise patients with diabetes to monitor glucose levels closely (may induce hyperglycemia).

Patient Education

- Discuss specific use of drug and side effects with patient as it relates to treatment. (HCAHPS: During this hospital stay, were you given any medicine that you had not taken before? Before giving you any new medicine, how often did

hospital staff tell you what the medicine was for? How often did hospital staff describe possible side effects in a way you could understand?)
- Patient may experience dyspepsia, diarrhea, constipation, sexual dysfunction, hot flashes, warmth sensation, hyperhidrosis, back pain, or pelvic pain. Have patient report immediately to prescriber signs of hyperglycemia, dyspnea, excessive weight gain, edema of extremities, ecchymosis, hemorrhaging, macromastia, mastalgia, melena, vision changes, osteodynia, urinary retention, oliguria, angina, hematuria, severe dizziness, syncope, arthralgia, depression, considerable asthenia, paresthesia, significant headache, or signs of hepatic impairment (HCAHPS).
- Educate patient about signs of a significant reaction (eg, wheezing; chest tightness; fever; itching; bad cough; blue skin color; seizures; or swelling of face, lips, tongue, or throat). **Note:** This is not a comprehensive list of all side effects. Patient should consult prescriber for additional questions.

Intended Use and Disclaimer: Should not be printed and given to patients. This information is intended to serve as a concise initial reference for healthcare professionals to use when discussing medications with a patient. You must ultimately rely on your own discretion, experience and judgment in diagnosing, treating and advising patients.

Related Information

Oral Medications That Should Not Be Crushed or Altered *on page 1712*

Bimatoprost (bi MAT oh prost)

Brand Names: U.S. Latisse; Lumigan
Pharmacologic Category Ophthalmic Agent, Antiglaucoma; Prostaglandin, Ophthalmic
Pregnancy Risk Factor C
Lactation Excretion in breast milk unknown/use caution
Breast-Feeding Considerations It is not known if bimatoprost is excreted in breast milk. The manufacturer recommends that caution be exercised when administering bimatoprost to nursing women.
Use Reduction of intraocular pressure (IOP) in patients with open-angle glaucoma or ocular hypertension; hypotrichosis treatment of the eyelashes
Mechanism of Action/Effect Decreases intraocular pressure by increasing outflow of aqueous humor. Increases the percent and duration of hairs in the growth phase, resulting in eyelash growth.
Contraindications
Latisse®: Hypersensitivity to bimatoprost or any component of the formulation
Lumigan®: There are no contraindications listed in the manufacturer's prescribing information.

Warnings/Precautions May cause permanent changes in eye color (increases the amount of brown pigment in the iris), the eyelid skin, and eyelashes. In addition, may increase the length and/or number of eyelashes (may vary between eyes). Use caution in patients with intraocular inflammation, aphakic patients, pseudophakic patients with a torn posterior lens capsule, or patients with risk factors for macular edema. Contains benzalkonium chloride (may be adsorbed by contact lenses). Safety and efficacy have not been determined for use in patients with angle-closure, inflammatory, or neovascular glaucoma. Not recommended for use in pediatrics <16 years of age due to potential concerns regarding long-term use and hyperpigmentation.

Latisse®: Additional warnings: Patients receiving medications to reduce intraocular pressure should consult their healthcare provider prior to using; may interfere with desired reduction of intraocular pressure. Unintentional hair growth may occur on skin that has repeated contact with solution; apply to upper eyelid only, blot away excess.

Drug Interactions

Avoid Concomitant Use There are no known interactions where it is recommended to avoid concomitant use.

Decreased Effect

The levels/effects of Bimatoprost may be decreased by: Nonsteroidal Anti-Inflammatory Agents

Increased Effect/Toxicity

The levels/effects of Bimatoprost may be increased by: Latanoprost

Adverse Reactions Adverse reactions and percentages are for Lumigan® unless noted:
>10%: Ocular: Conjunctival hyperemia (25% to 45%; Latisse®: <4%), growth of eyelashes, ocular pruritus (>10%; Latisse®: <4%)
1% to 10%:
Central nervous system: Headache (1% to 5%)
Dermatologic: Skin hyperpigmentation (Latisse®: <4%), abnormal hair growth
Hepatic: Liver function tests abnormal (1% to 5%)
Neuromuscular & skeletal: Weakness (1% to 5%)
Ocular: Dry eyes (1% to 10%; Latisse®: <4%), erythema (eyelid/periorbital region; 1% to 10%; Latisse®: <4%), irritation (1% to 10%; Latisse®: <4%), allergic conjunctivitis, asthenopia, blepharitis, burning, cataract, conjunctival edema, conjunctival hemorrhage, discharge, eyelash darkening, foreign body sensation, iris pigmentation increased (may be delayed), pain, photophobia, pigmentation of periocular skin, superficial punctate keratitis, tearing, visual disturbance
Miscellaneous: Infections (10% [primarily colds and upper respiratory tract infections])

Pharmacodynamics/Kinetics
  Onset of Action Reduction of IOP: ~4 hours;
  Peak effect: Maximum reduction of IOP: ~8-12
  hours
Available Dosage Forms
  Solution, External:
    Latisse: 0.03% (3 mL, 5 mL)
  Solution, Ophthalmic:
    Lumigan: 0.01% (2.5 mL, 5 mL, 7.5 mL)
General Dosage Range
  Ophthalmic: *Adults:* Instill 1 drop into affected
    eye(s) once daily
  Ophthalmic, topical: *Adults:* Place 1 drop on
    applicator and apply evenly along the skin of the
    upper eyelid at base of eyelashes once daily
Administration
  Other
    Latisse®: Remove make-up and contact lenses
    prior to application; ensure face is clean. Apply
    with the sterile applicator provided only; do not
    use other brushes or applicators. Use a tissue or
    cloth to blot any excess solution on the outside
    of the upper eyelid margin; do not apply to lower
    eyelash line. Do not reuse applicators; use new
    applicator for second eye. Applying more than
    once nightly will not increase eyelash growth;
    eyelash growth is expected to return to baseline
    when therapy is discontinued. May reinsert con-
    tacts 15 minutes after application.
    Lumigan®: May be used with other eye drops to
    lower intraocular pressure. If using more than
    one ophthalmic product, wait at least 5 minutes
    in between application of each medication.
    Remove contact lenses prior to administration
    and wait 15 minutes before reinserting.
Storage/Stability Store between 2°C to 25°C
  (36°F to 77°F).
Nursing Actions
  Patient Education
    • Discuss specific use of drug and side effects
      with patient as it relates to treatment. (HCAHPS:
      During this hospital stay, were you given any
      medicine that you had not taken before? Before
      giving you any new medicine, how often did
      hospital staff tell you what the medicine was
      for? How often did hospital staff describe possi-
      ble side effects in a way you could understand?)
    • Patient may experience blurred vision, lacrima-
      tion, sensitivity to light, foreign body sensation of
      eye, eyelid/eyelash changes. Have patient
      report immediately to prescriber severe eye irri-
      tation, ophthalmalgia, vision changes, eye dis-
      charge, asthenopia, or ocular discoloration
      (HCAHPS).
    • Educate patient about signs of a significant
      reaction (eg, wheezing; chest tightness; fever;
      itching; bad cough; blue skin color; seizures; or
      swelling of face, lips, tongue, or throat). **Note:**
      This is not a comprehensive list of all side
      effects. Patient should consult prescriber for
      additional questions.

Intended Use and Disclaimer: Should not be
printed and given to patients. This information is
intended to serve as a concise initial reference for
healthcare professionals to use when discussing
medications with a patient. You must ultimately
rely on your own discretion, experience and judgment in diagnosing, treating and advising
patients.

Bismuth (BIZ muth)

Brand Names: U.S. Bismatrol Maximum Strength
[OTC]; Bismatrol [OTC]; Diotame [OTC]; Kao-Tin
[OTC]; Peptic Relief [OTC]; Pepto-Bismol To-Go
[OTC]; Pepto-Bismol [OTC]; Pink Bismuth [OTC];
Stomach Relief Max St [OTC]; Stomach Relief Plus
[OTC]; Stomach Relief [OTC]
Index Terms Bismatrol; Bismuth Subsalicylate;
Pink Bismuth
Pharmacologic Category Antidiarrheal
Medication Safety Issues
  Sound-alike/look-alike issues:
    Kaopectate® may be confused with Kayexalate®
  Other safety concerns:
    Maalox® Total Relief® is a different formulation
      than other Maalox® liquid antacid products
      which contain aluminum hydroxide, magnesium
      hydroxide, and simethicone.
    Canadian formulation of Kaopectate® does not
      contain bismuth; the active ingredient in the
      Canadian formulation is attapulgite.
Use Subsalicylate formulation: Symptomatic treatment of mild, nonspecific diarrhea; control of traveler's diarrhea (enterotoxigenic *Escherichia coli*);
  as part of a multidrug regimen for *H. pylori* eradication to reduce the risk of duodenal ulcer recurrence
Available Dosage Forms
  Suspension, Oral:
    Bismatrol [OTC]: 262 mg/15 mL (236 mL)
    Bismatrol Maximum Strength [OTC]: 525 mg/15
      mL (236 mL)
    Kao-Tin [OTC]: 262 mg/15 mL (236 mL, 473 mL)
    Peptic Relief [OTC]: 262 mg/15 mL (237 mL)
    Pepto-Bismol [OTC]: 262 mg/15 mL (473 mL)
    Pink Bismuth [OTC]: 262 mg/15 mL (236 mL,
      237 mL)
    Stomach Relief [OTC]: 262 mg/15 mL (237 mL,
      355 mL); 527 mg/30 mL (240 mL, 480 mL)
    Stomach Relief Max St [OTC]: 525 mg/15 mL
      (237 mL)
    Stomach Relief Plus [OTC]: 525 mg/15 mL (240
      mL, 480 mL)
  Tablet Chewable, Oral:
    Bismatrol [OTC]: 262 mg
    Diotame [OTC]: 262 mg
    Peptic Relief [OTC]: 262 mg
    Pepto-Bismol To-Go [OTC]: 262 mg
    Pink Bismuth [OTC]: 262 mg
    Stomach Relief [OTC]: 262 mg
    Generic: 262 mg

General Dosage Range Oral:
Subsalicylate based on 262 mg/5 mL liquid or 262 mg tablet (diarrhea):
Children 3-6 years: 1/3 tablet **or** 5 mL every 30 minutes to 1 hour as needed (maximum: 8 doses/day)
Children 6-9 years: 2/3 tablet **or** 10 mL every 30 minutes to 1 hour as needed (maximum: 8 doses/day)
Children 9-12 years: 1 tablet **or** 15 mL every 30 minutes to 1 hour as needed (maximum: 8 doses/day)
Subsalicylate based on 262 mg/15 mL liquid or 262 mg tablet:
Children >12 years: Diarrhea: 2 tablets **or** 30 mL every 30 minutes to 1 hour as needed (maximum: 8 doses/day)
Adults:
Diarrhea: 2 tablets **or** 30 mL every 30 minutes to 1 hour as needed (maximum: 8 doses/day)
H. pylori eradication: 524 mg 4 times/day

Administration
Oral Liquids must be shaken prior to use. Chewable tablets should be chewed thoroughly. Nonchewable caplets should be swallowed whole with a full glass of water.

Nursing Actions
Physical Assessment Patient's history with aspirin products should be assessed prior to beginning treatment (contains ASA). Assess other drugs patient may be taking for potential interactions (eg, aspirin products). Monitor for CNS changes, impactions, and tinnitus.

Patient Education
• Discuss specific use of drug and side effects with patient as it relates to treatment. (HCAHPS: During this hospital stay, were you given any medicine that you had not taken before? Before giving you any new medicine, how often did hospital staff tell you what the medicine was for? How often did hospital staff describe possible side effects in a way you could understand?)
• Patient may experience tongue discoloration or stool discoloration. Have patient report immediately to prescriber illogical thinking, tinnitus, hearing impairment, severe constipation, ecchymosis, hemorrhaging, urine discoloration, melena, or hematemesis (HCAHPS).
• Educate patient about signs of a significant reaction (eg, wheezing; chest tightness; fever; itching; bad cough; blue skin color; seizures; or swelling of face, lips, tongue, or throat). **Note:** This is not a comprehensive list of all side effects. Patient should consult prescriber for additional questions.

Intended Use and Disclaimer: Should not be printed and given to patients. This information is intended to serve as a concise initial reference for healthcare professionals to use when discussing medications with a patient. You must ultimately rely on your own discretion, experience and judgment in diagnosing, treating and advising patients.

Bisoprolol (bis OH proe lol)

Brand Names: U.S. Zebeta
Index Terms Bisoprolol Fumarate
Pharmacologic Category Antihypertensive; Beta-Blocker, Beta-1 Selective
Medication Safety Issues
Sound-alike/look-alike issues:
Zebeta may be confused with DiaBeta, Zetia
Pregnancy Risk Factor C
Lactation Excretion unknown/use caution
Breast-Feeding Considerations It is not known if bisoprolol is excreted into breast milk. The manufacturer recommends that caution be exercised when administering bisoprolol to nursing women.
Use Treatment of hypertension, alone or in combination with other agents
Unlabeled Use
Chronic stable angina, supraventricular arrhythmias, PVCs, heart failure (HF)
Note: The ACCF/AHA 2013 heart failure guidelines recommend the use of 1 of the 3 beta blockers (ie, bisoprolol, carvedilol, or extended-release metoprolol succinate) for all patients with recent or remote history of MI or ACS and reduced ejection fraction (rEF) to reduce mortality, for all patients with rEF to prevent symptomatic HF (even if no history of MI), and for all patients with current or prior symptoms of HF with reduced ejection fraction (HFrEF), unless contraindicated, to reduce morbidity and mortality (Yancy, 2013).
Mechanism of Action/Effect Selective inhibitor of beta$_1$-adrenergic receptors; competitively blocks beta$_1$-receptors, with little or no effect on beta$_2$-receptors at doses ≤20 mg
Contraindications Cardiogenic shock; overt cardiac failure; marked sinus bradycardia or heart block greater than first-degree (except in patients with a functioning artificial pacemaker)
Warnings/Precautions Consider pre-existing conditions such as sick sinus syndrome before initiating. Use caution in patients with heart failure; use gradual and careful titration; monitor for symptoms of congestive heart failure. Use with caution in patients with myasthenia gravis, psychiatric disease, undergoing anesthesia; and in those with impaired hepatic function. Bradycardia may be observed more frequently in elderly patients (>65 years of age); dosage reductions may be necessary. Beta-blocker therapy should not be withdrawn abruptly (particularly in patients with CAD), but gradually tapered to avoid acute tachycardia, hypertension, and/or ischemia. Chronic beta-blocker therapy should not be routinely withdrawn prior to major surgery. Can precipitate or aggravate symptoms of arterial insufficiency in patients with

PVD and Raynaud's disease; use with caution and monitor for progression of arterial obstruction. Use caution with concurrent use of digoxin, verapamil, or diltiazem; bradycardia or heart block may occur. Use with caution in patients receiving inhaled anesthetic agents known to depress myocardial contractility. Bisoprolol, with beta$_1$-selectivity, may be used cautiously in bronchospastic disease with close monitoring. Use cautiously in patients with diabetes because it can mask prominent hypoglycemic symptoms. May mask signs of hyperthyroidism (eg, tachycardia); use caution if hyperthyroidism is suspected, abrupt withdrawal may precipitate thyroid storm. Dosage adjustment is required in patients with significant hepatic or renal dysfunction. Adequate alpha-blockade is required prior to use of any beta-blocker for patients with untreated pheochromocytoma. May induce or exacerbate psoriasis. Use caution with history of severe anaphylaxis to allergens; patients taking beta-blockers may become more sensitive to repeated challenges. Treatment of anaphylaxis (eg, epinephrine) in patients taking beta-blockers may be ineffective or promote undesirable effects.

Drug Interactions

Avoid Concomitant Use
Avoid concomitant use of Bisoprolol with any of the following: Conivaptan; Floctafenine; Fusidic Acid (Systemic); Methacholine

Decreased Effect
Bisoprolol may decrease the levels/effects of: Beta2-Agonists; Theophylline Derivatives

The levels/effects of Bisoprolol may be decreased by: Barbiturates; Bosentan; CYP3A4 Inducers (Strong); Dabrafenib; Deferasirox; Herbs (CYP3A4 Inducers); Herbs (Hypertensive Properties); Methylphenidate; Mitotane; Nonsteroidal Anti-Inflammatory Agents; Peginterferon Alfa-2b; Rifamycin Derivatives; Tocilizumab; Yohimbine

Increased Effect/Toxicity
Bisoprolol may increase the levels/effects of: Alpha-/Beta-Agonists (Direct-Acting); Alpha1-Blockers; Alpha2-Agonists; Amifostine; Antihypertensives; Antipsychotic Agents (Phenothiazines); Bupivacaine; Cardiac Glycosides; Cholinergic Agonists; DULoxetine; Ergot Derivatives; Fingolimod; Hypotensive Agents; Insulin; Lidocaine (Systemic); Lidocaine (Topical); Mepivacaine; Methacholine; Midodrine; Obinutuzumab; RiTUXimab; Sulfonylureas

The levels/effects of Bisoprolol may be increased by: Acetylcholinesterase Inhibitors; Alpha2-Agonists; Aminoquinolines (Antimalarial); Amiodarone; Anilidopiperidine Opioids; Antipsychotic Agents (Phenothiazines); Brimonidine (Topical); Calcium Channel Blockers (Dihydropyridine); Calcium Channel Blockers (Nondihydropyridine); Conivaptan; CYP3A4 Inhibitors (Moderate); CYP3A4 Inhibitors (Strong); Dasatinib; Diazoxide; Dipyridamole; Disopyramide; Dronedarone;

Floctafenine; Fusidic Acid (Systemic); Herbs (Hypotensive Properties); Ivacaftor; Luliconazole; MAO Inhibitors; Mifepristone; Pentoxifylline; Phosphodiesterase 5 Inhibitors; Propafenone; Prostacyclin Analogues; Regorafenib; Reserpine; Simeprevir; Stiripentol

Nutritional/Ethanol Interactions
Herb/Nutraceutical: Avoid dong quai if using for hypertension (has estrogenic activity). Avoid ephedra, yohimbe, ginseng (may worsen hypertension). Avoid garlic (may have increased antihypertensive effect).

Adverse Reactions 1% to 10%:
Cardiovascular: Chest pain (1% to 2%)

Central nervous system: Fatigue (dose related; 6% to 8%), insomnia (2% to 3%), hypoesthesia (1% to 2%)

Gastrointestinal: Diarrhea (dose related; 3% to 4%), nausea (2%), vomiting (1% to 2%)

Neuromuscular & skeletal: Arthralgia, weakness (dose related; ≤2%)

Respiratory: Upper respiratory infection (5%), rhinitis (3% to 4%), sinusitis (dose related; 2%), dyspnea (1% to 2%)

Pharmacodynamics/Kinetics
Onset of Action 1-2 hours

Available Dosage Forms
Tablet, Oral:
Zebeta: 5 mg, 10 mg
Generic: 5 mg, 10 mg

General Dosage Range Dosage adjustment recommended in patients with renal impairment
Oral: *Adults and Elderly:* Initial: 2.5-5 mg once daily; Maintenance: 2.5-20 mg once daily

Administration
Oral May be administered without regard to meals.
Storage/Stability Store at controlled room temperature 20°C to 25°C (68°F to 77°F). Protect from moisture.

Nursing Actions

Physical Assessment Monitor blood pressure and heart rate prior to and following first dose and with any change in dosage. Taper dosage slowly when discontinuing. Advise patients with diabetes to monitor glucose levels closely; beta-blockers may alter glucose tolerance. Teach patient how to handle orthostatic hypotension.

Patient Education
- Discuss specific use of drug and side effects with patient as it relates to treatment. (HCAHPS: During this hospital stay, were you given any medicine that you had not taken before? Before giving you any new medicine, how often did hospital staff tell you what the medicine was for? How often did hospital staff describe possible side effects in a way you could understand?)
- Patient may experience diarrhea, fatigue, asthenia, headache, dyspepsia, or insomnia. Have patient report immediately to prescriber signs of depression (ie, suicidal ideation, anxiety, emotional instability, illogical thinking), severe

dizziness, syncope, dyspnea, angina, bradycardia, or arrhythmia (HCAHPS).

• Educate patient about signs of a significant reaction (eg, wheezing; chest tightness; fever; itching; bad cough; blue skin color; seizures; or swelling of face, lips, tongue, or throat). **Note:** This is not a comprehensive list of all side effects. Patient should consult prescriber for additional questions.

Intended Use and Disclaimer: Should not be printed and given to patients. This information is intended to serve as a concise initial reference for healthcare professionals to use when discussing medications with a patient. You must ultimately rely on your own discretion, experience and judgment in diagnosing, treating and advising patients.

Dietary Considerations May be taken without regard to meals.

Bisoprolol and Hydrochlorothiazide
(bis OH proe lol & hye droe klor oh THYE a zide)

Brand Names: U.S. Ziac®

Index Terms Bisoprolol Fumarate and Hydrochlorothiazide; Hydrochlorothiazide and Bisoprolol

Pharmacologic Category Antihypertensive; Beta-Blocker, Beta-1 Selective; Diuretic, Thiazide

Medication Safety Issues

Sound-alike/look-alike issues:

Ziac® may be confused with Tiazac®, Zerit®

Pregnancy Risk Factor C

Use Treatment of hypertension

Unlabeled Use Treatment of hypertension in the pediatric patient

Available Dosage Forms

Tablet, oral: 2.5/6.25: Bisoprolol 2.5 mg and hydrochlorothiazide 6.25 mg; 5/6.25: Bisoprolol 5 mg and hydrochlorothiazide 6.25 mg; 10/6.25: Bisoprolol 10 mg and hydrochlorothiazide 6.25 mg

Ziac®: 2.5/6.25: Bisoprolol 2.5 mg and hydrochlorothiazide 6.25 mg; 5/6.25: Bisoprolol 5 mg and hydrochlorothiazide 6.25 mg; 10/6.25: Bisoprolol 10 mg and hydrochlorothiazide 6.25 mg

General Dosage Range Oral: *Adults:* Initial: Bisoprolol 2.5 mg and hydrochlorothiazide 6.25 mg once daily; Maintenance: Bisoprolol 2.5-20 mg and hydrochlorothiazide 6.25-12.5 mg once daily; Maximum dose (manufacturer recommended): Bisoprolol 20 mg and hydrochlorothiazide 12.5 mg once daily

Administration

Oral May be administered without regard to meals.

Nursing Actions

Physical Assessment See individual agents.

Patient Education

• Discuss specific use of drug and side effects with patient as it relates to treatment. (HCAHPS: During this hospital stay, were you given any

medicine that you had not taken before? Before giving you any new medicine, how often did hospital staff tell you what the medicine was for? How often did hospital staff describe possible side effects in a way you could understand?)

• Patient may experience signs of dizziness, diarrhea, headache, or asthenia. Have patient report immediately to prescriber signs of infection, signs of hyperglycemia, signs of hepatic impairment, signs of fluid and electrolyte imbalance, dyspnea, memory loss, hallucinations, angina, sensation of cold, akathisia, hearing impairment, severe dyspepsia, bradycardia, excessive weight gain, edema of extremities, ecchymosis, hemorrhaging, vision changes, or ophthalmalgia (HCAHPS).

• Educate patient about signs of a significant reaction (eg, wheezing; chest tightness; fever; itching; bad cough; blue skin color; seizures; or swelling of face, lips, tongue, or throat). **Note:** This is not a comprehensive list of all side effects. Patient should consult prescriber for additional questions.

Intended Use and Disclaimer: Should not be printed and given to patients. This information is intended to serve as a concise initial reference for healthcare professionals to use when discussing medications with a patient. You must ultimately rely on your own discretion, experience and judgment in diagnosing, treating and advising patients.

Related Information

Bisoprolol *on page 188*

Hydrochlorothiazide *on page 775*

Bleomycin (blee oh MYE sin)

Index Terms Blenoxane; Bleo; Bleomycin Sulfate; BLM

Pharmacologic Category Antineoplastic Agent, Antibiotic

Medication Safety Issues

Sound-alike/look-alike issues:

Bleomycin may be confused with Cleocin

High alert medication:

This medication is in a class the Institute for Safe Medication Practices (ISMP) includes among its list of drugs which have a heightened risk of causing significant patient harm when used in error.

International issues:

Some products available internationally may have vial strength and dosing expressed as international units or milligrams (instead of units or USP units). Refer to prescribing information for specific strength and dosing information.

Pregnancy Risk Factor D

Lactation Excretion in breast milk unknown/not recommended

Breast-Feeding Considerations It is not known if bleomycin is excreted in breast milk. Due to the potential for serious adverse reactions in the nursing infant, the manufacturer recommends against breast-feeding during treatment.

Use

Head and neck cancers: Treatment of squamous cell carcinomas of the head and neck

Hodgkin lymphoma: Treatment of Hodgkin lymphoma

Malignant pleural effusion: Sclerosing agent for malignant pleural effusion

Testicular cancer: Treatment of testicular cancer

Other malignancies: Approved for the treatment of squamous cell carcinomas of the penis, cervix, or vulva, and for non-Hodgkin lymphoma; however, decreased efficacy and possible increased toxicity may limit the use of bleomycin for these indications compared to other generally accepted treatments.

Unlabeled Use Treatment of ovarian germ cell tumors

Mechanism of Action/Effect Inhibits synthesis of DNA; also inhibits (to a lesser degree) RNA and protein synthesis

Contraindications Hypersensitivity to bleomycin or any component of the formulation

Warnings/Precautions Hazardous agent - use appropriate precautions for handling and disposal (NIOSH, 2012). **[U.S. Boxed Warning]: Occurrence of pulmonary fibrosis (commonly presenting as pneumonitis; occasionally progressing to pulmonary fibrosis) is the most severe toxicity. Risk is higher in elderly patients or patients receiving >400 units total lifetime dose;** other possible risk factors include smoking and patients with prior radiation therapy or receiving concurrent oxygen (especially high inspired oxygen doses). A review of patients receiving bleomycin for the treatment of germ cell tumors suggests risk for pulmonary toxicity is increased in patients >40 years of age, with glomerular filtration rate <80 mL/minute, advanced disease, and cumulative doses >300 units (O'Sullivan, 2003). Pulmonary toxicity may include bronchiolitis obliterans and organizing pneumonia (BOOP), eosinophilic hypersensitivity, and interstitial pneumonitis, progressing to pulmonary fibrosis (Sleijfer, 2001); pulmonary toxicity may be due to a lack of the enzyme which inactivates bleomycin (bleomycin hydrolase) in the lungs (Morgan, 2011; Sleijfer, 2001). If pulmonary changes occur, withhold treatment and investigate if drug-related. In children, a younger age at treatment, cumulative dose ≥400 units/m^2 (combined with chest irradiation), and renal impairment are associated with a higher incidence of pulmonary toxicity (Huang, 2011).

A severe idiosyncratic reaction consisting of hypotension, mental confusion, fever, chills, and wheezing (similar to anaphylaxis) has been reported in 1% of lymphoma patients treated with bleomycin. Since these reactions usually occur after the first or second dose, careful monitoring is essential after these doses. Use caution when administering O_2 during surgery to patients who have received bleomycin; the risk of bleomycin-related pulmonary toxicity is increased. Use caution with renal impairment (CrCl <50 mL/minute), may require dose adjustment. May cause renal or hepatic toxicity. **[U.S. Boxed Warning]: Should be administered under the supervision of an experienced cancer chemotherapy physician.** Potentially significant drug-drug interactions may exist, requiring dose or frequency adjustment, additional monitoring, and/or selection of alternative therapy. Some products available internationally may have vial strength and dosing expressed as international units or milligrams (instead of units or USP units); refer to prescribing information for specific dosing information.

Drug Interactions

Avoid Concomitant Use

Avoid concomitant use of Bleomycin with any of the following: BCG; Brentuximab Vedotin; Natalizumab; Pimecrolimus; Tacrolimus (Topical); Tofacitinib; Vaccines (Live)

Decreased Effect

Bleomycin may decrease the levels/effects of: BCG; Cardiac Glycosides; Coccidioidin Skin Test; Phenytoin; Sipuleucel-T; Vaccines (Inactivated); Vaccines (Live)

The levels/effects of Bleomycin may be decreased by: Echinacea

Increased Effect/Toxicity

Bleomycin may increase the levels/effects of: Leflunomide; Natalizumab; Tofacitinib; Vaccines (Live)

The levels/effects of Bleomycin may be increased by: Brentuximab Vedotin; Denosumab; Filgrastim; Gemcitabine; Pimecrolimus; Roflumilast; Sargramostim; Tacrolimus (Topical); Trastuzumab

Adverse Reactions

>10%:

Dermatologic: Pain at the tumor site, phlebitis. About 50% of patients develop erythema, rash, striae, induration, hyperkeratosis, vesiculation, and peeling of the skin, particularly on the palmar and plantar surfaces of the hands and feet. Hyperpigmentation (50%), alopecia, nailbed changes may also occur. These effects appear dose related and reversible with discontinuation.

Gastrointestinal: Stomatitis and mucositis (30%), anorexia, weight loss

Respiratory: Tachypnea, rales, acute or chronic interstitial pneumonitis, and pulmonary fibrosis (5% to 10%); hypoxia and death (1%). Symptoms include cough, dyspnea, and bilateral pulmonary infiltrates. The pathogenesis is not certain, but may be due to damage of pulmonary, vascular, or connective tissue. Response to steroid therapy is variable and somewhat controversial.

Miscellaneous: Acute febrile reactions (25% to 50%)

1% to 10%:

Dermatologic: Skin thickening, diffuse sclero-derma, onycholysis, pruritus

Miscellaneous: Anaphylactoid-like reactions (characterized by hypotension, confusion, fever, chills, and wheezing; onset may be immediate or delayed for several hours); idiosyncratic reactions (1% in lymphoma patients)

Available Dosage Forms

Solution Reconstituted, Injection:
Generic: 15 units (1 ea); 30 units (1 ea)

Solution Reconstituted, Injection [preservative free]:
Generic: 15 units (1 ea); 30 units (1 ea)

General Dosage Range Dosage adjustment recommended in patients with renal impairment or who develop toxicities.

I.V.: *Adults:* Dosage varies greatly depending on indication

Intrapleural: *Adults:* 60 units as a single instillation

Administration

I.M. May cause pain at injection site. Hazardous agent; use appropriate precautions for handling and disposal (NIOSH, 2012).

I.V. I.V. doses should be administered slowly over 10 minutes. Hazardous agent; use appropriate precautions for handling and disposal (NIOSH, 2012).

Injectable Detail pH: 4-6 (reconstituted solution, varies depending on diluent)

Subcutaneous May cause pain at injection site. Hazardous agent; use appropriate precautions for handling and disposal (NIOSH, 2012).

Other Intrapleural: 60 units in 50-100 mL NS; use of topical anesthetics or opioid analgesia is usually not necessary. Hazardous agent; use appropriate precautions for handling and disposal (NIOSH, 2012).

Preparation for Administration Hazardous agent; use appropriate precautions for handling and disposal (NIOSH, 2012). For I.V. use, reconstitute 15-unit vial with 5 mL with NS and the 30-unit vial with 10 mL NS; for I.M. or SubQ use, reconstitute 15-unit vial with 1-5 mL of SWFI, BWFI, or NS and the 30-unit vial with 2-10 mL of SWFI, BWFI, or NS. For intrapleural use, mix in 50-100 mL of NS.

Storage/Stability Refrigerate intact vials of powder. Intact vials are stable for up to 4 weeks at room temperature. Solutions reconstituted in NS are stable for up to 28 days refrigerated and 14 days at room temperature; however, the manufacturer recommends stability of 24 hours in NS at room temperature.

Nursing Actions

Physical Assessment Monitor pulmonary status for fine rales prior to each treatment (may be the first symptom of pulmonary toxicity) and notify physician of any changes. Lymphoma patients should be closely monitored (vital signs every 15 minutes) for 1 hour following test dose before remainder of dose is administered (for first and second dose). Infusion or injection site must be monitored closely to avoid extravasation. Monitor pulmonary, renal, and hepatic function regularly during therapy.

Patient Education

• Discuss specific use of drug and side effects with patient as it relates to treatment. (HCAHPS During this hospital stay, were you given any medicine that you had not taken before? Before giving you any new medicine, how often did hospital staff tell you what the medicine was for? How often did hospital staff describe possible side effects in a way you could understand?

• Patient may experience skin or nail discoloration, weight loss, lack of appetite, alopecia, or asthenia. Have patient report immediately to prescriber signs of hepatic impairment, signs of renal impairment, strength differences from one side to another, difficulty speaking or thinking, change in balance, blurred vision, angina, severe stomatitis, considerable skin irritation, or injection site edema or irritation (HCAHPS).

• Educate patient about signs of a significant reaction (eg, wheezing; chest tightness; fever; itching; bad cough; blue skin color; seizures; or swelling of face, lips, tongue, or throat). **Note:** This is not a comprehensive list of all side effects. Patient should consult prescriber for additional questions.

Intended Use and Disclaimer: Should not be printed and given to patients. This information is intended to serve as a concise initial reference for healthcare professionals to use when discussing medications with a patient. You must ultimately rely on your own discretion, experience and judgment in diagnosing, treating and advising patients.

Related Information

Management of Drug Extravasations *on page 1700*

Boceprevir (boe SE pre vir)

Brand Names: U.S. Victrelis

Index Terms SCH503034

Pharmacologic Category Antihepaciviral, Protease Inhibitor (Anti-HCV)

Medication Guide Available Yes

Pregnancy Risk Factor B / X (in combination with ribavirin)

Lactation Excretion in breast milk unknown/not recommended

Breast-Feeding Considerations It is not known if boceprevir is excreted into breast milk. According to the manufacturer, due to the potential for serious adverse reactions in the nursing infant, a decision should be made whether to discontinue nursing or to discontinue the drug, taking into account the importance of treatment to the mother.

Breast-feeding is not linked to the spread of hepatitis C virus; however, if nipples are cracked or bleeding, breast-feeding is not recommended (CDC, 2010).

Use Chronic hepatitis C: Treatment of chronic hepatitis C (CHC) genotype 1 (in combination with peginterferon alfa and ribavirin) in adult patients with compensated liver disease (including cirrhosis) who were previously untreated or have failed prior therapy with peginterferon alfa and ribavirin therapy including prior null responders, partial responders, and relapsers

Mechanism of Action/Effect Inhibits viral protein synthesis; direct-acting antiviral against the hepatitis C virus

Contraindications

Hypersensitivity to boceprevir or any component of the formulation; pregnancy; male partners of pregnant women

Coadministration with CYP3A4/5 highly-dependent substrates (alfuzosin, cisapride, doxazosin, drospirenone, ergot derivatives, lovastatin, midazolam [oral], pimozide, sildenafil/tadalafil [when used for treatment of pulmonary arterial hypertension], silodosin, simvastatin, tamsulosin, triazolam) or strong CYP3A4/5 inducers (carbamazepine, phenobarbital, phenytoin, rifampin, St John's wort)

Refer to Peginterferon Alfa and Ribavirin monographs for individual product contraindications.

Canadian labeling: Additional contraindications (not in U.S. labeling): Autoimmune hepatitis, hepatic decompensation (Child-Pugh class B or C); coadministration with amiodarone, astemizole, propafenone, quinidine, terfenadine

Warnings/Precautions Avoid pregnancy in female patients and female partners of male patients, during therapy, and for at least 6 months after treatment; two forms of contraception should be used. Serious acute hypersensitivity reactions, angioedema and urticaria have been reported with boceprevir, peginterferon alfa, and ribavirin combination therapy. Discontinuation of combination therapy and institution of supportive measures may be necessary. Safety and efficacy have not been established in patients who have uncompensated cirrhosis or have received organ transplants. Monotherapy is not effective for chronic hepatitis C infection. Patients who have less than 0.5-log_{10} HCV-RNA decline at treatment week 4 with peginterferon alfa and ribavirin when **initiating** boceprevir therapy are predicted to have less than a 2-log_{10} HCV-RNA decline by treatment week 12. Those poor responders treated with boceprevir will likely not have a sustained virologic response (SVR) and have a predisposition to viral resistance at treatment failure.

Anemia has been reported with peginterferon alfa and ribavirin; addition of boceprevir is associated with further hemoglobin decreases. With anemia management, average hemoglobin decrease in clinical trials was ~1 g/dL. Dose reduction of ribavirin therapy is recommended for the initial management of anemia if hemoglobin <10 g/dL; permanent discontinuation of ribavirin treatment is recommended if hemoglobin <8.5 g/dL. The addition of boceprevir to peginterferon alfa and ribavirin therapy is also associated with a higher incidence of neutropenia. May be severe or life-threatening (rare); discontinuation of therapy may be necessary. Dose reductions of peginterferon alfa and ribavirin were needed more often in patients also taking boceprevir. Serious cases of pancytopenia have been reported in patients receiving boceprevir in combination with peginterferon alfa and ribavirin. Complete blood counts with differential should be obtained pretreatment and at weeks 2, 4, 8, and 12, as well as other times during treatment. If ribavirin is permanently discontinued, boceprevir and peginterferon alfa must also be discontinued.

Drug Interactions

Avoid Concomitant Use

Avoid concomitant use of Boceprevir with any of the following: Ado-Trastuzumab Emtansine; Alfuzosin; Apixaban; Astemizole; Avanafil; Axitinib; Bosutinib; Cabozantinib; CarBAMazepine; Cisapride; Conivaptan; Crizotinib; CYP3A4 Inducers (Strong); Dihydroergotamine; Dronedarone; Drospirenone; Efavirenz; Eplerenone; Ergoloid Mesylates; Ergonovine; Ergotamine; Everolimus; Fosphenytoin; Halofantrine; Ibrutinib; Imatinib; Ivabradine; Lapatinib; Lomitapide; Lovastatin; Lurasidone; Macitentan; Methylergonovine; Midazolam; Nilotinib; Nisoldipine; PHENobarbital; Phenytoin; Pimozide; Pomalidomide; Primidone; Ranolazine; Red Yeast Rice; Regorafenib; Rifabutin; Rifampin; Rivaroxaban; Salmeterol; Sildenafil; Silodosin; Simeprevir; Simvastatin; St Johns Wort; Tamsulosin; Terfenadine; Ticagrelor; Tolvaptan; Toremifene; Triazolam; Ulipristal; Vemurafenib; VinCRIStine (Liposomal)

Decreased Effect

Boceprevir may decrease the levels/effects of: Buprenorphine; Contraceptives (Estrogens); Escitalopram; Ifosfamide; Methadone; Prasugrel; Protease Inhibitors; Ritonavir; Ticagrelor; Warfarin

The levels/effects of Boceprevir may be decreased by: Bosentan; CarBAMazepine; CYP3A4 Inducers (Strong); Dabrafenib; Deferasirox; Efavirenz; Fosphenytoin; PHENobarbital; Phenytoin; Primidone; Protease Inhibitors;

Rifabutin; Rifampin; Ritonavir; St Johns Wort; Tocilizumab

Increased Effect/Toxicity

Boceprevir may increase the levels/effects of: Ado-Trastuzumab Emtansine; Alfuzosin; Almotriptan; Alosetron; ALPRAZolam; Amiodarone; Apixaban; ARIPiprazole; Astemizole; AtorvaSTA-Tin; Avanafil; Axitinib; Bedaquiline; Bepridil [Off Market]; Bortezomib; Bosentan; Bosutinib; Brentuximab Vedotin; Brinzolamide; Budesonide (Nasal); Budesonide (Systemic, Oral Inhalation); Buprenorphine; Cabozantinib; Cisapride; Clarithromycin; Colchicine; Conivaptan; Contraceptives (Progestins); Corticosteroids (Orally Inhaled); Crizotinib; CycloSPORINE (Systemic); CYP3A4 Substrates; Desipramine; Dienogest; Digoxin; Dihydroergotamine; Dofetilide; DOXOrubicin (Conventional); Dronedarone; Drospirenone; Dutasteride; Efavirenz; Enzalutamide; Eplerenone; Ergoloid Mesylates; Ergonovine; Ergotamine; Everolimus; FentaNYL; Fesoterodine; Flecainide; Fluticasone (Nasal); Fluticasone (Oral Inhalation); Fluvastatin; GuanFACINE; Halofantrine; Ibrutinib; Iloperidone; Imatinib; Itraconazole; Ivabradine; Ivacaftor; Ixabepilone; Ketoconazole (Systemic); Lacosamide; Lapatinib; Levomilnacipran; Lomitapide; Lovastatin; Lumefantrine; Lurasidone; Macitentan; Maraviroc; Methadone; Methylergonovine; MethylPREDNISolone; Midazolam; Mifepristone; Nilotinib; Nisoldipine; Ospemifene; OxyCODONE; Paricalcitol; PAZOPanib; Pimecrolimus; Pimozide; Pitavastatin; Pomalidomide; PONATinib; Posaconazole; Pravastatin; PrednisoLONE (Systemic); PredniSONE; Propafenone; QUEtiapine; QuiNIDine; Ranolazine; Red Yeast Rice; Regorafenib; Repaglinide; Rifabutin; Rilpivirine; Rivaroxaban; RomiDEPsin; Rosuvastatin; Ruxolitinib; Salmeterol; Saxagliptin; Sildenafil; Silodosin; Simeprevir; Simvastatin; Sirolimus; SORAfenib; Tacrolimus (Systemic); Tadalafil; Tamsulosin; Terfenadine; Ticagrelor; Tofacitinib; Tolterodine; Tolvaptan; Toremifene; TraZODone; Triazolam; Ulipristal; Vardenafil; Vemurafenib; Vilazodone; VinCRIStine (Liposomal); Voriconazole; Warfarin; Zuclopenthixol

The levels/effects of Boceprevir may be increased by: Clarithromycin; CycloSPORINE (Systemic); Itraconazole; Ketoconazole (Systemic); Posaconazole; Voriconazole

Adverse Reactions

>10%:

Central nervous system: Fatigue (55% to 58%), chills (33% to 34%), insomnia (30% to 34%), irritability (21% to 22%), dizziness (16% to 19%), headache

Dermatologic: Alopecia (22% to 27%), dry skin (18% to 22%), rash (16% to 17%)

Gastrointestinal: Nausea (43% to 46%), abnormal taste (35% to 44%), appetite decreased (25% to 26%), diarrhea (24% to 25%), vomiting (15% to 20%), xerostomia (11% to 15%)

Hematologic: Anemia (45% to 50%), neutropenia (14% to 31%)

Neuromuscular & skeletal: Arthralgia (19% to 23%), weakness (15% to 21%)

Respiratory: Dyspnea (8% to 11%)

1% to 10%: Hematologic: Thrombocytopenia

Available Dosage Forms

Capsule, Oral:

Victrelis: 200 mg

General Dosage Range Oral: *Adults:* 800 mg 3 times daily

Administration

Oral Administer with food (a meal or light snack). Doses should be taken approximately every 7-9 hours. Administer concurrently with peginterferon alfa and ribavirin.

Storage/Stability Store refrigerated at 2°C to 8°C (36°F to 46°F). After dispensing, may be stored at room temperature of up to 25°C (77°F) for 3 months; keep container closed tightly; avoid excessive heat.

Nursing Actions

Physical Assessment Monitor for adherence to multidrug regimen. Educate women of childbearing years about risks of pregnancy; may require help with effective contraception options. Check results of CBC for anemia and/or neutropenia. Monitor for the most common side effects including fatigue, anemia, nausea, headache, and dysgeusia.

Patient Education

• Discuss specific use of drug and side effects with patient as it relates to treatment. (HCAHPS: During this hospital stay, were you given any medicine that you had not taken before? Before giving you any new medicine, how often did hospital staff tell you what the medicine was for? How often did hospital staff describe possible side effects in a way you could understand?)

• Patient may experience headache, dysgeusia, alopecia, diarrhea, lack of appetite, xerostomia, xeroderma, arthralgia, nausea, or insomnia. Have patient report immediately to prescriber signs of infection, signs of hemorrhaging, severe asthenia, pallor, significant dizziness, syncope, or dyspnea (HCAHPS).

• Educate patient about signs of a significant reaction (eg, wheezing; chest tightness; fever; itching; bad cough; blue skin color; seizures; or swelling of face, lips, tongue, or throat). **Note:** This is not a comprehensive list of all side effects. Patient should consult prescriber for additional questions.

Intended Use and Disclaimer: Should not be printed and given to patients. This information is intended to serve as a concise initial reference for

healthcare professionals to use when discussing medications with a patient. You must ultimately rely on your own discretion, experience and judgment in diagnosing, treating and advising patients.

Dietary Considerations Take with food. The type or timing of a meal is not important as long as dose is taken with food.

Bortezomib (bore TEZ oh mib)

Brand Names: U.S. Velcade

Index Terms LDP-341; MLN341; PS-341

Pharmacologic Category Antineoplastic Agent; Proteasome Inhibitor

Medication Safety Issues

Sound-alike/look-alike issues:

Bortezomib may be confused with carfilzomib

High alert medication:

This medication is in a class the Institute for Safe Medication Practices (ISMP) includes among its list of drug classes which have a heightened risk of causing significant patient harm when used in error.

Administration issues:

The reconstituted concentrations for I.V. and SubQ administration are different; use caution when calculating the volume for each dose. The manufacturer provides stickers to facilitate identification of the route for reconstituted vials.

For I.V. or SubQ administration only. Intrathecal administration is contraindicated; inadvertent intrathecal administration has resulted in death. Bortezomib should **NOT** be prepared during the preparation of any intrathecal medications. After preparation, keep bortezomib in a location **away** from the separate storage location recommended for intrathecal medications. Bortezomib should **NOT** be delivered to the patient at the same time with any medications intended for intrathecal administration.

Pregnancy Risk Factor D

Lactation Excretion in breast milk unknown/not recommended

Use

Mantle cell lymphoma: Treatment of relapsed or refractory mantle cell lymphoma

Multiple myeloma: Treatment of multiple myeloma

Unlabeled Use Treatment of relapsed/refractory cutaneous T-cell lymphomas (mycosis fungoides), relapsed/refractory follicular lymphoma, relapsed/refractory peripheral T-cell lymphoma, relapsed/refractory Waldenström's macroglobulinemia, systemic light-chain amyloidosis

Available Dosage Forms

Solution Reconstituted, Injection:

Velcade: 3.5 mg (1 ea)

General Dosage Range Dosage adjustment recommended in patients with hepatic impairment or who develop toxicities.

I.V., SubQ: *Adults:* Dosage varies greatly depending on indication

Administration

I.V.

Note: The reconstituted concentrations for I.V. and SubQ administration are different; use caution when calculating the volume for each dose. Consider SubQ administration in patients with pre-existing or at high risk for peripheral neuropathy.

Administer via rapid I.V. push (3-5 seconds).

For I.V. or SubQ administration only; fatalities have been reported with inadvertent intrathecal administration. Bortezomib should **NOT** be delivered to the patient at the same time with any medications intended for central nervous system administration.

Hazardous agent; use appropriate precautions for handling and disposal (NIOSH, 2012).

Injectable Detail pH: 2-6.5 (intact vial)

Subcutaneous Note: The reconstituted concentrations for I.V. and SubQ administration are different; use caution when calculating the volume for each dose.

Subcutaneous administration of bortezomib 1.3 mg/m^2 days 1, 4, 8, and 11 of a 21-day treatment cycle has been studied in a limited number of patients with relapsed multiple myeloma; doses were administered subcutaneously (concentration of 2.5 mg/mL) into the thigh or abdomen, rotating the injection site with each dose; injections at the same site within a single cycle were avoided (Moreau, 2010; Moreau, 2011). Response rates were similar to I.V. administration; decreased incidence of grade 3 or higher adverse events were observed with SubQ administration. Administer at least 1 inch from an old site and never administer to tender, bruised, erythematous, or indurated sites. If injection site reaction occurs, the more dilute 1 mg/mL concentration may be used SubQ (or I.V. administration of 1 mg/mL concentration may be considered).

For I.V. or SubQ administration only; fatalities have been reported with inadvertent intrathecal administration. Bortezomib should **NOT** be delivered to the patient at the same time with any medications intended for central nervous system administration.

Hazardous agent; use appropriate precautions for handling and disposal (NIOSH, 2012).

Nursing Actions

Physical Assessment Monitor for peripheral neuropathy, postural hypotension, dehydration, heart failure, and infections. Be alert to the potential for reactivation of herpes.

Patient Education
- Discuss specific use of drug and side effects with patient as it relates to treatment. (HCAHPS: During this hospital stay, were you given any medicine that you had not taken before? Before giving you any new medicine, how often did hospital staff tell you what the medicine was for? How often did hospital staff describe possible side effects in a way you could understand?)
- Patient may experience constipation, lack of appetite, or dyspepsia. Have patient report immediately to prescriber signs of infection, signs of hepatic impairment, strength differences from one side to another, difficulty speaking or thinking, change in balance, blurred vision, melena, hematemesis, severe dizziness, syncope, significant nausea, intolerable headache, considerable diarrhea, paresthesia, blindness, vision changes, inability to eat, severe asthenia, illogical thinking, ecchymosis, hemorrhaging, hyperhidrosis, dehydration, signs of injection site irritation, cardiac failure, signs of severe pulmonary disorder, or tumor lysis syndrome (TLS) (HCAHPS).
- Educate patient about signs of a significant reaction (eg, wheezing; chest tightness; fever; itching; bad cough; blue skin color; seizures; or swelling of face, lips, tongue, or throat). **Note:** This is not a comprehensive list of all side effects. Patient should consult prescriber for additional questions.

Intended Use and Disclaimer: Should not be printed and given to patients. This information is intended to serve as a concise initial reference for healthcare professionals to use when discussing medications with a patient. You must ultimately rely on your own discretion, experience and judgment in diagnosing, treating and advising patients.

Related Information
Management of Drug Extravasations *on page 1700*

Bosutinib (boe SUE ti nib)

Brand Names: U.S. Bosulif
Index Terms Bosutinib Monohydrate; SKI-606
Pharmacologic Category Antineoplastic Agent, BCR-ABL Tyrosine Kinase Inhibitor; Antineoplastic Agent, Tyrosine Kinase Inhibitor
Medication Safety Issues
Sound-alike/look-alike issues:
Bosutinib may be confused with bortezomib, bosentan, dasatinib, imatinib, nilotinib, PONATinib
High alert medication:
This medication is in a class the Institute for Safe Medical Practices (ISMP) includes among its list of drug classes which have a heightened risk of causing significant patient harm when used in error.

Pregnancy Risk Factor D
Lactation Excretion in breast milk unknown/not recommended
Use Chronic myelogenous leukemia (CML): Treatment of chronic, accelerated or blast phase Philadelphia chromosome-positive (Ph+) CML in patients resistant or intolerant to prior therapy
Available Dosage Forms
Tablet, Oral:
Bosulif: 100 mg, 500 mg
General Dosage Range Dosage adjustment recommended in patients with renal impairment, hepatic impairment or who develop toxicities.
Oral: *Adults:* 500-600 mg once daily
Administration
Oral Administer with food. Swallow tablet whole; do not crush or break.

Hazardous agent; use appropriate precautions for handling and disposal (meets NIOSH, 2012 criteria).

Nursing Actions
Physical Assessment Check results of blood counts and liver function monitoring regularly. Instruct patient on infection and bleeding precautions. Monitor for acute GI toxicities and severe allergic reactions. Evaluate hydration status based on GI toxicities; help patient to better manage if having difficulty.
Patient Education
- Discuss specific use of drug and side effects with patient as it relates to treatment. (HCAHPS: During this hospital stay, were you given any medicine that you had not taken before? Before giving you any new medicine, how often did hospital staff tell you what the medicine was for? How often did hospital staff describe possible side effects in a way you could understand?)
- Patient may experience headache, dizziness, lack of appetite, arthralgia, or back pain. Have patient report immediately to prescriber signs of infection, signs of hepatic impairment, signs of pancreatitis, dyspnea, excessive weight gain, edema or extremities, angina, arrhythmia, edema, severe dyspepsia, considerable nausea, significant diarrhea, ecchymosis, hemorrhaging, intolerable asthenia, urinary retention, oliguria, melena, hematemesis, xerostomia, or xeroderma (HCAHPS).
- Educate patient about signs of a significant reaction (eg, wheezing; chest tightness; fever; itching; bad cough; blue skin color; seizures; or swelling of face, lips, tongue, or throat). **Note:** This is not a comprehensive list of all side effects. Patient should consult prescriber for additional questions.

Intended Use and Disclaimer: Should not be printed and given to patients. This information is intended to serve as a concise initial reference for

healthcare professionals to use when discussing medications with a patient. You must ultimately rely on your own discretion, experience and judgment in diagnosing, treating and advising patients.

Related Information

Oral Medications That Should Not Be Crushed or Altered *on page 1712*

Brentuximab Vedotin
(bren TUX i mab ve DOE tin)

Brand Names: U.S. Adcetris

Index Terms Anti-CD30 ADC SGN-35; Anti-CD30 Antibody-Drug Conjugate SGN-35; Antibody-Drug Conjugate SGN-35; Brentuximab; SGN-35

Pharmacologic Category Antineoplastic Agent, Anti-CD30; Antineoplastic Agent, Antibody Drug Conjugate; Antineoplastic Agent, Monoclonal Antibody

Medication Safety Issues

Sound-alike/look-alike issues:

Brentuximab may be confused with bendamustine, bevacizumab, rituximab

High alert medication:

This medication is in a class the Institute for Safe Medication Practices (ISMP) includes among its list of drug classes which have a heightened risk of causing significant patient harm when used in error.

Pregnancy Risk Factor D

Lactation Excretion in breast milk unknown/not recommended

Use Treatment of Hodgkin lymphoma after failure of at least 2 prior chemotherapy regimens (in patients ineligible for transplant) or after stem cell transplant failure; treatment of systemic anaplastic large cell lymphoma (sALCL) after failure of at least 1 prior chemotherapy regimen

Available Dosage Forms

Solution Reconstituted, Intravenous [preservative free]:

Adcetris: 50 mg (1 ea)

General Dosage Range Dosage adjustment recommended in patients who develop toxicities.

I.V.: *Adults:* 1.8 mg/kg every 3 weeks (maximum dose: 180 mg)

Administration

I.V. Infuse over 30 minutes. Do not administer as I.V. push or bolus; do not mix or infuse with other medications. Hazardous agent; use appropriate precautions for handling and disposal (meets NIOSH, 2012 criteria).

Injectable Detail pH: 6.6

Nursing Actions

Physical Assessment Medication is given as an infusion. Inform of existing neuropathy or past infusion-related reaction. Monitor for symptoms of new or progressive neuropathy, symptoms of infection, mental status changes, balance issues, or vision problems. Educate patient regarding minimizing risk of infection and bleeding complications.

Patient Education

- Discuss specific use of drug and side effects with patient as it relates to treatment. (HCAHPS: During this hospital stay, were you given any medicine that you had not taken before? Before giving you any new medicine, how often did hospital staff tell you what the medicine was for? How often did hospital staff describe possible side effects in a way you could understand?)

- Patient may experience arthralgia, myalgia, headache, nausea, dyspepsia, constipation, diarrhea, back pain, xeroderma, alopecia, muscle spasms, lack of appetite, weight loss, night sweats, insomnia, or anxiety. Have patient report immediately to prescriber signs of infection, severe dizziness, syncope, significant asthenia, angina, hemoptysis, paresthesia, dyspnea, edema of extremities, ecchymosis, hemorrhaging, signs of tumor lysis syndrome, or signs of Stevens-Johnson syndrome/toxic epidermal necrolysis (HCAHPS).

- Educate patient about signs of a significant reaction (eg, wheezing; chest tightness; fever; itching; bad cough; blue skin color; seizures; or swelling of face, lips, tongue, or throat). **Note:** This is not a comprehensive list of all side effects. Patient should consult prescriber for additional questions.

Intended Use and Disclaimer: Should not be printed and given to patients. This information is intended to serve as a concise initial reference for healthcare professionals to use when discussing medications with a patient. You must ultimately rely on your own discretion, experience and judgment in diagnosing, treating and advising patients.

Brimonidine (Ophthalmic) (bri MOE ni deen)

Brand Names: U.S. Alphagan P

Index Terms Brimonidine Tartrate

Pharmacologic Category Alpha$_2$ Agonist, Ophthalmic; Ophthalmic Agent, Antiglaucoma

Medication Safety Issues

Sound-alike/look-alike issues:

Brimonidine may be confused with bromocriptine

Pregnancy Risk Factor B

Lactation Excretion in breast milk unknown/not recommended

Use Lowering of intraocular pressure (IOP) in patients with open-angle glaucoma or ocular hypertension

Available Dosage Forms

Solution, Ophthalmic:

Alphagan P: 0.1% (5 mL, 10 mL, 15 mL); 0.15% (5 mL, 10 mL, 15 mL)

Generic: 0.15% (5 mL, 10 mL, 15 mL); 0.2% (5 mL, 10 mL, 15 mL)

General Dosage Range Ophthalmic: *Children ≥2 years and Adults:* Instill 1 drop in affected eye(s) 3 times/day

Administration

Other Remove contact lenses prior to administration; wait 15 minutes before reinserting if using products containing benzalkonium chloride. Separate administration of other ophthalmic agents by 5 minutes.

Nursing Actions

Patient Education

• Discuss specific use of drug and side effects with patient as it relates to treatment. (HCAHPS: During this hospital stay, were you given any medicine that you had not taken before? Before giving you any new medicine, how often did hospital staff tell you what the medicine was for? How often did hospital staff describe possible side effects in a way you could understand?)

• Patient may experience blurred vision, xerophthalmia, xerostomia, headache, foreign body sensation of eye, fatigue, or light sensitivity. Have patient report immediately to prescriber severe dizziness, syncope, vision changes, ophthalmalgia, significant eye irritation, eyelid edema, depression, or arrhythmia (HCAHPS).

• Educate patient about signs of a significant reaction (eg, wheezing; chest tightness; fever; itching; bad cough; blue skin color; seizures; or swelling of face, lips, tongue, or throat). **Note:** This is not a comprehensive list of all side effects. Patient should consult prescriber for additional questions.

Intended Use and Disclaimer: Should not be printed and given to patients. This information is intended to serve as a concise initial reference for healthcare professionals to use when discussing medications with a patient. You must ultimately rely on your own discretion, experience and judgment in diagnosing, treating and advising patients.

Brimonidine (Topical) (bri MOE ni deen)

Brand Names: U.S. Mirvaso

Index Terms Brimonidine Tartrate

Pharmacologic Category Alpha$_2$-Adrenergic Agonist

Medication Safety Issues

Sound-alike/look-alike issues:

Brimonidine may be confused with bromocriptine

Pregnancy Risk Factor B

Lactation Excretion in breast milk unknown/not recommended

Use Rosacea: Topical treatment of persistent (nontransient) facial erythema of rosacea in adults

Available Dosage Forms

Gel, External:

Mirvaso: 0.33% (30 g)

General Dosage Range Topical: *Adults:* Apply a pea-size amount once daily as a thin layer across the entire face covering the central forehead, each cheek, nose, and chin. Do not apply to eyes or lips.

Administration

Topical Apply smoothly and evenly as a thin layer across the entire face avoiding the eyes and lips. Wash hands immediately after applying. Do not apply to open wounds or irritated skin.

Nursing Actions

Patient Education

• Discuss specific use of drug and side effects with patient as it relates to treatment. (HCAHPS: During this hospital stay, were you given any medicine that you had not taken before? Before giving you any new medicine, how often did hospital staff tell you what the medicine was for? How often did hospital staff describe possible side effects in a way you could understand?)

• Patient may experience flushing. Have patient report immediately to prescriber severe application site irritation (HCAHPS).

• Educate patient about signs of a significant reaction (eg, wheezing; chest tightness; fever; itching; bad cough; blue skin color; seizures; or swelling of face, lips, tongue, or throat). **Note:** This is not a comprehensive list of all side effects. Patient should consult prescriber for additional questions.

Intended Use and Disclaimer: Should not be printed and given to patients. This information is intended to serve as a concise initial reference for healthcare professionals to use when discussing medications with a patient. You must ultimately rely on your own discretion, experience and judgment in diagnosing, treating and advising patients.

Brinzolamide (brin ZOH la mide)

Brand Names: U.S. Azopt

Pharmacologic Category Carbonic Anhydrase Inhibitor (Ophthalmic); Ophthalmic Agent, Antiglaucoma

Pregnancy Risk Factor C

Lactation Excretion in breast milk unknown/not recommended

Use Treatment of elevated intraocular pressure in patients with ocular hypertension or open-angle glaucoma

Available Dosage Forms

Suspension, Ophthalmic:

Azopt: 1% (10 mL, 15 mL)

General Dosage Range Ophthalmic: *Adults:* Instill 1 drop in affected eye(s) 3 times/day

Administration

Other Remove contact lenses prior to administration; wait 15 minutes before reinserting. If more than one topical ophthalmic drug is being used, administer drugs at least 10 minutes apart. Shake well before use.

Nursing Actions

Patient Education

- Discuss specific use of drug and side effects with patient as it relates to treatment. (HCAHPS: During this hospital stay, were you given any medicine that you had not taken before? Before giving you any new medicine, how often did hospital staff tell you what the medicine was for? How often did hospital staff describe possible side effects in a way you could understand?)
- Patient may experience blurred vision, parageusia, xerophthalmia, eye discharge, headache, or rhinorrhea. Have patient report immediately to prescriber vision changes, ophthalmalgia, severe eye irritation, or signs of Stevens-Johnson syndrome/toxic epidermal necrolysis (HCAHPS).
- Educate patient about signs of a significant reaction (eg, wheezing; chest tightness; fever; itching; bad cough; blue skin color; seizures; or swelling of face, lips, tongue, or throat). **Note:** This is not a comprehensive list of all side effects. Patient should consult prescriber for additional questions.

Intended Use and Disclaimer: Should not be printed and given to patients. This information is intended to serve as a concise initial reference for healthcare professionals to use when discussing medications with a patient. You must ultimately rely on your own discretion, experience and judgment in diagnosing, treating and advising patients.

Bromfenac (BROME fen ak)

Brand Names: U.S. Bromday [DSC]; Prolensa
Index Terms Bromfenac Sodium
Pharmacologic Category Nonsteroidal Anti-inflammatory Drug (NSAID), Ophthalmic
Pregnancy Risk Factor C
Lactation Excretion in breast milk unknown/use caution
Use Treatment of postoperative inflammation and reduction in ocular pain following cataract removal
Available Dosage Forms
Solution, Ophthalmic:
Prolensa: 0.07% (1.6 mL, 3 mL)
Generic: 0.09% (1.7 mL, 2.5 mL, 5 mL)
General Dosage Range Ophthalmic: *Adults:* Instill 1 drop into affected eye(s) once daily
Administration
Ophthalmic Remove contact lenses prior to administration and wait 10 minutes before reinserting. May be used with other eye drops. If using more than 1 ophthalmic product, wait at least 5 minutes between application of each medication. Minimize contamination by not touching the eyelids or surrounding areas with the

dropper tip; keep bottle tightly closed when not in use. Also, to minimize the risk of infection following surgery of both eyes, two separate bottles of eye drops (one for each eye) should be used; instruct patients not to use the same bottle for both eyes.

Nursing Actions

Physical Assessment Assess for intraocular bleeding. Evaluate allergy history with aspirin or other NSAIDs.

Patient Education

- Discuss specific use of drug and side effects with patient as it relates to treatment. (HCAHPS: During this hospital stay, were you given any medicine that you had not taken before? Before giving you any new medicine, how often did hospital staff tell you what the medicine was for? How often did hospital staff describe possible side effects in a way you could understand?)
- Patient may experience headache. Have patient report immediately to prescriber vision changes, ophthalmalgia, severe eye irritation, or subconjunctival hemorrhage (HCAHPS).
- Educate patient about signs of a significant reaction (eg, wheezing; chest tightness; fever; itching; bad cough; blue skin color; seizures; or swelling of face, lips, tongue, or throat). **Note:** This is not a comprehensive list of all side effects. Patient should consult prescriber for additional questions.

Intended Use and Disclaimer: Should not be printed and given to patients. This information is intended to serve as a concise initial reference for healthcare professionals to use when discussing medications with a patient. You must ultimately rely on your own discretion, experience and judgment in diagnosing, treating and advising patients.

Bromocriptine (broe moe KRIP teen)

Brand Names: U.S. Cycloset; Parlodel
Index Terms Bromocriptine Mesylate; Cycloset®
Pharmacologic Category Anti-Parkinson's Agent, Dopamine Agonist; Antidiabetic Agent, Dopamine Agonist; Ergot Derivative
Medication Safety Issues
Sound-alike/look-alike issues:
Bromocriptine may be confused with benztropine, brimonidine
Cycloset® may be confused with Glyset®
Parlodel® may be confused with pindolol, Provera®
Pregnancy Risk Factor B
Lactation Enters breast milk/contraindicated
Breast-Feeding Considerations A previous indication for prevention of postpartum lactation was withdrawn voluntarily by the manufacturer following reports of serious adverse reactions, including stroke, MI, seizures, and severe hypertension.

Use during breast-feeding is specifically contraindicated in the product labeling for Cycloset®. Use in postpartum women with a history of coronary artery disease or other severe cardiovascular conditions is specifically contraindicated in the product labeling for Parlodel® (unless withdrawal of medication is medically contraindicated). Based on the risk/benefit assessment, other treatments should be considered for lactation suppression.

Use Treatment of hyperprolactinemia associated with amenorrhea with or without galactorrhea, infertility, or hypogonadism; treatment of prolactin-secreting adenomas; treatment of acromegaly; treatment of Parkinson's disease

Cycloset®: Management of type 2 diabetes mellitus (noninsulin dependent, NIDDM) as an adjunct to diet and exercise

Unlabeled Use Neuroleptic malignant syndrome

Mechanism of Action/Effect Semisynthetic ergot alkaloid derivative and a dopamine receptor agonist which activates postsynaptic dopamine receptors to decrease prolactin secretion (tuberoinfundibular pathway) and enhance coordinated motor control (nigrostriatal pathways).

In the treatment type 2 diabetes mellitus, bromocriptine's effect on improving glycemic control is unknown; however, when administered during the morning and released into the systemic circulation in a rapid, "pulse-like" dose, it is believed to affect circadian rhythms thought to play a role in obesity and insulin resistance.

Contraindications Hypersensitivity to bromocriptine, ergot alkaloids, or any component of the formulation

Additional contraindications:
Parlodel®: Uncontrolled hypertension; pregnancy (risk to benefit evaluation must be performed in women who become pregnant during treatment for acromegaly, prolactinoma, or Parkinson's disease - hypertension during treatment should generally result in efforts to withdraw); postpartum women with a history of coronary artery disease or other severe cardiovascular conditions (unless withdrawal of medication is medically contraindicated)

Cycloset®: Syncopal migraine; breast-feeding

Warnings/Precautions Complete evaluation of pituitary function should be completed prior to initiation of treatment of any hyperprolactinemia-associated dysfunction. Use caution in patients with a history of peptic ulcer disease, dementia, or cardiovascular disease (myocardial infarction, arrhythmia). Use with extreme caution or avoid in patients with psychosis. Symptomatic hypotension may occur in a significant number of patients. In addition, hypertension, seizures, MI, and stroke have been rarely associated with bromocriptine therapy. Severe headache or visual changes may precede events. The onset of reactions may be immediate or delayed (often may occur in the second week of therapy). Sudden sleep onset and somnolence have been reported with use, primarily in patients with Parkinson's disease. Patients must be cautioned about performing tasks which require mental alertness.

Use with caution in patients taking strong CYP3A4 inhibitors and/or major CYP3A4 substrates (includes protease inhibitors, azole antifungals, and some macrolide antibiotics); consider alternative agents that avoid or lessen the potential for CYP-mediated interactions. Concurrent antihypertensives or drugs which may alter blood pressure should be used with caution. Concurrent use with levodopa has been associated with an increased risk of hallucinations. Consider dosage reduction and/or discontinuation in patients with hallucinations. Hallucinations may require weeks to months before resolution.

Dopamine agonists have been associated with compulsive behaviors and/or loss of impulse control, which has manifested as pathological gambling/spending, libido increases (hypersexuality), and/or binge eating. Causality has not been established, and controversy exists as to whether this phenomenon is related to the underlying disease, prior behaviors/addictions and/or drug therapy. Dose reduction or discontinuation of therapy reverses these behaviors in some, but not all cases. Risk for melanoma development is increased in Parkinson's disease patients; drug causation or factors contributing to risk have not been established. Patients should be monitored closely and periodic skin examinations should be performed.

In the treatment of acromegaly, discontinuation is recommended if tumor expansion occurs during therapy. Digital vasospasm (cold sensitive) may occur in some patients with acromegaly; may require dosage reduction. Patients who receive bromocriptine during and immediately following pregnancy as a continuation of previous therapy (eg, acromegaly) should be closely monitored for cardiovascular effects. Should not be used postpartum in women with coronary artery disease or other cardiovascular disease. Use of bromocriptine to control or prevent lactation or in patients with uncontrolled hypertension is not recommended.

Monitoring and careful evaluation of visual changes during the treatment of hyperprolactinemia is recommended to differentiate between tumor shrinkage and traction on the optic chiasm; rapidly progressing visual field loss requires neurosurgical consultation. Discontinuation of bromocriptine in patients with macroadenomas has been associated with rapid regrowth of tumor and increased prolactin serum levels. Pleural and retroperitoneal fibrosis cases have been reported with prolonged daily use. Cardiac valvular fibrosis has also been associated with ergot alkaloids.

In the management of type 2 diabetes mellitus, Cycloset® ("quick-release" tablet) should not be interchanged with any other bromocriptine product due to formulation differences and resulting pharmacokinetics. Therapy is not appropriate in patients with diabetic ketoacidosis (DKA) or type 1 diabetes mellitus due to lack of efficacy in these patient populations. There is limited efficacy of use in combination with thiazolidinediones or in combination with insulin. Combination therapy with other hypoglycemic agents may increase risk for hypoglycemic events; dose reduction of concomitant hypoglycemics may be warranted.

Safety and efficacy have not been established in patients with hepatic or renal dysfunction. Safety and effectiveness in patients <11 years of age (for pituitary adenoma) have not been established. Safety has not been established for use >2 years in patients with Parkinson's disease. Dopaminergic agents have been associated with a syndrome resembling neuroleptic malignant syndrome on abrupt withdrawal or significant dosage reduction after long-term use; gradual dosage reduction is recommended when discontinuing therapy.

Drug Interactions

Avoid Concomitant Use

Avoid concomitant use of Bromocriptine with any of the following: Alpha-/Beta-Agonists; Alpha1-Agonists; Amisulpride; Conivaptan; Fusidic Acid (Systemic); Lorcaserin; Nitroglycerin; Protease Inhibitors; Serotonin 5-HT1D Receptor Agonists

Decreased Effect

Bromocriptine may decrease the levels/effects of: Amisulpride; Antipsychotics (Typical); Nitroglycerin

The levels/effects of Bromocriptine may be decreased by: Amisulpride; Antipsychotics (Atypical); Antipsychotics (Typical); Metoclopramide

Increased Effect/Toxicity

Bromocriptine may increase the levels/effects of: Alcohol (Ethyl); Alpha-/Beta-Agonists; Alpha1-Agonists; Antipsychotics; BuPROPion; CycloSPORINE (Systemic); Dofetilide; Lomitapide; Metoclopramide; Serotonin 5-HT1D Receptor Agonists; Serotonin Modulators

The levels/effects of Bromocriptine may be increased by: Alcohol (Ethyl); Antipsychotics; Beta-Blockers; Conivaptan; CYP3A4 Inhibitors (Moderate); CYP3A4 Inhibitors (Strong); Dasatinib; Fusidic Acid (Systemic); Ivacaftor; Lorcaserin; Luliconazole; Macrolide Antibiotics; MAO Inhibitors; Methylphenidate; Mifepristone; Nitroglycerin; Protease Inhibitors; Serotonin 5-HT1D Receptor Agonists; Simeprevir; Stiripentol

Nutritional/Ethanol Interactions

Ethanol: Avoid ethanol (may increase GI side effects or ethanol intolerance).

Herb/Nutraceutical: St John's wort may decrease bromocriptine levels.

Adverse Reactions Note: Frequency of adverse effects may vary by dose and/or indication.

>10%:

Central nervous system: Dizziness, fatigue, headache

Gastrointestinal: Constipation, nausea

Neuromuscular & skeletal: Weakness

Respiratory: Rhinitis

1% to 10%:

Cardiovascular: Hypotension (including postural/orthostatic), Raynaud's phenomenon, syncope, vasospasm (digital)

Central nervous system: Drowsiness, lightheadedness

Endocrine & metabolic: Hypoglycemia (4%; in combination with sulfonylureas or other antidiabetic agents: 7% to 9%)

Gastrointestinal: Abdominal cramps, anorexia, diarrhea, dyspepsia, gastrointestinal hemorrhage, vomiting, xerostomia

Infection: Increased susceptibility to infection

Ophthalmic: Amblyopia

Respiratory: Flu-like symptoms, nasal congestion, sinusitis

Pharmacodynamics/Kinetics

Onset of Action Parlodel®: Prolactin decreasing effect: 1-2 hours

Available Dosage Forms

Capsule, Oral:

Parlodel: 5 mg

Generic: 5 mg

Tablet, Oral:

Cycloset: 0.8 mg

Parlodel: 2.5 mg

Generic: 2.5 mg

General Dosage Range Oral:

Children 11-15 years: Initial: 1.25-2.5 mg daily; Maintenance: 2.5-10 mg/day

Children ≥16 years: Initial: 1.25-2.5 mg daily; Maintenance: 2.5-15 mg/day

Adults: Dosage varies greatly depending on indication

Administration

Oral Administer with food to decrease GI distress. Cycloset®: Administer within 2 hours of waking in the morning.

Storage/Stability Store at or below 25°C (77°F).

Nursing Actions

Physical Assessment Monitor blood pressure at beginning of therapy and periodically during course of treatment.

Patient Education

• Discuss specific use of drug and side effects with patient as it relates to treatment. (HCAHPS: During this hospital stay, were you given any

medicine that you had not taken before? Before giving you any new medicine, how often did hospital staff tell you what the medicine was for? How often did hospital staff describe possible side effects in a way you could understand?)

- Patient may experience nausea, insomnia, constipation, fatigue, asthenia, rhinorrhea, diarrhea, or lack of appetite. Have patient report immediately to prescriber significant severe dizziness, syncope, change in balance, vision changes, strength differences from one side to another, difficulty speaking or thinking, blurred vision, angina, depression, significant headache, dyspnea, uncontrollable urges, narcolepsy, back pain, melena, hematemesis, considerable dyspepsia, edema of extremities, hallucinations, urinary retention, oliguria, illogical thinking, or signs of hypoglycemia (HCAHPS).

- Educate patient about signs of a significant reaction (eg, wheezing; chest tightness; fever; itching; bad cough; blue skin color; seizures; or swelling of face, lips, tongue, or throat). **Note:** This is not a comprehensive list of all side effects. Patient should consult prescriber for additional questions.

Intended Use and Disclaimer: Should not be printed and given to patients. This information is intended to serve as a concise initial reference for healthcare professionals to use when discussing medications with a patient. You must ultimately rely on your own discretion, experience and judgment in diagnosing, treating and advising patients.

Dietary Considerations Should be taken with food to decrease GI distress.

Brompheniramine (brome fen IR a meen)

Brand Names: U.S. J-Tan PD [OTC]; Respa-BR
Index Terms Brompheniramine Maleate; Brompheniramine Tannate
Pharmacologic Category Alkylamine Derivative; Histamine H_1 Antagonist; Histamine H_1 Antagonist, First Generation
Medication Safety Issues
BEERS Criteria medication:
This drug may be potentially inappropriate for use in geriatric patients (Quality of evidence - moderate; Strength of recommendation - strong).
Pregnancy Risk Factor C
Lactation Excretion in breast milk unknown/contraindicated
Use Symptomatic relief of perennial and seasonal allergic rhinitis, vasomotor rhinitis, and other respiratory allergies
Available Dosage Forms
Liquid, Oral:
J-Tan PD [OTC]: 1 mg/mL (30 mL)
Tablet Extended Release 12 Hour, Oral:
Respa-BR: 11 mg

General Dosage Range Oral:
Children 2 to <6 years: J-Tan PD: 1 mg (1 mL) every 4-6 hours (maximum: 6 mg [6 mL]/24 hours)
Children 6-12 years:
J-Tan PD: 2 mg (2 mL) every 4-6 hours (maximum: 12 mg [12 mL]/24 hours)
LoHist-12: One tablet every 12 hours (maximum: 2 tablets/day)
Children >12 years and Adults:
Bromax: One tablet twice daily
LoHist-12: 1-2 tablets every 12 hours (maximum: 4 tablets/day)
Administration
Oral Extended release tablets are to be swallowed whole; do not crush or chew.
Nursing Actions
Patient Education
- Discuss specific use of drug and side effects with patient as it relates to treatment. (HCAHPS: During this hospital stay, were you given any medicine that you had not taken before? Before giving you any new medicine, how often did hospital staff tell you what the medicine was for? How often did hospital staff describe possible side effects in a way you could understand?)
- Patient may experience fatigue, mydriasis, headache, lack of appetite, anxiety, insomnia, constipation, xerostomia, or rhinitis. Have patient report immediately to prescriber angina, tachycardia, vision changes, change in balance, arrhythmia, dyspnea, mood changes, significant pharyngitis, difficult urination, ecchymosis, hemorrhaging, severe dizziness, syncope, or considerable asthenia (HCAHPS).
- Educate patient about signs of a significant reaction (eg, wheezing; chest tightness; fever; itching; bad cough; blue skin color; seizures; or swelling of face, lips, tongue, or throat). **Note:** This is not a comprehensive list of all side effects. Patient should consult prescriber for additional questions.

Intended Use and Disclaimer: Should not be printed and given to patients. This information is intended to serve as a concise initial reference for healthcare professionals to use when discussing medications with a patient. You must ultimately rely on your own discretion, experience and judgment in diagnosing, treating and advising patients.

Budesonide (Systemic, Oral Inhalation) (byoo DES oh nide)

Brand Names: U.S. Entocort EC; Pulmicort; Pulmicort Flexhaler; Uceris
Index Terms Uceris™
Pharmacologic Category Corticosteroid, Inhalant (Oral); Corticosteroid, Systemic

Pregnancy Risk Factor C (capsule, tablet)/B (inhalation)

Lactation Enters breast milk/use caution

Breast-Feeding Considerations Following use of the powder for oral inhalation, ~0.3% to 1% of the maternal dose was found in breast milk. The maximum concentration appeared within 45 minutes of dosing. Plasma budesonide levels obtained from infants ~90 minutes after breast-feeding (~140 minutes after maternal dose) were below the limit of quantification. Concentrations of budesonide in breast milk are expected to be higher following administration of oral capsules/tablets than after an inhaled dose.

Due to the potential for serious adverse reactions in the nursing infant, the manufacturers of the oral tablets and capsules recommend a decision be made whether to discontinue nursing or to discontinue the drug, taking into account the importance of treatment to the mother. If there is concern about exposure to the infant, some guidelines recommend waiting 4 hours after the maternal dose of an oral systemic corticosteroid before breast-feeding in order to decrease potential exposure to the nursing infant (based on a study using prednisolone) (Habal, 2012; Ost, 1985).

According to the manufacturer of the product for inhalation, the decision to continue or discontinue breast-feeding during therapy should take into account the risk of minimal exposure to the infant and the benefits of breast-feeding to the mother. The use of inhaled corticosteroids is not considered a contraindication to breast-feeding (NAEPP, 2005).

Use

Nebulization: Maintenance and prophylactic treatment of asthma

Oral capsule: Treatment of active Crohn's disease (mild-to-moderate) involving the ileum and/or ascending colon; maintenance of remission (for up to 3 months) of Crohn's disease (mild-to-moderate) involving the ileum and/or ascending colon

Oral inhalation: Maintenance and prophylactic treatment of asthma; includes patients who require oral corticosteroids and those who may benefit from systemic dose reduction/elimination

Oral tablet: Induction of remission in patients with active ulcerative colitis (mild-to-moderate)

Mechanism of Action/Effect Anti-inflammatory corticosteroid

Contraindications Hypersensitivity to budesonide or any component of the formulation; primary treatment of status asthmaticus, acute episodes of asthma; not for relief of acute bronchospasm

Canadian labeling: Additional contraindications (not in U.S. labeling): Moderate-to-severe bronchiectasis, pulmonary tuberculosis (active or quiescent), untreated respiratory infection (bacterial, fungal, or viral)

Warnings/Precautions May cause hypercorticism or suppression of hypothalamic-pituitary-adrenal (HPA) axis, particularly in younger children, in patients receiving high doses for prolonged periods, or with concomitant CYP3A4 inhibitor use. HPA axis suppression may lead to adrenal crisis. Withdrawal and discontinuation of a corticosteroid should be done slowly and carefully. Particular care is required when patients are transferred from systemic corticosteroids to inhaled products or corticosteroids with lower systemic effect due to possible adrenal insufficiency or withdrawal from steroids, including an increase in allergic symptoms. Patients receiving >20 mg per day of prednisone (or equivalent) may be most susceptible. Fatalities have occurred due to adrenal insufficiency in asthmatic patients during and after transfer from systemic corticosteroids to aerosol steroids; aerosol steroids do not provide the systemic steroid needed to treat patients having trauma, surgery, or infections. Do not use this product to transfer patients directly from oral corticosteroid therapy.

Bronchospasm may occur with wheezing after inhalation; if this occurs stop steroid and treat with a fast-acting bronchodilator (eg, albuterol). Supplemental steroids (oral or parenteral) may be needed during stress or severe asthma attacks. Not to be used in status asthmaticus or for the relief of acute bronchospasm. Acute myopathy has been reported with high-dose corticosteroids, usually in patients with neuromuscular transmission disorders; may involve ocular and/or respiratory muscles; monitor creatine kinase; recovery may be delayed. Corticosteroid use may cause psychiatric disturbances, including depression, euphoria, insomnia, mood swings, and personality changes. Pre-existing psychiatric conditions may be exacerbated by corticosteroid use. Prolonged use of corticosteroids may also increase the incidence of secondary infection, mask acute infection (including fungal infections), prolong or exacerbate viral infections, or limit response to vaccines. Exposure to chickenpox should be avoided; corticosteroids should not be used to treat ocular herpes simplex. Corticosteroids should not be used for viral hepatitis. Close observation is required in patients with latent tuberculosis and/or TB reactivity; restrict use in active TB (only in conjunction with antituberculosis treatment). *Candida albicans* infections may occur in the mouth and pharynx; rinsing (and spitting) with water after inhaler use may decrease risk. Prolonged treatment with corticosteroids has been associated with the development of Kaposi's sarcoma (case reports); if noted, discontinuation of therapy should be considered.

Use with caution in patients with thyroid disease, hepatic impairment, renal impairment, cardiovascular disease, diabetes, glaucoma, cataracts, myasthenia gravis, patients at risk for ▶

osteoporosis, patients at risk for seizures, or GI diseases (diverticulitis, peptic ulcer, ulcerative colitis) due to perforation risk. Use caution following acute MI (corticosteroids have been associated with myocardial rupture). Because of the risk of adverse effects, systemic corticosteroids should be used cautiously in the elderly in the smallest possible effective dose for the shortest duration.

Potentially significant interactions may exist, requiring dose or frequency adjustment, additional monitoring, and/or selection of alternative therapy. Consult drug interactions database for more detailed information.

Orally-inhaled corticosteroids may cause a reduction in growth velocity in pediatric patients (~1 centimeter per year [range: 0.3-1.8 cm per year] and related to dose and duration of exposure). To minimize the systemic effects of orally-inhaled corticosteroids, each patient should be titrated to the lowest effective dose. Growth should be routinely monitored in pediatric patients. Withdraw systemic therapy with gradual tapering of dose. There have been reports of systemic corticosteroid withdrawal symptoms (eg, joint/muscle pain, lassitude, depression) when withdrawing oral inhalation therapy. Pulmicort Flexhaler® contains lactose; very rare anaphylactic reactions have been reported in patients with severe milk protein allergy.

Drug Interactions

Avoid Concomitant Use

Avoid concomitant use of Budesonide (Systemic, Oral Inhalation) with any of the following: Aldesleukin; BCG; Fusidic Acid (Systemic); Grapefruit Juice; Natalizumab; Pimecrolimus; Tacrolimus (Topical); Tofacitinib

Decreased Effect

Budesonide (Systemic, Oral Inhalation) may decrease the levels/effects of: Aldesleukin; Antidiabetic Agents; BCG; Coccidioidin Skin Test; Corticorelin; Hyaluronidase; Sipuleucel-T; Vaccines (Inactivated)

The levels/effects of Budesonide (Systemic, Oral Inhalation) may be decreased by: Antacids; Bile Acid Sequestrants; Echinacea

Increased Effect/Toxicity

Budesonide (Systemic, Oral Inhalation) may increase the levels/effects of: Amphotericin B; Deferasirox; Leflunomide; Loop Diuretics; Natalizumab; Thiazide Diuretics; Tofacitinib

The levels/effects of Budesonide (Systemic, Oral Inhalation) may be increased by: CYP3A4 Inhibitors (Moderate); CYP3A4 Inhibitors (Strong); Dasatinib; Denosumab; Fusidic Acid (Systemic); Grapefruit Juice; Ivacaftor; Luliconazole; Mifepristone; Pimecrolimus; Simeprevir; Tacrolimus (Topical); Telaprevir; Trastuzumab

Nutritional/Ethanol Interactions

Food: Grapefruit juice may double systemic exposure of orally administered budesonide.

Administration of capsules with a high-fat meal delays peak concentration, but does not alter the extent of absorption; administration of tablets with a high-fat meal decreases peak concentration (~27%). Management: Avoid grapefruit juice when using oral capsules or tablets.

Herb/Nutraceutical: Echinacea may diminish the therapeutic effect of budesonide. Management: Avoid echinacea.

Adverse Reactions

Oral capsules:

>10%:

Central nervous system: Headache (21%)

Dermatologic: Bruising (5% to 15%), acne (<5% to 15%)

Gastrointestinal: Nausea (11%)

Respiratory: Respiratory infection (11%)

Miscellaneous: Fat redistribution (moon face, buffalo hump; 3% to 11%)

1% to 10%:

Cardiovascular: Edema (<5% to 7%), chest pain (<5%), facial edema (<5%), flushing (<5%), hypertension (<5%), palpitation (<5%), tachycardia (<5%)

Central nervous system: Dizziness (<5% to 7%), agitation (<5%), amnesia (<5%), confusion (<5%), fever (<5%), insomnia (<5%), malaise (<5%), nervousness (<5%), sleep disorder (<5%), somnolence (<5%), vertigo (<5%)

Dermatologic: Hirsutism (5%), alopecia (<5%), dermatitis (<5%), eczema (<5%), purpura (<5%), skin disorder (<5%), striae (2%)

Endocrine & metabolic: Hypokalemia (<5%), intermenstrual bleeding (<5%), menstrual disorder (<5%), adrenal insufficiency (≥1%)

Gastrointestinal: Diarrhea (10%), dyspepsia (6%), anus disorder (<5%), appetite increased (<5%), Crohn's disease exacerbation (<5%), enteritis (<5%), epigastric pain (<5%), gastrointestinal fistula (<5%), glossitis (<5%), hemorrhoids (<5%), intestinal obstruction (<5%), oral candidiasis (<5%), tongue edema (<5%), tooth disorder (<5%), weight gain (<5%)

Genitourinary: Dysuria (<5%), micturition frequency (<5%), nocturia (<5%), hematuria (≥1%), pyuria (≥1%), urinary tract infection (<5%)

Hematologic: Leukocytosis (<5%), anemia (≥1%), neutrophils abnormal (≥1%)

Hepatic: Alkaline phosphatase increased (≥1%)

Neuromuscular & skeletal: Arthralgia (5%), arthritis (<5%), hyperkinesia (<5%), muscle cramping (<5%), myalgia (<5%), paresthesia (<5%), tremor (<5%), weakness (<5%)

Ocular: Eye abnormality (<5%), vision abnormal (<5%)

Otic: Ear infection (<5%)

Respiratory: Sinusitis (8%), bronchitis (<5%), dyspnea (<5%), pharynx disorder (<5%), rhinitis (<5%)

Miscellaneous: Viral infection (6%), abscess (<5%), C-reactive protein increased (<5%), diaphoresis (<5%), flu-like syndrome (<5%), erythrocyte sedimentation rate increased (≥1%)

Postmarketing and/or case reports: Anaphylaxis, intracranial hypertension (benign), mood swings

Oral inhaler (Pulmicort Flexhaler®):

1% to 10%:

Cardiovascular: Syncope (1% to 3%)

Central nervous system: Fever (≥3%), headache (≥3%), pain (≥3%), insomnia (1% to 3%)

Dermatologic: Bruising (1% to 3%)

Gastrointestinal: Dyspepsia (≥5%), nausea (2% to ≥5%), abdominal pain (1% to 3%), taste perversion (1% to 3%), vomiting (1% to 3%), weight gain (1% to 3%), xerostomia (1% to 3%), gastroenteritis (viral; 2%), oral candidiasis (1%)

Neuromuscular & skeletal: Arthralgia (≥5%), weakness (≥5%), back pain (≥3%), fracture (1% to 3%), hypertonia (1% to 3%), myalgia (1% to 3%), neck pain (1% to 3%)

Otic: Otitis media (1%)

Respiratory: Nasopharyngitis (9%), cough (≥5%), rhinitis (≥5%), respiratory infection (≥3%), sinusitis (≥3%), nasal congestion (3%), pharyngitis (3%), allergic rhinitis (2%), upper respiratory tract infection (viral; 2%)

Miscellaneous: Infection (1% to 3%), voice alteration (1% to 3%)

Postmarketing and/or case reports: Aggressiveness, anxiety, cataracts, depression, glaucoma, hypercorticism, hypersensitivity reactions (immediate and delayed [includes rash, contact dermatitis, angioedema, bronchospasm, urticaria]), hypocorticism, intraocular pressure increased, irritability, nervousness, psychosis, restlessness, throat irritation, wheezing (patients with severe milk allergy)

Oral tablets:

>10%: Central nervous system: Headache (11%)

1% to 10%:

Central nervous system: Mood swings (7%), fatigue (3%)

Dermatologic: Acne (2% to 5%), hirsutism (<1% to 5%)

Endocrine & metabolic: Cortisol decreased (4%)

Gastrointestinal: Nausea (5%), upper abdominal pain (4%), flatulence (3%), abdominal distension (2%), constipation (2%)

Genitourinary: Urinary tract infection (2%)

Neuromuscular & skeletal: Arthralgia (2%)

Postmarketing and/or case reports: Anaphylaxis, intracranial hypertension (benign), mood swings

Suspension for nebulization:

>10%:

Otic: Otitis media (12%)

Respiratory: Respiratory infection (38%), rhinitis (11% to 12%)

1% to 10%:

Cardiovascular: Chest pain (1% to <3%)

Central nervous system: Dysphonia (1% to <3%), fatigue (1% to <3%), mood swings (1% to <3%)

Dermatologic: Rash (4%), contact dermatitis (1% to <3%), eczema (1% to <3%), pruritus (1% to <3%), purpura (1% to <3%), pustular rash (1% to <3%)

Gastrointestinal: Gastroenteritis (5%), diarrhea (4%), vomiting (4%), abdominal pain (3%), anorexia (1% to <3%)

Hematologic: Cervical lymphadenopathy (1% to <3%)

Neuromuscular & skeletal: Fracture (1% to <3%), hyperkinesia (1% to <3%), myalgia (1% to <3%)

Ocular: Conjunctivitis (4%), eye infection (1% to <3%)

Otic: Ear infection (5%), earache (1% to <3%), otitis externa (1% to <3%)

Respiratory: Cough (8% to 9%), epistaxis (2% to 4%), stridor (1% to <3%)

Miscellaneous: Viral infection (4% to 5%), moniliasis (4% to 5%), allergic reaction (1% to <3%), flu-like syndrome (1% to <3%), herpes simplex (1% to <3%), infection (1% to <3%)

Postmarketing and/or case reports: Aggressiveness, anxiety, avascular necrosis of the femoral head, bronchitis, bruising, cataracts, depression, facial skin irritation, fever, glaucoma, growth suppression, headache, hypercorticism, hypersensitivity reactions (immediate and delayed [includes angioedema, bronchospasm, urticaria]), hypocorticism, intraocular pressure increased, irritability, nervousness, osteoporosis, pain, pharyngitis, psychosis, restlessness, sinusitis, throat irritation

Pharmacodynamics/Kinetics

Onset of Action Nebulization: 2-8 days; Inhalation: 24 hours

Peak effect: Nebulization: 4-6 weeks; Inhalation: 1-2 weeks

Dosage Forms Considerations

Pulmicort Flexhaler 180 mcg/actuation canisters contain 120 actuations and the 90 mcg/actuation canisters contain 60 inhalations.

Available Dosage Forms

Aerosol Powder Breath Activated, Inhalation:

Pulmicort Flexhaler: 90 mcg/actuation (1 ea); 180 mcg/actuation (1 ea)

Capsule Extended Release 24 Hour, Oral:

Entocort EC: 3 mg

Generic: 3 mg

Suspension, Inhalation:

Pulmicort: 0.25 mg/2 mL (2 mL); 0.5 mg/2 mL (2 mL); 1 mg/2 mL (2 mL)

Generic: 0.25 mg/2 mL (2 mL); 0.5 mg/2 mL (2 mL)

Tablet Extended Release 24 Hour, Oral:

Uceris: 9 mg

◀ **General Dosage Range**

Inhalation:

Children ≥6 years: Initial: 180-360 mcg twice daily; Maintenance: 180->800 mcg/day in 2 divided doses

Adults: Initial: 180-720 mcg twice daily; Maintenance: 180-1440 mcg/day in 2 divided doses

Nebulization: *Children 12 months to 8 years:* 0.25-1 mg in 1-2 divided doses

Oral: *Adults:* Initial: (Crohn's disease, ulcerative colitis): 9 mg once daily; Maintenance (Crohn's disease): 6 mg once daily

Administration

Oral Oral capsule, tablet: May be administered without regard to meals. Swallow whole; do not crush, chew, or break.

Inhalation

Powder for inhalation:

Pulmicort Flexhaler®: Hold inhaler in upright position (mouthpiece up) to load dose. Do not shake prior to use. Unit should be primed prior to first use only. It will not need primed again, even if not used for a long time. Place mouthpiece between lips and inhale forcefully and deeply. Do not exhale through inhaler; do not use a spacer. Dose indicator does not move with every dose, usually only after 5 doses. Discard when dose indicator reads "0". Rinse mouth with water after each use to reduce incidence of candidiasis.

Pulmicort® Turbuhaler® [CAN, not available in the U.S.]: Hold inhaler in upright position (mouthpiece up) to load dose. Do not shake inhaler after dose is loaded. Unit should be primed prior to first use. Place mouthpiece between lips and inhale forcefully and deeply; mouthpiece should face up. Do not exhale through inhaler; do not use a spacer. When a red mark appears in the dose indicator window, 20 doses are left. When the red mark reaches the bottom of the window, the inhaler should be discarded. Rinse mouth with water after use to reduce incidence of candidiasis.

Suspension for nebulization: Shake well before using. Use Pulmicort Respules® with jet nebulizer connected to an air compressor; administer with mouthpiece or facemask. Do not use ultrasonic nebulizer. Do not mix with other medications in nebulizer. Rinse mouth following treatments to decrease risk of oral candidiasis (wash face if using face mask).

Storage/Stability

Oral capsules and tablets: Store at 25°C (77°F); excursions permitted to 15°C to 30°C (59°F to 86°F); keep container tightly closed.

Oral inhaler (Pulmicort Flexhaler®): Store at controlled room temperature of 20°C to 25°C (68°F to 77°F). Protect from moisture.

Suspension for nebulization: Store upright at 20°C to 25°C (68°F to 77°F). Protect from light. Do not refrigerate or freeze. Once aluminum package is opened, solution should be used within 2 weeks. Continue to protect from light.

Nursing Actions

Physical Assessment When changing from systemic steroids to inhalational steroids, taper reduction of systemic medication slowly (may take several months). Growth should be routinely monitored in pediatric patients.

Patient Education

• Discuss specific use of drug and side effects with patient as it relates to treatment. (HCAHPS: During this hospital stay, were you given any medicine that you had not taken before? Before giving you any new medicine, how often did hospital staff tell you what the medicine was for? How often did hospital staff describe possible side effects in a way you could understand?)

• Patient may experience headache, nausea, lipodystrophy, skin changes, insomnia, akathisia, hyperhidrosis, flatulence, constipation, bloating, back pain, dizziness, epistaxis, rhinitis, rhinorrhea, or pharyngitis. Have patient report immediately to prescriber signs of hyperglycemia, signs of infection, signs of hypokalemia, severe asthenia, irritability, tremors, tachycardia, confusion, hyperhidrosis, excessive weight gain, edema of extremities, intolerable headache, arrhythmia, angina, stomatitis, osteodynia, arthralgia, vision changes, mood changes, behavioral changes, depression, paresthesia, considerable dyspepsia, ecchymosis, hemorrhaging, melena, hematemesis, or intolerable dyspnea (HCAHPS).

• Educate patient about signs of a significant reaction (eg, wheezing; chest tightness; fever; itching; bad cough; blue skin color; seizures; or swelling of face, lips, tongue, or throat). **Note:** This is not a comprehensive list of all side effects. Patient should consult prescriber for additional questions.

Intended Use and Disclaimer: Should not be printed and given to patients. This information is intended to serve as a concise initial reference for healthcare professionals to use when discussing medications with a patient. You must ultimately rely on your own discretion, experience and judgment in diagnosing, treating and advising patients.

Dietary Considerations Oral capsules, tablets: Avoid grapefruit juice.

Related Information

Oral Medications That Should Not Be Crushed or Altered *on page 1712*

Budesonide (Nasal) (byoo DES oh nide)

Brand Names: U.S. Rhinocort Aqua

Pharmacologic Category Corticosteroid, Nasal

Pregnancy Risk Factor B

Lactation Enters breast milk

Use Management of symptoms of seasonal or perennial rhinitis

Canadian labeling: Additional use (not in U.S. labeling): Prevention and treatment of nasal polyps

Unlabeled Use Adjunct to antibiotics in empiric treatment of acute bacterial rhinosinusitis (ABRS) (Chow, 2012)

Dosage Forms Considerations
Rhinocort Aqua 8.6 g bottles contain 120 sprays.

Available Dosage Forms

Suspension, Nasal:
Rhinocort Aqua: 32 mcg/actuation (8.6 g)

General Dosage Range Intranasal inhalation:
Children ≥6 years and Adults: 64 mcg/day as a single 32 mcg spray in each nostril (maximum: 128 mcg/day [children <12 years]; 256 mcg/day [children ≥12 years and adults])

Administration

Inhalation
Powder for nasal inhalation: Rhinocort® Turbuhaler® [CAN, not available in the U.S.]: Hold inhaler in upright position and turn grey grip as far as it will go in one direction and then back to original position. Clicking sound means inhaler is loaded with dose and ready for use. Place nasal adapter into nostril and ensure firm fit. Cover opposite nostril with finger and inhale (sniff) quickly and forcefully. Do not exhale through inhaler. When a red mark appears in the dose indicator window, 20 doses are left. When the red mark reaches the bottom of the window, the inhaler should be discarded

Suspension for nasal inhalation: Shake gently before use. Prime before first use; discard after 120 sprays.

Nursing Actions

Patient Education
• Discuss specific use of drug and side effects with patient as it relates to treatment. (HCAHPS: During this hospital stay, were you given any medicine that you had not taken before? Before giving you any new medicine, how often did hospital staff tell you what the medicine was for? How often did hospital staff describe possible side effects in a way you could understand?)
• Patient may experience pharyngitis. Have patient report immediately to prescriber signs of infection, severe dizziness, considerable rhinitis, significant epistaxis, nasal sores, stomatitis, intolerable nausea, severe asthenia, or vision changes (HCAHPS).
• Educate patient about signs of a significant reaction (eg, wheezing; chest tightness; fever; itching; bad cough; blue skin color; seizures; or swelling of face, lips, tongue, or throat). **Note:** This is not a comprehensive list of all side effects. Patient should consult prescriber for additional questions.

Intended Use and Disclaimer: Should not be printed and given to patients. This information is intended to serve as a concise initial reference for healthcare professionals to use when discussing medications with a patient. You must ultimately rely on your own discretion, experience and judgment in diagnosing, treating and advising patients.

Budesonide and Formoterol
(byoo DES oh nide & for MOH te rol)

Brand Names: U.S. Symbicort®

Index Terms Budesonide and Eformoterol; Eformoterol and Budesonide; Formoterol and Budesonide; Formoterol Fumarate Dihydrate and Budesonide

Pharmacologic Category Beta$_2$ Agonist; Beta$_2$-Adrenergic Agonist, Long-Acting; Corticosteroid, Inhalant (Oral)

Medication Guide Available Yes

Pregnancy Risk Factor C

Breast-Feeding Considerations It is not known if formoterol is excreted into breast milk; budesonide is excreted in small amounts. The manufacturer does not recommend use of this combination product in breast-feeding women. Refer to individual agents.

Use Treatment of asthma in patients ≥12 years of age where combination therapy is indicated; maintenance treatment of airflow obstruction associated with chronic obstructive pulmonary disease (COPD; including chronic bronchitis and emphysema)

Unlabeled Use Treatment of asthma in children 5-11 years of age where combination therapy is indicated

Mechanism of Action/Effect Formoterol relaxes bronchial smooth muscle by selective action on beta$_2$ receptors with little effect on heart rate. Formoterol has a long-acting effect. Budesonide is a corticosteroid which controls the rate of protein synthesis, depresses the migration of polymorphonuclear leukocytes/fibroblasts, and reverses capillary permeability and lysosomal stabilization at the cellular level to prevent or control inflammation.

Contraindications Hypersensitivity to budesonide, formoterol, or any component of the formulation; need for acute bronchodilation in COPD or asthma (including status asthmaticus)

Canadian labeling: Additional contraindications (not in U.S. labeling): Hypersensitivity to inhaled lactose

Warnings/Precautions [U.S. Boxed Warning]: Long-acting beta$_2$-agonists (LABAs), such as formoterol, increase the risk of asthma-related deaths; budesonide and formoterol should only be used in patients not adequately controlled on a long-term asthma control medication (ie, inhaled corticosteroid) or whose disease severity requires initiation of two maintenance

therapies. In a large, randomized, placebo-controlled U.S. clinical trial (SMART, 2006), salmeterol was associated with an increase in asthma-related deaths (when added to usual asthma therapy); risk is considered a class effect among all LABAs. Data are not available to determine if the addition of an inhaled corticosteroid lessens this increased risk of death associated with LABA use. Assess patients at regular intervals once asthma control is maintained on combination therapy to determine if step-down therapy is appropriate (without loss of asthma control), and the patient can be maintained on an inhaled corticosteroid only. LABAs are not appropriate in patients whose asthma is adequately controlled on low- or medium-dose inhaled corticosteroids. **[U.S. Boxed Warning]: LABAs may increase the risk of asthma-related hospitalization in pediatric and adolescent patients.**

Do **not** use for acute bronchospasm or acute symptomatic COPD. Short-acting beta₂-agonist (eg, albuterol) should be used for acute symptoms and symptoms occurring between treatments. Do **not** initiate in patients with significantly worsening or acutely deteriorating asthma or COPD. Increased use and/or ineffectiveness of short-acting beta₂-agonists may indicate rapidly deteriorating disease and should prompt re-evaluation of the patient's condition. Patients must be instructed to seek medical attention in cases where acute symptoms are not relieved by short-acting beta-agonist (not formoterol) or a previous level of response is diminished. Medical evaluation must not be delayed. Patients using inhaled, short acting beta₂-agonists should be instructed to discontinue routine use of these medications prior to beginning treatment with Symbicort®; short acting agents should be reserved for symptomatic relief of acute symptoms. Data are not available to determine if LABA use increases the risk of death in patients with COPD.

Immediate hypersensitivity reactions (urticaria, angioedema, rash, bronchospasm) have been reported. Do not exceed recommended dose; serious adverse events, including fatalities, have been associated with excessive use of inhaled sympathomimetics. Rarely, paradoxical bronchospasm may occur with use of inhaled bronchodilating agents; this should be distinguished from inadequate response. Pneumonia and other lower respiratory tract infections have been reported in patients with COPD following the use of inhaled corticosteroids; monitor COPD patients closely since pneumonia symptoms may overlap symptoms of exacerbations.

Use caution in patients with cardiovascular disease (arrhythmia or hypertension or HF), seizure disorders, diabetes, hepatic impairment, ocular disease, osteoporosis, thyroid disease, or hypokalemia. Beta agonists may cause elevation in blood pressure, heart rate, and result in CNS stimulation/excitation. Beta₂-agonists may increase risk of arrhythmia, increase serum glucose, or decrease serum potassium. Long-term use may affect bone mineral density in adults. Infections with *Candida albicans* in the mouth and throat (thrush) have been reported with use. Use with caution in patients taking strong CYP3A4 inhibitors (see Drug Interactions); consider alternative agents that avoid or lessen the potential for CYP-mediated interactions.

Budesonide may cause hypercorticism and/or suppression of hypothalamic-pituitary-adrenal (HPA) axis, particularly in younger children or in patients receiving high doses for prolonged periods. Caution is required when patients are transferred from systemic corticosteroids to products with lower systemic bioavailability (ie, inhalation). May lead to possible adrenal insufficiency or withdrawal symptoms, including an increase in allergic symptoms. Patients receiving prolonged therapy ≥20 mg per day of prednisone (or equivalent) may be most susceptible. Aerosol steroids do **not** provide the systemic steroid needed to treat patients having trauma, surgery, or infections.

Orally-inhaled and intranasal corticosteroids may cause a reduction in growth velocity in pediatric patients (~1 centimeter per year [range 0.3-1.8 cm per year] and related to dose and duration of exposure). To minimize the systemic effects of orally-inhaled and intranasal corticosteroids, each patient should be titrated to the lowest effective dose. Growth should be routinely monitored in pediatric patients.

Prolonged use of corticosteroids may also increase the incidence of secondary infection, mask acute infection (including fungal infections), prolong or exacerbate viral infections, or limit response to vaccines. Exposure to chickenpox should be avoided; corticosteroids should not be used to treat ocular herpes simplex. Corticosteroids should not be used for cerebral malaria. Close observation is required in patients with latent tuberculosis and/or TB reactivity restrict use in active TB (only in conjunction with antituberculosis treatment).

Some products available in Canada contain lactose; very rare anaphylactic reactions have been reported in patients with severe milk protein allergy. Withdraw systemic therapy with gradual tapering of dose. There have been reports of systemic corticosteroid withdrawal symptoms (eg, joint/muscle pain, lassitude, depression) when withdrawing oral inhalation therapy.

Drug Interactions

Avoid Concomitant Use

Avoid concomitant use of Budesonide and Formoterol with any of the following: Aldesleukin; BCG; Beta-Blockers (Nonselective); Fusidic Acid

(Systemic); Grapefruit Juice; Highest Risk QTc-Prolonging Agents; Iobenguane I 123; Ivabradine; Long-Acting Beta2-Agonists; Mifepristone; Natalizumab; Pimecrolimus; Tacrolimus (Topical); Tofacitinib

Decreased Effect

Budesonide and Formoterol may decrease the levels/effects of: Aldesleukin; Antidiabetic Agents; BCG; Coccidioidin Skin Test; Corticorelin; Hyaluronidase; Iobenguane I 123; Sipuleucel-T; Vaccines (Inactivated)

The levels/effects of Budesonide and Formoterol may be decreased by: Antacids; Beta-Blockers (Beta1 Selective); Beta-Blockers (Nonselective); Betahistine; Bile Acid Sequestrants; Echinacea

Increased Effect/Toxicity

Budesonide and Formoterol may increase the levels/effects of: Amphotericin B; Atosiban; Deferasirox; Highest Risk QTc-Prolonging Agents; Leflunomide; Long-Acting Beta2-Agonists; Loop Diuretics; Moderate Risk QTc-Prolonging Agents; Natalizumab; Sympathomimetics; Thiazide Diuretics; Tofacitinib

The levels/effects of Budesonide and Formoterol may be increased by: AtoMOXetine; Caffeine; Cannabinoids; CYP3A4 Inhibitors (Moderate); CYP3A4 Inhibitors (Strong); Dasatinib; Denosumab; Fusidic Acid (Systemic); Grapefruit Juice; Inhalational Anesthetics; Ivabradine; Ivacaftor; Luliconazole; MAO Inhibitors; Mifepristone; Pimecrolimus; QTc-Prolonging Agents (Indeterminate Risk and Risk Modifying); Simeprevir; Tacrolimus (Topical); Telaprevir; Theophylline Derivatives; Trastuzumab; Tricyclic Antidepressants

Adverse Reactions Note: Percentage of adverse events may be dose related; causation not established. Also see individual agents.

>10%:
Central nervous system: Headache (7% to 11%)
Respiratory: Nasopharyngitis (7% to 11%), upper respiratory tract infections (4% to 11%)

1% to 10%:
Central nervous system: Dizziness (<3%)
Gastrointestinal: Stomach discomfort (1% to 7%), oral candidiasis (1% to 6%), vomiting (1% to 3%)
Neuromuscular & skeletal: Back pain (2% to 3%)
Respiratory: Pharyngolaryngeal pain (6% to 9%), lower respiratory tract infection (3% to 8%), sinusitis (4% to 6%), bronchitis (5%), nasal congestion (3%)
Miscellaneous: Influenza (2% to 3%)

Pharmacodynamics/Kinetics

Onset of Action Asthma: 15 minutes; maximum benefit: May take ≥2 weeks

Available Dosage Forms

Aerosol for oral inhalation:
Symbicort® 80/4.5: Budesonide 80 mcg and formoterol fumarate dihydrate 4.5 mcg per actuation (6.9 g) [60 metered inhalations]; budesonide 80 mcg and formoterol fumarate dihydrate 4.5 mcg per actuation (10.2 g) [120 metered inhalations]

Symbicort® 160/4.5: Budesonide 160 mcg and formoterol fumarate dihydrate 4.5 mcg per actuation (6 g) [60 metered inhalations]; budesonide 160 mcg and formoterol fumarate dihydrate 4.5 mcg per actuation (10.2 g) [120 metered inhalations]

General Dosage Range Inhalation:
Children 5-11 years: Symbicort® 80/4.5: Two inhalations twice daily (maximum: 4 inhalations/day)
Children ≥12 years: 2 inhalations once or twice daily (maximum: 4 inhalations/day)
Adults: 2 inhalations twice daily (maximum: 4 inhalations/day)

Administration

Inhalation
Symbicort® 80/4.5, Symbicort® 160/4.5: Prior to first use, inhaler must be primed by releasing 2 test sprays into the air; shake well for 5 seconds before each spray. Inhaler must be reprimed if not used for >7 days or if it has been dropped. Shake well for 5 seconds before each use. Discard inhaler after the labeled number of inhalations have been used or within 3 months after removal from foil pouch (do not use the "float test" to determine amount remaining in canister).

Symbicort® Turbuhaler® [CAN; not available in U.S.]:
To "load" inhaler: Turn grip on inhaler as far as it will move in one direction, then turn in opposite direction as far as it will go (inhaler is "loaded" with a dose, indicated by a "click"). Prior to first use, this procedure should be done twice, it does not need to be repeated with subsequent uses even when not used regularly.

Delivery of dose: Instruct patient to place mouthpiece gently between teeth, closing lips around inhaler. Instruct patient to inhale deeply and hold breath held for 5-10 seconds. The amount of drug delivered is small, and the individual will not sense the medication as it is inhaled. Remove mouthpiece prior to exhalation. Patient should not breathe out through the mouthpiece. After use of the inhaler, patient should rinse mouth/oropharynx with water and spit out rinse solution.

Storage/Stability
Symbicort® 80/4.5, Symbicort® 160/4.5: Store at room temperature of 20°C to 25°C (68°F to 77°F) with mouthpiece down. Do not puncture, incinerate, or store near heat or open flame. Discard inhaler after the labeled number of inhalations have been used or within 3 months after removal from foil pouch.

Symbicort® Turbuhaler®: Store at room temperature of 15°C to 30°C. Protect from heat and moisture.

◀ **Nursing Actions**
Physical Assessment See individual agents.
Patient Education
- Discuss specific use of drug and side effects with patient as it relates to treatment. (HCAHPS: During this hospital stay, were you given any medicine that you had not taken before? Before giving you any new medicine, how often did hospital staff tell you what the medicine was for? How often did hospital staff describe possible side effects in a way you could understand?)
- Patient may experience pharyngitis, dyspepsia, or rhinitis. Have patient report immediately to prescriber signs of infection, signs of hyperglycemia, signs of hypokalemia, angina, tachycardia, anxiety, stomatitis, osteodynia, severe dizziness, syncope, significant headache, considerable nausea, paresthesia, difficulty speaking, vision changes, or intolerable dyspnea (HCAHPS).
- Educate patient about signs of a significant reaction (eg, wheezing; chest tightness; fever; itching; bad cough; blue skin color; seizures; or swelling of face, lips, tongue, or throat). **Note:** This is not a comprehensive list of all side effects. Patient should consult prescriber for additional questions.

Intended Use and Disclaimer: Should not be printed and given to patients. This information is intended to serve as a concise initial reference for healthcare professionals to use when discussing medications with a patient. You must ultimately rely on your own discretion, experience and judgment in diagnosing, treating and advising patients.

Related Information
Budesonide (Systemic, Oral Inhalation) *on page 202*
Formoterol *on page 702*

Bumetanide (byoo MET a nide)

Index Terms Bumex
Pharmacologic Category Antihypertensive; Diuretic, Loop
Medication Safety Issues
Sound-alike/look-alike issues:
Bumetanide may be confused with Buminate
Bumex may be confused with Brevibloc, Buprenex
International issues:
Bumex [U.S.] may be confused with Permax brand name for pergolide [multiple international markets]
Pregnancy Risk Factor C
Lactation Excretion in breast milk unknown/not recommended
Breast-Feeding Considerations It is not known if bumetanide is excreted in breast milk. Breast-feeding is not recommended by the manufacturer.

Diuretics have the potential to decrease milk volume and suppress lactation. Breast-fed infants of mothers taking medications for hypertension should be monitored for adverse effects (Chobanian, 2003).

Use Management of edema secondary to heart failure or hepatic or renal disease (including nephrotic syndrome)
Unlabeled Use Treatment of hypertension
Mechanism of Action/Effect Inhibits reabsorption of sodium and chloride in the ascending loop of Henle and proximal renal tubule, causing increased excretion of water, sodium, chloride, magnesium, phosphate, and calcium
Contraindications Hypersensitivity to bumetanide or any component of the formulation; anuria; patients with hepatic coma or in states of severe electrolyte depletion until the condition improves or is corrected
Warnings/Precautions [U.S. Boxed Warning]: Excessive amounts can lead to profound diuresis with fluid and electrolyte loss; close medical supervision and dose evaluation are required. Potassium supplementation and/or use of potassium-sparing diuretics may be necessary to prevent hypokalemia. In cirrhosis, initiate bumetanide therapy with conservative dosing and close monitoring of electrolytes; avoid sudden changes in fluid and electrolyte balance and acid/base status which may lead to hepatic encephalopathy. *In vitro* studies using pooled sera from critically-ill neonates have shown bumetanide to be a potent displacer of bilirubin; avoid use in neonates at risk for kernicterus. Coadministration of antihypertensives may increase the risk of hypotension.

Monitor fluid status and renal function in an attempt to prevent oliguria, azotemia, and reversible increases in BUN and creatinine; close medical supervision of aggressive diuresis required. Bumetanide-induced ototoxicity (usually transient) may occur with rapid I.V. administration, renal impairment, excessive doses, and concurrent use of other ototoxins (eg, aminoglycosides). Asymptomatic hyperuricemia has been reported with use.

Chemical similarities are present among sulfonamides, sulfonylureas, carbonic anhydrase inhibitors, thiazides, and loop diuretics (except ethacrynic acid); the manufacturer's labeling states that bumetanide may be used in patients allergic to furosemide. Use in patients with sulfonylurea allergy is not specifically contraindicated in product labeling; however, a risk of cross-reaction exists in patients with allergy to any of these compounds; avoid use when previous reaction has been severe. Discontinue if signs of hypersensitivity are noted.

Drug Interactions
Avoid Concomitant Use There are no known interactions where it is recommended to avoid concomitant use.

Decreased Effect

Bumetanide may decrease the levels/effects of: Hypoglycemic Agents; Lithium; Neuromuscular-Blocking Agents

The levels/effects of Bumetanide may be decreased by: Bile Acid Sequestrants; Fosphenytoin; Herbs (Hypertensive Properties); Methotrexate; Methylphenidate; Nonsteroidal Anti-Inflammatory Agents; Phenytoin; Probenecid; Salicylates; Yohimbine

Increased Effect/Toxicity

Bumetanide may increase the levels/effects of: ACE Inhibitors; Allopurinol; Amifostine; Aminoglycosides; Antihypertensives; Cardiac Glycosides; CISplatin; Dofetilide; DULoxetine; Hypotensive Agents; Ivabradine; Lithium; Methotrexate; Neuromuscular-Blocking Agents; Obinutuzumab; RisperiDONE; RiTUXimab; Salicylates; Sodium Phosphates; Topiramate

The levels/effects of Bumetanide may be increased by: Alfuzosin; Analgesics (Opioid); Beta2-Agonists; Brimonidine (Topical); Corticosteroids (Orally Inhaled); Corticosteroids (Systemic); CycloSPORINE (Systemic); Diazoxide; Herbs (Hypotensive Properties); Licorice; MAO Inhibitors; Methotrexate; Pentoxifylline; Phosphodiesterase 5 Inhibitors; Probenecid; Prostacyclin Analogues

Nutritional/Ethanol Interactions

Food: Bumetanide serum levels may be decreased if taken with food. It has been recommended that bumetanide be administered without food (Bard, 2004).

Herb/Nutraceutical: Avoid ephedra, yohimbe, ginseng (may worsen hypertension). Avoid dong quai if using for hypertension (has estrogenic activity). Avoid garlic (may have increased antihypertensive effect).

Adverse Reactions

>10%:

Endocrine & metabolic: Hyperuricemia (18%), hypochloremia (15%), hypokalemia (15%)

Renal: Azotemia (11%)

1% to 10%:

Central nervous system: Dizziness (1%)

Endocrine & metabolic: Hyponatremia (9%), hyperglycemia (7%), phosphorus altered (5%), CO_2 content altered (4%), bicarbonate altered (3%), calcium altered (2%)

Neuromuscular & skeletal: Muscle cramps (1%)

Renal: Serum creatinine increased (7%)

Miscellaneous: LDH altered (1%)

Pharmacodynamics/Kinetics

Onset of Action Oral, I.M.: 0.5-1 hour; I.V.: 2-3 minutes

Peak effect: Oral: 1-2 hours; I.V.: 15-30 minutes

Duration of Action 4-6 hours

Available Dosage Forms

Solution, Injection:

Generic: 0.25 mg/mL (2 mL, 4 mL, 10 mL)

Tablet, Oral:

Generic: 0.5 mg, 1 mg, 2 mg

General Dosage Range

I.M., I.V.:

Infants and Children: 0.015-0.1 mg/kg/dose every 6-24 hours (maximum: 10 mg daily)

Adults: 0.5-1 mg/dose; may repeat in 2-3 hours for up to 2 doses (maximum: 10 mg daily)

Oral:

Infants and Children: 0.015-0.1 mg/kg/dose every 6-24 hours (maximum: 10 mg daily)

Adults: 0.5-2 mg 1-2 times daily; may repeat in 4-5 hours for up to 2 doses (maximum: 10 mg daily)

Administration

I.V. Administer slowly, over 1-2 minutes.

Injectable Detail pH: 6.8-7.8 (adjusted)

Oral An alternate-day schedule or a 3-4 daily dosing regimen with rest periods of 1-2 days in between may be the most tolerable and effective regimen for the continued control of edema.

Storage/Stability

I.V.: Store vials at 15°C to 30°C (59°F to 86°F). Infusion solutions should be used within 24 hours after preparation. Light sensitive; discoloration may occur when exposed to light.

Tablet: Store at 15°C to 30°C (59°F to 86°F).

Nursing Actions

Physical Assessment History of allergies and renal, electrolyte, hepatic, and pregnancy status should be assessed prior to beginning treatment. Monitor blood pressure, weight, and fluid status at beginning of therapy and periodically during therapy. Assess therapeutic effectiveness (reduced edema and cardiopulmonary symptoms). Monitor for hypotension, electrolyte imbalance, and ototoxicity.

Patient Education

• Discuss specific use of drug and side effects with patient as it relates to treatment. (HCAHPS: During this hospital stay, were you given any medicine that you had not taken before? Before giving you any new medicine, how often did hospital staff tell you what the medicine was for? How often did hospital staff describe possible side effects in a way you could understand?)

• Patient may experience headache or dyspepsia. Have patient report immediately to prescriber signs of fluid and electrolyte imbalance, signs of hyperglycemia, severe dizziness, syncope, significant diarrhea, hearing impairment, tinnitus, or injection site pain or irritation (HCAHPS).

• Educate patient about signs of a significant reaction (eg, wheezing; chest tightness; fever; itching; bad cough; blue skin color; seizures; or swelling of face, lips, tongue, or throat). **Note:** This is not a comprehensive list of all side effects. Patient should consult prescriber for additional questions.

Intended Use and Disclaimer: Should not be printed and given to patients. This information is intended to serve as a concise initial reference for healthcare professionals to use when discussing medications with a patient. You must ultimately rely on your own discretion, experience and judgment in diagnosing, treating and advising patients.

Dietary Considerations Administration with food slows the rate and reduces the extent of absorption and may reduce diuretic efficacy (Bard, 2004). May require increased intake of potassium-rich foods.

Bupivacaine (byoo PIV a kane)

Brand Names: U.S. Bupivacaine Spinal; Marcaine; Marcaine Preservative Free; Marcaine Spinal; Sensorcaine; Sensorcaine-MPF; Sensorcaine-MPF Spinal

Index Terms Bupivacaine Hydrochloride

Pharmacologic Category Local Anesthetic

Medication Safety Issues

Sound-alike/look-alike issues:

Bupivacaine may be confused with mepivacaine, ropivacaine

Marcaine® may be confused with Narcan®

High alert medication:

The Institute for Safe Medication Practices (ISMP) includes this medication (epidural administration) among its list of drug classes which have a heightened risk of causing significant patient harm when used in error.

Pregnancy Risk Factor C

Lactation Enters breast milk/not recommended

Use Local or regional anesthesia; spinal anesthesia; diagnostic and therapeutic procedures; obstetrical procedures (only 0.25% and 0.5% concentrations)

0.25%: Local infiltration, peripheral nerve block, sympathetic block, caudal or epidural block

0.5%: Peripheral nerve block, caudal and epidural block

0.75% **(not for obstetrical anesthesia)**: Retrobulbar block, epidural block. **Note:** Reserve for surgical procedures where a high degree of muscle relaxation and prolonged effect are necessary

Available Dosage Forms

Solution, Injection:

Marcaine: 0.25% (50 mL); 0.5% (50 mL)

Sensorcaine: 0.25% (50 mL); 0.5% (50 mL)

Sensorcaine-MPF: 0.25% (10 mL, 30 mL); 0.5% (10 mL, 30 mL); 0.75% (10 mL, 30 mL)

Generic: 0.25% (10 mL, 30 mL, 50 mL); 0.5% (10 mL, 30 mL, 50 mL); 0.75% (10 mL, 30 mL)

Solution, Injection [preservative free]:

Marcaine: 0.75% (10 mL, 30 mL)

Marcaine Preservative Free: 0.25% (10 mL, 30 mL); 0.5% (10 mL, 30 mL)

Generic: 0.25% (10 mL, 20 mL, 30 mL); 0.5% (10 mL, 20 mL, 30 mL); 0.75% (10 mL, 20 mL, 30 mL)

Solution, Intrathecal:

Marcaine Spinal: 0.75% [7.5 mg/mL] (2 mL)

Solution, Intrathecal [preservative free]:

Bupivacaine Spinal: 0.75% [7.5 mg/mL] (2 mL)

Sensorcaine-MPF Spinal: 0.75% [7.5 mg/mL] (2 mL)

General Dosage Range

Caudal block: *Children >12 years and Adults:* 15-30 mL of 0.25% or 0.5%

Epidural block: *Children >12 years and Adults:* 10-20 mL of 0.25% or 0.5% in 3-5 mL increments **or** 10-20 mL of 0.75% if high degree of muscle relaxation and prolonged effects needed

Infiltration (local): *Children >12 years and Adults:* 0.25% (maximum: 175 mg)

Nerve block: *Children >12 years and Adults:*

Peripheral: 5 mL of 0.25% or 0.5% (maximum: 400 mg/day)

Sympathetic: 20-50 mL of 0.25%

Retrobulbar anesthesia: *Children >12 years and Adults:* 2-4 mL of 0.75%

Spinal: *Adults:* Preservative free solution of 0.75% bupivacaine in 8.25% dextrose:

Cesarean section: 1-1.4 mL

Lower abdominal procedures: 1.6 mL

Lower extremity and perineal procedures: 1 mL

Normal vaginal delivery: 0.8 mL (higher doses may be required in some patients)

Administration

Injectable Detail pH: 4-6.5

Other Solutions containing preservatives should not be used for epidural or caudal blocks.

Nursing Actions

Physical Assessment Monitor for return of sensation. Teach patient appropriate interventions to promote safety.

Patient Education

• Discuss specific use of drug and side effects with patient as it relates to treatment. (HCAHPS: During this hospital stay, were you given any medicine that you had not taken before? Before giving you any new medicine, how often did hospital staff tell you what the medicine was for? How often did hospital staff describe possible side effects in a way you could understand?)

• Have patient report immediately to prescriber bradycardia, arrhythmia, angina, tachycardia, severe dizziness, syncope, change in balance, illogical thinking, akathisia, tremors, blurred vision, tinnitus, depression, dyspnea, or significant nausea (HCAHPS).

• Educate patient about signs of a significant reaction (eg, wheezing; chest tightness; fever; itching; bad cough; blue skin color; seizures; or swelling of face, lips, tongue, or throat). **Note:** This is not a comprehensive list of all side effects. Patient should consult prescriber for additional questions.

Intended Use and Disclaimer: Should not be printed and given to patients. This information is intended to serve as a concise initial reference for healthcare professionals to use when discussing medications with a patient. You must ultimately rely on your own discretion, experience and judgment in diagnosing, treating and advising patients.

Buprenorphine (byoo pre NOR feen)

Brand Names: U.S. Buprenex; Butrans

Index Terms Buprenorphine Hydrochloride

Pharmacologic Category Analgesic, Opioid; Analgesic, Opioid Partial Agonist

Medication Safety Issues

Sound-alike/look-alike issues:

Buprenex® may be confused with Brevibloc®, Bumex®

High alert medication:

The Institute for Safe Medication Practices (ISMP) includes this medication among its list of drug classes which have a heightened risk of causing significant patient harm when used in error.

Medication Guide Available Yes

Pregnancy Risk Factor C

Lactation Enters breast milk/not recommended

Breast-Feeding Considerations Buprenorphine is excreted in breast milk. Breast-feeding is not recommended by the manufacturer. Nursing infants exposed to large doses of opioids should be monitored for apnea and sedation (Montgomery, 2012).

When buprenorphine is used to treat opioid addiction in nursing women, most guidelines do not contraindicate breast-feeding as long as the infant is tolerant to the dose and other contraindications do not exist; caution should be used when nursing infants not previously exposed (ACOG, 2012; CSAT, 2004; Montgomery, 2012). If additional illicit substances are being abused, women treated with buprenorphine should pump and discard breast milk until sobriety is established (ACOG, 2012; Dow, 2012).

Use

Injection: Management of moderate-to-severe pain

Sublingual tablet: Treatment of opioid dependence

Transdermal patch: Management of moderate-to-severe chronic pain in patients requiring an around-the-clock opioid analgesic for an extended period of time

Unlabeled Use Injection: Management of opioid withdrawal in heroin-dependent hospitalized patients

Mechanism of Action/Effect Buprenorphine exerts its analgesic effect via high affinity binding to μ opiate receptors in the CNS; displays partial mu agonist and weak kappa antagonist activity

Contraindications Hypersensitivity to buprenorphine or any component of the formulation

Transdermal patch: Additional contraindications: Significant respiratory depression; acute or severe asthma; known or suspected paralytic ileus

Warnings/Precautions An opioid-containing analgesic regimen should be tailored to each patient's needs and based upon the type of pain being treated (acute versus chronic), the route of administration, degree of tolerance for opioids (naive versus chronic user), age, weight, and medical condition. The optimal analgesic dose varies widely among patients. Doses should be titrated to pain relief/prevention.

May cause CNS depression, which may impair physical or mental abilities; patients must be cautioned about performing tasks which require mental alertness (eg, operating machinery or driving). Effects with other sedative drugs or ethanol may be potentiated. Elderly may be more sensitive to CNS depressant and constipating effects. May cause respiratory depression - use caution in patients with respiratory disease or pre-existing respiratory depression. Hypersensitivity reactions, including bronchospasm, angioneurotic edema, and anaphylactic shock, have also been reported. Potential for drug dependency exists, abrupt cessation may precipitate withdrawal. Use caution in elderly, debilitated, cachectic, pediatric patients, depression or suicidal tendencies. Tolerance, psychological and physical dependence may occur with prolonged use. Partial antagonist activity may precipitate acute opioid withdrawal in opioid-dependent individuals.

After chronic maternal exposure to opioids, neonatal withdrawal syndrome may occur in the newborn; monitor neonate closely. Signs and symptoms include irritability, hyperactivity and abnormal sleep pattern, high pitched cry, tremor, vomiting, diarrhea and failure to gain weight. Onset, duration and severity depend on the drug used, duration of use, maternal dose, and rate of drug elimination by the newborn. Opioid withdrawal syndrome in the neonate, unlike in adults, may be life-threatening and should be treated according to protocols developed by neonatology experts.

Hepatitis has been reported with buprenorphine use; hepatic events ranged from transient, asymptomatic transaminase elevations to hepatic failure; in many cases, patients had pre-existing hepatic dysfunction. Monitor liver function tests in patients at increased risk for hepatotoxicity (eg, history of alcohol abuse, pre-existing hepatic dysfunction, I.V. drug abusers) prior to and during therapy. Use with caution in patients with hepatic impairment; dosage adjustments are recommended in hepatic impairment.

Use with caution in patients with pulmonary or renal function impairment. Also use caution in ▶

patients with head injury or increased ICP, biliary tract dysfunction, pancreatitis, patients with history of hyperthyroidism, morbid obesity, adrenal insufficiency, prostatic hyperplasia, urinary stricture, toxic psychosis, pancreatitis, alcoholism, delirium tremens, or kyphoscoliosis. Avoid use in patients with CNS depression or coma as these patients are susceptible to intracranial effects of CO_2 retention. May cause hypotension; use with caution in patients with hypovolemia, cardiovascular disease (including acute MI), or drugs which may exaggerate hypotensive effects (including phenothiazines or general anesthetics). May obscure diagnosis or clinical course of patients with acute abdominal conditions. Use with caution in patients with a history of ileus or bowel obstruction; use of transdermal patch is contraindicated in patients with known or suspected paralytic ileus. Opioid therapy may lower seizure threshold; use caution in patients with a history of seizure disorders. Potentially significant drug-drug interactions may exist, requiring dose or frequency adjustment, additional monitoring, and/or selection of alternative therapy.

Transdermal patch: Indicated for the management of chronic moderate-to-severe pain when around the clock pain control is needed for an extended time period; should not be used for as-needed pain relief or for the treatment of mild pain, acute pain, or postoperative pain requiring short-term opioid analgesia. **[U.S. Boxed Warning]: May cause potentially life-threatening respiratory depression even with therapeutic use. Ensure proper dosing and titration; monitor for respiratory depression, especially within the first 24-72 hours of initiation or dose escalation. Buprenorphine transdermal patches should only be prescribed by healthcare professionals familiar with the use of potent opioids for chronic pain.** Do not exceed one 20 **mcg**/hour transdermal patch due to the risk of QTc-interval prolongation. Avoid using in patients with history of long QT syndrome or in patients with predisposing factors increasing the risk of QT abnormalities (eg, concurrent medications such as antiarrhythmics, hypokalemia, unstable heart failure, unstable atrial fibrillation). **[U.S. Boxed Warning]: Healthcare provider should be alert to problems of abuse, misuse, and diversion.** Risk of opioid abuse is increased in patients with a history or family history of alcohol or drug abuse or mental illness. **[U.S. Boxed Warning]: Proper storage, handling, and disposal of used patches are essential to prevent accidental exposures, especially in children; accidental exposure may result in a fatal overdose.** To properly dispose of Butrans® patch, fold it over on itself and flush down the toilet; alternatively, seal the used patch in the provided Patch-Disposal Unit and dispose of in the trash. Avoid exposure of application site and surrounding area to direct external heat sources. Buprenorphine release from the patch is temperature-dependent and may result

in overdose. Patients who experience fever or increase in core temperature should be monitored closely. Application site reactions, including rare cases of severe reactions (eg, vesicles, discharge, "burns"), have been observed with use; onset varies from days to months after initiation; patients should be instructed to report severe reactions promptly. Therapy with the transdermal patch is not appropriate for use in the management of addictions.

Concurrent use of agonist/antagonist analgesics may precipitate withdrawal symptoms and/or reduced analgesic efficacy in patients following prolonged therapy with mu opioid agonists. Abrupt discontinuation following prolonged use may also lead to withdrawal symptoms and is not recommended; taper dose gradually when discontinuing.

Sublingual tablets, which are used for induction treatment of opioid dependence, should not be started until effects of withdrawal are evident.

Drug Interactions

Avoid Concomitant Use

Avoid concomitant use of Buprenorphine with any of the following: Atazanavir; Azelastine (Nasal); Conivaptan; Fusidic Acid (Systemic); MAO Inhibitors; Paraldehyde; Thalidomide

Decreased Effect

Buprenorphine may decrease the levels/effects of: Analgesics (Opioid); Atazanavir; Pegvisomant

The levels/effects of Buprenorphine may be decreased by: Ammonium Chloride; Boceprevir; Bosentan; CYP3A4 Inducers (Strong); Dabrafenib; Deferasirox; Efavirenz; Etravirine; Herbs (CYP3A4 Inducers); Mitotane; Mixed Agonist / Antagonist Opioids; Tocilizumab

Increased Effect/Toxicity

Buprenorphine may increase the levels/effects of: Alvimopan; ARIPiprazole; Azelastine (Nasal); Desmopressin; Diuretics; MAO Inhibitors; Metyrosine; Mirtazapine; Paraldehyde; Pramipexole; ROPINIRole; Rotigotine; Selective Serotonin Reuptake Inhibitors; Thalidomide; Zolpidem

The levels/effects of Buprenorphine may be increased by: Alcohol (Ethyl); Amphetamines; Anticholinergics; Antipsychotic Agents (Phenothiazines); Atazanavir; Boceprevir; Brimonidine (Topical); Cannabinoids; CNS Depressants; Conivaptan; CYP3A4 Inhibitors (Moderate); CYP3A4 Inhibitors (Strong); Dasatinib; Doxylamine; Droperidol; Fusidic Acid (Systemic); HydrOXYzine; Ivacaftor; Luliconazole; Magnesium Sulfate; Mifepristone; Perampanel; Simeprevir; Sodium Oxybate; Stiripentol; Succinylcholine

Nutritional/Ethanol Interactions

Ethanol: May increase CNS depression; monitor for increased effects with coadministration. Caution patients about effect.

Herb/Nutraceutical: Avoid valerian, St John's wort, kava kava, gotu kola (may increase CNS depression).

Adverse Reactions

Injection:

>10%: Central nervous system: Sedation (≤66%)

1% to 10%:

Cardiovascular: Hypotension (1% to 5%)

Central nervous system: Dizziness/vertigo (5% to 10%), headache (1% to 5%)

Gastrointestinal: Nausea (5% to 10%), vomiting (1% to 5%)

Ocular: Miosis (1% to 5%)

Respiratory: Respiratory depression (1% to 5%)

Miscellaneous: Diaphoresis (1% to 5%)

Tablet:

>10%:

Central nervous system: Headache (30%), pain (24%), insomnia (21% to 25%), anxiety (12%), depression (11%)

Gastrointestinal: Nausea (10% to 14%), abdominal pain (12%), constipation (8% to 11%)

Neuromuscular & skeletal: Back pain (14%), weakness (14%)

Respiratory: Rhinitis (11%)

Miscellaneous: Withdrawal syndrome (18% to 22%; placebo 37%), infection (12% to 20%), diaphoresis (12% to 13%)

1% to 10%:

Central nervous system: Chills (6%), nervousness (6%), somnolence (5%), dizziness (4%), fever (3%)

Gastrointestinal: Vomiting (5% to 8%), diarrhea (5%), dyspepsia (3%)

Local: Abscess formation (2%)

Ocular: Lacrimation (5%)

Respiratory: Cough (4%), pharyngitis (4%)

Miscellaneous: Flu-like syndrome (6%)

Transdermal patch:

>10%:

Central nervous system: Headache (3% to 14%), dizziness (2% to 15%), somnolence (2% to 13%)

Gastrointestinal: Nausea (6% to 23%), constipation (3% to 13%)

Local: Application site pruritus (4% to 15%)

1% to 10%:

Cardiovascular: Chest pain (1% to <5%), hypertension (1% to <5%), peripheral edema (1% to <5%)

Central nervous system: Anxiety (1% to <5%), depression (1% to <5%), fatigue (1% to 5%), fever (1% to <5%), hypoesthesia (1% to <5%), insomnia (1% to <5%), migraine (1% to <5%), pain (1% to <5%)

Dermatologic: Hyperhydrosis (1% to <5%), pruritus (1% to <5%), rash (1% to <5%)

Gastrointestinal: Vomiting (4% to 9%), xerostomia (6%), anorexia (1% to <5%), diarrhea (1% to <5%), dyspepsia (1% to <5%), upper abdominal pain (1% to <5%), abdominal discomfort (2%)

Genitourinary: Urinary tract infection (1% to <5%)

Local: Application site erythema (3% to 10%), application site irritation (1% to 6%), application site rash (3% to 8%)

Neuromuscular & skeletal: Arthralgia (1% to <5%), back pain (1% to <5%), joint swelling (1% to <5%), muscle spasms (1% to <5%), musculoskeletal pain (1% to <5%), myalgia (1% to <5%), neck pain (1% to <5%), pain in extremity (1% to <5%), paresthesia (1% to <5%), tremor (1% to <5%), weakness (1% to <5%)

Respiratory: Bronchitis (1% to <5%), cough (1% to <5%), dyspnea (1% to <5%), nasopharyngitis (1% to <5%), pharyngolaryngeal pain (1% to <5%), sinusitis (1% to <5%), upper respiratory tract infection (1% to <5%)

Miscellaneous: Flu-like syndrome (1% to <5%)

Pharmacodynamics/Kinetics

Onset of Action Analgesic: I.M: Within 15 minutes; Peak effect: I.M.: ~1 hour; Transdermal patch: Steady state achieved by day 3

Duration of Action I.M.: ≥6 hours

Controlled Substance C-III

Available Dosage Forms

Patch Weekly, Transdermal:

Butrans: 5 mcg/hr (4 ea); 10 mcg/hr (4 ea); 15 mcg/hr (4 ea); 20 mcg/hr (4 ea)

Solution, Injection:

Buprenex: 0.3 mg/mL (1 mL)

Generic: 0.3 mg/mL (1 mL)

Tablet Sublingual, Sublingual:

Generic: 2 mg, 8 mg

General Dosage Range Dosage adjustment recommended in patients with hepatic impairment.

I.M., I.V.:

Children 2-12 years: 2-6 **mcg**/kg every 4-6 hours

Children ≥13 years and Adults: Initial: 0.3 mg, may repeat once in 30-60 minutes then every 6-8 hours as needed; Maintenance: 0.15-0.6 mg every 4-8 hours as needed

Elderly: 0.15 mg every 6 hours

Sublingual: *Children ≥16 years and Adults:* Induction: 12-16 mg/day; Maintenance: 12-16 mg/day (target dose: 16 mg/day)

Transdermal: *Adults:* 5-20 **mcg**/hour applied once every 7 days (maximum: 20 **mcg**/hour once every 7 days)

Administration

I.M. Administer via deep I.M. injection.

I.V. Administer slowly, over at least 2 minutes. Administration over 20-30 minutes preferred when managing opioid withdrawal in heroin-dependent hospitalized patients (Welsh, 2002).

Injectable Detail pH: 3.5-5.5

Oral Sublingual: Tablet should be placed under the tongue until dissolved; should not be swallowed.

If two or more tablets are needed per dose, all may be placed under the tongue at once, or two at a time. To ensure consistent bioavailability, subsequent doses should always be taken the same way.

Topical Transdermal patch: Apply to patch to intact, nonirritated skin only. Apply to a hairless or nearly hairless skin site. If hairless site is not available, do not shave skin; hair at application site should be clipped. Prior to application, if the site must be cleaned, clean with clear water and allow to dry completely; do not use soaps, alcohol, lotions or abrasives due to potential for increased skin absorption. Do not use any patch that has been damaged, cut or manipulated in any way. Remove patch from protective pouch immediately before application. Remove the protective backing, and apply the sticky side of the patch to one of eight possible application sites (upper outer arm, upper chest, upper back, or the side of the chest [each site on either side of the body]). Firmly press patch in place and hold for ~15 seconds. Change patch every 7 days. Rotate patch application sites; wait ≥21 days before reapplying another patch to the same skin site. Avoid exposing application site to external heat sources (eg, heating pad, electric blanket, heat lamp, hot tub). If there is difficulty with patch adhesion, the edges of the system may be taped in place with first-aid tape. If the patch falls off during the 7-day dosing interval, dispose of the patch and apply a new patch to a different skin site.

Storage/Stability

Injection: Protect from excessive heat >40°C (>104°F). Protect from light.

Patch, tablet: Store at room temperature of 25°C (77°F); excursions permitted between 15°C to 30°C (59°F to 86°F).

Nursing Actions

Physical Assessment Monitor for effectiveness of pain relief. Monitor for possible respiratory depression. Monitor blood pressure, CNS and respiratory status, and degree of sedation prior to treatment and periodically throughout. For inpatients, implement safety measures (eg, side rails up, call light within reach, instructions to call for assistance). Assess patient's physical and/or psychological dependence. Discontinue slowly after prolonged use.

Patient Education

• Discuss specific use of drug and side effects with patient as it relates to treatment. (HCAHPS: During this hospital stay, were you given any medicine that you had not taken before? Before giving you any new medicine, how often did hospital staff tell you what the medicine was for? How often did hospital staff describe possible side effects in a way you could understand?)

• Patient may experience fatigue or nausea. Have patient report immediately to prescriber signs of hepatic impairment, severe dizziness, syncope, dyspnea, hyperhidrosis, tachycardia, bradycardia, arrhythmia, illogical thinking, severe constipation, significant asthenia, anxiety, chills, pharyngitis, change in balance, mood changes, intolerable dyspepsia, bradykinesia, dysarthria, edema of extremities, vision changes, paresthesia, difficulty speaking, angina, difficult urination, hallucinations, arthralgia, myalgia, memory loss, intolerable headache, tremors, injection site irritation, or severe application site irritation (HCAHPS).

• Educate patient about signs of a significant reaction (eg, wheezing; chest tightness; fever; itching; bad cough; blue skin color; seizures; or swelling of face, lips, tongue, or throat). **Note:** This is not a comprehensive list of all side effects. Patient should consult prescriber for additional questions.

Intended Use and Disclaimer: Should not be printed and given to patients. This information is intended to serve as a concise initial reference for healthcare professionals to use when discussing medications with a patient. You must ultimately rely on your own discretion, experience and judgment in diagnosing, treating and advising patients.

Buprenorphine and Naloxone
(byoo pre NOR feen & nal OKS one)

Brand Names: U.S. Suboxone; Zubsolv

Index Terms Buprenorphine Hydrochloride and Naloxone Hydrochloride Dihydrate; Naloxone and Buprenorphine; Naloxone Hydrochloride Dihydrate and Buprenorphine Hydrochloride

Pharmacologic Category Analgesic, Opioid; Analgesic, Opioid Partial Agonist

Medication Safety Issues

High alert medication:

The Institute for Safe Medication Practices (ISMP) includes this medication among its list of drug classes which have a heightened risk of causing significant patient harm when used in error.

Other safety concerns:

Potential for over- or underdosing when switching among various formulations and between strengths of the sublingual films: **Not all strengths of sublingual tablets and films are bioequivalent to one another.** In addition, systemic exposure between the various strengths of sublingual films may be different; pharmacists should not substitute one or more film strengths for another (eg, dispense three 4 mg films for one 12 mg film, or vice-versa) without physician approval. Any patient switching between sublingual tablet and sublingual film formulation or between one or more strengths of the sublingual films should be monitored for over- or underdosing.

Medication Guide Available Yes

Pregnancy Risk Factor C

Breast-Feeding Considerations Buprenorphine and its active metabolite, norbuprenorphine, are excreted in breast milk. It is not known if naloxone is excreted into breast milk, however, systemic absorption following oral administration is low (Smith, 2012) and any exposure of naloxone to a nursing infant would therefore be limited.

In general, breast-feeding is not recommended by the manufacturers of buprenorphine-containing products; the manufacturer of Zubsolv buprenorphine and naloxone sublingual tablets recommends that caution be exercised when administering this specific combination product to nursing women. See individual agents.

Use

Opioid dependence: For the maintenance treatment of opioid dependence.

General information: Buprenorphine/naloxone should be used as part of a complete treatment plan to include counseling and psychosocial support

Mechanism of Action/Effect See individual agents.

Contraindications Hypersensitivity to buprenorphine, naloxone, or any component of the formulation

Documentation of allergenic cross-reactivity for opioids is limited. However, because of similarities in chemical structure and/or pharmacologic actions, the possibility of cross-sensitivity cannot be ruled out with certainty.

Warnings/Precautions See individual agents.

Drug Interactions

Avoid Concomitant Use

Avoid concomitant use of Buprenorphine and Naloxone with any of the following: Atazanavir; Azelastine (Nasal); Conivaptan; Fusidic Acid (Systemic); MAO Inhibitors; Paraldehyde; Thalidomide

Decreased Effect

Buprenorphine and Naloxone may decrease the levels/effects of: Analgesics (Opioid); Atazanavir; Pegvisomant

The levels/effects of Buprenorphine and Naloxone may be decreased by: Ammonium Chloride; Boceprevir; Bosentan; CYP3A4 Inducers (Strong); Dabrafenib; Deferasirox; Efavirenz; Etravirine; Herbs (CYP3A4 Inducers); Mitotane; Mixed Agonist / Antagonist Opioids; Tocilizumab

Increased Effect/Toxicity

Buprenorphine and Naloxone may increase the levels/effects of: Alvimopan; ARIPiprazole; Azelastine (Nasal); Desmopressin; Diuretics; MAO Inhibitors; Metyrosine; Mirtazapine; Paraldehyde; Pramipexole; ROPINIRole; Rotigotine; Selective Serotonin Reuptake Inhibitors; Thalidomide; Zolpidem

The levels/effects of Buprenorphine and Naloxone may be increased by: Alcohol (Ethyl); Amphetamines; Anticholinergics; Antipsychotic Agents (Phenothiazines); Atazanavir; Boceprevir; Brimonidine (Topical); Cannabinoids; CNS Depressants; Conivaptan; CYP3A4 Inhibitors (Moderate); CYP3A4 Inhibitors (Strong); Dasatinib; Doxylamine; Droperidol; Fusidic Acid (Systemic); HydrOXYzine; Ivacaftor; Luliconazole; Magnesium Sulfate; Mifepristone; Perampanel; Simeprevir; Sodium Oxybate; Stiripentol; Succinylcholine

Nutritional/Ethanol Interactions

Ethanol: May increase CNS depression. Management: Avoid ethanol. Monitor for increased effects with coadministration. Caution patients about effect.

Herb/Nutraceutical: St John's wort may decrease the levels/effects of buprenorphine. Some herbal medications should be avoided due to the risk of increased CNS depression. Management: Avoid concomitant use of St John's wort, valerian, kava kava, and gotu kola.

Adverse Reactions Also see individual agents.

>10%:

Central nervous system: Headache (36%), pain (22%)

Gastrointestinal: Vomiting (8%), erythema (oral mucosa; film), glossodynia (film), oral hypoesthesia (film)

Miscellaneous: Withdrawal syndrome (25%; placebo 37%), diaphoresis (14%)

1% to 10%:

Cardiovascular: Vasodilation (9%)

Gastrointestinal: Vomiting (7%)

Controlled Substance C-III

Available Dosage Forms

Film, sublingual:

Suboxone: Buprenorphine 2 mg and naloxone 0.5 mg; buprenorphine 4 mg and naloxone 1 mg; buprenorphine 8 mg and naloxone 2 mg; buprenorphine 12 mg and naloxone 3 mg

Tablet, sublingual: Buprenorphine 2 mg and naloxone 0.5 mg; buprenorphine 8 mg and naloxone 2 mg

Zubsolv: Buprenorphine 1.4 mg and naloxone 0.36 mg; buprenorphine 5.7 mg and naloxone 1.4 mg

General Dosage Range Sublingual: *Children ≥16 years and Adults:* **Note:** Doses provided based on buprenorphine content: 2.8-24 mg daily (target dose: 11.4-16 mg daily)

Administration

Oral

Sublingual film: Film should be placed under the tongue. Keep under the tongue until film dissolves completely; film should not be chewed, swallowed or moved after placement. If more than one film is needed, the additional film should be placed under the tongue on the opposite side from the first film.

Sublingual tablet: Tablet should be placed under the tongue until dissolved; should not be swallowed. If two or more tablets are needed per dose, all may be placed under the tongue at once, or two at a time. In patients requiring more than one Zubsolv sublingual tablet, place all tablets in different places under the tongue at the same time. To ensure consistent bioavailability, subsequent doses should always be taken the same way. Patients should not eat or drink anything until the tablet(s) are completely dissolved. If a sequential mode of administration is preferred, patients should follow the same manner of dosing with continued use of the product, to ensure consistency in bioavailability.

Storage/Stability Store at 25°C (77°F); excursions are permitted between 15°C and 30°C (59°F and 86°F).

Nursing Actions

Physical Assessment Monitor for hypersensitivity reactions and signs of opioid withdrawal or drug abuse. Monitor liver function test. Caution use while driving or operating hazardous machinery.

Patient Education

- Discuss specific use of drug and side effects with patient as it relates to treatment. (HCAHPS: During this hospital stay, were you given any medicine that you had not taken before? Before giving you any new medicine, how often did hospital staff tell you what the medicine was for? How often did hospital staff describe possible side effects in a way you could understand?)
- Patient may experience fatigue, nausea, headache, insomnia, paresthesia of mouth, application site pain or irritation. Have patient report immediately to prescriber signs of hepatic impairment, severe dizziness, syncope, dyspnea, hyperhidrosis, illogical thinking, considerable constipation, vision changes, significant asthenia, anxiety, chills, pharyngitis, arrhythmia, change in balance, mood changes, intolerable dyspepsia, bradykinesia, dysarthria, or edema of extremities (HCAHPS).
- Educate patient about signs of a significant reaction (eg, wheezing; chest tightness; fever; itching; bad cough; blue skin color; seizures; or swelling of face, lips, tongue, or throat). **Note:** This is not a comprehensive list of all side effects. Patient should consult prescriber for additional questions.

Intended Use and Disclaimer: Should not be printed and given to patients. This information is intended to serve as a concise initial reference for healthcare professionals to use when discussing medications with a patient. You must ultimately rely on your own discretion, experience and judgment in diagnosing, treating and advising patients.

Related Information

Buprenorphine *on page 213*
Naloxone *on page 1098*

BuPROPion (byoo PROE pee on)

Brand Names: U.S. Aplenzin; Budeprion SR [DSC]; Buproban; Forfivo XL; Wellbutrin; Wellbutrin SR; Wellbutrin XL; Zyban

Index Terms Bupropion Hydrobromide; Bupropion Hydrochloride

Pharmacologic Category Antidepressant, Dopamine-Reuptake Inhibitor; Smoking Cessation Aid

Medication Safety Issues

Sound-alike/look-alike issues:

Aplenzin™ may be confused with Albenza®, Relenza®

BuPROPion may be confused with busPIRone

Forfivo™ XL may be confused with Forteo®

Wellbutrin XL® may be confused with Wellbutrin SR®

Zyban® may be confused with Diovan®

Medication Guide Available Yes

Pregnancy Risk Factor C

Lactation Enters breast milk

Breast-Feeding Considerations Bupropion and its metabolites are excreted into breast milk. The estimated dose to a nursing infant varies by study and has been reported as ~2% of the weight-adjusted maternal dose (range: 1.4% to 10.6%) (Davis, 2009; Haas, 2004). Adverse events have been reported with some antidepressants and a seizure was noted in one 6-month old nursing infant exposed to bupropion (a causal effect could not be confirmed) (Chaudron, 2004; Hale, 2010). Recommendations for use in nursing women vary by manufacturer labeling.

Use Treatment of major depressive disorder, including seasonal affective disorder (SAD); adjunct in smoking cessation (Buproban®, Zyban®)

Unlabeled Use Attention-deficit/hyperactivity disorder (ADHD); depression associated with bipolar disorder

Mechanism of Action/Effect Antidepressant structurally different from all other marketed antidepressants; like other antidepressants the mechanism of bupropion's activity is not fully understood; relatively weak inhibitor of the neuronal uptake of norepinephrine and dopamine

Contraindications Hypersensitivity to bupropion or any component of the formulation; seizure disorder; history of anorexia/bulimia; patients undergoing abrupt discontinuation of ethanol or sedatives, including benzodiazepines; use of MAO inhibitors or MAO inhibitors intended to treat psychiatric disorders (concurrently or within 14 days of discontinuing either bupropion or the MAO inhibitor); initiation of bupropion in a patient receiving linezolid or intravenous methylene blue; patients receiving other dosage forms of bupropion

Aplenzin™: Additional contraindications: Other conditions that increase seizure risk, including arteriovenous malformation, severe head injury, severe stroke, CNS tumor, CNS infection, or abrupt discontinuation of barbiturates or antiepileptics

Warnings/Precautions [U.S. Boxed Warning]: Use in treating psychiatric disorders: Antidepressants increase the risk of suicidal thinking and behavior in children, adolescents, and young adults (18-24 years of age) with major depressive disorder (MDD) and other psychiatric disorders; consider risk prior to prescribing. Short-term studies did not show an increased risk in patients >24 years of age and showed a decreased risk in patients ≥65 years. All patients must be closely monitored for clinical worsening, suicidality, or unusual changes in behavior, especially during the initiation of therapy (generally first 1-2 months) or following an increase or decrease in dosage. The patient's family or caregiver should be instructed to closely observe the patient and communicate condition with healthcare provider. A medication guide should be dispensed with each prescription. **Bupropion is not FDA approved for use in children.**

[U.S. Boxed Warning]: Use in smoking cessation: Serious neuropsychiatric events, including depression, suicidal thoughts, and suicide, have been reported with use; some cases may have been complicated by symptoms of nicotine withdrawal following smoking cessation. Smoking cessation (with or without treatment) is associated with nicotine withdrawal symptoms and the exacerbation of underlying psychiatric illness; however, some of the behavioral disturbances were reported in treated patients who continued to smoke. These neuropsychiatric symptoms (eg, mood disturbances, psychosis, hostility) have occurred in patients with and without pre-existing psychiatric disease; many cases resolved following therapy discontinuation although in some cases, symptoms persisted. Monitor all patients for behavioral changes and psychiatric symptoms (eg, agitation, depression, suicidal behavior, suicidal ideation); inform patients to discontinue treatment and contact their healthcare provider immediately if they experience any behavioral and/or mood changes.

The possibility of a suicide attempt is inherent in major depression and may persist until remission occurs. Use caution in high-risk patients. Worsening depression and severe abrupt suicidality that are not part of the presenting symptoms may require discontinuation or modification of drug therapy. The patient's family or caregiver should be alerted to monitor patients for the emergence of suicidality and associated behaviors (such as agitation, irritability, hostility, impulsivity, and hypomania) and notify the healthcare provider.

May worsen psychosis in some patients or precipitate a shift to mania or hypomania in patients with bipolar disorder. Patients presenting with depressive symptoms should be screened for bipolar disorder. Monotherapy in patients with bipolar disorder should be avoided. **Bupropion is not FDA approved for bipolar depression.**

May cause a dose-related risk of seizures. Use is contraindicated in patients with a history of seizures or certain conditions with high seizure risk (eg, arteriovenous malformation, severe head injury, severe stroke, CNS tumor, or CNS infection, history of anorexia/bulimia, or patients undergoing abrupt discontinuation of ethanol, benzodiazepines, barbiturates, or antiepileptic drugs). Use caution with concurrent use of antipsychotics, antidepressants, theophylline, systemic corticosteroids, stimulants (including cocaine), anorectants, or hypoglycemic agents, or with excessive use of ethanol, benzodiazepines, sedative/hypnotics, or opioids. Use with caution in seizure-potentiating metabolic disorders (hypoglycemia, hyponatremia, severe hepatic impairment, and hypoxia). The dose-dependent risk of seizures may be reduced by gradual dose increases and limiting the daily dose to bupropion hydrochloride ≤450 mg or bupropion hydrobromide ≤522 mg. Use of multiple bupropion formulations is contraindicated. Permanently discontinue if seizure occurs during therapy. Chewing, crushing, or dividing long-acting products may increase seizure risk.

May cause CNS stimulation (restlessness, anxiety, insomnia) or anorexia. May increase the risks associated with electroconvulsive therapy (ECT). Consider discontinuing, when possible, prior to ECT. May cause weight loss; use caution in patients where weight loss is not desirable. The incidence of sexual dysfunction with bupropion is generally lower than with SSRIs.

Use caution in patients with cardiovascular disease, history of hypertension, or coronary artery disease; treatment-emergent hypertension (including some severe cases) has been reported, both with bupropion alone and in combination with nicotine transdermal systems. All children diagnosed with ADHD who may be candidates for stimulant medications should have a thorough cardiovascular assessment to identify risk factors for sudden cardiac death prior to initiation of drug therapy. Use with caution in patients with hepatic or renal dysfunction and in elderly patients; reduced dose and/or frequency may be recommended. Elderly patients may be at greater risk of accumulation during chronic dosing. May cause motor or cognitive impairment in some patients; use with caution if tasks requiring alertness such as operating machinery or driving are undertaken. Anaphactoid/anaphylactic reactions have occurred, with symptoms of pruritus, urticaria, angioedema, and dyspnea. Serious reactions have been (rarely) reported, including Stevens-Johnson syndrome and anaphylactic shock. Arthralgia, myalgia, and fever with rash and other symptoms suggestive of delayed hypersensitivity resembling serum sickness have been reported. Potentially significant interactions may exist, requiring dose or frequency adjustment, additional monitoring, and/or selection of alternative therapy.

Extended release tablet: Insoluble tablet shell may remain intact and be visible in the stool.

Drug Interactions

Avoid Concomitant Use

Avoid concomitant use of BuPROPion with any of the following: MAO Inhibitors; Pimozide; Tamoxifen; Thioridazine

Decreased Effect

BuPROPion may decrease the levels/effects of: Codeine; Iloperidone; Ioflupane I 123; Tamoxifen; TraMADol

The levels/effects of BuPROPion may be decreased by: CYP2B6 Inducers (Strong); Dabrafenib; Efavirenz; Lopinavir; Peginterferon Alfa-2b; Ritonavir

Increased Effect/Toxicity

BuPROPion may increase the levels/effects of: Alcohol (Ethyl); ARIPiprazole; AtoMOXetine; CYP2D6 Substrates; DOXOrubicin (Conventional); Fesoterodine; FLUoxetine; FluvoxaMINE; Iloperidone; Lorcaserin; Metoprolol; Nebivolol; PARoxetine; Pimozide; Propafenone; Tetrabenazine; Thioridazine; Tricyclic Antidepressants; Vortioxetine

The levels/effects of BuPROPion may be increased by: Alcohol (Ethyl); Anti-Parkinson's Agents (Dopamine Agonist); CYP2B6 Inhibitors (Moderate); CYP2B6 Inhibitors (Strong); MAO Inhibitors; Mifepristone; Quazepam

Nutritional/Ethanol Interactions

Ethanol: May increase CNS depression; monitor for increased effects with coadministration. Caution patients about effects.

Herb/Nutraceutical: Avoid valerian, St John's wort, SAMe, gotu kola, kava kava (may increase CNS depression).

Adverse Reactions
Frequencies, when reported, reflect highest incidence reported with sustained release product.

>10%:
Cardiovascular: Tachycardia (11%)
Central nervous system: Headache (25% to 34%), insomnia (11% to 20%), dizziness (6% to 11%)
Gastrointestinal: Xerostomia (17% to 26%), weight loss (14% to 23%), nausea (1% to 18%)
Respiratory: Pharyngitis (3% to 13%)
1% to 10%:
Cardiovascular: Palpitation (2% to 6%), arrhythmias (5%), chest pain (3% to 4%), hypertension (2% to 4%; may be severe), flushing (1% to 4%), hypotension (3%)

Central nervous system: Agitation (2% to 9%), confusion (8%), anxiety (5% to 7%), hostility (6%), nervousness (3% to 5%), sleep disturbance (4%), sensory disturbance (4%), migraine (1% to 4%), abnormal dreams (3%), irritability (2% to 3%), somnolence (2% to 3%), pain (2% to 3%), memory decreased (≤3%), fever (1% to 2%), CNS stimulation (1% to 2%), depression
Dermatologic: Rash (1% to 5%), pruritus (2% to 4%), urticaria (1% to 2%)
Endocrine & metabolic: Menstrual complaints (2% to 5%), hot flashes (1% to 3%), libido decreased (3%)
Gastrointestinal: Constipation (5% to 10%), abdominal pain (2% to 9%), diarrhea (5% to 7%), flatulence (6%), anorexia (3% to 5%), appetite increased (4%), taste perversion (2% to 4%), vomiting (2% to 4%), dyspepsia (3%), dysphagia (≤2%)
Genitourinary: Polyuria (2% to 5%), urinary urgency (≤2%), vaginal hemorrhage (≤2%), UTI (≤1%)
Neuromuscular & skeletal: Tremor (3% to 6%), myalgia (2% to 6%), weakness (2% to 4%), arthralgia (1% to 4%), arthritis (2%), akathisia (≤2%), paresthesia (1% to 2%), twitching (1% to 2%), neck pain
Ocular: Blurred vision (2% to 3%), amblyopia (2%)
Otic: Tinnitus (3% to 6%), auditory disturbance (5%)
Respiratory: Upper respiratory infection (9%), cough increased (1% to 4%), sinusitis (1% to 5%)
Miscellaneous: Infection (8% to 9%), diaphoresis (5% to 6%), allergic reaction (including anaphylaxis, pruritus, urticaria)

Available Dosage Forms

Tablet, Oral:
Wellbutrin: 75 mg, 100 mg
Generic: 75 mg, 100 mg
Tablet Extended Release 12 Hour, Oral:
Buproban: 150 mg
Wellbutrin SR: 100 mg, 150 mg, 200 mg
Zyban: 150 mg
Generic: 100 mg, 150 mg, 200 mg
Tablet Extended Release 24 Hour, Oral:
Aplenzin: 174 mg, 348 mg, 522 mg
Forfivo XL: 450 mg
Wellbutrin XL: 150 mg, 300 mg
Generic: 150 mg, 300 mg

General Dosage Range
Dosage adjustment recommended in patients with hepatic impairment
Oral:
Extended release: *Adults:* Initial: Hydrochloride salt: Initial: 150 mg once daily; Maintenance: 300 mg once daily (maximum: 450 mg daily); Hydrobromide salt: Initial: 174 mg once daily (maximum: 522 mg daily)

Immediate release hydrochloride salt: *Adults:* Initial: 100 mg twice daily; Maintenance: 100 mg 3 times daily (maximum: 450 mg daily)

Sustained release hydrochloride salt: *Adults:* Initial: 150 mg once daily; Maintenance: 150 mg twice daily (maximum: 400 mg daily)

Administration

Oral May be taken without regard to meals. Sustained release and extended release tablets (hydrochloride and hydrobromide salt formulations) should be swallowed whole; do not crush, chew, or divide. The insoluble shell of the extended-release tablet may remain intact during GI transit and is eliminated in the feces.

Storage/Stability Store at controlled room temperature of 20°C to 25°C (68°F to 77°F). Aplenzin™, Wellbutrin XL®: Store at 15°C to 30°C (59°F to 86°F).

Nursing Actions

Physical Assessment Monitor blood pressure at beginning of therapy and periodically throughout treatment. Monitor mental status for clinical worsening, such as changes in behavior, hostility, agitation, paranoia, hallucinations, depression, and suicidality, especially at the beginning of therapy or when dose changes occur.

Patient Education

- Discuss specific use of drug and side effects with patient as it relates to treatment. (HCAHPS: During this hospital stay, were you given any medicine that you had not taken before? Before giving you any new medicine, how often did hospital staff tell you what the medicine was for? How often did hospital staff describe possible side effects in a way you could understand?)
- Patient may experience dizziness, fatigue, dyspepsia, tremors, nightmares, nausea, constipation, xerostomia, diarrhea, insomnia, rhinitis, pharyngitis, hyperhidrosis, lack of appetite, or tablet shell in stool. Have patient report immediately to prescriber signs of hepatic impairment, signs of depression (ie, suicidal ideation, considerable anxiety, emotional instability, illogical thinking), behavioral changes, hallucinations, akathisia, severe headache, excessive weight gain or loss, angina, arrhythmia, tinnitus, vision changes, polyuria, enlarged lymph nodes, bradykinesia, significant arthralgia, intolerable myalgia, or signs of Stevens-Johnson syndrome/toxic epidermal necrolysis (HCAHPS).
- Educate patient about signs of a significant reaction (eg, wheezing; chest tightness; fever; itching; bad cough; blue skin color; seizures; or swelling of face, lips, tongue, or throat). **Note:** This is not a comprehensive list of all side effects. Patient should consult prescriber for additional questions.

Intended Use and Disclaimer: Should not be printed and given to patients. This information is intended to serve as a concise initial reference for healthcare professionals to use when discussing medications with a patient. You must ultimately rely on your own discretion, experience and judgment in diagnosing, treating and advising patients.

Related Information

Oral Medications That Should Not Be Crushed or Altered *on page 1712*

BusPIRone (byoo SPYE rone)

Index Terms BuSpar; Buspirone Hydrochloride

Pharmacologic Category Antianxiety Agent, Miscellaneous

Medication Safety Issues

Sound-alike/look-alike issues:

BusPIRone may be confused with buPROPion

Pregnancy Risk Factor B

Lactation Excretion in breast milk unknown/not recommended

Breast-Feeding Considerations It is not known if buspirone is excreted in breast milk. Breast-feeding is not recommended by the manufacturer.

Use Management of generalized anxiety disorder (GAD)

Unlabeled Use Augmentation agent for antidepressants

Mechanism of Action/Effect The mechanism of action of buspirone is unknown. Buspirone has a high affinity for serotonin 5-HT$_{1A}$ and 5-HT$_2$ receptors, without affecting benzodiazepine-GABA receptors. Buspirone has moderate affinity for dopamine D$_2$ receptors.

Contraindications Hypersensitivity to buspirone or any component of the formulation

Warnings/Precautions Use in severe hepatic or renal impairment is not recommended. Low potential for cognitive or motor impairment; until effects on patient known, patients should be warned to use caution when performing tasks which require mental alertness (eg, operating machinery or driving). Use with MAO inhibitors may result in hypertensive reactions; concurrent use is not recommended. Restlessness syndrome has been reported in small number of patients; may be attributable to buspirone's antagonism of central dopamine receptors. Monitor for signs of any dopamine-related movement disorders (eg, dystonia, akathisia, pseudo-parkinsonism). Buspirone does not exhibit cross-tolerance with benzodiazepines or other sedative/hypnotic agents. If substituting buspirone for any of these agents, gradually withdraw the drug(s) prior to initiating buspirone.

Drug Interactions

Avoid Concomitant Use

Avoid concomitant use of BusPIRone with any of the following: Azelastine (Nasal); Conivaptan; Fusidic Acid (Systemic); MAO Inhibitors; Methylene Blue; Paraldehyde; Thalidomide

Decreased Effect

BusPIRone may decrease the levels/effects of: Ioflupane I 123

The levels/effects of BusPIRone may be decreased by: Bosentan; CYP3A4 Inducers (Strong); Dabrafenib; Deferasirox; Mitotane; Peginterferon Alfa-2b; Rifamycin Derivatives; Tocilizumab; Yohimbine

Increased Effect/Toxicity

BusPIRone may increase the levels/effects of: Alcohol (Ethyl); Antidepressants (Serotonin Reuptake Inhibitor/Antagonist); Antipsychotics; Azelastine (Nasal); Buprenorphine; CNS Depressants; Hydrocodone; MAO Inhibitors; Methylene Blue; Metoclopramide; Metyrosine; Paraldehyde; Pramipexole; ROPINIRole; Rotigotine; Selective Serotonin Reuptake Inhibitors; Serotonin Modulators; Thalidomide; Zolpidem

The levels/effects of BusPIRone may be increased by: Antifungal Agents (Azole Derivatives, Systemic); Antipsychotics; Brimonidine (Topical); Calcium Channel Blockers (Nondihydropyridine); Conivaptan; CYP3A4 Inhibitors (Moderate); CYP3A4 Inhibitors (Strong); Dasatinib; Doxylamine; Fusidic Acid (Systemic); Grapefruit Juice; HydrOXYzine; Ivacaftor; Luliconazole; Macrolide Antibiotics; Magnesium Sulfate; Mifepristone; Perampanel; Selective Serotonin Reuptake Inhibitors; Simeprevir; Sodium Oxybate; Stiripentol

Nutritional/Ethanol Interactions

Ethanol: Ethanol may increase CNS depression. Management: Monitor for increased effects with coadmiistration. Caution patients about effects.

Food: Food may decrease the absorption of buspirone, but it may also decrease the first-pass metabolism, thereby increasing the bioavailability of buspirone. Grapefruit juice may cause increased buspirone concentrations. Management: Administer with or without food, but must be consistent. Avoid intake of large quantities of grapefruit juice.

Herb/Nutraceutical: St John's wort may decrease buspirone levels or increase CNS depression. Kava kava, valerian, and gotu kola may increase CNS depression; yohimbe may diminish the therapeutic effect of buspirone. Management: Avoid St John's wort, kava kava, valerian, gotu kola, and yohimbe.

Adverse Reactions

>10%: Central nervous system: Dizziness (12%)

1% to 10%:

Cardiovascular: Chest pain (≥1%)

Central nervous system: Drowsiness (10%), headache (6%), nervousness (5%), lightheadedness (3%), anger/hostility (2%), confusion (2%), excitement (2%), dream disturbance (≥1%)

Dermatologic: Rash (1%)

Gastrointestinal: Nausea (8%), diarrhea (2%)

Neuromuscular & skeletal: Numbness (2%), weakness (2%), incoordination (1%), musculoskeletal pain (1%), paresthesia (1%), tremor (1%)

Ocular: Blurred vision (2%)

Otic: Tinnitus (≥1%)

Respiratory: Nasal congestion (≥1%), sore throat (≥1%)

Miscellaneous: Diaphoresis (1%)

Available Dosage Forms

Tablet, Oral:

Generic: 5 mg, 7.5 mg, 10 mg, 15 mg, 30 mg

General Dosage Range Oral: *Adults:* Initial: 7.5 mg twice daily; Maintenance: Up to 30 mg twice daily (usual dose: 10-15 mg twice daily)

Administration

Oral May be administered with or without food, but must be consistent.

Storage/Stability Store at 25°C (77°F); excursions permitted between 15°C to 30°C (59°F to 86°F). Protect from light.

Nursing Actions

Patient Education

- Discuss specific use of drug and side effects with patient as it relates to treatment. (HCAHPS: During this hospital stay, were you given any medicine that you had not taken before? Before giving you any new medicine, how often did hospital staff tell you what the medicine was for? How often did hospital staff describe possible side effects in a way you could understand?)

- Patient may experience dizziness, fatigue, anxiety, headache, or dyspepsia. Have patient report immediately to prescriber mood changes, depression, difficulty with motor activity, fasciculations, change in balance, dysphagia, difficulty speaking, illogical thinking, angina, nightmares, tinnitus, tachycardia, arrhythmia, or vision changes (HCAHPS).

- Educate patient about signs of a significant reaction (eg, wheezing; chest tightness; fever; itching; bad cough; blue skin color; seizures; or swelling of face, lips, tongue, or throat). **Note:** This is not a comprehensive list of all side effects. Patient should consult prescriber for additional questions.

Intended Use and Disclaimer: Should not be printed and given to patients. This information is intended to serve as a concise initial reference for healthcare professionals to use when discussing medications with a patient. You must ultimately rely on your own discretion, experience and judgment in diagnosing, treating and advising patients.

Dietary Considerations May be taken with or without food, but must be consistent. Avoid large quantities of grapefruit juice.

Busulfan (byoo SUL fan)

Brand Names: U.S. Busulfex; Myleran

Index Terms Bussulfam; Busulfanum; Busulphan

Pharmacologic Category Antineoplastic Agent, Alkylating Agent

Medication Safety Issues

Sound-alike/look-alike issues:
Myleran® may be confused with Alkeran®, Leukeran®, melphalan, Mylicon®

High alert medication:
This medication is in a class the Institute for Safe Medication Practices (ISMP) includes among its list of drug classes which have a heightened risk of causing significant patient harm when used in error.

Pregnancy Risk Factor D

Lactation Excretion in breast milk unknown/not recommended

Breast-Feeding Considerations According to the manufacturer, the decision to continue or discontinue breast-feeding during therapy should take into account the risk of exposure to the infant and the benefits of treatment to the mother.

Use Palliative treatment of chronic myelogenous leukemia (CML) (oral); conditioning regimen prior to allogeneic hematopoietic progenitor cell transplantation (I.V.) for CML

Unlabeled Use Conditioning regimen prior to hematopoietic stem cell transplant (HSCT) (oral); treatment of polycythemia vera and essential thrombocytosis

Mechanism of Action/Effect Alkylating agent which reacts with the N-7 position of guanosine and interferes with DNA replication and RNA transcription. Interferes with the normal function of DNA by alkylation and cross-linking the strands of DNA.

Contraindications Hypersensitivity to busulfan or any component of the formulation; oral busulfan is contraindicated in patients without a definitive diagnosis of CML

Warnings/Precautions Hazardous agent - use appropriate precautions for handling and disposal (NIOSH, 2012). **[U.S. Boxed Warning]: Severe bone marrow suppression is common; reduce dose or discontinue oral busulfan for unusual suppression; may require bone marrow biopsy.** May result in severe neutropenia, thrombocytopenia, anemia, bone marrow failure, and/or pancytopenia; pancytopenia may be prolonged (1 month up to 2 years) and may be reversible. Use with caution in patients with compromised bone marrow reserve (due to prior treatment or radiation therapy). Monitor closely for signs of infection (due to neutropenia) or bleeding (due to thrombocytopenia) Seizures have been reported with use; use caution in patients predisposed to seizures, history of seizures or head trauma; when using as a conditioning regimen for transplant, initiate prophylactic anticonvulsant therapy (eg, phenytoin) prior to treatment. Phenytoin increases busulfan clearance by ≥15%; busulfan kinetics and dosing recommendations for high-dose HSCT conditioning

were studied with concomitant phenytoin. If alternate anticonvulsants are used, busulfan clearance may be decreased and dosing should be monitored accordingly.

Bronchopulmonary dysplasia with pulmonary fibrosis ("busulfan lung") is associated with busulfan; onset is delayed with symptoms occurring at an average of 4 years (range: 4 months to 10 years) after treatment; may be fatal. Symptoms generally include a slow onset of cough, dyspnea, and fever (low-grade), although acute symptomatic onset may also occur. Diminished diffusion capacity and decreased pulmonary compliance have been noted with pulmonary function testing. Differential diagnosis should rule out opportunistic pulmonary infection or leukemic pulmonary infiltrates; may require lung biopsy. Discontinue busulfan if toxicity develops. Pulmonary toxicity may be additive if administered with other cytotoxic agents also associated with pulmonary toxicity. Cardiac tamponade as been reported in children with thalassemia treated with high-dose oral busulfan in combination with cyclophosphamide. Busulfan has been causally related to the development of secondary malignancies (tumors and acute leukemias); chromosomal alterations may also occur. Busulfan has been associated with ovarian failure (including failure to achieve puberty).

High busulfan area under the concentration versus time curve (AUC) values (>1500 micromolar•minute) are associated with increased risk of hepatic sinusoidal obstruction syndrome (SOS; formerly called veno-occlusive disease [VOD]) due to conditioning for allogenic HSCT; patients with a history of radiation therapy, prior chemotherapy (≥3 cycles), or prior stem cell transplantation are at increased risk; monitor liver function tests periodically. Oral busulfan doses above 16 mg/kg (based on IBW) and concurrent use with alkylating agents may also increase the risk for hepatic SOS. The solvent in I.V. busulfan, DMA, may impair fertility. DMA may also be associated with hepatotoxicity, hallucinations, somnolence, lethargy, and confusion. **[U.S. Boxed Warning]: Should be administered under the supervision of an experienced cancer chemotherapy physician; for the I.V. formulation, should be experienced in management of HSCT and management of patients with severe pancytopenia; according to the manufacturer, oral busulfan should not be used until CML diagnosis has been established.** Cellular dysplasia in many organs has been observed (in addition to lung dysplasia); giant hyperchromatic nuclei have been noted in adrenal glands, liver, lymph nodes, pancreas, thyroid, and bone marrow. May obscure routine diagnostic cytologic exams (eg, cervical smear).

Drug Interactions

Avoid Concomitant Use

Avoid concomitant use of Busulfan with any of the following: BCG; CloZAPine; Natalizumab; Pimecrolimus; Tacrolimus (Topical); Tofacitinib; Vaccines (Live)

Decreased Effect

Busulfan may decrease the levels/effects of: BCG; Coccidioidin Skin Test; Sipuleucel-T; Vaccines (Inactivated); Vaccines (Live); Vitamin K Antagonists

The levels/effects of Busulfan may be decreased by: Echinacea; Fosphenytoin; Phenytoin

Increased Effect/Toxicity

Busulfan may increase the levels/effects of: CloZAPine; Ifosfamide; Leflunomide; Natalizumab; Tofacitinib; Vaccines (Live); Vitamin K Antagonists

The levels/effects of Busulfan may be increased by: Acetaminophen; Antifungal Agents (Azole Derivatives, Systemic); Denosumab; MetroNIDAZOLE (Systemic); Pimecrolimus; Roflumilast; Tacrolimus (Topical); Trastuzumab

Nutritional/Ethanol Interactions

Ethanol: Avoid ethanol due to GI irritation.

Food: No clear or firm data on the effect of food on busulfan bioavailability.

Herb/Nutraceutical: Avoid St John's wort (may decrease busulfan levels).

Adverse Reactions

I.V.:

>10%:

Cardiovascular: Tachycardia (44%), hypertension (36%; grades 3/4: 7%), edema (28% to 79%), thrombosis (33%), chest pain (26%), vasodilation (25%), hypotension (11%; grades 3/4: 3%)

Central nervous system: Insomnia (84%), fever (80%), anxiety (72% to 75%), headache (69%), chills (46%), pain (44%), dizziness (30%), depression (23%), confusion (11%)

Dermatologic: Rash (57%), pruritus (28%), alopecia (17%)

Endocrine & metabolic: Hypomagnesemia (77%), hyperglycemia (66% to 67%; grades 3/4: 15%), hypokalemia (64%), hypocalcemia (49%), hypophosphatemia (17%)

Gastrointestinal: Vomiting (43% to 100%), nausea (83% to 98%), mucositis/stomatitis (79% to 97%; grades 3/4: 26%), anorexia (85%), diarrhea (84%; grades 3/4: 5%), abdominal pain (72%), dyspepsia (44%), constipation (38%), xerostomia (26%), rectal disorder (25%), abdominal fullness (23%)

Hematologic: Myelosuppression (≤100%), neutropenia (100%; onset: 4 days; median recovery: 13 days [with G-CSF support]), thrombocytopenia (98%; median onset: 5-6 days), lymphopenia (children: 79%), anemia (69%)

Hepatic: Hyperbilirubinemia (49%; grades 3/4: 30%), ALT increased (31%; grades 3/4: 7%), hepatic sinusoidal obstruction syndrome (SOS; veno-occlusive disease) (adults: 8% to 12%; children: 21%), alkaline phosphatase increased (15%), jaundice (12%)

Local: Injection site inflammation (25%), injection site pain (15%)

Neuromuscular & skeletal: Weakness (51%), back pain (23%), myalgia (16%), arthralgia (13%)

Renal: Creatinine increased (21%), oliguria (15%)

Respiratory: Rhinitis (44%), lung disorder (34%), cough (28%), epistaxis (25%), dyspnea (25%), pneumonia (children: 21%), hiccup (18%), pharyngitis (18%)

Miscellaneous: Infection (51%; includes severe bacterial, viral [CMV], and fungal infections), allergic reaction (26%)

1% to 10%:

Cardiovascular: Arrhythmia (5%), cardiomegaly (5%), atrial fibrillation (2%), ECG abnormal (2%), heart block (2%), heart failure (grade 3/4: 2%), pericardial effusion (2%), tamponade (children with thalassemia: 2%), ventricular extrasystoles (2%), hypervolemia

Central nervous system: Lethargy (7%), hallucination (5%), agitation (2%), delirium (2%), encephalopathy (2%), seizure (2%), somnolence (2%), cerebral hemorrhage (1%)

Dermatologic: Vesicular rash (10%), vesiculobullous rash (10%), skin discoloration (8%), maculopapular rash (8%), acne (7%), exfoliative dermatitis (5%), erythema nodosum (2%)

Endocrine & metabolic: Hyponatremia (2%)

Gastrointestinal: Ileus (8%), weight gain (8%), esophagitis (grade 3: 2%), hematemesis (2%), pancreatitis (2%)

Hematologic: Prothrombin time increased (2%)

Hepatic: Hepatomegaly (6%)

Renal: Hematuria (8%), dysuria (7%), hemorrhagic cystitis (grade 3/4: 7%), BUN increased (3%; grades 3/4: 2%)

Respiratory: Asthma (8%), alveolar hemorrhage (5%), hyperventilation (5%), hemoptysis (3%), pleural effusion (3%), sinusitis (3%), atelectasis (2%), hypoxia (2%)

Oral: Frequency not defined:

Dermatologic: Hyperpigmentation of skin (5% to 10%), rash

Endocrine & metabolic: Amenorrhea, ovarian suppression

Gastrointestinal: Xerostomia

Hematologic: Myelosuppression (anemia, leukopenia, thrombocytopenia)

Available Dosage Forms

Solution, Intravenous:

Busulfex: 6 mg/mL (10 mL)

Tablet, Oral:

Myleran: 2 mg

General Dosage Range
I.V.:
Children ≤12 kg: **HSCT:** 1.1 mg/kg (actual body weight) every 6 hours for 16 doses
Children >12 kg: **HSCT:** 0.8 mg/kg (actual body weight) every 6 hours for 16 doses
Adults: **HSCT:** 0.8 mg/kg every 6 hours for 16 doses (use ideal body weight or actual body weight, whichever is lower; use adjusted body weight if obese)
Oral: Dosage adjustment is recommended in patients who experience toxicity:
Children: Induction: 60 mcg/kg/day **or** 1.8 mg/m²/day; Maintenance: Resume induction dose **or** 1-3 mg/day
Adults: Induction: 60 mcg/kg/day **or** 1.8 mg/m²/day; usual range: 4-8 mg/day; Maintenance: Resume induction dose **or** 1-3 mg/day

Administration
I.V. Intravenous busulfan should be infused over 2 hours via central line. Flush line before and after each infusion with 5 mL D₅W or NS. Do not use polycarbonate syringes or filters for preparation or administration

Hazardous agent; use appropriate precautions for handling and disposal (NIOSH, 2012).

Oral HSCT only: To facilitate ingestion of high oral doses, may insert multiple tablets into gelatin capsules.

Hazardous agent; use appropriate precautions for handling and disposal (NIOSH, 2012).

Preparation for Administration Hazardous agent; use appropriate precautions for handling and disposal (NIOSH, 2012). Injection: Dilute NS or D₅W. The dilution volume should be 10 times the volume of busulfan injection, ensuring that the final concentration of busulfan is 0.5 mg/mL. Always add busulfan to the diluent, and not the diluent to the busulfan. Mix with several inversions. Do not use polycarbonate syringes or filters for preparation or administration.

Storage/Stability
Injection: Store intact vials under refrigeration at 2°C to 8°C (36°F to 46°F). Solutions diluted in sodium chloride (NS) injection or dextrose 5% in water (D₅W) for infusion are stable for up to 8 hours at room temperature (25°C [77°F]); the infusion must also be completed within that 8-hour timeframe. Dilution of busulfan injection in NS is stable for up to 12 hours at refrigeration (2°C to 8°C); the infusion must be completed within that 12-hour timeframe.
Tablet: Store at 25°C (77°F); excursions permitted to 15°C to 30°C (59°F to 86°F).

Nursing Actions
Physical Assessment HSCT: Phenytoin or clonazepam may be ordered prophylactically during and for at least 48 hours following completion of busulfan to reduce risk of seizures if patient is predisposed to seizures. Assess CBC with differential, platelet count, and LFTs. Monitor for pulmonary fibrosis or toxicity, adverse hematologic effects, pancytopenia, leukopenia, thrombocytopenia, anemia, and bone marrow suppression during therapy and for several months following therapy.

Patient Education
- Discuss specific use of drug and side effects with patient as it relates to treatment. (HCAHPS: During this hospital stay, were you given any medicine that you had not taken before? Before giving you any new medicine, how often did hospital staff tell you what the medicine was for? How often did hospital staff describe possible side effects in a way you could understand?)
- Patient may experience skin discoloration, xerostomia, anxiety, back pain, constipation, flushing, hiccups, arthralgia, myalgia, rhinorrhea, insomnia, stomatitis, lack of appetite, or diarrhea. Have patient report immediately to prescriber signs of infection, signs of hemorrhaging, signs of hepatic impairment, dyspepsia, severe nausea, ecchymosis, significant asthenia, angina, illogical thinking, dyspnea, vision changes, weight change, amenorrhea, signs of hyperglycemia, signs of electrolyte imbalance, urinary retention, oliguria, depression, intolerable dizziness, syncope, tachycardia, severe headache, edema of extremities, or edema (HCAHPS).
- Educate patient about signs of a significant reaction (eg, wheezing; chest tightness; fever; itching; bad cough; blue skin color; seizures; or swelling of face, lips, tongue, or throat). **Note:** This is not a comprehensive list of all side effects. Patient should consult prescriber for additional questions.

Intended Use and Disclaimer: Should not be printed and given to patients. This information is intended to serve as a concise initial reference for healthcare professionals to use when discussing medications with a patient. You must ultimately rely on your own discretion, experience and judgment in diagnosing, treating and advising patients.

Related Information
Management of Drug Extravasations *on page 1700*

Butalbital, Acetaminophen, and Caffeine (byoo TAL bi tal, a seet a MIN oh fen, & KAF een)

Brand Names: U.S. Alagesic LQ; Dolgic Plus; Esgic; Esgic-Plus; Fioricet; Margesic; Orbivan [DSC]; Repan; Zebutal

Index Terms Acetaminophen, Butalbital, and Caffeine

Pharmacologic Category Barbiturate

◀ **Medication Safety Issues**
Sound-alike/look-alike issues:
Fioricet may be confused with Fiorinal, Florinef, Lorcet, Percocet
Repan may be confused with Riopan
BEERS Criteria medication:
This drug may be potentially inappropriate for use in geriatric patients (Quality of evidence - high; Strength of recommendation - strong).
Other safety concerns:
Duplicate therapy issues: This product contains acetaminophen, which may be a component of other combination products. Do not exceed the maximum recommended daily dose of acetaminophen.
Pregnancy Risk Factor C
Lactation Enters breast milk/not recommended
Use Tension or muscle contraction headache:
Relief of symptom complex of tension or muscle contraction headache
Available Dosage Forms
Capsule, oral: Butalbital 50 mg, acetaminophen 300 mg, and caffeine 40 mg
Esgic: Butalbital 50 mg, acetaminophen 325 mg, and caffeine 40 mg
Esgic-Plus: Butalbital 50 mg, acetaminophen 500 mg, and caffeine 40 mg
Fioricet: Butalbital 50 mg, acetaminophen 300 mg, and caffeine 40 mg
Margesic: Butalbital 50 mg, acetaminophen 325 mg, and caffeine 40 mg
Zebutal: Butalbital 50 mg, acetaminophen 325 mg, and caffeine 40 mg; Butalbital 50 mg, acetaminophen 500 mg, and caffeine 40 mg
Liquid, oral:
Alagesic LQ: Butalbital 50 mg, acetaminophen 325 mg, and caffeine 40 mg per 15 mL
Tablet, oral: Butalbital 50 mg, acetaminophen 325 mg, and caffeine 40 mg; butalbital 50 mg, acetaminophen 500 mg, and caffeine 40 mg
Dolgic Plus: Butalbital 50 mg, acetaminophen 750 mg, and caffeine 40 mg
Esgic, Repan: Butalbital 50 mg, acetaminophen 325 mg, and caffeine 40 mg
Esgic-Plus: Butalbital 50 mg, acetaminophen 500 mg, and caffeine 40 mg
General Dosage Range Oral: *Adults:* 1-2 tablets/capsules or 15-30 mL solution every 4 hours (maximum: 6 tablets/capsules daily or 90 mL solution daily)
Nursing Actions
Physical Assessment See individual agents.
Patient Education
• Discuss specific use of drug and side effects with patient as it relates to treatment. (HCAHPS: During this hospital stay, were you given any medicine that you had not taken before? Before giving you any new medicine, how often did hospital staff tell you what the medicine was for? How often did hospital staff describe possible side effects in a way you could understand?)

• Patient may experience fatigue, dyspepsia, or nausea. Have patient report immediately to prescriber signs of hepatic impairment, illogical thinking, change in balance, considerable anxiety, severe dizziness, syncope, significant asthenia, tachycardia, chills, pharyngitis, mood changes, paresthesia, dyspnea, ecchymosis, hemorrhaging, urinary retention, oliguria, tremors, or signs of Stevens-Johnson syndrome/toxic epidermal necrolysis (HCAHPS).
• Educate patient about signs of a significant reaction (eg, wheezing; chest tightness; fever; itching; bad cough; blue skin color; seizures; or swelling of face, lips, tongue, or throat). **Note:** This is not a comprehensive list of all side effects. Patient should consult prescriber for additional questions.

Intended Use and Disclaimer: Should not be printed and given to patients. This information is intended to serve as a concise initial reference for healthcare professionals to use when discussing medications with a patient. You must ultimately rely on your own discretion, experience and judgment in diagnosing, treating and advising patients.
Related Information
Acetaminophen *on page 31*
Caffeine *on page 232*

Butalbital, Acetaminophen, Caffeine, and Codeine
(byoo TAL bi tal, a seet a MIN oh fen, KAF een, & KOE deen)

Brand Names: U.S. Fioricet with Codeine
Index Terms Acetaminophen, Caffeine, Codeine, and Butalbital; Caffeine, Acetaminophen, Butalbital, and Codeine; Codeine, Acetaminophen, Butalbital, and Caffeine
Pharmacologic Category Analgesic Combination (Opioid); Barbiturate
Medication Safety Issues
Sound-alike/look-alike issues:
Fioricet may be confused with Fiorinal, Florinef, Lorcet, Percocet
Phrenilin may be confused with Phenergan
High alert medication:
The Institute for Safe Medication Practices (ISMP) includes this medication among its list of drug classes which have a heightened risk of causing significant patient harm when used in error.
Other safety concerns:
Duplicate therapy issues: This product contains acetaminophen, which may be a component of other combination products. Do not exceed the maximum recommended daily dose of acetaminophen.
Pregnancy Risk Factor C
Lactation Enters breast milk/not recommended

Use Relief of symptoms of complex tension (muscle contraction) headache

Controlled Substance C-III

Available Dosage Forms

Capsule, oral: Butalbital 50 mg, acetaminophen 300 mg, caffeine 40 mg, and codeine phosphate 30 mg; Butalbital 50 mg, acetaminophen 325 mg, caffeine 40 mg, and codeine 30 mg

Fioricet with Codeine: Butalbital 50 mg, acetaminophen 300 mg, caffeine 40 mg, and codeine 30 mg

General Dosage Range Oral: *Adults:* 1-2 capsules every 4 hours (maximum: 6 capsules per day)

Nursing Actions

Physical Assessment See individual agents.

Patient Education

• Discuss specific use of drug and side effects with patient as it relates to treatment. (HCAHPS: During this hospital stay, were you given any medicine that you had not taken before? Before giving you any new medicine, how often did hospital staff tell you what the medicine was for? How often did hospital staff describe possible side effects in a way you could understand?)

• Patient may experience dyspepsia, fatigue, or nausea. Have patient report immediately to prescriber signs of hepatic impairment, severe dizziness, syncope, change in balance, illogical thinking, intolerable anxiety, significant asthenia, considerable constipation, urinary retention, oliguria, tachycardia, bradycardia, arrhythmia, chills, pharyngitis, mood changes, paresthesia, tinnitus, intolerable headache, dyspnea, tremors, ecchymosis, hemorrhaging, vision changes, or signs of Stevens-Johnson syndrome/toxic epidermal necrolysis (HCAHPS).

• Educate patient about signs of a significant reaction (eg, wheezing; chest tightness; fever; itching; bad cough; blue skin color; seizures; or swelling of face, lips, tongue, or throat). **Note:** This is not a comprehensive list of all side effects. Patient should consult prescriber for additional questions.

Intended Use and Disclaimer: Should not be printed and given to patients. This information is intended to serve as a concise initial reference for healthcare professionals to use when discussing medications with a patient. You must ultimately rely on your own discretion, experience and judgment in diagnosing, treating and advising patients.

Related Information

Acetaminophen *on page 31*
Caffeine *on page 232*
Codeine *on page 363*

Butalbital and Acetaminophen
(byoo TAL bi tal & a seet a MIN oh fen)

Brand Names: U.S. Bupap; Orviban CF; Phrenilin Forte; Promacet

Index Terms Acetaminophen and Butalbital

Pharmacologic Category Analgesic, Miscellaneous; Barbiturate

Medication Safety Issues

Other safety concerns:

Duplicate therapy issues: This product contains acetaminophen, which may be a component of other combination products. Do not exceed the maximum recommended daily dose of acetaminophen.

Pregnancy Risk Factor C

Lactation Enters breast milk/not recommended

Use Relief of the symptomatic complex of tension or muscle contraction headache

Available Dosage Forms

Tablet, oral: Butalbital 50 mg and acetaminophen 325 mg

Promacet: Butalbital 50 mg and acetaminophen 650 mg

Bupap, Orbivan CF: Butalbital 50 mg and acetaminophen 300 mg

Capsule, oral:

Phrenilin Forte: Butalbital 50 mg and acetaminophen 650 mg

General Dosage Range Oral: *Children ≥12 years and Adults:*

Butalbital 50 mg and acetaminophen 300-325 mg: 1-2 tablets every 4 hours as needed (maximum: 6 tablets/24 hours)

Butalbital 50 mg and acetaminophen 650 mg: One tablet/capsule every 4 hours as needed (maximum: 6 doses/24 hours)

Nursing Actions

Physical Assessment See individual agents.

Patient Education

• Discuss specific use of drug and side effects with patient as it relates to treatment. (HCAHPS: During this hospital stay, were you given any medicine that you had not taken before? Before giving you any new medicine, how often did hospital staff tell you what the medicine was for? How often did hospital staff describe possible side effects in a way you could understand?)

• Patient may experience fatigue, dyspepsia, or nausea. Have patient report immediately to prescriber signs of hepatic impairment, change in balance, illogical thinking, significant asthenia, severe dizziness, syncope, tachycardia, chills, pharyngitis, mood changes, paresthesia, dyspnea, ecchymosis, hemorrhaging, or signs of ▶

◄ Stevens-Johnson syndrome/toxic epidermal necrolysis (HCAHPS).
- Educate patient about signs of a significant reaction (eg, wheezing; chest tightness; fever; itching; bad cough; blue skin color; seizures; or swelling of face, lips, tongue, or throat). **Note:** This is not a comprehensive list of all side effects. Patient should consult prescriber for additional questions.

Intended Use and Disclaimer: Should not be printed and given to patients. This information is intended to serve as a concise initial reference for healthcare professionals to use when discussing medications with a patient. You must ultimately rely on your own discretion, experience and judgment in diagnosing, treating and advising patients.

Related Information
Acetaminophen *on page 31*
PHENobarbital *on page 1237*

Butalbital, Aspirin, and Caffeine
(byoo TAL bi tal, AS pir in, & KAF een)

Brand Names: U.S. Fiorinal®
Index Terms Aspirin, Caffeine, and Butalbital; Butalbital Compound
Pharmacologic Category Barbiturate
Medication Safety Issues
Sound-alike/look-alike issues:
Fiorinal® may be confused with Fioricet®, Florical®, Florinef®
Pregnancy Risk Factor C
Lactation Enters breast milk/not recommended
Use Relief of the symptomatic complex of tension or muscle contraction headache
Controlled Substance C-III
Available Dosage Forms
Capsule: Butalbital 50 mg, aspirin 325 mg, and caffeine 40 mg
Fiorinal®: Butalbital 50 mg, aspirin 325 mg, and caffeine 40 mg
General Dosage Range Oral: *Adults:* 1-2 tablets/capsules every 4 hours (maximum: 6 tablets/capsules daily)
Nursing Actions
Physical Assessment See individual agents.
Patient Education
- Discuss specific use of drug and side effects with patient as it relates to treatment. (HCAHPS: During this hospital stay, were you given any medicine that you had not taken before? Before giving you any new medicine, how often did hospital staff tell you what the medicine was for? How often did hospital staff describe possible side effects in a way you could understand?)
- Patient may experience fatigue, dizziness, flatulence, or nausea. Have patient report immediately to prescriber change in balance, illogical thinking, considerable anxiety, tachycardia,

ecchymosis, hemorrhaging, severe dyspepsia, melena, hematemesis, significant asthenia, tinnitus, hearing impairment, or signs of Stevens-Johnson syndrome/toxic epidermal necrolysis (HCAHPS).
- Educate patient about signs of a significant reaction (eg, wheezing; chest tightness; fever; itching; bad cough; blue skin color; seizures; or swelling of face, lips, tongue, or throat). **Note:** This is not a comprehensive list of all side effects. Patient should consult prescriber for additional questions.

Intended Use and Disclaimer: Should not be printed and given to patients. This information is intended to serve as a concise initial reference for healthcare professionals to use when discussing medications with a patient. You must ultimately rely on your own discretion, experience and judgment in diagnosing, treating and advising patients.

Related Information
Aspirin *on page 129*
Caffeine *on page 232*

Butalbital, Aspirin, Caffeine, and Codeine (byoo TAL bi tal, AS pir in, KAF een, & KOE deen)

Brand Names: U.S. Ascomp® with Codeine; Fiorinal® with Codeine
Index Terms Aspirin, Caffeine, Codeine, and Butalbital; Butalbital Compound and Codeine; Codeine and Butalbital Compound; Codeine, Butalbital, Aspirin, and Caffeine
Pharmacologic Category Analgesic Combination (Opioid); Barbiturate
Medication Safety Issues
Sound-alike/look-alike issues:
Fiorinal® may be confused with Fioricet®, Florical®, Florinef®
High alert medication:
The Institute for Safe Medication Practices (ISMP) includes this medication among its list of drug classes which have a heightened risk of causing significant patient harm when used in error.
Pregnancy Risk Factor C
Lactation Enters breast milk/not recommended
Use Relief of symptoms of complex tension (muscle contraction) headache
Controlled Substance C-III
Available Dosage Forms
Capsule: Butalbital 50 mg, aspirin 325 mg, caffeine 40 mg, and codeine 30 mg
Ascomp® with Codeine, Fiorinal® with Codeine: Butalbital 50 mg, aspirin 325 mg, caffeine 40 mg, and codeine 30 mg
General Dosage Range Oral: *Adults:* 1-2 capsules every 4 hours as needed (maximum: 6 capsules per day)

Nursing Actions

Physical Assessment See individual agents.

Patient Education

- Discuss specific use of drug and side effects with patient as it relates to treatment. (HCAHPS: During this hospital stay, were you given any medicine that you had not taken before? Before giving you any new medicine, how often did hospital staff tell you what the medicine was for? How often did hospital staff describe possible side effects in a way you could understand?)
- Patient may experience dizziness, fatigue, or dyspepsia. Have patient report immediately to prescriber dyspnea, illogical thinking, severe anxiety, ecchymosis, hemorrhaging, tinnitus, or signs of abdominal ulcers (HCAHPS).
- Educate patient about signs of a significant reaction (eg, wheezing; chest tightness; fever; itching; bad cough; blue skin color; seizures; or swelling of face, lips, tongue, or throat). **Note:** This is not a comprehensive list of all side effects. Patient should consult prescriber for additional questions.

Intended Use and Disclaimer: Should not be printed and given to patients. This information is intended to serve as a concise initial reference for healthcare professionals to use when discussing medications with a patient. You must ultimately rely on your own discretion, experience and judgment in diagnosing, treating and advising patients.

Related Information
Aspirin *on page 129*
Caffeine *on page 232*
Codeine *on page 363*

Butorphanol (byoo TOR fa nole)

Index Terms Butorphanol Tartrate; Stadol
Pharmacologic Category Analgesic, Opioid; Analgesic, Opioid Partial Agonist
Medication Safety Issues
  Sound-alike/look-alike issues:
  Stadol may be confused with Haldol®, sotalol
  High alert medication:
  The Institute for Safe Medication Practices (ISMP) includes this medication among its list of drug classes which have a heightened risk of causing significant patient harm when used in error.

Pregnancy Risk Factor C
Lactation Enters breast milk
Use
Parenteral: Management of pain when the use of an opioid analgesic is appropriate; preoperative or preanesthetic medication; supplement to balanced anesthesia; management of pain during labor.
Nasal spray: Management of pain when the use of an opioid analgesic is appropriate.

Controlled Substance C-IV
Available Dosage Forms
  Solution, Injection:
  Generic: 1 mg/mL (1 mL); 2 mg/mL (1 mL, 2 mL, 10 mL)
  Solution, Injection [preservative free]:
  Generic: 1 mg/mL (1 mL); 2 mg/mL (1 mL)
  Solution, Nasal:
  Generic: 10 mg/mL (2.5 mL)
General Dosage Range Dosage adjustment recommended in patients with hepatic or renal impairment
  I.M.:
  Adults: Initial: 2 mg, may repeat every 3-4 hours as needed; Usual range: 1-4 mg every 3-4 hours as needed **or** 2 mg prior to surgery
  Elderly: Initial: 1/2 of the recommended dose, repeated dosing generally should be at least 6 hours apart
  I.V.:
  Adults: Initial: 1 mg, may repeat every 3-4 hours as needed; Usual range: 0.5-2 mg every 3-4 hours as needed **or** 2 mg and/or an incremental dose of 0.5-1 mg (up to 0.06 mg/kg) as supplement to surgery
  Elderly: Initial: 1/2 of the recommended dose, repeated dosing generally should be at least 6 hours apart
  Intranasal:
  Adults: Initial: 1 spray (~1 mg) in 1 nostril, may repeat in 60-90 minutes, then repeat initial dose sequence in 3-4 hours after last dose as needed; may use initial dose of 1 spray in each nostril (2 mg) in patients who will remain recumbent
  Elderly: Initial: Should not exceed 1 mg, may repeat after 90-120 minutes

Administration
Injectable Detail pH: 3-5.5
Inhalation Prime pump prior to initial use and if it has not been used for ≥48 hours. Aim spray away from self and others when priming.

Nursing Actions
Physical Assessment Monitor for effectiveness of pain relief. Monitor blood pressure, CNS and respiratory status, and degree of sedation prior to treatment and periodically throughout. For inpatients, implement safety measures (eg, side rails up, call light within reach, instructions to call for assistance). Assess patient's physical and/or psychological dependence. Discontinue slowly after prolonged use.

Patient Education
- Discuss specific use of drug and side effects with patient as it relates to treatment. (HCAHPS: During this hospital stay, were you given any medicine that you had not taken before? Before giving you any new medicine, how often did hospital staff tell you what the medicine was for? How often did hospital staff describe possible side effects in a way you could understand?) ▶

• Patient may experience nausea, constipation, fatigue, rhinitis, or insomnia. Have patient report immediately to prescriber severe dizziness, syncope, dyspnea, illogical thinking, considerable asthenia, arrhythmia, tinnitus, urinary retention, significant headache, hallucinations, or vision changes (HCAHPS).

• Educate patient about signs of a significant reaction (eg, wheezing; chest tightness; fever; itching; bad cough; blue skin color; seizures; or swelling of face, lips, tongue, or throat). **Note:** This is not a comprehensive list of all side effects. Patient should consult prescriber for additional questions.

Intended Use and Disclaimer: Should not be printed and given to patients. This information is intended to serve as a concise initial reference for healthcare professionals to use when discussing medications with a patient. You must ultimately rely on your own discretion, experience and judgment in diagnosing, treating and advising patients.

Cabazitaxel (ca baz i TAKS el)

Brand Names: U.S. Jevtana
Index Terms RPR-116258A; XRP6258
Pharmacologic Category Antineoplastic Agent, Antimicrotubular; Antineoplastic Agent, Taxane Derivative
Medication Safety Issues
Sound-alike/look-alike issues:
Cabazitaxel may be confused with DOCEtaxel, PACLitaxel
Jevtana may be confused with Xgeva, Xofigo, Xtandi, Zometa, Zytiga
High alert medication:
This medication is in a class the Institute for Safe Medication Practices (ISMP) includes among its list of drug classes that have a heightened risk of causing significant patient harm when used in error.
Administration issues:
Cabazitaxel requires a two-step dilution process prior to administration.
Pregnancy Risk Factor D
Lactation Excretion in breast milk unknown/not recommended
Use Prostate cancer: Treatment of hormone-refractory metastatic prostate cancer (in combination with prednisone) in patients previously treated with a docetaxel-containing regimen
Available Dosage Forms
Solution, Intravenous:
Jevtana: 60 mg/1.5 mL (1.5 mL)
General Dosage Range Dosage adjustment recommended in patients with hepatic impairment or who develop toxicities
I.V.: *Adults:* 25 mg/m^2 once every 3 weeks

Administration
I.V. Infuse over 1 hour using a 0.22 micron inline filter. Do not use polyurethane-containing infusion sets for administration. Allow to reach room temperature prior to infusion. Premedicate with an antihistamine, a corticosteroid, and an H$_2$ antagonist at least 30 minutes prior to infusion. Observe closely during infusion (for hypersensitivity). Antiemetic prophylaxis (oral or I.V.) is also recommended.

Hazardous agent; use appropriate precautions for handling and disposal (meets NIOSH, 2012 criteria).

Nursing Actions
Physical Assessment Monitor patient closely for hypersensitivity reaction (rash, erythema, hypotension, bronchospasm); discontinue and notify prescriber. Monitor for hypersensitivity, hypotension, myelosuppression, and GI irritation (including severe diarrhea) prior to, during, and between each infusion.
Patient Education
• Discuss specific use of drug and side effects with patient as it relates to treatment. (HCAHPS: During this hospital stay, were you given any medicine that you had not taken before? Before giving you any new medicine, how often did hospital staff tell you what the medicine was for? How often did hospital staff describe possible side effects in a way you could understand?)

• Patient may experience headache, nausea, lack of appetite, back pain, arthralgia, alopecia, or dysgeusia. Have patient report immediately to prescriber signs of infection, signs of fluid and electrolyte imbalance, strength differences from one side to another, difficulty speaking or thinking, change in balance, blurred vision, severe dizziness, syncope, dyspnea, arrhythmia, considerable dyspepsia, melena, hematemesis, significant constipation, intolerable diarrhea, ecchymosis, hemorrhaging, paresthesia, considerable asthenia, edema of extremities, or signs of renal impairment (HCAHPS).

• Educate patient about signs of a significant reaction (eg, wheezing; chest tightness; fever; itching; bad cough; blue skin color; seizures; or swelling of face, lips, tongue, or throat). **Note:** This is not a comprehensive list of all side effects. Patient should consult prescriber for additional questions.

Intended Use and Disclaimer: Should not be printed and given to patients. This information is intended to serve as a concise initial reference for healthcare professionals to use when discussing medications with a patient. You must ultimately rely on your own discretion, experience and judgment in diagnosing, treating and advising patients.

Cabergoline (ca BER goe leen)

Pharmacologic Category Ergot Derivative
Pregnancy Risk Factor B
Lactation Excretion in breast milk unknown/not recommended
Use Treatment of hyperprolactinemic disorders, either idiopathic or due to pituitary adenomas
Canadian labeling: Additional use (not in U.S. labeling): Prevention of the onset of physiological lactation in the puerperium when clinically indicated (eg, still born baby or neonatal death, conditions that interfere with suckling, severe acute or chronic mental illness). **Note:** Not indicated for suppression of established postpartum lactation.

Available Dosage Forms
Tablet, Oral:
Generic: 0.5 mg
General Dosage Range Oral: *Adults:* Initial: 0.25 mg twice weekly; Maintenance: Up to 1 mg twice weekly

Administration
Oral Administer with meals (may increase tolerability).

Hazardous agent; use appropriate precautions for handling and disposal (NIOSH, 2012).

Nursing Actions
Patient Education
• Discuss specific use of drug and side effects with patient as it relates to treatment. (HCAHPS: During this hospital stay, were you given any medicine that you had not taken before? Before giving you any new medicine, how often did hospital staff tell you what the medicine was for? How often did hospital staff describe possible side effects in a way you could understand?)
• Patient may experience constipation, headache, nausea, or asthenia. Have patient report immediately to prescriber strength differences from one side to another, difficulty speaking or thinking, change in balance, blurred vision, dyspnea, angina, paresthesia, severe dizziness, syncope, behavioral changes, uncontrollable urges, back pain, urinary retention, oliguria, hallucinations, arrhythmia, mood changes, depression, significant dyspepsia, excessive weight gain, edema of extremities, vision changes, or heart valve injury (rare) (HCAHPS).
• Educate patient about signs of a significant reaction (eg, wheezing; chest tightness; fever; itching; bad cough; blue skin color; seizures; or swelling of face, lips, tongue, or throat). **Note:** This is not a comprehensive list of all side effects. Patient should consult prescriber for additional questions.

Intended Use and Disclaimer: Should not be printed and given to patients. This information is intended to serve as a concise initial reference for healthcare professionals to use when discussing medications with a patient. You must ultimately rely on your own discretion, experience and judgment in diagnosing, treating and advising patients.

Cabozantinib (ka boe ZAN ti nib)

Brand Names: U.S. Cometriq™
Index Terms BMS-907351; Cabozantinib s-Malate; XL184
Pharmacologic Category Antineoplastic Agent, Tyrosine Kinase Inhibitor; Antineoplastic Agent, Vascular Endothelial Growth Factor (VEGF) Inhibitor
Medication Safety Issues
Sound-alike/look-alike issues:
Cabozantinib may be confused with axitinib, bosutinib, cabazitaxel, crizotinib, dasatinib, imatinib, nilotinib, regorafenib, ruxolitinib, vandetanib, vemurafenib
Pregnancy Risk Factor D
Lactation Excretion in breast milk unknown/not recommended
Use Treatment of progressive, metastatic medullary thyroid cancer (MTC)
Available Dosage Forms
Capsule, oral:
Cometriq™: 60 mg daily-dose: 20 mg (21s)
Cometriq™: 100 mg daily-dose: 80 mg (7s) and 20 mg (7s)
Cometriq™: 140 mg daily-dose: 80 mg (7s) and 20 mg (21s)
General Dosage Range Dosage adjustment recommended in patients who develop toxicities or on concomitant therapy.
Oral: *Adults:* 140 mg once daily (maximum: 180 mg once daily)
Administration
Oral Administer on an empty stomach (1 hour before or 2 hours after eating). Swallow whole; do not open capsules.

Hazardous agent; use appropriate precautions for handling and disposal (meets NIOSH, 2012 criteria).

Nursing Actions
Physical Assessment Monitor for signs/symptoms of bleeding, fistulas and perforations, or RPLS. Monitor CBC and LFTs. Instruct patients to report signs of palmar-plantar erythema. Monitor blood pressure throughout treatment. Check urine for protein as recommended. Instruct patients to report symptoms of extremity swelling, redness, or pain. Report any shortness of breath due to increased risk of blood clots. Have patient visit dentist regularly.
Patient Education
• Discuss specific use of drug and side effects with patient as it relates to treatment. (HCAHPS: During this hospital stay, were you given any ▶

medicine that you had not taken before? Before giving you any new medicine, how often did hospital staff tell you what the medicine was for? How often did hospital staff describe possible side effects in a way you could understand?)

- Patient may experience leukopenia, thrombocytopenia, hypertension, alopecia, dysgeusia, constipation, or eczema hands and feet. Have patient report immediately to prescriber signs of infection, dyspnea, angina, severe dizziness, syncope, illogical thinking, edema or extremities, significant headache, considerable dyspepsia, intolerable nausea, severe diarrhea, ecchymosis, hemorrhaging, significant asthenia, melena, excessive weight loss, skin changes of hands and feet, poor wound healing, considerable jaw pain, intolerable stomatitis, or sudden vision changes (HCAHPS).
- Educate patient about signs of a significant reaction (eg, wheezing; chest tightness; fever; itching; bad cough; blue skin color; seizures; or swelling of face, lips, tongue, or throat). **Note:** This is not a comprehensive list of all side effects. Patient should consult prescriber for additional questions.

Intended Use and Disclaimer: Should not be printed and given to patients. This information is intended to serve as a concise initial reference for healthcare professionals to use when discussing medications with a patient. You must ultimately rely on your own discretion, experience and judgment in diagnosing, treating and advising patients.

Related Information
Oral Medications That Should Not Be Crushed or Altered *on page 1712*

Caffeine (KAF een)

Brand Names: U.S. Cafcit®; Enerjets [OTC]; No Doz® Maximum Strength [OTC]; Vivarin® [OTC]
Index Terms Caffeine and Sodium Benzoate; Caffeine Citrate; Caffeine Sodium Benzoate; Sodium Benzoate and Caffeine
Pharmacologic Category Central Nervous System Stimulant; Phosphodiesterase Enzyme Inhibitor, Nonselective
Pregnancy Risk Factor C
Lactation Enters breast milk
Use
Caffeine citrate: Treatment of idiopathic apnea of prematurity
Caffeine and sodium benzoate: Treatment of acute respiratory depression (not a preferred agent)
Caffeine [OTC labeling]: Restore mental alertness or wakefulness when experiencing fatigue
Unlabeled Use Caffeine and sodium benzoate: Treatment of spinal puncture headache; CNS stimulant; diuretic; augmentation of seizure induction during electroconvulsive therapy (ECT)

Available Dosage Forms
Caplet:
No Doz® Maximum Strength [OTC]: 200 mg
Injection, solution [preservative free]: 20 mg/mL (3 mL)
Cafcit®: 20 mg/mL (3 mL)
Lozenge:
Enerjets® [OTC]: 75 mg
Solution, oral [preservative free]: 20 mg/mL (3 mL)
Cafcit®: 20 mg/mL
Tablet: 200 mg
Vivarin® [OTC]: 200 mg
General Dosage Range
I.M. (caffeine and sodium benzoate):
Children: 8 mg/kg every 4 hours as needed
Adults: 250 mg as a single dose; may repeat as needed (maximum: 500 mg/dose; 2500 mg/day)
I.V.:
Neonates (caffeine citrate): Loading dose: 10-20 mg/kg; Maintenance: 5 mg/kg once daily
Children (caffeine and sodium benzoate): 8 mg/kg every 4 hours as needed
Adults (caffeine and sodium benzoate): 250 mg as a single dose; may repeat as needed (maximum: 500 mg/dose; 2500 mg/day) **or** 300-2000 mg (electroconvulsive therapy)
Oral:
Neonates (caffeine citrate): Loading dose: 10-20 mg/kg; Maintenance: 5 mg/kg once daily
Children ≥12 years and Adults: 100-200 mg every 3-4 hours as needed (OTC labeling)
SubQ (caffeine and sodium benzoate): *Children:* 8 mg/kg every 4 hours as needed
Administration
I.M. Parenteral: **Caffeine and sodium benzoate:** May administer I.M. undiluted
I.V. Parenteral:
Caffeine citrate: Infuse loading dose over at least 30 minutes; maintenance dose may be infused over at least 10 minutes. May administer without dilution.
Caffeine and sodium benzoate: I.V. as slow direct injection. For spinal headaches, infuse diluted solution over 1 hour. Follow with 1000 mL NS; infuse over 1 hour. May administer I.M. undiluted.
Oral May be administered without regard to feedings or meals. May administer injectable formulation (caffeine citrate) orally.
Nursing Actions
Patient Education
- Discuss specific use of drug and side effects with patient as it relates to treatment. (HCAHPS: During this hospital stay, were you given any medicine that you had not taken before? Before giving you any new medicine, how often did hospital staff tell you what the medicine was for? How often did hospital staff describe possible side effects in a way you could understand?)

- Patient may experience irritability or insomnia. Have patient report immediately to prescriber tachycardia or severe anxiety (HCAHPS).
- Educate patient about signs of a significant reaction (eg, wheezing; chest tightness; fever; itching; bad cough; blue skin color; seizures; or swelling of face, lips, tongue, or throat). **Note:** This is not a comprehensive list of all side effects. Patient should consult prescriber for additional questions.

Intended Use and Disclaimer: Should not be printed and given to patients. This information is intended to serve as a concise initial reference for healthcare professionals to use when discussing medications with a patient. You must ultimately rely on your own discretion, experience and judgment in diagnosing, treating and advising patients.

Calcipotriene (kal si POE try een)

Brand Names: U.S. Calcitrene; Dovonex; Sorilux
Pharmacologic Category Topical Skin Product; Vitamin D Analog
Pregnancy Risk Factor C
Lactation Excretion in breast milk unknown/use caution
Use Treatment of plaque psoriasis of the body (cream, foam, ointment) or of the scalp (foam, solution)
Available Dosage Forms
Cream, External:
Dovonex: 0.005% (60 g, 120 g)
Generic: 0.005% (60 g, 120 g)
Foam, External:
Sorilux: 0.005% (60 g, 120 g)
Ointment, External:
Calcitrene: 0.005% (60 g, 120 g)
Generic: 0.005% (60 g, 120 g)
Solution, External:
Generic: 0.005% (60 mL)
General Dosage Range Topical: *Adults:* Cream: Apply a thin film to affected area twice daily; Foam: Apply a thin film to the affected skin or scalp twice daily; Ointment: Apply a thin film to affected area 1-2 times daily; Solution: Apply to affected scalp twice daily
Administration
Topical For external use only.
Cream, foam, ointment: Apply to affected skin; rub in gently and completely. Wash hands thoroughly before and after use.
Foam, solution: Prior to using, comb hair to remove debris; apply only to scalp lesions. Rub in gently and completely.. Avoid contact with face and eyes (rinse thoroughly with water if contact occurs). Wash hands thoroughly before and after use. Foam should be applied when hair is dry.

Nursing Actions
Physical Assessment When applied to large areas of skin or for extensive periods of time, monitor for adverse skin or systemic reactions.
Patient Education
- Discuss specific use of drug and side effects with patient as it relates to treatment. (HCAHPS: During this hospital stay, were you given any medicine that you had not taken before? Before giving you any new medicine, how often did hospital staff tell you what the medicine was for? How often did hospital staff describe possible side effects in a way you could understand?)
- Patient may experience xeroderma or paresthesia. Have patient report immediately to prescriber signs of hypercalcemia or severe skin irritation (HCAHPS).
- Educate patient about signs of a significant reaction (eg, wheezing; chest tightness; fever; itching; bad cough; blue skin color; seizures; or swelling of face, lips, tongue, or throat). **Note:** This is not a comprehensive list of all side effects. Patient should consult prescriber for additional questions.

Intended Use and Disclaimer: Should not be printed and given to patients. This information is intended to serve as a concise initial reference for healthcare professionals to use when discussing medications with a patient. You must ultimately rely on your own discretion, experience and judgment in diagnosing, treating and advising patients.

Calcipotriene and Betamethasone
(kal si POE try een & bay ta METH a sone)

Brand Names: U.S. Taclonex®
Index Terms Betamethasone Dipropionate and Calcipotriene Hydrate; Calcipotriol and Betamethasone Dipropionate
Pharmacologic Category Corticosteroid, Topical; Vitamin D Analog
Pregnancy Risk Factor C
Lactation Excretion in breast milk unknown/use caution
Use Treatment of plaque psoriasis
Unlabeled Use Treatment of corticosteroid-responsive dermatoses
Available Dosage Forms
Ointment, topical:
Taclonex®: Calcipotriene 0.005% and betamethasone 0.064% (60 g, 100 g)
Suspension, topical:
Taclonex®: Calcipotriene 0.005% and betamethasone 0.064%
General Dosage Range Topical: *Adults:* Apply to affected area once daily (maximum: 100 g weekly)

Administration

Topical Wash hands before and after use.

Gel (Xamiol® [CAN]): Shake well before use. Avoid use of occlusive dressings over treated areas.

Ointment: Rub into affected area gently and completely. Do not apply to face, axillae, or groin.

Suspension: Shake well before use. Do not apply to face, axillae, or groin. If applying to the scalp, do not apply within 12 hours of chemical hair treatment. Do not wash hair directly after use.

Nursing Actions

Physical Assessment See individual agents.

Patient Education

- Discuss specific use of drug and side effects with patient as it relates to treatment. (HCAHPS: During this hospital stay, were you given any medicine that you had not taken before? Before giving you any new medicine, how often did hospital staff tell you what the medicine was for? How often did hospital staff describe possible side effects in a way you could understand?)
- Patient may experience xeroderma. Have patient report immediately to prescriber signs of hyperglycemia, skin changes, severe skin irritation, urinary retention, oliguria, constipation, polydipsia, arrhythmia, mood changes, myalgia, asthenia, nausea, or lack of appetite (HCAHPS).
- Educate patient about signs of a significant reaction (eg, wheezing; chest tightness; fever; itching; bad cough; blue skin color; seizures; or swelling of face, lips, tongue, or throat). **Note:** This is not a comprehensive list of all side effects. Patient should consult prescriber for additional questions.

Intended Use and Disclaimer: Should not be printed and given to patients. This information is intended to serve as a concise initial reference for healthcare professionals to use when discussing medications with a patient. You must ultimately rely on your own discretion, experience and judgment in diagnosing, treating and advising patients.

Related Information

Betamethasone on page 176
Calcipotriene on page 233

Calcitonin (kal si TOE nin)

Brand Names: U.S. Fortical; Miacalcin
Index Terms Calcitonin (Salmon)
Pharmacologic Category Antidote; Hormone
Medication Safety Issues

Sound-alike/look-alike issues:

Calcitonin may be confused with calcitriol
Miacalcin may be confused with Micatin

Administration issues:

Calcitonin nasal spray is administered as a single spray into **one** nostril daily, using alternate nostrils each day.

Pregnancy Risk Factor C
Lactation Excretion in breast milk unknown/not recommended
Use

U.S. labeling: Treatment of symptomatic Paget's disease of bone (osteitis deformans); adjunctive therapy for hypercalcemia; treatment of osteoporosis in women >5 years postmenopause

Canadian labeling: Injection: Treatment of symptomatic Paget's disease of bone (osteitis deformans) in patients who are nonresponsive or intolerant to alternative therapy; adjunctive therapy for hypercalcemia; Intranasal: Treatment of osteoporosis in women >5 years postmenopause

Available Dosage Forms

Solution, Injection:

Miacalcin: 200 units/mL (2 mL)

Solution, Nasal:

Fortical: 200 units/actuation (3.7 mL)
Miacalcin: 200 units/actuation (3.7 mL)
Generic: 200 units/actuation (3.7 mL)

General Dosage Range

I.M., SubQ: *Adults:* Paget's disease/osteoporosis: 50-100 units every 1-2 days; Hypercalcemia: 4-8 units/kg every 12 hours (maximum: 8 units/kg every 6 hours)

Intranasal: *Adults:* 200 units (1 spray) in one nostril daily

Administration

I.M. Injection: May be administered I.M. or SubQ; I.M route is preferred if the injection volume is >2 mL (use multiple injection sites if dose volume is >2 mL).

Subcutaneous Injection: May be administered I.M. or SubQ. SubQ route is preferred for outpatient self-administration unless the injection volume is >2 mL.

Inhalation Nasal spray: Before first use, allow bottle to reach room temperature, then prime pump by releasing at least 5 sprays until full spray is produced. To administer, place nozzle into nostril with head in upright position. Alternate nostrils daily. Do not prime pump before each daily use. Discard after 30 doses.

Nursing Actions

Physical Assessment Teach patient appropriate administration techniques. Monitor for allergic reaction if calcitonin solution (Miacalcin®) used.

Patient Education

- Discuss specific use of drug and side effects with patient as it relates to treatment. (HCAHPS: During this hospital stay, were you given any medicine that you had not taken before? Before giving you any new medicine, how often did hospital staff tell you what the medicine was for? How often did hospital staff describe possible side effects in a way you could understand?)
- Patient may experience rhinorrhea, headache, back pain, arthralgia, flushing, nausea, dyspepsia, parageusia, lack of appetite, polyuria,

CALCITRIOL

diarrhea, or injection site pain or irritation. Have patient report immediately to prescriber severe rhinitis, nasal sores, or epistaxis (HCAHPS).

- Educate patient about signs of a significant reaction (eg, wheezing; chest tightness; fever; itching; bad cough; blue skin color; seizures; or swelling of face, lips, tongue, or throat). **Note:** This is not a comprehensive list of all side effects. Patient should consult prescriber for additional questions.

Intended Use and Disclaimer: Should not be printed and given to patients. This information is intended to serve as a concise initial reference for healthcare professionals to use when discussing medications with a patient. You must ultimately rely on your own discretion, experience and judgment in diagnosing, treating and advising patients.

Calcitriol (kal si TRYE ole)

Brand Names: U.S. Rocaltrol; Vectical
Index Terms 1,25 Dihydroxycholecalciferol
Pharmacologic Category Vitamin D Analog
Medication Safety Issues
Sound-alike/look-alike issues:
Calcitriol may be confused with alfacalcidol, Calciferol™, calcitonin, calcium carbonate, captopril, colestipol, paricalcitol, ropinirole
Administration issues:
Dosage is expressed in mcg (micrograms), **not** mg (milligrams); rare cases of acute overdose have been reported
Pregnancy Risk Factor C
Lactation Enters breast milk/not recommended
Use
Management of hypocalcemia in patients on chronic renal dialysis (oral, injection); management of secondary hyperparathyroidism in patients with chronic kidney disease (CKD) (oral); management of hypocalcemia in patients with hypoparathyroidism and pseudohypoparathyroidism (oral); management of mild-to-moderate plaque psoriasis (topical)
Canadian labeling: Additional uses (not in U.S. labeling): Vitamin D-resistant rickets (oral)
Unlabeled Use Vitamin D-dependent rickets type I/ pseudovitamin D deficiency rickets (PDDR)
Available Dosage Forms
Capsule, Oral:
Rocaltrol: 0.25 mcg, 0.5 mcg
Generic: 0.25 mcg, 0.5 mcg
Ointment, External:
Vectical: 3 mcg/g (100 g)
Generic: 3 mcg/g (100 g)
Solution, Intravenous:
Generic: 1 mcg/mL (1 mL)
Solution, Oral:
Rocaltrol: 1 mcg/mL (15 mL)
Generic: 1 mcg/mL (15 mL)

General Dosage Range Dosage adjustment recommended in patients who develop toxicities
I.V.: *Adults:* 0.5-4 mcg 3 times weekly
Oral:
Children 1 to <3 years: 0.25-0.75 mcg daily **or** 0.01-0.015 mcg/kg/day (maximum: 0.5 mcg daily)
Children ≥3-5 years: 0.25-0.75 mcg daily
Children ≥6 years: 0.25-2 mcg daily
Adults: 0.25 mcg every other day to 2 mcg once daily
Topical: *Adults:* Apply to affected areas twice daily (maximum: 200 g weekly)
Administration
I.V. May be administered as a bolus dose I.V. through the catheter at the end of hemodialysis.
Injectable Detail pH: 5.9-7
Oral May be administered without regard to food. Administer with meals to reduce GI problems.
Topical Apply externally; not for ophthalmic, oral, or intravaginal use. Do not apply to eyes, lips, or facial skins. Rub in gently so that no medication remains visible. Limit application to only the areas of skin affected by psoriasis.
Nursing Actions
Physical Assessment Provide appropriate nutritional counseling.
Patient Education
- Discuss specific use of drug and side effects with patient as it relates to treatment. (HCAHPS: During this hospital stay, were you given any medicine that you had not taken before? Before giving you any new medicine, how often did hospital staff tell you what the medicine was for? How often did hospital staff describe possible side effects in a way you could understand?)
- Have patient report immediately to prescriber signs of hypercalcemia, severe skin irritation, illogical thinking, significant asthenia, behavioral changes, sexual dysfunction, diarrhea, difficult urination, dysuria, polyuria, dizziness, fatigue, xerostomia, eye irritation, flushing, polydipsia, arrhythmia, lack of appetite, mood changes, dysgeusia, myalgia, rhinorrhea, dyspepsia, or excessive weight loss (HCAHPS).
- Educate patient about signs of a significant reaction (eg, wheezing; chest tightness; fever; itching; bad cough; blue skin color; seizures; or swelling of face, lips, tongue, or throat). **Note:** This is not a comprehensive list of all side effects. Patient should consult prescriber for additional questions.

Intended Use and Disclaimer: Should not be printed and given to patients. This information is intended to serve as a concise initial reference for healthcare professionals to use when discussing medications with a patient. You must ultimately rely on your own discretion, experience and judgment in diagnosing, treating and advising patients.

Calcium Chloride (KAL see um KLOR ide)

Pharmacologic Category Calcium Salt; Electrolyte Supplement, Parenteral

Medication Safety Issues

Sound-alike/look-alike issues:
Calcium chloride may be confused with calcium gluconate

Administration issues:
Calcium chloride may be confused with calcium gluconate.

Confusion with the different intravenous salt forms of calcium has occurred. There is a threefold difference in the primary cation concentration between calcium chloride (in which 1 g = 14 mEq [270 mg] of elemental Ca++) and calcium gluconate (in which 1 g = 4.65 mEq [90 mg] of elemental Ca++).

Prescribers should specify which salt form is desired. Dosages should be expressed either as mEq, mg, or grams of the salt form.

Pregnancy Risk Factor C

Use Treatment of hypocalcemia and conditions secondary to hypocalcemia (eg, tetany, seizures, arrhythmias); emergent treatment of severe hypermagnesemia

Unlabeled Use Calcium channel blocker overdose; beta-blocker overdose (refractory to glucagon and high-dose vasopressors); severe hyperkalemia (K+ >6.5 mEq/L with toxic ECG changes) [ACLS guidelines]; malignant arrhythmias (including cardiac arrest) associated with hypermagnesemia [ACLS guidelines]

Dosage Forms Considerations
1 g calcium chloride = elemental calcium 273 mg = calcium 13.6 mEq = calcium 6.8 mmol

Available Dosage Forms

Solution, Intravenous:
Generic: 10% (10 mL)

Solution, Intravenous [preservative free]:
Generic: 10% (10 mL)

General Dosage Range I.V.: *Infants, Children, and Adults:* Dosage varies greatly depending on indication

Administration

I.V. For I.V. administration only. Not for I.M. or SubQ administration (severe necrosis and sloughing may occur). Avoid rapid administration (do not exceed 100 mg/minute except in emergency situations). For intermittent I.V. infusion, infuse diluted solution over 1 hour or no greater than 45-90 mg/kg/hour (0.6-1.2 mEq/kg/hour); administration via a central or deep vein is preferred; do not use scalp, small hand or foot veins for I.V. administration (severe necrosis and sloughing may occur). Monitor ECG if calcium is infused faster than 2.5 mEq/minute; **stop the infusion if the patient complains of pain or discomfort.** Warm solution to body temperature prior to administration. **Do not infuse calcium chloride in the same I.V. line as phosphate-containing solutions.**

Vesicant; ensure proper needle or catheter placement prior to and during I.V. infusion. Avoid extravasation.

Extravasation management: If extravasation occurs, stop infusion immediately and disconnect (leave needle/cannula in place); gently aspirate extravasated solution (do **NOT** flush the line); initiate hyaluronidase antidote; remove needle/cannula; apply dry cold compresses (Hurst, 2004); elevate extremity.

Hyaluronidase: Intradermal or SubQ: Inject a total of 1 mL (15 units/mL) as five separate 0.2 mL injections (using a 25-gauge needle) into area of extravasation at the leading edge in a clockwise manner (MacCara, 1983; Zenk, 1981).

Nursing Actions

Physical Assessment Infusion site should be monitored closely to prevent extravasation.

Patient Education
• Discuss specific use of drug and side effects with patient as it relates to treatment. (HCAHPS: During this hospital stay, were you given any medicine that you had not taken before? Before giving you any new medicine, how often did hospital staff tell you what the medicine was for? How often did hospital staff describe possible side effects in a way you could understand?)
• Patient may experience injection site irritation (HCAHPS).
• Educate patient about signs of a significant reaction (eg, wheezing; chest tightness; fever; itching; bad cough; blue skin color; seizures; or swelling of face, lips, tongue, or throat). **Note:** This is not a comprehensive list of all side effects. Patient should consult prescriber for additional questions.

Intended Use and Disclaimer: Should not be printed and given to patients. This information is intended to serve as a concise initial reference for healthcare professionals to use when discussing medications with a patient. You must ultimately rely on your own discretion, experience and judgment in diagnosing, treating and advising patients.

Related Information
Management of Drug Extravasations *on page 1700*

Calcium Gluconate (KAL see um GLOO koe nate)

Brand Names: U.S. Cal-Glu [OTC]

Pharmacologic Category Calcium Salt; Electrolyte Supplement, Oral; Electrolyte Supplement, Parenteral

Medication Safety Issues

Sound-alike/look-alike issues:

Calcium gluconate may be confused with calcium glubionate, cupric sulfate

Administration issues:

Calcium gluconate may be confused with calcium chloride.

Confusion with the different intravenous salt forms of calcium has occurred. There is a three-fold difference in the primary cation concentration between calcium gluconate (in which 1 g = 4.65 mEq [90 mg] of elemental Ca++) and calcium chloride (in which 1 g = 14 mEq [270 mg] of elemental Ca++).

Prescribers should specify which salt form is desired. Dosages should be expressed either as mEq, mg, or grams of the salt form.

Pregnancy Risk Factor C

Lactation Enters breast milk

Breast-Feeding Considerations Calcium is excreted in breast milk. The amount of calcium in breast milk is homeostatically regulated and not altered by maternal calcium intake. Calcium requirements are the same in lactating and non-lactating females (IOM, 2011).

Use

I.V.: Treatment of hypocalcemia and conditions secondary to hypocalcemia (eg, tetany, seizures, arrhythmias); treatment of cardiac disturbances secondary to hyperkalemia; adjunctive treatment of rickets, osteomalacia, and magnesium sulfate overdose; decrease capillary permeability in allergic conditions, nonthrombocytopenic purpura, and exudative dermatoses (eg, dermatitis herpetiformis, pruritus secondary to certain drugs)

Oral: Dietary calcium supplementation

Unlabeled Use Calcium channel blocker overdose; treatment of hydrofluoric acid exposure

Mechanism of Action/Effect Moderates nerve and muscle performance via action potential threshold regulation.

In hydrogen fluoride exposures, calcium gluconate provides a source of calcium ions to complex free fluoride ions and prevent or reduce toxicity; administration also helps to correct fluoride-induced hypocalcemia.

Contraindications Ventricular fibrillation; hypercalcemia; concomitant use of I.V. calcium gluconate and ceftriaxone in neonates (risk of precipitation of calcium-ceftriaxone)

Warnings/Precautions Avoid too rapid I.V. administration (do not exceed 200 mg/minute except in emergency situations);may result in vasodilation, hypotension, bradycardia, arrhythmias, and cardiac arrest. Vesicant; ensure proper catheter or needle position prior to and during infusion. Avoid extravasation; may result in necrosis. Monitor the I.V. site closely. Use with caution in digitalized patients, severe hyperphosphatemia, or severe hypokalemia. Hypercalcemia may occur in patients with renal failure; frequent determination of serum

calcium is necessary. Use caution with chronic renal disease. Use caution when administering calcium supplements to patients with a history of kidney stones. Hypomagnesemia is a common cause of hypocalcemia; therefore, correction of hypocalcemia may be difficult in patients with concomitant hypomagnesemia. Evaluate serum magnesium and correct hypomagnesemia (if necessary), particularly if initial treatment of hypocalcemia is refractory.

Solutions may contain aluminum; toxic levels may occur following prolonged administration in premature neonates or patients with renal dysfunction. Constipation, bloating, and gas are common with oral calcium supplements (especially carbonate salt). Taking calcium (≤500 mg) with food improves absorption. Calcium administration interferes with absorption of some minerals and drugs; use with caution. It is recommended to concomitantly administer vitamin D for optimal calcium absorption.

Ceftriaxone may complex with calcium causing precipitation. Fatal lung and kidney damage associated with calcium-ceftriaxone precipitates has been observed in premature and term neonates. Due to reports of precipitation reaction in neonates, do not coadminister ceftriaxone with calcium-containing solutions, even via separate infusion lines/sites or at different times in any neonate. Ceftriaxone should not be administered simultaneously with any calcium-containing solution via a Y-site in any patient. However, ceftriaxone and calcium-containing solutions may be administered sequentially of one another for use in patients **other than neonates** if infusion lines are thoroughly flushed (with a compatible fluid) between infusions.

Drug Interactions

Avoid Concomitant Use

Avoid concomitant use of Calcium Gluconate with any of the following: Calcium Acetate

Decreased Effect

Calcium Gluconate may decrease the levels/effects of: Bisphosphonate Derivatives; Calcium Channel Blockers; Deferiprone; DOBUTamine; Dolutegravir; Eltrombopag; Estramustine; Multivitamins/Fluoride (with ADE); Phosphate Supplements; Quinolone Antibiotics; Strontium Ranelate; Tetracycline Derivatives; Thyroid Products; Trientine

The levels/effects of Calcium Gluconate may be decreased by: Trientine

Increased Effect/Toxicity

Calcium Gluconate may increase the levels/effects of: Calcium Acetate; CefTRIAXone; Vitamin D Analogs

The levels/effects of Calcium Gluconate may be increased by: Multivitamins/Fluoride (with ADE); Multivitamins/Minerals (with ADEK, Folate, Iron); Thiazide Diuretics

◀ **Adverse Reactions** Frequency not defined.

I.V.:

Cardiovascular (with rapid I.V. injection): Arrhythmia, bradycardia, cardiac arrest, hypotension, syncope, vasodilation

Central nervous system: Sense of oppression (with rapid I.V. injection)

Endocrine & metabolic: Hypercalcemia

Gastrointestinal: Chalky taste

Neuromuscular & skeletal: Tingling sensation (with rapid I.V. injection)

Miscellaneous: Heat waves (with rapid I.V. injection)

Postmarketing and/or case reports: Calcinosis cutis

Oral: Gastrointestinal: Constipation

Dosage Forms Considerations

1 g calcium gluconate = elemental calcium 93 mg = calcium 4.65 mEq = calcium 2.33 mmol

Available Dosage Forms

Capsule, Oral [preservative free]:

Cal-Glu [OTC]: 500 mg

Solution, Intravenous:

Generic: 10% (10 mL, 50 mL, 100 mL)

Solution, Intravenous [preservative free]:

Generic: 10% (100 mL)

Tablet, Oral:

Generic: 50 mg, 500 mg

General Dosage Range

I.V.: *Children and Adults:* Dosage varies greatly depending on indication

Oral:

Children 1-6 months: Adequate intake: 200 mg **elemental calcium** daily

Children 7-12 months: Adequate intake: 260 mg **elemental calcium** daily

Children 1-3 years: RDA: 700 mg **elemental calcium** daily

Children 4-8 years: RDA: 1000 mg **elemental calcium** daily

Children 9-18 years: RDA: 1300 mg **elemental calcium** daily

Adults 19-50 years: RDA: 1000 mg **elemental calcium** daily

Adults ≥51 years, females: RDA: 1200 mg **elemental calcium** daily

Adults 51-70 years, males: RDA: 1000 mg **elemental calcium** daily

Adults >70 years, males: RDA: 1200 mg **elemental calcium** daily

Administration

I.V. Administer slowly (~1.5 mL calcium gluconate 10% per minute; not to exceed 200 mg/minute except in emergency situations) through a small needle into a large vein in order to avoid too rapid increases in the serum calcium and extravasation. **Note:** Due to the potential presence of particulates, American Regent, Inc recommends the use of a 0.22 micron inline filter for I.V. administration (1.2 micron filter if admixture contains lipids) (Important Drug Administration

Information, American Regent, 2013); a similar recommendation has not been noted by other manufacturers. Not for I.M. administration.

Vesicant; ensure proper needle or catheter placement prior to and during I.V. infusion. Avoid extravasation.

Extravasation management: If extravasation occurs, stop infusion immediately and disconnect (leave needle/cannula in place); gently aspirate extravasated solution (do **NOT** flush the line); initiate hyaluronidase antidote; remove needle/cannula; apply dry cold compresses (Hurst, 2004); elevate extremity.

Hyaluronidase: Intradermal or SubQ: Inject a total of 1 mL (15 units/mL) as five separate 0.2 mL injections (using a 25-gauge needle) into area of extravasation at the leading edge in a clockwise manner (MacCara, 1983; Zenk, 1981).

Subcutaneous Not for routine SubQ administration.

Treatment of hydrofluoric acid burns (unlabeled use): *SubQ infiltration (unlabeled route):* Using a 27- or 30-gauge needle, approach the wound from the distal point of injury and infiltrate directly into the affected dermis and subcutaneous tissue. The infiltration should be carried 0.5 cm away from the margin of the injured tissue into the surrounding uninjured areas (Dibbell, 1970). Avoid excessive administration as it can cause compartment syndrome and further exacerbate tissue damage. Following subungual exposure, administer to the affected area via the lateral or volar route through the fat pad (under digital nerve block); administration may also require removal of the nailbed, splitting the distal nail from the nailbed, or trimming the nail to the nailbed to reach the affected area (Kirkpatrick, 1995; Roberts, 1989).

Inhalation Treatment of hydrofluoric acid burns (unlabeled use): Dilute 10% calcium gluconate solution to 2.5% solution and administer via nebulization.

Intra-arterial Treatment of hydrofluoric acid burns (unlabeled use): *Intra-arterial (unlabeled route):* Requires radiology to place an arterial catheter in an artery supplying blood to the area of exposure; infuse over four hours (Vance, 1986). **This intervention should be used only by those accustomed to this technique. Care should be taken to avoid the extravasation.** A poison information center or clinical toxicologist should be consulted prior to implementation.

Preparation for Administration

I.V.: Observe the vial for the presence of particulates. If particulates are observed, place vial in a 60°C to 80°C water bath for 15-30 minutes (or until solution is clear); occasionally shake to dissolve; cool to body/room temperature before use. Do not use vial if particulates do not dissolve.

Note: Due to the potential presence of particulates, American Regent, Inc recommends the use of a 5 micron filter when preparing calcium gluconate-containing I.V. solutions (Important Drug Administration Information, American Regent, 2013); a similar recommendation has not been noted by other manufacturers.

Inhalation: Treatment of hydrofluoric acid burns (unlabeled use): Mix 1 mL of 10% calcium gluconate solution with 4 mL NS to make a 2.5% solution.

Storage/Stability I.V.: Store at 20°C to 25°C (68°F to 77°F); excursions permitted to 15°C to 30°C (59°F to 86°F).

Usual concentrations: 1 g/100 mL D_5W or NS; 2 g/ 100 mL D_5W or NS.

Maximum concentration in parenteral nutrition solutions is variable depending upon concentration and solubility (consult detailed reference).

Nursing Actions

Physical Assessment If administered I.V., monitor ECG, vital signs, and CNS. Observe infusion site closely. Avoid extravasation.

Patient Education

- Discuss specific use of drug and side effects with patient as it relates to treatment. (HCAHPS: During this hospital stay, were you given any medicine that you had not taken before? Before giving you any new medicine, how often did hospital staff tell you what the medicine was for? How often did hospital staff describe possible side effects in a way you could understand?)
- Patient may experience injection site irritation. Have patient report immediately to prescriber illogical thinking, severe nausea, or considerable constipation (HCAHPS).
- Educate patient about signs of a significant reaction (eg, wheezing; chest tightness; fever; itching; bad cough; blue skin color; seizures; or swelling of face, lips, tongue, or throat). **Note:** This is not a comprehensive list of all side effects. Patient should consult prescriber for additional questions.

Intended Use and Disclaimer: Should not be printed and given to patients. This information is intended to serve as a concise initial reference for healthcare professionals to use when discussing medications with a patient. You must ultimately rely on your own discretion, experience and judgment in diagnosing, treating and advising patients.

Related Information

Management of Drug Extravasations *on page 1700*

Calcium Phosphate (Tribasic)
(KAL see um FOS fate tri BAY sik)

Brand Names: U.S. Posture® [OTC]
Index Terms Tricalcium Phosphate
Pharmacologic Category Calcium Salt

Use Dietary supplement
Available Dosage Forms
Caplet:
Posture® [OTC]: Calcium 600 mg and phosphorus 280 mg

General Dosage Range Oral:
Children 1-6 months: Adequate intake: 200 mg/day
Children 7-12 months: Adequate intake: 260 mg/day
Children 1-3 years: RDA: 700 mg/day
Children 4-8 years: RDA: 1000 mg/day
Children 9-18 years: RDA: 1300 mg/day
Adults: 2 tablets daily
Adults 19-50 years: RDA: 1000 mg/day
Adults ≥51 years, females: RDA: 1200 mg/day
Adults 51-70 years, males: RDA: 1000 mg/day
Adults >70 years, males: RDA: 1200 mg/day

Nursing Actions
Patient Education

- Discuss specific use of drug and side effects with patient as it relates to treatment. (HCAHPS: During this hospital stay, were you given any medicine that you had not taken before? Before giving you any new medicine, how often did hospital staff tell you what the medicine was for? How often did hospital staff describe possible side effects in a way you could understand?)
- Patient may experience constipation. Have patient report immediately to prescriber severe nausea (HCAHPS).
- Educate patient about signs of a significant reaction (eg, wheezing; chest tightness; fever; itching; bad cough; blue skin color; seizures; or swelling of face, lips, tongue, or throat). **Note:** This is not a comprehensive list of all side effects. Patient should consult prescriber for additional questions.

Intended Use and Disclaimer: Should not be printed and given to patients. This information is intended to serve as a concise initial reference for healthcare professionals to use when discussing medications with a patient. You must ultimately rely on your own discretion, experience and judgment in diagnosing, treating and advising patients.

Canagliflozin (kan a gli FLOE zin)

Brand Names: U.S. Invokana
Pharmacologic Category Antidiabetic Agent, Sodium-Glucose Cotransporter 2 (SGLT2) Inhibitor; Sodium-Glucose Cotransporter 2 (SGLT2) Inhibitor
Medication Safety Issues
High alert medication:
The Institute for Safe Medication Practices (ISMP) includes this medication among its list of drugs which have a heightened risk of causing significant patient harm when used in error.
Medication Guide Available Yes

◄ **Pregnancy Risk Factor** C

Lactation Excretion in breast milk unknown/ not recommended

Breast-Feeding Considerations It is not known if canagliflozin is excreted in breast milk. Due to the potential for serious adverse reactions in the nursing infant, the manufacturer recommends a decision be made whether to discontinue nursing or to discontinue the drug, taking into account the importance of treatment to the mother.

Use Treatment of type 2 diabetes mellitus (non-insulin dependent, NIDDM) as an adjunct to diet and exercise as monotherapy or in combination therapy with other antidiabetic agents to improve glycemic control

Mechanism of Action/Effect Glucose reabsorption from the proximal renal tubules of the kidneys is reduced; urinary excretion of glucose is increased, thereby reducing plasma glucose concentrations.

Contraindications Hypersensitivity to canagliflozin or any component of the formulation; severe renal impairment (eGFR <30 mL/minute/1.73 m^2); end-stage renal disease or patients on dialysis.

Warnings/Precautions Potentially significant interactions may exist, requiring dose or frequency adjustment, additional monitoring, and/or selection of alternative therapy. Patients may experience hypersensitivity reactions (eg, urticaria) with some being severe; generally occurs within hours to days after therapy initiation. Discontinue canagliflozin if hypersensitivity occurs and treat as appropriate. May cause symptomatic hypotension due to intravascular volume depletion especially in patients with renal impairment (ie, eGFR <60 mL/minute/1.73 m^2), elderly, patients on other antihypertensives (eg, diuretics, ACE inhibitors, or angiotensin receptor blockers [ARBs]), or those with low systolic blood pressure. Assess volume status prior to initiation in patients at risk of hypotension and correct if depleted; monitor signs and symptoms of hypotension after initiation. May cause hyperkalemia. Patients predisposed to hyperkalemia (including patients with renal impairment or taking potassium-sparing diuretics, ACE inhibitors, and ARBs) are more likely to develop hyperkalemia; monitor serum potassium after initiation in those who are predisposed. May cause dose-related LDL-cholesterol (C) elevation; monitor LDL-C and treat as needed. May increase the risk of genital mycotic infections (eg, vulvovaginal mycotic infection, vulvovaginal candidiasis, vulvovaginitis, candida balanitis, balanoposthitis). Patients with a history of these infections or uncircumcised males are at greater risk.

Glycemic efficacy may be less and adverse reactions may be higher with moderate renal impairment (eGFR 30 to <50 mL/minute/1.73 m^2). Incidence of hyperkalemia may be higher with the 300 mg dose. Safety and efficacy in severe renal impairment (<30 mL/minute/1.73 m^2), ESRD, and in patients receiving dialysis are not established and canagliflozin should not be used in these patients. Abnormalities in renal function (decreased eGFR, increased serum creatinine) may occur upon initiation and are dose dependent. Renal function should be monitored frequently in patients with an eGFR <60 mL/minute/1.73 m^2 and canagliflozin should be discontinued if eGFR is persistently <45 mL/minute/1.73 m^2. Dosage adjustment may be necessary in patients with pre-existing renal impairment. Not recommended for use in severe hepatic impairment (has not been studied). Dose adjustment is not necessary in mild or moderate hepatic impairment.

Elderly patients may be predisposed to developing symptoms related to intravascular volume depletion (eg, hypotension, orthostatic hypotension, dizziness, syncope, and dehydration) during therapy, especially with the 300 mg dose. Hb A$_{1c}$ reductions may be less in patients >65 years compared to younger patients.

Canagliflozin should not be used to treat DKA. It has not been studied in patients with type 1 diabetes mellitus (insulin-dependent, IDDM) and should not be used in these patients.

Drug Interactions

Avoid Concomitant Use

Avoid concomitant use of Canagliflozin with any of the following: Pimozide

Decreased Effect

The levels/effects of Canagliflozin may be decreased by: Corticosteroids (Orally Inhaled); Corticosteroids (Systemic); Fosphenytoin; Loop Diuretics; Luteinizing Hormone-Releasing Hormone Analogs; PHENobarbital; Phenytoin; Primidone; Rifampin; Ritonavir; Somatropin; Thiazide Diuretics

Increased Effect/Toxicity

Canagliflozin may increase the levels/effects of: ACE Inhibitors; Aliskiren; Angiotensin II Receptor Blockers; ARIPiprazole; Dofetilide; DULoxetine; Eplerenone; Hypoglycemic Agents; Hypotensive Agents; Lomitapide; Pimozide; Potassium-Sparing Diuretics

The levels/effects of Canagliflozin may be increased by: Heparin; Heparin (Low Molecular Weight); Herbs (Hypoglycemic Properties); MAO Inhibitors; Pegvisomant; Salicylates; Selective Serotonin Reuptake Inhibitors

Nutritional/Ethanol Interactions Ethanol: May cause hypoglycemia. Management: Avoid ethanol.

Adverse Reactions Frequency not always defined.

>10%:

Endocrine & metabolic: Increased serum potassium (>5.4 mEq/mL: 12% to 27%, ≥6.5 mEq/mL: 2%; dose-related)

Genitourinary: Genitourinary infection (female) (10% to 11%; including vulvovaginal candidiasis, vulvovaginal mycotic infection, vulvovaginitis, vaginal infection, vulvitis)

Renal: Renal insufficiency (2% to 4%; 18% to 23% in patients with baseline eGFR 30 to <50 mL/minute/1.73 m^2)

1% to 10%:

Cardiovascular: Hypovolemia (2%), hypotension, orthostatic hypotension, syncope

Central nervous system: Fatigue (2%), orthostatic dizziness

Endocrine & metabolic: Hypoglycemia (3% to 4%; monotherapy), increased thirst (2% to 3%), dehydration, increased LDL cholesterol, increased serum cholesterol (non-HDL), increased serum magnesium, increased serum phosphate

Gastrointestinal: Abdominal pain (2%), constipation (2%)

Genitourinary: Urinary tract infection (4% to 6%; including cystitis, kidney infection, and urosepsis), polyuria (5%), genitourinary infection (male) (4%; including balanitis/balanoposthitis, balanitis candida, fungal genital infection), vulvovaginal pruritus (2% to 3%)

Hematologic & oncologic: Increased hemoglobin

Hypersensitivity: Hypersensitivity (4%; including erythema, rash, pruritus, urticaria, and angioedema)

Neuromuscular & skeletal: Weakness (1%)

Renal: Acute renal failure

Pharmacodynamics/Kinetics

Onset of Action Within 24 hours (dose-dependent)

Duration of Action Suppression of the renal threshold for glucose (RT_G) occurs throughout the 24-hour dosing interval; maximal RT_G suppression occurred with the 300 mg dose (RT_G decreased from baseline of ~240 mg/dL to a mean of 70-90 mg/dL over 24 hours).

Available Dosage Forms

Tablet, Oral:

Invokana: 100 mg, 300 mg

General Dosage Range Oral: *Adults:* 100-300 mg once daily

Administration

Oral May be administered with or without food. It is recommended to take before the first meal of the day (may reduce postprandial hyperglycemia via delayed intestinal glucose absorption).

Storage/Stability Store at 25°C (77°F); excursions permitted to 15°C to 30°C (59°F to 86°F).

Nursing Actions

Patient Education

• Discuss specific use of drug and side effects with patient as it relates to treatment. (HCAHPS: During this hospital stay, were you given any medicine that you had not taken before? Before giving you any new medicine, how often did hospital staff tell you what the medicine was

for? How often did hospital staff describe possible side effects in a way you could understand?)

• Patient may experience polyuria. Have patient report immediately to prescriber signs of hypoglycemia, signs of fluid and electrolyte imbalance, vaginal or penile yeast infection, dysuria, urinary retention, or oliguria (HCAHPS).

• Educate patient about signs of a significant reaction (eg, wheezing; chest tightness; fever; itching; bad cough; blue skin color; seizures; or swelling of face, lips, tongue, or throat). **Note:** This is not a comprehensive list of all side effects. Patient should consult prescriber for additional questions.

Intended Use and Disclaimer: Should not be printed and given to patients. This information is intended to serve as a concise initial reference for healthcare professionals to use when discussing medications with a patient. You must ultimately rely on your own discretion, experience and judgment in diagnosing, treating and advising patients.

Dietary Considerations Individualized medical nutrition therapy (MNT) based on ADA recommendations is an integral part of therapy.

Candesartan (kan de SAR tan)

Brand Names: U.S. Atacand

Index Terms Candesartan Cilexetil

Pharmacologic Category Angiotensin II Receptor Blocker; Antihypertensive

Medication Safety Issues

Sound-alike/look-alike issues:

Atacand may be confused with antacid

Pregnancy Risk Factor D

Lactation Excretion in breast milk unknown/not recommended

Breast-Feeding Considerations It is not known if candesartan is excreted into breast milk. Due to the potential for serious adverse reactions in the nursing infant, the manufacturer recommends a decision be made whether to discontinue nursing or to discontinue the drug, taking into account the importance of treatment to the mother. Breast-fed infants of mothers taking medications for hypertension should be monitored for adverse effects (Chobanian, 2003).

Use

Heart failure: Treatment of heart failure (NYHA class II-IV)

Note: The ACCF/AHA 2013 heart failure guidelines recommend the use of ARBs (ie, candesartan, losartan, and valsartan) in patients with HF with reduced ejection fraction who cannot tolerate ACE inhibitors (due to cough) to reduce morbidity and mortality. They also suggest that ARBs are reasonable first-line alternatives to ACE inhibitors in patients already maintained on an ARB for other indications (ACCF/AHA [Yancy, 2013]).

Hypertension: Alone or in combination with other antihypertensive agents in treating hypertension

Mechanism of Action/Effect Blocks the vasoconstrictor and aldosterone-secreting effects of angiotensin II by binding of angiotensin II at the AT1 receptor in many tissues, such as vascular smooth muscle and the adrenal gland. Independent of pathways for angiotensin II synthesis. Does not affect the response to bradykinin; does not bind to block other hormone receptors or ion channels known to be important in cardiovascular regulation.

Contraindications

Hypersensitivity to candesartan or any component of the formulation; concomitant use with aliskiren in patients with diabetes mellitus

Canadian labeling: Additional contraindications (not in U.S. labeling): Concomitant use with aliskiren in patients with moderate-to-severe renal impairment (GFR <60 mL/minute/1.73 m^2)

Warnings/Precautions [U.S. Boxed Warning]: Drugs that act on the renin-angiotensin system can cause injury and death to the developing fetus. Discontinue as soon as possible once pregnancy is detected. May cause hyperkalemia; avoid potassium supplementation unless specifically required by healthcare provider. Avoid use or use a smaller dose in patients who are volume depleted; correct depletion first. May be associated with deterioration of renal function and/or increases in serum creatinine, particularly in patients with low renal blood flow (eg, renal artery stenosis, heart failure) whose glomerular filtration rate (GFR) is dependent on efferent arteriolar vasoconstriction by angiotensin II; deterioration may result in oliguria, acute renal failure, and progressive azotemia. Small increases in serum creatinine may occur following initiation; consider discontinuation only in patients with progressive and/or significant deterioration in renal function. Use with caution in unstented unilateral/bilateral renal artery stenosis, pre-existing renal insufficiency, or significant aortic/mitral stenosis. Systemic exposure increases in hepatic impairment. Dosage adjustment recommended in patients with moderate hepatic impairment; pharmacokinetics have not been studied in severe hepatic impairment. Use caution when initiating in heart failure; may need to adjust dose, and/or concurrent diuretic therapy, because of candesartan-induced hypotension. Hypotension may occur during major surgery and anesthesia; use cautiously before, during, and immediately after such interventions. Potentially significant drug-drug interactions may exist, requiring dose or frequency adjustment, additional monitoring, and/or selection of alternative therapy. Pediatric patients with a GFR <30 mL/minute/1.73 m^2 should not receive candesartan; has not been evaluated. Children <1 year of age should not receive candesartan due to potential effects on the development of immature kidneys.

Angioedema has been reported rarely with some angiotensin II receptor antagonists (ARBs) and may occur at any time during treatment (especially following first dose). It may involve the head and neck (potentially compromising airway) or the intestine (presenting with abdominal pain). Patients with idiopathic or hereditary angioedema or previous angioedema associated with ACE-inhibitor therapy may be at an increased risk. Prolonged frequent monitoring may be required, especially if tongue, glottis, or larynx are involved, as they are associated with airway obstruction. Patients with a history of airway surgery may have a higher risk of airway obstruction. Discontinue therapy immediately if angioedema occurs. Aggressive early management is critical. Intramuscular (I.M.) administration of epinephrine may be necessary. Do not readminister to patients who have had angioedema with ARBs.

Drug Interactions

Avoid Concomitant Use There are no known interactions where it is recommended to avoid concomitant use.

Decreased Effect

The levels/effects of Candesartan may be decreased by: Herbs (Hypertensive Properties); Methylphenidate; Nonsteroidal Anti-Inflammatory Agents; Yohimbine

Increased Effect/Toxicity

Candesartan may increase the levels/effects of: ACE Inhibitors; Amifostine; Antihypertensives; CycloSPORINE (Systemic); DULoxetine; Hypotensive Agents; Lithium; Nonsteroidal Anti-Inflammatory Agents; Obinutuzumab; Potassium-Sparing Diuretics; RiTUXimab; Sodium Phosphates

The levels/effects of Candesartan may be increased by: Alfuzosin; Aliskiren; Brimonidine (Topical); Canagliflozin; Diazoxide; Eplerenone; Heparin; Heparin (Low Molecular Weight); Herbs (Hypotensive Properties); MAO Inhibitors; Pentoxifylline; Phosphodiesterase 5 Inhibitors; Potassium Salts; Prostacyclin Analogues; Tolvaptan; Trimethoprim

Nutritional/Ethanol Interactions

Food: Potassium supplements and/or potassium-containing salts may cause or worsen hyperkalemia. Management: Consult prescriber before consuming a potassium-rich diet, potassium supplements, or salt substitutes.

Herb/Nutraceutical: Dong quai has estrogenic activity. Ephedra, yohimbe, and ginseng may worsen hypertension. Garlic may increase antihypertensive effect of candesartan. Management: Avoid dong quai if using for hypertension. Avoid ephedra, yohimbe, ginseng, and garlic.

Adverse Reactions Frequency not always defined.

Cardiovascular: Hypotension (heart failure 19%), angina pectoris, myocardial infarction, palpitations, tachycardia

Central nervous system: Anxiety, depression, dizziness, drowsiness, headache, paresthesia, vertigo

Dermatologic: Diaphoresis, skin rash

Endocrine & metabolic: Hyperkalemia (heart failure <1% to 6%), hyperglycemia, hypertriglyceridemia, hyperuricemia

Gastrointestinal: Dyspepsia, gastroenteritis

Genitourinary: Hematuria

Neuromuscular & skeletal: Back pain, increased creatine phosphokinase, myalgia, weakness

Renal: Increased serum creatinine (≤13% in patients with heart failure with drug discontinuation required in 6%)

Respiratory: Dyspnea, epistaxis, pharyngitis, rhinitis, upper respiratory tract infection

Miscellaneous: Fever

Pharmacodynamics/Kinetics
Onset of Action 2-3 hours; Peak effect: 6-8 hours
Duration of Action >24 hours
Available Dosage Forms
Tablet, Oral:
Atacand: 4 mg, 8 mg, 16 mg, 32 mg
Generic: 4 mg, 8 mg, 16 mg, 32 mg
General Dosage Range Dosage adjustment recommended in patients with hepatic impairment.
Oral:
Children 1 to <6 years: Initial: 0.2 mg/kg/day in 1-2 divided doses; Maintenance: 0.05-0.4 mg/kg/day in 1-2 divided doses (maximum daily dose: 0.4 mg/kg/day)
Children ≥6 years and Adolescents <17 years: Initial: <50 kg: 4-8 mg daily in 1-2 divided doses; >50 kg: 8-16 mg daily in 1-2 divided doses; Maintenance: 2-32 mg daily in 1-2 divided doses (maximum daily dose: 32 mg daily)
Adults: Initial: 4-16 mg once daily; Maintenance: 4-32 mg daily in 1-2 divided doses
Administration
Oral Administer without regard to meals.
Storage/Stability Store at 25°C (77°F); excursions permitted to 15°C to 30°C (59°F to 86°F).
Nursing Actions
Physical Assessment Assess for potential interactions (eg, increased risk for hypotension, hyperkalemia). Monitor for reduced hypertension. Monitor for tachycardia, CNS changes, hyperglycemia, and hypotension prior to treatment, when changing dose, and throughout therapy.
Patient Education
• Discuss specific use of drug and side effects with patient as it relates to treatment. (HCAHPS: During this hospital stay, were you given any medicine that you had not taken before? Before giving you any new medicine, how often did hospital staff tell you what the medicine was

for? How often did hospital staff describe possible side effects in a way you could understand?)
• Patient may experience back pain, flu-like syndrome, pharyngitis, or rhinitis. Have patient report immediately to prescriber signs of renal impairment, signs of hyperkalemia, severe dizziness, or syncope (HCAHPS).
• Educate patient about signs of a significant reaction (eg, wheezing; chest tightness; fever; itching; bad cough; blue skin color; seizures; or swelling of face, lips, tongue, or throat). **Note:** This is not a comprehensive list of all side effects. Patient should consult prescriber for additional questions.

Intended Use and Disclaimer: Should not be printed and given to patients. This information is intended to serve as a concise initial reference for healthcare professionals to use when discussing medications with a patient. You must ultimately rely on your own discretion, experience and judgment in diagnosing, treating and advising patients.

Candesartan and Hydrochlorothiazide
(kan de SAR tan & hye droe klor oh THYE a zide)

Brand Names: U.S. Atacand HCT
Index Terms Candesartan Cilexetil and Hydrochlorothiazide; Hydrochlorothiazide and Candesartan
Pharmacologic Category Angiotensin II Receptor Blocker; Antihypertensive; Diuretic, Thiazide
Pregnancy Risk Factor D
Use Hypertension: Treatment of hypertension; combination product should not be used for initial therapy
Available Dosage Forms
Tablet, oral: 16/12.5: Candesartan cilexetil 16 mg and hydrochlorothiazide 12.5 mg; 32/12.5: Candesartan cilexetil 32 mg and hydrochlorothiazide 12.5 mg; 32/25: Candesartan cilexetil 32 mg and hydrochlorothiazide 25 mg
Atacand HCT: 16/12.5: Candesartan 16 mg and hydrochlorothiazide 12.5 mg; 32/12.5: Candesartan 32 mg and hydrochlorothiazide 12.5 mg; 32/25: Candesartan 32 mg and hydrochlorothiazide 25 mg
General Dosage Range Oral: *Adults:* Candesartan 8-32 mg daily in 1-2 divided doses and hydrochlorothiazide 12.5-50 mg once daily
Administration
Oral May administer with or without food.
Nursing Actions
Physical Assessment See individual agents.
Patient Education
• Discuss specific use of drug and side effects with patient as it relates to treatment. (HCAHPS: During this hospital stay, were you given any medicine that you had not taken before? Before

giving you any new medicine, how often did hospital staff tell you what the medicine was for? How often did hospital staff describe possible side effects in a way you could understand?)
- Have patient report immediately to prescriber signs of hyperglycemia, signs of fluid and electrolyte imbalance, signs of renal impairment, vision changes, or ophthalmalgia (HCAHPS).
- Educate patient about signs of a significant reaction (eg, wheezing; chest tightness; fever; itching; bad cough; blue skin color; seizures; or swelling of face, lips, tongue, or throat). **Note:** This is not a comprehensive list of all side effects. Patient should consult prescriber for additional questions.

Intended Use and Disclaimer: Should not be printed and given to patients. This information is intended to serve as a concise initial reference for healthcare professionals to use when discussing medications with a patient. You must ultimately rely on your own discretion, experience and judgment in diagnosing, treating and advising patients.

Related Information
Candesartan *on page 241*
Hydrochlorothiazide *on page 775*

Capecitabine (ka pe SITE a been)

Brand Names: U.S. Xeloda
Index Terms CAPE
Pharmacologic Category Antineoplastic Agent, Antimetabolite; Antineoplastic Agent, Antimetabolite (Pyrimidine Analog)
Medication Safety Issues
  Sound-alike/look-alike issues:
  Xeloda may be confused with Xenical
  High alert medication:
  This medication is in a class the Institute for Safe Medication Practices (ISMP) includes among its list of drug classes which have a heightened risk of causing significant patient harm when used in error.
Pregnancy Risk Factor D
Lactation Excretion in breast milk unknown/not recommended
Breast-Feeding Considerations Due to the potential for serious adverse reactions in the nursing infant, the decision to discontinue capecitabine or to discontinue breast-feeding should take into account the importance of treatment to the mother.
Use Treatment of metastatic colorectal cancer; adjuvant therapy of Dukes' C colon cancer; treatment of metastatic breast cancer
Unlabeled Use Treatment of CNS lesions from metastatic breast cancer, esophageal cancer, gastric cancer, hepatobiliary cancers (advanced), neuroendocrine (pancreatic/islet cell) tumors (metastatic or unresectable), ovarian cancer

(platinum-refractory), pancreatic cancer (metastatic), unknown primary cancer
Mechanism of Action/Effect Capecitabine is a prodrug of fluorouracil. It undergoes hydrolysis in the liver and tissues to form fluorouracil. It interferes with DNA (and to a lesser degree RNA) synthesis. Appears to be specific for G_1 and S phases of the cell cycle.
Contraindications Hypersensitivity to capecitabine, fluorouracil, or any component of the formulation; known deficiency of dihydropyrimidine dehydrogenase (DPD); severe renal impairment (CrCl <30 mL/minute)
Warnings/Precautions Hazardous agent - use appropriate precautions for handling and disposal (NIOSH, 2012). Bone marrow suppression may occur, hematologic toxicity is more common when used in combination therapy; use with caution; dosage adjustments may be required. Product labeling recommends that patients with baseline platelets <100,000/mm³ and/or neutrophils <1500/mm³ not receive capecitabine therapy and also to withhold for grade 3 or 4 hematologic toxicity during treatment. Rare and unexpected severe toxicity (stomatitis, diarrhea, neutropenia, neurotoxicity) may be attributed to dihydropyrimidine dehydrogenase (DPD) deficiency.

Capecitabine may cause diarrhea (may be severe); median time to first occurrence of grade 2-4 diarrhea was 34 days; median duration of grades 3 or 4 diarrhea was 5 days. Withhold treatment for grades 2-4 diarrhea; subsequent doses should be reduced after grade 3 or 4 diarrhea or recurrence of grade 2 diarrhea. Necrotizing enterocolitis (typhlitis) has been reported. Dehydration may occur rapidly in patients with diarrhea, nausea, vomiting, anorexia, and/or weakness; adequately hydrate prior to treatment initiation. Elderly patients may be a higher risk for dehydration. **Note:** Canadian labeling recommends treatment interruption for dehydration requiring I.V. hydration lasting <24 hours and dosage reduction if I.V hydration required for ≥24 hours; correct precipitating factors and ensure rehydration prior to resuming therapy.

Hand-and-foot syndrome is characterized by numbness, dysesthesia/paresthesia, tingling, painless or painful swelling, erythema, desquamation, blistering, and severe pain; median onset is 79 days (range: 11-360 days). If grade 2 or 3 hand-and-foot syndrome occurs, interrupt administration of capecitabine until decreases to grade 1. Following grade 3 hand-and-foot syndrome, decrease subsequent doses of capecitabine. In patients with colorectal cancer, treatment with capecitabine immediately following 6 weeks of fluorouracil/leucovorin (FU/LV) therapy has been associated with an increased incidence of grade ≥3 toxicity, when compared to patients receiving the reverse sequence, capecitabine (two 3-week courses) followed by FU/LV (Hennig, 2008).

Grade 3 and 4 hyperbilirubinemia have been observed in patients with and without hepatic metastases at baseline (median onset: 64 days). Transaminase and alkaline phosphatase elevations have also been reported. If capecitabine-related grade 3 or 4 hyperbilirubinemia occurs, Interrupt treatment until bilirubin ≤3 times ULN. Use with caution in patients with mild to moderate hepatic impairment due to liver metastases; effect of severe hepatic impairment has not been studied. Use with caution in patients with mild-to-moderate renal impairment; reduce dose with moderate impairment (exposure to capecitabine and metabolites is increased) and carefully monitor and reduce subsequent dose (with any grade 2 or higher adverse effect) with mild-to-moderate impairment; use is contraindicated in severe impairment. Use with caution in patients ≥60 years of age, the incidence of treatment-related adverse events may be higher.

Cardiotoxicity has been observed with capecitabine, including myocardial infarction, ischemia, angina, dysrhythmias, cardiac arrest, cardiac failure, sudden death, ECG changes, and cardiomyopathy; may be more common in patients with a history of coronary artery disease. **[U.S. Boxed Warning]: Capecitabine may increase the anticoagulant effects of warfarin; bleeding events, including death, have occurred with concomitant use. Increases in prothrombin time (PT) and INR may occur within several days to months after capecitabine initiation, and may continue up to 1 month after capecitabine discontinuation; may occur in patients with or without liver metastases. Monitor frequently and adjust anticoagulation dosing accordingly. An increased risk of coagulopathy is correlated with a cancer diagnosis and age >60 years.** Other potentially significant drug-drug interactions may exist, requiring dose or frequency adjustment, additional monitoring, and/or selection of alternative therapy.

Drug Interactions
Avoid Concomitant Use
Avoid concomitant use of Capecitabine with any of the following: BCG; CloZAPine; Gimeracil; Natalizumab; Pimecrolimus; Tacrolimus (Topical); Tofacitinib; Vaccines (Live)
Decreased Effect
Capecitabine may decrease the levels/effects of: BCG; Coccidioidin Skin Test; Sipuleucel-T; Vaccines (Inactivated); Vaccines (Live)

The levels/effects of Capecitabine may be decreased by: Echinacea
Increased Effect/Toxicity
Capecitabine may increase the levels/effects of: Bosentan; Carvedilol; CloZAPine; CYP2C9 Substrates; Diclofenac (Systemic); Fosphenytoin; Lacosamide; Leflunomide; Natalizumab; Ospemifene; Phenytoin; Tofacitinib; Vaccines (Live); Vitamin K Antagonists

The levels/effects of Capecitabine may be increased by: Cimetidine; Denosumab; Gimeracil; Leucovorin Calcium-Levoleucovorin; Pimecrolimus; Roflumilast; Tacrolimus (Topical); Trastuzumab
Nutritional/Ethanol Interactions Food: Food reduced the rate and extent of absorption of capecitabine.
Adverse Reactions Frequency listed derived from monotherapy trials.
>10%:
Cardiovascular: Edema (9% to 15%)
Central nervous system: Fatigue (16% to 42%), fever (7% to 18%), pain (12%)
Dermatologic: Palmar-plantar erythrodysesthesia (hand-and-foot syndrome) (54% to 60%; grade 3: 11% to 17%; may be dose limiting), dermatitis (27% to 37%)
Gastrointestinal: Diarrhea (47% to 57%; may be dose limiting; grade 3: 12% to 13%; grade 4: 2% to 3%), nausea (34% to 53%), vomiting (15% to 37%), abdominal pain (7% to 35%), stomatitis (22% to 25%), appetite decreased (26%), anorexia (9% to 23%), constipation (9% to 15%)
Hematologic: Lymphopenia (94%; grade 4: 14%), anemia (72% to 80%; grade 4: <1% to 1%), neutropenia (2% to 26%; grade 4: 2%), thrombocytopenia (24%; grade 4: 1%)
Hepatic: Bilirubin increased (22% to 48%; grades 3/4: 11% to 23%)
Neuromuscular & skeletal: Paresthesia (21%)
Ocular: Eye irritation (13% to 15%)
Respiratory: Dyspnea (14%)
5% to 10%:
Cardiovascular: Venous thrombosis (8%), chest pain (6%)
Central nervous system: Headache (5% to 10%), lethargy (10%), dizziness (6% to 8%), insomnia (7% to 8%), mood alteration (5%), depression (5%)
Dermatologic: Nail disorder (7%), rash (7%), skin discoloration (7%), alopecia (6%), erythema (6%)
Endocrine & metabolic: Dehydration (7%)
Gastrointestinal: Motility disorder (10%), oral discomfort (10%), dyspepsia (6% to 8%), upper GI inflammatory disorders (colorectal cancer: 8%), hemorrhage (6%), ileus (6%), taste perversion (colorectal cancer: 6%)
Neuromuscular & skeletal: Back pain (10%), weakness (10%), neuropathy (10%), myalgia (9%), arthralgia (8%), limb pain (6%)
Ocular: Abnormal vision (colorectal cancer: 5%), conjunctivitis (5%)
Respiratory: Cough (7%)
Miscellaneous: Viral infection (colorectal cancer: 5%)

Available Dosage Forms

Tablet, Oral:

Xeloda: 150 mg, 500 mg

Generic: 150 mg, 500 mg

General Dosage Range Dosage adjustment recommended in patients with renal impairment or who develop toxicities

Oral: *Adults:* 1250 mg/m² twice daily for 2 weeks, every 21 days

Administration

Oral Usually administered in 2 divided doses taken 12 hours apart. Doses should be taken with water within 30 minutes after a meal. Swallow tablets whole; do not cut or crush.

Hazardous agent; use appropriate precautions for handling and disposal (NIOSH, 2012).

Storage/Stability Store at room temperature of 25°C (77°F); excursions permitted between 15°C and 30°C (59°F and 86°F). Keep bottle tightly closed.

Nursing Actions

Physical Assessment Monitor for adverse reactions periodically during therapy. Teach sexually active female patients the necessity for contraception.

Patient Education

- Discuss specific use of drug and side effects with patient as it relates to treatment. (HCAHPS: During this hospital stay, were you given any medicine that you had not taken before? Before giving you any new medicine, how often did hospital staff tell you what the medicine was for? How often did hospital staff describe possible side effects in a way you could understand?)
- Patient may experience headache, dizziness, insomnia, nail changes, lack of appetite, constipation, asthenia, dyspepsia, back pain, arthralgia, or myalgia. Have patient report immediately to prescriber signs of infection, signs of fluid and electrolyte imbalance, signs of hepatic impairment, dyspnea, angina, arrhythmia, severe nausea, considerable diarrhea, paresthesia, ecchymosis, hemorrhaging, significant skin irritation, intolerable stomatitis, edema of extremities, vision changes, ophthalmalgia, severe eye irritation, or eczema of hands or feet (HCAHPS).
- Educate patient about signs of a significant reaction (eg, wheezing; chest tightness; fever; itching; bad cough; blue skin color; seizures; or swelling of face, lips, tongue, or throat). **Note:** This is not a comprehensive list of all side effects. Patient should consult prescriber for additional questions.

Intended Use and Disclaimer: Should not be printed and given to patients. This information is intended to serve as a concise initial reference for healthcare professionals to use when discussing medications with a patient. You must ultimately rely on your own discretion, experience and judgment in diagnosing, treating and advising patients.

Dietary Considerations Because current safety and efficacy data are based upon administration with food, it is recommended that capecitabine be administered with food. In all clinical trials, patients were instructed to take with water within 30 minutes after a meal.

Related Information

Oral Medications That Should Not Be Crushed or Altered *on page 1712*

Captopril (KAP toe pril)

Index Terms ACE

Pharmacologic Category Angiotensin-Converting Enzyme (ACE) Inhibitor; Antihypertensive

Medication Safety Issues

Sound-alike/look-alike issues:

Captopril may be confused with calcitriol, Capitrol®, carvedilol

International issues:

Acepril [Great Britain] may be confused with Accupril which is a brand name for quinapril in the U.S.

Acepril: Brand name for captopril [Great Britain], but also the brand name for enalapril [Hungary, Switzerland]; lisinopril [Malaysia]

Pregnancy Risk Factor D

Lactation Enters breast milk/not recommended

Breast-Feeding Considerations Captopril is excreted in breast milk. Breast-feeding is not recommended by the manufacturer.

Use Management of hypertension; treatment of heart failure (HF), left ventricular dysfunction after myocardial infarction, diabetic nephropathy

Note: The ACCF/AHA 2013 heart failure guidelines recommend the use of ACE inhibitors, along with other guideline directed medical therapies, to prevent heart failure in patients with a reduced ejection fraction who have a history of MI (Stage B HF), to prevent heart failure in any patient with a reduced ejection fraction (Stage B HF), or to treat those with heart failure and reduced ejection fraction (Stage C HFrEF) (ACCF/AHA [Yancy, 2013]).

Unlabeled Use To delay the progression of nephropathy and reduce risks of cardiovascular events in hypertensive patients with type 1 or 2 diabetes mellitus; treatment of hypertensive crisis, rheumatoid arthritis; diagnosis of anatomic renal artery stenosis, hypertension secondary to scleroderma renal crisis; diagnosis of aldosteronism, idiopathic edema, Bartter's syndrome, postmyocardial infarction for prevention of ventricular failure; increase circulation in Raynaud's phenomenon, hypertension secondary to Takayasu's disease

Mechanism of Action/Effect Competitive inhibitor of angiotensin-converting enzyme (ACE); prevents conversion of angiotensin I to angiotensin II, a potent vasoconstrictor; results in lower levels of angiotensin II which causes an increase in plasma renin activity and a reduction in aldosterone secretion

Contraindications Hypersensitivity to captopril, any other ACE inhibitor, or any component of the formulation; angioedema related to previous treatment with an ACE inhibitor; concomitant use with aliskiren in patients with diabetes mellitus

Warnings/Precautions Anaphylactic reactions may occur rarely with ACE inhibitors. At any time during treatment (especially following first dose) angioedema may occur rarely with ACE inhibitors; may involve the head and neck (potentially compromising airway) or the intestine (presenting with abdominal pain). African-Americans and patients with idiopathic or hereditary angioedema may be at an increased risk. Prolonged frequent monitoring may be required especially if tongue, glottis, or larynx are involved as they are associated with airway obstruction. Patients with a history of airway surgery may have a higher risk of airway obstruction. Aggressive early and appropriate management is critical. Use in patients with previous angioedema associated with ACE inhibitor therapy is contraindicated. Severe anaphylactoid reactions may be seen during hemodialysis (eg, CVVHD) with high-flux dialysis membranes (eg, AN69), and rarely, during low density lipoprotein apheresis with dextran sulfate cellulose. Rare cases of anaphylactoid reactions have been reported in patients undergoing sensitization treatment with hymenoptera (bee, wasp) venom while receiving ACE inhibitors.

Symptomatic hypotension with or without syncope can occur with ACE inhibitors (usually with the first several doses); effects are most often observed in volume depleted patients; close monitoring of patient is required especially with initial dosing and dosing increases; blood pressure must be lowered at a rate appropriate for the patient's clinical condition. Initiation of therapy in patients with ischemic heart disease or cerebrovascular disease warrants close observation due to the potential consequences posed by falling blood pressure (eg, MI, stroke). Use with caution in hypertrophic cardiomyopathy with outflow tract obstruction, severe aortic stenosis, or before, during, or immediately after major surgery. [U.S. Boxed Warning]: Drugs that act on the renin-angiotensin system can cause injury and death to the developing fetus. Discontinue as soon as possible once pregnancy is detected.

Hyperkalemia may occur with ACE inhibitors; risk factors include renal dysfunction, diabetes mellitus, concomitant use of potassium-sparing diuretics, potassium supplements and/or potassium containing salts. Use cautiously, if at all, with these agents and monitor potassium closely. Cough may occur with ACE inhibitors. Other causes of cough should be considered (eg, pulmonary congestion in patients with heart failure) and excluded prior to discontinuation.

May be associated with deterioration of renal function and/or increases in serum creatinine, particularly in patients with low renal blood flow (eg, renal artery stenosis, heart failure) whose glomerular filtration rate (GFR) is dependent on efferent arteriolar vasoconstriction by angiotensin II; deterioration may result in oliguria, acute renal failure, and progressive azotemia. Small increases in serum creatinine may occur following initiation; consider discontinuation only in patients with progressive and/or significant deterioration in renal function. Use with caution in patients with unstented unilateral/bilateral renal artery stenosis. When unstented bilateral renal artery stenosis is present, use is generally avoided due to the elevated risk of deterioration in renal function unless possible benefits outweigh risks. Concomitant use of an angiotensin receptor blocker (ARB) or renin inhibitor (eg, aliskiren) is associated with an increased risk of hypotension, hyperkalemia, and renal dysfunction; concomitant use with aliskiren should be avoided in patients with GFR <60 mL/minute and is contraindicated in patients with diabetes mellitus (regardless of GFR). Routine concomitant use of an ACE inhibitor, ARB, and aldosterone antagonist in the treatment of heart failure is not recommended (ACCF/AHA [Yancy, 2013]).

Rare toxicities associated with ACE inhibitors include cholestatic jaundice (which may progress to fulminant hepatic necrosis), agranulocytosis, neutropenia, or leukopenia with myeloid hypoplasia. Patients with collagen vascular diseases (especially with concomitant renal impairment) or renal impairment alone may be at increased risk for hematologic toxicity; closely monitor CBC with differential for the first 3 months of therapy and periodically thereafter in these patients.

Drug Interactions

Avoid Concomitant Use There are no known interactions where it is recommended to avoid concomitant use.

Decreased Effect

The levels/effects of Captopril may be decreased by: Antacids; Aprotinin; Herbs (Hypertensive Properties); Icatibant; Lanthanum; Methylphenidate; Nonsteroidal Anti-Inflammatory Agents; Peginterferon Alfa-2b; Salicylates; Yohimbine

Increased Effect/Toxicity

Captopril may increase the levels/effects of: Allopurinol; Amifostine; Antihypertensives; AzaTHIOprine; CycloSPORINE (Systemic); DULoxetine; Ferric Gluconate; Gold Sodium Thiomalate; Hypotensive Agents; Iron Dextran Complex; Lithium; Nonsteroidal Anti-Inflammatory Agents; Obinutuzumab; RiTUXimab; Sodium Phosphates

The levels/effects of Captopril may be increased by: Abiraterone Acetate; Alfuzosin; Aliskiren;

Angiotensin II Receptor Blockers; Brimonidine (Topical); Canagliflozin; CYP2D6 Inhibitors (Moderate); CYP2D6 Inhibitors (Strong); Darunavir; Diazoxide; DPP-IV Inhibitors; Eplerenone; Everolimus; Heparin; Heparin (Low Molecular Weight); Herbs (Hypotensive Properties); Loop Diuretics; MAO Inhibitors; Pentoxifylline; Phosphodiesterase 5 Inhibitors; Potassium Salts; Potassium-Sparing Diuretics; Prostacyclin Analogues; Sirolimus; Temsirolimus; Thiazide Diuretics; TiZANidine; Tolvaptan; Trimethoprim

Nutritional/Ethanol Interactions

Food: Captopril serum concentrations may be decreased if taken with food. Long-term use of captopril may lead to a zinc deficiency which can result in altered taste perception. Potassium supplements and/or potassium-containing salts may cause or worsen hyperkalemia. Management: Take on an empty stomach 1 hour before or 2 hours after meals. Consult prescriber before consuming a potassium-rich diet, potassium supplements, or salt substitutes.

Herb/Nutraceutical: Some herbal medications may worsen hypertension (eg, licorice); others may increase the antihypertensive effect of captopril (eg, shepherd's purse). Management: Avoid bayberry, blue cohosh, cayenne, ephedra, ginger, ginseng (American), kola, yohimbe, and licorice. Avoid black cohosh, california poppy, coleus, golden seal, hawthorn, mistletoe, periwinkle, quinine, and shepherd's purse.

Adverse Reactions

Frequency not defined:
Cardiovascular: Angioedema, cardiac arrest, cerebrovascular insufficiency, rhythm disturbances, orthostatic hypotension, syncope, flushing, pallor, angina, MI, Raynaud's syndrome, CHF
Central nervous system: Ataxia, confusion, depression, nervousness, somnolence
Dermatologic: Bullous pemphigus, erythema multiforme, Stevens-Johnson syndrome, exfoliative dermatitis
Endocrine & metabolic: Alkaline phosphatase increased, bilirubin increased, gynecomastia
Gastrointestinal: Pancreatitis, glossitis, dyspepsia
Genitourinary: Urinary frequency, impotence
Hematologic: Anemia, thrombocytopenia, pancytopenia, agranulocytosis, anemia
Hepatic: Jaundice, hepatitis, hepatic necrosis (rare), cholestasis, hyponatremia (symptomatic), transaminases increased
Neuromuscular & skeletal: Asthenia, myalgia, myasthenia
Ocular: Blurred vision
Renal: Renal insufficiency, renal failure, nephrotic syndrome, polyuria, oliguria
Respiratory: Bronchospasm, eosinophilic pneumonitis, rhinitis
Miscellaneous: Anaphylactoid reactions

1% to 10%:
Cardiovascular: Hypotension (1% to 3%), tachycardia (1%), chest pain (1%), palpitation (1%)
Dermatologic: Rash (maculopapular or urticarial) (4% to 7%), pruritus (2%); in patients with rash, a positive ANA and/or eosinophilia has been noted in 7% to 10%
Endocrine & metabolic: Hyperkalemia (1% to 11%)
Hematologic: Neutropenia may occur in up to 4% of patients with renal insufficiency or collagen-vascular disease
Renal: Proteinuria (1%), serum creatinine increased, worsening of renal function (may occur in patients with bilateral renal artery stenosis or hypovolemia)
Respiratory: Cough (<1% to 2%)
Miscellaneous: Hypersensitivity reactions (rash, pruritus, fever, arthralgia, and eosinophilia) have occurred in 4% to 7% of patients (depending on dose and renal function); dysgeusia - loss of taste or diminished perception (2% to 4%)

Pharmacodynamics/Kinetics

Onset of Action Peak effect: Blood pressure reduction: 1-1.5 hours after dose

Duration of Action Dose related, may require several weeks of therapy before full hypotensive effect

Available Dosage Forms

Tablet, Oral:
Generic: 12.5 mg, 25 mg, 50 mg, 100 mg

General Dosage Range Dosage adjustment recommended in patients with renal impairment

Oral:
Infants: Initial: 0.15-0.3 mg/kg/dose; Maximum: 6 mg/kg/day in 1-4 divided doses
Children: Initial: 0.3-0.5 mg/kg/dose; Maximum: 6 mg/kg/day in 2-4 divided doses
Older Children: Initial: 6.25-12.5 mg every 12-24 hours; Maximum: 6 mg/kg/day
Adolescents: Initial: 12.5-25 mg; Maximum: 450 mg/day
Adults: Initial: 6.25-25 mg 2-3 times/day; Maintenance: 25-450 mg/day in 2-3 divided doses

Administration

Oral Unstable in aqueous solutions; to prepare solution for oral administration, mix prior to administration and use within 10 minutes.

Nursing Actions

Physical Assessment Assess other pharmacological or herbal products patient may be taking that may impact renal function. When beginning therapy, monitor patient closely for anaphylactic reaction or severe angioedema. Monitor renal function tests and blood pressure. Monitor for hypovolemia, angioedema, and postural hypotension when beginning therapy, adjusting dosage, and on a regular basis throughout.

Patient Education

- Discuss specific use of drug and side effects with patient as it relates to treatment. (HCAHPS: During this hospital stay, were you given any medicine that you had not taken before? Before giving you any new medicine, how often did hospital staff tell you what the medicine was for? How often did hospital staff describe possible side effects in a way you could understand?)
- Have patient report immediately to signs of renal impairment, signs of hyperkalemia, severe dizziness, syncope, significant dyspepsia, considerable nausea, angina, tachycardia, ecchymosis, hemorrhaging, significant asthenia, or signs of hepatic impairment (HCAHPS).
- Educate patient about signs of a significant reaction (eg, wheezing; chest tightness; fever; itching; bad cough; blue skin color; seizures; or swelling of face, lips, tongue, or throat). **Note:** This is not a comprehensive list of all side effects. Patient should consult prescriber for additional questions.

Intended Use and Disclaimer: Should not be printed and given to patients. This information is intended to serve as a concise initial reference for healthcare professionals to use when discussing medications with a patient. You must ultimately rely on your own discretion, experience and judgment in diagnosing, treating and advising patients.

Dietary Considerations Should be taken at least 1 hour before or 2 hours after eating.

Captopril and Hydrochlorothiazide
(KAP toe pril & hye droe klor oh THYE a zide)

Index Terms Hydrochlorothiazide and Captopril

Pharmacologic Category Angiotensin-Converting Enzyme (ACE) Inhibitor; Antihypertensive; Diuretic, Thiazide

Pregnancy Risk Factor D

Use Management of hypertension

Available Dosage Forms

Tablet, oral: 25/15: Captopril 25 mg and hydrochlorothiazide 15 mg; 25/25: Captopril 25 mg and hydrochlorothiazide 25 mg; 50/15: Captopril 50 mg and hydrochlorothiazide 15 mg; 50/25: Captopril 50 mg and hydrochlorothiazide 25 mg

General Dosage Range Oral: *Adults:* Captopril 25-150 mg and hydrochlorothiazide 15-50 mg once daily

Nursing Actions

Physical Assessment See individual agents.

Patient Education

- Discuss specific use of drug and side effects with patient as it relates to treatment. (HCAHPS: During this hospital stay, were you given any medicine that you had not taken before? Before giving you any new medicine, how often did hospital staff tell you what the medicine was

for? How often did hospital staff describe possible side effects in a way you could understand?)
- Have patient report immediately to prescriber signs of hyperglycemia, signs of hepatic impairment, signs of fluid and electrolyte imbalance, signs of renal impairment, severe dyspepsia, dysphagia, considerable asthenia, angina, tachycardia, dyspnea, excessive weight gain, edema of extremities, ecchymosis, hemorrhaging, vision changes, or ophthalmalgia (HCAHPS).
- Patient may experience dizziness or abnormal taste. Have patient report immediately to prescriber signs of infection, signs of hyperglycemia, signs of renal or hepatic impairment, paresthesia, angina, fatigue, arthralgia, strength differences from one side to another, akathisia, dyspnea, significant weight gain, edema, bradycardia, severe headache, ecchymosis, bleeding, or vision changes (HCAHPS).
- Educate patient about signs of a significant reaction (eg, wheezing; chest tightness; fever; itching; bad cough; blue skin color; seizures; or swelling of face, lips, tongue, or throat). **Note:** This is not a comprehensive list of all side effects. Patient should consult prescriber for additional questions.

Intended Use and Disclaimer: Should not be printed and given to patients. This information is intended to serve as a concise initial reference for healthcare professionals to use when discussing medications with a patient. You must ultimately rely on your own discretion, experience and judgment in diagnosing, treating and advising patients.

Related Information

Captopril *on page 246*
Hydrochlorothiazide *on page 775*

CarBAMazepine (kar ba MAZ e peen)

Brand Names: U.S. Carbatrol; Epitol; Equetro; TEGretol; TEGretol-XR

Index Terms CBZ; SPD417

Pharmacologic Category Anticonvulsant, Miscellaneous

Medication Safety Issues

Sound-alike/look-alike issues:

CarBAMazepine may be confused with OXcarbazepine

Epitol may be confused with Epinal

TEGretol, TEGretol-XR may be confused with Mebaral, Toprol-XL, Toradol, TRENtal

BEERS Criteria medication:

This drug may be potentially inappropriate for use in geriatric patients (Quality of evidence - moderate; Strength of recommendation - strong).

Medication Guide Available Yes

Pregnancy Risk Factor D

Lactation Enters breast milk/not recommended

Breast-Feeding Considerations Carbamazepine and its active epoxide metabolite are found in breast milk. Carbamazepine can also be detected in the serum of nursing infants. Transient hepatic dysfunction has been observed in some case reports. Nursing should be discontinued if adverse events are observed. According to the manufacturer, the decision to continue or discontinue breast-feeding during therapy should take into account the risk of exposure to the infant and the benefits of treatment to the mother. Respiratory depression, seizures, nausea, vomiting, diarrhea, and/or decreased feeding have been observed in neonates exposed to carbamazepine *in utero* and may represent a neonatal withdrawal syndrome.

Use
Carbatrol, Tegretol, Tegretol-XR: Partial seizures with complex symptomatology (psychomotor, temporal lobe), generalized tonic-clonic seizures (grand mal), mixed seizure patterns, trigeminal neuralgia, glossopharyngeal neuralgia
Equetro: Acute manic or mixed episodes associated with bipolar 1 disorder

Unlabeled Use Treatment of restless leg syndrome and post-traumatic stress disorders

Mechanism of Action/Effect In addition to anticonvulsant effects, carbamazepine has anticholinergic, antineuralgic, antidiuretic, muscle relaxant, antimanic, antidepressive, and antiarrhythmic properties; chemically related to tricyclic antidepressants

Contraindications Hypersensitivity to carbamazepine, tricyclic antidepressants, or any component of the formulation; bone marrow depression; with or within 14 days of MAO inhibitor use; concurrent use of nefazodone; concomitant use of delavirdine or other non-nucleoside reverse transcriptase inhibitors

Warnings/Precautions Hazardous agent - use appropriate precautions for handling and disposal (NIOSH, 2012). **[U.S. Boxed Warning]: The risk of developing aplastic anemia or agranulocytosis is increased during treatment. Monitor CBC, platelets, and differential prior to and during therapy; discontinue if significant bone marrow suppression occurs.** A spectrum of hematologic effects has been reported with use (eg, agranulocytosis, aplastic anemia, neutropenia, leukopenia, thrombocytopenia, pancytopenia, and anemias); patients with a previous history of adverse hematologic reaction to any drug may be at increased risk. Early detection of hematologic change is important; advise patients of early signs and symptoms including fever, sore throat, mouth ulcers, infections, easy bruising, and petechial or purpuric hemorrhage.

[U.S. Boxed Warning]: Severe and sometimes fatal dermatologic reactions, including toxic epidermal necrolysis (TENS) and Stevens-Johnson syndrome (SJS), may occur during therapy. **The risk is increased in patients with the variant *HLA-B*1502* allele, found almost exclusively in patients of Asian ancestry. Patients of Asian descent should be screened prior to initiating therapy. Avoid use in patients testing positive for the allele; discontinue therapy in patients who have a serious dermatologic reaction.** The risk of SJS or TENS may also be increased if carbamazepine is used in combination with other antiepileptic drugs associated with these reactions. Presence of the *HLA-B*1502* allele has not been found to predict the risk of less serious dermatologic reactions such as anticonvulsant hypersensitivity syndrome or nonserious rash. The risk of developing a hypersensitivity reaction may be increased in patients with the variant *HLA-A*3101* allele. The *HLA-A*3101* allele may occur more frequently patients of African-American, Asian, European, Indian, Latin American, and Native American ancestry. Hypersensitivity has also been reported in patients experiencing reactions to other anticonvulsants; the history of hypersensitivity reactions in the patient or their immediate family members should be reviewed. Approximately 25% to 30% of patients allergic to carbamazepine will also have reactions with oxcarbazepine. Potentially serious, sometimes fatal multiorgan hypersensitivity reactions (also known as drug reaction with eosinophilia and systemic symptoms [DRESS]) have been reported with some antiepileptic drugs including carbamazepine; monitor for signs and symptoms of possible disparate manifestations associated with lymphatic, hepatic, renal, and/or hematologic organ systems; gradual discontinuation and conversion to alternate therapy may be required.

Antiepileptics are associated with an increased risk of suicidal behavior/thoughts with use (regardless of indication); patients should be monitored for signs/symptoms of depression, suicidal tendencies, and other unusual behavior changes during therapy and instructed to inform their healthcare provider immediately if symptoms occur.

Administer carbamazepine with caution to patients with history of cardiac damage, ECG abnormalities (or at risk for ECG abnormalities), hepatic or renal disease. When used to treat bipolar disorder, the smallest effective dose is suggested to reduce the risk for overdose/suicide; high-risk patients should be monitored for suicidal ideations. Prescription should be written for the smallest quantity consistent with good patient care. May activate latent psychosis and/or cause confusion or agitation; elderly patients may be at an increased risk for psychiatric effects.

Carbamazepine is not effective in absence, myoclonic, or akinetic seizures; exacerbation of certain seizure types have been seen after initiation of carbamazepine therapy in children with mixed seizure disorders. Abrupt discontinuation is not recommended in patients being treated for seizures. Dizziness or drowsiness may occur; caution should be used when performing tasks which require alertness until the effects are known. Effects with other sedative drugs or ethanol may be potentiated. Carbamazepine has a high potential for drug interactions; use caution in patients taking strong CYP3A4 inducers or inhibitors or medications significantly metabolized via CYP1A2, 2B6, 2C9, 2C19, and 3A4. Coadministration of carbamazepine and nefazodone may lead to insufficient plasma levels of nefazodone; combination is contraindicated. Coadministration yields insufficient plasma levels of delavirdine and other non-nucleoside reverse transcriptase inhibitors to achieve a therapeutic effect; concurrent use is contraindicated. Carbamazepine has mild anticholinergic activity; use with caution in patients with increased intraocular pressure, or sensitivity to anticholinergic effects. Hyponatremia caused by the syndrome of inappropriate antidiuretic hormone secretion (SIADH) may occur during therapy. Risk may be increased in the elderly or in patients also taking diuretics and may be dose-dependent. Use caution in elderly patients; may cause or exacerbate syndrome of inappropriate antidiuretic hormone secretion or hyponatremia; monitor sodium closely with initiation or dosage adjustments in older adults (Beers Criteria).

Administration of the suspension will yield higher peak and lower trough serum levels than an equal dose of the tablet form; consider a lower starting dose given more frequently (same total daily dose) when using the suspension. The suspension may contain sorbitol; avoid use in patents with hereditary fructose intolerance.

Drug Interactions

Avoid Concomitant Use

Avoid concomitant use of CarBAMazepine with any of the following: Abiraterone Acetate; Apixaban; Artemether; Axitinib; Azelastine (Nasal); Bedaquiline; Boceprevir; Bortezomib; Bosutinib; Cabozantinib; CloZAPine; Conivaptan; Crizotinib; Dabigatran Etexilate; Dienogest; Dolutegravir; Dronedarone; Enzalutamide; Everolimus; Fusidic Acid (Systemic); Ibrutinib; Itraconazole; Ivacaftor; Lapatinib; Lumefantrine; Lurasidone; Macitentan; MAO Inhibitors; Mifepristone; Nefazodone; NIFEdipine; Nilotinib; Nisoldipine; Paraldehyde; PAZOPanib; Pirfenidone; Pomalidomide; PONATinib; Praziquantel; Ranolazine; Regorafenib; Reverse Transcriptase Inhibitors (Non-Nucleoside); Rivaroxaban; Roflumilast; RomiDEPsin; Simeprevir; Sofosbuvir; SORAfenib; Stiripentol; Tasimelteon; Telaprevir; Thalidomide; Ticagrelor; Tofacitinib; Tolvaptan; Toremifene; TraMADol; Ulipristal; Vandetanib; Vemurafenib; VinCRIStine (Liposomal); Voriconazole

Decreased Effect

CarBAMazepine may decrease the levels/effects of: Abiraterone Acetate; Acetaminophen; Afatinib; Albendazole; Apixaban; ARIPiprazole; Artemether; Axitinib; Bazedoxifene; Bedaquiline; Bendamustine; Benzodiazepines (metabolized by oxidation); Boceprevir; Bortezomib; Bosutinib; Brentuximab Vedotin; Cabozantinib; Calcium Channel Blockers (Dihydropyridine); Calcium Channel Blockers (Nondihydropyridine); Caspofungin; Clarithromycin; CloZAPine; Cobicistat; Contraceptives (Estrogens); Contraceptives (Progestins); Crizotinib; CycloSPORINE (Systemic); CYP1A2 Substrates; CYP2B6 Substrates; CYP2C19 Substrates; CYP2C8 Substrates; CYP2C9 Substrates; CYP3A4 Substrates; Dabigatran Etexilate; Dasatinib; Diclofenac (Systemic); Dienogest; Dolutegravir; DOXOrubicin (Conventional); Doxycycline; Dronedarone; Elvitegravir; Enzalutamide; Eslicarbazepine; Everolimus; Exemestane; Ezogabine; Felbamate; Flunarizine; Fosphenytoin; Gefitinib; GuanFACINE; Haloperidol; Ibrutinib; Imatinib; Irinotecan; Itraconazole; Ivacaftor; Ixabepilone; Lacosamide; LamoTRIgine; Lapatinib; Linagliptin; Lopinavir; Lumefantrine; Lurasidone; Macitentan; Maraviroc; Mebendazole; Methadone; MethylPREDNISolone; Mifepristone; Nefazodone; NIFEdipine; Nilotinib; Nisoldipine; OXcarbazepine; Paliperidone; PAZOPanib; Perampanel; P-glycoprotein/ABCB1 Substrates; Phenytoin; Pirfenidone; Pomalidomide; PONATinib; Praziquantel; Protease Inhibitors; QUEtiapine; QuiNINE; Ranolazine; Regorafenib; Reverse Transcriptase Inhibitors (Non-Nucleoside); RisperiDONE; Rivaroxaban; Roflumilast; RomiDEPsin; Rufinamide; Saxagliptin; Selective Serotonin Reuptake Inhibitors; Simeprevir; Sofosbuvir; SORAfenib; SUNItinib; Tadalafil; Tasimelteon; Telaprevir; Temsirolimus; Theophylline Derivatives; Thyroid Products; Ticagrelor; Tofacitinib; Tolvaptan; Topiramate; Toremifene; TraMADol; Treprostinil; Tricyclic Antidepressants; Ulipristal; Valproic Acid and Derivatives; Vandetanib; Vecuronium; Vemurafenib; Vilazodone; VinCRIStine (Liposomal); Vitamin K Antagonists; Voriconazole; Vortioxetine; Ziprasidone; Zolpidem; Zuclopenthixol

The levels/effects of CarBAMazepine may be decreased by: Bosentan; CYP3A4 Inducers (Strong); Dabrafenib; Deferasirox; Felbamate; Fosphenytoin; Herbs (CYP3A4 Inducers); Ketorolac (Nasal); Ketorolac (Systemic); Mefloquine; Methylfolate; Mitotane; Orlistat; Phenytoin; Reverse Transcriptase Inhibitors (Non-Nucleoside); Rufinamide; Theophylline Derivatives; Tocilizumab; TraMADol; Valproic Acid and Derivatives

Increased Effect/Toxicity

CarBAMazepine may increase the levels/effects of: Adenosine; Alcohol (Ethyl); Azelastine (Nasal); Buprenorphine; Clarithromycin; ClomiPRAMINE;

CloZAPine; CNS Depressants; Desmopressin; Eslicarbazepine; Fosphenytoin; Hydrocodone; Ifosfamide; Lithium; MAO Inhibitors; Methotrimeprazine; Metyrosine; Mirtazapine; Paraldehyde; Phenytoin; Pramipexole; ROPINIRole; Rotigotine; Thalidomide

The levels/effects of CarBAMazepine may be increased by: Allopurinol; Brimonidine (Topical); Calcium Channel Blockers (Nondihydropyridine); Carbonic Anhydrase Inhibitors; Cimetidine; Clarithromycin; Conivaptan; CYP3A4 Inhibitors (Moderate); CYP3A4 Inhibitors (Strong); Danazol; Darunavir; Doxylamine; Droperidol; Fluconazole; Fusidic Acid (Systemic); Grapefruit Juice; HydrOXYzine; Isoniazid; LamoTRIgine; Luliconazole; Macrolide Antibiotics; Magnesium Sulfate; Methotrimeprazine; Nefazodone; Protease Inhibitors; QuiNINE; Selective Serotonin Reuptake Inhibitors; Sodium Oxybate; Stiripentol; Tapentadol; Telaprevir; Thiazide Diuretics; TraMADol; Zolpidem

Nutritional/Ethanol Interactions

Ethanol: Ethanol may increase CNS depression. Management: Avoid concurrent use of ethanol.

Food: Carbamazepine serum levels may be increased if taken with food and/or grapefruit juice. Management Avoid concurrent ingestion of grapefruit juice. Maintain adequate hydration, unless instructed to restrict fluid intake.

Herb/Nutraceutical: Evening primrose may decrease seizure threshold. Valerian, St John's wort, kava kava, and gotu kola may increase CNS depression. Management: Avoid evening primrose. Avoid valerian, St John's wort, kava kava, and gotu kola.

Adverse Reactions Frequency not defined, unless otherwise specified.

Cardiovascular: Hypertension (3%), aggravation of coronary artery disease, atrioventricular block, cardiac arrhythmia, cardiac failure, edema, hypotension, syncope, thromboembolism, thrombophlebitis

Central nervous system: Dizziness (44%), drowsiness (32%), headache (22%), ataxia (15%), speech disturbance (6%), abnormality in thinking (2%), paresthesia (2%), twitching (2%), vertigo (2%), agitation, amnesia, chills, confusion, depression, fatigue, hallucination, hyperacusis, neuroleptic malignant syndrome (NMS), peripheral neuritis, slurred speech, talkativeness

Dermatologic: Pruritus (8%), skin rash (7%), acute generalized exanthematous pustulosis, alopecia, diaphoresis, dyschromia, erythema multiforme, erythema nodosum, exfoliative dermatitis, onychomadesis, skin photosensitivity, Stevens-Johnson syndrome, toxic epidermal necrolysis, urticaria

Endocrine & metabolic: Abnormal thyroid function test, albuminuria, glycosuria, hypocalcemia, hyponatremia, porphyria, SIADH

Gastrointestinal: Nausea (29%), vomiting (18%) constipation (10%), xerostomia (8%), abdominal pain, anorexia, diarrhea, gastric distress, glossitis pancreatitis, stomatitis, vanishing bile duct syndrome

Genitourinary: Azotemia, impotence, oliguria, urinary frequency, urinary retention

Hematologic & oncologic: Agranulocytosis, anemia, aplastic anemia, bone marrow depression, eosinophilia, leukocytosis, leukopenia, lymphadenopathy, pancytopenia, purpura, thrombocytopenia

Hepatic: Abnormal hepatic function tests, hepatic failure, hepatitis, jaundice

Hypersensitivity: Hypersensitivity reaction, multiorgan hypersensitivity

Neuromuscular & skeletal: Weakness (8%), tremor (3%), arthralgia, exacerbation of systemic lupus erythematosus, leg cramps, myalgia, osteoporosis

Ophthalmic: Blurred vision (6%), cataract, conjunctivitis, diplopia, increased intraocular pressure, nystagmus, oculomotor disturbance

Otic: Tinnitus

Renal: Increased blood urea nitrogen, renal failure

Respiratory: Dry throat, pneumonia

Miscellaneous: Fever

Available Dosage Forms

Capsule Extended Release 12 Hour, Oral:
Carbatrol: 100 mg, 200 mg, 300 mg
Equetro: 100 mg, 200 mg, 300 mg
Generic: 100 mg, 200 mg, 300 mg

Suspension, Oral:
TEGretol: 100 mg/5 mL (450 mL)
Generic: 100 mg/5 mL (450 mL)

Tablet, Oral:
Epitol: 200 mg
TEGretol: 200 mg
Generic: 200 mg

Tablet Chewable, Oral:
Generic: 100 mg

Tablet Extended Release 12 Hour, Oral:
TEGretol-XR: 100 mg, 200 mg, 400 mg
Generic: 200 mg, 400 mg

General Dosage Range Dosage adjustment recommended in patients with renal impairment.

Oral:
Extended release:
Capsules:
Children <12 years: Receiving ≥400 mg/day of carbamazepine may be converted to extended release capsules (Carbatrol®) using the same total daily dosage divided twice daily
Children 12-15 years: Initial: 400 mg/day; Maintenance: 800-1000 mg/day in 2 divided doses (maximum: 1000 mg/day)
Adolescents >15 years: Initial: 400 mg/day; Maintenance: 800-1200 mg/day in 2 divided doses (maximum: 1200 mg/day)

Adults: Bipolar disorder (Equetro®): Initial: 400 mg/day in 2 divided doses: Maintenance: Adjust by 200 mg daily increments (maximum: 1600 mg/day); Epilepsy: Initial: 400 mg/day; Maintenance: 800-1200 mg/day in 2 divided doses (maximum: 2400 mg/day)

Tablets:

Children 6-12 years: Initial: 200 mg/day; Maintenance: 400-800 mg/day in 2 divided doses (maximum: 1000 mg/day)

Children 12-15 years: Initial: 400 mg/day; Maintenance: 800-1000 mg/day in 2 divided doses (maximum: 1000 mg/day)

Adolescents >15 years and Adults: Initial: 400 mg/day; Maintenance: 800-1200 mg/day in 2 divided doses (maximum: 1200 mg/day)

Immediate release:

Children <6 years: Initial: 10-20 mg/kg/day in 2-3 divided doses (tablets) **or** 4 divided doses (suspension); Maintenance: Up to 35 mg/kg/day in 3-4 divided doses

Children 6-12 years: Initial: 200 mg/day in 2 divided doses (tablets) **or** 4 divided doses (suspension); Maintenance: 400-800 mg/day in 2-4 divided doses (maximum: 1000 mg/day)

Children 12-15 years: Initial: 400 mg/day in 2 divided doses (tablets) **or** 4 divided doses (suspension); Maintenance: 800-1000 mg/day in 3-4 divided doses (maximum: 1000 mg/day)

Adolescents >15 years: Initial: 400 mg/day in 2 divided doses (tablets) **or** 4 divided doses (suspension); Maintenance: 800-1200 mg/day in 3-4 divided doses (maximum: 1200 mg/day)

Adults: Epilepsy: Initial: 400 mg/day in 2 divided doses (tablets) **or** 4 divided doses (suspension); Maintenance: 800-1200 mg/day in 3-4 divided doses (maximum: 2400 mg/day); Trigeminal or glossopharyngeal neuralgia: Initial: 200 mg/day in 2 divided doses; Maintenance: 400-800 mg/day in 2 divided doses (maximum: 1200 mg/day)

Administration

Oral

Suspension: Must be given on a 3-4 times/day schedule versus tablets which can be given 2-4 times/day. Since a given dose of suspension will produce higher peak and lower trough levels than the same dose given as the tablet form, patients given the suspension should be started on lower doses given more frequently (same total daily dose) and increased slowly to avoid unwanted side effects. When carbamazepine suspension has been combined with chlorpromazine or thioridazine solutions, a precipitate forms which may result in loss of effect. Therefore, it is recommended that the carbamazepine suspension dosage form not be administered at the same time with other liquid medicinal agents or diluents. Should be administered with meals.

Extended release capsule (Carbatrol®, Equetro®): Consists of three different types of beads: Immediate release, extended-release, and enteric release. The bead types are combined in a ratio to allow twice daily dosing. May be opened and contents sprinkled over food such as a teaspoon of applesauce; may be administered with or without food; do not crush or chew.

Extended release tablet: Should be inspected for damage. Damaged extended release tablets (without release portal) should not be administered. Should be administered with meals; swallow whole, do not crush or chew.

Hazardous agent; use appropriate precautions for handling and disposal (NIOSH, 2012).

Storage/Stability

Carbatrol®, Equetro®: Store at controlled room temperature (25°C [77°F]); excursions permitted to 15°C to 30°C (59°F to 86°F); protect from light and moisture.

Tegretol®-XR: Store at controlled room temperature, 15°C to 30°C (59°F to 86°F); protect from moisture.

Tegretol® tablets and chewable tablets: Store at ≤30°C (86°F); protect from light and moisture.

Tegretol® suspension: Store at ≤30°C (86°F); shake well before using.

Nursing Actions

Physical Assessment Monitor therapeutic response (seizure activity, type, duration) at beginning of therapy and periodically throughout. Observe and teach seizure/safety precautions. Monitor for mental and CNS changes, excessive sedation (especially when initiating or increasing therapy), suicide ideation, and mood changes.

Patient Education

- Discuss specific use of drug and side effects with patient as it relates to treatment. (HCAHPS: During this hospital stay, were you given any medicine that you had not taken before? Before giving you any new medicine, how often did hospital staff tell you what the medicine was for? How often did hospital staff describe possible side effects in a way you could understand?)
- Patient may experience fatigue or xerostomia. Have patient report immediately to prescriber significant change in balance, difficulty speaking, hallucinations, severe dizziness, syncope, considerable headache, bradycardia, tachycardia, arrhythmia, vision changes, intolerable nausea, ecchymosis, hemorrhaging, melena, edema of extremities, arthralgia, myalgia, urinary retention, oliguria, menstrual irregularities, signs of infection, signs of hepatic impairment, or signs of depression (ie, suicidal ideation, anxiety, emotional instability, illogical thinking) (HCAHPS).
- Educate patient about signs of a significant reaction (eg, wheezing; chest tightness; fever; itching; bad cough; blue skin color; seizures; or

swelling of face, lips, tongue, or throat). **Note:** This is not a comprehensive list of all side effects. Patient should consult prescriber for additional questions.

Intended Use and Disclaimer: Should not be printed and given to patients. This information is intended to serve as a concise initial reference for healthcare professionals to use when discussing medications with a patient. You must ultimately rely on your own discretion, experience and judgment in diagnosing, treating and advising patients.

Dietary Considerations Drug may cause GI upset, take with large amount of water or food to decrease GI upset. May need to split doses to avoid GI upset.

Related Information

Oral Medications That Should Not Be Crushed or Altered *on page 1712*

Peak and Trough Guidelines *on page 1710*

Carbidopa and Levodopa
(kar bi DOE pa & lee voe DOE pa)

Brand Names: U.S. Parcopa®; Sinemet®; Sinemet® CR

Index Terms Levodopa and Carbidopa

Pharmacologic Category Anti-Parkinson's Agent, Decarboxylase Inhibitor; Anti-Parkinson's Agent, Dopamine Precursor

Medication Safety Issues

Sound-alike/look-alike issues:

Sinemet® may be confused with Serevent®

International issues:

Zimox: Brand name for carbidopa and levodopa [Greece], but also the brand name for amoxicillin [Italy]

Zimox [Greece] may be confused with Diamox which is a brand name for acetazolamide [Canada and multiple international markets]

Pregnancy Risk Factor C

Breast-Feeding Considerations Levodopa is excreted into breast milk. A study was done in one lactating woman at 4.5 months postpartum who had been taking carbidopa/levodopa for several years. Regardless of the formulation (sustained release or immediate release) peak levodopa concentrations in the breast milk were found ~3 hours after the maternal dose and returned to baseline ~6 hours after the dose. The highest milk concentration (3.47 nmol/L) was found following the immediate release tablet and this was 27% of the peak maternal plasma concentration (occurring 30 minutes after the dose) and ~40% of the simultaneous plasma concentration. Carbidopa was not evaluated (Thulin, 1998). The manufacturer recommends that caution be used if administered to nursing women.

Use Idiopathic Parkinson's disease; postencephalitic parkinsonism; symptomatic parkinsonism

Duodopa™ intestinal gel: Canadian labeling (not available in U.S.): Treatment of advanced levodopa-responsive Parkinson's disease in which severe motor symptoms are not controlled by other Parkinson's agents

Unlabeled Use Restless leg syndrome

Mechanism of Action/Effect Parkinson's symptoms are due to a lack of striatal dopamine; levodopa circulates in the plasma to the blood-brain-barrier (BBB), where it crosses, to be converted by striatal enzymes to dopamine; carbidopa inhibits the peripheral plasma breakdown of levodopa by inhibiting its decarboxylation, and thereby increases available levodopa at the BBB

Contraindications Hypersensitivity to levodopa, carbidopa, or any component of the formulation; narrow-angle glaucoma; use of MAO inhibitors within prior 14 days (however, may be administered concomitantly with the manufacturer's recommended dose of an MAO inhibitor with selectivity for MAO type B); history of melanoma or undiagnosed skin lesions

Canadian labeling: Additional contraindications: Clinical or laboratory evidence of uncompensated cardiovascular, cerebrovascular, endocrine, renal, hepatic, hematologic or pulmonary disease; when administration of a sympathomimetic amine (eg, epinephrine, norepinephrine or isoproterenol) is contraindicated; intestinal gel therapy in patients with any condition preventing the required placement of a PEG tube for administration.

Warnings/Precautions Use with caution in patients with history of cardiovascular disease (including myocardial infarction and arrhythmias), pulmonary diseases (such as asthma), psychosis, wide-angle glaucoma, peptic ulcer disease, seizure disorder or prone to seizures, and in severe renal and hepatic dysfunction. Use with caution when interpreting plasma/urine catecholamine levels; falsely diagnosed pheochromocytoma has been rarely reported. Severe cases or rhabdomyolysis have been reported. Sudden discontinuation of levodopa may cause a worsening of Parkinson's disease. Elderly may be more sensitive to CNS effects of levodopa. May cause or exacerbate dyskinesias. Patients have reported falling asleep while engaging in activities of daily living; this has been reported to occur without significant warning signs. May cause orthostatic hypotension; Parkinson's disease patients appear to have an impaired capacity to respond to a postural challenge; use with caution in patients at risk of hypotension (such as those receiving antihypertensive drugs) or where transient hypotensive episodes would be poorly tolerated (cardiovascular disease or cerebrovascular disease). Observe patients closely for development of depression with concomitant suicidal tendencies.

Dopamine agonists have been associated with compulsive behaviors and/or loss of impulse control, which has manifested as pathological gambling, libido increases (hypersexuality), and/or binge eating. Causality has not been established, and controversy exists as to whether this phenomenon is related to the underlying disease, prior behaviors/addictions and/or drug therapy. Dose reduction or discontinuation of therapy has been reported to reverse these behaviors in some, but not all cases. Risk for melanoma development is increased in Parkinson's disease patients; drug causation or factors contributing to risk have not been established. Patients should be monitored closely and periodic skin examinations should be performed. Dopaminergic agents have been associated with a syndrome resembling neuroleptic malignant syndrome on abrupt withdrawal or significant dosage reduction after long-term use. Protein in the diet should be distributed throughout the day to avoid fluctuations in levodopa absorption.

Intestinal gel (available in Canada, not available in U.S.): Product should be prescribed only by neurologists experienced in the treatment of Parkinson's disease and who have completed the Duodopa™ Education Program. Response to levodopa/carbidopa intestinal gel therapy should be assessed with a test period (~3 days) of administration via a temporary nasoduodenal tube prior to placement of a percutaneous endoscopic gastrostomy (PEG) tube for permanent access and administration. Sudden deterioration in therapy response with recurring motor symptoms may indicate PEG tube complications (eg, displacement) or obstruction of the infusion device. Tube or infusion device complications may require initiation of oral levodopa/carbidopa therapy until complications are resolved. Discontinue therapy 2-3 hours prior to surgical procedures requiring general anesthesia, if possible. May resume therapy postoperatively when oral fluid intake is permitted.

Drug Interactions

Avoid Concomitant Use

Avoid concomitant use of Carbidopa and Levodopa with any of the following: Amisulpride; Sulpiride

Decreased Effect

Carbidopa and Levodopa may decrease the levels/effects of: Amisulpride; Antipsychotics (Typical); Droxidopa; Sulpiride

The levels/effects of Carbidopa and Levodopa may be decreased by: Amisulpride; Antipsychotics (Atypical); Antipsychotics (Typical); Fosphenytoin; Glycopyrrolate; Iron Salts; Methionine; Metoclopramide; Multivitamins/Fluoride (with ADE); Multivitamins/Minerals (with ADEK, Folate, Iron); Multivitamins/Minerals (with AE, No Iron); Phenytoin; Pyridoxine; Sulpiride

Increased Effect/Toxicity

Carbidopa and Levodopa may increase the levels/effects of: BuPROPion; Droxidopa; MAO Inhibitors

The levels/effects of Carbidopa and Levodopa may be increased by: MAO Inhibitors; Methylphenidate; Sapropterin

Nutritional/Ethanol Interactions

Ethanol: Avoid ethanol (due to CNS depression).

Food: Avoid high protein diets due to potential for impaired levodopa absorption; levodopa competes with certain amino acids for transport across the gut wall or across the blood-brain barrier.

Herb/Nutraceutical: Avoid kava kava (may decrease effects). Pyridoxine (vitamin B_6) in doses >10-25 mg (for levodopa alone) may decrease efficacy. Iron supplements or iron-containing multivitamins may reduce absorption of levodopa.

Adverse Reactions Frequency not defined.

Cardiovascular: Arrhythmia, chest pain, edema, flushing, hypotension, hypertension, MI, orthostatic hypotension, palpitation, phlebitis, syncope

Central nervous system: Agitation, anxiety, ataxia, confusion, delusions, dementia, depression (with or without suicidal tendencies), disorientation, dizziness, dreams abnormal, EPS, euphoria, faintness, falling, fatigue, gait abnormalities, headache, hallucinations, impulse control symptoms, insomnia, malaise, memory impairment, mental acuity decreased, nervousness, neuroleptic malignant syndrome, nightmares, on-off phenomena, paranoid ideation, pathological gambling, psychosis, seizure (causal relationship not established), somnolence

Dermatologic: Alopecia, malignant melanoma, rash

Endocrine & metabolic: Hot flashes, hyperglycemia, hypokalemia, libido increased (including hypersexuality), uric acid increased

Gastrointestinal: Abdominal pain, abdominal distress, anorexia, bruxism, constipation, diarrhea, discoloration of saliva, duodenal ulcer, dyspepsia, dysphagia, flatulence, GI bleeding, heartburn, nausea, sialorrhea, taste alterations, tongue burning sensation, weight gain/loss, vomiting, xerostomia

Genitourinary: Discoloration of urine, glycosuria, urinary frequency, priapism, proteinuria, urinary incontinence, urinary retention, urinary tract infection

Hematologic: Agranulocytosis, anemia, Coombs' test abnormal, hematocrit decreased, hemoglobin decreased, hemolytic anemia, leukopenia

Hepatic: Alkaline phosphatase abnormal, ALT abnormal, AST abnormal, bilirubin abnormal, LDH abnormal

Neuromuscular & skeletal: Back pain, dyskinesias (including choreiform, dystonic and other involuntary movements), leg pain, muscle cramps, muscle twitching, numbness, paresthesia, peripheral neuropathy, shoulder pain, tremor increased, trismus, weakness

Ocular: Blepharospasm, blurred vision, diplopia, Horner's syndrome reactivation, mydriasis, oculogyric crises (may be associated with acute dystonic reactions)

Renal: Difficult urination

Respiratory: Cough, dyspnea, hoarseness, pharyngeal pain, upper respiratory infection

Miscellaneous: Discoloration of sweat, diaphoresis increased, hiccups, hypersensitivity reactions (angioedema, pruritus, urticaria, bullous lesions [including pemphigus-like reactions], Henoch-Schönlein purpura [IgA vasculitis])

Available Dosage Forms

Tablet: 10/100: Carbidopa 10 mg and levodopa 100 mg; 25/100: Carbidopa 25 mg and levodopa 100 mg; 25/250: Carbidopa 25 mg and levodopa 250 mg

Sinemet®:

10/100: Carbidopa 10 mg and levodopa 100 mg

25/100: Carbidopa 25 mg and levodopa 100 mg

25/250: Carbidopa 25 mg and levodopa 250 mg

Tablet, extended release: 25/100: Carbidopa 25 mg and levodopa 100 mg; 50/200: Carbidopa 50 mg and levodopa 200 mg

Tablet, orally disintegrating: 10/100: Carbidopa 10 mg and levodopa 100 mg; 25/100: Carbidopa 25 mg and levodopa 100 mg; 25/250: Carbidopa 25 mg and levodopa 250 mg

Parcopa®:

10/100: Carbidopa 10 mg and levodopa 100 mg [contains phenylalanine 3.4 mg/tablet; mint flavor]

25/100: Carbidopa 25 mg and levodopa 100 mg [contains phenylalanine 3.4 mg/tablet; mint flavor]

25/250: Carbidopa 25 mg and levodopa 250 mg [contains phenylalanine 8.4 mg/tablet; mint flavor]

Tablet, sustained release: 25/100: Carbidopa 25 mg and levodopa 100 mg; 50/200: Carbidopa 50 mg and levodopa 200 mg

Sinemet® CR:

25/100: Carbidopa 25 mg and levodopa 100 mg

50/200: Carbidopa 50 mg and levodopa 200 mg

General Dosage Range Oral: Adults: Immediate release: Initial: Carbidopa 25 mg/levodopa 100 mg 3 times/day (maximum: 8 tablets of any strength/day **or** 200 mg of carbidopa and 2000 mg of levodopa); Controlled release: Adults: Initial: Carbidopa 50 mg/levodopa 200 mg 2 times/day, at intervals not <6 hours (maximum: 8 tablets/day)

Administration

Oral Tablet formulations: Space doses evenly over the waking hours. Give with meals to decrease GI upset. Controlled release product should not be chewed or crushed. Orally-disintegrating tablets do not require water; the tablet should disintegrate on the tongue's surface before swallowing.

Other Intestinal gel (Canadian labeling; not available in U.S.): Gel is administered directly to the duodenum via a portable infusion pump (CADD legacy Duodopa™ pump). Administer through a temporary nasoduodenal tube for at least 3 days to evaluate patient response and for dose optimization. Long-term administration requires placement of PEG tube for intestinal infusion. Continuous maintenance dose is infused throughout the day for up to 16 hours.

Storage/Stability

Tablet: Store at 20°C to 25°C (68°F to 77°F); excursions permitted between 15°C to 30°C (59°F to 86°F). Protect from light and moisture.

Intestinal gel (Canadian labeling; not available in U.S.): Store in refrigerator at 2°C to 8°C (36°F to 46°F). Keep in outer carton to protect from light. Cassettes are for single use only and should be discarded daily following infusion (up to 16 hours).

Nursing Actions

Physical Assessment Monitor therapeutic response (eg, activities of daily living, involuntary movements) at beginning of therapy and periodically throughout therapy.

Patient Education

• Discuss specific use of drug and side effects with patient as it relates to treatment. (HCAHPS. During this hospital stay, were you given any medicine that you had not taken before? Before giving you any new medicine, how often did hospital staff tell you what the medicine was for? How often did hospital staff describe possible side effects in a way you could understand?)

• Patient may experience constipation, fatigue, xerostomia, headache, lack of appetite, dysgeusia, insomnia, or body fluid discoloration. Have patient report immediately to prescriber signs of depression (ie, suicidal ideation, anxiety, emotional instability, illogical thinking), behavioral changes, hallucinations, uncontrollable urges, narcolepsy, skin growths, mole changes, difficulty with motor activity, fasciculations, change in balance, dysphagia, difficulty speaking, paresthesia, severe nausea, considerable diarrhea, hematemesis, melena, angina, severe dyspepsia, chills, pharyngitis, ecchymosis, hemorrhaging, significant dizziness, syncope, or signs of neuroleptic malignant syndrome (NMS) (HCAHPS).

• Educate patient about signs of a significant reaction (eg, wheezing; chest tightness; fever; itching; bad cough; blue skin color; seizures; or swelling of face, lips, tongue, or throat). **Note:** This is not a comprehensive list of all side effects. Patient should consult prescriber for additional questions.

Intended Use and Disclaimer: Should not be printed and given to patients. This information is intended to serve as a concise initial reference for healthcare professionals to use when discussing

medications with a patient. You must ultimately rely on your own discretion, experience and judgment in diagnosing, treating and advising patients.

Dietary Considerations Avoid high protein diets (>2 g/kg) which may decrease the efficacy of levodopa via competition with amino acids in crossing the blood-brain barrier. Some products may contain phenylalanine.

Related Information

Oral Medications That Should Not Be Crushed or Altered *on page 1712*

CARBOplatin (KAR boe pla tin)

Index Terms CBDCA; Paraplatin

Pharmacologic Category Antineoplastic Agent, Alkylating Agent; Antineoplastic Agent, Platinum Analog

Medication Safety Issues

Sound-alike/look-alike issues:

CARBOplatin may be confused with CISplatin, oxaliplatin

Paraplatin® may be confused with Platinol®

High alert medication:

This medication is in a class the Institute for Safe Medication Practices (ISMP) includes among its list of drug classes which have a heightened risk of causing significant patient harm when used in error.

BEERS Criteria medication:

This drug may be potentially inappropriate for use in geriatric patients (Quality of evidence - moderate; Strength of recommendation - strong).

Pregnancy Risk Factor D

Lactation Excretion in breast milk unknown/not recommended

Breast-Feeding Considerations Due to the potential for toxicity in nursing infants, breast-feeding is not recommended.

Use Initial treatment of advanced ovarian cancer in combination with other established chemotherapy agents; palliative treatment of recurrent ovarian cancer after prior chemotherapy, including cisplatin-based treatment

Unlabeled Use Treatment of bladder cancer, breast cancer (metastatic), central nervous system tumors, cervical cancer (recurrent or metastatic), endometrial cancer, esophageal cancer, head and neck cancer, Hodgkin's lymphoma (relapsed or refractory), malignant pleural mesothelioma, melanoma (advanced or metastatic), merkel cell carcinoma, neuroendocrine tumors (adrenal gland and carcinoid tumors), non-Hodgkin's lymphomas (relapsed or refractory), nonsmall cell lung cancer, retinoblastoma, sarcomas (Ewing's sarcoma and osteosarcoma), small-cell lung cancer, testicular cancer, thymic malignancies, unknown primary adenocarcinoma, and as a conditioning regimen prior to hematopoietic stem cell transplantation

Mechanism of Action/Effect Carboplatin is an alkylating agent which covalently binds to DNA; possible cross-linking and interference with the function of DNA

Contraindications History of severe allergic reaction to carboplatin, cisplatin, other platinum-containing formulations, mannitol, or any component of the formulation; should not be used in patients with severe bone marrow depression or significant bleeding

Warnings/Precautions Hazardous agent - use appropriate precautions for handling and disposal (NIOSH, 2012). High doses have resulted in severe abnormalities of liver function tests. **[U.S. Boxed Warning]: Bone marrow suppression, which may be severe, is dose related; may result in infection (due to neutropenia) or bleeding (due to thrombocytopenia); anemia may require blood transfusion;** reduce dosage in patients with bone marrow suppression; cycles should be delayed until WBC and platelet counts have recovered. Patients who have received prior myelosuppressive therapy and patients with renal dysfunction are at increased risk for bone marrow suppression. Anemia is cumulative.

When calculating the carboplatin dose using the Calvert formula and an estimated glomerular filtration rate (GFR), the laboratory method used to measure serum creatinine may impact dosing. Compared to other methods, standardized isotope dilution mass spectrometry (IDMS) may underestimate serum creatinine values in patients with low creatinine values (eg, ≤0.7 mg/dL) and may overestimate GFR in patients with normal renal function. This may result in higher calculated carboplatin doses and increased toxicities. If using IDMS, the Food and Drug Administration (FDA) recommends that clinicians consider capping estimated GFR at a maximum of 125 mL/minute to avoid potential toxicity.

[U.S. Boxed Warning]: Anaphylactic-like reactions have been reported with carboplatin; may occur within minutes of administration. Epinephrine, corticosteroids and antihistamines have been used to treat symptoms. The risk of allergic reactions (including anaphylaxis) is increased in patients previously exposed to platinum therapy. Skin testing and desensitization protocols have been reported (Confina-Cohen, 2005; Lee, 2004; Markman, 2003). When administered as sequential infusions, taxane derivatives (docetaxel, paclitaxel) should be administered before the platinum derivatives (carboplatin, cisplatin) to limit myelosuppression and to enhance efficacy. Ototoxicity may occur when administered concomitantly with aminoglycosides. Clinically significant hearing loss has been reported to occur in pediatric patients when carboplatin was administered at higher than recommended doses in combination with other ototoxic agents (eg, aminoglycosides).

In a study of children receiving carboplatin for the treatment of retinoblastoma, those <6 months of age at treatment initiation were more likely to experience ototoxicity; long-term audiology monitoring is recommended (Qaddoumi, 2012). Loss of vision (usually reversible within weeks of discontinuing) has been reported with higher than recommended doses.

Use caution in elderly patients; may cause or exacerbate syndrome of inappropriate antidiuretic hormone secretion or hyponatremia; monitor sodium closely with initiation or dosage adjustments in older adults (Beers Criteria). Peripheral neuropathy occurs infrequently, the incidence of peripheral neuropathy is increased patients >65 years of age and those who have previously received cisplatin treatment. Patients >65 years of age are more likely to develop severe thrombocytopenia.

Limited potential for nephrotoxicity unless administered concomitantly with aminoglycosides. **[U.S. Boxed Warning]: Vomiting may occur;** may be severe in patients who have received prior emetogenic therapy. **[U.S. Boxed Warning]: Should be administered under the supervision of an experienced cancer chemotherapy physician.**

Drug Interactions

Avoid Concomitant Use

Avoid concomitant use of CARBOplatin with any of the following: BCG; CloZAPine; Natalizumab; Pimecrolimus; SORAfenib; Tacrolimus (Topical); Tofacitinib; Vaccines (Live)

Decreased Effect

CARBOplatin may decrease the levels/effects of: BCG; Coccidioidin Skin Test; Fosphenytoin-Phenytoin; Sipuleucel-T; Vaccines (Inactivated); Vaccines (Live)

The levels/effects of CARBOplatin may be decreased by: Echinacea

Increased Effect/Toxicity

CARBOplatin may increase the levels/effects of: Bexarotene (Systemic); CloZAPine; Leflunomide; Natalizumab; Taxane Derivatives; Tofacitinib; Topotecan; Vaccines (Live)

The levels/effects of CARBOplatin may be increased by: Aminoglycosides; Denosumab; Pimecrolimus; Roflumilast; SORAfenib; Tacrolimus (Topical); Trastuzumab

Nutritional/Ethanol Interactions Herb/Nutraceutical: Avoid black cohosh, dong quai in estrogen-dependent tumors.

Adverse Reactions Percentages reported with single-agent therapy.

>10%:

Central nervous system: Pain (23%)

Endocrine & metabolic: Hyponatremia (29% to 47%), hypomagnesemia (29% to 43%), hypocalcemia(22% to 31%), hypokalemia (20% to 28%)

Gastrointestinal: Vomiting (65% to 81%), abdominal pain (17%), nausea (without vomiting: 10% to 15%)

Hematologic: Myelosuppression (dose related and dose limiting; nadir at ~21 days with single-agent therapy), anemia (71% to 90%; grades 3/4: 21%), leukopenia (85%; grades 3/4: 15% to 26%), neutropenia (67%; grades 3/4: 16% to 21%), thrombocytopenia (62%; grades 3/4: 25% to 35%)

Hepatic: Alkaline phosphatase increased (24% to 37%), AST increased (15% to 19%)

Neuromuscular & skeletal: Weakness (11%)

Renal: Creatinine clearance decreased (27%), BUN increased (14% to 22%)

Miscellaneous: Hypersensitivity/allergic reaction (2% to 16%)

1% to 10%:

Central nervous system: Neurotoxicity (5%)

Dermatologic: Alopecia (2% to 3%)

Gastrointestinal: Constipation (6%), diarrhea (6%), stomatitis/mucositis (1%), taste dysgeusia (1%)

Hematologic: Bleeding (5%), hemorrhagic complications (5%)

Hepatic: Bilirubin increased (5%)

Neuromuscular & skeletal: Peripheral neuropathy (4% to 6%)

Ocular: Visual disturbance (1%)

Otic: Ototoxicity (1%)

Renal: Creatinine increased (6% to 10%)

Miscellaneous: Infection (5%)

Available Dosage Forms

Solution, Intravenous:

Generic: 50 mg/5 mL (5 mL); 150 mg/15 mL (15 mL); 450 mg/45 mL (45 mL); 600 mg/60 mL (60 mL)

Solution, Intravenous [preservative free]:

Generic: 50 mg/5 mL (5 mL); 150 mg/15 mL (15 mL); 450 mg/45 mL (45 mL); 600 mg/60 mL (60 mL)

Solution Reconstituted, Intravenous:

Generic: 150 mg (1 ea)

General Dosage Range Dosage adjustment recommended in renal impairment or who develop toxicities

I.V.: *Adults:* 300-360 mg/m² every 4 weeks **or** AUC of 4-6 (using Calvert formula)

Administration

I.V. Usually infused over 15-60 minutes, although some protocols may require infusions up to 24 hours. When administered as a part of a combination chemotherapy regimen, sequence of administration may vary by regimen; refer to specific protocol for sequence recommendation.

Needles or I.V. administration sets that contain aluminum should not be used in the preparation or administration of carboplatin; aluminum can react with carboplatin resulting in precipitate formation and loss of potency.

Hazardous agent; use appropriate precautions for handling and disposal (NIOSH, 2012).

Preparation for Administration
Solution for injection: Manufacturer's labeling states solution can be further diluted to concentrations as low as 0.5 mg/mL in NS or D$_5$W; however, most clinicians generally dilute dose in either 100 mL or 250 mL of NS or D$_5$W.

Concentrations used for desensitization vary based on protocol.

Hazardous agent; use appropriate precautions for handling and disposal (NIOSH, 2012). Needles or I.V. administration sets that contain aluminum should not be used in the preparation or administration of carboplatin; aluminum can react with carboplatin resulting in precipitate formation and loss of potency.

Storage/Stability Store intact vials at room temperature at 25°C (77°F); excursions permitted to 15°C to 30°C (59°F to 86°F). Protect from light. Further dilution to a concentration as low as 0.5 mg/mL is stable at room temperature (25°C) for 8 hours in NS or D$_5$W. Stability has also been demonstrated for dilutions in D$_5$W in PVC bags at room temperature for 9 days (Benaji, 1994); however, the manufacturer recommends use within 8 hours due to lack of preservative.

Nursing Actions
Physical Assessment Patient allergy history must be assessed prior to therapy. Assess other drugs patient may be taking for potential interactions (especially products that may be ototoxic or nephrotoxic and need for sequencing with taxane derivatives). Assess hematology, electrolytes, and renal and hepatic function tests prior to treatment and on a regular basis during therapy. Monitor for nausea and vomiting (pretreatment with antiemetic may be required), ototoxicity (audiometry may be advisable), bone marrow depression, anemia, bleeding, and peripheral neuropathy.

Patient Education
• Discuss specific use of drug and side effects with patient as it relates to treatment. (HCAHPS: During this hospital stay, were you given any medicine that you had not taken before? Before giving you any new medicine, how often did hospital staff tell you what the medicine was for? How often did hospital staff describe possible side effects in a way you could understand?)
• Patient may experience constipation, alopecia, or lack of appetite. Have patient report immediately to prescriber signs of infection, severe dyspepsia, significant nausea, considerable diarrhea, ecchymosis, hemorrhaging, urine discoloration, jaundice, intolerable asthenia, urinary retention, oliguria, hearing impairment, paresthesia, stomatitis, tinnitus, or vision changes (HCAHPS).
• Educate patient about signs of a significant reaction (eg, wheezing; chest tightness; fever;

itching; bad cough; blue skin color; seizures; or swelling of face, lips, tongue, or throat). **Note:** This is not a comprehensive list of all side effects. Patient should consult prescriber for additional questions.

Intended Use and Disclaimer: Should not be printed and given to patients. This information is intended to serve as a concise initial reference for healthcare professionals to use when discussing medications with a patient. You must ultimately rely on your own discretion, experience and judgment in diagnosing, treating and advising patients.

Related Information
Management of Drug Extravasations *on page 1700*

Carboprost Tromethamine
(KAR boe prost tro METH a meen)

Brand Names: U.S. Hemabate
Index Terms Carboprost; Prostaglandin F$_2$ Alpha Analog; Prostaglandin F$_2$ Analog
Pharmacologic Category Abortifacient; Prostaglandin
Pregnancy Risk Factor C
Lactation Excretion in breast milk unknown
Use
Termination of pregnancy: For aborting pregnancy between week 13 and 20 of gestation as calculated from the first day of the last normal menstrual period and in the following conditions related to second trimester abortion: Failure of expulsion of the fetus during the course of treatment by another method; premature rupture of membranes in intrauterine methods with loss of drug and insufficient or absent uterine activity; requirement of a repeat intrauterine instillation of drug for expulsion of the fetus; inadvertent or spontaneous rupture of membranes in the presence of a previable fetus and absence of adequate activity for expulsion.

Refractory postpartum uterine hemorrhage: Treatment of postpartum hemorrhage due to uterine atony that has not responded to conventional methods of management. Prior treatment should include the use of intravenously (I.V.) administered oxytocin, manipulative techniques such as uterine massage and, unless contraindicated, intramuscular ergot preparations.

Available Dosage Forms
Solution, Intramuscular:
Hemabate: 250 mcg/mL (1 mL)
General Dosage Range I.M.: *Adults (females):* Termination of pregnancy: 250 mcg at 1.5- to 3.5-hour intervals, a 500 mcg dose may be given if uterine response is not adequate after several 250 mcg doses (maximum total dose: 12 mg); Postpartum bleeding: 250 mcg; may repeat if needed (maximum total dose: 2 mg [8 doses])

◄ **Administration**
I.M. Administer deep I.M. (use a tuberculin syringe for termination of pregnancy); rotate site if repeat injections are required.
I.V. Should only be administered deep I.M.; do not inject I.V.

Nursing Actions
Physical Assessment Note that nausea or vomiting may be significant; premedication with an antiemetic may be considered. Monitor for uterine contractions, hypertension, hemorrhage, respiratory effects, or prolonged or excessively elevated temperature. Report contractions lasting longer than 1 minute or absence of contractions to prescriber. Assess for complete expulsion of uterine contents (fetal tissue).

Patient Education
• Discuss specific use of drug and side effects with patient as it relates to treatment. (HCAHPS: During this hospital stay, were you given any medicine that you had not taken before? Before giving you any new medicine, how often did hospital staff tell you what the medicine was for? How often did hospital staff describe possible side effects in a way you could understand?)
• Patient may experience headache or diarrhea. Have patient report immediately to prescriber severe dizziness, syncope, significant nausea, or considerable dyspepsia (HCAHPS).
• Educate patient about signs of a significant reaction (eg, wheezing; chest tightness; fever; itching; bad cough; blue skin color; seizures; or swelling of face, lips, tongue, or throat). **Note:** This is not a comprehensive list of all side effects. Patient should consult prescriber for additional questions.

Intended Use and Disclaimer: Should not be printed and given to patients. This information is intended to serve as a concise initial reference for healthcare professionals to use when discussing medications with a patient. You must ultimately rely on your own discretion, experience and judgment in diagnosing, treating and advising patients.

Carfilzomib (kar FILZ oh mib)

Brand Names: U.S. Kyprolis
Index Terms PR-171
Pharmacologic Category Antineoplastic Agent; Proteasome Inhibitor
Medication Safety Issues
  Sound-alike/look-alike issues:
    Carfilzomib may be confused with bortezomib
  High alert medication:
    This medication is in a class the Institute for Safe Medication Practices (ISMP) includes among its list of drug classes which have a heightened risk of causing significant patient harm when used in error.

Pregnancy Risk Factor D
Lactation Excretion in breast milk unknown/not recommended
Use Treatment of multiple myeloma in patients who have received at least 2 prior treatment regimens (including a proteasome inhibitor and an immunomodulator) with disease progression within 60 days after the most recent treatment

Available Dosage Forms
  Solution Reconstituted, Intravenous:
    Kyprolis: 60 mg (1 ea)
General Dosage Range Dosage adjustment recommended in patients who develop toxicities.
  I.V.: *Adults:* 15-27 mg/m^2 on 2 consecutive days each week for 3 weeks (days 1, 2, 8, 9, 15, and 16) of a 28-day treatment cycle

Administration
I.V. Administer over 2-10 minutes. Flush line before and after carfilzomib with NS or D$_5$W.

Hazardous agent; use appropriate precautions for handling and disposal (meets NIOSH, 2012 criteria).
Injectable Detail pH: 3.5 (intact vial)

Nursing Actions
Physical Assessment Monitor vital signs, renal function, signs of infection or bleeding, new pulmonary symptoms, or infusion-related reactions. Check lab results, including creatinine, potassium, magnesium, AST, alkaline phosphatase, and CBC with differential. Monitor for symptoms of heart failure. Confirm patient adequately hydrated prior to treatment to prevent tumor lysis syndrome; educate patient about how to address if having problems with fluid intake.

Patient Education
• Discuss specific use of drug and side effects with patient as it relates to treatment. (HCAHPS: During this hospital stay, were you given any medicine that you had not taken before? Before giving you any new medicine, how often did hospital staff tell you what the medicine was for? How often did hospital staff describe possible side effects in a way you could understand?)
• Patient may experience constipation, lack of appetite, muscle spasms, arthralgia, back pain, or insomnia. Have patient report immediately to prescriber signs of infection, signs of renal impairment, signs of hypokalemia, signs of hyperglycemia, angina, severe dizziness, syncope, paresthesia, intolerable headache, illogical thinking, vision changes, considerable nausea, significant diarrhea, severe asthenia, ecchymosis, hemorrhaging, signs of tumor lysis syndrome (TLS), signs of cardiac failure, signs of severe pulmonary disorder, signs of hepatic impairment, chills, myalgia, arthralgia, facial flushing or edema, or dyspnea (HCAHPS).
• Educate patient about signs of a significant reaction (eg, wheezing; chest tightness; fever; itching; bad cough; blue skin color; seizures; or

swelling of face, lips, tongue, or throat). **Note:** This is not a comprehensive list of all side effects. Patient should consult prescriber for additional questions.

Intended Use and Disclaimer: Should not be printed and given to patients. This information is intended to serve as a concise initial reference for healthcare professionals to use when discussing medications with a patient. You must ultimately rely on your own discretion, experience and judgment in diagnosing, treating and advising patients.

Carisoprodol (kar eye soe PROE dole)

Brand Names: U.S. Soma
Index Terms Carisoprodate; Isobamate
Pharmacologic Category Skeletal Muscle Relaxant
Medication Safety Issues
  BEERS Criteria medication:
    This drug may be potentially inappropriate for use in geriatric patients (Quality of evidence - moderate; Strength of recommendation - strong).
Pregnancy Risk Factor C
Lactation Enters breast milk/use caution
Breast-Feeding Considerations Carisoprodol and its active metabolite, meprobamate are excreted into breast milk. Carisoprodol levels in breast milk may be 2-4 times that of maternal plasma levels. The estimated dose to the infant was reported as 6.9% of the weight adjusted maternal dose in one case report (Briggs, 2008) and ~4% of the weight-adjusted maternal dose in another (Nordeng, 2001). In both cases, breast milk production was decreased requiring supplemental formula or cessation of breast-feeding. Other than slight sedation reported in one infant, no symptoms of withdrawal or other adverse events were noted in these two cases. Effects on long-term development are not known. The manufacturer recommends caution be used if carisoprodol is administered to a nursing woman.
Use Short-term (2-3 weeks) treatment of acute musculoskeletal pain
Mechanism of Action/Effect Precise mechanism is not yet clear, but many effects have been ascribed to its central depressant actions. In animals, carisoprodol blocks interneuronal activity and depresses polysynaptic neuron transmission in the spinal cord and reticular formation of the brain. It is also metabolized to meprobamate, which has anxiolytic and sedative effects.
Contraindications Hypersensitivity to carisoprodol, carbamates (eg, meprobamate), or any component of the formulation; history of acute intermittent porphyria
Warnings/Precautions Can cause CNS depression, which may impair physical or mental abilities. Concomitant use of other CNS depressants may

enhance these effects. Patients must be cautioned about performing tasks which require mental alertness (eg, operating machinery or driving); postmarketing reports of motor vehicle accidents have been associated with use. Effects with other CNS-depressant drugs or ethanol may be potentiated. Use with caution in patients with hepatic/renal dysfunction. Tolerance or drug dependence may result from extended use. Limit use to 2-3 weeks; use caution in patients who may be prone to addiction. May precipitate withdrawal after abrupt cessation of prolonged use. Has been associated (rarely) with seizures in patients with and without seizure history.

Carisoprodol should be used with caution in patients who are poor CYP2C19 metabolizers; poor metabolizers have been shown to have a fourfold increase in exposure to carisoprodol and a 50% reduced exposure to the metabolite meprobamate compared to normal metabolizers. Prevalence of poor metabolizers in the Asian population is ~15% to 20% while that of Caucasians and African-Americans is ~3% to 5%. Potentially significant drug-drug interactions may exist, requiring dose or frequency adjustment, additional monitoring, and/or selection of alternative therapy. Muscle relaxants are poorly tolerated by the elderly due to potent anticholinergic effects, sedation, and risk of fracture. Efficacy is questionable at dosages tolerated by elderly patients; avoid use (Beers Criteria).
Drug Interactions
  Avoid Concomitant Use
    Avoid concomitant use of Carisoprodol with any of the following: Azelastine (Nasal); Paraldehyde; Thalidomide
  Decreased Effect
    The levels/effects of Carisoprodol may be decreased by: Aspirin; CYP2C19 Inducers (Strong); Dabrafenib; St Johns Wort
  Increased Effect/Toxicity
    Carisoprodol may increase the levels/effects of: Alcohol (Ethyl); Azelastine (Nasal); Buprenorphine; CNS Depressants; Hydrocodone; Methotrimeprazine; Metyrosine; Mirtazapine; Paraldehyde; Pramipexole; ROPINIRole; Rotigotine; Selective Serotonin Reuptake Inhibitors; Thalidomide; Zolpidem

    The levels/effects of Carisoprodol may be increased by: Aspirin; Brimonidine (Topical); CYP2C19 Inhibitors (Moderate); CYP2C19 Inhibitors (Strong); Doxylamine; Droperidol; HydrOXYzine; Luliconazole; Magnesium Sulfate; Methotrimeprazine; Perampanel; Sodium Oxybate; St Johns Wort; Tapentadol
Nutritional/Ethanol Interactions
  Ethanol: May increase CNS depression. Management: Instruct patients to avoid ethanol during therapy; monitor for increased effects with coadministration.

Herb/Nutraceutical: St John's wort may decrease exposure to carisoprodol and increase exposure to active metabolite (meprobamate). Kava kava, valerian, and gotu kola may increase CNS depression. Management: Avoid St John's wort, kava kava, valerian, and gotu kola.

Adverse Reactions
>10%: Central nervous system: Drowsiness (13% to 17%)
1% to 10%: Central nervous system: Dizziness (7% to 8%), headache (3% to 5%)

Pharmacodynamics/Kinetics
Onset of Action Rapid
Duration of Action 4-6 hours

Controlled Substance C-IV

Available Dosage Forms
Tablet, Oral:
Soma: 250 mg, 350 mg
Generic: 250 mg, 350 mg

General Dosage Range Oral: *Adolescents ≥16 years and Adults:* 250-350 mg 3 times daily and at bedtime

Administration
Oral Administer with or without food.

Storage/Stability Store at 20°C to 25°C (68°F to 77°F).

Nursing Actions
Physical Assessment Monitor for excessive drowsiness at beginning of therapy and periodically throughout. Do not discontinue abruptly; taper dosage slowly (withdrawal symptoms such as abdominal cramping, headache, and insomnia may occur). Teach patient postural hypotension precautions.

Patient Education
• Discuss specific use of drug and side effects with patient as it relates to treatment. (HCAHPS: During this hospital stay, were you given any medicine that you had not taken before? Before giving you any new medicine, how often did hospital staff tell you what the medicine was for? How often did hospital staff describe possible side effects in a way you could understand?)
• Patient may experience headache, dizziness, or fatigue. Have patient report immediately to prescriber severe asthenia (HCAHPS).
• Educate patient about signs of a significant reaction (eg, wheezing; chest tightness; fever; itching; bad cough; blue skin color; seizures; or swelling of face, lips, tongue, or throat). **Note:** This is not a comprehensive list of all side effects. Patient should consult prescriber for additional questions.

Intended Use and Disclaimer: Should not be printed and given to patients. This information is intended to serve as a concise initial reference for healthcare professionals to use when discussing medications with a patient. You must ultimately rely on your own discretion, experience and judgment in diagnosing, treating and advising patients.

Dietary Considerations May be taken with or without food.

Carisoprodol and Aspirin
(kar eye soe PROE dole & AS pir in)

Index Terms Aspirin and Carisoprodol; Soma Compound

Pharmacologic Category Skeletal Muscle Relaxant

Medication Safety Issues
BEERS Criteria medication:
This drug may be potentially inappropriate for use in geriatric patients (Quality of evidence - moderate; Strength of recommendation - strong).

Pregnancy Risk Factor C

Lactation Enters breast milk/not recommended

Use Relief of discomfort associated with acute, painful skeletal muscle conditions

Controlled Substance C-IV

Available Dosage Forms
Tablet: Carisoprodol 200 mg and aspirin 325 mg

General Dosage Range Oral: *Children ≥16 years and Adults:* 1-2 tablets 4 times/day (maximum: 8 tablets/24 hours)

Nursing Actions
Physical Assessment See individual agents.
Patient Education
• Discuss specific use of drug and side effects with patient as it relates to treatment. (HCAHPS: During this hospital stay, were you given any medicine that you had not taken before? Before giving you any new medicine, how often did hospital staff tell you what the medicine was for? How often did hospital staff describe possible side effects in a way you could understand?)
• Patient may experience fatigue, lack of appetite, nausea, or pyrosis. Have patient report immediately to prescriber strength differences from one side to another, difficulty speaking or thinking, change in balance, blurred vision, severe dizziness, syncope, tinnitus, ecchymosis, hemorrhaging, significant asthenia, considerable constipation, intolerable dyspepsia, melena, hematemesis, urinary retention, or oliguria (HCAHPS).
• Educate patient about signs of a significant reaction (eg, wheezing; chest tightness; fever; itching; bad cough; blue skin color; seizures; or swelling of face, lips, tongue, or throat). **Note:** This is not a comprehensive list of all side effects. Patient should consult prescriber for additional questions.

Intended Use and Disclaimer: Should not be printed and given to patients. This information is intended to serve as a concise initial reference for healthcare professionals to use when discussing medications with a patient. You must ultimately

rely on your own discretion, experience and judgment in diagnosing, treating and advising patients.

Related Information
Aspirin *on page 129*
Carisoprodol *on page 261*

Carmustine (kar MUS teen)

Brand Names: U.S. BiCNU; Gliadel Wafer
Index Terms BCNU; bis(chloroethyl) nitrosourea; bis-chloronitrosourea; Carmustine Polymer Wafer; Carmustinum; WR-139021
Pharmacologic Category Antineoplastic Agent, Alkylating Agent; Antineoplastic Agent, Alkylating Agent (Nitrosourea)
Medication Safety Issues
Sound-alike/look-alike issues:
Carmustine may be confused with bendamustine, lomustine
High alert medication:
This medication is in a class the Institute for Safe Medication Practices (ISMP) includes among its list of drug classes which have a heightened risk of causing significant patient harm when used in error.
Pregnancy Risk Factor D
Lactation Excretion in breast milk unknown/not recommended
Breast-Feeding Considerations Due to the potential for serious adverse reactions in the nursing infant, breast-feeding should be discontinued.
Use
Injection: Treatment of brain tumors (glioblastoma, brainstem glioma, medulloblastoma, astrocytoma, ependymoma, and metastatic brain tumors), multiple myeloma, Hodgkin's lymphoma (relapsed or refractory), non-Hodgkin's lymphomas (relapsed or refractory)
Wafer (implant): Adjunct to surgery in patients with recurrent glioblastoma multiforme; adjunct to surgery and radiation in patients with newly-diagnosed high-grade malignant glioma
Unlabeled Use Treatment of mycosis fungoides (topical)
Mechanism of Action/Effect Interferes with the normal function of DNA and RNA by alkylation and cross-linking the strands of DNA and RNA, and by possible protein modification; may also inhibit enzyme processes by carbamylation of amino acids in protein
Contraindications Hypersensitivity to carmustine or any component of the formulation
Warnings/Precautions Hazardous agent - use appropriate precautions for handling and disposal (NIOSH, 2012).

[U.S. Boxed Warning]: Injection: Bone marrow suppression (primarily thrombocytopenia and leukopenia) is the major carmustine toxicity; generally is delayed. Monitor blood counts weekly for at least 6 weeks after administration. Myelosuppression is cumulative. When given at the FDA-approved doses, treatment should not be administered less than 6 weeks apart. Consider nadir blood counts from prior dose for dosage adjustment. May cause bleeding (due to thrombocytopenia) or infections (due to neutropenia); monitor closely. Patients must have platelet counts >100,000/mm^3 and leukocytes >4000/mm^3 for a repeat dose. Anemia may occur (less common and less severe than leukopenia or thrombocytopenia). Long-term use is associated with the development of secondary malignancies (acute leukemias and bone marrow dysplasias).

[U.S. Boxed Warnings]: Injection: Dose-related pulmonary toxicity may occur; patients receiving cumulative doses >1400 mg/m^2 are at higher risk. Delayed onset of pulmonary fibrosis (may be fatal) has occurred in children up to 17 years after treatment; this occurred in ages 1-16 for the treatment of intracranial tumors; cumulative doses ranged from 770-1800 mg/m^2 (in combination with cranial radiotherapy). Pulmonary toxicity is characterized by pulmonary infiltrates and/or fibrosis and has been reported from 9 days to 43 months after nitrosourea treatment (including carmustine). Although pulmonary toxicity generally occurs in patients who have received prolonged treatment, pulmonary fibrosis has been reported with cumulative doses <1400 mg/m^2. In addition to high cumulative doses, other risk factors for pulmonary toxicity include history of lung disease and baseline predicted forced vital capacity (FVC) or carbon monoxide diffusing capacity (DL$_{CO}$) <70%. Baseline and periodic pulmonary function tests are recommended. For high-dose treatment (transplant; unlabeled dose), acute lung injury may occur ~1-3 months post transplant; advise patients to contact their transplant physician for dyspnea, cough, or fever; interstitial pneumonia may be managed with a course of corticosteroids. Children are at higher risk for delayed pulmonary toxicity.

Potentially significant drug-drug interactions may exist, requiring dose or frequency adjustment, additional monitoring, and/or selection of alternative therapy. Injection site burning and local tissue reactions, including swelling, pain, erythema, and necrosis have been reported. Monitor infusion site closely for infiltration or injection site reactions. Reversible increases in transaminases, bilirubin and alkaline phosphatase have been reported (rare); monitor liver function tests periodically during treatment. Renal failure, progressive azotemia, and decreased kidney size have been reported in patients who have received large cumulative doses or prolonged treatment (renal toxicity has also been reported in patients who have received lower cumulative doses); monitor renal function tests periodically during treatment. Unlabeled administration (intraarterial intracarotid route) has been associated with ocular toxicity. Consider initiating treatment at the lower end of the dose range in the elderly. Diluent contains ethanol. With wafer implantation, monitor closely for known craniotomy-related complications (seizure, intracranial infection, abnormal wound healing, brain edema); intracerebral mass effect (unresponsive to corticosteroids) has been reported; may lead to brain herniation; avoid communication between the resection cavity and the ventricular system to prevent wafer migration; communications larger than the wafer should be closed prior to implantation; wafer migration may cause obstructive hydrocephalus. **[U.S. Boxed Warning]: Injection: Should be administered under the supervision of an experienced cancer chemotherapy physician.**

Drug Interactions

Avoid Concomitant Use

Avoid concomitant use of Carmustine with any of the following: BCG; CloZAPine; Natalizumab; Pimecrolimus; Tacrolimus (Topical); Tofacitinib; Vaccines (Live)

Decreased Effect

Carmustine may decrease the levels/effects of: BCG; Cardiac Glycosides; Coccidioidin Skin Test; Sipuleucel-T; Vaccines (Inactivated); Vaccines (Live)

The levels/effects of Carmustine may be decreased by: Echinacea

Increased Effect/Toxicity

Carmustine may increase the levels/effects of: CloZAPine; Leflunomide; Natalizumab; Tofacitinib; Vaccines (Live)

The levels/effects of Carmustine may be increased by: Cimetidine; Denosumab; Melphalan; Pimecrolimus; Roflumilast; Tacrolimus (Topical); Trastuzumab

Adverse Reactions

I.V.: Frequency not defined:
Cardiovascular: Arrhythmia (with high doses), chest pain, flushing (with rapid infusion), hypotension, tachycardia
Central nervous system: Ataxia, dizziness
Central nervous system: Ethanol intoxication (with high doses), headache
Dermatologic: Hyperpigmentation/skin burning (after skin contact)
Gastrointestinal: Nausea (common; dose related), vomiting (common; dose related), mucositis (with high doses), toxic enterocolitis (with high doses)
Hematologic: Leukopenia (common; onset: 5-6 weeks; recovery: after 1-2 weeks), thrombocytopenia (common; onset: ~4 weeks; recovery: after 1-2 weeks), anemia, neutropenic fever, secondary malignancies (acute leukemia, bone marrow dysplasias)
Hepatic: Alkaline phosphatase increased, bilirubin increased, hepatic sinusoidal obstruction

syndrome (SOS; veno-occlusive disease; with high doses), transaminases increased
Local: Injection site reactions (burning, erythema, necrosis, pain, swelling)
Ocular: Conjunctival suffusion (with rapid infusion), neuroretinitis
Renal: Kidney size decreased, progressive azotemia, renal failure
Respiratory: Interstitial pneumonitis (with high doses), pulmonary fibrosis, pulmonary hypoplasia, pulmonary infiltrates
Miscellaneous: Allergic reaction, infection (with high doses)

Wafer: ≥4% (percentages reported only where incidence was greater compared to placebo):
Cardiovascular: Deep thrombophlebitis (10%), facial edema (6%), chest pain (5%)
Central nervous system: Brain edema (4% to 23%), confusion (10% to 23%), depression (16%), headache (15%), somnolence (14%), fever (12%), speech disorder (11%), intracranial hypertension (9%), anxiety (7%), facial paralysis (7%), pain (7%), ataxia (6%), hypesthesia (6%), hallucination (5%), seizure (grand mal 5%), meningitis (4%)
Dermatologic: Abnormal wound healing (14% to 16%), rash (5% to 12%)
Endocrine: Diabetes (5%)
Gastrointestinal: Nausea (8% to 22%), vomiting (8% to 21%), constipation (19%), abdominal pain (8%), diarrhea (5%)
Genitourinary: Urinary tract infection (21%)
Hematologic: Hemorrhage (7%)
Local: Abscess (4% to 8%)
Neuromuscular & skeletal: Weakness (22%), back pain (7%)

Available Dosage Forms

Solution Reconstituted, Intravenous:
BiCNU: 100 mg (1 ea)
Wafer, Implant:
Gliadel Wafer: 7.7 mg (8 ea)

General Dosage Range Dosage adjustment recommended in patients with renal impairment or who develop toxicity.
I.V.: *Adults:* 150-200 mg/m^2 every 6-8 weeks **or** 75-100 mg/m^2/day for 2 days every 6-8 weeks
Implantation: *Adults:* 8 wafers placed in the resection cavity (total dose: 61.6 mg)

Administration

I.V. Irritant (alcohol-based diluent). Significant absorption to PVC containers; should be prepared in either glass or polyolefin containers. Infuse over 2 hours (infusions <2 hours may lead to injection site pain or burning); infuse through a free-flowing saline or dextrose infusion, or administer through a central catheter to alleviate venous pain/irritation.

High-dose carmustine (transplant dose; unlabeled use): Infuse over a least 2 hours to avoid excessive flushing, agitation, and hypotension;

was infused over 1 hour in some trials (Chopra, 1993). **High-dose carmustine may be fatal if not followed by stem cell rescue.** Monitor vital signs frequently during infusion; patients should be supine during infusion and may require the Trendelenburg position, fluid support, and vasopressor support.

Hazardous agent; use appropriate precautions for handling and disposal (NIOSH, 2012).

Topical Hazardous agent; use appropriate precautions for handling and disposal (NIOSH, 2012). Topical (unlabeled use): Apply solution with brush or gauze pads; ointment and solution should be applied while wearing gloves to involved areas only; avoid contact with eyes or mouth (Zackheim, 2003).

Other Implant: Hazardous agent; use appropriate precautions for handling and disposal (NIOSH, 2012); double glove before handling; outer gloves should be discarded as chemotherapy waste after handling wafers. Any wafer or remnant that is removed upon repeat surgery should be discarded as chemotherapy waste. The outer surface of the external foil pouch is not sterile. Open pouch gently; avoid pressure on the wafers to prevent breakage. Wafer that are broken in half may be used, however, wafers broken into more than 2 pieces should be discarded in a biohazard container. Oxidized regenerated cellulose (Surgicel®) may be placed over the wafer to secure; irrigate cavity prior to closure.

Preparation for Administration Hazardous agent; use appropriate precautions for handling and disposal (NIOSH, 2012).

Injection: Reconstitute initially with 3 mL of supplied diluent (dehydrated alcohol injection, USP); then further dilute with SWFI (27 mL), this provides a concentration of 3.3 mg/mL in ethanol 10%; protect from light; further dilute for infusion with D_5W using a non-PVC container.

Storage/Stability

Injection: Store intact vials and provided diluent under refrigeration at 2°C to 8°C (36°F to 46°F). Reconstituted solutions are stable for 24 hours refrigerated (2°C to 8°C) and protected from light. Examine reconstituted vials for crystal formation prior to use. If crystals are observed, they may be redissolved by warming the vial to room temperature with agitation.

Solutions diluted to a concentration of 0.2 mg/mL in D_5W are stable for 8 hours at room temperature (25°C) in glass or polyolefin containers and protected from light.

Wafer: Store at or below -20°C (-4°F). Unopened foil pouches may be kept at room temperature for up to 6 hours.

Nursing Actions

Physical Assessment An antiemetic may be ordered prior to therapy. I.V.: Monitor infusion site closely to prevent extravasation. Monitor patient closely during and following high-dose BMT infusion; supine position (Trandelenburg position may be necessary), fluid support, and vasopressor support should be available. Assess results of hematology, pulmonary, hepatic, and renal function tests at baseline and periodically during therapy.

Patient Education
- Discuss specific use of drug and side effects with patient as it relates to treatment. (HCAHPS: During this hospital stay, were you given any medicine that you had not taken before? Before giving you any new medicine, how often did hospital staff tell you what the medicine was for? How often did hospital staff describe possible side effects in a way you could understand?)
- Patient may experience headache, nausea, flushing, anxiety, constipation, diarrhea, fatigue, or alopecia. Have patient report immediately to prescriber signs of infection; angina; ecchymosis; hemorrhaging; vision changes; illogical thinking; severe dizziness; syncope; memory loss; mood changes; myalgia; significant dyspepsia; neck stiffness; implant site pain, edema, or hemorrhaging; tremors; insomnia; difficulty speaking; paresthesia; dyspnea; urine discoloration; jaundice; considerable asthenia; urinary retention; oliguria; tachycardia; or injection site irritation (HCAHPS).
- Educate patient about signs of a significant reaction (eg, wheezing; chest tightness; fever; itching; bad cough; blue skin color; seizures; or swelling of face, lips, tongue, or throat). **Note:** This is not a comprehensive list of all side effects. Patient should consult prescriber for additional questions.

Intended Use and Disclaimer: Should not be printed and given to patients. This information is intended to serve as a concise initial reference for healthcare professionals to use when discussing medications with a patient. You must ultimately rely on your own discretion, experience and judgment in diagnosing, treating and advising patients.

Related Information
Management of Drug Extravasations on page 1700

Carvedilol (KAR ve dil ole)

Brand Names: U.S. Coreg; Coreg CR
Pharmacologic Category Antihypertensive; Beta-Blocker With Alpha-Blocking Activity
Medication Safety Issues
Sound-alike/look-alike issues:
Carvedilol may be confused with atenolol, captopril, carbidopa, carteolol
Coreg may be confused with Corgard, Cortef, Cozaar
Pregnancy Risk Factor C

Lactation Excretion in breast milk unknown/not recommended

Breast-Feeding Considerations It is not known if carvedilol is excreted into human milk. The manufacturer suggests that a decision should be made to either discontinue nursing or discontinue the medication.

Use Mild-to-severe heart failure (HF) of ischemic or cardiomyopathic origin (usually in addition to standard therapy); left ventricular dysfunction following myocardial infarction (MI) (clinically stable with LVEF ≤40%); management of hypertension

Note: The ACCF/AHA 2013 heart failure guidelines recommend the use of 1 of the 3 beta blockers (ie, bisoprolol, carvedilol, or extended-release metoprolol succinate) for all patients with recent or remote history of MI or ACS and reduced ejection fraction (rEF) to reduce mortality, for all patients with rEF to prevent symptomatic HF (even if no history of MI), and for all patients with current or prior symptoms of HF with reduced ejection fraction (HFrEF), unless contraindicated, to reduce morbidity and mortality (Yancy, 2013).

Unlabeled Use Angina pectoris

Mechanism of Action/Effect Nonselective beta-adrenoreceptor and alpha-adrenergic blocking agent, lowers heart rate and blood pressure. Has been shown to lower risk of hospitalization and increase survival in patients with mild to severe heart failure.

Contraindications Serious hypersensitivity to carvedilol or any component of the formulation; decompensated cardiac failure requiring intravenous inotropic therapy; bronchial asthma or related bronchospastic conditions; second- or third-degree AV block, sick sinus syndrome, and severe bradycardia (except in patients with a functioning artificial pacemaker); cardiogenic shock; severe hepatic impairment

Warnings/Precautions Consider pre-existing conditions such as sick sinus syndrome before initiating. Heart failure patients may experience a worsening of renal function (rare); risk factors include ischemic heart disease, diffuse vascular disease, underlying renal dysfunction, and systolic BP <100 mm Hg. Initiate cautiously and monitor for possible deterioration in patient status (eg, symptoms of HF). Worsening heart failure or fluid retention may occur during upward titration; dose reduction or temporary discontinuation may be necessary. Adjustment of other medications (ACE inhibitors and/or diuretics) may also be required. Bradycardia may be observed more frequently in elderly patients (>65 years of age); dosage reductions may be necessary.

Symptomatic hypotension with or without syncope may occur with carvedilol (usually within the first 30 days of therapy); close monitoring of patient is required especially with initial dosing and dosing increases; blood pressure must be lowered at a rate appropriate for the patient's clinical condition. Initiation with a low dose, gradual up-titration, and administration with food may help to decrease the occurrence of hypotension or syncope. Patients should be advised to avoid driving or other hazardous tasks during initiation of therapy due to the risk of syncope. Beta-blocker therapy should not be withdrawn abruptly (particularly in patients with CAD), but gradually tapered to avoid acute tachycardia, hypertension, and/or ischemia. Chronic beta-blocker therapy should not be routinely withdrawn prior to major surgery.

In general, patients with bronchospastic disease should not receive beta-blockers; if used at all, should be used cautiously with close monitoring. May precipitate or aggravate symptoms of arterial insufficiency in patients with PVD and Raynaud's disease; use with caution and monitor for progression of arterial obstruction. Use caution with concurrent use of digoxin, verapamil or diltiazem; bradycardia or heart block can occur. Use with caution in patients receiving inhaled anesthetic agents known to depress myocardial contractility. Use cautiously in patients with diabetes because it can mask prominent hypoglycemic symptoms. In patients with heart failure and diabetes, use of carvedilol may worsen hyperglycemia; may require adjustment of antidiabetic agents. May mask signs of hyperthyroidism (eg, tachycardia); if hyperthyroidism is suspected, carefully manage and monitor; abrupt withdrawal may exacerbate symptoms of hyperthyroidism or precipitate thyroid storm. May induce or exacerbate psoriasis. Use with caution in patients with myasthenia gravis or psychiatric disease (may cause CNS depression). Use with caution in patients with mild-to-moderate hepatic impairment; use is contraindicated in patients with severe impairment. Manufacturer recommends discontinuation of therapy if liver injury occurs (confirmed by laboratory testing). Adequate alpha-blockade is required prior to use of any beta-blocker for patients with untreated pheochromocytoma. Use caution with history of severe anaphylaxis to allergens; patients taking beta-blockers may become more sensitive to repeated challenges. Treatment of anaphylaxis (eg, epinephrine) in patients taking beta-blockers may be ineffective or promote undesirable effects.

Intraoperative floppy iris syndrome has been observed in cataract surgery patients who were on or were previously treated with alpha$_1$-blockers; causality has not been established and there appears to be no benefit in discontinuing alpha-blocker therapy prior to surgery. Instruct patients to inform ophthalmologist of carvedilol use when considering eye surgery.

Drug Interactions

Avoid Concomitant Use

Avoid concomitant use of Carvedilol with any of the following: Beta2-Agonists; Bosutinib;

Floctafenine; Methacholine; PAZOPanib; Pomalidomide; Topotecan; VinCRIStine (Liposomal)

Decreased Effect

Carvedilol may decrease the levels/effects of: Beta2-Agonists; Theophylline Derivatives

The levels/effects of Carvedilol may be decreased by: Barbiturates; Herbs (Hypertensive Properties); Methylphenidate; Nonsteroidal Anti-Inflammatory Agents; Peginterferon Alfa-2b; P-glycoprotein/ABCB1 Inducers; Rifamycin Derivatives; Yohimbine

Increased Effect/Toxicity

Carvedilol may increase the levels/effects of: Afatinib; Alpha-/Beta-Agonists (Direct-Acting); Alpha1-Blockers; Alpha2-Agonists; Amifostine; Antihypertensives; Antipsychotic Agents (Phenothiazines); Bosutinib; Bupivacaine; Cardiac Glycosides; Cholinergic Agonists; Colchicine; CycloSPORINE (Systemic); Dabigatran Etexilate; Digoxin; DOXOrubicin (Conventional); DULoxetine; Ergot Derivatives; Everolimus; Fingolimod; Hypotensive Agents; Insulin; Lidocaine (Systemic); Lidocaine (Topical); Mepivacaine; Methacholine; Midodrine; Obinutuzumab; PAZOPanib; P-glycoprotein/ABCB1 Substrates; Pomalidomide; Prucalopride; RiTUXimab; Rivaroxaban; Sulfonylureas; Topotecan; VinCRIStine (Liposomal)

The levels/effects of Carvedilol may be increased by: Abiraterone Acetate; Acetylcholinesterase Inhibitors; Alpha2-Agonists; Aminoquinolines (Antimalarial); Amiodarone; Anilidopiperidine Opioids; Antipsychotic Agents (Phenothiazines); Brimonidine (Topical); Calcium Channel Blockers (Dihydropyridine); Calcium Channel Blockers (Nondihydropyridine); Cimetidine; CYP2C9 Inhibitors (Moderate); CYP2C9 Inhibitors (Strong); CYP2D6 Inhibitors (Moderate); CYP2D6 Inhibitors (Strong); Darunavir; Diazoxide; Digoxin; Dipyridamole; Disopyramide; Dronedarone; Floctafenine; Herbs (Hypotensive Properties); MAO Inhibitors; NiCARdipine; Pentoxifylline; P-glycoprotein/ABCB1 Inhibitors; Phosphodiesterase 5 Inhibitors; Propafenone; Prostacyclin Analogues; Regorafenib; Reserpine; Selective Serotonin Reuptake Inhibitors

Nutritional/Ethanol Interactions

Food: Food decreases rate but not extent of absorption. Administration with food minimizes risks of orthostatic hypotension.

Herb/Nutraceutical: Avoid herbs with hypertensive properties (bayberry, blue cohosh, cayenne, ephedra, ginger, ginseng [American], kola, licorice); may diminish the antihypertensive effect of carvedilol. Avoid herbs with hypotensive properties (black cohosh, California poppy, coleus, golden seal, hawthorn, mistletoe, periwinkle, quinine, shepherd's purse); may enhance the hypotensive effect of carvedilol.

Adverse Reactions Note: Frequency ranges include data from hypertension and heart failure trials. Higher rates of adverse reactions have generally been noted in patients with heart failure. However, the frequency of adverse effects associated with placebo is also increased in this population.

>10%:
Cardiovascular: Hypotension (9% to 20%)
Central nervous system: Dizziness (2% to 32%), fatigue (4% to 24%)
Endocrine & metabolic: Hyperglycemia (5% to 12%)
Gastrointestinal: Diarrhea (1% to 12%), weight gain (10% to 12%)
Neuromuscular & skeletal: Weakness (7% to 11%)
1% to 10%:
Cardiovascular: Bradycardia (2% to 10%), syncope (3% to 8%), peripheral edema (1% to 7%), generalized edema (5% to 6%), angina (1% to 6%), dependent edema (≤4%), AV block, cerebrovascular accident, hypertension, hyper-/hypovolemia, orthostatic hypotension, palpitation
Central nervous system: Headache (5% to 8%), depression, fever, hypoesthesia, hypotonia, insomnia, malaise, somnolence, vertigo
Endocrine & metabolic: Hypercholesterolemia (1% to 4%), hypertriglyceridemia (1%), diabetes mellitus, gout, hyperkalemia, hyperuricemia, hypoglycemia, hyponatremia
Gastrointestinal: Nausea (2% to 9%), vomiting (1% to 6%), abdominal pain, melena, periodontitis, weight loss
Genitourinary: Impotence
Hematologic: Anemia, prothrombin decreased, purpura, thrombocytopenia
Hepatic: Alkaline phosphatase increased (1% to 3%), GGT increased, transaminases increased
Neuromuscular & skeletal: Back pain (2% to 7%), arthralgia (1% to 6%), arthritis, muscle cramps, paresthesia
Ocular: Blurred vision (1% to 5%)
Renal: BUN increased (≤6%), nonprotein nitrogen increased (6%), albuminuria, creatinine increased, glycosuria, hematuria, renal insufficiency
Respiratory: Cough (5% to 8%), nasopharyngitis (4%), rales (4%), dyspnea (>3%), pulmonary edema (>3%), rhinitis (2%), nasal congestion (1%), sinus congestion (1%)
Miscellaneous: Injury (3% to 6%), allergy, flu-like syndrome, sudden death

Pharmacodynamics/Kinetics

Onset of Action 1-2 hours; Peak antihypertensive effect: ~1-2 hours

Available Dosage Forms
Capsule Extended Release 24 Hour, Oral:
Coreg CR: 10 mg, 20 mg, 40 mg, 80 mg
Tablet, Oral:
Coreg: 3.125 mg, 6.25 mg, 12.5 mg, 25 mg
Generic: 3.125 mg, 6.25 mg, 12.5 mg, 25 mg
General Dosage Range Oral: *Adults:* Immediate release: Initial: 3.125-6.25 mg twice daily; Maintenance: 6.25-50 mg twice daily (maximum: 50 mg/day [<85 kg]; 100 mg/day [>85 kg]); Extended release: Initial: 10 mg once daily; range: 10-80 mg once daily

Administration
Oral Administer with food to minimize the risk of orthostatic hypotension. Extended release capsules should not be crushed or chewed. Capsules may be opened and sprinkled on applesauce for immediate use.

Storage/Stability
Coreg®: Store at <30°C (<86°F). Protect from moisture.
Coreg CR®: Store at 25°C (77°F); excursions permitted to 15°C to 30°C (59°F to 86°F).

Nursing Actions
Physical Assessment Take blood pressure and heart rate prior to and following first dose and with any change in dosage. Caution patients with diabetes to monitor glucose levels closely (beta-blockers may alter glucose tolerance).

Patient Education
• Discuss specific use of drug and side effects with patient as it relates to treatment. (HCAHPS: During this hospital stay, were you given any medicine that you had not taken before? Before giving you any new medicine, how often did hospital staff tell you what the medicine was for? How often did hospital staff describe possible side effects in a way you could understand?)
• Patient may experience asthenia, diarrhea, xerophthalmia, headache, or nausea. Have patient report immediately to prescriber severe dizziness, syncope, dyspnea, urinary retention, oliguria, angina, sensation of cold, bradycardia, arrhythmia, vision changes, excessive weight gain, edema of extremities, ecchymosis, hemorrhaging, painful extremities, or skin discoloration (HCAHPS).
• Educate patient about signs of a significant reaction (eg, wheezing; chest tightness; fever; itching; bad cough; blue skin color; seizures; or swelling of face, lips, tongue, or throat). **Note:** This is not a comprehensive list of all side effects. Patient should consult prescriber for additional questions.

Intended Use and Disclaimer: Should not be printed and given to patients. This information is intended to serve as a concise initial reference for healthcare professionals to use when discussing medications with a patient. You must ultimately rely on your own discretion, experience and judgment in diagnosing, treating and advising patients.

Dietary Considerations Should be taken with food to minimize the risk of orthostatic hypotension

Related Information
Oral Medications That Should Not Be Crushed or Altered *on page 1712*

Caspofungin (kas poe FUN jin)

Brand Names: U.S. Cancidas
Index Terms Caspofungin Acetate
Pharmacologic Category Antifungal Agent Parenteral; Echinocandin
Pregnancy Risk Factor C
Lactation Excretion in breast milk unknown/use caution
Breast-Feeding Considerations It is not known if caspofungin is excreted in breast milk. The manufacturer recommends that caution be exercised when administering caspofungin to nursing women.
Use Treatment of invasive *Aspergillus* infections in patients who are refractory or intolerant of other therapies; treatment of candidemia and other *Candida* infections (intra-abdominal abscesses, peritonitis, pleural space); treatment of esophageal candidiasis; empirical treatment for presumed fungal infections in febrile neutropenic patients
Unlabeled Use Alternate agent in the prophylaxis against *Candida* infection in neutropenic cancer patients with substantial risk (eg, allogeneic transplant or undergoing induction therapy for acute leukemia)
Mechanism of Action/Effect Blocks synthesis of a vital component of fungal cell walls, which limits their growth. The cell wall component is unique to specific fungi, limiting potential for toxicity in mammals.
Contraindications Hypersensitivity to caspofungin or any component of the formulation
Warnings/Precautions Anaphylaxis and histamine-related reactions (eg, angioedema, facial swelling, bronchospasm, rash, sensation of warmth) have been reported. Discontinue if anaphylaxis occurs; consider discontinuation if histamine-related reactions occur. Administer supportive treatment if needed. Concurrent use of cyclosporine should be limited to patients for whom benefit outweighs risk, due to a high frequency of hepatic transaminase elevations observed during concurrent use. Potentially significant drug-drug interactions may exist, requiring dose or frequency adjustment, additional monitoring, and/or selection of alternative therapy. Use caution in hepatic impairment; increased transaminases and rare cases of liver impairment (including failure and hepatitis) have been reported in pediatric and adult patients. Monitor liver function tests during therapy; if tests become abnormal or worsen, consider

discontinuation. Dosage reduction required in adults with moderate hepatic impairment; safety and efficacy have not been established in children with any degree of hepatic impairment and adults with severe hepatic impairment.

Drug Interactions

Avoid Concomitant Use There are no known interactions where it is recommended to avoid concomitant use.

Decreased Effect

Caspofungin may decrease the levels/effects of: Saccharomyces boulardii; Tacrolimus (Systemic)

The levels/effects of Caspofungin may be decreased by: Inducers of Drug Clearance; Rifampin

Increased Effect/Toxicity

The levels/effects of Caspofungin may be increased by: CycloSPORINE (Systemic)

Adverse Reactions

>10%:
Cardiovascular: Hypotension (3% to 20%), peripheral edema (6% to 11%), tachycardia (4% to 11%)
Central nervous system: Chills (9% to 23%), headache (5% to 15%)
Dermatologic: Skin rash (4% to 23%)
Endocrine & metabolic: Hypokalemia (5% to 23%)
Gastrointestinal: Diarrhea (6% to 27%), vomiting (6% to 17%), nausea (4% to 15%)
Hematologic & oncologic: Decreased hemoglobin (18% to 21%), decreased hematocrit (13% to 18%), decreased white blood cell count (12%), anemia (2% to 11%)
Hepatic: Increased serum alkaline phosphatase (9% to 22%), increased serum ALT (4% to 18%), increased serum AST (2% to 16%), increased serum bilirubin (5% to 13%)
Local: Localized phlebitis (18%)
Renal: Increased serum creatinine (3% to 11%)
Respiratory: Respiratory failure (2% to 20%), cough (6% to 11%), pneumonia (4% to 11%)
Miscellaneous: Infusion related reaction (20% to 35%), fever (6% to 30%), septic shock (11% to 14%)
5% to 10%:
Cardiovascular: Hypertension (5% to 10%)
Dermatologic: Erythema (4% to 9%), pruritus (6% to 7%)
Endocrine & metabolic: Hypomagnesemia (7%), hyperglycemia (6%)
Gastrointestinal: Gastric irritation (4% to 10%), abdominal pain (4% to 9%)
Hepatic: Decreased serum albumin (7%)
Immunologic: Graft versus host disease (infants, children, and adolescents 1% to 4%)
Infection: Sepsis (5% to 7%)
Local: Catheter infection (infants, children, and adolescents 1% to 9%)
Renal: Hematuria (10%), increased blood urea nitrogen (4% to 9%)

Respiratory: Dyspnea (9%), pleural effusion (9%), respiratory distress (≤8%), rales (7%)

Available Dosage Forms

Solution Reconstituted, Intravenous:
Cancidas: 50 mg (1 ea); 70 mg (1 ea)

General Dosage Range Dosage adjustment recommended in patients with hepatic impairment or on concomitant therapy

I.V.:

Infants ≥3 months, Children, and Adolescents ≤17 years: 70 mg/m² on day 1, subsequent dosing: 50-70 mg/m² once daily (maximum dose loading or maintenance: 70 mg daily)

Adults: Initial: 50-70 mg on day 1; subsequent dose: 50-70 mg once daily

Administration

I.V. Infuse slowly, over ~1 hour. Monitor during infusion; isolated cases of possible histamine-related reactions have occurred during clinical trials (rash, flushing, pruritus, facial edema).

Injectable Detail pH 6.6 (reconstituted solution in vial)

Preparation for Administration Bring refrigerated vial to room temperature. Reconstitute vials using 10.8 mL 0.9% sodium chloride for injection, SWFI, or bacteriostatic water for injection, resulting in a concentration of 5 mg/mL for the 50 mg vial, and 7 mg/mL for the 70 mg vial (vials contain overfill). Mix gently to dissolve until clear solution is formed; do not use if cloudy or contains particles. Solution should be further diluted with 0.9%, 0.45%, or 0.225% sodium chloride or LR (do not exceed final concentration of 0.5 mg/mL).

Storage/Stability Store intact vials at 2°C to 8°C (36°F to 46°F). Reconstituted solution may be stored at ≤25°C (≤77°F) for 1 hour prior to preparation of infusion solution. Solutions diluted for infusion should be used within 24 hours when stored at ≤25°C (≤77°F) or within 48 hours when stored at 2°C to 8°C (36°F to 46°F).

Nursing Actions

Patient Education

• Discuss specific use of drug and side effects with patient as it relates to treatment. (HCAHPS: During this hospital stay, were you given any medicine that you had not taken before? Before giving you any new medicine, how often did hospital staff tell you what the medicine was for? How often did hospital staff describe possible side effects in a way you could understand?)

• Patient may experience dyspepsia, nausea, or diarrhea. Have patient report immediately to prescriber signs of hepatic impairment, signs of renal impairment, signs of hypokalemia, signs of pancreatitis, severe dizziness, syncope, tachycardia, bradycardia, chills, pharyngitis, illogical thinking, mood changes, injection site pain or irritation, tachypnea, dyspnea, significant headache, blurred vision, edema of extremities, ecchymosis, hemorrhaging, or flushing (HCAHPS).

• Educate patient about signs of a significant reaction (eg, wheezing; chest tightness; fever; itching; bad cough; blue skin color; seizures; or swelling of face, lips, tongue, or throat). **Note:** This is not a comprehensive list of all side effects. Patient should consult prescriber for additional questions.

Intended Use and Disclaimer: Should not be printed and given to patients. This information is intended to serve as a concise initial reference for healthcare professionals to use when discussing medications with a patient. You must ultimately rely on your own discretion, experience and judgment in diagnosing, treating and advising patients.

Cefaclor (SEF a klor)

Pharmacologic Category Antibiotic, Cephalosporin (Second Generation)
Medication Safety Issues
Sound-alike/look-alike issues:
Cefaclor may be confused with cephalexin
Pregnancy Risk Factor B
Lactation Enters breast milk/use caution
Breast-Feeding Considerations Small amounts of cefaclor are excreted in breast milk. The manufacturer recommends that caution be exercised when administering cefaclor to nursing women. Nondose-related effects could include modification of bowel flora.
Use Treatment of susceptible bacterial infections including otitis media, lower respiratory tract infections, acute exacerbations of chronic bronchitis, pharyngitis and tonsillitis, urinary tract infections, skin and skin structure infections
Mechanism of Action/Effect Inhibits bacterial cell wall synthesis by binding to one or more of the penicillin-binding proteins (PBPs)
Contraindications Hypersensitivity to cefaclor, any component of the formulation, or other cephalosporins
Warnings/Precautions Modify dosage in patients with severe renal impairment. Prolonged use may result in fungal or bacterial superinfection, including C. difficile-associated diarrhea (CDAD) and pseudomembranous colitis; CDAD has been observed >2 months postantibiotic treatment. Use with caution in patients with a history of penicillin allergy, especially IgE-mediated reactions (eg, anaphylaxis, urticaria). Beta-lactamase-negative, ampicillin-resistant (BLNAR) strains of H. influenzae should be considered resistant to cefaclor. Extended release tablets are not approved for use in children <16 years of age.
Drug Interactions
Avoid Concomitant Use
Avoid concomitant use of Cefaclor with any of the following: BCG

Decreased Effect
Cefaclor may decrease the levels/effects of: BCG; Sodium Picosulfate; Typhoid Vaccine
Increased Effect/Toxicity
Cefaclor may increase the levels/effects of: Aminoglycosides; Vitamin K Antagonists

The levels/effects of Cefaclor may be increased by: Probenecid
Nutritional/Ethanol Interactions Food: Cefaclor serum levels may be decreased slightly if taken with food. The bioavailability of cefaclor extended release tablets is decreased 23% and the maximum concentration is decreased 67% when taken on an empty stomach.
Adverse Reactions
1% to 10%:
Dermatologic: Rash (maculopapular, erythematous, or morbilliform) (1% to 2%)
Gastrointestinal: Diarrhea (3%)
Genitourinary: Vaginitis (2%)
Hematologic: Eosinophilia (2%)
Hepatic: Transaminases increased (3%)
Miscellaneous: Moniliasis (2%)
Reactions reported with other cephalosporins: Fever, abdominal pain, superinfection, renal dysfunction, toxic nephropathy, hemorrhage, cholestasis
Available Dosage Forms
Capsule, Oral:
Generic: 250 mg, 500 mg
Suspension Reconstituted, Oral:
Generic: 125 mg/5 mL (150 mL); 250 mg/5 mL (150 mL); 375 mg/5 mL (100 mL)
Tablet Extended Release 12 Hour, Oral:
Generic: 500 mg
General Dosage Range Dosage adjustment recommended in patients with renal impairment
Oral:
Children >1 month: 20-40 mg/kg/day divided every 8-12 hours (maximum: 1 g/day)
Adults: 250-500 mg every 8 hours
Administration
Oral Administer around-the-clock to promote less variation in peak and trough serum levels.
Oral suspension: Shake well before using.
Storage/Stability Store at controlled room temperature. Refrigerate suspension after reconstitution. Discard after 14 days. Do not freeze.
Nursing Actions
Physical Assessment Results of culture/sensitivity tests and patient's allergy history should be assessed prior to therapy. Monitor for nephrotoxicity. Hypersensitivity can occur days after therapy is started. Advise patients with diabetes about use of Clinitest®. Teach patient to report hypersensitivity and opportunistic infections.
Patient Education
• Discuss specific use of drug and side effects with patient as it relates to treatment. (HCAHPS: During this hospital stay, were you given any

medicine that you had not taken before? Before giving you any new medicine, how often did hospital staff tell you what the medicine was for? How often did hospital staff describe possible side effects in a way you could understand?)
- Patient may experience nausea, diarrhea, asthenia, or headache. Have patient report immediately to prescriber ecchymosis, hemorrhaging, urinary retention, oliguria, vaginitis, or signs of pseudomembranous colitis (HCAHPS).
- Educate patient about signs of a significant reaction (eg, wheezing; chest tightness; fever; itching; bad cough; blue skin color; seizures; or swelling of face, lips, tongue, or throat). **Note:** This is not a comprehensive list of all side effects. Patient should consult prescriber for additional questions.

Intended Use and Disclaimer: Should not be printed and given to patients. This information is intended to serve as a concise initial reference for healthcare professionals to use when discussing medications with a patient. You must ultimately rely on your own discretion, experience and judgment in diagnosing, treating and advising patients.

Dietary Considerations Capsule and suspension may be taken with or without food.

Related Information
Oral Medications That Should Not Be Crushed or Altered *on page 1712*

Cefadroxil (sef a DROKS il)

Index Terms Cefadroxil Monohydrate; Duricef
Pharmacologic Category Antibiotic, Cephalosporin (First Generation)
Pregnancy Risk Factor B
Lactation Enters breast milk/use caution
Breast-Feeding Considerations Very small amounts of cefadroxil are excreted in breast milk. The manufacturer recommends that caution be exercised when administering cefadroxil to nursing women. Nondose-related effects could include modification of bowel flora.
Use
Pharyngitis and/or tonsillitis: Treatment of pharyngitis and/or tonsillitis caused by *Streptococcus pyogenes* (group A beta-hemolytic streptococci).
Skin and skin structure infections: Treatment of skin and skin structure infections caused by staphylococci and/or streptococci.
Urinary tract infection: Treatment of urinary tract infections caused by *Escherichia coli*, *Proteus mirabilis*, and *Klebsiella* species.
Unlabeled Use Chronic oral antimicrobial suppression of prosthetic joint infection with *Staphylococci* (oxacillin-susceptible) after completion of parenteral therapy

Mechanism of Action/Effect Inhibits bacterial cell wall synthesis by binding to one or more of the penicillin-binding proteins (PBPs)
Contraindications Hypersensitivity to cefadroxil, any component of the formulation, or other cephalosporins
Warnings/Precautions Modify dosage in patients with renal impairment (CrCl <50 mL/minute/1.73 m²). Use with caution in patients with a history of penicillin allergy, especially IgE-mediated reactions (eg, anaphylaxis, angioedema, urticaria). Use with caution in patients with a history of gastrointestinal disease, particularly colitis. Prolonged use may result in fungal or bacterial superinfection, including *C. difficile*-associated diarrhea (CDAD) and pseudomembranous colitis; CDAD has been observed >2 months postantibiotic treatment. Only I.M. penicillin has been shown to be effective in the prophylaxis of rheumatic fever. Cefadroxil is generally effective in the eradication of streptococci from the oropharynx; efficacy data for cefadroxil in the prophylaxis of subsequent rheumatic fever episodes are not available. Suspension may contain sulfur dioxide (sulfite); hypersensitivity reactions, including anaphylaxis and/or asthmatic exacerbations, may occur (may be life threatening).
Drug Interactions
Avoid Concomitant Use
Avoid concomitant use of Cefadroxil with any of the following: BCG
Decreased Effect
Cefadroxil may decrease the levels/effects of: BCG; Sodium Picosulfate; Typhoid Vaccine
Increased Effect/Toxicity
Cefadroxil may increase the levels/effects of: Vitamin K Antagonists

The levels/effects of Cefadroxil may be increased by: Probenecid
Nutritional/Ethanol Interactions Food: Concomitant administration with food, infant formula, or cow's milk does **not** significantly affect absorption.
Adverse Reactions 1% to 10%: Gastrointestinal: Diarrhea
Available Dosage Forms
Capsule, Oral:
Generic: 500 mg
Suspension Reconstituted, Oral:
Generic: 250 mg/5 mL (100 mL); 500 mg/5 mL (75 mL, 100 mL)
Tablet, Oral:
Generic: 1 g
General Dosage Range Dosage adjustment recommended in patients with renal impairment
Oral:
Children: 30 mg/kg/day in 2 divided doses (maximum: 2000 mg daily)
Adults: 1-2 g daily in a single dose or 2 divided doses

Administration

Oral Administer around-the-clock to promote less variation in peak and trough serum levels. Administer without regards to meals; administration with food may diminish GI complaints.

Preparation for Administration Powder for suspension: Refer to manufacturer's product labeling for reconstitution instructions. Shake vigorously until suspended.

Storage/Stability Store capsules, tablets and un-reconstituted oral suspension at 20°C to 25°C (68°F to 77F); excursions are permitted to 15°C to 30°C (59°F to 86°F). After reconstitution, oral suspension may be stored for 14 days under refrigeration (4°C).

Nursing Actions

Physical Assessment Results of culture/sensitivity tests and patient's allergy history should be assessed prior to therapy. Hypersensitivity can occur several days after therapy is started. Advise patients with diabetes about use of Clinitest®. Teach patient to report hypersensitivity, opportunistic infection, renal dysfunction, and anemia.

Patient Education

• Discuss specific use of drug and side effects with patient as it relates to treatment. (HCAHPS: During this hospital stay, were you given any medicine that you had not taken before? Before giving you any new medicine, how often did hospital staff tell you what the medicine was for? How often did hospital staff describe possible side effects in a way you could understand?)

• Patient may experience nausea or diarrhea. Have patient report immediately to prescriber signs of hepatic impairment, ecchymosis, hemorrhaging, chills, pharyngitis, severe asthenia, arthralgia, urinary retention, oliguria, vaginitis, or signs of pseudomembranous colitis (HCAHPS).

• Educate patient about signs of a significant reaction (eg, wheezing; chest tightness; fever; itching; bad cough; blue skin color; seizures; or swelling of face, lips, tongue, or throat). **Note:** This is not a comprehensive list of all side effects. Patient should consult prescriber for additional questions.

Intended Use and Disclaimer: Should not be printed and given to patients. This information is intended to serve as a concise initial reference for healthcare professionals to use when discussing medications with a patient. You must ultimately rely on your own discretion, experience and judgment in diagnosing, treating and advising patients.

Cefazolin (sef A zoe lin)

Index Terms Ancef; Cefazolin Sodium; Kefzol
Pharmacologic Category Antibiotic, Cephalosporin (First Generation)

Medication Safety Issues

Sound-alike/look-alike issues:
CeFAZolin may be confused with cefoTEtan, cefOXitin, cefprozil, cefTAZidime, cefTRIAXone, cephalexin

Pregnancy Risk Factor B
Lactation Enters breast milk/use caution
Breast-Feeding Considerations Small amounts of cefazolin are excreted in breast milk. The manufacturer recommends that caution be exercised when administering cefazolin to nursing women. Nondose-related effects could include modification of bowel flora.

Use

Biliary tract infections: Due to *Escherichia coli*, various strains of streptococci, *Proteus mirabilis*, *Klebsiella* species and *Staphylococcus aureus*.

Bone and joint infections: Due to *S. aureus*.

Endocarditis: Due to *S. aureus* (penicillin-sensitive and penicillin-resistant) and group A beta-hemolytic streptococci.

Genital infections (ie, prostatitis, epididymitis): Due to *E. coli*, *P. mirabilis*, and *Klebsiella* species.

Perioperative prophylaxis: The prophylactic administration of cefazolin preoperatively, intraoperatively, and postoperatively may reduce the incidence of certain postoperative infections in patients undergoing surgical procedures.

Respiratory tract infections: Due to *S. pneumoniae*, *Klebsiella* species, *Haemophilus influenzae*, *S. aureus* (penicillin-sensitive and penicillin-resistant) and group A beta-hemolytic streptococci.

Septicemia: Due to *Streptococcus pneumoniae*, *S. aureus* (penicillin-sensitive and penicillin-resistant), *P. mirabilis*, *E. coli* and *Klebsiella* species.

Skin and skin structure infections: Due to *S. aureus* (penicillin-sensitive and penicillin-resistant), group A beta-hemolytic streptococci and other strains of streptococci.

Urinary tract infections: Due to *E. coli*, *P. mirabilis*, *Klebsiella* species and some strains of enterobacter.

Unlabeled Use Prophylaxis against infective endocarditis

Mechanism of Action/Effect Inhibits bacterial cell wall synthesis by binding to one or more of the penicillin-binding proteins (PBPs)

Contraindications Known allergy to the cephalosporin group of antibiotics

Warnings/Precautions Modify dosage in patients with severe renal impairment. Use with caution in patients with a history of penicillin allergy, especially IgE-mediated reactions (eg, anaphylaxis, angioedema, urticaria). Prolonged use may result in fungal or bacterial superinfection, including *C. difficile*-associated diarrhea (CDAD) and pseudomembranous colitis; CDAD has been observed >2 months postantibiotic treatment. May be associated with increased INR, especially in nutritionally-deficient patients, prolonged treatment, hepatic or renal disease. Use with caution in patients with a history of seizure disorder; high levels, particularly in the presence of renal impairment, may increase risk of seizures. Potentially significant drug-drug interactions may exist, requiring dose or frequency adjustment, additional monitoring, and/or selection of alternative therapy.

Drug Interactions

Avoid Concomitant Use

Avoid concomitant use of CeFAZolin with any of the following: BCG

Decreased Effect

CeFAZolin may decrease the levels/effects of: BCG; Sodium Picosulfate; Typhoid Vaccine

Increased Effect/Toxicity

CeFAZolin may increase the levels/effects of: Fosphenytoin; Phenytoin; Vitamin K Antagonists

The levels/effects of CeFAZolin may be increased by: Probenecid

Adverse Reactions Frequency not defined.

Cardiovascular: Localized phlebitis

Central nervous system: Seizure

Dermatologic: Pruritus, skin rash, Stevens-Johnson syndrome

Gastrointestinal: Abdominal cramps, anorexia, diarrhea, nausea, oral candidiasis, pseudomembranous colitis, vomiting

Genitourinary: Vaginitis

Hepatic: Hepatitis, increased serum transaminases

Hematologic: Eosinophilia, leukopenia, neutropenia, thrombocythemia, thrombocytopenia

Hypersensitivity: Anaphylaxis

Local: Pain at injection site

Renal: Increased blood urea nitrogen, increased serum creatinine, renal failure

Miscellaneous: Fever

Available Dosage Forms

Solution, Intravenous:

Generic: 1 g (50 mL)

Solution Reconstituted, Injection:

Generic: 500 mg (1 ea); 1 g (1 ea); 10 g (1 ea); 20 g (1 ea); 100 g (1 ea); 300 g (1 ea)

Solution Reconstituted, Injection [preservative free]:

Generic: 500 mg (1 ea); 1 g (1 ea); 10 g (1 ea); 20 g (1 ea)

Solution Reconstituted, Intravenous:

Generic: 1 g (1 ea); 2 g (1 ea)

General Dosage Range Dosage adjustment recommended in patients with renal impairment

I.M., I.V.:

Children >1 month: 25-100 mg/kg/day divided every 6-8 hours (maximum: 6 **g** daily)

Adults: 250-1500 mg every 6-12 hours (maximum: 12 **g** daily)

Administration

I.M. Inject deep I.M. into large muscle mass.

I.V. Inject direct I.V. over 5 minutes or may infuse as an intermittent infusion over 30-60 minutes. Some penicillins (eg, carbenicillin, ticarcillin, and piperacillin) have been shown to inactivate

aminoglycosides in vitro. This has been observed to a greater extent with tobramycin and gentamicin, while amikacin has shown greater stability against inactivation. Concurrent use of these agents may pose a risk of reduced antibacterial efficacy in vivo, particularly in the setting of profound renal impairment. However, definitive clinical evidence is lacking. If combination penicillin/aminoglycoside therapy is desired in a patient with renal dysfunction, separation of doses (if feasible), and routine monitoring of aminoglycoside levels, CBC, and clinical response should be considered.

Injectable Detail pH: 4.5-6

Preparation for Administration Dilute 500 mg vial with 2 mL SWFI and 1 g vial with 2.5 mL SWFI; reconstituted solution may be directly injected after further dilution with 5 mL SWFI or further diluted for I.V. administration in 50-100 mL compatible solution; 10 g vial may be diluted with 45 mL to yield 1 g/5 mL or 96 mL to yield 1 g/10 mL.

Storage/Stability Store intact vials at room temperature and protect from temperatures exceeding 40°C. Reconstituted solutions of cefazolin are light yellow to yellow. Protection from light is recommended for the powder and for the reconstituted solutions. Reconstituted solutions are stable for 24 hours at room temperature and for 10 days under refrigeration. Stability of parenteral admixture at room temperature (25°C) is 48 hours. Stability of parenteral admixture at refrigeration temperature (4°C) is 14 days.

DUPLEX: Store at 20°C to 25°C (68°F to 77°F); excursions permitted to 15°C to 30°C (59°F to 86°F) prior to activation. Following activation, stable for 24 hours at room temperature and for 7 days under refrigeration.

Nursing Actions

Physical Assessment Assess results of culture/sensitivity tests and patient's allergy history prior to therapy. Teach patient to report hypersensitivity, opportunistic infection, renal dysfunction, and anemia. Monitor for diarrhea, oral thrush, rash, abdominal pain, difficulty breathing, unusual bleeding, or bruising.

Patient Education

• Discuss specific use of drug and side effects with patient as it relates to treatment. (HCAHPS: During this hospital stay, were you given any medicine that you had not taken before? Before giving you any new medicine, how often did hospital staff tell you what the medicine was for? How often did hospital staff describe possible side effects in a way you could understand?)

• Patient may experience nausea, diarrhea, or lack of appetite. Have patient report immediately to prescriber signs of hepatic impairment, severe nausea, ecchymosis, hemorrhaging, stomatitis, considerable asthenia, injection site pain or

irritation, urinary retention, oliguria, vaginitis, or signs of pseudomembranous colitis (HCAHPS).
• Educate patient about signs of a significant reaction (eg, wheezing; chest tightness; fever; itching; bad cough; blue skin color; seizures; or swelling of face, lips, tongue, or throat). **Note:** This is not a comprehensive list of all side effects. Patient should consult prescriber for additional questions.

Intended Use and Disclaimer: Should not be printed and given to patients. This information is intended to serve as a concise initial reference for healthcare professionals to use when discussing medications with a patient. You must ultimately rely on your own discretion, experience and judgment in diagnosing, treating and advising patients.

Dietary Considerations Some products may contain sodium.

Cefdinir (SEF di ner)

Index Terms CFDN; Omnicef
Pharmacologic Category Antibiotic, Cephalosporin (Third Generation)
Pregnancy Risk Factor B
Lactation Excretion in breast milk unknown
Breast-Feeding Considerations Cefdinir is not detectable in breast milk following a single cefdinir 600 mg dose. If present in breast milk, nondose-related effects could include modification of bowel flora.
Use Treatment of community-acquired pneumonia, acute exacerbations of chronic bronchitis, acute bacterial otitis media, acute maxillary sinusitis, pharyngitis/tonsillitis, and uncomplicated skin and skin structure infections.
Mechanism of Action/Effect Inhibits bacterial cell wall synthesis by binding to one or more of the penicillin-binding proteins (PBPs) which in turn inhibits the final transpeptidation step of peptidoglycan synthesis in bacterial cell walls, thus inhibiting cell wall biosynthesis. Bacteria eventually lyse due to ongoing activity of cell wall autolytic enzymes (autolysins and murein hydrolases) while cell wall assembly is arrested.
Contraindications Hypersensitivity to cefdinir, any component of the formulation, other cephalosporins, or related antibiotics
Warnings/Precautions Administer cautiously to penicillin-sensitive patients, especially IgE-mediated reactions (eg, anaphylaxis, urticaria). Prolonged use may result in fungal or bacterial superinfection, including C. difficile-associated diarrhea (CDAD) and pseudomembranous colitis; CDAD has been observed >2 months postantibiotic treatment. Use caution with renal dysfunction (CrCl <30 mL/minute); dose adjustment may be required.

Drug Interactions
Avoid Concomitant Use
Avoid concomitant use of Cefdinir with any of the following: BCG
Decreased Effect
Cefdinir may decrease the levels/effects of: BCG; Sodium Picosulfate; Typhoid Vaccine

The levels/effects of Cefdinir may be decreased by: Iron Salts; Multivitamins/Minerals (with ADEK, Folate, Iron)
Increased Effect/Toxicity
Cefdinir may increase the levels/effects of: Aminoglycosides; Vitamin K Antagonists

The levels/effects of Cefdinir may be increased by: Probenecid
Adverse Reactions
>10%: Gastrointestinal: Diarrhea (8% to 15%)
1% to 10%:
  Central nervous system: Headache (2%)
  Dermatologic: Rash (≤3%)
  Endocrine & metabolic: Bicarbonate decreased (≤1%), hyperglycemia (≤1%), hyperphosphatemia (≤1%)
  Gastrointestinal: Nausea (≤3%), abdominal pain (≤1%), vomiting (≤1%)
  Genitourinary: Vaginal moniliasis (≤4%), urine leukocytes increased (≤2%), urine pH increased (≤1%), urine specific gravity increased (≤1%), vaginitis (≤1%)
  Hematologic: Lymphocytes increased (≤2%), eosinophils increased (1%), lymphocytes decreased (1%), platelets increased (≤1%), PMN changes (≤1%), WBC decreased/increased (≤1%)
  Hepatic: Alkaline phosphatase increased (≤1%), ALT increased (≤1%)
  Renal: Proteinuria (1% to 2%), microhematuria (≤1%), glycosuria (≤1%)
  Miscellaneous: GGT increased (≤1%), lactate dehydrogenase increased (≤1%)
Additional reactions reported with other cephalosporins: Agranulocytosis, angioedema, aplastic anemia, asterixis, encephalopathy, hemorrhage, interstitial nephritis, neuromuscular excitability, PT prolonged, seizure, superinfection, and toxic nephropathy
Available Dosage Forms
Capsule, Oral:
  Generic: 300 mg
Suspension Reconstituted, Oral:
  Generic: 125 mg/5 mL (60 mL, 100 mL); 250 mg/5 mL (60 mL, 100 mL)
General Dosage Range Dosage adjustment recommended in patients with renal impairment
Oral:
  Children 6 months to 12 years: 14 mg/kg/day in 1-2 divided doses (maximum: 600 mg/day)
  Children >12 years and Adults: 600 mg/day in 1-2 divided doses

Administration

Oral Twice daily doses should be given every 12 hours. May be administered with or without food. Manufacturer recommends administering at least 2 hours before or after antacids or iron supplements. Shake suspension well before use.

Preparation for Administration Oral suspension should be mixed with 38 mL water for the 60 mL bottle and 63 mL of water for the 100 mL bottle.

Storage/Stability Capsules and unmixed powder should be stored at 25°C (77°F); excursions permitted to 15°C to 30°C (59°F to 86°F). Oral suspension should be mixed with 38 mL water for the 60 mL bottle and 63 mL of water for the 100 mL bottle. After mixing, the suspension can be stored at room temperature of 25°C (77°F) for 10 days.

Nursing Actions

Physical Assessment Results of culture/sensitivity tests and patient's allergy history should be assessed prior to therapy. Teach patient to report opportunistic infection and hypersensitivity.

Patient Education
- Discuss specific use of drug and side effects with patient as it relates to treatment. (HCAHPS: During this hospital stay, were you given any medicine that you had not taken before? Before giving you any new medicine, how often did hospital staff tell you what the medicine was for? How often did hospital staff describe possible side effects in a way you could understand?)
- Patient may experience diarrhea. Have patient report immediately to prescriber ecchymosis, hemorrhaging, urinary retention, oliguria, chills, pharyngitis, vaginitis, or signs of pseudomembranous colitis (HCAHPS).
- Educate patient about signs of a significant reaction (eg, wheezing; chest tightness; fever; itching; bad cough; blue skin color; seizures; or swelling of face, lips, tongue, or throat). **Note:** This is not a comprehensive list of all side effects. Patient should consult prescriber for additional questions.

Intended Use and Disclaimer: Should not be printed and given to patients. This information is intended to serve as a concise initial reference for healthcare professionals to use when discussing medications with a patient. You must ultimately rely on your own discretion, experience and judgment in diagnosing, treating and advising patients.

Cefditoren (sef de TOR en)

Brand Names: U.S. Spectracef
Index Terms Cefditoren Pivoxil
Pharmacologic Category Antibiotic, Cephalosporin (Third Generation)

Medication Safety Issues

International issues:
Spectracef [U.S., Great Britain, Mexico, Portugal, Spain] may be confused with Spectrocef brand name for cefotaxime [Italy]

Pregnancy Risk Factor B

Lactation Excretion in breast milk unknown/use caution

Breast-Feeding Considerations It is not known whether cefditoren is excreted in human milk. The manufacturer recommends caution when using cefditoren during breast-feeding. If cefditoren reaches the breast milk, the limited oral absorption may minimize the effect on the nursing infant. Nondose-related effects could include modification of bowel flora.

Use Treatment of acute bacterial exacerbation of chronic bronchitis or community-acquired pneumonia (due to susceptible organisms including *Haemophilus influenzae, Haemophilus parainfluenzae, Streptococcus pneumoniae*-penicillin susceptible only, *Moraxella catarrhalis*); pharyngitis or tonsillitis (*Streptococcus pyogenes*); and uncomplicated skin and skin-structure infections (*Staphylococcus aureus* - not MRSA, *Streptococcus pyogenes*)

Mechanism of Action/Effect Has bactericidal activity against susceptible gram-positive and gram-negative pathogens. Inhibits bacterial cell wall synthesis by binding to one or more of the penicillin-binding proteins (PBPs).

Contraindications Hypersensitivity to cefditoren, any component of the formulation, other cephalosporins, or milk protein; carnitine deficiency

Warnings/Precautions Use with caution in patients with a history of penicillin allergy, especially IgE-mediated reactions (eg, anaphylaxis, urticaria). Prolonged use may result in fungal or bacterial superinfection, including *C. difficile*-associated diarrhea (CDAD) and pseudomembranous colitis; CDAD has been observed >2 months postantibiotic treatment. Caution in individuals with seizure disorders; high levels, particularly in the presence of renal impairment, may increase risk of seizures. Use caution in patients with renal or hepatic impairment; modify dosage in patients with severe renal impairment. Cefditoren causes renal excretion of carnitine; do not use in patients with carnitine deficiency; not for long-term therapy due to the possible development of carnitine deficiency over time. May prolong prothrombin time; use with caution in patients with a history of bleeding disorder. Cefditoren tablets contain sodium caseinate, which may cause hypersensitivity reactions in patients with milk protein hypersensitivity; this does not affect patients with lactose intolerance.

Drug Interactions

Avoid Concomitant Use There are no known interactions where it is recommended to avoid concomitant use.

Decreased Effect

The levels/effects of Cefditoren may be decreased by: Antacids; H2-Antagonists; Proton Pump Inhibitors

Increased Effect/Toxicity

Cefditoren may increase the levels/effects of: Vitamin K Antagonists

The levels/effects of Cefditoren may be increased by: Probenecid

Nutritional/Ethanol Interactions Food: Moderate- to high-fat meals increase bioavailability and maximum plasma concentration. Management: Take with meals. Maintain adequate hydration, unless instructed to restrict fluid intake.

Adverse Reactions

>10%: Gastrointestinal: Diarrhea (11% to 15%)

1% to 10%:

Central nervous system: Headache (2% to 3%)

Endocrine & metabolic: Glucose increased (1% to 2%)

Gastrointestinal: Nausea (4% to 6%), abdominal pain (2%), dyspepsia (1% to 2%), vomiting (1%)

Genitourinary: Vaginal moniliasis (3% to 6%)

Hematologic: Hematocrit decreased (2%)

Renal: Hematuria (3%), urinary white blood cells increased (2%)

Reactions reported with other cephalosporins: Anaphylaxis, aplastic anemia, cholestasis, hemorrhage, hemolytic anemia, renal dysfunction, reversible hyperactivity, serum sickness-like reaction, toxic nephropathy

Available Dosage Forms

Tablet, Oral:

Spectracef: 200 mg, 400 mg

Generic: 200 mg, 400 mg

General Dosage Range Dosage adjustment recommended in patients with renal impairment

Oral: *Children ≥12 years and Adults:* 200-400 mg twice daily

Administration

Oral Administer with meals.

Storage/Stability Store at controlled room temperature of 15°C to 30°C (59°F to 86°F). Protect from light and moisture.

Nursing Actions

Physical Assessment Results of culture/sensitivity tests and patient's allergy history should be assessed prior to therapy. Teach patient to report hypersensitivity, opportunistic infection, gastrointestinal upset, and diarrhea.

Patient Education

• Discuss specific use of drug and side effects with patient as it relates to treatment. (HCAHPS: During this hospital stay, were you given any medicine that you had not taken before? Before giving you any new medicine, how often did hospital staff tell you what the medicine was for? How often did hospital staff describe possible side effects in a way you could understand?)

• Patient may experience headache or diarrhea. Have patient report immediately to prescriber signs of hepatic impairment, severe nausea, ecchymosis, hemorrhaging, stomatitis, considerable asthenia, urinary retention, oliguria, edema of extremities, vaginitis, or signs of pseudomembranous colitis (HCAHPS).

• Educate patient about signs of a significant reaction (eg, wheezing; chest tightness; fever; itching; bad cough; blue skin color; seizures; or swelling of face, lips, tongue, or throat). **Note:** This is not a comprehensive list of all side effects. Patient should consult prescriber for additional questions.

Intended Use and Disclaimer: Should not be printed and given to patients. This information is intended to serve as a concise initial reference for healthcare professionals to use when discussing medications with a patient. You must ultimately rely on your own discretion, experience and judgment in diagnosing, treating and advising patients.

Dietary Considerations Cefditoren should be taken with meals. Plasma carnitine levels are decreased during therapy (39% with 200 mg dosing, 63% with 400 mg dosing); normal concentrations return within 7-10 days after treatment is discontinued.

Cefepime (SEF e pim)

Brand Names: U.S. Maxipime

Index Terms Cefepime Hydrochloride

Pharmacologic Category Antibiotic, Cephalosporin (Fourth Generation)

Medication Safety Issues

Sound-alike/look-alike issues:

Cefepime may be confused with cefixime, cefTAZidime

Pregnancy Risk Factor B

Lactation Enters breast milk/use caution

Breast-Feeding Considerations Small amounts of cefepime are excreted in breast milk. The manufacturer recommends that caution be exercised when administering cefepime to nursing women. Nondose-related effects could include modification of bowel flora.

Use Treatment of uncomplicated and complicated urinary tract infections, including pyelonephritis caused by *Escherichia coli, Klebsiella pneumoniae,* or *Proteus mirabilis;* monotherapy for febrile neutropenia; uncomplicated skin and skin structure infections caused by *Streptococcus pyogenes* or methicillin-susceptible staphylococci; moderate-to-severe pneumonia caused by *Streptococcus pneumoniae, Pseudomonas aeruginosa, Klebsiella pneumoniae,* or *Enterobacter* species; complicated intra-abdominal infections (in combination with metronidazole) caused by *E. coli, P. aeruginosa, K. pneumoniae, Enterobacter* species, or

Bacteroides fragilis against methicillin-susceptible staphylococci, *Enterobacter* sp, and many other gram-negative bacilli.

Children 2 months to 16 years: Empiric therapy of febrile neutropenia patients, uncomplicated skin/ soft tissue infections, pneumonia, and uncomplicated/complicated urinary tract infections, including pyelonephritis.

Unlabeled Use Brain abscess (postneurosurgical prevention); malignant otitis externa; prosthetic joint infection; septic lateral/cavernous sinus thrombosis

Mechanism of Action/Effect Inhibits bacterial cell wall synthesis by binding to one or more of the penicillin-binding proteins (PBPs)

Contraindications Hypersensitivity to cefepime, other cephalosporins, penicillins, other beta-lactam antibiotics, or any component of the formulation

Warnings/Precautions Severe neurological reactions (some fatal) have been reported, including encephalopathy, myoclonus, seizures, and nonconvulsive status epilepticus; risk may be increased in the presence of renal impairment (CrCl ≤60 mL/minute); ensure dose adjusted for renal function or discontinue therapy if patient develops neurotoxicity; effects are often reversible upon discontinuation of cefepime. Use with caution in patients with a history of penicillin or cephalosporin allergy, especially IgE-mediated reactions (eg, anaphylaxis, urticaria). Prolonged use may result in fungal or bacterial superinfection, including *C. difficile*-associated diarrhea (CDAD) and pseudomembranous colitis; CDAD has been observed >2 months postantibiotic treatment. Use with caution in patients with a history of gastrointestinal disease, especially colitis. May be associated with increased INR, especially in nutritionally-deficient patients, prolonged treatment, hepatic or renal disease. Use with caution in patients with a history of seizure disorder; high levels, particularly in the presence of renal impairment, may increase risk of seizures.

Drug Interactions

Avoid Concomitant Use

Avoid concomitant use of Cefepime with any of the following: BCG

Decreased Effect

Cefepime may decrease the levels/effects of: BCG; Sodium Picosulfate; Typhoid Vaccine

Increased Effect/Toxicity

Cefepime may increase the levels/effects of: Aminoglycosides; Vitamin K Antagonists

The levels/effects of Cefepime may be increased by: Probenecid

Adverse Reactions

>10%: Hematologic & oncologic: Positive direct Coombs test (without hemolysis; 16%)

1% to 10%:

Cardiovascular: Localized phlebitis (1%)

Central nervous system: Headache (1%)

Dermatologic: Skin rash (1% to 4%), pruritus (1%)

Endocrine & metabolic: Hypophosphatemia (3%)

Gastrointestinal: Diarrhea (≤3%), nausea (≤2%), vomiting (≤1%)

Hematologic & oncologic: Eosinophilia (2%)

Hepatic: Increased serum ALT (3%), abnormal partial thromboplastin time (2%), increased serum AST (2%), abnormal prothrombin time (1%)

Local: Local pain (1%)

Miscellaneous: Fever (1%)

Available Dosage Forms

Solution, Intravenous:

Generic: 1 g/50 mL (50 mL); 2% (100 mL)

Solution Reconstituted, Injection:

Maxipime: 1 g (1 ea); 2 g (1 ea)

Generic: 1 g (1 ea); 2 g (1 ea)

Solution Reconstituted, Intravenous:

Maxipime: 1 g (1 ea); 2 g (1 ea)

Generic: 1 g/50 mL (1 ea); 2 g/50 mL (1 ea)

General Dosage Range Dosage adjustment recommended in patients with renal impairment

I.M.:

Children ≥2 months: 50 mg/kg/dose every 12 hours

Adults: 500-1000 mg every 12 hours

I.V.:

Children ≥2 months: 50 mg/kg/dose every 8-12 hours

Adults: 1-2 g every 8-12 hours

Administration

I.M. Inject deep I.M. into large muscle mass.

I.V. Inject direct I.V. over 5 minutes (Garrelts, 1999). Infuse intermittent infusion over 30 minutes.

Injectable Detail pH: 4-6

Storage/Stability

Vials: Store at 20°C to 25°C (68°F to 77°F). Protect from light. After reconstitution, stable in normal saline, D_5W, and a variety of other solutions for 24 hours at room temperature and 7 days refrigerated.

Premixed solution: Store frozen at -20°C (-4°F). Thawed solution is stable for 24 hours at room temperature or 7 days under refrigeration; do not refreeze.

Nursing Actions

Physical Assessment Results of culture/sensitivity tests and patient's allergy history should be assessed prior to therapy. Monitor prothrombin time. Teach patient to report hypersensitivity, nephrotoxicity, and opportunistic infection.

Patient Education

• Discuss specific use of drug and side effects with patient as it relates to treatment. (HCAHPS: During this hospital stay, were you given any medicine that you had not taken before? Before giving you any new medicine, how often did hospital staff tell you what the medicine was for? How often did hospital staff describe possible side effects in a way you could understand?)

◄ • Patient may experience diarrhea. Have patient report immediately to prescriber severe dizziness, syncope, considerable fatigue, ecchymosis, hemorrhaging, significant asthenia, chills, pharyngitis, urinary retention, oliguria, vaginitis, considerable injection site irritation, signs of pseudomembranous colitis, illogical thinking, or hallucinations (HCAHPS).
• Educate patient about signs of a significant reaction (eg, wheezing; chest tightness; fever; itching; bad cough; blue skin color; seizures; or swelling of face, lips, tongue, or throat). **Note:** This is not a comprehensive list of all side effects. Patient should consult prescriber for additional questions.

Intended Use and Disclaimer: Should not be printed and given to patients. This information is intended to serve as a concise initial reference for healthcare professionals to use when discussing medications with a patient. You must ultimately rely on your own discretion, experience and judgment in diagnosing, treating and advising patients.

Cefixime (sef IKS eem)

Brand Names: U.S. Suprax
Index Terms Cefixime Trihydrate
Pharmacologic Category Antibiotic, Cephalosporin (Third Generation)
Medication Safety Issues
Sound-alike/look-alike issues:
Cefixime may be confused with cefepime
Suprax® may be confused with Sporanox®
International issues:
Cefiton: Brand name for cefixime [Portugal] may be confused with Ceftim brand name for ceftazidime [Portugal]; Ceftime brand name for ceftazidime [Thailand]; Ceftin brand name for cefuroxime [U.S., Canada]
Pregnancy Risk Factor B
Lactation Excretion in breast milk unknown
Breast-Feeding Considerations It is not known if cefixime is excreted in breast milk. The manufacturer recommends that consideration be given to discontinuing nursing temporarily during treatment. If present in breast milk, nondose-related effects could include modification of bowel flora.
Use Treatment of uncomplicated urinary tract infections (due to *Escherichia coli* and *Proteus mirabilis*), otitis media (due to *Haemophilus influenzae, Moraxella catarrhalis,* and *Streptococcus pyogenes*), pharyngitis and tonsillitis (due to *Streptococcus pyogenes*), acute exacerbations of chronic bronchitis (due to *Streptococcus pneumoniae* and *Haemophilus influenzae*); uncomplicated cervical/urethral gonorrhea (due to *N. gonorrhoeae* [penicillinase- and nonpenicillinase-producing])

Note: Due to concerns of resistance, the CDC no longer recommends use of cefixime as a first-line

regimen in the treatment of uncomplicated gonorrhea in the U.S.; ceftriaxone is the preferred cephalosporin (CDC, 2012).
Unlabeled Use Acute bacterial rhinosinusitis (ABRS) (pediatric) in combination with clindamycin; typhoid fever
Mechanism of Action/Effect Inhibits bacterial cell wall synthesis by binding to one or more of the penicillin-binding proteins (PBPs)
Contraindications Hypersensitivity to cefixime, any component of the formulation, or other cephalosporins
Warnings/Precautions Prolonged use may result in fungal or bacterial superinfection, including *C. difficile*-associated diarrhea (CDAD) and pseudomembranous colitis; CDAD has been observed >2 months postantibiotic treatment. Modify dosage in patients with renal impairment. Use with caution in patients with a history of penicillin allergy, especially IgE-mediated reactions (eg, anaphylaxis, urticaria). Chewable tablets contain phenylalanine.
Drug Interactions
Avoid Concomitant Use
Avoid concomitant use of Cefixime with any of the following: BCG
Decreased Effect
Cefixime may decrease the levels/effects of: BCG; Sodium Picosulfate; Typhoid Vaccine
Increased Effect/Toxicity
Cefixime may increase the levels/effects of: Aminoglycosides; Vitamin K Antagonists

The levels/effects of Cefixime may be increased by: Probenecid
Nutritional/Ethanol Interactions Food: Delays cefixime absorption.
Adverse Reactions
>10%: Gastrointestinal: Diarrhea (16%)
2% to 10%: Gastrointestinal: Abdominal pain, nausea, dyspepsia, flatulence, loose stools
Reactions reported with other cephalosporins: Interstitial nephritis, aplastic anemia, hemolytic anemia, hemorrhage, pancytopenia, agranulocytosis, colitis, superinfection
Available Dosage Forms
Capsule, Oral:
Suprax: 400 mg
Suspension Reconstituted, Oral:
Suprax: 100 mg/5 mL (50 mL); 200 mg/5 mL (50 mL, 75 mL); 500 mg/5 mL (10 mL, 20 mL)
Tablet, Oral:
Suprax: 400 mg
Tablet Chewable, Oral:
Suprax: 100 mg, 200 mg
General Dosage Range Dosage adjustment recommended in patients with renal impairment
Oral:
Children ≥6 months to 12 years or ≤45 kg: 8 mg/kg/day divided every 12-24 hours (maximum: 400 mg daily)

Children >12 years or >45 kg, Adolescents, and Adults: 400 mg daily divided every 12-24 hours

Administration

Oral May be administered with or without food. Shake oral suspension well before use. Chewable tablets must be chewed or crushed before swallowing.

Preparation for Administration Powder for suspension: Refer to manufacturer's product labeling for reconstitution instructions.

Storage/Stability

Capsule, chewable tablet, tablet: Store at 20°C to 25°C (68°F to 77°F).

Powder for suspension: Prior to reconstitution, store at 20°C to 25°C (68°F to 77°F). After reconstitution, suspension may be stored for 14 days at room temperature or under refrigeration.

Nursing Actions

Physical Assessment Results of culture/sensitivity tests and patient's allergy history should be assessed prior to therapy. Teach patient adherence to therapy and to report hypersensitivity reactions and opportunistic infection.

Patient Education

- Discuss specific use of drug and side effects with patient as it relates to treatment. (HCAHPS: During this hospital stay, were you given any medicine that you had not taken before? Before giving you any new medicine, how often did hospital staff tell you what the medicine was for? How often did hospital staff describe possible side effects in a way you could understand?)
- Patient may experience dyspepsia, pyrosis, diarrhea, or flatulence. Have patient report immediately to prescriber severe nausea, ecchymosis, hemorrhaging, vaginal yeast infection, stomatitis, considerable asthenia, chills, pharyngitis, urinary retention, oliguria, signs of hepatic impairment, or signs of pseudomembranous colitis (HCAHPS).
- Educate patient about signs of a significant reaction (eg, wheezing; chest tightness; fever; itching; bad cough; blue skin color; seizures; or swelling of face, lips, tongue, or throat). **Note:** This is not a comprehensive list of all side effects. Patient should consult prescriber for additional questions.

Intended Use and Disclaimer: Should not be printed and given to patients. This information is intended to serve as a concise initial reference for healthcare professionals to use when discussing medications with a patient. You must ultimately rely on your own discretion, experience and judgment in diagnosing, treating and advising patients.

Dietary Considerations Chewable tablets contain phenylalanine.

Cefotaxime (sef oh TAKS eem)

Brand Names: U.S. Claforan; Claforan in D5W

Index Terms Cefotaxime Sodium

Pharmacologic Category Antibiotic, Cephalosporin (Third Generation)

Medication Safety Issues

Sound-alike/look-alike issues:

Cefotaxime may be confused with cefOXitin, cefuroxime

International issues:

Spectrocef [Italy] may be confused with Spectracef brand name for cefditoren [U.S., Great Britain, Mexico, Portugal, Spain]

Pregnancy Risk Factor B

Lactation Enters breast milk/use caution

Breast-Feeding Considerations Low concentrations of cefotaxime are found in breast milk. The manufacturer recommends that caution be exercised when administering cefotaxime to nursing women. Nondose-related effects could include modification of bowel flora. The pregnancy-related changes in cefotaxime pharmacokinetics continue into the early postpartum period.

Use Treatment of susceptible organisms in lower respiratory tract, skin and skin structure, bone and joint, urinary tract, intra-abdominal, gynecologic as well as bacteremia/septicemia, and documented or suspected central nervous system infections (eg, meningitis). Active against most gram-negative bacilli (not *Pseudomonas* spp) and gram-positive cocci (not enterococcus). Active against many penicillin-resistant pneumococci.

Unlabeled Use Acute bacterial rhinosinusitis (ABRS); surgical (perioperative) prophylaxis

Mechanism of Action/Effect Inhibits bacterial cell wall synthesis by binding to one or more of the penicillin-binding proteins (PBPs)

Contraindications Hypersensitivity to cefotaxime, any component of the formulation, or other cephalosporins

Warnings/Precautions Modify dosage in patients with severe renal impairment. Prolonged use may result in superinfection. A potentially life-threatening arrhythmia has been reported in patients who received a rapid (<1 minute) bolus injection via central venous catheter. Granulocytopenia and more rarely agranulocytosis may develop during prolonged treatment (>10 days). Minimize tissue inflammation by changing infusion sites when needed. Use with caution in patients with a history of penicillin allergy, especially IgE-mediated reactions (eg, anaphylaxis, urticaria). Prolonged use may result in fungal or bacterial superinfection, including *C. difficile*-associated diarrhea (CDAD) and pseudomembranous colitis; CDAD has been observed >2 months postantibiotic treatment.

◄ **Drug Interactions**

Avoid Concomitant Use

Avoid concomitant use of Cefotaxime with any of the following: BCG

Decreased Effect

Cefotaxime may decrease the levels/effects of: BCG; Sodium Picosulfate; Typhoid Vaccine

Increased Effect/Toxicity

Cefotaxime may increase the levels/effects of: Aminoglycosides; Vitamin K Antagonists

The levels/effects of Cefotaxime may be increased by: Probenecid

Adverse Reactions

1% to 10%:

Dermatologic: Pruritus, rash

Gastrointestinal: Colitis, diarrhea, nausea, vomiting

Local: Pain at injection site

Reactions reported with other cephalosporins: Aplastic anemia, hemorrhage, pancytopenia, renal dysfunction, seizure, superinfection, toxic nephropathy.

Available Dosage Forms

Solution, Intravenous:

Claforan in D$_5$W: 1 g/50 mL (50 mL); 2 g/50 mL (50 mL)

Solution Reconstituted, Injection:

Claforan: 500 mg (1 ea); 1 g (1 ea); 2 g (1 ea); 10 g (1 ea)

Generic: 500 mg (1 ea); 1 g (1 ea); 2 g (1 ea); 10 g (1 ea)

Solution Reconstituted, Intravenous:

Claforan: 1 g (1 ea); 2 g (1 ea)

General Dosage Range Dosage adjustment recommended in patients with hepatic or renal impairment

I.M.:

Infants and Children 1 month to 12 years and <50 kg: 50-200 mg/kg/day in divided doses every 6-8 hours (maximum: 12 g/day)

Children ≥50 kg, Children >12 years, and Adults: 1-2 g every 4-12 hours **or** 0.5-1 g as a single dose

I.V.:

Infants and Children 1 month to 12 years and <50 kg: 50-200 mg/kg/day in divided doses every 6-8 hours (maximum: 12 g/day)

Children ≥50 kg, Children >12 years, and Adults: 1-2 g every 4-12 hours

Administration

I.M. Inject deep I.M. into large muscle mass.

I.V. Inject direct I.V. over at least 3-5 minutes. Infuse intermittent infusion over 30 minutes.

Injectable Detail pH: 5-7.5 (injectable solution)

Preparation for Administration Reconstituted solution is stable for 12-24 hours at room temperature and 7-10 days when refrigerated and for 13 weeks when frozen. For I.V. infusion in NS or D$_5$W, solution is stable for 24 hours at room temperature, 5 days when refrigerated, or 13 weeks when frozen in Viaflex® plastic containers. Thawed solutions previously of frozen premixed bags are stable for 24 hours at room temperature or 10 days when refrigerated.

Nursing Actions

Physical Assessment Assess results of culture/sensitivity tests and patient's allergy history prior to therapy. Evaluate CBC with differential. Monitor for diarrhea, nausea/vomiting, and nephrotoxicity regularly during therapy. Teach patient to report hypersensitivity and opportunistic infection.

Patient Education

• Discuss specific use of drug and side effects with patient as it relates to treatment. (HCAHPS: During this hospital stay, were you given any medicine that you had not taken before? Before giving you any new medicine, how often did hospital staff tell you what the medicine was for? How often did hospital staff describe possible side effects in a way you could understand?)

• Patient may experience headache or diarrhea. Have patient report immediately to prescriber severe nausea, ecchymosis, hemorrhaging, stomatitis, urinary retention, oliguria, chills, pharyngitis, arrhythmia, injection site irritation, considerable asthenia, jaundice, vaginitis, or signs of pseudomembranous colitis (HCAHPS).

• Educate patient about signs of a significant reaction (eg, wheezing; chest tightness; fever; itching; bad cough; blue skin color; seizures; or swelling of face, lips, tongue, or throat). **Note:** This is not a comprehensive list of all side effects. Patient should consult prescriber for additional questions.

Intended Use and Disclaimer: Should not be printed and given to patients. This information is intended to serve as a concise initial reference for healthcare professionals to use when discussing medications with a patient. You must ultimately rely on your own discretion, experience and judgment in diagnosing, treating and advising patients.

Dietary Considerations Some products may contain sodium.

Cefotetan (SEF oh tee tan)

Index Terms Cefotan; Cefotetan Disodium

Pharmacologic Category Antibiotic, Cephalosporin (Second Generation)

Medication Safety Issues

Sound-alike/look-alike issues:

CefoTEtan may be confused with ceFAZolin, cefOXitin, cefTAZidime, Ceftin®, cefTRIAXone

Pregnancy Risk Factor B

Lactation Enters breast milk/use caution

Breast-Feeding Considerations Very small amounts of cefotetan are excreted in human milk. The manufacturer recommends caution when giving cefotetan to a breast-feeding mother. Nondose-related effects could include modification of bowel flora.

Use Surgical (perioperative) prophylaxis; intra-abdominal infections and other mixed infections; respiratory tract, skin and skin structure, bone and joint, urinary tract and gynecologic infections as well as septicemia; active against gram-negative enteric bacilli including *E. coli*, *Klebsiella*, and *Proteus*; less active against staphylococci and streptococci than first generation cephalosporins, but active against anaerobes including *Bacteroides fragilis*

Mechanism of Action/Effect Inhibits bacterial cell wall synthesis by binding to one or more of the penicillin-binding proteins (PBPs)

Contraindications Hypersensitivity to cefotetan, any component of the formulation, or other cephalosporins; previous cephalosporin-associated hemolytic anemia

Warnings/Precautions Modify dosage in patients with severe renal impairment. Although cefotetan contains the methyltetrazolethiol side chain, bleeding has not been a significant problem. Use with caution in patients with a history of penicillin allergy, especially IgE-mediated reactions (eg, anaphylaxis, urticaria). Cefotetan has been associated with a higher risk of hemolytic anemia relative to other cephalosporins (approximately threefold); monitor carefully during use and consider cephalosporin-associated immune anemia in patients who have received cefotetan within 2-3 weeks (either as treatment or prophylaxis). Prolonged use may result in fungal or bacterial superinfection, including *C. difficile*-associated diarrhea (CDAD) and pseudomembranous colitis; CDAD has been observed >2 months postantibiotic treatment. May be associated with increased INR, especially in nutritionally-deficient patients, prolonged treatment, hepatic or renal disease.

Drug Interactions

Avoid Concomitant Use
Avoid concomitant use of CefoTEtan with any of the following: BCG

Decreased Effect
CefoTEtan may decrease the levels/effects of: BCG; Sodium Picosulfate; Typhoid Vaccine

Increased Effect/Toxicity
CefoTEtan may increase the levels/effects of: Alcohol (Ethyl); Aminoglycosides; Carbocisteine; Vitamin K Antagonists

The levels/effects of CefoTEtan may be increased by: Probenecid

Nutritional/Ethanol Interactions Ethanol: Avoid ethanol (may cause a disulfiram-like reaction).

Adverse Reactions
1% to 10%:
Gastrointestinal: Diarrhea (1%)
Hepatic: Transaminases increased (1%)
Miscellaneous: Hypersensitivity reactions (1%)
Reactions reported with other cephalosporins: Seizure, Stevens-Johnson syndrome, toxic epidermal necrolysis, renal dysfunction, toxic nephropathy, cholestasis, aplastic anemia, hemolytic anemia, hemorrhage, pancytopenia, agranulocytosis, colitis, superinfection

Available Dosage Forms
Solution Reconstituted, Injection:
Generic: 1 g (1 ea); 2 g (1 ea); 10 g (1 ea)
Solution Reconstituted, Intravenous:
Generic: 1 g (1 ea); 2 g (1 ea)

General Dosage Range Dosage adjustment recommended in patients with renal impairment
I.M.: *Adults:* 1-6 g daily divided every 12 hours **or** 1-2 g every 24 hours **or** 1-2 g prior to surgery
I.V.:
Adolescents: PID: 2 g every 12 hours
Adults: 1-6 g daily divided every 12 hours **or** 1-2 g every 24 hours **or** 1-2 g prior to surgery

Administration
I.M. Inject deep I.M. into large muscle mass.
I.V. Inject direct I.V. over 3-5 minutes. Infuse intermittent infusion over 30 minutes.
Injectable Detail pH: 4.5-6.5 (reconstituted solution)

Preparation for Administration Reconstituted solution is stable for 24 hours at room temperature and 96 hours when refrigerated. For I.V. infusion in NS or D₅W solution and after freezing, thawed solution is stable for 24 hours at room temperature or 96 hours when refrigerated. Frozen solution is stable for 12 weeks.

Nursing Actions
Physical Assessment Assess results of culture/sensitivity tests and patient's allergy history prior to therapy. Assess prothrombin time. Advise patients with diabetes about use of Clinitest® (may cause false-positive test). Teach patient to report nephrotoxicity, opportunistic infection, and hypersensitivity reaction.

Patient Education
• Discuss specific use of drug and side effects with patient as it relates to treatment. (HCAHPS: During this hospital stay, were you given any medicine that you had not taken before? Before giving you any new medicine, how often did hospital staff tell you what the medicine was for? How often did hospital staff describe possible side effects in a way you could understand?)
• Patient may experience diarrhea. Have patient report immediately to prescriber signs of hepatic impairment, severe nausea, ecchymosis, hemorrhaging, injection site irritation, urinary retention, oliguria, significant asthenia, chills, pharyngitis, vaginitis, or signs of pseudomembranous colitis (HCAHPS).

• Educate patient about signs of a significant reaction (eg, wheezing; chest tightness; fever; itching; bad cough; blue skin color; seizures; or swelling of face, lips, tongue, or throat). **Note:** This is not a comprehensive list of all side effects. Patient should consult prescriber for additional questions.

Intended Use and Disclaimer: Should not be printed and given to patients. This information is intended to serve as a concise initial reference for healthcare professionals to use when discussing medications with a patient. You must ultimately rely on your own discretion, experience and judgment in diagnosing, treating and advising patients.

Dietary Considerations Some products may contain sodium.

Cefoxitin (se FOKS i tin)

Brand Names: U.S. Mefoxin
Index Terms Cefoxitin Sodium
Pharmacologic Category Antibiotic, Cephalosporin (Second Generation)
Medication Safety Issues
  Sound-alike/look-alike issues:
    CefOXitin may be confused with ceFAZolin, cefotaxime, cefoTEtan, cefTAZidime, cefTRIAXone, Cytoxan
    Mefoxin may be confused with Lanoxin
Pregnancy Risk Factor B
Lactation Enters breast milk/use caution
Breast-Feeding Considerations Very small amounts of cefoxitin are excreted in breast milk. The manufacturer recommends that caution be exercised when administering cefoxitin to nursing women. Nondose-related effects could include modification of bowel flora. Cefoxitin pharmacokinetics may be altered immediately postpartum.
Use
Bone and joint infections: Treatment of bone and joint infections caused by *Staphylococcus aureus* (including penicillinase-producing strains).
Gynecological infections: Treatment of endometritis, pelvic cellulitis, and pelvic inflammatory disease caused by *Escherichia coli*, *Neisseria gonorrhoeae* (including penicillinase-producing strains), *Bacteroides* species including *Bacteroides fragilis*, *Clostridium* species, *P. niger*, *Peptostreptococcus* species, and *Streptococcus agalactiae*.
Intra-abdominal infections: Treatment of peritonitis and intra-abdominal infections or abscess, caused by *E. coli*, *Klebsiella* species, *Bacteroides* species (including *B. fragilis*), and *Clostridium* species.
Lower respiratory tract infections: Treatment of pneumonia and lung abscess, caused by *Streptococcus pneumoniae*, other streptococci (excluding enterococci; eg, *Enterococcus faecalis*

[formerly *Streptococcus faecalis*]), *S. aureus* (including penicillinase-producing strains), *E. coli*, *Klebsiella* species, *Haemophilus influenzae*, and *Bacteroides* species.
Perioperative prophylaxis: Prophylaxis of infection in patients undergoing uncontaminated GI surgery, abdominal or vaginal hysterectomy, or cesarean section.
Septicemia: Treatment of septicemia caused by *S. pneumoniae*, *S. aureus* (including penicillinase-producing strains), *E. coli*, *Klebsiella* species, and *Bacteroides* species including *B. fragilis*.
Skin and skin structure infections: Treatment of skin and skin structure infections caused by *S. aureus* (including penicillinase-producing strains), *Staphylococcus epidermidis*, *Streptococcus pyogenes* and other streptococci (excluding enterococci [eg, *E. faecalis*] [formerly *S. faecalis*]), *E. coli*, *Proteus mirabilis*, *Klebsiella* species, *Bacteroides* species including *B. fragilis*, *Clostridium* species, *P. niger*, and *Peptostreptococcus* species.
Urinary tract infections: Treatment of UTIs caused by *E. coli*, *Klebsiella* species, *P. mirabilis*, *Morganella morganii*, *Proteus vulgaris*, and *Providencia* species (including *Providencia rettgeri*).

Limitations of use: Cefoxitin does not have activity against *Chlamydia trachomatis*. When cefoxitin is used to treat pelvic inflammatory disease, add appropriate antichlamydial coverage.

Mechanism of Action/Effect Inhibits bacterial cell wall synthesis by binding to one or more of the penicillin-binding proteins (PBPs)
Contraindications Hypersensitivity to cefoxitin, any component of the formulation, or other cephalosporins
Warnings/Precautions Modify dosage in patients with severe renal impairment. Prolonged use may result in superinfection. Use with caution in patients with a history of penicillin allergy, especially IgE-mediated hypersensitivity reactions (eg, anaphylaxis, urticaria). If a hypersensitivity reaction occurs, discontinue immediately. Use with caution in patients with a history of seizures or gastrointestinal disease (particularly colitis). Prolonged use may result in fungal or bacterial superinfection, including *C. difficile*-associated diarrhea (CDAD) and pseudomembranous colitis; CDAD has been observed >2 months postantibiotic treatment. For group A beta-hemolytic streptococcal infections, antimicrobial therapy should be given for at least 10 days to guard against the risk of rheumatic fever or glomerulonephritis. In pediatric patients ≥3 months of age, higher doses have been associated with an increased incidence of eosinophilia and elevated AST. Elderly patients are more likely to have decreased renal function; use care in dose selection and monitor renal function.

Drug Interactions

Avoid Concomitant Use
Avoid concomitant use of CefOXitin with any of the following: BCG

Decreased Effect
CefOXitin may decrease the levels/effects of: BCG; Sodium Picosulfate; Typhoid Vaccine

Increased Effect/Toxicity
CefOXitin may increase the levels/effects of: Aminoglycosides; Vitamin K Antagonists

The levels/effects of CefOXitin may be increased by: Probenecid

Adverse Reactions
1% to 10%: Gastrointestinal: Diarrhea

Reactions reported with other cephalosporins: Agranulocytosis, aplastic anemia, cholestasis, colitis, erythema multiforme, hemolytic anemia, hemorrhage, pancytopenia, renal dysfunction, serum-sickness reactions, seizure, Stevens-Johnson syndrome, superinfection, toxic nephropathy, vaginitis

Available Dosage Forms
Solution, Intravenous:
Mefoxin: 1 g (50 mL); 2 g (50 mL)
Solution Reconstituted, Injection:
Generic: 10 g (1 ea)
Solution Reconstituted, Injection [preservative free]:
Generic: 10 g (1 ea)
Solution Reconstituted, Intravenous:
Generic: 1 g (1 ea); 2 g (1 ea)
Solution Reconstituted, Intravenous [preservative free]:
Generic: 1 g (1 ea); 2 g (1 ea)

General Dosage Range Dosage adjustment recommended in patients with renal impairment
I.V.:
Children >3 months: 80-160 mg/kg/day divided every 4-6 hours (maximum: 12 **g daily**) **or** 30-40 mg/kg prior to surgery
Adolescents: 80-160 mg/kg/day divided every 4-6 hours (maximum: 12 **g daily) or** 1-2 g prior to surgery
Adults: 1-2 g every 4-8 hours (maximum: 12 g daily) **or** 2 g prior to surgery

Administration
I.M. Inject deep I.M. into large muscle mass. **Note:** I.M. injection is painful and this route of administration is not described in the manufacturer's information.

I.V. Can be administered IVP over 3-5 minutes or by I.V. intermittent infusion over 10-60 minutes

Injectable Detail pH: 4.2-7 (reconstituted solution); 6.5 (frozen premixed solution)

Preparation for Administration Reconstitute vials with SWFI, bacteriostatic water for injection, NS, or D₅W. For I.V. infusion, solutions may be further diluted in NS, $D_5^{1}/_4NS$, $D_5^{1}/_2NS$, D_5NS, D_5W, $D_{10}W$, LR, D_5LR, mannitol 5% or 10%, or sodium bicarbonate 5%.

Storage/Stability Prior to reconstitution store between 2°C and 25°C (36°F and 77°F). Avoid exposure to temperatures >50°C (122°F). Cefoxitin tends to darken depending on storage conditions; however, product potency is not adversely affected.

Reconstituted solutions of 1 g per 10 mL in sterile water for injection, bacteriostatic water for injection, sodium chloride 0.9% injection, or dextrose 5% injection are stable for 6 hours at room temperature or for 7 days under refrigeration (<5°C [43°F]).

Nursing Actions
Physical Assessment Results of culture/sensitivity tests and patient's allergy history should be assessed prior to therapy. Monitor for nephrotoxicity. Evaluate prothrombin time and CBC with differential. Monitor for diarrhea, nausea, vomiting, and nephrotoxicity. Advise patients with diabetes about use of Clinitest®. Teach patient to report hypersensitivity and opportunistic infection.

Patient Education
- Discuss specific use of drug and side effects with patient as it relates to treatment. (HCAHPS: During this hospital stay, were you given any medicine that you had not taken before? Before giving you any new medicine, how often did hospital staff tell you what the medicine was for? How often did hospital staff describe possible side effects in a way you could understand?)
- Patient may experience diarrhea. Have patient report immediately to prescriber signs of hepatic impairment, severe nausea, ecchymosis, hemorrhaging, stomatitis, urinary retention, oliguria, considerable asthenia, dizziness, injection site irritation, vaginitis, or signs of pseudomembranous colitis (HCAHPS).
- Educate patient about signs of a significant reaction (eg, wheezing; chest tightness; fever; itching; bad cough; blue skin color; seizures; or swelling of face, lips, tongue, or throat). **Note:** This is not a comprehensive list of all side effects. Patient should consult prescriber for additional questions.

Intended Use and Disclaimer: Should not be printed and given to patients. This information is intended to serve as a concise initial reference for healthcare professionals to use when discussing medications with a patient. You must ultimately rely on your own discretion, experience and judgment in diagnosing, treating and advising patients.

Dietary Considerations Some products may contain sodium.

Cefpodoxime (sef pode OKS eem)

Index Terms Cefpodoxime Proxetil; Vantin
Pharmacologic Category Antibiotic, Cephalosporin (Third Generation)

◄ **Medication Safety Issues**
Sound-alike/look-alike issues:
Vantin may be confused with Ventolin®
Pregnancy Risk Factor B
Lactation Enters breast milk/not recommended
Breast-Feeding Considerations Cefpodoxime is excreted in breast milk. The manufacturer recommends discontinuing nursing or discontinuing the medication in breast-feeding women. Nondose-related effects could include modification of bowel flora.
Use Treatment of susceptible acute, community-acquired pneumonia caused by *S. pneumoniae* or nonbeta-lactamase producing *H. influenzae*; acute uncomplicated gonorrhea caused by *N. gonorrhoeae*; uncomplicated skin and skin structure infections caused by *S. aureus* or *S. pyogenes*; acute otitis media caused by *S. pneumoniae*, *H. influenzae*, or *M. catarrhalis*; pharyngitis or tonsillitis; and uncomplicated urinary tract infections caused by *E. coli*, *Klebsiella*, and *Proteus*
Unlabeled Use Acute bacterial rhinosinusitis (ABRS) (pediatric) in combination with clindamycin
Mechanism of Action/Effect Inhibits bacterial cell wall synthesis by binding to one or more of the penicillin-binding proteins (PBPs)
Contraindications Hypersensitivity to cefpodoxime, any component of the formulation, or other cephalosporins
Warnings/Precautions Modify dosage in patients with severe renal impairment. Prolonged use may result in fungal or bacterial superinfection, including *C. difficile*-associated diarrhea (CDAD) and pseudomembranous colitis; CDAD has been observed >2 months postantibiotic treatment. Use with caution in patients with a history of penicillin allergy, especially IgE-mediated reactions (eg, anaphylaxis, urticaria).
Drug Interactions
Avoid Concomitant Use
Avoid concomitant use of Cefpodoxime with any of the following: BCG
Decreased Effect
Cefpodoxime may decrease the levels/effects of: BCG; Sodium Picosulfate; Typhoid Vaccine

The levels/effects of Cefpodoxime may be decreased by: Antacids; H2-Antagonists
Increased Effect/Toxicity
Cefpodoxime may increase the levels/effects of: Aminoglycosides; Vitamin K Antagonists

The levels/effects of Cefpodoxime may be increased by: Probenecid
Nutritional/Ethanol Interactions Food: Food and/or low gastric pH delays absorption and may increase serum levels. Management: Take with or without food at regular intervals on an around-the-clock schedule to promote less variation in peak and trough serum levels.

Adverse Reactions
>10%:
Dermatologic: Diaper rash (12%)
Gastrointestinal: Diarrhea in infants and toddlers (15%)
1% to 10%:
Central nervous system: Headache (1%)
Dermatologic: Rash (1%)
Gastrointestinal: Diarrhea (7%), nausea (4%), abdominal pain (2%), vomiting (1% to 2%)
Genitourinary: Vaginal infection (3%)
Reactions reported with other cephalosporins: Seizure, Stevens-Johnson syndrome, toxic epidermal necrolysis, erythema multiforme, urticaria, serum-sickness reactions, renal dysfunction, interstitial nephritis toxic nephropathy, cholestasis, aplastic anemia, hemolytic anemia, hemorrhage, pancytopenia, agranulocytosis, colitis, vaginitis, superinfection
Available Dosage Forms
Suspension Reconstituted, Oral:
Generic: 50 mg/5 mL (50 mL, 100 mL); 100 mg/5 mL (50 mL, 100 mL)
Tablet, Oral:
Generic: 100 mg, 200 mg
General Dosage Range Dosage adjustment recommended in patients with renal impairment
Oral:
Children 2 months to 12 years: 10 mg/kg/day divided every 12 hours (maximum: 200 mg/dose)
Children ≥12 years and Adults: 100-400 mg every 12 hours **or** 200 mg as a single dose
Administration
Oral Administer around-the-clock to promote less variation in peak and trough serum levels.
Preparation for Administration Shake well before using. After mixing, keep suspension in refrigerator. Discard unused portion after 14 days.
Nursing Actions
Physical Assessment Results of culture/sensitivity tests and patient's allergy history should be assessed prior to therapy. Monitor prothrombin time. Monitor for hemolytic anemia, hypoprothrombinemia, and bleeding. Teach patient to report nephrotoxicity, opportunistic infection, and hypersensitivity reaction.
Patient Education
• Discuss specific use of drug and side effects with patient as it relates to treatment. (HCAHPS: During this hospital stay, were you given any medicine that you had not taken before? Before giving you any new medicine, how often did hospital staff tell you what the medicine was for? How often did hospital staff describe possible side effects in a way you could understand?)
• Patient may experience headache or diarrhea. Have patient report immediately to prescriber severe nausea, ecchymosis, hemorrhaging, considerable asthenia, urinary retention,

oliguria, jaundice, vaginitis, or signs of pseudo-membranous colitis (HCAHPS).

- Educate patient about signs of a significant reaction (eg, wheezing; chest tightness; fever; itching; bad cough; blue skin color; seizures; or swelling of face, lips, tongue, or throat). **Note:** This is not a comprehensive list of all side effects. Patient should consult prescriber for additional questions.

Intended Use and Disclaimer: Should not be printed and given to patients. This information is intended to serve as a concise initial reference for healthcare professionals to use when discussing medications with a patient. You must ultimately rely on your own discretion, experience and judgment in diagnosing, treating and advising patients.

Dietary Considerations May be taken with food.

Cefprozil (sef PROE zil)

Index Terms Cefzil

Pharmacologic Category Antibiotic, Cephalosporin (Second Generation)

Medication Safety Issues

Sound-alike/look-alike issues:

Cefprozil may be confused with ceFAZolin, cefuroxime

Cefzil may be confused with Ceftin®

Pregnancy Risk Factor B

Lactation Enters breast milk/use caution

Breast-Feeding Considerations Small amounts of cefprozil are excreted in breast milk. The manufacturer recommends that caution be exercised when administering cefprozil to nursing women. Nondose-related effects could include modification of bowel flora.

Use Treatment of otitis media and infections involving the respiratory tract and skin and skin structure; active against methicillin-sensitive staphylococci, many streptococci, and various gram-negative bacilli including *E. coli*, some *Klebsiella*, *P. mirabilis*, *H. influenzae*, and *Moraxella*.

Mechanism of Action/Effect Inhibits bacterial cell wall synthesis by binding to one or more of the penicillin-binding proteins (PBPs)

Contraindications Hypersensitivity to cefprozil, any component of the formulation, or other cephalosporins

Warnings/Precautions Modify dosage in patients with severe renal impairment. Use with caution in patients with a history of penicillin allergy, especially IgE-mediated reactions (eg, anaphylaxis, urticaria). Prolonged use may result in fungal or bacterial superinfection, including *C. difficile*-associated diarrhea (CDAD) and pseudomembranous colitis; CDAD has been observed >2 months post-antibiotic treatment. Some products may contain phenylalanine.

Drug Interactions

Avoid Concomitant Use

Avoid concomitant use of Cefprozil with any of the following: BCG

Decreased Effect

Cefprozil may decrease the levels/effects of: BCG; Sodium Picosulfate; Typhoid Vaccine

Increased Effect/Toxicity

Cefprozil may increase the levels/effects of: Aminoglycosides; Vitamin K Antagonists

The levels/effects of Cefprozil may be increased by: Probenecid

Nutritional/Ethanol Interactions Food: Food delays cefprozil absorption.

Adverse Reactions

1% to 10%:

Central nervous system: Dizziness (1%)

Dermatologic: Diaper rash (2%)

Gastrointestinal: Diarrhea (3%), nausea (4%), vomiting (1%), abdominal pain (1%)

Genitourinary: Vaginitis, genital pruritus (2%)

Hepatic: Transaminases increased (2%)

Miscellaneous: Superinfection

Reactions reported with other cephalosporins: Seizure, toxic epidermal necrolysis, renal dysfunction, interstitial nephritis, toxic nephropathy, aplastic anemia, hemolytic anemia, hemorrhage, pancytopenia, agranulocytosis, colitis, vaginitis, superinfection

Available Dosage Forms

Suspension Reconstituted, Oral:

Generic: 125 mg/5 mL (50 mL, 75 mL, 100 mL); 250 mg/5 mL (50 mL, 75 mL, 100 mL)

Tablet, Oral:

Generic: 250 mg, 500 mg

General Dosage Range Dosage adjustment recommended in patients with renal impairment

Oral:

Children 6 months to 2 years: 7.5-30 mg/kg/day divided every 12 hours

Children 2-12 years: 7.5-30 mg/kg/day divided every 12 hours **or** 20 mg/kg every 24 hours (maximum: 1 g/day)

Adolescents >12 years and Adults: 250-500 mg every 12 hours **or** 500 mg every 24 hours

Administration

Oral Administer around-the-clock to promote less variation in peak and trough serum levels. Chilling the reconstituted oral suspension improves flavor (do not freeze).

Nursing Actions

Physical Assessment Results of culture/sensitivity tests and patient's allergy history should be assessed prior to therapy. Monitor prothrombin time. Advise patients with diabetes about use of Clinitest® (may cause false-positive test). Teach patient to report opportunistic infection and hypersensitivity reaction.

Patient Education

- Discuss specific use of drug and side effects with patient as it relates to treatment. (HCAHPS: During this hospital stay, were you given any medicine that you had not taken before? Before giving you any new medicine, how often did hospital staff tell you what the medicine was for? How often did hospital staff describe possible side effects in a way you could understand?)
- Patient may experience diarrhea or headache. Have patient report immediately to prescriber severe nausea, ecchymosis, hemorrhaging, considerable asthenia, urinary retention, oliguria, jaundice, vaginitis, or signs of pseudomembranous colitis (HCAHPS).
- Educate patient about signs of a significant reaction (eg, wheezing; chest tightness; fever; itching; bad cough; blue skin color; seizures; or swelling of face, lips, tongue, or throat). **Note:** This is not a comprehensive list of all side effects. Patient should consult prescriber for additional questions.

Intended Use and Disclaimer: Should not be printed and given to patients. This information is intended to serve as a concise initial reference for healthcare professionals to use when discussing medications with a patient. You must ultimately rely on your own discretion, experience and judgment in diagnosing, treating and advising patients.

Dietary Considerations May be taken with food. Oral suspension may contain phenylalanine; consult product labeling.

Ceftaroline Fosamil (sef TAR oh leen FOS a mil)

Brand Names: U.S. Teflaro
Index Terms PPI-0903; PPI-0903M; T-91825; TAK-599
Pharmacologic Category Antibiotic, Cephalosporin (Fifth Generation)
Pregnancy Risk Factor B
Lactation Excretion in breast milk unknown/use caution
Breast-Feeding Considerations It is not known if ceftaroline fosamil is excreted in breast milk. The manufacturer recommends that caution be exercised when administering ceftaroline fosamil to nursing women.
Use
Acute bacterial skin and skin structure infections: Treatment of acute bacterial skin and skin structure infections caused by susceptible isolates of the following gram-positive and gram-negative microorganisms: *Staphylococcus aureus* (including methicillin-susceptible and methicillin-resistant isolates), *Streptococcus pyogenes*, *Streptococcus agalactiae*, *Escherichia coli*, *Klebsiella pneumoniae*, and *Klebsiella oxytoca*.

Community-acquired bacterial pneumonia: Treatment of community-acquired bacterial pneumonia caused by susceptible isolates of the following gram-positive and gram-negative microorganisms: *Streptococcus pneumoniae* (including cases with concurrent bacteremia), *S. aureus* (methicillin-susceptible isolates only), *Haemophilus influenzae*, *K. pneumoniae*, *K. oxytoca*, and *E. coli*.

Mechanism of Action/Effect Inhibits bacterial cell wall synthesis by binding to 1 or more of the penicillin-binding proteins (PBPs)
Contraindications Known serious hypersensitivity to ceftaroline, other members of the cephalosporin class, or any component of the formulation
Warnings/Precautions Use with caution in patients with a history of penicillin cephalosporin, or carbapenem allergy, especially IgE-mediated reactions (eg, anaphylaxis, angioedema, urticaria). Seroconversion from a negative to a positive direct Coombs' test has been reported. Hemolytic anemia was not reported in clinical studies; however, if anemia develops during or after treatment, diagnostic tests should include a direct Coombs' test. If drug-induced hemolytic anemia is considered, discontinue the drug and institute supportive care as clinically indicated. Prolonged use may result in fungal or bacterial superinfection, including *C. difficile*-associated diarrhea (CDAD) and pseudomembranous colitis (including fatalities); CDAD has been observed >2 months postantibiotic treatment. Use with caution in patients with renal impairment (CrCl ≤50 mL/minute); dosage adjustments recommended. Use with caution in the elderly; dosage adjustment should be based on renal function. Potentially significant drug-drug interactions may exist, requiring dose or frequency adjustment, additional monitoring, and/or selection of alternative therapy.

Drug Interactions
Avoid Concomitant Use
Avoid concomitant use of Ceftaroline Fosamil with any of the following: BCG
Decreased Effect
Ceftaroline Fosamil may decrease the levels/effects of: BCG; Sodium Picosulfate; Typhoid Vaccine
Increased Effect/Toxicity
Ceftaroline Fosamil may increase the levels/effects of: Vitamin K Antagonists

The levels/effects of Ceftaroline Fosamil may be increased by: Probenecid
Adverse Reactions
>10%: Hematologic: Positive Coombs' test without hemolysis (~11%)
2% to 10%:
  Central nervous system: Headache (3% to 5%), insomnia (3% to 4%)
  Dermatologic: Pruritus (3% to 4%), rash (3%)
  Endocrine & metabolic: Hypokalemia (2%)

Gastrointestinal: Diarrhea (5%), nausea (4%), constipation (2%), vomiting (2%)

Hepatic: Transaminases increased (2%)

Local: Phlebitis (2%)

Available Dosage Forms

Solution Reconstituted, Intravenous:

Teflaro: 400 mg (1 ea); 600 mg (1 ea)

General Dosage Range Dosage adjustment recommended in patients with renal impairment.

I.V.: *Adults:* 600 mg every 12 hours

Administration

I.V. Administer by slow I.V. infusion over 60 minutes.

Injectable Detail pH: 4.8-6.5 (reconstituted solution)

Preparation for Administration Reconstitute 400 mg or 600 mg vial with 20 mL SWFI, NS, D_5W, or LR; mix gently. Reconstituted solution should be further diluted for I.V. administration in 50-250 mL of a compatible solution. Use the same solution as used for reconstitution (**Note:** If SWFI was used for reconstitution, then appropriate infusion solutions include NS, ½NS, D_5W, $D_{2.5}W$, or LR). Color of infusion solutions ranges from clear and light yellow to dark yellow depending on concentration and storage conditions; potency is not affected.

Storage/Stability Store unused vials at 25°C (77°F); excursions permitted between 15°C and 30°C (59°F and 86°F). Per the manufacturer, unused vials can also be stored at 2°C to 8°C (36°F to 46°F). Diluted solutions should be used within 6 hours when stored at room temperature or within 24 hours if refrigerated at 2°C to 8°C (36°F to 46°F).

Nursing Actions

Patient Education

- Discuss specific use of drug and side effects with patient as it relates to treatment. (HCAHPS: During this hospital stay, were you given any medicine that you had not taken before? Before giving you any new medicine, how often did hospital staff tell you what the medicine was for? How often did hospital staff describe possible side effects in a way you could understand?)
- Patient may experience diarrhea. Have patient report immediately to prescriber signs of hypoglycemia, bradycardia, severe nausea, ecchymosis, hemorrhaging, stomatitis, injection site irritation, urinary retention, oliguria, dizziness, considerable asthenia, chills, pharyngitis, jaundice, or signs of pseudomembranous colitis (HCAHPS).
- Educate patient about signs of a significant reaction (eg, wheezing; chest tightness; fever; itching; bad cough; blue skin color; seizures; or swelling of face, lips, tongue, or throat). **Note:** This is not a comprehensive list of all side effects. Patient should consult prescriber for additional questions.

Intended Use and Disclaimer: Should not be printed and given to patients. This information is intended to serve as a concise initial reference for healthcare professionals to use when discussing medications with a patient. You must ultimately rely on your own discretion, experience and judgment in diagnosing, treating and advising patients.

CefTAZidime (SEF tay zi deem)

Brand Names: U.S. Fortaz; Fortaz in D5W; Tazicef

Pharmacologic Category Antibiotic, Cephalosporin (Third Generation)

Medication Safety Issues

Sound-alike/look-alike issues:

CefTAZidime may be confused with ceFAZolin, cefepime, cefoTEtan, cefOXitin, cefTRIAXone

Ceptaz® may be confused with Septra®

Tazicef® may be confused with Tazidime®

International issues:

Ceftim [Portugal] and Ceftime [Thailand] brand names for ceftazidime may be confused with Ceftin brand name for cefuroxime [U.S., Canada]; Cefiton brand name for cefixime [Portugal]

Pregnancy Risk Factor B

Lactation Enters breast milk/use caution

Breast-Feeding Considerations Very small amounts of ceftazidime are excreted in breast milk. The manufacturer recommends that caution be exercised when administering ceftazidime to nursing women. Ceftazidime in not absorbed when given orally; therefore, any medication that is distributed to human milk should not result in systemic concentrations in the nursing infant. Nondose-related effects could include modification of bowel flora.

Use Treatment of documented susceptible *Pseudomonas aeruginosa* infection and infections due to other susceptible aerobic gram-negative organisms; empiric therapy of a febrile, granulocytopenic patient

Unlabeled Use Bacterial endophthalmitis

Mechanism of Action/Effect Inhibits bacterial cell wall synthesis by binding to one or more of the penicillin-binding proteins (PBPs)

Contraindications Hypersensitivity to ceftazidime, any component of the formulation, or other cephalosporins

Warnings/Precautions Modify dosage in patients with severe renal impairment. Use with caution in patients with a history of penicillin allergy, especially IgE-mediated reactions (eg, anaphylaxis, urticaria). Prolonged use may result in fungal or bacterial superinfection, including *C. difficile*-associated diarrhea (CDAD) and pseudomembranous colitis; CDAD has been observed >2 months post-antibiotic treatment. May be associated with increased INR, especially in nutritionally-deficient patients, prolonged treatment, hepatic or renal disease. Use with caution in patients with a history of seizure disorder; high levels, particularly in the presence of renal impairment, may increase risk of seizures.

Drug Interactions

Avoid Concomitant Use

Avoid concomitant use of CefTAZidime with any of the following: BCG

Decreased Effect

CefTAZidime may decrease the levels/effects of: BCG; Sodium Picosulfate; Typhoid Vaccine

Increased Effect/Toxicity

CefTAZidime may increase the levels/effects of: Aminoglycosides; Vitamin K Antagonists

The levels/effects of CefTAZidime may be increased by: Probenecid

Adverse Reactions

1% to 10%:

Gastrointestinal: Diarrhea (1%)

Local: Pain at injection site (1%)

Miscellaneous: Hypersensitivity reactions (2%)

Reactions reported with other cephalosporins: Seizure, urticaria, serum-sickness reactions, renal dysfunction, interstitial nephritis, toxic nephropathy, BUN increased, creatinine increased, cholestasis, aplastic anemia, hemolytic anemia, pancytopenia, agranulocytosis, colitis, prolonged PT, hemorrhage, superinfection

Available Dosage Forms

Solution, Intravenous:

Fortaz in D_5W: 1 g (50 mL); 2 g (50 mL)

Tazicef: 1 g/50 mL (50 mL)

Solution Reconstituted, Injection:

Fortaz: 500 mg (1 ea); 1 g (1 ea); 2 g (1 ea); 6 g (1 ea)

Tazicef: 1 g (1 ea); 2 g (1 ea); 6 g (1 ea)

Generic: 1 g (1 ea); 2 g (1 ea); 6 g (1 ea); 100 g (1 ea)

Solution Reconstituted, Injection [preservative free]:

Generic: 1 g (1 ea); 2 g (1 ea); 6 g (1 ea)

Solution Reconstituted, Intravenous:

Fortaz: 1 g (1 ea); 2 g (1 ea)

Tazicef: 1 g (1 ea); 2 g (1 ea)

Generic: 1 g/50 mL (1 ea); 2 g/50 mL (1 ea)

General Dosage Range Dosage adjustment recommended in patients with renal impairment

I.M.: *Adults:* 500 mg to 2 g every 8-12 hours

I.V.:

Children 1 month to 12 years: 30-50 mg/kg every 8 hours (maximum: 6 g daily)

Children ≥12 years and Adults: 500 mg to 2 g every 8-12 hours (maximum: 6 g daily)

Administration

I.M. Inject deep I.M. into large mass muscle.

I.V. Ceftazidime can be administered IVP over 3-5 minutes or I.V. intermittent infusion over 15-30 minutes.

Injectable Detail Any carbon dioxide bubbles that may be present in the withdrawn solution should be expelled prior to injection. Administer around-the-clock to promote less variation in peak and trough serum levels.

pH: 5-8 (Fortaz); 5-7.5 (Tazicef)

Intravitreal Ceftazidime may be administered intravitreally as 2-2.25 mg/0.1 mL NS in combination with vancomycin (separate syringes) (Jackson, 2003; Roth, 1997).

Preparation for Administration

I.M.: Using SWFI, bacteriostatic water, lidocaine 0.5%, or lidocaine 1%, reconstitute the 500 mg vials with 1.5 mL or the 1 g vials with 3 mL; final concentration of ~280 mg/mL

I.V.: Using SWFI, reconstitute as follows (**Note:** After reconstitution, may dilute further with a compatible solution to administer via I.V. infusion):

Fortaz®:

~100 mg/mL solution:

500 mg vial: 5.3 mL SWFI (withdraw 5 mL from the reconstituted vial to obtain a 500 mg dose)

1 g vial: 10 mL SWFI (withdraw 10 mL from the reconstituted vial to obtain a 1 g dose)

6 g vial: 56 mL SWFI (withdraw 10 mL from the reconstituted vial to obtain a 1 g dose)

~170 mg/mL solution: 2 g vial: 10 mL SWFI (withdraw 11.5 mL from the reconstituted vial to obtain a 2 g dose)

~200 mg/mL solution: 6 g vial: 26 mL SWFI (withdraw 5 mL from the reconstituted vial to obtain a 1 g dose)

Tazicef®:

~95 mg/mL solution: 1 g vial: 10 mL SWFI (withdraw 10.6 mL from the reconstituted vial to obtain a 1 g dose)

~180 mg/mL solution: 2 g vial: 10 mL SWFI (withdraw 11.2 mL from the reconstituted vial to obtain a 2 g dose)

Fortaz®, Tazicef®: ADD-Vantage® vials: Dilute in 50 or 100 mL of D_5W, NS, or 0.45% sodium chloride in an ADD-Vantage® flexible diluent container only.

Storage/Stability

Fortaz®: Store dry vials at 15°C to 30°C (59°F to 86°F). Protect from light. Reconstituted solution and solution further diluted for I.V. infusion are stable for 12 hours at room temperature, for 3 days when refrigerated, or for 12 weeks when frozen at -20°C (-4°F). After freezing, thawed solution in SWFI for I.M. administration is stable for 3 hours at room temperature or for 3 days when refrigerated; thawed solution in NS in a Viaflex® small volume container for I.V. administration is stable for 12 hours at room temperature or for 3 days when refrigerated; and thawed solution in SWFI in the original container is stable for 8 hours at room temperature or for 3 days when refrigerated.

Premixed frozen solution: Store frozen at -20°C (-4°F). Thawed solution is stable for 8 hours at room temperature or for 3 days under refrigeration; do not refreeze.

Fortaz®, Tazicef®: ADD-Vantage® vials: Following dilution, may be stored for up to 12 hours at room temperature or for 3 days under refrigeration. Freezing solutions in the ADD-Vantage® system is not recommended. Joined vials that have not been activated may be used within 14 days.

Tazicef® vials: Store dry vials at 20°C to 25°C (68°F to 77°F). Protect from light. Reconstituted vials and solution further diluted for I.V. infusion are stable for 24 hours at room temperature, for 7 days when refrigerated, or for 12 weeks when frozen at -20°C (-4°F). When thawed, solution is stable for 8 hours at room temperature and 4 days when refrigerated.

Nursing Actions

Physical Assessment Results of culture/sensitivity tests and patient's allergy history should be assessed prior to therapy. Monitor for nephrotoxicity. Assess prothrombin time. Monitor for hemolytic anemia, hypoprothrombinemia, and bleeding. Teach patient to report opportunistic infection and hypersensitivity reaction.

Patient Education
- Discuss specific use of drug and side effects with patient as it relates to treatment. (HCAHPS: During this hospital stay, were you given any medicine that you had not taken before? Before giving you any new medicine, how often did hospital staff tell you what the medicine was for? How often did hospital staff describe possible side effects in a way you could understand?)
- Patient may experience headache or diarrhea. Have patient report immediately to prescriber severe nausea, ecchymosis, hemorrhaging, stomatitis, injection site irritation, urinary retention, oliguria, difficulty with motor activity, considerable asthenia, jaundice, vaginitis, or signs of pseudomembranous colitis (HCAHPS).
- Educate patient about signs of a significant reaction (eg, wheezing; chest tightness; fever; itching; bad cough; blue skin color; seizures; or swelling of face, lips, tongue, or throat). **Note:** This is not a comprehensive list of all side effects. Patient should consult prescriber for additional questions.

Intended Use and Disclaimer: Should not be printed and given to patients. This information is intended to serve as a concise initial reference for healthcare professionals to use when discussing medications with a patient. You must ultimately rely on your own discretion, experience and judgment in diagnosing, treating and advising patients.

Dietary Considerations Some products may contain sodium.

Ceftibuten (sef TYE byoo ten)

Brand Names: U.S. Cedax

Pharmacologic Category Antibiotic, Cephalosporin (Third Generation)

Medication Safety Issues

Sound-alike/look-alike issues:
Cedax® may be confused with Cidex®

International issues:
Cedax [U.S. and multiple international markets] may be confused with Codex brand name for acetaminophen/codeine [Brazil] and *Saccharomyces boulardii* [Italy]

Pregnancy Risk Factor B

Lactation Excretion in breast milk unknown/use caution

Breast-Feeding Considerations Ceftibuten was not detectable in milk after a single 200 mg dose (limit of detection: 1 mcg/mL). It is not known if it would be detectable after a 400 mg dose or multiple doses. The manufacturer recommends that caution be exercised when administering ceftibuten to nursing women. If ceftibuten does reach the human milk, nondose-related effects could include modification of bowel flora.

Use Treatment of acute exacerbations of chronic bronchitis, acute bacterial otitis media, and pharyngitis/tonsillitis

Mechanism of Action/Effect Inhibits bacterial cell wall synthesis by binding to one or more of the penicillin-binding proteins (PBPs)

Contraindications Hypersensitivity to ceftibuten, any component of the formulation, or other cephalosporins

Warnings/Precautions Modify dosage in patients with moderate-to-severe renal impairment. Prolonged use may result in fungal or bacterial superinfection, including *C. difficile*-associated diarrhea (CDAD) and pseudomembranous colitis; CDAD has been observed >2 months postantibiotic treatment. Use with caution in patients with a history of colitis and other gastrointestinal diseases. Use with caution in patients with a history of penicillin allergy, especially IgE-mediated reactions (eg, anaphylaxis, urticaria). Oral suspension formulation contains sucrose.

Drug Interactions

Avoid Concomitant Use
Avoid concomitant use of Ceftibuten with any of the following: BCG

Decreased Effect
Ceftibuten may decrease the levels/effects of: BCG; Sodium Picosulfate; Typhoid Vaccine

The levels/effects of Ceftibuten may be decreased by: Multivitamins/Minerals (with ADEK, Folate, Iron); Multivitamins/Minerals (with AE, No Iron); Zinc Salts

Increased Effect/Toxicity

Ceftibuten may increase the levels/effects of: Aminoglycosides; Vitamin K Antagonists

The levels/effects of Ceftibuten may be increased by: Probenecid

Adverse Reactions

1% to 10%:

Central nervous system: Headache (≤3%), dizziness (≤1%)

Gastrointestinal: Nausea (≤4%), diarrhea (3% to 4%), dyspepsia (≤2%), loose stools (≤2%), abdominal pain (1% to 2%), vomiting (1% to 2%)

Hematologic: Eosinophils increased (3%), hemoglobin decreased (1% to 2%), platelets increased (≤1%)

Hepatic: ALT increased (≤1%), bilirubin increased (≤1%)

Renal: BUN increased (2% to 4%)

Additional reactions reported with other cephalosporins: Allergic reaction, agranulocytosis, angioedema, aplastic anemia, anaphylaxis, asterixis, cholestasis, drug fever, encephalopathy, erythema multiforme, hemolytic anemia, hemorrhage, interstitial nephritis, neuromuscular excitability, neutropenia, pancytopenia, prolonged PT, renal dysfunction, seizure, superinfection, toxic nephropathy

Available Dosage Forms

Capsule, Oral:

Cedax: 400 mg

Generic: 400 mg

Suspension Reconstituted, Oral:

Cedax: 90 mg/5 mL (60 mL, 90 mL, 120 mL); 180 mg/5 mL (30 mL, 60 mL)

Generic: 180 mg/5 mL (60 mL)

General Dosage Range Dosage adjustment recommended in patients with renal impairment

Oral:

Children 6 months to <12 years: 9 mg/kg/day (maximum: 400 mg/day)

Children ≥12 years and Adults: 400 mg once daily

Administration

Oral

Capsule: Administer without regard to food.

Suspension: Administer 2 hours before or 1 hour after meals. Shake well before use.

Storage/Stability Store capsules and powder for suspension at 2°C to 25°C (36°F to 77°F). Reconstituted suspension is stable for 14 days when refrigerated at 2°C to 8°C (36°F to 46°F).

Nursing Actions

Physical Assessment Results of culture/sensitivity tests and patient's allergy history should be assessed prior to therapy. Monitor for nephrotoxicity, hemolytic anemia, hypoprothrombinemia, and bleeding. Teach patient to report opportunistic infection and hypersensitivity reaction.

Patient Education

• Discuss specific use of drug and side effects with patient as it relates to treatment. (HCAHPS: During this hospital stay, were you given any medicine that you had not taken before? Before giving you any new medicine, how often did hospital staff tell you what the medicine was for? How often did hospital staff describe possible side effects in a way you could understand?)

• Patient may experience headache or diarrhea. Have patient report immediately to prescriber signs of hepatic impairment, severe nausea, ecchymosis, hemorrhaging, urinary retention, oliguria, chills, pharyngitis, arthralgia, mood changes, considerable asthenia, vaginitis, or signs of pseudomembranous colitis (HCAHPS).

• Educate patient about signs of a significant reaction (eg, wheezing; chest tightness; fever; itching; bad cough; blue skin color; seizures; or swelling of face, lips, tongue, or throat). **Note:** This is not a comprehensive list of all side effects. Patient should consult prescriber for additional questions.

Intended Use and Disclaimer: Should not be printed and given to patients. This information is intended to serve as a concise initial reference for healthcare professionals to use when discussing medications with a patient. You must ultimately rely on your own discretion, experience and judgment in diagnosing, treating and advising patients.

Dietary Considerations

Capsule: Take without regard to food.

Suspension: Take 2 hours before or 1 hour after meals.

CefTRIAXone (sef trye AKS one)

Brand Names: U.S. Rocephin

Index Terms Ceftriaxone Sodium

Pharmacologic Category Antibiotic, Cephalosporin (Third Generation)

Medication Safety Issues

Sound-alike/look-alike issues:

CefTRIAXone may be confused with CeFAZolin, cefoTEtan, cefOXitin, cefTAZidime, Cetraxal

Rocephin may be confused with Roferon

Pregnancy Risk Factor B

Lactation Enters breast milk/use caution

Breast-Feeding Considerations Low concentrations of ceftriaxone are excreted in breast milk. The manufacturer recommends that caution be exercised when administering ceftriaxone to nursing women. Nondose-related effects could include modification of bowel flora.

Use Treatment of lower respiratory tract infections, acute bacterial otitis media, skin and skin structure infections, bone and joint infections, intra-abdominal and urinary tract infections, pelvic inflammatory disease (PID), uncomplicated gonorrhea, bacterial septicemia, and meningitis; used in surgical (perioperative) prophylaxis

Unlabeled Use Treatment of chancroid, epididymitis, complicated gonococcal infections; sexually-transmitted diseases (STD); periorbital or buccal cellulitis; salmonellosis or shigellosis; atypical community-acquired pneumonia; acute bacterial rhinosinusitis (ABRS); epiglottitis, Lyme disease; used in chemoprophylaxis for high-risk contacts (close exposure to patients with invasive meningococcal disease); sexual assault; typhoid fever, Whipple's disease

Mechanism of Action/Effect Inhibits bacterial cell wall synthesis by binding to one or more of the penicillin-binding proteins (PBPs)

Contraindications Hypersensitivity to ceftriaxone sodium, any component of the formulation, or other cephalosporins; **do not use in hyperbilirubinemic neonates**, particularly those who are premature since ceftriaxone is reported to displace bilirubin from albumin binding sites; concomitant use with intravenous calcium-containing solutions/products in neonates (≤28 days)

Warnings/Precautions Use with caution in patients with a history of penicillin allergy, especially IgE-mediated reactions (eg, anaphylaxis, urticaria). Abnormal gallbladder sonograms have been reported, possibly due to cetriaxone-calcium precipitates; discontinue in patients who develop signs and symptoms of gallbladder disease. Secondary to biliary obstruction, pancreatitis has been reported rarely. Use with caution in patients with a history of GI disease, especially colitis. Severe cases (including some fatalities) of immune-related hemolytic anemia have been reported in patients receiving cephalosporins, including ceftriaxone. Prolonged use may result in fungal or bacterial superinfection, including *C. difficile*-associated diarrhea (CDAD) and pseudomembranous colitis; CDAD has been observed >2 months postantibiotic treatment.

Potentially significant interactions may exist, requiring dose or frequency adjustment, additional monitoring, and/or selection of alternative therapy. May be associated with increased INR (rarely), especially in nutritionally-deficient patients, prolonged treatment, hepatic or renal disease. No adjustment is generally necessary in patients with renal impairment; use with caution in patients with concurrent hepatic dysfunction and significant renal disease, dosage should not exceed 2 g/day. Ceftriaxone may complex with calcium causing precipitation. Fatal lung and kidney damage associated with calcium-ceftriaxone precipitates has been observed in premature and term neonates. Do not reconstitute, admix, or coadminister with calcium-containing solutions, even via separate infusion lines/sites or at different times in any neonatal patient. Ceftriaxone should not be diluted or administered simultaneously with any calcium-containing

solution via a Y-site in any patient. However, ceftriaxone and calcium-containing solution may be administered sequentially of one another for use in patients **other than neonates** if infusion lines are thoroughly flushed, with a compatible fluid, between infusions

Drug Interactions

Avoid Concomitant Use

Avoid concomitant use of CefTRIAXone with any of the following: BCG

Decreased Effect

CefTRIAXone may decrease the levels/effects of: BCG; Sodium Picosulfate; Typhoid Vaccine

Increased Effect/Toxicity

CefTRIAXone may increase the levels/effects of: Aminoglycosides; Vitamin K Antagonists

The levels/effects of CefTRIAXone may be increased by: Calcium Salts (Intravenous); Probenecid; Ringer's Injection (Lactated)

Adverse Reactions

>10%: Local: Induration (I.M. 5% to 17%), warmth (I.M.), tightness (I.M.)

1% to 10%:
Dermatologic: Rash (2%)
Gastrointestinal: Diarrhea (3%)
Hematologic: Eosinophilia (6%), thrombocytosis (5%), leukopenia (2%)
Hepatic: Transaminases increased (3%)
Local: Tenderness at injection site (I.V. 1%), pain
Renal: BUN increased (1%)

Reactions reported with other cephalosporins: Angioedema, allergic reaction, aplastic anemia, asterixis, cholestasis, encephalopathy, hemorrhage, hepatic dysfunction, hyperactivity (reversible), hypertonia, interstitial nephritis, LDH increased, neuromuscular excitability, pancytopenia, paresthesia, renal dysfunction, superinfection, toxic nephropathy

Available Dosage Forms

Solution, Intravenous:
Generic: 20 mg/mL (50 mL); 40 mg/mL (50 mL)

Solution Reconstituted, Injection:
Rocephin: 500 mg (1 ea); 1 g (1 ea)
Generic: 250 mg (1 ea); 500 mg (1 ea); 1 g (1 ea); 2 g (1 ea)

Solution Reconstituted, Intravenous:
Generic: 1 g (1 ea); 2 g (1 ea); 10 g (1 ea)

General Dosage Range Dosage adjustment recommended in patients with hepatic and renal impairment

I.M.:
Children: 50-100 mg/kg/day divided every 12-24 hours (maximum: 4000 mg daily) **or** 125 mg or 50 mg/kg as a single dose
Adults: 1-2 g every 12-24 hours **or** 125-250 mg as a single dose

I.V.:
Children: 50-100 mg/kg/day divided every 12-24 hours (maximum: 4000 mg daily)
Adults: 1-2 g every 12-24 hours

◀ **Administration**

I.M. Inject deep I.M. into large muscle mass; a concentration of 250 mg/mL or 350 mg/mL is recommended for all vial sizes except the 250 mg size (250 mg/mL is suggested); can be diluted with 1:1 water or 1% lidocaine for I.M. administration.

I.V. Do not reconstitute or coadminister with calcium-containing solutions. Infuse as an intermittent infusion over 30 minutes. I.V. push administration over 1-4 minutes has been reported in children ≥12 years, adolescents, and adults (concentration: 100 mg/mL), primarily in patients outside the hospital setting (Baumgartner, 1983; Garrelts, 1988; Poole, 1999), although a 2 g dose administered I.V. push over 5 minutes resulted in tachycardia, restlessness, diaphoresis, and palpitations in one patient (Lossos, 1994). I.V. push administration in young infants may also have been a contributing factor in risk of cardiopulmonary events occurring from interactions between ceftriaxone and calcium (Bradley, 2009).

Injectable Detail pH: 6.6 (premixed infusion solution); 6.7 (1% aqueous solution)

Preparation for Administration

I.M. injection: Vials should be reconstituted with appropriate volume of diluent (including D₅W, NS, SWFI, bacteriostatic water, or 1% lidocaine) to make a final concentration of 250 mg/mL or 350 mg/mL.

Volume to add to create a **250 mg/mL** solution:
250 mg vial: 0.9 mL
500 mg vial: 1.8 mL
1 g vial: 3.6 mL
2 g vial: 7.2 mL

Volume to add to create a **350 mg/mL** solution:
500 mg vial: 1.0 mL
1 g vial: 2.1 mL
2 g vial: 4.2 mL

I.V. infusion: Infusion is prepared in two stages: Initial reconstitution of powder, followed by dilution to final infusion solution.

Vials: Reconstitute powder with appropriate I.V. diluent (including SWFI, D₅W, D₁₀W, NS) to create an initial solution of ~100 mg/mL. Recommended volume to add:
250 mg vial: 2.4 mL
500 mg vial: 4.8 mL
1 g vial: 9.6 mL
2 g vial: 19.2 mL

Note: After reconstitution of powder, further dilution into a volume of compatible solution (eg, 50-100 mL of D₅W or NS) is recommended.

Piggyback bottle: Reconstitute powder with appropriate I.V. diluent (D₅W or NS) to create a resulting solution of ~100 mg/mL. Recommended initial volume to add:
1 g bottle:10 mL
2 g bottle: 20 mL

Note: After reconstitution, to prepare the final infusion solution, further dilution to 50 mL or 100 mL volumes with the appropriate I.V. diluent (including D₅W or NS) is recommended.

Storage/Stability

Powder for injection: Prior to reconstitution, store at room temperature ≤25°C (≤77°F). Protect from light.

Premixed solution (manufacturer premixed): Store at -20°C; once thawed, solutions are stable for 3 days at room temperature of 25°C (77°F) or for 21 days refrigerated at 5°C (41°F). Do not refreeze.

Stability of reconstituted solutions:

10-40 mg/mL: Reconstituted in D₅W, D₁₀W, NS, or SWFI: Stable for 2 days at room temperature of 25°C (77°F) or for 10 days when refrigerated at 4°C (39°F). Stable for 26 weeks when frozen at -20°C when reconstituted with D₅W or NS. Once thawed (at room temperature), solutions are stable for 2 days at room temperature of 25°C (77°F) or for 10 days when refrigerated at 4°C (39°F); does not apply to manufacturer's premixed bags. Do not refreeze.

100 mg/mL:
Reconstituted in D₅W, SWFI, or NS: Stable for 2 days at room temperature of 25°C (77°F) or for 10 days when refrigerated at 4°C (39°F).
Reconstituted in lidocaine 1% solution or bacteriostatic water: Stable for 24 hours at room temperature of 25°C (77°F) or for 10 days when refrigerated at 4°C (39°F).

250-350 mg/mL: Reconstituted in D₅W, NS, lidocaine 1% solution, bacteriostatic water, or SWFI: Stable for 24 hours at room temperature of 25°C (77°F) or for 3 days when refrigerated at 4°C (39°F).

Nursing Actions

Physical Assessment Culture/sensitivity tests should be performed and patient's allergy history should be assessed prior to beginning therapy. Monitor prothrombin times.

Patient Education

• Discuss specific use of drug and side effects with patient as it relates to treatment. (HCAHPS: During this hospital stay, were you given any medicine that you had not taken before? Before giving you any new medicine, how often did hospital staff tell you what the medicine was for? How often did hospital staff describe possible side effects in a way you could understand?)

• Patient may experience diarrhea. Have patient report immediately to prescriber signs of pancreatitis, severe nausea, ecchymosis, hemorrhaging, significant injection site irritation, vaginitis, signs of hemolytic anemia, or signs of pseudomembranous colitis (HCAHPS).

• Educate patient about signs of a significant reaction (eg, wheezing; chest tightness; fever; itching; bad cough; blue skin color; seizures; or swelling of face, lips, tongue, or throat). **Note:** This is not a comprehensive list of all side

effects. Patient should consult prescriber for additional questions.

Intended Use and Disclaimer: Should not be printed and given to patients. This information is intended to serve as a concise initial reference for healthcare professionals to use when discussing medications with a patient. You must ultimately rely on your own discretion, experience and judgment in diagnosing, treating and advising patients.

Dietary Considerations Some products may contain sodium.

Cefuroxime (se fyoor OKS eem)

Brand Names: U.S. Ceftin; Zinacef; Zinacef in D5W [DSC]; Zinacef in Sterile Water

Index Terms Cefuroxime Axetil; Cefuroxime Sodium

Pharmacologic Category Antibiotic, Cephalosporin (Second Generation)

Medication Safety Issues

Sound-alike/look-alike issues:

Cefuroxime may be confused with cefotaxime, cefprozil, deferoxamine

Ceftin may be confused with Cefzil, Cipro

Zinacef may be confused with Zithromax

International issues:

Ceftin [U.S., Canada] may be confused with Cefiton brand name for cefixime [Portugal]; Ceftim brand name for ceftazidime [Portugal]; Ceftime brand name for ceftazidime [Thailand]

Pregnancy Risk Factor B

Lactation Enters breast milk

Breast-Feeding Considerations Cefuroxime is excreted in breast milk. Manufacturer recommendations vary; caution is recommended if cefuroxime I.V. is given to a nursing woman and it is recommended to consider discontinuing nursing temporarily during treatment following oral cefuroxime. Nondose-related effects could include modification of bowel flora.

Use Treatment of infections caused by staphylococci, group B streptococci, *H. influenzae* (type A and B), *E. coli*, *Enterobacter*, *Salmonella*, and *Klebsiella*; treatment of susceptible infections of the upper and lower respiratory tract, otitis media, urinary tract, uncomplicated skin and soft tissue, bone and joint, sepsis, uncomplicated gonorrhea, and early Lyme disease; surgical (perioperative) prophylaxis

Mechanism of Action/Effect Inhibits bacterial cell wall synthesis by binding to one or more of the penicillin-binding proteins (PBPs)

Contraindications Hypersensitivity to cefuroxime, any component of the formulation, or other cephalosporins

Warnings/Precautions Modify dosage in patients with severe renal impairment. Use with caution in patients with a history of penicillin allergy, especially IgE-mediated reactions (eg, anaphylaxis, urticaria). Prolonged use may result in fungal or bacterial superinfection, including *C. difficile*-associated diarrhea (CDAD) and pseudomembranous colitis; CDAD has been observed >2 months postantibiotic treatment. May be associated with increased INR, especially in nutritionally-deficient patients, prolonged treatment, hepatic or renal disease. Tablets and oral suspension are not bioequivalent (do not substitute on a mg-per-mg basis). Some products may contain phenylalanine.

Drug Interactions

Avoid Concomitant Use

Avoid concomitant use of Cefuroxime with any of the following: BCG

Decreased Effect

Cefuroxime may decrease the levels/effects of: BCG; Sodium Picosulfate; Typhoid Vaccine

The levels/effects of Cefuroxime may be decreased by: Antacids; H2-Antagonists

Increased Effect/Toxicity

Cefuroxime may increase the levels/effects of: Aminoglycosides; Vitamin K Antagonists

The levels/effects of Cefuroxime may be increased by: Probenecid

Nutritional/Ethanol Interactions Food: Bioavailability is increased with food; cefuroxime serum levels may be increased if taken with food or dairy products.

Adverse Reactions

>10%: Gastrointestinal: Diarrhea (4% to 11%, duration-dependent)

1% to 10%:

Dermatologic: Diaper rash (3%)

Endocrine & metabolic: Alkaline phosphatase increased (2%), lactate dehydrogenase increased (1%)

Gastrointestinal: Nausea/vomiting (3% to 7%)

Genitourinary: Vaginitis (≤5%)

Hematologic: Eosinophilia (7%), hemoglobin and hematocrit decreased (10%)

Hepatic: Transaminases increased (2% to 4%)

Local: Thrombophlebitis (2%)

Reactions reported with other cephalosporins: Agranulocytosis, aplastic anemia, asterixis, encephalopathy, hemorrhage, neuromuscular excitability, serum-sickness reactions, superinfection, toxic nephropathy

Available Dosage Forms

Solution, Intravenous:

Zinacef in Sterile Water: 1.5 g (50 mL)

Solution Reconstituted, Injection:

Zinacef: 750 mg (1 ea); 1.5 g (1 ea); 7.5 g (1 ea)

Generic: 750 mg (1 ea); 1.5 g (1 ea); 7.5 g (1 ea); 75 g (1 ea); 225 g (1 ea)

Solution Reconstituted, Intravenous:

Zinacef: 750 mg (1 ea); 1.5 g (1 ea)

Generic: 750 mg (1 ea); 1.5 g (1 ea); 7.5 g (1 ea)

Suspension Reconstituted, Oral:
Ceftin: 125 mg/5 mL (100 mL); 250 mg/5 mL (50 mL, 100 mL)
Generic: 125 mg/5 mL (100 mL)
Tablet, Oral:
Ceftin: 250 mg, 500 mg
Generic: 250 mg, 500 mg
General Dosage Range Dosage adjustment recommended in patients with renal impairment
I.M., I.V.:
Children 3 months to 12 years: 75-150 mg/kg/day divided every 8 hours (maximum: 6 g daily)
Adolescents >12 years and Adults: 750 mg to 1.5 g every 6-8 hours (maximum: 6 g daily) **or** 1.5 g as a single dose
Oral:
Children 3 months to 12 years: 20-30 mg/kg/day in 2 divided doses **or** 125-250 mg every 12 hours (maximum: 1 g daily)
Adolescents >12 years and Adults: 250-500 mg every 12 hours **or** 1 g as a single dose
Administration
I.M. Inject deep I.M. into large muscle mass.
I.V. Inject direct I.V. over 3-5 minutes. Infuse intermittent infusion over 15-30 minutes.
Injectable Detail pH: 6-8.5 (reconstituted solution in vial); 5-7.5 (frozen premixed solution)
Oral
Suspension: Administer with food. Shake well before use.
Tablet: May administer without regard to meals.
Storage/Stability
Injection: Reconstituted solution is stable for 24 hours at room temperature and 48 hours when refrigerated. I.V. infusion in NS or D₅W solution is stable for 24 hours at room temperature, 7 days when refrigerated, or 26 weeks when frozen. After freezing, thawed solution is stable for 24 hours at room temperature or 21 days when refrigerated. Oral suspension: Prior to reconstitution, store at 2°C to 30°C (36°F to 86°F). Reconstituted suspension is stable for 10 days at 2°C to 8°C (36°F to 46°F).
Tablet: Store at 15°C to 30°C (59°F to 86°F).
Nursing Actions
Physical Assessment Results of culture/sensitivity tests and patient's allergy history should be assessed prior to therapy. Monitor for nephrotoxicity. Assess prothrombin times. Monitor for hemolytic anemia, hypoprothrombinemia, and bleeding. Advise patients with diabetes about use of Clinitest® (may cause false-positive test). Teach patient to report opportunistic infection and hypersensitivity reaction.
Patient Education
• Discuss specific use of drug and side effects with patient as it relates to treatment. (HCAHPS: During this hospital stay, were you given any medicine that you had not taken before? Before giving you any new medicine, how often did hospital staff tell you what the medicine was

for? How often did hospital staff describe possible side effects in a way you could understand?)
• Patient may experience diarrhea. Have patient report immediately to prescriber significant injection site irritation, signs of hepatic impairment, severe nausea, ecchymosis, hemorrhaging, urinary retention, oliguria, considerable asthenia, vaginitis, or signs of pseudomembranous colitis (HCAHPS).
• Educate patient about signs of a significant reaction (eg, wheezing; chest tightness; fever; itching; bad cough; blue skin color; seizures; or swelling of face, lips, tongue, or throat). **Note:** This is not a comprehensive list of all side effects. Patient should consult prescriber for additional questions.

Intended Use and Disclaimer: Should not be printed and given to patients. This information is intended to serve as a concise initial reference for healthcare professionals to use when discussing medications with a patient. You must ultimately rely on your own discretion, experience and judgment in diagnosing, treating and advising patients.
Dietary Considerations Some products may contain phenylalanine and/or sodium.
Oral suspension: May be taken with food.
Related Information
Oral Medications That Should Not Be Crushed or Altered *on page 1712*

Celecoxib (se le KOKS ib)

Brand Names: U.S. CeleBREX
Pharmacologic Category Nonsteroidal Anti-inflammatory Drug (NSAID), COX-2 Selective
Medication Safety Issues
Sound-alike/look-alike issues:
CeleBREX may be confused with CeleXA, Cerebyx, Cervarix, Clarinex
Medication Guide Available Yes
Pregnancy Risk Factor C (prior to 30 weeks gestation)/D (≥30 weeks gestation)
Lactation Enters breast milk/use caution
Breast-Feeding Considerations Small amounts of celecoxib are found in breast milk. The manufacturer recommends that caution be exercised when administering celecoxib to nursing women.
Use Relief of the signs and symptoms of osteoarthritis, ankylosing spondylitis, juvenile idiopathic arthritis (JIA), and rheumatoid arthritis; management of acute pain; treatment of primary dysmenorrhea
Mechanism of Action/Effect Inhibits prostaglandin synthesis by decreasing the activity of the enzyme, cyclooxygenase-2 (COX-2), which results in decreased formation of prostaglandin precursors; has antipyretic, analgesic, and anti-inflammatory properties. Celecoxib does not inhibit

cyclooxygenase-1 (COX-1) at therapeutic concentrations.

Contraindications Hypersensitivity to celecoxib, sulfonamides, aspirin, other NSAIDs, or any component of the formulation; perioperative pain in the setting of coronary artery bypass graft (CABG) surgery

Canadian labeling: Additional contraindications (not in U.S. labeling): Pregnancy (third trimester); women who are breast-feeding; severe, uncontrolled heart failure; active gastrointestinal ulcer (gastric, duodenal, peptic) or bleeding; inflammatory bowel disease; cerebrovascular bleeding; severe liver impairment or active hepatic disease; severe renal impairment (CrCl <30 mL/minute) or deteriorating renal disease; known hyperkalemia; use in children

Warnings/Precautions [U.S. Boxed Warning]: NSAIDs are associated with an increased risk of serious (and potentially fatal) adverse cardiovascular thrombotic events, including MI and stroke. Risk may be increased with duration of use or pre-existing cardiovascular risk factors or disease. Carefully evaluate individual cardiovascular risk profiles prior to prescribing. New-onset or exacerbation of hypertension may occur (NSAIDS may impair response to thiazide or loop diuretics); may contribute to cardiovascular events; monitor blood pressure; use with caution in patients with hypertension. May cause sodium and fluid retention; use with caution in patients with edema, cerebrovascular disease, or ischemic heart disease. Avoid use in patients with heart failure (ACCF/AHA [Yancy, 2013]). Long-term cardiovascular risk in children has not been evaluated.

[U.S. Boxed Warning]: Celecoxib is contraindicated for treatment of perioperative pain in the setting of coronary artery bypass graft (CABG) surgery. Risk of MI and stroke may be increased with use following CABG surgery.

[U.S. Boxed Warning]: NSAIDs may increase risk of serious gastrointestinal ulceration, bleeding, and perforation (may be fatal). These events may occur at any time during therapy and without warning. Use caution with a history of GI disease (bleeding or ulcers), concurrent therapy with aspirin, anticoagulants and/or corticosteroids, smoking, use of alcohol, the elderly or debilitated patients. When used concomitantly with aspirin, a substantial increase in the risk of gastrointestinal complications (eg, ulcer) occurs; concomitant gastroprotective therapy (eg, proton pump inhibitors) is recommended (Bhatt, 2008).

Use the lowest effective dose for the shortest duration of time, consistent with individual patient goals, to reduce risk of cardiovascular or GI adverse events. Alternate therapies should be considered for patients at high risk.

NSAIDs may cause serious skin adverse events including exfoliative dermatitis, Stevens-Johnson syndrome (SJS), and toxic epidermal necrolysis (TEN); may occur without warning and in patients without prior known sulfa allergy. Anaphylactoid reactions may occur, even without prior exposure; patients with "aspirin triad" (bronchial asthma, aspirin intolerance, rhinitis) may be at increased risk. Do not use in patients who experience bronchospasm, asthma, rhinitis, or urticaria with NSAID or aspirin therapy. Use with caution in other forms of asthma.

Use with caution in patients with decreased hepatic (dosage adjustments are recommended for moderate hepatic impairment; not recommended for patients with severe hepatic impairment) or renal function. Transaminase elevations have been reported with use; closely monitor patients with any abnormal LFT. Severe hepatic reactions (eg, fulminant hepatitis, liver failure) have occurred with NSAID use, rarely; discontinue if signs or symptoms of liver disease develop, if systemic manifestations occur, or with persistent or worsening abnormal hepatic function tests. NSAID use may compromise existing renal function; dose-dependent decreases in prostaglandin synthesis may result from NSAID use, causing a reduction in renal blood flow which may cause renal decompensation (usually reversible). Patients with impaired renal function, dehydration, heart failure, liver dysfunction, those taking diuretics, ACE inhibitors, angiotensin II receptor blockers, and the elderly are at greater risk for renal toxicity. Rehydrate patient before starting therapy; monitor renal function closely. Not recommended for use in patients with advanced renal disease or severe renal insufficiency; discontinue use with persistent or worsening abnormal renal function tests. Long-term NSAID use may result in renal papillary necrosis. Should not be considered a treatment or replacement of corticosteroid-dependent diseases.

Anaphylactoid reactions may occur, even with no prior exposure to celecoxib. Use with caution in patients with known or suspected deficiency of cytochrome P450 isoenzyme 2C9; poor metabolizers may have higher plasma levels due to reduced metabolism; consider reduced initial doses. Alternate therapies should be considered in patients with JIA who are poor metabolizers of CYP2C9.

Anemia may occur with use; monitor hemoglobin or hematocrit in patients on long-term treatment. Celecoxib does not affect PT, PTT or platelet counts; does not inhibit platelet aggregation at approved doses.

When used for juvenile idiopathic arthritis (JIA), celecoxib is not FDA-approved in children <2 years of age or in children <10 kg. Use caution with systemic onset JIA (may be at risk for ▶

disseminated intravascular coagulation). Safety and efficacy have not been established for use in children for indications other than JIA.

Drug Interactions

Avoid Concomitant Use

Avoid concomitant use of Celecoxib with any of the following: Floctafenine; Ketorolac (Nasal); Ketorolac (Systemic); Nonsteroidal Anti-Inflammatory Agents; NSAID (COX-2 Inhibitor); Omacetaxine; Thioridazine

Decreased Effect

Celecoxib may decrease the levels/effects of: ACE Inhibitors; Agents with Antiplatelet Properties; Aliskiren; Angiotensin II Receptor Blockers; Beta-Blockers; Codeine; Eplerenone; HydrALAZINE; Loop Diuretics; Potassium-Sparing Diuretics; Prostaglandins (Ophthalmic); Selective Serotonin Reuptake Inhibitors; Tamoxifen; Thiazide Diuretics; TraMADol

The levels/effects of Celecoxib may be decreased by: Bile Acid Sequestrants; CYP2C9 Inducers (Strong); Dabrafenib; Peginterferon Alfa-2b

Increased Effect/Toxicity

Celecoxib may increase the levels/effects of: 5-ASA Derivatives; Agents with Antiplatelet Properties; Aliskiren; Aminoglycosides; Anticoagulants; ARIPiprazole; Bisphosphonate Derivatives; CycloSPORINE (Systemic); CYP2C8 Substrates; CYP2D6 Substrates; Deferasirox; Desmopressin; Digoxin; DOXOrubicin (Conventional); Eplerenone; Estrogen Derivatives; Fesoterodine; Haloperidol; Lithium; Methotrexate; Metoprolol; Nebivolol; NSAID (COX-2 Inhibitor); Omacetaxine; Porfimer; Potassium-Sparing Diuretics; PRALAtrexate; Prilocaine; Quinolone Antibiotics; Sodium Nitrite; Tenofovir; Thioridazine; Vancomycin; Vitamin K Antagonists

The levels/effects of Celecoxib may be increased by: ACE Inhibitors; Angiotensin II Receptor Blockers; Antidepressants (Tricyclic, Tertiary Amine); Aspirin; Corticosteroids (Systemic); CycloSPORINE (Systemic); CYP2C9 Inhibitors (Moderate); CYP2C9 Inhibitors (Strong); Floctafenine; Herbs (Anticoagulant/Antiplatelet Properties); Ketorolac (Nasal); Ketorolac (Systemic); Mifepristone; Nitric Oxide; Nonsteroidal Anti-Inflammatory Agents; Probenecid; Propafenone; Selective Serotonin Reuptake Inhibitors; Sodium Phosphates; Treprostinil

Nutritional/Ethanol Interactions

Ethanol: Avoid ethanol (increased GI irritation).

Food: Peak concentrations are delayed and AUC is increased by 10% to 20% when taken with a high-fat meal.

Herb/Nutraceutical: Avoid concomitant use with herbs possessing anticoagulation/antiplatelet properties, including alfalfa, anise, bilberry, bladderwrack, bromelain, cat's claw, celery, chamomile, coleus, cordyceps, dong quai, evening primrose, fenugreek, feverfew, garlic, ginger, ginkgo biloba, ginseng (American, Panax, Siberian), grapeseed, green tea, guggul, horse chestnuts, horseradish, licorice, prickly ash, red clover, reishi, SAMe (S-adenosylmethionine), sweet clover, turmeric, white willow.

Adverse Reactions

≥2%

Cardiovascular: Peripheral edema

Central nervous system: Dizziness, fever, headache, insomnia

Dermatologic: Rash

Gastrointestinal: Abdominal pain, diarrhea, dyspepsia, flatulence, nausea, vomiting

Neuromuscular & skeletal: Arthralgia, back pain

Respiratory: Cough, nasopharyngitis, pharyngitis, rhinitis, sinusitis, upper respiratory tract infection

0.1% to 1.9%:

Cardiovascular: Angina, aortic valve incompetence, chest pain, coronary artery disorder, edema, facial edema, hypertension (aggravated), MI, palpitation, sinus bradycardia, tachycardia, ventricular hypertrophy

Central nervous system: Anxiety, depression, fatigue, hypoesthesia, migraine, nervousness, pain, somnolence, vertigo

Dermatologic: Alopecia, bruising, cellulitis, dermatitis, dry skin, photosensitivity, pruritus, rash (erythematous), rash (maculopapular), urticaria

Endocrine & metabolic: Hot flashes, hypercholesterolemia, hyperglycemia, hypokalemia, ovarian cyst, testosterone decreased

Gastrointestinal: Anorexia, appetite increased, constipation, diverticulitis, dysphagia, eructation, esophagitis, gastritis, gastroenteritis, gastroesophageal reflux, gastrointestinal ulcer, hemorrhoids, hiatal hernia, melena, stomatitis, tenesmus, weight gain, xerostomia

Genitourinary: Cystitis, dysuria, urinary frequency

Hematologic: Anemia, thrombocythemia

Hepatic: Alkaline phosphatase increased, transaminases increased

Neuromuscular & skeletal: Arthrosis, CPK increased, hypertonia, leg cramps, myalgia, paresthesia, synovitis, tendonitis

Ocular: Conjunctival hemorrhage, vitreous floaters

Otic: Deafness, labyrinthitis, tinnitus

Renal: Albuminuria, BUN increased, creatinine increased, hematuria, nonprotein nitrogen increased, renal calculi

Respiratory: Bronchitis, bronchospasm, dyspnea, epistaxis, laryngitis, pneumonia

Miscellaneous: Allergic reactions, allergy aggravated, cyst, diaphoresis, flu-like syndrome

Available Dosage Forms

Capsule, Oral:

CeleBREX: 50 mg, 100 mg, 200 mg, 400 mg

General Dosage Range Dosage adjustment recommended in patients with hepatic impairment

Oral:
Children ≥2 years and ≥10 kg to ≤25 kg: 50 mg twice daily
Children ≥2 years and >25 kg: 100 mg twice daily
Adults: 100-400 mg/day in 1-2 divided doses

Administration

Oral May be administered without regard to meals. Capsules may be swallowed whole or the entire contents emptied onto a teaspoon of cool or room temperature applesauce. The contents of the capsules sprinkled onto applesauce may be stored under refrigeration for up to 6 hours.

Storage/Stability Store at 25°C (77°F); excursions permitted to 15°C to 30°C (59°F to 86°F).

Nursing Actions

Physical Assessment Assess allergy history (aspirin, NSAIDs, salicylates). Monitor blood pressure at the beginning of therapy and periodically during use. Monitor effectiveness of therapy (pain, range of motion, mobility, ADL function, inflammation).

Patient Education

• Discuss specific use of drug and side effects with patient as it relates to treatment. (HCAHPS: During this hospital stay, were you given any medicine that you had not taken before? Before giving you any new medicine, how often did hospital staff tell you what the medicine was for? How often did hospital staff describe possible side effects in a way you could understand?)

• Patient may experience pyrosis, constipation, diarrhea, flatulence, pharyngitis, or rhinitis. Have patient report immediately to prescriber signs of hepatic impairment, dyspnea, excessive weight gain, edema of extremities, angina, tachycardia, strength differences from one side to another, difficulty speaking or thinking, change in balance, blurred vision, severe headache, considerable dizziness, syncope, significant asthenia, hearing impairment, tinnitus, mood changes, depression, arrhythmia, intolerable dyspepsia, severe nausea, considerable back pain, melena, hematemesis, ecchymosis, hemorrhaging, urinary retention, oliguria, chills, pharyngitis, significant myalgia, or intolerable arthralgia (HCAHPS).

• Educate patient about signs of a significant reaction (eg, wheezing; chest tightness; fever; itching; bad cough; blue skin color; seizures; or swelling of face, lips, tongue, or throat). **Note:** This is not a comprehensive list of all side effects. Patient should consult prescriber for additional questions.

Intended Use and Disclaimer: Should not be printed and given to patients. This information is intended to serve as a concise initial reference for healthcare professionals to use when discussing medications with a patient. You must ultimately rely on your own discretion, experience and judgment in diagnosing, treating and advising patients.

Dietary Considerations May be taken without regard to meals.

Cephalexin (sef a LEKS in)

Brand Names: U.S. Keflex
Index Terms Cephalexin Monohydrate
Pharmacologic Category Antibiotic, Cephalosporin (First Generation)
Medication Safety Issues
Sound-alike/look-alike issues:
Cephalexin may be confused with cefaclor, ceFAZolin, ciprofloxacin
Keflex may be confused with Keppra, Valtrex

Pregnancy Risk Factor B
Lactation Enters breast milk/use caution
Breast-Feeding Considerations Small amounts of cephalexin are excreted in breast milk. The manufacturer recommends that caution be exercised when administering cephalexin to nursing women. Maximum milk concentration occurs ~4 hours after a single oral dose and gradually disappears by 8 hours after administration. Nondose-related effects could include modification of bowel flora.

Use Treatment of susceptible bacterial infections including respiratory tract infections, otitis media, skin and skin structure infections, bone infections, and genitourinary tract infections, including acute prostatitis; alternative therapy for acute infective endocarditis prophylaxis

Unlabeled Use Chronic antimicrobial suppression of prosthetic joint infection

Mechanism of Action/Effect Inhibits bacterial cell wall synthesis by binding to one or more of the penicillin-binding proteins (PBPs)

Contraindications Hypersensitivity to cephalexin, any component of the formulation, or other cephalosporins

Warnings/Precautions Modify dosage in patients with severe renal impairment. Use with caution in patients with a history of penicillin allergy, especially IgE-mediated reactions (eg, anaphylaxis, urticaria). Prolonged use may result in fungal or bacterial superinfection, including *C. difficile*-associated diarrhea (CDAD) and pseudomembranous colitis; CDAD has been observed >2 months postantibiotic treatment. May be associated with increased INR, especially in nutritionally-deficient patients, prolonged treatment, hepatic or renal disease.

Drug Interactions
Avoid Concomitant Use
Avoid concomitant use of Cephalexin with any of the following: BCG
Decreased Effect
Cephalexin may decrease the levels/effects of: BCG; Sodium Picosulfate; Typhoid Vaccine

The levels/effects of Cephalexin may be decreased by: Multivitamins/Minerals (with ADEK, Folate, Iron); Multivitamins/Minerals (with AE, No Iron); Zinc Salts

Increased Effect/Toxicity

Cephalexin may increase the levels/effects of: MetFORMIN; Vitamin K Antagonists

The levels/effects of Cephalexin may be increased by: Probenecid

Nutritional/Ethanol Interactions Food: Peak antibiotic serum concentration is lowered and delayed, but total drug absorbed is not affected. Cephalexin serum levels may be decreased if taken with food.

Adverse Reactions Frequency not defined.

Central nervous system: Agitation, confusion, dizziness, fatigue, hallucinations, headache

Dermatologic: Angioedema, erythema multiforme (rare), rash, Stevens-Johnson syndrome (rare), toxic epidermal necrolysis (rare), urticaria

Gastrointestinal: Abdominal pain, diarrhea, dyspepsia, gastritis, nausea (rare), pseudomembranous colitis, vomiting (rare)

Genitourinary: Genital pruritus, genital moniliasis, vaginitis, vaginal discharge

Hematologic: Eosinophilia, hemolytic anemia, neutropenia, thrombocytopenia

Hepatic: ALT increased, AST increased, cholestatic jaundice (rare), transient hepatitis (rare)

Neuromuscular & skeletal: Arthralgia, arthritis, joint disorder

Renal: Interstitial nephritis (rare)

Miscellaneous: Allergic reactions, anaphylaxis

Available Dosage Forms

Capsule, Oral:

Keflex: 250 mg, 500 mg, 750 mg

Generic: 250 mg, 500 mg, 750 mg

Suspension Reconstituted, Oral:

Generic: 125 mg/5 mL (100 mL, 200 mL); 250 mg/5 mL (100 mL, 200 mL)

Tablet, Oral:

Generic: 250 mg, 500 mg

General Dosage Range Dosage adjustment recommended in patients with renal impairment

Oral:

Children >1-15 years: 25-100 mg/kg/day divided every 6-12 hours (maximum: 4 g/day) **or** 50 mg/kg prior to procedure (maximum: 2 g)

Adolescents >15 years: 25-100 mg/kg/day divided every 6-12 hours (maximum: 4 g/day) **or** 50 mg/kg prior to procedure (maximum: 2 g) **or** 500 mg every 12 hours

Adults: 250-1000 mg every 6 hours **or** 500 mg every 12 hours (maximum: 4 g/day) **or** 2 g prior to procedure

Administration

Oral Take without regard to food. If GI distress, take with food. Give around-the-clock to promote less variation in peak and trough serum levels.

Storage/Stability

Capsule: Store at 15°C to 30°C (59°F to 86°F). Powder for oral suspension: Refrigerate suspension after reconstitution; discard after 14 days.

Nursing Actions

Physical Assessment Assess results of culture/sensitivity tests and patient's allergy history prior to therapy. Monitor for nephrotoxicity. Advise patients with diabetes about use of Clinitest® (may cause false-positive test). Teach patient to report opportunistic infection and hypersensitivity reaction.

Patient Education

• Discuss specific use of drug and side effects with patient as it relates to treatment. (HCAHPS: During this hospital stay, were you given any medicine that you had not taken before? Before giving you any new medicine, how often did hospital staff tell you what the medicine was for? How often did hospital staff describe possible side effects in a way you could understand?)

• Patient may experience headache, nausea, diarrhea, dizziness, or arthralgia. Have patient report immediately to prescriber signs of hepatic impairment, ecchymosis, hemorrhaging, significant asthenia, mood changes, illogical thinking, hallucinations, urinary retention, oliguria, vaginitis, or signs of pseudomembranous colitis (HCAHPS).

• Educate patient about signs of a significant reaction (eg, wheezing; chest tightness; fever; itching; bad cough; blue skin color; seizures; or swelling of face, lips, tongue, or throat). **Note:** This is not a comprehensive list of all side effects. Patient should consult prescriber for additional questions.

Intended Use and Disclaimer: Should not be printed and given to patients. This information is intended to serve as a concise initial reference for healthcare professionals to use when discussing medications with a patient. You must ultimately rely on your own discretion, experience and judgment in diagnosing, treating and advising patients.

Dietary Considerations Take without regard to food. If GI distress, take with food.

Certolizumab Pegol (cer to LIZ u mab PEG ol)

Brand Names: U.S. Cimzia; Cimzia Prefilled; Cimzia Starter Kit

Index Terms CDP870

Pharmacologic Category Antirheumatic, Disease Modifying; Gastrointestinal Agent, Miscellaneous; Tumor Necrosis Factor (TNF) Blocking Agent

Medication Guide Available Yes

Pregnancy Risk Factor B

Lactation Excretion in breast milk unknown/not recommended

Breast-Feeding Considerations It is not known if certolizumab pegol is excreted in breast milk. Due to the potential for serious adverse reactions in the nursing infant, the manufacturer recommends a decision be made whether to discontinue nursing or to discontinue the drug, taking into account the importance of treatment to the mother.

Use

U.S. labeling:

Ankylosing spondylitis: Treatment of adults with active ankylosing spondylitis (AS)

Crohn disease: Treatment of moderately to severely active Crohn disease in patients who have inadequate response to conventional therapy

Psoriatic arthritis: Treatment of adult patients with active psoriatic arthritis

Rheumatoid arthritis: Treatment of adults with moderately to severely active rheumatoid arthritis (RA) (as monotherapy or in combination with nonbiological disease-modifying antirheumatic drugs [DMARDS])

Canadian labeling: **Rheumatoid arthritis:** Treatment of adults with moderately to severely active rheumatoid arthritis (in combination with methotrexate or as monotherapy if unable to tolerate methotrexate)

Mechanism of Action/Effect Elevated levels of TNF-alpha have a role in the inflammatory process associated with Crohn's disease and in joint destruction associated with rheumatoid arthritis. Certolizumab pegol binds to and selectively neutralizes human TNF-alpha activity, inhibiting the role of TNF-alpha as a mediator in the inflammatory process.

Contraindications There are no contraindications listed within the manufacturer's U.S. labeling.

Canadian labeling: Hypersensitivity to certolizumab pegol or any component of the formulation; active tuberculosis or other severe infections (eg, sepsis, abscesses, opportunistic infections); moderate to severe heart failure (NYHA Class III/IV)

Warnings/Precautions [U.S. Boxed Warning]: Patients receiving certolizumab are at increased risk for serious infections which may result in hospitalization and/or fatality; infections usually developed in patients receiving concomitant immunosuppressive agents (eg, methotrexate or corticosteroids) and may present as disseminated (rather than local) disease. Active tuberculosis (or reactivation of latent tuberculosis), invasive fungal (including aspergillosis, blastomycosis, candidiasis, coccidioidomycosis, histoplasmosis, and pneumocystosis) and bacterial, viral or other opportunistic infections (including legionellosis and listeriosis) have been reported in patients receiving TNF-blocking agents, including certolizumab. Monitor closely for signs/symptoms of infection. Discontinue for serious infection or sepsis. **Consider risks versus benefits prior to use in patients with a history of chronic or recurrent infection. Consider empiric antifungal therapy in patients who are at risk for invasive fungal infection and develop severe systemic illness.** Caution should be exercised when considering use in the elderly or in patients with conditions that predispose them to infections (eg, diabetes) or residence/travel from areas of endemic mycoses (blastomycosis, coccidioidomycosis, histoplasmosis), or with latent or localized infections. Do not initiate certolizumab therapy with active infection, including clinically important localized infection. Patients who develop a new infection while undergoing treatment should be monitored closely. **[U.S. Boxed Warning]: Lymphoma and other malignancies (some fatal) have been reported in children and adolescent patients receiving other TNF-blocking agents.** Approximately half of the malignancies reported in children were lymphomas (Hodgkin and non-Hodgkin) while other cases varied and included malignancies not typically observed in this population. The onset of malignancy was after a median of 30 months (range: 1-84 months) after the initiation of the TNF-blocking agent. Use of TNF blockers may affect defenses against malignancies; impact on the development and course of malignancies is not fully defined. Chronic immunosuppressant therapy use may be a predisposing factor for malignancy development; rheumatoid arthritis alone has been previously associated with an increased rate of lymphoma. Hepatosplenic T-cell lymphoma (HSTCL), a rare T-cell lymphoma, has also been associated with TNF-blocking agents, primarily reported in adolescent and young adult males with Crohn disease or ulcerative colitis, most of whom had received concurrent treatment with azathioprine and/or 6-mercaptopurine. Perform periodic skin examinations in all patients during therapy, particularly those at increased risk for skin cancer.

Tuberculosis has been reported with certolizumab treatment. **[U.S. Boxed Warnings]: Patients should be evaluated for tuberculosis risk factors and for latent tuberculosis infection (with a tuberculin skin test) prior to therapy. Treatment of latent tuberculosis should be initiated before use. Patients with initial negative tuberculin skin tests should receive continued monitoring for tuberculosis throughout treatment;** active tuberculosis has developed in this population during treatment. Use with caution in patients who have resided in regions where tuberculosis is endemic. Consider antituberculosis treatment (prior to certolizumab treatment) in patients with a history of latent or active tuberculosis if adequate treatment course cannot be confirmed, and for patients with risk factors for tuberculosis despite a negative test. Carefully consider benefits and risks of initiating certolizumab treatment in patients who have been exposed to tuberculosis.

Rare reactivation of hepatitis B virus (HBV) has occurred in chronic carriers of the virus, usually in patients receiving concomitant immunosuppressants; evaluate for HBV prior to initiation in all patients. Patients who test positive for HBV surface antigen should be referred for hepatitis B evaluation/treatment prior to certolizumab initiation. Monitor for clinical and laboratory signs of active infection during and for several months following discontinuation of treatment in HBV carriers; interrupt therapy if reactivation occurs and treat appropriately with antiviral therapy; if resumption of therapy is deemed necessary, exercise caution and monitor patient closely.

Hypersensitivity reactions, including angioedema, dyspnea, hypotension, rash, serum sickness and urticaria have been reported (rarely) with treatment; discontinue and do not resume therapy if hypersensitivity occurs. Some of these reactions have occurred after the first dose. Use with caution in patients who have experienced hypersensitivity with other TNF blockers. Use with caution in heart failure patients; worsening heart failure and new onset heart failure have been reported with TNF blockers, including certolizumab pegol; monitor closely. The Canadian labeling contraindicates use in moderate-to-severe heart failure (NYHA Class III/IV).

Rare cases of pancytopenia and other significant cytopenias, including aplastic anemia and have been reported with TNF-blocking agents. Leukopenia and thrombocytopenia have occurred with certolizumab; use with caution in patients with underlying hematologic disorders; consider discontinuing therapy with significant hematologic abnormalities. Autoantibody formation may develop; rarely resulting in autoimmune disorder, including lupus-like syndrome; monitor and discontinue if symptoms develop. A small number of patients (8%) develop antibodies to certolizumab during therapy. Antibody-positive patients may have an increased incidence of adverse events (including injection site pain/erythema, abdominal pain and erythema nodosum). Use with caution in patients with pre-existing or recent-onset CNS demyelinating disorders; rare cases of optic neuritis, seizure, peripheral neuropathy, and demyelinating disease (eg, multiple sclerosis, Guillain-Barré syndrome; new onset or exacerbation) have been reported.

Potentially significant drug-drug interactions may exist, requiring dose or frequency adjustment, additional monitoring, and/or selection of alternative therapy. Use caution when switching between biological disease modifying antirheumatic drugs (DMARDs); overlapping of biological activity may increase the risk for infection.

Patients should be up to date with all immunizations before initiating therapy; patients may receive vaccines other than live or live attenuated vaccines during therapy. There is no data available concerning the effects of therapy on vaccination or secondary transmission of live vaccines in patients receiving therapy. Use has not been studied in patients with renal impairment; however, the pharmacokinetics of the pegylated (polyethylene glycol) component may be dependent on renal function. Use with caution in the elderly, may be at higher risk for infections.

Drug Interactions

Avoid Concomitant Use

Avoid concomitant use of Certolizumab Pegol with any of the following: Abatacept; Anakinra; Anti-TNF Agents; BCG; Canakinumab; Natalizumab; Pimecrolimus; Rilonacept; RiTUXimab; Tacrolimus (Topical); Tocilizumab; Tofacitinib; Vaccines (Live)

Decreased Effect

Certolizumab Pegol may decrease the levels/effects of: BCG; Coccidioidin Skin Test; Sipuleucel-T; Vaccines (Inactivated); Vaccines (Live)

The levels/effects of Certolizumab Pegol may be decreased by: Echinacea; Pegloticase

Increased Effect/Toxicity

Certolizumab Pegol may increase the levels/effects of: Abatacept; Anakinra; Canakinumab; Leflunomide; Natalizumab; Rilonacept; Tofacitinib; Vaccines (Live)

The levels/effects of Certolizumab Pegol may be increased by: Anti-TNF Agents; Denosumab; Pimecrolimus; RiTUXimab; Roflumilast; Tacrolimus (Topical); Tocilizumab; Trastuzumab

Nutritional/Ethanol Interactions Herb/Nutraceutical: Echinacea may decrease the therapeutic effects of certolizumab. Management: Avoid concurrent use.

Adverse Reactions

>10%:

Gastrointestinal: Nausea (≤11%)

Respiratory: Upper respiratory infection (6% to 20%)

Miscellaneous: Infection (38%; serious: 3%)

1% to 10%:

Cardiovascular: Hypertension (≤5%)

Central nervous system: Headache (5%), fever (3%), fatigue (≤3%)

Dermatologic: Rash (≤9%)

Genitourinary: Urinary tract infection (≤8%)

Neuromuscular & skeletal: Arthralgia (6% to 7%), back pain (≤4%)

Respiratory: Cough (≤6%), nasopharyngitis (5%), bronchitis (≤3%), pharyngitis (≤3%)

Miscellaneous: Antibody formation (7% to 8%), positive ANA (≤4%)

Available Dosage Forms

Kit, Subcutaneous:

Cimzia: 200 mg

Kit, Subcutaneous [preservative free]:

Cimzia Prefilled: 200 mg/mL

Cimzia Starter Kit: 6 X 200 mg/mL

General Dosage Range SubQ: Adults: Initial: 400 mg, repeat dose 2 and 4 weeks after initial dose; Maintenance: 400 mg every 4 weeks **or** 200 mg every other week

Administration

Subcutaneous SubQ: Bring to room temperature prior to administration. After reconstitution (of vials), draw each vial into separate syringes (using 20-gauge needles).

Administer each syringe subcutaneously (using provided 23-gauge needle) to separate sites on abdomen or thigh. Rotate injections sites; do not administer to areas where skin is tender, bruised, red, or hard.

Preparation for Administration Vials: Allow to reach room temperature prior to reconstitution. Using aseptic technique, reconstitute each vial with 1 mL sterile water for injection (provided) to a concentration of ~200 mg/mL; the manufacturer recommends using a 20-gauge needle (provided). Gently swirl to facilitate wetting of powder; do not shake. Allow vials to set undisturbed (may take up to 30 minutes) until fully reconstituted. Reconstituted solutions should not contain visible particles or gels in the solution.

Storage/Stability

Store intact vials and syringes at 2°C to 8°C (36°F to 46°F); do not freeze. Do not separate contents of carton prior to use. Protect from light. Bring to room temperature prior to administration.

Reconstituted vials may be retained at room temperature for up to 2 hours or refrigerated (do not freeze) for up to 24 hours prior to administration. Discard unused portion of vial or syringe.

Nursing Actions

Physical Assessment Perform tuberculin skin test prior to initiating therapy. Monitor for signs of tuberculosis and other infections throughout therapy. Do not initiate therapy if active infection is present. Monitor for signs/symptoms of malignancy (eg, splenomegaly, hepatomegaly, abdominal pain, persistent fever, night sweats, weight loss). Assess results of PPD at regular intervals during treatment. Teach patient proper injection technique and syringe/needle disposal.

Patient Education

• Discuss specific use of drug and side effects with patient as it relates to treatment. (HCAHPS: During this hospital stay, were you given any medicine that you had not taken before? Before giving you any new medicine, how often did hospital staff tell you what the medicine was for? How often did hospital staff describe possible side effects in a way you could understand?)

• Patient may experience injection site pain or irritation. Have patient report immediately to prescriber signs of infection; signs of hepatic impairment; signs of depression (ie, suicidal ideation, anxiety, emotional instability, illogical thinking); angina; severe dizziness; syncope; significant headache; intolerable dyspepsia; vision changes; ecchymosis; hemorrhaging; arthralgia; excessive weight gain or loss; night sweats; skin irritation; paresthesia; dyspnea; edema of extremities; strength differences from one side to another; difficulty speaking or thinking; change in balance; blurred vision; myalgia; considerable asthenia; swollen lymph nodes; hyperhidrosis; or pallor (HCAHPS).

• Educate patient about signs of a significant reaction (eg, wheezing; chest tightness; fever; itching; bad cough; blue skin color; seizures; or swelling of face, lips, tongue, or throat). **Note:** This is not a comprehensive list of all side effects. Patient should consult prescriber for additional questions.

Intended Use and Disclaimer: Should not be printed and given to patients. This information is intended to serve as a concise initial reference for healthcare professionals to use when discussing medications with a patient. You must ultimately rely on your own discretion, experience and judgment in diagnosing, treating and advising patients.

Cetirizine (se TI ra zeen)

Brand Names: U.S. All Day Allergy Childrens [OTC]; All Day Allergy [OTC]; Cetirizine HCl Allergy Child [OTC]; Cetirizine HCl Childrens Alrgy [OTC]; Cetirizine HCl Childrens [OTC]; Cetirizine HCl Hives Relief [OTC]; ZyrTEC Allergy [OTC]; ZyrTEC Childrens Allergy [OTC]; ZyrTEC Childrens Hives Relief [OTC]; ZyrTEC Hives Relief [OTC]

Index Terms Cetirizine Hydrochloride; P-071; UCB-P071

Pharmacologic Category Histamine H_1 Antagonist; Histamine H_1 Antagonist, Second Generation; Piperazine Derivative

Medication Safety Issues

Sound-alike/look-alike issues:

Cetirizine may be confusd with sertraline

ZyrTEC may be confused with Lipitor, Serax, Xanax, Zantac, Zerit, Zocor, ZyPREXA, Zyr-TEC-D

ZyrTEC (cetirizine) may be confused with ZyrTEC Itchy Eye (ketotifen)

International issues:

Benadryl international brand name for cetirizine [Great Britain, Phillipines], but also the brand name for acrivastine and pseudoephedrine [Great Britain] and several products containing diphenhydramine [U.S., Canada]

Breast-Feeding Considerations Cetirizine is excreted into breast milk.

Use Perennial and seasonal allergic rhinitis and other allergic symptoms including urticaria; chronic idiopathic urticaria

Mechanism of Action/Effect Competes with histamine for H_1-receptor sites on effector cells in the GI tract, blood vessels, and respiratory tract

Contraindications Hypersensitivity to cetirizine, hydroxyzine, or any component of the formulation

Warnings/Precautions Cetirizine should be used cautiously in patients with hepatic or renal dysfunction; dosage adjustment recommended. Use with caution in the elderly; may be more sensitive to adverse effects. May cause drowsiness; use caution performing tasks which require alertness (eg, operating machinery or driving). Effects may be potentiated when used with other sedative drugs or ethanol.

Drug Interactions

Avoid Concomitant Use

Avoid concomitant use of Cetirizine with any of the following: Aclidinium; Azelastine (Nasal); Ipratropium (Oral Inhalation); Paraldehyde; Thalidomide; Tiotropium; Umeclidinium

Decreased Effect

Cetirizine may decrease the levels/effects of: Acetylcholinesterase Inhibitors (Central); Benzylpenicilloyl Polylysine; Betahistine; Hyaluronidase

The levels/effects of Cetirizine may be decreased by: Acetylcholinesterase Inhibitors (Central); Amphetamines; P-glycoprotein/ABCB1 Inducers

Increased Effect/Toxicity

Cetirizine may increase the levels/effects of: Alcohol (Ethyl); Analgesics (Opioid); Anticholinergics; Azelastine (Nasal); Buprenorphine; CNS Depressants; Hydrocodone; Methotrimeprazine; Metyrosine; Mirtazapine; Paraldehyde; Pramipexole; ROPINIRole; Rotigotine; Selective Serotonin Reuptake Inhibitors; Thalidomide; Tiotropium; Zolpidem

The levels/effects of Cetirizine may be increased by: Aclidinium; Brimonidine (Topical); Doxylamine; Droperidol; HydrOXYzine; Ipratropium (Oral Inhalation); Magnesium Sulfate; Methotrimeprazine; Perampanel; P-glycoprotein/ABCB1 Inhibitors; Pramlintide; Sodium Oxybate; Tapentadol; Umeclidinium

Nutritional/Ethanol Interactions Ethanol: May increase CNS depression; monitor for increased effects with coadministration. Caution patients about effects.

Adverse Reactions

>10%: Central nervous system: Headache (children 11% to 14%, placebo 12%), somnolence (adults 14%, children 2% to 4%)

2% to 10%:

Central nervous system: Insomnia (children 9%, adults <2%), fatigue (adults 6%), malaise (4%), dizziness (adults 2%)

Gastrointestinal: Abdominal pain (children 4% to 6%), dry mouth (adults 5%), diarrhea (children 2% to 3%), nausea (children 2% to 3%, placebo 2%), vomiting (children 2% to 3%)

Respiratory: Epistaxis (children 2% to 4%, placebo 3%), pharyngitis (children 3% to 6%, placebo 3%), bronchospasm (children 2% to 3%, placebo 2%)

Pharmacodynamics/Kinetics

Onset of Action Suppression of skin wheal and flare: 0.7 hours (Simons, 1999)

Duration of Action Suppression of skin wheal and flare: ≥24 hours (Simons, 1999)

Available Dosage Forms

Capsule, Oral:

ZyrTEC Allergy [OTC]: 10 mg

Solution, Oral:

All Day Allergy Childrens [OTC]: 1 mg/mL (118 mL); 5 mg/5 mL (118 mL)

Cetirizine HCl Allergy Child [OTC]: 5 mg/5 mL (120 mL)

Cetirizine HCl Childrens [OTC]: 1 mg/mL (118 mL)

Cetirizine HCl Hives Relief [OTC]: 5 mg/5 mL (120 mL)

Syrup, Oral:

Cetirizine HCl Childrens Alrgy [OTC]: 1 mg/mL (118 mL, 120 mL)

ZyrTEC Childrens Allergy [OTC]: 1 mg/mL (118 mL); 5 mg/5 mL (5 mL, 118 mL)

ZyrTEC Childrens Hives Relief [OTC]: 1 mg/mL (118 mL)

Generic: 1 mg/mL (120 mL, 480 mL); 5 mg/5 mL (5 mL, 120 mL)

Tablet, Oral:

All Day Allergy [OTC]: 10 mg

ZyrTEC Allergy [OTC]: 10 mg

ZyrTEC Hives Relief [OTC]: 10 mg

Generic: 5 mg, 10 mg

Tablet Chewable, Oral:

All Day Allergy Childrens [OTC]: 5 mg, 10 mg

ZyrTEC Childrens Allergy [OTC]: 5 mg, 10 mg

Generic: 5 mg, 10 mg

General Dosage Range Dosage adjustment recommended in patients with hepatic or renal impairment

Oral:

Children 6-12 months: 2.5 mg once daily

Children 12 months to <2 years: 2.5 mg once or twice daily

Children 2-5 years: 2.5-5 mg/day in 1-2 divided doses

Children ≥6 years and Adults: 5-10 mg once daily

Elderly: Initial: 5 mg once daily

Administration

Oral May be administered with or without food.

Storage/Stability Store at room temperature.

Syrup: Store at room temperature of 15°C to 30°C (59°F to 86°F), or under refrigeration at 2°C to 8°C (36°F to 46°F).

Nursing Actions

Patient Education

• Discuss specific use of drug and side effects with patient as it relates to treatment. (HCAHPS: During this hospital stay, were you given any medicine that you had not taken before? Before giving you any new medicine, how often did hospital staff tell you what the medicine was

for? How often did hospital staff describe possible side effects in a way you could understand?)
- Patient may experience increased susceptibility to erythema, fatigue, dyspepsia, xerostomia, or insomnia. Have patient report immediately to prescriber severe dizziness, syncope, significant asthenia, tachycardia, arrhythmia, mood changes, ecchymosis, hemorrhaging, or signs of hepatic impairment (HCAHPS).
- Educate patient about signs of a significant reaction (eg, wheezing; chest tightness; fever; itching; bad cough; blue skin color; seizures; or swelling of face, lips, tongue, or throat). **Note:** This is not a comprehensive list of all side effects. Patient should consult prescriber for additional questions.

Intended Use and Disclaimer: Should not be printed and given to patients. This information is intended to serve as a concise initial reference for healthcare professionals to use when discussing medications with a patient. You must ultimately rely on your own discretion, experience and judgment in diagnosing, treating and advising patients.

Dietary Considerations May be taken with or without food.

Cetuximab (se TUK see mab)

Brand Names: U.S. Erbitux
Index Terms C225; IMC-C225; MOAB C225
Pharmacologic Category Antineoplastic Agent, Epidermal Growth Factor Receptor (EGFR) Inhibitor; Antineoplastic Agent, Monoclonal Antibody
Medication Safety Issues
Sound-alike/look-alike issues:
Cetuximab may be confused with bevacizumab
Pregnancy Risk Factor C
Lactation Excretion in breast milk is unknown/not recommended
Breast-Feeding Considerations It is not known if cetuximab is excreted in breast milk. Due to the potential for serious adverse reactions in the nursing infant, the decision to discontinue cetuximab or discontinue breast-feeding should take into account the benefits of treatment to the mother. If breast-feeding is interrupted for cetuximab treatment, based on the half-life, breast-feeding should not be resumed for at least 60 days following the last cetuximab dose.
Use Treatment of *KRAS* mutation-negative (wild-type), EGFR-expressing metastatic colorectal cancer (in combination with FOLFIRI [irinotecan, fluorouracil, and leucovorin] as first-line treatment, in combination with irinotecan [in patients refractory to irinotecan-based chemotherapy], or as a single agent in patients who have failed oxaliplatin and irinotecan based chemotherapy or who are intolerant to irinotecan); treatment of squamous cell cancer of the head and neck (as a single agent

for recurrent or metastatic disease after platinum-based chemotherapy failure; in combination with radiation therapy as initial treatment of locally or regionally advanced disease; in combination with platinum and fluorouracil-based chemotherapy as first-line treatment of locoregional or metastatic disease)

Note: Cetuximab is not indicated for the treatment of *KRAS* mutation-positive colorectal cancer.
Unlabeled Use Treatment of EGFR-expressing advanced nonsmall cell lung cancer (NSCLC); treatment of unresectable squamous cell skin cancer; treatment of neurological symptoms of chordoma
Mechanism of Action/Effect EGFR inhibitor; inhibits cell growth, induces apoptosis and decreases matrix metalloproteinase and vascular endothelial growth factor production.
Contraindications There are no contraindications listed in the manufacturer's U.S. product labeling.
Canadian labeling: Severe hypersensitivity to cetuximab or any component of the formulation
Warnings/Precautions [U.S. Boxed Warning]: In clinical trials, serious infusion reactions have been reported in ~3% of patients; fatal outcome has been reported rarely (<1 in 1000); interrupt infusion promptly and permanently discontinue for serious infusion reactions. Reactions have included airway obstruction (bronchospasm, stridor, hoarseness), hypotension, loss of consciousness, shock, MI, and/or cardiac arrest. Premedicate with an I.V. H_1 antagonist 30-60 minutes prior to the first dose; premedication for subsequent doses is based on clinical judgement and with consideration of prior reaction to the initial infusion. The use of nebulized albuterol-based premedication to prevent infusion reaction has been reported (Tra, 2008). Approximately 90% of reactions occur with the first infusion despite the use of prophylactic antihistamines. Immediate treatment for anaphylactic/anaphylactoid reactions should be available during administration. The manufacturer recommends monitoring patients for at least 1 hour following completion of infusion, or longer if a reaction occurs. Mild-to-moderate infusion reactions are managed by slowing the infusion rate (by 50%) and administering antihistamines. Patients with pre-existing IgE antibody against cetuximab (specific for galactose-α-1,3-galactose) are reported to have a higher incidence of severe hypersensitivity reaction. Severe hypersensitivity reaction has been reported more frequently in patients living in the middle south area of the United States, including North Carolina and Tennessee (Chung, 2008; O'Neil, 2007).

[U.S. Boxed Warning]: In patients with squamous cell head and neck cancer, cardiopulmonary arrest and/or sudden death has occurred in 2% of patients receiving radiation therapy in combination with cetuximab and in 3% of

patients receiving combination chemotherapy (platinum and fluorouracil-based) with cetuximab. Closely monitor serum electrolytes (magnesium, potassium, calcium) during and after cetuximab treatment (monitor for at least 8 weeks after treatment). Use with caution in patients with history of coronary artery disease, HF, and arrhythmias; fatalities have been reported. Interstitial lung disease (ILD) has been reported; use with caution in patients with pre-existing lung disease; interrupt treatment for acute onset or worsening of pulmonary symptoms; permanently discontinue with confirmed ILD.

Acneiform rash has been reported in 76% to 88% of patients (severe in 1% to 17%), usually developing within the first 2 weeks of therapy; may require dose modification; generally resolved after discontinuation in most patients, although persisted beyond 28 days in some patients; monitor for dermatologic toxicity and corresponding infections. Acneiform rash should be treated with topical and/or oral antibiotics; topical corticosteroids are not recommended. In colorectal cancer, the presence of acneiform rash correlates with treatment response and prolonged survival (Cunningham, 2004). Other dermatologic toxicities, including dry skin, fissures, hypertrichosis, paronychial inflammation, and skin infections have been reported; related ocular toxicities (blepharitis, conjunctivitis, keratitis, ulcerative keratitis with decreased visual acuity) may also occur. Sunlight may exacerbate skin reactions (limit sun exposure). Hypomagnesemia is common (may be severe); the onset of electrolyte disturbance may occur within days to months after initiation of treatment; monitor magnesium, calcium, and potassium during treatment and for at least 8 weeks after completion; may require electrolyte replacement. Non-neutralizing anti-cetuximab antibodies were detected in 5% of evaluable patients. In a study of radiation therapy and cisplatin with or without cetuximab in patients with squamous cell head and neck cancer, an increase in the incidence of adverse reactions (eg, grade 3/4 mucositis, radiation recall, acneiform rash, and cardiac events including ischemia) was noted in patients receiving cetuximab, including fatal reactions; there was no improvement in the primary endpoint of progression-free survival.

In patients with colorectal cancer, cetuximab is only indicated for EGFR-expressing, KRAS mutation-negative metastatic colorectal cancer. Determine KRAS mutation status prior to treatment (the therascreen KRAS RGQ PCR Kit is approved in the U.S. to determine KRAS gene mutation information). Patients with a codon 12 or 13 (exon 2) KRAS mutation are unlikely to benefit from EGFR inhibitor therapy and should not receive cetuximab treatment; cetuximab is not effective for KRAS mutation-positive colorectal cancer. Cetuximab is also reported to be ineffective in patients with

BRAF V600E mutation (Di Nicolantonio, 2008). In trials for colorectal cancer, evidence of EGFR expression was required, although the response rate did not correlate with either the percentage of cells positive for EGFR or the intensity of expression. EGFR expression has been detected in nearly all patients with head and neck cancer, therefore laboratory evidence of EGFR expression is not necessary for head and neck cancers.

Drug Interactions

Avoid Concomitant Use There are no known interactions where it is recommended to avoid concomitant use.

Decreased Effect There are no known significant interactions involving a decrease in effect.

Increased Effect/Toxicity There are no known significant interactions involving an increase in effect.

Adverse Reactions Except where noted, percentages reported for studies with cetuximab monotherapy.

>10%:

Central nervous system: Fatigue (91%), pain (59%), sensory neuropathy (45%; grades 3/4: 1%), headache (38%), insomnia (27%), fever (25%), confusion (18%), anxiety (14%), chills/rigors (16%), depression (14%)

Dermatologic: Rash/desquamation (95%; grades 3/4: 16%), acneiform rash (all studies: 76% to 88%; grades 3/4: 1% to 17%; onset: ≤14 days), dry skin (57%), pruritus (47%), nail changes (31%)

Endocrine & metabolic: Hypomagnesemia (all studies: 55%; grades 3/4: 6% to 17%), dehydration (13%)

Gastrointestinal: Nausea (64%), abdominal pain (59%), constipation (53%), diarrhea (42%), vomiting (37% to 40%), stomatitis (32%), xerostomia (12%)

Neuromuscular & skeletal: Bone pain (15%), arthralgia (14%)

Respiratory: Dyspnea (48% to 49%), cough (30%)

Miscellaneous: Infection (all studies: 13% to 44%; grades 3/4: 11%), infusion reaction (all studies: 15% to 21%; grades 3/4: 2% to 5%; 90% of severe reactions occurred with first infusion)

1% to 10%:

Cardiovascular: Cardiopulmonary arrest (2%; with radiation therapy; 3% with platinum/fluorouracil-based chemotherapy)

Gastrointestinal: Taste disturbance (10%)

Renal: Renal failure (all studies: 1%)

Miscellaneous: Antibody formation (5%), sepsis (all studies: 1% to 4%)

Available Dosage Forms

Solution, Intravenous [preservative free]:

Erbitux: 100 mg/50 mL (50 mL); 200 mg/100 mL (100 mL)

General Dosage Range Dosage adjustment recommended in patients who develop toxicities

I.V.: *Adults:* Loading dose: 400 mg/m^2; Maintenance: 250 mg/m^2 weekly

Administration

I.V. I.V. infusion; loading dose over 2 hours, weekly maintenance dose over 1 hour. Do not administer as I.V. push or bolus. Do not shake or dilute. Administer via infusion pump or syringe pump. Following the infusion, an observation period (1 hour) is recommended; longer observation time (following an infusion reaction) may be required. Premedication with an H$_1$ antagonist prior to the initial dose is recommended. The maximum infusion rate is 10 mg/minute. Administer through a low protein-binding 0.22 micrometer in-line filter. Use 0.9% NaCl to flush line at the end of infusion.

For biweekly administration (unlabeled frequency and dose), the initial dose was infused over 120 minutes and subsequent doses infused over 60 minutes (Pfeiffer, 2007; Pfeiffer, 2008).

Injectable Detail pH: 7-7.4 (2 mg/mL solution in vial)

Preparation for Administration Reconstitution is not required. Appropriate dose should be added to empty sterile container (may contain a small amount of visible white, amorphous cetuximab particles); do not shake or dilute. Discard unused portion of the vial.

Storage/Stability Store intact vials refrigerated at 2°C to 8°C (36°F to 46°F); do not freeze. Preparations in infusion containers are stable for up to 12 hours refrigerated at 2°C to 8°C (36°F to 46°F) and up to 8 hours at room temperature of 20°C to 25°C (68°F to 77°F).

Nursing Actions

Physical Assessment Premedication with antihistamines may be prescribed. Monitor patient closely for airway obstruction, hives, and hypotension during and for at least 1 hour following infusion. Treatment for anaphylactic reactions should be available. In case of severe infusion reaction, stop infusion and notify prescriber. Instruct patient to report skin reactions, cough, dyspnea, gastrointestinal upset, and opportunistic infection. Monitor for skin reactions and signs of dermatologic toxicities. Monitor electrolytes up to 8 weeks after treatments.

Patient Education

- Discuss specific use of drug and side effects with patient as it relates to treatment. (HCAHPS: During this hospital stay, were you given any medicine that you had not taken before? Before giving you any new medicine, how often did hospital staff tell you what the medicine was for? How often did hospital staff describe possible side effects in a way you could understand?)
- Patient may experience flu-like syndrome, asthenia, dyspepsia, pyrosis, constipation, stomatitis, insomnia, xerostomia, xeroderma, skin or nail changes, osteodynia, or arthralgia. Have patient report immediately to prescriber signs of

infection, signs of depression (ie, suicidal ideation, anxiety, emotional instability, illogical thinking), signs of hypomagnesemia, urinary retention, oliguria, hemoptysis, dyspnea, eye irritation, angina, tachycardia, severe dizziness, syncope, intolerable headache, considerable nausea, significant diarrhea, severe skin irritation, hyperhidrosis, dehydration, paresthesia, or injection site irritation (HCAHPS).

- Educate patient about signs of a significant reaction (eg, wheezing; chest tightness; fever; itching; bad cough; blue skin color; seizures; or swelling of face, lips, tongue, or throat). **Note:** This is not a comprehensive list of all side effects. Patient should consult prescriber for additional questions.

Intended Use and Disclaimer: Should not be printed and given to patients. This information is intended to serve as a concise initial reference for healthcare professionals to use when discussing medications with a patient. You must ultimately rely on your own discretion, experience and judgment in diagnosing, treating and advising patients.

Cevimeline (se vi ME leen)

Brand Names: U.S. Evoxac
Index Terms Cevimeline Hydrochloride
Pharmacologic Category Cholinergic Agonist
Medication Safety Issues
  Sound-alike/look-alike issues:
    Cevimeline may be confused with Savella®
    Evoxac® may be confused with Eurax®
Pregnancy Risk Factor C
Lactation Excretion in breast milk unknown/not recommended
Use Treatment of symptoms of dry mouth in patients with Sjögren's syndrome
Available Dosage Forms
  Capsule, Oral:
    Evoxac: 30 mg
    Generic: 30 mg
General Dosage Range Oral: *Adults:* 30 mg 3 times/day
Administration
  Oral Administer with or without food.
Nursing Actions
Patient Education

- Discuss specific use of drug and side effects with patient as it relates to treatment. (HCAHPS: During this hospital stay, were you given any medicine that you had not taken before? Before giving you any new medicine, how often did hospital staff tell you what the medicine was for? How often did hospital staff describe possible side effects in a way you could understand?)
- Patient may experience rhinorrhea, rhinitis, or dyspepsia. Have patient report immediately to prescriber dyspnea, severe nausea,

considerable diarrhea, angina, tachycardia, bradycardia, arrhythmia, illogical thinking, vision changes, significant headache, tremors, dysuria, polyuria, hyperhidrosis, dehydration, lacrimation, edema of extremities, intolerable dizziness, or syncope (HCAHPS).
- Educate patient about signs of a significant reaction (eg, wheezing; chest tightness; fever; itching; bad cough; blue skin color; seizures; or swelling of face, lips, tongue, or throat). **Note:** This is not a comprehensive list of all side effects. Patient should consult prescriber for additional questions.

Intended Use and Disclaimer: Should not be printed and given to patients. This information is intended to serve as a concise initial reference for healthcare professionals to use when discussing medications with a patient. You must ultimately rely on your own discretion, experience and judgment in diagnosing, treating and advising patients.

Chenodiol (kee noe DYE ole)

Brand Names: U.S. Chenodal
Index Terms CDCA; Chenodeoxycholic Acid
Pharmacologic Category Bile Acid
Pregnancy Risk Factor X
Lactation Excretion in breast milk unknown/use caution
Use Oral dissolution of radiolucent cholesterol gallstones in selected patients as an alternative to surgery
Unlabeled Use Cerebrotendinous xanthomatosis (CTX)
Available Dosage Forms
Tablet, Oral:
Chenodal: 250 mg
General Dosage Range Oral: *Adults:* Initial: 250 mg twice daily; Maintenance: 13-16 mg/kg/day in 2 divided doses
Nursing Actions
Patient Education
- Discuss specific use of drug and side effects with patient as it relates to treatment. (HCAHPS: During this hospital stay, were you given any medicine that you had not taken before? Before giving you any new medicine, how often did hospital staff tell you what the medicine was for? How often did hospital staff describe possible side effects in a way you could understand?)
- Patient may experience nausea, dyspepsia, constipation, flatulence, pyrosis, or lack of appetite. Have patient report immediately to prescriber signs of hepatic impairment, significant diarrhea, or pharyngitis (HCAHPS).
- Educate patient about signs of a significant reaction (eg, wheezing; chest tightness; fever; itching; bad cough; blue skin color; seizures; or

swelling of face, lips, tongue, or throat). **Note:** This is not a comprehensive list of all side effects. Patient should consult prescriber for additional questions.

Intended Use and Disclaimer: Should not be printed and given to patients. This information is intended to serve as a concise initial reference for healthcare professionals to use when discussing medications with a patient. You must ultimately rely on your own discretion, experience and judgment in diagnosing, treating and advising patients.

Chloral Hydrate (KLOR al HYE drate)

Index Terms Chloral; Hydrated Chloral; Trichloroacetaldehyde Monohydrate
Pharmacologic Category Hypnotic, Miscellaneous
Medication Safety Issues
High alert medication:
The Institute for Safe Medication Practices (ISMP) includes this medication among its list of drugs which have a heightened risk of causing significant patient harm when used in error.
Lactation Enters breast milk/not recommended
Use
Pain control: Adjunct to opiates and analgesics for postoperative pain control.
Sedation: Short-term sedative and hypnotic (<2 weeks); sedative/hypnotic for diagnostic procedures; sedative prior to EEG evaluations.
Withdrawal: Monotherapy or concomitant with paraldehyde for prevention of alcohol withdrawal symptoms and/or to suppress syndrome once it develops; reduction of anxiety associated with withdrawal of opiates or barbiturates.
General Dosage Range Oral:
Children: Dosage varies greatly depending on indication
Adults: 250 mg 3 times daily **or** 500-1000 mg at bedtime or prior to procedure (maximum: 2000 mg daily)
Elderly: Hypnotic (oral): Initial: 250 mg at bedtime
Administration
Oral May dilute syrup in water or other oral liquid (eg, fruit juice or ginger ale) to minimize gastric irritation. Administer capsules after meals (when used as sedative).
Nursing Actions
Physical Assessment For short-term use. Assess for history of addiction; long-term use can result in dependence, abuse, or tolerance. Monitor for excessive sedation. For inpatient use, institute safety measures (side rails, night light, call bell, assistance with ambulation) to prevent falls.

Patient Education

- Discuss specific use of drug and side effects with patient as it relates to treatment. (HCAHPS: During this hospital stay, were you given any medicine that you had not taken before? Before giving you any new medicine, how often did hospital staff tell you what the medicine was for? How often did hospital staff describe possible side effects in a way you could understand?)
- Patient may experience dizziness, fatigue, nausea, or diarrhea. Have patient report immediately to prescriber urinary retention, oliguria, severe dyspepsia, change in balance, illogical thinking, or memory loss (HCAHPS).
- Educate patient about signs of a significant reaction (eg, wheezing; chest tightness; fever; itching; bad cough; blue skin color; seizures; or swelling of face, lips, tongue, or throat). **Note:** This is not a comprehensive list of all side effects. Patient should consult prescriber for additional questions.

Intended Use and Disclaimer: Should not be printed and given to patients. This information is intended to serve as a concise initial reference for healthcare professionals to use when discussing medications with a patient. You must ultimately rely on your own discretion, experience and judgment in diagnosing, treating and advising patients.

Related Information

Oral Medications That Should Not Be Crushed or Altered on page 1712

Chlorambucil (klor AM byoo sil)

Brand Names: U.S. Leukeran

Index Terms CB-1348; Chlorambucilum; Chloraminophene; Chlorbutinum; WR-139013

Pharmacologic Category Antineoplastic Agent, Alkylating Agent; Antineoplastic Agent, Alkylating Agent (Nitrogen Mustard)

Medication Safety Issues

Sound-alike/look-alike issues:

Chlorambucil may be confused with Chloromycetin®

Leukeran® may be confused with Alkeran®, leucovorin, Leukine®, Myleran®

High alert medication:

This medication is in a class the Institute for Safe Medication Practices (ISMP) includes among its list of drug classes which have a heightened risk of causing significant patient harm when used in error.

Pregnancy Risk Factor D

Lactation Excretion in breast milk unknown/not recommended

Use

Chronic lymphocytic leukemia (CLL): Management of CLL

Lymphomas: Management of Hodgkin lymphoma and non-Hodgkin lymphomas (NHL)

Canadian labeling: Additional uses (not in U.S. labeling): Management of Waldenström's macroglobulinemia

Unlabeled Use Treatment of nephrotic syndrome (steroid sensitive) in children; treatment of Waldenström's macroglobulinemia

Available Dosage Forms

Tablet, Oral:

Leukeran: 2 mg

General Dosage Range Dosage adjustment recommended in patients with hepatic impairment or who develop toxicities

Oral: *Adults:* 0.1-0.2 mg/kg/day for 3-6 weeks **or** 0.4 mg/kg intermittently, biweekly, or monthly (may increase by 0.1 mg/kg/dose)

Administration

Oral May be administered as a single daily dose; preferably on an empty stomach.

Hazardous agent; use appropriate precautions for handling and disposal (NIOSH, 2012).

Nursing Actions

Physical Assessment Monitor for hematologic myelosuppression, hypersensitivity rash, drug fever, seizures, gastrointestinal upset, and hepatotoxicity. Teach sexually-active female patients necessity for contraception.

Patient Education

- Discuss specific use of drug and side effects with patient as it relates to treatment. (HCAHPS: During this hospital stay, were you given any medicine that you had not taken before? Before giving you any new medicine, how often did hospital staff tell you what the medicine was for? How often did hospital staff describe possible side effects in a way you could understand?)
- Patient may experience stomatitis or diarrhea. Have patient report immediately to prescriber signs of infection, signs of hepatic impairment, illogical thinking, ecchymosis, hemorrhaging, mood changes, paresthesia, change in balance, hallucinations, dyspnea, tremors, significant asthenia, amenorrhea, nausea, skin growths, or signs of Stevens-Johnson syndrome/toxic epidermal necrolysis (HCAHPS).
- Educate patient about signs of a significant reaction (eg, wheezing; chest tightness; fever; itching; bad cough; blue skin color; seizures; or swelling of face, lips, tongue, or throat). **Note:** This is not a comprehensive list of all side effects. Patient should consult prescriber for additional questions.

Intended Use and Disclaimer: Should not be printed and given to patients. This information is intended to serve as a concise initial reference for healthcare professionals to use when discussing medications with a patient. You must ultimately rely on your own discretion, experience and

judgment in diagnosing, treating and advising patients.

Related Information

Oral Medications That Should Not Be Crushed or Altered *on page 1712*

ChlordiazePOXIDE (klor dye az e POKS ide)

Index Terms Librium; Methaminodiazepoxide Hydrochloride

Pharmacologic Category Benzodiazepine

Medication Safety Issues

Sound-alike/look-alike issues:

ChlordiazePOXIDE may be confused with chlorproMAZINE

Librium may be confused with Librax

BEERS Criteria medication:

This drug may be potentially inappropriate for use in geriatric patients (Quality of evidence - high; Strength of recommendation - strong).

Pregnancy Risk Factor D

Lactation Enters breast milk/not recommended

Use Management of anxiety disorder or for the short-term relief of symptoms of anxiety; withdrawal symptoms of acute alcoholism; preoperative apprehension and anxiety

Controlled Substance C-IV

Available Dosage Forms

Capsule, Oral:

Generic: 5 mg, 10 mg, 25 mg

General Dosage Range

Oral:

Children ≥6 years and Adolescents: 10-30 mg daily in 2-4 divided doses

Adults: 15-100 mg daily in 3-4 divided doses

Elderly: 10-20 mg daily in 2-4 divided doses

Administration

Oral Administer in divided doses.

Nursing Actions

Physical Assessment Assess for signs of CNS depression (sedation, dizziness, confusion, or ataxia). Assess for history of addiction; long-term use can result in dependence, abuse, or tolerance; periodically evaluate need for continued use. For inpatient use, institute safety measures to prevent falls. Taper dosage slowly when discontinuing.

Patient Education

• Discuss specific use of drug and side effects with patient as it relates to treatment. (HCAHPS: During this hospital stay, were you given any medicine that you had not taken before? Before giving you any new medicine, how often did hospital staff tell you what the medicine was for? How often did hospital staff describe possible side effects in a way you could understand?)

• Patient may experience presyncope, fatigue, blurred vision, dizziness, or headache. Have patient report immediately to prescriber significant change in balance, severe asthenia, signs of depression (ie, suicidal ideation, anxiety, emotional instability, illogical thinking), or jaundice (HCAHPS).

• Educate patient about signs of a significant reaction (eg, wheezing; chest tightness; fever; itching; bad cough; blue skin color; seizures; or swelling of face, lips, tongue, or throat). **Note:** This is not a comprehensive list of all side effects. Patient should consult prescriber for additional questions.

Intended Use and Disclaimer: Should not be printed and given to patients. This information is intended to serve as a concise initial reference for healthcare professionals to use when discussing medications with a patient. You must ultimately rely on your own discretion, experience and judgment in diagnosing, treating and advising patients.

Chloroquine (KLOR oh kwin)

Brand Names: U.S. Aralen

Index Terms Chloroquine Phosphate

Pharmacologic Category Aminoquinoline (Antimalarial)

Medication Safety Issues

International issues:

Aralen [U.S., Mexico] may be confused with Paralen brand name for acetaminophen [Czech Republic]

Lactation Enters breast milk/not recommended

Use

Malaria: Suppressive treatment and acute attacks of malaria due to *Plasmodium vivax, P. malariae, P. ovale*, and susceptible strains of *P. falciparum*.

Extraintestinal amebiasis: Treatment of extraintestinal amebiasis.

Unlabeled Use Rheumatoid arthritis; discoid lupus erythematosus

Available Dosage Forms

Tablet, Oral:

Aralen: 500 mg [equivalent to chloroquine base 300 mg]

Generic: 250 mg [equivalent to chloroquine base 150 mg], 500 mg [equivalent to chloroquine base 300 mg]

General Dosage Range Dosage adjustment recommended in patients with renal impairment

Oral: *Children and Adults:* Dosage varies greatly depending on indication

Nursing Actions

Physical Assessment Assess results of CBC and monitor for retinopathy, hearing loss, or myopathy regularly. Teach patient to report anemia, muscle weakness, or visual or auditory changes.

Patient Education

• Discuss specific use of drug and side effects with patient as it relates to treatment. (HCAHPS: During this hospital stay, were you given any medicine that you had not taken before? Before

giving you any new medicine, how often did hospital staff tell you what the medicine was for? How often did hospital staff describe possible side effects in a way you could understand?)
- Patient may experience dyspepsia or nausea. Have patient report immediately to prescriber dyspnea, sudden vision changes, ophthalmalgia, eye irritation, weight loss, ecchymosis, hemorrhaging, mood changes, hearing impairment, tinnitus, or signs of hepatic impairment (HCAHPS).
- Educate patient about signs of a significant reaction (eg, wheezing; chest tightness; fever; itching; bad cough; blue skin color; seizures; or swelling of face, lips, tongue, or throat). **Note:** This is not a comprehensive list of all side effects. Patient should consult prescriber for additional questions.

Intended Use and Disclaimer: Should not be printed and given to patients. This information is intended to serve as a concise initial reference for healthcare professionals to use when discussing medications with a patient. You must ultimately rely on your own discretion, experience and judgment in diagnosing, treating and advising patients.

ChlorproMAZINE (klor PROE ma zeen)

Index Terms Chlorpromazine Hydrochloride; CPZ; Thorazine
Pharmacologic Category Antimanic Agent; Antipsychotic Agent, Typical, Phenothiazine
Medication Safety Issues
Sound-alike/look-alike issues:
ChlorproMAZINE may be confused with chlordiazePOXIDE, chlorproPAMIDE, clomiPRAMINE, prochlorperazine, promethazine
Thorazine may be confused with thiamine, thioridazine
BEERS Criteria medication:
This drug may be potentially inappropriate for use in geriatric patients (Quality of evidence - moderate; Strength of recommendation - strong).
Lactation Enters breast milk/not recommended
Use Management of psychotic disorders (control of mania, treatment of schizophrenia); control of nausea and vomiting; relief of restlessness and apprehension before surgery; acute intermittent porphyria; adjunct in the treatment of tetanus; intractable hiccups; combativeness and/or explosive hyperexcitable behavior in children 1-12 years of age and in short-term treatment of hyperactive children
Unlabeled Use Behavioral symptoms associated with dementia (elderly); psychosis/agitation related to Alzheimer's dementia
Available Dosage Forms
Solution, Injection:
Generic: 25 mg/mL (1 mL, 2 mL)

Tablet, Oral:
Generic: 10 mg, 25 mg, 50 mg, 100 mg, 200 mg
General Dosage Range
I.M., I.V.:
Children ≥6 months: 0.5-1 mg/kg every 6-8 hours (maximum: <5 years [<22.7 kg]: 40 mg/day; 5-12 years [22.7-45.5 kg]: 75 mg/day)
Adults: Initial: 25 mg; may repeat (25-50 mg) in 1-4 hours; Usual dose: 300-800 mg/day (maximum: 400 mg every 4-6 hours)
Oral:
Children ≥6 months: 0.5-1 mg/ kg every 4-6 hours as needed
Adults: Dosage varies greatly depending on indication
Administration
I.V. Do not administer SubQ (tissue damage and irritation may occur); for direct I.V. injection, administer diluted solution slow I.V. at a rate not to exceed 0.5 mg/minute in children and 1 mg/minute in adults. To reduce the risk of hypotension, patients receiving I.V. chlorpromazine must remain lying down during and for 30 minutes after the injection. **Note:** Avoid skin contact with solution; may cause contact dermatitis.
Nursing Actions
Physical Assessment Review ophthalmic exam results. Monitor mental status, mood, affect, and gait. Monitor for suicide ideation, depression, excess sedation, extrapyramidal symptoms, and CNS changes at beginning of therapy and periodically throughout. I.V./I.M.: Significant hypotension may occur. Initiate at lower doses and taper dosage slowly when discontinuing.
Patient Education
- Discuss specific use of drug and side effects with patient as it relates to treatment. (HCAHPS: During this hospital stay, were you given any medicine that you had not taken before? Before giving you any new medicine, how often did hospital staff tell you what the medicine was for? How often did hospital staff describe possible side effects in a way you could understand?)
- Patient may experience anxiety, constipation, xerostomia, fatigue, rhinitis, mydriasis, and dyspepsia. Have patient report immediately to prescriber signs of infection, signs of hepatic impairment, signs of hypoglycemia or hyperglycemia, difficulty with motor activity, fasciculations, change in balance, dysphagia, difficulty speaking, severe dizziness, syncope, angina, tremors, bradykinesia, rigidity, sialorrhea, mood changes, edema of extremities, vision changes, ecchymosis, hemorrhaging, macromastia, nipple discharge, sexual dysfunction, amenorrhea, urinary retention, considerable asthenia, bradycardia, involuntary eye movements, pallor, significant constipation, insomnia, dyspnea, akathisia, signs of neuroleptic malignant syndrome (NMS), signs of tardive dyskinesia, or priapism (HCAHPS).

• Educate patient about signs of a significant reaction (eg, wheezing; chest tightness; fever; itching; bad cough; blue skin color; seizures; or swelling of face, lips, tongue, or throat). **Note:** This is not a comprehensive list of all side effects. Patient should consult prescriber for additional questions.

Intended Use and Disclaimer: Should not be printed and given to patients. This information is intended to serve as a concise initial reference for healthcare professionals to use when discussing medications with a patient. You must ultimately rely on your own discretion, experience and judgment in diagnosing, treating and advising patients.

Chlorthalidone (klor THAL i done)

Index Terms Hygroton
Pharmacologic Category Antihypertensive; Diuretic, Thiazide
Pregnancy Risk Factor B
Lactation Enters breast milk/not recommended
Use Management of mild-to-moderate hypertension when used alone or in combination with other agents; treatment of edema associated with heart failure, renal dysfunction, hepatic cirrhosis, or corticosteroid and estrogen therapy.
Unlabeled Use Pediatric hypertension
Available Dosage Forms
Tablet, Oral:
Generic: 25 mg, 50 mg, 100 mg
General Dosage Range Oral:
Adults: 25-100 mg/day (maximum: 200 mg/day)
Elderly: Initial: 12.5-25 mg once daily or every other day
Nursing Actions
Physical Assessment Allergy history should be assessed prior to beginning therapy. Monitor blood pressure, fluid status, and electrolyte balance regularly during long-term therapy. Caution patients with diabetes to monitor glucose levels; may reduce effect of oral hypoglycemics.
Patient Education
• Discuss specific use of drug and side effects with patient as it relates to treatment. (HCAHPS: During this hospital stay, were you given any medicine that you had not taken before? Before giving you any new medicine, how often did hospital staff tell you what the medicine was for? How often did hospital staff describe possible side effects in a way you could understand?)
• Patient may experience constipation or headache. Have patient report immediately to prescriber signs of fluid and electrolyte imbalance, signs of pancreatitis, severe dizziness, syncope, sexual dysfunction, akathisia, or jaundice (HCAHPS).
• Educate patient about signs of a significant reaction (eg, wheezing; chest tightness; fever; itching; bad cough; blue skin color; seizures; or swelling of face, lips, tongue, or throat). **Note:** This is not a comprehensive list of all side effects. Patient should consult prescriber for additional questions.

Intended Use and Disclaimer: Should not be printed and given to patients. This information is intended to serve as a concise initial reference for healthcare professionals to use when discussing medications with a patient. You must ultimately rely on your own discretion, experience and judgment in diagnosing, treating and advising patients.

Chlorzoxazone (klor ZOKS a zone)

Brand Names: U.S. Lorzone; Parafon Forte DSC
Pharmacologic Category Skeletal Muscle Relaxant
Medication Safety Issues
BEERS Criteria medication:
This drug may be potentially inappropriate for use in geriatric patients (Quality of evidence - moderate; Strength of recommendation - strong).
Use Symptomatic treatment of muscle spasm and pain associated with acute musculoskeletal conditions
Mechanism of Action/Effect Acts on the spinal cord and areas of the brain involved in causing and maintaining skeletal muscle spasms
Contraindications Hypersensitivity to chlorzoxazone or any component of the formulation
Warnings/Precautions Rare, serious (including fatal) idiosyncratic and unpredictable hepatocellular toxicity has been reported with use. Discontinue immediately if early signs/symptoms of hepatic toxicity arise (eg, fever, rash, anorexia, nausea, vomiting, fatigue, right upper quadrant pain, dark urine or jaundice). Also discontinue if elevated liver enzymes develop. May cause drowsiness, dizziness, or lightheadedness; effects may be potentiated by ethanol or other CNS depressants. Caution patients about performing tasks which require mental alertness (eg, operating machinery or driving) This class of medication is poorly tolerated by the elderly due to anticholinergic effects, sedation, and weakness. Efficacy is questionable at dosages tolerated by elderly patients (Beers Criteria).
Drug Interactions
Avoid Concomitant Use
Avoid concomitant use of Chlorzoxazone with any of the following: Azelastine (Nasal); Paraldehyde; Pimozide; Thalidomide
Decreased Effect
The levels/effects of Chlorzoxazone may be decreased by: Peginterferon Alfa-2b
Increased Effect/Toxicity
Chlorzoxazone may increase the levels/effects of: Alcohol (Ethyl); ARIPiprazole; Azelastine (Nasal); Buprenorphine; CNS Depressants; Dofetilide;

Hydrocodone; Lomitapide; Methotrimeprazine; Metyrosine; Mirtazapine; Paraldehyde; Pimozide; Pramipexole; ROPINIRole; Rotigotine; Selective Serotonin Reuptake Inhibitors; Thalidomide; Zolpidem

The levels/effects of Chlorzoxazone may be increased by: Brimonidine (Topical); Disulfiram; Doxylamine; Droperidol; HydrOXYzine; Isoniazid; Magnesium Sulfate; Methotrimeprazine; Perampanel; Sodium Oxybate; Tapentadol

Nutritional/Ethanol Interactions Ethanol: May increase CNS depression; monitor for increased effects with coadministration. Caution patients about effects.

Adverse Reactions Frequency not defined.
Central nervous system: Dizziness, drowsiness lightheadedness, paradoxical stimulation, malaise
Dermatologic: Rash (rare), petechiae (rare), ecchymoses (rare), angioedema (very rare)
Gastrointestinal: Diarrhea, GI bleeding (rare), nausea, vomiting
Genitourinary: Urine discoloration
Hepatic: Liver dysfunction
Miscellaneous: Anaphylaxis (very rare)

Pharmacodynamics/Kinetics
Onset of Action ~1 hour
Duration of Action Up to 6 hours (Desiraju, 1983)

Available Dosage Forms
Tablet, Oral:
Lorzone: 375 mg, 750 mg
Parafon Forte DSC: 500 mg
Generic: 500 mg

General Dosage Range Oral: *Adults:* 500-750 mg 3-4 times daily

Administration
Oral Administer with or without food.

Nursing Actions
Physical Assessment Monitor for effectiveness and CNS sedation.

Patient Education
• Discuss specific use of drug and side effects with patient as it relates to treatment. (HCAHPS: During this hospital stay, were you given any medicine that you had not taken before? Before giving you any new medicine, how often did hospital staff tell you what the medicine was for? How often did hospital staff describe possible side effects in a way you could understand?)
• Patient may experience fatigue, dizziness, asthenia, anxiety, or urine discoloration. Have patient report immediately to prescriber hematemesis, melena, severe dyspepsia, or signs of hepatic impairment (HCAHPS).
• Educate patient about signs of a significant reaction (eg, wheezing; chest tightness; fever; itching; bad cough; blue skin color; seizures; or swelling of face, lips, tongue, or throat). **Note:** This is not a comprehensive list of all side

effects. Patient should consult prescriber for additional questions.

Intended Use and Disclaimer: Should not be printed and given to patients. This information is intended to serve as a concise initial reference for healthcare professionals to use when discussing medications with a patient. You must ultimately rely on your own discretion, experience and judgment in diagnosing, treating and advising patients.

Cholestyramine Resin
(koe LES teer a meen REZ in)

Brand Names: U.S. Prevalite; Questran; Questran Light
Pharmacologic Category Antilipemic Agent, Bile Acid Sequestrant
Pregnancy Risk Factor C
Lactation Does not enter breast milk/use caution
Use Adjunct in the management of primary hypercholesterolemia; pruritus associated with elevated levels of bile acids; regression of arteriolosclerosis
Unlabeled Use Diarrhea associated with excess fecal bile acids (Westergaard, 2007); may be used to enhance elimination of digoxin when non-life-threatening toxicity occurs (Henderson, 1988)

Available Dosage Forms
Packet, Oral:
Prevalite: 4 g (1 ea, 42 ea, 60 ea)
Questran: 4 g (1 ea, 60 ea)
Generic: 4 g (1 ea, 60 ea)
Powder, Oral:
Prevalite: 4 g/dose (231 g)
Questran: 4 g/dose (378 g)
Questran Light: 4 g/dose (210 g)
Generic: 4 g/dose (210 g, 239.4 g, 378 g)

General Dosage Range Oral: *Adults:* 4-24 g/day in 1-6 divided doses

Administration
Oral Administer prepared suspension orally. Not to be taken in dry form. Suspension should not be sipped or held in mouth for prolonged periods (may cause tooth discoloration or enamel decay). Administration at mealtime is recommended. Twice-daily dosing is recommended, but may be administered in 1-6 doses daily.

Nursing Actions
Physical Assessment Monitor GI effects and nutritional status periodically throughout therapy.

Patient Education
• Discuss specific use of drug and side effects with patient as it relates to treatment. (HCAHPS: During this hospital stay, were you given any medicine that you had not taken before? Before giving you any new medicine, how often did hospital staff tell you what the medicine was for? How often did hospital staff describe possible side effects in a way you could understand?)

• Patient may experience nausea, flatulence, burping, bloating, or lack of appetite. Have patient report immediately to prescriber signs of hemorrhaging, severe dyspepsia, significant constipation, or considerable diarrhea (HCAHPS).

• Educate patient about signs of a significant reaction (eg, wheezing; chest tightness; fever; itching; bad cough; blue skin color; seizures; or swelling of face, lips, tongue, or throat). **Note:** This is not a comprehensive list of all side effects. Patient should consult prescriber for additional questions.

Intended Use and Disclaimer: Should not be printed and given to patients. This information is intended to serve as a concise initial reference for healthcare professionals to use when discussing medications with a patient. You must ultimately rely on your own discretion, experience and judgment in diagnosing, treating and advising patients.

Choline Magnesium Trisalicylate
(KOE leen mag NEE zhum trye sa LIS i late)

Index Terms Tricosal; Trilisate
Pharmacologic Category Salicylate
Pregnancy Risk Factor C/D (3rd trimester)
Lactation Enters breast milk/use caution
Use Management of osteoarthritis, rheumatoid arthritis, and other arthritis; acute painful shoulder
Available Dosage Forms
Liquid, Oral:
Generic: 500 mg/5 mL (240 mL)
Tablet, Oral:
Generic: 1000 mg
General Dosage Range Oral:
Children <37 kg: 50 mg/kg/day in 2 divided doses
Children ≥37 kg: 2250 mg/day in divided doses
Adults: 500 mg to 1.5 g 2-3 times/day **or** 3 g at bedtime
Elderly: 750 mg 3 times/day
Administration
Oral Liquid may be mixed with fruit juice just before drinking. Do not administer with antacids.
Nursing Actions
Physical Assessment Do not use for persons with allergic reaction to salicylates or other NSAIDs. Monitor for effectiveness of pain relief.
Patient Education
• Discuss specific use of drug and side effects with patient as it relates to treatment. (HCAHPS: During this hospital stay, were you given any medicine that you had not taken before? Before giving you any new medicine, how often did hospital staff tell you what the medicine was for? How often did hospital staff describe possible side effects in a way you could understand?)
• Patient may experience pyrosis, nausea, constipation, or diarrhea. Have patient report

immediately to prescriber signs of hepatic impairment, ecchymosis, hemorrhaging, severe dyspepsia, tinnitus, melena, hematemesis, hearing impairment, illogical thinking, or hallucinations (HCAHPS).

• Educate patient about signs of a significant reaction (eg, wheezing; chest tightness; fever; itching; bad cough; blue skin color; seizures; or swelling of face, lips, tongue, or throat). **Note:** This is not a comprehensive list of all side effects. Patient should consult prescriber for additional questions.

Intended Use and Disclaimer: Should not be printed and given to patients. This information is intended to serve as a concise initial reference for healthcare professionals to use when discussing medications with a patient. You must ultimately rely on your own discretion, experience and judgment in diagnosing, treating and advising patients.

Chorionic Gonadotropin (Human)
(kor ee ON ik goe NAD oh troe pin, HYU man)

Brand Names: U.S. Novarel; Pregnyl
Index Terms CG; hCG
Pharmacologic Category Gonadotropin; Ovulation Stimulator
Pregnancy Risk Factor X
Lactation Excretion in breast milk unknown/use caution
Use Induces ovulation and pregnancy in anovulatory, infertile females; treatment of hypogonadotropic hypogonadism, prepubertal cryptorchidism; spermatogenesis induction with follitropin alfa
Available Dosage Forms
Solution Reconstituted, Intramuscular:
Novarel: 10,000 units (1 ea)
Pregnyl: 10,000 units (1 ea)
Generic: 10,000 units (1 ea)
General Dosage Range I.M.:
Children: Dosage varies greatly depending on indication
Adults (females): 5000-10,000 units 1 day following last dose of menotropins
Adults (males): 1000-2000 units 2-3 times/week
Administration
I.M. I.M. administration only

Hazardous agent; use appropriate precautions for handling and disposal (NIOSH, 2012).
Nursing Actions
Physical Assessment If self-administered, teach patient appropriate injection technique and syringe/needle disposal.
Patient Education
• Discuss specific use of drug and side effects with patient as it relates to treatment. (HCAHPS: During this hospital stay, were you given any medicine that you had not taken before? Before giving you any new medicine, how often did

hospital staff tell you what the medicine was for? How often did hospital staff describe possible side effects in a way you could understand?)
- Patient may experience injection site irritation, headache, asthenia, or akathisia. Have patient report immediately to prescriber edema, strength changes from one side to another, difficulty speaking or thinking, change in balance, blurred vision, mastalgia, edema of extremities, angina, depression, signs of puberty, or signs of ovarian hyperstimulation syndrome (OHSS) (HCAHPS).
- Educate patient about signs of a significant reaction (eg, wheezing; chest tightness; fever; itching; bad cough; blue skin color; seizures; or swelling of face, lips, tongue, or throat). **Note:** This is not a comprehensive list of all side effects. Patient should consult prescriber for additional questions.

Intended Use and Disclaimer: Should not be printed and given to patients. This information is intended to serve as a concise initial reference for healthcare professionals to use when discussing medications with a patient. You must ultimately rely on your own discretion, experience and judgment in diagnosing, treating and advising patients.

Chorionic Gonadotropin (Recombinant)
(kor ee ON ik goe NAD oh troe pin ree KOM be nant)

Brand Names: U.S. Ovidrel
Index Terms Choriogonadotropin Alfa; r-hCG
Pharmacologic Category Gonadotropin; Ovulation Stimulator
Pregnancy Risk Factor X
Lactation Excretion in breast milk unknown/use caution
Breast-Feeding Considerations It is not known if chorionic gonadotropin (recombinant) is excreted in breast milk. The manufacturer recommends that caution be exercised when administering chorionic gonadotropin (recombinant) to nursing women.
Use As part of an assisted reproductive technology (ART) program, induces ovulation in infertile females who have been pretreated with follicle stimulating hormones (FSH); induces ovulation and pregnancy in infertile females when the cause of infertility is functional
Mechanism of Action/Effect Luteinizing hormone analogue produced by recombinant DNA techniques; stimulates late follicular maturation and intitates rupture of the ovarian follicle once follicular development has occurred
Contraindications Hypersensitivity to hCG preparations or any component of the formulation; primary ovarian failure; uncontrolled thyroid or adrenal dysfunction; uncontrolled organic intracranial lesion (ie, pituitary tumor); abnormal uterine bleeding, ovarian cyst or enlargement of undetermined origin; sex hormone dependent tumors; pregnancy

Warnings/Precautions Hazardous agent - use appropriate precautions for handling and disposal (NIOSH, 2012). Ovarian enlargement may occur; may be accompanied by abdominal distention or abdominal pain and generally regresses without treatment within 2-3 weeks. If ovaries are abnormally enlarged on the last day of treatment, withhold hCG to reduce the risk of ovarian hyperstimulation syndrome (OHSS). OHSS is characterized by severe ovarian enlargement, abdominal pain/distention, nausea, vomiting, diarrhea, dyspnea, and oliguria, and may be accompanied by ascites, pleural effusion, hypovolemia, electrolyte imbalance, hemoperitoneum, and thromboembolic events. If severe hyperstimulation occurs, stop treatment and hospitalize patient. This syndrome develops rapidly with 24 hours to several days and generally occurs during the 7-10 days immediately following treatment.

Arterial thromboembolic events have been reported in association with and separate from OHSS. These medications should only be used by healthcare providers who are thoroughly familiar with infertility problems and their management. Multiple births may result from the use of these medications; advise patients of the potential risk of multiple births before starting the treatment. Safety and efficacy have not been established in the elderly or in children.

Drug Interactions
Avoid Concomitant Use There are no known interactions where it is recommended to avoid concomitant use.
Decreased Effect There are no known significant interactions involving a decrease in effect.
Increased Effect/Toxicity There are no known significant interactions involving an increase in effect.

Adverse Reactions
2% to 10%:
  Endocrine & metabolic: Ovarian cyst (3%), ovarian hyperstimulation (<2% to 3%)
  Gastrointestinal: Abdominal pain (3% to 4%), nausea (3%), vomiting (3%)
  Local: Injection site: Pain (8%), bruising (3% to 5%), reaction (<2% to 3%), inflammation (<2% to 2%)
  Miscellaneous: Postoperative pain (5%)
<2%:
  Cardiovascular: Cardiac arrhythmia, heart murmur
  Central nervous system: Dizziness, emotional lability, fever, headache, insomnia, malaise
  Dermatologic: Pruritus, rash
  Endocrine & metabolic: Breast pain, hot flashes, hyperglycemia, intermenstrual bleeding, vaginal hemorrhage

Gastrointestinal: Abdominal enlargement, diarrhea, flatulence

Genitourinary: Cervical carcinoma, cervical lesion, dysuria, genital herpes, genital moniliasis, leukorrhea, urinary incontinence, urinary tract infection, vaginal discomfort, vaginal hemorrhage, vaginitis

Hematologic: Leukocytosis

Neuromuscular & skeletal: Back pain, paresthesia

Renal: Albuminuria

Respiratory: Cough, pharyngitis, upper respiratory tract infection

Miscellaneous: Ectopic pregnancy, hiccups

In addition, the following have been reported with menotropin therapy: Adnexal torsion, hemoperitoneum, mild-to-moderate ovarian enlargement, pulmonary and vascular complications. Ovarian neoplasms have also been reported (rare) with multiple drug regimens used for ovarian induction (relationship not established).

Available Dosage Forms

Injectable, Subcutaneous:

Ovidrel: 250 mcg/0.5 mL (0.5 mL)

General Dosage Range SubQ: *Adults (females):* 250 mcg given 1 day following last dose of follicle stimulating agent

Administration

Other For SubQ use only; inject into stomach area.

Hazardous agent; use appropriate precautions for handling and disposal (NIOSH, 2012).

Storage/Stability Prefilled syringe: Prior to dispensing, store at 2°C to 8°C (36°F to 46°F). Patient may store at 25°C (77°F) for up to 30 days. Protect from light.

Nursing Actions

Physical Assessment For use only under the supervision/direction of an infertility prescriber. If self-administered, teach patient proper storage, reconstitution, injection technique, and needle/syringe disposal.

Patient Education

• Discuss specific use of drug and side effects with patient as it relates to treatment. (HCAHPS: During this hospital stay, were you given any medicine that you had not taken before? Before giving you any new medicine, how often did hospital staff tell you what the medicine was for? How often did hospital staff describe possible side effects in a way you could understand?)

• Patient may experience injection site irritation. Have patient report immediately to prescriber strength changes from one side to another, difficulty speaking or thinking, change in balance, blurred vision, mastalgia, edema of extremities, angina, hematemesis, or signs of ovarian hyperstimulation syndrome (OHSS) (HCAHPS).

• Educate patient about signs of a significant reaction (eg, wheezing; chest tightness; fever; itching; bad cough; blue skin color; seizures; or swelling of face, lips, tongue, or throat). **Note:** This is not a comprehensive list of all side effects. Patient should consult prescriber for additional questions.

Intended Use and Disclaimer: Should not be printed and given to patients. This information is intended to serve as a concise initial reference for healthcare professionals to use when discussing medications with a patient. You must ultimately rely on your own discretion, experience and judgment in diagnosing, treating and advising patients.

Ciclesonide (Oral Inhalation)
(sye KLES oh nide)

Brand Names: U.S. Alvesco

Pharmacologic Category Corticosteroid, Inhalant (Oral)

Pregnancy Risk Factor C

Lactation Excretion in breast milk unknown/use caution

Breast-Feeding Considerations Systemic corticosteroids are excreted in human milk. It is not known if sufficient quantities of ciclesonide are absorbed following oral inhalation to produce detectable amounts in breast milk; however, oral absorption is limited (<1%). The manufacturer recommends that caution be exercised when administering ciclesonide to nursing women. The use of inhaled corticosteroids is not considered a contraindication to breast-feeding (NAEPP, 2005).

Use Prophylactic management of bronchial asthma

Mechanism of Action/Effect Ciclesonide is a nonhalogenated, glucocorticoid prodrug that is hydrolyzed to the pharmacologically active metabolite des-ciclesonide following administration. Des-ciclesonide has a high affinity for the glucocorticoid receptor and exhibits anti-inflammatory activity. The mechanism of action for corticosteroids is believed to be a combination of three important properties – anti-inflammatory activity, immunosuppressive properties, and antiproliferative actions.

Contraindications Hypersensitivity to ciclesonide or any component of the formulation; primary treatment of acute asthma or status asthmaticus

Canadian labeling: Additional contraindications (not in U.S. labeling): Untreated fungal, bacterial, or tuberculosis infections of the respiratory tract; moderate-to-severe bronchiectasis

Warnings/Precautions May cause hypercorticism or suppression of hypothalamic-pituitary-adrenal (HPA) axis, particularly in younger children or in patients receiving high doses for prolonged periods. HPA axis suppression may lead to adrenal crisis. Withdrawal and discontinuation of a corticosteroid should be done slowly and carefully. Particular care is required when patients are transferred from systemic corticosteroids to inhaled products due to possible adrenal insufficiency or withdrawal from steroids, including an increase in allergic symptoms. Patients receiving >20 mg per day of prednisone (or equivalent) may be most susceptible. Fatalities have occurred due to adrenal insufficiency in asthmatic patients during and after transfer from systemic corticosteroids to aerosol steroids; aerosol steroids do **not** provide the systemic steroid needed to treat patients having trauma, surgery, or infections.

Bronchospasm may occur with wheezing after inhalation; if this occurs stop steroid and treat with a fast-acting bronchodilator. Supplemental steroids (oral or parenteral) may be needed during stress or severe asthma attacks. Not to be used in status asthmaticus or for the relief of acute bronchospasm. Oropharyngeal thrush due to candida albicans infection may occur with use. Prolonged use of corticosteroids may also increase the incidence of secondary infection, mask acute infection (including fungal infections), prolong or exacerbate viral infections, or limit response to vaccines. Exposure to chickenpox and measles should be avoided; corticosteroids should not be used to treat ocular herpes simplex. Close observation is required in patients with latent tuberculosis and/or TB reactivity; restrict use in active TB (only in conjunction with antituberculosis treatment). Use in patients with TB is contraindicated in the Canadian labeling. Prolonged treatment with corticosteroids has been associated with the development of Kaposi's sarcoma (case reports); if noted, discontinuation of therapy should be considered.

Use with caution in patients with cardiovascular disease, diabetes, severe hepatic impairment, thyroid disease, psychiatric disturbances, myasthenia gravis, glaucoma, cataracts, patients at risk for osteoporosis, and patients at risk for seizures. Use in renally-impaired patients has not been studied; however, ≤20% of drug is eliminated renally. Use with caution in elderly patients.

Orally inhaled corticosteroids may cause a reduction in growth velocity in pediatric patients (~1 cm per year [range: 0.3-1.8 cm per year] and related to dose and duration of exposure). To minimize the systemic effects of orally inhaled corticosteroids, each patient should be titrated to the lowest effective dose. Growth should be routinely monitored in pediatric patients.

Drug Interactions

Avoid Concomitant Use

Avoid concomitant use of Ciclesonide (Oral Inhalation) with any of the following: Aldesleukin

Decreased Effect

Ciclesonide (Oral Inhalation) may decrease the levels/effects of: Aldesleukin; Antidiabetic Agents; Corticorelin; Hyaluronidase; Telaprevir

Increased Effect/Toxicity

Ciclesonide (Oral Inhalation) may increase the levels/effects of: Amphotericin B; Deferasirox; Loop Diuretics; Thiazide Diuretics

The levels/effects of Ciclesonide (Oral Inhalation) may be increased by: CYP3A4 Inhibitors (Strong); Telaprevir

Adverse Reactions

>10%:

Central nervous system: Headache (≤11%)

Respiratory: Nasopharyngitis (≤11%)

1% to 10%:

Cardiovascular: Facial edema (≥3%)

Central nervous system: Dizziness (≥3%), fatigue (≥3%), dysphonia (1%)

Dermatologic: Urticaria (≥3%)

Gastrointestinal: Gastroenteritis (≥3%), oral candidiasis (≥3%)

Neuromuscular & skeletal: Arthralgia (≥3%), musculoskeletal chest pain (≥3%), back pain (≥3%), extremity pain (≥3%)

Ocular: Conjunctivitis (≥3%)

Otic: Ear pain (2%)

Respiratory: Upper respiratory infection (≤9%), nasal congestion (≤6%), pharyngolaryngeal pain (≤5%), hoarseness (≥3%), pneumonia (≥3%), sinusitis (≥3%), paradoxical bronchospasm (2%)

Miscellaneous: Influenza (≥3%)

Dosage Forms Considerations Alvesco 6.1 g canisters contain 60 inhalations.

Available Dosage Forms

Aerosol Solution, Inhalation:

Alvesco: 80 mcg/actuation (6.1 g); 160 mcg/actuation (6.1 g)

General Dosage Range Oral inhalation: Children ≥12 years and Adults: 80-320 mcg twice daily (maximum: 640 mcg/day)

Administration

Inhalation Remove mouthpiece cover, place inhaler in mouth, close lips around mouthpiece, and inhale slowly and deeply. Press down on top of inhaler after slow inhalation has begun. Remove inhaler while holding breath for approximately 10 seconds. Breathe out slowly and replace mouthpiece on inhaler. Rinse mouth with water (and spit out) after inhalation. Do not wash or place inhaler in water. Clean mouthpiece using a dry cloth or tissue once weekly. Discard after the "discard by" date or after labeled number of doses has been used, even if container is not completely empty.

Shaking is not necessary since drug is formulated as a solution aerosol. Prime inhaler prior to initial use or if not in use for ≥7-10 days by releasing 3 puffs into the air.

Storage/Stability Store at 15°C to 30°C (59°F to 86°F); do not freeze.

◀ **Nursing Actions**

Physical Assessment Growth should be monitored periodically with long-term use in children. Do not discontinue abruptly after long-term use.

Patient Education

- Discuss specific use of drug and side effects with patient as it relates to treatment. (HCAHPS: During this hospital stay, were you given any medicine that you had not taken before? Before giving you any new medicine, how often did hospital staff tell you what the medicine was for? How often did hospital staff describe possible side effects in a way you could understand?)

- Patient may experience headache, rhinitis, pharyngitis, back pain, or painful extremities. Have patient report immediately to prescriber signs of infection, severe asthenia, irritability, tremors, tachycardia, confusion, dizziness, diaphoresis, stomatitis, angina, osteodynia, arthralgia, or vision changes (HCAHPS).

- Educate patient about signs of a significant reaction (eg, wheezing; chest tightness; fever; itching; bad cough; blue skin color; seizures; or swelling of face, lips, tongue, or throat). **Note:** This is not a comprehensive list of all side effects. Patient should consult prescriber for additional questions.

Intended Use and Disclaimer: Should not be printed and given to patients. This information is intended to serve as a concise initial reference for healthcare professionals to use when discussing medications with a patient. You must ultimately rely on your own discretion, experience and judgment in diagnosing, treating and advising patients.

Ciclesonide (Nasal) (sye KLES oh nide)

Brand Names: U.S. Omnaris; Zetonna
Pharmacologic Category Corticosteroid, Nasal
Pregnancy Risk Factor C
Lactation Excretion in breast milk unknown/use caution
Use Management of seasonal and perennial allergic rhinitis
Unlabeled Use Adjunct to antibiotics in empiric treatment of acute bacterial rhinosinusitis (ABRS) (Chow, 2012)

Dosage Forms Considerations
Omnaris 12.5 g bottles contain 120 actuations.
Zetonna 6.1 g canisters contain 60 actuations.

Available Dosage Forms
Aerosol Solution, Nasal:
Zetonna: 37 mcg/actuation (6.1 g)
Suspension, Nasal:
Omnaris: 50 mcg/actuation (12.5 g)

General Dosage Range Intranasal:
Omnaris®: *Children ≥6 years and Adults:* 2 sprays (50 mcg/spray) per nostril once daily (maximum: 200 mcg/day)

Zetonna™: *Children ≥12 years and Adults:* 1 spray (37 mcg/spray) per nostril once daily (maximum: 74 mcg/day)

Administration
Other Intranasal: Blow nose to clear nostrils. Insert applicator into nostril, keeping bottle upright, and close off the other nostril. Breathe in through nose. While inhaling, press pump to release spray. Avoid spraying directly onto the nasal septum or into eyes. Discard after the "discard by" date or after labeled number of doses has been used, even if bottle is not completely empty.

Omnaris®: Shake bottle gently before using. Prime pump prior to first use (press 8 times until fine mist appears) or if spray has not been used in 4 consecutive days (press 1 time or until a fine mist appears). Nasal applicator may be removed and rinsed with warm water to clean.

Zetonna™: Use nasal canister with supplied nasal actuator only. Prime pump prior to first use (press 3 times until fine mist appears) or if spray has not been used in 10 consecutive days (press 3 times or until a fine mist appears). If canister and actuator become separated, spray 1 test spray in air before using. Clean outside of nose piece with a clean, dry tissue or cloth weekly; do not wash or put in water.

Nursing Actions
Physical Assessment Monitor growth in pediatric patients.

Patient Education

- Discuss specific use of drug and side effects with patient as it relates to treatment. (HCAHPS: During this hospital stay, were you given any medicine that you had not taken before? Before giving you any new medicine, how often did hospital staff tell you what the medicine was for? How often did hospital staff describe possible side effects in a way you could understand?)

- Patient may experience headache. Have patient report immediately to prescriber signs of infection, severe dizziness, significant rhinitis, considerable epistaxis, nasal sores, stomatitis, intolerable nausea, severe asthenia, or vision changes (HCAHPS).

- Educate patient about signs of a significant reaction (eg, wheezing; chest tightness; fever; itching; bad cough; blue skin color; seizures; or swelling of face, lips, tongue, or throat). **Note:** This is not a comprehensive list of all side effects. Patient should consult prescriber for additional questions.

Intended Use and Disclaimer: Should not be printed and given to patients. This information is intended to serve as a concise initial reference for healthcare professionals to use when discussing medications with a patient. You must ultimately rely on your own discretion, experience and judgment in diagnosing, treating and advising patients.

Cidofovir (si DOF o veer)

Brand Names: U.S. Vistide
Pharmacologic Category Antiviral Agent
Pregnancy Risk Factor C
Lactation Excretion in breast milk unknown/contraindicated
Breast-Feeding Considerations The CDC recommends **not** to breast-feed if diagnosed with HIV to avoid postnatal transmission of the virus.
Use Treatment of cytomegalovirus (CMV) retinitis in patients with acquired immunodeficiency syndrome (AIDS). **Note:** Should be administered with probenecid.
Mechanism of Action/Effect Nucleotide analog that selectively inhibits viral DNA polymerase, suppressing viral DNA synthesis
Contraindications Hypersensitivity to cidofovir; history of clinically-severe hypersensitivity to probenecid or other sulfa-containing medications; serum creatinine >1.5 mg/dL; CrCl <55 mL/minute; urine protein ≥100 mg/dL (≥2+ proteinuria); use with or within 7 days of nephrotoxic agents; direct intraocular injection
Warnings/Precautions Hazardous agent - use appropriate precautions for handling and disposal (NIOSH, 2012). **[U.S. Boxed Warning]: Dose-dependent nephrotoxicity requires dose adjustment or discontinuation if changes in renal function occur during therapy (eg, proteinuria, glycosuria, decreased serum phosphate, uric acid or bicarbonate, and elevated creatinine).** Neutropenia has been reported; monitor counts during therapy. Cases of ocular hypotony have also occurred; monitor intraocular pressure. Monitor for signs of metabolic acidosis. Safety and efficacy have not been established in children or the elderly. Administration must be accompanied by oral probenecid and intravenous saline prehydration. **[U.S. Boxed Warning]: Indicated only for CMV retinitis treatment in HIV patients; possibly carcinogenic and teratogenic based on animal data. May cause hypospermia.**
Drug Interactions
Avoid Concomitant Use There are no known interactions where it is recommended to avoid concomitant use.
Decreased Effect There are no known significant interactions involving a decrease in effect.
Increased Effect/Toxicity
Cidofovir may increase the levels/effects of: Tenofovir
Adverse Reactions
>10%:
Central nervous system: Chills, fever, headache, pain
Dermatologic: Alopecia, rash
Gastrointestinal: Nausea, vomiting, diarrhea, anorexia
Hematologic: Anemia, neutropenia
Neuromuscular & skeletal: Weakness
Ocular: Intraocular pressure decreased, iritis, ocular hypotony, uveitis
Renal: Creatinine increased, proteinuria, renal toxicity
Respiratory: Cough, dyspnea
Miscellaneous: Infection, oral moniliasis, serum bicarbonate decreased
1% to 10%:
Renal: Fanconi syndrome
Respiratory: Pneumonia
Frequency not defined (limited to important or life-threatening reactions):
Cardiovascular: Cardiomyopathy, cardiovascular disorder, CHF, edema, orthostatic hypotension, shock, syncope, tachycardia
Central nervous system: Agitation, amnesia, anxiety, confusion, convulsion, dizziness, hallucinations, insomnia, malaise, vertigo
Dermatologic: Photosensitivity reaction, skin discoloration, urticaria
Endocrine & metabolic: Adrenal cortex insufficiency
Gastrointestinal: Abdominal pain, aphthous stomatitis, colitis, constipation, dysphagia, fecal incontinence, gastritis, GI hemorrhage, gingivitis, melena, proctitis, splenomegaly, stomatitis, tongue discoloration
Genitourinary: Urinary incontinence
Hematologic: Hypochromic anemia, leukocytosis, leukopenia, lymphadenopathy, lymphoma-like reaction, pancytopenia, thrombocytopenia, thrombocytopenic purpura
Hepatic: Hepatomegaly, hepatosplenomegaly, jaundice, liver function tests abnormal, liver damage, liver necrosis
Local: Injection site reaction
Neuromuscular & skeletal: Tremor
Ocular: Amblyopia, blindness, cataract, conjunctivitis, corneal lesion, diplopia, vision abnormal
Otic: Hearing loss
Miscellaneous: Allergic reaction, sepsis
Available Dosage Forms
Solution, Intravenous:
Vistide: 75 mg/mL (5 mL)
Solution, Intravenous [preservative free]:
Generic: 75 mg/mL (5 mL)
General Dosage Range Dosage adjustment recommended in patients with renal impairment
I.V.: *Adults:* Induction: 5 mg/kg once weekly for 2 consecutive weeks; Maintenance: 5 mg/kg once every 2 weeks
Administration
I.V. For I.V. infusion only. Infuse over 1 hour. Hydrate with 1 L of 0.9% NS I.V. prior to cidofovir infusion. A second liter may be administered over a 1- to 3-hour period immediately following infusion, if tolerated.

Hazardous agent; use appropriate precautions for handling and disposal (NIOSH, 2012).
Injectable Detail pH: 6.7-7.6

Preparation for Administration Hazardous agent; use appropriate precautions for handling and disposal (NIOSH, 2012). Dilute dose in NS 100 mL prior to infusion.

Storage/Stability Store at controlled room temperature 20°C to 25°C (68°F to 77°F). Store admixtures under refrigeration for ≤24 hours. Cidofovir infusion admixture should be administered within 24 hours of preparation at room temperature or refrigerated. Admixtures should be allowed to equilibrate to room temperature prior to use.

Nursing Actions

Physical Assessment Administration must be accompanied by oral probenecid and intravenous saline prehydration. Pretreatment with probenecid and both pre- and post-treatment hydration may be ordered. Monitor infusion site closely to avoid extravasation. Monitor for CNS changes, anemia, renal status, and visual acuity. Instruct patient to report any changes in vision or eye pain.

Patient Education

- Discuss specific use of drug and side effects with patient as it relates to treatment. (HCAHPS: During this hospital stay, were you given any medicine that you had not taken before? Before giving you any new medicine, how often did hospital staff tell you what the medicine was for? How often did hospital staff describe possible side effects in a way you could understand?)
- Patient may experience headache, diarrhea, lack of appetite, alopecia, or nausea. Have patient report immediately to prescriber signs of infection, signs of hepatic impairment, illogical thinking, urinary retention, oliguria, melena, angina, tachycardia, vision changes, ophthalmalgia, eye irritation, depression, hallucinations, change in balance, paresthesia, dyspnea, excessive weight gain, edema of extremities, bloating, tremors, brasdykinesia, rigidity, ecchymosis, hemorrhaging, severe asthenia, or stomatitis (HCAHPS).
- Educate patient about signs of a significant reaction (eg, wheezing; chest tightness; fever; itching; bad cough; blue skin color; seizures; or swelling of face, lips, tongue, or throat). **Note:** This is not a comprehensive list of all side effects. Patient should consult prescriber for additional questions.

Intended Use and Disclaimer: Should not be printed and given to patients. This information is intended to serve as a concise initial reference for healthcare professionals to use when discussing medications with a patient. You must ultimately rely on your own discretion, experience and judgment in diagnosing, treating and advising patients.

Cilostazol (sil OH sta zol)

Brand Names: U.S. Pletal
Index Terms OPC-13013
Pharmacologic Category Antiplatelet Agent; Phosphodiesterase-3 Enzyme Inhibitor
Medication Safety Issues
Sound-alike/look-alike issues:
Pletal® may be confused with Plendil®
Pregnancy Risk Factor C
Lactation Excretion in breast milk unknown/not recommended
Breast-Feeding Considerations It is not known if cilostazol is excreted in human milk. According to the manufacturer, the decision to continue or discontinue breast-feeding during therapy should take into account the risk of exposure to the infant and the benefits of treatment to the mother.
Use Symptomatic management of peripheral vascular disease, primarily intermittent claudication
Unlabeled Use Adjunct with aspirin and clopidogrel for prevention of stent thrombosis and restenosis after coronary stent placement; as an alternative agent to either aspirin or clopidogrel in a dual antiplatelet regimen when allergy or drug intolerance to either agent occurs in patients who have undergone elective PCI with bare metal or drug-eluting stent placement; secondary prevention of noncardioembolic ischemic stroke or transient ischemic attack (TIA)
Mechanism of Action/Effect Cilostazol and its metabolites are inhibitors of phosphodiesterase III. As a result, cyclic AMP is increased leading to reversible inhibition of platelet aggregation, vasodilation, and inhibition of vascular smooth muscle cell proliferation.
Contraindications Hypersensitivity to cilostazol or any component of the formulation; heart failure (HF) of any severity; hemostatic disorders or active bleeding
Warnings/Precautions [U.S. Boxed Warning]: The use of this drug is contraindicated in patients with heart failure. Use with caution in severe underlying heart disease. Use with caution in patients receiving other platelet aggregation inhibitors or in patients with thrombocytopenia. Discontinue therapy if thrombocytopenia or leukopenia occur; progression to agranulocytosis (reversible) has been reported when cilostazol was not immediately stopped. Withhold for at least 4-6 half-lives prior to elective surgical procedures. Use caution in moderate-to-severe hepatic impairment. Use cautiously in severe renal impairment (CrCl <25 mL/minute). Potentially significant drug-drug interactions may exist, requiring dose or frequency adjustment, additional monitoring, and/or selection of alternative therapy.

Drug Interactions
Avoid Concomitant Use
Avoid concomitant use of Cilostazol with any of the following: Conivaptan; Fusidic Acid (Systemic); Riociguat; Urokinase

Decreased Effect
The levels/effects of Cilostazol may be decreased by: Bosentan; CYP3A4 Inducers (Strong); Dabrafenib; Deferasirox; Herbs (CYP3A4 Inducers); Mitotane; Nonsteroidal Anti-Inflammatory Agents; Peginterferon Alfa-2b; Tocilizumab

Increased Effect/Toxicity
Cilostazol may increase the levels/effects of: Agents with Antiplatelet Properties; Anticoagulants; Collagenase (Systemic); Dabigatran Etexilate; Ibritumomab; Riociguat; Rivaroxaban; Salicylates; Thrombolytic Agents; Tositumomab and Iodine I 131 Tositumomab; Urokinase

The levels/effects of Cilostazol may be increased by: Anagrelide; Antifungal Agents (Azole Derivatives, Systemic); Conivaptan; CYP2C19 Inhibitors (Moderate); CYP2C19 Inhibitors (Strong); CYP3A4 Inhibitors (Moderate); CYP3A4 Inhibitors (Strong); Dasatinib; Esomeprazole; Fusidic Acid (Systemic); Glucosamine; Herbs (Anticoagulant/Antiplatelet Properties); Ibrutinib; Ivacaftor; Luliconazole; Macrolide Antibiotics; Mifepristone; Multivitamins/Fluoride (with ADE); Multivitamins/Minerals (with ADEK, Folate, Iron); Multivitamins/Minerals (with AE, No Iron); Nonsteroidal Anti-Inflammatory Agents; Omega-3 Fatty Acids; Omeprazole; Pentosan Polysulfate Sodium; Pentoxifylline; Prostacyclin Analogues; Simeprevir; Stiripentol; Tipranavir; Vitamin E

Nutritional/Ethanol Interactions
Food: Taking cilostazol with a high-fat meal may increase peak concentration by 90%. Grapefruit juice may increase serum levels of cilostazol and enhance toxic effects. Management: Administer cilostazol on an empty stomach 30 minutes before or 2 hours after meals. Avoid concurrent ingestion of grapefruit juice.

Herb/Nutraceutical: St John's wort may decrease the levels/effects of cilostazol. Other herbs/nutraceuticals have additional antiplatelet activity. Management: Avoid alfalfa, anise, bilberry, bladderwrack, bromelain, cat's claw, chamomile, coleus, cordyceps, dong quai, evening primrose oil, fenugreek, feverfew, garlic, ginger, ginkgo biloba, ginseng (American), ginseng (Panax), ginseng (Siberian), grapeseed, green tea, guggul, horse chestnut seed, horseradish, licorice, prickly ash, red clover, reishi, SAMe (S-adenosylmethionine), St John's wort, sweet clover, turmeric, and white willow.

Adverse Reactions
>10%:
Central nervous system: Headache (27% to 34%)
Gastrointestinal: Abnormal stools (12% to 15%), diarrhea (12% to 19%)
Infection: Increased susceptibility to infection (10% to 14%)
Respiratory: Rhinitis (7% to 12%)
2% to 10%:
Cardiovascular: Peripheral edema (7% to 9%), palpitations (5% to 10%), tachycardia (4%)
Central nervous system: Dizziness (9% to 10%), vertigo (≤3%)
Gastrointestinal: Dyspepsia (6%), nausea (6% to 7%), abdominal pain (4% to 5%), flatulence (2% to 3%)
Neuromuscular & skeletal: Back pain (6% to 7%), myalgia (2% to 3%)
Respiratory: Pharyngitis (7% to 10%), cough (3% to 4%)

Pharmacodynamics/Kinetics
Onset of Action 2-4 weeks; may require up to 12 weeks

Available Dosage Forms
Tablet, Oral:
Pletal: 50 mg, 100 mg
Generic: 50 mg, 100 mg

General Dosage Range Dosage adjustment recommended in patients on concomitant therapy
Oral: *Adults:* 100 mg twice daily

Administration
Oral Administer cilostazol 30 minutes before or 2 hours after meals (breakfast and dinner).

Storage/Stability Store at 20°C to 25°C (68°F to 77°F); protect from light.

Nursing Actions
Physical Assessment Monitor for signs of bleeding.

Patient Education
• Discuss specific use of drug and side effects with patient as it relates to treatment. (HCAHPS: During this hospital stay, were you given any medicine that you had not taken before? Before giving you any new medicine, how often did hospital staff tell you what the medicine was for? How often did hospital staff describe possible side effects in a way you could understand?)
• Patient may experience abnormal stools, dyspepsia, pharyngitis, rhinitis, or back pain. Have patient report immediately to prescriber signs of hemorrhaging, signs of infection, strength changes from one side to another, difficulty speaking or thinking, changed in balance, blurred vision, tachycardia, arrhythmia, or edema of extremities (HCAHPS).
• Educate patient about signs of a significant reaction (eg, wheezing; chest tightness; fever; itching; bad cough; blue skin color; seizures; or swelling of face, lips, tongue, or throat). **Note:** This is not a comprehensive list of all side effects. Patient should consult prescriber for additional questions.

Intended Use and Disclaimer: Should not be printed and given to patients. This information is intended to serve as a concise initial reference for

healthcare professionals to use when discussing medications with a patient. You must ultimately rely on your own discretion, experience and judgment in diagnosing, treating and advising patients.

Dietary Considerations It is best to take cilostazol 30 minutes before or 2 hours after meals (breakfast and dinner).

Cimetidine (sye MET i deen)

Brand Names: U.S. Cimetidine Acid Reducer [OTC]; Tagamet HB [OTC]

Pharmacologic Category Histamine H$_2$ Antagonist

Medication Safety Issues
Sound-alike/look-alike issues:
Cimetidine may be confused with simethicone

Pregnancy Risk Factor B

Lactation Enters breast milk/not recommended

Use Short-term treatment of active duodenal ulcers and benign gastric ulcers; maintenance therapy of duodenal ulcer; treatment of gastric hypersecretory states; treatment of gastroesophageal reflux disease (GERD)

OTC labeling: Prevention or relief of heartburn, acid indigestion, or sour stomach

Unlabeled Use Part of a multidrug regimen for *H. pylori* eradication to reduce the risk of duodenal ulcer recurrence

Available Dosage Forms
Solution, Oral:
Generic: 300 mg/5 mL (237 mL, 240 mL)
Tablet, Oral:
Cimetidine Acid Reducer [OTC]: 200 mg
Tagamet HB [OTC]: 200 mg
Generic: 200 mg, 300 mg, 400 mg, 800 mg

General Dosage Range Dosage adjustment recommended in patients with renal impairment

Oral:
Children <12 years: 20-40 mg/kg/day divided every 6 hours
Children ≥12 years: 20-40 mg/kg/day divided every 6 hours **or** 200 mg 1-2 times/day [OTC]
Adults: 300-600 mg 4 times/day **or** 400-800 mg 1-2 times/day **or** 200 mg 1-2 times/day [OTC]

Administration
Oral Administer with meals so that the drug's peak effect occurs at the proper time (peak inhibition of gastric acid secretion occurs at 1 and 3 hours after dosing in fasting subjects and approximately 2 hours in nonfasting subjects. This correlates well with the time food is no longer in the stomach offering a buffering effect). Stagger doses of antacids with cimetidine.

Nursing Actions
Physical Assessment Monitor for CNS changes, agitation, and gastric bleeding regularly during therapy.

Patient Education
• Discuss specific use of drug and side effects with patient as it relates to treatment. (HCAHPS During this hospital stay, were you given any medicine that you had not taken before? Before giving you any new medicine, how often did hospital staff tell you what the medicine was for? How often did hospital staff describe possible side effects in a way you could understand?
• Patient may experience fatigue, headache, or diarrhea. Have patient report immediately to prescriber angina, tachycardia, bradycardia, severe dizziness, syncope, illogical thinking, myalgia, arthralgia, ecchymosis, hemorrhaging, mood changes, hallucinations, male macromastia, sexual dysfunction, or injection site irritation (HCAHPS).
• Educate patient about signs of a significant reaction (eg, wheezing; chest tightness; fever; itching; bad cough; blue skin color; seizures; or swelling of face, lips, tongue, or throat). **Note:** This is not a comprehensive list of all side effects. Patient should consult prescriber for additional questions.

Intended Use and Disclaimer: Should not be printed and given to patients. This information is intended to serve as a concise initial reference for healthcare professionals to use when discussing medications with a patient. You must ultimately rely on your own discretion, experience and judgment in diagnosing, treating and advising patients.

Cinacalcet (sin a KAL cet)

Brand Names: U.S. Sensipar
Index Terms AMG 073; Cinacalcet Hydrochloride
Pharmacologic Category Calcimimetic
Pregnancy Risk Factor C
Lactation Excretion in breast milk unknown/not recommended
Use Treatment of secondary hyperparathyroidism in patients with chronic kidney disease (CKD) on dialysis; treatment of hypercalcemia in patients with parathyroid carcinoma; treatment of severe hypercalcemia in patients with primary hyperparathyroidism who are unable to undergo parathyroidectomy

Available Dosage Forms
Tablet, Oral:
Sensipar: 30 mg, 60 mg, 90 mg

General Dosage Range Dosage adjustment recommended in patients on concomitant therapy or who develop toxicities

Oral: *Adults:* Initial: 30 mg once or twice daily; Maintenance: Increase dose incrementally every 2-4 weeks to normalize calcium levels or maintain iPTH level (maximum: 360 mg/day [parathyroid cancer, primary hyperparathyroidism]; 180 mg/day [secondary hyperparathyroidism])

Administration

Oral Administer with food or shortly after a meal. Do not break or divide tablet; should be taken whole.

Nursing Actions

Physical Assessment Monitor for hypocalcemia (paresthesias, myalgia, cramping, tetany, seizures) at beginning of therapy and regularly thereafter.

Patient Education

- Discuss specific use of drug and side effects with patient as it relates to treatment. (HCAHPS: During this hospital stay, were you given any medicine that you had not taken before? Before giving you any new medicine, how often did hospital staff tell you what the medicine was for? How often did hospital staff describe possible side effects in a way you could understand?)
- Patient may experience constipation, diarrhea, or lack of appetite. Have patient report immediately to prescriber signs of hypocalcemia, angina, tachycardia, severe nausea, illogical thinking, urinary retention, oliguria, depression, significant dizziness, syncope, bradycardia, arrhythmia, arthralgia, myalgia, considerable asthenia, intolerable headache, dyspnea, edema of extremities, tremors, osteodynia, polydipsia, or xerostomia (HCAHPS).
- Educate patient about signs of a significant reaction (eg, wheezing; chest tightness; fever; itching; bad cough; blue skin color; seizures; or swelling of face, lips, tongue, or throat). **Note:** This is not a comprehensive list of all side effects. Patient should consult prescriber for additional questions.

Intended Use and Disclaimer: Should not be printed and given to patients. This information is intended to serve as a concise initial reference for healthcare professionals to use when discussing medications with a patient. You must ultimately rely on your own discretion, experience and judgment in diagnosing, treating and advising patients.

Related Information

Oral Medications That Should Not Be Crushed or Altered *on page 1712*

Ciprofloxacin (Systemic)
(sip roe FLOKS a sin)

Brand Names: U.S. Cipro; Cipro in D5W; Cipro XR

Index Terms Ciprofloxacin Hydrochloride

Pharmacologic Category Antibiotic, Fluoroquinolone

Medication Safety Issues

Sound-alike/look-alike issues:
Ciprofloxacin may be confused with cephalexin
Cipro may be confused with Ceftin

Medication Guide Available Yes

Pregnancy Risk Factor C

Lactation Enters breast milk/not recommended

Breast-Feeding Considerations Ciprofloxacin is excreted in breast milk. Due to the potential for serious adverse reactions in the nursing infant, the manufacturer recommends a decision be made whether to discontinue nursing or to discontinue the drug, taking into account the importance of treatment to the mother. However, due to the low concentrations in human milk, minimal toxicity would be expected in the nursing infant and infant serum levels were undetectable in one report (Gardner, 1992). Nondose-related effects could include modification of bowel flora. There has been a single case report of perforated pseudomembranous colitis in a breast-feeding infant whose mother was taking ciprofloxacin (Harmon, 1992).

Use

Children: Complicated urinary tract infections and pyelonephritis due to *E. coli*. **Note:** Although effective, ciprofloxacin is not the drug of first choice in children.

Children and Adults: To reduce incidence or progression of disease following exposure to aerolized *Bacillus anthracis*.

Adults: Treatment of the following infections when caused by susceptible bacteria: Urinary tract infections; acute uncomplicated cystitis in females; chronic bacterial prostatitis; lower respiratory tract infections (including acute exacerbations of chronic bronchitis); acute sinusitis; skin and skin structure infections; bone and joint infections; complicated intra-abdominal infections (in combination with metronidazole); infectious diarrhea; typhoid fever due to *Salmonella typhi* (eradication of chronic typhoid carrier state has not been proven); uncomplicated cervical and urethra gonorrhea (due to *N. gonorrhoeae*); nosocomial pneumonia; empirical therapy for febrile neutropenic patients (in combination with piperacillin)

Note: As of April 2007, the CDC no longer recommends the use of fluoroquinolones for the treatment of gonococcal disease.

Unlabeled Use Acute pulmonary exacerbations in cystic fibrosis (children); cutaneous/gastrointestinal/oropharyngeal anthrax (treatment, children and adults); disseminated gonococcal infection (adults); chancroid (adults); epididymitis (adults); prophylaxis to *Neisseria meningitidis* following close contact with an infected person; empirical therapy (oral) for febrile neutropenia in low-risk cancer patients; HACEK group endocarditis; infectious diarrhea (children); periodontitis; chronic oral antimicrobial suppression of prosthetic joint infection; surgical (preoperative) prophylaxis

Mechanism of Action/Effect Inhibits DNA-gyrase in susceptible organisms; inhibits relaxation of supercoiled DNA and promotes breakage of double-stranded DNA

Contraindications Hypersensitivity to ciprofloxacin, any component of the formulation, or other quinolones; concurrent administration of tizanidine

Warnings/Precautions [U.S. Boxed Warning]: There have been reports of tendon inflammation and/or rupture with quinolone antibiotics in all ages; risk may be increased with concurrent corticosteroids, solid organ transplant recipients, and in patients >60 years of age. Rupture of the Achilles tendon sometimes requiring surgical repair has been reported most frequently; but other tendon sites (eg, rotator cuff, biceps) have also been reported. Strenuous physical activity, rheumatoid arthritis, and renal impairment may be an independent risk factor for tendonitis. Inflammation and rupture may occur bilaterally. Cases have been reported within the first 48 hours, during, and up to several months after discontinuation of therapy. Discontinue at first sign of tendon inflammation or pain. Use with caution in patients with rheumatoid arthritis; may increase risk of tendon rupture. Use with caution in patients with a history of tendon disorders.

CNS effects may occur (tremor, restlessness, confusion, and hallucinations, increased intracranial pressure [including pseudotumor cerebri] or seizures). Reactions may occur following the first dose. Use with caution in patients with known or suspected CNS disorder or consider discontinuation if CNS effects develop. Potential for seizures, although very rare, may be increased with concomitant NSAID therapy. Use with caution in individuals at risk of seizures (CNS disorders or concurrent therapy with medications which may lower seizure threshold; status epilepticus has occurred) or if clinically appropriate, consider alternative antimicrobial therapy. Discontinue if seizures occur.

Fluoroquinolones may prolong QT_c interval; avoid use in patients with a history of or at risk for QT_c prolongation, torsade de pointes, uncorrected hypokalemia, hypomagnesemia, cardiac disease (heart failure, myocardial infarction, bradycardia) or concurrent administration of other medications known to prolong the QT interval (including Class Ia and Class III antiarrhythmics, cisapride, erythromycin, antipsychotics, and tricyclic antidepressants). Hepatocellular, cholestatic, or mixed liver injury has been reported, including hepatic necrosis, life-threatening hepatic events, and fatalities. Acute liver injury can be rapid onset (range: 1-39 days), often associated with hypersensitivity. Most fatalities occurred in patients >55 years of age. Discontinue immediately if signs/symptoms of hepatitis (abdominal tenderness, dark urine, jaundice, pruritus) occur. Additionally, temporary increases in transaminases or alkaline phosphatase or cholestatic jaundice may occur (highest risk in patients with previous liver damage).

Prolonged use may result in fungal or bacterial superinfection, including *C. difficile*-associated diarrhea (CDAD) and pseudomembranous colitis; CDAD has been observed >2 months postantibiotic treatment. Rarely crystalluria has occurred; urine alkalinity may increase the risk. Ensure adequate hydration during therapy. Adverse effects, including those related to joints and/or surrounding tissues, are increased in pediatric patients and therefore, ciprofloxacin should not be considered as drug of choice in children (exception is anthrax treatment). Peripheral neuropathy has been reported (rare); may occur soon after initiation of therapy and may be irreversible; discontinue if symptoms of sensory or sensorimotor neuropathy occur.

Fluoroquinolones have been associated with the development of serious, and sometimes fatal, hypoglycemia, most often in elderly diabetics but also in patients without diabetes. This occurred most frequently with gatifloxacin (no longer available systemically), but may occur at a lower frequency with other quinolones.

Severe hypersensitivity reactions, including anaphylaxis, have occurred with quinolone therapy. Reactions may present as typical allergic symptoms after a single dose, or may manifest as severe idiosyncratic dermatologic, vascular, pulmonary, renal, hepatic, and/or hematologic events, usually after multiple doses. Prompt discontinuation of drug should occur if skin rash or other symptoms arise. **[U.S. Boxed Warning]: Quinolones may exacerbate myasthenia gravis; avoid use (rare, potentially life-threatening weakness of respiratory muscles may occur).** Use caution in renal impairment. Avoid excessive sunlight and take precautions to limit exposure (eg, loose fitting clothing, sunscreen); may cause moderate-to-severe photosensitivity/phototoxicity reactions. Discontinue use if photosensitivity occurs. Since ciprofloxacin is ineffective in the treatment of syphilis and may mask symptoms, all patients should be tested for syphilis at the time of gonorrheal diagnosis and 3 months later. Hemolytic reactions may (rarely) occur with quinolone use in patients with latent or actual glucose-6-phosphate dehydrogenase (G6PD) deficiency.

Potentially significant interactions may exist, requiring dose or frequency adjustment, additional monitoring, and/or selection of alternative therapy. Serious and fatal reactions including seizures, status epilepticus, cardiac arrest and respiratory failure have been reported with concomitant administration of theophylline. If concurrent use is unavoidable, monitor serum theophylline levels and adjust theophylline dose as warranted.

Drug Interactions

Avoid Concomitant Use

Avoid concomitant use of Ciprofloxacin (Systemic) with any of the following: Agomelatine;

BCG; CloZAPine; Highest Risk QTc-Prolonging Agents; Ivabradine; Mifepristone; Pirfenidone; Pomalidomide; Strontium Ranelate; Tasimelteon; TiZANidine

Decreased Effect

Ciprofloxacin (Systemic) may decrease the levels/effects of: BCG; Didanosine; Fosphenytoin; Mycophenolate; Phenytoin; Sodium Picosulfate; Sulfonylureas; Typhoid Vaccine

The levels/effects of Ciprofloxacin (Systemic) may be decreased by: Antacids; Calcium Salts; Didanosine; Iron Salts; Lanthanum; Magnesium Salts; Multivitamins/Minerals (with ADEK, Folate, Iron); Multivitamins/Minerals (with AE, No Iron); P-glycoprotein/ABCB1 Inducers; Quinapril; Sevelamer; Strontium Ranelate; Sucralfate; Zinc Salts

Increased Effect/Toxicity

Ciprofloxacin (Systemic) may increase the levels/effects of: Agomelatine; ARIPiprazole; Bendamustine; Caffeine; CloZAPine; Corticosteroids (Systemic); CYP1A2 Substrates; Erlotinib; Highest Risk QTc-Prolonging Agents; Lomitapide; Methotrexate; Moderate Risk QTc-Prolonging Agents; Pentoxifylline; Pirfenidone; Pomalidomide; Porfimer; Roflumilast; ROPINIRole; Ropivacaine; Sulfonylureas; Tasimelteon; Theophylline Derivatives; TiZANidine; Varenicline; Vitamin K Antagonists

The levels/effects of Ciprofloxacin (Systemic) may be increased by: Fosphenytoin; Insulin; Ivabradine; Mifepristone; Nonsteroidal Anti-Inflammatory Agents; P-glycoprotein/ABCB1 Inhibitors; Probenecid; QTc-Prolonging Agents (Indeterminate Risk and Risk Modifying)

Nutritional/Ethanol Interactions

Food: Food decreases rate, but not extent, of absorption. Ciprofloxacin serum levels may be decreased if taken with divalent or trivalent cations. Ciprofloxacin may increase serum caffeine levels if taken concurrently. Rarely, crystalluria may occur. Enteral feedings may decrease plasma concentrations of ciprofloxacin probably by >30% inhibition of absorption. Management: May administer with food to minimize GI upset. Avoid or take ciprofloxacin 2 hours before or 6 hours after antacids, dairy products, or calcium-fortified juices alone or in a meal containing >800 mg calcium, oral multivitamins, or mineral supplements containing divalent and/or trivalent cations. Restrict caffeine intake if excessive cardiac or CNS stimulation occurs. Ensure adequate hydration during therapy. Ciprofloxacin should not be administered with enteral feedings. The feeding would need to be discontinued for 1-2 hours prior to and after ciprofloxacin administration. Nasogastric administration produces a greater loss of ciprofloxacin bioavailability than does nasoduodenal administration.

Herb/Nutraceutical: Dong quai and St John's wort may also cause photosensitization. Management: Avoid dong quai and St John's wort.

Adverse Reactions 1% to 10%:

Central nervous system: Neurologic events (children 2%, includes dizziness, insomnia, nervousness, somnolence); fever (children 2%); headache (I.V. administration); restlessness (I.V. administration)

Dermatologic: Rash (children 2%, adults 1%)

Gastrointestinal: Nausea (3%); diarrhea (children 5%, adults 2%); vomiting (children 5%, adults 1%); abdominal pain (children 3%, adults <1%); dyspepsia (children 3%)

Hepatic: ALT increased, AST increased (adults 1%)

Local: Injection site reactions (I.V. administration)

Respiratory: Rhinitis (children 3%)

Available Dosage Forms

Solution, Intravenous:

Cipro in D₅W: 200 mg/100 mL (100 mL)

Generic: 200 mg/100 mL (100 mL); 400 mg/200 mL (200 mL); 200 mg/20 mL (20 mL); 400 mg/40 mL (40 mL)

Solution, Intravenous [preservative free]:

Cipro in D₅W: 200 mg/100 mL (100 mL); 400 mg/200 mL (200 mL)

Generic: 200 mg/100 mL (100 mL); 400 mg/200 mL (200 mL); 200 mg/20 mL (20 mL); 400 mg/40 mL (40 mL)

Suspension Reconstituted, Oral:

Cipro: 250 mg/5 mL (100 mL); 500 mg/5 mL (100 mL)

Tablet, Oral:

Cipro: 250 mg, 500 mg

Generic: 100 mg, 250 mg, 500 mg, 750 mg

Tablet Extended Release 24 Hour, Oral:

Cipro XR: 500 mg, 1000 mg

Generic: 500 mg, 1000 mg

General Dosage Range Dosage adjustment recommended in patients with renal impairment

I.V.:

Children: 20-30 mg/kg/day divided every 12 hours (maximum: 800 mg daily)

Adults: 200-400 mg every 8-12 hours

Oral:

Extended release: *Adults:* 500-1000 mg every 24 hours

Immediate release:

Children: 20-40 mg/kg/day in 2 divided doses (maximum: 1.5 g daily)

Adults: 250-750 mg every 12 hours or 250 mg to 1 g as a single dose

Administration

I.V. Administer by slow I.V. infusion over 60 minutes into a large vein (reduces risk of venous irritation).

Injectable Detail pH: 3.3-3.9 (vials); 3.5-4.6 (PVC bags)

Oral May administer with food to minimize GI upset; avoid antacid use; maintain proper ▶

hydration and urine output. Administer immediate release ciprofloxacin and Cipro XR at least 2 hours before or 6 hours after antacids or other products containing calcium, iron, or zinc (including dairy products or calcium-fortified juices). Separate oral administration from drugs which may impair absorption (see Drug Interactions).

Oral suspension: Should not be administered through feeding tubes (suspension is oil-based and adheres to the feeding tube). Patients should avoid chewing on the microcapsules.

Nasogastric/orogastric tube: Crush immediate-release tablet and mix with water. Flush feeding tube before and after administration. Hold tube feedings at least 1 hour before and 2 hours after administration.

Tablet, extended release: Do not crush, split, or chew. May be administered with meals containing dairy products (calcium content <800 mg), but not with dairy products alone.

Preparation for Administration Injection, vial: May be diluted with NS, D_5W, SWFI, $D_{10}W$, $D_5^{1/4}NS$, $D_5^{1/2}NS$, LR.

Storage/Stability

Injection:

Premixed infusion: Store between 5°C to 25°C (41°F to 77°F); avoid freezing. Protect from light.

Vial: Store between 5°C to 30°C (41°F to 86°F); avoid freezing. Protect from light. Diluted solutions of 0.5-2 mg/mL are stable for up to 14 days refrigerated or at room temperature.

Microcapsules for oral suspension: Prior to reconstitution, store below 25°C (77°F). Protect from freezing. Following reconstitution, store below 30°C (86°F) for up to 14 days. Protect from freezing.

Tablet:

Immediate release: Store below 30°C (86°F).

Extended release: Store at room temperature of 15°C to 30°C (59°F to 86°F).

Nursing Actions

Physical Assessment Results of culture and sensitivity tests should be assessed prior to beginning therapy. I.V.: See Administration specifics. Monitor for hypersensitivity reactions (severe reactions, including anaphylaxis, have occurred with quinolone therapy), persistent diarrhea (*C. difficile*-associated colitis can occur post-treatment), and changes in CNS.

Patient Education

• Discuss specific use of drug and side effects with patient as it relates to treatment. (HCAHPS: During this hospital stay, were you given any medicine that you had not taken before? Before giving you any new medicine, how often did hospital staff tell you what the medicine was for? How often did hospital staff describe possible side effects in a way you could understand?)

• Patient may experience diarrhea or headache. Have patient report immediately to prescriber melena, angina, tachycardia, arrhythmia, severe dizziness, syncope, considerable nausea, ankle pain, arthralgia, significant myalgia, intolerable asthenia, vision changes, hallucinations, dyspnea, ecchymosis, hemorrhaging, tremors, urinary retention, oliguria, vaginitis, signs of depression (ie, suicidal ideation, anxiety, emotional instability, illogical thinking), signs of hepatic impairment, signs of severe neuropathy, or signs of pseudomembranous colitis (HCAHPS).

• Educate patient about signs of a significant reaction (eg, wheezing; chest tightness; fever; itching; bad cough; blue skin color; seizures; or swelling of face, lips, tongue, or throat). **Note:** This is not a comprehensive list of all side effects. Patient should consult prescriber for additional questions.

Intended Use and Disclaimer: Should not be printed and given to patients. This information is intended to serve as a concise initial reference for healthcare professionals to use when discussing medications with a patient. You must ultimately rely on your own discretion, experience and judgment in diagnosing, treating and advising patients.

Dietary Considerations Food: Drug may cause GI upset; take without regard to meals (manufacturer prefers that immediate release tablet is taken 2 hours after meals). Extended release tablet may be taken with meals that contain dairy products (calcium content <800 mg), but not with dairy products alone.

Dairy products, calcium-fortified juices, oral multivitamins, and mineral supplements: Absorption of ciprofloxacin is decreased by divalent and trivalent cations. The manufacturer states that the usual dietary intake of calcium (including meals which include dairy products) has not been shown to interfere with ciprofloxacin absorption. Immediate release ciprofloxacin and Cipro XR may be taken 2 hours before or 6 hours after any of these products.

Caffeine: Patients consuming regular large quantities of caffeinated beverages may need to restrict caffeine intake if excessive cardiac or CNS stimulation occurs.

Ciprofloxacin (Ophthalmic)
(sip roe FLOKS a sin)

Brand Names: U.S. Ciloxan

Index Terms Ciprofloxacin Hydrochloride

Pharmacologic Category Antibiotic, Fluoroquinolone; Antibiotic, Ophthalmic

Medication Safety Issues

Sound-alike/look-alike issues:

Ciprofloxacin may be confused with cephalexin

Ciloxan® may be confused with Cytoxan

Pregnancy Risk Factor C

Lactation Use caution

Use Treatment of superficial ocular infections (corneal ulcers, conjunctivitis) due to susceptible strains

Available Dosage Forms

Ointment, Ophthalmic:

Ciloxan: 0.3% (3.5 g)

Solution, Ophthalmic:

Ciloxan: 0.3% (5 mL)

Generic: 0.3% (2.5 mL, 5 mL, 10 mL)

General Dosage Range Ophthalmic:

Ointment: *Children ≥2 years and Adults:* Apply a ¹/₂ inch ribbon into the conjunctival sac 3 times/day for the first 2 days, followed by a ¹/₂ inch ribbon applied twice daily

Solution: *Children ≥1 year and Adults:* Conjunctivitis: Instill 1-2 drops into the conjunctival sac every 2 hours while awake for 2 days, then 1-2 drops every 4 hours while awake; Corneal ulcer: Instill 2 drops into affected eye every 15 minutes for the first 6 hours, then 2 drops every 30 minutes for the remainder of the first day; on day 2 instill 2 drops into the affected eye hourly; on days 3-14 instill 2 drops every 4 hours

Administration

Other For topical ophthalmic use only; avoid touching tip of applicator to eye or other surfaces.

Nursing Actions

Patient Education

• Discuss specific use of drug and side effects with patient as it relates to treatment. (HCAHPS: During this hospital stay, were you given any medicine that you had not taken before? Before giving you any new medicine, how often did hospital staff tell you what the medicine was for? How often did hospital staff describe possible side effects in a way you could understand?)

• Patient may experience subconjunctival hemorrhage, crusting of eyelid, short-term pain, or parageusia. Have patient report immediately to prescriber sudden vision changes, ophthalmalgia, severe eye irritation, eyelid edema, or crystalline eye deposits (HCAHPS).

• Educate patient about signs of a significant reaction (eg, wheezing; chest tightness; fever; itching; bad cough; blue skin color; seizures; or swelling of face, lips, tongue, or throat). **Note:** This is not a comprehensive list of all side effects. Patient should consult prescriber for additional questions.

Intended Use and Disclaimer: Should not be printed and given to patients. This information is intended to serve as a concise initial reference for healthcare professionals to use when discussing medications with a patient. You must ultimately rely on your own discretion, experience and judgment in diagnosing, treating and advising patients.

Ciprofloxacin (Otic) (sip roe FLOKS a sin)

Brand Names: U.S. Cetraxal

Index Terms Ciprofloxacin Hydrochloride

Pharmacologic Category Antibiotic, Fluoroquinolone; Antibiotic, Otic

Medication Safety Issues

Sound-alike/look-alike issues:

Cetraxal® may be confused with cefTRIAXone

Ciprofloxacin may be confused with cephalexin

Pregnancy Risk Factor C

Lactation Excretion unknown/Not recommended

Use Treatment of acute otitis externa due to susceptible strains of *Pseudomonas aeruginosa* or *Staphylococcus aureus*

Available Dosage Forms

Solution, Otic [preservative free]:

Cetraxal: 0.2% (1 ea)

Generic: 0.2% (1 ea)

General Dosage Range Otic: *Children ≥1 year and Adults:* 0.5 mg (0.25 mL) every 12 hours

Administration

Other For otic use only. Prior to use, warm solution by holding container in hands for at least 1 minute. Patient should lie down with affected ear upward and medication instilled. Patients should remain in the position for at least 1 minute to allow penetration of solution.

Nursing Actions

Patient Education

• Discuss specific use of drug and side effects with patient as it relates to treatment. (HCAHPS: During this hospital stay, were you given any medicine that you had not taken before? Before giving you any new medicine, how often did hospital staff tell you what the medicine was for? How often did hospital staff describe possible side effects in a way you could understand?)

• Patient may experience headache or short-term pain. Have patient report immediately to prescriber severe otalgia or significant ear irritation (HCAHPS).

• Educate patient about signs of a significant reaction (eg, wheezing; chest tightness; fever; itching; bad cough; blue skin color; seizures; or swelling of face, lips, tongue, or throat). **Note:** This is not a comprehensive list of all side effects. Patient should consult prescriber for additional questions.

Intended Use and Disclaimer: Should not be printed and given to patients. This information is intended to serve as a concise initial reference for healthcare professionals to use when discussing medications with a patient. You must ultimately rely on your own discretion, experience and judgment in diagnosing, treating and advising patients.

Ciprofloxacin and Dexamethasone
(sip roe FLOKS a sin & deks a METH a sone)

Brand Names: U.S. Ciprodex®
Index Terms Ciprofloxacin Hydrochloride and Dexamethasone; Dexamethasone and Ciprofloxacin
Pharmacologic Category Antibiotic, Otic; Antibiotic/Corticosteroid, Otic; Corticosteroid, Otic
Pregnancy Risk Factor C
Lactation Excretion in breast milk unknown/not recommended
Use Treatment of acute otitis media in pediatric patients with tympanostomy tubes or acute otitis externa in children and adults
Available Dosage Forms
Suspension, otic:
Ciprodex®: Ciprofloxacin 0.3% and dexamethasone 0.1% (7.5 mL)
General Dosage Range Otic: *Children and Adults:* Instill 4 drops into affected ear(s) twice daily
Administration
Other Otic: Prior to instillation, bottle should be warmed in hands for 1-2 minutes. Shake suspension well immediately before using. Patient should lie with affected ear upward and remain in this position for 60 seconds following application. Drops should be instilled directly into tympanostomy tube (if present) and tragus should be pumped 5 times to facilitate penetration into the middle ear.
Nursing Actions
Physical Assessment See individual agents.
Patient Education
• Discuss specific use of drug and side effects with patient as it relates to treatment. (HCAHPS: During this hospital stay, were you given any medicine that you had not taken before? Before giving you any new medicine, how often did hospital staff tell you what the medicine was for? How often did hospital staff describe possible side effects in a way you could understand?)
• Patient may experience otalgia. Have patient report immediately to prescriber severe ear irritation or hearing impairment (HCAHPS).
• Educate patient about signs of a significant reaction (eg, wheezing; chest tightness; fever; itching; bad cough; blue skin color; seizures; or swelling of face, lips, tongue, or throat). **Note:** This is not a comprehensive list of all side effects. Patient should consult prescriber for additional questions.

Intended Use and Disclaimer: Should not be printed and given to patients. This information is intended to serve as a concise initial reference for healthcare professionals to use when discussing medications with a patient. You must ultimately rely on your own discretion, experience and judgment in diagnosing, treating and advising patients.

Related Information
Ciprofloxacin (Otic) *on page 325*

Ciprofloxacin and Hydrocortisone
(sip roe FLOKS a sin & hye droe KOR ti sone)

Brand Names: U.S. Cipro® HC
Index Terms Ciprofloxacin Hydrochloride and Hydrocortisone; Hydrocortisone and Ciprofloxacin
Pharmacologic Category Antibiotic/Corticosteroid, Otic
Pregnancy Risk Factor C
Lactation Excretion in breast milk unknown/not recommended
Use Treatment of acute otitis externa, sometimes known as "swimmer's ear"
Available Dosage Forms
Suspension, otic:
Cipro® HC: Ciprofloxacin 0.2% and hydrocortisone 1% (10 mL)
General Dosage Range Otic: *Children >1 year and Adults:* 3 drops into affected ear(s) twice daily
Nursing Actions
Physical Assessment See individual agents.
Patient Education
• Discuss specific use of drug and side effects with patient as it relates to treatment. (HCAHPS: During this hospital stay, were you given any medicine that you had not taken before? Before giving you any new medicine, how often did hospital staff tell you what the medicine was for? How often did hospital staff describe possible side effects in a way you could understand?)
• Have patient report immediately to prescriber severe ear irritation (HCAHPS).
• Educate patient about signs of a significant reaction (eg, wheezing; chest tightness; fever; itching; bad cough; blue skin color; seizures; or swelling of face, lips, tongue, or throat). **Note:** This is not a comprehensive list of all side effects. Patient should consult prescriber for additional questions.

Intended Use and Disclaimer: Should not be printed and given to patients. This information is intended to serve as a concise initial reference for healthcare professionals to use when discussing medications with a patient. You must ultimately rely on your own discretion, experience and judgment in diagnosing, treating and advising patients.

Related Information
Ciprofloxacin (Otic) *on page 325*

Cisapride (SIS a pride)

Brand Names: U.S. Propulsid®
Pharmacologic Category Gastrointestinal Agent, Prokinetic

Medication Safety Issues

Sound-alike/look-alike issues:
Propulsid® may be confused with propranolol

Medication Guide Available Yes

Pregnancy Risk Factor C

Lactation Enters breast milk/use caution

Use Treatment of nocturnal symptoms of gastroesophageal reflux disease (GERD); has demonstrated effectiveness for gastroparesis, refractory constipation, and nonulcer dyspepsia

General Dosage Range

Oral:
Children: 0.15-0.3 mg/kg 3-4 times/day (maximum: 10 mg/dose)
Adults: Initial: 5-10 mg 4 times/day, may increase to 20 mg 4 times/day if needed

Nursing Actions

Physical Assessment Cardiac status must be evaluated prior to therapy (12-lead ECG). Monitor ECG, electrolyte balance, and renal function. Monitor for tachycardia, fatigue, diarrhea, and other abdominal symptoms.

Patient Education

• Discuss specific use of drug and side effects with patient as it relates to treatment. (HCAHPS: During this hospital stay, were you given any medicine that you had not taken before? Before giving you any new medicine, how often did hospital staff tell you what the medicine was for? How often did hospital staff describe possible side effects in a way you could understand?)

• Patient may experience headache or dyspepsia. Have patient report immediately to prescriber tachycardia, severe dizziness, syncope, or significant diarrhea (HCAHPS).

• Educate patient about signs of a significant reaction (eg, wheezing; chest tightness; fever; itching; bad cough; blue skin color; seizures; or swelling of face, lips, tongue, or throat). **Note:** This is not a comprehensive list of all side effects. Patient should consult prescriber for additional questions.

Intended Use and Disclaimer: Should not be printed and given to patients. This information is intended to serve as a concise initial reference for healthcare professionals to use when discussing medications with a patient. You must ultimately rely on your own discretion, experience and judgment in diagnosing, treating and advising patients.

Cisatracurium (sis a tra KYOO ree um)

Brand Names: U.S. Nimbex
Index Terms Cisatracurium Besylate
Pharmacologic Category Neuromuscular Blocker Agent, Nondepolarizing

Medication Safety Issues

Sound-alike/look-alike issues:
Nimbex may be confused with NovoLOG

High alert medication:
The Institute for Safe Medication Practices (ISMP) includes this medication among its list of drugs which have a heightened risk of causing significant patient harm when used in error.

Other safety concerns:
United States Pharmacopeia (USP) 2006: The Interdisciplinary Safe Medication Use Expert Committee of the USP has recommended the following:
- Hospitals, clinics, and other practice sites should institute special safeguards in the storage, labeling, and use of these agents and should include these safeguards in staff orientation and competency training.
- Healthcare professionals should be on high alert (especially vigilant) whenever a neuromuscular-blocking agent (NMBA) is stocked, ordered, prepared, or administered.

Pregnancy Risk Factor B

Lactation Excretion in breast milk unknown/use caution

Breast-Feeding Considerations It is not known if cisatracurium is excreted in breast milk. The manufacturer recommends that caution be exercised when administering cisatracurium to nursing women.

Use Adjunct to general anesthesia to facilitate endotracheal intubation and to relax skeletal muscles during surgery; to facilitate mechanical ventilation in ICU patients; does not relieve pain or produce sedation

Mechanism of Action/Effect Blocks neural transmission at the myoneural junction by binding with cholinergic receptor sites

Contraindications Hypersensitivity to cisatracurium besylate or any component of the formulation; use of the 10 mL multiple-dose vials in premature infants (formulation contains benzyl alcohol)

Warnings/Precautions Maintenance of an adequate airway and respiratory support is critical; certain clinical conditions may result in potentiation or antagonism of neuromuscular blockade:
Potentiation: Electrolyte abnormalities, severe hyponatremia, severe hypocalcemia, severe hypokalemia, hypermagnesemia, neuromuscular diseases, acidosis, acute intermittent porphyria, renal failure, hepatic failure
Antagonism: Alkalosis, hypercalcemia, demyelinating lesions, peripheral neuropathies, diabetes mellitus

Hypothermia may slow Hoffmann elimination thereby prolonging the duration of activity (Greenberg, 2013). Increased sensitivity in patients with myasthenia gravis, Eaton-Lambert syndrome; resistance in burn patients (>30% of body) for period of 5-70 days postinjury; resistance in patients with muscle trauma, denervation, immobilization, infection. Cross-sensitivity with other neuromuscular-blocking agents may occur; use extreme caution in patients with previous anaphylactic reactions to other neuromuscular-blocking agents. Bradycardia may be more common with cisatracurium than with other neuromuscular blocking agents since it has no clinically significant effects on heart rate to counteract the bradycardia produced by anesthetics. Use caution in the elderly. Should be administered by adequately trained individuals familiar with its use. Some dosage forms may contain benzyl alcohol which has been associated with "gasping syndrome" in neonates.

Drug Interactions

Avoid Concomitant Use

Avoid concomitant use of Cisatracurium with any of the following: QuiNINE

Decreased Effect

The levels/effects of Cisatracurium may be decreased by: Acetylcholinesterase Inhibitors; Fosphenytoin-Phenytoin; Loop Diuretics

Increased Effect/Toxicity

Cisatracurium may increase the levels/effects of: Cardiac Glycosides; Corticosteroids (Systemic); OnabotulinumtoxinA; RimabotulinumtoxinB

The levels/effects of Cisatracurium may be increased by: AbobotulinumtoxinA; Aminoglycosides; Calcium Channel Blockers; Capreomycin; Colistimethate; CycloSPORINE (Systemic); Fosphenytoin-Phenytoin; Inhalational Anesthetics; Ketorolac (Nasal); Ketorolac (Systemic); Lincosamide Antibiotics; Lithium; Loop Diuretics; Magnesium Salts; Polymyxin B; Procainamide; QuiNIDine; QuiNINE; Spironolactone; Tetracycline Derivatives; Vancomycin

Pharmacodynamics/Kinetics

Onset of Action I.V.: 2-3 minutes; Peak effect: 3-5 minutes

Duration of Action Recovery begins in 20-35 minutes when anesthesia is balanced; recovery is attained in 90% of patients in 25-93 minutes

Available Dosage Forms

Solution, Intravenous:
Nimbex: 10 mg/5 mL (5 mL); 20 mg/10 mL (10 mL); 10 mg/mL (20 mL)
Generic: 20 mg/10 mL (10 mL)

Solution, Intravenous [preservative free]:
Generic: 10 mg/5 mL (5 mL); 10 mg/mL (20 mL)

General Dosage Range I.V.:

Children 1-23 months: Intubating dose: 0.15 mg/kg
Children 2-12 years: Intubating dose: 0.1-0.15 mg/kg over 5-10 seconds; Infusion: Initial: 3 mcg/kg/minute; Maintenance: 1-2 mcg/kg/minute (surgery) or 0.5-10 mcg/kg/minute (ICU)
Children >12 years: Infusion: Initial: 3 mcg/kg/minute; Maintenance: 1-2 mcg/kg/minute (surgery) or 0.5-10 mcg/kg/minute (ICU)

Adults: Intubating dose: 0.1-0.2 mg/kg; Infusion: Initial: 3 mcg/kg/minute; Maintenance: 1-2 mcg/kg/minute (surgery) or 0.5-10 mcg/kg/minute (ICU)

Usual Infusion Concentrations: Adult I.V. infusion: 100 mg in 250 mL (total volume) (concentration: 400 mcg/mL) of D5W or NS

Administration

I.M. Do not administer I.M. (excessive tissue irritation).

I.V. Administer I.V. only; give undiluted as a bolus injection over 5-10 seconds. Continuous administration requires the use of an infusion pump. The use of a peripheral nerve stimulator will permit the most advantageous use of cisatracurium, minimize the possibility of overdosage or underdosage and assist in the evaluation of recovery.

Storage/Stability Refrigerate intact vials at 2°C to 8°C (36°F to 46°F). Use vials within 21 days upon removal from the refrigerator to room temperature of 25°C (77°F). Per the manufacturer, dilutions of 0.1 mg/mL in 0.9% sodium chloride (NS), dextrose 5% in water (D5W), or D5NS are stable for up to 24 hours at room temperature or under refrigeration; dilutions of 0.1-0.2 mg/mL in D5LR are stable for up to 24 hours in the refrigerator. *Additional stability data:* Dilutions of 0.1, 2, and 5 mg/mL in D5W or NS are stable in the refrigerator for up to 30 days; at room temperature (23°C), dilutions of 0.1 and 2 mg/mL began exhibiting substantial drug loss between 7-14 days; dilutions of 5 mg/mL in D5W or NS are stable for up to 30 days at room temperature (23°C) (Xu, 1998). Usual concentration: 0.1-0.4 mg/mL.

Nursing Actions

Physical Assessment Ventilatory support must be instituted and maintained until adequate respiratory muscle function and/or airway protection are assured. This drug is not an anesthetic or analgesic; pain must be treated with other agents. Continuous monitoring of vital signs, cardiac status, respiratory status, and degree of neuromuscular block (objective assessment with peripheral external nerve stimulator) is mandatory during infusion and until full muscle tone has returned. **Note:** It may take longer for return of muscle tone in obese or elderly patients or patients with renal or hepatic disease, myasthenia gravis, myopathy, other neuromuscular disease, dehydration, electrolyte imbalance, or severe acid/base imbalance.

Long-term use: Monitor level of neuromuscular blockade, skeletal muscle movement, and respiratory effort. Reposition patient and provide appropriate skin care, mouth care, and care of patient's eyes every 2-3 hours while sedated. Provide appropriate emotional and sensory support (auditory and environmental).

Patient Education

- Discuss specific use of drug and side effects with patient as it relates to treatment. (HCAHPS: During this hospital stay, were you given any medicine that you had not taken before? Before giving you any new medicine, how often did hospital staff tell you what the medicine was for? How often did hospital staff describe possible side effects in a way you could understand?)
- Have patient report immediately to prescriber bradycardia, severe dizziness, syncope, or flushing (HCAHPS).
- Educate patient about signs of a significant reaction (eg, wheezing; chest tightness; fever; itching; bad cough; blue skin color; seizures; or swelling of face, lips, tongue, or throat). **Note:** This is not a comprehensive list of all side effects. Patient should consult prescriber for additional questions.

Intended Use and Disclaimer: Should not be printed and given to patients. This information is intended to serve as a concise initial reference for healthcare professionals to use when discussing medications with a patient. You must ultimately rely on your own discretion, experience and judgment in diagnosing, treating and advising patients.

CISplatin (SIS pla tin)

Index Terms CDDP; cis-DDP; cis-Diamminedichloroplatinum; Platinol; Platinol-AQ

Pharmacologic Category Antineoplastic Agent, Alkylating Agent; Antineoplastic Agent, Platinum Analog

Medication Safety Issues

Sound-alike/look-alike issues:

CISplatin may be confused with CARBOplatin, oxaliplatin

High alert medication:

This medication is in a class the Institute for Safe Medication Practices (ISMP) includes among its list of drug classes which have a heightened risk of causing significant patient harm when used in error.

BEERS Criteria medication:

This drug may be potentially inappropriate for use in geriatric patients (Quality of evidence - moderate; Strength of recommendation - strong).

Administration issues:

Doses >100 mg/m^2 once every 3-4 weeks are rarely used and should be verified with the prescriber.

Pregnancy Risk Factor D

Lactation Enters breast milk/not recommended

Breast-Feeding Considerations Cisplatin is excreted in breast milk. Per the manufacturer, breast-feeding is not recommended.

Use Treatment of advanced bladder cancer, metastatic testicular cancer, and metastatic ovarian cancer

Unlabeled Use Treatment of breast cancer (metastatic), central nervous system tumors, cervical cancer, endometrial cancer, esophageal cancer, gastric cancer, germ cell tumors, gestational trophoblastic disease (refractory), head and neck cancer, hepatobiliary cancer, hepatoblastoma, Hodgkin lymphoma, malignant pleural mesothelioma, melanoma (metastatic), multiple myeloma, neuroblastoma, neuroendocrine tumors, non-Hodgkin lymphoma (NHL), nonsmall cell lung cancer (NSCLC), osteosarcoma, pancreatic cancer (advanced), prostate cancer, small cell lung cancer (SCLC), soft tissue sarcomas, and unknown primary cancers

Mechanism of Action/Effect Inhibits DNA synthesis

Contraindications Hypersensitivity to cisplatin, other platinum-containing compounds, or any component of the formulation (anaphylactic-like reactions have been reported); pre-existing renal impairment; myelosuppression; hearing impairment

Warnings/Precautions Hazardous agent - use appropriate precautions for handling and disposal (NIOSH, 2012). **[U.S. Boxed Warning]: Doses >100 mg/m^2 once every 3-4 weeks are rarely used; verify with the prescriber. Exercise caution to avoid potential sound-alike/look-alike confusion between CISplatin and CARBOplatin.** Patients should receive adequate hydration, with or without diuretics, prior to and for 24 hours after cisplatin administration. **[U.S. Boxed Warning]: Cumulative renal toxicity may be severe.** Monitor serum creatinine, blood urea nitrogen, creatinine clearance, and serum electrolytes closely. According to the manufacturer's labeling, use is contraindicated in patients with pre-existing renal impairment and renal function must return to normal prior to administering subsequent cycles; some literature recommends reduced doses with renal impairment. Nephrotoxicity may be potentiated by aminoglycosides.

Use caution in the elderly; may cause or exacerbate syndrome of inappropriate antidiuretic hormone secretion or hyponatremia; monitor sodium closely with initiation or dosage adjustments in older adults (Beers Criteria). Elderly patients may be more susceptible to nephrotoxicity and peripheral neuropathy; select dose cautiously and monitor closely.

[U.S. Boxed Warning]: Dose-related toxicities include myelosuppression, nausea, and vomiting. Nausea and vomiting may be immediate and/or delayed; antiemetics are recommended. Diarrhea may also occur. **[U.S. Boxed Warning]: Ototoxicity, especially pronounced in children, is manifested by tinnitus or loss of high**

frequency hearing and occasionally, deafness; may be significant. Pediatric patients with certain genetic variations in the thiopurine S-methyltransferase (TPMT) gene may be at increased risk of ototoxicity, even when conventional cisplatin doses are given. Ototoxicity is cumulative; audiometric testing should be performed at baseline and prior to each dose. Pediatric patients should receive audiometric testing for several years after discontinuing therapy. Severe (and possibly irreversible) neuropathies may occur with higher than recommended doses or more frequent administration; may require therapy discontinuation. Seizures, loss of motor function, loss of taste, leukoencephalopathy, and posterior reversible leukoencephalopathy syndrome (PRES [formerly RPLS]) have also been described. Serum electrolytes, particularly magnesium and potassium, should be monitored and replaced as needed during and after cisplatin therapy.

[U.S. Boxed Warning]: Anaphylactic-like reactions have been reported; may include facial edema, bronchoconstriction, tachycardia, and hypotension and may occur within minutes of administration; may be managed with epinephrine, corticosteroids, and/or antihistamines. Hyperuricemia has been reported with cisplatin use, and is more pronounced with doses >50 mg/m², consider allopurinol therapy to reduce uric acid levels. Local infusion site reactions may occur; monitor infusion site during administration; avoid extravasation. Secondary malignancies have been reported with cisplatin in combination with other chemotherapy agents. **[U.S. Boxed Warning]: Should be administered under the supervision of an experienced cancer chemotherapy physician.** Cisplatin is a vesicant at higher concentrations, and an irritant at lower concentrations; ensure proper needle or catheter placement prior to and during infusion; avoid extravasation.

Drug Interactions

Avoid Concomitant Use

Avoid concomitant use of CISplatin with any of the following: BCG; CloZAPine; Natalizumab; Pimecrolimus; Tacrolimus (Topical); Tofacitinib; Vaccines (Live)

Decreased Effect

CISplatin may decrease the levels/effects of: BCG; Coccidioidin Skin Test; Fosphenytoin-Phenytoin; Sipuleucel-T; Vaccines (Inactivated); Vaccines (Live)

The levels/effects of CISplatin may be decreased by: Echinacea

Increased Effect/Toxicity

CISplatin may increase the levels/effects of: Aminoglycosides; CloZAPine; Leflunomide; Natalizumab; Taxane Derivatives; Tofacitinib; Topotecan; Vaccines (Live); Vinorelbine

The levels/effects of CISplatin may be increased by: Denosumab; Loop Diuretics; Pimecrolimus; Roflumilast; Tacrolimus (Topical); Trastuzumab

Adverse Reactions

>10%:

Central nervous system: Neurotoxicity: Peripheral neuropathy is dose- and duration-dependent.

Gastrointestinal: Nausea and vomiting (76% to 100%)

Hematologic: Anemia (≤40%), leukopenia (25% to 30%; nadir: Day 18-23; recovery: By day 39; dose related), thrombocytopenia (25% to 30%; nadir: Day 18-23; recovery: By day 39; dose related)

Hepatic: Liver enzymes increased

Renal: Nephrotoxicity (28% to 36%; acute renal failure and chronic renal insufficiency)

Otic: Ototoxicity (children 40% to 60%; adults 10% to 31%; as tinnitus, high frequency hearing loss)

1% to 10%: Local: Tissue irritation

Available Dosage Forms

Solution, Intravenous:

Generic: 50 mg/50 mL (50 mL); 100 mg/100 mL (100 mL)

Solution, Intravenous [preservative free]:

Generic: 50 mg/50 mL (50 mL); 100 mg/100 mL (100 mL); 200 mg/200 mL (200 mL)

General Dosage Range Dosage adjustment recommended in patients with renal impairment

I.V.: *Adults:* 50-70 mg/m² every 3-4 weeks **or** 75-100 mg/m²/day every 3-4 weeks **or** 20 mg/m²/day for 5 days every 3 weeks

Administration

I.V. Pretreatment hydration with 1-2 L of fluid is recommended prior to cisplatin administration; adequate post hydration and urinary output (>100 mL/hour) should be maintained for 24 hours after administration.

I.V.: Infuse over 6-8 hours; has also been infused (unlabeled rates) over 30 minutes to 3 hours, at a rate of 1 mg/minute, or as a continuous infusion; infusion rate varies by protocol (refer to specific protocol for infusion details). Avoid extravasation.

Needles or I.V. administration sets that contain aluminum should not be used in the preparation or administration; aluminum may react with cisplatin resulting in precipitate formation and loss of potency.

Vesicant (at higher concentrations); ensure proper needle or catheter placement prior to and during infusion; avoid extravasation.

Extravasation management: If extravasation occurs, stop infusion immediately and disconnect (leave cannula/needle in place); gently aspirate extravasated solution (do **NOT** flush the line); initiate sodium thiosulfate antidote; elevate extremity.

Sodium thiosulfate 1/6 M solution: Inject 2 mL into existing I.V. line for each 100 mg of cisplatin extravasated; then consider also injecting 1 mL as 0.1 mL subcutaneous injections (clockwise) around the area of extravasation, may repeat subcutaneous injections several times over the next 3-4 hours (Ener, 2004).

Dimethyl sulfoxide (DMSO) may also be considered an option: Apply to a region covering twice the affected area every 8 hours for 7 days; begin within 10 minutes of extravasation; do not cover with a dressing (Perez Fidalgo, 2012).

Hazardous agent; use appropriate precautions for handling and disposal (NIOSH, 2012).

Injectable Detail pH: 3.7-6 (aqueous injection)

Preparation for Administration Hazardous agent; use appropriate precautions for handling and disposal (NIOSH, 2012). The infusion solution should have a final sodium chloride concentration ≥0.2%. Needles or I.V. administration sets that contain aluminum should not be used in the preparation or administration; aluminum can react with cisplatin resulting in precipitate formation and loss of potency.

Storage/Stability Store intact vials at room temperature 15°C to 25°C (59°F to 77°F). Protect from light. Do not refrigerate solution as a precipitate may form. Further dilution **stability is dependent on the chloride ion concentration** and should be mixed in solutions of NS (at least 0.3% NaCl). After initial entry into the vial, solution is stable for 28 days protected from light or for at least 7 days under fluorescent room light at room temperature. Further dilutions in NS, D_5/0.45% NaCl or D_5/NS to a concentration of 0.05-2 mg/mL are stable for 72 hours at 4°C to 25°C. The infusion solution should have a final sodium chloride concentration ≥0.2%.

Nursing Actions

Physical Assessment Verify any dose exceeding 100 mg/m^2 per course. Watch infusion site closely for any signs of malfunction or potential loss of access. Patient should be vigorously hydrated prior to and for 24 hours following infusion. Teach patient importance of adequate hydration and how to handle if significant nausea and vomiting occur. Assess adequacy of urine output, hearing, nausea, and vomiting after last infusion with relation to antiemetic use. Anaphylaxis-like reaction is possible; emergency equipment and medication should be readily available. Replacement of magnesium and potassium may be needed during therapy.

Patient Education

- Discuss specific use of drug and side effects with patient as it relates to treatment. (HCAHPS: During this hospital stay, were you given any medicine that you had not taken before? Before giving you any new medicine, how often did hospital staff tell you what the medicine was for? How often did hospital staff describe possible side effects in a way you could understand?)
- Patient may experience lack of appetite. Have patient report immediately to prescriber signs of infection, signs of hepatic impairment, severe dyspepsia, dyspnea, significant nausea, considerable diarrhea, hearing impairment, tinnitus, ecchymosis, hemorrhaging, urinary retention, oliguria, intolerable asthenia, hematuria, melena, paresthesia, angina, severe dizziness, syncope, tachycardia, arrhythmia, arthralgia, dysgeusia, strength differences from one side to another, difficulty speaking or thinking, change in balance, blurred eyesight, mood changes, myalgia, back pain, considerable headache, difficulty with motor activity, vision changes, or injection site irritation (HCAHPS).
- Educate patient about signs of a significant reaction (eg, wheezing; chest tightness; fever; itching; bad cough; blue skin color; seizures; or swelling of face, lips, tongue, or throat). **Note:** This is not a comprehensive list of all side effects. Patient should consult prescriber for additional questions.

Intended Use and Disclaimer: Should not be printed and given to patients. This information is intended to serve as a concise initial reference for healthcare professionals to use when discussing medications with a patient. You must ultimately rely on your own discretion, experience and judgment in diagnosing, treating and advising patients.

Dietary Considerations Some products may contain sodium.

Related Information
Management of Drug Extravasations *on page 1700*

Citalopram (sye TAL oh pram)

Brand Names: U.S. CeleXA

Index Terms Citalopram Hydrobromide; Nitalapram

Pharmacologic Category Antidepressant, Selective Serotonin Reuptake Inhibitor

Medication Safety Issues

Sound-alike/look-alike issues:
CeleXA® may be confused with CeleBREX®, Cerebyx®, Ranexa™, ZyPREXA®

BEERS Criteria medication:
This drug may be potentially inappropriate for use in geriatric patients (Quality of evidence - moderate; Strength of recommendation - strong).

Medication Guide Available Yes

Pregnancy Risk Factor C

Lactation Enters breast milk/consider risk:benefit

Breast-Feeding Considerations Citalopram and its metabolites are excreted in breast milk. According to the manufacturer, the decision to continue or discontinue breast-feeding during therapy should take into account the risk of exposure to the infant and the benefits of treatment to the mother. Excessive somnolence, decreased feeding, colic, irritability, restlessness, and weight loss have been reported in breast-fed infants. The long-term effects on development and behavior have not been studied; therefore, citalopram should be prescribed to a mother who is breast-feeding only when the benefits outweigh the potential risks. Maternal use of an SSRI during pregnancy may cause delayed milk secretion.

Use Treatment of depression

Unlabeled Use Obsessive-compulsive disorder (OCD)

Mechanism of Action/Effect A bicyclic phthalane derivative, citalopram selectively inhibits serotonin reuptake in the presynaptic neurons thus increasing serotonergic activity in the brain.

Contraindications Hypersensitivity to citalopram or any component of the formulation; use of MAO inhibitors intended to treat psychiatric disorders (concurrently or within 14 days of discontinuing either citalopram or the MAO inhibitor); initiation of citalopram in a patient receiving linezolid or intravenous methylene blue; concomitant use with pimozide

Warnings/Precautions [U.S. Boxed Warning]: Antidepressants increase the risk of suicidal thinking and behavior in children, adolescents, and young adults (18-24 years of age) with major depressive disorder (MDD) and other psychiatric disorders; consider risk prior to prescribing. Short-term studies did not show an increased risk in patients >24 years of age and showed a decreased risk in patients ≥65 years. Closely monitor patients for clinical worsening, suicidality, or unusual changes in behavior, particularly during the initial 1-2 months of therapy or during periods of dosage adjustments (increases or decreases); the patient's family or caregiver should be instructed to closely observe the patient and communicate condition with healthcare provider. A medication guide concerning the use of antidepressants should be dispensed with each prescription. **Citalopram is not FDA approved for use in children.**

The possibility of a suicide attempt is inherent in major depression and may persist until remission occurs. Use caution in high-risk patients. Worsening depression and severe abrupt suicidality that are not part of the presenting symptoms may require discontinuation or modification of drug therapy. The patient's family or caregiver should be alerted to monitor patients for the emergence of suicidality and associated behaviors (such as agitation, irritability, hostility, impulsivity, and hypomania) and call healthcare provider.

May worsen psychosis in some patients or precipitate a shift to mania or hypomania in patients with bipolar disorder. Patients presenting with depressive symptoms should be screened for bipolar disorder. Monotherapy in patients with bipolar disorder should be avoided. **Citalopram is not FDA approved for the treatment of bipolar depression.**

Potentially life-threatening serotonin syndrome (SS) has occurred with serotonergic agents (eg, SSRIs, SNRIs), particularly when used in combination with other serotonergic agents (eg, triptans, TCAs, fentanyl, lithium, tramadol, buspirone, St John's wort, tryptophan) or agents that impair metabolism of serotonin (eg, MAO inhibitors intended to treat psychiatric disorders, other MAO inhibitors [ie, linezolid and intravenous methylene blue]). Discontinue treatment (and any concomitant serotonergic agent) immediately if signs/symptoms arise. May increase the risks associated with electroconvulsive therapy. Has a low potential to impair cognitive or motor performance; caution operating hazardous machinery or driving. Bone fractures have been associated with antidepressant treatment. Consider the possibility of a fragility fracture if an antidepressant-treated patient presents with unexplained bone pain, point tenderness, swelling, or bruising (Rabenda, 2013; Rizzoli, 2012).

Citalopram causes dose-dependent QT_c prolongation; torsade de pointes, ventricular tachycardia, and sudden death have been reported. Use is not recommended in patients with congenital long QT syndrome, bradycardia, recent MI, uncompensated heart failure, hypokalemia, and/or hypomagnesemia, or patients receiving concomitant medications which prolong the QT interval; if use is essential and cannot be avoided in these patients, ECG monitoring is recommended. Discontinue therapy in any patient with persistent QT_c measurements >500 msec. Serum electrolytes, particularly potassium and magnesium, should be monitored prior to initiation and periodically during therapy in any patient at increased risk for significant electrolyte disturbances; hypokalemia and/or hypomagnesemia should be corrected prior to use. Due to the QT prolongation risk, doses >40 mg/day are not recommended. Additionally, the maximum daily dose should not exceed 20 mg/day in certain populations (eg, CYP2C19 poor metabolizers, patients with hepatic impairment, elderly patients). Potentially significant interactions may exist, requiring dose or frequency adjustment, additional monitoring, and/or selection of alternative therapy. Consult drug interactions database for more detailed information.

Use with caution in patients with a previous seizure disorder or condition predisposing to seizures such as brain damage or alcoholism. May cause or exacerbate sexual dysfunction. May cause hyponatremia/SIADH (elderly at increased risk); volume depletion and diuretics may increase risk. Monitor sodium closely with initiation or dosage adjustments in older adults (Beers Criteria). Citalopram is not FDA-approved for use in children; however, if used, monitor weight and growth regularly during therapy due to the potential for decreased appetite and weight loss with SSRI use.

Abrupt discontinuation or interruption of antidepressant therapy has been associated with a discontinuation syndrome. Symptoms arising may vary with antidepressant however commonly include nausea, vomiting, diarrhea, headaches, light-headedness, dizziness, diminished appetite, sweating, chills, tremors, paresthesias, fatigue, somnolence, and sleep disturbances (eg, vivid dreams, insomnia). Greater risks for developing a discontinuation syndrome have been associated with antidepressants with shorter half-lives, longer durations of treatment, and abrupt discontinuation. For antidepressants of short or intermediate half-lives, symptoms may emerge within 2-5 days after treatment discontinuation and last 7-14 days (APA, 2010; Fava, 2006; Haddad, 2001; Shelton, 2001; Warner, 2006).

Drug Interactions

Avoid Concomitant Use
Avoid concomitant use of Citalopram with any of the following: Conivaptan; Dosulepin; Fluconazole; Fusidic Acid (Systemic); Highest Risk QTc-Prolonging Agents; Iobenguane I 123; Ivabradine; Linezolid; MAO Inhibitors; Methylene Blue; Mifepristone; Moderate Risk QTc-Prolonging Agents; Pimozide; Tryptophan; Urokinase

Decreased Effect
Citalopram may decrease the levels/effects of: Iobenguane I 123; Ioflupane I 123; Thyroid Products

The levels/effects of Citalopram may be decreased by: Bosentan; CarBAMazepine; CYP2C19 Inducers (Strong); CYP3A4 Inducers (Strong); Cyproheptadine; Dabrafenib; Deferasirox; Mitotane; NSAID (COX-2 Inhibitor); NSAID (Nonselective); Peginterferon Alfa-2b; Rifampin; Tocilizumab

Increased Effect/Toxicity
Citalopram may increase the levels/effects of: Agents with Antiplatelet Properties; Anticoagulants; Antidepressants (Serotonin Reuptake Inhibitor/Antagonist); Antipsychotics; Aspirin; BusPIRone; CarBAMazepine; CloZAPine; Collagenase (Systemic); Dabigatran Etexilate; Desmopressin; Dextromethorphan; Dosulepin; Highest Risk QTc-Prolonging Agents; Hypoglycemic Agents; Ibritumomab; Methadone; Methylene Blue; Metoclopramide; Mexiletine; NSAID (COX-2 Inhibitor); NSAID (Nonselective); Pimozide; RisperiDONE; Rivaroxaban; Salicylates; Serotonin Modulators; Thiazide Diuretics; Thrombolytic Agents; Tositumomab and Iodine I 131 Tositumomab; TraMADol; Tricyclic Antidepressants; Urokinase; Vitamin K Antagonists

The levels/effects of Citalopram may be increased by: Alcohol (Ethyl); Analgesics (Opioid); Antipsychotics; BusPIRone; Cimetidine; CNS Depressants; Cobicistat; Conivaptan; CYP2C19 Inhibitors (Moderate); CYP2C19 Inhibitors (Strong); CYP3A4 Inhibitors (Moderate); CYP3A4 Inhibitors (Strong); Dasatinib; Fluconazole; Fusidic Acid (Systemic); Glucosamine; Herbs (Anticoagulant/Antiplatelet Properties); Ibrutinib; Ivabradine; Ivacaftor; Linezolid; Lithium; Luliconazole; Macrolide Antibiotics; MAO Inhibitors; Metoclopramide; Metyrosine; Mifepristone; Moderate Risk QTc-Prolonging Agents; Multivitamins/Fluoride (with ADE); Multivitamins/Minerals (with ADEK, Folate, Iron); Multivitamins/Minerals (with AE, No Iron); Omega-3 Fatty Acids; Pentosan Polysulfate Sodium; Pentoxifylline; Prostacyclin Analogues; QTc-Prolonging Agents (Indeterminate Risk and Risk Modifying); Simeprevir; Tipranavir; TraMADol; Tricyclic Antidepressants; Tryptophan; Vitamin E

Nutritional/Ethanol Interactions
Ethanol: May increase CNS depression; monitor for increased effects with coadministration. Caution patients about effects.

Herb/Nutraceutical: Avoid valerian, St John's wort, tryptophan, SAMe, kava kava, and gotu kola (may increase CNS depression).

Adverse Reactions
>10%:
Central nervous system: Somnolence (18%; dose related), insomnia (15%; dose related)
Gastrointestinal: Nausea (21%), xerostomia (20%)
Miscellaneous: Diaphoresis (11%; dose related)
1% to 10%:
Cardiovascular: QT prolongation (2%), hypotension (≥1%), orthostatic hypotension (≥1%), tachycardia (≥1%), bradycardia (1%)
Central nervous system: Fatigue (5%; dose related), anxiety (4%), agitation (3%), fever (2%), yawning (2%; dose related), amnesia (≥1%), apathy (≥1%), concentration impaired (≥1%), confusion (≥1%), depression (≥1%), migraine (≥1%), suicide attempt (≥1%)
Dermatologic: Rash (≥1%), pruritus (≥1%)
Endocrine & metabolic: Libido decreased (1% to 4%), dysmenorrhea (3%), amenorrhea (≥1%)
Gastrointestinal: Diarrhea (8%), dyspepsia (5%), anorexia (4%), vomiting (4%), abdominal pain (3%), appetite increased (≥1%), flatulence (≥1%), salivation increased (≥1%), taste perversion (≥1%), weight gain/loss (≥1%)
Genitourinary: Ejaculation disorder (6%), impotence (3%; dose related), polyuria (≥1%)
Neuromuscular & skeletal: Tremor (8%), arthralgia (2%), myalgia (2%), paresthesia (≥1%)
Ocular: Abnormal accommodation (≥1%)
Respiratory: Rhinitis (5%), upper respiratory tract infection (5%), sinusitis (3%), cough (≥1%)

◀ **Pharmacodynamics/Kinetics**
Onset of Action Depression: The onset of action is 1-4 weeks; however, individual response varies greatly and full response may not be seen until 8-12 weeks after initiation of treatment.

Available Dosage Forms
Solution, Oral:
Generic: 10 mg/5 mL (240 mL)
Tablet, Oral:
CeleXA: 10 mg, 20 mg, 40 mg
Generic: 10 mg, 20 mg, 40 mg

General Dosage Range Dosage adjustment recommended in patients with hepatic impairment
Oral:
Adults (<60 years): Initial: 20 mg daily; Maintenance: 40 mg daily; Maximum: 40 mg daily
Adults (≥60 years): Initial: 20 mg/day; Maximum: 20 mg/day

Administration
Oral May be administered without regard to food.

Storage/Stability Store at 25°C (77°F); excursions permitted to 15°C to 30°C (59°F to 86°F). Protect from moisture.

Nursing Actions
Physical Assessment Assess mental status: Mood (depression or mania), signs of clinical worsening, suicide ideation, anxiety, social functioning, sleep pattern, loss of appetite, or any new physical complaint. Assess gastrointestinal tolerance.

Patient Education
• Discuss specific use of drug and side effects with patient as it relates to treatment. (HCAHPS: During this hospital stay, were you given any medicine that you had not taken before? Before giving you any new medicine, how often did hospital staff tell you what the medicine was for? How often did hospital staff describe possible side effects in a way you could understand?)
• Patient may experience dyspepsia, fatigue, xerostomia, lack of appetite, asthenia, sexual dysfunction, insomnia, rhinorrhea, or oscitation. Have patient report immediately to prescriber signs of hyponatremia, signs of depression (ie, suicidal ideation, anxiety, emotional instability, illogical thinking), signs of hemorrhaging, behavioral changes, bradycardia, angina, dyspnea, syncope, vision changes, weight gain or loss, menstrual irregularities, serotonin syndrome (ie, dizziness, agitation, hallucinations, tachycardia, arrhythmia, flushing, tremors, hyperhidrosis, change in balance, severe nausea, significant diarrhea), or priapism (HCAHPS).
• Educate patient about signs of a significant reaction (eg, wheezing; chest tightness; fever; itching; bad cough; blue skin color; seizures; or swelling of face, lips, tongue, or throat). **Note:** This is not a comprehensive list of all side effects. Patient should consult prescriber for additional questions.

Intended Use and Disclaimer: Should not be printed and given to patients. This information is intended to serve as a concise initial reference for healthcare professionals to use when discussing medications with a patient. You must ultimately rely on your own discretion, experience and judgment in diagnosing, treating and advising patients.

Dietary Considerations May be taken without regard to food.

Cladribine (KLA dri been)

Index Terms 2-CdA; 2-Chlorodeoxyadenosine; Leustatin

Pharmacologic Category Antineoplastic Agent, Antimetabolite; Antineoplastic Agent, Antimetabolite (Purine Analog)

Medication Safety Issues
Sound-alike/look-alike issues:
Cladribine may be confused with clevidipine, clofarabine, cytarabine, fludarabine
Leustatin may be confused with lovastatin
High alert medication:
This medication is in a class the Institute for Safe Medication Practices (ISMP) includes among its list of drug classes which have a heightened risk of causing significant patient harm when used in error.

Pregnancy Risk Factor D

Lactation Excretion in breast milk unknown/not recommended

Use Treatment of active hairy cell leukemia

Unlabeled Use Treatment of acute myeloid leukemia (AML), chronic lymphocytic leukemia (CLL), non-Hodgkin's lymphomas (mantle cell), Waldenström's macroglobulinemia, refractory Langerhans cell histiocytosis

Available Dosage Forms
Solution, Intravenous [preservative free]:
Generic: 1 mg/mL (10 mL)

General Dosage Range Dosage adjustment recommended in patients with renal impairment
I.V.: Adults: Continuous infusion: 0.09 mg/kg/day for 7 days

Administration
I.V. Administer as a continuous infusion; may also be administered over 30 minutes or over 2 hours (unlabeled administration rates) depending on indication and/or protocol.

Hazardous agent; use appropriate precautions for handling and disposal (NIOSH, 2012).

Injectable Detail pH: 5.5-8 (solution in vial)

Subcutaneous May also be administered subcutaneously (unlabeled administration route; Laszlo, 2010)

Hazardous agent; use appropriate precautions for handling and disposal (NIOSH, 2012).

Nursing Actions

Physical Assessment Monitor for myelosup-pression, cardiac changes, and renal failure regularly during therapy and following therapy (patients should be considered immunosuppressed for up to 1 year after cladribine therapy).

Patient Education
- Discuss specific use of drug and side effects with patient as it relates to treatment. (HCAHPS: During this hospital stay, were you given any medicine that you had not taken before? Before giving you any new medicine, how often did hospital staff tell you what the medicine was for? How often did hospital staff describe possible side effects in a way you could understand?)
- Patient may experience dizziness, headache, myalgia, or lack of appetite. Have patient report immediately to prescriber signs of infection, signs of renal impairment, tachycardia, arrhythmia, ecchymosis, hemorrhaging, dyspnea, severe nausea, significant diarrhea, urine discoloration, jaundice, considerable skin irritation, intolerable asthenia, severe injection site irritation, or signs of tumor lysis syndrome (TLS) (HCAHPS).
- Educate patient about signs of a significant reaction (eg, wheezing; chest tightness; fever; itching; bad cough; blue skin color; seizures; or swelling of face, lips, tongue, or throat). **Note:** This is not a comprehensive list of all side effects. Patient should consult prescriber for additional questions.

Intended Use and Disclaimer: Should not be printed and given to patients. This information is intended to serve as a concise initial reference for healthcare professionals to use when discussing medications with a patient. You must ultimately rely on your own discretion, experience and judgment in diagnosing, treating and advising patients.

Related Information

Management of Drug Extravasations *on page 1700*

Clarithromycin (kla RITH roe mye sin)

Brand Names: U.S. Biaxin; Biaxin XL; Biaxin XL Pac

Pharmacologic Category Antibiotic, Macrolide

Medication Safety Issues

Sound-alike/look-alike issues:

Clarithromycin may be confused with Claritin, clindamycin, erythromycin

Pregnancy Risk Factor C

Lactation Excreted in breast milk/use caution

Breast-Feeding Considerations Clarithromycin and its active metabolite (14-hydroxy clarithromycin) are excreted into breast milk. The manufacturer recommends that caution be used if administered to nursing women. Decreased appetite, diarrhea, rash, and somnolence have been noted in nursing infants exposed to macrolide antibiotics (Goldstein, 2009).

Use

Infants and Children 6 months and older:

Acute maxillary sinusitis due to susceptible *H. influenzae, S. pneumoniae,* or *Moraxella catarrhalis*

Acute otitis media due to susceptible *H. influenzae, M. catarrhalis,* or *S. pneumoniae*

Community-acquired pneumonia due to susceptible *Mycoplasma pneumoniae, S. pneumoniae,* or *Chlamydophila pneumoniae* (TWAR)

Disseminated mycobacterial infections due to *M. avium* or *M. intracellulare*

Pharyngitis/tonsillitis due to susceptible *S. pyogenes*

Prevention of disseminated mycobacterial infections due to *M. avium* complex (MAC) disease in patients with advanced HIV infection (20 months of age and older)

Uncomplicated skin/skin structure infection due to susceptible *S. aureus* or *S. pyogenes*

Adults:

Pharyngitis/tonsillitis due to susceptible *S. pyogenes*

Acute maxillary sinusitis due to susceptible *H. influenzae, M. catarrhalis,* or *S. pneumoniae*

Acute exacerbation of chronic bronchitis due to susceptible *H. influenzae, H. parainfluenzae, M. catarrhalis,* or *S. pneumoniae*

Community-acquired pneumonia due to susceptible *H. influenzae, H. parainfluenzae, M. catarrhalis, Mycoplasma pneumoniae, S. pneumoniae,* or *Chlamydophila pneumoniae* (TWAR)

Uncomplicated skin/skin structure infections due to susceptible *S. aureus* or *S. pyogenes*

Disseminated mycobacterial infections due to *M. avium* or *M. intracellulare*

Prevention of disseminated mycobacterial infections due to MAC disease in patients with advanced HIV infection

Duodenal ulcer disease due to *H. pylori* in regimens with other drugs including amoxicillin and lansoprazole or omeprazole, or in combination with omeprazole or ranitidine bismuth citrate (no longer marketed in the U.S.). **Note:** Regimens that contain clarithromycin as the single antimicrobial agent are more likely to be associated with the development of clarithromycin resistance.

Unlabeled Use Pertussis (CDC guidelines); alternate antibiotic for prophylaxis of infective endocarditis in patients who are allergic to penicillin and undergoing dental procedures (ACC/AHA guidelines); alternate antibiotic for treatment and secondary prophylaxis of bartonellosis infection in HIV-exposed/-positive infants and children (CDC guidelines) and in HIV-positive adolescents and adults

(DHHS guidelines); Lyme disease (IDSA guidelines)

Mechanism of Action/Effect Exerts its antibacterial action by binding to 50S ribosomal subunit resulting in inhibition of protein synthesis. The 14-OH metabolite of clarithromycin is twice as active as the parent compound against some organisms.

Contraindications Hypersensitivity to clarithromycin, erythromycin, any of the macrolide antibiotics, or any component of the formulation; history of cholestatic jaundice/hepatic dysfunction associated with prior use of clarithromycin; history of QT prolongation or ventricular cardiac arrhythmia, including torsade de pointes; concomitant use with cisapride, pimozide, ergotamine, dihydroergotamine, HMG-CoA reductase inhibitors extensively metabolized by CYP3A4 (eg, lovastatin, simvastatin), astemizole or terfenadine (not available in the U.S.); concomitant use with colchicine in patients with renal or hepatic impairment

Warnings/Precautions Use has been associated with QT prolongation and infrequent cases of arrhythmias, including torsade de pointes; use is contraindicated in patients with a history of QT prolongation and ventricular arrhythmias, including torsade de pointes. Systemic exposure is increased in the elderly; may be at increased risk of torsade de pointes, particularly if concurrent severe renal impairment. Use with caution in patients at risk of prolonged cardiac repolarization. Avoid use in patients with uncorrected hypokalemia or hypomagnesemia, clinically significant bradycardia, and patients receiving Class IA (eg, quinidine, procainamide) or Class III (eg, amiodarone, dofetilide, sotalol) antiarrhythmic agents. Use caution in patients with coronary artery disease.

Elevated liver function tests and hepatitis (hepatocellular and/or cholestatic with or without jaundice) have been reported; usually reversible after discontinuation of clarithromycin. May lead to hepatic failure or death (rarely), especially in the presence of pre-existing diseases and/or concomitant use of medications. Discontinue immediately if symptoms of hepatitis occur. Dosage adjustment needed in severe renal impairment. Use with caution in patients with myasthenia gravis.

Potentially significant drug-drug interactions may exist, requiring dose or frequency adjustment, additional monitoring, and/or selection of alternative therapy. Colchicine toxicity (including fatalities) has been reported with concomitant use; concomitant use is contraindicated in patients with renal or hepatic impairment. Clarithromycin in combination with ranitidine bismuth citrate should not be used in patients with a history of acute porphyria. Prolonged use may result in fungal or bacterial superinfection, including *C. difficile*-associated diarrhea (CDAD) and pseudomembranous colitis; CDAD has been observed >2 months postantibiotic treatment. Decreased *H. pylori* eradication rates have been observed with short-term (≤7 days) combination therapy. The American College of Gastroenterology recommends 10-14 days of therapy (triple or quadruple) for eradication of *H. pylori* (Chey, 2007).

Severe acute reactions have (rarely) been reported, including anaphylaxis, Stevens-Johnson syndrome (SJS), toxic epidermal necrolysis (TEN), drug rash with eosinophilia and systemic symptoms (DRESS), and Henoch-Schönlein purpura (IgA vasculitis); discontinue therapy and initiate treatment immediately for severe acute hypersensitivity reactions. The presence of extended release tablets in the stool has been reported, particularly in patients with anatomic (eg, ileostomy, colostomy) or functional GI disorders with decreased transit times. Consider alternative dosage forms (eg, suspension) or an alternative antimicrobial for patients with tablet residue in the stool and no signs of clinical improvement.

Drug Interactions

Avoid Concomitant Use

Avoid concomitant use of Clarithromycin with any of the following: Ado-Trastuzumab Emtansine; Alfuzosin; Apixaban; Avanafil; Axitinib; BCG; Bosutinib; Cabozantinib; Cisapride; Conivaptan; Crizotinib; Dihydroergotamine; Disopyramide; Dronedarone; Eplerenone; Ergotamine; Everolimus; Fusidic Acid (Systemic); Halofantrine; Highest Risk QTc-Prolonging Agents; Ibrutinib; Imatinib; Ivabradine; Lapatinib; Lomitapide; Lovastatin; Lurasidone; Macitentan; Mifepristone; Nilotinib; Nisoldipine; Pimozide; Pomalidomide; QuiNIDine; QuiNINE; Ranolazine; Red Yeast Rice; Regorafenib; Salmeterol; Silodosin; Simeprevir; Simvastatin; Tamsulosin; Terfenadine; Ticagrelor; Tolvaptan; Topotecan; Toremifene; Ulipristal; Vemurafenib; VinCRIStine (Liposomal)

Decreased Effect

Clarithromycin may decrease the levels/effects of: BCG; Clopidogrel; Ifosfamide; Prasugrel; Sodium Picosulfate; Ticagrelor; Typhoid Vaccine; Zidovudine

The levels/effects of Clarithromycin may be decreased by: CYP3A4 Inducers (Strong); Dabrafenib; Deferasirox; Etravirine; Herbs (CYP3A4 Inducers); Protease Inhibitors; Tocilizumab

Increased Effect/Toxicity

Clarithromycin may increase the levels/effects of: Ado-Trastuzumab Emtansine; Afatinib; Alfentanil; Alfuzosin; Almotriptan; Alosetron; ALPRAZolam; Antifungal Agents (Azole Derivatives, Systemic); Antineoplastic Agents (Vinca Alkaloids); Apixaban; ARIPiprazole; AtorvaSTATin; Avanafil; Axitinib; Bedaquiline; Boceprevir; Bortezomib; Bosentan; Bosutinib; Brentuximab Vedotin; Brinzolamide; Budesonide (Nasal); Budesonide (Systemic, Oral Inhalation); BusPIRone; Cabozantinib; Calcium Channel Blockers; CarBAMazepine; Cardiac Glycosides; Cilostazol; Cisapride; CloZAPine; Cobicistat; Colchicine; Conivaptan;

Corticosteroids (Orally Inhaled); Corticosteroids (Systemic); Crizotinib; CycloSPORINE (Systemic); CYP3A4 Inducers (Strong); CYP3A4 Substrates; Dabigatran Etexilate; Dienogest; Dihydroergotamine; Disopyramide; Dofetilide; DOXOrubicin (Conventional); Dronedarone; Dutasteride; Eletriptan; Enzalutamide; Eplerenone; Ergot Derivatives; Ergotamine; Estazolam; Everolimus; FentaNYL; Fesoterodine; Fluticasone (Nasal); Fluticasone (Oral Inhalation); GlipiZIDE; GlyBURIDE; GuanFACINE; Halofantrine; Highest Risk QTc-Prolonging Agents; Ibrutinib; Iloperidone; Imatinib; Ivabradine; Ivacaftor; Ixabepilone; Lacosamide; Lapatinib; Levomilnacipran; Lomitapide; Lovastatin; Lumefantrine; Lurasidone; Macitentan; Maraviroc; MethylPREDNISolone; Midazolam; Mifepristone; Moderate Risk QTc-Prolonging Agents; Nilotinib; Nisoldipine; Ospemifene; OxyCODONE; Paricalcitol; PAZOPanib; P-glycoprotein/ABCB1 Substrates; Pimecrolimus; Pimozide; Pitavastatin; Pomalidomide; PONATinib; Pravastatin; Propafenone; Protease Inhibitors; Prucalopride; QUEtiapine; QuiNIDine; QuiNINE; Ranolazine; Red Yeast Rice; Regorafenib; Repaglinide; Rifamycin Derivatives; Rilpivirine; Rivaroxaban; RomiDEPsin; Ruxolitinib; Salmeterol; Saxagliptin; Selective Serotonin Reuptake Inhibitors; Sildenafil; Silodosin; Simeprevir; Simvastatin; Sirolimus; SORAfenib; Tacrolimus (Systemic); Tacrolimus (Topical); Tadalafil; Tamsulosin; Telaprevir; Temsirolimus; Terfenadine; Theophylline Derivatives; Ticagrelor; Tofacitinib; Tolterodine; Tolvaptan; Topotecan; Toremifene; Triazolam; Ulipristal; Vardenafil; Vemurafenib; Vilazodone; VinCRIStine (Liposomal); Vitamin K Antagonists; Zidovudine; Zopiclone; Zuclopenthixol

The levels/effects of Clarithromycin may be increased by: Antifungal Agents (Azole Derivatives, Systemic); Boceprevir; Cobicistat; CYP3A4 Inducers (Strong); CYP3A4 Inhibitors (Moderate); CYP3A4 Inhibitors (Strong); Dasatinib; Fusidic Acid (Systemic); Ivabradine; Luliconazole; Mifepristone; Protease Inhibitors; QTc-Prolonging Agents (Indeterminate Risk and Risk Modifying); Stiripentol; Telaprevir

Nutritional/Ethanol Interactions

Food: Immediate release: Food delays rate, but not extent of absorption; Extended release: Food increases clarithromycin AUC by ~30% relative to fasting conditions.

Herb/Nutraceutical: St John's wort may decrease clarithromycin levels; Management: Advise patient to avoid the use of St John's wort during clarithromycin therapy.

Adverse Reactions 1% to 10%:

Central nervous system: Headache (2%)

Dermatologic: Rash (children 3%)

Gastrointestinal: Abnormal taste (adults 3% to 7%), diarrhea (adults 3% to 6%; children 6%), vomiting (children 6%), nausea (adults 3%), abdominal pain (adults 2%; children 3%), dyspepsia (adults 2%)

Hepatic: Prothrombin time increased (adults 1%)

Renal: BUN increased (4%)

Available Dosage Forms

Suspension Reconstituted, Oral:

Biaxin: 250 mg/5 mL (50 mL, 100 mL)

Generic: 125 mg/5 mL (50 mL, 100 mL); 250 mg/5 mL (50 mL, 100 mL)

Tablet, Oral:

Biaxin: 250 mg, 500 mg

Generic: 250 mg, 500 mg

Tablet Extended Release 24 Hour, Oral:

Biaxin XL: 500 mg

Biaxin XL Pac: 500 mg

Generic: 500 mg

General Dosage Range

Dosage adjustment recommended in patients with renal impairment

Oral:

Extended release: *Adults:* 1000 mg once daily

Immediate release:

Children: 15 mg/kg/day divided every 12 hours (maximum: 1000 mg daily)

Adults: 250-500 mg every 8-12 hours

Administration

Oral Immediate release tablets and granules for suspension: Administer with or without meals. Administer every 12 hours rather than twice daily to avoid peak and trough variation. Shake suspension well before each use.

Extended release tablets: Administer with food. Do not crush or chew.

Storage/Stability

Extended release tablets: Store at 20°C to 25°C (68°F to 77°F); excursions are permitted between 15°C and 30°C (59°F and 86°F).

Immediate release tablets:

250 mg: Store at 15°C to 30°C (59°F to 86°F). Protect from light.

500 mg: Store at 20°C to 25°C (68°F to 77°F).

Granules for suspension: Store at 15°C to 30°C (59°F to 86°F) prior to and following reconstitution. Do not refrigerate. Use within 14 days of reconstitution.

Nursing Actions

Physical Assessment Results of culture and sensitivity tests and patient's allergy history should be evaluated prior to therapy.

Patient Education

• Discuss specific use of drug and side effects with patient as it relates to treatment. (HCAHPS: During this hospital stay, were you given any medicine that you had not taken before? Before giving you any new medicine, how often did hospital staff tell you what the medicine was for? How often did hospital staff describe possible side effects in a way you could understand?)

• Patient may experience dyspepsia, dysgeusia, nausea, or diarrhea. Have patient report ▶

immediately to prescriber tachycardia, severe dizziness, syncope, myalgia, dyspnea, chills, pharyngitis, hearing impairment, angina, tremors, signs of hepatic impairment, arrhythmia, signs of pseudomembranous colitis, signs of Stevens-Johnson syndrome/toxic epidermal necrolysis, or tablet shell in stool (HCAHPS).
- Educate patient about signs of a significant reaction (eg, wheezing; chest tightness; fever; itching; bad cough; blue skin color; seizures; or swelling of face, lips, tongue, or throat). **Note:** This is not a comprehensive list of all side effects. Patient should consult prescriber for additional questions.

Intended Use and Disclaimer: Should not be printed and given to patients. This information is intended to serve as a concise initial reference for healthcare professionals to use when discussing medications with a patient. You must ultimately rely on your own discretion, experience and judgment in diagnosing, treating and advising patients.

Dietary Considerations Extended release tablets should be taken with food.

Related Information
Oral Medications That Should Not Be Crushed or Altered *on page 1712*

Clevidipine (klev ID i peen)

Brand Names: U.S. Cleviprex
Index Terms Clevidipine Butyrate
Pharmacologic Category Antihypertensive; Calcium Channel Blocker; Calcium Channel Blocker, Dihydropyridine
Medication Safety Issues
Sound-alike/look-alike issues:
Clevidipine may be confused with cladribine, clofarabine, clomiPRAMINE
Cleviprex may be confused with Claravis

Pregnancy Risk Factor C
Lactation Excretion in breast milk unknown/not recommended
Breast-Feeding Considerations It is not known if clevidipine is excreted into breast milk. Per the manufacturer, the possibility of infant exposure should be considered. Breast-fed infants of mothers taking medications for hypertension should be monitored for adverse effects (Chobanian, 2003).
Use Management of hypertension
Mechanism of Action/Effect Dihydropyridine calcium channel blocker with potent arterial vasodilating activity. Inhibits calcium ion influx in arterial smooth muscle, producing a decrease in mean arterial pressure (MAP) by reducing systemic vascular resistance.
Contraindications Hypersensitivity to clevidipine or any component of the formulation (soybeans, soy products, eggs, egg products); hypertriglyceridemia or complications of hypertriglyceridemia

(eg, acute pancreatitis); lipoid nephrosis; severe aortic stenosis
Warnings/Precautions Symptomatic hypotension with or without syncope and reflex tachycardia may rarely occur. Blood pressure must be lowered at a rate appropriate for the patient's clinical condition; dosage reductions may be necessary. Treatment of clevidipine-induced tachycardia with beta-blockers is **not** recommended. After prolonged use, discontinuation may cause rebound hypertension; monitor closely for ≥8 hours after discontinuation. Dihydropyridine calcium channel blockers may cause negative inotropic effects and exacerbate HF. Avoid use in patients with HF due to lack of benefit and/or worse outcomes (ACCF/AHA [Yancy, 2013]). Clevidipine is formulated within a 20% fat emulsion (0.2 g/mL); hypertriglyceridemia is an expected side effect with high-dose or extended treatment periods; median infusion duration in clinical trials was approximately 6.5 hours (Aronson, 2008). Patients who develop hypertriglyceridemia (eg, >500 mg/dL) are at risk of developing pancreatitis. A reduction in the quantity of concurrently administered lipids may be necessary. Use is contraindicated in patients with hypertriglyceridemia or complications associated with hypertriglyceridemia (eg, acute pancreatitis) and lipoid nephrosis. Withdrawal from concomitant beta-blocker therapy should be done gradually. Initiate therapy at the low end of the dosage range in the elderly, with careful upward titration if needed. Use within 12 hours of puncturing vial; maintain aseptic technique while handling.

Drug Interactions
Avoid Concomitant Use There are no known interactions where it is recommended to avoid concomitant use.
Decreased Effect
Clevidipine may decrease the levels/effects of: QuiNIDine

The levels/effects of Clevidipine may be decreased by: Calcium Salts; Herbs (Hypertensive Properties); Melatonin; Methylphenidate; Yohimbine

Increased Effect/Toxicity
Clevidipine may increase the levels/effects of: Amifostine; Antihypertensives; Atosiban; Beta-Blockers; Calcium Channel Blockers (Nondihydropyridine); DULoxetine; Hypotensive Agents; Magnesium Salts; Neuromuscular-Blocking Agents (Nondepolarizing); Nitroprusside; Obinutuzumab; QuiNIDine; RiTUXimab

The levels/effects of Clevidipine may be increased by: Alpha1-Blockers; Brimonidine (Topical); Calcium Channel Blockers (Nondihydropyridine); Diazoxide; Herbs (Hypotensive Properties); Magnesium Salts; MAO Inhibitors; Pentoxifylline; Phosphodiesterase 5 Inhibitors; Prostacyclin Analogues; QuiNIDine

Nutritional/Ethanol Interactions Herb/Nutraceutical: Avoid bayberry, blue cohosh, cayenne, ephedra, ginger, ginseng (American), kola, licorice (may worsen hypertension). Avoid black cohosh, California poppy, coleus, golden seal, hawthorn, mistletoe, periwinkle, quinine, shepherd's purse (may have increased antihypertensive effect).

Adverse Reactions

>10%:

Cardiovascular: Atrial fibrillation (21%)

Central nervous system: Fever (19%), insomnia (12%)

Gastrointestinal: Nausea (5% to 21%)

1% to 10%:

Central nervous system: Headache (6%)

Gastrointestinal: Vomiting (3%)

Hematologic: Postprocedural hemorrhage (3%)

Renal: Acute renal failure (9%)

Respiratory: Pneumonia (3%), respiratory failure (3%)

Pharmacodynamics/Kinetics

Onset of Action 2-4 minutes after start of infusion

Duration of Action I.V.: 5-15 minutes

Available Dosage Forms

Emulsion, Intravenous:

Cleviprex: 0.5 mg/mL (50 mL, 100 mL)

General Dosage Range I.V.: *Adults:* Initial: 1-2 mg/hour; Usual maintenance: 4-6 mg/hour; Maximum: 21 mg/hour (1000 mL/24 hours)

Administration

I.V. I.V.: Maintain aseptic technique. Do not use if contamination is suspected. Do not dilute. Invert vial gently several times to ensure uniformity of emulsion prior to administration. Administer as a slow continuous infusion via central or peripheral line, using infusion device allowing for calibrated infusion rates. Use within 12 hours of puncturing vial; discard any tubing and unused portion, including that currently being infused.

Injectable Detail pH: 6-8

Storage/Stability Store in refrigerator at 2°C to 8°C (36°F to 46°F). Unopened vials are stable for 2 months at room temperature. Vials are stable for 12 hours once opened. Protect from light during storage. Do not freeze.

Nursing Actions

Physical Assessment Assess allergy history prior to treatment (soybeans or soy products, eggs or egg products). Monitor cardiac status and blood pressure closely during therapy and for a minimum of 8 hours after discontinuation (rebound hypertension may occur). Caution patient to call for assistance when rising or changing position until response to drug is known.

Patient Education

• Discuss specific use of drug and side effects with patient as it relates to treatment. (HCAHPS: During this hospital stay, were you given any medicine that you had not taken before? Before giving you any new medicine, how often did hospital staff tell you what the medicine was for? How often did hospital staff describe possible side effects in a way you could understand?)

• Patient may experience fatigue, headache, or nausea. Have patient report immediately to prescriber tachycardia, arrhythmia, severe dizziness, syncope, urinary retention, or oliguria (HCAHPS).

• Educate patient about signs of a significant reaction (eg, wheezing; chest tightness; fever; itching; bad cough; blue skin color; seizures; or swelling of face, lips, tongue, or throat). **Note:** This is not a comprehensive list of all side effects. Patient should consult prescriber for additional questions.

Intended Use and Disclaimer: Should not be printed and given to patients. This information is intended to serve as a concise initial reference for healthcare professionals to use when discussing medications with a patient. You must ultimately rely on your own discretion, experience and judgment in diagnosing, treating and advising patients.

Dietary Considerations Clevidipine is formulated in an oil-in-water emulsion containing 200 mg/mL of lipid (2 kcal/mL). If on parenteral nutrition, may need to adjust the amount of lipid infused. Emulsion contains soybean oil, egg yolk phospholipids, and glycerin.

Clidinium and Chlordiazepoxide
(kli DI nee um & klor dye az e POKS ide)

Brand Names: U.S. Librax®

Index Terms Chlordiazepoxide and Clidinium

Pharmacologic Category Antispasmodic Agent, Gastrointestinal; Benzodiazepine

Medication Safety Issues

Sound-alike/look-alike issues:

Librax® may be confused with Librium

BEERS Criteria medication:

This drug may be inappropriate for use in geriatric patients (Quality of evidence: moderate [clidinium]/high [chlordiazepoxide]; Strength of recommendation - strong).

Use Adjunct treatment of peptic ulcer; treatment of irritable bowel syndrome

Available Dosage Forms

Capsule: Clidinium 2.5 mg and chlordiazepoxide 5 mg

Librax®: Clidinium 2.5 mg and chlordiazepoxide 5 mg

General Dosage Range Oral: *Adults:* 1-2 capsules 3-4 times/day

Administration

Oral Administer before meals. **Caution:** Do not abruptly discontinue after prolonged use; taper dose gradually.

Nursing Actions

Physical Assessment See individual agents.

Patient Education

- Discuss specific use of drug and side effects with patient as it relates to treatment. (HCAHPS: During this hospital stay, were you given any medicine that you had not taken before? Before giving you any new medicine, how often did hospital staff tell you what the medicine was for? How often did hospital staff describe possible side effects in a way you could understand?)
- Patient may experience presyncope, fatigue, blurred vision, headache, xerostomia, or nausea. Have patient report immediately to prescriber severe dizziness, syncope, significant change in balance, signs of depression (ie, suicidal ideation, anxiety, emotional instability, illogical thinking), sexual dysfunction, urinary retention, oliguria, considerable constipation, intolerable asthenia, fasciculations, signs of hepatic impairment, chills, or pharyngitis (HCAHPS).
- Educate patient about signs of a significant reaction (eg, wheezing; chest tightness; fever; itching; bad cough; blue skin color; seizures; or swelling of face, lips, tongue, or throat). **Note:** This is not a comprehensive list of all side effects. Patient should consult prescriber for additional questions.

Intended Use and Disclaimer: Should not be printed and given to patients. This information is intended to serve as a concise initial reference for healthcare professionals to use when discussing medications with a patient. You must ultimately rely on your own discretion, experience and judgment in diagnosing, treating and advising patients.

Related Information

ChlordiazePOXIDE *on page 308*

Clindamycin (Systemic) (klin da MYE sin)

Brand Names: U.S. Cleocin; Cleocin in D5W; Cleocin Phosphate

Index Terms Clindamycin Hydrochloride; Clindamycin Palmitate

Pharmacologic Category Antibiotic, Lincosamide

Medication Safety Issues

Sound-alike/look-alike issues:

Cleocin may be confused with bleomycin, Clinoril, Cubicin, Lincocin

Clindamycin may be confused with clarithromycin, Claritin, vancomycin

Pregnancy Risk Factor B

Lactation Enters breast milk/not recommended

Breast-Feeding Considerations Clindamycin can be detected in breast milk; reported concentrations range from 0.7 to 3.8 mcg/mL following maternal doses of 150 mg orally to 600 mg I.V. Due to the potential for serious adverse reactions in neonates, breast-feeding is not recommended by the manufacturer. Nondose-related effects could include modification of bowel flora. One case of bloody stools in an infant occurred after a mother received clindamycin while breast-feeding; however, a causal relationship was not confirmed (Mann, 1980).

Use Treatment of susceptible bacterial infections, mainly those caused by anaerobes, streptococci, pneumococci, and staphylococci; pelvic inflammatory disease (I.V.)

Unlabeled Use May be useful in PCP; alternate treatment for toxoplasmosis; bacterial vaginosis (oral); alternate treatment for MRSA infections; alternate antibiotic for prophylaxis of infective endocarditis in patients who are allergic to penicillin and undergoing surgical or dental procedures (ACC/AHA guidelines); group B streptococcus (GBS) infection (maternal use for neonatal prophylaxis in penicillin-allergic women); treatment of severe or uncomplicated malaria; treatment of babesiosis; treatment of acute bacterial rhinosinusitis (ABRS) (pediatric) (in combination with a third-generation cephalosporin); chronic oral antimicrobial suppression of prosthetic joint infection

Mechanism of Action/Effect Reversibly binds to 50S ribosomal subunits preventing peptide bond formation thus inhibiting bacterial protein synthesis; bacteriostatic or bactericidal depending on drug concentration, infection site, and organism

Contraindications Hypersensitivity to clindamycin, lincomycin, or any component of the formulation

Warnings/Precautions Dosage adjustment may be necessary in patients with severe hepatic dysfunction. **[U.S. Boxed Warning]: Can cause severe and possibly fatal colitis.** Prolonged use may result in fungal or bacterial superinfection, including *C. difficile*-associated diarrhea (CDAD) and pseudomembranous colitis; CDAD has been observed >2 months postantibiotic treatment. Use with caution in patients with a history of gastrointestinal disease. Discontinue drug if significant diarrhea, abdominal cramps, or passage of blood and mucus occurs. Some dosage forms contain benzyl alcohol or tartrazine. Use caution in atopic patients. Not appropriate for use in the treatment of meningitis due to inadequate penetration into the CSF.

Drug Interactions

Avoid Concomitant Use

Avoid concomitant use of Clindamycin (Systemic) with any of the following: BCG; Erythromycin (Systemic)

Decreased Effect

Clindamycin (Systemic) may decrease the levels/effects of: BCG; Erythromycin (Systemic); Sodium Picosulfate; Typhoid Vaccine

The levels/effects of Clindamycin (Systemic) may be decreased by: Kaolin

Increased Effect/Toxicity

Clindamycin (Systemic) may increase the levels/effects of: Neuromuscular-Blocking Agents

Nutritional/Ethanol Interactions

Food: Peak concentrations may be delayed with food.

Herb/Nutraceutical: St John's wort may decrease clindamycin levels.

Adverse Reactions Frequency not defined.

Cardiovascular: Cardiac arrest (rare; I.V. administration), hypotension (rare; I.V. administration)

Dermatologic: Erythema multiforme (rare), exfoliative dermatitis (rare), pruritus, rash, Stevens-Johnson syndrome (rare), urticaria

Gastrointestinal: Abdominal pain, diarrhea, esophagitis, nausea, pseudomembranous colitis, vomiting

Genitourinary: Vaginitis

Hematologic: Agranulocytosis, eosinophilia (transient), neutropenia (transient), thrombocytopenia

Hepatic: Jaundice, liver function test abnormalities

Local: Induration/pain/sterile abscess (I.M.), thrombophlebitis (I.V.)

Neuromuscular & skeletal: Polyarthritis (rare)

Renal: Renal dysfunction (rare)

Miscellaneous: Anaphylactoid reactions (rare)

Available Dosage Forms

Capsule, Oral:

Cleocin: 75 mg, 150 mg, 300 mg

Generic: 75 mg, 150 mg, 300 mg

Solution, Injection:

Cleocin Phosphate: 300 mg/2 mL (2 mL); 600 mg/4 mL (4 mL); 900 mg/6 mL (6 mL); 9 g/60 mL (60 mL)

Generic: 300 mg/2 mL (2 mL); 600 mg/4 mL (4 mL); 900 mg/6 mL (6 mL); 9000 mg/60 mL (60 mL); 9 g/60 mL (60 mL)

Solution, Intravenous:

Cleocin in D_5W: 300 mg/50 mL (50 mL); 600 mg/50 mL (50 mL); 900 mg/50 mL (50 mL)

Cleocin Phosphate: 600 mg/4 mL (4 mL); 900 mg/6 mL (6 mL)

Generic: 300 mg/50 mL (50 mL); 600 mg/50 mL (50 mL); 900 mg/50 mL (50 mL); 300 mg/2 mL (2 mL); 600 mg/4 mL (4 mL); 900 mg/6 mL (6 mL)

Solution Reconstituted, Oral:

Cleocin: 75 mg/5 mL (100 mL)

Generic: 75 mg/5 mL (100 mL)

General Dosage Range

I.M., I.V.:

Children >1 month: 20-40 mg/kg/day in 3-4 divided doses

Adults: 1200-2700 mg daily in 2-4 divided doses (maximum: 4800 mg daily)

Oral:

Children: 8-20 mg/kg/day as hydrochloride or 8-25 mg/kg/day as palmitate in 3-4 divided doses (minimum dose of palmitate: 37.5 mg 3 times daily)

Adults: 150-450 mg every 6 hours (maximum: 1800 mg daily)

Administration

I.M. Deep I.M. sites, rotate sites. Do not exceed 600 mg in a single injection.

I.V. Never administer as bolus; administer by I.V. intermittent infusion over at least 10-60 minutes, at a rate **not** to exceed 30 mg/minute (do not exceed 1200 mg/hour). Final concentration for administration should not exceed 18 mg/mL.

Injectable Detail pH: 6-6.3 (usual); 5.5-7 (range)

Oral Administer oral dosage form with a full glass of water to minimize esophageal ulceration. Give around-the-clock to promote less variation in peak and trough serum levels.

Storage/Stability

Capsule: Store at room temperature of 20°C to 25°C (68°F to 77°F).

I.V.: Infusion solution in NS or D_5W solution is stable for 16 days at room temperature, 32 days refrigerated, or 8 weeks frozen. Prior to use, store vials and premixed bags at controlled room temperature 20°C to 25°C (68°F to 77°F). After initial use, discard any unused portion of vial after 24 hours.

Oral solution: Do not refrigerate reconstituted oral solution (it will thicken). Following reconstitution, oral solution is stable for 2 weeks at room temperature of 20°C to 25°C (68°F to 77°F).

Nursing Actions

Physical Assessment Previous allergy history should be assessed prior to beginning therapy. Monitor cardiac status and blood pressure and keep patient recumbent after infusion until blood pressure is stabilized.

Patient Education

- Discuss specific use of drug and side effects with patient as it relates to treatment. (HCAHPS: During this hospital stay, were you given any medicine that you had not taken before? Before giving you any new medicine, how often did hospital staff tell you what the medicine was for? How often did hospital staff describe possible side effects in a way you could understand?)
- Patient may experience dyspepsia, nausea, or diarrhea. Have patient report immediately to prescriber injection site pain or irritation, arthralgia, urinary retention, oliguria, jaundice, vaginitis, or signs of Stevens-Johnson syndrome/toxic epidermal necrolysis (HCAHPS).
- Educate patient about signs of a significant reaction (eg, wheezing; chest tightness; fever; itching; bad cough; blue skin color; seizures; or swelling of face, lips, tongue, or throat). **Note:** This is not a comprehensive list of all side effects. Patient should consult prescriber for additional questions.

Intended Use and Disclaimer: Should not be printed and given to patients. This information is intended to serve as a concise initial reference for healthcare professionals to use when discussing medications with a patient. You must ultimately

rely on your own discretion, experience and judgment in diagnosing, treating and advising patients.

Dietary Considerations May be taken with food.

Clindamycin (Topical) (klin da MYE sin)

Brand Names: U.S. Cleocin; Cleocin-T; Clindacin ETZ; Clindacin Pac; Clindacin-P; Clindagel; ClindaMax; Clindesse; Evoclin

Index Terms Clindamycin Phosphate

Pharmacologic Category Antibiotic, Lincosamide; Topical Skin Product, Acne

Medication Safety Issues

Sound-alike/look-alike issues:

Cleocin® may be confused with bleomycin, Clinoril®, Cubicin®, Lincocin®

Clindamycin may be confused with clarithromycin, Claritin®, vancomycin

Pregnancy Risk Factor B

Lactation Enters breast milk/not recommended

Use Treatment of bacterial vaginosis (vaginal cream, vaginal suppository); topically in treatment of severe acne

Available Dosage Forms

Cream, Vaginal:
Cleocin: 2% (40 g)
Clindesse: 2% (5.8 g)
Generic: 2% (40 g)

Foam, External:
Evoclin: 1% (50 g, 100 g)
Generic: 1% (50 g, 100 g)

Gel, External:
Cleocin-T: 1% (30 g, 60 g)
Clindagel: 1% (75 mL)
ClindaMax: 1% (30 g, 60 g)
Generic: 1% (30 g, 60 g)

Kit, External:
Clindacin ETZ: 1%
Clindacin Pac: 1%

Lotion, External:
Cleocin-T: 1% (60 mL)
ClindaMax: 1% (60 mL)
Generic: 1% (60 mL)

Solution, External:
Cleocin-T: 1% (30 mL, 60 mL)
Generic: 1% (30 mL, 60 mL)

Suppository, Vaginal:
Cleocin: 100 mg (3 ea)

Swab, External:
Cleocin-T: 1% (60 ea)
Clindacin ETZ: 1% (60 ea)
Clindacin-P: 1% (69 ea)
Generic: 1% (60 ea)

General Dosage Range

Intravaginal: *Adults:* Insert 1 ovule or applicatorful once daily **or** 1 applicatorful as a single dose (Clindesse®)

Topical: *Children ≥12 years and Adults:* Apply once or twice daily

Administration

Topical

Foam: Dispense directly into cap or onto a cool surface; do not dispense directly into hands or face (foam will melt on contact with warm skin). Wash skin with mild soap and allow to fully dry. Apply in small amounts to face using fingertips and gently massage into affected areas until foam disappears. Avoid contact with eyes, mouth, lips, mucous membranes, or broken skin.

Gel: Avoid contact with eyes.

Lotion: Shake well immediately before using.

Solution or pledget: Avoid contact with eyes, mouth or other mucous membranes; solution/pledget contains an alcohol base and if inadvertent contact with mucous membranes occurs, rinse with liberal amounts of water. Remove pledget from foil immediately before use; discard after single use. May use more than one pledget for each application to cover area.

Other Intravaginal:

Cream: Insertion with the applicator should be as far as possible into the vagina without causing discomfort.

Ovule: The foil should be removed; if the applicator is used for insertion, it should be washed for additional use.

Nursing Actions

Patient Education

• Discuss specific use of drug and side effects with patient as it relates to treatment. (HCAHPS: During this hospital stay, were you given any medicine that you had not taken before? Before giving you any new medicine, how often did hospital staff tell you what the medicine was for? How often did hospital staff describe possible side effects in a way you could understand?)

• Patient may experience application site irritation, xeroderma, or oily skin. Have patient report immediately to prescriber severe diarrhea, melena, dyspepsia, severe skin irritation, significant vaginitis, or dyspareunia (HCAHPS).

• Educate patient about signs of a significant reaction (eg, wheezing; chest tightness; fever; itching; bad cough; blue skin color; seizures; or swelling of face, lips, tongue, or throat). **Note:** This is not a comprehensive list of all side effects. Patient should consult prescriber for additional questions.

Intended Use and Disclaimer: Should not be printed and given to patients. This information is intended to serve as a concise initial reference for healthcare professionals to use when discussing medications with a patient. You must ultimately rely on your own discretion, experience and judgment in diagnosing, treating and advising patients.

Clindamycin and Benzoyl Peroxide

(klin da MYE sin & BEN zoe il peer OKS ide)

Brand Names: U.S. Acanya®; BenzaClin®; Duac®

Index Terms Benzoyl Peroxide and Clindamycin; Clindamycin Phosphate and Benzoyl Peroxide

Pharmacologic Category Acne Products; Topical Skin Product; Topical Skin Product, Acne

Pregnancy Risk Factor C

Use Topical treatment of acne vulgaris

Available Dosage Forms

Gel, topical: Clindamycin 1% and benzoyl peroxide 5% (50 g); Clindamycin phosphate 1.2% and benzoyl peroxide 5% (45 g)

Acanya®: Clindamycin 1.2% and benzoyl peroxide 2.5% (50 g)

BenzaClin®: Clindamycin 1% and benzoyl peroxide 5% (25 g, 35 g, 50 g)

Duac®: Clindamycin 1.2% and benzoyl peroxide 5% (45 g)

General Dosage Range Topical: *Children ≥12 years and Adults:* Apply once daily (Acanya®, Duac®) **or** twice daily (BenzaClin®) to affected areas

Administration

Topical Skin should be clean and dry before applying. For external use only; avoid applying to inside nose, mouth, eyes, and mucous membranes.

Nursing Actions

Physical Assessment See individual agents.

Patient Education

- Discuss specific use of drug and side effects with patient as it relates to treatment. (HCAHPS: During this hospital stay, were you given any medicine that you had not taken before? Before giving you any new medicine, how often did hospital staff tell you what the medicine was for? How often did hospital staff describe possible side effects in a way you could understand?)
- Patient may experience xeroderma. Have patient report immediately to prescriber severe skin irritation, significant diarrhea, melena, or dyspepsia (HCAHPS).
- Educate patient about signs of a significant reaction (eg, wheezing; chest tightness; fever; itching; bad cough; blue skin color; seizures; or swelling of face, lips, tongue, or throat). **Note:** This is not a comprehensive list of all side effects. Patient should consult prescriber for additional questions.

Intended Use and Disclaimer: Should not be printed and given to patients. This information is intended to serve as a concise initial reference for healthcare professionals to use when discussing medications with a patient. You must ultimately rely on your own discretion, experience and judgment in diagnosing, treating and advising patients.

Related Information

Clindamycin (Topical) *on page 342*

Clindamycin and Tretinoin

(klin da MYE sin & TRET i noyn)

Brand Names: U.S. Veltin™; Ziana®

Index Terms Clindamycin Phosphate and Tretinoin; Tretinoin and Clindamycin; Veltin™

Pharmacologic Category Acne Products; Retinoic Acid Derivative; Topical Skin Product; Topical Skin Product, Acne

Pregnancy Risk Factor C

Use Treatment of acne vulgaris

Available Dosage Forms

Gel, topical:

Veltin™: Clindamycin phosphate 1.2% and tretinoin 0.025% (30 g, 60 g)

Ziana®: Clindamycin phosphate 1.2% and tretinoin 0.025% (30 g, 60 g)

General Dosage Range Topical: *Children ≥12 years and Adults:* Apply pea-size amount to entire face once daily at bedtime

Administration

Topical At bedtime, clean face with a mild soap and pat dry before applying medication. A pea-size amount should be applied to one fingertip and then dotted on chin, cheeks, nose, and forehead. Gently rub over entire face or entire affected area while avoiding eyes, mouth, angles of nose, and mucous membranes.

Nursing Actions

Physical Assessment See individual agents.

Patient Education

- Discuss specific use of drug and side effects with patient as it relates to treatment. (HCAHPS: During this hospital stay, were you given any medicine that you had not taken before? Before giving you any new medicine, how often did hospital staff tell you what the medicine was for? How often did hospital staff describe possible side effects in a way you could understand?)
- Patient may experience xeroderma, skin irritation, or skin discoloration. Have patient report immediately to prescriber severe diarrhea, melena, or dyspepsia (HCAHPS).
- Educate patient about signs of a significant reaction (eg, wheezing; chest tightness; fever; itching; bad cough; blue skin color; seizures; or swelling of face, lips, tongue, or throat). **Note:** This is not a comprehensive list of all side effects. Patient should consult prescriber for additional questions.

Intended Use and Disclaimer: Should not be printed and given to patients. This information is intended to serve as a concise initial reference for healthcare professionals to use when discussing medications with a patient. You must ultimately rely on your own discretion, experience and

judgment in diagnosing, treating and advising patients.

CloBAZam (KLOE ba zam)

Brand Names: U.S. Onfi
Pharmacologic Category Benzodiazepine
Medication Safety Issues
Sound-alike/look-alike issues:
CloBAZam may be confused with clonazePAM
Medication Guide Available Yes
Lactation Enters breast milk/not recommended
Use Adjunctive treatment of seizures associated with Lennox-Gastaut syndrome
Canadian labeling: Adjunctive treatment of epilepsy
Unlabeled Use Catamenial epilepsy; epilepsy (monotherapy)
Controlled Substance C-IV
Available Dosage Forms
Suspension, Oral:
Onfi: 2.5 mg/mL (120 mL)
Tablet, Oral:
Onfi: 10 mg, 20 mg
General Dosage Range Dosage adjustment recommended in patients with hepatic impairment or CYP2C19 poor metabolizers.
Oral: *Children ≥2 years and Adults:* Initial: 5-10 mg/day; Maintenance: Up to 40 mg/day
Administration
Oral May be administered with or without food. Tablets can be crushed and mixed in applesauce. Shake suspension well before using; only use the oral dosing syringe supplied with the suspension.
Nursing Actions
Physical Assessment Evaluate tolerance of medication including CNS depression (ability to function without excessive sedation or coordination impairment). For inpatient use, institute safety measures to prevent falls.
Patient Education
• Discuss specific use of drug and side effects with patient as it relates to treatment. (HCAHPS: During this hospital stay, were you given any medicine that you had not taken before? Before giving you any new medicine, how often did hospital staff tell you what the medicine was for? How often did hospital staff describe possible side effects in a way you could understand?)
• Patient may experience presyncope, fatigue, blurred vision, sialorrhea, constipation, or emesis. Have patient report immediately to prescriber dyspnea, significant change in balance, severe asthenia, dysuria, dysarthria, insomnia, signs of depression (ie, suicidal ideation, anxiety, emotional instability, illogical thinking), or signs of Stevens-Johnson syndrome/toxic epidermal necrolysis (HCAHPS).
• Educate patient about signs of a significant reaction (eg, wheezing; chest tightness; fever; itching; bad cough; blue skin color; seizures; or swelling of face, lips, tongue, or throat). **Note:** This is not a comprehensive list of all side effects. Patient should consult prescriber for additional questions.

Intended Use and Disclaimer: Should not be printed and given to patients. This information is intended to serve as a concise initial reference for healthcare professionals to use when discussing medications with a patient. You must ultimately rely on your own discretion, experience and judgment in diagnosing, treating and advising patients.

ClomiPHENE (KLOE mi feen)

Brand Names: U.S. Clomid; Serophene
Index Terms Clomiphene Citrate
Pharmacologic Category Ovulation Stimulator; Selective Estrogen Receptor Modulator (SERM)
Medication Safety Issues
Sound-alike/look-alike issues:
ClomiPHENE may be confused with clomiPRAMINE, clonidine
Clomid® may be confused with clonidine
Serophene® may be confused with Sarafem®
Pregnancy Risk Factor X
Lactation Excretion in breast milk unknown/use caution
Breast-Feeding Considerations Clomiphene may decrease lactation.
Use Treatment of ovulatory dysfunction in patients desiring pregnancy
Mechanism of Action/Effect Clomiphene is a racemic mixture consisting of zuclomiphene (~38%) and enclomiphene (~62%) each with distinct pharmacologic properties. Zuclomiphene is more potent in inducing ovulation. Ovulation occurs by stimulating the release of pituitary gonadotropins, causing growth of the ovarian follicle followed by follicular rupture.
Contraindications Hypersensitivity to clomiphene citrate or any of its components; liver disease; abnormal uterine bleeding; enlargement or development of ovarian cyst (not due to polycystic ovarian syndrome); uncontrolled thyroid or adrenal dysfunction; presence of an organic intracranial lesion such as pituitary tumor; pregnancy
Warnings/Precautions Ovarian enlargement may occur with use; may be accompanied by abdominal distention or abdominal pain and generally regresses without treatment within 2-3 weeks. If ovaries are abnormally enlarged, withhold hCG to reduce the risk of ovarian hyperstimulation syndrome (OHSS). OHSS is characterized by severe ovarian enlargement, abdominal pain/distention, nausea, vomiting, diarrhea, dyspnea, and oliguria, and may be accompanied by ascites, pleural effusion, hypovolemia, electrolyte imbalance, hemoperitoneum, and thromboembolic events. If

severe hyperstimulation occurs, stop treatment and hospitalize patient. This syndrome develops rapidly within 24 hours to several days and generally occurs during the 7-10 days immediately following treatment. Use with caution in patients unusually sensitive to pituitary gonadotropins (eg, PCOS); a lower dose may be necessary. Blurring or other visual symptoms can occur; symptoms may increase with higher doses or duration of therapy; patients with visual disturbances should discontinue therapy and have an eye exam. Prolonged use may increase the risk of borderline or invasive ovarian cancer. Use caution in patients with uterine fibroids, may cause further enlargement. Multiple births may result from the use of these medications; advise patient of the potential risk of multiple births before starting the treatment. To minimize risks, use only at the lowest effective dose for the shortest duration of therapy (especially for the first course of therapy). Use should be supervised by physicians who are thoroughly familiar with infertility problems and their management.

Drug Interactions

Avoid Concomitant Use
Avoid concomitant use of ClomiPHENE with any of the following: Ospemifene

Decreased Effect
ClomiPHENE may decrease the levels/effects of: Ospemifene

Increased Effect/Toxicity
ClomiPHENE may increase the levels/effects of: Ospemifene

Adverse Reactions
>10%: Endocrine & metabolic: Ovarian enlargement (14%)

1% to 10%:
Central nervous system: Headache (1%)
Endocrine & metabolic: Hot flashes (10%), breast discomfort (2%), abnormal uterine bleeding (1%)
Gastrointestinal: Distention/bloating/discomfort (6%), nausea (2%), vomiting (2%)
Ocular: Visual symptoms (2%, includes blurred vision, diplopia, floaters, lights, phosphenes, photophobia, scotomata, waves)

Pharmacodynamics/Kinetics
Onset of Action Ovulation: 5-10 days following course of treatment

Duration of Action Effects are cumulative; ovulation may occur in the cycle following the last treatment

Available Dosage Forms
Tablet, Oral:
Clomid: 50 mg
Serophene: 50 mg
Generic: 50 mg

General Dosage Range Oral: *Adults (females):* 50-100 mg daily for 5 days

Administration
Oral The total daily dose should be taken at one time to maximize effectiveness.

Storage/Stability Store at room temperature of 15°C to 30°C (59°F to 86°F). Protect from light, heat, and excessive humidity.

Nursing Actions
Physical Assessment Teach patient proper use (eg, measuring basal body temperature and timing of intercourse).

Patient Education
• Discuss specific use of drug and side effects with patient as it relates to treatment. (HCAHPS: During this hospital stay, were you given any medicine that you had not taken before? Before giving you any new medicine, how often did hospital staff tell you what the medicine was for? How often did hospital staff describe possible side effects in a way you could understand?)
• Patient may experience hot flashes. Have patient report immediately to prescriber dyspnea, angina, hemoptysis, severe headache, depression, mood changes, edema of extremities, vaginal hemorrhaging, menstrual irregularities, significant back pain, vision changes, or signs of ovarian hyperstimulation (HCAHPS).
• Educate patient about signs of a significant reaction (eg, wheezing; chest tightness; fever; itching; bad cough; blue skin color; seizures; or swelling of face, lips, tongue, or throat). **Note:** This is not a comprehensive list of all side effects. Patient should consult prescriber for additional questions.

Intended Use and Disclaimer: Should not be printed and given to patients. This information is intended to serve as a concise initial reference for healthcare professionals to use when discussing medications with a patient. You must ultimately rely on your own discretion, experience and judgment in diagnosing, treating and advising patients.

ClomiPRAMINE (kloe MI pra meen)

Brand Names: U.S. Anafranil
Index Terms Clomipramine Hydrochloride
Pharmacologic Category Antidepressant, Tricyclic (Tertiary Amine)
Medication Safety Issues
Sound-alike/look-alike issues:
ClomiPRAMINE may be confused with chlorproMAZINE, clevidipine, clomiPHENE, desipramine, Norpramin®
Anafranil® may be confused with alfentanil, enalapril, nafarelin
BEERS Criteria medication:
This drug may be potentially inappropriate for use in geriatric patients (Quality of evidence - high [moderate for SIADH]; Strength of recommendation - strong).
Medication Guide Available Yes
Pregnancy Risk Factor C
Lactation Enters breast milk/not recommended

Breast-Feeding Considerations Clomipramine is excreted in breast milk. Based on information from three mother-infant pairs, following maternal use of clomipramine 75-150 mg/day, the estimated exposure to the breast-feeding infant would be 0.4% to 4% of the weight-adjusted maternal dose. Adverse events have not been reported in nursing infants (information from seven cases). Infants should be monitored for signs of adverse events; routine monitoring of infant serum concentrations is not recommended (Fortinguerra, 2009). Due to the potential for serious adverse reactions in the nursing infant, the decision to continue or discontinue breast-feeding during therapy should take into account the risk of exposure to the infant and the benefits of treatment to the mother.

Use Treatment of obsessive-compulsive disorder (OCD)

Unlabeled Use Depression, panic attacks

Mechanism of Action/Effect Clomipramine appears to affect serotonin uptake while its active metabolite, desmethylclomipramine, affects norepinephrine uptake

Contraindications Hypersensitivity to clomipramine, other tricyclic agents, or any component of the formulation; use of MAO inhibitors intended to treat psychiatric disorders (concurrently or within 14 days of discontinuing either clomipramine or the MAO inhibitor); initiation of clomipramine in a patient receiving linezolid or intravenous methylene blue; use in a patient during the acute recovery phase of MI

Warnings/Precautions [U.S. Boxed Warning]: Antidepressants increase the risk of suicidal thinking and behavior in children, adolescents, and young adults (18-24 years of age) with major depressive disorder (MDD) and other psychiatric disorders; consider risk prior to prescribing. Short-term studies did not show an increased risk in patients >24 years of age and showed a decreased risk in patients ≥65 years. Closely monitor for clinical worsening, suicidality, or unusual changes in behavior; the patient's family or caregiver should be instructed to closely observe the patient and communicate condition with healthcare provider. A medication guide should be dispensed with each prescription. **Clomipramine is FDA approved for the treatment of OCD in children ≥10 years of age.**

The possibility of a suicide attempt is inherent in major depression and may persist until remission occurs. Monitor for worsening of depression or suicidality, especially during initiation of therapy (generally first 1-2 months) or with dose increases or decreases. Use caution in high-risk patients. Worsening depression and severe abrupt suicidality that are not part of the presenting symptoms may require discontinuation or modification of drug therapy. The patient's family or caregiver should be alerted to monitor patients for the emergence of suicidality and associated behaviors (such as agitation, irritability, hostility, impulsivity, and hypomania) and notify the healthcare provider.

May worsen psychosis in some patients or precipitate a shift to mania or hypomania in patients with bipolar disorder. Patients presenting with depressive symptoms should be screened for bipolar disorder. Monotherapy in patients with bipolar disorder should be avoided. **Clomipramine is not FDA approved for bipolar depression.**

Potentially life-threatening serotonin syndrome (SS) has occurred with serotonergic agents (eg, SSRIs, SNRIs), particularly when used in combination with other serotonergic agents (eg, triptans, TCAs, fentanyl, lithium, tramadol, buspirone, St John's wort, tryptophan) or agents that impair metabolism of serotonin (eg, MAO inhibitors intended to treat psychiatric disorders, other MAO inhibitors [ie, linezolid and intravenous methylene blue]). Discontinue treatment (and any concomitant serotonergic agent) immediately if signs/symptoms arise. TCAs may rarely cause bone marrow suppression; monitor for any signs of infection and obtain CBC if symptoms (eg, fever, sore throat) evident. May cause seizures (relationship to dose and/or duration of therapy) - do not exceed maximum doses. Use caution in patients with a previous seizure disorder or condition predisposing to seizures such as brain damage, alcoholism, or concurrent therapy with other drugs which lower the seizure threshold. May increase the risks associated with electroconvulsive therapy. Bone fractures have been associated with antidepressant treatment. Consider the possibility of a fragility fracture if an antidepressant-treated patient presents with unexplained bone pain, point tenderness, swelling, or bruising (Rabenda, 2013; Rizzoli, 2012). Use with caution in patients with tumors of the adrenal medulla (eg, pheochromocytoma, neuroblastoma); may cause hypertensive crises. Has been associated with a high incidence of sexual dysfunction. Weight gain may occur.

The degree of sedation, anticholinergic effects, and conduction abnormalities are high relative to other antidepressants. Clomipramine often causes drowsiness/sedation, resulting in impaired performance of tasks requiring alertness (eg, operating machinery or driving). The risk of orthostasis is moderate to high relative to other antidepressants. Use with caution in patients with a history of cardiovascular disease (including previous MI, stroke, tachycardia, or conduction abnormalities). Use with caution in patients with urinary retention, benign prostatic hyperplasia, narrow-angle glaucoma, xerostomia, visual problems, constipation, or a history of bowel obstruction. Potentially significant drug-drug interactions may exist, requiring dose or frequency adjustment, additional monitoring, and/or selection of alternative therapy.

Recommended by the manufacturer to discontinue prior to elective surgery; risks exist for drug interactions with anesthesia and for cardiac arrhythmias. However, definitive drug interactions have not been widely reported in the literature and continuation of tricyclic antidepressants is generally recommended as long as precautions are taken to reduce the significance of any adverse events that may occur (Pass, 2004). Use with caution in hyperthyroid patients or those receiving thyroid supplementation. Use with caution in patients with hepatic impairment; increases in ALT/AST have occurred, including rare reports of severe hepatic injury (some fatal); monitor hepatic transaminases periodically in patients with hepatic impairment. Use with caution in patients with renal dysfunction. Avoid use in the elderly due to its potent anticholinergic and sedative properties, and potential to cause orthostatic hypotension. In addition, may also cause or exacerbate syndrome of inappropriate antidiuretic hormone secretion or hyponatremia; monitor sodium closely with initiation or dosage adjustments in older adults (Beers Criteria).

Abrupt discontinuation or interruption of antidepressant therapy has been associated with a discontinuation syndrome. Symptoms arising may vary with antidepressant however commonly include nausea, vomiting, diarrhea, headaches, light-headedness, dizziness, diminished appetite, sweating, chills, tremors, paresthesias, fatigue, somnolence, and sleep disturbances (eg, vivid dreams, insomnia). Greater risks for developing a discontinuation syndrome have been associated with antidepressants with shorter half-lives, longer durations of treatment, and abrupt discontinuation. For antidepressants of short or intermediate half-lives, symptoms may emerge within 2-5 days after treatment discontinuation and last 7-14 days (APA, 2010; Fava, 2006; Haddad, 2001; Shelton, 2001; Warner, 2006).

Drug Interactions
Avoid Concomitant Use
Avoid concomitant use of ClomiPRAMINE with any of the following: Aclidinium; Iobenguane I 123; Ipratropium (Oral Inhalation); Linezolid; MAO Inhibitors; Methylene Blue; Moxonidine; Thioridazine; Tiotropium; Umeclidinium

Decreased Effect
ClomiPRAMINE may decrease the levels/effects of: Acetylcholinesterase Inhibitors (Central); Alpha2-Agonists; Alpha2-Agonists (Ophthalmic); Codeine; Iobenguane I 123; Moxonidine; Tamoxifen

The levels/effects of ClomiPRAMINE may be decreased by: Acetylcholinesterase Inhibitors (Central); Barbiturates; CYP1A2 Inducers (Strong); CYP2C19 Inducers (Strong); Cyproterone; Dabrafenib; Peginterferon Alfa-2b; St Johns Wort

Increased Effect/Toxicity
ClomiPRAMINE may increase the levels/effects of: Alpha-/Beta-Agonists (Direct-Acting); Alpha1-Agonists; Amphetamines; Analgesics (Opioid); Anticholinergics; Antipsychotics; Aspirin; Beta2-Agonists; Citalopram; CYP2D6 Substrates; Desmopressin; DOXOrubicin (Conventional); Escitalopram; Fesoterodine; Highest Risk QTc-Prolonging Agents; Methylene Blue; Metoclopramide; Metoprolol; Milnacipran; Moderate Risk QTc-Prolonging Agents; Nebivolol; NSAID (COX-2 Inhibitor); NSAID (Nonselective); QuiNIDine; Serotonin Modulators; Sodium Phosphates; Sulfonylureas; Thioridazine; Tiotropium; TraMADol; Vitamin K Antagonists; Yohimbine

The levels/effects of ClomiPRAMINE may be increased by: Abiraterone Acetate; Aclidinium; Altretamine; Antipsychotics; BuPROPion; CarBAMazepine; Cimetidine; Cinacalcet; Citalopram; Cobicistat; CYP1A2 Inhibitors (Moderate); CYP1A2 Inhibitors (Strong); CYP2C19 Inhibitors (Moderate); CYP2C19 Inhibitors (Strong); CYP2D6 Inhibitors (Moderate); CYP2D6 Inhibitors (Strong); Deferasirox; Dexmethylphenidate; DULoxetine; Escitalopram; FLUoxetine; FluvoxaMINE; Grapefruit Juice; Ipratropium (Oral Inhalation); Linezolid; Lithium; Luliconazole; MAO Inhibitors; Methylphenidate; Metoclopramide; Metyrosine; Mifepristone; PARoxetine; Pramlintide; Propafenone; Protease Inhibitors; QuiNIDine; Sertraline; Terbinafine (Systemic); Thyroid Products; TraMADol; Umeclidinium; Valproic Acid and Derivatives; Vemurafenib

Nutritional/Ethanol Interactions
Ethanol: Ethanol may increase CNS depression. Management: Avoid ethanol.
Food: Serum concentrations/toxicity may be increased by grapefruit juice. Management: Avoid grapefruit juice.
Herb/Nutraceutical: St John's wort and tryptophan may increase the serotonergic effect of clomipramine, thus increasing the risk of serotonin syndrome. Clomipramine may increase the serum concentration of yohimbe. Management: Avoid valerian, St John's wort, tryptophan, SAMe, kava kava, and yohimbe.

Adverse Reactions
Data shown for children reflects both children and adolescents studied in clinical trials.
>10%:
Cardiovascular: Orthostatic hypotension (4% to 20%), tachycardia (2% to 20%)
Central nervous system: Somnolence (46% to 54%), dizziness (adults 54%; children 41%), headache (adults 52%; children 28%), fatigue (35% to 39%), insomnia (adults 25%; children 11%), nervousness (adults 18%; children 4%)
Endocrine & metabolic: Libido changes (adults 21%)

Gastrointestinal: Xerostomia (adults 84%, children 63%), constipation (adults 47%; children 22%), nausea (adults 33%; children 9%), dyspepsia (13% to 22%), anorexia (12% to 22%), weight gain (adults 18%; children 2%), diarrhea (7% to 13%), abdominal pain (11%), appetite increased (11%)

Genitourinary: Ejaculation failure (adults 42%, children 6%), impotence (adults 20%), micturition disorder (adults 14%; children 4%)

Neuromuscular & skeletal: Tremor (adults 54%; children 33%), myoclonus (adults 13%; children 2%), myalgia (adults 13%)

Ophthalmic: Abnormal vision (adults 18%; children 7%)

Respiratory: Pharyngitis (adults 14%), rhinitis (adults 12%)

Miscellaneous: Diaphoresis increased (adults 29%; children 9%)

1% to 10%:

Cardiovascular: Flushing (7% to 8%), chest pain (children 7%), palpitation (4%), ECG abnormality (2%), syncope (children 2%)

Central nervous system: Anxiety (adults 9%; children 2%), memory impairment (7% to 9%), sleep disorder (4% to 9%), twitching (adults 7%), concentration impaired (adults 5%), depression (adults 5%), fever (adults 4%), pain (3% to 4%), hypertonia (2% to 4%), abnormal dreaming (adults 3%), agitation (adults 3%), migraine (adults 3%), psychosomatic disorder (adults 3%), speech disorder (adults 3%), yawning (adults 3%), aggressiveness (children 2%), chills (adults 2%), depersonalization (2%), emotional lability (adults 2%), irritability (children 2%), myasthenia (1% to 2%), panic reaction (1% to 2%), abnormal thinking, vertigo

Dermatologic: Rash (4% to 8%), pruritus (adults 6%), purpura (adults 3%), body odor (children 2%), dermatitis (adults 2%), dry skin (adults 2%), urticaria (adults 1%)

Endocrine & metabolic: Hot flashes (2% to 5%), lactation (nonpuerperal; adults 4%), menstrual disorder (adults 4%), breast enlargement (adults 2%), amenorrhea (adults 1%), breast pain (adults 1%)

Gastrointestinal: Taste disturbance (4% to 8%), vomiting (7%), weight loss (children 7%), flatulence (adults 6%), tooth disorder (adults 5%), dysphagia (adults 2%), gastrointestinal disturbance (adults 2%), halitosis (children 2%), ulcerative stomatitis (children 2%), esophagitis (adults 1%)

Genitourinary: Urinary retention (children 7%; adults 2%), UTI (adults 6%), micturition frequency (adults 5%), cystitis (adults 2%), leukorrhea (adults 2%), vaginitis (adults 2%)

Hepatic: Increased serum ALT (>3 x ULN: 3%), increased serum AST (>3 x ULN: 1%)

Hypersensitivity: Hypersensitivity reaction (children 7%)

Neuromuscular & skeletal: Paresthesia (adults 9%; children 2%), paresis (children 2%), weakness (children 1%)

Ophthalmic: Lacrimation abnormal (adults 3%), anisocoria (children 2%), blepharospasm (children 2%), mydriasis (adults 2%), ocular allergy (children 2%), conjunctivitis (adults 1%)

Otic: Tinnitus (4% to 6%)

Respiratory: Bronchospasm (children 7%; adults 2%), sinusitis (adults 6%), dyspnea (children 2%), epistaxis (adults 2%), laryngitis (children 2%)

Available Dosage Forms

Capsule, Oral:

Anafranil: 25 mg, 50 mg, 75 mg

Generic: 25 mg, 50 mg, 75 mg

General Dosage Range Oral:

Children ≥10 years and Adolescents: Initial: 25 mg daily; Maintenance: Up to 3 mg/kg/day (maximum: 200 mg daily)

Adults: Initial: 25 mg daily; Maintenance: Up to 250 mg daily

Administration

Oral During titration, may divide doses and administer with meals to decrease gastrointestinal side effects. After titration, may administer total daily dose at bedtime to decrease daytime sedation.

Nursing Actions

Physical Assessment If history of cardiac problems, monitor cardiac status closely. Be alert to the potential of new or increased seizure activity. Observe for clinical worsening, suicidality, or unusual behavior changes, especially during the initial few months of therapy or during dosage changes. Instruct family or caregiver to observe the patient's behavior closely and communicate any changes to prescriber. Taper dosage slowly when discontinuing.

Patient Education

• Discuss specific use of drug and side effects with patient as it relates to treatment. (HCAHPS: During this hospital stay, were you given any medicine that you had not taken before? Before giving you any new medicine, how often did hospital staff tell you what the medicine was for? How often did hospital staff describe possible side effects in a way you could understand?)

• Patient may experience xerostomia, constipation, dyspepsia, anxiety, fatigue, polyphagia, lack of appetite, weight gain or loss, sexual dysfunction, or myalgia. Have patient report immediately to prescriber signs of hepatic impairment, signs of infection, suicidal ideation, syncope, illogical thinking, significant asthenia, tremors, bradykinesia, rigidity, vision changes, angina, difficult urination, ecchymosis, hemorrhaging, paresthesia, memory loss, serotonin syndrome (ie, dizziness, severe headache, agitation, hallucinations, tachycardia, arrhythmia, flushing, tremors, hyperhidrosis, change in balance, severe nausea, significant diarrhea), or signs of neuroleptic malignant syndrome (NMS) (HCAHPS).

- Educate patient about signs of a significant reaction (eg, wheezing; chest tightness; fever; itching; bad cough; blue skin color; seizures; or swelling of face, lips, tongue, or throat). **Note:** This is not a comprehensive list of all side effects. Patient should consult prescriber for additional questions.

Intended Use and Disclaimer: Should not be printed and given to patients. This information is intended to serve as a concise initial reference for healthcare professionals to use when discussing medications with a patient. You must ultimately rely on your own discretion, experience and judgment in diagnosing, treating and advising patients.

ClonazePAM (kloe NA ze pam)

Brand Names: U.S. KlonoPIN
Pharmacologic Category Benzodiazepine
Medication Safety Issues
Sound-alike/look-alike issues:
ClonazePAM may be confused with cloBAZam, cloNIDine, clorazepate, cloZAPine, LORazepam
KlonoPIN® may be confused with cloNIDine, clorazepate, cloZAPine, LORazepam

BEERS Criteria medication:
This drug may be potentially inappropriate for use in geriatric patients (Quality of evidence - high; Strength of recommendation - strong).

Medication Guide Available Yes
Pregnancy Risk Factor D
Lactation Enters breast milk/not recommended
Breast-Feeding Considerations Clonazepam enters breast milk. Drowsiness, lethargy, or weight loss in nursing infants have been observed in case reports following maternal use of some benzodiazepines (Iqbal, 2002). The manufacturer states that women taking clonazepam should not breast-feed their infants.

Use Alone or as an adjunct in the treatment of petit mal variant (Lennox-Gastaut), akinetic, and myoclonic seizures; petit mal (absence) seizures unresponsive to succimides; panic disorder with or without agoraphobia

Unlabeled Use Restless legs syndrome; neuralgia; multifocal tic disorder; parkinsonian dysarthria; bipolar disorder; adjunct therapy for schizophrenia; burning mouth syndrome; essential tremor

Mechanism of Action/Effect The exact mechanism is unknown, but believed to be related to its ability to enhance the activity of GABA; suppresses the spike-and-wave discharge in absence seizures by depressing nerve transmission in the motor cortex

Contraindications Hypersensitivity to clonazepam or any component of the formulation (cross-sensitivity with other benzodiazepines may exist);

significant liver disease; acute narrow-angle glaucoma

Warnings/Precautions Hazardous agent - use appropriate precautions for handling and disposal (NIOSH, 2012). Antiepileptics are associated with an increased risk of suicidal behavior/thoughts with use (regardless of indication); patients should be monitored for signs/symptoms of depression, suicidal tendencies, and other unusual behavior changes during therapy and instructed to inform their healthcare provider immediately if symptoms occur.

Use with caution in elderly or debilitated patients, patients with hepatic disease (including alcoholics), or renal impairment. Use with caution in patients with respiratory disease or impaired gag reflex or ability to protect the airway from secretions (salivation may be increased). Worsening of seizures may occur when added to patients with multiple seizure types. Concurrent use with valproic acid may result in absence status. Monitoring of CBC and liver function tests has been recommended during prolonged therapy.

Causes CNS depression (dose related) resulting in sedation, dizziness, confusion, or ataxia which may impair physical and mental capabilities. Patients must be cautioned about performing tasks which require mental alertness (eg, operating machinery or driving). Use with caution in patients receiving other CNS depressants or psychoactive agents. Effects with other sedative drugs or ethanol may be potentiated. Benzodiazepines have been associated with falls and traumatic injury and should be used with extreme caution in patients who are at risk of these events.

Use caution in patients with depression, particularly if suicidal risk may be present. Use with caution in patients with a history of drug dependence. Benzodiazepines have been associated with dependence and acute withdrawal symptoms, including seizures, on discontinuation or reduction in dose. Acute withdrawal, including seizures, may be precipitated in patients after administration of flumazenil to patients receiving long-term benzodiazepine therapy.

Benzodiazepines have been associated with anterograde amnesia. Paradoxical reactions, including hyperactive or aggressive behavior, have been reported with benzodiazepines, particularly in adolescent/pediatric or psychiatric patients. Does not have analgesic, antidepressant, or antipsychotic properties.

In older adults, benzodiazepines increase the risk of impaired cognition, delirium, falls, fractures, and motor vehicle accidents. Due to increased sensitivity in this age group and slower metabolism of long-acting agents (such as clonazepam), avoid use for treatment of insomnia, agitation, or delirium (Beers Criteria).

◄ **Drug Interactions**

Avoid Concomitant Use

Avoid concomitant use of ClonazePAM with any of the following: Azelastine (Nasal); Conivaptan; Fusidic Acid (Systemic); OLANZapine; Paraldehyde; Sodium Oxybate; Thalidomide

Decreased Effect

The levels/effects of ClonazePAM may be decreased by: Bosentan; CarBAMazepine; CYP3A4 Inducers (Strong); Dabrafenib; Deferasirox; Herbs (CYP3A4 Inducers); Mitotane; Rifamycin Derivatives; Theophylline Derivatives; Tocilizumab; Yohimbine

Increased Effect/Toxicity

ClonazePAM may increase the levels/effects of: Alcohol (Ethyl); Azelastine (Nasal); Buprenorphine; CloZAPine; CNS Depressants; Fosphenytoin; Hydrocodone; Methotrimeprazine; Metyrosine; Mirtazapine; Paraldehyde; Phenytoin; Pramipexole; ROPINIRole; Rotigotine; Selective Serotonin Reuptake Inhibitors; Sodium Oxybate; Thalidomide; Zolpidem

The levels/effects of ClonazePAM may be increased by: Antifungal Agents (Azole Derivatives, Systemic); Aprepitant; Brimonidine (Topical); Calcium Channel Blockers (Nondihydropyridine); Cimetidine; Cobicistat; Conivaptan; Contraceptives (Estrogens); Contraceptives (Progestins); Cosyntropin; CYP3A4 Inhibitors (Moderate); CYP3A4 Inhibitors (Strong); Dasatinib; Doxylamine; Droperidol; Fosaprepitant; Fusidic Acid (Systemic); Grapefruit Juice; HydrOXYzine; Isoniazid; Ivacaftor; Luliconazole; Magnesium Sulfate; Methotrimeprazine; Mifepristone; OLANZapine; Perampanel; Proton Pump Inhibitors; Selective Serotonin Reuptake Inhibitors; Simeprevir; Stiripentol; Tapentadol; Vigabatrin

Nutritional/Ethanol Interactions

Ethanol: May increase CNS depression; monitor for increased effects with coadministration. Caution patients about effects.

Food: Clonazepam serum concentration is unlikely to be increased by grapefruit juice because of clonazepam's high oral bioavailability.

Herb/Nutraceutical: St John's wort may decrease clonazepam levels. Avoid valerian, St John's wort, kava kava, gotu kola (may increase CNS depression).

Adverse Reactions Reactions reported in patients with seizure and/or panic disorder. Frequency not always defined.

Cardiovascular: Edema (ankle or facial), palpitation

Central nervous system: Amnesia, ataxia (seizure disorder ~30%; panic disorder 5%), behavior problems (seizure disorder ~25%), coma, confusion, coordination impaired, depression, dizziness, drowsiness (seizure disorder ~50%), emotional lability, fatigue, fever, hallucinations, headache, hysteria, insomnia, intellectual ability reduced, memory disturbance, nervousness; paradoxical reactions (including aggressive behavior, agitation, anxiety, excitability, hostility, irritability, nervousness, nightmares, sleep disturbance, vivid dreams); psychosis, slurred speech, somnolence (panic disorder 37%), vertigo

Dermatologic: Hair loss, hirsutism, skin rash

Endocrine & metabolic: Dysmenorrhea, libido increased/decreased

Gastrointestinal: Abdominal pain, anorexia, appetite increased/decreased, coated tongue, constipation, dehydration, diarrhea, encopresis, gastritis, gum soreness, nausea, weight changes (loss/gain), xerostomia

Genitourinary: Colpitis, dysuria, ejaculation delayed, enuresis, impotence, micturition frequency, nocturia, urinary retention, urinary tract infection

Hematologic: Anemia, eosinophilia, leukopenia, thrombocytopenia

Hepatic: Alkaline phosphatase increased (transient), hepatomegaly, transaminases increased (transient)

Neuromuscular & skeletal: Choreiform movements, coordination abnormal, dysarthria, hypotonia, muscle pain, muscle weakness, myalgia, tremor

Ocular: Blurred vision, eye movements abnormal, diplopia, nystagmus

Respiratory: Bronchitis, chest congestion, cough, hypersecretions, pharyngitis, respiratory depression, respiratory tract infection, rhinitis, rhinorrhea, shortness of breath, sinusitis

Miscellaneous: Allergic reaction, aphonia, dysdiadochokinesis, "glassy-eyed" appearance, hemiparesis, flu-like syndrome, lymphadenopathy

<1% (Limited to important or life-threatening): Apathy, burning skin, chest pain, depersonalization, dyspnea, excessive dreaming, hyperactivity, hypoesthesia, hypotension postural, infection, migraine, organic disinhibition, pain, paresthesia, paresis, periorbital edema, polyuria, suicidal attempt, suicide ideation, thick tongue, twitching, visual disturbance, xerophthalmia

Pharmacodynamics/Kinetics

Onset of Action ~20-40 minutes (Hanson, 1972)

Duration of Action Infants and young children: 6-8 hours (Hanson, 1972); Adults: ≤12 hours (Hanson, 1972)

Controlled Substance C-IV

Available Dosage Forms

Tablet, Oral:

KlonoPIN: 0.5 mg, 1 mg, 2 mg

Generic: 0.5 mg, 1 mg, 2 mg

Tablet Dispersible, Oral:

Generic: 0.125 mg, 0.25 mg, 0.5 mg, 1 mg, 2 mg

General Dosage Range Oral:

Children <10 years or <30 kg: Seizure disorders: Initial: 0.01-0.03 mg/kg/day in 2-3 divided doses (maximum: 0.05 mg/kg/day); Maintenance: 0.1-0.2 mg/kg/day in 3 divided doses (maximum: 0.2 mg/kg/day)

Children ≥10 years or ≥30 kg, Adolescents, and Adults: Seizure disorders: Initial: Up to 1.5 mg/day in 3 divided doses; Maintenance: 2-8 mg daily in 1-2 divided doses (Brodie, 1997) (maximum: 20 mg daily)
Adults: Panic disorders: Initial: 0.25 mg twice daily; Maintenance: 1-4 mg daily in 2 divided doses;

Administration
Oral
Orally-disintegrating tablet: Open pouch and peel back foil on the blister; do not push tablet through foil. Use dry hands to remove tablet and place in mouth. May be swallowed with or without water. Use immediately after removing from package.
Tablet: Swallow whole with water.

Hazardous agent; use appropriate precautions for handling and disposal (NIOSH, 2012).
Storage/Stability Store at 25°C (77°F); excursions permitted to 15°C to 30°C (59°F to 80°F)
Nursing Actions
Physical Assessment Assess for signs of CNS depression (sedation, dizziness, confusion, or ataxia). Assess history of addiction; long-term use can result in dependence, abuse, or tolerance; periodically evaluate need for continued use. For inpatient use, institute safety measures to prevent falls. Taper dosage slowly when discontinuing. Teach patient seizure precautions (if administered for seizures).
Patient Education
• Discuss specific use of drug and side effects with patient as it relates to treatment. (HCAHPS: During this hospital stay, were you given any medicine that you had not taken before? Before giving you any new medicine, how often did hospital staff tell you what the medicine was for? How often did hospital staff describe possible side effects in a way you could understand?)
• Patient may experience presyncope, fatigue, blurred vision, constipation, sialorrhea, or dizziness. Have patient report immediately to prescriber dyspnea, significant change in balance, considerable asthenia, memory loss, or signs of depression (ie, suicidal ideation, anxiety, emotional instability, illogical thinking) (HCAHPS).
• Educate patient about signs of a significant reaction (eg, wheezing; chest tightness; fever; itching; bad cough; blue skin color; seizures; or swelling of face, lips, tongue, or throat). **Note:** This is not a comprehensive list of all side effects. Patient should consult prescriber for additional questions.

Intended Use and Disclaimer: Should not be printed and given to patients. This information is intended to serve as a concise initial reference for healthcare professionals to use when discussing medications with a patient. You must ultimately rely on your own discretion, experience and judgment in diagnosing, treating and advising patients.

CloNIDine (KLON i deen)

Brand Names: U.S. Catapres; Catapres-TTS-1; Catapres-TTS-2; Catapres-TTS-3; Duraclon; Kapvay
Index Terms Clonidine Hydrochloride
Pharmacologic Category Alpha$_2$-Adrenergic Agonist; Antihypertensive
Medication Safety Issues
Sound-alike/look-alike issues:
CloNIDine may be confused with Clomid®, clomiPHENE, clonazePAM, cloZAPine, KlonoPIN®, quiNIDine
Catapres® may be confused with Cataflam®, Combipres
High alert medication:
The Institute for Safe Medication Practices (ISMP) includes this medication (epidural administration) among its list of drug classes which have a heightened risk of causing significant patient harm when used in error.
BEERS Criteria medication:
This drug may be potentially inappropriate for use in geriatric patients (Quality of evidence - low; Strength of recommendation - strong).
Administration issues:
Use caution when interpreting dosing information. Pediatric dose for epidural infusion expressed as mcg/kg/hour.
Other safety concerns:
Transdermal patch may contain conducting metal (eg, aluminum); remove patch prior to MRI. Errors have occurred when the inactive, optional adhesive cover has been applied instead of the active clonidine-containing patch.
Pregnancy Risk Factor C
Lactation Enters breast milk/use caution
Breast-Feeding Considerations Clonidine is excreted in breast milk. Concentrations have been noted as ~7% to 8% of those in the maternal plasma following oral dosing (Atkinson, 1988; Bunjes, 1993) and twice those in the maternal serum following epidural administration. The manufacturer recommends caution be used if administered to nursing women. Another source recommends avoiding use when nursing infants born <34 weeks gestation or when large maternal doses are needed (Atkinson, 1988). Breast-fed infants of mothers taking medications for hypertension should be monitored for adverse effects (Chobanian, 2003).
Use
Oral:
Immediate release: Management of hypertension (monotherapy or as adjunctive therapy)
Extended release (Kapvay™): Treatment of attention-deficit/hyperactivity disorder (ADHD) (monotherapy or as adjunctive therapy)

Epidural (Duraclon®): For continuous epidural administration as adjunctive therapy with opioids for treatment of severe cancer pain in patients tolerant to or unresponsive to opioids alone; epidural clonidine is generally more effective for neuropathic pain and less effective (or possibly ineffective) for somatic or visceral pain

Transdermal patch: Management of hypertension (monotherapy or as adjunctive therapy)

Unlabeled Use Heroin or nicotine withdrawal; severe pain; dysmenorrhea; vasomotor symptoms associated with menopause; ethanol dependence; prophylaxis of migraines; glaucoma; diabetes-associated diarrhea; impulse control disorder, clozapine-induced sialorrhea; aid in the diagnosis of growth hormone deficiency; attention-deficit/hyperactivity disorder (ADHD) and associated insomnia in children; Tourette's syndrome in children; aggression associated with conduct disorder

Mechanism of Action/Effect Stimulates alpha$_2$-adrenoceptors in the brain stem, thus activating an inhibitory neuron, resulting in reduced sympathetic outflow from the CNS, producing a decrease in peripheral resistance, renal vascular resistance, heart rate, and blood pressure; epidural clonidine may produce pain relief at spinal presynaptic and postjunctional alpha$_2$-adrenoceptors by preventing pain signal transmission; pain relief occurs only for the body regions innervated by the spinal segments where analgesic concentrations of clonidine exist; in the treatment of ADHD, the mechanism of action is unknown.

Contraindications Hypersensitivity to clonidine hydrochloride or any component of the formulation

Epidural administration: Injection site infection; concurrent anticoagulant therapy; bleeding diathesis; administration above the C4 dermatome

Warnings/Precautions May cause CNS depression, which may impair physical or mental abilities; patients must be cautioned about performing tasks which require mental alertness (eg, operating machinery or driving). Sedating effects may be potentiated when used with other CNS-depressant drugs or ethanol. Use with caution in patients with severe coronary insufficiency; conduction disturbances; recent MI, CVA, or chronic renal insufficiency. May cause dose dependent reductions in heart rate; use with caution in patients with pre-existing bradycardia or those predisposed to developing bradycardia. Caution in sinus node dysfunction. Use with caution in patients concurrently receiving agents known to reduce SA node function and/or AV nodal conduction (eg, digoxin, diltiazem, metoprolol, verapamil). May cause significant xerostomia. Clonidine may cause eye dryness in patients who wear contact lenses.

[U.S. Boxed Warning]: Must dilute concentrated epidural injectable (500 mcg/mL) solution prior to use. Epidural clonidine is not recommended for perioperative, obstetrical, or postpartum pain due to risk of hemodynamic instability. Clonidine injection should be administered via a continuous epidural infusion device. Monitor closely for catheter-related infection such as meningitis or epidural abscess. Epidural clonidine is not recommended for use in patients with severe cardiovascular disease or hemodynamic instability; may lead to cardiovascular instability (hypotension, bradycardia). Symptomatic hypotension may occur with use; in all patients, use epidural clonidine with caution due to the potential for severe hypotension especially in women and those of low body weight. Most hypotensive episodes occur within the first 4 days of initiation; however, episodes may occur throughout the duration of therapy.

Gradual withdrawal is needed (taper oral immediate release or epidural dose gradually over 2-4 days to avoid rebound hypertension) if drug needs to be stopped. Patients should be instructed about abrupt discontinuation (causes rapid increase in BP and symptoms of sympathetic overactivity). In patients on both a beta-blocker and clonidine where withdrawal of clonidine is necessary, withdraw the beta-blocker first and several days before clonidine withdrawal, then slowly decrease clonidine. In children and adolescents, extended release formulation (Kapvay™) should be tapered in decrements of no more than 0.1 mg every 3-7 days. Discontinue oral immediate release formulations within 4 hours of surgery then restart as soon as possible afterwards. Discontinue oral extended release formulations up to 28 hours prior to surgery, then restart the following day.

Oral formulations of clonidine (immediate release versus extended release) are not interchangeable on a mg:mg basis due to different pharmacokinetic profiles.

Transdermal patch may contain conducting metal (eg, aluminum); remove patch prior to MRI. Due to the potential for altered electrical conductivity, remove transdermal patch before cardioversion or defibrillation. Localized contact sensitization to the transdermal system has been reported; in these patients, allergic reactions (eg, generalized rash, urticaria, angioedema) have also occurred following subsequent substitution of oral therapy.

In the elderly, avoid use as first-line antihypertensive due to high risk of CNS adverse effects; may also cause orthostatic hypotension and bradycardia (Beers Criteria). In pediatric patients, epidural clonidine should be reserved for cancer patients with severe intractable pain, unresponsive to other analgesics or epidural or spinal opioids. Use oral formulations with caution in pediatric patients since children commonly have gastrointestinal illnesses with vomiting and are susceptible to hypertensive episodes due to abrupt inability to take oral medication.

Drug Interactions

Avoid Concomitant Use

Avoid concomitant use of CloNIDine with any of the following: Azelastine (Nasal); Iobenguane I 123; Paraldehyde; Thalidomide

Decreased Effect

CloNIDine may decrease the levels/effects of: Iobenguane I 123

The levels/effects of CloNIDine may be decreased by: Antidepressants (Alpha2-Antagonist); Herbs (Hypertensive Properties); Serotonin/Norepinephrine Reuptake Inhibitors; Tricyclic Antidepressants; Yohimbine

Increased Effect/Toxicity

CloNIDine may increase the levels/effects of: Alcohol (Ethyl); Amifostine; Antihypertensives; Azelastine (Nasal); Beta-Blockers; Buprenorphine; Calcium Channel Blockers (Nondihydropyridine); Cardiac Glycosides; CNS Depressants; Hydrocodone; Hypotensive Agents; Methotrimeprazine; Metyrosine; Obinutuzumab; Paraldehyde; Pramipexole; RiTUXimab; ROPINIRole; Rotigotine; Selective Serotonin Reuptake Inhibitors; Thalidomide; Zolpidem

The levels/effects of CloNIDine may be increased by: Alfuzosin; Beta-Blockers; Brimonidine (Topical); Diazoxide; Doxylamine; Droperidol; Herbs (Hypotensive Properties); HydrOXYzine; Magnesium Sulfate; MAO Inhibitors; Methotrimeprazine; Methylphenidate; Pentoxifylline; Perampanel; Phosphodiesterase 5 Inhibitors; Prostacyclin Analogues; Sodium Oxybate; Tapentadol

Nutritional/Ethanol Interactions

Ethanol: Avoid ethanol (may increase CNS depression).

Herb/Nutraceutical: Avoid dong quai if using for hypertension (has estrogenic activity). Avoid ephedra, yohimbe, ginseng (may worsen hypertension). Avoid valerian, St John's wort, kava kava, gotu kola (may increase CNS depression).

Adverse Reactions Frequency not always defined.

Oral, Transdermal: Incidence of adverse events may be less with transdermal compared to oral due to the lower peak/trough ratio.

Cardiovascular: Bradycardia (≤4%), palpitation (1%), tachycardia (1%), arrhythmia, atrioventricular block, chest pain, CHF, ECG abnormalities, flushing, orthostatic hypotension, pallor, Raynaud's phenomenon, syncope

Central nervous system: Drowsiness (12% to 38%), headache (1% to 29%), fatigue (4% to 16%), dizziness (2% to 16%), sedation (3% to 10%), insomnia (≤6%), lethargy (3%), nervousness (1% to 3%), mental depression (1%), aggression, agitation, anxiety, behavioral changes, CVA, delirium, delusional perception, fever, hallucinations (visual and auditory), irritability, malaise, nightmares, restlessness, vivid dreams

Dermatologic: Transient localized skin reactions characterized by pruritus and erythema (transdermal 15% to 50%), contact dermatitis (transdermal 8% to 34%), vesiculation (transdermal 7%), allergic contact sensitization (transdermal 5%), hyperpigmentation (transdermal 5%), burning (transdermal 3%), edema (3%), excoriation (transdermal 3%) blanching (transdermal 1%), generalized macular rash (1%), papules (transdermal 1%), throbbing (transdermal 1%), alopecia, angioedema, hives, localized hypopigmentation (transdermal), rash, urticaria

Endocrine & metabolic: Sexual dysfunction (3%), gynecomastia (1%), creatine phosphokinase increased (transient; oral), hyperglycemia (transient; oral), libido decreased

Gastrointestinal: Xerostomia (≤40%), constipation (2% to 10%), anorexia (1%), taste perversion (1%), weight gain (<1%), abdominal pain (oral), diarrhea, nausea, parotid gland pain (oral), parotitis (oral), pseudo-obstruction (oral), throat pain, vomiting

Genitourinary: Erectile dysfunction (2% to 3%), nocturia (1%), dysuria, enuresis, urinary retention

Hematologic: Thrombocytopenia (oral)

Hepatic: Liver function test (mild transient abnormalities; ≤1%), hepatitis

Neuromuscular & skeletal: Weakness (10%), arthralgia (1%), myalgia (1%), leg cramps (<1%), numbness (localized, transdermal), pain in extremities, paresthesia, tremor

Ocular: Accommodation disorder, blurred vision, burning eyes, dry eyes, lacrimation decreased, lacrimation increased

Otic: Ear pain, otitis media

Renal: Pollakiuria

Respiratory: Asthma, epistaxis, nasal congestion, nasal dryness, nasopharyngitis, respiratory tract infection, rhinorrhea

Miscellaneous: Withdrawal syndrome (1%), flu-like syndrome, thirst

Epidural: Note: The following adverse events occurred more often than placebo in cancer patients with intractable pain being treated with concurrent epidural morphine.

>10%:

Cardiovascular: Hypotension (45%), orthostatic hypotension (32%)

Central nervous system: Confusion (13%), dizziness (13%)

Gastrointestinal: Xerostomia (13%)

1% to 10%:

Cardiovascular: Chest pain (5%)

Central nervous system: Hallucinations (5%)

Gastrointestinal: Nausea/vomiting (8%)

Otic: Tinnitus (5%)

Miscellaneous: Diaphoresis (5%)

◀ **Pharmacodynamics/Kinetics**

Onset of Action Oral: Immediate release: 0.5-1 hour (maximum reduction in blood pressure: 2-4 hours); Transdermal: Initial application: 2-3 days

Duration of Action Oral: Immediate release: 6-10 hours

Available Dosage Forms

Patch Weekly, Transdermal:
Catapres-TTS-1: 0.1 mg/24 hr (4 ea)
Catapres-TTS-2: 0.2 mg/24 hr (4 ea)
Catapres-TTS-3: 0.3 mg/24 hr (4 ea)
Generic: 0.1 mg/24 hr (4 ea); 0.2 mg/24 hr (4 ea); 0.3 mg/24 hr (4 ea)

Solution, Epidural:
Duraclon: 100 mcg/mL (10 mL)
Generic: 100 mcg/mL (10 mL); 500 mcg/mL (10 mL)

Solution, Epidural [preservative free]:
Duraclon: 100 mcg/mL (10 mL); 500 mcg/mL (10 mL)
Generic: 100 mcg/mL (10 mL); 500 mcg/mL (10 mL)

Tablet, Oral:
Catapres: 0.1 mg, 0.2 mg, 0.3 mg
Generic: 0.1 mg, 0.2 mg, 0.3 mg

Tablet Extended Release 12 Hour, Oral:
Kapvay: 0.1 mg
Generic: 0.1 mg

General Dosage Range Note: Dosing is expressed as the salt (clonidine hydrochloride) unless otherwise noted.

Epidural:
Children: Initial: 0.5 mcg/kg/**hour**
Adults: Initial: 30 mcg/hour; Maintenance: Up to 40 mcg/hour

Oral, immediate release:
Adults: Initial: 0.1 mg twice daily; Maintenance: 0.1-0.8 mg/day in 2 divided doses (maximum: 2.4 mg/day)
Elderly: Initial: 0.1 mg once daily

Oral, extended release: *Children ≥6 years:* (Kapvay™): Initial: 0.1 mg at bedtime; maximum: 0.4 mg/day [ADHD use]

Transdermal: *Adults:* Initial: 0.1 mg/24 hour patch applied once every 7 days; Maintenance: 0.1-0.3 mg/24 hour patch applied once every 7 days (maximum: 0.6 mg/24 hours)

Administration

Oral May be taken with or without food. Do not discontinue clonidine abruptly. If needed, gradually reduce dose over 2-4 days to avoid rebound hypertension.
Extended release tablet: Kapvay™: Swallow whole; do not crush, split, or chew.

Topical Transdermal patch: Patches should be applied weekly at a consistent time to a clean, hairless area of the upper outer arm or chest. Rotate patch sites weekly. Redness under patch may be reduced if a topical corticosteroid spray is applied to the area before placement of the patch (Tom, 1994).

Other Epidural: Specialized techniques are required for continuous epidural administration; administration via this route should only be performed by qualified individuals familiar with the techniques of epidural administration and patient management problems associated with this route. Familiarization of the epidural infusion device is essential. Do not discontinue clonidine abruptly; if needed, gradually reduce dose over 2-4 days to avoid withdrawal symptoms.

Preparation for Administration Epidural formulation: Prior to administration, the 500 mcg/mL concentration must be diluted in 0.9% sodium chloride for injection (preservative-free) to a final concentration of 100 mcg/mL.

Storage/Stability
Epidural formulation: Store at 25°C (77°F); excursions permitted to 15°C to 30°C (59°F to 86°F). **Preservative free;** discard unused portion.
Tablets: Store at 25°C (77°F); excursions permitted to 15°C to 30°C (59°F to 86°F). Protect from light.
Extended release tablets: Store at 20°C to 25°C (68°F to 77°F). Protect from light.
Transdermal patches: Store below 30°C (86°F).

Nursing Actions

Physical Assessment Assess potential for interactions with other medications that may cause additive hypotension, bradycardia, or CNS depression. Monitor blood pressure and mental status throughout. Advise patients using oral hypoglycemic agents or insulin to check glucose levels closely; clonidine may decrease the symptoms of hypoglycemia. When discontinuing, monitor blood pressure and taper dose gradually (over 1 week for oral, 2-4 days for epidural).

Patient Education

• Discuss specific use of drug and side effects with patient as it relates to treatment. (HCAHPS: During this hospital stay, were you given any medicine that you had not taken before? Before giving you any new medicine, how often did hospital staff tell you what the medicine was for? How often did hospital staff describe possible side effects in a way you could understand?)

• Patient may experience xerostomia, constipation, fatigue, asthenia, insomnia, rhinitis, rhinorrhea, polyphagia, hyperhidrosis, emesis, or tinnitus. Have patient report immediately to prescriber severe dizziness, syncope, vision changes, angina, illogical thinking, urine discoloration, jaundice, sexual dysfunction, difficult urination, contact lens discomfort, bradycardia, tachycardia, arrhythmia, mood changes, depression, hallucinations, significant headache, dyspnea, significant weight gain, edema of extremities, dyspepsia, ecchymosis, hemorrhaging, otalgia, pharyngitis, chills, nightmares, epistaxis, polyuria, considerable skin irritation, or skin discoloration (HCAHPS).

• Educate patient about signs of a significant reaction (eg, wheezing; chest tightness; fever;

itching; bad cough; blue skin color; seizures; or swelling of face, lips, tongue, or throat). **Note:** This is not a comprehensive list of all side effects. Patient should consult prescriber for additional questions.

Intended Use and Disclaimer: Should not be printed and given to patients. This information is intended to serve as a concise initial reference for healthcare professionals to use when discussing medications with a patient. You must ultimately rely on your own discretion, experience and judgment in diagnosing, treating and advising patients.

Related Information
Oral Medications That Should Not Be Crushed or Altered *on page 1712*

Clopidogrel (kloh PID oh grel)

Brand Names: U.S. Plavix
Index Terms Clopidogrel Bisulfate
Pharmacologic Category Antiplatelet Agent; Antiplatelet Agent, Thienopyridine
Medication Safety Issues
Sound-alike/look-alike issues:
Plavix may be confused with Elavil, Paxil, Pradax (Canada), Pradaxa
Medication Guide Available Yes
Pregnancy Risk Factor B
Lactation Excretion in breast milk unknown/not recommended
Breast-Feeding Considerations It is not known if clopidogrel is excreted into breast milk. Due to the potential for serious adverse reactions in the nursing infant, the manufacturer recommends a decision be made whether to discontinue nursing or to discontinue the drug, taking into account the importance of treatment to the mother.
Use
Unstable angina/non-ST-segment elevation myocardial infarction: To decrease the rate of a combined end point of cardiovascular death, MI, or stroke, as well as the rate of a combined end point of cardiovascular death, MI, stroke, or refractory ischemia in patients with non-ST-segment elevation acute coronary syndrome (unstable angina/non-ST-elevation myocardial infarction [UA/NSTEMI]), including patients who are to be managed medically and those who are to be managed with coronary revascularization.
ST-segment elevation acute myocardial infarction: To reduce the rate of death from any cause and the rate of a combined end point of death, reinfarction, or stroke in patients with ST-elevation MI (STEMI).
Recent myocardial infarction, recent stroke, or established peripheral arterial disease: To reduce the rate of a combined end point of new ischemic stroke (fatal or nonfatal), new MI (fatal or nonfatal), and other vascular death in patients

with a history of recent MI, recent stroke, or established peripheral arterial disease.

Canadian labeling: Additional use (not in U.S. labeling): Prevention of atherothrombotic and thromboembolic events, including stroke, in patients with atrial fibrillation with at least 1 risk factor for vascular events who are not suitable for treatment with an anticoagulant and are at a low risk for bleeding.
Unlabeled Use In patients with allergy or major gastrointestinal intolerance to aspirin, initial treatment of acute coronary syndromes (ACS) or prevention of coronary artery bypass graft closure (saphenous vein); stable coronary artery disease (in combination with aspirin); adjunctive therapy to support reperfusion with primary percutaneous coronary intervention (PCI); in patients having undergone peripheral artery percutaneous transluminal angioplasty; symptomatic carotid artery stenosis (including recent carotid endarterectomy)
Mechanism of Action/Effect Irreversibly blocks platelet aggregation; platelets blocked by clopidogrel are affected for the remainder of their lifespan (~7-10 days).
Contraindications Hypersensitivity to clopidogrel or any component of the formulation; active pathological bleeding such as peptic ulcer or intracranial hemorrhage

Canadian labeling: Additional contraindications (not in U.S. labeling): Significant liver impairment or cholestatic jaundice
Warnings/Precautions [U.S. Boxed Warning]: Patients with one or more copies of the variant *CYP2C19*2* and/or *CYP2C19*3* alleles (and potentially other reduced-function variants) may have reduced conversion of clopidogrel to its active thiol metabolite. Lower active metabolite exposure may result in reduced platelet inhibition and, thus, a higher rate of cardiovascular events following MI or stent thrombosis following PCI. Although evidence is insufficient to recommend routine genetic testing, tests are available to determine CYP2C19 genotype and may be used to determine therapeutic strategy; alternative treatment or treatment strategies may be considered if patient is identified as a CYP2C19 poor metabolizer. Genetic testing may be considered prior to initiating clopidogrel in patients at moderate or high risk for poor outcomes (eg, PCI in patients with extensive and/or very complex disease). The optimal dose for CYP2C19 poor metabolizers has yet to be determined. After initiation of clopidogrel, functional testing (eg, VerifyNow® P2Y12 assay) may also be done to determine clopidogrel responsiveness (Holmes, 2010).

Use with caution in patients who may be at risk of increased bleeding, including patients with PUD, trauma, or surgery. In patients with coronary stents, premature interruption of therapy may result in stent thrombosis with subsequent fatal and non-fatal MI. Duration of therapy, in general, is determined by the type of stent placed (bare metal or drug eluting) and whether an ACS event was ongoing at the time of placement. Consider discontinuing 5 days before elective surgery (except in patients with cardiac stents that have not completed their full course of dual antiplatelet therapy; patient-specific situations need to be discussed with cardiologist; AHA/ACC/SCAI/ACS/ADA Science Advisory provides recommendations). Discontinue at least 5 days before elective CABG; when urgent CABG is necessary, the ACCF/AHA CABG guidelines recommend discontinuation for at least 24 hours prior to surgery (Hillis, 2011). The ACCF/AHA STEMI guidelines recommend discontinuation for at least 24 hours prior to *on-pump* CABG; *off-pump* CABG may be performed within 24 hours of clopidogrel administration if the benefits of prompt revascularization outweigh the risks of bleeding (O'Gara, 2013).

Because of structural similarities, cross-reactivity has been reported among the thienopyridines (clopidogrel, prasugrel, and ticlopidine); use with caution or avoid in patients with hypersensitivity or hematologic reactions to previous thienopyridine use. Use of clopidogrel is contraindicated in patients with hypersensitivity to clopidogrel, although desensitization may be considered for mild-to-moderate hypersensitivity.

Use caution in concurrent treatment with anticoagulants (eg, heparin, warfarin) or other antiplatelet drugs; bleeding risk is increased. Concurrent use with drugs known to inhibit CYP2C19 (eg, proton pump inhibitors) may reduce levels of active metabolite and subsequently reduce clinical efficacy and increase the risk of cardiovascular events; if possible, avoid concurrent use of moderate-to-strong CYP2C19 inhibitors. In patients requiring antacid therapy, consider use of an acid-reducing agent lacking (eg, ranitidine/famotidine) or with less CYP2C19 inhibition. According to the manufacturer, avoid concurrent use of omeprazole (even when scheduled 12 hours apart) or esomeprazole; if a PPI is necessary, the use of an agent with comparatively less effect on the antiplatelet activity of clopidogrel is recommended. Of the PPIs, pantoprazole has the lowest degree of CYP2C19 inhibition *in vitro* (Li, 2004) and has been shown to have has less effect on conversion of clopidogrel to its active metabolite compared to omeprazole (Angiolillo, 2011). Although lansoprazole exhibits the most potent CYP2C19 inhibition *in vitro* (Li, 2004; Ogilvie, 2012), an *in vivo* study of extensive CYP2C19 metabolizers showed less reduction of the active metabolite of clopidogrel by lansoprazole/dexlansoprazole compared to esomeprazole/omeprazole (Frelinger, 2012). Avoidance of rabeprazole appears prudent due to potent *in vitro* CYP2C19 inhibition and lack of sufficient comparative *in vivo* studies with other PPIs. In contrast to these warnings, others have recommended the continued use of PPIs, regardless of the degree of inhibition, in patients with multiple risk factors for GI bleeding who are also receiving clopidogrel since no evidence has established clinically meaningful differences in outcome; however, a clinically-significant interaction cannot be excluded in those who are poor metabolizers of clopidogrel. Staggering PPIs with clopidogrel is not recommended until further evidence is available (Abraham, 2010). Concurrent use of aspirin and clopidogrel is not recommended for secondary prevention of ischemic stroke or TIA in patients unable to take oral anticoagulants due to hemorrhagic risk (Furie, 2011).

Use with caution in patients with severe liver or renal disease (experience is limited). Cases of TTP (usually occurring within the first 2 weeks of therapy), resulting in some fatalities, have been reported; urgent plasmapheresis is required. Use in patients with severe hepatic impairment or cholestatic jaundice is contraindicated in the Canadian labeling. Cases of TTP (usually occurring within the first 2 weeks of therapy), resulting in some fatalities, have been reported; urgent plasmapheresis is required. In patients with recent lacunar stroke (within 180 days), the use of clopidogrel in addition to aspirin did not significantly reduce the incidence of the primary outcome of stroke recurrence (any ischemic stroke or intracranial hemorrhage) compared to aspirin alone; the use of clopidogrel in addition to aspirin did however increase the risk of major hemorrhage and the rate of all-cause mortality (SPS3 Investigators, 2012).

Assess bleeding risk carefully prior to initiating therapy in patients with atrial fibrillation (Canadian labeling; not an approved use in U.S. labeling); in clinical trials, a significant increase in major bleeding events (including intracranial hemorrhage and fatal bleeding events) were observed in patients receiving clopidogrel plus aspirin versus aspirin alone. Vitamin K antagonist (VKA) therapy (in suitable patients) has demonstrated a greater benefit in stroke reduction than aspirin (with or without clopidogrel).

Drug Interactions
Avoid Concomitant Use
Avoid concomitant use of Clopidogrel with any of the following: Esomeprazole; Omeprazole; Urokinase

Decreased Effect
The levels/effects of Clopidogrel may be decreased by: Amiodarone; Calcium Channel Blockers; CYP2C19 Inhibitors (Moderate); CYP2C19 Inhibitors (Strong); Dexlansoprazole; Esomeprazole; Grapefruit Juice; Lansoprazole; Macrolide Antibiotics; Morphine (Liposomal); Morphine (Systemic); Nonsteroidal Anti-Inflammatory

Agents; Omeprazole; Pantoprazole; RABEprazole

Increased Effect/Toxicity
Clopidogrel may increase the levels/effects of: Agents with Antiplatelet Properties; Anticoagulants; Collagenase (Systemic); CYP2B6 Substrates; Dabigatran Etexilate; Ibritumomab; Rivaroxaban; Salicylates; Thrombolytic Agents; Tositumomab and Iodine I 131 Tositumomab; Urokinase; Warfarin

The levels/effects of Clopidogrel may be increased by: Dasatinib; Glucosamine; Herbs (Anticoagulant/Antiplatelet Properties); Ibrutinib; Luliconazole; Multivitamins/Fluoride (with ADE); Multivitamins/Minerals (with ADEK, Folate, Iron); Multivitamins/Minerals (with AE, No Iron); Nonsteroidal Anti-Inflammatory Agents; Omega-3 Fatty Acids; Pentosan Polysulfate Sodium; Pentoxifylline; Prostacyclin Analogues; Rifamycin Derivatives; Tipranavir; Vitamin E

Nutritional/Ethanol Interactions
Food: Consumption of three 200 mL glasses of grapefruit juice a day may substantially reduce clopidogrel antiplatelet effects. Management: Avoid or minimize the consumption of grapefruit or grapefruit juice (Holmberg, 2013).

Herb/Nutraceutical: Avoid alfalfa, anise, bilberry, bladderwrack, bromelain, cat's claw, chamomile, coleus, cordyceps, dong quai, evening primrose oil, fenugreek, feverfew, garlic, ginger, ginkgo biloba, ginseng (American), ginseng (Panax), ginseng (Siberian), grape seed, green tea, guggul, horse chestnut seed, horseradish, licorice, prickly ash, red clover, reishi, SAMe (S-adenosylmethionine), sweet clover, turmeric, white willow (all have additional antiplatelet activity).

Adverse Reactions As with all drugs which may affect hemostasis, bleeding is associated with clopidogrel. Hemorrhage may occur at virtually any site. Risk is dependent on multiple variables, including the concurrent use of multiple agents which alter hemostasis and patient susceptibility.

3% to 10%:
Dermatologic: Rash (4%), pruritus (3%)
Hematologic: Bleeding (major 4%; minor 5%), purpura/bruising (5%), epistaxis (3%)
1% to 3%:
Gastrointestinal: GI hemorrhage (2%)
Hematologic: Hematoma

Pharmacodynamics/Kinetics
Onset of Action
Onset of action: Inhibition of platelet aggregation (IPA): Dose-dependent:
300-600 mg loading dose: Detected within 2 hours
50-100 mg/day: Detected by the second day of treatment

Peak effect: Time to maximal IPA: Dose-dependent: **Note:** Degree of IPA based on adenosine diphosphate (ADP) concentration used during light aggregometry:
300-600 mg loading dose:
ADP 5 micromole/L: 20% to 30% IPA at 6 hours post administration (Montelescot, 2006)
ADP 20 micromole/L: 30% to 37% IPA at 6 hours post administration (Montelescot, 2006)
50-100 mg/day: ADP 5 micromole/L: 50% to 60% IPA at 5-7 days (Herbert, 1993)

Available Dosage Forms
Tablet, Oral:
Plavix: 75 mg, 300 mg
Generic: 75 mg, 300 mg
General Dosage Range Oral: *Adults:* Loading dose: 300 mg (maximum: 600 mg); Maintenance: 75 mg once daily
Administration
Oral May be administered without regard to meals.
Storage/Stability Store at 25°C (77°F); excursions permitted to 15°C to 30°C (59°F to 86°F).
Nursing Actions
Physical Assessment Monitor for signs and symptoms of bleeding. Educate cardiac patients about adherence to therapy; avoid discontinuation for any procedures without consultation with patient's cardiologist.
Patient Education
• Discuss specific use of drug and side effects with patient as it relates to treatment. (HCAHPS: During this hospital stay, were you given any medicine that you had not taken before? Before giving you any new medicine, how often did hospital staff tell you what the medicine was for? How often did hospital staff describe possible side effects in a way you could understand?)
• Have patient report immediately to prescriber signs of hemorrhaging, signs of hepatic impairment, angina, severe headache, dyspnea, illogical thinking, skin discoloration, pharyngitis, arrhythmia, back pain, urinary retention, oliguria, weight loss, or signs of thrombotic thrombocytopenic purpura/hemolytic uremic syndrome (TTP/HUS) (HCAHPS).
• Educate patient about signs of a significant reaction (eg, wheezing; chest tightness; fever; itching; bad cough; blue skin color; seizures; or swelling of face, lips, tongue, or throat). **Note:** This is not a comprehensive list of all side effects. Patient should consult prescriber for additional questions.

Intended Use and Disclaimer: Should not be printed and given to patients. This information is intended to serve as a concise initial reference for healthcare professionals to use when discussing medications with a patient. You must ultimately rely on your own discretion, experience and judgment in diagnosing, treating and advising patients.

◀ **Dietary Considerations** May be taken without regard to meals. Avoid grapefruit juice (Holmberg, 2013).

Clorazepate (klor AZ e pate)

Brand Names: U.S. Tranxene-T
Index Terms Clorazepate Dipotassium; Tranxene T-Tab
Pharmacologic Category Benzodiazepine
Medication Safety Issues
Sound-alike/look-alike issues:
Clorazepate may be confused with clofibrate, clonazepam, KlonoPIN®
BEERS Criteria medication:
This drug may be potentially inappropriate for use in geriatric patients (Quality of evidence - high; Strength of recommendation - strong).
Medication Guide Available Yes
Lactation Enters breast milk/not recommended
Use Treatment of generalized anxiety disorder; management of ethanol withdrawal; adjunct anticonvulsant in management of partial seizures
Controlled Substance C-IV
Available Dosage Forms
Tablet, Oral:
Tranxene-T: 3.75 mg, 7.5 mg, 15 mg
Generic: 3.75 mg, 7.5 mg, 15 mg
General Dosage Range Oral:
Children 9-12 years: Initial: 3.75-7.5 mg twice daily; Maintenance: Up to 60 mg/day in 2-3 divided doses
Children >12 years: Initial: Up to 7.5 mg 2-3 times/day; Maintenance: Up to 90 mg/day
Adults: Initial: 7.5-15 mg 2-4 times/day; Maintenance: Up to 90 mg/day
Elderly: Anxiety: 7.5 mg 1-2 times/day
Nursing Actions
Physical Assessment Assess for signs of CNS depression (sedation, dizziness, confusion, ataxia, potential for suicide ideation). Assess for history of addiction; long-term use can result in dependence, abuse, or tolerance; periodically evaluate need for continued use. For inpatient use, institute safety measures to prevent falls. Taper dosage slowly when discontinuing.
Patient Education
• Discuss specific use of drug and side effects with patient as it relates to treatment. (HCAHPS: During this hospital stay, were you given any medicine that you had not taken before? Before giving you any new medicine, how often did hospital staff tell you what the medicine was for? How often did hospital staff describe possible side effects in a way you could understand?)
• Patient may experience presyncope, fatigue, blurred vision, dizziness, headache, nausea, or xerostomia. Have patient report immediately to prescriber significant change in balance, severe asthenia, urinary retention, oliguria, double vision, dysarthria, tremors, insomnia, or signs of depression (ie, suicidal ideation, anxiety, emotional instability, illogical thinking) (HCAHPS).
• Educate patient about signs of a significant reaction (eg, wheezing; chest tightness; fever; itching; bad cough; blue skin color; seizures; or swelling of face, lips, tongue, or throat). **Note:** This is not a comprehensive list of all side effects. Patient should consult prescriber for additional questions.

Intended Use and Disclaimer: Should not be printed and given to patients. This information is intended to serve as a concise initial reference for healthcare professionals to use when discussing medications with a patient. You must ultimately rely on your own discretion, experience and judgment in diagnosing, treating and advising patients.

Clotrimazole (Oral) (kloe TRIM a zole)

Index Terms Mycelex
Pharmacologic Category Antifungal Agent, Oral Nonabsorbed
Medication Safety Issues
Sound-alike/look-alike issues:
Clotrimazole may be confused with co-trimoxazole
Mycelex may be confused with Myoflex®
International issues:
Cloderm: Brand name for clotrimazole [Germany], but also brand name for alclometasone [Indonesia]; clobetasol [China, India, Malaysia, Singapore, Thailand]; clocortolone [U.S., Canada]
Canesten [multiple international markets] may be confused with Canesten Bifonazol Comp brand name for bifonazole/urea [Austria]; Canesten Extra brand name for bifonazole [China, Germany]; Canesten Extra Nagelset brand name for bifonazole/urea [Denmark]; Canesten Fluconazole brand name for fluconazole [New Zealand]; Canesten Oasis brand name for sodium citrate [Great Britain]; Canesten Once Daily brand name for bifonazole [Australia]; Canesten Oral brand name for fluconazole [United Kingdom]; Cenestin brand name for estrogens (conjugated A/synthetic) [U.S., Canada]
Mycelex: Brand name for clotrimazole [U.S.] may be confused with Mucolex brand name for bromhexine [Malaysia]; carbocisteine [Thailand]
Pregnancy Risk Factor C
Lactation Excretion in breast milk unknown
Use Treatment of susceptible fungal infections, including oropharyngeal candidiasis; limited data suggest that clotrimazole troches may be effective for prophylaxis against oropharyngeal candidiasis in neutropenic patients
Available Dosage Forms
Lozenge, Mouth/Throat:
Generic: 10 mg (70 ea, 140 ea)

Troche, Mouth/Throat:
Generic: 10 mg
General Dosage Range Oral: *Children >3 years and Adults:* Prophylaxis: 10 mg 3 times/day; Treatment: 10 mg 5 times/day
Administration
Oral Troche: Allow to dissolve slowly over 15-30 minutes.
Nursing Actions
Patient Education
- Discuss specific use of drug and side effects with patient as it relates to treatment. (HCAHPS: During this hospital stay, were you given any medicine that you had not taken before? Before giving you any new medicine, how often did hospital staff tell you what the medicine was for? How often did hospital staff describe possible side effects in a way you could understand?)
- Patient may experience nausea or dysgeusia. Have patient report immediately to prescriber signs of hepatic impairment (HCAHPS).
- Educate patient about signs of a significant reaction (eg, wheezing; chest tightness; fever; itching; bad cough; blue skin color; seizures; or swelling of face, lips, tongue, or throat). **Note:** This is not a comprehensive list of all side effects. Patient should consult prescriber for additional questions.

Intended Use and Disclaimer: Should not be printed and given to patients. This information is intended to serve as a concise initial reference for healthcare professionals to use when discussing medications with a patient. You must ultimately rely on your own discretion, experience and judgment in diagnosing, treating and advising patients.

Clozapine (KLOE za peen)

Brand Names: U.S. Clozaril; FazaClo; Versacloz
Pharmacologic Category Antipsychotic Agent, Atypical
Medication Safety Issues
Sound-alike/look-alike issues:
CloZAPine may be confused with clonazePAM, cloNIDine, KlonoPIN
Clozaril may be confused with Clinoril, Colazal
BEERS Criteria medication:
This drug may be potentially inappropriate for use in geriatric patients (Quality of evidence - moderate; Strength of recommendation - strong).
Pregnancy Risk Factor B
Lactation Enters breast milk/not recommended
Breast-Feeding Considerations Clozapine was found to accumulate in breast milk in concentrations higher than the maternal plasma (Barnas, 1994). Breast-feeding is not recommended by the manufacturer. Clozapine may theoretically cause agranulocytosis in the nursing infant and should

not routinely be used in women who are breast-feeding (NICE, 2007).
Use
Schizophrenia, treatment resistant: Treatment of severely ill patients with schizophrenia who fail to respond adequately to antipsychotic treatment
Suicidal behavior in schizophrenia or schizoaffective disorder: To reduce the risk of suicidal behavior in patients with schizophrenia or schizoaffective disorder
Unlabeled Use Treatment resistant schizophrenia in children and adolescents, schizoaffective disorder; treatment resistant bipolar disorder in adults and adolescents; treatment resistant psychosis/agitation related to Alzheimer dementia and Lewy body disease
Mechanism of Action/Effect The therapeutic efficacy of clozapine (dibenzodiazepine antipsychotic) is proposed to be mediated through antagonism of the dopamine type 2 (D_2) and serotonin type 2A ($5-HT_{2A}$) receptors. In addition, it acts as an antagonist at alpha-adrenergic, histamine H_1, cholinergic, and other dopaminergic and serotonergic receptors.
Contraindications Hypersensitivity to clozapine or any component of the formulation (eg, photosensitivity, vasculitis, erythema multiforme, or Stevens-Johnson syndrome [SJS]); history of clozapine-induced agranulocytosis or severe granulocytopenia

Canadian labeling: Additional contraindications (not in U.S. labeling): Active hepatic disease associated with nausea, anorexia, or jaundice; progressive hepatic disease or hepatic failure; severe renal impairment; severe cardiac disease (eg, myocarditis); patients unable to undergo blood testing

Warnings/Precautions [U.S. Boxed Warning]: Significant risk of potentially life-threatening agranulocytosis, defined as an ANC <500/mm³. Monitor ANC and WBC prior to and during treatment. ANC must be ≥2000/mm³ and WBC must be ≥3500/mm³ to begin treatment. Discontinue clozapine and do not rechallenge if ANC <1000/mm³ or WBC is <2000/mm³. Monitor for symptoms of agranulocytosis and infection (eg, fever, lethargy, or sore throat). Clozapine is only available through a restricted program requiring enrollment of prescribers, patients, and pharmacies to the Registry. Do not initiate in patients with a history of clozapine-induced agranulocytosis or granulocytopenia. Initial episodes of moderate leukopenia or granulopoietic suppression confer up to a 12-fold increased risk for subsequent episodes of agranulocytosis. Concurrent use with bone marrow suppressive agents or treatments also leads to an increased risk. WBCs must be monitored weekly for at least 4 weeks after therapy discontinuation or until WBC is ≥3500/mm³ and ANC is ≥2000/mm³. The restricted distribution system ensures appropriate ▶

WBC and ANC monitoring. Eosinophilia, defined as a blood eosinophil count of >700/mm^3, has been reported to occur with clozapine and usually occurs within the first month of treatment. If eosinophilia develops, evaluate for signs or symptoms of systemic reactions (eg, rash or other allergic symptoms), myocarditis, or organ-specific disease. If systemic disease is suspected, discontinue clozapine immediately. If an eosinophilia cause unrelated to clozapine is identified treat the underlying cause and continue clozapine. In the absence of organ involvement continue clozapine under careful monitoring. If the total eosinophil count continues to increase over several weeks in the absence of systemic disease, base interruption of treatment and rechallenge (after eosinophil count decreases) on overall clinical assessment and consultation with internist or hematologist (**Note:** The Canadian labeling recommends discontinuing therapy for eosinophil count >3000/mm^3; may resume therapy when eosinophil count <1000/mm^3).

[U.S. Boxed Warning]: Elderly patients with dementia-related psychosis treated with antipsychotics are at an increased risk of death compared to placebo. Most deaths appeared to be either cardiovascular (eg, heart failure, sudden death) or infectious (eg, pneumonia) in nature. Clozapine is not approved for the treatment of dementia-related psychosis. Avoid antipsychotic use for behavioral problems associated with dementia unless alternative nonpharmacologic therapies have failed and patient may harm self or others. May also be inappropriate in older adults depending on comorbidities (eg, dementia, delirium) due to its potent anticholinergic effects (Beers Criteria). The elderly are more susceptible to adverse effects (including agranulocytosis, cardiovascular, anticholinergic, and tardive dyskinesia). An increased incidence of cerebrovascular effects (eg, transient ischemic attack, stroke), including fatalities, has been reported in placebo-controlled trials of atypical antipsychotics in elderly patients with dementia-related psychosis.

Cognitive and/or motor impairment (sedation) is common with clozapine, resulting in impaired performance of tasks requiring alertness (eg, operating machinery or driving); use caution in patients receiving general anesthesia. **[U.S. Boxed Warning]: Seizures have been associated with clozapine use in a dose-dependent manner. Initiate treatment with no more than 12.5 mg, titrate gradually using divided dosing. Use with caution in patients at risk of seizures, including those with a history of seizures, head trauma, brain damage, alcoholism, or concurrent therapy with medications which may lower seizure threshold. Patients should be warned that a sudden loss of consciousness may occur with seizures.** Benign transient temperature elevation

(>100.4°F) may occur; peaking within the first 3 weeks of treatment. May be associated with an increase or decrease in WBC count. Rule out infection, agranulocytosis, and neuroleptic malignant syndrome (NMS) in patients presenting with fever. However, clozapine may also be associated with severe febrile reactions, including neuroleptic malignant syndrome (NMS). Clozapine's potential for extrapyramidal symptoms (including tardive dyskinesia) appears to be extremely low. Risk of dystonia (and probably other EPS) may be greater with increased doses, use of conventional antipsychotics, males, and younger patients.

[U.S. Boxed Warning]: Fatalities due to myocarditis and cardiomyopathy have been reported. Upon suspicion of these reactions discontinue clozapine and obtain a cardiac evaluation. Symptoms may include chest pain, tachycardia, palpitations, dyspenia, fever, flu-like symptoms, hypotension, or ECG changes. Patients with clozaril-related myocarditis or cardiomyopathy should generally not be rechallenged with clozapine. Myocarditis and cardiomyopathy may occur at any period during clozapine treatment, however, typically myocarditis presents within the first 2 months and cardiomyopathy after 8 weeks of treatment. Rare cases of thromboembolism, including pulmonary embolism and stroke resulting in fatalities, have been associated with clozapine. Clozapine is associated with QT prolongation and ventricular arrhythmias including torsade de pointes; cardiac arrest and sudden death may occur. Use caution in patients with a history of long QT syndrome, conditions which may increase the risk of QT prolongation (cardiovascular disease, recent MI, uncompensated heart failure, clinically significant arrhythmias, family history of long QT syndrome), concomitant use of medications known to prolong the QT interval, or treatment with medications that inhibit the metabolism of clozapine. Hypokalemia and/or hypomagnesemia may increase the risk. Consider obtaining a baseline ECG and serum chemistry panel. Correct electrolyte abnormalities prior to initiating therapy. Discontinue clozapine if QT$_c$ interval >500 msec. Undesirable changes in lipids have been observed with antipsychotic therapy; incidence varies with product. Periodically monitor total serum cholesterol, triglycerides, LDL, and HDL concentrations.

Potentially significant drug-drug interactions may exist, requiring dose or frequency adjustment, additional monitoring, and/or selection of alternative therapy.

May cause anticholinergic effects; use with caution in patients with urinary retention, benign prostatic hyperplasia, narrow-angle glaucoma, xerostomia, visual problems, constipation, or history of bowel obstruction. Because of its potential to significantly decreased GI motility, use is associated with increased risk of paralytic ileus, bowel obstruction, fecal impaction, bowel perforation, and in rare cases death. Bowel regimens and monitoring are recommended. May cause hyperglycemia; in some cases may be extreme and associated with ketoacidosis, hyperosmolar coma, or death. Monitor for symptoms of hyperglycemia including polydipsia, polyuria, polyphagia, and weakness. Use with caution in patients with diabetes or other disorders of glucose regulation; monitor for worsening of glucose control. Antipsychotic use has been associated with esophageal dysmotility and aspiration; use with caution in patients at risk of aspiration pneumonia (eg, Alzheimer disease). Use with caution in patients with hepatic disease or impairment; monitor hepatic function regularly. Hepatitis has been reported as a consequence of therapy. Discontinuation of therapy may be necessary with significant elevations in liver function tests; may reinitiate with close monitoring and if values return to normal. Use with caution in patients with renal disease.

Use caution with cardiovascular or pulmonary disease; gradually increase dose. **[U.S. Boxed Warning]: Orthostatic hypotension, bradycardia, syncope, and cardiac arrest have been reported with clozapine treatment. Risk is highest during the initial titration period and with rapid dose increases. Symptoms can develop with the first dose and with doses as low as 12.5 mg per day. Initiate treatment with no more than 12.5 mg once daily or twice daily, titrate slowly, and use divided doses. Use with caution in patients at risk for these effects (eg, cerebrovascular disease, cardiovascular disease) or with predisposing conditions for hypotensive episodes (eg, hypovolemia, concurrent antihypertensive medication);** reactions can be fatal. Consider dose reduction if hypotension occurs. May cause tachycardia (including sustained); sustained tachycardia is not limited to a reflex response to orthostatic hypotension, and is present in all positions.

The possibility of a suicide attempt is inherent in psychotic illness or bipolar disorder; use caution in high-risk patients during initiation of therapy. Prescriptions should be written for the smallest quantity consistent with good patient care. Medication should not be stopped abruptly; taper off over 1-2 weeks. If conditions warrant abrupt discontinuation (eg, leukopenia, myocarditis, cardiomyopathy), monitor patient for psychosis and cholinergic rebound (eg, headache, nausea, vomiting, diarrhea, profuse diaphoresis). Significant weight gain has been observed with antipsychotic therapy; incidence varies with product. Monitor waist circumference and BMI. Clozapine levels may be lower in patients who smoke. Smoking cessation may cause toxicity in a patient stabilized on clozapine. Monitor change in smoking. Clozapine concentrations may be increased in CYP2D6 poor

metabolizers; dose reduction may be necessary. FazaClo oral disintegrating tablets contain phenylalanine.

Drug Interactions

Avoid Concomitant Use

Avoid concomitant use of CloZAPine with any of the following: Aclidinium; Amisulpride; Azelastine (Nasal); CarBAMazepine; Ciprofloxacin (Systemic); CYP3A4 Inducers (Strong); Highest Risk QTc-Prolonging Agents; Ipratropium (Oral Inhalation); Ivabradine; Metoclopramide; Mifepristone; Myelosuppressive Agents; Paraldehyde; Sulpiride; Thioridazine; Tiotropium; Umeclidinium

Decreased Effect

CloZAPine may decrease the levels/effects of: Amphetamines; Anti-Parkinson's Agents (Dopamine Agonist); Codeine; Quinagolide; Tamoxifen

The levels/effects of CloZAPine may be decreased by: CarBAMazepine; CYP3A4 Inducers (Strong); Cyproterone; Lithium formulations; Omeprazole

Increased Effect/Toxicity

CloZAPine may increase the levels/effects of: Alcohol (Ethyl); Amisulpride; Analgesics (Opioid); Anticholinergics; ARIPiprazole; Azelastine (Nasal); Buprenorphine; CNS Depressants; CYP2D6 Substrates; Fesoterodine; Highest Risk QTc-Prolonging Agents; Hydrocodone; Lomitapide; Methotrimeprazine; Methylphenidate; Metoprolol; Moderate Risk QTc-Prolonging Agents; Nebivolol; Paraldehyde; Serotonin Modulators; Sulpiride; Thioridazine; Tiotropium; Zolpidem

The levels/effects of CloZAPine may be increased by: Abiraterone Acetate; Acetylcholinesterase Inhibitors (Central); Aclidinium; Benzodiazepines; Brimonidine (Topical); CarBAMazepine; Cimetidine; Ciprofloxacin (Systemic); CYP1A2 Inhibitors (Moderate); CYP1A2 Inhibitors (Strong); Deferasirox; Doxylamine; HydrOXYzine; Ipratropium (Oral Inhalation); Ivabradine; Lithium formulations; Macrolide Antibiotics; Magnesium Sulfate; MAO Inhibitors; Methotrimeprazine; Methylphenidate; Metoclopramide; Metyrosine; Mifepristone; Myelosuppressive Agents; Nefazodone; Omeprazole; Perampanel; Pramlintide; QTc-Prolonging Agents (Indeterminate Risk and Risk Modifying); Selective Serotonin Reuptake Inhibitors; Serotonin Modulators; Sodium Oxybate; Tetrabenazine; Umeclidinium

Nutritional/Ethanol Interactions

Ethanol: May increase CNS depression; monitor for increased effects with coadministration. Caution patients about effects.

Herb/Nutraceutical: St John's wort may decrease clozapine levels. Avoid kava kava, gotu kola, valerian, St John's wort (may increase CNS depression).

Adverse Reactions

>10%:

Cardiovascular: Tachycardia (25%)

Central nervous system: Drowsiness (39% to 46%), dizziness (19% to 27%), insomnia (2% to 20%)

Gastrointestinal: Sialorrhea (31% to 48%), weight gain (4% to 31%), constipation (14% to 25%), nausea/vomiting (3% to 17%), abdominal discomfort/heartburn (4% to 14%)

1% to 10%:

Cardiovascular: Hypotension (9%), syncope (6%), hypertension (4%), angina pectoris (1%), ECG changes (1%)

Central nervous system: Headache (7%), fever (5%), agitation (4%), akinesia (4%), nightmares (4%), restlessness (4%), akathisia (3%), confusion (3%), seizure (3%; dose related), fatigue (2%), anxiety (1%), ataxia (1%), depression (1%), lethargy (1%), myoclonic seizures (1%), pain (1%), slurred speech (1%)

Dermatologic: Skin rash (2%)

Gastrointestinal: Xerostomia (6%), diarrhea (2%), anorexia (1%), sore throat (1%)

Genitourinary: Urinary abnormalities (eg, abnormal ejaculation, retention, urgency, incontinence; 1% to 2%)

Hematologic: Leukopenia (3%), agranulocytosis (1%), eosinophilia (1%)

Hepatic: Abnormal liver function tests (1%)

Neuromuscular & skeletal: Tremor (6%), hypokinesia (4%), muscle rigidity (3%), hyperkinesia (1%), muscle spasm (1%), weakness (1%)

Ocular: Visual disturbances (5%)

Respiratory: Dyspnea (1%), nasal congestion (1%)

Miscellaneous: Diaphoresis (6%), numbness of tongue (1%)

Available Dosage Forms

Suspension, Oral:

Versacloz: 50 mg/mL (100 mL)

Tablet, Oral:

Clozaril: 25 mg, 100 mg

Generic: 25 mg, 50 mg, 100 mg, 200 mg

Tablet Dispersible, Oral:

FazaClo: 12.5 mg, 25 mg, 100 mg, 150 mg, 200 mg

Generic: 12.5 mg, 25 mg, 100 mg

General Dosage Range Dosage adjustment recommended in patients who develop toxicities

Oral: *Adults:* Initial: 12.5 mg once or twice daily; Usual maintenance: 300-450 mg daily (maximum: 900 mg daily)

Administration

Oral May be taken without regard to food. Total daily dose may be divided into uneven doses with larger dose administered at bedtime.

Canadian labeling: Maintenance dosing ≤200 mg daily may be administered as single dose in the evening.

Orally-disintegrating tablet: Should be removed from foil blister by peeling apart (do not push tablet through the foil). Remove immediately prior to use. Place tablet in mouth and chew or allow to dissolve; swallow with saliva. If dosing requires splitting tablet, throw unused portion away.

Suspension: Shake bottle prior to use. Using syringe adaptor and oral syringe provided withdrawal dose from bottle. Administer immediately after preparation using the oral syringe provided.

Storage/Stability

Suspension: Store at ≤25°C (77°F). Protect from light. Do not refrigerate or freeze. Suspension is stable for 100 days after initial bottle opening.

Tablet: Store at ≤30°C (86°F).

Tablet, dispersible: Store at 20°C to 25°C (68°F to 77°F); excursions permitted to 15°C to 30°C (59°F to 86°F). Protect from moisture; do not remove from package until ready to use.

Nursing Actions

Physical Assessment Educate patient about blood work monitoring and tie to dispensing. Monitor for orthostatic hypotension, tachycardia, weight gain, and metabolic syndrome. Educate patient about managing orthostasis: Making position changes slowly, maintain adequate hydration. Report to physician: Excessive dizziness, falls, palpitations, sudden fever, muscle rigidity, seizure, confusion. Development of excessive salivation increases risk for night time aspiration when supine; encourage elevation of head of bed or sleeping on pillows.

Patient Education

- Discuss specific use of drug and side effects with patient as it relates to treatment. (HCAHPS: During this hospital stay, were you given any medicine that you had not taken before? Before giving you any new medicine, how often did hospital staff tell you what the medicine was for? How often did hospital staff describe possible side effects in a way you could understand?)

- Patient may experience dizziness, fatigue, xerostomia, nausea, weight gain, insomnia, sialorrhea, or hyperhidrosis. Have patient report immediately to prescriber signs of infection, signs of hyperglycemia, difficulty with motor activity, fasciculations, change in balance, dysphagia, tremors, bradykinesia, rigidity, strength differences from one side to another, difficulty thinking or speaking, change in balance, blurred vision, edema of extremities, hemoptysis, discoloration of extremities, severe headache, significant asthenia, illogical thinking, bradycardia, considerable constipation, vision changes, signs of neuroleptic malignant syndrome (NMS), or signs of tardive dyskinesia (HCAHPS).

- Educate patient about signs of a significant reaction (eg, wheezing; chest tightness; fever; itching; bad cough; blue skin color; seizures; or

swelling of face, lips, tongue, or throat). **Note:** This is not a comprehensive list of all side effects. Patient should consult prescriber for additional questions.

Intended Use and Disclaimer: Should not be printed and given to patients. This information is intended to serve as a concise initial reference for healthcare professionals to use when discussing medications with a patient. You must ultimately rely on your own discretion, experience and judgment in diagnosing, treating and advising patients.

Dietary Considerations May be taken without regard to food. Some products may contain phenylalanine.

Codeine (KOE deen)

Index Terms Codeine Phosphate; Codeine Sulfate; Methylmorphine
Pharmacologic Category Analgesic, Opioid; Antitussive
Medication Safety Issues
Sound-alike/look-alike issues:
Codeine may be confused with Cardene®, Cordran®, iodine, Lodine
High alert medication:
The Institute for Safe Medication Practices (ISMP) includes this medication among its list of drug classes which have a heightened risk of causing significant patient harm when used in error.
Medication Guide Available Yes
Pregnancy Risk Factor C
Lactation Enters breast milk/use caution
Use Management of mild-to-moderately-severe pain
Unlabeled Use Short-term relief of cough in select patients
Controlled Substance C-II
Available Dosage Forms
Solution, Oral:
Generic: 30 mg/5 mL (500 mL)
Tablet, Oral:
Generic: 15 mg, 30 mg, 60 mg
General Dosage Range Dosage adjustment recommended in patients with renal and hepatic impairment
Oral: *Adults:* Initial: 15-60 mg every 4 hours as needed; maximum total daily dose: 360 mg/day
Administration
Oral May administer without regard to meals. Take with food or milk to decrease adverse GI effects. Controlled release tablets: Codeine Contin® (Canadian availability; not available in U.S.): Tablets should be swallowed whole; do not chew, dissolve, or crush. All strengths may be halved, **except** the 50 mg tablets; half tablets should also be swallowed intact.

Nursing Actions
Physical Assessment Monitor for effectiveness of pain relief. Monitor blood pressure, CNS and respiratory status, and degree of sedation prior to treatment and periodically throughout. May cause physical and/or psychological dependence. For inpatients, implement safety measures (eg, side rails up, call light within reach, instructions to call for assistance). Assess patient's physical and/or psychological dependence. Discontinue slowly after prolonged use.
Patient Education
• Discuss specific use of drug and side effects with patient as it relates to treatment. (HCAHPS: During this hospital stay, were you given any medicine that you had not taken before? Before giving you any new medicine, how often did hospital staff tell you what the medicine was for? How often did hospital staff describe possible side effects in a way you could understand?)
• Patient may experience fatigue or hyperhidrosis. Have patient report immediately to prescriber severe dizziness, syncope, angina, tachycardia, dyspnea, illogical thinking, arrhythmia, hallucinations, mood changes, significant dyspepsia, intolerable headache, difficult urination, tremors, vision changes, considerable nausea, severe constipation, or significant asthenia (HCAHPS).
• Educate patient about signs of a significant reaction (eg, wheezing; chest tightness; fever; itching; bad cough; blue skin color; seizures; or swelling of face, lips, tongue, or throat). **Note:** This is not a comprehensive list of all side effects. Patient should consult prescriber for additional questions.

Intended Use and Disclaimer: Should not be printed and given to patients. This information is intended to serve as a concise initial reference for healthcare professionals to use when discussing medications with a patient. You must ultimately rely on your own discretion, experience and judgment in diagnosing, treating and advising patients.

Colchicine (KOL chi seen)

Brand Names: U.S. Colcrys
Pharmacologic Category Antigout Agent
Medication Safety Issues
Sound-alike/look-alike issues:
Colchicine may be confused with Cortrosyn®
Medication Guide Available Yes
Pregnancy Risk Factor C
Lactation Enters breast milk/use caution
Breast-Feeding Considerations Colchicine enters breast milk; exclusively breast-fed infants are expected to receive <10% of the weight-adjusted maternal dose (limited data). The manufacturer recommends that caution be used if administered to a nursing woman.

Use Prevention and treatment of acute gout flares; treatment of familial Mediterranean fever (FMF)

Unlabeled Use Primary biliary cirrhosis; pericarditis

Mechanism of Action/Effect Reduces the deposition of urate crystals that perpetuates the inflammatory response

Contraindications Concomitant use of a P-glycoprotein (P-gp) or strong CYP3A4 inhibitor in presence of renal or hepatic impairment

Canadian labeling: Additional contraindications (not in U.S. labeling): Hypersensitivity to colchicine; serious gastrointestinal, hepatic, renal, and cardiac disease

Warnings/Precautions Hazardous agent - use appropriate precautions for handling and disposal (NIOSH, 2012). Myelosuppression (eg, thrombocytopenia, leukopenia, granulocytopenia, pancytopenia) and aplastic anemia have been reported in patients receiving therapeutic doses. Neuromuscular toxicity (including rhabdomyolysis) has been reported in patients receiving therapeutic doses; patients with renal dysfunction and elderly patients are at increased risk. Concomitant use of cyclosporine, diltiazem, verapamil, fibrates, and statins may increase the risk of myopathy. Clearance is decreased in renal or hepatic impairment; monitor closely for adverse effects/toxicity. Dosage adjustments may be required depending on degree of impairment or indication, and may be affected by the use of concurrent medication (CYP3A4 or P-gp inhibitors). Concurrent use of P-gp or strong CYP3A4 inhibitors is contraindicated in renal impairment; fatal toxicity has been reported. Colchicine does not have analgesic activity and should not be used to treat pain from other causes. Colchicine requires dosage adjustment when used concurrently with protease inhibitor regimens. Colchicine does not have analgesic activity and should not be used to treat pain from other causes. Canadian labeling does not include recommendations for use in children.

Drug Interactions

Avoid Concomitant Use

Avoid concomitant use of Colchicine with any of the following: Axitinib; Fusidic Acid (Systemic); Simeprevir

Decreased Effect

Colchicine may decrease the levels/effects of: ARIPiprazole; Axitinib; Cyanocobalamin; Ibrutinib; Multivitamins/Fluoride (with ADE); Multivitamins/Minerals (with ADEK, Folate, Iron); Multivitamins/Minerals (with AE, No Iron); Saxagliptin; Simeprevir

The levels/effects of Colchicine may be decreased by: P-glycoprotein/ABCB1 Inducers

Increased Effect/Toxicity

Colchicine may increase the levels/effects of: HMG-CoA Reductase Inhibitors

The levels/effects of Colchicine may be increased by: Cobicistat; CYP3A4 Inhibitors (Moderate); CYP3A4 Inhibitors (Strong); Dasatinib; Digoxin; Fibric Acid Derivatives; Fosamprenavir; Fusidic Acid (Systemic); Ivacaftor; Luliconazole; Mifepristone; P-glycoprotein/ABCB1 Inhibitors; Simeprevir; Telaprevir

Nutritional/Ethanol Interactions

Ethanol: Management: Avoid ethanol.

Food: Grapefruit juice may increase colchicine serum concentrations. Management: Administer orally with water and maintain adequate fluid intake. Dose adjustment may be required based on indication if ingesting grapefruit juice. Avoid grapefruit juice with hepatic or renal impairment.

Herb/Nutraceutical: Cyanocobalamin (vitamin B_{12}) absorption may be decreased by colchicine and result in macrocytic anemia or neurologic dysfunction. Management: Consider supplementing with vitamin B_{12}.

Adverse Reactions Frequency not always defined.

>10%: Gastrointestinal: Gastrointestinal disease (26% to 77%), diarrhea (23% to 77%), vomiting (17%), nausea (4% to 17%)

1% to 10%:

Central nervous system: Fatigue (1% to 4%), headache (1% to 2%)

Endocrine & metabolic: Gout (4%)

Gastrointestinal: Abdominal cramps, abdominal pain

Respiratory: Pharyngolaryngeal pain (3%)

Pharmacodynamics/Kinetics

Onset of Action Oral: Pain relief: ~18-24 hours

Available Dosage Forms

Tablet, Oral:

Colcrys: 0.6 mg

General Dosage Range Dosage adjustment recommended in patients with renal impairment or on concomitant therapy

Oral:

Children 4-6 years: 0.3-1.8 mg/day in 1-2 divided doses

Children 6-12 years: 0.9-1.8 mg/day in 1-2 divided doses

Children 12-16 years: 1.2-2.4 mg/day in 1-2 divided doses

Children >16 years and Adults: 0.6-2.4 mg/day in 1-2 divided doses **or** Initial: 1.2 mg; repeat with 0.6 mg in 1 hour (maximum total therapy: 1.8 mg)

Administration

Oral Administer orally with water and maintain adequate fluid intake. May be administered without regard to meals.

Hazardous agent; use appropriate precautions for handling and disposal (NIOSH, 2012).

Storage/Stability Store at 20°C to 25°C (68°F to 77°F). Protect from light.

Nursing Actions

Patient Education

- Discuss specific use of drug and side effects with patient as it relates to treatment. (HCAHPS: During this hospital stay, were you given any medicine that you had not taken before? Before giving you any new medicine, how often did hospital staff tell you what the medicine was for? How often did hospital staff describe possible side effects in a way you could understand?)
- Have patient report immediately to prescriber signs of infection, paresthesia, severe nausea, significant diarrhea, intolerable dyspepsia, severe asthenia, ecchymosis, hemorrhaging, pallor, myalgia, urinary retention, or oliguria (HCAHPS).
- Educate patient about signs of a significant reaction (eg, wheezing; chest tightness; fever; itching; bad cough; blue skin color; seizures; or swelling of face, lips, tongue, or throat). **Note:** This is not a comprehensive list of all side effects. Patient should consult prescriber for additional questions.

Intended Use and Disclaimer: Should not be printed and given to patients. This information is intended to serve as a concise initial reference for healthcare professionals to use when discussing medications with a patient. You must ultimately rely on your own discretion, experience and judgment in diagnosing, treating and advising patients.

Dietary Considerations May be taken without regard to meals. May need to supplement with vitamin B_{12}. Avoid grapefruit juice.

Colchicine and Probenecid

(KOL chi seen & proe BEN e sid)

Index Terms ColBenemid; Probenecid and Colchicine

Pharmacologic Category Anti-inflammatory Agent; Antigout Agent; Uricosuric Agent

Use Treatment of chronic gouty arthritis when complicated by frequent, recurrent acute attacks of gout

Available Dosage Forms

Tablet: Colchicine 0.5 mg and probenecid 0.5 g

General Dosage Range Dosage adjustment recommended in patients with renal impairment

Oral: *Adults:* Initial: One tablet daily; Maintenance: 1 tablet twice daily

Administration

Oral Do not initiate therapy until acute attack has subsided.

Nursing Actions

Physical Assessment See individual agents.

Patient Education

- Discuss specific use of drug and side effects with patient as it relates to treatment. (HCAHPS: During this hospital stay, were you given any medicine that you had not taken before? Before giving you any new medicine, how often did hospital staff tell you what the medicine was for? How often did hospital staff describe possible side effects in a way you could understand?)
- Patient may experience dizziness, headache, flushing, or lack of appetite. Have patient report immediately to prescriber signs of infection, signs of hepatic impairment, paresthesia, severe diarrhea, back pain, dyspepsia, hematuria, urinary retention, oliguria, ecchymosis, hemorrhaging, severe asthenia, or myalgia (HCAHPS).
- Educate patient about signs of a significant reaction (eg, wheezing; chest tightness; fever; itching; bad cough; blue skin color; seizures; or swelling of face, lips, tongue, or throat). **Note:** This is not a comprehensive list of all side effects. Patient should consult prescriber for additional questions.

Intended Use and Disclaimer: Should not be printed and given to patients. This information is intended to serve as a concise initial reference for healthcare professionals to use when discussing medications with a patient. You must ultimately rely on your own discretion, experience and judgment in diagnosing, treating and advising patients.

Related Information

Colchicine on page 363
Probenecid on page 1298

Colesevelam (koh le SEV a lam)

Brand Names: U.S. Welchol

Pharmacologic Category Antilipemic Agent, Bile Acid Sequestrant

Pregnancy Risk Factor B

Lactation Does not enter breast milk/use caution

Use

Diabetes mellitus, type 2: Improve glycemic control in adults with type 2 diabetes mellitus (non-insulin dependent, NIDDM) in conjunction with diet and exercise

Heterozygous familial hypercholesterolemia: Management of heterozygous familial hypercholesterolemia (heFH) in adolescent patients (males and postmenarcheal females 10-17 years of age) used alone or in combination with a 3-hydroxy-3-methylglutaryl coenzyme A (HMG-CoA) reductase inhibitor when after an adequate trial of dietary therapy patient continues to have low-density lipoprotein-cholesterol (LDL-C) ≥190 mg/dL or LDL-C ≥160 mg/dL with positive family history of premature cardiovascular disease (CVD) or with two or more CVD risk factors.

Hyperlipidemia:

U.S. labeling: Management of elevated LDL-C in adults with primary hyperlipidemia (Fredrickson type IIa) when used alone or in combination with an HMG-CoA reductase inhibitor in conjunction with diet and exercise

Canadian labeling (Lodalis): Adjunct to diet and lifestyle modifications in the management of primary hypercholesterolemia (Fredrickson type IIa) as monotherapy or in combination with an HMG-CoA reductase inhibitor

Limitations of use: Should not be used for the treatment of type 1 diabetes or diabetic ketoacidosis. Colesevelam has not been studied in Fredrickson Type I, III, IV, and V dyslipidemias; type 2 diabetes in combination with a dipeptidyl peptidase 4 inhibitor; pediatric patients with type 2 diabetes; children <10 years of age or in premenarchal girls. No effect on cardiovascular morbidity and mortality has been established. There is no evidence of macrovascular disease risk reduction with colesevelam use.

Available Dosage Forms
Packet, Oral:
Welchol: 1.875 g (60 ea), 3.75 g (30 ea)
Tablet, Oral:
Welchol: 625 mg
General Dosage Range Oral: *Children 10-17 years (males and postmenarchal females) and Adults:* 3.75 g daily in 1-2 divided doses
Administration
Oral Educate the patient on dietary guidelines.
Granules for oral suspension: Administer with meal(s). Powder is not to be taken in dry form (to avoid GI distress).
Tablets: Administer with meal(s) and a liquid. Due to tablet size, it is recommended that any patient who has trouble swallowing tablets should use the oral suspension form.
Nursing Actions
Physical Assessment Many other medications should not be administered with colesevelam.
Patient Education
• Discuss specific use of drug and side effects with patient as it relates to treatment. (HCAHPS: During this hospital stay, were you given any medicine that you had not taken before? Before giving you any new medicine, how often did hospital staff tell you what the medicine was for? How often did hospital staff describe possible side effects in a way you could understand?)
• Patient may experience rhinitis, rhinorrhea, asthenia, or myalgia. Have patient report immediately to prescriber signs of pancreatitis, severe constipation, considerable diarrhea, significant dyspepsia, dysphagia, pharyngitis, intolerable dizziness, significant headache, or signs of hypoglycemia (HCAHPS).
• Educate patient about signs of a significant reaction (eg, wheezing; chest tightness; fever; itching; bad cough; blue skin color; seizures; or swelling of face, lips, tongue, or throat). **Note:** This is not a comprehensive list of all side effects. Patient should consult prescriber for additional questions.

Intended Use and Disclaimer: Should not be printed and given to patients. This information is intended to serve as a concise initial reference for healthcare professionals to use when discussing medications with a patient. You must ultimately rely on your own discretion, experience and judgment in diagnosing, treating and advising patients.

Colestipol (koe LES ti pole)

Brand Names: U.S. Colestid; Colestid Flavored; Micronized Colestipol HCl
Index Terms Colestipol Hydrochloride
Pharmacologic Category Antilipemic Agent, Bile Acid Sequestrant
Medication Safety Issues
Sound-alike/look-alike issues:
Colestipol may be confused with calcitriol
Lactation Does not enter breast milk/use caution
Use Adjunct in management of primary hypercholesterolemia
Unlabeled Use Diarrhea associated with excess fecal bile acids (Westergaard, 2007); relief of pruritus associated with elevated levels of bile acids (Datta, 1963; Scaldaferri, 2011)
Dosage Forms Considerations
Colestid tablets contain micronized colestipol. Generic tablets are available in micronized and non-micronized formulations.
Available Dosage Forms
Granules, Oral:
Colestid: 5 g (300 g, 500 g)
Colestid Flavored: 5 g (450 g)
Generic: 5 g (500 g)
Packet, Oral:
Colestid: 5 g (30 ea, 90 ea)
Colestid Flavored: 5 g (60 ea)
Generic: 5 g (30 ea, 90 ea)
Tablet, Oral:
Colestid: 1 g
Micronized Colestipol HCl: 1 g
Generic: 1 g
General Dosage Range Oral: *Adults:* Granules: Initial: 5 g 1-2 times/day; Maintenance: 5-30 g/day once or in divided doses; Tablets: Initial: 2 g 1-2 times/day; Maintenance: 2-16 g/day once or in divided doses
Administration
Oral Other drugs should be administered at least 1 hour before or 4 hours after colestipol.
Granules: Do not administer in dry form (to avoid GI distress). After administration, rinse glass with a small amount of liquid to ensure all medication is taken.
Tablets: Administer tablets 1 at a time, swallowed whole, with plenty of liquid. Do not cut, crush, or chew tablets.

Nursing Actions

Physical Assessment Monitor bowel function. Be alert to potential for constipation or hemorrhoid problems.

Patient Education
- Discuss specific use of drug and side effects with patient as it relates to treatment. (HCAHPS: During this hospital stay, were you given any medicine that you had not taken before? Before giving you any new medicine, how often did hospital staff tell you what the medicine was for? How often did hospital staff describe possible side effects in a way you could understand?)
- Patient may experience nausea, pyrosis, headache, bloating, flatulence, diarrhea, or dizziness. Have patient report immediately to prescriber severe dyspepsia, considerable constipation, melena, dysphagia, angina, arrhythmia, myalgia, ecchymosis, or hemorrhaging (HCAHPS).
- Educate patient about signs of a significant reaction (eg, wheezing; chest tightness; fever; itching; bad cough; blue skin color; seizures; or swelling of face, lips, tongue, or throat). **Note:** This is not a comprehensive list of all side effects. Patient should consult prescriber for additional questions.

Intended Use and Disclaimer: Should not be printed and given to patients. This information is intended to serve as a concise initial reference for healthcare professionals to use when discussing medications with a patient. You must ultimately rely on your own discretion, experience and judgment in diagnosing, treating and advising patients.

Related Information

Oral Medications That Should Not Be Crushed or Altered *on page 1712*

Crizotinib (kriz OH ti nib)

Brand Names: U.S. Xalkori

Index Terms C-Met/Hepatocyte Growth Factor Receptor Tyrosine Kinase Inhibitor PF-02341066; C-Met/HGFR Tyrosine Kinase Inhibitor PF-02341066; MET Tyrosine Kinase Inhibitor PF-02341066; PF-02341066

Pharmacologic Category Antineoplastic Agent, Anaplastic Lymphoma Kinase Inhibitor; Antineoplastic Agent, Tyrosine Kinase Inhibitor

Medication Safety Issues

Sound-alike/look-alike issues:
Crizotinib may be confused with afatinib, cabozantinib, erlotinib, gefitinib, PONATinib

High alert medication:
This medication is in a class the Institute for Safe Medication Practices (ISMP) includes among its list of drug classes which have a heightened risk of causing significant patient harm when used in error.

Pregnancy Risk Factor D

Lactation Excretion in breast milk unknown/not recommended

Use Nonsmall cell lung cancer: Treatment of patients with metastatic nonsmall cell lung cancer (NSCLC) whose tumors are anaplastic lymphoma kinase (ALK)-positive (as detected by an approved test)

Available Dosage Forms

Capsule, Oral:
Xalkori: 200 mg, 250 mg

General Dosage Range Dosage adjustment recommended in patients with renal impairment or who develop toxicities.

Oral: *Adults:* 250 mg twice daily

Administration

Oral Swallow capsules whole (do not crush, dissolve, or open capsules). Administer with or without food. Crizotinib is associated with a moderate emetic potential; antiemetics may be needed to prevent nausea and vomiting. If vomiting occurs after dose, administer the next dose at the regularly scheduled time.

Hazardous agent; use appropriate precautions for handling and disposal (meets NIOSH, 2012 criteria).

Nursing Actions

Physical Assessment Obtain vital signs; can cause bradycardia. Monitor electrolytes (potassium, magnesium), especially in patients with heart disease. Evaluate EKG regularly for bradyarrhythmias and QT prolongation. Monitor LFTs. Patients may need ophthalmic evaluation in case of visual changes. Monitor for pulmonary symptoms such as cough, shortness of breath, or fluid retention. Instruct patients to report any abnormal bleeding, blood in the stool, petechia, jaundice, or dark-colored urine.

Patient Education
- Discuss specific use of drug and side effects with patient as it relates to treatment. (HCAHPS: During this hospital stay, were you given any medicine that you had not taken before? Before giving you any new medicine, how often did hospital staff tell you what the medicine was for? How often did hospital staff describe possible side effects in a way you could understand?)
- Patient may experience headache, dyspepsia, lack of appetite, stomatitis, constipation, arthralgia, back pain, or dysgeusia. Have patient report immediately to prescriber signs of infection, dyspnea, excessive weight gain, edema of extremities, angina, severe dizziness, syncope, tachycardia, arrhythmia, significant nausea, considerable diarrhea, intolerable asthenia, ecchymosis, hemorrhaging, vision changes, paresthesia, signs of hepatic impairment, or signs of severe pulmonary disorder (HCAHPS).
- Educate patient about signs of a significant reaction (eg, wheezing; chest tightness; fever; itching; bad cough; blue skin color; seizures; or

swelling of face, lips, tongue, or throat). **Note:** This is not a comprehensive list of all side effects. Patient should consult prescriber for additional questions.

Intended Use and Disclaimer: Should not be printed and given to patients. This information is intended to serve as a concise initial reference for healthcare professionals to use when discussing medications with a patient. You must ultimately rely on your own discretion, experience and judgment in diagnosing, treating and advising patients.

Related Information

Oral Medications That Should Not Be Crushed or Altered *on page 1712*

Crofelemer (kroe FEL e mer)

Brand Names: U.S. Fulyzaq
Index Terms *Croton lechleri*; Provir; SP-303
Pharmacologic Category Antidiarrheal
Medication Safety Issues
Sound-alike/look-alike issues:
Crofelemer may be confused with sevelamer
Pregnancy Risk Factor C
Lactation Excretion in breast milk unknown/not recommended
Use Symptomatic relief of noninfectious diarrhea in patients with HIV/AIDS on antiretroviral therapy
Available Dosage Forms
Tablet Delayed Release, Oral:
Fulyzaq: 125 mg
General Dosage Range Oral: *Adults:* 125 mg twice daily
Administration
Oral May be administered orally with or without food. Swallow whole; do not crush or chew.
Nursing Actions
Physical Assessment Monitor gastrointestinal function and side effects. Monitor for symptoms of bronchitis or other respiratory tract infections. Monitor liver function tests.
Patient Education
- Discuss specific use of drug and side effects with patient as it relates to treatment. (HCAHPS: During this hospital stay, were you given any medicine that you had not taken before? Before giving you any new medicine, how often did hospital staff tell you what the medicine was for? How often did hospital staff describe possible side effects in a way you could understand?)
- Patient may experience flatulence, dyspepsia, back pain, or arthralgia. Have patient report immediately to prescriber signs of infection (HCAHPS).
- Educate patient about signs of a significant reaction (eg, wheezing; chest tightness; fever; itching; bad cough; blue skin color; seizures; or swelling of face, lips, tongue, or throat). **Note:** This is not a comprehensive list of all side

effects. Patient should consult prescriber for additional questions.

Intended Use and Disclaimer: Should not be printed and given to patients. This information is intended to serve as a concise initial reference for healthcare professionals to use when discussing medications with a patient. You must ultimately rely on your own discretion, experience and judgment in diagnosing, treating and advising patients.

Related Information

Oral Medications That Should Not Be Crushed or Altered *on page 1712*

Cromolyn (Systemic, Oral Inhalation) (KROE moe lin)

Brand Names: U.S. Gastrocrom
Index Terms Cromoglicate; Cromoglycic Acid; Cromolyn Sodium; Disodium Cromoglycate; DSCG; Sodium Cromoglicate
Pharmacologic Category Mast Cell Stabilizer
Pregnancy Risk Factor B
Lactation Excretion in breast milk unknown/use caution
Breast-Feeding Considerations No data available on whether cromolyn enters into breast milk or clinical effects on the infant. Use of cromolyn is not considered a contraindication to breast-feeding.
Use
Inhalation: May be used as an adjunct in the prophylaxis of allergic disorders, including asthma; prevention of exercise-induced bronchospasm
Oral: Systemic mastocytosis
Unlabeled Use Oral: Food allergy, treatment of inflammatory bowel disease
Mechanism of Action/Effect Prevents the mast cell release of histamine, leukotrienes, and slow-reacting substance of anaphylaxis
Contraindications Hypersensitivity to cromolyn or any component of the formulation; acute asthma attacks
Warnings/Precautions Severe anaphylactic reactions may occur rarely; cromolyn is a prophylactic drug with no benefit for acute situations; caution should be used when withdrawing the drug or tapering the dose as symptoms may reoccur; use with caution in patients with a history of cardiac arrhythmias. Dosage of oral product should be decreased with hepatic or renal dysfunction.
Drug Interactions
Avoid Concomitant Use There are no known interactions where it is recommended to avoid concomitant use.
Decreased Effect There are no known significant interactions involving a decrease in effect.
Increased Effect/Toxicity There are no known significant interactions involving an increase in effect.

Adverse Reactions Frequency not defined.

Cardiovascular: Angioedema, chest pain, edema, flushing, palpitation, premature ventricular contractions, tachycardia

Central nervous system: Anxiety, behavior changes, convulsions, depression, dizziness, fatigue, hallucinations, headache, irritability, insomnia, lethargy, migraine, nervousness, hypoesthesia, postprandial lightheadedness, psychosis

Dermatologic: Erythema, photosensitivity, pruritus, purpura, rash, urticaria

Gastrointestinal: Abdominal pain, constipation, diarrhea, dyspepsia, dysphagia, esophagospasm, flatulence, glossitis, nausea, stomatitis, vomiting

Genitourinary: Dysuria, urinary frequency

Hematologic: Neutropenia, pancytopenia, polycythemia

Hepatic: Liver function test abnormal

Local: Burning

Neuromuscular & skeletal: Arthralgia, leg stiffness, leg weakness, myalgia, paresthesia

Otic: Tinnitus

Respiratory: Dyspnea, pharyngitis

Miscellaneous: Lupus erythematosus

Pharmacodynamics/Kinetics

Onset of Action Response to treatment: Oral: May occur within 2-6 weeks

Available Dosage Forms

Concentrate, Oral:
Gastrocrom: 100 mg/5 mL (5 mL)

Concentrate, Oral [preservative free]:
Generic: 100 mg/5 mL (5 mL)

Nebulization Solution, Inhalation:
Generic: 20 mg/2 mL (2 mL)

General Dosage Range

Inhalation: Nebulization: *Children ≥2 years and Adults:* Initial: 20 mg 4 times/day; Maintenance: 20 mg 3-4 times/day **or** 20 mg prior to exercise or allergen exposure

Oral:
Children 2-12 years: 100 mg 4 times/day (maximum: 40 mg/kg/day)
Children >12 years and Adults: 200 mg 4 times/day (maximum: 40 mg/kg/day)

Administration

Oral Oral solution: Open ampul and squeeze contents into glass of water; stir well. Administer at least 30 minutes before meals and at bedtime.

Storage/Stability Store at room temperature of 15°C to 30°C (59°F to 86°F). Protect from light. Do not use oral solution if solution becomes discolored or forms a precipitate.

Nursing Actions

Physical Assessment This is prophylactic therapy, not to be used for acute situations.

Patient Education

• Discuss specific use of drug and side effects with patient as it relates to treatment. (HCAHPS: During this hospital stay, were you given any medicine that you had not taken before? Before giving you any new medicine, how often did hospital staff tell you what the medicine was for? How often did hospital staff describe possible side effects in a way you could understand?)

• Patient may experience diarrhea, headache, sternutation, or parageusia. Have patient report immediately to prescriber dyspnea (HCAHPS).

• Educate patient about signs of a significant reaction (eg, wheezing; chest tightness; fever; itching; bad cough; blue skin color; seizures; or swelling of face, lips, tongue, or throat). **Note:** This is not a comprehensive list of all side effects. Patient should consult prescriber for additional questions.

Intended Use and Disclaimer: Should not be printed and given to patients. This information is intended to serve as a concise initial reference for healthcare professionals to use when discussing medications with a patient. You must ultimately rely on your own discretion, experience and judgment in diagnosing, treating and advising patients.

Dietary Considerations Oral: Should be taken at least 30 minutes before meals.

Cyanocobalamin (sye an oh koe BAL a min)

Brand Names: U.S. Nascobal; Physicians EZ Use B-12

Index Terms Vitamin B_{12}

Pharmacologic Category Vitamin, Water Soluble

Lactation Enters breast milk/compatible

Use Treatment of pernicious anemia; vitamin B_{12} deficiency due to dietary deficiencies or malabsorption diseases, inadequate secretion of intrinsic factor, and inadequate utilization of B_{12} (eg, during neoplastic treatment); increased B_{12} requirements due to pregnancy, thyrotoxicosis, hemorrhage, malignancy, liver or kidney disease

Available Dosage Forms

Kit, Injection:
Physicians EZ Use B-12: 1000 mcg/mL

Liquid, Sublingual:
Generic: 3000 mcg/mL (52 mL)

Lozenge, Oral:
Generic: 50 mcg (100 ea); 100 mcg (100 ea); 250 mcg (100 ea, 250 ea); 500 mcg (100 ea, 250 ea)

Solution, Injection:
Generic: 1000 mcg/mL (1 mL, 10 mL, 30 mL)

Solution, Nasal:
Nascobal: 500 mcg/0.1 mL (1.3 mL)

Tablet, Oral:
Generic: 100 mcg, 250 mcg, 500 mcg, 1000 mcg

Tablet, Oral [preservative free]:
Generic: 100 mcg, 500 mcg, 1000 mcg

Tablet Extended Release, Oral:
Generic: 1000 mcg
Tablet Sublingual, Sublingual:
Generic: 2500 mcg
Tablet Sublingual, Sublingual [preservative free]:
Generic: 2500 mcg
General Dosage Range
I.M., SubQ: *Children and Adults:* Dosage varies greatly depending on indication
Intranasal: *Adults:* Nascobal: 500 mcg in one nostril once weekly
Oral: *Adults:* 250-2000 mcg daily
Administration
I.M. I.M. or deep SubQ are preferred routes of administration.
I.V. Not recommended
Injectable Detail pH: 4.5-7
Oral Not recommended due to variable absorption; however, oral therapy of 1000-2000 mcg daily has been effective for anemia if I.M./SubQ routes refused or not tolerated.
Other Intranasal: Nasal spray (Nascobal): Prior to initial dose, activate (prime) spray nozzle by pumping unit quickly and firmly until first appearance of spray, then prime twice more. The unit must be reprimed once immediately before each subsequent use. Administer 1 hour before or after ingestion of hot foods/liquids.
Nursing Actions
Physical Assessment Provide patient appropriate nutritional counseling.
Patient Education
- Discuss specific use of drug and side effects with patient as it relates to treatment. (HCAHPS: During this hospital stay, were you given any medicine that you had not taken before? Before giving you any new medicine, how often did hospital staff tell you what the medicine was for? How often did hospital staff describe possible side effects in a way you could understand?)
- Patient may experience dizziness, headache, anxiety, or nausea. Have patient report immediately to prescriber edema of extremities, severe diarrhea, significant asthenia, angina, arrhythmia, myalgia, dyspnea, edema of extremities, ecchymosis, or hemorrhaging (HCAHPS).
- Educate patient about signs of a significant reaction (eg, wheezing; chest tightness; fever; itching; bad cough; blue skin color; seizures; or swelling of face, lips, tongue, or throat). **Note:** This is not a comprehensive list of all side effects. Patient should consult prescriber for additional questions.

Intended Use and Disclaimer: Should not be printed and given to patients. This information is intended to serve as a concise initial reference for healthcare professionals to use when discussing medications with a patient. You must ultimately rely on your own discretion, experience and judgment in diagnosing, treating and advising patients.

Cyclobenzaprine (sye kloe BEN za preen)

Brand Names: U.S. Amrix; EnovaRX-Cyclobenzaprine HCl; Fexmid; Flexeril [DSC]
Index Terms Cyclobenzaprine Hydrochloride
Pharmacologic Category Skeletal Muscle Relaxant
Medication Safety Issues
Sound-alike/look-alike issues:
Cyclobenzaprine may be confused with cycloSERINE, cyproheptadine
Flexeril may be confused with Floxin
BEERS Criteria medication:
This drug may be potentially inappropriate for use in geriatric patients (Quality of evidence - moderate; Strength of recommendation - strong).
International issues:
Flexin: Brand name for cyclobenzaprine [Chile], but also the brand name for diclofenac [Argentina] and orphenadrine [Israel]
Flexin [Chile] may be confused with Floxin brand name for flunarizine [Thailand], norfloxacin [South Africa], ofloxacin [U.S., Canada], and perfloxacin [Philippines]; Fluoxine brand name for fluoxetine [Thailand]; Flexinol brand name for methocarbamol and paracetamol [India]
Pregnancy Risk Factor B
Lactation Excretion in breast milk unknown/use caution
Breast-Feeding Considerations It is not known if cyclobenzaprine is excreted in breast milk. The manufacturer recommends that caution be exercised when administering cyclobenzaprine to nursing women.
Use Short-term (2-3 weeks) treatment of muscle spasm associated with acute, painful musculoskeletal conditions
Unlabeled Use Treatment of muscle spasm associated with acute temporomandibular joint pain (TMJ)
Mechanism of Action/Effect Centrally-acting skeletal muscle relaxant pharmacologically related to tricyclic antidepressants; reduces tonic somatic motor activity influencing both alpha and gamma motor neurons
Contraindications Hypersensitivity to cyclobenzaprine or any component of the formulation; during or within 14 days of MAO inhibitors; hyperthyroidism; congestive heart failure; arrhythmias; heart block or conduction disturbances; acute recovery phase of MI
Warnings/Precautions May cause CNS depression, which may impair physical or mental abilities; ethanol and/or other CNS depressants may enhance these effects. Patients must be cautioned about performing tasks which require mental alertness (eg, operating machinery or driving). Cyclobenzaprine shares the toxic potentials of the

tricyclic antidepressants (including arrhythmias, tachycardia, and conduction time prolongation) and the usual precautions of tricyclic antidepressant therapy should be observed; use with caution in patients with urinary hesitancy or retention, angle-closure glaucoma or increased intraocular pressure, hepatic impairment, or in the elderly.

Potentially life-threatening serotonin syndrome has occurred with cyclobenzaprine when used in combination with other serotonergic agents (eg, SSRIs, SNRIs, TCAs, meperidine, tramadol, buspirone, MAO inhibitors), bupropion, and verapamil. Monitor patients closely especially during initiation/dose titration for signs/symptoms of serotonin syndrome such as mental status changes (eg, agitation, hallucinations); autonomic instability (eg, tachycardia, labile blood pressure, diaphoresis); neuromuscular changes (eg, tremor, rigidity, myoclonus); GI symptoms (eg, nausea, vomiting, diarrhea); and/or seizures. Discontinue cyclobenzaprine and any concomitant serotonergic agent immediately if signs/symptoms arise. Concomitant use or use within 14 days of discontinuing an MAO inhibitor is contraindicated.

Muscle relaxants are poorly tolerated by the elderly due to potent anticholinergic effects, sedation, and risk of fracture. Efficacy is questionable at dosages tolerated by elderly patients; avoid use (Beers Criteria). Extended release capsules not recommended for use in mild-to-severe hepatic impairment or in the elderly. Potentially significant drug-drug interactions may exist, requiring dose or frequency adjustment, additional monitoring, and/or selection of alternative therapy. Effects may be potentiated when used with other CNS depressants or ethanol.

Drug Interactions
Avoid Concomitant Use
Avoid concomitant use of Cyclobenzaprine with any of the following: Aclidinium; Azelastine (Nasal); Ipratropium (Oral Inhalation); MAO Inhibitors; Paraldehyde; Thalidomide; Tiotropium; Umeclidinium

Decreased Effect
Cyclobenzaprine may decrease the levels/effects of: Acetylcholinesterase Inhibitors (Central)

The levels/effects of Cyclobenzaprine may be decreased by: Acetylcholinesterase Inhibitors (Central); Peginterferon Alfa-2b

Increased Effect/Toxicity
Cyclobenzaprine may increase the levels/effects of: Alcohol (Ethyl); Analgesics (Opioid); Anticholinergics; Antipsychotics; Azelastine (Nasal); Buprenorphine; CNS Depressants; Hydrocodone; MAO Inhibitors; Metoclopramide; Metyrosine; Paraldehyde; Pramipexole; ROPINIRole; Rotigotine; Serotonin Modulators; Thalidomide; Tiotropium; TraMADol; Zolpidem

The levels/effects of Cyclobenzaprine may be increased by: Abiraterone Acetate; Aclidinium; Antipsychotics; Brimonidine (Topical); CYP1A2 Inhibitors (Moderate); CYP1A2 Inhibitors (Strong); Deferasirox; Doxylamine; HydrOXYzine; Ipratropium (Oral Inhalation); Magnesium Sulfate; Perampanel; Pramlintide; Sodium Oxybate; Umeclidinium; Vemurafenib

Nutritional/Ethanol Interactions
Ethanol: May increase CNS depression. Management: Avoid ethanol during cyclobenzaprine therapy; monitor for increased effects with coadministration.

Food: Food increases bioavailability (peak plasma concentrations increased by 35% and area under the curve by 20%) of the extended release capsule. Management: Monitor for increased effects if taken with food.

Herb/Nutraceutical: Valerian, kava kava, gotu kola may increase CNS depression. Management: Avoid use during cyclobenzaprine therapy.

Adverse Reactions
>10%:
Central nervous system: Drowsiness (1% to 39%), dizziness (1% to 11%)
Gastrointestinal: Xerostomia (6% to 32%)
1% to 10%:
Central nervous system: Fatigue (1% to 6%), headache (1% to 5%), confusion (1% to 3%), decreased mental acuity (1% to 3%), irritability (1% to 3%), nervousness (1% to 3%)
Gastrointestinal: Dyspepsia (≤4%), abdominal pain (1% to 3%), acid regurgitation (1% to 3%), constipation (1% to 3%), diarrhea (1% to 3%), nausea (1% to 3%), unpleasant taste (1% to 3%)
Neuromuscular & skeletal: Weakness (1% to 3%)
Ophthalmic: Blurred vision (1% to 3%)
Respiratory: Pharyngitis (1% to 3%), upper respiratory tract infection (1% to 3%)

Dosage Forms Considerations
EnovaRX-Cyclobenzaprine is a compounding kit. Refer to manufacturer's package insert for compounding instructions.

Available Dosage Forms
Capsule Extended Release 24 Hour, Oral:
Amrix: 15 mg, 30 mg
Cream, Transdermal:
EnovaRX-Cyclobenzaprine HCl: 20 mg/g (120 g)
Tablet, Oral:
Fexmid: 7.5 mg
Generic: 5 mg, 7.5 mg, 10 mg
General Dosage Range Dosage adjustment recommended in patients with hepatic impairment
Oral capsule, extended release: *Adults:* Usual: 15 mg once daily (maximum: 30 mg once daily)
Oral tablet, immediate release:
Children ≥15 years and Adults: Initial: 5 mg 3 times daily; Maintenance: 5-10 mg 3 times daily
Elderly: Initial: 5 mg; titrate dose slowly and consider less frequent dosing

▶

Administration

Oral Extended release capsules: Administer at the same time each day. Do not crush or chew.

Storage/Stability

Amrix, Flexeril: Store at 25°C (77°F); excursions permitted to 15°C to 30°C (59°F to 86°F). Protect from light.

Fexmid: Store at 20°C to 25°C (68°F to 77°F).

Nursing Actions

Physical Assessment May cause significant CNS depression. Caution patients about sedation.

Patient Education

• Discuss specific use of drug and side effects with patient as it relates to treatment. (HCAHPS: During this hospital stay, were you given any medicine that you had not taken before? Before giving you any new medicine, how often did hospital staff tell you what the medicine was for? How often did hospital staff describe possible side effects in a way you could understand?)

• Patient may experience fatigue or xerostomia. Have patient report immediately to prescriber severe asthenia, anhidrosis, or serotonin syndrome (ie, dizziness, severe headache, agitation, hallucinations, tachycardia, arrhythmia, flushing, tremors, hyperhidrosis, change in balance, severe nausea, significant diarrhea) (HCAHPS).

• Educate patient about signs of a significant reaction (eg, wheezing; chest tightness; fever; itching; bad cough; blue skin color; seizures; or swelling of face, lips, tongue, or throat). **Note:** This is not a comprehensive list of all side effects. Patient should consult prescriber for additional questions.

Intended Use and Disclaimer: Should not be printed and given to patients. This information is intended to serve as a concise initial reference for healthcare professionals to use when discussing medications with a patient. You must ultimately rely on your own discretion, experience and judgment in diagnosing, treating and advising patients.

Related Information

Oral Medications That Should Not Be Crushed or Altered *on page 1712*

Cyclophosphamide (sye kloe FOS fa mide)

Index Terms CPM; CTX; CYT; Cytoxan; Neosar
Pharmacologic Category Antineoplastic Agent, Alkylating Agent; Antineoplastic Agent, Alkylating Agent (Nitrogen Mustard); Antirheumatic Miscellaneous; Immunosuppressant Agent
Medication Safety Issues
Sound-alike/look-alike issues:
Cyclophosphamide may be confused with cycloSPORINE, ifosfamide

Cytoxan may be confused with cefOXitin, Ciloxan®, cytarabine, CytoGam®, Cytosar®, Cytosar-U, Cytotec®

High alert medication:
This medication is in a class the Institute for Safe Medication Practices (ISMP) includes among its list of drug classes which have a heightened risk of causing significant patient harm when used in error.

Pregnancy Risk Factor D

Lactation Enters breast milk/not recommended

Breast-Feeding Considerations Cyclophosphamide is excreted into breast milk. Leukopenia and thrombocytopenia were noted in an infant exposed to cyclophosphamide while nursing. The mother was treated with one course of cyclophosphamide 6 weeks prior to delivery then cyclophosphamide I.V. 6 mg/kg (300 mg) once daily for 3 days beginning 20 days postpartum. Complete blood counts were obtained in the breast-feeding infant on each day of therapy; WBC and platelets decreased by day 3 (Durodola, 1979). Due to the potential for adverse effects and tumorigenicity, the manufacturer recommends that the decision to discontinue cyclophosphamide or to discontinue breast-feeding should take into account the benefits of treatment to the mother.

Use

Oncology-related uses: Treatment of Hodgkin lymphoma, non-Hodgkin lymphomas (including Burkitt lymphoma, chronic lymphocytic leukemia (CLL), chronic myelocytic leukemia (CML), acute myelocytic leukemia (AML), acute lymphoblastic leukemia (ALL), mycosis fungoides, multiple myeloma, neuroblastoma, retinoblastoma; breast cancer; ovarian adenocarcinoma

Canadian labeling: Additional use (not in U.S. labeling): Treatment of lung cancer

Nononcology uses: Treatment of refractory nephrotic syndrome in children who are unresponsive or intolerant to corticosteroid therapy

Unlabeled Use

Oncology-related uses: Ewing's sarcoma, rhabdomyosarcoma, Wilms tumor, ovarian germ cell tumors, gestational trophoblastic tumors (high-risk), small cell lung cancer, testicular cancer, pheochromocytoma, hematopoietic stem cell transplant (HSCT) conditioning regimen

Nononcology uses: Severe rheumatoid disorders, granulomatosis with polyangiitis (GPA; Wegener's granulomatosis), myasthenia gravis, multiple sclerosis, lupus nephritis, autoimmune hemolytic anemia, idiopathic thrombocytic purpura (ITP), antibody-induced pure red cell aplasia

Mechanism of Action/Effect Interferes with the normal function of DNA by alkylation and cross-linking the strands of DNA, and by possible protein modification; cyclophosphamide also possesses potent immunosuppressive activity; note that cyclophosphamide must be metabolized to its active form in the liver

Contraindications

U.S. labeling: Hypersensitivity to cyclophosphamide or any component of the formulation; severely depressed bone marrow function

Canadian labeling: Hypersensitivity to cyclophosphamide or its metabolites, urinary outflow obstructions, severe myelosuppression, severe renal or hepatic impairment, active infection (especially varicella zoster), severe immunosuppression

Warnings/Precautions Hazardous agent - use appropriate precautions for handling and disposal (NIOSH, 2012).

Cyclophosphamide is associated with the development of hemorrhagic cystitis; may rarely be severe and even fatal. Discontinue cyclophosphamide with severe hemorrhagic cystitis. Bladder injury is due to excretion of cyclophosphamide metabolites in the urine and appears to be dose- and treatment duration-dependent. Bladder fibrosis may also occur, either with or without cystitis. Increased hydration and frequent voiding is recommended to help prevent cystitis; some protocols utilize mesna to protect against hemorrhagic cystitis. Monitor urinalysis for hematuria. Severe or prolonged hemorrhagic cystitis may require medical or surgical treatment. Hematuria generally resolves within a few days after treatment is withheld, although it may persist. Cyclophosphamide may potentiate the cardiotoxicity of anthracyclines.

Cardiotoxicity has been reported, usually with high doses associated with transplant conditioning regimens, although may rarely occur with lower doses. Cardiac abnormalities do not appear to persist. Cardiotoxicities reported have included arrhythmia, congestive heart failure, heart block, hemorrhagic myocarditis, hemopericardium (secondary to hemorrhagic myocarditis and myocardial necrosis), pericarditis, and tachyarrhythmias. Cardiotoxicity is related to endothelial capillary damage; symptoms may be managed with diuretics, ACE inhibitors, beta blockers, or inotropics (Floyd, 2005). Use with caution in patients with pre-existing cardiovascular disease. For patients with multiple cardiac risk factors, considering monitoring during treatment (Floyd, 2005).

Pulmonary toxicities, including pneumonitis and acute respiratory distress syndrome, have been reported. Consider pulmonary function testing to assess the severity of pneumonitis (Morgan, 2011). Cyclophosphamide-induced pneumonitis is rare and may present as early (within 1-6 months) or late onset (several months to years); early onset has been reversible with discontinuation; late onset is associated with pleural thickening and may persist chronically (Malik, 1996).

Dose-related neutropenia is common; thrombocytopenia and anemia may also occur. Monitor for infections; immunosuppression and serious infections may occur; infections may require dose reduction, or interruption or discontinuation of treatment. Nausea and vomiting commonly occur; premedication with antiemetics is recommended. Stomatitis/mucositis may also occur. Anaphylactic reactions have been reported; cross-sensitivity with other alkylating agents may occur. May interfere with wound healing. Secondary malignancies (bladder cancer, myeloproliferative, and lymphoproliferative malignancies) have been reported with both single-agent and with combination chemotherapy regimens; onset may be delayed (up to several years after treatment); bladder malignancy usually occurs in patients previously experiencing hemorrhagic cystitis. May impair fertility; interferes with oogenesis and spermatogenesis; effect on fertility is generally dependent on dose and duration of treatment and may be irreversible. The age at treatment initiation and cumulative dose were determined to be risk factors for ovarian failure in cyclophosphamide use for the treatment of systemic lupus erythematosus (SLE) (Mok, 1998). Use with caution in patients with renal and hepatic impairment; dosage adjustment may be needed (use is contraindicated in severe impairment in the Canadian labeling).

Drug Interactions

Avoid Concomitant Use

Avoid concomitant use of Cyclophosphamide with any of the following: BCG; Belimumab; CloZAPine; Etanercept; Natalizumab; Pimecrolimus; Pimozide; Tacrolimus (Topical); Tofacitinib; Vaccines (Live)

Decreased Effect

Cyclophosphamide may decrease the levels/effects of: BCG; Cardiac Glycosides; Coccidioidin Skin Test; Sipuleucel-T; Vaccines (Inactivated); Vaccines (Live); Vitamin K Antagonists

The levels/effects of Cyclophosphamide may be decreased by: CYP2B6 Inducers (Strong); Dabrafenib; Echinacea

Increased Effect/Toxicity

Cyclophosphamide may increase the levels/effects of: Antineoplastic Agents (Anthracycline, Systemic); ARIPiprazole; CloZAPine; Dofetilide; Leflunomide; Lomitapide; Natalizumab; Pimozide; Succinylcholine; Tofacitinib; Vaccines (Live); Vitamin K Antagonists

The levels/effects of Cyclophosphamide may be increased by: Allopurinol; Belimumab; CYP2B6 Inhibitors (Moderate); CYP2B6 Inhibitors (Strong); Denosumab; Etanercept; Pentostatin; Pimecrolimus; Quazepam; Roflumilast; Tacrolimus (Topical); Trastuzumab

Nutritional/Ethanol Interactions Herb/Nutraceutical: Avoid black cohosh, dong quai in estrogen-dependent tumors.

Adverse Reactions Frequency not defined.

Dermatologic: Alopecia (reversible; onset: 3-6 weeks after start of treatment)

Endocrine & metabolic: Amenorrhea, azoospermia, gonadal suppression, oligospermia, oogenesis impaired, sterility

Gastrointestinal: Abdominal pain, anorexia, diarrhea, mucositis, nausea/vomiting (dose-related), stomatitis

Genitourinary: Hemorrhagic cystitis

Hematologic: Anemia, leukopenia (dose-related; recovery: 7-10 days after cessation), myelosuppression, neutropenia, neutropenic fever, thrombocytopenia

Miscellaneous: Infection

Product Availability Cyclophosphamide capsules: FDA approved September 2013; anticipated availability is currently unknown. Refer to the prescribing information for additional information.

Available Dosage Forms

Solution Reconstituted, Injection:

Generic: 500 mg (1 ea); 1 g (1 ea); 2 g (1 ea)

Tablet, Oral:

Generic: 25 mg, 50 mg

General Dosage Range Dosage adjustment recommended in patients with hepatic or renal impairment or who develop toxicities.

I.V.: *Children and Adults:* Dosage varies greatly depending on indication.

Oral: *Children and Adults:* Dosage varies greatly depending on indication.

Administration

I.V.

Infusion rate may vary based on protocol (refer to specific protocol for infusion rate). Administer by direct I.V. injection (if reconstituted in NS), IVPB, or continuous I.V. infusion

Bladder toxicity: To minimize bladder toxicity, increase normal fluid intake during and for 1-2 days after cyclophosphamide dose. Most adult patients will require a fluid intake of at least 2 L/day. High-dose regimens should be accompanied by vigorous hydration with or without mesna therapy.

Hematopoietic stem cell transplant: Approaches to reduction of hemorrhagic cystitis include infusion of 0.9% NaCl 3 L/m^2/24 hours, infusion of 0.9% NaCl 3 L/m^2/24 hours with continuous 0.9% NaCl bladder irrigation 300-1000 mL/hour, and infusion of 0.9% NaCl 1.5-3 L/m^2/24 hours with intravenous mesna. Hydration should begin at least 4 hours before cyclophosphamide and continue at least 24 hours after completion of cyclophosphamide. The dose of daily mesna used may be 67% to 100% of the daily dose of cyclophosphamide. Mesna can be administered as a continuous 24-hour intravenous infusion or be given in divided doses every 4 hours. Mesna should begin at the start of treatment, and continue at least 24 hours following the last dose of cyclophosphamide.

Hazardous agent; use appropriate precautions for handling and disposal (NIOSH, 2012).

Injectable Detail pH: 3-9 (reconstituted solution)

Oral Tablets are not scored and should not be cut or crushed. To minimize the risk of bladder irritation, do not administer tablets at bedtime.

Hazardous agent; use appropriate precautions for handling and disposal (NIOSH, 2012).

Preparation for Administration Hazardous agent; use appropriate precautions for handling and disposal (NIOSH, 2012).

Injection powder for reconstitution: Store intact vials of powder at room temperature of 25°C (77°F). For I.V. push, reconstitute with normal saline (NS) to a concentration of 20 mg/mL. For I.V. infusion, reconstitute with sterile water or NS to a concentration of 20 mg/mL; further dilute for infusion in D$_5$W, 1/2NS, or D$_5$NS.

Storage/Stability Hazardous agent; use appropriate precautions for handling and disposal (NIOSH, 2012).

Injection powder for reconstitution: Store intact vials of powder at room temperature of 25°C (77°F). Reconstituted solutions in normal saline (NS) are stable for 24 hours at room temperature and for 6 days refrigerated at 2°C to 8°C (36°F to 46°F). Solutions diluted for infusion in 1/2NS are stable for 24 hours at room temperature and for 6 days refrigerated; solutions diluted in D$_5$W or D$_5$NS are stable for 24 hours at room temperature and for 36 hours refrigerated.

Tablets: Store tablets at room temperature of 25°C (77°F); excursions permitted to 15°C to 30°C (59°F to 86°F).

Nursing Actions

Physical Assessment Note infusion specifics in administration. Pre- and posthydration are dose-dependent. Monitor infusion site for possible extravasation. Monitor for signs of infection and cystitis. Instruct patient to report hematuria or dysuria. Check UA per physician preference. Teach patient importance of adequate hydration, especially with oral tablet use.

Patient Education

• Discuss specific use of drug and side effects with patient as it relates to treatment. (HCAHPS: During this hospital stay, were you given any medicine that you had not taken before? Before giving you any new medicine, how often did hospital staff tell you what the medicine was for? How often did hospital staff describe possible side effects in a way you could understand?)

• Patient may experience lack of appetite, changes in skin or nails, diarrhea, alopecia, nausea, or amenorrhea. Have patient report immediately to prescriber signs of infection, dyspnea, severe dyspepsia, considerable back pain, ecchymosis, hemorrhaging, urine discoloration, jaundice, hematuria, significant asthenia, wound healing impairment, urinary retention, oliguria, dysuria, melena, angina, stomatitis, or edema of extremities (HCAHPS).

• Educate patient about signs of a significant reaction (eg, wheezing; chest tightness; fever; itching; bad cough; blue skin color; seizures; or swelling of face, lips, tongue, or throat). **Note:** This is not a comprehensive list of all side effects. Patient should consult prescriber for additional questions.

Intended Use and Disclaimer: Should not be printed and given to patients. This information is intended to serve as a concise initial reference for healthcare professionals to use when discussing medications with a patient. You must ultimately rely on your own discretion, experience and judgment in diagnosing, treating and advising patients.

Dietary Considerations Tablets should be administered during or after meals.

Related Information
Management of Drug Extravasations *on page 1700*

CycloSPORINE (Systemic)
(SYE kloe spor een)

Brand Names: U.S. Gengraf; Neoral; SandIMMUNE

Index Terms Ciclosporin; CsA; CyA; Cyclosporin A

Pharmacologic Category Calcineurin Inhibitor; Immunosuppressant Agent

Medication Safety Issues
Sound-alike/look-alike issues:
CycloSPORINE may be confused with cyclophosphamide, Cyklokapron, cycloSERINE
CycloSPORINE modified (Neoral, Gengraf) may be confused with cycloSPORINE non-modified (SandIMMUNE)
Gengraf may be confused with Prograf
Neoral may be confused with Neurontin, Nizoral
SandIMMUNE may be confused with SandoSTATIN

Pregnancy Risk Factor C

Lactation Enters breast milk/not recommended

Breast-Feeding Considerations Cyclosporine is excreted in breast milk. Concentrations of cyclosporine in milk vary widely and breast-feeding during therapy is generally not recommended (Bae, 2012; Cowan, 2012). Due to the potential for serious adverse in the nursing infant, the decision to discontinue cyclosporine or to discontinue breast-feeding should take into account the importance of treatment to the mother. Formulations may contain alcohol which may be present in breast milk and could be absorbed orally by the nursing infant.

Use
Cyclosporine modified:
Transplant rejection prophylaxis: Prophylaxis of organ rejection in kidney, liver, and heart

transplants (has been used with azathioprine and/or corticosteroids)

Rheumatoid arthritis: Treatment of severe, active rheumatoid arthritis (RA) not responsive to methotrexate alone

Psoriasis: Treatment of severe, recalcitrant plaque psoriasis in nonimmunocompromised adults unresponsive to or unable to tolerate other systemic therapy

Cyclosporine non-modified: Transplant rejection (prophylaxis/treatment): Prophylaxis of organ rejection in kidney, liver, and heart transplants (has been used with azathioprine and/or corticosteroids; treatment of chronic organ rejection)

Canadian labeling: Additional uses (not in U.S. labeling):

Cyclosporine modified: Nephrotic syndrome: Induction and maintenance of remission in steroid dependent/resistant nephrotic syndrome due to glomerular disease (eg, minimal change nephropathy, membranous glomerulonephritis, focal and segmental glomerulosclerosis); maintenance of steroid induced remission allowing for steroid dose reduction or withdrawal.

Cyclosporine modified/non-modified: Bone marrow transplant rejection (prophylaxis/treatment): Prophylaxis of graft rejection following bone marrow transplantation; prophylaxis or treatment of graft-versus-host disease (GVHD)

Unlabeled Use Prevention and treatment of acute graft-versus-host disease (GVHD) in allogeneic stem cell transplantation; treatment of chronic GVHD in allogeneic stem cell transplant; treatment of lupus nephritis; treatment of focal segmental glomerulosclerosis; treatment of severe refractory ulcerative colitis

Mechanism of Action/Effect Inhibits T-lymphocytes and lymphokine production and release in a reversible manner.

Contraindications
Hypersensitivity to cyclosporine or any component of the formulation. I.V. cyclosporine is contraindicated in hypersensitivity to polyoxyethylated castor oil (Cremophor EL).

Rheumatoid arthritis and psoriasis: Abnormal renal function, uncontrolled hypertension, malignancies. Concomitant treatment with PUVA or UVB therapy, methotrexate, other immunosuppressive agents, coal tar, or radiation therapy are also contraindications for use in patients with psoriasis.

Canadian labeling: Additional contraindications (not in U.S. labeling): Primary or secondary immunodeficiency excluding autoimmune disease; uncontrolled infection.

Warnings/Precautions Hazardous agent - use appropriate precautions for handling and disposal (NIOSH, 2012).

[U.S. Boxed Warning]: Increased risk of lymphomas and other malignancies (including fatal outcomes), particularly skin cancers; risk is related to intensity/duration of therapy and the use of more than one immunosuppressive agent; all patients should avoid excessive sun/UV light exposure. [U.S. Boxed Warning]: May cause hypertension; risk is increased with increasing doses/duration. Use caution when changing dosage forms.

[U.S. Boxed Warning]: Renal impairment, including structural kidney damage has occurred (when used at high doses); risk is increased with increasing doses/duration; monitor renal function closely. Elevations in serum creatinine and BUN generally respond to dosage reductions. Use caution with other potentially nephrotoxic drugs (eg, acyclovir, aminoglycoside antibiotics, amphotericin B, ciprofloxacin). Elevations in serum creatinine and BUN associated with nephrotoxicity generally respond to dosage reductions. In renal transplant patients with rapidly rising BUN and creatinine, carefully evaluate to differentiate between cyclosporine-associated nephrotoxicity and renal rejection episodes. In cases of severe rejection that fail to respond to pulse steroids and monoclonal antibodies, switching to an alternative immunosuppressant agent may be preferred to increasing cyclosporine to an excessive dosage.

[U.S. Boxed Warning]: Increased risk of infection with use; serious and fatal infections have been reported. Bacterial, viral, fungal, and protozoal infections (including opportunistic infections) have occurred. Polyoma virus infections, such as the JC virus and BK virus, may result in serious and sometimes fatal outcomes. The JC virus is associated with progressive multifocal leukoencephalopathy (PML), and PML has been reported in patients receiving cyclosporine. PML may be fatal and presents with hemiparesis, apathy, confusion, cognitive deficiencies, and ataxia; consider neurologic consultation as indicated. The BK virus is associated with nephropathy, and polyoma virus-associated nephropathy (PVAN) has been reported in patients receiving cyclosporine. PVAN is associated with serious adverse effects including renal dysfunction and renal graft loss. If PML or PVAN occur in transplant patients, consider reducing immunosuppression therapy as well as the risk that reduced immunosuppression poses to grafts.

Liver injury, including cholestasis, jaundice, hepatitis, and liver failure, has been reported. These events were mainly in patients with confounding factors including infections, coadministration with other potentially hepatotoxic medications, underlying conditions, and significant comorbidities. Fatalities have also been reported rarely, primarily in transplant patients. Increased hepatic enzymes and bilirubin have occurred (when used at high doses); improvement usually seen with dosage reduction.

Should be used initially with corticosteroids in transplant patients. Significant hyperkalemia (with or without hyperchloremic metabolic acidosis) and hyperuricemia have occurred with therapy. Syndromes of microangiopathic hemolytic anemia and thrombocytopenia have occurred and may result in graft failure; it is accompanied by platelet consumption within the graft. Syndrome may occur without graft rejection. Although management of the syndrome is unclear, discontinuation or reduction of cyclosporine, in addition to streptokinase and heparin administration or plasmapheresis, has been associated with syndrome resolution. However, resolution seems to be dependent upon early detection of the syndrome via indium 111 labeled platelet scans.

May cause seizures, particularly if used with high-dose corticosteroids. Encephalopathy (including posterior reversible encephalopathy syndrome [PRES]) has also been reported; predisposing factors include hypertension, hypomagnesemia, hypocholesterolemia, high-dose corticosteroids, high cyclosporine serum concentration, and graft-versus-host disease (GVHD). Encephalopathy may be more common in patients with liver transplant compared to kidney transplant. Other neurotoxic events, such as optic disc edema (including papilloedema and potential visual impairment), have been rarely reported primarily in transplant patients.

[U.S. Boxed Warning]: The modified/non-modified formulations are not bioequivalent; cyclosporine (modified) has increased bioavailability as compared to cyclosporine (non-modified) and the products cannot be used interchangeably without close monitoring. Cyclosporine (modified) refers to the oral solution and capsule dosage formulations of cyclosporine in an aqueous dispersion (previously referred to as "microemulsion"). Potentially significant drug-drug/drug-food interactions may exist, requiring dose or frequency adjustment, additional monitoring, and/or selection of alternative therapy. Gingival hyperplasia may occur; avoid concomitant nifedipine in patients who develop gingival hyperplasia (may increase frequency of hyperplasia). Monitor cyclosporine concentrations closely following the addition, modification, or deletion of other medication. Live, attenuated vaccines may be less effective; vaccination should be avoided. Make dose adjustments based on cyclosporine blood concentrations. [U.S. Boxed Warning]: Cyclosporine non-modified absorption is erratic; monitor blood concentrations closely. [U.S. Boxed Warning]: Prescribing and dosage adjustment should only be under the direct supervision of an experienced physician. Adequate laboratory/medical resources and follow-up are necessary. Anaphylaxis has been reported with I.V. use; reserve for patients who cannot take oral form. **[U.S. Boxed Warning]: Risk of skin cancer may be increased in transplant patients.** Due to the increased risk for nephrotoxicity in renal transplantation, avoid using standard doses of cyclosporine in combination with everolimus; reduced cyclosporine doses are recommended; monitor cyclosporine concentrations closely. Cyclosporine and everolimus combination therapy may increase the risk for proteinuria. Cyclosporine combined with either everolimus or sirolimus may increase the risk for thrombotic microangiopathy/thrombotic thrombocytopenic purpura/hemolytic uremic syndrome (TMA/TTP/HUS). Cyclosporine has extensive hepatic metabolism and exposure is increased in patients with severe hepatic impairment; may require dose reduction.

Patients with psoriasis should avoid excessive sun exposure. **[U.S. Boxed Warning]: Risk of skin cancer may be increased with a history of PUVA and possibly methotrexate or other immunosuppressants, UVB, coal tar, or radiation.**

Rheumatoid arthritis: If receiving other immunosuppressive agents, radiation or UV therapy, concurrent use of cyclosporine is not recommended.

Products may contain corn oil, ethanol (consider alcohol content in certain patient populations, including pregnant or breast feeding women, patients with liver disease, seizure disorders, alcohol dependency, or pediatrics), or propylene glycol; injection also contains the vehicle Cremophor EL (polyoxyethylated castor oil), which has been associated with hypersensitivity (anaphylactic) reactions.

Drug Interactions
Avoid Concomitant Use
Avoid concomitant use of CycloSPORINE (Systemic) with any of the following: Aliskiren; AtorvaSTATin; BCG; Bosentan; Bosutinib; Conivaptan; Crizotinib; Dronedarone; Enzalutamide; Eplerenone; Fusidic Acid (Systemic); Ibrutinib; Ivabradine; Lomitapide; Lovastatin; Mifepristone; Natalizumab; PAZOPanib; Pimecrolimus; Pimozide; Pitavastatin; Pomalidomide; Potassium-Sparing Diuretics; Rivaroxaban; Silodosin; Simvastatin; Sitaxentan; Tacrolimus (Systemic); Tacrolimus (Topical); Tofacitinib; Tolvaptan; Topotecan; Ulipristal; Vaccines (Live); VinCRIStine (Liposomal)

Decreased Effect
CycloSPORINE (Systemic) may decrease the levels/effects of: BCG; Coccidioidin Skin Test; GlyBURIDE; Ifosfamide; Mycophenolate; Sipuleucel-T; Vaccines (Inactivated); Vaccines (Live)

The levels/effects of CycloSPORINE (Systemic) may be decreased by: Adalimumab; Armodafinil; Ascorbic Acid; Barbiturates; Bosentan; CarBAMazepine; Colesevelam; CYP3A4 Inducers (Strong); Dabrafenib; Deferasirox; Dexamethasone (Systemic); Echinacea; Efavirenz; Enzalutamide; Fibric Acid Derivatives; Fosphenytoin; Griseofulvin; Imipenem; MethylPREDNISolone; Metreleptin; Mitotane; Modafinil; Multivitamins/Fluoride (with ADE); Multivitamins/Minerals (with ADEK, Folate, Iron); Multivitamins/Minerals (with AE, No Iron); Nafcillin; Orlistat; P-glycoprotein/ABCB1 Inducers; Phenytoin; PredniSOLONE (Systemic); PredniSONE; Rifamycin Derivatives; Somatostatin Analogs; St Johns Wort; Sulfinpyrazone [Off Market]; Sulfonamide Derivatives; Tocilizumab; Vitamin E

Increased Effect/Toxicity
CycloSPORINE (Systemic) may increase the levels/effects of: Afatinib; Aliskiren; Ambrisentan; ARIPiprazole; AtorvaSTATin; Avanafil; Boceprevir; Bosentan; Bosutinib; Budesonide (Systemic, Oral Inhalation); Calcium Channel Blockers (Dihydropyridine); Calcium Channel Blockers (Nondihydropyridine); Cardiac Glycosides; Caspofungin; Colchicine; CYP3A4 Substrates; Dabigatran Etexilate; Dexamethasone (Systemic); Dofetilide; DOXOrubicin (Conventional); Dronedarone; Etoposide; Etoposide Phosphate; Everolimus; Ezetimibe; FentaNYL; Fibric Acid Derivatives; Fluvastatin; Halofantrine; Ibrutinib; Imipenem; Ivabradine; Ivacaftor; Leflunomide; Lomitapide; Loop Diuretics; Lovastatin; Lurasidone; Methotrexate; MethylPREDNISolone; Minoxidil (Systemic); Minoxidil (Topical); MitoXANtrone; Natalizumab; Neuromuscular-Blocking Agents; Nonsteroidal Anti-Inflammatory Agents; OxyCODONE; PAZOPanib; P-glycoprotein/ABCB1 Substrates; Pimozide; Pitavastatin; Pomalidomide; Pravastatin; PrednisoLONE (Systemic); PredniSONE; Propafenone; Protease Inhibitors; Prucalopride; Ranolazine; Repaglinide; Rivaroxaban; Rosuvastatin; Salmeterol; Saxagliptin; Silodosin; Simvastatin; Sirolimus; Sitaxentan; Tacrolimus (Systemic); Tacrolimus (Topical); Ticagrelor; Tofacitinib; Tolvaptan; Topotecan; Ulipristal; Vaccines (Live); Vilazodone; VinCRIStine (Liposomal); Zuclopenthixol

The levels/effects of CycloSPORINE (Systemic) may be increased by: ACE Inhibitors; AcetaZOLAMIDE; Aminoglycosides; Amiodarone; Amphotericin B; Androgens; Angiotensin II Receptor Blockers; Antifungal Agents (Azole Derivatives, Systemic); Boceprevir; Bromocriptine; Calcium Channel Blockers (Nondihydropyridine); Carvedilol; Chloramphenicol; Conivaptan; Crizotinib; CYP3A4 Inhibitors (Moderate); CYP3A4 Inhibitors (Strong); Dasatinib; Denosumab; Dexamethasone (Systemic); Eplerenone; Ezetimibe; Fluconazole; Fusidic Acid (Systemic); GlyBURIDE; Grapefruit Juice; Imatinib; Imipenem; Ivacaftor; Luliconazole; Macrolide Antibiotics; Melphalan; Methotrexate; MethylPREDNISolone; Metoclopramide; Metreleptin; MetroNIDAZOLE ▶

(Systemic); Mifepristone; Nonsteroidal Anti-Inflammatory Agents; Norfloxacin; Omeprazole; P-glycoprotein/ABCB1 Inhibitors; Pimecrolimus; Potassium-Sparing Diuretics; Pravastatin; PrednisoLONE (Systemic); PredniSONE; Protease Inhibitors; Pyrazinamide; Quinupristin; Roflumilast; Sirolimus; Stiripentol; Sulfonamide Derivatives; Tacrolimus (Systemic); Tacrolimus (Topical); Telaprevir; Temsirolimus; Ticagrelor; Trastuzumab

Nutritional/Ethanol Interactions

Food: Grapefruit juice increases cyclosporine serum concentrations. Management: Avoid grapefruit juice.

Herb/Nutraceutical: St John's wort may increase the metabolism of and decrease plasma levels of cyclosporine; organ rejection and graft loss have been reported. Cat's claw and echinacea have immunostimulant properties. Management: Avoid St John's wort, cat's claw, and echinacea.

Adverse Reactions Adverse reactions reported with systemic use, including rheumatoid arthritis, psoriasis, and transplantation (kidney, liver, and heart). Percentages noted include the highest frequency regardless of indication/dosage. Frequencies may vary for specific conditions or formulation.

>10%:

Cardiovascular: Hypertension (8% to 53%), edema (5% to 14%)

Central nervous system: Headache (2% to 25%), paresthesia (1% to 11%)

Dermatologic: Hypertrichosis (5% to 19%)

Endocrine & metabolic: Hirsutism (21% to 45%), increased serum triglycerides (15%), female genital tract disease (9% to 11%)

Gastrointestinal: Nausea (2% to 23%), diarrhea (3% to 13%), gingival hyperplasia (2% to 16%), abdominal distress (<1% to 15%), dyspepsia (2% to 12%)

Genitourinary: Urinary tract infection (kidney transplant: 21%)

Infection: Increased susceptibility to infection (3% to 25%), viral infection (kidney transplant: 16%)

Neuromuscular & skeletal: Tremor (7% to 55%), leg cramps (2% to 12%)

Renal: Increased serum creatinine (16% to ≥50%), renal insufficiency (10% to 38%)

Respiratory: Upper respiratory tract infection (1% to 14%)

Kidney, liver, and heart transplant only (≤2% unless otherwise noted):

Cardiovascular: Chest pain (≤4%), flushing (<1% to 4%), glomerular capillary thrombosis, myocardial infarction

Central nervous system: Convulsions (1% to 5%), anxiety, confusion, lethargy, tingling sensation

Dermatologic: Skin infection (7%), acne vulgaris (1% to 6%), nail disease (brittle fingernails), hair breakage, night sweats, pruritus

Endocrine & metabolic: Gynecomastia (<1% to 4%), hyperglycemia, hypomagnesemia, weight loss

Gastrointestinal: Vomiting (2% to 10%), anorexia, aphthous stomatitis, constipation, dysphagia, gastritis, hiccups, pancreatitis

Genitourinary: Hematuria

Hematologic & oncologic: Leukopenia (<1% to 6%), lymphoma (<1% to 6%), anemia, thrombocytopenia, upper gastrointestinal hemorrhage

Hepatic: Hepatotoxicity (<1% to 7%)

Infection: Localized fungal infection (8%), cytomegalovirus disease (5%), septicemia (5%), abscess (4%), fungal infection (systemic: 2%)

Neuromuscular & skeletal: Arthralgia, myalgia, weakness

Ophthalmic: Conjunctivitis, visual disturbance

Otic: Hearing loss, tinnitus

Respiratory: Sinusitis (<1% to 7%), pneumonia (6%)

Miscellaneous: Fever

Rheumatoid arthritis only (1% to <3% unless otherwise noted):

Cardiovascular: Chest pain (4%), cardiac arrhythmia (2%), abnormal heart sounds, cardiac failure, myocardial infarction, peripheral ischemia

Central nervous system: Dizziness (8%), pain (6%), insomnia (4%), depression (3%), migraine (2% to 3%), anxiety, drowsiness, emotional lability, hypoesthesia, lack of concentration, malaise, neuropathy, nervousness, paranoia, vertigo

Dermatologic: Cellulitis, dermatological reaction, dermatitis, diaphoresis, dyschromia, eczema, enanthema, folliculitis, nail disease, pruritus, urticaria, xeroderma

Endocrine & metabolic: Menstrual disease (3%), decreased libido, diabetes mellitus, goiter, hot flash, hyperkalemia, hyperuricemia, hypoglycemia, increased libido, weight gain, weight loss

Gastrointestinal: Vomiting (9%), flatulence (5%), gingivitis (4%), constipation, dysgeusia, dysphagia, enlargement of salivary glands, eructation, esophagitis, gastric ulcer, gastritis, gastroenteritis, gingival hemorrhage, glossitis, peptic ulcer, tongue disease, xerostomia

Genitourinary: Leukorrhea (1%), breast fibroadenosis, hematuria, mastalgia, nocturia, urine abnormality, urinary incontinence, urinary urgency, uterine hemorrhage

Hematologic & oncologic: Purpura (3% to 4%), anemia, carcinoma, leukopenia, lymphadenopathy

Hepatic: Hyperbilirubinemia

Infection: Abscess (including renal), bacterial infection, candidiasis, fungal infection, herpes simplex infection, herpes zoster, viral infection

Neuromuscular & skeletal: Arthralgia, bone fracture, dislocation, myalgia, stiffness, synovial cyst, tendon disease, weakness

Ophthalmic: Cataract, conjunctivitis, eye pain, visual disturbance

Otic: Tinnitus, deafness, vestibular disturbance

Renal: Abscess (renal), increased blood urea nitrogen, polyuria, pyelonephritis

Respiratory: Cough (5%), dyspnea (5%), sinusitis (4%), abnormal breath sounds, bronchospasm, epistaxis, tonsillitis

Psoriasis only (1% to <3% unless otherwise noted):

Cardiovascular: Chest pain, flushing

Central nervous system: Psychiatric disturbance (4% to 5%), pain (3% to 4%), dizziness, insomnia, nervousness, vertigo

Dermatologic: Acne vulgaris, folliculitis, hyperkeratosis, pruritus, skin rash, xeroderma

Endocrine & metabolic: Hot flash

Gastrointestinal: Abdominal distention, constipation, gingival hemorrhage, increased appetite

Genitourinary: Urinary frequency

Hematologic & oncologic: Abnormal erythrocytes, altered platelet function, blood coagulation disorder, carcinoma, hemorrhagic diathesis

Hepatic: Hyperbilirubinemia

Neuromuscular & skeletal: Arthralgia (1% to 6%)

Ophthalmic: Visual disturbance

Respiratory: Flu-like symptoms (8% to 10%), bronchospasm (5%), cough (5%), dyspnea (5%), rhinitis (5%), respiratory tract infection

Miscellaneous: Fever

Dosage Forms Considerations

Cyclosporine (modified): Gengraf and Neoral

Cyclosporine (non-modified): SandIMMUNE

Available Dosage Forms

Capsule, Oral:

Gengraf: 25 mg, 100 mg

Neoral: 25 mg, 100 mg

SandIMMUNE: 25 mg, 100 mg

Generic: 25 mg, 50 mg, 100 mg

Solution, Intravenous:

SandIMMUNE: 50 mg/mL (5 mL)

Generic: 50 mg/mL (5 mL)

Solution, Oral:

Gengraf: 100 mg/mL (50 mL)

Neoral: 100 mg/mL (50 mL)

SandIMMUNE: 100 mg/mL (50 mL)

Generic: 100 mg/mL (50 mL)

General Dosage Range Dosage adjustment recommended in patients with renal impairment

I.V. (non-modified): *Children and Adults:* Initial dose: 5-6 mg/kg daily or one-third of the oral dose as a single dose; Maintenance: 3-7.5 mg/kg daily in 2-3 divided doses or give as continuous infusion over 24 hours

Oral:

Modified:

Children and Adults: Transplant: Heart: 7 ± 3 mg/kg daily in 2 divided doses; Liver: 8 ± 4 mg/kg daily in 2 divided doses; Renal: 9 ± 3 mg/kg daily in 2 divided doses

Adults: Initial: 2.5 mg/kg daily in 2 divided doses; Maintenance: Up to 4 mg/kg daily

Non-modified: *Children and Adults:* Initial: 10-14 mg/kg daily for 1-2 weeks; Maintenance: Taper by 5% per week to 3-10 mg/kg daily

Administration

I.V. The manufacturer recommends that following dilution, intravenous admixture be administered over 2-6 hours. However, many transplant centers administer as divided doses (2-3 doses/day) or as a 24-hour continuous infusion. Patients should be under continuous observation for at least the first 30 minutes of the infusion, and should be monitored frequently thereafter. To minimize leaching of DEHP, non-PVC sets should be used for administration.

Anaphylaxis has been reported with I.V. use; reserve for patients who cannot take oral form. Patients should be under continuous observation for at least the first 30 minutes of the infusion, and should be monitored frequently thereafter. Maintain patent airway; other supportive measures and agents for treating anaphylaxis should be present when I.V. drug is given. Discard solution after 24 hours.

Hazardous agent - use appropriate precautions for handling and disposal (NIOSH, 2012).

Oral Oral solution: Do not administer liquid from plastic or styrofoam cup. May dilute Neoral oral solution with orange juice or apple juice. May dilute Sandimmune oral solution with milk, chocolate milk, or orange juice. Avoid changing diluents frequently. Mix thoroughly and drink at once. Use syringe provided to measure dose. Mix in a glass container and rinse container with more diluent to ensure total dose is taken. Do not rinse syringe before or after use (may cause dose variation).

Combination therapy with renal transplantation:

Everolimus: Administer cyclosporine at the same time as everolimus

Sirolimus: Administer cyclosporine 4 hours prior to sirolimus

Hazardous agent - use appropriate precautions for handling and disposal (NIOSH, 2012).

Preparation for Administration Hazardous agent - use appropriate precautions for handling and disposal (NIOSH, 2012).

Injection: To minimize leaching of DEHP, non-PVC containers and sets should be used for preparation and administration.

Sandimmune injection: Injection should be further diluted (1 mL [50 mg] of concentrate in 20-100 mL of D_5W or NS) for administration by intravenous infusion.

Storage/Stability

Capsule: Store at controlled room temperature.

Injection: Store at controlled room temperature; do not refrigerate. Ampuls and vials should be protected from light. Stability of injection of parenteral admixture at room temperature (25°C) is 6 hours ▶

in PVC; 12-24 hours in Excel, PAB containers, or glass.

Oral solution: Store at controlled room temperature; do not refrigerate. Use within 2 months after opening; should be mixed in glass containers.

Nursing Actions

Physical Assessment Monitor kidney and hepatic function closely. Monitor blood pressure and assess for signs of fluid retention periodically. Monitor for infection (eg, fever, mouth, and vaginal sores or plaques, unhealed wounds). I.V: Monitor closely for first 30 minutes of infusion and frequently thereafter to assess for CNS changes or hypertension.

Patient Education

• Discuss specific use of drug and side effects with patient as it relates to treatment. (HCAHPS: During this hospital stay, were you given any medicine that you had not taken before? Before giving you any new medicine, how often did hospital staff tell you what the medicine was for? How often did hospital staff describe possible side effects in a way you could understand?)

• Patient may experience hair growth, acne vulgaris, or nausea. Have patient report immediately to prescriber signs of infection, signs of hepatic impairment, severe headache, significant diarrhea, melena, hematemesis, stomatitis, paresthesia, mole changes, skin growths, swollen lymph nodes, angina, tachycardia, arrhythmia, periodontal changes, behavioral changes, mood changes, myalgia, hearing impairment, considerable dizziness, dyspnea, dyspepsia, tremors, intolerable asthenia, ecchymosis; hemorrhaging; edema; vision changes; blindness; signs of progressive multifocal leukoencephalopathy (PML); or signs of renal impairment (HCAHPS).

• Educate patient about signs of a significant reaction (eg, wheezing; chest tightness; fever; itching; bad cough; blue skin color; seizures; or swelling of face, lips, tongue, or throat). **Note**: This is not a comprehensive list of all side effects. Patient should consult prescriber for additional questions.

Intended Use and Disclaimer: Should not be printed and given to patients. This information is intended to serve as a concise initial reference for healthcare professionals to use when discussing medications with a patient. You must ultimately rely on your own discretion, experience and judgment in diagnosing, treating and advising patients.

Dietary Considerations Administer this medication consistently with relation to time of day and meals. Avoid grapefruit juice with oral cyclosporine use.

Related Information

Oral Medications That Should Not Be Crushed or Altered *on page 1712*

Peak and Trough Guidelines *on page 1710*

CycloSPORINE (Ophthalmic)
(SYE kloe spor een)

Brand Names: U.S. Restasis

Index Terms Ciclosporin; CsA; CyA; Cyclosporin A

Pharmacologic Category Calcineurin Inhibitor Immunosuppressant Agent

Medication Safety Issues

Sound-alike/look-alike issues:

CycloSPORINE may be confused with cyclophosphamide, Cyklokapron®, cycloSERINE

Pregnancy Risk Factor C

Lactation Excretion unknown/use caution

Use Increase tear production when suppressed tear production is presumed to be due to keratoconjunctivitis sicca-associated ocular inflammation (in patients not already using topical anti-inflammatory drugs or punctal plugs)

Available Dosage Forms

Emulsion, Ophthalmic [preservative free]:

Restasis: 0.05% (1 ea)

General Dosage Range Ophthalmic: *Adolescents ≥16 years and Adults:* Instill 1 drop in each eye every 12 hours

Administration

Ophthalmic Prior to use, invert vial several times to obtain a uniform emulsion. Remove contact lenses prior to instillation of drops; may be reinserted 15 minutes after administration. May be used with artificial tears; allow 15 minute interval between products. To avoid contamination, do not touch vial tip to eyelids or other surfaces.

Hazardous agent; use appropriate precautions for handling and disposal (NIOSH, 2012).

Nursing Actions

Patient Education

• Discuss specific use of drug and side effects with patient as it relates to treatment. (HCAHPS: During this hospital stay, were you given any medicine that you had not taken before? Before giving you any new medicine, how often did hospital staff tell you what the medicine was for? How often did hospital staff describe possible side effects in a way you could understand?)

• Patient may experience blurred vision. Have patient report immediately to prescriber severe eye irritation, vision changes, ophthalmalgia, or eye discharge (HCAHPS).

• Educate patient about signs of a significant reaction (eg, wheezing; chest tightness; fever; itching; bad cough; blue skin color; seizures; or swelling of face, lips, tongue, or throat). **Note**: This is not a comprehensive list of all side effects. Patient should consult prescriber for additional questions.

Intended Use and Disclaimer: Should not be printed and given to patients. This information is intended to serve as a concise initial reference for healthcare professionals to use when discussing medications with a patient. You must ultimately rely on your own discretion, experience and judgment in diagnosing, treating and advising patients.

Cyproheptadine (si proe HEP ta deen)

Index Terms Cyproheptadine Hydrochloride; Periactin

Pharmacologic Category Histamine H_1 Antagonist; Histamine H_1 Antagonist, First Generation; Piperidine Derivative

Medication Safety Issues

Sound-alike/look-alike issues:
Cyproheptadine may be confused with cyclobenzaprine
Periactin may be confused with Percodan®, Persantine®

BEERS Criteria medication:
This drug may be potentially inappropriate for use in geriatric patients (Quality of evidence - moderate; Strength of recommendation - strong).

International issues:
Periactin brand name for cyproheptadine [U.S., multiple international markets] may be confused with Perative brand name for an enteral nutrition preparation [multiple international markets] and brand name for ketoconazole [Argentina]

Pregnancy Risk Factor B

Lactation Excretion in breast milk unknown/contraindicated

Use Perennial and seasonal allergic rhinitis and other allergic symptoms including urticaria

Unlabeled Use Migraine headache prophylaxis, pruritus, serotonin syndrome, spasticity associated with spinal cord damage

Available Dosage Forms

Syrup, Oral:
Generic: 2 mg/5 mL (10 mL, 473 mL)

Tablet, Oral:
Generic: 4 mg

General Dosage Range

Oral:
Children 2-6 years: 2 mg every 8-12 hours (not to exceed 12 mg daily)
Children 7-14 years: 4 mg every 8-12 hours (not to exceed 16 mg daily)
Adults: 4-20 mg daily divided every 8 hours (not to exceed 0.5 mg/kg/day)

Nursing Actions

Physical Assessment Monitor weight periodically. Monitor for excess anticholinergic effects at beginning of therapy and periodically throughout. Monitor for drowsiness, fatigue, dry mouth, nausea, and GI upset. Advise patient to use with caution while operating machinery or driving.

Patient Education
• Discuss specific use of drug and side effects with patient as it relates to treatment. (HCAHPS: During this hospital stay, were you given any medicine that you had not taken before? Before giving you any new medicine, how often did hospital staff tell you what the medicine was for? How often did hospital staff describe possible side effects in a way you could understand?)
• Patient may experience fatigue, headache, blurred vision, constipation, xerostomia, anxiety, dyspepsia, or akathisia. Have patient report immediately to prescriber signs of hepatic impairment, severe dizziness, syncope, tachycardia, arrhythmia, urinary retention, considerable asthenia, illogical thinking, hallucinations, mood changes, chills, pharyngitis, insomnia, ecchymosis, or hemorrhaging (HCAHPS).
• Educate patient about signs of a significant reaction (eg, wheezing; chest tightness; fever; itching; bad cough; blue skin color; seizures; or swelling of face, lips, tongue, or throat). **Note:** This is not a comprehensive list of all side effects. Patient should consult prescriber for additional questions.

Intended Use and Disclaimer: Should not be printed and given to patients. This information is intended to serve as a concise initial reference for healthcare professionals to use when discussing medications with a patient. You must ultimately rely on your own discretion, experience and judgment in diagnosing, treating and advising patients.

Cyproterone (sye PROE ter one)

Index Terms Cyproterone Acetate; SH 714

Pharmacologic Category Antiandrogen; Antineoplastic Agent, Antiandrogen

Use Palliative treatment of advanced prostate cancer

Unlabeled Use Treatment of paraphilia/hypersexuality

Product Availability Not available in U.S.

General Dosage Range

I.M.: *Adults (males):* 300 mg (3 mL) once weekly or every 2 weeks

Oral: *Adults (males):* 100-300 mg daily in 2-3 divided doses

Administration

I.M. Administer tablets at the same time each day, after meals and with liquids. Tablets may be divided into equal halves. Hazardous agent; use appropriate precautions for handling and disposal (meets NIOSH, 2012 criteria).

Oral Administer tablets at the same time each day, after meals and with liquids. Tablets may be divided into equal halves. Hazardous agent; use appropriate precautions for handling and disposal (meets NIOSH, 2012 criteria).

◄ **Nursing Actions**

Patient Education

- Discuss specific use of drug and side effects with patient as it relates to treatment. (HCAHPS: During this hospital stay, were you given any medicine that you had not taken before? Before giving you any new medicine, how often did hospital staff tell you what the medicine was for? How often did hospital staff describe possible side effects in a way you could understand?)
- Patient may experience flushing, decreased night vision, macromastia, mastalgia, alopecia, sexual dysfunction, or liver injury (rare). Have patient report immediately to prescriber signs of infection, severe nausea, considerable edema of hands or feet, significant dyspepsia, suicidal ideation, inability to eat, intolerable asthenia, urine discoloration, jaundice, or severe skin irritation (HCAHPS).
- Educate patient about signs of a significant reaction (eg, wheezing; chest tightness; fever; itching; bad cough; blue skin color; seizures; or swelling of face, lips, tongue, or throat). **Note:** This is not a comprehensive list of all side effects. Patient should consult prescriber for additional questions.

Intended Use and Disclaimer: Should not be printed and given to patients. This information is intended to serve as a concise initial reference for healthcare professionals to use when discussing medications with a patient. You must ultimately rely on your own discretion, experience and judgment in diagnosing, treating and advising patients.

Cytarabine (Conventional)
(sye TARE a been con VEN sha nal)

Index Terms Ara-C; Arabinosylcytosine; Conventional Cytarabine; Cytarabine; Cytarabine Hydrochloride; Cytosar-U; Cytosine Arabinosine Hydrochloride

Pharmacologic Category Antineoplastic Agent, Antimetabolite; Antineoplastic Agent, Antimetabolite (Pyrimidine Analog)

Medication Safety Issues

Sound-alike/look-alike issues:

Cytarabine may be confused with clofarabine, Cytosar®, Cytoxan, vidarabine

Cytarabine (conventional) may be confused with cytarabine liposomal

Cytosar-U may be confused with cytarabine, Cytovene®, Cytoxan, Neosar

High alert medication:

This medication is in a class the Institute for Safe Medication Practices (ISMP) includes among its list of drugs classes which have a heightened

risk of causing significant patient harm when used in error.

Administration issues:

Intrathecal medication safety: The American Society of Clinical Oncology (ASCO)/Oncology Nursing Society (ONS) chemotherapy administration safety standards (Jacobson, 2009) encourage the following safety measures for intrathecal chemotherapy:

- Intrathecal medication should not be prepared during the preparation of any other agents
- After preparation, store in an isolated location or container clearly marked with a label identifying as "intrathecal" use only
- Delivery to the patient should only be with other medications also intended for administration into the central nervous system

Pregnancy Risk Factor D

Lactation Excretion in breast milk unknown/not recommended

Breast-Feeding Considerations Due to the potential for serious adverse reactions in the nursing infant, breast-feeding is not recommended.

Use Remission induction in acute myeloid leukemia (AML), treatment of acute lymphocytic leukemia (ALL) and chronic myelocytic leukemia (CML; blast phase); prophylaxis and treatment of meningeal leukemia

Unlabeled Use AML consolidation treatment, AML salvage treatment; acute promyelocytic leukemia (APL) consolidation treatment; treatment of primary central nervous system (CNS) lymphoma; treatment of chronic lymphocytic leukemia (CLL); treatment of relapsed or refractory Hodgkin lymphoma; treatment of non-Hodgkin's lymphomas (NHL)

Mechanism of Action/Effect Inhibition of DNA synthesis in S Phase of cell division; degree of its cytotoxicity correlates linearly with its incorporation into DNA, therefore, incorporation into the DNA is responsible for drug activity and toxicity

Contraindications Hypersensitivity to cytarabine or any component of the formulation

Warnings/Precautions Hazardous agent - use appropriate precautions for handling and disposal (NIOSH, 2012). **[U.S. Boxed Warning]: Myelosuppression (leukopenia, thrombocytopenia and anemia) is the major toxicity of cytarabine.** Use with caution in patients with prior drug-induced bone marrow suppression. Monitor blood counts frequently; once blasts are no longer apparent in the peripheral blood, bone marrow should be monitored frequently. Monitor for signs of infection or neutropenic fever due to neutropenia or bleeding due to thrombocytopenia.

High-dose regimens are associated with CNS, gastrointestinal, ocular (reversible corneal toxicity and hemorrhagic conjunctivitis; prophylaxis with ophthalmic corticosteroid drops is recommended), pulmonary toxicities and cardiomyopathy. Neurotoxicity associated with high-dose treatment may present as acute cerebellar toxicity (with or without cerebral impairment), personality changes, or may be severe with seizure and/or coma; may be delayed, occurring up to 3-8 days after treatment has begun. Risk factors for neurotoxicity include cumulative cytarabine dose, prior CNS disease and renal impairment; high-dose therapy (>18 g/m^2 per cycle) and age >50 years also increase the risk for cerebellar toxicity (Herzig, 1987). Tumor lysis syndrome and subsequent hyperuricemia may occur with high dose cytarabine; monitor, consider allopurinol and hydrate accordingly. There have been case reports of fatal cardiomyopathy when high dose cytarabine was used in combination with cyclophosphamide as a preparation regimen for transplantation.

Use with caution in patients with impaired renal and hepatic function; may be at higher risk for CNS toxicities; dosage adjustments may be necessary. A sudden respiratory arrest syndrome is characterized by fever, myalgia, bone pain, chest pain, maculopapular rash, conjunctivitis, and malaise, and may occur 6-12 hours following administration; may be managed with corticosteroids. Anaphylaxis resulting in acute cardiopulmonary arrest has been reported (rare). There have been reports of acute pancreatitis in patients receiving continuous infusion and in patients previously treated with L-asparaginase. **[U.S. Boxed Warning]: Should be administered under the supervision of an experienced cancer chemotherapy physician. Due to the potential toxicities, induction treatment with cytarabine should be in a facility with sufficient laboratory and supportive resources.** Some products may contain benzyl alcohol; do not use products containing benzyl alcohol or products reconstituted with bacteriostatic diluent intrathecally or for high-dose cytarabine regimens. When used for intrathecal administration, should not be prepared during the preparation of any other agents; after preparation, store intrathecal medications in an isolated location or container clearly marked with a label identifying as "intrathecal" use only; delivery of intrathecal medications to the patient should only be with other medications also intended for administration into the central nervous system (Jacobson, 2009).

Drug Interactions
Avoid Concomitant Use
Avoid concomitant use of Cytarabine (Conventional) with any of the following: BCG; CloZAPine; Natalizumab; Pimecrolimus; Tacrolimus (Topical); Tofacitinib; Vaccines (Live)

Decreased Effect
Cytarabine (Conventional) may decrease the levels/effects of: BCG; Cardiac Glycosides; Coccidioidin Skin Test; Flucytosine; Sipuleucel-T; Vaccines (Inactivated); Vaccines (Live)

The levels/effects of Cytarabine (Conventional) may be decreased by: Echinacea

Increased Effect/Toxicity
Cytarabine (Conventional) may increase the levels/effects of: CloZAPine; Leflunomide; Natalizumab; Tofacitinib; Vaccines (Live)

The levels/effects of Cytarabine (Conventional) may be increased by: Denosumab; Pimecrolimus; Roflumilast; Tacrolimus (Topical); Trastuzumab

Adverse Reactions
Frequent:
Central nervous system: Fever

Dermatologic: Rash

Gastrointestinal: Anal inflammation, anal ulceration, anorexia, diarrhea, mucositis, nausea, vomiting

Hematologic: Myelosuppression, neutropenia (onset: 1-7 days; nadir [biphasic]: 7-9 days and at 15-24 days; recovery [biphasic]: 9-12 days and at 24-34 days), thrombocytopenia (onset: 5 days; nadir: 12-15 days; recovery 15-25 days), anemia, bleeding, leukopenia, megaloblastosis, reticulocytes decreased

Hepatic: Hepatic dysfunction, transaminases increased (acute)

Local: Thrombophlebitis

Less frequent:
Cardiovascular: Chest pain, pericarditis

Central nervous system: Dizziness, headache, neural toxicity, neuritis

Dermatologic: Alopecia, pruritus, skin freckling, skin ulceration, urticaria

Gastrointestinal: Abdominal pain, bowel necrosis, esophageal ulceration, esophagitis, pancreatitis, sore throat

Genitourinary: Urinary retention

Hepatic: Jaundice

Local: Injection site cellulitis

Ocular: Conjunctivitis

Renal: Renal dysfunction

Respiratory: Dyspnea

Miscellaneous: Allergic edema, anaphylaxis, sepsis

Infrequent and/or case reports: Acute respiratory distress syndrome, amylase increased, angina, aseptic meningitis, cardiopulmonary arrest (acute), cerebral dysfunction, cytarabine syndrome (bone pain, chest pain, conjunctivitis, fever, maculopapular rash, malaise, myalgia); exanthematous pustulosis, hepatic sinusoidal obstruction syndrome (SOS; veno-occlusive disease), hyperuricemia, injection site inflammation (SubQ injection), injection site pain (SubQ injection), interstitial pneumonitis, lipase increased, paralysis (intrathecal and I.V. combination therapy), reversible posterior leukoencephalopathy syndrome (RPLS), rhabdomyolysis, toxic megacolon

◀ **Adverse events associated with high-dose cytarabine** (CNS, gastrointestinal, ocular, and pulmonary toxicities are more common with high-dose regimens):

Cardiovascular: Cardiomegaly, cardiomyopathy (in combination with cyclophosphamide)

Central nervous system: Cerebellar toxicity, coma, neurotoxicity (up to 55% in patients with renal impairment), personality change, somnolence

Dermatologic: Alopecia (complete), desquamation, rash (severe)

Gastrointestinal: Gastrointestinal ulcer, pancreatitis, peritonitis, pneumatosis cystoides intestinalis

Hepatic: Hyperbilirubinemia, liver abscess, liver damage, necrotizing colitis

Neuromuscular & skeletal: Peripheral neuropathy (motor and sensory)

Ocular: Corneal toxicity, hemorrhagic conjunctivitis

Respiratory: Pulmonary edema, syndrome of sudden respiratory distress

Miscellaneous: Sepsis

Adverse events associated with intrathecal cytarabine administration:

Central nervous system: Accessory nerve paralysis, fever, necrotizing leukoencephalopathy (with concurrent cranial irradiation, I.T. methotrexate, and I.T. hydrocortisone), neurotoxicity, paraplegia

Gastrointestinal: Dysphagia, nausea, vomiting

Ocular: Blindness (with concurrent systemic chemotherapy and cranial irradiation), diplopia

Respiratory: Cough, hoarseness

Miscellaneous: Aphonia

Available Dosage Forms

Solution, Injection:

Generic: 20 mg/mL (25 mL); 100 mg/mL (20 mL)

Solution, Injection [preservative free]:

Generic: 20 mg/mL (5 mL, 50 mL); 100 mg/mL (20 mL)

Solution Reconstituted, Injection:

Generic: 100 mg (1 ea); 500 mg (1 ea); 1 g (1 ea)

General Dosage Range Dosage adjustment recommended in patients with hepatic or renal impairment

I.V.: *Children and Adults:* AML Induction: 100-200 mg/m^2/day for 7 days

Administration

I.V. Infuse standard dose therapy for AML (100-200 mg/m^2/day) as a continuous infusion. Infuse high-dose therapy (unlabeled) over 1-3 hours (usually). Other rates have been used, refer to specific reference.

Hazardous agent; use appropriate precautions for handling and disposal (NIOSH, 2012).

Subcutaneous May also be administered SubQ.

Hazardous agent; use appropriate precautions for handling and disposal (NIOSH, 2012).

Intrathecal Intrathecal doses should be administered as soon as possible after preparation.

Hazardous agent; use appropriate precautions for handling and disposal (NIOSH, 2012).

Preparation for Administration Hazardous agent; use appropriate precautions for handling and disposal (NIOSH, 2012). **Note:** Solutions containing bacteriostatic agents may be used for SubQ and standard-dose (100-200 mg/m^2) I.V. cytarabine preparations, but should not be used for the preparation of either intrathecal doses or high-dose I.V. therapies.

I.V.:

Powder for reconstitution: Reconstitute with bacteriostatic water for injection (for standard-dose)

For I.V. infusion: Further dilute in 250-1000 mL 0.9% NaCl or D$_5$W.

Intrathecal: Powder for reconstitution: Reconstitute with preservative free sodium chloride 0.9%; may further dilute to preferred final volume (volume generally based on institution or practitioner preference; may be up to 12 mL) with Elliott's B solution, sodium chloride 0.9% or lactated Ringer's. Intrathecal medications should not be prepared during the preparation of any other agents. Triple intrathecal therapy (TIT): Cytarabine 30-50 mg with hydrocortisone sodium succinate 15-25 mg and methotrexate 12 mg; compatible together for up to 24 hours in a syringe; however, should be administered administer as soon as possible after preparation because intrathecal preparations are preservative free

Storage/Stability Store intact vials of powder for injection at room temperature of 20°C to 25°C (68°F to 77°F); store intact vials of solution at room temperature of 15°C to 30°C (59°F to 86°F).

I.V.:

Powder for reconstitution: Reconstituted solutions should be stored at room temperature and used within 48 hours.

For I.V. infusion: Solutions for I.V. infusion diluted in D$_5$W or NS are stable for 7 days at room temperature, although the manufacturer recommends administration as soon as possible after preparation.

Intrathecal: Administer as soon as possible after preparation. After preparation, store intrathecal medications in an isolated location or container clearly marked with a label identifying as "intrathecal" use only.

Nursing Actions

Physical Assessment To be administered under the supervision of an experienced cancer chemotherapy physician. Ocular pain and conjunctivitis reactions may be reduced with ophthalmic corticosteroid premedication. Monitor patient closely throughout treatment, especially with high-dose regimens, for adverse gastrointestinal and pulmonary response, CNS toxicities, and cardiomyopathy.

Patient Education

- Discuss specific use of drug and side effects with patient as it relates to treatment. (HCAHPS: During this hospital stay, were you given any medicine that you had not taken before? Before giving you any new medicine, how often did hospital staff tell you what the medicine was for? How often did hospital staff describe possible side effects in a way you could understand?)
- Patient may experience lack of appetite, alopecia, or stomatitis. Have patient report immediately to prescriber signs of infection, dyspnea, severe dyspepsia, significant nausea, considerable diarrhea, ecchymosis, hemorrhaging, intolerable asthenia, signs of hepatic impairment, signs of renal impairment, signs of pancreatitis, or signs of tumor lysis syndrome (TLS) (HCAHPS).
- Educate patient about signs of a significant reaction (eg, wheezing; chest tightness; fever; itching; bad cough; blue skin color; seizures; or swelling of face, lips, tongue, or throat). **Note:** This is not a comprehensive list of all side effects. Patient should consult prescriber for additional questions.

Intended Use and Disclaimer: Should not be printed and given to patients. This information is intended to serve as a concise initial reference for healthcare professionals to use when discussing medications with a patient. You must ultimately rely on your own discretion, experience and judgment in diagnosing, treating and advising patients.

Cytomegalovirus Immune Globulin (Intravenous-Human)
(sye toe meg a low VYE rus i MYUN GLOB yoo lin in tra VEE nus HYU man)

Brand Names: U.S. CytoGam®

Index Terms CMV Hyperimmune Globulin; CMV-IGIV

Pharmacologic Category Blood Product Derivative; Immune Globulin

Medication Safety Issues
Sound-alike/look-alike issues:
CytoGam® may be confused with Cytoxan, Gamimune® N

Pregnancy Risk Factor C

Lactation Excretion in breast milk unknown

Use Prophylaxis of cytomegalovirus (CMV) disease associated with kidney, lung, liver, pancreas, and heart transplants; concomitant use with ganciclovir should be considered in organ transplants (other than kidney) from CMV seropositive donors to CMV seronegative recipients

Unlabeled Use Adjunctive therapy in the treatment of CMV pneumonitis in solid organ transplant and in hematopoietic stem cell transplant

Available Dosage Forms
Injection, solution [preservative free]:
CytoGam®: 50 mg (± 10 mg)/mL (50 mL)
General Dosage Range I.V.: *Children, Adolescents, and Adults:* Initial: 150 mg/kg within 72 hours of transplant; 2-, 4-, 6- and 8 weeks after transplant: 100 mg/kg (kidney) **or** 150 mg/kg (liver, lung, pancreas, heart); 12 and 16 weeks after transplant: 50 mg/kg (kidney) **or** 100 mg/kg (liver, lung, pancreas, heart)

Administration
I.V. Administer through an I.V. line containing an in-line 15 micron filter (a 0.2 micron filter is also acceptable) using an infusion pump. Do not mix with other infusions; do not use if turbid. Begin infusion within 6 hours of entering vial, complete infusion within 12 hours of vial entry.

Initial dose: Infuse at 15 mg/kg/hour. If no adverse reactions occur within 30 minutes, may increase rate to 30 mg/kg/hour. If no adverse reactions occur within the second 30 minutes, may increase rate to 60 mg/kg/hour; maximum rate of infusion: 75 mL/hour. Monitor closely after each rate change. If patient develops nausea, back pain, or flushing during infusion, slow the rate or temporarily stop the infusion. Discontinue if blood pressure drops or in case of anaphylactic reaction.

Subsequent doses: Infuse at 15 mg/kg/hour for 15 minutes; if no adverse reactions occur, may increase rate to 30 mg/kg/hour for 15 minutes; if no adverse reactions occur, may increase rate to 60 mg/kg/hour; maximum rate of infusion: 75 mL/hour.

Nursing Actions
Physical Assessment Assess for history of previous allergic reactions. Monitor vital signs during infusion and observe for adverse or allergic reactions.

Patient Education
- Discuss specific use of vaccine and side effects with patient as it relates to treatment. (HCAHPS: During this hospital stay, were you given any medicine that you had not taken before? Before giving you any new medicine, how often did hospital staff tell you what the medicine was for? How often did hospital staff describe possible side effects in a way you could understand?)
- Patient may experience flushing, injection site pain or irritation, arthralgia, back pain, muscle cramps, myalgia, or nausea. Have patient report immediately to prescriber signs of infection, signs of renal impairment, strength differences from one side to another, difficulty speaking or thinking, change in balance, blurred vision, edema of extremities, tachycardia, angina, hemoptysis, dyspnea, or signs of aseptic meningitis (HCAHPS).
- Educate patient about signs of a significant reaction (eg, wheezing; chest tightness; fever; itching; bad cough; blue skin color; seizures; or ▶

swelling of face, lips, tongue, or throat). **Note:** This is not a comprehensive list of all side effects. Patient should consult prescriber for additional questions.

Intended Use and Disclaimer: Should not be printed and given to patients. This information is intended to serve as a concise initial reference for healthcare professionals to use when discussing medications with a patient. You must ultimately rely on your own discretion, experience and judgment in diagnosing, treating and advising patients.

Related Information

Immunization Administration Recommendations *on page 1675*

Immunization Recommendations *on page 1680*

Dacarbazine (da KAR ba zeen)

Index Terms DIC; Dimethyl Triazeno Imidazole Carboxamide; DTIC; DTIC-Dome; Imidazole Carboxamide; Imidazole Carboxamide Dimethyltriazene; WR-139007

Pharmacologic Category Antineoplastic Agent, Alkylating Agent (Triazene)

Medication Safety Issues

Sound-alike/look-alike issues:

Dacarbazine may be confused with procarbazine

High alert medication:

This medication is in a class the Institute for Safe Medication Practices (ISMP) includes among its list of drugs which have a heightened risk of causing significant patient harm when used in error.

Pregnancy Risk Factor C

Lactation Excretion in breast milk unknown/not recommended

Use Treatment of malignant melanoma, Hodgkin's disease

Unlabeled Use Treatment of soft-tissue sarcomas, islet cell tumors, pheochromocytoma, medullary carcinoma of the thyroid

Available Dosage Forms

Solution Reconstituted, Intravenous:

Generic: 100 mg (1 ea); 200 mg (1 ea)

Solution Reconstituted, Intravenous [preservative free]:

Generic: 200 mg (1 ea)

General Dosage Range Dosage adjustment recommended in patients with renal impairment

I.V.:

Children: 375 mg/m^2 on days 1 and 15, repeat every 28 days

Adults: 375 mg/m^2 days 1 and 15 every 4 weeks or 250 mg/m^2 days 1-5 every 3 weeks

Administration

I.V. Irritant. Infuse over 30-60 minutes; may also be administered as a continuous infusion (unlabeled administration rate) depending on the protocol

Hazardous agent; use appropriate precautions for handling and disposal (NIOSH, 2012).

Injectable Detail Rapid infusion may cause severe venous irritation.

Extravasation management: Local pain, burning sensation, and irritation at the injection site may be relieved by local application of hot packs. If extravasation occurs, apply cold packs. Protect exposed tissue from light following extravasation.

pH: 3-4

Nursing Actions

Physical Assessment Antiemetic premedication may be ordered (emetic potential is moderately high). Monitor patient closely for anaphylactic reaction; emergency treatment should be available. Monitor infusion site closely; extravasation can cause severe cellulitis or tissue necrosis.

Patient Education

• Discuss specific use of drug and side effects with patient as it relates to treatment. (HCAHPS: During this hospital stay, were you given any medicine that you had not taken before? Before giving you any new medicine, how often did hospital staff tell you what the medicine was for? How often did hospital staff describe possible side effects in a way you could understand?)

• Patient may experience lack of appetite or alopecia. Have patient report immediately to prescriber signs of infection, severe dizziness, syncope, significant nausea, or injection site irritation (HCAHPS).

• Educate patient about signs of a significant reaction (eg, wheezing; chest tightness; fever; itching; bad cough; blue skin color; seizures; or swelling of face, lips, tongue, or throat). **Note:** This is not a comprehensive list of all side effects. Patient should consult prescriber for additional questions.

Intended Use and Disclaimer: Should not be printed and given to patients. This information is intended to serve as a concise initial reference for healthcare professionals to use when discussing medications with a patient. You must ultimately rely on your own discretion, experience and judgment in diagnosing, treating and advising patients.

DACTINomycin (dak ti noe MYE sin)

Brand Names: U.S. Cosmegen

Index Terms ACT-D; Actinomycin; Actinomycin Cl; Actinomycin D; DACT

Pharmacologic Category Antineoplastic Agent, Antibiotic

Medication Safety Issues
Sound-alike/look-alike issues:
DACTINomycin may be confused with Dacogen®, DAPTOmycin, DAUNOrubicin

Actinomycin may be confused with achromycin

High alert medication:
This medication is in a class the Institute for Safe Medication Practices (ISMP) includes among its list of drug classes which have a heightened risk of causing significant patient harm when used in error.

Pregnancy Risk Factor D

Lactation Excretion in breast milk unknown/not recommended

Use Treatment of Wilms' tumor, childhood rhabdomyosarcoma, Ewing's sarcoma, metastatic testicular tumors (nonseminomatous), gestational trophoblastic neoplasm; regional perfusion (palliative or adjunctive) of locally recurrent or locoregional solid tumors (sarcomas, carcinomas and adenocarcinomas)

Unlabeled Use Treatment of ovarian cancer (germ cell or stromal tumors), osteosarcoma, soft tissue sarcoma (other than rhabdomyosarcoma)

Available Dosage Forms
Solution Reconstituted, Intravenous:
Cosmegen: 0.5 mg (1 ea)

Generic: 0.5 mg (1 ea)

General Dosage Range
I.V.:
Children >6 months: 15 mcg/kg/day **or** 400-600 mcg/m^2/day for 5 days every 3-6 weeks

Adults: 12-15 mcg/kg/day **or** 400-600 mcg/m^2/day for 5 days every 3-6 weeks **or** 1000 mcg/m^2 on day 1 **or** 500 mcg/dose days 1 and 2

Regional perfusion: *Adults:* Lower extremity or pelvis: 50 mcg/kg; Upper extremity: 35 mcg/kg

Administration
I.V. Slow I.V. push or infuse over 10-15 minutes. Do not filter with cellulose ester membrane filters. Do not administer I.M. or SubQ.

Vesicant; ensure proper needle or catheter placement prior to and during infusion; avoid extravasation.

Extravasation management: If extravasation occurs, stop infusion immediately and disconnect (leave cannula/needle in place); gently aspirate extravasated solution (do **NOT** flush the line); remove needle/cannula; elevate extremity. Apply dry cold compresses for 20 minutes 4 times a day for 1-2 days (Perez Fildago, 2012).

Hazardous agent; use appropriate precautions for handling and disposal (NIOSH, 2012).

Injectable Detail pH: 5.5-7 (reconstituted solution)

Nursing Actions
Physical Assessment Monitor infusion site closely; extravasation can cause severe cellulitis or tissue necrosis. Monitor laboratory tests and patient response on a regular basis throughout (toxic effects may be delayed 2-4 days following a course of treatment and may take 1-2 weeks to reach maximum severity).

Patient Education
- Discuss specific use of drug and side effects with patient as it relates to treatment. (HCAHPS: During this hospital stay, were you given any medicine that you had not taken before? Before giving you any new medicine, how often did hospital staff tell you what the medicine was for? How often did hospital staff describe possible side effects in a way you could understand?)
- Patient may experience lack of appetite, alopecia, cheilitis, or acne vulgaris. Have patient report immediately to prescriber signs of infection, signs of hepatic impairment, severe dyspepsia, significant nausea, excessive weight loss, ecchymosis, hemorrhaging, considerable asthenia, diarrhea, stomatitis, dysphagia, or signs of Stevens-Johnson syndrome/toxic epidermal necrolysis (HCAHPS).
- Educate patient about signs of a significant reaction (eg, wheezing; chest tightness; fever; itching; bad cough; blue skin color; seizures; or swelling of face, lips, tongue, or throat). **Note:** This is not a comprehensive list of all side effects. Patient should consult prescriber for additional questions.

Intended Use and Disclaimer: Should not be printed and given to patients. This information is intended to serve as a concise initial reference for healthcare professionals to use when discussing medications with a patient. You must ultimately rely on your own discretion, experience and judgment in diagnosing, treating and advising patients.

Related Information
Management of Drug Extravasations *on page 1700*

Dalfampridine (dal FAM pri deen)

Brand Names: U.S. Ampyra

Index Terms 4-aminopyridine; 4-AP; EL-970; Fampridine; Fampridine-SR

Pharmacologic Category Potassium Channel Blocker

Medication Safety Issues
Sound-alike/look-alike issues:
Ampyra™ may be confused with anakinra

Dalfampridine may be confused with delavirdine, desipramine

Dalfampridine (U.S.) and fampridine (Canada) are different generic names for the same chemical entity (4-aminopyridine)

Medication Guide Available Yes

Pregnancy Risk Factor C

Lactation Excretion in breast milk unknown/not recommended

Use Treatment to improve walking in patients with multiple sclerosis (MS)

Available Dosage Forms

Tablet Extended Release 12 Hour, Oral:

Ampyra: 10 mg

General Dosage Range Oral: Extended release:

Adults: 10 mg every 12 hours

Administration

Oral May be administered with or without food. Do not chew, crush, dissolve, or divide tablet.

Nursing Actions

Physical Assessment If seizures occur, discontinue medication.

Patient Education

• Discuss specific use of drug and side effects with patient as it relates to treatment. (HCAHPS: During this hospital stay, were you given any medicine that you had not taken before? Before giving you any new medicine, how often did hospital staff tell you what the medicine was for? How often did hospital staff describe possible side effects in a way you could understand?)

• Patient may experience dyspepsia, headache, insomnia, back pain, rhinitis, pharyngitis, or constipation. Have patient report immediately to prescriber severe dizziness, syncope, significant asthenia, dysuria, change in balance, dyspnea, or parasthesia (HCAHPS).

• Educate patient about signs of a significant reaction (eg, wheezing; chest tightness; fever; itching; bad cough; blue skin color; seizures; or swelling of face, lips, tongue, or throat). **Note:** This is not a comprehensive list of all side effects. Patient should consult prescriber for additional questions.

Intended Use and Disclaimer: Should not be printed and given to patients. This information is intended to serve as a concise initial reference for healthcare professionals to use when discussing medications with a patient. You must ultimately rely on your own discretion, experience and judgment in diagnosing, treating and advising patients.

Related Information

Oral Medications That Should Not Be Crushed or Altered *on page 1712*

Dalteparin (dal TE pa rin)

Brand Names: U.S. Fragmin

Index Terms Dalteparin Sodium

Pharmacologic Category Anticoagulant; Anticoagulant, Low Molecular Weight Heparin

Medication Safety Issues

High alert medication:

The Institute for Safe Medication Practices (ISMP) includes this medication among its list of drugs which have a heightened risk of causing significant patient harm when used in error.

National Patient Safety Goals:

The Joint Commission (TJC) requires healthcare organizations that provide anticoagulant therapy to have a process in place to reduce the risk of anticoagulant-associated patient harm. Patients receiving anticoagulants should receive individualized care through a defined process that includes standardized ordering, dispensing, administration, monitoring, and education. This does not apply to routine short-term use of anticoagulants for prevention of venous thromboembolism when the expectation is that the patient's laboratory values will remain within or close to normal values (NPSG.03.05.01).

Pregnancy Risk Factor B

Lactation Enters breast milk/use caution

Breast-Feeding Considerations In lactating women receiving prophylactic doses of dalteparin, small amounts of anti-xa activity was noted in breast milk. The milk/plasma ratio was <0.025 to 0.224. Oral absorption of low molecular weight heparin is extremely low, and is therefore unlikely to cause adverse events in a nursing infant. Use of LMWH may be continued in breast-feeding women (Guyatt, 2012).

Use Prevention of deep vein thrombosis (DVT) which may lead to pulmonary embolism, in patients requiring abdominal surgery who are at risk for thromboembolism complications (eg, patients >40 years of age, obesity, patients with malignancy, history of DVT or pulmonary embolism, and surgical procedures requiring general anesthesia and lasting >30 minutes); prevention of DVT in patients undergoing hip-replacement surgery; patients immobile during an acute illness; prevention of ischemic complications in patients with unstable angina or non-Q-wave myocardial infarction on concurrent aspirin therapy; in patients with cancer, extended treatment (6 months) of acute symptomatic venous thromboembolism (DVT and/or PE) to reduce the recurrence of venous thromboembolism

Canadian labeling: Additional use (unlabeled use in U.S.): Treatment of acute DVT; prevention of venous thromboembolism (VTE) in patients at risk of VTE undergoing general surgery; anticoagulant in extracorporeal circuit during hemodialysis and hemofiltration

Unlabeled Use Active treatment of deep vein thrombosis (noncancer patients)

Mechanism of Action/Effect Low molecular weight heparin analog; the commercial product contains 3% to 15% heparin; has been shown to inhibit both factor Xa and factor IIa (thrombin), however, the antithrombotic effect of dalteparin is characterized by a higher ratio of antifactor Xa to antifactor IIa activity (ratio = 4)

Contraindications Hypersensitivity to dalteparin (eg, pruritus, rash, anaphylactic reactions) or any component of the formulation; history of heparin-induced thrombocytopenia (HIT) or HIT with thrombosis; hypersensitivity to heparin or pork products; active major bleeding; patients with unstable angina, non-Q-wave MI, or prolonged venous thromboembolism prophylaxis undergoing epidural/neuraxial anesthesia

Note: Use of dalteparin in patients with current HIT or HIT with thrombosis is **not** recommended and considered contraindicated due to high cross-reactivity to heparin-platelet factor-4 antibody (Guyatt [ACCP], 2012; Warkentin, 1999).

Canadian labeling: Additional contraindications (not in U.S. labeling): Septic endocarditis, major blood clotting disorders; acute gastroduodenal ulcer; cerebral hemorrhage; severe uncontrolled hypertension; diabetic or hemorrhagic retinopathy; other diseases that increase risk of hemorrhage; injuries to and operations on the CNS, eyes, and ears

Warnings/Precautions [U.S. Boxed Warning]: Spinal or epidural hematomas, including subsequent paralysis, may occur with recent or anticipated neuraxial anesthesia (epidural or spinal) or spinal puncture in patients anticoagulated with LMWH or heparinoids. Consider risk versus benefit prior to spinal procedures; risk is increased by the use of concomitant agents which may alter hemostasis, the use of indwelling epidural catheters for analgesia, a history of spinal deformity or spinal surgery, as well as traumatic or repeated epidural or spinal punctures. Use of dalteparin is contraindicated in patients undergoing epidural/neuraxial anesthesia. Patient should be observed closely for bleeding if enoxaparin is administered during or immediately following diagnostic lumbar puncture, epidural anesthesia, or spinal anesthesia.

Use with caution in patients with pre-existing thrombocytopenia, recent childbirth, subacute bacterial endocarditis, peptic ulcer disease, pericarditis or pericardial effusion, liver or renal function impairment, recent lumbar puncture, vasculitis, concurrent use of aspirin (increased bleeding risk), previous hypersensitivity to heparin, heparin-associated thrombocytopenia. Monitor platelet count closely. Cases of dalteparin-induced thrombocytopenia and thrombosis (similar to heparin-induced thrombocytopenia [HIT]), some complicated by organ infarction, limb ischemia, or death, have been observed. In patients with a history of HIT or HIT with thrombosis, dalteparin is contraindicated. Consider discontinuation of therapy in any patient developing significant thrombocytopenia (eg, <100,000/mm^3) and/or thrombosis related to initiation of dalteparin especially when associated with a positive *in vitro* test for antiplatelet antibodies. Use caution in patients with congenital or drug-induced thrombocytopenia or platelet defects.

Monitor patient closely for signs or symptoms of bleeding. Certain patients are at increased risk of bleeding. Risk factors include bacterial endocarditis; congenital or acquired bleeding disorders; active ulcerative or angiodysplastic GI diseases; severe uncontrolled hypertension; hemorrhagic stroke; or use shortly after brain, spinal, or ophthalmology surgery; in patients treated concomitantly with platelet inhibitors; recent GI bleeding; thrombocytopenia or platelet defects; severe liver disease; hypertensive or diabetic retinopathy; or in patients undergoing invasive procedures.

Use with caution in patients with severe renal impairment; accumulation may occur with repeated dosing increasing the risk for bleeding. Multidose vials contain benzyl alcohol and should not be used in pregnant women. In neonates, large amounts of benzyl alcohol (>100 mg/kg/day) have been associated with fatal toxicity (gasping syndrome). Heparin can cause hyperkalemia by affecting aldosterone. Similar reactions could occur with dalteparin. Monitor for hyperkalemia. Do **not** administer intramuscularly. Not to be used interchangeably (unit for unit) with heparin or any other low molecular weight heparins.

There is no consensus for adjusting/correcting the weight-based dosage of LMWH for patients who are morbidly obese (BMI ≥40 kg/m^2). The American College of Chest Physicians Practice Guidelines suggest consulting with a pharmacist regarding dosing in bariatric surgery patients and other obese patients who may require higher doses of LMWH (Gould, 2012).

Drug Interactions

Avoid Concomitant Use

Avoid concomitant use of Dalteparin with any of the following: Apixaban; Dabigatran Etexilate; Omacetaxine; Rivaroxaban; Urokinase

Decreased Effect

The levels/effects of Dalteparin may be decreased by: Estrogen Derivatives; Progestins

Increased Effect/Toxicity

Dalteparin may increase the levels/effects of: ACE Inhibitors; Aliskiren; Angiotensin II Receptor Blockers; Anticoagulants; Canagliflozin; Collagenase (Systemic); Deferasirox; Eplerenone; Ibritumomab; Omacetaxine; Palifermin; Potassium Salts; Potassium-Sparing Diuretics; Rivaroxaban; Tositumomab and Iodine I 131 Tositumomab

The levels/effects of Dalteparin may be increased by: 5-ASA Derivatives; Agents with Antiplatelet Properties; Apixaban; Dabigatran Etexilate; Dasatinib; Herbs (Anticoagulant/Antiplatelet Properties); Ibrutinib; Nonsteroidal Anti-Inflammatory Agents; Omega-3 Fatty Acids; Pentosan Polysulfate Sodium; Pentoxifylline; Prostacyclin

Analogues; Salicylates; Sugammadex; Thrombolytic Agents; Tibolone; Tipranavir; Urokinase; Vitamin E

Nutritional/Ethanol Interactions Herb/Nutraceutical: Alfalfa, anise, bilberry, bladderwrack, bromelain, cat's claw, celery, chamomile, coleus, cordyceps, dong quai, evening primrose oil, fenugreek, feverfew, garlic, ginger, ginkgo biloba, ginseng (American), ginseng (panax), ginseng (Siberian), grapeseed, green tea, guggul, horse chestnut seed, horseradish, licorice, prickly ash, red clover, reishi, SAMe (s-adenosylmethionine), sweet clover, turmeric, white willow (all have additional antiplatelet/anticoagulant activity)

Adverse Reactions Note: As with all anticoagulants, bleeding is the major adverse effect of dalteparin. Hemorrhage may occur at virtually any site. Risk is dependent on multiple variables.

>10%: Hematologic: Bleeding (3% to 14%), thrombocytopenia (including heparin-induced thrombocytopenia, <1%; cancer clinical trials: ~11%)

1% to 10%:
Hematologic: Major bleeding (up to 6%), wound hematoma (up to 3%)
Hepatic: AST >3 times upper limit of normal (5% to 9%), ALT >3 times upper limit of normal (4% to 10%)
Local: Pain at injection site (up to 12%), injection site hematoma (up to 7%)

Pharmacodynamics/Kinetics
Onset of Action Anti-Xa activity: Within 1-2 hours
Duration of Action >12 hours

Available Dosage Forms
Solution, Subcutaneous:
Fragmin: 25,000 units/mL (3.8 mL)
Solution, Subcutaneous [preservative free]:
Fragmin: 10,000 units/mL (1 mL); 2500 units/0.2 mL (0.2 mL); 5000 units/0.2 mL (0.2 mL); 7500 units/0.3 mL (0.3 mL); 12,500 units/0.5 mL (0.5 mL); 15,000 units/0.6 mL (0.6 mL); 18,000 units/0.72 mL (0.72 mL)

General Dosage Range SubQ: *Adults:* Prophylaxis: 2500-5000 units daily; Treatment: 120 units/kg every 12 hours (maximum: 10,000 units/dose) **or** ~150-200 units/kg (maximum: 18,000 units/dose) once daily

Administration
I.V. Canadian labeling (not an approved route in U.S. labeling): Administer as bolus I.V. injection or as continuous infusion. Recommended concentration for infusion: 20 units/mL.

Other For deep SubQ injection; may be injected in a U-shape to the area surrounding the navel, the upper outer side of the thigh, or the upper outer quadrangle of the buttock. Use thumb and forefinger to lift a fold of skin when injecting dalteparin to the navel area or thigh. Insert needle at a 45- to 90-degree angle. The entire length of needle should be inserted. Do not expel air bubble from fixed-dose syringe prior to injection. Air bubble (and extra solution, if applicable) may be expelled from graduated syringes. In order to minimize bruising, do not rub injection site.

To convert from I.V. unfractionated heparin (UFH) infusion to SubQ dalteparin (Nutescu, 2007): Calculate specific dose for dalteparin based on indication, discontinue UFH and begin dalteparin within 1 hour
To convert from SubQ dalteparin to I.V. UFH infusion (Nutescu, 2007): Discontinue dalteparin; calculate specific dose for I.V. UFH infusion based on indication; omit heparin bolus/loading dose
Converting from SubQ dalteparin dosed every 12 hours: Start I.V. UFH infusion 10-11 hours after last dose of dalteparin
Converting from SubQ dalteparin dosed every 24 hours: Start I.V. UFH infusion 22-23 hours after last dose of dalteparin

Preparation for Administration Canadian labeling: If necessary, may dilute in isotonic sodium chloride or dextrose solutions to a concentration of 20 units/mL. Use within 24 hours of mixing.

Storage/Stability Store at temperatures of 20°C to 25°C (68°F to 77°F). Multidose vials may be stored for up to 2 weeks at room temperature after entering.

Nursing Actions
Physical Assessment Bleeding precautions should be observed. Teach patient about bleeding precautions.

Patient Education
• Discuss specific use of drug and side effects with patient as it relates to treatment. (HCAHPS: During this hospital stay, were you given any medicine that you had not taken before? Before giving you any new medicine, how often did hospital staff tell you what the medicine was for? How often did hospital staff describe possible side effects in a way you could understand?)
• Patient may experience injection site irritation. Have patient report immediately to prescriber signs of hemorrhaging, severe dizziness, syncope, illogical thinking, significant headache, paresthesia, or asthenia (HCAHPS).
• Educate patient about signs of a significant reaction (eg, wheezing; chest tightness; fever; itching; bad cough; blue skin color; seizures; or swelling of face, lips, tongue, or throat). **Note:** This is not a comprehensive list of all side effects. Patient should consult prescriber for additional questions.

Intended Use and Disclaimer: Should not be printed and given to patients. This information is intended to serve as a concise initial reference for healthcare professionals to use when discussing medications with a patient. You must ultimately rely on your own discretion, experience and judgment in diagnosing, treating and advising patients.

Danazol (DA na zole)

Index Terms Danocrine
Pharmacologic Category Androgen
Medication Safety Issues
  Sound-alike/look-alike issues:
    Danazol may be confused with Dantrium®
Pregnancy Risk Factor X
Lactation Contraindicated
Use Treatment of endometriosis, fibrocystic breast disease, and hereditary angioedema
Available Dosage Forms
  Capsule, Oral:
    Generic: 50 mg, 100 mg, 200 mg
General Dosage Range Oral:
  Adults (females): 100-800 mg/day in 2 divided doses
  Adults (females/males): Hereditary angioedema: Initial: 200 mg 2-3 times/day; after favorable response decrease dosage by 50% or less
Administration
  Oral Endometriosis, fibrocystic breast disease: Initiate therapy during menstruation or ensure patient is not pregnant while on therapy. Symptoms may recur following discontinuation of therapy and treatment may need reinstated.
Nursing Actions
  Physical Assessment Monitor for hypertension, increased LDL, CNS changes, jaundice, and hematuria. Caution patients with diabetes to monitor glucose levels closely; may enhance the glucose-lowering effect of hypoglycemic agents. Teach patient good self-breast exam technique.
Patient Education
  • Discuss specific use of drug and side effects with patient as it relates to treatment. (HCAHPS: During this hospital stay, were you given any medicine that you had not taken before? Before giving you any new medicine, how often did hospital staff tell you what the medicine was for? How often did hospital staff describe possible side effects in a way you could understand?)
  • Patient may experience flushing, alopecia, nausea, emotional instability, acne vulgaris, sexual dysfunction, or signs of virilization. Have patient report immediately to prescriber angina, dyspnea, excessive weight gain, edema of extremities, strength differences from one side to another, difficulty speaking or thinking, change in balance, blurred vision, severe dizziness, syncope, significant headache, considerable anxiety, mood changes, sudden vision changes, ophthalmalgia, eye irritation, lump in breast, mastalgia, signs of hepatic impairment, or amenorrhea (HCAHPS).
  • Educate patient about signs of a significant reaction (eg, wheezing; chest tightness; fever; itching; bad cough; blue skin color; seizures; or swelling of face, lips, tongue, or throat). **Note:** This is not a comprehensive list of all side effects. Patient should consult prescriber for additional questions.

Intended Use and Disclaimer: Should not be printed and given to patients. This information is intended to serve as a concise initial reference for healthcare professionals to use when discussing medications with a patient. You must ultimately rely on your own discretion, experience and judgment in diagnosing, treating and advising patients.

Dantrolene (DAN troe leen)

Brand Names: U.S. Dantrium; Revonto
Index Terms Dantrolene Sodium
Pharmacologic Category Skeletal Muscle Relaxant
Medication Safety Issues
  Sound-alike/look-alike issues:
    Dantrium® may be confused with danazol, Daraprim®
    Revonto® may be confused with Revatio®
Pregnancy Risk Factor C
Lactation Enters breast milk/not recommended
Use Treatment of spasticity associated with upper motor neuron disorders (eg, spinal cord injury, stroke, cerebral palsy, or multiple sclerosis); management of malignant hyperthermia (MH); prevention of malignant hyperthermia in susceptible individuals (preoperative/postoperative administration)
Note: Dantrolene prophylaxis is not recommended for most MH-susceptible patients, provided nontriggering anesthetics are used and an adequate supply of dantrolene is available.
Unlabeled Use Neuroleptic malignant syndrome (NMS)
Available Dosage Forms
  Capsule, Oral:
    Dantrium: 25 mg, 50 mg, 100 mg
    Generic: 25 mg, 50 mg, 100 mg
  Solution Reconstituted, Intravenous:
    Dantrium: 20 mg (1 ea)
    Revonto: 20 mg (1 ea)
General Dosage Range
  I.V.: *Children and Adults:* 1-2.5 mg/kg; may repeat up to cumulative dose of 10 mg/kg **or** 2.5 mg/kg as a single dose
  Oral:
    Children: 4-8 mg/kg/day in 4 divided doses **or** 0.5-2 mg/kg/dose 1-4 times daily (maximum: 400 mg daily)
    Adults: 4-8 mg/kg/day in 4 divided doses **or** 25-100 mg 1-4 times daily (maximum: 400 mg daily)
Administration
  I.V. Therapeutic or emergency dose can be administered with rapid continuous I.V. push. Follow-up doses should be administered over at least 1 hour.

Vesicant; ensure proper needle or catheter placement prior to and during infusion; avoid extravasation.

Extravasation management: If extravasation occurs, stop infusion immediately and disconnect (leave cannula/needle in place); gently aspirate extravasated solution (do **NOT** flush the line); remove needle/cannula; elevate extremity.

Injectable Detail pH ~9.5 (after reconstitution)

Nursing Actions

Physical Assessment I.V.: Monitor vital signs, cardiac function, respiratory status, and I.V. site (extravasation very irritating to tissues) frequently during infusion.

Patient Education

- Discuss specific use of drug and side effects with patient as it relates to treatment. (HCAHPS: During this hospital stay, were you given any medicine that you had not taken before? Before giving you any new medicine, how often did hospital staff tell you what the medicine was for? How often did hospital staff describe possible side effects in a way you could understand?)
- Patient may experience fatigue or diarrhea. Have patient report immediately to prescriber signs of infection, severe asthenia, dyspnea, excessive weight gain, edema of extremities, angina, hematuria, melena, hematemesis, illogical thinking, depression, urinary retention, oliguria, tachycardia, significant dyspepsia, considerable headache, ecchymosis, hemorrhaging, vision changes, intolerable dizziness, syncope, severe constipation, signs of hepatic impairment, or injection site irritation (HCAHPS).
- Educate patient about signs of a significant reaction (eg, wheezing; chest tightness; fever; itching; bad cough; blue skin color; seizures; or swelling of face, lips, tongue, or throat). **Note:** This is not a comprehensive list of all side effects. Patient should consult prescriber for additional questions.

Intended Use and Disclaimer: Should not be printed and given to patients. This information is intended to serve as a concise initial reference for healthcare professionals to use when discussing medications with a patient. You must ultimately rely on your own discretion, experience and judgment in diagnosing, treating and advising patients.

Related Information

Management of Drug Extravasations *on page 1700*

Dapagliflozin (dap a gli FLOE zin)

Brand Names: U.S. Farxiga
Index Terms BMS-512148
Pharmacologic Category Antidiabetic Agent, Sodium-Glucose Cotransporter 2 (SGLT2) Inhibitor; Sodium-Glucose Cotransporter 2 (SGLT2) Inhibitor

Medication Safety Issues

High alert medication:

The Institute for Safe Medication Practices (ISMP) includes this medication among its list of drugs which have a heightened risk of causing significant patient harm when used in error.

Medication Guide Available Yes

Pregnancy Risk Factor C

Lactation Excretion in breast milk unknown/not recommended

Breast-Feeding Considerations It is not known if dapagliflozin is excreted into breast milk. Due to the potential for serious adverse reactions in the nursing infant, the manufacturer recommends a decision be made whether to discontinue nursing or to discontinue the drug, taking into account the importance of treatment to the mother.

Use Type 2 diabetes mellitus: As an adjunct to diet and exercise to improve glycemic control in adults with type 2 diabetes mellitus

Mechanism of Action/Effect Glucose reabsorption from the proximal renal tubules of the kidneys is reduced; urinary excretion of glucose is increased, thereby reducing plasma glucose concentrations.

Contraindications History of serious hypersensitivity to dapagliflozin or any component of the formulation; severe renal impairment, end-stage renal disease (ESRD), or patients on dialysis

Warnings/Precautions Potentially significant drug-drug interactions may exist, requiring dose or frequency adjustment, additional monitoring, and/or selection of alternative therapy. May increase the risk of genital mycotic infections (eg, vulvovaginal mycotic infection, vulvovaginal candidiasis, vulvovaginitis, candida balanitis, balanoposthitis). Patients with a history of these infections or uncircumcised males are at greater risk. Patients may experience hypersensitivity reactions (eg, angioedema, urticaria), with some being severe. Discontinue dapagliflozin if hypersensitivity occurs and treat as appropriate. May cause symptomatic hypotension due to intravascular volume depletion, especially in patients with renal impairment (ie, eGFR <60 mL/minute/1.73 m^2), elderly, patients on other antihypertensives (eg, diuretics, ACE inhibitors, or angiotensin receptor blockers [ARBs]), or those with low systolic blood pressure. Assess volume status prior to initiation in patients at risk of hypotension and correct if depleted; monitor signs and symptoms of hypotension after initiation. May cause dose-related LDL-cholesterol (C) elevation; monitor LDL-C and treat as needed.

Abnormalities in renal function (decreased eGFR, increased serum creatinine) may occur; elderly patients and patients with pre-existing renal impairment may be at greater risk. Glycemic efficacy may be less and adverse reactions (eg, renal-related adverse reactions, bone fractures) may be higher with moderate renal impairment (eGFR 30 to <60 mL/minute/1.73 m^2). Assess renal function prior to initiation and periodically during treatment; dapagliflozin should not be initiated if initial eGFR is <60 mL/minute/1.73 m^2 and should be discontinued when eGFR is persistently <60 mL/minute/1.73 m^2. Use is contraindicated in severe renal impairment (<30 mL/minute/1.73 m^2) and ESRD. Elderly patients may be predisposed to symptoms related to intravascular volume depletion (eg, hypotension, orthostatic hypotension, dizziness, syncope, and dehydration) and renal impairment or failure. Weigh benefits versus risk in patients with severe hepatic impairment (has not been studied).

Dapagliflozin should not be used in patients with DKA or in patients with type 1 diabetes mellitus (insulin-dependent, IDDM). Newly diagnosed bladder cancer occurred more frequently in dapagliflozin patients; causal relationship could not be established. Do not use in patients with active bladder cancer; weigh the benefits of glycemic control versus the unknown risks for cancer recurrence in patients with a history of bladder cancer.

Drug Interactions

Avoid Concomitant Use There are no known interactions where it is recommended to avoid concomitant use.

Decreased Effect
The levels/effects of Dapagliflozin may be decreased by: Corticosteroids (Orally Inhaled); Corticosteroids (Systemic); Loop Diuretics; Luteinizing Hormone-Releasing Hormone Analogs; Somatropin; Thiazide Diuretics

Increased Effect/Toxicity
Dapagliflozin may increase the levels/effects of: DULoxetine; Hypoglycemic Agents; Hypotensive Agents

The levels/effects of Dapagliflozin may be increased by: Herbs (Hypoglycemic Properties); MAO Inhibitors; Pegvisomant; Salicylates; Selective Serotonin Reuptake Inhibitors

Nutritional/Ethanol Interactions Ethanol: May cause hypoglycemia. Management: Avoid ethanol.

Adverse Reactions
1% to 10%:
Endocrine & metabolic: Mild hypoglycemia (plus insulin or other oral antidiabetic therapy: 40% to 43%), dyslipidemia (2% to 3%), hypovolemia (1%; includes dehydration, hypovolemia, orthostatic hypotension, hypotension)
Gastrointestinal: Nausea (3%), constipation (2%)
Genitourinary: Fungal vaginosis (7% to 8%; includes [in order of frequency] vulvovaginal mycotic infection, vaginal infection, vulvovaginal candidiasis, vulvovaginitis, genital infection, genital candidiasis, fungal genital infection, vulvitis, genitourinary tract infection, vulval abscess, vaginitis bacterial), urinary tract infection (4% to 6%: includes [in order of frequency] urinary tract infection, cystitis, Escherichia urinary tract infection, genitourinary tract infection, pyelonephritis, trigonitis, urethritis, kidney infection, prostatitis), increased urine output (3% to 4%: includes [in order of frequency] pollakiuria, polyuria, and urine output increased), genitourinary fungal infections (mycotic; in males: 3%; includes [in order of frequency] balanitis, fungal genital infection, balanitis candida, genital candidiasis, genital infection, penile infection, balanoposthitis, balanoposthitis infective, genital infection, posthitis), dysuria (2%)
Hematologic & oncologic: Increased hematocrit (1%, hematocrit >55%)
Infection: Influenza (2% to 3%)
Neuromuscular & skeletal: Back pain (3% to 4%), limb pain (2%)
Respiratory: Nasopharyngitis (6% to 7%)
Frequency not defined:
Dermatologic: Urticaria
Endocrine & metabolic: Increased LDL cholesterol, increased serum phosphate
Hypersensitivity: Hypersensitivity reaction (angioedema, urticaria, hypersensitivity)
Neuromuscular & skeletal: Bone fracture (in patients with moderate renal impairment)
Renal: Decreased estimated GFR, increased serum creatinine

Available Dosage Forms
Tablet, Oral:
Farxiga: 5 mg, 10 mg

General Dosage Range Oral: Adults: 5-10 mg once daily

Administration
Oral Administer in the morning, with or without food

Storage/Stability Store at 20°C to 25°C (68°F to 77°F); excursions are permitted between 15°C and 30°C (59°F and 86°F).

Nursing Actions
Patient Education
- Discuss specific use of drug and side effects with patient as it relates to treatment. (HCAHPS: During this hospital stay, were you given any medicine that you had not taken before? Before giving you any new medicine, how often did hospital staff tell you what the medicine was for? How often did hospital staff describe possible side effects in a way you could understand?)
- Patient may experience rhinitis, rhinorrhea, or pharyngitis. Have patient report immediately to prescriber signs of fluid and electrolyte imbalance, signs of renal impairment, vaginal yeast infection, penile yeast infection, hematuria, dysuria, polyuria, or signs of hypoglycemia (HCAHPS).

• Educate patient about signs of a significant reaction (eg, wheezing; chest tightness; fever; itching; bad cough; blue skin color; seizures; or swelling of face, lips, tongue, or throat). **Note:** This is not a comprehensive list of all side effects. Patient should consult prescriber for additional questions.

Intended Use and Disclaimer: Should not be printed and given to patients. This information is intended to serve as a concise initial reference for healthcare professionals to use when discussing medications with a patient. You must ultimately rely on your own discretion, experience and judgment in diagnosing, treating and advising patients.

Dietary Considerations Individualized medical nutrition therapy (MNT) based on ADA recommendations is an integral part of therapy.

Darbepoetin Alfa (dar be POE e tin AL fa)

Brand Names: U.S. Aranesp (Albumin Free)
Index Terms Erythropoiesis-Stimulating Agent (ESA); Erythropoiesis-Stimulating Protein; NESP; Novel Erythropoiesis-Stimulating Protein
Pharmacologic Category Colony Stimulating Factor; Erythropoiesis-Stimulating Agent (ESA); Hematopoietic Agent
Medication Safety Issues
Sound-alike/look-alike issues:
Aranesp may be confused with Aralast, Aricept
Darbepoetin alfa may be confused with dalteparin, epoetin alfa, epoetin beta
Medication Guide Available Yes
Pregnancy Risk Factor C
Lactation Excretion in breast milk unknown/use caution
Breast-Feeding Considerations It is not known if darbepoetin alfa is excreted in breast milk. The manufacturer recommends that caution be exercised when administering darbepoetin alfa to nursing women.
Use Anemia: Treatment of anemia due to concurrent myelosuppressive chemotherapy in patients with cancer (nonmyeloid malignancies) receiving chemotherapy (palliative intent) for a planned minimum of 2 additional months of chemotherapy; treatment of anemia due to chronic kidney disease (including patients on dialysis and not on dialysis)

Note: Darbepoetin is **not** indicated for use under the following conditions:
• Cancer patients receiving hormonal therapy, therapeutic biologic products, or radiation therapy unless also receiving concurrent myelosuppressive chemotherapy
• Cancer patients receiving myelosuppressive chemotherapy when the expected outcome is curative
• As a substitute for RBC transfusion in patients requiring immediate correction of anemia

Note: In clinical trials, darbepoetin has not demonstrated improved quality of life, fatigue, or well-being.

Unlabeled Use Treatment of symptomatic anemia in myelodysplastic syndrome (MDS)
Mechanism of Action/Effect Stimulates production of red blood cells within the bone marrow. There is a dose response relationship with this effect. This results in an increase in red blood cell counts followed by a rise in hematocrit and hemoglobin levels. When administered SubQ or I.V., darbepoetin's half-life is ~3 times that of epoetin alfa.
Contraindications Hypersensitivity to darbepoetin or any component of the formulation; uncontrolled hypertension; pure red cell aplasia (due to darbepoetin or other erythropoietin protein drugs)
Warnings/Precautions [U.S. Boxed Warning]: Erythropoiesis-stimulating agents (ESAs) increased the risk of serious cardiovascular events, thromboembolic events, stroke, and/or tumor progression in clinical studies when administered to target hemoglobin levels >11 g/dL (and provide no additional benefit); a rapid rise in hemoglobin (>1 g/dL over 2 weeks) may also contribute to these risks. **[U.S. Boxed Warning]: A shortened overall survival and/or increased risk of tumor progression or recurrence has been reported in studies with breast, cervical, head and neck, lymphoid, and non-small cell lung cancer patients.** It is of note that in these studies, patients received ESAs to a target hemoglobin of ≥12 g/dL; although risk has not been excluded when dosed to achieve a target hemoglobin of <12 g/dL. **[U.S. Boxed Warnings]: To decrease these risks, and risk of cardio- and thrombovascular events, use ESAs in cancer patients only for the treatment of anemia related to concurrent myelosuppressive chemotherapy and use the lowest dose needed to avoid red blood cell transfusions. Discontinue ESA following completion of the chemotherapy course. ESAs are not indicated for patients receiving myelosuppressive therapy when the anticipated outcome is curative.** A dosage modification is appropriate if hemoglobin levels rise >1 g/dL per 2-week time period during treatment (Rizzo, 2010). Use of ESAs has been associated with an increased risk of venous thromboembolism (VTE) without a reduction in transfusions in patients >65 years of age with cancer (Hershman, 2009). Improved anemia symptoms, quality of life, fatigue, or well-being have not been demonstrated in controlled clinical trials. **[U.S. Boxed Warning]: Because of the risks of decreased survival and increased risk of tumor growth or progression, all healthcare providers and hospitals are required to enroll and comply with the ESA APPRISE (Assisting Providers and Cancer Patients with Risk Information for the Safe use of ESAs) Oncology Program prior to**

prescribing or dispensing ESAs to cancer patients. Prescribers and patients will have to provide written documentation of discussed risks prior to each course.

[U.S. Boxed Warning]: An increased risk of death, serious cardiovascular events, and stroke was reported in patients with chronic kidney disease (CKD) administered ESAs to target hemoglobin levels ≥11 g/dL; use the lowest dose sufficient to reduce the need for RBC transfusions. An optimal target hemoglobin level, dose or dosing strategy to reduce these risks has not been identified in clinical trials. Hemoglobin rising >1 g/dL in a 2-week period may contribute to the risk (dosage reduction recommended). The American College of Physicians recommends against the use of ESAs in patients with mild to moderate anemia and heart failure or coronary heart disease (ACP [Qaseem, 2013]).

CKD patients who exhibit an inadequate hemoglobin response to ESA therapy may be at a higher risk for cardiovascular events and mortality compared to other patients. ESA therapy may reduce dialysis efficacy (due to increase in red blood cells and decrease in plasma volume); adjustments in dialysis parameters may be needed. Patients treated with epoetin may require increased heparinization during dialysis to prevent clotting of the extracorporeal circuit. CKD patients not requiring dialysis may have a better response to darbepoetin and may require lower doses. An increased risk of DVT has been observed in patients treated with epoetin undergoing surgical orthopedic procedures. Darbepoetin is **not** approved for reduction in allogeneic red blood cell transfusions in patients scheduled for surgical procedures. The risk for seizures is increased with darbepoetin use in patients with CKD; use with caution in patients with a history of seizures. Monitor closely for neurologic symptoms during the first several months of therapy. Use with caution in patients with hypertension; hypertensive encephalopathy has been reported. Use is contraindicated in patients with uncontrolled hypertension. If hypertension is difficult to control, reduce or hold darbepoetin alfa. Due to the delayed onset of erythropoiesis, darbepoetin alfa is **not** recommended for acute correction of severe anemia or as a substitute for emergency transfusion. Consider discontinuing in patients who receive a renal transplant.

Prior to treatment, correct or exclude deficiencies of iron, vitamin B_{12}, and/or folate, as well as other factors which may impair erythropoiesis (inflammatory conditions, infections, bleeding). Prior to and during therapy, iron stores must be evaluated. Supplemental iron is recommended if serum ferritin <100 mcg/L or serum transferrin saturation <20%; most patients with CKD will require iron supplementation. Poor response should prompt evaluation of these potential factors, as well as possible malignant processes and hematologic disease (thalassemia, refractory anemia, myelodysplastic disorder), occult blood loss, hemolysis, osteitis fibrosa cystic, and/or bone marrow fibrosis. Severe anemia and pure red cell aplasia (PRCA) with associated neutralizing antibodies to erythropoietin has been reported, predominantly in patients with CKD receiving SubQ darbepoetin (the I.V. route is preferred for hemodialysis patients). Cases have also been reported in patients with hepatitis C who were receiving ESAs, interferon, and ribavirin. Patients with a sudden loss of response to darbepoetin (with severe anemia and a low reticulocyte count) should be evaluated for PRCA with associated neutralizing antibodies to erythropoietin; discontinue treatment (permanently) in patients with PRCA secondary to neutralizing antibodies to erythropoietin. Antibodies may cross-react; do not switch to another ESA in patients who develop antibody-mediated anemia.

Potentially serious allergic reactions have been reported (rarely). Discontinue immediately (and permanently) in patients who experience serious allergic/anaphylactic reactions. Some products may contain albumin and the packaging of some formulations may contain latex.

Drug Interactions

Avoid Concomitant Use There are no known interactions where it is recommended to avoid concomitant use.

Decreased Effect There are no known significant interactions involving a decrease in effect.

Increased Effect/Toxicity There are no known significant interactions involving an increase in effect.

Nutritional/Ethanol Interactions Ethanol: Should be avoided due to adverse effects on erythropoiesis.

Adverse Reactions

>10%:

Cardiovascular: Hypertension (31%), peripheral edema (17%), edema (6% to 13%)

Gastrointestinal: Abdominal pain (10% to 13%)

Respiratory: Dyspnea (17%), cough (12%)

1% to 10%:

Cardiovascular: Angina, fluid overload, hypotension, MI, thromboembolic events

Central nervous system: Cerebrovascular disorder

Dermatologic: Rash/erythema

Local: AV graft thrombosis, vascular access complications

Respiratory: Pulmonary embolism

Pharmacodynamics/Kinetics

Onset of Action Increased hemoglobin levels not generally observed until 2-6 weeks after initiating treatment

Available Dosage Forms

Solution, Injection [preservative free]:

Aranesp (Albumin Free): 25 mcg/mL (1 mL); 40 mcg/mL (1 mL); 25 mcg/0.42 mL (0.42 mL); 60 mcg/mL (1 mL); 40 mcg/0.4 mL (0.4 mL); 100 mcg/mL (1 mL); 60 mcg/0.3 mL (0.3 mL); 100 mcg/0.5 mL (0.5 mL); 150 mcg/0.75 mL (0.75 mL); 200 mcg/mL (1 mL); 300 mcg/mL (1 mL); 150 mcg/0.3 mL (0.3 mL); 200 mcg/0.4 mL (0.4 mL); 300 mcg/0.6 mL (0.6 mL); 500 mcg/mL (1 mL)

General Dosage Range

I.V.:

Children 1-18 years: 6.25-200 mcg/week

Adults: 0.45 mcg/kg once weekly **or** every 4 weeks **or** 0.75 mcg/kg once every 2 weeks **or** 6.25-200 mcg/week

SubQ:

Children 1-18 years: 6.25-200 mcg/week

Adults: 0.45-4.5 mcg/kg/week **or** 0.45 mcg/kg every 4 weeks **or** 0.75 mcg/kg once every 2 weeks **or** 500 mcg once every 3 weeks **or** 6.25-200 mcg/week

Administration

I.V. May be administered by I.V. injection. The I.V. route is recommended in hemodialysis patients. Do not shake; vigorous shaking may denature darbepoetin alfa, rendering it biologically inactive. Do not dilute or administer in conjunction with other drug solutions. Discard any unused portion of the vial; do not pool unused portions.

Subcutaneous May be administered SubQ.

Storage/Stability Store at 2°C to 8°C (36°F to 46°F); do not freeze. Do not shake. Protect from light. Store in original carton until use. The following stability information has also been reported: May be stored at room temperature for up to 7 days (Cohen, 2007).

Nursing Actions

Physical Assessment Monitor blood pressure closely during therapy. If administered by intravenous infusion, lines should be monitored closely for possible clotting. Monitor for hyper-/hypotension, edema, thrombosis, stroke, TIA, and anemia. Teach patient proper SubQ injection technique and syringe/needle disposal. Evaluate history of hypertension or seizures and potential risk for thromboembolism prior to beginning therapy. Obtain baseline blood chemistries, hemoglobin/hematocrit, serum ferritin, and transferrin saturation prior to and on a regular basis during therapy.

Patient Education

- Discuss specific use of drug and side effects with patient as it relates to treatment. (HCAHPS: During this hospital stay, were you given any medicine that you had not taken before? Before giving you any new medicine, how often did hospital staff tell you what the medicine was for? How often did hospital staff describe possible side effects in a way you could understand?)
- Patient may experience injection site irritation or dyspepsia. Have patient report immediately to prescriber tachycardia, angina, arrhythmia, dyspnea, excessive weight gain, edema of extremities, strength differences from one side to another, difficulty speaking or thinking, change in balance, blurred vision, severe dizziness, syncope, significant headache, considerable asthenia, pallor, hemoptysis, or abnormal gait (HCAHPS).
- Educate patient about signs of a significant reaction (eg, wheezing; chest tightness; fever; itching; bad cough; blue skin color; seizures; or swelling of face, lips, tongue, or throat). **Note:** This is not a comprehensive list of all side effects. Patient should consult prescriber for additional questions.

Intended Use and Disclaimer: Should not be printed and given to patients. This information is intended to serve as a concise initial reference for healthcare professionals to use when discussing medications with a patient. You must ultimately rely on your own discretion, experience and judgment in diagnosing, treating and advising patients.

Dietary Considerations Supplemental iron intake may be required in patients with low iron stores.

Darifenacin (dar i FEN a sin)

Brand Names: U.S. Enablex

Index Terms Darifenacin Hydrobromide; UK-88,525

Pharmacologic Category Anticholinergic Agent

Medication Safety Issues

BEERS Criteria medication:

This drug may be potentially inappropriate for use in geriatric patients (Quality of evidence - varies based on comorbidity; Strength of recommendation - varies based on comorbidity)

Pregnancy Risk Factor C

Lactation Excretion in breast milk unknown/use caution

Breast-Feeding Considerations Although human data are not available, darifenacin is excreted in the breast milk in animals.

Use Management of symptoms of bladder overactivity (urge incontinence, urgency, and frequency)

Mechanism of Action/Effect Blocks muscarinic/cholinergic receptors (M3 subtype) on the smooth muscle of the urinary bladder to limit bladder contractions, reducing the symptoms of bladder irritability/overactivity (urge incontinence, urgency and frequency).

Contraindications Hypersensitivity to darifenacin or any component of the formulation; uncontrolled narrow-angle glaucoma; urinary retention, paralytic ileus, GI or GU obstruction

Warnings/Precautions Cases of angioedema involving the face, lips, tongue, and/or larynx have been reported during treatment; some cases have occurred after the first dose. May be life-threatening. Immediately discontinue and institute supportive care if tongue, hypopharynx, or larynx is involved. Central nervous system effects have been reported (eg, headache, confusion, hallucinations, somnolence); monitor, particularly at treatment initiation or dose increase, reduce dose or discontinue if necessary. May cause drowsiness and/or blurred vision, which may impair physical or mental abilities; patients must be cautioned about performing tasks which require mental alertness (eg, operating machinery or driving). May occur in the presence of increased environmental temperature; use caution in hot weather and/or exercise. Use with caution with hepatic impairment; dosage limitation is required in moderate hepatic impairment (Child-Pugh class B). Not recommended for use in severe hepatic impairment (Child-Pugh class C). Use with caution in patients with clinically-significant bladder outlet obstruction or prostatic hyperplasia (nonobstructive). Use caution in patients with decreased GI motility, constipation, hiatal hernia, reflux esophagitis, and ulcerative colitis. Use caution in patients with myasthenia gravis. In patients with controlled narrow-angle glaucoma, darifenacin should be used with extreme caution and only when the potential benefit outweighs risks of treatment. Use with caution in patients taking strong CYP3A4 inhibitors (see Drug Interactions); dosage limitation of darifenacin is required. This medication is associated with potent anticholinergic properties which may be inappropriate in older adults depending on comorbidities (eg, dementia, delirium) (Beers Criteria).

Drug Interactions
Avoid Concomitant Use
Avoid concomitant use of Darifenacin with any of the following: Aclidinium; Conivaptan; Fusidic Acid (Systemic); Ipratropium (Oral Inhalation); Pimozide; Potassium Chloride; Thioridazine; Tiotropium; Umeclidinium

Decreased Effect
Darifenacin may decrease the levels/effects of: Acetylcholinesterase Inhibitors (Central); Codeine; Secretin; Tamoxifen; TraMADol

The levels/effects of Darifenacin may be decreased by: Acetylcholinesterase Inhibitors (Central); Bosentan; CYP3A4 Inducers (Strong); Dabrafenib; Deferasirox; Herbs (CYP3A4 Inducers); Mitotane; Peginterferon Alfa-2b; Tocilizumab

Increased Effect/Toxicity
Darifenacin may increase the levels/effects of: AbobotulinumtoxinA; Analgesics (Opioid); Anticholinergics; ARIPiprazole; Cannabinoids; CYP2D6 Substrates; Dofetilide; DOXOrubicin (Conventional); Fesoterodine; Lomitapide; Metoprolol; Mirabegron; Nebivolol; OnabotulinumtoxinA; Pimozide; Potassium Chloride; RimabotulinumtoxinB; Thiazide Diuretics; Thioridazine; Tiotropium; Topiramate

The levels/effects of Darifenacin may be increased by: Aclidinium; Conivaptan; CYP3A4 Inhibitors (Moderate); CYP3A4 Inhibitors (Strong); Dasatinib; Fusidic Acid (Systemic); Ipratropium (Oral Inhalation); Ivacaftor; Luliconazole; Mifepristone; Pramlintide; Propafenone; Simeprevir; Stiripentol; Umeclidinium

Nutritional/Ethanol Interactions Herb/Nutraceutical: Darifenacin serum concentration may be decreased by St John's wort (avoid concurrent use.)

Adverse Reactions
>10%: Gastrointestinal: Xerostomia (19% to 35%), constipation (15% to 21%)

1% to 10%:
Cardiovascular: Hypertension (≥1%), peripheral edema (≥1%)
Central nervous system: Headache (7%), dizziness (<2%), pain (≥1%)
Dermatological: Dry skin (≥1%), pruritus (≥1%), rash (≥1%)
Gastrointestinal: Dyspepsia (3% to 8%), abdominal pain (2% to 4%), nausea (2% to 4%), vomiting (≥1%), weight gain (≥1%)
Genitourinary: Urinary tract infection (4% to 5%), vaginitis (≥1%), urinary retention (acute)
Neuromuscular & skeletal: Weakness (<3%), arthralgia (≥1%), back pain (≥1%)
Ocular: Dry eyes (2%), abnormal vision (≥1%)
Respiratory: Bronchitis (≥1%), pharyngitis (≥1%), rhinitis (≥1%), sinusitis (≥1%)
Miscellaneous: Flu-like syndrome (1% to 3%)

Available Dosage Forms
Tablet Extended Release 24 Hour, Oral:
Enablex: 7.5 mg, 15 mg

General Dosage Range Dosage adjustment recommended in patients with hepatic impairment or on concomitant therapy
Oral: *Adults:* Initial: 7.5 mg once daily; Maintenance: 7.5-15 mg once daily

Administration
Oral Tablet should be taken with liquid and swallowed whole; do not chew, crush, or split tablet. May be taken without regard to food.

Storage/Stability Store at 25°C (77°F); excursions permitted to 15°C to 30°C (59°F to 86°F). Protect from light.

Nursing Actions
Patient Education
• Discuss specific use of drug and side effects with patient as it relates to treatment. (HCAHPS: During this hospital stay, were you given any medicine that you had not taken before? Before giving you any new medicine, how often did hospital staff tell you what the medicine was

for? How often did hospital staff describe possible side effects in a way you could understand?)
- Patient may experience pyrosis or xerostomia. Have patient report immediately to prescriber signs of renal impairment, dyspnea, severe dizziness, syncope, illogical thinking, considerable dyspepsia, significant constipation, anhidrosis, intolerable nausea, or edema of hands or feet (HCAHPS).
- Educate patient about signs of a significant reaction (eg, wheezing; chest tightness; fever; itching; bad cough; blue skin color; seizures; or swelling of face, lips, tongue, or throat). **Note:** This is not a comprehensive list of all side effects. Patient should consult prescriber for additional questions.

Intended Use and Disclaimer: Should not be printed and given to patients. This information is intended to serve as a concise initial reference for healthcare professionals to use when discussing medications with a patient. You must ultimately rely on your own discretion, experience and judgment in diagnosing, treating and advising patients.

Dietary Considerations May be taken without regard to meals, with or without food.

Related Information

Oral Medications That Should Not Be Crushed or Altered *on page 1712*

Darunavir (dar OO na veer)

Brand Names: U.S. Prezista
Index Terms Darunavir Ethanolate; DRV; TMC-114
Pharmacologic Category Antiretroviral, Protease Inhibitor (Anti-HIV)
Pregnancy Risk Factor C
Lactation Excretion in breast milk unknown/not recommended
Breast-Feeding Considerations Maternal or infant antiretroviral therapy does not completely eliminate the risk of postnatal HIV transmission. In addition, multiclass-resistant virus has been detected in breast-feeding infants despite maternal therapy. Therefore, in the United States, where formula is accessible, affordable, safe, and sustainable, and the risk of infant mortality due to diarrhea and respiratory infections is low, complete avoidance of breast-feeding by HIV-infected women is recommended to decrease potential transmission of HIV (DHHS [perinatal], 2012).
Use Treatment of HIV-1 infections in combination with ritonavir and other antiretroviral agents
Mechanism of Action/Effect Blocks the site of HIV-1 protease activity, resulting in the formation of immature, noninfectious viral particles.
Contraindications Coadministration with medications highly dependent upon CYP3A4 for clearance and for which increased levels are associated with serious and/or life-threatening

events (includes alfuzosin, cisapride, ergot alkaloids [eg, dihydroergotamine, ergonovine, ergotamine, methylergonovine], lovastatin, midazolam [oral], pimozide, rifampin, sildenafil (when used for pulmonary artery hypertension [eg, Revatio®]), simvastatin, St John's wort, triazolam

Canadian labeling: Additional contraindications: Hypersensitivity to darunavir or any component of the formulation; coadministration with amiodarone, lidocaine (systemic), quinidine; severe (Child-Pugh class C) hepatic impairment

Warnings/Precautions Darunavir has a high potential for drug interactions requiring dose or frequency adjustment, additional monitoring, and/or selection of alternative therapy.

Use with caution in patients with hepatic impairment, including active chronic hepatitis; consider interruption or discontinuation with worsening hepatic function. Not recommended in severe hepatic impairment (contraindicated in Canadian labeling). Infrequent cases of drug-induced hepatitis (including acute and cytolytic) have been reported. Liver injury has been reported with use (including some fatalities), though generally in patients on multiple medications, with advanced HIV disease, hepatitis B/C coinfection, and/or immune reconstitution syndrome. Monitor patients closely; consider interrupting or discontinuing therapy if signs/symptoms of liver impairment occur.

May cause fat redistribution (buffalo hump, increased abdominal girth, breast engorgement, facial atrophy). Patients may develop immune reconstitution syndrome resulting in the occurrence of an inflammatory response to an indolent or residual opportunistic infection during initial HIV treatment or activation of autoimmune disorders (eg, Graves' disease, polymyositis, Guillain-Barré syndrome) later in therapy; further evaluation and treatment may be required. May increase cholesterol and/or triglycerides. Pancreatitis has been observed with use. Risk for pancreatitis may be increased in patients with elevated triglycerides, advanced HIV disease, or history of pancreatitis. Protease inhibitors have been associated with glucose dysregulation; use caution in patients with diabetes. Initiation or dose adjustments of antidiabetic agents may be required. Use with caution in patients with sulfonamide allergy (contains sulfa moiety) or hemophilia. Protease inhibitors have been associated with a variety of hypersensitivity events (some severe), including rash, anaphylaxis (rare), angioedema, bronchospasm, erythema multiforme, Stevens-Johnson syndrome (rare), acute generalized exanthematous pustulosis, and/or toxic epidermal necrolysis. Discontinue treatment if severe skin reactions develop. Severe skin reactions may be accompanied by fever, malaise, fatigue, arthralgias, hepatitis, oral lesion, blisters, conjunctivitis, and/or eosinophilia. Mild-to-moderate rash may occur early in treatment and resolve with continued therapy. Treatment history and resistance data should guide use of darunavir with ritonavir.

Drug Interactions

Avoid Concomitant Use

Avoid concomitant use of Darunavir with any of the following: Ado-Trastuzumab Emtansine; Alfuzosin; Amiodarone; Apixaban; Avanafil; Axitinib; Bosutinib; Cabozantinib; Cisapride; Conivaptan; Crizotinib; Dronedarone; Eplerenone; Ergot Derivatives; Everolimus; Fosphenytoin; Fusidic Acid (Systemic); Halofantrine; Ibrutinib; Imatinib; Ivabradine; Lapatinib; Lomitapide; Lopinavir; Lovastatin; Lurasidone; Macitentan; Midazolam; Nilotinib; Nisoldipine; PHENobarbital; Phenytoin; Pimozide; Pomalidomide; QuiNIDine; Ranolazine; Red Yeast Rice; Regorafenib; Rifampin; Rivaroxaban; Salmeterol; Saquinavir; Silodosin; Simeprevir; Simvastatin; St Johns Wort; Tamsulosin; Telaprevir; Ticagrelor; Tolvaptan; Topotecan; Toremifene; Triazolam; Uliprystal; Vemurafenib; VinCRIStine (Liposomal); Voriconazole

Decreased Effect

Darunavir may decrease the levels/effects of: Abacavir; Boceprevir; Clarithromycin; Contraceptives (Estrogens); Delavirdine; Didanosine; Etravirine; Ifosfamide; Meperidine; Methadone; Norethindrone; PARoxetine; Prasugrel; Sertraline; Telaprevir; Theophylline Derivatives; Ticagrelor; Valproic Acid and Derivatives; Voriconazole; Warfarin; Zidovudine

The levels/effects of Darunavir may be decreased by: Boceprevir; Bosentan; CYP3A4 Inducers (Strong); Dabrafenib; Deferasirox; Efavirenz; Fosphenytoin; Garlic; Lopinavir; Mitotane; PHENobarbital; Phenytoin; Rifampin; Saquinavir; St Johns Wort; Telaprevir; Tocilizumab

Increased Effect/Toxicity

Darunavir may increase the levels/effects of: Ado-Trastuzumab Emtansine; Afatinib; Alfuzosin; Almotriptan; Alosetron; ALPRAZolam; Amiodarone; Apixaban; ARIPiprazole; AtorvaSTATin; Avanafil; Axitinib; Bedaquiline; Bortezomib; Bosentan; Bosutinib; Brentuximab Vedotin; Brinzolamide; Budesonide (Nasal); Budesonide (Systemic, Oral Inhalation); Cabozantinib; Calcium Channel Blockers (Dihydropyridine); Calcium Channel Blockers (Nondihydropyridine); CarBAMazepine; Cisapride; Clarithromycin; Colchicine; Conivaptan; Corticosteroids (Orally Inhaled); Crizotinib; CycloSPORINE (Systemic); CYP2D6 Substrates; CYP3A4 Substrates; Dabigatran Etexilate; Dienogest; Digoxin; Dofetilide; DOXOrubicin (Conventional); Dronedarone; Dutasteride; Efavirenz; Enfuvirtide; Enzalutamide; Eplerenone; Ergot Derivatives; Everolimus; FentaNYL; Fesoterodine; Fluticasone (Nasal); Fluticasone (Oral Inhalation); GuanFACINE; Halofantrine; Ibrutinib; Iloperidone; Imatinib; Itraconazole; Ivabradine; Ivacaftor; Ixabepilone; Ketoconazole (Systemic); Lacosamide; Lapatinib; Levomilnacipran; Lomitapide; Lovastatin; Lumefantrine; Lurasidone; Macitentan; Maraviroc; Meperidine; Methyl-PREDNISolone; Midazolam; Mifepristone; Nefazodone; Nilotinib; Nisoldipine; Ospemifene; OxyCODONE; Paricalcitol; PAZOPanib; P-glycoprotein/ABCB1 Substrates; Pimecrolimus; Pimozide; Pomalidomide; PONATinib; Pravastatin; Propafenone; Protease Inhibitors; Prucalopride; QUEtiapine; QuiNIDine; Ranolazine; Red Yeast Rice; Regorafenib; Repaglinide; Rifabutin; Rilpivirine; Riociguat; Rivaroxaban; RomiDEPsin; Rosuvastatin; Ruxolitinib; Salmeterol; Saxagliptin; Sildenafil; Silodosin; Simeprevir; Simvastatin; SORAfenib; Tacrolimus (Systemic); Tacrolimus (Topical); Tadalafil; Tamsulosin; Temsirolimus; Tenofovir; Ticagrelor; Tofacitinib; Tolterodine; Tolvaptan; Topotecan; Toremifene; TraZODone; Triazolam; Tricyclic Antidepressants; Uliprystal; Vardenafil; Vemurafenib; Vilazodone; VinCRIStine (Liposomal); Zuclopenthixol

The levels/effects of Darunavir may be increased by: Clarithromycin; CycloSPORINE (Systemic); CYP3A4 Inhibitors (Moderate); CYP3A4 Inhibitors (Strong); Dasatinib; Delavirdine; Enfuvirtide; Etravirine; Fusidic Acid (Systemic); Itraconazole; Ketoconazole (Systemic); Luliconazole; Rifabutin; Simeprevir; Stiripentol; Tenofovir

Nutritional/Ethanol Interactions

Food: Absorption and bioavailability are increased when administered with food. Management: Take with meals.

Herb/Nutraceutical: St John's wort may decrease the plasma levels of darunavir. Garlic may decrease the serum concentration of darunavir. Management: Taking St John's wort concomitantly with darunavir is contraindicated. Use of garlic supplements with darunavir is not recommended.

Adverse Reactions As a class, protease inhibitors potentially cause dyslipidemias which includes elevated cholesterol and triglycerides and a redistribution of body fat centrally to cause increased abdominal girth, buffalo hump, facial atrophy, and breast enlargement. These agents also cause hyperglycemia. Frequency of adverse events is reported for darunavir/ritonavir. See also Ritonavir monograph.

>10%:

Endocrine & metabolic: Hypercholesterolemia (children: grade 3: 1%; adults: grade 2: 16% to 25%; grade 3: 1% to 10%), increased LDL cholesterol (children: grade 3: 3%; adults: grade 2: 14%; grade 3: 5% to 8%)

Gastrointestinal: Vomiting (children: 13% to 33%; adults 2% to 5%), nausea (4% to 25%), diarrhea (children: 11% to 24%; adults: 8% to 14%)

◄ 2% to 10%:

Central nervous system: Headache (children: 9%; adults: 3% to 6%), fatigue (children: 3%; adults: ≤2%)

Dermatologic: Skin rash (children: 5% to 10%; adults: 6% to 7%), pruritus (children: 8%)

Endocrine & metabolic: Hyperglycemia (grade 2: 7% to 10%; grade 3: ≤1%; grade 4: <1%), increased serum triglycerides (grade 2: 3% to 10%; grade 3: 1% to 7%; grade 4: ≤3%), increased amylase (children: grade 3: 4%, grade 4: 1%; adults: grade 2: 5% to 6%, grade 3: 3% to 7%), diabetes mellitus (2%)

Gastrointestinal: Abdominal pain (children: 8% to 10%; adults: 5% to 6%), decreased appetite (children: 8%; adults: 2%), increased serum lipase (children: grade 3: 1%; adults: grade 2: 2% to 3%, grade 3; ≤2%; grade 4: <1%), abdominal distention (2%), anorexia (2%), dyspepsia (2%)

Hepatic: Increased serum ALT (children: grade 3: 3%; grade 4: 1%; adults: grade 2: 7%, grade 3: 2% to 3%; grade 4: ≤1%), increased serum AST (children: grade 3: 1%; adults: grade 2: 6%; grade 3: 2% to 4%; grade 4: <1%), increased serum alkaline phosphatase (grade 2: ≤2%; grade 3: <1%)

Neuromuscular & skeletal: Weakness (≤3%)

Available Dosage Forms

Suspension, Oral:

Prezista: 100 mg/mL (200 mL)

Tablet, Oral:

Prezista: 75 mg, 150 mg, 600 mg, 800 mg

General Dosage Range Dosage adjustment recommended in patients on concomitant therapy or who develop toxicities.

Oral:

Children ≥3 years

≥10 kg to <11 kg: Darunavir 350 mg once daily with ritonavir 64 mg once daily **or** Darunavir 200 mg twice daily with ritonavir 32 mg twice daily

≥11 kg to <12 kg: Darunavir 385 mg once daily with ritonavir 64 mg once daily **or** Darunavir 220 mg twice daily with ritonavir 32 mg twice daily

≥12 kg to <13 kg: Darunavir 420 mg once daily with ritonavir 80 mg once daily **or** Darunavir 240 mg twice daily with ritonavir 40 mg twice daily

≥13 kg to <14 kg: Darunavir 455 mg once daily with ritonavir 80 mg once daily **or** Darunavir 260 mg twice daily with ritonavir 40 mg twice daily

≥14 kg to <15 kg: Darunavir 490 mg once daily with ritonavir 96 mg once daily **or** Darunavir 280 mg twice daily with ritonavir 48 mg twice daily

≥15 kg to <30 kg: Darunavir 600 mg once daily with ritonavir 100 mg once daily **or** Darunavir

375 mg twice daily with ritonavir 48 mg twice daily

≥30 kg to <40 kg: Darunavir 675 mg once daily with ritonavir 100 mg once daily **or** Darunavir 450 mg twice daily with ritonavir 60 mg twice daily

≥40 kg: Darunavir 800 mg once daily with ritonavir 100 mg once daily **or** Darunavir: 600 mg twice daily with ritonavir 100 mg twice daily

Adults: Darunavir: 600 mg twice daily; Ritonavir: 100 mg twice daily **or** Darunavir: 800 mg once daily; Ritonavir: 100 mg once daily

Administration

Oral Coadministration with ritonavir and food is required (bioavailability is increased). Shake suspension prior to each dose; use provided oral dosing syringe to measure dose.

Storage/Stability Store at 25°C (77°F); excursions permitted to 15°C to 30°C (59°F to 86°F).

Nursing Actions

Physical Assessment Monitor for adherence to regimen. Teach patient proper timing of multiple medications. Monitor for hypersensitivity reaction, gastrointestinal disturbance (nausea, vomiting, diarrhea) that can lead to dehydration and weight loss, hyperlipidemia, and redistribution of body fat. Caution patients with diabetes to monitor glucose levels closely; protease inhibitors may cause alterations in glucose regulation or new onset diabetes. Teach patient to test blood for glucose.

Patient Education

• Discuss specific use of drug and side effects with patient as it relates to treatment. (HCAHPS: During this hospital stay, were you given any medicine that you had not taken before? Before giving you any new medicine, how often did hospital staff tell you what the medicine was for? How often did hospital staff describe possible side effects in a way you could understand?)

• Patient may experience nausea, diarrhea, or dyspepsia. Have patient report immediately to prescriber signs of hepatic impairment, signs of hyperglycemia, signs of pancreatitis, severe dizziness, syncope, significant headache, considerable asthenia, lipodystrophy, signs of Stevens-Johnson syndrome/toxic epidermal necrolysis, or signs of infection (HCAHPS).

• Educate patient about signs of a significant reaction (eg, wheezing; chest tightness; fever; itching; bad cough; blue skin color; seizures; or swelling of face, lips, tongue, or throat). **Note:** This is not a comprehensive list of all side effects. Patient should consult prescriber for additional questions.

Intended Use and Disclaimer: Should not be printed and given to patients. This information is intended to serve as a concise initial reference for healthcare professionals to use when discussing medications with a patient. You must ultimately

rely on your own discretion, experience and judgment in diagnosing, treating and advising patients.

Dietary Considerations Absorption increased with food. Take with meals.

DAUNOrubicin (Conventional)
(daw noe ROO bi sin con VEN sha nal)

Brand Names: U.S. Cerubidine

Index Terms Conventional Daunomycin; Daunomycin; DAUNOrubicin Hydrochloride; Rubidomycin Hydrochloride

Pharmacologic Category Antineoplastic Agent, Anthracycline; Antineoplastic Agent, Topoisomerase II Inhibitor

Medication Safety Issues

Sound-alike/look-alike issues:

DAUNOrubicin may be confused with DACTINomycin, DOXOrubicin, DOXOrubicin liposomal, epirubicin, IDArubicin, valrubicin

Conventional formulation (Cerubidine®, DAUNOrubicin hydrochloride) may be confused with the liposomal formulation (DaunoXome®)

High alert medication:

The Institute for Safe Medication Practices (ISMP) includes this medication among its list of drug classes which have a heightened risk of causing significant patient harm when used in error.

Pregnancy Risk Factor D

Lactation Excretion in breast milk unknown/not recommended

Breast-Feeding Considerations It is not known if daunorubicin is excreted into breast milk. Due to the potential for serious adverse reactions in the nursing infant, the manufacturer recommends a decision be made whether to discontinue nursing or to discontinue the drug, taking into account the importance of treatment to the mother.

Use Treatment of acute lymphocytic leukemia (ALL) and acute myeloid leukemia (AML)

Mechanism of Action/Effect Inhibition of DNA and RNA synthesis by intercalation between DNA base pairs and by steric obstruction. Daunomycin intercalates at points of local uncoiling of the double helix. Although the exact mechanism is unclear, it appears that direct binding to DNA (intercalation) and inhibition of DNA repair (topoisomerase II inhibition) result in blockade of DNA and RNA synthesis and fragmentation of DNA.

Contraindications Hypersensitivity to daunorubicin or any component of the formulation

Warnings/Precautions Hazardous agent - use appropriate precautions for handling and disposal (NIOSH, 2012). **[U.S. Boxed Warning]: Potent vesicant; if extravasation occurs, severe local tissue damage leading to ulceration and necrosis, and pain may occur. For I.V. administration only. NOT for I.M. or SubQ administration. Administer through a rapidly flowing I.V. line.** Ensure proper needle or catheter placement prior to and during infusion. Avoid extravasation. **[U.S. Boxed Warning]: Severe bone marrow suppression may occur; may lead to infection or hemorrhage.**

[U.S. Boxed Warning]: May cause cumulative, dose-related myocardial toxicity; may lead to heart failure. The incidence of irreversible myocardial toxicity increases as the total cumulative (lifetime) dosages approach 550 mg/m² in adults, 400 mg/m² in adults receiving chest radiation, 300 mg/m² in children >2 years of age, or 10 mg/kg in children <2 years of age. Total cumulative dose should take into account previous or concomitant treatment with cardiotoxic agents or irradiation of chest. Although the risk increases with cumulative dose, irreversible cardiotoxicity may occur at any dose level. Cardiotoxicity may be delayed. Patients with pre-existing heart disease, hypertension, concurrent administration of other antineoplastic agents, prior or concurrent chest irradiation, advanced age; and infants and children are at increased risk. Monitor left ventricular (LV) function (baseline and periodic) with ECHO or MUGA scan; monitor ECG.

[U.S. Boxed Warning]: Dosage reductions are recommended in patients with renal or hepatic impairment; significant impairment may result in increased toxicities. Use with caution in patients who have received radiation therapy; reduce dosage in patients who are receiving radiation therapy simultaneously. Secondary leukemias may occur when used with combination chemotherapy or radiation therapy. **[U.S. Boxed Warning]: Should be administered under the supervision of an experienced cancer chemotherapy physician.**

Drug Interactions

Avoid Concomitant Use

Avoid concomitant use of DAUNOrubicin (Conventional) with any of the following: BCG; CloZAPine; Natalizumab; Pimecrolimus; Tacrolimus (Topical); Tofacitinib; Vaccines (Live)

Decreased Effect

DAUNOrubicin (Conventional) may decrease the levels/effects of: BCG; Cardiac Glycosides; Coccidioidin Skin Test; Sipuleucel-T; Vaccines (Inactivated); Vaccines (Live)

The levels/effects of DAUNOrubicin (Conventional) may be decreased by: Cardiac Glycosides; Echinacea; P-glycoprotein/ABCB1 Inducers

Increased Effect/Toxicity

DAUNOrubicin (Conventional) may increase the levels/effects of: CloZAPine; Leflunomide; Natalizumab; Tofacitinib; Vaccines (Live)

The levels/effects of DAUNOrubicin (Conventional) may be increased by: Bevacizumab; Cyclophosphamide; Denosumab; P-glycoprotein/ABCB1 Inhibitors; Pimecrolimus; Roflumilast; Tacrolimus (Topical); Taxane Derivatives; Trastuzumab

Nutritional/Ethanol Interactions Ethanol: Avoid ethanol (due to GI irritation).

Adverse Reactions

>10%:

Cardiovascular: Transient ECG abnormalities (supraventricular tachycardia, S-T wave changes, atrial or ventricular extrasystoles); generally asymptomatic and self-limiting. CHF, dose related, may be delayed for 7-8 years after treatment.

Dermatologic: Alopecia (reversible), radiation recall

Gastrointestinal: Mild nausea or vomiting, stomatitis

Genitourinary: Discoloration of urine (red)

Hematologic: Myelosuppression (onset: 7 days; nadir: 10-14 days; recovery: 21-28 days), primarily leukopenia; thrombocytopenia and anemia

1% to 10%:

Dermatologic: Skin "flare" at injection site; discoloration of saliva, sweat, or tears

Endocrine & metabolic: Hyperuricemia

Gastrointestinal: Abdominal pain, GI ulceration, diarrhea

Available Dosage Forms

Injectable, Intravenous:

Generic: 5 mg/mL (4 mL, 10 mL)

Injectable, Intravenous [preservative free]:

Generic: 5 mg/mL (4 mL)

Solution Reconstituted, Intravenous:

Cerubidine: 20 mg (1 ea)

Generic: 20 mg (1 ea)

General Dosage Range Dosage adjustment recommended in patients with hepatic or renal impairment

I.V.:

Children <2 years or BSA <0.5 m^2: 1 mg/kg/dose per protocol with frequency dependent on regimen employed (maximum cumulative dose: 10 mg/kg)

Children ≥2 years and BSA ≥0.5 m^2: 25 mg/m^2 on day 1 every week for 4 cycles **or** 30-60 mg/m^2/day for 3 days (maximum cumulative dose: 300 mg/m^2)

Adults <60 years: 30-60 mg/m^2/day for 2-3 days (maximum cumulative dose: 550 mg/m^2; 400 mg/m^2 with chest irradiation)

Adults ≥60 years: 30 mg/m^2/day for 2-3 days (maximum cumulative dose: 550 mg/m^2; 400 mg/m^2 with chest irradiation)

Administration

I.V. For I.V. administration only. Do not administer I.M. or SubQ. Administer as slow I.V. push over 1-5 minutes into the tubing of a rapidly infusing

I.V. solution of D$_5$W or NS or may dilute further and infuse over 15-30 minutes.

Vesicant; ensure proper needle or catheter placement prior to and during infusion; avoid extravasation.

Extravasation management: If extravasation occurs, stop infusion immediately and disconnect (leave cannula/needle in place); gently aspirate extravasated solution (do **NOT** flush the line); remove needle/cannula; elevate extremity. Initiate antidote (dexrazoxane or dimethyl sulfate [DMSO]). Apply dry cold compresses for 20 minutes 4 times daily for 1-2 days (Perez Fidalgo, 2012); withhold cooling beginning 15 minutes before dexrazoxane infusion; continue withholding cooling until 15 minutes after infusion is completed. Topical DMSO should not be administered in combination with dexrazoxane; may lessen dexrazoxane efficacy.

Dexrazoxane: Adults: 1000 mg/m^2 (maximum dose: 2000 mg) I.V. (administer in a large vein remote from site of extravasation) over 1-2 hours days 1 and 2, then 500 mg/m^2 (maximum dose: 1000 mg) I.V. over 1-2 hours day 3; begin within 6 hours of extravasation. Day 2 and day 3 doses should be administered at approximately the same time (± 3 hours) as the dose on day 1 (Mouridsen, 2007; Perez Fidalgo, 2012). **Note:** Reduce dexrazoxane dose by 50% in patients with moderate to severe renal impairment (CrCl <40 mL/minute).

DMSO: Children and Adults: Apply topically to a region covering twice the affected area every 8 hours for 7 days; begin within 10 minutes of extravasation; do not cover with a dressing (Perez Fidalgo, 2012).

Hazardous agent; use appropriate precautions for handling and disposal (NIOSH, 2012).

Injectable Detail pH: 3-6.5 (aqueous solution in vial)

Preparation for Administration Hazardous agent; use appropriate precautions for handling and disposal (NIOSH, 2012). Dilute vials of powder for injection with 4 mL SWFI for a final concentration of 5 mg/mL. May further dilute in 100 mL D$_5$W or NS.

Storage/Stability Store intact vials of powder for injection at room temperature of 15°C to 30°C (59°F to 86°F); intact vials of solution for injection should be refrigerated at 2°C to 8°C (36°F to 46°F). Protect from light. Reconstituted solution is stable for 4 days at 15°C to 25°C. Further dilution in D$_5$W, LR, or NS is stable at room temperature (25°C) for up to 4 weeks if protected from light.

Nursing Actions

Physical Assessment Monitor infusion site closely; extravasation can cause severe cellulitis or tissue necrosis (if drug is infiltrated, apply ice to the area, elevate the limb, and consult institutional policy immediately). Monitor for hypertension, tachycardia, cough, dyspnea, and gastrointestinal upset prior to each infusion and throughout therapy.

Patient Education
- Discuss specific use of drug and side effects with patient as it relates to treatment. (HCAHPS: During this hospital stay, were you given any medicine that you had not taken before? Before giving you any new medicine, how often did hospital staff tell you what the medicine was for? How often did hospital staff describe possible side effects in a way you could understand?)
- Patient may experience urine discoloration, stomatitis, cheilitis, or alopecia. Have patient report immediately to prescriber signs of infection, angina, syncope, severe dyspepsia, significant nausea, excessive weight loss, considerable diarrhea, ecchymosis, hemorrhaging, intolerable asthenia, osteodynia, or night sweats (HCAHPS).
- Educate patient about signs of a significant reaction (eg, wheezing; chest tightness; fever; itching; bad cough; blue skin color; seizures; or swelling of face, lips, tongue, or throat). **Note:** This is not a comprehensive list of all side effects. Patient should consult prescriber for additional questions.

Intended Use and Disclaimer: Should not be printed and given to patients. This information is intended to serve as a concise initial reference for healthcare professionals to use when discussing medications with a patient. You must ultimately rely on your own discretion, experience and judgment in diagnosing, treating and advising patients.

Related Information
Management of Drug Extravasations *on page 1700*

Decitabine (de SYE ta been)

Brand Names: U.S. Dacogen
Index Terms 5-Aza-2'-deoxycytidine; 5-Aza-dCyd; Deoxyazacytidine; Dezocitidine
Pharmacologic Category Antineoplastic Agent, Antimetabolite; Antineoplastic Agent, DNA Methylation Inhibitor
Medication Safety Issues
Sound-alike/look-alike issues:
Dacogen® may be confused with DACTINomycin
High alert medication:
This medication is in a class the Institute for Safe Medication Practices (ISMP) includes among its list of drug classes which have a heightened risk of causing significant patient harm when used in error.
Pregnancy Risk Factor D
Lactation Excretion in breast milk unknown/not recommended

Breast-Feeding Considerations Due to the potential for serious adverse reactions in the nursing infant, breast-feeding is not recommended.
Use Treatment of myelodysplastic syndrome (MDS)
Unlabeled Use Treatment of acute myelogenous leukemia (AML), sickle cell anemia
Mechanism of Action/Effect Hypomethylating agent
Contraindications There are no contraindications listed within the manufacturer's labeling.
Warnings/Precautions Hazardous agent - use appropriate precautions for handling and disposal (NIOSH, 2012). The dose-limiting toxicity is bone marrow suppression; worsening neutropenia is common in first two treatment cycles and may not correlate with progression of underlying MDS; may require dosage adjustment (after the first cycle), growth factor support and/or antimicrobial agents; monitor for infection. Not studied in hepatic and renal disease; use caution.
Drug Interactions
Avoid Concomitant Use
Avoid concomitant use of Decitabine with any of the following: CloZAPine
Decreased Effect There are no known significant interactions involving a decrease in effect.
Increased Effect/Toxicity
Decitabine may increase the levels/effects of: CloZAPine
Adverse Reactions
>10%:
Cardiovascular: Peripheral edema (25% to 27%), pallor (23%), edema (5% to 18%), cardiac murmur (16%), hypotension (6% to 11%)
Central nervous system: Fever (6% to 53%), fatigue (46%), headache (23% to 28%), insomnia (14% to 28%), dizziness (18% to 21%), chills (16%), pain (5% to 13%), confusion (8% to 12%), lethargy (12%), anxiety (9% to 11%), hypoesthesia (11%)
Dermatologic: Petechiae (12% to 39%), bruising (9% to 22%), rash (11% to 19%), erythema (5% to 14%), cellulitis (9% to 12%), lesions (5% to 11%), pruritus (9% to 11%)
Endocrine & metabolic: Hyperglycemia (6% to 33%), hypoalbuminemia (7% to 24%), hypomagnesemia (5% to 24%), hypokalemia (12% to 22%), hyperkalemia (13%), hyponatremia (19%)
Gastrointestinal: Nausea (40% to 42%), constipation (30% to 35%), diarrhea (28% to 34%), vomiting (16% to 25%), anorexia/appetite decreased (8% to 23%), abdominal pain (5% to 14%), oral mucosal petechiae (13%), stomatitis (11% to 12%), dyspepsia (10% to 12%)
Hematologic: Neutropenia (38% to 90%; grades 3/4: 37% to 87%; recovery 28-50 days), thrombocytopenia (27% to 89%; grades 3/4: 24% to 85%), anemia (31% to 82%; grades 3/4: 22%), febrile neutropenia (20% to 29%; grades 3/4: 23%), leukopenia (6% to 28%; grades 3/4: 22%), lymphadenopathy (12%)

Hepatic: Hyperbilirubinemia (6% to 14%), alkaline phosphatase increased (11%)

Local: Tenderness (11%)

Neuromuscular & skeletal: Rigors (22%), arthralgia (17% to 20%), limb pain (18% to 19%), back pain (17% to 18%), weakness (15%)

Respiratory: Cough (27% to 40%), dyspnea (29%), pneumonia (20% to 22%), pharyngitis (16%), lung crackles (14%), epistaxis (13%)

5% to 10%:

Cardiovascular: Tachycardia (8%), chest pain/discomfort (6% to 7%), facial edema (6%), hypertension (6%), heart failure (5%)

Central nervous system: Depression (9%), malaise (5%)

Dermatologic: Alopecia (8%), dry skin (8%), urticaria (6%)

Endocrine & metabolic: Hyperuricemia (10%), LDH increased (8%), bicarbonate increased (6%), dehydration (6% to 8%), hypochloremia (6%), bicarbonate decreased (5%), hypoproteinemia (5%)

Gastrointestinal: Mucosal inflammation (9%), weight loss (9%), gingival bleeding (8%), hemorrhoids (8%), loose stools (7%), tongue ulceration (7%), dysphagia (5% to 6%), oral candidiasis (6%), toothache (6%), abdominal distension (5%), gastroesophageal reflux (5%), glossodynia (5%), lip ulceration (5%), oral pain (5%), tooth abscess (5%)

Genitourinary: Urinary tract infection (7%), dysuria (6%), polyuria (5%)

Hematologic: Bacteremia (5% to 8%), hematoma (5%), pancytopenia (5%), thrombocythemia (5%)

Hepatic: Ascites (10%), AST increased (10%), hypobilirubinemia (5%)

Local: Catheter infection (8%), catheter site erythema (5%), catheter site pain (5%), injection site swelling (5%)

Neuromuscular & skeletal: Myalgia (5% to 9%), falling (8%), chest wall pain (7%), muscle spasm (7%), bone pain (6%), musculoskeletal pain/discomfort (5% to 6%), crepitation (5%)

Ocular: Blurred vision (6%)

Otic: Ear pain (6%)

Respiratory: Breath sounds abnormal (5% to 10%), hypoxia (10%), upper respiratory tract infection (10%), pharyngolaryngeal pain (8%), rales (8%), pulmonary edema (6%), sinusitis (5% to 6%), pleural effusion (5%), postnasal drip (5%), sinus congestion (5%)

Miscellaneous: Candidal infection (10%), staphylococcal infection (7%), transfusion reaction (7%), night sweats (5%)

Available Dosage Forms

Solution Reconstituted, Intravenous:

Dacogen: 50 mg (1 ea)

Generic: 50 mg (1 ea)

General Dosage Range Dosage adjustment recommended in patients who develop toxicities

I.V.: *Adults:* 15 mg/m^2 every 8 hours for 3 days every 6 weeks **or** 20 mg/m^2 daily for 5 days every 28 days

Administration

I.V. Infuse over 1-3 hours. Premedication with antiemetics is recommended.

Hazardous agent; use appropriate precautions for handling and disposal (NIOSH, 2012).

Injectable Detail pH: 6.7-7.3

Preparation for Administration Hazardous agent; use appropriate precautions for handling and disposal (NIOSH, 2012). Vials should be reconstituted with 10 mL SWFI to a concentration of 5 mg/mL. Immediately further dilute with 50-250 mL NS, D$_5$W, or lactated Ringer's to a final concentration of 0.1-1 mg/mL. Use appropriate precautions for handling and disposal. Solutions not administered within 15 minutes of preparation should be prepared with cold (2°C to 8°C [36°F to 46°F]) infusion solutions.

Storage/Stability Store vials at 25°C (77°F); excursions permitted to 15°C to 30°C (59°F to 86°F). Solutions diluted for infusion may be stored for up to 7 hours under refrigeration at 2°C to 8°C (36°F to 46°F) if prepared with cold infusion fluids.

Nursing Actions

Physical Assessment Premedication with antiemetic may be ordered. Monitor for worsening neutropenia, thrombocytopenia, anemia, pulmonary edema, gastrointestinal disturbance, CNS changes, hyperglycemia, and infection prior to each cycle and periodically as indicated during therapy. Advise patients with diabetes to monitor serum glucose closely (may cause hyperglycemia).

Patient Education

- Discuss specific use of drug and side effects with patient as it relates to treatment. (HCAHPS: During this hospital stay, were you given any medicine that you had not taken before? Before giving you any new medicine, how often did hospital staff tell you what the medicine was for? How often did hospital staff describe possible side effects in a way you could understand?)

- Patient may experience dizziness, asthenia, dyspepsia, stomatitis, insomnia, lack of appetite, headache, arthralgia, or back pain. Have patient report immediately to prescriber signs of infection, signs of hepatic impairment, dyspnea, severe nausea, considerable constipation, intolerable diarrhea, ecchymosis, hemorrhaging, significant edema, signs of hyperglycemia, or signs of fluid and electrolyte imbalance (HCAHPS).

- Educate patient about signs of a significant reaction (eg, wheezing; chest tightness; fever; itching; bad cough; blue skin color; seizures; or swelling of face, lips, tongue, or throat). **Note:** This is not a comprehensive list of all side effects. Patient should consult prescriber for additional questions.

Intended Use and Disclaimer: Should not be printed and given to patients. This information is intended to serve as a concise initial reference for healthcare professionals to use when discussing medications with a patient. You must ultimately rely on your own discretion, experience and judgment in diagnosing, treating and advising patients.

Deferasirox (de FER a sir ox)

Brand Names: U.S. Exjade
Index Terms ICL670
Pharmacologic Category Chelating Agent
Medication Safety Issues
  Sound-alike/look-alike issues:
  Deferasirox may be confused with deferiprone, deferoxamine
Pregnancy Risk Factor C
Lactation Excretion in breast milk unknown/not recommended
Use Chronic iron overload: Treatment of chronic iron overload due to blood transfusions (transfusional hemosiderosis) or due to non-transfusion-dependent thalassemia syndromes and with a liver iron concentration (LIC) of at least 5 mg iron per gram of liver dry weight (mg Fe/g dw) and serum ferritin >300 mcg/L.
Available Dosage Forms
Tablet Soluble, Oral:
  Exjade: 125 mg, 250 mg, 500 mg
General Dosage Range Dosage adjustment recommended in patients with renal or hepatic impairment or on concomitant therapy
  Oral: *Children ≥2 years, Adolescents, and Adults:*
  Initial: 20 mg/kg once daily; Maintenance (usual): 20-30 mg/kg once daily (maximum: 40 mg/kg/day)
Administration
  Oral Administer tablets by making an oral suspension; **do not chew or swallow tablets whole.** Completely disperse tablets in water, orange juice, or apple juice (use 3.5 ounces for total doses <1 g; 7 ounces for doses ≥1 g); stir to form a fine suspension and drink entire contents. Rinse remaining residue with more fluid; drink. Avoid dispersion of tablets in milk (due to slowed dissolution) or carbonated drinks (due to foaming) (Séchaud, 2008). Administer at same time each day on an empty stomach, at least 30 minutes before food. Do not take simultaneously with aluminum-containing antacids.
Nursing Actions
  Physical Assessment Assess hearing and vision prior to initiating therapy and periodically during treatment. Observe for skin rash. Mild-to-moderate rashes will usually resolve spontaneously. Assess for signs of liver dysfunction (eg, unusual fatigue, easy bruising or bleeding, jaundice), gastrointestinal bleeding (blood in vomitus

or stool), and renal dysfunction (eg, unusual weight gain, swelling of extremities, decrease in urine output).
Patient Education
• Discuss specific use of drug and side effects with patient as it relates to treatment. (HCAHPS: During this hospital stay, were you given any medicine that you had not taken before? Before giving you any new medicine, how often did hospital staff tell you what the medicine was for? How often did hospital staff describe possible side effects in a way you could understand?)
• Patient may experience dyspepsia or dizziness. Have patient report immediately to prescriber signs of infection, signs of renal impairment, signs of hepatic impairment, severe nausea, significant diarrhea, hearing impairment, vision changes, considerable asthenia, ecchymosis, hemorrhaging, melena, hematemesis, intolerable dyspepsia, severe skin irritation, or signs of Stevens-Johnson syndrome/toxic epidermal necrolysis (HCAHPS).
• Educate patient about signs of a significant reaction (eg, wheezing; chest tightness; fever; itching; bad cough; blue skin color; seizures; or swelling of face, lips, tongue, or throat). **Note:** This is not a comprehensive list of all side effects. Patient should consult prescriber for additional questions.

Intended Use and Disclaimer: Should not be printed and given to patients. This information is intended to serve as a concise initial reference for healthcare professionals to use when discussing medications with a patient. You must ultimately rely on your own discretion, experience and judgment in diagnosing, treating and advising patients.

Deferiprone (de FER i prone)

Brand Names: U.S. Ferriprox
Index Terms APO-066; Ferriprox®
Pharmacologic Category Chelating Agent
Medication Safety Issues
  Sound-alike/look-alike issues:
  Deferiprone may be confused with deferoxamine, deferasirox
Medication Guide Available Yes
Pregnancy Risk Factor D
Lactation Excretion in breast milk unknown/not recommended
Use Treatment of transfusional iron overload due to thalassemia syndromes with inadequate response to other chelation therapy
Available Dosage Forms
Tablet, Oral:
  Ferriprox: 500 mg
General Dosage Range Oral: *Adults:* 25-33 mg/kg 3 times/day (maximum: 99 mg/kg/day)

◄ **Administration**

Oral Administer in the morning, at mid day and in the evening. Administration with food may decrease nausea.

Nursing Actions

Physical Assessment Assess allergy history prior to beginning therapy. May monitor bloodwork for neutropenia or increased ALT or AST.

Patient Education

• Discuss specific use of drug and side effects with patient as it relates to treatment. (HCAHPS: During this hospital stay, were you given any medicine that you had not taken before? Before giving you any new medicine, how often did hospital staff tell you what the medicine was for? How often did hospital staff describe possible side effects in a way you could understand?)

• Patient may experience arthralgia, dyspepsia, or urine discoloration. Have patient report immediately to prescriber signs of infection, severe dizziness, syncope, tachycardia, arrhythmia, considerable nausea, ecchymosis, hemorrhaging, or signs of hepatic impairment (HCAHPS).

• Educate patient about signs of a significant reaction (eg, wheezing; chest tightness; fever; itching; bad cough; blue skin color; seizures; or swelling of face, lips, tongue, or throat). **Note:** This is not a comprehensive list of all side effects. Patient should consult prescriber for additional questions.

Intended Use and Disclaimer: Should not be printed and given to patients. This information is intended to serve as a concise initial reference for healthcare professionals to use when discussing medications with a patient. You must ultimately rely on your own discretion, experience and judgment in diagnosing, treating and advising patients.

Deferoxamine (de fer OKS a meen)

Brand Names: U.S. Desferal

Index Terms Deferoxamine Mesylate; Desferrioxamine; DFM

Pharmacologic Category Antidote; Chelating Agent

Medication Safety Issues

Sound-alike/look-alike issues:

Deferoxamine may be confused with cefuroxime, deferasirox, deferiprone

Desferal® may be confused with desflurane, Desyrel®, Dexferrum®

International issues:

Desferal [U.S., Canada, and multiple international markets] may be confused with Deseril brand name for methysergide [Australia, Belgium, Great Britain, Netherlands]; Disophrol brand name for dexbrompheniramine and pseudoephedrine [Czech Republic, Poland, Turkey]

Pregnancy Risk Factor C

Lactation Excretion in breast milk unknown/use caution

Use Adjunct in the treatment of acute iron intoxication; treatment of chronic iron overload secondary to multiple transfusions

Canadian labeling (unlabeled use in the U.S.): Diagnosis of aluminum overload; treatment of chronic aluminum overload in patients with end-stage renal failure undergoing maintenance dialysis

Unlabeled Use Diagnosis or treatment of aluminum induced toxicity associated with chronic kidney disease (CKD)

Available Dosage Forms

Solution Reconstituted, Injection:

Desferal: 500 mg (1 ea); 2 g (1 ea)

Generic: 500 mg (1 ea); 2 g (1 ea)

General Dosage Range Dosage adjustment recommended in patients with renal impairment

I.M.: *Adults:* Initial: 1000 mg, followed by 500 mg every 4 hours for 2 doses; Maintenance: 500 mg every 4-12 hours **or** 500-1000 mg once daily (maximum: 6000 mg/day)

I.V.:

Children ≥3 years: 20-40 mg/kg/day 5-7 days per week; dose should not exceed 40 mg/kg/day until growth has ceased

Adults: Initial: 1000 mg, followed by 500 mg every 4 hours for 2 doses; Maintenance: 500 mg every 4-12 hours (maximum: 6000 mg/day) **or** 40-50 mg/kg/day (maximum: 60 mg/kg/day) 5-7 days per week

SubQ:

Children ≥3 years: 20-40 mg/kg/day (maximum: 1000-2000 mg/day)

Adults: 1000-2000 mg/day **or** 20-40 mg/kg/day

Administration

I.M. I.M. administration may be used for patients with acute iron toxicity that do not exhibit severe symptoms (per the manufacturer); may also be used in the treatment of chronic iron toxicity.

I.V. Urticaria, flushing of the skin, hypotension, and shock have occurred following rapid I.V. administration; limiting infusion rate to 15mg/kg/hour may help avoid infusion-related adverse effects.

Acute iron toxicity: The manufacturer states that the I.M. route is preferred; however, the I.V. route is generally preferred in patients with severe toxicity (ie, patients in shock). For the first 1000 mg, infuse at 15 mg/kg/hour. Subsequent doses may be given over 4-12 hours at a rate not to exceed 125 mg/hour.

Chronic iron overload: Administer over 8-12 hours for 5-7 days per week; rate not to exceed 15 mg/kg/hour. In patients with poor compliance, deferoxamine may be administered on the same day of blood transfusion, either prior to or following transfusion; do not administer concurrently with transfusion. Longer infusion times (24 hours) and I.V. administration may be required in patients with severe cardiac iron deposition (Brittenham, 2011).

Diagnosis or treatment of aluminum-induced toxicity with CKD: Administer dose over 1 hour during the last hour of dialysis (K/DOQI guidelines, 2003).

Other SubQ: When administered for chronic iron overload, administration over 8-12 hours using a portable infusion pump is generally recommended; however, longer infusion times (24 hours) may also be used. Topical anesthetic or glucocorticoid creams may be used for induration or erythema (Brittenham, 2011).

Nursing Actions
Physical Assessment Infuse slowly and monitor infusion site. Monitor for acute reactions; urticaria, hypotension, and shock can occur following rapid I.V. administration. With chronic therapy, perform ophthalmologic exam (fundoscopy, slit-lamp exam) and audiometry. Teach patient proper injection technique and syringe/needle disposal. Monitor for adverse cardiac, respiratory, or CNS symptoms and teach patient importance of reporting adverse symptoms.

Patient Education
• Discuss specific use of drug and side effects with patient as it relates to treatment. (HCAHPS: During this hospital stay, were you given any medicine that you had not taken before? Before giving you any new medicine, how often did hospital staff tell you what the medicine was for? How often did hospital staff describe possible side effects in a way you could understand?)
• Patient may experience urine discoloration, headache, nausea, diarrhea, muscle spasms, arthralgia, or myalgia. Have patient report immediately to prescriber signs of infection, severe dizziness, syncope, dyspnea, signs of renal impairment, vision changes, hearing impairment, tinnitus, paresthesia, significant injection site irritation, or considerable skin irritation, or rash (HCAHPS).
• Educate patient about signs of a significant reaction (eg, wheezing; chest tightness; fever; itching; bad cough; blue skin color; seizures; or swelling of face, lips, tongue, or throat). **Note:** This is not a comprehensive list of all side effects. Patient should consult prescriber for additional questions.

Intended Use and Disclaimer: Should not be printed and given to patients. This information is intended to serve as a concise initial reference for healthcare professionals to use when discussing medications with a patient. You must ultimately rely on your own discretion, experience and judgment in diagnosing, treating and advising patients.

Degarelix (deg a REL ix)

Brand Names: U.S. Firmagon
Index Terms Degarelix Acetate; FE200486
Pharmacologic Category Antineoplastic Agent, Gonadotropin-Releasing Hormone Antagonist; Gonadotropin Releasing Hormone Antagonist

Medication Safety Issues
Sound-alike/look-alike issues:
Degarelix may be confused with cetrorelix, ganirelix

Pregnancy Risk Factor X
Lactation Excretion in breast milk unknown/not recommended
Use Treatment of advanced prostate cancer

Available Dosage Forms
Solution Reconstituted, Subcutaneous:
Firmagon: 80 mg (1 ea); 120 mg (1 ea)
General Dosage Range SubQ: *Adults:* Loading dose: 240 mg; Maintenance dose: 80 mg every 28 days

Administration
Subcutaneous Administer (deep) SubQ in the abdominal area by pinching skin and elevating SubQ tissue; insert needle deeply at a 45 degree angle. Avoid pressure exposed areas (eg, waistband, belt, or near ribs). Rotate injection site. Inject loading dose as two 3 mL injections (40 mg/mL) in different sites; maintenance dose should be administered as a single 4 mL injection (20 mg/mL); begin maintenance dose 28 days after initial loading dose.

Not for I.V. use; do not inject into a vein or into muscle.

Hazardous agent; use appropriate precautions for handling and disposal (NIOSH, 2012).

Nursing Actions
Physical Assessment Monitor PSA and serum testosterone levels, LFTs, electrolytes, and bone density on a regular basis during therapy. Supplemental calcium and vitamin D may be ordered to reduce risk of osteoporosis due to androgen deprivation.

Patient Education
• Discuss specific use of drug and side effects with patient as it relates to treatment. (HCAHPS: During this hospital stay, were you given any medicine that you had not taken before? Before giving you any new medicine, how often did hospital staff tell you what the medicine was for? How often did hospital staff describe possible side effects in a way you could understand?)
• Patient may experience weight gain, sexual dysfunction, asthenia, hot flashes, back pain, arthralgia, or chills. Have patient report immediately to prescriber arrhythmia, severe headache, significant dizziness, dysuria, difficult urination, osteodynia, or injection site irritation (HCAHPS).

• Educate patient about signs of a significant reaction (eg, wheezing; chest tightness; fever; itching; bad cough; blue skin color; seizures; or swelling of face, lips, tongue, or throat). **Note:** This is not a comprehensive list of all side effects. Patient should consult prescriber for additional questions.

Intended Use and Disclaimer: Should not be printed and given to patients. This information is intended to serve as a concise initial reference for healthcare professionals to use when discussing medications with a patient. You must ultimately rely on your own discretion, experience and judgment in diagnosing, treating and advising patients.

Delavirdine (de la VIR deen)

Brand Names: U.S. Rescriptor
Index Terms DLV; U-90152S
Pharmacologic Category Antiretroviral, Reverse Transcriptase Inhibitor, Non-nucleoside (Anti-HIV)
Medication Safety Issues
Sound-alike/look-alike issues:
Delavirdine may be confused with dalfampridine
Pregnancy Risk Factor C
Lactation Excretion in breast milk unknown/contraindicated
Breast-Feeding Considerations Maternal or infant antiretroviral therapy does not completely eliminate the risk of postnatal HIV transmission. In addition, multiclass-resistant virus has been detected in breast-feeding infants despite maternal therapy. Therefore, in the United States, where formula is accessible, affordable, safe, and sustainable, and the risk of infant mortality due to diarrhea and respiratory infections is low, complete avoidance of breast-feeding by HIV-infected women is recommended to decrease potential transmission of HIV (DHHS [perinatal], 2012).
Use Treatment of HIV-1 infection in combination with at least two additional antiretroviral agents
Mechanism of Action/Effect Delavirdine binds directly to reverse transcriptase, blocking RNA-dependent and DNA-dependent DNA polymerase activities
Contraindications Hypersensitivity to delavirdine or any component of the formulation; concurrent use of alprazolam, astemizole, cisapride, ergot alkaloids, midazolam, pimozide, rifampin, terfenadine, or triazolam
Warnings/Precautions Use with caution in patients with hepatic or renal dysfunction; due to rapid emergence of resistance, delavirdine should not be used as monotherapy or as a component of an initial antiretroviral regimen; cross-resistance may be conferred to other non-nucleoside reverse transcriptase inhibitors, although potential for cross-resistance with protease inhibitors is low. Long-term effects of delavirdine are not known.

May cause redistribution of fat (eg, buffalo hump, peripheral wasting with increased abdominal girth, cushingoid appearance). Patients may develop immune reconstitution syndrome resulting in the occurrence of an inflammatory response to an indolent or residual opportunistic infection during initial HIV treatment or activation of autoimmune disorders (eg, Graves' disease, polymyositis, Guillain-Barré syndrome) later in therapy; further evaluation and treatment may be required. Safety and efficacy have not been established in children. Rash, which occurs frequently, may require discontinuation of therapy; usually occurs within 1-3 weeks and lasts <2 weeks. Most patients may resume therapy following a treatment interruption. Use with caution in patients taking strong CYP3A4 inhibitors, moderate or strong CYP3A4 inducers and major CYP3A4 substrates (see Drug Interactions); consider alternative agents that avoid or lessen the potential for CYP-mediated interactions.

Drug Interactions
Avoid Concomitant Use
Avoid concomitant use of Delavirdine with any of the following: Ado-Trastuzumab Emtansine; Alfuzosin; Apixaban; Astemizole; Avanafil; Axitinib; Bosutinib; Cabozantinib; CarBAMazepine; Conivaptan; Crizotinib; Dronedarone; Eplerenone; Etravirine; Everolimus; Fosamprenavir; Fosphenytoin; H2-Antagonists; Halofantrine; Ibrutinib; Imatinib; Ivabradine; Lapatinib; Lomitapide; Lovastatin; Lurasidone; Macitentan; Nilotinib; Nisoldipine; Phenytoin; Pimozide; Pomalidomide; Proton Pump Inhibitors; Ranolazine; Red Yeast Rice; Regorafenib; Rilpivirine; Rivaroxaban; Salmeterol; Silodosin; Simeprevir; Simvastatin; St Johns Wort; Tamoxifen; Tamsulosin; Terfenadine; Thioridazine; Ticagrelor; Tolvaptan; Toremifene; Ulipristal; Vemurafenib; VinCRIStine (Liposomal)

Decreased Effect
Delavirdine may decrease the levels/effects of: CarBAMazepine; Clopidogrel; Codeine; Etravirine; Ifosfamide; Iloperidone; Prasugrel; Rilpivirine; Tamoxifen; Ticagrelor; TraMADol

The levels/effects of Delavirdine may be decreased by: Antacids; CarBAMazepine; CYP3A4 Inducers (Strong); Dabrafenib; Deferasirox; Fosamprenavir; Fosphenytoin; H2-Antagonists; Mitotane; Peginterferon Alfa-2b; Phenytoin; Protease Inhibitors; Proton Pump Inhibitors; Rifamycin Derivatives; St Johns Wort; Tocilizumab

Increased Effect/Toxicity
Delavirdine may increase the levels/effects of: Ado-Trastuzumab Emtansine; Alfuzosin; Almotriptan; Alosetron; Apixaban; ARIPiprazole; Astemizole; AtoMOXetine; Avanafil; Axitinib; Bedaquiline; Bortezomib; Bosentan; Bosutinib; Brentuximab Vedotin; Brinzolamide; Budesonide (Nasal); Budesonide (Systemic, Oral Inhalation); Cabozantinib; Carvedilol; Citalopram; Colchicine; Conivaptan; Corticosteroids (Orally Inhaled);

Crizotinib; CYP2C19 Substrates; CYP2C9 Substrates; CYP2D6 Substrates; CYP3A4 Substrates; Diclofenac (Systemic); Dienogest; Dofetilide; DOXOrubicin (Conventional); Dronedarone; Dutasteride; Enzalutamide; Eplerenone; Etravirine; Everolimus; FentaNYL; Fesoterodine; Fluticasone (Nasal); Fluticasone (Oral Inhalation); Fosamprenavir; Fosphenytoin; GuanFACINE; Halofantrine; Ibrutinib; Iloperidone; Imatinib; Ivabradine; Ivacaftor; Ixabepilone; Lacosamide; Lapatinib; Levomilnacipran; Lomitapide; Lovastatin; Lumefantrine; Lurasidone; Macitentan; Maraviroc; MethylPREDNISolone; Metoprolol; Mifepristone; Nebivolol; Nilotinib; Nisoldipine; Ospemifene; OxyCODONE; Paricalcitol; PAZOPanib; Phenytoin; Pimecrolimus; Pimozide; Pomalidomide; PONATinib; Propafenone; Protease Inhibitors; QUEtiapine; Ranolazine; Red Yeast Rice; Regorafenib; Repaglinide; Rifamycin Derivatives; Rilpivirine; Rivaroxaban; RomiDEPsin; Ruxolitinib; Salmeterol; Saxagliptin; Sildenafil; Silodosin; Simeprevir; Simvastatin; SORAfenib; Tadalafil; Tamsulosin; Terfenadine; Tetrabenazine; Thioridazine; Ticagrelor; Tofacitinib; Tolterodine; Tolvaptan; Toremifene; Ulipristal; Vardenafil; Vemurafenib; Vilazodone; VinCRIStine (Liposomal); Vortioxetine; Zuclopenthixol

Nutritional/Ethanol Interactions Herb/Nutraceutical: Delavirdine serum concentration may be decreased by St John's wort; avoid concurrent use.

Adverse Reactions

Frequency of adverse reactions reported from occurrence in clinical trials with delavirdine when used as part of combination antiretroviral therapy.

>10%:
Central nervous system: Headache (19% to 20%), depressive symptoms (10% to 15%), fever (4% to 12%)
Dermatologic: Rash (16% to 32%)
Gastrointestinal: Nausea (20% to 25%), vomiting (3% to 11%)
1% to 10%:
Central nervous system: Anxiety (6% to 8%)
Endocrine & metabolic: Transaminases increased (2% to 5%), amylase increased (3%), bilirubin increased (2%)
Gastrointestinal: Diarrhea, vomiting, abdominal pain (4% to 6%)
Hematologic: Prothrombin time increased (2%), hemoglobin decreased (1% to 3%)
Respiratory: Bronchitis (6% to 8%)
Frequency not defined (limited to important or life threatening): Abscess, adenopathy, alkaline phosphatase increased, allergic reaction, angioedema, anorexia, arrhythmia, bloody stool, bone pain, bruising, cardiac insufficiency, cardiac rate abnormal, cardiomyopathy, chest congestion, cognitive impairment, colitis, confusion, conjunctivitis, dermal leukocytoclastic vasculitis, desquamation, diverticulitis, dyspnea, emotional lability,

eosinophilia, erythema multiforme, fecal incontinence, fungal dermatitis, gamma glutamyl transpeptidase increased, gastroenteritis, gastrointestinal bleeding, granulocytosis, gum hemorrhage, hallucination, hematuria, hepatomegaly, hyperglycemia, hyperkalemia, hypertension, hypertriglyceridemia, hyperuricemia, hypocalcemia, hyponatremia, hypophosphatemia, infection, jaundice, kidney pain, leukopenia, lipase increased, menstrual irregularities, moniliasis (oral/vaginal), orthostatic hypotension, pancreatitis, pancytopenia, paralysis, peripheral vascular disorder, pneumonia, purpura, redistribution of body fat, renal calculi, serum creatinine increased, spleen disorder, Stevens-Johnson syndrome, tetany, thrombocytopenia, urinary tract infection, vertigo

Available Dosage Forms

Tablet, Oral:
Rescriptor: 100 mg, 200 mg
General Dosage Range Oral: *Children ≥16 years and Adults:* 400 mg 3 times/day

Administration

Oral Patients with achlorhydria should take the drug with an acidic beverage. Antacids and delavirdine should be separated by 1 hour. A dispersion of delavirdine may be prepared by adding four 100 mg tablets to at least 3 oz of water. Allow to stand for a few minutes and stir until uniform dispersion. Drink immediately. Rinse glass and mouth, then swallow the rinse to ensure total dose administered. The 200 mg tablets should be taken intact.

Storage/Stability Store at 20°C to 25°C (68°F to 77°F). Protect from humidity.

Nursing Actions

Physical Assessment Monitor for rash and gastrointestinal upset. Teach patient proper timing of multiple medications.

Patient Education

• Discuss specific use of drug and side effects with patient as it relates to treatment. (HCAHPS: During this hospital stay, were you given any medicine that you had not taken before? Before giving you any new medicine, how often did hospital staff tell you what the medicine was for? How often did hospital staff describe possible side effects in a way you could understand?)
• Patient may experience lipodystrophy, nausea, diarrhea, or dyspepsia. Have patient report immediately to prescriber signs of hepatic impairment, signs of pancreatitis, osteodynia, paresthesia, urinary retention, oliguria, illogical thinking, change in balance, tachycardia, bradycardia, arrhythmia, hallucinations, memory loss, moods changes, depression, myalgia, severe dizziness, syncope, considerable headache, dyspnea, edema of extremities, tremors, ecchymosis, hemorrhaging, significant asthenia, vision changes, signs of Stevens-Johnson

syndrome/toxic epidermal necrolysis, or signs of infection (HCAHPS).

- Educate patient about signs of a significant reaction (eg, wheezing; chest tightness; fever; itching; bad cough; blue skin color; seizures; or swelling of face, lips, tongue, or throat). **Note:** This is not a comprehensive list of all side effects. Patient should consult prescriber for additional questions.

Intended Use and Disclaimer: Should not be printed and given to patients. This information is intended to serve as a concise initial reference for healthcare professionals to use when discussing medications with a patient. You must ultimately rely on your own discretion, experience and judgment in diagnosing, treating and advising patients.

Dietary Considerations May be taken without regard to meals.

Related Information

Oral Medications That Should Not Be Crushed or Altered *on page 1712*

Demeclocycline (dem e kloe SYE kleen)

Index Terms Declomycin; Demeclocycline Hydrochloride; Demethylchlortetracycline

Pharmacologic Category Antibiotic, Tetracycline Derivative

Pregnancy Risk Factor D

Lactation Enters breast milk/not recommended

Use Treatment of susceptible bacterial infections (eg, acne, urinary tract infections, respiratory infections) caused by both gram-negative and gram-positive organisms

Note: Use of demeclocycline as an antibacterial agent is uncommon; alternative tetracycline agents (eg, doxycycline, minocycline, tetracycline) are generally preferred.

Unlabeled Use Treatment of chronic syndrome of inappropriate secretion of antidiuretic hormone (SIADH)

Available Dosage Forms

Tablet, Oral:

Generic: 150 mg, 300 mg

General Dosage Range Dosage adjustment recommended in patients with renal and hepatic impairment

Oral:

Children >8 years: 7-13 mg/kg/day (maximum: 600 mg/day) divided every 6-12 hours

Adults: 600 mg/day in 2 or 4 divided doses

Administration

Oral Administer 1 hour before or 2 hours after food or milk. Administer with adequate amounts of fluid to decrease the risk of esophageal irritation and ulceration.

Nursing Actions

Physical Assessment Results of culture and sensitivity tests and patient's allergy history

should be assessed prior to beginning therapy. Monitor for rash, anaphylactic reactions, anemia, and CNS changes.

Patient Education

- Discuss specific use of drug and side effects with patient as it relates to treatment. (HCAHPS: During this hospital stay, were you given any medicine that you had not taken before? Before giving you any new medicine, how often did hospital staff tell you what the medicine was for? How often did hospital staff describe possible side effects in a way you could understand?)
- Patient may experience diarrhea, dizziness, nausea, or lack of appetite. Have patient report immediately to prescriber signs of hepatic impairment, vision changes, urinary retention, oliguria, chills, pharyngitis, polydipsia, myalgia, severe headache, ecchymosis, hemorrhaging, considerable asthenia, vaginal yeast infection, or signs of pseudomembranous colitis (HCAHPS).
- Educate patient about signs of a significant reaction (eg, wheezing; chest tightness; fever; itching; bad cough; blue skin color; seizures; or swelling of face, lips, tongue, or throat). **Note:** This is not a comprehensive list of all side effects. Patient should consult prescriber for additional questions.

Intended Use and Disclaimer: Should not be printed and given to patients. This information is intended to serve as a concise initial reference for healthcare professionals to use when discussing medications with a patient. You must ultimately rely on your own discretion, experience and judgment in diagnosing, treating and advising patients.

Denosumab (den OH sue mab)

Brand Names: U.S. Prolia; Xgeva

Index Terms AMG-162

Pharmacologic Category Bone-Modifying Agent; Monoclonal Antibody

Medication Safety Issues

Sound-alike/look-alike issues:

Xgeva may be confused with Jevtana, Xofigo, Xtandi, Zometa, Zytiga

Other safety concerns:

Duplicate therapy issues: Prolia contains denosumab, which is the same ingredient contained in Xgeva; patients receiving Xgeva should not be treated with Prolia

Medication Guide Available Yes

Pregnancy Risk Factor D (Xgeva)/X (Prolia)

Lactation Excretion unknown/not recommended

Breast-Feeding Considerations It is not known if denosumab is excreted in breast milk. According to the manufacturer, the decision to discontinue denosumab or discontinue breast-feeding should take into account the benefits of treatment to the mother. In some animal studies, mammary gland development was impaired following exposure to denosumab during pregnancy, resulting in impaired lactation postpartum.

Use

Osteoporosis/bone loss (Prolia): Treatment of osteoporosis in postmenopausal women at high risk of fracture; treatment of osteoporosis (to increase bone mass) in men at high risk of fracture; treatment of bone loss in men receiving androgen-deprivation therapy (ADT) for nonmetastatic prostate cancer; treatment of bone loss in women receiving aromatase inhibitor (AI) therapy for breast cancer

Tumors (Xgeva): Prevention of skeletal-related events (eg, fracture, spinal cord compression, bone pain requiring surgery/radiation therapy) in patients with bone metastases from solid tumors; treatment of giant cell tumor of the bone in adults and skeletally mature adolescents that is unresectable or where surgical resection is likely to result in severe morbidity

Note: NOT indicated for prevention of skeletal-related events in patients with multiple myeloma

Unlabeled Use Treatment of bone destruction caused by rheumatoid arthritis

Mechanism of Action/Effect Denosumab is a monoclonal antibody which causes decreased bone resorption, increased bone mass, decreased skeletal-related events in solid tumors and inhibits tumor growth in giant cell tumor of the bone.

Contraindications Hypersensitivity to denosumab or any component of the formulation; pre-existing hypocalcemia; pregnancy (Prolia)

Warnings/Precautions Clinically significant hypersensitivity (including anaphylaxis) has been reported. May include throat tightness, facial edema, upper airway edema, dyspnea, pruritus, rash, urticaria, and hypotension. If anaphylaxis or clinically significant hypersensitivity occurs, initiate appropriate management and permanently discontinue. Denosumab may cause or exacerbate hypocalcemia; severe symptomatic cases (including fatalities) have been reported. Monitor calcium levels; correct pre-existing hypocalcemia prior to therapy. Use caution in patients with a history of hypoparathyroidism, thyroid surgery, parathyroid surgery, malabsorption syndromes, excision of small intestine, severe renal impairment/dialysis or other conditions which would predispose the patient to hypocalcemia; monitor calcium, phosphorus, and magnesium closely during therapy. Ensure adequate calcium and vitamin D intake; supplement with calcium and vitamin D; magnesium supplementation may also be necessary. Incidence of infections may be increased, including serious skin infections, abdominal, urinary, ear, or periodontal infections. Endocarditis has also been reported following use. Patients should be advised to contact their healthcare provider if signs or symptoms of severe infection or cellulitis develop.

Use with caution in patients with impaired immune systems or using concomitant immunosuppressive therapy; may be at increased risk for serious infections. Evaluate the need for continued treatment with serious infection.

Atypical femur fractures have been reported in patients receiving denosumab. The fractures may occur anywhere along the femoral shaft (may be bilateral) and commonly occur with minimal to no trauma to the area. Some patients experience prodromal pain weeks or months before the fracture occurs. Because these fractures also occur in osteoporosis patients not treated with denosumab, it is unclear if denosumab therapy is the cause for the fractures; concomitant glucocorticoids may contribute to fracture risk. Advise patients to report new/unusual hip, thigh, or groin pain; and if so, evaluate for atypical/incomplete fracture. Contralateral limb should be assessed if atypical fracture occurs. Consider interrupting therapy in patients who develop an atypical femoral fracture. Osteonecrosis of the jaw (ONJ) has been reported in patients receiving denosumab. ONJ may manifest as jaw pain, osteomyelitis, osteitis, bone erosion, tooth/periodontal infection, toothache, gingival ulceration/erosion. Risk factors include invasive dental procedures (eg, tooth extraction, dental implants, boney surgery); a diagnosis of cancer, concomitant chemotherapy or corticosteroids, poor oral hygiene, ill-fitting dentures; and comorbid disorders (anemia, coagulopathy, infection, pre-existing dental disease). In studies of patients with osseous metastasis, a longer duration of denosumab exposure was associated with a higher incidence of ONJ. Patients should maintain good oral hygiene during treatment. A dental exam and preventative dentistry should be performed prior to therapy. The benefit/risk must be assessed by the treating physician and/or dentist/surgeon prior to any invasive dental procedure; avoid invasive procedures in patients with bone metastases receiving therapy for prevention of skeletal-related events. Patients developing ONJ while on denosumab therapy should receive care by a dentist or oral surgeon; extensive dental surgery to treat ONJ may exacerbate ONJ; evaluate individually and consider discontinuing if extensive dental surgery is necessary.

Postmenopausal osteoporosis: For use in women at high risk for fracture which is defined as a history of osteoporotic fracture or multiple risk factors for fracture. May also be used in women who failed or did not tolerate other therapies.

Bone metastases: Denosumab is not indicated for the prevention of skeletal-related events in patients with multiple myeloma. In trials of with multiple myeloma patients, denosumab was noninferior to zoledronic acid in delaying time to first skeletal-related event and mortality was increased in a subset of the denosumab-treated group.

Denosumab therapy results in significant suppression of bone turnover; the long term effects of treatment are not known but may contribute to adverse outcomes such as ONJ, atypical fractures, or delayed fracture healing; monitor. Use with caution in patients with renal impairment (CrCl <30 mL/minute) or patients on dialysis; risk of hypocalcemia is increased. Dose adjustment is not needed when administered at 60 mg every 6 months (Prolia); once-monthly dosing has not been evaluated in patients with renal impairment (Xgeva). Dermatitis, eczema, and rash (which are not necessarily specific to the injection site) have been reported; consider discontinuing if severe symptoms occur. Packaging may contain natural latex rubber. May impair bone growth in children with open growth plates or inhibit eruption of dentition. In pediatrics, indicated only for the treatment of giant cell tumor of the bone in adolescents who are skeletally mature. Do not administer Prolia and Xgeva to the same patient for different indications.

Drug Interactions

Avoid Concomitant Use There are no known interactions where it is recommended to avoid concomitant use.

Decreased Effect There are no known significant interactions involving a decrease in effect.

Increased Effect/Toxicity
Denosumab may increase the levels/effects of: Immunosuppressants

Nutritional/Ethanol Interactions Ethanol: Ethanol may increase risk of osteoporosis. Management: Avoid ethanol.

Adverse Reactions A postmarketing safety program for Prolia is available to collect information on adverse events; more information is available at http://www.proliasafety.com. To report adverse events for either Prolia or Xgeva, prescribers may also call Amgen at 800-772-6436 or FDA at 800-332-1088.

Percentages noted with Prolia (60 mg every 6 months) unless specified as Xgeva (120 mg every 4 weeks):

>10%:
Central nervous system: Fatigue (Xgeva: 45%), headache (Xgeva: 13%)

Dermatologic: Dermatitis (4% to 11%), eczema (4% to 11%), skin rash (3% to 11%)

Endocrine & metabolic: Hypophosphatemia (Xgeva: 32%; grade 3: 10% to 15%), hypocalcemia (2%; Xgeva: 3% to 18%; grade 3: 3%)

Gastrointestinal: Nausea (Xgeva: 31%), diarrhea (Xgeva: 20%)

Neuromuscular & skeletal: Weakness (Xgeva: 45%), arthralgia (7% to 14%), limb pain (10% to 12%), back pain (8% to 12%)

Respiratory: Dyspnea (Xgeva: 21%), cough (Xgeva: 15%)

1% to 10%:
Cardiovascular: Peripheral edema (5%), angina pectoris (3%)

Central nervous system: Sciatica (5%)

Endocrine & metabolic: Hypercholesterolemia (7%)

Gastrointestinal: Flatulence (2%)

Hematologic & oncologic: Malignant neoplasm (new; 3% to 5%)

Infection: Serious infection (nonfatal; 4%)

Neuromuscular & skeletal: Musculoskeletal pain (6%), bone pain (4%), myalgia (3%), osteonecrosis (jaw; ≤2%; Xgeva ≤2%)

Ophthalmic: Cataract (≤5%)

Respiratory: Nasopharyngitis (7%), upper respiratory tract infection (5%)

Pharmacodynamics/Kinetics

Onset of Action Decreases markers of bone resorption by ~85% within 3 days; maximal reductions observed within 1 month

Duration of Action Markers of bone resorption return to baseline within 12 months of discontinuing therapy

Available Dosage Forms

Solution, Subcutaneous [preservative free]:
Prolia: 60 mg/mL (1 mL)
Xgeva: 120 mg/1.7 mL (1.7 mL)

General Dosage Range SubQ:

Adolescents (skeletally mature) 13-17 years: 120 mg every 4 weeks with an addition dose on days 8 and 15 in the first month only

Adults: Prolia: 60 mg every 6 months; Xgeva: 120 mg every 4 weeks **or** 120 mg every 4 weeks with additional doses on days 8 and 15 in the first month only

Administration

Subcutaneous Prior to administration, bring to room temperature in original container (allow to stand ~15-30 minutes); do not warm by any other method. Solution may contain trace amounts of translucent to white protein particles; do not use if cloudy, discolored (normal solution should be clear and colorless to pale yellow), or contains excessive particles or foreign matter. Avoid vigorous shaking. Administer via SubQ injection in the upper arm, upper thigh, or abdomen.

Prolia: If a dose is missed, administer as soon as possible, then continue dosing every 6 months from the date of the last injection.

Storage/Stability Prior to use, store in original carton under refrigeration, 2°C to 8°C (36°F to 46°F). Do not freeze. Prior to use, bring to room temperature of 25°C (77°F) in original container (usually takes 15-30 minutes); do not use any other methods for warming. Use within 14 days once at room temperature. Protect from direct heat and light; do not expose to temperatures >25°C (77°F). Avoid vigorous shaking.

Nursing Actions

Physical Assessment Assess for signs and symptoms of low calcium; provide education regarding need for dental exam prior to initiation of medication. Assess for and report increased pain in hips, groin, or thighs with long-term use of medication. Stress importance of good oral hygiene. Monitor lab results: Calcium, magnesium, phosphate. Instruct patient that drug should be taken along with vitamin D and calcium.

Patient Education

- Discuss specific use of drug and side effects with patient as it relates to treatment. (HCAHPS: During this hospital stay, were you given any medicine that you had not taken before? Before giving you any new medicine, how often did hospital staff tell you what the medicine was for? How often did hospital staff describe possible side effects in a way you could understand?)
- Patient may experience headache, nausea, diarrhea, back pain, arthralgia, pharyngitis, rhinorrhea, or painful extremities. Have patient report immediately to prescriber signs of hypocalcemia; stomatitis; groin, hip, or thigh pain; severe jaw bone pain; lack of appetite; considerable asthenia; myalgia; dyspnea; signs of infection; signs of pancreatitis; angina; arrhythmia; significant skin irritation; cystalgia; dysuria; oliguria; polyuria; or edema of extremities (HCAHPS).
- Educate patient about signs of a significant reaction (eg, wheezing; chest tightness; fever; itching; bad cough; blue skin color; seizures; or swelling of face, lips, tongue, or throat). **Note:** This is not a comprehensive list of all side effects. Patient should consult prescriber for additional questions.

Intended Use and Disclaimer: Should not be printed and given to patients. This information is intended to serve as a concise initial reference for healthcare professionals to use when discussing medications with a patient. You must ultimately rely on your own discretion, experience and judgment in diagnosing, treating and advising patients.

Dietary Considerations Ensure adequate calcium and vitamin D intake to prevent or treat hypocalcemia. Calcium 1000 mg/day and vitamin D ≥400 units/day is recommended in product labeling (Prolia). If dietary intake is inadequate, dietary supplementation is recommended. Women and men should consume:
Calcium: 1000 mg/day (men: 50-70 years) **or** 1200 mg/day (women ≥51 years and men ≥71 years) (IOM, 2011; NOF, 2013)
Vitamin D: 800-1000 IU/day (men and women ≥50 years) (NOF, 2013). Recommended Dietary Allowance (RDA): 600 IU/day (men and women ≤70 years) **or** 800 IU/day (men and women ≥71 years) (IOM, 2011).

Desipramine (des IP ra meen)

Brand Names: U.S. Norpramin
Index Terms Desipramine Hydrochloride; Desmethylimipramine Hydrochloride
Pharmacologic Category Antidepressant, Tricyclic (Secondary Amine)
Medication Safety Issues
Sound-alike/look-alike issues:
Desipramine may be confused with clomiPRAMINE, dalfampridine, diphenhydrAMINE, disopyramide, imipramine, nortriptyline
Norpramin® may be confused with clomiPRAMINE, imipramine, Normodyne®, Norpace®, nortriptyline, Tenormin®
BEERS Criteria medication:
This drug may be potentially inappropriate for use in geriatric patients (SIADH: Quality of evidence - moderate; Strength of recommendation - strong).
International issues:
Norpramin: Brand name for desipramine [U.S., Canada], but also the brand name for enalapril/hydrochlorothiazide [Portugal]; omeprazole [Spain]
Medication Guide Available Yes
Lactation Enters breast milk
Use Treatment of depression
Unlabeled Use Analgesic adjunct in chronic pain; peripheral neuropathies (including diabetic neuropathy); attention-deficit/hyperactivity disorder (ADHD); depression in children ≤12 years of age
Available Dosage Forms
Tablet, Oral:
Norpramin: 10 mg, 25 mg, 50 mg, 75 mg, 100 mg, 150 mg
Generic: 10 mg, 25 mg, 50 mg, 75 mg, 100 mg, 150 mg
General Dosage Range Oral:
Adolescents: 25-100 mg/day in single or divided doses (maximum: 150 mg/day)
Adults: 100-200 mg/day in single or divided doses (maximum: 300 mg/day)
Elderly: 25-100 mg/day in single or divided doses (maximum: 150 mg/day)
Nursing Actions
Physical Assessment Monitor CNS status. Assess cardiac and seizure history prior to initiating therapy. Assess for suicidal tendencies before beginning therapy, during initiation of therapy, or following an increase or decrease of dosage. Caution patients with diabetes to monitor glucose levels closely; may increase or decrease serum glucose levels. Taper dose slowly when discontinuing.

Patient Education
- Discuss specific use of drug and side effects with patient as it relates to treatment. (HCAHPS: During this hospital stay, were you given any medicine that you had not taken before? Before

giving you any new medicine, how often did hospital staff tell you what the medicine was for? How often did hospital staff describe possible side effects in a way you could understand?)
- Patient may experience xerostomia or fatigue. Have patient report immediately to prescriber suicidal ideation, syncope, illogical thinking, difficult urination, significant asthenia, vision changes, ecchymosis, hemorrhaging, angina, paresthesia, difficulty speaking, bradykinesia, rigidity, difficulty with motor activity, chills, pharyngitis, considerable constipation, signs of neuroleptic malignant syndrome, or serotonin syndrome (ie, dizziness, severe headache, agitation, hallucinations, tachycardia, arrhythmia, flushing, tremors, hyperhidrosis, change in balance, severe nausea, significant diarrhea) (HCAHPS).
- Educate patient about signs of a significant reaction (eg, wheezing; chest tightness; fever; itching; bad cough; blue skin color; seizures; or swelling of face, lips, tongue, or throat). **Note:** This is not a comprehensive list of all side effects. Patient should consult prescriber for additional questions.

Intended Use and Disclaimer: Should not be printed and given to patients. This information is intended to serve as a concise initial reference for healthcare professionals to use when discussing medications with a patient. You must ultimately rely on your own discretion, experience and judgment in diagnosing, treating and advising patients.

Desirudin (des i ROO din)

Brand Names: U.S. Iprivask
Index Terms CGP-39393; Desulfato-Hirudin; Desulfatohirudin; Desulphatohirudin; r-Hirudin; Recombinant Desulfatohirudin; Recombinant Hirudin
Pharmacologic Category Anticoagulant; Anticoagulant, Direct Thrombin Inhibitor
Medication Safety Issues
High alert medication:
  The Institute for Safe Medication Practices (ISMP) includes this medication among its list of drugs which have a heightened risk of causing significant patient harm when used in error.
Pregnancy Risk Factor C
Lactation Excretion in breast milk unknown/use caution
Breast-Feeding Considerations Due to the low enteral absorption of desirudin, it is unlikely to cause significant adverse events in a nursing infant, if it is present in breast milk. Use of desirudin may be continued in breast-feeding women (Guyatt, 2012).
Use Prophylaxis of deep vein thrombosis (DVT) in patients undergoing surgery for hip replacement

Mechanism of Action/Effect Desirudin is a direct, highly selective thrombin inhibitor. Reversibly binds to the active thrombin site of free and clot-associated thrombin. Inhibits fibrin formation, activation of coagulation factors V, VII, and XIII, and thrombin-induced platelet aggregation resulting in a dose-dependent prolongation of the activated partial thromboplastin time (aPTT).
Contraindications Hypersensitivity to natural or recombinant hirudins; active bleeding and/or irreversible coagulation disorders
Warnings/Precautions [U.S. Boxed Warning]: Patients with recent or anticipated neuraxial anesthesia (epidural or spinal anesthesia) are at risk of epidural or spinal hematoma and subsequent paralysis. Consider risk versus benefit prior to neuraxial anesthesia; risk is increased by concomitant agents which may alter hemostasis, as well as traumatic or repeated epidural or spinal puncture. Patient should be observed closely for bleeding and signs and symptoms of neurological impairment if therapy is administered during or immediately following diagnostic lumbar puncture, epidural anesthesia, or spinal anesthesia.

Allergic and hypersensitivity reactions, including anaphylaxis and fatal anaphylactoid reactions have been reported with other hirudin derivatives. Exercise caution when re-exposing patients (anaphylaxis has been reported). Monitor patient closely for signs or symptoms of bleeding. Certain patients are at increased risk of bleeding. Risk factors include bacterial endocarditis; congenital or acquired bleeding disorders; active ulcerative or angiodysplastic GI diseases; severe uncontrolled hypertension; history of hemorrhagic stroke; use shortly after brain, spinal, or ophthalmology surgery; patients treated concomitantly with platelet inhibitors; recent GI bleeding; thrombocytopenia or platelet defects; renal impairment; hepatic impairment; hypertensive or diabetic retinopathy; or in patients undergoing invasive procedures. Do not administer with other agents that increase the risk of hemorrhage unless coadministration cannot be avoided. Discontinue if bleeding occurs. Contraindicated with active bleeding and/or irreversible coagulation disorders.

Do **not** administer intramuscularly (I.M.). Do not use interchangeably (unit-for-unit) with other hirudins. Use with caution in patients with moderate-to-severe renal dysfunction (CrCl <60 mL/minute/1.73 m^2); dosage reduction is necessary; monitor aPTT and renal function daily.
Drug Interactions
Avoid Concomitant Use
  Avoid concomitant use of Desirudin with any of the following: Apixaban; Dabigatran Etexilate; Omacetaxine; Rivaroxaban; Urokinase

Decreased Effect

The levels/effects of Desirudin may be decreased by: Estrogen Derivatives; Progestins

Increased Effect/Toxicity

Desirudin may increase the levels/effects of: Anticoagulants; Collagenase (Systemic); Deferasirox; Ibritumomab; Omacetaxine; Rivaroxaban; Tositumomab and Iodine I 131 Tositumomab

The levels/effects of Desirudin may be increased by: Agents with Antiplatelet Properties; Apixaban; Dabigatran Etexilate; Dasatinib; Herbs (Anticoagulant/Antiplatelet Properties); Ibrutinib; Nonsteroidal Anti-Inflammatory Agents; Omega-3 Fatty Acids; Pentosan Polysulfate Sodium; Prostacyclin Analogues; Salicylates; Sugammadex; Thrombolytic Agents; Tibolone; Tipranavir; Urokinase; Vitamin E

Nutritional/Ethanol Interactions

Herb/Nutraceutical: Avoid alfalfa, anise, bilberry, bladderwrack, bromelain, cat's claw, celery, coleus, cordyceps, dong quai, evening primrose oil, fenugreek, feverfew, garlic, ginger, ginkgo biloba, ginseng (American/Panax/Siberian), grapeseed, green tea, guggul, horse chestnut seed, horseradish, licorice, prickly ash, red clover, reishi, sweet clover, turmeric, white willow (all possess anticoagulant or antiplatelet activity and as such, may enhance the anticoagulant effects of desirudin).

Adverse Reactions

As with all anticoagulants, bleeding is the major adverse effect. Hemorrhage may occur at any site.

2% to 10%:

Gastrointestinal: Nausea (2%)

Hematologic: Hematoma (6%), hemorrhage (major, <1% to 3%; may include cases of intracranial, retroperitoneal, intraocular, intraspinal, or prosthetic joint hemorrhage), anemia (3%)

Local: Injection site mass (4%), deep thrombophlebitis (2%)

Miscellaneous: Wound secretion (4%)

Available Dosage Forms

Solution Reconstituted, Subcutaneous:

Iprivask: 15 mg (1 ea)

General Dosage Range Dosage adjustment recommended in patients with renal impairment

SubQ: *Adults:* 15 mg every 12 hours

Administration

I.M. Do **not** administer I.M.

Other For SubQ administration only. Administration should be alternated between the left and right anterolateral and left and right posterolateral thigh or abdominal wall. Insert needle into a skin fold held between the thumb and forefinger; the skin fold should be held throughout the injection. Do not rub injection site. Do not mix with other injections or infusions. Administer according to recommended regimen.

Preparation for Administration Attach enclosed vial adapter to vial containing desirudin. Remove syringe cap and attach provided syringe containing diluent to adapter on vial. Slowly push plunger down to transfer entire contents of syringe into vial. Do not remove syringe from vial adapter. Gently swirl solution; round tablet in vial will dissolve within 10 seconds. Resultant solution concentration is 31.5 mg/mL (15.75 mg/0.5 mL provides a 15 mg dose). Turn vial upside down; withdraw appropriate dose amount back into syringe. Remove syringe from vial. Attach enclosed Eclipse™ needle (or any needle appropriate for subcutaneous administration); pull pink lever down and uncap needle; ready for injection. After injection, flip up pink lever to cover needle until it snaps into place; dispose of syringe appropriately.

Storage/Stability Store at 25°C (77°F); excursions permitted to 15°C to 30°C (59°F to 86°F). Protect from light. Following reconstitution, solution may be stored at room temperature for up to 24 hours. Discard unused solution after 24 hours.

Nursing Actions

Physical Assessment Monitor patient closely for anaphylactic reaction; treatment for anaphylactic reactions should be available. Bleeding precautions should be observed and patient monitored for signs or symptoms of bleeding (discontinue if bleeding occurs). Monitor for hypersensitivity reaction and bleeding regularly during therapy. Teach patient bleeding precautions.

Patient Education

- Discuss specific use of drug and side effects with patient as it relates to treatment. (HCAHPS: During this hospital stay, were you given any medicine that you had not taken before? Before giving you any new medicine, how often did hospital staff tell you what the medicine was for? How often did hospital staff describe possible side effects in a way you could understand?)
- Have patient report immediately to prescriber severe dizziness, syncope, strength differences from one side to another, difficulty speaking or thinking, change in balance, blurred vision, back pain, illogical thinking, significant headache, edema of extremities, ecchymosis, hemorrhaging, hematemesis, hematuria, melena, intolerable asthenia, or severe injection site irritation (HCAHPS).
- Educate patient about signs of a significant reaction (eg, wheezing; chest tightness; fever; itching; bad cough; blue skin color; seizures; or swelling of face, lips, tongue, or throat). **Note:** This is not a comprehensive list of all side effects. Patient should consult prescriber for additional questions.

Intended Use and Disclaimer: Should not be printed and given to patients. This information is intended to serve as a concise initial reference for healthcare professionals to use when discussing medications with a patient. You must ultimately rely on your own discretion, experience and

judgment in diagnosing, treating and advising patients.

Desloratadine (des lor AT a deen)

Brand Names: U.S. Clarinex; Clarinex Reditabs

Pharmacologic Category Histamine H_1 Antagonist; Histamine H_1 Antagonist, Second Generation; Piperidine Derivative

Medication Safety Issues

Sound-alike/look-alike issues:

Clarinex® may be confused with Celebrex®

Pregnancy Risk Factor C

Lactation Enters breast milk/not recommended

Breast-Feeding Considerations Desloratadine is excreted into breast milk. According to the manufacturer, the decision to continue or discontinue breast-feeding during therapy should take into account the risk of exposure to the infant and the benefits of treatment to the mother.

Use Relief of nasal and non-nasal symptoms of seasonal allergic rhinitis (SAR) and perennial allergic rhinitis (PAR); treatment of chronic idiopathic urticaria (CIU)

Mechanism of Action/Effect Desloratadine is a long-acting antihistamine with selective H_1 receptor antagonistic activity.

Contraindications Hypersensitivity to desloratadine, loratadine, or any component of the formulation

Warnings/Precautions Hypersensitivity reactions (including anaphylaxis) have been reported with use; discontinue therapy immediately with signs/symptoms of hypersensitivity. Dose should be adjusted in patients with liver or renal impairment. Use with caution in patients known to be slow metabolizers of desloratadine (incidence of side effects may be increased). Some products may contain phenylalanine.

Drug Interactions

Avoid Concomitant Use

Avoid concomitant use of Desloratadine with any of the following: Aclidinium; Azelastine (Nasal); Ipratropium (Oral Inhalation); Paraldehyde; Thalidomide; Tiotropium; Umeclidinium

Decreased Effect

Desloratadine may decrease the levels/effects of: Acetylcholinesterase Inhibitors (Central); Benzylpenicilloyl Polylysine; Betahistine; Hyaluronidase

The levels/effects of Desloratadine may be decreased by: Acetylcholinesterase Inhibitors (Central); Amphetamines; P-glycoprotein/ABCB1 Inducers

Increased Effect/Toxicity

Desloratadine may increase the levels/effects of: Alcohol (Ethyl); Analgesics (Opioid); Anticholinergics; Azelastine (Nasal); Buprenorphine; CNS Depressants; Hydrocodone; Methotrimeprazine; Metyrosine; Mirtazapine; Paraldehyde; Pramipexole; ROPINIRole; Rotigotine; Selective Serotonin Reuptake Inhibitors; Thalidomide; Tiotropium; Zolpidem

The levels/effects of Desloratadine may be increased by: Aclidinium; Brimonidine (Topical); Doxylamine; Droperidol; HydrOXYzine; Ipratropium (Oral Inhalation); Magnesium Sulfate; Methotrimeprazine; Perampanel; P-glycoprotein/ABCB1 Inhibitors; Pramlintide; Sodium Oxybate; Tapentadol; Umeclidinium

Nutritional/Ethanol Interactions

Ethanol: May increase CNS depression; monitor for increased effects with coadministration. Caution patients about effects.

Food: Does not affect bioavailability.

Adverse Reactions Note: Frequency reported in children, unless otherwise noted.

>10%:

Central nervous system: Fever (12% to 17%), headache (adults 14%), irritability (12%)

Gastrointestinal: Diarrhea (15% to 20%)

Respiratory: Upper respiratory tract infection (11% to 21%), cough (11%)

1% to 10%:

Central nervous system: Somnolence (children 9%; adults 2%), insomnia (5%), fatigue (adults 2% to 5%), dizziness (adults 4%), emotional lability (3%)

Dermatologic: Erythema (3%), maculopapular rash (3%)

Endocrine & metabolic: Dysmenorrhea (adults 2%)

Gastrointestinal: Vomiting (6%), anorexia (5%), nausea (children 3%; adults 5%), nausea (5%), appetite increased (3%), dyspepsia (adults 3%), xerostomia (adults 3%)

Genitourinary: Urinary tract infection (4%)

Neuromuscular & skeletal: Myalgia (adults 2% to 3%)

Otic: Otitis media (children 6%)

Respiratory: Bronchitis (6%), rhinorrhea (5%), pharyngitis (children 3% to 5%; adults 3% to 4%), epistaxis (3%)

Miscellaneous: Varicella infection (4%), parasitic infection (3%)

Pharmacodynamics/Kinetics

Onset of Action Within 1 hour

Duration of Action 24 hours

Available Dosage Forms

Syrup, Oral:

Clarinex: 0.5 mg/mL (473 mL)

Tablet, Oral:

Clarinex: 5 mg

Generic: 5 mg

Tablet Dispersible, Oral:

Clarinex Reditabs: 2.5 mg, 5 mg

Generic: 2.5 mg, 5 mg

General Dosage Range Dosage adjustment recommended in adult patients with hepatic or renal impairment. Dosage not established in children with hepatic or renal impairment.

Oral:
Children 6-11 months: 1 mg once daily
Children 1-5 years: 1.25 mg once daily
Children 6-11 years: 2.5 mg once daily
Children ≥12 years and Adults: 5 mg once daily

Administration

Oral May be taken with or without food.

RediTabs® should be placed on the tongue; tablet will disintegrate immediately. Take immediately after removing from blister package. Allow tablet to dissolve completely before swallowing. May be taken with or without water.

Syrup: A commercially-available measuring dropper or syringe calibrated to deliver 2 mL or 2.5 mL should be used to administer age-appropriate doses in children.

Storage/Stability Syrup, tablet, orally-disintegrating tablet: Store at 25°C (77°F); excursions permitted between 15°C to 30°C (59°F to 85°F). Protect from moisture and excessive heat. Use orally-disintegrating tablet immediately after opening blister package. Syrup should be protected from light.

Nursing Actions

Patient Education

- Discuss specific use of drug and side effects with patient as it relates to treatment. (HCAHPS: During this hospital stay, were you given any medicine that you had not taken before? Before giving you any new medicine, how often did hospital staff tell you what the medicine was for? How often did hospital staff describe possible side effects in a way you could understand?)
- Patient may experience headache, xerostomia, pharyngitis, myalgia, fatigue, or dysmenorrhea. Have patient report immediately to prescriber severe asthenia (HCAHPS).
- Educate patient about signs of a significant reaction (eg, wheezing; chest tightness; fever; itching; bad cough; blue skin color; seizures; or swelling of face, lips, tongue, or throat). **Note:** This is not a comprehensive list of all side effects. Patient should consult prescriber for additional questions.

Intended Use and Disclaimer: Should not be printed and given to patients. This information is intended to serve as a concise initial reference for healthcare professionals to use when discussing medications with a patient. You must ultimately rely on your own discretion, experience and judgment in diagnosing, treating and advising patients.

Dietary Considerations May be taken with or without food. Some products may contain phenylalanine.

Desmopressin (des moe PRES in)

Brand Names: U.S. DDAVP; DDAVP Rhinal Tube; Stimate

Index Terms 1-Deamino-8-D-Arginine Vasopressin; Desmopressin Acetate

Pharmacologic Category Antihemophilic Agent; Hemostatic Agent; Hormone, Posterior Pituitary; Vasopressin Analog, Synthetic

Pregnancy Risk Factor B

Lactation Excretion in breast milk unknown/use caution

Breast-Feeding Considerations It is not known if desmopressin is excreted in breast milk. The manufacturer recommends that caution be exercised when administering desmopressin to nursing women.

Use

Injection: Treatment of diabetes insipidus; maintenance of hemostasis and control of bleeding in hemophilia A with factor VIII coagulant activity levels >5% and mild-to-moderate classic von Willebrand's disease (type 1) with factor VIII coagulant activity levels >5%

Nasal solutions (DDAVP® Nasal Spray and DDAVP® Rhinal Tube): Treatment of central diabetes insipidus

Nasal spray (Stimate®): Maintenance of hemostasis and control of bleeding in hemophilia A with factor VIII coagulant activity levels >5% and mild-to-moderate classic von Willebrand's disease (type 1) with factor VIII coagulant activity levels >5%

Tablet: Treatment of central diabetes insipidus, temporary polyuria and polydipsia following pituitary surgery or head trauma, primary nocturnal enuresis

Unlabeled Use Uremic bleeding associated with acute or chronic renal failure; prevention of surgical bleeding in patients with uremia

Mechanism of Action/Effect Enhances reabsorption of water in the kidneys by increasing permeability of the collecting ducts; raises plasma levels of von Willebrand factor and factor VIII

Contraindications Hypersensitivity to desmopressin or any component of the formulation; hyponatremia or a history of hyponatremia; moderate-to-severe renal impairment (CrCl<50 mL/minute)

Canadian labeling: Additional contraindications (not in U.S. labeling): Type 2B or platelet-type (pseudo) von Willebrand's disease (injection, intranasal, oral, sublingual); known hyponatremia, habitual or psychogenic polydipsia, cardiac insufficiency or other conditions requiring diuretic therapy (intranasal, sublingual); nephrosis, severe hepatic dysfunction (sublingual); primary nocturnal enuresis (intranasal)

Warnings/Precautions Allergic reactions and anaphylaxis have been reported rarely with both the I.V. and intranasal formulations. Fluid intake should be adjusted downward in the elderly and very young patients to decrease the possibility of water intoxication and hyponatremia. Use may rarely lead to extreme decreases in plasma ▶

osmolality, resulting in seizures, coma, and death. Use caution with cystic fibrosis, heart failure, renal dysfunction, polydipsia (habitual or psychogenic [contraindicated in Canadian labeling]), or other conditions associated with fluid and electrolyte imbalance due to potential hyponatremia. Use caution with coronary artery insufficiency or hypertensive cardiovascular disease; may increase or decrease blood pressure leading to changes in heart rate. Consider switching from nasal to intravenous solution if changes in the nasal mucosa (scarring, edema) occur leading to unreliable absorption. Use caution in patients predisposed to thrombus formation; thrombotic events (acute cerebrovascular thrombosis, acute myocardial infarction) have occurred (rare).

Desmopressin (intranasal and I.V.), when used for hemostasis in hemophilia, is not for use in hemophilia B, type 2B von Willebrand disease, severe classic von Willebrand disease (type 1), or in patients with factor VIII antibodies. In general, desmopressin is also not recommended for use in patients with ≤5% factor VIII activity level, although it may be considered in selected patients with activity levels between 2% and 5%.

Consider switching from nasal to intravenous administration if changes in the nasal mucosa (scarring, edema) occur leading to unreliable absorption. Consider alternative rout of administration (I.V. or intranasal) with inadequate therapeutic response at maximum recommended oral doses. Therapy should be interrupted if patient experiences an acute illness (eg, fever, recurrent vomiting or diarrhea), vigorous exercise, or any condition associated with an increase in water consumption. Some patients may demonstrate a change in response after long-term therapy (>6 months) characterized as decreased response or a shorter duration of response.

Drug Interactions

Avoid Concomitant Use There are no known interactions where it is recommended to avoid concomitant use.

Decreased Effect

The levels/effects of Desmopressin may be decreased by: Demeclocycline; Lithium

Increased Effect/Toxicity

Desmopressin may increase the levels/effects of: Lithium

The levels/effects of Desmopressin may be increased by: Analgesics (Opioid); CarBAMazepine; ChlorproMAZINE; LamoTRIgine; Nonsteroidal Anti-Inflammatory Agents; Selective Serotonin Reuptake Inhibitors; Tricyclic Antidepressants

Nutritional/Ethanol Interactions Ethanol: Avoid ethanol (may decrease antidiuretic effect).

Adverse Reactions Frequency may not be defined (may be dose or route related).

Cardiovascular: Blood pressure increased/decreased (I.V.), facial flushing

Central nervous system: Headache (2% to 5%), dizziness (intranasal; ≤3%), chills (intranasal; 2%)

Dermatologic: Rash

Endocrine & metabolic: Hyponatremia, water intoxication

Gastrointestinal: Abdominal pain (intranasal; 2%), gastrointestinal disorder (intranasal; ≤2%), nausea (intranasal; ≤2%), abdominal cramps, sore throat

Hepatic: Transient increases in liver transaminases (associated primarily with tablets)

Local: Injection: Burning pain, erythema, and swelling at the injection site

Neuromuscular & Skeletal: Weakness (intranasal; ≤2%)

Ocular: Conjunctivitis (intranasal; ≤2%), eye edema (intranasal; ≤2%), lacrimation disorder (intranasal; ≤2%)

Respiratory: Rhinitis (intranasal; 3% to 8%), epistaxis (intranasal; ≤3%), nostril pain (intranasal; ≤2%), cough, nasal congestion, upper respiratory infection

Pharmacodynamics/Kinetics

Onset of Action

Intranasal: Antidiuretic: 15-30 minutes; Increased factor VIII and von Willebrand factor (vWF) activity (dose related): 30 minutes

Peak effect: Antidiuretic: 1 hour; Increased factor VIII and vWF activity: 1.5 hours

I.V. infusion: Increased factor VIII and vWF activity: 30 minutes (dose related)

Peak effect: 1.5-2 hours

Oral tablet: Antidiuretic: ~1 hour

Peak effect: 4-7 hours

Duration of Action Intranasal, I.V. infusion, Oral tablet: ~6-14 hours

Dosage Forms Considerations

DDAVP and Minirin 5 mL bottles contain 50 sprays. Stimate 2.5 mL bottles contain 25 sprays.

Available Dosage Forms

Solution, Injection:

DDAVP: 4 mcg/mL (1 mL, 10 mL)

Generic: 4 mcg/mL (1 mL, 10 mL)

Solution, Nasal:

DDAVP: 0.01% (5 mL)

DDAVP Rhinal Tube: 0.01% (2.5 mL)

Stimate: 1.5 mg/mL (2.5 mL)

Generic: 0.01% (2.5 mL, 5 mL)

Tablet, Oral:

DDAVP: 0.1 mg, 0.2 mg

Generic: 0.1 mg, 0.2 mg

General Dosage Range

I.V.:

Infants and Children ≥3 months: 0.3 mcg/kg as a single dose, may repeat dose if needed

Adults: 2-4 mcg/day in 2 divided doses **or** one-tenth (1/10) of the intranasal maintenance dose **or** 0.3 mcg/kg as a single dose

Intranasal:

Infants 3-11 months: Initial: 5 mcg/day (0.05 mL/day) in 1-2 divided doses; Maintenance: 5-30 mcg/day (0.05-0.3 mL/day) in 1-2 divided doses

Children 12 months to 12 years: Initial: 5 mcg/day (0.05 mL/day) in 1-2 divided doses; Maintenance: 5-30 mcg/day (0.05-0.3 mL/day) in 1-2 divided doses **or** 150 mcg (1 spray of high concentration) as a single dose

Children >12 years and Adults <50 kg: 10-40 mcg/day (0.1-0.4 mL) in 1-3 divided doses **or** 150 mcg (1 spray of high concentration spray) as a single dose

Children >12 years and Adults ≥50 kg: 10-40 mcg/day in 1-3 divided doses **or** 300 mcg (1 spray each nostril of high concentration spray) as a single dose

Oral:

Children 4-5 years: Initial: 0.05 mg twice daily; Maintenance: 0.1-1.2 mg/day in 2-3 divided doses

Children ≥6 years: Initial: 0.05 mg twice daily **or** 0.2 mg at bedtime; Maintenance: 0.1-1.2 mg/day in 2-3 divided doses **or** 0.2-0.6 mg at bedtime

Adults: 0.2-0.6 mg at bedtime **or** 0.1-1.2 mg/day in 2-3 divided doses

SubQ: *Adults:* 2-4 mcg/day in 2 divided doses **or** one-tenth (¹/₁₀) of the intranasal maintenance dose

Administration

I.M. Central diabetes insipidus: Withdraw dose from ampul into appropriate syringe size (eg, insulin syringe). Further dilution is not required. Administer as direct injection.

I.V.

I.V. push: Central diabetes insipidus: Withdraw dose from ampul into appropriate syringe size (eg, insulin syringe). Further dilution is not required. Administer as direct injection.

I.V. infusion:

Hemophilia A, von Willebrand disease (type 1), and prevention of surgical bleeding in patients with uremia (unlabeled) (Mannucci, 1983): Infuse over 15-30 minutes

Acute uremic bleeding (unlabeled) (Watson, 1984): May infuse over 10 minutes

Other

Intranasal:

DDAVP®: Nasal pump spray: Delivers 0.1 mL (10 mcg); for doses <10 mcg or for other doses which are not multiples, use rhinal tube. DDAVP® Nasal spray delivers fifty 10 mcg doses. For 10 mcg dose, administer in one nostril. Any solution remaining after 50 doses should be discarded. Pump must be primed prior to first use.

DDAVP® Rhinal tube: Insert top of dropper into tube (arrow marked end) in downward position. Squeeze dropper until solution reaches desired calibration mark. Disconnect dropper. Grasp the tube ³/₄ inch from the end and insert tube into nostril until the fingertips reach the nostril. Place opposite end of tube into the mouth (holding breath). Tilt head back and blow with a strong, short puff into the nostril (for very young patients, an adult should blow solution into the child's nose). Reseal dropper after use.

SubQ: Central diabetes insipidus: Withdraw dose from ampul into appropriate syringe size (eg, insulin syringe). Further dilution is not required. Administer as direct injection.

Preparation for Administration DDAVP®: Dilute solution for injection in 10-50 mL NS for I.V. infusion (10 mL for children ≤10 kg; 50 mL for adults and children >10 kg).

Storage/Stability

DDAVP®:

Nasal spray: Store at controlled room temperature of 20°C to 25°C (68°F to 77°F). Keep nasal spray in upright position.

Rhinal Tube solution: Store refrigerated at 2°C to 8°C (36°F to 46°F). May store at controlled room temperature of 20°C to 25°C (68°F to 77°F) for up to 3 weeks.

Solution for injection: Store refrigerated at 2°C to 8°C (36°F to 46°F).

Tablet: Store at controlled room temperature of 20°C to 25°C (68°F to 77°F).

DDAVP® Melt (CAN; not available in U.S.): Store at 15°C to 25°C (59°F to 77°F) in original container. Protect from moisture.

Stimate® nasal spray: Store at room temperature not to exceed 25°C (77°F). Discard 6 months after opening bottle.

Nursing Actions

Physical Assessment Monitor for thromboembolism, hyponatremia, and water intoxication regularly throughout therapy.

Patient Education

• Discuss specific use of drug and side effects with patient as it relates to treatment. (HCAHPS: During this hospital stay, were you given any medicine that you had not taken before? Before giving you any new medicine, how often did hospital staff tell you what the medicine was for? How often did hospital staff describe possible side effects in a way you could understand?)

• Patient may experience flushing, rhinitis, rhinorrhea, or pharyngitis. Have patient report immediately to prescriber signs of hyponatremia, nausea, mood changes, behavioral changes, hallucinations, asthenia, akathisia, myalgia, muscle spasms, excessive weight gain, lack of appetite, dyspnea, severe headache, considerable dizziness, syncope, edema, angina, hemoptysis, strength differences from one side to another, difficulty speaking or thinking, change in balance, blurred vision, vision changes, tachycardia, arrhythmia, significant epistaxis, or injection site pain or irritation (HCAHPS).

• Educate patient about signs of a significant reaction (eg, wheezing; chest tightness; fever; itching; bad cough; blue skin color; seizures; or swelling of face, lips, tongue, or throat). **Note:** This is not a comprehensive list of all side effects. Patient should consult prescriber for additional questions.

Intended Use and Disclaimer: Should not be printed and given to patients. This information is intended to serve as a concise initial reference for healthcare professionals to use when discussing medications with a patient. You must ultimately rely on your own discretion, experience and judgment in diagnosing, treating and advising patients.

Related Information
Diagnostics and Surgical Aids *on page 1670*

Desvenlafaxine (des ven la FAX een)

Brand Names: U.S. Khedezla; Pristiq
Index Terms O-desmethylvenlafaxine; ODV
Pharmacologic Category Antidepressant, Serotonin/Norepinephrine Reuptake Inhibitor
Medication Safety Issues
  BEERS Criteria medication:
  This drug may be potentially inappropriate for use in geriatric patients (Quality of evidence - moderate; Strength of recommendation - strong).
Medication Guide Available Yes
Pregnancy Risk Factor C
Lactation Enters breast milk/not recommended
Breast-Feeding Considerations Desvenlafaxine is excreted in human milk and can be detected in the serum of nursing infants. The manufacturer recommends breast-feeding during therapy only if the expected benefits to the mother outweigh any potential risk to the infant.
Use Treatment of major depressive disorder (acute and maintenance)
Mechanism of Action/Effect Desvenlafaxine is a serotonin and norepinephrine reuptake inhibitor.
Contraindications Hypersensitivity to desvenlafaxine, venlafaxine or any component of the formulation; use of MAO inhibitors intended to treat psychiatric disorders (concurrently or within 14 days of discontinuing the MAO inhibitor); initiation of MAO inhibitor intended to treat psychiatric disorders within 7 days of discontinuing desvenlafaxine; initiation of desvenlafaxine in a patient receiving linezolid or intravenous methylene blue
Warnings/Precautions [U.S. Boxed Warning]: Antidepressants increase the risk of suicidal thinking and behavior in children, adolescents, and young adults (18-24 years of age) with major depressive disorder (MDD) and other psychiatric disorders; consider risk prior to prescribing. Short-term studies did not show an increased risk in patients >24 years of age and showed a decreased risk in patients ≥65 years.

Closely monitor for clinical worsening, suicidality, or unusual changes in behavior; the patient's family or caregiver should be instructed to closely observe the patient and communicate condition with healthcare provider. A medication guide should be dispensed with each prescription. **Desvenlafaxine is not FDA approved for use in children.**

The possibility of a suicide attempt is inherent in major depression and may persist until remission occurs. Monitor for worsening of depression or suicidality, especially during initiation of therapy (generally first 1-2 months) or with dose increases or decreases. Use caution in high-risk patients. Worsening depression and severe abrupt suicidality that are not part of the presenting symptoms may require discontinuation or modification of drug therapy. The patient's family or caregiver should be alerted to monitor patients for the emergence of suicidality and associated behaviors (such as agitation, irritability, hostility, impulsivity, and hypomania) and call healthcare provider.

May worsen psychosis in some patients or precipitate a shift to mania or hypomania in patients with bipolar disorder. Patients presenting with depressive symptoms should be screened for bipolar disorder. Monotherapy in patients with bipolar disorder should be avoided. **Desvenlafaxine is not FDA approved for the treatment of bipolar depression.**

Potentially life-threatening serotonin syndrome (SS) has occurred with serotonergic agents (eg, SSRIs, SNRIs), particularly when used in combination with other serotonergic agents (eg, triptans, TCAs, fentanyl, lithium, tramadol, buspirone, St John's wort, tryptophan) or agents that impair metabolism of serotonin (eg, MAO inhibitors intended to treat psychiatric disorders, other MAO inhibitors [ie, linezolid and intravenous methylene blue]). Discontinue treatment (and any concomitant serotonergic agent) immediately if signs/symptoms arise. May cause sustained increase in blood pressure or heart rate; dose related. Control preexisting hypertension prior to initiation of desvenlafaxine. Use caution in patients with recent history of MI, unstable heart disease, or cerebrovascular disease; may cause increases in serum lipids (cholesterol, LDL, triglycerides). Use caution in patients with renal impairment; dose reduction required in severe renal impairment. Use caution in patients with hepatic impairment; clearance is decreased and average AUC is increased; dosage adjustment is recommended. May cause hyponatremia/SIADH (elderly at increased risk); volume depletion (diuretics may increase risk).

Interstitial lung disease and eosinophilic pneumonia have been rarely reported with venlafaxine (the parent drug of desvenlafaxine); may present as progressive dyspnea, cough, and/or chest pain. Prompt evaluation and possible discontinuation of therapy may be necessary. Use cautiously in patients with a history of seizures. The risks of cognitive or motor impairment are low. May cause or exacerbate sexual dysfunction. May impair platelet aggregation, resulting in bleeding. Bone fractures have been associated with antidepressant treatment. Consider the possibility of a fragility fracture if an antidepressant-treated patient presents with unexplained bone pain, point tenderness, swelling, or bruising (Rabenda, 2013; Rizzoli, 2012).

Use caution in elderly patients; may cause or exacerbate syndrome of inappropriate antidiuretic hormone secretion or hyponatremia; monitor sodium closely with initiation or dosage adjustments in older adults (Beers Criteria). In addition, the elderly are at increased risk for orthostatic hypotension with therapy compared to younger adults. Use caution in patients with increased intraocular pressure or at risk of acute narrow-angle glaucoma. Potentially significant drug-drug interactions may exist, requiring dose or frequency adjustment, additional monitoring, and/or selection of alternative therapy.

Abrupt discontinuation or interruption of antidepressant therapy has been associated with a discontinuation syndrome. Symptoms arising may vary with antidepressant however commonly include nausea, vomiting, diarrhea, headaches, light-headedness, dizziness, diminished appetite, sweating, chills, tremors, paresthesias, fatigue, somnolence, and sleep disturbances (eg, vivid dreams, insomnia). Greater risks for developing a discontinuation syndrome have been associated with antidepressants with shorter half-lives, longer durations of treatment, and abrupt discontinuation. For antidepressants of short or intermediate half-lives, symptoms may emerge within 2-5 days after treatment discontinuation and last 7-14 days (APA, 2010; Fava, 2006; Haddad, 2001; Shelton, 2001; Warner, 2006).

Drug Interactions
Avoid Concomitant Use
Avoid concomitant use of Desvenlafaxine with any of the following: Axitinib; Iobenguane I 123; Linezolid; MAO Inhibitors; Methylene Blue; Simeprevir; Urokinase

Decreased Effect
Desvenlafaxine may decrease the levels/effects of: Alpha2-Agonists; Axitinib; Ibrutinib; Iobenguane I 123; Ioflupane I 123; Saxagliptin; Simeprevir

The levels/effects of Desvenlafaxine may be decreased by: Nonsteroidal Anti-Inflammatory Agents

Increased Effect/Toxicity
Desvenlafaxine may increase the levels/effects of: Agents with Antiplatelet Properties; Alpha-/ Beta-Agonists; Anticoagulants; Antipsychotics; Aspirin; Collagenase (Systemic); Dabigatran Etexilate; Ibritumomab; Methylene Blue; Metoclopramide; NSAID (Nonselective); Rivaroxaban; Salicylates; Serotonin Modulators; Thrombolytic Agents; Tositumomab and Iodine I 131 Tositumomab; Urokinase; Vitamin K Antagonists

The levels/effects of Desvenlafaxine may be increased by: Alcohol (Ethyl); Antipsychotics; Dasatinib; Glucosamine; Herbs (Anticoagulant/ Antiplatelet Properties); Ibrutinib; Linezolid; MAO Inhibitors; Multivitamins/Fluoride (with ADE); Multivitamins/Minerals (with ADEK, Folate, Iron); Multivitamins/Minerals (with AE, No Iron); Nonsteroidal Anti-Inflammatory Agents; Omega-3 Fatty Acids; Pentosan Polysulfate Sodium; Pentoxifylline; Prostacyclin Analogues; Tipranavir; Vitamin E

Nutritional/Ethanol Interactions
Ethanol: May increase CNS depression; monitor for increased effects with coadministration. Caution patients about effects.
Herb/Nutraceutical: Avoid St John's wort, tryptophan (may increase risk of serotonin syndrome and/or excessive sedation).

Adverse Reactions Reported for 50-100 mg/day.
>10%:
Central nervous system: Dizziness (10% to 13%), insomnia (9% to 12%)
Dermatologic: Hyperhidrosis (10% to 11%)
Gastrointestinal: Nausea (22% to 26%), xerostomia (11% to 17%)
1% to 10%:
Cardiovascular: Orthostatic hypotension (elderly 8%), syncope (<2%), tachycardia (<2%), hypertension (dose related; ≤1% of patients taking 50-100 mg daily had sustained diastolic BP ≥90 mm Hg)
Central nervous system: Somnolence (≤9%), fatigue (7%), anxiety (3% to 5%), abnormal dreams (2% to 3%), vertigo (≤2%), feeling jittery (≤2%), depersonalization (<2%), seizures (<2%), attention disturbance (≤1%)
Dermatologic: Alopecia (<2%), angioedema (<2%), photosensitivity reaction (<2%), rash (<2%)
Endocrine & metabolic: Libido decreased (males 4% to 5%), cholesterol (increased by ≥50 mg/dL and ≥261 mg/dL: 3% to 4%), anorgasmia (females 1%; males ≤3%), prolactin increased (<2%), hot flushes (1%), low density lipoprotein cholesterol (increased by ≥50 mg/dL and ≥190 mg/dL: ≤1%), sexual dysfunction (males ≤1%)
Gastrointestinal: Constipation (9%), appetite decreased (5% to 8%), vomiting (≤4%), weight gain (<2%)
Genitourinary: Urinary retention (<2%), urinary hesitancy (≤1%)
Hepatic: Liver function tests abnormal (<2%)

Neuromuscular & skeletal: Tremor (≤3%), dystonia (<2%), stiffness (<2%), weakness (<2%)

Ocular: Blurred vision (3% to 4%), mydriasis (2%)

Otic: Tinnitus (≤2%)

Renal: Proteinuria (6% to 8%)

Miscellaneous: Ejaculation retarded (1% to 5%), erectile dysfunction (3% to 6%), bruxism (<2%), yawning (1%), ejaculation failure (≤1%)

Available Dosage Forms

Tablet Extended Release 24 Hour, Oral:

Khedezla: 50 mg, 100 mg

Pristiq: 50 mg, 100 mg

Generic: 50 mg, 100 mg

General Dosage Range Dosage adjustment recommended in patients with hepatic or renal impairment

Oral: *Adults:* Initial: 50 mg once daily

Administration

Oral Administer at approximately the same time each day. May be taken with or without food. Swallow tablet whole; do not crush, chew, break, or dissolve. When discontinuing therapy, extend dosing interval to taper.

Nursing Actions

Physical Assessment Observe for clinical worsening, suicidality, or unusual behavior changes; especially during the initial few months of therapy or during dosage changes. Monitor vital signs at the beginning and periodically throughout therapy. Taper dosage slowly when discontinuing.

Patient Education

• Discuss specific use of drug and side effects with patient as it relates to treatment. (HCAHPS: During this hospital stay, were you given any medicine that you had not taken before? Before giving you any new medicine, how often did hospital staff tell you what the medicine was for? How often did hospital staff describe possible side effects in a way you could understand?)

• Patient may experience constipation, xerostomia, sexual dysfunction, insomnia, hyperhidrosis, fatigue, lack of appetite, or tablet shell in stool. Have patient report immediately to prescriber signs of depression (ie, suicidal ideation, anxiety, emotional instability, illogical thinking), signs of hyponatremia, signs of hemorrhaging, angina, dyspnea, vision changes, significant asthenia, or serotonin syndrome (ie, dizziness, severe headache, agitation, hallucinations, tachycardia, arrhythmia, flushing, tremors, hyperhidrosis, change in balance, considerable nausea, intolerable diarrhea) (HCAHPS).

• Educate patient about signs of a significant reaction (eg, wheezing; chest tightness; fever; itching; bad cough; blue skin color; seizures; or swelling of face, lips, tongue, or throat). **Note:** This is not a comprehensive list of all side effects. Patient should consult prescriber for additional questions.

Intended Use and Disclaimer: Should not be printed and given to patients. This information is intended to serve as a concise initial reference for healthcare professionals to use when discussing medications with a patient. You must ultimately rely on your own discretion, experience and judgment in diagnosing, treating and advising patients.

Dietary Considerations May be taken with or without food.

Related Information

Oral Medications That Should Not Be Crushed or Altered *on page 1712*

Dexamethasone (Systemic)

(deks a METH a sone)

Brand Names: U.S. Baycadron; Dexamethasone Intensol; DexPak 10 Day; DexPak 13 Day; DexPak 6 Day

Index Terms Decadron; Dexamethasone Sodium Phosphate

Pharmacologic Category Anti-inflammatory Agent; Antiemetic; Corticosteroid, Systemic

Medication Safety Issues

Sound-alike/look-alike issues:

Dexamethasone may be confused with desoximetasone, dextroamphetamine

Decadron may be confused with Percodan

Pregnancy Risk Factor C

Lactation Excretion in breast milk unknown/not recommended

Breast-Feeding Considerations Corticosteroids are excreted in human milk; information specific to dexamethasone has not been located. The manufacturer notes that when used systemically, maternal use of corticosteroids have the potential to cause adverse events in a nursing infant (eg, growth suppression, interfere with endogenous corticosteroid production). Due to the potential for serious adverse reactions in the nursing infant, the manufacturer recommends a decision be made whether to discontinue nursing or to discontinue the drug, taking into account the importance of treatment to the mother. If there is concern about exposure to the infant, some guidelines recommend waiting 4 hours after the maternal dose of an oral systemic corticosteroid before breast feeding in order to decrease potential exposure to the nursing infant (based on a study using prednisolone) (Bae, 2011; Leachman, 2006; Makol, 2011; Ost, 1985).

Use Primarily as an anti-inflammatory or immunosuppressant agent in the treatment of a variety of diseases including those of allergic, dermatologic, endocrine, hematologic, inflammatory, neoplastic, nervous system, renal, respiratory, rheumatic, and autoimmune origin; may be used in management of cerebral edema, chronic swelling, as a diagnostic agent, diagnosis of Cushing's syndrome, antiemetic

Unlabeled Use Dexamethasone suppression test as an indicator of depression and/or risk of suicide; prevention and treatment of acute mountain sickness and high altitude cerebral edema; accelerate fetal lung maturation in patients with preterm labor

Mechanism of Action/Effect Decreases inflammation by suppression of neutrophil migration, decreased production of inflammatory mediators, and reversal of increased capillary permeability; suppresses normal immune response. Dexamethasone's mechanism of antiemetic activity is unknown.

Contraindications Hypersensitivity to dexamethasone or any component of the formulation; systemic fungal infections, cerebral malaria

Warnings/Precautions Use with caution in patients with thyroid disease, hepatic impairment, renal impairment, cardiovascular disease, diabetes, glaucoma, cataracts, myasthenia gravis, patients at risk for osteoporosis, patients at risk for seizures, or GI diseases (diverticulitis, peptic ulcer, ulcerative colitis) due to perforation risk. Use caution following acute MI (corticosteroids have been associated with myocardial rupture). Because of the risk of adverse effects, systemic corticosteroids should be used cautiously in the elderly in the smallest possible effective dose for the shortest duration. May affect growth velocity; growth should be routinely monitored in pediatric patients. Withdraw therapy with gradual tapering of dose.

May cause hypercorticism or suppression of hypothalamic-pituitary-adrenal (HPA) axis, particularly in younger children or in patients receiving high doses for prolonged periods. HPA axis suppression may lead to adrenal crisis. Withdrawal and discontinuation of a corticosteroid should be done slowly and carefully. Particular care is required when patients are transferred from systemic corticosteroids to inhaled products due to possible adrenal insufficiency or withdrawal from steroids, including an increase in allergic symptoms. Patients receiving >20 mg per day of prednisone (or equivalent) may be most susceptible. Fatalities have occurred due to adrenal insufficiency in asthmatic patients during and after transfer from systemic corticosteroids to aerosol steroids; aerosol steroids do not provide the systemic steroid needed to treat patients having trauma, surgery, or infections. Dexamethasone does not provide adequate mineralocorticoid activity in adrenal insufficiency (may be employed as a single dose while cortisol assays are performed). The lowest possible dose should be used during treatment; discontinuation and/or dose reductions should be gradual.

Acute myopathy has been reported with high dose corticosteroids, usually in patients with neuromuscular transmission disorders; may involve ocular and/or respiratory muscles; monitor creatine kinase; recovery may be delayed. Corticosteroid use may cause psychiatric disturbances, including depression, euphoria, insomnia, mood swings, and personality changes. Pre-existing psychiatric conditions may be exacerbated by corticosteroid use. Prolonged use of corticosteroids may also increase the incidence of secondary infection, mask acute infection (including fungal infections), prolong or exacerbate viral infections, or limit response to vaccines. Exposure to chickenpox should be avoided; corticosteroids should not be used to treat ocular herpes simplex. Corticosteroids should not be used for cerebral malaria or viral hepatitis. Close observation is required in patients with latent tuberculosis and/or TB reactivity; restrict use in active TB (only in conjunction with antituberculosis treatment). Prolonged treatment with corticosteroids has been associated with the development of Kaposi's sarcoma (case reports); if noted, discontinuation of therapy should be considered. High-dose corticosteroids should not be used to manage acute head injury.

Drug Interactions

Avoid Concomitant Use

Avoid concomitant use of Dexamethasone (Systemic) with any of the following: Abiraterone Acetate; Aldesleukin; Apixaban; Artemether; Axitinib; BCG; Bedaquiline; Boceprevir; Bosutinib; Cabozantinib; CloZAPine; Conivaptan; Crizotinib; Dabigatran Etexilate; Dienogest; Dronedarone; Enzalutamide; Everolimus; Fusidic Acid (Systemic); Ibrutinib; Indium 111 Capromab Pendetide; Itraconazole; Ivacaftor; Lapatinib; Lumefantrine; Lurasidone; Macitentan; Mifepristone; Natalizumab; NIFEdipine; Nilotinib; Nisoldipine; PAZOPanib; Perampanel; Pimecrolimus; Pomalidomide; PONATinib; Praziquantel; Ranolazine; Regorafenib; Rilpivirine; Rivaroxaban; Roflumilast; RomiDEPsin; Simeprevir; Sofosbuvir; SORAfenib; Tacrolimus (Topical); Tasimelteon; Telaprevir; Ticagrelor; Tofacitinib; Tolvaptan; Toremifene; Ulipristal; Vandetanib; Vemurafenib; VinCRIStine (Liposomal)

Decreased Effect

Dexamethasone (Systemic) may decrease the levels/effects of: Abiraterone Acetate; Afatinib; Aldesleukin; Antidiabetic Agents; Apixaban; ARIPiprazole; Artemether; Axitinib; BCG; Bedaquiline; Boceprevir; Bosutinib; Brentuximab Vedotin; Cabozantinib; Calcitriol; Caspofungin; Clarithromycin; CloZAPine; Cobicistat; Coccidioidin Skin Test; Corticorelin; Crizotinib; CycloSPORINE (Systemic); CYP3A4 Substrates; Dabigatran Etexilate; Dasatinib; Dienogest; DOXOrubicin (Conventional); Dronedarone; Elvitegravir; Enzalutamide; Everolimus; Exemestane; Gefitinib; GuanFACINE; Hyaluronidase; Ibrutinib; Imatinib; Indium 111 Capromab Pendetide; Isoniazid; Itraconazole; Ivacaftor; Ixabepilone; Lapatinib; Linagliptin; Lumefantrine; Lurasidone; Macitentan; Maraviroc; Mifepristone; NIFEdipine; Nilotinib;

Nisoldipine; PAZOPanib; Perampanel; P-glyco-protein/ABCB1 Substrates; Pomalidomide; PONATinib; Praziquantel; QUEtiapine; Ranolazine; Regorafenib; Rilpivirine; Rivaroxaban; Roflumilast; RomiDEPsin; Salicylates; Simeprevir; Sipuleucel-T; Sofosbuvir; SORAfenib; SUNItinib; Tadalafil; Tasimelteon; Telaprevir; Ticagrelor; Tofacitinib; Tolvaptan; Toremifene; Triazolam; Ulipristal; Urea Cycle Disorder Agents; Vaccines (Inactivated); Vandetanib; Vemurafenib; Vilazodone; VinCRIStine (Liposomal); Vortioxetine; Zuclopenthixol

The levels/effects of Dexamethasone (Systemic) may be decreased by: Aminoglutethimide; Antacids; Barbiturates; Bile Acid Sequestrants; Bosentan; CYP3A4 Inducers (Strong); Dabrafenib; Echinacea; Herbs (CYP3A4 Inducers); Mifepristone; Mitotane; P-glycoprotein/ABCB1 Inducers; Primidone; Rifamycin Derivatives; Tocilizumab

Increased Effect/Toxicity

Dexamethasone (Systemic) may increase the levels/effects of: Acetylcholinesterase Inhibitors; Amphotericin B; Clarithromycin; CycloSPORINE (Systemic); Deferasirox; Ifosfamide; Leflunomide; Lenalidomide; Loop Diuretics; Natalizumab; NSAID (COX-2 Inhibitor); NSAID (Nonselective); Thalidomide; Thiazide Diuretics; Tofacitinib; Vaccines (Live); Warfarin

The levels/effects of Dexamethasone (Systemic) may be increased by: Antifungal Agents (Azole Derivatives, Systemic); Aprepitant; Asparaginase (E. coli); Asparaginase (Erwinia); Calcium Channel Blockers (Nondihydropyridine); Clarithromycin; Conivaptan; CycloSPORINE (Systemic); CYP3A4 Inhibitors (Moderate); CYP3A4 Inhibitors (Strong); Denosumab; Estrogen Derivatives; Fluconazole; Fosaprepitant; Fusidic Acid (Systemic); Indacaterol; Luliconazole; Macrolide Antibiotics; Mifepristone; Neuromuscular-Blocking Agents (Nondepolarizing); P-glycoprotein/ABCB1 Inhibitors; Pimecrolimus; Quinolone Antibiotics; Roflumilast; Salicylates; Stiripentol; Tacrolimus (Topical); Telaprevir; Trastuzumab

Nutritional/Ethanol Interactions

Ethanol: Avoid ethanol (may enhance gastric mucosal irritation).

Food: Dexamethasone interferes with calcium absorption. Limit caffeine.

Herb/Nutraceutical: Avoid cat's claw, echinacea (have immunostimulant properties).

Adverse Reactions Frequency not defined.

Cardiovascular: Arrhythmia, bradycardia, cardiac arrest, cardiomyopathy, CHF, circulatory collapse, edema, hypertension, myocardial rupture (post-MI), syncope, thromboembolism, vasculitis

Central nervous system: Depression, emotional instability, euphoria, headache, intracranial pressure increased, insomnia, malaise, mood swings, neuritis, personality changes, pseudotumor cerebri (usually following discontinuation), psychic disorders, seizure, vertigo

Dermatologic: Acne, allergic dermatitis, alopecia, angioedema, bruising, dry skin, erythema, fragile skin, hirsutism, hyper-/hypopigmentation, hypertrichosis, perianal pruritus (following I.V. injection), petechiae, rash, skin atrophy, skin test reaction impaired, striae, urticaria, wound healing impaired

Endocrine & metabolic: Adrenal suppression, carbohydrate tolerance decreased, Cushing's syndrome, diabetes mellitus, glucose intolerance decreased, growth suppression (children), hyperglycemia, hypokalemic alkalosis, menstrual irregularities, negative nitrogen balance, pituitary-adrenal axis suppression, protein catabolism, sodium retention

Gastrointestinal: Abdominal distention, appetite increased, gastrointestinal hemorrhage, gastrointestinal perforation, nausea, pancreatitis, peptic ulcer, ulcerative esophagitis, weight gain

Genitourinary: Altered (increased or decreased) spermatogenesis

Hepatic: Hepatomegaly, transaminases increased

Local: Postinjection flare (intra-articular use), thrombophlebitis

Neuromuscular & skeletal: Arthropathy, aseptic necrosis (femoral and humoral heads), fractures, muscle mass loss, myopathy (particularly in conjunction with neuromuscular disease or neuromuscular-blocking agents), neuropathy, osteoporosis, parasthesia, tendon rupture, vertebral compression fractures, weakness

Ocular: Cataracts, exophthalmos, glaucoma, intraocular pressure increased

Renal: Glucosuria

Respiratory: Pulmonary edema

Miscellaneous: Abnormal fat deposition, anaphylactoid reaction, anaphylaxis, avascular necrosis, diaphoresis, hiccups, hypersensitivity, impaired wound healing, infections, Kaposi's sarcoma, moon face, secondary malignancy

Pharmacodynamics/Kinetics

Onset of Action Acetate: Prompt

Duration of Action Metabolic effect: 72 hours; acetate is a long-acting repository preparation

Available Dosage Forms

Concentrate, Oral:
Dexamethasone Intensol: 1 mg/mL (30 mL)

Elixir, Oral:
Baycadron: 0.5 mg/5 mL (237 mL)
Generic: 0.5 mg/5 mL (237 mL)

Solution, Injection:
Generic: 4 mg/mL (1 mL, 5 mL, 30 mL); 10 mg/mL (1 mL, 10 mL)

Solution, Injection [preservative free]:
Generic: 10 mg/mL (1 mL)

Solution, Oral:
Generic: 0.5 mg/5 mL (240 mL, 500 mL)

Tablet, Oral:
DexPak 10 Day: 1.5 mg
DexPak 13 Day: 1.5 mg

DexPak 6 Day: 1.5 mg
Generic: 0.5 mg, 0.75 mg, 1 mg, 1.5 mg, 2 mg, 4 mg, 6 mg

General Dosage Range

I.M.:
Children: 0.03-2 mg/kg/day or 0.6-10 mg/m^2/day divided every 6-12 hours
Adults: 0.75-9 mg/day or 0.03-2 mg/kg/day or 0.6-0.75 mg/m^2/day in divided doses every 6-12 hours **or** 4 mg every 4-6 hours

I.V.:
Children: 0.03-2 mg/kg/day or 0.6-10 mg/m^2/day divided every 6-12 hours **or** 10 mg/m^2/dose every 12-24 hours on days of chemotherapy
Adults: Dosage varies greatly depending on indication

Intra-articular, intralesional, or soft tissue:
Adults: 0.4-6 mg/day

Oral:
Children: 0.03-2 mg/kg/day or 0.6-10 mg/m^2/day divided every 6-12 hours
Adults: Dosage varies greatly depending on indication

Administration

I.M. Administer the 4 mg/mL or 10 mg/mL concentration deep IM.

I.V. Administer the 4 mg/mL or 10 mg/mL concentration intravenously as an undiluted or diluted solution.

Injectable Detail pH: 7-8.5

Oral Administer oral formulation with meals to decrease GI upset.

Topical Topical formulation is for external use. Do not use on open wounds.

Other
Intra-articular: Administer into affected joint using the 4 mg/mL concentration only.
Intralesional: Administer into affected area using the 4 mg/mL concentration only.
Soft tissue: Administer into affected tissue using the 4 mg/mL concentration only.

Preparation for Administration

Oral: Oral administration of dexamethasone for croup may be prepared using a parenteral dexamethasone formulation and mixing it with an oral flavored syrup (Bjornson, 2004).

I.V.: May be given undiluted or further diluted in NS or D$_5$W. Use preservative-free product when used in neonates, especially premature infants.

Storage/Stability Injection: Store intact vials at 20°C to 25°C (68°F to 77°F). Protect from light, heat, or freezing. Diluted solutions should be used within 24 hours.

Nursing Actions

Physical Assessment Caution patients with diabetes to monitor glucose levels closely (corticosteroids may alter glucose levels).

Patient Education

- Discuss specific use of drug and side effects with patient as it relates to treatment. (HCAHPS: During this hospital stay, were you given any medicine that you had not taken before? Before giving you any new medicine, how often did hospital staff tell you what the medicine was for? How often did hospital staff describe possible side effects in a way you could understand?)
- Patient may experience nausea, insomnia, or akathisia. Have patient report immediately to prescriber sings of infection, signs of hyperglycemia, signs of hypokalemia, signs of pancreatitis, severe asthenia, irritability, tremors, tachycardia, confusion, hyperhidrosis, dizziness, dyspnea, excessive weight gain, edema of extremities, skin changes, moon face, buffalo hump, significant headache, bradycardia, arrhythmia, angina, menstrual irregularities, osteodynia, arthralgia, vision changes, mood changes, behavioral changes, depression, paresthesia, ecchymosis, hemorrhaging, severe dyspepsia, melena, hematemesis, or injection site irritation (HCAHPS).
- Educate patient about signs of a significant reaction (eg, wheezing; chest tightness; fever; itching; bad cough; blue skin color; seizures; or swelling of face, lips, tongue, or throat). **Note:** This is not a comprehensive list of all side effects. Patient should consult prescriber for additional questions.

Intended Use and Disclaimer: Should not be printed and given to patients. This information is intended to serve as a concise initial reference for healthcare professionals to use when discussing medications with a patient. You must ultimately rely on your own discretion, experience and judgment in diagnosing, treating and advising patients.

Dietary Considerations May be taken with meals to decrease GI upset. May need diet with increased potassium, pyridoxine, vitamin C, vitamin D, folate, calcium, and phosphorus.

Dexamethasone (Ophthalmic)
(deks a METH a sone)

Brand Names: U.S. Maxidex; Ozurdex
Index Terms Dexamethasone Sodium Phosphate
Pharmacologic Category Anti-inflammatory Agent, Ophthalmic; Corticosteroid, Ophthalmic; Corticosteroid, Otic

Medication Safety Issues
Sound-alike/look-alike issues:
Dexamethasone may be confused with desoximetasone, dextroamphetamine
Maxidex® may be confused with Maxzide®

Pregnancy Risk Factor C
Lactation Excretion in breast milk unknown/use caution

◄ **Use** Management of steroid-responsive inflammatory conditions such as allergic conjunctivitis, iritis, or cyclitis; symptomatic treatment of corneal injury from chemical, radiation, or thermal burns, or penetration of foreign bodies. The ophthalmic solution is also indicated for otic use to treat steroid-responsive inflammatory conditions of the external auditory meatus.

Ophthalmic intravitreal implant (Ozurdex®): Treatment of macular edema following branch retinal vein occlusion (BRVO) or central retinal vein occlusion (CRVO); treatment of noninfective uveitis

Available Dosage Forms
Implant, Intraocular [preservative free]:
Ozurdex: 0.7 mg (1 ea)
Solution, Ophthalmic:
Generic: 0.1% (5 mL)
Suspension, Ophthalmic:
Maxidex: 0.1% (5 mL)

General Dosage Range
Intravitreal: *Adults:* 0.7 mg implant in affected eye
Ophthalmic:
Adults:
Solution: Instill 1-2 drops into conjunctival sac every hour during the day and every other hour during the night; gradually reduce dose to 1 drop every 4 hours, then to 3-4 times/day
Suspension: Instill 1-2 drops up to 4-6 times/day or hourly in severe cases
Otic: *Adults:* Initial: Instill 3-4 drops of the solution into the aural canal 2-3 times a day; reduce dose gradually. Alternately, pack the aural canal with a gauze wick saturated with the solution; remove from the ear after 12-24 hours.

Administration
Other
Ophthalmic solution, suspension: Remove soft contact lenses prior to using solutions containing benzalkonium chloride. Do not touch tip of container to eye. Shake suspension well prior to use.
Ophthalmic solution may also be administered otically. Prior to use, clean the aural canal thoroughly and sponge dry.
Ophthalmic implant (intravitreal injection): Ozurdex®: Administer under controlled aseptic conditions (eg, sterile gloves, sterile drape, sterile eyelid speculum). Adequate anesthesia and a broad-spectrum bactericidal agent should be administered prior to injection. In the sterile field, open foil pouch, remove applicator, and pull the safety tab straight off of the applicator (do not twist or flex the tab). If administration is required in the second eye, a new applicator should be used and the sterile field, syringe, gloves, drapes, and eyelid speculum should be changed.

Nursing Actions
Physical Assessment Monitor intraocular pressure if used >10 days.

Patient Education
• Discuss specific use of drug and side effects with patient as it relates to treatment. (HCAHPS: During this hospital stay, were you given any medicine that you had not taken before? Before giving you any new medicine, how often did hospital staff tell you what the medicine was for? How often did hospital staff describe possible side effects in a way you could understand?)
• Have patient report immediately to prescriber sudden vision changes, ophthalmalgia, or severe eye irritation (HCAHPS).
• Educate patient about signs of a significant reaction (eg, wheezing; chest tightness; fever; itching; bad cough; blue skin color; seizures; or swelling of face, lips, tongue, or throat). **Note:** This is not a comprehensive list of all side effects. Patient should consult prescriber for additional questions.

Intended Use and Disclaimer: Should not be printed and given to patients. This information is intended to serve as a concise initial reference for healthcare professionals to use when discussing medications with a patient. You must ultimately rely on your own discretion, experience and judgment in diagnosing, treating and advising patients.

Dexchlorpheniramine
(deks klor fen EER a meen)

Index Terms Dexchlorpheniramine Maleate
Pharmacologic Category Alkylamine Derivative; Histamine H$_1$ Antagonist; Histamine H$_1$ Antagonist, First Generation
Medication Safety Issues
BEERS Criteria medication:
This drug may be potentially inappropriate for use in geriatric patients (Quality of evidence - moderate; Strength of recommendation - strong).
Lactation Excretion in breast milk unknown/contraindicated
Use Perennial and seasonal allergic rhinitis and other allergic symptoms including urticaria
Available Dosage Forms
Syrup, Oral:
Generic: 2 mg/5 mL (473 mL)
General Dosage Range Oral:
Regular release:
Children 2-5 years: 0.5 mg every 4-6 hours
Children 6-11 years: 1 mg every 4-6 hours
Adults: 2 mg every 4-6 hours
Timed release:
Children 6-11 years: 4 mg at bedtime
Adults: 4-6 mg at bedtime **or** every 8-10 hours
Administration
Oral May be administered without regard to meals.

Nursing Actions

Patient Education

- Discuss specific use of drug and side effects with patient as it relates to treatment. (HCAHPS: During this hospital stay, were you given any medicine that you had not taken before? Before giving you any new medicine, how often did hospital staff tell you what the medicine was for? How often did hospital staff describe possible side effects in a way you could understand?)
- Patient may experience fatigue, diarrhea, constipation, xerostomia, anxiety, lack of appetite, nausea, or insomnia. Have patient report immediately to prescriber angina, tachycardia, arrhythmia, urinary retention, difficult urination, hallucinations, tremors, severe dizziness, syncope, significant headache, vision changes, change in balance, or considerable asthenia (HCAHPS).
- Educate patient about signs of a significant reaction (eg, wheezing; chest tightness; fever; itching; bad cough; blue skin color; seizures; or swelling of face, lips, tongue, or throat). **Note:** This is not a comprehensive list of all side effects. Patient should consult prescriber for additional questions.

Intended Use and Disclaimer: Should not be printed and given to patients. This information is intended to serve as a concise initial reference for healthcare professionals to use when discussing medications with a patient. You must ultimately rely on your own discretion, experience and judgment in diagnosing, treating and advising patients.

Dexlansoprazole (deks lan SOE pra zole)

Brand Names: U.S. Dexilant
Index Terms Kapidex; TAK-390MR
Pharmacologic Category Proton Pump Inhibitor; Substituted Benzimidazole
Medication Safety Issues
  Sound-alike/look-alike issues:
    Dexlansoprazole may be confused with aripiprazole, lansoprazole
    Kapidex [DSC] may be confused with Casodex®, Kadian®
  International issues:
    Kapidex [DSC] may be confused with Capadex which is a brand name for propoxyphene/acetaminophen combination product [Australia, New Zealand]
Medication Guide Available Yes
Pregnancy Risk Factor B
Lactation Excretion in breast milk unknown/not recommended
Breast-Feeding Considerations It is not known if dexlansoprazole is excreted into breast milk. Due to the potential for serious adverse reactions in the nursing infant, the manufacturer recommends a decision be made whether to discontinue nursing or to discontinue the drug, taking into account the importance of treatment to the mother.

Use
  Erosive esophagitis: For healing of all grades of erosive esophagitis for up to 8 weeks; to maintain healing of erosive esophagitis and relief of heartburn for up to 6 months.
  Gastroesophageal reflux disease: For the treatment of heartburn associated with symptomatic nonerosive gastroesophageal reflux disease (GERD) for 4 weeks.

Mechanism of Action/Effect A proton pump inhibitor which decreases acid secretion in gastric parietal cells

Contraindications Known hypersensitivity to any component of the formulation. Documentation of allergenic cross-reactivity for drugs in this class is limited. However, because of similarities in chemical structure and/or pharmacologic actions, the possibility of cross-sensitivity cannot be ruled out with certainty.

Warnings/Precautions Use of proton pump inhibitors (PPIs) may increase the risk of gastrointestinal infections (eg, *Salmonella, Campylobacter*). Relief of symptoms does not preclude the presence of a gastric malignancy. Atrophic gastritis (by biopsy) has been noted with long-term omeprazole therapy; this may also occur with dexlansoprazole. No occurrences of enterochromaffin-like (ECL) cell carcinoids, dysplasia, or neoplasia (such as those seen in studies of rodents exposed to lansoprazole) have been reported in humans. Use of PPIs may increase risk of CDAD, especially in hospitalized patients; consider CDAD diagnosis in patients with persistent diarrhea that does not improve. Use the lowest dose and shortest duration of PPI therapy appropriate for the condition being treated. Patients with moderate hepatic impairment (Child-Pugh class B) may require dosage reductions; no studies have been conducted in patients with severe hepatic impairment.

PPIs may diminish the therapeutic effect of clopidogrel, thought to be due to reduced formation of the active metabolite of clopidogrel. The manufacturer of clopidogrel recommends either avoidance of both omeprazole (even when scheduled 12 hours apart) and esomeprazole or use of a PPI with comparatively less effect on the active metabolite of clopidogrel (eg, pantoprazole). Although lansoprazole exhibits the most potent CYP2C19 inhibition *in vitro* (Li, 2004; Ogilvie, 2011), an *in vivo* study of extensive CYP2C19 metabolizers showed less reduction of the active metabolite of clopidogrel when administered with lansoprazole/dexlansoprazole compared to esomeprazole/omeprazole (Frelinger, 2012). The manufacturer of dexlansoprazole states that no dosage adjustment is necessary for clopidogrel when used concurrently with approved doses. In contrast to these ▶

warnings, others have recommended the continued use of PPIs, regardless of the degree of inhibition, in patients with a history of GI bleeding or multiple risk factors for GI bleeding who are also receiving clopidogrel since no evidence has established clinically meaningful differences in outcome; however, a clinically-significant interaction cannot be excluded in those who are poor metabolizers of clopidogrel (Abraham, 2010; Levine, 2011). Potentially significant drug-drug interactions may exist, requiring dose or frequency adjustment, additional monitoring, and/or selection of alternative therapy. Consult drug interactions database for more detailed information.

Increased incidence of osteoporosis-related bone fractures of the hip, spine, or wrist may occur with PPI therapy. Patients on high-dose (multiple daily doses) or long-term therapy (≥1 year) should be monitored. Use the lowest effective dose for the shortest duration of time, use vitamin D and calcium supplementation, and follow appropriate guidelines to reduce risk of fractures in patients at risk.

Hypomagnesemia, reported rarely, usually with prolonged PPI use of >3 months (most cases >1 year of therapy); may be symptomatic or asymptomatic; severe cases may cause tetany, seizures, and cardiac arrhythmias. Consider obtaining serum magnesium concentrations prior to beginning long-term therapy, especially if taking concomitant digoxin, diuretics, or other drugs known to cause hypomagnesemia; and periodically thereafter. Hypomagnesemia may be corrected by magnesium supplementation, although discontinuation of dexlansoprazole may be necessary; magnesium levels typically return to normal within 1 week of stopping.

Drug Interactions

Avoid Concomitant Use

Avoid concomitant use of Dexlansoprazole with any of the following: Dasatinib; Delavirdine; Erlotinib; Nelfinavir; PONATinib; Rilpivirine; Risedronate

Decreased Effect

Dexlansoprazole may decrease the levels/effects of: Atazanavir; Bisphosphonate Derivatives; Bosutinib; Cefditoren; Clopidogrel; Dabigatran Etexilate; Dabrafenib; Dasatinib; Delavirdine; Erlotinib; Gefitinib; Indinavir; Iron Salts; Itraconazole; Ketoconazole (Systemic); Mesalamine; Multivitamins/Minerals (with ADEK, Folate, Iron); Mycophenolate; Nelfinavir; Nilotinib; PONATinib; Posaconazole; Rilpivirine; Riociguat; Risedronate; Vismodegib

The levels/effects of Dexlansoprazole may be decreased by: Dabrafenib; Tipranavir

Increased Effect/Toxicity

Dexlansoprazole may increase the levels/effects of: Amphetamine; Benzodiazepines (metabolized by oxidation); Dexmethylphenidate; Dextroamphetamine; Methotrexate; Methylphenidate; Raltegravir; Risedronate; Saquinavir; Tacrolimus (Systemic); Voriconazole

The levels/effects of Dexlansoprazole may be increased by: Fluconazole; Ketoconazole (Systemic); Voriconazole

Nutritional/Ethanol Interactions
Ethanol: Avoid ethanol (may cause gastric mucosal irritation).

Adverse Reactions
2% to 10%:

Gastrointestinal: Diarrhea (5%), abdominal pain (4%), nausea (3%), flatulence (1% to 3%), vomiting (1% to 2%)

Respiratory: Upper respiratory tract infection (2% to 3%)

Available Dosage Forms

Capsule Delayed Release, Oral:

Dexilant: 30 mg, 60 mg

General Dosage Range
Dosage adjustment recommended in patients with hepatic impairment

Oral: *Adults:* 30-60 mg once daily

Administration

Oral May be administered without regard to meals; some patients may benefit from premeal administration if symptoms do not adequately respond to post-meal dosing. Capsules should be swallowed whole; alternatively, patients who are unable to swallow capsules may open the capsule, sprinkle the intact granules onto 1 tablespoon of applesauce, and swallow intact granules immediately (do not chew granules). Capsules may also be opened for administration via NG tube or oral syringe.

Oral syringe: Open capsules and mix intact granules (not crushed) with 20 mL water. Withdraw mixture into oral syringe; swirl syringe gently to prevent granules from settling and administer mixture immediately into the mouth. Refill syringe with 10 mL water, swirl gently, and administer; repeat. Do not save water and granule mixture for later use.

Other NG tube (≥16 French): Open capsules and mix intact granules (not crushed) with 20 mL of water. Withdraw mixture into catheter-tip syringe; swirl syringe gently to prevent granules from settling and administer mixture immediately through NG tube into the stomach. Refill syringe with 10 mL water, swirl gently, and flush NG tube; repeat. Do not save water and granule mixture for later use.

Storage/Stability
Store at 25°C (77°F); excursions are permitted to 15°C to 30°C (59°F to 86°F).

Nursing Actions

Patient Education

- Discuss specific use of drug and side effects with patient as it relates to treatment. (HCAHPS: During this hospital stay, were you given any medicine that you had not taken before? Before giving you any new medicine, how often did hospital staff tell you what the medicine was

for? How often did hospital staff describe possible side effects in a way you could understand?)
- Patient may experience nausea, flatulence, rhinitis, rhinorrhea, or sternutation. Have patient report immediately to prescriber signs of hypomagnesemia, severe dizziness, syncope, tachycardia, bradycardia, edema of extremities, significant dyspepsia, osteodynia, painful extremities, angina, depression, chills, pharyngitis, arthralgia, dyspnea, considerable asthenia, excessive weight loss, or intolerable diarrhea (HCAHPS).
- Educate patient about signs of a significant reaction (eg, wheezing; chest tightness; fever; itching; bad cough; blue skin color; seizures; or swelling of face, lips, tongue, or throat). **Note:** This is not a comprehensive list of all side effects. Patient should consult prescriber for additional questions.

Intended Use and Disclaimer: Should not be printed and given to patients. This information is intended to serve as a concise initial reference for healthcare professionals to use when discussing medications with a patient. You must ultimately rely on your own discretion, experience and judgment in diagnosing, treating and advising patients.

Dietary Considerations May be taken without regard to meals; some patients may benefit from premeal administration if symptoms do not adequately respond to post-meal dosing.

Related Information
Oral Medications That Should Not Be Crushed or Altered on page 1712

Dexmethylphenidate (dex meth il FEN i date)

Brand Names: U.S. Focalin; Focalin XR
Index Terms Dexmethylphenidate Hydrochloride
Pharmacologic Category Central Nervous System Stimulant
Medication Safety Issues
Sound-alike/look-alike issues:
Dexmethylphenidate may be confused with methadone
Focalin® may be confused with Folotyn®
Medication Guide Available Yes
Pregnancy Risk Factor C
Lactation Excretion in breast milk unknown/use caution
Breast-Feeding Considerations It is not known if dexmethylphenidate is excreted into breast milk. Dexmethylphenidate is the more active *d-threo*-enantiomer of racemic methylphenidate, and methylphenidate is excreted into breast milk. Refer to Methylphenidate monograph for additional information.
Use Treatment of attention-deficit/hyperactivity disorder (ADHD)
Mechanism of Action/Effect CNS stimulant

Contraindications Hypersensitivity to dexmethylphenidate, methylphenidate, or any component of the formulation; marked anxiety, tension, and agitation; glaucoma; motor tics, family history or diagnosis of Tourette's syndrome; use with or within 14 days following MAO inhibitor therapy

Warnings/Precautions CNS stimulant use has been associated with serious cardiovascular events including sudden death in patients with pre-existing structural cardiac abnormalities or other serious heart problems (sudden death in children and adolescents; sudden death, stroke, and MI in adults). These products should be avoided in patients with known serious structural cardiac abnormalities, cardiomyopathy, serious heart rhythm abnormalities, or other serious cardiac problems that could increase the risk of sudden death that these conditions alone carry. Patients should be carefully evaluated for cardiac disease prior to initiation of therapy. Use of stimulants can cause an increase in blood pressure (average 2-4 mm Hg) and increases in heart rate (average 3-6 bpm), although some patients may have larger than average increases. Use caution with hypertension, hyperthyroidism, or other cardiovascular conditions that might be exacerbated by increases in blood pressure or heart rate. Stimulants are associated with peripheral vasculopathy, including Raynaud's phenomenon; signs/symptoms are usually mild and intermittent, and generally improve with dose reduction or discontinuation. Digital ulceration and/or soft tissue breakdown have been observed rarely; monitor for digital changes during therapy and seek further evaluation (eg, rheumatology) if necessary.

Has demonstrated value as part of a comprehensive treatment program for ADHD. Use with caution in patients with bipolar disorder (may induce mixed/manic episode). May exacerbate symptoms of behavior and thought disorder in psychotic patients; new onset psychosis or mania may occur with stimulant use; observe for symptoms of aggression and/or hostility. Use caution with seizure disorders (may reduce seizure threshold). Use caution in patients with history of ethanol or drug abuse. May exacerbate symptoms of behavior and thought disorder in psychotic patients. **[U.S. Boxed Warning]: Potential for drug dependency exists - avoid abrupt discontinuation in patients who have received for prolonged periods.** Visual disturbances have been reported (rare). Stimulant use has been associated with growth suppression. Growth should be monitored during treatment. Prolonged and painful erections (priapism), sometimes requiring surgical intervention, have been reported with methylphenidate use in pediatric and adult patients. Priapism has been reported to develop after some time on the drug, often subsequent to an increase in dose and also during a period of drug withdrawal (drug holidays or discontinuation). Patients who develop abnormally sustained or frequent and painful erections should seek immediate medical attention.

Drug Interactions

Avoid Concomitant Use

Avoid concomitant use of Dexmethylphenidate with any of the following: Iobenguane I 123; MAO Inhibitors

Decreased Effect

Dexmethylphenidate may decrease the levels/ effects of: Iobenguane I 123; Ioflupane I 123

Increased Effect/Toxicity

Dexmethylphenidate may increase the levels/ effects of: Fosphenytoin; PHENobarbital; Phenytoin; Primidone; Sympathomimetics; Tricyclic Antidepressants; Vitamin K Antagonists

The levels/effects of Dexmethylphenidate may be increased by: Antacids; AtoMOXetine; Cannabinoids; H2-Antagonists; MAO Inhibitors; Proton Pump Inhibitors

Nutritional/Ethanol Interactions

Ethanol: Avoid ethanol (may cause CNS depression).

Food: High-fat meal may increase time to peak concentration.

Herb/Nutraceutical: Avoid ephedra (may cause hypertension or arrhythmias) and yohimbe (also has CNS stimulatory activity).

Adverse Reactions Actual frequency may be dependent upon dose and/or formulation.

>10%:

Central nervous system: Headache (25% to 39%), insomnia (children 5% to 17%), restlessness (adults 12%), anxiety (5% to 11%)

Gastrointestinal: Appetite decreased (children 30%), xerostomia (adults 7% to 20%), abdominal pain (children 15%)

1% to 10%:

Central nervous system: Dizziness (adults 6%), fever (children 5%), irritability (children ≤5%), depression (children ≤3%), mood swings (children ≤3%)

Dermatologic: Pruritus (children ≤3%)

Gastrointestinal: Nausea (children 9%), dyspepsia (5% to 9%), vomiting (children 2% to 9%), anorexia (children 5% to 7%), pharyngolaryngeal pain (adults 4% to 7%)

Respiratory: Nasal congestion (children ≤5%)

Also refer to Methylphenidate for adverse effects seen with other methylphenidate products.

Pharmacodynamics/Kinetics

Onset of Action Extended release: ≥0.5 hours

Duration of Action Extended release: 12 hours

Controlled Substance C-II

Available Dosage Forms

Capsule Extended Release 24 Hour, Oral:
Focalin XR: 5 mg, 10 mg, 15 mg, 20 mg, 25 mg, 30 mg, 35 mg, 40 mg
Generic: 15 mg, 30 mg, 40 mg

Tablet, Oral:
Focalin: 2.5 mg, 5 mg, 10 mg
Generic: 2.5 mg, 5 mg, 10 mg

General Dosage Range Oral:

Extended release:

Children ≥6 years: Initial: 5 mg once daily; Maintenance: Up to 30 mg/day

Adults: Initial: 10 mg once daily; Maintenance: Up to 40 mg/day

Immediate release: *Children ≥6 years and Adults:* Initial: 2.5 mg twice daily; Maintenance: Up to 20 mg/day in 2 divided doses (at least 4 hours apart)

Administration

Oral

Capsule: Should be administered once daily in the morning; do not crush or chew. Capsules may be opened and contents sprinkled over a spoonful of applesauce; consume immediately; do not store for future use.

Tablet: Should be administered at least 4 hours apart; may be taken with or without food.

Storage/Stability Store at 25°C (77°F); excursions permitted to 15°C to 30°C (59°F to 86°F). Protect from light and moisture.

Nursing Actions

Physical Assessment Perform careful cardiovascular assessment prior to initiating therapy. Monitor vital signs at beginning of therapy and periodically throughout. In children, monitor growth pattern. If growth/weight gain is not as expected, may need to discontinue medication. Taper dosage when discontinuing from long-term therapy.

Patient Education

• Discuss specific use of drug and side effects with patient as it relates to treatment. (HCAHPS: During this hospital stay, were you given any medicine that you had not taken before? Before giving you any new medicine, how often did hospital staff tell you what the medicine was for? How often did hospital staff describe possible side effects in a way you could understand?)

• Patient may experience dizziness, fatigue, dyspepsia, headache, weight loss, lack of appetite, insomnia, or xerostomia. Have patient report immediately to prescriber arthralgia, skin discoloration, bradycardia, tachycardia, arrhythmia, severe headache, considerable nausea, blurred vision, vision changes, urine discoloration, jaundice, chills, pharyngitis, tremors, difficulty with motor activity, hyperhidrosis, significant asthenia, paresthesia, temperature sensitivity, wounds on fingers or toes, priapism, signs of severe cardiac abnormalities, behavioral changes, mood changes, anger, hallucinations, or signs of depression (ie, suicidal ideation, anxiety, emotional instability, or illogical thinking) (HCAHPS).

• Educate patient about signs of a significant reaction (eg, wheezing; chest tightness; fever;

itching; bad cough; blue skin color; seizures; or swelling of face, lips, tongue, or throat). **Note:** This is not a comprehensive list of all side effects. Patient should consult prescriber for additional questions.

Intended Use and Disclaimer: Should not be printed and given to patients. This information is intended to serve as a concise initial reference for healthcare professionals to use when discussing medications with a patient. You must ultimately rely on your own discretion, experience and judgment in diagnosing, treating and advising patients.

Dietary Considerations May be taken without regard to meals.

Related Information

Oral Medications That Should Not Be Crushed or Altered *on page 1712*

Dexrazoxane (deks ray ZOKS ane)

Brand Names: U.S. Totect; Zinecard
Index Terms ICRF-187
Pharmacologic Category Antidote; Antidote, Extravasation; Chemoprotective Agent
Medication Safety Issues
Sound-alike/look-alike issues:
Zinecard may be confused with Gemzar

Pregnancy Risk Factor D
Lactation Excretion in breast milk unknown/not recommended
Use
Anthracycline extravasation (Totect): Treatment of anthracycline-induced extravasation
Cardioprotectant (Zinecard): Used to reduce the incidence and severity of cardiomyopathy associated with doxorubicin administration in women with metastatic breast cancer who have received a cumulative doxorubicin dose of 300 mg/m^2 and who would benefit from continuing therapy with doxorubicin. (Not recommended for use with initial doxorubicin therapy.)

Unlabeled Use Reduction of the incidence and severity of cardiomyopathy associated with doxorubicin administration (cumulative doses >300 mg/m^2) in patients with malignancies other than metastatic breast cancer who would benefit from continuing therapy with doxorubicin; reduction of the incidence and severity of cardiomyopathy associated with continued epirubicin administration for advanced breast cancer; prevention of doxorubicin cardiomyopathy associated with acute lymphoblastic leukemia treatment in children

Available Dosage Forms
Solution Reconstituted, Intravenous:
Totect: 500 mg (1 ea)
Zinecard: 250 mg (1 ea); 500 mg (1 ea)
Generic: 250 mg (1 ea); 500 mg (1 ea)

General Dosage Range Dosage adjustment recommended in patients with renal impairment and hepatic impairment

I.V.: *Adults:* A 10:1 ratio of dexrazoxane:doxorubicin (dexrazoxane 500 mg/m^2:doxorubicin 50 mg/m^2) (prevention of cardiomyopathy) **or** 1000 mg/m^2 on days 1 and 2 (maximum dose: 2000 mg), followed by 500 mg/m^2 on day 3 (maximum dose: 1000 mg) (anthracycline-induced extravasation)

Administration
I.V.
Prevention of doxorubicin cardiomyopathy: Administer doxorubicin within 30 minutes after beginning the infusion with dexrazoxane.

Zinecard: Administer by rapid drip infusion; do **not** administer by I.V. push

Dexrazoxane generic formulation (Bedford Laboratories, Mylan, Inc): Administer by slow I.V push or rapid drip infusion

Treatment of anthracycline extravasation: Stop vesicant infusion immediately and disconnect I.V. line (leave needle/cannula in place); gently aspirate extravasated solution from the I.V. line (do **NOT** flush the line); remove needle/cannula; elevate extremity. Administer dexrazoxane I.V. over 1-2 hours; begin infusion as soon as possible, within 6 hours of extravasation. Day 2 and 3 doses should be administered at approximately the same time (± 3 hours) as the dose on day 1. Infusion solution should be at room temperature prior to administration. Infuse in a large vein in an area remote from the extravasation. For I.V. administration only; not for local infiltration into extravasation.

Apply dry cold compresses for 20 minutes 4 times daily for 1-2 days (Pérez Fidalgo, 2012); withhold cooling beginning 15 minutes before dexrazoxane infusion; continue withholding cooling until 15 minutes after infusion is completed. Do not use DMSO in combination with dexrazoxane; may lessen efficacy.

Hazardous agent; use appropriate precautions for handling and disposal (meets NIOSH, 2012 criteria).

Nursing Actions
Physical Assessment Monitor cardiac function closely. Assess infusion site frequently. Avoid extravasation.
Patient Education
• Discuss specific use of drug and side effects with patient as it relates to treatment. (HCAHPS: During this hospital stay, were you given any medicine that you had not taken before? Before giving you any new medicine, how often did hospital staff tell you what the medicine was for? How often did hospital staff describe possible side effects in a way you could understand?)
• Patient may experience nausea. Have patient report immediately to prescriber signs of

infection, dyspnea, excessive weight gain, edema of extremities, ecchymosis, hemorrhaging, severe asthenia, or injection site irritation (HCAHPS).

- Educate patient about signs of a significant reaction (eg, wheezing; chest tightness; fever; itching; bad cough; blue skin color; seizures; or swelling of face, lips, tongue, or throat). **Note:** This is not a comprehensive list of all side effects. Patient should consult prescriber for additional questions.

Intended Use and Disclaimer: Should not be printed and given to patients. This information is intended to serve as a concise initial reference for healthcare professionals to use when discussing medications with a patient. You must ultimately rely on your own discretion, experience and judgment in diagnosing, treating and advising patients.

Related Information

Management of Drug Extravasations *on page 1700*

Dextranomer and Sodium Hyaluronate

(deks TRAN oh mer & SOW dee um hye al yoor ON ate)

Brand Names: U.S. Solesta®

Index Terms Sodium Hyaluronate and Dextranomer

Pharmacologic Category Skin and Mucous Membrane Agent, Miscellaneous

Use Treatment of fecal incontinence in patients who have failed to respond to conservative therapy (eg, diet, fiber therapy, antimotility medications)

Mechanism of Action/Effect Reduces frequency of fecal incontinence episodes; believed to work by building or bulking up tissue in the anal area to narrow the opening of the anus.

Contraindications Hypersensitivity to hyaluronic acid-based products or any component of the formulation; active inflammatory bowel disease; immunodeficiencies or immunosuppressive therapy; prior pelvic radiation; significant mucosal or full thickness rectal prolapse; active anorectal conditions (eg, abscess, fissure, sepsis, bleeding, proctitis, infection); anorectal atresia, tumors, stenosis, or malformation; rectocele; rectal varices; existing anorectal implant (other than Solesta®)

Warnings/Precautions Bleeding risk at injection site is increased in patients with bleeding diathesis or in patients using anticoagulant or antiplatelet agents. Avoid injection in the midline of the anterior rectal wall in men with enlarged prostate.

Should only be administered by a physician familiar with anorectal procedures and who has been trained and certified in the Solesta® injection procedure. Do not administer intravascularly; injection into blood vessels may cause vascular occlusion. Safety and efficacy have not been investigated in patients with complete external sphincter disruption, significant chronic anorectal pain, rectal anastomosis <12 cm from anal verge, anorectal surgery within past 12 months, hemorrhoid treatment with rubber band within 3 months, anorectal implants and previous injection therapy, stapled transanal rectal resection, or stapled hemorrhoidectomy.

Adverse Reactions

>10%: Gastrointestinal: Proctalgia (17%)

1% to 10%:

Central nervous system: Fever (7%), chills (2%), pain (1%)

Gastrointestinal: Rectal hemorrhage (8%), anal hemorrhage (4%), diarrhea (4%), rectal discharge (4%), proctitis (3%), anorectal discomfort (2%), anal prolapse (2%), anal pruritus (2%), constipation (2%), rectal abscess (2%), anal fissure (1%), defecation urgency (1%), lower abdominal pain (1%), painful defecation (1%), rectal obstruction (1%)

Genitourinary: Dyspareunia (1%)

Local: Injection site hemorrhage (8%), injection site pain (5%)

Available Dosage Forms

Injection, gel:

Solesta®: Dextranomer 50 mg and sodium hyaluronate 15 mg per 1 mL (1 mL)

General Dosage Range Submucosal: *Adults:* 4 mL given as 4 x 1mL injections in the anal canal

Administration

Other Submucosal injection: Do **not** administer intravascularly.

Administer enema immediately prior to evacuate the anorectum and cleanse injection site with antiseptic. Use of prophylactic antibiotics is recommended. Refer to product labeling for detailed administration instructions.

Storage/Stability Store at ≤25°C (≤77°F); do not freeze; protect from sunlight.

Nursing Actions

Patient Education

- Discuss specific use of drug and side effects with patient as it relates to treatment. (HCAHPS: During this hospital stay, were you given any medicine that you had not taken before? Before giving you any new medicine, how often did hospital staff tell you what the medicine was for? How often did hospital staff describe possible side effects in a way you could understand?)
- Educate patient about signs of a significant reaction (eg, wheezing; chest tightness; fever; itching; bad cough; blue skin color; seizures; or swelling of face, lips, tongue, or throat). **Note:** This is not a comprehensive list of all side effects. Patient should consult prescriber for additional questions.

Intended Use and Disclaimer: Should not be printed and given to patients. This information is intended to serve as a concise initial reference for healthcare professionals to use when discussing

medications with a patient. You must ultimately rely on your own discretion, experience and judgment in diagnosing, treating and advising patients.

Dextroamphetamine (deks troe am FET a meen)

Brand Names: U.S. Dexedrine; ProCentra; Zenzedi

Index Terms Dextroamphetamine Sulfate

Pharmacologic Category Central Nervous System Stimulant

Medication Safety Issues

Sound-alike/look-alike issues:

Dexedrine® may be confused with dextran, Excedrin®

Dextroamphetamine may be confused with dexamethasone

Medication Guide Available Yes

Pregnancy Risk Factor C

Lactation Enters breast milk/not recommended

Use Narcolepsy; attention-deficit/hyperactivity disorder (ADHD)

Controlled Substance C-II

Available Dosage Forms

Capsule Extended Release 24 Hour, Oral:
Dexedrine: 5 mg, 10 mg, 15 mg
Generic: 5 mg, 10 mg, 15 mg

Solution, Oral:
ProCentra: 5 mg/5 mL (473 mL)
Generic: 5 mg/5 mL (473 mL)

Tablet, Oral:
Zenzedi: 2.5 mg, 5 mg, 7.5 mg, 10 mg
Generic: 5 mg, 10 mg

General Dosage Range Oral:

Children 3-5 years: Initial: 2.5 mg once daily; Maintenance: 0.1-0.5 mg/kg once daily (maximum: 40 mg/day)

Children 6-12 years: Initial: 5 mg once or twice daily; Maintenance: 5-20 mg (0.1-0.5 mg/kg) once daily (maximum: 40 mg [ADHD]: 60 mg [narcolepsy])

Children >12 years: Initial: 5-10 mg/day in 1-2 divided doses; Maximum: Up to 40 mg/day [ADHD] or 60 mg/day [narcolepsy]

Adults: Initial: 10 mg once daily; Maximum: Up to 60 mg/day

Administration

Oral Administer initial dose upon awakening; do not administer doses late in the evening due to potential for insomnia.

Immediate release tablets and oral solution: If needed, 1-2 additional doses may be administered at intervals of 4-6 hours.

Extended release or sustained release capsules: Do not crush sustained release drug products. Formulations may be used for once-daily administration, if appropriate.

Nursing Actions

Physical Assessment Assess for history of suicidal tendencies. Monitor blood pressure and vital signs at start of therapy, when changing dosage, and at regular intervals throughout. Monitor serum glucose closely in patients with diabetes and monitor weight closely; weight loss may occur. Taper dosage slowly when discontinuing.

Patient Education

• Discuss specific use of drug and side effects with patient as it relates to treatment. (HCAHPS: During this hospital stay, were you given any medicine that you had not taken before? Before giving you any new medicine, how often did hospital staff tell you what the medicine was for? How often did hospital staff describe possible side effects in a way you could understand?)

• Patient may experience dizziness, xerostomia, lack of appetite, insomnia, constipation, diarrhea, dyspepsia, akathisia, or parageusia. Have patient report immediately to prescriber tachycardia, severe headache, sexual dysfunction, arrhythmia, excessive weight loss, significant nausea, difficulty with motor activity, asthenia, discoloration of hands or feet, paresthesia, temperature sensitivity, wounds on fingers or toes, strength differences from one side to another, difficulty speaking or thinking, change in balance, vision changes, dyspnea, intolerable dizziness, syncope, or signs of depression (ie, suicidal ideation, anxiety, emotional instability, illogical thinking) (HCAHPS).

• Educate patient about signs of a significant reaction (eg, wheezing; chest tightness; fever; itching; bad cough; blue skin color; seizures; or swelling of face, lips, tongue, or throat). **Note:** This is not a comprehensive list of all side effects. Patient should consult prescriber for additional questions.

Intended Use and Disclaimer: Should not be printed and given to patients. This information is intended to serve as a concise initial reference for healthcare professionals to use when discussing medications with a patient. You must ultimately rely on your own discretion, experience and judgment in diagnosing, treating and advising patients.

Related Information

Oral Medications That Should Not Be Crushed or Altered *on page 1712*

Dextroamphetamine and Amphetamine
(deks troe am FET a meen & am FET a meen)

Brand Names: U.S. Adderall; Adderall XR

Index Terms Amphetamine and Dextroamphetamine

Pharmacologic Category Central Nervous System Stimulant

Medication Safety Issues
Sound-alike/look-alike issues:
Adderall may be confused with Inderal
Medication Guide Available Yes
Pregnancy Risk Factor C
Lactation Enters breast milk/not recommended
Breast-Feeding Considerations The majority of human data is based on illicit amphetamine/meth-amphetamine exposure and not from therapeutic maternal use (Golub, 2005). Amphetamines are excreted into breast milk and use may decrease milk production. Increased irritability, agitation, and crying have been reported in nursing infants (ACOG, 2011). A case report describes maternal use of amphetamine 20 mg/day throughout pregnancy and while breast-feeding. Milk concentrations were higher in breast milk than the maternal serum. The milk/plasma ratio ranged from 2.8-7.5 when measured on days 10 and 42 following delivery (Steiner, 1984). The manufacturer recommends that mothers taking dextroamphetamine/amphetamine refrain from nursing.
Use Attention-deficit/hyperactivity disorder (ADHD); narcolepsy
Mechanism of Action/Effect Amphetamines release catecholamines from storage sites in the nerve terminals.
Contraindications Hypersensitivity or idiosyncrasy to the sympathomimetic amines; advanced arteriosclerosis; symptomatic cardiovascular disease; moderate-to-severe hypertension; hyperthyroidism; hypersensitivity or idiosyncrasy to the sympathomimetic amines; glaucoma; agitated states; patients with a history of drug abuse; during or within 14 days following MAO inhibitor (hypertensive crisis)
Warnings/Precautions [U.S. Boxed Warning]: Use has been associated with serious cardiovascular events including sudden death in patients with pre-existing structural cardiac abnormalities or other serious heart problems (sudden death in children and adolescents; sudden death, stroke and MI in adults. These products should be avoided in the patients with known serious structural cardiac abnormalities, cardiomyopathy, serious heart rhythm abnormalities, or other serious cardiac problems that could increase the risk of sudden death that these conditions alone carry. Patients should be carefully evaluated for cardiac disease prior to initiation of therapy. Patients who develop symptoms such as exertional chest pain, unexplained syncope, or other symptoms suggestive of cardiac disease during treatment should undergo a prompt cardiac evaluation. Use with caution in patients with hypertension and other cardiovascular conditions that might be exacerbated by increases in blood pressure or heart rate. Stimulants are associated with peripheral vasculopathy, including Raynaud's phenomenon; signs/symptoms are usually mild and intermittent, and generally improve with dose reduction or discontinuation. Digital ulceration and/or soft tissue breakdown have been observed rarely; monitor for digital changes during therapy and seek further evaluation (eg, rheumatology) if necessary. Amphetamines may impair the ability to engage in potentially hazardous activities. May cause visual disturbances.

Use with caution in patients with psychiatric or seizure disorders. May exacerbate symptoms of behavior and thought disorder in psychotic patients; new-onset psychosis or mania may occur with stimulant use; observe for symptoms of aggression and/or hostility. Screen patients with comorbid depressive symptoms prior to initiating treatment to determine if they are at risk for bipolar disorder. Stimulants may unmask tics in individuals with coexisting Tourette's syndrome. **[U.S. Boxed Warning]: Potential for drug dependency exists; prolonged use may lead to drug dependency.** Use is contraindicated in patients with history of drug abuse. Prescriptions should be written for the smallest quantity consistent with good patient care to minimize possibility of overdose. Abrupt discontinuation following high doses or for prolonged periods may result in symptoms for withdrawal.

Appetite suppression may occur; monitor weight during therapy, particularly in children. Use of stimulants has been associated with suppression of growth; monitor growth rate during treatment. Not recommended for children younger than 3 years.

Drug Interactions
Avoid Concomitant Use
Avoid concomitant use of Dextroamphetamine and Amphetamine with any of the following: Iobenguane I 123; MAO Inhibitors
Decreased Effect
Dextroamphetamine and Amphetamine may decrease the levels/effects of: Antihistamines; Ethosuximide; Iobenguane I 123; Ioflupane I 123; PHENobarbital; Phenytoin

The levels/effects of Dextroamphetamine and Amphetamine may be decreased by: Ammonium Chloride; Antipsychotics; Ascorbic Acid; Gastrointestinal Acidifying Agents; Lithium; Methenamine; Multivitamins/Fluoride (with ADE); Multivitamins/Minerals (with ADEK, Folate, Iron); Multivitamins/Minerals (with AE, No Iron); Peginterferon Alfa-2b; Urinary Acidifying Agents
Increased Effect/Toxicity
Dextroamphetamine and Amphetamine may increase the levels/effects of: Analgesics (Opioid); Sympathomimetics

The levels/effects of Dextroamphetamine and Amphetamine may be increased by: Alkalinizing Agents; Antacids; AtoMOXetine; Cannabinoids; Carbonic Anhydrase Inhibitors; MAO Inhibitors; Proton Pump Inhibitors; Tricyclic Antidepressants

Nutritional/Ethanol Interactions Food: Amphetamine serum levels may be reduced if taken with acidic food, juices, or vitamin C. Management: Monitor response when taken concurrently.

Adverse Reactions

As reported with Adderall XR:

>10%:

Central nervous system: Insomnia (12% to 27%), headache (adults ≤26%)

Gastrointestinal: Decreased appetite (22% to 36%), abdominal pain (11% to 14%), xerostomia (2% to 35%), weight loss (4% to 11%)

1% to 10%:

Cardiovascular: Tachycardia (adults ≤6%), palpitations (2% to 4%)

Central nervous system: Emotional lability (2% to 9%), agitation (adults ≤8%), anxiety (adults 8%), dizziness (2% to 7%), nervousness (6%), drowsiness (2% to 4%), speech disturbance (2% to 4%)

Dermatologic: Diaphoresis (2% to 4%), skin photosensitivity (2% to 4%)

Endocrine & metabolic: Dysmenorrhea (2% to 4%), decreased libido (2% to 4%)

Gastrointestinal: Nausea (2% to 8%), vomiting (2% to 7%), diarrhea (2% to 6%), constipation (2% to 4%), dyspepsia (2% to 4%), teeth clenching (2% to 4%), anorexia (2%)

Genitourinary: Urinary tract infection (5%), impotence (2% to 4%)

Infection: Increased susceptibility to infection (2% to 4%), tooth infection (2% to 4%)

Neuromuscular & skeletal: Twitching (2% to 4%)

Respiratory: Dyspnea (2% to 4%)

Miscellaneous: Fever (5%)

Controlled Substance C-II

Available Dosage Forms

Capsule, extended release, oral:

5 mg [dextroamphetamine sulfate 1.25 mg, dextroamphetamine saccharate 1.25 mg, amphetamine aspartate monohydrate 1.25 mg, amphetamine sulfate 1.25 mg]

10 mg [dextroamphetamine sulfate 2.5 mg, dextroamphetamine saccharate 2.5 mg, amphetamine aspartate monohydrate 2.5 mg, amphetamine sulfate 2.5 mg]

15 mg [dextroamphetamine sulfate 3.75 mg, dextroamphetamine saccharate 3.75 mg, amphetamine aspartate monohydrate 3.75 mg, amphetamine sulfate 3.75 mg]

20 mg [dextroamphetamine sulfate 5 mg, dextroamphetamine saccharate 5 mg, amphetamine aspartate monohydrate 5 mg, amphetamine sulfate 5 mg]

25 mg [dextroamphetamine sulfate 6.25 mg, dextroamphetamine saccharate 6.25 mg, amphetamine aspartate monohydrate 6.25 mg, amphetamine sulfate 6.25 mg]

30 mg [dextroamphetamine sulfate 7.5 mg, dextroamphetamine saccharate 7.5 mg, amphetamine aspartate monohydrate 7.5 mg, amphetamine sulfate 7.5 mg]

Adderall XR:

5 mg [dextroamphetamine 1.25 mg, dextroamphetamine saccharate 1.25 mg, amphetamine aspartate monohydrate 1.25 mg, amphetamine sulfate 1.25 mg]

10 mg [dextroamphetamine sulfate 2.5 mg, dextroamphetamine saccharate 2.5 mg, amphetamine aspartate monohydrate 2.5 mg, amphetamine sulfate 2.5 mg]

15 mg [dextroamphetamine sulfate 3.75 mg, dextroamphetamine saccharate 3.75 mg, amphetamine aspartate monohydrate 3.75 mg, amphetamine sulfate 3.75 mg]

20 mg [dextroamphetamine sulfate 5 mg, dextroamphetamine saccharate 5 mg, amphetamine aspartate monohydrate 5 mg, amphetamine sulfate 5 mg]

25 mg [dextroamphetamine sulfate 6.25 mg, dextroamphetamine saccharate 6.25 mg, amphetamine aspartate monohydrate 6.25 mg, amphetamine sulfate 6.25 mg]

30 mg [dextroamphetamine sulfate 7.5 mg, dextroamphetamine saccharate 7.5 mg, amphetamine aspartate monohydrate 7.5 mg, amphetamine sulfate 7.5 mg]

Tablet, oral: 5 mg, 7.5 mg, 10 mg, 12.5 mg, 15 mg, 20 mg, 30 mg

5 mg [dextroamphetamine sulfate 1.25 mg, dextroamphetamine saccharate 1.25 mg, amphetamine aspartate monohydrate 1.25 mg, amphetamine sulfate 1.25 mg]

7.5 mg [dextroamphetamine sulfate 1.875 mg, dextroamphetamine saccharate 1.875 mg, amphetamine aspartate monohydrate 1.875 mg, amphetamine sulfate 1.875 mg]

10 mg [dextroamphetamine sulfate 2.5 mg, dextroamphetamine saccharate 2.5 mg, amphetamine aspartate monohydrate 2.5 mg, amphetamine sulfate 2.5 mg]

12.5 mg [dextroamphetamine sulfate 3.125 mg, dextroamphetamine saccharate 3.125 mg, amphetamine aspartate monohydrate 3.125 mg, amphetamine sulfate 3.125 mg]

15 mg [dextroamphetamine sulfate 3.75 mg, dextroamphetamine saccharate 3.75 mg, amphetamine aspartate monohydrate 3.75 mg, amphetamine sulfate 3.75 mg]

20 mg [dextroamphetamine sulfate 5 mg, dextroamphetamine saccharate 5 mg, amphetamine aspartate monohydrate 5 mg, amphetamine sulfate 5 mg]

30 mg [dextroamphetamine sulfate 7.5 mg, dextroamphetamine saccharate 7.5 mg, amphetamine aspartate monohydrate 7.5 mg, amphetamine sulfate 7.5 mg]

Adderall:

5 mg [dextroamphetamine sulfate 1.25 mg, dextroamphetamine saccharate 1.25 mg, amphetamine aspartate monohydrate 1.25 mg, amphetamine sulfate 1.25 mg]

7.5 mg [dextroamphetamine sulfate 1.875 mg, dextroamphetamine saccharate 1.875 mg, amphetamine aspartate monohydrate 1.875 mg, amphetamine sulfate 1.875 mg]

10 mg [dextroamphetamine sulfate 2.5 mg, dextroamphetamine saccharate 2.5 mg, amphetamine aspartate monohydrate 2.5 mg, amphetamine sulfate 2.5 mg]

12.5 mg [dextroamphetamine sulfate 3.125 mg, dextroamphetamine saccharate 3.125 mg, amphetamine aspartate monohydrate 3.125 mg, amphetamine sulfate 3.125 mg]

15 mg [dextroamphetamine sulfate 3.75 mg, dextroamphetamine saccharate 3.75 mg, amphetamine aspartate monohydrate 3.75 mg, amphetamine sulfate 3.75 mg]

20 mg [dextroamphetamine sulfate 5 mg, dextroamphetamine saccharate 5 mg, amphetamine aspartate monohydrate 5 mg, amphetamine sulfate 5 mg]

30 mg [dextroamphetamine sulfate 7.5 mg, dextroamphetamine saccharate 7.5 mg, amphetamine aspartate monohydrate 7.5 mg, amphetamine sulfate 7.5 mg]

General Dosage Range Oral:

Extended release:

Children 6-12 years: Initial: 5-10 mg once daily (maximum: 30 mg daily)

Adolescents 13-17 years: Initial: 10 mg once daily; maintenance: 10-20 mg once daily

Adults: 20 mg once daily

Immediate release:

Children 3-5 years: Initial: 2.5 mg once daily (maximum: 40 mg daily)

Children 6-12 years: Initial: 5 mg once or twice daily (maximum: 40 mg daily [ADHD] or 60 mg daily [narcolepsy])

Children >12 years and Adults: Initial: 5 mg once or twice daily (maximum: 40 mg daily [ADHD]; 10 mg daily; maximum 60 mg daily [narcolepsy])

Administration

Oral May be administered without regard to meals. If possible, therapy should occasionally be interrupted to determine if continued therapy is needed.

Adderall: To avoid insomnia, late evening doses should be avoided.

Adderall XR: Administer first dose as soon as awake; should be given by noon. Capsule may be swallowed whole or it may be opened and the contents sprinkled on applesauce. Applesauce should be consumed immediately without chewing. Do not divide the contents of the capsule.

Storage/Stability Store at controlled room temperature of 15°C to 30°C (59°F to 86°F). Protect from light.

Nursing Actions

Physical Assessment See individual agents.

Patient Education

• Discuss specific use of drug and side effects with patient as it relates to treatment. (HCAHPS: During this hospital stay, were you given any medicine that you had not taken before? Before giving you any new medicine, how often did hospital staff tell you what the medicine was for? How often did hospital staff describe possible side effects in a way you could understand?)

• Patient may experience lack of appetite, insomnia, constipation, diarrhea, xerostomia, akathisia, or parageusia. Have patient report immediately to prescriber tachycardia, considerable headache, sexual dysfunction, arrhythmias, chills, pharyngitis, dysuria, polyuria, significant dyspepsia, excessive weight loss, intolerable nausea, difficulty with motor activity, severe asthenia, discoloration of hands or feet, paresthesia, temperature sensitivity, wounds on fingers or toes, strength differences from one side to another, difficulty speaking or thinking, change in balance, vision changes, dyspnea, intolerable dizziness, syncope, or signs of depression (ie, suicidal ideation, anxiety, emotional instability, illogical thinking) (HCAHPS).

• Educate patient about signs of a significant reaction (eg, wheezing; chest tightness; fever; itching; bad cough; blue skin color; seizures; or swelling of face, lips, tongue, or throat). **Note:** This is not a comprehensive list of all side effects. Patient should consult prescriber for additional questions.

Intended Use and Disclaimer: Should not be printed and given to patients. This information is intended to serve as a concise initial reference for healthcare professionals to use when discussing medications with a patient. You must ultimately rely on your own discretion, experience and judgment in diagnosing, treating and advising patients.

Related Information

Dextroamphetamine *on page 433*

Oral Medications That Should Not Be Crushed or Altered *on page 1712*

Dextromethorphan and Chlorpheniramine

(deks troe meth OR fan & klor fen IR a meen)

Brand Names: U.S. Coricidin® HBP Cough & Cold [OTC]; Dimetapp® Children's Long Acting Cough Plus Cold [OTC]; Robitussin® Children's Cough & Cold Long-Acting [OTC]; Scot-Tussin® DM Maximum Strength [OTC]; Triaminic® Children's Softchews® Cough & Runny Nose [OTC]

Index Terms Chlorpheniramine and Dextromethorphan; Chlorpheniramine Maleate and

Dextromethorphan Hydrobromide; Dextromethorphan Hydrobromide and Chlorpheniramine Maleate

Pharmacologic Category Alkylamine Derivative; Antitussive; Histamine H₁ Antagonist; Histamine H₁ Antagonist, First Generation

Use Symptomatic relief of runny nose, sneezing, itchy/watery eyes, cough, and other upper respiratory symptoms associated with hay fever, common cold, or upper respiratory allergies

Available Dosage Forms

Syrup, oral:

Dimetapp® Children's Long Acting Cough Plus Cold [OTC]: Dextromethorphan 7.5 mg and chlorpheniramine 1 mg per 5 mL (118 mL)

Robitussin® Children's Cough and Cold Long-Acting [OTC]: Dextromethorphan 7.5 mg and chlorpheniramine 1 mg per 5 mL (118 mL)

Scot-Tussin® DM Maximum Strength [OTC]: Dextromethorphan 15 mg and chlorpheniramine 2 mg per 5 mL (118 mL)

Tablet, oral:

Coricidin® HBP Cough and Cold [OTC]: Dextromethorphan 30 mg and chlorpheniramine 4 mg

Tablet, softchew, oral:

Triaminic® Children's Softchews® Cough & Runny Nose [OTC]: Dextromethorphan 5 mg and chlorpheniramine 1 mg

General Dosage Range Oral:

Children 6-11 years: Dextromethorphan 10-15 mg and chlorpheniramine 2 mg every 4-6 hours as needed (maximum: 60 mg dextromethorphan and 10 mg chlorpheniramine/24 hours)

Children ≥12 years and Adults: Dextromethorphan 30 mg and chlorpheniramine 4 mg every 6 hours as needed (maximum: 120 mg dextromethorphan and 16 mg chlorpheniramine/24 hours)

Administration

Oral Triaminic® Children's Softchews® Cough & Runny Nose: Dissolve in mouth or chew prior to swallowing.

Nursing Actions

Patient Education

• Discuss specific use of drug and side effects with patient as it relates to treatment. (HCAHPS: During this hospital stay, were you given any medicine that you had not taken before? Before giving you any new medicine, how often did hospital staff tell you what the medicine was for? How often did hospital staff describe possible side effects in a way you could understand?)

• Patient may experience fatigue or anxiety (HCAHPS).

• Educate patient about signs of a significant reaction (eg, wheezing; chest tightness; fever; itching; bad cough; blue skin color; seizures; or swelling of face, lips, tongue, or throat). **Note:** This is not a comprehensive list of all side effects. Patient should consult prescriber for additional questions.

Intended Use and Disclaimer: Should not be printed and given to patients. This information is intended to serve as a concise initial reference for healthcare professionals to use when discussing medications with a patient. You must ultimately rely on your own discretion, experience and judgment in diagnosing, treating and advising patients.

Dextromethorphan and Quinidine
(deks troe meth OR fan & KWIN i deen)

Brand Names: U.S. Nuedexta™

Index Terms Dextromethorphan Hydrobromide and Quinidine Sulfate; Quinidine and Dextromethorphan

Pharmacologic Category N-Methyl-D-Aspartate Receptor Antagonist

Medication Safety Issues

Sound-alike/look-alike issues:

Nuedexta™ may be confused with Neulasta®

Pregnancy Risk Factor C

Lactation Use caution

Use Treatment of pseudobulbar affect (PBA)

Available Dosage Forms

Capsule, oral:

Nuedexta™: Dextromethorphan hydrobromide 20 mg and quinidine sulfate 10 mg

General Dosage Range

Oral: *Adults:* Initial: Once capsule once daily for 7 days; Maintenance: One capsule twice daily

Administration

Oral May be administered with or without food. Administer twice-daily doses every 12 hours.

Nursing Actions

Physical Assessment See individual agents.

Patient Education

• Discuss specific use of drug and side effects with patient as it relates to treatment. (HCAHPS: During this hospital stay, were you given any medicine that you had not taken before? Before giving you any new medicine, how often did hospital staff tell you what the medicine was for? How often did hospital staff describe possible side effects in a way you could understand?)

• Have patient report immediately to prescriber signs of hemorrhaging, signs of hepatic impairment, syncope, significant asthenia, considerable nausea, chills, arthralgia, myalgia, enlarged lymph node, edema of extremities, depression, vision changes, or serotonin syndrome (ie, dizziness, severe headache, agitation, hallucinations, tachycardia, arrhythmia, flushing, tremors, hyperhidrosis, change in balance, severe nausea, significant diarrhea) (HCAHPS).

• Educate patient about signs of a significant reaction (eg, wheezing; chest tightness; fever; itching; bad cough; blue skin color; seizures; or swelling of face, lips, tongue, or throat). **Note:** This is not a comprehensive list of all side

effects. Patient should consult prescriber for additional questions.

Intended Use and Disclaimer: Should not be printed and given to patients. This information is intended to serve as a concise initial reference for healthcare professionals to use when discussing medications with a patient. You must ultimately rely on your own discretion, experience and judgment in diagnosing, treating and advising patients.

Diazepam (dye AZ e pam)

Brand Names: U.S. Diastat AcuDial; Diastat Pediatric; Diazepam Intensol; Valium
Pharmacologic Category Benzodiazepine
Medication Safety Issues
Sound-alike/look-alike issues:
Diazepam may be confused with diazoxide, diltiazem, Ditropan, LORazepam
Valium® may be confused with Valcyte®
BEERS Criteria medication:
This drug may be potentially inappropriate for use in geriatric patients (Quality of evidence - high; Strength of recommendation - strong).
Pregnancy Risk Factor D
Lactation Enters breast milk/not recommended
Breast-Feeding Considerations Diazepam and N-desmethyldiazepam can be found in breast milk; the oxazepam metabolite has also been detected in the urine of a nursing infant. Drowsiness, lethargy, or weight loss in nursing infants have been observed in case reports following maternal use of some benzodiazepines, including diazepam (Iqbal, 2002). Because diazepam and its metabolites may be present in breast milk for prolonged periods following administration, one manufacturer recommends discontinuing breast-feeding for an appropriate period of time.
Use Management of anxiety disorders, ethanol withdrawal symptoms; skeletal muscle relaxant; treatment of convulsive disorders; preoperative or preprocedural sedation and amnesia
Rectal gel: Management of selected, refractory epilepsy patients on stable regimens of antiepileptic drugs requiring intermittent use of diazepam to control episodes of increased seizure activity
Unlabeled Use Panic disorders; short-term treatment of spasticity in children with cerebral palsy; sedation for mechanically-ventilated patients in the intensive care unit
Mechanism of Action/Effect Binds to stereospecific benzodiazepine receptors on the postsynaptic GABA neuron at several sites within the central nervous system, including the limbic system, reticular formation. Enhancement of the inhibitory effect of GABA on neuronal excitability results by increased neuronal membrane permeability to chloride ions. This shift in chloride ions results in

hyperpolarization (a less excitable state) and stabilization.

Contraindications Hypersensitivity to diazepam or any component of the formulation (cross-sensitivity with other benzodiazepines may exist); myasthenia gravis; severe respiratory insufficiency; severe hepatic insufficiency; sleep apnea syndrome; acute narrow-angle glaucoma; not for use in children <6 months of age (oral)
Warnings/Precautions Withdrawal has also been associated with an increase in the seizure frequency. Use with caution with drugs which may decrease diazepam metabolism. Use with caution in debilitated patients, obese patients, patients with hepatic disease (including alcoholics), or renal impairment. Active metabolites with extended half-lives may lead to delayed accumulation and adverse effects. Use with caution in patients with respiratory disease or impaired gag reflex.

Acute hypotension, muscle weakness, apnea, and cardiac arrest have occurred with parenteral administration. Acute effects may be more prevalent in patients receiving concurrent barbiturates, opioids, or ethanol. Appropriate resuscitative equipment and qualified personnel should be available during administration and monitoring. Avoid use of the injection in patients with shock, coma, or acute ethanol intoxication. Intra-arterial injection or extravasation of the parenteral formulation should be avoided. Parenteral formulation contains propylene glycol, which has been associated with toxicity when administered in high dosages. Administration of rectal gel should only be performed by individuals trained to recognize characteristic seizure activity and monitor response.

Causes CNS depression (dose-related) resulting in sedation, dizziness, confusion, or ataxia which may impair physical and mental capabilities. Patients must be cautioned about performing tasks which require mental alertness (eg, operating machinery or driving). Use with caution in patients receiving other CNS depressants or psychoactive agents. Effects with other sedative drugs or ethanol may be potentiated. The dosage of opioids should be reduced by approximately one-third when diazepam is added. Benzodiazepines have been associated with falls and traumatic injury and should be used with extreme caution in patients who are at risk of these events. Benzodiazepines with long half-lives may produce prolonged sedation and increase the risk of falls and fracture. In older adults, benzodiazepines increase the risk of impaired cognition, delirium, falls, fractures, and motor vehicle accidents. Due to increased sensitivity in this age group and slower metabolism of long-acting agents (such as diazepam), avoid use for treatment of insomnia, agitation, or delirium (Beers Criteria).

Use with caution in patients taking strong CYP3A4 inhibitors, moderate or strong CYP3A4 and CYP2C19 inducers and major CYP3A4 substrates.

Use caution in patients with depression or anxiety associated with depression, particularly if suicidal risk may be present. Use with caution in patients with a history of drug dependence. Benzodiazepines have been associated with dependence and acute withdrawal symptoms on discontinuation or reduction in dose. Acute withdrawal, including seizures, may be precipitated in patients after administration of flumazenil to patients receiving long-term benzodiazepine therapy.

Diazepam has been associated with anterograde amnesia. Psychiatric and paradoxical reactions, including hyperactive or aggressive behavior, have been reported with benzodiazepines, particularly in adolescent/pediatric or elderly patients. Does not have analgesic, antidepressant, or antipsychotic properties.

Rectal gel: Safety and efficacy have not been established in children <2 years of age.

Oral: Safety and efficacy have not been established in children <6 months of age.

Injection: Safety and efficacy have not been established in children <30 days of age. Solution for injection may contain sodium benzoate, benzyl alcohol, or benzoic acid. Large amounts have been associated with "gasping syndrome" in neonates. I.V. administration: Vesicant; ensure proper needle or catheter placement prior to and during administration; avoid extravasation.

Drug Interactions

Avoid Concomitant Use

Avoid concomitant use of Diazepam with any of the following: Azelastine (Nasal); Conivaptan; Fusidic Acid (Systemic); OLANZapine; Paraldehyde; Pimozide; Sodium Oxybate; Thalidomide

Decreased Effect

The levels/effects of Diazepam may be decreased by: Bosentan; CarBAMazepine; CYP2C19 Inducers (Strong); CYP3A4 Inducers (Strong); Dabrafenib; Deferasirox; Etravirine; Herbs (CYP3A4 Inducers); Mitotane; Rifamycin Derivatives; Theophylline Derivatives; Tocilizumab; Yohimbine

Increased Effect/Toxicity

Diazepam may increase the levels/effects of: Alcohol (Ethyl); ARIPiprazole; Azelastine (Nasal); Buprenorphine; CloZAPine; CNS Depressants; Dofetilide; Fosphenytoin; Hydrocodone; Lomitapide; Methotrimeprazine; Metyrosine; Mirtazapine; Paraldehyde; Phenytoin; Pimozide; Pramipexole; ROPINIRole; Rotigotine; Selective Serotonin Reuptake Inhibitors; Sodium Oxybate; Thalidomide; Zolpidem

The levels/effects of Diazepam may be increased by: Antifungal Agents (Azole Derivatives, Systemic); Aprepitant; Brimonidine (Topical); Calcium Channel Blockers (Nondihydropyridine); Cimetidine; Conivaptan; Contraceptives (Estrogens); Contraceptives (Progestins); Cosyntropin; CYP2C19 Inhibitors (Moderate); CYP2C19 Inhibitors (Strong); CYP3A4 Inhibitors (Moderate); CYP3A4 Inhibitors (Strong); Dasatinib; Disulfiram; Doxylamine; Droperidol; Etravirine; Fosamprenavir; Fosaprepitant; Fusidic Acid (Systemic); Grapefruit Juice; HydrOXYzine; Isoniazid; Ivacaftor; Luliconazole; Magnesium Sulfate; Methotrimeprazine; Mifepristone; OLANZapine; Perampanel; Proton Pump Inhibitors; Ritonavir; Saquinavir; Selective Serotonin Reuptake Inhibitors; Simeprevir; Stiripentol; Tapentadol

Nutritional/Ethanol Interactions

Ethanol: Ethanol may increase CNS depression. Potential for drug dependency exists. Management: Avoid ethanol.

Food: Diazepam serum concentrations may be decreased if taken with food. Grapefruit juice may increase diazepam serum concentrations. Management: Avoid concurrent use of grapefruit juice. Maintain adequate hydration, unless instructed to restrict fluid intake.

Herb/Nutraceutical: St John's wort may decrease diazepam levels. Yohimbe may decrease the effectiveness of diazepam. Kava kava, valerian, and gotu kola may increase CNS depression. Avoid St John's wort, yohimbe, kava kava, valerian, and gotu kola.

Adverse Reactions Frequency not defined. Adverse reactions may vary by route of administration.

Cardiovascular: Hypotension, vasodilatation

Central nervous system: Amnesia, ataxia, confusion, depression, drowsiness, fatigue, headache, slurred speech, paradoxical reactions (eg, aggressiveness, agitation, anxiety, delusions, hallucinations, inappropriate behavior, increased muscle spasms, insomnia, irritability, psychoses, rage, restlessness, sleep disturbances, stimulation), vertigo

Dermatologic: Rash

Endocrine & metabolic: Libido changes

Gastrointestinal: Constipation, diarrhea, nausea, salivation changes (dry mouth or hypersalivation)

Genitourinary: Incontinence, urinary retention

Hepatic: Jaundice

Local: Phlebitis, pain with injection

Neuromuscular & skeletal: Dysarthria, tremor, weakness

Ocular: Blurred vision, diplopia

Respiratory: Apnea, asthma, respiratory rate decreased

Pharmacodynamics/Kinetics

Onset of Action I.V.: Almost immediate; Oral: Rapid

Duration of Action I.V.: 20-30 minutes; Oral: Variable (dose and frequency dependent)

Controlled Substance C-IV

Available Dosage Forms

Concentrate, Oral:
Diazepam Intensol: 5 mg/mL (30 mL)

Device, Intramuscular:
Generic: 10 mg/2 mL (2 mL)

Gel, Rectal:
Diastat AcuDial: 10 mg (1 ea); 20 mg (1 ea)
Diastat Pediatric: 2.5 mg (1 ea)
Generic: 2.5 mg (1 ea); 10 mg (1 ea); 20 mg (1 ea)

Solution, Injection:
Generic: 5 mg/mL (2 mL, 10 mL)

Solution, Oral:
Generic: 1 mg/mL (5 mL, 500 mL)

Tablet, Oral:
Valium: 2 mg, 5 mg, 10 mg
Generic: 2 mg, 5 mg, 10 mg

General Dosage Range

I.M.: *Children >30 days and Adults:* Dosage varies greatly depending on indication

I.V.: *Children >30 days and Adults:* Dosage varies greatly depending on indication

Oral:
Children: 0.12-1 mg/kg/day divided every 6-8 hours **or** 0.2-0.3 mg/kg (maximum: 10 mg) prior to procedures
Adolescents: 0.12-0.8 mg/kg/day divided every 6-8 hours **or** 10 mg prior to procedures
Adults: Dosage varies greatly depending on indication

Rectal:
Gel:
Children 2-5 years: Initial: 0.5 mg/kg (maximum dose: 20 mg); may repeat in 4-12 hours if needed
Children 6-11 years: Initial: 0.3 mg/kg (maximum dose: 20 mg); may repeat in 4-12 hours if needed
Children ≥12 years and Adults: Initial: 0.2 mg/kg (maximum dose: 20 mg); may repeat in 4-12 hours if needed

Administration

I.V. Continuous infusion is not recommended because of precipitation in I.V. fluids and absorption of drug into infusion bags and tubing. In children, do not exceed 1-2 mg/minute IVP; in adults 5 mg/minute.

Vesicant; ensure proper needle or catheter placement prior to and during infusion; avoid extravasation.

Extravasation management: If extravasation occurs, stop I.V. administration immediately and disconnect (leave cannula/needle in place); gently aspirate extravasated solution (do **NOT** flush the line); remove needle/cannula; elevate extremity. Apply dry cold compresses (Hurst, 2004).

Injectable Detail pH: 6.2-6.9 (5 mg/mL solution in vial)

Oral Oral solution (Intensol™) should be diluted before use.

Rectal Rectal gel: Prior to administration, confirm that prescribed dose is visible and correct, and that the green "ready" band is visible. Patient should be positioned on side (facing person responsible for monitoring), with top leg bent forward. Insert rectal tip (lubricated) into rectum and push in plunger gently over 3 seconds. Remove tip of rectal syringe after 3 additional seconds. Buttocks should be held together for 3 seconds after removal. Dispose of syringe appropriately.

Preparation for Administration
Per manufacturer, do not mix I.V. product with other medications.

Storage/Stability
Injection: Store at 20°C to 25°C (68°F to 77°F); excursions permitted to 15°C to 30°C (59°F to 86°F). Protect from light. Potency is retained for up to 3 months when kept at room temperature. Most stable at pH 4-8; hydrolysis occurs at pH <3. Rectal gel: Store at 25°C (77°F); excursion permitted to 15°C to 30°C (59°F to 86°F). Tablet: Store at 15°C to 30°C (59°F to 86°F).

Nursing Actions

Physical Assessment Assess for history of addiction; long-term use can result in dependence, abuse, or tolerance; periodically evaluate need for continued use. Monitor blood pressure and CNS status. For inpatient use, institute safety measures to prevent falls. Taper dosage slowly when discontinuing. Teach patient seizure precautions (if administered for seizures).

Patient Education
• Discuss specific use of drug and side effects with patient as it relates to treatment. (HCAHPS: During this hospital stay, were you given any medicine that you had not taken before? Before giving you any new medicine, how often did hospital staff tell you what the medicine was for? How often did hospital staff describe possible side effects in a way you could understand?)

• Patient may experience presyncope, fatigue, or blurred vision. Have patient report immediately to prescriber signs of depression (ie, suicidal ideation, anxiety, emotional instability, illogical thinking), dyspnea, significant change in balance, hallucinations, memory loss, severe dizziness, syncope, considerable asthenia, muscle spasms, fasciculations, insomnia, or intolerable injection site pain or irritation (HCAHPS).

• Educate patient about signs of a significant reaction (eg, wheezing; chest tightness; fever; itching; bad cough; blue skin color; seizures; or swelling of face, lips, tongue, or throat). **Note:** This is not a comprehensive list of all side effects. Patient should consult prescriber for additional questions.

Intended Use and Disclaimer: Should not be printed and given to patients. This information is intended to serve as a concise initial reference for

healthcare professionals to use when discussing medications with a patient. You must ultimately rely on your own discretion, experience and judgment in diagnosing, treating and advising patients.

Related Information
Management of Drug Extravasations *on page 1700*

Diclofenac (Systemic) (dye KLOE fen ak)

Brand Names: U.S. Cambia; Cataflam; Voltaren-XR; Zipsor; Zorvolex
Index Terms Diclofenac Potassium; Diclofenac Sodium; Voltaren; Zorvolex
Pharmacologic Category Nonsteroidal Anti-inflammatory Drug (NSAID); Nonsteroidal Anti-inflammatory Drug (NSAID), Oral
Medication Safety Issues
Sound-alike/look-alike issues:
Diclofenac may be confused with Diflucan
Cataflam may be confused with Catapres
Voltaren may be confused with traMADol, Ultram, Verelan
BEERS Criteria medication:
This drug may be potentially inappropriate for use in geriatric patients (Quality of evidence - moderate; Strength of recommendation - strong).
International issues:
Diclofenac may be confused with Duphalac brand name for lactulose [multiple international markets]
Flexin: Brand name for diclofenac [Argentina], but also the brand name for cyclobenzaprine [Chile] and orphenadrine [Israel]
Flexin [Argentina] may be confused with Floxin brand name for flunarizine [Thailand], norfloxacin [South Africa], and ofloxacin [U.S.]
Medication Guide Available Yes
Pregnancy Risk Factor C (oral)/D (≥30 weeks gestation [oral])
Lactation Excreted in breast milk/not recommended
Breast-Feeding Considerations Low concentrations of diclofenac can be found in breast milk. Breast-feeding is not recommended by most manufacturers. Use while breast-feeding is contraindicated in Canadian labeling.
Use
Analgesia (capsules/immediate-release tablets only): Relief of mild to moderate acute pain in adults
Ankylosing spondylitis (delayed-release tablets only): Acute or long-term use in the relief of signs and symptoms of ankylosing spondylitis
Arthritis (immediate-release, extended-release, and delayed-release tablets only): Relief of signs and symptoms of osteoarthritis and rheumatoid arthritis
Dysmenorrhea (immediate-release tablets only): Treatment of primary dysmenorrhea

Migraine (powder for oral solution only): Acute treatment of migraine attacks with or without aura in adults
Unlabeled Use Juvenile idiopathic arthritis (JIA)
Mechanism of Action/Effect Reversibly inhibits cyclooxygenase-1 and 2 (COX-1 and 2) enzymes, which results in decreased formation of prostaglandin precursors; has antipyretic, analgesic, and anti-inflammatory properties
Contraindications Hypersensitivity to diclofenac (eg, anaphylactoid reactions, serious skin reactions) or bovine protein (Zipsor only) or any component of the formulation; patients who have experienced asthma, urticaria, or other allergic-type reactions after taking aspirin or other NSAIDs; treatment of perioperative pain in the setting of CABG surgery

Canadian labeling: Additional contraindications (not in U.S. labeling): Uncontrolled heart failure, active gastric/duodenal/peptic ulcer; active GI bleed or perforation; regional ulcer, gastritis, or ulcerative colitis; cerebrovascular bleeding or other bleeding disorders; inflammatory bowel disease; severe hepatic impairment; active hepatic disease; severe renal impairment (CrCl <30 mL/minute) or deteriorating renal disease; known hyperkalemia; patients <16 years of age; breast-feeding; pregnancy (third trimester); use of diclofenac suppository if recent history of bleeding or inflammatory lesions of rectum/anus

Warnings/Precautions [U.S. Boxed Warning]: NSAIDs are associated with an increased risk of adverse cardiovascular thrombotic events, including MI and stroke. Risk may be increased with duration of use or pre-existing cardiovascular risk factors or disease. Carefully evaluate individual cardiovascular risk profiles prior to prescribing. May cause new-onset hypertension or worsening of existing hypertension. Monitor blood pressure closely. Use caution with fluid retention. Avoid use in heart failure (ACCF/AHA [Yancy, 2013]). Concurrent administration of ibuprofen, and potentially other nonselective NSAIDs, may interfere with aspirin's cardioprotective effect. **[U.S. Boxed Warning]: Use is contraindicated for treatment of perioperative pain in the setting of coronary artery bypass graft (CABG) surgery.** Risk of MI and stroke may be increased with use following CABG surgery.

NSAID use may compromise existing renal function; dose-dependent decreases in prostaglandin synthesis may result from NSAID use, reducing renal blood flow which may cause renal decompensation. NSAID use may increase the risk for hyperkalemia. Patients with impaired renal function, dehydration, heart failure, liver dysfunction, those taking diuretics and ACEI, and the elderly are at greater risk of renal toxicity and hyperkalemia. Rehydrate patient before starting therapy; monitor renal function closely. Not recommended for use in patients with advanced renal disease. Long-term NSAID use may result in renal papillary necrosis while persistent urinary symptoms (eg, dysuria, bladder pain), cystitis, or hematuria may occur anytime after initiating NSAID therapy. Discontinue therapy with symptom onset and evaluate for origin.

[U.S. Boxed Warning]: NSAIDs may increase risk of gastrointestinal irritation, inflammation, ulceration, bleeding, and perforation. These events may occur at any time during therapy and without warning. Use caution with a history of GI disease (bleeding or ulcers), concurrent therapy with aspirin, anticoagulants and/or corticosteroids, smoking, use of alcohol, the elderly or debilitated patients. When used concomitantly with aspirin, a substantial increase in the risk of gastrointestinal complications (eg, ulcer) occurs; concomitant gastroprotective therapy (eg, proton pump inhibitors) is recommended (Bhatt, 2008).

Use the lowest effective dose for the shortest duration of time, consistent with individual patient goals, to reduce risk of cardiovascular or GI adverse events. Alternate therapies should be considered for patients at high risk.

NSAIDs may cause photosensitivity or serious skin adverse events including exfoliative dermatitis, Stevens-Johnson syndrome (SJS), and toxic epidermal necrolysis (TEN); discontinue use at first sign of skin rash or hypersensitivity. Anaphylactoid reactions may occur, even without prior exposure; patients with "aspirin triad" (bronchial asthma, aspirin intolerance, rhinitis) may be at increased risk. Do not use in patients who experience bronchospasm, asthma, rhinitis, or urticaria with NSAID or aspirin therapy. Use caution in other forms of asthma. Platelet adhesion and aggregation may be decreased; may prolong bleeding time; patients with coagulation disorders or who are receiving anticoagulants should be monitored closely. Anemia may occur; patients on long-term NSAID therapy should be monitored for anemia. Rarely, NSAID use may cause severe blood dyscrasias (eg, agranulocytosis, aplastic anemia, thrombocytopenia).

Use with caution in patients with impaired hepatic function. Closely monitor patients with any abnormal LFT. Transaminase elevations have been observed with use, generally within the first 2 months of therapy, but may occur at any time. Risk may be higher with diclofenac than other NSAIDs (Laine, 2009; Rostom, 2005). Significant elevations in transaminases (eg, >3 x ULN) occur before patients become symptomatic; initiate monitoring 4-8 weeks into therapy. Rarely, severe hepatic reactions (eg, fulminant hepatitis, liver failure) have occurred; discontinue all formulations if signs or symptoms of liver disease develop, or if systemic manifestations occur. Use with caution in hepatic porphyria (may trigger attack; Jose, 2008).

NSAIDS may cause drowsiness, dizziness, blurred vision, and other neurologic effects which may impair physical or mental abilities; patients must be cautioned about performing tasks which require mental alertness (eg, operating machinery or driving). Discontinue use with blurred or diminished vision and perform ophthalmologic exam. Monitor vision with long-term therapy. May increase the risk of aseptic meningitis, especially in patients with systemic lupus erythematosus (SLE) and mixed connective tissue disorders. In the elderly, avoid chronic use (unless alternative agents ineffective and patient can receive concomitant gastroprotective agent); nonselective oral NSAID use is associated with an increased risk of GI bleeding and peptic ulcer disease in older adults in high risk category (eg, >75 years or age or receiving concomitant oral/parenteral corticosteroids, anticoagulants, or antiplatelet agents) (Beers Criteria).

Withhold for at least 4-6 half-lives prior to surgical or dental procedures.

Different formulations of oral diclofenac are not bioequivalent, even if the milligram strength is the same; do not interchange products. Zipsor (capsule) contains gelatin; use is contraindicated in patients with history of hypersensitivity to bovine protein. Oral solution is only indicated for the acute treatment of migraine; not indicated for migraine prophylaxis or cluster headache; contains phenylalanine.

Drug Interactions

Avoid Concomitant Use

Avoid concomitant use of Diclofenac (Systemic) with any of the following: Floctafenine; Ketorolac (Nasal); Ketorolac (Systemic); NSAID (COX-2 Inhibitor); Omacetaxine; Pimozide; Urokinase

Decreased Effect

Diclofenac (Systemic) may decrease the levels/ effects of: ACE Inhibitors; Agents with Antiplatelet Properties; Aliskiren; Angiotensin II Receptor Blockers; Beta-Blockers; Eplerenone; HydrALAZINE; Loop Diuretics; Potassium-Sparing Diuretics; Prostaglandins (Ophthalmic); Salicylates; Selective Serotonin Reuptake Inhibitors; Thiazide Diuretics

The levels/effects of Diclofenac (Systemic) may be decreased by: Bile Acid Sequestrants; CYP2C9 Inducers (Strong); Nonsteroidal Anti-Inflammatory Agents; Peginterferon Alfa-2b; Salicylates

Increased Effect/Toxicity

Diclofenac (Systemic) may increase the levels/ effects of: 5-ASA Derivatives; Agents with Antiplatelet Properties; Aliskiren; Aminoglycosides; Anticoagulants; ARIPiprazole; Bisphosphonate Derivatives; Collagenase (Systemic); CycloSPORINE (Systemic); Dabigatran Etexilate;

Deferasirox; Deferiprone; Desmopressin; Digoxin; Dofetilide; Eplerenone; Haloperidol; Ibritumomab; Lithium; Lomitapide; Methotrexate; Nonsteroidal Anti-Inflammatory Agents; NSAID (COX-2 Inhibitor); Omacetaxine; PEMEtrexed; Pimozide; Porfimer; Potassium-Sparing Diuretics; PRALAtrexate; Quinolone Antibiotics; Rivaroxaban; Salicylates; Tenofovir; Thrombolytic Agents; Tositumomab and Iodine I 131 Tositumomab; Urokinase; Vancomycin; Vitamin K Antagonists

The levels/effects of Diclofenac (Systemic) may be increased by: ACE Inhibitors; Angiotensin II Receptor Blockers; Antidepressants (Tricyclic, Tertiary Amine); Corticosteroids (Systemic); CycloSPORINE (Systemic); CYP2C9 Inhibitors (Strong); Dasatinib; Floctafenine; Glucosamine; Herbs (Anticoagulant/Antiplatelet Properties); Ibrutinib; Ketorolac (Nasal); Ketorolac (Systemic); Multivitamins/Fluoride (with ADE); Multivitamins/Minerals (with ADEK, Folate, Iron); Multivitamins/Minerals (with AE, No Iron); Nonsteroidal Anti-Inflammatory Agents; Omega-3 Fatty Acids; Pentosan Polysulfate Sodium; Pentoxifylline; Probenecid; Prostacyclin Analogues; Selective Serotonin Reuptake Inhibitors; Serotonin/Norepinephrine Reuptake Inhibitors; Sodium Phosphates; Tipranavir; Treprostinil; Vitamin E; Voriconazole

Nutritional/Ethanol Interactions

Ethanol: Avoid ethanol (may enhance gastric mucosal irritation).

Herb/Nutraceutical: Avoid alfalfa, anise, bilberry, bladderwrack, bromelain, cat's claw, celery, chamomile, coleus, cordyceps, dong quai, evening primrose, fenugreek, feverfew, garlic, ginger, ginkgo biloba, grapeseed, green tea, ginseng (Siberian), guggul, horse chestnut, horseradish, licorice, prickly ash, red clover, reishi, SAMe (s-adenosylmethionine), sweet clover, turmeric, white willow (all have additional antiplatelet activity).

Adverse Reactions

Oral:

1% to 10%:

Cardiovascular: Edema

Central nervous system: Dizziness, headache

Dermatologic: Pruritus, rash

Endocrine & metabolic: Fluid retention

Gastrointestinal: Abdominal distension, abdominal pain, constipation, diarrhea, dyspepsia, flatulence, GI perforation, heartburn, nausea, peptic ulcer/GI bleed, vomiting

Hematologic: Anemia, bleeding time increased

Hepatic: Liver enzyme abnormalities (>3 x ULN; ≤4%)

Otic: Tinnitus

Renal: Renal function abnormal

Miscellaneous: Diaphoresis increased

Rectal suppository [Canadian product]: Also refer to adverse reactions associated with oral formulations.

Pharmacodynamics/Kinetics

Onset of Action

Cataflam (potassium salt) is more rapid than the sodium salt because it dissolves in the stomach instead of the duodenum

Suppository [Canadian product]: more rapid onset, but slower rate of absorption when compared to enteric coated tablet

Available Dosage Forms

Capsule, Oral:

Zipsor: 25 mg

Zorvolex: 18 mg, 35 mg

Packet, Oral:

Cambia: 50 mg (1 ea, 9 ea)

Tablet, Oral:

Cataflam: 50 mg

Generic: 50 mg

Tablet Delayed Release, Oral:

Generic: 25 mg, 50 mg, 75 mg

Tablet Extended Release 24 Hour, Oral:

Voltaren-XR: 100 mg

Generic: 100 mg

General Dosage Range Oral:

Immediate release capsule: *Adults:* Zipsor: 100 mg daily in 4 divided doses; Zorvolex: 54 mg or 105 mg daily in 3 divided doses

Immediate release tablet: *Adults:* 100-200 mg daily in 2-4 divided doses

Delayed release tablet: *Adults:* 100-200 mg daily in 2-5 divided doses

Extended release tablet: *Adults:* 100-200 mg daily

Oral solution: *Adults:* 50 mg once

Administration

Oral Do not crush delayed or extended release tablets. Administer with food or milk to avoid gastric distress.

Cambia, Zorvolex: Taking with food may cause a reduction in effectiveness.

Rectal Rectal suppository [Canadian product]: Remove entire plastic wrapping prior to inserting rectally.

Preparation for Administration Oral solution: Empty contents of packet into 1-2 ounces (30-60 mL) of water (do not use other liquids); mix well and administer immediately.

Storage/Stability

Capsule, powder for oral solution: Store at 25°C (77°F); excursions permitted to 15°C to 30°C (59°F to 86°F). Protect from moisture.

Suppository [Canadian product]: Store at 15°C to 30°C (59°F to 86°F); protect from heat.

Tablet: Store immediate-release and ER tablets below 30°C (86°F); store delayed-release tablets at 20°C to 25°C (68°F to 77°F). Protect from moisture.

Nursing Actions

Physical Assessment Monitor blood pressure at the beginning of therapy and periodically during use. Schedule ophthalmic evaluations for patients who develop eye complaints during long-term NSAID therapy.

Patient Education

- Discuss specific use of drug and side effects with patient as it relates to treatment. (HCAHPS: During this hospital stay, were you given any medicine that you had not taken before? Before giving you any new medicine, how often did hospital staff tell you what the medicine was for? How often did hospital staff describe possible side effects in a way you could understand?)
- Patient may experience pyrosis, constipation, diarrhea, flatulence, or fatigue. Have patient report immediately to prescriber signs of hepatic impairment, dyspnea, excessive weight gain, edema of extremities, angina, tachycardia, strength differences from one side to another, difficulty speaking or thinking, change in balance, blurred vision, severe headache, significant dizziness, syncope, considerable asthenia, tinnitus, mood changes, depression, arrhythmia, intolerable nausea, severe dyspepsia, significant back pain, melena, hematemesis, ecchymosis, hemorrhaging, urinary retention, oliguria, chills, pharyngitis, considerable arthralgia, or intolerable myalgia (HCAHPS).
- Educate patient about signs of a significant reaction (eg, wheezing; chest tightness; fever; itching; bad cough; blue skin color; seizures; or swelling of face, lips, tongue, or throat). **Note:** This is not a comprehensive list of all side effects. Patient should consult prescriber for additional questions.

Intended Use and Disclaimer: Should not be printed and given to patients. This information is intended to serve as a concise initial reference for healthcare professionals to use when discussing medications with a patient. You must ultimately rely on your own discretion, experience and judgment in diagnosing, treating and advising patients.

Dietary Considerations Oral formulations may be taken with food to decrease GI distress. Food may reduce effectiveness of oral solution. Some products may contain phenylalanine.

Related Information

Oral Medications That Should Not Be Crushed or Altered *on page 1712*

Diclofenac (Topical) (dye KLOE fen ak)

Brand Names: U.S. Flector; Pennsaid; Solaraze; Voltaren

Index Terms Diclofenac Diethylamine [CAN]; Diclofenac Epolamine; Diclofenac Sodium

Pharmacologic Category Nonsteroidal Anti-inflammatory Drug (NSAID); Nonsteroidal Anti-inflammatory Drug (NSAID), Topical

Medication Safety Issues

Sound-alike/look-alike issues:

Diclofenac may be confused with Diflucan

Voltaren may be confused with traMADol, Ultram, Verelan

Other safety concerns:

Transdermal patch (Flector) contains conducting metal (eg, aluminum); remove patch prior to MRI.

International issues:

Diclofenac may be confused with Duphalac brand name for lactulose [multiple international markets]

Flexin: Brand name for diclofenac [Argentina], but also the brand name for cyclobenzaprine [Chile] and orphenadrine [Israel]

Flexin [Argentina] may be confused with Floxin brand name for flunarizine [Thailand], norfloxacin [South Africa], ofloxacin [U.S., Canada], and perfloxacin [Philippines]

Medication Guide Available Yes

Pregnancy Risk Factor B (topical gel 3%) / C (topical gel 1%, topical solution, topical patch) / D (topical solution ≥30 weeks gestation)

Lactation Not recommended

Use

Topical gel 1%: Relief of osteoarthritis pain in joints amenable to topical therapy (eg, ankle, elbow, foot, hand, knee, wrist)

Canadian labeling (not in U.S. labeling): Relief of pain associated with acute, localized joint/muscle injuries (eg, sports injuries, strains) in patients ≥16 years of age

Topical gel 3%: Actinic keratosis (AK) in conjunction with sun avoidance

Topical patch: Acute pain due to minor strains, sprains, and contusions

Topical solution: Relief of osteoarthritis pain of the knee

Available Dosage Forms

Gel, Transdermal:

Solaraze: 3% (100 g)

Voltaren: 1% (100 g)

Generic: 3% (100 g)

Patch, Transdermal:

Flector: 1.3% (5 ea, 30 ea)

Solution, Transdermal:

Pennsaid: 1.5% (150 mL); 2% (112 g)

General Dosage Range Topical: *Adults:*

1% gel: Apply 2-4 g to affected joint 4 times/day (maximum: 16 g/day single joint of lower extremity, 8 g/day single joint of upper extremity); Maximum total body dose of 1% gel should not exceed 32 g per day.

3% gel: Apply to lesion area twice daily

Patch: Apply 1 patch twice daily

Solution: Apply 40 drops to each affected knee 4 times/day

Administration

Topical

Topical gel: Do not cover with occlusive dressings or apply sunscreens, cosmetics, lotions, moisturizers, insect repellents or other topical medications to affected area. Do not wash area for 1 hour following application. Wash hands immediately after application (unless hands are treated joint). Avoid sunlight to exposure areas.

1% formulation: Apply gel to affected area or joint and rub into skin gently, making sure to apply to entire affected area or joint.

3% formulation: Apply to lesion with gel and smooth into skin gently.

Topical solution: Apply to clean, dry, intact skin; do not apply to eyes, mucous membranes, or open wounds. Wash hands before and after use. Apply 10 drops at a time either directly onto knee **or** into hand then onto knee (helps avoid spillage). Repeat procedure until total dose applied. Spread evenly around knee (front, back, sides). Allow knee to dry before applying clothing. Do not shower or bathe for at least 30 minutes after applying. Do not apply heat or occlusive dressing to treated knee; protect treated knee from sunlight. Cosmetics, insect repellant, lotion, moisturizer, sunscreens, or other topical medication may be applied to treated knee once solution has dried.

Transdermal patch: Apply to intact, nondamaged skin. Remove transparent liner prior to applying to skin. Wash hands after applying as well as after removal of patch. May tape down edges of patch, if peeling occurs. Should not be worn while bathing or showering. Fold used patches so the adhesive side sticks to itself; dispose of used patches out of reach of children and pets.

Nursing Actions

Patient Education

- Discuss specific use of drug and side effects with patient as it relates to treatment. (HCAHPS: During this hospital stay, were you given any medicine that you had not taken before? Before giving you any new medicine, how often did hospital staff tell you what the medicine was for? How often did hospital staff describe possible side effects in a way you could understand?)
- Patient may experience xeroderma or flu-like syndrome. Have patient report immediately to prescriber signs of Stevens-Johnson syndrome/toxic epidermal necrolysis, paresthesia, angina, severe application site irritation, dyspnea, signs of hepatic impairment, tachycardia, strength differences from one side to another, difficulty speaking or thinking, change in balance, blurred vision, ecchymosis, hemorrhaging, significant dyspepsia, considerable back pain, melena, hematemesis, excessive weight gain, edema of extremities, urinary retention, oliguria, severe dizziness, syncope, intolerable

headache, significant nausea, or considerable asthenia (HCAHPS).

- Educate patient about signs of a significant reaction (eg, wheezing; chest tightness; fever; itching; bad cough; blue skin color; seizures; or swelling of face, lips, tongue, or throat). **Note:** This is not a comprehensive list of all side effects. Patient should consult prescriber for additional questions.

Intended Use and Disclaimer: Should not be printed and given to patients. This information is intended to serve as a concise initial reference for healthcare professionals to use when discussing medications with a patient. You must ultimately rely on your own discretion, experience and judgment in diagnosing, treating and advising patients.

Diclofenac and Misoprostol
(dye KLOE fen ak & mye soe PROST ole)

Brand Names: U.S. Arthrotec

Index Terms Misoprostol and Diclofenac

Pharmacologic Category Nonsteroidal Anti-inflammatory Drug (NSAID), Oral; Prostaglandin

Medication Guide Available Yes

Pregnancy Risk Factor X

Lactation Enters breast milk/use caution

Use Treatment of osteoarthritis and rheumatoid arthritis in patients at high risk for NSAID-induced gastric and duodenal ulceration

Available Dosage Forms

Tablet, oral: Diclofenac 50 mg and misoprostol 200 mcg; Diclofenac 75 mg and misoprostol 200 mcg

Arthrotec 50: Diclofenac 50 mg and misoprostol 200 mcg

Arthrotec 75: Diclofenac 75 mg and misoprostol 200 mcg

General Dosage Range Oral: *Adults:* Arthrotec® 50: One tablet 2-4 times/day; Arthrotec® 75: One tablet twice daily

Administration

Oral Incidence of diarrhea may be lessened by having patient take dose right after meals and avoiding magnesium containing antacids. Tablets should not be crushed or chewed. Therapy is usually begun on the second or third day of the next normal menstrual period in women of child bearing potential.

Nursing Actions

Physical Assessment See individual agents.

Patient Education

- Discuss specific use of drug and side effects with patient as it relates to treatment. (HCAHPS: During this hospital stay, were you given any medicine that you had not taken before? Before giving you any new medicine, how often did hospital staff tell you what the medicine was

for? How often did hospital staff describe possible side effects in a way you could understand?)
- Patient may experience flatulence. Have patient report immediately to prescriber signs of hemorrhaging, angina, tachycardia, strength differences from one side to another, difficulty speaking or thinking, change in balance, blurred vision, severe headache, considerable nausea, significant dyspepsia, dyspnea, excessive weight gain, edema of extremities, intolerable diarrhea, urinary retention, oliguria, severe asthenia, signs of hepatic impairment, signs of Stevens-Johnson syndrome/toxic epidermal necrolysis, or signs of aseptic meningitis (HCAHPS).
- Educate patient about signs of a significant reaction (eg, wheezing; chest tightness; fever; itching; bad cough; blue skin color; seizures; or swelling of face, lips, tongue, or throat). **Note:** This is not a comprehensive list of all side effects. Patient should consult prescriber for additional questions.

Intended Use and Disclaimer: Should not be printed and given to patients. This information is intended to serve as a concise initial reference for healthcare professionals to use when discussing medications with a patient. You must ultimately rely on your own discretion, experience and judgment in diagnosing, treating and advising patients.

Related Information
Diclofenac (Systemic) *on page 441*
Misoprostol *on page 1066*
Oral Medications That Should Not Be Crushed or Altered *on page 1712*

Dicloxacillin (dye kloks a SIL in)

Index Terms Dicloxacillin Sodium
Pharmacologic Category Antibiotic, Penicillin
Pregnancy Risk Factor B
Lactation Excretion in breast milk unknown/use caution
Use Treatment of systemic infections such as pneumonia, skin and soft tissue infections, and osteomyelitis caused by penicillinase-producing staphylococci
Available Dosage Forms
Capsule, Oral:
Generic: 250 mg, 500 mg
General Dosage Range Oral:
Children <40 kg: 12.5-100 mg/kg/day divided every 6 hours
Children >40 kg: 125-250 mg every 6 hours
Adults: 125-1000 mg every 6-8 hours
Administration
Oral Administer 1 hour before or 2 hours after meals. Administer around-the-clock to promote less variation in peak and trough serum levels.

Nursing Actions
Physical Assessment Assess allergy history prior to beginning therapy.
Patient Education
- Discuss specific use of drug and side effects with patient as it relates to treatment. (HCAHPS: During this hospital stay, were you given any medicine that you had not taken before? Before giving you any new medicine, how often did hospital staff tell you what the medicine was for? How often did hospital staff describe possible side effects in a way you could understand?)
- Patient may experience diarrhea. Have patient report immediately to prescriber dyspnea, severe nausea, stomatitis, tongue discoloration, ecchymosis, hemorrhaging, chills, pharyngitis, arthralgia, considerable dizziness, syncope, vaginitis, or signs of pseudomembranous colitis (HCAHPS).
- Educate patient about signs of a significant reaction (eg, wheezing; chest tightness; fever; itching; bad cough; blue skin color; seizures; or swelling of face, lips, tongue, or throat). **Note:** This is not a comprehensive list of all side effects. Patient should consult prescriber for additional questions.

Intended Use and Disclaimer: Should not be printed and given to patients. This information is intended to serve as a concise initial reference for healthcare professionals to use when discussing medications with a patient. You must ultimately rely on your own discretion, experience and judgment in diagnosing, treating and advising patients.

Didanosine (dye DAN oh seen)

Brand Names: U.S. Videx; Videx EC
Index Terms ddl; Dideoxyinosine
Pharmacologic Category Antiretroviral, Reverse Transcriptase Inhibitor, Nucleoside (Anti-HIV)
Medication Safety Issues
Sound-alike/look-alike issues:
Videx® may be confused with Lidex®
Medication Guide Available Yes
Pregnancy Risk Factor B
Lactation Excretion in breast milk unknown/contraindicated
Breast-Feeding Considerations Maternal or infant antiretroviral therapy does not completely eliminate the risk of postnatal HIV transmission. In addition, multiclass-resistant virus has been detected in breast-feeding infants despite maternal therapy. Therefore, in the United States, where formula is accessible, affordable, safe, and sustainable, and the risk of infant mortality due to diarrhea and respiratory infections is low, complete avoidance of breast-feeding by HIV-infected women is recommended to decrease potential transmission of HIV (DHHS [perinatal], 2012).

Use Treatment of HIV infection; always to be used in combination with at least two other antiretroviral agents

Mechanism of Action/Effect Didanosine, a purine nucleoside (adenosine) analog and the deamination product of dideoxyadenosine (ddA), inhibits HIV replication *in vitro* in both T cells and monocytes. Didanosine is converted within the cell to the mono-, di-, and triphosphates of ddA. These ddA triphosphates act as substrate and inhibitor of HIV reverse transcriptase substrate and inhibitor of HIV reverse transcriptase thereby blocking viral DNA synthesis and suppressing HIV replication.

Contraindications Concurrent administration with allopurinol or ribavirin

Warnings/Precautions [U.S. Boxed Warning]: Pancreatitis (sometimes fatal) has been reported; incidence is dose related. Risk factors for developing pancreatitis may include a previous history of the condition, concurrent cytomegalovirus or *Mycobacterium avium-intracellulare* infection, renal impairment, advanced age, and concomitant use of stavudine, pentamidine, or hydroxyurea. Discontinue didanosine if clinical signs of pancreatitis occur. **[U.S. Boxed Warning]: Lactic acidosis, symptomatic hyperlactatemia, and severe hepatomegaly with steatosis (sometimes fatal) have occurred with antiretroviral nucleoside analogues, including didanosine.** Hepatotoxicity may occur even in the absence of marked transaminase elevations; suspend therapy in any patient developing clinical/laboratory findings which suggest hepatotoxicity. Hepatotoxicity and hepatic failure (including fatal cases) have been reported in HIV patients receiving combination drug therapy with didanosine and stavudine or hydroxyurea, or didanosine, stavudine, and hydroxyurea; avoid these combinations. Not currently recommended in combination with tenofovir due to failure and resistance. Noncirrhotic portal hypertension may develop within months to years of starting didanosine therapy. Signs may include elevated liver enzymes, esophageal varices, hematemesis, ascites, and splenomegaly. Noncirrhotic portal hypertension may lead to liver failure and/or death. Discontinue use in patients with evidence of this condition. Pregnant women may be at increased risk of lactic acidosis and liver damage. Use with caution in patients with hepatic impairment; safety and efficacy have not been established in patients with significant hepatic disease. Patients on combination antiretroviral therapy with hepatic impairment may be at increased risk of potentially severe and fatal hepatic toxicity; consider interruption or discontinuation of therapy if hepatic impairment worsens.

Peripheral neuropathy occurs in ~20% of patients receiving the drug. If symptomatic, discontinue therapy; after resolution of symptoms, reinitiation of therapy at a reduced dose may be tolerated.

Permanently discontinue if neuropathy recurs. Retinal changes (including retinal depigmentation) and optic neuritis have been reported in adults and children using didanosine. Patients should undergo retinal examination every 6-12 months. Use caution in renal impairment; dose reduction recommended for CrCl <60 mL/minute. May cause redistribution of fat (eg, buffalo hump, peripheral wasting with increased abdominal girth, cushingoid appearance). Patients may develop immune reconstitution syndrome resulting in the occurrence of an inflammatory response to an indolent or residual opportunistic infection during initial HIV treatment or activation of autoimmune disorders (eg, Graves' disease, polymyositis, Guillain-Barré syndrome) later in therapy; further evaluation and treatment may be required. Didanosine delayed release capsules are indicated for once-daily use.

Drug Interactions

Avoid Concomitant Use

Avoid concomitant use of Didanosine with any of the following: Alcohol (Ethyl); Allopurinol; Febuxostat; Hydroxyurea; Ribavirin; Tenofovir

Decreased Effect

Didanosine may decrease the levels/effects of: Antifungal Agents (Azole Derivatives, Systemic); Atazanavir; Indinavir; Quinolone Antibiotics; Rilpivirine

The levels/effects of Didanosine may be decreased by: Atazanavir; Darunavir; Lopinavir; Methadone; Quinolone Antibiotics; Rilpivirine; Tenofovir; Tipranavir

Increased Effect/Toxicity

Didanosine may increase the levels/effects of: Hydroxyurea

The levels/effects of Didanosine may be increased by: Alcohol (Ethyl); Allopurinol; Febuxostat; Ganciclovir-Valganciclovir; Hydroxyurea; Ribavirin; Stavudine; Tenofovir

Nutritional/Ethanol Interactions

Ethanol: Ethanol increases risk of pancreatitis. Management: Avoid ethanol.

Food: Food decreases AUC and C_{max}; serum levels may be decreased by 55%. Management: Administer on an empty stomach at least 30 minutes before or 2 hours after eating depending on dosage form.

Adverse Reactions As reported in monotherapy studies; risk of toxicity may increase when combined with other agents.

>10%:

Gastrointestinal: Diarrhea (19% to 28%), amylase increased (15% to 17%), abdominal pain (7% to 13%)

Neuromuscular & skeletal: Peripheral neuropathy (17% to 20%)

1% to 10%:

Dermatologic: Rash/pruritus (7% to 9%)

Endocrine & metabolic: Uric acid increased (2% to 3%)

Gastrointestinal: Pancreatitis (1% to 7% dose dependent); patients >65 years of age had a higher frequency of pancreatitis than younger patients patients (10% vs 5% in younger patients)

Hepatic: AST increased (7% to 9%), ALT increased (6% to 9%), alkaline phosphatase increased (1% to 4%)

Available Dosage Forms

Capsule Delayed Release, Oral:

Videx EC: 125 mg, 200 mg, 250 mg, 400 mg

Generic: 125 mg, 200 mg, 250 mg, 400 mg

Solution Reconstituted, Oral:

Videx: 2 g (100 mL); 4 g (200 mL)

General Dosage Range Dosage adjustment recommended in patients with renal impairment

Oral:

Delayed release:

Children ≥6 years and 20 kg to <25 kg: 200 mg once daily

Children ≥6 years and 25 kg to <60 kg and Adults <60 kg: 250 mg once daily

Children and Adults ≥60 kg: 400 mg once daily

Pediatric powder for oral solution (Videx®):

Infants 2 weeks to 8 months: 100 mg/m² twice daily

Children >8 months to 18 years: 120 mg/m² twice daily

Adolescents and Adults <60 kg: 125 mg twice daily **or** 250 mg once daily

Adolescents and Adults ≥60 kg: 200 mg twice daily **or** 400 mg once daily

Administration

Oral Pediatric powder for oral solution: Administer on an empty stomach at least 30 minutes before or 2 hours after eating. Shake well prior to use.

Videx® EC: Administer on an empty stomach at least 1 hour before or 2 hours after eating; swallow capsule whole.

Preparation for Administration Pediatric powder for oral solution: Prior to dispensing, add 100 mL or 200 mL purified water, USP to the 2 g or 4 g container, respectively, to achieve a 20 mg/mL solution. Immediately mix the resulting solution with an equal volume of Mylanta® Maximum Strength (or equivalent) to achieve a final concentration of 10 mg/mL.

Storage/Stability Delayed release capsules should be stored in tightly closed bottles at controlled room temperature of 25°C (77°F). Unreconstituted powder should be stored at 15°C to 30°C (59°F to 86°F); reconstituted pediatric solution is stable for 30 days if refrigerated.

Nursing Actions

Physical Assessment Monitor for hepatotoxicity, peripheral neuropathy, gastrointestinal pain, and vision changes regularly during therapy. Teach patient proper timing of multiple medications.

Patient Education

• Discuss specific use of drug and side effects with patient as it relates to treatment. (HCAHPS: During this hospital stay, were you given any medicine that you had not taken before? Before giving you any new medicine, how often did hospital staff tell you what the medicine was for? How often did hospital staff describe possible side effects in a way you could understand?)

• Patient may experience headache, dyspepsia, nausea, diarrhea, or lipodystrophy. Have patient report immediately to prescriber signs of hepatic impairment, signs of lactic acidosis, signs of pancreatitis, severe dizziness, syncope, bradycardia, paresthesia or hands or feet, ecchymosis, hemorrhaging, hematemesis, melena, vision changes, angina, illogical thinking, or signs of infection (HCAHPS).

• Educate patient about signs of a significant reaction (eg, wheezing; chest tightness; fever; itching; bad cough; blue skin color; seizures; or swelling of face, lips, tongue, or throat). **Note:** This is not a comprehensive list of all side effects. Patient should consult prescriber for additional questions.

Intended Use and Disclaimer: Should not be printed and given to patients. This information is intended to serve as a concise initial reference for healthcare professionals to use when discussing medications with a patient. You must ultimately rely on your own discretion, experience and judgment in diagnosing, treating and advising patients.

Dietary Considerations Take on an empty stomach; administer at least 30 minutes before or 2 hours after eating

Related Information

Oral Medications That Should Not Be Crushed or Altered *on page 1712*

Dienogest (dye EN oh jest)

Pharmacologic Category Antiandrogen

Medication Safety Issues

Sound-alike/look-alike issues:

Visanne® may be confused with Vyvanse®

Lactation Excretion in breast milk unknown/contraindicated

Breast-Feeding Considerations It is not known whether dienogest is excreted into human breast milk. The risk of thromboembolism may be increased immediately postpartum.

Use Management of pelvic pain associated with endometriosis

Mechanism of Action/Effect Dienogest is a steroid with antiandrogen properties that lacks androgen, mineralocorticoid or glucocorticoid activity. Decreases estradiol production and thus suppresses estradiol's trophic effects on eutopic and ectopic endometrium. Inhibits cellular proliferation via direct antiproliferative, immunologic, and anti-angiogenic effects.

Contraindications Hypersensitivity to dienogest or any component of the formulation; undiagnosed abnormal vaginal bleeding; active venous thromboembolic disorder; history of or current arterial and cardiovascular disease (eg, MI, CVA); diabetes mellitus with vascular involvement; history of or current severe hepatic disease where liver function tests remain abnormal; history of or current hepatic neoplasia (benign or malignant); known or suspected sex-hormone-dependent malignancy; ocular lesions due to ophthalmic vascular disease, such as partial or complete vision loss or defect in visual fields; current or history of migraine with focal aura; breast-feeding; known or suspected pregnancy

Warnings/Precautions Use is associated with irregular menstrual bleeding (eg, amenorrhea, infrequent or frequent bleeding, prolonged bleeding) and may be aggravated in some women (eg, those with fibroids). Bleeding patterns generally show a reduced intensity over time. If bleeding irregularities continue with prolonged use, appropriate diagnostic measures should be taken to rule out endometrial pathology (eg, endometrial sampling, pelvic ultrasound). Consider discontinuation of therapy with prolonged heavy bleeding. Pretreatment menstrual bleeding patterns return within 2 months of therapy discontinuation. The use of combination hormonal contraceptives has been associated with a slight increase in the frequency of breast cancer however studies are not consistent. Data is insufficient to determine if progestin only contraceptives also increase this risk. Routine breast examinations are recommended during therapy. Persistent ovarian cysts which are often asymptomatic may occur during therapy. Use is associated with a moderate decrease in endogenous estrogen levels; in a small study, a reduction in mean bone mineral density was not observed 6 months after initiating therapy though long term data are not available.

Use with caution in women with diabetes. Use with caution in patients with depression; discontinue use with onset of clinically relevant depression or with aggravation of pre-existing depression. Use is contraindicated in patients with a history of or current severe hepatic disease. Patients with a prior history of cholestatic jaundice during pregnancy or due to the use of sex steroids should discontinue use of dienogest if cholestatic jaundice reoccurs during therapy. Rare cases of benign and malignant hepatic tumors have been reported with use.

Progestin-only therapy has been associated with a slight but non-significant increase risk of VTE in some studies; discontinue therapy promptly with suspicion or symptoms of a thrombotic event. Discontinue use in patients with prolonged immobilization and at least 4 weeks prior to elective surgery; may resume therapy 2 weeks after complete remobilization. The risk of stroke may be increased in women with hypertension. Discontinue if clinically significant hypertension develops during therapy. The risk of cardiovascular side effects is increased in women who smoke cigarettes. Women should be advised not to smoke.

Progestin use has been associated with retinal vascular lesions; discontinue pending examination in case of sudden vision loss, complete loss of vision, sudden onset of proptosis, diplopia, or migraine. Chloasma may occur occasionally; women with a history of chloasma should avoid sun or ultraviolet radiation exposure during therapy. Patients with a prior history of pruritus during pregnancy or due to use of sex steroids should discontinue dienogest therapy if pruritus reoccurs during therapy. Not indicated for use prior to menarche or in the geriatric population. Not intended for use as a contraceptive.

Drug Interactions

Avoid Concomitant Use

Avoid concomitant use of Dienogest with any of the following: CYP3A4 Inducers (Strong); Griseofulvin; Tranexamic Acid; Ulipristal

Decreased Effect

Dienogest may decrease the levels/effects of: Anticoagulants; Vitamin K Antagonists

The levels/effects of Dienogest may be decreased by: Acitretin; Aminoglutethimide; Aprepitant; Artemether; Barbiturates; Bexarotene (Systemic); Bile Acid Sequestrants; Bosentan; CarBAMazepine; CloBAZam; CYP3A4 Inducers (Strong); Dabrafenib; Deferasirox; Eslicarbazepine; Felbamate; Fosaprepitant; Fosphenytoin; Griseofulvin; LamoTRIgine; Metreleptin; Mifepristone; Mycophenolate; Nelfinavir; Nevirapine; OXcarbazepine; Perampanel; Phenytoin; Primidone; Prucalopride; Retinoic Acid Derivatives; Rifamycin Derivatives; St Johns Wort; Sugammadex; Telaprevir; Tocilizumab; Topiramate; Ulipristal

Increased Effect/Toxicity

Dienogest may increase the levels/effects of: Benzodiazepines (metabolized by oxidation); Selegiline; Thalidomide; Tranexamic Acid; Voriconazole

The levels/effects of Dienogest may be increased by: Atazanavir; Boceprevir; Cobicistat; CYP3A4 Inhibitors (Strong); Herbs (Progestogenic Properties); Metreleptin; Mifepristone; Voriconazole

Nutritional/Ethanol Interactions Herb/Nutraceutical: St John's wort may induce dienogest hepatic metabolism and decrease its systemic exposure.

Adverse Reactions 1% to 10%:

Central nervous system: Headache (7%), depression (3%), sleep disturbance (2%), irritability (1%), migraine (1%), nervousness (1%)

Dermatologic: Acne (2%), alopecia (1%)

Endocrine & metabolic: Breast discomfort (5%), ovarian cyst (3%), libido decreased (2%)

Gastrointestinal: Nausea (4%), weight gain (4%), abdominal pain (2%)

Genitourinary: Vaginal bleeding (1%)

Neuromuscular & skeletal: Weakness (2%)

Product Availability Not available in the U.S.

General Dosage Range Oral: *Adult females:* 2 mg once daily

Administration

Oral Administer without regard to meals. If a dose is not absorbed due to vomiting and/or diarrhea within 3-4 hours of administration, repeat dose.

Storage/Stability Store in original packaging at 15°C to 30°C (59°F to 86°F).

Nursing Actions

Physical Assessment

Monitor for possible side effects such as headache, depression, breast soreness, nausea, vomiting, and weight gain. If patient immobilized or having surgery, be sure to notify their prescriber or have them call their prescriber to discuss as medication should be temporarily stopped.

Patient Education

• Discuss specific use of drug and side effects with patient as it relates to treatment. (HCAHPS: During this hospital stay, were you given any medicine that you had not taken before? Before giving you any new medicine, how often did hospital staff tell you what the medicine was for? How often did hospital staff describe possible side effects in a way you could understand?)

• Patient may experience headache, depression, mastalgia, or weight gain. Have patient report immediately to prescriber signs of infection, hypertension, severe nausea, significant edema of hands or feet, considerable dyspepsia, suicidal ideation, inability to eat, intolerable asthenia, urine discoloration, jaundice, severe skin irritation, or sudden vision changes (HCAHPS).

• Educate patient about signs of a significant reaction (eg, wheezing; chest tightness; fever; itching; bad cough; blue skin color; seizures; or swelling of face, lips, tongue, or throat). **Note:** This is not a comprehensive list of all side effects. Patient should consult prescriber for additional questions.

Intended Use and Disclaimer: Should not be printed and given to patients. This information is intended to serve as a concise initial reference for healthcare professionals to use when discussing medications with a patient. You must ultimately rely on your own discretion, experience and judgment in diagnosing, treating and advising patients.

Diethylpropion (dye eth il PROE pee on)

Index Terms Amfepramone; Diethylpropion Hydrochloride; Tenuate; Tenuate Dospan

Pharmacologic Category Anorexiant; Central Nervous System Stimulant; Sympathomimetic

Pregnancy Risk Factor B

Lactation Enters breast milk/use caution

Use Short-term (few weeks) adjunct in the management of exogenous obesity

Pharmacotherapy for weight loss is recommended only for obese patients with a body mass index ≥30 kg/m², or ≥27 kg/m² in the presence of other risk factors such as hypertension, diabetes, and/or dyslipidemia or a high waist circumference; therapy should be used in conjunction with a comprehensive weight management program.

Controlled Substance C-IV

Available Dosage Forms

Tablet, Oral:
Generic: 25 mg

Tablet Extended Release 24 Hour, Oral:
Generic: 75 mg

General Dosage Range Oral:

Controlled release: *Children >16 years and Adults:* 75 mg once daily

Immediate release: *Children >16 years and Adults:* 25 mg 3 times daily

Administration

Oral Dose should not be administered in evening or at bedtime.

Immediate release: Administer 1 hour before meals.

Controlled release: Do not crush tablet; administer at midmorning.

Nursing Actions

Physical Assessment Assess for history of psychopathology, homicidal or suicidal tendencies, or addiction; long-term use can result in dependence, abuse, or tolerance. Periodically evaluate the need for continued use. Monitor blood pressure and vital signs prior to treatment, when changing dosage, and at regular intervals during therapy. Monitor serum glucose closely in patients with diabetes (amphetamines may alter antidiabetic requirements). Taper dosage slowly when discontinuing.

Patient Education

• Discuss specific use of drug and side effects with patient as it relates to treatment. (HCAHPS: During this hospital stay, were you given any medicine that you had not taken before? Before giving you any new medicine, how often did hospital staff tell you what the medicine was for? How often did hospital staff describe possible side effects in a way you could understand?)

• Patient may experience xerostomia, lack of appetite, insomnia, parageusia, constipation, diarrhea, headache, or nausea. Have patient

report immediately to prescriber strength differences from one side to another, difficulty speaking or thinking, change in balance, blurred vision, angina, tachycardia, arrhythmia, behavioral changes, mood changes, depression, severe dizziness, syncope, considerable anxiety, significant headache, vision changes, sexual dysfunction, chills, pharyngitis, dysuria, polyuria, dyspnea, edema of extremities, difficulty with motor activity, intolerable asthenia, akathisia, macromastia, or dysmenorrhea (HCAHPS).
- Educate patient about signs of a significant reaction (eg, wheezing; chest tightness; fever; itching; bad cough; blue skin color; seizures; or swelling of face, lips, tongue, or throat). **Note:** This is not a comprehensive list of all side effects. Patient should consult prescriber for additional questions.

Intended Use and Disclaimer: Should not be printed and given to patients. This information is intended to serve as a concise initial reference for healthcare professionals to use when discussing medications with a patient. You must ultimately rely on your own discretion, experience and judgment in diagnosing, treating and advising patients.

Difenoxin and Atropine
(dye fen OKS in & A troe peen)

Brand Names: U.S. Motofen®
Index Terms Atropine and Difenoxin
Pharmacologic Category Antidiarrheal
Pregnancy Risk Factor C
Lactation Not recommended
Use Treatment of diarrhea
Controlled Substance C-IV
Available Dosage Forms
Tablet, oral:
Motofen®: Difenoxin 1 mg and atropine 0.025 mg
General Dosage Range Oral: *Adults:* 2 tablets (each tablet contains difenoxin hydrochloride 1 mg and atropine sulfate 0.025 mg) initially, then 1 tablet after each loose stool (maximum: 8 tablets/day)
Nursing Actions
Physical Assessment See individual agents.
Patient Education
- Discuss specific use of drug and side effects with patient as it relates to treatment. (HCAHPS: During this hospital stay, were you given any medicine that you had not taken before? Before giving you any new medicine, how often did hospital staff tell you what the medicine was for? How often did hospital staff describe possible side effects in a way you could understand?)
- Patient may experience fatigue or dizziness. Have patient report immediately to prescriber signs of fluid and electrolyte imbalance, signs

of pancreatitis, dyspnea, tachycardia, difficult urination, illogical thinking, vision changes, mood changes, severe constipation, or intolerable dyspepsia (HCAHPS).
- Educate patient about signs of a significant reaction (eg, wheezing; chest tightness; fever; itching; bad cough; blue skin color; seizures; or swelling of face, lips, tongue, or throat). **Note:** This is not a comprehensive list of all side effects. Patient should consult prescriber for additional questions.

Intended Use and Disclaimer: Should not be printed and given to patients. This information is intended to serve as a concise initial reference for healthcare professionals to use when discussing medications with a patient. You must ultimately rely on your own discretion, experience and judgment in diagnosing, treating and advising patients.
Related Information
Atropine *on page 144*

Difluprednate (dye floo PRED nate)

Brand Names: U.S. Durezol
Pharmacologic Category Corticosteroid, Ophthalmic
Medication Safety Issues
Sound-alike/look-alike issues:
Durezol may be confused with Durasal
Pregnancy Risk Factor C
Lactation Excretion in breast milk unknown/use caution
Use Treatment of inflammation and pain following ocular surgery; treatment of endogenous anterior uveitis
Available Dosage Forms
Emulsion, Ophthalmic:
Durezol: 0.05% (5 mL)
General Dosage Range Ophthalmic: *Children, Adolescents, and Adults:* Instill 1 drop in affected eye(s) 2-4 times daily (ocular surgery) or 4 times daily for 14 days (uveitis); taper to discontinue
Administration
Other Wash hands prior to use and avoid touching tip of dropper. Remove contact lenses prior to use. Do not reinsert contact lenses within 10 minutes of difluprednate eye drops. The use of the same bottle for both eyes is not recommended in surgical patients.
Nursing Actions
Patient Education
- Discuss specific use of drug and side effects with patient as it relates to treatment. (HCAHPS: During this hospital stay, were you given any medicine that you had not taken before? Before giving you any new medicine, how often did hospital staff tell you what the medicine was for? How often did hospital staff describe possible side effects in a way you could understand?) ▶

- Have patient report immediately to prescriber vision changes, ophthalmalgia, or severe eye irritation (HCAHPS).
- Educate patient about signs of a significant reaction (eg, wheezing; chest tightness; fever; itching; bad cough; blue skin color; seizures; or swelling of face, lips, tongue, or throat). **Note:** This is not a comprehensive list of all side effects. Patient should consult prescriber for additional questions.

Intended Use and Disclaimer: Should not be printed and given to patients. This information is intended to serve as a concise initial reference for healthcare professionals to use when discussing medications with a patient. You must ultimately rely on your own discretion, experience and judgment in diagnosing, treating and advising patients.

Digoxin (di JOKS in)

Brand Names: U.S. Digox; Lanoxin; Lanoxin Pediatric

Index Terms Digitalis

Pharmacologic Category Antiarrhythmic Agent, Miscellaneous; Cardiac Glycoside

Medication Safety Issues

Sound-alike/look-alike issues:

Digoxin may be confused with Desoxyn, doxepin Lanoxin may be confused with Lasix, levothyroxine, Levoxyl, Levsinex, Lomotil, Mefoxin, naloxone, Xanax

High alert medication:

The Institute for Safe Medication Practices (ISMP) includes this medication among its list of drugs which have a heightened risk of causing significant patient harm when used in error.

BEERS Criteria medication:

This drug may be potentially inappropriate for use in geriatric patients (Quality of evidence - moderate; Strength of recommendation - strong).

International issues:

Lanoxin [U.S., Canada, and multiple international markets] may be confused with Limoxin brand name for ambroxol [Indonesia] and amoxicillin [Mexico]

Pregnancy Risk Factor C

Lactation Enters breast milk/use caution

Breast-Feeding Considerations Digoxin is excreted into breast milk and similar concentrations are found within mother's serum and milk. The manufacturer recommends that caution be used when administered to nursing women.

Use

Atrial fibrillation: For the control of ventricular response rate in adults with chronic atrial fibrillation.

Heart failure: For the treatment of mild-to-moderate (or stage C as recommended by the ACCF/AHA) heart failure (HF) in adults; to increase myocardial contractility in pediatric patients with heart failure

Note: In treatment of atrial fibrillation (AF), use is not considered first-line unless AF coexistent with heart failure or in sedentary patients (Anderson, 2013). In the treatment of heart failure, digoxin should be considered for use only in HF with reduced ejection fraction (HFrEF) when symptoms remain despite guideline-directed medical therapy or as initial therapy in patients with severe symptoms yet to respond to guideline-directed medical therapy (Yancy, 2013).

Unlabeled Use Fetal tachycardia with or without hydrops; to slow ventricular rate in supraventricular tachyarrhythmias such as supraventricular tachycardia (SVT) excluding atrioventricular reciprocating tachycardia (AVRT)

Mechanism of Action/Effect

Heart failure: Inhibition of the sodium/potassium ATPase pump in myocardial cells results in a transient increase of intracellular sodium, which in turn promotes calcium influx via the sodium-calcium exchange pump leading to increased contractility.

Supraventricular arrhythmias: Direct suppression of the AV node conduction to increase effective refractory period and decrease conduction velocity - positive inotropic effect, enhanced vagal tone, and decreased ventricular rate to fast atrial arrhythmias. Atrial fibrillation may decrease sensitivity and increase tolerance to higher serum digoxin concentrations.

Contraindications Hypersensitivity to digoxin (rare) or other forms of digitalis, or any component of the formulation; ventricular fibrillation

Warnings/Precautions Watch for proarrhythmic effects (especially with digoxin toxicity). Withdrawal in clinically stable patients with HF may lead to recurrence of HF symptoms. During an episode of atrial fibrillation or flutter in patients with an accessory bypass tract (eg, Wolff-Parkinson-White syndrome), use has been associated with increased anterograde conduction down the accessory pathway leading to ventricular fibrillation; avoid use in such patients (Anderson, 2013; Neumar, 2010). Because digoxin slows sinoatrial and AV conduction, the drug commonly prolongs the PR interval. Digoxin may cause severe sinus bradycardia or sinoatrial block in patients with pre-existing sinus node disease. Avoid use in patients with second- or third-degree heart block (except in patients with a functioning artificial pacemaker) (Yancy, 2013); incomplete AV block (eg, Stokes-Adams attack) may progress to complete block with digoxin administration. Digoxin should be considered for use only in heart failure (HF) with reduced ejection fraction (HFrEF) when symptoms remain despite guideline-directed medical therapy. It may also be considered in patients with both HF and atrial fibrillation; however, beta blockers may offer better ventricular rate control than digoxin (ACCF/AHA

[Yancy, 2013]). Avoid use in patients with hypertrophic cardiomyopathy (HCM) and outflow tract obstruction unless used to control ventricular response with atrial fibrillation; outflow obstruction may worsen due to the positive inotropic effects of digoxin. Digoxin is potentially harmful in the treatment of dyspnea in patients with HCM in the absence of atrial fibrillation (Gersh, 2011). In a murine model of viral myocarditis, digoxin in high doses was shown to be detrimental (Matsumori, 1999). If used in humans, therefore, digoxin should be used with caution and only at low doses (Frishman, 2007). The manufacturer recommends avoiding the use of digoxin in patients with myocarditis.

Use with caution in patients with hyperthyroidism (increased digoxin clearance) and hypothyroidism (reduced digoxin clearance). Atrial arrhythmias associated with hypermetabolic (eg, hyperthyroidism) or hyperdynamic (hypoxia, arteriovenous shunt) states are very difficult to treat; treat underlying condition first. Use with caution in patients with an acute MI; may increase myocardial oxygen demand. During the immediate post-MI period, digoxin administered I.V. may be used to slow a rapid ventricular response and improve left ventricular (LV) function in the acute treatment of atrial fibrillation associated with severe LV function and heart failure (Anderson, 2013). Reduce dose with renal impairment and when amiodarone, propafenone, quinidine, or verapamil are added to a patient on digoxin; use with caution in patients taking strong inducers or inhibitors of P-glycoprotein (eg, cyclosporine). Avoid rapid I.V. administration of calcium in digitalized patients; may produce serious arrhythmias.

Atrial arrhythmias associated with hypermetabolic states are very difficult to treat; treat underlying condition first; if digoxin is used, ensure digoxin toxicity does not occur. Patients with beri beri heart disease may fail to adequately respond to digoxin therapy; treat underlying thiamine deficiency concomitantly. Correct electrolyte disturbances, especially hypokalemia or hypomagnesemia, prior to use and throughout therapy; toxicity may occur despite therapeutic digoxin concentrations. Hypercalcemia may increase the risk of digoxin toxicity; maintain normocalcemia. It is not necessary to routinely reduce or hold digoxin therapy prior to elective electrical cardioversion for atrial fibrillation; however, exclusion of digoxin toxicity (eg, clinical and ECG signs) is necessary prior to cardioversion. If signs of digoxin excess exist, withhold digoxin and delay cardioversion until toxicity subsides (Anderson, 2013). I.V. administration: Vesicant; ensure proper needle or catheter placement prior to and during administration; avoid extravasation. Use with caution in the elderly; decreases in renal clearance may result in toxic effects; in general, avoid doses >0.125 mg/day; in heart failure, higher doses may increase the risk of potential toxicity and have not been shown to provide additional benefit (Beers Criteria).

Drug Interactions

Avoid Concomitant Use There are no known interactions where it is recommended to avoid concomitant use.

Decreased Effect

Digoxin may decrease the levels/effects of: Antineoplastic Agents (Anthracycline, Systemic)

The levels/effects of Digoxin may be decreased by: 5-ASA Derivatives; Acarbose; Aminoglycosides; Antineoplastic Agents; Antineoplastic Agents (Anthracycline, Systemic); Bile Acid Sequestrants; Kaolin; PenicillAMINE; P-glycoprotein/ABCB1 Inducers; Potassium-Sparing Diuretics; St Johns Wort; Sucralfate

Increased Effect/Toxicity

Digoxin may increase the levels/effects of: Adenosine; Carvedilol; Colchicine; Dronedarone; Midodrine

The levels/effects of Digoxin may be increased by: Aminoquinolines (Antimalarial); Amiodarone; Antithyroid Agents; AtorvaSTATin; Beta-Blockers; Boceprevir; Brimonidine (Topical); Calcium Channel Blockers (Nondihydropyridine); Calcium Polystyrene Sulfonate; Carvedilol; CloNIDine; Conivaptan; CycloSPORINE (Systemic); Dronedarone; Etravirine; Ezogabine; Flecainide; Glycopyrrolate; Itraconazole; Lenalidomide; Loop Diuretics; Macrolide Antibiotics; Mifepristone; Milnacipran; Mirabegron; Multivitamins/Fluoride (with ADE); Multivitamins/Minerals (with ADEK, Folate, Iron); Multivitamins/Minerals (with AE, No Iron); Nefazodone; Neuromuscular-Blocking Agents; NIFEdipine; Nonsteroidal Anti-Inflammatory Agents; Paricalcitol; P-glycoprotein/ABCB1 Inhibitors; Posaconazole; Potassium-Sparing Diuretics; Propafenone; Protease Inhibitors; QuiNIDine; QuiNINE; Ranolazine; Regorafenib; Reserpine; Simeprevir; SitaGLIPtin; Sodium Polystyrene Sulfonate; Spironolactone; Telaprevir; Telmisartan; Ticagrelor; Tolvaptan; Trimethoprim; Vitamin D Analogs

Nutritional/Ethanol Interactions

Food: Digoxin peak serum concentrations may be decreased if taken with food. Meals containing increased fiber (bran) or foods high in pectin may decrease oral absorption of digoxin.

Herb/Nutraceutical: Avoid ephedra (risk of cardiac stimulation). Avoid natural licorice (causes sodium and water retention and increases potassium loss).

Adverse Reactions Incidence not always reported.

Cardiovascular: Accelerated junctional rhythm, asystole, atrial tachycardia with or without block, AV dissociation, first-, second- (Wenckebach), or third-degree heart block, facial edema, PR prolongation, PVCs (especially bigeminy or trigeminy), ST segment depression, ventricular tachycardia or ventricular fibrillation

Central nervous system: Dizziness (6%), mental disturbances (5%), headache (4%), apathy, anxiety, confusion, delirium, depression, fever, hallucinations

Dermatologic: Rash (erythematous, maculopapular [most common], papular, scarlatiniform, vesicular or bullous), pruritus, urticaria, angioneurotic edema

Gastrointestinal: Nausea (4%), vomiting (2%), diarrhea (4%), abdominal pain, anorexia

Neuromuscular & skeletal: Weakness

Ocular: Visual disturbances (blurred or yellow vision)

Respiratory: Laryngeal edema

Pharmacodynamics/Kinetics

Onset of Action

Heart rate control: Oral: 1-2 hours; I.V.: 5-60 minutes

Peak effect: Heart rate control: Oral: 2-8 hours; I.V.: 1-6 hours; **Note:** In patients with atrial fibrillation, median time to ventricular rate control in one study was 6 hours (range: 3-15 hours) (Siu, 2009)

Duration of Action Adults: 3-4 days

Available Dosage Forms

Solution, Injection:

Lanoxin: 0.25 mg/mL (2 mL)

Lanoxin Pediatric: 0.1 mg/mL (1 mL)

Generic: 0.25 mg/mL (1 mL, 2 mL)

Solution, Oral:

Generic: 0.05 mg/mL (60 mL)

Tablet, Oral:

Digox: 0.125 mg, 0.25 mg

Lanoxin: 187.5 mcg, 0.0625 mg, 0.125 mg, 0.25 mg

Generic: 0.125 mg, 0.25 mg

General Dosage Range Dosage adjustment recommended in patients with renal impairment

I.M., I.V.:

Preterm infants: Digitalizing dose: 15-25 mcg/kg; Maintenance: 4-6 mcg/kg/day in divided doses every 12 hours

Full-term infants: Digitalizing dose: 20-30 mcg/kg; Maintenance: 5-8 mcg/kg/day in divided doses every 12 hours

Children 1 month to 2 years: Digitalizing dose: 30-50 mcg/kg; Maintenance: 7.5-12 mcg/kg/day in divided doses every 12 hours

Children 2-5 years: Digitalizing dose: 25-35 mcg/kg; Maintenance: 6-9 mcg/kg/day in divided doses every 12 hours

Children 5-10 years: Digitalizing dose: 15-30 mcg/kg; Maintenance: 4-8 mcg/kg/day in divided doses every 12 hours

Children >10 years: Digitalizing dose: 8-12 mcg/kg; Maintenance: 2-3 mcg/kg once daily

Adults: Digitalizing dose: 0.5-1 mg; Maintenance: 0.1-0.4 mg once daily

Oral:

Preterm infants: Digitalizing dose: 20-30 mcg/kg; Maintenance: 5-7.5 mcg/kg/day in divided doses every 12 hours

Full-term infants: Digitalizing dose: 25-35 mcg/kg; Maintenance: 6-10 mcg/kg/day in divided doses every 12 hours

Children 1 month to 2 years: Digitalizing dose: 35-60 mcg/kg; Maintenance: 10-15 mcg/kg/day in divided doses every 12 hours

Children 2-5 years: Digitalizing dose: 30-40 mcg/kg; Maintenance: 7.5-10 mcg/kg/day in divided doses every 12 hours

Children 5-10 years: Digitalizing dose: 20-35 mcg/kg; Maintenance: 5-10 mcg/kg/day in divided doses every 12 hours

Children >10 years: Digitalizing dose: 10-15 mcg/kg; Maintenance: 2.5-5 mcg/kg once daily

Adults: Digitalizing dose: 0.75-1.5 mg; Maintenance: 0.125-0.5 mg once daily

Administration

I.M. I.V. route preferred. If I.M. injection necessary, administer by deep injection followed by massage at the injection site. Inject no more than 2 mL per injection site. May cause intense pain.

Vesicant; ensure proper needle or catheter placement prior to and during administration; avoid extravasation.

Extravasation management: If extravasation occurs, stop I.V. administration immediately and disconnect (leave cannula/needle in place); gently aspirate extravasated solution (do **NOT** flush the line); remove needle/cannula; elevate extremity.

I.V. May be administered undiluted or diluted. Inject slowly over ≥5 minutes

Injectable Detail pH: 6.8-7.2 (0.25 mg/mL undiluted solution)

Preparation for Administration

I.M.: No dilution required.

I.V.: May be administered undiluted or diluted fourfold in D_5W, NS, or SWFI for direct injection. Less than fourfold dilution may lead to drug precipitation.

Storage/Stability Store at 25°C (77°F); excursions permitted to 15°C to 30°C (59°F to 86°F). Protect elixir, injection, and tablets from light.

Nursing Actions

Physical Assessment Monitor laboratory tests when beginning or changing dosage, especially with I.V. administration. I.V.: Monitor ECG continuously. Oral: Monitor apical pulse before administering any dose. Teach patient to report noncardiac signs of toxicity (eg, anorexia, blurred vision, "yellow" vision, confusion).

Patient Education

• Discuss specific use of drug and side effects with patient as it relates to treatment. (HCAHPS: During this hospital stay, were you given any medicine that you had not taken before? Before giving you any new medicine, how often did

hospital staff tell you what the medicine was for? How often did hospital staff describe possible side effects in a way you could understand?)

- Patient may experience headache. Have patient report immediately to prescriber severe dizziness, syncope, considerable nausea, significant diarrhea, sudden vision changes, lack of appetite, intolerable asthenia, melena, illogical thinking, bradycardia, tachycardia, arrhythmia, hallucinations, mood changes, severe dyspepsia, abdominal swelling, ecchymosis, hemorrhaging, or hematemesis (HCAHPS).

- Educate patient about signs of a significant reaction (eg, wheezing; chest tightness; fever; itching; bad cough; blue skin color; seizures; or swelling of face, lips, tongue, or throat). **Note:** This is not a comprehensive list of all side effects. Patient should consult prescriber for additional questions.

Intended Use and Disclaimer: Should not be printed and given to patients. This information is intended to serve as a concise initial reference for healthcare professionals to use when discussing medications with a patient. You must ultimately rely on your own discretion, experience and judgment in diagnosing, treating and advising patients.

Dietary Considerations Maintain adequate amounts of potassium in diet to decrease risk of hypokalemia (hypokalemia may increase risk of digoxin toxicity).

Related Information

Management of Drug Extravasations *on page 1700*

Peak and Trough Guidelines *on page 1710*

Digoxin Immune Fab (di JOKS in i MYUN fab)

Brand Names: U.S. DigiFab

Index Terms Antidigoxin Fab Fragments, Ovine; Digibind

Pharmacologic Category Antidote

Pregnancy Risk Factor C

Lactation Excretion in breast milk unknown/use caution

Use Treatment of life-threatening or potentially life-threatening digoxin intoxication, including:

- acute digoxin ingestion (ie, >10 mg in adults; >0.1 mg/kg or >4 mg in children; ingestions resulting in serum concentrations >10 ng/mL)
- chronic ingestions leading to steady-state digoxin concentrations >6 ng/mL in adults or >4 ng/mL in children
- manifestations of digoxin toxicity due to overdose (eg, life-threatening ventricular arrhythmias, progressive bradycardia, second- or third-degree heart block not responsive to atropine, serum potassium >5.5 mEq/L in adults or >6 mEq/L in children)

Available Dosage Forms

Solution Reconstituted, Intravenous [preservative free]:

DigiFab: 40 mg (1 ea)

General Dosage Range I.V.:

Acute ingestion of known amount: *Children and Adults:* Digoxin Immune Fab Dose (vials) = Total body load (mg) / (0.5)

Based on steady-state digoxin concentration:

Infants and Children ≤20 kg: Digoxin Immune Fab Dose (mg) = [(serum digoxin concentration [ng/mL] x weight [kg]) / 100] x (digoxin immune Fab amount per vial [mg/vial])

Note: Digoxin immune Fab amount per vial: 40 mg/vial.

Children >20 kg and Adults: Digoxin Immune Fab Dose (vials) = (serum digoxin concentration [ng/mL] x weight [kg]) / 100

Amount ingested and blood level unknown:

Children ≤20 kg: Acute toxicity: 20 vials total in 2 divided doses; Chronic toxicity: 1 vial may be sufficient

Children >20 kg and Adults: Acute toxicity: 20 vials total in 2 divided doses; Chronic toxicity: 6 vials

Administration

I.V. I.V. infusion over at least 30 minutes is preferred. May also be given by bolus injection if cardiac arrest is imminent (infusion-related reaction may occur). Small doses (eg, those required in infants or small children) may be administered using a tuberculin syringe as undiluted digoxin immune Fab or diluted with NS to a concentration of 1 mg/mL digoxin immune Fab. Stopping the infusion and restarting at a slower rate may help if an infusion-related reaction occurs.

Nursing Actions

Physical Assessment Assess allergy history prior to administration. Monitor lab values, cardiac status, vital signs, and blood pressure during and following infusion. Monitor for signs of reoccurrence of cardiac toxicity.

Patient Education

- Discuss specific use of drug and side effects with patient as it relates to treatment. (HCAHPS: During this hospital stay, were you given any medicine that you had not taken before? Before giving you any new medicine, how often did hospital staff tell you what the medicine was for? How often did hospital staff describe possible side effects in a way you could understand?)

- Have patient report immediately to prescriber severe dizziness, syncope, tachycardia, or signs of hypokalemia (HCAHPS).

- Educate patient about signs of a significant reaction (eg, wheezing; chest tightness; fever; itching; bad cough; blue skin color; seizures; or swelling of face, lips, tongue, or throat). **Note:** This is not a comprehensive list of all side effects. Patient should consult prescriber for additional questions.

◀ **Intended Use and Disclaimer:** Should not be printed and given to patients. This information is intended to serve as a concise initial reference for healthcare professionals to use when discussing medications with a patient. You must ultimately rely on your own discretion, experience and judgment in diagnosing, treating and advising patients.

Dihydrocodeine, Aspirin, and Caffeine (dye hye droe KOE deen, AS pir in, & KAF een)

Brand Names: U.S. Synalgos®-DC
Index Terms Aspirin, Dihydrocodeine, and Caffeine; Caffeine, Dihydrocodeine, and Aspirin; Dihydrocodeine Compound; Dihydrocodeine, Aspirin, and Caffeine
Pharmacologic Category Analgesic, Opioid
Medication Safety Issues
Sound-alike/look-alike issues:
Synalgos®-DC may be confused with Synagis®
High alert medication:
The Institute for Safe Medication Practices (ISMP) includes this medication among its list of drug classes which have a heightened risk of causing significant patient harm when used in error.
Use Management of mild-to-moderate pain
Controlled Substance C-III
Available Dosage Forms
Capsule, oral:
Synalgos®-DC: Dihydrocodeine 16 mg, aspirin 356.4 mg, and caffeine 30 mg
Generic: Dihydrocodeine bitartrate 16 mg, aspirin 356.4 mg, and caffeine 30 mg
General Dosage Range Oral: *Adults:* 1-2 capsules every 4-6 hours as needed
Nursing Actions
Physical Assessment See individual agents.
Patient Education
• Discuss specific use of drug and side effects with patient as it relates to treatment. (HCAHPS: During this hospital stay, were you given any medicine that you had not taken before? Before giving you any new medicine, how often did hospital staff tell you what the medicine was for? How often did hospital staff describe possible side effects in a way you could understand?)
• Patient may experience constipation, dizziness, fatigue, or nausea. Have patient report immediately to prescriber dyspnea, illogical thinking, severe anxiety, ecchymosis, hemorrhaging, tinnitus, dysphagia, hearing impairment, mood changes, hyperhidrosis, or signs of abdominal ulcers (HCAHPS).
• Educate patient about signs of a significant reaction (eg, wheezing; chest tightness; fever; itching; bad cough; blue skin color; seizures; or swelling of face, lips, tongue, or throat). **Note:** This is not a comprehensive list of all side

effects. Patient should consult prescriber for additional questions.

Intended Use and Disclaimer: Should not be printed and given to patients. This information is intended to serve as a concise initial reference for healthcare professionals to use when discussing medications with a patient. You must ultimately rely on your own discretion, experience and judgment in diagnosing, treating and advising patients.
Related Information
Aspirin *on page 129*
Caffeine *on page 232*

Dihydroergotamine (dye hye droe er GOT a meen)

Brand Names: U.S. D.H.E. 45; Migranal
Index Terms DHE; Dihydroergotamine Mesylate
Pharmacologic Category Antimigraine Agent; Ergot Derivative
Pregnancy Risk Factor X
Lactation Enters breast milk/contraindicated
Use Treatment of migraine headache with or without aura; injection also indicated for treatment of cluster headaches
Unlabeled Use Adjunct for DVT prophylaxis for hip surgery, for orthostatic hypotension, xerostomia secondary to antidepressant use, and pelvic congestion with pain
Dosage Forms Considerations
Migranal nasal solution contains caffeine 10 mg/mL
Available Dosage Forms
Solution, Injection:
D.H.E. 45: 1 mg/mL (1 mL)
Generic: 1 mg/mL (1 mL)
Solution, Nasal:
Migranal: 4 mg/mL (1 mL)
Generic: 4 mg/mL (1 mL)
General Dosage Range
I.M., SubQ: *Adults:* 1 mg initially, may repeat hourly up to 3 mg total (maximum: 6 mg/week)
I.V.: *Adults:* 1 mg initially, may repeat hourly up to 2 mg total (maximum: 6 mg/week)
Intranasal: *Adults:* 1 spray (0.5 mg) in each nostril initially, may repeat after 15 minutes up to 4 sprays total (maximum: 6 sprays/24 hours; 8 sprays/week)
Administration
I.M. May administer by intramuscular injection. Hazardous agent; use appropriate precautions for handling and disposal (meets NIOSH, 2012 criteria).
I.V. Administer slowly over 2-3 minutes (Raskin protocol). Hazardous agent; use appropriate precautions for handling and disposal (meets NIOSH, 2012 criteria).
Subcutaneous May administer by subcutaneous injection. Hazardous agent; use appropriate

precautions for handling and disposal (meets NIOSH, 2012 criteria).

Inhalation Intranasal: Prior to administration of nasal spray, the nasal spray applicator must be primed (pumped 4 times); in order to let the drug be absorbed through the skin in the nose, patients should not inhale deeply through the nose while spraying or immediately after spraying; for best results, treatment should be initiated at the first symptom or sign of an attack; however, nasal spray can be used at any stage of a migraine attack

Hazardous agent; use appropriate precautions for handling and disposal (meets NIOSH, 2012 criteria).

Nursing Actions

Physical Assessment Monitor for hypertension and cardiac events. Teach patient proper use (treatment of acute migraine). Teach patient proper storage, administration, injection technique, and syringe/needle disposal.

Patient Education
- Discuss specific use of drug and side effects with patient as it relates to treatment. (HCAHPS: During this hospital stay, were you given any medicine that you had not taken before? Before giving you any new medicine, how often did hospital staff tell you what the medicine was for? How often did hospital staff describe possible side effects in a way you could understand?)
- Patient may experience nausea, rhinitis, pharyngitis, dysgeusia, epistaxis, or rhinorrhea. Have patient report immediately to prescriber strength differences from one side to another, difficulty speaking and thinking, change in balance, blurred vision, angina, tachycardia, paresthesia, severe dizziness, syncope, myalgia, asthenia, muscle cramps, arrhythmia, discoloration of hands or feet, sensation of cold, bradycardia, edema, or considerable dyspepsia (HCAHPS).
- Educate patient about signs of a significant reaction (eg, wheezing; chest tightness; fever; itching; bad cough; blue skin color; seizures; or swelling of face, lips, tongue, or throat). **Note:** This is not a comprehensive list of all side effects. Patient should consult prescriber for additional questions.

Intended Use and Disclaimer: Should not be printed and given to patients. This information is intended to serve as a concise initial reference for healthcare professionals to use when discussing medications with a patient. You must ultimately rely on your own discretion, experience and judgment in diagnosing, treating and advising patients.

Diltiazem (dil TYE a zem)

Brand Names: U.S. Cardizem; Cardizem CD; Cardizem LA; Cartia XT; Dilacor XR; Dilt-CD [DSC]; Dilt-XR; Diltiazem HCl CD; Diltzac [DSC]; Matzim LA; Taztia XT; Tiazac

Index Terms Diltiazem Hydrochloride

Pharmacologic Category Antianginal Agent; Antiarrhythmic Agent, Class IV; Antihypertensive; Calcium Channel Blocker; Calcium Channel Blocker, Nondihydropyridine

Medication Safety Issues

Sound-alike/look-alike issues:

Cardizem may be confused with Cardene, Cardene SR, Cardizem CD, Cardizem SR, cortisone

Cartia XT may be confused with Procardia XL

Diltiazem may be confused with Calan, diazepam, Dilantin

Tiazac may be confused with Tigan, Tiazac XC [CAN], Ziac

High alert medication:

The Institute for Safe Medication Practices (ISMP) includes this medication (I.V. formulation) among its list of drug classes which have a heightened risk of causing significant patient harm when used in error.

Administration issues:

Significant differences exist between oral and I.V. dosing. Use caution when converting from one route of administration to another.

International issues:

Cardizem [U.S., Canada, and multiple international markets] may be confused with Cardem brand name for celiprolol [Spain]

Cartia XT [U.S.] may be confused with Cartia brand name for aspirin [multiple international markets]

Dilacor XR [U.S.] may be confused with Dilacor brand name for verapamil [Brazil]

Dipen [Greece] may be confused with Depen brand name for penicillamine [U.S.]; Depin brand name for nifedipine [India]; Depon brand name for acetaminophen [Greece]

Tiazac: Brand name for diltiazem [U.S, Canada], but also the brand name for pioglitazone [Chile]

Pregnancy Risk Factor C

Lactation Enters breast milk/not recommended

Breast-Feeding Considerations Diltiazem is excreted into breastmilk in concentrations similar to those in the maternal plasma (Okada, 1985). Breast-feeding is not recommended by the manufacturer. Breast-fed infants of mothers taking medications for hypertension should be monitored for adverse effects (Chobanian, 2003).

Use

Oral: Primary hypertension; chronic stable angina or angina from coronary artery spasm

Injection: Control of rapid ventricular rate in patients with atrial fibrillation or atrial flutter; conversion of paroxysmal supraventricular tachycardia (PSVT)

Unlabeled Use

ACLS guidelines: Injection: Stable narrow-complex tachycardia uncontrolled or unconverted by adenosine or vagal maneuvers or if SVT is recurrent

Hypertrophic cardiomyopathy; pediatric hypertension

Mechanism of Action/Effect Nondihydropyridine calcium channel blocker which inhibits calcium ion from entering the "slow channels" or select voltage-sensitive areas of vascular smooth muscle and myocardium during depolarization, producing a relaxation of coronary vascular smooth muscle and coronary vasodilation; increases myocardial oxygen delivery in patients with vasospastic angina

Contraindications

Oral: Hypersensitivity to diltiazem or any component of the formulation; sick sinus syndrome (except in patients with a functioning artificial pacemaker); second- or third-degree AV block (except in patients with a functioning artificial pacemaker); severe hypotension (systolic <90 mm Hg); acute MI and pulmonary congestion

Intravenous (I.V.): Hypersensitivity to diltiazem or any component of the formulation; sick sinus syndrome (except in patients with a functioning artificial pacemaker); second- or third-degree AV block (except in patients with a functioning artificial pacemaker); severe hypotension (systolic <90 mm Hg); cardiogenic shock; administration concomitantly or within a few hours of the administration of I.V. beta-blockers; atrial fibrillation or flutter associated with accessory bypass tract (eg, Wolff-Parkinson-White syndrome); ventricular tachycardia (with wide-complex tachycardia, must determine whether origin is supraventricular or ventricular)

Canadian labeling: Additional contraindications (not in U.S. labeling): I.V. and Oral: Pregnancy; use in women of childbearing potential

Warnings/Precautions Can cause first-, second-, and third-degree AV block or sinus bradycardia and risk increases with agents known to slow cardiac conduction. The most common side effect is peripheral edema; occurs within 2-3 weeks of starting therapy. Symptomatic hypotension with or without syncope can rarely occur; blood pressure must be lowered at a rate appropriate for the patient's clinical condition. Use caution when using diltiazem together with a beta-blocker; may result in conduction disturbances, hypotension, and worsened LV function. Simultaneous administration of I.V. diltiazem and an I.V. beta-blocker or administration within a few hours of each other may result in asystole and is contraindicated. Use with other agents known to either reduce SA node function and/or AV nodal conduction (eg, digoxin) or reduce sympathetic outflow (eg, clonidine) may increase the risk of serious bradycardia. Use caution in left ventricular dysfunction (may exacerbate condition). The ACCF/AHA heart failure guidelines recommend to avoid use in patients with heart failure due to lack of benefit and/or worse outcomes with calcium channel blockers in general (ACCF/AHA [Yancy, 2013]). Use with caution with

hypertrophic obstructive cardiomyopathy; routine use is currently not recommended due to insufficient evidence (Maron, 2003). Use with caution in hepatic or renal dysfunction. Transient dermatologic reactions have been observed with use; if reaction persists, discontinue. May (rarely) progress to erythema multiforme or exfoliative dermatitis.

Drug Interactions

Avoid Concomitant Use

Avoid concomitant use of Diltiazem with any of the following: Bosutinib; Conivaptan; Dantrolene; Fusidic Acid (Systemic); Ibrutinib; Ivabradine; Lomitapide; Pimozide; Rivaroxaban; Simeprevir; Tolvaptan; Ulipristal

Decreased Effect

Diltiazem may decrease the levels/effects of: Clopidogrel; Ifosfamide

The levels/effects of Diltiazem may be decreased by: Barbiturates; Bosentan; Calcium Salts; CarBAMazepine; Colestipol; CYP3A4 Inducers (Strong); Dabrafenib; Deferasirox; Herbs (CYP3A4 Inducers); Herbs (Hypertensive Properties); Methylphenidate; Mitotane; Nafcillin; Peginterferon Alfa-2b; P-glycoprotein/ABCB1 Inducers; Rifamycin Derivatives; Tocilizumab; Yohimbine

Increased Effect/Toxicity

Diltiazem may increase the levels/effects of: Alfentanil; Amifostine; Amiodarone; Antihypertensives; Aprepitant; ARIPiprazole; AtorvaSTATin; Atosiban; Avanafil; Benzodiazepines (metabolized by oxidation); Beta-Blockers; Bosentan; Bosutinib; Budesonide (Systemic, Oral Inhalation); BusPIRone; Calcium Channel Blockers (Dihydropyridine); CarBAMazepine; Cardiac Glycosides; Colchicine; Corticosteroids (Systemic); CycloSPORINE (Systemic); CYP3A4 Substrates; Dofetilide; DOXOrubicin (Conventional); Dronedarone; DULoxetine; Eletriptan; Eplerenone; Everolimus; Fingolimod; Fosaprepitant; Fosphenytoin; Halofantrine; Hypotensive Agents; Ibrutinib; Imatinib; Ivabradine; Ivacaftor; Lithium; Lomitapide; Lovastatin; Lurasidone; Magnesium Salts; Midodrine; Neuromuscular-Blocking Agents (Nondepolarizing); Nitroprusside; Obinutuzumab; OxyCODONE; Phenytoin; Pimecrolimus; Pimozide; Propafenone; QuiNIDine; Ranolazine; Red Yeast Rice; RiTUXimab; Rivaroxaban; Salicylates; Salmeterol; Saxagliptin; Simeprevir; Simvastatin; Tacrolimus (Systemic); Tacrolimus (Topical); Tolvaptan; Ulipristal; Vilazodone; Zuclopenthixol

The levels/effects of Diltiazem may be increased by: Alpha1-Blockers; Anilidopiperidine Opioids; Antifungal Agents (Azole Derivatives, Systemic); Aprepitant; AtorvaSTATin; Brimonidine (Topical); Calcium Channel Blockers (Dihydropyridine); Cimetidine; CloNIDine; Conivaptan; CycloSPORINE (Systemic); CYP3A4 Inhibitors (Moderate); CYP3A4 Inhibitors (Strong); Dantrolene;

Dasatinib; Diazoxide; Dronedarone; Fluconazole; Fosaprepitant; Fusidic Acid (Systemic); Grapefruit Juice; Herbs (Hypotensive Properties); Ivabradine; Ivacaftor; Lovastatin; Luliconazole; Macrolide Antibiotics; Magnesium Salts; MAO Inhibitors; Mifepristone; Pentoxifylline; P-glycoprotein/ABCB1 Inhibitors; Phosphodiesterase 5 Inhibitors; Prostacyclin Analogues; Protease Inhibitors; Regorafenib; Simeprevir; Simvastatin; Stiripentol

Nutritional/Ethanol Interactions

Ethanol: Ethanol may increase risk of hypotension or vasodilation. Management: Avoid ethanol.

Food: Diltiazem serum levels may be elevated if taken with food. Serum concentrations were not altered by grapefruit juice in small clinical trials.

Herb/Nutraceutical: St John's wort may decrease diltiazem levels. Some herbal medications may worsen hypertension (eg, licorice); others may increase the antihypertensive effect of diltiazem (eg, shepherd's purse). Management: Avoid St John's wort, bayberry, blue cohosh, cayenne, ephedra, ginger, ginseng (American), kola, licorice, and yohimbe. Avoid black cohosh, California poppy, coleus, golden seal, hawthorn, mistletoe, periwinkle, quinine, and shepherd's purse.

Adverse Reactions Note: Frequencies represent ranges for various dosage forms. Patients with impaired ventricular function and/or conduction abnormalities may have higher incidence of adverse reactions.

>10%:

Cardiovascular: Edema (2% to 15%)

Central nervous system: Headache (5% to 12%)

2% to 10%:

Cardiovascular: AV block (first degree 2% to 8%), edema (lower limb 2% to 8%), pain (6%), bradycardia (2% to 6%), hypotension (<2% to 4%), vasodilation (2% to 3%), extrasystoles (2%), flushing (1% to 2%), palpitation (1% to 2%)

Central nervous system: Dizziness (3% to 10%), nervousness (2%)

Dermatologic: Rash (1% to 4%)

Endocrine & metabolic: Gout (1% to 2%)

Gastrointestinal: Dyspepsia (1% to 6%), constipation (<2% to 4%), vomiting (2%), diarrhea (1% to 2%)

Local: Injection site reactions: Burning, itching (4%)

Neuromuscular & skeletal: Weakness (1% to 4%), myalgia (2%)

Respiratory: Rhinitis (<2% to 10%), pharyngitis (2% to 6%), dyspnea (1% to 6%), bronchitis (1% to 4%), cough (≤3%), sinus congestion (1% to 2%)

Pharmacodynamics/Kinetics

Onset of Action Oral: Immediate release tablet: 30-60 minutes; I.V.: 3 minutes

Duration of Action I.V.: Bolus: 1-3 hours; Continuous infusion (after discontinuation): 0.5-10 hours

Available Dosage Forms

Capsule Extended Release 12 Hour, Oral:

Generic: 60 mg, 90 mg, 120 mg

Capsule Extended Release 24 Hour, Oral:

Cardizem CD: 120 mg, 180 mg, 240 mg, 300 mg, 360 mg

Cartia XT: 120 mg, 180 mg, 240 mg, 300 mg

Dilacor XR: 240 mg

Dilt-XR: 120 mg, 180 mg, 240 mg

Diltiazem HCl CD: 360 mg

Taztia XT: 120 mg, 180 mg, 240 mg, 300 mg, 360 mg

Tiazac: 120 mg, 180 mg, 240 mg, 300 mg, 360 mg, 420 mg

Generic: 120 mg, 180 mg, 240 mg, 300 mg, 360 mg, 420 mg

Solution, Intravenous:

Generic: 25 mg/5 mL (5 mL); 50 mg/10 mL (10 mL); 125 mg/25 mL (25 mL)

Solution, Intravenous [preservative free]:

Generic: 25 mg/5 mL (5 mL); 50 mg/10 mL (10 mL); 125 mg/25 mL (25 mL)

Solution Reconstituted, Intravenous:

Generic: 100 mg (1 ea)

Tablet, Oral:

Cardizem: 30 mg, 60 mg, 120 mg

Generic: 30 mg, 60 mg, 90 mg, 120 mg

Tablet Extended Release 24 Hour, Oral:

Cardizem LA: 120 mg, 180 mg, 240 mg, 300 mg, 360 mg, 420 mg

Matzim LA: 180 mg, 240 mg, 300 mg, 360 mg, 420 mg

General Dosage Range

I.V.: *Adults:* Bolus: 0.25 mg/kg, may repeat 0.35 mg/kg after 15 minutes; Infusion: 5-15 mg/hour

Oral:

Extended release: *Adults:* Initial: 120-240 mg once daily **or** 60-120 mg twice daily; Maintenance: 120-540 mg once daily **or** 240-360 mg/day in 2 divided doses

Immediate release: *Adults:* Initial: 30 mg 4 times/day; Maintenance: 120-320 mg/day in divided doses

Usual Infusion Concentrations: Pediatric I.V. infusion: 1 mg/mL

Usual Infusion Concentrations: Adult I.V. infusion: 125 mg in 125 mL (total volume) (concentration: 1 mg/mL) of D_5W or NS

Administration

I.V. Bolus doses given over 2 minutes with continuous ECG and blood pressure monitoring. Continuous infusion should be via infusion pump.

Injectable Detail Response to bolus may require several minutes to reach maximum. Response may persist for several hours after infusion is discontinued.

pH: 3.7-4.1

Oral

Immediate release tablet (Cardizem®): Administer before meals and at bedtime.

Long acting dosage forms: Do not open, chew, or crush; swallow whole.

Cardizem® CD, Cardizem® LA, Cartia XT®, Dilt-CD, Matzim® LA: May be administered without regards to meals.

Dilacor XR®, Dilt-XR, Diltia XT®: Administer on an empty stomach.

Taztia XT™, Tiazac®: Capsules may be opened and sprinkled on a spoonful of applesauce. Applesauce should not be hot and should be swallowed without chewing, followed by drinking a glass of water.

Tiazac® XC [CAN; not available in U.S.]: Administer at bedtime

Storage/Stability

Capsule, tablet: Store at room temperature. Protect from light.

Solution for injection: Store in refrigerator at 2°C to 8°C (36°F to 46°F); do not freeze. May be stored at room temperature for up to 1 month. Following dilution to ≤1 mg/mL with $D_5^{1/2}NS$, D_5W, or NS, solution is stable for 24 hours at room temperature or under refrigeration.

Nursing Actions

Physical Assessment Assess potential for interactions with other agents that may cause increased risk of bradycardia, conduction delays, or decreased cardiac output. I.V. requires use of infusion pump and continuous cardiac and hemodynamic monitoring. Monitor therapeutic effectiveness according to use (hypertension, angina, atrial fib/flutter, or PSVT).

Patient Education

- Discuss specific use of drug and side effects with patient as it relates to treatment. (HCAHPS: During this hospital stay, were you given any medicine that you had not taken before? Before giving you any new medicine, how often did hospital staff tell you what the medicine was for? How often did hospital staff describe possible side effects in a way you could understand?)
- Have patient report immediately to prescriber signs of hepatic impairment, severe dizziness, syncope, or signs of Stevens-Johnson syndrome/toxic epidermal necrolysis (HCAHPS).
- Educate patient about signs of a significant reaction (eg, wheezing; chest tightness; fever; itching; bad cough; blue skin color; seizures; or swelling of face, lips, tongue, or throat). **Note:** This is not a comprehensive list of all side effects. Patient should consult prescriber for additional questions.

Intended Use and Disclaimer: Should not be printed and given to patients. This information is intended to serve as a concise initial reference for healthcare professionals to use when discussing medications with a patient. You must ultimately rely on your own discretion, experience and judgment in diagnosing, treating and advising patients.

Related Information

Oral Medications That Should Not Be Crushed or Altered *on page 1712*

Dimethyl Fumarate (dye meth il FYOO ma rate)

Brand Names: U.S. Tecfidera

Index Terms BG-12; Dimethylfumarate; DMF; FAG-201

Pharmacologic Category Fumaric Acid Derivative; Immunomodulator, Systemic

Medication Safety Issues

Sound-alike/look-alike issues:

Dimethyl fumarate may be confused with dimethyl sulfoxide

Pregnancy Risk Factor C

Lactation Excretion in breast milk unknown/use caution

Use Treatment of relapsing forms of multiple sclerosis (MS)

Available Dosage Forms

Capsule Delayed Release, Oral:

Tecfidera: 120 mg, 240 mg

Miscellaneous, Oral:

Tecfidera: Capsule, delayed release: 120 mg (14s) and Capsule, delayed release: 240 mg (46s) (60 ea)

General Dosage Range Oral: *Adults:* Initial: 120 mg twice daily; Maintenance: 240 mg twice daily

Administration

Oral Swallow capsules whole (delayed release); do not crush, chew, open the capsule, or sprinkle contents on food. May administer orally with or without food however administering with food may decrease the incidence of flushing. Canadian labeling suggests that short-term (≤4 days) administration of aspirin (non-enteric coated) 30 minutes prior to dimethyl fumarate may reduce the incidence and severity of flushing. Missed doses may be taken if ≥4 hours lapse between the morning and evening doses.

Nursing Actions

Physical Assessment Monitor for signs of weight loss, GI side effects, infection, skin changes.

Patient Education

- Discuss specific use of drug and side effects with patient as it relates to treatment. (HCAHPS: During this hospital stay, were you given any medicine that you had not taken before? Before giving you any new medicine, how often did hospital staff tell you what the medicine was for? How often did hospital staff describe possible side effects in a way you could understand?)
- Patient may experience flushing, dyspepsia, diarrhea, or nausea. Have patient report

immediately to prescriber signs of infection (HCAHPS).

• Educate patient about signs of a significant reaction (eg, wheezing; chest tightness; fever; itching; bad cough; blue skin color; seizures; or swelling of face, lips, tongue, or throat). **Note:** This is not a comprehensive list of all side effects. Patient should consult prescriber for additional questions.

Intended Use and Disclaimer: Should not be printed and given to patients. This information is intended to serve as a concise initial reference for healthcare professionals to use when discussing medications with a patient. You must ultimately rely on your own discretion, experience and judgment in diagnosing, treating and advising patients.

Related Information

Oral Medications That Should Not Be Crushed or Altered *on page 1712*

Dinoprostone (dye noe PROST one)

Brand Names: U.S. Cervidil; Prepidil; Prostin E2
Index Terms PGE$_2$; Prostaglandin E$_2$
Pharmacologic Category Abortifacient; Prostaglandin
Medication Safety Issues
International issues:
Cervidil brand name for dinoprostone [U.S., Canada, Australia, New Zealand], but also the brand name for gemeprost [Italy]

Pregnancy Risk Factor C
Lactation Excretion in breast milk unknown
Use
Endocervical gel (Prepidil®): Promote cervical ripening in patients at or near term in whom there is a medical or obstetrical indication for the induction of labor

Suppositories (Prostin E$_2$®): Terminate pregnancy from 12th through 20th week of gestation; evacuate uterus in cases of missed abortion or intrauterine fetal death up to 28 weeks of gestation; manage benign hydatidiform mole (nonmetastatic gestational trophoblastic disease)

Tablet (oral) (Prostin E$_2$®; Canadian availability): Elective induction of labor; when indications for induction of labor exist (eg, premature rupture of amniotic membranes, toxemia of pregnancy, Rh incompatibility, diabetes mellitus, hypertension, postmaturity, intrauterine death or fetal growth retardation)

Vaginal gel (Prostin E$_2$®; Canadian availability): Induction of labor in patients at or near term with singleton pregnancy, vertex presentation, and favorable induction features

Vaginal insert (Cervidil®): Initiation and/or continuation of cervical ripening in patients at or near term in whom there is a medical or obstetrical indication for the induction of labor

Available Dosage Forms

Gel, Vaginal:
Prepidil: 0.5 mg/3 g (3 g)
Insert, Vaginal:
Cervidil: 10 mg (1 ea)
Suppository, Vaginal:
Prostin E2: 20 mg (5 ea)

General Dosage Range

Endocervical: *Children (females of reproductive age) and Adults (females):* 0.5 mg; may repeat every 6 hours if needed. Maximum cumulative dose: 1.5 mg/24 hours

Intravaginal: *Children (females of reproductive age) and Adults (females):* Insert: 10 mg; remove at onset of active labor or after 12 hours; Suppository: 20 mg every 3-5 hours until abortion occurs

Administration

Oral Tablet (oral) (Canadian availability): Administer with small amount of water. Use of oxytocin should be avoided until ≥1 hour after administration of the last oral tablet.

Hazardous agent; use appropriate precautions for handling and disposal (NIOSH, 2012).

Other Endocervical gel: Bring to room temperature just prior to use. Do not force the warming process (eg, water bath, microwave). Avoid contact with skin while handling; wash hands thoroughly with soap and water after administration. For cervical ripening, patient should be supine in the dorsal position. The appropriate catheter length should be based on degree of effacement; 20 mm for no effacement; 10 mm if 50% effaced. Patient should remain supine for 15-30 minutes following administration. The manufacturer recommends waiting 6-12 hours after dinoprostone gel administration before initiating oxytocin.

Hazardous agent; use appropriate precautions for handling and disposal (NIOSH, 2012).

Intravaginal

Vaginal gel: (Canadian availability): Using prefilled syringe, dose is placed in the posterior fornix of the vagina. Patient should remain in lateral or supine position for 30 minutes to prevent leakage. Syringe contains overfill. Syringe is for single use only. Use of oxytocin should be avoided for 12-24 hours after administration of vaginal gel

Vaginal insert: One vaginal insert is placed transversely in the posterior fornix of the vagina immediately after removal from its foil package. Patients should remain in the recumbent position for 2 hours after insertion, but thereafter may be ambulatory. Do not use without retrieval system. Product does not need warmed prior to use. A water miscible lubricant may be used to facilitate insertion (avoid excessive use of lubricant). Ensure complete removal of system at completion of therapy. The manufacturer recommends waiting ≥30 minutes after removing the dinoprostone vaginal insert before initiating oxytocin.

Vaginal suppository: Insert high into vagina after removal from its foil package. Bring to room temperature just prior to use. Patient should remain supine for 10 minutes following insertion.

Hazardous agent; use appropriate precautions for handling and disposal (NIOSH, 2012).

Nursing Actions

Physical Assessment Monitor temperature closely. Monitor uterine tone and vaginal discharge closely throughout procedure and post-procedure. Monitor abortion for completeness (other measures may be necessary if incomplete).

Patient Education

• Discuss specific use of drug and side effects with patient as it relates to treatment. (HCAHPS: During this hospital stay, were you given any medicine that you had not taken before? Before giving you any new medicine, how often did hospital staff tell you what the medicine was for? How often did hospital staff describe possible side effects in a way you could understand?)

• Have patient report immediately to prescriber severe dizziness, syncope, ecchymosis, hemorrhaging, considerable nausea, or significant dyspepsia (HCAHPS).

• Educate patient about signs of a significant reaction (eg, wheezing; chest tightness; fever; itching; bad cough; blue skin color; seizures; or swelling of face, lips, tongue, or throat). **Note:** This is not a comprehensive list of all side effects. Patient should consult prescriber for additional questions.

Intended Use and Disclaimer: Should not be printed and given to patients. This information is intended to serve as a concise initial reference for healthcare professionals to use when discussing medications with a patient. You must ultimately rely on your own discretion, experience and judgment in diagnosing, treating and advising patients.

DiphenhydrAMINE (Systemic)
(dye fen HYE dra meen)

Brand Names: U.S. Aler-Dryl [OTC]; Allergy Relief Childrens [OTC]; Allergy Relief [OTC]; Altaryl [OTC]; Anti-Hist Allergy [OTC]; Anti-Hist [OTC]; Banophen [OTC]; Benadryl Allergy Childrens [OTC]; Benadryl Allergy [OTC]; Benadryl Dye-Free Allergy [OTC]; Benadryl [OTC]; Complete Allergy Medication [OTC]; Complete Allergy Relief [OTC]; Diphen [OTC]; Diphenhist [OTC]; Genahist [OTC]; Geri-Dryl [OTC]; Nighttime Sleep Aid [OTC]; Nytol Maximum Strength [OTC]; Nytol [OTC]; PediaCare Childrens Allergy [OTC]; Pharbedryl [OTC]; Q-Dryl [OTC]; Quenalin [OTC]; Scot-Tussin Allergy Relief [OTC]; Siladryl Allergy [OTC]; Silphen Cough [OTC]; Simply Allergy [OTC]; Simply Sleep [OTC]; Sleep Tabs [OTC]; Sominex Maximum Strength [OTC]; Sominex [OTC]; Tetra-Formula Nighttime Sleep [OTC]; Total Allergy Medicine [OTC]; Total Allergy [OTC]; Triaminic Cough/Runny Nose [OTC]; ZzzQuil [OTC]

Index Terms Diphenhydramine Citrate; Diphenhydramine Hydrochloride; Diphenhydramine Tannate

Pharmacologic Category Ethanolamine Derivative; Histamine H_1 Antagonist; Histamine H_1 Antagonist, First Generation

Medication Safety Issues

Sound-alike/look-alike issues:

DiphenhydrAMINE may be confused with desipramine, dicyclomine, dimenhyDRINATE

Benadryl® may be confused with benazepril, Bentyl®, Benylin®, Caladryl®

BEERS Criteria medication:

This drug may be potentially inappropriate for use in geriatric patients (Quality of evidence - moderate; Strength of recommendation - strong).

International issues:

Benadryl brand name for diphenhydramine [U.S., Canada], but also the brand name for cetirizine [Great Britain, Phillipines] and acrivastine and pseudoephedrine [Great Britain]

Sominex brand name for diphenhydramine [U.S., Canada], but also the brand name for promethazine [Great Britain]; valerian [Chile]

Pregnancy Risk Factor B

Lactation Enters breast milk/contraindicated

Breast-Feeding Considerations Diphenhydramine is excreted into breast milk; drowsiness has been reported in a breast-feeding infant. Premature infants and newborns have a higher risk of intolerance to antihistamines. Breast-feeding is contraindicated by the manufacturer. Antihistamines may decrease maternal serum prolactin concentrations when administered prior to the establishment of nursing.

Use Symptomatic relief of allergic symptoms caused by histamine release including nasal allergies and allergic dermatosis; adjunct to epinephrine in the treatment of anaphylaxis; nighttime sleep aid; prevention or treatment of motion sickness; antitussive; management of Parkinsonian syndrome including drug-induced extrapyramidal symptoms

Mechanism of Action/Effect Competes with histamine for H_1-receptor sites on effector cells in the gastrointestinal tract, blood vessels, and respiratory tract; anticholinergic and sedative effects are also seen

Contraindications Hypersensitivity to diphenhydramine or any component of the formulation; acute asthma; neonates or premature infants; breast-feeding; use as a local anesthetic (injection)

Warnings/Precautions Causes sedation, caution must be used in performing tasks which require alertness (eg, operating machinery or driving).

Sedative effects of CNS depressants or ethanol are potentiated. Antihistamines may cause excitation in young children. Use with caution in patients with angle-closure glaucoma, pyloroduodenal obstruction (including stenotic peptic ulcer), urinary tract obstruction (including bladder neck obstruction and symptomatic prostatic hyperplasia), asthma, hyperthyroidism, increased intraocular pressure, and cardiovascular disease (including hypertension and tachycardia). Some preparations contain soy protein; avoid use in patients with soy protein or peanut allergies. Some products may contain phenylalanine.

Oral products: In the elderly, avoid use of this potent anticholinergic agent due to increased risk of confusion, dry mouth, constipation, and other anticholinergic effects; clearance decreases in patients of advanced age; tolerance develops to hypnotic effects; when used for severe allergic reaction, use may be appropriate (Beers Criteria).

Self-medication (OTC use): Do not use with other products containing diphenhydramine, even ones used on the skin. Oral products are not for OTC use in children <6 years of age.

Drug Interactions
Avoid Concomitant Use
Avoid concomitant use of DiphenhydrAMINE (Systemic) with any of the following: Aclidinium; Azelastine (Nasal); Ipratropium (Oral Inhalation); Paraldehyde; Thalidomide; Thioridazine; Tiotropium; Umeclidinium

Decreased Effect
DiphenhydrAMINE (Systemic) may decrease the levels/effects of: Acetylcholinesterase Inhibitors (Central); Benzylpenicilloyl Polylysine; Betahistine; Codeine; Hyaluronidase; Tamoxifen; TraMADol

The levels/effects of DiphenhydrAMINE (Systemic) may be decreased by: Acetylcholinesterase Inhibitors (Central); Amphetamines

Increased Effect/Toxicity
DiphenhydrAMINE (Systemic) may increase the levels/effects of: Alcohol (Ethyl); Analgesics (Opioid); Anticholinergics; ARIPiprazole; Azelastine (Nasal); Buprenorphine; CNS Depressants; CYP2D6 Substrates; DOXOrubicin (Conventional); Fesoterodine; Highest Risk QTc-Prolonging Agents; Hydrocodone; Methotrimeprazine; Metoprolol; Metyrosine; Mirtazapine; Moderate Risk QTc-Prolonging Agents; Nebivolol; Paraldehyde; Pramipexole; ROPINIRole; Rotigotine; Selective Serotonin Reuptake Inhibitors; Thalidomide; Thioridazine; Tiotropium; Zolpidem

The levels/effects of DiphenhydrAMINE (Systemic) may be increased by: Aclidinium; Brimonidine (Topical); Doxylamine; Droperidol; HydrOXYzine; Ipratropium (Oral Inhalation); Magnesium Sulfate; Methotrimeprazine; Mifepristone; Perampanel; Pramlintide; Propafenone; Sodium Oxybate; Tapentadol; Umeclidinium

Nutritional/Ethanol Interactions
Ethanol: May increase CNS depression; monitor for increased effects with coadministration. Caution patients about effects.

Herb/Nutraceutical: Avoid valerian, St John's wort, kava kava, gotu kola (may increase CNS depression).

Adverse Reactions Frequency not defined.
Cardiovascular: Chest tightness, extrasystoles, hypotension, palpitation, tachycardia

Central nervous system: Chills, confusion, convulsion, disturbed coordination, dizziness, euphoria, excitation, fatigue, headache, insomnia, irritability, nervousness, paradoxical excitement, restlessness, sedation, sleepiness, vertigo

Endocrine & metabolic: Menstrual irregularities (early menses)

Gastrointestinal: Anorexia, constipation, diarrhea, dry mucous membranes, epigastric distress, nausea, throat tightness, vomiting, xerostomia

Genitourinary: Difficult urination, urinary frequency, urinary retention

Hematologic: Agranulocytosis, hemolytic anemia, thrombocytopenia

Neuromuscular & skeletal: Neuritis, paresthesia, tremor

Ocular: Blurred vision, diplopia

Otic: Labyrinthitis (acute), tinnitus

Respiratory: Nasal stuffiness, thickening of bronchial secretions, wheezing

Miscellaneous: Anaphylactic shock, diaphoresis

Pharmacodynamics/Kinetics
Duration of Action
Histamine-induced wheal suppression: ≤10 hours (Simons, 1990)

Histamine-induced flare suppression: ≤12 hours (Simons, 1990)

Available Dosage Forms
Capsule, Oral:
Allergy Relief [OTC]: 25 mg
Anti-Hist [OTC]: 25 mg
Banophen [OTC]: 25 mg, 50 mg
Benadryl [OTC]: 25 mg
Benadryl Allergy [OTC]: 25 mg
Benadryl Dye-Free Allergy [OTC]: 25 mg
Diphenhist [OTC]: 25 mg
Genahist [OTC]: 25 mg
Geri-Dryl [OTC]: 25 mg
Pharbedryl [OTC]: 25 mg, 50 mg
Q-Dryl [OTC]: 25 mg
ZzzQuil [OTC]: 25 mg
Generic: 25 mg, 50 mg

Elixir, Oral:
Altaryl [OTC]: 12.5 mg/5 mL (120 mL, 480 mL, 3840 mL)
Generic: 12.5 mg/5 mL (5 mL, 10 mL)

Liquid, Oral:
Allergy Relief Childrens [OTC]: 12.5 mg/5 mL (118 mL, 480 mL)

Banophen [OTC]: 12.5 mg/5 mL (118 mL, 473 mL)

Benadryl Allergy Childrens [OTC]: 12.5 mg/5 mL (5 mL, 118 mL, 236 mL)

Diphenhist [OTC]: 12.5 mg/5 mL (118 mL, 473 mL)

PediaCare Childrens Allergy [OTC]: 12.5 mg/5 mL (118 mL)

Q-Dryl [OTC]: 12.5 mg/5 mL (118 mL, 237 mL, 473 mL)

Scot-Tussin Allergy Relief [OTC]: 12.5 mg/5 mL (118.3 mL, 240 mL, 480 mL, 3780 mL)

Siladryl Allergy [OTC]: 12.5 mg/5 mL (118 mL, 237 mL, 473 mL)

Total Allergy Medicine [OTC]: 12.5 mg/5 mL (118 mL)

ZzzQuil [OTC]: 50 mg/30 mL (177 mL, 354 mL)

Solution, Injection:
Generic: 50 mg/mL (1 mL, 10 mL)

Solution, Injection [preservative free]:
Generic: 50 mg/mL (1 mL)

Strip, Oral:
Triaminic Cough/Runny Nose [OTC]: 12.5 mg (14 ea, 16 ea)

Syrup, Oral:
Altaryl [OTC]: 12.5 mg/5 mL (120 mL, 480 mL, 3785 mL)

Quenalin [OTC]: 12.5 mg/5 mL (120 mL)

Silphen Cough [OTC]: 12.5 mg/5 mL (118 mL, 237 mL, 473 mL)

Tablet, Oral:
Aler-Dryl [OTC]: 50 mg
Allergy Relief [OTC]: 25 mg
Anti-Hist Allergy [OTC]: 25 mg
Banophen [OTC]: 25 mg
Benadryl [OTC]: 25 mg
Benadryl Allergy [OTC]: 25 mg
Complete Allergy Medication [OTC]: 25 mg
Complete Allergy Relief [OTC]: 25 mg
Diphen [OTC]: 25 mg
Diphenhist [OTC]: 25 mg
Geri-Dryl [OTC]: 25 mg
Nighttime Sleep Aid [OTC]: 25 mg, 50 mg
Nytol [OTC]: 25 mg
Nytol Maximum Strength [OTC]: 50 mg
Simply Allergy [OTC]: 25 mg
Simply Sleep [OTC]: 25 mg
Sleep Tabs [OTC]: 25 mg
Sominex [OTC]: 25 mg
Sominex Maximum Strength [OTC]: 50 mg
Tetra-Formula Nighttime Sleep [OTC]: 50 mg
Total Allergy [OTC]: 25 mg
Generic: 25 mg

Tablet Chewable, Oral:
Benadryl Allergy Childrens [OTC]: 12.5 mg

General Dosage Range

I.M., I.V.:
Children: 5 mg/kg/day or 150 mg/m^2/day in divided every 6-8 hours (maximum: 300 mg/day)
Adults: 10-100 per dose (maximum: 400 mg/day)
Elderly: Initial: 25 mg 2-3 times/day

Oral:
Children 2 to <6 years: 5 mg/kg/day or 150 mg/m^2/day in divided every 6-8 hours (maximum: 300 mg/day) or 6.25 mg every 4-6 hours (maximum: 37.5 mg/day)
Children 6 to <12 years: 5 mg/kg/day or 150 mg/m^2/day in divided every 6-8 hours (maximum: 300 mg/day) or 12.5-25 mg every 4-6 hours (maximum: 150 mg/day)
Children ≥12 years: 5 mg/kg/day or 150 mg/m^2/day in divided doses every 6-8 hours or 25-50 mg every 4-6 hours (maximum: 300 mg/day) or 50 mg at bedtime
Adults: 25-50 mg every 4-6 hours (maximum: 400 mg/day) or 50 mg at bedtime
Elderly: Initial: 25 mg 2-3 times/day

Administration

I.V. Injection solution: For I.V. or I.M. administration only. Local necrosis may result with SubQ or intradermal use. For I.V. administration, inject at a rate ≤25 mg/minute.

Injectable Detail pH: 5-6

Oral When used to prevent motion sickness, first dose should be given 30 minutes prior to exposure.

Storage/Stability Injection: Store at room temperature of 15°C to 30°C (59°F to 86°F); protect from freezing. Protect from light.

Nursing Actions

Physical Assessment Monitor for excess anticholinergic effects at beginning of therapy and periodically throughout.

Patient Education

• Discuss specific use of drug and side effects with patient as it relates to treatment. (HCAHPS: During this hospital stay, were you given any medicine that you had not taken before? Before giving you any new medicine, how often did hospital staff tell you what the medicine was for? How often did hospital staff describe possible side effects in a way you could understand?)

• Patient may experience fatigue, dizziness, xerostomia, or thickening of mucus. Have patient report immediately to prescriber urinary retention, severe asthenia, anhidrosis, considerable anxiety, angina, tachycardia, hallucinations, tremors, or injection site pain or irritation (HCAHPS).

• Educate patient about signs of a significant reaction (eg, wheezing; chest tightness; fever; itching; bad cough; blue skin color; seizures; or swelling of face, lips, tongue, or throat). **Note:** This is not a comprehensive list of all side effects. Patient should consult prescriber for additional questions.

Intended Use and Disclaimer: Should not be printed and given to patients. This information is intended to serve as a concise initial reference for healthcare professionals to use when discussing medications with a patient. You must ultimately

rely on your own discretion, experience and judgment in diagnosing, treating and advising patients.

Dietary Considerations Some products may contain sodium and/or phenylalanine.

DiphenhydrAMINE (Topical)
(dye fen HYE dra meen)

Brand Names: U.S. Allergy [OTC]; Anti-Itch Maximum Strength [OTC]; Anti-Itch [OTC]; Banophen [OTC]; Benadryl Itch Relief [OTC]; Benadryl Itch Stopping [OTC]; Benadryl Maximum Strength [OTC]; Itch Relief [OTC]

Index Terms Diphenhydramine Hydrochloride

Pharmacologic Category Ethanolamine Derivative; Histamine H_1 Antagonist; Histamine H_1 Antagonist, First Generation; Topical Skin Product

Medication Safety Issues

Sound-alike/look-alike issues:

DiphenhydrAMINE may be confused with desipramine, dicyclomine, dimenhyDRINATE

Benadryl® may be confused with benazepril, Bentyl®, Benylin®, Caladryl®

Administration issues:

Institute for Safe Medication Practices (ISMP) has reported cases of patients mistakenly *swallowing* Benadryl® Itch Stopping [OTC] gel intended for topical application. Unclear labeling and similar packaging of the topical gel in containers resembling an oral liquid are factors believed to be contributing to the administration errors. The topical gel contains camphor which can be toxic if swallowed. ISMP has requested the manufacturer to make the necessary changes to prevent further confusion.

Use Topically for relief of pain and itching associated with insect bites, minor cuts and burns, or rashes due to poison ivy, poison oak, and poison sumac

Available Dosage Forms

Cream, External:

Allergy [OTC]: 2% (28.4 g)

Anti-Itch [OTC]: 2% (28.4 g)

Anti-Itch Maximum Strength [OTC]: 2% (30 g)

Banophen [OTC]: 2% (28 g)

Benadryl Itch Stopping [OTC]: 1% (28.3 g)

Itch Relief [OTC]: 2% (15 g, 30 g, 56.8 g)

Gel, External:

Benadryl Itch Stopping [OTC]: 2% (118 mL)

Solution, External:

Benadryl Maximum Strength [OTC]: 2% (60 mL)

Stick, External:

Benadryl Itch Relief [OTC]: 2% (14 mL)

General Dosage Range Topical: *Children ≥2 years and Adults:* Apply 1% or 2% up to 3-4 times/day

Nursing Actions

Patient Education

- Discuss specific use of drug and side effects with patient as it relates to treatment. (HCAHPS: During this hospital stay, were you given any medicine that you had not taken before? Before giving you any new medicine, how often did hospital staff tell you what the medicine was for? How often did hospital staff describe possible side effects in a way you could understand?)
- Have patient report immediately to prescriber severe application site irritation (HCAHPS).
- Educate patient about signs of a significant reaction (eg, wheezing; chest tightness; fever; itching; bad cough; blue skin color; seizures; or swelling of face, lips, tongue, or throat). **Note:** This is not a comprehensive list of all side effects. Patient should consult prescriber for additional questions.

Intended Use and Disclaimer: Should not be printed and given to patients. This information is intended to serve as a concise initial reference for healthcare professionals to use when discussing medications with a patient. You must ultimately rely on your own discretion, experience and judgment in diagnosing, treating and advising patients.

Diphenhydramine and Phenylephrine (dye fen HYE dra meen & fen il EF rin)

Brand Names: U.S. Aldex® CT; Benadryl-D® Allergy & Sinus [OTC]; Benadryl-D® Children's Allergy & Sinus [OTC]; Dimetapp® Children's Nighttime Cold & Congestion [OTC]; Triaminic® Children's Night Time Cold & Cough [OTC]

Index Terms Diphenhydramine Hydrochloride and Phenylephrine Hydrochloride; Diphenhydramine Tannate and Phenylephrine Tannate; Phenylephrine and Diphenhydramine; Phenylephrine Hydrochloride and Diphenhydramine Hydrochloride; Phenylephrine Tannate and Diphenhydramine Tannate

Pharmacologic Category Alpha-Adrenergic Agonist; Decongestant; Ethanolamine Derivative; Histamine H_1 Antagonist; Histamine H_1 Antagonist, First Generation

Medication Safety Issues

International issues:

Benadryl-D brand name for diphenhydramine and phenylephrine [U.S.] may be confused with Benadryl brand name for cetirizine [Great Britain, Phillipines] and Benadryl brand name for acrivastine and pseudoephedrine [Great Britain]

Use Temporary relief of symptoms of allergic rhinitis, sinusitis, and other upper respiratory conditions, including sinus/nasal congestion, sneezing, stuffy/runny nose, itchy/watery eyes, and cough

Available Dosage Forms

Liquid, oral:

Benadryl-D® Children's Allergy & Sinus [OTC]: Diphenhydramine 12.5 mg and phenylephrine 5 mg per 5 mL (118 mL)

Syrup, oral:

Dimetapp® Children's Nighttime Cold and Congestion [OTC]: Diphenhydramine 6.25 mg and phenylephrine 2.5 mg per 5 mL (120 mL)

Triaminic® Children's Night Time Cold & Cough [OTC]: Diphenhydramine 6.25 mg and phenylephrine 2.5 mg per 5 mL (118 mL)

Tablet, oral:

Benadryl-D® Allergy & Sinus [OTC]: Diphenhydramine 25 mg and phenylephrine 10 mg

Tablet, chewable, oral:

Aldex® CT: Diphenhydramine 12.5 mg and phenylephrine 5 mg

General Dosage Range Oral:

Children 6-11 years: Aldex® CT: 1/2 to 1 tablet every 6 hours; OTC labeling: 5-10 mL every 4 hours as needed (maximum: 6 doses/24 hours)

Children ≥12 years and Adults: Aldex® CT: 1-2 tablets every 6 hours; OTC labeling: 10-20 mL every 4 hours as needed or 1 tablet every 4 hours as needed (maximum: 6 doses/24 hours)

Nursing Actions

Physical Assessment See individual agents.

Patient Education

- Discuss specific use of drug and side effects with patient as it relates to treatment. (HCAHPS: During this hospital stay, were you given any medicine that you had not taken before? Before giving you any new medicine, how often did hospital staff tell you what the medicine was for? How often did hospital staff describe possible side effects in a way you could understand?)
- Patient may experience anxiety, insomnia, or fatigue. Have patient report immediately to prescriber severe dizziness, syncope, arrhythmia, tachycardia, considerable asthenia, ecchymosis, hemorrhaging, change in balance, illogical thinking, tremors, vision changes, or difficult urination (HCAHPS).
- Educate patient about signs of a significant reaction (eg, wheezing; chest tightness; fever; itching; bad cough; blue skin color; seizures; or swelling of face, lips, tongue, or throat). **Note:** This is not a comprehensive list of all side effects. Patient should consult prescriber for additional questions.

Intended Use and Disclaimer: Should not be printed and given to patients. This information is intended to serve as a concise initial reference for healthcare professionals to use when discussing medications with a patient. You must ultimately rely on your own discretion, experience and judgment in diagnosing, treating and advising patients.

Related Information

DiphenhydrAMINE (Systemic) *on page 462*

Phenylephrine (Systemic) *on page 1240*

Diphenoxylate and Atropine

(dye fen OKS i late & A troe peen)

Brand Names: U.S. Lomotil®

Index Terms Atropine and Diphenoxylate

Pharmacologic Category Antidiarrheal

Medication Safety Issues

Sound-alike/look-alike issues:

Lomotil® may be confused with LaMICtal®, LamISIL®, lamoTRIgine, Lanoxin®, Lasix®, loperamide

International issues:

Lomotil [U.S., Canada, and multiple international markets] may be confused with Ludiomil brand name for maprotiline [multiple international markets]

Lomotil: Brand name for diphenoxylate [U.S., Canada, and multiple international markets], but also the brand name for loperamide [Mexico, Philippines]

Pregnancy Risk Factor C

Lactation Enters breast milk/use caution

Use Treatment of diarrhea

Controlled Substance C-V

Available Dosage Forms

Solution, oral: Diphenoxylate 2.5 mg and atropine 0.025 mg per 5 mL

Tablet, oral: Diphenoxylate 2.5 mg and atropine 0.025 mg

General Dosage Range Oral:

Children 2-12 years: Initial: Diphenoxylate 0.3-0.4 mg/kg/day in 4 divided doses (maximum: 10 mg/day); Maintenance: Reduce as needed, may be as low as 25% of the initial daily dose

Adults: Initial: Diphenoxylate 5 mg 4 times/day (maximum: 20 mg/day); Maintenance: Reduce as needed, may be as low as 5 mg/day

Administration

Oral If there is no response within 48 hours of continuous therapy, this medication is unlikely to be effective and should be discontinued; if chronic diarrhea is not improved symptomatically within 10 days at maximum dosage, control is unlikely with further use. Use of the liquid preparation is recommended in children <13 years of age; use plastic dropper provided when measuring liquid.

Nursing Actions

Physical Assessment See individual agents.

Patient Education

- Discuss specific use of drug and side effects with patient as it relates to treatment. (HCAHPS: During this hospital stay, were you given any medicine that you had not taken before? Before giving you any new medicine, how often did hospital staff tell you what the medicine was

for? How often did hospital staff describe possible side effects in a way you could understand?)
- Patient may experience xerostomia, fatigue, dizziness, or headache. Have patient report immediately to prescriber signs of pancreatitis, signs of fluid and electrolyte imbalance, dyspnea, paresthesia, tachycardia, difficult urination, mood changes, vision changes, illogical thinking, severe constipation, intolerable dyspepsia, or abdominal edema (HCAHPS).
- Educate patient about signs of a significant reaction (eg, wheezing; chest tightness; fever; itching; bad cough; blue skin color; seizures; or swelling of face, lips, tongue, or throat). **Note:** This is not a comprehensive list of all side effects. Patient should consult prescriber for additional questions.

Intended Use and Disclaimer: Should not be printed and given to patients. This information is intended to serve as a concise initial reference for healthcare professionals to use when discussing medications with a patient. You must ultimately rely on your own discretion, experience and judgment in diagnosing, treating and advising patients.

Related Information
Atropine *on page 144*

Diphtheria and Tetanus Toxoids, Acellular Pertussis, and Poliovirus Vaccine

(dif THEER ee a & TET a nus TOKS oyds, ay CEL yoo lar per TUS sis & POE lee oh VYE rus vak SEEN)

Brand Names: U.S. Kinrix®

Index Terms Diphtheria and Tetanus Toxoids and Acellular Pertussis Adsorbed, and Inactivated Poliovirus Vaccine Combined; Diphtheria, Tetanus Toxoids, Acellular Pertussis (DTaP); DTaP-IPV; Poliovirus, Inactivated (IPV)

Pharmacologic Category Vaccine, Inactivated (Bacterial); Vaccine, Inactivated (Viral)

Medication Safety Issues
Sound-alike/look-alike issues:
Adacel® (trade name for Diphtheria and Tetanus Toxoids, and Acellular Pertussis Vaccine) should not be confused with Adacel®-Polio (trade name for Diphtheria and Tetanus Toxoids, Acellular Pertussis, and Poliovirus Vaccine in Canada)

Pregnancy Risk Factor C

Use Kinrix®: Active immunization against diphtheria, tetanus, pertussis, and poliomyelitis, used as the fifth dose in the DTaP series and the 4th dose in the IPV series

The Advisory Committee on Immunization Practices (ACIP) recommends routine vaccination for use as the fifth dose in the DTaP series and the fourth dose in the IPV series in children who received DTaP (Infanrix®) and/or DTaP-Hepatitis B-IPV (Pediarix®) as the first 3 doses and DTaP

(Infanrix®) as the fourth dose. Whenever feasible, the same manufacturer should be used to provide the pertussis component; however, vaccination should not be deferred if a specific brand is not known or is not available.

Adacel®-Polio (Canadian availability): Active booster immunization against diphtheria, tetanus, pertussis, and poliomyelitis; alternative to fifth dose of DTaP-IPV; May be used for wound management when a tetanus toxoid-containing vaccine is needed for wound management [refer to current National Advisory Committee on Immunization (NACI) guidelines]

Available Dosage Forms
Injection, suspension [preservative free]:
Kinrix®: Diphtheria toxoid 25 Lf, tetanus toxoid 10 Lf, acellular pertussis antigens [inactivated pertussis toxin 25 mcg, filamentous hemagglutinin 25 mcg, pertactin 8 mcg], type 1 poliovirus 40 D-antigen units, type 2 poliovirus 8 D-antigen units, and type 3 poliovirus 32 D-antigen units per 0.5 mL (0.5 mL)

General Dosage Range I.M.: *Children 4-6 years:* 0.5 mL

Administration
I.M. For I.M. use only, preferably in the deltoid; Adacel®-Polio (Canadian availability) label recommends avoiding administration into the buttocks. Do not administer intradermally, I.V., or SubQ. Shake well prior to use; do not use unless a homogeneous, turbid, white suspension forms. Discard if the suspension is discolored or if there are cracks in the vial or syringe. Administer in the deltoid muscle of the upper arm. Do not administer additional vaccines or immunoglobulins at the same site, or using the same syringe.

For patients at risk of hemorrhage following intramuscular injection, the ACIP recommends "it should be administered intramuscularly if, in the opinion of the physician familiar with the patient's bleeding risk, the vaccine can be administered by this route with reasonable safety. If the patient receives antihemophilia or other similar therapy, intramuscular vaccination can be scheduled shortly after such therapy is administered. A fine needle (23 gauge or smaller) can be used for the vaccination and firm pressure applied to the site (without rubbing) for at least 2 minutes. The patient should be instructed concerning the risk of hematoma from the injection." Patients on anticoagulant therapy should be considered to have the same bleeding risks and treated as those with clotting factor disorders (CDC, 2011).

Simultaneous administration of vaccines helps ensure the patients will be fully vaccinated by the appropriate age. Simultaneous administration of vaccines is defined as administering >1 vaccine on the same day at different anatomic sites. The use of licensed combination vaccines is generally preferred over separate injections of the equivalent components. Separate vaccines should not be combined in the same syringe unless indicated by product specific labeling. Separate needles and syringes should be used for each injection. The ACIP prefers each dose of a specific vaccine in a series come from the same manufacturer when possible. Adolescents and adults should be vaccinated while seated or lying down. In general, preterm infants should be vaccinated at the same chronological age as full-term infants (CDC, 2011).

Antipyretics have not been shown to prevent febrile seizures. Antipyretics may be used to treat fever or discomfort following vaccination (CDC, 2011). One study reported that routine prophylactic administration of acetaminophen to prevent fever prior to vaccination decreased the immune response of some vaccines; the clinical significance of this reduction in immune response has not been established (Prymula, 2009).

Nursing Actions

Physical Assessment Treatment for anaphylactic reactions should be immediately available during vaccine use. For I.M. use only. U.S. federal law requires entry into the patient's medical record.

Patient Education

• Discuss specific use of vaccine and side effects with caregiver as it relates to treatment. (HCAHPS: During this hospital stay, were you given any medicine that you had not taken before? Before giving you any new medicine, how often did hospital staff tell you what the medicine was for? How often did hospital staff describe possible side effects in a way you could understand?)

• Educate caregiver about signs of a significant reaction (eg, wheezing; chest tightness; fever; itching; bad cough; blue skin color; seizures; or swelling of face, lips, tongue, or throat). **Note:** This is not a comprehensive list of all side effects. Caregiver should consult prescriber for additional questions.

Intended Use and Disclaimer: Should not be printed and given to patients. This information is intended to serve as a concise initial reference for healthcare professionals to use when discussing medications with a patient. You must ultimately rely on your own discretion, experience and judgment in diagnosing, treating and advising patients.

Related Information

Immunization Administration Recommendations *on page 1675*
Immunization Recommendations *on page 1680*

Diphtheria and Tetanus Toxoids, Acellular Pertussis, Hepatitis B (Recombinant), Poliovirus (Inactivated), and *Haemophilus influenzae* B Conjugate (Adsorbed) Vaccine

(dif THEER ee a & TET a nus TOKS oyds, ay CEL yoo lar per TUS sis, hep a TYE tis bee ree KOM be nant, POE lee oh VYE rus in ak ti VAY ted, & hem OF fi lus in floo EN za bee KON joo gate ad SORBED vak SEEN)

Index Terms Diphtheria and Tetanus Toxoids and Acellular Pertussis, Hepatitis B (Recombinant), Inactivated Poliovirus Vaccine, and *Haemophilus influenzae* Type B Combined; DTaP-HepB-IPV-Hib

Pharmacologic Category Vaccine, Inactivated (Bacterial, Viral)

Medication Safety Issues

Sound-alike/look-alike issues:

Infanrix Hexa™ may be confused with Infanrix®

Use Active primary immunization against diphtheria, tetanus, pertussis, hepatitis B, poliomyelitis and disease caused by *Haemophilus influenzae* type b in infants and children 6 weeks to 2 years of age; booster immunization (at 18 months) in infants who previously received a full primary vaccination course of each component of the vaccine

Product Availability Not available in U.S.

General Dosage Range I.M.: *Children 6 weeks to 2 years:* Primary immunization: 0.5 mL every 8 weeks for a total of 3 doses; booster dose: 0.5 mL

Administration

I.M. Administer by I.M. injection only, preferably in the anterolateral aspects of the thigh or the deltoid muscle of the upper arm. Do not administer intravenously or subcutaneously. Do not inject into the gluteal area (suboptimal hepatitis B immune response) or areas where major nerve trunks may be located. Fractional dosing (use of reduced volume) is not recommended. If more than one vaccine is to be given by IM injection use separate limbs. Rotate injection sites when completing vaccination series.

Acetaminophen may be used when needed to provide comfort; however, routine prophylactic administration of acetaminophen to prevent fever due to vaccine use is not recommended. There is evidence of a decreased immune response to some vaccines associated with acetaminophen administration; the clinical significance of this reduction in immune response has not been established.

Nursing Actions

Physical Assessment See individual agents.

Patient Education

• Discuss specific use of vaccine and side effects with caregiver as it relates to treatment. (HCAHPS: During this hospital stay, were you given any medicine that you had not taken before? Before giving you any new medicine, how often did hospital staff tell you what the medicine was for? How often did hospital staff describe possible side effects in a way you could understand?)

• Educate caregiver about signs of a significant reaction (eg, wheezing; chest tightness; fever; itching; bad cough; blue skin color; seizures; or swelling of face, lips, tongue, or throat). **Note:** This is not a comprehensive list of all side effects. Caregiver should consult prescriber for additional questions.

Intended Use and Disclaimer: Should not be printed and given to patients. This information is intended to serve as a concise initial reference for healthcare professionals to use when discussing medications with a patient. You must ultimately rely on your own discretion, experience and judgment in diagnosing, treating and advising patients.

Related Information

Immunization Administration Recommendations *on page 1675*

Immunization Recommendations *on page 1680*

Diphtheria and Tetanus Toxoids, Acellular Pertussis, Poliovirus and *Haemophilus* b Conjugate Vaccine

(dif THEER ee a & TET a nus TOKS oyds ay CEL yoo lar per TUS sis POE lee oh VYE rus & hem OF fi lus bee KON joo gate vak SEEN)

Brand Names: U.S. Pentacel®

Index Terms *Haemophilus* B Conjugate (Hib); *Haemophilus* B Polysaccharide; Diphtheria Toxoid; Diphtheria, Tetanus Toxoids, Acellular Pertussis (DTaP); DTaP-IPV/Hib; Pertussis, Acellular (Adsorbed); Poliovirus, Inactivated (IPV); Tetanus Toxoid

Pharmacologic Category Vaccine, Inactivated (Bacterial); Vaccine, Inactivated (Viral)

Medication Safety Issues

Administration issues:

Pentacel® is supplied in two vials, one containing DTaP-IPV liquid and one containing Hib powder, which must be mixed together in order to administer the recommended vaccine components.

Pregnancy Risk Factor C

Use Active immunization against diphtheria, tetanus, pertussis, poliomyelitis, and invasive disease caused by *H. influenzae* type b in children 6 weeks through 4 years of age

Advisory Committee on Immunization Practices (ACIP) recommends that Pentacel® (DTaP-IPV/Hib) may be used to provide the recommended DTaP, IPV, and Hib immunization in children <5 years of age. Whenever feasible, the same manufacturer should be used to provide the pertussis component; however, vaccination should not be deferred if a specific brand is not known or is not available. The Hib component in Pentacel® contains a tetanus toxoid conjugate. A Hib vaccine containing the PRP-OMP conjugate (PedvaxHIB®) may provide a more rapid seroconversion following the first dose and may be preferable to use in certain populations (eg, American Indian or Alaska Native children).

Available Dosage Forms

Injection, suspension:

Pentacel®: Diphtheria toxoid 15 Lf, tetanus toxoid 5 Lf, acellular pertussis antigens, poliovirus, and *Haemophilus* b capsular polysaccharide 10 mcg per 0.5 mL (0.5 mL)

General Dosage Range I.M.: *Children 6 weeks to ≤4 years:* 0.5 mL

Administration

I.M. For I.M. administration only. Do not administer I.V. or SubQ. Administer in the anterolateral aspect of thigh in children <1 year of age or deltoid muscle of upper arm in older children. Do not administer to gluteal area or areas near a major nerve trunk. Do not administer additional vaccines or immunoglobulins at the same site or using the same syringe.

For patients at risk of hemorrhage following intramuscular injection, the ACIP recommends: "It should be administered intramuscularly if, in the opinion of the physician familiar with the patient's bleeding risk, the vaccine can be administered by this route with reasonable safety. If the patient receives antihemophilia or other similar therapy, intramuscular vaccination can be scheduled shortly after such therapy is administered. A fine needle (23-gauge or smaller) can be used for the vaccination and firm pressure applied to the site (without rubbing) for at least 2 minutes. The patient should be instructed concerning the risk of hematoma from the injection." Patients on anticoagulant therapy should be considered to have the same bleeding risks and treated as those with clotting factor disorders (CDC, 2011).

Simultaneous administration of vaccines helps ensure the patients will be fully vaccinated by the appropriate age. Simultaneous administration of vaccines is defined as administering >1 vaccine on the same day at different anatomic sites. The use of licensed combination vaccines is generally preferred over separate injections of the equivalent components. Separate vaccines should not be combined in the same syringe unless indicated by product specific labeling. Separate needles and syringes should be used

▶

for each injection. The ACIP prefers each dose of a specific vaccine in a series come from the same manufacturer when possible. Adolescents and adults should be vaccinated while seated or lying down. In general, preterm infants should be vaccinated at the same chronological age as full-term infants (CDC, 2011).

Antipyretics have not been shown to prevent febrile seizures. Antipyretics may be used to treat fever or discomfort following vaccination (CDC, 2011). One study reported that routine prophylactic administration of acetaminophen to prevent fever prior to vaccination decreased the immune response of some vaccines; the clinical significance of this reduction in immune response has not been established (Prymula, 2009).

Nursing Actions
Physical Assessment U.S. federal law requires entry into the patient's medical record.

Patient Education
- Discuss specific use of vaccine and side effects with patient as it relates to treatment. (HCAHPS: During this hospital stay, were you given any medicine that you had not taken before? Before giving you any new medicine, how often did hospital staff tell you what the medicine was for? How often did hospital staff describe possible side effects in a way you could understand?)
- Educate patient about signs of a significant reaction (eg, wheezing; chest tightness; fever; itching; bad cough; blue skin color; seizures; or swelling of face, lips, tongue, or throat). **Note:** This is not a comprehensive list of all side effects. Patient should consult prescriber for additional questions.

Intended Use and Disclaimer: Should not be printed and given to patients. This information is intended to serve as a concise initial reference for healthcare professionals to use when discussing medications with a patient. You must ultimately rely on your own discretion, experience and judgment in diagnosing, treating and advising patients.

Related Information
Immunization Administration Recommendations *on page 1675*
Immunization Recommendations *on page 1680*

Diphtheria and Tetanus Toxoids, and Acellular Pertussis Vaccine
(dif THEER ee a & TET a nus TOKS oyds & ay CEL yoo lar per TUS sis vak SEEN)

Brand Names: U.S. Adacel; Boostrix; Daptacel; Infanrix

Index Terms DTaP; Tdap; Tetanus Toxoid, Reduced Diphtheria Toxoid, and Acellular Pertussis, Adsorbed; Tripedia

Pharmacologic Category Vaccine, Inactivated (Bacterial)

Medication Safety Issues
Sound-alike/look-alike issues:
Adacel (Tdap) may be confused with Daptacel (DTaP)
Tdap (Adacel, Boostrix) may be confused with DTaP (Daptacel, Infanrix, Tripedia)

Administration issues:
Carefully review product labeling to prevent inadvertent administration of Tdap when DTaP is indicated. Tdap contains lower amounts of diphtheria toxoid and some pertussis antigens than DTaP.
Tdap is not indicated for use in children <10 years of age
DTaP is not indicated for use in persons ≥7 years of age
Guidelines are available in case of inadvertent administration of these products; refer to ACIP recommendations, February 2006 available at http://www.cdc.gov/mmwr/preview/mmwrhtml/rr55e223a1.htm

Other safety concerns:
DTaP: Diphtheria and tetanus toxoids and acellular pertussis vaccine
DTP: Diphtheria and tetanus toxoids and pertussis vaccine (unspecified pertussis antigens)
DTwP: Diphtheria and tetanus toxoids and whole-cell pertussis vaccine (no longer available on U.S. market)
Tdap: Tetanus toxoid, reduced diphtheria toxoid, and acellular pertussis vaccine

Pregnancy Risk Factor B/C (manufacturer specific)

Lactation Excretion in breast milk unknown/use caution

Use
Daptacel®, Infanrix® (DTaP): Active immunization against diphtheria, tetanus, and pertussis from age 6 weeks through 6 years of age (prior to seventh birthday)
Adacel®, Boostrix® (Tdap): Active booster immunization against diphtheria, tetanus, and pertussis

The Advisory Committee on Immunization Practices (ACIP) recommends routine vaccination for the following:
Children 6 weeks to <7 years (DTaP):
- For primary immunization against diphtheria, tetanus and pertussis
- Pediatric patients who are wounded in bombings or similar mass casualty events and who have penetrating injuries or nonintact skin exposure, and have an uncertain vaccination history should receive a tetanus booster with DTaP (if no contraindications exist) (CDC, 57 [RR6], 2008)
Children 7-10 years (Tdap):
- Children not fully vaccinated against pertussis should receive a single dose of Tdap (if no contraindications exist) (CDC, 60[1], 2011)

- Children never vaccinated against diphtheria, tetanus, or pertussis, or whose vaccination status is not known should receive a series of three vaccinations containing tetanus and diphtheria toxoids and the first dose should be with Tdap (CDC, 60[1], 2011)

Adolescents 11-18 years (Tdap):
- A single dose of Tdap as a booster dose in adolescents who have completed the recommended childhood DTaP vaccination series (preferred age of administration is 11-12 years) (CDC, 60[1], 2011)

Adolescents ≥11 years and Adults (Tdap):
- Persons wounded in bombings or similar mass casualty events and who cannot confirm receipt of a tetanus booster within the previous 5 years and who have penetrating injuries or nonintact skin exposure should receive a single dose of Tdap (CDC, 57 [RR6] 2008; CDC, 61[25], 2012)

Adolescent and Adult females (Tdap): Pregnant females should receive a single dose with each pregnancy, preferably between 27-36 weeks gestation (CDC, 62 [7], 2013)

Adults ≥19 years (including adults ≥65 years) (Tdap): A single dose of Tdap should be given to all patients who have not previously received Tdap or for whom their vaccine status is unknown (CDC, 62[1], 2013). Following administration of Tdap, Td vaccine should be used for routine boosters. (CDC, 61[25], 2012). The following patients, who have not yet received Tdap or for whom vaccine status is not known, should receive a single dose of Tdap as soon as feasible:
- Close contacts of children <12 months of age; Tdap should ideally be administered at least 2 weeks prior to beginning close contact (CDC, 55 [RR17], 2006; CDC, 60[41], 2011)
- Healthcare providers with direct patient contact (CDC, 55[RR17], 2006)

Note: Tdap is currently recommended for a single dose only (all age groups) (CDC, 60[1], 2011; CDC, 61[25], 2012), except pregnant females (CDC, 62 [7], 2013

Available Dosage Forms

Injection, suspension [Tdap, booster formulation]:
Adacel®: Diphtheria 2 Lf units, tetanus 5 Lf units, and acellular pertussis antigens per 0.5 mL (0.5 mL)
Boostrix®: Diphtheria 2.5 Lf units, tetanus 5 Lf units, and acellular pertussis antigens per 0.5 mL (0.5 mL)

Injection, suspension [DTaP, active immunization formulation]:
Daptacel®: Diphtheria 15 Lf units, tetanus 5 Lf units, and acellular pertussis antigens per 0.5 mL (0.5 mL)
Infanrix®: Diphtheria 25 Lf units, tetanus 10 Lf units, and acellular pertussis antigens per 0.5 mL (0.5 mL) [preservative free]

General Dosage Range I.M.:
Children 6 weeks to <7 years: Primary immunization: 0.5 mL per dose, total of 5 doses
Children ≥10 years and Adults: Booster immunization: 0.5 mL as a single dose

Administration
I.M. Shake suspension well.
Adacel®, Boostrix®: Administer only I.M. in deltoid muscle of upper arm.
Daptacel®, Infanrix®: Administer only I.M. in anterolateral aspect of thigh or deltoid muscle of upper arm.
If feasible, the same brand of DTaP should be used for all doses in the series (CDC, 60 [2], 2011).

For patients at risk of hemorrhage following intramuscular injection, the ACIP recommends "it should be administered intramuscularly if, in the opinion of the physician familiar with the patient's bleeding risk, the vaccine can be administered by this route with reasonable safety. If the patient receives antihemophilia or other similar therapy, intramuscular vaccination can be scheduled shortly after such therapy is administered. A fine needle (23 gauge or smaller) can be used for the vaccination and firm pressure applied to the site (without rubbing) for at least 2 minutes. The patient should be instructed concerning the risk of hematoma from the injection." Patients on anticoagulant therapy should be considered to have the same bleeding risks and treated as those with clotting factor disorders (CDC, 60[2], 2011).

Simultaneous administration of vaccines helps ensure the patients will be fully vaccinated by the appropriate age. Simultaneous administration of vaccines is defined as administering >1 vaccine on the same day at different anatomic sites. The use of licensed combination vaccines is generally preferred over separate injections of the equivalent components. Separate vaccines should not be combined in the same syringe unless indicated by product specific labeling. Separate needles and syringes should be used for each injection. The ACIP prefers each dose of a specific vaccine in a series come from the same manufacturer when possible. Adolescents and adults should be vaccinated while seated or lying down. In general, preterm infants should be vaccinated at the same chronological age as full-term infants (CDC, 60[2], 2011).

Antipyretics have not been shown to prevent febrile seizures. Antipyretics may be used to treat fever or discomfort following vaccination (CDC, 2011). One study reported that routine prophylactic administration of acetaminophen to prevent fever prior to vaccination decreased the immune response of some vaccines; the clinical significance of this reduction in immune response has not been established (Prymula, 2009).

◀ **Nursing Actions**

Physical Assessment U.S. federal law requires entry into the patient's medical record. Monitor for immediate anaphylactoid or hypersensitivity reaction.

Patient Education

• Discuss specific use of vaccine and side effects with patient as it relates to treatment. (HCAHPS: During this hospital stay, were you given any medicine that you had not taken before? Before giving you any new medicine, how often did hospital staff tell you what the medicine was for? How often did hospital staff describe possible side effects in a way you could understand?)

• Educate patient about signs of a significant reaction (eg, wheezing; chest tightness; fever; itching; bad cough; blue skin color; seizures; or swelling of face, lips, tongue, or throat). **Note:** This is not a comprehensive list of all side effects. Patient should consult prescriber for additional questions.

Intended Use and Disclaimer: Should not be printed and given to patients. This information is intended to serve as a concise initial reference for healthcare professionals to use when discussing medications with a patient. You must ultimately rely on your own discretion, experience and judgment in diagnosing, treating and advising patients.

Related Information

Immunization Administration Recommendations *on page 1675*

Immunization Recommendations *on page 1680*

Diphtheria, Tetanus Toxoids, Acellular Pertussis, Hepatitis B (Recombinant), and Poliovirus (Inactivated) Vaccine

(dif THEER ee a, TET a nus TOKS oyds, ay CEL yoo lar per TUS sis, hep a TYE tis bee ree KOM be nant, & POE lee oh VYE rus in ak ti VAY ted vak SEEN)

Brand Names: U.S. Pediarix®

Index Terms Diphtheria and Tetanus Toxoids and Acellular Pertussis Adsorbed, Hepatitis B (Recombinant) and Inactivated Poliovirus Vaccine Combined; Diphtheria, Tetanus Toxoids, Acellular Pertussis, Hepatitis B (Recombinant), and Poliovirus (Inactivated) Vaccine; Diphtheria, Tetanus Toxoids, Acellular Pertussis, Hepatitis B (Recombinant), and Poliovirus Vaccine; DTaP-HepB-IPV

Pharmacologic Category Vaccine, Inactivated (Bacterial); Vaccine, Inactivated (Viral)

Pregnancy Risk Factor C

Use Combination vaccine for the active immunization against diphtheria, tetanus, pertussis, hepatitis B virus (all known subtypes), and poliomyelitis (caused by poliovirus types 1, 2, and 3)

The Advisory Committee on Immunization Practices (ACIP) recommends Pediarix® for the following:

- Primary vaccination for DTaP, Hep B, and IPV in children at 2, 4, and 6 months of age.

- To complete the primary vaccination series in children who have received DTaP (Infanrix®) and who are scheduled to receive the other components of the vaccine. Whenever feasible, the same manufacturer should be used to provide the pertussis component; however, vaccination should not be deferred if a specific brand is not known or is not available. HepB and IPV from different manufacturers are interchangeable.

Available Dosage Forms

Injection, suspension [preservative free]:

Pediarix®: Diphtheria toxoid 25 Lf, tetanus toxoid 10 Lf, acellular pertussis antigens per 0.5 mL (0.5 mL)

General Dosage Range I.M.: *Children 6 weeks to <7 years:* 0.5 mL/dose for a total of 3 doses

Administration

I.M. For I.M. use only; do not administer I.V., SubQ, or intradermally. Shake well prior to use; do not use unless a homogeneous, turbid, white suspension forms. Administer in the anterolateral aspects of the thigh or the deltoid muscle of the upper arm. Do not inject in the gluteal area (suboptimal hepatitis B immune response) or where there may be a major nerve trunk. Do not administer additional vaccines or immunoglobulins at the same site, or using the same syringe.

For patients at risk of hemorrhage following intramuscular injection, the ACIP recommends "it should be administered intramuscularly if, in the opinion of the physician familiar with the patient's bleeding risk, the vaccine can be administered by this route with reasonable safety. If the patient receives antihemophilia or other similar therapy, intramuscular vaccination can be scheduled shortly after such therapy is administered. A fine needle (23 gauge or smaller) can be used for the vaccination and firm pressure applied to the site (without rubbing) for at least 2 minutes. The patient should be instructed concerning the risk of hematoma from the injection." Patients on anticoagulant therapy should be considered to have the same bleeding risks and treated as those with clotting factor disorders (CDC, 2011).

Simultaneous administration of vaccines helps ensure the patients will be fully vaccinated by the appropriate age. Simultaneous administration of vaccines is defined as administering >1 vaccine on the same day at different anatomic sites. The use of licensed combination vaccines is generally preferred over separate injections of the equivalent components. Separate vaccines should not be combined in the same syringe unless indicated by product specific labeling.

Separate needles and syringes should be used for each injection. The ACIP prefers each dose of a specific vaccine in a series come from the same manufacturer when possible. Adolescents and adults should be vaccinated while seated or lying down. In general, preterm infants should be vaccinated at the same chronological age as full-term infants (CDC, 2011).

Antipyretics have not been shown to prevent febrile seizures. Antipyretics may be used to treat fever or discomfort following vaccination (CDC, 2011). One study reported that routine prophylactic administration of acetaminophen to prevent fever prior to vaccination decreased the immune response of some vaccines; the clinical significance of this reduction in immune response has not been established (Prymula, 2009).

Nursing Actions

Physical Assessment Children who are moderately-to-severely ill should not get this vaccination until they have recovered. Assess any hypersensitivity history prior to administering. Treatment for anaphylactic/anaphylactoid reaction should be available. Antipyretics should be administered at time of and for 24 hours following vaccination to patients at high-risk for seizures. U.S. federal law requires entry into the patient's medical record.

Patient Education

• Discuss specific use of vaccine and side effects with patient as it relates to treatment. (HCAHPS: During this hospital stay, were you given any medicine that you had not taken before? Before giving you any new medicine, how often did hospital staff tell you what the medicine was for? How often did hospital staff describe possible side effects in a way you could understand?)

• Educate patient about signs of a significant reaction (eg, wheezing; chest tightness; fever; itching; bad cough; blue skin color; seizures; or swelling of face, lips, tongue, or throat). **Note:** This is not a comprehensive list of all side effects. Patient should consult prescriber for additional questions.

Intended Use and Disclaimer: Should not be printed and given to patients. This information is intended to serve as a concise initial reference for healthcare professionals to use when discussing medications with a patient. You must ultimately rely on your own discretion, experience and judgment in diagnosing, treating and advising patients.

Related Information

Immunization Administration Recommendations on page 1675
Immunization Recommendations on page 1680

Dipyridamole (dye peer ID a mole)

Brand Names: U.S. Persantine

Pharmacologic Category Antiplatelet Agent; Vasodilator

Medication Safety Issues

Sound-alike/look-alike issues:

Dipyridamole may be confused with disopyramide

Persantine® may be confused with Periactin

BEERS Criteria medication:

This drug may be potentially inappropriate for use in geriatric patients (Quality of evidence - moderate; Strength of recommendation - strong).

International issues:

Persantine [U.S., Canada, Belgium, Denmark, France] may be confused with Permitil brand name for sildenafil [Argentina]

Pregnancy Risk Factor B

Lactation Enters breast milk/use caution

Use

Oral: Used with warfarin to decrease thrombosis in patients after artificial heart valve replacement

I.V.: Diagnostic agent in CAD

Unlabeled Use Stroke prevention (in combination with aspirin); **Note:** For this indication, the use of aspirin/extended release dipyridamole is recommended (Guyatt, 2012).

Available Dosage Forms

Solution, Intravenous:

Generic: 5 mg/mL (2 mL, 10 mL)

Tablet, Oral:

Persantine: 25 mg, 50 mg, 75 mg

Generic: 25 mg, 50 mg, 75 mg

General Dosage Range

I.V.: Adults: 0.14 mg/kg/minute for 4 minutes (maximum: 60 mg)

Oral: Children ≥12 years and Adults: 75-100 mg 4 times/day

Administration

I.V. I.V.: Infuse diluted solution over 4 minutes.

Oral Administer with water 1 hour before meals.

Nursing Actions

Physical Assessment Observe bleeding precautions. Oral: Monitor blood pressure on a regular basis. I.V.: Continuous ECG and blood pressure monitoring necessary during infusion.

Patient Education

• Discuss specific use of drug and side effects with patient as it relates to treatment. (HCAHPS: During this hospital stay, were you given any medicine that you had not taken before? Before giving you any new medicine, how often did hospital staff tell you what the medicine was for? How often did hospital staff describe possible side effects in a way you could understand?)

• Patient may experience dizziness or dyspepsia. Have patient report immediately to prescriber changes in angina, tachycardia, severe headache, considerable diarrhea, ecchymosis, hemorrhaging, or jaundice (HCAHPS).

• Educate patient about signs of a significant reaction (eg, wheezing; chest tightness; fever; itching; bad cough; blue skin color; seizures; or

swelling of face, lips, tongue, or throat). **Note:** This is not a comprehensive list of all side effects. Patient should consult prescriber for additional questions.

Intended Use and Disclaimer: Should not be printed and given to patients. This information is intended to serve as a concise initial reference for healthcare professionals to use when discussing medications with a patient. You must ultimately rely on your own discretion, experience and judgment in diagnosing, treating and advising patients.

Disulfiram (dye SUL fi ram)

Brand Names: U.S. Antabuse
Pharmacologic Category Aldehyde Dehydrogenase Inhibitor
Medication Safety Issues
Sound-alike/look-alike issues:
Disulfiram may be confused with Diflucan®
Lactation Excretion in breast milk unknown/not recommended
Use Management of chronic alcoholism
Available Dosage Forms
Tablet, Oral:
Antabuse: 250 mg, 500 mg
Generic: 250 mg, 500 mg
General Dosage Range Oral: *Adults:* Initial: 500 mg once daily; Maintenance: 125-500 mg once daily (maximum: 500 mg daily)
Administration
Oral Administration of any medications containing alcohol, including topicals, is contraindicated. Do not administer disulfiram if ethanol has been consumed within the prior 12 hours. Morning administration is preferred, but may be given at bedtime if sedation is experienced.
Nursing Actions
Physical Assessment Do not administer until the patient has abstained from ethanol for 12 hours. Monitor laboratory tests and for CNS changes (eg, sedation, restlessness, peripheral neuropathy, and optic or retrobulbar neuritis) prior to treatment and periodically. Advise patient about disulfiram reaction if alcohol is ingested.
Patient Education
• Discuss specific use of drug and side effects with patient as it relates to treatment. (HCAHPS: During this hospital stay, were you given any medicine that you had not taken before? Before giving you any new medicine, how often did hospital staff tell you what the medicine was for? How often did hospital staff describe possible side effects in a way you could understand?)
• Patient may experience fatigue, asthenia, sexual dysfunction, acne vulgaris, headache, or dysgeusia. Have patient report immediately to prescriber vision changes, paresthesia, mood

changes, behavioral changes, or signs of hepatic impairment (HCAHPS).
• Educate patient about signs of a significant reaction (eg, wheezing; chest tightness; fever; itching; bad cough; blue skin color; seizures; or swelling of face, lips, tongue, or throat). **Note:** This is not a comprehensive list of all side effects. Patient should consult prescriber for additional questions.

Intended Use and Disclaimer: Should not be printed and given to patients. This information is intended to serve as a concise initial reference for healthcare professionals to use when discussing medications with a patient. You must ultimately rely on your own discretion, experience and judgment in diagnosing, treating and advising patients.

DOBUTamine (doe BYOO ta meen)

Index Terms Dobutamine Hydrochloride
Pharmacologic Category Adrenergic Agonist Agent; Inotrope
Medication Safety Issues
Sound-alike/look-alike issues:
DOBUTamine may be confused with DOPamine
High alert medication:
The Institute for Safe Medication Practices (ISMP) includes this medication among its list of drugs which have a heightened risk of causing significant patient harm when used in error.
Pregnancy Risk Factor B
Lactation Excretion in breast milk unknown/use caution
Breast-Feeding Considerations It is not known if dobutamine is excreted in breast milk. The manufacturer recommends that caution be exercised when administering dobutamine to nursing women.
Use
Short-term management of patients with cardiac decompensation

American College of Cardiology/American Heart Association heart failure (HF) guideline recommendations (ACCF/AHA [Yancy, 2013]): To maintain systemic perfusion and preserve end-organ performance in patients with cardiogenic shock; bridge therapy in stage D HF unresponsive to guideline-directed medical therapy and device therapy in patients awaiting heart transplant or mechanical circulatory support; short-term management of hospitalized patients with severe systolic dysfunction presenting with low blood pressure and significantly depressed cardiac output; long-term management (palliative therapy) in select patients with stage D HF unresponsive to guideline-directed medical therapy and device therapy who are not candidates for heart transplant or mechanical circulatory support.

Unlabeled Use Positive inotropic agent for use in myocardial dysfunction related to sepsis; stress echocardiography

Mechanism of Action/Effect Stimulates $beta_1$-adrenergic receptors, causing increased contractility and heart rate, with little effect on $beta_2$- or alpha-receptors

Contraindications Hypersensitivity to dobutamine or sulfites (some contain sodium metabisulfate), or any component of the formulation; idiopathic hypertrophic subaortic stenosis (IHSS)

Warnings/Precautions May increase heart rate. Patients with atrial fibrillation may experience an increase in ventricular response. An increase in blood pressure is more common, but occasionally a patient may become hypotensive. May exacerbate ventricular ectopy. If needed, correct hypovolemia first to optimize hemodynamics. Ineffective therapeutically in the presence of mechanical obstruction such as severe aortic stenosis. Use caution post-MI (can increase myocardial oxygen demand). Use cautiously in the elderly starting at lower end of the dosage range. Use with extreme caution in patients taking MAO inhibitors. Dobutamine in combination with stress echo may be used diagnostically. The ACCF/AHA 2013 heart failure guidelines do not recommend long-term use of intravenous inotropic therapy except for palliative purposes in end-stage disease (ACCF/AHA [Yancy, 2013]). Product may contain sodium sulfite.

Drug Interactions

Avoid Concomitant Use
Avoid concomitant use of DOBUTamine with any of the following: Iobenguane I 123

Decreased Effect
DOBUTamine may decrease the levels/effects of: Iobenguane I 123

The levels/effects of DOBUTamine may be decreased by: Calcium Salts

Increased Effect/Toxicity
DOBUTamine may increase the levels/effects of: Sympathomimetics

The levels/effects of DOBUTamine may be increased by: AtoMOXetine; Cannabinoids; COMT Inhibitors; Linezolid

Adverse Reactions Incidence of adverse events is not always reported.

Cardiovascular: Increased heart rate, increased blood pressure, increased ventricular ectopic activity, hypotension, premature ventricular beats (5%, dose related), anginal pain (1% to 3%), nonspecific chest pain (1% to 3%), palpitation (1% to 3%)

Central nervous system: Fever (1% to 3%), headache (1% to 3%), paresthesia

Endocrine & metabolic: Slight decrease in serum potassium

Gastrointestinal: Nausea (1% to 3%)

Hematologic: Thrombocytopenia (isolated cases)

Local: Phlebitis, local inflammatory changes and pain from infiltration, cutaneous necrosis (isolated cases)

Neuromuscular & skeletal: Mild leg cramps

Respiratory: Dyspnea (1% to 3%)

Pharmacodynamics/Kinetics

Onset of Action I.V.: 1-10 minutes; Peak effect: 10-20 minutes

Available Dosage Forms

Solution, Intravenous:
Generic: 1 mg/mL (250 mL); 2 mg/mL (250 mL); 4 mg/mL (250 mL); 250 mg/20 mL (20 mL); 500 mg/40 mL (40 mL)

Solution, Intravenous [preservative free]:
Generic: 250 mg/20 mL (20 mL)

General Dosage Range I.V.: *Children and Adults:* 0.5-20 mcg/kg/minute (maximum: 40 mcg/kg/minute)

Usual Infusion Concentrations: Pediatric Note: Premixed solutions available.
I.V. infusion: 1000 **mcg**/mL, 2000 **mcg**/mL, or 4000 **mcg**/mL

Usual Infusion Concentrations: Adult Note: Premixed solutions available.
I.V. infusion: 250 mg in 500 mL (concentration: 500 **mcg**/mL), 500 mg in 250 mL (concentration: 2000 **mcg**/mL), **or** 1000 mg in 250 mL (concentration: 4000 **mcg**/mL) of D_5W or NS

Administration

I.V. Always administer via infusion device; administer into large vein.

Injectable Detail pH: 2.5-5.5

Storage/Stability Store reconstituted solution under refrigeration for 48 hours or 6 hours at room temperature. Stability of parenteral admixture at room temperature (25°C) is 48 hours; at refrigeration (4°C) stability is 7 days. Remix solution every 24 hours. Pink discoloration of solution indicates slight oxidation but no significant loss of potency.

Nursing Actions

Physical Assessment Infusion pump and frequent cardiac monitoring are required.

Patient Education

• Discuss specific use of drug and side effects with patient as it relates to treatment. (HCAHPS: During this hospital stay, were you given any medicine that you had not taken before? Before giving you any new medicine, how often did hospital staff tell you what the medicine was for? How often did hospital staff describe possible side effects in a way you could understand?)

• Have patient report immediately to prescriber dyspnea, angina, tachycardia, arrhythmia, severe dizziness, syncope, significant asthenia, or considerable headache (HCAHPS).

• Educate patient about signs of a significant reaction (eg, wheezing; chest tightness; fever; itching; bad cough; blue skin color; seizures; or swelling of face, lips, tongue, or throat). **Note:** This is not a comprehensive list of all side

effects. Patient should consult prescriber for additional questions.

Intended Use and Disclaimer: Should not be printed and given to patients. This information is intended to serve as a concise initial reference for healthcare professionals to use when discussing medications with a patient. You must ultimately rely on your own discretion, experience and judgment in diagnosing, treating and advising patients.

Docetaxel (doe se TAKS el)

Brand Names: U.S. Docefrez; Taxotere
Index Terms RP-6976
Pharmacologic Category Antineoplastic Agent, Antimicrotubular; Antineoplastic Agent, Taxane Derivative
Medication Safety Issues
Sound-alike/look-alike issues:
DOCEtaxel may be confused with cabazitaxel, PACLitaxel
Taxotere may be confused with Taxol
High alert medication:
This medication is in a class the Institute for Safe Medication Practices (ISMP) includes among its list of drug classes which have a heightened risk of causing significant patient harm when used in error.
Administration issues:
Multiple concentrations: Docetaxel is available as a one-vial formulation at concentrations of 10 mg/mL (generic formulation) and 20 mg/mL (concentrate; Taxotere), and as a lyophilized powder (Docefrez) which is reconstituted (with provided diluent) to 20 mg/0.8 mL (20 mg vial) or 24 mg/mL (80 mg vial). Docetaxel was previously available as a two-vial formulation (a concentrated docetaxel solution vial and a diluent vial) resulting in a reconstituted concentration of 10 mg/mL. The two-vial formulation has been discontinued by the Taxotere manufacturer (available generically). Admixture errors have occurred due to the availability of various docetaxel concentrations.
Pregnancy Risk Factor D
Lactation Excretion in breast milk unknown/not recommended
Use
U.S. labeling:
Docefrez: Treatment of breast cancer (locally-advanced/metastatic) after prior chemotherapy failure; treatment of locally-advanced or metastatic nonsmall cell lung cancer (NSCLC) after failure of prior platinum-based chemotherapy; treatment of hormone-refractory metastatic prostate cancer

Taxotere: Treatment of breast cancer (locally-advanced/metastatic) after prior chemotherapy failure, or adjuvant treatment of operable node-positive); locally-advanced or metastatic non-small cell lung cancer (NSCLC); hormone refractory, metastatic prostate cancer; advanced gastric adenocarcinoma; locally-advanced squamous cell head and neck cancer
Canadian labeling: Treatment of breast cancer (locally-advanced/metastatic or adjuvant treatment of operable node-positive); locally-advanced or metastatic nonsmall cell lung cancer (NSCLC); hormone refractory, metastatic prostate cancer; recurrent and/or metastatic squamous cell head and neck cancer; treatment of metastatic ovarian cancer following failure of first-line or subsequent chemotherapy
Unlabeled Use Treatment of bladder cancer (metastatic), ovarian cancer, cervical cancer (recurrent), esophageal cancer, small cell lung cancer (relapsed), soft tissue sarcoma, Ewing's sarcoma, osteosarcoma, and unknown-primary adenocarcinoma
Available Dosage Forms
Concentrate, Intravenous:
Taxotere: 20 mg/mL (1 mL); 80 mg/4 mL (4 mL)
Generic: 20 mg/mL (1 mL); 80 mg/4 mL (4 mL); 160 mg/8 mL (8 mL); 20 mg/0.5 mL (0.5 mL); 80 mg/2 mL (2 mL)
Concentrate, Intravenous [preservative free]:
Generic: 20 mg/mL (1 mL); 80 mg/4 mL (4 mL); 140 mg/7 mL (7 mL)
Solution, Intravenous:
Generic: 20 mg/2 mL (2 mL); 80 mg/8 mL (8 mL); 160 mg/16 mL (16 mL)
Solution Reconstituted, Intravenous:
Docefrez: 20 mg (1 ea); 80 mg (1 ea)
General Dosage Range Dosage adjustment recommended in patients with hepatic impairment, on concomitant therapy, or who develop toxicities.
I.V.: *Adults:* 60-100 mg/m^2 every 3 weeks
Administration
I.V. Administer I.V. infusion over 1-hour through nonsorbing polyethylene lined (non-DEHP) tubing; in-line filter is not necessary (the use of a filter during administration is not recommended by the manufacturer). Infusion should be completed within 4 hours of final preparation. **Note:** Premedication with corticosteroids for 3 days, beginning the day before docetaxel administration, is recommended to reduce the incidence and severity of hypersensitivity reactions and fluid retention.

Irritant with vesicant-like properties; avoid extravasation. Assure proper needle or catheter position prior to administration.

Extravasation management: If extravasation occurs, stop infusion immediately and disconnect (leave cannula/needle in place); gently aspirate extravasated solution (do **NOT** flush the line); remove needle/cannula; elevate extremity.

Information conflicts regarding the use of warm or cold compresses (Perez Fidalgo, 2012; Polovich, 2009).

Hazardous agent; use appropriate precautions for handling and disposal (NIOSH, 2012).

Nursing Actions

Physical Assessment Severe hypersensitivity reactions have been reported; premedication with dexamethasone may be advisable. Assess vital signs and weight prior to administration and monitor patient continuously during infusion (dosing adjustment may be necessary). Monitor for neutropenia, severe fluid retention, pleural effusion, and opportunistic infections prior to each infusion and on a regular basis.

Patient Education
- Discuss specific use of drug and side effects with patient as it relates to treatment. (HCAHPS: During this hospital stay, were you given any medicine that you had not taken before? Before giving you any new medicine, how often did hospital staff tell you what the medicine was for? How often did hospital staff describe possible side effects in a way you could understand?)
- Patient may experience diarrhea, stomatitis, alopecia, nail changes, dysgeusia, constipation, lack of appetite, arthralgia, or lacrimation. Have patient report immediately to prescriber signs of infection, signs of hepatic impairment, dyspnea, excessive weight gain, edema of extremities, severe dizziness, syncope, significant nausea, paresthesia, ecchymosis, hemorrhaging, considerable asthenia, intolerable eye irritation, angina, tachycardia, arrhythmia, severe headache, myalgia, or injection site irritation (HCAHPS).
- Educate patient about signs of a significant reaction (eg, wheezing; chest tightness; fever; itching; bad cough; blue skin color; seizures; or swelling of face, lips, tongue, or throat). **Note:** This is not a comprehensive list of all side effects. Patient should consult prescriber for additional questions.

Intended Use and Disclaimer: Should not be printed and given to patients. This information is intended to serve as a concise initial reference for healthcare professionals to use when discussing medications with a patient. You must ultimately rely on your own discretion, experience and judgment in diagnosing, treating and advising patients.

Related Information
Management of Drug Extravasations *on page 1700*

Dofetilide (doe FET il ide)

Brand Names: U.S. Tikosyn
Pharmacologic Category Antiarrhythmic Agent, Class III

Medication Safety Issues
Sound-alike/look-alike issues:
Dofetilide may be confused with defibrotide
Medication Guide Available Yes
Pregnancy Risk Factor C
Lactation Excretion in breast milk unknown/not recommended
Use Maintenance of normal sinus rhythm in patients with chronic atrial fibrillation/atrial flutter of longer than 1-week duration who have been converted to normal sinus rhythm; conversion of atrial fibrillation and atrial flutter to normal sinus rhythm
Unlabeled Use Alternative antiarrhythmic for the treatment of atrial fibrillation in patients with hypertrophic cardiomyopathy (HCM)
Available Dosage Forms
Capsule, Oral:
Tikosyn: 125 mcg, 250 mcg, 500 mcg
General Dosage Range Dosage adjustment recommended in patients with renal impairment
Oral: *Adults:* Initial: 500 mcg twice daily; Maintenance: 125-500 mcg twice daily **or** 125 mcg once daily

Nursing Actions
Physical Assessment Must be initiated or reinitiated by a cardiologist in a setting with continuous ECG monitoring for a period of time at beginning or adjustment of therapy. Monitor for signs of electrolyte imbalance (muscle weakness, spasms, twitching, numbness, lethargy, irregular heartbeat, and seizures).

Patient Education
- Discuss specific use of drug and side effects with patient as it relates to treatment. (HCAHPS: During this hospital stay, were you given any medicine that you had not taken before? Before giving you any new medicine, how often did hospital staff tell you what the medicine was for? How often did hospital staff describe possible side effects in a way you could understand?)
- Patient may experience headache or dyspepsia. Have patient report immediately to prescriber signs of hepatic impairment, paresthesia, angina, severe dizziness, syncope, strength differences from one side to another, difficulty speaking or thinking, change in balance, blurred vision, bradycardia, tachycardia, arrhythmia, dyspnea, or edema of extremities (HCAHPS).
- Educate patient about signs of a significant reaction (eg, wheezing; chest tightness; fever; itching; bad cough; blue skin color; seizures; or swelling of face, lips, tongue, or throat). **Note:** This is not a comprehensive list of all side effects. Patient should consult prescriber for additional questions.

Intended Use and Disclaimer: Should not be printed and given to patients. This information is intended to serve as a concise initial reference for healthcare professionals to use when discussing medications with a patient. You must ultimately

rely on your own discretion, experience and judgment in diagnosing, treating and advising patients.

Dolasetron (dol A se tron)

Brand Names: U.S. Anzemet
Index Terms Dolasetron Mesylate; MDL 73,147EF
Pharmacologic Category Antiemetic; Selective 5-HT₃ Receptor Antagonist
Medication Safety Issues
Sound-alike/look-alike issues:
Anzemet may be confused with Aldomet, Antivert, Avandamet
Dolasetron may be confused with granisetron, ondansetron, palonosetron
Pregnancy Risk Factor B
Lactation Excretion in breast milk unknown/use caution
Use
U.S. labeling:
Injection: Prevention and treatment of postoperative nausea and vomiting
Oral: Prevention of nausea and vomiting associated with emetogenic cancer chemotherapy (initial and repeat courses)
Canadian labeling: Oral: Prevention of nausea and vomiting associated with emetogenic cancer chemotherapy (initial and repeat courses)
Available Dosage Forms
Solution, Intravenous:
Anzemet: 20 mg/mL (0.625 mL, 5 mL, 25 mL)
Tablet, Oral:
Anzemet: 50 mg, 100 mg
General Dosage Range
I.V.:
Children 2-16 years: 0.35 mg/kg as a single dose (maximum: 12.5 mg/dose)
Adults: 12.5 mg as a single dose (maximum: 12.5 mg)
Oral:
Children 2-16 years: 1.2 or 1.8 mg/kg as a single dose (maximum: 100 mg/dose)
Adults: 100 mg as single dose
Administration
I.V. I.V. injection may be given either undiluted as an I.V. push over 30 seconds or diluted in 50 mL of compatible fluid and infused over 15 minutes. Flush line before and after dolasetron administration.
Injectable Detail pH: 3.2-3.8 (in vial)
Oral When unable to administer in tablet form, dolasetron injection may be diluted in apple or apple-grape juice and taken orally; this dilution is stable for 2 hours at room temperature (Anzemet prescribing information, 2013).
Nursing Actions
Physical Assessment I.V.: Follow infusion specifics. Oral and I.V. doses have different schedules and should not be administered on "PRN"

basis. Educate patients about how to take for prevention of chemotherapy-associated nausea and vomiting.
Patient Education
• Discuss specific use of drug and side effects with patient as it relates to treatment. (HCAHPS: During this hospital stay, were you given any medicine that you had not taken before? Before giving you any new medicine, how often did hospital staff tell you what the medicine was for? How often did hospital staff describe possible side effects in a way you could understand?)
• Patient may experience asthenia, diarrhea, chills, or pyrosis. Have patient report immediately to prescriber severe headache, significant dizziness, syncope, bradycardia, tachycardia, arrhythmia, angina, painful extremities, dyspnea, considerable dyspepsia, sudden vision changes, urinary retention, or oliguria (HCAHPS).
• Educate patient about signs of a significant reaction (eg, wheezing; chest tightness; fever; itching; bad cough; blue skin color; seizures; or swelling of face, lips, tongue, or throat). **Note:** This is not a comprehensive list of all side effects. Patient should consult prescriber for additional questions.

Intended Use and Disclaimer: Should not be printed and given to patients. This information is intended to serve as a concise initial reference for healthcare professionals to use when discussing medications with a patient. You must ultimately rely on your own discretion, experience and judgment in diagnosing, treating and advising patients.

Dolutegravir (doe loo TEG ra vir)

Brand Names: U.S. Tivicay
Index Terms 572; Dolutegravir Sodium; S/GSK1349572
Pharmacologic Category Antiretroviral, Integrase Inhibitor (Anti-HIV)
Medication Guide Available Yes
Pregnancy Risk Factor B
Lactation Excretion in breast milk unknown/contraindicated
Use HIV infection:
Adults: In combination with other antiretroviral agents for the treatment of HIV-1 infection
Children: In combination with other antiretroviral agents for the treatment of HIV-1 infection in children and adolescents ≥12 years of age and weighing ≥40 kg
Available Dosage Forms
Tablet, Oral:
Tivicay: 50 mg
General Dosage Range Dosage adjustment recommended in patients on concomitant therapy.

Oral: *Adolescents ≥12 years (and ≥40 kg):* 50 mg daily

Adults: 50-100 mg daily

Administration

Oral May be administered without regard to meals.

Nursing Actions

Patient Education

- Discuss specific use of drug and side effects with patient as it relates to treatment. (HCAHPS: During this hospital stay, were you given any medicine that you had not taken before? Before giving you any new medicine, how often did hospital staff tell you what the medicine was for? How often did hospital staff describe possible side effects in a way you could understand?)
- Patient may experience headache or insomnia. Have patient report immediately to prescriber signs of hepatic impairment, myalgia, arthralgia, stomatitis, eye irritation, dyspnea, severe asthenia, lipodystrophy, or signs of infection (HCAHPS).
- Educate patient about signs of a significant reaction (eg, wheezing; chest tightness; fever; itching; bad cough; blue skin color; seizures; or swelling of face, lips, tongue, or throat). **Note:** This is not a comprehensive list of all side effects. Patient should consult prescriber for additional questions.

Intended Use and Disclaimer: Should not be printed and given to patients. This information is intended to serve as a concise initial reference for healthcare professionals to use when discussing medications with a patient. You must ultimately rely on your own discretion, experience and judgment in diagnosing, treating and advising patients.

Donepezil (doh NEP e zil)

Brand Names: U.S. Aricept; Aricept ODT
Index Terms E2020
Pharmacologic Category Acetylcholinesterase Inhibitor (Central)
Medication Safety Issues
Sound-alike/look-alike issues:
Aricept® may be confused with AcipHex®, Ascriptin®, and Azilect®
Pregnancy Risk Factor C
Lactation Excretion in breast milk unknown/use caution
Breast-Feeding Considerations It is not known if donepezil is excreted in breast milk. The manufacturer recommends that caution be used if administered to a nursing woman.
Use Treatment of mild, moderate, or severe dementia of the Alzheimer's type
Unlabeled Use Behavioral syndromes in dementia; mild-to-moderate dementia associated with Parkinson's disease; Lewy body dementia

Mechanism of Action/Effect Alzheimer's disease is characterized by cholinergic deficiency in the cortex and basal forebrain, which contributes to cognitive deficits. Donepezil reversibly and noncompetitively inhibits centrally-active acetylcholinesterase, the enzyme responsible for hydrolysis of acetylcholine. This appears to result in increased concentrations of acetylcholine available for synaptic transmission in the central nervous system.

Contraindications Hypersensitivity to donepezil, piperidine derivatives, or any component of the formulation

Warnings/Precautions Cholinesterase inhibitors may have vagotonic effects which may cause bradycardia and/or heart block with or without a history of cardiac disease; syncopal episodes have been associated with donepezil. Alzheimer's treatment guidelines consider bradycardia to be a relative contraindication for use of centrally-active cholinesterase inhibitors. Use with caution with sick sinus syndrome or other supraventricular cardiac conduction abnormalities, COPD, or asthma. Use with caution in patients with a history of seizure disorder; cholinomimetics may potentially cause generalized seizures, although seizure activity may also result from Alzheimer's disease. Use with caution in patients at risk of ulcer disease (eg, previous history or NSAID use), or in patients with bladder outlet obstruction. May cause dose-related diarrhea, nausea, and/or vomiting, which usually resolves in 1-3 weeks. May cause anorexia and/or weight loss (dose-related). Patients weighing <55 kg may experience more nausea, vomiting, and weight loss than patients ≥55 kg. May exaggerate neuromuscular blockade effects of depolarizing neuromuscular-blocking agents (eg, succinylcholine). Potentially significant interactions may exist, requiring dose or frequency adjustment, additional monitoring, and/or selection of alternative therapy. Consult drug interactions database for more detailed information.

Drug Interactions

Avoid Concomitant Use There are no known interactions where it is recommended to avoid concomitant use.

Decreased Effect

Donepezil may decrease the levels/effects of: Anticholinergics; Neuromuscular-Blocking Agents (Nondepolarizing)

The levels/effects of Donepezil may be decreased by: Anticholinergics; Dipyridamole; Peginterferon Alfa-2b

Increased Effect/Toxicity

Donepezil may increase the levels/effects of: Antipsychotics; Beta-Blockers; Cholinergic Agonists; Succinylcholine

The levels/effects of Donepezil may be increased by: Corticosteroids (Systemic)

Nutritional/Ethanol Interactions

Ethanol: Avoid ethanol (may increase CNS adverse events).

Herb/Nutraceutical: St John's wort may decrease donepezil levels. Ginkgo biloba may increase adverse effects/toxicity of acetylcholinesterase inhibitors.

Adverse Reactions

>10%:

Central nervous system: Insomnia (2% to 14%)

Gastrointestinal: Nausea (3% to 19%; dose related), diarrhea (5% to 15%; dose related)

Miscellaneous: Accident (7% to 13%), infection (11%)

1% to 10%:

Cardiovascular: Hypertension (3%), chest pain (2%), hemorrhage (2%), syncope (2%), hypotension, atrial fibrillation, bradycardia, ECG abnormal, edema, heart failure, hot flashes, peripheral edema, vasodilation

Central nervous system: Headache (3% to 10%), pain (3% to 9%), fatigue (1% to 8%), dizziness (2% to 8%), abnormal dreams (3%), hostility (3%), nervousness (1% to 3%), hallucinations (3%), depression (2% to 3%), confusion (2%), emotional lability (2%), personality disorder (2%), fever (2%), somnolence (2%), abnormal crying, aggression, agitation, anxiety, aphasia, delusions, irritability, restlessness, seizure, vertigo

Dermatologic: Bruising (4% to 5%), eczema (3%), pruritus, rash, skin ulcer, urticaria

Endocrine & metabolic: Dehydration (1% to 2%), hyperlipemia (2%), libido increased

Gastrointestinal: Anorexia (2% to 8%), vomiting (3% to 9%; dose related), weight loss (3% to 5%; dose related), abdominal pain, bloating, constipation, dyspepsia, epigastric pain, fecal incontinence, gastroenteritis, GI bleeding, toothache

Genitourinary: Urinary frequency (2%), urinary incontinence (1% to 3%), cystitis, hematuria, glycosuria, nocturia, UTI

Hematologic: Contusion (≤2%), anemia

Hepatic: Alkaline phosphatase increased

Neuromuscular & skeletal: Muscle cramps (3% to 8%), back pain (3%), CPK increased (3%), arthritis (1% to 2%), ataxia, bone fracture, gait abnormal, lactate dehydrogenase increased, paresthesia, tremor, weakness (1% to 2%)

Ocular: Blurred vision, cataract, eye irritation

Respiratory: Bronchitis, cough increased, dyspnea, pharyngitis, pneumonia, sore throat

Miscellaneous: Diaphoresis, fungal infection, flu symptoms, wandering

Available Dosage Forms

Tablet, Oral:

Aricept: 5 mg, 10 mg, 23 mg

Generic: 5 mg, 10 mg, 23 mg

Tablet Dispersible, Oral:

Aricept ODT: 5 mg, 10 mg

Generic: 5 mg, 10 mg

General Dosage Range Oral: *Adults:* 5 mg once daily; Maintenance: 5-23 mg once daily

Administration

Oral Administer at bedtime without regard to food.

Aricept® 5 mg or 10 mg tablet: Swallow whole with water.

Aricept® 23 mg tablet: Swallow whole with water; do NOT crush or chew due to an increased rate of absorption. The 23 mg strength is provided in a unique film-coated formulation different from the 5 mg or 10 mg tablet strengths, which results in an altered pharmacokinetic profile.

Aricept® ODT: Allow tablet to dissolve completely on tongue and follow with water.

Storage/Stability Store at 15°C to 30°C (59°F to 86°F).

Nursing Actions

Physical Assessment Assess bladder adequacy prior to treatment. Monitor for cholinergic crisis (DUMBELS - **d**iarrhea, **u**rination, **m**iosis, **b**ronchospasm/**b**radycardia, **e**xcitability, **l**acrimation, and **s**alivation/excessive **s**weating). Monitor pulse.

Patient Education

• Discuss specific use of drug and side effects with patient as it relates to treatment. (HCAHPS: During this hospital stay, were you given any medicine that you had not taken before? Before giving you any new medicine, how often did hospital staff tell you what the medicine was for? How often did hospital staff describe possible side effects in a way you could understand?)

• Patient may experience nausea, diarrhea, insomnia, cramps, lack of appetite, or weight loss. Have patient report immediately to prescriber signs of depression (ie, suicidal ideation, anxiety, emotional instability, illogical thinking), severe dizziness, syncope, ecchymosis, hemorrhaging, bradycardia, arrhythmia, angina, difficult urination, dysuria, urinary retention, pyrosis, hematemesis, melena, edema of hands or feet, flu-like syndrome, dyspnea, considerable headache, tremors, or significant asthenia (HCAHPS).

• Educate patient about signs of a significant reaction (eg, wheezing; chest tightness; fever; itching; bad cough; blue skin color; seizures; or swelling of face, lips, tongue, or throat). **Note:** This is not a comprehensive list of all side effects. Patient should consult prescriber for additional questions.

Intended Use and Disclaimer: Should not be printed and given to patients. This information is intended to serve as a concise initial reference for healthcare professionals to use when discussing medications with a patient. You must ultimately rely on your own discretion, experience and judgment in diagnosing, treating and advising patients.

Dietary Considerations May take with or without food.

Related Information
Oral Medications That Should Not Be Crushed or Altered *on page 1712*

DOPamine (DOE pa meen)

Index Terms Dopamine Hydrochloride; Intropin
Pharmacologic Category Adrenergic Agonist Agent; Inotrope
Medication Safety Issues
Sound-alike/look-alike issues:
DOPamine may be confused with DOBUTamine, Dopram
High alert medication:
The Institute for Safe Medication Practices (ISMP) includes this medication among its list of drugs which have a heightened risk of causing significant patient harm when used in error.
Pregnancy Risk Factor C
Lactation Excretion in breast milk unknown/use caution
Breast-Feeding Considerations It is not known if dopamine is excreted in breast milk. The manufacturer recommends that caution be exercised when administering dopamine to nursing women.
Use Adjunct in the treatment of shock (eg, MI, open heart surgery, renal failure, cardiac decompensation) which persists after adequate fluid volume replacement

American College of Cardiology/American Heart Association heart failure (HF) guideline recommendations (ACCF/AHA [Yancy, 2013]): To maintain systemic perfusion and preserve end-organ performance in patients with cardiogenic shock; bridge therapy in stage D HF unresponsive to guideline-directed medical therapy and device therapy in patients awaiting heart transplant or mechanical circulatory support; short-term management of hospitalized patients with severe systolic dysfunction presenting with low blood pressure and significantly depressed cardiac output; long-term management (palliative therapy) in select patients with stage D HF unresponsive to guideline-directed medical therapy and device therapy who are not candidates for heart transplant or mechanical circulatory support.

Unlabeled Use Symptomatic bradycardia or heart block unresponsive to atropine or pacing
Mechanism of Action/Effect Stimulates both adrenergic and dopaminergic receptors, lower doses are mainly dopaminergic stimulating and produce renal and mesenteric vasodilation, higher doses also are both dopaminergic and beta$_1$-adrenergic stimulating and produce cardiac stimulation and renal vasodilation; large doses stimulate alpha-adrenergic receptors

Contraindications Hypersensitivity to sulfites (commercial preparation contains sodium bisulfite); pheochromocytoma; ventricular fibrillation
Warnings/Precautions Use with caution in patients with cardiovascular disease or cardiac arrhythmias or patients with occlusive vascular disease. Correct hypovolemia and electrolytes when used in hemodynamic support. May cause increases in HR increasing the risk of tachycardia and other tachyarrhythmia. Use with caution in patients with recent myocardial infarction; may increase myocardial oxygen consumption. Use has been associated with a higher incidence of adverse events (eg, tachyarrhythmias) in patients with shock compared to norepinephrine. Higher 28-day mortality was also seen in patients with septic shock; the use of norepinephrine in patients with shock may be preferred. The 2012 Surviving Sepsis Campaign (SSC) guidelines suggest dopamine use as an alternative to norepinephrine only in patients with low risk of tachyarrhythmias and absolute or relative bradycardia (SCCM [Dellinger, 2013]). Use with extreme caution in patients taking MAO inhibitors.

Vesicant; ensure proper needle or catheter placement prior to and during infusion. Avoid extravasation; infuse into a large vein if possible. Avoid infusion into leg veins. Watch I.V. site closely. **[U.S. Boxed Warning]: If extravasation occurs, infiltrate the area with diluted phentolamine (5-10 mg in 10-15 mL of saline) with a fine hypodermic needle. Phentolamine should be administered as soon as possible after extravasation is noted to prevent sloughing/necrosis.** Product may contain sodium metabisulfite.
Drug Interactions
Avoid Concomitant Use
Avoid concomitant use of DOPamine with any of the following: Inhalational Anesthetics; Iobenguane I 123; Lurasidone
Decreased Effect
DOPamine may decrease the levels/effects of: Iobenguane I 123
Increased Effect/Toxicity
DOPamine may increase the levels/effects of: Lurasidone; Sympathomimetics

The levels/effects of DOPamine may be increased by: AtoMOXetine; Cannabinoids; COMT Inhibitors; Hyaluronidase; Inhalational Anesthetics; Linezolid
Adverse Reactions Frequency not defined.
Cardiovascular: Anginal pain, ectopic beats, hypotension, palpitation, tachycardia, vasoconstriction
Central nervous system: Headache
Gastrointestinal: Nausea and vomiting
Respiratory: Dyspnea
Pharmacodynamics/Kinetics
Onset of Action Adults: Within 5 minutes
Duration of Action Adults: <10 minutes

Available Dosage Forms

Solution, Intravenous:

Generic: 0.8 mg/mL (250 mL, 500 mL); 1.6 mg/mL (250 mL, 500 mL); 3.2 mg/mL (250 mL); 40 mg/mL (5 mL, 10 mL); 80 mg/mL (5 mL); 160 mg/mL (5 mL)

General Dosage Range I.V.:

Children: 1-20 mcg/kg/minute (maximum: 50 mcg/kg/minute)

Adults: 1-50 mcg/kg/minute

Usual Infusion Concentrations: Pediatric

Note: Premixed solutions available.

I.V. infusion: 1600 **mcg**/mL or 3200 **mcg**/mL

Usual Infusion Concentrations: Adult Note:

Premixed solutions available.

I.V. infusion: 400 mg in 250 mL (concentration: 1600 **mcg**/mL) or 800 mg in 250 mL (concentration: 3200 **mcg**/mL) of D$_5$W or NS

Administration

I.V. Administer as a continuous infusion with the use of an infusion pump. Administer into large vein to prevent the possibility of extravasation (central line administration); monitor continuously for free flow; use infusion device to control rate of flow; administration into an umbilical arterial catheter is not recommended; when discontinuing the infusion, gradually decrease the dose of dopamine (sudden discontinuation may cause hypotension). Vials (concentrated solution) must be diluted prior to use.

Vesicant; ensure proper needle or catheter placement prior to and during infusion; avoid extravasation.

Extravasation management: If extravasation occurs, stop infusion immediately and disconnect (leave cannula/needle in place); gently aspirate extravasated solution (do **NOT** flush the line); remove needle/cannula; elevate extremity. Initiate phentolamine (or alternative) antidote. Apply dry warm compresses (Hurst, 2004).

Phentolamine: Dilute 5-10 mg in 10-15 mL NS and administer into extravasation site as soon as possible after extravasation (AHA [Peberdy, 2010])

Alternatives to phentolamine:

Nitroglycerin topical 2% ointment (based on limited case reports in neonates/infants): Apply 4 mm/kg as a thin ribbon to the affected areas; may repeat after 8 hours if needed (Wong, 1992) **or** apply a 1-inch strip on the affected site (Denkler, 1989)

Terbutaline (based on limited case reports): Infiltrate extravasation area using a solution of terbutaline 1 mg diluted to 10 mL in NS (large extravasation site; administration volume varied from 3-10 mL) **or** 1 mg diluted in 1 mL NS (small/distal extravasation site; administration volume varied from 0.5-1 mL) (Stier, 1999)

Injectable Detail pH: 2.5-5 (undiluted vials); 2.5-4.5 (premixed solution in D$_5$W)

Storage/Stability Protect from light. Solutions that are darker than slightly yellow should not be used.

Nursing Actions

Physical Assessment Infusion pump and continuous cardiac and hemodynamic monitoring are required for inpatient therapy. Assess I.V. site frequently. Monitor cardiac status and renal function. Monitor for peripheral ischemia.

Patient Education

- Discuss specific use of drug and side effects with patient as it relates to treatment. (HCAHPS: During this hospital stay, were you given any medicine that you had not taken before? Before giving you any new medicine, how often did hospital staff tell you what the medicine was for? How often did hospital staff describe possible side effects in a way you could understand?)
- Patient may experience nausea or anxiety. Have patient report immediately to prescriber dyspnea, angina, bradycardia, tachycardia, arrhythmia, severe dizziness, syncope, significant headache, considerable asthenia, urinary retention, oliguria, or intolerable injection site irritation (HCAHPS).
- Educate patient about signs of a significant reaction (eg, wheezing; chest tightness; fever; itching; bad cough; blue skin color; seizures; or swelling of face, lips, tongue, or throat). **Note:** This is not a comprehensive list of all side effects. Patient should consult prescriber for additional questions.

Intended Use and Disclaimer: Should not be printed and given to patients. This information is intended to serve as a concise initial reference for healthcare professionals to use when discussing medications with a patient. You must ultimately rely on your own discretion, experience and judgment in diagnosing, treating and advising patients.

Related Information

Management of Drug Extravasations *on page 1700*

Doripenem (dore i PEN em)

Brand Names: U.S. Doribax

Index Terms S-4661

Pharmacologic Category Antibiotic, Carbapenem

Medication Safety Issues

Sound-alike/look-alike issues:

Doripenem may be confused with ertapenem

Doribax may be confused with Zovirax

Pregnancy Risk Factor B

Lactation Excretion in breast milk unknown/use caution

Breast-Feeding Considerations It is not known if doripenem is excreted into breast milk. The manufacturer recommends that caution be exercised when administering doripenem to nursing women.

Use Treatment of complicated intra-abdominal infections and complicated urinary tract infections (including pyelonephritis) due to susceptible aerobic gram-positive, aerobic gram-negative (including *Pseudomonas aeruginosa*), and anaerobic bacteria

Unlabeled Use Treatment of intravascular catheter-related bloodstream infection due to extended-spectrum β-lactamase (ESBL)-producing *Escherichia coli* and *Klebsiella* spp

Mechanism of Action/Effect Inhibits cell wall synthesis in susceptible bacteria

Contraindications Known serious hypersensitivity to doripenem or other carbapenems (eg, ertapenem, imipenem, meropenem) or any component of the formulation; anaphylactic reactions to beta-lactam antibiotics

Warnings/Precautions Serious hypersensitivity reactions, including anaphylaxis, and skin reactions have been reported in patients receiving beta-lactams. Use may result in fungal or bacterial superinfection, including *C. difficile*-associated diarrhea (CDAD) and pseudomembranous colitis; CDAD has been observed >2 months postantibiotic treatment. Not indicated for the treatment of pneumonia including ventilator-associated pneumonia; decreased efficacy and increased mortality observed in a phase 3 study using a higher dose and fixed 7-day administration (Kollef, 2012). Use with caution in patients with renal impairment; dosage adjustment required in patients with moderate-to-severe renal dysfunction. Carbapenems have been associated with CNS adverse effects, including confusional states and seizures (myoclonic); use caution with CNS disorders (eg, brain lesions, stroke, or history of seizures) and adjust dose in renal impairment to avoid drug accumulation, which may increase seizure risk. Patients receiving doses >500 mg every 8 hours may also be at increased risk of seizures. Potentially significant interactions may exist, requiring dose or frequency adjustment, additional monitoring, and/or selection of alternative therapy. Administer via intravenous infusion only. Per manufacturer's labeling, investigational experience of doripenem via inhalation resulted in pneumonitis.

Drug Interactions

Avoid Concomitant Use

Avoid concomitant use of Doripenem with any of the following: BCG; Probenecid

Decreased Effect

Doripenem may decrease the levels/effects of: BCG; Sodium Picosulfate; Typhoid Vaccine; Valproic Acid and Derivatives

Increased Effect/Toxicity

The levels/effects of Doripenem may be increased by: Probenecid

Adverse Reactions

>10%:

Central nervous system: Headache (3% to 16%)

Gastrointestinal: Diarrhea (6% to 12%), nausea (4% to 12%)

1% to 10%:

Cardiovascular: Phlebitis (2% to 8%)

Dermatologic: Skin rash (2% to 7%; includes allergic/bullous dermatitis, erythema, macular/papular eruptions, urticaria, and erythema multiforme), pruritus (1% to 3%)

Gastrointestinal: Oral candidiasis (1% to 3%), pseudomembranous colitis (≤1%)

Hematologic & oncologic: Anemia (2% to 10%)

Hepatic: Increased serum transaminases (2% to 7%)

Renal: Renal insufficiency (≤1%)

Miscellaneous: Vaginal infection (1% to 2%)

Available Dosage Forms

Solution Reconstituted, Intravenous:

Doribax: 250 mg (1 ea); 500 mg (1 ea)

General Dosage Range Dosage adjustment recommended in patients with renal impairment

I.V.: *Adults:* 500 mg every 8 hours

Administration

I.V. Infuse intravenously over 1 hour. Use of 4-hour infusion has been studied in the treatment of VAP (unlabeled use) (Chastre, 2008).

Injectable Detail pH: 4.5-5.5 (infusion solution)

Preparation for Administration Reconstitute 250 mg vial with 10 mL of SWFI or NS; further dilute for infusion with 50 mL or 100 mL of NS or D_5W. Shake gently until clear. Reconstitute 500 mg vial with 10 mL of SWFI or NS; further dilute for infusion with 100 mL of NS or D_5W. Shake gently until clear. Reconstituted vial may be stored for up to 1 hour prior to preparation of infusion solution. To prepare a 250 mg dose using a 500 mg vial, reconstitute the 500 mg vial with 10 mL of SWFI or NS and further dilute with 100 mL of compatible solution as above, but remove and discard 55 mL from the infusion bag to leave the remaining solution containing the 250 mg dose.

Storage/Stability Store dry powder vials at 15°C to 30°C (59°F to 86°F). Stability of solution when diluted in NS is 12 hours at room temperature or 72 hours under refrigeration; stability in D_5W is 4 hours at room temperature and 24 hours under refrigeration.

Nursing Actions

Physical Assessment Results of culture and sensitivity tests and patient history of previous allergies should be assessed prior to beginning treatment. Monitor closely for adverse reactions.

Patient Education

• Discuss specific use of drug and side effects with patient as it relates to treatment. (HCAHPS: During this hospital stay, were you given any medicine that you had not taken before? Before giving you any new medicine, how often did hospital staff tell you what the medicine was

for? How often did hospital staff describe possible side effects in a way you could understand?)
• Patient may experience headache, nausea, diarrhea, or injection site irritation. Have patient report immediately to prescriber illogical thinking, severe asthenia, vaginitis, signs of pseudomembranous colitis, or signs of Stevens-Johnson syndrome/toxic epidermal necrolysis (HCAHPS).
• Educate patient about signs of a significant reaction (eg, wheezing; chest tightness; fever; itching; bad cough; blue skin color; seizures; or swelling of face, lips, tongue, or throat). **Note:** This is not a comprehensive list of all side effects. Patient should consult prescriber for additional questions.

Intended Use and Disclaimer: Should not be printed and given to patients. This information is intended to serve as a concise initial reference for healthcare professionals to use when discussing medications with a patient. You must ultimately rely on your own discretion, experience and judgment in diagnosing, treating and advising patients.

Dornase Alfa (DOOR nase AL fa)

Brand Names: U.S. Pulmozyme
Index Terms Recombinant Human Deoxyribonuclease; rhDNase
Pharmacologic Category Enzyme; Mucolytic Agent
Pregnancy Risk Factor B
Lactation Excretion in breast milk unknown/use caution
Use Management of cystic fibrosis patients to reduce the frequency of respiratory infections that require parenteral antibiotics in patients with FVC ≥40% of predicted; in conjunction with standard therapies, to improve pulmonary function in patients with cystic fibrosis
Unlabeled Use Infected parapneumonic effusion (following alteplase administration)
Available Dosage Forms
Solution, Inhalation:
Pulmozyme: 1 mg/mL (2.5 mL)
General Dosage Range Inhalation: *Children >5 years and Adults:* 2.5 mg once daily
Administration
Inhalation Nebulization: Prior to use, squeeze each ampul to check for leaks. Should not be diluted or mixed with any other drugs in the nebulizer, this may inactivate the drug
Other Parapneumonic effusion (unlabeled use): Intrapleural: **Note:** Each dose must be diluted in 30 mL of sterile water. Stability of dornase alfa diluted in sterile water has not been formally evaluated; use immediately after preparation. Instill dose into chest tube and clamp drain. After

1 hour dwell time, release clamp and connect chest tube to continuous suction (Rahman, 2011).
Nursing Actions
Physical Assessment Teach patient appropriate use of nebulizer.
Patient Education
• Discuss specific use of drug and side effects with patient as it relates to treatment. (HCAHPS: During this hospital stay, were you given any medicine that you had not taken before? Before giving you any new medicine, how often did hospital staff tell you what the medicine was for? How often did hospital staff describe possible side effects in a way you could understand?)
• Patient may experience voice changes, rhinitis, rhinorrhea, dyspepsia, pharyngitis, or eye irritation. Have patient report immediately to prescriber angina or dyspnea (HCAHPS).
• Educate patient about signs of a significant reaction (eg, wheezing; chest tightness; fever; itching; bad cough; blue skin color; seizures; or swelling of face, lips, tongue, or throat). **Note:** This is not a comprehensive list of all side effects. Patient should consult prescriber for additional questions.

Intended Use and Disclaimer: Should not be printed and given to patients. This information is intended to serve as a concise initial reference for healthcare professionals to use when discussing medications with a patient. You must ultimately rely on your own discretion, experience and judgment in diagnosing, treating and advising patients.

Dorzolamide (dor ZOLE a mide)

Brand Names: U.S. Trusopt
Index Terms Dorzolamide Hydrochloride
Pharmacologic Category Carbonic Anhydrase Inhibitor (Ophthalmic); Ophthalmic Agent, Antiglaucoma
Pregnancy Risk Factor C
Lactation Excretion in breast milk unknown/not recommended
Use Treatment of elevated intraocular pressure in patients with ocular hypertension or open-angle glaucoma
Available Dosage Forms
Solution, Ophthalmic:
Trusopt: 2% (10 mL)
Generic: 2% (10 mL)
General Dosage Range Ophthalmic: *Children and Adults:* Instill 1 drop into affected eye(s) 3 times/day
Administration
Other If more than one topical ophthalmic drug is being used, administer the drugs at least 5 minutes apart. Remove contact lens prior to administration and wait 15 minutes before reinserting. Instruct patients to avoid allowing the tip

of the dispensing container to contact the eye or surrounding structures. Ocular solutions can become contaminated by common bacteria known to cause ocular infections. Serious damage to the eye and subsequent loss of vision may occur from using contaminated solutions.

Nursing Actions

Patient Education

- Discuss specific use of drug and side effects with patient as it relates to treatment. (HCAHPS: During this hospital stay, were you given any medicine that you had not taken before? Before giving you any new medicine, how often did hospital staff tell you what the medicine was for? How often did hospital staff describe possible side effects in a way you could understand?)
- Patient may experience blurred vision, parageusia, xerophthalmia, lacrimation, or light sensitivity. Have patient report immediately to prescriber vision changes, ophthalmalgia, severe eye irritation, edema of eye or eyelid, or signs of Stevens-Johnson syndrome/toxic epidermal necrolysis (HCAHPS).
- Educate patient about signs of a significant reaction (eg, wheezing; chest tightness; fever; itching; bad cough; blue skin color; seizures; or swelling of face, lips, tongue, or throat). **Note:** This is not a comprehensive list of all side effects. Patient should consult prescriber for additional questions.

Intended Use and Disclaimer: Should not be printed and given to patients. This information is intended to serve as a concise initial reference for healthcare professionals to use when discussing medications with a patient. You must ultimately rely on your own discretion, experience and judgment in diagnosing, treating and advising patients.

Doxazosin (doks AY zoe sin)

Brand Names: U.S. Cardura; Cardura XL
Index Terms Doxazosin Mesylate
Pharmacologic Category Alpha$_1$ Blocker; Antihypertensive
Medication Safety Issues
  Sound-alike/look-alike issues:
  Doxazosin may be confused with doxapram, doxepin, DOXOrubicin
  Cardura® may be confused with Cardene®, Cordarone®, Cordran®, Coumadin®, K-Dur®, Ridaura®

  BEERS Criteria medication:
  This drug may be potentially inappropriate for use in geriatric patients (Quality of evidence - moderate; Strength of recommendation - strong).

Pregnancy Risk Factor C
Lactation Enters breast milk/use caution
Breast-Feeding Considerations Doxazosin is excreted into breast milk. Information is available

from a single case report following a maternal dose of doxazosin 4 mg every 24 hours for 2 doses. Milk samples were obtained at various intervals over 24 hours, beginning ~17 hours after the first dose. Maternal serum samples were obtained at nearly the same times, beginning ~1 hour later. The highest serum and milk concentrations of doxazosin were observed ~1 hour after the dose. Using the highest milk concentration (4.15 mcg/L), the estimated dose to the nursing infant was calculated to be <1% of the weight-adjusted maternal dose (Jensen, 2013). The manufacturer recommends that caution be used if administered to nursing women.

Use
Immediate release formulation: Treatment of hypertension as monotherapy or in conjunction with diuretics, ACE inhibitors, beta-blockers, or calcium antagonists; treatment of urinary outflow obstruction and/or obstructive and irritative symptoms associated with benign prostatic hyperplasia (BPH)

Extended release formulation: Treatment of urinary outflow obstruction and/or obstructive and irritative symptoms associated with BPH

Unlabeled Use Pediatric hypertension; facilitation of distal ureteral stone expulsion; erectile dysfunction in patients with concomitant BPH

Mechanism of Action/Effect
Hypertension: Competitively inhibits postsynaptic alpha$_1$-adrenergic receptors which results in vasodilation of veins and arterioles and a decrease in total peripheral resistance and blood pressure; ~50% as potent on a weight by weight basis as prazosin.

BPH: Competitively inhibits postsynaptic alpha$_1$-adrenergic receptors in prostatic stromal and bladder neck tissues. This reduces the sympathetic tone-induced urethral stricture causing BPH symptoms.

Contraindications Hypersensitivity to quinazolines (prazosin, terazosin), doxazosin, or any component of the formulation

Warnings/Precautions Can cause significant orthostatic hypotension and syncope, especially with first dose; anticipate a similar effect if therapy is interrupted for a few days, if dosage is rapidly increased, or if another antihypertensive drug (particularly vasodilators) or a PDE-5 inhibitor is introduced. Discontinue if symptoms of angina occur or worsen. Patients should be cautioned about performing hazardous tasks when starting new therapy or adjusting dosage upward. Priapism has been associated with use (rarely). Prostate cancer should be ruled out before starting for BPH. Use with caution in mild-to-moderate hepatic impairment; not recommended in severe dysfunction. Intraoperative floppy iris syndrome has been observed in cataract surgery patients who were on or were previously treated with alpha$_1$-blockers.

Causality has not been established and there appears to be no benefit in discontinuing alpha-blocker therapy prior to surgery. In the elderly, avoid use as an antihypertensive due to high risk of orthostatic hypotension; alternative agents preferred due to a more favorable risk/benefit profile (Beers Criteria).

The extended release formulation consists of drug within a nondeformable matrix; following drug release/absorption, the matrix/shell is expelled in the stool. The use of nondeformable products in patients with known stricture/narrowing of the GI tract has been associated with symptoms of obstruction. Use caution in patients with increased GI retention (eg, chronic constipation) as doxazosin exposure may be increased. Extended release formulation is not indicated for use in women or for the treatment of hypertension.

Drug Interactions

Avoid Concomitant Use

Avoid concomitant use of Doxazosin with any of the following: Alpha1-Blockers; Conivaptan; Fusidic Acid (Systemic)

Decreased Effect

Doxazosin may decrease the levels/effects of: Alpha-/Beta-Agonists; Alpha1-Agonists

The levels/effects of Doxazosin may be decreased by: Bosentan; CYP3A4 Inducers (Strong); Dabrafenib; Deferasirox; Herbs (CYP3A4 Inducers); Herbs (Hypertensive Properties); Methylphenidate; Mitotane; Peginterferon Alfa-2b; Tocilizumab; Yohimbine

Increased Effect/Toxicity

Doxazosin may increase the levels/effects of: Alpha1-Blockers; Amifostine; Antihypertensives; Calcium Channel Blockers; DULoxetine; Hypotensive Agents; Obinutuzumab; RiTUXimab

The levels/effects of Doxazosin may be increased by: Beta-Blockers; Brimonidine (Topical); Conivaptan; CYP3A4 Inhibitors (Moderate); CYP3A4 Inhibitors (Strong); Dasatinib; Diazoxide; Fusidic Acid (Systemic); Herbs (Hypotensive Properties); Ivacaftor; Luliconazole; MAO Inhibitors; Mifepristone; Pentoxifylline; Phosphodiesterase 5 Inhibitors; Prostacyclin Analogues; Simeprevir; Stiripentol

Nutritional/Ethanol Interactions Herb/Nutraceutical: Avoid dong quai if using for hypertension (has estrogenic activity). Avoid ephedra, yohimbe, ginseng (may worsen hypertension). Avoid saw palmetto when used for BPH (due to limited experience with this combination). Avoid garlic (may have increased antihypertensive effect).

Adverse Reactions Note: Type and frequency of adverse reactions reflect combined data from BPH and hypertension trials and immediate release and extended release products.

>10%: Central nervous system: Dizziness (5% to 19%), malaise (12%), fatigue (8% to 12%), headache (6% to 10%)

1% to 10%:

Cardiovascular: Edema (3% to 4%), hypotension (1% to 2%), orthostatic hypotension (dose related; 0.3% up to 2%), arrhythmia (1%), facial edema (1%), flushing (1%)

Central nervous system: Vertigo (2% to 4%), somnolence (1% to 5%), pain (2%), anxiety (1%), ataxia (1%), hypertonia (1%), insomnia (1%), movement disorder (1%)

Endocrine & metabolic: Sexual dysfunction (2%)

Gastrointestinal: Abdominal pain (2%), nausea (1% to 2%), dyspepsia (1%), xerostomia (1%)

Genitourinary: Polyuria (2%), impotence (1%), incontinence (1%), urinary tract infection (1%)

Neuromuscular & skeletal: Weakness (4% to 7%), arthritis (1%), muscle cramps (1%), muscle weakness (1%), myalgia (1%)

Ocular: Abnormal vision (2%)

Otic: Tinnitus (1%)

Respiratory: Respiratory tract infection (5%), rhinitis (3%), dyspnea (1% to 3%), epistaxis (1%)

Pharmacodynamics/Kinetics

Duration of Action >24 hours

Available Dosage Forms

Tablet, Oral:

Cardura: 1 mg, 2 mg, 4 mg, 8 mg

Generic: 1 mg, 2 mg, 4 mg, 8 mg

Tablet Extended Release 24 Hour, Oral:

Cardura XL: 4 mg, 8 mg

General Dosage Range Oral:

Extended release: *Adults:* Initial: 4 mg once daily; Maintenance: 4-8 mg daily (maximum: 8 mg daily)

Immediate release:

Adults: Initial: 1-4 mg once daily; Maintenance: 4-8 mg daily (maximum: 8 mg daily [BPH]; 16 mg daily [Hypertension])

Elderly: Initial: 0.5 mg once daily

Administration

Oral Cardura® XL: Tablets should be swallowed whole; do not crush, chew, or divide. Administer with morning meal.

Storage/Stability Store at 25°C (77°F); excursions permitted between 15°C to 30°C (59°F to 86°F).

Nursing Actions

Physical Assessment Assess blood pressure and monitor for hypotension, CNS changes, and urinary retention prior to treatment and on a regular basis. When discontinuing, monitor blood pressure and taper dose slowly over 1 week or more.

Patient Education

• Discuss specific use of drug and side effects with patient as it relates to treatment. (HCAHPS: During this hospital stay, were you given any medicine that you had not taken before? Before giving you any new medicine, how often did hospital staff tell you what the medicine was

for? How often did hospital staff describe possible side effects in a way you could understand?)
• Patient may experience fatigue, rhinitis, asthenia, or dyspepsia. Have patient report immediately to prescriber severe dizziness, syncope, significant headache, angina, tachycardia, arrhythmia, dyspnea, edema of extremities, vision changes, urinary retention, dysuria, or priapism (HCAHPS).
• Educate patient about signs of a significant reaction (eg, wheezing; chest tightness; fever; itching; bad cough; blue skin color; seizures; or swelling of face, lips, tongue, or throat). **Note:** This is not a comprehensive list of all side effects. Patient should consult prescriber for additional questions.

Intended Use and Disclaimer: Should not be printed and given to patients. This information is intended to serve as a concise initial reference for healthcare professionals to use when discussing medications with a patient. You must ultimately rely on your own discretion, experience and judgment in diagnosing, treating and advising patients.

Dietary Considerations Cardura® XL: Take with morning meal.

Related Information
Oral Medications That Should Not Be Crushed or Altered *on page 1712*

Doxepin (Systemic) (DOKS e pin)

Brand Names: U.S. Silenor
Index Terms Doxepin Hydrochloride
Pharmacologic Category Antidepressant, Tricyclic (Tertiary Amine)
Medication Safety Issues
Sound-alike/look-alike issues:
Doxepin may be confused with digoxin, doxapram, doxazosin, Doxidan®, doxycycline
SINEquan® may be confused with saquinavir, SEROquel®, Singulair®, Zonegran®
BEERS Criteria medication:
This drug may be potentially inappropriate for use in geriatric patients (Quality of evidence - high [moderate for SIADH]; Strength of recommendation - strong).
International issues:
Doxal [Finland] may be confused with Doxil brand name for doxorubicin (liposomal) [U.S., Israel]
Doxal brand name for doxepin [Finland] but also brand name for pyridoxine/thiamine [Brazil]
Medication Guide Available Yes
Pregnancy Risk Factor C
Lactation Enters breast milk/use caution
Use Depression; treatment of insomnia (with difficulty of sleep maintenance)
Unlabeled Use Analgesic for certain chronic and neuropathic pain; anxiety

Available Dosage Forms
Capsule, Oral:
Generic: 10 mg, 25 mg, 50 mg, 75 mg, 100 mg, 150 mg
Concentrate, Oral:
Generic: 10 mg/mL (118 mL, 120 mL)
Tablet, Oral:
Silenor: 3 mg, 6 mg
General Dosage Range Dosage adjustment recommended for oral route in patients with hepatic impairment
Oral:
Adults: Initial: 25-150 mg/day in 2-3 divided doses; Maintenance: Up to 300 mg/day in single (≤150 mg) or divided doses; 3-6 mg once daily prior to bedtime (insomnia)
Elderly: Initial: 10-25 mg at bedtime; Maintenance: Up to 75 mg at bedtime

Administration
Oral Do not mix oral concentrate with carbonated beverages (physically incompatible).
Silenor®: Administer within 30 minutes prior to bedtime; do not take within 3 hours of food

Nursing Actions
Physical Assessment Monitor CNS status. Be alert for signs of clinical worsening, suicidal ideation, or other changes in behavior. Taper dosage slowly when discontinuing.

Patient Education
• Discuss specific use of drug and side effects with patient as it relates to treatment. (HCAHPS: During this hospital stay, were you given any medicine that you had not taken before? Before giving you any new medicine, how often did hospital staff tell you what the medicine was for? How often did hospital staff describe possible side effects in a way you could understand?)
• Patient may experience fatigue, nausea, constipation, or xerostomia. Have patient report immediately to prescriber suicidal ideation, tachycardia, severe dizziness, syncope, illogical thinking, difficult urination, considerable asthenia, significant anxiety, ecchymosis, hemorrhaging, chills, hallucinations, paresthesia, difficulty with motor activity, fasciculations, change in balance, dysphagia, difficulty speaking, vision changes, jaundice, intolerable headache, or sexual dysfunction (HCAHPS).
• Educate patient about signs of a significant reaction (eg, wheezing; chest tightness; fever; itching; bad cough; blue skin color; seizures; or swelling of face, lips, tongue, or throat). **Note:** This is not a comprehensive list of all side effects. Patient should consult prescriber for additional questions.

Intended Use and Disclaimer: Should not be printed and given to patients. This information is intended to serve as a concise initial reference for healthcare professionals to use when discussing medications with a patient. You must ultimately

rely on your own discretion, experience and judgment in diagnosing, treating and advising patients.

Doxepin (Topical) (DOKS e pin)

Brand Names: U.S. Prudoxin; Zonalon
Index Terms Doxepin Hydrochloride
Pharmacologic Category Topical Skin Product
Medication Safety Issues
  Sound-alike/look-alike issues:
    Doxepin may be confused with digoxin, doxapram, doxazosin, Doxidan®, doxycycline
    Zonalon® may be confused with Zone-A®
  International issues:
    Doxal [Finland] may be confused with Doxil brand name for doxorubicin (liposomal) [U.S., Israel]
    Doxal brand name for doxepin [Finland] but also brand name for pyridoxine/thiamine [Brazil]
Pregnancy Risk Factor B
Lactation Enters breast milk/not recommended
Use Short-term (<8 days) management of moderate pruritus in adults with atopic dermatitis or lichen simplex chronicus
Unlabeled Use Cream: Treatment of burning mouth syndrome and neuropathic pain
Available Dosage Forms
  Cream, External:
    Prudoxin: 5% (45 g)
    Zonalon: 5% (30 g, 45 g)
General Dosage Range
  Dental: *Adults:* Apply 3-4 times/day
  Topical: *Adults:* Apply a thin film 4 times/day (maximum total therapy: 8 days)
Administration
  Topical Apply thin film to affected area; use of occlusive dressings is not recommended.
Nursing Actions
  Patient Education
- Discuss specific use of drug and side effects with patient as it relates to treatment. (HCAHPS: During this hospital stay, were you given any medicine that you had not taken before? Before giving you any new medicine, how often did hospital staff tell you what the medicine was for? How often did hospital staff describe possible side effects in a way you could understand?)
- Patient may experience dizziness, fatigue, xeroderma, xerostomia, headache, dysgeusia, or polydipsia. Have patient report immediately to prescriber paresthesia, mood changes, illogical thinking, edema, blurred vision, tachycardia, arrhythmia, severe asthenia, or considerable application site irritation (HCAHPS).
- Educate patient about signs of a significant reaction (eg, wheezing; chest tightness; fever; itching; bad cough; blue skin color; seizures; or swelling of face, lips, tongue, or throat). **Note:** This is not a comprehensive list of all side effects. Patient should consult prescriber for additional questions.

Intended Use and Disclaimer: Should not be printed and given to patients. This information is intended to serve as a concise initial reference for healthcare professionals to use when discussing medications with a patient. You must ultimately rely on your own discretion, experience and judgment in diagnosing, treating and advising patients.

Doxercalciferol (doks er kal si fe FEER ole)

Brand Names: U.S. Hectorol
Index Terms 1α-Hydroxyergocalciferol
Pharmacologic Category Vitamin D Analog
Pregnancy Risk Factor B
Lactation Excretion in breast milk unknown/not recommended
Use Treatment of secondary hyperparathyroidism in patients with chronic kidney disease
Available Dosage Forms
  Capsule, Oral:
    Hectorol: 0.5 mcg, 1 mcg, 2.5 mcg
    Generic: 0.5 mcg, 1 mcg, 2.5 mcg
  Solution, Intravenous:
    Hectorol: 2 mcg/mL (1 mL); 4 mcg/2 mL (2 mL)
    Generic: 4 mcg/2 mL (2 mL)
General Dosage Range
  I.V.: *Adults:* Initial: 4 mcg 3 times/week after dialysis; Maintenance: Up to 18 mcg/week
  Oral:
    Adults (dialysis patients): Initial: 10 mcg 3 times/week at dialysis; Maintenance: Up to 60 mcg/week
    Adults (predialysis patients): Initial: 1 mcg/day; Maintenance: Up to 3.5 mcg/day
Nursing Actions
  Physical Assessment Provide appropriate nutritional counseling.

  Patient Education
- Discuss specific use of drug and side effects with patient as it relates to treatment. (HCAHPS: During this hospital stay, were you given any medicine that you had not taken before? Before giving you any new medicine, how often did hospital staff tell you what the medicine was for? How often did hospital staff describe possible side effects in a way you could understand?)
- Patient may experience headache, dizziness, insomnia, nausea, pyrosis, arthralgia, or weight gain. Have patient report immediately to prescriber signs of hypercalcemia, xerostomia, polydipsia, polyuria, arrhythmia, lack of appetite, dysgeusia, myalgia, bradycardia, or edema (HCAHPS).

- Educate patient about signs of a significant reaction (eg, wheezing; chest tightness; fever; itching; bad cough; blue skin color; seizures; or swelling of face, lips, tongue, or throat). **Note:** This is not a comprehensive list of all side effects. Patient should consult prescriber for additional questions.

Intended Use and Disclaimer: Should not be printed and given to patients. This information is intended to serve as a concise initial reference for healthcare professionals to use when discussing medications with a patient. You must ultimately rely on your own discretion, experience and judgment in diagnosing, treating and advising patients.

DOXOrubicin (Conventional)
(doks oh ROO bi sin con VEN sha nal)

Brand Names: U.S. Adriamycin
Index Terms ADR (error-prone abbreviation); Adria; Conventional Doxorubicin; Doxorubicin HCl; Doxorubicin Hydrochloride; Hydroxydaunomycin Hydrochloride; Hydroxyldaunorubicin Hydrochloride
Pharmacologic Category Antineoplastic Agent, Anthracycline; Antineoplastic Agent, Topoisomerase II Inhibitor
Medication Safety Issues
Sound-alike/look-alike issues:
DOXOrubicin may be confused with DACTINomycin, DAUNOrubicin, DAUNOrubicin liposomal, doxapram, doxazosin, DOXOrubicin liposomal, epirubicin, IDArubicin, valrubicin
Adriamycin PFS may be confused with achromycin, Aredia, Idamycin
Conventional formulation (Adriamycin PFS, Adriamycin RDF) may be confused with the liposomal formulation (Doxil)
High alert medication:
This medication is in a class the Institute for Safe Medication Practices (ISMP) includes among its list of drug classes which have a heightened risk of causing significant patient harm when used in error.
Administration issues:
Use caution when selecting product for preparation and dispensing; indications, dosages and adverse event profiles differ between conventional DOXOrubicin hydrochloride solution and DOXOrubicin liposomal. Both formulations are the same concentration. As a result, serious errors have occurred.
Other safety concerns:
ADR is an error-prone abbreviation
International issues:
Doxil may be confused with Doxal which is a brand name for doxepin in Finland, a brand name for doxycycline in Austria, and a brand name for pyridoxine/thiamine combination in Brazil

Rubex, a discontinued brand name for DOXOrubicin in the U.S, is a brand name for ascorbic acid in Ireland
Pregnancy Risk Factor D
Lactation Enters breast milk/not recommended
Breast-Feeding Considerations Doxorubicin and its metabolites are excreted in breast milk. Due to the potential for serious adverse reactions in the nursing infant, the manufacturer recommends a decision be made whether to discontinue nursing or to discontinue the drug, taking into account the importance of treatment to the mother. Per the NCCN guidelines (v3.2013), breast-feeding after breast-conserving treatment for breast cancer is not contraindicated; however, the quantity and quality of breast milk may not be sufficient or may be lacking some nutrients needed.
Use
Breast cancer: Treatment component of adjuvant therapy in women with evidence of axillary lymph node involvement following resection of primary breast cancer
Metastatic cancers or disseminated neoplastic conditions: Treatment of acute lymphoblastic leukemia, acute myeloid leukemia, Wilms tumor, neuroblastoma, soft tissue and bone sarcomas, breast cancer, ovarian cancer, transitional cell bladder carcinoma, thyroid carcinoma, gastric carcinoma, Hodgkin lymphoma, non-Hodgkin lymphoma, and bronchogenic carcinoma in which the small cell histologic type is the most responsive compared with other cell types
Unlabeled Use Treatment of multiple myeloma, endometrial carcinoma, uterine sarcoma, head and neck cancer, liver cancer, kidney cancer, thymomas and thymic malignancies, Waldenström's macroglobulinemia
Mechanism of Action/Effect Inhibits DNA and RNA synthesis, active throughout cell cycle, results in cell death.
Contraindications Hypersensitivity (including anaphylaxis) to doxorubicin, any component of the formulation, or to other anthracyclines or anthracenediones; recent MI (within past 4-6 weeks), severe myocardial insufficiency, severe arrhythmia; previous therapy with high cumulative doses of doxorubicin, daunorubicin, idarubicin, or other anthracycline and anthracenediones; severe persistent drug-induced myelosuppression or baseline neutrophil count <1500/mm³; severe hepatic impairment (Child-Pugh class C or bilirubin >5 mg/dL)
Warnings/Precautions Hazardous agent - use appropriate precautions for handling and disposal (NIOSH, 2012). **[U.S. Boxed Warning]: May cause cumulative, dose-related, myocardial toxicity (early or delayed, including acute left ventricular failure and HF). The risk of cardiomyopathy increases with cumulative exposure and with concomitant cardiotoxic therapy; the incidence of irreversible myocardial toxicity**

increases as the total cumulative (lifetime) dosages approach 300-500 mg/m². Assess left ventricular ejection fraction (LVEF) with either an echocardiogram or MUGA scan before, during, and after therapy; increase the frequency of assessments as the cumulative dose exceeds 300 mg/m². Cardiotoxicity is dose-limiting. Delayed cardiotoxicity may occur late in treatment or within months to years after completion of therapy, and is typically manifested by LVEF reduction and/or heart failure (may be life threatening). Subacute effects such as pericarditis and myocarditis may also occur. Early toxicity may consist of tachyarrhythmias, including sinus tachycardia, premature ventricular contractions, and ventricular tachycardia, as well as bradycardia. Electrocardiographic changes including ST-T wave changes, atrioventricular and bundle-branch block have also been reported. These effects are not necessarily predictive of subsequent delayed cardiotoxicity. Total cumulative dose should take into account prior treatment with other anthracyclines or anthracenediones, previous or concomitant treatment with other cardiotoxic agents or irradiation of chest. Although the risk increases with cumulative dose, irreversible cardiotoxicity may occur at any dose level. Patients with active or dominant cardiovascular disease, concurrent administration of cardiotoxic drugs, prior therapy with other anthracyclines or anthracenediones, prior or concurrent chest irradiation, advanced age, and infants and children are at increased risk. Alternative administration schedules (weekly or continuous infusions) are associated with less cardiotoxicity.

[U.S. Boxed Warning]: Vesicant; if extravasation occurs, severe local tissue damage leading to tissue injury, blistering, ulceration, and necrosis may occur. Discontinue infusion immediately and apply ice to the affected area. For I.V. administration only. Do not administer I.M. or SubQ. Ensure proper needle or catheter placement prior to and during infusion. Avoid extravasation.

[U.S. Boxed Warning]: May cause severe myelosuppression, which may result in serious infection, septic shock, transfusion requirements, hospitalization, and death. Myelosuppression may be dose-limiting and primarily manifests as leukopenia and neutropenia; anemia and thrombocytopenia may also occur. The nadir typically occurs 10 to 14 days after administration with cell count recovery around day 21. Monitor blood counts at baseline and regularly during therapy.

[U.S. Boxed Warning]: Secondary acute myelogenous leukemia (AML) and myelodysplastic syndrome (MDS) have been reported following treatment. AML and MDS typically occur within one to three years of treatment; risk factors for development of secondary AML or MDS include treatment with anthracyclines in combination with DNA-damaging antineoplastics (eg, alkylating agents) and/or radiation therapy, heavily pretreated patients, and escalated anthracycline doses. May cause tumor lysis syndrome and hyperuricemia (in patients with rapidly growing tumors). Urinary alkalinization and prophylaxis with an antihyperuricemic agent may be necessary. Monitor electrolytes, renal function, and hydration status. [U.S. Boxed Warning]: Dosage modification is recommended in patients with impaired hepatic function; toxicities may be increased in patients with hepatic impairment. Use is contraindicated in patients with severe impairment (Child-Pugh class C or bilirubin >5 mg/dL). Monitor hepatic function tests (eg, transaminases, alkaline phosphatase, and bilirubin) closely. Use with caution in patients who have received radiation therapy; radiation recall may occur. May increase radiation-induced toxicity to the myocardium, mucosa, skin, and liver. Doxorubicin is associated with a moderate or high emetic potential (depending on dose or regimen); antiemetics are recommended to prevent nausea and vomiting (Basch, 2011). Potentially significant drug-drug interactions may exist, requiring dose or frequency adjustment, additional monitoring, and/or selection of alternative therapy.

In men, doxorubicin may damage spermatozoa and testicular tissue, resulting in possible genetic fetal abnormalities; may also result in oligospermia, azoospermia, and permanent loss of fertility (sperm counts have been reported to return to normal levels in some men, occurring several years after the end of therapy). In females of reproductive potential, doxorubicin may cause infertility and result in amenorrhea; premature menopause can occur. Children are at increased risk for developing delayed cardiotoxicity; long-term cardiac function monitoring is recommended. Doxorubicin may contribute to prepubertal growth failure in children; may also contribute to gonadal impairment (usually temporary). Radiation recall pneumonitis has been reported in children receiving concomitant dactinomycin and doxorubicin. [U.S. Boxed Warning]: Should be administered under the supervision of an experienced cancer chemotherapy physician. Use caution when selecting product for preparation and dispensing; indications, dosages and adverse event profiles differ between conventional doxorubicin hydrochloride solution and doxorubicin liposomal. Both formulations are the same concentration. As a result, serious errors have occurred.

Drug Interactions

Avoid Concomitant Use

Avoid concomitant use of DOXOrubicin (Conventional) with any of the following: BCG; CloZAPine; Dabigatran Etexilate; Fusidic Acid (Systemic); Natalizumab; Pimecrolimus; Pimozide; Pomalidomide; Sofosbuvir; Tacrolimus (Topical); Tofacitinib; Vaccines (Live); VinCRIStine (Liposomal)

Decreased Effect

DOXOrubicin (Conventional) may decrease the levels/effects of: Afatinib; BCG; Cardiac Glycosides; Coccidioidin Skin Test; Dabigatran Etexilate; Linagliptin; P-glycoprotein/ABCB1 Substrates; Pomalidomide; Sipuleucel-T; Sofosbuvir; Stavudine; Vaccines (Inactivated); Vaccines (Live); VinCRIStine (Liposomal); Vitamin K Antagonists; Zidovudine

The levels/effects of DOXOrubicin (Conventional) may be decreased by: Bosentan; Cardiac Glycosides; CYP3A4 Inducers (Strong); Dabrafenib; Deferasirox; Dexrazoxane; Echinacea; Herbs (CYP3A4 Inducers); Peginterferon Alfa-2b; P-glycoprotein/ABCB1 Inducers; Tocilizumab

Increased Effect/Toxicity

DOXOrubicin (Conventional) may increase the levels/effects of: ARIPiprazole; CloZAPine; CYP2B6 Substrates; Dofetilide; Leflunomide; Lomitapide; Mercaptopurine; Natalizumab; Pimozide; Tofacitinib; Vaccines (Live); Vitamin K Antagonists; Zidovudine

The levels/effects of DOXOrubicin (Conventional) may be increased by: Abiraterone Acetate; Bevacizumab; Cyclophosphamide; CycloSPORINE (Systemic); CYP2D6 Inhibitors (Moderate); CYP2D6 Inhibitors (Strong); CYP3A4 Inhibitors (Moderate); CYP3A4 Inhibitors (Strong); Dasatinib; Denosumab; Fusidic Acid (Systemic); Ivacaftor; Luliconazole; Mifepristone; P-glycoprotein/ABCB1 Inhibitors; Pimecrolimus; Roflumilast; Simeprevir; SORAfenib; Tacrolimus (Topical); Taxane Derivatives; Trastuzumab

Nutritional/Ethanol Interactions Herb/Nutraceutical: Avoid St John's wort (may decrease doxorubicin levels). Avoid black cohosh, dong quai in estrogen-dependent tumors.

Adverse Reactions Frequency not defined.

Cardiovascular:

Acute cardiotoxicity: Atrioventricular block, bradycardia, bundle branch block, ECG abnormalities, extrasystoles (atrial or ventricular), sinus tachycardia, ST-T wave changes, supraventricular tachycardia, tachyarrhythmia, ventricular tachycardia

Delayed cardiotoxicity: LVEF decreased, CHF (manifestations include ascites, cardiomegaly, dyspnea, edema, gallop rhythm, hepatomegaly, oliguria, pleural effusion, pulmonary edema, tachycardia); myocarditis, pericarditis

Central nervous system: Malaise

Dermatologic: Alopecia, itching, photosensitivity, radiation recall, rash; discoloration of saliva, sweat, or tears

Endocrine & metabolic: Amenorrhea, dehydration, infertility (may be temporary), hyperuricemia

Gastrointestinal: Abdominal pain, anorexia, colon necrosis, diarrhea, GI ulceration, mucositis, nausea, vomiting

Genitourinary: Discoloration of urine

Hematologic: Leukopenia/neutropenia (75%; nadir: 10-14 days; recovery: by day 21); thrombocytopenia and anemia

Local: Skin "flare" at injection site, urticaria

Neuromuscular & skeletal: Weakness

Available Dosage Forms

Solution, Intravenous:

Adriamycin: 2 mg/mL (5 mL, 10 mL, 25 mL, 100 mL)

Generic: 2 mg/mL (5 mL, 10 mL, 25 mL, 100 mL)

Solution, Intravenous [preservative free]:

Generic: 2 mg/mL (5 mL, 10 mL, 25 mL, 75 mL, 100 mL)

Solution Reconstituted, Intravenous:

Adriamycin: 10 mg (1 ea); 20 mg (1 ea); 50 mg (1 ea)

Generic: 50 mg (1 ea)

Solution Reconstituted, Intravenous [preservative free]:

Generic: 10 mg (1 ea)

General Dosage Range Dosage adjustment recommended in patients with hepatic impairment or who develop toxicities

I.V.: *Children, Adolescents, and Adults:* Dosage varies greatly depending on indication

Administration

I.V. Administer I.V. push over at least 3-10 minutes or by continuous infusion (infusion via central venous line recommended). Do not administer I.M. or SubQ. Rate of administration varies by protocol, refer to individual protocol for details. Protect from light until completion of infusion. Avoid contact with alkaline solutions. Monitor for local erythematous streaking along vein and/or facial flushing (may indicate rapid infusion rate); decrease rate if occurs. Doxorubicin is associated with a moderate to high emetic potential (depending on dose or regimen); antiemetics are recommended to prevent nausea and vomiting (Basch, 2011).

Vesicant; ensure proper needle or catheter placement prior to and during infusion; avoid extravasation.

Extravasation management: If extravasation occurs, stop infusion immediately and disconnect (leave cannula/needle in place); gently aspirate extravasated solution (do **NOT** flush the line); remove needle/cannula; elevate extremity. Initiate antidote (dexrazoxane or dimethyl sulfate [DMSO]). Apply dry cold compresses for 20 minutes 4 times daily for 1-2 days (Perez Fidalgo, 2012); withhold cooling beginning 15 minutes before dexrazoxane infusion; continue withholding cooling until 15 minutes after infusion is completed. Topical DMSO should not be administered in combination with dexrazoxane; may lessen dexrazoxane efficacy.

Dexrazoxane: Adults: 1000 mg/m^2 (maximum dose: 2000 mg) I.V. (administer in a large vein remote from site of extravasation) over 1-2 hours days 1 and 2, then 500 mg/m^2 (maximum dose: 1000 mg) I.V. over 1-2 hours day 3; begin within 6 hours of extravasation. Day 2 and day 3 doses should be administered at approximately the same time (± 3 hours) as the dose on day 1 (Mouridsen, 2007; Perez Fidalgo, 2012). **Note:** Reduce dexrazoxane dose by 50% in patients with moderate to severe renal impairment (CrCl <40 mL/minute).

DMSO: Children and Adults: Apply topically to a region covering twice the affected area every 8 hours for 7 days; begin within 10 minutes of extravasation; do not cover with a dressing (Perez Fidalgo, 2012).

Hazardous agent; use appropriate precautions for handling and disposal (NIOSH, 2012).

Injectable Detail pH: 3.8-6.5 (lyophilized doxorubicin HCl reconstituted with sodium chloride 0.9%); 2.5-4.5 (adjusted solution)

Preparation for Administration Hazardous agent; use appropriate precautions for handling and disposal (NIOSH, 2012). Reconstitute lyophilized powder with NS (using 5 mL for the 10 mg vial; 10 mL for the 20 mg vial; or 25 mL for the 50 mg vial) to a final concentration of 2 mg/mL; gently shake until contents are dissolved. May further dilute doxorubicin solution or reconstituted doxorubicin solution in 50-1000 mL D$_5$W or NS for infusion. Unstable in solutions with a pH <3 or >7.

Storage/Stability
Lyophilized powder: Store powder at 20°C to 25°C (68°F to 77°F). Protect from light. Retain in carton until time of use. Discard unused portion from single-dose vials. Reconstituted doxorubicin is stable for 7 days at room temperature under normal room lighting and for 15 days when refrigerated at 2°C to 8°C (36°F to 46°F). Protect reconstituted solution from light.

Solution: Store refrigerated at 2°C to 8°C (36°F to 46°F). Protect from light. Retain in carton until time of use. Discard unused portion. Storage of vials of solution under refrigeration may result in formation of a gelled product; if gelling occurs, place vials at room temperature for 2-4 hours to return the product to a slightly viscous, mobile solution.

Nursing Actions
Physical Assessment Premedication with antiemetic may be ordered (especially with larger doses). Monitor infusion site closely; extravasation can cause sloughing or tissue necrosis (do not apply heat or sodium bicarbonate). Teach patient importance of adequate hydration.

Patient Education
• Discuss specific use of drug and side effects with patient as it relates to treatment. (HCAHPS: During this hospital stay, were you given any

medicine that you had not taken before? Before giving you any new medicine, how often did hospital staff tell you what the medicine was for? How often did hospital staff describe possible side effects in a way you could understand?)
• Patient may experience diarrhea, lack of appetite, stomatitis, alopecia, or urine discoloration. Have patient report immediately to prescriber signs of infection, severe nausea, ecchymosis, hemorrhaging, considerable asthenia, or paresthesia (HCAHPS).
• Educate patient about signs of a significant reaction (eg, wheezing; chest tightness; fever; itching; bad cough; blue skin color; seizures; or swelling of face, lips, tongue, or throat). **Note:** This is not a comprehensive list of all side effects. Patient should consult prescriber for additional questions.

Intended Use and Disclaimer: Should not be printed and given to patients. This information is intended to serve as a concise initial reference for healthcare professionals to use when discussing medications with a patient. You must ultimately rely on your own discretion, experience and judgment in diagnosing, treating and advising patients.

Related Information
Management of Drug Extravasations *on page 1700*

DOXOrubicin (Liposomal)
(doks oh ROO bi sin lye po SO mal)

Brand Names: U.S. Doxil; Lipodox; Lipodox 50
Index Terms DOXOrubicin Hydrochloride (Liposomal); DOXOrubicin Hydrochloride Encapsulated Liposomes (Myocet™); DOXOrubicin Hydrochloride Liposome; DOXOrubicin Hydrochloride Liposomes (Myocet™); Lipodox; Liposomal DOXOrubicin; Pegylated DOXOrubicin Liposomal; Pegylated Liposomal DOXOrubicin; Pegylated Liposomal DOXOrubicin Hydrochloride (Doxil®, Caelyx®)
Pharmacologic Category Antineoplastic Agent, Anthracycline; Antineoplastic Agent, Topoisomerase II Inhibitor
Medication Safety Issues
Sound-alike/look-alike issues:
DOXOrubicin liposomal may be confused with DACTINomycin, DAUNOrubicin, DAUNOrubicin liposomal, doxapram, doxazosin, DOXOrubicin, epirubicin, IDArubicin, valrubicin
DOXOrubicin liposomal may be confused with DAUNOrubicin liposomal
Doxil® may be confused with Doxy 100™, Paxil®
Liposomal formulation (Doxil®) may be confused with the conventional formulation (Adriamycin PFS®, Adriamycin RDF®)
High alert medication:
This medication is in a class the Institute for Safe Medication Practices (ISMP) includes among its

list of drug classes which have a heightened risk of causing significant patient harm when used in error.

Administration issues:
Use caution when selecting product for preparation and dispensing; indications, dosages and adverse event profiles differ between conventional DOXOrubicin hydrochloride solution and DOXOrubicin liposomal. Both formulations are the same concentration. As a result, serious errors have occurred. Liposomal formulation of doxorubicin should NOT be substituted for doxorubicin hydrochloride on a mg-per-mg basis.

International issues:
Caelyx® [Canada] may be confused with Myocet™ [Canada]; product formulations and indications differ

Doxil [U.S., Israel] may be confused with Doxal brand name for doxepin [Finland] and pyridoxine/thiamine [Brazil]

Pregnancy Risk Factor D

Lactation Excretion in breast milk unknown/not recommended

Breast-Feeding Considerations Due to the potential for serious adverse reactions in the nursing infant, breast-feeding should be discontinued during treatment.

Use
U.S. labeling: Treatment of ovarian cancer (progressive or recurrent after platinum-based treatment); multiple myeloma (in combination with bortezomib in patients who are bortezomib naïve and after failure of at least 1 prior therapy); AIDS-related Kaposi's sarcoma (after failure of or intolerance to prior systemic therapy)

Canadian labeling: Treatment of metastatic breast cancer (as monotherapy [Caelyx®] or in combination with cyclophosphamide [Myocet™]); advanced ovarian cancer (after failure of first-line treatment [Caelyx®]); AIDS-related Kaposi's sarcoma (after failure of or intolerance to prior systemic therapy [Caelyx®])

Unlabeled Use Treatment of metastatic breast cancer, Hodgkin lymphoma (salvage treatment), cutaneous T-cell lymphomas (mycosis fungoides and Sézary syndrome), advanced soft tissue sarcomas; advanced or recurrent uterine sarcoma

Mechanism of Action/Effect Inhibits DNA and RNA synthesis of susceptible bacteria, active throughout cell cycle, results in cell death

Contraindications Hypersensitivity to doxorubicin liposomal, conventional doxorubicin, or any component of the formulation

Canadian labeling (Caelyx®): Additional contraindications (not in U.S. labeling): Breast-feeding

Warnings/Precautions Hazardous agent - use appropriate precautions for handling and disposal (NIOSH, 2012).

[U.S. Boxed Warning]: Doxorubicin may cause cumulative, dose-related myocardial toxicity

may lead to congestive heart failure as the cumulative (lifetime) dose of pegylated doxorubicin liposomal approaches 550 mg/m^2. When calculating cumulative doses, also include prior dose of other anthracyclines and anthracenediones. Cardiotoxicity may occur at lower cumulative doses (400 mg/m^2) in patients who have received prior mediastinal irradiation or are receiving concurrent cyclophosphamide treatment. For Myocet™ (Canadian availability), cardiotoxicity may occur as the cumulative (lifetime) dose approaches 750 mg/m^2. Anthracycline-induced cardiotoxicity may be delayed (after discontinuation of anthracycline treatment). Use only if potential benefits outweigh cardiovascular risk in patients with a history of cardiovascular disease. Monitor cardiac function with biopsy, echocardiography, or MUGA scan; evaluate left ventricular ejection fraction (LVEF) prior to treatment and periodically during treatment; if results indicate possible heart failure, carefully evaluate the potential effects of continued treatment.

[U.S. Boxed Warning]: Acute infusion reactions may occur, some may be serious/life-threatening (eg, allergic or anaphylactoid reactions). Reactions may include flushing, dyspnea, facial swelling, headache, chills, back pain, hypotension, and/or chest/throat tightness. Infusion reactions typically occur with the first dose and usually resolve with within several hours to a day after terminating the infusion; some have resolved with slowing the infusion rate. To minimize the risk of infusion reactions, infuse at an initial rate of 1 mg/minute. Medications for the treatment of reactions should be readily available in the event of severe reaction.

[U.S. Boxed Warning]: Use with caution in patients with hepatic impairment; dosage reduction is recommended. Use in patients with hepatic impairment has not been adequately studied; no dosing adjustment recommendations are available for multiple myeloma patients with hepatic impairment. **[U.S. Boxed Warning]: Severe myelosuppression may occur.** Monitor blood counts. Treatment delay, dosage modification, or discontinuation may be required. Leukopenia is usually transient, although persistent or severe neutropenia may result in superinfection or neutropenic fever; sepsis due to neutropenia has resulted in discontinuation (may rarely be fatal). Hemorrhage due to thrombocytopenia may occur. Hematologic toxicity may be more severe with combination chemotherapy. Palmar-plantar erythrodysesthesia (hand-foot syndrome) has been reported, more commonly in patients with ovarian cancer and multiple myeloma, and less commonly in patients with Kaposi's sarcoma. May occur early in treatment, but is usually seen after 2-3 treatment cycles. Dosage modification may be required; mild cases resolve within 1-2 weeks; in severe cases, treatment discontinuation may be required. Use of Caelyx® (Canadian availability) in splenectomized patients with AIDS-related Kaposi's sarcoma is not recommended (has not been studied). **[U.S. Boxed Warning]: Liposomal formulations of doxorubicin should NOT be substituted for conventional doxorubicin hydrochloride on a mg-per-mg basis.**

Cases of secondary oral cancers (primarily squamous cell carcinoma) have been reported with long-term (>1 year) doxorubicin liposomal exposure; these secondary oral malignancies have occurred during treatment and up to 6 years after treatment. The development of oral ulceration or discomfort should be monitored and further evaluated in patients with past or present use of doxorubicin liposomal. Tissue distribution of the liposomal doxorubicin compared to free doxorubicin may play a role in the development of oral secondary malignancies associated with long-term use.

Doxorubicin may potentiate the toxicity of cyclophosphamide (hemorrhagic cystitis) and mercaptopurine (hepatotoxicity). Radiation recall reaction has been reported with doxorubicin liposomal treatment after radiation therapy. Radiation-induced toxicity (to the myocardium, mucosa, skin, and liver) may be increased by doxorubicin.

Drug Interactions

Avoid Concomitant Use
Avoid concomitant use of DOXOrubicin (Liposomal) with any of the following: BCG; CloZAPine; Conivaptan; Fusidic Acid (Systemic); Natalizumab; Pimecrolimus; Tacrolimus (Topical); Tofacitinib; Vaccines (Live)

Decreased Effect
DOXOrubicin (Liposomal) may decrease the levels/effects of: BCG; Cardiac Glycosides; Coccidioidin Skin Test; Sipuleucel-T; Stavudine; Vaccines (Inactivated); Vaccines (Live); Zidovudine

The levels/effects of DOXOrubicin (Liposomal) may be decreased by: Bosentan; Cardiac Glycosides; CYP3A4 Inducers (Strong); Dabrafenib; Deferasirox; Echinacea; Herbs (CYP3A4 Inducers); Mitotane; Peginterferon Alfa-2b; Tocilizumab

Increased Effect/Toxicity
DOXOrubicin (Liposomal) may increase the levels/effects of: CloZAPine; CYP2B6 Substrates; Leflunomide; Natalizumab; Tofacitinib; Vaccines (Live); Zidovudine

The levels/effects of DOXOrubicin (Liposomal) may be increased by: Abiraterone Acetate; Bevacizumab; Conivaptan; Cyclophosphamide; CYP2D6 Inhibitors (Moderate); CYP2D6 Inhibitors (Strong); CYP3A4 Inhibitors (Moderate); CYP3A4 Inhibitors (Strong); Darunavir; Dasatinib; Denosumab; Fusidic Acid (Systemic); Ivacaftor; Luliconazole; Mifepristone; Pimecrolimus; Roflumilast; Simeprevir; Stiripentol; Tacrolimus (Topical); Taxane Derivatives; Trastuzumab

Nutritional/Ethanol Interactions
Ethanol: Avoid ethanol (due to GI irritation).
Herb/Nutraceutical: St John's wort may decrease doxorubicin levels.

Adverse Reactions
>10%:
Cardiovascular: Peripheral edema (≤11%)
Central nervous system: Fever (8% to 21%), headache (≤11%), pain (≤21%)
Dermatologic: Palmar-plantar erythrodysesthesia/hand-foot syndrome (≤51% in ovarian cancer [grades 3/4: 24%]; 3% in Kaposi's sarcoma), rash (≤29% in ovarian cancer, ≤5% in Kaposi's sarcoma), alopecia (9% to 19%)
Gastrointestinal: Nausea (17% to 46%), stomatitis (5% to 41%), vomiting (8% to 33%), constipation (≤30%), diarrhea (5% to 21%), anorexia (≤20%), mucositis (≤14%), dyspepsia (≤12%), intestinal obstruction (≤11%)
Hematologic: Myelosuppression (onset: 7 days; nadir: 10-14 days; recovery: 21-28 days), thrombocytopenia (13% to 65%; grades 3/4: 1%), neutropenia (12% to 62%; grade 4: 4%), leukopenia (36%), anemia (6% to 74%; grade 4: <1%)
Neuromuscular & skeletal: Weakness (7% to 40%), back pain (≤12%)
Respiratory: Pharyngitis (≤16%), dyspnea (≤15%)
Miscellaneous: Infection (≤12%)
1% to 10%:
Cardiovascular: Cardiac arrest, chest pain, deep thrombophlebitis, edema, hypotension, pallor, tachycardia, vasodilation
Central nervous system: Agitation, anxiety, chills, confusion, depression, dizziness, emotional lability, insomnia, somnolence, vertigo
Dermatologic: Acne, bruising, dry skin (6%), exfoliative dermatitis, fungal dermatitis, furunculosis, maculopapular rash, pruritus, skin discoloration, vesiculobullous rash
Endocrine & metabolic: Dehydration, hypercalcemia, hyperglycemia, hypokalemia, hyponatremia
Gastrointestinal: Abdomen enlarged, anorexia, ascites, cachexia, dyspepsia, dysphagia, esophagitis, flatulence, gingivitis, glossitis, ileus, mouth ulceration, oral moniliasis, rectal bleeding, taste perversion, weight loss, xerostomia
Genitourinary: Cystitis, dysuria, leukorrhea, pelvic pain, polyuria, urinary incontinence, urinary tract infection, urinary urgency, vaginal bleeding, vaginal moniliasis
Hematologic: Hemolysis, prothrombin time increased
Hepatic: ALT increased, alkaline phosphatase increased, hyperbilirubinemia
Local: Thrombophlebitis
Neuromuscular & skeletal: Arthralgia, hypertonia, myalgia, neuralgia, neuritis (peripheral), neuropathy, paresthesia (≤10%), pathological fracture

Ocular: Conjunctivitis, dry eyes, retinitis

Otic: Ear pain

Renal: Albuminuria, hematuria

Respiratory: Apnea, cough (≤10%), epistaxis, pleural effusion, pneumonia, rhinitis, sinusitis

Miscellaneous: Allergic reaction; infusion-related reactions (7%; includes bronchospasm, chest tightness, chills, dyspnea, facial edema, flushing, headache, herpes simplex/zoster, hypotension, pruritus); moniliasis, diaphoresis

Available Dosage Forms

Injectable, Intravenous:

Doxil: 2 mg/mL (10 mL, 25 mL)

Lipodox: 2 mg/mL (10 mL)

Lipodox 50: 2 mg/mL (25 mL)

Generic: 2 mg/mL (10 mL, 25 mL)

General Dosage Range Dosage adjustment recommended in patients with hepatic impairment or who develop toxicities

I.V.: *Adults:* 20-30 mg/m^2 every 3 weeks **or** 50 mg/m^2 every 4 weeks

Administration

I.V. Do not administer as a bolus injection or I.M. or SubQ. Avoid extravasation (irritant); monitor infusion site; extravasation may occur without stinging or burning. Monitor for infusion reaction.

Doxil®, Caelyx®: Administer IVPB over 60 minutes; manufacturer recommends administering at initial rate of 1 mg/minute to minimize risk of infusion reactions until the absence of a reaction has been established, then increase the infusion rate for completion over 1 hour. Do **NOT** administer undiluted. Do **NOT** infuse with in-line filters. Incompatible with heparin flushes; flush with 5-10 mL of D$_5$W solution before and after drug administration (do not rapidly flush through the I.V. line). Monitor for local erythematous streaking along vein and/or facial flushing (may indicate rapid infusion rate).

Myocet™: Infuse over 1 hour.

Hazardous agent; use appropriate precautions for handling and disposal (NIOSH, 2012).

Preparation for Administration Hazardous agent; use appropriate precautions for handling and disposal (NIOSH, 2012).

Doxil®, Caelyx®: Doses ≤90 mg must be diluted in D$_5$W 250 mL prior to administration. Doses >90 mg should be diluted in D$_5$W 500 mL. Solution is not clear, but has a red, translucent appearance due to the liposomal dispersion. Dilute only in D$_5$W; do not use bacteriostatic agents; do not mix with other medications.

Myocet™: Refer to product labeling for detailed reconstitution and preparation information.

Storage/Stability Store intact vials refrigerated at 2°C to 8°C (36°F to 46°F); avoid freezing.

Doxil®, Caelyx®: Prolonged freezing may adversely affect liposomal drug products, however, short-term freezing (<1 month) does not appear to have a deleterious effect (Doxil®). Solutions diluted for infusion should be refrigerated at 2°C to 8°C (36°F to 46°F); administer within 24 hours. **Do not infuse with in-line filters.**

Myocet™: Refer to product labeling for detailed reconstitution and preparation information. Following reconstitution, may be stored up to 8 hours at room temperature or up to 72 hours refrigerated at 2°C to 8°C (36°F to 46°F); do not freeze.

Nursing Actions

Physical Assessment Radiation recall may be experienced with this drug, noted by a reddened, burned appearance over the area radiated. Note and be aware of past cumulative doxorubicin dose, as patients can develop cardiotoxicity. Obtain MUGA scan or ECHO prior to doxorubicin (liposomal) therapy to evaluate for ejection fraction. Verify drug is mixed in D$_5$W solution. If patient is at home and needs help with ADLs, thorough instruction on handling body fluids should be reviewed. This drug has a potential for hypersensitivity reactions and patients should be prescribed Benadryl® as a premedication. Monitor closely throughout infusion for HSR, as these have the potential to be fatal.

Patient Education

- Discuss specific use of drug and side effects with patient as it relates to treatment. (HCAHPS: During this hospital stay, were you given any medicine that you had not taken before? Before giving you any new medicine, how often did hospital staff tell you what the medicine was for? How often did hospital staff describe possible side effects in a way you could understand?)

- Patient may experience constipation, diarrhea, flu-like syndrome, lack of appetite, stomatitis, cheilitis, back pain, headache, alopecia, or urine or body fluid discoloration. Have patient report immediately to prescriber signs of infection, angina, severe nausea, excessive weight loss, osteodynia, night sweats, ecchymosis, hemorrhaging, paresthesia, eczema of hands or feet, considerable asthenia, significant skin irritation, or hematuria (HCAHPS).

- Educate patient about signs of a significant reaction (eg, wheezing; chest tightness; fever; itching; bad cough; blue skin color; seizures; or swelling of face, lips, tongue, or throat). **Note:** This is not a comprehensive list of all side effects. Patient should consult prescriber for additional questions.

Intended Use and Disclaimer: Should not be printed and given to patients. This information is intended to serve as a concise initial reference for healthcare professionals to use when discussing medications with a patient. You must ultimately rely on your own discretion, experience and judgment in diagnosing, treating and advising patients.

Related Information
Management of Drug Extravasations *on page 1700*

Doxycycline (doks i SYE kleen)

Brand Names: U.S. Adoxa; Adoxa Pak 1/100; Adoxa Pak 1/150; Adoxa Pak 2/100; Alodox Convenience; Avidoxy; Doryx; Doxy 100; Monodox; Morgidox; NicAzelDoxy 30; NicAzelDoxy 60; Ocudox; Oracea; Oraxyl [DSC]; Vibramycin

Index Terms Doxycycline Calcium; Doxycycline Hyclate; Doxycycline Monohydrate

Pharmacologic Category Antibiotic, Tetracycline Derivative

Medication Safety Issues
Sound-alike/look-alike issues:
Doxycycline may be confused with dicyclomine, doxepin, doxylamine
Doxy100 may be confused with Doxil
Monodox may be confused with Maalox
Oracea may be confused with Orencia
Vibramycin may be confused with vancomycin, Vibativ
International issues:
Oracea (U.S brand name) is marketed in Canada under the brand name Aprilon

Pregnancy Risk Factor D

Lactation Enters breast milk/not recommended

Breast-Feeding Considerations Doxycycline is excreted in breast milk (Chung, 2002). According to the manufacturer, the decision to continue or discontinue breast-feeding during therapy should take into account the risk of exposure to the infant and the benefits of treatment to the mother. Although nursing is not specifically contraindicated, the effects of long-term exposure via breast milk are not known. Oral absorption of doxycycline is not markedly influenced by simultaneous ingestion of milk; therefore, oral absorption of doxycycline by the breast-feeding infant would not be expected to be diminished by the calcium in the maternal milk. Nondose-related effects could include modification of bowel flora.

Use Principally in the treatment of infections caused by susceptible *Rickettsia*, *Chlamydia*, *Chlamydophila*, and *Mycoplasma*; malaria prophylaxis (areas with chloroquine- or pyrimethamine-sulfadoxine resistant strains) for short-term travel (<4 months); treatment for syphilis, uncomplicated *Neisseria gonorrhoeae* (alternative agent), *Listeria*, *Actinomyces israelii*, and *Clostridium* infections in penicillin-allergic patients; used for community-acquired pneumonia and other common infections due to susceptible organisms; anthrax due to *Bacillus anthracis,* including inhalational anthrax (postexposure); treatment of infections caused by uncommon susceptible gram-negative and gram-positive organisms including *Borrelia recurrentis, Ureaplasma urealyticum, Haemophilus ducreyi, Yersinia pestis, Francisella tularensis, Vibrio cholerae, Campylobacter fetus, Brucella* spp, *Bartonella bacilliformis,* and *Klebsiella granulomatis,* Q fever, Lyme disease; intestinal amebiasis; severe acne

Oracea® (U.S. labeling), Aprilon™ (Canadian labeling): Treatment of inflammatory lesions associated with rosacea

Periostat® (Canadian labeling; not available in U.S.): Adjunctive periodontitis treatment to scaling and root planing to promote attachment level gain and reduce pocket depth

Unlabeled Use Sclerosing agent for pleural effusion (injection); vancomycin-resistant enterococci (VRE); alternate treatment for MRSA infections; treatment of periodontitis (refractory); localized juvenile periodontitis (LJP); treatment of acute bacterial rhinosinusitis (ABRS) (adults); oral phase treatment of prosthetic joint infection; chronic oral antimicrobial suppression of prosthetic joint infection; anorectal gonococcal infections

Mechanism of Action/Effect Inhibits protein synthesis by binding with the 30S and possibly the 50S ribosomal subunit(s) of susceptible bacteria; may also cause alterations in the cytoplasmic membrane

Doxycycline inhibits collagenase *in vitro* and has been shown to inhibit collagenase in the gingival crevicular fluid in adults with periodontitis

Contraindications
U.S. labeling: Hypersensitivity to doxycycline, tetracycline or any component of the formulation
Canadian labeling: Hypersensitivity to doxycycline, tetracycline or any component of the formulation; myasthenia gravis

Periostat®, Aprilon™: Additional contraindications: Use in infants and children <8 years of age or during second or third trimester of pregnancy; breast-feeding

Warnings/Precautions Photosensitivity reaction may occur with this drug; avoid prolonged exposure to sunlight or tanning equipment. Antianabolic effects of tetracyclines can increase BUN (dose-related). Hypersensitivity syndromes have been reported, including drug rash with eosinophilia and systemic symptoms (DRESS), urticaria, angioneurotic edema, anaphylaxis, anaphylactoid purpura, serum sickness, pericarditis, and systemic lupus erythematosus exacerbation. Hepatotoxicity rarely occurs; if symptomatic, conduct LFT and discontinue drug. Intracranial hypertension (headache, blurred vision, diplopia, vision loss, and/or papilledema) has been associated with use. Women of childbearing age who are overweight or have a history of intracranial hypertension are at greater risk. Concomitant use of isotretinoin (known to cause pseudotumor cerebri) and doxycycline should be avoided. Intracranial hypertension typically resolves after discontinuation of treatment; however, permanent visual loss is possible. If visual symptoms develop during treatment, prompt ophthalmologic evaluation is warranted. Intracranial pressure can remain elevated for weeks after drug discontinuation; monitor patients until they stabilize. Prolonged use may result in fungal or bacterial superinfection, including *C. difficile*-associated diarrhea (CDAD) and pseudomembranous colitis; CDAD has been observed >2 months postantibiotic treatment. May cause tissue hyperpigmentation, tooth enamel hypoplasia, or permanent tooth discoloration; use of tetracyclines should be avoided during tooth development (last half or pregnancy, infancy, and children <8 years of age) unless other drugs are not likely to be effective or are contraindicated. However, recommended in treatment of anthrax exposure, tickborne rickettsial diseases, and Q fever. Do not use during pregnancy. In addition to affecting tooth development, tetracycline use has been associated with retardation of skeletal development and reduced bone growth. When used for malaria prophylaxis, does not completely suppress asexual blood stages of *Plasmodium* strains. Doxycycline does not suppress *Plasmodium falciparum*'s sexual blood stage gametocytes. Patients completing a regimen may still transmit the infection to mosquitoes outside endemic areas.

Oracea® (U.S. labeling) or Apprilon™ (Canadian labeling): Additional specific warnings: Should not be used for the treatment or prophylaxis of bacterial infections, since the lower dose of drug per capsule may be subefficacious and promote resistance. Syrup contains sodium metabisulfite. Effectiveness of products intended for use in periodontitis has not been established in patients with coexistent oral candidiasis; use with caution in patients with a history or predisposition to oral candidiasis.

Drug Interactions

Avoid Concomitant Use

Avoid concomitant use of Doxycycline with any of the following: BCG; Pimozide; Retinoic Acid Derivatives; Strontium Ranelate

Decreased Effect

Doxycycline may decrease the levels/effects of: BCG; Penicillins; Sodium Picosulfate; Typhoid Vaccine

The levels/effects of Doxycycline may be decreased by: Antacids; Barbiturates; Bile Acid Sequestrants; Bismuth; Bismuth Subsalicylate; Calcium Salts; CarBAMazepine; Fosphenytoin; Iron Salts; Lanthanum; Magnesium Salts; Multivitamins/Minerals (with ADEK, Folate, Iron); Multivitamins/Minerals (with AE, No Iron); Phenytoin; Quinapril; Rifampin; Strontium Ranelate; Sucralfate; Sucroferric Oxyhydroxide

Increased Effect/Toxicity

Doxycycline may increase the levels/effects of: ARIPiprazole; Dofetilide; Lomitapide; Mipomersen; Neuromuscular-Blocking Agents;

Pimozide; Porfimer; Retinoic Acid Derivatives; Vitamin K Antagonists

Nutritional/Ethanol Interactions

Ethanol: Chronic ethanol ingestion may reduce the serum concentration of doxycycline.

Food: Doxycycline serum levels may be slightly decreased if taken with food or milk. Doryx® tablets can be administered without regard to meals. Administration with iron or calcium may decrease doxycycline absorption. May decrease absorption of calcium, iron, magnesium, zinc, and amino acids.

Herb/Nutraceutical: St John's wort may decrease doxycycline levels. Avoid dong quai, St John's wort (may also cause photosensitization).

Adverse Reactions Frequency not always defined.

Central nervous system: Headache (2%), bulging fontanel (infants), intracranial hypertension (adults), pericarditis

Dermatologic: Discoloration of thyroid gland (brown/black, no dysfunction reported), erythema multiforme, erythematous rash, exfoliative dermatitis, maculopapular rash, skin hyperpigmentation, skin photosensitivity, Stevens-Johnson syndrome, toxic epidermal necrolysis, urticaria

Endocrine & metabolic: Hypoglycemia

Gastrointestinal: Nausea (13%), vomiting (8%), diarrhea (3%), upper abdominal pain (2%), anorexia, *Clostridium difficile* associated diarrhea, dental discoloration (children), dysphagia, enterocolitis, esophageal ulcer, esophagitis, glossitis

Genitourinary: Vaginitis (bacterial, 3%), vulvovaginal disease (mycotic infection, 2%), inflammatory anogenital lesion

Hematologic & oncologic: Anaphylactoid purpura, eosinophilia, hemolytic anemia, neutropenia, thrombocytopenia

Hepatic: Hepatotoxicity (rare)

Hypersensitivity: Anaphylaxis, angioedema, serum sickness

Neuromuscular & skeletal: Exacerbation of systemic lupus erythematosus

Renal: Increased blood urea nitrogen (dose related)

Note: Additional adverse reactions not listed above that have been reported with Oracea or Periostat (Canadian availability; not available in the U.S.):

Periostat: Arthralgia (6%), dyspepsia (6%), dysmenorrhea (4%), pain (4%), bronchitis (3%)

Oracea: Nasopharyngitis (5%), hypertension (3%), sinusitis (3%), anxiety (2%), fungal infection (2%), increased blood pressure (2%), increased lactate dehydrogenase (2%), increased serum AST (2%), influenza (2%), pain (2%), abdominal pain (1% to 2%), back pain (1%), hyperglycemia (1%), sinus headache (1%), xerostomia (1%)

◄ **Dosage Forms Considerations**

NizAzel Doxy kits contain doxycycline tablets 100 mg, plus NicAzel FORTE dietary supplement tablets

Available Dosage Forms

Capsule, Oral:
Adoxa: 150 mg
Monodox: 75 mg, 100 mg
Morgidox: 100 mg
Vibramycin: 100 mg
Generic: 50 mg, 75 mg, 100 mg, 150 mg

Capsule Delayed Release, Oral:
Oracea: 40 mg

Capsule Delayed Release Particles, Oral:
Generic: 100 mg

Kit, Combination:
Alodox Convenience: 20 mg
Morgidox: 1 x 100 mg, 2 x 100 mg
Ocudox: 50 mg

Kit, Oral:
NicAzelDoxy 30: 100 mg
NicAzelDoxy 60: 100 mg

Solution Reconstituted, Intravenous:
Generic: 100 mg (1 ea)

Solution Reconstituted, Intravenous [preservative free]:
Doxy 100: 100 mg (1 ea)
Generic: 100 mg (1 ea)

Suspension Reconstituted, Oral:
Vibramycin: 25 mg/5 mL (60 mL)
Generic: 25 mg/5 mL (60 mL)

Syrup, Oral:
Vibramycin: 50 mg/5 mL (473 mL)

Tablet, Oral:
Adoxa: 50 mg, 75 mg, 100 mg
Adoxa Pak 1/100: 100 mg
Adoxa Pak 2/100: 100 mg
Adoxa Pak 1/150: 150 mg
Avidoxy: 100 mg
Generic: 20 mg, 50 mg, 75 mg, 100 mg, 150 mg

Tablet Delayed Release, Oral:
Doryx: 150 mg, 200 mg
Generic: 75 mg, 100 mg, 150 mg

General Dosage Range

I.V.:
Children ≤8 years: 2.2 mg/kg every 12 hours
Children >8 years and ≤45 kg: 2-5 mg/kg/day in 1-2 divided doses (maximum: 200 mg/day)
Children >8 years and >45 kg and Adults: 100-200 mg/day in 1-2 divided doses

Oral:
Children ≤8 years: 2.2 mg/kg every 12 hours
Children >8 years and ≤45 kg: 2-5 mg/kg/day in 1-2 divided doses (maximum: 200 mg/day)
Children >8 years and >45 kg: 100-200 mg/day in 1-2 divided doses
Adults: 100-200 mg/day in 1-2 divided doses **or** 300 mg as a single dose **or** 40 mg/day in 1-2 divided doses

Administration

I.V. Infuse slowly, usually over 1-4 hours. Avoid extravasation. Oral administration is preferable unless patient has significant nausea and vomiting; I.V. and oral routes are bioequivalent.

Injectable Detail Avoid extravasation. Very irritating to vein; use central line if possible.

pH: 1.8-3.3 (reconstituted solution)

Oral Oral administration is preferable unless patient has significant nausea and vomiting; I.V. and oral routes are bioequivalent. May give with meals to decrease GI upset. Capsule and tablet: Administer with at least 8 ounces of water and have patient sit up for at least 30 minutes after taking to reduce the risk of esophageal irritation and ulceration.

Oracea® (U.S. labeling), Apprilon™ (Canadian labeling): Administer on an empty stomach 1 hour before or 2 hours after meals.

Doryx®: Administer without regard to meals; nausea occurs more frequently when taken on an empty stomach. May be administered by carefully breaking up the tablet and sprinkling tablet contents on a spoonful of cold applesauce. The delayed release pellets must not be crushed or damaged when breaking up tablet. Should be administered immediately after preparation and without chewing.

Periostat® (Canadian availability; not available in the U.S.): Administer 1 hour before breakfast and evening meal.

Other Intrapleural (unlabeled route): Add to 100 mL NS and instill into chest tube (Porcel, 2006)

Preparation for Administration I.V. infusion: Following reconstitution with sterile water for injection, dilute to a final concentration of 0.1-1 mg/mL using a compatible solution.

Storage/Stability

Syrup, oral suspension: All products are to be stored below 30°C (86°F) and dispensed in tight, light-resistant containers.

Capsule, tablet: Store at 20°C to 25°C (68°F to 77°F); excursions are permitted between 15°C and 30°C (59°F and 86°F). Dispense in a tight, light-resistant container.

I.V. infusion: Protect from light. Stability varies based on solution.

Nursing Actions

Physical Assessment Results of culture and sensitivity test and patient's allergy history should be assessed prior to beginning therapy. I.V.: Infusion site may be closely monitored; extravasation can be very irritating to veins (use of central line is preferable). Teach patient importance of adequate hydration and photosensitivity precautions.

Patient Education
• Discuss specific use of drug and side effects with patient as it relates to treatment. (HCAHPS: During this hospital stay, were you given any

medicine that you had not taken before? Before giving you any new medicine, how often did hospital staff tell you what the medicine was for? How often did hospital staff describe possible side effects in a way you could understand?)

• Patient may experience nausea, diarrhea, or lack of appetite. Have patient report immediately to prescriber signs of hepatic impairment, severe headache, angina, urinary retention, oliguria, chills, pharyngitis, dysphagia, ecchymosis, hemorrhaging, arthralgia, considerable asthenia, vaginal yeast infection, vision changes, erythema, or signs of pseudomembranous colitis (HCAHPS).

• Educate patient about signs of a significant reaction (eg, wheezing; chest tightness; fever; itching; bad cough; blue skin color; seizures; or swelling of face, lips, tongue, or throat). **Note:** This is not a comprehensive list of all side effects. Patient should consult prescriber for additional questions.

Intended Use and Disclaimer: Should not be printed and given to patients. This information is intended to serve as a concise initial reference for healthcare professionals to use when discussing medications with a patient. You must ultimately rely on your own discretion, experience and judgment in diagnosing, treating and advising patients.

Dietary Considerations
Tetracyclines (in general): Take with food if gastric irritation occurs. While administration with food may decrease GI absorption of doxycycline by up to 20%, administration on an empty stomach is not recommended due to GI intolerance. Of currently available tetracyclines, doxycycline has the least affinity for calcium.

Doryx® tablets: May be taken without regard to meals; nausea occurs more frequently when taken on an empty stomach.

Oracea® (U.S. labeling), Apprilon™ (Canadian labeling): Take on an empty stomach 1 hour before or 2 hours after meals.

Periostat® (Canadian availability; not available in the U.S.): Take at least 1 hour before morning and evening meals.

Some products may contain sodium.

Related Information
Oral Medications That Should Not Be Crushed or Altered *on page 1712*

Dronabinol (droe NAB i nol)

Brand Names: U.S. Marinol

Index Terms Delta-9 THC; Delta-9-tetrahydro-cannabinol; Tetrahydrocannabinol; THC

Pharmacologic Category Antiemetic; Appetite Stimulant

Medication Safety Issues
Sound-alike/look-alike issues:
Dronabinol may be confused with droperidol

Pregnancy Risk Factor C

Lactation Enters breast milk/not recommended

Use Chemotherapy-associated nausea and vomiting refractory to other antiemetic(s); AIDS-related anorexia

Unlabeled Use Cancer-related anorexia

Controlled Substance C-III

Available Dosage Forms
Capsule, Oral:
Marinol: 2.5 mg, 5 mg, 10 mg
Generic: 2.5 mg, 5 mg, 10 mg

General Dosage Range Oral:
Children: Initial: 5 mg/m^2 as a single dose; Maintenance: 5 mg/m^2/dose every 2-4 hours for a total of 4-6 doses/day (maximum: 15 mg/m^2/dose)
Adults: Initial: 5 mg/m^2 as a single dose; Maintenance: 5 mg/m^2/dose every 2-4 hours for a total of 4-6 doses/day (maximum: 15 mg/m^2/dose) **or** Initial: 2.5 mg twice daily; Maintenance: Titrate up to 20 mg/day in 2 divided doses

Nursing Actions
Physical Assessment Monitor for CNS changes, psychotic reactions; this drug is the psychoactive substance in marijuana.

Patient Education
• Discuss specific use of drug and side effects with patient as it relates to treatment. (HCAHPS: During this hospital stay, were you given any medicine that you had not taken before? Before giving you any new medicine, how often did hospital staff tell you what the medicine was for? How often did hospital staff describe possible side effects in a way you could understand?)

• Patient may experience fatigue, dyspepsia, nausea, or asthenia. Have patient report immediately to prescriber illogical thinking, severe dizziness, syncope, behavioral changes, mood changes, tachycardia, arrhythmia, hallucinations, memory loss, vision changes, or significant change in balance (HCAHPS).

• Educate patient about signs of a significant reaction (eg, wheezing; chest tightness; fever; itching; bad cough; blue skin color; seizures; or swelling of face, lips, tongue, or throat). **Note:** This is not a comprehensive list of all side effects. Patient should consult prescriber for additional questions.

Intended Use and Disclaimer: Should not be printed and given to patients. This information is intended to serve as a concise initial reference for healthcare professionals to use when discussing medications with a patient. You must ultimately rely on your own discretion, experience and judgment in diagnosing, treating and advising patients.

Dronedarone (droe NE da rone)

Brand Names: U.S. Multaq

Index Terms Dronedarone Hydrochloride; SR33589

Pharmacologic Category Antiarrhythmic Agent, Class III

Medication Safety Issues

BEERS Criteria medication:

This drug may be potentially inappropriate for use in geriatric patients (Quality of evidence - moderate/high; Strength of recommendation - strong).

Medication Guide Available Yes

Pregnancy Risk Factor X

Lactation Excretion in breast milk unknown/contraindicated

Breast-Feeding Considerations It is not known if dronedarone is excreted in breast milk. Due to the potential for serious adverse reactions in the nursing infant, breast-feeding contraindicated by the manufacturer.

Use Paroxysmal or persistent atrial fibrillation: To reduce the risk of hospitalization for atrial fibrillation (AF) in patients in sinus rhythm with a history of paroxysmal or persistent AF

Unlabeled Use Alternative antiarrhythmic for the treatment of atrial fibrillation in patients with hypertrophic cardiomyopathy (HCM)

Mechanism of Action/Effect A noniodinated antiarrhythmic agent structurally related to amiodarone exhibiting properties of all 4 antiarrhythmic classes. Dronedarone prolongs the action potential and refractory period in myocardial tissue, and slows heart rate through inhibition of calcium channels and beta$_1$-receptors.

Contraindications

Hypersensitivity to dronedarone or any component of the formulation; permanent AF (patients in whom normal sinus rhythm will not or cannot be restored); symptomatic heart failure (heart failure with recent decompensation requiring hospitalization or NYHA Class IV symptoms); liver or lung toxicity related to previous amiodarone use; second-degree or third-degree atrioventricular block or sick sinus syndrome (except when used in conjunction with a functioning artificial pacemaker); bradycardia <50 bpm; concomitant use of strong CYP3A4 inhibitors (eg, ketoconazole, itraconazole, voriconazole, cyclosporine, telithromycin, clarithromycin, nefazodone, ritonavir); concomitant use of drugs or herbal products known to prolong the QT interval increasing the risk for torsade de pointes (eg, phenothiazine antipsychotics, tricyclic antidepressants, certain oral macrolide antibiotics, class I and III antiarrhythmics); QT$_c$ (Bazett) interval ≥500 msec or PR interval >280 msec; severe hepatic impairment; pregnancy; breast-feeding

Canadian labeling: Additional contraindications (not in U.S. labeling): Permanent atrial fibrillation of any duration where sinus rhythm cannot be restored and further attempts to restore it are no longer considered; history of or current heart failure regardless of NYHA class; left ventricular systolic dysfunction; complete bundle branch block, distal block, sinus node dysfunction, or atrial conduction defects (except when used in conjunction with a functioning pacemaker); unstable hemodynamic condition

Warnings/Precautions Hazardous agent - use appropriate precautions for handling and disposal (NIOSH, 2012). **[U.S. Boxed Warning]: The risk of death is doubled when used in patients with symptomatic heart failure with recent decompensation requiring hospitalization or NYHA Class IV symptoms; use is contraindicated in these patients.** New-onset or worsening HF symptoms have been observed. If patient develops new or worsening HF symptoms (eg, weight gain, dependent edema, or increasing shortness of breath) requiring hospitalization while on therapy, discontinue dronedarone. Canadian labeling contraindicates use of dronedarone in patients with a history of or current heart failure, regardless of NYHA class.

[U.S. Boxed Warning]: Use in patients with permanent atrial fibrillation doubles the risk of death, stroke (especially within the first 2 weeks of therapy) and hospitalization for heart failure. Use is contraindicated in patients with AF who will not or cannot be converted to normal sinus rhythm. Monitor ECG at least every 3 months. Cardiovert patients who are in AF (if clinically indicated) or discontinue dronedarone. Initiate only in patients in sinus rhythm who are receiving appropriate antithrombotic therapy. Assess defibrillation threshold when initiating dronedarone and during therapy.

In the treatment of atrial fibrillation in the elderly, avoid antiarrhythmics as first-line treatment. In older adults, data suggests rate control may provide more benefits than risks compared to rhythm control for most patients. Avoid use in patients with permanent atrial fibrillation or heart failure (Beers Criteria).

Dronedarone induces a moderate prolongation of the QT interval (average ~10 msec); much greater effects have been observed. Use in patients with QT$_c$ (Bazett) interval ≥500 msec is contraindicated; discontinue use of dronedarone if this occurs during therapy. May produce a slight increase in serum creatinine (~0.1 mg/dL) within 7 days of initiation due to inhibition of tubular secretion; glomerular filtration rate is not affected; effect is reversible upon discontinuation. Marked increase in serum creatinine, pre-renal azotemia and acute renal failure have been reported; usually in the setting of heart failure or hypovolemia. The effects appear to be reversible upon drug discontinuation and with appropriate medical treatment; monitor renal function periodically. Discontinue use in the setting of heart failure as this is a contraindication. Interstitial lung disease (including pulmonary fibrosis and pneumonitis) has been reported. Evaluate patients with onset of dyspnea or nonproductive cough for pulmonary toxicity. Discontinue therapy with confirmed pulmonary toxicity. Use is contraindicated in patients with previous pulmonary toxicity with amiodarone.

Severe liver injury, including acute liver failure leading to liver transplant, has been reported. If liver injury is suspected, discontinue therapy and evaluate liver enzymes/bilirubin. Appropriate treatment should be started and therapy should not be reinitiated if liver injury is confirmed. Advise patients to report any signs or symptoms of hepatic injury (fatigue, jaundice, nausea, vomiting, abdominal pain, and/or fever). Consider periodic monitoring of serum liver enzymes and bilirubin, especially during the first 6 months of therapy. Use with caution in patients with mild-to-moderate hepatic impairment; use is contraindicated in severe hepatic impairment. Use is also contraindicated in patients with previous liver toxicity with amiodarone.

Potentially significant drug-drug interactions may exist, requiring dose or frequency adjustment, additional monitoring, and/or selection of alternative therapy. Correct electrolyte disturbances, especially hypokalemia or hypomagnesemia, prior to use and throughout therapy. Women of childbearing potential should use effective contraceptive methods during treatment.

Drug Interactions

Avoid Concomitant Use

Avoid concomitant use of Dronedarone with any of the following: Bosutinib; CycloSPORINE (Systemic); CYP3A4 Inducers (Strong); CYP3A4 Inhibitors (Strong); Fingolimod; Fusidic Acid (Systemic); Grapefruit Juice; Highest Risk QTc-Prolonging Agents; Ibrutinib; Ivabradine; Lomitapide; Mifepristone; Moderate Risk QTc-Prolonging Agents; Pomalidomide; Propafenone; Rivaroxaban; Silodosin; Simeprevir; St Johns Wort; Thioridazine; Tolvaptan; Topotecan; Ulipristal; VinCRIStine (Liposomal)

Decreased Effect

Dronedarone may decrease the levels/effects of: Codeine; Ifosfamide; Tamoxifen; TraMADol

The levels/effects of Dronedarone may be decreased by: Bosentan; CYP3A4 Inducers (Strong); Dabrafenib; Deferasirox; St Johns Wort; Tocilizumab

Increased Effect/Toxicity

Dronedarone may increase the levels/effects of: Afatinib; ARIPiprazole; AtorvaSTATin; Avanafil; Beta-Blockers; Bosentan; Bosutinib; Budesonide (Systemic, Oral Inhalation); Calcium Channel Blockers (Nondihydropyridine); Colchicine; CYP2D6 Substrates; CYP3A4 Substrates; Dabigatran Etexilate; Digoxin; DOCEtaxel; DOXOrubicin (Conventional); Eplerenone; Everolimus; FentaNYL; Fesoterodine; Highest Risk QTc-Prolonging Agents; Ibrutinib; Imatinib; Ivacaftor; Lidocaine (Topical); Lomitapide; Lovastatin; Lurasidone; Metoprolol; OxyCODONE; P-glycoprotein/ABCB1 Substrates; Pimecrolimus; Pomalidomide; Prucalopride; Red Yeast Rice; Rivaroxaban; Rosuvastatin; Salmeterol; Saxagliptin; Silodosin; Simeprevir; Simvastatin; Thioridazine; Tolvaptan; Topotecan; Ulipristal; Vilazodone; VinCRIStine (Liposomal); Vitamin K Antagonists

The levels/effects of Dronedarone may be increased by: Calcium Channel Blockers (Nondihydropyridine); CycloSPORINE (Systemic); CYP3A4 Inhibitors (Moderate); CYP3A4 Inhibitors (Strong); Dasatinib; Digoxin; Fingolimod; Fusidic Acid (Systemic); Grapefruit Juice; Ivabradine; Ivacaftor; Lidocaine (Topical); Luliconazole; Mifepristone; Moderate Risk QTc-Prolonging Agents; Propafenone; QTc-Prolonging Agents (Indeterminate Risk and Risk Modifying); Simeprevir

Nutritional/Ethanol Interactions

Food: Food increases the rate and extent of absorption of dronedarone; bioavailability is increased ~15% with a high-fat meal. Grapefruit/grapefruit juice increases bioavailability of dronedarone significantly; altered effects are possible. Management: Administer with food. Avoid grapefruit/grapefruit juice.

Herb/Nutraceutical: St John's wort may decrease dronedarone levels. Management: Avoid St John's wort.

Adverse Reactions

>10%:

Cardiovascular: Prolonged Q-T interval on ECG (Bazett; 28% [placebo: 19%]; defined as >450 msec in males or >470 msec in female)

Renal: Increased serum creatinine (51%; increased >10%; occurred 5 days after initiation)

1% to 10%:

Cardiovascular: Bradycardia (3%)

Dermatologic: Allergic dermatitis (≤5%), dermatitis (≤5%), eczema (≤5%), pruritus (≤5%), skin rash (≤5%; described as generalized, macular, maculopapular, erythematous)

Gastrointestinal: Diarrhea (9%), nausea (5%), abdominal pain (4%), dyspepsia (2%), vomiting (2%)

Neuromuscular & skeletal: Weakness (7%)

Available Dosage Forms

Tablet, Oral:

Multaq: 400 mg

General Dosage Range Oral: *Adults:* 400 mg twice daily

Administration

Oral Administer with morning and evening meal. Avoid coadministration with grapefruit/grapefruit juice.

Hazardous agent; use appropriate precautions for handling and disposal (NIOSH, 2012).

Storage/Stability Store at 25°C (77°F); excursions permitted to 15°C to 30°C (59°F to 86°F).

Nursing Actions

Patient Education
- Discuss specific use of drug and side effects with patient as it relates to treatment. (HCAHPS: During this hospital stay, were you given any medicine that you had not taken before? Before giving you any new medicine, how often did hospital staff tell you what the medicine was for? How often did hospital staff describe possible side effects in a way you could understand?)
- Patient may experience diarrhea, nausea, asthenia, or dyspepsia. Have patient report immediately to prescriber signs of hepatic impairment, dyspnea, excessive weight gain, edema of extremities, bradycardia, arrhythmia, or renal impairment (HCAHPS).
- Educate patient about signs of a significant reaction (eg, wheezing; chest tightness; fever; itching; bad cough; blue skin color; seizures; or swelling of face, lips, tongue, or throat). **Note:** This is not a comprehensive list of all side effects. Patient should consult prescriber for additional questions.

Intended Use and Disclaimer: Should not be printed and given to patients. This information is intended to serve as a concise initial reference for healthcare professionals to use when discussing medications with a patient. You must ultimately rely on your own discretion, experience and judgment in diagnosing, treating and advising patients.

Dietary Considerations Take with a meal. Avoid coadministration with grapefruit/grapefruit juice.

Related Information

Oral Medications That Should Not Be Crushed or Altered *on page 1712*

Droperidol (droe PER i dole)

Index Terms Dehydrobenzperidol

Pharmacologic Category Antiemetic; Antipsychotic Agent, Typical

Medication Safety Issues

Sound-alike/look-alike issues:
Droperidol may be confused with dronabinol

Pregnancy Risk Factor C

Lactation Excretion in breast milk unknown/use caution

Use Prevention and/or treatment of nausea and vomiting from surgical and diagnostic procedures

Available Dosage Forms

Solution, Injection:
Generic: 2.5 mg/mL (2 mL)

General Dosage Range I.M., I.V.:
Children 2-12 years: Maximum: 0.1 mg/kg; additional doses may be repeated
Adults: Maximum initial dose: 2.5 mg; additional doses of 1.25 mg may be administered

Administration

I.M. May administer I.M.

I.V. According to the manufacturer, I.V. push administration should be slow. For I.V. infusion, further dilute. May also administer I.M.

Injectable Detail pH: 3-3.8

Nursing Actions

Physical Assessment Monitor vital signs and cardiac and respiratory status on a frequent basis and especially immediately following administration and for several hours afterward. Monitor for extrapyramidal symptoms for 24-48 hours after therapy. Monitor for orthostatic hypotension until the patient is stable.

Patient Education
- Discuss specific use of drug and side effects with patient as it relates to treatment. (HCAHPS: During this hospital stay, were you given any medicine that you had not taken before? Before giving you any new medicine, how often did hospital staff tell you what the medicine was for? How often did hospital staff describe possible side effects in a way you could understand?)
- Patient may experience anxiety, fatigue, or akathisia. Have patient report immediately to prescriber difficulty with motor activity, fasciculations, change in balance, dysphagia, or difficulty speaking, tachycardia, arrhythmia, severe dizziness, syncope, hallucinations, angina, illogical thinking, or signs of neuroleptic malignant syndrome (NMS) (HCAHPS).
- Educate patient about signs of a significant reaction (eg, wheezing; chest tightness; fever; itching; bad cough; blue skin color; seizures; or swelling of face, lips, tongue, or throat). **Note:** This is not a comprehensive list of all side effects. Patient should consult prescriber for additional questions.

Intended Use and Disclaimer: Should not be printed and given to patients. This information is intended to serve as a concise initial reference for healthcare professionals to use when discussing medications with a patient. You must ultimately rely on your own discretion, experience and judgment in diagnosing, treating and advising patients.

Drospirenone and Estradiol
(droh SPYE re none & es tra DYE ole)

Brand Names: U.S. Angeliq®

Index Terms E2 and DRSP; Estradiol and Drospirenone

Pharmacologic Category Estrogen and Progestin Combination

Medication Safety Issues

BEERS Criteria medication:
This drug may be potentially inappropriate for use in geriatric patients (Quality of evidence - high [oral and transdermal patch]; Strength of recommendation - strong [oral and transdermal patch]).

Lactation Enters breast milk/use caution

Use Treatment of moderate-to-severe vasomotor symptoms associated with menopause; treatment of vulvar and vaginal atrophy associated with menopause

Available Dosage Forms

Tablet:
Angeliq®: Drospirenone 0.25 mg and estradiol 0.5 mg; drospirenone 0.5 mg and estradiol 1 mg

General Dosage Range Oral: *Adults (females):* 1 tablet daily

Administration

Oral Tablets should be swallowed whole and taken at the same time each day. Bleeding may occur if several doses are missed. Women who are not taking estrogen or who are changing from a continuous combination product may start therapy at any time. Women who are switching from sequential or cyclic hormone therapy should complete the current cycle before switching to this product.

Hazardous agent; use appropriate precautions for handling and disposal (NIOSH, 2012).

Nursing Actions

Physical Assessment See individual agents.

Patient Education
• Discuss specific use of drug and side effects with patient as it relates to treatment. (HCAHPS: During this hospital stay, were you given any medicine that you had not taken before? Before giving you any new medicine, how often did hospital staff tell you what the medicine was for? How often did hospital staff describe possible side effects in a way you could understand?)
• Patient may experience diarrhea, cramps, bloating, edema, mastalgia, macromastia, vaginal hemorrhaging, or skin discoloration. Have patient report immediately to prescriber signs of hepatic impairment, angina, dyspnea, hemoptysis, strength differences from one side to another, difficulty speaking or thinking, change in balance, blurred vision, edema of extremities, severe headache, considerable nausea, significant dyspepsia, intolerable dizziness, syncope, exophthalmos, contact lens discomfort, vision changes, ophthalmalgia, severe eye irritation, lump in breast, mastalgia, nipple discharge, vaginitis, vaginal hemorrhaging, depression, mood changes, memory loss,

edema of hands or feet, or arrhythmia (HCAHPS).
• Educate patient about signs of a significant reaction (eg, wheezing; chest tightness; fever; itching; bad cough; blue skin color; seizures; or swelling of face, lips, tongue, or throat). **Note:** This is not a comprehensive list of all side effects. Patient should consult prescriber for additional questions.

Intended Use and Disclaimer: Should not be printed and given to patients. This information is intended to serve as a concise initial reference for healthcare professionals to use when discussing medications with a patient. You must ultimately rely on your own discretion, experience and judgment in diagnosing, treating and advising patients.

DULoxetine (doo LOX e teen)

Brand Names: U.S. Cymbalta

Index Terms (+)-(S)-N-Methyl-γ-(1-naphthyloxy)-2-thiophenepropylamine Hydrochloride; Duloxetine Hydrochloride; LY248686

Pharmacologic Category Antidepressant, Serotonin/Norepinephrine Reuptake Inhibitor

Medication Safety Issues

Sound-alike/look-alike issues:
Cymbalta® may be confused with Symbyax®
DULoxetine may be confused with FLUoxetine, vortioxetine

BEERS Criteria medication:
This drug may be potentially inappropriate for use in geriatric patients (Quality of evidence - moderate; Strength of recommendation - strong).

Medication Guide Available Yes

Pregnancy Risk Factor C

Lactation Enters breast milk/not recommended

Breast-Feeding Considerations Duloxetine is excreted in human milk and has been detected in the serum of a nursing infant. Breast-feeding is not recommended by the manufacturer. The long-term effects on neurobehavior have not been studied, thus one should prescribe duloxetine to a mother who is breast-feeding only when the benefits outweigh the potential risks.

Use Acute and maintenance treatment of major depressive disorder (MDD); treatment of generalized anxiety disorder (GAD); management of diabetic peripheral neuropathic pain (DPNP); management of fibromyalgia (FM); chronic musculoskeletal pain (eg, chronic low back pain, osteoarthritis)

Unlabeled Use Treatment of stress incontinence

Mechanism of Action/Effect Inhibits reuptake of both norepinephrine and serotonin (SNRI); improves symptoms of depression and chronic pain

Contraindications Concomitant use or within 14 days of discontinuing MAO inhibitor (intended to ▶

treat psychiatric disorders); concomitant use with linezolid or intravenous methylene blue; uncontrolled narrow-angle glaucoma

Note: Treatment with MAO inhibitors for psychiatric disorders should not be initiated until 5 days after the discontinuation of duloxetine. Although acceptable alternatives should be considered, there may be circumstances when it is necessary to initiate an MAO inhibitor (eg, linezolid or intravenous methylene blue) in a patient taking duloxetine; in this case, discontinue duloxetine prior to administering the MAO inhibitor.

Canadian labeling: Additional contraindications (not in U.S. labeling): Hypersensitivity to duloxetine or any component of the formulation; hepatic impairment; severe renal impairment (eg, CrCl <30 mL/minute) or end-stage renal disease (ESRD); concomitant use with thioridazine or with CYP1A2 inhibitors

Warnings/Precautions [U.S. Boxed Warning]: Antidepressants increase the risk of suicidal thinking and behavior in children, adolescents, and young adults (18-24 years of age) with major depressive disorder (MDD) and other psychiatric disorders; consider risk prior to prescribing. Short-term studies did not show an increased risk in patients >24 years of age and showed a decreased risk in patients ≥65 years. Closely monitor for clinical worsening, suicidality, or unusual changes in behavior; the patient's family or caregiver should be instructed to closely observe the patient and communicate condition with healthcare provider. A medication guide concerning the use of antidepressants in children and teenagers should be dispensed with each prescription. **Duloxetine is not FDA approved for use in children.**

The possibility of a suicide attempt is inherent in major depression and may persist until remission occurs. Patients treated with antidepressants should be observed for clinical worsening and suicidality, especially during the initial (generally first 1-2 months) few months of a course of drug therapy, or at times of dose changes, either increases or decreases. Use caution in high-risk patients. Worsening depression and severe abrupt suicidality that are not part of the presenting symptoms may require discontinuation or modification of drug therapy. The patient's family or caregiver should be alerted to monitor patients for the emergence of suicidality and associated behaviors (such as agitation, irritability, hostility, impulsivity, and hypomania) and call healthcare provider.

May worsen psychosis in some patients or precipitate a shift to mania or hypomania in patients with bipolar disorder. Patients presenting with depressive symptoms should be screened for bipolar disorder. Monotherapy in patients with bipolar disorder should be avoided. **Duloxetine is not FDA approved for the treatment of bipolar depression.**

May cause orthostatic hypotension/syncope at therapeutic doses especially within the first week of therapy and after dose increases. Monitor blood pressure with initiation of therapy, dose increases (especially in patients receiving >60 mg/day), or with concomitant use of vasodilators, CYP2D6 inhibitors/substrates, or CYP1A2 inhibitors. Use caution in patients with hypertension. May increase blood pressure. Rare cases of hypertensive crisis have been reported in patients with pre-existing hypertension; evaluate blood pressure prior to initiating therapy and periodically thereafter; consider dose reduction or gradual discontinuation of therapy in individuals with sustained hypertension during therapy.

Modest increases in serum glucose and hemoglobin A_{1c} (HbA_{1c}) levels have been observed in some diabetic patients receiving duloxetine therapy for diabetic peripheral neuropathic pain (DPNP). Duloxetine may cause increased urinary resistance; advise patient to report symptoms of urinary hesitation/difficulty. Has a low potential to impair cognitive or motor performance. Use caution with a previous seizure disorder or condition predisposing to seizures such as brain damage or alcoholism. Avoid use in patients with substantial ethanol intake, evidence of chronic liver disease, or hepatic impairment (contraindicated in Canadian labeling). Rare cases of hepatic failure (including fatalities) have been reported with use. Hepatitis with abdominal pain, hepatomegaly, elevated transaminase levels >20 times the upper limit of normal (ULN) with and without jaundice have all been observed. Discontinue therapy with the presentation of jaundice or other signs of hepatic dysfunction and do not reinitiate therapy unless another source or cause is identified. Use caution in patients with impaired gastric motility (eg, some diabetics) may affect stability of the capsule's enteric coating.

Severe skin reactions (including Stevens-Johnson syndrome and erythema multiforme) have been reported; discontinue immediately if hypersensitivity reaction suspected. May cause hyponatremia/SIADH (elderly at increased risk); volume depletion (diuretics may increase risk). Use with caution in patients with controlled narrow angle glaucoma. May cause or exacerbate sexual dysfunction. Use caution with renal impairment (contraindicated in Canadian labeling for severe renal impairment or ESRD). Use caution with concomitant CNS depressants. May impair platelet aggregation; use caution with concomitant use of NSAIDs, ASA, or other drugs that affect coagulation; the risk of bleeding may be potentiated. Bone fractures have been associated with antidepressant treatment. Consider the possibility of a fragility fracture if an antidepressant-treated patient presents with unexplained bone pain, point tenderness, swelling, or bruising (Rabenda, 2013; Rizzoli, 2012).

Serotonin syndrome (SS) reactions have occurred with duloxetine when used alone and particularly when used in combination with other serotonergic agents (eg, triptans, tricyclic antidepressants, fentanyl, lithium, tramadol, tryptophan, buspirone, and St John's wort) and drugs that inhibit serotonin metabolism (eg, MAO inhibitors, specifically linezolid, methylene blue, and others used for psychiatric disorders). The diagnosis of SS can be made using the Hunter Serotonin Toxicity Criteria (Dunkley, 2003). Monitor patients closely for signs/symptoms of SS which may include mental status changes (eg, agitation, hallucinations, delirium), seizures, autonomic instability (eg, tachycardia, dizziness, diaphoresis), neuromuscular symptoms (eg, tremor, rigidity, myoclonus), or gastrointestinal symptoms (eg, nausea, vomiting, diarrhea). Discontinue treatment (and any concomitant serotonergic agents) immediately if signs/symptoms of SS arise. Concurrent use of serotonergic agents is not recommended; however, if clinically indicated, use with caution and advise patients of increased SS risk especially during initiation and dose increases.

Concurrent use with or within 14 days of MAO inhibitors is contraindicated. Allow 5 days to elapse after discontinuation of duloxetine before initiating an MAO inhibitor for psychiatric disorders. If already receiving duloxetine and urgent treatment with MAO inhibitors (eg, linezolid or I.V. methylene blue) is required, stop duloxetine and initiate linezolid or I.V. methylene blue if the potential benefits outweigh the risk of SS. Monitor for serotonin syndrome for 5 days or for 24 hours after the last dose of linezolid or methylene blue, whichever occurs first; may resume duloxetine 24 hours after the last dose of linezolid or methylene blue. The risks associated with methylene blue doses <1 mg/kg or when administered nonparenterally are unknown.

Use caution during concurrent therapy with drugs which lower the seizure threshold. May increase the risks associated with electroconvulsive therapy. Use caution in elderly patients; may cause or exacerbate syndrome of inappropriate antidiuretic hormone secretion or hyponatremia; monitor sodium closely with initiation or dosage adjustments in older adults (Beers Criteria). Formulation contains sucrose; patients with fructose intolerance, glucose-galactose malabsorption, or sucrase-isomaltase deficiency should avoid use.

Abrupt discontinuation or interruption of antidepressant therapy has been associated with a discontinuation syndrome. Symptoms arising may vary with antidepressant however commonly include nausea, vomiting, diarrhea, headaches, light-headedness, dizziness, diminished appetite, sweating, chills, tremors, paresthesias, fatigue, somnolence, and sleep disturbances (eg, vivid dreams, insomnia). Greater risks for developing a discontinuation syndrome have been associated with antidepressants with shorter half-lives, longer durations of treatment, and abrupt discontinuation. For antidepressants of short or intermediate half-lives, symptoms may emerge within 2-5 days after treatment discontinuation and last 7-14 days (APA, 2010; Fava, 2006; Haddad, 2001; Shelton, 2001; Warner, 2006).

Drug Interactions

Avoid Concomitant Use
Avoid concomitant use of DULoxetine with any of the following: Iobenguane I 123; Linezolid; MAO Inhibitors; Methylene Blue; Thioridazine; Urokinase

Decreased Effect
DULoxetine may decrease the levels/effects of: Alpha2-Agonists; Codeine; Iobenguane I 123; Ioflupane I 123; Tamoxifen

The levels/effects of DULoxetine may be decreased by: CYP1A2 Inducers (Strong); Cyproterone; Nonsteroidal Anti-Inflammatory Agents; Peginterferon Alfa-2b

Increased Effect/Toxicity
DULoxetine may increase the levels/effects of: Agents with Antiplatelet Properties; Alpha-/Beta-Agonists; Anticoagulants; Antipsychotics; ARIPiprazole; Aspirin; Collagenase (Systemic); CYP2D6 Substrates; Dabigatran Etexilate; DOXOrubicin (Conventional); Fesoterodine; FluvoxaMINE; Ibritumomab; Methylene Blue; Metoclopramide; Metoprolol; Nebivolol; NSAID (Nonselective); PARoxetine; Rivaroxaban; Salicylates; Serotonin Modulators; Thioridazine; Thrombolytic Agents; Tositumomab and Iodine I 131 Tositumomab; Tricyclic Antidepressants; Urokinase

The levels/effects of DULoxetine may be increased by: Abiraterone Acetate; Alcohol (Ethyl); Antipsychotics; ARIPiprazole; CYP1A2 Inhibitors (Moderate); CYP1A2 Inhibitors (Strong); CYP2D6 Inhibitors (Moderate); CYP2D6 Inhibitors (Strong); Darunavir; Dasatinib; Deferasirox; FluvoxaMINE; Glucosamine; Herbs (Anticoagulant/Antiplatelet Properties); Hypotensive Agents; Ibrutinib; Linezolid; MAO Inhibitors; Multivitamins/Fluoride (with ADE); Multivitamins/Minerals (with ADEK, Folate, Iron); Multivitamins/Minerals (with AE, No Iron); Nonsteroidal Anti-Inflammatory Agents; Omega-3 Fatty Acids; PARoxetine; Pentosan Polysulfate Sodium; Pentoxifylline; Propafenone; Prostacyclin Analogues; Tipranavir; Vemurafenib; Vitamin E

Nutritional/Ethanol Interactions
Ethanol: Ethanol may increase hepatotoxic potential of duloxetine and increase CNS depression. Management: Avoid ethanol.

Herb/Nutraceutical: Some herbal medications may increase CNS depression. Management: Avoid valerian, St John's wort, SAMe, kava kava, and gotu kola.

Adverse Reactions

>10%:

Central nervous system: Headache (13% to 14%), somnolence (10% to 12%; dose related), fatigue (10% to 11%)

Gastrointestinal: Nausea (23% to 25%), xerostomia (11% to 15%; dose related)

1% to 10%:

Cardiovascular: Palpitation (1% to 2%)

Central nervous system: Dizziness (10%), insomnia (10%; dose related), agitation (3% to 5%), anxiety (3%), dreams abnormal (1% to 2%), yawning (1% to 2%), hypoesthesia (≥1%), lethargy (≥1%), vertigo (≥1%), chills (1%), sleep disorder (1%)

Dermatologic: Hyperhydrosis (6% to 7%)

Endocrine & metabolic: Libido decreased (2% to 4%), hot flushes (1% to 3%), orgasm abnormality (1% to 3%)

Gastrointestinal: Constipation (10%; dose related), diarrhea (9% to 10%), appetite decreased (7% to 9%; dose related), abdominal pain (4% to 6%), vomiting (3% to 5%), dyspepsia (2%), weight loss (2%), flatulence (≥1%), taste abnormal (≥1%), weight gain (≥1%)

Genitourinary: Erectile dysfunction (4% to 5%), ejaculation delayed (3%; dose related), ejaculatory dysfunction (2%)

Hepatic: ALT >3x ULN (1%)

Neuromuscular & skeletal: Muscle spasms (3%), tremor (2% to 3%; dose related), musculoskeletal pain (≥1%), paresthesia (≥1%), rigors (≥1%)

Ocular: Blurred vision (1% to 3%)

Respiratory: Nasopharyngitis (5%), cough (3%)

Miscellaneous: Influenza (3%)

Available Dosage Forms

Capsule Delayed Release Particles, Oral:

Cymbalta: 20 mg, 30 mg, 60 mg

Generic: 20 mg, 30 mg, 60 mg

General Dosage Range Oral:

Adults: 30-60 mg/day in 1-2 divided doses (maximum: 120 mg/day)

Elderly: Initial: 20 mg 1-2 times/day

Administration

Oral Capsule should be swallowed whole; do not crush or chew. Although the manufacturer does not recommend opening the capsule to facilitate administration; the contents of capsule may be sprinkled on applesauce or in apple juice and swallowed (without chewing) immediately. Do not sprinkle contents on chocolate pudding (Wells, 2008). Administer without regard to meals.

Storage/Stability Store at 25°C (77°F); excursions permitted to 15°C to 30°C (59°F to 86°F)

Nursing Actions

Physical Assessment Monitor blood pressure (can cause elevation or orthostatic hypotension)

at the beginning of treatment and periodically throughout. Monitor for worsening of depression and suicide ideation. Taper dosage slowly when discontinuing. Do not discontinue abruptly.

Patient Education

• Discuss specific use of drug and side effects with patient as it relates to treatment. (HCAHPS: During this hospital stay, were you given any medicine that you had not taken before? Before giving you any new medicine, how often did hospital staff tell you what the medicine was for? How often did hospital staff describe possible side effects in a way you could understand?)

• Patient may experience anxiety, constipation, xerostomia, sexual dysfunction, insomnia, fatigue, lack of appetite, or dyspepsia. Have patient report immediately to prescriber signs of depression (ie, suicidal ideation, anxiety, emotional instability, illogical thinking), signs of hyponatremia, signs of hemorrhaging, behavioral changes, blurred vision, syncope, memory loss, tinnitus, considerable asthenia, urinary retention, oliguria, excessive weight gain or loss, serotonin syndrome (ie, severe dizziness, significant headache, agitation, hallucinations, tachycardia, arrhythmia, flushing, tremors, hyperhidrosis, change in balance, severe nausea, significant diarrhea), signs of hepatic impairment, or signs of Stevens-Johnson syndrome/toxic epidermal necrolysis (HCAHPS).

• Educate patient about signs of a significant reaction (eg, wheezing; chest tightness; fever; itching; bad cough; blue skin color; seizures; or swelling of face, lips, tongue, or throat). **Note:** This is not a comprehensive list of all side effects. Patient should consult prescriber for additional questions.

Intended Use and Disclaimer: Should not be printed and given to patients. This information is intended to serve as a concise initial reference for healthcare professionals to use when discussing medications with a patient. You must ultimately rely on your own discretion, experience and judgment in diagnosing, treating and advising patients.

Dietary Considerations May be taken without regard to meals.

Related Information

Oral Medications That Should Not Be Crushed or Altered *on page 1712*

Dutasteride (doo TAS teer ide)

Brand Names: U.S. Avodart

Pharmacologic Category 5 Alpha-Reductase Inhibitor

Pregnancy Risk Factor X

Lactation Excretion in breast milk unknown/contraindicated in women of childbearing potential

Breast-Feeding Considerations It is not known if dutasteride is excreted in breast milk. Use is contraindicated in women of childbearing potential.

Use Treatment of symptomatic benign prostatic hyperplasia (BPH) as monotherapy or combination therapy with tamsulosin

Unlabeled Use Treatment of male pattern baldness

Mechanism of Action/Effect Inhibits the conversion of testosterone to dihydrotestosterone (DHT) via 5α-reductase DHT stimulates prostatic cell hyperplasia.

Contraindications Hypersensitivity to dutasteride, other 5α-reductase inhibitors (eg, finasteride), or any component of the formulation; children; women of childbearing potential; pregnancy

Warnings/Precautions Hazardous agent - use appropriate precautions for handling and disposal (NIOSH, 2012). Pregnant women or women trying to conceive should not handle the product; active ingredient can be absorbed through the skin and may negatively impact fetal development. Urological diseases, including prostate cancer, and/or obstructive uropathy should be ruled out before initiating. Avoid donating blood during or for 6 months following treatment due to risk of administration to a pregnant female transfusion recipient. Use caution in hepatic impairment and with concurrent use of potent, chronic CYP3A4 inhibitors. Reduces PSA by ~50% within 3-6 months of use; if following serial PSAs, re-establish a new baseline ≥3 months after treatment initiation and monitor PSA periodically thereafter. If interpreting an isolated PSA value in a patient treated for ≥3 months, then double the PSA value for comparison to a normal PSA value in an untreated man. Failure to demonstrate a meaningful PSA decrease (<50%) or a PSA increase while on this medication may be associated with an increased risk for prostate cancer (NCCN Prostate Cancer Early Detection Guidelines, v.1.2011). Patients on a 5-alpha-reductase inhibitor (5-ARI) with any increase in PSA levels, even if within normal limits, should be evaluated; may indicate presence of prostate cancer. When compared to placebo, 5-ARIs have been shown to reduce the overall incidence of prostate cancer, although an increase in the incidence of high-grade prostate cancers has been observed; 5-ARIs are not approved in the U.S. or Canada for the prevention of prostate cancer.

Drug Interactions

Avoid Concomitant Use There are no known interactions where it is recommended to avoid concomitant use.

Decreased Effect There are no known significant interactions involving a decrease in effect.

Increased Effect/Toxicity

The levels/effects of Dutasteride may be increased by: CYP3A4 Inhibitors (Strong)

Nutritional/Ethanol Interactions

Ethanol: No effect or interaction noted.

Food: Maximum serum concentrations reduced by 10% to 15% when taken with food; not clinically significant.

Herb/Nutraceutical: St John's wort may decrease dutasteride levels. Avoid saw palmetto (concurrent use has not been adequately studied).

Adverse Reactions

1% to 10%:

Endocrine & metabolic: Decreased libido (≤3%; incidence highest during first 6 months of therapy), ejaculatory disorder (≤1%), gynecomastia (including breast tenderness, breast enlargement; ≤1%)

Genitourinary: Impotence (1% to 5%; incidence highest during first 6 months of therapy)

Note: Frequency of adverse events (except gynecomastia) tends to decrease with continued use (>6 months).

Available Dosage Forms

Capsule, Oral:

Avodart: 0.5 mg

General Dosage Range Oral: *Adults (males):* 0.5 mg once daily

Administration

Oral May be administered without regard to meals. Capsule should be swallowed whole; do not chew or open; contact with opened capsule can cause oropharyngeal irritation. Should not be touched or handled by women who are pregnant or are of childbearing age.

Hazardous agent; use appropriate precautions for handling and disposal (NIOSH, 2012).

Storage/Stability Store at controlled room temperature of 25°C (77°F); excursions permitted to 15°C to 30°C (59°F to 86°F).

Nursing Actions

Patient Education

• Discuss specific use of drug and side effects with patient as it relates to treatment. (HCAHPS: During this hospital stay, were you given any medicine that you had not taken before? Before giving you any new medicine, how often did hospital staff tell you what the medicine was for? How often did hospital staff describe possible side effects in a way you could understand?)

• Patient may experience sexual dysfunction. Have patient report immediately to prescriber lump in breast, mastalgia, macromastia, or depression (HCAHPS).

• Educate patient about signs of a significant reaction (eg, wheezing; chest tightness; fever; itching; bad cough; blue skin color; seizures; or swelling of face, lips, tongue, or throat). **Note:** This is not a comprehensive list of all side effects. Patient should consult prescriber for additional questions.

Intended Use and Disclaimer: Should not be printed and given to patients. This information is ▶

intended to serve as a concise initial reference for healthcare professionals to use when discussing medications with a patient. You must ultimately rely on your own discretion, experience and judgment in diagnosing, treating and advising patients.

Dietary Considerations May be taken without regard to meals.

Related Information

Oral Medications That Should Not Be Crushed or Altered *on page 1712*

Dutasteride and Tamsulosin
(doo TAS teer ide & tam SOO loe sin)

Brand Names: U.S. Jalyn

Index Terms Tamsulosin and Dutasteride; Tamsulosin Hydrochloride and Dutasteride

Pharmacologic Category 5 Alpha-Reductase Inhibitor; Alpha$_1$ Blocker

Pregnancy Risk Factor X

Use Benign prostatic hyperplasia: Treatment of symptomatic benign prostatic hyperplasia (BPH) in men with an enlarged prostate

Available Dosage Forms

Capsule, oral:

Jalyn™: Dutasteride 0.5 mg and tamsulosin hydrochloride 0.4 mg

General Dosage Range Oral: *Adults (males):* 1 capsule (0.5 mg dutasteride/0.4 mg tamsulosin) once daily

Administration

Oral Administer 30 minutes after the same meal each day. Capsules should be swallowed whole; do not crush, chew, or open. Oropharyngeal contact with capsule contents may result in irritation of the mucosa.

Hazardous agent; use appropriate precautions for handling and disposal (NIOSH, 2012).

Nursing Actions

Physical Assessment See individual agents.

Patient Education

- Discuss specific use of drug and side effects with patient as it relates to treatment. (HCAHPS: During this hospital stay, were you given any medicine that you had not taken before? Before giving you any new medicine, how often did hospital staff tell you what the medicine was for? How often did hospital staff describe possible side effects in a way you could understand?)
- Patient may experience rhinorrhea, dizziness, headache, rhinitis, or sexual dysfunction. Have patient report immediately to prescriber severe dizziness, syncope, lump in breast, mastalgia, macromastia, nipple discharge, blurred vision, angina, depression, tachycardia, arrhythmia, chills, pharyngitis, dyspnea, or priapism (HCAHPS).
- Educate patient about signs of a significant reaction (eg, wheezing; chest tightness; fever;

itching; bad cough; blue skin color; seizures; or swelling of face, lips, tongue, or throat). **Note:** This is not a comprehensive list of all side effects. Patient should consult prescriber for additional questions.

Intended Use and Disclaimer: Should not be printed and given to patients. This information is intended to serve as a concise initial reference for healthcare professionals to use when discussing medications with a patient. You must ultimately rely on your own discretion, experience and judgment in diagnosing, treating and advising patients.

Related Information

Dutasteride *on page 506*
Oral Medications That Should Not Be Crushed or Altered *on page 1712*
Tamsulosin *on page 1471*

Edrophonium (ed roe FOE nee um)

Brand Names: U.S. Enlon

Index Terms Edrophonium Chloride

Pharmacologic Category Acetylcholinesterase Inhibitor; Antidote; Diagnostic Agent

Lactation Excretion in breast milk unknown

Use Diagnosis of myasthenia gravis; differentiation of cholinergic crises from myasthenia crises; reversal of nondepolarizing neuromuscular blockers

Available Dosage Forms

Solution, Injection:

Enlon: 10 mg/mL (15 mL)

General Dosage Range

I.M.:

Infants: 0.5-1 mg

Children ≤34 kg: 1 mg

Children >34 kg: 5 mg

Adults: 10 mg, followed by 2 mg if no response

I.V.:

Infants: 0.1 mg, followed by 0.4 mg if no response (maximum total dose: 0.5 mg)

Children ≤34 kg: 0.04 mg/kg as single dose or followed by 0.16 mg/kg if no response **or** 1 mg, followed by 1mg every 30-45 seconds if no response (maximum total dose: 5 mg)

Children >34 kg: 0.04 mg/kg as single dose or followed by 0.16 mg/kg if no response **or** 2 mg, followed by 1 mg every 30-45 seconds if no response (maximum total dose: 10 mg)

Adults: 2 mg test dose, followed by 8 mg if no response **or** 1-10 mg as a single dose **or** 10 mg every 5-10 minutes up to 40 mg **or** 1 mg; may repeat after 1 minute

Administration

Injectable Detail pH: 5.4

Nursing Actions

Physical Assessment Administration of edrophonium for MG diagnosis is supervised by a neurologist and use as a neuromuscular blocking agent is supervised by an anesthesiologist.

Nursing responsibilities include careful monitoring of the patient during and following procedure for cholinergic crisis; keep atropine at hand for antidote. Ascertain that patients receiving the medication for MG testing will have been advised by their neurologist about drug effects. Patient should never be left alone until all drug effects and the possibility of cholinergic crisis have passed.

Patient Education

• Discuss specific use of drug and side effects with patient as it relates to treatment. (HCAHPS: During this hospital stay, were you given any medicine that you had not taken before? Before giving you any new medicine, how often did hospital staff tell you what the medicine was for? How often did hospital staff describe possible side effects in a way you could understand?)

• Educate patient about signs of a significant reaction (eg, wheezing; chest tightness; fever; itching; bad cough; blue skin color; seizures; or swelling of face, lips, tongue, or throat). **Note:** This is not a comprehensive list of all side effects. Patient should consult prescriber for additional questions.

Intended Use and Disclaimer: Should not be printed and given to patients. This information is intended to serve as a concise initial reference for healthcare professionals to use when discussing medications with a patient. You must ultimately rely on your own discretion, experience and judgment in diagnosing, treating and advising patients.

Efavirenz (e FAV e renz)

Brand Names: U.S. Sustiva
Pharmacologic Category Antiretroviral, Reverse Transcriptase Inhibitor, Non-nucleoside (Anti-HIV)
Pregnancy Risk Factor D
Lactation Enters breast milk/contraindicated
Breast-Feeding Considerations Efavirenz is excreted into breast milk. Although breast-feeding is not recommended, plasma concentrations of efavirenz in nursing infants have been reported as ~13% of maternal plasma concentrations.

Maternal or infant antiretroviral therapy does not completely eliminate the risk of postnatal HIV transmission. In addition, multiclass-resistant virus has been detected in breast-feeding infants despite maternal therapy. Therefore, in the United States, where formula is accessible, affordable, safe, and sustainable, and the risk of infant mortality due to diarrhea and respiratory infections is low, complete avoidance of breast-feeding by HIV-infected women is recommended to decrease potential transmission of HIV (DHHS [perinatal], 2012).

Use Treatment of HIV-1 infections in combination with at least two other antiretroviral agents

Mechanism of Action/Effect As a non-nucleoside reverse transcriptase inhibitor, efavirenz has activity against HIV-1 by binding to reverse transcriptase. It consequently blocks the RNA-dependent and DNA-dependent DNA polymerase activities including HIV-1 replication. It does not require intracellular phosphorylation for antiviral activity.

Contraindications Previous significant hypersensitivity (eg, Stevens-Johnson syndrome, erythema multiforme, toxic skin eruptions) to efavirenz or any component of the formulation; concurrent use of bepridil, cisapride, midazolam, pimozide, triazolam, St. John's wort, or ergot alkaloids (includes dihydroergotamine, ergotamine, ergonovine, methylergonovine)

Warnings/Precautions Do not use as single-agent therapy. Avoid pregnancy; women of childbearing potential should undergo pregnancy testing prior to initiation of therapy. Use caution with other agents metabolized by cytochrome P450 isoenzyme 3A4 (see Contraindications); concomitant use of other efavirenz-containing products should be avoided (unless needed for dosage adjustment with concomitant rifampin treatment). Use caution with history of mental illness/drug abuse (predisposition to psychological reactions); may cause CNS and psychiatric symptoms, which include impaired concentration, dizziness or drowsiness (avoid potentially hazardous tasks such as driving or operating machinery if these effects are noted); CNS effects may be potentiated when used with other sedative drugs or ethanol. Serious psychiatric side effects have been associated with efavirenz, including severe depression, suicide, paranoia, and mania; instruct patients to contact healthcare provider if serious psychiatric effects occur. May cause mild-to-moderate maculopapular rash; usually occurs within 2 weeks of starting therapy; discontinue if severe rash (involving blistering, desquamation, mucosal involvement, or fever) develops; contraindicated in patients with a history of a severe cutaneous reaction (eg, Stevens-Johnson syndrome). Children are more susceptible.

Caution in patients with known or suspected hepatitis B or C infection (monitoring of liver function is recommended) or Child-Pugh class A hepatic impairment; not recommended in Child-Pugh class B or C hepatic impairment. Persistent elevations of serum transaminases >5 times the upper limit of normal should prompt evaluation - benefit of continued therapy should be weighed against possible risk of hepatotoxicity. Increases in total cholesterol and triglycerides have been reported; screening should be done prior to therapy and periodically throughout treatment. May cause redistribution of fat (eg, buffalo hump, peripheral wasting with increased abdominal girth, cushingoid appearance). Patients may develop immune reconstitution syndrome resulting in the occurrence of an inflammatory response to an indolent or residual opportunistic infection during initial HIV treatment or activation of autoimmune disorders (eg, Graves' disease, polymyositis, Guillain-Barré syndrome) later in therapy; further evaluation and treatment may be required. Use with caution in patients with a history of seizure disorder; seizures have been associated with use. Efavirenz administered as monotherapy or added on to a failing regimen may result in rapid viral resistance to efavirenz. Consider cross-resistance when adding antiretroviral agents on to efavirenz therapy.

Drug Interactions

Avoid Concomitant Use

Avoid concomitant use of Efavirenz with any of the following: Atovaquone; Axitinib; Azelastine (Nasal); Bepridil [Off Market]; Boceprevir; Bosutinib; CarBAMazepine; Cisapride; Dihydroergotamine; Ergoloid Mesylates; Ergonovine; Ergotamine; Etravirine; Ibrutinib; Ivabradine; Lomitapide; Methylergonovine; Midazolam; Nevirapine; Paraldehyde; Pimozide; Posaconazole; Rilpivirine; Rivaroxaban; Simeprevir; St Johns Wort; Thalidomide; Tolvaptan; Triazolam; Ulipristal

Decreased Effect

Efavirenz may decrease the levels/effects of: Alcohol (Ethyl); ARIPiprazole; Atazanavir; AtorvaSTATin; Atovaquone; Axitinib; Boceprevir; Buprenorphine; BuPROPion; CarBAMazepine; Caspofungin; Clopidogrel; CycloSPORINE (Systemic); Darunavir; Dolutegravir; Etonogestrel; Etravirine; Everolimus; Fosamprenavir; Ibrutinib; Ifosfamide; Indinavir; Itraconazole; Lopinavir; Lovastatin; Methadone; Norgestimate; Posaconazole; Pravastatin; Proguanil; Raltegravir; Rifabutin; Rilpivirine; Saquinavir; Saxagliptin; Sertraline; Simeprevir; Simvastatin; Sirolimus; Tacrolimus (Systemic); Telaprevir; Vitamin K Antagonists; Voriconazole

The levels/effects of Efavirenz may be decreased by: Bosentan; CarBAMazepine; CYP3A4 Inducers (Strong); Dabrafenib; Deferasirox; Fosphenytoin; Mitotane; Nevirapine; Phenytoin; Rifabutin; Rifampin; St Johns Wort; Telaprevir; Tocilizumab

Increased Effect/Toxicity

Efavirenz may increase the levels/effects of: Alcohol (Ethyl); ARIPiprazole; Avanafil; Azelastine (Nasal); Bepridil [Off Market]; Bosentan; Bosutinib; Budesonide (Systemic, Oral Inhalation); Carvedilol; Cisapride; Citalopram; CNS Depressants; Colchicine; CYP2C19 Substrates; CYP2C9 Substrates; CYP3A4 Substrates; Dihydroergotamine; Dofetilide; DOXOrubicin (Conventional); Eplerenone; Ergoloid Mesylates; Ergonovine; Ergotamine; Etravirine; FentaNYL; Fosphenytoin; Halofantrine; Hydrocodone; Ibrutinib; Imatinib; Ivabradine; Ivacaftor; Lomitapide; Lurasidone;

Methotrimeprazine; Methylergonovine; Metyrosine; Midazolam; Mirtazapine; Nevirapine; OxyCODONE; Paraldehyde; Phenytoin; Pimecrolimus; Pimozide; Pramipexole; Propafenone; Ranolazine; Rilpivirine; Ritonavir; Rivaroxaban; ROPINIRole; Rotigotine; Salmeterol; Saxagliptin; Selective Serotonin Reuptake Inhibitors; Simeprevir; Thalidomide; Tolvaptan; Triazolam; Ulipristal; Vilazodone; Vitamin K Antagonists; Zolpidem; Zuclopenthixol

The levels/effects of Efavirenz may be increased by: Boceprevir; Brimonidine (Topical); CYP2B6 Inhibitors (Moderate); CYP2B6 Inhibitors (Strong); Darunavir; Doxylamine; Droperidol; HydrOXYzine; Magnesium Sulfate; Methotrimeprazine; Mifepristone; Nevirapine; Perampanel; Quazepam; Ritonavir; Saquinavir; Sodium Oxybate; Tapentadol; Voriconazole

Nutritional/Ethanol Interactions

Ethanol: Ethanol may increase hepatotoxic potential of efavirenz and increase CNS depression. Management: Limit or avoid ethanol.

Food: High-fat meals increase the absorption of efavirenz. CNS effects are possible. Management: Avoid high-fat meals. Administer at or before bedtime on an empty stomach unless using capsule sprinkle method in patients unable to swallow capsules or tablets. If capsule sprinkle method is used, patient should not consume additional food for 2 hours after administration.

Herb/Nutraceutical: St John's wort may decrease efavirenz serum levels. Management: Avoid concurrent use.

Adverse Reactions Unless otherwise noted, frequency of adverse events is as reported in adults receiving combination antiretroviral therapy.

>10%:

Central nervous system: Dizziness (2% to 28%; children 16%), fever (children 21%), depression (≤19%; severe: 1% to 2%), insomnia (≤16%), anxiety (2% to 13%), pain (1% to 13%; children 14%), headache (2% to 8%; children 11%)

Dermatologic: Rash (5% to 26%, grade 3/4: <1%; children ≤46%, grade 3/4: 2% to 4%)

Endocrine & metabolic: HDL increased (25% to 35%), total cholesterol increased (20% to 40%), triglycerides increased (≥751 mg/dL: 6% to 11%)

Gastrointestinal: Diarrhea (3% to 14%; children: ≤39%), nausea (2% to 10%; children 12%), vomiting (3% to 6%; children 12%)

Respiratory: Cough (children 16%)

1% to 10%:

Central nervous system: Impaired concentration (≤8%), somnolence (≤7%), fatigue (≤8%), abnormal dreams (1% to 6%), nervousness (2% to 7%), hallucinations (1%)

Dermatologic: Pruritus (≤9%)

Endocrine & metabolic: Hyperglycemia (>250 mg/dL: 2% to 5%)

Gastrointestinal: Dyspepsia (≤4%), abdominal pain (2% to 3%), anorexia (≤2%), amylase increased (grade 3/4: ≤6%)

Hematologic: Neutropenia (grade 3/4: 2% to 10%)

Hepatic: Incidence higher with hepatitis B and/or C coinfection: ALT increased (grades 3/4: 2% to 8%), AST increased (grades 3/4: 5% to 8%)

Available Dosage Forms
Capsule, Oral:
Sustiva: 50 mg, 200 mg
Tablet, Oral:
Sustiva: 600 mg

General Dosage Range Dosage adjustment recommended in patients on concomitant therapy
Oral:
Children ≥3 months and 3.5 kg to <5 kg: 100 mg once daily
Children ≥3 months and 5 kg to <7.5 kg: 150 mg once daily
Children ≥3 months and 7.5 kg to <15 kg: 200 mg once daily
Children ≥3 months and 15 kg to <20 kg: 250 mg once daily
Children ≥3 months and 20 kg to <25 kg: 300 mg once daily
Children ≥3 months and 25 kg to <32.5 kg: 350 mg once daily
Children ≥3 months and 32.5 kg to <40 kg: 400 mg once daily
Children ≥3 months and ≥40 kg and Adults: 600 mg once daily

Administration
Oral Administer on an empty stomach. Dosing at or before bedtime is recommended to limit central nervous system effects (DHHS, 2013). Tablets should not be broken.

Capsule contents may be sprinkled onto a small amount of soft food (eg, applesauce, grape jelly, yogurt) for pediatric or adult patients who cannot swallow capsules. Place 1-2 teaspoonfuls of food in a small container. Hold capsule horizontally over container and carefully twist in opposite directions to open, sprinkling contents over food. If more than 1 capsule is needed for a dose, add contents of all capsules needed to 1-2 teaspoonfuls of food; do not add more food. Use a small spoon to gently mix capsule contents with food and administer all of mixture to patient. To ensure entire capsule contents are administered, add another 2 teaspoonfuls of food to the container, mix to incorporate any drug residue, and administer.

Capsule contents may also be mixed with infant formula only for pediatric patients who cannot reliably consume solid foods. Combine entire contents of capsule(s) with 10 mL of reconstituted, room temperature infant formula in a 30 mL medicine cup, stir carefully, then draw up mixture in a 10 mL oral syringe for administration. If more than 1 capsule is needed for a dose, add contents of all capsules needed to 10 mL of formula; do not add more formula. To ensure entire capsule contents are administered, add another 10 mL of formula to the cup, stir to incorporate any drug residue, draw up in oral syringe and administer.

Administer within 30 minutes of mixing. Patient should not consume any additional food or administer additional formula for 2 hours after administration.

Storage/Stability Store at 25°C (77°F); excursion permitted to 15°C to 30°C (59°F to 86°F).

Nursing Actions
Physical Assessment Assess adherence with regimen and progression of disease. Teach patient proper timing of multiple medications. Monitor for CNS changes, rash, seizure, mood changes, suicidal ideation, and gastrointestinal upset.

Patient Education
- Discuss specific use of drug and side effects with patient as it relates to treatment. (HCAHPS: During this hospital stay, were you given any medicine that you had not taken before? Before giving you any new medicine, how often did hospital staff tell you what the medicine was for? How often did hospital staff describe possible side effects in a way you could understand?)
- Patient may experience nausea, diarrhea, headache, lipodystrophy, asthenia, dizziness, fatigue, insomnia, difficulty focusing, or abnormal dreams. Have patient report immediately to prescriber signs of depression (ie, suicidal ideation, anxiety, emotional instability, illogical thinking), behavioral changes, hallucinations, memory loss, signs of infection, signs of Stevens-Johnson syndrome/toxic epidermal necrolysis, or signs of hepatic impairment (HCAHPS).
- Educate patient about signs of a significant reaction (eg, wheezing; chest tightness; fever; itching; bad cough; blue skin color; seizures; or swelling of face, lips, tongue, or throat). **Note:** This is not a comprehensive list of all side effects. Patient should consult prescriber for additional questions.

Intended Use and Disclaimer: Should not be printed and given to patients. This information is intended to serve as a concise initial reference for healthcare professionals to use when discussing medications with a patient. You must ultimately rely on your own discretion, experience and judgment in diagnosing, treating and advising patients.

Dietary Considerations Should be taken on an empty stomach unless using capsule sprinkle method in patients unable to swallow capsules or tablets. If capsule sprinkle method is used, do not consume additional food for 2 hours after administration.

Related Information

Oral Medications That Should Not Be Crushed or Altered *on page 1712*

Efavirenz, Emtricitabine, and Tenofovir

(e FAV e renz, em trye SYE ta been, & ten OF oh vir)

Brand Names: U.S. Atripla

Index Terms Emtricitabine, Efavirenz, and Tenofovir; FTC, TDF, and EFV; Tenofovir Disoproxil Fumarate, Efavirenz, and Emtricitabine

Pharmacologic Category Antiretroviral, Reverse Transcriptase Inhibitor, Non-nucleoside (Anti-HIV); Antiretroviral, Reverse Transcriptase Inhibitor, Nucleoside (Anti-HIV); Antiretroviral, Reverse Transcriptase Inhibitor, Nucleotide (Anti-HIV)

Pregnancy Risk Factor D

Lactation See individual agents.

Breast-Feeding Considerations See individual agents.

Use Treatment of HIV-1 infection

Mechanism of Action/Effect See individual agents.

Contraindications

History of clinically-significant hypersensitivity (eg, Stevens-Johnson syndrome, erythema multiforme, or toxic skin reactions) to efavirenz; concurrent use of bepridil, cisapride, midazolam, triazolam, voriconazole, ergot alkaloids (includes dihydroergotamine, ergotamine, ergonovine, methylergonovine), St John's wort, pimozide

Canadian labeling: Additional contraindications (not in U.S. labeling): Concomitant use with astemizole or terfenadine (not marketed in Canada)

Warnings/Precautions [U.S. Boxed Warning]: Lactic acidosis and severe hepatomegaly with steatosis have been reported with nucleoside analogues, including fatal cases. Not recommended in patients with moderate or severe hepatic impairment (Child-Pugh class B, C). Use caution in patients with mild hepatic impairment (Child-Pugh class A), HBV or HCV coinfection, elevated transaminases or use of concomitant hepatotoxic drugs. Use caution in hepatic impairment. Use with caution in patients with risk factors for liver disease (risk may be increased in obese patients or prolonged exposure) and suspend treatment in any patient who develops clinical or laboratory findings suggestive of lactic acidosis or hepatotoxicity (transaminase elevation may/may not accompany hepatomegaly and steatosis). Persistent elevations of serum transaminases >5 times the upper limit of normal should prompt evaluation - benefit of continued therapy should be weighed against possible risk of hepatotoxicity. May cause redistribution of fat (eg, buffalo hump, peripheral wasting with increased abdominal girth, cushingoid appearance).

[U.S. Boxed Warning]: Safety and efficacy during coinfection of HIV and HBV have not been established; acute, severe exacerbations of HBV have been reported following discontinuation of antiretroviral therapy. All patients with HIV should be tested for HBV prior to initiation of treatment. Caution in patients with known or suspected hepatitis B or C infection (monitoring of liver function is recommended). In HBV coinfected patients, monitor hepatic function closely for several months following discontinuation.

Potentially significant drug-drug interactions may exist, requiring dose or frequency adjustment, additional monitoring, and/or selection of alternative therapy. Patients may develop immune reconstitution syndrome resulting in the occurrence of an inflammatory response to an indolent or residual opportunistic infection during initial HIV treatment or activation of autoimmune disorders (eg, Graves' disease, polymyositis, Guillain-Barré syndrome) later in therapy; further evaluation and treatment may be required. Discontinue if severe rash (involving blistering, desquamation, mucosal involvement or fever) develops. Consider alternative therapy in the case of life-threatening cutaneous reactions (see Contraindications). Children are more susceptible to development of rash (median time to onset: 8 days); prophylactic antihistamines may be used. To avoid duplicate therapy, do not use concurrently with efavirenz, emtricitabine, tenofovir, or any combination of these drugs; however, coadministration with efavirenz may be required for dose-adjustment with concomitant rifampin therapy.

Use caution with history of mental illness/drug abuse (predisposition to psychological reactions); may cause CNS and psychiatric symptoms, which include impaired concentration, dizziness or drowsiness (avoid potentially hazardous tasks such as driving or operating machinery if these effects are noted); serious psychiatric side effects have been associated with efavirenz, including severe depression, suicidal ideation, paranoia, and mania. Seizures have been associated with efavirenz use; use caution in patients with a history of seizure disorder.

May cause osteomalacia with proximal renal tubulopathy. Bone pain, extremity pain, fractures, arthralgias, weakness and muscle pain have been reported. In patients at risk for renal dysfunction, persistent or worsening bone or muscle symptoms should be evaluated for hypophosphatemia and osteomalacia. May cause acute renal failure or Fanconi syndrome; use caution with other nephrotoxic agents (including high dose or multiple NSAID use or those which compete for active tubular secretion). Acute renal failure has occurred in HIV-infected patients with risk factors for renal impairment who were on a stable tenofovir regimen to which a high dose or multiple NSAID therapy was added. Consider alternatives to NSAIDS in patients taking tenofovir and at risk for renal impairment.

Product is a fixed-dose combination and is not appropriate for use in renal impairment (CrCl <50 mL/minute).

In clinical trials, use has been associated with decreases in bone mineral density in HIV-1 infected adults and increases in bone metabolism markers. Serum parathyroid hormone and 1,25 vitamin D levels were also higher. Decreases in bone mineral density have also been observed in clinical trials of HIV-1 infected pediatric patients. Observations in chronic hepatitis B infected pediatric patients (aged 12-18 years) were similar.

Avoid pregnancy; women of childbearing potential should undergo pregnancy testing prior to initiation of therapy. Two forms of contraception should be used during and for 12 weeks after discontinuation of therapy. Fixed-dose combination product; safety and efficacy have not been established in pediatric patients <12 years of age and <40 kg. In children <40 kg, the dose of efavirenz would be excessive.

Drug Interactions
Avoid Concomitant Use
Avoid concomitant use of Efavirenz, Emtricitabine, and Tenofovir with any of the following: Adefovir; Atovaquone; Axitinib; Azelastine (Nasal); Bepridil [Off Market]; Boceprevir; Bosutinib; CarBAMazepine; Cisapride; Dabigatran Etexilate; Didanosine; Dihydroergotamine; Ergoloid Mesylates; Ergonovine; Ergotamine; Etravirine; Ibrutinib; Ivabradine; LamiVUDine; Lomitapide; Methylergonovine; Midazolam; Nevirapine; Paraldehyde; Pimozide; Pomalidomide; Posaconazole; Rilpivirine; Rivaroxaban; St Johns Wort; Thalidomide; Tolvaptan; Triazolam; Ulipristal; VinCRIStine (Liposomal)

Decreased Effect
Efavirenz, Emtricitabine, and Tenofovir may decrease the levels/effects of: Afatinib; Alcohol (Ethyl); ARIPiprazole; Atazanavir; AtorvaSTATin; Atovaquone; Axitinib; Boceprevir; Buprenorphine; BuPROPion; CarBAMazepine; Caspofungin; Clopidogrel; CycloSPORINE (Systemic); Dabigatran Etexilate; Darunavir; Didanosine; Dolutegravir; DOXOrubicin (Conventional); Etonogestrel; Etravirine; Everolimus; Fosamprenavir; Ibrutinib; Ifosfamide; Indinavir; Itraconazole; Linagliptin; Lopinavir; Lovastatin; Methadone; Norgestimate; P-glycoprotein/ABCB1 Substrates; Pomalidomide; Posaconazole; Pravastatin; Proguanil; Raltegravir; Rifabutin; Rilpivirine; Saquinavir; Saxagliptin; Sertraline; Simeprevir; Simvastatin; Sirolimus; Tacrolimus (Systemic); Telaprevir; Tipranavir; VinCRIStine (Liposomal); Vitamin K Antagonists; Voriconazole

The levels/effects of Efavirenz, Emtricitabine, and Tenofovir may be decreased by: Adefovir; Bosentan; CarBAMazepine; CYP3A4 Inducers (Strong); Dabrafenib; Deferasirox; Fosphenytoin; Mitotane; Nevirapine; Phenytoin; Rifabutin; Rifampin; St Johns Wort; Telaprevir; Tipranavir; Tocilizumab

Increased Effect/Toxicity
Efavirenz, Emtricitabine, and Tenofovir may increase the levels/effects of: Adefovir; Alcohol (Ethyl); Aminoglycosides; ARIPiprazole; Avanafil; Azelastine (Nasal); Bepridil [Off Market]; Bosentan; Bosutinib; Budesonide (Systemic, Oral Inhalation); Carvedilol; Cisapride; Citalopram; CNS Depressants; Colchicine; CYP2C19 Substrates; CYP2C9 Substrates; CYP3A4 Substrates; Darunavir; Didanosine; Dihydroergotamine; Dofetilide; DOXOrubicin (Conventional); Eplerenone; Ergoloid Mesylates; Ergonovine; Ergotamine; Etravirine; FentaNYL; Fosphenytoin; Ganciclovir-Valganciclovir; Halofantrine; Hydrocodone; Ibrutinib; Imatinib; Ivabradine; Ivacaftor; Lomitapide; Lurasidone; Methotrimeprazine; Methylergonovine; Metyrosine; Midazolam; Mirtazapine; Nevirapine; OxyCODONE; Paraldehyde; Phenytoin; Pimecrolimus; Pimozide; Pramipexole; Propafenone; Ranolazine; Rilpivirine; Ritonavir; Rivaroxaban; ROPINIRole; Rotigotine; Salmeterol; Saxagliptin; Selective Serotonin Reuptake Inhibitors; Thalidomide; Tolvaptan; Triazolam; Ulipristal; Vilazodone; Vitamin K Antagonists; Zolpidem; Zuclopenthixol

The levels/effects of Efavirenz, Emtricitabine, and Tenofovir may be increased by: Acyclovir-Valacyclovir; Adefovir; Aminoglycosides; Atazanavir; Boceprevir; Brimonidine (Topical); Cidofovir; CYP2B6 Inhibitors (Moderate); CYP2B6 Inhibitors (Strong); Darunavir; Diclofenac (Systemic); Doxylamine; Droperidol; Ganciclovir-Valganciclovir; HydrOXYzine; LamiVUDine; Lopinavir; Magnesium Sulfate; Methotrimeprazine; Mifepristone; Nevirapine; Nonsteroidal Anti-Inflammatory Agents; Perampanel; Quazepam; Ribavirin; Ritonavir; Saquinavir; Simeprevir; Sodium Oxybate; Tapentadol; Telaprevir; Voriconazole

Nutritional/Ethanol Interactions
Ethanol: Ethanol may increase hepatotoxic potential of efavirenz. Ethanol may also increase CNS depression. Management: Monitor for increased effects with coadministration. Caution patients about effects.

Food: High-fat meals increase the absorption of efavirenz. Food decreases peak plasma concentrations of emtricitabine, but does not alter the extent of absorption or overall systemic exposure. Fatty meals may increase the bioavailability of tenofovir. Management: Avoid high-fat meals.

Herb/Nutraceutical: St John's wort may decrease efavirenz serum levels. Management: Concurrent use is contraindicated.

◀ **Adverse Reactions** The complete adverse reaction profile of combination therapy has not been established. **See individual agents.** The following adverse effects were noted in clinical trials with combination therapy:

>10%: Endocrine & metabolic: Hypercholesterolemia (22%)

1% to 10%:

Central nervous system: Depression (9%), fatigue (9%), dizziness (8%), headache (6%), anxiety (5%), insomnia (5%), somnolence (4%), abnormal dreams

Dermatologic: Rash (7%)

Endocrine & metabolic: Triglycerides increased (4%), hyperglycemia (2%)

Gastrointestinal: Nausea (9%), diarrhea (9%), serum amylase increased (8%), vomiting (2%)

Hematologic: Neutropenia (3%)

Hepatic: AST increased (3%), ALT increased (2%), alkaline phosphatase increased (1%)

Neuromuscular & skeletal: Creatine increased (9%)

Renal: Hematuria (3%)

Respiratory: Sinusitis (8%), upper respiratory infection (8%), nasopharyngitis (5%)

Available Dosage Forms

Tablet, oral:

Atripla®: Efavirenz 600 mg, emtricitabine 200 mg, and tenofovir disoproxil fumarate 300 mg

General Dosage Range Oral: *Children ≥12 years and ≥40 kg, Adolescents, and Adults:* 1 tablet (efavirenz 600 mg/emtricitabine 200 mg/tenofovir 300 mg) once daily

Administration

Oral Should be taken on an empty stomach, normally at bedtime to increase gastrointestinal tolerance and decrease nervous system manifestations.

Storage/Stability Store at 25°C (77°F); excursions permitted between 15°C to 30°C (59°F to 86°F). Dispense only in original container.

Nursing Actions

Physical Assessment See individual agents.

Patient Education

• Discuss specific use of drug and side effects with patient as it relates to treatment. (HCAHPS: During this hospital stay, were you given any medicine that you had not taken before? Before giving you any new medicine, how often did hospital staff tell you what the medicine was for? How often did hospital staff describe possible side effects in a way you could understand?)

• Patient may experience headache, fatigue, nightmares, dizziness, insomnia, or lipodystrophy. Have patient report immediately to prescriber signs of infection, signs of renal impairment, signs of depression (ie, suicidal ideation, anxiety, emotional instability, illogical thinking), severe nausea, considerable diarrhea, osteodynia, arthralgia, asthenia, painful extremities, skin discoloration, significant skin irritation, signs of hepatic impairment, or signs of lactic acidosis (HCAHPS).

• Educate patient about signs of a significant reaction (eg, wheezing; chest tightness; fever; itching; bad cough; blue skin color; seizures; or swelling of face, lips, tongue, or throat). **Note:** This is not a comprehensive list of all side effects. Patient should consult prescriber for additional questions.

Intended Use and Disclaimer: Should not be printed and given to patients. This information is intended to serve as a concise initial reference for healthcare professionals to use when discussing medications with a patient. You must ultimately rely on your own discretion, experience and judgment in diagnosing, treating and advising patients.

Dietary Considerations Should be taken on an empty stomach. In patients with history of bone fracture or osteopenia, consider calcium and vitamin D supplementation.

Related Information

Efavirenz *on page 509*

Emtricitabine *on page 521*

Tenofovir *on page 1490*

Eletriptan (el e TRIP tan)

Brand Names: U.S. Relpax

Index Terms Eletriptan Hydrobromide

Pharmacologic Category Antimigraine Agent; Serotonin 5-HT$_{1B, 1D}$ Receptor Agonist

Pregnancy Risk Factor C

Lactation Enters breast milk/use caution

Breast-Feeding Considerations Eletriptan is excreted in breast milk. Eight women were given a single dose of eletriptan 80 mg. The amount of drug detected in breast milk over 24 hours was ~0.02% of the maternal dose and the milk-to-plasma ratio was variable. The presence of the active metabolite was not measured. The manufacturer recommends that caution be exercised when administering eletriptan to nursing women.

Use Migraines: Acute treatment of migraine, with or without aura in adults

Mechanism of Action/Effect Selective agonist for serotonin receptor in cranial arteries; causes vasoconstriction and relief of migraine

Contraindications

Ischemic coronary artery disease (eg, angina pectoris, history of myocardial infarction, documented silent ischemia); coronary artery vasospasm, including Prinzmetal's angina; Wolff-Parkinson-White syndrome or arrhythmias associated with other cardiac accessory conduction pathway disorders; history of stroke, transient ischemic attack, or history or current evidence of hemiplegic or basilar migraine; peripheral vascular disease; ischemic bowel disease; uncontrolled hypertension; recent use (within 24 hours) of treatment with another 5-HT$_1$ agonist, or an ergotamine-containing or ergot-type medication (eg, dihydroergotamine or methysergide); recent use (within at least 72 hours) of the following potent CYP3A4 inhibitors: ketoconazole, itraconazole, nefazodone, troleandomycin, clarithromycin, ritonavir, or nelfinavir; known hypersensitivity to eletriptan or any component of the formulation.

Canadian labeling: Additional contraindications (not in U.S. labeling): Cardiac arrhythmias (especially tachycardias), valvular heart disease, congenital heart disease, atherosclerotic disease; management of ophthalmoplegic migraine; Raynaud's syndrome; severe hepatic impairment.

Documentation of allergenic cross-reactivity for serotonin 5-HT$_1$ receptor agonists (triptans) in this class is limited. However, because of similarities in chemical structure and/or pharmacologic actions, the possibility of cross-sensitivity cannot be ruled out with certainty.

Warnings/Precautions Only indicated for treatment of acute migraine; not indicated for migraine prophylaxis, or for the treatment of cluster headache, hemiplegic or basilar migraine. If a patient does not respond to the first dose, the diagnosis of migraine should be reconsidered. Acute migraine agents (eg, triptans, opioids, ergotamine, or a combination of the agents) used for 10 or more days per month may lead to worsening of headaches (medication overuse headache); withdrawal treatment may be necessary in the setting of overuse. Do not give to patients with risk factors for CAD until a cardiovascular evaluation has been performed; if evaluation is satisfactory, the health care provider should administer the first dose (consider ECG monitoring) and cardiovascular status should be periodically evaluated. Cardiac events (coronary artery vasospasm, transient ischemia, MI, ventricular tachycardia/fibrillation, cardiac arrest, and death), cerebral/subarachnoid hemorrhage, stroke (some fatal), peripheral vascular ischemia, gastrointestinal vascular ischemia/infarction, and Raynaud's syndrome have been reported with 5-HT$_1$ agonist administration. Patients who experience sensations of chest pain/pressure/tightness or symptoms suggestive of angina following dosing should be evaluated for coronary artery disease or Prinzmetal's angina before receiving additional doses; if dosing is resumed and similar symptoms recur, monitor with ECG. Significant elevation in blood pressure, including hypertensive crisis with acute impairment of organ systems, has been reported on rare occasions in patients with and without a history of hypertension; monitor blood pressure.

Not recommended for use in patients with severe hepatic impairment; the Canadian labeling contraindicates use in patients with severe impairment. Symptoms of agitation, confusion, hallucinations, hyper-reflexia, myoclonus, shivering, and tachycardia (serotonin syndrome) may occur with concomitant proserotonergic drugs (ie, SSRIs/SNRIs or triptans) or agents which reduce eletriptan's metabolism. Concurrent use of serotonin precursors (eg, tryptophan) is not recommended. If concomitant administration with SSRIs is warranted, monitor closely, especially at initiation and with dose increases. Discontinue eletriptan if serotonin syndrome is suspected. Potentially significant drug-drug interactions may exist, requiring dose or frequency adjustment, additional monitoring, and/or selection of alternative therapy. Use is contraindicated within 72 hours of patients taking strong CYP3A4 inhibitors. Anaphylaxis, anaphylactoid, and hypersensitivity reactions (including angioedema) have occurred; may be life-threatening or fatal.

Drug Interactions

Avoid Concomitant Use

Avoid concomitant use of Eletriptan with any of the following: Conivaptan; Ergot Derivatives; Fusidic Acid (Systemic); Itraconazole; Ketoconazole (Systemic); Posaconazole; Voriconazole

Decreased Effect There are no known significant interactions involving a decrease in effect.

Increased Effect/Toxicity

Eletriptan may increase the levels/effects of: Antipsychotics; Droxidopa; Ergot Derivatives; Metoclopramide; Serotonin Modulators

The levels/effects of Eletriptan may be increased by: Antipsychotics; Calcium Channel Blockers (Nondihydropyridine); Conivaptan; CYP3A4 Inhibitors (Moderate); CYP3A4 Inhibitors (Strong); Dasatinib; Ergot Derivatives; Fluconazole; Fusidic Acid (Systemic); Itraconazole; Ivacaftor; Ketoconazole (Systemic); Luliconazole; Macrolide Antibiotics; Mifepristone; Posaconazole; Simeprevir; Stiripentol; Voriconazole

Nutritional/Ethanol Interactions Food: High-fat meal increases bioavailability.

Adverse Reactions 1% to 10%:

Cardiovascular: Chest pain/tightness (1% to 4%; placebo 1%), palpitation

Central nervous system: Dizziness (3% to 7%; placebo 3%), somnolence (3% to 7%; placebo 4%), headache (3% to 4%; placebo 3%), chills, pain, vertigo

Gastrointestinal: Nausea (4% to 8%; placebo 5%), xerostomia (2% to 4%, placebo 2%), dysphagia (1% to 2%), abdominal pain/discomfort (1% to 2%; placebo 1%), dyspepsia (1% to 2%; placebo 1%)

Neuromuscular & skeletal: Weakness (4% to 10%), paresthesia (3% to 4%), back pain, hypertonia, hypoesthesia

Respiratory: Pharyngitis

Miscellaneous: Diaphoresis

Available Dosage Forms

Tablet, Oral:

Relpax: 20 mg, 40 mg

General Dosage Range Oral: *Adults:* 20-40 mg as a single dose, may repeat after 2 hours have elapsed (maximum: 80 mg daily)

Administration

Oral Administer as soon as symptoms appear. May take with or without food.

Storage/Stability Store at 20°C to 25°C (68°F to 77°F); excursions are permitted between 15°C and 30°C (59°F and 86°F).

Nursing Actions

Physical Assessment Monitor for hypertension and cardiac events. Teach patient proper use (treatment of acute migraine).

Patient Education

• Discuss specific use of drug and side effects with patient as it relates to treatment. (HCAHPS: During this hospital stay, were you given any medicine that you had not taken before? Before giving you any new medicine, how often did hospital staff tell you what the medicine was for? How often did hospital staff describe possible side effects in a way you could understand?)

• Patient may experience asthenia or fatigue. Have patient report immediately to prescriber constipation, considerable dyspepsia, melena, paresthesia, weight loss, leg cramps, leg pain, sensation of cold, paresthesia of feet, dyspnea, serotonin syndrome (ie, dizziness, severe headache, agitation, hallucinations, tachycardia, arrhythmia, flushing, tremors, hyperhidrosis, change in balance, illogical thinking, severe nausea, significant diarrhea), signs of severe cardiac abnormalities, strength differences from one side to another, difficulty speaking or thinking, or vision changes (HCAHPS).

• Educate patient about signs of a significant reaction (eg, wheezing; chest tightness; fever; itching; bad cough; blue skin color; seizures; or swelling of face, lips, tongue, or throat). **Note:** This is not a comprehensive list of all side effects. Patient should consult prescriber for additional questions.

Intended Use and Disclaimer: Should not be printed and given to patients. This information is intended to serve as a concise initial reference for healthcare professionals to use when discussing medications with a patient. You must ultimately rely on your own discretion, experience and judgment in diagnosing, treating and advising patients.

Eltrombopag (el TROM boe pag)

Brand Names: U.S. Promacta
Index Terms Eltrombopag Olamine; Revolade; SB-497115; SB-497115-GR
Pharmacologic Category Colony Stimulating Factor; Hematopoietic Agent; Thrombopoietic Agent
Medication Guide Available Yes

Pregnancy Risk Factor C
Lactation Excretion in breast milk unknown/not recommended
Breast-Feeding Considerations It is not known if eltrombopag is excreted in breast milk. Due to the potential for serious adverse effects in the nursing infant, the decision to discontinue therapy or to discontinue breast-feeding should take into account the importance of treatment to the mother.

Use

Chronic immune (idiopathic) thrombocytopenia: Treatment of thrombocytopenia in patients with chronic immune (idiopathic) thrombocytopenia (ITP) who have had insufficient response to corticosteroids, immune globulin, or splenectomy.

Chronic hepatitis C infection-associated thrombocytopenia: Treatment of thrombocytopenia in patients with chronic hepatitis C (CHC) to allow the initiation and maintenance of interferon-based therapy.

Limitations of use: Eltrombopag should not be used to normalize platelet counts. For ITP, use eltrombopag only if the degree of thrombocytopenia and clinical condition increase the risk for bleeding. For chronic hepatitis C (CHC), use eltrombopag only if the degree of thrombocytopenia prevents initiation of or limits the ability to maintain interferon-based therapy. For CHC, safety and efficacy have not been established when used in combination with direct-acting antiviral agents approved for CHC genotype 1 infection.

Unlabeled Use Treatment of refractory aplastic anemia

Mechanism of Action/Effect Thrombopoietin (TPO) nonpeptide agonist which increases platelet counts by binding to and activating the human TPO receptor.

Contraindications There are no contraindications listed in the manufacturer's labeling.

Warnings/Precautions Liver enzyme elevations may occur; obtain ALT, AST, and bilirubin prior to treatment initiation, every 2 weeks during adjustment phase, then monthly (after stable dose established); obtain fractionation for elevated bilirubin levels. Repeat abnormal liver function tests within 3-5 days; if confirmed abnormal, monitor weekly until resolves, stabilizes, or returns to baseline. Discontinue treatment for ALT levels ≥3 times the upper limit of normal (ULN) in patients with normal hepatic function, or ≥3 times baseline in those with pre-existing transaminase elevations and which are progressive, or persistent (≥4 weeks), or accompanied by increased direct bilirubin, or accompanied by clinical signs of liver injury or evidence of hepatic decompensation. Hepatotoxicity may reoccur with retreatment after therapy interruption; however, if the benefit of treatment outweighs the hepatotoxicity risk, initiate carefully, and monitor liver function tests weekly during the dose adjustment phase; permanently discontinue if liver abnormalities persist, worsen, or recur with rechallenge. Use with caution in patients with pre-existing hepatic impairment (clearance may be reduced); dosage reductions are recommended in patients with ITP who have hepatic dysfunction (no initial dose reductions are necessary in patients with chronic hepatitis C-related thrombocytopenia); monitor closely.

[U.S. Boxed Warning]: May increase risk of hepatic decompensation when used in combination with interferon and ribavirin in patients with chronic hepatitis C. In clinical trials, patients with low albumin (<3.5 g/dL) or a Model for End-Stage Liver Disease (MELD) score ≥10 at baseline had an increased risk of hepatic decompensation; closely monitor these patients during therapy. If antiviral therapy is discontinued for hepatic decompensation according to interferon/ribavirin recommendations, eltrombopag should also be discontinued. Indirect hyperbilirubinemia is commonly observed with eltrombopag when used in combination with peginterferon and ribavirin. In addition, ascites, encephalopathy, and thrombotic events were reported more frequently than placebo in chronic hepatitis C trials.

May increase the risk for bone marrow reticulin formation or progression (Canadian labeling). Monitor peripheral blood smear for cellular morphologic abnormalities; analyze CBC monthly; discontinue treatment with onset of new or worsening abnormalities (eg, teardrop and nucleated RBC, immature WBC) or cytopenias and consider bone marrow biopsy (with staining for fibrosis).

Thromboembolism may occur with excess increases in platelet levels. Use with caution in patients with known risk factors for thromboembolism (eg, Factor V Leiden, ATIII deficiency, antiphospholipid syndrome, chronic liver disease). Thrombotic events, primarily involving the portal venous system, were more commonly seen in eltrombopag-treated chronic hepatitis C patients with thrombocytopenia (when compared to placebo). In addition, portal venous thrombosis was reported in a study of non-ITP thrombocytopenic patients with chronic liver disease undergoing elective invasive procedures receiving eltrombopag 75 mg once daily for 14 days as a preparative regimen to reduce platelet transfusions (not an FDA-approved indication). Stimulation of cell surface thrombopoietin (TPO) receptors may increase the risk for hematologic malignancies (Canadian labeling).

Cataract formation or worsening was observed in clinical trials. Monitor regularly for signs and symptoms of cataracts; obtain ophthalmic exam at baseline and during therapy. Use with caution in patients at risk for cataracts (eg, advanced age, long-term glucocorticoid use). Potentially significant drug-drug interactions may exist, requiring dose or frequency adjustment, additional monitoring, and/or selection of alternative therapy. Allow at least 4 hours between dosing of eltrombopag and antacids, minerals (eg, iron, calcium, aluminum, magnesium, selenium, zinc), or foods high in calcium; may reduce eltrombopag levels. Patients of East-Asian ethnicity (eg, Chinese, Japanese, Korean, Taiwanese) may have greater drug exposure (compared to non-East Asians); therapy should be initiated with lower starting doses in ITP patients. Use with caution in renal impairment (any degree) and monitor closely; initial dosage adjustment is not necessary.

Do not use to normalize platelet counts. *ITP:* Indicated only when the degree of thrombocytopenia and clinical conditions increase the risk for bleeding in patients with chronic immune ITP; use the lowest dose necessary to achieve and maintain platelet count ≥50,000/mm^3. Discontinue if platelet count does not respond to a level to avoid clinically important bleeding after 4 weeks at the maximum recommended dose. *Chronic hepatitis C-associated thrombocytopenia:* Use only when thrombocytopenia prevents the initiation and maintenance of interferon-based therapy; discontinue if antiviral therapy is discontinued. Safety and efficacy have not been established when combined with direct acting antiviral medications approved for chronic hepatitis C genotype 1 infection therapy.

Drug Interactions

Avoid Concomitant Use There are no known interactions where it is recommended to avoid concomitant use.

Decreased Effect
The levels/effects of Eltrombopag may be decreased by: Aluminum Hydroxide; Calcium Salts; Iron Salts; Magnesium Salts; Multivitamins/Minerals (with ADEK, Folate, Iron); Multivitamins/Minerals (with AE, No Iron); Selenium; Sucralfate; Zinc Salts

Increased Effect/Toxicity
Eltrombopag may increase the levels/effects of: CYP2C8 Substrates; Deferiprone; OATP1B1/SLCO1B1 Substrates; Rosuvastatin

Nutritional/Ethanol Interactions Food: Food, especially dairy products, may decrease the absorption of eltrombopag. Management: Take on an empty stomach at least 1 hour before or 2 hours after a meal. Separate intake from antacids, foods high in calcium, or minerals (eg, iron, calcium, aluminum, magnesium, selenium, zinc) by at least 4 hours.

Adverse Reactions Adverse reactions and incidences reported are associated with ITP unless otherwise indicated.

>10%:

Central nervous system: Fever (chronic hepatitis C 30%), fatigue (4%; chronic hepatitis C 28%), headache (10%; chronic hepatitis C 21%), insomnia (chronic hepatitis C 16%), chills (chronic hepatitis C 14%)

Dermatologic: Pruritus (chronic hepatitis C 15%)
Gastrointestinal: Diarrhea (9%; chronic hepatitis C 19%), nausea (4% to 9%; chronic hepatitis C 19%), appetite decreased (chronic hepatitis C 18%)
Hematologic: Myelofibrosis (bone marrow biopsy: Grade ≤1: 93%; grade 2: 7%; grade 3: <3%) anemia (chronic hepatitis C 40%)
Hepatic: Liver function tests abnormal (11%)
Neuromuscular & skeletal: Weakness (chronic hepatitis C 16%), myalgia (5% to 12%)
Respiratory: Cough (chronic hepatitis C 15%)
Miscellaneous: Flu-like syndrome (3%; chronic hepatitis C 18%)
1% to 10%:
Cardiovascular: Peripheral edema (chronic hepatitis C 10%), thrombosis (chronic hepatitis C 3%)
Dermatologic: Alopecia (2%; chronic hepatitis C 10%), rash (3%)
Gastrointestinal: Vomiting (6%), xerostomia (2%)
Genitourinary: Urinary tract infection (5%)
Hematologic: Rebound thrombocytopenia (8%)
Hepatic: Ascites and encephalopathy (chronic hepatitis C 7%), hyperbilirubinemia (6% to 8%), ALT increased (5% to 6%), AST increased (4%), alkaline phosphatase increased (2%)
Neuromuscular & skeletal: Back pain (3%), paresthesia (3%), musculoskeletal pain (2%)
Ocular: Cataract (4% to 8%)
Respiratory: Upper respiratory infection (7%), oropharyngeal pain (4%), pharyngitis (4%)

Pharmacodynamics/Kinetics
Onset of Action Platelet count increase: Within 1-2 weeks; Peak platelet count increase: 14-16 days
Duration of Action Platelets return to baseline: 1-2 weeks after last dose

Available Dosage Forms
Tablet, Oral:
Promacta: 12.5 mg, 25 mg, 50 mg, 75 mg
General Dosage Range Dosage adjustment recommended in patients with hepatic impairment, of East-Asian ethnicity, or who develop toxicities
Oral: *Adults:* Initial: 25-50 mg once daily (maximum: 75 mg once daily for ITP; 100 mg once daily for chronic hepatitis C-associated thrombocytopenia)

Administration
Oral Administer on an empty stomach, 1 hour before or 2 hours after a meal. Do not administer concurrently with antacids, foods high in calcium, or minerals (eg, iron, calcium, aluminum, magnesium, selenium, zinc); separate by at least 4 hours. Do not administer more than one dose within 24 hours.
Storage/Stability Store at 20°C to 25°C (68°F to 77°F); excursions are permitted between 15°C and 30°C (59°F and 86°F). If present, do not remove desiccant. Dispense in original bottle.

Nursing Actions
Physical Assessment Check liver function test and platelet results. Evaluate for signs and symptoms of DVT or pulmonary embolism. Monitor for GI intolerance, fever, and fatigue. Hepatitis C patients seem to have more side effects. Ensure patient gets yearly eye examination; cataracts can form.
Patient Education
• Discuss specific use of drug and side effects with patient as it relates to treatment. (HCAHPS: During this hospital stay, were you given any medicine that you had not taken before? Before giving you any new medicine, how often did hospital staff tell you what the medicine was for? How often did hospital staff describe possible side effects in a way you could understand?)
• Patient may experience headache, insomnia, lack of appetite, flu-like symptoms, myalgia, rhinorrhea, rhinitis, sternutation, back pain, or alopecia. Have patient report immediately to prescriber signs of hepatic impairment, severe asthenia, considerable dyspepsia, angina, dyspnea, hemoptysis, strength differences from one side to another, difficulty speaking or thinking, change in balance, blurred vision, edema of extremities, vision changes, ophthalmalgia, significant eye irritation, paresthesia, intolerable nausea, severe diarrhea, ecchymosis, hemorrhaging, stomatitis, dysuria, polyuria, illogical thinking, or abdominal edema (HCAHPS).
• Educate patient about signs of a significant reaction (eg, wheezing; chest tightness; fever; itching; bad cough; blue skin color; seizures; or swelling of face, lips, tongue, or throat). **Note:** This is not a comprehensive list of all side effects. Patient should consult prescriber for additional questions.

Intended Use and Disclaimer: Should not be printed and given to patients. This information is intended to serve as a concise initial reference for healthcare professionals to use when discussing medications with a patient. You must ultimately rely on your own discretion, experience and judgment in diagnosing, treating and advising patients.
Dietary Considerations Food, especially dairy products, may decrease the absorption of eltrombopag; allow at least 4 hours between dosing of eltrombopag and polyvalent cation intake (eg, dairy products, calcium-rich foods, multivitamins with minerals).

Elvitegravir, Cobicistat, Emtricitabine, and Tenofovir
(el vi TEG ra vir, koe BIK i stat, em trye SYE ta been, & ten OF oh vir)

Brand Names: U.S. Stribild
Index Terms Cobicistat, Emtricitabine, Tenofovir, and Elvitegravir; Elvitegravir, Cobicistat,

Emtricitabine, and Tenofovir Disoproxil Fumarate; Emtricitabine, Tenofovir, Elvitegravir, and Cobicistat; EVG/COBI/FTC/TDF; Quad Pill; Tenofovir, Elvitegravir, Cobicistat, and Emtricitabine

Pharmacologic Category Antiretroviral, Integrase Inhibitor (Anti-HIV); Antiretroviral, Reverse Transcriptase Inhibitor, Nucleoside (Anti-HIV); Antiretroviral, Reverse Transcriptase Inhibitor, Nucleotide (Anti-HIV); Cytochrome P-450 Inhibitor

Pregnancy Risk Factor B

Lactation See individual agents.

Breast-Feeding Considerations Maternal or infant antiretroviral therapy does not completely eliminate the risk of postnatal HIV transmission. In addition, multiclass-resistant virus has been detected in breast-feeding infants despite maternal therapy. Therefore, in the United States, where formula is accessible, affordable, safe, and sustainable, and the risk of infant mortality due to diarrhea and respiratory infections is low, complete avoidance of breast-feeding by HIV-infected women is recommended to decrease potential transmission of HIV (DHHS [perinatal], 2012).

Use Treatment of human immunodeficiency virus type 1 (HIV-1) infection in antiretroviral treatment-naive adult patients

Mechanism of Action/Effect Inhibits the production of new HIV virus by blocking the viral enzymes responsible for the replication process.

Contraindications Concurrent use of alfuzosin, cisapride, ergot derivatives (eg, dihydroergotamine, ergotamine, methylergonovine); lovastatin, midazolam (oral), pimozide, rifampin, sildenafil (when used for pulmonary arterial hypertension), simvastatin, St John's wort, triazolam

Warnings/Precautions [U.S. Boxed Warning]: Lactic acidosis and severe hepatomegaly with steatosis have been reported with nucleoside and nucleotide analogues (eg, tenofovir), including fatal cases. Use with caution in patients with risk factors for liver disease (risk may be increased in obese patients or prolonged exposure) and suspend treatment in any patient who develops clinical or laboratory findings suggestive of lactic acidosis (transaminase elevation may/may not accompany hepatomegaly and steatosis). Use is not recommended in severe hepatic impairment (Child-Pugh Class C) and has not been studied in this population; no dosage adjustment is required in mild or moderate (Child-Pugh Class A or B) hepatic impairment.

Do not initiate therapy in patients with CrCl <70 mL/minute. Continued use is not recommended in patients with CrCl <50 mL/minute. May cause acute renal failure or Fanconi syndrome; use caution with other nephrotoxic agents (including high dose or multiple NSAID use or those which compete for active tubular secretion). Acute renal failure has occurred in HIV-infected patients with risk factors for renal impairment who were on a stable tenofovir regimen to which a high dose or multiple NSAID therapy was added. Consider alternatives to NSAIDS in patients taking tenofovir and at risk for renal impairment. Calculate creatinine clearance prior to initiation in all patients; monitor renal function during therapy (including recalculation of creatinine clearance, urine glucose, and protein and serum phosphorus) in patients at risk for renal impairment. Cobicistat component may cause modest declines in renal function without affecting glomerular filtration; closely monitor patients with >0.4 mg/dL increase of serum creatinine from baseline. In clinical trials, use has been associated with decreases in bone mineral density in HIV-1 infected adults and increases in bone metabolism markers. Serum parathyroid hormone and 1,25 vitamin D levels were also higher. Decreases in bone mineral density have also been observed in clinical trials of HIV-1 infected pediatric patients. Observations in chronic hepatitis B infected pediatric patients (aged 12-18 years) were similar. May cause osteomalacia with proximal renal tubulopathy. Bone pain, extremity pain, fractures, arthralgias, weakness and muscle pain have been reported. In patients at risk for renal dysfunction, persistent or worsening bone or muscle symptoms should be evaluated for hypophosphatemia and osteomalacia.

All patients with HIV should be tested for HBV prior to initiation of treatment. **[U.S. Boxed Warning]: Safety and efficacy during coinfection of HIV and HBV have not been established; acute, severe exacerbations of HBV have been reported following discontinuation of antiretroviral therapy. Not indicated for the treatment of chronic hepatitis B.** In HBV-coinfected patients, monitor hepatic function closely for several months following discontinuation. May cause redistribution of fat (eg, buffalo hump, peripheral wasting with increased abdominal girth, cushingoid appearance). Patients may develop immune reconstitution syndrome resulting in the occurrence of an inflammatory response to an indolent or residual opportunistic infection during initial HIV treatment or activation of autoimmune disorders (eg, Graves' disease, polymyositis, Guillain-Barré syndrome) later in therapy; further evaluation and treatment may be required.

Drug Interactions

Avoid Concomitant Use

Avoid concomitant use of Elvitegravir, Cobicistat, Emtricitabine, and Tenofovir with any of the following: Adefovir; Ado-Trastuzumab Emtansine; Alfuzosin; Apixaban; Avanafil; Axitinib; Bosutinib; Cabozantinib; Cisapride; Conivaptan; Crizotinib; Dabigatran Etexilate; Didanosine; Dihydroergotamine; Dronedarone; Eplerenone; Ergotamine; Everolimus; Fluticasone (Oral Inhalation); Halofantrine; Ibrutinib; Imatinib; Ivabradine; LamiVUDine; Lapatinib; Lomitapide; Lovastatin;

Lurasidone; Macitentan; Methylergonovine; Midazolam; Nilotinib; Nisoldipine; PAZOPanib; Pimozide; Pomalidomide; Ranolazine; Red Yeast Rice; Regorafenib; Rifabutin; Rifampin; Rifapentine; Rivaroxaban; Salmeterol; Sildenafil; Silodosin; Simeprevir; Simvastatin; St Johns Wort; Tamsulosin; Ticagrelor; Tolvaptan; Toremifene; Triazolam; Ulipristal; Vardenafil; Vemurafenib; VinCRIStine (Liposomal)

Decreased Effect

Elvitegravir, Cobicistat, Emtricitabine, and Tenofovir may decrease the levels/effects of: Afatinib; Atazanavir; Contraceptives (Estrogens); Dabigatran Etexilate; Didanosine; Ifosfamide; Linagliptin; P-glycoprotein/ABCB1 Substrates; Prasugrel; Simeprevir; Ticagrelor; Tipranavir; Warfarin

The levels/effects of Elvitegravir, Cobicistat, Emtricitabine, and Tenofovir may be decreased by: Adefovir; Antacids; CarBAMazepine; CYP3A4 Inducers (Strong); Dabrafenib; Deferasirox; Dexamethasone (Systemic); Fosphenytoin-Phenytoin; Mitotane; OXcarbazepine; PHENobarbital; Rifabutin; Rifampin; Rifapentine; St Johns Wort; Tipranavir; Tocilizumab

Increased Effect/Toxicity

Elvitegravir, Cobicistat, Emtricitabine, and Tenofovir may increase the levels/effects of: Adefovir; Ado-Trastuzumab Emtansine; Afatinib; Alfuzosin; Almotriptan; Alosetron; Aminoglycosides; Apixaban; ARIPiprazole; AtorvaSTATin; Avanafil; Axitinib; Bedaquiline; Bortezomib; Bosentan; Bosutinib; Brentuximab Vedotin; Brinzolamide; Budesonide (Nasal); Budesonide (Systemic, Oral Inhalation); Cabozantinib; Cisapride; Clarithromycin; ClonazePAM; Colchicine; Conivaptan; Contraceptives (Progestins); Corticosteroids (Orally Inhaled); Crizotinib; CYP3A4 Substrates; Dabigatran Etexilate; Darunavir; Didanosine; Dienogest; Dihydroergotamine; Dofetilide; DOXOrubicin (Conventional); Dronedarone; Dutasteride; Enzalutamide; Eplerenone; Ergotamine; Ethosuximide; Everolimus; FentaNYL; Fesoterodine; Fluticasone (Nasal); Fluticasone (Oral Inhalation); Ganciclovir-Valganciclovir; GuanFACINE; Halofantrine; Ibrutinib; Iloperidone; Imatinib; Itraconazole; Ivabradine; Ivacaftor; Ixabepilone; Ketoconazole (Systemic); Lacosamide; Lapatinib; Levomilnacipran; Lomitapide; Lovastatin; Lumefantrine; Lurasidone; Macitentan; Maraviroc; Methylergonovine; MethylPREDNISolone; Midazolam; Mifepristone; Nilotinib; Nisoldipine; Ospemifene; OxyCODONE; Paricalcitol; PAZOPanib; P-glycoprotein/ABCB1 Substrates; Pimecrolimus; Pimozide; Pomalidomide; PONATinib; Propafenone; Prucalopride; QUEtiapine; Ranolazine; Red Yeast Rice; Regorafenib; Repaglinide; Rilpivirine; Riociguat; Rivaroxaban; RomiDEPsin; Ruxolitinib; Salmeterol; Saxagliptin; Selective Serotonin Reuptake Inhibitors; Sildenafil; Silodosin; Simeprevir; Simvastatin; SORAfenib;

Tadalafil; Tamsulosin; Telithromycin; Ticagrelor; Tofacitinib; Tolterodine; Tolvaptan; Topotecan; Toremifene; TraZODone; Triazolam; Tricyclic Antidepressants; Ulipristal; Vardenafil; Vemurafenib; Vilazodone; VinCRIStine (Liposomal); Voriconazole; Warfarin; Zuclopenthixol

The levels/effects of Elvitegravir, Cobicistat, Emtricitabine, and Tenofovir may be increased by: Acyclovir-Valacyclovir; Adefovir; Aminoglycosides; Atazanavir; Cidofovir; Clarithromycin; Darunavir; Diclofenac (Systemic); Ganciclovir-Valganciclovir; Itraconazole; Ketoconazole (Systemic); LamiVUDine; Lopinavir; Nonsteroidal Anti-Inflammatory Agents; Ribavirin; Simeprevir; Telaprevir; Telithromycin; Voriconazole

Adverse Reactions Percentages as reported for combination product.

>10%:

Gastrointestinal: Nausea (16%), diarrhea (12%)

Renal: Proteinuria (39% to 46%)

1% to 10%:

Central nervous system: Abnormal dreams (9%), headache (7%), fatigue (4% to 5%), dizziness (3%), insomnia (3%), somnolence (1%)

Dermatologic: Rash (3%)

Endocrine & metabolic: Cholesterol increased (grades 3/4: ≤1%), triglycerides increased (grades 3/4: ≤1%)

Gastrointestinal: Amylase increased (2% to 3%), flatulence (2%)

Hepatic: AST increased (2%)

Neuromuscular & skeletal: Increased creatine phosphokinase (5% to 7%), bone fracture (1% to 2%)

Renal: Increased serum creatinine (7% to 10%), hematuria (3%)

Available Dosage Forms

Tablet, oral:

Stribild™: Elvitegravir 150 mg, cobicistat 150 mg, emtricitabine 200 mg, and tenofovir disoproxil fumarate 300 mg

General Dosage Range Oral: *Adults:* One tablet once daily

Administration

Oral Administer with food.

Storage/Stability Store tablets at 25°C (77°F); excursions permitted to 15°C to 30°C (59°F to 86°F). Keep container tightly closed. Dispense in original container.

Nursing Actions

Physical Assessment Monitor for lactic acidosis, osteomalacia, gastrointestinal disturbance, neutropenia, myalgia, and peripheral neuropathy periodically during therapy.

Patient Education

• Discuss specific use of drug and side effects with patient as it relates to treatment. (HCAHPS: During this hospital stay, were you given any medicine that you had not taken before? Before giving you any new medicine, how often did

hospital staff tell you what the medicine was for? How often did hospital staff describe possible side effects in a way you could understand?)

- Patient may experience nightmares, headache, nausea, diarrhea, or lipodystrophy. Have patient report immediately to prescriber signs of renal impairment, signs of hepatic impairment, signs of lactic acidosis, signs of pancreatitis, osteodynia, asthenia, myalgia, painful extremities, polydipsia, dyspnea, or signs of infection (HCAHPS).
- Educate patient about signs of a significant reaction (eg, wheezing; chest tightness; fever; itching; bad cough; blue skin color; seizures; or swelling of face, lips, tongue, or throat). **Note:** This is not a comprehensive list of all side effects. Patient should consult prescriber for additional questions.

Intended Use and Disclaimer: Should not be printed and given to patients. This information is intended to serve as a concise initial reference for healthcare professionals to use when discussing medications with a patient. You must ultimately rely on your own discretion, experience and judgment in diagnosing, treating and advising patients.

Dietary Considerations Take with a meal. Consider calcium and vitamin D supplementation in patients with history of bone fracture or osteopenia.

Related Information

Emtricitabine *on page 521*
Tenofovir *on page 1490*

Emtricitabine (em trye SYE ta been)

Brand Names: U.S. Emtriva
Index Terms BW524W91; Coviracil; FTC
Pharmacologic Category Antiretroviral, Reverse Transcriptase Inhibitor, Nucleoside (Anti-HIV)
Pregnancy Risk Factor B
Lactation Enters breast milk/contraindicated
Breast-Feeding Considerations Emtricitabine is excreted into breast milk. Maternal or infant antiretroviral therapy does not completely eliminate the risk of postnatal HIV transmission. In addition, multiclass-resistant virus has been detected in breast-feeding infants despite maternal therapy. Therefore, in the United States, where formula is accessible, affordable, safe, and sustainable, and the risk of infant mortality due to diarrhea and respiratory infections is low, complete avoidance of breast-feeding by HIV-infected women is recommended to decrease potential transmission of HIV (DHHS [perinatal], 2012).
Use Treatment of HIV infection in combination with at least two other antiretroviral agents
Mechanism of Action/Effect Nucleoside reverse transcriptase inhibitor which interferes with viral RNA-dependent DNA synthesis, resulting in inhibition of viral replication.

Contraindications Hypersensitivity to emtricitabine or any component of the formulation

Warnings/Precautions [U.S. Boxed Warning]: Lactic acidosis, severe hepatomegaly with steatosis, and hepatic failure have occurred rarely with emtricitabine (similar to other nucleoside analogues). Some cases have been fatal; stop treatment if lactic acidosis or hepatotoxicity occur. Prior liver disease, obesity, extended duration of therapy, and female gender may represent risk factors for severe hepatic reactions. Testing for hepatitis B is recommended prior to the initiation of therapy; **[U.S. Boxed Warnings]: Hepatitis B may be exacerbated following discontinuation of emtricitabine; not indicated for treatment of chronic hepatitis B; safety and efficacy in HIV/HBV coinfected patients not established.** May be associated with fat redistribution (buffalo hump, increased abdominal girth, breast engorgement, facial atrophy, and dyslipidemia). Immune reconstitution syndrome may develop resulting in the occurrence of an inflammatory response to an indolent or residual opportunistic infection during initial HIV treatment or activation of autoimmune disorders (eg, Graves' disease, polymyositis, Guillain-Barré syndrome) later in therapy; further evaluation and treatment may be required. Use caution in patients with renal impairment (dosage adjustment required). Concomitant use of other emtricitabine-containing products should be avoided. Concomitant use of lamivudine or lamivudine-containing products should be avoided; cross-resistance may develop.

Drug Interactions

Avoid Concomitant Use

Avoid concomitant use of Emtricitabine with any of the following: LamiVUDine

Decreased Effect There are no known significant interactions involving a decrease in effect.

Increased Effect/Toxicity

The levels/effects of Emtricitabine may be increased by: Ganciclovir-Valganciclovir; LamiVUDine; Ribavirin

Nutritional/Ethanol Interactions Food: Food decreases peak plasma concentrations, but does not alter the extent of absorption or overall systemic exposure.

Adverse Reactions Clinical trials were conducted in patients receiving other antiretroviral agents, and it is not possible to correlate frequency of adverse events with emtricitabine alone. The range of frequencies of adverse events is generally comparable to comparator groups, with the exception of hyperpigmentation, which occurred more frequently in patients receiving emtricitabine. Unless otherwise noted, percentages are as reported in adults.

>10%:

Central nervous system: Dizziness (4% to 25%), headache (6% to 22%), fever (children 18%), insomnia (5% to 16%), abnormal dreams (2% to 11%)

Dermatologic: Hyperpigmentation (children 32%; adults 2% to 4%; primarily of palms and/or soles but may include tongue, arms, lip and nails; generally mild and nonprogressive without associated local reactions such as pruritus or rash); rash (17% to 30%; includes pruritus, maculopapular rash, vesiculobullous rash, pustular rash, and allergic reaction)

Gastrointestinal: Diarrhea (children 20%; adults 9% to 23%), vomiting (children 23%; adults 9%), nausea (13% to 18%), abdominal pain (8% to 14%), gastroenteritis (children 11%)

Neuromuscular & skeletal: Weakness (12% to 16%), CPK increased (grades 3/4: 11% to 12%)

Otic: Otitis media (children 23%)

Respiratory: Cough (children 28%; adults 14%), rhinitis (children 20%; adults 12% to 18%), pneumonia (children 15%)

Miscellaneous: Infection (children 44%)

1% to 10%:

Central nervous system: Depression (6% to 9%), neuropathy/neuritis (4%)

Endocrine & metabolic: Serum triglycerides increased (grades 3/4: 4% to 10%), disordered glucose homeostasis (grades 3/4: 2% to 3%), serum amylase increased (grades 3/4: children 9%; adults 2% to 5%), serum lipase increased (grades 3/4: ≤1%)

Gastrointestinal: Dyspepsia (4% to 8%), serum amylase increased (grades 3/4: 8%)

Genitourinary: Hematuria (grades 3/4: 3%)

Hematologic: Anemia (children: 7%), neutropenia (grades 3/4: children 2%; adults 5%)

Hepatic: Transaminases increased (grades 3/4: 2% to 6%), alkaline phosphatase increased (>550 units/L: 1%), bilirubin increased (grades 3/4: 1%)

Neuromuscular & skeletal: Creatinine kinase increased (grades 3/4: 9%), myalgia (4% to 6%), paresthesia (5% to 6%), arthralgia (3% to 5%)

Respiratory: Upper respiratory tract infection (8%), sinusitis (8%), pharyngitis (5%)

Available Dosage Forms

Capsule, Oral:

Emtriva: 200 mg

Solution, Oral:

Emtriva: 10 mg/mL (170 mL)

General Dosage Range Dosage adjustment recommended in patients with renal impairment

Oral:

Capsule: *Children 3 months to 17 years and >33 kg and Adults:* 200 mg once daily

Solution:

Children <3 months: 3 mg/kg/day

Children 3 months to 17 years: 6 mg/kg once daily (maximum: 240 mg/day)

Adults: 240 mg once daily

Administration

Oral May be administered with or without food.

Storage/Stability Store capsules at 15°C to 30°C (59°F to 86°F). Solution should be stored under refrigeration at 2°C to 8°C (36°F to 46°F). Once dispensed, may be stored at 15°C to 30°C (59°F to 86°F) if used within 3 months.

Nursing Actions

Physical Assessment Assess viral load and CD4 count. Monitor for lactic acidosis periodically during therapy. Teach patient proper timing of multiple medications.

Patient Education

• Discuss specific use of drug and side effects with patient as it relates to treatment. (HCAHPS: During this hospital stay, were you given any medicine that you had not taken before? Before giving you any new medicine, how often did hospital staff tell you what the medicine was for? How often did hospital staff describe possible side effects in a way you could understand?)

• Patient may experience dizziness, headache, insomnia, dyspepsia, rhinorrhea, or lipodystrophy. Have patient report immediately to prescriber signs of infection, depression, severe nausea, significant diarrhea, considerable asthenia, skin discoloration, intolerable skin irritation, signs of hepatic impairment, or signs of lactic acidosis (HCAHPS).

• Educate patient about signs of a significant reaction (eg, wheezing; chest tightness; fever; itching; bad cough; blue skin color; seizures; or swelling of face, lips, tongue, or throat). **Note:** This is not a comprehensive list of all side effects. Patient should consult prescriber for additional questions.

Intended Use and Disclaimer: Should not be printed and given to patients. This information is intended to serve as a concise initial reference for healthcare professionals to use when discussing medications with a patient. You must ultimately rely on your own discretion, experience and judgment in diagnosing, treating and advising patients.

Dietary Considerations May be taken with or without food.

Emtricitabine and Tenofovir
(em trye SYE ta been & ten OF oh vir)

Brand Names: U.S. Truvada

Index Terms Tenofovir and Emtricitabine

Pharmacologic Category Antiretroviral, Reverse Transcriptase Inhibitor, Nucleoside (Anti-HIV); Antiretroviral, Reverse Transcriptase Inhibitor, Nucleotide (Anti-HIV)

Medication Guide Available Yes

Pregnancy Risk Factor B

Lactation Use in combination with safer sex practices for preexposure prophylaxis (PrEP) in lactating women who are HIV-uninfected is limited (DHHS [perinatal], 2012). Use is not recommended (CDC, 2012).

Breast-Feeding Considerations See individual agents.

Use

Treatment of HIV-1 infection in combination with other antiretroviral agents in adults and pediatric patients ≥12 years of age

Pre-exposure prophylaxis (PrEP) for prevention of HIV-1 infection in adults who are at high risk for acquiring HIV

High risk individuals include those with partners known to be HIV-1 infected or who engage in sexual activity within a high prevalence area or social network, and one or more of the following:
- Inconsistent or no condom use
- Diagnosis of sexually-transmitted infections
- Exchange of sex for commodities
- Use of illicit drugs or alcohol dependence
- Incarceration
- Partner of unknown HIV-1 status with any of the above risk factors

When prescribing PrEP healthcare providers **MUST**:
- Include PrEP as part of a comprehensive prevention strategy because PrEP alone is not always effective in preventing HIV-1 infection
- Counsel all uninfected patients to strictly adhere to the dosing schedule, because adherence was strongly correlated with effectiveness in clinical trials
- Confirm a negative HIV-1 test prior to starting PrEP; if a candidate has acute viral infection symptoms and unprotected exposure events <1 month prior, delay PrEP for at least 1 month and retest HIV-1 status or use an Food and Drug Administration (FDA) test approved for HIV-1 diagnosis, including acute or primary HIV-1 infection
- Retest for HIV-1 infection at least every 3 months while the patient receives PrEP

Unlabeled Use Treatment of hepatitis B in patients with antiviral-resistant HBV or coinfection with HIV; pre-exposure prophylaxis (PrEP) for prevention of HIV-1 infection in injecting drug users (IDU) who are at risk for parenteral acquisition of HIV but not at risk for sexual acquisition of HIV; postexposure prophylaxis (PEP) for occupational exposure to HIV

Mechanism of Action/Effect Inhibits the production of new HIV virus by blocking the viral enzyme responsible for making DNA from viral RNA.

Contraindications

U.S. labeling: Do not use for preexposure prophylaxis in patients with unknown or HIV-1 positive status. For HIV-1 treatment, use only in HIV-1-infected patients in combination with other antiretrovirals.

Canadian labeling: Previously demonstrated hypersensitivity to any component of the formulation.

Warnings/Precautions Not recommended as a component of a triple nucleoside regimen.

[U.S. Boxed Warning]: Lactic acidosis and severe hepatomegaly with steatosis have been reported with nucleoside and nucleotide analogues (eg, tenofovir), including fatal cases. Use with caution in patients with risk factors for liver disease (risk may be increased in obese patients or prolonged exposure) and suspend treatment in any patient who develops clinical or laboratory findings suggestive of lactic acidosis (transaminase elevation may/may not accompany hepatomegaly and steatosis). Use caution in hepatic impairment; no dosage adjustment is required; limited studies indicate the pharmacokinetics of tenofovir are not altered in hepatic dysfunction.

HIV-1 treatment: Use caution in moderate renal impairment (CrCl <50 mL/minute); dosage adjustment required. May cause acute renal failure or Fanconi syndrome; use caution with other nephrotoxic agents (including high dose or multiple NSAID use or those which compete for active tubular secretion). Acute renal failure has occurred in HIV-infected patients with risk factors for renal impairment who were on a stable tenofovir regimen to which a high dose or multiple NSAID therapy was added. Consider alternatives to NSAIDS in patients taking tenofovir and at risk for renal impairment. Calculate creatinine clearance prior to initiation in all patients; monitor renal function during therapy (including recalculation of creatinine clearance and serum phosphorus) in patients at risk for renal impairment, including those with previous renal decline on adefovir. In clinical trials, use has been associated with decreases in bone mineral density in HIV-1 infected adults and increases in bone metabolism markers. Serum parathyroid hormone and 1,25 vitamin D levels were also higher. Decreases in bone mineral density have also been observed in clinical trials of HIV-1 infected pediatric patients. Observations in chronic hepatitis B infected pediatric patients (aged 12-18 years) were similar. Consider monitoring of bone density in adult and pediatric patients with a history of pathologic fractures or with other risk factors for bone loss or osteoporosis. Consider calcium and vitamin D supplementation for all patients; effect of supplementation has not been studied but may be beneficial. Long-term bone health and fracture risk unknown. Skeletal growth (height) appears to be unaffected in tenofovir-treated children and adolescents. May cause osteomalacia with proximal renal tubulopathy. Bone pain, extremity pain, fractures, arthralgias, weakness and muscle pain have been reported. In patients at risk for renal dysfunction, persistent or worsening bone or muscle symptoms should be evaluated for hypophosphatemia and osteomalacia. Avoid use in patients with CrCl <30 mL/minute; monitor for possible bone abnormalities during therapy. All patients with HIV should be tested for HBV prior to initiation of treatment.

Pre-exposure prophylaxis (PrEP): Routinely monitor patients with mild renal impairment. Calculate creatinine clearance prior to initiation in all patients; monitor renal function during therapy (including recalculation of creatinine clearance and serum phosphorus). Do not use in CrCl <60 mL/minute. PrEP should be accompanied by a comprehensive HIV-1 prevention program (eg, risk reduction counseling, access to condoms), with particular emphasis on medication adherence. In addition, regular monitoring (eg, HIV status of patient and partner(s), risk behavior, adherence, adverse effects, sexually transmitted infections that facilitate HIV-1 transmission) is highly recommended.

[U.S. Boxed Warning]: Safety and efficacy during coinfection of HIV and HBV have not been established; acute, severe exacerbations of HBV have been reported following discontinuation of antiretroviral therapy. In HBV coinfected patients, monitor hepatic function closely for several months following discontinuation. May cause redistribution of fat (eg, buffalo hump, peripheral wasting with increased abdominal girth, cushingoid appearance). Patients may develop immune reconstitution syndrome resulting in the occurrence of an inflammatory response to an indolent or residual opportunistic infection during initial HIV treatment or activation of autoimmune disorders (eg, Graves' disease, polymyositis, Guillain-Barré syndrome) later in therapy; further evaluation and treatment may be required. Do not use concurrently with adefovir, emtricitabine, tenofovir, lamivudine, or lamivudine-combination products.

[U.S. Boxed Warning]: Confirm HIV-1 negative status immediately before and at least every 3 months during therapy. Risk of drug resistant HIV-1 variants with PrEP use if patient had undetected acute HIV-1 infection. Some HIV-1 tests (eg, rapid tests) do not detect acute HIV-1 infection. Screen PrEP candidates for acute viral infections and potential exposure events ≤1 month of starting PrEP. If infections or events exist, wait 1 month to start PrEP and reconfirm HIV-1 negative status. Do not start PrEP if signs or symptoms of acute HIV-1 infection are present unless HIV-1 negative status is confirmed by a test approved by the Food and Drug Administration (FDA) as an aid to detect HIV-1 infection (including acute or primary infection).

Drug Interactions
Avoid Concomitant Use
Avoid concomitant use of Emtricitabine and Tenofovir with any of the following: Adefovir; Dabigatran Etexilate; Didanosine; LamiVUDine; Pomalidomide; VinCRIStine (Liposomal)

Decreased Effect
Emtricitabine and Tenofovir may decrease the levels/effects of: Afatinib; Atazanavir; Dabigatran Etexilate; Didanosine; DOXOrubicin (Conventional); Linagliptin; P-glycoprotein/ABCB1 Substrates; Pomalidomide; Simeprevir; Tipranavir; VinCRIStine (Liposomal)

The levels/effects of Emtricitabine and Tenofovir may be decreased by: Adefovir; Tipranavir

Increased Effect/Toxicity
Emtricitabine and Tenofovir may increase the levels/effects of: Adefovir; Aminoglycosides; Darunavir; Didanosine; Ganciclovir-Valganciclovir

The levels/effects of Emtricitabine and Tenofovir may be increased by: Acyclovir-Valacyclovir; Adefovir; Aminoglycosides; Atazanavir; Cidofovir; Darunavir; Diclofenac (Systemic); Ganciclovir-Valganciclovir; LamiVUDine; Lopinavir; Nonsteroidal Anti-Inflammatory Agents; Ribavirin; Simeprevir; Telaprevir

Nutritional/Ethanol Interactions Food: Food decreases peak plasma concentrations, but does not alter the extent of absorption or overall systemic exposure.

Adverse Reactions The adverse reaction profile of combination therapy has not been established. See individual agents.

Available Dosage Forms
Tablet:
Truvada: Emtricitabine 200 mg and tenofovir 300 mg

General Dosage Range Dosage adjustment recommended in patients with renal impairment

Oral: Children ≥12 (and >35 kg), Adolescents (≥35 kg), and Adults: 1 tablet (emtricitabine 200 mg and tenofovir 300 mg) once daily

Administration
Oral May be administered with or without food.

Storage/Stability Store tablets at 25°C (77°F); excursions permitted to 15°C to 30°C (59°F to 86°F).

Nursing Actions
Physical Assessment Monitor hepatic and renal functions. Test for HBV prior to treatment.

Patient Education
- Discuss specific use of drug and side effects with patient as it relates to treatment. (HCAHPS: During this hospital stay, were you given any medicine that you had not taken before? Before giving you any new medicine, how often did hospital staff tell you what the medicine was for? How often did hospital staff describe possible side effects in a way you could understand?)

- Patient may experience diarrhea, insomnia, headache, dyspepsia, nightmares, weight loss, or lipodystrophy. Have patient report immediately to prescriber signs of infection, signs of renal impairment, signs of hepatic impairment, signs of lactic acidosis, dyspnea, severe dizziness, syncope, considerable nausea, depression, osteodynia, myalgia, asthenia, painful extremities, polydipsia, or paresthesia (HCAHPS).
- Educate patient about signs of a significant reaction (eg, wheezing; chest tightness; fever; itching; bad cough; blue skin color; seizures; or swelling of face, lips, tongue, or throat). **Note:** This is not a comprehensive list of all side effects. Patient should consult prescriber for additional questions.

Intended Use and Disclaimer: Should not be printed and given to patients. This information is intended to serve as a concise initial reference for healthcare professionals to use when discussing medications with a patient. You must ultimately rely on your own discretion, experience and judgment in diagnosing, treating and advising patients.

Dietary Considerations May be taken without regard to meals. Consider calcium and vitamin D supplementation in patients with history of bone fracture or osteopenia.

Related Information

Emtricitabine *on page 521*
Tenofovir *on page 1490*

Emtricitabine, Rilpivirine, and Tenofovir

(em trye SYE ta been, ril pi VIR een, & ten OF oh vir)

Brand Names: U.S. Complera

Index Terms FTC/RPV/TDF; Rilpivirine, Emtricitabine, and Tenofovir; Tenofovir Disoproxil Fumarate, Rilpivirine, and Emtricitabine; Tenofovir, Emtricitabine, and Rilpivirine

Pharmacologic Category Antiretroviral, Reverse Transcriptase Inhibitor, Non-nucleoside (Anti-HIV); Antiretroviral, Reverse Transcriptase Inhibitor, Nucleoside (Anti-HIV); Antiretroviral, Reverse Transcriptase Inhibitor, Nucleotide (Anti-HIV)

Pregnancy Risk Factor B

Lactation See individual agents.

Use

Treatment of human immunodeficiency virus type 1 (HIV-1) infection in antiretroviral treatment-naive patients with HIV-1 RNA ≤100,000 copies/mL at the start of therapy

Treatment (replacement of a current antiretroviral treatment regimen) in virologically-suppressed (HIV-1 RNA <50 copies/mL) patients who meet all of the following parameters:

- are on a stable antiretroviral regimen at start of therapy

- have no history of virologic failure
- prior to regimen replacement, have been suppressed for at least 6 months
- are currently on their first or second antiretroviral regimen
- have no history of resistance to emtricitabine, rilpivirine, or tenofovir.

Available Dosage Forms

Tablet, oral:

Complera: Emtricitabine 200 mg, rilpivirine 25 mg, and tenofovir 300 mg

General Dosage Range Oral: *Adults:* One tablet once daily

Administration

Oral Administer with food.

Nursing Actions

Physical Assessment Monitor renal function and bone density in patients at risk for osteopenia. Assess patient for depression.

Patient Education

- Discuss specific use of drug and side effects with patient as it relates to treatment. (HCAHPS: During this hospital stay, were you given any medicine that you had not taken before? Before giving you any new medicine, how often did hospital staff tell you what the medicine was for? How often did hospital staff describe possible side effects in a way you could understand?)
- Patient may experience headache, insomnia, diarrhea, dyspepsia, skin discoloration, nightmares, or lipodystrophy. Have patient report immediately to prescriber signs of infection, signs of renal impairment, signs of hepatic impairment, signs of lactic acidosis, signs of depression (ie, suicidal ideation, anxiety, emotional instability, illogical thinking), severe dizziness, syncope, significant nausea, polydipsia, angina, arrhythmia, paresthesia, dyspnea, osteodynia, myalgia, asthenia, or painful extremities (HCAHPS).
- Educate patient about signs of a significant reaction (eg, wheezing; chest tightness; fever; itching; bad cough; blue skin color; seizures; or swelling of face, lips, tongue, or throat). **Note:** This is not a comprehensive list of all side effects. Patient should consult prescriber for additional questions.

Intended Use and Disclaimer: Should not be printed and given to patients. This information is intended to serve as a concise initial reference for healthcare professionals to use when discussing medications with a patient. You must ultimately rely on your own discretion, experience and judgment in diagnosing, treating and advising patients.

Related Information

Emtricitabine *on page 521*
Rilpivirine *on page 1355*
Tenofovir *on page 1490*

Enalapril (e NAL a pril)

Brand Names: U.S. Epaned; Vasotec
Index Terms Enalapril Maleate
Pharmacologic Category Angiotensin-Converting Enzyme (ACE) Inhibitor; Antihypertensive
Medication Safety Issues
Sound-alike/look-alike issues:
Enalapril may be confused with Anafranil, Elavil, Eldepryl, ramipril
Administration issues:
Significant differences exist between oral and I.V. dosing. Use caution when converting from one route of administration to another.
International issues:
Acepril [Hungary, Switzerland] may be confused with Accupril which is a brand name for quinapril [U.S., Canada, multiple international markets]
Acepril: Brand name for enalapril [Hungary, Switzerland], but also brand name for captopril [Great Britain]; lisinopril [Malaysia]
Pregnancy Risk Factor D
Lactation Enters breast milk/not recommended
Breast-Feeding Considerations Enalapril and enalaprilat are excreted in breast milk. Breastfeeding is not recommended by the manufacturer.
Use Treatment of hypertension; treatment of symptomatic heart failure (HF); treatment of asymptomatic left ventricular dysfunction
Note: The ACCF/AHA 2013 heart failure guidelines recommend the use of ACE inhibitors, along with other guideline directed medical therapies, to prevent heart failure in patients with a reduced ejection fraction who have a history of MI (Stage B HF), to prevent heart failure in any patient with a reduced ejection fraction (Stage B HF), or to treat those with heart failure and reduced ejection fraction (Stage C HFrEF) (ACCF/AHA [Yancy, 2013]).
Unlabeled Use To delay the progression of nephropathy and reduce risks of cardiovascular events in hypertensive patients with type 1 or 2 diabetes mellitus; hypertensive crisis, diabetic nephropathy, hypertension secondary to scleroderma renal crisis, diagnosis of aldosteronism, idiopathic edema, Bartter's syndrome, postmyocardial infarction for prevention of ventricular failure
Mechanism of Action/Effect Competitive inhibitor of angiotensin-converting enzyme (ACE); prevents conversion of angiotensin I to angiotensin II, a potent vasoconstrictor; results in lower levels of angiotensin II which causes an increase in plasma renin activity and a reduction in aldosterone secretion

Contraindications

Hypersensitivity to enalapril or enalaprilat; angioedema related to previous treatment with an ACE inhibitor; patients with idiopathic or hereditary angioedema; concomitant use with aliskiren in patients with diabetes mellitus
Canadian labeling: Additional contraindications (not in U.S. labeling): Concomitant use with aliskiren-containing drugs in patients with moderate-to-severe renal impairment (GFR <60 mL/minute/1.73m^2)

Warnings/Precautions Anaphylactic reactions may occur rarely with ACE inhibitors. At any time during treatment (especially following first dose) angioedema may occur rarely with ACE inhibitors; it may involve the head and neck (potentially compromising airway) or the intestine (presenting with abdominal pain). African-Americans may be at an increased risk. Prolonged frequent monitoring may be required especially if tongue, glottis, or larynx are involved as they are associated with airway obstruction. Patients with a history of airway surgery may have a higher risk of airway obstruction. Aggressive early and appropriate management is critical. Use in patients with idiopathic or hereditary angioedema or previous angioedema associated with ACE inhibitor therapy is contraindicated. Severe anaphylactoid reactions may be seen during hemodialysis (eg, CVVHD) with high-flux dialysis membranes (eg, AN69), and rarely, during low density lipoprotein apheresis with dextran sulfate cellulose. Rare cases of anaphylactoid reactions have been reported in patients undergoing sensitization treatment with hymenoptera (bee, wasp) venom while receiving ACE inhibitors.

Symptomatic hypotension with or without syncope can occur with ACE inhibitors (usually with the first several doses); effects are most often observed in volume depleted patients; correct volume depletion prior to initiation; close monitoring of patient is required especially with initial dosing and dosing increases; blood pressure must be lowered at a rate appropriate for the patient's clinical condition. Initiation of therapy in patients with ischemic heart disease or cerebrovascular disease warrants close observation due to the potential consequences posed by falling blood pressure (eg, MI, stroke). Use with caution in hypertrophic cardiomyopathy with outflow tract obstruction, severe aortic stenosis, or before, during, or immediately after major surgery. **[U.S. Boxed Warning]: Drugs that act on the renin-angiotensin system can cause injury and death to the developing fetus. Discontinue as soon as possible once pregnancy is detected.**

Hyperkalemia may occur with ACE inhibitors; risk factors include renal dysfunction, diabetes mellitus, concomitant use of potassium-sparing diuretics, potassium supplements, and/or potassium-containing salts. Use cautiously, if at all, with these agents and monitor potassium closely. Cough may occur with ACE inhibitors. Other causes of cough should be considered (eg, pulmonary congestion in patients with heart failure) and excluded prior to discontinuation.

May be associated with deterioration of renal function and/or increases in serum creatinine, particularly in patients with low renal blood flow (eg, renal artery stenosis, heart failure) whose glomerular filtration rate (GFR) is dependent on efferent arteriolar vasoconstriction by angiotensin II; deterioration may result in oliguria, acute renal failure, and progressive azotemia. Small increases in serum creatinine may occur following initiation; consider discontinuation only in patients with progressive and/or significant deterioration in renal function. Use with caution in patients with unstented unilateral/bilateral renal artery stenosis. When unstented bilateral renal artery stenosis is present, use is generally avoided due to the elevated risk of deterioration in renal function unless possible benefits outweigh risks. Potentially significant drug-drug interactions may exist, requiring dose or frequency adjustment, additional monitoring, and/or selection of alternative therapy.

Rare toxicities associated with ACE inhibitors include cholestatic jaundice (which may progress to fulminant hepatic necrosis), agranulocytosis, neutropenia or leukopenia with myeloid hypoplasia. Patients with collagen vascular diseases (especially with concomitant renal impairment) or renal impairment alone may be at increased risk for hematologic toxicity; periodically monitor CBC with differential in these patients.

Drug Interactions

Avoid Concomitant Use There are no known interactions where it is recommended to avoid concomitant use.

Decreased Effect
The levels/effects of Enalapril may be decreased by: Antacids; Aprotinin; Herbs (Hypertensive Properties); Icatibant; Lanthanum; Methylphenidate; Nonsteroidal Anti-Inflammatory Agents; Salicylates; Yohimbine

Increased Effect/Toxicity
Enalapril may increase the levels/effects of: Allopurinol; Amifostine; Antihypertensives; AzaTHIOprine; CycloSPORINE (Systemic); DULoxetine; Ferric Gluconate; Gold Sodium Thiomalate; Hypotensive Agents; Iron Dextran Complex; Lithium; Nonsteroidal Anti-Inflammatory Agents; Obinutuzumab; RiTUXimab; Sodium Phosphates

The levels/effects of Enalapril may be increased by: Alfuzosin; Aliskiren; Angiotensin II Receptor Blockers; Brimonidine (Topical); Canagliflozin; Diazoxide; DPP-IV Inhibitors; Eplerenone; Everolimus; Heparin; Heparin (Low Molecular Weight); Herbs (Hypotensive Properties); Loop Diuretics; MAO Inhibitors; Pentoxifylline; Phosphodiesterase 5 Inhibitors; Potassium Salts; Potassium-Sparing Diuretics; Prostacyclin Analogues; Sirolimus; Temsirolimus; Thiazide Diuretics; TiZANidine; Tolvaptan; Trimethoprim

Nutritional/Ethanol Interactions
Food: Potassium supplements and/or potassium-containing salts may cause or worsen hyperkalemia. Management: Consult prescriber before consuming a potassium-rich diet, potassium supplements, or salt substitutes.

Herb/Nutraceutical: Some herbal medications may worsen hypertension (eg, licorice); others may increase the antihypertensive effect of enalapril (eg, shepherd's purse). Management: Avoid bayberry, blue cohosh, cayenne, ephedra, ginger, ginseng (American), kola, licorice, and yohimbe. Avoid black cohosh, California poppy, coleus, golden seal, hawthorn, mistletoe, periwinkle, quinine, and shepherd's purse.

Adverse Reactions Note: Frequency ranges include data from hypertension and heart failure trials. Higher rates of adverse reactions have generally been noted in patients with CHF. However, the frequency of adverse effects associated with placebo is also increased in this population.

>10%: Renal: Increased serum creatinine (≤20%)
1% to 10%:
  Cardiovascular: Hypotension (1% to 7%), chest pain (2%), orthostatic effect (1% to 2%), orthostatic hypotension (2%), syncope (≤2%)
  Central nervous system: Dizziness (4% to 8%), headache (2% to 5%), fatigue (2% to 3%)
  Dermatologic: Skin rash (1% to 2%)
  Gastrointestinal: Abdominal pain, anorexia, constipation, diarrhea, dysgeusia, nausea, vomiting
  Neuromuscular & skeletal: Weakness
  Renal: Renal insufficiency (in patients with bilateral renal artery stenosis or hypovolemia)
  Respiratory: Bronchitis (1% to 2%), cough (1% to 2%), dyspnea (1% to 2%)

Pharmacodynamics/Kinetics
Onset of Action ~1 hour; Peak effect: 4-6 hours
Duration of Action 12-24 hours

Available Dosage Forms
Solution Reconstituted, Oral:
  Epaned: 1 mg/mL (150 mL)
Tablet, Oral:
  Vasotec: 2.5 mg, 5 mg, 10 mg, 20 mg
  Generic: 2.5 mg, 5 mg, 10 mg, 20 mg
General Dosage Range Dosage adjustment recommended in patients with renal impairment.
Oral:
  Children ≥1 month and Adolescents Initial: 0.08 mg/kg (up to 5 mg) once daily; Maintenance: Up to 0.58 mg/kg (40 mg)
  Adults: Initial: 2.5-5 mg daily in 1-2 divided doses; Maintenance: 2.5-40 mg daily in 1-2 divided doses

Preparation for Administration Epaned: Solution kit (for 150 mL, enalapril solution 1 mg/mL): Kit contains 1 bottle of enalapril powder and 1 bottle of Ora-Sweet SF dilution to be added to the enalapril powder prior to dispensing. Firmly tap the enalapril powder for oral solution bottle on a hard surface 5 times. Add approximately one-half (75 mL) of the Ora-Sweet SF diluent to the enalapril 150 mL oral solution bottle and shake well for 30 seconds. Add the remainder of the Ora-Sweet SF diluent and shake well for an additional 30 seconds. May be used for 60 days after reconstitution.

Storage/Stability

Solution kit: Store at 25°C (77°F); excursions are permitted between 15°C and 30°C (59°F and 86°F). Do not freeze. Protect from moisture. Once reconstituted, the solution should be stored at room temperature [(15°C to 30°C (59°F to 86°F)] and can be stored for up to 60 days.

Tablet: Store below 30°C (86°F); avoid temperatures >50°C (122°F). Protect from moisture.

Nursing Actions

Physical Assessment Assess potential for interactions with other pharmacological agents or herbal products that may impact fluid balance or cardiac status. Monitor blood pressure closely with first dose or change in dose. Monitor laboratory tests closely during first 3 months and regularly thereafter. Monitor for anaphylactic reaction, hypovolemia, angioedema, and postural hypotension.

Patient Education

• Discuss specific use of drug and side effects with patient as it relates to treatment. (HCAHPS: During this hospital stay, were you given any medicine that you had not taken before? Before giving you any new medicine, how often did hospital staff tell you what the medicine was for? How often did hospital staff describe possible side effects in a way you could understand?)

• Have patient report immediately to prescriber signs of renal impairment, signs of hyperkalemia, severe dizziness, syncope, angina, significant dyspepsia, considerable nausea, or signs of hepatic impairment (HCAHPS).

• Educate patient about signs of a significant reaction (eg, wheezing; chest tightness; fever; itching; bad cough; blue skin color; seizures; or swelling of face, lips, tongue, or throat). **Note:** This is not a comprehensive list of all side effects. Patient should consult prescriber for additional questions.

Intended Use and Disclaimer: Should not be printed and given to patients. This information is intended to serve as a concise initial reference for healthcare professionals to use when discussing medications with a patient. You must ultimately rely on your own discretion, experience and judgment in diagnosing, treating and advising patients.

Dietary Considerations Limit salt substitutes or potassium-rich diet.

Enalapril and Hydrochlorothiazide
(e NAL a pril & hye droe klor oh THYE a zide)

Brand Names: U.S. Vaseretic

Index Terms Enalapril Maleate and Hydrochlorothiazide; Hydrochlorothiazide and Enalapril

Pharmacologic Category Angiotensin-Converting Enzyme (ACE) Inhibitor; Antihypertensive; Diuretic, Thiazide

Medication Safety Issues
International issues:
Norpramin: Brand name for enalapril/hydrochlorothiazide [Portugal], but also the brand name for desipramine [U.S., Canada]; omeprazole [Spain]

Pregnancy Risk Factor D

Use Treatment of hypertension

Available Dosage Forms
Tablet: 5/12.5: Enalapril 5 mg and hydrochlorothiazide 12.5 mg; 10/25: Enalapril 10 mg and hydrochlorothiazide 25 mg
Vaseretic: 10/25: enalapril 10 mg and hydrochlorothiazide 25 mg

General Dosage Range Oral: *Adults:* Enalapril 5-10 mg and hydrochlorothiazide 12.5-25 mg once daily (maximum: 40 mg/day [enalapril]; 50 mg/day [hydrochlorothiazide])

Nursing Actions

Physical Assessment See individual agents.

Patient Education

• Discuss specific use of drug and side effects with patient as it relates to treatment. (HCAHPS: During this hospital stay, were you given any medicine that you had not taken before? Before giving you any new medicine, how often did hospital staff tell you what the medicine was for? How often did hospital staff describe possible side effects in a way you could understand?)

• Patient may experience dizziness, headache, or asthenia. Have patient report immediately to prescriber signs of hyperglycemia, signs of fluid and electrolyte imbalance, signs of renal impairment, paresthesia, angina, tachycardia, dyspnea, severe dyspepsia, vision changes, ophthalmalgia, or signs of hepatic impairment (HCAHPS).

• Educate patient about signs of a significant reaction (eg, wheezing; chest tightness; fever; itching; bad cough; blue skin color; seizures; or swelling of face, lips, tongue, or throat). **Note:** This is not a comprehensive list of all side effects. Patient should consult prescriber for additional questions.

Intended Use and Disclaimer: Should not be printed and given to patients. This information is intended to serve as a concise initial reference for

healthcare professionals to use when discussing medications with a patient. You must ultimately rely on your own discretion, experience and judgment in diagnosing, treating and advising patients.

Related Information

Enalapril *on page 526*

Hydrochlorothiazide *on page 775*

Enalaprilat (en AL a pril at)

Pharmacologic Category Angiotensin-Converting Enzyme (ACE) Inhibitor; Antihypertensive

Medication Safety Issues

Administration issues:

Significant differences exist between oral and I.V. dosing. Use caution when converting from one route of administration to another.

Pregnancy Risk Factor C (1st trimester); D (2nd and 3rd trimesters)

Lactation Enters breast milk/not recommended

Breast-Feeding Considerations Enalapril and enalaprilat are excreted in breast milk. Breast-feeding is not recommended by the manufacturer.

Use Treatment of hypertension when oral therapy is not practical

Unlabeled Use Severe congestive heart failure in infants, acute cardiogenic pulmonary edema

Mechanism of Action/Effect Competitive inhibitor of angiotensin-converting enzyme (ACE); prevents conversion of angiotensin I to angiotensin II, a potent vasoconstrictor; results in lower levels of angiotensin II which causes an increase in plasma renin activity and a reduction in aldosterone secretion

Contraindications Hypersensitivity to enalapril or enalaprilat; angioedema related to previous treatment with an ACE inhibitor; patients with idiopathic or hereditary angioedema; concomitant use with aliskiren in patients with diabetes mellitus

Warnings/Precautions Anaphylactic reactions may occur rarely with ACE inhibitors. At any time during treatment (especially following first dose) angioedema may occur rarely with ACE inhibitors; it may involve the head and neck (potentially compromising airway) or the intestine (presenting with abdominal pain). African-Americans may be at an increased risk. Prolonged frequent monitoring may be required especially if tongue, glottis, or larynx are involved as they are associated with airway obstruction. Patients with a history of airway surgery may have a higher risk of airway obstruction. Aggressive early and appropriate management is critical. Use in patients with idiopathic or hereditary angioedema or previous angioedema associated with ACE inhibitor therapy is contraindicated. Severe anaphylactoid reactions may be seen during hemodialysis (eg, CVVHD) with high-flux dialysis membranes (eg, AN69), and rarely, during low density lipoprotein apheresis with dextran sulfate cellulose. Rare cases of anaphylactoid reactions have been reported in patients undergoing sensitization treatment with hymenoptera (bee, wasp) venom while receiving ACE inhibitors.

Symptomatic hypotension with or without syncope can occur with ACE inhibitors (usually with the first several doses); effects are most often observed in volume-depleted patients; correct volume depletion prior to initiation; close monitoring of patient is required especially with initial dosing and dosing increases; blood pressure must be lowered at a rate appropriate for the patient's clinical condition. Initiation of therapy in patients with ischemic heart disease or cerebrovascular disease warrants close observation due to the potential consequences posed by falling blood pressure (eg, MI, stroke). Use with caution in hypertrophic cardiomyopathy with outflow tract obstruction, severe aortic stenosis, or before, during, or immediately after major surgery. **[U.S. Boxed Warning]: Based on human data, ACEIs can cause injury and death to the developing fetus when used in the second and third trimesters. ACEIs should be discontinued as soon as possible once pregnancy is detected.** Injection contains benzyl alcohol which has been associated with "gasping syndrome" in neonates.

Hyperkalemia may occur with ACE inhibitors; risk factors include renal dysfunction, diabetes mellitus, concomitant use of potassium-sparing diuretics, potassium supplements, and/or potassium-containing salts. Use cautiously, if at all, with these agents and monitor potassium closely. Cough may occur with ACE inhibitors. Other causes of cough should be considered (eg, pulmonary congestion in patients with heart failure) and excluded prior to discontinuation.

May be associated with deterioration of renal function and/or increases in serum creatinine, particularly in patients with low renal blood flow (eg, renal artery stenosis, heart failure) whose glomerular filtration rate (GFR) is dependent on efferent arteriolar vasoconstriction by angiotensin II; deterioration may result in oliguria, acute renal failure, and progressive azotemia. Small increases in serum creatinine may occur following initiation; consider discontinuation only in patients with progressive and/or significant deterioration in renal function. Use with caution in patients with unstented unilateral/bilateral renal artery stenosis. When unstented bilateral renal artery stenosis is present, use is generally avoided due to the elevated risk of deterioration in renal function unless possible benefits outweigh risks. Concomitant use of an angiotensin receptor blocker (ARB) or renin inhibitor (eg, aliskiren) is associated with an increased risk of hypotension, hyperkalemia, and renal dysfunction; concomitant use with aliskiren should be avoided in patients with GFR <60 mL/minute and is ▶

contraindicated in patients with diabetes mellitus (regardless of GFR).

Rare toxicities associated with ACE inhibitors include cholestatic jaundice (which may progress to fulminant hepatic necrosis), agranulocytosis, neutropenia, or leukopenia with myeloid hypoplasia. Patients with collagen vascular diseases (especially with concomitant renal impairment) or renal impairment alone may be at increased risk for hematologic toxicity; periodically monitor CBC with differential in these patients.

Drug Interactions

Avoid Concomitant Use There are no known interactions where it is recommended to avoid concomitant use.

Decreased Effect

The levels/effects of Enalaprilat may be decreased by: Aprotinin; Herbs (Hypertensive Properties); Icatibant; Methylphenidate; Nonsteroidal Anti-Inflammatory Agents; Salicylates; Yohimbine

Increased Effect/Toxicity

Enalaprilat may increase the levels/effects of: Allopurinol; Amifostine; Antihypertensives; Aza-THIOprine; CycloSPORINE (Systemic); DULoxetine; Ferric Gluconate; Gold Sodium Thiomalate; Hypotensive Agents; Iron Dextran Complex; Lithium; Nonsteroidal Anti-Inflammatory Agents; Obinutuzumab; RiTUXimab; Sodium Phosphates

The levels/effects of Enalaprilat may be increased by: Alfuzosin; Aliskiren; Angiotensin II Receptor Blockers; Brimonidine (Topical); Canagliflozin; Diazoxide; DPP-IV Inhibitors; Eplerenone; Everolimus; Heparin; Heparin (Low Molecular Weight); Herbs (Hypotensive Properties); Loop Diuretics; MAO Inhibitors; Pentoxifylline; Phosphodiesterase 5 Inhibitors; Potassium Salts; Potassium-Sparing Diuretics; Prostacyclin Analogues; Sirolimus; Temsirolimus; Thiazide Diuretics; TiZANidine; Tolvaptan; Trimethoprim

Nutritional/Ethanol Interactions Herb/Nutraceutical: Avoid bayberry, blue cohosh, cayenne, ephedra, ginger, ginseng (American), kola, licorice (may worsen hypertension). Avoid black cohosh, California poppy, coleus, golden seal, hawthorn, mistletoe, periwinkle, quinine, shepherd's purse (may have increased antihypertensive effect).

Adverse Reactions Note: Since enalapril is converted to enalaprilat, adverse reactions associated with enalapril may also occur with enalaprilat (also refer to Enalapril monograph). Frequency ranges include data from hypertension and heart failure trials. Higher rates of adverse reactions have generally been noted in patients with CHF. However, the frequency of adverse effects associated with placebo is also increased in this population.

1% to 10%:

Cardiovascular: Hypotension (2% to 5%)

Central nervous system: Headache (3%)

Gastrointestinal: Nausea (1%)

Pharmacodynamics/Kinetics

Onset of Action I.V.: ≤15 minutes; Peak effect: I.V.: 1-4 hours

Duration of Action I.V.: ~6 hours

Available Dosage Forms

Injectable, Intravenous:

Generic: 1.25 mg/mL (1 mL, 2 mL)

General Dosage Range Dosage adjustment recommended in patients with renal impairment.

I.V.: *Adults:* 0.625-5 mg every 6 hours

Administration

I.V. Administer I.V. push undiluted over at least 5 minutes or as an infusion with a diluted solution; discontinue diuretic, if possible, for 2-3 days before beginning enalaprilat therapy.

Preparation for Administration No dilution required, but may dilute in up to 50 mL of a compatible solution.

Storage/Stability Enalaprilat is a clear, colorless solution which should be stored at <30°C (86°F). I.V. is stable for 24 hours at room temperature in D_5W, NS, D_5NS, or D_5LR.

Nursing Actions

Physical Assessment Assess potential for interactions with other pharmacological agents or herbal products that may impact fluid balance or cardiac status. Monitor blood pressure closely with first dose or change in dose. Monitor laboratory tests closely during first 3 months and regularly thereafter. Monitor for anaphylactic reaction, hypovolemia, angioedema, and postural hypotension.

Patient Education

• Discuss specific use of drug and side effects with patient as it relates to treatment. (HCAHPS: During this hospital stay, were you given any medicine that you had not taken before? Before giving you any new medicine, how often did hospital staff tell you what the medicine was for? How often did hospital staff describe possible side effects in a way you could understand?)

• Have patient report immediately to prescriber signs of renal impairment, signs of hyperkalemia, severe dizziness, syncope, angina, significant dyspepsia, considerable nausea, or signs of hepatic impairment (HCAHPS).

• Educate patient about signs of a significant reaction (eg, wheezing; chest tightness; fever; itching; bad cough; blue skin color; seizures; or swelling of face, lips, tongue, or throat). **Note:** This is not a comprehensive list of all side effects. Patient should consult prescriber for additional questions.

Intended Use and Disclaimer: Should not be printed and given to patients. This information is intended to serve as a concise initial reference for healthcare professionals to use when discussing medications with a patient. You must ultimately rely on your own discretion, experience and

judgment in diagnosing, treating and advising patients.

Dietary Considerations Limit salt substitutes or potassium-rich diet.

Enfuvirtide (en FYOO vir tide)

Brand Names: U.S. Fuzeon
Index Terms T-20
Pharmacologic Category Antiretroviral, Fusion Protein Inhibitor (Anti-HIV)
Pregnancy Risk Factor B
Lactation Excretion in breast milk unknown/contraindicated
Breast-Feeding Considerations Maternal or infant antiretroviral therapy does not completely eliminate the risk of postnatal HIV transmission. In addition, multiclass-resistant virus has been detected in breast-feeding infants despite maternal therapy. Therefore, in the United States, where formula is accessible, affordable, safe, and sustainable, and the risk of infant mortality due to diarrhea and respiratory infections is low, complete avoidance of breast-feeding by HIV-infected women is recommended to decrease potential transmission of HIV (DHHS [perinatal], 2012).
Use Treatment of HIV-1 infection in combination with other antiretroviral agents in treatment-experienced patients with evidence of HIV-1 replication despite ongoing antiretroviral therapy
Mechanism of Action/Effect Inhibits the fusion of HIV-1 virus with CD4 cells
Contraindications Hypersensitivity to enfuvirtide or any component of the formulation
Warnings/Precautions Use is not recommended in antiretroviral therapy-naive patients (DHHS, 2013). Monitor closely for signs/symptoms of pneumonia; associated with an increased incidence during clinical trials, particularly in patients with a low CD4 cell count, high initial viral load, I.V. drug use, smoking, or a history of lung disease. May cause hypersensitivity reactions (symptoms may include rash, fever, nausea, vomiting, hypotension, and elevated transaminases). In addition, local injection site reactions are common. Patients may develop immune reconstitution syndrome resulting in the occurrence of an inflammatory response to an indolent or residual opportunistic infection during initial HIV treatment or activation of autoimmune disorders (eg, Graves' disease, polymyositis, Guillain-Barré syndrome) later in therapy; further evaluation and treatment may be required. Administration using a needle-free device has been associated with nerve pain (including neuralgia and/or paresthesia lasting up to 6 months), bruising, and hematomas when administered at sites where large nerves are close to the skin; only administer medication in recommended sites and use caution in patients with coagulation disorders (eg, hemophilia) or receiving anticoagulants. Safety and efficacy have not been established in children <6 years of age.

Drug Interactions
Avoid Concomitant Use There are no known interactions where it is recommended to avoid concomitant use.
Decreased Effect There are no known significant interactions involving a decrease in effect.
Increased Effect/Toxicity
Enfuvirtide may increase the levels/effects of: Protease Inhibitors

The levels/effects of Enfuvirtide may be increased by: Protease Inhibitors
Adverse Reactions
>10%:
  Gastrointestinal: Diarrhea (32%), nausea (23%)
  Local: Injection site infection (children 11%), injection site reactions (98%; may include pain, erythema, induration, pruritus, ecchymosis, nodule or cyst formation)
1% to 10%:
  Dermatologic: Folliculitis (2%)
  Gastrointestinal: Weight loss (7%), abdominal pain (4%), appetite decreased (3%), pancreatitis (3%), anorexia (2%), xerostomia (2%)
  Hematologic: Eosinophilia (2% to 9%)
  Hepatic: Transaminases increased (4%, grade 4: 1%)
  Local: Injection site infection (adults 2%)
  Neuromuscular & skeletal: CPK increased (3% to 7%), limb pain (3%), myalgia (3%)
  Ocular: Conjunctivitis (2%)
  Respiratory: Sinusitis (6%), cough (4%), bacterial pneumonia (3%)
  Miscellaneous: Infections (4% to 6%), herpes simplex (4%), flu-like syndrome (2%)
Available Dosage Forms
Solution Reconstituted, Subcutaneous:
  Fuzeon: 90 mg (1 ea)
General Dosage Range Dosage adjustment recommended in patients with renal impairment
SubQ:
  Children 6-16 years: 2 mg/kg twice daily (maximum: 90 mg/dose)
  Adolescents ≥16 years and Adults: 90 mg twice daily
Administration
Subcutaneous Inject subcutaneously into upper arm, abdomen, or anterior thigh. Do not inject into moles, the navel, over a blood vessel or skin abnormalities such as scar tissue, surgical scars, bruises, or tattoos. In addition, do not inject in or near sites where large nerves are close to the skin including the elbow, knee, groin, or buttocks. Rotate injection site, give injections at a site different from the preceding injection site; do not inject into any site where an injection site reaction is evident. Bioequivalence was found to be similar in a study comparing standard administration using a needle versus a needle-free device.

Preparation for Administration Reconstitute with 1.1 mL SWFI; tap vial for 10 seconds and roll gently to ensure contact with diluent; then allow to stand until solution is completed; may require up to 45 minutes to form solution (108 mg/1.2 mL).

Storage/Stability Store powder at 15°C to 30°C (59°F to 86°F). Reconstituted solutions should be refrigerated and must be used within 24 hours.

Nursing Actions

Physical Assessment Monitor for pneumonia, neuropathy, and CNS changes on a regular basis throughout therapy. Teach patient or caregiver proper use (eg, reconstitution, injection procedure, needle/syringe disposal, and proper timing of mediations). Teach patient to report hypersensitivity reaction and injection site infection.

Patient Education

• Discuss specific use of drug and side effects with patient as it relates to treatment. (HCAHPS: During this hospital stay, were you given any medicine that you had not taken before? Before giving you any new medicine, how often did hospital staff tell you what the medicine was for? How often did hospital staff describe possible side effects in a way you could understand?)

• Patient may experience insomnia, short-term pain, diarrhea, or dyspepsia. Have patient report immediately to prescriber signs of infection, signs of depression (ie, suicidal ideation, anxiety, emotional instability, illogical thinking), signs of pancreatitis, flu-like syndrome, severe injection site irritation, hematuria, paresthesia, urinary retention, oliguria, angina, significant dizziness, syncope, asthenia, dyspnea, edema of extremities, enlarged lymph nodes, ecchymosis, or hemorrhaging (HCAHPS).

• Educate patient about signs of a significant reaction (eg, wheezing; chest tightness; fever; itching; bad cough; blue skin color; seizures; or swelling of face, lips, tongue, or throat). **Note:** This is not a comprehensive list of all side effects. Patient should consult prescriber for additional questions.

Intended Use and Disclaimer: Should not be printed and given to patients. This information is intended to serve as a concise initial reference for healthcare professionals to use when discussing medications with a patient. You must ultimately rely on your own discretion, experience and judgment in diagnosing, treating and advising patients.

Enoxaparin (ee noks a PA rin)

Brand Names: U.S. Lovenox

Index Terms Enoxaparin Sodium

Pharmacologic Category Anticoagulant; Anticoagulant, Low Molecular Weight Heparin

Medication Safety Issues

Sound-alike/look-alike issues:

Lovenox may be confused with Lasix, Levaquin, Lotronex, Protonix

High alert medication:

The Institute for Safe Medication Practices (ISMP) includes this medication among its list of drugs which have a heightened risk of causing significant patient harm when used in error.

National Patient Safety Goals:

The Joint Commission (TJC) requires healthcare organizations that provide anticoagulant therapy to have a process in place to reduce the risk of anticoagulant-associated patient harm. Patients receiving anticoagulants should receive individualized care through a defined process that includes standardized ordering, dispensing, administration, monitoring and education. This does not apply to routine short-term use of anticoagulants for prevention of venous thromboembolism when the expectation is that the patient's laboratory values will remain within or close to normal values (NPSG.03.05.01).

Pregnancy Risk Factor B

Lactation Excretion in breast milk unknown/not recommended

Breast-Feeding Considerations Small amounts of LMWH have been detected in breast milk; however, because it has a low oral bioavailability, it is unlikely to cause adverse events in a nursing infant. Enoxaparin product labeling does not recommend use in nursing women; however, antithrombotic guidelines state that use of LMWH may be continued in breast-feeding women (Guyatt, 2012).

Use

Acute coronary syndromes: Unstable angina (UA), non-ST-elevation (NSTEMI), and ST-elevation myocardial infarction (STEMI)

DVT prophylaxis: Following hip or knee replacement surgery, abdominal surgery, or in medical patients with severely-restricted mobility during acute illness who are at risk for thromboembolic complications. **Note:** Patients at risk of thromboembolic complications who undergo abdominal surgery include those with one or more of the following risk factors: >40 years of age, obesity, general anesthesia lasting >30 minutes, malignancy, history of deep vein thrombosis or pulmonary embolism

DVT treatment (acute): Inpatient treatment (patients with or without pulmonary embolism) and outpatient treatment (patients without pulmonary embolism)

Unlabeled Use Prophylaxis and treatment of thromboembolism in children; anticoagulant bridge therapy during temporary interruption of vitamin K antagonist therapy in patients at high risk for thromboembolism; DVT prophylaxis following moderate-risk general surgery, major gynecologic surgery and following higher-risk general surgery for cancer; management of venous thromboembolism (VTE) during pregnancy; anticoagulant used during percutaneous coronary intervention (PCI)

Mechanism of Action/Effect Low molecular weight heparin that blocks factor Xa and IIa to prevent thrombus and clot formation

Contraindications

Hypersensitivity to enoxaparin, heparin, pork products, or any component of the formulation (including benzyl alcohol in multiple-dose vials); thrombocytopenia associated with a positive *in vitro* test for antiplatelet antibodies in the presence of enoxaparin; active major bleeding

Canadian labeling: Additional contraindications (not in U.S. labeling): Use of multiple-dose vials in newborns or premature neonates; history of confirmed or suspected immunologically-mediated heparin-induced thrombocytopenia; acute or subacute bacterial endocarditis; major blood clotting disorders; active gastric or duodenal ulcer; hemorrhagic cerebrovascular accident (except if there are systemic emboli); severe uncontrolled hypertension; diabetic or hemorrhagic retinopathy; other conditions or diseases involving an increased risk of hemorrhage; injuries to and operations on the brain, spinal cord, eyes, and ears; spinal/epidural anesthesia when repeated dosing of enoxaparin (1 mg/kg every 12 hours or 1.5 mg/kg daily) is required, due to increased risk of bleeding.

Note: Use of enoxaparin in patients with current heparin-induced thrombocytopenia (HIT) or HIT with thrombosis is **not** recommended and considered contraindicated due to high cross-reactivity to heparin-platelet factor-4 antibody (Guyatt [ACCP], 2012; Warkentin, 1999).

Warnings/Precautions [U.S. Boxed Warning]: Spinal or epidural hematomas, including subsequent long-term or permanent paralysis, may occur with recent or anticipated neuraxial anesthesia (epidural or spinal anesthesia) or spinal puncture in patients anticoagulated with LMWH or heparinoids. Consider risk versus benefit prior to spinal procedures; risk is increased by the use of concomitant agents which may alter hemostasis, the use of indwelling epidural catheters, a history of spinal deformity or spinal surgery, as well as a history of traumatic or repeated epidural or spinal punctures. Optimal timing between neuraxial procedures and enoxaparin administration is not known. Delay placement or removal of catheter for at least 12 hours after administration of low-dose enoxaparin (eg, 30-60 mg/day) and at least 24 hours after high-dose enoxaparin (eg, 0.75-1 mg/kg twice daily or 1.5 mg/kg once daily) and consider doubling these times in patients with creatinine clearance <30 mL/minute; risk of neuraxial hematoma may still exist since anti-factor Xa levels are still detectable at these time points. Patients receiving twice daily high-dose enoxaparin should have the second dose withheld to allow a longer time period prior to catheter placement or removal. Upon removal of catheter, consider withholding enoxaparin for at least 4 hours. **Patient should be observed closely for bleeding and signs and symptoms of neurological impairment if therapy is administered during or immediately following diagnostic lumbar puncture, epidural anesthesia, or spinal anesthesia. If neurological compromise is noted, urgent treatment is necessary.** If spinal hematoma is suspected, diagnose and treat immediately; spinal cord decompression may be considered although it may not prevent or reverse neurological sequelae.

Do not administer intramuscularly. Discontinue use 12-24 hours prior to CABG and dose with unfractionated heparin per institutional practice (Jneid, 2012). Not recommended for thromboprophylaxis in patients with prosthetic heart valves (especially pregnant women). Not to be used interchangeably (unit for unit) with heparin or any other low molecular weight heparins. Monitor patient closely for signs or symptoms of bleeding. Certain patients are at increased risk of bleeding. Risk factors include bacterial endocarditis; congenital or acquired bleeding disorders; active ulcerative or angiodysplastic GI diseases; severe uncontrolled hypertension; hemorrhagic stroke; use shortly after brain, spinal, or ophthalmic surgery; patients treated concomitantly with platelet inhibitors; recent GI bleeding or ulceration; renal dysfunction and hemorrhage; thrombocytopenia or platelet defects or history of heparin-induced thrombocytopenia; severe liver disease; hypertensive or diabetic retinopathy; or in patients undergoing invasive procedures. To minimize risk of bleeding following PCI, achieve hemostasis at the puncture site after PCI. If a closure device is used, sheath can be removed immediately. If manual compression is used, remove sheath 6 hours after the last I.V./SubQ dose of enoxaparin. Do not administer further doses until 6-8 hours after sheath removal; observe for signs of bleeding/hematoma formation. Cases of enoxaparin-induced thrombocytopenia and thrombosis (similar to heparin-induced thrombocytopenia [HIT]), some complicated by organ infarction, limb ischemia, or death, have been observed. Use with extreme caution or avoid in patients with history of HIT, especially if administered within 100 days of HIT episode (Warkentin, 2001); monitor platelet count closely. Use is contraindicated in patients with thrombocytopenia associated with a positive *in vitro* test for antiplatelet antibodies in the presence of enoxaparin. Discontinue therapy and consider alternative treatment if platelets are <100,000/mm^3 and/or thrombosis develops. Use caution in patients with congenital or drug-induced thrombocytopenia or platelet defects. Risk of bleeding may be increased in women <45 kg and in men <57 kg. Use caution in patients with renal failure; dosage adjustment needed if CrCl <30 mL/minute. Use with caution in the elderly (delayed elimination may occur); dosage alteration/adjustment may be required (eg, omission of I.V. bolus in acute STEMI in patients ≥75 years of age). Monitor for hyperkalemia; can cause hyperkalemia possibly by suppressing aldosterone production. Multiple-dose vials contain benzyl alcohol (use caution in pregnant women). In neonates, large amounts of benzyl alcohol (>100 mg/kg/day) have been associated with fatal toxicity (gasping syndrome). Use of multiple-dose vials is contraindicated in patients who have hypersensitivity to benzyl alcohol.

Safety and efficacy of prophylactic dosing of enoxaparin has not been established in patients who are obese (>30 kg/m^2) nor is there a consensus regarding dosage adjustments. The American College of Chest Physicians Practice Guidelines suggest consulting with a pharmacist regarding dosing in bariatric surgery patients and other obese patients who may require higher doses of LMWH (Gould, 2012).

Drug Interactions

Avoid Concomitant Use

Avoid concomitant use of Enoxaparin with any of the following: Apixaban; Dabigatran Etexilate; Omacetaxine; Rivaroxaban; Urokinase

Decreased Effect

The levels/effects of Enoxaparin may be decreased by: Estrogen Derivatives; Progestins

Increased Effect/Toxicity

Enoxaparin may increase the levels/effects of: ACE Inhibitors; Aliskiren; Angiotensin II Receptor Blockers; Anticoagulants; Canagliflozin; Collagenase (Systemic); Deferasirox; Eplerenone; Ibritumomab; Omacetaxine; Palifermin; Potassium Salts; Potassium-Sparing Diuretics; Rivaroxaban; Tositumomab and Iodine I 131 Tositumomab

The levels/effects of Enoxaparin may be increased by: 5-ASA Derivatives; Agents with Antiplatelet Properties; Apixaban; Dabigatran Etexilate; Dasatinib; Herbs (Anticoagulant/Antiplatelet Properties); Ibrutinib; Nonsteroidal Anti-Inflammatory Agents; Omega-3 Fatty Acids; Pentosan Polysulfate Sodium; Pentoxifylline; Prostacyclin Analogues; Salicylates; Sugammadex; Thrombolytic Agents; Tibolone; Tipranavir; Urokinase; Vitamin E

Nutritional/Ethanol Interactions Herb/Nutraceutical: Avoid cat's claw, dong quai, evening primrose, feverfew, garlic, ginger, ginkgo, red clover, horse chestnut, green tea, ginseng (all have additional antiplatelet activity).

Adverse Reactions As with all anticoagulants, bleeding is the major adverse effect of enoxaparin. Hemorrhage may occur at virtually any site. Risk is dependent on multiple variables. At the recommended doses, single injections of enoxaparin do not significantly influence platelet aggregation or affect global clotting time (ie, PT or aPTT).

1% to 10%:
Central nervous system: Confusion (2%), pain
Gastrointestinal: Nausea (3%), diarrhea (2%)
Hematologic & oncologic: Major hemorrhage (<1% to 4%; includes cases of intracranial, retroperitoneal, or intraocular hemorrhage; incidence varies with indication/population), thrombocytopenia (moderate 1%; severe 0.1%), anemia (<2%), bruise
Hepatic: Increased serum ALT (6%), increased serum AST (6%)
Local: Hematoma at injection site (9%), irritation at injection site, bruising at injection site, erythema at injection site, pain at injection site
Renal: Hematuria (≤2%)
Miscellaneous: Fever (5% to 8%)

Pharmacodynamics/Kinetics

Onset of Action Peak effect: SubQ: Antifactor Xa and antithrombin (antifactor IIa): 3-5 hours

Duration of Action 40 mg dose: Antifactor Xa activity: ~12 hours

Available Dosage Forms

Solution, Injection:
Lovenox: 300 mg/3 mL (3 mL)
Generic: 300 mg/3 mL (3 mL)

Solution, Subcutaneous:
Lovenox: 30 mg/0.3 mL (0.3 mL); 40 mg/0.4 mL (0.4 mL); 60 mg/0.6 mL (0.6 mL); 80 mg/0.8 mL (0.8 mL); 100 mg/mL (1 mL); 120 mg/0.8 mL (0.8 mL); 150 mg/mL (1 mL)
Generic: 30 mg/0.3 mL (0.3 mL); 40 mg/0.4 mL (0.4 mL); 60 mg/0.6 mL (0.6 mL); 80 mg/0.8 mL (0.8 mL); 100 mg/mL (1 mL); 120 mg/0.8 mL (0.8 mL); 150 mg/mL (1 mL)

Solution, Subcutaneous [preservative free]:
Lovenox: 30 mg/0.3 mL (0.3 mL); 40 mg/0.4 mL (0.4 mL); 60 mg/0.6 mL (0.6 mL); 80 mg/0.8 mL (0.8 mL); 100 mg/mL (1 mL); 120 mg/0.8 mL (0.8 mL); 150 mg/mL (1 mL)
Generic: 30 mg/0.3 mL (0.3 mL); 40 mg/0.4 mL (0.4 mL); 60 mg/0.6 mL (0.6 mL); 80 mg/0.8 mL (0.8 mL); 100 mg/mL (1 mL); 120 mg/0.8 mL (0.8 mL); 150 mg/mL (1 mL)

General Dosage Range Dosage varies greatly depending on indication.

Administration

I.V. STEMI and PCI only: The U.S. labeling recommends using the multiple-dose vial to prepare I.V. doses. The Canadian labeling recommends either the multiple-dose vial or a prefilled syringe. Do not mix or coadminister with other medications; may be administered with NS or D$_5$W. Flush I.V. access site with a sufficient amount of NS or D$_5$W prior to and following I.V. bolus administration. **Note:** Enoxaparin is available in 100 mg/mL and 150 mg/mL concentrations. When used prior to percutaneous coronary intervention or as part of treatment for ST-elevation myocardial infarction

(STEMI), a single dose may be administered I.V. except when the patient is ≥75 years of age and is experiencing STEMI then only administer by SubQ injection.

Injectable Detail pH: 5.5-7.5

Subcutaneous Administer by deep SubQ injection alternating between the left or right anterolateral and left or right posterolateral abdominal wall. Do not mix with other infusions or injections. In order to minimize bruising, do not rub injection site. To avoid loss of drug from the 30 mg and 40 mg prefilled syringes, do not expel the air bubble from the syringe prior to injection. **Note:** Enoxaparin is available in 100 mg/mL and 150 mg/mL concentrations.

Storage/Stability Store at 25°C (77°F); excursions permitted to 15°C to 30°C (59°F to 86°F); do not freeze. Do not store multiple-dose vials for >28 days after first use.

Nursing Actions

Physical Assessment Do **not** administer via I.M. route. Monitor for signs and symptoms of bleeding.

Patient Education

• Discuss specific use of drug and side effects with patient as it relates to treatment. (HCAHPS: During this hospital stay, were you given any medicine that you had not taken before? Before giving you any new medicine, how often did hospital staff tell you what the medicine was for? How often did hospital staff describe possible side effects in a way you could understand?)

• Patient may experience dyspepsia, injection site irritation, or diarrhea. Have patient report immediately to prescriber signs of hemorrhaging, severe dizziness, syncope, illogical thinking, considerable headache, paresthesia, or asthenia (HCAHPS).

• Educate patient about signs of a significant reaction (eg, wheezing; chest tightness; fever; itching; bad cough; blue skin color; seizures; or swelling of face, lips, tongue, or throat). **Note:** This is not a comprehensive list of all side effects. Patient should consult prescriber for additional questions.

Intended Use and Disclaimer: Should not be printed and given to patients. This information is intended to serve as a concise initial reference for healthcare professionals to use when discussing medications with a patient. You must ultimately rely on your own discretion, experience and judgment in diagnosing, treating and advising patients.

Entacapone (en TA ka pone)

Brand Names: U.S. Comtan
Pharmacologic Category Anti-Parkinson's Agent, COMT Inhibitor
Pregnancy Risk Factor C

Lactation Excretion in breast milk unknown/use caution

Breast-Feeding Considerations It is not known if entacapone is excreted in breast milk. The manufacturer recommends that caution be exercised when administering entacapone to nursing women.

Use Adjunct to levodopa/carbidopa therapy in patients with idiopathic Parkinson's disease who experience "wearing-off" symptoms at the end of a dosing interval

Mechanism of Action/Effect Entacapone inhibits COMT peripherally and alters the pharmacokinetics of levodopa so serum levels of levodopa become more sustained when used with levodopa/carbidopa combinations.

Contraindications

Hypersensitivity to entacapone or any component of the formulation

Canadian labeling: Additional contraindications (not in U.S. labeling): Clinical or laboratory evidence of uncompensated cardiovascular, endocrine, hematologic, pulmonary (including bronchial asthma), or renal disease; history of neuroleptic malignant syndrome (NMS) and/or nontraumatic rhabdomyolysis; hepatic impairment; narrow-angle glaucoma; pheochromocytoma; in the presence of a suspicious, undiagnosed skin lesion or history of melanoma; concomitant use with a nonselective monoamine oxidase (MAO) inhibitor (eg, tranylcypromine, phenelzine) or concomitant use with both a selective MAO-A and selective MAO-B inhibitor; when administration of a sympathomimetic amine is contraindicated

Warnings/Precautions Use with caution in patients with cardiovascular disease, including a history of myocardial infarction (MI) and arrhythmias; MI and other ischemic adverse events have been observed in clinical trials (Comtan Canadian product monograph, 2013). May cause orthostatic hypotension and syncope; Parkinson's disease patients appear to have an impaired capacity to respond to a postural challenge; use with caution in patients at risk of hypotension (such as those receiving antihypertensive drugs) or where transient hypotensive episodes would be poorly tolerated (cardiovascular disease or cerebrovascular disease). Parkinson's patients being treated with dopaminergic agonists ordinarily require careful monitoring for signs and symptoms of postural hypotension, especially during dose escalation, and should be informed of this risk. May cause hallucinations, which may improve with reduction in levodopa therapy. Use with caution in patients with pre-existing dyskinesias; exacerbation of pre-existing dyskinesia and severe rhabdomyolysis has been reported. Levodopa dosage reduction may be required, particularly in patients with levodopa dosages >600 mg daily or with moderate-to-severe dyskinesia prior to initiation. Entacapone, in conjunction with other drug therapy that alters brain

▶

biogenic amine concentrations (eg, MAO inhibitors, SSRIs), has been associated with a syndrome resembling neuroleptic malignant syndrome (hyperpyrexia and confusion - some fatal) on abrupt withdrawal or dosage reduction. Concomitant use of entacapone and nonselective MAO inhibitors should be avoided.

Dopaminergic agents have been associated with compulsive behaviors and/or loss of impulse control, which has manifested as pathological gambling, libido increases (hypersexuality), and/or binge eating. Causality has not been established, and controversy exists as to whether this phenomenon is related to the underlying disease, prior behaviors/addictions and/or drug therapy. Dose reduction or discontinuation of therapy has been reported to reverse these behaviors in some, but not all cases. Risk for melanoma development is increased in Parkinson's disease patients; drug causation or factors contributing to risk have not been established. Patients should be monitored closely and periodic skin examinations should be performed. The Canadian labeling contraindicates use in patients with suspicious, undiagnosed skin lesions or history of melanoma. Dopaminergic agents from the ergot class have also been associated with fibrotic complications, such as retroperitoneal fibrosis, pulmonary infiltrates or effusion and pleural thickening. It is unknown whether nonergot, pro-dopaminergic agents like entacapone confer this risk. Use caution in patients with hepatic impairment (Canadian labeling contraindicates use in hepatic impairment) or severe renal impairment. Do not withdraw therapy abruptly. Discoloration of urine, saliva, or sweat to dark colors (red, brown, black) may be observed during therapy. Use with caution in patients with lower gastrointestinal disease or an increased risk of dehydration; has been associated with delayed development of diarrhea (usual onset after 4-12 weeks). Diarrhea may be a sign of drug-induced colitis. Monitor for weight loss. Discontinue use with prolonged diarrhea. Potentially significant drug-drug interactions may exist, requiring dose or frequency adjustment, additional monitoring, and/or selection of alternative therapy.

Drug Interactions

Avoid Concomitant Use

Avoid concomitant use of Entacapone with any of the following: Azelastine (Nasal); Paraldehyde; Pimozide; Thalidomide

Decreased Effect There are no known significant interactions involving a decrease in effect.

Increased Effect/Toxicity

Entacapone may increase the levels/effects of: Alcohol (Ethyl); ARIPiprazole; Azelastine (Nasal); Buprenorphine; CNS Depressants; COMT Substrates; Dofetilide; Hydrocodone; Lomitapide; MAO Inhibitors; Methotrimeprazine; Metyrosine; Mirtazapine; Paraldehyde; Pimozide;

Pramipexole; ROPINIRole; Rotigotine; Selective Serotonin Reuptake Inhibitors; Thalidomide; Zolpidem

The levels/effects of Entacapone may be increased by: Brimonidine (Topical); Doxylamine; Droperidol; HydrOXYzine; Magnesium Sulfate; Methotrimeprazine; Perampanel; Sodium Oxybate; Tapentadol

Nutritional/Ethanol Interactions

Ethanol: May increase CNS depression; monitor for increased effects with coadministration. Caution patients about effects.

Food: Entacapone has been reported to chelate iron and decreasing serum iron levels were noted in clinical trials; however, clinically significant anemia has not been observed.

Adverse Reactions

>10%:

Gastrointestinal: Nausea (14%)

Neuromuscular & skeletal: Dyskinesia (25%), placebo (15%)

1% to 10%:

Cardiovascular: Orthostatic hypotension (4%), syncope (1%)

Central nervous system: Dizziness (8%), fatigue (6%), hallucinations (4%), anxiety (2%), somnolence (2%), agitation (1%)

Dermatologic: Purpura (2%)

Gastrointestinal: Diarrhea (10%), abdominal pain (8%), constipation (6%), vomiting (4%), dry mouth (3%), dyspepsia (2%), flatulence (2%), gastritis (1%), taste perversion (1%)

Genitourinary: Brown-orange urine discoloration (10%)

Neuromuscular & skeletal: Hyperkinesia (10%), hypokinesia (9%), back pain (4%), weakness (2%)

Respiratory: Dyspnea (3%)

Miscellaneous: Diaphoresis increased (2%), bacterial infection (1%)

Pharmacodynamics/Kinetics

Onset of Action Rapid; Peak effect: 1 hour

Available Dosage Forms

Tablet, Oral:

Comtan: 200 mg

Generic: 200 mg

General Dosage Range Oral: *Adults:* 200 mg with each dose of levodopa/carbidopa (maximum: 1600 mg daily)

Administration

Oral Always administer in association with levodopa/carbidopa; can be combined with both the immediate and sustained release formulations of levodopa/carbidopa. May be administered without regard to meals. Should not be abruptly withdrawn from patient's therapy due to significant worsening of symptoms.

Nursing Actions

Physical Assessment Monitor for postural hypotension, increased dyskinesias, and CNS changes (hallucinations, compulsive behaviors). Dose should be tapered slowly when discontinued. Teach patient proper timing of multiple medications.

Patient Education
- Discuss specific use of drug and side effects with patient as it relates to treatment. (HCAHPS: During this hospital stay, were you given any medicine that you had not taken before? Before giving you any new medicine, how often did hospital staff tell you what the medicine was for? How often did hospital staff describe possible side effects in a way you could understand?)
- Patient may experience asthenia, fatigue, dyspepsia, constipation, xerostomia, or urine discoloration. Have patient report immediately to prescriber severe dizziness, syncope, illogical thinking, considerable nausea, significant diarrhea, angina, uncontrollable urges, difficulty with motor activity, dyspnea, myalgia, hallucinations, mood changes, skin growth, or mole changes (HCAHPS).
- Educate patient about signs of a significant reaction (eg, wheezing; chest tightness; fever; itching; bad cough; blue skin color; seizures; or swelling of face, lips, tongue, or throat). **Note:** This is not a comprehensive list of all side effects. Patient should consult prescriber for additional questions.

Intended Use and Disclaimer: Should not be printed and given to patients. This information is intended to serve as a concise initial reference for healthcare professionals to use when discussing medications with a patient. You must ultimately rely on your own discretion, experience and judgment in diagnosing, treating and advising patients.

Dietary Considerations May be taken without regard to meals.

Enzalutamide (en za LOO ta mide)

Brand Names: U.S. Xtandi
Index Terms MDV3100
Pharmacologic Category Antineoplastic Agent, Antiandrogen
Medication Safety Issues
Sound-alike/look-alike issues:
Enzalutamide may be confused with bicalutamide, flutamide, nilutamide
Xtandi may be confused with Jevtana, Xgeva, Xofigo, Zometa, Zytiga
High alert medication:
This medication is in a class the Institute for Safe Medication Practices (ISMP) includes among its list of drug classes which have a heightened risk of causing significant patient harm when used in error.

Pregnancy Risk Factor X
Lactation Excretion unknown/not recommended

Use Prostate cancer: Treatment of metastatic, castration-resistant prostate cancer in patients previously treated with docetaxel

Available Dosage Forms
Capsule, Oral:
Xtandi: 40 mg
General Dosage Range Dosage adjustment recommended in patients on concomitant therapy or who develop toxicities.
Oral: *Adults:* 160 mg once daily

Administration
Oral May be administered with or without food; take at the same time each day. Swallow capsules whole; do not chew, dissolve, or open the capsules.

Hazardous agent; use appropriate precautions for handling and disposal (meets NIOSH, 2012 criteria).

Nursing Actions
Physical Assessment Monitor for signs/symptoms of seizures. Monitor for hypertension; drug may cause gradual increase in blood pressure.
Patient Education
- Discuss specific use of drug and side effects with patient as it relates to treatment. (HCAHPS: During this hospital stay, were you given any medicine that you had not taken before? Before giving you any new medicine, how often did hospital staff tell you what the medicine was for? How often did hospital staff describe possible side effects in a way you could understand?)
- Patient may experience dizziness, asthenia, back pain, myalgia, arthralgia, diarrhea, hot flashes, headache, insomnia, anxiety, rhinitis, rhinorrhea, or sternutation. Have patient report immediately to prescriber severe headache, dyspnea, illogical thinking, paresthesia, urine discoloration, edema of extremities, osteodynia, chills, pharyngitis, hallucinations, memory loss, urinary retention, or oliguria (HCAHPS).
- Educate patient about signs of a significant reaction (eg, wheezing; chest tightness; fever; itching; bad cough; blue skin color; seizures; or swelling of face, lips, tongue, or throat). **Note:** This is not a comprehensive list of all side effects. Patient should consult prescriber for additional questions.

Intended Use and Disclaimer: Should not be printed and given to patients. This information is intended to serve as a concise initial reference for healthcare professionals to use when discussing medications with a patient. You must ultimately rely on your own discretion, experience and judgment in diagnosing, treating and advising patients.

◀ **Related Information**
Oral Medications That Should Not Be Crushed or Altered *on page 1712*

Epinastine (ep i NAS teen)

Brand Names: U.S. Elestat
Index Terms Epinastine Hydrochloride
Pharmacologic Category Histamine H$_1$ Antagonist; Histamine H$_1$ Antagonist, Second Generation
Pregnancy Risk Factor C
Lactation Excretion in breast milk unknown/use caution
Use Treatment of allergic conjunctivitis
Available Dosage Forms
 Solution, Ophthalmic:
  Elestat: 0.05% (5 mL)
  Generic: 0.05% (5 mL)
General Dosage Range Ophthalmic: *Children ≥2 years and Adults:* Instill 1 drop into each eye twice daily
Administration
 Other For ophthalmic use only; avoid touching tip of applicator to eye or other surfaces. Contact lenses should be removed prior to application, may be reinserted after 10 minutes. Do not wear contact lenses if eyes are red.
Nursing Actions
 Physical Assessment For ophthalmic use only.
 Patient Education
  • Discuss specific use of drug and side effects with patient as it relates to treatment. (HCAHPS: During this hospital stay, were you given any medicine that you had not taken before? Before giving you any new medicine, how often did hospital staff tell you what the medicine was for? How often did hospital staff describe possible side effects in a way you could understand?)
  • Patient may experience signs of infection or rhinorrhea. Have patient report immediately to prescriber vision changes, ophthalmalgia, or severe eye irritation (HCAHPS).
  • Educate patient about signs of a significant reaction (eg, wheezing; chest tightness; fever; itching; bad cough; blue skin color; seizures; or swelling of face, lips, tongue, or throat). **Note:** This is not a comprehensive list of all side effects. Patient should consult prescriber for additional questions.

Intended Use and Disclaimer: Should not be printed and given to patients. This information is intended to serve as a concise initial reference for healthcare professionals to use when discussing medications with a patient. You must ultimately rely on your own discretion, experience and judgment in diagnosing, treating and advising patients.

EPINEPHrine (Systemic, Oral Inhalation) (ep i NEF rin)

Brand Names: U.S. Adrenaclick; Adrenalin; Asthmanefrin Refill [OTC]; Asthmanefrin Starter Kit [OTC]; Auvi-Q; EpiPen 2-Pak; EpiPen Jr 2-Pak; Micronefrin [OTC]; S2 [OTC]
Index Terms Adrenaline; Auvi-Q; Epinephrine Bitartrate; Epinephrine Hydrochloride; Racemic Epinephrine; Racepinephrine
Pharmacologic Category Alpha/Beta Agonist
Medication Safety Issues
 Sound-alike/look-alike issues:
  EPINEPHrine may be confused with ePHEDrine
  Epifrin may be confused with ephedrine, EpiPen
 High alert medication:
  The Institute for Safe Medication Practices (ISMP) includes this medication among its list of drugs which have a heightened risk of causing significant patient harm when used in error.
 Administration issues:
  Medication errors have occurred due to confusion with epinephrine products expressed as ratio strengths (eg, 1:1000 vs 1:10,000).
  Epinephrine 1:1000 = 1 mg/mL and is most commonly used I.M.
  Epinephrine 1:10,000 = 0.1 mg/mL and is used I.V.
  Medication errors have occurred when topical epinephrine 1 mg/mL (1:1000) has been inadvertently injected. Vials of injectable and topical epinephrine look very similar. Epinephrine should always be appropriately labeled with the intended administration.
 International issues:
  EpiPen [U.S., Canada, and multiple international markets] may be confused with Epigen brand name for glycyrrhizinic acid [Argentina, Mexico, Russia] and Epopen brand name for epoetin alfa [Spain]
Pregnancy Risk Factor C
Lactation Excretion in breast milk unknown/use caution
Breast-Feeding Considerations It is not known if epinephrine is excreted in breast milk. The manufacturer recommends that caution be exercised when administering epinephrine to nursing women.
Use Treatment of bronchospasms, bronchial asthma, viral croup, anaphylactic reactions, cardiac arrest; added to local anesthetics to decrease systemic absorption of intraspinal and local anesthetics and increase duration of action; decrease superficial hemorrhage; induction and maintenance of mydriasis during intraocular surgery
Unlabeled Use ACLS guidelines: Ventricular fibrillation (VF) or pulseless ventricular tachycardia (VT) unresponsive to initial defibrillatory shocks; pulseless electrical activity; asystole; hypotension/ shock unresponsive to volume resuscitation;

symptomatic bradycardia unresponsive to atropine or pacing; inotropic support

Mechanism of Action/Effect Stimulates alpha-, beta$_1$-, and beta$_2$-adrenergic receptors resulting in relaxation of smooth muscle of the bronchial tree, cardiac stimulation (increasing myocardial oxygen consumption), and dilation of skeletal muscle vasculature; small doses can cause vasodilation via beta$_2$-vascular receptors; large doses may produce constriction of skeletal and vascular smooth muscle

Contraindications There are no absolute contraindications to the use of injectable epinephrine (including Adrenaclick, Auvi-Q, EpiPen, EpiPen Jr, and Twinject) in a life-threatening situation.

Oral inhalation: Concurrent use or within 2 weeks of MAO inhibitors

Injectable solution: There are no contraindications listed in the manufacturer's labeling.

Warnings/Precautions Use with caution in elderly patients, patients with diabetes mellitus, cardiovascular diseases (eg, coronary artery disease, hypertension), thyroid disease, cerebrovascular disease, Parkinson's disease, or patients taking tricyclic antidepressants. Some products contain sulfites as preservatives; the presence of sulfites in some products should not deter administration during a serious allergic or other emergency situation even if the patient is sulfite-sensitive.

I.V. administration: Vesicant; ensure proper needle or catheter placement prior to and during infusion; avoid extravasation. Accidental injection into digits, hands, or feet may result in local reactions, including injection site pallor, coldness and hypoesthesia or injury, resulting in bruising, bleeding, discoloration, erythema or skeletal injury; patient should seek immediate medical attention if this occurs. Rapid I.V. administration may cause death from cerebrovascular hemorrhage or cardiac arrhythmias; however, rapid I.V. administration during pulseless arrest is necessary. Prior to intraocular use, must dilute 1:**1000** (1 mg/mL) solution to a concentration of 1:**100,000** to 1:**1,000,000** (10 **mcg**/mL to 1 **mcg**/mL) prior to intraocular use. When used undiluted, has been associated with corneal endothelial damage.

Oral inhalation: Use with caution in patients with prostate enlargement or urinary retention; may cause temporary worsening of symptoms.

Self medication (OTC use): Oral inhalation: Prior to self-medication, patients should contact healthcare provider. The product should only be used in persons with a diagnosis of asthma. If symptoms are not relieved in 20 minutes or become worse do not continue to use the product - seek immediate medical assistance. The product should not be used more frequently or at higher doses than recommended unless directed by a healthcare provider. This product should not be used in patients who have required hospitalization for asthma or if a patient is taking prescription medication for asthma. Do not use if you have taken a MAO inhibitor (certain drugs used for depression, Parkinson's disease, or other conditions) within 2 weeks.

Drug Interactions

Avoid Concomitant Use

Avoid concomitant use of EPINEPHrine (Systemic, Oral Inhalation) with any of the following: Ergot Derivatives; Iobenguane I 123; Lurasidone

Decreased Effect

EPINEPHrine (Systemic, Oral Inhalation) may decrease the levels/effects of: Benzylpenicilloyl Polylysine; Iobenguane I 123

The levels/effects of EPINEPHrine (Systemic, Oral Inhalation) may be decreased by: Alpha1-Blockers; Promethazine; Spironolactone

Increased Effect/Toxicity

EPINEPHrine (Systemic, Oral Inhalation) may increase the levels/effects of: Lurasidone; Sympathomimetics

The levels/effects of EPINEPHrine (Systemic, Oral Inhalation) may be increased by: Antacids; AtoMOXetine; Beta-Blockers; Cannabinoids; Carbonic Anhydrase Inhibitors; COMT Inhibitors; Ergot Derivatives; Hyaluronidase; Inhalational Anesthetics; MAO Inhibitors; Serotonin/Norepinephrine Reuptake Inhibitors; Tricyclic Antidepressants

Nutritional/Ethanol Interactions Herb/Nutraceutical: Avoid ephedra, yohimbe (may cause CNS stimulation).

Adverse Reactions Frequency not defined.

Cardiovascular: Angina, cardiac arrhythmia, chest pain, flushing, hypertension, pallor, palpitation, sudden death, tachycardia (parenteral), vasoconstriction, ventricular ectopy, ventricular fibrillation

Central nervous system: Anxiety (transient), apprehensiveness, cerebral hemorrhage, dizziness, headache, insomnia, lightheadedness, nervousness, restlessness

Gastrointestinal: Dry throat, loss of appetite, nausea, vomiting, xerostomia

Genitourinary: Acute urinary retention in patients with bladder outflow obstruction

Neuromuscular & skeletal: Tremor, weakness

Ocular: Allergic lid reaction, burning, corneal endothelial damage (intraocular use), eye pain, ocular irritation, precipitation of or exacerbation of narrow-angle glaucoma, transient stinging

Respiratory: Dyspnea, pulmonary edema

Miscellaneous: Diaphoresis

Pharmacodynamics/Kinetics

Onset of Action Bronchodilation: SubQ: ~5-10 minutes; Inhalation: ~1 minute

Available Dosage Forms
Device, Injection:
Adrenaclick: 0.15 mg/0.15 mL (2 ea); 0.3 mg/0.3 mL (2 ea)
Auvi-Q: 0.15 mg/0.15 mL (2 ea); 0.3 mg/0.3 mL (2 ea)
EpiPen 2-Pak: 0.3 mg/0.3 mL (2 ea)
EpiPen Jr 2-Pak: 0.15 mg/0.3 mL (2 ea)
Generic: 0.15 mg/0.15 mL (2 ea); 0.3 mg/0.3 mL (1 ea, 2 ea)

Nebulization Solution, Inhalation:
Asthmanefrin Refill [OTC]: 2.25% (1 ea)
Asthmanefrin Starter Kit [OTC]: 2.25% (1 ea)
Micronefrin [OTC]: 2.25% (15 mL, 30 mL)

Nebulization Solution, Inhalation [preservative free]:
S2 [OTC]: 2.25% (1 ea)

Solution, Injection:
Adrenalin: 1 mg/mL (1 mL)
Generic: 0.1 mg/mL (10 mL); 1 mg/mL (1 mL, 30 mL)

General Dosage Range
I.M.:
Adults: 0.3-0.5 mg (**1:1000** [1 mg/mL] solution) every 15-20 minutes
Adrenaclick, Auvi-Q, EpiPen Jr., Twinject: *Children 15-29 kg:* 0.15 mg as single dose; may repeat if needed
Adrenaclick, Auvi-Q, EpiPen, Twinject: *Children ≥30 kg and Adults:* 0.3 mg as single dose; may repeat if needed

Inhalation: *Children ≥4 years and Adults:* 1 inhalation; may repeat once after 1 minute, then do not use again for at least 3 hours

I.V. (1:10,000 [0.1 mg/mL] solution):
Children: 0.01 mg/kg kg (maximum single dose: 1 mg) every 3-5 minutes as needed **or** 0.1-1 mcg/kg/minute as a continuous infusion **or** 0.01 mg/kg every 20 minutes (hypersensitivity reaction)
Adults: 1 mg every 3-5 minutes (up to 0.2 mg/kg) **or** 1-10 mcg/minute as a continuous infusion

Intraocular: *Children and Adults:* Irrigation as a 1:**100,000** to 1:**1,000,000** (10 **mcg**/mL to 1 **mcg**/mL) solution or 0.1 mL of a 1:**100,000** to 1:**400,000** (10 **mcg**/mL to 2.5 **mcg**/mL) dilution

Nebulization (S2 Racepinephrine, OTC):
Children <4 years: Jet nebulizer: 0.05 mL/kg (maximum dose: 0.5 mL) diluted in 3 mL NS up to every 2 hours
Children ≥4 years and Adults:
Hand-bulb nebulizer: Add 0.5 mL (~10 drops) to nebulizer; 1-3 inhalations up to every 3 hours if needed
Jet nebulizer: Add 0.5 mL (~10 drops) to nebulizer and dilute with 3 mL of NS. Administer over ~15 minutes every 3-4 hours as needed.

SubQ:
Children: 0.01 mg/kg (**1:1000** [1 mg/mL] solution) every 20 minutes for 3 doses or as condition requires (maximum: 0.3 mg/dose)

Adults: 0.3-0.5 mg (**1:1000** [1 mg/mL] solution) every 15-20 minutes for 3 doses or as condition requires
Adrenaclick, EpiPen Jr, Twinject: *Children 15-29 kg:* 0.15 mg as single dose; may repeat if needed
Adrenaclick, EpiPen, Twinject: *Children ≥30 kg and Adults:* 0.3 mg as single dose; may repeat if needed

Usual Infusion Concentrations: Pediatric I.V. infusion: 16 **mcg**/mL, 32 **mcg**/mL, or 64 **mcg**/mL
Usual Infusion Concentrations: Adult I.V. infusion: 1 mg in 250 mL (concentration: 4 **mcg**/mL) or 4 mg in 250 mL (concentration: 16 **mcg**/mL) of D_5W or NS

Administration
I.M. I.M. administration in the anterolateral aspect of the middle third of the thigh is preferred in the setting of anaphylaxis (ACLS guidelines, 2010; Kemp, 2008). I.M. administration into the buttocks should be avoided. Adrenaclick, Auvi-Q, EpiPen, EpiPen Jr, and Twinject Auto-Injectors should only be injected into the anterolateral aspect of the thigh, through clothing if necessary.

Note: Adrenaclick, Auvi-Q, EpiPen and EpiPen Jr Auto-Injectors contain a single, fixed-dose of epinephrine and may only be administered I.M. (preferred) or SubQ. Twinject Auto-Injectors contain two doses; the first fixed-dose is available for auto-injection; the second dose is available for manual injection following partial disassembly of device.

Obesity: In overweight or obese children, because skin surface to muscle depth is greater in the upper half of the thigh, administration into the lower half of the thigh may be preferred. In very obese children, injection into the calf will provide an even greater chance of intramuscular administration (Arkwright, 2013).

I.V. When administering as a continuous infusion, central line administration is preferred. I.V. infusions require an infusion pump.

Vesicant; ensure proper needle or catheter placement prior to and during infusion; avoid extravasation.

Extravasation management: If extravasation occurs, stop infusion immediately and disconnect (leave cannula/needle in place); gently aspirate extravasated solution (do **NOT** flush the line); remove needle/cannula; elevate extremity. Initiate phentolamine (or alternative antidote). Apply dry warm compresses (Hurst, 2004).

Phentolamine: Dilute 5-10 mg in 10-15 mL NS and administer into extravasation site as soon as possible after extravasation (Peberdy, 2010).

Alternatives to phentolamine (due to shortage):
Nitroglycerin topical 2% ointment (based on limited case reports in neonates/infants): Apply 4 mm/kg as a thin ribbon to the affected areas; may repeat after 8 hours if needed (Wong, 1992) **or** apply a 1-inch strip on the affected site (Denkler, 1989).

Terbutaline (based on limited case reports): Infiltrate extravasation area using a solution of terbutaline 1 mg diluted to 10 mL in NS (large extravasation site; administration volume varied from 3-10 mL) **or** 1 mg diluted in 1 mL NS (small/distal extravasation site; administration volume varied from 0.5-1 mL) (Stier, 1999).

Injectable Detail
pH: 2.2-5 (0.1 mg/mL syringe; 1 mg/mL solution in ampul/vial)

Subcutaneous SubQ administration results in slower absorption and is less reliable. I.M. administration in the anterolateral aspect of the middle third of the thigh is preferred in the setting of anaphylaxis (ACLS guidelines, 2010; Kemp, 2008). I.M. administration into the buttocks should be avoided. Adrenaclick, Auvi-Q, EpiPen, EpiPen Jr, and Twinject Auto-Injectors should only be injected into the anterolateral aspect of the thigh, through clothing if necessary.

Note: Adrenaclick, Auvi-Q, EpiPen and EpiPen Jr Auto-Injectors contain a single, fixed-dose of epinephrine and may only be administered I.M. (preferred) or SubQ. Twinject Auto-Injectors contain two doses; the first fixed-dose is available for auto-injection; the second dose is available for manual injection following partial disassembly of device.

Inhalation S2: If using jet nebulizer: Administer diluted over ~15 minutes. If using handheld rubber bulb nebulizer, dilution is not required.

Endotracheal Cardiac arrest: Dilute in NS or sterile water. Absorption may be greater with sterile water (Naganobu, 2000). Stop compressions, spray drug quickly down tube. Follow immediately with several quick insufflations and continue chest compressions. May cause false-negative reading with exhaled CO_2 detectors; use second method to confirm tube placement if CO_2 is not detected (Neumar, 2010)

Preparation for Administration
Endotracheal (unlabeled route): Dilute in NS or sterile water.

Intraocular: Dilute 1 mL of 1 mg/mL (1:**1000**) solution in 100 mL to 1000 mL of an ophthalmic irrigation fluid for a final concentration of 1:**100,000** to 1:**1,000,000** (10 **mcg**/mL to 1 **mcg**/mL); may use this solution as an irrigation as needed during the procedure. May also prepare a dilution of 1:**100,000** to 1:**400,000** (10 **mcg**/mL to 2.5 **mcg**/mL) for intracameral administration.

Oral inhalation: S2: If using jet nebulizer,must be diluted with 3-5 mL NS. If using handheld rubber bulb nebulizer, dilution is not required.

Storage/Stability Epinephrine is sensitive to light and air. Protection from light is recommended. Oxidation turns drug pink, then a brown color. **Solutions should not be used if they are discolored or contain a precipitate.**

Adrenaclick: Store between 20°C to 25°C (68°F to 77°F); excursions permitted to 15°C to 30°C (59°F to 86°F); do not freeze or refrigerate. Protect from light.

Adrenalin: Store between 20°C to 25°C (68°F to 77°F); do not freeze. Protect from light.

Auvi-Q: Store between 20°C to 25°C (68°F to 77°F); excursions permitted to 15°C to 30°C (59°F to 86°F); do not refrigerate. Protect from light by storing in outer case provided.

EpiPen and EpiPen Jr: Store at 25°C (77°F); excursions permitted to 15°C to 30°C (59°F to 86°F); do not freeze or refrigerate. Protect from light by storing in carrier tube provided.

Twinject: Store between 20°C to 25°C (68°F to 77°F); excursions permitted to 15°C to 30°C (59°F to 86°F); do not freeze or refrigerate. Protect from light.

Primatene Mist: Store between 20°C to 25°C (68°F to 77°F).

S2: Store between 2°C to 20°C (36°F to 68°F). Protect from light.

Stability of injection of parenteral admixture at room temperature (25°C) or refrigeration (4°C) is 24 hours.

Nursing Actions

Physical Assessment Monitor for hypertension, CNS excitability, urinary retention, and dysrhythmias. I.V. (cardiovascular therapy): Central line with infusion pump and continuous cardiac/hemodynamic monitoring is necessary.

Patient Education
• Discuss specific use of drug and side effects with patient as it relates to treatment. (HCAHPS: During this hospital stay, were you given any medicine that you had not taken before? Before giving you any new medicine, how often did hospital staff tell you what the medicine was for? How often did hospital staff describe possible side effects in a way you could understand?)

• Patient may experience dizziness, anxiety, tremors, nausea, anxiety, akathisia, hyperhidrosis, pallor, or insomnia. Have patient report immediately to prescriber angina, tachycardia, arrhythmia, dyspnea, severe asthenia, strength differences from one side to another, difficulty speaking or thinking, change in balance, blurred vision, considerable headache, or injection site pain or irritation (HCAHPS).

• Educate patient about signs of a significant reaction (eg, wheezing; chest tightness; fever; itching; bad cough; blue skin color; seizures; or

swelling of face, lips, tongue, or throat). **Note:** This is not a comprehensive list of all side effects. Patient should consult prescriber for additional questions.

Intended Use and Disclaimer: Should not be printed and given to patients. This information is intended to serve as a concise initial reference for healthcare professionals to use when discussing medications with a patient. You must ultimately rely on your own discretion, experience and judgment in diagnosing, treating and advising patients.

Related Information

Management of Drug Extravasations *on page 1700*

EPINEPHrine (Nasal) (ep i NEF rin)

Brand Names: U.S. Adrenalin
Index Terms Adrenaline; Epinephrine Hydrochloride
Pharmacologic Category Alpha/Beta Agonist
Medication Safety Issues
Sound-alike/look-alike issues:
EPINEPHrine may be confused with ePHEDrine
Use Treatment of nasal congestion
Available Dosage Forms
Solution, Nasal:
Adrenalin: 0.1% (30 mL)
General Dosage Range Intranasal: *Children ≥6 years and Adults:* Apply **1:1000** (1 mg/mL) solution locally as drops, spray, or with sterile swab
Nursing Actions
Physical Assessment Monitor for hypertension, CNS excitability, urinary retention, dysrhythmias, and respiratory depression.
Patient Education
• Discuss specific use of drug and side effects with patient as it relates to treatment. (HCAHPS: During this hospital stay, were you given any medicine that you had not taken before? Before giving you any new medicine, how often did hospital staff tell you what the medicine was for? How often did hospital staff describe possible side effects in a way you could understand?)
• Patient may experience dizziness or xerostomia. Have patient report immediately to prescriber severe headache or considerable nausea (HCAHPS).
• Educate patient about signs of a significant reaction (eg, wheezing; chest tightness; fever; itching; bad cough; blue skin color; seizures; or swelling of face, lips, tongue, or throat). **Note:** This is not a comprehensive list of all side effects. Patient should consult prescriber for additional questions.

Intended Use and Disclaimer: Should not be printed and given to patients. This information is intended to serve as a concise initial reference for healthcare professionals to use when discussing medications with a patient. You must ultimately rely on your own discretion, experience and judgment in diagnosing, treating and advising patients.

Epirubicin (ep i ROO bi sin)

Brand Names: U.S. Ellence
Index Terms Epidoxorubicin; Epirubicin Hydrochloride; Pidorubicin; Pidorubicin Hydrochloride
Pharmacologic Category Antineoplastic Agent, Anthracycline; Antineoplastic Agent, Topoisomerase II Inhibitor
Medication Safety Issues
Sound-alike/look-alike issues:
EPIrubicin may be confused with DOXOrubicin, DAUNOrubicin, eriBULin, idarubicin
International issues:
Ellence [U.S.] may be confused with Elase brand name for dornase alfa [Chile, France, Malaysia]
High alert medication:
This drug is in a class the Institute for Safe Medication Practices (ISMP) includes among its list of drug classes which have a heightened risk of causing significant patient harm when used in error.
Pregnancy Risk Factor D
Lactation Excretion in breast milk unknown/not recommended
Breast-Feeding Considerations Excretion in human breast milk is unknown, however, other anthracyclines are excreted. According to the manufacturers, the decision to continue or discontinue breast-feeding during therapy should take into account the risk of exposure to the infant and the benefits of treatment to the mother.
Use Adjuvant therapy component for primary breast cancer
Unlabeled Use Treatment of esophageal cancer, gastric cancer, soft tissue sarcoma, uterine sarcoma
Mechanism of Action/Effect Epirubicin is an anthracycline agent which inhibits DNA and RNA synthesis throughout the cell cycle.
Contraindications Hypersensitivity to epirubicin or any component of the formulation, other anthracyclines, or anthracenediones; previous anthracycline treatment up to maximum cumulative dose; cardiomyopathy and/or heart failure, severe arrhythmias, recent myocardial infarction
Warnings/Precautions Hazardous agent - use appropriate precautions for handling and disposal (NIOSH, 2012).

[U.S. Boxed Warning]: Myocardial toxicity, including heart failure (HF) may occur, particularly in patients who have received prior anthracyclines, prior or concomitant radiotherapy to the mediastinal/pericardial area, who have pre-existing cardiac disease (active or dormant), or with concomitant cardiotoxic

medications. Cardiotoxicity may be concurrent or delayed (months to years after treatment). The risk of HF is ~0.9% at a cumulative dose of 550 mg/m^2, ~1.6% at a cumulative dose of 700 mg/m^2, and ~3.3% at a cumulative dose of 900 mg/m^2. Cardiotoxicity may also occur at lower cumulative doses or without risk factors. The risk of delayed cardiotoxicity increases more steeply with cumulative doses >900 mg/m^2 and this dose should be exceeded only with extreme caution. Acute toxicity, primarily sinus tachycardia and/or ECG abnormalities, including arrhythmia, and delayed toxicity, including decreased left ventricular ejection fraction (LVEF) and HF, have been described. Delayed toxicity usually develops late in the course of therapy or within 2-3 months after completion. Toxicity may be additive with other anthracyclines or anthracenediones, and may be increased in pediatric patients. Regular monitoring of LVEF and discontinuation at the first sign of impairment is recommended especially in patients with cardiac risk factors or impaired cardiac function. Discontinue treatment with signs of decreased LVEF. The half life of other cardiotoxic agents must be considered in sequential therapy; avoid epirubicin for up to 24 weeks after completing trastuzumab treatment.

[U.S. Boxed Warning]: May cause severe myelosuppression; neutropenia is the dose-limiting toxicity; severe thrombocytopenia or anemia may occur; obtain baseline and periodic blood counts. Patients should recover from myelosuppression due to prior chemotherapy treatment before beginning treatments. Thrombophlebitis and thromboembolic phenomena (including pulmonary embolism) have occurred.

[U.S. Boxed Warning]: Reduce dosage in patients with mild-to-moderate hepatic impairment (not recommended in severe hepatic impairment; predominantly hepatically eliminated) and in patients with serum creatinine >5 mg/dL (has not been studied in patients on dialysis); monitor hepatic and renal function at baseline and during treatment. May cause tumor lysis syndrome (TLS), although generally generally does not occur in patients with breast cancer; if TLS risk is suspected, consider monitoring serum uric acid, potassium, calcium, phosphate, and serum creatinine after initial administration; hydration and allopurinol prophylaxis may minimize potential TLS complications. Radiation recall (inflammatory) has been reported; epirubicin may have radiosensitizing activity. **[U.S. Boxed Warning]: Treatment with anthracyclines (including epirubicin) may increase the risk of secondary acute myelogenous leukemia (AML).** AML is more common when given in combination with other antineoplastic agents, in patients who have received multiple courses of previous chemotherapy, or

with escalated cumulative anthracycline doses (>720 mg/m^2 for epirubicin). In breast cancer patients, the risk for treatment-related AML or myelodysplastic syndrome (MDS) was estimated at 0.3% at 3 years, 0.5% at 5 years, and 0.6% at 8 years after treatment. The latency period for secondary leukemias may be short (1-3 years).

[U.S. Boxed Warning]: For I.V. administration only, severe local tissue damage and necrosis will result if extravasation occurs (vesicant); not for I.M. or SubQ use. Injection in to a small vein or repeated administration in the same vein may result in venous sclerosis. Ensure proper needle or catheter placement prior to and during infusion. Avoid extravasation. Women ≥70 years of age should be closely monitored for toxicity. **[U.S. Boxed Warning]: Should be administered under the supervision of an experienced cancer chemotherapy physician.** Epirubicin is emetogenic; consider prophylactic antiemetics prior to administration. Patients should recover from acute toxicities (stomatitis, myelosuppression, infections) prior to initiating treatment. Assess baseline labs (blood counts, bilirubin, ALT, AST, serum creatinine) and cardiac function (with LVEF). Prophylactic antibiotics should be administered with the CDF-120 regimen. Patients should not be immunized with live viral vaccines during or shortly after treatment. Inactivated vaccines may be administered (response may be diminished).

Drug Interactions
Avoid Concomitant Use
Avoid concomitant use of EPIrubicin with any of the following: BCG; Cimetidine; CloZAPine; Natalizumab; Pimecrolimus; Tacrolimus (Topical); Tofacitinib; Vaccines (Live)

Decreased Effect
EPIrubicin may decrease the levels/effects of: BCG; Cardiac Glycosides; Coccidioidin Skin Test; Sipuleucel-T; Vaccines (Inactivated); Vaccines (Live)

The levels/effects of EPIrubicin may be decreased by: Cardiac Glycosides; Echinacea

Increased Effect/Toxicity
EPIrubicin may increase the levels/effects of: CloZAPine; Leflunomide; Natalizumab; Tofacitinib; Vaccines (Live)

The levels/effects of EPIrubicin may be increased by: Bevacizumab; Cimetidine; Cyclophosphamide; Denosumab; Pimecrolimus; Roflumilast; Tacrolimus (Topical); Taxane Derivatives; Trastuzumab

Nutritional/Ethanol Interactions
Ethanol: Avoid ethanol (due to GI irritation).
Herb/Nutraceutical: Avoid black cohosh, dong quai in estrogen-dependent tumors.

Adverse Reactions Percentages reported as part of combination chemotherapy regimens.

>10%:
Central nervous system: Lethargy (1% to 46%)
Dermatologic: Alopecia (70% to 96%)
Endocrine & metabolic: Amenorrhea (69% to 72%), hot flashes (5% to 39%)
Gastrointestinal: Nausea/vomiting (83% to 92%; grades 3/4: 22% to 25%), mucositis (9% to 59%; grades 3/4: ≤9%), diarrhea (7% to 25%)
Hematologic: Leukopenia (50% to 80%; grades 3/4: 2% to 59%), neutropenia (54% to 80%; grades 3/4: 11% to 67%; nadir: 10-14 days; recovery: by day 21), anemia (13% to 72%; grades 3/4: ≤6%), thrombocytopenia (5% to 49%; grades 3/4: ≤5%)
Local: Injection site reactions (3% to 20%; grades 3/4: <1%)
Ocular: Conjunctivitis (1% to 15%)
Miscellaneous: Infection (15% to 22%; grades 3/4: ≤2%)
1% to 10%:
Cardiovascular: LVEF decreased (asymptomatic; delayed: 1% to 2%), HF (0.4% to 1.5%)
Central nervous system: Fever (1% to 5%)
Dermatologic: Rash (1% to 9%), skin changes (1% to 5%)
Gastrointestinal: Anorexia (2% to 3%)
Hematologic: Neutropenic fever (grades 3/4: ≤6%)

Available Dosage Forms
Solution, Intravenous [preservative free]:
Ellence: 50 mg/25 mL (25 mL); 200 mg/100 mL (100 mL)
Generic: 50 mg/25 mL (25 mL); 200 mg/100 mL (100 mL)
Solution Reconstituted, Intravenous:
Generic: 50 mg (1 ea)

General Dosage Range Dosage adjustment recommended in patients with hepatic or renal impairment or who develop toxicities
I.V.: *Adults:* 100 mg/m² on day 1 every 3 weeks **or** 60 mg/m² on days 1 and 8 every 4 weeks

Administration
I.V. Infuse over 15-20 minutes or slow I.V. push; if lower doses due to dose reduction are administered, may reduce infusion time proportionally. Do not infuse over <3 minutes. Infuse into a free-flowing I.V. solution. Avoid the use of veins over joints or in extremities with compromised venous or lymphatic drainage.

Vesicant; ensure proper needle or catheter placement prior to and during infusion; avoid extravasation.

Extravasation management: If extravasation occurs, stop infusion immediately and disconnect (leave cannula/needle in place); gently aspirate extravasated solution (do **NOT** flush the line); remove needle/cannula; elevate extremity. Initiate antidote (dexrazoxane or dimethyl sulfate [DMSO]). Apply dry cold compresses for 20 minutes 4 times daily for 1-2 days (Perez Fidalgo,

2012); withhold cooling beginning 15 minutes before dexrazoxane infusion; continue withholding cooling until 15 minutes after infusion is completed. Topical DMSO should not be administered in combination with dexrazoxane; may lessen dexrazoxane efficacy.
Dexrazoxane: Adults: 1000 mg/m² (maximum dose: 2000 mg) I.V. (administer in a large vein remote from site of extravasation) over 1-2 hours days 1 and 2, then 500 mg/m² (maximum dose: 1000 mg) I.V. over 1-2 hours day 3; begin within 6 hours of extravasation. Day 2 and day 3 doses should be administered at approximately the same time (± 3 hours) as the dose on day 1 (Mouridsen, 2007; Perez Fidalgo, 2012). **Note:** Reduce dexrazoxane dose by 50% in patients with moderate to severe renal impairment (CrCl <40 mL/minute).
DMSO: Children and Adults: Apply topically to a region covering twice the affected area every 8 hours for 7 days; begin within 10 minutes of extravasation; do not cover with a dressing (Perez Fidalgo, 2012).

Hazardous agent; use appropriate precautions for handling and disposal (NIOSH, 2012).
Preparation for Administration Hazardous agent; use appropriate precautions for handling and disposal (NIOSH, 2012). Reconstitute lyophilized powder with SWFI (25 mL for the 50 mg vial or 100 mL for the 200 mg vial) to a final concentration of 2 mg/mL.
Storage/Stability Protect from light.
Solution: Store intact vials refrigerated at 2°C to 8°C (36°F to 46°F); do not freeze. Product may "gel" at refrigerated temperatures; will return to slightly viscous solution after 2-4 hours at room temperature (15°C to 30°C). Discard unused solution from single dose vials within 24 hours of entry.
Lyophilized powder: Store at room temperature of 25°C (77°F); excursions permitted to 15°C to 30°C (59°F to 86°F). Reconstituted solutions are stable for 24 hours when stored at 2°C to 8°C (36°F to 46°F) or at room temperature.
Nursing Actions
Physical Assessment Note specific infusion instructions. Premedication with an antiemetic may be ordered (emetogenic). Monitor infusion site closely to prevent extravasation; severe local tissue necrosis will result if extravasation occurs. Monitor for acute nausea and vomiting, anemia, cardiotoxicity, infection, and bleeding. Teach patient importance of adequate hydration.
Patient Education
• Discuss specific use of drug and side effects with patient as it relates to treatment. (HCAHPS: During this hospital stay, were you given any medicine that you had not taken before? Before giving you any new medicine, how often did hospital staff tell you what the medicine was

for? How often did hospital staff describe possible side effects in a way you could understand?)

• Patient may experience urine discoloration, hot flashes, lack of appetite, stomatitis, cheilitis, alopecia, amenorrhea, or eye irritation. Have patient report immediately to prescriber signs of infection, severe dizziness, syncope, considerable nausea, significant diarrhea, excessive weight loss, osteodynia, night sweats, ecchymosis, hemorrhaging, intolerable asthenia, or signs of blood clots (HCAHPS).

• Educate patient about signs of a significant reaction (eg, wheezing; chest tightness; fever; itching; bad cough; blue skin color; seizures; or swelling of face, lips, tongue, or throat). **Note:** This is not a comprehensive list of all side effects. Patient should consult prescriber for additional questions.

Intended Use and Disclaimer: Should not be printed and given to patients. This information is intended to serve as a concise initial reference for healthcare professionals to use when discussing medications with a patient. You must ultimately rely on your own discretion, experience and judgment in diagnosing, treating and advising patients.

Related Information

Management of Drug Extravasations *on page 1700*

Eplerenone (e PLER en one)

Brand Names: U.S. Inspra

Pharmacologic Category Antihypertensive; Diuretic, Potassium-Sparing; Selective Aldosterone Blocker

Medication Safety Issues

Sound-alike/look-alike issues:

Inspra may be confused with Spiriva

Pregnancy Risk Factor B

Lactation Excretion in breast milk unknown/not recommended

Breast-Feeding Considerations It is not known if eplerenone is excreted in breast milk. Due to the potential for serious adverse reactions in the nursing infant, the manufacturer recommends a a decision be made whether to discontinue nursing or to discontinue the drug, taking into account the importance of treatment to the mother.

Use

U.S. labeling: Treatment of hypertension (may be used alone or in combination with other antihypertensive agents); treatment of heart failure (HF) (LVEF ≤40%) following acute MI

Note: The ACCF/AHA 2013 heart failure guidelines recommend the use of aldosterone antagonists, along with other guideline directed medical therapies, to reduce morbidity and mortality in patients with an LVEF ≤40% following

acute MI who develop symptoms of HF or have a history of diabetes mellitus (Yancy, 2013).

Canadian labeling: Treatment of NYHA class II chronic heart failure (HF) with left ventricular systolic dysfunction; treatment of HF following acute MI

Unlabeled Use The ACCF/AHA 2013 heart failure (HF) guidelines recommend the use of aldosterone antagonists, along with other guideline directed medical therapies, to reduce morbidity and mortality in patients with HF (NYHA class II-IV) with LVEF ≤35%. Patients with NYHA class II HF should have a history of prior cardiovascular hospitalization or elevated plasma natriuretic peptide levels to reduce morbidity and mortality (ACCF/AHA [Yancy, 2013]).

Mechanism of Action/Effect Aldosterone increases blood pressure primarily by inducing sodium reabsorption. Eplerenone reduces blood pressure by blocking aldosterone binding at mineralocorticoid receptors found in the kidney, heart, blood vessels and brain.

Contraindications

U.S. labeling: Serum potassium >5.5 mEq/L at initiation; CrCl ≤30 mL/minute; concomitant use of strong CYP3A4 inhibitors (see Drug Interactions for details)

The following additional contraindications apply to patients with hypertension: Type 2 diabetes mellitus (noninsulin dependent, NIDDM) with microalbuminuria; serum creatinine >2.0 mg/dL in males or >1.8 mg/dL in females; CrCl <50 mL/minute; concomitant use with potassium supplements or potassium-sparing diuretics

Canadian labeling: Hypersensitivity to eplerenone or any component of the formulation; serum potassium >5 mEq/L at initiation; severe hepatic impairment (Child-Pugh class C); severe renal impairment (eGFR <30 mL/minute/1.73 m^2); clinically significant hyperkalemia; concomitant use with potassium supplements, potassium-sparing diuretics or strong CYP3A4 inhibitors

Warnings/Precautions Monitor closely for hyperkalemia; increases in serum potassium were dose related during clinical trials and rates of hyperkalemia also increased with declining renal function. The concurrent use of larger doses of ACE inhibitors (eg, ≥ lisinopril 10 mg daily) also increases the risk of hyperkalemia (ACCF/AHA [Yancy, 2013]). Dose reduction or interruption of therapy may be necessary with development of hyperkalemia. Use is contraindicated in patients with potassium >5.5 mEq/L (U.S. labeling) or >5 mEq/L (Canadian labeling) at initiation of therapy. Safety and efficacy have not been established in patients with severe hepatic impairment (Canadian labeling contraindicates use in severe hepatic impairment). Use with caution in HF patients post-MI with diabetes (especially if patient has proteinuria); risk of hyperkalemia is increased. Risk of hyperkalemia is increased with declining renal function. Use with caution in patients with mild renal impairment; contraindicated with moderate-severe impairment (hypertension: CrCl <50 mL/minute; heart failure post-MI: CrCl ≤30 mL/minute). Canadian labeling contraindicates use in all patients with severe renal impairment. Potentially significant drug-drug interactions may exist, requiring dose or frequency adjustment, additional monitoring, and/or selection of alternative therapy. Avoid potassium supplements, potassium-containing salt substitutes, a diet rich in potassium, or other drugs that can cause hyperkalemia (eg, other potassium-sparing diuretics, NSAIDS). For the treatment of hypertension, the use of potassium supplements or potassium-sparing diuretics is contraindicated.

When evaluating a heart failure patient for eplerenone treatment, eGFR should be >30 mL/minute/1.73 m^2 or creatinine should be ≤2.5 mg/dL (men) or ≤2 mg/dL (women) with no recent worsening and potassium <5 mEq/L with no history of severe hyperkalemia (ACCF/AHA [Yancy, 2013]). Serum potassium levels require close monitoring and management if elevated. The manufacturer recommends to withhold therapy if serum potassium >6 mEq/L. The ACCF/AHA recommends considering discontinuation upon the development of serum potassium >5.5 mEq/L or worsening renal function with careful evaluation of the entire medical regimen. Avoid routine triple therapy with the combined use of an ACE inhibitor, ARB, and eplerenone. Instruct patients with heart failure to discontinue use during an episode of diarrhea or dehydration or when loop diuretic therapy is interrupted (ACCF/AHA [Yancy, 2013]).

Drug Interactions

Avoid Concomitant Use

Avoid concomitant use of Eplerenone with any of the following: CycloSPORINE (Systemic); CYP3A4 Inhibitors (Strong); Fusidic Acid (Systemic); Itraconazole; Ketoconazole (Systemic); Posaconazole; Tacrolimus (Systemic); Voriconazole

Decreased Effect

The levels/effects of Eplerenone may be decreased by: Bosentan; CYP3A4 Inducers (Strong); Dabrafenib; Deferasirox; Herbs (CYP3A4 Inducers); Herbs (Hypertensive Properties); Methylphenidate; Mitotane; Nonsteroidal Anti-Inflammatory Agents; Tocilizumab; Yohimbine

Increased Effect/Toxicity

Eplerenone may increase the levels/effects of: ACE Inhibitors; Amifostine; Angiotensin II Receptor Blockers; Antihypertensives; CycloSPORINE (Systemic); DULoxetine; Hypotensive Agents; Lithium; Obinutuzumab; Potassium Salts; Potassium-Sparing Diuretics; RiTUXimab; Tacrolimus (Systemic)

The levels/effects of Eplerenone may be increased by: Alfuzosin; Brimonidine (Topical); Canagliflozin; CYP3A4 Inhibitors (Moderate); CYP3A4 Inhibitors (Strong); Dasatinib; Diazoxide; Fluconazole; Fusidic Acid (Systemic); Heparin; Heparin (Low Molecular Weight); Herbs (Hypotensive Properties); Itraconazole; Ivacaftor; Ketoconazole (Systemic); Luliconazole; MAO Inhibitors; Mifepristone; Nitrofurantoin; Nonsteroidal Anti-Inflammatory Agents; Pentoxifylline; Phosphodiesterase 5 Inhibitors; Posaconazole; Prostacyclin Analogues; Simeprevir; Trimethoprim; Voriconazole

Nutritional/Ethanol Interactions

Food: Grapefruit juice increases eplerenone AUC ~25%.

Herb/Nutraceutical: St John's wort may decrease levels of eplerenone. Avoid black cohosh, California poppy, coleus, golden seal, hawthorn, mistletoe, periwinkle, quinine, shepherd's purse (may have increased antihypertensive effect). Avoid bayberry, blue cohosh, cayenne, ephedra, ginger, ginseng (American), kola, licorice (may diminish the antihypertensive effect).

Adverse Reactions

>10%: Endocrine & metabolic: Hyperkalemia ([HF post-MI: K >5.5 mEq/L: 16%; K ≥6 mEq/L: 6%] [HTN: K >5.5 mEq/L at doses ≤200 mg: ≤1%; dose of 400 mg: 9%]), hypertriglyceridemia (1% to 15%, dose related)

1% to 10%:

Central nervous system: Dizziness (3%), fatigue (2%)

Endocrine & metabolic: Hyponatremia (2%, dose related), breast pain (males <1% to 1%), gynecomastia (males <1% to 1%), hypercholesterolemia (<1% to 1%)

Gastrointestinal: Diarrhea (2%), abdominal pain (1%)

Genitourinary: Abnormal vaginal bleeding (<1% to 2%)

Renal: Creatinine increased (HF post-MI: 6%), albuminuria (1%)

Respiratory: Cough (2%)

Miscellaneous: Flu-like syndrome (2%)

Available Dosage Forms

Tablet, Oral:

Inspra: 25 mg, 50 mg

Generic: 25 mg, 50 mg

General Dosage Range Dosage adjustment recommended in patients on concomitant therapy or based on potassium concentrations

Oral: *Adults:* Initial: 25-50 mg once daily; Maintenance: 50 mg once or twice daily (maximum daily dose: 100 mg)

Administration

Oral May be administered with or without food.

Storage/Stability Store at controlled room temperature of 25°C (77°F); excursions permitted to 15°C to 30°C (59°F to 86°F).

Nursing Actions

Physical Assessment Monitor potassium levels, blood pressure, and renal function prior to and periodically during therapy. Monitor for hypotension and hyperkalemia at beginning of and at regular intervals during therapy.

Patient Education

- Discuss specific use of drug and side effects with patient as it relates to treatment. (HCAHPS: During this hospital stay, were you given any medicine that you had not taken before? Before giving you any new medicine, how often did hospital staff tell you what the medicine was for? How often did hospital staff describe possible side effects in a way you could understand?)
- Have patient report immediately to prescriber severe dizziness, syncope, considerable asthenia, angina, tachycardia, arrhythmia, significant diarrhea, edema of extremities, emesis, or dyspnea (HCAHPS).
- Educate patient about signs of a significant reaction (eg, wheezing; chest tightness; fever; itching; bad cough; blue skin color; seizures; or swelling of face, lips, tongue, or throat). **Note:** This is not a comprehensive list of all side effects. Patient should consult prescriber for additional questions.

Intended Use and Disclaimer: Should not be printed and given to patients. This information is intended to serve as a concise initial reference for healthcare professionals to use when discussing medications with a patient. You must ultimately rely on your own discretion, experience and judgment in diagnosing, treating and advising patients.

Dietary Considerations May be taken with or without food. Do not use salt substitutes containing potassium.

Epoetin Alfa (e POE e tin AL fa)

Brand Names: U.S. Epogen; Procrit

Index Terms rHuEPO; rHuEPO-α; EPO; Erythropoiesis-Stimulating Agent (ESA); Erythropoietin

Pharmacologic Category Colony Stimulating Factor; Erythropoiesis-Stimulating Agent (ESA); Hematopoietic Agent

Medication Safety Issues

Sound-alike/look-alike issues:

Epoetin alfa may be confused with darbepoetin alfa, epoetin beta

Epogen may be confused with Neupogen

International issues:

Epopen [Spain] may be confused with EpiPen brand name for epinephrine [U.S., Canada, and multiple international markets]

Medication Guide Available Yes

Pregnancy Risk Factor C

Lactation Excretion in breast milk unknown/use caution

Breast-Feeding Considerations Endogenous erythropoietin is found in breast milk (Semba, 2002). It is not known if recombinant erythropoietin alfa is excreted into breast milk. The manufacturer recommends caution be used if the single dose vial preparation is administered to nursing women; use of the multiple dose vials containing benzyl alcohol is contraindicated in breast-feeding women. When administered enterally to neonates (mixed with human milk or infant formula), recombinant erythropoietin did not significantly increase serum EPO concentrations. If passage via breast milk does occur, risk to a nursing infant appears low (Juul, 2003).

Use Treatment of anemia due to concurrent myelosuppressive chemotherapy in patients with cancer (nonmyeloid malignancies) receiving chemotherapy (palliative intent) for a planned minimum of 2 additional months of chemotherapy; treatment of anemia due to chronic kidney disease (including patients on dialysis and not on dialysis) to decrease the need for RBC transfusion; treatment of anemia associated with HIV (zidovudine) therapy when endogenous erythropoietin levels ≤500 mUnits/mL; reduction of allogeneic RBC transfusion for elective, noncardiac, nonvascular surgery when perioperative hemoglobin is >10 to ≤13 g/dL and there is a high risk for blood loss

Note: Epoetin is **not** indicated for use under the following conditions:

- Cancer patients receiving hormonal therapy, therapeutic biologic products, or radiation therapy unless also receiving concurrent myelosuppressive chemotherapy
- Cancer patients receiving myelosuppressive chemotherapy when the expected outcome is curative
- Surgery patients who are willing to donate autologous blood
- Surgery patients undergoing cardiac or vascular surgery
- As a substitute for RBC transfusion in patients requiring immediate correction of anemia

Note: In clinical trials (and one meta-analysis), epoetin has not demonstrated improved quality of life, fatigue, or well-being.

Unlabeled Use Treatment of symptomatic anemia in myelodysplastic syndrome (MDS)

Mechanism of Action/Effect Induces red blood cell production in the bone marrow to be released into the blood stream where they mature to erythrocytes; results in rise in hematocrit and hemoglobin levels

Contraindications Hypersensitivity to epoetin or any component of the formulation; uncontrolled hypertension; pure red cell aplasia (due to epoetin or other epoetin protein drugs); multidose vials contain benzyl alcohol and are contraindicated in neonates, infants, pregnant women, and nursing women

Warnings/Precautions [U.S. Boxed Warning]: Erythropoiesis-stimulating agents (ESAs) increased the risk of serious cardiovascular events, thromboembolic events, stroke, mortality, and/or tumor progression in clinical studies when administered to target hemoglobin levels >11 g/dL (and provide no additional benefit); a rapid rise in hemoglobin (>1 g/dL over 2 weeks) may also contribute to these risks. **[U.S. Boxed Warning]: A shortened overall survival and/or increased risk of tumor progression or recurrence has been reported in studies with breast, cervical, head and neck, lymphoid, and non-small cell lung cancer patients.** It is of note that in these studies, patients received ESAs to a target hemoglobin of ≥12 g/dL; although risk has not been excluded when dosed to achieve a target hemoglobin of <12 g/dL. **[U.S. Boxed Warnings]: To decrease these risks, and risk of cardio- and thrombovascular events, use the lowest dose needed to avoid red blood cell transfusions. Use ESAs in cancer patients only for the treatment of anemia related to concurrent myelosuppressive chemotherapy; discontinue ESA following completion of the chemotherapy course. ESAs are not indicated for patients receiving myelosuppressive therapy when the anticipated outcome is curative.** A dosage modification is appropriate if hemoglobin levels rise >1 g/dL per 2-week time period during treatment (Rizzo, 2010). Use of ESAs has been associated with an increased risk of venous thromboembolism (VTE) without a reduction in transfusions in patients with cancer (Hershman, 2009). Improved anemia symptoms, quality of life, fatigue, or well-being have not been demonstrated in controlled clinical trials. **[U.S. Boxed Warning]: Because of the risks of decreased survival and increased risk of tumor growth or progression, all health-care providers and hospitals are required to enroll and comply with the ESA APPRISE (Assisting Providers and Cancer Patients with Risk Information for the Safe use of ESAs) Oncology Program prior to prescribing or dispensing ESAs to cancer patients.** Prescribers and patients will have to provide written documentation of discussed risks prior to each new course.

[U.S. Boxed Warning]: An increased risk of death, serious cardiovascular events, and stroke was reported in chronic kidney disease (CKD) patients administered ESAs to target hemoglobin levels ≥11 g/dL; use the lowest dose sufficient to reduce the need for RBC transfusions. An optimal target hemoglobin level, dose or dosing strategy to reduce these risks has not been identified in clinical trials. Hemoglobin rising >1 g/dL in a 2-week period may contribute to the risk (dosage reduction recommended). The American College of Physicians recommends against the use of ESAs in patients with mild to moderate anemia and heart failure or coronary heart disease (ACP [Qaseem, 2013]).

Chronic kidney disease patients who exhibit an inadequate hemoglobin response to ESA therapy may be at a higher risk for cardiovascular events and mortality compared to other patients. ESA therapy may reduce dialysis efficacy (due to increase in red blood cells and decrease in plasma volume); adjustments in dialysis parameters may be needed. Patients treated with epoetin may require increased heparinization during dialysis to prevent clotting of the extracorporeal circuit. **[U.S. Boxed Warning]: DVT prophylaxis is recommended in perisurgery patients due to the risk of DVT.** Increased mortality was also observed in patients undergoing coronary artery bypass surgery who received epoetin alfa; these deaths were associated with thrombotic events. Epoetin is **not** approved for reduction of red blood cell transfusion in patients undergoing cardiac or vascular surgery and is **not** indicated for surgical patients willing to donate autologous blood.

Use with caution in patients with hypertension (contraindicated in uncontrolled hypertension) or with a history of seizures; hypertensive encephalopathy and seizures have been reported. If hypertension is difficult to control, reduce or hold epoetin alfa. An excessive rate of rise of hemoglobin is associated with hypertension or exacerbation of hypertension; decrease the epoetin dose if the hemoglobin increase exceeds 1 g/dL in any 2-week period. Blood pressure should be controlled prior to start of therapy and monitored closely throughout treatment. The risk for seizures is increased with epoetin use in patients with CKD; monitor closely for neurologic symptoms during the first several months of therapy. Due to the delayed onset of erythropoiesis, epoetin alfa is **not** recommended for acute correction of severe anemia or as a substitute for emergency transfusion.

Prior to treatment, correct or exclude deficiencies of iron, vitamin B_{12}, and/or folate, as well as other factors which may impair erythropoiesis (inflammatory conditions, infections). Prior to and periodically during therapy, iron stores must be evaluated. Supplemental iron is recommended if serum ferritin <100 mcg/L or serum transferrin saturation <20%; most patients with chronic kidney disease will require iron supplementation. Poor response should prompt evaluation of these potential factors, as well as possible malignant processes and hematologic disease (thalassemia, refractory anemia, myelodysplastic disorder), occult blood loss, hemolysis, ostetis fibrosa cystic, and/or bone marrow fibrosis. Severe anemia and pure red cell aplasia (PRCA) with associated neutralizing antibodies to erythropoietin has been reported, predominantly in patients with CKD receiving SubQ epoetin (the I.V. route is preferred for hemodialysis patients). Cases have also been reported in patients with hepatitis C who were receiving ESAs, interferon, and ribavirin. Patients with a sudden loss of response to epoetin alfa (with severe anemia and a low reticulocyte count) should be evaluated for PRCA with associated neutralizing antibodies to erythropoietin; discontinue treatment (permanently) in patients with PRCA secondary to neutralizing antibodies to epoetin.

Potentially serious allergic reactions have been reported (rarely). Discontinue immediately (and permanently) in patients who experience serious allergic/anaphylactic reactions. Some products may contain albumin. Multidose vials contain benzyl alcohol; do not use in premature infants.

Drug Interactions

Avoid Concomitant Use There are no known interactions where it is recommended to avoid concomitant use.

Decreased Effect There are no known significant interactions involving a decrease in effect.

Increased Effect/Toxicity There are no known significant interactions involving an increase in effect.

Adverse Reactions

>10%:
Cardiovascular: Hypertension (3% to 28%)
Central nervous system: Fever (10% to 42%), headache (5% to 18%)
Dermatologic: Pruritus (12% to 21%), rash (2% to 19%)
Gastrointestinal: Nausea (35% to 56%), vomiting (12% to 28%)
Local: Injection site reaction (7% to 13%)
Neuromuscular & skeletal: Arthralgia (10% to 16%)
Respiratory: Cough (4% to 26%)
1% to 10%:
Cardiovascular: Deep vein thrombosis, edema, thrombosis
Central nervous system: Chills, depression, dizziness, insomnia
Dermatologic: Urticaria
Endocrine & metabolic: Hyperglycemia, hypokalemia
Gastrointestinal: Dysphagia, stomatitis, weight loss
Hematologic: Leukopenia
Local: Clotted vascular access
Neuromuscular & skeletal: Bone pain, muscle spasm, myalgia
Respiratory: Pulmonary embolism, respiratory congestion, upper respiratory infection

Pharmacodynamics/Kinetics

Onset of Action Several days; Peak effect: Hemoglobin level: 2-6 weeks

Available Dosage Forms

Solution, Injection:
Epogen: 10,000 units/mL (2 mL); 20,000 units/mL (1 mL)

Procrit: 10,000 units/mL (2 mL); 20,000 units/mL (1 mL)
Solution, Injection [preservative free]:
Epogen: 2000 units/mL (1 mL); 3000 units/mL (1 mL); 4000 units/mL (1 mL); 10,000 units/mL (1 mL)
Procrit: 2000 units/mL (1 mL); 3000 units/mL (1 mL); 4000 units/mL (1 mL); 10,000 units/mL (1 mL); 40,000 units/mL (1 mL)

General Dosage Range I.V., SubQ: Children and Adults: Dosage varies greatly depending on indication

Administration

I.V. Patients with CKD on hemodialysis: I.V. route preferred; it may be administered into the venous line at the end of the dialysis procedure
Note: SubQ administration is the preferred route in other patient populations.
Injectable Detail pH: 6.6-7.2 (single dose vial); 5.8-6.4 (multidose vial)
Subcutaneous SubQ: SubQ is the preferred route of administration **except** in patients with CKD on hemodialysis; 1:1 dilution with bacteriostatic NS (containing benzyl alcohol) acts as a local anesthetic to reduce pain at the injection site
Preparation for Administration Prior to SubQ administration, preservative free solutions may be mixed with bacteriostatic NS containing benzyl alcohol 0.9% in a 1:1 ratio.
Storage/Stability Vials should be stored at 2°C to 8°C (36°F to 46°F); **do not freeze or shake.** Protect from light.
Single-dose 1 mL vial contains no preservative: Use one dose per vial. Do not re-enter vial; discard unused portions.
Single-dose vials (except 40,000 units/mL vial) are stable for 2 weeks at room temperature (Cohen, 2007). Single-dose 40,000 units/mL vial is stable for 1 week at room temperature.
Multidose 1 mL or 2 mL vial contains preservative. Store at 2°C to 8°C after initial entry and between doses. Discard 21 days after initial entry. Multidose vials (with preservative) are stable for 1 week at room temperature (Cohen, 2007).
Prefilled syringes containing the 20,000 units/mL formulation with preservative are stable for 6 weeks refrigerated (2°C to 8°C) (Naughton, 2003).
Dilutions of 1:10 and 1:20 (1 part epoetin:19 parts sodium chloride) are stable for 18 hours at room temperature (Ohls, 1996).
Prior to SubQ administration, preservative free solutions may be mixed with bacteriostatic NS containing benzyl alcohol 0.9% in a 1:1 ratio (Corbo, 1992).
Dilutions of 1:10 in $D_{10}W$ with human albumin 0.05% or 0.1% are stable for 24 hours.

Nursing Actions

Physical Assessment Evaluate history of hypertension or seizures and potential risk for thromboembolism prior to beginning therapy. Blood pressure should be monitored closely and controlled during therapy. If administered by intravenous infusion, lines should be monitored closely for possible clotting. Assess blood chemistries, hemoglobin/hematocrit, serum ferritin, and transferrin saturation prior to and on a regular basis during therapy; dosage adjustment and iron supplements may be necessary. Monitor for hypertension, thrombotic events, edema, and anemia. Serious allergic or anaphylactic reactions may occur. Teach patient proper SubQ injection technique and syringe/needle disposal.

Patient Education
- Discuss specific use of drug and side effects with patient as it relates to treatment. (HCAHPS: During this hospital stay, were you given any medicine that you had not taken before? Before giving you any new medicine, how often did hospital staff tell you what the medicine was for? How often did hospital staff describe possible side effects in a way you could understand?)
- Patient may experience injection site irritation, headache, nausea, osteodynia, arthralgia, myalgia, muscle spasms, stomatitis, weight loss, or insomnia. Have patient report immediately to prescriber angina, tachycardia, arrhythmia, dyspnea, excessive weight gain, edema of extremities, strength differences from one side to another, difficulty speaking or thinking, change in balance, blurred vision, severe dizziness, syncope, painful extremities, considerable headache, significant asthenia, pallor, hemoptysis, or abnormal gait (HCAHPS).
- Educate patient about signs of a significant reaction (eg, wheezing; chest tightness; fever; itching; bad cough; blue skin color; seizures; or swelling of face, lips, tongue, or throat). **Note:** This is not a comprehensive list of all side effects. Patient should consult prescriber for additional questions.

Intended Use and Disclaimer: Should not be printed and given to patients. This information is intended to serve as a concise initial reference for healthcare professionals to use when discussing medications with a patient. You must ultimately rely on your own discretion, experience and judgment in diagnosing, treating and advising patients.

Epoprostenol (e poe PROST en ole)

Brand Names: U.S. Flolan; Veletri
Index Terms Epoprostenol Sodium; PGI_2; PGX; Prostacyclin
Pharmacologic Category Prostacyclin; Prostaglandin; Vasodilator
Medication Safety Issues
High alert medication:
The Institute for Safe Medication Practices (ISMP) includes this medication among its list of drugs which have a heightened risk of causing significant patient harm when used in error.

Pregnancy Risk Factor B
Lactation Excretion in breast milk unknown/use caution
Use Treatment of pulmonary arterial hypertension (PAH) (WHO Group I) in patients with NYHA Class III or IV symptoms to improve exercise capacity
Unlabeled Use Acute vasodilator testing in pulmonary arterial hypertension (PAH)

Inhalation: Intraoperative treatment of pulmonary hypertension in patients undergoing cardiac surgery with cardiopulmonary bypass; post-cardiothoracic surgery pulmonary hypertension, right ventricular dysfunction, or refractory hypoxemia

Available Dosage Forms
Solution Reconstituted, Intravenous:
Flolan: 0.5 mg (1 ea); 1.5 mg (1 ea)
Veletri: 0.5 mg (1 ea); 1.5 mg (1 ea)
Generic: 0.5 mg (1 ea); 1.5 mg (1 ea)
General Dosage Range I.V.: *Adults:* Initial: 1-2 ng/kg/minute; increase dose in increments of 1-2 ng/kg/minute every 15 minutes until response
Administration
I.V. Use infusion sets with an in-line 0.22 micron filter for Veletri or Caripul infusions. Flolan labeling does not specifically recommend filtering; however, the use of an in-line 0.22 micron filter was used during clinical trials. The ambulatory infusion pump should be small and lightweight, be able to adjust infusion rates in 2 ng/kg/minute increments, have occlusion, end of infusion, and low battery alarms, have ± 6% accuracy of the programmed rate, and have positive continuous or pulsatile pressure with intervals ≤3 minutes between pulses. The reservoir should be made of polyvinyl chloride, polypropylene, or glass. Immediate access to back up pump, infusion sets and medication is essential to prevent treatment interruptions.

When administered on an ongoing basis, must be infused through a central venous catheter. Peripheral infusion may be used temporarily until central line is established. Infuse using an infusion pump. Avoid abrupt withdrawal (including interruptions in delivery) or sudden large reductions in dosing.

Injectable Detail
pH: 10.2-10.8
Inhalation Inhalation is an unlabeled route of administration.
Intraoperative administration: Administer via jet nebulizer connected to the inspiratory limb of the ventilator near the endotracheal tube with a bypass oxygen flow of 8 L/minute to achieve administration of a high proportion of small particles (Fattouch, 2006; Hache, 2003).
Post-cardiothoracic surgery: May also be administered via jet nebulizer connected to the inspiratory limb of the ventilator near the endotracheal tube or via face mask with a Venturi attachment

for aerosolization with a bypass oxygen flow of 2-3 L/minute (De Wet, 2004). **Note:** Glycine buffer diluent may cause ventilator valve malfunction; it has been recommended that filters be changed on the ventilator every 2 hours; may also use a ventilator heating coil (De Wet, 2004).

Nursing Actions

Physical Assessment Monitor patient's ability to manage a central venous catheter in the home setting. Review with patient the importance of infection control practices for the management of a central venous catheter. **Institutional:** Continuous pulmonary and hemodynamic arterial monitoring, protimes. **Home therapy:** Avoid sudden rate reduction or abrupt withdrawal or interruption of therapy. When adjustment in rate is made, monitor blood pressure (standing and supine) and pulse for several hours to ensure tolerance to new rate. Monitor for bleeding. Monitor vital signs daily. Monitor for improved pulmonary function (decreased exertional dyspnea, fatigue, syncope, chest pain) and improved quality of life. Be alert for any infusion pump malfunction.

Patient Education

- Discuss specific use of drug and side effects with patient as it relates to treatment. (HCAHPS: During this hospital stay, were you given any medicine that you had not taken before? Before giving you any new medicine, how often did hospital staff tell you what the medicine was for? How often did hospital staff describe possible side effects in a way you could understand?)
- Patient may experience anxiety, back pain, diarrhea, flushing, lack of appetite, jaw pain, osteodynia, arthralgia, myalgia, nausea, flu-like syndrome, or anxiety. Have patient report immediately to prescriber signs of infection, dyspnea, severe dizziness, syncope, significant headache, ecchymosis, hemorrhaging, hematuria, urine discoloration, angina, melena, tachycardia, bradycardia, arrhythmia, pallor, tremors, intolerable asthenia, paresthesia, or injection site pain or irritation (HCAHPS).
- Educate patient about signs of a significant reaction (eg, wheezing; chest tightness; fever; itching; bad cough; blue skin color; seizures; or swelling of face, lips, tongue, or throat). **Note:** This is not a comprehensive list of all side effects. Patient should consult prescriber for additional questions.

Intended Use and Disclaimer: Should not be printed and given to patients. This information is intended to serve as a concise initial reference for healthcare professionals to use when discussing medications with a patient. You must ultimately rely on your own discretion, experience and judgment in diagnosing, treating and advising patients.

Eprosartan (ep roe SAR tan)

Brand Names: U.S. Teveten
Pharmacologic Category Angiotensin II Receptor Blocker; Antihypertensive
Pregnancy Risk Factor D
Lactation Excretion unknown/Not recommended
Breast-Feeding Considerations It is not known if eprosartan is excreted into breast milk. Due to the potential for serious adverse reactions in the nursing infant, the manufacturer recommends a decision be made whether to discontinue nursing or to discontinue the drug, taking into account the importance of treatment to the mother. Breast-fed infants of mothers taking medications for hypertension should be monitored for adverse effects (Chobanian, 2003).
Use Treatment of hypertension; may be used alone or in combination with other antihypertensives
Mechanism of Action/Effect Eprosartan is an angiotensin receptor antagonist which blocks the vasoconstriction and aldosterone-secreting effects of angiotensin II.
Contraindications Hypersensitivity to eprosartan or any component of the formulation; concomitant use with aliskiren in patients with diabetes mellitus
Warnings/Precautions [U.S. Boxed Warning]: Drugs that act on the renin-angiotensin system can cause injury and death to the developing fetus. Discontinue as soon as possible once pregnancy is detected. May cause hyperkalemia; avoid potassium supplementation unless specifically required by healthcare provider. Avoid use or use a smaller dose in patients who are volume depleted; correct depletion first. May be associated with deterioration of renal function and/or increases in serum creatinine, particularly in patients with low renal blood flow (eg, renal artery stenosis, heart failure) whose glomerular filtration rate (GFR) is dependent on efferent arteriolar vasoconstriction by angiotensin II. Use with caution in unstented unilateral/bilateral renal artery stenosis. When unstented bilateral renal artery stenosis is present, use is generally avoided due to the elevated risk of deterioration in renal function unless possible benefits outweigh risks. Use with caution in pre-existing renal insufficiency; significant aortic/mitral stenosis. Concomitant use of an angiotensin-converting enzyme (ACE) inhibitor or renin inhibitor (eg, aliskiren) is associated with an increased risk of hypotension, hyperkalemia, and renal dysfunction; concomitant use with aliskiren should be avoided in patients with GFR <60 mL/minute and is contraindicated in patients with diabetes mellitus (regardless of GFR).

Angioedema has been reported rarely with some angiotensin II receptor antagonists (ARBs) and may occur at any time during treatment (especially following first dose). It may involve the head and neck (potentially compromising airway) or the intestine (presenting with abdominal pain). Patients with idiopathic or hereditary angioedema or previous angioedema associated with ACE-inhibitor therapy may be at an increased risk. Prolonged frequent monitoring may be required, especially if tongue, glottis, or larynx are involved, as they are associated with airway obstruction. Patients with a history of airway surgery may have a higher risk of airway obstruction. Discontinue therapy immediately if angioedema occurs. Aggressive early management is critical. Intramuscular (I.M.) administration of epinephrine may be necessary. Do not readminister to patients who have had angioedema with ARBs.

Drug Interactions

Avoid Concomitant Use There are no known interactions where it is recommended to avoid concomitant use.

Decreased Effect

The levels/effects of Eprosartan may be decreased by: Herbs (Hypertensive Properties); Methylphenidate; Nonsteroidal Anti-Inflammatory Agents; Yohimbine

Increased Effect/Toxicity

Eprosartan may increase the levels/effects of: ACE Inhibitors; Amifostine; Antihypertensives; CycloSPORINE (Systemic); DULoxetine; Hypotensive Agents; Lithium; Nonsteroidal Anti-Inflammatory Agents; Obinutuzumab; Potassium-Sparing Diuretics; RiTUXimab; Sodium Phosphates

The levels/effects of Eprosartan may be increased by: Alfuzosin; Aliskiren; Brimonidine (Topical); Canagliflozin; Diazoxide; Eplerenone; Heparin; Heparin (Low Molecular Weight); Herbs (Hypotensive Properties); MAO Inhibitors; Pentoxifylline; Phosphodiesterase 5 Inhibitors; Potassium Salts; Prostacyclin Analogues; Tolvaptan; Trimethoprim

Nutritional/Ethanol Interactions Herb/Nutraceutical: Dong quai has estrogenic activity. Some herbal medications may worsen hypertension (eg, ephedra); garlic may have additional antihypertensive effects. Management: Avoid dong quai if using for hypertension. Avoid ephedra, yohimbe, ginseng, and garlic.

Adverse Reactions 1% to 10%:

Central nervous system: Fatigue (2%), depression (1%)

Endocrine & metabolic: Hypertriglyceridemia (1%)

Gastrointestinal: Abdominal pain (2%)

Genitourinary: Urinary tract infection (1%)

Respiratory: Upper respiratory tract infection (8%), rhinitis (4%), pharyngitis (4%), cough (4%)

Miscellaneous: Viral infection (2%), injury (2%)

Available Dosage Forms

Tablet, Oral:

Teveten: 600 mg

Generic: 600 mg

General Dosage Range Oral: *Adults:* Initial: 400-600 mg once daily; Maintenance: 400-800 mg/day in 1-2 divided doses

Nursing Actions

Physical Assessment Monitor for hypotension on a regular basis during therapy.

Patient Education

• Discuss specific use of drug and side effects with patient as it relates to treatment. (HCAHPS: During this hospital stay, were you given any medicine that you had not taken before? Before giving you any new medicine, how often did hospital staff tell you what the medicine was for? How often did hospital staff describe possible side effects in a way you could understand?)

• Patient may experience rhinitis or pharyngitis. Have patient report immediately to prescriber signs of renal impairment, signs of hyperkalemia, severe dizziness, syncope, myalgia, or asthenia (HCAHPS).

• Educate patient about signs of a significant reaction (eg, wheezing; chest tightness; fever; itching; bad cough; blue skin color; seizures; or swelling of face, lips, tongue, or throat). **Note:** This is not a comprehensive list of all side effects. Patient should consult prescriber for additional questions.

Intended Use and Disclaimer: Should not be printed and given to patients. This information is intended to serve as a concise initial reference for healthcare professionals to use when discussing medications with a patient. You must ultimately rely on your own discretion, experience and judgment in diagnosing, treating and advising patients.

Eprosartan and Hydrochlorothiazide
(ep roe SAR tan & hye droe klor oh THYE a zide)

Brand Names: U.S. Teveten® HCT

Index Terms Eprosartan Mesylate and Hydrochlorothiazide; Hydrochlorothiazide and Eprosartan

Pharmacologic Category Angiotensin II Receptor Blocker; Antihypertensive; Diuretic, Thiazide

Pregnancy Risk Factor D

Use Treatment of hypertension (not indicated for initial treatment)

Available Dosage Forms

Tablet:

Teveten® HCT: 600 mg/12.5 mg: Eprosartan 600 mg and hydrochlorothiazide 12.5 mg; 600 mg/25 mg: Eprosartan 600 mg and hydrochlorothiazide 25 mg

General Dosage Range Oral: *Adults:* Eprosartan 600 mg and hydrochlorothiazide 12.5-25 mg once daily

Administration

Oral May be administered without regard to meals.

Nursing Actions

Physical Assessment See individual agents.

Patient Education

- Discuss specific use of drug and side effects with patient as it relates to treatment. (HCAHPS: During this hospital stay, were you given any medicine that you had not taken before? Before giving you any new medicine, how often did hospital staff tell you what the medicine was for? How often did hospital staff describe possible side effects in a way you could understand?)
- Patient may experience dizziness. Have patient report immediately to prescriber signs of hyperglycemia, signs of fluid and electrolyte imbalance, signs of renal impairment, vision changes, or ophthalmalgia (HCAHPS).
- Educate patient about signs of a significant reaction (eg, wheezing; chest tightness; fever; itching; bad cough; blue skin color; seizures; or swelling of face, lips, tongue, or throat). **Note:** This is not a comprehensive list of all side effects. Patient should consult prescriber for additional questions.

Intended Use and Disclaimer: Should not be printed and given to patients. This information is intended to serve as a concise initial reference for healthcare professionals to use when discussing medications with a patient. You must ultimately rely on your own discretion, experience and judgment in diagnosing, treating and advising patients.

Related Information

Eprosartan *on page 551*
Hydrochlorothiazide *on page 775*

Eptifibatide (ep TIF i ba tide)

Brand Names: U.S. Integrilin
Index Terms Intrifiban
Pharmacologic Category Antiplatelet Agent, Glycoprotein IIb/IIIa Inhibitor
Medication Safety Issues
High alert medication:
  The Institute for Safe Medication Practices (ISMP) includes this medication among its list of drugs which have a heightened risk of causing significant patient harm when used in error.
Pregnancy Risk Factor B
Lactation Excretion in breast milk unknown/use caution
Breast-Feeding Considerations It is not known if eptifibatide is excreted in breast milk. The manufacturer recommends that caution be exercised when administering eptifibatide to nursing women.
Use Treatment of patients with acute coronary syndrome (unstable angina/non-ST-segment elevation myocardial infarction [UA/NSTEMI]), including patients who are to be managed medically and those undergoing percutaneous coronary intervention (PCI including angioplasty, intracoronary stenting)

Unlabeled Use To support PCI during ST-elevation myocardial infarction (administered at the time of primary PCI); elective PCI for stable ischemic heart disease (in combination with unfractionated heparin)

Mechanism of Action/Effect Eptifibatide is a glycoprotein IIb/IIIa receptor antagonist that reversibly blocks platelet aggregation and prevents thrombosis.

Contraindications Hypersensitivity to eptifibatide or any component of the product; active abnormal bleeding within the previous 30 days or a history of bleeding diathesis; history of stroke within 30 days or a history of hemorrhagic stroke; severe hypertension (systolic blood pressure >200 mm Hg or diastolic blood pressure >110 mm Hg) not adequately controlled on antihypertensive therapy; major surgery within the preceding 6 weeks; current or planned administration of another parenteral GP IIb/IIIa inhibitor; dependency on hemodialysis

Canadian labeling: Additional contraindications (not in U.S. labeling): PT >1.2 times control or INR ≥2.0; known history of intracranial disease (eg, neoplasm, arteriovenous malformation, aneurysm); severe renal impairment (CrCl <30 mL/minute); thrombocytopenia (<100,000 cells/mm^3); clinically significant liver disease

Warnings/Precautions Bleeding is the most common complication. Most major bleeding occurs at the arterial access site where the cardiac catheterization was done. When bleeding can not be controlled with pressure, discontinue infusion and heparin. Patients <70 kg may be at greater risk for major and minor bleeding. Discontinue ≥2-4 hours prior to coronary artery bypass graft surgery (Hillis, 2011). Use caution in patients with hemorrhagic retinopathy or with other drugs that affect hemostasis. Use with extreme caution in patients with platelet counts <100,000/mm^3 (contraindicated in the Canadian labeling). If platelet count decreases to <100,000/mm^3 during therapy, discontinue eptifibatide and heparin if administered concurrently.

Minimize invasive procedures, including arterial and venous punctures, I.M. injections, and nasogastric tube insertion. Prior to sheath removal, the aPTT or ACT should be checked (do not remove unless aPTT is <45 seconds or the ACT <150 seconds). Use caution in renal dysfunction (estimated CrCl <50 mL/minute, using Cockcroft-Gault equation); dosage adjustment required. Use is contraindicated in patients dependent upon hemodialysis.

Drug Interactions
Avoid Concomitant Use
  Avoid concomitant use of Eptifibatide with any of the following: Urokinase

Decreased Effect

The levels/effects of Eptifibatide may be decreased by: Nonsteroidal Anti-Inflammatory Agents

Increased Effect/Toxicity

Eptifibatide may increase the levels/effects of: Agents with Antiplatelet Properties; Anticoagulants; Collagenase (Systemic); Dabigatran Etexilate; Ibritumomab; Rivaroxaban; Salicylates; Thrombolytic Agents; Tositumomab and Iodine I 131 Tositumomab; Urokinase

The levels/effects of Eptifibatide may be increased by: Dasatinib; Glucosamine; Herbs (Anticoagulant/Antiplatelet Properties); Ibrutinib; Multivitamins/Fluoride (with ADE); Multivitamins/Minerals (with ADEK, Folate, Iron); Multivitamins/Minerals (with AE, No Iron); Nonsteroidal Anti-Inflammatory Agents; Omega-3 Fatty Acids; Pentosan Polysulfate Sodium; Pentoxifylline; Prostacyclin Analogues; Tipranavir; Vitamin E

Nutritional/Ethanol Interactions Herb/Nutraceutical: Avoid alfalfa, anise, bilberry, bladderwrack, bromelain, cat's claw, celery, coleus, cordyceps, dong quai, evening primrose oil, fenugreek, feverfew, garlic, ginger, ginkgo biloba, ginseng (American), ginseng (Panax), ginseng (Siberian), grapeseed, green tea, guggul, horse chestnut seed, horseradish, licorice, prickly ash, red clover, reishi, same (s-adenosylmethionine), sweet clover, turmeric, and white willow (all have additional antiplatelet activity).

Adverse Reactions Bleeding is the major drug-related adverse effect. Access site is often primary source of bleeding complications. Incidence of bleeding is also related to heparin intensity. Patients weighing <70 kg may have an increased risk of major bleeding.

>10%: Hematologic: Bleeding (major: 1% to 11%; minor: 3% to 14%; transfusion required: 2% to 13%)

1% to 10%:
Cardiovascular: Hypotension (up to 7%)
Hematologic: Thrombocytopenia (1% to 3%)
Local: Injection site reaction

Pharmacodynamics/Kinetics

Onset of Action Within 1 hour

Duration of Action Platelet function restored ~4 hours following discontinuation

Available Dosage Forms

Solution, Intravenous:
Integrilin: 0.75 mg/mL (100 mL); 2 mg/mL (10 mL, 100 mL)

General Dosage Range Dosage adjustment recommended in patients with renal impairment

I.V.: *Adults:* Bolus: 180 mcg/kg (maximum: 22.6 mg), repeat once for PCI; Infusion: 2 mcg/kg/minute (maximum: 15 mg/hour)

Administration

I.V. Do not shake vial. Administer bolus doses by I.V. push over 1-2 minutes. Begin continuous infusion immediately following bolus administration; administer directly from the 100 mL vial.

Injectable Detail Visually inspect for discoloration or particulate matter prior to administration. The bolus dose should be withdrawn from the 10 mL vial into a syringe. The 100 mL vial should be spiked with a vented infusion set.

Storage/Stability Vials should be stored refrigerated at 2°C to 8°C (36°F to 46°F). Vials can be kept at room temperature for 2 months, after which they must be discarded. Protect from light until administration. Do not use beyond the expiration date. Discard any unused portion left in the vial.

Nursing Actions

Physical Assessment Monitor vital signs prior to, during, and after therapy. Assess infusion insertion site during and after therapy (every 15 minutes or as institutional policy). Observe and teach patient bleeding precautions. Monitor closely for signs of excessive bleeding (CNS changes; blood in urine, stool, or vomitus; unusual bruising or bleeding).

Patient Education

- Discuss specific use of drug and side effects with patient as it relates to treatment. (HCAHPS: During this hospital stay, were you given any medicine that you had not taken before? Before giving you any new medicine, how often did hospital staff tell you what the medicine was for? How often did hospital staff describe possible side effects in a way you could understand?)
- Have patient report immediately to prescriber strength differences from one side to another, difficulty speaking or thinking, change in balance, blurred vision, severe dizziness, syncope, considerable headache, ecchymosis, hemorrhaging, melena, hematuria, hemoptysis, hematemesis, intolerable dyspepsia, abdominal edema, or injection site irritation (HCAHPS).
- Educate patient about signs of a significant reaction (eg, wheezing; chest tightness; fever; itching; bad cough; blue skin color; seizures; or swelling of face, lips, tongue, or throat). **Note:** This is not a comprehensive list of all side effects. Patient should consult prescriber for additional questions.

Intended Use and Disclaimer: Should not be printed and given to patients. This information is intended to serve as a concise initial reference for healthcare professionals to use when discussing medications with a patient. You must ultimately rely on your own discretion, experience and judgment in diagnosing, treating and advising patients.

Ergocalciferol (er goe kal SIF e role)

Brand Names: U.S. Calcidol [OTC]; Calciferol [OTC]; Drisdol; Drisdol [OTC]

Index Terms Activated Ergosterol; D2; Viosterol; Vitamin D2

Pharmacologic Category Vitamin D Analog

Medication Safety Issues

Sound-alike/look-alike issues:

Calciferol™ may be confused with calcitriol

Drisdol® may be confused with Drysol™

Ergocalciferol may be confused with alfacalcidol, cholecalciferol

Administration issues:

Liquid vitamin D preparations have the potential for dosing errors when administered to infants. Droppers should be clearly marked to easily provide 400 international units. For products intended for infants, the FDA recommends that accompanying droppers deliver no more than 400 international units per dose.

Pregnancy Risk Factor C (manufacturer); A/C (dose exceeding RDA recommendation; per expert analysis)

Lactation Enters breast milk/use caution

Use Treatment of refractory rickets, hypophosphatemia, hypoparathyroidism; dietary supplement

Unlabeled Use Prevention and treatment of vitamin D deficiency in patients with chronic kidney disease (CKD); osteoporosis prevention

Available Dosage Forms

Capsule, Oral:

Drisdol: 50,000 units

Generic: 50,000 units

Solution, Oral:

Calcidol [OTC]: 8000 units/mL (60 mL)

Calciferol [OTC]: 8000 units/mL (60 mL)

Drisdol [OTC]: 8000 units/mL (60 mL)

Generic: 8000 units/mL (60 mL)

Tablet, Oral:

Generic: 400 units, 2000 units

General Dosage Range Oral:

Children 0-12 months: Adequate intake: 400 units/day

Children 1 year to Adults ≤70 years: RDA: 600 units/day

Elderly >70 years: RDA: 800 units/day

Nursing Actions

Physical Assessment Provide patient appropriate nutritional counseling.

Patient Education

• Discuss specific use of drug and side effects with patient as it relates to treatment. (HCAHPS: During this hospital stay, were you given any medicine that you had not taken before? Before giving you any new medicine, how often did hospital staff tell you what the medicine was for? How often did hospital staff describe possible side effects in a way you could understand?)

• Have patient report immediately to prescriber signs of hypercalcemia, significant asthenia, severe dizziness, intolerable headache, urinary retention, oliguria, polyuria, lack of appetite, polydipsia, or weight loss (HCAHPS).

• Educate patient about signs of a significant reaction (eg, wheezing; chest tightness; fever; itching; bad cough; blue skin color; seizures; or swelling of face, lips, tongue, or throat). **Note:** This is not a comprehensive list of all side effects. Patient should consult prescriber for additional questions.

Intended Use and Disclaimer: Should not be printed and given to patients. This information is intended to serve as a concise initial reference for healthcare professionals to use when discussing medications with a patient. You must ultimately rely on your own discretion, experience and judgment in diagnosing, treating and advising patients.

Related Information

Oral Medications That Should Not Be Crushed or Altered *on page 1712*

Ergonovine (er goe NOE veen)

Index Terms Ergometrine Maleate; Ergonovine Maleate

Pharmacologic Category Ergot Derivative

Lactation Enters breast milk/contraindicated

Use Prevention and treatment of postpartum and postabortion hemorrhage caused by uterine atony

Unlabeled Use Diagnostically to identify Prinzmetal's angina

Product Availability Not available in the U.S.

General Dosage Range I.M., I.V.: *Adults:* 0.2 mg, may repeat in 2-4 hours if needed, up to maximum of 5 total doses

Administration

I.M. May be administered by I.M injection. Hazardous agent; use appropriate precautions for handling and disposal (NIOSH, 2012).

I.V. I.V. use should be limited to patients with severe uterine bleeding or other life-threatening emergency situations. I.V. doses should be administered over a period of not <1 minute.

Hazardous agent; use appropriate precautions for handling and disposal (NIOSH, 2012).

Nursing Actions

Physical Assessment Blood pressure should be monitored, especially with I.V. use. For postpartum use, monitor character and amount of vaginal bleeding. Monitor patient response, including ergotamine toxicity (eg, headache, ringing in ears, nausea and vomiting, diarrhea, numbness or coldness of extremities, confusion, hallucinations, dyspnea, chest pain, convulsions). When used to test for Prinzmetal's angina during coronary arteriography, emergency equipment, including nitroglycerin, must be on hand. When used at any time other than postpartum, determine that patient is not pregnant.

Patient Education

- Discuss specific use of drug and side effects with patient as it relates to treatment. (HCAHPS: During this hospital stay, were you given any medicine that you had not taken before? Before giving you any new medicine, how often did hospital staff tell you what the medicine was for? How often did hospital staff describe possible side effects in a way you could understand?)
- Patient may experience hypertension. Have patient report immediately to prescriber angina, tachycardia, paresthesia of hands or feet, severe dizziness, syncope, dyspnea, considerable headache, significant dyspepsia, or intolerable nausea (HCAHPS).
- Educate patient about signs of a significant reaction (eg, wheezing; chest tightness; fever; itching; bad cough; blue skin color; seizures; or swelling of face, lips, tongue, or throat). **Note:** This is not a comprehensive list of all side effects. Patient should consult prescriber for additional questions.

Intended Use and Disclaimer: Should not be printed and given to patients. This information is intended to serve as a concise initial reference for healthcare professionals to use when discussing medications with a patient. You must ultimately rely on your own discretion, experience and judgment in diagnosing, treating and advising patients.

Eribulin (er i BUE lin)

Brand Names: U.S. Halaven
Index Terms B1939; E7389; ER-086526; Eribulin Mesylate; Halichondrin B Analog
Pharmacologic Category Antineoplastic Agent, Antimicrotubular
Medication Safety Issues
Sound-alike/look-alike issues:
EriBULin may be confused with EPIrubicin, erlotinib
High alert medication:
This medication is in a class the Institute for Safe Medication Practices (ISMP) includes among its list of drug classes which have a heightened risk of causing significant patient harm when used in error.
International Issues:
Some products available internationally may have vial strength and dosing expressed as the base (instead of as the salt). Refer to prescribing information for specific strength and dosing information.
Pregnancy Risk Factor D
Lactation Excretion in breast milk unknown/not recommended
Use Breast cancer: Treatment of metastatic breast cancer in patients who have received at least 2 prior chemotherapy regimens for the treatment of

metastatic disease (prior treatment should have included an anthracycline and a taxane either in adjuvant or metastatic setting)
Available Dosage Forms
Solution, Intravenous:
Halaven: 1 mg/2 mL (2 mL)
General Dosage Range Dosage adjustment recommended in patients with renal or hepatic impairment or who develop toxicities
I.V.: *Adults:* Eribulin mesylate: 1.4 mg/m^2/dose days 1 and 8 every 3 weeks
Administration
I.V. Infuse over 2-5 minutes. May be administered undiluted or diluted.
Hazardous agent; use appropriate precautions for handling and disposal (meets NIOSH, 2012 criteria).
Nursing Actions
Patient Education
- Discuss specific use of drug and side effects with patient as it relates to treatment. (HCAHPS: During this hospital stay, were you given any medicine that you had not taken before? Before giving you any new medicine, how often did hospital staff tell you what the medicine was for? How often did hospital staff describe possible side effects in a way you could understand?)
- Patient may experience headache, alopecia, nausea, constipation, diarrhea, stomatitis, lack of appetite, weight loss, arthralgia, myalgia, osteodynia, or back pain. Have patient report immediately to prescriber signs of infection, paresthesia, tachycardia, arrhythmia, severe dizziness, syncope, dyspnea, edema of extremities, ecchymosis, hemorrhaging, or considerable asthenia (HCAHPS).
- Educate patient about signs of a significant reaction (eg, wheezing; chest tightness; fever; itching; bad cough; blue skin color; seizures; or swelling of face, lips, tongue, or throat). **Note:** This is not a comprehensive list of all side effects. Patient should consult prescriber for additional questions.

Intended Use and Disclaimer: Should not be printed and given to patients. This information is intended to serve as a concise initial reference for healthcare professionals to use when discussing medications with a patient. You must ultimately rely on your own discretion, experience and judgment in diagnosing, treating and advising patients.

Erlotinib (er LOE tye nib)

Brand Names: U.S. Tarceva
Index Terms CP358774; Erlotinib Hydrochloride; OSI-774
Pharmacologic Category Antineoplastic Agent, Epidermal Growth Factor Receptor (EGFR) Inhibitor; Antineoplastic Agent, Tyrosine Kinase Inhibitor

Medication Safety Issues

Sound-alike/look-alike issues:

Erlotinib may be confused with afatinib, crizotinib, eribulin, gefitinib, imatinib, regorafenib, SUNItinib, vandetanib

High alert medication:

This medication is in a class the Institute for Safe Medication Practices (ISMP) includes among its list of drug classes which have a heightened risk of causing significant patient harm when used in error.

Pregnancy Risk Factor D

Lactation Excretion in breast milk unknown/not recommended

Breast-Feeding Considerations It is not known if erlotinib is excreted in breast milk. Due to the potential for serious adverse reactions in the nursing infant, the decision to discontinue breast-feeding or discontinue erlotinib should take into account the benefits of treatment to the mother.

Use

Nonsmall cell lung cancer (NSCLC): First-line treatment of metastatic NSCLC in patients with known EGFR exon 19 deletions or exon 21 (L858R) substitution mutations; treatment (as monotherapy) of locally-advanced or metastatic NSCLC refractory to at least 1 prior chemotherapy regimen; maintenance treatment of locally-advanced or metastatic NCSLC which has not progressed after 4 cycles of first-line platinum-based chemotherapy

Note: Use in combination with platinum-based chemotherapy is not recommended. First-line treatment in patients with metastatic NSCLC with EGFR mutations other than exon 19 deletion or exon 21 (L858R) substitution has not been evaluated.

Pancreatic cancer (not an approved use in Canada): First-line treatment of locally-advanced, unresectable or metastatic pancreatic cancer (combination with gemcitabine)

Mechanism of Action/Effect Inhibits the intracellular phosphorylation of tyrosine kinase associated with epidermal growth factor receptor (EGFR) which is located on both normal and cancer cells causing cell death. In nonsmall cell lung cancer, erlotinib has higher binding affinity for certain EGFR mutations.

Contraindications There are no contraindications listed within the manufacturer's U.S. labeling.

Canadian labeling: Hypersensitivity to erlotinib or any component of the formulation

Warnings/Precautions Hazardous agent - use appropriate precautions for handling and disposal (meets NIOSH, 2012 criteria). Rare, sometimes fatal, interstitial lung disease (ILD) has occurred; symptoms include acute respiratory distress syndrome, interstitial pneumonia, obliterative bronchiolitis, pneumonitis (including radiation and hypersensitivity), pulmonary fibrosis, and pulmonary infiltrates. The onset of symptoms has been within 5 days to more than 9 months after treatment initiation (median: 39 days). Interrupt treatment for unexplained new or worsening pulmonary symptoms (dyspnea, cough, and fever); discontinue for confirmed ILD.

Liver enzyme elevations have been reported. Hepatic failure and hepatorenal syndrome have also been reported, particularly in patients with baseline hepatic impairment. Monitor liver function; patients with any hepatic impairment (total bilirubin >ULN; Child-Pugh class A, B, or C) should be closely monitored, including those with hepatic disease due to tumor burden; use with extreme caution in patients with total bilirubin >3 times ULN. Increased monitoring of liver function is required in patients with pre-existing hepatic impairment or biliary obstruction. Dosage reduction, interruption or discontinuation may be recommended for changes in hepatic function. Acute renal failure, renal insufficiency, and hepatorenal syndrome have been reported, either secondary to hepatic impairment at baseline or due to severe dehydration; use with caution in patients with or at risk for renal impairment. Monitor closely for dehydration; monitor renal function and electrolytes in patients at risk for dehydration. Gastrointestinal perforation has been reported with use; risk for perforation is increased with concurrent anti-angiogenic agents, corticosteroids, NSAIDs, and/or taxane based-therapy, and patients with history of peptic ulcers or diverticular disease; permanently discontinue in patients who develop perforation.

Bullous, blistering, or exfoliating skin conditions, some suggestive of Stevens-Johnson or toxic epidermal necrolysis (TEN) have been reported. An acne-like rash commonly appears on the face, back, and upper chest. Generalized or severe acneiform, erythematous or maculopapular rash may occur. Skin rash may correlate with treatment response and prolonged survival (Saif, 2008); management of skin rashes that are not serious should include alcohol-free lotions, topical antibiotics, or topical corticosteroids, or if necessary, oral antibiotics and systemic corticosteroids; avoid sunlight. Reduce dose or temporarily interrupt treatment for severe skin reactions; discontinue treatment for bullous, blistering or exfoliative skin toxicity. Corneal perforation and ulceration have been reported with use; abnormal eyelash growth, keratoconjunctivitis sicca, or keratitis have also been reported and are known risk factors for corneal ulceration/perforation. Interrupt or discontinue treatment in patients presenting with eye pain or other acute or worsening ocular symptoms.

MI, CVA, and microangiopathic hemolytic anemia with thrombocytopenia have been reported. Elevated INR and bleeding events (including fatal hemorrhage) have been reported; monitor for INR changes. Erlotinib levels may be lower in patients who smoke; advise patients to stop smoking. Smokers treated with 300 mg/day exhibited steady-state erlotinib levels comparable to former- and never-smokers receiving 150 mg/day (Hughes, 2009). Potentially significant drug-drug interactions may exist, requiring dose or frequency adjustment, additional monitoring, and/or selection of alternative therapy. Avoid concomitant use with proton pump inhibitors. If taken with an H_2-receptor antagonist (eg, ranitidine), administer erlotinib 10 hours after the H_2-receptor antagonist dose and at least 2 hours prior to the next H_2-receptor dose. If an antacid is necessary, separate dosing by several hours. In patients with NSCLC, EGFR mutations, specifically exon 19 deletions and exon 21 mutation (L858R), are associated with better response to erlotinib (Riely, 2006); erlotinib treatment is not recommended in patients with K-ras mutations; they are not likely to benefit from erlotinib treatment (Eberhard, 2005; Miller, 2008). Concurrent erlotinib plus platinum-based chemotherapy is not recommended for first line treatment of locally advanced or metastatic NSCLC due to a lack of clinical benefit. The cobas® EGFR mutation test has been approved to detect EGFR mutation for first-line NSCLC treatment. Product may contain lactose; avoid use in patients with Lapp lactase deficiency, glucose-galactose malabsorption, or glucose intolerance.

Drug Interactions

Avoid Concomitant Use

Avoid concomitant use of Erlotinib with any of the following: Conivaptan; Fusidic Acid (Systemic); Proton Pump Inhibitors

Decreased Effect

Erlotinib may decrease the levels/effects of: Cardiac Glycosides; Vitamin K Antagonists

The levels/effects of Erlotinib may be decreased by: Antacids; Bosentan; CYP3A4 Inducers (Strong); Dabrafenib; Deferasirox; H2-Antagonists; Herbs (CYP3A4 Inducers); Mitotane; Proton Pump Inhibitors; Rifampin; Tocilizumab

Increased Effect/Toxicity

Erlotinib may increase the levels/effects of: Vitamin K Antagonists

The levels/effects of Erlotinib may be increased by: Ciprofloxacin (Systemic); Conivaptan; CYP3A4 Inhibitors (Moderate); CYP3A4 Inhibitors (Strong); Dasatinib; FluvoxaMINE; Fusidic Acid (Systemic); Ivacaftor; Luliconazole; Mifepristone; Simeprevir; Stiripentol

Nutritional/Ethanol Interactions

Food: Erlotinib bioavailability is increased with food. Grapefruit or grapefruit juice may decrease metabolism and increase erlotinib plasma concentrations. Management: Take on an empty stomach at least 1 hour before or 2 hours after the ingestion of food. Avoid grapefruit and grapefruit juice. Maintain adequate nutrition and hydration, unless instructed to restrict fluid intake.

Herb/Nutraceutical: St John's wort may increase metabolism and decrease erlotinib concentrations. Management: Avoid St John's wort.

Adverse Reactions

Adverse reactions reported with monotherapy:

>10%:

Cardiovascular: Chest pain (≤18%)

Central nervous system: Fatigue (9% to 52%)

Dermatologic: Skin rash (49% to 85%; grade 3: 5% to 13%; grade 4: <1%; median onset: 8 days), xeroderma (4% to 21%), pruritus (7% to 16%), paronychia (4% to 16%), alopecia (14% to 15%), acne vulgaris (6% to 12%)

Gastrointestinal: Diarrhea (20% to 62%; grade 3: 2% to 6%; grade 4: <1%; median onset: 12 days), anorexia (9% to 52%), nausea (23% to 33%), decreased appetite (≤28%), vomiting (13% to 23%), mucositis (≤18%), stomatitis (11% to 17%), abdominal pain (3% to 11%), constipation (≤8%)

Genitourinary: Urinary tract infection (≤4%)

Hematologic & oncologic: Anemia (≤11%; grade 4: 1%)

Infection: Increased susceptibility to infection (4% to 24%)

Miscellaneous: Fever (≤11%)

Neuromuscular & skeletal: Weakness (≤53%), back pain (19%), arthralgia (≤13%), musculoskeletal pain (11%)

Ophthalmic: Conjunctivitis (12% to 18%), keratoconjunctivitis sicca (12%)

Respiratory: Cough (33% to 48%), dyspnea (41% to 45%; grades 3/4: 8% to 28%)

1% to 10%:

Cardiovascular: Peripheral edema (≤5%)

Central nervous system: Pain (≤9%), headache (≤7%), anxiety (≤5%), dizziness (≤4%), insomnia (≤4%), neurotoxicity (≤4%), voice disorder (≤4%)

Dermatologic: Folliculitis (≤8%), nail disease (≤7%), exfoliative dermatitis (5%), hypertrichosis (5%), skin fissure (5%), acneiform eruption (4% to 5%), erythema (≤5%), dermatitis (4%), erythematous rash (≤4%), palmar-plantar erythrodysesthesia (≤4%), bullous dermatitis

Endocrine & metabolic: Weight loss (4% to 5%)

Gastrointestinal: Dyspepsia (≤5%), xerostomia (≤3%), taste disorder (≤1%)

Hematologic & oncologic: Lymphocytopenia (≤4%; grade 3: 1%), leukopenia (≤3%), thrombocytopenia (≤1%)

Hepatic: Hyperbilirubinemia (7%; grade 3: ≤1%), increased serum ALT (grade 2: 2% to 4%; grade 3: 1% to 3%), increased gamma-glutamyl transferase (≤4%), hepatic failure (≤1%)

Neuromuscular & skeletal: Muscle spasm (≤4%), musculoskeletal chest pain (≤4%), ostealgia (≤4%), paresthesia (≤4%)

Otic: Tinnitus (≤1%)

Renal: Increased serum creatinine (≤1%), renal failure (≤1%)

Respiratory: Nasopharyngitis (≤7%), epistaxis (≤4%), pulmonary embolism (≤4%), respiratory tract infection (≤4%), pneumonitis (3%), pulmonary fibrosis (3%)

<1%: Interstitial pulmonary disease

Adverse reactions reported with combination (erlotinib plus gemcitabine) therapy:

>10%:

Cardiovascular: Edema (37%), thrombosis (grades 3/4: 11%)

Central nervous system: Fatigue (73% to 79%), depression (19%), dizziness (15%), headache (15%), anxiety (13%)

Dermatologic: Skin rash (70%), alopecia (14%)

Gastrointestinal: Nausea (60%), anorexia (52%), diarrhea (48%), abdominal pain (46%), vomiting (42%), weight loss (39%), stomatitis (22%), dyspepsia (17%), flatulence (13%)

Hepatic: Increased serum ALT (grade 2: 31%, grade 3: 13%, grade 4: <1%), increased serum AST (grade 2: 24%, grade 3: 10%, grade 4 <1%), hyperbilirubinemia (grade 2: 17%, grade 3: 10%, grade 4: <1%)

Infection: Increased susceptibility to infection (39%)

Miscellaneous: Fever (36%)

Neuromuscular & skeletal: Ostealgia (25%), myalgia (21%), neuropathy (13%), rigors (12%)

Respiratory: Dyspnea (24%), cough (16%)

1% to 10%:

Cardiovascular: Cardiac arrhythmia (<5%), syncope (<5%), deep vein thrombosis (4%), cerebrovascular accident (3%; including cerebral hemorrhage), myocardial infarction (2%)

Gastrointestinal: Intestinal obstruction (<5%), pancreatitis (<5%)

Hematologic: Hemolytic anemia (<5%; microangiopathic with thrombocytopenia: 1%)

Renal: Renal insufficiency (<5%), renal failure (1%)

Respiratory: Interstitial pulmonary disease (<3%)

<1%: Bullous dermatitis, exfoliative dermatitis, hepatic failure

Available Dosage Forms

Tablet, Oral:

Tarceva: 25 mg, 100 mg, 150 mg

General Dosage Range Dosage adjustment recommended in patients with hepatic impairment, on concomitant therapy, who smoke, or who develop toxicities

Oral: *Adults:* 100-150 mg daily

Administration

Oral The manufacturer recommends administration on an empty stomach (at least 1 hour before or 2 hours after the ingestion of food). Avoid concomitant use with proton pump inhibitors. If taken with an H₂-receptor antagonist (eg, ranitidine), administer erlotinib 10 hours after the H₂-receptor antagonist dose and at least 2 hours prior to the next H₂- receptor dose. If an antacid is necessary, separate dosing by several hours.

For patients unable to swallow whole, tablets may be dissolved in 100 mL water and administered orally or via feeding tube (silicone-based); to ensure full dose is received, rinse container with 40 mL water, administer residue and repeat rinse (data on file, Genentech; Siu, 2007; Soulieres, 2004).

Hazardous agent; use appropriate precautions for handling and disposal (meets NIOSH, 2012 criteria).

Storage/Stability Store at room temperature of 25°C (77°F); excursions permitted to 15°C and 30°C (59°F and 86°F).

Nursing Actions

Physical Assessment Monitor for gastrointestinal perforation, diarrhea, ocular reactions, severe skin reactions, urine output, signs and symptoms of liver disease, and interstitial lung disease; notify prescriber if any occur. Monitor for acute or progressive shortness of breath. Educate patient about proper hydration including antidiarrheal use and significant diarrhea.

Patient Education

• Discuss specific use of drug and side effects with patient as it relates to treatment. (HCAHPS: During this hospital stay, were you given any medicine that you had not taken before? Before giving you any new medicine, how often did hospital staff tell you what the medicine was for? How often did hospital staff describe possible side effects in a way you could understand?)

• Patient may experience acne vulgaris, lack of appetite, stomatitis, headache, back pain, arthralgia, myalgia, hair or nail changes, or xeroderma. Have patient report immediately to prescriber signs of infection, signs of hepatic impairment, signs of renal impairment, signs of pulmonary disorder, strength differences from one side to another, difficulty speaking or thinking, change in balance, blurred vision, angina, severe nausea, considerable diarrhea, ecchymosis, hemorrhaging, intolerable asthenia, vision changes, ophthalmalgia, significant eye irritation, excessive weight loss, depression, severe dyspepsia, hematemesis, melena, or signs of Stevens-Johnson syndrome/toxic epidermal necrolysis (HCAHPS).

• Educate patient about signs of a significant reaction (eg, wheezing; chest tightness; fever; itching; bad cough; blue skin color; seizures; or swelling of face, lips, tongue, or throat). **Note:** This is not a comprehensive list of all side effects. Patient should consult prescriber for additional questions.

Intended Use and Disclaimer: Should not be printed and given to patients. This information is intended to serve as a concise initial reference for ▶

healthcare professionals to use when discussing medications with a patient. You must ultimately rely on your own discretion, experience and judgment in diagnosing, treating and advising patients.

Dietary Considerations Take this medicine an empty stomach, 1 hour before or 2 hours after a meal. Avoid grapefruit juice.

Ertapenem (er ta PEN em)

Brand Names: U.S. INVanz

Index Terms Ertapenem Sodium; L-749,345; MK0826

Pharmacologic Category Antibiotic, Carbapenem

Medication Safety Issues
Sound-alike/look-alike issues:
Ertapenem may be confused with doripenem, imipenem, meropenem
INVanz may be confused with AVINza, I.V. vancomycin

Pregnancy Risk Factor B

Lactation Enters breast milk/use caution

Breast-Feeding Considerations Ertapenem is excreted in breast milk. The low concentrations in milk and low oral bioavailability suggest minimal exposure risk to the infant. The manufacturer recommends that caution be exercised when administering ertapenem to nursing women. Nondose-related effects could include modification of bowel flora.

Use Moderate-to-severe infections:
Acute pelvic infections: For the treatment of acute pelvic infections, including postpartum endomyometritis, septic abortion, and postsurgical gynecologic infections caused by *Streptococcus agalactiae*, *Escherichia coli*, *Bacteroides fragilis*, *Porphyromonas asaccharolytica*, *Peptostreptococcus* spp, or *Prevotella bivia*.

Community-acquired pneumonia: For the treatment of community-acquired pneumonia (CAP) caused by *Streptococcus pneumoniae* (penicillin-susceptible isolates only), including cases with concurrent bacteremia; *Haemophilus influenzae* (beta-lactamase-negative isolates only); or *Moraxella catarrhalis*.

Complicated intra-abdominal infections: For the treatment of complicated intra-abdominal infections caused by *E. coli*, *Clostridium clostridioforme*, *Eubacterium lentum*, *Peptostreptococcus* spp, *B. fragilis*, *Bacteroides distasonis*, *Bacteroides ovatus*, *Bacteroides thetaiotaomicron*, or *Bacteroides uniformis*.

Complicated skin and skin structure infections: For the treatment of complicated skin and skin structure infections, including diabetic foot infections without osteomyelitis caused by *Staphylococcus aureus* (methicillin-susceptible isolates only), *S. agalactiae*, *Streptococcus pyogenes*, *E. coli*, *Klebsiella pneumoniae*, *Proteus mirabilis*, *B.*

fragilis, *Peptostreptococcus* spp, *P. asaccharolytica*, or *P. bivia*. Ertapenem has not been studied in diabetic foot infections with concomitant osteomyelitis.

Complicated urinary tract infections: For the treatment of complicated urinary tract infections (UTIs), including pyelonephritis caused by *E. coli*, including cases with concurrent bacteremia or *K. pneumoniae*.

Prophylaxis of surgical-site infection in colorectal surgery: For the prophylaxis of surgical-site infection in adults following elective colorectal surgery.

Note: Methicillin-resistant *Staphylococcus aureus*, *Enterococcus* spp, penicillin-resistant strains of *Streptococcus pneumoniae*, *Acinetobacter*, and *Pseudomonas aeruginosa*, are **resistant** to ertapenem while most extended-spectrum beta-lactamase (ESBL)-producing bacteria remain sensitive to ertapenem.

Unlabeled Use Treatment of intravenous catheter-related bloodstream infection; treatment of prosthetic joint infection

Mechanism of Action/Effect Inhibits cell wall biosynthesis; cell wall assembly is arrested and the bacteria eventually lyse.

Contraindications Known hypersensitivity to any component of this product or to other drugs in the same class or in patients who have demonstrated anaphylactic reactions to beta-lactams; known hypersensitivity to local anesthetics of the amide type due to the use of lidocaine as a diluent (I.M. use only).

Warnings/Precautions Use caution with renal impairment. Dosage adjustment required in patients with moderate-to-severe renal dysfunction; elderly patients often require lower doses (based upon renal function). Use may result in fungal or bacterial superinfection, including *C. difficile*-associated diarrhea (CDAD) and pseudomembranous colitis; CDAD has been observed >2 months postantibiotic treatment. Carbapenems have been associated with CNS adverse effects, including confusional states and seizures (myoclonic); use caution with CNS disorders (eg, brain lesions and history of seizures) and adjust dose in renal impairment to avoid drug accumulation, which may increase seizure risk. Serious hypersensitivity reactions, including anaphylaxis, have been reported (some without a history of previous allergic reactions to beta-lactams). Doses for I.M. administration are mixed with lidocaine; consult Lidocaine (Systemic) information for associated Warnings/Precautions. May decrease divalproex sodium/valproic acid concentrations leading to breakthrough seizures; concomitant use not recommended. Safety and efficacy have not been established in children <3 months of age.

Drug Interactions

Avoid Concomitant Use
Avoid concomitant use of Ertapenem with any of the following: BCG

Decreased Effect
Ertapenem may decrease the levels/effects of: BCG; Sodium Picosulfate; Typhoid Vaccine; Valproic Acid and Derivatives

Increased Effect/Toxicity
Ertapenem may increase the levels/effects of: Tacrolimus (Systemic)

The levels/effects of Ertapenem may be increased by: Probenecid

Adverse Reactions
>10%: Gastrointestinal: Diarrhea (2% to 12%)
1% to 10%:
Cardiovascular: Edema (3%), chest pain (1% to 2%), hypertension (1% to 2%), hypotension (1% to 2%), tachycardia (1% to 2%)
Central nervous system: Headache (4% to 7%); altered mental status (eg, agitation, confusion, disorientation, mental acuity decreased, somnolence, stupor) (3% to 5%); fever (2% to 5%), insomnia (3%), dizziness (2%), hypothermia (infants, children, and adolescents <2%), anxiety (1%), fatigue (1%)
Dermatologic: Diaper rash (infants and children 5%), skin rash (2% to 3%), erythema (1% to 2%), pruritus (1% to 2%), genital rash (infants, children, and adolescents <2%), skin lesions (infants, children, and adolescents <2%)
Endocrine & metabolic: Hypokalemia (2%), hyperglycemia (1% to 2%), hyperkalemia (≤1%)
Gastrointestinal: Vomiting (2% to 10%), nausea (6% to 9%), abdominal pain (4% to 5%), constipation (2% to 4%), acid regurgitation (1% to 2%), decreased appetite (infants, children, and adolescents <2%), dyspepsia (1%), oral candidiasis (≤1%)
Genitourinary: Urine WBCs increased (2% to 3%), urine RBCs increased (1% to 3%), vaginitis (1% to 3%)
Hematologic: Thrombocytosis (4% to 7%), decreased hematocrit/hemoglobin (3% to 5%), decreased neutrophils (1% to 2%), eosinophilia (1% to 2%), leukopenia (1% to 2%), thrombocytopenia (1%), prolonged prothrombin time (≤1%)
Hepatic: Increased liver enzymes (7% to 9%), increased serum alkaline (4% to 7%), decreased serum albumin (1% to 2%), increased serum bilirubin (total) (1% to 2%)
Local: Infused vein complications (5% to 7%), phlebitis/thrombophlebitis (2%), extravasation (1% to 2%)
Neuromuscular & skeletal: Arthralgia (infants, children, and adolescents <2%), weakness (1%), leg pain (≤1%)
Otic: Otitis media (infants, children, and adolescents <2%)
Renal: Increased serum creatinine (1%)

Respiratory: Cough (1% to 4%), dyspnea (1% to 3%), nasopharyngitis (infants, children, and adolescents <2%), rhinitis (infants, children, and adolescents <2%), rhinorrhea (infants, children, and adolescents <2%), upper respiratory tract infection (infants, children, and adolescents <2%), wheezing (infants, children, and adolescents <2%), pharyngitis (1%), rales/rhonchi (1%), respiratory distress (≤1%)
Miscellaneous: Herpes simplex (infants, children, and adolescents <2%)

Available Dosage Forms

Solution Reconstituted, Injection:
INVanz: 1 g (1 ea)

Solution Reconstituted, Intravenous:
INVanz: 1 g (1 ea)

General Dosage Range
Dosage adjustment recommended in patients with renal impairment

I.M., I.V.:
Infants ≥3 months and Children: 15 **mg**/kg twice daily (maximum: 1 g daily)
Adolescents and Adults: 1 g once daily or as single dose

Administration

I.M. Avoid injection into a blood vessel. Make sure patient does not have an allergy to lidocaine or another anesthetic of the amide type. Administer by deep I.M. injection into a large muscle mass (eg, gluteal muscle or lateral part of the thigh). Do not administer I.M. preparation or drug reconstituted for I.M. administration intravenously.

I.V. Infuse over 30 minutes

Injectable Detail pH 7.5

Preparation for Administration
I.M.: Reconstitute 1 g vial with 3.2 mL of 1% lidocaine HCl injection (without epinephrine). Shake well.
I.V.: Reconstitute 1 g vial with 10 mL of sterile water for injection, 0.9% sodium chloride injection, or bacteriostatic water for injection. Shake well. For adults, transfer dose to 50 mL of 0.9% sodium chloride injection; for children, dilute dose with NS to a final concentration ≤20 mg/mL.

Storage/Stability
Prior to reconstitution, store vials at ≤25°C (77°F). The reconstituted I.M. solution should be used within 1 hour after preparation. The reconstituted I.V. solution may be stored at room temperature (25°C [77°F]) and used within 6 hours, or stored for 24 hours under refrigeration (5°C [41°F]) and used within 4 hours after removal from refrigeration. Do not freeze.

Nursing Actions

Physical Assessment Results of culture and sensitivity tests and patient history of previous allergies should be assessed prior to beginning treatment. Monitor closely for adverse reactions, especially CNS adverse effects (history of seizures, head injuries, or other CNS events increases risk).

Patient Education
- Discuss specific use of drug and side effects with patient as it relates to treatment. (HCAHPS: During this hospital stay, were you given any medicine that you had not taken before? Before giving you any new medicine, how often did hospital staff tell you what the medicine was for? How often did hospital staff describe possible side effects in a way you could understand?)
- Patient may experience nausea, diarrhea, headache, or injection site irritation. Have patient report immediately to prescriber severe dizziness, syncope, illogical thinking, considerable asthenia, mood changes, dyspnea, excessive weight gain, edema, vaginitis, or signs of pseudomembranous colitis (HCAHPS).
- Educate patient about signs of a significant reaction (eg, wheezing; chest tightness; fever; itching; bad cough; blue skin color; seizures; or swelling of face, lips, tongue, or throat). **Note:** This is not a comprehensive list of all side effects. Patient should consult prescriber for additional questions.

Intended Use and Disclaimer: Should not be printed and given to patients. This information is intended to serve as a concise initial reference for healthcare professionals to use when discussing medications with a patient. You must ultimately rely on your own discretion, experience and judgment in diagnosing, treating and advising patients.

Dietary Considerations Some products may contain sodium.

Erythromycin (Systemic) (er ith roe MYE sin)

Brand Names: U.S. E.E.S. 400; E.E.S. Granules; Ery-Tab; EryPed 200; EryPed 400; Erythrocin Lactobinate; Erythrocin Stearate; PCE

Index Terms Erythromycin Base; Erythromycin Ethylsuccinate; Erythromycin Lactobionate; Erythromycin Stearate

Pharmacologic Category Antibiotic, Macrolide

Medication Safety Issues

Sound-alike/look-alike issues:

Erythromycin may be confused with azithromycin, clarithromycin

Eryc may be confused with Emcyt, Ery-Tab

Pregnancy Risk Factor B

Lactation Enters breast milk/use caution

Breast-Feeding Considerations Erythromycin is excreted in breast milk; therefore, the manufacturer recommends that caution be exercised when administering erythromycin to breast-feeding women. Decreased appetite, diarrhea, rash, and somnolence have been reported in nursing infants exposed to macrolide antibiotics (Goldstein, 2009).

One case report and a cohort study raise the possibility for a connection with pyloric stenosis in neonates exposed to erythromycin via breast milk and an alternative antibiotic may be preferred for breast-feeding mothers of infants in this age group (Sorensen, 2003; Stang, 1986).

Use Treatment of susceptible bacterial infections including *S. pyogenes*, some *S. pneumoniae*, some *S. aureus*, *M. pneumoniae*, *Legionella pneumophila*, diphtheria, pertussis, *Chlamydia*, erythrasma, *N. gonorrhoeae*, *E. histolytica*, syphilis and nongonococcal urethritis, and *Campylobacter* gastroenteritis; used in conjunction with neomycin for decontaminating the bowel

Unlabeled Use Management of gastroparesis, chancroid; treatment of *Bartonella* spp infections

Mechanism of Action/Effect Inhibits RNA-dependent protein synthesis

Contraindications Hypersensitivity to erythromycin, any macrolide antibiotics, or any component of the formulation

Concomitant use with pimozide, cisapride, ergotamine or dihydroergotamine, terfenadine, astemizole, lovastatin, or simvastatin

Warnings/Precautions Use caution with hepatic impairment with or without jaundice has occurred, it may be accompanied by malaise, nausea, vomiting, abdominal colic, and fever; discontinue use if these occur. Use caution with other medication relying on CYP3A4 metabolism; high potential for drug interactions exists. Prolonged use may result in fungal or bacterial superinfection, including *C. difficile*-associated diarrhea (CDAD) and pseudomembranous colitis; CDAD has been observed >2 months postantibiotic treatment. Use in infants has been associated with infantile hypertrophic pyloric stenosis (IHPS). Macrolides have been associated with rare QT_c prolongation and ventricular arrhythmias, including torsade de pointes; avoid use in patients with prolonged QT interval, uncorrected hypokalemia or hypomagnesemia, clinically significant bradycardia, or concurrent use of Class IA (eg, quinidine, procainamide) or Class III (eg, amiodarone, dofetilide, sotalol) antiarrhythmic agents. Avoid concurrent use with strong CYP3A inhibitors; may increase the risk of sudden cardiac death (Ray, 2004). Use caution in elderly patients, as risk of adverse events may be increased. Use caution in myasthenia gravis patients; erythromycin may aggravate muscular weakness.

Drug Interactions

Avoid Concomitant Use
Avoid concomitant use of Erythromycin (Systemic) with any of the following: BCG; Bosutinib; Cisapride; Conivaptan; Disopyramide; Fusidic Acid (Systemic); Highest Risk QTc-Prolonging Agents; Ibrutinib; Ivabradine; Lincosamide Antibiotics; Lomitapide; Lovastatin; Mifepristone; Pimozide; Pomalidomide; QuiNIDine; QuiNINE; Silodosin; Simeprevir; Simvastatin; Terfenadine; Tolvaptan; Topotecan; Uliprisal

Decreased Effect

Erythromycin (Systemic) may decrease the levels/effects of: BCG; Clopidogrel; Ifosfamide; Sodium Picosulfate; Typhoid Vaccine; Zafirlukast

The levels/effects of Erythromycin (Systemic) may be decreased by: Bosentan; CYP3A4 Inducers (Strong); Dabrafenib; Deferasirox; Etravirine; Herbs (CYP3A4 Inducers); Lincosamide Antibiotics; Mitotane; P-glycoprotein/ABCB1 Inducers; Tocilizumab

Increased Effect/Toxicity

Erythromycin (Systemic) may increase the levels/effects of: Afatinib; Alfentanil; ALPRAZolam; Antifungal Agents (Azole Derivatives, Systemic); Antineoplastic Agents (Vinca Alkaloids); ARIPiprazole; AtorvaSTATin; Avanafil; Bosentan; Bosutinib; Budesonide (Systemic, Oral Inhalation); BusPIRone; Calcium Channel Blockers; CarBAMazepine; Cardiac Glycosides; Cilostazol; Cisapride; CloZAPine; Colchicine; Corticosteroids (Systemic); CycloSPORINE (Systemic); CYP3A4 Substrates; Dabigatran Etexilate; Disopyramide; DOXOrubicin (Conventional); Eletriptan; Eplerenone; Ergot Derivatives; Estazolam; Everolimus; FentaNYL; Fexofenadine; Highest Risk QTc-Prolonging Agents; Ibrutinib; Imatinib; Ivacaftor; Lomitapide; Lovastatin; Lurasidone; Midazolam; Moderate Risk QTc-Prolonging Agents; OxyCODONE; P-glycoprotein/ABCB1 Substrates; Pimecrolimus; Pimozide; Pitavastatin; Pomalidomide; Pravastatin; QuiNIDine; QuiNINE; Repaglinide; Rifamycin Derivatives; Rilpivirine; Rivaroxaban; Salmeterol; Saxagliptin; Selective Serotonin Reuptake Inhibitors; Sildenafil; Silodosin; Simeprevir; Simvastatin; Sirolimus; Tacrolimus (Systemic); Tacrolimus (Topical); Telaprevir; Temsirolimus; Terfenadine; Theophylline Derivatives; Tolvaptan; Topotecan; Triazolam; Ulipristal; Vardenafil; Vitamin K Antagonists; Zopiclone

The levels/effects of Erythromycin (Systemic) may be increased by: Antifungal Agents (Azole Derivatives, Systemic); Conivaptan; CYP3A4 Inhibitors (Moderate); CYP3A4 Inhibitors (Strong); Dasatinib; Fusidic Acid (Systemic); Ivabradine; Ivacaftor; Luliconazole; Mifepristone; P-glycoprotein/ABCB1 Inhibitors; QTc-Prolonging Agents (Indeterminate Risk and Risk Modifying); Stiripentol; Telaprevir

Nutritional/Ethanol Interactions

Ethanol: Ethanol may decrease absorption of erythromycin or enhance effects of ethanol. Management: Avoid ethanol.

Food: Erythromycin serum levels may be altered if taken with food (formulation-dependent). GI upset, including diarrhea, is common. Management: May be taken with food to decrease GI upset, otherwise take around-the-clock with a full glass of water. Do not give with milk or acidic beverages (eg, soda, juice).

Herb/Nutraceutical: St John's wort may decrease erythromycin levels. Management: Avoid St John's wort.

Adverse Reactions
Frequency not defined. Incidence may vary with formulation.

Cardiovascular: QT_c prolongation, torsade de pointes, ventricular arrhythmia, ventricular tachycardia

Central nervous system: Seizure

Dermatologic: Erythema multiforme, pruritus, rash, Stevens-Johnson syndrome, toxic epidermal necrolysis

Gastrointestinal: Abdominal pain, anorexia, diarrhea, infantile hypertrophic pyloric stenosis, nausea, oral candidiasis, pancreatitis, pseudomembranous colitis, vomiting

Hepatic: Cholestatic jaundice (most common with estolate), hepatitis, liver function tests abnormal

Local: Phlebitis at the injection site, thrombophlebitis

Neuromuscular & skeletal: Weakness

Otic: Hearing loss

Miscellaneous: Allergic reactions, anaphylaxis, hypersensitivity reactions, interstitial nephritis, urticaria

Available Dosage Forms

Capsule Delayed Release Particles, Oral:
Generic: 250 mg

Solution Reconstituted, Intravenous:
Erythrocin Lactobionate: 500 mg (1 ea); 1000 mg (1 ea)

Suspension Reconstituted, Oral:
E.E.S. Granules: 200 mg/5 mL (100 mL, 200 mL)
EryPed 200: 200 mg/5 mL (100 mL)
EryPed 400: 400 mg/5 mL (100 mL)

Tablet, Oral:
E.E.S. 400: 400 mg
Erythrocin Stearate: 250 mg
Generic: 250 mg, 400 mg, 500 mg

Tablet Delayed Release, Oral:
Ery-Tab: 250 mg, 333 mg, 500 mg
PCE: 333 mg, 500 mg

General Dosage Range

I.V.:
Children: 15-50 mg/kg/day divided every 6 hours (maximum: 4 g daily)
Adults: 15-20 mg/kg/day divided every 6 hours **or** 500 mg to 1 g every 6 hours or as a continuous infusion over 24 hours (maximum: 4 g daily)

Oral:
Children: 30-50 mg/kg/day in 2-4 divided doses (maximum base or stearate: 2 g daily; maximum ethylsuccinate: 3.2 g daily)
Adults: Base: 250-500 mg every 6-12 hours (maximum: 4 g daily); Ethylsuccinate: 400-800 mg every 6-12 hours (maximum: 4 g daily)

Administration

I.V. Infuse 1 g over 20-60 minutes.

Injectable Detail I.V. infusion may be very irritating to the vein. If phlebitis/pain occurs with used ▶

dilution, consider diluting further (eg, 1:5) if fluid status of the patient will tolerate, or consider administering in larger available vein. The addition of lidocaine or bicarbonate does not decrease the irritation of erythromycin infusions.

pH: Erythromycin lactobionate: 6.5-7.5 (reconstituted with sterile water for injection or D_5W to a 50 mg/mL concentration)

Oral Do not crush enteric coated drug product. GI upset, including diarrhea, is common. May be administered with food to decrease GI upset. Do not give with milk or acidic beverages.

Preparation for Administration Erythromycin lactobionate should be reconstituted with sterile water for injection without preservatives to avoid gel formation. I.V. form has the longest stability in NS and should be prepared in this base solution whenever possible. Do not use D_5W as a diluent unless sodium bicarbonate is added to solution. If I.V. must be prepared in D_5W, 0.5 mL of the 8.4% sodium bicarbonate solution should be added per each 100 mL of D_5W.

Standard diluent: 500 mg/250 mL D_5W/NS; 750 mg/250 mL D_5W/NS; 1 g/250 mL D_5W/NS.

Storage/Stability

Injection: Store unreconstituted vials at 15°C to 30°C (59°F to 86°F). Reconstituted solution is stable for 2 weeks when refrigerated or for 8 hours at room temperature. Erythromycin I.V. infusion solution is stable at pH 6-8; stability of lactobionate is pH dependent; I.V. form has longest stability in NS. Stability of parenteral admixture at room temperature (25°C) and at refrigeration temperature (4°C) is 24 hours.

Oral suspension:

Granules: Prior to mixing, store at <30°C (86°F). After mixing, store under refrigeration and use within 10 days.

Powder: Prior to mixing, store at <30°C (86°F). After mixing, store at ≤25°C (77°F) and use within 35 days.

Tablet and capsule formulations: Store at <30°C (86°F).

Nursing Actions

Physical Assessment Results of culture and sensitivity tests and patient's previous allergy history should be assessed prior to therapy. Most common side effects: Nausea, vomiting, abdominal pain, diarrhea (assess frequency), and anorexia.

Patient Education

• Discuss specific use of drug and side effects with patient as it relates to treatment. (HCAHPS: During this hospital stay, were you given any medicine that you had not taken before? Before giving you any new medicine, how often did hospital staff tell you what the medicine was for? How often did hospital staff describe possible side effects in a way you could understand?)

• Patient may experience dyspepsia, nausea, diarrhea, lack of appetite, or injection site irritation. Have patient report immediately to prescriber signs of hepatic impairment, urinary retention, oliguria, signs of pancreatitis, arrhythmia, signs of Stevens-Johnson syndrome/toxic epidermal necrolysis, signs of pseudomembranous colitis, hearing impairment, or signs of myasthenia gravis (HCAHPS).

• Educate patient about signs of a significant reaction (eg, wheezing; chest tightness; fever; itching; bad cough; blue skin color; seizures; or swelling of face, lips, tongue, or throat). **Note:** This is not a comprehensive list of all side effects. Patient should consult prescriber for additional questions.

Intended Use and Disclaimer: Should not be printed and given to patients. This information is intended to serve as a concise initial reference for healthcare professionals to use when discussing medications with a patient. You must ultimately rely on your own discretion, experience and judgment in diagnosing, treating and advising patients.

Dietary Considerations Drug may cause GI upset; may take with food. Some products may contain sodium.

Related Information

Oral Medications That Should Not Be Crushed or Altered *on page 1712*

Erythromycin (Topical) (er ith roe MYE sin)

Brand Names: U.S. Akne-Mycin; Ery; Erygel

Pharmacologic Category Acne Products; Antibiotic, Macrolide; Antibiotic, Topical; Topical Skin Product; Topical Skin Product, Acne

Medication Safety Issues

Sound-alike/look-alike issues:

Erythromycin may be confused with azithromycin, clarithromycin

Pregnancy Risk Factor B

Lactation Use caution

Use Treatment of acne vulgaris

Available Dosage Forms

Gel, External:

Erygel: 2% (30 g, 60 g)

Generic: 2% (30 g, 60 g)

Ointment, External:

Akne-Mycin: 2% (25 g)

Pad, External:

Ery: 2% (60 ea)

Generic: 2% (60 ea)

Solution, External:

Generic: 2% (60 mL)

General Dosage Range Topical: *Adolescents and Adults:* Apply over the affected area twice daily

Administration

Topical Prior to treatment, area should be washed with mild soap and warm water, rinsed and patted dry. Ointment and gel should be rubbed in gently. Ery pledgets should be discarded after single use. Additional pledgets may be used if necessary. Wash hands after use. Avoid contact with the eyes, nose, mouth and other mucous membranes, and broken skin.

Nursing Actions

Patient Education

- Discuss specific use of drug and side effects with patient as it relates to treatment. (HCAHPS: During this hospital stay, were you given any medicine that you had not taken before? Before giving you any new medicine, how often did hospital staff tell you what the medicine was for? How often did hospital staff describe possible side effects in a way you could understand?)
- Patient may experience xeroderma, eye irritation, or peeling. Have patient report immediately to prescriber severe application site irritation or signs of pseudomembranous colitis (HCAHPS).
- Educate patient about signs of a significant reaction (eg, wheezing; chest tightness; fever; itching; bad cough; blue skin color; seizures; or swelling of face, lips, tongue, or throat). **Note:** This is not a comprehensive list of all side effects. Patient should consult prescriber for additional questions.

Intended Use and Disclaimer: Should not be printed and given to patients. This information is intended to serve as a concise initial reference for healthcare professionals to use when discussing medications with a patient. You must ultimately rely on your own discretion, experience and judgment in diagnosing, treating and advising patients.

Escitalopram (es sye TAL oh pram)

Brand Names: U.S. Lexapro
Index Terms Escitalopram Oxalate; Lu-26-054; S-Citalopram
Pharmacologic Category Antidepressant, Selective Serotonin Reuptake Inhibitor
Medication Safety Issues
Sound-alike/look-alike issues:
Lexapro may be confused with Loxitane
BEERS Criteria medication:
This drug may be potentially inappropriate for use in geriatric patients (Quality of evidence - moderate; Strength of recommendation - strong).
International issues:
Zavesca: Brand name for escitalopram [in multiple international markets; ISMP April 21, 2010], but also brand name for miglustat [Canada, U.S., and multiple international markets]
Medication Guide Available Yes
Pregnancy Risk Factor C
Lactation Enters breast milk/consider risk:benefit
Breast-Feeding Considerations Escitalopram and its metabolite are excreted into breast milk.

Limited data is available concerning the effects escitalopram may have in the nursing infant and the long-term effects on development and behavior have not been studied. Adverse effects have been reported in nursing infants exposed to some SSRIs. According to the manufacturer, the decision to continue or discontinue breast-feeding during therapy should take into account the risk of exposure to the infant and the benefits of treatment to the mother. Maternal use of an SSRI during pregnancy may cause delayed milk secretion. Escitalopram is the S-enantiomer of the racemic derivative citalopram; also refer to the Citalopram monograph.

Use Treatment of major depressive disorder; generalized anxiety disorders (GAD)
Canadian labeling: Additional use (not in U.S. labeling): Treatment of obsessive-compulsive disorder (OCD)

Unlabeled Use Treatment of vasomotor symptoms associated with menopause

Mechanism of Action/Effect Escitalopram is the S-enantiomer of the racemic derivative citalopram, which selectively inhibits the reuptake of serotonin with little to no effect on norepinephrine or dopamine reuptake. It has no or very low affinity for 5-HT$_{1-7}$, alpha- and beta-adrenergic, D$_{1-5}$, H$_{1-3}$, M$_{1-5}$, and benzodiazepine receptors. Escitalopram does not bind to or has low affinity for Na$^+$, K$^+$, Cl$^-$, and Ca^{++} ion channels.

Contraindications Hypersensitivity to escitalopram, citalopram, or any component of the formulation; use of MAO inhibitors intended to treat psychiatric disorders (concurrently or within 14 days of discontinuing either escitalopram or the MAO inhibitor); initiation of escitalopram in a patient receiving linezolid or intravenous methylene blue; concurrent use of pimozide

Canadian labeling: Additional contraindications (not in U.S. labeling): Known QT-interval prolongation or congenital long QT syndrome

Warnings/Precautions [U.S. Boxed Warning]: Antidepressants increase the risk of suicidal thinking and behavior in children, adolescents, and young adults (18-24 years of age) with major depressive disorder (MDD) and other psychiatric disorders; consider risk prior to prescribing. Short-term studies did not show an increased risk in patients >24 years of age and showed a decreased risk in patients ≥65 years. Closely monitor patients for clinical worsening, suicidality, or unusual changes in behavior, particularly during the initial 1-2 months of therapy or during periods of dosage adjustments (increases or decreases); the patient's family or caregiver should be instructed to closely observe the patient and communicate condition with healthcare provider. A medication guide concerning the use of antidepressants should be dispensed with each ▶

prescription. **Escitalopram is not FDA approved for use in children <12 years of age.**

The possibility of a suicide attempt is inherent in major depression and may persist until remission occurs. Use caution in high-risk patients. Worsening depression and severe abrupt suicidality that are not part of the presenting symptoms may require discontinuation or modification of drug therapy. The patient's family or caregiver should be alerted to monitor patients for the emergence of suicidality and associated behaviors (such as agitation, irritability, hostility, impulsivity, and hypomania) and call healthcare provider.

May precipitate a shift to mania or hypomania in patients with bipolar disorder. Patients presenting with depressive symptoms should be screened for bipolar disorder. Monotherapy in patients with bipolar disorder should be avoided. Escitalopram is not FDA approved for the treatment of bipolar depression.

Potentially life-threatening serotonin syndrome (SS) has occurred with serotonergic agents (eg, SSRIs, SNRIs), particularly when used in combination with other serotonergic agents (eg, triptans, TCAs, fentanyl, lithium, tramadol, buspirone, St John's wort, tryptophan) or agents that impair metabolism of serotonin (eg, MAO inhibitors intended to treat psychiatric disorders, other MAO inhibitors [ie, linezolid and intravenous methylene blue]). Discontinue treatment (and any concomitant serotonergic agent) immediately if signs/symptoms arise. May increase the risks associated with electroconvulsive therapy. Has a low potential to impair cognitive or motor performance; caution operating hazardous machinery or driving. Bone fractures have been associated with antidepressant treatment. Consider the possibility of a fragility fracture if an antidepressant-treated patient presents with unexplained bone pain, point tenderness, swelling, or bruising (Rabenda, 2013; Rizzoli, 2012).

Use with caution in patients with a recent history of MI or unstable heart disease. Use has been associated with dose-dependent QT-interval prolongation with doses of 10 mg and 30 mg/day in healthy subjects (mean change from baseline: 4.3 msec and 10.7 msec, respectively); prolongation of QT interval and ventricular arrhythmia (including torsade de pointes) have been reported, particularly in females with pre-existing QT prolongation or other risk factors (eg, hypokalemia, other cardiac disease).

Use caution with a previous seizure disorder or condition predisposing to seizures such as brain damage, alcoholism, or concurrent therapy with other drugs which lower the seizure threshold. May cause hyponatremia/SIADH (elderly at increased risk); volume depletion (diuretics may increase risk) may occur. Use caution in patients with metabolic disease. May cause or exacerbate sexual dysfunction. Use caution in elderly patients; may cause or exacerbate syndrome of inappropriate antidiuretic hormone secretion or hyponatremia; monitor sodium closely with initiation or dosage adjustments in older adults (Beers Criteria). Bioavailability and half-life are increased by 50% in the elderly. Use caution with severe renal impairment or liver impairment; concomitant CNS depressants. May cause mydriasis; use caution in patients at risk of acute narrow-angle glaucoma or with increased intraocular pressure. Use with caution in patients who are hemodynamically unstable. Potentially significant interactions may exist, requiring dose or frequency adjustment, additional monitoring, and/or selection of alternative therapy. Consult drug interactions database for more detailed information. Escitalopram systemic exposure may be increased in CYP2C19 poor metabolizers; Canadian labeling recommends a dosage adjustment in this patient population.

Abrupt discontinuation or interruption of antidepressant therapy has been associated with a discontinuation syndrome. Symptoms arising may vary with antidepressant however commonly include nausea, vomiting, diarrhea, headaches, light-headedness, dizziness, diminished appetite, sweating, chills, tremors, paresthesias, fatigue, somnolence, and sleep disturbances (eg, vivid dreams, insomnia). Greater risks for developing a discontinuation syndrome have been associated with antidepressants with shorter half-lives, longer durations of treatment, and abrupt discontinuation. For antidepressants of short or intermediate half-lives, symptoms may emerge within 2-5 days after treatment discontinuation and last 7-14 days (APA, 2010; Fava, 2006; Haddad, 2001; Shelton, 2001; Warner, 2006).

Drug Interactions

Avoid Concomitant Use

Avoid concomitant use of Escitalopram with any of the following: Conivaptan; Dosulepin; Fusidic Acid (Systemic); Highest Risk QTc-Prolonging Agents; Iobenguane I 123; Ivabradine; Linezolid; MAO Inhibitors; Methylene Blue; Mifepristone; Moderate Risk QTc-Prolonging Agents; Pimozide; Tryptophan; Urokinase

Decreased Effect

Escitalopram may decrease the levels/effects of: Iobenguane I 123; Ioflupane I 123; Simeprevir; Thyroid Products

The levels/effects of Escitalopram may be decreased by: Boceprevir; Bosentan; CarBAMazepine; CYP2C19 Inducers (Strong); CYP3A4 Inducers (Strong); Cyproheptadine; Dabrafenib; Deferasirox; Mitotane; NSAID (COX-2 Inhibitor); NSAID (Nonselective); Telaprevir; Tocilizumab

Increased Effect/Toxicity

Escitalopram may increase the levels/effects of: Agents with Antiplatelet Properties; Anticoagulants; Antidepressants (Serotonin Reuptake

Inhibitor/Antagonist); Antipsychotics; Aspirin; BusPIRone; CarBAMazepine; CloZAPine; Collagenase (Systemic); Dabigatran Etexilate; Desmopressin; Dextromethorphan; Dosulepin; Highest Risk QTc-Prolonging Agents; Hypoglycemic Agents; Ibritumomab; Methadone; Methylene Blue; Metoclopramide; Mexiletine; NSAID (COX-2 Inhibitor); NSAID (Nonselective); Pimozide; RisperiDONE; Rivaroxaban; Salicylates; Serotonin Modulators; Thiazide Diuretics; Thrombolytic Agents; Tositumomab and Iodine I 131 Tositumomab; TraMADol; Tricyclic Antidepressants; Urokinase; Vitamin K Antagonists

The levels/effects of Escitalopram may be increased by: Alcohol (Ethyl); Analgesics (Opioid); Antipsychotics; BusPIRone; Cimetidine; CNS Depressants; Cobicistat; Conivaptan; CYP2C19 Inhibitors (Moderate); CYP2C19 Inhibitors (Strong); CYP3A4 Inhibitors (Moderate); CYP3A4 Inhibitors (Strong); Dasatinib; Fusidic Acid (Systemic); Glucosamine; Herbs (Anticoagulant/Antiplatelet Properties); Ibrutinib; Ivabradine; Ivacaftor; Linezolid; Lithium; Luliconazole; Macrolide Antibiotics; MAO Inhibitors; Metoclopramide; Metyrosine; Mifepristone; Moderate Risk QTc-Prolonging Agents; Multivitamins/Fluoride (with ADE); Multivitamins/Minerals (with ADEK, Folate, Iron); Multivitamins/Minerals (with AE, No Iron); Omega-3 Fatty Acids; Omeprazole; Pentosan Polysulfate Sodium; Pentoxifylline; Prostacyclin Analogues; QTc-Prolonging Agents (Indeterminate Risk and Risk Modifying); Stiripentol; Tipranavir; TraMADol; Tricyclic Antidepressants; Tryptophan; Vitamin E

Nutritional/Ethanol Interactions

Ethanol: Concurrent use with ethanol may increase CNS depression. Management: Monitor for increased effects with coadministration; caution patients about effects.

Herb/Nutraceutical: Concurrent use with some herbal medications may increase the risk of CNS depression and/or serotonin syndrome. Management: Avoid valerian, St John's wort, tryptophan, SAMe, kava kava, and gotu kola.

Adverse Reactions

>10%:
Central nervous system: Headache (24%), somnolence (4% to 13%), insomnia (7% to 12%)
Gastrointestinal: Diarrhea (6% to 14%), nausea (15% to 18%)
Genitourinary: Ejaculation disorder (9% to 14%)
1% to 10%:
Central nervous system: Fatigue (2% to 8%), dizziness (4% to 7%), abnormal dreaming (3%), lethargy (3%), yawning (2%)
Endocrine & metabolic: Libido decreased (3% to 7%), anorgasmia (2% to 6%), menstrual disorder (2%)
Gastrointestinal: Xerostomia (4% to 9%), constipation (3% to 6%), indigestion (2% to 6%),

appetite decreased (3%), vomiting (3%), abdominal pain (2%), flatulence (2%), toothache (2%)
Genitourinary: Impotence (2% to 3%), urinary tract infection (children ≥2%)
Neuromuscular & skeletal: Neck/shoulder pain (3%), back pain (children ≥2%), paresthesia (2%)
Respiratory: Rhinitis (5%), sinusitis (3%), nasal congestion (children ≥2%)
Miscellaneous: Diaphoresis (3% to 8%), flu-like syndrome (5%)

Pharmacodynamics/Kinetics

Onset of Action Depression: The onset of action is within a week; however, individual response varies greatly and full response may not be seen until 8-12 weeks after initiation of treatment.

Available Dosage Forms

Solution, Oral:
Lexapro: 5 mg/5 mL (240 mL)
Generic: 5 mg/5 mL (240 mL)
Tablet, Oral:
Lexapro: 5 mg, 10 mg, 20 mg
Generic: 5 mg, 10 mg, 20 mg

General Dosage Range Dosage adjustment recommended in patients with hepatic impairment
Oral:
Children ≥12 years and Adults: Initial: 10 mg once daily; Maintenance: 10-20 mg once daily
Elderly: 10 mg once daily

Administration

Oral
Administer once daily (morning or evening), with or without food.
Cipralex MELTZ [Canadian product] should be dissolved on the tongue and swallowed without water.

Endotracheal Mental status for depression, suicidal ideation (especially at the beginning of therapy or when doses are increased or decreased), anxiety, social functioning, mania, panic attacks; akathisia; signs/symptoms of serotonin syndrome

Storage/Stability Store at 25°C (77°F); excursions permitted to 15°C to 30°C (59°F to 86°F). Cipralex MELTZ [Canadian product] should be stored in original package and protected from light.

Nursing Actions

Physical Assessment Assess therapeutic effectiveness (mental status for depression, suicide ideation, social functioning, mania, or panic attacks). Monitor for signs of clinical worsening or hypomania. Taper dosage slowly when discontinuing.

Patient Education
• Discuss specific use of drug and side effects with patient as it relates to treatment. (HCAHPS: During this hospital stay, were you given any medicine that you had not taken before? Before giving you any new medicine, how often did hospital staff tell you what the medicine was

for? How often did hospital staff describe possible side effects in a way you could understand?)

• Patient may experience dyspepsia, constipation, xerostomia, sexual dysfunction, insomnia, asthenia, fatigue, rhinorrhea, or oscitation. Have patient report immediately to prescriber signs of hyponatremia, signs of hemorrhaging, signs of depression (ie, suicidal ideation, anxiety, emotional instability, illogical thinking), behavioral changes, bradycardia, syncope, angina, vision changes, menstrual irregularities, signs of serotonin syndrome (ie, dizziness, severe headache, agitation, hallucinations, tachycardia, arrhythmia, flushing, tremors, hyperhidrosis, change in balance, severe nausea, significant diarrhea), or priapism (HCAHPS).

• Educate patient about signs of a significant reaction (eg, wheezing; chest tightness; fever; itching; bad cough; blue skin color; seizures; or swelling of face, lips, tongue, or throat). **Note:** This is not a comprehensive list of all side effects. Patient should consult prescriber for additional questions.

Intended Use and Disclaimer: Should not be printed and given to patients. This information is intended to serve as a concise initial reference for healthcare professionals to use when discussing medications with a patient. You must ultimately rely on your own discretion, experience and judgment in diagnosing, treating and advising patients.

Dietary Considerations May be taken with or without food.

Eslicarbazepine (es li kar BAZ e peen)

Brand Names: U.S. Aptiom
Index Terms Aptiom; Eslicarbazepine Acetate
Pharmacologic Category Anticonvulsant, Miscellaneous
Medication Guide Available Yes
Pregnancy Risk Factor C
Lactation Enters breast milk/not recommended
Breast-Feeding Considerations Eslicarbazepine is excreted into breast milk. Due to the potential for serious adverse reactions in the nursing infant, the manufacturer recommends a decision be made whether to discontinue nursing or to discontinue the drug, taking into account the importance of treatment to the mother.
Use Partial-onset seizures (epilepsy): Adjunctive therapy in the treatment of partial-onset seizures
Mechanism of Action/Effect Eslicarbazepine acetate is extensively converted to eslicarbazepine, which is considered responsible for therapeutic effects. A precise mechanism has not been defined, but is thought to involve inhibition of voltage-gated sodium channels.

Contraindications Hypersensitivity to eslicarbazepine, oxcarbazepine, or any component of the formulation

Warnings/Precautions Antiepileptics are associated with an increased risk of suicidal thoughts/behavior with use, regardless of indication. Monitor all patients for notable changes in behavior that might indicate suicidal thoughts or depression; patients should be instructed to notify their healthcare provider immediately if symptoms occur.

Potentially serious, sometimes fatal, dermatologic reactions (eg, Stevens-Johnson syndrome) and drug reaction with eosinophilia and systemic symptoms (DRESS), also known as multiorgan hypersensitivity reactions, have been reported. Monitor for signs and symptoms of skin reactions and DRESS (eg, fever, rash, lymphadenopathy, eosinophilia) in association with other organ involvement. In addition, rare cases of anaphylaxis and angioedema have been reported. Avoid use in patients with prior dermatologic, DRESS, or anaphylactic-type reactions with either oxcarbazepine or eslicarbazepine.

Clinically significant hyponatremia (serum sodium <125 mmol/L) and concurrent hypochloremia may develop during use. Consider monitoring serum sodium and chloride levels during maintenance treatment, especially in patients at risk for hyponatremia and measure if symptoms of hyponatremia develop.

Use has been associated with dose-dependent CNS-related adverse events; most significant of these were cognitive symptoms, somnolence or fatigue, dizziness and coordination abnormalities, and visual changes. There was an increased risk of visual changes and dizziness and coordination abnormalities during the titration period, in patients >60 years of age, and with concomitant carbamazepine use; consider dosage modifications in patients using eslicarbazepine and carbamazepine concomitantly. Caution patients about performing tasks which require mental alertness (eg, operating machinery or driving).

Dosage adjustment is necessary with impaired renal function (CrCl <50 mL/minute). Hepatic effects ranging from mild to moderate elevations in transaminases (>3 times the upper limit of normal) to rare cases of concomitant elevations of total bilirubin (>2 times the upper limit of normal have been reported. Perform baseline liver laboratory tests. Avoid use in patients with severe hepatic impairment. Dose-dependent decreases in serum T_3 and T_4 (free and total) values have been observed; changes were not associated with other abnormal thyroid function tests suggesting hypothyroidism. Anticonvulsants should not be discontinued abruptly because of the possibility of increasing seizure frequency; therapy should be withdrawn gradually to minimize the potential of increased seizure frequency, unless safety concerns require a more rapid withdrawal.

Drug Interactions

Avoid Concomitant Use

Avoid concomitant use of Eslicarbazepine with any of the following: Axitinib; Simeprevir

Decreased Effect

Eslicarbazepine may decrease the levels/effects of: ARIPiprazole; Axitinib; Clopidogrel; Contraceptives (Estrogens); Contraceptives (Progestins); Ibrutinib; Oral Contraceptive (Progestins); Rosuvastatin; Saxagliptin; Simeprevir; Simvastatin; Warfarin

The levels/effects of Eslicarbazepine may be decreased by: CarBAMazepine; Fosphenytoin; Ketorolac (Nasal); Ketorolac (Systemic); Mefloquine; Orlistat; PHENobarbital; Phenytoin; Primidone

Increased Effect/Toxicity

Eslicarbazepine may increase the levels/effects of: Citalopram; CYP2C19 Substrates; Fosphenytoin; Phenytoin

The levels/effects of Eslicarbazepine may be increased by: CarBAMazepine

Nutritional/Ethanol Interactions

Ethanol: Concomitant use with ethanol may increase CNS depression. Management: Advise patient that ethanol may enhance CNS depression; monitor for increased effects.

Herb/Nutraceutical: Some herbal medications should be avoided due to the risk of CNS depression with concomitant use. Evening primrose may decrease seizure threshold. Management: Avoid kava kava, valerian, St John's wort, gotu kola, and evening primrose.

Adverse Reactions

>10%:

Central nervous system: Dizziness (20% to 28%), drowsiness (16% to 28%, including fatigue, hypersomnia, sedation, lethargy, and malaise), headache (13% to 15%)

Gastrointestinal: Nausea (10% to 16%)

Ophthalmic: Diplopia (9% to 11%)

1% to 10%:

Cardiovascular: Hypertension (2%), peripheral edema (2%)

Central nervous system: Fatigue (7%), ataxia (4% to 6%), cognitive dysfunction (4% to 7%, including aphasia, lack of concentration, psychomotor retardation, speech disturbance), vertigo (2% to 6%), depression (3%), equilibrium disturbance (3%), falling (3%), abnormal gait (2%), insomnia (2%), dysarthria (1% to 2%), memory impairment (1% to 2%)

Dermatologic: Skin rash (3%)

Endocrine & metabolic: Decreased serum sodium (>10 mEq/L: 5%), hyponatremia (serum sodium <125 mEq/L: 1% to 2%)

Gastrointestinal: Vomiting (6% to 10%), diarrhea (4%), abdominal pain (2%), constipation (2%), gastritis (2%)

Genitourinary: Urinary tract infection (2%)

Neuromuscular & skeletal: Tremor (2% to 4%), weakness (3%)

Ophthalmic: Blurred vision (5% to 6%), decreased visual acuity (2%), nystagmus (1% to 2%)

Respiratory: Cough (2%)

Product Availability Aptiom: FDA approved November 2013; anticipated availability is second quarter of 2014.

Available Dosage Forms

Tablet, Oral:

Aptiom: 200 mg, 400 mg, 600 mg, 800 mg

Administration

Oral Administer with or with food; tablets may be swallowed whole or crushed.

Storage/Stability Store at 20°C to 25°C (68°F to 77°F); excursions are permitted between 15°C and 30°C (59°F and 86°F).

Nursing Actions

Patient Education

• Discuss specific use of drug and side effects with patient as it relates to treatment. (HCAHPS: During this hospital stay, were you given any medicine that you had not taken before? Before giving you any new medicine, how often did hospital staff tell you what the medicine was for? How often did hospital staff describe possible side effects in a way you could understand?)

• Patient may experience headache, nausea, fatigue, or tremors. Have patient report immediately to prescriber signs of hyponatremia, signs of infection, signs of hepatic impairment, signs of renal impairment, enlarged lymph nodes, dyspnea, significant weight gain, edema of extremities, angina, intolerable dizziness, syncope, considerable myalgia, vision changes, severe asthenia, ecchymosis, hemorrhaging, uncontrollable eye movements, change in balance, inability to focus, abnormal gait, signs of depression (ie, suicidal ideation, anxiety, emotional instability, illogical thinking), or signs of Stevens-Johnson syndrome/toxic epidermal necrolysis (HCAHPS).

• Educate patient about signs of a significant reaction (eg, wheezing; chest tightness; fever; itching; bad cough; blue skin color; seizures; or swelling of face, lips, tongue, or throat). **Note:** This is not a comprehensive list of all side effects. Patient should consult prescriber for additional questions.

Intended Use and Disclaimer: Should not be printed and given to patients. This information is intended to serve as a concise initial reference for healthcare professionals to use when discussing medications with a patient. You must ultimately rely on your own discretion, experience and

judgment in diagnosing, treating and advising patients.

Esmolol (ES moe lol)

Brand Names: U.S. Brevibloc; Brevibloc in NaCl

Index Terms Esmolol Hydrochloride

Pharmacologic Category Antiarrhythmic Agent, Class II; Antihypertensive; Beta-Blocker, Beta-1 Selective

Medication Safety Issues

Sound-alike/look-alike issues:

Esmolol may be confused with Osmitrol®

Brevibloc® may be confused with Brevital®, Bumex®, Buprenex®

High alert medication:

The Institute for Safe Medication Practices (ISMP) includes this medication among its list of drugs which have a heightened risk of causing significant patient harm when used in error.

Pregnancy Risk Factor C

Lactation Excretion in breast milk unknown/not recommended

Breast-Feeding Considerations It is not known if esmolol is excreted into breast milk. Due to the potential for serious adverse reactions in the nursing infant, the manufacturer recommends a decision be made whether to discontinue nursing or to discontinue the drug, taking into account the importance of treatment to the mother. The short half-life and the fact that it is not intended for chronic use should limit any potential exposure to the nursing infant.

Use Treatment of supraventricular tachycardia (SVT) and atrial fibrillation/flutter (control ventricular rate); treatment of intraoperative and postoperative tachycardia and/or hypertension; treatment of noncompensatory sinus tachycardia

Unlabeled Use

Children: SVT and postoperative hypertension

Adults: Arrhythmia/rate control during acute coronary syndrome (eg, acute myocardial infarction, unstable angina), aortic dissection, intubation, thyroid storm, pheochromocytoma, electroconvulsive therapy

Mechanism of Action/Effect Class II antiarrhythmic: Beta$_1$-adrenergic receptor blocking agent that competes with beta$_1$-adrenergic agonists for available beta-receptor sites; it is a selective beta$_1$-antagonist with a very short duration of action; has little if any intrinsic sympathomimetic activity; and lacks membrane stabilizing action; it is administered intravenously and is used when beta-blockade of short duration is desired or in critically-ill patients in whom adverse effects of bradycardia, heart failure, or hypotension may necessitate rapid withdrawal of the drug

Contraindications Hypersensitivity to esmolol or any component of the formulation; severe sinus bradycardia; heart block greater than first degree (except in patients with a functioning artificial ventricular pacemaker); sick sinus syndrome; cardiogenic shock; decompensated heart failure; I.V. administration of calcium channel blockers (eg, verapamil) in close proximity to esmolol (ie, while effects of other drug are still present); pulmonary hypertension

Canadian labeling: Additional contraindications (not in U.S. labeling): Patients requiring inotropic agents and/or vasopressors to maintain cardiac output and systolic blood pressure; hypotension; right ventricular failure secondary to pulmonary hypertension; untreated pheochromocytoma

Warnings/Precautions Can cause bradycardia including sinus pause, heart block, severe bradycardia, and cardiac arrest. Consider pre-existing conditions such as first degree AV block, sick sinus syndrome, or other conduction disorders before initiating; use is contraindicated in patients with sick sinus syndrome or second- or third-degree AV block (except in patients with a functioning artificial ventricular pacemaker). Bradycardia may be observed more frequently in elderly patients (>65 years of age); dosage reductions may be necessary. Hypotension is common; patients need close blood pressure monitoring. If an unacceptable drop in blood pressure occurs, reduction in dose or discontinuation may reverse hypotension (usually within 30 minutes). Avoid use in patients with hypovolemia; treat hypovolemia first, otherwise, use of esmolol may attenuate reflex tachycardia and further increase the risk of hypotension. Administer cautiously in compensated heart failure and monitor for a worsening of the condition; use is contraindicated in patients with decompensated heart failure.

Esmolol has been associated with elevations in serum potassium and development of hyperkalemia especially in patients with risk factors (eg, renal impairment); monitor serum potassium during therapy. Use with caution in patients with myasthenia gravis. Use caution in patients with renal dysfunction (active metabolite retained). Adequate alpha-blockade is required prior to use of any beta-blocker for patients with untreated pheochromocytoma; Canadian labeling contraindicates use in this patient population. Use beta-blockers cautiously in patients with bronchospastic disease; monitor pulmonary status closely. Use cautiously in patients with diabetes because it can mask prominent hypoglycemic symptoms. May mask signs of hyperthyroidism (eg, tachycardia); if hyperthyroidism is suspected, carefully manage and monitor; abrupt withdrawal may exacerbate symptoms of hyperthyroidism or precipitate thyroid storm. Use esmolol with caution in patients with hypertension associated with hypothermia; monitor vital signs closely and titrate esmolol slowly. Use caution with history of severe anaphylaxis to allergens; patients taking beta-blockers may become more sensitive to repeated challenges. Treatment of anaphylaxis (eg, epinephrine) in patients taking beta-blockers may be ineffective or promote undesirable effects. Can precipitate or aggravate symptoms of arterial insufficiency in patients with PVD and Raynaud's disease; use with caution and monitor for progression of arterial obstruction.

Use caution with concurrent use of digoxin, verapamil or diltiazem; bradycardia or heart block can occur (may be fatal). Use is contraindicated when I.V. calcium channel blockers have been administered in close proximity to esmolol (ie, while effects of other drug are still present). Beta-blocker therapy should not be withdrawn abruptly (particularly in patients with CAD), but gradually tapered to avoid acute tachycardia, hypertension, and/or ischemia. Vesicant; ensure proper needle or catheter placement prior to and during infusion; avoid extravasation. Extravasation can lead to skin necrosis and sloughing; avoid infusions into small veins or through a butterfly catheter.

Drug Interactions

Avoid Concomitant Use

Avoid concomitant use of Esmolol with any of the following: Floctafenine; Methacholine

Decreased Effect

Esmolol may decrease the levels/effects of: Beta2-Agonists; Theophylline Derivatives

The levels/effects of Esmolol may be decreased by: Barbiturates; Herbs (Hypertensive Properties); Methylphenidate; Nonsteroidal Anti-Inflammatory Agents; Rifamycin Derivatives; Yohimbine

Increased Effect/Toxicity

Esmolol may increase the levels/effects of: Alpha-/Beta-Agonists (Direct-Acting); Alpha1-Blockers; Alpha2-Agonists; Amifostine; Antihypertensives; Antipsychotic Agents (Phenothiazines); Bupivacaine; Cardiac Glycosides; Cholinergic Agonists; DULoxetine; Ergot Derivatives; Fingolimod; Hypotensive Agents; Insulin; Lidocaine (Systemic); Lidocaine (Topical); Mepivacaine; Methacholine; Midodrine; Obinutuzumab; RiTUXimab; Sulfonylureas

The levels/effects of Esmolol may be increased by: Acetylcholinesterase Inhibitors; Alpha2-Agonists; Aminoquinolines (Antimalarial); Amiodarone; Anilidopiperidine Opioids; Antipsychotic Agents (Phenothiazines); Brimonidine (Topical); Calcium Channel Blockers (Dihydropyridine); Calcium Channel Blockers (Nondihydropyridine); Diazoxide; Dipyridamole; Disopyramide; Dronedarone; Floctafenine; Herbs (Hypotensive Properties); MAO Inhibitors; Pentoxifylline; Phosphodiesterase 5 Inhibitors; Propafenone; Prostacyclin Analogues; Regorafenib; Reserpine

Adverse Reactions

>10%: Cardiovascular: Blood pressure decreased (20% to 50%), asymptomatic hypotension (dose related: 25%), symptomatic hypotension (dose related: 12%)

1% to 10%:
Cardiovascular: Peripheral ischemia (1%)
Central nervous system: Dizziness (3%), somnolence (3%), confusion (2%), headache (2%), agitation (2%)
Gastrointestinal: Nausea (7%), vomiting (1%)
Local: Infusion site reaction (8%; including irritation, inflammation, and severe reactions associated with extravasation [eg, thrombophlebitis, necrosis, and blistering])

Pharmacodynamics/Kinetics

Onset of Action Beta-blockade: I.V.: 2-10 minutes (quickest when loading doses are administered)

Duration of Action Hemodynamic effects: 10-30 minutes; prolonged following higher cumulative doses, extended duration of use

Available Dosage Forms

Solution, Intravenous:
Brevibloc: 10 mg/mL (10 mL)
Brevibloc in NaCl: 2000 mg (100 mL); 2500 mg (250 mL)
Generic: 10 mg/mL (10 mL)
Solution, Intravenous [preservative free]:
Generic: 10 mg/mL (10 mL); 100 mg/10 mL (10 mL)

General Dosage Range I.V.: *Adults:* Bolus: 0.5 mg/kg or 1 mg/kg; Infusion: 50-200 mcg/kg/minute (maximum: 300 mcg/kg/minute)

Usual Infusion Concentrations: Pediatric

Note: Premixed solutions available.
I.V. infusion: 10,000 mcg/mL or 20,000 mcg/mL

Usual Infusion Concentrations: Adult Note:

Premixed solutions available.
I.V. infusion: 2500 mg in 250 mL (concentration: 10,000 mcg/mL) or 2000 mg in 100 mL (concentration: 20,000 mcg/mL) of D_5W or NS

Administration

I.V. Loading doses (eg, 0.5 mg/kg) may be administered over 30 seconds to 1 minute depending on how urgent the need for effect. Infusion into small veins or through a butterfly catheter should be avoided (can cause thrombophlebitis). Medication port of premixed bags should be used to withdraw only the initial bolus, if necessary (not to be used for withdrawal of additional bolus doses).

Vesicant; ensure proper needle or catheter placement prior to and during infusion; avoid extravasation.

Extravasation management: If extravasation occurs, stop infusion immediately and disconnect (leave cannula/needle in place); gently aspirate extravasated solution (do **NOT** flush the line); remove needle/cannula; elevate extremity.

Injectable Detail pH: 4.5-5.5

Storage/Stability Clear, colorless to light yellow solution which should be stored at 25°C (77°F); excursions permitted to 15°C to 30°C (59°F to 86°F); do not freeze. Protect from excessive heat.

Nursing Actions

Physical Assessment Requires continuous cardiac, hemodynamic, and infusion site monitoring (to prevent extravasation). Taper dosage slowly when discontinuing. Advise patients with diabetes to monitor glucose levels closely; beta-blockers may alter glucose tolerance.

Patient Education
- Discuss specific use of drug and side effects with patient as it relates to treatment. (HCAHPS: During this hospital stay, were you given any medicine that you had not taken before? Before giving you any new medicine, how often did hospital staff tell you what the medicine was for? How often did hospital staff describe possible side effects in a way you could understand?)
- Patient may experience fatigue or dyspepsia. Have patient report immediately to prescriber dyspnea, severe dizziness, syncope, considerable asthenia, angina, illogical thinking, bradycardia, arrhythmia, mood changes, injection site pain or irritation, significant nausea, or hyperhidrosis (HCAHPS).
- Educate patient about signs of a significant reaction (eg, wheezing; chest tightness; fever; itching; bad cough; blue skin color; seizures; or swelling of face, lips, tongue, or throat). **Note:** This is not a comprehensive list of all side effects. Patient should consult prescriber for additional questions.

Intended Use and Disclaimer: Should not be printed and given to patients. This information is intended to serve as a concise initial reference for healthcare professionals to use when discussing medications with a patient. You must ultimately rely on your own discretion, experience and judgment in diagnosing, treating and advising patients.

Related Information
Management of Drug Extravasations *on page 1700*

Esomeprazole (es oh ME pray zol)

Brand Names: U.S. NexIUM; NexIUM I.V.

Index Terms Esomeprazole Magnesium; Esomeprazole Sodium; Esomeprazole Strontium

Pharmacologic Category Proton Pump Inhibitor; Substituted Benzimidazole

Medication Safety Issues
Sound-alike/look-alike issues:
Esomeprazole may be confused with ARIPiprazole, omeprazole
NexIUM may be confused with NexAVAR

Medication Guide Available Yes

Pregnancy Risk Factor B/C (product specific)

Lactation Enters breast milk/not recommended

Breast-Feeding Considerations Limited data indicate esomeprazole and strontium are excreted in breast milk. Esomeprazole is the s-isomer of omeprazole and omeprazole is excreted in breast milk; refer to the Omeprazole monograph for additional information. Due to the potential for serious adverse reactions in the nursing infant, the manufacturer recommends a decision be made whether to discontinue nursing or to discontinue the drug, taking into account the importance of treatment to the mother.

Use
Oral: Esomeprazole magnesium, esomeprazole strontium: Short-term (4-8 weeks) treatment of erosive esophagitis; maintaining symptom resolution and healing of erosive esophagitis; short-term (4-8 weeks) treatment of symptomatic gastroesophageal reflux disease (GERD); as part of a multidrug regimen for *Helicobacter pylori* eradication in patients with duodenal ulcer disease (active or history of within the past 5 years); prevention of gastric ulcers associated with continuous NSAID therapy in patients at risk (age ≥60 years and/or history of gastric ulcer); long-term treatment of pathological hypersecretory conditions including Zollinger-Ellison syndrome
Canadian labeling: Additional use (not in U.S. labeling): Oral: Treatment of nonerosive reflux disease (NERD); treatment of NSAID-induced gastric ulcers

I.V.: Esomeprazole sodium: Short-term (≤10 days) treatment of gastroesophageal reflux disease (GERD) when oral therapy is not possible or appropriate

Unlabeled Use I.V.: Esomeprazole sodium: Prevention of recurrent peptic ulcer bleeding postendoscopy

Mechanism of Action/Effect Prevents gastric acid secretion

Contraindications Hypersensitivity to esomeprazole, other substituted benzimidazole proton pump inhibitors, or any component of the formulation

Warnings/Precautions Use of proton pump inhibitors (PPIs) may increase the risk of gastrointestinal infections (eg, *Salmonella, Campylobacter*). Relief of symptoms does not preclude the presence of a gastric malignancy. Atrophic gastritis (by biopsy) has been noted with long-term omeprazole therapy; this may also occur with esomeprazole. No reports of enterochromaffin-like (ECL) cell carcinoids, dysplasia, or neoplasia have occurred. Use of PPIs may increase risk of CDAD, especially in hospitalized patients; consider CDAD diagnosis in patients with persistent diarrhea that does not improve. Use the lowest dose and shortest duration of PPI therapy appropriate for the condition being treated. Safety and efficacy of I.V. therapy >10 days have not been established; transition from I.V. to oral therapy as soon possible. Bioavailability may be increased in Asian populations, the elderly, and patients with hepatic dysfunction. Decreased *H. pylori* eradication rates have been observed with short-term (≤7 days) combination therapy. The American College of Gastroenterology recommends 10-14 days of therapy (triple or quadruple) for eradication of *H. pylori* (Chey, 2007).

PPIs may diminish the therapeutic effect of clopidogrel, thought to be due to reduced formation of the active metabolite of clopidogrel. The manufacturer of clopidogrel recommends either avoidance of both omeprazole (even when scheduled 12 hours apart) and esomeprazole or use of a PPI with comparatively less effect on the active metabolite of clopidogrel (eg, pantoprazole). In contrast to these warnings, others have recommended the continued use of PPIs, regardless of the degree of inhibition, in patients with a history of GI bleeding or multiple risk factors for GI bleeding who are also receiving clopidogrel since no evidence has established clinically meaningful differences in outcome; however, a clinically-significant interaction cannot be excluded in those who are poor metabolizers of clopidogrel (Abraham, 2010; Levine, 2011). Additionally, potentially significant drug-drug interactions may exist, requiring dose or frequency adjustment, additional monitoring, and/or selection of alternative therapy.

Increased incidence of osteoporosis-related bone fractures of the hip, spine, or wrist may occur with PPI therapy. Patients on high-dose or long-term therapy should be monitored. Use the lowest effective dose for the shortest duration of time, use vitamin D and calcium supplementation, and follow appropriate guidelines to reduce risk of fractures in patients at risk.

Hypomagnesemia, reported rarely, usually with prolonged PPI use of >3 months (most cases >1 year of therapy); may be symptomatic or asymptomatic; severe cases may cause tetany, seizures, and cardiac arrhythmias. Consider obtaining serum magnesium concentrations prior to beginning long-term therapy, especially if taking concomitant digoxin, diuretics, or other drugs known to cause hypomagnesemia; and periodically thereafter. Hypomagnesemia may be corrected by magnesium supplementation, although discontinuation of esomeprazole may be necessary; magnesium levels typically return to normal within 1 week of stopping. Serum chromogranin A levels may be increased if assessed while patient on esomeprazole; may lead to diagnostic errors related to neuroendocrine tumors.

Severe liver dysfunction may require dosage reductions. Dosage adjustments are not necessary for any degree of renal impairment when using esomeprazole magnesium or esomeprazole sodium; however, since pharmacokinetics of the strontium may be reduced in mild to moderate renal impairment, esomeprazole strontium is not recommended for use in severe impairment (has not been studied). Esomeprazole strontium competes with calcium for intestinal absorption and is incorporated into bone; use of esomeprazole strontium in pediatric patients is not recommended.

Drug Interactions

Avoid Concomitant Use

Avoid concomitant use of Esomeprazole with any of the following: Clopidogrel; Dasatinib; Delavirdine; Erlotinib; Nelfinavir; PONATinib; Rifampin; Rilpivirine; Risedronate; St Johns Wort

Decreased Effect

Esomeprazole may decrease the levels/effects of: Atazanavir; Bisphosphonate Derivatives; Bosutinib; Cefditoren; Clopidogrel; Dabigatran Etexilate; Dabrafenib; Dasatinib; Delavirdine; Erlotinib; Gefitinib; Indinavir; Iron Salts; Itraconazole; Ketoconazole (Systemic); Mesalamine; Multivitamins/Minerals (with ADEK, Folate, Iron); Mycophenolate; Nelfinavir; Nilotinib; PONATinib; Posaconazole; Rilpivirine; Riociguat; Risedronate; Vismodegib

The levels/effects of Esomeprazole may be decreased by: CYP2C19 Inducers (Strong); Dabrafenib; Rifampin; St Johns Wort; Tipranavir

Increased Effect/Toxicity

Esomeprazole may increase the levels/effects of: Amphetamine; Benzodiazepines (metabolized by oxidation); Cilostazol; Citalopram; CYP2C19 Substrates; Dexmethylphenidate; Dextroamphetamine; Methotrexate; Methylphenidate; Raltegravir; Risedronate; Saquinavir; Tacrolimus (Systemic); Vitamin K Antagonists; Voriconazole

The levels/effects of Esomeprazole may be increased by: Fluconazole; Ketoconazole (Systemic); Voriconazole

Nutritional/Ethanol Interactions

Food: Absorption is decreased by 43% to 53% when taken with food. Management: Take at least 1 hour before meals at the same time each day, best if before breakfast.

Herb/Nutraceutical: St John's wort may decrease the efficacy of esomeprazole. Management: Avoid St John's wort.

Adverse Reactions

Unless otherwise specified, percentages represent adverse reactions identified in clinical trials evaluating the oral formulation.

>10%: Central nervous system: Headache (I.V. 11%; oral 2% to 8%)

1% to 10%:

Central nervous system: Dizziness (I.V. 3%; oral <1%), somnolence (adults <1%; children 2%)

Dermatologic: Pruritus (I.V. 1%; oral <1%)

Gastrointestinal: Flatulence (I.V. 10%; oral ≤5%), diarrhea (I.V. 4%; oral 2% to <7%), abdominal pain (I.V. 6%; oral 1% to ≤6%), nausea (I.V. 6%; oral 2% to ≤6%), xerostomia (I.V. 4%; oral 3%), constipation (I.V. 3%; oral 2%)

Local: Injection site reaction (I.V. 2%)

Dosage Forms Considerations

Esomeprazole strontium 24.65 mg is equivalent to 20 mg of esomeprazole base; esomeprazole strontium 49.3 mg is equivalent to 40 mg of esomeprazole base.

Available Dosage Forms

Capsule Delayed Release, Oral:
NexIUM: 20 mg, 40 mg
Generic: 24.65 mg, 49.3 mg

Packet, Oral:
NexIUM: 2.5 mg (30 ea); 5 mg (30 ea); 10 mg (30 ea); 20 mg (30 ea); 40 mg (30 ea)

Solution Reconstituted, Intravenous:
NexIUM I.V.: 20 mg (1 ea); 40 mg (1 ea)
Generic: 20 mg (1 ea); 40 mg (1 ea)

General Dosage Range

Dosage adjustment recommended in patients with hepatic impairment.

I.V.:
Children 1 month to <1 year: 0.5 mg/kg once daily
Children ≥1 year and Adolescents ≤17 years: <55 kg: 10 mg once daily; ≥55 kg: 20 mg once daily
Adults: 20-40 mg once daily

Oral:
Children 1 month to <1 year: Esomeprazole magnesium: 3-5 kg: 2.5 mg once daily; >5-7.5 kg: 5 mg once daily; >7.5 kg: 10 mg once daily
Children 1-11 years: Esomeprazole magnesium: <20 kg: 10 mg once daily; ≥20 kg: 10-20 mg once daily
Adolescents 12-17 years: Esomeprazole magnesium: 20-40 mg once daily
Adults: Esomeprazole magnesium, esomeprazole strontium: 20-40 mg (esomeprazole base) once daily **or** 80-240 mg (esomeprazole base) daily in divided doses (hypersecretory conditions)

Usual Infusion Concentrations: Pediatric I.V.

infusion: 0.4 mg/mL **or** 0.8 mg/mL

Usual Infusion Concentrations: Adult I.V. infusion:

20 mg in 50 mL (concentration: 0.4 mg/mL) **or** 40 mg in 50 mL (concentration: 0.8 mg/mL) of D_5W, LR, or NS

Administration

I.V. Flush line prior to and after administration with NS, LR, or D_5W.

Children: Administer by intermittent infusion (10-30 minutes); the manufacturer recommends that children receive intravenous esomeprazole by intermittent infusion only.

Adults: May be administered by injection (≥3 minutes), intermittent infusion (10-30 minutes), or continuous infusion for up to 72 hours (Sung, 2009).

Injectable Detail pH: 9-11

Oral

Capsule: Should be swallowed whole and taken at least 1 hour before eating (best if taken before breakfast). Capsule can be opened and contents mixed with 1 tablespoon of applesauce. Swallow immediately; mixture should not be chewed or warmed. For patients with difficulty swallowing, use of granules may be more appropriate.

Granules: Empty the 2.5 mg or 5 mg packet into a container with 5 mL of water or the 10 mg, 20 mg, or 40 mg packet into a container with 15 mL of water and stir; leave 2-3 minutes to thicken. Stir and drink within 30 minutes. If any medicine remains after drinking, add more water, stir and drink immediately.

Tablet (Canadian formulation, not available in U.S.): Swallow whole or may be dispersed in a half a glass of noncarbonated water. Stir until tablets disintegrate, leaving a liquid containing pellets. Drink contents within 30 minutes. Do not chew or crush pellets. After drinking, rinse glass with water and drink.

Other Nasogastric tube:

Capsule: Open capsule and place intact granules into a 60 mL catheter-tip syringe; mix with 50 mL of water. Replace plunger and shake vigorously for 15 seconds. Ensure that no granules remain in syringe tip. Do not administer if pellets dissolve or disintegrate. Use immediately after preparation. After administration, flush nasogastric tube with additional water.

Granules: Delayed release oral suspension granules can also be given by nasogastric or gastric tube. If using a 2.5 mg or 5 mg packet, first add 5 mL of water to a catheter-tipped syringe, then add granules from packet. If using a 10 mg, 20 mg, or 40 mg packet, first add 15 mL of water to a catheter-tipped syringe, then add granules from packet. Shake the syringe, leave 2-3 minutes to thicken. Shake the syringe and administer through nasogastric or gastric tube (size 6 French or greater) within 30 minutes. Refill the syringe with equal amount (5 mL or 15 mL) of water, shake and flush nasogastric/gastric tube.

Tablet (Canadian formulation, not available in U.S.): Disperse tablets in 50 mL of noncarbonated water. Stir until tablets disintegrate leaving a liquid containing pellets. After administration, flush with additional 25-50 mL of water to clear the syringe and tube.

Preparation for Administration

Granules for oral administration: Empty the 2.5 mg or 5 mg packet into a container with 5 mL of water or empty the 10 mg, 20 mg, or 40 mg packet into a container with 15 mL of water and stir; leave 2-3 minutes to thicken.

Powder for injection:

For I.V. injection: Adults: Reconstitute powder with 5 mL NS.

For I.V. infusion:

Children: Initially reconstitute powder (20 mg or 40 mg) with 5 mL of NS, then further dilute to a final volume of 50 mL; withdraw the appropriate amount of the final solution to administer the intended dose.

Adults: Initially reconstitute powder with 5 mL of NS, LR, or D$_5$W, then further dilute to a final volume of 50 mL.

Storage/Stability

Capsules: Keep container tightly closed.

Esomeprazole magnesium: Store at 25°C (77°F); excursions permitted to 15°C to 30°C (59°F to 86°F).

Esomeprazole strontium: Store at 20°C to 25°C (68°F to 77°F); excursions permitted to 15°C to 30°C (59°F to 86°F).

Granules: Store at 25°C (77°F); excursions permitted to 15°C to 30°C (59°F to 86°F).

Powder for injection: Store at 25°C (77°F); excursions permitted to 15°C to 30°C (59°F to 86°F). Protect from light. Per the manufacturer, following reconstitution, solution for injection prepared in NS, and solution for infusion prepared in NS or LR should be used within 12 hours. Following reconstitution, solution for infusion prepared in D$_5$W should be used within 6 hours. Refrigeration is not required following reconstitution.

Additional stability data: Following reconstitution, solutions for infusion prepared in D$_5$W, NS, or LR in PVC bags are chemically and physically stable for 48 hours at room temperature (25°C) and for at least 120 hours under refrigeration (4°C) (Kupiec, 2008).

Nursing Actions

Physical Assessment Monitor for rebleeding; ongoing diarrhea related to *C. difficile*; fractures in patients with a history of osteoporosis, tetany, arrhythmias; and seizures related to hypomagnesemia. Monitor for common side effects including headache, nausea, abdominal discomfort, dry mouth, diarrhea, gas, constipation, and drowsiness.

Patient Education

• Discuss specific use of drug and side effects with patient as it relates to treatment. (HCAHPS: During this hospital stay, were you given any medicine that you had not taken before? Before giving you any new medicine, how often did hospital staff tell you what the medicine was for? How often did hospital staff describe possible side effects in a way you could understand?)

• Patient may experience headache, fatigue, constipation, flatulence, or xerostomia. Have patient report immediately to prescriber signs of hypomagnesemia, severe dizziness, syncope, considerable dyspepsia, osteodynia, chills, pharyngitis, dyspnea, excessive weight loss, significant diarrhea, signs of Stevens-Johnson syndrome/toxic epidermal necrolysis, or injection site irritation (HCAHPS).

• Educate patient about signs of a significant reaction (eg, wheezing; chest tightness; fever; itching; bad cough; blue skin color; seizures; or swelling of face, lips, tongue, or throat). **Note:** This is not a comprehensive list of all side effects. Patient should consult prescriber for additional questions.

Intended Use and Disclaimer: Should not be printed and given to patients. This information is intended to serve as a concise initial reference for healthcare professionals to use when discussing medications with a patient. You must ultimately rely on your own discretion, experience and judgment in diagnosing, treating and advising patients.

Dietary Considerations Take at least 1 hour before meals; best if taken before breakfast.

Related Information

Oral Medications That Should Not Be Crushed or Altered *on page 1712*

Estradiol (Systemic) (es tra DYE ole)

Brand Names: U.S. Alora; Climara; Delestrogen; Depo-Estradiol; Divigel; Elestrin; Estrace; Estrasorb; Estrogel; Evamist; Femring; Menostar; Minivelle; Vivelle-Dot

Index Terms Estradiol; Estradiol Acetate; Estradiol Transdermal; Estradiol Valerate

Pharmacologic Category Estrogen Derivative

Medication Safety Issues

Sound-alike/look-alike issues:

Alora may be confused with Aldara

Elestrin may be confused with alosetron

BEERS Criteria medication:

This drug may be potentially inappropriate for use in geriatric patients (Quality of evidence - high [oral and transdermal patch]; Strength of recommendation - strong [oral and transdermal patch]).

Other safety issues:

Transdermal patch may contain conducting metal (eg, aluminum); remove patch prior to MRI.

International issues:

Vivelle: Brand name for estradiol [U.S. and multiple international markets, but also the brand name for ethinyl estradiol and norgestimate [Austria]

Pregnancy Risk Factor X

Lactation Enters breast milk/use caution

Use Treatment of moderate-to-severe vasomotor symptoms associated with menopause; treatment of moderate-to-severe vulvar and vaginal atrophy associated with menopause; hypoestrogenism (due to hypogonadism, castration, or primary ovarian failure); advanced prostatic cancer (palliation); metastatic breast cancer (palliation) in men and postmenopausal women; postmenopausal osteoporosis (prophylaxis)

Available Dosage Forms

Emulsion, Transdermal:
Estrasorb: 4.35 mg/1.74 g (1.74 g)

Gel, Transdermal:
Divigel: 0.25 mg/0.25 g (1 ea); 0.5 mg/0.5 g (1 ea); 1 mg/g (1 g)
Elestrin: 0.06% (26 g)
Estrogel: 0.06% (50 g)

Oil, Intramuscular:
Delestrogen: 10 mg/mL (5 mL); 20 mg/mL (5 mL); 40 mg/mL (5 mL)
Depo-Estradiol: 5 mg/mL (5 mL)
Generic: 10 mg/mL (5 mL); 20 mg/mL (5 mL); 40 mg/mL (5 mL)

Patch Biweekly, Transdermal:
Alora: 0.025 mg/24 hr (1 ea, 8 ea); 0.05 mg/24 hr (1 ea, 8 ea); 0.075 mg/24 hr (1 ea, 8 ea); 0.1 mg/24 hr (1 ea, 8 ea)
Minivelle: 0.0375 mg/24 hr (8 ea); 0.05 mg/24 hr (8 ea); 0.075 mg/24 hr (8 ea); 0.1 mg/24 hr (8 ea)
Vivelle-Dot: 0.025 mg/24 hr (8 ea); 0.0375 mg/24 hr (1 ea, 8 ea); 0.05 mg/24 hr (1 ea, 8 ea); 0.075 mg/24 hr (1 ea, 8 ea); 0.1 mg/24 hr (1 ea, 8 ea)

Patch Weekly, Transdermal:
Climara: 0.025 mg/24 hr (4 ea); 0.0375 mg/24 hr (4 ea); 0.05 mg/24 hr (4 ea); 0.06 mg/24 hr (4 ea); 0.075 mg/24 hr (4 ea); 0.1 mg/24 hr (1 ea, 4 ea)
Menostar: 14 mcg/24 hr (4 ea)
Generic: 0.025 mg/24 hr (4 ea); 0.0375 mg/24 hr (4 ea); 0.05 mg/24 hr (4 ea); 0.06 mg/24 hr (4 ea); 0.075 mg/24 hr (4 ea); 0.1 mg/24 hr (4 ea)

Ring, Vaginal:
Femring: 0.05 mg/24 hr (1 ea); 0.1 mg/24 hr (1 ea)

Solution, Transdermal:
Evamist: 1.53 mg/spray (8.1 mL)

Tablet, Oral:
Estrace: 0.5 mg, 1 mg, 2 mg
Generic: 0.5 mg, 1 mg, 2 mg

General Dosage Range

I.M.:
Cypionate:
Adults (females): Hypoestrogenism: 1.5-2 mg monthly
Adults (females): Menopause: 1-5 mg every 3-4 weeks
Valerate:
Adults (females): Menopause: 10-20 mg every 4 weeks
Adults (males): Prostate cancer: 30 mg or more every 1-2 weeks

Oral:
Adults (females): Estrace: Breast cancer: 10 mg 3 times/day; Hypoestrogenism: 1-2 mg/day; Menopause: 0.5-2 mg/day
Adults (males): Estrace: Prostate cancer: 1-2 mg 3 times/day; Breast cancer: 10 mg 3 times/day

Intravaginal: *Adults (females):* (Femring): 0.05-0.1 mg, leave in place for 3 months

Topical: *Adults (females):*
Emulsion (Estrasorb): 3.48 g applied once daily in the morning
Gel: 1.25 g/day (EstroGel) or 0.87-1.7 g/day (Elestrin) or 0.25-1 g/day (Divigel) applied at the same time each day
Spray (Evamist): 1 spray (1.53 mg) per day; dosing range: 1-3 sprays/day

Transdermal: *Adults (females):*
Alora, Estraderm, Minivelle, Vivelle-Dot: Apply twice weekly continuously or cyclically (3 weeks on, 1 week off)
Climara: Apply once weekly continuously or cyclically (3 weeks on, 1 week off)
Menostar: Apply once weekly continuously

Administration

I.M. The use of a progestin should be considered when administering estrogens to postmenopausal women with an intact uterus.
Injection for intramuscular administration only. Estradiol valerate should be injected into the upper outer quadrant of the gluteal muscle; administer with a dry needle (solution may become cloudy with wet needle).

Hazardous agent; use appropriate precautions for handling and disposal (NIOSH, 2012).

Topical The use of a progestin should be considered when administering estrogens to postmenopausal women with an intact uterus.
Emulsion (Estrasorb): Apply to clean, dry skin while in a sitting position. Contents of two pouches (total 3.48 g) are to be applied individually, once daily in the morning. Apply contents of first pouch to left thigh; massage into skin of left thigh and calf until thoroughly absorbed (~3 minutes). Apply excess from both hands to the buttocks. Apply contents of second pouch to the right thigh; massage into skin of right thigh and calf until thoroughly absorbed (~3 minutes). Apply excess from both hands to buttocks. Wash hands with soap and water. Allow skin to dry before covering legs with clothing. Do not apply to other areas of body. Do not apply to red or irritated skin.
Gel: Apply to clean, dry, unbroken skin at the same time each day. Allow to dry for 5 minutes prior to dressing. Gel is flammable; avoid fire or flame until dry. After application, wash hands with soap and water. Prior to the first use, pump must be primed. Do not apply gel to breast.
Divigel: Apply entire contents of packet to right or left upper thigh each day (alternate sites). Do not apply to face, breasts, vaginal area or irritated skin. Apply over an area ~5x7 inches. Do not wash application site for 1 hour. Allow gel to dry before dressing
Elestrin: Apply to upper arm and shoulder area using two fingers to spread gel. Apply after

bath or shower; allow at least 2 hours between applying gel and going swimming. Wait at least 25 minutes before applying sunscreen to application area. Do not apply sunscreen to application area for ≥7 days (may increase absorption of gel).

EstroGel: Apply gel to the arm, from the wrist to the shoulder. Spread gel as thinly as possible over one arm.

Spray: Evamist: Prior to first use, prime pump by spraying 3 sprays with the cover on. To administer dose, hold container upright and vertical and rest the plastic cone flat against the skin while spraying. Spray to the inner surface of the forearm, starting near the elbow. If more than one spray is needed, apply to adjacent but not overlapping areas. Apply at the same time each day. Allow spray to dry for ~2 minutes; do not rub into skin; do not cover with clothing until dry. Do not wash application site for at least 60 minutes. Apply to clean, dry, unbroken skin. Do not apply to skin other than that of the forearm. Make sure that children do not come in contact with any skin area where the drug was applied. If contact with children is unavoidable, wear a garment with long sleeves that covers the site of application. If direct exposure should occur, wash the child in the area of exposure with soap and water as soon as possible. Solution contained in the spray is flammable; avoid fire, flame, or smoking until spray has dried. If needed, sunscreen should be applied ~1 hour prior to application of Evamist.

Transdermal patch: Do not apply transdermal system to breasts, but place on trunk of body (preferably abdomen). Rotate application sites allowing a 1-week interval between applications at a particular site. Do not apply to oily, damaged or irritated skin; avoid waistline or other areas where tight clothing may rub the patch off. Apply patch immediately after removing from protective pouch. In general, if patch falls off, the same patch may be reapplied or a new system may be used for the remainder of the dosing interval (not recommended with all products) When replacing patch, reapply to a new site. Swimming, bathing or showering are not expected to affect use of the patch. Note the following exceptions:

Estraderm: Do not apply to an area exposed to direct sunlight.

Climara, Menostar, Minivelle: Swimming, bathing, or wearing patch while in a sauna have not been studied; adhesion of patch may be decreased or delivery of estradiol may be affected. Showering is not expected to cause the Minivelle patch to fall off. Remove patch slowly after use to avoid skin irritation. If any adhesive remains on the skin after removal, first allow skin to dry for 15 minutes, then gently rub area with an oil-based cream or lotion. If

patch falls off, a new patch should be applied for the remainder of the dosing interval.

Hazardous agent; use appropriate precautions for handling and disposal (NIOSH, 2012).

Other Vaginal ring: Exact positioning is not critical for efficacy; however, patient should not feel anything once inserted. In case of discomfort, ring should be pushed further into vagina. If ring is expelled prior to 90 days, it may be rinsed off and reinserted. Ensure proper vaginal placement of the ring to avoid inadvertent urinary bladder insertion. If vaginal infection develops, Femring may remain in place during local treatment of a vaginal infection.

Hazardous agent; use appropriate precautions for handling and disposal (NIOSH, 2012).

Nursing Actions

Physical Assessment Monitor for CNS changes, hypertension, thromboembolism, fluid retention, edema, CHF, and respiratory changes on a regular basis during therapy. Caution patients with diabetes to monitor glucose levels closely (may impair glucose tolerance). Remind patient about the importance of frequent self-breast exams and the need for annual gynecological exam.

Patient Education

• Discuss specific use of drug and side effects with patient as it relates to treatment. (HCAHPS: During this hospital stay, were you given any medicine that you had not taken before? Before giving you any new medicine, how often did hospital staff tell you what the medicine was for? How often did hospital staff describe possible side effects in a way you could understand?)

• Patient may experience alopecia, cramps, bloating, macromastia, or injection site irritation. Have patient report immediately to prescriber angina, dyspnea, hemoptysis, edema, skin discoloration, painful extremities, severe headache, considerable dizziness, syncope, strength differences from one side to another, difficulty speaking or thinking, change in balance, blurred vision, significant nausea, intolerable dyspepsia, back pain, exophthalmos, contact lens discomfort, vision changes, lump in breast, mastalgia, nipple discharge, vaginitis, vaginal hemorrhaging, depression, mood changes, memory loss, urinary retention, oliguria, dysuria, signs of hepatic impairment, severe skin irritation, or signs of toxic shock syndrome (TSS) (HCAHPS).

• Educate patient about signs of a significant reaction (eg, wheezing; chest tightness; fever; itching; bad cough; blue skin color; seizures; or swelling of face, lips, tongue, or throat). **Note:** This is not a comprehensive list of all side effects. Patient should consult prescriber for additional questions.

Intended Use and Disclaimer: Should not be printed and given to patients. This information is intended to serve as a concise initial reference for healthcare professionals to use when discussing medications with a patient. You must ultimately rely on your own discretion, experience and judgment in diagnosing, treating and advising patients.

Estradiol and Dienogest
(es tra DYE ole & dye EN oh jest)

Brand Names: U.S. Natazia®

Index Terms Dienogest and Estradiol; Estradiol Valerate and Dienogest

Pharmacologic Category Contraceptive; Estrogen and Progestin Combination

Lactation Enters breast milk/not recommended

Use Prevention of pregnancy; treatment of heavy menstrual bleeding

Unlabeled Use Pain associated with endometriosis; dysmenorrhea; treatment of polycystic ovary syndrome (PCOS) in women with menstrual irregularities and hirsutism/acne

Available Dosage Forms

Tablet, oral [four-phasic formulation]:
Natazia®:
Days 1-2: Estradiol valerate 3 mg [2 dark yellow tablets]
Days 3-7: Estradiol valerate 2 mg and dienogest 2 mg [5 medium red tablets]
Days 8-24: Estradiol valerate 2 mg and dienogest 3 mg [17 light yellow tablets]
Days 25-26: Estradiol valerate 1 mg [2 dark red tablets]
Days 27-28: 2 white inactive tablets (28s)

General Dosage Range Oral: *Children and Adults (females, postmenarche):* 1 tablet daily

Administration

Oral Tablets should be taken at the same time each day in the order presented in the blister pack. Do not delay administration by >12 hours. In case of vomiting or diarrhea within 3-4 hours of taking a colored tablet, treat as if the dose was missed (or can take another tablet of the same color from an extra blister pack). Patients should be instructed not to take more than 2 tablets in any one day. A nonhormonal contraceptive (eg, condom or spermicide) should be used for the first 9 days of therapy. If patient is unsure of number of tablets missed, they should continue taking one tablet each day and use a back-up form of contraception.

Hazardous agent; use appropriate precautions for handling and disposal (NIOSH, 2012).

Nursing Actions

Physical Assessment Monitor blood pressure on a regular basis. Teach importance of regular (monthly) blood pressure checks and annual physical assessment; Pap smear; and vision assessment.

Patient Education

• Discuss specific use of drug and side effects with patient as it relates to treatment. (HCAHPS: During this hospital stay, were you given any medicine that you had not taken before? Before giving you any new medicine, how often did hospital staff tell you what the medicine was for? How often did hospital staff describe possible side effects in a way you could understand?)

• Patient may experience acne vulgaris, weight gain, cramps, bloating, macromastia, menstrual irregularities, or sexual dysfunction. Have patient report immediately to prescriber hemoptysis, dyspnea, angina, severe dizziness, syncope, considerable nausea, strength differences from one side to another, difficulty speaking or thinking, change in balance, blurred vision, edema, skin discoloration, painful extremities, significant headache, depression, intolerable asthenia, severe dyspepsia, signs of hepatic impairment, lump in breast, mastalgia, nipple discharge, vaginitis, vaginal hemorrhaging, exophthalmos, vision changes, or contact lens discomfort (HCAHPS).

• Educate patient about signs of a significant reaction (eg, wheezing; chest tightness; fever; itching; bad cough; blue skin color; seizures; or swelling of face, lips, tongue, or throat). **Note:** This is not a comprehensive list of all side effects. Patient should consult prescriber for additional questions.

Intended Use and Disclaimer: Should not be printed and given to patients. This information is intended to serve as a concise initial reference for healthcare professionals to use when discussing medications with a patient. You must ultimately rely on your own discretion, experience and judgment in diagnosing, treating and advising patients.

Related Information
Dienogest *on page 448*

Estradiol and Norethindrone
(es tra DYE ole & nor eth IN drone)

Brand Names: U.S. Activella; CombiPatch; Mimvey

Index Terms Norethindrone and Estradiol

Pharmacologic Category Estrogen and Progestin Combination

Use Women with an intact uterus:

Tablet: Treatment of moderate-to-severe vasomotor symptoms associated with menopause; treatment of moderate-to-severe symptoms of vulvar and vaginal atrophy associated with menopause; prophylaxis for postmenopausal osteoporosis

Transdermal patch: Treatment of moderate-to-severe vasomotor symptoms associated with menopause; treatment of moderate-to-severe symptoms of vulvar and vaginal atrophy associated with menopause; treatment of hypoestrogenism due to hypogonadism, castration, or primary ovarian failure

Available Dosage Forms

Patch, transdermal:

CombiPatch:

0.05/0.14: Estradiol 0.05 mg and norethindrone 0.14 mg per day (8s) [9 sq cm]

0.05/0.25: Estradiol 0.05 mg and norethindrone 0.25 mg per day (8s) [16 sq cm]

Tablet, oral: 0.5/0.1: Estradiol 0.5 mg and norethindrone acetate 0.1 mg (28s); Estradiol 1 mg and norethindrone acetate 0.5 mg (28s)

Activella 0.5/0.1: Estradiol 0.5 mg and norethindrone acetate 0.1 mg (28s)

Activella 1/0.5, Mimvey: Estradiol 1 mg and norethindrone acetate 0.5 mg (28s)

General Dosage Range

Oral: *Adults (females):* 1 tablet daily

Transdermal: *Adults (females):* Apply 1 patch twice weekly

Administration

Topical Transdermal patch: Apply to smooth (fold free), clean, dry skin. Do not apply transdermal patch to breasts; apply to lower abdomen, avoiding waistline (Estalis [Canadian product] may be applied to lower abdomen or buttocks). Do not apply to oily, damaged or irritated skin. Rotate application sites; allow at least a 1-week interval before applying to the same site. Hold system firmly in place for ≥10 seconds. If system falls off, the same system may be applied to another area of the lower abdomen or a new system may be applied if necessary. Only 1 system should be worn during the dosing interval. Do not expose the applied transdermal system to the sun for long periods of time. Following removal of the system, allow area to dry for 15 minutes, then gently rub with an oil-based cream or lotion if needed to remove any remaining adhesive. Women not previously using oral estrogen or estrogen/progestin therapy may initially start the patch at any time. Women on oral therapy should complete the current cycle of therapy prior to starting the patch. If bleeding occurs when the oral cycle is completed, the first day of bleeding is an appropriate time to start the patch.

Hazardous agent; use appropriate precautions for handling and disposal (NIOSH, 2012).

Nursing Actions

Physical Assessment See individual agents.

Patient Education

- Discuss specific use of drug and side effects with patient as it relates to treatment. (HCAHPS: During this hospital stay, were you given any medicine that you had not taken before? Before giving you any new medicine, how often did hospital staff tell you what the medicine was for? How often did hospital staff describe possible side effects in a way you could understand?)

- Patient may experience alopecia, cramps, bloating, or macromastia. Have patient report immediately to prescriber angina, dyspnea, hemoptysis, strength differences from one side to another, difficulty speaking or thinking, change in balance, blurred vision, edema, skin discoloration, painful extremities, severe headache, considerable nausea, significant dyspepsia, intolerable dizziness, syncope, vision changes, exophthalmos, contact lens discomfort, lump in breast, mastalgia, nipple discharge, vaginitis, vaginal hemorrhaging, depression, memory loss, signs of hepatic impairment, or severe skin irritation (HCAHPS).

- Educate patient about signs of a significant reaction (eg, wheezing; chest tightness; fever; itching; bad cough; blue skin color; seizures; or swelling of face, lips, tongue, or throat). **Note:** This is not a comprehensive list of all side effects. Patient should consult prescriber for additional questions.

Intended Use and Disclaimer: Should not be printed and given to patients. This information is intended to serve as a concise initial reference for healthcare professionals to use when discussing medications with a patient. You must ultimately rely on your own discretion, experience and judgment in diagnosing, treating and advising patients.

Related Information

Estradiol (Systemic) *on page 575*

Norethindrone *on page 1139*

Estramustine (es tra MUS teen)

Brand Names: U.S. Emcyt

Index Terms Estramustine Phosphate; Estramustine Phosphate Sodium

Pharmacologic Category Antineoplastic Agent, Alkylating Agent; Antineoplastic Agent, Antimicrotubular; Antineoplastic Agent, Hormone (Estrogen/Nitrogen Mustard)

Medication Safety Issues

Sound-alike/look-alike issues:

Emcyt may be confused with Eryc

Estramustine may be confused with exemestane.

High alert medication:

This medication is in a class the Institute for Safe Medication Practices (ISMP) includes among its list of drug classes which have a heightened risk of causing significant patient harm when used in error.

Breast-Feeding Considerations Estramustine is not indicated for use in women.

Use Prostate cancer: Treatment (palliative) of progressive or metastatic prostate cancer

Mechanism of Action/Effect Estradiol and nornitrogen mustard combination which has antiandrogen effects.

Contraindications Hypersensitivity to estramustine, estradiol, nitrogen mustard, or any component of the formulation; active thrombophlebitis or thromboembolic disorders (except where tumor mass is the cause of thromboembolic disorder and the benefit may outweigh the risk)

Canadian labeling: Additional contraindications (not in the U.S. labeling): Severe hepatic or cardiac disease

Warnings/Precautions Hazardous agent - use appropriate precautions for handling and disposal (NIOSH, 2012). Glucose tolerance may be decreased; use with caution in patients with diabetes. Hypertension (monitor blood pressure periodically), peripheral edema (new-onset or exacerbation), or congestive heart disease may occur; use with caution in patients where fluid accumulation may be poorly tolerated, including cardiovascular disease (HF or hypertension), migraine, seizure disorder or renal dysfunction. Estrogen treatment for prostate cancer is associated with an increased risk of thrombosis and MI; (including fatalities); use caution with history of thrombophlebitis, thrombosis, or thromboembolic disease or history of cerebrovascular or coronary artery disease. Liver enzyme and bilirubin abnormalities may occur; monitor during and for 2 months after treatment. Use with caution in patients with hepatic impairment (may be metabolized poorly) or with metabolic bone diseases. Allergic reactions and angioedema, including airway involvement, have been reported with use. Patients with prostate cancer and osteoblastic metastases are at risk for hypocalcemia; monitor calcium. Estrogenic effects may decrease testosterone levels; may cause gynecomastia and/or impotence. Potentially significant drug-drug/drug-food interactions may exist, requiring dose or frequency adjustment, additional monitoring, and/or selection of alternative therapy. Avoid vaccination with live vaccines during treatment (risk of infection may be increased due to immunosuppression). Although the response to vaccines may be diminished, inactivated vaccines may be administered during treatment. Estramustine is moderately emetogenic; antiemetics may be needed to prevent nausea and vomiting.

Drug Interactions

Avoid Concomitant Use

Avoid concomitant use of Estramustine with any of the following: BCG; Natalizumab; Pimecrolimus; Tacrolimus (Topical); Tofacitinib; Vaccines (Live)

Decreased Effect

Estramustine may decrease the levels/effects of: BCG; Coccidioidin Skin Test; Sipuleucel-T; Vaccines (Inactivated); Vaccines (Live)

The levels/effects of Estramustine may be decreased by: Calcium Salts; Echinacea

Increased Effect/Toxicity

Estramustine may increase the levels/effects of: Leflunomide; Natalizumab; Tofacitinib; Vaccines (Live)

The levels/effects of Estramustine may be increased by: Clodronate; Denosumab; Pimecrolimus; Roflumilast; Tacrolimus (Topical); Trastuzumab

Nutritional/Ethanol Interactions Food: Estramustine serum levels may be decreased if taken with milk or other dairy products, calcium supplements, and vitamins containing calcium. Management: Take on an empty stomach at least 1 hour before or 2 hours after eating.

Adverse Reactions

>10%:
Cardiovascular: Edema (20%)
Endocrine & metabolic: Gynecomastia (75%), breast tenderness (71%), libido decreased
Gastrointestinal: Nausea (16%), diarrhea (13%), gastrointestinal upset (12%)
Hepatic: LDH increased (2% to 33%), AST increased (2% to 33%)
Respiratory: Dyspnea (12%)

1% to 10%:
Cardiovascular: CHF (3%), MI (3%), cerebrovascular accident (2%), chest pain (1%), flushing (1%)
Central nervous system: Lethargy (4%), insomnia (3%), emotional lability (2%), anxiety (1%), headache (1%)
Dermatologic: Bruising (3%), dry skin (2%), pruritus (2%), hair thinning (1%), rash (1%), skin peeling (1%)
Gastrointestinal: Anorexia (4%), flatulence (2%), burning throat (1%), gastrointestinal bleeding (1%), thirst (1%), vomiting (1%)
Hematologic: Leukopenia (4%), thrombocytopenia (1%)
Hepatic: Bilirubin increased (1% to 2%)
Local: Thrombophlebitis (3%)
Neuromuscular & skeletal: Leg cramps (9%)
Ocular: Tearing (1%)
Respiratory: Pulmonary embolism (2%), upper respiratory discharge (1%), hoarseness (1%)

Available Dosage Forms

Capsule, Oral:
Emcyt: 140 mg

General Dosage Range Oral: *Adults (males):* 14 mg/kg/day (range: 10-16 mg/kg/day) in 3 or 4 divided doses

Administration

Oral Administer on an empty stomach, at least 1 hour before or 2 hours after eating. Administer with water; do not administer with milk, milk-based products, or calcium products.

Hazardous agent; use appropriate precautions for handling and disposal (NIOSH, 2012).

Storage/Stability Store refrigerated at 2°C to 8°C (36°F to 46°F).

Nursing Actions

Physical Assessment Monitor for CNS changes, hypertension, and thromboembolism on a regular basis. Caution patients with diabetes to monitor glucose carefully; glucose tolerance may be decreased.

Patient Education

- Discuss specific use of drug and side effects with patient as it relates to treatment. (HCAHPS: During this hospital stay, were you given any medicine that you had not taken before? Before giving you any new medicine, how often did hospital staff tell you what the medicine was for? How often did hospital staff describe possible side effects in a way you could understand?)
- Patient may experience dyspepsia, diarrhea, macromastia, mastalgia, or sexual dysfunction. Have patient report immediately to prescriber strength differences from one side to another, difficulty speaking or thinking, change in balance, blurred vision, angina, tachycardia, severe dizziness, syncope, dyspnea, excessive weight gain, edema of extremities, painful extremities, significant headache, melena, hematemesis, ecchymosis, hemorrhaging, or considerable skin irritation (HCAHPS).
- Educate patient about signs of a significant reaction (eg, wheezing; chest tightness; fever; itching; bad cough; blue skin color; seizures; or swelling of face, lips, tongue, or throat). **Note:** This is not a comprehensive list of all side effects. Patient should consult prescriber for additional questions.

Intended Use and Disclaimer: Should not be printed and given to patients. This information is intended to serve as a concise initial reference for healthcare professionals to use when discussing medications with a patient. You must ultimately rely on your own discretion, experience and judgment in diagnosing, treating and advising patients.

Dietary Considerations Should be taken at least 1 hour before or 2 hours after eating. Milk products and calcium-rich foods or supplements may impair the oral absorption of estramustine phosphate sodium.

Estrogens (Conjugated/Equine) and Bazedoxifene

(ES troe jenz, KON joo gate ed/EE kwine & ba ze DOX i feen)

Brand Names: U.S. Duavee

Index Terms Bazedoxifene and Estrogens (Conjugated/Equine); Duavee; Estrogens (Conjugated/Equine) and Bazedoxifene Acetate

Pharmacologic Category Estrogen Derivative; Selective Estrogen Receptor Modulator (SERM); Tissue-Selective Estrogen Complex (TSEC)

Pregnancy Risk Factor X

Breast-Feeding Considerations Estrogens can be detected in breast milk; excretion of bazedoxifene is not known. Use of this combination product is contraindicated in women who are nursing.

Use

Postmenopausal osteoporosis prophylaxis: Prevention of postmenopausal osteoporosis in women with a uterus

Vasomotor symptoms: Treatment of moderate-to-severe vasomotor symptoms associated with menopause in women with a uterus

Mechanism of Action/Effect The combination of conjugated estrogens and bazedoxifene provides relief of vasomotor symptoms and maintenance of bone mineral density in postmenopausal women with a uterus, while reducing the risk of endometrial hyperplasia observed with estrogen use alone.

Contraindications Angioedema or anaphylactic reaction to estrogens, bazedoxifene, or any component of the formulation; undiagnosed abnormal uterine bleeding; active or past history of venous thromboembolism (VTE) (eg, PE, DVT); active or history of arterial thromboembolic disease (eg, stroke, MI); carcinoma of the breast (known, suspected or history of); estrogen-dependent tumor; hepatic impairment or disease; known protein C, protein S, or antithrombin deficiency or other known thrombophilic disorders; pregnancy or women who may become pregnant; breast-feeding

Warnings/Precautions Hazardous agent: Use appropriate precautions for handling and disposal (NIOSH, 2012).

[U.S. Boxed Warning]: Estrogens should not be used to prevent cardiovascular disease. Using data from the Women's Health Initiative (WHI) studies, an increased risk of deep vein thrombosis (DVT) and stroke has been reported with conjugated estrogens (CE) in postmenopausal women 50-79 years of age. Estrogens and bazedoxifene are known to increase the risk of venous thromboembolism (VTE). Additional risk factors include diabetes mellitus, hypercholesterolemia, hypertension, SLE, obesity, tobacco use, and/or history of VTE. Risk factors should be managed appropriately; discontinue use if adverse cardiovascular events occur or are suspected. Women with inherited thrombophilias (eg, protein C or S deficiency) may have increased risk of venous thromboembolism (DeSancho, 2010; van Vlijmen, 2011). Use is contraindicated in women with protein C, protein S, antithrombin deficiency, or other known thrombophilic disorders. Whenever possible, estrogens should be discontinued at least 4-6 weeks prior to elective surgery associated with an increased risk of thromboembolism or during periods of prolonged immobilization.

[U.S. Boxed Warning]: In the Women's Health Initiative Memory Study (WHIMS), an increased incidence of probable dementia was observed

in women ≥65 years of age taking CE alone. It is not known if this finding applies to younger postmenopausal women. Estrogens should not be used for the prevention of dementia.

[U.S. Boxed Warning]: The use of unopposed estrogen in women with an intact uterus is associated with an increased risk of endometrial cancer. Estrogens (conjugated/equine) in combination with bazedoxifene has been shown to decrease the risk of endometrial hyperplasia, a precursor to endometrial cancer. Adequate diagnostic measures, including endometrial sampling if indicated, should be performed to rule out malignancy in postmenopausal women with undiagnosed abnormal vaginal bleeding. Women taking this combination should not take additional estrogen (may increase the risk of endometrial hyperplasia). Based on data from the Women's Health Initiative (WHI) studies, an increased risk of invasive breast cancer was not observed in postmenopausal women using conjugated estrogens (CE) alone. An increase in abnormal mammogram findings has been reported with estrogen alone. Postmenopausal estrogen therapy may increase the risk of ovarian cancer; however, studies are not consistent, and the effects of this combination product on the risk of ovarian cancer are not known. Although the risk of ovarian cancer is rare, women who are at an increased risk (eg, family history) should be counseled about the association (NAMS, 2012).

[U.S. Boxed Warning]: Women taking estrogens (conjugated/equine) in combination with bazedoxifene should not take additional estrogen. Estrogens should be used for the shortest duration possible at the lowest effective dose consistent with treatment goals. Women taking this combination should also not take progestins or additional estrogen agonists/antagonists. Patients should be reevaluated as clinically appropriate to determine if treatment is still necessary. Available data related to treatment risks are from Women's Health Initiative (WHI) studies, which evaluated oral CE 0.625 mg relative to placebo in postmenopausal women. Other combinations and dosage forms of estrogens were not studied; outcomes should be assumed to be similar for other doses and other dosage forms of estrogens until comparable data becomes available. When used for osteoporosis prevention, use only in women at significant risk of osteoporosis and for who other nonestrogen medications are not considered appropriate.

Estrogens are poorly metabolized in patients with hepatic dysfunction. Use caution with a history of cholestatic jaundice associated with prior estrogen use or pregnancy. Discontinue if jaundice develops or if acute or chronic hepatic disturbances occur. Use is contraindicated with hepatic disease. Estrogens may cause retinal vascular thrombosis;

discontinue pending examination if migraine, loss of vision, proptosis, diplopia, or other visual disturbances occur; discontinue permanently if papilledema or retinal vascular lesions are observed on examination. Use caution in patients with asthma, epilepsy, hepatic hemangiomas, hereditary angioedema, migraine, porphyria, SLE; may exacerbate disease. May have adverse effects on glucose tolerance; use caution in women with diabetes. Use with caution in patients with diseases which may be exacerbated by fluid retention, including cardiac or renal dysfunction. Use of postmenopausal estrogen may be associated with an increased risk of gallbladder disease requiring surgery.

The use of estrogens and/or progestins may change the results of some laboratory tests (eg, coagulation factors, lipids, glucose tolerance, binding proteins). The dose, route, and the specific estrogen/progestin influences these changes. In addition, personal risk factors (eg, cardiovascular disease, smoking, diabetes, age) also contribute to adverse events; use of specific products may be contraindicated in women with certain risk factors. Estrogen compounds are generally associated with lipid effects such as increased HDL-cholesterol and decreased LDL-cholesterol. Triglycerides may also be increased; discontinue if pancreatitis occurs. Use caution in patients with hypoparathyroidism; estrogen-induced hypocalcemia may occur. Estrogens may increase thyroid-binding globulin (TBG) levels leading to increased circulating total thyroid hormone levels. Women on thyroid replacement therapy may require higher doses of thyroid hormone while receiving estrogens.

Bazedoxifene exposure is decreased in women with a BMI >27 kg/m2 which may be associated with an increased risk of endometrial hyperplasia. Women with a BMI >34 kg/m^2 or >32.2 kg/m^2 were excluded from some initial vasomotor or osteoporosis studies, respectively (Lindsay, 2009; Pinkerton, 2009). Regardless of BMI, monitoring should be done to rule out malignancy in postmenopausal women with undiagnosed persistent or recurrent abnormal genital bleeding.

Drug Interactions

Avoid Concomitant Use

Avoid concomitant use of Estrogens (Conjugated/Equine) and Bazedoxifene with any of the following: Anastrozole; Axitinib; Dehydroepiandrosterone; Indium 111 Capromab Pendetide; Ospemifene; Simeprevir

Decreased Effect

Estrogens (Conjugated/Equine) and Bazedoxifene may decrease the levels/effects of: Anastrozole; Anticoagulants; ARIPiprazole; Axitinib; Chenodiol; Hyaluronidase; Ibrutinib; Indium 111 Capromab Pendetide; Ospemifene; Saxagliptin; Simeprevir; Somatropin; Thyroid Products; Ursodiol

The levels/effects of Estrogens (Conjugated/ Equine) and Bazedoxifene may be decreased by: Bosentan; CarBAMazepine; CYP3A4 Inducers (Strong); Cyproterone; Dabrafenib; Deferasirox; Fosphenytoin; Herbs (CYP3A4 Inducers); Mitotane; Peginterferon Alfa-2b; PHE-Nobarbital; Primidone; Rifampin; Tipranavir; Tocilizumab

Increased Effect/Toxicity

Estrogens (Conjugated/Equine) and Bazedoxifene may increase the levels/effects of: Corticosteroids (Systemic); Ospemifene; ROPINIRole; Theophylline Derivatives; Tipranavir

The levels/effects of Estrogens (Conjugated/ Equine) and Bazedoxifene may be increased by: Ascorbic Acid; Dehydroepiandrosterone; Herbs (Estrogenic Properties); NSAID (COX-2 Inhibitor)

Adverse Reactions Percentages as reported with combination product.

1% to 10%:

Central nervous system: Dizziness (5%)

Gastrointestinal: Diarrhea (8%), nausea (8%), dyspepsia (7%), upper abdominal pain (7%)

Neuromuscular & skeletal: Muscle spasm (9%), neck pain (5%)

Respiratory: Oropharyngeal pain (7%)

Pharmacodynamics/Kinetics

Onset of Action

Relief of vasomotor symptoms: A significant reduction in the number and severity of moderate/severe hot flashes was observed after 4 weeks of therapy (Pinkerton, 2009).

Osteoporosis: A significant increase in BMD measured at the lumbar spine and hip was observed at 12 months of therapy (Lindsay, 2009).

Product Availability Duavee: FDA approved October 2013; anticipated availability is first quarter of 2014. Consult prescribing information for additional information.

Available Dosage Forms

Tablet, oral:

Duavee: Conjugated estrogens 0.45 mg and bazedoxifene 20 mg

General Dosage Range Oral: *Adults: Females:* One tablet daily

Administration

Oral Administer once daily, without regard to meals. Patient should swallow tablets whole.

Hazardous agent; use appropriate precautions for handling and disposal (NIOSH, 2012).

Storage/Stability Store at 20°C to 25°C (68°F to 77°F); excursions are permitted between 15°C and 30°C (59°F and 86°F). Dispense in original package. Protect from moisture. After opening foil pouch, product must be used within 60 days.

Nursing Actions

Physical Assessment Monitor blood pressure. Assess for side effects including hypertension, migraines, blood clots.

Patient Education

• Discuss specific use of drug and side effects with patient as it relates to treatment. (HCAHPS: During this hospital stay, were you given any medicine that you had not taken before? Before giving you any new medicine, how often did hospital staff tell you what the medicine was for? How often did hospital staff describe possible side effects in a way you could understand?)

• Patient may experience dizziness, muscle spasms, diarrhea, throat pain, cervicalgia, cramps, or bloating. Have patient report immediately to prescriber signs of hepatic impairment, angina, dyspnea, hemoptysis, edema, severe headache, significant dizziness, syncope, strength differences from one side to another, difficulty speaking or thinking, change in balance, blurred vision, considerable nausea, intolerable dyspepsia, vaginitis, vaginal hemorrhaging, exophthalmos, contact lens discomfort, vision changes, lump in breast, mastalgia, nipple discharge, depression, or memory loss (HCAHPS).

• Educate patient about signs of a significant reaction (eg, wheezing; chest tightness; fever; itching; bad cough; blue skin color; seizures; or swelling of face, lips, tongue, or throat). **Note:** This is not a comprehensive list of all side effects. Patient should consult prescriber for additional questions.

Intended Use and Disclaimer: Should not be printed and given to patients. This information is intended to serve as a concise initial reference for healthcare professionals to use when discussing medications with a patient. You must ultimately rely on your own discretion, experience and judgment in diagnosing, treating and advising patients.

Dietary Considerations Ensure adequate calcium and vitamin D intake when used for the prevention of osteoporosis.

Related Information

Oral Medications That Should Not Be Crushed or Altered *on page 1712*

Estrogens (Conjugated A/Synthetic)
(ES troe jenz, KON joo gate ed, aye, sin THET ik)

Brand Names: U.S. Cenestin

Pharmacologic Category Estrogen Derivative

◀ **Medication Safety Issues**
Sound-alike/look-alike issues:
Cenestin® may be confused with Senexon®
BEERS Criteria medication:
This drug may be potentially inappropriate for use in geriatric patients (Quality of evidence - high; Strength of recommendation - strong).
International issues:
Cenestin [U.S., Canada] may be confused with Canesten which is a brand name for clotrimazole [multiple international markets]
Lactation Enters breast milk/use caution
Use Treatment of moderate-to-severe vasomotor symptoms of menopause; treatment of vulvar and vaginal atrophy
Available Dosage Forms
Tablet, Oral:
Cenestin: 0.3 mg, 0.45 mg, 0.625 mg, 0.9 mg
General Dosage Range Oral: *Adults (females):* 0.3-1.25 mg once daily
Administration
Oral Hazardous agent; use appropriate precautions for handling and disposal (NIOSH, 2012).
Nursing Actions
Physical Assessment Monitor annual gynecological exam. Monitor for thromboembolism, hypertension, edema, and CNS changes on a regular basis during therapy. Caution patients with diabetes to monitor glucose levels closely (may impair glucose tolerance). Remind patient about the importance of frequent self-breast exams and the need for annual gynecological exam.
Patient Education
• Discuss specific use of drug and side effects with patient as it relates to treatment. (HCAHPS: During this hospital stay, were you given any medicine that you had not taken before? Before giving you any new medicine, how often did hospital staff tell you what the medicine was for? How often did hospital staff describe possible side effects in a way you could understand?)
• Patient may experience flatulence, alopecia, bloating, diarrhea, or leg cramps. Have patient report immediately to prescriber signs of hepatic impairment, angina, dyspnea, hemoptysis, strength differences from one side to another, difficulty speaking or thinking, change in balance, blurred vision, edema, skin discoloration, painful extremities, severe headache, considerable nausea, significant dizziness, syncope, vision changes, exophthalmos, contact lens discomfort, lump in breast, mastalgia, nipple discharge, vaginal hemorrhaging, vaginitis, depression, mood changes, or memory loss (HCAHPS).
• Educate patient about signs of a significant reaction (eg, wheezing; chest tightness; fever; itching; bad cough; blue skin color; seizures; or swelling of face, lips, tongue, or throat). **Note:** This is not a comprehensive list of all side effects. Patient should consult prescriber for additional questions.

Intended Use and Disclaimer: Should not be printed and given to patients. This information is intended to serve as a concise initial reference for healthcare professionals to use when discussing medications with a patient. You must ultimately rely on your own discretion, experience and judgment in diagnosing, treating and advising patients.

Estrogens (Conjugated B/Synthetic)
(ES troe jenz, KON joo gate ed, bee, sin THET ik)

Brand Names: U.S. Enjuvia
Pharmacologic Category Estrogen Derivative
Medication Safety Issues
Sound-alike/look-alike issues:
Enjuvia™ may be confused with Januvia®
BEERS Criteria medication:
This drug may be potentially inappropriate for use in geriatric patients (Quality of evidence - high; Strength of recommendation - strong).
Lactation Enters breast milk/use caution
Use Treatment of moderate-to-severe vasomotor symptoms of menopause; treatment of vulvar and vaginal atrophy associated with menopause; treatment of moderate-to-severe vaginal dryness and pain with intercourse associated with menopause
Available Dosage Forms
Tablet, Oral:
Enjuvia: 0.3 mg, 0.45 mg, 0.9 mg, 1.25 mg
General Dosage Range Oral: *Adults (females):* 0.3-1.25 mg once daily
Administration
Oral Hazardous agent; use appropriate precautions for handling and disposal (NIOSH, 2012).
Nursing Actions
Physical Assessment Monitor annual gynecological exam. Monitor for thromboembolism, hypertension, edema, and CNS changes on a regular basis during therapy. Caution patients with diabetes to monitor glucose levels closely (may impair glucose tolerance). Remind patient about the importance of frequent self-breast exams and the need for annual gynecological exam.
Patient Education
• Discuss specific use of drug and side effects with patient as it relates to treatment. (HCAHPS: During this hospital stay, were you given any medicine that you had not taken before? Before giving you any new medicine, how often did hospital staff tell you what the medicine was for? How often did hospital staff describe possible side effects in a way you could understand?)
• Patient may experience flatulence, cramps, bloating, or diarrhea. Have patient report immediately to prescriber angina, dyspnea, hemoptysis, strength differences from one side to

another, difficulty speaking or thinking, change in balance, blurred vision, edema, skin discoloration, painful extremities, severe headache, considerable nausea, significant dizziness, syncope, vision changes, exophthalmos, contact lens discomfort, lump in breast, mastalgia, nipple discharge, vaginitis, vaginal hemorrhaging, depression, memory loss, or signs of hepatic impairment (HCAHPS).

• Educate patient about signs of a significant reaction (eg, wheezing; chest tightness; fever; itching; bad cough; blue skin color; seizures; or swelling of face, lips, tongue, or throat). **Note:** This is not a comprehensive list of all side effects. Patient should consult prescriber for additional questions.

Intended Use and Disclaimer: Should not be printed and given to patients. This information is intended to serve as a concise initial reference for healthcare professionals to use when discussing medications with a patient. You must ultimately rely on your own discretion, experience and judgment in diagnosing, treating and advising patients.

Estrogens (Conjugated/Equine, Systemic) (ES troe jenz KON joo gate ed, EE kwine)

Brand Names: U.S. Premarin

Index Terms C.E.S.; CE; CEE; Conjugated Estrogen; Estrogenic Substances, Conjugated

Pharmacologic Category Estrogen Derivative

Medication Safety Issues

Sound-alike/look-alike issues:

Premarin® may be confused with Primaxin®, Provera®, Remeron®

BEERS Criteria medication:

This drug may be potentially inappropriate for use in geriatric patients (Quality of evidence - high [oral]; Strength of recommendation - strong [oral]).

Lactation Enters breast milk/use caution

Breast-Feeding Considerations Estrogen has been shown to decrease the quantity and quality of human milk. Use only if clearly needed. Monitor the growth of the infant closely.

Use Treatment of moderate-to-severe vasomotor symptoms associated with menopause; treatment of vulvar and vaginal atrophy due to menopause; hypoestrogenism (due to hypogonadism, castration, or primary ovarian failure); prostatic cancer (palliation); breast cancer (palliation); postmenopausal osteoporosis (prophylaxis); abnormal uterine bleeding

Unlabeled Use Uremic bleeding

Mechanism of Action/Effect Estrogens modulate the pituitary secretion of gonadotropins, luteinizing hormone, and follicle-stimulating hormone through a negative feedback system; estrogen replacement reduces elevated levels of these hormones in postmenopausal women

Contraindications Angioedema or anaphylactic reaction to estrogens or any component of the formulation; undiagnosed abnormal vaginal bleeding; history of or current thrombophlebitis or venous thromboembolic disorders (including DVT, PE); active or history of arterial thromboembolic disease (eg, stroke, MI); carcinoma of the breast (except in appropriately selected patients being treated for metastatic disease); estrogen-dependent tumor; hepatic dysfunction or disease; known protein C, protein S, antithrombin deficiency or other known thrombophilic disorders; pregnancy

Canadian labeling: Additional contraindications (not in U.S. labeling): Endometrial hyperplasia; partial or complete vision loss due to ophthalmic vascular disease; migraine with aura

Warnings/Precautions

Hazardous agent - use appropriate precautions for handling and disposal (NIOSH, 2012). Anaphylaxis requiring emergency medical management has been reported within minutes to hours of taking conjugated estrogen (CE) tablets. Angioedema involving the face, feet, hands, larynx, and tongue has also been reported. Exogenous estrogens may exacerbate symptoms in women with hereditary angioedema.

[U.S. Boxed Warning]: Based on data from the Women's Health Initiative (WHI) studies, an increased risk of invasive breast cancer was observed in postmenopausal women using conjugated estrogens (CE) in combination with medroxyprogesterone acetate (MPA). This risk may be associated with duration of use and declines once combined therapy is discontinued (Chlebowski, 2009). The risk of invasive breast cancer was decreased in postmenopausal women with a hysterectomy using CE only, regardless of weight. However, the risk was not significantly decreased in women at high risk for breast cancer (family history of breast cancer, personal history of benign breast disease) (Anderson, 2012). An increase in abnormal mammogram findings has also been reported with estrogen alone or in combination with progestin therapy. Estrogen use may lead to severe hypercalcemia in patients with breast cancer and bone metastases; discontinue estrogen if hypercalcemia occurs. **[U.S. Boxed Warning]: The use of unopposed estrogen in women with an intact uterus is associated with an increased risk of endometrial cancer. The addition of a progestin to estrogen therapy may decrease the risk of endometrial hyperplasia, a precursor to endometrial cancer. Adequate diagnostic measures, including endometrial sampling if indicated, should be performed to rule out malignancy in postmenopausal women with undiagnosed abnormal vaginal bleeding.** Estrogens may exacerbate endometriosis. ▶

Malignant transformation of residual endometrial implants has been reported posthysterectomy with unopposed estrogen therapy. Consider adding a progestin in women with residual endometriosis posthysterectomy. Postmenopausal estrogen therapy and combined estrogen/progesterone therapy may increase the risk of ovarian cancer; however, the absolute risk to an individual woman is small. Although results from various studies are not consistent, risk does not appear to be significantly associated with the duration, route, or dose of therapy. In one study, the risk decreased after 2 years following discontinuation of therapy (Mørch, 2009). Although the risk of ovarian cancer is rare, women who are at an increased risk (eg, family history) should be counseled about the association (NAMS, 2012).

[U.S. Boxed Warning]: Estrogens with or without progestin should not be used to prevent cardiovascular disease. Using data from the Women's Health Initiative (WHI) studies, an increased risk of deep vein thrombosis (DVT) and stroke has been reported with CE and an increased risk of DVT, stroke, pulmonary emboli (PE) and myocardial infarction (MI) has been reported with CE with MPA in postmenopausal women. Additional risk factors include diabetes mellitus, hypercholesterolemia, hypertension, SLE, obesity, tobacco use, and/or history of venous thromboembolism (VTE). Adverse cardiovascular events have also been reported in males taking estrogens for prostate cancer. Risk factors should be managed appropriately; discontinue use if adverse cardiovascular events occur or are suspected. Women with inherited thrombophilias (eg, protein C or S deficiency) may have increased risk of venous thromboembolism (DeSancho, 2010; van Vlijmen, 2011). Use is contraindicated in women with protein C, protein S, antithrombin deficiency, or other known thrombophilic disorders.

[U.S. Boxed Warning]: Estrogens with or without progestin should not be used to prevent dementia. In the Women's Health Initiative Memory Study (WHIMS), an increased incidence of dementia was observed in women ≥65 years of age taking CE alone or in combination with MPA.

Estrogen compounds are generally associated with lipid effects such as increased HDL-cholesterol and decreased LDL-cholesterol. Triglycerides may also be increased; discontinue if pancreatitis occurs. Use with caution in patients with familial defects of lipoprotein metabolism. Estrogens may increase thyroid-binding globulin (TBG) levels leading to increased circulating total thyroid hormone levels. Women on thyroid replacement therapy may require higher doses of thyroid hormone while receiving estrogens. Use caution in patients with hypoparathyroidism; estrogen-induced hypocalcemia may occur. May have adverse effects on glucose tolerance; use caution in women with diabetes. Use caution in patients with asthma, epilepsy, hepatic hemangiomas, porphyria, or SLE; may exacerbate disease. Use with caution in patients with diseases which may be exacerbated by fluid retention, including cardiac or renal dysfunction. Use of postmenopausal estrogen may be associated with an increased risk of gallbladder disease requiring surgery. Use caution with migraine; may exacerbate disease. Canadian labeling contraindicates use in migraine with aura. Estrogens may cause retinal vascular thrombosis; discontinue if migraine, loss of vision, proptosis, diplopia, or other visual disturbances occur; discontinue permanently if papilledema or retinal vascular lesions are observed on examination.

Estrogens are poorly metabolized in patients with hepatic dysfunction. Use caution with a history of cholestatic jaundice associated with prior estrogen use or pregnancy. Discontinue if jaundice develops or if acute or chronic hepatic disturbances occur. Use is contraindicated with hepatic disease.

Whenever possible, estrogens should be discontinued at least 4-6 weeks prior to elective surgery associated with an increased risk of thromboembolism or during periods of prolonged immobilization. Avoid use of oral estrogen (with or without progestins) in the elderly due to potential of increased risk of breast and endometrial cancers, and lack of proven cardioprotection and cognitive protection (Beers Criteria). Prior to puberty, estrogens may cause premature closure of the epiphyses, premature breast development in girls or gynecomastia in boys. Vaginal bleeding and vaginal cornification may also be induced in girls. The use of estrogens and/or progestins may change the results of some laboratory tests (eg, coagulation factors, lipids, glucose tolerance, binding proteins). The dose, route, and the specific estrogen/progestin influences these changes. In addition, personal risk factors (eg, cardiovascular disease, smoking, diabetes, age) also contribute to adverse events; use of specific products may be contraindicated in women with certain risk factors.

[U.S. Boxed Warning]: Estrogens with or without progestin should be used for the shortest duration possible at the lowest effective dose consistent with treatment goals. Before prescribing estrogen therapy to postmenopausal women, the risks and benefits must be weighed for each patient. Women should be informed of these risks and benefits, as well as possible effects of progestin when added to estrogen therapy. Patients should be reevaluated as clinically appropriate to determine if treatment is still necessary. Available data related to treatment risks are from Women's Health Initiative (WHI) studies, which evaluated oral CE 0.625 mg with or without MPA 2.5 mg relative to placebo in postmenopausal women. Other combinations and dosage forms of estrogens and progestins were not studied. **Outcomes reported from clinical trials using CE with or without MPA should be assumed to be similar for other doses and other dosage forms of estrogens and progestins until comparable data becomes available.**

Vulvar and vaginal atrophy use: Moderate-to-severe symptoms of vulvar and vaginal atrophy include vaginal dryness, dyspareunia, and atrophic vaginitis. When used solely for the treatment of vulvar and vaginal atrophy, topical vaginal products should be considered (NAMS, 2007).

Osteoporosis use: For use only in women at significant risk of osteoporosis and for who other nonestrogen medications are not considered appropriate.

Drug Interactions

Avoid Concomitant Use

Avoid concomitant use of Estrogens (Conjugated/ Equine, Systemic) with any of the following: Anastrozole; Axitinib; Dehydroepiandrosterone; Indium 111 Capromab Pendetide; Ospemifene; Simeprevir

Decreased Effect

Estrogens (Conjugated/Equine, Systemic) may decrease the levels/effects of: Anastrozole; Anticoagulants; ARIPiprazole; Axitinib; Chenodiol; Hyaluronidase; Ibrutinib; Indium 111 Capromab Pendetide; Ospemifene; Saxagliptin; Simeprevir; Somatropin; Thyroid Products; Ursodiol

The levels/effects of Estrogens (Conjugated/ Equine, Systemic) may be decreased by: Bosentan; CYP1A2 Inducers (Strong); CYP3A4 Inducers (Strong); Cyproterone; Dabrafenib; Deferasirox; Herbs (CYP3A4 Inducers); Mitotane; Peginterferon Alfa-2b; Tipranavir; Tocilizumab

Increased Effect/Toxicity

Estrogens (Conjugated/Equine, Systemic) may increase the levels/effects of: Corticosteroids (Systemic); Ospemifene; ROPINIRole; Theophylline Derivatives; Tipranavir

The levels/effects of Estrogens (Conjugated/ Equine, Systemic) may be increased by: Ascorbic Acid; Dehydroepiandrosterone; Herbs (Estrogenic Properties); NSAID (COX-2 Inhibitor)

Nutritional/Ethanol Interactions

Ethanol: Avoid ethanol (routine use increases estrogen plasma concentrations and risk of breast cancer). Ethanol may also increase the risk of osteoporosis.

Food: Folic acid absorption may be decreased.

Herb/Nutraceutical: St John's wort may decrease levels. Herbs with estrogenic properties may enhance the adverse/toxic effect of estrogen derivatives; examples include alfalfa, black cohosh, bloodroot, hops, kudzu, licorice, red clover, saw palmetto, soybean, thyme, wild yam, yucca.

Adverse Reactions

Note: Percentages reported in postmenopausal women following oral use.

>10%:

Central nervous system: Headache (26% to 32%; placebo 28%), pain (17% to 20%; placebo 18%)

Endocrine & metabolic: Breast pain (7% to 12%; placebo 9%)

Gastrointestinal: Abdominal pain (15% to 17%), diarrhea (6% to 7%; placebo 6%)

Genitourinary: Vaginal hemorrhage (2% to 14%)

Neuromuscular & skeletal: Back pain (13% to 14%), arthralgia (7% to 14%; placebo 12%)

Respiratory: Pharyngitis (10% to 12%; placebo 11%), sinusitis: (6% to 11%; placebo 7%)

1% to 10%:

Central nervous system: Depression (5% to 8%), dizziness (4% to 6%), nervousness (2% to 5%)

Dermatologic: Pruritus (4% to 5%)

Gastrointestinal: Flatulence (6% to 7%)

Genitourinary: Vaginitis (5% to 7%), leukorrhea (4% to 7%), vaginal moniliasis (5% to 6%)

Neuromuscular & skeletal: Weakness (7% to 8%), leg cramps (3% to 7%)

Respiratory: Cough increased (4% to 7%)

Additional adverse reactions reported with injection; frequency not defined: Local: injection site: Edema, pain, phlebitis

Available Dosage Forms

Solution Reconstituted, Injection:

Premarin: 25 mg (1 ea)

Tablet, Oral:

Premarin: 0.3 mg, 0.45 mg, 0.625 mg, 0.9 mg, 1.25 mg

General Dosage Range

I.M., I.V.: *Children (postmenarche) and Adults (females):* Abnormal uterine bleeding: 25 mg, may repeat in 6-12 hours if needed

Oral:

Adolescents and Adult (females): 0.3-1.25 mg daily or cyclically **or** 10 mg 3 times/day [breast cancer]

Adults (males): Breast cancer: 10 mg 3 times/ day; Prostate cancer: 1.25-2.5 mg 3 times/day

Administration

I.M. May be administered intramuscularly.

Hazardous agent; use appropriate precautions for handling and disposal (NIOSH, 2012).

I.V. Administer I.V. doses slowly to avoid a flushing reaction.

Hazardous agent; use appropriate precautions for handling and disposal (NIOSH, 2012).

Oral Administer at bedtime to minimize adverse effects. May be administered without regard to meals.

Abnormal uterine bleeding: High-dose therapy (eg, 10-20 mg/day) may cause nausea; consider concomitant use of an antiemetic

Hazardous agent; use appropriate precautions for handling and disposal (NIOSH, 2012).

Preparation for Administration Injection: Reconstitute with sterile water for injection; slowly inject diluent against side wall of the vial. Agitate gently; do not shake violently.

Hazardous agent; use appropriate precautions for handling and disposal (NIOSH, 2012).

Storage/Stability

Injection: Refrigerate at 2°C to 8°C (36°F to 46°F) prior to reconstitution. Use immediately following reconstitution.

Tablets: Store at room temperature 20°C to 25°C (68°F to 77°F).

Nursing Actions

Physical Assessment Monitor results of annual gynecological exam. Monitor for thromboembolism, hypertension, edema, and CNS changes on a regular basis during therapy. Caution patients with diabetes to monitor glucose levels closely (may impair glucose tolerance). Remind patient about the importance of frequent self-breast exams and the need for annual gynecological exam. Determine that patient is not pregnant before starting therapy. Do not give to females of childbearing age unless patient is capable of complying with contraceptive use. Advise patient about appropriate contraceptive measures as appropriate.

Patient Education

- Discuss specific use of drug and side effects with patient as it relates to treatment. (HCAHPS: During this hospital stay, were you given any medicine that you had not taken before? Before giving you any new medicine, how often did hospital staff tell you what the medicine was for? How often did hospital staff describe possible side effects in a way you could understand?)
- Patient may experience alopecia, mastalgia, macromastia, cramps, bloating, or injection site irritation. Have patient report immediately to prescriber signs of hepatic impairment, signs of pancreatitis, angina, dyspnea, hemoptysis, strength differences from one side to another, difficulty speaking or thinking, change in balance, blurred vision, edema, skin discoloration, painful extremities, severe headache, considerable nausea, significant dizziness, syncope, pelvic pain, vision changes, exophthalmos, contact lens discomfort, lump in breast, mastalgia, nipple discharge, vaginal hemorrhaging, vaginitis, depression, mood changes, or memory loss (HCAHPS).
- Educate patient about signs of a significant reaction (eg, wheezing; chest tightness; fever; itching; bad cough; blue skin color; seizures; or swelling of face, lips, tongue, or throat). **Note:** This is not a comprehensive list of all side effects. Patient should consult prescriber for additional questions.

Intended Use and Disclaimer: Should not be printed and given to patients. This information is intended to serve as a concise initial reference for healthcare professionals to use when discussing medications with a patient. You must ultimately rely on your own discretion, experience and judgment in diagnosing, treating and advising patients.

Dietary Considerations Ensure adequate calcium and vitamin D intake when used for the prevention of osteoporosis. Powder for reconstitution for injection (25 mg) contains lactose 200 mg.

Estrogens (Conjugated/Equine, Topical) (ES troe jenz KON joo gate ed, EE kwine)

Brand Names: U.S. Premarin

Index Terms C.E.S.; CE; CEE; Conjugated Estrogen; Estrogenic Substances, Conjugated

Pharmacologic Category Estrogen Derivative

Medication Safety Issues

Sound-alike/look-alike issues:

Premarin® may be confused with Primaxin®, Provera®, Remeron®

BEERS Criteria medication:

This drug may be potentially inappropriate for use in geriatric patients (Quality of evidence - moderate [topical]; Strength of recommendation - weak [topical]).

Lactation Enters breast milk/use caution

Use Treatment of atrophic vaginitis and kraurosis vulvae; moderate-to-severe dyspareunia (pain during intercourse) due to vaginal/vulvar atrophy of menopause

Available Dosage Forms

Cream, Vaginal:

Premarin: 0.625 mg/g (30 g)

General Dosage Range Intravaginal: *Adults (females):*

Atrophic vaginitis, kraurosis vulvae: 0.5-2 g/day given cyclically

Moderate-to-severe dyspareunia due to menopause: 0.5 g twice weekly (eg, Monday and Thursday) **or** once daily cyclically

Administration

Intravaginal Administer at bedtime to minimize adverse effects. Applicator calibrated in 0.5 g increments up to 2 g. To clean applicator, remove plunger from barrel. Wash with mild soap and warm water; do not boil or use hot water.

Hazardous agent; use appropriate precautions for handling and disposal (NIOSH, 2012).

Nursing Actions

Physical Assessment Monitor results of annual gynecological exam. Monitor for thromboembolism, hypertension, edema, and CNS changes on a regular basis during therapy. Caution patients with diabetes to monitor glucose levels closely (may impair glucose tolerance). Remind patient about the importance of frequent self-breast exams and the need for annual gynecological exam. Determine that patient is not pregnant before starting therapy.

Patient Education
- Discuss specific use of drug and side effects with patient as it relates to treatment. (HCAHPS: During this hospital stay, were you given any medicine that you had not taken before? Before giving you any new medicine, how often did hospital staff tell you what the medicine was for? How often did hospital staff describe possible side effects in a way you could understand?)
- Patient may experience alopecia, macromastia, cramps, or bloating. Have patient report immediately to prescriber signs of hepatic impairment, signs of pancreatitis, angina, dyspnea, hemoptysis, strength differences from one side to another, difficulty speaking or thinking, change in balance, blurred vision, edema, skin discoloration, painful extremities, severe headache, considerable nausea, significant dizziness, syncope, pelvic pain, vision changes, exophthalmos, contact lens discomfort, lump in breast, mastalgia, nipple discharge, vaginal hemorrhaging, vaginitis, significant vaginal irritation, depression, mood changes, or memory loss (HCAHPS).
- Educate patient about signs of a significant reaction (eg, wheezing; chest tightness; fever; itching; bad cough; blue skin color; seizures; or swelling of face, lips, tongue, or throat). **Note:** This is not a comprehensive list of all side effects. Patient should consult prescriber for additional questions.

Intended Use and Disclaimer: Should not be printed and given to patients. This information is intended to serve as a concise initial reference for healthcare professionals to use when discussing medications with a patient. You must ultimately rely on your own discretion, experience and judgment in diagnosing, treating and advising patients.

Estrogens (Conjugated/Equine) and Medroxyprogesterone
(ES troe jenz KON joo gate ed/EE kwine & me DROKS ee proe JES te rone)

Brand Names: U.S. Premphase®; Prempro®
Index Terms Medroxyprogesterone and Estrogens (Conjugated); MPA and Estrogens (Conjugated)
Pharmacologic Category Estrogen and Progestin Combination
Medication Safety Issues
 BEERS Criteria medication:
 This drug may be potentially inappropriate for use in geriatric patients (Quality of evidence - high [oral]; Strength of recommendation - strong [oral]).
Lactation Enters breast milk/use caution

Use Women with an intact uterus: Treatment of moderate-to-severe vasomotor symptoms associated with menopause; treatment of moderate-to-severe vulvar and vaginal atrophy due to menopause; postmenopausal osteoporosis (prophylaxis)

Available Dosage Forms
 Tablet:
 Premphase® [therapy pack contains two separate tablet formulations]: Conjugated estrogens 0.625 mg [14 maroon tablets] and conjugated estrogen 0.625 mg/medroxyprogesterone 5 mg [14 light blue tablets] (28s)
 Prempro®:
 0.3/1.5: Conjugated estrogens 0.3 mg and medroxyprogesterone 1.5 mg (28s)
 0.45/1.5: Conjugated estrogens 0.45 mg and medroxyprogesterone 1.5 mg (28s)
 0.625/2.5: Conjugated estrogens 0.625 mg and medroxyprogesterone 2.5 mg (28s)
 0.625/5: Conjugated estrogens 0.625 mg and medroxyprogesterone 5 mg (28s)

General Dosage Range Oral: *Adults (females):* Prempro®: Conjugated estrogen 0.3-0.625 mg/mPA 1.5-5 mg once daily **or** Premphase®: One 0.625 mg tablet daily on days 1 through 14 and 1 conjugated estrogen 0.625 mg/mPA 5 mg tablet daily on days 15 through 28

Administration
 Oral Hazardous agent; use appropriate precautions for handling and disposal (NIOSH, 2012).

Nursing Actions
 Physical Assessment See individual agents.
 Patient Education
- Discuss specific use of drug and side effects with patient as it relates to treatment. (HCAHPS: During this hospital stay, were you given any medicine that you had not taken before? Before giving you any new medicine, how often did hospital staff tell you what the medicine was for? How often did hospital staff describe possible side effects in a way you could understand?)
- Patient may experience cramps, bloating, macromastia, or alopecia. Have patient report immediately to prescriber angina, dyspnea, strength differences from one side to another, difficulty speaking or thinking, change in balance, blurred vision, edema, skin discoloration, painful extremities, severe headache, considerable nausea, significant dizziness, syncope, exophthalmos, contact lens discomfort, vision changes, ophthalmalgia, intolerable eye irritation, lump in breast, mastalgia, nipple discharge, vaginal hemorrhaging, vaginitis, depression, memory loss, or signs of hepatic impairment (HCAHPS).

• Educate patient about signs of a significant reaction (eg, wheezing; chest tightness; fever; itching; bad cough; blue skin color; seizures; or swelling of face, lips, tongue, or throat). **Note:** This is not a comprehensive list of all side effects. Patient should consult prescriber for additional questions.

Intended Use and Disclaimer: Should not be printed and given to patients. This information is intended to serve as a concise initial reference for healthcare professionals to use when discussing medications with a patient. You must ultimately rely on your own discretion, experience and judgment in diagnosing, treating and advising patients.

Related Information

Estrogens (Conjugated/Equine, Systemic) *on page 585*

MedroxyPROGESTERone *on page 987*

Estrogens (Esterified)
(ES troe jenz, es TER i fied)

Brand Names: U.S. Menest

Index Terms Esterified Estrogens

Pharmacologic Category Estrogen Derivative

Medication Safety Issues

BEERS Criteria medication:

This drug may be potentially inappropriate for use in geriatric patients (Quality of evidence - high [oral]; Strength of recommendation - strong [oral]).

Lactation Enters breast milk/use caution

Use Treatment of moderate-to-severe vasomotor symptoms associated with menopause; treatment of moderate-to-severe vulvar and vaginal atrophy associated with menopause; hypoestrogenism (due to hypogonadism, castration, or primary ovarian failure); advanced prostatic cancer (palliation), metastatic breast cancer (palliation) in men and postmenopausal women

Available Dosage Forms

Tablet, Oral:

Menest: 0.3 mg, 0.625 mg, 1.25 mg, 2.5 mg

General Dosage Range

Oral:

Adults (females): Hypogonadism: 2.5-7.5 mg/day for 20 days followed by a 10-day rest, repeat until response; Castration or ovarian failure: 1.25 mg/day, cyclically; Menopause 0.3-1.25 mg/day given cyclically; Breast cancer: 10 mg 3 times/day

Adults (males): Breast cancer: 10 mg 3 times/day; Prostate cancer: 1.25-2.5 mg 3 times/day

Administration

Oral Administer with food at same time each day.

Hazardous agent; use appropriate precautions for handling and disposal (NIOSH, 2012).

Nursing Actions

Physical Assessment Assess results of annual gynecological exam. Monitor for thromboembolism, hypertension, edema, and CNS changes on a regular basis during therapy. Caution patients with diabetes to monitor glucose levels closely (may impair glucose tolerance). Remind patient about the importance of frequent self-breast exams and the need for annual gynecological exam.

Patient Education

• Discuss specific use of drug and side effects with patient as it relates to treatment. (HCAHPS: During this hospital stay, were you given any medicine that you had not taken before? Before giving you any new medicine, how often did hospital staff tell you what the medicine was for? How often did hospital staff describe possible side effects in a way you could understand?)

• Patient may experience headache, alopecia, mastalgia, leg cramps, bloating, or nausea. Have patient report immediately to prescriber signs of hepatic impairment, signs of pancreatitis, angina, dyspnea, hemoptysis, strength differences from one side to another, difficulty speaking or thinking, change in balance, blurred vision, edema, skin discoloration, painful extremities, severe headache, significant dizziness, syncope, vision changes, exophthalmos, contact lens discomfort, lump in breast, mastalgia, nipple discharge, vaginal hemorrhaging, vaginitis, depression, mood changes, or memory loss (HCAHPS).

• Educate patient about signs of a significant reaction (eg, wheezing; chest tightness; fever; itching; bad cough; blue skin color; seizures; or swelling of face, lips, tongue, or throat). **Note:** This is not a comprehensive list of all side effects. Patient should consult prescriber for additional questions.

Intended Use and Disclaimer: Should not be printed and given to patients. This information is intended to serve as a concise initial reference for healthcare professionals to use when discussing medications with a patient. You must ultimately rely on your own discretion, experience and judgment in diagnosing, treating and advising patients.

Eszopiclone (es zoe PIK lone)

Brand Names: U.S. Lunesta

Pharmacologic Category Hypnotic, Miscellaneous

Medication Safety Issues
Sound-alike/look-alike issues:
 Lunesta® may be confused with Neulasta®
BEERS Criteria medication:
 This drug may be potentially inappropriate for use in geriatric patients (Quality of evidence - moderate; Strength of recommendation - strong).
Medication Guide Available Yes
Pregnancy Risk Factor C
Lactation Excretion in breast milk unknown
Breast-Feeding Considerations It is not known if eszopiclone is excreted in breast milk. Eszopiclone is the S-isomer of the racemic derivative zopiclone. Zopiclone is excreted in human milk and is not recommended for use while breast-feeding.
Use Treatment of insomnia (with difficulty of sleep onset and/or sleep maintenance)
Mechanism of Action/Effect Interact with the GABA-receptor complex to promote sleep.
Contraindications Hypersensitivity to eszopiclone or any component of the formulation.
Warnings/Precautions Symptomatic treatment of insomnia should be initiated only after careful evaluation of potential causes of sleep disturbance. Failure of sleep disturbance to resolve after 7-10 days may indicate psychiatric and/or medical illness. Administer only when the patient is able to stay in bed a full night (7-8 hours) before being active again. Tolerance did not develop over 6 months of use. May cause CNS depression impairing physical and mental capabilities; patients must be cautioned about performing tasks which require mental alertness (operating machinery or driving); dose adjustment may be necessary if taking concomitant CNS depressants. Potentially significant interactions may exist, requiring dose or frequency adjustment, additional monitoring, and/or selection of alternative therapy.

Use with caution in patients with depression; worsening of depression, including suicidal ideation has been reported with the use of hypnotics. Intentional overdose may be an issue with this population. The minimum dose that will effectively treat the individual patient should be used. Prescriptions should be written for the smallest quantity consistent with good patient care. Use caution in patients with a history of drug dependence. Hypnotics/sedatives have been associated with abnormal thinking and behavior changes including decreased inhibition, aggression, bizarre behavior, agitation, hallucinations, and depersonalization. These changes may occur unpredictably and may indicate previously unrecognized psychiatric disorders; evaluate appropriately. An increased risk for hazardous sleep-related activities such as sleep-driving, cooking and eating food, and making phone calls while asleep has also been noted; amnesia may also occur. The use of alcohol, other CNS depressants, and exceeding the recommended maximum dose may increase the risk of

these activities. Discontinue treatment in patients who report any sleep-related episodes. Use caution in patients with respiratory compromise, COPD, sleep apnea, and hepatic dysfunction (dose adjustment recommended with severe impairment). Because of the rapid onset of action, administer immediately prior to bedtime or after the patient has gone to bed and is having difficulty falling asleep. Abrupt discontinuance may lead to withdrawal symptoms. Hypersensitivity reactions including anaphylaxis as well as angioedema have been reported, in some cases following initial dosing. Patients who develop severe reactions should not be rechallenged.

Use with caution in debilitated and elderly patients; dosage adjustment recommended. Closely monitor elderly or debilitated patients for impaired cognitive and/or motor performance, confusion, and potential for falling. Avoid chronic use (>90 days) in older adults; adverse events, including delirium, falls, fractures, have been observed with nonbenzodiazepine hypnotic use in the elderly similar to events observed with benzodiazepines. Data suggests improvements in sleep duration and latency are minimal (Beers Criteria).
Drug Interactions
Avoid Concomitant Use
 Avoid concomitant use of Eszopiclone with any of the following: Azelastine (Nasal); Conivaptan; Fusidic Acid (Systemic); Paraldehyde; Sodium Oxybate; Thalidomide
Decreased Effect
 The levels/effects of Eszopiclone may be decreased by: Bosentan; CYP3A4 Inducers (Strong); Dabrafenib; Deferasirox; Flumazenil; Herbs (CYP3A4 Inducers); Mitotane; Tocilizumab
Increased Effect/Toxicity
 Eszopiclone may increase the levels/effects of: Alcohol (Ethyl); Azelastine (Nasal); Buprenorphine; CNS Depressants; Hydrocodone; Methotrimeprazine; Metyrosine; Mirtazapine; Paraldehyde; Pramipexole; ROPINIRole; Rotigotine; Selective Serotonin Reuptake Inhibitors; Sodium Oxybate; Thalidomide; Zolpidem

The levels/effects of Eszopiclone may be increased by: Brimonidine (Topical); Conivaptan; CYP3A4 Inhibitors (Moderate); CYP3A4 Inhibitors (Strong); Dasatinib; Doxylamine; Droperidol; Fusidic Acid (Systemic); HydrOXYzine; Ivacaftor; Luliconazole; Magnesium Sulfate; Methotrimeprazine; Mifepristone; Perampanel; Simeprevir; Stiripentol; Tapentadol
Nutritional/Ethanol Interactions
 Ethanol: Ethanol may increase CNS depression. Management: Avoid ethanol.
 Food: Onset of action may be reduced if taken with or immediately after a heavy meal. Management: Take immediately prior to bedtime, not with or immediately after a heavy or high-fat meal.

Herb/Nutraceutical: Some herbal medications may increase CNS depression. Management: Avoid valerian, St John's wort, kava kava, and gotu kola.

Adverse Reactions

>10%:

Central nervous system: Headache (15% to 21%)

Gastrointestinal: Unpleasant taste (8% to 34%)

1% to 10%:

Cardiovascular: Cardiovascular: Chest pain (≥1%), peripheral edema (≥1%)

Central nervous system: Somnolence (8% to 10%), dizziness (5% to 7%), pain (4% to 5%), nervousness (up to 5%), depression (1% to 4%), confusion (up to 3%), hallucinations (1% to 3%), anxiety (1% to 3%), abnormal dreams (1% to 3%), migraine

Dermatologic: Rash (3% to 4%), pruritus (1% to 4%)

Endocrine & metabolic: Libido decreased (up to 3%), dysmenorrhea (up to 3%), gynecomastia (males up to 3%)

Gastrointestinal: Xerostomia (3% to 7%), dyspepsia (2% to 6%), nausea (4% to 5%), diarrhea (2% to 4%), vomiting (up to 3%)

Genitourinary: Urinary tract infection (up to 3%)

Neuromuscular & skeletal: Neuralgia (up to 3%)

Miscellaneous: Infection (5% to 10%), viral infection (3%), accidental injury (up to 3%)

Controlled Substance C-IV

Available Dosage Forms

Tablet, Oral:

Lunesta: 1 mg, 2 mg, 3 mg

General Dosage Range Dosage adjustment recommended in patients with hepatic impairment or on concomitant therapy

Oral:

Adults: Initial: 1-2 mg immediately before bedtime (maximum: 3 mg daily)

Elderly: 1-2 mg immediately before bedtime (maximum: 2 mg daily)

Administration

Oral Because of the rapid onset of action, eszopiclone should be administered immediately prior to bedtime or after the patient has gone to bed and is having difficulty falling asleep. Do not take with, or immediately following, a high-fat meal.

Storage/Stability Store at 25°C (77°F); excursions permitted to 15°C to 30°C (59°F to 86°F).

Nursing Actions

Physical Assessment Evaluate potential causes of insomnia prior to initiating medication. Monitor for excessive CNS depression, abnormal thinking, and behavior changes. For inpatient use, institute safety measures (side rails, night light, call bell, assistance with ambulation).

Patient Education

• Discuss specific use of drug and side effects with patient as it relates to treatment. (HCAHPS: During this hospital stay, were you given any medicine that you had not taken before? Before giving you any new medicine, how often did hospital staff tell you what the medicine was for? How often did hospital staff describe possible side effects in a way you could understand?)

• Patient may experience parageusia, xerostomia, headache, or fatigue. Have patient report immediately to prescriber signs of depression (ie, suicidal ideation, anxiety, emotional instability, illogical thinking), hallucinations, memory loss, severe dizziness, change in balance, or significant asthenia (HCAHPS).

• Educate patient about signs of a significant reaction (eg, wheezing; chest tightness; fever; itching; bad cough; blue skin color; seizures; or swelling of face, lips, tongue, or throat). **Note:** This is not a comprehensive list of all side effects. Patient should consult prescriber for additional questions.

Intended Use and Disclaimer: Should not be printed and given to patients. This information is intended to serve as a concise initial reference for healthcare professionals to use when discussing medications with a patient. You must ultimately rely on your own discretion, experience and judgment in diagnosing, treating and advising patients.

Dietary Considerations Avoid taking after a heavy meal; may delay onset.

Etanercept (et a NER sept)

Brand Names: U.S. Enbrel; Enbrel SureClick

Pharmacologic Category Antirheumatic, Disease Modifying; Tumor Necrosis Factor (TNF) Blocking Agent

Medication Safety Issues

Sound-alike/look-alike issues:

Enbrel may be confused with Levbid

Medication Guide Available Yes

Pregnancy Risk Factor B

Lactation Enters breast milk/use caution.

Breast-Feeding Considerations Etanercept is excreted into breast milk in low concentrations and is minimally absorbed by a nursing infant (limited data). The manufacturer recommends that caution be used if administered to a nursing woman, taking into account the importance of the drug to the mother and potential effects to the nursing infant. A lactation surveillance program has been established to monitor outcomes of breastfed infants exposed to etanercept (800-772-6436).

Use

Ankylosing spondylitis: For reducing signs and symptoms in patients with active ankylosing spondylitis.

Plaque psoriasis: For treatment of adults ≥18 years of age with chronic moderate to severe plaque psoriasis who are candidates for systemic therapy or phototherapy.

Polyarticular juvenile idiopathic arthritis: For reducing signs and symptoms of moderately to severely active polyarticular juvenile idiopathic arthritis in patients ≥2 years of age.

Psoriatic arthritis: For reducing signs and symptoms, inhibiting the progression of structural damage of active arthritis, and improving physical function in patients with psoriatic arthritis. Etanercept can be used in combination with methotrexate in patients who do not respond adequately to methotrexate alone.

Rheumatoid arthritis: For reducing signs and symptoms, inducing major clinical response, inhibiting the progression of structural damage, and improving physical function in patients with moderately to severely active rheumatoid arthritis (RA). Etanercept can be initiated in combination with methotrexate or used alone.

Unlabeled Use Treatment of acute graft-versus-host disease (GVHD).

Mechanism of Action/Effect Etanercept is a recombinant DNA-derived protein composed of tumor necrosis factor receptor (TNFR) linked to the Fc portion of human IgG1. Etanercept binds tumor necrosis factor (TNF) and blocks its interaction with cell surface receptors. TNF plays an important role in the inflammatory processes and the resulting joint pathology of rheumatoid arthritis (RA), polyarticular-course juvenile idiopathic arthritis (JIA), ankylosing spondylitis (AS), and plaque psoriasis.

Contraindications Sepsis

Warnings/Precautions [U.S. Boxed Warning]: Patients receiving etanercept are at increased risk for serious infections which may result in hospitalization and/or fatality; infections usually developed in patients receiving concomitant immunosuppressive agents (eg, methotrexate or corticosteroids) and may present as disseminated (rather than local) disease. Active tuberculosis (or reactivation of latent tuberculosis), invasive fungal (including aspergillosis, blastomycosis, candidiasis, coccidioidomycosis, histoplasmosis, and pneumocystosis) and bacterial, viral or other opportunistic infections (including legionellosis and listeriosis) have been reported in patients receiving TNF-blocking agents, including etanercept. Monitor closely for signs/symptoms of infection. Discontinue for serious infection or sepsis. Consider risks versus benefits prior to use in patients with a history of chronic or recurrent infection. Consider empiric antifungal therapy in patients who are at risk for invasive fungal infection and develop severe systemic illness. Caution should be exercised when considering use in the elderly or in patients with conditions that predispose them to infections (eg, diabetes) or residence/travel from areas of endemic mycoses (blastomycosis, coccidioidomycosis, histoplasmosis), or with latent or localized infections. Do not initiate etanercept therapy with clinically important active infection. Patients who develop a new infection while undergoing treatment should be monitored closely. **[U.S. Boxed Warning]: Tuberculosis (disseminated or extrapulmonary) has been reported in patients receiving etanercept; both reactivation of latent infection and new infections have been reported.** Patients should be evaluated for tuberculosis risk factors and for latent tuberculosis infection with a tuberculin skin test prior to starting therapy. Treatment of latent tuberculosis should be initiated before etanercept therapy; consider antituberculosis treatment if adequate course of treatment cannot be confirmed in patients with a history of latent or active tuberculosis or with risk factors despite negative skin test. Some patients who tested negative prior to therapy have developed active infection; tests for latent tuberculosis infection may be falsely negative while on etanercept therapy. Monitor for signs and symptoms of tuberculosis in all patients. Rare reactivation of hepatitis B virus (HBV) has occurred in chronic virus carriers, usually in patients receiving concomitant immunosuppressants; evaluate for HBV prior to initiation in all patients. Monitor during and for several months following discontinuation of treatment in HBV carriers; interrupt therapy if reactivation occurs and treat appropriately with antiviral therapy; if resumption of therapy is deemed necessary, exercise caution and monitor patient closely. Patients should be brought up to date with all immunizations before initiating therapy. Live vaccines should not be given concurrently with etanercept; there is no data available concerning secondary transmission of live vaccines in patients receiving therapy. Patients with a significant exposure to varicella virus should temporarily discontinue etanercept. Treatment with varicella zoster immune globulin should be considered.

[U.S. Boxed Warning]: Lymphoma and other malignancies have been reported in children and adolescent patients receiving TNF-blocking agents, including etanercept. Half of the malignancies reported in children were lymphomas (Hodgkin and non-Hodgkin) while other cases varied and included malignancies not typically observed in this population. The impact of etanercept on the development and course of malignancy is not fully defined. Compared to the general population, an increased risk of lymphoma has been noted in clinical trials; however, rheumatoid arthritis alone has been previously associated with an increased rate of lymphoma. Lymphomas and other malignancies were also observed (at rates higher than expected for the general population) in adult patients receiving etanercept. Etanercept is not recommended for use in patients with Wegener's granulomatosis who are receiving immunosuppressive therapy due to higher incidence of noncutaneous solid malignancies. Hepatosplenic

T-cell lymphoma (HSTCL), a rare T-cell lymphoma, has also been associated with TNF-blocking agents, primarily reported in adolescent and young adult males with Crohn's disease or ulcerative colitis. Melanoma, nonmelanoma skin cancer, and Merkel cell carcinoma have been reported in patients receiving TNF-blocking agents, including etanercept. Perform periodic skin examinations in all patients during therapy, particularly those at increased risk of skin cancer. Positive antinuclear antibody titers have been detected in patients (with negative baselines). Rare cases of autoimmune disorder, including lupus-like syndrome or auto-immune hepatitis, have been reported; monitor and discontinue if symptoms develop.

Allergic reactions may occur; if an anaphylactic reaction or other serious allergic reaction occurs, administration should be discontinued immediately and appropriate therapy initiated. Use with caution in patients with pre-existing or recent onset CNS demyelinating disorders; rare cases of new-onset or exacerbation of CNS demyelinating disorders have occurred; may present with mental status changes and some may be associated with perma-nent disability. Optic neuritis, transverse myelitis, multiple sclerosis, Guillain-Barré syndrome, other peripheral demyelinating neuropathies, and new-onset or exacerbation of seizures have been reported. Use with caution in patients with heart failure or decreased left ventricular function; wor-sening and new-onset heart failure has been reported, including in patients without known pre-existing cardiovascular disease. Use caution in patients with a history of significant hematologic abnormalities; has been associated with pancyto-penia and aplastic anemia (rare). Patients must be advised to seek medical attention if they develop signs and symptoms suggestive of blood dyscra-sias; discontinue if significant hematologic abnor-malities are confirmed. Use with caution in patients with moderate to severe alcoholic hepatitis. Com-pared to placebo, the mortality rate in patients treated with etanercept was similar at one month but significantly higher after 6 months.

Due to a higher incidence of serious infections, concomitant use with anakinra is not recom-mended. Hypoglycemia has been reported in patients receiving concomitant therapy with etaner-cept and antidiabetic medications; dose reduction of antidiabetic medication may be necessary. Use with caution in patient with diabetes; monitor blood glucose as clinically necessary. Some dosage forms may contain dry natural rubber (latex). Some dosage forms may contain benzyl alcohol which has been associated with "gasping syndrome" in neonates.

Drug Interactions

Avoid Concomitant Use

Avoid concomitant use of Etanercept with any of the following: Abatacept; Anakinra; BCG; Belimumab; Canakinumab; Certolizumab Pegol; Cyclophosphamide; InFLIXimab; Natalizumab; Pimecrolimus; Rilonacept; Tacrolimus (Topical); Tocilizumab; Tofacitinib; Vaccines (Live)

Decreased Effect

Etanercept may decrease the levels/effects of: BCG; Coccidioidin Skin Test; Sipuleucel-T; Vac-cines (Inactivated); Vaccines (Live)

The levels/effects of Etanercept may be decreased by: Echinacea

Increased Effect/Toxicity

Etanercept may increase the levels/effects of: Abatacept; Anakinra; Belimumab; Canakinumab; Certolizumab Pegol; Cyclophosphamide; InFLIX-imab; Leflunomide; Natalizumab; Rilonacept; Tofacitinib; Vaccines (Live)

The levels/effects of Etanercept may be increased by: Denosumab; Pimecrolimus; Roflu-milast; Tacrolimus (Topical); Tocilizumab; Trastu-zumab

Nutritional/Ethanol Interactions Herb/Nutra-ceutical: Echinacea may decrease the therapeutic effects of etanercept (avoid concurrent use).

Adverse Reactions

>10%:
Central nervous system: Headache (17% to 19%)
Dermatologic: Skin rash (3% to 13%)
Gastrointestinal: Abdominal pain (5%; children 19%), diarrhea (3% to 16%), vomiting (3%; children 13%)
Infection: Infection (50% to 81%; children 62%)
Local: Injection site reaction (14% to 43%; bleed-ing, bruising, erythema, itching, pain, or swelling)
Respiratory: Upper respiratory tract infection (38% to 65%), respiratory tract infection (21% to 54%), rhinitis (12%)
Miscellaneous: Antibody development (positive antidouble-stranded DNA antibodies 15% by RIA, 3% by *Crithidia luciliae* assay), positive ANA titer (11%)
≥3% to 10%:
Central nervous system: Dizziness (7%)
Dermatologic: Pruritus (2% to 5%)
Gastrointestinal: Nausea (children 9%), dyspep-sia (4%)
Neuromuscular & skeletal: Weakness (5%)
Respiratory: Pharyngitis (7%), cough (6%), respi-ratory distress (5%), sinusitis (3%)
Miscellaneous: Fever (2% to 3%)

Pharmacodynamics/Kinetics

Onset of Action ~2-3 weeks; RA: 1-2 weeks

Available Dosage Forms

Kit, Subcutaneous [preservative free]:
Enbrel: 25 mg
Solution, Subcutaneous [preservative free]:
Enbrel: 25 mg/0.5 mL (0.51 mL); 50 mg/mL (0.98 mL)
Enbrel SureClick: 50 mg/mL (0.98 mL)

General Dosage Range SubQ:

Children ≥2 years: 0.8 mg/kg (maximum: 50 mg/dose) once weekly

Adults: 50 mg once weekly **or** 25-50 mg twice weekly; maximum dose (rheumatoid arthritis): 50 mg weekly

Administration

Subcutaneous Administer subcutaneously. Rotate injection sites; may inject into the thigh (preferred), abdomen (avoiding the 2-inch area around the navel), or upper arm. New injections should be given at least one inch from an old site and never into areas where the skin is tender, bruised, red, or hard or into any raised thick, red or scaly skin patches or lesions. For a more comfortable injection, autoinjectors, prefilled syringes, and dose trays may be allowed to reach room temperature by removing from the refrigerator 15-30 minutes prior to injection. **Note:** If the physician determines that it is appropriate, patients may self-inject after proper training in injection technique.

Preparation for Administration Reconstitute lyophilized powder aseptically with 1 mL sterile bacteriostatic water for injection, USP (supplied); swirl gently, do not shake. Do not filter reconstituted solution during preparation or administration.

Storage/Stability

Refrigerate at 2°C to 8°C (36°F to 46°F). Do not freeze. Do not store in extreme heat or cold. Store in the original carton to protect from light or physical damage until the time of use.

For convenience and a more comfortable injection, autoinjectors, prefilled syringes, or individual dose trays (containing multi-use vials and diluent syringes) may be stored at room temperature for a maximum single period of 14 days with protection from light and sources of heat, and humidity. Once an autoinjector, prefilled syringe or dose tray has been stored at room temperature, it should not be placed back into the refrigerator; discard after 14 days.

Once the multi-use vial has been reconstituted, use the reconstituted solution immediately or refrigerate at 2°C to 8°C (36°F to 46°F). Reconstituted solution must be used within 14 days; discard after 14 days.

Nursing Actions

Physical Assessment Monitor for signs and symptoms of infection, especially respiratory infections (fever, night sweats, weight loss, excessive fatigue, pallor, dry or productive cough, or shortness of breath). Monitor for symptoms of local fungal infections (red or white patches, drainage, itching, pain, or burning). Monitor for signs/symptoms of malignancy (eg, splenomegaly, hepatomegaly, abdominal pain, persistent fever, night sweats, weight loss). Perform tuberculin skin test prior to initiating therapy; monitor for signs of tuberculosis throughout therapy. Assess for liver dysfunction (unusual fatigue,

easy bruising or bleeding, jaundice). Monitor effectiveness of therapy (eg, pain, range of motion, mobility, ADL function, inflammation). Report abnormal hematology lab results. If self-administered, teach patient appropriate injection technique and needle disposal. Monitor injection site for local reaction which should lessen after a few days or after the first month. Observe for continued injection site irritation which may indicate a latex or rubber allergy from the prefilled syringe.

Patient Education

- Discuss specific use of drug and side effects with patient as it relates to treatment. (HCAHPS: During this hospital stay, were you given any medicine that you had not taken before? Before giving you any new medicine, how often did hospital staff tell you what the medicine was for? How often did hospital staff describe possible side effects in a way you could understand?)
- Patient may experience headache, rhinitis, rhinorrhea, or pharyngitis. Have patient report immediately to prescriber signs of infection, paresthesia, severe asthenia, vision changes, dizziness, dyspnea, excessive weight gain, edema of extremities, ecchymosis, hemorrhaging, pallor, skin eczema, rash exacerbated by sun exposure, night sweats, skin growths, mole changes, significant injection site irritation, or signs of hepatic impairment (HCAHPS).
- Educate patient about signs of a significant reaction (eg, wheezing; chest tightness; fever; itching; bad cough; blue skin color; seizures; or swelling of face, lips, tongue, or throat). **Note:** This is not a comprehensive list of all side effects. Patient should consult prescriber for additional questions.

Intended Use and Disclaimer: Should not be printed and given to patients. This information is intended to serve as a concise initial reference for healthcare professionals to use when discussing medications with a patient. You must ultimately rely on your own discretion, experience and judgment in diagnosing, treating and advising patients.

Ethacrynic Acid (eth a KRIN ik AS id)

Brand Names: U.S. Edecrin; Sodium Edecrin

Index Terms Ethacrynate Sodium

Pharmacologic Category Diuretic, Loop

Medication Safety Issues

Sound-alike/look-alike issues:

Edecrin may be confused with Eulexin, Ecotrin

Pregnancy Risk Factor B

Lactation Excretion unknown/not recommended

Use Management of edema associated with congestive heart failure; hepatic cirrhosis or renal disease; short-term management of ascites due to malignancy, idiopathic edema, and lymphedema ▸

Available Dosage Forms

Solution Reconstituted, Intravenous:

Sodium Edecrin: 50 mg (1 ea)

Tablet, Oral:

Edecrin: 25 mg

General Dosage Range

I.V.: *Adults:* 0.5-1 mg/kg/dose (maximum: 100 mg/dose)

Oral:

Children: 1-3 mg/kg/day

Adults: 50-400 mg/day in 1-2 divided doses

Elderly: Initial: 25-50 mg/day

Administration

I.V. Injection should **not** be given SubQ or I.M. due to local pain and irritation. Single I.V. doses should not exceed 100 mg. Administer each 10 mg over a minute.

Injectable Detail If a second dose is needed, it is recommended to use a new injection site to avoid possible thrombophlebitis.

pH: 6.3-7.7

Nursing Actions

Physical Assessment Monitor for dehydration and electrolyte imbalance on a regular basis.

Patient Education

- Discuss specific use of drug and side effects with patient as it relates to treatment. (HCAHPS: During this hospital stay, were you given any medicine that you had not taken before? Before giving you any new medicine, how often did hospital staff tell you what the medicine was for? How often did hospital staff describe possible side effects in a way you could understand?)
- Patient may experience asthenia, headache, lack of appetite, or nausea. Have patient report immediately to prescriber signs of fluid and electrolyte imbalance, signs of hyperglycemia, severe dizziness, syncope, hearing impairment, tinnitus, vision changes, significant arthralgia, ecchymosis, hemorrhaging, jaundice, or considerable diarrhea (HCAHPS).
- Educate patient about signs of a significant reaction (eg, wheezing; chest tightness; fever; itching; bad cough; blue skin color; seizures; or swelling of face, lips, tongue, or throat). **Note:** This is not a comprehensive list of all side effects. Patient should consult prescriber for additional questions.

Intended Use and Disclaimer: Should not be printed and given to patients. This information is intended to serve as a concise initial reference for healthcare professionals to use when discussing medications with a patient. You must ultimately rely on your own discretion, experience and judgment in diagnosing, treating and advising patients.

Ethambutol (e THAM byoo tole)

Brand Names: U.S. Myambutol

Index Terms Ethambutol Hydrochloride

Pharmacologic Category Antitubercular Agent

Medication Safety Issues

Sound-alike/look-alike issues:

Myambutol® may be confused with Nembutal®

Pregnancy Risk Factor C

Lactation Enters breast milk/use caution

Breast-Feeding Considerations The manufacturer suggests use during breast-feeding only if benefits to the mother outweigh the possible risk to the infant. Some references suggest that exposure to the infant is low and does not produce toxicity, and breast-feeding should not be discouraged. Other references recommend if breast-feeding, monitor the infant for rash, malaise, nausea, and vomiting.

Use Treatment of pulmonary tuberculosis in conjunction with other antituberculosis agents

Unlabeled Use Other mycobacterial diseases in conjunction with other antimycobacterial agents

Mechanism of Action/Effect Inhibits arabinosyl transferase resulting in impaired mycobacterial cell wall synthesis

Contraindications Hypersensitivity to ethambutol or any component of the formulation; optic neuritis (risk vs benefit decision); use in young children, unconscious patients, or any other patient who may be unable to discern and report visual changes

Warnings/Precautions May cause optic neuritis (unilateral or bilateral), resulting in decreased visual acuity or other vision changes. Discontinue promptly in patients with changes in vision, color blindness, or visual defects (effects normally reversible, but reversal may require up to a year). Irreversible blindness has been reported. Monitor visual acuity prior to and during therapy. Evaluation of visual acuity changes may be more difficult in patients with cataracts, optic neuritis, diabetic retinopathy, and inflammatory conditions of the eye; consideration should be given to whether or not visual changes are related to disease progression or effects of therapy. Use only in children whose visual acuity can accurately be determined and monitored (not recommended for use in children <13 years of age unless the benefit outweighs the risk). Dosage modification is required in patients with renal insufficiency; monitor renal function prior to and during treatment. Hepatic toxicity has been reported, possibly due to concurrent therapy; monitor liver function prior to and during treatment.

Drug Interactions

Avoid Concomitant Use There are no known interactions where it is recommended to avoid concomitant use.

Decreased Effect

The levels/effects of Ethambutol may be decreased by: Aluminum Hydroxide

Increased Effect/Toxicity There are no known significant interactions involving an increase in effect.

Adverse Reactions Frequency not defined.

Cardiovascular: Myocarditis, pericarditis

Central nervous system: Confusion, disorientation, dizziness, fever, hallucinations, headache, malaise

Dermatologic: Dermatitis, erythema multiforme, exfoliative dermatitis, pruritus, rash

Endocrine & metabolic: Acute gout or hyperuricemia

Gastrointestinal: Abdominal pain, anorexia, GI upset, nausea, vomiting

Hematologic: Eosinophilia, leukopenia, lymphadenopathy, neutropenia, thrombocytopenia

Hepatic: Hepatitis, hepatotoxicity (possibly related to concurrent therapy), LFTs abnormal

Neuromuscular & skeletal: Arthralgia, peripheral neuritis

Ocular: Optic neuritis; symptoms may include decreased acuity, scotoma, color blindness, or visual defects (usually reversible with discontinuation, irreversible blindness has been described)

Renal: Nephritis

Respiratory: Infiltrates (with or without eosinophilia), pneumonitis

Miscellaneous: Anaphylaxis, anaphylactoid reaction; hypersensitivity syndrome (cutaneous reactions, eosinophilia, and organ-specific inflammation)

Available Dosage Forms

Tablet, Oral:

Myambutol: 100 mg, 400 mg

Generic: 100 mg, 400 mg

General Dosage Range Dosage adjustment recommended in patients with renal impairment

Oral:

Children: 15-20 mg/kg/day (maximum: 1 g/day) or 50 mg/kg twice weekly (maximum: 2.5 g/dose)

Adults: Daily therapy: 1.5-2.5 g/kg/day (maximum dose: 1.5-2.5 g); 3 times/week DOT: 25-30 mg/kg/dose (maximum dose: 2.4 g/dose); Twice weekly DOT: 50 mg/kg/dose (maximum dose: 4 g/dose)

Storage/Stability Store at controlled room temperature of 20°C to 25°C (68°F to 77°F).

Nursing Actions

Physical Assessment Monitor for CNS changes, neuritis, and ocular changes on a regular basis during therapy. Teach patient need to adhere to dosing program and importance of regular laboratory tests and ophthalmic evaluations.

Patient Education

• Discuss specific use of drug and side effects with patient as it relates to treatment. (HCAHPS: During this hospital stay, were you given any medicine that you had not taken before? Before giving you any new medicine, how often did

hospital staff tell you what the medicine was for? How often did hospital staff describe possible side effects in a way you could understand?)

• Patient may experience nausea, lack of appetite, dizziness, headache, or dyspepsia. Have patient report immediately to prescriber illogical thinking, hallucinations, arthralgia, paresthesia, ecchymosis, hemorrhaging, signs of hepatic impairment, or vision changes (HCAHPS).

• Educate patient about signs of a significant reaction (eg, wheezing; chest tightness; fever; itching; bad cough; blue skin color; seizures; or swelling of face, lips, tongue, or throat). **Note:** This is not a comprehensive list of all side effects. Patient should consult prescriber for additional questions.

Intended Use and Disclaimer: Should not be printed and given to patients. This information is intended to serve as a concise initial reference for healthcare professionals to use when discussing medications with a patient. You must ultimately rely on your own discretion, experience and judgment in diagnosing, treating and advising patients.

Dietary Considerations May be taken with food as absorption is not affected, may cause gastric irritation.

Ethinyl Estradiol and Desogestrel
(ETH in il es tra DYE ole & des oh JES trel)

Brand Names: U.S. Apri; Azurette; Caziant; Cyclessa; Desogen; Emoquette; Enskyce; Kariva; Mircette; Ortho-Cept; Pimtrea; Reclipsen; Velivet; Viorele

Index Terms Desogestrel and Ethinyl Estradiol; Ortho Cept

Pharmacologic Category Contraceptive; Estrogen and Progestin Combination

Medication Safety Issues

Sound-alike/look-alike issues:

Apri may be confused with Apriso

Ortho-Cept may be confused with Ortho-Cyclen

Pregnancy Risk Factor X

Lactation Enters breast milk/not recommended

Use Contraception: For the prevention of pregnancy.

Unlabeled Use Treatment of heavy (excessive) menstrual bleeding (menorrhagia); dysmenorrhea; abnormal uterine bleeding; treatment of polycystic ovary syndrome (PCOS) in women with menstrual irregularities and hirsutism/acne

Available Dosage Forms

Tablet, oral [low dose formulation]:

Azurette:

Day 1-21: Ethinyl estradiol 0.02 mg and desogestrel 0.15 mg [21 white tablets]

Day 22-23: 2 inactive green tablets

Day 24-28: Ethinyl estradiol 0.01 mg [5 blue tablets] (28s)

Kariva:
Day 1-21: Ethinyl estradiol 0.02 mg and desogestrel 0.15 mg [21 white tablets]
Day 22-23: 2 inactive light green tablets
Day 24-28: Ethinyl estradiol 0.01 mg [5 light blue tablets] (28s)
Mircette:
Day 1-21: Ethinyl estradiol 0.02 mg and desogestrel 0.15 mg [21 white tablets]
Day 22-23: 2 inactive green tablets
Day 24-28: Ethinyl estradiol 0.01 mg [5 yellow tablets] (28s)
Pimtrea:
Day 1-21: Ethinyl estradiol 0.02 mg and desogestrel 0.15 mg [21 dark blue tablets]
Day 22-23: 2 inactive white tablets
Day 24-28: Ethinyl estradiol 0.01 mg [5 green tablets] (28s)
Viorele:
Day 1-21: Ethinyl estradiol 0.02 mg and desogestrel 0.15 mg [21 white tablets]
Day 22-23: 2 inactive green tablets
Day 24-28: Ethinyl estradiol 0.01 mg [5 yellow tablets] (28s)

Tablet, oral [monophasic formulation]:
Apri 28: Ethinyl estradiol 0.03 mg and desogestrel 0.15 mg [21 rose tablets and 7 white inactive tablets] (28s)
Desogen, Reclipsen: Ethinyl estradiol 0.03 mg and desogestrel 0.15 mg [21 white tablets and 7 green inactive tablets] (28s)
Emoquette: Ethinyl estradiol 0.03 mg and desogestrel 0.15 mg [21 white tablets and 7 light green inactive tablets] (28s)
Enskyce: Ethinyl estradiol 0.03 mg and desogestrel 0.15 mg [21 light orange tablets and 7 green inactive tablets] (28s)
Ortho-Cept 28: Ethinyl estradiol 0.03 mg and desogestrel 0.15 mg [21 light orange tablets and 7 green inactive tablets] (28s)

Tablet, oral [triphasic formulation]:
Caziant:
Day 1-7: Ethinyl estradiol 0.025 mg and desogestrel 0.1 mg [7 white tablets]
Day 8-14: Ethinyl estradiol 0.025 mg and desogestrel 0.125 mg [7 light blue tablets]
Day 15-21: Ethinyl estradiol 0.025 mg and desogestrel 0.15 mg [7 blue tablets]
Day 22-28: 7 green inactive tablets (28s)
Cyclessa:
Day 1-7: Ethinyl estradiol 0.025 mg and desogestrel 0.1 mg [7 light yellow tablets]
Day 8-14: Ethinyl estradiol 0.025 mg and desogestrel 0.125 mg [7 orange tablets]
Day 15-21: Ethinyl estradiol 0.025 mg and desogestrel 0.15 mg [7 red tablets]
Day 22-28: 7 green inactive tablets (28s)
Velivet:
Day 1-7: Ethinyl estradiol 0.025 mg and desogestrel 0.1 mg [7 beige tablets]

Day 8-14: Ethinyl estradiol 0.025 mg and desogestrel 0.125 mg [7 orange tablets]
Day 15-21: Ethinyl estradiol 0.025 mg and desogestrel 0.15 mg [7 pink tablets]
Day 22-28: 7 white inactive tablets (28s)

General Dosage Range Oral: *Children and Adults (females, postmenarche):* 1 tablet daily

Administration

Oral Administer at the same time each day at intervals not >24 hours. Hazardous agent; use appropriate precautions for handling and disposal (NIOSH, 2012).

Nursing Actions

Physical Assessment Monitor blood pressure on a regular basis. Teach importance of regular (monthly) blood pressure checks and annual physical assessment, Pap smear, and vision assessment. Teach importance of maintaining prescribed schedule of dosing.

Patient Education
• Discuss specific use of drug and side effects with patient as it relates to treatment. (HCAHPS: During this hospital stay, were you given any medicine that you had not taken before? Before giving you any new medicine, how often did hospital staff tell you what the medicine was for? How often did hospital staff describe possible side effects in a way you could understand?)
• Patient may experience lack of appetite, polyphagia, weight gain, bloating, menstrual irregularities, macromastia, sexual dysfunction, or alopecia. Have patient report immediately to prescriber angina, dyspnea, hemoptysis, severe dizziness, syncope, considerable nausea, strength differences from one side to another, difficulty speaking or thinking, change in balance, blurred vision, edema, skin discoloration, painful extremities, severe headache, depression, intolerable asthenia, severe dyspepsia, signs of hepatic impairment, vision changes, exophthalmos, contact lens discomfort, urinary retention, oliguria, lump in breast, mastalgia, nipple discharge, vaginal hemorrhaging, or vaginitis (HCAHPS).
• Educate patient about signs of a significant reaction (eg, wheezing; chest tightness; fever; itching; bad cough; blue skin color; seizures; or swelling of face, lips, tongue, or throat). **Note:** This is not a comprehensive list of all side effects. Patient should consult prescriber for additional questions.

Intended Use and Disclaimer: Should not be printed and given to patients. This information is intended to serve as a concise initial reference for healthcare professionals to use when discussing medications with a patient. You must ultimately rely on your own discretion, experience and judgment in diagnosing, treating and advising patients.

Ethinyl Estradiol and Drospirenone
(ETH in il es tra DYE ole & droh SPYE re none)

Brand Names: U.S. Gianvi™; Loryna™; Ocella™; Syeda™; Vestura™; Yasmin®; Yaz®; Zarah®

Index Terms Drospirenone and Ethinyl Estradiol

Pharmacologic Category Contraceptive; Estrogen and Progestin Combination

Medication Safety Issues

Sound-alike/look-alike issues:

Yaz® may be confused with Beyaz™, Yasmin®

Pregnancy Risk Factor X

Lactation Enters breast milk/not recommended

Use Prevention of pregnancy; treatment of premenstrual dysphoric disorder (PMDD); treatment of acne

Unlabeled Use Treatment of hypermenorrhea (menorrhagia); pain associated with endometriosis; dysmenorrhea; dysfunctional uterine bleeding; treatment of polycystic ovary syndrome (PCOS) in women with menstrual irregularities and hirsutism/acne

Available Dosage Forms

Tablet, oral: Ethinyl estradiol 0.03 mg and drospirenone 3 mg [21 active tablets and 7 inactive tablets] (28s)

Gianvi™: Ethinyl estradiol 0.03 mg and drospirenone 3 mg [24 light pink active tablets and 4 white inactive tablets] (28s)

Loryna™: Ethinyl estradiol 0.02 mg and drospirenone 3 mg [24 peach active tablets and 4 white inactive tablets] (28s)

Ocella™, Syeda™, Yasmin®: Ethinyl estradiol 0.03 mg and drospirenone 3 mg [21 yellow active tablets and 7 white inactive tablets] (28s)

Vestura™: Ethinyl estradiol 0.02 mg and drospirenone 3 mg [24 pink active tablets and 4 peach inactive tablets] (28s)

Yaz®: Ethinyl estradiol 0.02 mg and drospirenone 3 mg [24 light pink active tablets and 4 white inactive tablets] (28s)

Zarah®: Ethinyl estradiol 0.03 mg and drospirenone 3 mg [21 blue active tablets and 7 peach inactive tablets] (28s)

General Dosage Range Oral: *Children and Adults (females, postmenarche):* 1 tablet daily

Administration

Oral Dose should be taken at the same time each day, either after the evening meal or at bedtime. If severe vomiting or diarrhea occurs, additional contraception (nonhormonal) should be used. If vomiting occurs within 3-4 hours of dosing, consider the dose to be missed.

Hazardous agent; use appropriate precautions for handling and disposal (NIOSH, 2012).

Nursing Actions

Physical Assessment Monitor blood pressure on a regular (monthly) basis. Teach patient the importance of annual physical examinations (including Pap smear and vision exam) and the importance of maintaining prescribed schedule of dosing.

Patient Education

- Discuss specific use of drug and side effects with patient as it relates to treatment. (HCAHPS: During this hospital stay, were you given any medicine that you had not taken before? Before giving you any new medicine, how often did hospital staff tell you what the medicine was for? How often did hospital staff describe possible side effects in a way you could understand?)
- Patient may experience lack of appetite, polyphagia, weight gain, cramps, bloating, menstrual irregularities, macromastia, or sexual dysfunction. Have patient report immediately to prescriber angina, arrhythmia, dyspnea, hemoptysis, severe dizziness, syncope, considerable nausea, strength differences from one side to another, difficulty speaking or thinking, change in balance, blurred vision, edema, skin discoloration, painful extremities, severe headache, depression, intolerable asthenia, signs of hepatic impairment, urinary retention, oliguria, lump in breast, mastalgia, nipple discharge, vaginal hemorrhaging, vaginitis, vision changes, or exophthalmos (HCAHPS).
- Educate patient about signs of a significant reaction (eg, wheezing; chest tightness; fever; itching; bad cough; blue skin color; seizures; or swelling of face, lips, tongue, or throat). **Note:** This is not a comprehensive list of all side effects. Patient should consult prescriber for additional questions.

Intended Use and Disclaimer: Should not be printed and given to patients. This information is intended to serve as a concise initial reference for healthcare professionals to use when discussing medications with a patient. You must ultimately rely on your own discretion, experience and judgment in diagnosing, treating and advising patients.

Ethinyl Estradiol and Ethynodiol Diacetate
(ETH in il es tra DYE ole & e thye noe DYE ole dye AS e tate)

Brand Names: U.S. Kelnor™; Zovia®

Index Terms Ethynodiol Diacetate and Ethinyl Estradiol

Pharmacologic Category Contraceptive; Estrogen and Progestin Combination

Medication Safety Issues

Sound-alike/look-alike issues:

Demulen® may be confused with Dalmane®, Demerol®

Pregnancy Risk Factor X

Lactation Enters breast milk/not recommended

Use Prevention of pregnancy

Unlabeled Use Treatment of hypermenorrhea (menorrhagia); pain associated with endometriosis;

dysmenorrhea; dysfunctional uterine bleeding; treatment of polycystic ovary syndrome (PCOS) in women with menstrual irregularities and hirsutism/acne

Available Dosage Forms

Tablet, oral [monophasic formulation]:

Kelnor™ 1/35: Ethinyl estradiol 0.035 mg and ethynodiol diacetate 1 mg [21 light yellow tablets and 7 white inactive tablets] (28s)

Zovia® 1/35-28: Ethinyl estradiol 0.035 mg and ethynodiol diacetate 1 mg [21 light pink tablets and 7 white inactive tablets] (28s)

Zovia® 1/50-28: Ethinyl estradiol 0.05 mg and ethynodiol diacetate 1 mg [21 pink tablets and 7 white inactive tablets] (28s)

General Dosage Range Oral: *Children and Adults (females, postmenarche):* 1 tablet daily

Administration

Oral Administer at the same time each day. Hazardous agent; use appropriate precautions for handling and disposal (NIOSH, 2012)

Nursing Actions

Physical Assessment Assess blood pressure on a regular basis. Monitor for thromboembolic disease, visual changes, and neuromuscular weakness. Teach importance of regular (monthly) blood pressure checks and annual physical assessment, Pap smear, and vision assessment. Teach importance of maintaining prescribed schedule of dosing.

Patient Education

• Discuss specific use of drug and side effects with patient as it relates to treatment. (HCAHPS: During this hospital stay, were you given any medicine that you had not taken before? Before giving you any new medicine, how often did hospital staff tell you what the medicine was for? How often did hospital staff describe possible side effects in a way you could understand?)

• Patient may experience lack of appetite, polyphagia, weight gain, cramps, bloating, menstrual irregularities, macromastia, alopecia, or sexual dysfunction. Have patient report immediately to prescriber angina, dyspnea, hemoptysis, severe dizziness, syncope, considerable nausea, strength differences from one side to another, difficulty speaking or thinking, change in balance, blurred vision, edema, skin discoloration, painful extremities, severe headache, depression, intolerable asthenia, severe dyspepsia, urinary retention, oliguria, signs of hepatic impairment, lump in breast, mastalgia, nipple discharge, vaginal hemorrhaging, vaginitis, vision changes, contact lens discomfort, or exophthalmos (HCAHPS).

• Educate patient about signs of a significant reaction (eg, wheezing; chest tightness; fever; itching; bad cough; blue skin color; seizures; or swelling of face, lips, tongue, or throat). **Note:** This is not a comprehensive list of all side effects. Patient should consult prescriber for additional questions.

Intended Use and Disclaimer: Should not be printed and given to patients. This information is intended to serve as a concise initial reference for healthcare professionals to use when discussing medications with a patient. You must ultimately rely on your own discretion, experience and judgment in diagnosing, treating and advising patients.

Ethinyl Estradiol and Levonorgestrel

(ETH in il es tra DYE ole & LEE voe nor jes trel)

Brand Names: U.S. Altavera; Amethia; Amethia Lo; Amethyst; Aubra; Aviane; camrese; Chateal; Daysee; Enpresse; Falmina; Introvale; Jolessa; Kurvelo; Lessina; Levonest; Levora; LoSeasonique; Lutera; Lybrel; Marlissa; Myzilra; Nordette 28 [DSC]; Orsythia; Portia; Quartette; Quasense; Seasonique; Sronyx; Trivora

Index Terms Levonorgestrel and Ethinyl Estradiol

Pharmacologic Category Contraceptive; Estrogen and Progestin Combination

Medication Safety Issues

Sound-alike/look-alike issues:

Nordette may be confused with Nicorette

Portia may be confused with Potiga

Seasonale may be confused with Seasonique

Tri-Levlen may be confused with Trilafon

Pregnancy Risk Factor X

Lactation Enters breast milk/not recommended

Use Prevention of pregnancy; postcoital contraception

Unlabeled Use Treatment of hypermenorrhea (menorrhagia); pain associated with endometriosis; dysmenorrhea; dysfunctional uterine bleeding; treatment of polycystic ovary syndrome (PCOS) in women with menstrual irregularities and hirsutism/acne

Available Dosage Forms

Tablet, oral [low-dose formulation]: Ethinyl estradiol 0.02 mg and levonorgestrel 0.1 mg [21 tablets and 7 inactive tablets] (28s)

Aubra: Ethinyl estradiol 0.02 mg and levonorgestrel 0.1 mg [21 light yellow tablets and 7 brown inactive tablets] (28s)

Aviane: Ethinyl estradiol 0.02 mg and levonorgestrel 0.1 mg [21 orange tablets and 7 light green inactive tablets] (28s)

Falmina: Ethinyl estradiol 0.02 mg and levonorgestrel 0.1 mg [21 orange tablets and 7 white inactive tablets] (28s)

Lessina: Ethinyl estradiol 0.02 mg and levonorgestrel 0.1 mg [21 pink tablets and 7 white inactive tablets] (28s)

Lutera, Sronyx: Ethinyl estradiol 0.02 mg and levonorgestrel 0.1 mg [21 white tablets and 7 peach inactive tablets] (28s)

Orsythia: Ethinyl estradiol 0.02 mg and levonorgestrel 0.1 mg [21 pink tablets and 7 light green inactive tablets] (28s)

Tablet, oral [monophasic formulation]: Ethinyl estradiol 0.03 mg and levonorgestrel 0.15 mg [21 tablets and 7 inactive tablets] (28s)

Altavera: Ethinyl estradiol 0.03 mg and levonorgestrel 0.15 mg [21 peach tablets and 7 white inactive tablets] (28s)

Chateal: Ethinyl estradiol 0.03 mg and levonorgestrel 0.15 mg [21 white tablets and 7 green inactive tablets] (28s)

Kurvelo: Ethinyl estradiol 0.03 mg and levonorgestrel 0.15 mg [21 light orange tablets and 7 pink inactive tablets] (28s)

Levora: Ethinyl estradiol 0.03 mg and levonorgestrel 0.15 mg [21 white tablets and 7 peach inactive tablets] (28s)

Marlissa: Ethinyl estradiol 0.03 mg and levonorgestrel 0.15 mg [21 light orange tablets and 7 pink inactive tablets] (28s)

Portia 28: Ethinyl estradiol 0.03 mg and levonorgestrel 0.15 mg [21 pink tablets and 7 white inactive tablets] (28s)

Tablet, oral [extended cycle regimen]: Ethinyl estradiol 0.02 mg and levonorgestrel 0.1 mg [84 tablets] and ethinyl estradiol 0.01 mg [7 tablets] (91s); Ethinyl estradiol 0.03 mg and levonorgestrel 0.15 mg [84 tablets and 7 inactive tablets] (91s)

Amethia:Ethinyl estradiol 0.03 mg and levonorgestrel 0.15 mg [84 white tablets] and ethinyl estradiol 0.01 mg [7 light blue tablets] (91s)

Amethia Lo: Ethinyl estradiol 0.02 mg and levonorgestrel 0.1 mg [84 white tablets] and ethinyl estradiol 0.01 mg [7 blue tablets] (91s)

camrese: Ethinyl estradiol 0.03 mg and levonorgestrel 0.15 mg [84 light blue-green tablets] and ethinyl estradiol 0.01 mg [7 yellow tablets] (91s)

Daysee: Ethinyl estradiol 0.03 mg and levonorgestrel 0.15 mg [84 light blue tablets] and ethinyl estradiol 0.01 mg [7 mustard tablets] (91s)

Introvale: Ethinyl estradiol 0.03 mg and levonorgestrel 0.15 mg [84 peach tablets and 7 white inactive tablets] (91s)

Jolessa: Ethinyl estradiol 0.03 mg and levonorgestrel 0.15 mg [84 pink tablets and 7 white inactive tablets] (91s)

LoSeasonique: Ethinyl estradiol 0.02 mg and levonorgestrel 0.1 mg [84 orange tablets] and ethinyl estradiol 0.01 mg [7 yellow tablets] (91s)

Quartette:
Day 1-42: Ethinyl estradiol 0.02 mg and levonorgestrel 0.15 mg [42 light pink tablets]
Day 43-63: Ethinyl estradiol 0.025 mg and levonorgestrel 0.15 mg [21 pink tablets]
Day 64-84: Ethinyl estradiol 0.03 mg and levonorgestrel 0.15 mg [21 purple tablets]
Day 85-91: Ethinyl estradiol 0.01 mg [7 yellow tablets] (91s)

Quasense: Ethinyl estradiol 0.03 mg and levonorgestrel 0.15 mg] [84 white tablets and 7 peach inactive tablets] (91s)

Seasonique: Ethinyl estradiol 0.03 mg and levonorgestrel 0.15 mg [84 light blue-green tablets] and ethinyl estradiol 0.01 mg [7 yellow tablets] (91s)

Tablet, oral [noncyclic regimen]:
Amethyst: Ethinyl estradiol 0.02 mg and levonorgestrel 0.09 mg [28 white tablets] (28s)

Lybrel: Ethinyl estradiol 0.02 mg and levonorgestrel 0.09 mg [28 yellow tablets] (28s)

Tablet, oral [triphasic formulation]:
Enpresse:
Day 1-6: Ethinyl estradiol 0.03 mg and levonorgestrel 0.05 mg [6 pink tablets]
Day 7-11: Ethinyl estradiol 0.04 mg and levonorgestrel 0.075 mg [5 white tablets]
Day 12-21: Ethinyl estradiol 0.03 mg and levonorgestrel 0.125 mg [10 orange tablets]
Day 22-28: 7 light green inactive tablets (28s)

Levonest:
Day 1-6: Ethinyl estradiol 0.03 mg and levonorgestrel 0.05 mg [6 yellow tablets]
Day 7-11: Ethinyl estradiol 0.04 mg and levonorgestrel 0.075 mg [5 green tablets]
Day 12-21: Ethinyl estradiol 0.03 mg and levonorgestrel 0.125 mg [10 light brown tablets]
Day 22-28: 7 white inactive tablets (28s)

Myzilra:
Day 1-6: Ethinyl estradiol 0.03 mg and levonorgestrel 0.05 mg [6 beige tablets]
Day 7-11: Ethinyl estradiol 0.04 mg and levonorgestrel 0.075 mg [5 white tablets]
Day 12-21: Ethinyl estradiol 0.03 mg and levonorgestrel 0.125 mg [10 light yellow tablets]
Day 22-28: 7 light green inactive tablets (28s)

Trivora:
Day 1-6: Ethinyl estradiol 0.03 mg and levonorgestrel 0.05 mg [6 blue tablets]
Day 7-11: Ethinyl estradiol 0.04 mg and levonorgestrel 0.075 mg [5 white tablets]
Day 12-21: Ethinyl estradiol 0.03 mg and levonorgestrel 0.125 mg [10 pink tablets]
Day 22-28: 7 peach inactive tablets (28s)

General Dosage Range Oral: *Children and Adults (females, postmenarche):* 1 tablet daily **or** 2 tablets as soon as possible (but within 72 hours of unprotected intercourse), followed by 2 tablets 12 hours later

Administration

Oral Administer at the same time each day.

Quartette: If severe diarrhea or vomiting occur within 3-4 hours after taking a light pink, pink, or purple tablet, it should be considered a missed dose; additional contraceptive measures are recommended.

Hazardous agent; use appropriate precautions for handling and disposal (NIOSH, 2012)

◀ **Nursing Actions**

Physical Assessment See individual agents.

Patient Education

- Discuss specific use of drug and side effects with patient as it relates to treatment. (HCAHPS: During this hospital stay, were you given any medicine that you had not taken before? Before giving you any new medicine, how often did hospital staff tell you what the medicine was for? How often did hospital staff describe possible side effects in a way you could understand?)
- Patient may experience lack of appetite, polyphagia, weight gain, cramps, bloating, menstrual irregularities, macromastia, alopecia, acne vulgaris, or sexual dysfunction. Have patient report immediately to prescriber signs of hepatic impairment, angina, dyspnea, hemoptysis, severe dizziness, syncope, considerable nausea, strength differences from one side to another, difficulty speaking or thinking, change in balance, blurred vision, edema, skin discoloration, painful extremities, severe headache, depression, intolerable asthenia, considerable dyspepsia, urinary retention, oliguria, lump in breast, mastalgia, nipple discharge, vaginal hemorrhaging, vaginitis, vision changes, exophthalmos, or contact lens discomfort (HCAHPS).
- Educate patient about signs of a significant reaction (eg, wheezing; chest tightness; fever; itching; bad cough; blue skin color; seizures; or swelling of face, lips, tongue, or throat). **Note:** This is not a comprehensive list of all side effects. Patient should consult prescriber for additional questions.

Intended Use and Disclaimer: Should not be printed and given to patients. This information is intended to serve as a concise initial reference for healthcare professionals to use when discussing medications with a patient. You must ultimately rely on your own discretion, experience and judgment in diagnosing, treating and advising patients.

Related Information

Levonorgestrel on page 933

Ethinyl Estradiol and Norethindrone
(ETH in il es tra DYE ole & nor eth IN drone)

Brand Names: U.S. Alyacen 1/35; Alyacen 7/7/7; Aranelle; Balziva; Brevicon; Briellyn; Cyclafem 1/35; Cyclafem 7/7/7; Dasetta 1/35; Dasetta 7/7/7; Estrostep Fe; Femcon Fe; femhrt; Generess Fe; Gildess FE 1.5/30; Gildess FE 1/20; Jinteli; Junel 1.5/30; Junel 1/20; Junel Fe 1.5/30; Junel Fe 1/20; Larin Fe 1.5/30; Larin Fe 1/20; Leena; Lo Loestrin Fe; Lo Minastrin Fe [DSC]; Loestrin 21 1.5/30; Loestrin 21 1/20; Loestrin 24 Fe; Loestrin Fe 1.5/30; Loestrin Fe 1/20; Lomedia 24 Fe; Microgestin 1.5/30; Microgestin 1/20; Microgestin Fe 1.5/30; Microgestin Fe 1/20; Minastrin 24 Fe; Modicon; Necon 0.5/35; Necon 1/35; Necon 10/11;

Necon 7/7/7; Norinyl 1+35; Nortrel 0.5/35; Nortrel 1/35; Nortrel 7/7/7; Ortho-Novum 1/35; Ortho-Novum 7/7/7; Ovcon 35; Philith; Pirmella 1/35; Tilia Fe; Tri-Legest Fe; Tri-Norinyl; Vyfemla; Wera; Wymzya Fe; Zenchent; Zenchent Fe

Index Terms Norethindrone Acetate and Ethinyl Estradiol; Ortho Novum

Pharmacologic Category Contraceptive; Estrogen and Progestin Combination

Medication Safety Issues

Sound-alike/look-alike issues:

femhrt may be confused with Femara

Lo Loestrin Fe may be confused with Loestrin Fe

Modicon may be confused with Mylicon

Norinyl may be confused with Nardil

Pregnancy Risk Factor X

Lactation Enters breast milk/not recommended

Use

Acne vulgaris: For the treatment of moderate acne vulgaris in females at least 15 years of age. Limitations of Use: When used for acne, use only in females ≥15 years of age who have achieved menarche, who also desire combination hormonal contraceptive therapy, are unresponsive to topical treatments, have no contraindications to combination hormonal contraceptive use, and plan to stay on therapy for ≥6 months.

Contraception: For the prevention of pregnancy.

Moderate to severe vasomotor symptoms: Treatment of moderate to severe vasomotor symptoms associated with menopause.

Osteoporosis prevention: For prevention of postmenopausal osteoporosis.

Limitations of use: For use only in women at significant risk of osteoporosis and for whom other nonestrogen medications are not considered appropriate.

Unlabeled Use Treatment of heavy (excessive) menstrual bleeding (menorrhagia); dysmenorrhea; abnormal uterine bleeding; treatment of polycystic ovary syndrome (PCOS) in women with menstrual irregularities and hirsutism/acne

Available Dosage Forms

Tablet, oral:

femhrt 0.5/2.5: Ethinyl estradiol 0.0025 mg and norethindrone acetate 0.5 mg [white tablets] (28s)

Jinteli: Ethinyl estradiol 0.005 mg and norethindrone acetate 1 mg [white tablets] (28s, 90s)

Tablet, oral [monophasic formulation]:

Alyacen 1/35: Ethinyl estradiol 0.035 mg and norethindrone 1 mg [21 peach tablets and 7 light green inactive tablets] (28s)

Balziva: Ethinyl estradiol 0.035 mg and norethindrone 0.4 mg [21 light peach tablets and 7 white inactive tablets] (28s)

Brevicon: Ethinyl estradiol 0.035 mg and norethindrone 0.5 mg [21 blue tablets and 7 orange inactive tablets] (28s)

Briellyn: Ethinyl estradiol 0.035 mg and norethindrone 0.4 mg [21 light peach tablets and 7 white-off-white inactive tablets] (28s)

Cyclafem 1/35: Ethinyl estradiol 0.035 mg and norethindrone 1 mg [21 pink tablets and 7 light green inactive tablets] (28s)

Dasetta 1/35: Ethinyl estradiol 0.035 mg and norethindrone 1 mg [21 orange tablets and 7 white inactive tablets] (28s)

Gildess FE 1/20: Ethinyl estradiol 0.02 mg and norethindrone acetate 1 mg [21 white tablets] and ferrous fumarate 75 mg [7 white-speckled brown tablets] (28s)

Gildess FE 1.5/30: Ethinyl estradiol 0.03 mg and norethindrone acetate 1.5 mg [21 light green tablets] and ferrous fumarate 75 mg [7 white-speckled brown tablets] (28s)

Junel 1/20: Ethinyl estradiol 0.02 mg and norethindrone acetate 1 mg [yellow tablets] (21s)

Junel 1.5/30, Loestrin 21 1.5/30: Ethinyl estradiol 0.03 mg and norethindrone acetate 1.5 mg [pink tablets] (21s)

Junel Fe 1/20: Ethinyl estradiol 0.02 mg and norethindrone acetate 1 mg [21 yellow tablets] and ferrous fumarate 75 mg [7 brown tablets] (28s)

Junel Fe 1.5/30, Loestrin Fe 21 1.5/30: Ethinyl estradiol 0.03 mg and norethindrone acetate 1.5 mg [21 pink tablets] and ferrous fumarate 75 mg [7 brown tablets] (28s)

Larin Fe 1/20: Ethinyl estradiol 0.02 mg and norethindrone acetate 1 mg [21 pale yellow tablets] and ferrous fumarate 75 mg [7 brown tablets] (28s)

Larin Fe 1.5/30: Ethinyl estradiol 0.03 mg and norethindrone acetate 1.5 mg [21 green tablets] and ferrous fumarate 75 mg [7 brown tablets] (28s) [contains soya lecithin]

Loestrin 21 1/20: Ethinyl estradiol 0.02 mg and norethindrone acetate 1 mg [light yellow tablets] (21s)

Loestrin 24 Fe: Ethinyl estradiol 0.02 mg and norethindrone acetate 1 mg [24 white tablets] and ferrous fumarate 75 mg [4 brown tablets] (28s)

Loestrin Fe 1/20: Ethinyl estradiol 0.02 mg and norethindrone acetate 1 mg [21 light yellow tablets] and ferrous fumarate 75 mg [7 brown tablets] (28s)

Loestrin Fe 1.5/30: Ethinyl estradiol 0.03 mg and norethindrone acetate 1.5 mg [21 pink tablets] and ferrous fumarate 75 mg [7 brown tablets] (28s)

Lomedia 24 Fe: Ethinyl estradiol 0.02 mg and norethindrone acetate 1 mg [24 white tablets] and ferrous fumarate 75 mg [4 brown tablets] (28s)

Microgestin 1/20: Ethinyl estradiol 0.02 mg and norethindrone acetate 1 mg [white tablets] (21s)

Microgestin 1.5/30: Ethinyl estradiol 0.03 mg and norethindrone acetate 1.5 mg [green tablets] (21s)

Microgestin Fe 1/20: Ethinyl estradiol 0.02 mg and norethindrone acetate 1 mg [21 white tablets] and ferrous fumarate 75 mg [7 brown tablets] (28s)

Microgestin Fe 1.5/30: Ethinyl estradiol 0.03 mg and norethindrone acetate 1.5 mg [21 green tablets] and ferrous fumarate 75 mg [7 brown tablets] (28s)

Modicon: Ethinyl estradiol 0.035 mg and norethindrone 0.5 mg [21 white tablets and 7 green inactive tablets] (28s)

Necon 0.5/35, Nortrel 0.5/35: Ethinyl estradiol 0.035 mg and norethindrone 0.5 mg [21 light yellow tablets and 7 white inactive tablets] (28s)

Necon 1/35: Ethinyl estradiol 0.035 mg and norethindrone 1 mg [21 dark yellow tablets and 7 white inactive tablets] (28s)

Norinyl 1+35: Ethinyl estradiol 0.035 mg and norethindrone 1 mg [21 yellow-green tablets and 7 orange inactive tablets] (28s)

Nortrel 1/35:
Ethinyl estradiol 0.035 mg and norethindrone 1 mg [yellow tablets] (21s)
Ethinyl estradiol 0.035 mg and norethindrone 1 mg [21 yellow tablets and 7 white inactive tablets] (28s)

Ortho-Novum 1/35: Ethinyl estradiol 0.035 mg and norethindrone 1 mg [21 peach tablets and 7 green inactive tablets] (28s)

Ovcon 35: Ethinyl estradiol 0.035 mg and norethindrone 0.4 mg [21 light peach tablets and 7 green inactive tablets] (28s)

Philith: Ethinyl estradiol 0.035 mg and norethindrone 0.4 mg [21 tan tablets and 7 white inactive tablets] (28s)

Pirmella 1/35: Ethinyl estradiol 0.035 mg and norethindrone 1 mg [21 peach tablets and 7 green inactive tablets] (28s)

Vyfemla: Ethinyl estradiol 0.035 mg and norethindrone 0.4 mg [21 light peach tablets and 7 white inactive tablets] (28s)

Wera: Ethinyl estradiol 0.035 mg and norethindrone 0.5 mg [21 light peach tablets and 7 white inactive tablets] (28s)

Zenchent: Ethinyl estradiol 0.035 mg and norethindrone 0.4 mg [21 orange tablets and 7 white inactive tablets] (28s)

Tablet, chewable, oral [monophasic formulation]: Ethinyl estradiol 0.035 mg and norethindrone 0.4 mg [21 tablets] and ferrous fumarate 75 mg [7 tablets] (28s)

Femcon Fe, Wymzya Fe: Ethinyl estradiol 0.035 mg and norethindrone 0.4 mg [21 white tablets] and ferrous fumarate 75 mg [7 brown tablets] (28s)

Generess Fe: Ethinyl estradiol 0.025 mg and norethindrone 0.8 mg [24 light green tablets] and ferrous fumarate 75 mg [4 brown tablets] (28s)

Minastrin 24 Fe: Ethinyl estradiol 0.02 mg and norethindrone 1 mg [24 white tablets] and ferrous fumarate 75 mg [4 brown tablets] (28s)

Zenchent Fe: Ethinyl estradiol 0.035 mg and norethindrone 0.4 mg [21 light yellow tablets] and ferrous fumarate 75 mg [7 brown tablets] (28s)

Tablet, oral [biphasic formulation]:

Lo Loestrin Fe:

Day 1-24: Ethinyl estradiol 0.01 mg and norethindrone acetate 1 mg [24 blue tablets]

Day 25-26: Ethinyl estradiol 0.01 mg [2 white tablets]

Day 27-28: Ferrous fumarate 75 mg [2 brown tablets] (28s)

Necon 10/11:

Day 1-10: Ethinyl estradiol 0.035 mg and norethindrone 0.5 mg [10 light yellow tablets]

Day 11-21: Ethinyl estradiol 0.035 mg and norethindrone 1 mg [11 dark yellow tablets]

Day 22-28: 7 white inactive tablets (28s)

Tablet, oral [triphasic formulation]:

Alyacen 7/7/7:

Day 1-7: Ethinyl estradiol 0.035 mg and norethindrone 0.5 mg [7 white-off-white tablets]

Day 8-14: Ethinyl estradiol 0.035 mg and norethindrone 0.75 mg [7 light peach tablets]

Day 15-21: Ethinyl estradiol 0.035 mg and norethindrone 1 mg [7 peach tablets]

Day 22-28: 7 light green inactive tablets (28s)

Aranelle:

Day 1-7: Ethinyl estradiol 0.035 mg and norethindrone 0.5 mg [7 light yellow tablets]

Day 8-16: Ethinyl estradiol 0.035 mg and norethindrone 1 mg [9 white tablets]

Day 17-21: Ethinyl estradiol 0.035 mg and norethindrone 0.5 mg [5 light yellow tablets]

Day 22-28: 7 peach inactive tablets (28s)

Cyclafem 7/7/7:

Day 1-7: Ethinyl estradiol 0.035 mg and norethindrone 0.5 mg [7 white tablets]

Day 8-14: Ethinyl estradiol 0.035 mg and norethindrone 0.75 mg [7 light pink tablets]

Day 15-21: Ethinyl estradiol 0.035 mg and norethindrone 1 mg [7 pink tablets]

Day 22-28: 7 light green inactive tablets (28s)

Dasetta 7/7/7:

Day 1-7: Ethinyl estradiol 0.035 mg and norethindrone 0.5 mg [7 light peach tablets]

Day 8-14: Ethinyl estradiol 0.035 mg and norethindrone 0.75 mg [7 peach tablets]

Day 15-21: Ethinyl estradiol 0.035 mg and norethindrone 1 mg [7 orange tablets]

Day 22-28: 7 white inactive tablets (28s)

Estrostep Fe, Tilia Fe:

Day 1-5: Ethinyl estradiol 0.02 mg and norethindrone acetate 1 mg [5 white triangular tablets]

Day 6-12: Ethinyl estradiol 0.03 mg and norethindrone acetate 1 mg [7 white square tablets]

Day 13-21: Ethinyl estradiol 0.035 mg and norethindrone acetate 1 mg [9 white round tablets]

Day 22-28: Ferrous fumarate 75 mg [7 brown tablets] (28s)

Leena:

Day 1-7: Ethinyl estradiol 0.035 mg and norethindrone 0.5 mg [7 light blue tablets]

Day 8-16: Ethinyl estradiol 0.035 mg and norethindrone 1 mg [9 light yellow-green tablets]

Day 17-21: Ethinyl estradiol 0.035 mg and norethindrone 0.5 mg [5 light blue tablets]

Day 22-28: 7 orange inactive tablets (28s)

Necon 7/7/7, Ortho-Novum 7/7/7:

Day 1-7: Ethinyl estradiol 0.035 mg and norethindrone 0.5 mg [7 white tablets]

Day 8-14: Ethinyl estradiol 0.035 mg and norethindrone 0.75 mg [7 light peach tablets]

Day 15-21: Ethinyl estradiol 0.035 mg and norethindrone 1 mg [7 peach tablets]

Day 22-28: 7 green inactive tablets (28s)

Nortrel 7/7/7:

Day 1-7: Ethinyl estradiol 0.035 mg and norethindrone 0.5 mg [7 light yellow tablets]

Day 8-14: Ethinyl estradiol 0.035 mg and norethindrone 0.75 mg [7 blue tablets]

Day 15-21: Ethinyl estradiol 0.035 mg and norethindrone 1 mg [7 peach tablets]

Day 22-28: 7 white inactive tablets (28s)

Tri-Legest Fe:

Day 1-5: Ethinyl estradiol 0.02 mg and norethindrone acetate 1 mg [5 light pink tablets]

Day 6-12: Ethinyl estradiol 0.03 mg and norethindrone acetate 1 mg [7 light yellow tablets]

Day 13-21: Ethinyl estradiol 0.035 mg and norethindrone acetate 1 mg [9 light blue tablets]

Day 22-28: Ferrous fumarate 75 mg [7 brown tablets] (28s)

Tri-Norinyl:

Day 1-7: Ethinyl estradiol 0.035 mg and norethindrone 0.5 mg [7 blue tablets]

Day 8-16: Ethinyl estradiol 0.035 mg and norethindrone 1 mg [9 yellow-green tablets]

Day 17-21: Ethinyl estradiol 0.035 mg and norethindrone 0.5 mg [5 blue tablets]

Day 22-28: 7 orange inactive tablets (28s)

General Dosage Range Oral: *Children and Adults (females, postmenarche):* 1 tablet daily

Administration

Oral Administer at the same time each day at intervals not >24 hours; without regard to meals.

For some products (eg, Generess Fe, Lo Loestrin Fe, Lo Minastrin Fe): If vomiting or diarrhea occurs within 3-4 hours of a dose, consider the dose to be missed.

Hazardous agent; use appropriate precautions for handling and disposal (NIOSH, 2012).

Nursing Actions

Physical Assessment See individual agents.

Patient Education

- Discuss specific use of drug and side effects with patient as it relates to treatment. (HCAHPS: During this hospital stay, were you given any medicine that you had not taken before? Before giving you any new medicine, how often did hospital staff tell you what the medicine was for? How often did hospital staff describe possible side effects in a way you could understand?)
- Patient may experience lack of appetite, polyphagia, weight gain, cramps, bloating, macromastia, alopecia, sexual dysfunction, menstrual irregularities, or diarrhea. Have patient report immediately to prescriber signs of hepatic impairment, angina, dyspnea, hemoptysis, severe dizziness, syncope, considerable nausea, strength differences from one side to another, difficulty speaking or thinking, change in balance, blurred vision, edema, skin discoloration, painful extremities, severe headache, depression, intolerable asthenia, considerable dyspepsia, urinary retention, oliguria, lump in breast, mastalgia, nipple discharge, vaginal hemorrhaging, vaginitis, vision changes, exophthalmos, or contact lens discomfort (HCAHPS).
- Educate patient about signs of a significant reaction (eg, wheezing; chest tightness; fever; itching; bad cough; blue skin color; seizures; or swelling of face, lips, tongue, or throat). **Note:** This is not a comprehensive list of all side effects. Patient should consult prescriber for additional questions.

Intended Use and Disclaimer: Should not be printed and given to patients. This information is intended to serve as a concise initial reference for healthcare professionals to use when discussing medications with a patient. You must ultimately rely on your own discretion, experience and judgment in diagnosing, treating and advising patients.

Related Information
Norethindrone *on page 1139*

Ethinyl Estradiol and Norgestimate
(ETH in il es tra DYE ole & nor JES ti mate)

Brand Names: U.S. Estarylla; MonoNessa; Ortho Tri-Cyclen; Ortho Tri-Cyclen Lo; Ortho-Cyclen; Previfem; Sprintec; Tri-Estarylla; Tri-Previfem; Tri-Sprintec; TriNessa

Index Terms Ethinyl Estradiol and NGM; Norgestimate and Ethinyl Estradiol; Ortho Cyclen; Ortho Tri Cyclen

Pharmacologic Category Contraceptive; Estrogen and Progestin Combination

Medication Safety Issues
Sound-alike/look-alike issues:
Ortho-Cyclen may be confused with Ortho-Cept

Ortho Tri-Cyclen may be confused with Ortho Tri-Cyclen Lo

International issues:
Vivelle: Brand name for ethinyl estradiol/norgestimate [Austria], but also a brand name for estradiol [U.S. (discontinued), Belgium]

Pregnancy Risk Factor X

Lactation Enters breast milk/not recommended

Use
Acne vulgaris: For the treatment of moderate acne vulgaris in females at least 15 years of age
Limitations of use: When used for acne, use only in females ≥15 years of age who achieved menarche, who also desire combination hormonal contraceptive therapy, are unresponsive to topical treatments, have no contraindications to combination hormonal contraceptive use, and plan to stay on therapy for ≥6 months
Contraception: For the prevention of pregnancy.

Unlabeled Use Treatment of heavy (excessive) menstrual bleeding (menorrhagia); dysmenorrhea; abnormal uterine bleeding; treatment of polycystic ovary syndrome (PCOS) in women with menstrual irregularities and hirsutism/acne

Available Dosage Forms
Tablet, oral [monophasic formulation]:
Estarylla: Ethinyl estradiol 0.035 mg and norgestimate 0.25 mg [21 blue tablets and 7 green inactive tablets] (28s)
MonoNessa, Ortho-Cyclen: Ethinyl estradiol 0.035 mg and norgestimate 0.25 mg [21 blue tablets and 7 dark green inactive tablets] (28s)
Previfem: Ethinyl estradiol 0.035 mg and norgestimate 0.25 mg [21 blue tablets and 7 light green inactive tablets] (28s)
Sprintec: Ethinyl estradiol 0.035 mg and norgestimate 0.25 mg [21 blue tablets and 7 white inactive tablets] (28s)

Tablet, oral [triphasic formulation]:
Ortho Tri-Cyclen, TriNessa:
Day 1-7: Ethinyl estradiol 0.035 mg and norgestimate 0.18 mg [7 white tablets]
Day 8-14: Ethinyl estradiol 0.035 mg and norgestimate 0.215 mg [7 light blue tablets]
Day 15-21: Ethinyl estradiol 0.035 mg and norgestimate 0.25 mg [7 blue tablets]
Day 22-28: 7 dark green inactive tablets (28s)
Tri-Estarylla
Day 1-7: Ethinyl estradiol 0.035 mg and norgestimate 0.18 mg [7 white tablets]
Day 8-14: Ethinyl estradiol 0.035 mg and norgestimate 0.215 mg [7 light blue tablets]
Day 15-21: Ethinyl estradiol 0.035 mg and norgestimate 0.25 mg [7 blue tablets]
Day 22-28: 7 green inactive tablets (28s)
Tri-Previfem::
Day 1-7: Ethinyl estradiol 0.035 mg and norgestimate 0.18 mg [7 white tablets]
Day 8-14: Ethinyl estradiol 0.035 mg and norgestimate 0.215 mg [7 light blue tablets]

Day 15-21: Ethinyl estradiol 0.035 mg and nor-gestimate 0.25 mg [7 blue tablets]

Day 22-28: 7 light green inactive tablets (28s)

Tri-Sprintec:

Day 1-7: Ethinyl estradiol 0.035 mg and norges-timate 0.18 mg [7 gray tablets]

Day 8-14: Ethinyl estradiol 0.035 mg and nor-gestimate 0.215 mg [7 light blue tablets]

Day 15-21: Ethinyl estradiol 0.035 mg and nor-gestimate 0.25 mg [7 blue tablets]

Day 22-28: 7 white inactive tablets (28s)

Ortho Tri-Cyclen Lo:

Day 1-7: Ethinyl estradiol 0.025 mg and norges-timate 0.18 mg [7 white tablets]

Day 8-14: Ethinyl estradiol 0.025 mg and nor-gestimate 0.215 mg [7 light blue tablets]

Day 15-21: Ethinyl estradiol 0.025 mg and nor-gestimate 0.25 mg [7 dark blue tablets]

Day 22-28: 7 dark green inactive tablets (28s)

General Dosage Range Oral: *Children and Adults (females, postmenarche):* 1 tablet daily

Administration

Oral Administer at the same time each day at intervals not >24 hours. Hazardous agent; use appropriate precautions for handling and disposal (NIOSH, 2012).

Nursing Actions

Physical Assessment Emphasize importance of regular (monthly) blood pressure checks and annual physical assessment, Pap smear, and vision assessment. Teach importance of maintaining prescribed schedule of dosing.

Patient Education

• Discuss specific use of drug and side effects with patient as it relates to treatment. (HCAHPS: During this hospital stay, were you given any medicine that you had not taken before? Before giving you any new medicine, how often did hospital staff tell you what the medicine was for? How often did hospital staff describe possible side effects in a way you could understand?)

• Patient may experience lack of appetite, poly-phagia, weight gain, abdominal cramps, bloating, macromastia, alopecia, acne vulgaris, sexual dysfunction, or menstrual irregularities. Have patient report immediately to prescriber signs of hepatic impairment, angina, dyspnea, hemoptysis, severe dizziness, syncope, considerable nausea, strength differences from one side to another, difficulty speaking or thinking, change in balance, blurred vision, edema, skin discoloration, painful extremities, severe headache, depression, intolerable asthenia, considerable dyspepsia, urinary retention, oliguria, lump in breast, mastalgia, nipple discharge, vaginal hemorrhaging, vaginitis, vision changes, exophthalmos, or contact lens discomfort (HCAHPS).

• Educate patient about signs of a significant reaction (eg, wheezing; chest tightness; fever; itching; bad cough; blue skin color; seizures; or swelling of face, lips, tongue, or throat). **Note:** This is not a comprehensive list of all side effects. Patient should consult prescriber for additional questions.

Intended Use and Disclaimer: Should not be printed and given to patients. This information is intended to serve as a concise initial reference for healthcare professionals to use when discussing medications with a patient. You must ultimately rely on your own discretion, experience and judgment in diagnosing, treating and advising patients.

Ethinyl Estradiol, Drospirenone, and Levomefolate

(ETH in il es tra DYE ole, droh SPYE re none, & lee voe me FOE late)

Brand Names: U.S. Beyaz; Safyral

Index Terms Drospirenone, Ethinyl Estradiol, and Levomefolate Calcium; Ethinyl Estradiol, Drospirenone, and Levomefolate Calcium; Levomefolate Calcium, Drospirenone, and Ethinyl Estradiol; Levomefolate, Drospirenone, and Ethinyl Estradiol

Pharmacologic Category Contraceptive; Estrogen and Progestin Combination

Medication Safety Issues

Sound-alike/look-alike issues:

Beyaz may be confused with Yaz

Lactation Enters breast milk/not recommended

Use Prevention of pregnancy; treatment of premenstrual dysphoric disorder (PMDD); treatment of acne; folate supplementation

Unlabeled Use Treatment of hypermenorrhea (menorrhagia); pain associated with endometriosis; dysmenorrhea; dysfunctional uterine bleeding; treatment of polycystic ovary syndrome (PCOS) in women with menstrual irregularities and hirsutism/acne

Available Dosage Forms

Tablet, oral:

Beyaz: Ethinyl estradiol 0.02 mg, drospirenone 3 mg, and levomefolate calcium 0.451 mg [24 pink tablets] and levomefolate calcium 0.451 mg [4 light orange tablets] (28s)

Safyral: Ethinyl estradiol 0.03 mg, drospirenone 3 mg, and levomefolate calcium 0.451 mg [21 orange tablets] and levomefolate calcium 0.451 mg [7 light orange tablets] (28s)

General Dosage Range Oral: *Children ≥14 years and Adults:* 1 tablet daily

Administration

Oral May be administered with or without food, but must be taken at the same time each day, preferably after the evening meal or at bedtime. If severe vomiting or diarrhea occurs, additional contraception (nonhormonal) should be used. If vomiting occurs within 3-4 hours of dosing, consider the dose to be missed.

Hazardous agent; use appropriate precautions for handling and disposal (NIOSH, 2012).

Nursing Actions

Patient Education

• Discuss specific use of drug and side effects with patient as it relates to treatment. (HCAHPS: During this hospital stay, were you given any medicine that you had not taken before? Before giving you any new medicine, how often did hospital staff tell you what the medicine was for? How often did hospital staff describe possible side effects in a way you could understand?)

• Patient may experience lack of appetite, polyphagia, weight gain, cramps, bloating, macromastia, sexual dysfunction, or menstrual irregularities. Have patient report immediately to prescriber signs of hepatic impairment, arrhythmia, angina, dyspnea, hemoptysis, severe dizziness, syncope, considerable nausea, strength differences from one side to another, difficulty speaking or thinking, change in balance, blurred vision, edema, skin discoloration, painful extremities, severe headache, depression, intolerable asthenia, urinary retention, oliguria, lump in breast, mastalgia, nipple discharge, vaginal hemorrhaging, vaginitis, vision changes, exophthalmos, or contact lens discomfort (HCAHPS).

• Educate patient about signs of a significant reaction (eg, wheezing; chest tightness; fever; itching; bad cough; blue skin color; seizures; or swelling of face, lips, tongue, or throat). **Note:** This is not a comprehensive list of all side effects. Patient should consult prescriber for additional questions.

Intended Use and Disclaimer: Should not be printed and given to patients. This information is intended to serve as a concise initial reference for healthcare professionals to use when discussing medications with a patient. You must ultimately rely on your own discretion, experience and judgment in diagnosing, treating and advising patients.

Etodolac (ee toe DOE lak)

Index Terms Etodolic Acid; Lodine
Pharmacologic Category Nonsteroidal Anti-inflammatory Drug (NSAID), Oral
Medication Safety Issues
Sound-alike/look-alike issues:
Lodine may be confused with codeine, iodine, Lopid®
BEERS Criteria medication:
This drug may be potentially inappropriate for use in geriatric patients (Quality of evidence - moderate; Strength of recommendation - strong).
Medication Guide Available Yes
Pregnancy Risk Factor C

Lactation Excretion in breast milk unknown/not recommended
Use Acute and long-term use in the management of signs and symptoms of osteoarthritis; rheumatoid arthritis and juvenile idiopathic arthritis (JIA); management of acute pain
Available Dosage Forms
Capsule, Oral:
Generic: 200 mg, 300 mg
Tablet, Oral:
Generic: 400 mg, 500 mg
Tablet Extended Release 24 Hour, Oral:
Generic: 400 mg, 500 mg, 600 mg
General Dosage Range Oral:
Extended release:
Children 6-16 years and 20-30 kg: 400 mg once daily
Children 6-16 years and 31-45 kg: 600 mg once daily
Children 6-16 years and 46-60 kg: 800 mg once daily
Children 6-16 years and >60 kg: 1000 mg once daily
Adults: 400-1000 mg once daily
Regular release: *Adults:* 200-400 mg every 6-12 hours as needed **or** 500 mg 2 times/day (maximum: 1 g/day)
Administration
Oral May be administered with food to decrease GI upset.
Nursing Actions
Physical Assessment Monitor blood pressure at the beginning of therapy and periodically during use. Monitor for adverse gastrointestinal effects, cardiovascular complaints, and ototoxicity at beginning of therapy and periodically throughout.
Patient Education
• Discuss specific use of drug and side effects with patient as it relates to treatment. (HCAHPS: During this hospital stay, were you given any medicine that you had not taken before? Before giving you any new medicine, how often did hospital staff tell you what the medicine was for? How often did hospital staff describe possible side effects in a way you could understand?)
• Patient may experience pyrosis, constipation, flatulence, diarrhea, or rhinitis. Have patient report immediately to prescriber signs of hepatic impairment, dyspnea, excessive weight gain, edema of extremities, angina, tachycardia, strength differences from one side to another, difficulty speaking or thinking, change in balance, blurred vision, severe headache, considerable dizziness, syncope, significant asthenia, tinnitus, mood changes, depression, arrhythmia, intolerable nausea, severe dyspepsia, considerable back pain, melena, hematemesis, ecchymosis, hemorrhaging, urinary retention, oliguria, chills, pharyngitis, significant arthralgia, or intolerable myalgia (HCAHPS).

• Educate patient about signs of a significant reaction (eg, wheezing; chest tightness; fever; itching; bad cough; blue skin color; seizures; or swelling of face, lips, tongue, or throat). **Note:** This is not a comprehensive list of all side effects. Patient should consult prescriber for additional questions.

Intended Use and Disclaimer: Should not be printed and given to patients. This information is intended to serve as a concise initial reference for healthcare professionals to use when discussing medications with a patient. You must ultimately rely on your own discretion, experience and judgment in diagnosing, treating and advising patients.

Etonogestrel (e toe noe JES trel)

Brand Names: U.S. Implanon; Nexplanon

Index Terms 3-Keto-desogestrel; ENG

Pharmacologic Category Contraceptive; Progestin

Lactation Enters breast milk/use caution

Breast-Feeding Considerations Etonogestrel was not found to affect the quality or quantity of breast milk. Do not insert <21 days postpartum. Levels of etonogestrel are highest during the first month following insertion (~2.2% of the weight-adjusted maternal daily dose). Breast-fed infants of mothers with an etonogestrel implant were not found to have adverse physical or psychomotor development in comparison to those infants of mothers using nonhormonal contraception.

Use Prevention of pregnancy; for use in women who request long-acting (up to 3 years) contraception

Mechanism of Action/Effect Etonogestrel is the active metabolite of desogestrel. It prevents pregnancy by suppressing ovulation, increasing the viscosity of cervical mucous, and inhibiting endometrial proliferation.

Contraindications Hypersensitivity to etonogestrel or any component of the formulation; undiagnosed abnormal genital bleeding; active hepatic disease or tumors; thrombosis or thromboembolic disorders (current or history of); known/suspected or history of carcinoma of the breast; pregnancy

Warnings/Precautions Hazardous agent - use appropriate precautions for handling and disposal (NIOSH, 2012).

Use does not protect against HIV infection or other sexually-transmitted diseases. Insert intradermally; should be palpable after implanted. Improper insertion may lead to unintended pregnancy or may cause difficult or impossible removal. Failure to properly remove may lead to infertility, ectopic pregnancy, or continued adverse reactions. Following removal of the implant, alternative contraception should be initiated immediately. Pregnancies have been observed as early as 7-14 days following implant removal. A nonhormonal contraceptive should be used until the presence of the implant has been confirmed. Menstrual bleeding patterns are likely to be altered; patients should be counseled prior to implant insertion. Abnormal bleeding should be evaluated as required to exclude pathologic conditions or pregnancy. Ectopic pregnancy (rare) may occur more commonly than in women using no contraception. Follicular development may occur and may continue to increase in size beyond what may occur in a normal cycle; generally ovarian cysts resolve spontaneously without intervention; however, surgery may rarely be required. Contraceptive therapy with etonogestrel commonly results in an average weight gain of ~2.8 pounds after 1 year and ~3.7 pounds after 2 years of treatment. Use caution in overweight women; women >130% of ideal body weight were not included in clinical studies.

May increase the risk of thromboembolism; prior to implantation, carefully consider use in women with known risk factors for arterial/venous thromboembolism. Consider removal during periods of prolonged immobilization due to surgery or illness. Due to risk of thromboembolism associated with pregnancy and the postpartum period, do not use etonogestrel prior to 21 days postpartum. Women with a history of hypertension-related diseases should be encouraged to use a nonhormonal form of contraception. In women with hypertension that is well-controlled, use may be considered; monitor blood pressure closely. Estrogens may cause retinal vascular thrombosis; discontinue if migraine, loss of vision, proptosis, diplopia, or other visual disturbances occur; discontinue permanently if papilledema or retinal vascular lesions are observed on examination. Not for use prior to menarche.

Hormonal contraception should be avoided in women with active or a history of breast cancer. Combination hormonal contraception use has been associated with a slight increase in frequency of breast cancer; however, studies are not consistent. Use with caution in patients with diabetes, patients treated for hyperlipidemia, a history of depression, or in patients with diseases which may be exacerbated by fluid retention, including asthma, epilepsy, migraine, diabetes, or renal dysfunction. Use with caution in patients with renal impairment; women with renal disease should be encouraged to use a nonhormonal form of contraception. Use is contraindicated active hepatic disease; remove implant if jaundice develops or if liver function becomes abnormal. Extremely rare hepatic adenomas have been reported in association with long-term combination oral contraceptive use; risk with progestin only contraceptives is not known. The manufacturer does not recommend use in women chronically taking hepatic enzyme inducers. Etonogestrel serum levels and contraceptive efficacy may be significantly decreased by potent hepatic enzyme inducers. Any changes with lens tolerance or vision in contact lens wearers should be evaluated by an ophthalmologist. The use of estrogens and/or progestins may change the results of some laboratory tests (eg, coagulation factors, lipids, glucose tolerance, binding proteins). The dose, route, and the specific estrogen/progestin influences these changes. In addition, personal risk factors (eg, cardiovascular disease, smoking, diabetes, age) also contribute to adverse events; use of specific products may be contraindicated in women with certain risk factors.

Additional warnings based on combination hormonal (estrogen and progestin) contraceptives: The risk of cardiovascular side effects increases in women who smoke cigarettes, especially those who are >35 years of age; women who use combination hormonal contraceptives should be strongly advised not to smoke. Combination hormonal contraceptives may lead to increased risk of myocardial infarction; use with caution in patients with risk factors for coronary artery disease. Combination hormonal contraceptives may have a dose-related risk of gallbladder disease.

Drug Interactions

Avoid Concomitant Use

Avoid concomitant use of Etonogestrel with any of the following: Griseofulvin; Tranexamic Acid; Ulipristal

Decreased Effect

Etonogestrel may decrease the levels/effects of: Anticoagulants; Vitamin K Antagonists

The levels/effects of Etonogestrel may be decreased by: Acitretin; Aminoglutethimide; Aprepitant; Artemether; Barbiturates; Bexarotene (Systemic); Bile Acid Sequestrants; Bosentan; CarBAMazepine; CloBAZam; Dabrafenib; Efavirenz; Eslicarbazepine; Exenatide; Felbamate; Fosaprepitant; Fosphenytoin; Griseofulvin; LamoTRIgine; Metreleptin; Mifepristone; Mycophenolate; Nelfinavir; Nevirapine; OXcarbazepine; Perampanel; Phenytoin; Primidone; Prucalopride; Retinoic Acid Derivatives; Rifamycin Derivatives; St Johns Wort; Sugammadex; Telaprevir; Topiramate; Uliprsital

Increased Effect/Toxicity

Etonogestrel may increase the levels/effects of: Benzodiazepines (metabolized by oxidation); Selegiline; Thalidomide; Tranexamic Acid; Voriconazole

The levels/effects of Etonogestrel may be increased by: Atazanavir; Boceprevir; Cobicistat; Herbs (Progestogenic Properties); Metreleptin; Mifepristone; Voriconazole

Nutritional/Ethanol Interactions

Herb/Nutraceutical: St John's wort (an enzyme inducer) may decrease serum levels of etonogestrel. Concomitant use is not recommended.

Bloodroot, chasteberry, damiana, oregano, and yucca may enhance the adverse/toxic effect of progestins.

Adverse Reactions

>10%:

Central nervous system: Headache (25%)

Dermatologic: Acne (14%)

Endocrine & metabolic: Infrequent menstrual bleeding (<3 episodes/90 days: 34%), amenorrhea (no bleeding in 90 days: 22%), prolonged menstrual bleeding (lasting >14 days: 18%), breast pain (13%), menstrual bleeding irregularities requiring discontinuation (11%)

Gastrointestinal: Weight gain (14%), abdominal pain (11%)

Genitourinary: Vaginitis (15%)

Respiratory: Pharyngitis (11%)

1% to 10%:

Central nervous system: Dizziness (7%), emotional lability (7%), depression (6%), nervousness (6%), pain (6%)

Endocrine & metabolic: Dysmenorrhea (7%), frequent menstrual bleeding (>5 episodes/90 days: 7%)

Gastrointestinal: Nausea (6%)

Genitourinary: Leukorrhea (10%)

Local: Implant site reactions (9%), insertion site pain (3% to 5%)

Neuromuscular & skeletal: Back pain (7%)

Miscellaneous: Flu-like syndrome (8%), hypersensitivity reactions (5%)

Pharmacodynamics/Kinetics

Onset of Action Serum levels sufficient to inhibit ovulation: ≤8 hours of implant

Duration of Action Implant: Each rod maintains etonogestrel levels sufficient to inhibit ovulation for 3 years

Available Dosage Forms

Implant, Subcutaneous:

Implanon: 68 mg (1 ea)

Nexplanon: 68 mg (1 ea)

General Dosage Range Subdermal: *Adults (females, postmenarche):* Implant 1 rod for up to 3 years

Administration

Other Subdermal: For insertion under local anesthesia by healthcare providers trained in the insertion and removal procedure. Rod should be inserted ~8-10 cm (3-4 inches) above the medial epicondyle of the humerus just under the skin. Rod must be palpable after insertion. Deep insertion may require surgery to remove. A pressure bandage should be applied and left in place for 24 hours after insertion to decrease bruising; a small bandage placed over the insertion site should remain in place for 3-5 days.

If rod is impalpable:

Implanon®: Ultrasound should be used to locate the rod; MRI may also be useful if ultrasound is not successful. Implanon® is not radiopaque and cannot be visualized by x-ray or CT scan. If ultrasound and MRI are unsuccessful, call 1-877-467-5266 for more information.

Nexplanon®: Two-dimensional x-ray should be used to locate the rod; other methods for localization include x-ray computer tomography (CT), ultrasound scanning (USS) with a high-frequency linear array transducer (≥10 MHz), or MRI. If these methods are unsuccessful, call 1-877-467-5266.

Hazardous agent; use appropriate precautions for handling and disposal (NIOSH, 2012).

Storage/Stability Store at controlled room temperature of 25°C (77°F); excursions permitted to 15°C to 30°C (59°F to 86°F). Implanon®: Protect from light.

Nursing Actions

Physical Assessment Assess insertion site.

Patient Education

• Discuss specific use of drug and side effects with patient as it relates to treatment. (HCAHPS: During this hospital stay, were you given any medicine that you had not taken before? Before giving you any new medicine, how often did hospital staff tell you what the medicine was for? How often did hospital staff describe possible side effects in a way you could understand?)

• Patient may experience weight gain, headache, acne vulgaris, mood changes, vaginal irritation, menstrual irregularities, or vascular diseases (ie, gallbladder disease, blood clots, heart attacks, other blood vessel problems) (rare). Have patient report immediately to prescriber angina, dyspnea, edema of extremities, skin discoloration, painful extremities, signs of depression (ie, suicidal ideation, anxiety, emotional instability, illogical thinking), severe vaginal hemorrhaging, significant dyspepsia, considerable nausea, vision changes, ophthalmalgia, eye irritation, lump in breast, mastalgia, intolerable skin irritation, or pregnancy (HCAHPS).

• Educate patient about signs of a significant reaction (eg, wheezing; chest tightness; fever; itching; bad cough; blue skin color; seizures; or swelling of face, lips, tongue, or throat). **Note:** This is not a comprehensive list of all side effects. Patient should consult prescriber for additional questions.

Intended Use and Disclaimer: Should not be printed and given to patients. This information is intended to serve as a concise initial reference for healthcare professionals to use when discussing medications with a patient. You must ultimately rely on your own discretion, experience and judgment in diagnosing, treating and advising patients.

Etoposide (e toe POE side)

Brand Names: U.S. Toposar

Index Terms EPEG; Epipodophyllotoxin; VePesid; VP-16; VP-16-213

Pharmacologic Category Antineoplastic Agent, Podophyllotoxin Derivative; Antineoplastic Agent, Topoisomerase II Inhibitor

Medication Safety Issues

Sound-alike/look-alike issues:

Etoposide may be confused with teniposide

Etoposide may be confused with etoposide phosphate (a prodrug of etoposide which is rapidly converted in the plasma to etoposide)

VePesid may be confused with Versed

High alert medication:

This medication is in a class the Institute for Safe Medication Practices (ISMP) includes among its list of drug classes which have a heightened risk of causing significant patient harm when used in error.

Pregnancy Risk Factor D

Lactation Excretion in breast milk unknown/not recommended

Breast-Feeding Considerations Due to the potential for serious adverse reactions in the nursing infant, the decision to discontinue etoposide or to discontinue breast-feeding during treatment should take into account the benefits of treatment to the mother.

Use Treatment of refractory testicular tumors (injectable formulation); treatment of small cell lung cancer (SCLC)

Canadian labeling: Treatment of small cell lung cancer (SCLC; first- and second-line); treatment of nonsmall cell lung cancer (NSCLC); treatment of non-Hodgkin lymphomas (first-line); treatment of testicular cancer (first-line [injectable formulation] and refractory)

Unlabeled Use Treatment of acute lymphocytic leukemia (ALL), refractory acute myeloid leukemia (AML), recurrent or metastatic breast cancer, central nervous system tumors, Ewing's sarcoma, gestational trophoblastic disease, Hodgkin lymphoma, merkel cell cancer, refractory multiple myeloma, neuroblastoma, neuroendocrine tumors (adrenal gland and carcinoid tumors), non-Hodgkin lymphomas, nonsmall cell lung cancer (NSCLC), osteosarcoma, ovarian cancer (refractory), prostate cancer, retinoblastoma, metastatic soft tissue sarcoma, thymic malignancies (locally advanced or metastatic), unknown-primary adenocarcinoma, Wilms' tumor; conditioning regimen for hematopoietic cell transplantation

Mechanism of Action/Effect Inhibits DNA synthesis leading to cell death.

Contraindications Hypersensitivity to etoposide or any component of the formulation

Canadian labeling: Additional contraindications (not in U.S. labeling): Severe leukopenia or thrombocytopenia; severe hepatic impairment; severe renal impairment

Warnings/Precautions Hazardous agent – use appropriate precautions for handling and disposal

(NIOSH, 2012). **[U.S. Boxed Warning]: Severe dose-limiting and dose-related myelosuppression with resulting infection or bleeding may occur.** Treatment should be withheld for platelets <50,000/mm^3 or absolute neutrophil count (ANC) <500/mm^3. May cause anaphylactic-like reactions manifested by chills, fever, tachycardia, bronchospasm, dyspnea, and hypotension. In addition, facial/tongue swelling, coughing, chest tightness, cyanosis, laryngospasm, diaphoresis, hypertension, back pain, loss of consciousness, and flushing have also been reported less commonly. Incidence is primarily associated with intravenous administration (up to 2%) compared to oral administration (<1%). Infusion should be interrupted and medications for the treatment of anaphylaxis should be available for immediate use. High drug concentration and rate of infusion, as well as presence of polysorbate 80 and benzyl alcohol in the etoposide intravenous formulation have been suggested as contributing factors to the development of hypersensitivity reactions. Etoposide intravenous formulations may contain polysorbate 80 and/or benzyl alcohol, while etoposide phosphate (the water soluble prodrug of etoposide) intravenous formulation does not contain either vehicle. Case reports have suggested that etoposide phosphate has been used successfully in patients with previous hypersensitivity reactions to etoposide (Collier, 2008; Siderov, 2002). The use of concentrations higher than recommended were associated with higher rates of anaphylactic-like reactions in children.

Secondary acute leukemias have been reported with etoposide, either as monotherapy or in combination with other chemotherapy agents. Must be diluted; do not give I.V. push, infuse over at least 30-60 minutes; hypotension is associated with rapid infusion. If hypotension occurs, interrupt infusion and administer I.V. hydration and supportive care; decrease infusion upon reinitiation. Tissue irritation and inflammation have occurred following extravasation. Do not administer I.M. or SubQ. Dosage should be adjusted in patients with hepatic or renal impairment (Canadian labeling contraindicates use in severe hepatic and/or renal impairment). Use with caution in patients with low serum albumin; may increase risk for toxicities. Use with caution in elderly patients; may be more likely to develop severe myelosuppression and/or GI effects (eg, nausea/vomiting). **[U.S. Boxed Warning]: Should be administered under the supervision of an experienced cancer chemotherapy physician.** Injectable formulation contains polysorbate 80; do not use in premature infants. May contain benzyl alcohol; do not use in newborn infants. Injectable formulation also contains alcohol (~33% v/v); may contribute to adverse reactions, especially with higher etoposide doses.

Drug Interactions

Avoid Concomitant Use

Avoid concomitant use of Etoposide with any of the following: BCG; CloZAPine; Conivaptan; Fusidic Acid (Systemic); Natalizumab; Pimecrolimus; Pimozide; Tacrolimus (Topical); Tofacitinib; Vaccines (Live)

Decreased Effect

Etoposide may decrease the levels/effects of: BCG; Coccidioidin Skin Test; Sipuleucel-T; Vaccines (Inactivated); Vaccines (Live); Vitamin K Antagonists

The levels/effects of Etoposide may be decreased by: Barbiturates; Bosentan; CYP3A4 Inducers (Strong); Dabrafenib; Deferasirox; Fosphenytoin; Herbs (CYP3A4 Inducers); Mitotane; P-glycoprotein/ABCB1 Inducers; Phenytoin; Tocilizumab

Increased Effect/Toxicity

Etoposide may increase the levels/effects of: ARIPiprazole; CloZAPine; Dofetilide; Leflunomide; Lomitapide; Natalizumab; Pimozide; Tofacitinib; Vaccines (Live); Vitamin K Antagonists

The levels/effects of Etoposide may be increased by: Atovaquone; Conivaptan; CycloSPORINE (Systemic); CYP3A4 Inhibitors (Moderate); CYP3A4 Inhibitors (Strong); Dasatinib; Denosumab; Fusidic Acid (Systemic); Ivacaftor; Luliconazole; Mifepristone; P-glycoprotein/ABCB1 Inhibitors; Pimecrolimus; Roflumilast; Simeprevir; Stiripentol; Tacrolimus (Topical); Trastuzumab

Nutritional/Ethanol Interactions

Ethanol: Avoid ethanol (may increase GI irritation). Herb/Nutraceutical: Avoid concurrent St John's wort; may decrease etoposide levels.

Adverse Reactions Note: The following may occur with higher doses used in stem cell transplantation: Alopecia, ethanol intoxication, hepatitis, hypotension (infusion-related), metabolic acidosis, mucositis, nausea and vomiting (severe), secondary malignancy, skin lesions (resembling Stevens-Johnson syndrome).

>10%:

Dermatologic: Alopecia (8% to 66%)

Gastrointestinal: Nausea/vomiting (31% to 43%), anorexia (10% to 13%), diarrhea (1% to 13%)

Hematologic: Leukopenia (60% to 91%; grade 4: 3% to 17%; nadir: 7-14 days; recovery: by day 20), thrombocytopenia (22% to 41%; grades 3/4: 1% to 20%; nadir 9-16 days; recovery: by day 20), anemia (≤33%)

1% to 10%:

Cardiovascular: Hypotension (1% to 2%; due to rapid infusion)

Gastrointestinal: Stomatitis (1% to 6%), abdominal pain (up to 2%)

Hepatic: Hepatic toxicity (up to 3%)

Neuromuscular & skeletal: Peripheral neuropathy (1% to 2%)

◀

Miscellaneous: Anaphylactic-like reaction (I.V. infusion 1% to 2%; oral capsules <1%; including chills, fever, tachycardia, bronchospasm, dyspnea)

Available Dosage Forms

Capsule, Oral:

Generic: 50 mg

Solution, Intravenous:

Toposar: 20 mg/mL (5 mL); 500 mg/25 mL (25 mL); 1 g/50 mL (50 mL)

Generic: 20 mg/mL (5 mL); 500 mg/25 mL (25 mL); 1 g/50 mL (50 mL)

General Dosage Range Dosage adjustment recommended in patients with hepatic impairment, renal impairment, or who develop toxicities.

I.V., oral: *Adults:* Dosage varies greatly depending on indication

Administration

I.V. Administer standard doses over at least 30-60 minutes to minimize the risk of hypotension. Higher (unlabeled) doses used in transplantation may be infused over longer time periods depending on the protocol. Etoposide injection contains polysorbate 80 which may cause leaching of diethylhexyl phthalate (DEHP), a plasticizer contained in polyvinyl chloride (PVC) tubing. Administration through non-PVC (low sorbing) tubing will minimize patient exposure to DEHP. Tissue irritation and inflammation have occurred following extravasation.

Concentrations >0.4 mg/mL are very unstable and may precipitate within a few minutes. For large doses, where dilution to ≤0.4 mg/mL is not feasible, consideration should be given to slow infusion of the undiluted drug through a running normal saline, dextrose or saline/dextrose infusion; or use of etoposide phosphate. Etoposide solutions of 0.1-0.4 mg/mL may be filtered through a 0.22 micron filter without damage to the filter; etoposide solutions of 0.2 mg/mL may be filtered through a 0.22 micron filter without significant loss of drug.

Hazardous agent; use appropriate precautions for handling and disposal (NIOSH, 2012).

Oral Doses ≤200 mg/day as a single once daily dose; doses >200 mg should be given in 2-4 divided doses. If necessary, the injection may be used for oral administration. Canadian labeling recommends administering capsule on an empty stomach.

Hazardous agent; use appropriate precautions for handling and disposal (NIOSH, 2012).

Preparation for Administration Hazardous agent; use appropriate precautions for handling and disposal (NIOSH, 2012). Etoposide should be diluted to a concentration of 0.2-0.4 mg/mL in D_5W or NS for administration. Diluted solutions have concentration-dependent stability: More concentrated solutions have shorter stability times.

Precipitation may occur with concentrations >0.4 mg/mL.

Storage/Stability

Capsules: Store oral capsules under refrigeration at 2°C to 8°C (36°F to 46°F); do not freeze.

Injection: Store intact vials of injection at room temperature of 25°C (77°F); do not freeze. Protect from light. Diluted solutions for infusion, at room temperature, in D_5W or NS in polyvinyl chloride, are stable as follows, depending on the concentration:

0.2 mg/mL: 96 hours

0.4 mg/mL: 24 hours

Etoposide injection contains polysorbate 80 which may cause leaching of diethylhexyl phthalate (DEHP), a plasticizer contained in polyvinyl chloride (PVC) bags and tubing. Higher concentrations and longer storage time after preparation in PVC bags may increase DEHP leaching. Preparation in glass or polyolefin containers will minimize patient exposure to DEHP. When undiluted etoposide injection is stored in acrylic or ABS (acrylonitrile, butadiene and styrene) plastic containers, the containers may crack and leak.

Nursing Actions

Physical Assessment Patient should be monitored closely for anaphylactic reaction (chills, fever, tachycardia, bronchospasm, dyspnea, hypotension). Emergency equipment should be available. Assess renal and hepatic function prior to each treatment and on a regular basis.

Patient Education

- Discuss specific use of drug and side effects with patient as it relates to treatment. (HCAHPS: During this hospital stay, were you given any medicine that you had not taken before? Before giving you any new medicine, how often did hospital staff tell you what the medicine was for? How often did hospital staff describe possible side effects in a way you could understand?)

- Patient may experience lack of appetite, stomatitis, or alopecia. Have patient report immediately to prescriber signs of infection, signs of hepatic impairment, paresthesia, severe dyspepsia, dyspnea, significant nausea, considerable diarrhea, ecchymosis, hemorrhaging, intolerable asthenia, vision changes, severe dizziness, syncope, tachycardia, considerable headache, flushing, signs of Stevens-Johnson syndrome/toxic epidermal necrolysis, or injection site irritation (HCAHPS).

- Educate patient about signs of a significant reaction (eg, wheezing; chest tightness; fever; itching; bad cough; blue skin color; seizures; or swelling of face, lips, tongue, or throat). **Note:** This is not a comprehensive list of all side effects. Patient should consult prescriber for additional questions.

Intended Use and Disclaimer: Should not be printed and given to patients. This information is

intended to serve as a concise initial reference for healthcare professionals to use when discussing medications with a patient. You must ultimately rely on your own discretion, experience and judgment in diagnosing, treating and advising patients.

Related Information

Management of Drug Extravasations *on page 1700*

Oral Medications That Should Not Be Crushed or Altered *on page 1712*

Etoposide Phosphate (e toe POE side FOS fate)

Brand Names: U.S. Etopophos
Index Terms Epipodophyllotoxin; ETOP
Pharmacologic Category Antineoplastic Agent, Podophyllotoxin Derivative; Antineoplastic Agent, Topoisomerase II Inhibitor
Medication Safety Issues
Sound-alike/look-alike issues:
Etoposide phosphate may be confused with etoposide, teniposide
Etoposide phosphate is a prodrug of etoposide and is rapidly converted in the plasma to etoposide. To avoid confusion or dosing errors, equivalent doses should be used when converting from etoposide to etoposide phosphate. Each 100 mg vial of etoposide phosphate is equivalent to 100 mg of etoposide.

High alert medication:
This medication is in a class the Institute for Safe Medication Practices (ISMP) includes among its list of drug classes which have a heightened risk of causing significant patient harm when used in error.

Pregnancy Risk Factor D
Lactation Excretion in breast milk unknown/not recommended
Breast-Feeding Considerations Due to the potential for serious adverse reactions in the nursing infant, breast feeding is not recommended.
Use Treatment of refractory testicular tumors; treatment of small cell lung cancer
Mechanism of Action/Effect Etoposide phosphate is converted *in vivo* to the active moiety, etoposide, by dephosphorylation. Etoposide inhibits mitotic activity; inhibits cells from entering prophase; inhibits DNA synthesis. Initially thought to be mitotic inhibitors similar to podophyllotoxin, but actually have no effect on microtubule assembly. However, later shown to induce DNA strand breakage and inhibition of topoisomerase II (an enzyme which breaks and repairs DNA); etoposide acts in late S or early G2 phases.
Contraindications Hypersensitivity to etoposide, etoposide phosphate, or any component of the formulation
Warnings/Precautions Hazardous agent - use appropriate precautions for handling and disposal

(NIOSH, 2012). **[U.S. Boxed Warning]: Severe dose-limiting and dose-related myelosuppression with resulting infection or bleeding may occur.** Treatment should be withheld for platelets <50,000/mm^3 or absolute neutrophil count (ANC) <500/mm^3. May cause anaphylactic-like reactions manifested by chills, fever, tachycardia, bronchospasm, dyspnea, and hypotension. In addition, facial/tongue swelling, coughing, throat tightness, cyanosis, laryngospasm, diaphoresis, back pain, hypertension, flushing, apnea and loss of consciousness have also been reported less commonly. Anaphylactic-type reactions have occurred with the first infusion. Infusion should be interrupted and medications for the treatment of anaphylaxis should be available for immediate use. Underlying mechanisms behind the development of hypersensitivity reactions is unknown, but have been attributed to high drug concentration and rate of infusion. Another possible mechanism may be due to the differences between available etoposide intravenous formulations. Etoposide intravenous formulation contains polysorbate 80 and benzyl alcohol, while etoposide phosphate (the water soluble prodrug of etoposide) intravenous formulation does not contain either vehicle. Case reports have suggested that etoposide phosphate has been used successfully in patients with previous hypersensitivity reactions to etoposide (Collier, 2008; Siderov, 2002).

Secondary acute leukemias have been reported with etoposide, either as monotherapy or in combination with other chemotherapy agents. Dosage should be adjusted in patients with hepatic or renal impairment. Use with caution in patients with low serum albumin; may increase risk for toxicities. Doses of etoposide phosphate >175 mg/m^2 have not been evaluated. Use caution in elderly patients (may be more likely to develop severe myelosuppression and/or GI effects. Administer by slow I.V. infusion; hypotension has been reported with etoposide phosphate administration, generally associated with rapid I.V. infusion. Injection site reactions may occur; monitor infusion site closely. **[U.S. Boxed Warning]: Should be administered under the supervision of an experienced cancer chemotherapy physician.**

Drug Interactions
Avoid Concomitant Use
Avoid concomitant use of Etoposide Phosphate with any of the following: BCG; CloZAPine; Conivaptan; Fusidic Acid (Systemic); Natalizumab; Pimecrolimus; Pimozide; Tacrolimus (Topical); Tofacitinib; Vaccines (Live)
Decreased Effect
Etoposide Phosphate may decrease the levels/ effects of: BCG; Coccidioidin Skin Test; Sipuleucel-T; Vaccines (Inactivated); Vaccines (Live)

The levels/effects of Etoposide Phosphate may be decreased by: Barbiturates; Bosentan; ▶

CYP3A4 Inducers (Strong); Dabrafenib; Deferasirox; Echinacea; Fosphenytoin; Herbs (CYP3A4 Inducers); Mitotane; P-glycoprotein/ABCB1 Inducers; Phenytoin; Tocilizumab

Increased Effect/Toxicity

Etoposide Phosphate may increase the levels/ effects of: ARIPiprazole; CloZAPine; Dofetilide; Leflunomide; Lomitapide; Natalizumab; Pimozide; Tofacitinib; Vaccines (Live)

The levels/effects of Etoposide Phosphate may be increased by: Conivaptan; CycloSPORINE (Systemic); CYP3A4 Inhibitors (Moderate); CYP3A4 Inhibitors (Strong); Dasatinib; Denosumab; Fusidic Acid (Systemic); Ivacaftor; Luliconazole; Mifepristone; P-glycoprotein/ABCB1 Inhibitors; Pimecrolimus; Roflumilast; Simeprevir; Stiripentol; Tacrolimus (Topical); Trastuzumab

Nutritional/Ethanol Interactions

Ethanol: Avoid ethanol (may increase GI irritation).
Herb/Nutraceutical: Avoid St John's wort (may decrease etoposide levels).

Adverse Reactions Note: Also see adverse reactions for **etoposide**; etoposide phosphate is converted to etoposide, adverse reactions experienced with etoposide would also be expected with etoposide phosphate.

>10%:
Central nervous system: Chills/fever (24%)
Dermatologic: Alopecia (33% to 44%)
Gastrointestinal: Nausea/vomiting (37%), anorexia (16%), mucositis (11%)
Hematologic: Leukopenia (91%; grade 4: 17%; nadir: day 15-22; recovery: usually by day 21), neutropenia (88%; grade 4: 37%; nadir: day 12-19; recovery: usually by day 21), anemia (72%; grades 3/4: 19%), thrombocytopenia (23%; grade 4: 9%; nadir: day 10-15; recovery: usually by day 21)
Neuromuscular & skeletal: Weakness/ malaise (39%)
1% to 10%:
Cardiovascular: Hypotension (1% to 5%), hypertension (3%), facial flushing (2%)
Central nervous system: Dizziness (5%)
Dermatologic: Skin rash (3%)
Gastrointestinal: Constipation (8%), abdominal pain (7%), diarrhea (6%), taste perversion (6%)
Local: Extravasation/phlebitis (5%; including swelling, pain, cellulitis, necrosis, and/or skin necrosis at site of infiltration)
Miscellaneous: Anaphylactic-type reactions (3%; including chills, diaphoresis, fever, rigor, tachycardia, bronchospasm, dyspnea, pruritus)

Available Dosage Forms

Solution Reconstituted, Intravenous:
Etopophos: 100 mg (1 ea)

General Dosage Range Dosage adjustment recommended in patients with hepatic or renal impairment

I.V.: *Adults:* Dosage varies greatly depending on indication

Administration

I.V. Infuse by slow I.V. infusion over 5-210 minutes; risk of hypotension may increase with rate of infusion. Do not administer as a bolus injection.

Hazardous agent; use appropriate precautions for handling and disposal (NIOSH, 2012).

Injectable Detail pH: 2.9 (reconstituted with sterile water for injection)

Preparation for Administration Hazardous agent; use appropriate precautions for handling and disposal (NIOSH, 2012). Reconstitute vials with 5 mL or 10 mL SWFI, D_5W, NS, bacteriostatic SWFI, or bacteriostatic NS to a concentration of 20 mg/mL or 10 mg/mL etoposide equivalent. These solutions may be administered without further dilution or may be diluted in 50-500 mL of D_5W or NS to a concentration as low as 0.1 mg/mL.

Storage/Stability Store intact vials under refrigeration at 2°C to 8°C (36°F to 46°F). Protect from light. Reconstituted solution is stable refrigerated at 2°C to 8°C (36°F to 46°F) for 7 days. At room temperature of 20°C to 25°C (68°F to 77°F), reconstituted solutions are stable for 24 hours when reconstituted with SWFI, D_5W, or NS, or for 48 hours when reconstituted with bacteriostatic SWFI or bacteriostatic NS. Further diluted solutions for infusion are stable at room temperature 20°C to 25°C (68°F to 77°F) or under refrigeration 2°C to 8°C (36°F to 46°F) for up to 24 hours.

Nursing Actions

Physical Assessment Use caution in presence of hepatic or renal impairment. Assess renal function prior to each treatment and on a regular basis.

Patient Education
- Discuss specific use of drug and side effects with patient as it relates to treatment. (HCAHPS: During this hospital stay, were you given any medicine that you had not taken before? Before giving you any new medicine, how often did hospital staff tell you what the medicine was for? How often did hospital staff describe possible side effects in a way you could understand?)
- Patient may experience anemia, stomatitis, cheilitis, injection site irritation, alopecia, or infertility. Have patient report immediately to prescriber signs of infection, dyspnea, significant nausea, ecchymosis, hemorrhaging, urine discoloration, jaundice, inability to eat, or considerable asthenia (HCAHPS).
- Educate patient about signs of a significant reaction (eg, wheezing; chest tightness; fever; itching; bad cough; blue skin color; seizures; or swelling of face, lips, tongue, or throat). **Note:** This is not a comprehensive list of all side effects. Patient should consult prescriber for additional questions.

Intended Use and Disclaimer: Should not be printed and given to patients. This information is intended to serve as a concise initial reference for healthcare professionals to use when discussing medications with a patient. You must ultimately rely on your own discretion, experience and judgment in diagnosing, treating and advising patients.

Related Information

Management of Drug Extravasations *on page 1700*

Etravirine (et ra VIR een)

Brand Names: U.S. Intelence

Index Terms ETR; TMC125

Pharmacologic Category Antiretroviral, Reverse Transcriptase Inhibitor, Non-nucleoside (Anti-HIV)

Medication Safety Issues

International issues:

Etravirine [U.S. and multiple international markets] may be confused with ethaverine [multiple international markets]

Pregnancy Risk Factor B

Lactation Excretion in breast milk unknown/contraindicated

Breast-Feeding Considerations Maternal or infant antiretroviral therapy does not completely eliminate the risk of postnatal HIV transmission. In addition, multiclass-resistant virus has been detected in breast-feeding infants despite maternal therapy. Therefore, in the United States, where formula is accessible, affordable, safe, and sustainable, and the risk of infant mortality due to diarrhea and respiratory infections is low, complete avoidance of breast-feeding by HIV-infected women is recommended to decrease potential transmission of HIV (DHHS [perinatal], 2012).

Use Treatment of HIV-1 infection in combination with at least two additional antiretroviral agents in treatment-experienced patients exhibiting viral replication with documented non-nucleoside reverse transcriptase inhibitor (NNRTI) resistance

Mechanism of Action/Effect As a non-nucleoside reverse transcriptase inhibitor, etravirine has activity against HIV-1 by binding to reverse transcriptase. It consequently blocks the RNA-dependent and DNA-dependent DNA polymerase activities, including HIV-1 replication. It does not require intracellular phosphorylation for antiviral activity.

Contraindications There are no contraindications listed in the manufacturer's U.S. labeling.

Canadian labeling: Hypersensitivity to etravirine or any component of the formulation.

Warnings/Precautions Severe and possibly life-threatening skin reactions (including Stevens-Johnson syndrome, toxic epidermal necrolysis, and erythema multiforme) and hypersensitivity reactions ranging from rash (including drug rash with eosinophilia and systemic symptoms [DRESS]) and/or constitutional symptoms to occasional organ dysfunction (including hepatic failure) have been reported; discontinue immediately with signs or symptoms of severe skin reaction or hypersensitivity. Self-limiting (with continued therapy) mild-to-moderate rashes (higher incidence in females) were also observed in clinical trials (pediatric and adult), usually during second week of therapy initiation. Not for use in treatment-naive patients, or experienced patients without evidence of viral mutations conferring resistance to NNRTIs and PIs. May cause redistribution of fat (eg, buffalo hump, peripheral wasting with increased abdominal girth, cushingoid appearance). Patients may develop immune reconstitution syndrome resulting in the occurrence of an inflammatory response to an indolent or residual opportunistic infection during initial HIV treatment or activation of autoimmune disorders (eg, Graves' disease, polymyositis, Guillain-Barré syndrome) later in therapy; further evaluation and treatment may be required.

High potential for drug interactions; concomitant use of etravirine with some drugs may require cautious use, may not be recommended, or may require dosage adjustments.

Drug Interactions

Avoid Concomitant Use

Avoid concomitant use of Etravirine with any of the following: Atazanavir; Axitinib; CarBAMazepine; Fosamprenavir; Fosphenytoin; PHENobarbital; Phenytoin; Primidone; Reverse Transcriptase Inhibitors (Non-Nucleoside); Rifamycin Derivatives; Rilpivirine; Ritonavir; Simeprevir; St Johns Wort; Tipranavir

Decreased Effect

Etravirine may decrease the levels/effects of: Amiodarone; Antifungal Agents (Azole Derivatives, Systemic); ARIPiprazole; Artemether; Atazanavir; Axitinib; Bepridil [Off Market]; Buprenorphine; CarBAMazepine; Clopidogrel; Diazepam; Disopyramide; Dolutegravir; Flecainide; HMG-CoA Reductase Inhibitors; Ibrutinib; Lidocaine (Systemic); Macrolide Antibiotics; Methadone; Mexiletine; Phosphodiesterase 5 Inhibitors; Propafenone; QuiNIDine; Rilpivirine; Saxagliptin; Simeprevir; Telaprevir

The levels/effects of Etravirine may be decreased by: Bosentan; CarBAMazepine; CYP2C19 Inducers (Strong); CYP2C9 Inducers (Strong); CYP3A4 Inducers (Strong); Dabrafenib; Deferasirox; Fosphenytoin; Mitotane; Peginterferon Alfa-2b; PHENobarbital; Phenytoin; Primidone; Protease Inhibitors; Reverse Transcriptase Inhibitors (Non-Nucleoside); Rifabutin; Rifamycin Derivatives; Ritonavir; St Johns Wort; Tipranavir; Tocilizumab

◀ **Increased Effect/Toxicity**
Etravirine may increase the levels/effects of: Antifungal Agents (Azole Derivatives, Systemic); Artemether; Bosentan; Carvedilol; Citalopram; CYP2C19 Substrates; CYP2C9 Substrates; Diazepam; Digoxin; Fosamprenavir; Protease Inhibitors; Rilpivirine

The levels/effects of Etravirine may be increased by: Antifungal Agents (Azole Derivatives, Systemic); Artemether; Atazanavir; Reverse Transcriptase Inhibitors (Non-Nucleoside)

Nutritional/Ethanol Interactions
Food: Food increases absorption of etravirine by ~50%. Management: Take after meals and maintain adequate hydration, unless instructed to restrict fluid intake.
Herb/Nutraceutical: St John's wort may decrease the levels/effects of etravirine. Management: Avoid St John's wort.

Adverse Reactions
>10%:
Dermatologic: Rash (≥grade 2: 10% to 15%)
Endocrine & metabolic: Cholesterol (total) increased (≤300 mg/dL: 20%; >300 mg/dL: 8%), hyperglycemia (≤250 mg/dL: 15%; 251-500 mg/dL: 4%), LDL increased (≤190 mg/dL: 13%)
Gastrointestinal: Nausea
2% to 10%:
Endocrine & metabolic: Triglycerides increased (≤750 mg/dL: 9%; >750 mg/dL: 4% to 6%)
Gastrointestinal: Diarrhea (children and adolescents ≥2%), amylase increased (>5 x ULN: 2%)
Hepatic: ALT increased (≤5 x ULN: 6%; >5 x ULN: 3%), AST increased (≤5 x ULN: 6%; >5 x ULN: 3%)
Neuromuscular & skeletal: Peripheral neuropathy (≥ grade 2: 4%)
Renal: Creatinine increased (≤1.8 x ULN: 6%; >1.8 x ULN: 2%)

Available Dosage Forms
Tablet, Oral:
Intelence: 25 mg, 100 mg, 200 mg
General Dosage Range Oral:
Children ≥6 years and ≥16 kg to <20 kg: 100 mg twice daily
Children ≥6 years and ≥20 kg to <25 kg: 125 mg twice daily
Children ≥6 years and ≥25 kg to <30 kg: 150 mg twice daily
Children ≥6 years and ≥30 kg and Adults: 200 mg twice daily
Administration
Oral Administer after meals. If unable to swallow tablets, may disperse tablets in water (≥1 teaspoonful [enough to cover tablets]); stir well (until milky), add additional water (or may add milk or orange juice), and drink immediately. Rinse glass several times (with water, milk or orange juice) and swallow entire contents to ensure administration of dose. Do not use grapefruit juice, carbonated beverages or warm (>40°C) water.

Storage/Stability Store at USP controlled room temperature of 25°C (77°F); excursions permitted to 15°C to 30°C (59°F to 86°F). Protect from moisture.
Nursing Actions
Physical Assessment Assess adherence to therapy. Monitor for rash and gastrointestinal upset. Teach patient proper timing of multiple medications.
Patient Education
• Discuss specific use of drug and side effects with patient as it relates to treatment. (HCAHPS: During this hospital stay, were you given any medicine that you had not taken before? Before giving you any new medicine, how often did hospital staff tell you what the medicine was for? How often did hospital staff describe possible side effects in a way you could understand?)
• Patient may experience nausea, diarrhea, or lipodystrophy. Have patient report immediately to prescriber signs of hepatic impairment, signs of pancreatitis, signs of hyperglycemia, severe asthenia, paresthesia, hematemesis, vision changes, urinary retention, oliguria, angina, considerable dizziness, syncope, arrhythmia, arthralgia, illogical thinking, memory loss, myalgia, significant headache, dyspnea, tremors, ecchymosis, hemorrhaging, hyperhidrosis, signs of Stevens-Johnson syndrome/toxic epidermal necrolysis, or signs of infection (HCAHPS).
• Educate patient about signs of a significant reaction (eg, wheezing; chest tightness; fever; itching; bad cough; blue skin color; seizures; or swelling of face, lips, tongue, or throat). **Note:** This is not a comprehensive list of all side effects. Patient should consult prescriber for additional questions.

Intended Use and Disclaimer: Should not be printed and given to patients. This information is intended to serve as a concise initial reference for healthcare professionals to use when discussing medications with a patient. You must ultimately rely on your own discretion, experience and judgment in diagnosing, treating and advising patients.
Dietary Considerations Take after meals.
Related Information
Oral Medications That Should Not Be Crushed or Altered *on page 1712*

Everolimus (e ver OH li mus)

Brand Names: U.S. Afinitor; Afinitor Disperz; Zortress
Index Terms RAD001

Pharmacologic Category Antineoplastic Agent, mTOR Kinase Inhibitor; Immunosuppressant Agent; mTOR Kinase Inhibitor

Medication Safety Issues

Sound-alike/look-alike issues:

Everolimus may be confused with sirolimus, tacrolimus, temsirolimus

Afinitor may be confused with afatinib

High alert medication:

This medication is in a class the Institute for Safe Medication Practices (ISMP) includes among its list of drug classes which have a heightened risk of causing significant patient harm when used in error.

Administration issues:

Tablets (Afinitor, Zortress) and tablets for oral suspension (Afinitor Disperz) are not interchangeable; do not combine formulations to achieve total desired dose.

Medication Guide Available Yes

Pregnancy Risk Factor D (Afinitor) / C (Zortress)

Lactation Excretion in breast milk unknown/not recommended

Breast-Feeding Considerations It is not known if everolimus is excreted in breast milk. Due to the potential for serious adverse reactions in the nursing infant, breast-feeding should be avoided.

Use

Breast cancer, advanced (Afinitor only): Treatment of advanced hormone receptor-positive, HER2-negative breast cancer in postmenopausal women (in combination with exemestane and after letrozole or anastrozole failure)

Pancreatic neuroendocrine tumors (Afinitor only): Treatment of advanced, metastatic or unresectable pancreatic neuroendocrine tumors (PNET)

Limitations of use: Afinitor is not indicated for the treatment of functional carcinoid tumors.

Renal angiomyolipoma with tuberous sclerosis complex (Afinitor only): Treatment of renal angiomyolipoma with tuberous sclerosis complex (TSC) not requiring immediate surgery

Renal cell carcinoma, advanced (Afinitor only): Treatment of advanced renal cell cancer (RCC) after sunitinib or sorafenib failure

Subependymal giant cell astrocytoma (Afinitor or Afinitor Disperz only): Treatment of subependymal giant cell astrocytoma (SEGA) associated with TSC which requires intervention, but cannot be curatively resected

Liver transplantation (Zortress only): Prophylaxis of organ rejection in liver transplantation (in combination with corticosteroids and reduced doses of tacrolimus)

Renal transplantation (Zortress only): Prophylaxis of organ rejection in renal transplant patients at low to moderate immunologic risk (in combination with basiliximab induction and concurrent with corticosteroids and reduced doses of cyclosporine)

Unlabeled Use Treatment of relapsed or refractory Waldenström's macroglobulinemia (WM); treatment of progressive advanced carcinoid tumors

Mechanism of Action/Effect Everolimus is a macrolide immunosuppressant and an mTOR inhibitor which has antiproliferative and antiangiogenic properties; everolimus also reduces lipoma volume in patients with angiomyolipoma

Contraindications Hypersensitivity to everolimus, sirolimus, other rapamycin derivatives, or any component of the formulation.

Warnings/Precautions Hazardous agent - use appropriate precautions for handling and disposal (NIOSH, 2012). To avoid potential contact with everolimus, caregivers should wear gloves when preparing suspension from tablets for oral suspension. Noninfectious pneumonitis (sometimes fatal) has been observed with mTOR inhibitors including everolimus; symptoms include dyspnea, cough, hypoxia and/or pleural effusion; promptly evaluate worsening respiratory symptoms; may require treatment interruption followed by dose reduction (pneumonitis has developed even with reduced doses) and/or corticosteroid therapy; discontinue for grade 4 pneumonitis. Imaging may overestimate the incidence of clinical pneumonitis. **[U.S. Boxed Warning]: Everolimus has immunosuppressant properties which may result in infection;** the risk of developing bacterial (including mycobacterial), viral, fungal and protozoal infections and for local, opportunistic (including polyomavirus infection), and/or systemic infections is increased; may lead to sepsis, respiratory failure, hepatic failure, or fatality. Polyomavirus infection in transplant patients may be serious and/or fatal. Polyoma virus-associated nephropathy (due to BK virus), which may result in serious cases of deteriorating renal function and renal graft loss, has been observed with use. JC virus-associated progressive multiple leukoencephalopathy (PML) may also be associated with everolimus use in transplantation. Reduced immunosuppression (taking into account the risks of rejection) should be considered with evidence of polyoma virus infection or PML. Reactivation of hepatitis B has been observed in patients receiving everolimus. Resolve pre-existing invasive fungal infections prior to treatment initiation. Transplant recipient patients should receive prophylactic therapy for pneumocystis jiroveci pneumonia (PCP) and for cytomegalovirus (CMV). Monitor for signs and symptoms of infection during treatment. Discontinue if invasive systemic fungal infection is diagnosed (and manage with appropriate antifungal therapy).

[U.S. Boxed Warning]: Immunosuppressant use may result in the development of malignancy, including lymphoma and skin cancer. The risk is associated with treatment intensity and the duration of therapy. To minimize the risk for skin cancer, limit exposure to sunlight and ultraviolet light; wear protective clothing and use effective sunscreen.

[U.S. Boxed Warning]: Due to the increased risk for nephrotoxicity in renal transplantation, avoid standard doses of cyclosporine in combination with everolimus; reduced cyclosporine doses are recommended when everolimus is used in combination with cyclosporine. Therapeutic monitoring of cyclosporine and everolimus concentrations is recommended. Monitor for proteinuria; the risk of proteinuria is increased when everolimus is used in combination with cyclosporine, and with higher serum everolimus concentrations. Everolimus and cyclosporine combination therapy may increase the risk for thrombotic microangiopathy/thrombotic thrombocytopenic purpura/hemolytic uremic syndrome (TMA/TTP/HUS); monitor blood counts. Elevations in serum creatinine (generally mild), renal failure, and proteinuria have been also observed with everolimus use; monitor renal function (BUN, creatinine, and/or urinary protein). Risk of nephrotoxicity may be increased when administered with calcineurin inhibitors (eg, cyclosporine, tacrolimus); dosage adjustment of calcineurin inhibitor is necessary. An increased incidence of rash, infection and dose interruptions have been reported in patients with renal insufficiency (CrCl ≤60 mL/minute) who received mTOR inhibitors for the treatment of renal cell cancer (Gupta, 2011); serum creatinine elevations and proteinuria have been reported. Monitor renal function (BUN, serum creatinine, urinary protein) at baseline and periodically, especially if risk factors for further impairment exist; pharmacokinetic studies have not been conducted; dosage adjustments are not required based on renal impairment. **[U.S. Boxed Warning]: An increased risk of renal arterial and venous thrombosis has been reported with use in renal transplantation, generally within the first 30 days after transplant; may result in graft loss.** MTOR inhibitors are associated with an increase in hepatic artery thrombosis, most cases have been reported within 30 days after transplant and usually proceeded to graft loss or death; do not use everolimus prior to 30 days post liver transplant.

Potentially significant drug-drug/drug-food interactions may exist, requiring dose or frequency adjustment, additional monitoring, and/or selection of alternative therapy. In transplant patients, avoid the use of certain HMG-CoA reductase inhibitors (eg, simvastatin, lovastatin); may increase the risk for rhabdomyolysis due to the potential interaction with cyclosporine (which may be given in combination with everolimus for transplantation).

Use is associated with mouth ulcers, mucositis and stomatitis; manage with topical therapy; avoid the use of alcohol-, hydrogen peroxide-, iodine-, or thyme-based mouthwashes (due to the high potential for drug interactions, avoid the use of systemic antifungals unless fungal infection has been diagnosed). Everolimus is associated with the development of angioedema; concomitant use with other agents known to cause angioedema (eg, ACE inhibitors) may increase the risk. Everolimus use may delay wound healing and increase the occurrence of wound-related complications (eg, wound dehiscence, infection, incisional hernia, lymphocele, seroma); may require surgical intervention; use with caution in the peri-surgical period. Generalized edema, including peripheral edema and lymphedema, and local fluid accumulation (eg, pericardial effusion, pleural effusion, ascites) may also occur.

Everolimus exposure is increased in patients with hepatic impairment. For patients with breast cancer, PNET, RCC, or renal angiomyolipoma with mild and moderate hepatic impairment, reduced doses are recommended; in patients with severe hepatic impairment, use is recommended (at reduced doses) if the potential benefit outweighs risks. Reduced doses are recommended in transplant patients with hepatic impairment; pharmacokinetic information does not exist for renal transplant patients with severe impairment (Child-Pugh class B or C); monitor whole blood trough levels closely for patients with SEGA, reduced doses may be needed for mild and moderate hepatic impairment (based on therapeutic drug monitoring), and are recommended in severe hepatic impairment; monitor whole blood trough levels. The Canadian labeling recommends against the use of everolimus in patients <18 years of age with SEGA and hepatic impairment.

[U.S. Boxed Warning]: Increased mortality (usually associated with infections) within the first 3 months after transplant was noted in a study of patients with *de novo* heart transplant receiving immunosuppressive regimens containing everolimus (with or without induction therapy). Use in heart transplantation is not recommended. Hyperglycemia, hyperlipidemia, and hypertriglyceridemia have been reported. Higher serum everolimus concentrations are associated with an increased risk for hyperlipidemia. Use has not been studied in patients with baseline cholesterol >350 mg/dL. Monitor fasting glucose and lipid profile prior to treatment initiation and periodically thereafter; monitor more frequently in patients with concomitant medications affecting glucose. Manage with appropriate medical therapy (if possible, optimize glucose control and lipids prior to treatment initiation). Antihyperlipidemic therapy may not normalize levels. May alter insulin and/or oral hypoglycemic therapy requirements in patients with diabetes; the risk for new onset diabetes is increased with everolimus use after transplantation. Decreases in hemoglobin, neutrophils, platelets, and lymphocytes have been reported; monitor blood counts at baseline and periodically. Patients should not be immunized with live viral vaccines during or shortly after treatment and should avoid close contact with recently vaccinated (live vaccine) individuals; consider the timing of routine immunizations prior to the start of therapy in pediatric patients treated for SEGA. Continue treatment with everolimus for renal cell cancer as long as clinical benefit is demonstrated or until occurrence of unacceptable toxicity. Safety and efficacy have not been established for the use of everolimus in the treatment of carcinoid tumors. Decreases in hemoglobin, neutrophils, platelets, and lymphocytes have been reported with use. Increases in serum glucose are common; may alter insulin and/or oral hypoglycemic therapy requirements in patients with diabetes; the risk for new onset diabetes is increased with everolimus use after transplantation. Patients should not be immunized with live viral vaccines during or shortly after treatment and should avoid close contact with recently vaccinated (live vaccine) individuals. In pediatric patients treated for SEGA, complete recommended series of live virus childhood vaccinations prior to treatment (if immediate everolimus treatment is not indicated); an accelerated vaccination schedule may be appropriate. Continue treatment with everolimus for renal cell cancer as long as clinical benefit is demonstrated or until occurrence of unacceptable toxicity.

Tablets (Afinitor, Zortress) and tablets for oral suspension (Afinitor Disperz) are not interchangeable; Afinitor Disperz is only indicated in conjunction with therapeutic monitoring for the treatment of SEGA. Do not combine formulations to achieve total desired dose. May cause infertility; in females, menstrual irregularities, secondary amenorrhea, and increases in luteinizing hormone and follicle-stimulating hormone have occurred; azoospermia and oligospermia have been observed in males. Avoid use in patients with hereditary galactose intolerance, Lapp lactase deficiency, or glucose-galactose malabsorption; may result in diarrhea and malabsorption. The safety and efficacy of everolimus in renal transplantation patients with high-immunologic risk or in solid organ transplant other than renal or liver have not been established. **[U.S. Boxed Warning]: In transplantation, everolimus should only be used by physicians experienced in immunosuppressive therapy and management of transplant patients. Adequate laboratory and supportive medical resources must be readily available.** For indications requiring whole blood trough concentrations to determine dosage adjustments, a consistent method should be used; concentration values from different assay methods may not be interchangeable.

Drug Interactions

Avoid Concomitant Use

Avoid concomitant use of Everolimus with any of the following: BCG; CloZAPine; CYP3A4 Inducers (Strong); CYP3A4 Inhibitors (Strong); Fusidic Acid (Systemic); Grapefruit Juice; Natalizumab; Pimecrolimus; St Johns Wort; Tacrolimus (Topical); Tofacitinib; Vaccines (Live)

Decreased Effect

Everolimus may decrease the levels/effects of: BCG; Coccidioidin Skin Test; Sipuleucel-T; Vaccines (Inactivated); Vaccines (Live)

The levels/effects of Everolimus may be decreased by: Bosentan; CYP3A4 Inducers (Strong); Dabrafenib; Deferasirox; Echinacea; Efavirenz; P-glycoprotein/ABCB1 Inducers; St Johns Wort; Tocilizumab

Increased Effect/Toxicity

Everolimus may increase the levels/effects of: ACE Inhibitors; CloZAPine; Leflunomide; Natalizumab; Tofacitinib; Vaccines (Live)

The levels/effects of Everolimus may be increased by: CycloSPORINE (Systemic); CYP3A4 Inhibitors (Moderate); CYP3A4 Inhibitors (Strong); Dasatinib; Denosumab; Fusidic Acid (Systemic); Grapefruit Juice; Ivacaftor; Luliconazole; Mifepristone; P-glycoprotein/ABCB1 Inhibitors; Pimecrolimus; Roflumilast; Simeprevir; Tacrolimus (Topical); Trastuzumab

Nutritional/Ethanol Interactions

Food: Grapefruit juice may increase levels of everolimus. Absorption with food may be variable. Management: Avoid grapefruit juice. Take with or without food, but be consistent with regard to food.

Herb/Nutraceutical: St John's wort may decrease the levels of everolimus. Management: Avoid St John's wort.

Adverse Reactions

>10%:

Cardiovascular: Peripheral edema (4% to 45%), hypertension (4% to 30%; hypertensive crisis: 1%)

Central nervous system: Fatigue (7% to 45%), fever (13% to 32%), headache (18% to 30%), seizure (5% to 29%), behavioral changes (anxiety/aggression/behavioral disturbance; SEGA: 21%), insomnia (6% to 17%), dizziness (7% to 14%)

Dermatologic: Skin rash (18% to 59%), cellulitis (SEGA: 29%), acneiform eruption (3% to 25%), nail disease (including onychoclasis, 4% to 22%), acne vulgaris (3% to 22%), pruritus (13% to 21%), xeroderma (9% to 18%), contact dermatitis (14%), excoriation (14%)

Endocrine & metabolic: Hypercholesterolemia (17% to 85%), hyperglycemia (12% to 75%; grades 3/4: <1% to 17%), hypertriglyceridemia (≤73%), decreased serum bicarbonate (≤56%), hypophosphatemia (9% to 49%), hypocalcemia (17% to 37%), decreased serum albumin (≤33%), diabetes mellitus ([new onset] <10%; liver transplant: 32%), hypoglycemia (≤32%), hypokalemia (12% to 29%), hyperlipidemia (renal, liver transplant: 21% to 24%), hyperkalemia (renal transplant: 18%), amenorrhea (≤17%), hyponatremia (≤16%), lipid metabolism disorder (renal transplant: 15%), hypomagnesemia (renal transplant: 14%)

Gastrointestinal: Stomatitis (oncology uses: 44% to 86%; grade 3: 4% to 9%; grade 4: <1%; renal transplant: 8%), diarrhea (14% to 50%; grade 3: ≤5%; grade 4: <1%), constipation (10% to 38%), abdominal pain (3% to 36%), nausea (8% to 32%; grade 3: ≤2%; grade 4: <1%), decreased appetite (6% to 30%), anorexia (1% to 30%), vomiting (15% to 29%; grade 3: ≤2%; grade 4: <1%), weight loss (9% to 28%), dysgeusia (1% to 22%), gastroenteritis (1% to 18%), xerostomia (8% to 11%)

Genitourinary: Urinary tract infection (5% to 22%), hematuria (renal transplant: 12%), dysuria (renal transplant: 11%)

Hematologic & oncologic: Anemia (26% to 92%; grades 3/4: ≤15%; grade 4: <1%), prolonged partial thromboplastin time (SEGA: 72%), leukopenia (oncology uses: 26% to 58%; renal, liver transplant: 3% to 12%), lymphocytopenia (20% to 54%; grades 3/4: ≤18%), thrombocytopenia (oncology uses: 19% to 54%; grade 3: ≤3%; renal transplant: <10%), neutropenia (≤46%; grades 3/4: ≤9%)

Hepatic: Increased serum AST (23% to 89%; grade 3: ≤4%; grade 4: <1%), increased serum alkaline phosphatase (oncology uses: 32% to 74%; renal, liver transplant: <10%), increased serum ALT (18% to 51%; grade 3: ≤4%; grade 4: 1%)

Infection: Infection (13% to 62%; grade 3: 4% to 7%; grade 4: 1% to 3%)

Neuromuscular & skeletal: Weakness (13% to 33%), arthralgia (≤20%), back pain (11% to 15%), limb pain (8% to 14%)

Otic: Otitis (6% to 36%)

Renal: Increased serum creatinine (11% to 50%)

Respiratory: Upper respiratory tract infection (11% to 82%), sinusitis (3% to 39%), cough (7% to 30%), dyspnea (20% to 24%; grade 3: 2% to 6%; grade 4: ≤1%), epistaxis (≤22%), pneumonitis (including alveolitis, interstitial lung disease, lung infiltrate, pulmonary alveolar hemorrhage, pulmonary toxicity, 1% to 19%; grade 3: 3% to 4%; grade 4: <1%), nasal congestion (14%), rhinitis (14%), pharyngitis (4% to 11%)

Miscellaneous: Wound healing impairment (liver transplant: 11%; oncology uses: <1%)

1% to 10%:

Cardiovascular: Chest pain (5%), tachycardia (3%), cardiac failure (1%), angina pectoris, atrial fibrillation, chest discomfort, deep vein thrombosis, edema (generalized), hypotension, palpitations, syncope, venous thromboembolism

Central nervous system: Depression (5%), migraine (5%), paresthesia (5%), chills (4%), agitation, drowsiness, hallucination, hemiparesis, hypoesthesia, lethargy, malaise, neuralgia

Dermatologic: Eczema (10%), alopecia (≤10%), palmar-plantar erythrodysesthesia ([hand-foot syndrome] 5%), papule (5%), erythema (4%), pityriasis rosea (4%), skin lesion (4%), hirsutism, hyperhidrosis, hypertrichosis

Endocrine & metabolic: Hypermenorrhea (6% to 10%), menstrual disease (6% to 10%), dysmenorrhea (6%), irregular menses (6%), exacerbation of diabetes mellitus (2%), cushingoid appearance, cyanocobalamin deficiency, dehydration, gout, hypercalcemia, hyperparathyroidism, hyperphosphatemia, hyperuricemia, iron deficiency, ovarian cyst, scrotal edema

Gastrointestinal: Gastritis (7%), hemorrhoids (5%), dyspepsia (4%), dysphagia (4%), ageusia (1%), abdominal distention, epigastric distress, flatulence, gastroesophageal reflux disease, gingival hyperplasia, hematemesis, intestinal obstruction, oral herpes

Genitourinary: Vaginal hemorrhage (8%), bladder spasm, erectile dysfunction, pollakiuria, pyuria, urinary retention, urinary urgency

Hematologic & oncologic: Neoplasm (liver transplant: 4%), hemorrhage (3%), leukocytosis, lymphadenopathy, pancytopenia (renal, liver transplant)

Hepatic: Increased serum bilirubin (3% to 10%; grades 3/4: ≤1%), abnormal hepatic function tests (liver transplant: 7%), ascites (liver transplant: 4%), increased serum transaminases

Hypersensitivity: Hypersensitivity (including anaphylaxis, dyspnea, flushing, chest pain, angioedema, 3%)

Infection: BK virus infection, candidiasis, herpes infection, sepsis

Neuromuscular & skeletal: Muscle spasm (≤10%), tremor (8% to 9%), jaw pain (3%), joint swelling, musculoskeletal pain, myalgia, osteonecrosis, osteopenia, osteoporosis, spondylitis

Ophthalmic: Eyelid edema (4%), ocular hyperemia (4%), conjunctivitis (2%), blurred vision, cataract

Renal: Renal failure (3%), hydronephrosis, increased blood urea nitrogen, interstitial nephritis, polyuria, proteinuria, renal artery thrombosis, renal insufficiency

Respiratory: Pleural effusion (5% to 7%), nasopharyngitis (6%), pneumonia (6%), bronchitis (4%), pharyngolaryngeal pain (4%), rhinorrhea (3%), atelectasis, lower respiratory tract infection, oropharyngeal pain, pulmonary edema, pulmonary embolism, sinus congestion, wheezing

Miscellaneous: Night sweats, peritonitis, postoperative wound complication (including incisional hernia)

Available Dosage Forms

Tablet, Oral:

Afinitor: 2.5 mg, 5 mg, 7.5 mg, 10 mg

Zortress: 0.25 mg, 0.5 mg, 0.75 mg

Tablet Soluble, Oral:

Afinitor Disperz: 2 mg, 3 mg, 5 mg

General Dosage Range Dosage adjustment recommended in patients with hepatic impairment, on concomitant therapy, or who develop toxicities

Oral: *Children ≥1 year and Adults:* Dosage varies greatly depending on indication

Administration

Oral May be taken with or without food; to reduce variability, take consistently with regard to food. Afinitor missed doses may be taken up to 6 hours after regularly scheduled time; if >6 hours, resume at next regularly scheduled time.

Tablets: Swallow whole with a glass of water. Do not break, chew, or crush (do not administer tablets that are crushed or broken). Avoid contact with or exposure to crushed or broken tablets.

Tablets for oral suspension: Administer as a suspension only. Administer immediately after preparation; discard if not administered within 60 minutes after preparation. Prepare suspension in water only. Do not break or crush tablets.

Preparation in an oral syringe: Place dose into 10 mL oral syringe (maximum: 10 mg/syringe; use an additional syringe for doses >10 mg). Draw ~5 mL of water and ~4 mL of air into oral syringe; allow to sit (tip up) in a container until tablets are in suspension (3 minutes). Gently invert syringe 5 times immediately prior to administration; administer contents, then add ~5 mL water and ~4 mL of air to same syringe, swirl to suspend remaining particles and administer entire contents.

Preparation in a small glass: Place dose into a small glass (≤100 mL) containing ~25 mL water (maximum: 10 mg/glass; use an additional glass for doses >10 mg); allow to sit until tablets are in suspension (3 minutes). Stir gently with spoon immediately prior to administration; administer contents, then add ~25 mL water to same glass, swirl with same spoon to suspend remaining particles and administer entire contents.

Breast cancer, pancreatic neuroendocrine tumors, renal cell cancer, renal angiolipoma, SEGA: Administer at the same time each day.

Liver transplantation: Administer consistently ~12 hours apart; administer at the same time as tacrolimus.

Renal transplantation: Administer consistently ~12 hours apart; administer at the same time as cyclosporine.

Hazardous agent; use appropriate precautions for handling and disposal (NIOSH, 2012). To avoid potential contact with everolimus, caregivers should wear gloves when preparing suspension from tablets for oral suspension.

Storage/Stability Tablets and tablets for suspension: Store at room temperature of 25°C (77°F); excursions permitted to 15°C to 30°C (59°F to 86°F). Protect from light; protect from moisture.

Nursing Actions

Physical Assessment Check results of blood work for elevated cholesterol, triglycerides, hepatic and renal function, and glucose. Encourage patient to monitor home glucose levels, especially during initiation of drug therapy and record insulin and/or oral hypoglycemic therapy requirements. Instruct patient to report signs of hyperglycemia (eg, increased thirst, increased urination, sleepiness).

Patients are at increased risk for renal toxicities; monitor creatinine and instruct patient to report any decrease in urination or change in color of urine. Patients are at increased risk for bacterial, fungal, and viral infections. Instruct patients to monitor for symptoms of infections, including temperature >100.4°F (38°C). Monitor labs and evaluate for neutropenia risk. Instruct patient on good hand washing. Patients should avoid being around those who have received live vaccines. Monitor for angioedema, CNS toxicities, fatigue, headaches, seizures, or behavioral changes. Monitor wound healing; patients are at risk for impaired wound healing.

Make patients aware that drug increases risk of secondary malignancies of lymphoma or skin cancers; will need lifelong monitoring. Instruct women of childbearing age about the need for birth control while taking this drug and for a period of time after discontinuation.

Patient Education

• Discuss specific use of drug and side effects with patient as it relates to treatment. (HCAHPS: During this hospital stay, were you given any medicine that you had not taken before? Before giving you any new medicine, how often did hospital staff tell you what the medicine was for? How often did hospital staff describe possible side effects in a way you could understand?)

• Patient may experience acne vulgaris, insomnia, nausea, diarrhea, constipation, dysgeusia, lack of appetite, weight loss, xerostomia, xeroderma, nail changes, alopecia, arthralgia, back pain, painful extremities, muscle spasms, epistaxis, or dyspepsia. Have patient report immediately to prescriber signs of infection, signs of hyperglycemia, signs of hepatic impairment, eczema of hands or feet, paresthesia, angina, ecchymosis, hemorrhaging, severe stomatitis, tachycardia, arrhythmia, considerable dizziness, syncope, significant headache, intolerable asthenia, myalgia, menstrual irregularities, mood changes, behavioral changes, edema, signs of pulmonary disorder, signs of renal impairment, mole changes, skin growths, enlarged lymph nodes, night sweats, poor wound healing, or signs of progressive multifocal leukoencephalopathy (PML) (HCAHPS).

- Educate patient about signs of a significant reaction (eg, wheezing; chest tightness; fever; itching; bad cough; blue skin color; seizures; or swelling of face, lips, tongue, or throat). **Note:** This is not a comprehensive list of all side effects. Patient should consult prescriber for additional questions.

Intended Use and Disclaimer: Should not be printed and given to patients. This information is intended to serve as a concise initial reference for healthcare professionals to use when discussing medications with a patient. You must ultimately rely on your own discretion, experience and judgment in diagnosing, treating and advising patients.

Dietary Considerations Avoid grapefruit juice.

Related Information

Oral Medications That Should Not Be Crushed or Altered *on page 1712*

Exemestane (ex e MES tane)

Brand Names: U.S. Aromasin

Pharmacologic Category Antineoplastic Agent, Aromatase Inhibitor

Medication Safety Issues

Sound-alike/look-alike issues:

Aromasin may be confused with Arimidex

Exemestane may be confused with estramustine.

Pregnancy Risk Factor X

Lactation Excretion in breast milk unknown/not recommended

Breast-Feeding Considerations Exemestane is indicated for use only in postmenopausal women. Due to the potential for serious adverse reactions in the nursing infant, the manufacturer recommends a decision be made whether to discontinue nursing or to discontinue the drug, taking into account the importance of treatment to the mother.

Use Breast cancer: Treatment of advanced breast cancer in postmenopausal women whose disease has progressed following tamoxifen therapy; adjuvant treatment of postmenopausal women with estrogen receptor-positive early breast cancer following 2-3 years of tamoxifen (for a total of 5 consecutive years of adjuvant therapy).

Unlabeled Use Risk reduction for invasive breast cancer in postmenopausal women; first-line adjuvant treatment of estrogen receptor-positive early breast cancer in postmenopausal women

Mechanism of Action/Effect Exemestane prevents conversion of androgens to estrogens (aromatase inhibitor) and significantly lowers circulating estrogen levels in postmenopausal breast cancers.

Contraindications Hypersensitivity to exemestane or any component of the formulation; women who are or may become pregnant; premenopausal women

Warnings/Precautions Hazardous agent - use appropriate precautions for handling and disposal (NIOSH, 2012). Due to decreased circulating estrogen levels, exemestane is associated with a reduction in bone mineral density over time; decreases (from baseline) in lumbar spine and femoral neck density have been observed; assess bone mineral density at baseline in patients with, or at risk for osteoporosis; monitor exemestane therapy and initiate osteoporosis treatment if indicated. Due to high prevalence of vitamin D deficiency in women with breast cancer, assess 25-hydroxy vitamin D levels at baseline and supplement accordingly. Grade 3 or 4 lymphopenia has been observed with exemestane, although most patients had preexisting lower grade lymphopenia; some patients improved or recovered while continuing exemestane; lymphopenia did not result in a significant increase in viral infections, and no opportunistic infections were observed. Elevations of AST, ALT, alkaline phosphatase, and gamma glutamyl transferase >5 times ULN have been observed (rarely) in patients with advanced breast cancer; may be attributable to underlying liver and/or bone metastases. In patients with early breast cancer, elevations of bilirubin, alkaline phosphatase, and serum creatinine were more common with exemestane treatment than with tamoxifen or placebo. Potentially significant drug-drug interactions may exist, requiring dose or frequency adjustment, additional monitoring, and/or selection of alternative therapy. Not to be given with estrogen-containing agents. Dose adjustment recommended with concomitant strong CYP3A4 inducers.

Drug Interactions

Avoid Concomitant Use

Avoid concomitant use of Exemestane with any of the following: Axitinib; Simeprevir

Decreased Effect

Exemestane may decrease the levels/effects of: ARIPiprazole; Axitinib; Ibrutinib; Saxagliptin; Simeprevir

The levels/effects of Exemestane may be decreased by: Bosentan; CYP3A4 Inducers (Strong); Dabrafenib; Deferasirox; Herbs (CYP3A4 Inducers); Tocilizumab

Increased Effect/Toxicity There are no known significant interactions involving an increase in effect.

Nutritional/Ethanol Interactions

Food: Plasma levels increased by 40% when exemestane was taken with a fatty meal.

Herb/Nutraceutical: St John's wort may decrease exemestane levels. Avoid black cohosh, dong quai in estrogen-dependent tumors.

Adverse Reactions

>10%:

Cardiovascular: Hypertension (5% to 15%)

Central nervous system: Fatigue (8% to 22%), insomnia (11% to 14%), pain (13%), headache (7% to 13%), depression (6% to 13%)

Dermatological: Hyperhidrosis (4% to 18%), alopecia (15%)

Endocrine & metabolic: Hot flashes (13% to 33%)

Gastrointestinal: Nausea (9% to 18%), abdominal pain (6% to 11%)

Hepatic: Alkaline phosphatase increased (14% to 15%)

Neuromuscular & skeletal: Arthralgia (15% to 29%)

1% to 10%:

Cardiovascular: Edema (6% to 7%); cardiac ischemic events (2%: MI, angina, myocardial ischemia); chest pain

Central nervous system: Dizziness (8% to 10%), anxiety (4% to 10%), fever (5%), confusion, hypoesthesia

Dermatologic: Dermatitis (8%), itching, rash

Endocrine & metabolic: Weight gain (8%)

Gastrointestinal: Diarrhea (4% to 10%), vomiting (7%), anorexia (6%), constipation (5%), appetite increased (3%), dyspepsia

Genitourinary: Urinary tract infection (2% to 5%)

Hepatic: Bilirubin increased (5% to 7%)

Neuromuscular & skeletal: Back pain (9%), limb pain (9%), myalgia (6%), osteoarthritis (6%), weakness (6%), osteoporosis (5%), pathological fracture (4%), paresthesia (3%), carpal tunnel syndrome (2%), cramps (2%)

Ocular: Visual disturbances (5%)

Renal: Creatinine increased (6%)

Respiratory: Dyspnea (10%), cough (6%), bronchitis, pharyngitis, rhinitis, sinusitis, upper respiratory infection

Miscellaneous: Flu-like syndrome (6%), lymphedema, infection

A dose-dependent decrease in sex hormone-binding globulin has been observed with daily doses of ≥2.5 mg. Serum luteinizing hormone and follicle-stimulating hormone levels have increased with this medicine.

Available Dosage Forms

Tablet, Oral:

Aromasin: 25 mg

Generic: 25 mg

General Dosage Range Dosage adjustment recommended in patients on concomitant therapy

Oral: *Adults (postmenopausal females):* 25 mg once daily

Administration

Oral Administer after a meal.

Hazardous agent; use appropriate precautions for handling and disposal (NIOSH, 2012).

Storage/Stability Store at 25°C (77°F); excursions permitted to 15°C to 30°C (59°F to 86°F).

Nursing Actions

Physical Assessment Monitor for new or unusual bone pain and swelling of face, lips, or throat. Monitor blood pressure; may cause hypertension.

Patient Education

- Discuss specific use of drug and side effects with patient as it relates to treatment. (HCAHPS: During this hospital stay, were you given any medicine that you had not taken before? Before giving you any new medicine, how often did hospital staff tell you what the medicine was for? How often did hospital staff describe possible side effects in a way you could understand?)

- Patient may experience hot flashes, arthralgia, alopecia, asthenia, hyperhidrosis, back pain, diarrhea, or anxiety. Have patient report immediately to prescriber angina, strength differences from one side to another, difficulty speaking or thinking, change in balance, blurred vision, dyspnea, excessive weight gain, edema of extremities, skin discoloration, painful extremities, paresthesia, osteodynia, vision changes, depression, severe headache, considerable dizziness, syncope, significant dyspepsia, jaundice, or intolerable nausea (HCAHPS).

- Educate patient about signs of a significant reaction (eg, wheezing; chest tightness; fever; itching; bad cough; blue skin color; seizures; or swelling of face, lips, tongue, or throat). **Note:** This is not a comprehensive list of all side effects. Patient should consult prescriber for additional questions.

Intended Use and Disclaimer: Should not be printed and given to patients. This information is intended to serve as a concise initial reference for healthcare professionals to use when discussing medications with a patient. You must ultimately rely on your own discretion, experience and judgment in diagnosing, treating and advising patients.

Dietary Considerations Patients on aromatase inhibitor therapy should receive vitamin D and calcium supplements.

Exenatide (ex EN a tide)

Brand Names: U.S. Bydureon; Byetta 10 MCG Pen; Byetta 5 MCG Pen

Index Terms AC 2993; AC002993; Exendin-4; LY2148568

Pharmacologic Category Antidiabetic Agent, Glucagon-Like Peptide-1 (GLP-1) Receptor Agonist

Medication Guide Available Yes

Pregnancy Risk Factor C

Lactation Excretion in breast milk unknown/not recommended

Breast-Feeding Considerations It is not known if exenatide is present in breast milk. According to the manufacturer, the decision to continue or discontinue breast-feeding during therapy should take into account the risk of exposure to the infant and the benefits of treatment to the mother; use caution if administering exenatide to nursing women.

Use Treatment of type 2 diabetes mellitus (non-insulin dependent, NIDDM) to improve glycemic control

Mechanism of Action/Effect Exenatide is an analog of the hormone incretin (glucagon-like peptide 1 or GLP-1) which increases glucose-dependent insulin secretion, decreases inappropriate glucagon secretion, increases B-cell growth/replication, slows gastric emptying, and decreases food intake. Exenatide administration results in decreases in hemoglobin A_{1c} by approximately 0.5% to 1% (immediate release) or 1.5% to 1.9% (extended release).

Contraindications Hypersensitivity to exenatide or any component of the formulation

Bydureon: Additional contraindications: History of or family history of medullary thyroid carcinoma (MTC); patients with multiple endocrine neoplasia syndrome type 2 (MEN2)

Byetta: Canadian labeling: Additional contraindications (not in U.S. labeling): End-stage renal disease or severe renal impairment (CrCl <30 mL/minute) including dialysis patients; diabetic ketoacidosis, diabetic coma/precoma or type 1 diabetes mellitus

Warnings/Precautions Bydureon™: **[U.S. Boxed Warning] Dose- and duration- dependent thyroid C-cell tumors have developed in animal studies with exenatide extended release therapy; relevance in humans unknown.** Patients should be counseled on the risk and symptoms (eg, neck mass, dysphagia, dyspnea, persistent hoarseness) of thyroid tumors. Consultation with an endocrinologist is recommended in patients who develop elevated calcitonin concentrations or have thyroid nodules detected during imaging studies or physical exam. Use is contraindicated in patients with a personal or a family history of medullary thyroid cancer and in patients with multiple endocrine neoplasia syndrome type 2 (MEN2). All cases of MTC should be reported to the applicable state cancer registry.

Mechanism requires the presence of insulin, therefore use in type 1 diabetes (insulin dependent, IDDM) or diabetic ketoacidosis is not recommended (use is contraindicated in the Canadian labeling); it is not a substitute for insulin in insulin-requiring patients. Concurrent use with insulin therapy has not been evaluated and is not recommended. (Exception: Safety and efficacy of concurrent insulin glargine and immediate release exenatide has been demonstrated in a clinical trial.) May increase the risk of hypoglycemia in patients receiving concomitant insulin secretagogues (eg, sulfonylureas, meglitinides); dosage reduction of sulfonylureas may be required. Clinicians should note that the risk of hypoglycemia is not increased when exenatide is added to metformin monotherapy. Avoid concurrent use of extended release (weekly) and immediate release (daily) exenatide formulations. Bydureon™ is not recommended for first-line therapy in patients inadequately controlled on diet and exercise alone.

Exenatide is frequently associated with gastrointestinal adverse effects and is not recommended for use in patients with gastroparesis or severe gastrointestinal disease. Gastrointestinal effects may be dose-related and may decrease in frequency/severity with gradual titration and continued use. Due to its effects on gastric emptying, exenatide may reduce the rate and extent of absorption of orally-administered drugs; use with caution in patients receiving medications with a narrow therapeutic window or require rapid absorption from the GI tract. Administer medications 1 hour prior to the use of immediate release (daily) exenatide when optimal drug absorption and peak levels are important to the overall therapeutic effect (eg, antibiotics, oral contraceptives); effects of extended release (weekly) exenatide on drug absorption have not been evaluated; use caution. Cases of acute pancreatitis (including hemorrhagic and necrotizing with some fatalities) have been reported; monitor for unexplained severe abdominal pain and if pancreatitis suspected, discontinue use. Do not resume unless an alternative etiology of pancreatitis is confirmed. Consider alternative antidiabetic therapy in patients with a history of pancreatitis. Use may be associated with the development of anti-exenatide antibodies. Low titers are not associated with a loss of efficacy; however, high titers (observed in 6% to 12% of patients in clinical studies) may result in an attenuation of response. May be associated with weight loss (due to reduced intake) independent of the change in hemoglobin A_{1c}.

Not recommended in severe renal impairment (CrCl <30 mL/minute) or end-stage renal disease (ESRD) (use in these patients and in dialysis patients is contraindicated in the Canadian labeling). Patients with ESRD receiving dialysis may be more susceptible to GI effects (eg, nausea, vomiting) which may result in hypovolemia and further reductions in renal function. Use with caution in patients with renal transplantation or in patients with moderate renal impairment (CrCl 30-50 mL/minute). Cases of acute renal failure and chronic renal failure exacerbation, including severe cases requiring hemodialysis, have been reported, predominately in patients with nausea/vomiting/diarrhea or dehydration; renal dysfunction was usually reversible with appropriate corrective measures, including discontinuation of exenatide. Risk may be increased in patients receiving concomitant medications affecting renal function and/or hydration status.

According to the Centers for Disease Control and Prevention (CDC), pen-shaped injection devices should never be used for more than one person (even when the needle is changed) because of the risk of infection. The injection device should be clearly labeled with individual patient information to ensure that the correct pen is used (CDC, 2012).

Drug Interactions

Avoid Concomitant Use There are no known interactions where it is recommended to avoid concomitant use.

Decreased Effect
Exenatide may decrease the levels/effects of: Contraceptives (Estrogens); Oral Contraceptive (Progestins)

The levels/effects of Exenatide may be decreased by: Corticosteroids (Orally Inhaled); Corticosteroids (Systemic); Luteinizing Hormone-Releasing Hormone Analogs; Somatropin; Thiazide Diuretics

Increased Effect/Toxicity
Exenatide may increase the levels/effects of: Sulfonylureas; Vitamin K Antagonists

The levels/effects of Exenatide may be increased by: Pegvisomant

Nutritional/Ethanol Interactions

Ethanol: Ethanol may cause hypoglycemia. Management: Consume ethanol with caution.

Food: Administer Byetta® within 60 minutes of meals, not after meals. May administer Bydureon™ without regard to meals or time of day.

Adverse Reactions

>10%:
Endocrine & metabolic: Hypoglycemia (monotherapy 2% to 5%; combination therapy with sulfonylurea 14% to 36%, with metformin ≤4%, with thiazolidinedione 11%)

Gastrointestinal: Nausea (monotherapy 8% to 11%; combination therapy 13% to 44%; dose-dependent), vomiting (monotherapy 4%; combination therapy 11% to 13%), diarrhea (monotherapy <2% to 11%; combination therapy 6% to 20%), constipation (monotherapy 9%; combination therapy 6% to 10%)

Local: Injection site nodule (Bydureon™ 6% to 77%), injection site reactions (2% to 18%; includes erythema, hematoma, pruritus)

Miscellaneous: Anti-exenatide antibodies (low titers 38% to 49%, high titers 6% to 12%)

1% to 10%:
Central nervous system: Nervousness (9%), dizziness (monotherapy <2%; combination therapy 9%), headache (5% to 9%), fatigue (3% to 6%)

Dermatologic: Hyperhidrosis (3%)

Gastrointestinal: Viral gastroenteritis (6% to 9%), dyspepsia (monotherapy 3% to 7%; combination

therapy 5% to 7%), GERD (3% to 7%), appetite decreased (1% to 5%)

Neuromuscular & skeletal: Weakness (4%)

Product Availability Bydureon Pen: FDA approved February 2014; availability anticipated later this year.

Available Dosage Forms

Solution, Subcutaneous:
Byetta 10 MCG Pen: 10 mcg/0.04 mL (2.4 mL)
Byetta 5 MCG Pen: 5 mcg/0.02 mL (1.2 mL)

Suspension Reconstituted, Subcutaneous:
Bydureon: 2 mg (1 ea)

General Dosage Range SubQ: *Adults:*
Immediate release: Initial: 5 mcg twice daily; Maintenance: 5-10 mcg twice daily
Extended release: 2 mg once weekly

Administration

Other SubQ:
Immediate release: Use only if clear, colorless, and free of particulate matter. Administer via injection in the upper arm, thigh, or abdomen. Administer within 60 minutes prior to morning and evening meal (or prior to the 2 main meals of the day, approximately ≥6 hours apart). Set up each new pen before the first use by priming it. See pen user manual for further details. Dial the dose into the dose window before each administration.

Extended release: Administer via injection in the upper arm, thigh, or abdomen; rotate injection sites weekly. Administer immediately after reconstitution. May administer without regard to meals or time of day.

Preparation for Administration Bydureon™: Reconstitute vial using provided diluent; use immediately.

Storage/Stability

Bydureon™: Store under refrigeration at 2°C to 8°C (36°F to 46°F); vials may be stored at ≤25°C (≤77°F) for up to 4 weeks. Do not freeze (discard if freezing occurs). Protect from light.

Byetta®: Prior to initial use, store under refrigeration at 2°C to 8°C (36°F to 46°F); after initial use, may store at ≤25°C (≤77°F). Do not freeze (discard if freezing occurs). Protect from light. Pen should be discarded 30 days after initial use.

Nursing Actions

Physical Assessment Monitor for signs and symptoms of hyperglycemia. Teach appropriate subcutaneous injection technique and disposal of needles. Assess gastrointestinal side effects of medication; can improve with use or with lower dose.

Patient Education
• Discuss specific use of drug and side effects with patient as it relates to treatment. (HCAHPS: During this hospital stay, were you given any medicine that you had not taken before? Before giving you any new medicine, how often did hospital staff tell you what the medicine was

for? How often did hospital staff describe possible side effects in a way you could understand?)

- Patient may experience weight loss, constipation, diarrhea, lack of appetite, nausea, or asthenia. Have patient report immediately to prescriber signs of pancreatitis, severe dizziness, syncope, considerable headache, urinary retention, oliguria, significant injection site pain or irritation, or signs of hypoglycemia (HCAHPS).
- Educate patient about signs of a significant reaction (eg, wheezing; chest tightness; fever; itching; bad cough; blue skin color; seizures; or swelling of face, lips, tongue, or throat). **Note:** This is not a comprehensive list of all side effects. Patient should consult prescriber for additional questions.

Intended Use and Disclaimer: Should not be printed and given to patients. This information is intended to serve as a concise initial reference for healthcare professionals to use when discussing medications with a patient. You must ultimately rely on your own discretion, experience and judgment in diagnosing, treating and advising patients.

Ezetimibe (ez ET i mibe)

Brand Names: U.S. Zetia
Pharmacologic Category Antilipemic Agent, 2-Azetidinone
Medication Safety Issues
Sound-alike/look-alike issues:
Ezetimibe may be confused with ezogabine
Zetia may be confused with Zebeta, Zestril
Pregnancy Risk Factor C
Lactation Excretion in breast milk unknown/not recommended
Breast-Feeding Considerations It is not known if ezetimibe is excreted in breast milk. According to the manufacturer, the decision to continue or discontinue breast-feeding during therapy should take into account the risk of exposure to the infant and the benefits of treatment to the mother. Use is contraindicated in nursing women who require combination therapy with an HMG-CoA reductase inhibitor.
Use Use in combination with dietary therapy for the treatment of primary hypercholesterolemia (as monotherapy or in combination with HMG-CoA reductase inhibitors); homozygous sitosterolemia; homozygous familial hypercholesterolemia (in combination with atorvastatin or simvastatin); mixed hyperlipidemia (in combination with fenofibrate)
Mechanism of Action/Effect Inhibits absorption of cholesterol at the brush border of the small intestine, leading to a decreased delivery of cholesterol to the liver, reduction of hepatic cholesterol stores and an increased clearance of cholesterol

from the blood; decreases total C, LDL-C, ApoB, and triglycerides while increasing HDL-C
Contraindications Hypersensitivity to ezetimibe or any component of the formulation; concomitant use with an HMG-CoA reductase inhibitor in patients with active hepatic disease, unexplained persistent elevations in serum transaminases; pregnancy; breast-feeding
Warnings/Precautions Secondary causes of hyperlipidemia should be ruled out prior to therapy. Use caution with severe renal (CrCl <30 mL/minute); if using concurrent simvastatin in patients with moderate-to-severe renal impairment, the manufacturer of ezetimibe recommends that simvastatin doses exceeding 20 mg be used with caution and close monitoring for adverse events (eg, myopathy). Use caution with mild hepatic impairment (Child-Pugh class A); not recommended for use with moderate or severe hepatic impairment (Child-Pugh classes B and C). Concurrent use of ezetimibe and fibric acid derivatives may increase the risk of cholelithiasis.
Drug Interactions
Avoid Concomitant Use There are no known interactions where it is recommended to avoid concomitant use.
Decreased Effect
The levels/effects of Ezetimibe may be decreased by: Bile Acid Sequestrants
Increased Effect/Toxicity
Ezetimibe may increase the levels/effects of: CycloSPORINE (Systemic)

The levels/effects of Ezetimibe may be increased by: CycloSPORINE (Systemic); Eltrombopag; Fibric Acid Derivatives
Nutritional/Ethanol Interactions Food: Ezetimibe did not cause meaningful reductions in fat-soluble vitamin concentrations during a 2-week clinical trial. Effects of long-term therapy have not been evaluated.
Adverse Reactions 1% to 10%:
Central nervous system: Fatigue (2%)
Gastrointestinal: Diarrhea (4%)
Hepatic: Transaminases increased (with HMG-CoA reductase inhibitors) (≥3 x ULN, 1%)
Neuromuscular & skeletal: Arthralgia (3%), pain in extremity (3%)
Respiratory: Upper respiratory tract infection (4%), sinusitis (3%)
Miscellaneous: Influenza (2%)
Available Dosage Forms
Tablet, Oral:
Zetia: 10 mg
General Dosage Range Oral: *Children ≥10 years and Adults:* 10 mg once daily
Administration
Oral May be administered without regard to meals. May be taken at the same time as HMG-CoA reductase inhibitors. Administer ≥2 hours before or ≥4 hours after bile acid sequestrants.

Storage/Stability Store at controlled room temperature of 25°C (77°F). Protect from moisture.

Nursing Actions

Physical Assessment Assess lipid profile at beginning of and at regular intervals during therapy. Teach patient to report signs of hepatic or muscle reactions. Consider dietary assessment and plan for teaching.

Patient Education

- Discuss specific use of drug and side effects with patient as it relates to treatment. (HCAHPS: During this hospital stay, were you given any medicine that you had not taken before? Before giving you any new medicine, how often did hospital staff tell you what the medicine was for? How often did hospital staff describe possible side effects in a way you could understand?)
- Patient may experience arthralgia, diarrhea, rhinitis, rhinorrhea, or pharyngitis. Have patient report immediately to prescriber myalgia or asthenia (HCAHPS).
- Educate patient about signs of a significant reaction (eg, wheezing; chest tightness; fever; itching; bad cough; blue skin color; seizures; or swelling of face, lips, tongue, or throat). **Note:** This is not a comprehensive list of all side effects. Patient should consult prescriber for additional questions.

Intended Use and Disclaimer: Should not be printed and given to patients. This information is intended to serve as a concise initial reference for healthcare professionals to use when discussing medications with a patient. You must ultimately rely on your own discretion, experience and judgment in diagnosing, treating and advising patients.

Dietary Considerations May be taken without regard to meals. Before initiation of therapy, patients should be placed on a standard cholesterol-lowering diet for 6 weeks and the diet should be continued during drug therapy.

Ezetimibe and Atorvastatin
(ez ET i mibe & a TORE va sta tin)

Brand Names: U.S. Liptruzet™

Index Terms Atorvastatin and Ezetimibe

Pharmacologic Category Antilipemic Agent, 2-Azetidinone; Antilipemic Agent, HMG-CoA Reductase Inhibitor

Pregnancy Risk Factor X

Lactation Excretion in breast milk unknown/contraindicated

Use

Homozygous familial hypercholesterolemia: For the reduction of elevated total cholesterol (total-C) and low-density lipoprotein cholesterol (LDL-C) in patients with homozygous familial hypercholesterolemia, as an adjunct to other lipid-lowering treatments (eg, LDL apheresis), or if such treatments are unavailable.

Primary hyperlipidemia: For the reduction of elevated total-C, LDL-C, apolipoprotein B (apo B), triglycerides, and non–high-density lipoprotein cholesterol (non HDL-C), and to increase HDL-C in patients with primary (heterozygous familial and nonfamilial) hyperlipidemia or mixed hyperlipidemia

Available Dosage Forms

Tablet, oral:
Liptruzet™ 10/10: Ezetimibe 10 mg and atorvastatin 10 mg
Liptruzet™ 10/20: Ezetimibe 10 mg and atorvastatin 20 mg
Liptruzet™ 10/40: Ezetimibe 10 mg and atorvastatin 40 mg
Liptruzet™ 10/80: Ezetimibe 10 mg and atorvastatin 80 mg

General Dosage Range Dosage adjustment recommended in patients on concomitant therapy.

Oral: *Adults:* Ezetimibe 10 mg and atorvastatin 10-80 mg once daily

Administration

Oral May be administered without regard to meals. Swallow tablets whole; do not crush, dissolve, or chew. Administer ≥2 hours before or ≥4 hours after bile acid sequestrants.

Nursing Actions

Physical Assessment Monitor for muscle weakness, pain, or fatigue. If these symptoms develop, draw CPK. If elevated, discontinue medication. Educate patient about signs and symptoms of muscle weakness, tenderness, and fatigue and when to call provider. Check results of LFTs, lipid panel.

Patient Education

- Discuss specific use of drug and side effects with patient as it relates to treatment. (HCAHPS: During this hospital stay, were you given any medicine that you had not taken before? Before giving you any new medicine, how often did hospital staff tell you what the medicine was for? How often did hospital staff describe possible side effects in a way you could understand?)
- Patient may experience dyspepsia or arthralgia. Have patient report immediately to prescriber severe myalgia, significant asthenia, flu-like syndrome, ecchymosis, hemorrhaging, or signs of hepatic impairment (HCAHPS).
- Educate patient about signs of a significant reaction (eg, wheezing; chest tightness; fever; itching; bad cough; blue skin color; seizures; or swelling of face, lips, tongue, or throat). **Note:** This is not a comprehensive list of all side effects. Patient should consult prescriber for additional questions.

Intended Use and Disclaimer: Should not be printed and given to patients. This information is

intended to serve as a concise initial reference for healthcare professionals to use when discussing medications with a patient. You must ultimately rely on your own discretion, experience and judgment in diagnosing, treating and advising patients.

Related Information
AtorvaSTATin *on page 139*
Ezetimibe *on page 626*

Ezetimibe and Simvastatin
(ez ET i mibe & SIM va stat in)

Brand Names: U.S. Vytorin
Index Terms Simvastatin and Ezetimibe
Pharmacologic Category Antilipemic Agent, 2-Azetidinone; Antilipemic Agent, HMG-CoA Reductase Inhibitor
Medication Safety Issues
Sound-alike/look-alike issues:
Vytorin may be confused with Vyvanse
Pregnancy Risk Factor X
Use
Homozygous familial hypercholesterolemia: As an adjunct to diet for the reduction of elevated total cholesterol (total-C) and low-density lipoprotein cholesterol (LDL-C) in patients with homozygous familial hypercholesterolemia, as an adjunct to other lipid-lowering treatments (eg, LDL apheresis), or if such treatments are unavailable
Primary hyperlipidemia: As an adjunct to diet for the reduction of elevated total-C, LDL-C, apolipoprotein B (apo B), triglycerides, and non-high-density lipoprotein cholesterol (HDL-C), and to increase HDL-C in patients with primary (heterozygous familial and nonfamilial) hyperlipidemia or mixed hyperlipidemia
Limitations of use: No incremental benefit of ezetimibe/simvastatin on cardiovascular morbidity and mortality over and above that demonstrated for simvastatin has been established. Ezetimibe/simvastatin has not been studied in Fredrickson type I, III, IV, and V dyslipidemias.
Available Dosage Forms
Tablet:
Vytorin®:
10/10: Ezetimibe 10 mg and simvastatin 10 mg
10/20: Ezetimibe 10 mg and simvastatin 20 mg
10/40: Ezetimibe 10 mg and simvastatin 40 mg
10/80: Ezetimibe 10 mg and simvastatin 80 mg
General Dosage Range Dosage adjustment recommended in patients with renal impairment or on concomitant therapy
Oral: *Adults:* Ezetimibe 10 mg and simvastatin 10-40 mg once daily
Administration
Oral May be administered without regard to meals. Administer in the evening for maximal efficacy. Ezetimibe/simvastatin should be taken ≥2 hours before or ≥4 hours after administration of a bile acid sequestrant.

Nursing Actions
Physical Assessment See individual agents.
Patient Education
• Discuss specific use of drug and side effects with patient as it relates to treatment. (HCAHPS: During this hospital stay, were you given any medicine that you had not taken before? Before giving you any new medicine, how often did hospital staff tell you what the medicine was for? How often did hospital staff describe possible side effects in a way you could understand?)
• Patient may experience headache, diarrhea, rhinorrhea, or rhinitis. Have patient report immediately to prescriber signs of hepatic impairment, signs of pancreatitis, myalgia, arthralgia, dyspnea, chills, pharyngitis, paresthesia, ecchymosis, hemorrhaging, dizziness, sexual dysfunction, arrhythmia, depression, illogical thinking, memory loss, edema of hands or feet, severe asthenia, urinary retention, oliguria, dysuria, polyuria, emesis, or insomnia (HCAHPS).
• Educate patient about signs of a significant reaction (eg, wheezing; chest tightness; fever; itching; bad cough; blue skin color; seizures; or swelling of face, lips, tongue, or throat). **Note:** This is not a comprehensive list of all side effects. Patient should consult prescriber for additional questions.

Intended Use and Disclaimer: Should not be printed and given to patients. This information is intended to serve as a concise initial reference for healthcare professionals to use when discussing medications with a patient. You must ultimately rely on your own discretion, experience and judgment in diagnosing, treating and advising patients.
Related Information
Ezetimibe *on page 626*
Simvastatin *on page 1414*

Ezogabine (e ZOG a been)

Brand Names: U.S. Potiga
Index Terms D-23129; EZG; Retigabine; RTG
Pharmacologic Category Anticonvulsant, Neuronal Potassium Channel Opener
Medication Safety Issues
Sound-alike/look-alike issues:
Ezogabine may be confused with ezetimibe.
Potiga™ may be confused with Portia®
Medication Guide Available Yes
Pregnancy Risk Factor C
Lactation Excretion in breast milk unknown/not recommended
Breast-Feeding Considerations According to the manufacturer, due to the potential for serious adverse reactions in the nursing infant, the decision to continue or discontinue breast-feeding during therapy should take into account the risk of

exposure to the infant and the benefits to the mother.

Use Adjuvant treatment of partial-onset seizures in patients ≥18 years of age who have responded inadequately to several alternative treatments and for whom the benefits outweigh the risk of retinal abnormalities and potential decline in visual acuity.

Mechanism of Action/Effect Ezogabine binds the KCNQ (Kv7.2-7.5) voltage-gated potassium channels. As a result, neuronal excitability is regulated and epileptiform activity is suppressed.

Contraindications There are no contraindications listed in the manufacturer's labeling.

Warnings/Precautions [U.S. Boxed Warning]: Retinal abnormalities that may progress to vision loss have been reported and were seen in about one-third of patients after approximately 4 years of treatment. These retinal abnormalities exhibited fundoscopic features similar to those of retinal pigment dystrophies. The rate of progression and reversibility of these retinal abnormalities is unknown. Limit use to patients who have responded inadequately to other treatments and in whom the benefits of therapy exceed the risk of vision loss. Visual monitoring (at least visual acuity and dilated fundus photography) by an ophthalmic professional is recommended at baseline and at 6-month intervals. Other visual tests may include fluorescein angiograms, ocular coherence tomography, perimetry, and electroretinograms. Discontinue use if there is no substantial benefit after adequate titration or if retinal pigmentary abnormalities or vision changes are detected. If no other treatment options are available and the benefits of treatment outweigh the potential risk of vision loss, then may cautiously continue treatment with ezogabine.

Skin discoloration has been reported; typically blue in color (but may also be grey-blue or brown) and is predominantly located on or around the lips, nail beds of the fingers or toes, face and legs; and discoloration of the palate, sclera, and conjunctiva may also occur. Skin discoloration developed in ~10% of patients, generally after ≥2 years of treatment and at higher doses (≥900 mg). If detected, consider other treatment options or discontinue use.

Urinary retention, including retention requiring catheterization, has been reported, generally within the first 6 months of treatment. All patients should be monitored for urologic symptoms; close monitoring is recommended in patients with other risk factors for urinary retention (eg, benign prostatic hyperplasia), patients unable to communicate clinical symptoms, or patients who use concomitant medications that may affect voiding (eg, anticholinergics). Dose-related neuropsychiatric disorders, including confusion, psychotic symptoms, and hallucinations, have been reported, generally within the first 8 weeks of treatment; some patients required hospitalization. Symptoms resolved in most patients within 7 days of discontinuation of ezogabine. The risk appears to be greatest with rapid titration at greater than the recommended doses. Dose-related dizziness and somnolence (generally mild-to-moderate) have been reported; effects generally occur during dose titration and appear to diminish with continued use. Patients must be cautioned about performing tasks which require mental alertness (eg, operating machinery or driving). QT prolongation has been observed; monitor ECG in patients with electrolyte abnormalities (eg, hypokalemia, hypomagnesemia), hypothyroidism, familial long QT syndrome, concomitant medications which may augment QT prolongation, or any underlying cardiac abnormality which may also potentiate risk (eg, heart failure, ventricular hypertrophy). Pooled analysis of trials involving various antiepileptics (regardless of indication) showed an increased risk of suicidal thoughts/behavior (incidence rate: 0.43% treated patients compared to 0.24% of patients receiving placebo); risk observed as early as 1 week after initiation and continued through duration of trials (most trials ≤24 weeks). Monitor all patients for notable changes in behavior that might indicate suicidal thoughts or depression; notify healthcare provider immediately if symptoms occur.

Dosage adjustment recommended in hepatic impairment; ezogabine exposure increases in moderate-to-severe impairment. Dosage adjustment recommended in renal impairment; ezogabine undergoes significant renal elimination. Use caution in elderly due to potential for urinary retention, particularly in older men with symptomatic BPH. Systemic exposure is increased in the elderly; dosage adjustment is recommended in patients ≥65 years of age.

Anticonvulsants should not be discontinued abruptly because of the possibility of increasing seizure frequency; therapy should be withdrawn gradually over a period of ≥3 weeks to minimize the potential of increased seizure frequency, unless safety concerns require a more rapid withdrawal.

Drug Interactions

Avoid Concomitant Use

Avoid concomitant use of Ezogabine with any of the following: Azelastine (Nasal); Highest Risk QTc-Prolonging Agents; Ivabradine; Mifepristone; Paraldehyde; Thalidomide

Decreased Effect

Ezogabine may decrease the levels/effects of: LamoTRIgine

The levels/effects of Ezogabine may be decreased by: CarBAMazepine; Ketorolac (Nasal); Ketorolac (Systemic); Mefloquine; Orlistat; Phenytoin

Increased Effect/Toxicity

Ezogabine may increase the levels/effects of: Azelastine (Nasal); Buprenorphine; CNS Depressants; Digoxin; Highest Risk QTc-Prolonging Agents; Hydrocodone; Methotrimeprazine; Metyrosine; Mirtazapine; Moderate Risk QTc-Prolonging Agents; Paraldehyde; Pramipexole; ROPINIRole; Rotigotine; Selective Serotonin Reuptake Inhibitors; Thalidomide; Zolpidem

The levels/effects of Ezogabine may be increased by: Alcohol (Ethyl); Brimonidine (Topical); Doxylamine; HydrOXYzine; Ivabradine; Magnesium Sulfate; Methotrimeprazine; Mifepristone; Perampanel; QTc-Prolonging Agents (Indeterminate Risk and Risk Modifying); Sodium Oxybate; Tapentadol

Adverse Reactions

>10%: Central nervous system: Dizziness (dose related; 23%), drowsiness (dose related; 22%), fatigue (15%)

2% to 10%:

Central nervous system: Confusion (dose related; 9%), vertigo (8%), coordination impaired (dose related; 7%), lack of concentration (6%), memory impairment (dose related; 6%), abnormal gait (dose related; 4%), aphasia (dose related; 4%), dysarthria (4%), equilibrium disturbance (dose related; 4%), anxiety (3%), paresthesia (3%), amnesia (2%), disorientation (2%), dysphasia (2%), hallucination (2%)

Endocrine & metabolic: Weight gain (dose related; 3%)

Gastrointestinal: Nausea (7%), constipation (dose related; 3%), dysphagia (2%)

Genitourinary: Dysuria (dose related; 2%), hematuria (2%), urinary hesitancy (2%), urinary retention (2%), urine discoloration (dose related; 2%)

Infection: Influenza (3%)

Ophthalmic: Diplopia (7%), blurred vision (dose related; 5%)

Neuromuscular & skeletal: Tremor (dose related; 8%), weakness (5%)

Controlled Substance C-V

Available Dosage Forms

Tablet, Oral:

Potiga: 50 mg, 200 mg, 300 mg, 400 mg

General Dosage Range Dosage adjustment recommended in patients with renal impairment or hepatic impairment.

Oral:

Adults: Initial: 100 mg 3 times daily; Maintenance: 200-400 mg 3 times daily (maximum: 1200 mg daily)

Elderly: Initial: 50 mg 3 times daily; Maintenance: 250 mg 3 times daily (maximum: 750 mg daily)

Administration

Oral Swallow tablets whole. If therapy is discontinued, gradually reduce dose over ≥3 weeks unless safety concerns require abrupt withdrawal.

Storage/Stability Store at 25°C (77°F); excursions permitted to 15°C to 30°C (59°F to 86°F).

Nursing Actions

Physical Assessment Monitor for efficacy; ECG in patients with electrolyte abnormalities, hypothyroidism, or familial long QT syndrome.

Patient Education

• Discuss specific use of drug and side effects with patient as it relates to treatment. (HCAHPS: During this hospital stay, were you given any medicine that you had not taken before? Before giving you any new medicine, how often did hospital staff tell you what the medicine was for? How often did hospital staff describe possible side effects in a way you could understand?)

• Patient may experience fatigue, dizziness, tremors, dyspepsia, or constipation. Have patient report immediately to prescriber arrhythmia, difficulty speaking, change in balance, difficulty with motor activity, difficulty focusing, memory loss, hallucinations, paresthesia, severe asthenia, urinary retention, oliguria, dysuria, or signs of depression (ie, suicidal ideation, anxiety, emotional instability, illogical thinking) (HCAHPS).

• Educate patient about signs of a significant reaction (eg, wheezing; chest tightness; fever; itching; bad cough; blue skin color; seizures; or swelling of face, lips, tongue, or throat). **Note:** This is not a comprehensive list of all side effects. Patient should consult prescriber for additional questions.

Intended Use and Disclaimer: Should not be printed and given to patients. This information is intended to serve as a concise initial reference for healthcare professionals to use when discussing medications with a patient. You must ultimately rely on your own discretion, experience and judgment in diagnosing, treating and advising patients.

Factor VIIa (Recombinant)

(FAK ter SEV en aye ree KOM be nant)

Brand Names: U.S. NovoSeven RT

Index Terms Coagulation Factor VIIa; Eptacog Alfa (Activated); rFVIIa

Pharmacologic Category Antihemophilic Agent

Pregnancy Risk Factor C

Lactation Excretion in breast milk unknown/not recommended

Use Treatment of bleeding episodes and prevention of bleeding in surgical interventions in patients with either hemophilia A or B with inhibitors to factor VIII or factor IX, acquired hemophilia, or congenital factor VII deficiency

Unlabeled Use Warfarin-related intracerebral hemorrhage; treatment of refractory bleeding after cardiac surgery in nonhemophiliac patients

Available Dosage Forms

Solution Reconstituted, Intravenous [preservative free]:

NovoSeven RT: 1 mg (1 ea); 2 mg (1 ea); 5 mg (1 ea); 8 mg (1 ea)

General Dosage Range I.V.: *Children and Adults:* Dosage varies greatly depending on indication

Administration

I.V. I.V. administration only; bolus over 2-5 minutes. Administer within 3 hours after reconstitution.

Injectable Detail pH: 5.5

Nursing Actions

Physical Assessment Monitor patient closely (eg, vital signs, cardiac and CNS status, hemolytic status, hypersensitivity) during and after infusion.

Patient Education

• Discuss specific use of drug and side effects with patient as it relates to treatment. (HCAHPS: During this hospital stay, were you given any medicine that you had not taken before? Before giving you any new medicine, how often did hospital staff tell you what the medicine was for? How often did hospital staff describe possible side effects in a way you could understand?)

• Patient may experience injection site irritation, nausea, or chills. Have patient report immediately to prescriber severe dizziness, syncope, tachycardia, mouth discoloration, or significant headache (HCAHPS).

• Educate patient about signs of a significant reaction (eg, wheezing; chest tightness; fever; itching; bad cough; blue skin color; seizures; or swelling of face, lips, tongue, or throat). **Note:** This is not a comprehensive list of all side effects. Patient should consult prescriber for additional questions.

Intended Use and Disclaimer: Should not be printed and given to patients. This information is intended to serve as a concise initial reference for healthcare professionals to use when discussing medications with a patient. You must ultimately rely on your own discretion, experience and judgment in diagnosing, treating and advising patients.

Factor IX (Human) (FAK ter nyne HYU man)

Brand Names: U.S. AlphaNine SD; Mononine

Index Terms Factor IX Concentrate

Pharmacologic Category Antihemophilic Agent; Blood Product Derivative

Medication Safety Issues

Sound-alike/look-alike issues:

Factor IX may be confused with Factor IX Complex

Pregnancy Risk Factor C

Use Prevention and control of bleeding in patients with hemophilia B (congenital factor IX deficiency or Christmas disease)

NOTE: Contains **nondetectable levels of factors II, VII, and X.** Therefore, **NOT INDICATED** for replacement therapy of any other clotting factor besides factor IX or for reversal of anticoagulation due to either vitamin K antagonists or other anticoagulants (eg, dabigatran), for hemophilia A patients with factor VIII inhibitors, or for patients in a hemorrhagic state caused by reduced production of liver-dependent coagulation factors (eg, hepatitis, cirrhosis).

Mechanism of Action/Effect Replaces deficient clotting factor IX. Hemophilia B, or Christmas disease, is an X-linked inherited disorder of blood coagulation characterized by insufficient or abnormal synthesis of the clotting protein factor IX. Factor IX is a vitamin K-dependent coagulation factor which is synthesized in the liver. Factor IX is activated by factor XIa in the intrinsic coagulation pathway. Activated factor IX (IXa), in combination with factor VII:C activates factor X to Xa, resulting ultimately in the conversion of prothrombin to thrombin and the formation of a fibrin clot. The infusion of exogenous factor IX to replace the deficiency present in hemophilia B temporarily restores hemostasis.

Contraindications

AlphaNine SD®: There are no contraindications listed in the manufacturer's labeling.

Mononine®: Hypersensitivity to mouse protein

Warnings/Precautions Hypersensitivity and anaphylactic reactions have been reported with use. Delayed reactions (up to 20 days after infusion) in previously untreated patients may also occur. Due to potential for allergic reactions, the initial ~10-20 administrations should be performed under appropriate medical supervision. Hypersensitivity reactions may be associated with factor IX inhibitor development; patients experiencing allergic reactions should be evaluated for factor IX inhibitors. The development of factor IX antibodies (or inhibitors) has been reported with factor IX therapy (usually occurs within the first 10-20 exposure days); the risk of severe hypersensitivity reactions occurring may be greater in these patients. When clinical response is suboptimal, the patient has reached a specified number of exposure days, or patient is to undergo surgical procedure, screen for inhibitors. Patients with severe hemophilia compared to those with mild or moderate hemophilia are more likely to develop inhibitors (WFH, 2012).

Observe closely for signs or symptoms of intravascular coagulation or thrombosis; risk is generally associated with the use of factor IX complex concentrates (containing therapeutic amounts of additional factors); however, potential risk exists with use of factor IX products (containing only factor IX). Use with caution when administering to patients with liver disease, postoperatively, neonates, or patients at risk of thromboembolic phenomena, disseminated intravascular coagulation or

◄ patients with signs of fibrinolysis due to the potential risk of thromboembolic complications.

Contains **nondetectable levels of factors II, VII, and X**. Therefore, **NOT INDICATED** for replacement therapy of any other clotting factor besides factor IX. In addition, factor IX concentrate is **NOT INDICATED** for reversal of anticoagulation due to either vitamin K antagonists or other anticoagulants (eg, dabigatran), hemophilia A patients with factor VIII inhibitors, or patients in a hemorrhagic state caused by reduced production of liver-dependent coagulation factors (eg, hepatitis, cirrhosis). Product of human plasma; despite purification methods (AlphaNine® SD - solvent detergent treated/virus filtered; Mononine® - virus filtered); products may potentially contain infectious agents which could transmit disease. Screening of donors, as well as testing and/or inactivation or removal of certain viruses, reduces the risk. Infections thought to be transmitted by this product should be reported to the manufacturer. Safety and efficacy have not been established with factor IX products in immune tolerance induction. Nephrotic syndrome has occurred following immune tolerance induction in patients with factor IX inhibitors and a history of allergic reactions to therapy.

Drug Interactions

Avoid Concomitant Use

Avoid concomitant use of Factor IX (Human) with any of the following: Aminocaproic Acid

Decreased Effect There are no known significant interactions involving a decrease in effect.

Increased Effect/Toxicity

The levels/effects of Factor IX (Human) may be increased by: Aminocaproic Acid

Adverse Reactions Frequency not defined.

Cardiovascular: Chest tightness, flushing, hypotension, thrombosis

Central nervous system: Burning sensation (in jaw/skull), chills, dizziness, drowsiness, headache, lethargy, paresthesia, rigors

Dermatologic: Skin photosensitivity, skin rash, urticaria

Gastrointestinal: Diarrhea, dysgeusia, nausea, vomiting

Hematologic & Oncologic: Disseminated intravascular coagulation, factor IX inhibitor development

Hepatic: Increased serum alkaline phosphatase, increased serum ALT, increased serum AST

Hypersensitivity: Anaphylaxis, angioedema, hypersensitivity reaction

Local: Injection site reaction: Cellulitis at injection site, discomfort at injection site, injection site phlebitis, pain at injection site

Miscellaneous: Fever (including transient fever following rapid administration)

Neuromuscular & skeletal: Neck tightness

Ophthalmic: Visual disturbance

Respiratory: Allergic rhinitis, asthma, cough, cyanosis, dyspnea, hypoxia, laryngeal edema, pulmonary disease

Available Dosage Forms

Solution Reconstituted, Intravenous [preservative free]:

AlphaNine SD: 500 units (1 ea); 1000 units (1 ea); 1500 units (1 ea)

Mononine: 250 units (1 ea); 500 units (1 ea)

General Dosage Range I.V.: *Infants, Children, Adolescents, and Adults:* Dosage varies greatly depending on indication

Administration

I.V. Solution should be infused at room temperature.

I.V. administration only: Should be infused **slowly over several minutes**: Rate of administration should be determined by the response and comfort of the patient.

AlphaNine® SD: Administer I.V. at a rate not exceeding 10 mL/minute

Mononine®: Administer I.V. at a rate of ~2 mL/minute. Administration rates of up to 225 **units**/minute have been regularly tolerated without incident (when reconstituted as directed to ~100 units/mL).

World Federation of Hemophilia (WFH) recommendations: Infuse at rate of 3 mL/minute for adults or 100 **units**/minute for young children; may also administer as a continuous infusion in select patients. With patients who have had allergic reactions during factor IX infusion, administration of hydrocortisone prior to infusion may be necessary (WFH, 2012).

Preparation for Administration Refer to instructions for individual products. Exact potency labeled on each vial. Diluent and factor IX should come to room temperature before combining.

Storage/Stability When stored at refrigerator temperature, 2°C to 8°C (36°F to 46°F), factor IX is stable for the period indicated by the expiration date on its label. Avoid freezing which may damage container for the diluent.

AlphaNine® SD: May also be stored at room temperature not to exceed 30°C (86°F) for up to 1 month. Reconstituted solution should be used within 3 hours of preparation.

Mononine®: May also be stored at room temperature not to exceed 25°C (77°F) for up to 1 month. Reconstituted solution should be at room temperature and used within 3 hours of preparation.

Nursing Actions

Patient Education

• Discuss specific use of drug and side effects with patient as it relates to treatment. (HCAHPS: During this hospital stay, were you given any medicine that you had not taken before? Before giving you any new medicine, how often did hospital staff tell you what the medicine was

for? How often did hospital staff describe possible side effects in a way you could understand?)

• Patient may experience headache, dyspepsia, injection site irritation, or chills. Have patient report immediately to prescriber signs of infection, dyspnea, severe dizziness, syncope, tachycardia, mouth discoloration, angina, hemoptysis, strength differences from one side to another, difficulty speaking or thinking, change in balance, blurred vision, edema of extremities, extremity discoloration, or painful extremities (HCAHPS).

• Educate patient about signs of a significant reaction (eg, wheezing; chest tightness; fever; itching; bad cough; blue skin color; seizures; or swelling of face, lips, tongue, or throat). **Note:** This is not a comprehensive list of all side effects. Patient should consult prescriber for additional questions.

Intended Use and Disclaimer: Should not be printed and given to patients. This information is intended to serve as a concise initial reference for healthcare professionals to use when discussing medications with a patient. You must ultimately rely on your own discretion, experience and judgment in diagnosing, treating and advising patients.

Factor IX (Recombinant)
(FAK ter nyne ree KOM be nant)

Brand Names: U.S. BeneFIX; Rixubis
Index Terms Factor IX Concentrate
Pharmacologic Category Antihemophilic Agent
Medication Safety Issues
Sound-alike/look-alike issues:
Factor IX may be confused with Factor IX Complex
Pregnancy Risk Factor C
Lactation Excretion in breast milk unknown/use caution
Breast-Feeding Considerations It is not known if factor IX (recombinant) is excreted in breast milk. The manufacturer recommends that caution be exercised when administering factor IX (recombinant) to nursing women.
Use Prevention and control of bleeding episodes in patients with hemophilia B (congenital factor IX deficiency or Christmas disease); perioperative management in patients with hemophilia B; routine prophylaxis in adults with hemophilia B to prevent or reduce the frequency of bleeding episodes (Rixubis)

NOTE: Contains **only factor IX.** Therefore, **NOT INDICATED** for replacement therapy of any other clotting factor besides factor IX or for reversal of anticoagulation due to either vitamin K antagonists or other anticoagulants (eg, dabigatran), for hemophilia A patients with factor VIII inhibitors, or for patients in a hemorrhagic state caused by reduced

production of liver-dependent coagulation factors (eg, hepatitis, cirrhosis).

Mechanism of Action/Effect Replaces deficient clotting factor IX. Hemophilia B, or Christmas disease, is an X-linked inherited disorder of blood coagulation characterized by insufficient or abnormal synthesis of the clotting protein factor IX. Factor IX is a vitamin K-dependent coagulation factor which is synthesized in the liver. Factor IX is activated by factor XIa in the intrinsic coagulation pathway. Activated factor IX (IXa) in combination with factor VII:C activates factor X to Xa, resulting ultimately in the conversion of prothrombin to thrombin and the formation of a fibrin clot. The infusion of exogenous factor IX to replace the deficiency present in hemophilia B temporarily restores hemostasis.

Contraindications Life-threatening, immediate hypersensitivity reactions (including anaphylaxis) to factor IX, hamster protein, or any component of the formulation; disseminated intravascular coagulation (Rixubis); signs of fibrinolysis (Rixubis)

Warnings/Precautions Contains **only factor IX.** Therefore, **NOT INDICATED** for replacement therapy of any other clotting factor besides factor IX or for reversal of anticoagulation due to either vitamin K antagonists or other anticoagulants (eg, dabigatran), for hemophilia A patients with factor VIII inhibitors, or for patients in a hemorrhagic state caused by reduced production of liver-dependent coagulation factors (eg, hepatitis, cirrhosis).

Hypersensitivity and anaphylactic reactions have been reported with use. Risk is highest during the early phases of initial exposure in previously untreated patients, especially those with high-risk gene mutations. Delayed reactions (up to 20 days after infusion) in previously untreated patients may also occur. Due to potential for allergic reactions, the initial ~10-20 administrations should be performed under appropriate medical supervision. Hypersensitivity reactions may be associated with factor IX inhibitor development; patients experiencing allergic reactions should be evaluated for factor IX inhibitors. If severe hypersensitivity reactions occur, consider the use of alternative hemostatic measures.

The development of factor IX antibodies (or inhibitors) has been reported with factor IX therapy (usually occurs within the first 10-20 exposure days); the risk of severe hypersensitivity reactions occurring may be greater in these patients. When clinical response is suboptimal, the patient has reached a specified number of exposure days, or patient is to undergo surgical procedure, screen for inhibitors. Patients with severe hemophilia compared to those with mild or moderate hemophilia are more likely to develop inhibitors (WFH, 2012).

Observe closely for signs or symptoms of intravascular coagulation or thrombosis; risk is generally associated with the use of factor IX complex concentrates (containing therapeutic amounts of additional factors); however, potential risk exists with use of factor IX products (containing only factor IX). Use with caution when administering to patients with liver disease, postoperatively, neonates, patients at risk of thromboembolic phenomena or disseminated intravascular coagulation, or patients with signs of fibrinolysis due to the potential risk of thromboembolic complications.

Safety and efficacy have not been established with factor IX products in immune tolerance induction. Nephrotic syndrome has occurred following immune tolerance induction in patients with factor IX inhibitors and a history of allergic reactions to therapy.

Drug Interactions

Avoid Concomitant Use

Avoid concomitant use of Factor IX (Recombinant) with any of the following: Aminocaproic Acid

Decreased Effect There are no known significant interactions involving a decrease in effect.

Increased Effect/Toxicity

The levels/effects of Factor IX (Recombinant) may be increased by: Aminocaproic Acid

Adverse Reactions

>10%: Central nervous system: Headache (11%)

1% to 10%:

Cardiovascular: Flushing (3%), chest tightness (2%)

Central nervous system: Dizziness (8%), drowsiness (2%), chills (2%)

Dermatologic: Skin rash (2% to 6%), urticaria (3% to 5%)

Gastrointestinal: Nausea (6%), dysgeusia (1% to 5%), vomiting (2%)

Immunologic: Factor IX inhibitor development (2% to 3%), antibody development (furin: 1%)

Local: Injection site reaction (2% to 8%; including cellulitis, pain, phlebitis)

Neuromuscular & skeletal: Tremor (2%), limb pain (1%)

Ophthalmic: Blurred vision (2%)

Renal: Renal infarction (2%)

Respiratory: Dyspnea (3%), cough (2%), hypoxia (2%)

Miscellaneous: Fever (3%; including transient fever following rapid administration)

Available Dosage Forms

Solution Reconstituted, Intravenous [preservative free]:

BeneFIX: 250 units (1 ea); 500 units (1 ea); 1000 units (1 ea); 2000 units (1 ea)

Rixubis: 250 units (1 ea); 500 units (1 ea); 1000 units (1 ea); 2000 units (1 ea); 3000 units (1 ea)

General Dosage Range I.V.: *Infants, Children, Adolescents, and Adults:* Dosage varies greatly depending on indication

Administration

I.V. Solution should be infused at room temperature. Safety and efficacy of continuous infusion administration have not been determined.

I.V. administration only:

BeneFIX: Should be infused **slowly over several minutes.** Rate of administration should be determined by the response and comfort of the patient.

Rixubis: Bolus infusion; maximum rate of administration is 10 mL/minute

Per the WFH, infuse at rate of 3 mL/minute for adults or 100 **units**/minute for young children; may also administer as a continuous infusion in select patients. With patients who have had allergic reactions during factor IX infusion, administration of hydrocortisone prior to infusion may be necessary (WFH, 2012).

Preparation for Administration Refer to instructions provided by the manufacturer. Diluent and factor IX should come to room temperature (if refrigerated) before combining.

Storage/Stability

BeneFIX:

Product labeled for room temperature storage: May either store at 2°C to 30°C (36°F to 86°F) or refrigerated at 2°C to 8°C (36°F to 46°F). Avoid freezing which may damage the diluent syringe. Reconstituted solution should be at room temperature and used within 3 hours of preparation.

Product labeled for refrigerated storage: Store at 2°C to 8°C (36°F to 46°F). May be stored at room temperature (not to exceed 30°C [86°F]) for up to 6 months; do not use after this 6-month period has elapsed even if the expiration date on the carton has not been exceeded. If date of removal from refrigeration is not recorded on the carton, the assigned expiration date (printed on the end flap of the carton) **must be reduced by 12 months.** Avoid freezing which may damage the diluent syringe. Reconstituted solution should be at room temperature and used within 3 hours of preparation.

Rixubis: Store at 2°C to 8°C (36°F to 46°F) for up to 18 months; do not freeze. After removal from refrigeration, may store at room temperature not to exceed 30°C (86°F) for up to 6 months within the 18-month time period; do not return to refrigerator. Following reconstitution, use within 3 hours and do not refrigerate.

Nursing Actions

Physical Assessment Assess for signs of hypersensitivity reactions including anaphylaxis (difficulty breathing, chest tightness, tachycardia, edema, rash, or hives). Have equipment and treatment available in the event of a severe hypersensitivity reaction. Headache or dizziness may occur; observe patient to assure safety with ambulation. Monitor injection site for pain and local reaction. Monitor I.V. site for signs of phlebitis or cellulitis and change sites as necessary. Observe patient and report signs of excess bleeding (bruising, bleeding from nose or mouth, abdominal or chest pain) or signs of clotting (shortness of breath, chest pain, numbness, tingling, pain, duskiness, or discoloration to extremity). Monitor and report abnormal lab results, including plasma albumin, urinalysis results, cholesterol levels.

Patient Education

• Discuss specific use of drug and side effects with patient as it relates to treatment. (HCAHPS: During this hospital stay, were you given any medicine that you had not taken before? Before giving you any new medicine, how often did hospital staff tell you what the medicine was for? How often did hospital staff describe possible side effects in a way you could understand?)

• Patient may experience headache, dyspepsia, or injection site irritation. Have patient report immediately to prescriber signs of renal impairment, severe dizziness, syncope, tachycardia, angina, illogical thinking, hemoptysis, strength differences from one side to another, difficulty speaking or thinking, change in balance, blurred vision, edema of extremities, extremity discoloration, painful extremities, or mouth discoloration (HCAHPS).

• Educate patient about signs of a significant reaction (eg, wheezing; chest tightness; fever; itching; bad cough; blue skin color; seizures; or swelling of face, lips, tongue, or throat). **Note:** This is not a comprehensive list of all side effects. Patient should consult prescriber for additional questions.

Intended Use and Disclaimer: Should not be printed and given to patients. This information is intended to serve as a concise initial reference for healthcare professionals to use when discussing medications with a patient. You must ultimately rely on your own discretion, experience and judgment in diagnosing, treating and advising patients.

Related Information

Diagnostics and Surgical Aids *on page 1670*

Famciclovir (fam SYE kloe veer)

Brand Names: U.S. Famvir
Pharmacologic Category Antiviral Agent
Medication Safety Issues
  Sound-alike/look-alike issues:
    Famvir® may be confused with Femara®
Pregnancy Risk Factor B
Lactation Excretion in breast milk unknown/not recommended
Breast-Feeding Considerations There is no specific data describing the excretion of famciclovir in breast milk. Breast-feeding is not recommended by the manufacturer unless the potential benefits

outweigh any possible risk. If herpes lesions are on breast, breast-feeding should be avoided in order to avoid transmission to infant.

Use Treatment of acute herpes zoster (shingles) in immunocompetent patients; treatment and suppression of recurrent episodes of genital herpes in immunocompetent patients; treatment of herpes labialis (cold sores) in immunocompetent patients; treatment of recurrent orolabial/genital (mucocutaneous) herpes simplex in HIV-infected patients

Mechanism of Action/Effect The prodrug famciclovir undergoes rapid biotransformation to the active compound, penciclovir, then intracellular conversion to triphosphate which is active against HSV-1, HSV-2, VZV, and EBV infected cells.

Contraindications Hypersensitivity to famciclovir, penciclovir, or any component of the formulation

Warnings/Precautions Has not been established for use in immunocompromised patients (except HIV-infected patients with orolabial or genital herpes, patients with ophthalmic or disseminated zoster or with initial episode of genital herpes, and in Black and African American patients with recurrent episodes of genital herpes. Acute renal failure has been reported with use of inappropriate high doses in patients with underlying renal disease. Dosage adjustment is required in patients with renal insufficiency. Tablets contain lactose; do not use with galactose intolerance, severe lactase deficiency, or glucose-galactose malabsorption syndromes.

Drug Interactions

Avoid Concomitant Use

Avoid concomitant use of Famciclovir with any of the following: Zoster Vaccine

Decreased Effect

Famciclovir may decrease the levels/effects of: Zoster Vaccine

Increased Effect/Toxicity There are no known significant interactions involving an increase in effect.

Nutritional/Ethanol Interactions Food: Rate of absorption and/or conversion to penciclovir and peak concentration are reduced with food, but bioavailability is not affected.

Adverse Reactions Note: Frequencies vary with dose and duration.

>10%:
  Central nervous system: Headache (9% to 39%)
  Gastrointestinal: Nausea (2% to 13%)
1% to 10%:
  Central nervous system: Fatigue (1% to 5%), migraine (1% to 3%)
  Dermatologic: Pruritus (≤4%), rash (≤3%)
  Endocrine & metabolic: Dysmenorrhea (≤8%)
  Gastrointestinal: Diarrhea (2% to 9%), abdominal pain (≤8%), vomiting (1% to 5%), flatulence (≤5%)

Hematologic: Neutropenia (3%)

Hepatic: Transaminases increased (2% to 3%), bilirubin increased (2%)

Neuromuscular & skeletal: Paresthesia (≤3%)

Available Dosage Forms

Tablet, Oral:

Famvir: 125 mg, 250 mg, 500 mg

Generic: 125 mg, 250 mg, 500 mg

General Dosage Range

Dosage adjustment recommended in patients with renal impairment

Oral: *Adults:* 250-1000 mg twice daily **or** 500 mg every 8 hours **or** 1500 mg once

Administration

Oral May be administered without regard to meals.

Storage/Stability Store at 25°C (77°F); excursions permitted to 15°C to 30°C (59°F to 86°F).

Nursing Actions

Physical Assessment Monitor for persistent fatigue and gastrointestinal upset.

Patient Education

• Discuss specific use of drug and side effects with patient as it relates to treatment. (HCAHPS: During this hospital stay, were you given any medicine that you had not taken before? Before giving you any new medicine, how often did hospital staff tell you what the medicine was for? How often did hospital staff describe possible side effects in a way you could understand?)

• Patient may experience headache, nausea, or diarrhea (HCAHPS).

• Educate patient about signs of a significant reaction (eg, wheezing; chest tightness; fever; itching; bad cough; blue skin color; seizures; or swelling of face, lips, tongue, or throat). **Note:** This is not a comprehensive list of all side effects. Patient should consult prescriber for additional questions.

Intended Use and Disclaimer: Should not be printed and given to patients. This information is intended to serve as a concise initial reference for healthcare professionals to use when discussing medications with a patient. You must ultimately rely on your own discretion, experience and judgment in diagnosing, treating and advising patients.

Dietary Considerations May be taken without regard to meals.

Famotidine (fa MOE ti deen)

Brand Names: U.S. Acid Reducer Maximum Strength [OTC]; Acid Reducer [OTC]; Heartburn Relief Max St [OTC]; Heartburn Relief [OTC]; Pepcid

Pharmacologic Category Histamine H_2 Antagonist

Medication Safety Issues

Sound-alike/look-alike issues:

Famotidine may be confused with FLUoxetine, furosemide

Pregnancy Risk Factor B

Lactation Enters breast milk/not recommended

Breast-Feeding Considerations Famotidine is excreted into breast milk with peak concentrations occurring ~6 hours after the maternal dose. According to the manufacturer, the decision to continue or discontinue breast-feeding during therapy should take into account the risk of exposure to the infant and the benefits of treatment to the mother.

Use Maintenance therapy and treatment of duodenal ulcer; treatment of gastroesophageal reflux disease (GERD), active benign gastric ulcer; pathological hypersecretory conditions

OTC labeling: Relief of heartburn, acid indigestion, and sour stomach

Unlabeled Use Part of a multidrug regimen for *H. pylori* eradication to reduce the risk of duodenal ulcer recurrence; stress ulcer prophylaxis in critically-ill patients; symptomatic relief in gastritis

Mechanism of Action/Effect Competitive inhibition of histamine at H_2 receptors at the gastric parietal cells, which inhibits gastric acid secretion

Contraindications Hypersensitivity to famotidine, other H_2 antagonists, or any component of the formulation

Warnings/Precautions Modify dose in patients with moderate-to-severe renal impairment. Prolonged QT interval has been reported in patients with renal dysfunction. The FDA has received reports of torsade de pointes occurring with famotidine (Poluzzi, 2009). Relief of symptoms does not preclude the presence of a gastric malignancy. Reversible confusional states, usually clearing within 3-4 days after discontinuation, have been linked to use. Increased age (>50 years) and renal or hepatic impairment are thought to be associated. Multidose vials for injection contain benzyl alcohol.

OTC labeling: When used for self-medication, patients should be instructed not to use if they have difficulty swallowing, are vomiting blood, or have bloody or black stools. Not for use with other acid reducers.

Drug Interactions

Avoid Concomitant Use

Avoid concomitant use of Famotidine with any of the following: Dasatinib; Delavirdine; PONATinib; Risedronate

Decreased Effect

Famotidine may decrease the levels/effects of: Atazanavir; Bosutinib; Cefditoren; Cefpodoxime; Cefuroxime; Dabrafenib; Dasatinib; Delavirdine; Erlotinib; Fosamprenavir; Gefitinib; Indinavir; Iron Salts; Itraconazole; Ketoconazole (Systemic); Mesalamine; Multivitamins/Minerals (with ADEK,

Folate, Iron); Nelfinavir; Nilotinib; PONATinib; Posaconazole; Rilpivirine; Vismodegib

Increased Effect/Toxicity

Famotidine may increase the levels/effects of: Dexmethylphenidate; Highest Risk QTc-Prolonging Agents; Methylphenidate; Moderate Risk QTc-Prolonging Agents; Risedronate; Saquinavir; Varenicline

The levels/effects of Famotidine may be increased by: Mifepristone

Nutritional/Ethanol Interactions

Ethanol: Avoid ethanol (may cause gastric mucosal irritation).

Food: Famotidine bioavailability may be increased if taken with food.

Adverse Reactions

Note: Agitation and vomiting have been reported in up to 14% of pediatric patients <1 year of age.

1% to 10%:

Central nervous system: Headache (5%), dizziness (1%)

Gastrointestinal: Diarrhea (2%), constipation (1%), necrotizing enterocolitis (VLBW neonates; Guillet, 2006)

Pharmacodynamics/Kinetics

Onset of Action Antisecretory effect: Oral: Within 1 hour; I.V.: Within 30 minutes

Peak effect: Antisecretory effect: Oral: Within 1-3 hours (dose-dependent)

Duration of Action Antisecretory effect: I.V., Oral: 10-12 hours

Available Dosage Forms

Solution, Intravenous:

Generic: 20 mg (50 mL); 10 mg/mL (2 mL, 4 mL, 20 mL, 50 mL)

Solution, Intravenous [preservative free]:

Generic: 10 mg/mL (2 mL)

Suspension Reconstituted, Oral:

Pepcid: 40 mg/5 mL (50 mL)

Generic: 40 mg/5 mL (50 mL)

Tablet, Oral:

Acid Reducer [OTC]: 10 mg

Acid Reducer Maximum Strength [OTC]: 20 mg

Heartburn Relief [OTC]: 10 mg

Heartburn Relief Max St [OTC]: 20 mg

Pepcid: 20 mg, 40 mg

Generic: 10 mg, 20 mg, 40 mg

General Dosage Range Dosage adjustment recommended in patients with renal impairment

I.V.:

Children 1-16 years: 0.25 mg/kg every 12 hours (maximum: 40 mg/day)

Adults: 20 mg every 12 hours

Oral:

Children <3 months: 0.5 mg/kg once daily

Children 3-12 months: 0.5 mg/kg twice daily

Children 1-11 years: 0.5-1 mg/kg/day in 1-2 divided doses (maximum: 80 mg/day)

Children 12-16 years: 0.5-1 mg/kg/day in 1-2 divided doses (maximum: 80 mg/day) **or** 10-20 mg every 12 hours (OTC dosing)

Adults: 20-40 mg/day in 1-2 divided doses **or** 20-160 mg every 6 hours [hypersecretory conditions]

Administration

I.V.

I.V. push: Inject over at least 2 minutes.

Solution for infusion: Administer over 15-30 minutes.

Injectable Detail pH: 5.7-6.4 (premixed solution); 5-5.6 (injection)

Oral May administer with antacids.

Suspension: Shake vigorously before use. May be taken without regard to meals.

Tablet: May be taken without regard to meals.

Preparation for Administration Solution for injection:

I.V. push: Dilute famotidine with NS (or another compatible solution) to a total of 5-10 mL (may also administer undiluted [Lipsy, 1995])

Infusion: Dilute with D_5W 100 mL or another compatible solution.

Storage/Stability

Oral:

Powder for oral suspension: Prior to mixing, dry powder should be stored at controlled room temperature of 25°C (77°F). Reconstituted oral suspension is stable for 30 days at room temperature; do not freeze.

Tablet: Store controlled room temperature. Protect from moisture.

I.V.:

Solution for injection: Prior to use, store at 2°C to 8°C (36°F to 46°F). If solution freezes, allow to solubilize at controlled room temperature. May be stored at room temperature for up to 3 months (data on file [Bedford Laboratories, 2011]).

I.V. push: Following preparation, solutions for I.V. push should be used immediately, or may be stored in refrigerator and used within 48 hours.

Infusion: Following preparation, the manufacturer states may be stored for up to 48 hours under refrigeration; however, solutions for infusion have been found to be physically and chemically stable for 7 days at room temperature.

Solution for injection, premixed bags: Store at controlled room temperature of 25°C (77°F); avoid excessive heat.

Nursing Actions

Physical Assessment Teach patient proper timing of administration.

Patient Education

• Discuss specific use of drug and side effects with patient as it relates to treatment. (HCAHPS: During this hospital stay, were you given any medicine that you had not taken before? Before giving you any new medicine, how often did hospital staff tell you what the medicine was

for? How often did hospital staff describe possible side effects in a way you could understand?)
• Patient may experience headache, diarrhea, or constipation. Have patient report immediately to prescriber dysphagia, difficulty speaking, severe nausea, considerable dizziness, syncope, illogical thinking, angina, tachycardia, ecchymosis, hemorrhaging, or injection site irritation (HCAHPS).
• Educate patient about signs of a significant reaction (eg, wheezing; chest tightness; fever; itching; bad cough; blue skin color; seizures; or swelling of face, lips, tongue, or throat). **Note:** This is not a comprehensive list of all side effects. Patient should consult prescriber for additional questions.

Intended Use and Disclaimer: Should not be printed and given to patients. This information is intended to serve as a concise initial reference for healthcare professionals to use when discussing medications with a patient. You must ultimately rely on your own discretion, experience and judgment in diagnosing, treating and advising patients.

Dietary Considerations May be taken without regard to meals.

Fat Emulsion (Fish Oil Based)
(fat e MUL shun fish oyl baste)

Index Terms Intravenous Fat Emulsion (Fish-Oil Based)
Pharmacologic Category Caloric Agent
Use Caloric/fatty acid source: Source of calories, essential fatty acids, and omega-3 fatty acids for patients requiring parenteral nutrition
Product Availability Not available in the U.S.
General Dosage Range I.V.: *Adults:* 1-2 g lipid/kg daily or 5-10 mL/kg daily
Administration
I.V. Gently invert bag prior to use. Do not use if discolored or if the emulsion contains a precipitate, phase separation, or there are leaks in the bag. Infuse I.V. through peripheral or central venous line using DEHP-free administration sets and lines. Do not exceed a rate of 0.15 g lipid/kg/ hour (equivalent to 0.75 mL/kg/hour). Change tubing after each infusion. May be simultaneously infused with amino acid dextrose mixtures by means of Y-connector located near infusion site. Peripheral administration of parenteral nutrition is dependent upon osmolality of solution (ie, should not exceed 900 mOsm/L; Mirtello, 2004).
Injectable Detail pH: ~8
Osmolality: 380 mOsm/kg water
Nursing Actions
Patient Education
• Discuss specific use of drug and side effects with patient as it relates to treatment. (HCAHPS: During this hospital stay, were you given any

medicine that you had not taken before? Before giving you any new medicine, how often did hospital staff tell you what the medicine was for? How often did hospital staff describe possible side effects in a way you could understand?)
• Patient may experience headache. Have patient report immediately to prescriber signs of hepatic impairment, severe asthenia, ecchymosis, hemorrhaging, paresthesia, or injection site irritation (HCAHPS).
• Educate patient about signs of a significant reaction (eg, wheezing; chest tightness; fever; itching; bad cough; blue skin color; seizures; or swelling of face, lips, tongue, or throat). **Note:** This is not a comprehensive list of all side effects. Patient should consult prescriber for additional questions.

Intended Use and Disclaimer: Should not be printed and given to patients. This information is intended to serve as a concise initial reference for healthcare professionals to use when discussing medications with a patient. You must ultimately rely on your own discretion, experience and judgment in diagnosing, treating and advising patients.

Fat Emulsion (Plant Based)
(fat e MUL shun plant baste)

Brand Names: U.S. Clinolipid; Intralipid; Liposyn II; Liposyn III
Index Terms Clinolipid; Intravenous Fat Emulsion
Pharmacologic Category Caloric Agent
Medication Safety Issues
Sound-alike/look-alike issues:
Intralipid may be confused with ViperSlide (lubricant used during atherectomy procedures)
Pregnancy Risk Factor C
Lactation Enters breast milk/use with caution
Use Caloric/fatty acid source: Source of calories and essential fatty acids for patients requiring parenteral nutrition for extended periods of time (usually for longer than 5 days) or when oral or enteral nutrition is not possible, insufficient, or contraindicated; to prevent and treat essential fatty acid deficiency (except Clinolipid)
Unlabeled Use Treatment of local anesthetic-induced cardiac arrest unresponsive to conventional resuscitation
Dosage Forms Considerations
Product oil components:
Soybean oil: Intralipid 20%, 30%; Liposyn III 10%, 20%, 30%
Soybean and safflower oil: Liposyn II 20% (10% each)
Available Dosage Forms
Emulsion, Intravenous:
Intralipid: 20% (100 mL, 250 mL, 500 mL, 1000 mL); 30% (500 mL)
Liposyn II: 20% (200 mL, 250 mL)

Liposyn III: 10% (200 mL, 250 mL, 500 mL); 20% (200 mL, 250 mL, 500 mL); 30% (500 mL)

General Dosage Range I.V.:

Infants: Initial: 1-2 g/kg/day; Maintenance: Up to 3 g/kg/day

Children: 1-2 g/kg/day; Maintenance: Up to 2-3 g/kg/day **or** 8% to 10% of caloric intake given up to once daily

Adolescents: Initial: 1 g/kg/day; Maintenance: Up to 2.5 g/kg/day **or** 8% to 10% of caloric intake given up to once daily

Adults: Initial: 1-1.5 g/kg/day; Maintenance: Up to 2.5 g/kg/day **or** 8% to 10% of caloric intake given up to once daily

Administration

I.V. Administer via peripheral line or by central venous infusion. At the onset of therapy, the patient should be observed for any immediate allergic reactions such as dyspnea, cyanosis, and fever. Change tubing after each infusion. May be simultaneously infused with carbohydrate/amino acid solutions by means of Y-connector located near infusion site or administered in total nutrient mixtures (3-in-1) with amino acids, dextrose, and other nutrients. Fat emulsions of 30% should only be administered in total nutrient mixtures (3-in-1) with amino acids, dextrose, and other nutrients. Hang fat emulsion higher than other fluids (has low specific gravity and could run up into other lines).

Clinolipid: Do not use <1.2 micron filter. Prior to opening the overwrap of Clinolipid, check the color of the oxygen indicator and compare to the reference color next to the OK symbol. If the color of the oxygen absorber/indicator does not correspond to the reference color, do not use. After opening the bag, use the contents immediately and do not store for a subsequent infusion. Do not connect flexible bags in series to avoid air embolism due to possible residual gas contained in the primary bag. When preparing total parenteral nutrition admixture, do not use the EXACTAMIX Inlet H938173 with an EXACTAMIX compounder to transfer Clinolipid injection; associated with dislodgement of the administration port membrane into the Clinolipid injection bag.

Intralipid: Do not use <1.2 micron filter. Prior to opening the overwrap the integrity indicator should be inspected. If the indicator is black, the overwrap is damaged; do not use.

Liposyn III: Do not use a filter.

Caloric source/EFAD:

Children: Initiate infusions of 10% emulsions at ≤0.1 mL/minute for 10-15 minutes; if no untoward effects occur, the infusion rate may be increased to 1 mL/kg/hour (maximum rate: 100 mL/hour). Initiate infusions of 20% emulsions at ≤0.05 mL/minute for 10-15 minutes; if no untoward effects occur, the infusion rate may be increased to 0.5 mL/kg/hour. Liposyn II 20%

should be started at a rate of 0.1 mL/minute for the first 15 minutes; if no untoward effects occur, the rate can be increased to allow no more 50 mL of Liposyn II 20% per hour. **Note:** Premature and/or septic infants may require reduced infusion rates. Do not exceed 1 g fat/kg in 4 hours in this population.

Adults: Initiate infusions of 10% emulsions at 1 mL/minute for 15-30 minutes; if no untoward effects occur, the infusion rate may be increased to 2 mL/minute. Initiate infusions of 20% emulsions at 0.5 mL/minute for 15-30 minutes; if no untoward effects occur, the infusion rate may be increased to 1 mL/minute.

Local anesthetic toxicity (unlabeled use): Administer initial bolus over 1 minute followed by a continuous infusion. Chest compressions should continue during administration if patient is in cardiac arrest. The infusion rate may be increased if hemodynamic instability persists or recurs. Continue the infusion for at least 10 minutes after hemodynamic stability is restored (ACMT, 2010; Neal, 2012).

Injectable Detail

pH: ~6-9

Osmolality: ~300-350 mOsmol/kg water

Nursing Actions

Physical Assessment Assess for allergy to eggs prior to initiating therapy. Inspect emulsion before administering. Do not administer if oil separation or oiliness is noted. Monitor closely for allergic reactions or fluid overload.

Patient Education

• Discuss specific use of drug and side effects with patient as it relates to treatment. (HCAHPS: During this hospital stay, were you given any medicine that you had not taken before? Before giving you any new medicine, how often did hospital staff tell you what the medicine was for? How often did hospital staff describe possible side effects in a way you could understand?)

• Have patient report immediately to prescriber signs of hepatic impairment, dyspnea, angina, severe asthenia, ecchymosis, hemorrhaging, or application site irritation (HCAHPS).

• Educate patient about signs of a significant reaction (eg, wheezing; chest tightness; fever; itching; bad cough; blue skin color; seizures; or swelling of face, lips, tongue, or throat). **Note:** This is not a comprehensive list of all side effects. Patient should consult prescriber for additional questions.

Intended Use and Disclaimer: Should not be printed and given to patients. This information is intended to serve as a concise initial reference for healthcare professionals to use when discussing medications with a patient. You must ultimately rely on your own discretion, experience and judgment in diagnosing, treating and advising patients.

Febuxostat (feb UX oh stat)

Brand Names: U.S. Uloric
Index Terms TEI-6720; TMX-67
Pharmacologic Category Antigout Agent; Xanthine Oxidase Inhibitor
Pregnancy Risk Factor C
Lactation Excretion in breast milk unknown/use caution
Breast-Feeding Considerations It is not known if febuxostat is excreted in breast milk.. The manufacturer recommends that caution be exercised when administering febuxostat to nursing women.
Use Chronic management of hyperuricemia in patients with gout
Mechanism of Action/Effect Selectively inhibits xanthine oxidase, the enzyme responsible for the conversion of hypoxanthine to xanthine to uric acid thereby decreasing uric acid.
Contraindications Concurrent use with azathioprine or mercaptopurine

Canadian labeling: Additional contraindications (not in U.S. labeling): Hypersensitivity to febuxostat or any component of the formulation; concomitant administration with theophylline
Warnings/Precautions Administer concurrently with an NSAID or colchicine (up to 6 months) to prevent gout flare upon initiation of therapy. Do not use to treat asymptomatic or secondary hyperuricemia. Postmarketing cases of hepatic failure (both fatal and nonfatal) have been reported (causal relationship has not been established). Significant hepatic transaminase elevations (>3 x ULN), MI, stroke and cardiovascular deaths have been reported in controlled trials (causal relationship not established). Monitor patients for signs/symptoms of MI and stroke. Liver function tests should be evaluated at baseline, 2 and 4 months after initiation of therapy, and periodically thereafter; evaluate liver function tests in patients experiencing signs and symptoms of hepatic injury (eg, fatigue, anorexia, right upper quadrant pain, dark urine, jaundice). Interrupt therapy in patients who develop abnormal liver function tests (eg, ALT >3 x ULN); permanently discontinue use if no other explanation for the abnormalities is elucidated and in patients who develop ALT >3 x ULT and serum total bilirubin >2 x ULN. All other patients may be cautiously restarted on febuxostat. All other patients may be cautiously restarted on febuxostat. Use with caution in patients with severe renal impairment (CrCl <30 mL/minute); insufficient data.

Drug Interactions

Avoid Concomitant Use

Avoid concomitant use of Febuxostat with any of the following: AzaTHIOprine; Didanosine; Mercaptopurine; Pegloticase

Decreased Effect There are no known significant interactions involving a decrease in effect.

Increased Effect/Toxicity

Febuxostat may increase the levels/effects of AzaTHIOprine; Didanosine; Mercaptopurine; Pegloticase; Theophylline Derivatives
Adverse Reactions 1% to 10%:
Dermatologic: Rash (1% to 2%)
Gastrointestinal: Nausea (1%)
Hepatic: Liver function abnormalities (5% to 7%)
Neuromuscular & skeletal: Arthralgia (1%)
Available Dosage Forms
Tablet, Oral:
Uloric: 40 mg, 80 mg
General Dosage Range Oral: Adults: 40-80 mg once daily
Administration
Oral Administer with or without meals or antacids.
Storage/Stability Store at 25°C (77°F); excursions permitted to 15°C to 30°C (59°F to 86°F). Protect from light.
Nursing Actions

Patient Education

- Discuss specific use of drug and side effects with patient as it relates to treatment. (HCAHPS: During this hospital stay, were you given any medicine that you had not taken before? Before giving you any new medicine, how often did hospital staff tell you what the medicine was for? How often did hospital staff describe possible side effects in a way you could understand?)
- Patient may experience arthralgia or dyspepsia. Have patient report immediately to prescriber strength differences from one side to another, difficulty speaking or thinking, change in balance, blurred vision, angina, dysuria, hematuria, severe asthenia, considerable dizziness, syncope, significant headache, intolerable nausea, ecchymosis, hemorrhaging, hyperhidrosis, melena, hemoptysis, hematemesis, urinary retention, oliguria, tachycardia, bradycardia, arrhythmia, chills, pharyngitis, hearing impairment, mood changes, myalgia, dyspnea, or signs of hepatic impairment (HCAHPS).
- Educate patient about signs of a significant reaction (eg, wheezing; chest tightness; fever; itching; bad cough; blue skin color; seizures; or swelling of face, lips, tongue, or throat). **Note:** This is not a comprehensive list of all side effects. Patient should consult prescriber for additional questions.

Intended Use and Disclaimer: Should not be printed and given to patients. This information is intended to serve as a concise initial reference for healthcare professionals to use when discussing medications with a patient. You must ultimately rely on your own discretion, experience and judgment in diagnosing, treating and advising patients.

Dietary Considerations Take with or without meals or antacids.

Felodipine (fe LOE di peen)

Index Terms Plendil

Pharmacologic Category Antihypertensive; Calcium Channel Blocker; Calcium Channel Blocker, Dihydropyridine

Medication Safety Issues

Sound-alike/look-alike issues:

Plendil may be confused with Isordil®, pindolol, Pletal, PriLOSEC, Prinivil

Pregnancy Risk Factor C

Lactation Excretion in breast milk unknown/not recommended

Breast-Feeding Considerations It is not known if felodipine is excreted in breast milk. Due to the potential for serious adverse reactions in the nursing infant, the manufacturer recommends a decision be made whether to discontinue nursing or to discontinue the drug, taking into account the importance of treatment to the mother. Breast-fed infants of mothers taking medications for hypertension should be monitored for adverse effects (Chobanian, 2003).

Use Treatment of hypertension

Unlabeled Use Pediatric hypertension

Mechanism of Action/Effect Inhibits calcium ions from entering the "slow channels" or select voltage-sensitive areas of vascular smooth muscle and myocardium during depolarization

Contraindications Hypersensitivity to felodipine, any component of the formulation, or other calcium channel blocker

Warnings/Precautions Increased angina and/or MI has occurred with initiation or dosage titration of dihydropyridine calcium channel blockers, reflex tachycardia may occur resulting in angina and/or MI in patients with obstructive coronary disease especially in the absence of concurrent beta-blockade. Use with extreme caution in patients with severe aortic stenosis. Use caution in patients with hypertrophic cardiomyopathy with outflow tract obstruction. The ACCF/AHA heart failure guidelines recommend to avoid use in patients with heart failure due to lack of benefit and/or worse outcomes with calcium channel blockers in general (Yancy, 2013). Elderly patients and patients with hepatic impairment should start off with a lower dose. Peripheral edema (dose dependent) is the most common side effect (occurs within 2-3 weeks of starting therapy). Symptomatic hypotension with or without syncope can rarely occur; blood pressure must be lowered at a rate appropriate for the patient's clinical condition. Dosage titration should occur after 14 days on a given dose.

Drug Interactions

Avoid Concomitant Use

Avoid concomitant use of Felodipine with any of the following: Conivaptan; Fusidic Acid (Systemic); Itraconazole; Pimozide

Decreased Effect

Felodipine may decrease the levels/effects of: Clopidogrel

The levels/effects of Felodipine may be decreased by: Barbiturates; Bosentan; Calcium Salts; CarBAMazepine; CYP3A4 Inducers (Strong); Dabrafenib; Deferasirox; Herbs (CYP3A4 Inducers); Herbs (Hypertensive Properties); Melatonin; Methylphenidate; Mitotane; Nafcillin; Rifamycin Derivatives; Tocilizumab; Yohimbine

Increased Effect/Toxicity

Felodipine may increase the levels/effects of: Amifostine; Antihypertensives; ARIPiprazole; Atosiban; Beta-Blockers; Calcium Channel Blockers (Nondihydropyridine); CYP2C8 Substrates; Dofetilide; DULoxetine; Fosphenytoin; Hypotensive Agents; Lomitapide; Magnesium Salts; Neuromuscular-Blocking Agents (Nondepolarizing); Nitroprusside; Obinutuzumab; Phenytoin; Pimozide; RiTUXimab; Tacrolimus (Systemic)

The levels/effects of Felodipine may be increased by: Alpha1-Blockers; Antifungal Agents (Azole Derivatives, Systemic); Brimonidine (Topical); Calcium Channel Blockers (Nondihydropyridine); Cimetidine; Conivaptan; CycloSPORINE (Systemic); CYP3A4 Inhibitors (Moderate); CYP3A4 Inhibitors (Strong); Dasatinib; Diazoxide; Fluconazole; Fusidic Acid (Systemic); Grapefruit Juice; Herbs (Hypotensive Properties); Itraconazole; Ivacaftor; Luliconazole; Macrolide Antibiotics; Magnesium Salts; MAO Inhibitors; Mifepristone; Pentoxifylline; Phosphodiesterase 5 Inhibitors; Prostacyclin Analogues; Protease Inhibitors; Simeprevir; Stiripentol

Nutritional/Ethanol Interactions

Ethanol: Ethanol increases felodipine absorption. Management: Monitor for a greater hypotensive effect if ethanol is consumed.

Food: Compared to a fasted state, felodipine peak plasma concentrations are increased up to twofold when taken after a meal high in fat or carbohydrates. Grapefruit juice similarly increases felodipine C_{max} by twofold. Increased therapeutic and vasodilator side effects, including severe hypotension and myocardial ischemia, may occur. Management: May be taken with a small meal that is low in fat and carbohydrates; avoid grapefruit juice during therapy.

Herb/Nutraceutical: St John's wort may decrease felodipine levels. Dong quai has estrogenic activity. Some herbal medications may worsen hypertension (eg, ephedra); garlic may have additional antihypertensive effects. Management: Avoid dong quai if using for hypertension. Avoid ephedra, yohimbe, ginseng, and garlic.

Adverse Reactions

>10%: Central nervous system: Headache (11% to 15%)

2% to 10%: Cardiovascular: Peripheral edema (2% to 17%), tachycardia (0.4% to 2.5%), flushing (4% to 7%)

Pharmacodynamics/Kinetics
Onset of Action Antihypertensive: 2-5 hours
Duration of Action Antihypertensive effect: 24 hours

Available Dosage Forms
Tablet Extended Release 24 Hour, Oral:
Generic: 2.5 mg, 5 mg, 10 mg

General Dosage Range Dosage adjustment recommended in patients with hepatic impairment
Oral:
Adults: Initial: 2.5-10 mg once daily; Maintenance: 2.5-20 mg once daily (maximum: 20 mg/day)
Elderly: Initial: 2.5 mg/day

Administration
Oral Swallow tablet whole; tablet should not be divided, crushed, or chewed. May be administered without food or with a small meal that is low in fat and carbohydrates.

Nursing Actions
Physical Assessment When discontinuing, taper dose gradually.

Patient Education
- Discuss specific use of drug and side effects with patient as it relates to treatment. (HCAHPS: During this hospital stay, were you given any medicine that you had not taken before? Before giving you any new medicine, how often did hospital staff tell you what the medicine was for? How often did hospital staff describe possible side effects in a way you could understand?)
- Patient may experience headache or gum changes. Have patient report immediately to prescriber tachycardia, arrhythmia, severe dizziness, syncope, angina, or edema of extremities (HCAHPS).
- Educate patient about signs of a significant reaction (eg, wheezing; chest tightness; fever; itching; bad cough; blue skin color; seizures; or swelling of face, lips, tongue, or throat). **Note:** This is not a comprehensive list of all side effects. Patient should consult prescriber for additional questions.

Intended Use and Disclaimer: Should not be printed and given to patients. This information is intended to serve as a concise initial reference for healthcare professionals to use when discussing medications with a patient. You must ultimately rely on your own discretion, experience and judgment in diagnosing, treating and advising patients.

Dietary Considerations May be taken with a small meal that is low in fat and carbohydrates.

Related Information
Oral Medications That Should Not Be Crushed or Altered *on page 1712*

Fenofibrate and Derivatives
(fen oh FYE brate & dah RIV ah tives)

Brand Names: U.S. Antara; Fenoglide; Fibricor; Lipofen; Lofibra; Tricor; Triglide; Trilipix
Index Terms ABT-335; Choline Fenofibrate; Fenofibric Acid; Procetofene; Proctofene
Pharmacologic Category Antilipemic Agent, Fibric Acid

Medication Safety Issues
Sound-alike/look-alike issues:
Fibricor may be confused with Tricor
TriCor may be confused with Fibricor, Tracleer
TriLipix may be confused with Trileptal, TriLyte

Medication Guide Available Yes
Pregnancy Risk Factor C
Lactation Excretion in breast milk unknown/contraindicated

Breast-Feeding Considerations It is not known if fenofibrate is excreted into breast milk. Use is contraindicated in nursing women. The manufacturer recommends a decision be made whether to discontinue nursing or to discontinue the drug, taking into account the importance of treatment to the mother.

Use
Hypercholesterolemia or mixed dyslipidemia: Adjunctive therapy to diet for the reduction of low-density lipoprotein cholesterol (LDL-C), total cholesterol (total-C), triglycerides, and apolipoprotein B (apo B), and to increase high-density lipoprotein cholesterol (HDL-C) in adults with primary hypercholesterolemia or mixed dyslipidemia (Fredrickson types IIa and IIb). Use lipid-altering agents in addition to a diet restricted in saturated fat and cholesterol when response to diet and nonpharmacological interventions alone has been inadequate.
Trilipix is also indicated as an adjunct to diet in combination with a statin to reduce triglycerides and increase HDL-C in patients with mixed dyslipidemia and coronary heart disease (CHD) or a CHD risk equivalent who are on optimal statin therapy.

Hypertriglyceridemia: Adjunctive therapy to diet for treatment of adult patients with severe hypertriglyceridemia (Fredrickson types IV and V hyperlipidemia).

Unlabeled Use Adjunctive therapy for the treatment of hyperuricemia in patients with gout

Mechanism of Action/Effect Fenofibric acid increases VLDL catabolism by enhancing the synthesis of lipoprotein lipase; as a result of a decrease in VLDL levels, total plasma triglycerides are reduced by 30% to 60%. Modest increase in HDL occurs in some hypertriglyceridemic patients.

Contraindications

Active liver disease, including primary biliary cirrhosis and unexplained, persistent liver function abnormality; severe renal dysfunction, including those receiving dialysis; preexisting gallbladder disease; breast-feeding; hypersensitivity to fenofibrate or fenofibric acid.

Documentation of allergenic cross-reactivity for fibrates is limited. However, because of similarities in chemical structure and/or pharmacologic actions, the possibility of cross-sensitivity cannot be ruled out with certainty.

Canadian labeling: Additional contraindications (not in U.S. labeling): Pregnancy; known photoallergy or phototoxic reaction during treatment with fibrates or ketoprofen

Lipidil EZ, Lipidil Micro, Lipidil Supra: Additional contraindications: Allergy to soya lecithin or peanut or arachis oil; chronic or acute pancreatitis; patients <18 years of age; coadministration with HMG-CoA reductase inhibitors in patients with a predisposition for myopathy.

Warnings/Precautions

Secondary causes of hyperlipidemia should be ruled out prior to therapy. Hepatic transaminases can become significantly elevated (dose-related); hepatocellular, chronic active, and cholestatic hepatitis have been reported. Regular monitoring of liver function tests is required; discontinue therapy in patients whose enzyme levels persist above 3 times the upper limit of normal. Use with caution in patients with mild-to-moderate renal impairment; dosage adjustment may be required. Contraindicated with severe renal impairment including those receiving dialysis. Contraindicated active liver disease, including primary biliary cirrhosis and unexplained persistent liver function abnormalities. Increases in serum creatinine (>2 mg/dL) have been observed with use; clinical significance unknown. Fenofibrate has been shown to increase creatinine production (unknown mechanism) resulting in an equal increase of creatinuria thereby demonstrating that the increase does not reflect a reduction in creatinine clearance (Hottelart, 2002). Monitor renal function in patients with renal impairment and consider monitoring patients with increased risk for developing renal impairment. May cause cholelithiasis.

Therapy should be discontinued in patients who develop markedly elevated CPK concentrations or if myopathy/myositis is suspected or diagnosed. No incremental benefit of combination therapy on cardiovascular morbidity and mortality over statin monotherapy has been established. In patients with type 2 diabetes mellitus, neither fenofibrate monotherapy nor the addition of fenofibrate to simvastatin compared to placebo has been shown to reduce cardiovascular disease morbidity and mortality in patients with type 2 diabetes. Potentially significant drug-drug interactions may exist, requiring dose or frequency adjustment, additional monitoring, and/or selection of alternative therapy. In combination with HMG-CoA reductase inhibitors, fenofibrate is generally regarded as safer than gemfibrozil due to limited pharmacokinetic interaction with statins. According to the 2013 ACC/AHA Blood Cholesterol Guidelines, fenofibrate may be considered in patients on low- or moderate-intensity statin therapy (ie, statin therapy intended to lower LDL-C by <30% or ~30% to 50%, respectively) only if the benefits from atherosclerotic cardiovascular disease (ASCVD) risk reduction or triglyceride lowering when triglycerides are >500 mg/dL, outweigh the potential risk for adverse effects (Stone, 2013). Therapy should be withdrawn if an adequate response is not obtained after 2-3 months of therapy at the maximal daily dose. In patients with severe hypertriglyceridemia, the occurrence of pancreatitis may represent a failure of efficacy, a direct effect of the drug, or obstruction of the common bile duct due to biliary tract stone or sludge formation. A paradoxical, severe, and reversible decrease in HDL-C (as low as 2 mg/dL) with a simultaneous decrease in apolipoprotein A1 has been reported within 2 weeks to years after initiation of fibrate therapy; clinical significance unknown. Monitor HDL-C within a few months of initiation of therapy and discontinue if HDL-C becomes severely depressed; do not restart therapy. The occurrence of pancreatitis may represent a failure of efficacy in patients with severely elevated triglycerides. May cause mild-to-moderate decreases in hemoglobin, hematocrit, and WBC upon initiation of therapy which usually stabilizes with long-term therapy. Agranulocytosis and thrombocytopenia have been reported (rare). Periodic monitoring of blood counts is recommended during the first year of therapy.

Rare hypersensitivity reactions may occur. Use has been associated with pulmonary embolism (PE) and deep vein thrombosis (DVT). Use with caution in patients with risk factors for VTE. Dose adjustment may be required for elderly patients.

Some products may contain soya lecithin or peanut or arachis oil; use is contraindicated in patients with a soya lecithin allergy or a peanut or arachis allergy for applicable formulations.

Drug Interactions

Avoid Concomitant Use There are no known interactions where it is recommended to avoid concomitant use.

Decreased Effect

Fenofibrate and Derivatives may decrease the levels/effects of: Chenodiol; CycloSPORINE (Systemic); Ursodiol

The levels/effects of Fenofibrate and Derivatives may be decreased by: Bile Acid Sequestrants

Increased Effect/Toxicity

Fenofibrate and Derivatives may increase the levels/effects of: Colchicine; Ezetimibe; HMG-CoA Reductase Inhibitors; Sulfonylureas; Vitamin K Antagonists; Warfarin

The levels/effects of Fenofibrate and Derivatives may be increased by: CycloSPORINE (Systemic); Raltegravir; Tacrolimus (Systemic)

Nutritional/Ethanol Interactions

Food:

Antara (micronized): When administered under fasted conditions or with a low-fat meal, the extent of absorption and the time to peak did not change; however peak concentrations were increased in the presence of a low-fat meal. When administered with a high fat meal, a 26% increase in the AUC and 108% increase in the peak concentration were seen in comparison to the fasted state. Management: Administer with or without food.

Fenoglide: When administered with a high-fat meal, the peak concentration was increased by 44% as compared to fasting conditions. Management: Administer with meals.

Fibricor: When administered with a high-fat meal, the peak concentration was decreased by ~35% while AUC remained unchanged as compared to fasting conditions. Management: Administer with or without food.

Lipidil EZ [Canadian product]: Bioavailability was not significantly different when administered under fasting and nonfasting conditions. Management: Administer with or without food.

Lipidil Micro [Canadian product]: In comparison with nonmicronized fenofibrate formulations, micronized fenofibrate is better absorbed when administered with a low-fat meal; absorption is less influenced by a higher fat content meal. Management: Administer with meals.

Lipidil Supra [Canadian product]: In general, fenofibrate absorption is low and variable when administered under fasting conditions; absorption is increased when administered with food. Management: Administer with meals.

Lipofen: When administered with a low-fat and high-fat meal, the extent of absorption is increased by ~25% and ~58%, respectively, as compared to fasting conditions. Management: Administer with meals.

Lofibra (micronized) capsules: Absorption is increased by ~35% under fed as compared to fasting conditions. Management: Administer with meals.

Lofibra tablets: Peak concentrations and AUC were not significantly different when a single dose was administered under fasting and non-fasting conditions. Management: Administer with or without food.

TriCor: Peak concentrations and AUC were not significantly different when a single dose was administered under fasting and nonfasting conditions. Management: Administer with or without food.

Triglide: When administered with food, the rate of absorption was increased ~55% as compared to fasting conditions; the AUC remained unchanged. Management: Administer with or without food.

Trilipix: Peak concentrations and AUC were not significantly different when a single dose was administered under fasting and nonfasting conditions. Management: Administer with or without food.

Adverse Reactions

>10%: Hepatic: Liver function tests increased (dose related; 3% to 13%; ALT/AST increased >3 x ULN: 5% to 13%)

1% to 10%:

Central nervous system: Headache (3%)

Dermatologic: Urticaria (1%)

Gastrointestinal: Abdominal pain (5%), constipation (2%), nausea (2%)

Neuromuscular & skeletal: Back pain (3%), CPK increased (3%)

Respiratory: Respiratory disorder (6%), rhinitis (2%)

Dosage Forms Considerations

Micronized formulations: Antara, Lofibra capsules Strength of choline fenofibrate products are expressed in terms of fenofibric acid.

Available Dosage Forms

Capsule, Oral:

Antara: 30 mg, 43 mg, 90 mg, 130 mg

Lipofen: 50 mg, 150 mg

Lofibra: 67 mg, 134 mg, 200 mg

Generic: 43 mg, 67 mg, 130 mg, 134 mg, 200 mg

Capsule Delayed Release, Oral:

Trilipix: 45 mg, 135 mg

Generic: 45 mg, 135 mg

Tablet, Oral:

Fenoglide: 40 mg, 120 mg

Fibricor: 35 mg, 105 mg

Lofibra: 54 mg, 160 mg

Tricor: 48 mg, 145 mg

Triglide: 160 mg

Generic: 35 mg, 48 mg, 54 mg, 105 mg, 145 mg, 160 mg

General Dosage Range Dosage adjustment recommended in patients with renal impairment and in patients who develop toxicities.

Oral: *Adults and Elderly:* Dosage varies greatly depending on product

Administration

Oral

Antara, Fibricor, Lipidil EZ [Canadian product], Lofibra tablets, TriCor, Triglide, Trilipix: Administer with or without food. Swallow whole; do not open (capsules), crush, dissolve, or chew.

Lipidil Micro [Canadian product]; Lofibra (micronized) capsules: Administer with meals.

Fenoglide, Lipofen, Lipidil Supra [Canadian product]: Administer with meals. Swallow whole; do not open (capsules), crush, dissolve, or chew.

Storage/Stability Store at 25°C (77°F); excursions are permitted between 15°C and 30°C (59°F and 86°F). Protect Fibricor, Lipofen, Lofibra, TriCor, Triglide, and Trilipix from moisture. Protect Fibricor, Lofibra tablets, Lipofen, and Triglide from light. Canadian products: Lipidil EZ, Lipidil Micro, Lipidil Supra: Store at 15°C to 25°C (59°F to 77°F). Protect Lipidil EZ, Lipidil Micro, and Lipidil Supra from moisture. Protect Lipidil EZ and Lipidil Supra from light.

Nursing Actions

Physical Assessment Monitor for signs/symptoms of myopathy (muscular pain, weakness, fatigue). Obtain baseline liver function tests and monitor throughout therapy. Increased risk of cholelithiasis due to increased cholesterol excretion in the bile.

Patient Education

• Discuss specific use of drug and side effects with patient as it relates to treatment. (HCAHPS: During this hospital stay, were you given any medicine that you had not taken before? Before giving you any new medicine, how often did hospital staff tell you what the medicine was for? How often did hospital staff describe possible side effects in a way you could understand?)

• Patient may experience headache, back pain, or dyspepsia. Have patient report immediately to prescriber signs of hepatic impairment, signs of pancreatitis, myalgia, considerable asthenia, severe arthralgia, angina, chills, edema of extremities, extremity discoloration, painful extremities, urinary retention, oliguria, ecchymosis, hemorrhaging, or Stevens-Johnson syndrome/toxic epidermal necrolysis (HCAHPS).

• Educate patient about signs of a significant reaction (eg, wheezing; chest tightness; fever; itching; bad cough; blue skin color; seizures; or swelling of face, lips, tongue, or throat). **Note:** This is not a comprehensive list of all side effects. Patient should consult prescriber for additional questions.

Intended Use and Disclaimer: Should not be printed and given to patients. This information is intended to serve as a concise initial reference for healthcare professionals to use when discussing medications with a patient. You must ultimately rely on your own discretion, experience and judgment in diagnosing, treating and advising patients.

Dietary Considerations

Antara, Fibricor, Lipidil EZ [Canadian product], Lofibra tablets, TriCor, Triglide, Trilipix: May be taken with or without food.

Fenoglide, Lipidil Micro [Canadian product], Lipidil Supra [Canadian product], Lipofen, Lofibra (micronized capsules): Take with meals.

Fenoprofen (fen oh PROE fen)

Brand Names: U.S. Nalfon

Index Terms Fenoprofen Calcium

Pharmacologic Category Nonsteroidal Anti-inflammatory Drug (NSAID), Oral

Medication Safety Issues

Sound-alike/look-alike issues:

Fenoprofen may be confused with flurbiprofen

BEERS Criteria medication:

This drug may be potentially inappropriate for use in geriatric patients (Quality of evidence - moderate; Strength of recommendation - strong).

Medication Guide Available Yes

Pregnancy Risk Factor C

Lactation Enters breast milk/not recommended

Use Symptomatic treatment of acute and chronic rheumatoid arthritis and osteoarthritis; relief of mild-to-moderate pain

Unlabeled Use Migraine prophylaxis

Available Dosage Forms

Capsule, Oral:

Nalfon: 400 mg

Tablet, Oral:

Generic: 600 mg

General Dosage Range Oral: *Adults:* 200 mg every 4-6 hours as needed **or** 300-600 mg 3-4 times/day (maximum: 3.2 g/day)

Administration

Oral Do not crush tablets. Swallow whole with a full glass of water. Take with food to minimize stomach upset.

Nursing Actions

Physical Assessment Monitor blood pressure at the beginning of therapy and periodically during use. Monitor for adverse gastrointestinal effects or ototoxicity at beginning of therapy and periodically throughout.

Patient Education

• Discuss specific use of drug and side effects with patient as it relates to treatment. (HCAHPS: During this hospital stay, were you given any medicine that you had not taken before? Before giving you any new medicine, how often did hospital staff tell you what the medicine was for? How often did hospital staff describe possible side effects in a way you could understand?)

• Patient may experience dyspepsia, pyrosis, constipation, diarrhea, flatulence, or fatigue. Have patient report immediately to prescriber signs of hepatic impairment, dyspnea, excessive weight gain, edema of extremities, angina, tachycardia, strength differences from one side to another, difficulty speaking or thinking, change in balance, blurred vision, severe headache, considerable dizziness, syncope, significant asthenia, tinnitus, hearing impairment, mood changes, depression, arrhythmia, intolerable nausea, severe dyspepsia, considerable back pain, melena, hematemesis, ecchymosis, hemorrhaging, urinary retention, oliguria, chills, pharyngitis, significant myalgia, or severe arthralgia (HCAHPS).

- Educate patient about signs of a significant reaction (eg, wheezing; chest tightness; fever; itching; bad cough; blue skin color; seizures; or swelling of face, lips, tongue, or throat). **Note:** This is not a comprehensive list of all side effects. Patient should consult prescriber for additional questions.

Intended Use and Disclaimer: Should not be printed and given to patients. This information is intended to serve as a concise initial reference for healthcare professionals to use when discussing medications with a patient. You must ultimately rely on your own discretion, experience and judgment in diagnosing, treating and advising patients.

FentaNYL (FEN ta nil)

Brand Names: U.S. Abstral; Actiq; Duragesic; Fentora; Lazanda; Onsolis; Subsys

Index Terms Fentanyl Citrate; Fentanyl Hydrochloride; Fentanyl Patch; OTFC (Oral Transmucosal Fentanyl Citrate)

Pharmacologic Category Analgesic, Opioid; Anilidopiperidine Opioid; General Anesthetic

Medication Safety Issues

Sound-alike/look-alike issues:

FentaNYL may be confused with alfentanil, SUFentanil

High alert medication:

The Institute for Safe Medication Practices (ISMP) includes this medication among its list of drug classes which have a heightened risk of causing significant patient harm when used in error.

Administration issues:

Fentanyl transdermal system patches: Leakage of fentanyl gel from the patch has been reported; patch may be less effective; do not use. Thoroughly wash any skin surfaces coming into direct contact with gel with water (do not use soap). May contain conducting metal (eg, aluminum); remove patch prior to MRI.

Other safety concerns:

Fentanyl transdermal system patches:

Dosing of transdermal fentanyl patches may be confusing. Transdermal fentanyl patches should always be prescribed in mcg/hour, not size. Patch dosage form of Duragesic-12 actually delivers 12.5 mcg/hour of fentanyl. Use caution, as orders may be written as "Duragesic 12.5" which can be erroneously interpreted as a 125 mcg dose.

Patches should be stored and disposed of with care to avoid accidental exposure to children. The FDA has issued numerous safety advisories to warn users of the possible consequences (including hospitalization and death) of inappropriate storage or disposal of patches.

Abstral, Actiq, Fentora, Onsolis, and Subsys are not interchangeable; do not substitute doses on a mcg-per-mcg basis.

Medication Guide Available Yes

Pregnancy Risk Factor C

Lactation Enters breast milk/not recommended

Breast-Feeding Considerations Fentanyl is excreted in low concentrations into breast milk and breast-feeding is not recommended by the manufacturers.

Parenteral opioids used during labor have the potential to interfere with a newborn's natural reflex to nurse within the first few hours after birth. When needed, a short-acting opioid, such as fentanyl, is preferred for women who will be nursing (Montgomery, 2012)

Breast-feeding is considered acceptable following single doses to the mother; however, limited information is available when used long-term (Spigset, 2000). Nursing infants exposed to large doses of opioids should be monitored for apnea and sedation (Montgomery, 2012).

Note: Transdermal patch, transmucosal lozenge, sublingual tablet, sublingual spray (Subsys), buccal tablet (Fentora), and buccal film (Onsolis) are not recommended in nursing women due to potential for sedation and/or respiratory depression.

Use

Injection: Relief of pain, preoperative medication, adjunct to general or regional anesthesia

Transdermal patch (eg, Duragesic): Management of persistent moderate-to-severe chronic pain in opioid-tolerant patients when around-the-clock analgesia is needed for an extended period of time

Transmucosal lozenge (eg, Actiq), buccal tablet (Fentora), buccal film (Onsolis), nasal spray (Lazanda), sublingual tablet (Abstral), sublingual spray (Subsys): Management of breakthrough cancer pain in opioid-tolerant patients who are already receiving and who are tolerant to around-the-clock opioid therapy for their underlying persistent cancer pain.

Note: "Opioid-tolerant" patients are defined as patients who are taking at least:

Oral morphine 60 mg/day, **or**

Transdermal fentanyl 25 mcg/hour, **or**

Oral oxycodone 30 mg/day, **or**

Oral hydromorphone 8 mg/day, **or**

Oral oxymorphone 25 mg/day, **or**

Equianalgesic dose of another opioid for at least 1 week

Mechanism of Action/Effect Binds with stereospecific receptors at many sites within the CNS, increases pain threshold, alters pain reception, inhibits ascending pain pathways

Contraindications Hypersensitivity to fentanyl or any component of the formulation

Additional contraindications for transdermal patches (eg, Duragesic): Severe respiratory disease or depression including acute asthma (unless patient is mechanically ventilated); paralytic ileus; patients requiring short-term therapy, management of acute or intermittent pain, postoperative or mild pain, and in patients who are **not** opioid tolerant

Additional contraindications for transmucosal buccal tablets (Fentora), buccal films (Onsolis), lozenges (eg, Actiq), sublingual tablets (Abstral), sublingual spray (Subsys), nasal spray (Lazanda): Contraindicated in the management of acute or postoperative pain (including headache, migraine, or dental pain), and in patients who are **not** opioid tolerant. Abstral and Onsolis also are contraindicated for acute pain management in the emergency room.

Canadian labeling: Additional contraindication (not in U.S. labeling): Sublingual tablets (Abstral): Severe respiratory depression or severe obstructive lung disease

Warnings/Precautions An opioid-containing analgesic regimen should be tailored to each patient's needs and based upon the type of pain being treated (acute versus chronic), the route of administration, degree of tolerance for opioids (naive versus chronic user), age, weight, and medical condition. The optimal analgesic dose varies widely among patients. Doses should be titrated to pain relief/prevention. May cause CNS depression, which may impair physical or mental abilities; patients must be cautioned about performing tasks which require mental alertness (eg, operating machinery or driving). Fentanyl shares the toxic potentials of opioid agonists, and precautions of opioid agonist therapy should be observed; use with caution in patients with bradycardia or bradyarrhythmias; rapid I.V. infusion may result in skeletal muscle and chest wall rigidity leading to respiratory distress and/or apnea, bronchoconstriction, laryngospasm; inject slowly over 3-5 minutes. **[U.S. Boxed Warning]: Healthcare provider should be alert to problems of abuse, misuse, and diversion.** Tolerance or drug dependence may result from extended use. The elderly may be particularly susceptible to the CNS depressant and constipating effects of opioids. Use extreme caution in patients with COPD or other chronic respiratory conditions. Use caution with biliary tract impairment, pancreatitis, head injuries, morbid obesity, renal impairment, or hepatic dysfunction. **[U.S. Boxed Warning]: Use with strong or moderate CYP3A4 inhibitors may result in increased effects and potentially fatal respiratory depression.** Concurrent use of agonist/antagonist analgesics may precipitate withdrawal symptoms and/or reduced analgesic efficacy in patients following prolonged therapy with mu opioid agonists. Abrupt discontinuation following prolonged use may also lead to withdrawal symptoms. Potentially significant interactions may exist, requiring dose or frequency adjustment, additional monitoring, and/or selection of alternative therapy.

Pediatric patients: **[U.S. Boxed Warning]: Buccal film, buccal tablet, nasal spray, sublingual tablet, sublingual spray, transdermal patch, and lozenge preparations contain an amount of medication that can be fatal to children. Keep all used and unused products out of the reach of children at all times and discard products properly.** Patients and caregivers should be counseled on the dangers to children including the risk of exposure to partially-consumed products. After chronic maternal exposure to opioids, neonatal withdrawal syndrome may occur in the newborn; monitor neonate closely. Signs and symptoms include irritability, hyperactivity and abnormal sleep pattern, high pitched cry, tremor, vomiting, diarrhea and failure to gain weight. Onset, duration and severity depend on the drug used, duration of use, maternal dose, and rate of drug elimination by the newborn. Opioid withdrawal syndrome in the neonate, unlike in adults, may be life-threatening and should be treated according to protocols developed by neonatology experts.

[U.S. Boxed Warning] Abstral, Actiq, Duragesic, Fentora, Lazanda, Onsolis, Subsys: May cause potentially life-threatening hypoventilation, respiratory depression, and/or death; Abstral, Actiq, Duragesic, Fentora, Lazanda, Onsolis, or Subsys should only be prescribed for opioid-tolerant patients. Risk of respiratory depression increased in elderly patients, debilitated patients, and patients with conditions associated with hypoxia or hypercapnia; usually occurs after administration of initial dose in nontolerant patients or when given with other drugs that depress respiratory function.

Transmucosal (buccal film/tablet, sublingual spray/tablet, lozenge) and nasal spray: **[U.S. Boxed Warning]: Transmucosal and nasal fentanyl formulations are contraindicated in the management of acute or postoperative pain and in opioid nontolerant patients.** Should be used only for the care of opioid-tolerant cancer patients with breakthrough pain and is intended for use by specialists who are knowledgeable in treating cancer pain. **[U.S. Boxed Warning]: Substantial differences exist in the pharmacokinetic profile of fentanyl products. Do not convert patients on a mcg-per-mcg basis from one fentanyl product to another fentanyl product; the substitution of one fentanyl product for another fentanyl product may result in a fatal overdose. [U.S. Boxed Warning]: Available only through the TIRF REMS ACCESS program, a restricted distribution program with outpatients, prescribers who prescribe to outpatients, pharmacies (inpatient and outpatient), and distributor-required**

enrollment. Avoid use of topical nasal decongestants (eg, oxymetazoline) during episodes of rhinitis when using fentanyl nasal spray; response to fentanyl may be delayed or reduced. Avoid use of sublingual spray in cancer patients with grade 2 or higher mucositis (fentanyl exposure increased); use with caution in patients with grade 1 mucositis, and closely monitor for respiratory and CNS depression.

Transdermal patch: **[U.S. Boxed Warning]: Transdermal patch is contraindicated in the management of short-term analgesia, or in the management of postoperative pain, and in patients who are opioid nontolerant. Should only be prescribed by healthcare professionals who are knowledgeable in the use of potent opioids in the management of chronic pain. Monitor closely for respiratory depression during use, particularly during first two applications after initiation of therapy or after dose increases. [U.S. Boxed Warning]: Avoid exposure of application site and surrounding area to direct external heat sources. Patients who experience fever or increase in core body temperature should be monitored closely.** Serum fentanyl concentrations may increase by approximately one-third for patients with a body temperature of 40°C (104°F) secondary to a temperature-dependent increase in fentanyl release from the patch and increased skin permeability. **[U.S. Boxed Warning]: Accidental exposure may lead to severe respiratory depression, including death, in children and adults; proper procedures for handling and disposal of patches should be followed.** Avoid unclothed/unwashed application site exposure, inadvertent person-to-person patch transfer (eg, while hugging), incidental exposure (eg, sharing same bed, sitting on patch), intentional exposure (eg, chewing), or accidental exposure by caregivers when applying/removing patch. Should be applied only to intact skin. Use of a patch that has been cut, damaged, or altered in any way may result in overdosage. Patients who experience adverse reactions should be monitored for at least 24 hours after removal of the patch. May contain conducting metal (eg, aluminum); remove patch prior to MRI.

Drug Interactions
Avoid Concomitant Use
Avoid concomitant use of FentaNYL with any of the following: Azelastine (Nasal); Crizotinib; Enzalutamide; Fusidic Acid (Systemic); MAO Inhibitors; Mifepristone; Paraldehyde; Pimozide; Thalidomide

Decreased Effect
FentaNYL may decrease the levels/effects of: Ioflupane I 123; Pegvisomant

The levels/effects of FentaNYL may be decreased by: Alpha-/Beta-Agonists (Indirect-Acting); Alpha1-Agonists; Ammonium Chloride; Enzalutamide; Mixed Agonist / Antagonist Opioids; Rifamycin Derivatives

Increased Effect/Toxicity
FentaNYL may increase the levels/effects of: Alcohol (Ethyl); Alvimopan; ARIPiprazole; Azelastine (Nasal); Beta-Blockers; Calcium Channel Blockers (Nondihydropyridine); CNS Depressants; Desmopressin; Diuretics; Dofetilide; Hydrocodone; Lomitapide; MAO Inhibitors; Metyrosine; Mirtazapine; Paraldehyde; Pimozide; Pramipexole; ROPINIRole; Rotigotine; Selective Serotonin Reuptake Inhibitors; Thalidomide; Zolpidem

The levels/effects of FentaNYL may be increased by: Amphetamines; Anticholinergics; Antipsychotic Agents (Phenothiazines); Brimonidine (Topical); Cannabinoids; Crizotinib; CYP3A4 Inhibitors (Moderate); CYP3A4 Inhibitors (Strong); Dasatinib; Doxylamine; Droperidol; Fusidic Acid (Systemic); HydrOXYzine; Ivacaftor; Luliconazole; Magnesium Sulfate; MAO Inhibitors; Mifepristone; Perampanel; Simeprevir; Sodium Oxybate; Succinylcholine; Tapentadol

Nutritional/Ethanol Interactions
Ethanol: Ethanol may increase CNS depression. Management: Monitor for increased effects with coadministration. Caution patients about effects.

Food: Fentanyl concentrations may be increased by grapefruit juice. Management: Avoid concurrent intake of large quantities (>1 quart/day) of grapefruit juice.

Herb/Nutraceutical: St John's wort may decrease fentanyl levels; gotu kola, valerian, and kava kava may increase CNS depression. Management: Avoid St John's wort, gotu kola, valerian, and kava kava.

Adverse Reactions
>10%:
Cardiovascular: Bradycardia, edema
Central nervous system: CNS depression, confusion, dizziness, drowsiness, fatigue, headache, sedation
Endocrine & metabolic: Dehydration
Gastrointestinal: Constipation, nausea, vomiting, xerostomia
Local: Application-site reaction erythema
Neuromuscular & skeletal: Chest wall rigidity (high dose I.V.), muscle rigidity, weakness
Ocular: Miosis
Respiratory: Dyspnea, respiratory depression
Miscellaneous: Diaphoresis
1% to 10%:
Cardiovascular: Cardiac arrhythmia, cardiorespiratory arrest, chest pain, DVT, flushing, hyper-/hypotension, orthostatic hypotension, pallor, palpitation, peripheral edema, sinus tachycardia, syncope, tachycardia, vasodilation
Central nervous system: Abnormal dreams, abnormal thinking, agitation, amnesia, anxiety, attention disturbance, chills, depression, disorientation, dysphoria, euphoria, fever,

hallucinations, hypoesthesia, insomnia, irritability, lethargy, malaise, mental status change, migraine, nervousness, paranoid reaction, restlessness, somnolence, stupor, vertigo

Dermatologic: Alopecia, bruising, cellulitis, decubitus ulcer, erythema, hyperhidrosis, papules, pruritus, rash

Endocrine & metabolic: Breast pain, dehydration, hot flashes, hyper-/hypocalcemia, hyper-/hypoglycemia, hypoalbuminemia, hypokalemia, hypomagnesemia, hyponatremia

Gastrointestinal: Abdominal distension, abdominal pain, abnormal taste, anorexia, appetite decreased, biliary tract spasm, diarrhea, dyspepsia, dysphagia (buccal tablet/film/sublingual spray), flatulence, gastritis, gastroenteritis, gastroesophageal reflux, GI hemorrhage, gingival pain (buccal tablet), gingivitis (lozenge), glossitis (lozenge), hematemesis, ileus, intestinal obstruction (buccal film), periodontal abscess (lozenge/buccal tablet), proctalgia, stomatitis (lozenge/buccal tablet/sublingual tablet/sublingual spray), tongue disorder (sublingual tablet), ulceration (gingival, lip, mouth; transmucosal use/nasal spray), weight loss

Genitourinary: Dysuria, erectile dysfunction, urinary incontinence, urinary retention, urinary tract infection, vaginitis, vaginal hemorrhage

Hematologic: Anemia, leukopenia, neutropenia, thrombocytopenia

Hepatic: Alkaline phosphatase increased, ascites, AST increased, jaundice

Local: Application site pain, application site irritation

Neuromuscular & skeletal: Abnormal coordination, abnormal gait, arthralgia, back pain, limb pain, myalgia, neuropathy, paresthesia, rigors, tremor

Ocular: Blurred vision, diplopia, dry eye, swelling, ptosis, strabismus

Renal: Renal failure

Respiratory: Apnea, asthma, bronchitis, cough, dyspnea (exertional), epistaxis, hemoptysis, hypoventilation, hypoxia, laryngitis, nasal congestion (nasal spray), nasal discomfort (nasal spray), nasopharyngitis, pharyngolaryngeal pain, pharyngitis, pneumonia, postnasal drip (nasal spray), pulmonary embolism (nasal spray), rhinitis, rhinorrhea (nasal spray), sinusitis, upper respiratory infection, wheezing

Miscellaneous: Flu-like syndrome, hiccups, hypersensitivity, lymphadenopathy, night sweats, parosmia, speech disorder, withdrawal syndrome

Pharmacodynamics/Kinetics

Onset of Action Analgesic: I.M.: 7-8 minutes; I.V.: Almost immediate (maximal analgesic and respiratory depressant effects may not be seen for several minutes); Transdermal (initial placement): 6 hours; Transmucosal: 5-15 minutes

Duration of Action I.M.: 1-2 hours; I.V.: 0.5-1 hour; Transdermal (removal of patch/no replacement): Related to blood level; some effects may last 72-96 hours due to extended half-life and absorption from the skin, fentanyl concentrations decrease by ~50% in 20-27 hours; Transmucosal: Related to blood level; respiratory depressant effect may last longer than analgesic effect

Controlled Substance C-II

Available Dosage Forms

Film, for buccal application:
Onsolis: 200 mcg (30s); 400 mcg (30s); 600 mcg (30s); 800 mcg (30s); 1200 mcg (30s)

Injection, solution [preservative free]: 0.05 mg/mL (2 mL, 5 mL, 10 mL, 20 mL, 30 mL, 50 mL)

Liquid, sublingual, [spray]:
Subsys: 100 mcg (30s); 200 mcg (30s); 400 mcg (30s); 600 mcg (30s); 800 mcg (30s)

Lozenge, oral: 200 mcg (30s); 400 mcg (30s); 600 mcg (30s); 800 mcg (30s); 1200 mcg (30s); 1600 mcg (30s)
Actiq: 200 mcg (30s); 400 mcg (30s); 600 mcg (30s); 800 mcg (30s); 1200 mcg (30s); 1600 mcg (30s)

Patch, transdermal: 12 [delivers 12.5 mcg/hr] (5s); 25 [delivers 25 mcg/hr] (5s); 50 [delivers 50 mcg/hr] (5s); 75 [delivers 75 mcg/hr] (5s); 100 [delivers 100 mcg/hr] (5s)
Duragesic: 12 [delivers 12.5 mcg/hr] (5s); 25 [delivers 25 mcg/hr] (5s); 50 [delivers 50 mcg/hr] (5s); 75 [delivers 75 mcg/hr] (5s); 100 [delivers 100 mcg/hr] (5s)

Powder, for prescription compounding: USP: 100% (1 g)

Solution, intranasal, as citrate [spray]:
Lazanda: 100 mcg/spray (5 mL); 400 mcg/spray (5 mL) [delivers 8 metered sprays]

Tablet, for buccal application:
Fentora: 100 mcg (28s); 200 mcg (28s); 400 mcg (28s); 600 mcg (28s); 800 mcg (28s)

Tablet, sublingual:
Abstral: 100 mcg (12s, 32s); 200 mcg (12s, 32s); 300 mcg (12s, 32s); 400 mcg (12s, 32s); 600 mcg (32s); 800 mcg (32s)

General Dosage Range

I.M.: *Adults:* 50-100 mcg as a single dose

I.V.:
Children 2-12 years: 2-3 mcg/kg/dose every 1-2 hours
Children >12 years and Adults: 25-100 mcg as a single dose
Adults: Mechanically-ventilated patients (based on 70 kg patient) (unlabeled): 0.35-1.5 mcg/kg every 30-60 minutes as needed; Infusion: 0.7-10 mcg/kg/**hour**

Nasal: *Adults:* Initial 100 mcg; Maintenance dose range: 100-800 mcg; maximum single dose: 800 mcg; maximum frequency: 4 administrations per day

◄ **Transmucosal:**
Buccal film (Onsolis): *Adults:* Initial: 200 mcg; Maintenance dose range: 200-1200 mcg; maximum dose: 1200 mcg film; maximum frequency: 4 applications per day

Buccal tablet (Fentora): *Adults:* Initial: 100 mcg; may repeat (maximum: 2 doses per breakthrough pain episode every 4 hours)

Lozenge (Actiq): *Children ≥16 years and Adults:* Initial: 200 mcg; may repeat (maximum: 2 doses per breakthrough pain episode every 4 hours; maximum daily dose: 4 units per day)

Sublingual spray (Subsys): Adults: Initial: 100 mcg; may repeat (maximum: 2 doses per breakthrough pain every 4 hours); maintenance dose range: 100-1600 mcg per breakthrough pain episode; maximum 4 breakthrough doses per day

Sublingual tablet (Abstral): *Adults:* Initial: 100 mcg; may repeat (maximum: 2 doses per breakthrough pain episode every 2 hours); usual maximum: 800 mcg per dose

Transdermal: Dosage adjustment recommended in patients with renal or hepatic impairment. *Children ≥2 years and Adults:* 12.5-300 mcg/hour applied every 72 hours

Usual Infusion Concentrations: Pediatric I.V. infusion: 10 mcg/mL

Usual Infusion Concentrations: Adult I.V. infusion: 10 mcg/mL

Administration

I.V. Administer as slow I.V. infusion over 1-2 minutes. May also be administered as continuous infusion or PCA (unlabeled use) routes. Muscular rigidity may occur with rapid I.V. administration.

Injectable Detail pH: 4-7.5

Oral
Lozenge: Foil overwrap should be removed just prior to administration. Place the unit in mouth between the cheek and gum and allow it to dissolve. Do not chew. Lozenge may be moved from one side of the mouth to the other. The unit should be consumed over a period of 15 minutes. Handle should be removed after the lozenge is consumed; early removal should be considered if the patient has achieved an adequate response and/or shows signs of respiratory depression.

Buccal film: Foil overwrap should be removed just prior to administration. Prior to placing film, wet inside of cheek using tongue or by rinsing with water. Place film inside mouth with the pink side of the unit against the inside of the moistened cheek. With finger, press the film against cheek and hold for 5 seconds. The film should stick to the inside of cheek after 5 seconds. The film should be left in place until it dissolves (usually within 15-30 minutes after application). Liquids may be consumed after 5 minutes of application. Food can be eaten after film dissolves. If using more than 1 film simultaneously (during titration

period), apply films on either side of mouth (do not apply on top of each other). Do not chew or swallow film. Do not cut or tear the film. All patients must initiate therapy using the 200 mcg film.

Buccal tablet: Patient should not open blister until ready to administer. The blister backing should be peeled back to expose the tablet; tablet should not be pushed out through the blister. Immediately use tablet once removed from blister. Place entire tablet in the buccal cavity (above a rear molar, between the upper cheek and gum) or under the tongue (maintenance dosing only); should dissolve in about 14-25 minutes. If remnants remain after 30 minutes, they may be swallowed with water. Tablet should not be split, crushed, sucked, chewed, or swallowed whole. When possible, alternate sides of mouth with each dose.

Sublingual spray: Open sealed blister unit with scissors immediately prior to administration. Contents of unit should be sprayed into mouth under the tongue.

Sublingual tablet: Remove from the blister unit immediately prior to administration. Place tablet directly under the tongue on the floor of the mouth and allow to completely dissolve; do not chew, suck, or swallow. Do not eat or drink anything until tablet is completely dissolved. In patients with a dry mouth, water may be used to moisten the buccal mucosa just before administration. All patients must initiate therapy using the 100 mcg tablet.

Topical
Nasal spray: Prior to initial use, prime device by spraying 4 sprays into the provided pouch (the counting window will show a green bar when the bottle is ready for use). Insert nozzle a short distance into the nose (~1/2 inch or 1 cm) and point towards the bridge of the nose (while closing off the other nostril using 1 finger). Press on finger grips until a "click" sound is heard and the number in the counting window advances by one. The "click" sound and dose counter are the only reliable methods for ensuring a dose has been administered (spray is not always felt on the nasal mucosa). Patient should remain seated for at least 1 minute following administration. Do not blow nose for ≥30 minutes after administration. Wash hands before and after use. There are 8 full therapeutic sprays in each bottle; do not continue to use bottle after "8" sprays have been used. Dispose of bottle and contents if ≥5 days have passed since last use or if it has been ≥4 days since bottle was primed. Spray the remaining contents into the provided pouch, seal in the child-resistant container, and dispose of in the trash.

Transdermal patch (eg, Duragesic): Apply to nonirritated and nonirradiated skin, such as chest, back, flank, or upper arm. Do not shave skin;

hair at application site should be clipped. Prior to application, clean site with clear water and allow to dry completely. Do not use damaged, cut or leaking patches; patch may be less effective. Skin exposure from fentanyl gel leaking from patch may lead to serious adverse effects; thoroughly wash affected skin surfaces with water (do not use soap). Firmly press in place and hold for 30 seconds. Change patch every 72 hours. Do **not** use soap, alcohol, or other solvents to remove transdermal gel if it accidentally touches skin; use copious amounts of water. Avoid exposing application site to external heat sources (eg, heating pad, electric blanket, heat lamp, hot tub). If there is difficulty with patch adhesion, the edges of the system may be taped in place with first-aid tape. If there is continued difficulty with adhesion, an adhesive film dressing (eg, Bioclusive, Tegaderm) may be applied over the system.

Storage/Stability
Injection formulation: Store at controlled room temperature of 20°C to 25°C (68°F to 77°F). Protect from light.

Nasal spray: Do not store above 25°C (77°F); do not freeze. Protect from light. Bottle should be stored in the provided child-resistant container when not in use and kept out of the reach of children at all times.

Transdermal patch: Do not store above 25°C (77°F). Keep out of the reach of children.

Transmucosal (buccal film, buccal tablet, lozenge, sublingual spray, sublingual tablet): Store at controlled room temperature of 20°C to 25°C (68°F to 77°F). Protect from freezing and moisture. Keep out of the reach of children.

Nursing Actions

Physical Assessment Monitor effectiveness of pain relief. Monitor blood pressure, CNS and respiratory status, and degree of sedation prior to treatment and periodically throughout. Monitor closely for signs of withdrawal for 24 hours after transdermal product is removed. For inpatients, implement safety measures (eg, side rails up, call light within reach, instructions to call for assistance). Assess patient's physical and/or psychological dependence. Discontinue slowly after prolonged use.

Patient Education
• Discuss specific use of drug and side effects with patient as it relates to treatment. (HCAHPS: During this hospital stay, were you given any medicine that you had not taken before? Before giving you any new medicine, how often did hospital staff tell you what the medicine was for? How often did hospital staff describe possible side effects in a way you could understand?)
• Patient may experience xerostomia, diarrhea, headache, fatigue, cold sensation, lack of appetite, insomnia, hyperhidrosis, application site irritation, tongue irritation, or mouth paresthesia.

Have patient report immediately to prescriber severe dizziness, syncope, illogical thinking, considerable nausea, significant constipation, intolerable asthenia, dyspnea, angina, tachycardia, bradycardia, severe stomatitis, edema of extremities, or edema of hands or feet (HCAHPS).
• Educate patient about signs of a significant reaction (eg, wheezing; chest tightness; fever; itching; bad cough; blue skin color; seizures; or swelling of face, lips, tongue, or throat). **Note:** This is not a comprehensive list of all side effects. Patient should consult prescriber for additional questions.

Intended Use and Disclaimer: Should not be printed and given to patients. This information is intended to serve as a concise initial reference for healthcare professionals to use when discussing medications with a patient. You must ultimately rely on your own discretion, experience and judgment in diagnosing, treating and advising patients.

Dietary Considerations Transmucosal lozenge contains 2 g sugar per unit.

Related Information
Oral Medications That Should Not Be Crushed or Altered *on page 1712*

Ferrous Gluconate (FER us GLOO koe nate)

Brand Names: U.S. Ferate [OTC]; Fergon [OTC]
Index Terms Iron Gluconate
Pharmacologic Category Iron Salt
Lactation Enters breast milk
Use Prevention and treatment of iron-deficiency anemias

Available Dosage Forms
Tablet, Oral:
Fergon [OTC]: 240 (27 Fe) mg
Generic: 240 (27 Fe) mg, 324 (37.5 Fe) mg, 324 (38 Fe) mg, 325 (36 Fe) mg
Tablet, Oral [preservative free]:
Ferate [OTC]: 256 (28 Fe) mg

General Dosage Range Oral:
Children: 1-6 mg Fe/kg/day in 1-3 divided doses
Adults: 60 mg 1-4 times/day

Administration
Oral Administer 2 hours before or 4 hours after antacids. Administration of iron preparations to premature infants with vitamin E deficiency may cause increased red cell hemolysis and hemolytic anemia, therefore, vitamin E deficiency should be corrected if possible.

Nursing Actions
Patient Education
• Discuss specific use of drug and side effects with patient as it relates to treatment. (HCAHPS: During this hospital stay, were you given any medicine that you had not taken before? Before giving you any new medicine, how often did

hospital staff tell you what the medicine was for? How often did hospital staff describe possible side effects in a way you could understand?)

• Patient may experience diarrhea, constipation, stool discoloration, or lack of appetite. Have patient report immediately to prescriber melena, severe nausea, considerable dyspepsia, or hematemesis (HCAHPS).

• Educate patient about signs of a significant reaction (eg, wheezing; chest tightness; fever; itching; bad cough; blue skin color; seizures; or swelling of face, lips, tongue, or throat). **Note:** This is not a comprehensive list of all side effects. Patient should consult prescriber for additional questions.

Intended Use and Disclaimer: Should not be printed and given to patients. This information is intended to serve as a concise initial reference for healthcare professionals to use when discussing medications with a patient. You must ultimately rely on your own discretion, experience and judgment in diagnosing, treating and advising patients.

Related Information

Oral Medications That Should Not Be Crushed or Altered *on page 1712*

Ferrous Sulfate (FER us SUL fate)

Brand Names: U.S. BProtected Pedia Iron [OTC]; Fer-In-Sol [OTC]; Fer-Iron [OTC]; FeroSul [OTC]; Ferro-Bob [OTC]; FerrouSul [OTC]; Iron Supplement Childrens [OTC]; Slow Fe [OTC]; Slow Iron [OTC]; Slow Release Iron [OTC] [DSC]

Index Terms $FeSO_4$; Iron Sulfate

Pharmacologic Category Iron Salt

Medication Safety Issues

Sound-alike/look-alike issues:

Feosol® may be confused with Fer-In-Sol®

Fer-In-Sol® may be confused with Feosol®

Slow FE® may be confused with Slow-K®

Administration issues:

Multiple concentrations of liquid iron preparations exist. Fer-In-Sol® drops (manufactured by Mead Johnson) and a limited number of generic products are available at a concentration of 15 mg/mL. However, a suspension product, MyKidz Iron 10™ drops, is available at a concentration of 15 mg/1.5 mL. Check concentration closely prior to dispensing. Prescriptions written in milliliters (mL) should be clarified.

Lactation Enters breast milk

Use Prevention and treatment of iron-deficiency anemias

Available Dosage Forms

Elixir, Oral:

FeroSul [OTC]: 220 (Fe) mg/5 mL (473 mL)

Generic: 220 (44 Fe) mg/5 mL (5 mL, 473 mL)

Liquid, Oral:

Generic: 220 (44 Fe) mg/5 mL (473 mL)

Solution, Oral:

BProtected Pedia Iron [OTC]: 75 (15 Fe) mg/mL (50 mL)

Fer-In-Sol [OTC]: 75 (15 Fe) mg/mL (50 mL)

Fer-Iron [OTC]: 75 (15 Fe) mg/mL (50 mL)

Iron Supplement Childrens [OTC]: 75 (15 Fe) mg/mL (50 mL)

Generic: 75 (15 Fe) mg/mL (50 mL)

Syrup, Oral:

Generic: 300 (60 Fe) mg/5 mL (5 mL)

Tablet, Oral:

Ferro-Bob [OTC]: 325 (65 Fe) mg

Generic: 325 (65 Fe) mg

Tablet, Oral [preservative free]:

FerrouSul [OTC]: 325 (65 Fe) mg

Generic: 325 (65 Fe) mg

Tablet Delayed Release, Oral:

Generic: 324 (65 Fe) mg, 325 (65 Fe) mg

Tablet Extended Release, Oral:

Slow Fe [OTC]: 142 (45 Fe) mg, 160 (50 Fe) mg

Tablet Extended Release, Oral [preservative free]:

Slow Iron [OTC]: 160 (50 Fe) mg

Generic: 140 (45 Fe) mg

General Dosage Range Oral:

Extended release: *Adults:* 250 mg 1-2 times/day

Immediate release:

Children: 1-6 mg Fe/kg/day in 1-3 divided doses (maximum: 15 mg/day [prophylaxis dosing])

Adults: 300 mg 1-4 times/day

Administration

Oral Should be taken with water or juice on an empty stomach; administer ferrous sulfate 2 hours prior to, or 4 hours after antacids

Nursing Actions

Physical Assessment May cause GI irritation. Monitor GI function (observe for epigastric pain, nausea, dark stools, vomiting, stomach cramping, constipation).

Patient Education

• Discuss specific use of drug and side effects with patient as it relates to treatment. (HCAHPS: During this hospital stay, were you given any medicine that you had not taken before? Before giving you any new medicine, how often did hospital staff tell you what the medicine was for? How often did hospital staff describe possible side effects in a way you could understand?)

• Patient may experience diarrhea; constipation; stool discoloration; lack of appetite; or staining of mouth, teeth, or fillings. Have patient report immediately to prescriber melena, severe nausea, significant dyspepsia, or hematemesis (HCAHPS).

• Educate patient about signs of a significant reaction (eg, wheezing; chest tightness; fever; itching; bad cough; blue skin color; seizures; or swelling of face, lips, tongue, or throat). **Note:** This is not a comprehensive list of all side effects. Patient should consult prescriber for additional questions.

Intended Use and Disclaimer: Should not be printed and given to patients. This information is intended to serve as a concise initial reference for healthcare professionals to use when discussing medications with a patient. You must ultimately rely on your own discretion, experience and judgment in diagnosing, treating and advising patients.

Related Information

Oral Medications That Should Not Be Crushed or Altered *on page 1712*

Ferumoxytol (fer ue MOX i tol)

Brand Names: U.S. Feraheme
Pharmacologic Category Iron Salt
Medication Safety Issues
  Sound-alike/look-alike issues:
  Ferumoxytol may be confused with ferric carboxymaltose, ferric gluconate, iron dextran complex, iron sucrose
Pregnancy Risk Factor C
Lactation Excretion in breast milk unknown/not recommended
Use Treatment of iron-deficiency anemia in chronic kidney disease
Dosage Forms Considerations
  Strength of ferumoxytol is expressed as elemental iron
Available Dosage Forms
  Solution, Intravenous [preservative free]:
  Feraheme: 510 mg/17 mL (17 mL)
General Dosage Range I.V.: *Adults:* 510 mg (17 mL) as a single dose; repeat once 3-8 days later
Administration
  I.V. Administer intravenously as an undiluted injection at a rate ≤1 mL/second (30 mg of elemental iron/second). Do not administer if solution has particulate matter or is discolored (solution is black to reddish-brown).
  Hemodialysis patients should receive injection after at least 1 hour of hemodialysis has been completed and once blood pressure has stabilized.
Nursing Actions
  Physical Assessment Monitor closely during administration and for at least 30 minutes following for hypersensitive reactions. Resuscitation equipment should be available. Monitor blood pressure closely; can cause hypotension.
  Patient Education
  • Discuss specific use of drug and side effects with patient as it relates to treatment. (HCAHPS: During this hospital stay, were you given any medicine that you had not taken before? Before giving you any new medicine, how often did hospital staff tell you what the medicine was for? How often did hospital staff describe possible side effects in a way you could understand?)

• Patient may experience diarrhea, nausea, or constipation. Have patient report immediately to prescriber angina, tachycardia, severe dizziness, syncope, arrhythmia, skin or nail discoloration, dyspnea, urinary retention, oliguria, considerable headache, injection site irritation, or edema of extremities (HCAHPS).

• Educate patient about signs of a significant reaction (eg, wheezing; chest tightness; fever; itching; bad cough; blue skin color; seizures; or swelling of face, lips, tongue, or throat). **Note:** This is not a comprehensive list of all side effects. Patient should consult prescriber for additional questions.

Intended Use and Disclaimer: Should not be printed and given to patients. This information is intended to serve as a concise initial reference for healthcare professionals to use when discussing medications with a patient. You must ultimately rely on your own discretion, experience and judgment in diagnosing, treating and advising patients.

Fesoterodine (fes oh TER oh deen)

Brand Names: U.S. Toviaz
Index Terms FESO; Fesoterodine Fumarate
Pharmacologic Category Anticholinergic Agent
Medication Safety Issues
  Sound-alike/look-alike issues:
  Fesoterodine may be confused with fexofenadine, tolterodine
  BEERS Criteria medication:
  This drug may be potentially inappropriate for use in geriatric patients (Quality of evidence - varies based on comorbidity; Strength of recommendation - varies based on comorbidity)
Pregnancy Risk Factor C
Lactation Excretion in breast milk unknown/not recommended
Use Treatment of patients with an overactive bladder with symptoms of urinary frequency, urgency, or urge incontinence.
Available Dosage Forms
  Tablet Extended Release 24 Hour, Oral:
  Toviaz: 4 mg, 8 mg
General Dosage Range Dosage adjustment recommended in patients with renal impairment or on concomitant therapy
  Oral: *Adults:* 4-8 mg once daily
Administration
  Oral May be administered with or without food. Swallow whole; do not chew, crush, or divide.
Nursing Actions
  Patient Education
  • Discuss specific use of drug and side effects with patient as it relates to treatment. (HCAHPS: During this hospital stay, were you given any medicine that you had not taken before? Before giving you any new medicine, how often did

hospital staff tell you what the medicine was for? How often did hospital staff describe possible side effects in a way you could understand?)
- Patient may experience xerostomia or xerophthalmia. Have patient report immediately to prescriber signs of renal impairment, severe headache, considerable dizziness, syncope, illogical thinking, significant dyspepsia, intolerable constipation, anhidrosis, or edema of extremities (HCAHPS).
- Educate patient about signs of a significant reaction (eg, wheezing; chest tightness; fever; itching; bad cough; blue skin color; seizures; or swelling of face, lips, tongue, or throat). **Note:** This is not a comprehensive list of all side effects. Patient should consult prescriber for additional questions.

Intended Use and Disclaimer: Should not be printed and given to patients. This information is intended to serve as a concise initial reference for healthcare professionals to use when discussing medications with a patient. You must ultimately rely on your own discretion, experience and judgment in diagnosing, treating and advising patients.

Related Information
Oral Medications That Should Not Be Crushed or Altered *on page 1712*

Fexofenadine (feks oh FEN a deen)

Brand Names: U.S. Allegra Allergy Childrens [OTC]; Allegra Allergy [OTC]
Index Terms Fexofenadine Hydrochloride
Pharmacologic Category Histamine H_1 Antagonist; Histamine H_1 Antagonist, Second Generation; Piperidine Derivative
Medication Safety Issues
Sound-alike/look-alike issues:
Fexofenadine may be confused with fesoterodine
Allegra® may be confused with Viagra®
International issues:
Allegra [U.S, Canada, and multiple international markets] may be confused with Allegro brand name for fluticasone [Israel] and frovatriptan [Germany]
Pregnancy Risk Factor C
Lactation Excretion in breast milk unknown/use caution
Breast-Feeding Considerations It is not known if fexofenadine is excreted in breast milk. The manufacturer recommends that caution be exercised when administering fexofenadine to nursing women.
Use Relief of symptoms associated with seasonal allergic rhinitis; treatment of chronic idiopathic urticaria
OTC labeling: Relief of symptoms associated with allergic rhinitis

Mechanism of Action/Effect Fexofenadine is an active metabolite of terfenadine and like terfenadine it competes with histamine for H_1-receptor sites on effector cells in the GI tract, blood vessels, and respiratory tract; binds to lung receptors significantly greater than it binds to cerebellar receptors, resulting in a greatly reduced sedative potential
Contraindications Hypersensitivity to fexofenadine or any component of the formulation
Warnings/Precautions Use with caution in patients with renal impairment; dosage adjustment recommended. Safety and efficacy in children <6 months of age have not been established; orally disintegrating tablet not recommended for use in children <6 years of age. Orally disintegrating tablet contains phenylalanine.
Drug Interactions
Avoid Concomitant Use
Avoid concomitant use of Fexofenadine with any of the following: Aclidinium; Azelastine (Nasal); Ipratropium (Oral Inhalation); Paraldehyde; Thalidomide; Tiotropium; Umeclidinium
Decreased Effect
Fexofenadine may decrease the levels/effects of: Acetylcholinesterase Inhibitors (Central); Benzylpenicilloyl Polylysine; Betahistine; Hyaluronidase

The levels/effects of Fexofenadine may be decreased by: Acetylcholinesterase Inhibitors (Central); Amphetamines; Antacids; Grapefruit Juice; P-glycoprotein/ABCB1 Inducers; Rifampin
Increased Effect/Toxicity
Fexofenadine may increase the levels/effects of: Alcohol (Ethyl); Analgesics (Opioid); Anticholinergics; ARIPiprazole; Azelastine (Nasal); Buprenorphine; CNS Depressants; Hydrocodone; Methotrimeprazine; Metyrosine; Mirtazapine; Paraldehyde; Pramipexole; ROPINIRole; Rotigotine; Selective Serotonin Reuptake Inhibitors; Thalidomide; Tiotropium; Zolpidem

The levels/effects of Fexofenadine may be increased by: Aclidinium; Brimonidine (Topical); Doxylamine; Droperidol; Eltrombopag; Erythromycin (Systemic); HydrOXYzine; Ipratropium (Oral Inhalation); Itraconazole; Ketoconazole (Systemic); Magnesium Sulfate; Methotrimeprazine; Perampanel; P-glycoprotein/ABCB1 Inhibitors; Pramlintide; Rifampin; Sodium Oxybate; Tapentadol; Umeclidinium; Verapamil
Nutritional/Ethanol Interactions
Ethanol: Ethanol may increase CNS depression. Management: Avoid ethanol.
Food: Fruit juice (apple, grapefruit, orange) may decrease bioavailability of fexofenadine by ~36%. Management: Administer with water only, avoid fruit juice.
Herb/Nutraceutical: St John's wort may decrease fexofenadine levels.

Adverse Reactions

>10%:

Central nervous system: Headache (5% to 11%)

Gastrointestinal: Vomiting (children 6 months to 5 years: 4% to 12%)

1% to 10%:

Central nervous system: Fatigue (1% to 3%), somnolence (1% to 3%), dizziness (2%), fever (2%), pain (2%), drowsiness (1%)

Endocrine & metabolic: Dysmenorrhea (2%)

Gastrointestinal: Diarrhea (3% to 4%), nausea (2%), dyspepsia (1% to 2%)

Neuromuscular & skeletal: Myalgia (3%), back pain (2% to 3%), pain in extremities (2%)

Otic: Otitis media (2% to 4%)

Respiratory: Upper respiratory tract infection (3% to 4%), cough (2% to 4%), rhinorrhea (1% to 2%)

Miscellaneous: Viral infection (3%)

Pharmacodynamics/Kinetics

Onset of Action 60 minutes

Duration of Action Antihistaminic effect: ≥12 hours

Available Dosage Forms

Suspension, Oral:

Allegra Allergy Childrens [OTC]: 30 mg/5 mL (120 mL)

Tablet, Oral:

Allegra Allergy [OTC]: 60 mg, 180 mg

Allegra Allergy Childrens [OTC]: 30 mg

Generic: 60 mg, 180 mg

Tablet Dispersible, Oral:

Allegra Allergy Childrens [OTC]: 30 mg

General Dosage Range Dosage adjustment recommended in patients with renal impairment

Oral:

Children 6 months to <2 years: 15 mg twice daily

Children 2-11 years: 30 mg twice daily

Children ≥12 years and Adults: 60 mg twice daily or 180 mg once daily

Administration

Oral

Suspension, tablet: Administer with water only; do not administer with fruit juices. Shake suspension well before use.

Orally disintegrating tablet: Take on an empty stomach. Do not remove from blister pack until administered. Using dry hands, place immediately on tongue. Tablet will dissolve within seconds, and may be swallowed with or without liquid (do not administer with fruit juices). Do not split or chew.

Storage/Stability Store at controlled room temperature of 20°C to 25°C (68°F to 77°F). Protect from excessive moisture.

Nursing Actions

Patient Education

• Discuss specific use of drug and side effects with patient as it relates to treatment. (HCAHPS: During this hospital stay, were you given any medicine that you had not taken before? Before giving you any new medicine, how often did hospital staff tell you what the medicine was for? How often did hospital staff describe possible side effects in a way you could understand?)

• Patient may experience headache, back pain, or dyspepsia. Have patient report immediately to prescriber severe dizziness, syncope, significant asthenia, considerable nausea, or otalgia (HCAHPS).

• Educate patient about signs of a significant reaction (eg, wheezing; chest tightness; fever; itching; bad cough; blue skin color; seizures; or swelling of face, lips, tongue, or throat). **Note:** This is not a comprehensive list of all side effects. Patient should consult prescriber for additional questions.

Intended Use and Disclaimer: Should not be printed and given to patients. This information is intended to serve as a concise initial reference for healthcare professionals to use when discussing medications with a patient. You must ultimately rely on your own discretion, experience and judgment in diagnosing, treating and advising patients.

Dietary Considerations Some products may contain phenylalanine and/or sodium. Take suspension and tablets with water only; do not administer with fruit juices.

Fexofenadine and Pseudoephedrine

(feks oh FEN a deen & soo doe e FED rin)

Brand Names: U.S. Allegra-D® 12 Hour; Allegra-D® 24 Hour

Index Terms Pseudoephedrine and Fexofenadine

Pharmacologic Category Alpha/Beta Agonist; Decongestant; Histamine H₁ Antagonist; Histamine H₁ Antagonist, Second Generation; Piperidine Derivative

Medication Safety Issues

Sound-alike/look-alike issues:

Allegra-D® may be confused with Viagra®

International issues:

Allegra-D [U.S, Canada, and multiple international markets] may be confused with Allegro brand name for fluticasone [Israel] and frovatriptan [Germany]

Pregnancy Risk Factor C

Lactation Enters breast milk/use caution

Use Relief of symptoms associated with seasonal allergic rhinitis in adults and children ≥12 years of age

Available Dosage Forms

Tablet, extended release: Fexofenadine 60 mg [immediate release] and pseudoephedrine 120 mg [extended release]; fexofenadine 180 mg [immediate release] and pseudoephedrine 240 mg [extended release]

Allegra-D® 12 Hour: Fexofenadine 60 mg [immediate release] and pseudoephedrine 120 mg [extended release]

Allegra-D® 24 Hour: Fexofenadine 180 mg [immediate release] and pseudoephedrine 240 mg [extended release]

General Dosage Range Dosage adjustment recommended in patients with renal impairment

Oral: *Children ≥12 years and Adults:* 1 tablet (fexofenadine 60 mg/pseudoephedrine 120 mg) twice daily **or** 1 tablet (fexofenadine 180 mg/ pseudoephedrine 240 mg) once daily

Administration

Oral Tablets should be swallowed whole; do not crush or chew. Administer on an empty stomach with water; avoid administration with food. The inactive ingredients may be eliminated in the feces in a form resembling the original tablet.

Nursing Actions

Physical Assessment See individual agents.

Patient Education

- Discuss specific use of drug and side effects with patient as it relates to treatment. (HCAHPS: During this hospital stay, were you given any medicine that you had not taken before? Before giving you any new medicine, how often did hospital staff tell you what the medicine was for? How often did hospital staff describe possible side effects in a way you could understand?)
- Patient may experience dizziness, anxiety, insomnia, or fatigue (HCAHPS).
- Educate patient about signs of a significant reaction (eg, wheezing; chest tightness; fever; itching; bad cough; blue skin color; seizures; or swelling of face, lips, tongue, or throat). **Note:** This is not a comprehensive list of all side effects. Patient should consult prescriber for additional questions.

Intended Use and Disclaimer: Should not be printed and given to patients. This information is intended to serve as a concise initial reference for healthcare professionals to use when discussing medications with a patient. You must ultimately rely on your own discretion, experience and judgment in diagnosing, treating and advising patients.

Related Information

Fexofenadine *on page 654*

Oral Medications That Should Not Be Crushed or Altered *on page 1712*

Pseudoephedrine *on page 1311*

Fidaxomicin (fye DAX oh mye sin)

Brand Names: U.S. Dificid

Index Terms Difimicin; Lipiarrmycin; OPT-80; PAR-101; Tiacumicin B

Pharmacologic Category Antibiotic, Macrolide

Pregnancy Risk Factor B

Lactation Excretion in breast milk unknown/use caution

Breast-Feeding Considerations It is not known if fidaxomicin is excreted in breast milk. The manufacturer recommends that caution be exercised when administering fidaxomicin to nursing women.

Use Treatment of *Clostridium difficile*-associated diarrhea (CDAD)

Mechanism of Action/Effect Inhibits protein synthesis in susceptible organisms including *C. difficile*; bactericidal

Contraindications Hypersensitivity to fidaxomicin

Warnings/Precautions Do not use for systemic infections; fidaxomicin systemic absorption is negligible. Hypersensitivity reactions (angioedema [mouth, face, throat], dyspnea, pruritus, and rash) to fidaxomicin have been reported. Patients with a history of macrolide allergy may be at increased risk. If a severe reaction occurs, discontinue drug and institute supportive care. Use only in patients with proven or strongly suspected *Clostridium difficile (C. difficile)* infections.

Drug Interactions

Avoid Concomitant Use There are no known interactions where it is recommended to avoid concomitant use.

Decreased Effect
Fidaxomicin may decrease the levels/effects of: Sodium Picosulfate

Increased Effect/Toxicity
Fidaxomicin may increase the levels/effects of: Rilpivirine

Adverse Reactions

>10%: Gastrointestinal: Nausea (11%)

2% to 10%:

Gastrointestinal: Gastrointestinal hemorrhage (4%), abdominal pain, vomiting

Hematologic: Anemia (2%), neutropenia (2%)

Available Dosage Forms

Tablet, Oral:

Dificid: 200 mg

General Dosage Range

Oral: *Adults:* 200 mg twice daily

Administration

Oral May be administered with or without food.

Storage/Stability Store at 20°C to 25°C (68°F to 77°F); excursions permitted to 15°C to 30°C (59°F to 86°F).

Nursing Actions

Patient Education

- Discuss specific use of drug and side effects with patient as it relates to treatment. (HCAHPS: During this hospital stay, were you given any medicine that you had not taken before? Before giving you any new medicine, how often did hospital staff tell you what the medicine was for? How often did hospital staff describe possible side effects in a way you could understand?)
- Patient may experience nausea. Have patient report immediately to prescriber melena, hematemesis, chills, pharyngitis, significant constipation, considerable dyspepsia, or severe asthenia (HCAHPS).

- Educate patient about signs of a significant reaction (eg, wheezing; chest tightness; fever; itching; bad cough; blue skin color; seizures; or swelling of face, lips, tongue, or throat). **Note:** This is not a comprehensive list of all side effects. Patient should consult prescriber for additional questions.

Intended Use and Disclaimer: Should not be printed and given to patients. This information is intended to serve as a concise initial reference for healthcare professionals to use when discussing medications with a patient. You must ultimately rely on your own discretion, experience and judgment in diagnosing, treating and advising patients.

Filgrastim (fil GRA stim)

Brand Names: U.S. Granix; Neupogen
Index Terms G-CSF; Granulocyte Colony Stimulating Factor; Tbo-Filgrastim; Tevagrastim
Pharmacologic Category Colony Stimulating Factor; Hematopoietic Agent
Medication Safety Issues
Sound-alike/look-alike issues:
Neupogen may be confused with Epogen, Neulasta, Neumega, Nutramigen
International issues:
Neupogen [U.S., Canada, and multiple international markets] may be confused with Neupro brand name for rotigotine [multiple international markets]
Pregnancy Risk Factor C
Lactation Excretion in breast milk unknown/use caution
Breast-Feeding Considerations It is not known if filgrastim or tbo-filgrastim are is excreted in breast milk. The manufacturers recommend that caution be exercised when administering filgrastim or tbo-filgrastim to nursing women.

Women who are nursing during Neupogen treatment are encouraged to enroll in the manufacturer's Lactation Surveillance program (1-800-772-6436).

Use
Myelosuppressive chemotherapy recipients with nonmyeloid malignancies:
Neupogen: To decrease the incidence of infection (neutropenic fever) in patients with nonmyeloid malignancies receiving myelosuppressive chemotherapy associated with a significant incidence of neutropenia with fever.
Granix: To decrease the duration of severe neutropenia in patients with nonmyeloid malignancies receiving myelosuppressive chemotherapy associated with a clinically significant incidence of neutropenic fever.
Acute myeloid leukemia (AML) patients following induction or consolidation chemotherapy (Neupogen): To reduce the time to neutrophil

recovery and reduce the duration of fever following induction or consolidation chemotherapy in adults with AML.
Bone marrow transplantation (Neupogen): To reduce the duration of neutropenia and neutropenia-related events (eg, neutropenic fever) in patients with nonmyeloid malignancies receiving myeloablative chemotherapy followed by marrow transplantation.
Peripheral blood progenitor cell collection and therapy (Neupogen): Mobilization of hematopoietic progenitor cells into peripheral blood for apheresis collection (mobilization allows for collection of increased numbers of progenitor cells capable of engraftment, which may lead to more rapid engraftment).
Severe chronic neutropenia (Neupogen): Long-term administration to reduce the incidence and duration of neutropenic complications (eg, fever, infections, oropharyngeal ulcers) in symptomatic patients with congenital, cyclic, or idiopathic neutropenia.
Unlabeled Use Treatment of anemia in myelodysplastic syndrome (in combination with epoetin); mobilization of hematopoietic stem cells (HSC) for collection and subsequent autologous transplantation (in combination with plerixafor) in patients with non-Hodgkin's lymphoma (NHL) and multiple myeloma (MM); treatment of neutropenia in HIV-infected patients receiving zidovudine; hepatitis C treatment-associated neutropenia; treatment of radiation-induced myelosuppression of the bone marrow
Mechanism of Action/Effect Filgrastim and tbo-filgrastim are granulocyte colony stimulating factors (G-CSF) produced by recombinant DNA technology. G-CSFs stimulate the production, maturation, and activation of neutrophils to increase both their migration and cytotoxicity.
Contraindications
Neupogen: Hypersensitivity to filgrastim, *E. coli*-derived proteins, or any component of the formulation
Granix: There are no contraindications listed in the manufacturer's labeling
Warnings/Precautions Anaphylaxis, rash, urticaria, facial edema, wheezing, dyspnea, tachycardia, and/or hypotension have occurred with first or subsequent doses. Reactions tended to involve two or more body systems and occur more frequently with intravenous administration and generally within 30 minutes of administration. Symptoms recurred in >50% of patients when rechallenged. Management may include administration of antihistamines, steroids, bronchodilators, and/or epinephrine. Do not administer tbo-filgrastim to patients who experienced allergic reaction to filgrastim or pegfilgrastim. Permanently discontinue tbo-filgrastim in patients with serious allergic reactions. Rare cases of splenic rupture have been reported (may be fatal); in patients with left upper

quadrant pain or shoulder tip pain, withhold treatment and evaluate for enlarged spleen or splenic rupture. Cutaneous vasculitis has been reported with filgrastim, generally occurring in patients with severe chronic neutropenia on chronic therapy; symptoms generally developed with increasing absolute neutrophil count (ANC) and subsided when the ANC decreased; dose reductions may improve symptoms to allow for continued therapy.

White blood cell counts of ≥100,000/mm³ have been reported with filgrastim doses >5 mcg/kg/day. Monitor CBC twice weekly during therapy. Thrombocytopenia has also been reported with filgrastim; monitor platelet counts. Although the incidence of antibody development has not been determined, there is a potential for immunogenicity, which may result in cytopenias. Filgrastim should not be routinely used in the treatment of established neutropenic fever. Colony-stimulating factors may be considered in cancer patients with febrile neutropenia who are at high risk for infection-associated complications or who have prognostic factors indicative of a poor clinical outcome (eg, prolonged and severe neutropenia, age ≥65 years, pneumonia, sepsis syndrome, presence of invasive fungal infection) (Freifeld, 2011; Smith, 2006). Do not use filgrastim in the period 24 hours before to 24 hours after administration of cytotoxic chemotherapy because of the potential sensitivity of rapidly dividing myeloid cells to cytotoxic chemotherapy. Transient increase in neutrophil count is seen 1-2 days after filgrastim initiation; however, for sustained neutrophil response, continue until post-nadir ANC reaches 10,000/mm³. Avoid simultaneous use of filgrastim with chemotherapy and radiation therapy. Safety and efficacy have not been established with patients receiving chemotherapy associated with delayed myelosuppression (eg, nitrosoureas, mitomycin). Avoid concurrent radiation therapy with filgrastim; safety and efficacy have not been established with patients receiving radiation therapy. May potentially act as a growth factor for any tumor type; caution should be exercised when using in any malignancy with myeloid characteristics. When used for stem cell mobilization, may release tumor cells from marrow which could be collected in leukapheresis product; potential effect of tumor cell reinfusion is unknown.

May precipitate severe sickle cell crises, sometimes resulting in fatalities, in patients with sickle cell disorders; carefully evaluate potential risks and benefits. Discontinue in patients undergoing sickle cell crisis. Cytogenic abnormalities and transformation to AML or myelodysplastic syndrome (MDS) have been reported in patients with severe chronic neutropenia (SCN), including patients receiving cytokine therapy; carefully consider the risks of continued filgrastim treatment if abnormal cytogenetics or myelodysplasia develop. Establish diagnosis prior to filgrastim initiation; use prior to appropriate diagnosis of SCN may impair or delay proper evaluation and treatment for neutropenia due to conditions other than SCN. Acute respiratory distress syndrome (ARDS) has been reported (possibly due to influx of neutrophils to sites of lung inflammation); patients must be instructed to report respiratory distress; monitor for fever, infiltrates, or respiratory distress; discontinue in patients with ARDS. Reports of alveolar hemorrhage, manifested as pulmonary infiltrates and hemoptysis, have occurred in healthy donors undergoing PBPC mobilization (unlabeled for use in healthy donors); hemoptysis resolved upon discontinuation. The packaging of some dosage forms may contain latex.

Drug Interactions

Avoid Concomitant Use There are no known interactions where it is recommended to avoid concomitant use.

Decreased Effect There are no known significant interactions involving a decrease in effect.

Increased Effect/Toxicity

Filgrastim may increase the levels/effects of: Bleomycin; Topotecan

Adverse Reactions

>10%:

Dermatologic: Skin rash (≤12%)

Endocrine & metabolic: Increased lactate dehydrogenase, increased uric acid

Hematologic & oncologic: Splenomegaly (severe chronic neutropenia: 30%; rare in other patients), petechiae (≤17%), thrombocytopenia (6% to 12%)

Hepatic: Increased serum alkaline phosphatase (21%)

Miscellaneous: Fever (12%)

Neuromuscular & skeletal: Ostealgia (22% to 33%; dose related), commonly in the lower back, posterior iliac crest, and sternum

Respiratory: Epistaxis (9% to 15%)

1% to 10%:

Cardiovascular: Hypertension (4%), cardiac arrhythmia (3%), myocardial infarction

Central nervous system: Headache (7%)

Gastrointestinal: Nausea (10%), vomiting (7%), peritonitis (≤2%)

Hematologic & oncologic: Leukocytosis (2%)

Hypersensitivity: Transfusion reaction (≤10%)

Pharmacodynamics/Kinetics

Onset of Action

Filgrastim: ~24 hours; plateaus in 3-5 days

Tbo-filgrastim: Time to maximum ANC: 3-5 days

Duration of Action

Filgrastim: Neutrophil counts generally return to baseline within 4 days

Tbo-filgrastim: ANC returned to baseline by 21 days after completion of chemotherapy

Dosage Forms Considerations

Prefilled syringes: Granix, Neupogen: 300 mcg/0.5 mL (0.5 mL); 480 mcg/0.8 mL (0.8 mL)

Vials: Neupogen: 300 mcg/mL (1 mL); 480 mcg/1.6 mL (1.6 mL)

Available Dosage Forms
Solution, Injection:
Neupogen: 300 mcg/mL (1 mL); 480 mcg/1.6 mL (1.6 mL)
Solution, Injection [preservative free]:
Neupogen: 300 mcg/0.5 mL (0.5 mL); 480 mcg/0.8 mL (0.8 mL)
Solution Prefilled Syringe, Subcutaneous [preservative free]:
Granix: 300 mcg/0.5 mL (0.5 mL); 480 mcg/0.8 mL (0.8 mL)

General Dosage Range
I.V.: *Children and Adults:* 5-10 mcg/kg/day
SubQ: *Children and Adults:* 1.2-10 mcg/kg/day

Administration
I.V. Neupogen: May be administered I.V. as a short infusion over 15-30 minutes (chemotherapy-induced neutropenia) or by continuous infusion (chemotherapy-induced neutropenia) or as a 4- or 24-hour infusion (bone marrow transplantation). Do not administer earlier than 24 hours after or in the 24 hours prior to cytotoxic chemotherapy.
Injectable Detail pH: 4
Subcutaneous May be administered by SubQ, either as a bolus injection (chemotherapy-induced neutropenia, peripheral blood progenitor cell collection, severe chronic neutropenia) or as a continuous infusion (chemotherapy-induced neutropenia, bone marrow transplantation, and peripheral blood progenitor cell collection). Administer into the outer upper arm, abdomen (except within 2 inches of navel), front middle thigh, or the upper outer buttocks area. Do not administer earlier than 24 hours after or in the 24 hours prior to cytotoxic chemotherapy.

Preparation for Administration Visually inspect prior to use; discard if discolored or if particulates are present.
Neupogen: **Do not dilute with saline at any time; product may precipitate.** Filgrastim may be diluted with D$_5$W to a concentration of 5-15 mcg/mL for I.V. infusion administration (minimum concentration: 5 mcg/mL). Concentrations of 5-15 mcg/mL require addition of albumin (final albumin concentration of 2 mg/mL) to prevent adsorption to plastics. Dilution to <5 mcg/mL is not recommended. Do not shake. Discard unused portion of vial/prefilled syringe.
Granix: Remove needle shield and expel extra volume if needed (depending on dose). Prefilled syringe is single use; discard unused portion.

Storage/Stability
Neupogen: Store intact vials/prefilled syringes at 2°C to 8°C (36°F to 46°F). Do not shake. Protect from direct sunlight. Prior to injection, allow to reach room temperature for a maximum of 24 hours. Discard any vial or prefilled syringe left at room temperature for more than 24 hours.

Extended storage information may be available for undiluted filgrastim; contact product manufacturer to obtain current recommendations. Sterility has been assessed and maintained for up to 7 days when prepared under strict aseptic conditions (Jacobson, 1996; Singh, 1994). The manufacturer recommends using syringes within 24 hours due to the potential for bacterial contamination.
Granix: Store prefilled syringes at 2°C to 8°C (36°F to 46°F). Protect from light. Do not shake. May be removed from 2°C to 8°C (36°F to 46°F) storage for a single period of up to 5 days between 23°C to 27°C (73°F to 81°F). If not used within 5 days, the product may be returned to 2°C to 8°C (36°F to 46°F) up to the expiration date. Exposure to -1°C to -5°C (23°F to 30°F) for up to 72 hours and temperatures as low as -15°C to -25°C (5°F to -13°F) for up to 24 hours do not adversely affect stability. Discard unused product.

Nursing Actions
Physical Assessment Hypersensitivity to *E. coli* products should be assessed prior to beginning therapy. Allergic-type reactions have occurred within 30 minutes of administration. Prepare for such an event with equipment and medications for treatment (antihistamines, steroids, bronchodilators, and/or epinephrine). Assess for history of latex allergy. If self-administered, teach patient proper storage, administration, and syringe/needle disposal. Instruct patient to report upper quadrant pain, shoulder tip pain, or respiratory distress in addition to fever, chills, swelling, or redness at injection site. Instruct patient to inform radiologist if receiving Neupogen for any bone-imaging test. Bone, joint, or muscle pain may be experienced. Instruct patient to keep lab appointments. Do not give within 24 hours of receiving chemotherapy or while undergoing radiation therapy.

Patient Education
• Discuss specific use of drug and side effects with patient as it relates to treatment. (HCAHPS: During this hospital stay, were you given any medicine that you had not taken before? Before giving you any new medicine, how often did hospital staff tell you what the medicine was for? How often did hospital staff describe possible side effects in a way you could understand?)
• Patient may experience osteodynia, myalgia, stomatitis, or nausea. Have patient report immediately to prescriber tachycardia, arrhythmia, severe dizziness, syncope, dyspnea, tachypnea, hemoptysis, significant asthenia, ecchymosis, hemorrhaging, considerable injection site irritation, abdominal pain, or shoulder pain (HCAHPS).
• Educate patient about signs of a significant reaction (eg, wheezing; chest tightness; fever; itching; bad cough; blue skin color; seizures; or swelling of face, lips, tongue, or throat). **Note:** This is not a comprehensive list of all side

effects. Patient should consult prescriber for additional questions.

Intended Use and Disclaimer: Should not be printed and given to patients. This information is intended to serve as a concise initial reference for healthcare professionals to use when discussing medications with a patient. You must ultimately rely on your own discretion, experience and judgment in diagnosing, treating and advising patients.

Dietary Considerations Some products may contain sodium.

Finasteride (fi NAS teer ide)

Brand Names: U.S. Propecia; Proscar
Pharmacologic Category 5 Alpha-Reductase Inhibitor
Medication Safety Issues
Sound-alike/look-alike issues:
Finasteride may be confused with furosemide
Proscar® may be confused with ProSom, Provera®, PROzac®
Pregnancy Risk Factor X
Lactation Excretion in breast milk unknown/contraindicated in women of childbearing potential
Breast-Feeding Considerations It is not known if finasteride is excreted in breast milk. Use is contraindicated in women of childbearing potential.
Use
Propecia®: Treatment of male pattern hair loss in **men only**. Safety and efficacy were demonstrated in men between 18-41 years of age.
Proscar®: Treatment of symptomatic benign prostatic hyperplasia (BPH); can be used in combination with an alpha-blocker, doxazosin
Unlabeled Use Treatment of female hirsutism
Mechanism of Action/Effect Finasteride inhibits conversion of testosterone to dihydrotestosterone and markedly suppresses serum dihydrotestosterone levels
Contraindications Hypersensitivity to finasteride or any component of the formulation; women of childbearing potential
Warnings/Precautions Hazardous agent - use appropriate precautions for handling and disposal (NIOSH, 2012). Other urological diseases (including prostate cancer) should be ruled out before initiating. For BPH, a minimum of 6 months of treatment may be necessary to determine whether an individual will respond to finasteride; for male pattern hair loss, daily use for 3 months or longer may be required before benefit is observed. Reduces prostate specific antigen (PSA) by ~50%; in patients treated for ≥6 months the PSA value should be doubled when comparing to normal ranges in untreated patients (for interpretation of serial PSAs, a new PSA baseline should be established ≥6 months after treatment initiation and PSA monitored periodically thereafter). Failure

to demonstrate a meaningful PSA decrease (<50%) or a PSA increase while on this medication may be associated with an increased risk for prostate cancer (NCCN prostate cancer early detection guidelines, v.1.2011). Patients on a 5-alpha-reductase inhibitor (5-ARI) with any increase in PSA levels, even if within normal limits, should be evaluated; may indicate presence of prostate cancer. Use with caution in patients with hepatic dysfunction; finasteride is extensively metabolized in the liver. When compared to placebo, 5-ARIs have been shown to reduce the overall incidence of prostate cancer, although an increase in the incidence of high-grade prostate cancers has been observed; 5-ARIs are not approved in the U.S. or Canada for the prevention of prostate cancer. Carefully monitor patients with a large residual urinary volume or severely diminished urinary flow for obstructive uropathy; these patients may not be candidates for finasteride therapy. Rare reports of male breast cancer have been observed with finasteride use. Patients should promptly report any breast changes, including breast enlargement, lumps, tenderness, pain, or nipple discharge to their healthcare provider. Active ingredient of crushed or broken tablets can be absorbed through the skin; unbroken tablets are coated which prevents contact with the active ingredient during normal handling. Women should avoid contact with crushed or broken tablets and the semen from a male partner exposed to finasteride; finasteride may negatively impact fetal development.

Drug Interactions
Avoid Concomitant Use There are no known interactions where it is recommended to avoid concomitant use.
Decreased Effect There are no known significant interactions involving a decrease in effect.
Increased Effect/Toxicity There are no known significant interactions involving an increase in effect.
Nutritional/Ethanol Interactions Herb/Nutraceutical: St John's wort may decrease finasteride levels. Avoid saw palmetto (concurrent use has not been adequately studied).
Adverse Reactions Note: "Combination therapy" refers to finasteride and doxazosin.
Cardiovascular: Orthostatic hypotension (combination therapy 18%; monotherapy 9%)
Central nervous system: Dizziness (combination therapy 23%; monotherapy 7%)
Endocrine & metabolic: Decreased libido (combination therapy 12%; monotherapy 2% to 10%)
Genitourinary: Impotence (combination therapy 23%; monotherapy 5% to 19%), ejaculatory disorder (combination therapy 14%; monotherapy <1% to 7%)
Neuromuscular & skeletal: Weakness (combination therapy 17%; monotherapy 5%)

1% to 10%:
  Cardiovascular: Edema (combination therapy 3%; monotherapy 1%)
  Central nervous system: Drowsiness (combination therapy 3%; monotherapy 2%)
  Dermatologic: Skin rash (monotherapy 1%)
  Endocrine & metabolic: Gynecomastia (monotherapy 1% to 2%)
  Genitourinary: Decreased ejaculate volume (monotherapy 2% to 4%), breast tenderness (monotherapy ≤1%)
  Respiratory: Dyspnea (combination therapy 2%; monotherapy 1%), rhinitis (combination therapy 2%; monotherapy 1%)

Pharmacodynamics/Kinetics
Onset of Action BPH: 6 months; Male pattern hair loss: ≥3 months of daily use.
Duration of Action
  After a single oral dose as small as 0.5 mg: 65% depression of plasma dihydrotestosterone levels persists 5-7 days
  After 6 months of treatment with 5 mg/day: Circulating dihydrotestosterone levels are reduced to castrate levels without significant effects on circulating testosterone; levels return to normal within 14 days of discontinuation of treatment

Available Dosage Forms
Tablet, Oral:
  Propecia: 1 mg
  Proscar: 5 mg
  Generic: 1 mg, 5 mg
General Dosage Range Oral: *Adults:* 1 mg or 5 mg once daily

Administration
Oral May be administered without regard to meals. Women of childbearing age should not touch or handle broken tablets.

  Hazardous agent; use appropriate precautions for handling and disposal (NIOSH, 2012).

Storage/Stability
Propecia®: Store at 15°C to 30°C (59°F to 86°F). Protect from moisture.
Proscar®: Store below 30°C (86°F). Protect from light.

Nursing Actions
Physical Assessment Assess urinary pattern prior to therapy and periodically during therapy. A minimum of 6 months of treatment may be necessary to evaluate response.
Patient Education
• Discuss specific use of drug and side effects with patient as it relates to treatment. (HCAHPS: During this hospital stay, were you given any medicine that you had not taken before? Before giving you any new medicine, how often did hospital staff tell you what the medicine was for? How often did hospital staff describe possible side effects in a way you could understand?)
• Patient may experience sexual dysfunction. Have patient report immediately to prescriber lump in breast, mastalgia, or nipple discharge (HCAHPS).
• Educate patient about signs of a significant reaction (eg, wheezing; chest tightness; fever; itching; bad cough; blue skin color; seizures; or swelling of face, lips, tongue, or throat). **Note:** This is not a comprehensive list of all side effects. Patient should consult prescriber for additional questions.

Intended Use and Disclaimer: Should not be printed and given to patients. This information is intended to serve as a concise initial reference for healthcare professionals to use when discussing medications with a patient. You must ultimately rely on your own discretion, experience and judgment in diagnosing, treating and advising patients.
Dietary Considerations May be taken without regard to meals.
Related Information
Oral Medications That Should Not Be Crushed or Altered *on page 1712*

Fingolimod (fin GOL i mod)

Brand Names: U.S. Gilenya
Index Terms FTY720
Pharmacologic Category Sphingosine 1-Phosphate (S1P) Receptor Modulator
Medication Guide Available Yes
Pregnancy Risk Factor C
Lactation Excretion in breast milk unknown/not recommended
Use Treatment of relapsing forms of multiple sclerosis (MS) to reduce the frequency of clinical exacerbations and delay disability progression
Available Dosage Forms
Capsule, Oral:
  Gilenya: 0.5 mg
General Dosage Range Oral: *Adults:* 0.5 mg once daily
Administration
Oral May be administered with or without food.
Nursing Actions
Patient Education
• Discuss specific use of drug and side effects with patient as it relates to treatment. (HCAHPS: During this hospital stay, were you given any medicine that you had not taken before? Before giving you any new medicine, how often did hospital staff tell you what the medicine was for? How often did hospital staff describe possible side effects in a way you could understand?)
• Patient may experience headache, flu-like syndrome, diarrhea, or back pain. Have patient report immediately to prescriber signs of infection, signs of hepatic impairment, severe dizziness, syncope, considerable headache, bradycardia, arrhythmia, angina, dyspnea, significant asthenia, vision changes, ophthalmalgia, ▶

intolerable eye irritation, light sensitivity, paresthesia, or depression (HCAHPS).

- Educate patient about signs of a significant reaction (eg, wheezing; chest tightness; fever; itching; bad cough; blue skin color; seizures; or swelling of face, lips, tongue, or throat). **Note:** This is not a comprehensive list of all side effects. Patient should consult prescriber for additional questions.

Intended Use and Disclaimer: Should not be printed and given to patients. This information is intended to serve as a concise initial reference for healthcare professionals to use when discussing medications with a patient. You must ultimately rely on your own discretion, experience and judgment in diagnosing, treating and advising patients.

Flecainide (fle KAY nide)

Brand Names: U.S. Tambocor [DSC]
Index Terms Flecainide Acetate
Pharmacologic Category Antiarrhythmic Agent, Class Ic
Medication Safety Issues
Sound-alike/look-alike issues:
Flecainide may be confused with fluconazole
Tambocor™ may be confused with Pamelor™, Temodar®, tamoxifen, Tamiflu®
BEERS Criteria medication:
This drug may be potentially inappropriate for use in geriatric patients (Quality of evidence - high; Strength of recommendation - strong).
Pregnancy Risk Factor C
Lactation Enters breast milk/compatible
Use Prevention and suppression of documented life-threatening ventricular arrhythmias (eg, sustained ventricular tachycardia); controlling symptomatic, disabling supraventricular tachycardias in patients without structural heart disease in whom other agents fail
Available Dosage Forms
Tablet, Oral:
Generic: 50 mg, 100 mg, 150 mg
General Dosage Range Dosage adjustment recommended in patients with renal impairment
Oral:
Children: Initial: 3 mg/kg/day **or** 50-100 mg/m²/day in 3 divided doses; Maintenance: 3-6 mg/kg/day **or** 100-150 mg/m²/day in 3 divided doses (maximum: 11 mg/kg/day; 200 mg/m²/day)
Adults: Initial: 50-100 mg every 12 hours; Maintenance: 100-400 mg/day in 2 divided doses (maximum: 400 mg/day)
Administration
Oral Administer around-the-clock to promote less variation in peak and trough serum levels.

Nursing Actions
Physical Assessment Monitor cardiac status. Flecainide has a low toxic:therapeutic ratio and overdose may easily produce severe and life-threatening reactions.
Patient Education
- Discuss specific use of drug and side effects with patient as it relates to treatment. (HCAHPS: During this hospital stay, were you given any medicine that you had not taken before? Before giving you any new medicine, how often did hospital staff tell you what the medicine was for? How often did hospital staff describe possible side effects in a way you could understand?)
- Patient may experience headache, or blurred vision. Have patient report immediately to prescriber signs of hepatic impairment, angina, tachycardia, severe dizziness, syncope, arrhythmia, dyspnea, tremors, vision changes (HCAHPS).
- Educate patient about signs of a significant reaction (eg, wheezing; chest tightness; fever; itching; bad cough; blue skin color; seizures; or swelling of face, lips, tongue, or throat). **Note:** This is not a comprehensive list of all side effects. Patient should consult prescriber for additional questions.

Intended Use and Disclaimer: Should not be printed and given to patients. This information is intended to serve as a concise initial reference for healthcare professionals to use when discussing medications with a patient. You must ultimately rely on your own discretion, experience and judgment in diagnosing, treating and advising patients.

Floctafenine (flok ta FEN een)

Index Terms Floctafenina; Floctafeninum
Pharmacologic Category Nonsteroidal Anti-inflammatory Drug (NSAID), Oral
Lactation Enters breast milk/not recommended
Use Short-term management of acute, mild-to-moderate pain
Product Availability Not available in U.S.
General Dosage Range Dosage adjustment recommended in patients with renal impairment
Oral: *Adults:* 200-400 mg every 6-8 hours as needed (maximum: 1200 mg/day)
Administration
Oral Administer after food or meal with glass of water.
Nursing Actions
Physical Assessment Assess for allergic reactions to salicylates or other NSAIDs. Monitor blood pressure at the beginning of therapy and periodically throughout. With long-term therapy, periodic ophthalmic exams are recommended.

Patient Education

- Discuss specific use of drug and side effects with patient as it relates to treatment. (HCAHPS: During this hospital stay, were you given any medicine that you had not taken before? Before giving you any new medicine, how often did hospital staff tell you what the medicine was for? How often did hospital staff describe possible side effects in a way you could understand?)
- Patient may experience headache. Have patient report immediately to prescriber angina, strength differences from one side to another, difficulty speaking or thinking, change in balance, blurred vision, considerable nausea, severe dyspepsia, significant edema or pain of hands or feet, excessive weight gain, melena, hematuria, intolerable diarrhea, ecchymosis, or hemorrhaging (HCAHPS).
- Educate patient about signs of a significant reaction (eg, wheezing; chest tightness; fever; itching; bad cough; blue skin color; seizures; or swelling of face, lips, tongue, or throat). **Note:** This is not a comprehensive list of all side effects. Patient should consult prescriber for additional questions.

Intended Use and Disclaimer: Should not be printed and given to patients. This information is intended to serve as a concise initial reference for healthcare professionals to use when discussing medications with a patient. You must ultimately rely on your own discretion, experience and judgment in diagnosing, treating and advising patients.

Floxuridine (floks YOOR i deen)

Index Terms 5-FUDR; FdUrD; Floxuridin; Fluorodeoxyuridine; FUDR

Pharmacologic Category Antineoplastic Agent, Antimetabolite; Antineoplastic Agent, Antimetabolite (Pyrimidine Analog)

Medication Safety Issues
Sound-alike/look-alike issues:
Floxuridine may be confused with Fludara, fludarabine, fluorouracil
FUDR may be confused with Fludara

High alert medication:
This medication is in a class the Institute for Safe Medication Practices (ISMP) includes among its list of drug classes which have a heightened risk of causing significant patient harm when used in error.

Pregnancy Risk Factor D

Lactation Excretion in breast milk unknown/not recommended

Use Colorectal cancer, hepatic metastases: Palliative management of hepatic metastases of colorectal cancer (administered by continuous regional intra-arterial infusion) in select patients considered incurable by surgical resection or other means.

Available Dosage Forms
Solution Reconstituted, Injection:
Generic: 0.5 g (1 ea)

General Dosage Range Dosage adjustment recommended in patients with hepatic impairment or who develop toxicities
Intra-arterial: *Adults:* 0.1-0.6 mg/kg/day

Administration
Injectable Detail pH: 4-5.5
Intra-arterial Administer as a continuous intra-arterial infusion using an infusion pump.

Hazardous agent; use appropriate precautions for handling and disposal (NIOSH, 2012).

Nursing Actions
Physical Assessment Inform physician immediately with trouble swallowing, mouth sores, chest pain, stomach pain, difficulty walking, or abnormal bleeding. Report any skin changes such as unusual sunburn appearance, or blistered or dark peeling skin. Monitor for CNS changes and acute gastrointestinal reactions (intractable vomiting or diarrhea may be dose limiting). Instruct patient to report use of any NSAIDS or anticoagulants as may increase bleeding risk. Teach patient or caregiver use and care of implantable pump. Routine laboratory monitoring is needed; instruct patient on keeping all lab appointments.

Patient Education

- Discuss specific use of drug and side effects with patient as it relates to treatment. (HCAHPS: During this hospital stay, were you given any medicine that you had not taken before? Before giving you any new medicine, how often did hospital staff tell you what the medicine was for? How often did hospital staff describe possible side effects in a way you could understand?)
- Patient may experience alopecia or lack of appetite. Have patient report immediately to prescriber signs of infection, angina, stomatitis, significant diarrhea, severe nausea, signs of hemorrhaging, urine discoloration, jaundice, intolerable asthenia, or injection site irritation (HCAHPS).
- Educate patient about signs of a significant reaction (eg, wheezing; chest tightness; fever; itching; bad cough; blue skin color; seizures; or swelling of face, lips, tongue, or throat). **Note:** This is not a comprehensive list of all side effects. Patient should consult prescriber for additional questions.

Intended Use and Disclaimer: Should not be printed and given to patients. This information is intended to serve as a concise initial reference for healthcare professionals to use when discussing medications with a patient. You must ultimately rely on your own discretion, experience and judgment in diagnosing, treating and advising patients.

Fluconazole (floo KOE na zole)

Brand Names: U.S. Diflucan

Pharmacologic Category Antifungal Agent, Oral; Antifungal Agent, Parenteral

Medication Safety Issues

Sound-alike/look-alike issues:

Fluconazole may be confused with flecainide, FLUoxetine, furosemide, itraconazole, voriconazole

Diflucan may be confused with diclofenac, Diprivan, disulfiram

International issues:

Canesten (oral capsules) [Great Britain] may be confused with Canesten brand name for clotrimazole (various dosage forms) [multiple international markets]; Cenestin brand name estrogens (conjugated A/synthetic) [U.S., Canada]

Pregnancy Risk Factor C (single dose for vaginal candidiasis)/D (all other indications)

Lactation Enters breast milk/use caution

Breast-Feeding Considerations Fluconazole is excreted in breast milk. The manufacturer recommends that caution be exercised when administering fluconazole to nursing women. Fluconazole is found in breast milk at concentrations similar to maternal plasma.

Use Treatment of candidiasis (esophageal, oropharyngeal, peritoneal, urinary tract, vaginal); systemic candida infections (eg, candidemia, disseminated candidiasis, and pneumonia); cryptococcal meningitis; antifungal prophylaxis in allogeneic bone marrow transplant recipients

Unlabeled Use Cryptococcal pneumonia; candidal intertrigo; surgical (perioperative) prophylaxis in high-risk patients undergoing liver, pancreas, kidney, or pancreas-kidney transplantation

Mechanism of Action/Effect Interferes with cytochrome P450 activity, decreasing ergosterol synthesis (principal sterol in fungal cell membrane) and inhibiting cell membrane formation

Contraindications Hypersensitivity to fluconazole or any component of the formulation (cross-reaction with other azole antifungal agents may occur, but has not been established; use caution); coadministration of terfenadine in patients receiving multiple doses of 400 mg or higher or with CYP3A4 substrates which may lead to QT_c prolongation (eg, astemizole, cisapride, pimozide, or quinidine)

Warnings/Precautions Serious (and sometimes fatal) hepatic toxicity (eg, hepatitis, cholestasis, fulminant hepatic failure) has been observed. Use with caution in patients with renal and hepatic dysfunction or previous hepatotoxicity from other azole derivatives. Patients who develop abnormal liver function tests during fluconazole therapy should be monitored closely and discontinued if symptoms consistent with liver disease develop. Rare exfoliative skin disorders have been observed; monitor closely if rash develops and discontinue if lesions progress. Cases of QT_c prolongation and torsade de pointes associated with fluconazole use have been reported (usually high dose or in combination with agents known to prolong the QT interval); use caution in patients with concomitant medications or conditions which are arrhythmogenic. Potentially significant drug-drug interactions may exist, requiring dose or frequency adjustment, additional monitoring, and/or selection of alternative therapy. May occasionally cause dizziness or seizures; use caution driving or operating machines. Powder for oral suspension contains sucrose; use caution with fructose intolerance, sucrose-isomaltase deficiency, or glucose-galactose malabsorption.

Drug Interactions

Avoid Concomitant Use

Avoid concomitant use of Fluconazole with any of the following: Bosutinib; Cisapride; Citalopram; Conivaptan; Dofetilide; Highest Risk QTc-Prolonging Agents; Ibrutinib; Ivabradine; Lomitapide; Mifepristone; Ospemifene; Pimozide; QuiNIDine; Ranolazine; Rivaroxaban; Simeprevir; Tolvaptan; Ulipristal; Voriconazole

Decreased Effect

Fluconazole may decrease the levels/effects of: Amphotericin B; Clopidogrel; Ifosfamide; Saccharomyces boulardii

The levels/effects of Fluconazole may be decreased by: Didanosine; Etravirine; Rifamycin Derivatives

Increased Effect/Toxicity

Fluconazole may increase the levels/effects of: Alfentanil; ARIPiprazole; AtorvaSTATin; Avanafil; Benzodiazepines (metabolized by oxidation); Bosentan; Bosutinib; Budesonide (Systemic, Oral Inhalation); BusPIRone; Busulfan; Calcium Channel Blockers; CarBAMazepine; Carvedilol; Cilostazol; Cisapride; Citalopram; Colchicine; Conivaptan; Corticosteroids (Systemic); CycloSPORINE (Systemic); CYP2C19 Substrates; CYP2C9 Substrates; CYP3A4 Substrates; DOCEtaxel; Dofetilide; DOXOrubicin (Conventional); Eletriptan; Eplerenone; Etravirine; Everolimus; FentaNYL; Fluvastatin; Fosphenytoin; Highest Risk QTc-Prolonging Agents; Ibrutinib; Imatinib; Irbesartan; Irinotecan; Ivacaftor; Lomitapide; Losartan; Lovastatin; Lurasidone; Macrolide Antibiotics; Methadone; Moderate Risk QTc-Prolonging Agents; Nevirapine; Ospemifene; OxyCODONE; Phenytoin; Pimecrolimus; Pimozide; Proton Pump Inhibitors; QuiNIDine; Ramelteon; Ranolazine; Red Yeast Rice; Rifamycin Derivatives; Rivaroxaban; Salmeterol; Saxagliptin; Sildenafil; Simeprevir; Simvastatin; Sirolimus; Solifenacin; Sulfonylureas; SUNItinib; Tacrolimus (Systemic); Tacrolimus (Topical); Tadalafil; Temsirolimus; Tipranavir; Tofacitinib; Tolterodine; Tolvaptan; Ulipristal; Vardenafil; Vilazodone; Vitamin

K Antagonists; Voriconazole; Zidovudine; Zolpidem

The levels/effects of Fluconazole may be increased by: Etravirine; Ivabradine; Macrolide Antibiotics; Mifepristone; QTc-Prolonging Agents (Indeterminate Risk and Risk Modifying)

Adverse Reactions Frequency not always defined.

Cardiovascular: Angioedema (rare)

Central nervous system: Headache (2% to 13%), dizziness (1%)

Dermatologic: Rash (2%)

Gastrointestinal: Nausea (2% to 7%), abdominal pain (2% to 6%), vomiting (2% to 5%), diarrhea (2% to 3%), dysgeusia (1%), dyspepsia (1%)

Hepatic: Alkaline phosphatase increased, ALT increased, AST increased, hepatic failure (rare), hepatitis, jaundice

Miscellaneous: Anaphylactic reactions (rare)

Available Dosage Forms

Solution, Intravenous:
Generic: 100 mg (50 mL); 200 mg (100 mL); 400 mg (200 mL)

Solution, Intravenous [preservative free]:
Generic: 200 mg (100 mL); 400 mg (200 mL)

Suspension Reconstituted, Oral:
Diflucan: 10 mg/mL (35 mL); 40 mg/mL (35 mL)
Generic: 10 mg/mL (35 mL); 40 mg/mL (35 mL)

Tablet, Oral:
Diflucan: 50 mg, 100 mg, 150 mg, 200 mg
Generic: 50 mg, 100 mg, 150 mg, 200 mg

General Dosage Range Dosage adjustment recommended in patients with renal impairment

Oral, I.V.:
Children: Loading dose: 6-12 mg/kg/dose; maintenance: 3-12 mg/kg/dose once daily; duration and dosage depend on location and severity of infection

Adults: 150 mg once **or** Loading dose: 200-800 mg; maintenance: 200-800 mg once daily; duration and dosage depend on location and severity of infection

Administration

I.V. Do not use if cloudy or precipitated. Infuse over ~1-2 hours; do not exceed 200 mg/hour.

Injectable Detail Premixed solutions: pH: 4-8 (sodium chloride diluent); 3.5-6.5 (dextrose diluent)

Oral May be administered without regard to meals.

Storage/Stability

Tablet: Store at <30°C (86°F).

Powder for oral suspension: Store dry powder at <30°C (86°F). Following reconstitution, store at 5°C to 30°C (41°F to 86°F). Discard unused portion after 2 weeks. Do not freeze.

Injection: Store injection in glass at 5°C to 30°C (41°F to 86°F). Store injection in plastic flexible containers at 5°C to 25°C (41°F to 77°F). Brief exposure of up to 40°C (104°F) does not adversely affect the product. Do not freeze. Do not unwrap unit until ready for use.

Nursing Actions

Physical Assessment Cultures should be obtained and allergy history assessed prior to beginning therapy. Assess renal and hepatic function. Monitor for hepatotoxicity (jaundice), skin disorders, and abdominal pain on a regular basis.

Patient Education

• Discuss specific use of drug and side effects with patient as it relates to treatment. (HCAHPS: During this hospital stay, were you given any medicine that you had not taken before? Before giving you any new medicine, how often did hospital staff tell you what the medicine was for? How often did hospital staff describe possible side effects in a way you could understand?)

• Patient may experience headache, dyspepsia, or dysgeusia. Have patient report immediately to prescriber signs of hypokalemia, signs of hepatic impairment, severe dizziness, syncope, considerable nausea, significant diarrhea, paresthesia, chills, pharyngitis, ecchymosis, or hemorrhaging (HCAHPS).

• Educate patient about signs of a significant reaction (eg, wheezing; chest tightness; fever; itching; bad cough; blue skin color; seizures; or swelling of face, lips, tongue, or throat). **Note:** This is not a comprehensive list of all side effects. Patient should consult prescriber for additional questions.

Intended Use and Disclaimer: Should not be printed and given to patients. This information is intended to serve as a concise initial reference for healthcare professionals to use when discussing medications with a patient. You must ultimately rely on your own discretion, experience and judgment in diagnosing, treating and advising patients.

Flucytosine (floo SYE toe seen)

Brand Names: U.S. Ancobon

Index Terms 5-FC; 5-Fluorocytosine; 5-Flurocytosine

Pharmacologic Category Antifungal Agent, Oral

Medication Safety Issues

Sound-alike/look-alike issues:
Flucytosine may be confused with fluorouracil
Ancobon® may be confused with Oncovin

High alert medication:
The Institute for Safe Medication Practices (ISMP) includes this medication among its list of drugs which have a heightened risk of causing significant patient harm when used in error.

Pregnancy Risk Factor C

Lactation Excretion in breast milk unknown/not recommended

Breast-Feeding Considerations It is not known if flucytosine is excreted in breast milk. Due to the potential for serious adverse reactions in the nursing infant, a decision should be made whether to discontinue nursing or to discontinue the drug, taking into account the importance of treatment to the mother.

Use Adjunctive treatment of systemic fungal infections (eg, septicemia, endocarditis, UTI, meningitis, or pulmonary) caused by susceptible strains of *Candida* or *Cryptococcus*

Mechanism of Action/Effect Penetrates fungal cells and interferes with fungal RNA and protein synthesis

Contraindications Hypersensitivity to flucytosine or any component of the formulation

Warnings/Precautions [U.S. Boxed Warning]: Use with extreme caution in patients with renal dysfunction; dosage adjustment required. Avoid use as monotherapy; resistance rapidly develops. Use with caution in patients with bone marrow depression; patients with hematologic disease or who have been treated with radiation or drugs that suppress the bone marrow may be at greatest risk. Bone marrow toxicity may be irreversible. **[U.S. Boxed Warning]: Closely monitor hematologic, renal, and hepatic status.** Hepatotoxicity and bone marrow toxicity appear to be dose related; monitor levels closely and adjust dose accordingly.

Drug Interactions

Avoid Concomitant Use

Avoid concomitant use of Flucytosine with any of the following: CloZAPine; Gimeracil

Decreased Effect

Flucytosine may decrease the levels/effects of: Saccharomyces boulardii

The levels/effects of Flucytosine may be decreased by: Cytarabine (Conventional)

Increased Effect/Toxicity

Flucytosine may increase the levels/effects of: CloZAPine

The levels/effects of Flucytosine may be increased by: Amphotericin B; Gimeracil

Nutritional/Ethanol Interactions Food: Food decreases the rate, but not the extent of absorption.

Adverse Reactions Frequency not defined.

Cardiovascular: Cardiac arrest, myocardial toxicity, ventricular dysfunction, chest pain

Central nervous system: Ataxia, confusion, fatigue, hallucinations, headache, parkinsonism, psychosis, pyrexia, sedation, seizure, vertigo

Dermatologic: Rash, photosensitivity, pruritus, toxic epidermal necrolysis, urticaria

Endocrine & metabolic: Hypoglycemia, hypokalemia

Gastrointestinal: Abdominal pain, anorexia, diarrhea, duodenal ulcer, enterocolitis, hemorrhage, nausea, ulcerative colitis, vomiting, xerostomia

Hematologic: Agranulocytosis, anemia, aplastic anemia, bone marrow aplasia, eosinophilia, leukopenia, pancytopenia, thrombocytopenia

Hepatic: Acute hepatic injury, bilirubin increased, hepatic dysfunction, jaundice, liver enzymes increased

Neuromuscular & skeletal: Paresthesia, peripheral neuropathy, weakness

Otic: Hearing loss

Renal: Azotemia, BUN increased, crystalluria, renal failure, serum creatinine increased

Respiratory: Dyspnea, respiratory arrest

Miscellaneous: Allergic reaction

Available Dosage Forms

Capsule, Oral:

Ancobon: 250 mg, 500 mg

Generic: 250 mg, 500 mg

General Dosage Range Dosage adjustment recommended in patients with renal impairment

Oral: *Adults:* 50-150 mg/kg daily in 3 or 4 divided doses

Administration

Oral Administer around-the-clock to promote less variation in peak and trough serum levels. To avoid nausea and vomiting, administer a few capsules at a time over 15 minutes until full dose is taken.

Storage/Stability Store at room temperature of 25°C (77°F); excursions permitted to 15°C to 30°C (59°F to 86°F).

Nursing Actions

Physical Assessment Hematologic, renal, and hepatic status must be closely monitored; dose adjustments may be necessary. Monitor for cardiac incidents, CNS changes, bone marrow suppression, jaundice, skin reactions, and hearing loss on a regular basis.

Patient Education

• Discuss specific use of drug and side effects with patient as it relates to treatment. (HCAHPS: During this hospital stay, were you given any medicine that you had not taken before? Before giving you any new medicine, how often did hospital staff tell you what the medicine was for? How often did hospital staff describe possible side effects in a way you could understand?)

• Patient may experience fatigue, xerostomia, dyspepsia, nausea, diarrhea, or lack of appetite. Have patient report immediately to prescriber signs of renal impairment, signs of hypokalemia, melena, hematemesis, angina, tachycardia, illogical thinking, mood changes, hearing impairment, change in balance, paresthesia, dyspnea, hallucinations, signs of hepatic impairment, signs of infection, or signs of hypoglycemia (HCAHPS).

• Educate patient about signs of a significant reaction (eg, wheezing; chest tightness; fever; itching; bad cough; blue skin color; seizures; or swelling of face, lips, tongue, or throat). **Note:** This is not a comprehensive list of all side effects. Patient should consult prescriber for additional questions.

Intended Use and Disclaimer: Should not be printed and given to patients. This information is intended to serve as a concise initial reference for healthcare professionals to use when discussing medications with a patient. You must ultimately rely on your own discretion, experience and judgment in diagnosing, treating and advising patients.

Fludarabine (floo DARE a been)

Brand Names: U.S. Fludara
Index Terms 2F-ara-AMP; Fludarabine Phosphate
Pharmacologic Category Antineoplastic Agent, Antimetabolite; Antineoplastic Agent, Antimetabolite (Purine Analog)
Medication Safety Issues
Sound-alike/look-alike issues:
Fludarabine may be confused with cladribine, floxuridine, Flumadine
Fludara may be confused with FUDR
High alert medication:
This medication is in a class the Institute for Safe Medication Practices (ISMP) includes among its list of drug classes which have a heightened risk of causing significant patient harm when used in error.
Pregnancy Risk Factor D
Lactation Excretion in breast milk unknown/not recommended
Breast-Feeding Considerations Due to the potential for serious adverse reactions in the nursing infant, breast-feeding is not recommended.
Use Treatment of progressive or refractory B-cell chronic lymphocytic leukemia (CLL)
Canadian labeling: Second-line treatment of chronic lymphocytic leukemia (CLL); second-line treatment of low-grade, refractory non-Hodgkin lymphoma (NHL)
Unlabeled Use Treatment of non-Hodgkin lymphomas (NHL); acute myeloid leukemia (AML), either refractory or in poor risk patients; relapsed acute lymphocytic leukemia (ALL) or AML in pediatric patients; Waldenström's macroglobulinemia (WM); reduced-intensity conditioning regimens prior to allogeneic hematopoietic stem cell transplantation (generally administered in combination with busulfan or cyclophosphamide and antithymocyte globulin or lymphocyte immune globulin, or in combination with melphalan and alemtuzumab)
Mechanism of Action/Effect Inhibits DNA synthesis by inhibition of DNA polymerase and ribonucleotide reductase; also inhibits DNA primase and DNA ligase I
Contraindications Hypersensitivity of fludarabine or any component of the formulation
Canadian labeling: Additional contraindications (not in U.S. labeling): Severe renal impairment (CrCl <30 mL/minute); decompensated hemolytic anemia; concurrent use with pentostatin

Warnings/Precautions Hazardous agent - use appropriate precautions for handling and disposal (NIOSH, 2012). Use with caution in patients with renal insufficiency (clearance of the primary metabolite 2-fluoro-ara-A is reduced); dosage reductions are recommended (monitor closely for excessive toxicity); use of the I.V. formulation is not recommended if CrCl <30 mL/minute. Canadian labeling contraindicates use of oral and I.V. formulations if CrCl <30 mL/minute. Use with caution in patients with pre-existing hematological disorders (particularly granulocytopenia) or pre-existing central nervous system disorder (epilepsy), spasticity, or peripheral neuropathy. **[U.S. Boxed Warning]: Higher than recommended doses are associated with severe neurologic toxicity (delayed blindness, coma, death); similar neurotoxicity (agitation, coma, confusion and seizure) has been reported with standard CLL doses.** Neurotoxicity symptoms due to high doses appear from 21-60 days following the last fludarabine dose, although neurotoxicity has been reported as early as 7 days and up to 225 days. Possible neurotoxic effects of chronic administration are unknown. Caution patients about performing tasks which require mental alertness (eg, operating machinery or driving).

[U.S. Boxed Warning]: Life-threatening (and sometimes fatal) autoimmune effects, including hemolytic anemia, autoimmune thrombocytopenia/thrombocytopenic purpura (ITP), Evans syndrome, and acquired hemophilia have occurred; monitor closely for hemolysis; discontinue fludarabine if hemolysis occurs; the hemolytic effects usually recur with fludarabine rechallenge. **[U.S. Boxed Warning]: Severe bone marrow suppression (anemia, thrombocytopenia, and neutropenia) may occur;** may be cumulative. Severe myelosuppression (trilineage bone marrow hypoplasia/aplasia) has been reported (rare) with a duration of significant cytopenias ranging from 2 months to 1 year. First-line combination therapy is associated with prolonged cytopenias, with anemia lasting up to 7 months, neutropenia up to 9 months, and thrombocytopenia up to 10 months; increased age is predictive for prolonged cytopenias (Gill, 2010).

Use with caution in patients with documented infection, fever, immunodeficiency, or with a history of opportunistic infection; prophylactic anti-infectives should be considered for patients with an increased risk for developing opportunistic infections. Progressive multifocal leukoencephalopathy (PML) due to JC virus (usually fatal) has been reported with use; usually in patients who had received prior and/or other concurrent chemotherapy; onset ranges from a few weeks to 1 year; evaluate any neurological change promptly. Avoid vaccination with live vaccines during and after fludarabine treatment. May cause tumor lysis ▶

syndrome; risk is increased in patients with large tumor burden prior to treatment. Patients receiving blood products should only receive irradiated blood products due to the potential for transfusion related GVHD. **[U.S. Boxed Warnings]: Do not use in combination with pentostatin; may lead to severe, even fatal pulmonary toxicity. Should be administered under the supervision of an experienced cancer chemotherapy physician.**

Drug Interactions

Avoid Concomitant Use
Avoid concomitant use of Fludarabine with any of the following: BCG; CloZAPine; Natalizumab; Pentostatin; Pimecrolimus; Tacrolimus (Topical); Tofacitinib; Vaccines (Live)

Decreased Effect
Fludarabine may decrease the levels/effects of: BCG; Coccidioidin Skin Test; Sipuleucel-T; Vaccines (Inactivated); Vaccines (Live)

The levels/effects of Fludarabine may be decreased by: Echinacea; Imatinib

Increased Effect/Toxicity
Fludarabine may increase the levels/effects of: CloZAPine; Leflunomide; Natalizumab; Pentostatin; Tofacitinib; Vaccines (Live)

The levels/effects of Fludarabine may be increased by: Denosumab; Pentostatin; Pimecrolimus; Roflumilast; Tacrolimus (Topical); Trastuzumab

Nutritional/Ethanol Interactions Ethanol: Avoid ethanol (due to GI irritation).

Adverse Reactions
>10%:
Cardiovascular: Edema (8% to 19%)
Central nervous system: Fever (60% to 69%), fatigue (10% to 38%), pain (20% to 22%), chills (11% to 19%)
Dermatologic: Rash (15%)
Gastrointestinal: Nausea/vomiting (31% to 36%), anorexia (7% to 34%), diarrhea (13% to 15%), gastrointestinal bleeding (3% to 13%)
Genitourinary: Urinary tract infection (2% to 15%)
Hematologic: Myelosuppression (nadir: 10-14 days; recovery: 5-7 weeks; dose-limiting toxicity), anemia (60%), neutropenia (grade 4: 59%; nadir: ~13 days), thrombocytopenia (55%; nadir: ~16 days)
Neuromuscular & skeletal: Weakness (9% to 65%), myalgia (4% to 16%), paresthesia (4% to 12%)
Ocular: Visual disturbance (3% to 15%)
Respiratory: Cough (10% to 44%), pneumonia (16% to 22%), dyspnea (9% to 22%), upper respiratory infection (2% to 16%)
Miscellaneous: Infection (33% to 44%), diaphoresis (1% to 13%)
1% to 10%:
Cardiovascular: Angina (≤6%), arrhythmia (≤3%), cerebrovascular accident (≤3%), heart failure (≤3%), MI (≤3%), supraventricular tachycardia

(≤3%), deep vein thrombosis (1% to 3%), phlebitis (1% to 3%), aneurysm (≤1%), transient ischemic attack (≤1%)
Central nervous system: Malaise (6% to 8%), headache (≤3%), sleep disorder (1% to 3%), cerebellar syndrome (≤1%), depression (≤1%), mentation impaired (≤1%)
Dermatologic: Alopecia (≤3%), pruritus (1% to 3%), seborrhea (≤1%)
Endocrine & metabolic: Hyperglycemia (1% to 6%), dehydration (≤1%)
Gastrointestinal: Stomatitis (≤9%), esophagitis (≤3%), constipation (1% to 3%), mucositis (≤2%), dysphagia (≤1%)
Genitourinary: Dysuria (3% to 4%), hesitancy (≤3%)
Hematologic: Hemorrhage (≤1%)
Hepatic: Cholelithiasis (≤3%), liver function tests abnormal (1% to 3%), liver failure (≤1%)
Neuromuscular & skeletal: Osteoporosis (≤2%), arthralgia (≤1%)
Otic: Hearing loss (2% to 6%)
Renal: Hematuria (2% to 3%), renal failure (≤1%), renal function test abnormal (≤1%), proteinuria (≤1%)
Respiratory: Pharyngitis (≤9%), allergic pneumonitis (≤6%), hemoptysis (1% to 6%), sinusitis (≤5%), bronchitis (≤1%), epistaxis (≤1%), hypoxia (≤1%)
Miscellaneous: Anaphylaxis (≤1%), tumor lysis syndrome (≤1%)

Available Dosage Forms
Solution, Intravenous:
Generic: 50 mg/2 mL (2 mL)
Solution Reconstituted, Intravenous:
Fludara: 50 mg (1 ea)
Generic: 50 mg (1 ea)
Solution Reconstituted, Intravenous [preservative free]:
Generic: 50 mg (1 ea)
General Dosage Range Dosage adjustment recommended in patients with renal impairment or who develop toxicities.
I.V.: *Adults:* 25 mg/m^2/day for 5 days every 28 days

Administration
I.V. Administer I.V. over 30 minutes; continuous infusions (unlabeled administration rate) are occasionally used

Hazardous agent; use appropriate precautions for handling and disposal (NIOSH, 2012).

Injectable Detail pH: 7.2-8.2
Oral Tablet may be administered with or without food; should be swallowed whole with water; do not chew, break, or crush.

Hazardous agent; use appropriate precautions for handling and disposal (NIOSH, 2012).

Preparation for Administration Hazardous agent; use appropriate precautions for handling and disposal (NIOSH, 2012).

Lyophilized vials: Reconstitute with 2 mL SWFI; further dilute in 100-125 mL D$_5$W or NS.

Solution for injection: Dilute in 100-125 mL D$_5$W or NS.

Storage/Stability

I.V.: Store intact vials under refrigeration or at room temperature, as specified according to each manufacturer's labeling. Reconstituted solution or vials of the solution for injection that have been punctured (in use) should be used within 8 hours.

Tablet: Store at 15°C to 30°C (59°F to 86°F); should be kept within packaging until use.

Nursing Actions

Patient Education

- Discuss specific use of drug and side effects with patient as it relates to treatment. (HCAHPS: During this hospital stay, were you given any medicine that you had not taken before? Before giving you any new medicine, how often did hospital staff tell you what the medicine was for? How often did hospital staff describe possible side effects in a way you could understand?)

- Patient may experience lack of appetite, chills, hyperhidrosis, or myalgia. Have patient report immediately to prescriber signs of infection, signs of hemorrhaging, dyspnea, angina, mood changes, illogical thinking, severe nausea, considerable diarrhea, urinary retention, significant asthenia, paresthesia of hands or feet, inability to eat, vision changes, edema of extremities, signs of tumor lysis syndrome (TLS), or signs of Stevens-Johnson syndrome/toxic epidermal necrolysis (HCAHPS).

- Educate patient about signs of a significant reaction (eg, wheezing; chest tightness; fever; itching; bad cough; blue skin color; seizures; or swelling of face, lips, tongue, or throat). **Note:** This is not a comprehensive list of all side effects. Patient should consult prescriber for additional questions.

Intended Use and Disclaimer: Should not be printed and given to patients. This information is intended to serve as a concise initial reference for healthcare professionals to use when discussing medications with a patient. You must ultimately rely on your own discretion, experience and judgment in diagnosing, treating and advising patients.

Fludrocortisone (floo droe KOR ti sone)

Index Terms 9α-Fluorohydrocortisone Acetate; Florinef; Fludrocortisone Acetate; Fluohydrisone Acetate; Fluohydrocortisone Acetate

Pharmacologic Category Corticosteroid, Systemic

Medication Safety Issues

Sound-alike/look-alike issues:

Florinef® may be confused with Fioricet®, Fiorinal®

Pregnancy Risk Factor C

Lactation Excretion in breast milk unknown/use caution

Breast-Feeding Considerations Corticosteroids are excreted in human milk; information specific to fludrocortisone has not been located. The manufacturer recommends that caution be exercised when administering fludrocortisone to nursing women.

Use Partial replacement therapy for primary and secondary adrenocortical insufficiency in Addison's disease; treatment of salt-losing adrenogenital syndrome (or congenital adrenal hyperplasia)

Unlabeled Use Treatment of idiopathic orthostatic hypotension in conjunction with increased sodium intake

Mechanism of Action/Effect Very potent mineralocorticoid with high glucocorticoid activity; used primarily for its mineralocorticoid effects. Promotes increased reabsorption of sodium and loss of potassium from renal distal tubules.

Contraindications Hypersensitivity to fludrocortisone, hypersensitivity to other corticosteroids, or any component of the formulation; systemic fungal infections

Warnings/Precautions May cause hypercorticism or suppression of hypothalamic-pituitary-adrenal (HPA) axis, particularly in younger children or in patients receiving high doses for prolonged periods. HPA axis suppression may lead to adrenal crisis. Withdrawal and discontinuation of a corticosteroid should be done slowly and carefully. Fludrocortisone is primarily a mineralocorticoid agonist, but may also inhibit the HPA axis. Prolonged use may increase risk of infection, mask acute infection, prolong or exacerbate viral infections, or limit response to vaccinations. Exposure to chickenpox should be avoided. Corticosteroids should not be used to treat ocular herpes simplex, cerebral malaria, or viral hepatitis. Close observation is required in patients with latent tuberculosis (TB) and/or TB reactivity. Restrict use in active TB (only in conjunction with antituberculosis treatment). Prolonged treatment with corticosteroids has been associated with the development of Kaposi's sarcoma (case reports); if noted, discontinuation of therapy should be considered. Acute myopathy has been reported with high-dose corticosteroids, usually in patients with neuromuscular transmission disorders; may involve ocular and/or respiratory muscles; monitor creatine kinase; recovery may be delayed.

Corticosteroid use may cause psychiatric disturbances, including depression, euphoria, insomnia, mood swings, and personality changes. Pre-existing psychiatric conditions may be exacerbated by corticosteroid use. Use with caution in patients with HF; use may be associated with fluid retention, edema, weight gain and hypertension. Use with caution in patients with sodium retention and potassium loss, diabetes mellitus, GI diseases (diverticulitis, peptic ulcer, ulcerative colitis), hepatic impairment, myasthenia gravis, post- myocardial infarction, osteoporosis, and/or renal impairment. Use with caution in patients with cataracts and/or glaucoma; increased intraocular pressure, open-angle glaucoma, and cataracts have occurred with prolonged use. Consider routine eye exams in chronic users. Use with caution in patients with a history of seizure disorder; seizures have been reported with adrenal crisis. Changes in thyroid status may necessitate dosage adjustments; metabolic clearance of corticosteroids increases in hyperthyroid patients and decreases in hypothyroid ones. Use with caution in the elderly. May affect growth velocity in pediatric patients. Withdraw therapy with gradual tapering of dose.

Drug Interactions

Avoid Concomitant Use

Avoid concomitant use of Fludrocortisone with any of the following: Aldesleukin; BCG; Indium 111 Capromab Pendetide; Mifepristone; Natalizumab; Pimecrolimus; Tacrolimus (Topical); Tofacitinib

Decreased Effect

Fludrocortisone may decrease the levels/effects of: Aldesleukin; Antidiabetic Agents; BCG; Calcitriol; Coccidioidin Skin Test; Corticorelin; Hyaluronidase; Indium 111 Capromab Pendetide; Isoniazid; Salicylates; Sipuleucel-T; Telaprevir; Urea Cycle Disorder Agents; Vaccines (Inactivated)

The levels/effects of Fludrocortisone may be decreased by: Aminoglutethimide; Antacids; Barbiturates; Bile Acid Sequestrants; Echinacea; Mifepristone; Mitotane; Primidone; Rifamycin Derivatives

Increased Effect/Toxicity

Fludrocortisone may increase the levels/effects of: Acetylcholinesterase Inhibitors; Amphotericin B; Deferasirox; Leflunomide; Loop Diuretics; Natalizumab; NSAID (COX-2 Inhibitor); NSAID (Nonselective); Thiazide Diuretics; Tofacitinib; Vaccines (Live); Warfarin

The levels/effects of Fludrocortisone may be increased by: Antifungal Agents (Azole Derivatives, Systemic); Aprepitant; Calcium Channel Blockers (Nondihydropyridine); Denosumab; Estrogen Derivatives; Fluconazole; Fosaprepitant; Indacaterol; Macrolide Antibiotics; Mifepristone; Neuromuscular-Blocking Agents (Nondepolarizing); Pimecrolimus; Quinolone Antibiotics; Roflumilast; Salicylates; Tacrolimus (Topical); Telaprevir; Trastuzumab

Adverse Reactions Frequency not defined.

Cardiovascular: Cardiac enlargement, CHF, edema, hypertension

Central nervous system: Delirium, depression, emotional instability, euphoria, hallucinations, headache, insomnia, intracranial pressure increased, malaise, mood swings, nervousness, personality changes, pseudotumor cerebri, psychiatric disorders, psychoses, seizure, vertigo

Dermatologic: Acne, bruising, erythema, hirsutism, hives, hyperpigmentation, maculopapular rash, petechiae, purpura, rash, skin test reaction impaired, striae, subcutaneous fat atrophy, thin fragile skin, urticaria, wound healing (impaired)

Endocrine & metabolic: Cushing's syndrome, diabetes mellitus, glucose intolerance, growth suppression, hyperglycemia, hypokalemia, hypokalemic alkalosis, menstrual irregularities, negative nitrogen balance, pituitary-adrenal axis suppression

Gastrointestinal: Abdominal distention, esophagitis ulceration, pancreatitis, peptic ulcer

Neuromuscular & skeletal: Fractures, necrosis (femoral and humeral heads), muscle mass loss, muscle weakness, myopathy, osteoporosis, vertebral compression fractures

Ocular: Cataracts, exophthalmos, glaucoma, increased intraocular pressure

Renal: Glycosuria

Miscellaneous: Anaphylaxis (generalized), diaphoresis

Available Dosage Forms

Tablet, Oral:

Generic: 0.1 mg

General Dosage Range Oral:

Children: 0.05-0.2 mg daily

Adults: 0.05-0.2 mg daily (range: 0.1 mg 3 times weekly to 0.2 mg daily)

Administration

Oral May be administered without regard to food.

Storage/Stability Store at controlled room temperature at 20°C to 25°C (68°F 77°F); avoid excessive heat.

Nursing Actions

Physical Assessment Teach patients to report opportunistic infection and adrenal suppression. Instruct patients with diabetes to monitor serum glucose levels closely; corticosteroids can alter glycemic response. Dose may need to be increased if patient is experiencing higher than normal levels of stress. When discontinuing, taper dose and frequency slowly.

Patient Education

- Discuss specific use of drug and side effects with patient as it relates to treatment. (HCAHPS: During this hospital stay, were you given any medicine that you had not taken before? Before giving you any new medicine, how often did hospital staff tell you what the medicine was for? How often did hospital staff describe possible side effects in a way you could understand?)
- Patient may experience nausea, insomnia, or akathisia. Have patient report immediately to prescriber signs of infection, signs of hyperglycemia, signs of hypokalemia, severe asthenia, irritability, tremors, tachycardia, confusion, hyperhidrosis, dizziness, dyspnea, excessive

weight gain, edema of extremities, skin changes, moon face, buffalo hump, considerable headache, bradycardia, arrhythmia, angina, extremity discoloration, painful extremities, menstrual irregularities, osteodynia, arthralgia, vision changes, mood changes, behavioral changes, depression, paresthesia, ecchymosis, hemorrhaging, intolerable dyspepsia, melena, or hematemesis (HCAHPS).

- Educate patient about signs of a significant reaction (eg, wheezing; chest tightness; fever; itching; bad cough; blue skin color; seizures; or swelling of face, lips, tongue, or throat). **Note:** This is not a comprehensive list of all side effects. Patient should consult prescriber for additional questions.

Intended Use and Disclaimer: Should not be printed and given to patients. This information is intended to serve as a concise initial reference for healthcare professionals to use when discussing medications with a patient. You must ultimately rely on your own discretion, experience and judgment in diagnosing, treating and advising patients.

Dietary Considerations Systemic use of mineralocorticoids/corticosteroids may require a diet with increased potassium, vitamins A, B_6, C, D, folate, calcium, zinc, and phosphorus, and decreased sodium. With fludrocortisone, a decrease in dietary sodium is often not required as the increased retention of sodium is usually the desired therapeutic effect.

Flumazenil (FLOO may ze nil)

Pharmacologic Category Antidote
Medication Safety Issues
  Sound-alike/look-alike issues:
  Flumazenil may be confused with influenza virus vaccine
Pregnancy Risk Factor C
Lactation Excretion in breast milk unknown/use caution
Breast-Feeding Considerations It is not known if flumazenil is excreted in breast milk. The manufacturer recommends that caution be used if administering to breast-feeding women.
Use Benzodiazepine antagonist; reverses sedative effects of benzodiazepines used in conscious sedation and general anesthesia; treatment of benzodiazepine overdose
Mechanism of Action/Effect Competitively inhibits the activity at the benzodiazepine receptor site on the GABA/benzodiazepine receptor complex. Flumazenil does not antagonize the CNS effect of drugs affecting GABA-ergic neurons by means other than the benzodiazepine receptor (ethanol, barbiturates, general anesthetics) and does not reverse the effects of opioids.

Contraindications Hypersensitivity to flumazenil, benzodiazepines, or any component of the formulation; patients given benzodiazepines for control of potentially life-threatening conditions (eg, control of intracranial pressure or status epilepticus); patients who are showing signs of serious cyclic-antidepressant overdosage

Warnings/Precautions [U.S. Boxed Warning]: Benzodiazepine reversal may result in seizures; seizures may occur more frequently in patients on benzodiazepines for long-term sedation or following tricyclic antidepressant overdose. Dose should be individualized and practitioners should be prepared to manage seizures. Seizures may also develop in patients with concurrent major sedative-hypnotic drug withdrawal, recent therapy with repeated doses of parenteral benzodiazepines, myoclonic jerking or seizure activity prior to flumazenil administration. Use with caution in patients relying on a benzodiazepine for seizure control. May cause CNS depression, which may impair physical or mental abilities; patients must be cautioned about performing tasks which require mental alertness (eg, operating machinery or driving) for 24 hours after discharge.

Flumazenil may not reliably reverse respiratory depression/hypoventilation. Flumazenil is not a substitute for evaluation of oxygenation; establishing an airway and assisting ventilation, as necessary, is always the initial step in overdose management. Resedation occurs more frequently in patients where a large single dose or cumulative dose of a benzodiazepine is administered along with a neuromuscular-blocking agent and multiple anesthetic agents. Flumazenil should be used with caution in the intensive care unit because of increased risk of unrecognized benzodiazepine dependence in such settings. Should not be used to diagnose benzodiazepine-induced sedation. Reverse neuromuscular blockade before considering use. Flumazenil does not antagonize the CNS effects of other GABA agonists (such as ethanol, barbiturates, or general anesthetics); nor does it reverse opioids. Flumazenil does not consistently reverse amnesia; patient may not recall verbal instructions after procedure.

Use with caution in patients with a history of panic disorder; may provoke panic attacks. Use caution in drug and ethanol-dependent patients; these patients may also be dependent on benzodiazepines. Not recommended for treatment of benzodiazepine dependence. Use with caution in patients with a head injury; may alter cerebral blood flow or precipitate convulsions in patients receiving benzodiazepines. Use caution in patients with mixed drug overdoses; toxic effects of other drugs taken may emerge once benzodiazepine effects are reversed. Use caution in hepatic dysfunction; repeated doses of the drug should be reduced in frequency or amount.

Drug Interactions

Avoid Concomitant Use There are no known interactions where it is recommended to avoid concomitant use.

Decreased Effect

Flumazenil may decrease the levels/effects of:
Hypnotics (Nonbenzodiazepine)

Increased Effect/Toxicity There are no known significant interactions involving an increase in effect.

Adverse Reactions

>10%: Gastrointestinal: Vomiting (11%)

1% to 10%:

Cardiovascular: Palpitation (3% to 9%), flushing (1% to 3%), vasodilation (1% to 3%)

Central nervous system: Ataxia (10%), dizziness (10%), vertigo (10%), agitation (3% to 9%), anxiety (3% to 9%), insomnia (3% to 9%), nervousness (3% to 9%), abnormal crying (1% to 3%), depersonalization (1% to 3%), depression (1% to 3%), dysphoria (1% to 3%), emotional lability (1% to 3%), euphoria (1% to 3%), fatigue (1% to 3%), headache (1% to 3%), malaise (1% to 3%), paranoia (1% to 3%)

Endocrine & metabolic: Hot flashes (1% to 3%)

Gastrointestinal: Xerostomia (3% to 9%), nausea (1% to 3%)

Local: Pain at injection site (3% to 9%), injection site reaction (1% to 3%), rash (1% to 3%), skin abnormality (1% to 3%), thrombophlebitis (1% to 3%)

Neuromuscular & skeletal: Hypoesthesia (1% to 3%), paresthesia (1% to 3%), weakness (1% to 3%), tremor

Ocular: Blurred vision (3% to 9%), abnormal vision (1% to 3%), lacrimation (1% to 3%)

Respiratory: Dyspnea (3% to 9%), hyperventilation (3% to 9%)

Miscellaneous: Diaphoresis (1% to 3%)

Pharmacodynamics/Kinetics

Onset of Action 1-2 minutes; 80% response within 3 minutes; Peak effect: 6-10 minutes

Duration of Action Resedation occurs after ~1 hour (range: 19-50 minutes); duration related to dose given and benzodiazepine plasma concentrations; reversal effects of flumazenil may wear off before effects of benzodiazepine

Available Dosage Forms

Solution, Intravenous:

Generic: 0.5 mg/5 mL (5 mL); 1 mg/10 mL (10 mL)

General Dosage Range I.V.:

Children ≥1 year: Initial: 0.01 mg/kg (maximum dose: 0.2 mg), may repeat 0.01 mg/kg (maximum dose: 0.2 mg) as needed (maximum cumulative total: 1 mg or 0.05 mg/kg, whichever is lower)

Adults: Benzodiazepine overdose: Initial: 0.2 mg, may repeat with 0.3 mg, then 0.5 mg (maximum cumulative total dose: 5 mg); Reversal of conscious sedation/general anesthesia: Initial: 0.2 mg, may repeat (maximum total dose: 1 mg)

Administration

I.V. Administer in freely-running I.V. into large vein. Inject over 15 seconds for reversal of conscious sedation and general anesthesia and over 30 seconds for benzodiazepine overdose.

Injectable Detail pH: ~4 (solution in vial)

Storage/Stability Store at 20°C to 25°C (68°F to 77°F). For I.V. use only. Once drawn up in the syringe or mixed with solution use within 24 hours. Discard any unused solution after 24 hours.

Nursing Actions

Physical Assessment Assess level of consciousness frequently. Monitor vital signs and airway closely. Observe continually for resedation, respiratory depression, seizure activity, or other residual benzodiazepine effects.

Patient Education

- Discuss specific use of drug and side effects with patient as it relates to treatment. (HCAHPS: During this hospital stay, were you given any medicine that you had not taken before? Before giving you any new medicine, how often did hospital staff tell you what the medicine was for? How often did hospital staff describe possible side effects in a way you could understand?)

- Patient may experience dizziness, nausea, blurred vision, xerostomia, application site irritation, headache, hyperhidrosis, anxiety, tremors, or insomnia. Have patient report immediately to prescriber dyspnea, tachypnea, tachycardia, arrhythmia, bradycardia, severe headache, angina, considerable asthenia, vision changes, mood changes, change in balance, or paresthesia (HCAHPS).

- Educate patient about signs of a significant reaction (eg, wheezing; chest tightness; fever; itching; bad cough; blue skin color; seizures; or swelling of face, lips, tongue, or throat). **Note:** This is not a comprehensive list of all side effects. Patient should consult prescriber for additional questions.

Intended Use and Disclaimer: Should not be printed and given to patients. This information is intended to serve as a concise initial reference for healthcare professionals to use when discussing medications with a patient. You must ultimately rely on your own discretion, experience and judgment in diagnosing, treating and advising patients.

Dietary Considerations Avoid alcohol for the first 24 hours after administration or as long as the effects of benzodiazepines exist.

Flunisolide (Nasal) (floo NISS oh lide)

Pharmacologic Category Corticosteroid, Nasal

Medication Safety Issues

Sound-alike/look-alike issues:

Flunisolide may be confused with Flumadine®, fluocinonide

Pregnancy Risk Factor C

Lactation Excretion in breast milk unknown/use caution

Use Seasonal or perennial rhinitis

Unlabeled Use Adjunct to antibiotics in empiric treatment of acute bacterial rhinosinusitis (ABRS) (Chow, 2012)

Available Dosage Forms

Solution, Nasal:

Generic: 25 mcg/actuation (0.025%) (25 mL)

General Dosage Range Intranasal:

Children 6-14 years: 1-2 sprays 2-3 times/day (maximum: 4 sprays/day in each nostril)

Children ≥15 years and Adults: 2 sprays twice daily (maximum: 8 sprays/day in each nostril)

Administration

Inhalation Before first use, prime by pressing pump 5-6 times or until a fine spray appears. Repeat priming if ≥5 days between use, or if dissembled for cleaning. Administer at regular intervals. Blow nose to clear nostrils. Insert applicator into nostril, keeping bottle upright, and close off the other nostril. Breathe in through nose. While inhaling, press pump to release spray.

Nursing Actions

Patient Education

- Discuss specific use of drug and side effects with patient as it relates to treatment. (HCAHPS: During this hospital stay, were you given any medicine that you had not taken before? Before giving you any new medicine, how often did hospital staff tell you what the medicine was for? How often did hospital staff describe possible side effects in a way you could understand?)
- Patient may experience sinusitis. Have patient report immediately to prescriber signs of infection, considerable rhinitis, significant epistaxis, nasal sores, severe dizziness, stomatitis, pharyngitis, intolerable nausea, severe asthenia, or vision changes (HCAHPS).
- Educate patient about signs of a significant reaction (eg, wheezing; chest tightness; fever; itching; bad cough; blue skin color; seizures; or swelling of face, lips, tongue, or throat). **Note:** This is not a comprehensive list of all side effects. Patient should consult prescriber for additional questions.

Intended Use and Disclaimer: Should not be printed and given to patients. This information is intended to serve as a concise initial reference for healthcare professionals to use when discussing medications with a patient. You must ultimately rely on your own discretion, experience and judgment in diagnosing, treating and advising patients.

Flunisolide (Oral Inhalation)
(floo NISS oh lide)

Brand Names: U.S. Aerospan

Index Terms AeroBid; Flunisolide Hemihydrate

Pharmacologic Category Corticosteroid, Inhalant (Oral)

Medication Safety Issues

Sound-alike/look-alike issues:

Flunisolide may be confused with Flumadine®, fluocinonide

Pregnancy Risk Factor C

Lactation Excretion in breast milk unknown/use caution

Breast-Feeding Considerations Other corticosteroids have been found in breast milk. It is not known if sufficient quantities of flunisolide are absorbed following inhalation to produce detectable amounts in breast milk. The manufacturer recommends that caution be exercised when administering flunisolide to nursing women. The use of inhaled corticosteroids is not considered a contraindication to breast-feeding (NAEPP, 2005).

Use Maintenance treatment and prophylactic therapy for asthma; to reduce or eliminate the need for oral corticosteroids in steroid-dependent asthma patients

Mechanism of Action/Effect Decreases airway inflammation by suppression of endogenous inflammatory mediators, inhibits inflammatory cell migration, and reverses increased capillary permeability to decrease access of inflammatory cells to the site of inflammation; does not depress hypothalamus

Contraindications Hypersensitivity to flunisolide or any component of the formulation; acute status asthmaticus or other acute asthma episodes

Warnings/Precautions May cause hypercorticism or suppression of hypothalamic-pituitary-adrenal (HPA) axis, particularly in younger children, in patients receiving high doses for prolonged periods, or when used with inhaled or systemic corticosteroids (even alternate-day dosing). HPA axis suppression may lead to adrenal crisis. Withdrawal and discontinuation of a corticosteroid should be done slowly, carefully, and may require several months. Particular care is required when patients are transferred from systemic corticosteroids to inhaled products due to possible adrenal insufficiency or withdrawal from steroids, including an increase in allergic symptoms. Patients receiving >20 mg per day of prednisone (or equivalent) may be most susceptible. Fatalities have occurred due to adrenal insufficiency in asthmatic patients during and after transfer from systemic corticosteroids to aerosol steroids; aerosol steroids do **not** provide the systemic effects needed to treat patients having trauma, surgery, or infections. Do **not** use flunisolide to transfer patients from oral corticosteroid therapy.

Bronchospasm may occur with wheezing after inhalation; if this occurs, treat with a fast-acting bronchodilator. Stop flunisolide therapy and select an alternative agent. Supplemental steroids (oral or parenteral) may be needed during stress or severe asthma attacks. Not to be used in status asthmaticus or for the relief of acute bronchospasm. Corticosteroid use may cause psychiatric disturbances, including depression, euphoria, insomnia, mood swings, and personality changes. Pre-existing psychiatric conditions may be exacerbated by corticosteroid use. Prolonged use of corticosteroids may also increase the incidence of secondary infection, mask acute infection (including fungal infections), prolong or exacerbate viral infections, or limit response to vaccines. Exposure to chickenpox and measles should be avoided; use with caution in patients with ocular herpes simplex. Close observation is required in patients with latent tuberculosis and/or TB reactivity; restrict use in active TB (only in conjunction with antituberculosis treatment). Prolonged treatment with corticosteroids has been associated with the development of Kaposi's sarcoma (case reports); if noted, discontinuation of therapy should be considered.

Use with caution in patients with thyroid disease, hepatic impairment, renal impairment, cardiovascular disease, diabetes, glaucoma, cataracts, myasthenia gravis, patients at risk for osteoporosis, patients at risk for seizures, or GI diseases (diverticulitis, peptic ulcer, ulcerative colitis) due to perforation risk. Use caution following acute MI (corticosteroids have been associated with myocardial rupture). Because of the risk of adverse effects, systemic corticosteroids should be used cautiously in the elderly in the smallest possible effective dose for the shortest duration.

Orally-inhaled corticosteroids may cause a reduction in growth velocity in pediatric patients (~1 centimeter per year [range 0.3-1.8 cm per year] and related to dose and duration of exposure). To minimize the systemic effects of orally-inhaled corticosteroids, each patient should be titrated to the lowest effective dose. Growth should be routinely monitored in pediatric patients. There have been reports of systemic corticosteroid withdrawal symptoms (eg, joint/muscle pain, lassitude, depression) when withdrawing oral inhalation therapy.

Drug Interactions
Avoid Concomitant Use
Avoid concomitant use of Flunisolide (Oral Inhalation) with any of the following: Aldesleukin
Decreased Effect
Flunisolide (Oral Inhalation) may decrease the levels/effects of: Aldesleukin; Antidiabetic Agents; Corticorelin; Hyaluronidase; Telaprevir
Increased Effect/Toxicity
Flunisolide (Oral Inhalation) may increase the levels/effects of: Amphotericin B; Deferasirox; Loop Diuretics; Thiazide Diuretics

The levels/effects of Flunisolide (Oral Inhalation) may be increased by: CYP3A4 Inhibitors (Strong); Telaprevir

Adverse Reactions
>10%:
Central nervous system: Headache (9% to 14%)
Respiratory: Pharyngitis (17% to 18%), rhinitis (4% to 16%)
1% to 10%:
Cardiovascular: Chest pain (1% to 3%), edema (1% to 3%)
Central nervous system: Fever (1% to 7%), pain (2% to 5%), dizziness (1% to 3%), insomnia (1% to 3%), migraine (1% to 3%)
Dermatologic: Rash (2% to 4%), erythema multiforme (1% to 3%)
Endocrine & metabolic: Dysmenorrhea (1% to 3%)
Gastrointestinal: Vomiting (≤5%), dyspepsia (2% to 4%), abdominal pain (1% to 3%), diarrhea (1% to 3%), gastroenteritis (1% to 3%), nausea (1% to 3%), oral moniliasis (1% to 3%), taste perversion (1% to 3%)
Genitourinary: Urinary tract infection (1% to 4%), vaginitis (1% to 3%)
Neuromuscular & skeletal: Back pain (1% to 3%), myalgia (1% to 3%), neck pain (1% to 3%)
Ocular: Conjunctivitis (1% to 3%)
Otic: Ear pain (1% to 3)
Respiratory: Sinusitis (4% to 9%), cough increased (2% to 9%), bronchitis (1% to 3%), laryngitis (1% to 3%), epistaxis (≤3%)
Miscellaneous: Allergic reaction (4% to 5%), bacterial infection (1% to 4%), infection (1% to 3%), voice alteration (1% to 3%)

Product Availability Aerospan®: FDA approved September 2012; availability anticipated in March 2014.

Dosage Forms Considerations
Aerospan 5.1 g canisters contain 60 inhalations and the 8.9 g canisters contain 120 inhalations.

Available Dosage Forms
Aerosol Solution, Inhalation:
Aerospan: 80 mcg/actuation (8.9 g)
General Dosage Range Oral inhalation:
Children 6-11 years: 80 mcg twice daily (maximum: 160 mcg twice daily)
Children ≥12 years, Adolescents, and Adults: 160 mcg twice daily (maximum: 320 mcg twice daily)

Administration
Inhalation Shake well before using. Prime inhaler prior to first use and when the inhaler has not been used for >2 weeks by releasing 2 test sprays away from the face. Rinse mouth following use of oral inhalers. Do not immerse the canister into water to determine remaining amount in the canister (ie, "float test").

Storage/Stability Store at 25°C (77°F); excursions permitted between 15°C to 30°C (59°F to 86°F). Do not puncture; do not use or store near heat or flame. Protect from prolonged sunlight exposure.

Nursing Actions

Physical Assessment Not to be used to treat status asthmaticus. When changing from systemic steroids to inhalational steroid, taper reduction of systemic medication slowly.

Patient Education
- Discuss specific use of drug and side effects with patient as it relates to treatment. (HCAHPS: During this hospital stay, were you given any medicine that you had not taken before? Before giving you any new medicine, how often did hospital staff tell you what the medicine was for? How often did hospital staff describe possible side effects in a way you could understand?)
- Patient may experience rhinitis or rhinorrhea. Have patient report immediately to prescriber signs of infection, fatigue, irritability, tremors, tachycardia, confusion, diaphoresis, dizziness, stomatitis, pharyngitis, dyspnea, excessive weight gain, edema of extremities, severe headache, arrhythmia, angina, tachycardia, menstrual irregularities, arthralgia, osteodynia, considerable asthenia, vision changes, mood changes, behavioral changes, or depression (HCAHPS).
- Educate patient about signs of a significant reaction (eg, wheezing; chest tightness; fever; itching; bad cough; blue skin color; seizures; or swelling of face, lips, tongue, or throat). **Note:** This is not a comprehensive list of all side effects. Patient should consult prescriber for additional questions.

Intended Use and Disclaimer: Should not be printed and given to patients. This information is intended to serve as a concise initial reference for healthcare professionals to use when discussing medications with a patient. You must ultimately rely on your own discretion, experience and judgment in diagnosing, treating and advising patients.

Fluocinolone (Otic) (floo oh SIN oh lone)

Brand Names: U.S. DermOtic
Index Terms Fluocinolone Acetonide
Pharmacologic Category Corticosteroid, Otic
Medication Safety Issues
  Sound-alike/look-alike issues:
  Fluocinolone may be confused with fluocinonide
Pregnancy Risk Factor C
Lactation Excretion in breast milk unknown/use caution
Use Relief of chronic eczematous external otitis
Available Dosage Forms
  Oil, Otic:
    DermOtic: 0.01% (20 mL)
    Generic: 0.01% (20 mL)
General Dosage Range Otic: *Children ≥2 years and Adults:* 5 drops into affected ear twice daily

Nursing Actions

Patient Education
- Discuss specific use of drug and side effects with patient as it relates to treatment. (HCAHPS: During this hospital stay, were you given any medicine that you had not taken before? Before giving you any new medicine, how often did hospital staff tell you what the medicine was for? How often did hospital staff describe possible side effects in a way you could understand?)
- Have patient report immediately to prescriber signs of hyperglycemia or severe skin irritation (HCAHPS).
- Educate patient about signs of a significant reaction (eg, wheezing; chest tightness; fever; itching; bad cough; blue skin color; seizures; or swelling of face, lips, tongue, or throat). **Note:** This is not a comprehensive list of all side effects. Patient should consult prescriber for additional questions.

Intended Use and Disclaimer: Should not be printed and given to patients. This information is intended to serve as a concise initial reference for healthcare professionals to use when discussing medications with a patient. You must ultimately rely on your own discretion, experience and judgment in diagnosing, treating and advising patients.

Fluocinolone (Topical) (floo oh SIN oh lone)

Brand Names: U.S. Capex; Derma-Smoothe/FS Body; Derma-Smoothe/FS Scalp; Fluocinolone Acetonide Body; Fluocinolone Acetonide Scalp; Synalar; Synalar (Cream); Synalar (Ointment); Synalar TS
Index Terms Fluocinolone Acetonide
Pharmacologic Category Corticosteroid, Topical
Medication Safety Issues
  Sound-alike/look-alike issues:
  Fluocinolone may be confused with fluocinonide
Pregnancy Risk Factor C
Lactation Excretion in breast milk unknown/use caution
Use Relief of susceptible inflammatory dermatosis (low, medium corticosteroid); dermatitis or psoriasis of the scalp; atopic dermatitis in adults and children ≥3 months of age
Available Dosage Forms
  Cream, External:
    Synalar: 0.025% (120 g)
    Generic: 0.01% (15 g, 60 g); 0.025% (15 g, 60 g)
  Kit, External:
    Synalar (Cream): 0.025%
    Synalar (Ointment): 0.025%
    Synalar TS: 0.01%

◀ **Oil, External**:
Derma-Smoothe/FS Body: 0.01% (118.28 mL)
Derma-Smoothe/FS Scalp: 0.01% (118.28 mL)
Fluocinolone Acetonide Body: 0.01% (118.28 mL)
Fluocinolone Acetonide Scalp: 0.01% (118.28 mL)

Ointment, External:
Synalar: 0.025% (120 g)
Generic: 0.025% (15 g, 60 g)

Shampoo, External:
Capex: 0.01% (120 mL)

Solution, External:
Synalar: 0.01% (60 mL, 90 mL)
Generic: 0.01% (60 mL)

General Dosage Range Topical:
Children ≥3 months: Apply a thin layer to affected area 2-4 times/day
Adults: Body: Apply thin layer to affected area 2-4 times/day; Scalp: 1 ounce daily (Capex®) **or** massage into wet hair and leave on for at least 4 hours (Derma-Smoothe/FS®)

Administration
Topical Apply thin film to affected area; avoid eyes.

Nursing Actions
Patient Education
• Discuss specific use of drug and side effects with patient as it relates to treatment. (HCAHPS: During this hospital stay, were you given any medicine that you had not taken before? Before giving you any new medicine, how often did hospital staff tell you what the medicine was for? How often did hospital staff describe possible side effects in a way you could understand?)
• Patient may experience xeroderma. Have patient report immediately to prescriber signs of hyperglycemia, skin changes, or severe skin irritation (HCAHPS).
• Educate patient about signs of a significant reaction (eg, wheezing; chest tightness; fever; itching; bad cough; blue skin color; seizures; or swelling of face, lips, tongue, or throat). **Note:** This is not a comprehensive list of all side effects. Patient should consult prescriber for additional questions.

Intended Use and Disclaimer: Should not be printed and given to patients. This information is intended to serve as a concise initial reference for healthcare professionals to use when discussing medications with a patient. You must ultimately rely on your own discretion, experience and judgment in diagnosing, treating and advising patients.

Fluocinonide (floo oh SIN oh nide)

Brand Names: U.S. Vanos
Index Terms Lidex
Pharmacologic Category Corticosteroid, Topical

Medication Safety Issues
Sound-alike/look-alike issues:
Fluocinonide may be confused with flunisolide, fluocinolone
Lidex® may be confused with Lasix®, Videx®

Pregnancy Risk Factor C
Lactation Excretion unknown/not recommended
Use Anti-inflammatory, antipruritic; treatment of plaque-type psoriasis (up to 10% of body surface area) [high-potency topical corticosteroid]

Available Dosage Forms
Cream, External:
Vanos: 0.1% (30 g, 60 g, 120 g)
Generic: 0.05% (15 g, 30 g, 60 g, 120 g); 0.1% (30 g, 60 g, 120 g)

Gel, External:
Generic: 0.05% (15 g, 30 g, 60 g)

Ointment, External:
Generic: 0.05% (15 g, 30 g, 60 g)

Solution, External:
Generic: 0.05% (20 mL, 60 mL)

General Dosage Range Topical:
Children <12 years: Apply thin layer of 0.05% cream to affected area 2-4 times/day
Children ≥12 years and Adults: Apply thin layer of 0.05% cream to affected area 2-4 times/day **or** apply a thin layer of 0.1% cream once or twice daily to affected area

Nursing Actions
Patient Education
• Discuss specific use of drug and side effects with patient as it relates to treatment. (HCAHPS: During this hospital stay, were you given any medicine that you had not taken before? Before giving you any new medicine, how often did hospital staff tell you what the medicine was for? How often did hospital staff describe possible side effects in a way you could understand?)
• Patient may experience xeroderma. Have patient report immediately to prescriber signs of hyperglycemia, skin changes, severe skin irritation, signs of weak adrenal gland, or signs of Cushing's disease (HCAHPS).
• Educate patient about signs of a significant reaction (eg, wheezing; chest tightness; fever; itching; bad cough; blue skin color; seizures; or swelling of face, lips, tongue, or throat). **Note:** This is not a comprehensive list of all side effects. Patient should consult prescriber for additional questions.

Intended Use and Disclaimer: Should not be printed and given to patients. This information is intended to serve as a concise initial reference for healthcare professionals to use when discussing medications with a patient. You must ultimately rely on your own discretion, experience and judgment in diagnosing, treating and advising patients.

Fluorometholone (flure oh METH oh lone)

Brand Names: U.S. Flarex; FML; FML Forte; FML Liquifilm

Pharmacologic Category Corticosteroid, Ophthalmic

Medication Safety Issues

International issues:

Flarex [U.S., Canada, and multiple international markets] may be confused with Fluarix brand name for influenza virus vaccine (inactivated) [U.S. and multiple international markets] and Fluorex brand name for fluoride [France]

Pregnancy Risk Factor C

Lactation Excretion in breast milk unknown/not recommended

Use Treatment of steroid-responsive inflammatory conditions of the eye

Available Dosage Forms

Ointment, Ophthalmic:

FML: 0.1% (3.5 g)

Suspension, Ophthalmic:

Flarex: 0.1% (5 mL)

FML Forte: 0.25% (5 mL, 10 mL)

FML Liquifilm: 0.1% (5 mL, 10 mL)

Generic: 0.1% (5 mL, 10 mL, 15 mL)

General Dosage Range Ophthalmic:

Ointment: *Children ≥2 years, Adolescents, and Adults:* Apply small amount (~1/2" ribbon) every 4 hours (initial: 24-48 hours) **or** 1-3 times daily

Suspension:

Children ≥2 years, Adolescents, and Adults (FML®, FML® Forte): Instill 1 drop every 4 hours (initial: 24-48 hours) **or** 1 drop 2-4 times daily

Adults (Flarex®): Instill 2 drops (initial: 24-48 hours) **or** 1-2 drops 2-4 times daily

Administration

Ophthalmic Wash hands prior to use. Do not touch tip of container to eye. Contact lenses should be removed before instillation; do not reinsert contact lenses within 15 minutes of fluorometholone eye drops. Shake suspension well before use.

Nursing Actions

Physical Assessment Monitor intraocular pressure in patients with glaucoma or when used for ≥10 days; monitor for presence of secondary infections (including the development of fungal infections and exacerbation of viral infections).

Patient Education

• Discuss specific use of drug and side effects with patient as it relates to treatment. (HCAHPS: During this hospital stay, were you given any medicine that you had not taken before? Before giving you any new medicine, how often did hospital staff tell you what the medicine was for? How often did hospital staff describe possible side effects in a way you could understand?)

• Have patient report immediately to prescriber vision changes, ophthalmalgia, or severe eye irritation (HCAHPS).

• Educate patient about signs of a significant reaction (eg, wheezing; chest tightness; fever; itching; bad cough; blue skin color; seizures; or swelling of face, lips, tongue, or throat). **Note:** This is not a comprehensive list of all side effects. Patient should consult prescriber for additional questions.

Intended Use and Disclaimer: Should not be printed and given to patients. This information is intended to serve as a concise initial reference for healthcare professionals to use when discussing medications with a patient. You must ultimately rely on your own discretion, experience and judgment in diagnosing, treating and advising patients.

Fluorouracil (Systemic) (flure oh YOOR a sil)

Brand Names: U.S. Adrucil

Index Terms 5-Fluorouracil; 5-Fluracil; 5-FU; Fluoro Uracil; Fluouracil; FU

Pharmacologic Category Antineoplastic Agent, Antimetabolite; Antineoplastic Agent, Antimetabolite (Pyrimidine Analog)

Medication Safety Issues

Sound-alike/look-alike issues:

Fluorouracil may be confused with floxuridine, flucytosine

High alert medication:

This medication is in a class the Institute for Safe Medication Practices (ISMP) includes among its list of drug classes which have a heightened risk of causing significant patient harm when used in error.

Pregnancy Risk Factor D

Lactation Excretion in breast milk unknown/not recommended

Breast-Feeding Considerations Based on the mechanism of action, the manufacturer's labeling recommends against breast-feeding if receiving fluorouracil.

Use Treatment of breast cancer, colon cancer, rectal cancer, pancreatic cancer, and stomach (gastric) cancer

Unlabeled Use Treatment of anal cancer, bladder cancer, cervical cancer, esophageal cancer, head and neck cancer, hepatobiliary cancers, neuroendocrine tumors, penile cancer (metastatic), thymic cancers, and unknown primary cancer

Mechanism of Action/Effect A pyrimidine analog antimetabolite that interferes with DNA and RNA synthesis; active metabolite F-UMP is incorporated into RNA to replace uracil and inhibit cell growth; active metabolite F-dUMP inhibits thymidylate synthetase, depleting thymidine triphosphate (a necessary component of DNA synthesis).

▶

Contraindications Hypersensitivity to fluorouracil or any component of the formulation; poor nutritional states; depressed bone marrow function; potentially serious infections

Warnings/Precautions Hazardous agent - use appropriate precautions for handling and disposal (NIOSH, 2012). Use with caution in patients with impaired kidney or liver function. Discontinue if intractable vomiting or diarrhea, precipitous falls in leukocyte or platelet counts, gastrointestinal ulcer or bleeding, stomatitis, or esophagopharyngitis, hemorrhage, or myocardial ischemia occurs. Use with caution in poor-risk patients who have had high-dose pelvic radiation or previous use of alkylating agents and in patients with widespread metastatic marrow involvement. Palmar-plantar erythrodysesthesia (hand-foot) syndrome has been associated with use (symptoms include a tingling sensation, which may progress to pain, and then to symmetrical swelling and erythema with tenderness; desquamation may occur; with treatment interruption, generally resolves over 5-7 days).

Administration to patients with a genetic deficiency of dihydropyrimidine dehydrogenase (DPD) has been associated with prolonged clearance and increased toxicity (diarrhea, neutropenia, and neurotoxicity) following administration; rechallenge has resulted in recurrent toxicity (despite dose reduction). **[U.S. Boxed Warning]: Should be administered under the supervision of an experienced cancer chemotherapy physician; the manufacturer's labeling recommends hospitalizing patients during the first treatment course due to the potential for severe toxicity.**

Drug Interactions

Avoid Concomitant Use
Avoid concomitant use of Fluorouracil (Systemic) with any of the following: BCG; CloZAPine; Gimeracil; Natalizumab; Pimecrolimus; Tacrolimus (Topical); Tofacitinib; Vaccines (Live)

Decreased Effect
Fluorouracil (Systemic) may decrease the levels/effects of: BCG; Coccidioidin Skin Test; Sipuleucel-T; Vaccines (Inactivated); Vaccines (Live); Vitamin K Antagonists

The levels/effects of Fluorouracil (Systemic) may be decreased by: Echinacea; SORAfenib

Increased Effect/Toxicity
Fluorouracil (Systemic) may increase the levels/effects of: Bosentan; Carvedilol; CloZAPine; CYP2C9 Substrates; Diclofenac (Systemic); Fosphenytoin; Lacosamide; Leflunomide; Natalizumab; Ospemifene; Phenytoin; Tofacitinib; Vaccines (Live); Vitamin K Antagonists

The levels/effects of Fluorouracil (Systemic) may be increased by: Cimetidine; Denosumab; Gemcitabine; Gimeracil; Leucovorin Calcium-Levoleucovorin; MetroNIDAZOLE (Systemic); Pimecrolimus; Roflumilast; SORAfenib; Tacrolimus (Topical); Trastuzumab

Nutritional/Ethanol Interactions
Ethanol: Avoid ethanol (due to GI irritation).
Herb/Nutraceutical: Avoid black cohosh, dong quai in estrogen-dependent tumors.

Adverse Reactions Toxicity depends on duration of treatment and/or rate of administration
Cardiovascular: Angina, arrhythmia, heart failure, MI, myocardial ischemia, vasospasm, ventricular ectopy
Central nervous system: Acute cerebellar syndrome, confusion, disorientation, euphoria, headache, nystagmus, stroke
Dermatologic: Alopecia, dermatitis, dry skin, fissuring, nail changes (nail loss), palmar-plantar erythrodysesthesia syndrome, pruritic maculopapular rash, photosensitivity, Stevens-Johnson syndrome, toxic epidermal necrolysis, vein pigmentation
Gastrointestinal: Anorexia, bleeding, diarrhea, esophagopharyngitis, mesenteric ischemia (acute), nausea, sloughing, stomatitis, ulceration, vomiting
Hematologic: Agranulocytosis, anemia, leukopenia (nadir: days 9-14; recovery by day 30), pancytopenia, thrombocytopenia
Local: Thrombophlebitis
Ocular: Lacrimation, lacrimal duct stenosis, photophobia, visual changes
Respiratory: Epistaxis
Miscellaneous: Anaphylaxis, generalized allergic reactions

Available Dosage Forms
Solution, Intravenous:
Adrucil: 500 mg/10 mL (10 mL); 2.5 g/50 mL (50 mL); 5 g/100 mL (100 mL)
Generic: 500 mg/10 mL (10 mL); 1 g/20 mL (20 mL); 2.5 g/50 mL (50 mL); 5 g/100 mL (100 mL)

General Dosage Range Dosage adjustment recommended in patients with hepatic or renal impairment or who develop toxicities
I.V.: *Adults:* Dosage varies greatly depending on indication

Administration
I.V. Administration rate varies by protocol; refer to specific reference for protocol. May be administered by I.V. push, I.V. bolus, or as a continuous infusion. Avoid extravasation (may be an irritant).

Hazardous agent; use appropriate precautions for handling and disposal (NIOSH, 2012).

Injectable Detail pH: 8.6-9.4 (50 mg/mL solution in vial)

Preparation for Administration Hazardous agent; use appropriate precautions for handling and disposal (NIOSH, 2012). May dispense in a syringe or dilute in 50-1000 mL NS or D_5W for infusion.

Storage/Stability Store intact vials at room temperature. Do not refrigerate or freeze. Protect from light. Slight discoloration may occur during storage; does not usually denote decomposition. If exposed to cold, a precipitate may form; **gentle** heating to 60°C (140°F) will dissolve the precipitate without impairing the potency. According to the manufacturer, pharmacy bulk vials should be used within 4 hours of initial entry. Solutions for infusion should be used promptly. Fluorouracil 50 mg/mL in NS was stable in polypropylene infusion pump syringes for 7 days when stored at 30°C (86°F) (Stiles, 1996). Stability of fluorouracil 1 mg/mL or 10 mg/mL in NS or D$_5$W in PVC bags was demonstrated for up to 14 days at 4°C (39.2°F) and 21°C (69.8°F) (Martel, 1996). Stability of undiluted fluorouracil (50 mg/mL) in ethylene-vinyl acetate ambulatory pump reservoirs was demonstrated for 3 days at 4°C (39.2°F) (precipitate formed after 3 days) and for 14 days at 33°C (91.4°F) (Martel, 1996). Stability of undiluted fluorouracil (50 mg/mL) in PVC ambulatory pump reservoirs was demonstrated for 5 days at 4°C (39.2°F) (precipitate formed after 5 days) and for 14 days at 33°C (91.4°F) (Martel, 1996).

Nursing Actions

Physical Assessment Instruct patient to report symptoms of mouth sores, nausea, vomiting, diarrhea, or numbness, pain, or tingling in hands or feet. Patients need to have labs monitored frequently. Oral cryotherapy may help in preventing oral mucositis with bolus fluorouracil. Instruct patients in the importance of good oral hygiene and hydration. Monitor patients for palmar-plantar erythema. Use good emollient to help decrease friction. Teach patients to report diarrhea as GI side effects may be dose-limiting. Instruct patients to avoid lengthy sun exposure; wear appropriate clothing and sunscreen. Patients should not receive live vaccinations.

Patient Education

• Discuss specific use of drug and side effects with patient as it relates to treatment. (HCAHPS: During this hospital stay, were you given any medicine that you had not taken before? Before giving you any new medicine, how often did hospital staff tell you what the medicine was for? How often did hospital staff describe possible side effects in a way you could understand?)

• Patient may experience lack of appetite, alopecia, or nail changes. Have patient report immediately to prescriber signs of infection, arrhythmia, angina, severe dyspepsia, considerable nausea, significant diarrhea, intolerable edema of hands or feet, signs of hemorrhaging, stomatitis, urine discoloration, jaundice, severe asthenia, inability to eat, vision changes, injection site irritation, or eczema of hands or feet. (HCAHPS).

• Educate patient about signs of a significant reaction (eg, wheezing; chest tightness; fever; itching; bad cough; blue skin color; seizures; or swelling of face, lips, tongue, or throat). **Note:** This is not a comprehensive list of all side effects. Patient should consult prescriber for additional questions.

Intended Use and Disclaimer: Should not be printed and given to patients. This information is intended to serve as a concise initial reference for healthcare professionals to use when discussing medications with a patient. You must ultimately rely on your own discretion, experience and judgment in diagnosing, treating and advising patients.

Dietary Considerations Increase dietary intake of thiamine.

Related Information

Management of Drug Extravasations *on page 1700*

FLUoxetine (floo OKS e teen)

Brand Names: U.S. PROzac; PROzac Weekly; Sarafem

Index Terms Fluoxetine Hydrochloride

Pharmacologic Category Antidepressant, Selective Serotonin Reuptake Inhibitor

Medication Safety Issues

Sound-alike/look-alike issues:

FLUoxetine may be confused with DULoxetine, famotidine, Feldene, fluconazole, fluvastatin, fluvoxaMINE, fosinopril, furosemide, PARoxetine, thiothixene, vortioxetine

PROzac may be confused with Paxil, Prelone, PriLOSEC, Prograf, Proscar, ProSom, Provera

Sarafem may be confused with Serophene

BEERS Criteria medication:

This drug may be potentially inappropriate for use in geriatric patients (Quality of evidence - moderate; Strength of recommendation - strong).

International issues:

Reneuron [Spain] may be confused with Remeron brand name for mirtazapine [U.S., Canada, and multiple international markets]

Medication Guide Available Yes

Pregnancy Risk Factor C

Lactation Enters breast milk/not recommended

Breast-Feeding Considerations Fluoxetine and its metabolite are excreted into breast milk and can be detected in the serum of breast-feeding infants. Concentrations in breast milk are variable. In comparison to other SSRIs, fluoxetine concentrations in breast milk are higher and adverse events have been observed in nursing infants. Maternal use of an SSRI during pregnancy may cause delayed milk secretion. Breast-feeding is not recommended by the manufacturer. Long-term effects on development and behavior have not been studied.

Use Treatment of major depressive disorder (MDD); treatment of binge-eating and vomiting in patients with moderate-to-severe bulimia nervosa;

obsessive-compulsive disorder (OCD); premenstrual dysphoric disorder (PMDD); panic disorder with or without agoraphobia; in combination with olanzapine for treatment-resistant or bipolar I depression

Unlabeled Use Selective mutism; post-traumatic stress disorder (PTSD); social anxiety disorder; fibromyalgia; Raynaud phenomenon

Mechanism of Action/Effect Inhibits CNS neuron serotonin reuptake; minimal or no effect on reuptake of norepinephrine or dopamine; does not significantly bind to alpha-adrenergic, histamine or cholinergic receptors

Contraindications Hypersensitivity to fluoxetine or any component of the formulation; use of MAO inhibitors intended to treat psychiatric disorders (concurrently, within 5 weeks of discontinuing fluoxetine, or within 2 weeks of discontinuing the MAO inhibitor); initiation of fluoxetine in a patient receiving linezolid or intravenous methylene blue; use with pimozide or thioridazine (**Note:** Thioridazine should not be initiated until 5 weeks after the discontinuation of fluoxetine)

Warnings/Precautions [U.S. Boxed Warning]: Antidepressants increase the risk of suicidal thinking and behavior in children, adolescents, and young adults (18-24 years of age) with major depressive disorder (MDD) and other psychiatric disorders; consider risk prior to prescribing. Short-term studies did not show an increased risk in patients >24 years of age and showed a decreased risk in patients ≥65 years. Closely monitor all patients for clinical worsening, suicidality, or unusual changes in behavior, particularly during the initial 1-2 months of therapy or during periods of dosage adjustments (increases or decreases); the patient's family or caregiver should be instructed to closely observe the patient and communicate condition with healthcare provider. A medication guide concerning the use of antidepressants should be dispensed with each prescription. **Fluoxetine is FDA approved for the treatment of OCD in children ≥7 years of age and MDD in children ≥8 years of age.**

The possibility of a suicide attempt is inherent in major depression and may persist until remission occurs. Use caution in high-risk patients. Worsening depression and severe abrupt suicidality that are not part of the presenting symptoms may require discontinuation or modification of drug therapy. Prescriptions should be written for the smallest quantity consistent with good patient care. The patient's family or caregiver should be alerted to monitor patients for the emergence of suicidality and associated behaviors (such as agitation, irritability, hostility, impulsivity, and hypomania) and call healthcare provider.

May worsen psychosis in some patients or precipitate a shift to mania or hypomania in patients with bipolar disorder. Patients presenting with depressive symptoms should be screened for bipolar disorder. Monotherapy in patients with bipolar disorder should be avoided. **Fluoxetine monotherapy is not FDA approved for the treatment of bipolar depression.** May cause insomnia, anxiety, nervousness, or anorexia. Use with caution in patients where weight loss is undesirable. May impair cognitive or motor performance; caution operating hazardous machinery or driving.

QT prolongation and ventricular arrhythmia including torsade de pointes has occurred. Use with caution in patients with risk factors for QT prolongation, under conditions that predispose to arrhythmias, or increased fluoxetine exposure. Consider discontinuation of fluoxetine if ventricular arrhythmia suspected and initiate cardiac evaluation. Avoid concurrent use with other medications that increase QT interval.

Potentially life-threatening serotonin syndrome (SS) has occurred with serotonergic agents (eg, SSRIs, SNRIs), particularly when used in combination with other serotonergic agents (eg, triptans, TCAs, fentanyl, lithium, tramadol, buspirone, St John's wort, tryptophan) or agents that impair metabolism of serotonin (eg, MAO inhibitors intended to treat psychiatric disorders, other MAO inhibitors [ie, linezolid and intravenous methylene blue]). Discontinue treatment (and any concomitant serotonergic agent) immediately if signs/symptoms arise. Fluoxetine use has been associated with occurrences of significant rash and allergic events, including vasculitis, lupus-like syndrome, laryngospasm, anaphylactoid reactions, and pulmonary inflammatory disease. Discontinue if underlying cause of rash cannot be identified.

Use caution in patients with a previous seizure disorder or condition predisposing to seizures such as brain damage, alcoholism, or concurrent therapy with other drugs which lower the seizure threshold. Use with caution in patients with hepatic or severe renal dysfunction and in elderly patients. Use caution in elderly patients; may cause or exacerbate syndrome of inappropriate antidiuretic hormone secretion or hyponatremia; monitor sodium closely with initiation or dosage adjustments in older adults (Beers Criteria). May also cause agitation, sleep disturbances, and excessive CNS stimulation. May cause hyponatremia/SIADH (elderly at increased risk); volume depletion (diuretics may increase risk). May increase the risks associated with electroconvulsive treatment. Use caution with history of MI or unstable heart disease; use in these patients is limited. May alter glycemic control in patients with diabetes. Due to the long half-life of fluoxetine and its metabolites, the effects and interactions noted may persist for prolonged periods following discontinuation. May cause or exacerbate sexual dysfunction. May cause mydriasis; use caution in patients at risk of acute narrow-angle glaucoma or with increased intraocular pressure. Bone fractures have been associated with antidepressant treatment. Consider the possibility of a fragility fracture if an antidepressant-treated patient presents with unexplained bone pain, point tenderness, swelling, or bruising (Rabenda, 2013; Rizzoli, 2012). Potentially significant drug-drug interactions may exist, requiring dose or frequency adjustment, additional monitoring, and/or selection of alternative therapy.

Abrupt discontinuation or interruption of antidepressant therapy has been associated with a discontinuation syndrome. Symptoms arising may vary with antidepressant however commonly include nausea, vomiting, diarrhea, headaches, light-headedness, dizziness, diminished appetite, sweating, chills, tremors, paresthesias, fatigue, somnolence, and sleep disturbances (eg, vivid dreams, insomnia). Greater risks for developing a discontinuation syndrome have been associated with antidepressants with shorter half-lives, longer durations of treatment, and abrupt discontinuation. For antidepressants of short or intermediate half-lives, symptoms may emerge within 2-5 days after treatment discontinuation and last 7-14 days (APA, 2010; Fava, 2006; Haddad, 2001; Shelton, 2001; Warner, 2006).

Drug Interactions

Avoid Concomitant Use

Avoid concomitant use of FLUoxetine with any of the following: Dosulepin; Haloperidol; Highest Risk QTc-Prolonging Agents; Iobenguane I 123; Ivabradine; Linezolid; MAO Inhibitors; Methylene Blue; Mifepristone; Moderate Risk QTc-Prolonging Agents; Pimozide; Propafenone; Tamoxifen; Thioridazine; Tryptophan; Urokinase; Ziprasidone

Decreased Effect

FLUoxetine may decrease the levels/effects of: Clopidogrel; Codeine; Iloperidone; Iobenguane I 123; Ioflupane I 123; Tamoxifen; Thyroid Products; TraMADol

The levels/effects of FLUoxetine may be decreased by: CarBAMazepine; CYP2C9 Inducers (Strong); Cyproheptadine; Dabrafenib; NSAID (COX-2 Inhibitor); NSAID (Nonselective); Peginterferon Alfa-2b

Increased Effect/Toxicity

FLUoxetine may increase the levels/effects of: Agents with Antiplatelet Properties; Anticoagulants; Antidepressants (Serotonin Reuptake Inhibitor/Antagonist); Antipsychotics; ARIPiprazole; Aspirin; AtoMOXetine; Benzodiazepines (metabolized by oxidation); Beta-Blockers; BusPIRone; CarBAMazepine; CloZAPine; Collagenase (Systemic); CYP2C19 Substrates; CYP2D6 Substrates; Dabigatran Etexilate; Desmopressin; Dextromethorphan; Dosulepin; DOXOrubicin (Conventional); Fesoterodine; Fosphenytoin; Galantamine; Haloperidol; Highest Risk QTc-Prolonging Agents; Hypoglycemic Agents; Ibritumomab; Iloperidone; Methadone;

Methylene Blue; Metoclopramide; Metoprolol; Mexiletine; Nebivolol; NIFEdipine; NiMODipine; NSAID (COX-2 Inhibitor); NSAID (Nonselective); Phenytoin; Pimozide; Propafenone; QuiNIDine; RisperiDONE; Rivaroxaban; Salicylates; Serotonin Modulators; Tetrabenazine; Thiazide Diuretics; Thioridazine; Thrombolytic Agents; Tositumomab and Iodine I 131 Tositumomab; TraMADol; Tricyclic Antidepressants; Urokinase; Vitamin K Antagonists; Vortioxetine; Ziprasidone

The levels/effects of FLUoxetine may be increased by: Abiraterone Acetate; Alcohol (Ethyl); Analgesics (Opioid); Antipsychotics; ARIPiprazole; BuPROPion; BusPIRone; Cimetidine; CNS Depressants; Cobicistat; CYP2C9 Inhibitors (Moderate); CYP2C9 Inhibitors (Strong); CYP2D6 Inhibitors (Moderate); CYP2D6 Inhibitors (Strong); Darunavir; Dasatinib; Fosphenytoin; Glucosamine; Herbs (Anticoagulant/Antiplatelet Properties); Ibrutinib; Ivabradine; Linezolid; Lithium; Macrolide Antibiotics; MAO Inhibitors; Metoclopramide; Metyrosine; Mifepristone; Moderate Risk QTc-Prolonging Agents; Multivitamins/Fluoride (with ADE); Multivitamins/Minerals (with ADEK, Folate, Iron); Multivitamins/Minerals (with AE, No Iron); Omega-3 Fatty Acids; Pentosan Polysulfate Sodium; Pentoxifylline; Propafenone; Prostacyclin Analogues; QTc-Prolonging Agents (Indeterminate Risk and Risk Modifying); Tipranavir; TraMADol; Tryptophan; Vitamin E; Ziprasidone

Nutritional/Ethanol Interactions

Ethanol: May increase CNS depression; monitor for increased effects with coadministration. Caution patients about effects.

Herb/Nutraceutical: Avoid valerian, St John's wort, tryptophan, kava kava, gotu kola (may increase CNS depression and/or risk of serotonin syndrome).

Adverse Reactions

Percentages listed for adverse effects as reported in placebo-controlled trials and were generally similar in adults and children; actual frequency may be dependent upon diagnosis and in some cases the range presented may be lower than or equal to placebo for a particular disorder.

>10%:

Central nervous system: Insomnia (10% to 33%), headache (21%), somnolence (5% to 17%), anxiety (6% to 15%), nervousness (8% to 14%)

Endocrine & metabolic: Libido decreased (1% to 11%)

Gastrointestinal: Nausea (12% to 29%), diarrhea (8% to 18%), anorexia (4% to 17%), xerostomia (4% to 12%)

Neuromuscular & skeletal: Weakness (7% to 21%), tremor (3% to 13%)

Respiratory: Pharyngitis (3% to 11%), yawn (≤11%)

1% to 10%:
Cardiovascular: Vasodilation (1% to 5%), chest pain, hemorrhage, hypertension, palpitation
Central nervous system: Dizziness (9%), abnormal dreams (1% to 5%), abnormal thinking (2%), agitation, amnesia, chills, confusion, emotional lability, sleep disorder
Dermatologic: Rash (2% to 6%), pruritus (4%)
Endocrine & metabolic: Ejaculation abnormal (≤7%), impotence (≤7%), menorrhagia (≥2%)
Gastrointestinal: Dyspepsia (6% to 10%), constipation (5%), flatulence (3%), vomiting (3%), thirst (≥2%), weight loss (2%), appetite increased, taste perversion, weight gain
Genitourinary: Urinary frequency
Neuromuscular & skeletal: Hyperkinesia (≥2%)
Ocular: Vision abnormal (2%)
Otic: Ear pain, tinnitus
Respiratory: Sinusitis (1% to 6%)
Miscellaneous: Flu-like syndrome (3% to 10%), diaphoresis (2% to 8%), epistaxis (≥2%)

Pharmacodynamics/Kinetics

Onset of Action Depression: The onset of action is within a week; however, individual response varies greatly and full response may not be seen until 8-12 weeks after initiation of treatment.

Available Dosage Forms

Capsule, Oral:
PROzac: 10 mg, 20 mg, 40 mg
Generic: 10 mg, 20 mg, 40 mg
Capsule Delayed Release, Oral:
PROzac Weekly: 90 mg
Generic: 90 mg
Solution, Oral:
Generic: 20 mg/5 mL (5 mL, 120 mL)
Tablet, Oral:
Sarafem: 10 mg, 20 mg
Generic: 10 mg, 20 mg, 60 mg

General Dosage Range Dosage adjustment recommended in patients with hepatic impairment

Oral:
Children 7-18 years: Initial: 10-20 mg once daily; Maintenance: 10-60 mg once daily
Adults: 10-80 mg once daily **or** 90 mg once weekly
Elderly: 10 mg/day

Administration

Oral Administer without regard to meals.
Bipolar I disorder and treatment-resistant depression: Take once daily in the evening.
Major depressive disorder and obsessive compulsive disorder: Once daily doses should be taken in the morning, or twice daily (morning and noon).
Bulimia: Take once daily in the morning.

Storage/Stability All dosage forms should be stored at controlled room temperature. Protect from light.

Nursing Actions

Physical Assessment Assess therapeutic response (eg, mental status, mode, affect) at beginning of therapy and periodically throughout. Monitor for CNS and gastrointestinal disturbances. Taper dosage slowly when discontinuing. Assess mental status for depression, signs of clinical worsening, suicide ideation, anxiety, social functioning, mania, or panic attack.

Patient Education
• Discuss specific use of drug and side effects with patient as it relates to treatment. (HCAHPS: During this hospital stay, were you given any medicine that you had not taken before? Before giving you any new medicine, how often did hospital staff tell you what the medicine was for? How often did hospital staff describe possible side effects in a way you could understand?)
• Patient may experience dyspepsia, lack of appetite, xerostomia, fatigue, sexual dysfunction, nightmares, insomnia, asthenia, flu-like syndrome, or oscitation. Have patient report immediately to prescriber signs of hyponatremia, signs of hemorrhaging, signs of depression (ie, suicidal ideation, anxiety, emotional instability, illogical thinking), behavioral changes, syncope, vision changes, excessive weight gain or loss, serotonin syndrome (ie, considerable dizziness, severe headache, agitation, hallucinations, tachycardia, arrhythmia, flushing, tremors, hyperhidrosis, change in balance, illogical thinking, severe nausea, significant diarrhea), priapism, oliguria, urine discoloration, stool discoloration, jaundice, or dyspnea (HCAHPS).
• Educate patient about signs of a significant reaction (eg, wheezing; chest tightness; fever; itching; bad cough; blue skin color; seizures; or swelling of face, lips, tongue, or throat). **Note:** This is not a comprehensive list of all side effects. Patient should consult prescriber for additional questions.

Intended Use and Disclaimer: Should not be printed and given to patients. This information is intended to serve as a concise initial reference for healthcare professionals to use when discussing medications with a patient. You must ultimately rely on your own discretion, experience and judgment in diagnosing, treating and advising patients.

Dietary Considerations May be taken without regard to meals.

Related Information
Oral Medications That Should Not Be Crushed or Altered *on page 1712*

Fluphenazine (floo FEN a zeen)

Index Terms Fluphenazine Decanoate; Fluphenazine Hydrochloride

Pharmacologic Category Antipsychotic Agent, Typical, Phenothiazine

Medication Safety Issues

Sound-alike/look-alike issues:
FluPHENAZine may be confused with fluvox-aMINE

BEERS Criteria medication:
This drug may be potentially inappropriate for use in geriatric patients (Quality of evidence - moderate; Strength of recommendation - strong).

International issues:
Prolixin [Turkey] may be confused with Prolixan brand name for azapropazone [Greece]

Use Management of manifestations of psychotic disorders and schizophrenia; depot formulation may offer improved outcome in individuals with psychosis who are nonadherent with oral antipsychotics

Unlabeled Use Psychosis/agitation related to Alzheimer's dementia

Available Dosage Forms

Concentrate, Oral:
Generic: 5 mg/mL (120 mL)

Elixir, Oral:
Generic: 2.5 mg/5 mL (60 mL, 473 mL)

Solution, Injection:
Generic: 2.5 mg/mL (10 mL); 25 mg/mL (5 mL)

Tablet, Oral:
Generic: 1 mg, 2.5 mg, 5 mg, 10 mg

General Dosage Range

I.M. (hydrochloride): *Adults:* Initial: 1.25 mg as a single dose; Maintenance: 2.5-10 mg/day in divided doses every 6-8 hours

I.M., SubQ (Depot): *Adults:* Initial: 6.25-25 mg every 2-4 weeks (maximum: 100 mg)

Oral: *Adults:* 1-20 mg/day in divided doses every 6-8 hours (maximum: 40 mg/day)

Administration

I.M. The hydrochloride or decanoate formulation may be administered intramuscularly. Watch for hypotension when administering I.M. Use a dry syringe and needle of ≥21 gauge to administer the fluphenazine decanoate; a wet needle/syringe may cause the solution to become cloudy.

Injectable Detail pH: 4.8-5.2

Oral Avoid contact of oral solution or injection with skin (contact dermatitis). Oral liquid concentrate should be diluted immediately prior to administration.

Subcutaneous Only the decanoate formulation may be administered subcutaneously. Use a dry syringe and needle of ≥21 gauge to administer the fluphenazine decanoate; a wet needle/syringe may cause the solution to become cloudy.

Nursing Actions

Physical Assessment Monitor for anticholinergic and extrapyramidal symptoms. With I.M. or SubQ use, monitor closely for hypotension. Avoid skin contact with oral or injection medication; may cause contact dermatitis (wash immediately with warm, soapy water). Initiate at lower doses and taper dosage slowly when discontinuing.

Patient Education

• Discuss specific use of drug and side effects with patient as it relates to treatment. (HCAHPS: During this hospital stay, were you given any medicine that you had not taken before? Before giving you any new medicine, how often did hospital staff tell you what the medicine was for? How often did hospital staff describe possible side effects in a way you could understand?)

• Patient may experience anxiety, akathisia, nightmares, constipation, xerostomia, fatigue, lack of appetite. Have patient report immediately to prescriber signs of infection; signs of hepatic impairment; severe dizziness; syncope; significant headache; angina; dyspnea; dysphagia; difficulty speaking; fasciculations; considerable change in balance; sialorrhea; edema of hands or feet; vision changes; involuntary eye movements; ecchymosis; hemorrhaging; urinary retention; oliguria; intolerable asthenia; macromastia; sexual dysfunction; amenorrhea; severe diarrhea; considerable dyspepsia; signs of neuroleptic malignant syndrome (NMS); difficulty with motor activity; or signs of muscle problems with tongue, face, mouth, or jaw (HCAHPS).

• Educate patient about signs of a significant reaction (eg, wheezing; chest tightness; fever; itching; bad cough; blue skin color; seizures; or swelling of face, lips, tongue, or throat). **Note:** This is not a comprehensive list of all side effects. Patient should consult prescriber for additional questions.

Intended Use and Disclaimer: Should not be printed and given to patients. This information is intended to serve as a concise initial reference for healthcare professionals to use when discussing medications with a patient. You must ultimately rely on your own discretion, experience and judgment in diagnosing, treating and advising patients.

Flurandrenolide (flure an DREN oh lide)

Brand Names: U.S. Cordran; Cordran SP

Index Terms Flurandrenolone

Pharmacologic Category Corticosteroid, Topical

Medication Safety Issues

Sound-alike/look-alike issues:
Cordran may be confused with Cardura, codeine, Cordarone

Pregnancy Risk Factor C

Lactation Enters breast milk/use caution

Use Dermatoses: Relief of inflammatory and pruritic manifestations of corticosteroid-responsive dermatoses

Available Dosage Forms

Cream, External:
Cordran SP: 0.05% (15 g, 30 g, 60 g, 120 g)

Lotion, External:
Cordran: 0.05% (15 mL, 60 mL, 120 mL)

Tape, External:
Cordran: 4 mcg/cm^2 (1 ea)
General Dosage Range Topical: *Children, Adolescents, and Adults:* Cream, lotion: Apply thin film to affected area 2-3 times per day; Tape: Apply 1-2 times per day.

Administration

Topical

Cream, lotion: For external use only. Apply a thin film to clean, dry skin and rub in gently. Avoid contact with eyes; generally not for routine use on the face, underarms, or groin area. Use of occlusive dressings is not recommended unless directed by the healthcare provider. Do not use tight-fitting diapers or plastic pants on children being treated in the diaper area. Shake lotion well before use.

Tape: Apply to clean, dry skin (allow skin to dry 1 hour before applying new tape). Shave or clip hair in the treatment area to promote adherence and easy removal. Do not tear tape; always cut. Use of occlusive dressings is not recommended unless used for management of psoriasis or recalcitrant conditions. Replacement of tape every 12 hours is best tolerated, but may be left in place for 24 hours if well tolerated. May be used just at night and removed during the day.

Nursing Actions

Physical Assessment Monitor for improvement in skin reaction. Educate patient to return if concurrent skin infection does not resolve.

Patient Education

• Discuss specific use of drug and side effects with patient as it relates to treatment. (HCAHPS: During this hospital stay, were you given any medicine that you had not taken before? Before giving you any new medicine, how often did hospital staff tell you what the medicine was for? How often did hospital staff describe possible side effects in a way you could understand?)
• Patient may experience xeroderma. Have patient report immediately to prescriber signs of hyperglycemia, skin changes, or severe skin irritation (HCAHPS).
• Educate patient about signs of a significant reaction (eg, wheezing; chest tightness; fever; itching; bad cough; blue skin color; seizures; or swelling of face, lips, tongue, or throat). **Note:** This is not a comprehensive list of all side effects. Patient should consult prescriber for additional questions.

Intended Use and Disclaimer: Should not be printed and given to patients. This information is intended to serve as a concise initial reference for healthcare professionals to use when discussing medications with a patient. You must ultimately rely on your own discretion, experience and judgment in diagnosing, treating and advising patients.

Flurazepam (flure AZ e pam)

Index Terms Flurazepam Hydrochloride
Pharmacologic Category Hypnotic, Benzodiazepine
Medication Safety Issues
Sound-alike/look-alike issues:
Flurazepam may be confused with temazepam
Dalmane® may be confused with Demulen®
BEERS Criteria medication:
This drug may be potentially inappropriate for use in geriatric patients (Quality of evidence - high; Strength of recommendation - strong).
Medication Guide Available Yes
Lactation Excretion in breast milk unknown
Use Short-term treatment of insomnia
Controlled Substance C-IV
Available Dosage Forms
Capsule, Oral:
Generic: 15 mg, 30 mg
General Dosage Range Oral:
Children ≥15 years and Elderly: 15 mg at bedtime
Adults: 15-30 mg at bedtime
Nursing Actions
Physical Assessment For short-term use. Assess for history of addiction; long-term use can result in dependence, abuse, or tolerance. Be alert to possibility of anaphylaxis any time during therapy. Evaluate periodically need for continued use. Monitor for CNS changes. For inpatient use, institute safety measures to prevent falls.

Patient Education

• Discuss specific use of drug and side effects with patient as it relates to treatment. (HCAHPS: During this hospital stay, were you given any medicine that you had not taken before? Before giving you any new medicine, how often did hospital staff tell you what the medicine was for? How often did hospital staff describe possible side effects in a way you could understand?)
• Patient may experience headache or fatigue. Have patient report immediately to prescriber signs of depression (ie, suicidal ideation, anxiety, emotional instability, illogical thinking), hallucinations, memory loss, severe dizziness, change in balance, illogical thinking, or significant asthenia (HCAHPS).
• Educate patient about signs of a significant reaction (eg, wheezing; chest tightness; fever; itching; bad cough; blue skin color; seizures; or swelling of face, lips, tongue, or throat). **Note:** This is not a comprehensive list of all side effects. Patient should consult prescriber for additional questions.

Intended Use and Disclaimer: Should not be printed and given to patients. This information is intended to serve as a concise initial reference for healthcare professionals to use when discussing

medications with a patient. You must ultimately rely on your own discretion, experience and judgment in diagnosing, treating and advising patients.

Flutamide (FLOO ta mide)

Index Terms Eulexin; Flucinom; Flugerel; Niftolid; SCH 13521
Pharmacologic Category Antineoplastic Agent, Antiandrogen
Medication Safety Issues
Sound-alike/look-alike issues:
Flutamide may be confused with Flumadine, thalidomide
Eulexin may be confused with Edecrin, Eurax
Pregnancy Risk Factor D
Use Prostate cancer: Management of locally confined metastatic prostatic cancer (in combination with an LHRH agonist)
Available Dosage Forms
Capsule, Oral:
Generic: 125 mg
General Dosage Range Oral: *Adults (males):* 250 mg 3 times daily
Administration
Oral May be administered with or without food. Administer in 3 divided doses (every 8 hours). Hazardous agent; use appropriate precautions for handling and disposal (NIOSH, 2012).
Nursing Actions
Physical Assessment Assess serum transaminase levels prior to and periodically during therapy. Monitor for galactorrhea, CNS changes, ataxia, anorexia, vomiting, lacrimation, and anemia on a regular basis. Monitor liver function. Teach patient to report chest pain, respiratory difficulty, abdominal pain, and signs of liver dysfunction.
Patient Education
• Discuss specific use of drug and side effects with patient as it relates to treatment. (HCAHPS: During this hospital stay, were you given any medicine that you had not taken before? Before giving you any new medicine, how often did hospital staff tell you what the medicine was for? How often did hospital staff describe possible side effects in a way you could understand?)
• Patient may experience hot flashes, nausea, macromastia, or sexual dysfunction. Have patient report immediately to prescriber signs of infection, signs of depression (ie, suicidal ideation, anxiety, emotional instability, illogical thinking), hematuria, rectal pain, hematochezia, severe headache, considerable asthenia, ecchymosis, hemorrhaging, edema of extremities, or significant diarrhea (HCAHPS).

• Educate patient about signs of a significant reaction (eg, wheezing; chest tightness; fever; itching; bad cough; blue skin color; seizures; or swelling of face, lips, tongue, or throat). **Note:** This is not a comprehensive list of all side effects. Patient should consult prescriber for additional questions.

Intended Use and Disclaimer: Should not be printed and given to patients. This information is intended to serve as a concise initial reference for healthcare professionals to use when discussing medications with a patient. You must ultimately rely on your own discretion, experience and judgment in diagnosing, treating and advising patients.

Fluticasone (Oral Inhalation)
(floo TIK a sone)

Brand Names: U.S. Flovent Diskus; Flovent HFA
Index Terms Flovent; Fluticasone Propionate
Pharmacologic Category Corticosteroid, Inhalant (Oral)
Medication Safety Issues
Sound-alike/look-alike issues:
Flovent® may be confused with Flonase®
International issues:
Allegro: Brand name for fluticasone [Israel], but also the brand name for frovatriptan [Germany]
Allegro [Israel] may be confused with Allegra and Allegra-D brand names for fexofenadine and fexofenadine/pseudoephedrine, respectively [U.S., Canada, and multiple international markets]
Flovent [U.S., Canada] may be confused with Flogen brand name for naproxen [Mexico]; Flogene brand name for piroxicam [Brazil]
Pregnancy Risk Factor C
Lactation Excretion in breast milk unknown/use caution
Breast-Feeding Considerations Systemic corticosteroids are excreted in human milk. It is not known if sufficient quantities of fluticasone are absorbed following inhalation to produce detectable amounts in breast milk. The manufacturer recommends that caution be exercised when administering fluticasone to nursing women. The use of inhaled corticosteroids is not considered a contraindication to breast-feeding (NAEPP, 2005).
Use Maintenance treatment of asthma as prophylactic therapy; also indicated for patients requiring oral corticosteroid therapy for asthma to assist in total discontinuation or reduction of total oral dose
Mechanism of Action/Effect Fluticasone belongs to a group of corticosteroids which utilizes a fluorocarbothioate ester linkage at the 17 carbon position; extremely potent vasoconstrictive and anti-inflammatory activity. The effectiveness of inhaled fluticasone is due to its direct local effect.
Contraindications Hypersensitivity to fluticasone or any component of the formulation; severe

hypersensitivity to milk proteins or lactose (Flovent® Diskus®); primary treatment of status asthmaticus or other acute episodes of asthma requiring intensive measures

Canadian labeling: Additional contraindications (not in U.S. labeling): Moderate-to-severe bronchiectasis; untreated fungal, bacterial or tubercular infections of the respiratory tract

Warnings/Precautions May cause hypercorticism or suppression of hypothalamic-pituitary-adrenal (HPA) axis, particularly in younger children or in patients receiving high doses for prolonged periods. HPA axis suppression may lead to adrenal crisis. Withdrawal and discontinuation of a corticosteroid should be done slowly and carefully. Particular care is required when patients are transferred from systemic corticosteroids to inhaled products due to possible adrenal insufficiency or withdrawal from steroids, including an increase in allergic symptoms. Patients receiving ≥20 mg per day of prednisone (or equivalent) may be most susceptible. Fatalities have occurred due to adrenal insufficiency in asthmatic patients during and after transfer from systemic corticosteroids to aerosol steroids; aerosol steroids do **not** provide the systemic steroid needed to treat patients having trauma, surgery, or infections.

Bronchospasm may occur with wheezing after inhalation; if this occurs, stop steroid and treat with a fast-acting bronchodilator. Supplemental steroids (oral or parenteral) may be needed during stress or severe asthma attacks. Corticosteroid use may cause psychiatric disturbances, including depression, euphoria, insomnia, mood swings, and personality changes. Pre-existing psychiatric conditions may be exacerbated by corticosteroid use. Prolonged use of corticosteroids may also increase the incidence of secondary infection, mask acute infection (including fungal infections), prolong or exacerbate viral infections, or limit response to vaccines. Avoid use in patients with ocular herpes or untreated viral, fungal, parasitic or bacterial systemic infections (Canadian labeling contraindicates use with untreated respiratory infections). Exposure to chickenpox should be avoided. Close observation is required in patients with latent tuberculosis and/or TB reactivity; restrict use in active TB (only in conjunction with antituberculosis treatment). Rare cases of vasculitis (Churg-Strauss syndrome) or other eosinophilic conditions can occur. Prolonged treatment with corticosteroids has been associated with the development of Kaposi's sarcoma (case reports); if noted, discontinuation of therapy should be considered.

Use with caution in patients with thyroid disease, hepatic impairment, renal impairment, cardiovascular disease, diabetes, glaucoma, cataracts, myasthenia gravis, patients at risk for osteoporosis, patients at risk for seizures, or GI diseases

(diverticulitis, peptic ulcer, ulcerative colitis) due to perforation risk. Use caution following acute MI (corticosteroids have been associated with myocardial rupture). Because of the risk of adverse effects, systemic corticosteroids should be used cautiously in the elderly in the smallest possible effective dose for the shortest duration.

Orally-inhaled corticosteroids may cause a reduction in growth velocity in pediatric patients (~1 centimeter per year [range: 0.3-1.8 cm per year] and related to dose and duration of exposure). To minimize the systemic effects of orally-inhaled corticosteroids, each patient should be titrated to the lowest effective dose. Growth should be routinely monitored in pediatric patients.

Use with strong CYP3A4 inhibitors is not recommended (see Drug Interactions). Not to be used in status asthmaticus or for the relief of acute bronchospasm. Flovent® Diskus® contains lactose; very rare anaphylactic reactions have been reported in patients with severe milk protein allergy. There have been reports of systemic corticosteroid withdrawal symptoms (eg, joint/muscle pain, lassitude, depression) when withdrawing oral inhalation therapy. Local yeast infections (eg, oral pharyngeal candidiasis) may occur.

Drug Interactions

Avoid Concomitant Use

Avoid concomitant use of Fluticasone (Oral Inhalation) with any of the following: Aldesleukin; BCG; Cobicistat; Fusidic Acid (Systemic); Natalizumab; Pimecrolimus; Tacrolimus (Topical); Tofacitinib

Decreased Effect

Fluticasone (Oral Inhalation) may decrease the levels/effects of: Aldesleukin; Antidiabetic Agents; BCG; Coccidioidin Skin Test; Corticorelin; Hyaluronidase; Sipuleucel-T; Telaprevir; Vaccines (Inactivated)

The levels/effects of Fluticasone (Oral Inhalation) may be decreased by: Echinacea

Increased Effect/Toxicity

Fluticasone (Oral Inhalation) may increase the levels/effects of: Amphotericin B; Deferasirox; Leflunomide; Loop Diuretics; Natalizumab; Thiazide Diuretics; Tofacitinib

The levels/effects of Fluticasone (Oral Inhalation) may be increased by: Cobicistat; CYP3A4 Inhibitors (Moderate); CYP3A4 Inhibitors (Strong); Dasatinib; Denosumab; Fusidic Acid (Systemic); Ivacaftor; Luliconazole; Mifepristone; Pimecrolimus; Simeprevir; Tacrolimus (Topical); Telaprevir; Trastuzumab

Nutritional/Ethanol Interactions Herb/Nutraceutical: In theory, St John's wort may decrease serum levels of fluticasone by inducing CYP3A4 isoenzymes.

Adverse Reactions

>10%:

Central nervous system: Malaise/fatigue (16%), headache (2% to 14%)

Gastrointestinal: Oral candidiasis (≤31%)

Neuromuscular & skeletal: Arthralgia/articular rheumatism (17%), musculoskeletal pain (2% to 12%)

Respiratory: Sinusitis/sinus infection (≤33%), upper respiratory tract infection (≤31%), throat irritation (3% to 22%), nasal congestion/blockage (16%), rhinitis (≤13%)

1% to 10%:

Central nervous system: Pain (10%), fever (1% to 7%)

Dermatologic: Rash (8%), pruritus (6%)

Gastrointestinal: Nausea/vomiting (1% to 9%), gastrointestinal infection (including viral; 1% to 5%), gastrointestinal discomfort/pain (1% to 4%)

Neuromuscular & skeletal: Muscle injury (≤5%)

Respiratory: Hoarseness/dysphonia (2% to 9%), cough (1% to 9%), viral respiratory infection (1% to 9%), bronchitis (≤8%), upper respiratory tract inflammation (≤5%)

Miscellaneous: Viral infection (≤5%)

Pharmacodynamics/Kinetics

Onset of Action Maximal benefit may take 1-2 weeks or longer

Dosage Forms Considerations

Flovent HFA 10.6 g and 12 g canisters contain 120 inhalations.

Available Dosage Forms

Aerosol, Inhalation:

Flovent HFA: 44 mcg/actuation (10.6 g); 110 mcg/actuation (12 g); 220 mcg/actuation (12 g)

Aerosol Powder Breath Activated, Inhalation:

Flovent Diskus: 50 mcg/blister (60 ea); 100 mcg/blister (28 ea, 60 ea); 250 mcg/blister (28 ea, 60 ea)

General Dosage Range Inhalation:

Flovent® HFA:

Children 4-11 years: 88 mcg twice daily

Children ≥12 years and Adults: 88-880 mcg twice daily

Flovent® Diskus®:

Children 4-11 years: 50-100 mcg twice daily

Children ≥12 years and Adults: 100-1000 mcg twice daily

Administration

Inhalation

Aerosol inhalation: Flovent® HFA: Shake container thoroughly before using. Take 3-5 deep breaths. Use inhaler on inspiration. Allow 1 full minute between inhalations. Rinse mouth with water after use to reduce aftertaste and incidence of candidiasis; do not swallow. Flovent® HFA inhaler must be primed before first use, when not used for 7 days, or if dropped. To prime the first time, release 4 sprays into air; shake well before each spray and spray away from face. If dropped or not used for 7 days,

prime by releasing a single test spray. Patient should contact pharmacy for refill when the dose counter reads "020". Discard device when the dose counter reads "000". Do not use "float" test to determine contents.

Powder for oral inhalation: Flovent® Diskus®: Do not use with a spacer device. Do not exhale into Diskus®. Do not wash or take apart. Use in horizontal position. Mouth should be rinsed with water after use (do not swallow). Discard after 6 weeks (50 mcg diskus) or after 2 months (100 mcg and 250 mcg diskus) once removed from protective pouch or when the dose counter reads "0", whichever comes first (device is not reusable).

Storage/Stability

Flovent® HFA: Store at 15°C to 30°C (59°F to 86°F). Discard device when the dose counter reads "000". Store with mouthpiece down.

Flovent® Diskus®: Store at 20°C to 25°C (68°F to 77°F) in a dry place away from direct heat or sunlight. Discard after 6 weeks (50 mcg diskus) or after 2 months (100 mcg and 250 mcg diskus) from removal from protective foil pouch or when the dose counter reads "0" (whichever comes first); device is not reusable.

Nursing Actions

Physical Assessment May take as long as 2 weeks before full benefit of medication is known. Encourage regular eye exams with long-term use. Monitor for possible eosinophilic conditions (including Churg-Strauss syndrome) and signs/symptoms of HPA axis suppression/adrenal insufficiency. Assess growth in adolescents and children.

Patient Education

• Discuss specific use of drug and side effects with patient as it relates to treatment. (HCAHPS: During this hospital stay, were you given any medicine that you had not taken before? Before giving you any new medicine, how often did hospital staff tell you what the medicine was for? How often did hospital staff describe possible side effects in a way you could understand?)

• Patient may experience headache or rhinitis. Have patient report immediately to prescriber signs of infection, severe asthenia, irritability, tremors, tachycardia, confusion, dizziness, diaphoresis, stomatitis, dyspnea, excessive weight gain, edema of extremities, bradycardia, arrhythmia, angina, osteodynia, arthralgia, vision changes, or paresthesia (HCAHPS).

• Educate patient about signs of a significant reaction (eg, wheezing; chest tightness; fever; itching; bad cough; blue skin color; seizures; or swelling of face, lips, tongue, or throat). **Note:** This is not a comprehensive list of all side effects. Patient should consult prescriber for additional questions.

Intended Use and Disclaimer: Should not be printed and given to patients. This information is intended to serve as a concise initial reference for healthcare professionals to use when discussing medications with a patient. You must ultimately rely on your own discretion, experience and judgment in diagnosing, treating and advising patients.

Dietary Considerations Flovent® Diskus® contains lactose; very rare anaphylactic reactions have been reported in patients with severe milk protein allergy.

Fluticasone (Nasal) (floo TIK a sone)

Brand Names: U.S. Flonase; Veramyst

Index Terms Fluticasone Furoate; Fluticasone Propionate

Pharmacologic Category Corticosteroid, Nasal

Medication Safety Issues

Sound-alike/look-alike issues:

Flonase® may be confused with Flovent®

International issues:

Allegro: Brand name for fluticasone [Israel], but also the brand name for frovatriptan [Germany]

Allegro [Israel] may be confused with Allegra and Allegra-D brand names for fexofenadine and fexofenadine/pseudoephedrine, respectively, [U.S., Canada, and multiple international markets]

Pregnancy Risk Factor C

Lactation Excretion in breast milk unknown/use caution

Use

Flonase®: Management of seasonal and perennial allergic rhinitis and nonallergic rhinitis

Veramyst®, Avamys® (Canadian availability; not available in the U.S.): Management of seasonal and perennial allergic rhinitis

Unlabeled Use Adjunct to antibiotics in empiric treatment of acute bacterial rhinosinusitis (ABRS) (Chow, 2012)

Dosage Forms Considerations

Flonase 16 g bottles and Veramyst 10 g bottles contain 120 sprays each.

Available Dosage Forms

Suspension, Nasal:

Flonase: 50 mcg/actuation (16 g)

Veramyst: 27.5 mcg/spray (10 g)

Generic: 50 mcg/actuation (16 g); 50 mcg/actuation (16 g)

General Dosage Range Intranasal:

Propionate (Flonase®):

Children ≥4 years: Initial: 1 spray (50 mcg/spray) per nostril once daily (100 mcg/day); Maintenance: 1-2 sprays per nostril once daily (100-200 mcg/day); (maximum: 2 sprays in each nostril [200 mcg]/day)

Adults: Initial: 2 sprays (50 mcg/spray) per nostril once daily (200 mcg/day); Maintenance: 1-2 sprays per nostril once daily (100-200 mcg/day)

Furoate (Veramyst®):

Children 2-11 years: Initial: 1 spray (27.5 mcg/spray) per nostril once daily (55 mcg/day); Maintenance 1-2 sprays per nostril once daily (55-110 mcg/day) (maximum: 2 sprays in each nostril [110 mcg]/day)

Children ≥12 years and Adults: Initial: 2 sprays (27.5 mcg/spray) per nostril once (110 mcg/day); Maintenance 1-2 sprays per nostril once daily (55-110 mcg/day) (maximum: 2 sprays in each nostril [110 mcg]/day)

Administration

Inhalation Nasal spray: Administer at regular intervals. Shake bottle gently before using. Blow nose to clear nostrils. Insert applicator into nostril, keeping bottle upright, and close off the other nostril. Breathe in through nose. While inhaling, press pump to release spray. Discard after labeled number of doses has been used, even if bottle is not completely empty.

Flonase®: Prime pump (press 6 times until fine spray appears) prior to first use or if spray unused for ≥7 days. Once weekly, nasal applicator may be removed and rinsed with warm water to clean.

Veramyst®, Avamys® (Canadian availability; not available in the U.S.): Prime pump (press 6 times until fine spray appears) prior to first use, if spray unused for ≥30 days, or if cap left off bottle for ≥5 days. After each use, nozzle should be wiped with a clean, dry tissue. Once weekly, inside of cap should be cleaned with a clean, dry tissue.

Nursing Actions

Physical Assessment May take as long as 2 weeks before full benefit of medication is known. Encourage regular eye exams with long-term use. Monitor growth in adolescents and children. Assess signs/symptoms of HPA axis suppression/adrenal insufficiency.

Patient Education

• Discuss specific use of drug and side effects with patient as it relates to treatment. (HCAHPS: During this hospital stay, were you given any medicine that you had not taken before? Before giving you any new medicine, how often did hospital staff tell you what the medicine was for? How often did hospital staff describe possible side effects in a way you could understand?)

• Patient may experience headache or pharyngitis. Have patient report immediately to prescriber signs of infection, severe dizziness, considerable rhinitis, nasal sores, considerable epistaxis, stomatitis, intolerable nausea, severe asthenia, or vision changes (HCAHPS).

• Educate patient about signs of a significant reaction (eg, wheezing; chest tightness; fever; itching; bad cough; blue skin color; seizures; or

swelling of face, lips, tongue, or throat). **Note:** This is not a comprehensive list of all side effects. Patient should consult prescriber for additional questions.

Intended Use and Disclaimer: Should not be printed and given to patients. This information is intended to serve as a concise initial reference for healthcare professionals to use when discussing medications with a patient. You must ultimately rely on your own discretion, experience and judgment in diagnosing, treating and advising patients.

Fluticasone (Topical) (floo TIK a sone)

Brand Names: U.S. Cutivate
Index Terms Fluticasone Propionate
Pharmacologic Category Corticosteroid, Topical
Medication Safety Issues
  Sound-alike/look-alike issues:
    Cutivate® may be confused with Ultravate®
  International issues:
    Allegro: Brand name for fluticasone [Israel], but also the brand name for frovatriptan [Germany]
    Allegro [Israel] may be confused with Allegra and Allegra-D brand names for fexofenadine and fexofenadine/pseudoephedrine, respectively, [U.S., Canada, and multiple international markets]
Pregnancy Risk Factor C
Lactation Excretion in breast milk unknown/use caution
Use Relief of inflammation and pruritus associated with corticosteroid-responsive dermatoses; atopic dermatitis
Available Dosage Forms
  Cream, External:
    Cutivate: 0.05% (30 g, 60 g)
    Generic: 0.05% (15 g, 30 g, 60 g)
  Lotion, External:
    Cutivate: 0.05% (120 mL)
    Generic: 0.05% (60 mL, 120 mL)
  Ointment, External:
    Cutivate: 0.005% (30 g, 60 g)
    Generic: 0.005% (15 g, 30 g, 60 g)
General Dosage Range Topical:
  Cream: *Children ≥3 months and Adults:* Apply sparingly to affected area once or twice daily
  Lotion:
    Children ≥1 year: Apply sparingly to affected area once daily
    Adults: Apply sparingly to affected area once or twice daily
Administration
  Topical Apply sparingly in a thin film. Rub in lightly. Unless otherwise directed by healthcare professional, do not use with occlusive dressing; do not use on children's skin covered by diapers or plastic pants.

Nursing Actions
  Physical Assessment May take as long as 2 weeks before full benefit of medication is known. Monitor for possible eosinophilic conditions (including Churg-Strauss syndrome) and signs/symptoms of HPA axis suppression/adrenal insufficiency. Assess growth in adolescents and children.
Patient Education
  • Discuss specific use of drug and side effects with patient as it relates to treatment. (HCAHPS: During this hospital stay, were you given any medicine that you had not taken before? Before giving you any new medicine, how often did hospital staff tell you what the medicine was for? How often did hospital staff describe possible side effects in a way you could understand?)
  • Patient may experience xeroderma. Have patient report immediately to prescriber signs of hyperglycemia, skin changes, severe skin irritation (HCAHPS).
  • Educate patient about signs of a significant reaction (eg, wheezing; chest tightness; fever; itching; bad cough; blue skin color; seizures; or swelling of face, lips, tongue, or throat). **Note:** This is not a comprehensive list of all side effects. Patient should consult prescriber for additional questions.

Intended Use and Disclaimer: Should not be printed and given to patients. This information is intended to serve as a concise initial reference for healthcare professionals to use when discussing medications with a patient. You must ultimately rely on your own discretion, experience and judgment in diagnosing, treating and advising patients.

Fluticasone and Salmeterol
(floo TIK a sone & sal ME te role)

Brand Names: U.S. Advair Diskus®; Advair® HFA
Index Terms Fluticasone Propionate and Salmeterol Xinafoate; Salmeterol and Fluticasone
Pharmacologic Category Beta$_2$ Agonist; Beta$_2$-Adrenergic Agonist, Long-Acting; Corticosteroid, Inhalant (Oral)
Medication Safety Issues
  Sound-alike/look-alike issues:
    Advair® may be confused with Adcirca®, Advicor®
Medication Guide Available Yes
Pregnancy Risk Factor C
Use Maintenance treatment of asthma; maintenance treatment of COPD
Available Dosage Forms
  Aerosol, for oral inhalation:
    Advair® HFA:
      45/21: Fluticasone propionate 45 mcg and salmeterol 21 mcg (8 g, 12 g) [chlorofluorocarbon free]

115/21: Fluticasone propionate 115 mcg and salmeterol 21 mcg (8 g, 12 g) [chlorofluorocarbon free]

230/21: Fluticasone propionate 230 mcg and salmeterol 21 mcg (8 g, 12 g) [chlorofluorocarbon free]

Powder, for oral inhalation:

Advair Diskus®:

100/50: Fluticasone propionate 100 mcg and salmeterol 50 mcg (14s, 60s)

250/50: Fluticasone propionate 250 mcg and salmeterol 50 mcg (14s, 60s)

500/50: Fluticasone propionate 500 mcg and salmeterol 50 mcg (14s, 60s)

General Dosage Range Oral inhalation:

Children 4-11 years: Advair Diskus®: Fluticasone 100 mcg/salmeterol 50 mcg/inhalation: One inhalation twice daily (maximum dose)

Children ≥12 years:

Advair Diskus®: Fluticasone 100-500 mcg/salmeterol 50 mcg/inhalation: One inhalation twice daily. Maximum: Fluticasone 500 mcg/salmeterol 50 mcg/inhalation twice daily

Advair® HFA: Fluticasone 45-230 mcg/salmeterol 21 mcg/inhalation: Two inhalations twice daily

Adults:

Advair Diskus®: Initial, maximum: Fluticasone 250 mcg/salmeterol 50 mcg twice daily [COPD]; maximum dose: Fluticasone 500 mcg/salmeterol 50 mcg/inhalation twice daily [Asthma]

Advair® HFA: Fluticasone 45-230 mcg/salmeterol 50 mcg/inhalation: Two inhalations twice daily

Administration

Inhalation

Advair Diskus®: After removing from box and foil pouch, write the "Pouch opened" and "Use by" dates on the label on top of the Diskus®. The "Use by" date is 1 month from date of opening the pouch. Every time the lever is pushed back, a dose is ready to be inhaled. Do not close or tilt the Diskus® after the lever is pushed back. Do not play with the lever or move the lever more than once. The dose indicator tells you how many doses are left. When the numbers 5 to 0 appear in red, only a few doses remain. Discard device 1 month after you remove it from the foil pouch or when the dose counter reads "0" (whichever comes first). Rinse mouth with water after use and spit to reduce risk of oral candidiasis.

Advair® HFA: Shake well for 5 seconds before each spray. Prime with 4 test sprays (into air and away from face) before using for the first time. If canister is dropped or not used for >4 weeks, prime with 2 sprays. Patient should contact pharmacy for refill when the dose counter reads "020". Discard device when the dose counter reads "000". Do not spray in eyes. Rinse mouth with water after use and spit to reduce risk of oral candidiasis.

Nursing Actions

Physical Assessment See individual agents.

Patient Education

• Discuss specific use of drug and side effects with patient as it relates to treatment. (HCAHPS: During this hospital stay, were you given any medicine that you had not taken before? Before giving you any new medicine, how often did hospital staff tell you what the medicine was for? How often did hospital staff describe possible side effects in a way you could understand?)

• Patient may experience nausea or pharyngitis. Have patient report immediately to prescriber signs of infection, signs of hyperglycemia, signs of hypokalemia, angina, tachycardia, anxiety, behavioral changes, vision changes, paresthesia, choking, dysphonia, osteodynia, severe dizziness, considerable headache, insomnia, significant asthenia, vaginitis, weight gain, stomatitis, or dyspnea (HCAHPS).

• Educate patient about signs of a significant reaction (eg, wheezing; chest tightness; fever; itching; bad cough; blue skin color; seizures; or swelling of face, lips, tongue, or throat). **Note:** This is not a comprehensive list of all side effects. Patient should consult prescriber for additional questions.

Intended Use and Disclaimer: Should not be printed and given to patients. This information is intended to serve as a concise initial reference for healthcare professionals to use when discussing medications with a patient. You must ultimately rely on your own discretion, experience and judgment in diagnosing, treating and advising patients.

Related Information

Fluticasone (Oral Inhalation) *on page 685*

Salmeterol *on page 1394*

Fluticasone and Vilanterol
(floo TIK a sone & VYE lan ter ol)

Brand Names: U.S. Breo Ellipta

Index Terms Fluticasone Furoate and Vilanterol; Vilanterol and Fluticasone; Vilanterol and Fluticasone Furoate

Pharmacologic Category Beta$_2$ Agonist; Beta$_2$-Adrenergic Agonist, Long-Acting; Corticosteroid, Inhalant (Oral)

Medication Guide Available Yes

Pregnancy Risk Factor C

Use Maintenance treatment of airflow obstruction in patients with chronic obstructive pulmonary disease (COPD), including chronic bronchitis and/or emphysema; reduce exacerbations of COPD in patients with a history of exacerbations

Available Dosage Forms Powder, for oral inhalation:

Breo Ellipta: Fluticasone furoate 100 mcg and vilanterol 25 mcg per actuation [contains lactose; blister pack]

General Dosage Range

Oral inhalation: *Adults:* Fluticasone 100 mcg/ vilanterol 25 mcg: One inhalation once daily; maximum: 1 inhalation once daily

Administration

Inhalation Administer at the same time each day. Discard device 6 weeks after it is removed from the foil tray or when the dose counter reads "0" (whichever comes first). Rinse mouth with water after use and spit.

Nursing Actions

Physical Assessment Ensure proper use. After administration, encourage patient to rinse mouth out with water to reduce the potential of developing oropharyngeal candidiasis.

Patient Education

- Discuss specific use of drug and side effects with patient as it relates to treatment. (HCAHPS: During this hospital stay, were you given any medicine that you had not taken before? Before giving you any new medicine, how often did hospital staff tell you what the medicine was for? How often did hospital staff describe possible side effects in a way you could understand?)
- Patient may experience headache, rhinorrhea, or pharyngitis. Have patient report immediately to prescriber signs of infection, severe asthenia, irritability, tremors, tachycardia, confusion, diaphoresis, dizziness, angina, arrhythmia, decreased peak flow measurement, anxiety, or sudden vision changes (HCAHPS).
- Educate patient about signs of a significant reaction (eg, wheezing; chest tightness; fever; itching; bad cough; blue skin color; seizures; or swelling of face, lips, tongue, or throat). **Note:** This is not a comprehensive list of all side effects. Patient should consult prescriber for additional questions.

Intended Use and Disclaimer: Should not be printed and given to patients. This information is intended to serve as a concise initial reference for healthcare professionals to use when discussing medications with a patient. You must ultimately rely on your own discretion, experience and judgment in diagnosing, treating and advising patients.

Related Information

Fluticasone (Oral Inhalation) *on page 685*

Fluvastatin (FLOO va sta tin)

Brand Names: U.S. Lescol; Lescol XL
Pharmacologic Category Antilipemic Agent, HMG-CoA Reductase Inhibitor

Medication Safety Issues

Sound-alike/look-alike issues:

Fluvastatin may be confused with fluoxetine, nystatin, pitavastatin

Pregnancy Risk Factor X

Lactation Excretion unknown/contraindicated

Use To be used as a component of multiple risk factor intervention in patients at risk for atherosclerosis vascular disease due to hypercholesterolemia

Adjunct to dietary therapy to reduce elevated total cholesterol (total-C), LDL-C, triglyceride, and apolipoprotein B (apo-B) levels and to increase HDL-C in primary hypercholesterolemia and mixed dyslipidemia (Fredrickson types IIa and IIb); to slow the progression of coronary atherosclerosis in patients with coronary heart disease; reduce risk of coronary revascularization procedures in patients with coronary heart disease

Primary and secondary prevention of atherosclerotic cardiovascular disease (ASCVD) according to the American College of Cardiology/American Heart Association: To reduce the risk of ASCVD in patients with clinical ASCVD (eg, coronary heart disease, stroke/TIA, or peripheral arterial disease presumed to be of atherosclerotic origin) who are greater than 75 years of age or not a candidate for high-intensity statin therapy; in patients without clinical ASCVD if LDL-C is 190 mg/dL or greater and not a candidate for high-intensity statin therapy; in patients without clinical ASCVD who have type 1 or type 2 diabetes and are between 40 and 75 years of age; in patients with an estimated 10-year ASCVD risk 7.5% or greater and who are between 40 and 75 years of age (Stone, 2013).

Available Dosage Forms

Capsule, Oral:

Lescol: 20 mg, 40 mg

Generic: 20 mg, 40 mg

Tablet Extended Release 24 Hour, Oral:

Lescol XL: 80 mg

General Dosage Range Oral:

Extended release: *Adolescents 10-16 years (females 1 year postmenarche) and Adults:* 80 mg once daily

Immediate release:

Adolescents 10-16 years (females 1 year postmenarche): Initial: 20 mg once daily; Maintenance: Up to 80 mg/day in 2 divided doses

Adults: Initial: 20-40 mg once daily; Maintenance: Up to 80 mg/day in 2 divided doses

Administration

Oral Patient should be placed on a standard cholesterol-lowering diet before and during treatment. Fluvastatin may be taken without regard to meals. Adjust dosage as needed in response to periodic lipid determinations during the first 4 weeks after a dosage change; lipid-lowering effects are additive when fluvastatin is combined with a bile-acid binding resin or niacin, however, it must be administered at least 2 hours following these drugs. Do not break, chew, or crush extended release tablets; do not open capsules.

Nursing Actions

Physical Assessment Monitor for signs and symptoms of myopathy including muscle tenderness, pain, or weakness. Assess LFTs and cholesterol panel prior to treatment and at regular intervals. Consider dietary assessment and plan for education.

Patient Education

• Discuss specific use of drug and side effects with patient as it relates to treatment. (HCAHPS: During this hospital stay, were you given any medicine that you had not taken before? Before giving you any new medicine, how often did hospital staff tell you what the medicine was for? How often did hospital staff describe possible side effects in a way you could understand?)

• Patient may experience dyspepsia, diarrhea, insomnia, or flu-like syndrome. Have patient report immediately to prescriber severe headache, edema of extremities, angina, urinary retention, oliguria, dysuria, myalgia, asthenia, or signs of hepatic impairment (HCAHPS).

• Educate patient about signs of a significant reaction (eg, wheezing; chest tightness; fever; itching; bad cough; blue skin color; seizures; or swelling of face, lips, tongue, or throat). **Note:** This is not a comprehensive list of all side effects. Patient should consult prescriber for additional questions.

Intended Use and Disclaimer: Should not be printed and given to patients. This information is intended to serve as a concise initial reference for healthcare professionals to use when discussing medications with a patient. You must ultimately rely on your own discretion, experience and judgment in diagnosing, treating and advising patients.

Related Information

Oral Medications That Should Not Be Crushed or Altered on page 1712

Fluvoxamine (floo VOKS a meen)

Brand Names: U.S. Luvox CR
Index Terms Luvox
Pharmacologic Category Antidepressant, Selective Serotonin Reuptake Inhibitor

Medication Safety Issues

Sound-alike/look-alike issues:

FluvoxaMINE may be confused with flavoxATE, FLUoxetine, fluPHENAZine

Luvox may be confused with Lasix, Levoxyl, Lovenox

BEERS Criteria medication:

This drug may be potentially inappropriate for use in geriatric patients (Quality of evidence - moderate; Strength of recommendation - strong).

Medication Guide Available Yes

Pregnancy Risk Factor C
Lactation Enters breast milk/consider risk:benefit
Breast-Feeding Considerations Fluvoxamine is excreted in breast milk. Based on case reports, the dose the infant receives is relatively small and adverse events have not been observed. Adverse events have been reported in nursing infants exposed to some SSRIs. According to the manufacturer, the decision to continue or discontinue breast-feeding during therapy should take into account the risk of exposure to the infant and the benefits of treatment to the mother.

The long-term effects on development and behavior have not been studied; therefore, fluvoxamine should be prescribed to a mother who is breast-feeding only when the benefits outweigh the potential risks. Maternal use of an SSRI during pregnancy may cause delayed milk secretion.

Use Treatment of obsessive-compulsive disorder (OCD)

Unlabeled Use Treatment of major depression; panic disorder; anxiety disorders in children; post-traumatic stress disorder (PTSD); social anxiety disorder (SAD)

Mechanism of Action/Effect Inhibits CNS neuron serotonin uptake; minimal or no effect on reuptake of norepinephrine or dopamine; does not significantly bind to alpha-adrenergic, histamine or cholinergic receptors

Contraindications Concurrent use with alosetron, pimozide, ramelteon, thioridazine, or tizanidine; use of MAO inhibitors intended to treat psychiatric disorders (concurrently or within 14 days of discontinuing either fluvoxamine or the MAO inhibitor); initiation of fluvoxamine in a patient receiving linezolid or intravenous methylene blue

Warnings/Precautions [U.S. Boxed Warning]: Antidepressants increase the risk of suicidal thinking and behavior in children, adolescents, and young adults (18-24 years of age) with major depressive disorder (MDD) and other psychiatric disorders; consider risk prior to prescribing. Short-term studies did not show an increased risk in patients >24 years of age and showed a decreased risk in patients ≥65 years. Closely monitor patients for clinical worsening, suicidality, or unusual changes in behavior, particularly during the initial 1-2 months of therapy or during periods of dosage adjustments (increases or decreases); the patient's family or caregiver should be instructed to closely observe the patient and communicate condition with healthcare provider. A medication guide concerning the use of antidepressants should be dispensed with each prescription. **Fluvoxamine is FDA approved for the treatment of OCD in children ≥8 years of age; extended release capsules are not FDA approved for use in children.**

The possibility of a suicide attempt is inherent in major depression and may persist until remission occurs. Use caution in high-risk patients. Worsening depression and severe abrupt suicidality that are not part of the presenting symptoms may require discontinuation or modification of drug therapy. The patient's family or caregiver should be alerted to monitor patients for the emergence of suicidality and associated behaviors (such as agitation, irritability, hostility, impulsivity, and hypomania) and call healthcare provider.

May worsen psychosis in some patients or precipitate a shift to mania or hypomania in patients with bipolar disorder. Patients presenting with depressive symptoms should be screened for bipolar disorder. Monotherapy in patients with bipolar disorder should be avoided. **Fluvoxamine is not FDA approved for the treatment of bipolar depression.**

Potentially life-threatening serotonin syndrome (SS) has occurred with serotonergic agents (eg, SSRIs, SNRIs), particularly when used in combination with other serotonergic agents (eg, triptans, TCAs, fentanyl, lithium, tramadol, buspirone, St John's wort, tryptophan) or agents that impair metabolism of serotonin (eg, MAO inhibitors intended to treat psychiatric disorders, other MAO inhibitors [ie, linezolid and intravenous methylene blue]). Discontinue treatment (and any concomitant serotonergic agent) immediately if signs/symptoms arise. Fluvoxamine has a low potential to impair cognitive or motor performance; caution operating hazardous machinery or driving. Use caution in patients with a previous seizure disorder or condition predisposing to seizures such as brain damage, alcoholism, or concurrent therapy with other drugs which lower the seizure threshold. Potentially significant drug-drug interactions may exist, requiring dose or frequency adjustment, additional monitoring, and/or selection of alternative therapy. Fluvoxamine levels may be lower in patients who smoke.

May increase the risks associated with electroconvulsive therapy. Bone fractures have been associated with antidepressant treatment. Consider the possibility of a fragility fracture if an antidepressant-treated patient presents with unexplained bone pain, point tenderness, swelling, or bruising (Rabenda, 2013; Rizzoli, 2012). Use with caution in patients with hepatic dysfunction and in elderly patients. May cause hyponatremia/SIADH (elderly at increased risk); volume depletion (diuretics may increase risk). Use with caution in patients at risk of bleeding or receiving concurrent anticoagulant therapy, although not consistently noted, fluvoxamine may cause impairment in platelet function. May cause or exacerbate sexual dysfunction. Use caution in elderly patients; monitor sodium closely with initiation or dosage adjustments in older adults (Beers Criteria).

Abrupt discontinuation or interruption of antidepressant therapy has been associated with a discontinuation syndrome. Symptoms arising may vary with antidepressant however commonly include nausea, vomiting, diarrhea, headaches, light-headedness, dizziness, diminished appetite, sweating, chills, tremors, paresthesias, fatigue, somnolence, and sleep disturbances (eg, vivid dreams, insomnia). Greater risks for developing a discontinuation syndrome have been associated with antidepressants with shorter half-lives, longer durations of treatment, and abrupt discontinuation. For antidepressants of short or intermediate half-lives, symptoms may emerge within 2-5 days after treatment discontinuation and last 7-14 days (APA, 2010; Fava, 2006; Haddad, 2001; Shelton, 2001; Warner, 2006).

Drug Interactions

Avoid Concomitant Use

Avoid concomitant use of FluvoxaMINE with any of the following: Agomelatine; Alosetron; Dosulepin; Iobenguane I 123; Linezolid; MAO Inhibitors; Methylene Blue; Pimozide; Pirfenidone; Pomalidomide; Ramelteon; Tasimelteon; Thioridazine; TiZANidine; Tryptophan; Urokinase

Decreased Effect

FluvoxaMINE may decrease the levels/effects of: Clopidogrel; Iobenguane I 123; Ioflupane I 123; Thyroid Products

The levels/effects of FluvoxaMINE may be decreased by: CarBAMazepine; CYP1A2 Inducers (Strong); Cyproheptadine; Cyproterone; NSAID (COX-2 Inhibitor); NSAID (Nonselective); Peginterferon Alfa-2b

Increased Effect/Toxicity

FluvoxaMINE may increase the levels/effects of: Agents with Antiplatelet Properties; Agomelatine; Alosetron; Anticoagulants; Antidepressants (Serotonin Reuptake Inhibitor/Antagonist); Antipsychotics; Asenapine; Aspirin; Bendamustine; Benzodiazepines (metabolized by oxidation); Bromazepam; BusPIRone; CarBAMazepine; Citalopram; CloZAPine; Collagenase (Systemic); CYP1A2 Substrates; CYP2C19 Substrates; Dabigatran Etexilate; Desmopressin; Dofetilide; Dosulepin; DULoxetine; Erlotinib; Fosphenytoin; Haloperidol; Hypoglycemic Agents; Ibritumomab; Lomitapide; Methadone; Methylene Blue; Metoclopramide; Mexiletine; NSAID (COX-2 Inhibitor); NSAID (Nonselective); OLANZapine; Phenytoin; Pimozide; Pirfenidone; Pomalidomide; Propafenone; Propranolol; QuiNIDine; Ramelteon; Rivaroxaban; Roflumilast; Ropivacaine; Salicylates; Serotonin Modulators; Tasimelteon; Theophylline Derivatives; Thiazide Diuretics; Thioridazine; Thrombolytic Agents; TiZANidine; Tositumomab and Iodine I 131 Tositumomab; TraMADol; Tricyclic Antidepressants; Urokinase; Vitamin K Antagonists; Zolpidem

The levels/effects of FluvoxaMINE may be increased by: Abiraterone Acetate; Alcohol (Ethyl); Analgesics (Opioid); Antipsychotics; BuPROPion; BusPIRone; Cimetidine; CNS Depressants; Cobicistat; CYP1A2 Inhibitors (Moderate); CYP1A2 Inhibitors (Strong); CYP2D6 Inhibitors (Moderate); CYP2D6 Inhibitors (Strong); Darunavir; Dasatinib; Deferasirox; DULoxetine; Glucosamine; Grapefruit Juice; Herbs (Anticoagulant/Antiplatelet Properties); Ibrutinib; Linezolid; Lithium; MAO Inhibitors; Metoclopramide; Metyrosine; Multivitamins/Fluoride (with ADE); Multivitamins/Minerals (with ADEK, Folate, Iron); Multivitamins/Minerals (with AE, No Iron); Omega-3 Fatty Acids; Pentosan Polysulfate Sodium; Pentoxifylline; Prostacyclin Analogues; Tipranavir; TraMADol; Tryptophan; Vemurafenib; Vitamin E

Nutritional/Ethanol Interactions

Ethanol: May increase CNS depression; monitor for increased effects with coadministration. Caution patients about effects.

Herb/Nutraceutical: Avoid valerian, St John's wort, tryptophan, SAMe, kava kava (may increase risk of serotonin syndrome and/or excessive sedation). Avoid alfalfa, anise, bilberry, bladderwrack, bromelain, cat's claw, celery, chamomile, coleus, cordyceps, dong quai, evening primrose, fenugreek, feverfew, garlic, ginger, ginkgo biloba, ginseng (American), ginseng (Panax), ginseng (Siberian), grape seed, green tea, guggul, horse chestnuts, horseradish, licorice, prickly ash, red clover, reishi, SAMe (S-adenosylmethionine), sweet clover, turmeric, white willow (all have additional antiplatelet activity). Bioavailability of melatonin may be increased by fluvoxamine.

Adverse Reactions

Frequency varies by dosage form and indication. Adverse reactions reported as a composite of all indications.

>10%:

Central nervous system: Headache (22% to 35%), insomnia (21% to 35%), somnolence (22% to 27%), dizziness (11% to 15%), nervousness (10% to 12%)

Gastrointestinal: Nausea (34% to 40%), diarrhea (11% to 18%), xerostomia (10% to 14%), anorexia (6% to 14%)

Genitourinary: Ejaculation abnormal (8% to 11%)

Neuromuscular & skeletal: Weakness (14% to 26%)

1% to 10%:

Cardiovascular: Chest pain (3%), palpitation (3%), vasodilation (2% to 3%), hypertension (1% to 2%), edema (≤1%), hypotension (≤1%), syncope (≤1%), tachycardia (≤1%)

Central nervous system: Pain (10%), anxiety (5% to 8%), abnormal dreams (3%), abnormal thinking (3%), agitation (2% to 3%), apathy (≥1% to 3%), chills (2%), CNS stimulation (2%), depression (2%), neurosis (2%), amnesia, malaise, manic reaction, psychotic reaction

Dermatologic: Bruising (4%), acne (2%)

Endocrine & metabolic: Libido decreased (2% to 10%; incidence higher in males), anorgasmia (2% to 5%), sexual function abnormal (2% to 4%), menorrhagia (3%)

Gastrointestinal: Dyspepsia (8% to 10%), constipation (4% to 10%), vomiting (4% to 6%), abdominal pain (5%), flatulence (4%), taste perversion (2% to 3%), toothache and dental caries (2% to 3%), dysphagia (2%), gingivitis (2%), weight loss (≤1% to 2%), weight gain

Genitourinary: Polyuria (2% to 3%), impotence (2%), urinary tract infection (2%), urinary retention (1%)

Hepatic: Liver function tests abnormal (≥1% to 2%)

Neuromuscular & skeletal: Tremor (5% to 8%), myalgia (5%), paresthesia (3%), hypertonia (2%), twitching (2%), hyper-/hypokinesia, myoclonus

Ocular: Amblyopia (2% to 3%)

Respiratory: Upper respiratory infection (9%), pharyngitis (6%), yawn (2% to 5%), laryngitis (3%), bronchitis (2%), dyspnea (2%), epistaxis (2%), cough increased, sinusitis

Miscellaneous: Diaphoresis (6% to 7%), flu-like syndrome (3%), viral infection (2%)

Pharmacodynamics/Kinetics

Onset of Action Depression: The onset of action is within a week; however, individual response varies greatly and full response may not be seen until 8-12 weeks after initiation of treatment.

Available Dosage Forms

Capsule Extended Release 24 Hour, Oral:

Luvox CR: 100 mg, 150 mg

Generic: 100 mg, 150 mg

Tablet, Oral:

Generic: 25 mg, 50 mg, 100 mg

General Dosage Range Dosage adjustment recommended in patients with hepatic impairment

Oral:

Children 8-11 years: Initial: 25 mg at bedtime; Maintenance: 50-200 mg/day (maximum: 200 mg/day)

Children 12-17 years: Initial: 25 mg at bedtime; Maintenance: 50-200 mg/day (maximum: 300 mg/day)

Adults: Initial: 50-100 mg at bedtime; Maintenance: 100-300 mg/day in 1-2 divided doses

Administration

Oral May be administered with or without food. Do not crush, open, or chew extended release capsules.

Storage/Stability Protect from high humidity and store at controlled room temperature 25°C (77°F).

Nursing Actions

Physical Assessment Monitor for CNS and gastrointestinal disturbances. Taper dosage slowly when discontinuing. Assess mental status for depression, signs of clinical worsening, suicide ideation, anxiety, social functioning, mania, or panic attack.

Patient Education

- Discuss specific use of drug and side effects with patient as it relates to treatment. (HCAHPS: During this hospital stay, were you given any medicine that you had not taken before? Before giving you any new medicine, how often did hospital staff tell you what the medicine was for? How often did hospital staff describe possible side effects in a way you could understand?)
- Patient may experience anxiety, xerostomia, fatigue, sexual dysfunction, insomnia, asthenia, lack of appetite, rhinorrhea, constipation, flatulence, or dysgeusia. Have patient report immediately to prescriber signs of hyponatremia, signs of hemorrhaging, suicidal ideation, syncope, irritability, fasciculations, muscle rigidity, angina, memory loss, vision changes, polyuria, serotonin syndrome (ie, severe dizziness, severe headache, agitation, hallucinations, tachycardia, arrhythmia, flushing, tremors, hyperhidrosis, change in balance, severe nausea, significant diarrhea), or priapism (HCAHPS).
- Educate patient about signs of a significant reaction (eg, wheezing; chest tightness; fever; itching; bad cough; blue skin color; seizures; or swelling of face, lips, tongue, or throat). **Note:** This is not a comprehensive list of all side effects. Patient should consult prescriber for additional questions.

Intended Use and Disclaimer: Should not be printed and given to patients. This information is intended to serve as a concise initial reference for healthcare professionals to use when discussing medications with a patient. You must ultimately rely on your own discretion, experience and judgment in diagnosing, treating and advising patients.

Dietary Considerations May be taken with or without food.

Related Information

Oral Medications That Should Not Be Crushed or Altered *on page 1712*

Folic Acid (FOE lik AS id)

Brand Names: U.S. FA-8 [OTC]

Index Terms Folacin; Folate; Pteroylglutamic Acid

Pharmacologic Category Vitamin, Water Soluble

Medication Safety Issues

Sound-alike/look-alike issues:

Folic acid may be confused with folinic acid

Pregnancy Risk Factor A

Lactation Enters breast milk/compatible

Use Treatment of megaloblastic and macrocytic anemias due to folate deficiency; dietary supplement to prevent neural tube defects

Unlabeled Use Adjunctive cofactor therapy in methanol toxicity (alternative to leucovorin calcium)

Available Dosage Forms

Capsule, Oral [preservative free]:

FA-8 [OTC]: 0.8 mg

Generic: 5 mg, 20 mg

Solution, Injection:

Generic: 5 mg/mL (10 mL)

Tablet, Oral:

Generic: 400 mcg, 800 mcg, 1 mg

Tablet, Oral [preservative free]:

FA-8 [OTC]: 800 mcg

Generic: 400 mcg, 800 mcg

General Dosage Range

I.M., I.V., SubQ:

Infants: 0.1 mg/day

Children <4 years: Up to 0.3 mg/day

Children ≥4 years and Adults: 0.4 mg/day

Pregnant and lactating women: 0.8 mg/day (anemia)

Oral:

Infants: 0.1 mg/day

Children <4 years: Up to 0.3 mg/day

Children ≥4 years and Adults: 0.4 mg/day

Pregnant and lactating women: 0.8 mg/day (anemia) **or** 4 mg/day (prevention of neural tube defects)

Females of childbearing potential: Prevention of neural tube defects: 0.4-0.8 mg/day

Administration

I.M. May also be administered by deep I.M. injection.

I.V. May administer ≤5 mg dose undiluted over ≥1 minute **or** may dilute ≤5 mg in 50 mL of NS or D_5W and infuse over 30 minutes. May also be added to I.V. maintenance solutions and given as an infusion.

Injectable Detail pH: 8-11

Nursing Actions

Patient Education

- Discuss specific use of drug and side effects with patient as it relates to treatment. (HCAHPS: During this hospital stay, were you given any medicine that you had not taken before? Before giving you any new medicine, how often did hospital staff tell you what the medicine was for? How often did hospital staff describe possible side effects in a way you could understand?)
- Have patient report immediately to prescriber injection site pain or irritation (HCAHPS).
- Educate patient about signs of a significant reaction (eg, wheezing; chest tightness; fever; itching; bad cough; blue skin color; seizures; or swelling of face, lips, tongue, or throat). **Note:** This is not a comprehensive list of all side effects. Patient should consult prescriber for additional questions.

Intended Use and Disclaimer: Should not be printed and given to patients. This information is intended to serve as a concise initial reference for

healthcare professionals to use when discussing medications with a patient. You must ultimately rely on your own discretion, experience and judgment in diagnosing, treating and advising patients.

Follitropin Alfa (foe li TRO pin AL fa)

Brand Names: U.S. Gonal-f; Gonal-f RFF; Gonal-f RFF Pen; Gonal-f RFF Rediject
Index Terms Follicle Stimulating Hormone, Recombinant; FSH; rFSH-alpha; rhFSH-alpha
Pharmacologic Category Gonadotropin; Ovulation Stimulator
Pregnancy Risk Factor X
Lactation Excretion in breast milk unknown/not recommended
Breast-Feeding Considerations It is not known if follitropin alfa is excreted in breast milk. Due to the potential for serious adverse reactions in the nursing infant, a decision should be made whether to discontinue nursing or to discontinue the drug, taking into account the importance of treatment to the mother.
Use
Multifollicular development during Assisted Reproductive Technology (ART): To stimulate the development of multiple follicles with ART
Ovulation induction: Induction of ovulation in oligo-anovulatory infertile patients in whom the cause of infertility is functional and not caused by primary ovarian failure; induction of spermatogenesis in men with primary and secondary hypogonadotropic hypogonadism in whom the cause of infertility is not due to primary testicular failure
Spermatogenesis induction (Gonal-f only): Induction of spermatogenesis in men with primary and secondary hypogonadotropic hypogonadism in whom the cause of infertility is not due to primary testicular failure
Mechanism of Action/Effect Follitropin alfa is a human FSH preparation of recombinant DNA origin. Follitropins stimulate ovarian follicular growth in women who do not have primary ovarian failure, and stimulate spermatogenesis in men with hypogonadotrophic hypogonadism. FSH is required for normal follicular growth, maturation, gonadal steroid production, and spermatogenesis.
Contraindications Hypersensitivity to follitropins or any component of the formulation; high levels of FSH indicating primary gonadal failure (ovarian or testicular); sex hormone dependent tumors of the reproductive tract and accessory organs; intracranial lesions (eg, pituitary or hypothalamus tumor); uncontrolled thyroid, pituitary or adrenal dysfunction; abnormal uterine bleeding of undetermined origin; ovarian cysts or enlargement of undetermined origin not due to polycystic ovary syndrome; pregnancy
Warnings/Precautions The risk of spontaneous abortion is increased with the use of

gonadotropins; causal effect has not been established. These medications should only be used by physicians who are thoroughly familiar with infertility problems and their management. To minimize risks, use only at the lowest effective dose. Monitor ovarian response with serum estradiol and vaginal ultrasound on a regular basis. Risk for ectopic pregnancy may be increased in women with tubal abnormalities; intrauterine pregnancy should be confirmed early with hCG testing and transvaginal ultrasound.

Ovarian enlargement, which may be accompanied by abdominal distention or abdominal pain, occurs in ~20% of those treated with urofollitropin and hCG, and generally regresses without treatment within 2-3 weeks. If ovaries are abnormally enlarged on the last day of treatment, withhold hCG to reduce the risk of ovarian hyperstimulation syndrome (OHSS). OHSS is reported in about 7% of patients; it is characterized by severe ovarian enlargement, abdominal pain/distention, nausea, vomiting, diarrhea, dyspnea, and oliguria, and may be accompanied by ascites, pleural effusion, hypovolemia, electrolyte imbalance, hemoperitoneum, and thromboembolic events. If hyperstimulation occurs, stop treatment and hospitalize patient. This syndrome develops rapidly within 24 hours to several days and generally occurs after treatment has ended and reaches its maximum on days 7-10 days following treatment. Hemoconcentration associated with fluid loss into the abdominal cavity has occurred and should be assessed by fluid intake and output, weight, hematocrit, serum and urinary electrolytes, urine specific gravity, BUN and creatinine, and abdominal girth. Determinations should be performed daily or more often if the need arises. Treatment is primarily symptomatic and consists of bedrest, fluid and electrolyte replacement, and analgesics. The ascitic, pleural, and pericardial fluids should not be removed unless needed to relieve symptoms of cardiopulmonary distress.

Ovarian torsion has been reported following gonadotropin treatment; may be related to OHSS, prior ovarian torsion, prior or current ovarian cyst, polycystic ovaries, pregnancy, or prior abdominal surgery. Early diagnosis and prompt detorsion may limit the extent of ovarian damage. Benign and malignant neoplasms have been reported (infrequently) in women receiving multiple-drug therapy for controlled ovarian stimulation; causal effect has not been established. Serious hypersensitivity reactions including anaphylaxis have been reported; discontinue use for serious reactions and treat appropriately. Serious pulmonary conditions (atelectasis, acute respiratory distress syndrome, and exacerbation of asthma) have been reported. Thromboembolic events, both in association with and separate from ovarian hyperstimulation syndrome, have been reported.

Multiple births may result from the use of these medications; advise patient of the potential risk of multiple births before starting the treatment.

According to the Centers for Disease Control and Prevention (CDC), pen-shaped injection devices should never be used for more than one person (even when the needle is changed) because of the risk of infection. The injection device should be clearly labeled with individual patient information to ensure that the correct pen is used (CDC, 2012).

Drug Interactions

Avoid Concomitant Use There are no known interactions where it is recommended to avoid concomitant use.

Decreased Effect There are no known significant interactions involving a decrease in effect.

Increased Effect/Toxicity There are no known significant interactions involving an increase in effect.

Adverse Reactions Percentage may vary by indication, product formulation

>10%:

Central nervous system: Headache

Dermatologic: Acne (males)

Endocrine & metabolic: Breast pain (males), ovarian cyst

Gastrointestinal: Abdomen enlarged, abdominal pain, nausea

Miscellaneous: Upper respiratory infection

1% to 10%:

Cardiovascular: Chest pain, hypotension, palpitation

Central nervous system: Anxiety, dizziness, emotional lability, fatigue, fever, malaise, migraine, nervousness, pain, somnolence

Dermatologic: Acne (females), pruritus

Endocrine & metabolic: Breast pain (females), cervix lesion, dysmenorrhea, gynecomastia, hot flashes, intermenstrual bleeding, menstrual disorder, ovarian disorder, ovarian hyperstimulation

Gastrointestinal: Anorexia, constipation, diarrhea, dyspepsia, flatulence, stomatitis (ulcerative), toothache, vomiting, weight gain

Genitourinary: Cystitis, leukorrhea, micturition frequency, pelvic pain, urinary tract infection, uterine hemorrhage, vaginal hemorrhage

Local: Injection site bruising, edema, inflammation, pain, reaction

Neuromuscular & skeletal: Back pain, myalgia, paresthesia

Respiratory: Asthma, cough, dyspnea, pharyngitis, rhinitis, sinusitis

Miscellaneous: Flu-like syndrome, infection, moniliasis, thirst increased

Pharmacodynamics/Kinetics

Onset of Action Peak effect:

Spermatogenesis, median: 6.8-12.4 months (range: 2.7-18.1 months)

Follicle development: Within cycle

Available Dosage Forms

Solution, Subcutaneous:

Gonal-f RFF Pen: 300 units/0.5 mL (0.5 mL); 450 units/0.75 mL (0.75 mL); 900 units/1.5 mL (1.5 mL)

Gonal-f RFF Rediject: 300 units/0.5 mL (0.5 mL); 450 units/0.75 mL (0.75 mL); 900 units/1.5 mL (1.5 mL)

Solution Reconstituted, Injection:

Gonal-f: 450 units (1 ea); 1050 units (1 ea)

Solution Reconstituted, Subcutaneous:

Gonal-f RFF: 75 units (1 ea)

General Dosage Range SubQ

Adults (females): Initial: 75-225 units daily; Maximum: Up to 300-450 units daily

Adults (males): Gonal-f: Initial: 150 units 3 times weekly; Maximum: Up to 300 units 3 times weekly

Administration

Other Administer SubQ. Contents of multidose vials (Gonal-f or Gonal-f RFF) should be administered using the calibrated syringes provided by the manufacturer. Do not shake solution; allow any bubbles to settle prior to administration. Allow Gonal-f RFF Rediject and Gonal-f RFF Pen to warm to room temperature prior to administration.

Preparation for Administration

Gonal-f: Dissolve the contents of vial by slowly injecting provided diluent; do not shake. If bubbles appear, allow to settle prior to use. Final concentration: 600 units/mL.

Gonal-f RFF: Powder: Dissolve contents of one or more vials using diluent provided in prefilled syringe. Total concentration should not exceed 450 units/mL. Slowly inject diluent into vial, and gently rotate vial until powder is dissolved; do not shake vial. If bubbles appear, allow to settle prior to use. Use immediately after reconstitution.

Gonal-f RFF Pen: Allow to warm to room temperature prior to use. Pen must be primed before initial use only. Refer to manufacturer's labeling for instructions on needle assembly.

Gonal-f RFF Rediject: Allow to warm to room temperature prior to use. Do not attempt to mix any other medications inside of the device.

Storage/Stability

Gonal-f: Store powder refrigerated or at room temperature of 2°C to 25°C (36°F to 77°F). Protect from light; do not freeze. Following reconstitution, multidose vials may be stored under refrigeration or at room temperature for up to 28 days.

Gonal-f RFF:

Powder: Store at room temperature or under refrigeration of 2°C to 25°C (36°F to 77°F). Protect from light. Discard unused drug.

Solution (pen): Prior to dispensing, store under refrigeration at 2°C to 8°C (36°F to 46°F). Upon dispensing, patient may store under refrigeration until product expiration date or at room temperature of 20°C to 25°C (68°F to 77°F) for up to 3 months. Do not freeze. Protect from light. After first use, store pen in the refrigerator (2°C to 8°C

[36°F to 46°F]) or at room temperature (20°C to 25°C [68°F to 77°F]); discard unused portion after 28 days.

Nursing Actions

Physical Assessment This medication should only be prescribed by a fertility specialist. Teach patient appropriate injection technique and syringe disposal.

Patient Education

- Discuss specific use of drug and side effects with patient as it relates to treatment. (HCAHPS: During this hospital stay, were you given any medicine that you had not taken before? Before giving you any new medicine, how often did hospital staff tell you what the medicine was for? How often did hospital staff describe possible side effects in a way you could understand?)
- Patient may experience injection site irritation, dyspepsia, acne vulgaris, headache, flatulence, asthenia, or mood changes. Have patient report immediately to prescriber mastalgia, male macromastia, arrhythmia, skin discoloration, pallor, vaginal hemorrhaging, vaginitis, signs of ovarian hyperstimulation syndrome (OHSS), or signs of blood clots (HCAHPS).
- Educate patient about signs of a significant reaction (eg, wheezing; chest tightness; fever; itching; bad cough; blue skin color; seizures; or swelling of face, lips, tongue, or throat). **Note:** This is not a comprehensive list of all side effects. Patient should consult prescriber for additional questions.

Intended Use and Disclaimer: Should not be printed and given to patients. This information is intended to serve as a concise initial reference for healthcare professionals to use when discussing medications with a patient. You must ultimately rely on your own discretion, experience and judgment in diagnosing, treating and advising patients.

Follitropin Beta (foe li TRO pin BAY ta)

Brand Names: U.S. Follistim AQ

Index Terms Follicle Stimulating Hormone, Recombinant; FSH; rFSH-beta; rhFSH-beta

Pharmacologic Category Gonadotropin; Ovulation Stimulator

Pregnancy Risk Factor X

Lactation Excretion in breast milk unknown/not recommended

Breast-Feeding Considerations It is not known if follitropin beta is excreted in breast milk. Due to the potential for serious adverse reactions in the nursing infant, a decision should be made whether to discontinue nursing or to discontinue the drug, taking into account the importance of treatment to the mother.

Use

Females: Induction of ovulation and pregnancy in anovulatory infertile patients in whom the cause of infertility is functional and not caused by primary ovarian failure; induction of pregnancy in normal ovulatory women undergoing Assisted Reproductive Technology (ART) (eg, *in vitro* fertilization [IVF], intracytoplasmic sperm injection [ICSI])

Males: Induction of spermatogenesis in men with primary and secondary hypogonadotropic hypogonadism in whom the cause of infertility is not due to primary testicular failure.

Mechanism of Action/Effect Follitropin beta is a human FSH preparation of recombinant DNA origin. Follitropins stimulate ovarian follicular growth in women who do not have primary ovarian failure and stimulate spermatogenesis in men with hypogonadotrophic hypogonadism. FSH is required for normal follicular growth, maturation, gonadal steroid production, and spermatogenesis.

Contraindications Hypersensitivity to follitropins or any component of the formulation; high levels of FSH indicating primary gonadal failure; uncontrolled nongonadal endocrinopathies (eg, adrenal, pituitary, or thyroid disorders); tumor of the ovary, breast, uterus, testis, hypothalamus, or pituitary gland

Females: Additional contraindications: Abnormal vaginal bleeding of undetermined origin; ovarian cysts or enlargement not due to polycystic ovary syndrome; pregnancy

Warnings/Precautions These medications should only be used by physicians who are thoroughly familiar with infertility problems and their management. To minimize risks, use only at the lowest effective dose. Monitor ovarian response with serum estradiol and vaginal ultrasound on a regular basis.

If ovaries are abnormally enlarged on the last day of treatment, withhold hCG to reduce the risk of ovarian hyperstimulation syndrome (OHSS). OHSS is characterized by severe ovarian enlargement, abdominal pain/distention, nausea, vomiting, diarrhea, dyspnea, and oliguria, and may be accompanied by ascites, pleural effusion, hypovolemia, electrolyte imbalance, hemoperitoneum, and thromboembolic events. If hyperstimulation occurs, stop treatment and hospitalize patient. This syndrome develops rapidly within 24 hours to several days and generally occurs after treatment has ended and reaches its maximum on days 7-10 following treatment. Hemoconcentration associated with fluid loss into the abdominal cavity has occurred and should be assessed by fluid intake and output, weight, hematocrit, serum and urinary electrolytes, urine specific gravity, BUN and creatinine, and abdominal girth. Determinations should be performed daily or more often if the need arises. Treatment is primarily symptomatic and consists of bedrest, fluid and electrolyte replacement, and analgesics. The ascitic, pleural, and pericardial fluids should not be removed unless needed to relieve symptoms of cardiopulmonary distress. Ovarian torsion may occur in relation to OHSS, pregnancy, previous or current ovarian cyst and polycystic ovaries, previous abdominal surgery, and previous history of ovarian torsion

Serious pulmonary conditions (atelectasis, acute respiratory distress syndrome, and exacerbation of asthma) have been reported. Thromboembolic events, both in association with and separate from ovarian hyperstimulation syndrome, have been reported.

Multiple births may result from the use of these medications; advise patient of the potential risk of multiple births before starting the treatment. May contain trace amounts of neomycin or streptomycin.

According to the Centers for Disease Control and Prevention (CDC), pen-shaped injection devices should never be used for more than one person (even when the needle is changed) because of the risk of infection. The injection device should be clearly labeled with individual patient information to ensure that the correct pen is used (CDC, 2012).

Drug Interactions

Avoid Concomitant Use There are no known interactions where it is recommended to avoid concomitant use.

Decreased Effect There are no known significant interactions involving a decrease in effect.

Increased Effect/Toxicity There are no known significant interactions involving an increase in effect.

Adverse Reactions Frequency may vary based on indication.

Central nervous system: Headache (7%), fatigue (2%)

Dermatologic: Acne (7%), rash (3%)

Endocrine & metabolic: Pelvic discomfort (8%), ovarian hyperstimulation (6% to 8%), pelvic pain (6%), gynecomastia (3%), ovarian cyst (3%)

Gastrointestinal: Nausea (4%), abdominal pain/discomfort (2% to 3%)

Local: Injection site pain (7%), injection site reaction (7%)

Postmarketing and/or case reports: Abdominal distension, breast tenderness, constipation, diarrhea, metrorrhagia, miscarriage, ovarian enlargement, ovarian neoplasm, ovarian torsion, thromboembolism, vaginal hemorrhage

Pharmacodynamics/Kinetics

Onset of Action Peak effect: Females: Follicle development: Within cycle

Available Dosage Forms

Solution, Injection:

Follistim AQ: 75 units/0.5 mL (0.5 mL); 150 units/ 0.5 mL (0.5 mL)

Solution, Subcutaneous:

Follistim AQ: 300 units/0.36 mL (0.42 mL); 600 units/0.72 mL (0.78 mL); 900 units/1.08 mL (1.17 mL)

General Dosage Range

I.M., SubQ: *Adults (females):* Initial: 75-225 units/ day; Maintenance: Up to 175-600 units/day

SubQ: *Adults (males):* 450 units/week

Administration

I.M. Follistim® AQ may be administered by I.M. or SubQ injection.

Other

Follistim® AQ may be administered by I.M. or SubQ injection. Follistim® AQ cartridge may be administered only by SubQ injection using the Follistim Pen® which can be set to deliver the appropriate dose.

Storage/Stability Prior to dispensing, store refrigerated at 2°C to 8°C (36°F to 46°F). After dispensed, may be stored under refrigeration or ≤25°C (77°F) for up to 3 months. Once cartridge is pierced, must be stored at 2°C to 25°C (36°F to 77°F) and used within 28 days. Do not freeze. Protect from light.

Nursing Actions

Physical Assessment This medication should only be prescribed by a fertility specialist. Teach patient appropriate injection technique and syringe disposal.

Patient Education

- Discuss specific use of drug and side effects with patient as it relates to treatment. (HCAHPS: During this hospital stay, were you given any medicine that you had not taken before? Before giving you any new medicine, how often did hospital staff tell you what the medicine was for? How often did hospital staff describe possible side effects in a way you could understand?)
- Patient may experience dyspepsia, acne vulgaris, headache, or asthenia. Have patient report immediately to prescriber mastalgia, macromastia, vaginal hemorrhaging, severe injection site irritation, pallor, skin discoloration, signs of ovarian hyperstimulation syndrome (OHSS), or signs of blood clots (HCAHPS).
- Educate patient about signs of a significant reaction (eg, wheezing; chest tightness; fever; itching; bad cough; blue skin color; seizures; or swelling of face, lips, tongue, or throat). **Note:** This is not a comprehensive list of all side effects. Patient should consult prescriber for additional questions.

Intended Use and Disclaimer: Should not be printed and given to patients. This information is intended to serve as a concise initial reference for healthcare professionals to use when discussing medications with a patient. You must ultimately rely on your own discretion, experience and judgment in diagnosing, treating and advising patients.

Fondaparinux (fon da PARE i nuks)

Brand Names: U.S. Arixtra
Index Terms Fondaparinux Sodium
Pharmacologic Category Anticoagulant; Anticoagulant, Factor Xa Inhibitor
Medication Safety Issues
Sound-alike/look-alike issues:
Arixtra® may be confused with Arista® AH (hemostatic device)
High alert medication:
The Institute for Safe Medication Practices (ISMP) includes this medication among its list of drugs which have a heightened risk of causing significant patient harm when used in error.
Pregnancy Risk Factor B
Lactation Excretion in breast milk unknown/use caution
Breast-Feeding Considerations It is not known if fondaparinux is excreted into breast milk. The manufacturer recommends caution be used if administered to nursing women. The use of alternative anticoagulants is preferred (Guyatt, 2012).
Use Prophylaxis of deep vein thrombosis (DVT) in patients undergoing surgery for hip replacement, knee replacement, hip fracture (including extended prophylaxis following hip fracture surgery), or abdominal surgery (in patients at risk for thromboembolic complications); treatment of acute pulmonary embolism (PE); treatment of acute DVT without PE

Canadian labeling: Additional uses (not approved in U.S.): Unstable angina or non-ST segment elevation myocardial infarction (UA/NSTEMI) for the prevention of death and subsequent MI; ST segment elevation MI (STEMI) for the prevention of death and myocardial reinfarction
Unlabeled Use Prophylaxis of DVT in patients with a history of heparin-induced thrombocytopenia (HIT); treatment of acute thrombosis (unrelated to HIT) in patients with a past history of HIT; acute symptomatic superficial vein thrombosis (≥5 cm in length) of the legs
Mechanism of Action/Effect Fondaparinux prevents factor Xa from binding with antithrombin III and inhibits thrombin formation and thrombus development.
Contraindications Serious hypersensitivity (eg, angioedema, anaphylactoid/anaphylactic reactions) to fondaparinux or any component of the formulation; severe renal impairment (CrCl <30 mL/minute); body weight <50 kg (prophylaxis); active major bleeding; bacterial endocarditis; thrombocytopenia associated with a positive *in vitro* test for antiplatelet antibody in the presence of fondaparinux
Warnings/Precautions [U.S. Boxed Warning]: Spinal or epidural hematomas, including subsequent paralysis, may occur with recent or anticipated neuraxial anesthesia (epidural or spinal anesthesia) or spinal puncture in patients anticoagulated with LMWH, heparinoids, or fondaparinux. Consider risk versus benefit prior to spinal procedures; risk is increased by the use of concomitant agents which may alter hemostasis, the use of indwelling epidural catheters for analgesia, a history of spinal deformity or spinal surgery, as well as a history of traumatic or repeated epidural or spinal punctures. Patient should be observed closely for bleeding and signs and symptoms of neurological impairment if therapy is administered during or immediately following diagnostic lumbar puncture, epidural anesthesia, or spinal anesthesia.

Discontinue use 24 hours prior to CABG and dose with unfractionated heparin per institutional practice (Jneid, 2012). Use caution in patients with moderate renal dysfunction (CrCl 30-50 mL/minute); contraindicated in patients with CrCl <30 mL/minute. Discontinue if severe dysfunction or labile function develops.

Use caution in congenital or acquired bleeding disorders; bacterial endocarditis; renal impairment; hepatic impairment; active ulcerative or angiodysplastic gastrointestinal disease; hemorrhagic stroke; shortly after brain, spinal, or ophthalmologic surgery; or in patients taking platelet inhibitors. Risk of major bleeding may be increased if initial dose is administered earlier than recommended (initiation recommended at 6-8 hours following surgery). Discontinue agents that may enhance the risk of hemorrhage if possible. Although considered an insensitive measure of fondaparinux activity, there have been postmarketing reports of bleeding associated with elevated aPTT. Has occurred with administration, including very rare reports of thrombocytopenia with thrombosis similar to heparin-induced thrombocytopenia (HIT); however, has been used in patients with current or history of HIT due to a lack of an immune-mediated effect on platelets (Guyatt [ACCP], 2012; Savi, 2005). Use is contraindicated in patients with thrombocytopenia associated with a positive *in vitro* test for antiplatelet antibodies in the presence of fondaparinux. Monitor patients closely and discontinue therapy if platelets fall to <100,000/mm^3 and/or thrombosis develops.

For subcutaneous administration; not for I.M. administration. Do not use interchangeably (unit for unit) with low molecular weight heparins, heparin, or heparinoids. Use caution in patients <50 kg who are being treated for DVT/PE; dosage reduction recommended. Contraindicated in patients <50 kg when used for prophylactic therapy. Use with caution in the elderly. The needle guard contains natural latex rubber.

The administration of fondaparinux as the sole anticoagulant is **not recommended** during PCI due to an increased risk for guiding-catheter thrombosis. Use of an anticoagulant with antithrombin activity (eg, unfractionated heparin) is recommended as adjunctive therapy to PCI even if prior treatment with fondaparinux (must take into account whether GP IIb/IIIa antagonists have been administered) (Levine, 2011). Do not administer with other agents that increase the risk of hemorrhage unless they are essential for the management of the underlying condition (eg, warfarin for treatment of VTE).

Drug Interactions

Avoid Concomitant Use

Avoid concomitant use of Fondaparinux with any of the following: Apixaban; Dabigatran Etexilate; Omacetaxine; Rivaroxaban; Urokinase

Decreased Effect

The levels/effects of Fondaparinux may be decreased by: Estrogen Derivatives; Progestins

Increased Effect/Toxicity

Fondaparinux may increase the levels/effects of: Anticoagulants; Collagenase (Systemic); Deferasirox; Ibritumomab; Omacetaxine; Rivaroxaban; Tositumomab and Iodine I 131 Tositumomab

The levels/effects of Fondaparinux may be increased by: Agents with Antiplatelet Properties; Apixaban; Dabigatran Etexilate; Dasatinib; Herbs (Anticoagulant/Antiplatelet Properties); Ibrutinib; Nonsteroidal Anti-Inflammatory Agents; Omega-3 Fatty Acids; Pentosan Polysulfate Sodium; Prostacyclin Analogues; Salicylates; Sugammadex; Thrombolytic Agents; Tibolone; Tipranavir; Urokinase; Vitamin E

Nutritional/Ethanol Interactions Herb/Nutraceutical: Avoid alfalfa, anise, bilberry, bladderwrack, bromelain, cat's claw, celery, coleus, cordyceps, dong quai, evening primrose oil, fenugreek, feverfew, garlic, ginger, ginkgo biloba, ginseng (American/Panax/Siberian), grapeseed, green tea, guggul, horse chestnut seed, horseradish, licorice, prickly ash, red clover, reishi, sweet clover, turmeric, white willow (all possess anticoagulant or antiplatelet activity and as such, may enhance the anticoagulant effects of fondaparinux).

Adverse Reactions As with all anticoagulants, bleeding is the major adverse effect. Hemorrhage may occur at any site. Risk appears increased by a number of factors including renal dysfunction, age (>75 years), and weight (<50 kg).

>10%:
Central nervous system: Fever (4% to 14%)
Gastrointestinal: Nausea (11%)
Hematologic: Anemia (20%)

1% to 10%:
Cardiovascular: Edema (9%), hypotension (4%), thrombosis PCI catheter (without heparin 1%)
Central nervous system: Insomnia (5%), dizziness (4%), headache (2% to 5%), confusion (3%), pain (2%)

Dermatologic: Rash (8%), purpura (4%), bullous eruption (3%)
Endocrine & metabolic: Hypokalemia (1% to 4%)
Gastrointestinal: Constipation (5% to 9%), nausea (3%), vomiting (6%), diarrhea (3%), dyspepsia (2%)
Genitourinary: Urinary tract infection (4%), urinary retention (3%)
Hematologic: Moderate thrombocytopenia ($50,000\text{-}100,000/\text{mm}^3$: 3%), major bleeding (1% to 3%), minor bleeding (2% to 4%), hematoma (3%); risk of major bleeding increased as high as 5% in patients receiving initial dose <6 hours following surgery
Hepatic: ALT increased (≤3%), AST increased (≤2%)
Local: Injection site reaction (bleeding, rash, pruritus)
Miscellaneous: Wound drainage increased (5%)

Available Dosage Forms

Solution, Subcutaneous:
Generic: 2.5 mg/0.5 mL (0.5 mL); 5 mg/0.4 mL (0.4 mL); 7.5 mg/0.6 mL (0.6 mL); 10 mg/0.8 mL (0.8 mL)

Solution, Subcutaneous [preservative free]:
Arixtra: 2.5 mg/0.5 mL (0.5 mL); 5 mg/0.4 mL (0.4 mL); 7.5 mg/0.6 mL (0.6 mL); 10 mg/0.8 mL (0.8 mL)
Generic: 2.5 mg/0.5 mL (0.5 mL); 5 mg/0.4 mL (0.4 mL); 7.5 mg/0.6 mL (0.6 mL); 10 mg/0.8 mL (0.8 mL)

General Dosage Range SubQ:

Adults <50 kg: Treatment: 5 mg once daily
Adults 50-100 kg: Prophylaxis: 2.5 mg once daily; Treatment: 7.5 mg once daily
Adults >100 kg: Prophylaxis: 2.5 mg once daily; Treatment: 10 mg once daily

Administration

I.M. Do **not** administer I.M.

I.V. For STEMI patients (Canadian labeling; unlabeled use in U.S.) may administer initial dose as I.V. push or mix in 25-50 mL of NS (do not mix with other agents) and infuse over 2 minutes; flush tubing with NS after infusion to ensure complete administration for fondaparinux.

Subcutaneous Intended for SubQ administration. Do not mix with other injections or infusions. Do not expel air bubble from syringe before injection. Administer according to recommended regimen; when used for DVT prophylaxis, early initiation (before 6 hours after orthopedic surgery) has been associated with increased bleeding.

To convert from I.V. unfractionated heparin (UFH) infusion to SubQ fondaparinux (Nutescu, 2007): Calculate specific dose for fondaparinux based on indication, discontinue UFH, and begin fondaparinux within 1 hour

To convert from SubQ fondaparinux to I.V. UFH infusion (Nutescu, 2007): Discontinue fondaparinux; calculate specific dose for I.V. UFH infusion based on indication; omit heparin bolus/loading dose

For subQ fondaparinux dosed every 24 hours: Start I.V. UFH infusion 22-23 hours after last dose of fondaparinux

Preparation for Administration Canadian labeling: For I.V. administration: May mix with 25 mL or 50 mL NS

Storage/Stability Store at 25°C (77°F); excursions permitted to 15°C to 30°C (59°F to 86°F).

Canadian labeling: For I.V. administration: Manufacturer recommends immediate use once diluted in NS, but is stable for up to 24 hours at 15°C to 30°C (59°F to 86°F).

Nursing Actions

Physical Assessment Monitor renal function and signs or symptoms of bleeding.

Patient Education

• Discuss specific use of drug and side effects with patient as it relates to treatment. (HCAHPS: During this hospital stay, were you given any medicine that you had not taken before? Before giving you any new medicine, how often did hospital staff tell you what the medicine was for? How often did hospital staff describe possible side effects in a way you could understand?)

• Patient may experience injection site irritation or insomnia. Have patient report immediately to prescriber signs of hemorrhaging, severe dizziness, syncope, illogical thinking, considerable headache, paresthesia, myalgia, or significant asthenia (HCAHPS).

• Educate patient about signs of a significant reaction (eg, wheezing; chest tightness; fever; itching; bad cough; blue skin color; seizures; or swelling of face, lips, tongue, or throat). **Note:** This is not a comprehensive list of all side effects. Patient should consult prescriber for additional questions.

Intended Use and Disclaimer: Should not be printed and given to patients. This information is intended to serve as a concise initial reference for healthcare professionals to use when discussing medications with a patient. You must ultimately rely on your own discretion, experience and judgment in diagnosing, treating and advising patients.

Formoterol (for MOH te rol)

Brand Names: U.S. Foradil Aerolizer; Perforomist

Index Terms Formoterol Fumarate; Formoterol Fumarate Dihydrate

Pharmacologic Category Beta$_2$ Agonist; Beta$_2$-Adrenergic Agonist, Long-Acting

Medication Safety Issues

Sound-alike/look-alike issues:

Foradil® may be confused with Toradol®

Administration issues:

Foradil® capsules for inhalation are for administration via Aerolizer® inhaler and are **not** for oral use.

International issues:

Foradil [U.S., Canada, and multiple international markets] may be confused with Theradol brand name for tramadol [Netherlands]

Medication Guide Available Yes

Pregnancy Risk Factor C

Lactation Excretion in breast milk unknown/use caution

Breast-Feeding Considerations It is not known if formoterol is excreted into breast milk. The manufacturer recommends that caution be exercised when administering formoterol to nursing women. The use of beta$_2$-receptor agonists are not considered a contraindication to breast-feeding (NAEPP, 2005).

Use U.S. labeling: Treatment of asthma (only as concomitant therapy with an inhaled corticosteroid) in patients with reversible obstructive airway disease, including patients with symptoms of nocturnal asthma (Foradil® Aerolizer®); maintenance treatment of bronchoconstriction in patients with COPD (Foradil® Aerolizer®, Perforomist®); prevention of exercise-induced bronchospasm when administered on an as-needed basis (monotherapy may be indicated in patients without persistent asthma) (Foradil® Aerolizer®)

Canadian labeling: Treatment of asthma (only as concomitant therapy with an inhaled corticosteroid) in patients with reversible obstructive airway disease, including patients with symptoms of nocturnal asthma (Foradil®, Oxeze® Turbuhaler®); maintenance treatment of COPD (Foradil®); prevention of exercise-induced bronchospasm when administered on an as-needed basis (monotherapy may be indicated in patients without persistent asthma) (Oxeze® Turbuhaler®)

Mechanism of Action/Effect Relaxes bronchial smooth muscle

Contraindications Hypersensitivity to formoterol or any component of the formulation (Foradil® Aerolizer® only); treatment of status asthmaticus or other acute episodes of asthma or COPD (Foradil® Aerolizer® only); monotherapy in the treatment of asthma (ie, use without a concomitant long-term asthma control medication, such as an inhaled corticosteroid)

Canadian labeling: Additional contraindications (not in U.S. labeling): Presence of tachyarrhythmias

Warnings/Precautions [U.S. Boxed Warning]: Long-acting beta$_2$-agonists (LABAs) increase the risk of asthma-related deaths. Formoterol

should only be used in asthma patients as adjuvant therapy in patients who are currently receiving but are not adequately controlled on a long-term asthma control medication (ie, an inhaled corticosteroid). Monotherapy with an LABA is contraindicated in the treatment of asthma. In a large, randomized, placebo-controlled U.S. clinical trial (SMART, 2006), salmeterol was associated with an increase in asthma-related deaths (when added to usual asthma therapy); risk is considered a class effect among all LABAs. Data are not available to determine if the addition of an inhaled corticosteroid lessens this increased risk of death associated with LABA use. Assess patients at regular intervals once asthma control is maintained on combination therapy to determine if step-down therapy is appropriate and the LABA can be discontinued (without loss of asthma control), and the patient can be maintained on an inhaled corticosteroid. LABAs are not appropriate in patients whose asthma is adequately controlled on low- or medium-dose inhaled corticosteroids. Do **not** use for acute bronchospasm. Short-acting beta$_2$-agonist (eg, albuterol) should be used for acute symptoms and symptoms occurring between treatments. Do **not** initiate in patients with significantly worsening or acutely deteriorating asthma; reports of severe (sometimes fatal) respiratory events have been reported when formoterol has been initiated in this situation. Corticosteroids should not be stopped or reduced when formoterol is initiated. Formoterol is not a substitute for inhaled or systemic corticosteroids and should not be used as monotherapy. During initiation, watch for signs of worsening asthma. **[U.S. Boxed Warning] (Foradil® Aerolizer®): LABAs may increase the risk of asthma-related hospitalization in pediatric and adolescent patients**. In general, a combination product containing a LABA and an inhaled corticosteroid is preferred in patients <18 years of age to ensure compliance.

Because LABAs may disguise poorly controlled persistent asthma, frequent or chronic use of LABAs for exercise-induced bronchospasm is discouraged by the NIH Asthma Guidelines (NIH, 2007). The safety and efficacy of Perforomist® in asthma patients have not been established and is not FDA approved for the treatment of asthma.

Do **not** use for acute episodes of COPD. Do **not** initiate in patients with significantly worsening or acutely deteriorating COPD. Data are not available to determine if LABA use increases the risk of death in patients with COPD. Increased use and/or ineffectiveness of short-acting beta$_2$-agonists may indicate rapidly deteriorating disease and should prompt re-evaluation of the patient's condition.

Immediate hypersensitivity reactions (urticaria, angioedema, rash, bronchospasm) have been reported. Do not exceed recommended dose or frequency; serious adverse events (including serious asthma exacerbations and fatalities) have been associated with excessive use of inhaled sympathomimetics. Beta$_2$-agonists may increase risk of arrhythmias, decrease serum potassium, prolong QT$_c$ interval, or increase serum glucose. These effects may be exacerbated in hypoxemia. Use caution in patients with cardiovascular disease (arrhythmia, coronary insufficiency, hypertension, HF, or aneurysm), seizures, diabetes, hyperthyroidism, pheochromocytoma, or hypokalemia. Beta-agonists may cause elevation in blood pressure and heart rate, and result in CNS stimulation/excitation. Tolerance to the bronchodilator effect, measured by FEV$_1$, has been observed in studies.

Powder for oral inhalation contains lactose; very rare anaphylactic reactions have been reported in patients with severe milk protein allergy. The contents of the Foradil® Aerolizer® capsules are for inhalation only via the Aerolizer® device. There have been reports of incorrect administration (swallowing of the capsules).

Drug Interactions

Avoid Concomitant Use

Avoid concomitant use of Formoterol with any of the following: Beta-Blockers (Nonselective); Highest Risk QTc-Prolonging Agents; Iobenguane I 123; Ivabradine; Long-Acting Beta2-Agonists; Mifepristone

Decreased Effect

Formoterol may decrease the levels/effects of: Iobenguane I 123

The levels/effects of Formoterol may be decreased by: Beta-Blockers (Beta1 Selective); Beta-Blockers (Nonselective); Betahistine

Increased Effect/Toxicity

Formoterol may increase the levels/effects of: Atosiban; Highest Risk QTc-Prolonging Agents; Long-Acting Beta2-Agonists; Loop Diuretics; Moderate Risk QTc-Prolonging Agents; Sympathomimetics; Thiazide Diuretics

The levels/effects of Formoterol may be increased by: AtoMOXetine; Caffeine; Cannabinoids; Inhalational Anesthetics; Ivabradine; MAO Inhibitors; Mifepristone; QTc-Prolonging Agents (Indeterminate Risk and Risk Modifying); Theophylline Derivatives; Tricyclic Antidepressants

Adverse Reactions

1% to 10%:

Cardiovascular: Chest pain (2% to 3%), palpitation

Central nervous system: Anxiety (2%), dizziness (2%), fever (2%), insomnia (2%), dysphonia (1%), headache

Dermatologic: Pruritus (2%), rash (1%)

Gastrointestinal: Diarrhea (5%), nausea (5%), xerostomia (1% to 3%), vomiting (2%), abdominal pain, dyspepsia, gastroenteritis

Neuromuscular & skeletal: Muscle cramps (2%), tremor

Respiratory: Infection (3% to 7%), asthma exacerbation (age 5-12 years: 5% to 6%; age >12 years: <4%), bronchitis (5%), pharyngitis (3% to 4%), sinusitis (3%), dyspnea (2%), tonsillitis (1%)

Pharmacodynamics/Kinetics

Onset of Action Powder for inhalation: Within 3 minutes

Peak effect: Powder for inhalation: 80% of peak effect within 15 minutes; Solution for nebulization: 2 hours

Duration of Action Improvement in FEV_1 observed for 12 hours in most patients

Available Dosage Forms

Capsule, Inhalation:

Foradil Aerolizer: 12 mcg

Nebulization Solution, Inhalation:

Perforomist: 20 mcg/2 mL (2 mL)

General Dosage Range Inhalation:

Powder for inhalation: *Children ≥5 years, Adolescents, and Adults:* 12 mcg every 12 hours (maximum: 24 mcg daily) **or** 12 mcg inhaled prior to exercise

Solution for nebulization: *Adults:* 20 mcg twice daily (maximum: 40 mcg daily)

Administration

Inhalation

Foradil® Aerolizer®: Remove capsule from foil blister **immediately** before use. Place capsule in the capsule-chamber in the base of the Aerolizer® Inhaler. Capsules must not be swallowed whole; must only use the Aerolizer® Inhaler. Press both buttons **once only** and then release. Keep inhaler in a level, horizontal position. Exhale fully. Do not exhale into inhaler. Tilt head slightly back and inhale (rapidly, steadily, and deeply). Hold breath as long as possible. If any powder remains in capsule, exhale and inhale again. Repeat until capsule is empty. Throw away empty capsule; do not leave in inhaler. Do not use a spacer with the Aerolizer® Inhaler. Always keep capsules and inhaler dry.

Perforomist®: Remove unit-dose vial from foil pouch **immediately** before use. Solution does not require dilution prior to administration; do not mix other medications with formoterol solution. Place contents of unit-dose vial into the reservoir of a standard jet nebulizer connected to an air compressor; assemble nebulizer based on the manufacturer's instructions and turn nebulizer on; breathe deeply and evenly until all of the medication has been inhaled. Discard any unused medication immediately; do not ingest contents of vial. Clean nebulizer after use.

Oxeze® Turbuhaler® (Canadian availability): Hold inhaler upright. Turn colored grip as far as it will go in one direction and then turn back to original position; a clicking sound should be heard which means the inhaler is ready for use. Exhale fully. Do not exhale into mouthpiece of inhaler. Place mouthpiece to lips and inhale forcefully and deeply. Do not chew or bite on mouthpiece. Clean outside of mouthpiece once weekly with a dry tissue. Avoid getting inhaler wet. If the inhaler is accidently dropped or shaken, or if the patient exhales into the inhaler, the dose will be lost and a new dose should be loaded.

Storage/Stability

Foradil® Aerolizer®: Prior to dispensing, store in refrigerator at 2°C to 8°C (36°F to 46°F). After dispensing, store at room temperature at 20°C to 25°C (68°F to 77°F). Protect from heat and moisture. Capsules should always be stored in the blister and only removed immediately before use.

Perforomist®: Prior to dispensing, store in refrigerator at 2°C to 8°C (36°F to 46°F). After dispensing, store at 2°C to 25°C (36°F to 77°F) for up to 3 months. Protect from heat. Unit-dose vials should always be stored in the foil pouch and only removed immediately before use.

Nursing Actions

Physical Assessment Monitor for signs of worsening asthma when initiating therapy. Patient should always be on at least one other drug to treat asthma with this drug. Monitor heart rate, blood pressure, peak-flow measurements, and blood glucose and potassium levels. Assessment and monitoring of lung exam should be on-going.

Monitor insulin and/or oral hypoglycemic therapy requirements in diabetics. Encourage patient to keep good records of home glucose monitoring, especially during initiation of drug therapy. Instruct patient to report if home glucose consistently high or if signs of hyperglycemia (eg, increased thirst, increased urination, sleepiness) occur.

Patient Education

- Discuss specific use of drug and side effects with patient as it relates to treatment. (HCAHPS: During this hospital stay, were you given any medicine that you had not taken before? Before giving you any new medicine, how often did hospital staff tell you what the medicine was for? How often did hospital staff describe possible side effects in a way you could understand?)
- Patient may experience diarrhea. Have patient report immediately to prescriber signs of hyperglycemia, signs of hypokalemia, angina, tachycardia, anxiety, severe dizziness, syncope, tachypnea, chills, pharyngitis, considerable headache, significant nausea, intolerable dyspepsia, voice changes, or dyspnea (HCAHPS).
- Educate patient about signs of a significant reaction (eg, wheezing; chest tightness; fever; itching; bad cough; blue skin color; seizures; or swelling of face, lips, tongue, or throat). **Note:** This is not a comprehensive list of all side effects. Patient should consult prescriber for additional questions.

Intended Use and Disclaimer: Should not be printed and given to patients. This information is intended to serve as a concise initial reference for healthcare professionals to use when discussing medications with a patient. You must ultimately rely on your own discretion, experience and judgment in diagnosing, treating and advising patients.

Fosamprenavir (FOS am pren a veer)

Brand Names: U.S. Lexiva
Index Terms Fosamprenavir Calcium; GW433908G
Pharmacologic Category Antiretroviral, Protease Inhibitor (Anti-HIV)
Medication Safety Issues
Sound-alike/look-alike issues:
Lexiva® may be confused with Levitra®
Pregnancy Risk Factor C
Lactation Excretion in breast milk unknown/contraindicated
Breast-Feeding Considerations Maternal or infant antiretroviral therapy does not completely eliminate the risk of postnatal HIV transmission. In addition, multiclass-resistant virus has been detected in breast-feeding infants despite maternal therapy. Therefore, in the United States, where formula is accessible, affordable, safe, and sustainable, and the risk of infant mortality due to diarrhea and respiratory infections is low, complete avoidance of breast-feeding by HIV-infected women is recommended to decrease potential transmission of HIV (DHHS [perinatal], 2012).
Use Treatment of HIV infections in combination with at least two other antiretroviral agents
Mechanism of Action/Effect Fosamprenavir is rapidly and almost completely converted to amprenavir in vivo. Amprenavir blocks the site of HIV-1 protease activity, resulting in the formation of immature, noninfectious viral particles.
Contraindications Clinically-significant hypersensitivity (eg, Stevens-Johnson syndrome) to fosamprenavir, amprenavir, or any component of the formulation; concurrent therapy with CYP3A4 substrates with a narrow therapeutic window; concomitant use with alfuzosin, cisapride, delavirdine, ergot derivatives, lovastatin, midazolam, pimozide, rifampin, simvastatin, St John's wort, and triazolam; use of flecainide and propafenone with concomitant ritonavir therapy; sildenafil (when used for pulmonary artery hypertension [eg, Revatio®])
Warnings/Precautions Concomitant use of fosamprenavir with some drugs may require cautious use, may not be recommended, may require dosage adjustments, or may be contraindicated. Do not use with hormonal contraceptives. Do not coadminister colchicine in patient with renal or hepatic impairment.

Use with caution in patients with diabetes mellitus or sulfonamide allergy. Use caution with hepatic impairment (dosage adjustment required) or underlying hepatitis B or C. Redistribution of fat may occur (eg, buffalo hump, peripheral wasting, cushingoid appearance). Dosage adjustment is required for combination therapies (ritonavir and/or efavirenz); in addition, the risk of hyperlipidemia may be increased during concurrent therapy. Protease inhibitors have been associated with a variety of hypersensitivity events (some severe), including rash, anaphylaxis (rare), angioedema, bronchospasm, erythema multiforme, and/or Stevens-Johnson syndrome (rare). It is generally recommended to discontinue treatment if severe rash or moderate symptoms accompanied by other systemic symptoms occur. Acute hemolytic anemia has been reported in association with amprenavir use. Cases of nephrolithiasis have been reported in postmarketing surveillance; temporary or permanent discontinuation of therapy should be considered if symptoms develop. Spontaneous bleeding has been reported in patients with hemophilia A or B following treatment with protease inhibitors; use caution. Immune reconstitution syndrome may develop, resulting in the occurrence of an inflammatory response to an indolent or residual opportunistic infection during initial HIV treatment or activation of autoimmune disorders (eg, Graves' disease, polymyositis, Guillain-Barré syndrome) later in therapy; further evaluation and treatment may be required.

Drug Interactions
Avoid Concomitant Use
Avoid concomitant use of Fosamprenavir with any of the following: Ado-Trastuzumab Emtansine; Alfuzosin; Amiodarone; Apixaban; Avanafil; Axitinib; Bosutinib; Cabozantinib; Cisapride; Conivaptan; Crizotinib; Delavirdine; Dronedarone; Eplerenone; Ergot Derivatives; Etravirine; Everolimus; Flecainide; Halofantrine; Ibrutinib; Imatinib; Ivabradine; Lapatinib; Lomitapide; Lovastatin; Lurasidone; Macitentan; Midazolam; Nilotinib; Nisoldipine; Pimozide; Pomalidomide; Propafenone; QuiNIDine; Ranolazine; Red Yeast Rice; Regorafenib; Rifampin; Rivaroxaban; Salmeterol; Silodosin; Simeprevir; Simvastatin; St Johns Wort; Tamsulosin; Telaprevir; Ticagrelor; Tolvaptan; Toremifene; Triazolam; Ulipristal; Vemurafenib; VinCRIStine (Liposomal)

Decreased Effect
Fosamprenavir may decrease the levels/effects of: Abacavir; Boceprevir; Clarithromycin; Contraceptives (Estrogens); Delavirdine; Dolutegravir; Fosphenytoin; Ifosfamide; Lopinavir; Meperidine; Methadone; PARoxetine; Phenytoin; Posaconazole; Prasugrel; Raltegravir; Telaprevir; Ticagrelor; Valproic Acid and Derivatives; Zidovudine

The levels/effects of Fosamprenavir may be decreased by: Antacids; Boceprevir; Bosentan;

705

CarBAMazepine; CYP3A4 Inducers (Strong); Dabrafenib; Deferasirox; Efavirenz; Garlic; H2-Antagonists; Methadone; Mitotane; Nevirapine; Peginterferon Alfa-2b; P-glycoprotein/ABCB1 Inducers; Raltegravir; Rifampin; St Johns Wort; Telaprevir; Tocilizumab

Increased Effect/Toxicity

Fosamprenavir may increase the levels/effects of: Ado-Trastuzumab Emtansine; Alfuzosin; Almotriptan; Alosetron; ALPRAZolam; Amiodarone; Apixaban; ARIPiprazole; AtorvaSTATin; Avanafil; Axitinib; Bedaquiline; Bortezomib; Bosentan; Bosutinib; Brentuximab Vedotin; Brinzolamide; Budesonide (Nasal); Budesonide (Systemic, Oral Inhalation); Cabozantinib; Calcium Channel Blockers (Dihydropyridine); Calcium Channel Blockers (Nondihydropyridine); CarBAMazepine; Cisapride; Clarithromycin; Clorazepate; Colchicine; Conivaptan; Corticosteroids (Orally Inhaled); Crizotinib; CycloSPORINE (Systemic); CYP3A4 Substrates; Diazepam; Dienogest; Digoxin; Dofetilide; DOXOrubicin (Conventional); Dronedarone; Dutasteride; Enfuvirtide; Enzalutamide; Eplerenone; Ergot Derivatives; Everolimus; FentaNYL; Fesoterodine; Flecainide; Flurazepam; Fluticasone (Nasal); Fluticasone (Oral Inhalation); GuanFACINE; Halofantrine; Ibrutinib; Iloperidone; Imatinib; Itraconazole; Ivabradine; Ivacaftor; Ixabepilone; Ketoconazole (Systemic); Lacosamide; Lapatinib; Levomilnacipran; Lomitapide; Lovastatin; Lumefantrine; Lurasidone; Macitentan; Maraviroc; Meperidine; MethylPREDNISolone; Midazolam; Mifepristone; Nefazodone; Nilotinib; Nisoldipine; Ospemifene; OxyCODONE; Paricalcitol; PAZOPanib; Pimecrolimus; Pimozide; Pomalidomide; PONATinib; Propafenone; Protease Inhibitors; QUEtiapine; QuiNIDine; Ranolazine; Red Yeast Rice; Regorafenib; Repaglinide; Rifabutin; Rilpivirine; Riociguat; Rivaroxaban; RomiDEPsin; Rosuvastatin; Ruxolitinib; Salmeterol; Saxagliptin; Sildenafil; Silodosin; Simeprevir; Simvastatin; SORAfenib; Tacrolimus (Systemic); Tacrolimus (Topical); Tadalafil; Tamsulosin; Temsirolimus; Ticagrelor; Tofacitinib; Tolterodine; Tolvaptan; Toremifene; TraZODone; Triazolam; Tricyclic Antidepressants; Ulipristal; Vardenafil; Vemurafenib; Vilazodone; VinCRIStine (Liposomal); Voriconazole; Warfarin; Zuclopenthixol

The levels/effects of Fosamprenavir may be increased by: Clarithromycin; CycloSPORINE (Systemic); Delavirdine; Enfuvirtide; Etravirine; Fosphenytoin; Itraconazole; Ketoconazole (Systemic); P-glycoprotein/ABCB1 Inhibitors; Phenytoin; Posaconazole; Rifabutin; Simeprevir; Voriconazole

Nutritional/Ethanol Interactions

Food: Management:
Oral suspension: Administer without food to adults or with food to pediatric patients.

Tablet: Administer with food if taken with ritonavir. May be administered without regard to food if not taken with ritonavir.

Herb/Nutraceutical: Serum concentration may be decreased by St John's wort. Management: Avoid St John's wort; concurrent use is contraindicated.

Adverse Reactions

>10%:
Dermatologic: Rash (≤19%; onset: ~11 days; duration: ~13 days)
Endocrine & metabolic: Hypertriglyceridemia (>750 mg/dL: ≤11%)
Gastrointestinal: Diarrhea (moderate-to-severe; 5% to 13%)

1% to 10%:
Central nervous system: Headache (moderate-to-severe; 2% to 4%), fatigue (moderate-to-severe; 2% to 4%)
Dermatologic: Pruritus (7% to 8%)
Endocrine & metabolic: Hyperglycemia (>251 mg/dL: ≤2%)
Gastrointestinal: Serum lipase increased (>2 times ULN: 5% to 8%), nausea (moderate-to-severe; 3% to 7%), vomiting (moderate-to-severe; 2% to 6%), abdominal pain (moderate-to-severe; ≤2%)
Hematologic: Neutropenia (<750 cells/mm^3: 3%)
Hepatic: Transaminases increased (>5 times ULN: 4% to 8%)

Frequency not defined: Diabetes mellitus, fat redistribution, and immune reconstitution syndrome have been associated with protease inhibitor therapy. Spontaneous bleeding has been reported in patients with hemophilia A or B following treatment with protease inhibitors. Acute hemolytic anemia has been reported in association with amprenavir use.

Available Dosage Forms

Suspension, Oral:
Lexiva: 50 mg/mL (225 mL)
Tablet, Oral:
Lexiva: 700 mg

General Dosage Range Dosage adjustment recommended in patients with hepatic impairment or on concomitant therapy

Oral:
Infants ≥4 weeks (PI-naive patients) or Infants ≥6 months (PI-experienced patients): Ritonavir-boosted regimen:
<11 kg: 45 mg/kg/dose twice daily (plus ritonavir); maximum: 700 mg/dose
11 to <15 kg: 30 mg/kg/dose twice daily (plus ritonavir); maximum: 700 mg/dose
15 to <20 kg: 23 mg/kg/dose twice daily (plus ritonavir); maximum: 700 mg/dose
≥20 kg: 18 mg/kg/dose twice daily (plus ritonavir); maximum: 700 mg/dose

Children ≥2 years (PI-naive patients): Unboosted regimen:

<47 kg: 30 mg/kg/dose twice daily; maximum: 1400 mg/dose

≥47 kg: 1400 mg twice daily

Adults:

Ritonavir-boosted regimen: 700 mg twice daily **or** 1400 mg once daily

Unboosted regimen: 1400 mg twice daily

Administration
Oral
Oral suspension: Administer **without** food to adults; administer **with** food to pediatric patients. Readminister dose of suspension if emesis occurs within 30 minutes after dosing. Shake suspension vigorously prior to use.

Tablet: Administer with food if taken with ritonavir. May be administered without regard to food if not taken with ritonavir.

Storage/Stability
Lexiva®: Store tablets at 25°C (77°F); excursions permitted to 15°C to 30°C (59°F to 86°F). Store oral suspension at 5°C to 30°C (41°F to 86°F). Do not freeze.

Telzir®: Store tablets 2°C to 30°C; do not freeze and discard 25 days after opening.

Nursing Actions
Physical Assessment Monitor for adherence to regimen. Monitor for hypersensitivity, gastrointestinal disturbance (nausea, vomiting, diarrhea) that can lead to dehydration and weight loss, hyperglycemia, and cardiac status. Caution patients to monitor glucose levels closely; protease inhibitors may cause hyperglycemia or new-onset diabetes. Teach patient proper timing of multiple medications and drugs that should not be used concurrently. Instruct patient on glucose testing (protease inhibitors may cause hyperglycemia), exacerbation or new-onset diabetes.

Patient Education
- Discuss specific use of drug and side effects with patient as it relates to treatment. (HCAHPS: During this hospital stay, were you given any medicine that you had not taken before? Before giving you any new medicine, how often did hospital staff tell you what the medicine was for? How often did hospital staff describe possible side effects in a way you could understand?)
- Patient may experience headache or diarrhea. Have patient report immediately to prescriber signs of hepatic impairment, signs of hyperglycemia, angina, severe nausea, abdominal pain, polyuria, polydipsia, weight loss, dysuria, back pain, hematuria, paresthesia of mouth, significant dizziness, syncope, dyspnea, hyperhidrosis, considerable asthenia, lipodystrophy, signs of Stevens-Johnson syndrome/toxic epidermal necrolysis, or signs of infection (HCAHPS).
- Educate patient about signs of a significant reaction (eg, wheezing; chest tightness; fever; itching; bad cough; blue skin color; seizures; or swelling of face, lips, tongue, or throat). **Note:** This is not a comprehensive list of all side effects. Patient should consult prescriber for additional questions.

Intended Use and Disclaimer: Should not be printed and given to patients. This information is intended to serve as a concise initial reference for healthcare professionals to use when discussing medications with a patient. You must ultimately rely on your own discretion, experience and judgment in diagnosing, treating and advising patients.

Dietary Considerations Tablets may be taken with or without food. Adults should take oral suspension **without** food; however, children should take oral suspension **with** food.

Fosaprepitant (fos a PRE pi tant)

Brand Names: U.S. Emend

Index Terms Aprepitant Injection; Fosaprepitant Dimeglumine; L-758,298; MK 0517

Pharmacologic Category Antiemetic; Substance P/Neurokinin 1 Receptor Antagonist

Medication Safety Issues

Sound-alike/look-alike issues:

Fosaprepitant may be confused with aprepitant, fosamprenavir, fospropofol

Emend® for Injection (fosaprepitant) may be confused with Emend® (aprepitant) which is an oral capsule formulation.

Pregnancy Risk Factor B

Lactation Excretion in breast milk unknown/not recommended

Breast-Feeding Considerations It is not known if fosaprepitant is excreted in breast milk. Due to the potential for serious adverse reactions in the nursing infant, a decision should be made whether to discontinue nursing or to discontinue the drug, taking into account the importance of treatment to the mother.

Use Prevention of acute and delayed nausea and vomiting associated with moderately- and highly-emetogenic chemotherapy (in combination with other antiemetics)

Mechanism of Action/Effect Fosaprepitant is a prodrug of aprepitant, a substance P/neurokinin 1 (NK1) receptor antagonist. It is rapidly converted to aprepitant which prevents acute and delayed vomiting by inhibiting the substance P/neurokinin 1 (NK1) receptor; augments the antiemetic activity of the 5-HT$_3$ receptor antagonist and corticosteroid activity and inhibits chemotherapy-induced emesis.

Contraindications Hypersensitivity to fosaprepitant, aprepitant, polysorbate 80, or any component of the formulation; concurrent use with pimozide or cisapride

Canadian labeling: Additional contraindications (not in U.S. labeling): Concurrent use with astemizole or terfenadine

Warnings/Precautions Fosaprepitant is rapidly converted to aprepitant, which has a high potential for drug interactions. Potentially significant drug-drug interactions may exist, requiring dose or frequency adjustment, additional monitoring, and/or selection of alternative therapy. Immediate hypersensitivity has been reported (rarely) with fosaprepitant; stop infusion with hypersensitivity symptoms (dyspnea, erythema, flushing, or anaphylaxis); do not reinitiate. Contains polysorbate 80, which is associated with hypersensitivity reactions. Use caution with hepatic impairment; has not been studied in patients with severe hepatic impairment (Child-Pugh class C). Not studied for treatment of existing nausea and vomiting. Chronic continuous administration of fosaprepitant is not recommended.

Drug Interactions

Avoid Concomitant Use

Avoid concomitant use of Fosaprepitant with any of the following: Astemizole; Axitinib; Bosutinib; Cisapride; Conivaptan; Fusidic Acid (Systemic); Ibrutinib; Ivabradine; Lomitapide; Pimozide; Rivaroxaban; Simeprevir; Terfenadine; Tolvaptan; Ulipristal

Decreased Effect

Fosaprepitant may decrease the levels/effects of: ARIPiprazole; Axitinib; Contraceptives (Estrogens); Contraceptives (Progestins); Ibrutinib; Ifosfamide; PARoxetine; Saxagliptin; Simeprevir; TOLBUTamide; Warfarin

The levels/effects of Fosaprepitant may be decreased by: Bosentan; CYP3A4 Inducers (Strong); Dabrafenib; Deferasirox; Herbs (CYP3A4 Inducers); Mitotane; PARoxetine; Rifampin; Tocilizumab

Increased Effect/Toxicity

Fosaprepitant may increase the levels/effects of: ARIPiprazole; Astemizole; Avanafil; Benzodiazepines (metabolized by oxidation); Bosentan; Bosutinib; Budesonide (Systemic, Oral Inhalation); Cisapride; Colchicine; Corticosteroids (Systemic); CYP3A4 Substrates; Diltiazem; Dofetilide; DOXOrubicin (Conventional); Eplerenone; Everolimus; FentaNYL; Halofantrine; Ibrutinib; Imatinib; Ivabradine; Ivacaftor; Lomitapide; Lurasidone; OxyCODONE; Pimecrolimus; Pimozide; Propafenone; Ranolazine; Rivaroxaban; Salmeterol; Saxagliptin; Simeprevir; Terfenadine; Tolvaptan; Ulipristal; Vilazodone; Zuclopenthixol

The levels/effects of Fosaprepitant may be increased by: Conivaptan; CYP3A4 Inhibitors (Moderate); CYP3A4 Inhibitors (Strong); Dasatinib; Diltiazem; Fusidic Acid (Systemic); Ivacaftor; Luliconazole; Mifepristone; Simeprevir; Stiripentol

Nutritional/Ethanol Interactions

Food: Aprepitant serum concentration may be increased when taken with grapefruit juice; avoid concurrent use.

Herb/Nutraceutical: Avoid St John's wort (may decrease aprepitant levels).

Adverse Reactions Adverse reactions reported with aprepitant and fosaprepitant (as part of a combination chemotherapy regimen) occurring at a higher frequency than standard antiemetic therapy:

1% to 10%:

Central nervous system: Fatigue (1% to 3%), headache (2%)

Gastrointestinal: Anorexia (2%), constipation (2%), dyspepsia (2%), diarrhea (1%), eructation (1%)

Hepatic: ALT increased (1% to 3%), AST increased (1%)

Local: Injection site reactions (3%; includes erythema, induration, pain, pruritus, or thrombophlebitis)

Neuromuscular & skeletal: Weakness (3%)

Miscellaneous: Hiccups (5%)

Available Dosage Forms

Solution Reconstituted, Intravenous:

Emend: 150 mg (1 ea)

General Dosage Range I.V.: *Adults:* 150 mg as a single dose

Administration

I.V. 150 mg: Infuse over 20-30 minutes ~30 minutes prior to chemotherapy

Preparation for Administration Reconstitute vial with 5 mL of sodium chloride 0.9%, directing diluent down side of vial to avoid foaming; swirl gently. Add reconstituted contents of the 150 mg vial to 145 mL sodium chloride 0.9%, resulting in a final concentration of 1 mg/mL; gently invert bag to mix. Solutions may be diluted to a final volume of 250 mL (0.6 mg/mL) (data on file [Merck, 2013]).

Storage/Stability Store intact vials at 2°C to 8°C (36°F to 46°F). Solutions diluted to 1 mg/mL for infusion are stable for 24 hours at room temperature or at ≤25°C (≤77°F). Solutions diluted to a final volume of 250 mL (0.6 mg/mL) should be administered within 24 hours (data on file [Merck, 2013]).

Nursing Actions

Physical Assessment Monitor patient closely for immediate hypersensitivity reaction (dyspnea, erythema, and/or flushing); if reaction occurs, stop infusion (do not restart) and notify prescriber. Assess efficacy. Monitor infusion site for adverse events including pain, itching, and signs of phlebitis.

Patient Education

• Discuss specific use of drug and side effects with patient as it relates to treatment. (HCAHPS: During this hospital stay, were you given any medicine that you had not taken before? Before giving you any new medicine, how often did hospital staff tell you what the medicine was for? How often did hospital staff describe possible side effects in a way you could understand?)

- Patient may experience asthenia, diarrhea, constipation, lack of appetite, hiccups, belching, dizziness, headache, nausea, or pyrosis. Have patient report immediately to prescriber signs of infection, flushing, injection site pain or irritation, or Stevens-Johnson syndrome/toxic epidermal necrolysis (HCAHPS).
- Educate patient about signs of a significant reaction (eg, wheezing; chest tightness; fever; itching; bad cough; blue skin color; seizures; or swelling of face, lips, tongue, or throat). **Note:** This is not a comprehensive list of all side effects. Patient should consult prescriber for additional questions.

Intended Use and Disclaimer: Should not be printed and given to patients. This information is intended to serve as a concise initial reference for healthcare professionals to use when discussing medications with a patient. You must ultimately rely on your own discretion, experience and judgment in diagnosing, treating and advising patients.

Foscarnet (fos KAR net)

Brand Names: U.S. Foscavir
Index Terms PFA; Phosphonoformate; Phosphonoformic Acid
Pharmacologic Category Antiviral Agent
Pregnancy Risk Factor C
Lactation Excretion in breast milk unknown/contraindicated
Use Treatment of acyclovir-resistant mucocutaneous herpes simplex virus (HSV) infections in immunocompromised persons (eg, with advanced AIDS); treatment of CMV retinitis in persons with HIV
Unlabeled Use Other CMV infections (eg, colitis, esophagitis, neurological disease); CMV prophylaxis for cancer patients receiving alemtuzumab therapy or allogeneic stem cell transplant
Available Dosage Forms
Solution, Intravenous:
Foscavir: 24 mg/mL (250 mL)
Generic: 24 mg/mL (500 mL)
General Dosage Range Dosage adjustment recommended in patients with renal impairment
I.V.: *Children >12 years and Adults:* Induction: CMV: 180 mg/kg/day in 2-3 evenly divided doses; HSV: 40 mg/kg/dose every 8-12 hours; Maintenance: CMV: 90-120 mg/kg once daily
Administration
I.V. Use an infusion pump, at a rate not exceeding 1 mg/kg/minute. Adult induction doses of 60 mg/kg are administered over 1 hour. Adult maintenance doses of 90-120 mg/kg are infused over 2 hours. The manufacturer recommends 750-1000 mL of NS or D_5W be administered prior to first infusion to establish diuresis. With subsequent infusions of 90-120 mg/kg, this volume would be repeated. If the dose were 40-60 mg/kg, then the volume could be reduced to 500 mL. After the first dose, the hydration fluid should be administered concurrently with foscarnet.
Injectable Detail Undiluted (24 mg/mL) solution can be administered without further dilution when using a central venous catheter for infusion. For peripheral vein administration, the solution **must** be diluted to a final concentration **not to exceed** 12 mg/mL. The recommended dosage, frequency, and rate of infusion should not be exceeded.

pH: 7.4 (adjusted)
Nursing Actions
Physical Assessment Evaluate electrolytes, renal status, and dental status prior to beginning therapy. Monitor for nephrotoxicity, electrolyte imbalance, and seizures. Teach patient need for regular dental evaluations.
Patient Education
- Discuss specific use of drug and side effects with patient as it relates to treatment. (HCAHPS: During this hospital stay, were you given any medicine that you had not taken before? Before giving you any new medicine, how often did hospital staff tell you what the medicine was for? How often did hospital staff describe possible side effects in a way you could understand?)
- Patient may experience diarrhea, headache, anxiety, nausea, asthenia, dizziness, lack of appetite, or dyspepsia. Have patient report immediately to prescriber signs of infection, signs of fluid and electrolyte imbalance, paresthesia, difficulty with motor activity, depression, dyspnea, hyperhidrosis, rigidity, vision changes, angina, or injection site irritation (HCAHPS).
- Educate patient about signs of a significant reaction (eg, wheezing; chest tightness; fever; itching; bad cough; blue skin color; seizures; or swelling of face, lips, tongue, or throat). **Note:** This is not a comprehensive list of all side effects. Patient should consult prescriber for additional questions.

Intended Use and Disclaimer: Should not be printed and given to patients. This information is intended to serve as a concise initial reference for healthcare professionals to use when discussing medications with a patient. You must ultimately rely on your own discretion, experience and judgment in diagnosing, treating and advising patients.

Fosinopril (foe SIN oh pril)

Index Terms Fosinopril Sodium; Monopril
Pharmacologic Category Angiotensin-Converting Enzyme (ACE) Inhibitor; Antihypertensive

Medication Safety Issues

Sound-alike/look-alike issues:

Fosinopril may be confused with FLUoxetine, Fosamax®, furosemide, lisinopril

Monopril may be confused with Accupril®, minoxidil, moexipril, Monoket®, Monurol®, ramipril

Pregnancy Risk Factor D

Lactation Enters breast milk/not recommended

Breast-Feeding Considerations Fosinoprilat is excreted in breast milk. Breast-feeding is not recommended by the manufacturer.

Use

Hypertension: Treatment of hypertension, either alone or in combination with other antihypertensive agents

Heart failure: Adjunctive treatment of heart failure (HF)

Note: The ACCF/AHA 2013 heart failure guidelines recommend the use of ACE inhibitors, along with other guideline directed medical therapies, to prevent heart failure in patients with a reduced ejection fraction who have a history of MI (Stage B HF), to prevent HF in any patient with a reduced ejection fraction (Stage B HF), or to treat those with HF and reduced ejection fraction (Stage C HFrEF) (ACCF/AHA [Yancy, 2013]).

Mechanism of Action/Effect Competitive inhibitor of angiotensin-converting enzyme (ACE); prevents conversion of angiotensin I to angiotensin II, a potent vasoconstrictor; results in lower levels of angiotensin II which causes an increase in plasma renin activity and a reduction in aldosterone secretion; a CNS mechanism may also be involved in hypotensive effect as angiotensin II increases adrenergic outflow from CNS; vasoactive kallikreins may be decreased in conversion to active hormones by ACE inhibitors, thus reducing blood pressure

Contraindications Hypersensitivity to fosinopril, any other ACE inhibitor, or any component of the formulation; angioedema related to previous treatment with an ACE inhibitor; concomitant use with aliskiren in patients with diabetes mellitus

Warnings/Precautions Anaphylactic reactions may occur rarely with ACE inhibitors. At any time during treatment (especially following first dose), angioedema may occur rarely with ACE inhibitors; it may involve the head and neck (potentially compromising airway) or the intestine (presenting with abdominal pain). African-Americans may be at an increased risk and patients with idiopathic or hereditary angioedema may be at an increased risk. Prolonged frequent monitoring may be required especially if tongue, glottis, or larynx are involved as they are associated with airway obstruction. Patients with a history of airway surgery may have a higher risk of airway obstruction. Aggressive early and appropriate management is critical. Use in patients with previous angioedema associated with ACE inhibitor therapy is contraindicated. Severe anaphylactoid reactions may be seen during hemodialysis (eg, CVVHD) with high-flux dialysis membranes (eg, AN69), and rarely, during low density lipoprotein apheresis with dextran sulfate cellulose. Rare cases of anaphylactoid reactions have been reported in patients undergoing sensitization treatment with hymenoptera (bee, wasp) venom while receiving ACE inhibitors.

Symptomatic hypotension with or without syncope can occur with ACE inhibitors (usually with the first several doses); effects are most often observed in volume-depleted patients; correct volume depletion prior to initiation; close monitoring of patient is required especially with initial dosing and dosing increases; blood pressure must be lowered at a rate appropriate for the patient's clinical condition. Initiation of therapy in patients with ischemic heart disease or cerebrovascular disease warrants close observation due to the potential consequences posed by falling blood pressure (eg, MI, stroke). Use with caution in hypertrophic cardiomyopathy with outflow tract obstruction, severe aortic stenosis, or before, during, or immediately after major surgery. **[U.S. Boxed Warning]: Drugs that act on the renin-angiotensin system can cause injury and death to the developing fetus. Discontinue as soon as possible once pregnancy is detected.**

Hyperkalemia may occur with ACE inhibitors; risk factors include renal dysfunction, diabetes mellitus, concomitant use of potassium-sparing diuretics, potassium supplements, and/or potassium-containing salts. Use cautiously, if at all, with these agents and monitor potassium closely. Cough may occur with ACE inhibitors. Other causes of cough should be considered (eg, pulmonary congestion in patients with heart failure) and excluded prior to discontinuation. Use with caution in hepatic impairment; fosinopril undergoes hepatic and gut wall metabolism to its active form (fosinoprilat) and may accumulate in hepatic impairment. In patients with alcoholic or biliary cirrhosis, the rate of fosinoprilat formation is slowed, its total body clearance decreased and its AUC ~doubled.

May be associated with deterioration of renal function and/or increases in serum creatinine, particularly in patients with low renal blood flow (eg, renal artery stenosis, heart failure) whose glomerular filtration rate (GFR) is dependent on efferent arteriolar vasoconstriction by angiotensin II; deterioration may result in oliguria, acute renal failure, and progressive azotemia. Small increases in serum creatinine may occur following initiation; consider discontinuation only in patients with progressive and/or significant deterioration in renal function. Use with caution in patients with unstented unilateral/bilateral renal artery stenosis. When unstented bilateral renal artery stenosis is present, use is generally avoided due to the elevated risk of deterioration in renal function unless possible benefits outweigh risks. Potentially significant drug-drug interactions may exist, requiring dose or frequency adjustment, additional monitoring, and/or selection of alternative therapy.

Rare toxicities associated with ACE inhibitors include cholestatic jaundice (which may progress to fulminant hepatic necrosis), agranulocytosis, neutropenia or leukopenia with myeloid hypoplasia. Patients with collagen vascular diseases (especially with concomitant renal impairment) or renal impairment alone may be at increased risk for hematologic toxicity; periodically monitor CBC with differential in these patients.

Drug Interactions

Avoid Concomitant Use There are no known interactions where it is recommended to avoid concomitant use.

Decreased Effect
The levels/effects of Fosinopril may be decreased by: Antacids; Aprotinin; Herbs (Hypertensive Properties); Icatibant; Lanthanum; Methylphenidate; Nonsteroidal Anti-Inflammatory Agents; Salicylates; Yohimbine

Increased Effect/Toxicity
Fosinopril may increase the levels/effects of: Allopurinol; Amifostine; Antihypertensives; AzaTHIOprine; CycloSPORINE (Systemic); DULoxetine; Ferric Gluconate; Gold Sodium Thiomalate; Hypotensive Agents; Iron Dextran Complex; Lithium; Nonsteroidal Anti-Inflammatory Agents; Obinutuzumab; RiTUXimab; Sodium Phosphates

The levels/effects of Fosinopril may be increased by: Alfuzosin; Aliskiren; Angiotensin II Receptor Blockers; Brimonidine (Topical); Canagliflozin; Diazoxide; DPP-IV Inhibitors; Eplerenone; Everolimus; Heparin; Heparin (Low Molecular Weight); Herbs (Hypotensive Properties); Loop Diuretics; MAO Inhibitors; Pentoxifylline; Phosphodiesterase 5 Inhibitors; Potassium Salts; Potassium-Sparing Diuretics; Prostacyclin Analogues; Sirolimus; Temsirolimus; Thiazide Diuretics; TiZANidine; Tolvaptan; Trimethoprim

Nutritional/Ethanol Interactions

Food: Potassium supplements and/or potassium-containing salts may cause or worsen hyperkalemia. Management: Advise patient to consult prescriber before consuming a potassium-rich diet, potassium supplements, or salt substitutes.

Herb/Nutraceutical: Some herbal medications may worsen hypertension (eg, licorice); others may increase the antihypertensive effect of fosinopril (eg, shepherd's purse). Management: Avoid bayberry, blue cohosh, cayenne, ephedra, ginger, ginseng (American), kola, licorice, and yohimbe. Avoid black cohosh, california poppy, coleus, golden seal, hawthorn, mistletoe, periwinkle, quinine, and shepherd's purse.

Adverse Reactions Note: Frequency ranges include data from hypertension and heart failure trials. Higher rates of adverse reactions have generally been noted in patients with CHF. However, the frequency of adverse effects associated with placebo is also increased in this population.

>10%: Central nervous system: Dizziness (2% to 12%)

1% to 10%:
Cardiovascular: Orthostatic hypotension (1% to 2%), palpitation (1%)
Central nervous system: Dizziness (1% to 2%; up to 12% in CHF patients), headache (3%), fatigue (1% to 2%)
Endocrine & metabolic: Hyperkalemia (2.6%)
Gastrointestinal: Diarrhea (2%), nausea/vomiting (1.2% to 2.2%)
Hepatic: Transaminases increased
Neuromuscular & skeletal: Musculoskeletal pain (<1% to 3%), noncardiac chest pain (<1% to 2%), weakness (1%)
Renal: Serum creatinine increased, renal function worsening (in patients with bilateral renal artery stenosis or hypovolemia)
Respiratory: Cough (2% to 10%)
Miscellaneous: Upper respiratory infection (2%)

>1% but ≤ frequency in patients receiving placebo: Sexual dysfunction, fever, flu-like syndrome, dyspnea, rash, headache, insomnia

Other events reported with ACE inhibitors: Neutropenia, agranulocytosis, eosinophilic pneumonitis, cardiac arrest, pancytopenia, hemolytic anemia, anemia, aplastic anemia, thrombocytopenia, acute renal failure, hepatic failure, jaundice, symptomatic hyponatremia, bullous pemphigus, exfoliative dermatitis, Stevens-Johnson syndrome. In addition, a syndrome which may include fever, myalgia, arthralgia, interstitial nephritis, vasculitis, rash, eosinophilia and positive ANA, and elevated ESR has been reported for other ACE inhibitors.

Pharmacodynamics/Kinetics
Onset of Action 1 hour
Duration of Action 24 hours

Available Dosage Forms
Tablet, Oral:
Generic: 10 mg, 20 mg, 40 mg

General Dosage Range Oral:
Children ≥6 years and Adolescents >50 kg: Initial: 5-10 mg once daily (maximum: 40 mg once daily)
Adults: Initial: 10 mg once daily; Maintenance: 10-40 mg daily in 1-2 divided doses (maximum: 80 mg daily)

Storage/Stability Store at 20°C to 25°C (68°F to 77°F). Protect from moisture.

Nursing Actions
Physical Assessment Assess potential for interactions with other pharmacological agents or herbal products that may impact fluid balance or cardiac status. Monitor for anaphylactic reactions, hypovolemia, angioedema, and postural hypotension.

Patient Education

- Discuss specific use of drug and side effects with patient as it relates to treatment. (HCAHPS: During this hospital stay, were you given any medicine that you had not taken before? Before giving you any new medicine, how often did hospital staff tell you what the medicine was for? How often did hospital staff describe possible side effects in a way you could understand?)
- Have patient report immediately to prescriber signs of renal impairment, signs of hyperkalemia, severe dizziness, syncope, angina, considerable dyspepsia, significant nausea, or signs of hepatic impairment (HCAHPS).
- Educate patient about signs of a significant reaction (eg, wheezing; chest tightness; fever; itching; bad cough; blue skin color; seizures; or swelling of face, lips, tongue, or throat). **Note:** This is not a comprehensive list of all side effects. Patient should consult prescriber for additional questions.

Intended Use and Disclaimer: Should not be printed and given to patients. This information is intended to serve as a concise initial reference for healthcare professionals to use when discussing medications with a patient. You must ultimately rely on your own discretion, experience and judgment in diagnosing, treating and advising patients.

Dietary Considerations Should not take a potassium salt supplement without the advice of healthcare provider.

Fosphenytoin (FOS fen i toyn)

Brand Names: U.S. Cerebyx
Index Terms Cerebyx; Fosphenytoin Sodium
Pharmacologic Category Anticonvulsant, Hydantoin
Medication Safety Issues
Sound-alike/look-alike issues:
Cerebyx may be confused with CeleBREX®, CeleXA®, Cerezyme®, Cervarix®
Fosphenytoin may be confused with fospropofol
Administration issues:
Overdoses have occurred due to confusion between the **mg per mL concentration** of fosphenytoin (50 mg phenytoin equivalent (PE)/mL) and **total drug content per vial** (either 100 mg PE/2 mL vial or 500 mg PE/10 mL vial). ISMP recommends that the total drug content per container is identified instead of the concentration in mg per mL to avoid confusion and potential overdoses. Additionally, since most errors have occurred with overdoses in children, ISMP recommends that pediatric hospitals consider stocking only the 2 mL vial.
Pregnancy Risk Factor D
Lactation Excretion in breast milk unknown/not recommended

Breast-Feeding Considerations Fosphenytoin is the prodrug of phenytoin. It is not known if fosphenytoin is excreted in breast milk prior to conversion to phenytoin. Refer to Phenytoin monograph for additional information.

Use Used for the control of generalized convulsive status epilepticus and prevention and treatment of seizures occurring during neurosurgery; indicated for short-term parenteral administration when other means of phenytoin administration are unavailable, inappropriate, or deemed less advantageous (the safety and effectiveness of fosphenytoin use for more than 5 days has not been systematically evaluated)

Mechanism of Action/Effect Diphosphate ester salt of phenytoin which acts as a water soluble prodrug of phenytoin; after administration, plasma esterases convert fosphenytoin to phosphate, formaldehyde, and phenytoin as the active moiety; phenytoin works by stabilizing neuronal membranes and decreasing seizure activity by increasing efflux or decreasing influx of sodium ions across cell membranes in the motor cortex during generation of nerve impulses

Contraindications Hypersensitivity to phenytoin, other hydantoins, or any component of the formulation; patients with sinus bradycardia, sinoatrial block, second- and third-degree AV block, or Adams-Stokes syndrome; occurrence of rash during treatment (should not be resumed if rash is exfoliative, purpuric, or bullous); treatment of absence seizures; concurrent use of delavirdine (due to loss of virologic response and possible resistance to delavirdine or other non-nucleoside reverse transcriptase inhibitors [NNRTIs])

Warnings/Precautions [U.S. Boxed Warning]: Fosphenytoin administration should not exceed 150 mg phenytoin equivalents (PE)/ minute in adult patients. Hypotension and severe cardiac arrhythmias (eg, heart block, ventricular tachycardia, ventricular fibrillation) may occur with rapid administration; adverse cardiac events have been reported at or below the recommended infusion rate. In the treatment of status epilepticus, the rate of administration is 150 mg PE/minute. In a nonemergent situation, administer more slowly or use oral phenytoin. Cardiac monitoring is necessary during and after administration of intravenous fosphenytoin; reduction in rate of administration or discontinuation of infusion may be necessary.

Doses of fosphenytoin are always expressed as their phenytoin sodium equivalent (PE). 1 mg PE is equivalent to 1 mg phenytoin sodium. Do not change the recommended doses when substituting fosphenytoin for phenytoin or vice versa as they are not equivalent on a mg to mg basis. Dosing errors have also occurred due to misinterpretation of vial concentrations resulting in two- or tenfold overdoses (some fatal); ensure correct volume of fosphenytoin is withdrawn from vial. Severe burning or itching, and/or paresthesias, mostly perineal, may occur upon administration, usually at the maximum administration rate and last from minutes to hours; occurrence and intensity may be lessened by slowing or temporarily stopping the infusion. Antiepileptic drugs should not be abruptly discontinued. Acute hepatotoxicity associated with a hypersensitivity syndrome characterized by fever, skin eruptions, and lymphadenopathy has been reported to occur within the first 2 months of treatment. Discontinue if skin rash or lymphadenopathy occurs. A spectrum of hematologic effects have been reported with use (eg, neutropenia, leukopenia, thrombocytopenia, pancytopenia, and anemias). Use with caution in patients with hypotension, severe myocardial insufficiency, diabetes mellitus, porphyria, hypoalbuminemia, hypothyroidism, fever, or hepatic dysfunction. Use with caution in patients with renal impairment; also consider the phosphate load of fosphenytoin (0.0037 mmol phosphate/mg PE fosphenytoin). Effects with other sedative drugs or ethanol may be potentiated. Severe reactions, including toxic epidermal necrolysis (TEN) and Stevens-Johnson syndromes, although rarely reported, have resulted in fatalities; drug should be discontinued if there are any signs of rash and patient should be evaluated for signs and symptoms of drug reaction with eosinophilia and systemic symptoms (DRESS). Patients of Asian descent with the variant HLA-B*1502 may be at an increased risk of developing Stevens-Johnson syndrome and/or TEN.

The "purple glove syndrome" (ie, discoloration with edema and pain of distal limb) may occur following peripheral I.V. administration of fosphenytoin. This syndrome may or may not be associated with drug extravasation. Symptoms may resolve spontaneously; however, skin necrosis and limb ischemia may occur. In general, fosphenytoin has significantly less venous irritation and phlebitis compared with an equimolar dose of phenytoin (Jamerson, 1994). Sedation, confusional states, or cerebellar dysfunction (loss of motor coordination) may occur at higher total serum concentrations or at lower total serum concentrations when the free fraction of phenytoin is increased.

Drug Interactions

Avoid Concomitant Use

Avoid concomitant use of Fosphenytoin with any of the following: Abiraterone Acetate; Apixaban; Artemether; Axitinib; Azelastine (Nasal); Bedaquiline; Boceprevir; Bortezomib; Bosutinib; Cabozantinib; CloZAPine; Crizotinib; Dabigatran Etexilate; Darunavir; Delavirdine; Dienogest; Dolutegravir; Dronedarone; Enzalutamide; Etravirine; Everolimus; Ibrutinib; Itraconazole; Ivacaftor; Lapatinib; Lumefantrine; Lurasidone; Macitentan; Mifepristone; NIFEdipine; Nilotinib; Nisoldipine; Paraldehyde; PAZOPanib;

Pomalidomide; PONATinib; Praziquantel; Ranolazine; Regorafenib; Rilpivirine; Rivaroxaban; Roflumilast; RomiDEPsin; Simeprevir; Sofosbuvir; SORAfenib; Tasimelteon; Telaprevir; Thalidomide; Ticagrelor; Tofacitinib; Tolvaptan; Toremifene; Ulipristal; Vandetanib; Vemurafenib; VinCRIStine (Liposomal)

Decreased Effect

Fosphenytoin may decrease the levels/effects of: Abiraterone Acetate; Acetaminophen; Afatinib; Amiodarone; Antifungal Agents (Azole Derivatives, Systemic); Apixaban; ARIPiprazole; Artemether; Axitinib; Bazedoxifene; Bedaquiline; Boceprevir; Bortezomib; Bosutinib; Brentuximab Vedotin; Busulfan; Cabozantinib; Canagliflozin; CarBAMazepine; Chloramphenicol; Clarithromycin; CloZAPine; Cobicistat; Contraceptives (Estrogens); Contraceptives (Progestins); Crizotinib; CycloSPORINE (Systemic); CYP2B6 Substrates; CYP2C19 Substrates; CYP2C8 Substrates; CYP2C9 Substrates; CYP3A4 Substrates; Dabigatran Etexilate; Darunavir; Dasatinib; Deferasirox; Delavirdine; Diclofenac (Systemic); Dienogest; Disopyramide; Dolutegravir; DOXOrubicin (Conventional); Doxycycline; Dronedarone; Efavirenz; Elvitegravir; Enzalutamide; Eslicarbazepine; Ethosuximide; Etoposide; Etoposide Phosphate; Etravirine; Everolimus; Exemestane; Felbamate; Flunarizine; Gefitinib; GuanFACINE; HMG-CoA Reductase Inhibitors; Ibrutinib; Imatinib; Irinotecan; Itraconazole; Ivacaftor; Ixabepilone; Lacosamide; LamoTRIgine; Lapatinib; Levodopa; Linagliptin; Loop Diuretics; Lopinavir; Lumefantrine; Lurasidone; Macitentan; Maraviroc; Mebendazole; Meperidine; Methadone; MethylPREDNISolone; MetroNIDAZOLE (Systemic); Metyrapone; Mexiletine; Mifepristone; Nelfinavir; Neuromuscular-Blocking Agents (Nondepolarizing); NIFEdipine; Nilotinib; Nisoldipine; Omeprazole; OXcarbazepine; PAZOPanib; Perampanel; P-glycoprotein/ABCB1 Substrates; Pomalidomide; PONATinib; Praziquantel; PrednisoLONE (Systemic); PredniSONE; Primidone; QUEtiapine; QuiNIDine; QuiNINE; Ranolazine; Regorafenib; Rilpivirine; Ritonavir; Rivaroxaban; Roflumilast; RomiDEPsin; Rufinamide; Saxagliptin; Sertraline; Simeprevir; Sirolimus; Sofosbuvir; SORAfenib; SUNItinib; Tacrolimus (Systemic); Tadalafil; Tasimelteon; Telaprevir; Temsirolimus; Teniposide; Theophylline Derivatives; Thyroid Products; Ticagrelor; Tipranavir; Tofacitinib; Tolvaptan; Topiramate; Topotecan; Toremifene; TraZODone; Treprostinil; Trimethoprim; Ulipristal; Valproic Acid and Derivatives; Vandetanib; Vemurafenib; Vilazodone; VinCRIStine; VinCRIStine (Liposomal); Vortioxetine; Zonisamide; Zuclopenthixol

The levels/effects of Fosphenytoin may be decreased by: Alcohol (Ethyl); Antacids; CarBAMazepine; Ciprofloxacin (Systemic); CYP2C19 Inducers (Strong); CYP2C9 Inducers (Strong);

Dabrafenib; Diazoxide; Enzalutamide; Folic Acid; Fosamprenavir; Ketorolac (Nasal); Ketorolac (Systemic); Leucovorin Calcium-Levoleucovorin; Levomefolate; Lopinavir; Mefloquine; Methotrexate; Methylfolate; Multivitamins/Minerals (with ADEK, Folate, Iron); Nelfinavir; Orlistat; Peginterferon Alfa-2b; PHENobarbital; Platinum Derivatives; Pyridoxine; Rifampin; Ritonavir; Theophylline Derivatives; Tipranavir; Valproic Acid and Derivatives; Vigabatrin; VinCRIStine

Increased Effect/Toxicity

Fosphenytoin may increase the levels/effects of: Amiodarone; Azelastine (Nasal); Buprenorphine; Ciprofloxacin (Systemic); Clarithromycin; CNS Depressants; FLUoxetine; Fosamprenavir; Highest Risk QTc-Prolonging Agents; Hydrocodone; Ifosfamide; Lithium; Methotrimeprazine; Metyrosine; Mirtazapine; Moderate Risk QTc-Prolonging Agents; Neuromuscular-Blocking Agents (Nondepolarizing); Paraldehyde; PHENobarbital; Pramipexole; QuiNIDine; ROPINIRole; Rotigotine; Selective Serotonin Reuptake Inhibitors; Thalidomide; Vitamin K Antagonists; Zolpidem

The levels/effects of Fosphenytoin may be increased by: Alcohol (Ethyl); Allopurinol; Amiodarone; Antifungal Agents (Azole Derivatives, Systemic); Benzodiazepines; Brimonidine (Topical); Calcium Channel Blockers; Capecitabine; CarBAMazepine; Carbonic Anhydrase Inhibitors; CeFAZolin; Chloramphenicol; Cimetidine; Clarithromycin; CYP2C19 Inhibitors (Moderate); CYP2C19 Inhibitors (Strong); CYP2C9 Inhibitors (Moderate); CYP2C9 Inhibitors (Strong); Delavirdine; Dexmethylphenidate; Disopyramide; Disulfiram; Doxylamine; Droperidol; Efavirenz; Eslicarbazepine; Ethosuximide; Felbamate; Floxuridine; Fluconazole; Fluorouracil (Systemic); Fluorouracil (Topical); FLUoxetine; FluvoxaMINE; Halothane; HydrOXYzine; Isoniazid; Luliconazole; Magnesium Sulfate; Methotrimeprazine; Methylphenidate; MetroNIDAZOLE (Systemic); Omeprazole; OXcarbazepine; Rufinamide; Sertraline; Sodium Oxybate; Tacrolimus (Systemic); Tapentadol; Tegafur; Telaprevir; Ticlopidine; Topiramate; TraZODone; Trimethoprim; Vitamin K Antagonists

Nutritional/Ethanol Interactions Ethanol:

Acute use: Avoid or limit ethanol (inhibits metabolism of phenytoin). Ethanol may also increase CNS depression; monitor for increased effects with coadministration. Caution patients about effects.

Chronic use: Avoid or limit ethanol (stimulates metabolism of phenytoin).

Adverse Reactions The more important adverse clinical events caused by the I.V. use of fosphenytoin or phenytoin are cardiovascular collapse and/or central nervous system depression. Hypotension can occur when either drug is administered rapidly by the I.V. route.

The adverse clinical events most commonly observed with the use of fosphenytoin in clinical trials were nystagmus, dizziness, pruritus, paresthesia, headache, somnolence, and ataxia. Paresthesia and pruritus were seen more often following fosphenytoin (versus phenytoin) administration and occurred more often with I.V. fosphenytoin than with I.M. administration. These events were dose and rate related (adult doses ≥15 mg/kg at a rate of 150 mg PE/minute) and occurred in up to 64% of patients. These sensations, generally described as itching, burning, or tingling are usually not at the infusion site. The location of the discomfort varied with the groin mentioned most frequently. The paresthesia and pruritus were transient events that occurred within several minutes of the start of infusion and generally resolved within 10 minutes after completion of infusion.

Transient pruritus, tinnitus, nystagmus, somnolence, and ataxia occurred 2-3 times more often at adult doses ≥15 mg/kg and rates ≥150 mg PE/minute.

Also refer to Phenytoin monograph for additional adverse reactions.

I.V. and I.M. administration (as reported in clinical trials):

1% to 10%:

Cardiovascular: Facial edema, hypertension

Central nervous system: Chills, fever, intracranial hypertension, nervousness

Endocrine & metabolic: Hypokalemia

Neuromuscular & skeletal: Hyperreflexia, myasthenia

I.V. administration (maximum dose/rate):

>10%:

Central nervous system: Paresthesia (4% to 64%), nystagmus (44%), dizziness (31%), somnolence (20%), ataxia (11%)

Dermatologic: Pruritus (49% to 64%)

1% to 10%:

Cardiovascular: Hypotension (7%), vasodilation (6%), tachycardia (2%)

Central nervous system: Stupor (7%), extrapyramidal syndrome (4%), incoordination (4%), agitation (3%), tremor (3%), brain edema (2%), headache (2%), hypoesthesia (2%), vertigo (2%)

Gastrointestinal: Nausea (9%), tongue disorder (4%), xerostomia (4%), taste perversion (3%), vomiting (2%)

Neuromuscular & skeletal: Pelvic pain (4%), back pain (2%), dysarthria (2%), weakness (2%)

Ocular: Diplopia (3%), amblyopia (2%)

Otic: Tinnitus (9%), deafness (2%)

I.M. administration (substitute for oral phenytoin):

>10%: Central nervous system: Nystagmus (15%)

1% to 10%:

Central nervous system: Tremor (10%), headache (9%), ataxia (8%), incoordination (8%), somnolence (7%), dizziness (5%), paresthesia (4%), reflexes decreased (3%)

Dermatologic: Bruising (7%), pruritus (3%)

Gastrointestinal: Nausea (5%), vomiting (3%)

Neuromuscular & skeletal: Weakness (4%)

Available Dosage Forms

Solution, Injection:

Cerebyx: 100 mg PE/2 mL (2 mL); 500 mg PE/10 mL (10 mL)

Generic: 100 mg PE/2 mL (2 mL); 500 mg PE/10 mL (10 mL)

General Dosage Range

I.M.: *Adults:* Loading: 10-20 mg PE/kg; Maintenance: 4-6 mg PE/kg/day

I.V.: *Adults:* Loading: 10-20 mg PE/kg; Maintenance: 4-6 mg PE/kg/day

Administration

I.M. May be administered as a single daily dose using 1-4 injection sites (up to 20 mL per site well tolerated in adults) (Meek, 1999; Pryor, 2001).

I.V. Rates of infusion:

Children: 1-3 mg PE/kg/minute (**maximum rate: 150 mg PE/minute**) (Pellock, 1996)

Adults: **Do not exceed 150 mg PE/minute.** Slower administration reduces incidence of cardiovascular events (eg, hypotension, arrhythmia) as well as severity of paresthesias and pruritus. For nonemergent situations, may administer loading dose more slowly (eg, over 30 minutes [~33 mg PE/minute for 1000 mg PE] **or** 50-100 mg PE/minute [Fischer, 2003]). Highly-sensitive patients (eg, elderly, patients with pre-existing cardiovascular conditions) should receive fosphenytoin more slowly (eg, 25-50 mg PE/minute) (Meek, 1999).

Preparation for Administration Must be diluted to concentrations of 1.5-25 mg PE/mL, in normal saline or D_5W, for I.V. infusion.

Storage/Stability Refrigerate at 2°C to 8°C (36°F to 46°F). Do not store at room temperature for more than 48 hours. Do not use vials that develop particulate matter. Has been shown to be stable at 1, 8, and 20 mg PE/mL in normal saline or D_5W at 25°C (77°F) for 30 days in glass container and at 4°C to 20°C (39°F to 68°F) for 30 days in PVC bag (Fischer, 1997).

Nursing Actions

Physical Assessment Continuous hemodynamic monitoring and respiratory status are essential during infusion and for 30 minutes following infusion. Monitor closely for adverse reactions during and following infusion; most commonly nystagmus, dizziness, itching, paresthesia, sedation, and ataxia. Educate patient that most side effects are transient and resolve within 10 minutes postinfusion.

Patient Education

• Discuss specific use of drug and side effects with patient as it relates to treatment. (HCAHPS: During this hospital stay, were you given any medicine that you had not taken before? Before giving you any new medicine, how often did hospital staff tell you what the medicine was for? How often did hospital staff describe possible side effects in a way you could understand?)

• Patient may experience xerostomia or headache. Have patient report immediately to prescriber hyperglycemia, signs of depression (ie, suicidal ideation, anxiety, emotional instability, illogical thinking), signs of hypokalemia, signs of infection, severe dizziness, syncope, tachycardia, bradycardia, arrhythmia, difficulty with motor activity, fasciculations, change in balance, dysphagia, difficulty speaking, tinnitus, hearing impairment, gum changes, tremors, ecchymosis, hemorrhaging, involuntary eye movements, considerable asthenia, injection site irritation, skin discoloration, paresthesia, signs of Stevens-Johnson syndrome/toxic epidermal necrolysis, enlarged lymph nodes, angina, urinary retention, oliguria, signs of hepatic impairment, fatigue, lack of appetite, nausea, dyspepsia, stool discoloration, or jaundice (HCAHPS).

• Educate patient about signs of a significant reaction (eg, wheezing; chest tightness; fever; itching; bad cough; blue skin color; seizures; or swelling of face, lips, tongue, or throat). **Note:** This is not a comprehensive list of all side effects. Patient should consult prescriber for additional questions.

Intended Use and Disclaimer: Should not be printed and given to patients. This information is intended to serve as a concise initial reference for healthcare professionals to use when discussing medications with a patient. You must ultimately rely on your own discretion, experience and judgment in diagnosing, treating and advising patients.

Dietary Considerations Provides phosphate 0.0037 mmol/mg PE fosphenytoin

Frovatriptan (froe va TRIP tan)

Brand Names: U.S. Frova

Index Terms Frovatriptan Succinate

Pharmacologic Category Antimigraine Agent; Serotonin 5-HT$_{1B, 1D}$ Receptor Agonist

Medication Safety Issues

International issues:

Allegro: Brand name for frovatriptan [Germany], but also the brand name for fluticasone [Israel]

Allegro [Germany] may be confused with Allegra and Allegra-D brand names for fexofenadine and fexofenadine/pseudoephedrine, respectively, in the [U.S., Canada, and multiple international markets]

◀ **Pregnancy Risk Factor** C

Lactation Excretion in breast milk unknown/use caution

Breast-Feeding Considerations It is not known if frovatriptan is excreted in breast milk. Due to the potential for serious adverse reactions in the nursing infant, the manufacturer recommends a decision be made whether to discontinue nursing or to discontinue the drug, taking into account the importance of treatment to the mother.

Use Migraines: Acute treatment of migraine with or without aura in adults.

Unlabeled Use Short-term prevention of menstrually-associated migraines (MAMs)

Mechanism of Action/Effect Selective agonist for serotonin receptor in cranial arteries; causes vasoconstriction and relief of migraine

Contraindications

Ischemic coronary artery disease (eg, angina pectoris, history of MI, documented silent ischemia); coronary artery vasospasm, including Prinzmetal's angina; Wolff-Parkinson-White syndrome or arrhythmias associated with other cardiac accessory conduction pathway disorders; history of stroke, transient ischemic attack, or history of hemiplegic or basilar migraine; peripheral vascular disease; ischemic bowel disease; uncontrolled hypertension; recent use (within 24 hours) of another 5-HT$_1$ agonist, an ergotamine containing or ergot-type medication (eg, dihydroergotamine, methysergide); hypersensitivity to frovatriptan or any component of the formulation.

Canadian labeling: Additional contraindications (not in U.S. labeling): Cardiac arrhythmias, valvular heart disease (especially tachycardia), congenital heart disease, atherosclerotic disease; management of ophthalmoplegic migraine; severe hepatic impairment; Raynaud's syndrome Documentation of allergenic cross-reactivity for triptans is limited. However, because of similarities in chemical structure and/or pharmacologic actions, the possibility of cross-sensitivity cannot be ruled out with certainty.

Warnings/Precautions Not intended for migraine prophylaxis, or treatment of cluster headaches, hemiplegic or basilar migraines. Rule out underlying neurologic disease in patients with atypical headache, migraine (with no prior history of migraine) or inadequate clinical response to initial dosing. Cardiac events (coronary artery vasospasm, transient ischemia, MI, ventricular tachycardia/fibrillation, cardiac arrest, and death), cerebral/subarachnoid hemorrhage, stroke (some fatal), peripheral vascular ischemia, gastrointestinal vascular ischemia and infarction, splenic infarction, and Raynaud's syndrome have been reported with 5-HT$_1$ agonist administration. Partial vision loss and blindness (transient and permanent) have been reported with use of 5-HT$_1$ agonists; a causal relationship between these events and 5-HT$_1$ agonist administration has not been clearly

determined. Patients who experience sensations of chest pain/pressure/tightness or symptoms suggestive of angina following dosing should be evaluated for coronary artery disease or Prinzmetal's angina before receiving additional doses; if dosing is resumed and similar symptoms recur, monitor with ECG. Do not give to patients with risk factors for CAD until a cardiovascular evaluation has been performed; if evaluation is satisfactory, the healthcare provider should administer the first dose (consider ECG monitoring) and cardiovascular status should be periodically evaluated. Significant elevation in blood pressure, including hypertensive crisis with acute impairment of organ systems, has been reported on rare occasions in patients using other 5-HT$_{1D}$ agonists with and without a history of hypertension; monitor blood pressure. Blood pressure was increased to a greater extent in elderly.

Use with caution in severe hepatic impairment (has not been studied) (Canadian labeling contraindicates use in severe impairment). Potentially significant drug-drug interactions may exist, requiring dose or frequency adjustment, additional monitoring, and/or selection of alternative therapy. Symptoms of agitation, confusion, hallucinations, hyperreflexia, myoclonus, shivering, and tachycardia (serotonin syndrome) may occur with concomitant proserotonergic drugs (ie, SSRIs/SNRIs or triptans) or agents which reduce frovatriptan's metabolism. Concurrent use of serotonin precursors (eg, tryptophan) is not recommended. If concomitant administration with SSRIs is warranted, monitor closely, especially at initiation and with dose increases. Discontinue frovatriptan if serotonin syndrome is suspected. Anaphylaxis, anaphylactoid, and hypersensitivity reactions (including angioedema) have occurred; may be life-threatening or fatal.

Drug Interactions

Avoid Concomitant Use

Avoid concomitant use of Frovatriptan with any of the following: Ergot Derivatives

Decreased Effect There are no known significant interactions involving a decrease in effect.

Increased Effect/Toxicity

Frovatriptan may increase the levels/effects of: Antipsychotics; Droxidopa; Ergot Derivatives; Metoclopramide; Serotonin Modulators

The levels/effects of Frovatriptan may be increased by: Antipsychotics; Ergot Derivatives

Nutritional/Ethanol Interactions Food: Food does not affect frovatriptan bioavailability.

Adverse Reactions

1% to 10%:

Cardiovascular: Flushing (4%), hot or cold flashes (3%), chest pain (2%), palpitations (1%)

Central nervous system: Dizziness (8%), fatigue (5%), headache (4%), paresthesia (4%), drowsiness (≥2%), anxiety (1%), dysesthesia (1%), hypoesthesia (1%), insomnia (1%), pain (1%)

Dermatologic: Diaphoresis (1%)
Gastrointestinal: Xerostomia (3%), nausea (≥2%), dyspepsia (2%), abdominal pain (1%), diarrhea (1%), vomiting (1%)
Neuromuscular & skeletal: Musculoskeletal pain (3%)
Ophthalmic: Visual disturbance (1%)
Otic: Tinnitus (1%)
Respiratory: Rhinitis (1%), sinusitis (1%)

Available Dosage Forms

Tablet, Oral:

Frova: 2.5 mg

General Dosage Range Oral: *Adults:* 2.5 mg as a single dose, may repeat after 2 hours (maximum: 7.5 mg daily)

Administration

Oral Administer with fluids as soon as symptoms appear.

Storage/Stability Store at 25°C (77°F); excursions are permitted between 15°C and 30°C (59°F and 86°F). Protect from moisture.

Nursing Actions

Physical Assessment Monitor cardiovascular status periodically; monitor for hypertension and cardiac events. Teach patient proper use (treatment of acute migraine).

Patient Education

- Discuss specific use of drug and side effects with patient as it relates to treatment. (HCAHPS: During this hospital stay, were you given any medicine that you had not taken before? Before giving you any new medicine, how often did hospital staff tell you what the medicine was for? How often did hospital staff describe possible side effects in a way you could understand?)
- Patient may experience asthenia, xerostomia, flushing, warmth sensation, head heaviness or pressure, osteodynia, or arthralgia. Have patient report immediately to prescriber constipation, significant dyspepsia, melena, weight loss, leg cramps, leg pain, cold sensation, paresthesia, dyspnea, serotonin syndrome (ie, dizziness, severe headache, agitation, hallucinations, tachycardia, arrhythmia, flushing, tremors, hyperhidrosis, change in balance, illogical thinking, severe nausea, significant diarrhea), signs of severe cardiac abnormalities, strength differences from one side to another, difficulty speaking or thinking, change in balance, or vision changes (HCAHPS).
- Educate patient about signs of a significant reaction (eg, wheezing; chest tightness; fever; itching; bad cough; blue skin color; seizures; or swelling of face, lips, tongue, or throat). **Note:** This is not a comprehensive list of all side effects. Patient should consult prescriber for additional questions.

Intended Use and Disclaimer: Should not be printed and given to patients. This information is intended to serve as a concise initial reference for healthcare professionals to use when discussing medications with a patient. You must ultimately rely on your own discretion, experience and judgment in diagnosing, treating and advising patients.

Fulvestrant (fool VES trant)

Brand Names: U.S. Faslodex
Index Terms ICI-182,780; ZD9238
Pharmacologic Category Antineoplastic Agent, Estrogen Receptor Antagonist
Pregnancy Risk Factor D
Lactation Excretion in breast milk unknown/not recommended
Breast-Feeding Considerations Approved for use only in postmenopausal women.
Use Treatment of hormone receptor positive metastatic breast cancer in postmenopausal women with disease progression following antiestrogen therapy
Mechanism of Action/Effect Estrogen receptor antagonist; competitively binds to estrogen receptors on tumors and other tissue targets, producing a nuclear complex that causes a dose-related down-regulation of estrogen receptors and inhibits tumor growth.
Contraindications Hypersensitivity to fulvestrant or any component of the formulation
Warnings/Precautions Hazardous agent - use appropriate precautions for handling and disposal (NIOSH, 2012). Use caution in hepatic impairment; dosage adjustment is recommended in patients with moderate hepatic impairment. Safety and efficacy have not been established in severe hepatic impairment. Use with caution in patients with a history of bleeding disorders (including thrombocytopenia) and/or patients on anticoagulant therapy; bleeding/hematoma may occur from I.M. administration.

Drug Interactions

Avoid Concomitant Use There are no known interactions where it is recommended to avoid concomitant use.

Decreased Effect There are no known significant interactions involving a decrease in effect.

Increased Effect/Toxicity There are no known significant interactions involving an increase in effect.

Adverse Reactions Adverse reactions reported with 500 mg dose.

>10%:

Endocrine & metabolic: Hot flushes (7% to 13%)
Hepatic: Alkaline phosphatase increased (>15%; grades 3/4: 1% to 2%), transaminases increased (>15%; grades 3/4: 1% to 2%)
Local: Injection site pain (12% to 14%)
Neuromuscular & skeletal: Joint disorders (14% to 19%)

1% to 10%:
Cardiovascular: Ischemic disorder (1%)
Central nervous system: Fatigue (8%), headache (8%)
Gastrointestinal: Nausea (10%), anorexia (6%), vomiting (6%), constipation (5%), weight gain (≤1%)
Genitourinary: Urinary tract infection (2% to 4%)
Neuromuscular & skeletal: Bone pain (9%), arthralgia (8%), back pain (8%), extremity pain (7%), musculoskeletal pain (6%), weakness (6%)
Respiratory: Cough (5%), dyspnea (4%)

Pharmacodynamics/Kinetics
Duration of Action I.M.: Steady state concentrations reached within first month, when administered with additional dose given 2 weeks following the initial dose; plasma levels maintained for at least 1 month

Available Dosage Forms
Solution, Intramuscular:
Faslodex: 250 mg/5 mL (5 mL)

General Dosage Range Dosage adjustment recommended in patients with hepatic impairment
I.M.: *Adults (postmenopausal women):* Initial: 500 mg on days 1, 15, and 29; Maintenance: 500 mg once monthly

Administration
I.M. For I.M. administration only; do not administer I.V., SubQ, or intra-arterially. Administer 500 mg dose as two 5 mL injections (one in each buttock) slowly over 1-2 minutes per injection.

Hazardous agent; use appropriate precautions for handling and disposal (NIOSH, 2012).

Storage/Stability Store in original carton under refrigeration at 2°C to 8°C (36°F to 46°F). Protect from light.

Nursing Actions
Physical Assessment Monitor for thromboembolism, vasodilation, edema, gastrointestinal disturbances, dyspnea, and pain on a regular basis throughout.

Patient Education
• Discuss specific use of drug and side effects with patient as it relates to treatment. (HCAHPS: During this hospital stay, were you given any medicine that you had not taken before? Before giving you any new medicine, how often did hospital staff tell you what the medicine was for? How often did hospital staff describe possible side effects in a way you could understand?)
• Patient may experience hot flashes, nausea, headache, back pain, constipation, lack of appetite, pharyngitis, or injection site pain or irritation. Have patient report immediately to prescriber paresthesia, depression, severe arthralgia, significant myalgia, considerable osteodynia, angina, dyspnea, intolerable asthenia, dysuria, or difficult urination (HCAHPS).

• Educate patient about signs of a significant reaction (eg, wheezing; chest tightness; fever; itching; bad cough; blue skin color; seizures; or swelling of face, lips, tongue, or throat). **Note:** This is not a comprehensive list of all side effects. Patient should consult prescriber for additional questions.

Intended Use and Disclaimer: Should not be printed and given to patients. This information is intended to serve as a concise initial reference for healthcare professionals to use when discussing medications with a patient. You must ultimately rely on your own discretion, experience and judgment in diagnosing, treating and advising patients.

Furosemide (fyoor OH se mide)

Brand Names: U.S. Lasix
Index Terms Frusemide
Pharmacologic Category Antihypertensive; Diuretic, Loop
Medication Safety Issues
Sound-alike/look-alike issues:
Furosemide may be confused with famotidine, finasteride, fluconazole, FLUoxetine, fosinopril, loperamide, torsemide
Lasix may be confused with Lanoxin, Lidex, Lomotil, Lovenox, Luvox, Luxiq
International issues:
Lasix [U.S., Canada, and multiple international markets] may be confused with Esidrex brand name for hydrochlorothiazide [multiple international markets]; Esidrix brand name for hydrochlorothiazide [Germany]
Urex [Australia, Hong Kong, Turkey] may be confused with Eurax brand name for crotamiton [U.S., Canada, and multiple international markets]

Pregnancy Risk Factor C
Lactation Enters breast milk/use caution
Breast-Feeding Considerations Crosses into breast milk; may suppress lactation
Use Management of edema associated with heart failure and hepatic or renal disease; acute pulmonary edema; treatment of hypertension (alone or in combination with other antihypertensives)
Canadian labeling: Additional use: Furosemide Special Injection and Lasix Special (products not available in the U.S.): Adjunctive treatment of oliguria in patients with severe renal impairment
Mechanism of Action/Effect Inhibits reabsorption of sodium and chloride in the ascending loop of Henle and distal renal tubule, interfering with the chloride-binding cotransport system, thus causing increased excretion of water, sodium, chloride, magnesium, and calcium
Contraindications Hypersensitivity to furosemide or any component of the formulation; anuria

Canadian labeling: Additional contraindications (not in U.S. labeling): Hypersensitivity to sulfonamide-derived drugs; complete renal shutdown; hepatic coma and precoma; uncorrected states of electrolyte depletion, hypovolemia, or hypotension; jaundiced newborn infants or infants with disease(s) capable of causing hyperbilirubinemia and possibly kernicterus; breast-feeding. **Note:** manufacturer's labeling for Lasix® Special and Furosemide Special Injection also includes: GFR <5 mL/minute or GFR >20 mL/minute; hepatic cirrhosis; renal failure accompanied by hepatic coma and precoma; renal failure due to poisoning with nephrotoxic or hepatotoxic substances.

Warnings/Precautions [U.S. Boxed Warning]: If given in excessive amounts, furosemide, similar to other loop diuretics, can lead to profound diuresis, resulting in fluid and electrolyte depletion; close medical supervision and dose evaluation are required. Watch for and correct electrolyte disturbances; adjust dose to avoid dehydration. When electrolyte depletion is present, therapy should not be initiated unless serum electrolytes, especially potassium, are normalized. In cirrhosis, avoid electrolyte and acid/base imbalances that might lead to hepatic encephalopathy; correct electrolyte and acid/base imbalances prior to initiation when hepatic coma is present. Coadministration of antihypertensives may increase the risk of hypotension.

Monitor fluid status and renal function in an attempt to prevent oliguria, azotemia, and reversible increases in BUN and creatinine; close medical supervision of aggressive diuresis is required. May increase risk of contrast-induced nephropathy. Rapid I.V. administration, renal impairment, excessive doses, hypoproteinemia, and concurrent use of other ototoxins is associated with ototoxicity. Asymptomatic hyperuricemia has been reported with use; rarely, gout may precipitate. Photosensitization may occur.

Use with caution in patients with prediabetes or diabetes mellitus; may see a change in glucose control. Use with caution in patients with systemic lupus erythematosus (SLE); may cause SLE exacerbation or activation. Use with caution in patients with prostatic hyperplasia/urinary stricture; may cause urinary retention. May lead to nephrocalcinosis or nephrolithiasis in premature infants or in children <4 years of age with chronic use. May prevent closure of patent ductus arteriosus in premature infants. Chemical similarities are present among sulfonamides, sulfonylureas, carbonic anhydrase inhibitors, thiazides, and loop diuretics (except ethacrynic acid). A risk of cross-reaction exists in patients with allergy to any of these compounds; avoid use when previous reaction has been severe. Discontinue if signs of hypersensitivity are noted.

Drug Interactions
Avoid Concomitant Use
Avoid concomitant use of Furosemide with any of the following: Chloral Hydrate; Ethacrynic Acid
Decreased Effect
Furosemide may decrease the levels/effects of: Hypoglycemic Agents; Lithium; Neuromuscular-Blocking Agents

The levels/effects of Furosemide may be decreased by: Aliskiren; Bile Acid Sequestrants; Fosphenytoin; Herbs (Hypertensive Properties); Methotrexate; Methylphenidate; Nonsteroidal Anti-Inflammatory Agents; Phenytoin; Probenecid; Salicylates; Sucralfate; Yohimbine
Increased Effect/Toxicity
Furosemide may increase the levels/effects of: ACE Inhibitors; Allopurinol; Amifostine; Aminoglycosides; Antihypertensives; Cardiac Glycosides; Chloral Hydrate; CISplatin; Dofetilide; DULoxetine; Ethacrynic Acid; Hypotensive Agents; Ivabradine; Lithium; Methotrexate; Neuromuscular-Blocking Agents; Obinutuzumab; RisperiDONE; RiTUXimab; Salicylates; Sodium Phosphates; Topiramate

The levels/effects of Furosemide may be increased by: Alfuzosin; Analgesics (Opioid); Beta2-Agonists; Brimonidine (Topical); Corticosteroids (Orally Inhaled); Corticosteroids (Systemic); CycloSPORINE (Systemic); Diazoxide; Herbs (Hypotensive Properties); Licorice; MAO Inhibitors; Methotrexate; Pentoxifylline; Phosphodiesterase 5 Inhibitors; Probenecid; Prostacyclin Analogues
Nutritional/Ethanol Interactions
Food: Furosemide serum levels may be decreased if taken with food.
Herb/Nutraceutical: Avoid bayberry, blue cohosh, cayenne, ephedra, ginger, ginseng (American), kola, licorice (may worsen hypertension). Avoid black cohosh, California poppy, coleus, golden seal, hawthorn, mistletoe, periwinkle, quinine, shepherd's purse (may increase antihypertensive effect). Licorice may also cause or worsen hypokalemia.
Adverse Reactions Frequency not defined.
Cardiovascular: Acute hypotension, chronic aortitis, necrotizing angiitis, orthostatic hypotension, vasculitis
Central nervous system: Dizziness, fever, headache, hepatic encephalopathy, lightheadedness, restlessness, vertigo
Dermatologic: Bullous pemphigoid, cutaneous vasculitis, drug rash with eosinophilia and systemic symptoms (DRESS), erythema multiforme, exanthematous pustulosis (generalized), exfoliative dermatitis, photosensitivity, pruritus, purpura, rash, Stevens-Johnson syndrome, toxic epidermal necrolysis, urticaria
Endocrine & metabolic: Cholesterol and triglycerides increased, glucose tolerance test altered,

gout, hyperglycemia, hyperuricemia, hypocalcemia, hypochloremia, hypokalemia, hypomagnesemia, hyponatremia, metabolic alkalosis

Gastrointestinal: Anorexia, constipation, cramping, diarrhea, nausea, oral and gastric irritation, pancreatitis, vomiting

Genitourinary: Urinary bladder spasm, urinary frequency

Hematological: Agranulocytosis (rare), anemia, aplastic anemia (rare), eosinophilia, hemolytic anemia, leukopenia, thrombocytopenia

Hepatic: Intrahepatic cholestatic jaundice, ischemic hepatitis, liver enzymes increased

Local: Injection site pain (following I.M. injection), thrombophlebitis

Neuromuscular & skeletal: Muscle spasm, paresthesia, weakness

Ocular: Blurred vision, xanthopsia

Otic: Hearing impairment (reversible or permanent with rapid I.V. or I.M. administration), tinnitus

Renal: Allergic interstitial nephritis, fall in glomerular filtration rate and renal blood flow (due to overdiuresis), glycosuria, transient rise in BUN

Miscellaneous: Anaphylaxis (rare), exacerbate or activate systemic lupus erythematosus

Pharmacodynamics/Kinetics

Onset of Action Diuresis: Oral, S.L.: 30-60 minutes; I.M.: 30 minutes; I.V.: ~5 minutes

Symptomatic improvement with acute pulmonary edema: Within 15-20 minutes; occurs prior to diuretic effect

Peak effect: Oral: 1-2 hours

Duration of Action Oral, S.L.: 6-8 hours; I.V.: 2 hours

Available Dosage Forms

Solution, Injection:
Generic: 10 mg/mL (2 mL, 4 mL, 10 mL)

Solution, Injection [preservative free]:
Generic: 10 mg/mL (2 mL, 4 mL, 10 mL)

Solution, Oral:
Generic: 8 mg/mL (5 mL, 500 mL); 10 mg/mL (60 mL, 120 mL)

Tablet, Oral:
Lasix: 20 mg, 40 mg, 80 mg
Generic: 20 mg, 40 mg, 80 mg

General Dosage Range

I.M.:
Children: Initial: 1 mg/kg/dose; Maintenance: Up to 6 mg/kg/dose every 6-12 hours
Adults: Initial: 20-40 mg/dose; Usual maintenance dose interval: 6-12 hours (maximum: 200 mg/dose)
Elderly: Initial: 20 mg/day

I.V.:
Children: Initial: 1 mg/kg/dose; Maintenance: Up to 6 mg/kg/dose every 6-12 hours
Adults: Initial: 20-40 mg/dose; Usual maintenance dose interval: 6-12 hours (maximum: 200 mg/dose) **or** 40 mg, followed by 80 mg within 1 hour if inadequate response
Elderly: Initial: 20 mg daily

Oral:
Children: Initial: 2 mg/kg/dose every 6-8 hours (maximum: 6 mg/kg/dose)
Adults: Initial: 20-80 mg/dose every 6-8 hours; Usual maintenance dose interval: Once or twice daily (maximum: 600 mg daily)
Elderly: Initial: 20 mg daily

Usual Infusion Concentrations: Pediatric I.V. infusion: 1 mg/mL **or** 2 mg/mL **or** undiluted as 10 mg/mL

Usual Infusion Concentrations: Adult I.V. infusion: 1 mg/mL **or** 2 mg/mL **or** undiluted as 10 mg/mL

Administration

I.V. I.V. injections should be given slowly. In adults, undiluted direct I.V. injections may be administered at a rate of 20-40 mg per minute; maximum rate of administration for short-term intermittent infusion is 4 mg/minute; exceeding this rate increases the risk of ototoxicity. In children, a maximum rate of 0.5 mg/kg/minute has been recommended.

Injectable Detail pH: 8-9.3

Oral Administer on an empty stomach (Bard, 2004). May be administered with food or milk if GI distress occurs; however, this may reduce diuretic efficacy.

Other When I.V. or oral administration is not possible, the sublingual route may be used. Place 1 tablet under tongue for at least 5 minutes to allow for maximal absorption. Patients should be advised not to swallow during disintegration time (Haegeli, 2007).

Preparation for Administration I.V. infusion solution mixed in NS or D$_5$W solution is stable for 24 hours at room temperature. May also be diluted for infusion to 1-2 mg/mL (maximum: 10 mg/mL).

Storage/Stability

Injection: Store at room temperature of 15°C to 30°C (59°F to 86°F). Protect from light. Exposure to light may cause discoloration; do not use furosemide solutions if they have a yellow color. Furosemide solutions are unstable in acidic media, but very stable in basic media. Refrigeration may result in precipitation or crystallization; however, resolubilization at room temperature or warming may be performed without affecting the drug's stability.

Tablet: Store at 25°C (77°F); excursions permitted to 15°C to 30°C (59°F to 89°F). Protect from light.

Nursing Actions

Physical Assessment Allergy history should be assessed before beginning therapy. Monitor for dehydration, electrolyte imbalance, and postural hypotension on a regular basis during therapy.

Patient Education

• Discuss specific use of drug and side effects with patient as it relates to treatment. (HCAHPS: During this hospital stay, were you given any medicine that you had not taken before? Before

giving you any new medicine, how often did hospital staff tell you what the medicine was for? How often did hospital staff describe possible side effects in a way you could understand?)
- Patient may experience constipation or diarrhea. Have patient report immediately to prescriber signs of fluid and electrolyte imbalance, signs of hyperglycemia, signs of hepatic impairment, signs of pancreatitis, arthralgia, severe dizziness, syncope, paresthesia, hearing impairment, or Stevens-Johnson syndrome/toxic epidermal necrolysis (HCAHPS).
- Educate patient about signs of a significant reaction (eg, wheezing; chest tightness; fever; itching; bad cough; blue skin color; seizures; or swelling of face, lips, tongue, or throat). **Note:** This is not a comprehensive list of all side effects. Patient should consult prescriber for additional questions.

Intended Use and Disclaimer: Should not be printed and given to patients. This information is intended to serve as a concise initial reference for healthcare professionals to use when discussing medications with a patient. You must ultimately rely on your own discretion, experience and judgment in diagnosing, treating and advising patients.

Dietary Considerations May cause potassium loss; potassium supplement or dietary changes may be required.

Gabapentin (GA ba pen tin)

Brand Names: U.S. Gralise; Gralise Starter; Neurontin

Pharmacologic Category Anticonvulsant, Miscellaneous; GABA Analog

Medication Safety Issues

Sound-alike/look-alike issues:

Neurontin may be confused with Motrin, Neoral, nitrofurantoin, Noroxin, Zarontin

Medication Guide Available Yes

Pregnancy Risk Factor C

Lactation Enters breast milk/use caution

Breast-Feeding Considerations Gabapentin is excreted in human breast milk. Per the manufacturer, a nursed infant could be exposed to ~1 mg/kg/day of gabapentin; the effect on the child is not known. Use in breast-feeding women only if the benefits to the mother outweigh the potential risk to the infant.

In a small study of breast-feeding women (n=6), the estimated exposure of gabapentin to the nursing infants was ~1% to 4% of the weight-adjusted maternal dose (sampling occurred from 12-97 days after delivery and maternal doses ranged from 600-2100 mg daily). Gabapentin was detected in the serum of 2 nursing infants 2-3 weeks after delivery and in 1 infant after 3 months of breast-feeding. Serum concentrations were <12% of the maternal plasma concentrations and <5% of those measured in the umbilical cord. Adverse events were not reported in the breast-fed infants (Ohman, 2005).

Use Adjunct for treatment of partial seizures with and without secondary generalized seizures in patients >12 years of age with epilepsy; adjunct for treatment of partial seizures in pediatric patients 3-12 years of age; management of postherpetic neuralgia (PHN) in adults

Unlabeled Use Neuropathic pain, diabetic peripheral neuropathy, fibromyalgia, postoperative pain (adjunct), restless legs syndrome (RLS), vasomotor symptoms

Mechanism of Action/Effect Although structurally related to GABA, it does not interact with GABA receptors. Interacts with calcium channels to inhibit neurotransmission related to seizure activity and pain perception.

Contraindications Hypersensitivity to gabapentin or any component of the formulation

Warnings/Precautions Antiepileptics are associated with an increased risk of suicidal behavior/thoughts with use (regardless of indication); patients should be monitored for signs/symptoms of depression, suicidal tendencies, and other unusual behavior changes during therapy and instructed to inform their healthcare provider immediately if symptoms occur. Avoid abrupt withdrawal, may precipitate seizures; Gralise™ should be withdrawn over ≥1 week. Use cautiously in patients with severe renal dysfunction; male rat studies demonstrated an association with pancreatic adenocarcinoma (clinical implication unknown). May cause CNS depression, which may impair physical or mental abilities. Patients must be cautioned about performing tasks which require mental alertness (eg, operating machinery or driving). Effects with other sedative drugs or ethanol may be potentiated. Pediatric patients (3-12 years of age) have shown increased incidence of CNS-related adverse effects, including emotional lability, hostility, thought disorder, and hyperkinesia. Gabapentin immediate release and extended release (Gralise™) products are not interchangeable with each other **or** with gabapentin enacarbil (Horizant™). The safety and efficacy of extended release gabapentin (Gralise™) has not been studied in patients with epilepsy. Potentially serious, sometimes fatal multiorgan hypersensitivity (also known as drug reaction with eosinophilia and systemic symptoms [DRESS]) has been reported with some antiepileptic drugs, including gabapentin; may affect lymphatic, hepatic, renal, cardiac, and/or hematologic systems; fever, rash, and eosinophilia may also be present. Discontinue immediately if suspected.

▶

Drug Interactions
Avoid Concomitant Use
Avoid concomitant use of Gabapentin with any of the following: Azelastine (Nasal); Paraldehyde; Thalidomide
Decreased Effect
The levels/effects of Gabapentin may be decreased by: Antacids; Ketorolac (Nasal); Ketorolac (Systemic); Magnesium Salts; Mefloquine; Orlistat
Increased Effect/Toxicity
Gabapentin may increase the levels/effects of: Alcohol (Ethyl); Azelastine (Nasal); Buprenorphine; CNS Depressants; Hydrocodone; Methotrimeprazine; Metyrosine; Mirtazapine; Paraldehyde; Pramipexole; ROPINIRole; Rotigotine; Selective Serotonin Reuptake Inhibitors; Thalidomide; Zolpidem

The levels/effects of Gabapentin may be increased by: Brimonidine (Topical); Doxylamine; Droperidol; HydrOXYzine; Methotrimeprazine; Perampanel; Sodium Oxybate; Tapentadol

Nutritional/Ethanol Interactions
Ethanol: May increase CNS depression; monitor for increased effects with coadministration. Caution patients about effects.

Food: Tablet, solution (immediate release): No significant effect on rate or extent of absorption; tablet (extended release): Increases rate and extent of absorption.

Herb/Nutraceutical: Avoid evening primrose (seizure threshold decreased). Avoid valerian, St John's wort, kava kava, gotu kola (may increase CNS depression).

Adverse Reactions
As reported for immediate release (IR) formulations in patients >12 years of age, unless otherwise noted in children (3-12 years) or with use of extended release (ER) formulation

>10%:
- Central nervous system: Dizziness (IR: 17% to 28%; children 3%; ER: 11%), drowsiness (IR: 19% to 21%; children 8%; ER: 5%), ataxia (1% to 13%), fatigue (11%; children 3%)
- Infection: Viral infection (children 11%)

1% to 10%:
- Cardiovascular: Peripheral edema (IR: 2% to 8%; ER: 4%), vasodilatation (1%)
- Central nervous system: Hostility (children 5% to 8%), tremor (7%), emotional lability (children 4% to 6%), hyperkinesia (children 3% to 5%), headache (ER: 4%; IR: 3%), abnormality in thinking (2% to 3%; children 2%), abnormal gait (2%), amnesia (2%), depression (2%), nervousness (2%), pain (ER: 1% to 2%), hyperesthesia (1%), lethargy (ER: 1%), twitching (1%), vertigo (ER: 1%)
- Dermatologic: Pruritus (1%), skin rash (1%)
- Endocrine & metabolic: Weight gain (IR: Adults and children 2% to 3%; ER: 2%), hyperglycemia (1%)
- Gastrointestinal: Diarrhea (IR: 6%; ER: 3%), nausea and vomiting (3% to 4%; children 8%), xerostomia (IR: 2% to 5%; ER: 3%), constipation (IR: 1% to 4%; ER: 1%), abdominal pain (3%), dyspepsia (IR: 2%; ER: 1%), dry throat (2%), dental disease (2%), flatulence (2%), increased appetite (1%)
- Genitourinary: Impotence (2%), urinary tract infection (ER: 2%)
- Hematologic & oncologic: Decreased white blood cell count (1%), leukopenia (1%)
- Infection: Infection (5%)
- Neuromuscular & skeletal: Weakness (6%), back pain (IR: 2%; ER: 2%), dysarthria (2%), limb pain (ER: 2%), myalgia (2%), bone fracture (1%)
- Ophthalmic: Nystagmus (8%), diplopia (1% to 6%), blurred vision (3% to 4%), conjunctivitis (1%)
- Otic: Otitis media (1%)
- Respiratory: Rhinitis (4%), bronchitis (children 3%), nasopharyngitis (ER: 3%), respiratory tract infection (children 3%), pharyngitis (1% to 3%), cough (2%)
- Miscellaneous: Fever (children 10%)

Available Dosage Forms
Capsule, Oral:
Neurontin: 100 mg, 300 mg, 400 mg
Generic: 100 mg, 300 mg, 400 mg
Miscellaneous, Oral:
Gralise Starter: 300 & 60 mg (78 ea)
Solution, Oral:
Neurontin: 250 mg/5 mL (470 mL)
Generic: 250 mg/5 mL (5 mL, 6 mL, 470 mL, 473 mL)
Tablet, Oral:
Gralise: 300 mg, 600 mg
Neurontin: 600 mg, 800 mg
Generic: 600 mg, 800 mg

General Dosage Range
Dosage adjustment recommended in patients with renal impairment
Oral:
Children 3-4 years: Initial: 10-15 mg/kg/day in 3 divided doses; Usual dose: 40 mg/kg/day in 3 divided doses (maximum: 50 mg/kg/day)
Children 5-12 years: Initial: 10-15 mg/kg/day in 3 divided doses; Usual dose: 25-35 mg/kg/day in 3 divided doses (maximum: 50 mg/kg/day)
Children >12 years: Initial: 300 mg 3 times/day; Usual dose: 900-1800 mg/day in 3 divided doses (maximum: 3600 mg/day [short-term])
Adults:
Immediate release: Initial: 300 mg 1-3 times/day; Maintenance: 900-3600 mg/day in 3 divided doses (maximum: 3600 mg/day [short-term])
Extended release: Initial: 300 mg; Maintenance: 1800 mg once daily

Administration

Oral

Tablet, solution (immediate release): Administer first dose on first day at bedtime to avoid somnolence and dizziness. Dosage must be adjusted for renal function; when given 3 times daily, the maximum time between doses should not exceed 12 hours.

Tablet (extended release): Take with evening meal. Swallow whole; do not chew, crush, or split.

Storage/Stability

Capsules and tablets: Store at 25°C (77°F); excursions permitted to 15°C to 30°C (59°F to 86°F). Oral solution: Store refrigerated at 2°C to 8°C (36°F to 46°F).

Nursing Actions

Physical Assessment Monitor therapeutic response (seizure activity, force, type, duration) at beginning of therapy and periodically throughout. Assess for CNS depression. Monitor for multiorgan sensitivity (lymphatic, hepatic, renal, cardiac, hematologic symptoms, fever, rash, eosinophilia). Taper dosage slowly when discontinuing. If treating seizures, observe and teach seizure/safety precautions.

Patient Education

- Discuss specific use of drug and side effects with patient as it relates to treatment. (HCAHPS: During this hospital stay, were you given any medicine that you had not taken before? Before giving you any new medicine, how often did hospital staff tell you what the medicine was for? How often did hospital staff describe possible side effects in a way you could understand?)
- Patient may experience dyspraxia, fatigue, weight gain, diarrhea, constipation, or xerostomia. Have patient report immediately to prescriber edema of extremities, behavioral changes, emotional instability, hostility, memory loss, vision changes, signs of infection, illogical thinking, tremors, angina, severe dizziness, syncope, dyspnea, hyperhidrosis, significant asthenia, considerable headache, intolerable nausea, bradycardia, tachycardia, arrhythmia, strength differences from one side to another, difficulty speaking or thinking, change in balance, blurred vision, involuntary eye movements, fasciculations, ecchymosis, hemorrhaging, jaundice, or signs of depression (ie, suicidal ideation, anxiety, emotional instability, illogical thinking) (HCAHPS).
- Educate patient about signs of a significant reaction (eg, wheezing; chest tightness; fever; itching; bad cough; blue skin color; seizures; or swelling of face, lips, tongue, or throat). **Note:** This is not a comprehensive list of all side effects. Patient should consult prescriber for additional questions.

Intended Use and Disclaimer: Should not be printed and given to patients. This information is intended to serve as a concise initial reference for healthcare professionals to use when discussing medications with a patient. You must ultimately rely on your own discretion, experience and judgment in diagnosing, treating and advising patients.

Dietary Considerations Immediate release tablet and solution may be taken without regard to meals; extended release tablet should be taken with food.

Related Information

Oral Medications That Should Not Be Crushed or Altered *on page 1712*

Gabapentin Enacarbil
(gab a PEN tin en a KAR bil)

Brand Names: U.S. Horizant

Index Terms GSK 1838262; Solzira; XP13512

Pharmacologic Category Anticonvulsant, Miscellaneous

Medication Guide Available Yes

Pregnancy Risk Factor C

Lactation Excretion in breast milk unknown/not recommended

Breast-Feeding Considerations It is not known if gabapentin enacarbil is excreted in human breast milk; however, other gabapentin products are excreted in human breast milk. Refer to Gabapentin monograph for additional information.

Use Treatment of moderate-to-severe restless leg syndrome (RLS); management of postherpetic neuralgia (PHN)

Mechanism of Action/Effect Gabapentin enacarbil is a prodrug of gabapentin. Although gabapentin is structurally related to GABA, it does not interact with GABA receptors. Interacts with calcium channels to inhibit neurotransmission. These effects on RLS are unknown.

Contraindications There are no contraindications listed within the manufacturer's labeling.

Warnings/Precautions Potentially serious, sometimes fatal multiorgan hypersensitivity (also known as drug reaction with eosinophilia and systemic symptoms [DRESS]) has been reported with some antiepileptic drugs, including gabapentin. Monitor for signs and symptoms of possible disparate manifestations associated with lymphatic, hepatic, renal, cardiac, and/or hematologic systems; fever, rash, and eosinophilia may also be present. Discontinue immediately if suspected. Gabapentin and other antiepileptics are associated with an increased risk of suicidal behavior/thoughts with use (regardless of indication); gabapentin enacarbil is a prodrug of gabapentin and may also increase patient's risk. Patients should be monitored for signs/symptoms of depression, suicidal tendencies, and other unusual behavior changes during therapy and instructed to inform their healthcare provider immediately if symptoms occur. To avoid the potential for withdrawal seizure, dose reduction is recommended for patients with post-herpetic neuralgia (PHN) receiving twice daily doses or patients with restless legs syndrome (RLS) receiving daily doses >600 mg (daily doses of ≤600 mg can be discontinued without tapering in patients with RLS). Rat studies demonstrated an association with pancreatic adenocarcinoma (clinical implication unknown). May cause CNS depression, which may impair physical or mental abilities. Patients must be cautioned about performing tasks which require mental alertness (eg, operating machinery or driving). Effects with other sedative drugs or ethanol may be potentiated. Use with caution in patients with renal impairment; dose adjustment is needed. Gabapentin enacarbil (Horizant®) and other gabapentin products are not interchangeable due to differences in formulation, indications, and pharmacokinetics.

Restless legs syndrome (RLS): Not recommended for use in patients who are required to sleep during the day and remain awake during the night.

Drug Interactions

Avoid Concomitant Use
Avoid concomitant use of Gabapentin Enacarbil with any of the following: Alcohol (Ethyl); Azelastine (Nasal); Paraldehyde; Thalidomide

Decreased Effect
The levels/effects of Gabapentin Enacarbil may be decreased by: Ketorolac (Nasal); Ketorolac (Systemic); Mefloquine; Orlistat

Increased Effect/Toxicity
Gabapentin Enacarbil may increase the levels/effects of: Azelastine (Nasal); Buprenorphine; CNS Depressants; Hydrocodone; Methotrimeprazine; Metyrosine; Mirtazapine; Paraldehyde; Pramipexole; ROPINIRole; Rotigotine; Selective Serotonin Reuptake Inhibitors; Thalidomide; Zolpidem

The levels/effects of Gabapentin Enacarbil may be increased by: Alcohol (Ethyl); Brimonidine (Topical); Doxylamine; Droperidol; HydrOXYzine; Magnesium Sulfate; Methotrimeprazine; Perampanel; Sodium Oxybate; Tapentadol

Nutritional/Ethanol Interactions
Ethanol: May increase CNS depression and cause rapid release of gabapentin enacarbil from the extended release tablet. Management: Avoid ethanol.

Herb/Nutraceutical: Avoid evening primrose (seizure threshold decreased). Avoid valerian, St John's wort, kava kava, gotu kola (may increase CNS depression).

Adverse Reactions Percentages reported are for restless leg syndrome (RLS) 600 mg daily and postherpetic neuralgia (PHN) 1200 mg daily.

>10%: Central nervous system: Sedation/somnolence (PHN 10%; RLS 20%), dizziness (13% to 17%), headache (10% to 12%)

1% to 10%:
Cardiovascular: Peripheral edema (PHN 6%; RLS <1%)

Central nervous system: Fatigue (6%), irritability (≤4%), insomnia (PHN 3%), balance disorder (<2%), depression (<2%), disorientation (<2%), lethargy (<2%), drunk feeling (<2%), vertigo (<2%)

Gastrointestinal: Nausea (6% to 8%), flatulence (≤3%), xerostomia (≤3%), weight gain (2% to 3%), appetite increased (≤2%)

Ocular: Blurred vision (≤2%)

Available Dosage Forms
Tablet Extended Release 24 Hour, Oral:
Horizant: 300 mg, 600 mg

General Dosage Range Dosage adjustment recommended in patients with renal impairment.

Oral: *Adults:* 600 mg once daily (RLS) **or** 600 mg once daily for 3 days, then 600 mg twice daily (PHN)

Administration
Oral Tablet should be swallowed whole; do not break, chew, cut, or crush. Administer with food. Restless leg syndrome: Administer at ~5:00 pm daily.

Storage/Stability Store at 25°C (77°F); excursions permitted to 15°C to 30°C (59°F to 86°F). Protect from moisture. Do not remove from original container.

Nursing Actions
Physical Assessment Monitor for efficacy.

Patient Education
• Discuss specific use of drug and side effects with patient as it relates to treatment. (HCAHPS: During this hospital stay, were you given any medicine that you had not taken before? Before giving you any new medicine, how often did hospital staff tell you what the medicine was for? How often did hospital staff describe possible side effects in a way you could understand?)

• Patient may experience fatigue, headache, dyspepsia, or insomnia. Have patient report immediately to prescriber signs of hepatic impairment, signs of renal impairment, signs of infection, severe asthenia, myalgia, considerable dizziness, syncope, blurred vision, change in balance, angina, dyspnea, excessive weight gain, edema of extremities, ecchymosis, hemorrhaging, chills, pharyngitis, enlarged lymph nodes, or signs of depression (ie, suicidal ideation, anxiety, emotional instability, illogical thinking) (HCAHPS).

• Educate patient about signs of a significant reaction (eg, wheezing; chest tightness; fever; itching; bad cough; blue skin color; seizures; or swelling of face, lips, tongue, or throat). **Note:** This is not a comprehensive list of all side effects. Patient should consult prescriber for additional questions.

Intended Use and Disclaimer: Should not be printed and given to patients. This information is intended to serve as a concise initial reference for healthcare professionals to use when discussing medications with a patient. You must ultimately rely on your own discretion, experience and judgment in diagnosing, treating and advising patients.

Dietary Considerations Take with food.

Related Information

Oral Medications That Should Not Be Crushed or Altered *on page 1712*

Galantamine (ga LAN ta meen)

Brand Names: U.S. Razadyne; Razadyne ER
Index Terms Galantamine Hydrobromide
Pharmacologic Category Acetylcholinesterase Inhibitor (Central)

Medication Safety Issues

Sound-alike/look-alike issues:

Razadyne® may be confused with Rozerem®

International issues:

Reminyl [Canada and multiple international markets] may be confused with Amarel brand name for glimepiride [France]; Amaryl brand name for glimepiride [U.S., Canada, and multiple international markets]; Robinul brand name for glycopyrrolate [U.S. and multiple international markets]

Pregnancy Risk Factor B

Lactation Excretion in breast milk unknown/not recommended

Breast-Feeding Considerations It is not known if galantamine is excreted in breast milk. Galantamine is not indicated in nursing mothers.

Use Treatment of mild-to-moderate dementia of Alzheimer's disease

Unlabeled Use Severe dementia associated with Alzheimer's disease; mild-to-moderate dementia associated with Parkinson's disease; Lewy body dementia

Mechanism of Action/Effect Increases the concentration of acetylcholine in the brain by slowing its metabolism.

Contraindications Hypersensitivity to galantamine or any component of the formulation

Warnings/Precautions Use caution in patients with supraventricular conduction delays (without a functional pacemaker in place); Alzheimer's treatment guidelines consider bradycardia to be a relative contraindication for use of centrally-active cholinesterase inhibitors. Use caution in patients taking medicines that slow conduction through SA or AV node. Use caution in peptic ulcer disease (or in patients at risk); seizure disorder; asthma; COPD; mild-to-moderate liver dysfunction; moderate renal dysfunction. May cause bladder outflow obstruction. May exaggerate neuromuscular blockade effects of succinylcholine and like agents.

Drug Interactions

Avoid Concomitant Use There are no known interactions where it is recommended to avoid concomitant use.

Decreased Effect

Galantamine may decrease the levels/effects of: Anticholinergics; Neuromuscular-Blocking Agents (Nondepolarizing)

The levels/effects of Galantamine may be decreased by: Anticholinergics; Dipyridamole; Peginterferon Alfa-2b

Increased Effect/Toxicity

Galantamine may increase the levels/effects of: Antipsychotics; Beta-Blockers; Cholinergic Agonists; Highest Risk QTc-Prolonging Agents; Moderate Risk QTc-Prolonging Agents; Succinylcholine

The levels/effects of Galantamine may be increased by: Corticosteroids (Systemic); Mifepristone; Selective Serotonin Reuptake Inhibitors

Nutritional/Ethanol Interactions

Ethanol: Avoid ethanol (may increase CNS adverse events).

Herb/Nutraceutical: St John's wort may decrease galantamine serum levels; avoid concurrent use.

Adverse Reactions

>10%: Gastrointestinal: Nausea (13% to 24%), vomiting (6% to 13%), diarrhea (6% to 12%)

1% to 10%:

Cardiovascular: Bradycardia (2% to 3%), hypertension (≥2%), peripheral edema (≥2%), syncope (0.4% to 2.2%: dose related), chest pain (≥1% to 2%)

Central nervous system: Dizziness (9%), headache (8%), depression (7%), fatigue (5%), insomnia (5%), somnolence (4%), agitation (≥2%), anxiety (≥2%), confusion (≥2%), hallucination (≥2%), fever (≥1%), malaise (≥1%)

Dermatologic: Purpura (≥2%)

Gastrointestinal: Anorexia (7% to 9%), weight loss (5% to 7%), abdominal pain (5%), dyspepsia (5%), constipation (≥2%), flatulence (≥1%)

Genitourinary: Urinary tract infection (8%), hematuria (<1% to 3%), incontinence (≥1% to 2%)

Hematologic: Anemia (3%)

Neuromuscular & skeletal: Tremor (3%), back pain (≥2%), fall (≥2%), weakness (≥1% to 2%)

Respiratory: Rhinitis (4%), bronchitis (≥2%), cough (≥2%), upper respiratory tract infection (≥2%)

Pharmacodynamics/Kinetics

Duration of Action 3 hours; maximum inhibition of erythrocyte acetylcholinesterase ~40% at 1 hour post 8 mg oral dose; levels return to baseline at 30 hours

Available Dosage Forms

Capsule Extended Release 24 Hour, Oral:

Razadyne ER: 8 mg, 16 mg, 24 mg

Generic: 8 mg, 16 mg, 24 mg

Solution, Oral:
Razadyne: 4 mg/mL (100 mL)
Generic: 4 mg/mL (100 mL)
Tablet, Oral:
Razadyne: 4 mg, 8 mg, 12 mg
Generic: 4 mg, 8 mg, 12 mg
General Dosage Range Dosage adjustment recommended in patients with hepatic or renal impairment
Oral:
Extended-release: *Adults:* Initial: 8 mg once daily; Maintenance: 16-24 mg once daily
Immediate release: *Adults:* Initial: 4 mg twice daily; Maintenance: 16-24 mg/day in 2 divided doses

Administration

Oral Administer oral solution or tablet with breakfast and dinner; administer extended release capsule with breakfast. If therapy is interrupted for ≥3 days, restart at the lowest dose and increase to current dose. If using oral solution, mix dose with 3-4 ounces of any nonalcoholic beverage; mix well and drink immediately.

Storage/Stability Store at 25°C (77°F); excursions permitted to 15°C to 30°C (59°F to 86°F). Do not freeze oral solution.

Nursing Actions

Physical Assessment Assess bladder and sphincter adequacy prior to treatment. Monitor for cholinergic crisis.

Patient Education
• Discuss specific use of drug and side effects with patient as it relates to treatment. (HCAHPS: During this hospital stay, were you given any medicine that you had not taken before? Before giving you any new medicine, how often did hospital staff tell you what the medicine was for? How often did hospital staff describe possible side effects in a way you could understand?)
• Patient may experience headache, lack of appetite, or insomnia. Have patient report immediately to prescriber signs of depression (ie, suicidal ideation, anxiety, emotional instability, illogical thinking), severe dizziness, syncope, strength differences from one side to another, difficulty speaking or thinking, change in balance, blurred vision, difficult urination, arrhythmia, bradycardia, melena, hematemesis, considerable asthenia, angina, edema of hands or feet, paresthesia, hallucinations, dyspnea, significant nausea, intolerable diarrhea, severe dyspepsia, tremors, or urinary retention (HCAHPS).
• Educate patient about signs of a significant reaction (eg, wheezing; chest tightness; fever; itching; bad cough; blue skin color; seizures; or swelling of face, lips, tongue, or throat). **Note:** This is not a comprehensive list of all side effects. Patient should consult prescriber for additional questions.

Intended Use and Disclaimer: Should not be printed and given to patients. This information is intended to serve as a concise initial reference for healthcare professionals to use when discussing medications with a patient. You must ultimately rely on your own discretion, experience and judgment in diagnosing, treating and advising patients.

Dietary Considerations Administration with food is preferred, but not required; should be taken with breakfast and dinner (tablet or solution) or with breakfast (capsule).

Related Information
Oral Medications That Should Not Be Crushed or Altered *on page 1712*

Ganciclovir (Systemic) (gan SYE kloe veer)

Brand Names: U.S. Cytovene
Index Terms DHPG Sodium; GCV Sodium; Nordeoxyguanosine
Pharmacologic Category Antiviral Agent
Medication Safety Issues
Sound-alike/look-alike issues:
Cytovene® may be confused with Cytosar®, Cytosar-U
Ganciclovir may be confused with acyclovir

Pregnancy Risk Factor C
Lactation Excretion in breast milk unknown/not recommended

Breast-Feeding Considerations Due to the carcinogenic and teratogenic effects observed in animal studies, the possibility of adverse events in a nursing infant is considered likely. Therefore, nursing should be discontinued during therapy. In addition, the CDC recommends **not** to breast-feed if diagnosed with HIV to avoid postnatal transmission of the virus.

Use Treatment of CMV retinitis in immunocompromised individuals, including patients with acquired immunodeficiency syndrome; prophylaxis of CMV infection in transplant patients

Unlabeled Use CMV retinitis: May be given in combination with foscarnet in patients who relapse after monotherapy with either drug

Mechanism of Action/Effect Ganciclovir is phosphorylated to a substrate which competitively inhibits the binding of deoxyguanosine triphosphate to DNA polymerase resulting in inhibition of viral DNA synthesis.

Contraindications Hypersensitivity to ganciclovir, acyclovir, or any component of the formulation

Warnings/Precautions Hazardous agent - use appropriate precautions for handling and disposal (NIOSH, 2012). **[U.S. Boxed Warning]: Granulocytopenia (neutropenia), anemia, and thrombocytopenia may occur.** Dosage adjustment or interruption of ganciclovir therapy may be necessary in patients with neutropenia and/or thrombocytopenia and patients with impaired renal function. **[U.S. Boxed Warning]: Animal studies have demonstrated carcinogenic and teratogenic effects, and inhibition of spermatogenesis;** contraceptive precautions for female and male patients need to be followed during and for at least 90 days after therapy with the drug; take care to administer only into veins with good blood flow. **[U.S. Boxed Warning]: Indicated only for treatment of CMV retinitis in the immunocompromised patient and CMV prevention in transplant patients at risk.**

Drug Interactions

Avoid Concomitant Use

Avoid concomitant use of Ganciclovir (Systemic) with any of the following: Imipenem

Decreased Effect There are no known significant interactions involving a decrease in effect.

Increased Effect/Toxicity

Ganciclovir (Systemic) may increase the levels/ effects of: Imipenem; Mycophenolate; Reverse Transcriptase Inhibitors (Nucleoside); Tenofovir

The levels/effects of Ganciclovir (Systemic) may be increased by: Mycophenolate; Probenecid; Tenofovir

Adverse Reactions

>10%:

Central nervous system: Fever (48%)

Gastrointestinal: Diarrhea (44%), anorexia (14%), vomiting (13%)

Hematologic: Thrombocytopenia (57%), leukopenia (41%), anemia (16% to 26%), neutropenia with ANC <500/mm^3 (12% to 14%)

Ocular: Retinal detachment (11%; relationship to ganciclovir not established)

Renal: Serum creatinine increased (2% to 14%)

Miscellaneous: Sepsis (15%), diaphoresis (12%)

1% to 10%:

Central nervous system: Chills (10%), neuropathy (9%)

Dermatologic: Pruritus (5%)

<1%, postmarketing, and/or case reports (limited to important or life-threatening): Allergic reaction (including anaphylaxis), alopecia, arrhythmia, bronchospasm, cardiac arrest, cataracts, cholestasis, coma, dyspnea, edema, encephalopathy, exfoliative dermatitis, extrapyramidal symptoms, hepatitis, hepatic failure, pancreatitis, pancytopenia, pulmonary fibrosis, psychosis, rhabdomyolysis, seizure, alopecia, urticaria, eosinophilia, hemorrhage, Stevens-Johnson syndrome, torsade de pointes, renal failure, SIADH, visual loss

Available Dosage Forms

Solution Reconstituted, Intravenous:

Cytovene: 500 mg (1 ea)

Generic: 500 mg (1 ea)

General Dosage Range Dosage adjustment recommended in patients with renal impairment

I.V.: *Children and Adults:* Induction: 30-35 mg/kg/ week, given as once-daily dose for 5-7 days per week

Administration

I.V. Should not be administered by I.M., SubQ, or rapid IVP. Administer by slow I.V. infusion over at least 1 hour. Too rapid infusion can cause increased toxicity and excessive plasma levels. Flush line well with NS before and after administration.

Hazardous agent; use appropriate precautions for handling and disposal (NIOSH, 2012).

Injectable Detail pH: 11

Preparation for Administration Hazardous agent; use appropriate precautions for handling and disposal (NIOSH, 2012). Reconstitute 500 mg vial with 10 mL unpreserved sterile water **not** bacteriostatic water because parabens may cause precipitation. Typically, dilute in 100 mL D$_5$W or NS to a concentration ≤10 mg/mL for infusion.

Storage/Stability Store intact vials at temperatures below 40°C (104°F). Reconstituted solution is stable for 12 hours at room temperature, however, conflicting data indicates that reconstituted solution is stable for 60 days under refrigeration (4°C). Stability of parenteral admixture at room temperature (25°C) and at refrigeration temperature (4°C) for 35 days has been reported. However, the manufacturer recommends use within 24 hours of preparation.

Nursing Actions

Physical Assessment I.V.: Monitor for paresthesia, neutropenia, anemia, and nephrotoxicity throughout therapy. Teach patient importance of contraceptive precautions during and for 90 days following therapy.

Patient Education

• Discuss specific use of drug and side effects with patient as it relates to treatment. (HCAHPS: During this hospital stay, were you given any medicine that you had not taken before? Before giving you any new medicine, how often did hospital staff tell you what the medicine was for? How often did hospital staff describe possible side effects in a way you could understand?)

• Patient may experience dizziness, fatigue, lack of appetite, nausea, or diarrhea. Have patient report immediately to prescriber signs of infection, ecchymosis, hemorrhaging, severe asthenia, hyperhidrosis, illogical thinking, urinary retention, oliguria, change in balance, hallucinations, depression, melena, paresthesia, considerable dyspepsia, vision changes, hematemesis, or injection site irritation (HCAHPS).

• Educate patient about signs of a significant reaction (eg, wheezing; chest tightness; fever; itching; bad cough; blue skin color; seizures; or swelling of face, lips, tongue, or throat). **Note:** This is not a comprehensive list of all side effects. Patient should consult prescriber for additional questions.

◄ **Intended Use and Disclaimer:** Should not be printed and given to patients. This information is intended to serve as a concise initial reference for healthcare professionals to use when discussing medications with a patient. You must ultimately rely on your own discretion, experience and judgment in diagnosing, treating and advising patients.

Dietary Considerations Some products may contain sodium.

Ganirelix (ga ni REL ix)

Index Terms Antagon; Ganirelix Acetate

Pharmacologic Category Gonadotropin Releasing Hormone Antagonist

Medication Safety Issues

International issues:

Antagon former U.S. brand name for ganirelix, but also the brand name for ranitidine in Brazil

Pregnancy Risk Factor X

Lactation Excretion in breast milk unknown/not recommended

Breast-Feeding Considerations It is not known if ganirelix is excreted in breast milk. Breast-feeding is not recommended by the manufacturer.

Use Inhibits premature luteinizing hormone (LH) surges in women undergoing controlled ovarian hyperstimulation

Mechanism of Action/Effect Suppresses gonadotropin secretion and luteinizing hormone secretion to prevent ovulation until the follicles are of adequate size.

Contraindications Hypersensitivity to ganirelix or any component of the formulation; hypersensitivity to gonadotropin-releasing hormone (GnRH) or any other GnRH analog; known or suspected pregnancy

Warnings/Precautions Hazardous agent - use appropriate precautions for handling and disposal (NIOSH, 2012). Should only be prescribed by fertility specialists. Hypersensitivity reactions, including anaphylactoid reactions, have been reported; may occur with the first dose; risk may be increased in patients with other allergic conditions; use with caution. The packaging contains natural rubber latex (may cause allergic reactions). Pregnancy must be excluded before starting medication.

Drug Interactions

Avoid Concomitant Use

Avoid concomitant use of Ganirelix with any of the following: Indium 111 Capromab Pendetide

Decreased Effect

Ganirelix may decrease the levels/effects of: Indium 111 Capromab Pendetide

Increased Effect/Toxicity There are no known significant interactions involving an increase in effect.

Adverse Reactions 1% to 10%:

Central nervous system: Headache (3%)

Endocrine & metabolic: Ovarian hyperstimulation syndrome (2%)

Gastrointestinal: Abdominal pain (1%), nausea (1%)

Genitourinary: Pelvic pain (5%), vaginal bleeding (2%)

Local: Injection site reaction (1%)

Pharmacodynamics/Kinetics

Duration of Action <48 hours

Available Dosage Forms

Solution, Subcutaneous:

Generic: 250 mcg/0.5 mL (0.5 mL)

General Dosage Range SubQ: *Adults:* 250 mcg/day

Administration

Other Administer SubQ in abdomen (around upper navel) or upper thigh; rotate injection site.

Hazardous agent; use appropriate precautions for handling and disposal (NIOSH, 2012).

Storage/Stability Store at controlled room temperature of 25°C (77°F); excursions permitted to 15°C to 30°C (59°F to 86°F). Protect from light.

Nursing Actions

Physical Assessment This medication should only be prescribed by a fertility specialist. Teach patient proper injection procedures and syringe disposal.

Patient Education

• Discuss specific use of drug and side effects with patient as it relates to treatment. (HCAHPS: During this hospital stay, were you given any medicine that you had not taken before? Before giving you any new medicine, how often did hospital staff tell you what the medicine was for? How often did hospital staff describe possible side effects in a way you could understand?)

• Patient may experience injection site irritation. Have patient report immediately to prescriber severe vaginal hemorrhaging or signs of ovarian hyperstimulation syndrome (OHSS) (HCAHPS).

• Educate patient about signs of a significant reaction (eg, wheezing; chest tightness; fever; itching; bad cough; blue skin color; seizures; or swelling of face, lips, tongue, or throat). **Note:** This is not a comprehensive list of all side effects. Patient should consult prescriber for additional questions.

Intended Use and Disclaimer: Should not be printed and given to patients. This information is intended to serve as a concise initial reference for healthcare professionals to use when discussing medications with a patient. You must ultimately rely on your own discretion, experience and judgment in diagnosing, treating and advising patients.

Gatifloxacin (gat i FLOKS a sin)

Brand Names: U.S. Zymaxid
Pharmacologic Category Antibiotic, Fluoroquinolone; Antibiotic, Ophthalmic
Pregnancy Risk Factor C
Lactation Excretion in breast milk unknown/use caution
Breast-Feeding Considerations Other quinolones are known to be excreted in breast milk. The manufacturer recommends using caution if gatifloxacin is administered while nursing.
Use Treatment of bacterial conjunctivitis
Mechanism of Action/Effect Inhibits bacterial DNA
Contraindications
Zymaxid: There are no contraindications listed in the manufacturer's labeling.
Zymar: Hypersensitivity to gatifloxacin, other quinolones, or any component of the formulation
Warnings/Precautions Severe hypersensitivity reactions, including anaphylaxis, have occurred with systemic quinolone therapy. Reactions may present as typical allergic symptoms after a single dose, or may manifest as severe idiosyncratic dermatologic, vascular, pulmonary, renal, hepatic, and/or hematologic events, usually after multiple doses. Prompt discontinuation of drug should occur if skin rash or other symptoms arise. Prolonged use may result in fungal or bacterial superinfection. For topical ophthalmic use only. Do not inject ophthalmic solution subconjunctivally or introduce directly into the anterior chamber of the eye. Contact lenses should not be worn during treatment of ophthalmic infections.
Drug Interactions
Avoid Concomitant Use There are no known interactions where it is recommended to avoid concomitant use.
Decreased Effect There are no known significant interactions involving a decrease in effect.
Increased Effect/Toxicity There are no known significant interactions involving an increase in effect.
Adverse Reactions 1% to 10%:
Cardiovascular: Edema
Dermatologic: Contact dermatitis, erythema
Gastrointestinal: Taste disturbance
Ocular: Conjunctival irritation, discharge, dry eye, edema, irritation, keratitis, lacrimation increased, pain, papillary conjunctivitis, visual acuity decreased
Respiratory: Rhinorrhea
Available Dosage Forms
Solution, Ophthalmic:
Zymaxid: 0.5% (2.5 mL)
Generic: 0.5% (2.5 mL)
General Dosage Range Ophthalmic: *Children ≥1 year and Adults:* 1 drop into affected eye(s) every 2 hours while awake (maximum: 8 times/day) for 1 day; followed by 1 drop into affected eye(s) 2-4 times/day for 6 days
Administration
Other For topical ophthalmic use only; avoid touching tip of applicator to eye, fingers, or other surfaces.
Storage/Stability Store between 15°C to 25°C (59°F to 77°F); do not freeze.
Nursing Actions
Patient Education
• Discuss specific use of drug and side effects with patient as it relates to treatment. (HCAHPS: During this hospital stay, were you given any medicine that you had not taken before? Before giving you any new medicine, how often did hospital staff tell you what the medicine was for? How often did hospital staff describe possible side effects in a way you could understand?)
• Patient may experience parageusia, headache, or short-term change in vision. Have patient report immediately to prescriber sudden vision changes, ophthalmalgia, eye irritation, or eye or eyelid edema (HCAHPS).
• Educate patient about signs of a significant reaction (eg, wheezing; chest tightness; fever; itching; bad cough; blue skin color; seizures; or swelling of face, lips, tongue, or throat). **Note:** This is not a comprehensive list of all side effects. Patient should consult prescriber for additional questions.

Intended Use and Disclaimer: Should not be printed and given to patients. This information is intended to serve as a concise initial reference for healthcare professionals to use when discussing medications with a patient. You must ultimately rely on your own discretion, experience and judgment in diagnosing, treating and advising patients.

Gefitinib (ge FI tye nib)

Brand Names: U.S. Iressa®
Index Terms ZD1839
Pharmacologic Category Antineoplastic Agent, Epidermal Growth Factor Receptor (EGFR) Inhibitor; Antineoplastic Agent, Tyrosine Kinase Inhibitor
Medication Safety Issues
Sound-alike/look-alike issues:
Gefitinib may be confused with afatinib, axitinib, crizotinib, erlotinib, imatinib, SORAfenib, SUNItinib, vandetanib
High alert medication:
This medication is in a class the Institute for Safe Medication Practices (ISMP) includes among its list of drug classes which have a heightened risk of causing significant patient harm when used in error.
Pregnancy Risk Factor D
Lactation Excretion in breast milk unknown/not recommended

Use Treatment of locally advanced or metastatic nonsmall cell lung cancer (NSCLC) after failure of platinum-based and docetaxel therapies. Treatment is limited to patients who are benefiting or have benefited from treatment with gefitinib.

Note: Due to the lack of improved survival data from clinical trials of gefitinib, and in response to positive survival data with another EGFR inhibitor, according to the U.S. labeling, physicians are advised to use treatment options other than gefitinib in patients with advanced nonsmall cell lung cancer following one or two prior chemotherapy regimens when they are refractory/intolerant to their most recent regimen.

Canada labeling: First-line treatment of locally advanced or metastatic NSCLC with activating mutations of EGFR-TK

Unlabeled Use First-line treatment of NSCLC with known EGFR mutation

Available Dosage Forms

Tablet, oral:

Iressa®: 250 mg

General Dosage Range Dosage adjustment recommended in patients on concomitant therapy or who develop toxicities.

Oral: *Adults:* 250 mg once daily

Administration

Oral May administer with or without food.

For patients unable to swallow tablets or for administration via NG tube: Tablets may be dispersed in noncarbonated drinking water. Drop whole tablet (do not crush) into 1/2 glass of water; stir until tablet is dispersed (~10 minutes). Drink immediately. Rinse glass with 1/2 glass of water and drink.

Hazardous agent; use appropriate precautions for handling and disposal (meets NIOSH, 2012 criteria).

Nursing Actions

Physical Assessment Assess results of liver function tests on a regular basis.

Patient Education

• Discuss specific use of drug and side effects with patient as it relates to treatment. (HCAHPS: During this hospital stay, were you given any medicine that you had not taken before? Before giving you any new medicine, how often did hospital staff tell you what the medicine was for? How often did hospital staff describe possible side effects in a way you could understand?)

• Patient may experience acne vulgaris, xeroderma, or lung injury (rare). Have patient report immediately to prescriber dyspnea, severe nausea, considerable diarrhea, excessive weight loss, ecchymosis, hemorrhaging, urine discoloration, jaundice, intolerable asthenia, sudden vision changes, ophthalmalgia, considerable eye irritation, or significant edema (HCAHPS).

• Educate patient about signs of a significant reaction (eg, wheezing; chest tightness; fever; itching; bad cough; blue skin color; seizures; or swelling of face, lips, tongue, or throat). **Note:** This is not a comprehensive list of all side effects. Patient should consult prescriber for additional questions.

Intended Use and Disclaimer: Should not be printed and given to patients. This information is intended to serve as a concise initial reference for healthcare professionals to use when discussing medications with a patient. You must ultimately rely on your own discretion, experience and judgment in diagnosing, treating and advising patients.

Gemcitabine (jem SITE a been)

Brand Names: U.S. Gemzar

Index Terms dFdC; dFdCyd; Difluorodeoxycytidine Hydrochlorothiazide; Gemcitabine Hydrochloride; LY-188011

Pharmacologic Category Antineoplastic Agent, Antimetabolite; Antineoplastic Agent, Antimetabolite (Pyrimidine Analog)

Medication Safety Issues

Sound-alike/look-alike issues:

Gemcitabine may be confused with gemtuzumab

Gemzar may be confused with Zinecard

High alert medication:

This medication is in a class the Institute for Safe Medication Practices (ISMP) includes among its list of drug classes which have a heightened risk of causing significant patient harm when used in error.

International issues:

In Canada, gemcitabine is available as a concentrated solution for injection in different strengths (38 mg/mL and 40 mg/mL), and a powder for reconstitution (final concentration of 38 mg/mL after reconstitution). Verify product concentration prior to preparation for administration.

Pregnancy Risk Factor D

Lactation Excretion in breast milk unknown/not recommended

Breast-Feeding Considerations It is not known if gemcitabine is excreted in breast milk. Due to the potential for serious adverse reactions in the nursing infant, the decision to discontinue gemcitabine or to discontinue breast-feeding should take into account the benefits of treatment to the mother.

Use

Breast cancer: First-line treatment of metastatic breast cancer (in combination with paclitaxel) after failure of adjuvant chemotherapy which contained an anthracycline (unless contraindicated)

Nonsmall cell lung cancer (NSCLC): First-line treatment of inoperable, locally-advanced (stage IIIA or IIIB) or metastatic (stage IV) NSCLC (in combination with cisplatin)

Ovarian cancer: Treatment of advanced ovarian cancer (in combination with carboplatin) that has relapsed at least 6 months following completion of platinum-based chemotherapy

Pancreatic cancer: First-line treatment of locally-advanced (nonresectable stage II or III) or metastatic (stage IV) pancreatic adenocarcinoma

Unlabeled Use Treatment of bladder cancer, cervical cancer (recurrent or persistent), Ewing's sarcoma (refractory), head and neck cancer (nasopharyngeal), hepatobiliary cancers (advanced), Hodgkin lymphoma (relapsed), non-Hodgkin lymphomas (refractory), malignant pleural mesothelioma, osteosarcoma (refractory), renal cell cancer (metastatic), small cell lung cancer (refractory or relapsed), soft tissue sarcoma (advanced), testicular cancer (refractory germ cell tumors), thymic malignancies, uterine sarcoma, and unknown-primary adenocarcinoma

Mechanism of Action/Effect A pyrimidine antimetabolite that inhibits DNA synthesis by inhibition of DNA polymerase and ribonucleotide reductase, cell cycle-specific for the S-phase of the cycle (also blocks cellular progression at G1/S-phase).

Contraindications Hypersensitivity to gemcitabine or any component of the formulation

Warnings/Precautions Hazardous agent - use appropriate precautions for handling and disposal (NIOSH, 2012). Gemcitabine may suppress bone marrow function (neutropenia, thrombocytopenia, and anemia); myelosuppression is usually the dose-limiting toxicity; toxicity is increased when used in combination with other chemotherapy; monitor blood counts; dosage adjustments are frequently required.

Hemolytic uremic syndrome (HUS) has been reported; may lead to renal failure and dialysis (including fatalities); monitor for evidence of anemia with microangiopathic hemolysis (elevation of bilirubin or LDH, reticulocytosis, severe thrombocytopenia, and/or renal failure) and monitor renal function at baseline and periodically during treatment. Permanently discontinue if HUS or severe renal impairment occurs; renal failure may not be reversible despite discontinuation. Serious hepatotoxicity (including liver failure and death) has been reported (when used alone or in combination with other hepatotoxic medications); use in patients with hepatic impairment (history of cirrhosis, hepatitis, or alcoholism) or in patients with hepatic metastases may lead to exacerbation of hepatic impairment. Monitor hepatic function at baseline and periodically during treatment; consider dose adjustments with elevated bilirubin; discontinue if severe liver injury develops. Capillary leak syndrome (CLS) with serious consequences has been reported, both with single-agent gemcitabine and with combination chemotherapy; discontinue if CLS develops.

Pulmonary toxicity, including adult respiratory distress syndrome, interstitial pneumonitis, pulmonary edema, and pulmonary fibrosis, has been observed; may lead to respiratory failure (some fatal) despite discontinuation. Onset for symptoms of pulmonary toxicity may be delayed up to 2 weeks beyond the last dose. Discontinue for unexplained dyspnea (with or without bronchospasm) or other evidence of pulmonary toxicity. Not indicated for use with concurrent radiation therapy; radiation toxicity, including tissue injury, severe mucositis, esophagitis, or pneumonitis, has been reported with concurrent and nonconcurrent administration; may have radiosensitizing activity when gemcitabine and radiation therapy are given ≤7 days apart; radiation recall may occur when gemcitabine and radiation therapy are given >7 days apart. Potentially significant drug-drug interactions may exist, requiring dose or frequency adjustment, additional monitoring, and/or selection of alternative therapy.

Prolongation of the infusion duration >60 minutes or more frequent than weekly dosing have been shown to alter the half-life and increase toxicity (hypotension, flu-like symptoms, myelosuppression, weakness); a fixed-dose rate (FDR) infusion rate of 10 mg/m²/minute has been studied in order to optimize the pharmacokinetics (unlabeled); prolonged infusion times increase the intracellular accumulation of the active metabolite, gemcitabine triphosphate (Ko, 2006; Tempero, 2003); patients who receive gemcitabine FDR experience more grade 3/4 hematologic toxicity (Ko, 2006; Poplin, 2009).

Drug Interactions

Avoid Concomitant Use

Avoid concomitant use of Gemcitabine with any of the following: BCG; CloZAPine; Natalizumab; Pimecrolimus; Tacrolimus (Topical); Tofacitinib; Vaccines (Live)

Decreased Effect

Gemcitabine may decrease the levels/effects of: BCG; Coccidioidin Skin Test; Sipuleucel-T; Vaccines (Inactivated); Vaccines (Live); Vitamin K Antagonists

The levels/effects of Gemcitabine may be decreased by: Echinacea

Increased Effect/Toxicity

Gemcitabine may increase the levels/effects of: Bleomycin; CloZAPine; Fluorouracil (Systemic); Fluorouracil (Topical); Leflunomide; Natalizumab; Tofacitinib; Vaccines (Live); Vitamin K Antagonists

The levels/effects of Gemcitabine may be increased by: Denosumab; Pimecrolimus; Roflumilast; Tacrolimus (Topical); Trastuzumab

Adverse Reactions Frequency of adverse reactions reported for single-agent use of gemcitabine only.

>10%:
Cardiovascular: Peripheral edema (20%), edema (13%)
Central nervous system: Drowsiness (11%)

Dermatologic: Skin rash (28% to 30%), alopecia (15% to 16%), pruritus (13%)

Gastrointestinal: Nausea/vomiting (69% to 71%), diarrhea (19% to 30%), stomatitis (10% to 11%)

Genitourinary: Proteinuria (32% to 45%), hematuria (23% to 35%), increased blood urea nitrogen (15% to 16%)

Hematologic & oncologic: Anemia (68% to 73%; grade 4: 1% to 3%), leukopenia (62% to 64%; grade 4: ≤1%), neutropenia (61% to 63%; grade 4: 6% to 7%), thrombocytopenia (24% to 36%; grade 4: 1%), hemorrhage (4% to 17%; grade 3: <1%; grade 4: <1%); bone marrow depression is the dose-limiting toxicity

Hepatic: Increased serum AST (67%; grade 3: 6%; grade 4: 2%), increased serum alkaline phosphatase (55%; grade 3: 7%; grade 4: 2%), increased serum ALT (68%; grade 3: 8%, grade 4: 2%), increased serum bilirubin (13%; grade 3: 2%, grade 4: <1%)

Infection: Localized infection (10% to 16%)

Respiratory: Dyspnea (10% to 23%; grade 3: 3%; grade 4: <1%)

Miscellaneous: Fever (16% to 41%), flu-like symptoms (19%)

1% to 10%:

Central nervous system: Paresthesia (10%; grade 3: <1%)

Local: Injection site reaction (4%)

Renal: Increased serum creatinine (6% to 8%)

Respiratory: Bronchospasm (<2%)

Available Dosage Forms

Solution, Intravenous:

Generic: 200 mg/5.26 mL (5.26 mL); 1 g/26.3 mL (26.3 mL); 2 g/52.6 mL (52.6 mL)

Solution Reconstituted, Intravenous:

Gemzar: 200 mg (1 ea); 1 g (1 ea)

Generic: 200 mg (1 ea); 1 g (1 ea); 2 g (1 ea)

Solution Reconstituted, Intravenous [preservative free]:

Generic: 200 mg (1 ea); 1 g (1 ea)

General Dosage Range Dosage adjustment recommended in patients with hepatic impairment or who develop toxicities

I.V.: *Adults:* Dosage varies greatly depending on indication

Administration

I.V. Infuse over 30 minutes; for unlabeled uses, infusion times may vary (refer to specific references). **Note:** Prolongation of the infusion time >60 minutes has been shown to increase toxicity. Gemcitabine has been administered at a fixed-dose rate (FDR) infusion rate of 10 mg/m²/minute to optimize the pharmacokinetics (unlabeled); prolonged infusion times increase the intracellular accumulation of the active metabolite, gemcitabine triphosphate (Ko, 2006; Tempero, 2003). Patients who receive gemcitabine FDR experience more grade 3/4 hematologic toxicity (Ko, 2006; Poplin, 2009).

Hazardous agent; use appropriate precautions for handling and disposal (NIOSH, 2012).

Other For intravesicular (bladder) instillation (unlabeled route), gemcitabine was diluted in 50-100 mL normal saline; patients were instructed to retain in the bladder for 1 hour (Addeo, 2010; Dalbaghi, 2006)

Hazardous agent; use appropriate precautions for handling and disposal (NIOSH, 2012).

Preparation for Administration

Hazardous agent; use appropriate precautions for handling and disposal (NIOSH, 2012).

Reconstitute lyophilized powder with preservative free NS; add 5 mL to the 200 mg vial, add 25 mL to the 1000 mg vial, or add 50 mL to the 2000 mg vial, resulting in a reconstituted concentration of 38 mg/mL (solutions must be reconstituted to ≤40 mg/mL to completely dissolve). **Note:** In Canada, gemcitabine is also supplied as a concentrated solution for injection in different concentrations (38 mg/mL and 40 mg/mL); verify product concentration prior to preparation for administration.

Further dilute for infusion in NS 50-500 mL injection; to concentrations as low as 0.1 mg/mL.

Storage/Stability

Lyophilized powder: Store intact vials at room temperature of 20°C to 25°C (68°F to 77°F); excursions permitted to 15°C to 30°C (59°F to 86°F). Reconstituted vials are stable for 24 hours at room temperature. Do not refrigerate (may form crystals).

Solution for injection: Store intact vials refrigerated at 2°C to 8°C (36°F to 46°F); do not freeze.

Solutions diluted for infusion in NS are stable for 24 hours at room temperature. Do not refrigerate.

Nursing Actions

Physical Assessment Monitor hepatic and renal function. Monitor for fever, CNS changes, rash, gastrointestinal upset, myelosuppression, anemia, dyspnea, and infection prior to each treatment and on a regular basis.

Patient Education

- Discuss specific use of drug and side effects with patient as it relates to treatment. (HCAHPS: During this hospital stay, were you given any medicine that you had not taken before? Before giving you any new medicine, how often did hospital staff tell you what the medicine was for? How often did hospital staff describe possible side effects in a way you could understand?)

- Patient may experience flu-like syndrome, stomatitis, alopecia, or fatigue. Have patient report immediately to prescriber signs of infection, signs of hemorrhaging, severe dizziness, syncope, arrhythmia, dyspnea, angina, considerable nausea, significant asthenia, illogical thinking, paresthesia, edema, intolerable diarrhea, signs of hemolytic uremic syndrome

(HUS), signs of hepatic impairment, or injection site irritation (HCAHPS).

• Educate patient about signs of a significant reaction (eg, wheezing; chest tightness; fever; itching; bad cough; blue skin color; seizures; or swelling of face, lips, tongue, or throat). **Note:** This is not a comprehensive list of all side effects. Patient should consult prescriber for additional questions.

Intended Use and Disclaimer: Should not be printed and given to patients. This information is intended to serve as a concise initial reference for healthcare professionals to use when discussing medications with a patient. You must ultimately rely on your own discretion, experience and judgment in diagnosing, treating and advising patients.

Related Information

Management of Drug Extravasations *on page 1700*

Gemfibrozil (jem FI broe zil)

Brand Names: U.S. Lopid
Index Terms Cl-719
Pharmacologic Category Antilipemic Agent, Fibric Acid
Medication Safety Issues
Sound-alike/look-alike issues:
Lopid may be confused with Levbid, Lipitor, Lodine

Pregnancy Risk Factor C
Lactation Excretion in breast milk unknown/not recommended
Breast-Feeding Considerations It is not known if gemfibrozil is excreted in breast milk. Due to the potential for serious adverse reactions in the nursing infant, a decision should be made whether to discontinue nursing or to discontinue the drug, taking into account the importance of treatment to the mother. The Canadian product labeling specifically contraindicates use during breast-feeding.
Use Treatment of hypertriglyceridemia in Fredrickson types IV and V hyperlipidemia for patients who are at greater risk for pancreatitis and who have not responded to dietary intervention; to reduce the risk of CHD development in Fredrickson type IIb patients without a history or symptoms of existing CHD who have not responded to dietary and other interventions (including pharmacologic treatment) and who have decreased HDL, increased LDL, and increased triglycerides
Mechanism of Action/Effect Inhibits lipolysis and decreases subsequent hepatic fatty acid uptake and hepatic secretion of VLDL; decreases serum levels of VLDL and increases HDL levels
Contraindications Hypersensitivity to gemfibrozil or any component of the formulation; hepatic or severe renal dysfunction; primary biliary cirrhosis;

pre-existing gallbladder disease; concurrent use with repaglinide
Warnings/Precautions Secondary causes of hyperlipidemia should be ruled out prior to therapy. Possible increased risk of malignancy and cholelithiasis. Anemia, leukopenia, thrombocytopenia, and bone marrow hypoplasia have rarely been reported. Periodic monitoring recommended during the first year of therapy. Elevations in serum transaminases can be seen. Discontinue if lipid response not seen. Be careful in patient selection; this is not a first- or second-line choice. Other agents may be more suitable. Has been associated with rare myositis or rhabdomyolysis; patients should be monitored closely. Patients should be instructed to report unexplained muscle pain, tenderness, weakness, or brown urine. Potentially significant drug-drug interactions may exist, requiring dose or frequency adjustment, additional monitoring, and/or selection of alternative therapy. Use with caution in patients with mild-to-moderate renal impairment; contraindicated in patients with severe renal impairment. Renal function deterioration has been seen when used in patients with a serum creatinine >2 mg/dL.
Drug Interactions
Avoid Concomitant Use
Avoid concomitant use of Gemfibrozil with any of the following: AtorvaSTATin; Bexarotene (Systemic); Enzalutamide; Fluvastatin; Lovastatin; Pirfenidone; Pitavastatin; Pravastatin; Repaglinide; Rosuvastatin; Simvastatin
Decreased Effect
Gemfibrozil may decrease the levels/effects of: Chenodiol; Clopidogrel; CycloSPORINE (Systemic); Imatinib; Ursodiol

The levels/effects of Gemfibrozil may be decreased by: Bile Acid Sequestrants
Increased Effect/Toxicity
Gemfibrozil may increase the levels/effects of: Agomelatine; Antidiabetic Agents (Thiazolidinedione); AtorvaSTATin; Bexarotene (Systemic); Bosentan; Carvedilol; Citalopram; Colchicine; CYP1A2 Substrates; CYP2C19 Substrates; CYP2C8 Substrates; CYP2C9 Substrates; Diclofenac (Systemic); Enzalutamide; Ezetimibe; Fluvastatin; Lacosamide; Lovastatin; Ospemifene; Pirfenidone; Pitavastatin; Pravastatin; Repaglinide; Rosuvastatin; Simvastatin; Sulfonylureas; Treprostinil; Vitamin K Antagonists

The levels/effects of Gemfibrozil may be increased by: CycloSPORINE (Systemic); Raltegravir
Nutritional/Ethanol Interactions
Ethanol: Avoid ethanol to decrease triglycerides.
Food: When given after meals, the AUC of gemfibrozil is decreased.

◀ **Adverse Reactions**
>10%: Gastrointestinal: Dyspepsia (20%)
1% to 10%:
Cardiovascular: Atrial fibrillation (1%)
Central nervous system: Fatigue (4%), vertigo (2%)
Dermatologic: Eczema (2%), rash (2%)
Gastrointestinal: Abdominal pain (10%), nausea/vomiting (3%)

Reports where causal relationship has not been established: Alopecia, anaphylaxis, cataracts, colitis, confusion, decreased fertility (male), drug-induced lupus-like syndrome, extrasystoles, hepatoma, intracranial hemorrhage, pancreatitis, peripheral vascular disease, photosensitivity, positive ANA, renal dysfunction, retinal edema, seizure, syncope, thrombocytopenia, vasculitis, weight loss

Pharmacodynamics/Kinetics
Onset of Action May require several days
Available Dosage Forms
Tablet, Oral:
Lopid: 600 mg
Generic: 600 mg
General Dosage Range Oral: *Adults:* 600 mg twice daily
Administration
Oral Administer 30 minutes prior to breakfast and dinner.
Storage/Stability Store at controlled room temperature of 20°C to 25°C (68°F to 77°F). Protect from light and moisture.
Nursing Actions
Physical Assessment Assess serum cholesterol and LFTs. Monitor for signs of myopathy (muscular pain, weakness, fatigue). If myopathy is suspected or diagnosed, discontinue therapy. If inadequate response to therapy in 3 months, discontinue. Caution when on concomitant anticoagulants. Monitor PT/INR closely.

Patient Education
• Discuss specific use of drug and side effects with patient as it relates to treatment. (HCAHPS: During this hospital stay, were you given any medicine that you had not taken before? Before giving you any new medicine, how often did hospital staff tell you what the medicine was for? How often did hospital staff describe possible side effects in a way you could understand?)
• Patient may experience pyrosis. Have patient report immediately to prescriber severe dyspepsia, considerable nausea, significant diarrhea, myalgia, arthralgia, urine discoloration, jaundice, paresthesia, blurred vision, intolerable headache, arrhythmia, depression, sexual dysfunction, chills, pharyngitis, dysuria, hematuria, polyuria, ecchymosis, hemorrhaging, severe asthenia, significant dizziness, or syncope (HCAHPS).

• Educate patient about signs of a significant reaction (eg, wheezing; chest tightness; fever; itching; bad cough; blue skin color; seizures; or swelling of face, lips, tongue, or throat). **Note:** This is not a comprehensive list of all side effects. Patient should consult prescriber for additional questions.

Intended Use and Disclaimer: Should not be printed and given to patients. This information is intended to serve as a concise initial reference for healthcare professionals to use when discussing medications with a patient. You must ultimately rely on your own discretion, experience and judgment in diagnosing, treating and advising patients.

Dietary Considerations Before initiation of therapy, patients should be placed on a standard cholesterol-lowering diet for 3-6 months and the diet should be continued during drug therapy. Should be taken 30 minutes prior to breakfast and dinner

Gemifloxacin (je mi FLOKS a sin)

Brand Names: U.S. Factive
Index Terms DW286; Gemifloxacin Mesylate; LA 20304a; SB-265805
Pharmacologic Category Antibiotic, Fluoroquinolone; Antibiotic, Respiratory Fluoroquinolone
Medication Guide Available Yes
Pregnancy Risk Factor C
Lactation Excretion in breast milk unknown/not recommended
Breast-Feeding Considerations It is not known if gemifloxacin is excreted in breast milk. Breast-feeding is not recommended by the manufacturer. Nondose-related effects could include modification of bowel flora.
Use Treatment of acute exacerbation of chronic bronchitis; treatment of community-acquired pneumonia (CAP), including pneumonia caused by multidrug-resistant strains of *S. pneumoniae* (MDRSP)
Unlabeled Use Acute sinusitis
Mechanism of Action/Effect Gemifloxacin is a DNA gyrase inhibitor and also inhibits topoisomerase IV. These enzymes are required for DNA replication and transcription, DNA repair, recombination, and transposition; quinolones are bactericidal
Contraindications Hypersensitivity to gemifloxacin, other fluoroquinolones, or any component of the formulation
Warnings/Precautions [U.S. Boxed Warning]: There have been reports of tendon inflammation and/or rupture with quinolone antibiotics; risk may be increased with concurrent corticosteroids, organ transplant recipients, and in patients >60 years of age. Rupture of the Achilles tendon sometimes requiring surgical repair has

been reported most frequently; but other tendon sites (eg, rotator cuff, biceps) have also been reported. Strenuous physical activity, rheumatoid arthritis, and renal impairment may be an independent risk factor for tendonitis. Discontinue at first sign of tendon inflammation or pain. May occur even after discontinuation of therapy. Use with caution in patients with rheumatoid arthritis; may increase risk of tendon rupture. Fluoroquinolones may prolong QT_c interval; avoid use of gemifloxacin in patients with a history of QT_c prolongation, uncorrected hypokalemia, hypomagnesemia, or concurrent administration of other medications known to prolong the QT interval (including Class Ia and Class III antiarrhythmics, cisapride, erythromycin, antipsychotics, and tricyclic antidepressants). Use with caution in patients with significant bradycardia or acute myocardial ischemia. CNS effects may occur (tremor, restlessness, confusion, and very rarely hallucinations, increased intracranial pressure [including pseudotumor cerebri] or seizures). Use with caution in patients with known or suspected CNS disorder. Potential for seizures, although very rare, may be increased with concomitant NSAID therapy. Use with caution in individuals at risk of seizures. Use caution in renal dysfunction; dosage adjustment required for CrCl ≤40 mL/minute.

Fluoroquinolones have been associated with the development of serious, and sometimes fatal, hypoglycemia, most often in elderly diabetics, but also in patients without diabetes. This occurred most frequently with gatifloxacin (no longer available systemically) but may occur at a lower frequency with other quinolones.

Severe hypersensitivity reactions, including anaphylaxis, have occurred with quinolone therapy. Reactions may present as typical allergic symptoms after a single dose, or may manifest as severe idiosyncratic dermatologic, vascular, pulmonary, renal, hepatic, and/or hematologic events, usually after multiple doses. May cause maculopapular rash, usually 8-10 days after treatment initiation; risk factors may include age <40 years, female gender (including postmenopausal women on HRT), and treatment duration >7 days. Prompt discontinuation of drug should occur if skin rash or other symptoms arise. **[U.S. Boxed Warning]: Quinolones may exacerbate myasthenia gravis; avoid use (rare, potentially life-threatening weakness of respiratory muscles may occur).** Avoid excessive sunlight and take precautions to limit exposure (eg, loose fitting clothing, sunscreen); may cause moderate-to-severe phototoxicity reactions. Discontinue use if photosensitivity occurs. Prolonged use may result in fungal or bacterial superinfection, including *C. difficile*-associated diarrhea (CDAD) and pseudomembranous colitis; CDAD has been observed >2 months post-antibiotic treatment. Peripheral neuropathy has

been reported (rare); may occur soon after initiation of therapy and may be irreversible; discontinue if symptoms of sensory or sensorimotor neuropathy occur. Hemolytic reactions may (rarely) occur with quinolone use in patients with latent or actual G6PD deficiency.

Drug Interactions
Avoid Concomitant Use
Avoid concomitant use of Gemifloxacin with any of the following: BCG; Highest Risk QTc-Prolonging Agents; Ivabradine; Mifepristone; Strontium Ranelate

Decreased Effect
Gemifloxacin may decrease the levels/effects of: BCG; Didanosine; Mycophenolate; Sodium Picosulfate; Sulfonylureas; Typhoid Vaccine

The levels/effects of Gemifloxacin may be decreased by: Antacids; Calcium Salts; Didanosine; Iron Salts; Magnesium Salts; Multivitamins/Minerals (with ADEK, Folate, Iron); Multivitamins/Minerals (with AE, No Iron); Quinapril; Sevelamer; Strontium Ranelate; Sucralfate; Zinc Salts

Increased Effect/Toxicity
Gemifloxacin may increase the levels/effects of: Corticosteroids (Systemic); Highest Risk QTc-Prolonging Agents; Moderate Risk QTc-Prolonging Agents; Porfimer; Sulfonylureas; Varenicline; Vitamin K Antagonists

The levels/effects of Gemifloxacin may be increased by: Insulin; Ivabradine; Mifepristone; Nonsteroidal Anti-Inflammatory Agents; Probenecid; QTc-Prolonging Agents (Indeterminate Risk and Risk Modifying)

Nutritional/Ethanol Interactions Herb/Nutraceutical: Avoid dong quai, St John's wort (may also cause photosensitization).

Adverse Reactions 1% to 10%:
Central nervous system: Headache (4%), dizziness (2%)
Dermatologic: Rash (4%)
Gastrointestinal: Diarrhea (5%), nausea (4%), abdominal pain (2%), vomiting (2%)
Hepatic: Transaminases increased (1% to 4%)

Important adverse effects reported with other agents in this drug class include (not reported for gemifloxacin): Allergic reactions, CNS stimulation, hepatitis, jaundice, peripheral neuropathy, pneumonitis (eosinophilic), seizure; sensorimotor-axonal neuropathy (paresthesia, hypoesthesias, dysesthesias, weakness); severe dermatologic reactions (toxic epidermal necrolysis, Stevens-Johnson syndrome); torsade de pointes, vasculitis

Available Dosage Forms
Tablet, Oral:
Factive: 320 mg
General Dosage Range Dosage adjustment recommended in patients with renal impairment
Oral: *Adults:* 320 mg once daily

◀ **Administration**

Oral May be administered with or without food, milk, or calcium supplements. Gemifloxacin should be taken 3 hours before or 2 hours after supplements (including multivitamins) containing iron, zinc, or magnesium.

Storage/Stability Store at 25°C (77°F). Protect from light.

Nursing Actions

Physical Assessment Allergy history should be ascertained prior to initiating therapy. Monitor for hypersensitivity, opportunistic infection, pseudomembranous colitis, and tendon inflammation. Teach patient proper use (timing of meals, supplements, or other medications).

Patient Education

- Discuss specific use of drug and side effects with patient as it relates to treatment. (HCAHPS: During this hospital stay, were you given any medicine that you had not taken before? Before giving you any new medicine, how often did hospital staff tell you what the medicine was for? How often did hospital staff describe possible side effects in a way you could understand?)
- Patient may experience diarrhea, headache, nausea, or dyspepsia. Have patient report immediately to prescriber signs of depression (ie, suicidal ideation, anxiety, emotional instability, illogical thinking), signs of hyperglycemia, signs of hepatic impairment, angina, tachycardia, arrhythmia, severe dizziness, syncope, chills, nightmares, insomnia, dyspnea, ecchymosis, hemorrhaging, hallucinations, significant asthenia, tremors, abnormal gait, urinary retention, oliguria, vaginitis, vision changes, signs of neuropathy, or signs of pseudomembranous colitis (HCAHPS).
- Educate patient about signs of a significant reaction (eg, wheezing; chest tightness; fever; itching; bad cough; blue skin color; seizures; or swelling of face, lips, tongue, or throat). **Note:** This is not a comprehensive list of all side effects. Patient should consult prescriber for additional questions.

Intended Use and Disclaimer: Should not be printed and given to patients. This information is intended to serve as a concise initial reference for healthcare professionals to use when discussing medications with a patient. You must ultimately rely on your own discretion, experience and judgment in diagnosing, treating and advising patients.

Dietary Considerations May take tablets with or without food, milk, or calcium supplements. Gemifloxacin should be taken 3 hours before or 2 hours after supplements (including multivitamins) containing iron, zinc, or magnesium.

Gentamicin (Systemic) (jen ta MYE sin)

Index Terms Gentamicin Sulfate

Pharmacologic Category Antibiotic, Aminoglycoside

Medication Safety Issues

Sound-alike/look-alike issues:

Gentamicin may be confused with gentian violet, kanamycin, vancomycin

High alert medication:

The Institute for Safe Medication Practices (ISMP) includes this medication (intrathecal administration) among its list of drug classes which have a heightened risk of causing significant patient harm when used in error.

Pregnancy Risk Factor D

Lactation Enters breast milk/use caution

Breast-Feeding Considerations Gentamicin is excreted into breast milk; however, it is not well absorbed when taken orally. This limited oral absorption may minimize exposure to the nursing infant. Nondose-related effects could include modification of bowel flora.

Use Treatment of susceptible bacterial infections, normally gram-negative organisms, including *Pseudomonas*, *Proteus*, *Serratia*, and gram-positive *Staphylococcus*; treatment of bone infections, respiratory tract infections, skin and soft tissue infections, as well as abdominal and urinary tract infections, and septicemia; treatment of infective endocarditis

Unlabeled Use Surgical (preoperative) prophylaxis

Mechanism of Action/Effect Bactericidal; interferes with bacterial protein synthesis resulting in cell death

Contraindications Hypersensitivity to gentamicin or other aminoglycosides

Warnings/Precautions [U.S. Boxed Warning]: Aminoglycosides may cause neurotoxicity and/or nephrotoxicity; usual risk factors include pre-existing renal impairment, concomitant neuro-/nephrotoxic medications, advanced age and dehydration. Ototoxicity may be directly proportional to the amount of drug given and the duration of treatment; tinnitus or vertigo are indications of vestibular injury and impending hearing loss; renal damage is usually reversible. May cause neuromuscular blockade and respiratory paralysis; especially when given soon after anesthesia or muscle relaxants.

Not intended for long-term therapy due to toxic hazards associated with extended administration; use caution in pre-existing renal insufficiency, vestibular or cochlear impairment, myasthenia gravis, hypocalcemia, conditions which depress neuromuscular transmission. Dosage modification required in patients with impaired renal function. Prolonged use may result in fungal or bacterial superinfection, including *C. difficile*-associated diarrhea (CDAD) and pseudomembranous colitis;

CDAD has been observed >2 months postantibiotic treatment.

Drug Interactions

Avoid Concomitant Use

Avoid concomitant use of Gentamicin (Systemic) with any of the following: Agalsidase Alfa; Agalsidase Beta; BCG; Gallium Nitrate

Decreased Effect

Gentamicin (Systemic) may decrease the levels/effects of: Agalsidase Alfa; Agalsidase Beta; BCG; Sodium Picosulfate; Typhoid Vaccine

The levels/effects of Gentamicin (Systemic) may be decreased by: Penicillins

Increased Effect/Toxicity

Gentamicin (Systemic) may increase the levels/effects of: AbobotulinumtoxinA; Bisphosphonate Derivatives; CARBOplatin; Colistimethate; CycloSPORINE (Systemic); Gallium Nitrate; Neuromuscular-Blocking Agents; OnabotulinumtoxinA; RimabotulinumtoxinB; Tenofovir

The levels/effects of Gentamicin (Systemic) may be increased by: Amphotericin B; Capreomycin; Cephalosporins (2nd Generation); Cephalosporins (3rd Generation); Cephalosporins (4th Generation); CISplatin; Loop Diuretics; Nonsteroidal Anti-Inflammatory Agents; Tenofovir; Vancomycin

Adverse Reactions Frequency not defined.

Cardiovascular: Edema, hyper/hypotension

Central nervous system: Ataxia, confusion, depression, dizziness, drowsiness, encephalopathy, fever, headache, lethargy, pseudomotor cerebri, seizures, vertigo

Dermatologic: Alopecia, erythema, itching, purpura, rash, urticaria

Endocrine & metabolic: Hypocalcemia, hypokalemia, hypomagnesemia, hyponatremia

Gastrointestinal: Anorexia, appetite decreased, *C. difficile*-associated diarrhea, enterocolitis, nausea, salivation increased, splenomegaly, stomatitis, vomiting, weight loss

Hematologic: Agranulocytosis, anemia, eosinophilia, granulocytopenia, leukopenia, reticulocytes increased/decreased, thrombocytopenia

Hepatic: Hepatomegaly, LFTs increased

Local: Injection site reactions, pain at injection site, phlebitis/thrombophlebitis

Neuromuscular & skeletal: Arthralgia, gait instability, muscle cramps, muscle twitching, muscle weakness, myasthenia gravis-like syndrome, numbness, paresthesia, peripheral neuropathy, tremor, weakness

Ocular: Visual disturbances

Otic: Hearing impairment, hearing loss (associated with persistently increased serum concentrations; early toxicity usually affects high-pitched sound), tinnitus

Renal: BUN increased, casts (hyaline, granular) in urine, creatinine clearance decreased, distal tubular dysfunction, Fanconi-like syndrome (high dose, prolonged course) (infants and adults), oliguria, renal failure (high trough serum concentrations), polyuria, proteinuria, serum creatinine increased, tubular necrosis, urine specific gravity decreased

Respiratory: Dyspnea, laryngeal edema, pulmonary fibrosis, respiratory depression

Miscellaneous: Allergic reaction, anaphylaxis, anaphylactoid reactions

Available Dosage Forms

Solution, Injection:
Generic: 10 mg/mL (2 mL); 40 mg/mL (2 mL, 20 mL)

Solution, Injection [preservative free]:
Generic: 10 mg/mL (2 mL)

Solution, Intravenous:
Generic: 60 mg (50 mL); 70 mg (50 mL); 80 mg (50 mL, 100 mL); 90 mg (100 mL); 100 mg (50 mL, 100 mL); 120 mg (100 mL); 10 mg/mL (6 mL, 8 mL, 10 mL)

General Dosage Range Dosage adjustment recommended for the I.M. and I.V. routes in patients with renal impairment

I.M., I.V.:
Children <5 years: 2.5 mg/kg/dose every 8 hours
Children ≥5 years: 2-2.5 mg/kg/dose every 8 hours
Adults: 1-2.5 mg/kg/dose every 8-12 hours **or** 4-7 mg/kg once daily

Intrathecal: *Adults:* 4-8 mg/day

Administration

I.M. Administer by deep I.M. route if possible. Slower absorption and lower peak concentrations, probably due to poor circulation in the atrophic muscle, may occur following I.M. injection; in paralyzed patients, suggest I.V. route.

I.V. Infuse over 30-120 minutes.

Some penicillins (eg, carbenicillin, ticarcillin, and piperacillin) have been shown to inactivate aminoglycosides *in vitro*. This has been observed to a greater extent with tobramycin and gentamicin, while amikacin has shown greater stability against inactivation. Concurrent use of these agents may pose a risk of reduced antibacterial efficacy *in vivo*, particularly in the setting of profound renal impairment. However, definitive clinical evidence is lacking. If combination penicillin/aminoglycoside therapy is desired in a patient with renal dysfunction, separation of doses (if feasible), and routine monitoring of aminoglycoside levels, CBC, and clinical response should be considered.

Injectable Detail pH: 3-5.5 (I.V./I.M. injection); pH: 4 (premixed infusion in sodium chloride)

Storage/Stability Gentamicin is a colorless to slightly yellow solution which should be stored between 2°C to 30°C, but refrigeration is not recommended. I.V. infusion solutions mixed in NS or D_5W solution are stable for 48 hours at room temperature and refrigeration (Goodwin, 1991). Premixed bag: Manufacturer expiration date; remove from overwrap stability: 30 days.

◀ **Nursing Actions**

Physical Assessment Assess patient's hearing level before, during, and following therapy; report changes to prescriber immediately. Monitor for neurotoxicity (vertigo, ataxia), ototoxicity, decreased renal function, and opportunistic infection (eg, fever, mouth, and vaginal sores or plaques).

Patient Education

- Discuss specific use of drug and side effects with patient as it relates to treatment. (HCAHPS: During this hospital stay, were you given any medicine that you had not taken before? Before giving you any new medicine, how often did hospital staff tell you what the medicine was for? How often did hospital staff describe possible side effects in a way you could understand?)
- Have patient report immediately to prescriber significant change in balance, urinary retention, oliguria, severe dizziness, hearing impairment, asthenia, paresthesia, tinnitus, vaginal yeast infection, or signs of pseudomembranous colitis (HCAHPS).
- Educate patient about signs of a significant reaction (eg, wheezing; chest tightness; fever; itching; bad cough; blue skin color; seizures; or swelling of face, lips, tongue, or throat). **Note:** This is not a comprehensive list of all side effects. Patient should consult prescriber for additional questions.

Intended Use and Disclaimer: Should not be printed and given to patients. This information is intended to serve as a concise initial reference for healthcare professionals to use when discussing medications with a patient. You must ultimately rely on your own discretion, experience and judgment in diagnosing, treating and advising patients.

Dietary Considerations Calcium, magnesium, potassium: Renal wasting may cause hypocalcemia, hypomagnesemia, and/or hypokalemia.

Related Information

Peak and Trough Guidelines *on page 1710*

Gentamicin (Ophthalmic) (jen ta MYE sin)

Brand Names: U.S. Garamycin; Gentak

Index Terms Gentamicin Sulfate

Pharmacologic Category Antibiotic, Aminoglycoside; Antibiotic, Ophthalmic

Medication Safety Issues

Sound-alike/look-alike issues:

Gentamicin may be confused with gentian violet, kanamycin, vancomycin

Pregnancy Risk Factor C

Use Treatment of ophthalmic infections caused by susceptible bacteria

---

Available Dosage Forms

Ointment, Ophthalmic:

Garamycin: 0.3% (3.5 g)

Gentak: 0.3% (3.5 g)

Generic: 0.3% (3.5 g)

Solution, Ophthalmic:

Garamycin: 0.3% (5 mL)

Generic: 0.3% (5 mL, 15 mL)

General Dosage Range Ophthalmic: *Children and Adults:* Ointment: Instill 1/2" (1.25 cm) 2-3 times/day to every 3-4 hours; Solution: Instill 1-2 drops every 4 hours, up to 2 drops every hour for severe infections

Administration

Other Avoid contaminating tip of the solution container or ointment tube.

Nursing Actions

Patient Education

- Discuss specific use of drug and side effects with patient as it relates to treatment. (HCAHPS: During this hospital stay, were you given any medicine that you had not taken before? Before giving you any new medicine, how often did hospital staff tell you what the medicine was for? How often did hospital staff describe possible side effects in a way you could understand?)
- Have patient report immediately to prescriber sudden vision changes, ophthalmalgia, eye irritation, hallucinations, ecchymosis, or hemorrhaging (HCAHPS).
- Educate patient about signs of a significant reaction (eg, wheezing; chest tightness; fever; itching; bad cough; blue skin color; seizures; or swelling of face, lips, tongue, or throat). **Note:** This is not a comprehensive list of all side effects. Patient should consult prescriber for additional questions.

Intended Use and Disclaimer: Should not be printed and given to patients. This information is intended to serve as a concise initial reference for healthcare professionals to use when discussing medications with a patient. You must ultimately rely on your own discretion, experience and judgment in diagnosing, treating and advising patients.

Glatiramer Acetate (gla TIR a mer AS e tate)

Brand Names: U.S. Copaxone

Index Terms Copolymer-1

Pharmacologic Category Biological, Miscellaneous

Medication Safety Issues

Sound-alike/look-alike issues:

Copaxone may be confused with Compazine

Pregnancy Risk Factor B

Lactation Excretion in breast milk unknown/use caution

Breast-Feeding Considerations It is not known if glatiramer acetate is excreted in breast milk. The manufacturer recommends that caution be exercised when administering glatiramer acetate to nursing women.

Use Multiple sclerosis: Treatment of relapsing forms of multiple sclerosis

Mechanism of Action/Effect Glatiramer is a mixture of random polymers of four amino acids; L-alanine, L-glutamic acid, L-lysine, and L-tyrosine, the resulting mixture is antigenically similar to myelin basic protein, which is an important component of the myelin sheath of nerves; glatiramer is thought to induce and activate T-lymphocyte suppressor cells specific for a myelin antigen, it is also proposed that glatiramer interferes with the antigen-presenting function of certain immune cells opposing pathogenic T-cell function

Contraindications Hypersensitivity to glatiramer acetate, mannitol, or any component of the formulation

Warnings/Precautions Glatiramer acetate is antigenic, and may interfere with recognition of foreign antigens affecting tumor surveillance and infection defense systems. Immediate postinjection systemic reactions occur in a substantial percentage of patients (~16% [20 mg/mL] and ~2% [40 mg/mL] in studies); symptoms (anxiety, chest pain, dyspnea, dysphagia, flushing, palpitations, urticaria) are usually self-limited and transient. These symptoms generally occur several months after initiation of glatiramer. Chest pain may or may not occur with the immediate postinjection reaction; described as a transient pain usually resolving in a few minutes; often unassociated with other symptoms. Episodes usually begin ≥1 month after initiation of glatiramer. Lipoatrophy may occur locally at injection site at various times after treatment and may not resolve; advise patient to follow proper injection technique and rotate site daily. Skin necrosis has been observed rarely.

Drug Interactions

Avoid Concomitant Use

Avoid concomitant use of Glatiramer Acetate with any of the following: BCG; Natalizumab; Pimecrolimus; Tacrolimus (Topical); Tofacitinib; Vaccines (Live)

Decreased Effect

Glatiramer Acetate may decrease the levels/effects of: BCG; Coccidioidin Skin Test; Sipuleucel-T; Vaccines (Inactivated); Vaccines (Live)

The levels/effects of Glatiramer Acetate may be decreased by: Echinacea

Increased Effect/Toxicity

Glatiramer Acetate may increase the levels/effects of: Leflunomide; Natalizumab; Tofacitinib; Vaccines (Live)

The levels/effects of Glatiramer Acetate may be increased by: Denosumab; Pimecrolimus; Roflumilast; Tacrolimus (Topical); Trastuzumab

Adverse Reactions

>10%:

Cardiovascular: Vasodilatation (3% to 20%), chest pain (2% to 13%)

Central nervous system: Pain (20%), anxiety (13%)

Dermatologic: Skin rash (2% to 19%), diaphoresis (15%)

Gastrointestinal: Nausea (2% to 15%)

Hypersensitivity: Immediate hypersensitivity (2% to 16%; postinjection, including flushing, chest pain, palpitations, anxiety, dyspnea, throat constriction, and/or urticaria)

Immunologic: Development of IgG antibodies (3 months: ≥3 x baseline: 80%; 12 months: 90%; ≥3 x baseline: 30%)

Infection: Infection (30%)

Local: Inflammation at injection site (2% to 49%), erythema at injection site (22% to 43%), pain at injection site (10% to 40%), itching at injection site (6% to 27%), residual mass at injection site (6% to 27%), swelling (1% to 19%)

Neuromuscular & skeletal: Weakness (22%), back pain (12%)

Respiratory: Dyspnea (3% to 14%), flu-like symptoms (3% to 14%), nasopharyngitis (11%)

1% to 10%:

Cardiovascular: Palpitations (7% to 9%), edema (8%), tachycardia (5%), facial edema (3%), peripheral edema (3%), syncope (3%), hypertension (1%)

Central nervous system: Migraine (4%), chills (2% to 3%), nervousness (2%), speech disturbance (2%), abnormal dreams (1%), emotional lability (1%), stupor (1%)

Dermatologic: Hyperhidrosis (7%), pruritus (5%), erythema (2% to 4%), urticaria (3%), skin atrophy (≥1%), warts (≥1%), eczema (1%), pustular rash (1%)

Endocrine & metabolic: Weight gain (3%), amenorrhea (1%), hypermenorrhea (1%)

Gastrointestinal: Vomiting (7%), gastroenteritis (6%), dysphagia (2%), aphthous stomatitis (≥1%), bowel urgency (≥1%), dental caries (≥1%), enlargement of salivary glands (≥1%), oral candidiasis (≥1%)

Genitourinary: Urinary urgency (5%), volvovaginal candidiasis (4%), abnormal Pap smear (≥1%), hematuria (≥1%), vaginal hemorrhage (≥1%), impotence (1%)

Hematologic & oncologic: Bruise (8%), lymphadenopathy (7%), benign skin neoplasm (2%)

Hypersensitivity: Hypersensitivity (3%)

Infection: Abscess (≥1%), herpes zoster (≥1%)

Local: Bleeding at injection site (5%), hypersensitivity reaction at injection site (4%), fibrosis at injection site (2%), lipoatrophy at injection site (≤2%), abscess at injection site (1%)

Neuromuscular & skeletal: Neck pain (8%), tremor (4%), laryngospasm (2%)

Ophthalmic: Diplopia (3%), visual field defect (1%)

Respiratory: Rhinitis (7%), bronchitis (6%), cough (6%), laryngismus (5%), viral respiratory tract infection (3%), hyperventilation (1%)

Miscellaneous: Fever (3% to 6%)

Available Dosage Forms

Kit, Subcutaneous:

Copaxone: 20 mg/mL

Solution Prefilled Syringe, Subcutaneous:

Copaxone: 40 mg/mL (1 mL)

General Dosage Range SubQ: *Adults:* 20 mg daily or 40 mg 3 times weekly

Administration

Subcutaneous For SubQ administration in the arms, abdomen, hips, or thighs; rotate injection sites to prevent lipoatrophy. Administer the 40 mg dose on the same 3 days each week (eg, Monday, Wednesday, Friday) at least 48 hours apart. Allow syringe to stand at room temperature for 20 minutes prior to injection. Solution in the syringe should appear clear and colorless to slightly yellow; discard if solution is cloudy or contains any particulate matter. Discard unused portions.

Storage/Stability Store refrigerated at 2°C to 8°C (36°F to 46°F). If needed, may store at 15°C to 30°C (59°F to 86°F) for up to 1 month (refrigeration is preferred). Avoid exposure to high temperatures; protect from intense light. Do not freeze. Discard if syringe freezes.

Nursing Actions

Physical Assessment Monitor for postinjection reactions (eg, self-resolving flushing, chest tightness, dyspnea, and palpitations). Teach patient proper use (reconstitution, injection technique, and syringe/needle disposal).

Patient Education

• Discuss specific use of drug and side effects with patient as it relates to treatment. (HCAHPS: During this hospital stay, were you given any medicine that you had not taken before? Before giving you any new medicine, how often did hospital staff tell you what the medicine was for? How often did hospital staff describe possible side effects in a way you could understand?)

• Patient may experience flushing, nausea, asthenia, or back pain. Have patient report immediately to prescriber signs of infection, angina, tachycardia, syncope, arrhythmia, anxiety, hyperhidrosis, dizziness, dyspnea, enlarged lymph nodes, tremors, or significant injection site irritation (HCAHPS).

• Educate patient about signs of a significant reaction (eg, wheezing; chest tightness; fever; itching; bad cough; blue skin color; seizures; or swelling of face, lips, tongue, or throat). **Note:** This is not a comprehensive list of all side effects. Patient should consult prescriber for additional questions.

Intended Use and Disclaimer: Should not be printed and given to patients. This information is intended to serve as a concise initial reference for healthcare professionals to use when discussing medications with a patient. You must ultimately rely on your own discretion, experience and judgment in diagnosing, treating and advising patients.

Glimepiride (GLYE me pye ride)

Brand Names: U.S. Amaryl

Pharmacologic Category Antidiabetic Agent, Sulfonylurea

Medication Safety Issues

Sound-alike/look-alike issues:

Glimepiride may be confused with glipiZIDE

Amaryl may be confused with Altace, Amerge

High alert medication:

The Institute for Safe Medication Practices (ISMP) includes this medication among its list of drugs which have a heightened risk of causing significant patient harm when used in error.

International issues:

Amarel [France], Amaryl [U.S., Canada, and multiple international markets] may be confused with Reminyl brand name for galantamine [multiple international markets]

Amaryl [U.S., Canada, and multiple international markets] may be confused with Almarl brand name for arotinolol [Japan]

Pregnancy Risk Factor C

Lactation Excretion in breast milk unknown/not recommended

Breast-Feeding Considerations It is not known if glimepiride is excreted in breast milk. According to the manufacturer, due to the potential for hypoglycemia in the nursing infant, a decision should be made whether to discontinue nursing or to discontinue the drug, taking into account the importance of treatment to the mother.

Use Type 2 diabetes mellitus: As an adjunct to diet and exercise to improve glycemic control in adults with type 2 diabetes mellitus

Mechanism of Action/Effect Stimulates insulin release from the pancreatic beta cells; reduces glucose output from the liver; insulin sensitivity is increased at peripheral target sites

Contraindications

Hypersensitivity to glimepiride, any component of the formulation, or sulfonamides; diabetic ketoacidosis (with or without coma)

Documentation of allergenic cross-reactivity for drugs in this class is limited. However, because of similarities in chemical structure and/or pharmacologic actions, the possibility of cross-sensitivity cannot be ruled out with certainty.

Canadian labeling: Additional contraindications (not in U.S. labeling): Pregnancy; breast-feeding; type 1 diabetes; severe renal or hepatic impairment

Warnings/Precautions All sulfonylurea drugs are capable of producing severe hypoglycemia. Hypoglycemia is more likely to occur when caloric intake is deficient, after severe or prolonged exercise, when ethanol is ingested, or when more than one glucose-lowering drug is used. It is also more likely in elderly patients, malnourished patients and in patients with impaired renal or hepatic function; use with caution. Reduce dosage in patients with renal impairment.

Loss of efficacy may be observed following prolonged use as a result of the progression of type 2 diabetes mellitus which results in continued beta cell destruction. In patients who were previously responding to sulfonylurea therapy, consider additional factors which may be contributing to decreased efficacy (eg, inappropriate dose, nonadherence to diet and exercise regimen). If no contributing factors can be identified, consider discontinuing use of the sulfonylurea due to secondary failure of treatment. Additional antidiabetic therapy (eg, insulin) will be required. It may be necessary to discontinue therapy and administer insulin if the patient is exposed to stress (fever, trauma, infection, surgery).

Chemical similarities are present among sulfonamides, sulfonylureas, carbonic anhydrase inhibitors, thiazides, and loop diuretics (except ethacrynic acid); a risk of cross-reaction exists in patients with allergy to any of these compounds. Use in patients with sulfonamide allergy is contraindicated. Patients with G6PD deficiency may be at an increased risk of sulfonylurea-induced hemolytic anemia; however, cases have also been described in patients without G6PD deficiency during postmarketing surveillance. Use with caution and consider a nonsulfonylurea alternative in patients with G6PD deficiency. Systemic exposure of glimepiride is increased in patients with CYP2C9*3 allele; dose reductions may be necessary (Niemi, 2002).

Product labeling states oral hypoglycemic drugs may be associated with an increased cardiovascular mortality as compared to treatment with diet alone or diet plus insulin. Data to support this association are limited, and several studies, including a large prospective trial (UKPDS) have not supported an association.

Drug Interactions

Avoid Concomitant Use There are no known interactions where it is recommended to avoid concomitant use.

Decreased Effect

The levels/effects of Glimepiride may be decreased by: Colesevelam; Corticosteroids (Orally Inhaled); Corticosteroids (Systemic); CYP2C9 Inducers (Strong); Dabrafenib; Loop Diuretics; Luteinizing Hormone-Releasing Hormone Analogs; Peginterferon Alfa-2b; Quinolone Antibiotics; Rifampin; Somatropin; Thiazide Diuretics

Increased Effect/Toxicity

Glimepiride may increase the levels/effects of: Alcohol (Ethyl); Carbocisteine; Hypoglycemic Agents; Porfimer; Vitamin K Antagonists

The levels/effects of Glimepiride may be increased by: Beta-Blockers; Chloramphenicol; Cimetidine; Cyclic Antidepressants; CYP2C9 Inhibitors (Moderate); CYP2C9 Inhibitors (Strong); Fibric Acid Derivatives; Fluconazole; GLP-1 Agonists; Herbs (Hypoglycemic Properties); MAO Inhibitors; Metreleptin; Miconazole (Oral); Mifepristone; Pegvisomant; Probenecid; Quinolone Antibiotics; Ranitidine; Salicylates; Selective Serotonin Reuptake Inhibitors; Sulfonamide Derivatives; Vitamin K Antagonists; Voriconazole

Nutritional/Ethanol Interactions

Ethanol: Caution with ethanol (may cause hypoglycemia).

Herb/Nutraceutical: Caution with chromium, garlic, gymnema (may cause hypoglycemia).

Adverse Reactions

>10%: Endocrine & metabolic: Hypoglycemia (4% to 20%)

1% to 10%:

Central nervous system: Dizziness (2%), headache

Gastrointestinal: Nausea (5%)

Hepatic: Increased serum ALT (2%)

Respiratory: Flu-like symptoms (5%)

Miscellaneous: Accidental injury (6%)

Pharmacodynamics/Kinetics

Onset of Action Peak effect: Blood glucose reductions: 2-3 hours

Duration of Action 24 hours

Available Dosage Forms

Tablet, Oral:

Amaryl: 1 mg, 2 mg, 4 mg

Generic: 1 mg, 2 mg, 4 mg

General Dosage Range Dosage adjustment recommended in patients with renal impairment

Oral:

Adults: Initial: 1-2 mg once daily; (maximum: 8 mg daily)

Elderly: Initial: 1 mg once daily

Administration

Oral Administer once daily with breakfast or first main meal of the day. Patients that are NPO or require decreased caloric intake may need doses held to avoid hypoglycemia.

Storage/Stability Store at 25°C (77°F); excursions permitted between 20°C and 25°C (68°F and 77°F)

Nursing Actions

Physical Assessment Allergy history should be assessed prior to beginning therapy.

◀ **Patient Education**
- Discuss specific use of drug and side effects with patient as it relates to treatment. (HCAHPS: During this hospital stay, were you given any medicine that you had not taken before? Before giving you any new medicine, how often did hospital staff tell you what the medicine was for? How often did hospital staff describe possible side effects in a way you could understand?)
- Patient may experience dyspepsia. Have patient report immediately to prescriber signs of infection, illogical thinking, arrhythmia, severe dizziness, syncope, vision changes, ecchymosis, hemorrhaging, considerable asthenia, angina, urine discoloration, jaundice, or hypoglycemia (HCAHPS).
- Educate patient about signs of a significant reaction (eg, wheezing; chest tightness; fever; itching; bad cough; blue skin color; seizures; or swelling of face, lips, tongue, or throat). **Note:** This is not a comprehensive list of all side effects. Patient should consult prescriber for additional questions.

Intended Use and Disclaimer: Should not be printed and given to patients. This information is intended to serve as a concise initial reference for healthcare professionals to use when discussing medications with a patient. You must ultimately rely on your own discretion, experience and judgment in diagnosing, treating and advising patients.

Dietary Considerations Take with breakfast or the first main meal of the day. Individualized medical nutrition therapy (MNT) based on ADA recommendations is an integral part of therapy.

GlipiZIDE (GLIP i zide)

Brand Names: U.S. GlipiZIDE XL; Glucotrol; Glucotrol XL

Index Terms Glydiazinamide

Pharmacologic Category Antidiabetic Agent, Sulfonylurea

Medication Safety Issues

Sound-alike/look-alike issues:

GlipiZIDE may be confused with glimepiride, glyBURIDE

Glucotrol® may be confused with Glucophage®, Glucotrol® XL, glyBURIDE, GlycoTrol (dietary supplement)

High alert medication:

The Institute for Safe Medication Practices (ISMP) includes this medication among its list of drugs which have a heightened risk of causing significant patient harm when used in error.

Pregnancy Risk Factor C

Lactation Not recommended

Breast-Feeding Considerations Data from two mother-infant pairs note that glipizide was not detected in breast milk (Feig, 2005). Breast-feeding is encouraged for all women including those with diabetes; all types of insulin may be used while breast-feeding and some oral agents, including glipizide, may be acceptable for use as well (Metzger 2007). According to the manufacturer, due to the potential for hypoglycemia in the nursing infant, a decision should be made whether to discontinue nursing or to discontinue the drug, taking into account the importance of treatment to the mother.

Use Management of type 2 diabetes mellitus (non-insulin dependent, NIDDM) as an adjunct to diet and exercise to lower blood glucose; may be used in combination with metformin or insulin in patients whose hyperglycemia cannot be controlled by diet and exercise in conjunction with a single oral hypoglycemic agent

Mechanism of Action/Effect Stimulates insulin release from the pancreatic beta cells; reduces glucose output from the liver; insulin sensitivity is increased at peripheral target sites

Contraindications Hypersensitivity to glipizide or any component of the formulation; type 1 diabetes mellitus (insulin dependent, IDDM); diabetic ketoacidosis (with or without coma)

Warnings/Precautions All sulfonylurea drugs are capable of producing severe hypoglycemia. Hypoglycemia is more likely to occur when caloric intake is deficient, after severe or prolonged exercise, when ethanol is ingested, or when more than one glucose-lowering drug is used. It is also more likely in elderly patients, malnourished patients and in patients with impaired renal or hepatic function; use with caution. Autonomic neuropathy, advanced age, and concomitant use of beta-blockers or other sympatholytic agents may impair the patient's ability to recognize the signs and symptoms of hypoglycemia; use with caution.

Use with caution in patients with hepatic or renal impairment. It may be necessary to discontinue therapy and administer insulin if the patient is exposed to stress (fever, trauma, infection, surgery). Loss of efficacy may be observed following prolonged use as a result of the progression of type 2 diabetes mellitus which results in continued beta cell destruction. In patients who were previously responding to sulfonylurea therapy, consider additional factors which may be contributing to decreased efficacy (eg, inappropriate dose, nonadherence to diet and exercise regimen). If no contributing factors can be identified, consider discontinuing use of the sulfonylurea due to secondary failure of treatment. Additional antidiabetic therapy (eg, insulin) will be required.

Chemical similarities are present among sulfonamides, sulfonylureas, carbonic anhydrase inhibitors, thiazides, and loop diuretics (except ethacrynic acid). Use in patients with sulfonamide allergy is not specifically contraindicated in product labeling; however, a risk of cross-reaction exists in patients with allergy to any of these compounds; avoid use when previous reaction has been severe. Patients with G6PD deficiency may be at an increased risk of sulfonylurea-induced hemolytic anemia; however, cases have also been described in patients without G6PD deficiency during postmarketing surveillance. Use with caution and consider a nonsulfonylurea alternative in patients with G6PD deficiency.

Product labeling states oral hypoglycemic drugs may be associated with an increased cardiovascular mortality as compared to treatment with diet alone or diet plus insulin. Data to support this association are limited, and several studies, including a large prospective trial (UKPDS) have not supported an association. Avoid use of extended release tablets (Glucotrol XL®) in patients with known stricture/narrowing of the GI tract.

Drug Interactions

Avoid Concomitant Use There are no known interactions where it is recommended to avoid concomitant use.

Decreased Effect

The levels/effects of GlipiZIDE may be decreased by: Colesevelam; Corticosteroids (Orally Inhaled); Corticosteroids (Systemic); CYP2C9 Inducers (Strong); Dabrafenib; Loop Diuretics; Luteinizing Hormone-Releasing Hormone Analogs; Peginterferon Alfa-2b; Quinolone Antibiotics; Rifampin; Somatropin; Thiazide Diuretics

Increased Effect/Toxicity

GlipiZIDE may increase the levels/effects of: Alcohol (Ethyl); Carbocisteine; Hypoglycemic Agents; Porfimer; Vitamin K Antagonists

The levels/effects of GlipiZIDE may be increased by: Beta-Blockers; Chloramphenicol; Cimetidine; Clarithromycin; Cyclic Antidepressants; CYP2C9 Inhibitors (Moderate); CYP2C9 Inhibitors (Strong); Fibric Acid Derivatives; Fluconazole; GLP-1 Agonists; Herbs (Hypoglycemic Properties); MAO Inhibitors; Metreleptin; Miconazole (Oral); Mifepristone; Pegvisomant; Posaconazole; Probenecid; Quinolone Antibiotics; Ranitidine; Salicylates; Selective Serotonin Reuptake Inhibitors; Sulfonamide Derivatives; Vitamin K Antagonists; Voriconazole

Nutritional/Ethanol Interactions

Ethanol: Caution with ethanol (may cause hypoglycemia or rare disulfiram reaction).

Food: A delayed release of insulin may occur if glipizide is taken with food. Immediate release tablets should be administered 30 minutes before meals to avoid erratic absorption.

Herb/Nutraceutical: Herbs with hypoglycemic properties may enhance the hypoglycemic effect of glipizide. This includes alfalfa, aloe, bilberry, bitter melon, burdock, celery, damiana, fenugreek, garcinia, garlic, ginger, ginseng (American), gymnema, marshmallow, stinging nettle

Adverse Reactions Frequency not always defined.

Cardiovascular: Syncope (<3%)

Central nervous system: Dizziness (2% to 7%), nervousness (4%), anxiety (<3%), depression (<3%), hypoesthesia (<3%), insomnia (<3%), pain (<3%), drowsiness (2%), headache (2%)

Dermatologic: Pruritus (1% to <3%), eczema (1%), erythema (1%), maculopapular eruptions (1%), morbilliform eruptions (1%), rash (1%), urticaria (1%)

Endocrine & metabolic: Hypoglycemia (<3%)

Gastrointestinal: Diarrhea (1% to 5%), flatulence (3%), constipation (1% to <3%), nausea (1% to <3%), dyspepsia (<3%), vomiting (<3%), abdominal pain (1%)

Hepatic: Alkaline phosphatase increased, AST increased, LDH increased

Neuromuscular & skeletal: Tremor (4%), arthralgia (<3%), leg cramps (<3%), myalgia (<3%), paresthesia (<3%)

Ocular: Blurred vision (<3%)

Renal: Blood urea nitrogen increased, creatinine increased

Respiratory: Rhinitis (<3%)

Miscellaneous: Diaphoresis (<3%)

Pharmacodynamics/Kinetics

Duration of Action 12-24 hours

Available Dosage Forms

Tablet, Oral:

Glucotrol: 5 mg, 10 mg

Generic: 5 mg, 10 mg

Tablet Extended Release 24 Hour, Oral:

GlipiZIDE XL: 2.5 mg, 5 mg, 10 mg

Glucotrol XL: 2.5 mg, 5 mg, 10 mg

Generic: 2.5 mg, 5 mg, 10 mg

General Dosage Range Dosage adjustment recommended in patients with hepatic impairment

Oral:

Immediate release:

Adults: Initial: 5 mg once daily; Maintenance: Up to 40 mg/day

Elderly: Initial: 2.5 mg once daily

Extended release: *Adults:* Initial: 5 mg once daily; Maintenance: Up to 20 mg/day

Administration

Oral Administer immediate release tablets 30 minutes before a meal (preferably before breakfast if once-daily dosing) to achieve greatest reduction in postprandial hyperglycemia. Extended release tablets should be given with breakfast. Patients that are NPO or require decreased caloric intake may need doses held to avoid hypoglycemia.

Storage/Stability Store below 30°C (86°F) ▶

◄ **Nursing Actions**

Physical Assessment Monitor for hypoglycemia during therapy.

Patient Education

- Discuss specific use of drug and side effects with patient as it relates to treatment. (HCAHPS: During this hospital stay, were you given any medicine that you had not taken before? Before giving you any new medicine, how often did hospital staff tell you what the medicine was for? How often did hospital staff describe possible side effects in a way you could understand?)
- Patient may experience flatulence, fatigue, headache, diarrhea, dyspepsia, or shell tablet in stool. Have patient report immediately to prescriber signs of infection, signs of hepatic impairment, illogical thinking, arrhythmia, severe dizziness, syncope, vision changes, ecchymosis, hemorrhaging, significant asthenia, considerable abdominal pain, intolerable back pain, or signs of hypoglycemia (HCAHPS).
- Educate patient about signs of a significant reaction (eg, wheezing; chest tightness; fever; itching; bad cough; blue skin color; seizures; or swelling of face, lips, tongue, or throat). **Note:** This is not a comprehensive list of all side effects. Patient should consult prescriber for additional questions.

Intended Use and Disclaimer: Should not be printed and given to patients. This information is intended to serve as a concise initial reference for healthcare professionals to use when discussing medications with a patient. You must ultimately rely on your own discretion, experience and judgment in diagnosing, treating and advising patients.

Dietary Considerations Take immediate release tablets 30 minutes before meals (preferably before breakfast if once-daily dosing); extended release tablets should be taken with breakfast. Individualized medical nutrition therapy (MNT) based on ADA recommendations is an integral part of therapy.

Related Information

Oral Medications That Should Not Be Crushed or Altered *on page 1712*

Glipizide and Metformin
(GLIP i zide & met FOR min)

Index Terms Glipizide and Metformin Hydrochloride; Metformin and Glipizide

Pharmacologic Category Antidiabetic Agent, Biguanide; Antidiabetic Agent, Sulfonylurea

Medication Safety Issues

High alert medication:

The Institute for Safe Medication Practices (ISMP) includes this medication among its list of drugs which have a heightened risk of causing significant patient harm when used in error.

Pregnancy Risk Factor C

Use Indicated as an adjunct to diet and exercise to improve glycemic control in adults with type 2 diabetes mellitus (noninsulin dependent, NIDDM)

Available Dosage Forms

Tablet, oral: 2.5/250: Glipizide 2.5 mg and metformin 250 mg; 2.5/500: Glipizide 2.5 mg and metformin 500 mg; 5/500: Glipizide 5 mg and metformin 500 mg

General Dosage Range Oral: *Adults:* Initial: Glipizide 2.5 mg and metformin 250 mg once daily; Maintenance: Up to glipizide 20 mg/day and metformin 2000 mg/day in divided doses

Administration

Oral All doses should be administered with a meal. Twice-daily dosing should be administered with the morning and evening meals. Patients that are NPO or require decreased caloric intake may need doses held to avoid hypoglycemia.

Nursing Actions

Physical Assessment See individual agents.

Patient Education

- Discuss specific use of drug and side effects with patient as it relates to treatment. (HCAHPS: During this hospital stay, were you given any medicine that you had not taken before? Before giving you any new medicine, how often did hospital staff tell you what the medicine was for? How often did hospital staff describe possible side effects in a way you could understand?)
- Patient may experience headache, nausea, diarrhea, or flatulence. Have patient report immediately to prescriber signs of hepatic impairment, vision changes, signs of hypoglycemia, or signs of lactic acidosis (HCAHPS).
- Educate patient about signs of a significant reaction (eg, wheezing; chest tightness; fever; itching; bad cough; blue skin color; seizures; or swelling of face, lips, tongue, or throat). **Note:** This is not a comprehensive list of all side effects. Patient should consult prescriber for additional questions.

Intended Use and Disclaimer: Should not be printed and given to patients. This information is intended to serve as a concise initial reference for healthcare professionals to use when discussing medications with a patient. You must ultimately rely on your own discretion, experience and judgment in diagnosing, treating and advising patients.

Related Information

GlipiZIDE *on page 742*

MetFORMIN *on page 1014*

Glucagon (GLOO ka gon)

Brand Names: U.S. GlucaGen; GlucaGen Hypo-Kit; Glucagon Emergency

Index Terms Glucagon Hydrochloride

Pharmacologic Category Antidote; Antidote, Hypoglycemia; Diagnostic Agent

Pregnancy Risk Factor B

Lactation Excretion in breast milk unknown/use caution

Breast-Feeding Considerations Glucagon is not absorbed from the GI tract and therefore, it is unlikely adverse effects would occur in a breast-feeding infant.

Use Management of hypoglycemia; diagnostic aid in radiologic examinations to temporarily inhibit GI tract movement

Unlabeled Use Beta-blocker- or calcium channel blocker-induced myocardial depression (with or without hypotension) unresponsive to standard measures; suspected or documented hypoglycemia secondary to insulin or sulfonylurea overdose (as adjunct to dextrose)

Mechanism of Action/Effect Stimulates adenylate cyclase to produce increased cyclic AMP, which promotes hepatic glycogenolysis and gluconeogenesis, causing a raise in blood glucose levels

Contraindications Hypersensitivity to glucagon or any component of the formulation; insulinoma; pheochromocytoma

Warnings/Precautions Use of glucagon is contraindicated in insulinoma; exogenous glucagon may cause an initial rise in blood glucose followed by rebound hypoglycemia. Use of glucagon is contraindicated in pheochromocytoma; exogenous glucagon may cause the release of catecholamines, resulting in an increase in blood pressure. Use caution with prolonged fasting, starvation, adrenal insufficiency or chronic hypoglycemia; levels of glucose stores in liver may be decreased. Supplemental carbohydrates should be given to patients who respond to glucagon for severe hypoglycemia to prevent secondary hypoglycemia. Monitor blood glucose levels closely.

In patients with hypoglycemia secondary to insulin or sulfonylurea overdose, dextrose should be immediately administered; if I.V. access cannot be established or if dextrose is not available, glucagon may be considered as alternative acute treatment until dextrose can be administered.

May contain lactose; avoid administration in hereditary galactose intolerance, Lapp lactase deficiency, or glucose-galactose malabsorption.

Drug Interactions

Avoid Concomitant Use There are no known interactions where it is recommended to avoid concomitant use.

Decreased Effect There are no known significant interactions involving a decrease in effect.

Increased Effect/Toxicity
Glucagon may increase the levels/effects of: Vitamin K Antagonists

Nutritional/Ethanol Interactions Glucagon depletes glycogen stores.

Adverse Reactions Frequency not defined.
Cardiovascular: Hypotension (up to 2 hours after GI procedures), hypertension, tachycardia
Gastrointestinal: Nausea, vomiting (high incidence with rapid administration of high doses)
Miscellaneous: Hypersensitivity reactions, anaphylaxis

Pharmacodynamics/Kinetics
Onset of Action Peak effect: Blood glucose levels: Parenteral: I.V.: 5-20 minutes; I.M.: 30 minutes; SubQ: 30-45 minutes

Duration of Action Glucose elevation: SubQ: 60-90 minutes; I.V.: 30 minutes

Available Dosage Forms
Kit, Injection:
Glucagon Emergency: 1 mg
Solution Reconstituted, Injection:
GlucaGen: 1 mg (1 ea)
GlucaGen HypoKit: 1 mg (1 ea)

General Dosage Range
I.M.:
Children <20 kg: 0.5 mg or 20-30 mcg/kg/dose, may repeat
Children ≥20 kg: 1 mg, may repeat
Adults: 1 mg, may repeat or 1-2 mg prior to gastrointestinal procedure
I.V.:
Children <20 kg: 0.5 mg or 20-30 mcg/kg/dose, may repeat
Children ≥20 kg: 1 mg, may repeat
Adults: 1 mg, may repeat in 20 minutes or 0.25-2 mg 10 minutes prior to gastrointestinal procedure
SubQ:
Children <20 kg: 0.5 mg or 20-30 mcg/kg/dose, may repeat
Children ≥20 kg and Adults: 1 mg, may repeat
Usual Infusion Concentrations: Adult I.V. infusion: 4 mg in 50 mL (concentration: 0.08 mg/mL) of D_5W

Administration
I.V. Bolus may be associated with nausea and vomiting.
Beta-blocker/calcium channel blocker toxicity: Administer bolus over 3-5 minutes; continuous infusions may be used. Ensure adequate supply available to continue therapy.

Preparation for Administration Reconstitute powder for injection by adding 1 mL of sterile diluent to a vial containing 1 unit of the drug, to provide solutions containing 1 mg of glucagon/mL. Gently roll vial to dissolve. Solution for infusion may be prepared by reconstitution with and further dilution in NS or D_5W (Love, 1998).

Storage/Stability Prior to reconstitution, store at controlled room temperature of 20°C to 25°C (69°F to 77°F); do not freeze. Use reconstituted solution immediately. May be kept at 5°C for up to 48 hours if necessary.

Nursing Actions

Physical Assessment Arouse patient from hypoglycemic or insulin shock as soon as possible and administer carbohydrates. Instruct patient (or significant other) in appropriate administration procedures for emergency use of glucagon.

Patient Education
- Discuss specific use of drug and side effects with patient as it relates to treatment. (HCAHPS: During this hospital stay, were you given any medicine that you had not taken before? Before giving you any new medicine, how often did hospital staff tell you what the medicine was for? How often did hospital staff describe possible side effects in a way you could understand?)
- Patient may experience nausea. Have patient report immediately to prescriber severe dizziness, syncope, significant headache, tachycardia, or bradycardia (HCAHPS).
- Educate patient about signs of a significant reaction (eg, wheezing; chest tightness; fever; itching; bad cough; blue skin color; seizures; or swelling of face, lips, tongue, or throat). **Note:** This is not a comprehensive list of all side effects. Patient should consult prescriber for additional questions.

Intended Use and Disclaimer: Should not be printed and given to patients. This information is intended to serve as a concise initial reference for healthcare professionals to use when discussing medications with a patient. You must ultimately rely on your own discretion, experience and judgment in diagnosing, treating and advising patients.

Dietary Considerations Administer carbohydrates to patient as soon as possible after response to treatment.

Related Information
Diagnostics and Surgical Aids *on page 1670*

Glucarpidase (gloo KAR pid ase)

Brand Names: U.S. Voraxaze
Index Terms Carboxypeptidase-G2; CPDG2; CPG2; Voraxaze
Pharmacologic Category Antidote; Enzyme
Pregnancy Risk Factor C
Lactation Excretion in breast milk unknown/use caution
Use Treatment of toxic plasma methotrexate concentrations (>1 micromole/L) in patients with delayed clearance due to renal impairment

Note: Due to the risk of subtherapeutic methotrexate exposure, glucarpidase is **NOT** indicated when methotrexate clearance is within expected range (plasma methotrexate concentration ≤2 standard deviations of mean methotrexate excretion curve specific for dose administered) **or** with normal renal function or mild renal impairment.

Unlabeled Use Rescue agent to reduce methotrexate toxicity in patients with accidental intrathecal methotrexate overdose
Available Dosage Forms
Solution Reconstituted, Intravenous [preservative free]:
Voraxaze: 1000 units (1 ea)
General Dosage Range I.V.: *Children and Adults:* 50 units/kg
Administration
I.V. Infuse over 5 minutes. Flush I.V. line before and after glucarpidase administration.

Other Intrathecal (for intrathecal methotrexate overdose; unlabeled route/use): Glucarpidase was administered within 3-9 hours of accidental intrathecal methotrexate overdose in conjunction with lumbar drainage or ventriculolumbar perfusion (Widemann, 2004). Administered over 5 minutes via lumbar route, ventriculostomy, Ommaya reservoir, or lumbar and ventriculostomy (O'Marcaigh, 1996; Widemann, 2004). In one case report, 1000 units was administered through the ventricular catheter over 5 minutes and another 1000 units was administered through the lumbar catheter (O'Marcaigh, 1996).

Nursing Actions

Physical Assessment Assess patient tolerance during infusion.

Patient Education
- Discuss specific use of drug and side effects with patient as it relates to treatment. (HCAHPS: During this hospital stay, were you given any medicine that you had not taken before? Before giving you any new medicine, how often did hospital staff tell you what the medicine was for? How often did hospital staff describe possible side effects in a way you could understand?)
- Patient may experience nausea. Have patient report immediately to prescriber severe dizziness, syncope, flushing, or paresthesia (HCAHPS).
- Educate patient about signs of a significant reaction (eg, wheezing; chest tightness; fever; itching; bad cough; blue skin color; seizures; or swelling of face, lips, tongue, or throat). **Note:** This is not a comprehensive list of all side effects. Patient should consult prescriber for additional questions.

Intended Use and Disclaimer: Should not be printed and given to patients. This information is intended to serve as a concise initial reference for healthcare professionals to use when discussing medications with a patient. You must ultimately rely on your own discretion, experience and judgment in diagnosing, treating and advising patients.

GlyBURIDE (GLYE byoor ide)

Brand Names: U.S. Diabeta; Glynase

Index Terms Diabeta; Glibenclamide; Glybenclamide; Glybenzcyclamide; Micronase

Pharmacologic Category Antidiabetic Agent, Sulfonylurea

Medication Safety Issues

Sound-alike/look-alike issues:

GlyBURIDE may be confused with glipiZIDE, Glucotrol

Diaβeta may be confused with Zebeta

High alert medication:

The Institute for Safe Medication Practices (ISMP) includes this medication among its list of drugs which have a heightened risk of causing significant patient harm when used in error.

BEERS Criteria medication:

This drug may be potentially inappropriate for use in geriatric patients (Quality of evidence - high; Strength of recommendation - strong).

Pregnancy Risk Factor B/C (manufacturer dependent)

Lactation Not recommended

Breast-Feeding Considerations Data from initial studies note that glyburide was not detected in breast milk (Feig, 2005). According to the manufacturer, due to the potential for hypoglycemia in the nursing infant, a decision should be made whether to discontinue nursing or to discontinue the drug, taking into account the importance of treatment to the mother. Current guidelines note that breast-feeding is encouraged for all women, including those with diabetes; all types of insulin may be used while breast-feeding and some oral agents, including glyburide, may be acceptable for use as well (Metzger, 2007).

Use Type 2 diabetes mellitus: Adjunct to diet and exercise to improve glycemic control in adults with type 2 diabetes mellitus (noninsulin dependent, NIDDM)

Unlabeled Use Alternative to insulin in women for the treatment of gestational diabetes mellitus (GDM) (11-33 weeks' gestation)

Mechanism of Action/Effect Stimulates insulin release from the pancreatic beta cells; reduces glucose output from the liver; insulin sensitivity is increased at peripheral target sites

Contraindications

Hypersensitivity to glyburide or any component of the formulation; type 1 diabetes mellitus or diabetic ketoacidosis, with or without coma; concomitant use with bosentan.

Canadian labeling: Additional contraindications (not in U.S. labeling): Diabetic precoma or coma, stress conditions (eg, severe infections, trauma, surgery); liver disease or frank jaundice; renal impairment; pregnancy; breast-feeding.

Documentation of allergenic cross-reactivity for sulfonylureas is limited. However, because of similarities in chemical structure and/or pharmacologic actions, the possibility of cross-sensitivity cannot be ruled out with certainty.

Warnings/Precautions All sulfonylurea drugs are capable of producing severe hypoglycemia. Hypoglycemia is more likely to occur when caloric intake is deficient, after severe or prolonged exercise, when ethanol is ingested, or when more than one glucose-lowering drug is used. It is also more likely in elderly patients, malnourished, or debilitated patients and in patients with severe renal or hepatic impairment; adrenal and/or pituitary insufficiency; use with caution.

It may be necessary to discontinue therapy and administer insulin if the patient is exposed to stress (fever, trauma, infection, surgery). Loss of efficacy may be observed following prolonged use as a result of the progression of type 2 diabetes mellitus which results in continued beta cell destruction. In patients who were previously responding to sulfonylurea therapy, consider additional factors which may be contributing to decreased efficacy (eg, inappropriate dose, nonadherence to diet and exercise regimen). If no contributing factors can be identified, consider discontinuing use of the sulfonylurea due to secondary failure of treatment. Additional antidiabetic therapy (eg, insulin) will be required.

Avoid use in elderly patients due to increased risk of prolonged hypoglycemia (Beers Criteria). If therapy is initiated, dosing should be conservative; monitor closely for hypoglycemia.

Chemical similarities are present among sulfonamides, sulfonylureas, carbonic anhydrase inhibitors, thiazides, and loop diuretics (except ethacrynic acid). Use in patients with sulfonamide allergy is not specifically contraindicated in product labeling, however, a risk of cross-reaction exists in patients with allergy to any of these compounds; avoid use when previous reaction has been severe.

Product labeling states oral hypoglycemic drugs may be associated with an increased cardiovascular mortality as compared to treatment with diet alone or diet plus insulin. Data to support this association are limited, and several studies, including a large prospective trial (UKPDS) have not supported an association.

Patients with G6PD deficiency may be at an increased risk of sulfonylurea-induced hemolytic anemia; however, cases have also been described in patients without G6PD deficiency during postmarketing surveillance. Use with caution and consider a nonsulfonylurea alternative in patients with G6PD deficiency.

Micronized glyburide tablets are **not** bioequivalent to conventional glyburide tablets; retitration should occur if patients are being transferred to a different glyburide formulation (eg, micronized-to-conventional or vice versa) or from other hypoglycemic agents.

Drug Interactions

Avoid Concomitant Use

Avoid concomitant use of GlyBURIDE with any of the following: Bosentan; Pimozide

Decreased Effect

GlyBURIDE may decrease the levels/effects of: Bosentan

The levels/effects of GlyBURIDE may be decreased by: Bosentan; Colesevelam; Corticosteroids (Orally Inhaled); Corticosteroids (Systemic); CycloSPORINE (Systemic); CYP2C9 Inducers (Strong); Dabrafenib; Loop Diuretics; Luteinizing Hormone-Releasing Hormone Analogs; Peginterferon Alfa-2b; Quinolone Antibiotics; Rifampin; Somatropin; Thiazide Diuretics

Increased Effect/Toxicity

GlyBURIDE may increase the levels/effects of: Alcohol (Ethyl); ARIPiprazole; Bosentan; Carbocisteine; CycloSPORINE (Systemic); Dofetilide; Hypoglycemic Agents; Lomitapide; Pimozide; Porfimer; Vitamin K Antagonists

The levels/effects of GlyBURIDE may be increased by: Beta-Blockers; Chloramphenicol; Cimetidine; Clarithromycin; Cyclic Antidepressants; CYP2C9 Inhibitors (Moderate); CYP2C9 Inhibitors (Strong); Fibric Acid Derivatives; Fluconazole; GLP-1 Agonists; Herbs (Hypoglycemic Properties); MAO Inhibitors; Metreleptin; Miconazole (Oral); Mifepristone; Pegvisomant; Probenecid; Quinolone Antibiotics; Ranitidine; Salicylates; Selective Serotonin Reuptake Inhibitors; Sulfonamide Derivatives; Vitamin K Antagonists; Voriconazole

Nutritional/Ethanol Interactions

Ethanol: Caution with ethanol (may cause hypoglycemia).

Herb/Nutraceutical: Herbs with hypoglycemic properties may enhance the hypoglycemic effect of glyburide. This includes alfalfa, aloe, bilberry, bitter melon, burdock, celery, damiana, fenugreek, garcinia, garlic, ginger, ginseng (American), gymnema, marshmallow, stinging nettle

Adverse Reactions Frequency not defined.

Cardiovascular: Vasculitis

Central nervous system: Dizziness, headache

Dermatologic: Angioedema, erythema, maculopapular eruptions, morbilliform eruptions, photosensitivity reaction, pruritus, purpura, rash, urticaria

Endocrine & metabolic: Disulfiram-like reaction, hypoglycemia, hyponatremia (SIADH reported with other sulfonylureas)

Gastrointestinal: Anorexia, constipation, diarrhea, epigastric fullness, heartburn, nausea

Genitourinary: Nocturia

Hematologic: Agranulocytosis, aplastic anemia, hemolytic anemia, leukopenia, pancytopenia, porphyria cutanea tarda, thrombocytopenia

Hepatic: Cholestatic jaundice, hepatitis, liver failure, transaminase increased

Neuromuscular & skeletal: Arthralgia, myalgia, paresthesia

Ocular: Blurred vision

Renal: Diuretic effect (minor)

Miscellaneous: Allergic reaction

Pharmacodynamics/Kinetics

Onset of Action Serum insulin levels begin to increase 15-60 minutes after a single dose

Duration of Action ≤24 hours

Dosage Forms Considerations

Micronized formulation: Glynase

Available Dosage Forms

Tablet, Oral:

Diabeta: 1.25 mg, 2.5 mg, 5 mg

Glynase: 1.5 mg, 3 mg, 6 mg

Generic: 1.25 mg, 1.5 mg, 2.5 mg, 3 mg, 5 mg, 6 mg

General Dosage Range Oral:

Conventional tablets (Diaβeta): *Adults:* Initial: 1.25-5 mg once daily; Maintenance: 1.25-20 mg daily as single or divided doses (maximum: 20 mg daily)

Micronized tablets (Glynase PresTab): *Adults:* Initial: 0.75-3 mg once daily; Maintenance: 0.75-12 mg daily as single or divided doses (maximum: 12 mg daily)

Administration

Oral Administer with meals at the same time each day (twice-daily dosing may be beneficial if conventional glyburide doses are >10 mg or micronized glyburide doses are >6 mg). Patients that are NPO or require decreased caloric intake may need doses held to avoid hypoglycemia.

Storage/Stability

Conventional tablets (Diaβeta): Store at 25°C (77°F); excursions are permitted between 15°C and 30°C (59°F and 86°F).

Micronized tablets (Glynase PresTab): Store at 20°C to 25°C (68°F to 77°F).

Nursing Actions

Physical Assessment Allergy history should be evaluated prior to beginning therapy. Monitor for hypoglycemia during therapy.

Patient Education

- Discuss specific use of drug and side effects with patient as it relates to treatment. (HCAHPS: During this hospital stay, were you given any medicine that you had not taken before? Before giving you any new medicine, how often did hospital staff tell you what the medicine was for? How often did hospital staff describe possible side effects in a way you could understand?)

- Patient may experience dyspepsia, pyrosis, or bloating. Have patient report immediately to prescriber signs of infection, signs of hepatic impairment, illogical thinking, arrhythmia, severe dizziness, syncope, vision changes, ecchymosis, hemorrhaging, considerable asthenia, or hypoglycemia (HCAHPS).

- Educate patient about signs of a significant reaction (eg, wheezing; chest tightness; fever; itching; bad cough; blue skin color; seizures; or swelling of face, lips, tongue, or throat). **Note:** This is not a comprehensive list of all side effects. Patient should consult prescriber for additional questions.

Intended Use and Disclaimer: Should not be printed and given to patients. This information is intended to serve as a concise initial reference for healthcare professionals to use when discussing medications with a patient. You must ultimately rely on your own discretion, experience and judgment in diagnosing, treating and advising patients.

Dietary Considerations Should be taken with meals at the same time each day (twice-daily dosing may be beneficial if conventional glyburide doses are >10 mg or micronized glyburide doses are >6 mg). Individualized medical nutrition therapy (MNT) based on ADA recommendations is an integral part of therapy.

Glyburide and Metformin
(GLYE byoor ide & met FOR min)

Brand Names: U.S. Glucovance
Index Terms Glyburide and Metformin Hydrochloride; Metformin and Glyburide
Pharmacologic Category Antidiabetic Agent, Biguanide; Antidiabetic Agent, Sulfonylurea
Medication Safety Issues
  Sound-alike/look-alike issues:
    Glucovance may be confused with Vyvanse
  High alert medication:
    This medication is in a class the Institute for Safe Medication Practices (ISMP) includes among its list of drug classes that have a heightened risk of causing significant patient harm when used in error.
Pregnancy Risk Factor B
Use Type 2 diabetes mellitus: As an adjunct to diet and exercise, to improve glycemic control in adults with type 2 diabetes (noninsulin dependent, NIDDM)
Available Dosage Forms
  Tablet, oral: Glyburide 1.25 mg and metformin 250 mg; glyburide 2.5 mg and metformin 500 mg; glyburide 5 mg and metformin 500 mg
    Glucovance®: 2.5 mg/500 mg: Glyburide 2.5 mg and metformin 500 mg; 5 mg/500 mg: Glyburide 5 mg and metformin 500 mg
General Dosage Range Oral: *Adults:* Initial: Glyburide 1.25-5 mg and metformin 250-500 mg once or twice daily; Maintenance: Up to glyburide 20 mg/day and metformin 2000 mg/day
Administration
  Oral All doses should be administered with a meal. Twice-daily dosing should be administered with the morning and evening meals. Patients that are

NPO or require decreased caloric intake may need doses held to avoid hypoglycemia.
Nursing Actions
  Physical Assessment See individual agents.
  Patient Education
- Discuss specific use of drug and side effects with patient as it relates to treatment. (HCAHPS: During this hospital stay, were you given any medicine that you had not taken before? Before giving you any new medicine, how often did hospital staff tell you what the medicine was for? How often did hospital staff describe possible side effects in a way you could understand?)
- Patient may experience headache, dyspepsia, nausea, diarrhea, or flatulence. Have patient report immediately to prescriber signs of hepatic impairment, signs of hypoglycemia, or signs of lactic acidosis (HCAHPS).
- Educate patient about signs of a significant reaction (eg, wheezing; chest tightness; fever; itching; bad cough; blue skin color; seizures; or swelling of face, lips, tongue, or throat). **Note:** This is not a comprehensive list of all side effects. Patient should consult prescriber for additional questions.

Intended Use and Disclaimer: Should not be printed and given to patients. This information is intended to serve as a concise initial reference for healthcare professionals to use when discussing medications with a patient. You must ultimately rely on your own discretion, experience and judgment in diagnosing, treating and advising patients.
Related Information
  GlyBURIDE *on page 746*
  MetFORMIN *on page 1014*

Glycopyrrolate (glye koe PYE roe late)

Brand Names: U.S. Cuvposa; Glycate; Robinul; Robinul-Forte
Index Terms Glycopyrronium Bromide; NVA237
Pharmacologic Category Anticholinergic Agent
Medication Safety Issues
  International issues:
    Robinul [U.S. and multiple international markets] may be confused with Reminyl brand name for galantamine [Canada and multiple international markets]
Pregnancy Risk Factor B (injection) / C (oral solution)
Lactation Excretion in breast milk unknown/use caution
Use Inhibit salivation and excessive secretions of the respiratory tract preoperatively; control of upper airway secretions; intraoperatively to counteract drug-induced or vagal mediated bradyarrhythmias; adjunct in treatment of peptic ulcer (indication listed in product labeling but currently has no place in management of peptic ulcer disease)

Cuvposa: Reduce chronic, severe drooling in those with neurologic conditions (eg, cerebral palsy) associated with drooling

Seebri Breezhaler [Canadian product]: Maintenance treatment of chronic obstructive pulmonary disease (COPD) including chronic bronchitis and emphysema

Unlabeled Use Adjunct with acetylcholinesterase inhibitors (eg, neostigmine, edrophonium, pyridostigmine) to antagonize cholinergic effects

Available Dosage Forms

Solution, Injection:
Robinul: 0.2 mg/mL (1 mL); 0.4 mg/2 mL (2 mL); 1 mg/5 mL (5 mL); 4 mg/20 mL (20 mL)
Generic: 0.2 mg/mL (1 mL); 0.4 mg/2 mL (2 mL); 1 mg/5 mL (5 mL); 4 mg/20 mL (20 mL)

Solution, Oral:
Cuvposa: 1 mg/5 mL (473 mL)

Tablet, Oral:
Glycate: 1.5 mg
Robinul: 1 mg
Robinul-Forte: 2 mg
Generic: 1 mg, 2 mg

General Dosage Range

I.M.:
Children <2 years: 4-9 mcg/kg once **or** 4-10 mcg/kg every 3-4 hours (maximum: 0.2 mg/dose; 0.8 mg/day)
Children ≥2 years: 4 mcg/kg once **or** 4-10 mcg/kg every 3-4 hours (maximum: 0.2 mg/dose; 0.8 mg/day)
Adults: 4 mcg/kg once **or** 0.1-0.2 mg 3-4 times/day

I.V.:
Children: 4-10 mcg/kg every 3-4 hours (maximum: 0.2 mg/dose; 0.8 mg/day) **or** 4 mcg/kg (maximum: 0.1 mg); repeat as needed
Adults: 0.1-0.2 mg 3-4 times/day **or** 0.1 mg repeated as needed

Oral: *Children 3-16 years:* 0.02-0.1 mg/kg/dose 3 times/day (maximum: 3 mg/dose)

Administration

I.M. Administer undiluted.

I.V. Administer at a rate of 0.2 mg over 1-2 minutes.

Injectable Detail May administer undiluted. May also be administered via the tubing of a running I.V. infusion of a compatible solution. May be administered in the same syringe with neostigmine or pyridostigmine.

pH: 2-3

Oral Administer oral solution on an empty stomach, 1 hour before or 2 hours after meals

Inhalation Oral inhalation [Canadian product]: Administer once daily preferably at the same time each day using the Seebri® Breezhaler® only. Remove capsule from foil blister immediately before use. Do not swallow capsule. Avoid getting powder into eyes. Place capsule in the capsule-chamber in the base of the Seebri® Breezhaler®.

A click is heard as it fully closes. Hold inhaler with mouthpiece in upright position and pierce capsule within chamber by simultaneously pressing piercing buttons on base of inhaler (click is heard as capsule is pierced). Release buttons. Exhale fully. Do not exhale into inhaler. Tilt head slightly back and place mouthpiece in mouth with piercing buttons on base of inhaler in horizontal position and not up and down. Do not press piercing buttons. Inhale (rapidly, steadily and deeply); the capsule vibration should be heard within the device. Hold breath for at least 5-10 seconds or as long as possible. Remove mouthpiece prior to exhalation. Patient should not breathe out through the mouthpiece. If any powder remains in capsule, exhale and inhale again. Repeat until capsule is empty. Throw away empty capsule; do not leave in inhaler. Always keep capsules and inhaler dry. **Note:** If a dose is missed, take as soon as possible on that day; do not take 2 doses on the same day.

Nursing Actions

Physical Assessment Assess potential for interactions with any drugs that may add to anticholinergic effects.

Patient Education

• Discuss specific use of drug and side effects with patient as it relates to treatment. (HCAHPS: During this hospital stay, were you given any medicine that you had not taken before? Before giving you any new medicine, how often did hospital staff tell you what the medicine was for? How often did hospital staff describe possible side effects in a way you could understand?)

• Patient may experience fatigue, asthenia, constipation, blurred vision, flushing, xerostomia, xeroderma, dysgeusia, nausea, rhinitis, rhinorrhea, pharyngitis, or injection site irritation. Have patient report immediately to prescriber severe dizziness, syncope, illogical thinking, urinary retention, angina, tachycardia, arrhythmia, diarrhea, abdominal edema, dyspepsia, vision changes, considerable headache, tachypnea, significant asthenia, mood changes, or sexual dysfunction (HCAHPS).

• Educate patient about signs of a significant reaction (eg, wheezing; chest tightness; fever; itching; bad cough; blue skin color; seizures; or swelling of face, lips, tongue, or throat). **Note:** This is not a comprehensive list of all side effects. Patient should consult prescriber for additional questions.

Intended Use and Disclaimer: Should not be printed and given to patients. This information is intended to serve as a concise initial reference for healthcare professionals to use when discussing medications with a patient. You must ultimately rely on your own discretion, experience and judgment in diagnosing, treating and advising patients.

Golimumab (goe LIM ue mab)

Brand Names: U.S. Simponi; Simponi Aria
Index Terms CNTO-148
Pharmacologic Category Antipsoriatic Agent; Antirheumatic, Disease Modifying; Monoclonal Antibody; Tumor Necrosis Factor (TNF) Blocking Agent
Medication Guide Available Yes
Pregnancy Risk Factor B
Lactation Excretion in breast milk unknown/not recommended
Breast-Feeding Considerations It is not known whether golimumab is secreted in human milk. Because many immunoglobulins are secreted in milk and the potential for serious adverse reactions exists, a decision should be made whether to discontinue nursing or discontinue the drug, taking into account the importance of the drug to the mother.

Use

Ankylosing spondylitis (Simponi): Treatment of active ankylosing spondylitis

Psoriatic arthritis (Simponi): Treatment of active psoriatic arthritis (either alone or in combination with methotrexate)

Rheumatoid arthritis (Simponi, Simponi Aria): Treatment of moderately-to-severely active rheumatoid arthritis (in combination with methotrexate)

Ulcerative colitis (Simponi): Treatment of moderately-to-severely active ulcerative colitis in patients with corticosteroid dependence or who are refractory or intolerant to oral aminosalicylates, oral corticosteroids, azathioprine, or 6-mercaptopurine (to induce and maintain clinical response, improve mucosal appearance during induction, induce clinical remission, and achieve and sustain remission in induction responders)

Mechanism of Action/Effect Monoclonal antibody that binds to human tumor necrosis factor alpha (TNFα), thereby decreasing inflammatory and other responses

Contraindications There are no contraindications listed in the manufacturer's U.S. labeling.

Canadian labeling: Hypersensitivity to golimumab, latex, or any other component of formulation or packaging; patients with severe infections (eg, sepsis, tuberculosis, opportunistic infections); moderate or severe heart failure (NYHA class III/IV)

Warnings/Precautions [U.S. Boxed Warning]: Patients receiving golimumab are at increased risk for serious infections which may result in hospitalization and/or fatality; infections usually developed in patients receiving concomitant immunosuppressive agents (eg, methotrexate or corticosteroids). Active tuberculosis (or reactivation of latent tuberculosis), invasive fungal (including aspergillosis, blastomycosis, candidiasis, coccidioidomycosis, histoplasmosis, and pneumocystosis) and other bacterial, viral or other opportunistic infections (including legionellosis and listeriosis) have been reported in patients receiving TNF-blocking agents, including golimumab. May present as disseminated (rather than local) disease. Histoplasmosis testing (antigen or antibody) may be negative in some patients with active infection. Monitor closely for signs/symptoms of infection. Discontinue for serious infection or sepsis. Consider risks versus benefits prior to use in patients with a history of chronic or recurrent infection. Consider empiric antifungal therapy in patients who are at risk for invasive fungal infection and develop severe systemic illness. Discontinue in patients who develop a serious infection or an opportunistic infection. Caution should be exercised when considering use in the elderly, patients taking concomitant immunosuppressants, patients with a history of opportunistic infection, patients with comorbid conditions that predispose them to infections (eg, diabetes), or residence/travel from areas of endemic mycoses (blastomycosis, coccidioidomycosis, histoplasmosis). Do not initiate golimumab therapy in patients with with active infection, including localized infection which is clinically important. Patients who develop a new infection while undergoing treatment should be monitored closely.

[U.S. Boxed Warning]: Tuberculosis (disseminated or extrapulmonary) has been reported in patients receiving golimumab; both reactivation of latent infection and new infections have been reported. Patients should be evaluated for tuberculosis risk factors and latent tuberculosis infection (with a tuberculin skin test) prior to and during therapy. Treatment of latent tuberculosis should be initiated before use. Patients with initial negative tuberculin skin tests should receive continued monitoring for tuberculosis throughout treatment; active tuberculosis has developed in this population during treatment with TNF-blocking agents. Use with caution in patients who have resided in regions where tuberculosis is endemic. Consider antituberculosis therapy if an adequate course of treatment cannot be confirmed in patients with a history of latent or active tuberculosis or for patients with risk factors despite negative skin test.

Rare reactivation of hepatitis B virus (HBV) has occurred in chronic virus carriers (usually in patients receiving concomitant immunosuppressants); evaluate prior to initiation in all patients. Patients who test positive for HBV surface antigen should be referred for hepatitis B evaluation/treatment prior to golimumab initiation. Monitor during and for several months following discontinuation of treatment in HBV carriers; interrupt therapy if reactivation occurs and treat appropriately with antiviral therapy; if resumption of therapy is deemed necessary, exercise caution and monitor patient closely.

Patients should be brought up to date with all immunizations before initiating therapy. Live vaccines should not be given concurrently. In clinical trials, humoral response to pneumococcal vaccine was not suppressed in psoriatic arthritis patients.

[U.S. Boxed Warning]: Lymphoma and other malignancies (some fatal) have been reported in children and adolescent patients receiving TNF-blocking agents. Half of the malignancies reported in children were lymphomas (Hodgkin's and non-Hodgkin's) while other cases varied and included malignancies not typically observed in this population. The onset of malignancy was after a median of 30 months (range: 1-84 months) after the initiation of the TNF-blocking agent. The impact of golimumab on the development and course of malignancy is not fully defined. Compared to the general population, an increased risk of lymphoma has been noted in clinical trials; however, rheumatoid arthritis alone has been previously associated with an increased rate of lymphoma. Lymphomas and other malignancies were also observed (at rates higher than expected for the general population) in adult patients receiving TNF-blocking agents. Hepatosplenic T-cell lymphoma (HSTCL), a rare T-cell lymphoma, has also been associated with TNF-blocking agents, primarily reported in adolescent and young adult males with Crohn's disease (or in some cases ulcerative colitis) treated with a TNF-blocking agent and concurrent or prior azathioprine or mercaptopurine. Melanoma and Merkel cell carcinoma have been reported in patients receiving TNF-blocking agents including golimumab. Perform periodic skin examinations in all patients during therapy, particularly those at increased risk for skin cancer. Consider risks versus benefits in patients with a known malignancy (other than a successfully treated nonmelanoma skin cancer) and if considering continuing treatment in a patient who develops a malignancy. Rare cases of pancytopenia and other significant cytopenias, including aplastic anemia, have been reported with TNF-blocking agents. Pancytopenia, leukopenia, neutropenia and thrombocytopenia have occurred with golimumab; use with caution in patients with underlying hematologic disorders. Consider discontinuing therapy with significant hematologic abnormalities. Treatment may result in the formation of autoimmune antibodies; cases of autoimmune disease have not been described.

Use with caution in patients with pre-existing or recent onset central or peripheral nervous system demyelinating disorders; rare cases of new-onset or exacerbation of demyelinating disorders (eg, multiple sclerosis, optic neuritis, Guillain-Barré syndrome, polyneuropathy) have been reported. Consider discontinuing use in patients who develop peripheral or central nervous system demyelinating disorders during treatment. Use with caution in patients with heart failure or decreased left ventricular function; monitor closely and discontinue with new-onset or worsening of symptoms. Canadian labeling contraindicates use in moderate or severe heart failure (NYHA class III/IV). Severe systemic hypersensitivity reactions (including anaphylaxis), have been reported (some have occurred with the first dose) following subcutaneous administration; discontinue immediately if signs develop and initiate appropriate treatment.

Avoid concomitant use with abatacept (increased incidence of serious infections) or anakinra (increased incidence of neutropenia and serious infection). Potentially significant drug-drug interactions may exist, requiring dose or frequency adjustment, additional monitoring, and/or selection of alternative therapy. Use caution when switching between biological disease-modifying antirheumatic drugs (DMARDs); overlapping of biological activity may increase the risk for infection. Use with caution in the elderly (general incidence of infection is higher). Packaging (prefilled syringe and needle cover) contains dry natural rubber (latex). Some dosage forms may contain dry natural rubber (latex) and/or polysorbate 80. The safety and efficacy of switching between the I.V. and SubQ formulations and routes have not been studied.

Drug Interactions

Avoid Concomitant Use
Avoid concomitant use of Golimumab with any of the following: Abatacept; Anakinra; BCG; Belimumab; Canakinumab; Certolizumab Pegol; InFLIXimab; Natalizumab; Pimecrolimus; Rilonacept; Tacrolimus (Topical); Tocilizumab; Tofacitinib; Vaccines (Live)

Decreased Effect
Golimumab may decrease the levels/effects of: BCG; Coccidioidin Skin Test; Sipuleucel-T; Vaccines (Inactivated); Vaccines (Live)

The levels/effects of Golimumab may be decreased by: Echinacea

Increased Effect/Toxicity
Golimumab may increase the levels/effects of: Abatacept; Anakinra; Belimumab; Canakinumab; Certolizumab Pegol; InFLIXimab; Leflunomide; Natalizumab; Rilonacept; Tofacitinib; Vaccines (Live)

The levels/effects of Golimumab may be increased by: Abciximab; Denosumab; Pimecrolimus; Roflumilast; Tacrolimus (Topical); Tocilizumab; Trastuzumab

Adverse Reactions
>10%:

Hematologic & oncologic: Positive ANA titer (≥1:160 titer, newly positive; 17% intravenous, 4% subcutaneous)

Miscellaneous: Infection (27% to 28%)

Respiratory: Upper respiratory tract infection (includes laryngitis, nasopharyngitis, pharyngitis, and rhinitis; 13% to 16%)

1% to 10%:

Cardiovascular: Hypertension (3%)

Central nervous system: Dizziness (<1% to 2%), paresthesia (<1% to 2%)

Dermatologic: Skin rash (<1% to 3%)

Gastrointestinal: Constipation (≤1%)

Hematologic & oncologic: Leukopenia (≤1%)

Hepatic: Increased serum ALT (subcutaneous 4%; ≥3 x ULN: subcutaneous 2%; ≥5 x ULN: intravenous <1%), increased serum AST (<1% to 3%)

Immunologic: Antibody development (3% to 7%)

Infection: Viral infection (4% to 5%; includes herpes and influenza), fungal infection (superficial; <1% to 2%), bacterial infection (intravenous 1%)

Local: Injection site reaction (subcutaneous 3% to 6%)

Miscellaneous: Fever (1% to 2%), infusion related reaction (intravenous 1%)

Respiratory: Bronchitis (2% to 3%), sinusitis (<1% to 2%)

Available Dosage Forms

Solution, Intravenous [preservative free]:

Simponi Aria: 50 mg/4 mL (4 mL)

Solution, Subcutaneous [preservative free]:

Simponi: 50 mg/0.5 mL (0.5 mL); 100 mg/mL (1 mL)

General Dosage Range

I.V.: *Adults:* 2 mg/kg at weeks 0 and 4 and then every 8 weeks thereafter

SubQ: *Adults:* Induction: 200 mg at week 0, then 100 mg at week 2; maintenance: 100 mg every 4 weeks (ulcerative colitis) **or** 50 mg once per month

Administration

I.V. Dilute prior to use. Infuse over 30 minutes, using an infusion set with an in-line low protein-binding 0.22 micron filter. Do not infuse in the same line with other medications.

Injectable Detail pH: 5.5 (solution in intact vial or syringe)

Subcutaneous Hold autoinjector firmly against skin and inject subcutaneously into thigh, lower abdomen (below navel), or upper arm. A loud click is heard when injection has begun. Continue to hold autoinjector against skin until second click is heard (may take 3-15 seconds). Following second click, lift autoinjector from injection site. Rotate injection sites and avoid injecting into tender, red, hard, or bruised skin. If multiple injections are required for a single dose, administer at different sites on body.

Preparation for Administration Intact solution should be colorless to light yellow.

SubQ: Bring to room temperature by allowing syringe/autoinjector to sit at room temperature outside the carton for 30 minutes prior to administration (do not warm in any other way). Do not use if discolored, cloudy, or if foreign particles are present.

I.V.: Do not use if solution in vial is discolored, or contains opaque or foreign particles. Dilute for infusion by slowly adding calculated dose/volume to sodium chloride 0.9% to a total volume of 100 mL. Gently mix. Visually inspect; do not use if particulate matter exists or if discolored.

Discard unused portion of vial/syringe/autoinjector.

Storage/Stability Store intact vials and syringes refrigerated at 2°C to 8°C (36°F to 46°F); do not freeze. Do not shake. Protect from light.

I.V.: Solutions diluted for infusion may be stored at room temperature for 4 hours.

Nursing Actions

Physical Assessment Monitor closely for signs and symptoms of infection; malignancy (eg, splenomegaly, hepatomegaly, abdominal pain, persistent fever, night sweats, weight loss); liver dysfunction. Assess results of laboratory tests (PDD) at regular intervals during treatment. If self-injected, teach patient appropriate injection technique and syringe/needle disposal.

Patient Education

• Discuss specific use of drug and side effects with patient as it relates to treatment. (HCAHPS: During this hospital stay, were you given any medicine that you had not taken before? Before giving you any new medicine, how often did hospital staff tell you what the medicine was for? How often did hospital staff describe possible side effects in a way you could understand?)

• Patient may experience injection site irritation. Have patient report immediately to prescriber signs of infection, signs of hepatic impairment, signs of lupus, angina, significant asthenia, paresthesia, vision changes, enlarged lymph nodes, night sweats, excessive weight gain or loss, ecchymosis, hemorrhaging, pallor, considerable headache, dyspnea, edema of extremities, or eczema (HCAHPS).

• Educate patient about signs of a significant reaction (eg, wheezing; chest tightness; fever; itching; bad cough; blue skin color; seizures; or swelling of face, lips, tongue, or throat). **Note:** This is not a comprehensive list of all side effects. Patient should consult prescriber for additional questions.

Intended Use and Disclaimer: Should not be printed and given to patients. This information is intended to serve as a concise initial reference for healthcare professionals to use when discussing medications with a patient. You must ultimately rely on your own discretion, experience and judgment in diagnosing, treating and advising patients.

Goserelin (GOE se rel in)

Brand Names: U.S. Zoladex

Index Terms Goserelin Acetate; ICI-118630; ZDX ▶

Pharmacologic Category Antineoplastic Agent, Gonadotropin-Releasing Hormone Agonist; Gonadotropin Releasing Hormone Agonist

Pregnancy Risk Factor X (endometriosis, endometrial thinning); D (advanced breast cancer)

Lactation Excretion in breast milk unknown/not recommended

Breast-Feeding Considerations Goserelin is inactivated when used orally. Breast-feeding is not recommended by the manufacturer.

Use Treatment of locally confined prostate cancer; palliative treatment of advanced prostate cancer; palliative treatment of advanced breast cancer in pre- and perimenopausal women; treatment of endometriosis, including pain relief and reduction of endometriotic lesions; endometrial thinning agent as part of treatment for dysfunctional uterine bleeding

Mechanism of Action/Effect LHRH synthetic analog of luteinizing hormone-releasing hormone also known as gonadotropin-releasing hormone (GnRH)

Contraindications Hypersensitivity to goserelin, GnRH, GnRH agonist analogues, or any component of the formulation; pregnancy (except if using for palliative treatment of advanced breast cancer)

Warnings/Precautions Hazardous agent - use appropriate precautions for handling and disposal (NIOSH, 2012). Allergic hypersensitivity reactions (including anaphylaxis) and antibody formation may occur; monitor. Androgen-deprivation therapy may increase the risk for cardiovascular disease (Levine, 2010). Transient increases in serum testosterone (in men with prostate cancer) and estrogen (in women with breast cancer) may result in a worsening of disease signs and symptoms (tumor flare) during the first few weeks of treatment. Urinary tract obstruction or spinal cord compression have been reported when used for prostate cancer; closely observe patients for weakness, paresthesias, and urinary tract obstruction in first few weeks of therapy. Decreased bone density has been reported in women and may be irreversible; use caution if other risk factors are present; evaluate and institute preventative treatment if necessary.

Women of childbearing potential should not receive therapy until pregnancy has been excluded. Nonhormonal contraception is recommended for premenopausal women during therapy and for 12 weeks after therapy is discontinued. Cervical resistance may be increased; use caution when dilating the cervix. The 3-month implant currently has no approved indications for use in women. Rare cases of pituitary apoplexy (frequently secondary to pituitary adenoma) have been observed with GnRH agonist administration (onset from 1 hour to usually <2 weeks); may present as sudden headache, vomiting, visual or mental status changes, and infrequently cardiovascular collapse;

immediate medical attention required. Hyperglycemia has been reported in males and may manifest as diabetes or worsening of pre-existing diabetes. Decreased AUC may be observed when using the 3-month implant in obese patients. Monitor testosterone levels if desired clinical response is not observed. Safety and efficacy have not been established in pediatric patients.

Drug Interactions

Avoid Concomitant Use

Avoid concomitant use of Goserelin with any of the following: Indium 111 Capromab Pendetide

Decreased Effect

Goserelin may decrease the levels/effects of: Antidiabetic Agents; Indium 111 Capromab Pendetide

Increased Effect/Toxicity There are no known significant interactions involving an increase in effect.

Adverse Reactions Percentages reported with the 1-month implant:

>10%:

Cardiovascular: Vasodilatation (female 57%), peripheral edema (female 21%),

Central nervous system: Headache (female 32% to 75%; male 1% to 5%), emotional lability (female 60%), depression (female 54%; male 1% to 5%), pain (8% to 17%), dyspareunia (female 14%), insomnia (5% to 11%)

Dermatologic: Diaphoresis (female 16% to 45%; male 6%), acne vulgaris (female 42%; usually within 1 month after starting treatment), seborrhea (female 26%)

Endocrine & metabolic: Hot flash (female 57% to 96%; male 62%), decreased libido (female 48% to 61%), increased libido (female 12%)

Gastrointestinal: Abdominal pain (female 7% to 11%), nausea (5% to 11%)

Genitourinary: Vaginitis (75%), breast atrophy (female 33%), sexual disorder (male 21%), breast hypertrophy (female 18%), decrease in erectile frequency (18%), pelvic symptoms (female 9% to 18%), genitourinary signs and symptoms (lower; male 13%)

Hematologic & oncologic: Tumor flare (female 23%; male: Incidence not reported)

Infection: Infection (female 13%; male: Incidence not reported)

Neuromuscular & skeletal: Decreased bone mineral density (female 23%; ~4% decrease from baseline in 6 months; male: Incidence not reported), weakness (female 11%)

1% to 10%:

Cardiovascular: Cardiac arrhythmia, cardiac failure, cerebrovascular accident, chest pain, edema, hypertension, myocardial infarction, palpitations, peripheral vascular disease, tachycardia

Central nervous system: Abnormality in thinking, anxiety, chills, dizziness, drowsiness, lethargy, malaise, migraine, nervousness, paresthesia, voice disorder

Dermatologic: Alopecia, hair disease, pruritus, skin discoloration, skin rash, xeroderma

Endocrine & metabolic: Gout, hirsutism, hyperglycemia, weight gain, weight loss

Gastrointestinal: Anorexia, constipation, diarrhea, dyspepsia, flatulence, gastric ulcer, increased appetite, vomiting, xerostomia

Genitourinary: Breast swelling, breast tenderness, dysmenorrhea, mastalgia, urinary frequency, urinary tract infection, urinary tract obstruction, uterine hemorrhage, vaginal hemorrhage, vulvovaginitis

Hematologic & oncologic: Anemia, bruise, hemorrhage

Hypersensitivity: Hypersensitivity reaction

Local: Application site reaction

Neuromuscular & skeletal: Arthralgia, arthropathy, back pain, hypertonia, leg cramps, myalgia

Ophthalmic: Amblyopia, dry eye syndrome

Renal: Renal insufficiency

Respiratory: Bronchitis, chronic obstructive pulmonary disease, cough, epistaxis, flu-like symptoms, pharyngitis, rhinitis, sinusitis, upper respiratory tract infection

Miscellaneous: Fever

Pharmacodynamics/Kinetics

Onset of Action

Females: Estradiol suppression reaches postmenopausal levels within 3 weeks and FSH and LH are suppressed to follicular phase levels within 4 weeks of initiation.

Males: Testosterone suppression reaches castrate levels within 2-4 weeks after initiation.

Duration of Action

Females: Estradiol, LH and FSH generally return to baseline levels within 12 weeks following the last monthly implant.

Males: Testosterone levels maintained at castrate levels throughout the duration of therapy.

Available Dosage Forms

Implant, Subcutaneous:

Zoladex: 3.6 mg (1 ea); 10.8 mg (1 ea)

General Dosage Range SubQ: *Adults:* 3.6 mg every 28 days **or** 10.8 mg every 12 weeks

Administration

Other SubQ: Administer implant by inserting needle at a 30-45 degree angle into the anterior abdominal wall below the navel line. Goserelin is an implant; therefore, do not attempt to eliminate air bubbles prior to injection (may displace implant). Do not attempt to aspirate prior to injection; if a large vessel is penetrated, blood will be visualized in the syringe chamber (if vessel is penetrated, withdraw needle and inject elsewhere with a new syringe). Do not penetrate into muscle or peritoneum. Implant may be detected by ultrasound if removal is required.

Hazardous agent; use appropriate precautions for handling and disposal (NIOSH, 2012).

Storage/Stability Zoladex® should be stored at room temperature not to exceed 25°C (77°F). Protect from light.

Nursing Actions

Physical Assessment Observe patients for weakness and paresthesias in the first few weeks of therapy. Monitor for symptoms of hypoglycemia.

Patient Education

- Discuss specific use of drug and side effects with patient as it relates to treatment. (HCAHPS: During this hospital stay, were you given any medicine that you had not taken before? Before giving you any new medicine, how often did hospital staff tell you what the medicine was for? How often did hospital staff describe possible side effects in a way you could understand?)
- Patient may experience acne vulgaris, mastalgia, headache, sexual dysfunction, diarrhea, hot flashes, lack of appetite, hyperhidrosis, insomnia, or vaginal irritation. Have patient report immediately to prescriber signs of hyperglycemia, signs of hypercalcemia, signs of depression (ie, suicidal ideation, anxiety, emotional instability, illogical thinking), dyspnea, excessive weight gain, edema of extremities, significant asthenia, urinary retention, dysuria, injection site irritation, back pain, dyspepsia, hematuria, urine discoloration, hematemesis, osteodynia, mastalgia, paresthesia, tachycardia, arrhythmia, chills, pharyngitis, severe dizziness, signs of pituitary apoplexy, angina, strength differences from one side to another, difficulty speaking or thinking, change in balance, or vision changes (HCAHPS).
- Educate patient about signs of a significant reaction (eg, wheezing; chest tightness; fever; itching; bad cough; blue skin color; seizures; or swelling or face, lips, tongue, or throat). **Note:** This is not a comprehensive list of all side effects. Patient should consult prescriber for additional questions.

Intended Use and Disclaimer: Should not be printed and given to patients. This information is intended to serve as a concise initial reference for healthcare professionals to use when discussing medications with a patient. You must ultimately rely on your own discretion, experience and judgment in diagnosing, treating and advising patients.

Granisetron (gra NI se tron)

Brand Names: U.S. Granisol; Sancuso
Index Terms BRL 43694; Kytril
Pharmacologic Category Antiemetic; Selective 5-HT₃ Receptor Antagonist

◄ **Medication Safety Issues**
Sound-alike/look-alike issues:
Granisetron may be confused with dolasetron, ondansetron, palonosetron

Pregnancy Risk Factor B

Lactation Excretion in breast milk unknown/use caution

Breast-Feeding Considerations It is not known if granisetron is excreted in breast milk. The manufacturer recommends that caution be exercised when administering granisetron to nursing women.

Use Prophylaxis of nausea and vomiting associated with emetogenic chemotherapy and radiation therapy; prophylaxis and treatment of postoperative nausea and vomiting (PONV)

Unlabeled Use Breakthrough treatment of nausea and vomiting associated with chemotherapy

Mechanism of Action/Effect Selective 5-HT$_3$ receptor antagonist, blocking serotonin, both peripherally on vagal nerve terminals and centrally in the chemoreceptor trigger zone.

Contraindications Hypersensitivity to granisetron or any component of the formulation

Warnings/Precautions Use with caution in patients with congenital long QT syndrome or other risk factors for QT prolongation (eg, medications known to prolong QT interval, electrolyte abnormalities, and cumulative high-dose anthracycline therapy). 5-HT$_3$ antagonists have been associated with a number of dose-dependent increases in ECG intervals (eg, PR, QRS duration, QT/QT$_c$, JT), usually occurring 1-2 hours after I.V. administration. In general, these changes are not clinically relevant, however, when used in conjunction with other agents that prolong these intervals, arrhythmia may occur. When used with agents that prolong the QT interval (eg, Class I and III antiarrhythmics), clinically relevant QT interval prolongation may occur resulting in torsade de pointes. I.V. formulations of 5-HT$_3$ antagonists have more association with ECG interval changes, compared to oral formulations.

For chemotherapy-related emesis, **granisetron should be used on a scheduled basis, not on an "as needed" (PRN) basis**, since data support the use of this drug in the prevention of nausea and vomiting and not in the rescue of nausea and vomiting. Granisetron should be used only in the first 24-48 hours of receiving chemotherapy or radiation. Data do not support any increased efficacy of granisetron in delayed nausea and vomiting.

Use with caution in patients allergic to other 5-HT$_3$ receptor antagonists; cross-reactivity has been reported. Routine prophylaxis for PONV is not recommended in patients where there is little expectation of nausea and vomiting postoperatively. In patients where nausea and vomiting must be avoided postoperatively, administer to all patients even when expected incidence of nausea and vomiting is low. Use caution following abdominal surgery or in chemotherapy-induced nausea and vomiting; may mask progressive ileus or gastric distention. Application site reactions, generally mild, have occurred with transdermal patch use; if skin reaction is severe or generalized, remove patch. Cover patch application site with clothing to protect from natural or artificial sunlight exposure while patch is applied and for 10 days following removal; granisetron may potentially be affected by natural or artificial sunlight. Do not apply patch to red, irritated, or damaged skin. Injection contains benzyl alcohol (1 mg/mL) and should not be used in neonates.

Drug Interactions

Avoid Concomitant Use
Avoid concomitant use of Granisetron with any of the following: Apomorphine; Highest Risk QTc-Prolonging Agents; Ivabradine; Mifepristone

Decreased Effect
Granisetron may decrease the levels/effects of: Tapentadol; TraMADol

Increased Effect/Toxicity
Granisetron may increase the levels/effects of: Apomorphine; Highest Risk QTc-Prolonging Agents; Moderate Risk QTc-Prolonging Agents

The levels/effects of Granisetron may be increased by: Ivabradine; Mifepristone; QTc-Prolonging Agents (Indeterminate Risk and Risk Modifying)

Adverse Reactions
>10%:
Central nervous system: Headache (3% to 21%; transdermal patch: 1%)
Gastrointestinal: Constipation (3% to 18%)
Neuromuscular & skeletal: Weakness (5% to 18%)
1% to 10%:
Cardiovascular: QT$_c$ prolongation (1% to 3%), hypertension (1% to 2%)
Central nervous system: Pain (10%), fever (3% to 9%), dizziness (4% to 5%), insomnia (<2% to 5%), somnolence (1% to 4%), anxiety (2%), agitation (<2%), CNS stimulation (<2%)
Dermatologic: Rash (1%)
Gastrointestinal: Diarrhea (3% to 9%), abdominal pain (4% to 6%), dyspepsia (3% to 6%), taste perversion (2%)
Hepatic: Liver enzymes increased (5% to 6%)
Renal: Oliguria (2%)
Respiratory: Cough (2%)
Miscellaneous: Infection (3%)

Pharmacodynamics/Kinetics
Duration of Action Oral, I.V.: Generally up to 24 hours

Available Dosage Forms
Patch, Transdermal:
Sancuso: 3.1 mg/24 hr (1 ea)

Solution, Intravenous:
Generic: 0.1 mg/mL (1 mL); 1 mg/mL (1 mL); 4 mg/4 mL (4 mL)
Solution, Intravenous [preservative free]:
Generic: 0.1 mg/mL (1 mL); 1 mg/mL (1 mL)
Solution, Oral:
Granisol: 2 mg/10 mL (30 mL)
Tablet, Oral:
Generic: 1 mg

General Dosage Range

I.V.:
Children ≥2 years: 10 mcg/kg/dose (maximum: 1 mg/dose) as a single dose or every 12 hours
Adults: 10 mcg/kg/dose (maximum: 1 mg/dose) as a single dose or every 12 hours **or** 1 mg as a single dose
Oral: *Adults:* 2 mg/day in 1-2 divided dose
Transdermal: *Adults:* 1 patch prior to chemotherapy; Maximum duration: Patch may be worn up to 7 days

Administration

I.V. Administer I.V. push over 30 seconds or as a 5- to 10-minute infusion
Prevention of PONV: Administer before induction of anesthesia or immediately before reversal of anesthesia.
Treatment of PONV: Administer undiluted over 30 seconds.

Injectable Detail pH: 4.7-7.3

Oral Doses should be given up to 1 hour prior to initiation of chemotherapy/radiation

Topical Transdermal (Sancuso®): Apply patch to clean, dry, intact skin on upper outer arm. Do not use on red, irritated or damaged skin. Remove patch from pouch immediately before application. Do not cut patch.

Storage/Stability
I.V.: Store at 15°C to 30°C (59°F to 86°F). Protect from light. Do not freeze vials. Stable when mixed in NS or D$_5$W for 7 days under refrigeration and for 3 days at room temperature.
Oral: Store tablet or oral solution at 15°C to 30°C (59°F to 86°F). Protect from light.
Transdermal patch: Store at 20°C to 25°C (68°F to 77°F). Keep patch in original packaging until immediately prior to use.

Nursing Actions

Physical Assessment Allergy history to selective 5-HT$_3$ receptor antagonists should be assessed prior to administering. Assess other drugs patient may be taking that may prolong QT interval. I.V.: Follow infusion specifics. Oral, I.V., and transdermal formulations have different doses and schedules and should not be administered on a PRN basis.

Patient Education
• Discuss specific use of drug and side effects with patient as it relates to treatment. (HCAHPS: During this hospital stay, were you given any medicine that you had not taken before? Before giving you any new medicine, how often did hospital staff tell you what the medicine was for? How often did hospital staff describe possible side effects in a way you could understand?)
• Patient may experience headache, constipation, diarrhea, or injection site pain or irritation. Have patient report immediately to prescriber tachycardia, arrhythmia, severe dizziness, syncope, angina, considerable asthenia, chills, pharyngitis, dyspepsia, difficulty with motor activity, abdominal edema, or significant skin irritation (HCAHPS).
• Educate patient about signs of a significant reaction (eg, wheezing; chest tightness; fever; itching; bad cough; blue skin color; seizures; or swelling of face, lips, tongue, or throat). **Note:** This is not a comprehensive list of all side effects. Patient should consult prescriber for additional questions.

Intended Use and Disclaimer: Should not be printed and given to patients. This information is intended to serve as a concise initial reference for healthcare professionals to use when discussing medications with a patient. You must ultimately rely on your own discretion, experience and judgment in diagnosing, treating and advising patients.

Griseofulvin (gri see oh FUL vin)

Brand Names: U.S. Grifulvin V; Gris-PEG
Index Terms Griseofulvin Microsize; Griseofulvin Ultramicrosize
Pharmacologic Category Antifungal Agent, Oral
Pregnancy Risk Factor X
Lactation Excretion in breast milk unknown/not recommended
Use Treatment of tinea infections of the skin, hair, and nails caused by susceptible species of *Microsporum, Epidermophyton,* or *Trichophyton*
Dosage Forms Considerations
Microsized formulations: Suspensions, Grifulvin V tablets
Ultramicrosize formulation: Gris-PEG tablets
Available Dosage Forms
Suspension, Oral:
Generic: 125 mg/5 mL (118 mL, 120 mL)
Tablet, Oral:
Grifulvin V: 500 mg
Gris-PEG: 125 mg, 250 mg
Generic: 125 mg, 250 mg, 500 mg
General Dosage Range Oral:
Microsize:
Children >2 years: 10-20 mg/kg/day in single or divided doses (maximum: 1000 mg daily)
Adults: 500-1000 mg daily in single or divided doses
Ultramicrosize:
Children >2 years: 5-15 mg/kg/day in single dose or 2 divided doses (maximum: 750 mg daily)

Adults: 375 mg daily in single or divided doses or up to 750 mg daily in divided doses

Administration

Oral Administer with a fatty meal (peanut butter or ice cream) to increase absorption, or with food or milk to avoid GI upset (*Red Book*, 2012)

Gris-PEG® tablets: May be swallowed whole or crushed and sprinkled onto 1 tablespoonful of applesauce and swallowed immediately without chewing.

Suspension: Shake well before use.

Nursing Actions

Physical Assessment Assess renal and hepatic function with long-term use. Monitor for CNS changes, gastrointestinal upset, rash, and opportunistic infection periodically during therapy.

Patient Education

- Discuss specific use of drug and side effects with patient as it relates to treatment. (HCAHPS: During this hospital stay, were you given any medicine that you had not taken before? Before giving you any new medicine, how often did hospital staff tell you what the medicine was for? How often did hospital staff describe possible side effects in a way you could understand?)
- Patient may experience asthenia. Have patient report immediately to prescriber signs of hepatic impairment, severe dizziness, syncope, illogical thinking, considerable headache, significant dyspepsia, intolerable nausea, chills, pharyngitis, flu-like syndrome, mood changes, paresthesia, or stomatitis (HCAHPS).
- Educate patient about signs of a significant reaction (eg, wheezing; chest tightness; fever; itching; bad cough; blue skin color; seizures; or swelling of face, lips, tongue, or throat). **Note:** This is not a comprehensive list of all side effects. Patient should consult prescriber for additional questions.

Intended Use and Disclaimer: Should not be printed and given to patients. This information is intended to serve as a concise initial reference for healthcare professionals to use when discussing medications with a patient. You must ultimately rely on your own discretion, experience and judgment in diagnosing, treating and advising patients.

GuaiFENesin (gwye FEN e sin)

Brand Names: U.S. Altarussin [OTC]; Bidex [OTC]; Buckleys Chest Congestion [OTC]; Cough Syrup [OTC]; Diabetic Siltussin DAS-Na [OTC]; Diabetic Tussin Mucus Relief [OTC]; Diabetic Tussin [OTC]; Fenesin IR [OTC]; Geri-Tussin [OTC]; GoodSense Mucus Relief [OTC]; Iophen-NR [OTC]; Liquibid [OTC]; Liquituss GG [OTC]; Mucinex Chest Congestion Child [OTC]; Mucinex For Kids [OTC]; Mucinex Maximum Strength [OTC]; Mucinex [OTC]; Mucosa [OTC]; Mucus Relief

Childrens [OTC]; Mucus Relief [OTC]; Mucus-ER [OTC]; Organ-I NR [OTC]; Q-Tussin [OTC]; Refenesen 400 [OTC]; Refenesen [OTC]; Robafen [OTC]; Robitussin Chest Congestion [OTC]; Robitussin Mucus+Chest Congest [OTC]; Scot-Tussin Expectorant [OTC]; Siltussin DAS [OTC]; Siltussin SA [OTC]; Tussin [OTC]; Xpect [OTC]

Index Terms Cheratussin; GG; Glycerol Guaiacolate

Pharmacologic Category Expectorant

Medication Safety Issues

Sound-alike/look-alike issues:

GuaiFENesin may be confused with guanFACINE

Mucinex® may be confused with Mucomyst®

Lactation Excretion in breast milk unknown

Use Help loosen phlegm and thin bronchial secretions to make coughs more productive

Available Dosage Forms

Liquid, Oral:

Buckleys Chest Congestion [OTC]: 100 mg/5 mL (118 mL)

Diabetic Siltussin DAS-Na [OTC]: 100 mg/5 mL (118 mL)

Diabetic Tussin [OTC]: 100 mg/5 mL (118 mL)

Diabetic Tussin Mucus Relief [OTC]: 200 mg/5 mL (118 mL)

Iophen-NR [OTC]: 100 mg/5 mL (473 mL)

Liquituss GG [OTC]: 200 mg/5 mL (118 mL, 473 mL)

Mucinex Chest Congestion Child [OTC]: 100 mg/5 mL (118 mL)

Mucus Relief Childrens [OTC]: 100 mg/5 mL (118 mL)

Robitussin Mucus+Chest Congest [OTC]: 100 mg/5 mL (118 mL)

Scot-Tussin Expectorant [OTC]: 100 mg/5 mL (30 mL, 118 mL, 240 mL, 480 mL, 3780 mL)

Siltussin DAS [OTC]: 100 mg/5 mL (118 mL)

Packet, Oral:

Mucinex For Kids [OTC]: 50 mg (12 ea); 100 mg (12 ea)

Solution, Oral:

Generic: 100 mg/5 mL (5 mL, 10 mL, 15 mL); 200 mg/10 mL (10 mL); 300 mg/15 mL (15 mL)

Syrup, Oral:

Altarussin [OTC]: 100 mg/5 mL (120 mL, 236 mL, 240 mL, 473 mL, 480 mL, 3840 mL)

Cough Syrup [OTC]: 100 mg/5 mL (118 mL, 473 mL)

Geri-Tussin [OTC]: 100 mg/5 mL (473 mL)

Q-Tussin [OTC]: 100 mg/5 mL (118 mL, 240 mL, 473 mL)

Robafen [OTC]: 100 mg/5 mL (118 mL, 473 mL)

Robitussin Chest Congestion [OTC]: 100 mg/5 mL (118 mL, 237 mL)

Siltussin SA [OTC]: 100 mg/5 mL (118 mL, 237 mL, 473 mL)

Tussin [OTC]: 100 mg/5 mL (118 mL, 237 mL)

Generic: 100 mg/5 mL (480 mL)

Tablet, Oral:
Bidex [OTC]: 400 mg
Diabetic Tussin Mucus Relief [OTC]: 400 mg
Fenesin IR [OTC]: 400 mg
GoodSense Mucus Relief [OTC]: 400 mg
Liquibid [OTC]: 400 mg
Mucosa [OTC]: 400 mg
Mucus Relief [OTC]: 400 mg
Organ-I NR [OTC]: 200 mg
Refenesen [OTC]: 200 mg
Refenesen 400 [OTC]: 400 mg
Xpect [OTC]: 400 mg
Generic: 200 mg, 400 mg
Tablet Extended Release 12 Hour, Oral:
Mucinex [OTC]: 600 mg
Mucinex Maximum Strength [OTC]: 1200 mg
Mucus-ER [OTC]: 600 mg
Generic: 600 mg

General Dosage Range Oral:
Extended release: *Children ≥12 years and Adults:* 600-1200 mg every 12 hours (maximum: 2.4 g/day)
Immediate release:
Children 6 months to 2 years: 25-50 mg every 4 hours (maximum: 300 mg/day)
Children 2-5 years: 50-100 mg every 4 hours (maximum: 600 mg/day)
Children 6-11 years: 100-200 mg every 4 hours (maximum: 1.2 g/day)
Children ≥12 years and Adults: 200-400 mg every 4 hours (maximum: 2.4 g/day)

Administration
Oral Do not crush, chew, or break extended release tablets. Administer with a full glass of water.

Nursing Actions
Patient Education
• Discuss specific use of drug and side effects with patient as it relates to treatment. (HCAHPS: During this hospital stay, were you given any medicine that you had not taken before? Before giving you any new medicine, how often did hospital staff tell you what the medicine was for? How often did hospital staff describe possible side effects in a way you could understand?)
• Patient may experience nausea (HCAHPS).
• Educate patient about signs of a significant reaction (eg, wheezing; chest tightness; fever; itching; bad cough; blue skin color; seizures; or swelling of face, lips, tongue, or throat). **Note:** This is not a comprehensive list of all side effects. Patient should consult prescriber for additional questions.

Intended Use and Disclaimer: Should not be printed and given to patients. This information is intended to serve as a concise initial reference for healthcare professionals to use when discussing medications with a patient. You must ultimately rely on your own discretion, experience and judgment in diagnosing, treating and advising patients.

Related Information
Oral Medications That Should Not Be Crushed or Altered *on page 1712*

Guaifenesin and Codeine
(gwye FEN e sin & KOE deen)

Brand Names: U.S. Allfen CD; Allfen CDX; Codar® GF; Dex-Tuss; Guaiatussin AC; Iophen C-NR; M-Clear; M-Clear WC; Mar-Cof® CG; Robafen AC; Virtussin A/C

Index Terms Codeine and Guaifenesin; Robitussin AC

Pharmacologic Category Antitussive; Cough Preparation; Expectorant

Use Temporary control of cough due to minor throat and bronchial irritation

Controlled Substance Capsule: C-V; Liquid products: C-V; Tablet: C-III

Available Dosage Forms
Capsule, oral:
M-Clear: Guaifenesin 200 mg and codeine 9 mg
Liquid, oral:
Codar® GF: Guaifenesin 200 mg and codeine 8 mg per 5 mL
Dex-Tuss: Guaifenesin 300 mg and codeine 10 mg per 5 mL
Iophen C-NR: Guaifenesin 100 mg and codeine 10 mg per 5 mL
M-Clear WC: Guaifenesin 100 mg and codeine 6.33 mg per 5 mL
Solution, oral: Guaifenesin 100 mg and codeine 10 mg per 5 mL
Mar-Cof® CG: Guaifenesin 225 mg and codeine 7.5 mg per 5 mL
Virtussin A/C: Guaifenesin 100 mg and codeine phosphate 10 mg per 5 mL
Syrup, oral: Guaifenesin 100 mg and codeine 10 mg per 5 mL (473 mL)
Guaiatussin AC, Robafen AC: Guaifenesin 100 mg and codeine 10 mg per 5 mL
Tablet, oral:
Allfen CD: Guaifenesin 400 mg and codeine 10 mg
Allfen CDX: Guaifenesin 400 mg and codeine 20 mg

General Dosage Range Oral: *Children ≥6 years and Adults:* Dosage varies greatly depending on product

Nursing Actions
Physical Assessment See individual agents.
Patient Education
• Discuss specific use of drug and side effects with patient as it relates to treatment. (HCAHPS: During this hospital stay, were you given any medicine that you had not taken before? Before giving you any new medicine, how often did hospital staff tell you what the medicine was

for? How often did hospital staff describe possible side effects in a way you could understand?)
- Patient may experience fatigue or hyperhidrosis. Have patient report immediately to prescriber severe dizziness, syncope, angina, tachycardia, dyspnea, illogical thinking, arrhythmia, hallucinations, mood changes, considerable dyspepsia, significant headache, difficult urination, tremors, vision changes, intolerable nausea, considerable constipation, or severe asthenia (HCAHPS).
- Educate patient about signs of a significant reaction (eg, wheezing; chest tightness; fever; itching; bad cough; blue skin color; seizures; or swelling of face, lips, tongue, or throat). **Note:** This is not a comprehensive list of all side effects. Patient should consult prescriber for additional questions.

Intended Use and Disclaimer: Should not be printed and given to patients. This information is intended to serve as a concise initial reference for healthcare professionals to use when discussing medications with a patient. You must ultimately rely on your own discretion, experience and judgment in diagnosing, treating and advising patients.

Related Information
Codeine *on page 363*
GuaiFENesin *on page 758*

Haemophilus b Conjugate and Hepatitis B Vaccine
(he MOF i lus bee KON joo gate & hep a TYE tis bee vak SEEN)

Brand Names: U.S. Comvax®
Index Terms *Haemophilus* b (meningococcal protein conjugate) Conjugate Vaccine; Hepatitis B Vaccine (Recombinant); Hib Conjugate Vaccine; Hib-HepB
Pharmacologic Category Vaccine, Inactivated (Bacterial); Vaccine, Inactivated (Viral)
Medication Safety Issues
Sound-alike/look-alike issues:
Comvax® may be confused with Recombivax [Recombivax HB®]
Pregnancy Risk Factor C
Use
Immunization against invasive disease caused by *H. influenzae* type b and against infection caused by all known subtypes of hepatitis B virus in infants 6 weeks to 15 months of age born of hepatitis B surface antigen (HBsAg)-negative mothers
Infants born of HBsAg-positive mothers or mothers of unknown HBsAg status should receive hepatitis B vaccine (recombinant) at birth and should complete the hepatitis B vaccination series given according to a particular schedule (refer to current ACIP recommendations).

Available Dosage Forms
Injection, suspension [preservative free]:
Comvax®: *Haemophilus* b capsular polysaccharide 7.5 mcg and hepatitis B surface antigen 5 mcg per 0.5 mL (0.5 mL)
General Dosage Range I.M.: *Infants ≥6 weeks:* 0.5 mL (series includes 3 doses)
Administration
I.M. Shake well prior to use. Administer 0.5 mL I.M. into anterolateral thigh [data suggests that injections given in the buttocks frequently are given into fatty tissue instead of into muscle and result in lower seroconversion rates]; **do not administer intravenously, intradermally, or subcutaneously.**

For patients at risk of hemorrhage following intramuscular injection, the ACIP recommends "it should be administered intramuscularly if, in the opinion of the physician familiar with the patient's bleeding risk, the vaccine can be administered with by this route with reasonable safety. If the patient receives antihemophilia or other similar therapy, intramuscular vaccination can be scheduled shortly after such therapy is administered. A fine needle (23 gauge or smaller) can be used for the vaccination and firm pressure applied to the site (without rubbing) for at least 2 minutes. The patient should be instructed concerning the risk of hematoma from the injection." Patients on anticoagulant therapy should be considered to have the same bleeding risks and treated as those with clotting factor disorders (CDC, 2011).

Simultaneous administration of vaccines helps ensure the patients will be fully vaccinated by the appropriate age. Simultaneous administration of vaccines is defined as administering >1 vaccine on the same day at different anatomic sites. The use of licensed combination vaccines is generally preferred over separate injections of the equivalent components. Separate vaccines should not be combined in the same syringe unless indicated by product specific labeling. Separate needles and syringes should be used for each injection. The ACIP prefers each dose of a specific vaccine in a series come from the same manufacturer when possible. Adolescents and adults should be vaccinated while seated or lying down. In general, preterm infants should be vaccinated at the same chronological age as full-term infants (CDC, 2011).

Antipyretics have not been shown to prevent febrile seizures. Antipyretics may be used to treat fever or discomfort following vaccination (CDC, 2011). One study reported that routine prophylactic administration of acetaminophen to prevent fever prior to vaccination decreased the immune response of some vaccines; the clinical significance of this reduction in immune response has not been established (Prymula, 2009).

Nursing Actions

Physical Assessment U.S. federal law requires entry into the patient's medical record.

Patient Education

• Discuss specific use of vaccine and side effects with patient as it relates to treatment. (HCAHPS: During this hospital stay, were you given any medicine that you had not taken before? Before giving you any new medicine, how often did hospital staff tell you what the medicine was for? How often did hospital staff describe possible side effects in a way you could understand?)

• Patient may experience fatigue, lack of appetite, nausea, or edema (HCAHPS).

• Educate patient about signs of a significant reaction (eg, wheezing; chest tightness; fever; itching; bad cough; blue skin color; seizures; or swelling of face, lips, tongue, or throat). **Note:** This is not a comprehensive list of all side effects. Patient should consult prescriber for additional questions.

Intended Use and Disclaimer: Should not be printed and given to patients. This information is intended to serve as a concise initial reference for healthcare professionals to use when discussing medications with a patient. You must ultimately rely on your own discretion, experience and judgment in diagnosing, treating and advising patients.

Related Information

Immunization Administration Recommendations *on page 1675*
Immunization Recommendations *on page 1680*

Haemophilus b Conjugate Vaccine
(he MOF fi lus bee KON joo gate vak SEEN)

Brand Names: U.S. ActHIB; Hiberix; PedvaxHIB

Index Terms *Haemophilus influenzae* Type b; Hib; PRP-OMP (PedvaxHIB); PRP-T (ActHIB); PRP-T (Hiberix)

Pharmacologic Category Vaccine, Inactivated (Bacterial)

Pregnancy Risk Factor C

Use

Active immunization for the prevention of invasive disease caused by *Haemophilus influenzae* type b (Hib):

ActHIB: Immunization of infants and children 2 months to 5 years of age.

Hiberix: Booster dose in children 15 months to 4 years of age (prior to fifth birthday).

PedvaxHIB: Routine vaccination of infants and children 2 to 71 months of age.

The Advisory Committee on Immunization Practices (ACIP) recommends routine vaccination of all children through age 59 months (CDC, 1993). Efficacy data are not available for use in older children and adults with chronic conditions associated with an increased risk of Hib disease.

However, a single dose may also be considered for older children, adolescents, and adults who did not receive the childhood series and who have a chronic condition associated with an increased risk of Hib disease (eg, splenectomy, sickle cell disease, leukemia, HIV infection) (CDC, 2012).

Available Dosage Forms

Injection, powder for reconstitution [preservative free]:

ActHIB: *Haemophilus* b capsular polysaccharide 10 mcg per 0.5 mL

Hiberix: *Haemophilus* b capsular polysaccharide 10 mcg per 0.5 mL

Injection, suspension:

PedvaxHIB: *Haemophilus* b capsular polysaccharide 7.5 mcg

General Dosage Range I.M.: *Infants and Children:* 0.5 mL (number of doses determined by age at first dose)

Administration

I.M. For I.M. administration; do not inject I.V., intradermally, or subcutaneously. Shake well prior to use. Administer into the anterolateral thigh or deltoid. Do not administer into buttocks due to potential risk of injury to sciatic nerve.

ActHIB, PedvaxHIB: If the primary series is delayed or interrupted, there is no need to start the series over, regardless of the interval between doses.

Hiberix: If Hiberix is inadvertently administered during the primary vaccination series, the dose can be counted as a valid PRP-T dose that does not need to be repeated if administered according to schedule. In this case, a total of 3 doses completes the primary series (CDC, 2009).

For patients at risk of hemorrhage following intramuscular injection, the ACIP recommends "it should be administered intramuscularly if, in the opinion of the physician familiar with the patient's bleeding risk, the vaccine can be administered by this route with reasonable safety. If the patient receives antihemophilia or other similar therapy, intramuscular vaccination can be scheduled shortly after such therapy is administered. A fine needle (23 gauge or smaller) can be used for the vaccination and firm pressure applied to the site (without rubbing) for at least 2 minutes. The patient should be instructed concerning the risk of hematoma from the injection." Patients on anticoagulant therapy should be considered to have the same bleeding risks and treated as those with clotting factor disorders (CDC, 2011).

Simultaneous administration of vaccines helps ensure the patients will be fully vaccinated by the appropriate age. Simultaneous administration of vaccines is defined as administering >1 vaccine on the same day at different anatomic sites. The use of licensed combination vaccines is generally preferred over separate injections of the equivalent components. Separate vaccines should not be combined in the same syringe unless indicated by product specific labeling. Separate needles and syringes should be used for each injection. The ACIP prefers each dose of a specific vaccine in a series come from the same manufacturer when possible. Adolescents and adults should be vaccinated while seated or lying down. In general, preterm infants should be vaccinated at the same chronological age as full-term infants (CDC, 2011).

Antipyretics have not been shown to prevent febrile seizures. Antipyretics may be used to treat fever or discomfort following vaccination (CDC, 2011). One study reported that routine prophylactic administration of acetaminophen to prevent fever prior to vaccination decreased the immune response of some vaccines; the clinical significance of this reduction in immune response has not been established (Prymula, 2009).

Nursing Actions

Physical Assessment U.S. federal law requires entry into the patient's medical record.

Patient Education

• Discuss specific use of vaccine and side effects with patient as it relates to treatment. (HCAHPS: During this hospital stay, were you given any medicine that you had not taken before? Before giving you any new medicine, how often did hospital staff tell you what the medicine was for? How often did hospital staff describe possible side effects in a way you could understand?)

• Patient may experience pain, redness or swelling at injection site, headache, fatigue, nausea, emesis, diarrhea, or dyspepsia. Have patient report immediately to prescriber severe injection site reaction (HCAHPS).

• Educate patient about signs of a significant reaction (eg, wheezing; chest tightness; fever; itching; bad cough; blue skin color; seizures; or swelling of face, lips, tongue, or throat). **Note:** This is not a comprehensive list of all side effects. Patient should consult prescriber for additional questions.

Intended Use and Disclaimer: Should not be printed and given to patients. This information is intended to serve as a concise initial reference for healthcare professionals to use when discussing medications with a patient. You must ultimately rely on your own discretion, experience and judgment in diagnosing, treating and advising patients.

Related Information

Immunization Administration Recommendations *on page 1675*

Immunization Recommendations *on page 1680*

Halcinonide (hal SIN oh nide)

Brand Names: U.S. Halog

Pharmacologic Category Corticosteroid, Topical

Medication Safety Issues

Sound-alike/look-alike issues:

Halcinonide may be confused with Halcion®

Halog® may be confused with Haldol®

Pregnancy Risk Factor C

Lactation Excretion in breast milk unknown/use caution

Use Relief of inflammatory and pruritic effects of corticosteroid-responsive dermatoses [high potency topical corticosteroid]

Available Dosage Forms

Cream, External:

Halog: 0.1% (30 g, 60 g, 216 g)

Ointment, External:

Halog: 0.1% (30 g, 60 g)

General Dosage Range Topical: *Children and Adults:* Apply sparingly 2-3 times daily

Administration

Topical For external use only; not for oral, ophthalmic, or intravaginal use. Wash hands before and after use. Apply a thin film to clean, dry skin and rub in gently. Avoid use of topical preparations on weeping or exudative lesions; occlusive dressings may be used on severe or resistant dermatoses.

Nursing Actions

Patient Education

• Discuss specific use of drug and side effects with patient as it relates to treatment. (HCAHPS: During this hospital stay, were you given any medicine that you had not taken before? Before giving you any new medicine, how often did hospital staff tell you what the medicine was for? How often did hospital staff describe possible side effects in a way you could understand?)

• Patient may experience xeroderma. Have patient report immediately to prescriber signs of hyperglycemia, skin changes, or severe skin irritation (HCAHPS).

• Educate patient about signs of a significant reaction (eg, wheezing; chest tightness; fever; itching; bad cough; blue skin color; seizures; or swelling of face, lips, tongue, or throat). **Note:** This is not a comprehensive list of all side effects. Patient should consult prescriber for additional questions.

Intended Use and Disclaimer: Should not be printed and given to patients. This information is intended to serve as a concise initial reference for healthcare professionals to use when discussing medications with a patient. You must ultimately rely on your own discretion, experience and judgment in diagnosing, treating and advising patients.

Haloperidol (ha loe PER i dole)

Brand Names: U.S. Haldol; Haldol Decanoate

Index Terms Haloperidol Decanoate; Haloperidol Lactate

Pharmacologic Category Antipsychotic Agent, Typical

Medication Safety Issues

Sound-alike/look-alike issues:

Haldol may be confused with Halcion, Halog, Stadol

BEERS Criteria medication:

This drug may be potentially inappropriate for use in geriatric patients (Quality of evidence - moderate; Strength of recommendation - strong).

International issues:

Haldol [U.S. and multiple international markets] may be confused with Halotestin brand name for fluoxymesterone [Great Britain]

Pregnancy Risk Factor C

Lactation Enters breast milk/not recommended

Breast-Feeding Considerations Haloperidol is found in breast milk and has been detected in the plasma and urine of nursing infants (Whalley, 1981; Yoshida, 1999). Breast engorgement, gynecomastia, and lactation are known side effects with the use of haloperidol. Breast-feeding is not recommended by the manufacturer.

Use Management of schizophrenia; control of tics and vocal utterances of Tourette's disorder in children and adults; severe behavioral problems in children

Unlabeled Use Treatment of nonschizophrenia psychosis; may be used for the emergency sedation of severely-agitated or delirious patients; treatment of ICU delirium; adjunctive treatment of ethanol dependence; postoperative nausea and vomiting (alternative therapy); psychosis/agitation related to Alzheimer's dementia

Mechanism of Action/Effect Haloperidol is a butyrophenone antipsychotic which blocks postsynaptic mesolimbic dopaminergic D_1 and D_2 receptors in the brain; depresses the release of hypothalamic and hypophyseal hormones; believed to depress the reticular activating system thus affecting basal metabolism, body temperature, wakefulness, vasomotor tone, and emesis

Contraindications Hypersensitivity to haloperidol or any component of the formulation; Parkinson's disease; severe CNS depression; coma

Warnings/Precautions [U.S. Boxed Warning]: Elderly patients with dementia-related psychosis treated with antipsychotics are at an increased risk of death compared to placebo. Most deaths appeared to be either cardiovascular (eg, heart failure, sudden death) or infectious (eg, pneumonia) in nature. Haloperidol is not approved for the treatment of dementia-related psychosis. Hypotension may occur, particularly with parenteral administration. Although the short-acting form (lactate) is used clinically, the I.V. use of the injection is not an FDA-approved route of administration; the decanoate form should never be administered intravenously.

May alter cardiac conduction and prolong QT interval; life-threatening arrhythmias have occurred with therapeutic doses of antipsychotics but risk may be increased with doses exceeding recommendations and/or intravenous administration (unlabeled route). Use caution or avoid use in patients with electrolyte abnormalities (eg, hypokalemia, hypomagnesemia), hypothyroidism, familial long QT syndrome, concomitant medications which may augment QT prolongation, or any underlying cardiac abnormality which may also potentiate risk. Monitor ECG closely for dose-related QT effects. Adverse effects of decanoate may be prolonged. Avoid in thyrotoxicosis.

Leukopenia, neutropenia, and agranulocytosis (sometimes fatal) have been reported in clinical trials and postmarketing reports with antipsychotic use; presence of risk factors (eg, pre-existing low WBC or history of drug-induced leuko-/neutropenia) should prompt periodic blood count assessment. Discontinue therapy at first signs of blood dyscrasias or if absolute neutrophil count <1000/mm^3.

May be sedating, use with caution in disorders where CNS depression is a feature. Effects may be potentiated when used with other sedative drugs or ethanol. Caution in patients with severe cardiovascular disease, predisposition to seizures, subcortical brain damage, or renal disease. Esophageal dysmotility and aspiration have been associated with antipsychotic use - use with caution in patients at risk of pneumonia (eg, Alzheimer's disease). Use associated with increased prolactin levels; clinical significance of hyperprolactinemia in patients with breast cancer or other prolactin-dependent tumors is unknown. May alter temperature regulation or mask toxicity of other drugs due to antiemetic effects. May cause orthostatic hypotension; use with caution in patients at risk of this effect or those who would tolerate transient hypotensive episodes (cerebrovascular disease, cardiovascular disease, or other medications which may predispose). Some tablets contain tartrazine. Antipsychotics have been associated with pigmentary retinopathy.

May cause anticholinergic effects (confusion, agitation, constipation, xerostomia, blurred vision, urinary retention). Therefore, they should be used with caution in patients with decreased gastrointestinal motility, urinary retention, BPH, xerostomia, visual problems, or narrow-angle glaucoma (screening is recommended). Relative to other neuroleptics, haloperidol has a low potency of cholinergic blockade.

May cause extrapyramidal symptoms (EPS), including pseudoparkinsonism, acute dystonic reactions, akathisia, and tardive dyskinesia. Risk of dystonia (and possibly other EPS) may be greater with increased doses, use of conventional antipsychotics, males, and younger patients. May be associated with neuroleptic malignant syndrome (NMS). Use in elderly patients with dementia is associated with an increased risk of mortality and cerebrovascular accidents; avoid antipsychotic use for behavioral problems associated with dementia unless alternative nonpharmacologic therapies have failed and patient may harm self or others. In addition, use may cause or exacerbate syndrome of inappropriate antidiuretic hormone secretion or hyponatremia; monitor sodium closely with initiation or dosage adjustments in older adults (Beers Criteria). Increased risk for developing tardive dyskinesia, particularly elderly women.

Drug Interactions

Avoid Concomitant Use

Avoid concomitant use of Haloperidol with any of the following: Aclidinium; Amisulpride; Azelastine (Nasal); Bosutinib; Conivaptan; FLUoxetine; Fusidic Acid (Systemic); Highest Risk QTc-Prolonging Agents; Ibrutinib; Ipratropium (Oral Inhalation); Ivabradine; Lomitapide; Metoclopramide; Mifepristone; Paraldehyde; QuiNIDine; Rivaroxaban; Simeprevir; Sulpiride; Thalidomide; Thioridazine; Tiotropium; Tolvaptan; Ulipristal; Umeclidinium

Decreased Effect

Haloperidol may decrease the levels/effects of: Amphetamines; Anti-Parkinson's Agents (Dopamine Agonist); Codeine; Ifosfamide; Quinagolide; Tamoxifen; Urea Cycle Disorder Agents

The levels/effects of Haloperidol may be decreased by: Anti-Parkinson's Agents (Dopamine Agonist); ARIPiprazole; Bosentan; CarBAMazepine; CYP3A4 Inducers (Strong); Dabrafenib; Deferasirox; Glycopyrrolate; Lithium formulations; Mitotane; Peginterferon Alfa-2b; Tocilizumab

Increased Effect/Toxicity

Haloperidol may increase the levels/effects of: Alcohol (Ethyl); Amisulpride; Analgesics (Opioid); Anticholinergics; ARIPiprazole; Avanafil; Azelastine (Nasal); Bosentan; Bosutinib; Budesonide (Systemic, Oral Inhalation); Buprenorphine; ChlorproMAZINE; CNS Depressants; Colchicine; CYP2D6 Substrates; CYP3A4 Substrates; DOXOrubicin (Conventional); Eplerenone; Everolimus; FentaNYL; Fesoterodine; Highest Risk QTc-Prolonging Agents; Hydrocodone; Ibrutinib; Imatinib; Ivacaftor; Lomitapide; Lurasidone; Methotrimeprazine; Methylphenidate; Metoprolol; Moderate Risk QTc-Prolonging Agents; Nebivolol; OxyCODONE; Paraldehyde; Pimecrolimus; QuiNIDine; Rivaroxaban; Salmeterol; Saxagliptin; Serotonin Modulators; Simeprevir; Sulpiride; Thalidomide; Thioridazine; Tiotropium; Tolvaptan; Ulipristal; Zolpidem

The levels/effects of Haloperidol may be increased by: Abiraterone Acetate; Acetylcholinesterase Inhibitors (Central); Aclidinium; ARIPiprazole; Brimonidine (Topical); ChlorproMAZINE; Conivaptan; CYP2D6 Inhibitors (Moderate); CYP2D6 Inhibitors (Strong); CYP3A4 Inhibitors (Moderate); CYP3A4 Inhibitors (Strong); Darunavir; Dasatinib; Doxylamine; FLUoxetine; FluvoxaMINE; Fusidic Acid (Systemic); HydrOXYzine; Ipratropium (Oral Inhalation); Ivabradine; Ivacaftor; Lithium formulations; Luliconazole; Magnesium Sulfate; Methotrimeprazine; Methylphenidate; Metoclopramide; Metyrosine; Mifepristone; Nonsteroidal Anti-Inflammatory Agents; Perampanel; Pramlintide; QTc-Prolonging Agents (Indeterminate Risk and Risk Modifying); QuiNIDine; Serotonin Modulators; Simeprevir; Sodium Oxybate; Stiripentol; Tetrabenazine; Umeclidinium

Nutritional/Ethanol Interactions

Ethanol: May increase CNS depression; monitor for increased effects with coadministration. Caution patients about effects.

Herb/Nutraceutical: Avoid valerian, St John's wort, kava kava, gotu kola (may increase CNS depression).

Adverse Reactions Frequency not defined.

Cardiovascular: Abnormal T waves with prolonged ventricular repolarization, arrhythmia, hyper-/hypotension, QT prolongation, sudden death, tachycardia, torsade de pointes

Central nervous system: Agitation, akathisia, altered central temperature regulation, anxiety, confusion, depression, drowsiness, dystonic reactions, euphoria, extrapyramidal reactions, headache, insomnia, lethargy, neuroleptic malignant syndrome (NMS), pseudoparkinsonian signs and symptoms, restlessness, seizure, tardive dyskinesia, tardive dystonia, vertigo

Dermatologic: Alopecia, contact dermatitis, hyperpigmentation, photosensitivity (rare), pruritus, rash

Endocrine & metabolic: Amenorrhea, breast engorgement, galactorrhea, gynecomastia, hyper-/hypoglycemia, hyponatremia, lactation, mastalgia, menstrual irregularities, sexual dysfunction

Gastrointestinal: Anorexia, constipation, diarrhea, dyspepsia, hypersalivation, nausea, vomiting, xerostomia

Genitourinary: Priapism, urinary retention

Hematologic: Agranulocytosis (rare), leukopenia, leukocytosis, neutropenia, anemia, lymphomonocytosis

Hepatic: Cholestatic jaundice, obstructive jaundice

Ocular: Blurred vision

Respiratory: Bronchospasm, laryngospasm

Miscellaneous: Diaphoresis, heat stroke

Pharmacodynamics/Kinetics

Onset of Action Sedation: I.M., I.V.: 30-60 minutes

Duration of Action Decanoate: ~3 weeks

Available Dosage Forms

Concentrate, Oral:

Generic: 2 mg/mL (5 mL, 15 mL, 120 mL)

Solution, Injection:
Haldol: 5 mg/mL (1 mL)
Generic: 5 mg/mL (1 mL, 10 mL)
Solution, Injection [preservative free]:
Generic: 5 mg/mL (1 mL)
Solution, Intramuscular:
Haldol Decanoate: 50 mg/mL (1 mL); 100 mg/mL (1 mL)
Generic: 50 mg/mL (1 mL, 5 mL); 100 mg/mL (1 mL, 5 mL)
Tablet, Oral:
Generic: 0.5 mg, 1 mg, 2 mg, 5 mg, 10 mg, 20 mg

General Dosage Range

I.M.:
Decanoate: *Adults:* Initial: 10-20 times daily oral dose at 4-week intervals; Maintenance: 10-15 times initial oral dose
Lactate:
Children 6-12 years: 1-3 mg/dose every 4-8 hours (maximum: 0.15 mg/kg/day)
Adults: 2-5 mg every 4-8 hours as needed
Oral:
Children 3-12 years (15-40 kg): Initial: 0.5 mg/day in 2-3 divided doses; Maintenance: 0.05-0.15 mg/kg/day in 2-3 divided doses
Adults: Initial: 0.5-5 mg 2-3 times/day; Maintenance: Up to 30 mg/day in 2-3 divided doses

Administration

I.M. The decanoate injectable formulation should be administered I.M. only; **do not give decanoate I.V.**

I.V.
Decanoate: Do **not** administer I.V.
Lactate: May be administered I.M. or I.V. (unlabeled route). Rate of I.V. administration not well defined; rates of a maximum of 5 mg/minute (Lerner, 1979) and 0.125 mg/kg (in 10 mL NS) over 1-2 minutes (Magliozzi, 1985) have been reported. **Note:** I.V. administration has been associated with QT prolongation and the manufacturer recommends ECG monitoring for QT prolongation and arrhythmias. Consult individual institutional policies and procedures prior to administration.

Injectable Detail
pH: 3-3.6

Oral Dilute the oral concentrate with water or juice before administration. **Note:** Avoid skin contact with oral medication; may cause contact dermatitis.

Preparation for Administration Haloperidol lactate may be administered IVPB or I.V. infusion in D_5W solutions. NS solutions should not be used due to reports of decreased stability and incompatibility.

Usual concentration range: 0.5-100 mg/50-100 mL D_5W.

Storage/Stability Protect oral dosage forms from light. Haloperidol lactate injection should be stored at controlled room temperature; do not freeze or expose to temperatures >40°C. Protect from light; exposure to light may cause discoloration and the development of a grayish-red precipitate over several weeks. Stability of standardized solutions is 38 days at room temperature (24°C).

Nursing Actions

Physical Assessment Monitor for sedation, anticholinergic and extrapyramidal symptoms, and QT_c prolongation with high doses. With I.M. or I.V. use, monitor closely for hypotension and cardiac irregularities. Initiate at lower doses and taper dosage slowly when discontinuing. Avoid skin contact with oral medication; may cause contact dermatitis (wash immediately with warm, soapy water).

Patient Education

- Discuss specific use of drug and side effects with patient as it relates to treatment. (HCAHPS: During this hospital stay, were you given any medicine that you had not taken before? Before giving you any new medicine, how often did hospital staff tell you what the medicine was for? How often did hospital staff describe possible side effects in a way you could understand?)
- Patient may experience presyncope, fatigue, blurred vision, illogical thinking, dizziness, nervousness and anxiety, constipation, xerostomia, weight gain, or impotence. Have patient report immediately to prescriber tachycardia, significant change in balance, tremors, urinary retention, severe asthenia, or pregnancy (HCAHPS).
- Educate patient about signs of a significant reaction (eg, wheezing; chest tightness; fever; itching; bad cough; blue skin color; seizures; or swelling of face, lips, tongue, or throat). **Note:** This is not a comprehensive list of all side effects. Patient should consult prescriber for additional questions.

Intended Use and Disclaimer: Should not be printed and given to patients. This information is intended to serve as a concise initial reference for healthcare professionals to use when discussing medications with a patient. You must ultimately rely on your own discretion, experience and judgment in diagnosing, treating and advising patients.

Heparin (HEP a rin)

Brand Names: U.S. Hep Flush-10
Index Terms Heparin Calcium; Heparin Lock Flush; Heparin Sodium; Heparinized Saline
Pharmacologic Category Anticoagulant; Anticoagulant, Heparin

Medication Safety Issues

Sound-alike/look-alike issues:

Heparin may be confused with Hespan®

High alert medication:

The Institute for Safe Medication Practices (ISMP) includes this medication among its list of drugs which have a heightened risk of causing significant patient harm when used in error.

National Patient Safety Goals:

The Joint Commission (TJC) requires healthcare organizations that provide anticoagulant therapy to have a process in place to reduce the risk of anticoagulant-associated patient harm. Patients receiving anticoagulants should receive individualized care through a defined process that includes standardized ordering, dispensing, administration, monitoring and education. This does not apply to routine short-term use of anticoagulants for prevention of venous thromboembolism when the expectation is that the patient's laboratory values will remain within or close to normal values (NPSG.03.05.01).

Administration issues:

The 100 unit/mL concentration should not be used to flush heparin locks, I.V. lines, or intra-arterial lines in neonates or infants <10 kg (systemic anticoagulation may occur). The 10 unit/mL flush concentration may inadvertently cause systemic anticoagulation in infants <1 kg who receive frequent flushes.

Other safety concerns:

Heparin sodium injection 10,000 units/mL and Hep-Lock U/P 10 units/mL have been confused with each other. Fatal medication errors have occurred between the two whose labels are both blue. **Never rely on color as a sole indicator to differentiate product identity.**

Labeling changes: Effective May 1st, 2013, heparin labeling is required to include the total amount of heparin per vial (rather than only including the amount of heparin per mL). During the transition, hospitals should consider only stocking the newly labeled heparin to avoid potential errors and confusion with the older labeling.

Heparin lock flush solution is intended only to maintain patency of I.V. devices and is **not** to be used for anticoagulant therapy.

Pregnancy Risk Factor C

Lactation Does not enter breast milk

Breast-Feeding Considerations Heparin is not excreted into breast milk and can be used in breast-feeding women (Guyatt, 2012). Some products contain benzyl alcohol as a preservative; their use in breast-feeding women is contraindicated by some manufacturers due to the association of gasping syndrome in premature infants.

Use Prophylaxis and treatment of thromboembolic disorders; as an anticoagulant for extracorporeal and dialysis procedures

Note: Heparin lock flush solution is intended only to maintain patency of I.V. devices and is **not** to be used for systemic anticoagulant therapy.

Unlabeled Use ST-elevation myocardial infarction (STEMI) as an adjunct to thrombolysis; unstable angina/non-STEMI (UA/NSTEMI); anticoagulant used during percutaneous coronary intervention (PCI)

Mechanism of Action/Effect Potentiates the action of antithrombin III and thereby inactivates thrombin (as well as activated coagulation factors IX, X, XI, XII, and plasmin) and prevents the conversion of fibrinogen to fibrin; heparin also stimulates release of lipoprotein lipase (lipoprotein lipase hydrolyzes triglycerides to glycerol and free fatty acids)

Contraindications Hypersensitivity to heparin or any component of the formulation (unless a life-threatening situation necessitates use and use of an alternative anticoagulant is not possible); severe thrombocytopenia; uncontrolled active bleeding except when due to disseminated intravascular coagulation (DIC); not for use when appropriate blood coagulation tests cannot be obtained at appropriate intervals (applies to full-dose heparin only)

Note: Some products contain benzyl alcohol as a preservative; their use in neonates, infants, or pregnant or nursing mothers is contraindicated by some manufacturers.

Warnings/Precautions Hypersensitivity reactions can occur. Only in life-threatening situations when use of an alternative anticoagulant is not possible should heparin be cautiously used in patients with a documented hypersensitivity reaction. Hemorrhage is the most common complication. Monitor for signs and symptoms of bleeding. Certain patients are at increased risk of bleeding. Risk factors for bleeding include bacterial endocarditis; congenital or acquired bleeding disorders; active ulcerative or angiodysplastic GI diseases; continuous GI tube drainage; severe uncontrolled hypertension; history of hemorrhagic stroke; or use shortly after brain, spinal, or ophthalmology surgery; patient treated concomitantly with platelet inhibitors; conditions associated with increased bleeding tendencies (hemophilia, vascular purpura); recent GI bleeding; thrombocytopenia or platelet defects; severe liver disease; hypertensive or diabetic retinopathy; renal failure; or in patients undergoing invasive procedures including spinal tap or spinal anesthesia. Many concentrations of heparin are available ranging from 1 unit/mL to 20,000 units/mL. Clinicians **must** carefully examine each prefilled syringe or vial prior to use ensuring that the correct concentration is chosen; fatal hemorrhages have occurred related to heparin overdose especially in pediatric patients. A higher incidence of bleeding has been reported in patients >60 years of age, particularly women. They are also more sensitive to the dose. Discontinue heparin if hemorrhage occurs; severe hemorrhage or overdosage may require protamine.

May cause thrombocytopenia; monitor platelet count closely. Patients who develop HIT may be at risk of developing a new thrombus (heparin-induced thrombocytopenia and thrombosis [HITT]). Discontinue therapy and consider alternatives if platelets are <100,000/mm^3 and/or thrombosis develops. HIT or HITT may be delayed and can occur up to several weeks after discontinuation of heparin. Use with extreme caution (for a limited duration) or avoid in patients with history of HIT, especially if administered within 100 days of HIT episode (Dager, 2007; Warkentin, 2001); monitor platelet count closely. Osteoporosis may occur with prolonged use (>6 months) due to a reduction in bone mineral density. Monitor for hyperkalemia; can cause hyperkalemia by suppressing aldosterone production. Patients >60 years of age may require lower doses of heparin.

[U.S. Boxed Warning]: Some products contain benzyl alcohol as a preservative; use of these products is contraindicated in neonates. In neonates, large amounts of benzyl alcohol (>100 mg/kg/day) have been associated with fatal toxicity (gasping syndrome). Use in neonates, infants, or pregnant or nursing mothers is contraindicated by some manufacturers; the use of preservative-free heparin is, therefore, recommended in these populations. Some preparations contain sulfite which may cause allergic reactions.

Heparin resistance may occur in patients with antithrombin deficiency, increased heparin clearance, elevations in heparin-binding proteins, elevations in factor VIII and/or fibrinogen; frequently encountered in patients with fever, thrombosis, thrombophlebitis, infections with thrombosing tendencies, MI, cancer, and in postsurgical patients; measurement of anticoagulant effects using anti-factor Xa levels may be of benefit.

Drug Interactions

Avoid Concomitant Use

Avoid concomitant use of Heparin with any of the following: Apixaban; Corticorelin; Dabigatran Etexilate; Omacetaxine; Palifermin; Rivaroxaban; Streptokinase [Off Market]; Urokinase

Decreased Effect

The levels/effects of Heparin may be decreased by: Estrogen Derivatives; Nitroglycerin; Progestins

Increased Effect/Toxicity

Heparin may increase the levels/effects of: ACE Inhibitors; Aliskiren; Angiotensin II Receptor Blockers; Anticoagulants; Canagliflozin; Collagenase (Systemic); Corticorelin; Deferasirox; Eplerenone; Ibritumomab; Omacetaxine; Palifermin; Potassium Salts; Potassium-Sparing Diuretics;

Rivaroxaban; Tositumomab and Iodine I 131 Tositumomab

The levels/effects of Heparin may be increased by: 5-ASA Derivatives; Agents with Antiplatelet Properties; Apixaban; Aspirin; Dabigatran Etexilate; Dasatinib; Herbs (Anticoagulant/Antiplatelet Properties); Ibrutinib; Nonsteroidal Anti-Inflammatory Agents; Omega-3 Fatty Acids; Pentosan Polysulfate Sodium; Pentoxifylline; Prostacyclin Analogues; Salicylates; Streptokinase [Off Market]; Sugammadex; Thrombolytic Agents; Tibolone; Tipranavir; Urokinase; Vitamin E

Nutritional/Ethanol Interactions Herb/Nutraceutical: Avoid cat's claw, dong quai, evening primrose, feverfew, red clover, horse chestnut, garlic, green tea, ginseng, ginkgo (all have additional antiplatelet activity).

Adverse Reactions Note: Thrombocytopenia has been reported to occur at an incidence between 0% and 30%. It is often of no clinical significance. However, immunologically mediated heparin-induced thrombocytopenia (HIT) has been estimated to occur in 1% to 2% of patients, and is marked by a progressive fall in platelet counts and, in some cases, thromboembolic complications (skin necrosis, pulmonary embolism, gangrene of the extremities, stroke, or MI).

Frequency not defined.

Cardiovascular: Allergic vasospastic reaction (possibly related to thrombosis), chest pain, hemorrhagic shock, shock, thrombosis

Central nervous system: Chills, fever, headache

Dermatologic: Alopecia (delayed, transient), bruising (unexplained), cutaneous necrosis, dysesthesia pedis, erythematous plaques (case reports), eczema, urticaria, purpura

Endocrine & metabolic: Adrenal hemorrhage, hyperkalemia (suppression of aldosterone synthesis), ovarian hemorrhage, rebound hyperlipidemia on discontinuation

Gastrointestinal: Constipation, hematemesis, nausea, tarry stools, vomiting

Genitourinary: Frequent or persistent erection

Hematologic: Bleeding from gums, epistaxis, hemorrhage, ovarian hemorrhage, retroperitoneal hemorrhage, thrombocytopenia (see note)

Hepatic: Liver enzymes increased

Local: Irritation, erythema, pain, hematoma, and ulceration have been rarely reported with deep SubQ injections; I.M. injection (not recommended) is associated with a high incidence of these effects

Neuromuscular & skeletal: Peripheral neuropathy, osteoporosis (chronic therapy effect)

Ocular: Conjunctivitis (allergic reaction), lacrimation

Renal: Hematuria

Respiratory: Asthma, bronchospasm (case reports), hemoptysis, pulmonary hemorrhage, rhinitis

Miscellaneous: Allergic reactions, anaphylactoid reactions, heparin resistance, hypersensitivity (including chills, fever, and urticaria)

Pharmacodynamics/Kinetics

Onset of Action Anticoagulation: I.V.: Immediate; SubQ: ~20-30 minutes

Available Dosage Forms

Solution, Injection:

Generic: 1000 units (500 mL); 2000 units (1000 mL); 25,000 units (250 mL, 500 mL); 1000 units/mL (1 mL, 10 mL, 30 mL); 2500 units/mL (10 mL); 5000 units/mL (1 mL, 10 mL); 10,000 units/mL (1 mL, 4 mL, 5 mL); 20,000 units/mL (1 mL)

Solution, Injection [preservative free]:

Generic: 1000 units/mL (2 mL); 5000 units/0.5 mL (0.5 mL)

Solution, Intravenous:

Hep Flush-10: 10 units/mL (10 mL)

Generic: 10,000 units (250 mL); 12,500 units (250 mL); 20,000 units (500 mL); 25,000 units (250 mL, 500 mL); 1 units/mL (1 mL, 2 mL, 2.5 mL, 3 mL, 5 mL, 10 mL); 2 units/mL (3 mL); 10 units/mL (1 mL, 2 mL, 2.5 mL, 3 mL, 5 mL, 10 mL, 30 mL); 100 units/mL (1 mL, 2 mL, 2.5 mL, 3 mL, 5 mL, 10 mL, 30 mL); 2000 units/mL (5 mL)

Solution, Intravenous [preservative free]:

Generic: 1 units/mL (3 mL); 10 units/mL (1 mL, 3 mL, 5 mL); 100 units/mL (1 mL, 3 mL, 5 mL)

General Dosage Range

I.V.:

Children: Bolus: 50-100 units/kg; Initial infusion: 15-25 units/kg/hour; Maintenance: Increase dose by 2-4 units/kg/hour every 6-8 hours as needed **or** 50-100 units/kg every 4 hours intermittently

Adults: Bolus: 60-80 units/kg; Infusion: 10-30 units/kg/hour **or** 10,000 units (initially), then 50-70 units/kg (5000-10,000 units) every 4-6 hours intermittently

SubQ: *Adults:* Thromboprophylaxis: 5000 units every 8-12 hours; Treatment: 17,500 units every 12 hours

Usual Infusion Concentrations: Pediatric

Note: Premixed solutions available

I.V. infusion: 100 units/mL

Usual Infusion Concentrations: Adult Note: Premixed solutions available

I.V. infusion: 25,000 units in 250 mL (concentration: 100 units/mL) of D$_5$W, 1/2NS, or NS

Administration

I.M. Do not administer I.M. due to pain, irritation, and hematoma formation.

I.V.

Continuous I.V. infusion: Infuse via infusion pump. If preparing solution, mix thoroughly prior to administration.

Heparin lock: Inject via injection cap using positive pressure flushing technique. Heparin lock flush solution is intended only to maintain patency of I.V. devices and is **not** to be used for anticoagulant therapy.

Other SubQ: Inject in subcutaneous tissue only (not muscle tissue). Injection sites should be rotated (usually left and right portions of the abdomen, above iliac crest).

Storage/Stability Heparin solutions are colorless to slightly yellow. Minor color variations do not affect therapeutic efficacy. Heparin should be stored at controlled room temperature. Protect from freezing and temperatures >40°C.

Stability at room temperature and refrigeration:

Prepared bag: 24-72 hours (specific to solution, concentration, and/or study conditions)

Premixed bag: After seal is broken, 4 days.

Out of overwrap stability: 30 days.

Nursing Actions

Physical Assessment Assess potential for interactions with any drugs that will affect coagulation or platelet function. Note specific infusion directions in Administration. Bleeding precautions must be observed at all times during heparin therapy. Monitor laboratory tests regularly (dosing adjustments may be necessary). Monitor patient closely for hypersensitivity reaction, bleeding, chest pain, hyperkalemia, and peripheral neuropathy. For I.V. bolus, emergency treatment for hypersensitivity reactions should be immediately available. Teach patient bleeding precautions.

Patient Education

• Discuss specific use of drug and side effects with patient as it relates to treatment. (HCAHPS: During this hospital stay, were you given any medicine that you had not taken before? Before giving you any new medicine, how often did hospital staff tell you what the medicine was for? How often did hospital staff describe possible side effects in a way you could understand?)

• Patient may experience bleeding problems, injection site irritation, or osteopenia. Have patient report immediately to prescriber severe dizziness, imbalance, illogical thinking, significant headache, edema, ecchymosis, or rash (HCAHPS).

• Educate patient about signs of a significant reaction (eg, wheezing; chest tightness; fever; itching; bad cough; blue skin color; seizures; swelling of face, lips, tongue, or throat). **Note:** This is not a comprehensive list of all side effects. Patient should consult prescriber for additional questions.

Intended Use and Disclaimer: Should not be printed and given to patients. This information is intended to serve as a concise initial reference for healthcare professionals to use when discussing medications with a patient. You must ultimately rely on your own discretion, experience and judgment in diagnosing, treating and advising patients.

Hepatitis A and Hepatitis B Recombinant Vaccine

(hep a TYE tis aye & hep a TYE tis bee ree KOM be nant vak SEEN)

Brand Names: U.S. Twinrix®

Index Terms Engerix-B® and Havrix®; Havrix® and Engerix-B®; HepA-HepB; Hepatitis B and Hepatitis A Vaccine

Pharmacologic Category Vaccine, Inactivated (Viral)

Pregnancy Risk Factor C

Lactation Excretion in breast milk unknown/use caution

Use Active immunization against disease caused by hepatitis A virus and hepatitis B virus (all known subtypes) in populations desiring protection against or at high risk of exposure to these viruses.

Populations include travelers or people living in or relocating to areas of intermediate/high endemicity for **both** HAV and HBV and are at increased risk of HBV infection due to behavioral or occupational factors; patients with chronic liver disease; laboratory workers who handle live HAV and HBV; healthcare workers, police, and other personnel who render first-aid or medical assistance; workers who come in contact with sewage; employees of day care centers and correctional facilities; patients/staff of hemodialysis units; men who have sex with men; patients frequently receiving blood products; military personnel; users of injectable illicit drugs; close household contacts of patients with hepatitis A and hepatitis B infection; residents of drug and alcohol treatment centers

Available Dosage Forms

Injection, suspension [preservative free]:

Twinrix®: Hepatitis A virus antigen 720 ELISA units and hepatitis B surface antigen 20 mcg per mL (1 mL)

General Dosage Range I.M.: *Adults:* 3 doses (1 mL each) given on a 0-, 1-, and 6-month schedule

Administration

I.M. Shake well prior to use. Do not dilute prior to administration. Discard if the suspension is discolored or does not appear homogenous after shaking or if there are cracks in the vial or syringe. Administer in the deltoid region; do not administer in the gluteal region (may give suboptimal response). Administer in the anterolateral thigh in infants (Canadian labeling). Do not administer at the same site, or using the same syringe, as additional vaccines or immunoglobulins.

For patients at risk of hemorrhage following intramuscular injection, the ACIP recommends "it should be administered intramuscularly if, in the opinion of the physician familiar with the patient's bleeding risk, the vaccine can be administered by this route with reasonable safety. If the patient receives antihemophilia or other similar therapy, intramuscular vaccination can be scheduled shortly after such therapy is administered. A fine needle (23 gauge or smaller) can be used for the vaccination and firm pressure applied to the site (without rubbing) for at least 2 minutes. The patient should be instructed concerning the risk of hematoma from the injection." Patients on anticoagulant therapy should be considered to have the same bleeding risks and treated as those with clotting factor disorders (CDC, 2011). Subcutaneous administration is not recommended; antibody response may be suboptimal. The Canadian product labeling recommends subcutaneous administration in patients with thrombocytopenia or at risk for hemorrhage.

Simultaneous administration of vaccines helps ensure the patients will be fully vaccinated by the appropriate age. Simultaneous administration of vaccines is defined as administering >1 vaccine on the same day at different anatomic sites. The use of licensed combination vaccines is generally preferred over separate injections of the equivalent components. Separate vaccines should not be combined in the same syringe unless indicated by product specific labeling. Separate needles and syringes should be used for each injection. The ACIP prefers each dose of a specific vaccine in a series come from the same manufacturer when possible. Adolescents and adults should be vaccinated while seated or lying down. In general, preterm infants should be vaccinated at the same chronological age as full-term infants (CDC, 2011).

Antipyretics have not been shown to prevent febrile seizures. Antipyretics may be used to treat fever or discomfort following vaccination (CDC, 2011). One study reported that routine prophylactic administration of acetaminophen to prevent fever prior to vaccination decreased the immune response of some vaccines; the clinical significance of this reduction in immune response has not been established (Prymula, 2009).

Subcutaneous Subcutaneous administration is not recommended; antibody response may be suboptimal. The Canadian product labeling recommends subcutaneous administration in patients with thrombocytopenia or at risk for hemorrhage.

Nursing Actions

Physical Assessment Have emergency treatment for anaphylactoid or hypersensitivity reaction available. Observe patient for 15 minutes following administration. All serious adverse reactions must be reported to the U.S. DHHS. U.S. federal law also requires entry into the patient's medical record.

Patient Education

• Discuss specific use of vaccine and side effects with patient as it relates to treatment. (HCAHPS: During this hospital stay, were you given any medicine that you had not taken before? Before

giving you any new medicine, how often did hospital staff tell you what the medicine was for? How often did hospital staff describe possible side effects in a way you could understand?)

• Patient may experience pain, redness or swelling at injection site, headache, fatigue, nausea, emesis, diarrhea, or dyspepsia. Have patient report immediately to prescriber severe injection site reaction (HCAHPS).

• Educate patient about signs of a significant reaction (eg, wheezing; chest tightness; fever; itching; bad cough; blue skin color; seizures; or swelling of face, lips, tongue, or throat). **Note:** This is not a comprehensive list of all side effects. Patient should consult prescriber for additional questions.

Intended Use and Disclaimer: Should not be printed and given to patients. This information is intended to serve as a concise initial reference for healthcare professionals to use when discussing medications with a patient. You must ultimately rely on your own discretion, experience and judgment in diagnosing, treating and advising patients.

Related Information

Immunization Administration Recommendations *on page 1675*

Immunization Recommendations *on page 1680*

Hepatitis A Vaccine (hep a TYE tis aye vak SEEN)

Brand Names: U.S. Havrix; VAQTA

Index Terms HepA

Pharmacologic Category Vaccine, Inactivated (Viral)

Medication Safety Issues

International issues:

Avaxim [Canada and multiple international markets] may be confused with Avastin brand name for bevacizumab [U.S., Canada, and multiple international markets]

Pregnancy Risk Factor C

Lactation Excretion in breast milk unknown/use caution

Use Hepatitis A virus vaccination:

For active immunization of persons 12 months and older against disease caused by hepatitis A virus (HAV).

The Advisory Committee on Immunization Practices (ACIP) recommends routine vaccination for:

- All children ≥12 months of age (CDC, 2006)

- All unvaccinated adults requesting protection from HAV infection (CDC, 2006)

- Unvaccinated persons with any of the following conditions: Men who have sex with men; injection and non-injection illicit drug users; persons who work with HAV-infected primates or with HAV in a research laboratory setting; persons with chronic liver disease; patients who receive clotting-factor concentrates; persons traveling to

or working in countries with high or intermediate levels of endemic HAV infection (CDC, 2006)

- Unvaccinated persons who anticipate close personal contact with international adoptee from a country of intermediate to high endemicity of HAV, during their first 60 days of arrival into the United States (eg, household contacts, babysitters) (CDC, 2009)

-Vaccination can be a component of hepatitis A outbreak response or as postexposure prophylaxis, as determined by local public health authorities (CDC, 2006; CDC, 2007)

Available Dosage Forms

Injection, suspension [preservative free]:

Havrix: Hepatitis A virus antigen 720 ELISA units/ 0.5 mL (0.5 mL); Hepatitis A virus antigen 1440 ELISA units/mL (1 mL)

VAQTA: Hepatitis A virus antigen 25 units/0.5 mL (0.5 mL); Hepatitis A virus antigen 50 units/mL (1 mL)

General Dosage Range I.M.:

Children ≥12 years and Adolescents: 0.5 mL

Adults: 1 mL

Administration

I.M. For I.M. administration. The deltoid muscle is the preferred site for injection for older children and adults; administer to the anterolateral aspect of the thigh in infants and young children. Do not administer to the gluteal region; may decrease efficacy. Do not administer intravenously, intradermally, or subcutaneously. Shake well prior to use; discard if the suspension is discolored or does not appear homogenous after shaking, or if there are cracks in the vial or syringe. Do not dilute. When used for primary immunization, the vaccine should be given at least 2 weeks prior to expected HAV exposure. When used for postexposure prophylaxis, the vaccine should be given as soon as possible.

For patients at risk of hemorrhage following intramuscular injection, the ACIP recommends "it should be administered intramuscularly if, in the opinion of the physician familiar with the patient's bleeding risk, the vaccine can be administered by this route with reasonable safety. If the patient receives antihemophilia or other similar therapy, intramuscular vaccination can be scheduled shortly after such therapy is administered. A fine needle (23 gauge or smaller) can be used for the vaccination and firm pressure applied to the site (without rubbing) for at least 2 minutes. The patient should be instructed concerning the risk of hematoma from the injection." Patients on anticoagulant therapy should be considered to have the same bleeding risks and treated as those with clotting factor disorders (CDC, 2011). **Note:** Canadian product labeling suggests that subcutaneous administration may be considered in exceptional circumstances (eg, patients with thrombocytopenia or at risk for hemorrhage), although this may convey a higher risk for local reactions (eg, injection site nodule). In healthy adults, seroconversion following an initial subcutaneous dose of VAQTA was slower than that historically observed following intramuscular administration (Linglöf, 2001).

Simultaneous administration of vaccines helps ensure the patients will be fully vaccinated by the appropriate age. Simultaneous administration of vaccines is defined as administering >1 vaccine on the same day at different anatomic sites. The use of licensed combination vaccines is generally preferred over separate injections of the equivalent components. Separate vaccines should not be combined in the same syringe unless indicated by product specific labeling. Separate needles and syringes should be used for each injection. The ACIP prefers each dose of a specific vaccine in a series come from the same manufacturer when possible. Adolescents and adults should be vaccinated while seated or lying down. In general, preterm infants should be vaccinated at the same chronological age as full-term infants (CDC, 2011).

Antipyretics have not been shown to prevent febrile seizures. Antipyretics may be used to treat fever or discomfort following vaccination (CDC, 2011). One study reported that routine prophylactic administration of acetaminophen to prevent fever prior to vaccination decreased the immune response of some vaccines; the clinical significance of this reduction in immune response has not been established (Prymula, 2009).

Subcutaneous Subcutaneous administration is not recommended. The Canadian product labeling suggests that subcutaneous administration may be considered in exceptional circumstances (eg, patients with thrombocytopenia or at risk for hemorrhage), although this may convey a higher risk for local reactions (eg, injection site nodule). In healthy adults, seroconversion following an initial subcutaneous dose of Vaqta was slower than that historically observed following intramuscular administration (Linglöf, 2001).

Nursing Actions

Physical Assessment All serious adverse reactions must be reported to the U.S. DHHS. U.S. federal law also requires entry into the patient's medical record. Educate patient about need to complete vaccine series.

Patient Education
• Discuss specific use of vaccine and side effects with patient as it relates to treatment. (HCAHPS: During this hospital stay, were you given any medicine that you had not taken before? Before giving you any new medicine, how often did hospital staff tell you what the medicine was for? How often did hospital staff describe possible side effects in a way you could understand?)

• Patient may experience pain, redness or swelling at injection site, headache, fatigue, nausea, emesis, diarrhea, or dyspepsia. Have patient report immediately to prescriber severe injection site reaction (HCAHPS).

• Educate patient about signs of a significant reaction (eg, wheezing; chest tightness; fever; itching; bad cough; blue skin color; seizures; or swelling of face, lips, tongue, or throat). **Note:** This is not a comprehensive list of all side effects. Patient should consult prescriber for additional questions.

Intended Use and Disclaimer: Should not be printed and given to patients. This information is intended to serve as a concise initial reference for healthcare professionals to use when discussing medications with a patient. You must ultimately rely on your own discretion, experience and judgment in diagnosing, treating and advising patients.

Related Information

Immunization Administration Recommendations on page 1675
Immunization Recommendations on page 1680

Hepatitis B Vaccine (Recombinant)
(hep a TYE tis bee vak SEEN ree KOM be nant)

Brand Names: U.S. Engerix-B; Recombivax HB

Index Terms Hepatitis B Inactivated Virus Vaccine (recombinant DNA); HepB

Pharmacologic Category Vaccine, Inactivated (Viral)

Medication Safety Issues
Sound-alike/look-alike issues:
  Engerix-B adult may be confused with Engerix-B pediatric/adolescent
  Recombivax HB may be confused with Comvax

Pregnancy Risk Factor C

Lactation Excretion in breast milk unknown/use caution

Use Immunization against infection caused by all known subtypes of hepatitis B virus (HBV)

The Advisory Committee on Immunization Practices (ACIP) recommends routine vaccination for the following:
- All infants at birth (CDC, 2005)
- All infants and children not previously vaccinated (CDC, 2005) (post-birth dose; refer to recommended vaccination schedule)
- All unvaccinated adults requesting protection from HBV infection (CDC, 2006)
- All unvaccinated adults at risk for HBV infection such as those with:
  Behavioral risks: Sexually-active persons with >1 partner in a 6-month period; persons seeking evaluation or treatment for a sexually-transmitted disease; men who have sex with men; injection drug users (CDC, 2006)

Occupational risks: Healthcare personnel (HCP) and public safety workers with reasonably anticipated risk for exposure to blood or blood contaminated body fluids (CDC, 2006)

Medical risks: Persons with end-stage renal disease (including predialysis, hemodialysis, peritoneal dialysis, and home dialysis); persons with HIV infection; persons with chronic liver disease (CDC, 2006). Adults (19 through 59 years of age) with diabetes mellitus type 1 or type 2 should be vaccinated as soon as possible following diagnosis. Adults ≥60 years with diabetes mellitus may also be vaccinated at the discretion of their treating clinician (CDC 60 [50], 2011).

Other risks: Household contacts and sex partners of persons with chronic HBV infection; residents and staff of facilities for developmentally disabled persons; international travelers to regions with high or intermediate levels of endemic HBV infection (CDC, 2006)

In addition, the ACIP recommends vaccination for any persons who are wounded in bombings or similar mass casualty events who have penetrating injuries or nonintact skin exposure, or who have contact with mucous membranes (exception - superficial contact with intact skin), and who cannot confirm receipt of a hepatitis B vaccination (CDC, 2008).

Available Dosage Forms

Injection, suspension [preservative free]:

Engerix-B®: Hepatitis B surface antigen 10 mcg/0.5 mL (0.5 mL); Hepatitis B surface antigen 20 mcg/mL (1 mL)

Recombivax HB®: Hepatitis B surface antigen 5 mcg/0.5 mL (0.5 mL); Hepatitis B surface antigen 10 mcg/mL (1 mL); Hepatitis B surface antigen 40 mcg/mL (1 mL)

General Dosage Range Dosage adjustment recommended in patients with renal impairment.

I.M.: Note: Various dosing regimens available

Birth to 19 years: 0.5 mL

Adults ≥20 years: 1 mL

Administration

I.M. Pediatric/adolescent formulations of hepatitis B vaccine products differ by concentration (mcg/mL). However, when dosed in terms of volume (mL), the dose of Engerix-B and Recombivax HB are the same (both 0.5 mL). Adult formulations of hepatitis B vaccine products also differ by concentration (mcg/mL), but when dosed in terms of volume (mL), the dose of Engerix-B and Recombivax HB are the same (both 1 mL). It is possible to interchange the vaccines for completion of a series or for booster doses; the antibody produced in response to each type of vaccine is comparable, however, the quantity of the vaccine will vary.

I.M. injection only; in adults, the deltoid muscle is the preferred site; the anterolateral thigh is the recommended site in infants and young children. Not for gluteal administration. Shake well prior to withdrawal and use. Obese patients may require an adjustment of needle length (CDC 62 [10], 2013).

For patients at risk of hemorrhage following intramuscular injection, hepatitis B vaccine may be administered subcutaneously although lower titers and/or increased incidence of local reactions may result. The ACIP recommends "it should be administered intramuscularly if, in the opinion of the physician familiar with the patient's bleeding risk, the vaccine can be administered by this route with reasonable safety. If the patient receives antihemophilia or other similar therapy, intramuscular vaccination can be scheduled shortly after such therapy is administered. A fine needle (23 gauge or smaller) can be used for the vaccination and firm pressure applied to the site (without rubbing) for at least 2 minutes. The patient should be instructed concerning the risk of hematoma from the injection." Patients on anticoagulant therapy should be considered to have the same bleeding risks and treated as those with clotting factor disorders (CDC 60 [2], 2011).

Simultaneous administration of vaccines helps ensure the patients will be fully vaccinated by the appropriate age. Simultaneous administration of vaccines is defined as administering >1 vaccine on the same day at different anatomic sites. The use of licensed combination vaccines is generally preferred over separate injections of the equivalent components. Separate vaccines should not be combined in the same syringe unless indicated by product specific labeling. Separate needles and syringes should be used for each injection. The ACIP prefers each dose of a specific vaccine in a series come from the same manufacturer when possible. Adolescents and adults should be vaccinated while seated or lying down. In general, preterm infants should be vaccinated at the same chronological age as full-term infants (CDC 60 [2], 2011).

Antipyretics have not been shown to prevent febrile seizures. Antipyretics may be used to treat fever or discomfort following vaccination (CDC 60 [2], 2011). One study reported that routine prophylactic administration of acetaminophen to prevent fever prior to vaccination decreased the immune response of some vaccines; the clinical significance of this reduction in immune response has not been established (Prymula, 2009).

Vaccination at the time of HB$_s$Ag testing: For persons in whom vaccination is recommended, the first dose of hepatitis B vaccine can be given after blood is drawn to test for HB$_s$Ag.

Nursing Actions

Physical Assessment All serious adverse reactions must be reported to the U.S. DHHS. U.S. federal law also requires entry into the patient's medical record.

Patient Education

• Discuss specific use of vaccine and side effects with patient as it relates to treatment. (HCAHPS: During this hospital stay, were you given any medicine that you had not taken before? Before giving you any new medicine, how often did hospital staff tell you what the medicine was for? How often did hospital staff describe possible side effects in a way you could understand?)

• Patient may experience pain, redness or swelling at injection site, headache, fatigue, nausea, emesis, diarrhea, or dyspepsia. Have patient report immediately to prescriber severe injection site reaction (HCAHPS).

• Educate patient about signs of a significant reaction (eg, wheezing; chest tightness; fever; itching; bad cough; blue skin color; seizures; or swelling of face, lips, tongue, or throat). **Note:** This is not a comprehensive list of all side effects. Patient should consult prescriber for additional questions.

Intended Use and Disclaimer: Should not be printed and given to patients. This information is intended to serve as a concise initial reference for healthcare professionals to use when discussing medications with a patient. You must ultimately rely on your own discretion, experience and judgment in diagnosing, treating and advising patients.

Related Information

Immunization Administration Recommendations *on page 1675*

Immunization Recommendations *on page 1680*

Hetastarch (HET a starch)

Brand Names: U.S. Hespan; Hextend

Index Terms HES; HES 450/0.7; Hydroxyethyl Starch

Pharmacologic Category Plasma Volume Expander, Colloid

Medication Safety Issues

Sound-alike/look-alike issues:

Hespan may be confused with heparin

Pregnancy Risk Factor C

Lactation Excretion in· breast milk unknown/use caution

Use

Granulocyte yield increase (Hespan): Used as an adjunct in leukapheresis to improve harvesting and increase the yield of granulocytes by centrifugation

Hypovolemia: Blood volume expander used in treatment of hypovolemia

Available Dosage Forms

Solution, Intravenous:

Hespan: 6% (500 mL)

Hextend: 6% (500 mL)

Generic: 6% (500 mL)

General Dosage Range

I.V.: *Adults:* 500-1500 mL/day **or** 20 mL/kg/day (up to 1500 mL/day)

Leukapheresis: *Adults:* 250-700 mL

Administration

I.V. Do not use if crystalline precipitate forms or is turbid deep brown.

Volume expansion: Administer I.V. only; may be administered via infusion pump or pressure infusion. Administration rates vary depending upon the extent of blood loss, age, and clinical condition of patient, but, *in general*, should not exceed 1.2 g/kg/hour (20 mL/kg/hour); *however,* **rates up to 1000 mL over 7-8 minutes via pressure infusion have been studied in otherwise healthy subjects (McIlroy, 2003).** Anaphylactoid reactions can occur, have epinephrine and resuscitative equipment available. If administered by pressure infusion, air should be withdrawn or expelled from bag prior to infusion to prevent air embolus. Do not administer Hextend with blood through the same administration set. Change I.V. tubing or flush copiously with normal saline before administering blood through the same line. Change I.V. tubing at least every 24 hours.

Injectable Detail pH: 5.9

Other Leukapheresis: Mix Hespan and citrate well. Administer to the input line of the centrifuge apparatus at a ratio of 1:8 to 1:13 to venous whole blood.

Nursing Actions

Physical Assessment Patient's allergy history must be assessed prior to therapy (patients allergic to corn may have a cross allergy to hetastarch). Monitor patient closely for hypersensitivity reaction and circulatory overload. Vital signs, CVP, and urine output should be monitored frequently (every 5-15 minutes) during first hour and at regular intervals thereafter.

Patient Education

• Discuss specific use of drug and side effects with patient as it relates to treatment. (HCAHPS: During this hospital stay, were you given any medicine that you had not taken before? Before giving you any new medicine, how often did hospital staff tell you what the medicine was for? How often did hospital staff describe possible side effects in a way you could understand?)

• Patient may experience edema. Have patient report immediately to prescriber dyspnea, ecchymosis, bleeding, or rash (HCAHPS).

• Educate patient about signs of a significant reaction (eg, wheezing; chest tightness; fever; itching; bad cough; blue skin color; seizures; or swelling of face, lips, tongue, or throat). **Note:** This is not a comprehensive list of all side effects. Patient should consult prescriber for additional questions.

Intended Use and Disclaimer: Should not be printed and given to patients. This information is intended to serve as a concise initial reference for healthcare professionals to use when discussing medications with a patient. You must ultimately rely on your own discretion, experience and judgment in diagnosing, treating and advising patients.

HydrALAZINE (hye DRAL a zeen)

Index Terms Apresoline; Hydralazine Hydrochloride

Pharmacologic Category Antihypertensive; Vasodilator

Medication Safety Issues

Sound-alike/look-alike issues:

HydrALAZINE may be confused with hydrOXYzine

Pregnancy Risk Factor C

Lactation Enters breast milk/use caution

Breast-Feeding Considerations Hydralazine is excreted into breast milk. In a case report, following a maternal dose of hydralazine 50 mg three times daily, exposure to the infant was calculated to be 0.013 mg per 75 mL breast milk (Liedholm, 1982). The manufacturer recommends that caution be used if administered to a nursing woman.

Use Management of moderate-to-severe hypertension

Unlabeled Use Patients with heart failure with reduced ejection fraction (HFrEF) who do not tolerate an ACE inhibitor or an angiotensin receptor blocker (ARB) (in combination with isosorbide dinitrate); African-American (self-identified) patients with HFrEF NYHA Class III-IV remaining symptomatic despite optimal guideline directed medical therapy (in combination with isosorbide dinitrate); hypertensive emergency (with or without pre-eclampsia/eclampsia) in pregnancy; postoperative hypertension.

Mechanism of Action/Effect Direct vasodilation of arterioles (with little effect on veins) with decreased systemic resistance

Contraindications Hypersensitivity to hydralazine or any component of the formulation; mitral valve rheumatic heart disease

Warnings/Precautions May cause peripheral neuritis or a drug-induced lupus-like syndrome (more likely on larger doses, longer duration). Discontinue hydralazine in patients who develop SLE-like syndrome or positive ANA. Use with caution in patients with severe renal disease or

cerebral vascular accidents or with known or suspected coronary artery disease; monitor blood pressure closely with I.V. use. Slow acetylators, patients with decreased renal function, and patients receiving >200 mg/day (chronically) are at higher risk for SLE. Titrate dosage cautiously to patient's response. Hypotensive effect after I.V. administration may be delayed and unpredictable in some patients. Usually administered with diuretic and a beta-blocker to counteract side effects of sodium and water retention and reflex tachycardia.

Adjust dose in severe renal dysfunction. Use with caution in CAD (increase in tachycardia may increase myocardial oxygen demand). Use with caution in pulmonary hypertension (may cause hypotension). Patients may be poorly compliant because of frequent dosing. Hydralazine-induced fluid and sodium retention may require addition or increased dosage of a diuretic.

Drug Interactions

Avoid Concomitant Use

Avoid concomitant use of HydrALAZINE with any of the following: Pimozide

Decreased Effect

The levels/effects of HydrALAZINE may be decreased by: Herbs (Hypertensive Properties); Methylphenidate; Nonsteroidal Anti-Inflammatory Agents; Yohimbine

Increased Effect/Toxicity

HydrALAZINE may increase the levels/effects of: Amifostine; Antihypertensives; ARIPiprazole; Dofetilide; DULoxetine; Hypotensive Agents; Lomitapide; Obinutuzumab; Pimozide; RiTUXimab

The levels/effects of HydrALAZINE may be increased by: Alfuzosin; Brimonidine (Topical); Diazoxide; Herbs (Hypotensive Properties); MAO Inhibitors; Pentoxifylline; Phosphodiesterase 5 Inhibitors; Prostacyclin Analogues

Nutritional/Ethanol Interactions

Ethanol: Avoid ethanol (may increase CNS depression).

Food: Food enhances bioavailability of hydralazine.

Herb/Nutraceutical: Avoid dong quai if using for hypertension (has estrogenic activity). Avoid ephedra, yohimbe, ginseng (may worsen hypertension). Avoid garlic (may have increased antihypertensive effect).

Adverse Reactions Frequency not defined.

Cardiovascular: Angina pectoris, flushing, orthostatic hypotension, palpitations, paradoxical hypertension, peripheral edema, tachycardia, vascular collapse

Central nervous system: Anxiety, chills, depression, disorientation, dizziness, fever, headache, increased intracranial pressure (I.V.; in patient with pre-existing increased intracranial pressure), psychotic reaction

Dermatologic: Pruritus, rash, urticaria

Gastrointestinal: Anorexia, constipation, diarrhea, nausea, paralytic ileus, vomiting

Genitourinary: Dysuria, impotence

Hematologic: Agranulocytosis, eosinophilia, erythrocyte count reduced, hemoglobin decreased, hemolytic anemia, leukopenia, thrombocytopenia (rare)

Neuromuscular & skeletal: Muscle cramps, peripheral neuritis, rheumatoid arthritis, tremor, weakness

Ocular: Conjunctivitis, lacrimation

Respiratory: Dyspnea, nasal congestion

Miscellaneous: Diaphoresis, drug-induced lupuslike syndrome (dose related; fever, arthralgia, splenomegaly, lymphadenopathy, asthenia, myalgia, malaise, pleuritic chest pain, edema, positive ANA, positive LE cells, maculopapular facial rash, positive direct Coombs' test, pericarditis, pericardial tamponade)

Pharmacodynamics/Kinetics

Onset of Action Oral: 20-30 minutes; I.V.: 5-20 minutes

Duration of Action Oral: Up to 8 hours; I.V.: 1-4 hours; **Note:** May vary depending on acetylator status of patient

Available Dosage Forms

Solution, Injection:
Generic: 20 mg/mL (1 mL)

Tablet, Oral:
Generic: 10 mg, 25 mg, 50 mg, 100 mg

General Dosage Range Dosage adjustment recommended in patients with renal impairment

I.M., I.V.:
Children: 0.1-0.2 mg/kg/dose (not to exceed 20 mg) every 4-6 hours as needed (maximum: 3.5 mg/kg/day in 4-6 divided doses)

Adults: Initial: 10-20 mg/dose every 4-6 hours as needed

Oral:
Children: Initial: 0.75-1 mg/kg/day in 2-4 divided doses; Maintenance: Up to 7.5 mg/kg/day in 2-4 divided doses (maximum: 200 mg/day)

Adults: Initial: 10 mg 4 times daily; Maintenance: Up to 50 mg 4 times daily (maximum: 300 mg daily in divided doses)

Elderly: Refer to adult dosing.

Administration

I.V. Solution for injection: Administer as a slow I.V. push; maximum rate: 5 mg/minute

Injectable Detail pH: 3.4-4

Preparation for Administration Hydralazine should be diluted in NS for IVPB administration due to decreased stability in D_5W. Stability of IVPB solution in NS is 4 days at room temperature.

Storage/Stability Intact ampuls/vials of hydralazine should not be stored under refrigeration because of possible precipitation or crystallization.

Nursing Actions

Physical Assessment Orthostatic precautions should be observed and patient monitored closely during and following infusion. Monitor for hypotension and fluid retention periodically during therapy.

Patient Education

- Discuss specific use of drug and side effects with patient as it relates to treatment. (HCAHPS: During this hospital stay, were you given any medicine that you had not taken before? Before giving you any new medicine, how often did hospital staff tell you what the medicine was for? How often did hospital staff describe possible side effects in a way you could understand?)
- Patient may experience dizziness, headache, or nausea. Have patient report immediately to prescriber significant weight gain, arthralgia, edema, or rash (HCAHPS).
- Educate patient about signs of a significant reaction (eg, wheezing; chest tightness; fever; itching; bad cough; blue skin color; seizures; or swelling of face, lips, tongue, or throat). **Note:** This is not a comprehensive list of all side effects. Patient should consult prescriber for additional questions.

Intended Use and Disclaimer: Should not be printed and given to patients. This information is intended to serve as a concise initial reference for healthcare professionals to use when discussing medications with a patient. You must ultimately rely on your own discretion, experience and judgment in diagnosing, treating and advising patients.

Dietary Considerations Administer tablet with meals.

Hydrochlorothiazide
(hye droe klor oh THYE a zide)

Brand Names: U.S. Microzide

Index Terms HCTZ (error-prone abbreviation); Hydrodiuril

Pharmacologic Category Antihypertensive; Diuretic, Thiazide

Medication Safety Issues

Sound-alike/look-alike issues:

HCTZ is an error-prone abbreviation (mistaken as hydrocortisone)

Hydrochlorothiazide may be confused with hydrocortisone, Viskazide

Microzide may be confused with Maxzide, Micronase

International issues:

Esidrex [multiple international markets] may be confused with Lasix brand name for furosemide [U.S., Canada, and multiple international markets]

Esidrix [Germany] may be confused with Lasix brand name for furosemide [U.S., Canada, and multiple international markets]

Pregnancy Risk Factor B

Lactation Enters breast milk/not recommended

▶

Breast-Feeding Considerations Thiazide diuretics are found in breast milk. Following a single oral maternal dose of hydrochlorothiazide 50 mg, the mean breast milk concentration was 80 ng/mL (samples collected over 24 hours) and hydrochlorothiazide was not detected in the blood of the breast feeding infant (limit of detection 20 ng/mL) (Miller, 1982). Peak plasma concentrations reported in adults following hydrochlorothiazide 12.5-100 mg are 70-490 ng/mL. Due to the potential for serious adverse reactions in the nursing infant, the manufacturer recommends a decision be made whether to discontinue nursing or to discontinue the drug, taking into account the importance of treatment to the mother. Breast-fed infants of mothers taking medications for hypertension should be monitored for adverse effects (Chobanian, 2003). Diuretics have the potential to decrease milk volume and suppress lactation.

Use Management of mild-to-moderate hypertension; treatment of edema due to heart failure, hepatic cirrhosis (see "**Note**"), various forms of renal dysfunction (eg, nephrotic syndrome, acute glomerulosclerosis, chronic renal failure) (see "**Note**"), corticosteroid and estrogen therapy

Note: The use of hydrochlorothiazide in the treatment of edema for hepatic cirrhosis has largely been replaced by spironolactone. The use of hydrochlorothiazide in the management of edema in patients with renal dysfunction has largely been replaced by the use of loop diuretics (eg, furosemide).

Unlabeled Use Treatment of lithium-induced diabetes insipidus

Mechanism of Action/Effect Inhibits sodium reabsorption in the distal tubules causing increased excretion of sodium and water as well as potassium and hydrogen ions

Contraindications Hypersensitivity to hydrochlorothiazide, any component of the formulation, or sulfonamide-derived drugs; anuria

Warnings/Precautions Hypersensitivity reactions may occur with hydrochlorothiazide. Risk is increased in patients with a history of allergy or bronchial asthma. Avoid in severe renal disease (ineffective as a diuretic). Electrolyte disturbances (hypokalemia, hypochloremic alkalosis, hypomagnesemia, hyponatremia) can occur. Development of electrolyte disturbances can be minimized when used in combination with other electrolyte sparing antihypertensives (eg, ACE inhibitors or angiotensin receptor blockers). (Sica, 2011) Use with caution in severe hepatic dysfunction; hepatic encephalopathy can be caused by electrolyte disturbances. Gout may be precipitated in certain patients with a history of gout, a familial predisposition to gout, or chronic renal failure. Thiazide diuretics reduce calcium excretion; pathologic changes in the parathyroid glands with hypercalcemia and hypophosphatemia have been observed with prolonged use. Should be discontinued prior to testing for parathyroid function. Use with caution in patients with prediabetes and diabetes; may alter glucose control. May cause SLE exacerbation or activation. Use with caution in patients with moderate or high cholesterol concentrations. Photosensitization may occur. Correct hypokalemia before initiating therapy. Thiazide diuretics may decrease renal calcium excretion; consider avoiding use in patients with hypercalcemia. May cause acute transient myopia and acute angle-closure glaucoma, typically occurring within hours to weeks following initiation; discontinue therapy immediately in patients with acute decreases in visual acuity or ocular pain. Risk factors may include a history of sulfonamide or penicillin allergy. Cumulative effects may develop, including azotemia, in patients with impaired renal function.

Chemical similarities are present among sulfonamides, sulfonylureas, carbonic anhydrase inhibitors, thiazides, and loop diuretics (except ethacrynic acid). Use in patients with sulfonamide allergy is specifically contraindicated in product labeling, however, a risk of cross-reaction exists in patients with allergy to any of these compounds; avoid use when previous reaction has been severe. Discontinue if signs of hypersensitivity are noted.

Drug Interactions

Avoid Concomitant Use

Avoid concomitant use of Hydrochlorothiazide with any of the following: Dofetilide

Decreased Effect

Hydrochlorothiazide may decrease the levels/effects of: Antidiabetic Agents

The levels/effects of Hydrochlorothiazide may be decreased by: Benazepril; Bile Acid Sequestrants; Herbs (Hypertensive Properties); Methylphenidate; Nonsteroidal Anti-Inflammatory Agents; Yohimbine

Increased Effect/Toxicity

Hydrochlorothiazide may increase the levels/effects of: ACE Inhibitors; Allopurinol; Amifostine; Antihypertensives; Benazepril; Calcium Salts; CarBAMazepine; Diazoxide; Dofetilide; DULoxetine; Hypotensive Agents; Ivabradine; Lithium; Multivitamins/Minerals (with ADEK, Folate, Iron); Multivitamins/Minerals (with AE, No Iron); Obinutuzumab; OXcarbazepine; Porfimer; RiTUXimab; Sodium Phosphates; Topiramate; Toremifene; Valsartan; Vitamin D Analogs

The levels/effects of Hydrochlorothiazide may be increased by: Alcohol (Ethyl); Alfuzosin; Analgesics (Opioid); Anticholinergic Agents; Barbiturates; Beta2-Agonists; Brimonidine (Topical); Corticosteroids (Orally Inhaled); Corticosteroids (Systemic); Herbs (Hypotensive Properties); Licorice; MAO Inhibitors; Multivitamins/Fluoride (with ADE); Pentoxifylline; Phosphodiesterase 5

Inhibitors; Prostacyclin Analogues; Selective Serotonin Reuptake Inhibitors; Valsartan

Nutritional/Ethanol Interactions

Food: Hydrochlorothiazide peak serum levels may be decreased if taken with food. This product may deplete potassium, sodium, and magnesium.

Herb/Nutraceutical: Avoid herbs with *hypertensive* properties (bayberry, blue cohosh, cayenne, ephedra, ginger, ginseng [American], kola, licorice); may diminish the antihypertensive effect of hydrochlorothiazide. Avoid herbs with *hypotensive* properties (black cohosh, California poppy, coleus, golden seal, hawthorn, mistletoe, periwinkle, quinine, shepherd's purse); may enhance the hypotensive effect of hydrochlorothiazide.

Adverse Reactions Frequency not defined; the occurrence of adverse events are dose related, with the majority occurring with doses ≥25 mg.

Cardiovascular: Hypotension, necrotizing angiitis, orthostatic hypotension

Central nervous system: Dizziness, headache, paresthesia, restlessness, vertigo

Dermatologic: Alopecia, erythema multiforme, exfoliative dermatitis, skin photosensitivity, skin rash, Stevens-Johnson syndrome, toxic epidermal necrolysis, urticaria

Endocrine & metabolic: Glycosuria, hypercalcemia, hyperglycemia, hyperuricemia, hypochloremic alkalosis, hypokalemia, hypomagnesemia, hyponatremia

Gastrointestinal: Abdominal cramps, anorexia, constipation, diarrhea, gastric irritation, nausea, pancreatitis, sialadenitis, vomiting

Genitourinary: Impotence

Hematologic & oncologic: Agranulocytosis, aplastic anemia, hemolytic anemia, leukopenia, purpura, thrombocytopenia

Hepatic: Jaundice

Hypersensitivity: Anaphylaxis

Neuromuscular & skeletal: Muscle spasm, weakness

Ophthalmic: Blurred vision (transient), xanthopsia

Renal: Interstitial nephritis, renal failure, renal insufficiency

Respiratory: Respiratory distress, pneumonitis, pulmonary edema

Miscellaneous: Fever

Pharmacodynamics/Kinetics

Onset of Action Diuresis: ~2 hours; Peak effect: 4-6 hours

Duration of Action 6-12 hours

Available Dosage Forms

Capsule, Oral:

Microzide: 12.5 mg

Generic: 12.5 mg

Tablet, Oral:

Generic: 12.5 mg, 25 mg, 50 mg

General Dosage Range Oral:

Children <6 months: 1-3 mg/kg/day in 2 divided doses

Children >6 months to 2 years: 1-3 mg/kg/day in 2 divided doses (maximum: 37.5 mg daily)

Children >2-17 years: Initial: 1 mg/kg/day (maximum: 3 mg/kg/day [100 mg daily])

Adults: 12.5-100 mg daily in 1-2 divided doses (maximum: 200 mg daily)

Administration

Oral May be administered with or without food. Take early in day to avoid nocturia. Take the last dose of multiple doses no later than 6 PM unless instructed otherwise.

Storage/Stability Store at 20°C to 25°C (68°F to 77°F) (USP Controlled Room Temperature). Protect from light and moisture.

Nursing Actions

Physical Assessment Allergy history should be identified prior to beginning therapy. Monitor for hypotension, hyponatremia, hypokalemia, and hypercalcemia.

Patient Education

• Discuss specific use of drug and side effects with patient as it relates to treatment. (HCAHPS: During this hospital stay, were you given any medicine that you had not taken before? Before giving you any new medicine, how often did hospital staff tell you what the medicine was for? How often did hospital staff describe possible side effects in a way you could understand?)

• Patient may experience hypokalemia, dizziness, nausea, or xerostomia. Have patient report immediately to prescriber urinary retention, sudden vision changes, eye pain, eye irritation, or rash (HCAHPS).

• Educate patient about signs of a significant reaction (eg, wheezing; chest tightness; fever; itching; bad cough; blue skin color; seizures; or swelling of face, lips, tongue, or throat). **Note:** This is not a comprehensive list of all side effects. Patient should consult prescriber for additional questions.

Intended Use and Disclaimer: Should not be printed and given to patients. This information is intended to serve as a concise initial reference for healthcare professionals to use when discussing medications with a patient. You must ultimately rely on your own discretion, experience and judgment in diagnosing, treating and advising patients.

Dietary Considerations May be taken with or without food.

Hydrochlorothiazide and Spironolactone
(hye droe klor oh THYE a zide & speer on oh LAK tone)

Brand Names: U.S. Aldactazide

Index Terms Spironolactone and Hydrochlorothiazide

Pharmacologic Category Antihypertensive; Diuretic, Thiazide; Selective Aldosterone Blocker

◀ **Medication Safety Issues**

Sound-alike/look-alike issues:

Aldactazide may be confused with Aldactone

Pregnancy Risk Factor C

Use Management of mild-to-moderate hypertension; treatment of edema in congestive heart failure and nephrotic syndrome, and cirrhosis of the liver accompanied by edema and/or ascites

Available Dosage Forms

Tablet: Hydrochlorothiazide 25 mg and spironolactone 25 mg

Aldactazide: 25/25: Hydrochlorothiazide 25 mg and spironolactone 25 mg; 50/50: Hydrochlorothiazide 50 mg and spironolactone 50 mg

General Dosage Range Oral: *Adults:* 12.5-50 mg hydrochlorothiazide and 12.5-50 mg spironolactone daily in single or divided doses

Administration

Oral Administer in the morning; administer the last dose of multiple doses before 6 PM unless instructed otherwise.

Nursing Actions

Physical Assessment See individual agents.

Patient Education

• Discuss specific use of drug and side effects with patient as it relates to treatment. (HCAHPS: During this hospital stay, were you given any medicine that you had not taken before? Before giving you any new medicine, how often did hospital staff tell you what the medicine was for? How often did hospital staff describe possible side effects in a way you could understand?)

• Patient may experience dizziness, nausea, xerostomia, or signs of virilization. Have patient report immediately to prescriber urinary retention, macromastia, sudden vision changes, eye pain, eye irritation, or pregnancy (HCAHPS).

• Educate patient about signs of a significant reaction (eg, wheezing; chest tightness; fever; itching; bad cough; blue skin color; seizures; or swelling of face, lips, tongue, or throat). **Note:** This is not a comprehensive list of all side effects. Patient should consult prescriber for additional questions.

Intended Use and Disclaimer: Should not be printed and given to patients. This information is intended to serve as a concise initial reference for healthcare professionals to use when discussing medications with a patient. You must ultimately rely on your own discretion, experience and judgment in diagnosing, treating and advising patients.

Related Information

Hydrochlorothiazide *on page 775*

Spironolactone *on page 1444*

Hydrochlorothiazide and Triamterene

(hye droe klor oh THYE a zide & trye AM ter een)

Brand Names: U.S. Dyazide; Maxzide; Maxzide-25

Index Terms Triamterene and Hydrochlorothiazide

Pharmacologic Category Antihypertensive; Diuretic, Potassium-Sparing; Diuretic, Thiazide

Medication Safety Issues

Sound-alike/look-alike issues:

Dyazide may be confused with diazoxide, Dynacin

Maxzide may be confused with Maxidex, Microzide

Pregnancy Risk Factor C

Use Treatment of hypertension or edema (not recommended for initial treatment) when hypokalemia has developed on hydrochlorothiazide alone or when the development of hypokalemia must be avoided

Available Dosage Forms

Capsule: Hydrochlorothiazide 25 mg and triamterene 37.5 mg; hydrochlorothiazide 25 mg and triamterene 50 mg

Dyazide: Hydrochlorothiazide 25 mg and triamterene 37.5 mg

Tablet: Hydrochlorothiazide 25 mg and triamterene 37.5 mg; hydrochlorothiazide 50 mg and triamterene 75 mg

Maxzide: Hydrochlorothiazide 50 mg and triamterene 75 mg [scored]

Maxzide-25: Hydrochlorothiazide 25 mg and triamterene 37.5 mg [scored]

General Dosage Range Oral: *Adults:* 25-50 mg hydrochlorothiazide and 37.5-75 mg triamterene once daily

Nursing Actions

Physical Assessment See individual agents.

Patient Education

• Discuss specific use of drug and side effects with patient as it relates to treatment. (HCAHPS: During this hospital stay, were you given any medicine that you had not taken before? Before giving you any new medicine, how often did hospital staff tell you what the medicine was for? How often did hospital staff describe possible side effects in a way you could understand?)

• Patient may experience diarrhea, dizziness, headache, lack of appetite, or dyspepsia. Have patient report immediately to prescriber signs of fluid and electrolyte imbalance, signs of hyperglycemia, signs of hepatic impairment, paresthesia, bradycardia, chills, pharyngitis, akathisia, dyspnea, tremors, ecchymosis, hemorrhaging, change in vision, or ophthalmalgia (HCAHPS).

- Educate patient about signs of a significant reaction (eg, wheezing; chest tightness; fever; itching; bad cough; blue skin color; seizures; or swelling of face, lips, tongue, or throat). **Note:** This is not a comprehensive list of all side effects. Patient should consult prescriber for additional questions.

Intended Use and Disclaimer: Should not be printed and given to patients. This information is intended to serve as a concise initial reference for healthcare professionals to use when discussing medications with a patient. You must ultimately rely on your own discretion, experience and judgment in diagnosing, treating and advising patients.

Related Information
Hydrochlorothiazide *on page 775*

Hydrocodone (hye droe KOE done)

Brand Names: U.S. Zohydro ER
Index Terms Hydrocodone Bitartrate; Zohydro ER
Pharmacologic Category Analgesic, Opioid
Medication Safety Issues
  Sound-alike/look-alike issues:
    HYDROcodone may be confused with oxyCO-DONE, oxymorphone
  High alert medication:
    The Institute for Safe Medication Practices (ISMP) includes this medication among its list of drug classes which have a heightened risk of causing significant patient harm when used in error.

Medication Guide Available Yes
Pregnancy Risk Factor C
Lactation Enters breast milk/not recommended
Use Pain: Management of pain severe enough to require daily around-the-clock opioid, long-term treatment and for which alternative treatment options (eg, nonopioid analgesics or immediate release opioids) are inadequate
Product Availability Zohydro ER: FDA approved October 2013; anticipated availability is first quarter of 2014. Consult prescribing information for additional information.
Controlled Substance C-II
Available Dosage Forms
  Capsule Extended Release 12 Hour, Oral:
    Zohydro ER: 10 mg, 15 mg, 20 mg, 30 mg, 40 mg, 50 mg
General Dosage Range Dosage adjustment recommended in patients with renal or severe hepatic impairment.
  Oral: *Adults:* Initial: 10 mg every 12 hours; Maintenance: Titrate upward to desired response
Administration
  Oral Administer whole; do not crush, chew or dissolve the capsules. Capsules should be administered one at a time, with enough water to ensure complete swallowing immediately after placing in the mouth. Crushing, chewing, or dissolving the capsules will result in uncontrolled delivery of hydrocodone and can lead to overdose or death.

Nursing Actions
  Patient Education
- Discuss specific use of drug and side effects with patient as it relates to treatment. (HCAHPS: During this hospital stay, were you given any medicine that you had not taken before? Before giving you any new medicine, how often did hospital staff tell you what the medicine was for? How often did hospital staff describe possible side effects in a way you could understand?)
- Patient may experience constipation, fatigue, nausea, asthenia, dyspepsia, headache, or dizziness. Have patient report immediately to prescriber signs of hypokalemia, angina, dyspnea, edema of extremities, paresthesia, tachycardia, illogical thinking, mood changes, memory impairment, or dysuria (HCAHPS).
- Educate patient about signs of a significant reaction (eg, wheezing; chest tightness; fever; itching; bad cough; blue skin color; seizures; or swelling of face, lips, tongue, or throat). **Note:** This is not a comprehensive list of all side effects. Patient should consult prescriber for additional questions.

Intended Use and Disclaimer: Should not be printed and given to patients. This information is intended to serve as a concise initial reference for healthcare professionals to use when discussing medications with a patient. You must ultimately rely on your own discretion, experience and judgment in diagnosing, treating and advising patients.

Related Information
Oral Medications That Should Not Be Crushed or Altered *on page 1712*

Hydrocodone and Acetaminophen
(hye droe KOE done & a seet a MIN oh fen)

Brand Names: U.S. hycet®; Lorcet® 10/650; Lorcet® Plus; Lortab®; Margesic® H; Maxidone® [DSC]; Norco®; Stagesic™; Vicodin ES®; Vicodin HP®; Vicodin®; Xodol® 10/300; Xodol® 5/300; Xodol® 7.5/300; Zamicet™; Zolvit®; Zydone®
Index Terms Acetaminophen and Hydrocodone
Pharmacologic Category Analgesic Combination (Opioid)
Medication Safety Issues
  Sound-alike/look-alike issues:
    Hydrocodone and Acetaminophen may be confused with Oxycodone and Acetaminophen
    Lorcet® may be confused with Fioricet®
    Lortab® may be confused with Cortef®

◀ Vicodin® may be confused with Hycodan, Indocin®

Zydone® may be confused with Vytone

High alert medication:

The Institute for Safe Medication Practices (ISMP) includes this medication among its list of drug classes which have a heightened risk of causing significant patient harm when used in error.

Other safety concerns:

Duplicate therapy issues: This product contains acetaminophen, which may be a component of other combination products. Do not exceed the maximum recommended daily dose of acetaminophen.

Pregnancy Risk Factor C

Use Relief of moderate-to-severe pain

Controlled Substance C-III

Available Dosage Forms

Capsule, oral: Hydrocodone 5 mg and acetaminophen 500 mg

Margesic® H, Stagesic™: Hydrocodone 5 mg and acetaminophen 500 mg

Elixir, oral:

Lortab®: Hydrocodone 10 mg and acetaminophen 300 mg per 15 mL

Solution, oral: Hydrocodone 7.5 mg and acetaminophen 325 mg per 15 mL; hydrocodone 7.5 mg and acetaminophen 500 mg per 15 mL; hydrocodone 10 mg and acetaminophen 325 mg per 15 mL

hycet®: Hydrocodone 7.5 mg and acetaminophen 325 mg per 15 mL

Zamicet™: Hydrocodone 10 mg and acetaminophen 325 mg per 15 mL

Zolvit®: Hydrocodone 10 mg and acetaminophen 300 mg per 15 mL (480 mL)

Tablet, oral:

Generics:

Hydrocodone 2.5 mg and acetaminophen 325 mg

Hydrocodone 2.5 mg and acetaminophen 500 mg

Hydrocodone 5 mg and acetaminophen 300 mg

Hydrocodone 5 mg and acetaminophen 325 mg

Hydrocodone 5 mg and acetaminophen 500 mg

Hydrocodone 7.5 mg and acetaminophen 300 mg

Hydrocodone 7.5 mg and acetaminophen 325 mg

Hydrocodone 7.5 mg and acetaminophen 500 mg

Hydrocodone 7.5 mg and acetaminophen 650 mg

Hydrocodone 7.5 mg and acetaminophen 750 mg

Hydrocodone 10 mg and acetaminophen 300 mg

Hydrocodone 10 mg and acetaminophen 325 mg

Hydrocodone 10 mg and acetaminophen 500 mg

Hydrocodone 10 mg and acetaminophen 650 mg

Hydrocodone 10 mg and acetaminophen 660 mg

Hydrocodone 10 mg and acetaminophen 750 mg

Brands:

Lorcet® 10/650: Hydrocodone 10 mg and acetaminophen 650 mg

Lorcet® Plus: Hydrocodone 7.5 mg and acetaminophen 650 mg

Lortab®: 5/500: Hydrocodone 5 mg and acetaminophen 500 mg; 7.5/500: Hydrocodone 7.5 mg and acetaminophen 500 mg; 10/500: Hydrocodone 10 mg and acetaminophen 500 mg

Norco®: Hydrocodone 5 mg and acetaminophen 325 mg; hydrocodone 7.5 mg and acetaminophen 325 mg; hydrocodone 10 mg and acetaminophen 325 mg

Vicodin®: Hydrocodone 5 mg and acetaminophen 300 mg

Vicodin ES®: Hydrocodone 7.5 mg and acetaminophen 300 mg

Vicodin HP®: Hydrocodone 10 mg and acetaminophen 300 mg

Xodol®: 5/300: Hydrocodone 5 mg and acetaminophen 300 mg; 7.5/300: Hydrocodone 7.5 mg and acetaminophen 300 mg; 10/300: Hydrocodone 10 mg and acetaminophen 300 mg

Zydone®: Hydrocodone 5 mg and acetaminophen 400 mg; hydrocodone 7.5 mg and acetaminophen 400 mg; hydrocodone 10 mg and acetaminophen 400 mg

General Dosage Range Oral:

Children 2-13 years or <50 kg: Hydrocodone 0.1-0.2 mg/kg/dose every 4-6 hours (maximum: 6 doses/day or maximum recommended dose of acetaminophen for age/weight)

Children ≥50 kg and Adults: Hydrocodone 2.5-10 mg every 4-6 hours (maximum: 4 g/day [acetaminophen])

Elderly: Hydrocodone 2.5-5 mg every 4-6 hours

Nursing Actions

Physical Assessment Assess patient for history of liver disease or ethanol abuse (acetaminophen and any ethanol may have adverse liver effects). Ensure adult patients keep daily dose to ≤4 g/day. Monitor for effectiveness of pain relief. Monitor blood pressure, CNS and respiratory status, and degree of sedation prior to treatment and periodically throughout. For inpatients, implement safety measures (eg, side rails up, call light within reach, instructions to call for assistance). Assess patient's physical and/or psychological dependence. Discontinue slowly after prolonged use.

Patient Education

- Discuss specific use of drug and side effects with patient as it relates to treatment. (HCAHPS: During this hospital stay, were you given any medicine that you had not taken before? Before giving you any new medicine, how often did hospital staff tell you what the medicine was for? How often did hospital staff describe possible side effects in a way you could understand?)
- Patient may experience fatigue or nausea. Have patient report immediately to prescriber signs of hepatic impairment, severe dizziness, syncope, dyspnea, illogical thinking, significant constipation, considerable asthenia, urinary retention, oliguria, hearing impairment, angina, chills, pharyngitis, mood changes, significant headache, difficult urination, ecchymosis, hemorrhaging, vision changes, or Stevens-Johnson syndrome/toxic epidermal necrolysis (HCAHPS).
- Educate patient about signs of a significant reaction (eg, wheezing; chest tightness; fever; itching; bad cough; blue skin color; seizures; or swelling of face, lips, tongue, or throat). **Note:** This is not a comprehensive list of all side effects. Patient should consult prescriber for additional questions.

Intended Use and Disclaimer: Should not be printed and given to patients. This information is intended to serve as a concise initial reference for healthcare professionals to use when discussing medications with a patient. You must ultimately rely on your own discretion, experience and judgment in diagnosing, treating and advising patients.

Related Information

Acetaminophen on page 31

Hydrocodone and Ibuprofen
(hye droe KOE done & eye byoo PROE fen)

Brand Names: U.S. Ibudone; Reprexain; Vicoprofen

Index Terms Hydrocodone Bitartrate and Ibuprofen; Ibuprofen and Hydrocodone

Pharmacologic Category Analgesic Combination (Opioid); Nonsteroidal Anti-inflammatory Drug (NSAID), Oral

Medication Safety Issues
Sound-alike/look-alike issues:
Reprexain may be confused with ZyPREXA
High alert medication:
The Institute for Safe Medication Practices (ISMP) includes this medication among its list of drug classes which have a heightened risk of causing significant patient harm when used in error.

Medication Guide Available Yes

Pregnancy Risk Factor C

Use Short-term (generally <10 days) management of moderate-to-severe acute pain; is not indicated for treatment of such conditions as osteoarthritis or rheumatoid arthritis

Controlled Substance C-III

Available Dosage Forms
Tablet: Hydrocodone 2.5 mg and ibuprofen 200 mg; Hydrocodone 5 mg and ibuprofen 200 mg; Hydrocodone 7.5 mg and ibuprofen 200 mg; Hydrocodone bitartrate 10 mg and ibuprofen 200 mg
Ibudone: 5/200: Hydrocodone 5 mg and ibuprofen 200 mg; 10/200: Hydrocodone 10 mg and ibuprofen 200 mg
Reprexain: 2.5/200: Hydrocodone 2.5 mg and ibuprofen 200 mg; 5/200: Hydrocodone 5 mg and ibuprofen 200 mg; 10/200: Hydrocodone 10 mg and ibuprofen 200 mg
Vicoprofen: 7.5/200: Hydrocodone 7.5 mg and ibuprofen 200 mg

General Dosage Range Oral: *Adults:* 1 tablet every 4-6 hours (maximum: 5 tablets/day; <10 days total therapy)

Nursing Actions
Physical Assessment Assess patient for allergic reaction to salicylates or other NSAIDs. Monitor blood pressure and for adverse gastrointestinal response prior to treatment and periodically throughout. Monitor for effectiveness of pain relief. Monitor CNS and respiratory status and degree of sedation prior to treatment and periodically throughout. For inpatients, implement safety measures (eg, side rails up, call light within reach, instructions to call for assistance). Assess patient's physical and/or psychological dependence. Discontinue slowly after prolonged use.

Patient Education

- Discuss specific use of drug and side effects with patient as it relates to treatment. (HCAHPS: During this hospital stay, were you given any medicine that you had not taken before? Before giving you any new medicine, how often did hospital staff tell you what the medicine was for? How often did hospital staff describe possible side effects in a way you could understand?)
- Patient may experience constipation, insomnia, diarrhea, or flatulence. Have patient report immediately to prescriber severe dizziness, syncope, dyspnea, angina, tachycardia, strength differences from one side to another, difficulty speaking or thinking, change in balance, blurred vision, significant nausea, considerable dyspepsia, ecchymosis, hemorrhaging, intolerable asthenia, urinary retention, oliguria, jaundice, mood changes, arrhythmia, chills, pharyngitis, tinnitus, severe headache, neck rigidity, arthralgia, myalgia, melena, hematemesis, excessive weight gain, or edema of extremities (HCAHPS).
- Educate patient about signs of a significant reaction (eg, wheezing; chest tightness; fever; itching; bad cough; blue skin color; seizures; or swelling of face, lips, tongue, or throat). **Note:** This is not a comprehensive list of all side

effects. Patient should consult prescriber for additional questions.

Intended Use and Disclaimer: Should not be printed and given to patients. This information is intended to serve as a concise initial reference for healthcare professionals to use when discussing medications with a patient. You must ultimately rely on your own discretion, experience and judgment in diagnosing, treating and advising patients.

Related Information
Ibuprofen on page 798

Hydrocortisone (Systemic)
(hye droe KOR ti sone)

Brand Names: U.S. A-Hydrocort; Cortef; Solu-CORTEF

Index Terms A-hydroCort; Compound F; Cortisol; Hydrocortisone Sodium Succinate

Pharmacologic Category Corticosteroid, Systemic

Medication Safety Issues
Sound-alike/look-alike issues:
Hydrocortisone may be confused with hydrocodone, hydroxychloroquine, hydrochlorothiazide
Cortef® may be confused with Coreg®, Lortab®
HCT (occasional abbreviation for hydrocortisone) is an error-prone abbreviation (mistaken as hydrochlorothiazide)
Solu-CORTEF® may be confused with Solu-MEDROL®

Pregnancy Risk Factor C

Lactation Enters breast milk/use caution

Breast-Feeding Considerations Corticosteroids are excreted in breast milk. The manufacturer notes that when used systemically, maternal use of corticosteroids have the potential to cause adverse events in a nursing infant (eg, growth suppression, interfere with endogenous corticosteroid production). If there is concern about exposure to the infant, some guidelines recommend waiting 4 hours after the maternal dose of an oral systemic corticosteroid before breast-feeding in order to decrease potential exposure to the nursing infant (based on a study using prednisolone) (Bae, 2011; Leachman, 2006; Makol, 2011; Ost, 1985).

Use Management of adrenocortical insufficiency; anti-inflammatory or immunosuppressive

Unlabeled Use Management of septic shock when blood pressure is poorly responsive to fluid resuscitation and vasopressor therapy; treatment of thyroid storm

Mechanism of Action/Effect Decreases inflammation by suppression of migration of polymorphonuclear leukocytes and reversal of increased capillary permeability

Contraindications Hypersensitivity to hydrocortisone or any component of the formulation; serious infections, except septic shock or tuberculous meningitis; viral, fungal, or tubercular skin lesions; I.M. administration contraindicated in idiopathic thrombocytopenia purpura; intrathecal administration of injection

Warnings/Precautions Use with caution in patients with thyroid disease, hepatic impairment, renal impairment, heart failure, hypertension, diabetes, glaucoma, cataracts, myasthenia gravis, patients at risk for osteoporosis, patients at risk for seizures, or GI diseases (diverticulitis, peptic ulcer, ulcerative colitis) due to perforation risk. Use caution following acute MI (corticosteroids have been associated with myocardial rupture). Because of the risk of adverse effects, systemic corticosteroids should be used cautiously in the elderly in the smallest possible effective dose for the shortest duration. May affect growth velocity; growth should be routinely monitored in pediatric patients. Withdraw therapy with gradual tapering of dose.

May cause hypercorticism or suppression of hypothalamic-pituitary-adrenal (HPA) axis, particularly in younger children or in patients receiving high doses for prolonged periods. HPA axis suppression may lead to adrenal crisis. Withdrawal and discontinuation of a corticosteroid should be done slowly and carefully. Particular care is required when patients are transferred from systemic corticosteroids to inhaled products due to possible adrenal insufficiency or withdrawal from steroids, including an increase in allergic symptoms. Patients receiving >20 mg per day of prednisone (or equivalent) may be most susceptible. Fatalities have occurred due to adrenal insufficiency in asthmatic patients during and after transfer from systemic corticosteroids to aerosol steroids; aerosol steroids do not provide the systemic steroid needed to treat patients having trauma, surgery, or infections.

Acute myopathy has been reported with high dose corticosteroids, usually in patients with neuromuscular transmission disorders; may involve ocular and/or respiratory muscles; monitor creatine kinase; recovery may be delayed. Corticosteroid use may cause psychiatric disturbances, including depression, euphoria, insomnia, mood swings, and personality changes. Pre-existing psychiatric conditions may be exacerbated by corticosteroid use. Prolonged use of corticosteroids may also increase the incidence of secondary infection, mask acute infection (including fungal infections), prolong or exacerbate viral infections, or limit response to vaccines. Exposure to chickenpox should be avoided; corticosteroids should not be used to treat ocular herpes simplex. Corticosteroids should not be used for cerebral malaria or viral hepatitis. Oral steroid treatment is not recommended for the treatment of acute optic neuritis. Close observation is required in patients with latent tuberculosis and/or TB reactivity; restrict use in active TB (only in conjunction with antituberculosis treatment). Prolonged treatment with corticosteroids has been associated with the development of Kaposi's sarcoma (case reports); if noted, discontinuation of therapy should be considered. High-dose corticosteroids should not be used to manage acute head injury. Some dosage forms contain benzyl alcohol which has been associated with "gasping syndrome" in neonates.

Drug Interactions

Avoid Concomitant Use

Avoid concomitant use of Hydrocortisone (Systemic) with any of the following: Aldesleukin; Axitinib; BCG; Indium 111 Capromab Pendetide; Mifepristone; Natalizumab; Pimecrolimus; Simeprevir; Tacrolimus (Topical); Tofacitinib

Decreased Effect

Hydrocortisone (Systemic) may decrease the levels/effects of: Aldesleukin; Antidiabetic Agents; ARIPiprazole; Axitinib; BCG; Calcitriol; Coccidioidin Skin Test; Corticorelin; Hyaluronidase; Ibrutinib; Indium 111 Capromab Pendetide; Isoniazid; Salicylates; Simeprevir; Sipuleucel-T; Telaprevir; Urea Cycle Disorder Agents; Vaccines (Inactivated)

The levels/effects of Hydrocortisone (Systemic) may be decreased by: Aminoglutethimide; Antacids; Barbiturates; Bile Acid Sequestrants; Echinacea; Mifepristone; Mitotane; P-glycoprotein/ABCB1 Inducers; Primidone; Rifamycin Derivatives

Increased Effect/Toxicity

Hydrocortisone (Systemic) may increase the levels/effects of: Acetylcholinesterase Inhibitors; Amphotericin B; Deferasirox; Leflunomide; Loop Diuretics; Natalizumab; NSAID (COX-2 Inhibitor); NSAID (Nonselective); Thiazide Diuretics; Tofacitinib; Vaccines (Live); Warfarin

The levels/effects of Hydrocortisone (Systemic) may be increased by: Antifungal Agents (Azole Derivatives, Systemic); Aprepitant; Calcium Channel Blockers (Nondihydropyridine); Denosumab; Estrogen Derivatives; Fluconazole; Fosaprepitant; Indacaterol; Macrolide Antibiotics; Mifepristone; Neuromuscular-Blocking Agents (Nondepolarizing); P-glycoprotein/ABCB1 Inhibitors; Pimecrolimus; Quinolone Antibiotics; Roflumilast; Salicylates; Tacrolimus (Topical); Telaprevir; Trastuzumab

Nutritional/Ethanol Interactions

Ethanol: Avoid ethanol (may enhance gastric mucosal irritation).

Food: Hydrocortisone interferes with calcium absorption.

Herb/Nutraceutical: St John's wort may decrease hydrocortisone levels. Avoid cat's claw, echinacea (have immunostimulant properties).

Adverse Reactions Frequency not defined.

Cardiovascular: Arrhythmias, bradycardia, cardiac arrest, cardiomegaly, circulatory collapse, congestive heart failure, edema, fat embolism, hypertension, hypertrophic cardiomyopathy (premature infants), myocardial rupture (post MI), syncope, tachycardia, thromboembolism, vasculitis

Central nervous system: Delirium, depression, emotional instability, euphoria, hallucinations, headache, insomnia, intracranial pressure increased, malaise, mood swings, nervousness, neuritis, neuropathy, personality changes, pseudotumor cerebri, psychic disorders, psychoses, seizure, vertigo

Dermatologic: Acne, allergic dermatitis, alopecia, bruising, burning/tingling, dry scaly skin, edema, erythema, hirsutism, hyper-/hypopigmentation, impaired wound healing, petechiae, rash, skin atrophy, skin test reaction impaired, sterile abscess, striae, urticaria

Endocrine & metabolic: Adrenal suppression, alkalosis, amenorrhea, carbohydrate intolerance increased, Cushing's syndrome, diabetes mellitus, glucose intolerance, growth suppression, hyperglycemia, hyperlipidemia, hypokalemia, hypokalemic alkalosis, menstrual irregularities, negative nitrogen balance, pituitary-adrenal axis suppression, potassium loss, protein catabolism, sodium and water retention, sperm motility increased/decreased, spermatogenesis increased/decreased

Gastrointestinal: Abdominal distention, appetite increased, bowel dysfunction (intrathecal administration), indigestion, nausea, pancreatitis, peptic ulcer, gastrointestinal perforation, ulcerative esophagitis, vomiting, weight gain

Genitourinary: Bladder dysfunction (intrathecal administration)

Hematologic: Leukocytosis (transient)

Hepatic: Hepatomegaly, transaminases increased

Local: Atrophy (at injection site), postinjection flare (intra-articular use), thrombophlebitis

Neuromuscular & skeletal: Arthralgia, necrosis (femoral and humoral heads), Charcot-like arthropathy, fractures, muscle mass loss, muscle weakness, myopathy, osteoporosis, tendon rupture, vertebral compression fractures

Ocular: Cataracts, exophthalmoses, glaucoma, intraocular pressure increased

Miscellaneous: Abnormal fat deposits, anaphylaxis, avascular necrosis, diaphoresis, hiccups, hypersensitivity reactions, infection, secondary malignancy

Pharmacodynamics/Kinetics

Onset of Action Hydrocortisone sodium succinate (water soluble): Rapid

Available Dosage Forms

Solution Reconstituted, Injection:

A-Hydrocort: 100 mg (1 ea)

Solu-CORTEF: 100 mg (1 ea)

Solution Reconstituted, Injection [preservative free]:

Solu-CORTEF: 100 mg (1 ea); 250 mg (1 ea); 500 mg (1 ea); 1000 mg (1 ea)

Tablet, Oral:

Cortef: 5 mg, 10 mg, 20 mg

Generic: 5 mg, 10 mg, 20 mg

General Dosage Range

I.M., I.V.: *Children and Adults:* Dosage varies greatly depending on indication

Oral:

Children: 0.5-10 mg/kg/day **or** 10-300 mg/m²/day divided every 6-8 hours

Adolescents: 0.5-10 mg/kg/day **or** 10-300 mg/m²/day divided every 6-8 hours **or** 15-240 mg every 12 hours

Adults: 20-480 mg/day in divided doses every 8-12 hours **or** 10-20 mg/m²/day in 3 divided doses

Administration

I.V. Hydrocortisone sodium succinate may be administered by I.M. or I.V. routes. Dermal and/or subdermal skin depression may occur at the site of injection. Avoid injection into deltoid muscle (high incidence of subcutaneous atrophy).

I.V. bolus: Administer over 30 seconds or over 10 minutes for doses ≥500 mg.

I.V. intermittent infusion: Administer over 20-30 minutes.

Note: Should be administered in a 0.1-1 mg/mL concentration due to stability problems.

Injectable Detail pH: Hydrocortisone sodium succinate: 7-8

Oral Administer with food or milk to decrease GI upset.

Preparation for Administration

Sodium succinate: I.V. bolus or I.M. administration: Reconstitute 100 mg vials with bacteriostatic water (not >2 mL). Act-O-Vial (self-contained powder for injection plus diluent) may be reconstituted by pressing the activator to force diluent into the powder compartment. Following gentle agitation, solution may be withdrawn via syringe through a needle inserted into the center of the stopper. May be administered (I.V. or I.M.) without further dilution.

Solutions for I.V. infusion: Reconstituted solutions may be added to an appropriate volume of compatible solution for infusion. Concentration should generally not exceed 1 mg/mL. However, in cases where administration of a small volume of fluid is desirable, 100-3000 mg may be added to 50 mL of D₅W or NS (stability limited to 4 hours).

Storage/Stability Store at controlled room temperature 20°C to 25°C (68°F to 77°F). Protect from light. Hydrocortisone sodium phosphate and hydrocortisone sodium succinate are clear, light yellow solutions which are heat labile.

Sodium succinate: After initial reconstitution, hydrocortisone sodium succinate solutions are stable for 3 days at room temperature or under refrigeration when protected from light. Stability of parenteral admixture (Solu-Cortef®) at room temperature (25°C) and at refrigeration temperature (4°C) is concentration-dependent:

Stability of concentration 1 mg/mL: 24 hours

Stability of concentration 2 mg/mL to 60 mg/mL: At least 4 hours

Nursing Actions

Physical Assessment Assess for signs of fluid retention, signs of hyperglycemia, or infection. Taper dosage slowly when discontinuing if patient has been on for a period of time; assess tolerance of taper (BP, pulse, mentation, energy level). Do not use with existing fungal infections.

Patient Education

• Discuss specific use of drug and side effects with patient as it relates to treatment. (HCAHPS: During this hospital stay, were you given any medicine that you had not taken before? Before giving you any new medicine, how often did hospital staff tell you what the medicine was for? How often did hospital staff describe possible side effects in a way you could understand?)

• Patient may experience nausea, insomnia, akathisia, or hyperhidrosis. Have patient report immediately to prescriber signs of infection, signs of hyperglycemia, signs of hypokalemia, signs of pancreatitis, severe asthenia, irritability, tremors, tachycardia, confusion, dizziness, dyspnea, excessive weight gain, edema of extremities, skin changes, moon face, buffalo hump, significant headache, osteodynia, arthralgia, menstrual irregularities, angina, vision changes, mood changes, behavioral changes, depression, paresthesia, ecchymosis, hemorrhaging, considerable dyspepsia, melena, hematemesis, or injection site irritation (HCAHPS).

• Educate patient about signs of a significant reaction (eg, wheezing; chest tightness; fever; itching; bad cough; blue skin color; seizures; or swelling of face, lips, tongue, or throat). **Note:** This is not a comprehensive list of all side effects. Patient should consult prescriber for additional questions.

Intended Use and Disclaimer: Should not be printed and given to patients. This information is intended to serve as a concise initial reference for healthcare professionals to use when discussing medications with a patient. You must ultimately rely on your own discretion, experience and judgment in diagnosing, treating and advising patients.

Dietary Considerations Systemic use of corticosteroids may require a diet with increased potassium, vitamins A, B₆, C, D, folate, calcium, zinc, phosphorus, and decreased sodium. Some products may contain sodium.

Hydrocortisone (Topical)
(hye droe KOR ti sone)

Brand Names: U.S. Ala Cort; Ala Scalp; Anti-Itch Maximum Strength [OTC]; Anucort-HC; Anusol-HC; Aquanil HC [OTC]; Beta HC [OTC]; Colocort; CortAlo; Cortenema; Corticool [OTC]; Cortifoam; Dermasorb HC; First-Hydrocortisone; GRx HiCort 25; Hemril-30; Hydro Skin Maximum Strength [OTC]; Hydrocortisone Max St [OTC]; Hydrocortisone Max St/12 Moist [OTC]; HydroSKIN [OTC]; Instacort 10 [OTC]; Instacort 5 [OTC]; Locoid; Locoid Lipocream; Med-Derm Hydrocortisone [OTC]; Medi-First Hydrocortisone [OTC]; NuCort; NuZon; Pandel; Pediaderm HC; Preparation H Hydrocortisone [OTC]; Procto-Pak; Proctocort; Proctocream HC [DSC]; Proctosol HC; Proctozone-HC; Recort Plus [OTC]; Rectacort-HC; Rederm [OTC]; Sarnol-HC [OTC]; Scalacort; Scalacort DK; Scalpicin Maximum Strength [OTC]; Texacort; TheraCort [OTC]; U-Cort; Westcort

Index Terms A-hydroCort; Compound F; Cortisol; Hemorrhoidal HC; Hydrocortisone Acetate; Hydrocortisone Butyrate; Hydrocortisone Probutate; Hydrocortisone Valerate; Nutracort

Pharmacologic Category Antihemorrhoidal Agent; Corticosteroid, Rectal; Corticosteroid, Topical

Medication Safety Issues
Sound-alike/look-alike issues:
Hydrocortisone may be confused with hydrocodone, hydroxychloroquine, hydrochlorothiazide
Anusol® may be confused with Anusol-HC®, Aplisol®, Aquasol®
Cortizone® may be confused with cortisone
HCT (occasional abbreviation for hydrocortisone) is an error-prone abbreviation (mistaken as hydrochlorothiazide)
Hytone® may be confused with Vytone®
Proctocort® may be confused with ProctoCream®

International issues:
Nutracort [multiple international markets] may be confused with Nitrocor brand name of nitroglycerin [Italy, Russia, and Venezuela]

Pregnancy Risk Factor C

Lactation Enters breast milk/use caution

Use Relief of inflammation of corticosteroid-responsive dermatoses (low and medium potency topical corticosteroid); adjunctive treatment of ulcerative colitis; mild-to-moderate atopic dermatitis; inflamed hemorrhoids, postirradiation (factitial) proctitis, and other inflammatory conditions of anorectum and pruritus ani

Available Dosage Forms
Cream, External:
Ala Cort: 1% (28.4 g, 85.2 g)
Anti-Itch Maximum Strength [OTC]: 1% (28 g)
Hydrocortisone Max St [OTC]: 1% (28.4 g)
Hydrocortisone Max St/12 Moist [OTC]: 1% (28.4 g)

HydroSKIN [OTC]: 1% (28 g)
Instacort 5 [OTC]: 0.5% (28.4 g)
Locoid: 0.1% (15 g, 45 g)
Locoid Lipocream: 0.1% (45 g, 60 g)
Med-Derm Hydrocortisone [OTC]: 0.5% (30 g); 1% (30 g)
Medi-First Hydrocortisone [OTC]: 1% (1 ea)
Pandel: 0.1% (15 g, 45 g, 80 g)
Preparation H Hydrocortisone [OTC]: 1% (26 g)
Recort Plus [OTC]: 1% (30 g)
U-Cort: 1% (28.35 g)
Generic: 0.1% (15 g, 45 g, 60 g); 0.2% (15 g, 45 g, 60 g); 0.5% (15 g, 28.35 g, 28.4 g, 30 g); 1% (1 g, 1.5 g, 15 g, 20 g, 28 g, 28.35 g, 28.4 g, 30 g, 120 g, 453.6 g, 454 g); 2.5% (20 g, 28 g, 28.35 g, 30 g, 453.6 g)

Cream, Rectal:
Anusol-HC: 2.5% (30 g)
Procto-Pak: 1% (28.4 g)
Proctocort: 1% (28.35 g)
Proctosol HC: 2.5% (28.35 g)
Proctozone-HC: 2.5% (30 g)

Enema, Rectal:
Colocort: 100 mg/60 mL (60 mL)
Cortenema: 100 mg/60 mL (60 mL)
Generic: 100 mg/60 mL (60 mL)

Foam, Rectal:
Cortifoam: 90 mg (15 g)

Gel, External:
CortAlo: 2% (43 g)
Corticool [OTC]: 1% (42.53 g)
First-Hydrocortisone: 10% (60 g)
Instacort 10 [OTC]: 1% (30 g)
NuZon: 2% (43 g)
Generic: 2% (43 g)

Kit, External:
Dermasorb HC: 2%
Pediaderm HC: 2%
Scalacort DK: Hydrocortisone lotion 2% and Sal Acid 2% and sulfur 2%

Lotion, External:
Ala Scalp: 2% (29.6 mL)
Aquanil HC [OTC]: 1% (120 mL)
Beta HC [OTC]: 1% (60 mL)
Hydro Skin Maximum Strength [OTC]: 1% (118 mL)
Locoid: 0.1% (59 mL, 118 mL)
NuCort: 2% (60 g)
Rederm [OTC]: 1% (120 mL)
Sarnol-HC [OTC]: 1% (59 mL)
Scalacort: 2% (29.6 mL)
TheraCort [OTC]: 1% (118 mL)
Generic: 1% (114 g); 2.5% (59 mL, 118 mL)

Ointment, External:
Locoid: 0.1% (15 g, 45 g)
Westcort: 0.2% (15 g, 45 g, 60 g)
Generic: 0.1% (15 g, 45 g); 0.2% (15 g, 45 g, 60 g); 0.5% (28.35 g, 30 g); 1% (25 g, 28 g, 28.35 g, 28.4 g, 30 g, 110 g, 430 g, 453.6 g); 2.5% (20 g, 28.35 g, 453.6 g, 454 g)

Solution, External:
Locoid: 0.1% (60 mL)
Scalpicin Maximum Strength [OTC]: 1% (44 mL)
Texacort: 2.5% (30 mL)
Generic: 0.1% (20 mL, 60 mL)

Suppository, Rectal:
Anucort-HC: 25 mg (12 ea, 24 ea, 100 ea)
Anusol-HC: 25 mg (12 ea, 24 ea)
GRx HiCort 25: 25 mg (12 ea)
Hemril-30: 30 mg (12 ea, 24 ea)
Proctocort: 30 mg (12 ea)
Rectacort-HC: 25 mg (12 ea, 24 ea)
Generic: 25 mg (12 ea, 24 ea); 30 mg (12 ea)

General Dosage Range

Rectal: *Adults:* Foam: One applicatorful 1-2 times/
day; Suppository: 1-2 suppositories 2-3 times/
day; Suspension: One enema at bedtime

Topical: *Children and Adults:* Apply thin film to
affected area 2-4 times/day

Administration

Topical
Topical cream, lotion, ointment: Apply a thin film to
clean, dry skin and rub in gently.

Rectal foam: Shake vigorously for 5-10 seconds
prior to use. Do not remove cap during use. Hold
container upright to fill applicator. Gently insert
applicator tip into anus. Only use applicator provided by manufacturer; do not insert any part of
the aerosol container in the anus. Clean applicator after each use.

Rectal suppository: Remove foil from rectal suppository and insert pointed end first. Avoid handling unwrapped suppository for too long.

Rectal suspension: Shake bottle well. Remove
protective sheath from applicator tip. Lie on left
side with left leg extended and right leg flexed
forward. Gently insert lubricated applicator tip into
rectum, pointed slightly toward navel. Grasp bottle firmly and squeeze slowly to instill the medication. After administering, withdraw and discard
the used unit. Remain in position for at least 30
minutes. Retain the enema all night if possible.

Nursing Actions

Physical Assessment Topical absorption may
be minimal.

Patient Education
• Discuss specific use of drug and side effects
with patient as it relates to treatment. (HCAHPS:
During this hospital stay, were you given any
medicine that you had not taken before? Before
giving you any new medicine, how often did
hospital staff tell you what the medicine was
for? How often did hospital staff describe possible side effects in a way you could understand?)
• Patient may experience xeroderma or rectal
irritation. Have patient report immediately to
prescriber signs of hyperglycemia, weight gain,
vision changes, severe headache, skin
changes, considerable skin irritation, significant

hematochezia, or intolerable rectal pain
(HCAHPS).
• Educate patient about signs of a significant
reaction (eg, wheezing; chest tightness; fever;
itching; bad cough; blue skin color; seizures; or
swelling of face, lips, tongue, or throat). **Note:**
This is not a comprehensive list of all side
effects. Patient should consult prescriber for
additional questions.

Intended Use and Disclaimer: Should not be
printed and given to patients. This information is
intended to serve as a concise initial reference for
healthcare professionals to use when discussing
medications with a patient. You must ultimately
rely on your own discretion, experience and judgment in diagnosing, treating and advising
patients.

HYDROmorphone (hye droe MOR fone)

Brand Names: U.S. Dilaudid; Dilaudid-HP; Exalgo
Index Terms Dihydromorphinone; Hydromorphone
Hydrochloride
Pharmacologic Category Analgesic, Opioid

Medication Safety Issues

Sound-alike/look-alike issues:
Dilaudid may be confused with Demerol, Dilantin
HYDROmorphone may be confused with morphine; significant overdoses have occurred
when hydromorphone products have been inadvertently administered instead of morphine sulfate. Commercially available prefilled syringes of
both products looks similar and are often stored
in close proximity to each other. **Note:** Hydromorphone 1 mg oral is approximately equal to
morphine 4 mg oral; hydromorphone 1 mg I.V. is
approximately equal to morphine 5 mg I.V.

High alert medication:
The Institute for Safe Medication Practices
(ISMP) includes this medication among its list
of drug classes which have a heightened risk of
causing significant patient harm when used in
error.

Administration issues:
Dilaudid, Dilaudid-HP: Extreme caution should be
taken to avoid confusing the highly-concentrated
(Dilaudid-HP) injection with the less-concentrated (Dilaudid) injectable product.
Exalgo: Extreme caution should be taken to avoid
confusing the extended release Exalgo 8 mg
tablets with immediate release hydromorphone
8 mg tablets.
Significant differences exist between oral and I.V.
dosing. Use caution when converting from one
route of administration to another.

Medication Guide Available Yes
Pregnancy Risk Factor C
Lactation Enters breast milk/not recommended
Breast-Feeding Considerations Low concentra-
tions of hydromorphone can be found in breast

milk. Withdrawal symptoms may be observed in breast-feeding infants when opioid analgesics are discontinued. Breast-feeding is not recommended by the manufacturer. Parenteral opioids used during labor have the potential to interfere with a newborn's natural reflex to nurse within the first few hours after birth. Nursing infants exposed to large doses of opioids should be monitored for apnea and sedation (Montgomery, 2012).

Use Management of moderate-to-severe pain

Exalgo: Management of moderate-to-severe pain in opioid-tolerant patients (requiring around-the-clock analgesia for an extended period of time)

Mechanism of Action/Effect Binds to opioid receptors in the CNS, causing inhibition of ascending pain pathways, altering the perception of and response to pain; causes cough supression by direct central action in the medulla; produces generalized CNS depression

Contraindications Hypersensitivity to hydromorphone, any component of the formulation; acute or severe asthma, severe respiratory depression (in absence of resuscitative equipment or ventilatory support)

Additional product-specific contraindications:

Dilaudid liquid and tablets: Obstetrical analgesia

Dilaudid injection, Dilaudid-HP injection: Opioid nontolerant patients (Dilaudid-HP injection only); patients with risk of developing GI obstruction, especially paralytic ileus

Exalgo: Opioid nontolerant patients, paralytic ileus (known or suspected), pre-existing GI surgery or diseases resulting in narrowing of GI tract, loops in the GI tract or GI obstruction

Suppository: Intracranial lesion associated with increased intracranial pressure; whenever ventilatory function is depressed (COPD, cor pulmonale, emphysema, kyphoscoliosis, status asthmaticus)

Warnings/Precautions [U.S. Boxed Warning]: May cause potentially life-threatening respiratory depression even with therapeutic use, especially with initiation or dose increases; instruct patients on proper administration of extended release tablets. The use of ethanol, other opioids, and other CNS depressants may increase the risk of adverse outcomes, including death. Critical respiratory depression may occur, even at therapeutic dosages, particularly in elderly, cachectic, or debilitated patients or in patients with pre-existing respiratory compromise (hypoxia and/or hypercapnia). Use caution in COPD or other obstructive pulmonary disease.

Use with caution in patients with hypersensitivity reactions to other phenanthrene derivative opioid agonists (codeine, hydrocodone, levorphanol, oxycodone, oxymorphone). Hydromorphone shares toxic potential of opioid agonists, including CNS depression and respiratory depression. Precautions associated with opioid agonist therapy should

be observed. May cause CNS depression, which may impair physical or mental abilities; patients must be cautioned about performing tasks which require mental alertness (eg, operating machinery or driving). Myoclonus and seizures have been reported with high doses; use with caution in patients with a history of seizure disorder. Use with caution in patients with kyphoscoliosis, cardiovascular disease, morbid obesity, adrenocortical insufficiency, hypothyroidism, acute alcoholism, delirium tremens, toxic psychoses, prostatic hyperplasia and/or urinary stricture, or severe liver or renal failure. Avoid use in patients with CNS depression or coma as these patients are susceptible to intracranial effects of CO_2 retention. Use with caution in patients with biliary tract dysfunction. Hydromorphone may increase biliary tract pressure following spasm in sphincter of Oddi. Use caution in patients with inflammatory or obstructive bowel disorder, acute pancreatitis secondary to biliary tract disease, and patients undergoing biliary surgery. Use extreme caution in patients with head injury, intracranial lesions, or elevated intracranial pressure; exaggerated elevation of ICP may occur (in addition, hydromorphone may complicate neurologic evaluation due to pupillary dilation and CNS depressant effects). Use with caution in patients with depleted blood volume or drugs which may exaggerate hypotensive effects (including phenothiazines or general anesthetics). May obscure diagnosis or clinical course of patients with acute abdominal conditions. Severe and unpredictable potentiation by MAO inhibitors has been reported with opioid analgesics; use within 14 days of MAO inhibitors is not recommended.

[U.S. Boxed Warning]: Hydromorphone has a high potential for abuse; health care provider should be alert to problems of abuse, misuse, and diversion. Risk of opioid abuse is increased in patients with a history or family history of alcohol or drug abuse or mental illness. Tolerance or drug dependence may result from extended use; however, concerns for abuse should not prevent effective management of pain. In general, abrupt discontinuation of therapy in dependent patients should be avoided. After chronic maternal exposure to opioids, neonatal withdrawal syndrome may occur in the newborn; monitor neonate closely. Signs and symptoms include irritability, hyperactivity and abnormal sleep pattern, high pitched cry, tremor, vomiting, diarrhea and failure to gain weight. Onset, duration and severity depend on the drug used, duration of use, maternal dose, and rate of drug elimination by the newborn. Opioid withdrawal syndrome in the neonate, unlike in adults, may be life-threatening and should be treated according to protocols developed by neonatology experts.

An opioid-containing analgesic regimen should be tailored to each patient's needs and based upon the type of pain being treated (acute versus chronic), the route of administration, degree of tolerance for opioids (naive versus chronic user), age, weight, and medical condition. The optimal analgesic dose varies widely among patients. Doses should be titrated to pain relief/prevention. I.M. use may result in variable absorption and a lag time to peak effect.

Dosage form specific warnings:

[U.S. Boxed Warning]: Dilaudid-HP: Extreme caution should be taken to avoid confusing the highly-concentrated (Dilaudid-HP) injection with the less-concentrated (Dilaudid) injectable product. Dilaudid-HP should only be used in patients who are opioid-tolerant.

Controlled release: Capsules should only be used when continuous analgesia is required over an extended period of time. Controlled release products are not to be used on an "as needed" (PRN) basis.

Extended release tablets (Exalgo): **[U.S. Boxed Warning]: For use in opioid tolerant patients only; fatal respiratory depression may occur in patient who are not opioid tolerant. The highest risk of fatal respiratory depression is at initiation and with dose increases. Indicated for the management of moderate-to-severe pain when around the clock pain control is needed for an extended time period. Not for use as an as-needed analgesic or for the management of acute or post-operative pain. Tablets should be swallowed whole; do not crush, break, chew, dissolve or inject; doing so may lead to rapid release and absorption of a potentially fatal dose of hydromorphone. Accidental consumption may lead to fatal overdose, especially in children.** Exalgo tablets are nondeformable; do not administer to patients with pre-existing severe gastrointestinal narrowing (eg, esophageal motility, small bowel inflammatory disease, short gut syndrome, history of peritonitis, cystic fibrosis, chronic intestinal pseudo-obstruction, Meckel's diverticulum); obstruction may occur.

Some dosage forms contain trace amounts of sodium metabisulfite which may cause allergic reactions in susceptible individuals. Vial stoppers of single-dose injectable vials may contain latex.

Drug Interactions

Avoid Concomitant Use

Avoid concomitant use of HYDROmorphone with any of the following: Azelastine (Nasal); MAO Inhibitors; Paraldehyde; Thalidomide

Decreased Effect

HYDROmorphone may decrease the levels/effects of: Pegvisomant

The levels/effects of HYDROmorphone may be decreased by: Ammonium Chloride; Mixed Agonist / Antagonist Opioids

Increased Effect/Toxicity

HYDROmorphone may increase the levels/effects of: Alcohol (Ethyl); Alvimopan; Azelastine (Nasal); CNS Depressants; Desmopressin; Diuretics; Hydrocodone; Metyrosine; Mirtazapine; Paraldehyde; Pramipexole; ROPINIRole; Rotigotine; Selective Serotonin Reuptake Inhibitors; Thalidomide; Zolpidem

The levels/effects of HYDROmorphone may be increased by: Amphetamines; Anticholinergics; Antipsychotic Agents (Phenothiazines); Brimonidine (Topical); Cannabinoids; Doxylamine; Droperidol; HydrOXYzine; Magnesium Sulfate; MAO Inhibitors; Perampanel; Sodium Oxybate; Succinylcholine; Tapentadol

Nutritional/Ethanol Interactions

Ethanol: Ethanol may increase CNS depression. Management: Monitor for increased effects with coadministration. Caution patients about effects.

Herb/Nutraceutical: Gotu kola, valerian, and kava kava may increase CNS depression. Management: Avoid gotu kola, valerian, and kava kava.

Adverse Reactions Frequency not defined.

Cardiovascular: Bradycardia, extrasystoles, flushing (facial), hypertension, hypotension, palpitations, peripheral edema, peripheral vasodilation, syncope, tachycardia

Central nervous system: Abnormal dreams, abnormal gait, abnormality in thinking, aggressive behavior, agitation, apprehension, ataxia, brain disease, burning sensation of skin (Exalgo), central nervous system depression, chills, cognitive dysfunction, confusion, decreased body temperature (Exalgo), depression, disruption of body temperature regulation (Exalgo), dizziness, drowsiness, drug dependence, dysarthria, dysphoria, equilibrium disturbance, euphoria, fatigue, hallucination, headache, hyperesthesia, hyperreflexia, hypoesthesia, hypothermia, increased intracranial pressure, insomnia, lack of concentration, lethargy, malaise, memory impairment, mood changes, myoclonus, nervousness, painful defecation, panic attack, paranoia, paresthesia, psychomotor agitation, restlessness, sedation, seizure, sleep disorder (Exalgo), suicidal ideation, uncontrolled crying, vertigo

Dermatologic: Diaphoresis, erythema (Exalgo), hyperhidrosis, pruritus, skin rash, urticaria

Endocrine & metabolic: Antidiuretic effect, decreased amylase, decreased libido, decreased plasma testosterone, dehydration, fluid retention, hyperuricemia, hypokalemia, weight loss

Gastrointestinal: Abdominal distention, anal fissure, anorexia, bezoar formation (Exalgo), biliary tract spasm, constipation, decreased appetite, decreased gastrointestinal motility (Exalgo), delayed gastric emptying, diarrhea, diverticulitis, diverticulosis, duodenitis, dysgeusia, dysphagia, eructation, flatulence, gastroenteritis, gastroesophageal reflux disease (aggravated; Exalgo), hematochezia, increased appetite, intestinal perforation (large intestine; Exalgo), nausea, paralytic ileus, stomach cramps, vomiting, xerostomia

Genitourinary: Bladder spasm, decreased urine output, difficulty in micturition, dysuria, erectile dysfunction, hypogonadism, sexual disorder, ureteral spasm, urinary frequency, urinary hesitancy, urinary retention

Hematologic & oncologic: Oxygen desaturation

Hepatic: Increased liver enzymes

Hypersensitivity: Histamine release

Local: Pain at injection site, post-injection flare

Neuromuscular & skeletal: Arthralgia, dyskinesia, laryngospasm, muscle rigidity, muscle spasm, myalgia, tremor, weakness

Ophthalmic: Blurred vision, diplopia, dry eye syndrome, miosis, nystagmus

Otic: Tinnitus

Respiratory: Apnea, bronchospasm, dyspnea, flu-like symptoms (Exalgo), hyperventilation, hypoxia, respiratory depression, respiratory distress, rhinorrhea

Pharmacodynamics/Kinetics

Onset of Action Analgesic:

Immediate release formulations:

Oral: 15-30 minutes; Peak effect: 30-60 minutes

I.V.: 5 minutes; Peak effect: 10-20 minutes

Extended release tablet: 6 hours; Peak effect: ~9 hours (Angst, 2001)

Duration of Action

Immediate release formulations: Oral, I.V.: 3-4 hours

Extended release tablet: ~13 hours (Angst, 2001)

Controlled Substance C-II

Available Dosage Forms

Liquid, Oral:

Dilaudid: 1 mg/mL (473 mL)

Generic: 1 mg/mL (473 mL)

Solution, Injection:

Dilaudid: 1 mg/mL (1 mL); 2 mg/mL (1 mL); 4 mg/mL (1 mL)

Dilaudid-HP: 10 mg/mL (1 mL, 5 mL, 50 mL)

Generic: 1 mg/mL (0.5 mL, 1 mL); 2 mg/mL (1 mL, 20 mL); 4 mg/mL (1 mL); 10 mg/mL (1 mL); 50 mg/5 mL (5 mL); 500 mg/50 mL (50 mL)

Solution, Injection [preservative free]:

Generic: 10 mg/mL (1 mL); 50 mg/5 mL (5 mL); 500 mg/50 mL (50 mL)

Solution Reconstituted, Injection:

Dilaudid-HP: 250 mg (1 ea)

Suppository, Rectal:

Generic: 3 mg (6 ea)

Tablet, Oral:

Dilaudid: 2 mg, 4 mg, 8 mg

Generic: 2 mg, 4 mg, 8 mg

Tablet ER 24 Hour Abuse-Deterrent, Oral:

Exalgo: 8 mg, 12 mg, 16 mg, 32 mg

General Dosage Range Dosage adjustment recommended in patients with hepatic or renal impairment

I.M., SubQ: *Children >50 kg and Adults:* 0.8-1 mg every 3-4 hours

I.V.: *Children >50 kg and Adults:* 0.2-0.6 mg every 2-3 hours as needed

Oral:

Children >50 kg: 2-4 mg every 4 hours as needed

Adults: 2-4 mg every 4 hours as needed; Extended release: 8-64 mg every 24 hours

Elderly: Initiation at the low end of dosage range is recommended

Rectal: *Children >50 kg and Adults:* 3 mg every 6-8 hours as needed

Administration

I.M. Note: Vial stopper may contain latex. May be given I.M; however, this route is not recommended (APS, 2008)

I.V. Note: Vial stopper may contain latex. For IVP, must be given slowly over 2-3 minutes (rapid IVP has been associated with an increase in side effects, especially respiratory depression and hypotension)

Injectable Detail pH: 4-5.5

Oral Hydromorphone is available in an 8 mg immediate release tablet and an 8 mg extended release tablet. Extreme caution should be taken to avoid confusing dosage forms.

Exalgo: Tablets should be swallowed whole; do not crush, break, chew, dissolve or inject. May be taken with or without food.

Hydromorph Contin: Capsule should be swallowed whole; do not crush or chew; contents may be sprinkled on soft food and swallowed

Subcutaneous Note: Vial stopper may contain latex. May be given SubQ.

Storage/Stability

Injection: Store at 15°C to 30°C (59°F to 86°F). A slightly yellowish discoloration has not been associated with a loss of potency.

Oral dosage forms: Store at 15°C to 30°C (59°F to 86°F). Protect tablets from light.

Suppository: Store in refrigerator. Protect from light.

Nursing Actions

Physical Assessment Monitor for effectiveness of pain relief. Monitor blood pressure, CNS and respiratory status, and degree of sedation prior to treatment and periodically throughout. Assess patient's physical and/or psychological dependence. For inpatients, implement safety measures (eg, side rails up, call light within reach, instructions to call for assistance). Discontinue slowly after prolonged use.

Patient Education

• Discuss specific use of drug and side effects with patient as it relates to treatment. (HCAHPS: During this hospital stay, were you given any medicine that you had not taken before? Before giving you any new medicine, how often did

hospital staff tell you what the medicine was for? How often did hospital staff describe possible side effects in a way you could understand?)

- Patient may experience fatigue, xerostomia, flushing, hyperhidrosis, arthralgia, or tablet shell in stool. Have patient report immediately to prescriber severe dizziness, syncope, illogical thinking, significant nausea, considerable constipation, tachycardia, bradycardia, arrhythmia, hallucinations, mood changes, intolerable headache, severe dyspepsia, tremors, difficult urination, difficulty with eye movements, difficulty with motor activity, vision changes, angina, change in balance, memory loss, suicidal ideation, or edema of extremities (HCAHPS).
- Educate patient about signs of a significant reaction (eg, wheezing; chest tightness; fever; itching; bad cough; blue skin color; seizures; or swelling of face, lips, tongue, or throat). **Note:** This is not a comprehensive list of all side effects. Patient should consult prescriber for additional questions.

Intended Use and Disclaimer: Should not be printed and given to patients. This information is intended to serve as a concise initial reference for healthcare professionals to use when discussing medications with a patient. You must ultimately rely on your own discretion, experience and judgment in diagnosing, treating and advising patients.

Related Information

Oral Medications That Should Not Be Crushed or Altered *on page 1712*

Hydroquinone (HYE droe kwin one)

Brand Names: U.S. Aclaro; Aclaro PD; Alphaquin HP; Eldopaque Forte [DSC]; Eldopaque [OTC] [DSC]; Eldoquin Forte [DSC]; Eldoquin [OTC] [DSC]; EpiQuin Micro; Esoterica Daytime [OTC]; Esoterica Facial [OTC]; Esoterica Fade Nighttime [OTC]; Esoterica Sensitive Skin [OTC]; Exuviance Lightening Complex [OTC]; Hydroquinone Time Release; Lustra; Lustra-AF; Lustra-Ultra; Melpaque HP; Melquin 3; Melquin HP; NAVA-SC; NeoCeuticals Post-Acne Fade [OTC]; NeoStrata HQ Skin Lightening [OTC]; Nuquin HP; Remergent HQ; Skin Bleaching; Skin Bleaching-Sunscreen; TL Hydroquinone

Index Terms Hydroquinol; Quinol

Pharmacologic Category Depigmenting Agent

Medication Safety Issues

Sound-alike/look-alike issues:

Eldopaque® may be confused with Eldoquin® Eldopaque Forte® may be confused with Eldoquin Forte®

Pregnancy Risk Factor C

Lactation Excretion in breast milk unknown/use caution

Use Gradual bleaching of hyperpigmented skin conditions

Available Dosage Forms

Cream, External:

Alphaquin HP: 4% (28.4 g, 56.7 g)

EpiQuin Micro: 4% (30 g)

Esoterica Daytime [OTC]: 2% (70 g)

Esoterica Facial [OTC]: 2% (85 g)

Esoterica Fade Nighttime [OTC]: 2% (70 g)

Esoterica Sensitive Skin [OTC]: 1.5% (85 g)

Hydroquinone Time Release: 4% (30 g)

Lustra: 4% (56.8 g)

Lustra-AF: 4% (56.8 g)

Lustra-Ultra: 4% (28.4 g, 56.8 g)

Melpaque HP: 4% (28.4 g)

Melquin HP: 4% (28.4 g)

NAVA-SC: 4% (28.4 g)

Nuquin HP: 4% (28.4 g, 56.7 g)

Remergent HQ: 4% (30 mL)

Skin Bleaching: 4% (28.35 g)

Skin Bleaching-Sunscreen: 4% (28.35 g)

TL Hydroquinone: 4% (30 g)

Generic: 4% (28.35 g)

Emulsion, External:

Aclaro: 4% (48.2 g)

Aclaro PD: 4% (42.5 g)

Gel, External:

Exuviance Lightening Complex [OTC]: 2% (30 g)

NeoCeuticals Post-Acne Fade [OTC]: 2% (30 g)

NeoStrata HQ Skin Lightening [OTC]: 2% (30 g)

Nuquin HP: 4% (28.4 g)

Solution, External:

Melquin 3: 3% (29.57 mL)

General Dosage Range Topical: *Children >12 years and Adults:* Apply thin layer and rub in twice daily

Administration

Topical For external use only; avoid contact with eyes

Nursing Actions

Physical Assessment When applied to large areas or for extensive periods of time, monitor for skin irritation.

Patient Education

- Discuss specific use of drug and side effects with patient as it relates to treatment. (HCAHPS: During this hospital stay, were you given any medicine that you had not taken before? Before giving you any new medicine, how often did hospital staff tell you what the medicine was for? How often did hospital staff describe possible side effects in a way you could understand?)
- Patient may experience short-term pain, xeroderma, or skin irritation. Have patient report immediately to prescriber rash (HCAHPS).
- Educate patient about signs of a significant reaction (eg, wheezing; chest tightness; fever; itching; bad cough; blue skin color; seizures; or swelling of face, lips, tongue, or throat). **Note:** This is not a comprehensive list of all side

effects. Patient should consult prescriber for additional questions.

Intended Use and Disclaimer: Should not be printed and given to patients. This information is intended to serve as a concise initial reference for healthcare professionals to use when discussing medications with a patient. You must ultimately rely on your own discretion, experience and judgment in diagnosing, treating and advising patients.

Hydroxocobalamin (hye droks oh koe BAL a min)

Brand Names: U.S. Cyanokit
Index Terms Vitamin B_{12a}
Pharmacologic Category Antidote; Vitamin, Water Soluble
Pregnancy Risk Factor C
Lactation Excretion in breast milk unknown/use caution
Use
I.M. injection: Treatment of pernicious anemia; treatment of vitamin B_{12} deficiency due to dietary deficiencies or malabsorption diseases, inadequate secretion of intrinsic factor, competition for vitamin B_{12} by intestinal parasites/bacteria, or inadequate utilization of B_{12} (eg, during neoplastic treatment)
I.V. infusion (Cyanokit®): Treatment of cyanide poisoning (known or suspected)
Available Dosage Forms
Solution, Intramuscular:
Generic: 1000 mcg/mL (30 mL)
Solution Reconstituted, Intravenous:
Cyanokit: 5 g (1 ea)
General Dosage Range
I.M.:
Children: Initial: 100 mcg once daily for ≥2 weeks (total dose: 1-5 **mg**); maintenance: 30-50 mcg once per month
Adults: Initial: 30 mcg once daily for 5-10 days; maintenance: 100-200 mcg once per month **or** 1000 mcg once
I.V.: *Adults:* 5 **g** as a single infusion; may repeat if needed (maximum: 10 **g** cumulative dose)
Administration
I.M. Administer 1000 mcg/mL solution I.M. only
I.V. Cyanokit®: Administer initial dose by I.V. infusion over 15 minutes; if a second dose is needed, administer the second dose over 15 minutes to 2 hours; hydroxocobalamin is chemically incompatible with sodium thiosulfate and sodium nitrite and separate I.V. lines must be used if concomitant administration is desired **(the safety of coadministration is not established)**
Nursing Actions
Physical Assessment Teach patient appropriate injection technique and needle disposal and appropriate nutrition. Cyanide toxicity: Monitor blood pressure and heart rate during infusion.

Patient Education
• Discuss specific use of drug and side effects with patient as it relates to treatment. (HCAHPS: During this hospital stay, were you given any medicine that you had not taken before? Before giving you any new medicine, how often did hospital staff tell you what the medicine was for? How often did hospital staff describe possible side effects in a way you could understand?)
• Patient may experience diarrhea, injection site irritation, hypertension, hematuria, flushing, rash, headache, or nausea. Have patient report immediately to prescriber edema or severe asthenia (HCAHPS).
• Educate patient about signs of a significant reaction (eg, wheezing; chest tightness; fever; itching; bad cough; blue skin color; seizures; or swelling of face, lips, tongue, or throat). **Note:** This is not a comprehensive list of all side effects. Patient should consult prescriber for additional questions.

Intended Use and Disclaimer: Should not be printed and given to patients. This information is intended to serve as a concise initial reference for healthcare professionals to use when discussing medications with a patient. You must ultimately rely on your own discretion, experience and judgment in diagnosing, treating and advising patients.

Hydroxychloroquine
(hye droks ee KLOR oh kwin)

Brand Names: U.S. Plaquenil
Index Terms Hydroxychloroquine Sulfate
Pharmacologic Category Aminoquinoline (Antimalarial)
Medication Safety Issues
Sound-alike/look-alike issues:
Hydroxychloroquine may be confused with hydrocortisone
Plaquenil may be confused with Platinol
Lactation Enters breast milk
Use Suppression and treatment of acute attacks of malaria; treatment of systemic lupus erythematosus (SLE) and rheumatoid arthritis
Unlabeled Use Porphyria cutanea tarda, polymorphous light eruptions, treatment of Q fever (*Coxiella burnetti*)
Available Dosage Forms
Tablet, Oral:
Plaquenil: 200 mg
Generic: 200 mg
General Dosage Range Oral:
Children: 13 mg/kg for 1-2 doses, followed by 6.5 mg/kg for 3 doses or once weekly
Adults: Initial: 400-800 mg/day divided 1-2 times/day; Maintenance: 200-400 mg/day **or** 800 mg for 1-2 doses, followed by 400 mg for 3 doses or once weekly

Administration

Oral Administer with food or milk.

Nursing Actions

Physical Assessment Evaluate results of CBC, liver function tests, and ophthalmic exam prior to treatment and periodically throughout. Monitor for dermatologic, neuromuscular [deep tendon reflexes, muscle weakness], and ocular changes throughout.

Patient Education

- Discuss specific use of drug and side effects with patient as it relates to treatment. (HCAHPS: During this hospital stay, were you given any medicine that you had not taken before? Before giving you any new medicine, how often did hospital staff tell you what the medicine was for? How often did hospital staff describe possible side effects in a way you could understand?)
- Patient may experience anemia, dyspepsia, or nausea. Have patient report immediately to prescriber dyspnea; sudden vision changes, eye pain, or eye irritation; or rash (HCAHPS).
- Educate patient about signs of a significant reaction (eg, wheezing; chest tightness; fever; itching; bad cough; blue skin color; seizures; or swelling of face, lips, tongue, or throat). **Note:** This is not a comprehensive list of all side effects. Patient should consult prescriber for additional questions.

Intended Use and Disclaimer: Should not be printed and given to patients. This information is intended to serve as a concise initial reference for healthcare professionals to use when discussing medications with a patient. You must ultimately rely on your own discretion, experience and judgment in diagnosing, treating and advising patients.

Hydroxyprogesterone Caproate
(hye droks ee proe JES te rone CAP ro ate)

Brand Names: U.S. Makena

Index Terms 17OHPC

Pharmacologic Category Progestin

Medication Safety Issues

Sound-alike/look-alike issues:

Hydroxyprogesterone caproate may be confused with medroxyPROGESTERone

Pregnancy Risk Factor B

Use To reduce the risk of preterm birth in women with singleton pregnancies who have a history of spontaneous preterm birth (delivery <37 weeks gestation) with previous singleton pregnancies

Available Dosage Forms

Oil, Intramuscular:

Makena: 250 mg/mL (5 mL)

General Dosage Range I.M.: *Pregnant females:* 250 mg every 7 days

Administration

I.M. For I.M. administration into the upper outer quadrant of the gluteus maximus. Withdraw dose using an 18 gauge needle; inject dose using a 21 gauge 1½ inch needle. Administer by slow injection (≥1 minute). Solution is viscous and oily; do not use if solution is cloudy or contains solid particles. Apply pressure to injection site to decrease bruising and swelling.

Hazardous agent; use appropriate precautions for handling and disposal (NIOSH, 2012).

Nursing Actions

Patient Education

- Discuss specific use of drug and side effects with patient as it relates to treatment. (HCAHPS: During this hospital stay, were you given any medicine that you had not taken before? Before giving you any new medicine, how often did hospital staff tell you what the medicine was for? How often did hospital staff describe possible side effects in a way you could understand?)
- Patient may experience injection site irritation, diarrhea, or nausea. Have patient report immediately to prescriber depression, nervousness, emotional instability, illogical thinking, anxiety, angina, dyspnea, edema, sudden vision changes, eye pain, eye irritation, jaundice, or rash (HCAHPS).
- Educate patient about signs of a significant reaction (eg, wheezing; chest tightness; fever; itching; bad cough; blue skin color; seizures; or swelling of face, lips, tongue, or throat). **Note:** This is not a comprehensive list of all side effects. Patient should consult prescriber for additional questions.

Intended Use and Disclaimer: Should not be printed and given to patients. This information is intended to serve as a concise initial reference for healthcare professionals to use when discussing medications with a patient. You must ultimately rely on your own discretion, experience and judgment in diagnosing, treating and advising patients.

Hydroxyurea (hye droks ee yoor EE a)

Brand Names: U.S. Droxia; Hydrea

Index Terms HU; Hydroxycarbamide; Hydurea

Pharmacologic Category Antineoplastic Agent, Miscellaneous

Medication Safety Issues

Sound-alike/look-alike issues:

Hydroxyurea may be confused with hydrOXYzine

High alert medication:
This medication is in a class the Institute for Safe Medication Practices (ISMP) includes among its list of drug classes which have a heightened risk of causing significant patient harm when used in error.

International issues:
Hydrea [U.S., Canada, and multiple international markets] may be confused with Hydra brand name for isoniazid [Japan]

Pregnancy Risk Factor D

Lactation Enters breast milk/not recommended

Breast-Feeding Considerations Hydroxyurea is excreted in breast milk. Due to the potential for serious adverse reactions in the nursing infant, the decision to discontinue hydroxyurea or to discontinue breast-feeding should take into account the importance of treatment to the mother.

Use Treatment of melanoma, refractory chronic myelocytic leukemia (CML); recurrent, metastatic, or inoperable ovarian cancer; management (with concomitant radiation therapy) of squamous cell head and neck cancer (excluding lip cancer); management of sickle cell patients who have had at least three painful crises in the previous 12 months (to reduce frequency of these crises and the need for blood transfusions)

Unlabeled Use Treatment of essential thrombocythemia, polycythemia vera, hypereosinophilic syndrome; management of hyperleukocytosis due to acute myeloid leukemia (AML); treatment of AML in poor-risk patients; treatment of meningiomas

Mechanism of Action/Effect Antimetabolite which selectively inhibits ribonucleoside diphosphate reductase, preventing the conversion of ribonucleotides to deoxyribonucleotides, halting the cell cycle at the G1/S phase and therefore has radiation sensitizing activity by maintaining cells in the G_1 phase and interfering with DNA repair. In sickle cell anemia, hydroxyurea increases red blood cell (RBC) hemoglobin F levels, RBC water content, deformability of sickled cells, and alters adhesion of RBCs to endothelium.

Contraindications Hypersensitivity to hydroxyurea or any component of the formulation

Hydrea: Marked bone marrow suppression (WBC <2500/mm^3 or platelet count <100,000/mm^3) or severe anemia

Warnings/Precautions Hazardous agent - use appropriate precautions for handling and disposal (NIOSH, 2012); to decrease risk of exposure, wear gloves when handling and wash hands before and after contact. Leukopenia and neutropenia commonly occur (thrombocytopenia and anemia are less common); leukopenia/neutropenia occur first. Hematologic toxicity reversible (rapid) with treatment interruption. Correct severe anemia prior to initiating treatment. Hydrea® use is contraindicated in marked bone marrow suppression; should not be used in sickle cell anemia with severe bone marrow suppression (neutrophils <2000/mm^3, platelets <80,000/mm^3, hemoglobin <4.5 g/dL, or reticulocytes <80,000/mm^3 when hemoglobin <9 g/dL). Use with caution in patients with a history of prior chemotherapy or radiation therapy; myelosuppression is more common. Patients with a history of radiation therapy are also at risk for exacerbation of post irradiation erythema. Self-limiting megaloblastic erythropoiesis may be seen early in treatment (may resemble pernicious anemia, but is unrelated to vitamin B_{12} or folic acid deficiency). Plasma iron clearance may be delayed and iron utilization rate (by erythrocytes) may be reduced. Potentially significant drug-drug interactions may exist, requiring dose or frequency adjustment, additional monitoring, and/or selection of alternative therapy. When treated concurrently with hydroxyurea and antiretroviral agents (including didanosine and stavudine), HIV-infected patients are at higher risk for potentially fatal pancreatitis, hepatotoxicity, hepatic failure, and severe peripheral neuropathy; discontinue immediately if signs of these toxicities develop. Hyperuricemia may occur with antineoplastic treatment; adequate hydration and initiation or dosage adjustment of uricosuric agents (eg, allopurinol) may be necessary.

In patients with sickle cell anemia, use is not recommended if neutrophils <2000/mm^3, platelets <80,000/mm^3, hemoglobin <4.5 g/dL, or reticulocytes <80,000/mm^3 when hemoglobin <9 g/dL. May cause macrocytosis, which can mask folic acid deficiency; prophylactic fold acid supplementation is recommended. **[U.S. Boxed Warning]: Hydroxyurea is mutagenic and clastogenic; causes cellular transformation resulting in tumorigenicity; also considered genotoxic and may be carcinogenic. Treatment of myeloproliferative disorders (eg, polycythemia vera, thrombocythemia) with long-term hydroxyurea is associated with secondary leukemia;** it is unknown if this is drug-related or disease-related. Skin cancer has been reported with long-term hydroxyurea use. Cutaneous vasculitic toxicities (vasculitic ulceration and gangrene) have been reported with hydroxyurea treatment, most often in patients with a history of or receiving concurrent interferon therapy; discontinue hydroxyurea and consider alternate cytoreductive therapy if cutaneous vasculitic toxicity develops. Use caution with renal dysfunction; may require dose reductions. Elderly patients may be more sensitive to the effects of hydroxyurea; may require lower doses. **[U.S. Boxed Warning]: Should be administered under the supervision of a physician experienced in the treatment of sickle cell anemia** or in cancer chemotherapy.

Drug Interactions

Avoid Concomitant Use
Avoid concomitant use of Hydroxyurea with any of the following: BCG; CloZAPine; Didanosine; ▶

Natalizumab; Pimecrolimus; Stavudine; Tacrolimus (Topical); Tofacitinib; Vaccines (Live)

Decreased Effect

Hydroxyurea may decrease the levels/effects of: BCG; Coccidioidin Skin Test; Sipuleucel-T; Vaccines (Inactivated); Vaccines (Live)

The levels/effects of Hydroxyurea may be decreased by: Echinacea

Increased Effect/Toxicity

Hydroxyurea may increase the levels/effects of: CloZAPine; Didanosine; Leflunomide; Natalizumab; Stavudine; Tofacitinib; Vaccines (Live)

The levels/effects of Hydroxyurea may be increased by: Denosumab; Didanosine; Pimecrolimus; Roflumilast; Stavudine; Tacrolimus (Topical); Trastuzumab

Adverse Reactions Frequency not defined.

Cardiovascular: Edema

Central nervous system: Chills, disorientation, dizziness, drowsiness (dose-related), fever, hallucinations, headache, malaise, seizure

Dermatologic: Alopecia, cutaneous vasculitic toxicities, dermatomyositis-like skin changes, facial erythema, gangrene, hyperpigmentation, maculopapular rash, nail atrophy, nail discoloration, peripheral erythema, scaling, skin atrophy, skin cancer, skin ulcer, vasculitis ulcerations, violet papules

Endocrine & metabolic: Hyperuricemia

Gastrointestinal: Anorexia, constipation, diarrhea, gastrointestinal irritation and mucositis, (potentiated with radiation therapy), nausea, pancreatitis, stomatitis, vomiting

Genitourinary: Dysuria

Hematologic: Myelosuppression (anemia, leukopenia/neutropenia [common], thrombocytopenia; hematologic recovery: within 2 weeks); macrocytosis, megaloblastic erythropoiesis, secondary leukemias (long-term use)

Hepatic: Hepatic enzymes increased, hepatotoxicity

Neuromuscular & skeletal: Peripheral neuropathy, weakness

Renal: BUN increased, creatinine increased, renal tubular dysfunction

Respiratory: Acute diffuse pulmonary infiltrates (rare), dyspnea, pulmonary fibrosis (rare)

Pharmacodynamics/Kinetics

Onset of Action Sickle cell anemia: Fetal hemoglobin increase: 4-12 weeks

Available Dosage Forms

Capsule, Oral:

Droxia: 200 mg, 300 mg, 400 mg

Hydrea: 500 mg

Generic: 500 mg

General Dosage Range Dosage adjustment recommended in patients with renal impairment or who develop toxicities.

Oral: *Adults:* 15-35 mg/kg/day or 500-3000 mg/day as single or divided dose or 80 mg/kg as a single dose every third day

Administration

Oral The manufacturer does not recommend opening the capsules.

Hazardous agent; use appropriate precautions for handling and disposal (NIOSH, 2012). Impervious gloves should be worn when handling; avoid exposure to crushed or open capsules.

Storage/Stability Store at room temperature of 25°C (77°F); excursions permitted between 15°C and 30°C (59°F and 86°F).

Nursing Actions

Physical Assessment Teach proper use and safe handling. Instruct patients to wash hands before and after touching medication. Teach patient to have lab work monitored frequently. Monitor for CNS changes and peripheral neuropathy. Instruct patient to call with fever, chills, severe nausea/vomiting, dysuria, hallucinations, seizures, any bleeding, or yellowing of skin and eyes.

Patient Education

- Discuss specific use of drug and side effects with patient as it relates to treatment. (HCAHPS: During this hospital stay, were you given any medicine that you had not taken before? Before giving you any new medicine, how often did hospital staff tell you what the medicine was for? How often did hospital staff describe possible side effects in a way you could understand?)
- Patient may experience anemia, leukopenia, thrombocytopenia, headache, dyspepsia, emesis, lack of appetite, constipation, diarrhea, stomatitis, edema, or changes in skin. Have patient report immediately to prescriber illogical thinking, ecchymosis, bleeding, severe asthenia, or rash (HCAHPS).
- Educate patient about signs of a significant reaction (eg, wheezing; chest tightness; fever; itching; bad cough; blue skin color; seizures; or swelling of face, lips, tongue, or throat). **Note:** This is not a comprehensive list of all side effects. Patient should consult prescriber for additional questions.

Intended Use and Disclaimer: Should not be printed and given to patients. This information is intended to serve as a concise initial reference for healthcare professionals to use when discussing medications with a patient. You must ultimately rely on your own discretion, experience and judgment in diagnosing, treating and advising patients.

Dietary Considerations In sickle cell patients, supplemental administration of folic acid is recommended; hydroxyurea may mask development of folic acid deficiency.

Related Information
Oral Medications That Should Not Be Crushed or Altered *on page 1712*

HydrOXYzine (hye DROKS i zeen)

Brand Names: U.S. Vistaril
Index Terms Hydroxyzine Hydrochloride; Hydroxyzine Pamoate
Pharmacologic Category Antiemetic; Histamine H_1 Antagonist; Histamine H_1 Antagonist, First Generation; Piperazine Derivative
Medication Safety Issues
Sound-alike/look-alike issues:
HydrOXYzine may be confused with hydrALAZINE, hydroxyurea
Atarax may be confused with Ativan
Vistaril may be confused with Restoril, Versed, Zestril®
BEERS Criteria medication:
This drug may be potentially inappropriate for use in geriatric patients (Quality of evidence - high; Strength of recommendation - strong).
International issues:
Vistaril [U.S. and Turkey] may be confused with Vastarel brand name for trimetazidine [multiple international markets]
Lactation Excretion in breast milk unknown/not recommended
Use Treatment of anxiety/agitation (including adjunctive therapy in alcoholism); adjunct to pre- and postoperative analgesia and anesthesia; antipruritic; antiemetic
Available Dosage Forms
Capsule, Oral:
Vistaril: 25 mg, 50 mg
Generic: 25 mg, 50 mg, 100 mg
Solution, Intramuscular:
Generic: 25 mg/mL (1 mL); 50 mg/mL (1 mL, 2 mL, 10 mL)
Solution, Oral:
Generic: 10 mg/5 mL (473 mL)
Syrup, Oral:
Generic: 10 mg/5 mL (118 mL, 473 mL)
Tablet, Oral:
Generic: 10 mg, 25 mg, 50 mg
General Dosage Range Dosage adjustment recommended in patients with hepatic impairment
I.M.:
Children: 1.1 mg/kg/dose
Adults: 25-100 mg/dose
Oral:
Children: 0.6 mg/kg/dose (sedation)
Children <6 years: 50 mg/day in divided doses
Children ≥6 years: 50-100 mg/day in divided doses
Adults: 25-100 mg/dose
Administration
I.M. For I.M. use only. Do **NOT** administer I.V., SubQ, or intra-arterially. Administer I.M. deep in large muscle. In adults, the preferred site is the upper outer quadrant of the buttock or midlateral thigh. In children, the preferred site is the midlateral thigh. The upper outer quadrant of the gluteal region should be used only when necessary to minimize potential damage to the sciatic nerve.
Oral Shake suspension vigorously prior to use.
Nursing Actions
Physical Assessment Ensure patient safety to prevent falls (side rails up, call light within reach).
Patient Education
• Discuss specific use of drug and side effects with patient as it relates to treatment. (HCAHPS: During this hospital stay, were you given any medicine that you had not taken before? Before giving you any new medicine, how often did hospital staff tell you what the medicine was for? How often did hospital staff describe possible side effects in a way you could understand?)
• Patient may experience presyncope, fatigue, blurred vision, illogical thinking, dizziness, xerostomia, or headache. Have patient report immediately to prescriber urinary retention, significant change in balance, severe asthenia, nervousness and anxiety, or rash (HCAHPS).
• Educate patient about signs of a significant reaction (eg, wheezing; chest tightness; fever; itching; bad cough; blue skin color; seizures; or swelling of face, lips, tongue, or throat). **Note:** This is not a comprehensive list of all side effects. Patient should consult prescriber for additional questions.

Intended Use and Disclaimer: Should not be printed and given to patients. This information is intended to serve as a concise initial reference for healthcare professionals to use when discussing medications with a patient. You must ultimately rely on your own discretion, experience and judgment in diagnosing, treating and advising patients.
Related Information
Management of Drug Extravasations *on page 1700*

Ibandronate (eye BAN droh nate)

Brand Names: U.S. Boniva
Index Terms Ibandronate Sodium; Ibandronic Acid
Pharmacologic Category Bisphosphonate Derivative
Medication Guide Available Yes
Pregnancy Risk Factor C
Lactation Excretion in breast milk unknown/use caution
Breast-Feeding Considerations It is not known if ibandronate is excreted into breast milk. The manufacturer recommends caution be exercised when administering ibandronate to nursing women.
Use Treatment and prevention of osteoporosis in postmenopausal females

◄ **Unlabeled Use** Hypercalcemia of malignancy; reduce bone pain and skeletal complications from metastatic bone disease due to breast cancer

Mechanism of Action/Effect A bisphosphonate which inhibits bone resorption via actions on osteoclasts or on osteoclast precursors; decreases the rate of bone resorption, leading to an indirect increase in bone mineral density.

Contraindications Hypersensitivity to ibandronate or any component of the formulation; hypocalcemia; oral tablets are also contraindicated in patients unable to stand or sit upright for at least 60 minutes and in patients with abnormalities of the esophagus which delay esophageal emptying, such as stricture or achalasia

Warnings/Precautions Hypocalcemia must be corrected before therapy initiation. Ensure adequate calcium and vitamin D intake. Osteonecrosis of the jaw (ONJ) has been reported in patients receiving bisphosphonates. Risk factors include invasive dental procedures (eg, tooth extraction, dental implants, boney surgery); a diagnosis of cancer, with concomitant chemotherapy or corticosteroids; poor oral hygiene, ill-fitting dentures; and comorbid disorders (anemia, coagulopathy, infection, pre-existing dental disease); risk may increase with duration of bisphosphonate use. Most reported cases occurred after I.V. bisphosphonate therapy; however, cases have been reported following oral therapy. A dental exam and preventative dentistry should be performed prior to placing patients with risk factors on chronic bisphosphonate therapy. The manufacturer's labeling states that discontinuing bisphosphonates in patients requiring invasive dental procedures may reduce the risk of ONJ. However, other experts suggest that there is no evidence that discontinuing therapy reduces the risk of developing ONJ (Assael, 2009). The benefit/risk must be assessed by the treating physician and/or dentist/surgeon prior to any invasive dental procedure. Patients developing ONJ while on bisphosphonates should receive care by an oral surgeon.

Atypical femur fractures have been reported in patients receiving bisphosphonates for treatment/prevention of osteoporosis. The fractures include subtrochanteric femur (bone just below the hip joint) and diaphyseal femur (long segment of the thigh bone). Some patients experience prodromal pain weeks or months before the fracture occurs. It is unclear if bisphosphonate therapy is the cause for these fractures, although the majority of cases have been reported in patients taking bisphosphonates. Patients receiving long-term (>3-5 years) therapy may be at an increased risk. Discontinue bisphosphonate therapy in patients who develop a femoral shaft fracture.

Infrequently, severe (and occasionally debilitating) bone, joint, and/or muscle pain have been reported during bisphosphonate treatment. The onset of pain ranged from a single day to several months. Discontinue intravenous ibandronate therapy in patients who experience severe symptoms; symptoms usually resolve upon discontinuation. Some patients experienced recurrence when rechallenged with same drug or another bisphosphonate; avoid use in patients with a history of these symptoms in association with bisphosphonate therapy.

Oral bisphosphonates may cause dysphagia, esophagitis, esophageal or gastric ulcer; risk may increase in patients unable to comply with dosing instructions; discontinue use if new or worsening symptoms develop. Intravenous bisphosphonates may cause transient decreases in serum calcium and have also been associated with renal toxicity.

Use not recommended with severe renal impairment (CrCl <30 mL/minute). In the management of osteoporosis, re-evaluate the need for continued therapy periodically; the optimal duration of treatment has not yet been determined. Consider discontinuing after 3-5 years of use in patients at low-risk for fracture; following discontinuation, re-evaluate fracture risk periodically. Potentially significant drug-drug interactions may exist, requiring dose or frequency adjustment, additional monitoring, and/or selection of alternative therapy.

Drug Interactions

Avoid Concomitant Use There are no known interactions where it is recommended to avoid concomitant use.

Decreased Effect

The levels/effects of Ibandronate may be decreased by: Antacids; Calcium Salts; Iron Salts; Magnesium Salts; Multivitamins/Minerals (with ADEK, Folate, Iron); Multivitamins/Minerals (with AE, No Iron); Proton Pump Inhibitors; Sucroferric Oxyhydroxide

Increased Effect/Toxicity

Ibandronate may increase the levels/effects of: Deferasirox; Phosphate Supplements

The levels/effects of Ibandronate may be increased by: Aminoglycosides; Nonsteroidal Anti-Inflammatory Agents; Systemic Angiogenesis Inhibitors

Nutritional/Ethanol Interactions

Ethanol: Ethanol may increase risk of osteoporosis. Management: Avoid ethanol.

Food: May reduce absorption; mean oral bioavailability is decreased up to 90% when given with food. Management: Take with a full glass (6-8 oz) of plain water, at least 60 minutes prior to any food, beverages, or medications. Mineral water with a high calcium content should be avoided. Wait at least 60 minutes after taking ibandronate before taking anything else.

Adverse Reactions Percentages vary based on frequency of administration (daily vs monthly). Unless specified, percentages are reported with oral use.

>10%:

Gastrointestinal: Dyspepsia (6% to 12%)

Neuromuscular & skeletal: Back pain (4% to 14%)

1% to 10%:

Cardiovascular: Hypertension (6% to 7%)

Central nervous system: Headache (3% to 7%), dizziness (1% to 4%), insomnia (1% to 2%)

Dermatologic: Rash (1% to 2%)

Endocrine & metabolic: Hypercholesterolemia (5%)

Gastrointestinal: Abdominal pain (5% to 8%), diarrhea (4% to 7%), nausea (5%), constipation (3% to 4%), vomiting (3%)

Genitourinary: Urinary tract infection (2% to 6%)

Hepatic: Alkaline phosphatase decreased (frequency not defined)

Local: Injection site reaction (<2%)

Neuromuscular & skeletal: Pain in extremity (1% to 8%), arthralgia (4% to 6%), myalgia (1% to 6%), joint disorder (4%), osteonecrosis of the jaw (4%), weakness (4%), osteoarthritis (localized; 1% to 3%), muscle cramp (2%)

Respiratory: Bronchitis (3% to 10%), pneumonia (6%), pharyngitis/nasopharyngitis (3% to 4%), upper respiratory infection (2%)

Miscellaneous: Acute phase reaction (I.V. 10%; oral 3% to 9%), infection (4%), flu-like syndrome (1% to 4%), allergic reaction (3%)

Available Dosage Forms

Solution, Intravenous:

Boniva: 3 mg/3 mL (3 mL)

Generic: 3 mg/3 mL (3 mL)

Tablet, Oral:

Boniva: 150 mg

Generic: 150 mg

General Dosage Range

I.V.: *Adults:* 3 mg every 3 months

Oral: *Adults:* 150 mg once a month

Administration

I.V. Administer as a 15-30 second bolus intravenously; avoid paravenous or intraarterial administration (may cause tissue damage). Do not mix with calcium-containing solutions or other drugs. For osteoporosis, do not administer more frequently than every 3 months. Infuse over 1 hour for metastatic bone disease due to breast cancer (Diel, 2004) and over 1-2 hours for hypercalcemia of malignancy (Pecherstorfer, 2003; Ralston, 1997).

Oral Administer 60 minutes before the first food or drink of the day (other than water) and prior to taking any oral medications or supplements (eg, calcium, antacids, vitamins). Ibandronate should be taken in an upright position with a full glass (6-8 oz) of plain water and the patient should avoid lying down for 60 minutes to minimize the possibility of GI side effects. Mineral water with a high calcium content should be avoided. The tablet should be swallowed whole; do not chew or suck. Do not eat or drink anything (except water) for 60 minutes following administration of ibandronate.

Storage/Stability Store at controlled room temperature of 25°C (77°F); excursions permitted to 15°C to 30°C (59°F to 86°F).

Nursing Actions

Physical Assessment Monitor for unusual or acute musculoskeletal pain. Teach patient appropriate administration of medication. Instruct patient in lifestyle and dietary changes that may optimize bone strength.

Patient Education

- Discuss specific use of drug and side effects with patient as it relates to treatment. (HCAHPS: During this hospital stay, were you given any medicine that you had not taken before? Before giving you any new medicine, how often did hospital staff tell you what the medicine was for? How often did hospital staff describe possible side effects in a way you could understand?)
- Patient may experience dyspepsia, pyrosis, nausea, diarrhea, arthralgia, myalgia, osteodynia, or injection site irritation. Have patient report immediately to prescriber angina; dysphagia; severe jaw, groin, or thigh pain; paresthesia; fasciculations; or rash (HCAHPS).
- Educate patient about signs of a significant reaction (eg, wheezing; chest tightness; fever; itching; bad cough; blue skin color; seizures; or swelling of face, lips, tongue, or throat). **Note:** This is not a comprehensive list of all side effects. Patient should consult prescriber for additional questions.

Intended Use and Disclaimer: Should not be printed and given to patients. This information is intended to serve as a concise initial reference for healthcare professionals to use when discussing medications with a patient. You must ultimately rely on your own discretion, experience and judgment in diagnosing, treating and advising patients.

Dietary Considerations

Ensure adequate calcium and vitamin D intake; if dietary intake is inadequate, dietary supplementation is recommended. Women and men should consume:

Calcium: 1000 mg/day (men: 50-70 years) **or** 1200 mg/day (women ≥51 years and men ≥71 years) (IOM, 2011; NOF, 2013)

Vitamin D: 800-1000 IU/day (men and women ≥50 years) (NOF, 2013). Recommended Dietary Allowance (RDA): 600 IU/day (men and women ≤70 years) **or** 800 IU/day (men and women ≥71 years) (IOM, 2011).

Ibandronate tablet should be taken with a full glass (6-8 oz) of plain water, at least 60 minutes prior to any food, beverages, or medications. Mineral water with a high calcium content should be avoided.

◀ **Related Information**
Oral Medications That Should Not Be Crushed or
Altered *on page 1712*

Ibuprofen (eye byoo PROE fen)

Brand Names: U.S. Addaprin [OTC]; Advil Junior
Strength [OTC]; Advil Migraine [OTC]; Advil [OTC];
Caldolor; Childrens Advil [OTC]; Childrens Ibupro-
fen [OTC]; Childrens Motrin Jr Strength [OTC];
Childrens Motrin [OTC]; Dyspel [OTC]; EnovaRX-
Ibuprofen; Genpril [OTC]; I-Prin [OTC]; IBU-200
[OTC]; Ibuprofen Childrens [OTC]; Ibuprofen Com-
fort Pac; Ibuprofen Junior Strength [OTC]; Infants
Advil [OTC]; Infants Ibuprofen [OTC]; KS Ibuprofen
[OTC]; Motrin IB [OTC]; Motrin Infants Drops
[OTC]; Motrin Junior Strength [OTC]; Motrin
[OTC]; NeoProfen; Provil [OTC]

Index Terms p-Isobutylhydratropic Acid; Ibuprofen
Lysine

Pharmacologic Category Nonsteroidal Anti-
inflammatory Drug (NSAID), Oral; Nonsteroidal
Anti-inflammatory Drug (NSAID), Parenteral

Medication Safety Issues
Sound-alike/look-alike issues:
Haltran may be confused with Halfprin
Motrin may be confused with Neurontin

BEERS Criteria medication:
This drug may be potentially inappropriate for use
in geriatric patients (Quality of evidence - moderate; Strength of recommendation - strong).

Administration issues:
Injectable formulations: Both ibuprofen and ibuprofen lysine are available for parenteral use.
Ibuprofen lysine is **only** indicated for closure of a
clinically-significant patent ductus arteriosus.

Medication Guide Available Yes
Pregnancy Risk Factor C/D ≥30 weeks gestation
Lactation Enters breast milk/not recommended
Use

Oral: Inflammatory diseases and rheumatoid disorders including juvenile idiopathic arthritis (JIA),
mild-to-moderate pain, fever, dysmenorrhea,
osteoarthritis

Ibuprofen injection (Caldolor): Management of
mild-to-moderate pain; management moderate-
to-severe pain when used concurrently with an
opioid analgesic; reduction of fever

Ibuprofen lysine injection (NeoProfen): Patent ductus arteriosus (PDA): To close a clinically significant PDA in premature infants weighing between
500-1500 g who are no more than 32 weeks of
gestational age when usual medical management
(eg, diuretics, fluid restriction, respiratory support)
is ineffective.

Unlabeled Use Ankylosing spondylitis, cystic fibrosis, gout, acute migraine headache, migraine
prophylaxis, pericarditis

Dosage Forms Considerations
EnovaRX-Ibuprofen is a compounding kit. Refer to
manufacturer's package insert for compounding
instructions.

Available Dosage Forms
Capsule, Oral:
Advil [OTC]: 200 mg
Advil Migraine [OTC]: 200 mg
KS Ibuprofen [OTC]: 200 mg
Generic: 200 mg
Cream, External:
EnovaRX-Ibuprofen: 10% (60 g)
Kit, Combination:
Ibuprofen Comfort Pac: 800 mg
Solution, Intravenous:
Caldolor: 400 mg/4 mL (4 mL); 800 mg/8 mL
(8 mL)
Solution, Intravenous [preservative free]:
NeoProfen: 10 mg/mL (2 mL)
Suspension, Oral:
Childrens Advil [OTC]: 100 mg/5 mL (30 mL, 120
mL); 50 mg/1.25 mL (15 mL)
Childrens Ibuprofen [OTC]: 100 mg/5 mL (118
mL, 120 mL, 240 mL); 40 mg/mL (15 mL)
Childrens Motrin [OTC]: 100 mg/5 mL (60 mL,
120 mL); 40 mg/mL (15 mL)
Ibuprofen Childrens [OTC]: 100 mg/5 mL (120
mL, 240 mL)
Infants Advil [OTC]: 50 mg/1.25 mL (15 mL)
Infants Ibuprofen [OTC]: 50 mg/1.25 mL (15 mL,
30 mL)
Motrin [OTC]: 40 mg/mL (15 mL)
Motrin Infants Drops [OTC]: 50 mg/1.25 mL (15
mL, 30 mL)
Generic: 100 mg/5 mL (5 mL, 118 mL, 120 mL,
473 mL)
Tablet, Oral:
Addaprin [OTC]: 200 mg
Advil [OTC]: 200 mg
Advil Junior Strength [OTC]: 100 mg
Dyspel [OTC]: 200 mg
Genpril [OTC]: 200 mg
I-Prin [OTC]: 200 mg
IBU-200 [OTC]: 200 mg
Motrin IB [OTC]: 200 mg
Motrin Junior Strength [OTC]: 100 mg
Provil [OTC]: 200 mg
Generic: 200 mg, 400 mg, 600 mg, 800 mg
Tablet Chewable, Oral:
Advil Junior Strength [OTC]: 100 mg
Childrens Motrin [OTC]: 50 mg
Childrens Motrin Jr Strength [OTC]: 100 mg
Ibuprofen Junior Strength [OTC]: 100 mg
Motrin Junior Strength [OTC]: 100 mg

General Dosage Range
I.V. (ibuprofen [Caldolor]): *Adults:* 100-400 mg
every 4-6 hours or 400-800 mg every 6 hours
(maximum: 3.2 g/day)

I.V. (ibuprofen lysine [NeoProfen]): *Infants between 500-1500 g and ≤32 weeks GA:* Initial: 10 mg/kg, followed by two doses of 5 mg/kg at 24 and 48 hours; **Note:** Dose should be based on birth weight.

Oral:

Analgesic/antipyretic:

Children 6-11 months and 12-17 lbs: 50 mg every 6-8 hours (maximum: 4 doses/day) **or** 4-10 mg/kg every 6-8 hours (maximum: 40 mg/kg/day)

Children 12-23 months and 18-23 lbs: 75 mg every 6-8 hours (maximum: 4 doses/day) **or** 4-10 mg/kg every 6-8 hours (maximum: 40 mg/kg/day)

Children 2-3 years and 24-35 lbs: 100 mg every 6-8 hours (maximum: 4 doses/day) **or** 4-10 mg/kg every 6-8 hours (maximum: 40 mg/kg/day)

Children 4-5 years and 36-47 lbs: 150 mg every 6-8 hours (maximum: 4 doses/day) **or** 4-10 mg/kg every 6-8 hours (maximum: 40 mg/kg/day)

Children 6-8 years and 48-59 lbs: 200 mg every 6-8 hours (maximum: 4 doses/day) **or** 4-10 mg/kg every 6-8 hours (maximum: 40 mg/kg/day)

Children 9-10 years and 60-71 lbs: 250 mg every 6-8 hours (maximum: 4 doses/day) **or** 4-10 mg/kg every 6-8 hours (maximum: 40 mg/kg/day)

Children 11-12 years and 72-95 lbs: 300 mg every 6-8 hours (maximum: 4 doses/day) **or** 4-10 mg/kg every 6-8 hours (maximum: 40 mg/kg/day)

Children >12 years: 200 mg every 4-6 hours as needed (maximum: 1200 mg/day) **or** 4-10 mg/kg every 6-8 hours (maximum: 40 mg/kg/day)

Adults: 200-400 mg every 4-6 hours

Inflammatory disease: *Adults:* 400-800 mg 3-4 times/day (maximum: 3200 mg/day)

JIA: *Children >6 months:* 30-50 mg/kg/day divided every 8 hours (maximum: 2.4 g/day)

Administration

I.V.

Caldolor: For I.V. administration only; infuse over at least 30 minutes

NeoProfen (ibuprofen lysine): For I.V. administration only; administration via umbilical arterial line has not been evaluated. Infuse over 15 minutes through port closest to insertion site. Avoid extravasation. Do not administer simultaneously via same line with TPN. If needed, interrupt TPN for 15 minutes prior to and after ibuprofen administration, keeping line open with dextrose or saline.

Injectable Detail

Caldolor: pH: 7.4

NeoProfen: pH: 7

Oral Administer with food.

Nursing Actions

Physical Assessment Assess patient for allergic reaction to salicylates or other NSAIDs. Monitor blood pressure prior to treatment and periodically throughout. Monitor for adverse gastrointestinal response prior to treatment and periodically throughout.

Patient Education

• Discuss specific use of drug and side effects with patient as it relates to treatment. (HCAHPS: During this hospital stay, were you given any medicine that you had not taken before? Before giving you any new medicine, how often did hospital staff tell you what the medicine was for? How often did hospital staff describe possible side effects in a way you could understand?)

• Patient may experience dyspepsia, nausea, diarrhea, or constipation. Have patient report immediately to prescriber angina, strength differences from one side to another, severe edema, significant weight gain, sudden vision changes, eye pain, eye irritation, melena, hematuria, ecchymosis, or bleeding (HCAHPS).

• Educate patient about signs of a significant reaction (eg, wheezing; chest tightness; fever; itching; bad cough; blue skin color; seizures; or swelling of face, lips, tongue, or throat). **Note:** This is not a comprehensive list of all side effects. Patient should consult prescriber for additional questions.

Intended Use and Disclaimer: Should not be printed and given to patients. This information is intended to serve as a concise initial reference for healthcare professionals to use when discussing medications with a patient. You must ultimately rely on your own discretion, experience and judgment in diagnosing, treating and advising patients.

Related Information

Oral Medications That Should Not Be Crushed or Altered *on page 1712*

Ibuprofen and Famotidine
(eye byoo PROE fen & fa MOE ti deen)

Brand Names: U.S. Duexis

Index Terms Famotidine and Ibuprofen; HZT-501

Pharmacologic Category Histamine H_2 Antagonist; Nonsteroidal Anti-inflammatory Drug (NSAID), Oral

Medication Guide Available Yes

Pregnancy Risk Factor C

Lactation Enters breast milk/not recommended

Use Reduction of the risk of NSAID-associated gastric ulcers in patients who require an NSAID for the treatment of rheumatoid arthritis or osteoarthritis

Available Dosage Forms

Tablet, oral:

Duexis®: Ibuprofen 800 mg and famotidine 26.6 mg

General Dosage Range Oral: *Adults:* One tablet (800 mg ibuprofen/26.6 mg famotidine) 3 times daily

Administration

Oral Administer with or without food. Tablets should be swallowed whole; do not chew, crush, or split.

Nursing Actions

Physical Assessment See individual agents.

Patient Education

- Discuss specific use of drug and side effects with patient as it relates to treatment. (HCAHPS: During this hospital stay, were you given any medicine that you had not taken before? Before giving you any new medicine, how often did hospital staff tell you what the medicine was for? How often did hospital staff describe possible side effects in a way you could understand?)
- Patient may experience dyspepsia, pyrosis, diarrhea, headache, nausea, or constipation. Have patient report immediately to prescriber angina, strength differences from one side to another, significant weight gain, melena, hematuria, ecchymosis, bleeding, severe edema, inability to eat, discolored urine, jaundice, considerable asthenia, significant skin irritation, sudden vision changes, or rash (HCAHPS).
- Educate patient about signs of a significant reaction (eg, wheezing; chest tightness; fever; itching; bad cough; blue skin color; seizures; or swelling of face, lips, tongue, or throat). **Note:** This is not a comprehensive list of all side effects. Patient should consult prescriber for additional questions.

Intended Use and Disclaimer: Should not be printed and given to patients. This information is intended to serve as a concise initial reference for healthcare professionals to use when discussing medications with a patient. You must ultimately rely on your own discretion, experience and judgment in diagnosing, treating and advising patients.

Related Information

Famotidine *on page 636*

Ibuprofen *on page 798*

Ibutilide (i BYOO ti lide)

Brand Names: U.S. Corvert

Index Terms Ibutilide Fumarate

Pharmacologic Category Antiarrhythmic Agent, Class III

Medication Safety Issues

High alert medication:

The Institute for Safe Medication Practices (ISMP) includes this medication among its list of drugs which have a heightened risk of causing significant patient harm when used in error.

BEERS Criteria medication:

This drug may be potentially inappropriate for use in geriatric patients (Quality of evidence - high; Strength of recommendation - strong).

Pregnancy Risk Factor C

Lactation Enters breast milk/contraindicated

Breast-Feeding Considerations It is not known if ibutilide is excreted in breast milk. The manufacturer does not recommend use in nursing women.

Use Acute termination of atrial fibrillation or flutter of recent onset; the effectiveness of ibutilide has not been determined in patients with arrhythmias >90 days in duration

Mechanism of Action/Effect Exact mechanism of action is unknown; prolongs the action potential in cardiac tissue

Contraindications Hypersensitivity to ibutilide or any component of the formulation; QT_c >440 msec

Warnings/Precautions [U.S. Boxed Warning]: Potentially fatal arrhythmias (eg, polymorphic ventricular tachycardia) can occur with ibutilide, usually in association with torsade de pointes (QT prolongation). Studies indicate a 1.7% incidence of arrhythmias in treated patients. The drug should be given in a setting of continuous ECG monitoring and by personnel trained in treating arrhythmias particularly polymorphic ventricular tachycardia. **[U.S. Boxed Warning]: Patients with chronic atrial fibrillation may not be the best candidates for ibutilide since they often revert after conversion and the risks of treatment may not be justified when compared to alternative management.** Dosing adjustments are not required in patients with renal or hepatic dysfunction. Safety and efficacy in children have not been established. In the treatment of atrial fibrillation in the elderly, avoid antiarrhythmics as first-line treatment. In older adults, data suggests rate control may provide more benefits than risks compared to rhythm control for most patients (Beers Criteria). Avoid concurrent use of any drug that can prolong QT interval. Correct hyperkalemia and hypomagnesemia before using. Monitor for heart block.

Drug Interactions

Avoid Concomitant Use

Avoid concomitant use of Ibutilide with any of the following: Fingolimod; Highest Risk QTc-Prolonging Agents; Ivabradine; Mifepristone; Moderate Risk QTc-Prolonging Agents; Propafenone

Decreased Effect There are no known significant interactions involving a decrease in effect.

Increased Effect/Toxicity

Ibutilide may increase the levels/effects of: Highest Risk QTc-Prolonging Agents; Lidocaine (Topical)

The levels/effects of Ibutilide may be increased by: Fingolimod; Ivabradine; Lidocaine (Topical); Mifepristone; Moderate Risk QTc-Prolonging

Agents; Propafenone; QTc-Prolonging Agents (Indeterminate Risk and Risk Modifying)

Adverse Reactions 1% to 10%:

Cardiovascular: Ventricular extrasystoles (5.1%), nonsustained monomorphic ventricular tachycardia (4.9%), nonsustained polymorphic ventricular tachycardia (2.7%), tachycardia/supraventricular tachycardia (2.7%), hypotension (2%), bundle branch block (1.9%), sustained polymorphic ventricular tachycardia (eg, torsade de pointes) (1.7%, often requiring cardioversion), AV block (1.5%), bradycardia (1.2%), QT segment prolongation, hypertension (1.2%), palpitation (1%)

Central nervous system: Headache (3.6%)

Gastrointestinal: Nausea (>1%)

Pharmacodynamics/Kinetics

Onset of Action ~90 minutes after start of infusion ($1/2$ of conversions to sinus rhythm occur during infusion)

Available Dosage Forms

Solution, Intravenous:

Corvert: 1 mg/10 mL (10 mL)

Generic: 1 mg/10 mL (10 mL)

General Dosage Range I.V.:

Adults <60 kg: 0.01 mg/kg; may repeat once

Adults ≥60 kg: 1 mg; may repeat once

Administration

I.V. Infuse undiluted or diluted over 10 minutes. Observe patient with continuous ECG monitoring for at least 4 hours (>4 hours in patients with abnormal hepatic function) following infusion or until QT_c has returned to baseline. Skilled personnel and proper equipment should be available during administration of ibutilide and subsequent monitoring of the patient.

Preparation for Administration No dilution required. May dilute in 50 mL diluent (0.9% NS or D_5W).

Storage/Stability Admixtures are chemically and physically stable for 24 hours at room temperature and for 48 hours at refrigerated temperatures.

Nursing Actions

Physical Assessment Requires infusion pump and continuous cardiac and hemodynamic monitoring during and for 4 hours following infusion.

Patient Education

- Discuss specific use of drug and side effects with patient as it relates to treatment. (HCAHPS: During this hospital stay, were you given any medicine that you had not taken before? Before giving you any new medicine, how often did hospital staff tell you what the medicine was for? How often did hospital staff describe possible side effects in a way you could understand?)
- Patient may experience headache or tachycardia. Have patient report immediately to prescriber severe dizziness or rash (HCAHPS).
- Educate patient about signs of a significant reaction (eg, wheezing; chest tightness; fever; itching; bad cough; blue skin color; seizures; or swelling of face, lips, tongue, or throat). **Note:** This is not a comprehensive list of all side effects. Patient should consult prescriber for additional questions.

Intended Use and Disclaimer: Should not be printed and given to patients. This information is intended to serve as a concise initial reference for healthcare professionals to use when discussing medications with a patient. You must ultimately rely on your own discretion, experience and judgment in diagnosing, treating and advising patients.

Icatibant (eye KAT i bant)

Brand Names: U.S. Firazyr

Index Terms HOE 140; Icatibant Acetate

Pharmacologic Category Selective Bradykinin B2 Receptor Antagonist

Pregnancy Risk Factor C

Lactation Excretion unknown/use caution

Breast-Feeding Considerations It is not known if icatibant is excreted in breast milk. The manufacturer recommends that caution be exercised when administering icatibant to nursing women.

Use Treatment of acute attacks of hereditary angioedema (HAE)

Mechanism of Action/Effect Icatibant is a selective competitive antagonist for the bradykinin B_2 receptor. Icatibant inhibits bradykinin from binding at the B_2 receptor, thereby treating the symptoms associated with acute attack.

Contraindications There are no contraindications listed in the manufacturer's labeling.

Warnings/Precautions Airway obstruction may occur during acute laryngeal attacks of HAE. Patients with laryngeal attacks should be instructed to seek medical attention immediately in addition to treatment with icatibant. Icatibant may potentially attenuate the antihypertensive effect of ACE inhibitors; patients taking ACE inhibitors were excluded from initial clinical trials.

Drug Interactions

Avoid Concomitant Use There are no known interactions where it is recommended to avoid concomitant use.

Decreased Effect

Icatibant may decrease the levels/effects of: ACE Inhibitors

Increased Effect/Toxicity There are no known significant interactions involving an increase in effect.

Adverse Reactions

>10%: Local: Injection site reaction (97%)

1% to 10%:

Central nervous system: Pyrexia (4%), dizziness (3%)

Hepatic: Transaminase increased (4%)

Pharmacodynamics/Kinetics

Onset of Action Median time to 50% decrease of symptoms: ~2 hours

Duration of Action Inhibits symptoms caused by bradykinin for ~6 hours

Available Dosage Forms

Solution, Subcutaneous [preservative free]: Firazyr: 30 mg/3 mL (3 mL)

General Dosage Range SubQ: *Adults:* 30 mg/dose; maximum: 3 doses/24 hours

Administration

Other For SubQ injection only. Inject into the abdomen over ≥30 seconds, using the 25 gauge needle provided. Inject 2-4 inches below belly button and away from any scars; do not inject into an area that is bruised, swollen, or painful.

Storage/Stability Store between 2°C to 25°C (36°F to 77°F); do not freeze. Store in original container until time of administration.

Nursing Actions

Physical Assessment Monitor for laryngeal symptoms or airway obstruction. Report adverse reactions to the FDA at 1-866-880-0660.

Patient Education

• Discuss specific use of drug and side effects with patient as it relates to treatment. (HCAHPS: During this hospital stay, were you given any medicine that you had not taken before? Before giving you any new medicine, how often did hospital staff tell you what the medicine was for? How often did hospital staff describe possible side effects in a way you could understand?)

• Patient may experience injection site irritation, dizziness, headache, or dyspepsia. Have patient report immediately to prescriber dyspnea or rash (HCAHPS).

• Educate patient about signs of a significant reaction (eg, wheezing; chest tightness; fever; itching; bad cough; blue skin color; seizures; or swelling of face, lips, tongue, or throat). **Note:** This is not a comprehensive list of all side effects. Patient should consult prescriber for additional questions.

Intended Use and Disclaimer: Should not be printed and given to patients. This information is intended to serve as a concise initial reference for healthcare professionals to use when discussing medications with a patient. You must ultimately rely on your own discretion, experience and judgment in diagnosing, treating and advising patients.

Icosapent Ethyl (eye KOE sa pent ETH il)

Brand Names: U.S. Vascepa

Index Terms AMR101; Ethyl Eicosapentaenoate; Ethyl Icosapentate; Ethyl-Eicosapentaenoic Acid; Ethyl-EPA

Pharmacologic Category Antilipemic Agent, Omega-3 Fatty Acids

Pregnancy Risk Factor C

Lactation Excreted in breast milk/use caution

Breast-Feeding Considerations Maternal dietary consumption of omega-3-fatty acids (containing eicosapentaenoic acid [EPA] and docosahexaenoic acid [DHA]) influences milk concentrations (Coletta, 2010; Miles, 2011). Information specific to the therapeutic use of this product by nursing women has not been located.

Use Adjunct to dietary therapy in the treatment of hypertriglyceridemia (≥500 mg/dL)

Mechanism of Action/Effect Lowers serum triglycerides; possibly by increased clearance or decreased synthesis of triglycerides

Contraindications Hypersensitivity to icosapent ethyl or any component of the formulation

Warnings/Precautions Should be used as an adjunct to diet therapy and exercise and only in those with very high triglyceride levels (≥500 mg/dL). The effect, if any, of icosapent ethyl on the risk of pancreatitis or cardiovascular mortality or morbidity in patients with severe hypertriglyceridemia is not known. Treatment of primary metabolic disorders (eg, diabetes, thyroid disease) and/or evaluation of the patient's medication regimen for possible etiologic agents should be completed prior to a decision to initiate therapy. Secondary causes of hyperlipidemia should be ruled out prior to therapy. Medications known to worsen hypertriglyceridemia (eg, beta-blockers, thiazides, estrogens) should be discontinued or changed prior to initiation of triglyceride-lowering therapy if possible.

Use with caution in patients with known allergy or sensitivity to fish and/or shellfish. Studies have not been conducted in patients with hepatic impairment; however, ALT/AST levels should be monitored periodically during therapy in hepatically impaired patients. Prolongation of bleeding time not exceeding normal limits has been observed in some clinical studies of omega-3 fatty acids; clinically significant bleeding episodes did not occur. Use with caution in patients with coagulopathy or in those receiving therapeutic anticoagulation; monitor for changes in INR (with warfarin) or signs/symptoms of bleeding following initiation and dosage changes of icosapent ethyl and in patients receiving concomitant anticoagulant or antiplatelet therapy.

Drug Interactions

Avoid Concomitant Use There are no known interactions where it is recommended to avoid concomitant use.

Decreased Effect There are no known significant interactions involving a decrease in effect.

Increased Effect/Toxicity

Icosapent Ethyl may increase the levels/effects of: Agents with Antiplatelet Properties; Anticoagulants

Nutritional/Ethanol Interactions Ethanol: Monitor ethanol use (alcohol use may increase triglycerides).

Adverse Reactions 1% to 10%: Neuromuscular & skeletal: Arthralgia (2%)

Available Dosage Forms .

Capsule, Oral:

Vascepa: 1 g

General Dosage Range

Oral: *Adults:* 2 g twice daily

Administration

Oral Administer with food. Swallow whole; do not chew, crush, or divide.

Storage/Stability Store at 20°C to 25°C (68°F to 77°F); excursions permitted to 15°C to 30°C (59°F to 86°F).

Nursing Actions

Physical Assessment Make sure patient gets liver function tests periodically during treatment. Monitor for any bleeding problems. Review patient's medications to ensure patient not taking another source of omega-3 fatty acids.

Patient Education

• Discuss specific use of drug and side effects with patient as it relates to treatment. (HCAHPS: During this hospital stay, were you given any medicine that you had not taken before? Before giving you any new medicine, how often did hospital staff tell you what the medicine was for? How often did hospital staff describe possible side effects in a way you could understand?)

• Patient may experience arthralgia. Have patient report immediately to prescriber dyspepsia, emesis, significant weight gain, or rash (HCAHPS).

• Educate patient about signs of a significant reaction (eg, wheezing; chest tightness; fever; itching; bad cough; blue skin color; seizures; or swelling of face, lips, tongue, or throat). **Note:** This is not a comprehensive list of all side effects. Patient should consult prescriber for additional questions.

Intended Use and Disclaimer: Should not be printed and given to patients. This information is intended to serve as a concise initial reference for healthcare professionals to use when discussing medications with a patient. You must ultimately rely on your own discretion, experience and judgment in diagnosing, treating and advising patients.

Dietary Considerations Take with food. Dietary modification is important in the control of severe hypertriglyceridemia. Maintain standard cholesterol-lowering diet during therapy.

Related Information

Oral Medications That Should Not Be Crushed or Altered *on page 1712*

IDArubicin (eye da ROO bi sin)

Brand Names: U.S. Idamycin PFS

Index Terms 4-Demethoxydaunorubicin; 4-DMDR; Idarubicin Hydrochloride; IDR; IMI 30; SC 33428

Pharmacologic Category Antineoplastic Agent, Anthracycline; Antineoplastic Agent, Topoisomerase II Inhibitor

Medication Safety Issues

Sound-alike/look-alike issues:

IDArubicin may be confused with DOXOrubicin, DAUNOrubicin, epirubicin

Idamycin PFS® may be confused with Adriamycin

High alert medication:

The Institute for Safe Medication Practices (ISMP) includes this medication among its list of drugs which have a heightened risk of causing significant patient harm when used in error.

Pregnancy Risk Factor D

Lactation Excretion in breast milk unknown/not recommended

Breast-Feeding Considerations It is not known if idarubicin is excreted in breast milk. Breast-feeding is not recommended by the manufacturer.

Use Treatment of acute myeloid leukemia (AML)

Unlabeled Use Acute lymphocytic leukemia (ALL)

Mechanism of Action/Effect Similar to daunorubicin, idarubicin exhibits inhibitory effects on DNA and RNA polymerase.

Contraindications Hypersensitivity to idarubicin, other anthracyclines, or any component of the formulation; bilirubin >5 mg/dL

Warnings/Precautions Hazardous agent - use appropriate precautions for handling and disposal (NIOSH, 2012). **[U.S. Boxed Warning]: May cause myocardial toxicity; may lead to heart failure. Cardiotoxicity is more common in patients who have previously received anthracyclines or have pre-existing cardiac disease.** The risk of myocardial toxicity is also increased in patients with concomitant or prior mediastinal/pericardial irradiation, patients with anemia, bone marrow depression, infections, leukemic pericarditis or myocarditis. Acute arrhythmias (may be life-threatening) or other cardiomyopathies may also occur. Monitor cardiac function during treatment.

[U.S. Boxed Warning]: Vesicant; may cause severe local tissue damage and necrosis if extravasation occurs. For I.V. administration only. NOT for I.M. or SubQ administration. Administer through a rapidly flowing I.V. line. Ensure proper needle or catheter placement prior to and during infusion. Avoid extravasation.

[U.S. Boxed Warning]: May cause severe mye-losuppression; use caution in patients with pre-existing myelosuppression from prior treat-ment or radiation. [U.S. Boxed Warning]: Dos-age reductions are recommended in patients with renal or hepatic impairment. Rapid lysis of leukemic cells may lead to hyperuricemia. Sys-temic infections should be managed prior to initia-tion of treatment. [U.S. Boxed Warning]: Should be administered under the supervision of an experienced cancer chemotherapy physician.

Drug Interactions

Avoid Concomitant Use

Avoid concomitant use of IDArubicin with any of the following: BCG; CloZAPine; Natalizumab; Pimecrolimus; Tacrolimus (Topical); Tofacitinib; Vaccines (Live)

Decreased Effect

IDArubicin may decrease the levels/effects of: BCG; Cardiac Glycosides; Coccidioidin Skin Test; Sipuleucel-T; Vaccines (Inactivated); Vaccines (Live)

The levels/effects of IDArubicin may be decreased by: Cardiac Glycosides; Echinacea; P-glycoprotein/ABCB1 Inducers

Increased Effect/Toxicity

IDArubicin may increase the levels/effects of: CloZAPine; Leflunomide; Natalizumab; Tofaciti-nib; Vaccines (Live)

The levels/effects of IDArubicin may be increased by: Bevacizumab; Cyclophosphamide; Denosu-mab; P-glycoprotein/ABCB1 Inhibitors; Pimecroli-mus; Roflumilast; Tacrolimus (Topical); Taxane Derivatives; Trastuzumab

Adverse Reactions

>10%:

Cardiovascular: Transient ECG abnormalities (supraventricular tachycardia, S-T wave changes, atrial or ventricular extrasystoles); gen-erally asymptomatic and self-limiting. CHF, dose related. The relative cardiotoxicity of idarubicin compared to doxorubicin is unclear. Some inves-tigators report no increase in cardiac toxicity for adults at cumulative oral idarubicin doses up to 540 mg/m^2; other reports suggest a maximum cumulative intravenous dose of 150 mg/m^2.

Central nervous system: Headache

Dermatologic: Alopecia (25% to 30%), radiation recall, skin rash (11%), urticaria

Gastrointestinal: Nausea, vomiting (30% to 60%); diarrhea (9% to 22%); stomatitis (11%); GI hem-orrhage (30%)

Genitourinary: Discoloration of urine (darker yellow)

Hematologic: Myelosuppression (nadir: 10-15 days; recovery: 21-28 days), primarily leukope-nia; thrombocytopenia and anemia. Effects are generally less severe with oral dosing.

Hepatic: Bilirubin and transaminases increased (44%)

1% to 10%:

Central nervous system: Seizure

Neuromuscular & skeletal: Peripheral neuropathy

Available Dosage Forms

Solution, Intravenous [preservative free]:

Idamycin PFS: 5 mg/5 mL (5 mL); 10 mg/10 mL (10 mL); 20 mg/20 mL (20 mL)

Generic: 5 mg/5 mL (5 mL); 10 mg/10 mL (10 mL); 20 mg/20 mL (20 mL)

General Dosage Range

Dosage adjustment rec-ommended in patients with hepatic or renal impair-ment

I.V.: *Adults:* Induction: 12 mg/m^2/day for 3 days; Consolidation: 10-12 mg/m^2/day for 2 days

Administration

I.V. For I.V. administration only. Do not administer I.M. or SubQ; administer as slow push over 3-5 minutes, preferably into the side of a freely-run-ning saline or dextrose infusion **or** as intermittent infusion over 10-15 minutes into a free-flowing I.V. solution of NS or D$_5$W; also occasionally admin-istered as a bladder lavage.

Vesicant; ensure proper needle or catheter place-ment prior to and during infusion; avoid extrava-sation.

Extravasation management: If extravasation occurs, stop infusion immediately and disconnect (leave cannula/needle in place); gently aspirate extravasated solution (do **NOT** flush the line); remove needle/cannula; elevate extremity. Initiate antidote (dexrazoxane or dimethyl sulfate [DMSO]). Apply dry cold compresses for 20 minutes 4 times daily for 1-2 days (Perez Fidalgo, 2012); withhold cooling beginning 15 minutes before dexrazoxane infusion; continue withhold-ing cooling until 15 minutes after infusion is com-pleted. Topical DMSO should not be administered in combination with dexrazoxane; may lessen dexrazoxane efficacy.

Dexrazoxane: Adults: 1000 mg/m^2 (maximum dose: 2000 mg) I.V. (administer in a large vein remote from site of extravasation) over 1-2 hours days 1 and 2, then 500 mg/m^2 (maxi-mum dose: 1000 mg) I.V. over 1-2 hours day 3; begin within 6 hours of extravasation. Day 2 and day 3 doses should be administered at approximately the same time (± 3 hours) as the dose on day 1 (Mouridsen, 2007; Perez Fidalgo, 2012). **Note:** Reduce dexrazoxane dose by 50% in patients with moderate to severe renal impairment (CrCl <40 mL/minute).

DMSO: Children and Adults: Apply topically to a region covering twice the affected area every 8 hours for 7 days; begin within 10 minutes of extravasation; do not cover with a dressing (Perez Fidalgo, 2012).

Hazardous agent; use appropriate precautions for handling and disposal (NIOSH, 2012).

Injectable Detail pH: ~3.5 (1 mg/mL solution in vial)

Storage/Stability Store intact vials of solution under refrigeration at 2°C to 8°C (36°F to 46°F). Protect from light. Solutions diluted in D₅W or NS for infusion are stable for 4 weeks at room temperature, protected from light. Syringe and IVPB solutions are stable for 72 hours at room temperature and 7 days under refrigeration.

Nursing Actions

Physical Assessment Infusion site must be closely monitored; extravasation can cause severe cellulitis or tissue necrosis (eg, do not apply heat). Monitor for cardiac toxicity, myelosuppression, and peripheral neuropathy frequently during therapy.

Patient Education

• Discuss specific use of drug and side effects with patient as it relates to treatment. (HCAHPS: During this hospital stay, were you given any medicine that you had not taken before? Before giving you any new medicine, how often did hospital staff tell you what the medicine was for? How often did hospital staff describe possible side effects in a way you could understand?)

• Patient may experience headache, stomatitis, cheilitis, or alopecia. Have patient report immediately to prescriber signs of infection, severe dizziness, syncope, significant nausea, considerable diarrhea, excessive weight loss, osteodynia, night sweats, intolerable dyspepsia, melena, hematemesis, paresthesia, ecchymosis, hemorrhaging, severe asthenia, or eczema of hands or feet (HCAHPS).

• Educate patient about signs of a significant reaction (eg, wheezing; chest tightness; fever; itching; bad cough; blue skin color; seizures; or swelling of face, lips, tongue, or throat). **Note:** This is not a comprehensive list of all side effects. Patient should consult prescriber for additional questions.

Intended Use and Disclaimer: Should not be printed and given to patients. This information is intended to serve as a concise initial reference for healthcare professionals to use when discussing medications with a patient. You must ultimately rely on your own discretion, experience and judgment in diagnosing, treating and advising patients.

Related Information

Management of Drug Extravasations *on page 1700*

Ifosfamide (eye FOSS fa mide)

Brand Names: U.S. Ifex

Index Terms Isophosphamide; Z4942

Pharmacologic Category Antineoplastic Agent, Alkylating Agent; Antineoplastic Agent, Alkylating Agent (Nitrogen Mustard)

Medication Safety Issues

Sound-alike/look-alike issues:
Ifosfamide may be confused with cyclophosphamide

High alert medication:
This medication is in a class the Institute for Safe Medication Practices (ISMP) includes its list of drug classes which have a heightened risk of causing significant patient harm when used in error.

Pregnancy Risk Factor D

Lactation Enters breast milk/not recommended

Breast-Feeding Considerations Breast-feeding should be avoided during ifosfamide treatment. According to the manufacturer, the decision to discontinue ifosfamide or discontinue breast-feeding should take into account the risk of exposure to the infant and the benefits of treatment to the mother.

Use

U.S. labeling: Treatment (third-line) of germ cell testicular cancer (in combination with other chemotherapy drugs and with concurrent mesna)

Canadian labeling (not approved indications in the U.S.): Treatment of soft tissue sarcoma, pancreatic cancer (relapsed or refractory), cervical cancer (advanced or recurrent; as monotherapy or in combination with cisplatin and bleomycin)

Unlabeled Use Treatment of bladder cancer (metastatic), cervical cancer (recurrent or metastatic), head and neck cancers (recurrent or metastatic), ovarian cancer, small cell lung cancer (relapsed), Hodgkin lymphoma (relapsed or refractory), non-Hodgkin lymphomas, thymomas and thymic cancers (advanced), sarcomas (Ewing's sarcoma, osteosarcoma, and soft tissue sarcoma)

Mechanism of Action/Effect Inhibits protein synthesis and DNA synthesis

Contraindications Hypersensitivity to ifosfamide or any component of the formulation; urinary outflow obstruction

Canadian labeling: Additional contraindications (not in U.S. labeling): Severe myelosuppression; severe renal or hepatic impairment; active infection (bacterial, fungal, viral); severe immunosuppression; urinary tract disease (eg, cystitis); advanced cerebral arteriosclerosis

Warnings/Precautions Hazardous agent: Use appropriate precautions for handling and disposal (NIOSH, 2012). **[U.S. Boxed Warning]: Hemorrhagic cystitis may occur; concomitant mesna reduces the risk of hemorrhagic cystitis.** Hydration (at least 2 L/day), dose fractionation, and/or mesna administration will reduce the incidence of hematuria and protect against hemorrhagic cystitis. Obtain urinalysis prior to each dose; if microscopic hematuria is detected, withhold until complete resolution. Exclude or correct urinary tract obstructions prior to treatment. Use with caution (if at all) in patients with active urinary tract infection. Hemorrhagic cystitis is dose-dependent and is ▶

increased with high single doses (compared with fractionated doses); past or concomitant bladder radiation or busulfan treatment may increase the risk for hemorrhagic cystitis. **[U.S. Boxed Warning]: May cause severe nephrotoxicity, resulting in renal failure.** Acute and chronic renal failure as well as renal parenchymal and tubular necrosis (including acute) have been reported; tubular damage may be delayed and may persist. Renal manifestations include decreased glomerular rate, increased creatinine, proteinuria, enzymuria, cylindruria, aminoaciduria, phosphaturia, and glycosuria. Syndrome of inappropriate antidiuretic hormone (SIADH), renal rickets, and Fanconi syndrome have been reported. Evaluate renal function prior to and during treatment; monitor urine for erythrocytes and signs of urotoxicity.

[U.S. Boxed Warning]: May cause CNS toxicity which may be severe, resulting in encephalopathy and death; monitor for CNS toxicity; discontinue for encephalopathy. Symptoms of CNS toxicity (somnolence, confusion, dizziness, disorientation, hallucinations, cranial nerve dysfunction, psychotic behavior, extrapyramidal symptoms, seizures, coma blurred vision, and/or incontinence) have been observed within a few hours to a few days after initial dose and generally resolve within 2-3 days of treatment discontinuation (although may persist longer); maintain supportive care until complete resolution. Risk factors may include hypoalbuminemia, renal dysfunction, and prior history of ifosfamide-induced encephalopathy. Concomitant centrally-acting medications may result in additive CNS effects. Peripheral neuropathy has been reported.

[U.S. Boxed Warning]: Severe bone marrow suppression may occur (dose-limiting toxicity); monitor blood counts before and after each cycle. Leukopenia, neutropenia, thrombocytopenia and anemia are associated with ifosfamide. Myelosuppression is dose dependent, increased with single high doses (compared to fractionated doses) and increased with decreased renal function. Severe myelosuppression may occur when administered in combination with other chemotherapy agents or radiation therapy. Use with caution in patients with compromised bone marrow reserve. Unless clinically necessary, avoid administering to patients with WBC <2000/mm^3 and platelets <50,000/mm^3. Antimicrobial prophylaxis may be necessary in some neutropenic patients; Administer antibiotics and/or antifungal agents for neutropenic fever. May cause significant suppression of the immune responses; may lead to serious infection, sepsis or septic shock; reported infections have included bacterial, viral, fungal, and parasitic; latent infections may be reactivated; use with caution with other immunosuppressants or in patients with infection.

Arrhythmias, ST-segment or T-wave changes, cardiomyopathy, pericardial effusion, pericarditis, and epicardial fibrosis have been observed; the risk for cardiotoxicity is dose-dependent; concomitant cardiotoxic agents (eg, anthracyclines), irradiation of the cardiac region, and renal impairment may also increase the risk; use with caution in patients with cardiac risk factors or pre-existing cardiac disease. Interstitial pneumonitis, pulmonary fibrosis, and pulmonary toxicity leading to respiratory failure have been reported; monitor for signs and symptoms of pulmonary toxicity.

Anaphylactic/anaphylactoid reactions have been associated with ifosfamide; cross sensitivity with similar agents may occur. Hepatic sinusoidal obstruction syndrome (SOS), formerly called veno-occlusive disease (VOD), has been reported with ifosfamide-containing regimens. Secondary malignancies may occur; the risk for myelodysplastic syndrome (which may progress to acute leukemia) is increased with treatment. May interfere with wound healing. Use with caution in patients with prior radiation therapy.

Drug Interactions

Avoid Concomitant Use

Avoid concomitant use of Ifosfamide with any of the following: BCG; CloZAPine; Natalizumab; Pimecrolimus; Pimozide; Tacrolimus (Topical); Tofacitinib; Vaccines (Live)

Decreased Effect

Ifosfamide may decrease the levels/effects of: BCG; Coccidioidin Skin Test; Sipuleucel-T; Vaccines (Inactivated); Vaccines (Live); Vitamin K Antagonists

The levels/effects of Ifosfamide may be decreased by: CYP2A6 Inducers (Strong); CYP2C19 Inducers (Strong); CYP3A4 Inhibitors (Moderate); CYP3A4 Inhibitors (Strong); Dabrafenib; Echinacea

Increased Effect/Toxicity

Ifosfamide may increase the levels/effects of: ARIPiprazole; CloZAPine; Dofetilide; Leflunomide; Lomitapide; Natalizumab; Pimozide; Tofacitinib; Vaccines (Live); Vitamin K Antagonists

The levels/effects of Ifosfamide may be increased by: Busulfan; CYP2A6 Inhibitors (Moderate); CYP2A6 Inhibitors (Strong); CYP2C19 Inhibitors (Moderate); CYP2C19 Inhibitors (Strong); CYP3A4 Inducers (Strong); Denosumab; Luliconazole; Pimecrolimus; Roflumilast; Tacrolimus (Topical); Trastuzumab

Nutritional/Ethanol Interactions
Herb/Nutraceutical: St John's wort may decrease ifosfamide levels.

Adverse Reactions
>10%:

Central nervous system: CNS toxicity or encephalopathy (12% to 15%)

Dermatologic: Alopecia (83% to 90%; 100% with combination therapy)

Endocrine & metabolic: Metabolic acidosis (31%)

Gastrointestinal: Nausea/vomiting (47% to 58%)

Hematologic: Leukopenia (50% to ≤100%; grade 4: ≤50%; nadir: 8-14 days), anemia (38%), thrombocytopenia (20%; grades 3/4: ≤8%)

Renal: Hematuria (6% to 92%; reduced with mesna; grade 2 [gross hematuria]: 8% to 12%)

1% to 10%:

Central nervous system: Fever (1%)

Gastrointestinal: Anorexia (1%)

Hematologic: Neutropenic fever (1%)

Hepatic: Bilirubin increased (2% to 3%), liver dysfunction (2% to 3%), transaminases increased (2% to 3%)

Local: Phlebitis (2% to 3%)

Renal: Renal impairment (6%)

Miscellaneous: Infection (8% to 10%)

Available Dosage Forms

Kit, Intravenous:

Generic: 1-1 g

Solution, Intravenous:

Generic: 1 g/20 mL (20 mL); 3 g/60 mL (60 mL)

Solution, Intravenous [preservative free]:

Generic: 1 g/20 mL (20 mL); 3 g/60 mL (60 mL)

Solution Reconstituted, Intravenous:

Ifex: 1 g (1 ea); 3 g (1 ea)

Generic: 1 g (1 ea); 3 g (1 ea)

General Dosage Range Dosage adjustment recommended in patients with hepatic or renal impairment or who develop toxicities.

I.V.: *Adults:* 1200 mg/m^2/day for 5 days every 21 days

Administration

I.V. Administer I.V. over at least 30 minutes (infusion times may vary by protocol; refer to specific protocol for infusion duration)

Hazardous agent; use appropriate precautions for handling and disposal (NIOSH, 2012).

Preparation for Administration Hazardous agent; use appropriate precautions for handling and disposal (NIOSH, 2012). Reconstitute powder with SWFI or bacteriostatic SWFI (1 g in 20 mL or 3 g in 60 mL) to a concentration of 50 mg/mL. Further dilution in 50-1000 mL D$_5$W, NS, or lactated Ringer's (to a final concentration of 0.6-20 mg/mL) is recommended for I.V. infusion (may also dilute in D$_{2.5}$W, 1/2NS, or D$_5$NS).

Storage/Stability Store intact vials of powder for injection at room temperature of 20°C to 25°C (68°F to 77°F); avoid temperatures >30°C (86°F). Store intact vials of solution under refrigeration at 2°C to 8°C (36°F to 46°F). Reconstituted solutions and solutions diluted for administration are stable for 24 hours refrigerated.

Nursing Actions

Physical Assessment Ensure patient is adequately hydrating before treatment to minimize risk of hemorrhagic cystitis. Instruct patient on importance of hydration and help to provide directions that may help when home. Obtain baseline urinalysis prior to each dose. Premedicate with appropriate antiemetic. Educate patient about how to take antiemetic and when to call provider if not adequately addressing nausea and vomiting. Monitor vital signs prior to each infusion and regularly during therapy. Monitor for CNS depression or psychoses, hematuria, and infection throughout therapy.

Patient Education

• Discuss specific use of drug and side effects with patient as it relates to treatment. (HCAHPS: During this hospital stay, were you given any medicine that you had not taken before? Before giving you any new medicine, how often did hospital staff tell you what the medicine was for? How often did hospital staff describe possible side effects in a way you could understand?)

• Patient may experience leukopenia, thrombocytopenia, presyncope, fatigue, blurred vision, illogical thinking, asthenia, confusion, nausea, stomatitis, alopecia, hematuria, or bleeding problems. Have patient report immediately to prescriber signs of infection, dyspnea, severe dyspepsia, significant back pain, diarrhea, urinary retention, ecchymosis, or rash (HCAHPS).

• Educate patient about signs of a significant reaction (eg, wheezing; chest tightness; fever; itching; bad cough; blue skin color; seizures; or swelling of face, lips, tongue, or throat). **Note:** This is not a comprehensive list of all side effects. Patient should consult prescriber for additional questions.

Intended Use and Disclaimer: Should not be printed and given to patients. This information is intended to serve as a concise initial reference for healthcare professionals to use when discussing medications with a patient. You must ultimately rely on your own discretion, experience and judgment in diagnosing, treating and advising patients.

Related Information

Management of Drug Extravasations *on page 1700*

Iloperidone (eye loe PER i done)

Brand Names: U.S. Fanapt; Fanapt Titration Pack

Pharmacologic Category Antipsychotic Agent, Atypical

Medication Safety Issues

Sound-alike/look-alike issues:

Fanapt® may be confused with Xanax®

Iloperidone may be confused with domperidone

BEERS Criteria medication:

This drug may be potentially inappropriate for use in geriatric patients (Quality of evidence - moderate; Strength of recommendation - strong).

Pregnancy Risk Factor C

Lactation Excretion in breast milk unknown/not recommended

Breast-Feeding Considerations It is not known if iloperidone is excreted into breast milk. Breast-feeding is not recommended by the manufacturer.

Use Acute treatment of schizophrenia

Mechanism of Action/Effect Iloperidone is an atypical antipsychotic which blocks serotonin and dopamine receptors. Results in improvement of psychoses with lower incidence of extrapyramidal side effects.

Contraindications Hypersensitivity to iloperidone or any component of the formulation

Warnings/Precautions [U.S. Boxed Warning]: Elderly patients with dementia-related psychosis treated with antipsychotics are at an increased risk of death compared to placebo. Most deaths appeared to be either cardiovascular (eg, heart failure, sudden death) or infectious (eg, pneumonia) in nature. In addition, an increased incidence of cerebrovascular effects (eg, transient ischemic attack, cerebrovascular accidents) has been reported in studies of placebo-controlled trials of antipsychotics in elderly patients with dementia-related psychosis. Iloperidone is not approved for the treatment of dementia-related psychosis.

May be sedating; use with caution in disorders where CNS depression is a feature. Caution in patients with predisposition to seizures. Use is not recommended in patients with hepatic impairment. Esophageal dysmotility and aspiration have been associated with antipsychotic use; use with caution in patients at risk of aspiration pneumonia (ie, Alzheimer's disease). Use is associated with increased prolactin levels; clinical significance of hyperprolactinemia in patients with breast cancer or other prolactin-dependent tumors is unknown. May alter temperature regulation. Leukopenia, neutropenia, and agranulocytosis (sometimes fatal) have been reported in clinical trials and postmarketing reports; presence of risk factors (eg, pre-existing low WBC or history of drug-induced leuko-/neutropenia) should prompt periodic blood count assessment and discontinuation at first signs of blood dyscrasias.

May alter cardiac conduction and prolong the QT_c interval; life-threatening arrhythmias have occurred with therapeutic doses of antipsychotics. Risks may be increased by conditions or concomitant medications which cause bradycardia, hypokalemia, and/or hypomagnesemia. Avoid use in combination with QT_c-prolonging drugs and in patients with congenital long QT syndrome, history of cardiac arrhythmia, recent MI, or uncompensated heart failure. Discontinue treatment in patients found to have persistent QT_c intervals >500 msec. Further cardiac evaluation is warranted in patients with symptoms of dizziness, palpitations, or syncope. May cause orthostatic hypotension; use with caution in patients at risk of this effect (eg, concurrent medication use which may predispose to hypotension/bradycardia or presence of hypovolemia) or in those who would not tolerate transient hypotensive episodes. Use with caution in patients with cardiovascular diseases (eg, heart failure, history of myocardial infarction or ischemia, cerebrovascular disease, conduction abnormalities).

May cause anticholinergic effects (confusion, agitation, constipation, xerostomia, blurred vision, urinary retention); therefore, use with caution in patients with decreased gastrointestinal motility, urinary retention, BPH, xerostomia, or visual problems (including narrow-angle glaucoma). May cause extrapyramidal symptoms (EPS), including pseudoparkinsonism, acute dystonic reactions, akathisia, and tardive dyskinesia. Risk of dystonia (and probably other EPS) may be greater with increased doses, use of conventional antipsychotics, males, and younger patients. Risk of neuroleptic malignant syndrome (NMS) may be increased in patients with Parkinson's disease or Lewy body dementia. May cause hyperglycemia; in some cases may be extreme and associated with ketoacidosis, hyperosmolar coma, or death. Use with caution in patients with diabetes or other disorders of glucose regulation; monitor for worsening of glucose control. Dyslipidemia has been reported with atypical antipsychotics; risk profile may differ between agents. In clinical trials, changes in triglyceride and total cholesterol levels observed with iloperidone were similar to those observed with placebo or were clinically insignificant. Small reductions in cholesterol and triglycerides have been observed in longer term iloperidone trials.

Significant weight gain has been observed with antipsychotic therapy; incidence varies with product. Monitor waist circumference and BMI. Rare cases of priapism have been reported.

Use in elderly patients with dementia is associated with an increased risk of mortality and cerebrovascular accidents; avoid antipsychotic use for behavioral problems associated with dementia unless alternative nonpharmacologic therapies have failed and patient may harm self or others. In addition, use may cause or exacerbate syndrome of inappropriate antidiuretic hormone secretion or hyponatremia; monitor sodium closely with initiation or dosage adjustments in older adults (Beers Criteria).

Dosage adjustments are recommended for iloperidone when given concomitantly with strong CYP2D6 or CYP3A4 inhibitors or in poor metabolizers of CYP2D6. The possibility of a suicide attempt is inherent in psychotic illness; use caution in high-risk patients during initiation of therapy. Prescriptions should be written for the smallest quantity consistent with good patient care. Continued use for >6 weeks has not been evaluated.

Drug Interactions

Avoid Concomitant Use

Avoid concomitant use of Iloperidone with any of the following: Amisulpride; Azelastine (Nasal); Bosutinib; Highest Risk QTc-Prolonging Agents; Ibrutinib; Ivabradine; Lomitapide; Metoclopramide; Mifepristone; Moderate Risk QTc-Prolonging Agents; Paraldehyde; Rivaroxaban; Simeprevir; Sulpiride; Thalidomide; Tolvaptan; Ulipristal

Decreased Effect

Iloperidone may decrease the levels/effects of: Amphetamines; Anti-Parkinson's Agents (Dopamine Agonist); Ifosfamide; Quinagolide

The levels/effects of Iloperidone may be decreased by: CYP2D6 Inhibitors (Strong); Lithium formulations; Peginterferon Alfa-2b

Increased Effect/Toxicity

Iloperidone may increase the levels/effects of: Alcohol (Ethyl); Amisulpride; ARIPiprazole; Avanafil; Azelastine (Nasal); Bosentan; Bosutinib; Budesonide (Systemic, Oral Inhalation); Buprenorphine; CNS Depressants; Colchicine; CYP3A4 Substrates; DOXOrubicin (Conventional); Eplerenone; Everolimus; FentaNYL; Highest Risk QTc-Prolonging Agents; Hydrocodone; Ibrutinib; Imatinib; Ivacaftor; Lomitapide; Lurasidone; Methylphenidate; OxyCODONE; Paraldehyde; Pimecrolimus; Rivaroxaban; Salmeterol; Saxagliptin; Serotonin Modulators; Simeprevir; Sulpiride; Thalidomide; Tolvaptan; Ulipristal; Zolpidem

The levels/effects of Iloperidone may be increased by: Abiraterone Acetate; Acetylcholinesterase Inhibitors (Central); Brimonidine (Topical); CYP2D6 Inhibitors (Moderate); CYP2D6 Inhibitors (Strong); CYP3A4 Inhibitors (Strong); Doxylamine; HydrOXYzine; Ivabradine; Lithium formulations; Magnesium Sulfate; MAO Inhibitors; Methylphenidate; Metoclopramide; Metyrosine; Mifepristone; Moderate Risk QTc-Prolonging Agents; Perampanel; QTc-Prolonging Agents (Indeterminate Risk and Risk Modifying); Serotonin Modulators; Sodium Oxybate; Tetrabenazine

Nutritional/Ethanol Interactions

Ethanol: May increase CNS depression; monitor for increased effects with coadministration. Caution patients about effects.

Herb/Nutraceutical: Avoid St John's wort (may decrease serum levels of iloperidone). Avoid kava kava, gotu kola, valerian, St John's wort (may increase CNS depression).

Adverse Reactions

>10%:
- Cardiovascular: Tachycardia (3% to 12%; dose related)
- Central nervous system: Dizziness (10% to 20%; dose related), somnolence (9% to 15%)

1% to 10%:
- Cardiovascular: Orthostatic hypotension (3% to 5%), hypotension (<1% to 3%; dose related), palpitations (≥1%)
- Central nervous system: Fatigue (4% to 6%), extrapyramidal symptoms (4% to 5%), tremor (3%), lethargy (1% to 3%), akathisia (2%), aggression (≥1%), delusion (≥1%), restlessness (≥1%)
- Dermatologic: Rash (2% to 3%)
- Gastrointestinal: Nausea (≤10%), xerostomia (8% to 10%), weight gain (1% to 9%; dose related), diarrhea (5% to 7%), abdominal discomfort (≤3%; dose related), weight loss (≥1%)
- Genitourinary: Ejaculation failure (2%), erectile dysfunction (≥1%), urinary incontinence (≥1%)
- Neuromuscular & skeletal: Arthralgia (3%), stiffness (1% to 3%; dose related), dyskinesia (<2%), muscle spasm (≥1%), myalgia (≥1%)
- Ocular: Blurred vision (≤3%), conjunctivitis (≥1%)
- Respiratory: Nasal congestion (5% to 8%), nasopharyngitis (≤4%), upper respiratory tract infection (2% to 3%), dyspnea (2%)

Available Dosage Forms

Tablet, Oral:
Fanapt: 1 mg, 2 mg, 4 mg, 6 mg, 8 mg, 10 mg, 12 mg
Fanapt Titration Pack: 1 mg (2s), 2 mg (2s), 4 mg, (2s), and 6 mg (2s)

General Dosage Range Oral: *Adults:* Initial: 1 mg twice daily; Dosage range: 6-12 mg twice daily (maximum: 24 mg daily)

Administration

Oral May be administered with or without food.

Storage/Stability Store at 25°C (77°F); excursions permitted to 15°C to 30°C (59°F to 86°F). Protect from light and moisture.

Nursing Actions

Physical Assessment Monitor weight prior to initiating therapy and at least monthly; can cause weight gain. Be alert to the potential for suicide ideation and orthostatic hypotension, especially during the titration phase. Initiate at lower doses and titrate to target dose. Taper dosage slowly when discontinuing.

Patient Education
- Discuss specific use of drug and side effects with patient as it relates to treatment. (HCAHPS: During this hospital stay, were you given any medicine that you had not taken before? Before giving you any new medicine, how often did hospital staff tell you what the medicine was for? How often did hospital staff describe possible side effects in a way you could understand?)
- Patient may experience dizziness, presyncope, fatigue, blurred vision, illogical thinking, nausea, weight gain, xerostomia, rhinitis, or diarrhea. Have patient report immediately to prescriber angina, tachycardia, tremors, nervousness and anxiety, significant change in balance, considerable asthenia, polyuria, polydipsia, weight loss, or rash (HCAHPS).

• Educate patient about signs of a significant reaction (eg, wheezing; chest tightness; fever; itching; bad cough; blue skin color; seizures; or swelling of face, lips, tongue, or throat). **Note:** This is not a comprehensive list of all side effects. Patient should consult prescriber for additional questions.

Intended Use and Disclaimer: Should not be printed and given to patients. This information is intended to serve as a concise initial reference for healthcare professionals to use when discussing medications with a patient. You must ultimately rely on your own discretion, experience and judgment in diagnosing, treating and advising patients.

Dietary Considerations May be given with or without food.

Imatinib (eye MAT eh nib)

Brand Names: U.S. Gleevec
Index Terms CGP-57148B; Glivec; Imatinib Mesylate; STI-571
Pharmacologic Category Antineoplastic Agent, BCR-ABL Tyrosine Kinase Inhibitor; Antineoplastic Agent, Tyrosine Kinase Inhibitor
Medication Safety Issues
Sound-alike/look-alike issues:
Imatinib may be confused with axitinib, dasatinib, erlotinib, gefitinib, ibrutinib, nilotinib, PONATinib, SORAfenib, SUNItinib, vandetanib
High alert medication:
This medication is in a class the Institute for Safe Medication Practices (ISMP) includes among its list of drug classes which have a heightened risk of causing significant patient harm when used in error.
Pregnancy Risk Factor D
Lactation Enters breast milk/not recommended
Breast-Feeding Considerations Imatinib and its active metabolite are found in human breast milk; the milk/plasma ratio is 0.5 for imatinib and 0.9 for the active metabolite. Based on body weight, up to 10% of a therapeutic maternal dose could potentially be received by a breastfed infant, the decision to discontinue breast-feeding during therapy or to discontinue imatinib should take into account the benefits of treatment to the mother.
Use Treatment of:
Gastrointestinal stromal tumors (GIST) kit-positive (CD117), including unresectable and/or metastatic malignant and adjuvant treatment following complete resection
Philadelphia chromosome-positive (Ph+) chronic myeloid leukemia (CML) in chronic phase (newly-diagnosed) in children and adults
Ph+ CML in blast crisis, accelerated phase, or chronic phase after failure of interferon therapy
Ph+ acute lymphoblastic leukemia (ALL) (relapsed or refractory)

Ph+ ALL (newly diagnosed; in combination with chemotherapy) in children
Aggressive systemic mastocytosis (ASM) without D816V c-Kit mutation (or c-Kit mutation status unknown)
Dermatofibrosarcoma protuberans (DFSP) (unresectable, recurrent and/or metastatic)
Hypereosinophilic syndrome (HES) and/or chronic eosinophilic leukemia (CEL)
Myelodysplastic/myeloproliferative disease (MDS/MPD) associated with platelet-derived growth factor receptor (PDGFR) gene rearrangements

Canadian labeling (not an approved indication in the U.S.): Ph+ ALL induction therapy (newly diagnosed; as a single agent)
Unlabeled Use Treatment of desmoid tumors or chordoma (soft tissue sarcomas); post-stem cell transplant (allogeneic) follow-up treatment for recurrence in CML; treatment of advanced or metastatic melanoma (C-KIT mutated tumors)
Mechanism of Action/Effect Inhibits a specific enzyme (Bcr-Abl tyrosine kinase) produced by the Philadelphia chromosome found in many patients with chronic myeloid leukemia (CML). Inhibition of this enzyme blocks proliferation and induces cell death in leukemic cells. Also inhibits tyrosine kinase for platelet-derived growth factor (SCF), c-Kit, and cellular events mediated by PDGF and SCF.
Contraindications There are no contraindications listed within the FDA-approved manufacturer's labeling.
Canadian labeling: Hypersensitivity to imatinib or any component of the formulation
Warnings/Precautions Hazardous agent - use appropriate precautions for handling and disposal (NIOSH, 2012). Often associated with fluid retention, weight gain, and edema (risk increases with higher doses and age >65 years); occasionally serious and may lead to significant complications, including pleural effusion, pericardial effusion, pulmonary edema, and ascites. Monitor regularly for rapid weight gain or other signs/symptoms of fluid retention. Use with caution in patients where fluid accumulation may be poorly tolerated, such as in cardiovascular disease (heart failure [HF] or hypertension) and pulmonary disease. Severe HF and left ventricular dysfunction (LVD) have been reported occasionally, usually in patients with comorbidities and/or risk factors; carefully monitor patients with pre-existing cardiac disease or risk factors for HF or history of renal failure. With initiation of imatinib treatment, cardiogenic shock and/or LVD have been reported in patients with hypereosinophilic syndrome and cardiac involvement (reversible with systemic steroids, circulatory support and temporary cessation of imatinib). Patients with high eosinophil levels and an abnormal echocardiogram or abnormal serum troponin

level may benefit from prophylactic systemic steroids (for 1-2 weeks) with the initiation of imatinib.

Severe bullous dermatologic reactions (including erythema multiforme and Stevens-Johnson syndrome) have been reported; recurrence has been described with rechallenge. Case reports of successful resumption at a lower dose (with corticosteroids and/or antihistamine) have been described; however, some patients may experience recurrent reactions.

Hepatotoxicity may occur (may be severe); fatal hepatic failure and severe hepatic injury requiring liver transplantation have been reported with both short- and long-term use; monitor liver function prior to initiation and monthly or as needed thereafter; therapy interruption or dose reduction may be necessary. Transaminase and bilirubin elevations, and acute liver failure have been observed with imatinib in combination with chemotherapy. Use with caution in patients with pre-existing hepatic impairment; dosage adjustment recommended in patients with severe impairment. Use with caution in renal impairment; dosage adjustment recommended for moderate and severe impairment. Tumor lysis syndrome (TLS), including fatalities, has been reported in patients with ALL, CML eosinophilic leukemias, and GIST; risk for TLS is higher in patients with a high tumor burden or high proliferation rate; monitor closely; correct clinically significant dehydration and treat high uric acid levels prior to initiation of imatinib.

May cause GI irritation, severe hemorrhage (grades 3 and 4; including gastrointestinal hemorrhage and/or tumor hemorrhage; hemorrhage incidence is higher in patients with GIST [gastrointestinal tumors may have been hemorrhage source]), or hematologic toxicity (anemia, neutropenia, and thrombocytopenia; usually occurring within the first several months of treatment); monitor blood counts weekly for the first month, biweekly for the second month, and as clinically necessary thereafter; median duration of neutropenia is 2-3 weeks; median duration of thrombocytopenia is 3-4 weeks; in CML, cytopenias are more common in accelerated or blast phase than in chronic phase. Hypothyroidism has been reported in patients who were receiving thyroid hormone replacement therapy prior to the initiation of imatinib; monitor thyroid function; the average onset for imatinib-induced hypothyroidism is 2 weeks; consider doubling levothyroxine doses upon initiation of imatinib (Hamnvik, 2011). Potentially significant drug-drug interactions may exist, requiring dose or frequency adjustment, additional monitoring, and/or selection of alternative therapy. Imatinib exposure may be reduced in patients who have had gastric surgery (eg, bypass, major gastrectomy, or resection); monitor imatinib trough concentrations (Liu, 2011; Pavlovsky, 2009; Yoo, 2010). Growth retardation has been reported in children receiving

imatinib for the treatment of CML; generally where treatment was initiated in prepubertal children; growth velocity was usually restored as pubertal age was reached (Shima, 2010); monitor growth closely. Reports of accidents have been received but it is unclear if imatinib has been the direct cause in any case; advise patients regarding side effects such as dizziness, blurred vision, or somnolence; use caution when driving/operating motor vehicles and heavy machinery.

Drug Interactions

Avoid Concomitant Use

Avoid concomitant use of Imatinib with any of the following: BCG; Bosutinib; CloZAPine; CYP3A4 Inhibitors (Strong); Ibrutinib; Ivabradine; Lomitapide; Natalizumab; PAZOPanib; Pimecrolimus; Pimozide; Rivaroxaban; Simeprevir; Tacrolimus (Topical); Tofacitinib; Tolvaptan; Ulipristal; Vaccines (Live)

Decreased Effect

Imatinib may decrease the levels/effects of: BCG; Cardiac Glycosides; Coccidioidin Skin Test; Fludarabine; Ifosfamide; Sipuleucel-T; Vaccines (Inactivated); Vaccines (Live); Vitamin K Antagonists

The levels/effects of Imatinib may be decreased by: Bosentan; CYP3A4 Inducers (Strong); Dabrafenib; Deferasirox; Echinacea; Gemfibrozil; Ibuprofen; Peginterferon Alfa-2b; P-glycoprotein/ABCB1 Inducers; Rifamycin Derivatives; St Johns Wort; Tocilizumab

Increased Effect/Toxicity

Imatinib may increase the levels/effects of: ARIPiprazole; Avanafil; Bosentan; Bosutinib; Budesonide (Systemic, Oral Inhalation); CloZAPine; Colchicine; CycloSPORINE (Systemic); CYP3A4 Substrates; Dofetilide; DOXOrubicin (Conventional); Eplerenone; Everolimus; FentaNYL; Halofantrine; Ibrutinib; Ivabradine; Ivacaftor; Leflunomide; Lomitapide; Lurasidone; Natalizumab; OxyCODONE; PAZOPanib; Pimozide; Propafenone; Ranolazine; Rivaroxaban; Salmeterol; Saxagliptin; Simeprevir; Simvastatin; Tofacitinib; Tolvaptan; Topotecan; Ulipristal; Vaccines (Live); Vilazodone; Vitamin K Antagonists; Warfarin; Zuclopenthixol

The levels/effects of Imatinib may be increased by: Acetaminophen; CYP3A4 Inhibitors (Moderate); CYP3A4 Inhibitors (Strong); Denosumab; Lansoprazole; P-glycoprotein/ABCB1 Inhibitors; Pimecrolimus; Roflumilast; Tacrolimus (Topical); Trastuzumab

Nutritional/Ethanol Interactions

Ethanol: Management: Avoid ethanol.

Food: Food may reduce GI irritation. Grapefruit juice may increase imatinib plasma concentration. Management: Take with a meal and a large glass of water. Avoid grapefruit juice. Maintain adequate hydration, unless instructed to restrict fluid intake. ▶

Herb/Nutraceutical: St John's wort may increase metabolism and decrease imatinib plasma concentration. Management: Avoid St John's wort.

Adverse Reactions Note: Adverse reactions listed as a composite of data across many trials, except where noted for a specific indication.

>10%:

Cardiovascular: Edema/fluid retention (11% to 86%; grades 3/4: 3% to 13%; includes aggravated edema, anasarca, ascites, pericardial effusion, peripheral edema, pulmonary edema, and superficial edema); facial edema (≤17%), chest pain (7% to 11%), hypotension (Ph+ ALL [pediatric] grades 3/4: 11%)

Central nervous system: Fatigue (29% to 75%), pain (≤47%), fever (6% to 41%), headache (8% to 37%), dizziness (5% to 19%), insomnia (10% to 15%), depression (≤15%), anxiety (8% to 12%), chills (≤11%)

Dermatologic: Rash (9% to 50%; grades 3/4: 1% to 9%), dermatitis (GIST ≤39%), pruritus (8% to 26%), alopecia (GIST 10% to 15%)

Endocrine & metabolic: LDH increased (GIST ≤60%), hypokalemia (6% to 13%; Ph+ ALL [pediatric] grades 3/4: 34%), hypoproteinemia (≤32%), albumin decreased (≤21%; grade 3: ≤4%)

Gastrointestinal: Nausea (42% to 73%; Ph+ ALL [pediatric] grades 3/4: 16%), diarrhea (25% to 59%; Ph+ ALL [pediatric] grades 3/4: 9%), vomiting (11% to 58%), abdominal pain (3% to 57%), anorexia (≤36%), weight gain (5% to 32%), dyspepsia (11% to 27%), flatulence (≤25%), abdominal distension (≤19%), stomatitis/mucositis (≤10% to 16%), constipation (9% to 16%), taste disturbance (≤13%)

Hematologic: Anemia (25% to 80%; grade 3: 1% to 42%; grade 4: ≤11%), leukopenia (GIST 5% to 47%; grades 3/4: 2%), hemorrhage (3% to 53%; grades 3/4: ≤19%), neutropenia (12% to 16%, grade 3: 7% to 27%; grade 4: 3% to 48%), thrombocytopenia (grade 3: 1% to 31%; grade 4: <1% to 33%)

Hepatic: Transaminases and/or bilirubin increased (Ph+ ALL [pediatric] grades 3/4: 57%), AST increased (≤38%; grade 3: 2% to 5%; grade 4: ≤3%), ALT increased (≤34%; grade 3: 2% to 7%; grade 4: <3%), alkaline phosphatase increased (≤17%; grade 3: ≤6%; grade 4: <1%), bilirubin increased (≤13%; grade 3: 1% to 4%; grade 4: ≤3%)

Neuromuscular & skeletal: Muscle cramps (16% to 62%), arthralgia (≤40%), musculoskeletal pain (children 21%; adults 38% to 49%), myalgia (9% to 32%), joint pain (11% to 31%), weakness (≤21%), rigors (10% to 12%), paresthesia (≤12%), bone pain (≤11%)

Ocular: Periorbital edema (29% to ≤74%), lacrimation increased (DFSP 25%; GIST ≤18%), blurred vision (≤11%)

Renal: Serum creatinine increased (≤44%; grade 3: ≤3%; DFSP: grade 4: 8%)

Respiratory: Nasopharyngitis (1% to 31%), cough (11% to 27%), dyspnea (≤21%), upper respiratory tract infection (3% to 21%), pharyngolaryngeal pain (≤18%), rhinitis (DFSP 17%), pharyngitis (CML 10% to 15%), pneumonia (CML 4% to 13%), sinusitis (4% to 11%)

Miscellaneous: Infection (Ph+ ALL [pediatric] grades 3/4: 53%; GIST ≤28%), night sweats (CML 13% to 17%), flu-like syndrome (1% to 14%), diaphoresis (GIST ≤13%)

1% to 10%:

Cardiovascular: Pleural effusion (Ph+ ALL [pediatric] grades 3/4: 7%), palpitation (≤5%), flushing

Central nervous system: CNS/cerebral hemorrhage (≤9%), depression (≤8%), hypoesthesia

Dermatologic: Photosensitivity reaction (4% to 7%), dry skin (≤7%), erythema

Endocrine & metabolic: Hyperglycemia (≤10%), hypocalcemia (GIST ≤6%)

Gastrointestinal: Appetite decreased (10%), weight loss (≤10%), gastrointestinal hemorrhage (2% to 8%), gastritis, gastroesophageal reflux, xerostomia

Hematologic: Lymphopenia (GIST ≤10%; grades 3/4: 1% to 2%), neutropenic fever, pancytopenia

Neuromuscular & skeletal: Back pain (GIST ≤7%), limb pain (GIST ≤7%), peripheral neuropathy, joint swelling

Ocular: Conjunctivitis (5% to 8%), conjunctival hemorrhage, dry eyes

Respiratory: Hypoxia (9%), pneumonitis (Ph+ ALL [pediatric] grades 3/4: 8%), epistaxis

Available Dosage Forms

Tablet, Oral:

Gleevec: 100 mg, 400 mg

General Dosage Range Dosage adjustment recommended in patients with hepatic or renal impairment, on concomitant therapy, and/or who develop toxicities

Oral:

Children ≥1 year and Adolescents: 340 mg/m^2/day in 1-2 divided doses (maximum: 600 mg daily)

Adults: 100-800 mg daily in 1-2 divided doses

Administration

Oral Should be administered with a meal and a large glass of water; do not crush tablets. In adults, doses ≤600 mg may be given once daily; 800 mg dose should be administered as 400 mg twice daily. Dosing in children may be once or twice daily for CML and once daily for Ph+ ALL. Tablets may be dispersed in water or apple juice (using ~50 mL for 100 mg tablet, ~200 mL for 400 mg tablet); stir until dissolved and administer immediately. For daily dosing ≥800 mg, the 400 mg tablets should be used in order to reduce iron exposure.

Hazardous agent; use appropriate precautions for handling and disposal (NIOSH, 2012).

Storage/Stability Store at 25°C (77°F); excursions permitted between 15°C to 30°C (59°F to 86°F). Protect from moisture.

Nursing Actions

Physical Assessment Much laboratory monitoring required. Monitor weight and fluid status, especially in patients with underlying heart failure or those with risk factors for heart disease. Monitor for hemorrhage, paresthesia, and respiratory or CNS changes. Monitor growth in pediatric patients.

Patient Education

- Discuss specific use of drug and side effects with patient as it relates to treatment. (HCAHPS: During this hospital stay, were you given any medicine that you had not taken before? Before giving you any new medicine, how often did hospital staff tell you what the medicine was for? How often did hospital staff describe possible side effects in a way you could understand?)

- Patient may experience fatigue, dizziness, insomnia, lack of appetite, flatulence, alopecia, nausea, diarrhea, constipation, dysgeusia, rhinitis, pharyngitis, arthralgia, myalgia, muscle cramps, or night sweats. Have patient report immediately to prescriber signs of infection, signs of hepatic impairment, signs of hypokalemia, dyspnea, excessive weight gain, edema of extremities, angina, paresthesia, severe headache, significant dyspepsia, ecchymosis, hemorrhaging, considerable asthenia, melena, hematemesis, vision changes, depression, osteodynia, Stevens-Johnson syndrome/toxic epidermal necrolysis, or tumor lysis syndrome (TLS) (HCAHPS).

- Educate patient about signs of a significant reaction (eg, wheezing; chest tightness; fever; itching; bad cough; blue skin color; seizures; or swelling of face, lips, tongue, or throat). **Note:** This is not a comprehensive list of all side effects. Patient should consult prescriber for additional questions.

Intended Use and Disclaimer: Should not be printed and given to patients. This information is intended to serve as a concise initial reference for healthcare professionals to use when discussing medications with a patient. You must ultimately rely on your own discretion, experience and judgment in diagnosing, treating and advising patients.

Dietary Considerations Should be taken with food and a large glass of water to decrease gastrointestinal irritation. Avoid grapefruit juice.

Related Information

Oral Medications That Should Not Be Crushed or Altered *on page 1712*

Imipenem and Cilastatin
(i mi PEN em & sye la STAT in)

Brand Names: U.S. Primaxin® I.V.

Index Terms Cilastatin and Imipenem; Imipemide; Primaxin I.M. [DSC]

Pharmacologic Category Antibiotic, Carbapenem

Medication Safety Issues

Sound-alike/look-alike issues:

Imipenem may be confused with ertapenem, meropenem

Primaxin® may be confused with Premarin, Primacor

Pregnancy Risk Factor C

Lactation Enters breast milk/use caution

Use Treatment of lower respiratory tract, urinary tract, intra-abdominal, gynecologic, bone and joint, skin and skin structure, endocarditis (caused by *Staphylococcus aureus*) and polymicrobic infections as well as bacterial septicemia. Antibacterial activity includes gram-positive bacteria (methicillin-sensitive *S. aureus* and *Streptococcus* spp), resistant gram-negative bacilli (including extended spectrum beta-lactamase-producing *Escherichia coli* and *Klebsiella* spp, *Enterobacter* spp, and *Pseudomonas aeruginosa*), and anaerobes.

Unlabeled Use Hepatic abscess; neutropenic fever; melioidosis

Available Dosage Forms

Injection, powder for reconstitution: Imipenem 250 mg and cilastatin 250 mg; imipenem 500 mg and cilastatin 500 mg

Primaxin® I.V.: Imipenem 250 mg and cilastatin 250 mg; imipenem 500 mg and cilastatin 500 mg

General Dosage Range Dosage adjustment recommended in patients with renal impairment

I.V.:

Children >3 months: 15-25 mg/kg every 6 hours (maximum: 4 g/day)

Adults 30 to <70 kg: 125 mg every 12 hours up to 1000 mg every 8 hours

Adults ≥70 kg: 250-1000 mg every 6-8 hours (maximum: 50 mg/kg/day; 4 g/day)

Administration

I.V. Do not administer I.V. push. Infuse doses ≤500 mg over 20-30 minutes; infuse doses ≥750 mg over 40-60 minutes.

Injectable Detail Vial contents must be transferred to 100 mL of infusion solution. If nausea and/or vomiting occur during administration, decrease the rate of I.V. infusion. Do not mix with or physically add to other antibiotics; however, may administer concomitantly.

pH: 6.5-8.5 (buffered)

Nursing Actions

Physical Assessment Results of culture and sensitivity tests and patient's allergy history should be assessed prior to beginning therapy. Advise patients with diabetes about use of Clinitest®.

Patient Education

• Discuss specific use of drug and side effects with patient as it relates to treatment. (HCAHPS: During this hospital stay, were you given any medicine that you had not taken before? Before giving you any new medicine, how often did hospital staff tell you what the medicine was for? How often did hospital staff describe possible side effects in a way you could understand?)

• Patient may experience nausea, diarrhea, or vaginal yeast infection. Have patient report immediately to prescriber dizziness, syncope, illogical thinking, asthenia, or rash (HCAHPS).

• Educate patient about signs of a significant reaction (eg, wheezing; chest tightness; fever; itching; bad cough; blue skin color; seizures; or swelling of face, lips, tongue, or throat). **Note:** This is not a comprehensive list of all side effects. Patient should consult prescriber for additional questions.

Intended Use and Disclaimer: Should not be printed and given to patients. This information is intended to serve as a concise initial reference for healthcare professionals to use when discussing medications with a patient. You must ultimately rely on your own discretion, experience and judgment in diagnosing, treating and advising patients.

Imipramine (im IP ra meen)

Brand Names: U.S. Tofranil; Tofranil-PM

Index Terms Imipramine Hydrochloride; Imipramine Pamoate

Pharmacologic Category Antidepressant, Tricyclic (Tertiary Amine)

Medication Safety Issues

Sound-alike/look-alike issues:

Imipramine may be confused with amitriptyline, desipramine, Norpramin®

BEERS Criteria medication:

This drug may be potentially inappropriate for use in geriatric patients (Quality of evidence - high [moderate for SIADH]; Strength of recommendation - strong).

Medication Guide Available Yes

Lactation Enters breast milk/not recommended

Use

Childhood enuresis: As temporary adjunctive therapy in reducing enuresis in children ≥6 years of age, after possible organic causes have been excluded by appropriate tests

Depression: Treatment of depression

Unlabeled Use Analgesic for certain chronic and neuropathic pain (including diabetic neuropathy); panic disorder; attention-deficit/hyperactivity disorder (ADHD); post-traumatic stress disorder (PTSD)

Available Dosage Forms

Capsule, Oral:

Tofranil-PM: 75 mg, 100 mg, 125 mg, 150 mg

Generic: 75 mg, 100 mg, 125 mg, 150 mg

Tablet, Oral:

Tofranil: 10 mg, 25 mg, 50 mg

Generic: 10 mg, 25 mg, 50 mg

General Dosage Range Oral:

Children ≥6-12 years: Initial: 25 mg at bedtime, may increase to 50 mg at bedtime if no response (maximum: 2.5 mg/kg/day; 50 mg daily)

Children >12 years: Initial: 25 mg at bedtime, may increase to 75 mg at bedtime if not response (maximum: 75 mg daily) **or** 30-40 mg daily, increase gradually, to a maximum of 100 mg daily in single or divided doses

Adults: Initial: 75-150 mg daily, increase gradually to a maximum of 200 mg daily (outpatients) or 300 mg daily (inpatients) in divided doses or a single dose at bedtime

Elderly: Initial: 25-50 mg at bedtime (maximum: 100 mg daily)

Nursing Actions

Physical Assessment Monitor orthostatic vital signs, signs of anticholinergic side effects, or overload. Monitor mental status for worsening of mood, confusion, suicidal ideations.

Patient Education

• Discuss specific use of drug and side effects with patient as it relates to treatment. (HCAHPS: During this hospital stay, were you given any medicine that you had not taken before? Before giving you any new medicine, how often did hospital staff tell you what the medicine was for? How often did hospital staff describe possible side effects in a way you could understand?)

• Patient may experience presyncope, fatigue, blurred vision, illogical thinking, dizziness, constipation, or xerostomia. Have patient report immediately to prescriber tachycardia, urinary retention, severe asthenia, nervousness and anxiety, or rash (HCAHPS).

• Educate patient about signs of a significant reaction (eg, wheezing; chest tightness; fever; itching; bad cough; blue skin color; seizures; or swelling of face, lips, tongue, or throat). **Note:** This is not a comprehensive list of all side effects. Patient should consult prescriber for additional questions.

Intended Use and Disclaimer: Should not be printed and given to patients. This information is intended to serve as a concise initial reference for healthcare professionals to use when discussing medications with a patient. You must ultimately rely on your own discretion, experience and

judgment in diagnosing, treating and advising patients.

Imiquimod (i mi KWI mod)

Brand Names: U.S. Aldara; Zyclara; Zyclara Pump

Pharmacologic Category Skin and Mucous Membrane Agent; Topical Skin Product

Medication Safety Issues

Sound-alike/look-alike issues:

Aldara® may be confused with Alora®, Lialda®

Pregnancy Risk Factor C

Lactation Excretion in breast milk unknown/use caution

Use

Aldara®: Treatment of external genital and perianal warts/condyloma acuminata; nonhyperkeratotic, nonhypertrophic actinic keratosis on face or scalp; superficial basal cell carcinoma (sBCC) with a maximum tumor diameter of 2 cm located on the trunk (excluding anogenital skin), neck, or extremities (excluding hands or feet)

Vyloma™ (Canadian availability; not available in the U.S.): Treatment of external genital and perianal warts/condyloma acuminata

Zyclara®:

U.S. labeling: Treatment of external genital and perianal warts/condyloma acuminata (3.75% formulation); treatment of clinically typical visible or palpable, actinic keratoses on face or scalp (2.5% or 3.75% formulation)

Canadian labeling: Treatment of clinically typical visible or palpable, actinic keratoses on face or scalp

Unlabeled Use Treatment of common warts

Available Dosage Forms

Cream, External:

Aldara: 5% (12 ea)

Zyclara: 3.75% (28 ea)

Zyclara Pump: 2.5% (7.5 g); 3.75% (7.5 g)

Generic: 5% (1 ea, 12 ea, 24 ea)

General Dosage Range Topical:

Children ≥12 years: Apply a thin layer 3 times/week on alternate days, leave on for 6-10 hours

Adults:

Actinic keratosis: Apply twice weekly or once daily at bedtime for 2 treatment cycles (14 days each) separated by a 14-day rest period with no treatment; leave on for ~8 hours

External genital and/or perianal warts/condyloma acuminata: Apply a thin layer 3 times/week on alternate days; leave on for 6-10 hours

Superficial basal cell carcinoma: Apply once daily at bedtime 5 days/week; leave on for 8 hours before washing

Administration

Topical Topical: For all products, wash hands prior to and following application. Zyclara® pump should be primed prior to first use only by pressing top of pump completely down repeatedly until

cream appears; discard cream obtained during priming. No further priming is required throughout therapy. Zyclara® pump should be discarded after a full course of therapy has been completed. Partially used packets of imiquimod cream should be discarded and not reused. Do not occlude the application site.

Actinic keratosis: The treatment area should be washed and thoroughly dried prior to application. Apply Aldara® over a single contiguous area (approximately 25 cm^2) on the face or scalp or Zyclara® over an area <200 cm^2 on the face or scalp. Both areas should not be treated concurrently. Apply a thin layer to the affected area and rub in until the cream is no longer visible. Avoid contact with the eyes, lips, and nostrils.

External genital warts: Instruct patients to apply to external or perianal warts; not for vaginal use. Apply a thin layer to the wart area and rub in until the cream is no longer visible. Avoid use of excessive amounts of cream. Nonocclusive dressings (such as cotton gauze or cotton underwear) may be used in the management of skin reactions.

Superficial basal cell carcinoma: Aldara®: Treatment area should have a maximum diameter no more than 2 cm on the trunk, neck, or extremities (excluding the hands, feet, and anogenital skin). Treatment area should include a 1 cm margin around the tumor. Wash and thoroughly dry treatment area prior to application; apply a thin layer to the affected area (and margin) and rub in until the cream is no longer visible. Avoid contact with the eyes, lips, and nostrils.

Nursing Actions

Patient Education

- Discuss specific use of drug and side effects with patient as it relates to treatment. (HCAHPS: During this hospital stay, were you given any medicine that you had not taken before? Before giving you any new medicine, how often did hospital staff tell you what the medicine was for? How often did hospital staff describe possible side effects in a way you could understand?)
- Patient may experience skin irritation, scleroderma, change in skin color, or edema. Have patient report immediately to prescriber rash (HCAHPS).
- Educate patient about signs of a significant reaction (eg, wheezing; chest tightness; fever; itching; bad cough; blue skin color; seizures; or swelling of face, lips, tongue, or throat). **Note:** This is not a comprehensive list of all side effects. Patient should consult prescriber for additional questions.

Intended Use and Disclaimer: Should not be printed and given to patients. This information is intended to serve as a concise initial reference for healthcare professionals to use when discussing medications with a patient. You must ultimately

◄ rely on your own discretion, experience and judgment in diagnosing, treating and advising patients.

Immune Globulin (i MYUN GLOB yoo lin)

Brand Names: U.S. Bivigam; Carimune NF; Flebogamma; Flebogamma DIF; GamaSTAN S/D; Gammagard; Gammagard S/D; Gammagard S/D Less IgA; Gammaked; Gammaplex; Gamunex-C; Hizentra; Hizentra 20%; Octagam; Privigen

Index Terms Gamma Globulin; IG; IGIM; IGIV; IGSC; Immune Globulin Subcutaneous (Human); Immune Serum Globulin; ISG; IV Immune Globulin; IVIG; Panglobulin; SCIG

Pharmacologic Category Blood Product Derivative; Immune Globulin

Medication Safety Issues

Sound-alike/look-alike issues:

Gamimune N may be confused with CytoGam

Immune globulin (intravenous) may be confused with hepatitis B immune globulin

Pregnancy Risk Factor C

Lactation Excretion in breast milk unknown/use caution

Breast-Feeding Considerations It is not known if immune globulin from these preparations is excreted in breast milk. The manufacturer recomends that caution be exercised when administering immune globulin to nursing women.

Use

Treatment of primary humoral immunodeficiency syndromes (congenital agammaglobulinemia, severe combined immunodeficiency syndromes [SCIDS], common variable immunodeficiency, X-linked immunodeficiency, Wiskott-Aldrich syndrome) (Bivigam, Carimune NF, Flebogamma DIF, Gammagard Liquid, Gammagard S/D, Gammaked, Gammaplex, Gamunex-C, Hizentra, Octagam, Privigen)

Treatment of acute and chronic immune thrombocytopenia (ITP) (Carimune NF, Gammagard S/D, Gammaked, Gammaplex [chronic only], Gamunex-C, Privigen [chronic only])

Treatment of chronic inflammatory demyelinating polyneuropathy (CIDP) (Gammaked, Gamunex-C)

Treatment of multifocal motor neuropathy (MMN) (Gammagard Liquid)

Prevention of coronary artery aneurysms associated with Kawasaki syndrome (in combination with aspirin) (Gammagard S/D)

Prevention of bacterial infection in patients with hypogammaglobulinemia and/or recurrent bacterial infections with B-cell chronic lymphocytic leukemia (CLL) (Gammagard S/D)

Prevention of serious infection in immunoglobulin deficiency (select agammaglobulinemias) (GamaSTAN S/D)

Provision of passive immunity in the following susceptible individuals (GamaSTAN S/D):

Hepatitis A: Pre-exposure prophylaxis; postexposure: within 14 days and/or prior to manifestation of disease

Measles: For use within 6 days of exposure in an unvaccinated person, who has not previously had measles

Rubella: Postexposure prophylaxis to reduce the risk of infection and fetal damage in exposed pregnant women who will not consider therapeutic abortion

Varicella: For immunosuppressed patients when varicella zoster immune globulin is not available

Unlabeled Use Acquired hypogammaglobulinemia secondary to malignancy; Guillain-Barré syndrome; hematopoietic stem cell transplantation (HSCT), to prevent bacterial infections among allogeneic recipients with severe hypogammaglobulinemia (IgG <400 mg/dL) at <100 days post transplant (CDC guidelines); HIV-associated thrombocytopenia; multiple sclerosis (relapsing, remitting when other therapies cannot be used); Lambert-Eaton myasthenic syndrome (LEMS); myasthenia gravis; refractory dermatomyositis/polymyositis

Mechanism of Action/Effect Replacement therapy for primary and secondary immunodeficiencies, and IgG antibodies against bacteria, viral, parasitic and mycoplasma antigens; interference with F_c receptors on the cells of the reticuloendothelial system for autoimmune cytopenias and ITP; provides passive immunity by increasing the antibody titer and antigen-antibody reaction potential

Contraindications Hypersensitivity to immune globulin or any component of the formulation; IgA deficiency (with antibodies against IgA and history of hypersensitivity); hyperprolinemia (Hizentra, Privigen); isolated IgA deficiency (GamaSTAN S/D); severe thrombocytopenia or coagulation disorders where I.M. injections are contraindicated (GamaSTAN S/D)

Warnings/Precautions [U.S. Boxed Warning]: I.V. administration only: Acute renal dysfunction (increased serum creatinine, oliguria, acute renal failure, osmotic nephrosis) can rarely occur and has been associated with fatalities; usually within 7 days of use (more likely with products stabilized with sucrose). Use with caution in the elderly, patients with renal disease, diabetes mellitus, volume depletion, sepsis, paraproteinemia, and nephrotoxic medications due to risk of renal dysfunction. In patients at risk of renal dysfunction, the rate of infusion and concentration of solution should be minimized. Discontinue if renal function deteriorates.

[U.S. Boxed Warning]: Thrombosis may occur with immune globulin products even in the absence of risk factors for thrombosis. For

patients at risk of thrombosis (eg, advanced age, history of atherosclerosis, impaired cardiac output, prolonged immobilization, hypercoagulable conditions, history of venous or arterial thrombosis, use of estrogens, indwelling central vascular catheters, hyperviscosity, and cardiovascular risk factors), administer at the minimum dose and infusion rate practicable. Ensure adequate hydration before administration. Monitor for signs and symptoms of thrombosis and assess blood viscosity in patients at risk for hyperviscosity such as those with cryoglobulins, fasting chylomicronemia/severe hypertriglyceridemia, or monoclonal gammopathies.

High-dose regimens (1 g/kg for 1-2 days) are not recommended for individuals with fluid overload or where fluid volume may be of concern. Hypersensitivity and anaphylactic reactions can occur; a severe fall in blood pressure may rarely occur with anaphylactic reaction; immediate treatment (including epinephrine 1:1000) should be available. Product of human plasma; may potentially contain infectious agents which could transmit disease. Screening of donors, as well as testing and/or inactivation or removal of certain viruses, reduces the risk. Infections thought to be transmitted by this product should be reported to the manufacturer. Aseptic meningitis may occur with high doses (≥1-2 g/kg [product-dependent]) and/or rapid infusion; syndrome usually appears within several hours to 2 days following treatment; usually resolves within several days after product is discontinued; patients with a migraine history may be at higher risk for AMS. Increased risk of hypersensitivity, especially in patients with anti-IgA antibodies; use is contraindicated in patients with IgA deficiency (with antibodies against IgA and history of hypersensitivity) or isolated IgA deficiency (GamaSTAN S/D). Increased risk of hematoma formation when administered subcutaneously for the treatment of ITP.

Intravenous immune globulin has been associated with antiglobulin hemolysis (acute or delayed); monitor for signs of hemolytic anemia. Cases of hemolysis-related renal dysfunction/failure or disseminated intravascular coagulation (DIC) have been reported. Risk factors include high doses (≥2 g/kg) and non-O blood type. In chronic ITP, assess risk versus benefit of high-dose regimen in patients with increased risk of thrombosis, hemolysis, acute kidney injury, or volume overload.

Patients should be adequately hydrated prior to initiation of therapy. Hyperproteinemia, increased serum viscosity and hyponatremia may occur; distinguish hyponatremia from pseudohyponatremia to prevent volume depletion, a further increase in serum viscosity, and a higher risk of thrombotic events. Patients should be monitored for adverse events during and after the infusion. Stop administration with signs of infusion reaction (fever, chills, nausea, vomiting, and rarely shock). Risk may be increased with initial treatment, when switching brands of immune globulin, and with treatment interruptions of >8 weeks. Monitor for transfusion-related acute lung injury (TRALI); non-cardiogenic pulmonary edema has been reported with immune globulin use. TRALI is characterized by severe respiratory distress, pulmonary edema, hypoxemia, and fever (in the presence of normal left ventricular function) and usually occurs within 1-6 hours after infusion. Response to live vaccinations may be impaired. Some clinicians may administer intravenous immune globulin products as a subcutaneous infusion based on patient tolerability and clinical judgment. SubQ infusion should begin 1 week after the last I.V. dose; dose should be individualized based on clinical response and serum IgG trough concentrations; consider premedicating with acetaminophen and diphenhydramine.

Some products may contain maltose, which may result in falsely-elevated blood glucose readings; maltose-containing products are contraindicated in patients with an allergy to corn. Some products may contain polysorbate 80, sodium, and/or sucrose. Some products may contain sorbitol; do not use in patients with fructose intolerance. Hizentra and Privigen contain the stabilizer L-proline and are contraindicated in patients with hyperprolinemia. Packaging of some products may contain natural latex/natural rubber; skin testing should not be performed with GamaSTAN S/D as local irritation can occur and be misinterpreted as a positive reaction.

Drug Interactions

Avoid Concomitant Use There are no known interactions where it is recommended to avoid concomitant use.

Decreased Effect

Immune Globulin may decrease the levels/effects of: Vaccines (Live)

Increased Effect/Toxicity There are no known significant interactions involving an increase in effect.

Adverse Reactions Frequency not always defined.

Cardiovascular: Chest tightness (7%), hypertension (5% to 6%), angioedema, edema, flushing of the face, hypotension, palpitation, tachycardia

Central nervous system: Headache (16% to 48%), fever (6% to 16%), chills (3% to 6%), dizziness (1% to 6%), malaise (1%), anxiety, aseptic meningitis syndrome, drowsiness, fatigue, irritability, lethargy, lightheadedness, migraine, pain

Dermatologic: Bruising, contact dermatitis, eczema, erythema, hyperhidrosis, petechiae, pruritus, purpura, rash, urticaria

Endocrine & metabolic: Hyperglycemia (neuromuscular disease: 1%) dehydration

Gastrointestinal: Nausea (3% to 18%), anorexia (neuromuscular disease: 1%), abdominal cramps, abdominal pain, diarrhea, discomfort, dyspepsia, gastroenteritis, sore throat, toothache, vomiting

Hematologic: Anemia, autoimmune hemolytic anemia, hematocrit decreased, hematoma, hemolysis (mild), hemorrhage, thrombocytopenia

Hepatic: Bilirubin increased, LDH increased, liver function test increased

Local: Muscle stiffness at I.M. site; pain, swelling, redness or irritation at the infusion site

Neuromuscular & skeletal: Muscle spasm (MMN 7%), weakness (1%; MMN: 7%), arthralgia (1%), back or hip pain, leg cramps, muscle cramps, myalgia, neck pain, rigors

Ocular: Conjunctivitis

Otic: Ear pain

Renal: Acute renal failure, acute tubular necrosis, anuria, BUN increased, creatinine increased, oliguria, proximal tubular nephropathy, osmotic nephrosis

Respiratory: Oropharyngeal pain (7%), asthma aggravated, bronchitis, cough, dyspnea, epistaxis, nasal congestion, pharyngeal pain, pharyngitis, rhinitis, rhinorrhea, sinus headache, sinusitis, upper respiratory infection, wheezing

Miscellaneous: Anaphylaxis, diaphoresis, flu-like syndrome, hypersensitivity reactions, infusion reaction, thermal burn

Pharmacodynamics/Kinetics

Onset of Action I.V.: Provides immediate antibody levels

Duration of Action I.M., I.V.: Immune effects: 3-4 weeks (variable)

Available Dosage Forms

Injectable, Intramuscular [preservative free]:
GamaSTAN S/D: 15% to 18% [150 to 180 mg/mL] (2 mL, 10 mL)

Solution, Injection:
Gamunex-C: 1 g/10 mL (10 mL); 2.5 g/25 mL (25 mL); 5 g/50 mL (50 mL); 10 g/100 mL (100 mL); 20 g/200 mL (200 mL)

Solution, Injection [preservative free]:
Gammagard: 1 g/10 mL (10 mL); 2.5 g/25 mL (25 mL); 5 g/50 mL (50 mL); 10 g/100 mL (100 mL); 20 g/200 mL (200 mL); 30 g/300 mL (300 mL)
Gammaked: 1 g/10 mL (10 mL); 2.5 g/25 mL (25 mL); 5 g/50 mL (50 mL); 10 g/100 mL (100 mL); 20 g/200 mL (200 mL)

Solution, Intravenous:
Flebogamma: 0.5 g/10 mL (10 mL)
Flebogamma DIF: 0.5 g/10 mL (10 mL); 2.5 g/50 mL (50 mL); 5 g/50 mL (50 mL); 5 g/100 mL (100 mL); 10 g/100 mL (100 mL); 10 g/200 mL (200 mL); 20 g/200 mL (200 mL); 20 g/400 mL (400 mL)
Octagam: 1 g/20 mL (20 mL); 2.5 g/50 mL (50 mL); 5 g/100 mL (100 mL); 10 g/200 mL (200 mL); 25 g/500 mL (500 mL)

Solution, Intravenous [preservative free]:
Bivigam: 5 g/50 mL (50 mL); 10 g/100 mL (100 mL)
Gammaplex: 2.5 g/50 mL (50 mL); 5 g/100 mL (100 mL); 10 g/200 mL (200 mL)
Privigen: 5 g/50 mL (50 mL); 10 g/100 mL (100 mL); 20 g/200 mL (200 mL); 40 g/400 mL (400 mL)

Solution, Subcutaneous [preservative free]:
Hizentra 20%: 1 g/5 mL (5 mL); 2 g/10 mL (10 mL); 4 g/20 mL (20 mL); 10 g/50 mL (50 mL)

Solution Reconstituted, Intravenous:
Carimune NF: 3 g (1 ea); 6 g (1 ea); 12 g (1 ea)
Gammagard S/D: 2.5 g (1 ea); 5 g (1 ea); 10 g (1 ea)

Solution Reconstituted, Intravenous [preservative free]:
Gammagard S/D Less IgA: 5 g (1 ea); 10 g (1 ea)

General Dosage Range

I.M.: *Children and Adults:*

Hepatitis A:
Pre-exposure prophylaxis upon travel into endemic areas:
0.02 **mL**/kg for anticipated risk of exposure <3 months
0.06 **mL**/kg for anticipated risk of exposure ≥3 months
Postexposure prophylaxis: 0.02 **mL**/kg

Measles:
Postexposure, immunocompetent: 0.25 **mL**/kg
Postexposure, immunocompromised: 0.5 **mL**/kg (maximum dose: 15 **mL**)

Rubella: Prophylaxis during pregnancy: 0.55 **mL**/kg

Varicella: Prophylaxis: 0.6-1.2 **mL**/kg

Immune globulin deficiency: 0.66 **mL**/kg; administer a double dose at onset of therapy

I.V.:

Children and Adults:

B-cell chronic lymphocytic leukemia (CLL): 400 mg/kg

Chronic inflammatory demyelinating polyneuropathy (CIDP): Loading dose: 2000 mg/kg; Maintenance: 500-1000 mg/kg

Immune thrombocytopenia (ITP): Dosage varies greatly depending on product

Kawasaki syndrome: 400-2000 mg/kg

Measles: >400 mg/kg

Primary humoral immunodeficiency disorders: 200-800 mg/kg

Adults: Multifocal motor neuropathy (MMN): 500-2400 mg/kg/month

SubQ: *Children and Adults:*

Measles: ≥200-≥400 mg/kg

Primary humoral immunodeficiency disorders: Dosage varies greatly depending on product

Administration

I.M. Note: If plasmapheresis employed for treatment of condition, administer immune globulin **after** completion of plasmapheresis session.

Administer I.M. in the anterolateral aspects of the upper thigh or deltoid muscle of the upper arm. Avoid gluteal region due to risk of injury to sciatic nerve. Divide doses >10 mL and inject in multiple sites. GamaSTAN S/D is for I.M. administration only.

I.V. **Note:** If plasmapheresis employed for treatment of condition, administer immune globulin **after** completion of plasmapheresis session.

Infuse over 2-24 hours; administer in separate infusion line from other medications; if using primary line, flush with NS or D₅W (product specific; consult product prescribing information) prior to administration. Decrease dose, rate and/or concentration of infusion in patients who may be at risk of renal failure. Decreasing the rate or stopping the infusion may help relieve some adverse effects (flushing, changes in pulse rate, changes in blood pressure). Epinephrine should be available during administration.

For initial treatment or in the elderly, a lower concentration and/or a slower rate of infusion should be used. Initial rate of administration and titration is specific to each IVIG product. Refrigerated product should be warmed to room temperature prior to infusion. Some products require filtration; refer to individual product labeling. Antecubital veins should be used, especially with concentrations ≥10% to prevent injection site discomfort.

Bivigam 10%: Primary humoral immunodeficiency: Initial (first 10 minutes): 0.5 mg/kg/minute (0.3 **mL**/kg/**hour**); Maintenance: Increase every 20 minutes (if tolerated) by 0.8 mg/kg/minute (0.48 **mL**/kg/**hour**) up to 6 mg/kg/minute (3.6 **mL**/kg/**hour**)

Carimune NF: Refer to product labeling.

Flebogamma DIF 10%: Primary humoral immunodeficiency: Initial: 1 mg/kg/minute (0.6 **mL**/kg/**hour**); Maintenance: Increase slowly (if tolerated) up to 8 mg/kg/minute (4.8 **mL**/kg/**hour**)

Gammagard Liquid 10%:
Multifocal motor neuropathy (MMN): Initial: 0.8 mg/kg/minute (0.5 **mL**/kg/**hour**); Maintenance: Increase gradually (if tolerated) up to 9 mg/kg/minute (5.4 **mL**/kg/**hour**)
Primary humoral immunodeficiency: Initial (first 30 minutes): 0.8 mg/kg/minute (0.5 **mL**/kg/**hour**); Maintenance: Increase every 30 minutes (if tolerated) up to: 8 mg/kg/minute (5 **mL**/kg/**hour**)

Gammagard S/D: 5% solution: Initial: 0.5 **mL**/kg/**hour**; may increase (if tolerated) to a maximum rate of 4 **mL**/kg/**hour**. If 5% solution is tolerated at maximum rate, may administer 10% solution with an initial rate of 0.5 **mL**/kg/**hour**; may increase (if tolerated) to a maximum rate of 8 **mL**/kg/**hour**

Gammaked 10%:
CIDP: Initial (first 30 minutes): 2 mg/kg/minute (1.2 **mL**/kg/**hour**); Maintenance: Increase

gradually (if tolerated) up to 8 mg/kg/minute (**4.8 mL/kg/hour**)
Primary humoral immunodeficiency or ITP: Initial (first 30 minutes): 1 mg/kg/minute (0.6 **mL**/kg/**hour**); Maintenance: Increase gradually (if tolerated) up to 8 mg/kg/minute (4.8 **mL**/kg/**hour**)

Gammaplex 5%: Primary humoral immunodeficiency or ITP: Initial (first 15 minutes): 0.5 mg/kg/minute (0.6 **mL**/kg/**hour**); Maintenance: Increase every 15 minutes (if tolerated) up to 4 mg/kg/minute (4.8 **mL**/kg/**hour**)

Gamunex-C 10%:
CIDP: Initial (first 30 minutes): 2 mg/kg/minute (1.2 **mL**/kg/**hour**); Maintenance: Increase gradually (if tolerated) up to 8 mg/kg/minute (**4.8 mL**/kg/**hour**)
Primary humoral immunodeficiency or ITP: Initial (first 30 minutes): 1 mg/kg/minute (0.6 **mL**/kg/**hour**); Maintenance: Increase gradually (if tolerated) up to 8 mg/kg/minute (4.8 **mL**/kg/**hour**)

Octagam 5%: Primary humoral immunodeficiency: Initial (first 30 minutes): 0.5 mg/kg/minute (0.6 **mL**/kg/**hour**); Maintenance: Double infusion rate (if tolerated) every 30 minutes up to a maximum rate of <3.33 mg/kg/minute (4.2 **mL**/kg/**hour**)

Privigen 10%
ITP: Initial: 0.5 mg/kg/minute (0.3 **mL**/kg/**hour**); Maintenance: Increase gradually (if tolerated) up to 4 mg/kg/minute (2.4 **mL**/kg/**hour**)
Primary humoral immunodeficiency: Initial: 0.5 mg/kg/minute (0.3 **mL**/kg/**hour**); Maintenance: Increase gradually (if tolerated) up to 8 mg/kg/minute (4.8 **mL**/kg/**hour**)

Injectable Detail
Bivigam: pH 4-4.6
Carimune NF: pH 6.4-6.8
Flebogamma DIF: pH 5-6
GamaSTAN S/D: pH 6.4-7.2
Gammagard Liquid: pH 4.6-5.1
Gammagard S/D 5%: pH 6.4-7.2
Gammaked: pH 4-4.5
Gammaplex: pH 4.8-5.1
Gamunex-C: pH 4-4.5
Hizentra: pH: 4.6-5.2
Octagam: pH 5.1-6
Privigen: pH 4.6-5

Subcutaneous SubQ infusion: Initial dose should be administered in a healthcare setting capable of providing monitoring and treatment in the event of hypersensitivity. Using aseptic technique, follow the infusion device manufacturer's instructions for filling the reservoir and preparing the pump. Remove air from administration set and needle by priming. Appropriate injection sites include the abdomen, thigh, upper arm, lower back, and/or lateral hip; dose may be infused into multiple sites (spaced ≥2 inches apart) simultaneously. After the sites are clean and dry, insert subcutaneous needle and prime administration set. Attach sterile needle to administration set, gently pull back on the syringe to assure a blood vessel has not been inadvertently accessed (do not use needle and tubing if blood present). Repeat for each injection site; deliver the dose following instructions for the infusion device. Rotate the site(s) weekly. Treatment may be transitioned to the home/home care setting in the absence of adverse reactions.

Gammagard Liquid:
Injection sites: ≤8 simultaneous injection sites
Initial infusion rate:
<40 kg: 15 mL/hour per injection site (maximum volume: 20 mL per injection site)
≥40 kg: 20 mL/hour per injection site (maximum volume: 30 mL per injection site)
Maintenance infusion rate:
<40 kg: 15-20 mL/hour per injection site (maximum volume: 20 mL per injection site)
≥40 kg: 20-30 mL/hour per injection site (maximum volume: 30 mL per injection site)
Gammaked, Gamunex-C:
Injection sites: ≤8 simultaneous injection sites
Recommended infusion rate: 20 mL/hour per injection site
Hizentra:
Weekly dosing: Injection sites: ≤4 simultaneous injection sites or ≤12 sites consecutively per infusion.
Biweekly dosing: Increase the number of injection sites as needed.
Maximum infusion rate: First infusion: 15 mL/hour per injection site; subsequent infusions: 25 mL/hour per injection site
Maximum infusion volume: First 4 infusions: 15 mL per injection site; subsequent infusions: 20 mL per injection site (maximum: 25 mL per site as tolerated)

Preparation for Administration Dilution is dependent upon the manufacturer and brand. Gently swirl; do not shake; avoid foaming. Do not heat. Do not mix products from different manufacturers together. Discard unused portion of vials.

Bivigam: Dilution is not recommended.
Carimune NF: In a sterile laminar air flow environment, reconstitute with NS, D_5W, or SWFI. Complete dissolution may take up to 20 minutes. Begin infusion within 24 hours.
Flebogamma DIF: Dilution is not recommended.
Gammagard Liquid: May dilute in D_5W only.
Gammagard S/D: Reconstitute with SWFI.
Gammaked: May dilute in D_5W only.
Gamunex-C: May dilute in D_5W only.
Privigen: If necessary to further dilute, D_5W may be used.

Storage/Stability Stability is dependent upon the manufacturer and brand. Do not freeze (do not use if previously frozen). Do not shake. Do not heat (do not use if previously heated).

Bivigam: Store under refrigeration at 2°C to 8°C (36°F to 46°F). Dilution is not recommended.
Carimune NF: Prior to reconstitution, store at or below 30°C (86°F). Reconstitute with NS, D_5W, or SWFI. Following reconstitution in a sterile laminar air flow environment, store under refrigeration. Begin infusion within 24 hours.
Flebogamma DIF: Store at 2°C to 25°C (36°F to 77°F).
GamaSTAN S/D: Store under refrigeration at 2°C to 8°C (36°F to 46°F). The following stability information has also been reported for GamaSTAN S/D: May be exposed to room temperature for a cumulative 7 days (Cohen, 2007).
Gammagard Liquid: Prior to use, store at 2°C to 8°C (36°F to 46°F). May store at room temperature of 25°C (77°F) within the first 24 months of manufacturing. Storage time at room temperature varies with length of time previously refrigerated; refer to product labeling for details.
Gammagard S/D: Store at ≤25°C (≤77°F). May store diluted solution under refrigeration at 2°C to 8°C (36°F to 46°F) for up to 24 hours if originally prepared in a sterile laminar air flow environment.
Gammaked: Store at 2°C to 8°C (36°F to 46°F); may be stored at ≤25°C (≤77°F) for up to 6 months.
Gammaplex: Store at 2°C to 25°C (36°F to 77°F). Protect from light.
Gamunex-C: Store at 2°C to 8°C (36°F to 46°F); may be stored at ≤25°C (≤77°F) for up to 6 months.
Hizentra: Store at ≤25°C (≤77°F). Keep in original carton to protect from light.
Octagam: Store at 2°C to 25°C (36°F to 77°F).
Privigen: Store at ≤25°C (≤77°F). Protect from light.

Nursing Actions

Physical Assessment Monitor vital signs during infusion or injection and observe for adverse or allergic reactions. Hypersensitivity and anaphylaxis can occur. Monitor rate of infusion for those with pre-existing renal dysfunction, diabetes mellitus, or volume depletion.

Instruct patient to avoid receiving live vaccines (eg, some flu shots, smallpox immunizations, measles-mumps-rubella vaccine, varicella and zoster vaccines). Instruct patient to report signs of decreased urination, jaundice, sudden weight gain, or shortness of breath.

Patient Education

• Discuss specific use of vaccine and side effects with patient as it relates to treatment. (HCAHPS: During this hospital stay, were you given any medicine that you had not taken before? Before giving you any new medicine, how often did hospital staff tell you what the medicine was for? How often did hospital staff describe possible side effects in a way you could understand?)

• Patient may experience application site irritation, dyspepsia, emesis, headache, diarrhea, asthenia, back pain, pharyngitis, or hypertension. Have patient report immediately to prescriber dyspnea; angina; significant weight gain; swelling, warmth, or painful extremities; sudden changes in vision, eye pain, or irritation; inability to urinate; or discolored urine, skin, or eyes (HCAHPS).

• Educate patient about signs of a significant reaction (eg, wheezing; chest tightness; fever; itching; bad cough; blue skin color; seizures; or swelling of face, lips, tongue, or throat). **Note:** This is not a comprehensive list of all side effects. Patient should consult prescriber for additional questions.

Intended Use and Disclaimer: Should not be printed and given to patients. This information is intended to serve as a concise initial reference for healthcare professionals to use when discussing medications with a patient. You must ultimately rely on your own discretion, experience and judgment in diagnosing, treating and advising patients.

Dietary Considerations Some products may contain sodium.

Related Information
Immunization Administration Recommendations *on page 1675*
Immunization Recommendations *on page 1680*

Indacaterol (in da KA ter ol)

Brand Names: U.S. Arcapta Neohaler
Index Terms Indacaterol Maleate; QAB149
Pharmacologic Category Beta$_2$ Agonist; Beta$_2$-Adrenergic Agonist, Long-Acting
Medication Guide Available Yes
Pregnancy Risk Factor C
Lactation Excretion unknown/use caution
Breast-Feeding Considerations It is not known if indacaterol is excreted into breast milk. The manufacturer recommends that caution be exercised when administering indacaterol to nursing women. The use of beta$_2$-receptor agonists are not considered a contraindication to breast-feeding (NAEPP, 2005).
Use Long-term maintenance treatment of airflow obstruction in chronic obstructive pulmonary disease (COPD) including chronic bronchitis and/or emphysema
Mechanism of Action/Effect Relaxes bronchial smooth muscle by selective action on beta$_2$-receptors with little effect on heart rate; acts locally in the lung.
Contraindications Hypersensitivity to indacaterol or any component of the formulation; monotherapy in the treatment of asthma (ie, use without a concomitant long-term asthma control medication,

such as an inhaled corticosteroid). **Note:** Indacaterol is not FDA approved for treatment of asthma.
Warnings/Precautions Asthma-related deaths: **[U.S. Boxed Warning]: Long-acting beta$_2$-agonists (LABAs) increase the risk of asthma-related deaths. Indacaterol is not indicated for treatment of asthma and should not be used.** In a large, randomized, placebo-controlled U.S. clinical trial (SMART, 2006), salmeterol was associated with an increase in asthma-related deaths (when added to usual asthma therapy); risk is considered a class effect among all LABAs. It is unknown if indacaterol increases asthma-related deaths. Do not use for acutely deteriorating COPD or as rescue therapy in acute episodes. Short-acting beta$_2$-agonists (eg, albuterol) should be used for acute symptoms and symptoms occurring between treatments. If deterioration develops, prompt evaluation of the COPD regimen is warranted. Do not increase the dose or frequency of indacaterol. Data are not available to determine if LABA use increases the risk of death in patients with COPD. Do not use more than once daily or at a higher dose than indicated; do not combine use with other long-acting beta$_2$-agonists. Deaths and significant cardiovascular effects have been reported with excessive sympathomimetic use. Rarely, paradoxical bronchospasm may occur with use of inhaled bronchodilators; this should be distinguished from inadequate response. Hypersensitivity reactions may occur; discontinue therapy if patient develops an allergic reaction.

Use caution in patients with cardiovascular disease (eg, arrhythmias, coronary insufficiency, hypertension), diabetes mellitus, hyperthyroidism, seizure disorders, or hypokalemia. Beta-agonists may cause elevation in blood pressure, heart rate, CNS stimulation/excitation, increased risk of arrhythmia, increase serum glucose, or decrease serum potassium.

Drug Interactions

Avoid Concomitant Use
Avoid concomitant use of Indacaterol with any of the following: Beta-Blockers (Nonselective); Highest Risk QTc-Prolonging Agents; Iobenguane I 123; Ivabradine; Long-Acting Beta2-Agonists; Mifepristone

Decreased Effect
Indacaterol may decrease the levels/effects of: Iobenguane I 123

The levels/effects of Indacaterol may be decreased by: Beta-Blockers (Beta1 Selective); Beta-Blockers (Nonselective); Betahistine; Peginterferon Alfa-2b

Increased Effect/Toxicity

Indacaterol may increase the levels/effects of: Atosiban; Corticosteroids (Systemic); Highest Risk QTc-Prolonging Agents; Long-Acting Beta2-Agonists; Loop Diuretics; Moderate Risk QTc-Prolonging Agents; Sympathomimetics; Thiazide Diuretics

The levels/effects of Indacaterol may be increased by: AtoMOXetine; Caffeine; Cannabinoids; Ivabradine; MAO Inhibitors; Mifepristone; QTc-Prolonging Agents (Indeterminate Risk and Risk Modifying; Theophylline Derivatives; Tricyclic Antidepressants

Adverse Reactions

>10%: Respiratory: Cough (post inhalation 7% to 24%)

1% to 10%:

Central nervous system: Headache (5%)

Gastrointestinal: Nausea (2%)

Respiratory: Nasopharyngitis (5%), oropharyngeal pain (2%)

Pharmacodynamics/Kinetics

Onset of Action 5 minutes; Peak effect: 1-4 hours

Duration of Action 24 hours

Available Dosage Forms

Capsule, Inhalation:

Arcapta Neohaler: 75 mcg

General Dosage Range Inhalation: *Adults:* One inhalation once daily

Administration

Inhalation For inhalation using Neohaler™ inhaler (U.S.) or Onbrez® Breezhaler® (Canada) only. Do **not** swallow indacaterol capsules. Use the new inhaler included with each prescription. Do not remove capsules from blister until immediately before use. Use at the same time each day. Not to be used for the relief of acute attacks. Not for use with a spacer device. Do not wash mouthpiece; inhalation device should be kept dry. Discard any capsules that are exposed to air and not used immediately.

Storage/Stability Store capsules at controlled room temperature of 25°C (77°F); excursions permitted to 15°C to 30°C (59°F to 86°F). Protect from direct sunlight and moisture. Remove from blister pack immediately before use; discard capsule if not used immediately.

Nursing Actions

Physical Assessment Monitor pulmonary function tests regularly. Instruct patient to expect a mild cough up to 15 seconds after use. Report immediately hives; difficulty breathing; wheezing; swelling of the face, lips, tongue, or throat; or development of chest pain. Other symptoms to report include tremors or lower extremity swelling. Monitor blood sugars and electrolytes. Instruct patient to monitor for symptoms of hyperglycemia.

Patient Education

• Discuss specific use of drug and side effects with patient as it relates to treatment. (HCAHPS: During this hospital stay, were you given any medicine that you had not taken before? Before giving you any new medicine, how often did hospital staff tell you what the medicine was for? How often did hospital staff describe possible side effects in a way you could understand?)

• Patient may experience headache, dyspepsia, rhinorrhea, or pharyngitis. Have patient report immediately to prescriber uncontrollable breathing attack, frequent use of inhaler, angina, tachycardia, dyspnea, nervousness and anxiety, severe asthenia, polyuria, polydipsia, weight loss, or rash (HCAHPS).

• Educate patient about signs of a significant reaction (eg, wheezing; chest tightness; fever; itching; bad cough; blue skin color; seizures; or swelling of face, lips, tongue, or throat). **Note:** This is not a comprehensive list of all side effects. Patient should consult prescriber for additional questions.

Intended Use and Disclaimer: Should not be printed and given to patients. This information is intended to serve as a concise initial reference for healthcare professionals to use when discussing medications with a patient. You must ultimately rely on your own discretion, experience and judgment in diagnosing, treating and advising patients.

Indapamide (in DAP a mide)

Pharmacologic Category Antihypertensive; Diuretic, Thiazide-Related

Medication Safety Issues

Sound-alike/look-alike issues:

Indapamide may be confused with Iopidine

International issues:

Pretanix [Hungary] may be confused with Protonix brand name for pantoprazole [U.S., Canada]

Pregnancy Risk Factor B

Lactation Excretion in breast milk unknown/not recommended

Use Management of mild-to-moderate hypertension; treatment of edema in heart failure

Unlabeled Use Nephrotic syndrome (Tanaka, 2005)

Available Dosage Forms

Tablet, Oral:

Generic: 1.25 mg, 2.5 mg

General Dosage Range Oral: *Adults:* 1.25-5 mg once daily

Administration

Oral May be administered without regard to meals (Caruso, 1983); however, administration with food or milk may to decrease GI adverse effects. Administer early in day to avoid nocturia.

Nursing Actions

Physical Assessment Allergy history should be assessed prior to beginning therapy (sulfonamides, thiazides). Monitor for hypotension, hypokalemia, and photosensitivity at regular intervals during therapy.

Patient Education

- Discuss specific use of drug and side effects with patient as it relates to treatment. (HCAHPS: During this hospital stay, were you given any medicine that you had not taken before? Before giving you any new medicine, how often did hospital staff tell you what the medicine was for? How often did hospital staff describe possible side effects in a way you could understand?)
- Patient may experience hypokalemia, dizziness, nausea, or asthenia. Have patient report immediately to prescriber rash (HCAHPS).
- Educate patient about signs of a significant reaction (eg, wheezing; chest tightness; fever; itching; bad cough; blue skin color; seizures; or swelling of face, lips, tongue, or throat). **Note:** This is not a comprehensive list of all side effects. Patient should consult prescriber for additional questions.

Intended Use and Disclaimer: Should not be printed and given to patients. This information is intended to serve as a concise initial reference for healthcare professionals to use when discussing medications with a patient. You must ultimately rely on your own discretion, experience and judgment in diagnosing, treating and advising patients.

Indinavir (in DIN a veer)

Brand Names: U.S. Crixivan
Index Terms IDV; Indinavir Sulfate
Pharmacologic Category Antiretroviral, Protease Inhibitor (Anti-HIV)
Medication Safety Issues
   Sound-alike/look-alike issues:
   Indinavir may be confused with Denavir®
Pregnancy Risk Factor C
Lactation Excretion in breast milk unknown/contraindicated
Breast-Feeding Considerations Maternal or infant antiretroviral therapy does not completely eliminate the risk of postnatal HIV transmission. In addition, multiclass-resistant virus has been detected in breast-feeding infants despite maternal therapy. Therefore, in the United States, where formula is accessible, affordable, safe, and sustainable, and the risk of infant mortality due to diarrhea and respiratory infections is low, complete avoidance of breast-feeding by HIV-infected women is recommended to decrease potential transmission of HIV (DHHS [perinatal], 2012).

Use Treatment of HIV infection; should always be used as part of a multidrug regimen (at least three antiretroviral agents)
Mechanism of Action/Effect Blocks the site of HIV-1 protease activity, resulting in the formation of immature, noninfectious viral particles.
Contraindications Hypersensitivity to indinavir or any component of the formulation; concurrent use of alfuzosin, alprazolam, amiodarone, cisapride, ergot alkaloids, lovastatin, midazolam (oral), pimozide, simvastatin, St John's wort, or triazolam; sildenafil (when used for pulmonary artery hypertension [eg, Revatio®])
Warnings/Precautions Because indinavir may cause nephrolithiasis/urolithiasis the drug should be discontinued if signs and symptoms occur. Adequate hydration is recommended. May cause tubulointerstitial nephritis (rare); severe asymptomatic leukocyturia may warrant evaluation. Indinavir has a high potential for drug interactions; concomitant use of indinavir with some drugs may require cautious use, may not be recommended, may require dosage adjustments, or may be contraindicated.

Patients with hepatic insufficiency due to cirrhosis should have dose reduction. Warn patients about fat redistribution that can occur. Indinavir has been associated with hemolytic anemia (discontinue if diagnosed), hepatitis, hyperbilirubinemia, and hyperglycemia (exacerbation or new-onset diabetes).

Patients may develop immune reconstitution syndrome resulting in the occurrence of an inflammatory response to an indolent or residual opportunistic infection during initial HIV treatment or activation of autoimmune disorders (eg, Graves' disease, polymyositis, Guillain-Barré syndrome) later in therapy; further evaluation and treatment may be required.

Use caution in patients with hemophilia; spontaneous bleeding has been reported.
Drug Interactions
Avoid Concomitant Use
Avoid concomitant use of Indinavir with any of the following: Ado-Trastuzumab Emtansine; Alfuzosin; ALPRAZolam; Amiodarone; Apixaban; Atazanavir; Avanafil; Axitinib; Bosutinib; Cabozantinib; Cisapride; Conivaptan; Crizotinib; Dronedarone; Eplerenone; Ergot Derivatives; Everolimus; Halofantrine; Ibrutinib; Imatinib; Ivabradine; Lapatinib; Lomitapide; Lovastatin; Lurasidone; Macitentan; Midazolam; Nilotinib; Nisoldipine; Pimozide; Pomalidomide; QuiNIDine; Ranolazine; Red Yeast Rice; Regorafenib; Rifampin; Rivaroxaban; Salmeterol; Silodosin; Simeprevir; Simvastatin; St Johns Wort; Tamsulosin; Ticagrelor; Tolvaptan; Toremifene; Triazolam; Ulipristal; Vemurafenib; VinCRIStine (Liposomal)

Decreased Effect

Indinavir may decrease the levels/effects of: Abacavir; Boceprevir; Clarithromycin; Delavirdine; Etravirine; Ifosfamide; Meperidine; Prasugrel; Theophylline Derivatives; Ticagrelor; Valproic Acid and Derivatives; Zidovudine

The levels/effects of Indinavir may be decreased by: Antacids; Atovaquone; Boceprevir; Bosentan; CarBAMazepine; CYP3A4 Inducers (Strong); Dabrafenib; Deferasirox; Didanosine; Efavirenz; Garlic; H2-Antagonists; Mitotane; Nevirapine; Peginterferon Alfa-2b; P-glycoprotein/ABCB1 Inducers; Proton Pump Inhibitors; Rifabutin; Rifampin; St Johns Wort; Tocilizumab; Venlafaxine

Increased Effect/Toxicity

Indinavir may increase the levels/effects of: Ado-Trastuzumab Emtansine; Alfuzosin; Almotriptan; Alosetron; ALPRAZolam; Amiodarone; Apixaban; ARIPiprazole; Atazanavir; AtorvaSTATin; Avanafil; Axitinib; Bedaquiline; Bortezomib; Bosentan; Bosutinib; Brentuximab Vedotin; Brinzolamide; Budesonide (Nasal); Budesonide (Systemic, Oral Inhalation); Cabozantinib; Calcium Channel Blockers (Dihydropyridine); Calcium Channel Blockers (Nondihydropyridine); CarBAMazepine; Cisapride; Clarithromycin; Colchicine; Conivaptan; Corticosteroids (Orally Inhaled); Crizotinib; CycloSPORINE (Systemic); CYP3A4 Substrates; Dienogest; Digoxin; Dofetilide; DOXOrubicin (Conventional); Dronedarone; Dutasteride; Enfuvirtide; Enzalutamide; Eplerenone; Ergot Derivatives; Everolimus; FentaNYL; Fesoterodine; Fluticasone (Nasal); Fluticasone (Oral Inhalation); GuanFACINE; Halofantrine; Ibrutinib; Iloperidone; Imatinib; Itraconazole; Ivabradine; Ivacaftor; Ixabepilone; Ketoconazole (Systemic); Lacosamide; Lapatinib; Levomilnacipran; Lomitapide; Lovastatin; Lumefantrine; Lurasidone; Macitentan; Maraviroc; Meperidine; MethylPREDNISolone; Midazolam; Mifepristone; Nefazodone; Nilotinib; Nisoldipine; Ospemifene; OxyCODONE; Paricalcitol; PAZOPanib; Pimecrolimus; Pimozide; Pomalidomide; PONATinib; Propafenone; Protease Inhibitors; QUEtiapine; QuiNIDine; Ranolazine; Red Yeast Rice; Regorafenib; Repaglinide; Rifabutin; Rilpivirine; Riociguat; Rivaroxaban; RomiDEPsin; Rosuvastatin; Ruxolitinib; Salmeterol; Saxagliptin; Sildenafil; Silodosin; Simeprevir; Simvastatin; SORAfenib; Tacrolimus (Systemic); Tacrolimus (Topical); Tadalafil; Tamsulosin; Temsirolimus; Ticagrelor; Tofacitinib; Tolterodine; Tolvaptan; Toremifene; TraZODone; Triazolam; Tricyclic Antidepressants; Uliprital; Vardenafil; Vemurafenib; Vilazodone; VinCRIStine (Liposomal); Zuclopenthixol

The levels/effects of Indinavir may be increased by: Atazanavir; Clarithromycin; CycloSPORINE (Systemic); Delavirdine; Enfuvirtide; Etravirine;

Itraconazole; Ketoconazole (Systemic); P-glycoprotein/ABCB1 Inhibitors; Simeprevir

Nutritional/Ethanol Interactions

Food: Indinavir bioavailability may be decreased if taken with food. Meals high in calories, fat, and protein result in a significant decrease in drug levels. Indinavir serum concentrations may be decreased by grapefruit juice. Management: Administer with water 1 hour before or 2 hours after a meal. May also be administered with other liquids (eg, skim milk, juice, coffee, tea) or a light meal (eg, toast, corn flakes). Administer around-the-clock to avoid significant fluctuation in serum levels. Drink at least 48 oz of water daily. May be taken with food when administered in combination with ritonavir.

Herb/Nutraceutical: Garlic may decrease the levels/effects of protease inhibitors. St John's wort appears to induce CYP3A enzymes and has lead to 57% reductions in indinavir AUCs and 81% reductions in trough serum concentrations, which may lead to treatment failures. Management: Avoid garlic and St John's wort while taking indinavir.

Adverse Reactions

>10%:

Gastrointestinal: Abdominal pain (17%), nausea (12%)

Hepatic: Hyperbilirubinemia (14%; dose dependent)

Renal: Nephrolithiasis/urolithiasis, including flank pain with/without hematuria (29%, pediatric patients; 12% adult patients; dose dependent)

1% to 10%:

Central nervous system: Headache (5%), dizziness (3%), somnolence (2%), fever (2%), malaise (2%), fatigue (2%)

Dermatologic: Pruritus (4%), rash (1%)

Endocrine & metabolic: Hyperglycemia (1%)

Gastrointestinal: Vomiting (8%), diarrhea (3%), taste perversion (3%), acid reflux (3%), anorexia (3%), appetite increased (2%), dyspepsia (2%), serum amylase increased (2%)

Hematologic: Neutropenia (2%), anemia (1%), thrombocytopenia (1%)

Hepatic: Transaminases increased (4% to 5%), jaundice (2%)

Neuromuscular & skeletal: Back pain (8%), weakness (2%)

Renal: Dysuria (2%)

Respiratory: Cough (2%)

Available Dosage Forms

Capsule, Oral:

Crixivan: 200 mg, 400 mg

General Dosage Range Dosage adjustment recommended in patients with hepatic impairment or on concomitant therapy

Oral: *Adults:* 800 mg every 8 hours; Boosted regimen: 800 mg every 12 hours

Administration

Oral Drink at least 48 oz of water daily. Administer with water, 1 hour before or 2 hours after a meal. May also be administered with other liquids (eg, skim milk, juice, coffee, tea) or a light meal (eg, toast, corn flakes). Administer around-the-clock to avoid significant fluctuation in serum levels. May be taken with food when administered in combination with ritonavir.

Storage/Stability Medication should be stored at 15°C to 30°C (59°F to 86°F), and used in the original container and the desiccant should remain in the bottle. Capsules are sensitive to moisture.

Nursing Actions

Physical Assessment Monitor for adherence to regimen. Monitor for gastrointestinal disturbance (nausea, vomiting, diarrhea) that can lead to dehydration and weight loss, hyperlipidemia and redistribution of body fat, rash, CNS effects (malaise, insomnia, abnormal thinking), and electrolyte imbalance at regular intervals during therapy. Teach patient proper timing of multiple medications. Instruct patient on glucose testing (protease inhibitors may cause hyperglycemia, exacerbation or new-onset diabetes).

Patient Education
- Discuss specific use of drug and side effects with patient as it relates to treatment. (HCAHPS: During this hospital stay, were you given any medicine that you had not taken before? Before giving you any new medicine, how often did hospital staff tell you what the medicine was for? How often did hospital staff describe possible side effects in a way you could understand?)
- Patient may experience hyperlipidemia, hypertriglyceridemia, headache, dyspepsia, nausea, diarrhea, lipodystrophy, or asthenia. Have patient report immediately to prescriber back pain, hematuria, chills, polydipsia, polyuria, weight loss, or rash (HCAHPS).
- Educate patient about signs of a significant reaction (eg, wheezing; chest tightness; fever; itching; bad cough; blue skin color; seizures; or swelling of face, lips, tongue, or throat). **Note:** This is not a comprehensive list of all side effects. Patient should consult prescriber for additional questions.

Intended Use and Disclaimer: Should not be printed and given to patients. This information is intended to serve as a concise initial reference for healthcare professionals to use when discussing medications with a patient. You must ultimately rely on your own discretion, experience and judgment in diagnosing, treating and advising patients.

Dietary Considerations Should be taken without food but with water 1 hour before or 2 hours after a meal. Administration with lighter meals (eg, dry toast, skim milk, corn flakes) resulted in little/no change in indinavir concentration. If taking with ritonavir, may take with food. Patient should drink at least 48 oz of water daily.

Related Information

Oral Medications That Should Not Be Crushed or Altered *on page 1712*

Indomethacin (in doe METH a sin)

Brand Names: U.S. Indocin

Index Terms Indometacin; Indomethacin Sodium Trihydrate; Tivorbex

Pharmacologic Category Nonsteroidal Anti-inflammatory Drug (NSAID), Oral; Nonsteroidal Anti-inflammatory Drug (NSAID), Parenteral

Medication Safety Issues

Sound-alike/look-alike issues:

Indocin® may be confused with Imodium®, Lincocin®, Minocin®, Vicodin®

BEERS Criteria medication:

This drug may be potentially inappropriate for use in geriatric patients (Quality of evidence - moderate; Strength of recommendation - strong).

Medication Guide Available Yes

Pregnancy Risk Factor C

Lactation Enters breast milk/not recommended

Breast-Feeding Considerations Indomethacin is excreted into breast milk and low amounts have been measured in the plasma of nursing infants. Seizures in a nursing infant were observed in one case report, although adverse events have not been noted in other cases. Breast-feeding is not recommended by the manufacturer. (The therapeutic use of indomethacin is contraindicated in neonates with significant renal failure.) Hypertensive crisis and psychiatric side effects have been noted in case reports following use of indomethacin for analgesia in postpartum women. Use with caution in nursing women with hypertensive disorders of pregnancy or pre-existing renal disease.

Use Acute gouty arthritis, acute bursitis/tendonitis, moderate-to-severe osteoarthritis, rheumatoid arthritis, ankylosing spondylitis; I.V. form used as alternative to surgery for closure of patent ductus arteriosus in neonates

Unlabeled Use Management of preterm labor; prevention of pancreatitis post-endoscopic retrograde cholangiopancreatography (ERCP)

Mechanism of Action/Effect Reversibly inhibits cyclooxygenase-1 and 2 (COX-1 and 2) enzymes, which results in decreased formation of prostaglandin precursors; has antipyretic, analgesic, and anti-inflammatory properties

Contraindications Hypersensitivity to indomethacin, aspirin, other NSAIDs, or any component of the formulation; perioperative pain in the setting of coronary artery bypass graft (CABG) surgery; patients with a history of proctitis or recent rectal bleeding (suppositories)

Neonates: Necrotizing enterocolitis; impaired renal function; active bleeding (including intracranial hemorrhage and gastrointestinal bleeding), thrombocytopenia, coagulation defects; untreated infection; congenital heart disease where patent ductus arteriosus is necessary

Warnings/Precautions [U.S. Boxed Warning]: NSAIDs are associated with an increased risk of adverse cardiovascular thrombotic events, including MI and stroke. Risk may be increased with duration of use or pre-existing cardiovascular risk factors or disease. May cause new-onset hypertension or worsening of existing hypertension. Use caution with fluid retention. Avoid use in heart failure (ACCF/AHA [Yancy, 2013]). Concurrent administration of ibuprofen, and potentially other nonselective NSAIDs, may interfere with aspirin's cardioprotective effect. **[U.S. Boxed Warning]: Use is contraindicated for treatment of perioperative pain in the setting of coronary artery bypass graft (CABG) surgery.** Risk of MI and stroke may be increased with use following CABG surgery.

Platelet adhesion and aggregation may be decreased; may prolong bleeding time; patients with coagulation disorders or who are receiving anticoagulants should be monitored closely. Anemia may occur; patients on long-term NSAID therapy should be monitored for anemia. Rarely, NSAID use may cause severe blood dyscrasias (eg, agranulocytosis, aplastic anemia, thrombocytopenia).

NSAID use may compromise existing renal function; dose-dependent decreases in prostaglandin synthesis may result from NSAID use, reducing renal blood flow which may cause renal decompensation. NSAID use may increase the risk for hyperkalemia. Patients with impaired renal function, dehydration, heart failure, liver dysfunction, those taking diuretics, and ACE inhibitors are at greater risk of renal toxicity and hyperkalemia. Rehydrate patient before starting therapy; monitor renal function closely. Not recommended for use in patients with advanced renal disease. Long-term NSAID use may result in renal papillary necrosis.

[U.S. Boxed Warning]: NSAIDs may increase risk of gastrointestinal irritation, inflammation, ulceration, bleeding, and perforation. Use caution with a history of GI disease (bleeding or ulcers), concurrent therapy with aspirin, anticoagulants and/or corticosteroids, smoking, use of alcohol, the elderly or debilitated patients. When used concomitantly with aspirin, a substantial increase in the risk of gastrointestinal complications (eg, ulcer) occurs; concomitant gastroprotective therapy (eg, proton pump inhibitors) is recommended (Bhatt, 2008).

Use the lowest effective dose for the shortest duration of time, consistent with individual patient goals, to reduce risk of cardiovascular or GI adverse events. Alternate therapies should be considered for patients at high risk.

NSAIDS may cause drowsiness, dizziness, blurred vision and other neurologic effects which may impair physical or mental abilities; patients must be cautioned about performing tasks which require mental alertness (eg, operating machinery or driving). Discontinue use with blurred or diminished vision and perform ophthalmologic exam. Monitor vision with long-term therapy.

NSAIDs may cause serious skin adverse events including exfoliative dermatitis, Stevens-Johnson syndrome (SJS) and toxic epidermal necrolysis (TEN); discontinue use at first sign of skin rash or hypersensitivity. Anaphylactoid reactions may occur, even without prior exposure; patients with "aspirin triad" (bronchial asthma, aspirin intolerance, rhinitis) may be at increased risk. Do not use in patients who experience bronchospasm, asthma, rhinitis, or urticaria with NSAID or aspirin therapy. Use caution in other forms of asthma.

Use with caution in patients with decreased hepatic function. Closely monitor patients with any abnormal LFT. Severe hepatic reactions (eg, fulminant hepatitis, liver failure) have occurred with NSAID use, rarely; discontinue if signs or symptoms of liver disease develop, or if systemic manifestations occur. The elderly are at increased risk for adverse effects (especially peptic ulceration, CNS effects, renal toxicity) from NSAIDs even at low doses. Prolonged use may cause corneal deposits and retinal disturbances; discontinue if visual changes are observed. Use caution with depression, epilepsy, or Parkinson's disease.

Withhold for at least 4-6 half-lives prior to surgical or dental procedures.

Elderly: Nonselective oral NSAID use is associated with an increased risk of GI bleeding and peptic ulcer disease in older adults in high risk category (eg, >75 years or age or receiving concomitant oral/parenteral corticosteroids, anticoagulants, or antiplatelet agents). Risk of adverse events may be higher with indomethacin compared to other NSAIDs; avoid use in this age group (Beers Criteria).

Oral: Safety and efficacy have not been established in children <14 years of age. Hepatotoxicity has been reported in younger children treated for juvenile idiopathic arthritis (JIA). Closely monitor if use is needed in children ≥2 years of age.

Drug Interactions

Avoid Concomitant Use

Avoid concomitant use of Indomethacin with any of the following: Floctafenine; Ketorolac (Nasal); Ketorolac (Systemic); NSAID (COX-2 Inhibitor); Omacetaxine; Urokinase

Decreased Effect

Indomethacin may decrease the levels/effects of: ACE Inhibitors; Agents with Antiplatelet Properties; Aliskiren; Angiotensin II Receptor Blockers; Beta-Blockers; Eplerenone; HydrALAZINE; Loop Diuretics; Potassium-Sparing Diuretics; Prostaglandins (Ophthalmic); Salicylates; Selective Serotonin Reuptake Inhibitors; Thiazide Diuretics

The levels/effects of Indomethacin may be decreased by: Bile Acid Sequestrants; Nonsteroidal Anti-Inflammatory Agents; Salicylates

Increased Effect/Toxicity

Indomethacin may increase the levels/effects of: 5-ASA Derivatives; Agents with Antiplatelet Properties; Aliskiren; Aminoglycosides; Anticoagulants; Bisphosphonate Derivatives; Collagenase (Systemic); CycloSPORINE (Systemic); Dabigatran Etexilate; Deferasirox; Desmopressin; Digoxin; Eplerenone; Haloperidol; Ibritumomab; Lithium; Methotrexate; Nonsteroidal Anti-Inflammatory Agents; NSAID (COX-2 Inhibitor); Omacetaxine; PEMEtrexed; Porfimer; Potassium-Sparing Diuretics; PRALAtrexate; Quinolone Antibiotics; Rivaroxaban; Salicylates; Tenofovir; Thrombolytic Agents; Tiludronate; Tositumomab and Iodine I 131 Tositumomab; Triamterene; Urokinase; Vancomycin; Vitamin K Antagonists

The levels/effects of Indomethacin may be increased by: ACE Inhibitors; Angiotensin II Receptor Blockers; Antidepressants (Tricyclic, Tertiary Amine); Corticosteroids (Systemic); CycloSPORINE (Systemic); Dasatinib; Floctafenine; Glucosamine; Herbs (Anticoagulant/Antiplatelet Properties); Ibrutinib; Ketorolac (Nasal); Ketorolac (Systemic); Multivitamins/Fluoride (with ADE); Multivitamins/Minerals (with ADEK, Folate, Iron); Multivitamins/Minerals (with AE, No Iron); Nonsteroidal Anti-Inflammatory Agents; Omega-3 Fatty Acids; Pentosan Polysulfate Sodium; Pentoxifylline; Probenecid; Prostacyclin Analogues; Selective Serotonin Reuptake Inhibitors; Serotonin/Norepinephrine Reuptake Inhibitors; Sodium Phosphates; Tipranavir; Treprostinil; Vitamin E

Nutritional/Ethanol Interactions

Ethanol: Avoid ethanol (may enhance gastric mucosal irritation).

Food: Food may decrease the rate but not the extent of absorption. Indomethacin peak serum levels may be delayed if taken with food.

Herb/Nutraceutical: Avoid alfalfa, anise, bilberry, bladderwrack, bromelain, cat's claw, celery, chamomile, coleus, cordyceps, dong quai, evening primrose, fenugreek, feverfew, garlic, ginger, ginkgo biloba, ginseng (American, Panax, Siberian), grapeseed, green tea, guggul, horse chestnut seed, horseradish, licorice, prickly ash, red clover, reishi, SAMe (S-adenosylmethionine), sweet clover, turmeric, white willow (all have additional antiplatelet activity).

Adverse Reactions

>10%: Central nervous system: Headache (12%)

1% to 10%:

Central nervous system: Dizziness (3% to 9%), depression (<3%), fatigue (<3%), malaise (<3%), somnolence (<3%), vertigo (<3%)

Gastrointestinal: Dyspepsia (3% to 9%), epigastric pain (3% to 9%), heartburn (3% to 9%), indigestion (3% to 9%), nausea (3% to 9%), abdominal pain/cramps/distress (<3%), constipation (<3%), diarrhea (<3%), rectal irritation (suppository), tenesmus (suppository), vomiting

Otic: Tinnitus (<3%)

Pharmacodynamics/Kinetics

Onset of Action ~30 minutes

Duration of Action 4-6 hours

Product Availability Tivorbex: FDA approved February 2014; anticipated availability currently unknown. Refer to the prescribing information for additional information.

Available Dosage Forms

Capsule, Oral:

Generic: 25 mg, 50 mg

Capsule Extended Release, Oral:

Generic: 75 mg

Solution Reconstituted, Intravenous:

Indocin: 1 mg (1 ea)

Generic: 1 mg (1 ea)

Suppository, Rectal:

Indocin: 50 mg (30 ea)

Suspension, Oral:

Indocin: 25 mg/5 mL (237 mL)

General Dosage Range

I.V.:

Neonates <48 hours old at time of first dose: Initial: 0.2 mg/kg, followed by 2 doses of 0.1 mg/kg at 12- to 24-hour intervals

Neonates 2-7 days old at time of first dose: Initial: 0.2 mg/kg, followed by 2 doses of 0.2 mg/kg at 12- to 24-hour intervals

Neonates >7 days old at time of first dose: Initial: 0.2 mg/kg, followed by 2 doses of 0.25 mg/kg at 12- to 24-hour intervals

Oral:

Extended release: *Children >14 years and Adults:* 75-150 mg/day in 1-2 divided doses (maximum: 150 mg/day)

Immediate release:

Children ≥2 years: 1-2 mg/kg/day in 2-4 divided doses (maximum: 4 mg/kg/day; 200 mg/day)

Adults: 50-150 mg/day in 2-4 divided doses (maximum: 200 mg/day)

Rectal: *Children >14 years and Adults:* 50-150 mg/day in 2-4 divided doses (maximum: 200 mg/day)

Administration

I.V. Administer over 20-30 minutes. Reconstitute I.V. formulation just prior to administration; discard any unused portion; avoid I.V. bolus administration or infusion via an umbilical catheter into vessels near the superior mesenteric artery as these may cause vasoconstriction and can compromise blood flow to the intestines. Do not administer intra-arterially.

Injectable Detail pH: 6-7.5

Oral Administer with food, milk, or antacids to decrease GI adverse effects. Extended release capsules must be swallowed whole; do not crush.

Preparation for Administration I.V.: Reconstitute with 1-2 mL preservative free NS or SWFI just prior to administration. Discard any unused portion. Do not use preservative-containing diluents for reconstitution.

Storage/Stability

Capsules: Store at controlled room temperature.

I.V.: Store below 30°C (86°F). Protect from light.

Suppositories: Store refrigerated at 2°C to 8°C (36°F to 46°F).

Suspension: Store at controlled room temperature.

Nursing Actions

Physical Assessment Monitor blood pressure prior to treatment and periodically throughout. Regular ophthalmic evaluations are recommended.

Patient Education

- Discuss specific use of drug and side effects with patient as it relates to treatment. (HCAHPS: During this hospital stay, were you given any medicine that you had not taken before? Before giving you any new medicine, how often did hospital staff tell you what the medicine was for? How often did hospital staff describe possible side effects in a way you could understand?)
- Patient may experience headache, dyspepsia, nausea, diarrhea, or constipation. Have patient report immediately to prescriber angina, strength differences from one side to another, edema or pain of hands or feet, significant weight gain, melena, hematuria, ecchymosis, or rash (HCAHPS).
- Educate patient about signs of a significant reaction (eg, wheezing; chest tightness; fever; itching; bad cough; blue skin color; seizures; or swelling of face, lips, tongue, or throat). **Note:** This is not a comprehensive list of all side effects. Patient should consult prescriber for additional questions.

Intended Use and Disclaimer: Should not be printed and given to patients. This information is intended to serve as a concise initial reference for healthcare professionals to use when discussing medications with a patient. You must ultimately rely on your own discretion, experience and judgment in diagnosing, treating and advising patients.

Dietary Considerations May cause GI upset; take with food or milk to minimize

Related Information

Oral Medications That Should Not Be Crushed or Altered *on page 1712*

InFLIXimab (in FLIKS e mab)

Brand Names: U.S. Remicade

Index Terms Avakine; Infliximab, Recombinant

Pharmacologic Category Antirheumatic, Disease Modifying; Gastrointestinal Agent, Miscellaneous; Immunosuppressant Agent; Monoclonal Antibody; Tumor Necrosis Factor (TNF) Blocking Agent

Medication Safety Issues

Sound-alike/look-alike issues:

InFLIXimab may be confused with riTUXimab

Remicade® may be confused with Renacidin®, Rituxan®

Medication Guide Available Yes

Pregnancy Risk Factor B

Lactation Excreted in breast milk/not recommended

Breast-Feeding Considerations Small amounts of infliximab have been detected in breast milk. Information is available from three postpartum women who were administered infliximab 5 mg/kg 1-24 weeks after delivery. Infliximab was detected within 12 hours and the highest milk concentrations (0.09-0.105 mcg/mL) were seen 2-3 days after the dose. Corresponding maternal serum concentrations were 18-64 mcg/mL (Ben-Horin, 2011). Due to the potential for serious adverse reactions in the nursing infant, the manufacturer recommends a decision be made whether to discontinue nursing or to discontinue the drug, taking into account the importance of treatment to the mother.

Use

Treatment of moderately- to severely-active rheumatoid arthritis (with methotrexate) (to reduce signs/symptoms of active arthritis and inhibit progression of structural damage and improve physical function)

Treatment of moderately- to severely-active Crohn's disease with inadequate response to conventional therapy (to reduce signs/symptoms and induce and maintain clinical remission) or to reduce the number of draining enterocutaneous and rectovaginal fistulas and maintain fistula closure

Treatment of psoriatic arthritis (to reduce signs/symptoms of active arthritis and inhibit progression of structural damage and improve physical function)

Treatment of chronic severe (extensive and/or disabling) plaque psoriasis as an alternative to other systemic therapy

Treatment of active ankylosing spondylitis (to reduce signs/symptoms)

Treatment of moderately- to severely-active ulcerative colitis with inadequate response to conventional therapy (to reduce signs/symptoms and induce and maintain clinical remission, mucosal healing and eliminate corticosteroid use)

Mechanism of Action/Effect Infliximab is a monoclonal antibody that binds to human tumor necrosis factor alpha (TNFα), thereby decreasing inflammatory and other responses.

Contraindications Hypersensitivity to infliximab, murine proteins or any component of the formulation; doses >5 mg/kg in patients with moderate or severe heart failure (NYHA Class III/IV)

Canadian labeling: Additional contraindications (not in U.S. labeling): Severe infections (eg, sepsis, abscesses, tuberculosis, and opportunistic infections)

Warnings/Precautions [U.S. Boxed Warning]: Patients receiving infliximab are at increased risk for serious infections which may result in hospitalization and/or fatality; infections usually developed in patients receiving concomitant immunosuppressive agents (eg, methotrexate or corticosteroids) and may present as disseminated (rather than local) disease. Active tuberculosis (or reactivation of latent tuberculosis), invasive fungal (including aspergillosis, blastomycosis, candidiasis, coccidioidomycosis, histoplasmosis, and pneumocystosis) and bacterial, viral or other opportunistic infections (including legionellosis and listeriosis) have been reported in patients receiving TNF-blocking agents, including infliximab. Monitor closely for signs/symptoms of infection. Discontinue for serious infection or sepsis. Consider risks versus benefits prior to use in patients with a history of chronic or recurrent infection. Consider empiric antifungal therapy in patients who are at risk for invasive fungal infection and develop severe systemic illness. Caution should be exercised when considering use the elderly or in patients with conditions that predispose them to infections (eg, diabetes) or residence/travel from areas of endemic mycoses (blastomycosis, coccidioidomycosis, histoplasmosis), or with latent or localized infections. Do not initiate infliximab therapy with an active infection, including clinically important localized infection. Patients who develop a new infection while undergoing treatment should be monitored closely. Serious infections and neutropenia have been reported when anakinra or abatacept have been used concurrently with other TNF-blocking agents; concurrent use of infliximab with anakinra or abatacept is not recommended. Concurrent use of infliximab and other biologic agents is not recommended due to possible increased risk of infection. Use caution when switching from one biologic disease-modifying antirheumatic drug (DMARD) to another; overlapping biological activities may further increase the risk of infection. Potentially significant drug interactions may exist, requiring dose or frequency adjustment, additional monitoring, and/or selection of alternative therapy.

[U.S. Boxed Warning]: Infliximab treatment has been associated with active tuberculosis (may be disseminated or extrapulmonary) or reactivation of latent infections; evaluate patients for tuberculosis risk factors and latent tuberculosis infection (with a tuberculin skin test) prior to and during therapy; treatment of latent tuberculosis should be initiated before use. Patients with initial negative tuberculin skin tests should receive continued monitoring for tuberculosis throughout treatment. Most cases of reactivation have been reported within the first 3-6 months of treatment. Caution should be exercised when considering the use of infliximab in patients who have been exposed to tuberculosis.

Patients should be brought up to date with all immunizations before initiating therapy. Live vaccines should not be given concurrently; there is no data available concerning secondary transmission of live vaccines in patients receiving therapy. Use caution when administering live vaccines to infants born to female patients who received infliximab therapy while pregnant; infliximab crosses the placenta and has been detected in infants' serum for up to 6 months. Rare reactivation of hepatitis B virus (HBV) has occurred in chronic virus carriers; use with caution; evaluate prior to initiation and during treatment.

[U.S. Boxed Warning]: Lymphoma and other malignancies have been reported in children and adolescent patients receiving TNF-blocking agents including infliximab. Half the cases are lymphomas (Hodgkin's and non-Hodgkin's). **[U.S. Boxed Warning]: Hepatosplenic T-cell lymphoma has been reported in patients with Crohn's disease or ulcerative colitis treated with infliximab and concurrent or prior azathioprine or mercaptopurine use, usually reported in adolescent and young adult males.** The impact of infliximab on the development and course of malignancies is not fully defined, but may be dose dependent. As compared to the general population, an increased risk of lymphoma has been noted in clinical trials; however, rheumatoid arthritis alone has been previously associated with an increased rate of lymphoma. Use caution in patients with a history of COPD, higher rates of malignancy were reported in COPD patients treated with infliximab. Psoriasis patients with a history of phototherapy had a higher incidence of nonmelanoma skin cancers. Melanoma and Merkel cell carcinoma have been reported in patients receiving TNF-blocking agents including infliximab. Perform periodic skin examinations in all patients during therapy, particularly those at increased risk for skin cancer.

Severe hepatic reactions (including hepatitis, jaundice, acute hepatic failure, and cholestasis) have been reported during treatment; discontinue with jaundice or marked increase in liver enzymes (≥5 times ULN). Use caution with heart failure; if a decision is made to use with heart failure, monitor closely and discontinue if exacerbated or new symptoms occur. Doses >5 mg/kg should not be administered in patients with moderate-to-severe heart failure (NYHA Class III/IV). Use caution with history of hematologic abnormalities; hematologic toxicities (eg, leukopenia, neutropenia, thrombocytopenia, pancytopenia) have been reported; discontinue if significant abnormalities occur. Autoimmune antibodies and a lupus-like syndrome have been reported. If antibodies to double-stranded DNA are confirmed in a patient with lupus-like symptoms, infliximab should be discontinued. Rare cases of optic neuritis and demyelinating disease (including multiple sclerosis, systemic vasculitis, and Guillain-Barré syndrome) have been reported; use with caution in patients with pre-existing or recent onset CNS demyelinating disorders, or seizures; discontinue if significant CNS adverse reactions develop.

Acute infusion reactions may occur. Hypersensitivity reaction may occur within 2 hours of infusion. Medication and equipment for management of hypersensitivity reaction should be available for immediate use. Interruptions and/or reinstitution at a slower rate may be required (consult protocols). Pretreatment may be considered, and may be warranted in all patients with prior infusion reactions. Serum sickness-like reactions have occurred; may be associated with a decreased response to treatment. The development of antibodies to infliximab may increase the risk of hypersensitivity and/or infusion reactions; concomitant use of immunosuppressants may lessen the development of anti-infliximab antibodies. The risk of infusion reactions may be increased with retreatment after an interruption or discontinuation of prior maintenance therapy. Retreatment in psoriasis patients should be resumed as a scheduled maintenance regimen without any induction doses; use of an induction regimen should be used cautiously for retreatment of all other patients.

Efficacy was not established in a study to evaluate infliximab use in juvenile idiopathic arthritis (JIA). Safety and efficacy for use in pediatric plaque psoriasis or pediatric ulcerative colitis have not been established. **Note:** For use in Crohn's disease: Safety and efficacy have not been established in children <6 years of age (U.S. labeling) and in children <9 years of age (Canadian labeling).

Drug Interactions
Avoid Concomitant Use
Avoid concomitant use of InFLIXimab with any of the following: Abatacept; Adalimumab; Anakinra; BCG; Belimumab; Canakinumab; Certolizumab Pegol; Etanercept; Golimumab; Natalizumab; Pimecrolimus; Rilonacept; Tacrolimus (Topical); Tocilizumab; Tofacitinib; Ustekinumab; Vaccines (Live)

Decreased Effect
InFLIXimab may decrease the levels/effects of: BCG; Coccidioidin Skin Test; Sipuleucel-T; Vaccines (Inactivated); Vaccines (Live)

The levels/effects of InFLIXimab may be decreased by: Echinacea

Increased Effect/Toxicity
InFLIXimab may increase the levels/effects of: Abatacept; Anakinra; Belimumab; Canakinumab; Certolizumab Pegol; Leflunomide; Natalizumab; Rilonacept; Tofacitinib; Vaccines (Live)

The levels/effects of InFLIXimab may be increased by: Abciximab; Adalimumab; Denosumab; Etanercept; Golimumab; Pimecrolimus; Roflumilast; Tacrolimus (Topical); Tocilizumab; Trastuzumab; Ustekinumab

Nutritional/Ethanol Interactions Herb/Nutraceutical: Avoid echinacea (may diminish the therapeutic effect of infliximab).

Adverse Reactions Although profile is similar, frequency of adverse effects may vary with disease state. Except where noted, percentages reported in adults with rheumatoid arthritis:

>10%:
Central nervous system: Headache (18%)
Gastrointestinal: Nausea (21%), diarrhea (12%), abdominal pain (Crohn's: 26%; other indications: 12%)
Hepatic: Increased serum ALT (risk increased with concomitant methotrexate)
Immunologic: Increased ANA titer (~50%), antibody development (double-stranded DNA, 20%), antibody development (anti-infliximab; variable; ~10% to 15% [range: 6% to 61%]; Mayer, 2006)
Infection: Infection (36%), abscess (Crohn's patients with fistulizing disease: 15%)
Respiratory: Upper respiratory tract infection (32%), sinusitis (14%), cough (12%), pharyngitis (12%)
Miscellaneous: Infusion related reaction (20%; severe <1%)
5% to 10%:
Cardiovascular: Hypertension (7%)
Central nervous system: Fatigue (9%), pain (8%)
Dermatologic: Skin rash (1% to 10%), pruritus (7%)
Gastrointestinal: Dyspepsia (10%)
Genitourinary: Urinary tract infection (8%)
Infection: Candidiasis (5%)
Neuromuscular & skeletal: Arthralgia (1% to 8%), back pain (8%)

Respiratory: Bronchitis (10%), rhinitis (8%), dyspnea (6%)

Miscellaneous: Fever (7%)

<5%: Abscess, adult respiratory distress syndrome, anemia, basal cell carcinoma, biliary colic, bradycardia, cardiac arrest, cardiac arrhythmia, cardiac failure, cellulitis, cerebral infarction, cholecystitis, cholelithiasis, circulatory shock, confusion, constipation, dehydration, delayed hypersensitivity (plaque psoriasis), diaphoresis, dizziness, edema, gastrointestinal hemorrhage, hemolytic anemia, hepatitis, herniated disk, hypersensitivity reaction, hypotension, intestinal obstruction, intestinal perforation, intestinal stenosis, leukopenia, lupus-like syndrome, lymphadenopathy, malignant lymphoma, malignant neoplasm, malignant neoplasm of breast, meningitis, menstrual disease, myalgia, myocardial infarction, nephrolithiasis, neuritis, pancreatitis, pancytopenia, peripheral neuropathy, peritonitis, pleural effusion, pleurisy, pulmonary edema, pulmonary embolism, rectal pain, renal failure, respiratory insufficiency, sarcoidosis, seizure, sepsis, serum sickness, suicidal tendencies, syncope, tachycardia, tendon disease, thrombocytopenia, thrombophlebitis (deep), ulcer

The following adverse events were reported in children with Crohn's disease and were found more frequently in children than adults:

>10%:

Hepatic: Increased liver enzymes (18%; ≥5 times ULN: 1%)

Hematologic & oncologic: Anemia (11%)

Infection: Infection (56%; more common with every 8-week vs every 12-week infusions)

1% to 10%:

Cardiovascular: Flushing (9%)

Gastrointestinal: Bloody stools (10%)

Hematologic & oncologic: Leukopenia (9%), neutropenia (7%)

Hypersensitivity: Hypersensitivity reaction (respiratory, 6%)

Immunologic: Antibody development (anti-infliximab, 3%)

Infection: Viral infection (8%), bacterial infection (6%)

Neuromuscular & skeletal: Bone fracture (7%)

Pharmacodynamics/Kinetics

Onset of Action Crohn's disease: ~2 weeks

Available Dosage Forms

Solution Reconstituted, Intravenous [preservative free]:

Remicade: 100 mg (1 ea)

General Dosage Range Dosage adjustment is required in heart failure patients.

I.V.:

Children ≥6 years and Adolescents: Initial: 5 mg/kg at 0, 2, and 6 weeks; Maintenance: 5 mg/kg every 8 weeks

Adults: Initial: 3-10 mg/kg at 0, 2, and 6 weeks; Maintenance: 3-10 mg/kg every 8 weeks **or** 5 mg/kg every 6 weeks

Administration

I.V. The infusion should begin within 3 hours of reconstitution and dilution. Infuse over at least 2 hours; do not infuse with other agents; use in-line low protein binding filter (≤1.2 micron). Temporarily discontinue or decrease infusion rate with infusion-related reactions. Antihistamines (H$_1$-antagonist +/- H$_2$-antagonist), acetaminophen and/or corticosteroids may be used to manage reactions. Infusion may be reinitiated at a lower rate upon resolution of mild-to-moderate symptoms.

Canadian labeling (not approved in U.S. labeling): Infusion of doses ≤6 mg/kg over not less than 1 hour may be considered in patients treated for rheumatoid arthritis who have initially tolerated 3 infusions each over 2 hours. Safety of shortened infusion has not been studied with doses >6 mg/kg.

Guidelines for the treatment and prophylaxis of infusion reactions: (**Note:** Limited to adult patients and dosages used in Crohn's; prospective data for other populations [pediatrics, other indications/dosing] are not available).

A protocol for the treatment of infusion reactions, as well as prophylactic therapy for repeat infusions, has been published (Mayer, 2006).

Treatment of infusion reactions: Medications for the treatment of hypersensitivity reactions should be available for immediate use. For mild reactions, the rate of infusion should be decreased to 10 mL/hour. Initiate a normal saline infusion (500-1000 mL/hour) and appropriate symptomatic treatment (eg, acetaminophen and diphenhydramine); monitor vital signs every 10 minutes until normal. After 20 minutes, the infusion may be increased at 15-minute intervals, as tolerated, to completion (initial increase to 20 mL/hour, then 40 mL/hour, then 80 mL/hour, etc [maximum of 125 mL/hour]). For moderate reactions, the infusion should be stopped or slowed. Initiate a normal saline infusion (500-1000 mL/hour) and appropriate symptomatic treatment. Monitor vital signs every 5 minutes until normal. After 20 minutes, the infusion may be reinstituted at 10 mL/hour; then increased at 15-minute intervals, as tolerated, to completion (initial increase 20 mL/hour, then 40 mL/hour, then 80 mL/hour, etc [maximum of 125 mL/hour]). For severe reactions, the infusion should be stopped with administration of appropriate symptomatic treatment (eg, hydrocortisone/methylprednisolone, diphenhydramine and epinephrine) and frequent monitoring of vitals (consult institutional policies, if available). Retreatment after a severe reaction should only ▶

be done if the benefits outweigh the risks and with appropriate prophylaxis. Delayed infusion reactions typically occur 1-7 days after an infusion. Treatment should consist of appropriate symptomatic treatment (eg, acetaminophen, antihistamine, methylprednisolone).

Prophylaxis of infusion reactions: Premedication with acetaminophen and diphenhydramine 90 minutes prior to infusion may be considered in all patients with prior infusion reactions, and in patients with severe reactions corticosteroid administration is recommended. Steroid dosing may be oral (prednisone 50 mg orally every 12 hours for 3 doses prior to infusion) or intravenous (a single dose of hydrocortisone 100 mg or methylprednisolone 20-40 mg administered 20 minutes prior to the infusion). On initiation of the infusion, begin with a test dose at 10 mL/hour for 15 minutes. Thereafter, the infusion may be increased at 15-minute intervals, as tolerated, to completion (initial increase 20 mL/hour, then 40 mL/hour, then 80 mL/hour, etc). A maximum rate of 125 mL/hour is recommended in patients who experienced prior mild-moderate reactions and 100 mL/hour is recommended in patients who experienced prior severe reactions. In patients with cutaneous flushing, aspirin may be considered (Becker, 2004). For delayed infusion reactions, premedicate with acetaminophen and diphenhydramine 90 minutes prior to infusion. On initiation of the infusion, begin with a test dose at 10 mL/hour for 15 minutes. Thereafter, the infusion may be increased to infuse over 3 hours. Postinfusion therapy with acetaminophen for 3 days and an antihistamine for 7 days is recommended.

Injectable Detail pH ~7.2 (reconstituted vial)

Preparation for Administration Reconstitute vials with 10 mL sterile water for injection. Swirl vial gently to dissolve powder; do not shake. Allow solution to stand for 5 minutes. Total dose of reconstituted product should be further diluted to 250 mL of 0.9% sodium chloride injection to a final concentration of 0.4-4 mg/mL. Infusion of dose should begin within 3 hours of preparation.

Storage/Stability Store vials at 2°C to 8°C (36°F to 46°F).

Nursing Actions

Physical Assessment Monitor for hypersensitivity and respiratory effects. Infusion reactions may occur. Premedication may be helpful. Treatment for hypersensitivity reactions should be available. Monitor for signs or symptoms of infection. Assess for signs of liver dysfunction (eg, unusual fatigue, dark urine, decreased urine output, abdominal pain, easy bruising or bleeding, jaundice). Report immediately chest pain; bloody or mucus-producing cough; or neck stiffness. Monitor labs throughout treatment. Do not use with live vaccines, such as BCG or influenza, or past allergies to mouse proteins.

Patient Education

• Discuss specific use of drug and side effects with patient as it relates to treatment. (HCAHPS: During this hospital stay, were you given any medicine that you had not taken before? Before giving you any new medicine, how often did hospital staff tell you what the medicine was for? How often did hospital staff describe possible side effects in a way you could understand?)

• Patient may experience headache, dyspepsia, nausea, diarrhea, hepatic impairment, or abscess. Have patient report immediately to prescriber signs of infection, dyspnea, edema, angina, severe asthenia, paresthesia, significant back pain, sudden vision changes, ecchymosis, bleeding, discolored urine, jaundice, night sweats, significant weight gain or loss, or rash (HCAHPS).

• Educate patient about signs of a significant reaction (eg, wheezing; chest tightness; fever; itching; bad cough; blue skin color; seizures; or swelling of face, lips, tongue, or throat). **Note:** This is not a comprehensive list of all side effects. Patient should consult prescriber for additional questions.

Intended Use and Disclaimer: Should not be printed and given to patients. This information is intended to serve as a concise initial reference for healthcare professionals to use when discussing medications with a patient. You must ultimately rely on your own discretion, experience and judgment in diagnosing, treating and advising patients.

Influenza A Virus Vaccine (H5N1)
(in floo EN za aye VYE rus vak SEEN H5N1)

Index Terms Avian Influenza Virus Vaccine; Bird Flu Vaccine; H5N1 Influenza Vaccine; Highly Pathogenic Avian Influenza (HPAI) A (H5N1) Virus Vaccine; Influenza Virus Vaccine (H5N1); Influenza Virus Vaccine (Monovalent); Q-Pan H5N1 Influenza Vaccine

Pharmacologic Category Vaccine, Inactivated (Viral)

Medication Safety Issues

Sound-alike/look-alike issues:

Influenza A virus vaccine (H5N1) may be confused with the nonavian or avian strains of influenza virus vaccine

Pregnancy Risk Factor B/C (product specific)

Lactation Excretion in breast milk unknown/use caution

Use Influenza A (H5N1) immunization:

GlaxoSmithKline product (adjuvanted): For active immunization of persons ≥18 years of age at increased risk of exposure to the influenza A (H5N1) virus subtype contained in the vaccine

Sanofi Pasteur product: For active immunization of persons 18-64 years of age at increased risk of exposure to the influenza A (H5N1) virus subtype contained in the vaccine

Product Availability Products will not be commercially available; distribution will be limited as part of the U.S. Strategic National Stockpile.

GlaxoSmithKline product (adjuvanted) product, (also referred to as Q-Pan H5N1 influenza vaccine): FDA approved November 2013.

Available Dosage Forms

Injection, emulsion [monovalent]: GlaxoSmithKline product: Adjuvanted Hemagglutinin [A/Indonesia/05/2005 (H5N1)] 3.75 mcg/0.5 mL (5 mL)

Injection, suspension [monovalent]: Sanofi Pasteur product: Hemagglutinin [A/Vietnam/1203/2004 (H5N1)] 90 mcg/mL (5 mL)

General Dosage Range I.M.:

Adults ≥18 years: GlaxoSmithKline product (adjuvanted): 0.5 mL, followed by a second 0.5 mL dose given 21 days later

Adults 18-64 years: Sanofi Pasteur product: 1 mL, followed by second 1 mL dose given 28 days later

Administration

I.M. For I.M. administration only. Inspect for particulate matter and discoloration prior to administration. Vaccinate in the deltoid muscle using a ≥1 inch needle length. Suspension should be shaken well prior to use.

GlaxoSmithKline product (adjuvanted): If vaccine is stored under refrigeration after mixing, bring to room temperature prior to administration (minimum 15 minutes).

Note: For patients at risk of hemorrhage following intramuscular injection, the ACIP recommends "it should be administered intramuscularly if, in the opinion of the physician familiar with the patient's bleeding risk, the vaccine can be administered by this route with reasonable safety. If the patient receives antihemophilia or other similar therapy, intramuscular vaccination can be scheduled shortly after such therapy is administered. A fine needle (23 gauge or smaller) can be used for the vaccination and firm pressure applied to the site (without rubbing) for at least 2 minutes. The patient should be instructed concerning the risk of hematoma from the injection." Patients on anticoagulant therapy should be considered to have the same bleeding risks and treated as those with clotting factor disorders (CDC, 2011).

Simultaneous administration of vaccines helps ensure the patients will be fully vaccinated by the appropriate age. Simultaneous administration of vaccines is defined as administering >1 vaccine on the same day at different anatomic sites. Separate vaccines should not be combined in the same syringe unless indicated by product specific labeling. Separate needles and syringes should be used for each injection. The ACIP prefers each

dose of a specific vaccine in a series come from the same manufacturer when possible. Adolescents and adults should be vaccinated while seated or lying down. In general, preterm infants should be vaccinated at the same chronological age as full-term infants (CDC, 2011).

Antipyretics have not been shown to prevent febrile seizures. Antipyretics may be used to treat fever or discomfort following vaccination (CDC, 2011). One study reported that routine prophylactic administration of acetaminophen to prevent fever prior to vaccination decreased the immune response of some vaccines; the clinical significance of this reduction in immune response has not been established (Prymula, 2009).

Nursing Actions

Physical Assessment Patient should be evaluated for contraindications prior to treatment. Treatment for anaphylactic/anaphylactoid reaction should be immediately available during vaccine use. All serious adverse reactions must be reported to the U.S. DHHS. U.S. federal law also requires entry into the patient's medical record.

Patient Education

• Discuss specific use of vaccine and side effects with patient as it relates to treatment. (HCAHPS: During this hospital stay, were you given any medicine that you had not taken before? Before giving you any new medicine, how often did hospital staff tell you what the medicine was for? How often did hospital staff describe possible side effects in a way you could understand?)

• Patient may experience pain, redness or swelling at injection site, headache, fatigue, nausea, emesis, diarrhea, or dyspepsia. Have patient report immediately to prescriber severe injection site reaction (HCAHPS).

• Educate patient about signs of a significant reaction (eg, wheezing; chest tightness; fever; itching; bad cough; blue skin color; seizures; or swelling of face, lips, tongue, or throat). **Note:** This is not a comprehensive list of all side effects. Patient should consult prescriber for additional questions.

Intended Use and Disclaimer: Should not be printed and given to patients. This information is intended to serve as a concise initial reference for healthcare professionals to use when discussing medications with a patient. You must ultimately rely on your own discretion, experience and judgment in diagnosing, treating and advising patients.

Related Information
Immunization Administration Recommendations *on page 1675*
Immunization Recommendations *on page 1680*

Influenza Virus Vaccine (Inactivated)
(in floo EN za VYE rus vak SEEN, in ak ti VAY ted)

Brand Names: U.S. Afluria; Afluria Preservative Free; Fluarix; Fluarix Quadrivalent; Flucelvax; Flulaval; Flulaval Quadrivalent; Fluvirin; Fluvirin Preservative Free; Fluzone; Fluzone High-Dose; Fluzone Pediatric PF; Fluzone Preservative Free; Fluzone Quadrivalent; Medical Provider EZ Flu PF; Physicians EZ Use Flu

Index Terms ccIIV3 [Flucelvax]; Cell Culture Inactivated Influenza Vaccine, Trivalent [Flucelvax]; H1N1 Influenza Vaccine; IIV; IIV3; IIV4; Inactivated Influenza Vaccine, Quadrivalent; Inactivated Influenza Vaccine, Trivalent; Influenza Vaccine; Influenza Virus Vaccine (Purified Surface Antigen); Influenza Virus Vaccine (Split-Virus); TIV (Trivalent Inactivated Influenza Vaccine)

Pharmacologic Category Vaccine, Inactivated (Viral)

Medication Safety Issues
Sound-alike/look-alike issues:
Fluarix may be confused with Flarex
Influenza virus vaccine may be confused with flumazenil
Influenza virus vaccine may be confused with tetanus toxoid and tuberculin products. Medication errors have occurred when tuberculin skin tests (PPD) have been inadvertently administered instead of tetanus toxoid products and influenza virus vaccine. These products are refrigerated and often stored in close proximity to each other.

International issues:
Fluarix [U.S., Canada, and multiple international markets] may be confused with Flarex brand name for fluorometholone [U.S. and multiple international markets] and Fluorex brand name for fluoride [France]

Pregnancy Risk Factor B/C (manufacturer specific)

Lactation Excretion in breast milk unknown/use caution

Use For active immunization against influenza disease caused by influenza virus subtypes A and type B contained in the vaccine

The Advisory Committee on Immunization Practices (ACIP) recommends routine annual vaccination with the seasonal influenza vaccine for all persons ≥6 months of age who do not otherwise have contraindications to the vaccine (CDC, 2013c).

The ACIP recommends use of any age and risk factor appropriate product and does not have a preferential recommendation for use of the trivalent inactivated influenza vaccine (IIV₃) or the quadrivalent inactivated influenza vaccine (IIV₄). In addition to the IIV products, other alternative products are available for certain patient populations: Healthy nonpregnant persons aged 2-49 years may receive vaccination with the live attenuated influenza vaccine (LAIV), and persons 18-49 years may receive vaccination with the recombinant influenza vaccine (RIV) (CDC, 2013c).

When vaccine supply is limited, target groups for vaccination (those at higher risk of complications from influenza infection and their close contacts) include the following:
• Children 6-59 months of age
• Persons ≥50 years of age
• Residents of nursing homes and other long-term care facilities
• Adults and children with chronic pulmonary disorders (including asthma) or cardiovascular systems disorders (except hypertension), renal, hepatic, neurologic, or metabolic disorders (including diabetes mellitus)
• Persons who have immunosuppression (including immunosuppression caused by medications or HIV)
• Children and adolescents (6 months to 18 years of age) who are receiving long-term aspirin therapy, and therefore, may be at risk for developing Reye's syndrome after influenza
• Women who are or will be pregnant during the influenza season
• Healthcare personnel
• Household contacts (including children) and caregivers of children <5 years (particularly children <6 months) and adults ≥50 years
• Household contacts (including children) and caregivers of persons with medical conditions which put them at high risk of complications from influenza infection
• American Indians/Alaska Natives
• Morbidly obese (BMI ≥40)

Available Dosage Forms
Device, Intradermal [preservative free]:
Fluzone: 9 mcg/strain (0.1 mL); 9 mcg/strain (0.1 mL)
Injectable, Intramuscular:
Flulaval: (5 mL)
Fluvirin: (5 mL)
Fluzone: (5 mL)
Kit, Intramuscular:
Physicians EZ Use Flu:
Kit, Intramuscular [preservative free]:
Medical Provider EZ Flu PF:
Suspension, Intramuscular:
Afluria: (5 mL)
Flulaval Quadrivalent: (5 mL)
Suspension, Intramuscular [preservative free]:
Afluria Preservative Free: (0.5 mL)
Fluarix: (0.5 mL)
Fluarix Quadrivalent: 0.5 mL (0.5 mL)

Flucelvax: (0.5 mL)

Fluvirin Preservative Free: (0.5 mL)

Fluzone High-Dose: (0.5 mL)

Fluzone Pediatric PF: (0.25 mL)

Fluzone Preservative Free: (0.5 mL)

Fluzone Quadrivalent: 0.25 mL (0.25 mL); 0.5 mL (0.5 mL)

General Dosage Range

I.M.:

Children 6-35 months: 0.25 mL/dose (1 or 2 doses per season)

Children 3-9 years: 0.5 mL/dose (1 or 2 doses per season)

Children ≥9 years, Adolescents, and Adults: 0.5 mL/dose (1 dose per season)

Intradermal: *Adults:* 18-64 years: 0.1 mL/dose (1 dose per season)

Administration

I.M. *Afluria, Fluarix, Fluarix Quadrivalent, Flucelvax, FluLaval, FluLaval Quadrivalent, Fluvirin, Fluzone, Fluzone High-Dose, Fluzone Quadrivalent, Agriflu (Canadian availability), Fluad (Canadian availability), Fluviral (Canadian availability), Vaxigrip (Canadian availability):* For I.M. administration only. Inspect for particulate matter and discoloration prior to administration. Adults and older children should be vaccinated in the deltoid muscle using a ≥1 inch needle length. Young children (≥6 months to <12 months of age) of age should be vaccinated in the anterolateral aspect of the thigh using a 1 inch needle length. Children ≥1 years with adequate deltoid muscle mass should be vaccinated using a 1 inch needle. A ⅝-inch needle may be adequate in younger children (refer to guidelines) (CDC, 2011a; CDC, 2013c). Do not inject into the gluteal region or areas where there may be a major nerve trunk. Suspensions should be shaken well prior to use. Some manufacturers recommend avoiding use if visible particles are present in the suspension after shaking. See manufacturer's labeling for specific recommendations.

Influvac (Canadian availability): May be administered by I.M. injection. Shake well prior to use.

Unless otherwise indicated in product labeling, jet injectors should **not** be used to administer inactivated influenza vaccines. Currently, there are no influenza vaccines licensed in the United States that can be given by a jet-injector device (2013c).

If a pediatric vaccine (0.25 mL) is inadvertently administered to an adult, an additional 0.25 mL should be administered to provide the full adult dose (0.5 mL). If the error is discovered after the patient has left, an adult dose should be given as soon as the patient can return. If an adult vaccine (0.5 mL) is inadvertently given to a child, no action needs to be taken (CDC, 2013c). *Agriflu (Canadian availability):* If 0.25 mL dose is to be given, discard half the contained syringe volume prior to administration.

Note: For patients at risk of hemorrhage following intramuscular injection, the ACIP recommends "it should be administered intramuscularly if, in the opinion of the physician familiar with the patient's bleeding risk, the vaccine can be administered by this route with reasonable safety. If the patient receives antihemophilia or other similar therapy, intramuscular vaccination can be scheduled shortly after such therapy is administered. A fine needle (23 gauge or smaller) can be used for the vaccination and firm pressure applied to the site (without rubbing) for at least 2 minutes. The patient should be instructed concerning the risk of hematoma from the injection." Patients on anti-coagulant therapy should be considered to have the same bleeding risks and treated as those with clotting factor disorders (CDC, 2011a).

Simultaneous administration of vaccines helps ensure the patients will be fully vaccinated by the appropriate age. Simultaneous administration of vaccines is defined as administering >1 vaccine on the same day at different anatomic sites. Separate vaccines should not be combined in the same syringe unless indicated by product specific labeling. Separate needles and syringes should be used for each injection. However, in general, vaccination should not be deferred if the brand name or route of the previous dose is not available or not known (CDC, 2011a). Adolescents and adults should be vaccinated while seated or lying down. In general, preterm infants should be vaccinated at the same chronological age as full-term infants (CDC, 2011a).

Antipyretics have not been shown to prevent febrile seizures. Antipyretics may be used to treat fever or discomfort following vaccination (CDC, 2011b). One study reported that routine prophylactic administration of acetaminophen to prevent fever prior to vaccination decreased the immune response of some vaccines; the clinical significance of this reduction in immune response has not been established (Prymula, 2009).

Subcutaneous

Influvac (Canadian availability): May be administered by deep subcutaneous injection. Shake well prior to use.

Unless otherwise indicated in product labeling, jet injectors should **not** be used to administer inactivated influenza vaccines. Currently, there are no influenza vaccines licensed in the United States that can be given by a jet-injector device (2013c).

Simultaneous administration of vaccines helps ensure the patients will be fully vaccinated by the appropriate age. Simultaneous administration of vaccines is defined as administering >1 vaccine on the same day at different anatomic sites. Separate vaccines should not be combined in the same syringe unless indicated by product specific labeling. Separate needles and syringes should be used for each injection. However, in general, vaccination should not be deferred if the brand name or route of the previous dose is not available or not known (CDC, 2011a). Adolescents and adults should be vaccinated while seated or lying down. In general, preterm infants should be vaccinated at the same chronological age as full-term infants (CDC, 2011a).

Antipyretics have not been shown to prevent febrile seizures. Antipyretics may be used to treat fever or discomfort following vaccination (CDC, 2011b). One study reported that routine prophylactic administration of acetaminophen to prevent fever prior to vaccination decreased the immune response of some vaccines; the clinical significance of this reduction in immune response has not been established (Prymula, 2009).

Intradermal

Fluzone Intradermal, Intanza (Canadian availability): For intradermal administration over the deltoid muscle only. Fluzone Intradermal should be shaken gently prior to use. Intanza should not be shaken prior to use. Hold system using the thumb and middle finger (do not place fingers on windows). Insert needle perpendicular to the skin; inject using index finger to push on plunger. Do not aspirate.

Unless otherwise indicated in product labeling, jet injectors should **not** be used to administer inactivated influenza vaccines. Currently, there are no influenza vaccines licensed in the United States that can be given by a jet-injector device (2013c).

Simultaneous administration of vaccines helps ensure the patients will be fully vaccinated by the appropriate age. Simultaneous administration of vaccines is defined as administering >1 vaccine on the same day at different anatomic sites. Separate vaccines should not be combined in the same syringe unless indicated by product specific labeling. Separate needles and syringes should be used for each injection. However, in general, vaccination should not be deferred if the brand name or route of the previous dose is not available or not known (CDC, 2011a). Adolescents and adults should be vaccinated while seated or lying down. In general, preterm infants should be vaccinated at the same chronological age as full-term infants (CDC, 2011a).

Antipyretics have not been shown to prevent febrile seizures. Antipyretics may be used to treat fever or discomfort following vaccination (CDC, 2011a). One study reported that routine prophylactic administration of acetaminophen to prevent fever prior to vaccination decreased the immune response of some vaccines; the clinical significance of this reduction in immune response has not been established (Prymula, 2009).

Nursing Actions

Physical Assessment Have emergency treatment for anaphylactoid or hypersensitivity reaction available. Evaluate for allergies (some products are manufactured with chicken egg protein, gentamicin, neomycin, polymyxin, and/or thimerosal), previous adverse reactions (especially Guillain-Barré syndrome), bleeding disorders, presence of acute illness, and immunosuppressed status. All serious adverse reactions must be reported to the U.S. DHHS. U.S. federal law also requires entry into the patient's medical record. Monitor for mild side effects (soreness, redness, or swelling at injection site; fever; aches; itching; fatigue; or headache).

Patient Education

• Discuss specific use of vaccine and side effects with patient as it relates to treatment. (HCAHPS: During this hospital stay, were you given any medicine that you had not taken before? Before giving you any new medicine, how often did hospital staff tell you what the medicine was for? How often did hospital staff describe possible side effects in a way you could understand?)

• Patient may experience pain, redness or swelling at injection site, headache, fatigue, nausea, emesis, diarrhea, or dyspepsia. Have patient report immediately to prescriber severe injection site reaction (HCAHPS).

• Educate patient about signs of a significant reaction (eg, wheezing; chest tightness; fever; itching; bad cough; blue skin color; seizures; or swelling of face, lips, tongue, or throat). **Note:** This is not a comprehensive list of all side effects. Patient should consult prescriber for additional questions.

Intended Use and Disclaimer: Should not be printed and given to patients. This information is intended to serve as a concise initial reference for healthcare professionals to use when discussing medications with a patient. You must ultimately rely on your own discretion, experience and judgment in diagnosing, treating and advising patients.

Related Information

Immunization Administration Recommendations *on page 1675*

Immunization Recommendations *on page 1680*

Influenza Virus Vaccine (Live/ Attenuated)

(in floo EN za VYE rus vak SEEN live ah TEN yoo aye ted)

Brand Names: U.S. FluMist; FluMist Quadrivalent

Index Terms H1N1 Influenza Vaccine; Influenza Vaccine; Influenza Virus Vaccine (Trivalent, Live); LAIV; LAIV$_4$; Live Attenuated Influenza Vaccine; Live Attenuated Influenza Vaccine (Quadrivalent)

Pharmacologic Category Vaccine, Live (Viral)

Medication Safety Issues

Sound-alike/look-alike issues:

Influenza virus vaccine may be confused with flumazenil

Pregnancy Risk Factor B

Lactation Excretion in breast milk unknown/use caution

Use For the active immunization against influenza disease caused by influenza virus subtypes A and type B contained in the vaccine.

The Advisory Committee on Immunization Practices (ACIP) recommends routine annual vaccination with seasonal influenza vaccine for all persons who do not otherwise have contraindications to the vaccine. ACIP recommends use of any age and risk factor appropriate product. Healthy, nonpregnant persons aged 2-49 years may receive vaccination with the seasonal live, attenuated influenza vaccine (LAIV) (nasal spray). In addition, other alternative products are available for certain patient populations: Persons ≥6 months of age may receive the trivalent inactivated influenza vaccine (IIV$_3$) or the quadrivalent inactivated influenza vaccine (IIV$_4$). Persons 18-49 years may also receive vaccination with the recombinant influenza vaccine (RIV) (CDC, 2013c).

Available Dosage Forms

Liquid, Nasal [preservative free]:

FluMist: (1 ea)

Suspension, Nasal [preservative free]:

FluMist Quadrivalent: (1 ea)

General Dosage Range Intranasal:

Children 2-8 years: 0.2 mL/dose (1 or 2 doses per season)

Children ≥9 years, Adolescents, and Adults ≤49 years: 0.2 mL/dose (1 dose per season)

Administration

Other LAIV: Intranasal: For intranasal administration; do not inject. Half the dose (0.1 mL) is administered to each nostril; patient should be in upright position. A dose divider clip is provided to allow administration of 0.1 mL into each nostril. Place the tip of the sprayer inside the nostril and depress plunger as rapidly as possible to deliver the dose. Remove dose divider clip and repeat into opposite nostril. The patient does not need to inhale during administration (may breath normally). Severely immunocompromised persons should not administer the live vaccine. If recipient sneezes following administration, the dose should not be repeated. Defer immunization if nasal congestion is present which may impede delivery of vaccine (CDC, 2013c).

Simultaneous administration of vaccines helps ensure the patients will be fully vaccinated by the appropriate age. Simultaneous administration of vaccines is defined as administering >1 vaccine on the same day at different anatomic sites. The ACIP prefers each dose of a specific vaccine in a series come from the same manufacturer when possible. However, in general, vaccination should not be deferred if the brand name or route of the previous dose is not available or not known (CDC, 2011).

Antipyretics have not been shown to prevent febrile seizures. Antipyretics may be used to treat fever or discomfort following vaccination (CDC, 2011). One study reported that routine prophylactic administration of acetaminophen to prevent fever prior to vaccination decreased the immune response of some vaccines; the clinical significance of this reduction in immune response has not been established (Prymula, 2009). Aspirin-containing products should be avoided for 4 weeks following vaccination in children and adolescents ≤17 years of age.

Vaccine administration with oral influenza antiviral medications: Live influenza virus vaccine (LAIV) should not be given until 48 hours after the completion of influenza antiviral therapy (influenza A and B). Influenza antiviral therapy (influenza A and B) should not be administered for 2 weeks after receiving LAIV. If influenza antiviral therapy (influenza A and B) and LAIV are administered concomitantly, revaccination should be considered.

Nursing Actions

Physical Assessment Monitor for side effects including runny nose, headache, wheezing, vomiting, muscle aches, sore throat, cough, or fever.

Patient Education

- Discuss specific use of vaccine and side effects with patient as it relates to treatment. (HCAHPS: During this hospital stay, were you given any medicine that you had not taken before? Before giving you any new medicine, how often did hospital staff tell you what the medicine was for? How often did hospital staff describe possible side effects in a way you could understand?)
- Patient may experience headache, nausea, diarrhea, or rhinitis. Have patient report immediately to prescriber severe asthenia or rash (HCAHPS).
- Educate patient about signs of a significant reaction (eg, wheezing; chest tightness; fever; itching; bad cough; blue skin color; seizures; or swelling of face, lips, tongue, or throat). **Note:** This is not a comprehensive list of all side effects. Patient should consult prescriber for additional questions.

Intended Use and Disclaimer: Should not be printed and given to patients. This information is intended to serve as a concise initial reference for healthcare professionals to use when discussing medications with a patient. You must ultimately rely on your own discretion, experience and judgment in diagnosing, treating and advising patients.

◀ **Related Information**
Immunization Administration Recommendations *on page 1675*
Immunization Recommendations *on page 1680*

Influenza Virus Vaccine (Recombinant)
(in floo EN za VYE rus vak SEEN ree KOM be nant)

Brand Names: U.S. Flublok
Index Terms Recombinant Influenza Vaccine, Trivalent; RIV; RIV_3; Trivalent Recombinant Hemagglutinin (rHA) Vaccine
Pharmacologic Category Vaccine, Recombinant
Medication Safety Issues
Sound-alike/look-alike issues:
Influenza virus vaccine may be confused with tetanus toxoid and tuberculin products. Medication errors have occurred when tuberculin skin tests (PPD) have been inadvertently administered instead of tetanus toxoid products and influenza virus vaccine. These products are refrigerated and often stored in close proximity to each other.
Pregnancy Risk Factor B
Lactation Excretion in breast milk unknown/use caution
Breast-Feeding Considerations It is not known if this vaccine is excreted into breast milk. The manufacturer recommends that caution be used if administered to breast-feeding women. Recombinant vaccines do not affect the safety of breast-feeding for the mother or the infant. Breast-feeding infants should be vaccinated according to the recommended schedules (CDC, 2011). When vaccine supply is limited, focus on delivering the vaccine should be given to women who are pregnant or will be pregnant during the flu season, as well as mothers of newborns and contacts or caregivers of children <5 years of age (CDC, 2013).
Use For active immunization against influenza disease caused by influenza virus subtypes A and type B contained in the vaccine

The Advisory Committee on Immunization Practices (ACIP) recommends routine annual vaccination with seasonal influenza vaccine for all persons who do not otherwise have contraindications to the vaccine. ACIP recommends use of any age and risk factor appropriate product. Persons 18-49 years of age may receive vaccination with the recombinant influenza vaccine (RIV). In addition to RIV, other products are available for certain patient populations: Healthy nonpregnant persons aged 2-49 years may receive vaccination with the live attenuated influenza vaccine (LAIV). Persons ≥6 months of age may receive the trivalent inactivated influenza vaccine (IIV_3) or the quadrivalent inactivated influenza vaccine (IIV_4) (CDC, 2013c).
Mechanism of Action/Effect Promotes immunity to seasonal influenza virus by inducing specific

antibody production. Each year the formulation is standardized according to the U.S. Public Health Service. Preparations from previous seasons must not be used.
Contraindications Severe allergic reaction (eg, anaphylaxis) to any component of the vaccine
Warnings/Precautions Immediate treatment (including epinephrine 1:1000) for anaphylactoid and/or hypersensitivity reactions should be available during vaccine use. Syncope has been reported with use of injectable vaccines and may be accompanied by transient visual disturbances, weakness, or tonic-clonic movements. Procedures should be in place to avoid injuries from falling and to restore cerebral perfusion if syncope occurs (CDC, 2011). May consider deferring administration in patients with moderate or severe acute illness (with or without fever); may administer to patients with mild acute illness (with or without fever) (CDC, 2011). Use with caution in patients with a history of bleeding disorders (including thrombocytopenia) and/or patients on anticoagulant therapy; bleeding/hematoma may occur from I.M. administration (CDC, 2011). Use with caution in patients with history of Guillain-Barré syndrome (GBS); patients with history of GBS have a greater likelihood of developing GBS than those without. As a precaution, the ACIP recommends that patients with a history of GBS and who are at low risk for severe influenza complications, and patients known to have experienced GBS within 6 weeks following previous vaccination should generally not be vaccinated (consider influenza antiviral chemoprophylaxis in these patients). The benefits of vaccination may outweigh the potential risks in persons with a history of GBS who are also at high risk for complications of influenza. Influenza infection itself may cause Guillain-Barré syndrome (CDC, 2013c). Use with caution in severely-immunocompromised patients (eg, patients receiving chemo/radiation therapy or other immunosuppressive therapy [including high-dose corticosteroid]); may have a reduced response to vaccination. Inactivated vaccine (IIV or RIV) is preferred over live virus vaccine for household members, healthcare workers and others coming in close contact with severely immunosuppressed persons requiring care in a protected environment (CDC, 2011a; CDC, 2013c).

Children 6 months to <3 years of age showed a decreased response to Flublok suggesting that it would not be effective. Flublok is not currently approved for children <18 years of age. Flublok is a trivalent influenza vaccine produced using continuous insect cell lines. It is a recombinant hemagglutinin (rHA) vaccine; it does not use the influenza virus or eggs in its production process. ACIP states it may be used in persons with an egg allergy of any severity if otherwise appropriate (CDC, 2013c).

In order to maximize vaccination rates, the ACIP recommends simultaneous administration of all age-appropriate vaccines (live or inactivated) for which a person is eligible at a single clinic visit, unless contraindications exist (CDC, 2011). Vaccination may not result in effective immunity in all patients. Response depends upon multiple factors (eg, type of vaccine, age of patient) and may be improved by administering the vaccine at the recommended dose, route, and interval. Vaccines may not be effective if administered during periods of altered immune competence (CDC, 2011). Influenza vaccines from previous seasons must not be used (CDC, 2013c). Use of this vaccine for specific medical and/or other indications (eg, immunocompromising conditions, hepatic or kidney disease, diabetes) is also addressed in the ACIP Recommended Immunization Schedule (CDC, 2013a; CDC, 2013b).

Adverse Reactions All serious adverse reactions must be reported to the U.S. Department of Health and Human Services (DHHS) Vaccine Adverse Event Reporting System (VAERS) 1-800-822-7967 or online at https://vaers.hhs. gov/esub/index. In Canada, adverse reactions may be reported to local provincial/territorial health agencies or to the Vaccine Safety Section at Public Health Agency of Canada (1-866-844-0018).

>10%:
  Central nervous system: Fatigue (15%)
  Local: Injection site reactions: Pain (37%)
  Neuromuscular & skeletal: Muscle pain (11%)
1% to 10%:
  Central nervous system: Headache (1% to 2%)
  Gastrointestinal: Nausea (6%)
  Local: Injection site reactions: Redness (4%), Swelling (3%)
  Respiratory: Cough (1% to 2%), nasal congestion (1% to 2%), nasopharyngitis (1% to 2%), pharyngolaryngeal pain (1% to 2%), rhinorrhea (1% to 2%), upper respiratory tract infection (1% to 2%)

Pharmacodynamics/Kinetics
  Onset of Action Most adults have antibody protection within 2 weeks of vaccination (CDC, 2013c)
  Duration of Action ≥6-8 months when vaccine is antigenically similar to circulating virus; response may be diminished in persons ≥65 years and limited evidence suggests titers may decline significantly 6 months following vaccination in this population (CDC, 2013c)

Available Dosage Forms
  Solution, Intramuscular [preservative free]:
  Flublok: (0.5 mL)

General Dosage Range
  I.M.: *Adults 18-49 years:* 0.5 mL/dose (1 per season)

Administration
  I.M. For I.M. administration only. Inspect for particulate matter and discoloration prior to administration. Adults should be vaccinated in the deltoid muscle. Do not inject into the gluteal region or areas where there may be a major nerve trunk. Shake gently prior to use. Avoiding use if visible particles are present in the solution after shaking.

Unless otherwise indicated in product labeling, jet injectors should **not** be used to administer inactivated influenza vaccines. Currently, there are no influenza vaccines licensed in the United States that can be given by a jet-injector device (CDC, 2013c).

Note: For patients at risk of hemorrhage following intramuscular injection, the ACIP recommends "it should be administered intramuscularly if, in the opinion of the physician familiar with the patient's bleeding risk, the vaccine can be administered by this route with reasonable safety. If the patient receives antihemophilia or other similar therapy, intramuscular vaccination can be scheduled shortly after such therapy is administered. A fine needle (23 gauge or smaller) can be used for the vaccination and firm pressure applied to the site (without rubbing) for at least 2 minutes. The patient should be instructed concerning the risk of hematoma from the injection." Patients on anticoagulant therapy should be considered to have the same bleeding risks and treated as those with clotting factor disorders (CDC, 2011).

Simultaneous administration of vaccines helps ensure the patients will be fully vaccinated by the appropriate age. Simultaneous administration of vaccines is defined as administering >1 vaccine on the same day at different anatomic sites. Separate vaccines should not be combined in the same syringe unless indicated by product specific labeling. Separate needles and syringes should be used for each injection. However, in general, vaccination should not be deferred if the brand name or route of the previous dose is not available or not known (CDC, 2011). Adults should be vaccinated while seated or lying down (CDC, 2011).

Antipyretics have not been shown to prevent febrile seizures. Antipyretics may be used to treat fever or discomfort following vaccination (CDC, 2011). One study reported that routine prophylactic administration of acetaminophen to prevent fever prior to vaccination decreased the immune response of some vaccines; the clinical significance of this reduction in immune response has not been established (Prymula, 2009).

Storage/Stability Store between 2°C to 8°C (36°F to 46°F). Protect from light. Do not freeze. Discard if frozen.

Nursing Actions

Physical Assessment Monitor for most common side effects; pain at injection site, headache, fatigue, myalgia, and malaise.

Patient Education

- Discuss specific use of vaccine and side effects with patient as it relates to treatment. (HCAHPS: During this hospital stay, were you given any medicine that you had not taken before? Before giving you any new medicine, how often did hospital staff tell you what the medicine was for? How often did hospital staff describe possible side effects in a way you could understand?)
- Patient may experience pain, redness, or swelling at injection site; headache; fatigue; nausea; emesis; diarrhea; or dyspepsia. Have patient report immediately to prescriber severe injection site reaction (HCAHPS).
- Educate patient about signs of a significant reaction (eg, wheezing; chest tightness; fever; itching; bad cough; blue skin color; seizures; or swelling of face, lips, tongue, or throat). **Note:** This is not a comprehensive list of all side effects. Patient should consult prescriber for additional questions.

Intended Use and Disclaimer: Should not be printed and given to patients. This information is intended to serve as a concise initial reference for healthcare professionals to use when discussing medications with a patient. You must ultimately rely on your own discretion, experience and judgment in diagnosing, treating and advising patients.

Related Information

Immunization Administration Recommendations *on page 1675*
Immunization Recommendations *on page 1680*

Ingenol Mebutate (IN je nol MEB u tate)

Brand Names: U.S. Picato
Index Terms *Euphorbia peplus* Derivative; PEP005
Pharmacologic Category Topical Skin Product
Pregnancy Risk Factor C
Use Topical treatment of actinic keratosis
Available Dosage Forms

Gel, External:
Picato: 0.015% (3 ea); 0.05% (2 ea)

General Dosage Range Topical: *Adults:* Apply once daily for 2 days (0.05%) or 3 days (0.015%)

Administration

Topical Apply to one contiguous affected area of skin using one unit-dose tube; one unit-dose tube will cover ~5 cm x 5 cm (~25 cm^2 or ~2 inch x 2 inch). Spread evenly then allow gel to dry for 15 minutes. Do not cover with bandages or occlusive dressings. Wash hands immediately after applying and avoid transferring gel to any other areas. Avoid washing or touching the treatment area for at least 6 hours, and following this period of time, patients may wash the area with a mild soap. Not for oral, ophthalmic, or intravaginal use.

Nursing Actions

Physical Assessment Educate patient about sun avoidance and ways to protect skin against further sun damage.

Patient Education

- Discuss specific use of drug and side effects with patient as it relates to treatment. (HCAHPS: During this hospital stay, were you given any medicine that you had not taken before? Before giving you any new medicine, how often did hospital staff tell you what the medicine was for? How often did hospital staff describe possible side effects in a way you could understand?)
- Patient may experience skin irritation, scleroderma, edema, or headache. Have patient report immediately to prescriber rash (HCAHPS).
- Educate patient about signs of a significant reaction (eg, wheezing; chest tightness; fever; itching; bad cough; blue skin color; seizures; or swelling of face, lips, tongue, or throat). **Note:** This is not a comprehensive list of all side effects. Patient should consult prescriber for additional questions.

Intended Use and Disclaimer: Should not be printed and given to patients. This information is intended to serve as a concise initial reference for healthcare professionals to use when discussing medications with a patient. You must ultimately rely on your own discretion, experience and judgment in diagnosing, treating and advising patients.

Insulin Aspart (IN soo lin AS part)

Brand Names: U.S. NovoLOG; NovoLOG FlexPen; NovoLOG PenFill
Index Terms Aspart Insulin
Pharmacologic Category Insulin, Rapid-Acting
Medication Safety Issues

Sound-alike/look-alike issues:

NovoLOG® may be confused with HumaLOG®, HumuLIN® R, Nimbex®, NovoLIN® N, Novo-LIN® R, NovoLOG® Mix 70/30

High alert medication:

The Institute for Safe Medication Practices (ISMP) includes this medication among its list of drugs which have a heightened risk of causing significant patient harm when used in error. *Due to the number of insulin preparations, it is essential to identify/clarify the type of insulin to be used.*

Other safety concerns:

Cross-contamination may occur if insulin pens are shared among multiple patients. Steps should be taken to prohibit sharing of insulin pens.

Pregnancy Risk Factor B

Lactation Excretion in breast milk unknown/compatible

Breast-Feeding Considerations It is not known if insulin aspart distributes into breast milk. Endogenous insulin can be found in breast milk. Plasma glucose concentrations in the mother affect glucose concentrations in breast milk. The gastrointestinal tract destroys insulin when administered orally; therefore, insulin is not expected to be absorbed intact by the breast-feeding infant. All types of insulin are safe for use while breast-feeding. Due to increased calorie expenditure, women with diabetes may require less insulin while nursing.

Use Treatment of type 1 diabetes mellitus (insulin dependent, IDDM) and type 2 diabetes mellitus (noninsulin dependent, NIDDM) to improve glycemic control

Unlabeled Use Diabetic ketoacidosis (DKA) (mild-to-moderate); gestational diabetes mellitus (GDM); hyperglycemia during critical illness; hyperosmolar hyperglycemic state (HHS) (mild-to-moderate)

Mechanism of Action/Effect Insulin acts via specific membrane-bound receptors on target tissues to regulate metabolism of carbohydrate, protein, and fats. Target organs for insulin include the liver, skeletal muscle, and adipose tissue.

Within the liver, insulin stimulates hepatic glycogen synthesis. Insulin promotes hepatic synthesis of fatty acids, which are released into the circulation as lipoproteins. Skeletal muscle effects of insulin include increased protein synthesis and increased glycogen synthesis. Within adipose tissue, insulin stimulates the processing of circulating lipoproteins to provide free fatty acids, facilitating triglyceride synthesis and storage by adipocytes; it also directly inhibits the hydrolysis of triglycerides. In addition, insulin stimulates the cellular uptake of amino acids and increases cellular permeability to several ions, including potassium, magnesium, and phosphate. By activating sodium-potassium ATPases, insulin promotes the intracellular movement of potassium.

Insulins are categorized based on the onset, peak, and duration of effect (eg, rapid-, short-, intermediate-, and long-acting insulin). Insulin aspart is a rapid-acting insulin analog.

Contraindications Hypersensitivity to insulin aspart or any component of the formulation; during episodes of hypoglycemia

Warnings/Precautions Hypoglycemia is the most common adverse effect of insulin. The timing of hypoglycemia differs among various insulin formulations. Hypoglycemia may result from increased work or exercise without eating; use of long-acting insulin preparations (eg, insulin detemir, insulin glargine) may delay recovery from hypoglycemia. Profound and prolonged episodes of hypoglycemia may result in convulsions, unconsciousness, temporary or permanent brain damage, or even death.

Insulin requirements may be altered during illness, emotional disturbances, or other stressors. Insulin may produce hypokalemia which, if left untreated, may result in respiratory paralysis, ventricular arrhythmia, and even death. Use with caution in patients at risk for hypokalemia (eg, I.V. insulin use). Use with caution in renal or hepatic impairment. In the elderly, avoid use of sliding scale insulin in this population due to increased risk of hypoglycemia without benefits in management of hyperglycemia regardless of care setting (Beers Criteria).

Due to the short duration of action of insulin aspart, a longer acting insulin or CSII via an external insulin pump is needed to maintain adequate glucose control in patients with type 1 diabetes mellitus. In both type 1 and type 2 diabetes, preprandial administration of insulin aspart should be immediately followed by a meal within 5-10 minutes. May also be administered via CSII; do not dilute or mix with other insulin formulations when using an external insulin pump. Rule out pump failure if unexplained hyperglycemia or ketosis occurs; temporary SubQ insulin administration may be required until the problem is identified and corrected. Insulin aspart may also be administered I.V. in selected clinical situations to control hyperglycemia; close monitoring of blood glucose and serum potassium as well as medical supervision is required. According to the Centers for Disease Control and Prevention (CDC), pen-shaped injection devices should never be used for more than one person (even when the needle is changed) because of the risk of infection. The injection device should be clearly labeled with individual patient information to ensure that the correct pen is used (CDC, 2012).

The general objective of exogenous insulin therapy is to approximate the physiologic pattern of insulin secretion which is characterized by two distinct phases. Phase 1 insulin secretion suppresses hepatic glucose production and phase 2 insulin secretion occurs in response to carbohydrate ingestion; therefore, exogenous insulin therapy may consist of basal insulin (eg, intermediate- or long-acting insulin or via continuous subcutaneous insulin infusion [CSII]) and/or preprandial insulin (eg, short- or rapid-acting insulin [eg, insulin aspart]) (see Related Information: Insulin Regular). Patients with type 1 diabetes do not produce endogenous insulin; therefore, these patients require both basal and preprandial insulin administration. Patients with type 2 diabetes retain some beta-cell function in the early stages of their disease; however, as the disease progresses, phase 1 insulin secretion may become completely impaired and phase 2 insulin secretion becomes delayed and/or inadequate in response to meals. Therefore, patients with type 2 diabetes may be treated with oral antidiabetic agents, basal insulin, and/or prandial insulin depending on the stage of disease and current glycemic control. Since treatment regimens often consist of multiple agents, dosage adjustments must address the specific phase of insulin release that is primarily contributing to the patient's impaired glycemic control. Diabetes self-management education (DSME) is essential to maximize the effectiveness of therapy. Treatment and monitoring regimens must be individualized.

Potentially significant drug-drug interactions may exist, requiring dose or frequency adjustment, additional monitoring, and/or selection of alternative therapy.

Drug Interactions

Avoid Concomitant Use There are no known interactions where it is recommended to avoid concomitant use.

Decreased Effect

The levels/effects of Insulin Aspart may be decreased by: Corticosteroids (Orally Inhaled); Corticosteroids (Systemic); Loop Diuretics; Luteinizing Hormone-Releasing Hormone Analogs; Somatropin; Thiazide Diuretics

Increased Effect/Toxicity

Insulin Aspart may increase the levels/effects of: Antidiabetic Agents (Thiazolidinedione); Hypoglycemic Agents; Quinolone Antibiotics

The levels/effects of Insulin Aspart may be increased by: Beta-Blockers; Edetate CALCIUM Disodium; Edetate Disodium; Herbs (Hypoglycemic Properties); MAO Inhibitors; Metreleptin; Pegvisomant; Salicylates; Selective Serotonin Reuptake Inhibitors

Nutritional/Ethanol Interactions

Ethanol: Use caution with ethanol; may increase risk of hypoglycemia.

Herb/Nutraceutical: Use caution with alfalfa, aloe, bilberry, bitter melon, burdock, celery, damiana, fenugreek, garcinia, garlic, ginger, ginseng (American), gymnema, marshmallow, stinging nettle; may increase risk of hypoglycemia.

Pharmacodynamics/Kinetics

Onset of Action 0.2-0.3 hours; Peak effect: 1-3 hours

Duration of Action 3-5 hours

Available Dosage Forms

Solution, Subcutaneous:

NovoLOG: 100 units/mL (10 mL)

NovoLOG FlexPen: 100 units/mL (3 mL)

NovoLOG PenFill: 100 units/mL (3 mL)

General Dosage Range SubQ: *Children ≥2 years, Adolescents, and Adults:* Daily doses are expressed as the **total units/kg/day of all insulin formulations combined.** Diabetes mellitus, type 1: Initial: 0.2-0.6 units/kg/day in divided doses; usual maintenance: 0.5-1 units/kg/day in divided doses.

Administration

I.V. Do not use if solution is viscous or cloudy; use only if clear and colorless. May be administered I.V. with close monitoring of blood glucose and serum potassium; appropriate medical supervision is required. **Do not administer insulin mixtures intravenously.**

I.V. infusions: To minimize insulin adsorption to I.V. tubing: Flush the I.V. tubing with a priming infusion of 20 mL from the insulin infusion, whenever a new I.V. tubing set is added to the insulin infusion container (Jacobi, 2012; Thompson, 2012).

Note: Also refer to institution-specific protocols where appropriate.

Because of insulin adsorption to I.V. tubing or infusion bags, the actual amount of insulin being administered via I.V. infusion could be substantially less than the apparent amount. Therefore, adjustment of the I.V. infusion rate should be based on effect and not solely on the apparent insulin dose. The apparent dose may be used as a starting point for determining the subsequent SubQ dosing regimen (Moghissi, 2009); however, the transition to SubQ administration requires continuous medical supervision, frequent monitoring of blood glucose, and careful adjustment of therapy. In addition, SubQ insulin should be given 1-4 hours prior to the discontinuation of I.V. insulin to prevent hyperglycemia (Moghissi, 2009).

Injectable Detail pH: 7.2-7.6

Subcutaneous

SubQ administration: Do not use if solution is viscous or cloudy; use only if clear and colorless. Insulin aspart should be administered immediately (within 5-10 minutes) before a meal. Cold injections should be avoided. SubQ administration is usually made into the thighs, arms, buttocks, or abdomen; rotate injection sites. When mixing insulin aspart with other preparations of insulin (eg, insulin NPH), insulin aspart should be drawn into syringe first. Do not dilute or mix other insulin formulations with insulin aspart contained in a cartridge or prefilled pen.

CSII administration: Do not use if solution is viscous or cloudy; use only if clear and colorless. Patients should be trained in the proper use of their external insulin pump and in intensive insulin therapy. Infusion sets and infusion set insertion sites should be changed at least every 3 days; rotate infusion sites. Do not dilute or mix other insulin formulations with insulin aspart that is to be used in an external insulin pump.

Preparation for Administration

For SubQ administration: *NovoLog® vials:* May be diluted with Insulin Diluting Medium for NovoLog® to a concentration of 10 units/mL (U-10) or 50 units/mL (U-50). Do not dilute insulin contained in a cartridge, prefilled pen, or external insulin pump.

For I.V. infusion: May be diluted in NS, D$_5$W, or D$_{10}$W to concentrations of 0.05-1 unit/mL.

Storage/Stability Unopened vials, cartridges, and prefilled pens may be stored under refrigeration between 2°C and 8°C (36°F to 46°F) until the expiration date or at room temperature <30°C (<86°F) for 28 days; do not freeze; keep away from heat and sunlight. Once punctured (in use), vials may be stored under refrigeration or at room temperature <30°C (<86°F); use within 28 days. Cartridges and prefilled pens that have been punctured (in use) should be stored at temperatures <30°C (<86°F) and used within 28 days; do not freeze or refrigerate. When used for CSII, insulin aspart contained within an external insulin pump reservoir should be replaced at least every 6 days; discard if exposed to temperatures >37°C (>98.6°F).

For SubQ administration: *NovoLog® vials:* According to the manufacturer, diluted insulin should be stored at temperatures <30°C (<86°F) and used within 28 days.

For I.V. infusion: Stable for 24 hours at room temperature.

Nursing Actions

Physical Assessment Monitor for hypoglycemia at regular intervals during therapy. Teach patient proper use, including appropriate injection technique and syringe/needle disposal, and monitoring requirements.

Patient Education

- Discuss specific use of drug and side effects with patient as it relates to treatment. (HCAHPS: During this hospital stay, were you given any medicine that you had not taken before? Before giving you any new medicine, how often did hospital staff tell you what the medicine was for? How often did hospital staff describe possible side effects in a way you could understand?)
- Patient may experience hypoglycemia, nausea, weight gain, or application site irritation. Have patient report immediately to prescriber rash, signs of infection, or severe hyperglycemia (HCAHPS).
- Educate patient about signs of a significant reaction (eg, wheezing; chest tightness; fever; itching; bad cough; blue skin color; seizures; or swelling of face, lips, tongue, or throat). **Note:** This is not a comprehensive list of all side effects. Patient should consult prescriber for additional questions.

Intended Use and Disclaimer: Should not be printed and given to patients. This information is intended to serve as a concise initial reference for healthcare professionals to use when discussing medications with a patient. You must ultimately rely on your own discretion, experience and judgment in diagnosing, treating and advising patients.

Dietary Considerations Individualized medical nutrition therapy (MNT) based on ADA recommendations is an integral part of therapy.

Related Information

Insulin Regular *on page 855*

Insulin Aspart Protamine and Insulin Aspart (IN soo lin AS part PROE ta meen & IN soo lin AS part)

Brand Names: U.S. NovoLOG® Mix 70/30; NovoLOG® Mix 70/30 FlexPen®

Index Terms Insulin Aspart and Insulin Aspart Protamine; NovoLog 70/30

Pharmacologic Category Insulin, Combination

Medication Safety Issues

Sound-alike/look-alike issues:

NovoLOG® Mix 70/30 may be confused with HumaLOG® Mix 75/25™, HumuLIN® 70/30, NovoLIN® 70/30, NovoLOG®

High alert medication:

The Institute for Safe Medication Practices (ISMP) includes this medication among its list of drugs which have a heightened risk of causing significant patient harm when used in error. *Due to the number of insulin preparations, it is essential to identify/clarify the type of insulin to be used.*

Other safety concerns:

Cross-contamination may occur if insulin pens are shared among multiple patients. Steps should be taken to prohibit sharing of insulin pens.

Pregnancy Risk Factor B

Lactation Excretion in breast milk unknown

Use Treatment of type 1 diabetes mellitus (insulin dependent, IDDM) and type 2 diabetes mellitus (noninsulin dependent, NIDDM) to improve glycemic control

Available Dosage Forms

Injection, suspension:

NovoLOG® Mix 70/30: Insulin aspart protamine suspension 70% [intermediate acting] and insulin aspart solution 30% [rapid acting]: 100 units/mL (10 mL)

NovoLOG® Mix 70/30 FlexPen®: Insulin aspart protamine suspension 70% [intermediate acting] and insulin aspart solution 30% [rapid acting]: 100 units/mL (3 mL)

General Dosage Range SubQ: *Adults:* Diabetes mellitus, type 1 or 2: **Not** intended for initial therapy; basal insulin requirements should be established **first** to direct dosing of combination insulin products.

Administration

Other SubQ administration: In order to properly resuspend the insulin, vials and prefilled pens should be gently rolled between the palms ten times; in addition, prefilled pens should be inverted 180° ten times. Properly resuspended insulin should look uniformly cloudy or milky; do not use if any white insulin substance remains at ▶

the bottom of the container, if any clumps are present, if the insulin remains clear after adequate mixing, or if white particles are stuck to the bottom or wall of the container. Cold injections should be avoided. Insulin aspart protamine and insulin aspart combination products should be administered within 15 minutes before a meal (type 1 diabetes) or 15 minutes before or after a meal (type 2 diabetes); typically given twice daily. SubQ administration is usually made into the thighs, arms, buttocks, or abdomen; rotate injection sites. Do not dilute or mix with any other insulin formulation or solution; not recommended for use in external SubQ insulin infusion pump.

Nursing Actions
Physical Assessment See individual agents.
Patient Education
- Discuss specific use of drug and side effects with patient as it relates to treatment. (HCAHPS: During this hospital stay, were you given any medicine that you had not taken before? Before giving you any new medicine, how often did hospital staff tell you what the medicine was for? How often did hospital staff describe possible side effects in a way you could understand?)
- Patient may experience hypoglycemia, nausea, weight gain, or injection site irritation. Have patient report immediately to prescriber signs of infection, dyspnea, edema, or severe hyperglycemia (HCAHPS).
- Educate patient about signs of a significant reaction (eg, wheezing; chest tightness; fever; itching; bad cough; blue skin color; seizures; or swelling of face, lips, tongue, or throat). **Note:** This is not a comprehensive list of all side effects. Patient should consult prescriber for additional questions.

Intended Use and Disclaimer: Should not be printed and given to patients. This information is intended to serve as a concise initial reference for healthcare professionals to use when discussing medications with a patient. You must ultimately rely on your own discretion, experience and judgment in diagnosing, treating and advising patients.

Related Information
Insulin Regular *on page 855*

Insulin Detemir (IN soo lin DE te mir)

Brand Names: U.S. Levemir; Levemir FlexPen
Index Terms Detemir Insulin
Pharmacologic Category Insulin, Intermediate-to Long-Acting
Medication Safety Issues
High alert medication:
The Institute for Safe Medication Practices (ISMP) includes this medication among its list of drugs which have a heightened risk of causing significant patient harm when used in error. *Due*

to the number of insulin preparations, it is essential to identify/clarify the type of insulin to be used.
Administration issues:
Insulin detemir is a clear solution, but it is NOT intended for I.V. or I.M. administration.
Other safety concerns:
Cross-contamination may occur if insulin pens are shared among multiple patients. Steps should be taken to prohibit sharing of insulin pens.
Pregnancy Risk Factor B
Lactation Excretion in breast milk unknown/use caution
Breast-Feeding Considerations It is not known if insulin detemir distributes into breast milk. Endogenous insulin can be found in breast milk. Plasma glucose concentrations in the mother affect glucose concentrations in breast milk. The gastrointestinal tract destroys insulin when administered orally; therefore, insulin is not expected to be absorbed intact by the breast-feeding infant. All types of insulin are safe for use while breast-feeding. Although use of insulin detemir is compatible with breast-feeding, the manufacturer recommends that caution be used when insulin detemir is used by nursing women. Due to increased calorie expenditure, women with diabetes may require less insulin while nursing.
Use Treatment of type 1 diabetes mellitus (insulin dependent, IDDM) and type 2 diabetes mellitus (noninsulin dependent, NIDDM) to improve glycemic control
Mechanism of Action/Effect Insulin acts via specific membrane-bound receptors on target tissues to regulate metabolism of carbohydrate, protein, and fats. Target organs for insulin include the liver, skeletal muscle, and adipose tissue.

Within the liver, insulin stimulates hepatic glycogen synthesis. Insulin promotes hepatic synthesis of fatty acids, which are released into the circulation as lipoproteins. Skeletal muscle effects of insulin include increased protein synthesis and increased glycogen synthesis. Within adipose tissue, insulin stimulates the processing of circulating lipoproteins to provide free fatty acids, facilitating triglyceride synthesis and storage by adipocytes; also directly inhibits the hydrolysis of triglycerides. In addition, insulin stimulates the cellular uptake of amino acids and increases cellular permeability to several ions, including potassium, magnesium, and phosphate. By activating sodium-potassium ATPases, insulin promotes the intracellular movement of potassium.

Insulins are categorized based on the onset, peak, and duration of effect (eg, rapid-, short-, intermediate-, and long-acting insulin). Insulin detemir is an intermediate- to long-acting insulin analog.
Contraindications Hypersensitivity to insulin detemir or any component of the formulation
Warnings/Precautions Hypoglycemia is the most common adverse effect of insulin. The timing of

hypoglycemia differs among various insulin formulations. Hypoglycemia may result from increased work or exercise without eating; use of long-acting insulin preparations (eg, insulin detemir, insulin glargine) may delay recovery from hypoglycemia. Profound and prolonged episodes of hypoglycemia may result in convulsions, unconsciousness, temporary or permanent brain damage or even death. Insulin requirements may be altered during illness, emotional disturbances or other stressors. Insulin may produce hypokalemia which, if left untreated, may result in respiratory paralysis, ventricular arrhythmia and even death. Use with caution in renal or hepatic impairment.

The duration of action of insulin detemir is dose-dependent; consider this factor during dosage adjustment and titration. Insulin detemir, although a clear solution, is **NOT** intended for I.V. or I.M. administration. According to the Centers for Disease Control and Prevention (CDC), pen-shaped injection devices should never be used for more than one person (even when the needle is changed) because of the risk of infection. The injection device should be clearly labeled with individual patient information to ensure that the correct pen is used (CDC, 2012).

The general objective of exogenous insulin therapy is to approximate the physiologic pattern of insulin secretion which is characterized by two distinct phases. Phase 1 insulin secretion suppresses hepatic glucose production and phase 2 insulin secretion occurs in response to carbohydrate ingestion; therefore, exogenous insulin therapy may consist of basal insulin (eg, intermediate- or long-acting insulin [eg, insulin detemir] or via continuous subcutaneous insulin infusion [CSII]) and/or preprandial insulin (eg, short- or rapid-acting insulin) (see Related Information: Insulin Regular). Patients with type 1 diabetes do not produce endogenous insulin; therefore, these patients require both basal and preprandial insulin administration. Patients with type 2 diabetes retain some beta-cell function in the early stages of their disease; however, as the disease progresses, phase 1 insulin secretion may become completely impaired and phase 2 insulin secretion becomes delayed and/or inadequate in response to meals. Therefore, patients with type 2 diabetes may be treated with oral antidiabetic agents, basal insulin, and/or preprandial insulin depending on the stage of disease and current glycemic control. Since treatment regimens often consist of multiple agents, dosage adjustments must address the specific phase of insulin release that is primarily contributing to the patient's impaired glycemic control. Diabetes self-management education (DSME) is essential to maximize the effectiveness of therapy. Treatment and monitoring regimens must be individualized.

Potentially significant drug-drug interactions may exist, requiring dose or frequency adjustment, additional monitoring, and/or selection of alternative therapy.

Drug Interactions

Avoid Concomitant Use There are no known interactions where it is recommended to avoid concomitant use.

Decreased Effect

The levels/effects of Insulin Detemir may be decreased by: Corticosteroids (Orally Inhaled); Corticosteroids (Systemic); Loop Diuretics; Luteinizing Hormone-Releasing Hormone Analogs; Somatropin; Thiazide Diuretics

Increased Effect/Toxicity

Insulin Detemir may increase the levels/effects of: Antidiabetic Agents (Thiazolidinedione); Hypoglycemic Agents; Quinolone Antibiotics

The levels/effects of Insulin Detemir may be increased by: Beta-Blockers; Edetate CALCIUM Disodium; Edetate Disodium; Herbs (Hypoglycemic Properties); MAO Inhibitors; Metreleptin; Pegvisomant; Salicylates; Selective Serotonin Reuptake Inhibitors

Nutritional/Ethanol Interactions

Ethanol: Use caution with ethanol; may increase risk of hypoglycemia.

Herb/Nutraceutical: Use caution with alfalfa, aloe, bilberry, bitter melon, burdock, celery, damiana, fenugreek, garcinia, garlic, ginger, ginseng (American), gymnema, marshmallow, stinging nettle; may increase risk of hypoglycemia.

Adverse Reactions Primarily symptoms of hypoglycemia

Cardiovascular: Pallor, palpitation, tachycardia

Central nervous system: Fatigue, headache, hypothermia, loss of consciousness, mental confusion

Dermatologic: Redness, urticaria

Endocrine & metabolic: Hypoglycemia, hypokalemia

Gastrointestinal: Hunger, nausea, numbness of mouth

Local: Atrophy or hypertrophy of SubQ fat tissue; edema, itching, pain or warmth at injection site; stinging

Neuromuscular & skeletal: Muscle weakness, paresthesia, tremor

Ocular: Transient presbyopia or blurred vision

Miscellaneous: Anaphylaxis, diaphoresis, local and/or systemic hypersensitivity reactions

Pharmacodynamics/Kinetics

Onset of Action 3-4 hours; Peak effect: 3-9 hours (Plank, 2005)

Duration of Action Dose dependent: 6-23 hours; **Note:** Duration is dose-dependent. At lower dosages (0.1-0.2 units/kg), mean duration is variable (5.7-12.1 hours). At 0.4 units/kg, the mean duration was 19.9 hours. At high dosages (≥0.8 units/kg) the duration is longer and less variable (mean of 22-23 hours) (Plank, 2005).

Available Dosage Forms
Solution, Subcutaneous:
Levemir: 100 units/mL (10 mL)
Levemir FlexPen: 100 units/mL (3 mL)
General Dosage Range SubQ:
Children ≥2 years, Adolescents, and Adults: Diabetes mellitus, type 1: Initial dose: Approximately one-third of the total daily insulin requirement administered in 1-2 divided doses.
Adults: Diabetes mellitus, type 2: Initial: 10 units **or** 0.1-0.2 units/kg in 1-2 divided doses

Administration
Other Do **not** administer I.M or I.V.; for SubQ administration only: Do not use if solution is viscous or cloudy; use only if clear and colorless with no visible particles. Insulin detemir should be administered once or twice daily. When given once daily, administer with the evening meal or at bedtime. When given twice daily, administer the evening dose with the evening meal, at bedtime, or 12 hours following the morning dose. Cold injections should be avoided. SubQ administration is usually made into the thighs, arms, or abdomen; rotate injection sites. Do not dilute or mix insulin detemir with any other insulin formulation or solution; **not** recommended for use in external SubQ insulin infusion pump.

Storage/Stability Unopened vials, cartridges, and prefilled pens may be stored under refrigeration between 2°C and 8°C (36°F to 46°F) until the expiration date or at room temperature <30°C (<86°F) for 42 days; do not freeze; keep away from heat and sunlight. Once punctured (in use), vials may be stored under refrigeration or at room temperature <30°C (<86°F); use within 42 days. Cartridges and prefilled pens that have been punctured (in use) should be stored at temperatures <30°C (<86°F) and used within 42 days; do not freeze or refrigerate.

Nursing Actions
Physical Assessment Monitor for hypoglycemia at regular intervals during therapy. Teach patient proper use, including appropriate injection technique and syringe/needle disposal, and monitoring requirements.

Patient Education
• Discuss specific use of drug and side effects with patient as it relates to treatment. (HCAHPS: During this hospital stay, were you given any medicine that you had not taken before? Before giving you any new medicine, how often did hospital staff tell you what the medicine was for? How often did hospital staff describe possible side effects in a way you could understand?)
• Patient may experience hypoglycemia, nausea, weight gain, or application site irritation. Have patient report immediately to prescriber rash, signs of infection, or severe hyperglycemia (HCAHPS).
• Educate patient about signs of a significant reaction (eg, wheezing; chest tightness; fever; itching; bad cough; blue skin color; seizures; or swelling of face, lips, tongue, or throat). **Note:** This is not a comprehensive list of all side effects. Patient should consult prescriber for additional questions.

Intended Use and Disclaimer: Should not be printed and given to patients. This information is intended to serve as a concise initial reference for healthcare professionals to use when discussing medications with a patient. You must ultimately rely on your own discretion, experience and judgment in diagnosing, treating and advising patients.

Dietary Considerations Individualized medical nutrition therapy (MNT) based on ADA recommendations is an integral part of therapy.

Related Information
Insulin Regular *on page 855*

Insulin Glargine (IN soo lin GLAR jeen)

Brand Names: U.S. Lantus; Lantus SoloStar
Index Terms Glargine Insulin
Pharmacologic Category Insulin, Long-Acting
Medication Safety Issues
Sound-alike/look-alike issues:
Insulin glargine may be confused with insulin glulisine
Lantus® may be confused with latanoprost, Latuda®, Xalatan®
High alert medication:
The Institute for Safe Medication Practices (ISMP) includes this medication among its list of drugs which have a heightened risk of causing significant patient harm when used in error. *Due to the number of insulin preparations, it is essential to identify/clarify the type of insulin to be used.*
Administration issues:
Insulin glargine is a clear solution, but it is NOT intended for I.V. or I.M. administration.
Other safety concerns:
Cross-contamination may occur if insulin pens are shared among multiple patients. Steps should be taken to prohibit sharing of insulin pens.
International issues:
Lantus [U.S., Canada, and multiple international markets] may be confused with Lanvis brand name for thioguanine [Canada and multiple international markets]

Pregnancy Risk Factor C
Lactation Excretion in breast milk unknown/use caution
Breast-Feeding Considerations It is not known if significant amounts of insulin glargine distributes into breast milk. Endogenous insulin can be found in breast milk. Plasma glucose concentrations in the mother affect glucose concentrations in breast milk. The gastrointestinal tract destroys insulin when administered orally; therefore, insulin is not

expected to be absorbed intact by the breast-feeding infant. All types of insulin are safe for use while breast-feeding. Due to increased calorie expenditure, women with diabetes may require less insulin while nursing.

Use Treatment of type 1 diabetes mellitus (insulin dependent, IDDM) and type 2 diabetes mellitus (noninsulin dependent, NIDDM) to improve glycemic control

Mechanism of Action/Effect Insulin acts via specific membrane-bound receptors on target tissues to regulate metabolism of carbohydrate, protein, and fats. Target organs for insulin include the liver, skeletal muscle, and adipose tissue.

Within the liver, insulin stimulates hepatic glycogen synthesis. Insulin promotes hepatic synthesis of fatty acids, which are released into the circulation as lipoproteins. Skeletal muscle effects of insulin include increased protein synthesis and increased glycogen synthesis. Within adipose tissue, insulin stimulates the processing of circulating lipoproteins to provide free fatty acids, facilitating triglyceride synthesis and storage by adipocytes; also directly inhibits the hydrolysis of triglycerides. In addition, insulin stimulates the cellular uptake of amino acids and increases cellular permeability to several ions, including potassium, magnesium, and phosphate. By activating sodium-potassium ATPases, insulin promotes the intracellular movement of potassium.

Insulins are categorized based on the onset, peak, and duration of effect (eg, rapid-, short-, intermediate-, and long-acting insulin). Insulin glargine is a long-acting insulin analog.

Contraindications Hypersensitivity to insulin glargine or any component of the formulation

Warnings/Precautions Hypoglycemia is the most common adverse effect of insulin. The timing of hypoglycemia differs among various insulin formulations. Hypoglycemia may result from increased work or exercise without eating; use of long-acting insulin preparations (eg, insulin detemir, insulin glargine) may delay recovery from hypoglycemia. Profound and prolonged episodes of hypoglycemia may result in convulsions, unconsciousness, temporary or permanent brain damage or even death. Insulin requirements may be altered during illness, emotional disturbances or other stressors. Insulin may produce hypokalemia which, if left untreated, may result in respiratory paralysis, ventricular arrhythmia and even death. Use with caution in renal or hepatic impairment.

Insulin glargine is a clear solution, but it is **NOT** intended for I.V. or I.M. administration. According to the Centers for Disease Control and Prevention (CDC), pen-shaped injection devices should never be used for more than one person (even when the needle is changed) because of the risk of infection. The injection device should be clearly labeled with individual patient information to ensure that the correct pen is used (CDC, 2012).

The general objective of exogenous insulin therapy is to approximate the physiologic pattern of insulin secretion which is characterized by two distinct phases. Phase 1 insulin secretion suppresses hepatic glucose production and phase 2 insulin secretion occurs in response to carbohydrate ingestion; therefore, exogenous insulin therapy may consist of basal insulin (eg, intermediate- or long-acting insulin [eg, insulin glargine] or via continuous subcutaneous insulin infusion [CSII]) and/or preprandial insulin (eg, short- or rapid-acting insulin) (see Related Information: Insulin Regular). Patients with type 1 diabetes do not produce endogenous insulin; therefore, these patients require both basal and preprandial insulin administration. Patients with type 2 diabetes retain some beta-cell function in the early stages of their disease; however, as the disease progresses, phase 1 insulin secretion may become completely impaired and phase 2 insulin secretion becomes delayed and/or inadequate in response to meals. Therefore, patients with type 2 diabetes may be treated with oral antidiabetic agents, basal insulin, and/or preprandial insulin depending on the stage of disease and current glycemic control. Since treatment regimens often consist of multiple agents, dosage adjustments must address the specific phase of insulin release that is primarily contributing to the patient's impaired glycemic control. Diabetes self-management education (DSME) is essential to maximize the effectiveness of therapy. Treatment and monitoring regimens must be individualized.

Potentially significant drug-drug interactions may exist, requiring dose or frequency adjustment, additional monitoring, and/or selection of alternative therapy.

Drug Interactions

Avoid Concomitant Use There are no known interactions where it is recommended to avoid concomitant use.

Decreased Effect

The levels/effects of Insulin Glargine may be decreased by: Corticosteroids (Orally Inhaled); Corticosteroids (Systemic); Loop Diuretics; Luteinizing Hormone-Releasing Hormone Analogs; Somatropin; Thiazide Diuretics

Increased Effect/Toxicity

Insulin Glargine may increase the levels/effects of: Antidiabetic Agents (Thiazolidinedione); Hypoglycemic Agents; Quinolone Antibiotics

The levels/effects of Insulin Glargine may be increased by: Beta-Blockers; Edetate CALCIUM Disodium; Edetate Disodium; Herbs (Hypoglycemic Properties); MAO Inhibitors; Metreleptin; Pegvisomant; Salicylates; Selective Serotonin Reuptake Inhibitors

Nutritional/Ethanol Interactions

Ethanol: Use caution with ethanol; may increase risk of hypoglycemia.

Herb/Nutraceutical: Use caution with alfalfa, aloe, bilberry, bitter melon, burdock, celery, damiana, fenugreek, garcinia, garlic, ginger, ginseng (American), gymnema, marshmallow, stinging nettle; may increase risk of hypoglycemia.

Adverse Reactions Primarily symptoms of hypoglycemia

Cardiovascular: Pallor, palpitation, tachycardia

Central nervous system: Fatigue, headache, hypothermia, loss of consciousness, mental confusion

Dermatologic: Redness, urticaria

Endocrine & metabolic: Hypoglycemia, hypokalemia

Gastrointestinal: Hunger, nausea, numbness of mouth

Local: Atrophy or hypertrophy of SubQ fat tissue; edema, itching, pain or warmth at injection site; stinging

Neuromuscular & skeletal: Muscle weakness, paresthesia, tremor

Ocular: Transient presbyopia or blurred vision

Miscellaneous: Anaphylaxis, diaphoresis, local and/or systemic hypersensitivity reactions

Pharmacodynamics/Kinetics

Onset of Action 3-4 hours; Peak effect: No pronounced peak

Duration of Action Generally 24 hours or longer; reported range: 10.8 to >24 hours (up to 32 hours documented in some studies)

Available Dosage Forms

Solution, Subcutaneous:

Lantus: 100 units/mL (10 mL)

Lantus SoloStar: 100 units/mL (3 mL)

General Dosage Range SubQ:

Children ≥6 years, Adolescents, and Adults: Diabetes mellitus, type 1: Initial dose: Approximately one-third of the total daily insulin requirement administered once daily

Adults: Diabetes mellitus, type 2: Initial: 10 units or 0.2 units/kg once daily

Administration

Other SubQ administration: Do not use if solution is viscous or cloudy; use only if clear and colorless with no visible particles. Insulin glargine should be administered once daily, at any time of day; however, administer at the same time each day. Cold injections should be avoided. SubQ administration is usually made into the thighs, arms, buttocks, or abdomen; rotate injection sites. Do not dilute or mix insulin glargine with any other insulin formulation or solution.

Storage/Stability Unopened vials, cartridges, and prefilled pens may be stored under refrigeration between 2°C and 8°C (36°F to 46°F) until the expiration date or at room temperature <30°C (<86°F) for 28 days; do not freeze; keep away from heat and sunlight. Once punctured (in use), vials may be stored under refrigeration or at room temperature <30°C (<86°F); use within 28 days. Cartridges within the OptiClik® system and pre-filled pens (SoloStar®) that have been punctured (in use) should be stored at temperatures <30°C (<86°F) and used within 28 days; do not freeze or refrigerate.

Nursing Actions

Physical Assessment Monitor for hypoglycemia at regular intervals during therapy. Teach patient proper use, including appropriate injection technique and syringe/needle disposal, and monitoring requirements.

Patient Education

• Discuss specific use of drug and side effects with patient as it relates to treatment. (HCAHPS: During this hospital stay, were you given any medicine that you had not taken before? Before giving you any new medicine, how often did hospital staff tell you what the medicine was for? How often did hospital staff describe possible side effects in a way you could understand?)

• Patient may experience hypoglycemia, nausea, weight gain, or application site irritation. Have patient report immediately to prescriber rash, signs of infection, or severe hyperglycemia (HCAHPS).

• Educate patient about signs of a significant reaction (eg, wheezing; chest tightness; fever; itching; bad cough; blue skin color; seizures; or swelling of face, lips, tongue, or throat). **Note:** This is not a comprehensive list of all side effects. Patient should consult prescriber for additional questions.

Intended Use and Disclaimer: Should not be printed and given to patients. This information is intended to serve as a concise initial reference for healthcare professionals to use when discussing medications with a patient. You must ultimately rely on your own discretion, experience and judgment in diagnosing, treating and advising patients.

Dietary Considerations Individualized medical nutrition therapy (MNT) based on ADA recommendations is an integral part of therapy.

Related Information

Insulin Regular *on page 855*

Insulin Glulisine (IN soo lin gloo LIS een)

Brand Names: U.S. Apidra; Apidra SoloStar

Index Terms Glulisine Insulin

Pharmacologic Category Insulin, Rapid-Acting

Medication Safety Issues

Sound-alike/look-alike issues:

Insulin glulisine may be confused with insulin glargine

High alert medication:

The Institute for Safe Medication Practices (ISMP) includes this medication among its list of drugs which have a heightened risk of causing significant patient harm when used in error. *Due to the number of insulin preparations, it is essential to identify/clarify the type of insulin to be used.*

Other safety concerns:

Cross-contamination may occur if insulin pens are shared among multiple patients. Steps should be taken to prohibit sharing of insulin pens.

Pregnancy Risk Factor C

Lactation Excretion in breast milk unknown/use caution

Use Treatment of type 1 diabetes mellitus (insulin dependent, IDDM) and type 2 diabetes mellitus (noninsulin dependent, NIDDM) to improve glycemic control

Unlabeled Use Hyperglycemia during critical illness

Available Dosage Forms

Solution, Injection:

Apidra: 100 units/mL (10 mL)

Solution, Subcutaneous:

Apidra SoloStar: 100 units/mL (3 mL)

General Dosage Range SubQ: *Children ≥4 years, Adolescents and Adults:* Diabetes mellitus, type 1: **Note:** Multiple daily doses or continuous subcutaneous infusions guided by blood glucose monitoring are the standard of diabetes care. Combinations of insulin formulations are commonly used. The daily doses presented below are expressed as the **total units/kg/day of all insulin formulations combined.**

Initial: 0.2-0.6 units/kg/day in divided doses; usual maintenance: 0.5-1 units/kg/day in divided doses.

Administration

I.V.

Do not use if solution is viscous or cloudy; use only if clear and colorless. May be administered I.V. with close monitoring of blood glucose and serum potassium; appropriate medical supervision is required. **Do not administer insulin mixtures intravenously.**

I.V. infusions: To minimize insulin adsorption to I.V. tubing: Flush the I.V. tubing with a priming infusion of 20 mL from the insulin infusion, whenever a new I.V. tubing set is added to the insulin infusion container (Jacobi, 2012; Thompson, 2012).

Note: Also refer to institution-specific protocols where appropriate.

Because of insulin adsorption to I.V. tubing or infusion bags, the actual amount of insulin being administered via I.V. infusion could be substantially less than the apparent amount. Therefore, adjustment of the I.V. infusion rate should be based on effect and not solely on the apparent insulin dose. The apparent dose may be used as a starting point for determining the subsequent SubQ dosing regimen (Moghissi, 2009); however, the transition to SubQ administration requires continuous medical supervision, frequent monitoring of blood glucose, and careful adjustment of therapy. In addition, SubQ insulin should be given 1-4 hours prior to the discontinuation of I.V. insulin to prevent hyperglycemia (Moghissi, 2009).

Injectable Detail pH: ~7.3

Subcutaneous

SubQ administration: Do not use if solution is viscous or cloudy; use only if clear and colorless. Insulin glulisine should be administered within 15 minutes before or within 20 minutes after starting a meal. Cold injections should be avoided. SubQ administration is usually made into the thighs, arms, buttocks, or abdomen; rotate injection sites. When mixing insulin glulisine with other preparations of insulin (eg, insulin NPH), insulin glulisine should be drawn into syringe first. Do not mix other insulin formulations with insulin glulisine contained in a cartridge or prefilled pen.

CSII administration: Do not use if solution is viscous or cloudy; use only if clear and colorless. Patients should be trained in the proper use of their external insulin pump and in intensive insulin therapy. Infusion sets, reservoirs, and infusion set insertion sites should be changed every 48 hours; rotate infusion sites. Do not dilute or mix other insulin formulations with insulin glulisine that is to be used in an external insulin pump.

Nursing Actions

Physical Assessment Monitor for hypoglycemia at regular intervals during therapy. Teach patient proper use, including appropriate injection technique and syringe/needle disposal, and monitoring requirements.

Patient Education

• Discuss specific use of drug and side effects with patient as it relates to treatment. (HCAHPS: During this hospital stay, were you given any medicine that you had not taken before? Before giving you any new medicine, how often did hospital staff tell you what the medicine was for? How often did hospital staff describe possible side effects in a way you could understand?)

• Patient may experience hypoglycemia, nausea, weight gain, or application site irritation. Have patient report immediately to prescriber rash, signs of infection, or severe hyperglycemia (HCAHPS).

• Educate patient about signs of a significant reaction (eg, wheezing; chest tightness; fever; itching; bad cough; blue skin color; seizures; or swelling of face, lips, tongue, or throat). **Note:** This is not a comprehensive list of all side effects. Patient should consult prescriber for additional questions.

Intended Use and Disclaimer: Should not be printed and given to patients. This information is intended to serve as a concise initial reference for healthcare professionals to use when discussing ▶

medications with a patient. You must ultimately rely on your own discretion, experience and judgment in diagnosing, treating and advising patients.

Related Information
Insulin Regular *on page 855*

Insulin Lispro (IN soo lin LYE sproe)

Brand Names: U.S. HumaLOG; HumaLOG KwikPen
Index Terms Lispro Insulin
Pharmacologic Category Insulin, Rapid-Acting
Medication Safety Issues
Sound-alike/look-alike issues:
HumaLOG® may be confused with HumaLOG® Mix 50/50, Humira®, HumuLIN® N, HumuLIN® R, NovoLOG®
High alert medication:
The Institute for Safe Medication Practices (ISMP) includes this medication among its list of drugs which have a heightened risk of causing significant patient harm when used in error. *Due to the number of insulin preparations, it is essential to identify/clarify the type of insulin to be used.*
Other safety concerns:
Cross-contamination may occur if insulin pens are shared among multiple patients. Steps should be taken to prohibit sharing of insulin pens.
Pregnancy Risk Factor B
Lactation Excretion in breast milk unknown/compatible
Breast-Feeding Considerations It is not known if insulin lispro distributes into breast milk. Endogenous insulin can be found in breast milk. Plasma glucose concentrations in the mother affect glucose concentrations in breast milk. The gastrointestinal tract destroys insulin when administered orally; therefore, insulin is not expected to be absorbed intact by the breast-feeding infant. All types of insulin are safe for use while breast-feeding. Due to increased calorie expenditure, women with diabetes may require less insulin while nursing.
Use Treatment of type 1 diabetes mellitus (insulin dependent, IDDM) and type 2 diabetes mellitus (noninsulin dependent, NIDDM) to improve glycemic control
Unlabeled Use Gestational diabetes mellitus (GDM); mild-to-moderate diabetic ketoacidosis (DKA); mild-to-moderate hyperosmolar hyperglycemic state (HHS)
Mechanism of Action/Effect Insulin acts via specific membrane-bound receptors on target tissues to regulate metabolism of carbohydrate, protein, and fats. Target organs for insulin include the liver, skeletal muscle, and adipose tissue.

Within the liver, insulin stimulates hepatic glycogen synthesis. Insulin promotes hepatic synthesis of fatty acids, which are released into the circulation as lipoproteins. Skeletal muscle effects of insulin include increased protein synthesis and increased glycogen synthesis. Within adipose tissue, insulin stimulates the processing of circulating lipoproteins to provide free fatty acids, facilitating triglyceride synthesis and storage by adipocytes; also directly inhibits the hydrolysis of triglycerides. In addition, insulin stimulates the cellular uptake of amino acids and increases cellular permeability to several ions, including potassium, magnesium, and phosphate. By activating sodium-potassium ATPases, insulin promotes the intracellular movement of potassium.

Insulins are categorized based on the onset, peak, and duration of effect (eg, rapid-, short-, intermediate-, and long-acting insulin). Insulin lispro is a rapid-acting insulin analog.
Contraindications Hypersensitivity to insulin lispro or any component of the formulation; during episodes of hypoglycemia
Warnings/Precautions Hypoglycemia is the most common adverse effect of insulin. The timing of hypoglycemia differs among various insulin formulations. Hypoglycemia may result from increased work or exercise without eating; use of long-acting insulin preparations (eg, insulin detemir, insulin glargine) may delay recovery from hypoglycemia. Profound and prolonged episodes of hypoglycemia may result in convulsions, unconsciousness, temporary or permanent brain damage, or even death. Insulin requirements may be altered during illness, emotional disturbances, or other stressors. Insulin may produce hypokalemia which, if left untreated, may result in respiratory paralysis, ventricular arrhythmia, and even death. Use with caution in patients at risk for hypokalemia (eg, I.V. insulin use). Use with caution in renal or hepatic impairment. In the elderly, avoid use of sliding scale insulin in this population due to increased risk of hypoglycemia without benefits in management of hyperglycemia regardless of care setting (Beers Criteria).

Due to the short duration of action of insulin lispro, a longer acting insulin or CSII via an external insulin pump is needed to maintain adequate glucose control in patients with type 1 diabetes mellitus. In both type 1 and type 2 diabetes, preprandial administration of insulin lispro should be immediately followed by a meal within 15 minutes. May also be administered via CSII; do not dilute or mix with other insulin formulations when using an external insulin pump. Rule out pump failure if unexplained hyperglycemia or ketosis occurs; temporary SubQ insulin administration may be required until the problem is identified and corrected. Insulin lispro may also be administered I.V. in selected clinical situations to control hyperglycemia; close monitoring of blood glucose and serum potassium as well as medical supervision is required. According to the Centers for Disease

Control and Prevention (CDC), pen-shaped injection devices should never be used for more than one person (even when the needle is changed) because of the risk of infection. The injection device should be clearly labeled with individual patient information to ensure that the correct pen is used (CDC, 2012).

The general objective of exogenous insulin therapy is to approximate the physiologic pattern of insulin secretion which is characterized by two distinct phases. Phase 1 insulin secretion suppresses hepatic glucose production and phase 2 insulin secretion occurs in response to carbohydrate ingestion; therefore, exogenous insulin therapy may consist of basal insulin (eg, intermediate- or long-acting insulin or via continuous subcutaneous insulin infusion [CSII]) and/or preprandial insulin (eg, short- or rapid-acting insulin [insulin lispro]) (see Related Information: Insulin Regular). Patients with type 1 diabetes do not produce endogenous insulin; therefore, these patients require both basal and preprandial insulin administration. Patients with type 2 diabetes retain some beta-cell function in the early stages of their disease; however, as the disease progresses, phase 1 insulin secretion may become completely impaired and phase 2 insulin secretion becomes delayed and/or inadequate in response to meals. Therefore, patients with type 2 diabetes may be treated with oral antidiabetic agents, basal insulin, and/or preprandial insulin depending on the stage of disease and current glycemic control. Since treatment regimens often consist of multiple agents, dosage adjustments must address the specific phase of insulin release that is primarily contributing to the patient's impaired glycemic control. Diabetes self-management education (DSME) is essential to maximize the effectiveness of therapy. Treatment and monitoring regimens must be individualized.

Potentially significant drug-drug interactions may exist, requiring dose or frequency adjustment, additional monitoring, and/or selection of alternative therapy.

Drug Interactions

Avoid Concomitant Use There are no known interactions where it is recommended to avoid concomitant use.

Decreased Effect

The levels/effects of Insulin Lispro may be decreased by: Corticosteroids (Orally Inhaled); Corticosteroids (Systemic); Loop Diuretics; Luteinizing Hormone-Releasing Hormone Analogs; Somatropin; Thiazide Diuretics

Increased Effect/Toxicity

Insulin Lispro may increase the levels/effects of: Antidiabetic Agents (Thiazolidinedione); Hypoglycemic Agents; Quinolone Antibiotics

The levels/effects of Insulin Lispro may be increased by: Beta-Blockers; Edetate CALCIUM Disodium; Edetate Disodium; Herbs (Hypoglycemic Properties); MAO Inhibitors; Metreleptin; Pegvisomant; Salicylates; Selective Serotonin Reuptake Inhibitors

Nutritional/Ethanol Interactions

Ethanol: Use caution with ethanol; may increase risk of hypoglycemia.

Herb/Nutraceutical: Use caution with alfalfa, aloe, bilberry, bitter melon, burdock, celery, damiana, fenugreek, garcinia, garlic, ginger, ginseng (American), gymnema, marshmallow, stinging nettle; may increase risk of hypoglycemia.

Adverse Reactions Primarily symptoms of hypoglycemia

Cardiovascular: Pallor, palpitation, tachycardia

Central nervous system: Fatigue, headache, hypothermia, loss of consciousness, mental confusion

Dermatologic: Redness, urticaria

Endocrine & metabolic: Hypoglycemia, hypokalemia

Gastrointestinal: Hunger, nausea, numbness of mouth

Local: Atrophy or hypertrophy of SubQ fat tissue; edema, itching, pain or warmth at injection site; stinging

Neuromuscular & skeletal: Muscle weakness, paresthesia, tremor

Ocular: Transient presbyopia or blurred vision

Miscellaneous: Anaphylaxis, diaphoresis, local and/or systemic hypersensitivity reactions

Pharmacodynamics/Kinetics

Onset of Action SubQ: 0.25-0.5 hours; Peak effect: SubQ: 0.5-2.5 hours

Duration of Action SubQ: ≤5 hours

Available Dosage Forms

Solution, Subcutaneous:

HumaLOG: 100 units/mL (3 mL, 10 mL)

HumaLOG KwikPen: 100 units/mL (3 mL)

General Dosage Range SubQ: *Children ≥3 years, Adolescents and Adults:* Daily doses are expressed as the **total units/kg/day of all insulin formulations combined.** Diabetes mellitus, type 1: Initial: 0.2-0.6 units/kg/day in divided doses; usual maintenance: 0.5-1 units/kg/day in divided doses.

Administration

I.V. I.V. administration: Do not use if solution is viscous or cloudy; use only if clear and colorless. May be administered I.V. with close monitoring of blood glucose and serum potassium; appropriate medical supervision is required. Do not administer insulin mixtures intravenously.

I.V. infusions: To minimize adsorption to I.V. solution bag: **Note:** Refer to institution-specific protocols where appropriate.

If new tubing is not needed: Wait a minimum of 30 minutes between the preparation of the solution and the initiation of the infusion. Wait a minimum of 30 minutes between the preparation of the solution and the initiation of the infusion.

If new tubing is needed: After receiving the insulin drip solution, the administration set should be attached to the I.V. container and the entire line should be flushed with a priming infusion of 20-50 mL of the insulin solution (Goldberg, 2006; Hirsch, 2006). Wait 30 minutes, and then flush the line again with the insulin solution prior to initiating the infusion. Because of adsorption, the actual amount of insulin being administered via I.V. infusion could be substantially less than the apparent amount. Therefore, adjustment of the I.V. infusion rate should be based on effect and not solely on the apparent insulin dose. The apparent dose may be used as a starting point for determining the subsequent SubQ dosing regimen (Moghissi, 2009); however, the transition to SubQ administration requires continuous medical supervision, frequent monitoring of blood glucose, and careful adjustment of therapy. In addition, SubQ insulin should be given 1-4 hours prior to the discontinuation of I.V. insulin to prevent hyperglycemia (Moghissi, 2009).

Injectable Detail pH: 7-7.8

Subcutaneous Do not use if solution is viscous or cloudy; use only if clear and colorless. Insulin lispro should be administered within 15 minutes before or immediately after a meal. Cold injections should be avoided. SubQ administration is usually made into the thighs, arms, buttocks, or abdomen; rotate injection sites. When mixing insulin lispro with other preparations of insulin (eg, insulin NPH), insulin lispro should be drawn into syringe first. Do not dilute or mix other insulin formulations with insulin lispro contained in a cartridge or prefilled pen.

Other CSII administration: Do not use if solution is viscous or cloudy; use only if clear and colorless. Patients should be trained in the proper use of their external insulin pump and in intensive insulin therapy. Infusion sets and infusion set insertion sites should be changed every 3 days; rotate infusion sites. Insulin in reservoir should be changed every 7 days. Do not dilute or mix other insulin formulations with insulin lispro contained in an external insulin pump.

Preparation for Administration

For SubQ administration: *Humalog® vials:* May be diluted with the universal diluent, Sterile Diluent for Humalog®, Humulin® N, Humulin® R, Humulin® 70/30, and Humulin® R U-500, to a concentration of 10 units/mL (U-10) or 50 units/mL (U-50). Do not dilute insulin contained in a cartridge, prefilled pen, or external insulin pump.

For I.V. infusion: May be diluted in NS to concentrations of 0.1-1 units/mL.

Storage/Stability Unopened vials, cartridges, and prefilled pens may be stored under refrigeration between 2°C and 8°C (36°F to 46°F) until the expiration date or at room temperature <30°C (<86°F) for 28 days; do not freeze; keep away from heat and sunlight. Once punctured (in use), vials may be stored under refrigeration or at room temperature <30°C (<86°F); use within 28 days. Cartridges and prefilled pens that have been punctured (in use) should be stored at temperatures <30°C (<86°F) and used within 28 days; do not freeze or refrigerate. When used for CSII, insulin lispro contained within an external insulin pump reservoir should be changed every 7 days and insulin lispro contained within a 3 mL cartridge should be discarded after 7 days; discard if exposed to temperatures >37°C (>98.6°F).

For SubQ administration: *Humalog® vials:* According to the manufacturer, diluted insulin should be stored at 30°C (86°F) and used within 14 days or 5°C (41°F) and used within 28 days.

For I.V. infusion: Stable for 48 hours when stored under refrigeration between 2°C and 8°C (36°F to 46°F); may then be used at room temperature for an additional 48 hours.

Nursing Actions

Physical Assessment Monitor for hypoglycemia at regular intervals during therapy. Teach patient proper use, including appropriate injection technique and syringe/needle disposal, and monitoring requirements.

Patient Education

- Discuss specific use of drug and side effects with patient as it relates to treatment. (HCAHPS: During this hospital stay, were you given any medicine that you had not taken before? Before giving you any new medicine, how often did hospital staff tell you what the medicine was for? How often did hospital staff describe possible side effects in a way you could understand?)
- Patient may experience hypoglycemia, nausea, weight gain, or application site irritation. Have patient report immediately to prescriber rash, signs of infection, or severe hyperglycemia (HCAHPS).
- Educate patient about signs of a significant reaction (eg, wheezing; chest tightness; fever; itching; bad cough; blue skin color; seizures; or swelling of face, lips, tongue, or throat). **Note:** This is not a comprehensive list of all side effects. Patient should consult prescriber for additional questions.

Intended Use and Disclaimer: Should not be printed and given to patients. This information is intended to serve as a concise initial reference for healthcare professionals to use when discussing medications with a patient. You must ultimately rely on your own discretion, experience and judgment in diagnosing, treating and advising patients.

Dietary Considerations Individualized medical nutrition therapy (MNT) based on ADA recommendations is an integral part of therapy.

Related Information

Insulin Regular *on page 855*

Insulin Lispro Protamine and Insulin Lispro

(IN soo lin LYE sproe PROE ta meen & IN soo lin LYE sproe)

Brand Names: U.S. HumaLOG® Mix 50/50™; HumaLOG® Mix 50/50™ KwikPen™; HumaLOG® Mix 75/25™; HumaLOG® Mix 75/25™ KwikPen™

Index Terms Insulin Lispro and Insulin Lispro Protamine

Pharmacologic Category Insulin, Combination

Medication Safety Issues

Sound-alike/look-alike issues:

HumaLOG® Mix 50/50™ may be confused with HumaLOG®

HumaLOG® Mix 75/25™ may be confused with HumuLIN® 70/30, NovoLIN® 70/30, and Novo-LOG® Mix 70/30

High alert medication:

The Institute for Safe Medication Practices (ISMP) includes this medication among its list of drugs which have a heightened risk of causing significant patient harm when used in error. *Due to the number of insulin preparations, it is essential to identify/clarify the type of insulin to be used.*

Other safety concerns:

Cross-contamination may occur if insulin pens are shared among multiple patients. Steps should be taken to prohibit sharing of insulin pens.

Pregnancy Risk Factor B

Lactation Excretion in breast milk unknown/compatible

Use Treatment of type 1 diabetes mellitus (insulin dependent, IDDM) and type 2 diabetes mellitus (noninsulin dependent, NIDDM) to improve glycemic control

Available Dosage Forms

Injection, suspension:

HumaLOG® Mix 50/50™: Insulin lispro protamine suspension 50% [intermediate acting] and insulin lispro solution 50% [rapid acting]: 100 units/mL (10 mL)

HumaLOG® Mix 50/50™ KwikPen™: Insulin lispro protamine suspension 50% [intermediate acting] and insulin lispro solution 50% [rapid acting]: 100 units/mL (3 mL)

HumaLOG® Mix 75/25™: Insulin lispro protamine suspension 75% [intermediate acting] and insulin lispro solution 25% [rapid acting]: 100 units/mL (10 mL)

HumaLOG® Mix 75/25™ KwikPen™: Insulin lispro protamine suspension 75% [intermediate acting] and insulin lispro solution 25% [rapid acting]: 100 units/mL (3 mL)

General Dosage Range SubQ: *Adults:* Diabetes mellitus, type 1 or 2: **Not** intended for initial therapy; basal insulin requirements should be established **first** to direct dosing of combination insulin products.

Administration

Other SubQ administration: In order to properly resuspend the insulin, vials should be carefully shaken or rolled several times and prefilled pens should be rolled between the palms ten times and inverted 180° ten times. Properly resuspended insulin should look uniformly cloudy or milky; do not use if any white insulin substance remains at the bottom of the container, if any clumps are present, if the insulin remains clear after adequate mixing, or if white particles are stuck to the bottom or wall of the container. Cold injections should be avoided. Insulin lispro protamine and insulin lispro combination products should be administered within 15 minutes before a meal; typically given once- or twice daily. SubQ administration is usually made into the thighs, arms, buttocks, or abdomen; rotate injection sites. Do not dilute or mix with any other insulin formulation or solution; **not** recommended for use in external SubQ insulin infusion pump.

Nursing Actions

Physical Assessment See individual agents.

Patient Education

- Discuss specific use of drug and side effects with patient as it relates to treatment. (HCAHPS: During this hospital stay, were you given any medicine that you had not taken before? Before giving you any new medicine, how often did hospital staff tell you what the medicine was for? How often did hospital staff describe possible side effects in a way you could understand?)

- Patient may experience hypoglycemia, nausea, weight gain, or injection site irritation. Have patient report immediately to prescriber signs of infection, dyspnea, edema, or severe hyperglycemia (HCAHPS).

- Educate patient about signs of a significant reaction (eg, wheezing; chest tightness; fever; itching; bad cough; blue skin color; seizures; or swelling of face, lips, tongue, or throat). **Note:** This is not a comprehensive list of all side effects. Patient should consult prescriber for additional questions.

Intended Use and Disclaimer: Should not be printed and given to patients. This information is intended to serve as a concise initial reference for healthcare professionals to use when discussing medications with a patient. You must ultimately rely on your own discretion, experience and judgment in diagnosing, treating and advising patients.

Related Information
Insulin Regular *on page 855*

Insulin NPH (IN soo lin N P H)

Brand Names: U.S. HumuLIN N KwikPen; Humu-LIN N Pen [OTC]; HumuLIN N [OTC]; NovoLIN N ReliOn [OTC]; NovoLIN N [OTC]
Index Terms Isophane Insulin; NPH Insulin
Pharmacologic Category Insulin, Intermediate-Acting
Medication Safety Issues
Sound-alike/look-alike issues:
HumuLIN® N may be confused with HumuLIN® R, HumaLOG®, Humira®
NovoLIN® N may be confused with NovoLIN® R, NovoLOG®
High alert medication:
The Institute for Safe Medication Practices (ISMP) includes this medication among its list of drugs which have a heightened risk of causing significant patient harm when used in error. *Due to the number of insulin preparations, it is essential to identify/clarify the type of insulin to be used.*
Other safety concerns:
Cross-contamination may occur if insulin pens are shared among multiple patients. Steps should be taken to prohibit sharing of insulin pens.
Lactation Excretion in breast milk unknown
Use Treatment of type 1 diabetes mellitus (insulin dependent, IDDM) and type 2 diabetes mellitus (noninsulin dependent, NIDDM) to improve glycemic control
Unlabeled Use Gestational diabetes mellitus (GDM)
Available Dosage Forms
Suspension, Subcutaneous:
HumuLIN N [OTC]: 100 units/mL (3 mL, 10 mL)
HumuLIN N KwikPen: 100 units/mL (3 mL)
HumuLIN N Pen [OTC]: 100 units/mL (3 mL)
NovoLIN N [OTC]: 100 units/mL (10 mL)
NovoLIN N ReliOn [OTC]: 100 units/mL (10 mL)
General Dosage Range SubQ:
Children ≥2 years, Adolescents, and Adults: Daily doses are expressed as the **total units/kg/day of all insulin formulations combined.** Diabetes mellitus, type 1: Initial: 0.2-0.6 units/kg/day in divided doses; usual maintenance: 0.5-1 units/kg/day in divided doses.
Adults: Diabetes mellitus, type 2: Initial: 0.2 units/kg/day or 10 units/day in divided doses before meals.
Administration
Other SubQ administration: In order to properly resuspend the insulin, vials should be carefully shaken or rolled several times, prefilled pens should be rolled between the palms ten times and inverted 180° ten times, and cartridges should be inverted 180° at least ten times.

Properly resuspended insulin NPH should look uniformly cloudy or milky; do not use if any white insulin substance remains at the bottom of the container, if any clumps are present, or if white particles are stuck to the bottom or wall of the container. Cold injections should be avoided. SubQ administration is usually made into the thighs, arms, buttocks, or abdomen; rotate injection sites. When mixing insulin NPH with other preparations of insulin (eg, insulin aspart, insulin glulisine, insulin lispro, insulin regular), insulin NPH should be drawn into the syringe **after** the other insulin preparations. Do not dilute or mix other insulin formulations with insulin NPH contained in a cartridge or prefilled pen. Insulin NPH is **not** recommended for use in external SubQ insulin infusion pump.
Nursing Actions
Physical Assessment Monitor for hypoglycemia at regular intervals during therapy. Teach patient proper use, including appropriate injection technique and syringe/needle disposal, and monitoring requirements.
Patient Education
• Discuss specific use of drug and side effects with patient as it relates to treatment. (HCAHPS: During this hospital stay, were you given any medicine that you had not taken before? Before giving you any new medicine, how often did hospital staff tell you what the medicine was for? How often did hospital staff describe possible side effects in a way you could understand?)
• Patient may experience hypoglycemia, nausea, weight gain, or application site irritation. Have patient report immediately to prescriber rash, signs of infection, or severe hyperglycemia (HCAHPS).
• Educate patient about signs of a significant reaction (eg, wheezing; chest tightness; fever; itching; bad cough; blue skin color; seizures; or swelling of face, lips, tongue, or throat). **Note:** This is not a comprehensive list of all side effects. Patient should consult prescriber for additional questions.

Intended Use and Disclaimer: Should not be printed and given to patients. This information is intended to serve as a concise initial reference for healthcare professionals to use when discussing medications with a patient. You must ultimately rely on your own discretion, experience and judgment in diagnosing, treating and advising patients.
Related Information
Insulin Regular *on page 855*

Insulin NPH and Insulin Regular
(IN soo lin N P H & IN soo lin REG yoo ler)

Brand Names: U.S. HumuLIN® 70/30; HumuLIN® 70/30 KwikPen; NovoLIN® 70/30

Index Terms Insulin Regular and Insulin NPH; Isophane Insulin and Regular Insulin; NPH Insulin and Regular Insulin

Pharmacologic Category Insulin, Combination

Medication Safety Issues

Sound-alike/look-alike issues:

HumuLIN® 70/30 may be confused with Huma-LOG® Mix 75/25, HumuLIN® R, NovoLIN® 70/30, NovoLOG® Mix 70/30

NovoLIN® 70/30 may be confused with Huma-LOG® Mix 75/25, HumuLIN® 70/30, HumuLIN® R, NovoLIN® R, and NovoLOG® Mix 70/30

High alert medication:

The Institute for Safe Medication Practices (ISMP) includes this medication among its list of drugs which have a heightened risk of causing significant patient harm when used in error. *Due to the number of insulin preparations, it is essential to identify/clarify the type of insulin to be used.*

Other safety concerns:

Cross-contamination may occur if insulin pens are shared among multiple patients. Steps should be taken to prohibit sharing of insulin pens.

Use Treatment of type 1 diabetes mellitus (insulin dependent, IDDM) and type 2 diabetes mellitus (noninsulin dependent, NIDDM) to improve glycemic control

Unlabeled Use Gestational diabetes mellitus (GDM)

Available Dosage Forms

Injection, suspension:

HumuLIN® 70/30: Insulin NPH suspension 70% [intermediate acting] and insulin regular solution 30% [short acting]: 100 units/mL (3 mL, 10 mL)

HumuLIN® 70/30 KwikPen: Insulin NPH suspension 70% [intermediate acting] and insulin regular solution 30% [short acting]: 100 units/mL (3 mL)

NovoLIN® 70/30: Insulin NPH suspension 70% [intermediate acting] and insulin regular solution 30% [short acting]: 100 units/mL (10 mL)

General Dosage Range SubQ:

Children, Adolescents, and Adults: Daily doses are expressed as the **total units/kg/day of all insulin formulations combined.** Diabetes mellitus, type 1: Initial: 0.2-0.6 units/kg/day in divided doses; usual maintenance: 0.5-1 units/kg/day in divided doses.

Adults: Diabetes mellitus, type 2: **Not** intended for initial therapy; basal insulin requirements should be established **first** to direct dosing of combination insulin products.

Administration

Other SubQ administration: In order to properly resuspend the insulin, vials should be carefully shaken or rolled several times, prefilled pens should be rolled between the palms ten times and inverted 180° ten times, and cartridges should be inverted 180° at least ten times. Properly resuspended insulin should look uniformly cloudy or milky; do not use if any white insulin substance remains at the bottom of the container, if any clumps are present, if the insulin remains clear after adequate mixing, or if white particles are stuck to the bottom or wall of the container. Cold injections should be avoided. Insulin NPH and insulin regular combination products should be administered within 30 minutes before a meal; typically given once- or twice daily. SubQ administration is usually made into the thighs, arms, buttocks, or abdomen; rotate injection sites. Do not mix with any other insulin formulation. Do not dilute combination product (insulin NPH and insulin regular) contained in a cartridge or prefilled pen. Combination insulin products are not recommended for use in an external SubQ insulin infusion pump.

Nursing Actions

Physical Assessment See individual agents.

Patient Education

• Discuss specific use of drug and side effects with patient as it relates to treatment. (HCAHPS: During this hospital stay, were you given any medicine that you had not taken before? Before giving you any new medicine, how often did hospital staff tell you what the medicine was for? How often did hospital staff describe possible side effects in a way you could understand?)

• Patient may experience hypoglycemia, nausea, weight gain, or injection site irritation. Have patient report immediately to prescriber signs of infection, dyspnea, edema, or severe hyperglycemia (HCAHPS).

• Educate patient about signs of a significant reaction (eg, wheezing; chest tightness; fever; itching; bad cough; blue skin color; seizures; or swelling of face, lips, tongue, or throat). **Note:** This is not a comprehensive list of all side effects. Patient should consult prescriber for additional questions.

Intended Use and Disclaimer: Should not be printed and given to patients. This information is intended to serve as a concise initial reference for healthcare professionals to use when discussing medications with a patient. You must ultimately rely on your own discretion, experience and judgment in diagnosing, treating and advising patients.

Related Information

Insulin Regular *on page 855*

Insulin Regular (IN soo lin REG yoo ler)

Brand Names: U.S. HumuLIN R U-500 (CONCENTRATED); HumuLIN R [OTC]; NovoLIN R ReliOn [OTC]; NovoLIN R [OTC]

Index Terms Regular Insulin

Pharmacologic Category Insulin, Short-Acting

Medication Safety Issues

Sound-alike/look-alike issues:

HumuLIN® R may be confused with HumaLOG®, Humira®, HumuLIN® 70/30, HumuLIN® N, NovoLIN® 70/30, NovoLIN® R, NovoLOG®

NovoLIN® R may be confused with HumuLIN® R, NovoLIN® 70/30, NovoLIN® N, NovoLOG®

High alert medication:

The Institute for Safe Medication Practices (ISMP) includes this medication among its list of drugs which have a heightened risk of causing significant patient harm when used in error. *Due to the number of insulin preparations, it is essential to identify/clarify the type of insulin to be used.*

BEERS Criteria medication:

This drug may be potentially inappropriate for use in geriatric patients (Quality of evidence - moderate; Strength of recommendation - strong).

Administration issues:

Concentrated solutions (eg, U-500) should not be available in patient care areas. U-500 regular insulin should be stored, dispensed, and administered separately from U-100 regular insulin. For patients who receive U-500 insulin in the hospital setting, highlighting the strength prominently on the patient's medical chart and medication record may help to reduce dispensing errors.

Other safety concerns:

Cross-contamination may occur if insulin pens are shared among multiple patients. Steps should be taken to prohibit sharing of insulin pens.

Pregnancy Risk Factor B

Lactation Excretion in breast milk unknown

Breast-Feeding Considerations Endogenous insulin can be found in breast milk. Plasma glucose concentrations in the mother affect glucose concentrations in breast milk. The gastrointestinal tract destroys insulin when administered orally; therefore, insulin is not expected to be absorbed intact by the breast-feeding infant. All types of insulin are safe for use while breast-feeding. Due to increased calorie expenditure, women with diabetes may require less insulin while nursing.

Use Treatment of type 1 diabetes mellitus (insulin dependent, IDDM) and type 2 diabetes mellitus (noninsulin dependent, NIDDM) to improve glycemic control

Unlabeled Use Adjunct of parenteral nutrition; diabetic ketoacidosis (DKA); gestational diabetes mellitus (GDM); hyperglycemia during critical illness; hyperkalemia; hyperosmolar hyperglycemic state (HHS)

Mechanism of Action/Effect Insulin acts via specific membrane-bound receptors on target tissues to regulate metabolism of carbohydrate, protein, and fats. Target organs for insulin include the liver, skeletal muscle, and adipose tissue.

Within the liver, insulin stimulates hepatic glycogen synthesis. Insulin promotes hepatic synthesis of fatty acids, which are released into the circulation as lipoproteins. Skeletal muscle effects of insulin include increased protein synthesis and increased glycogen synthesis. Within adipose tissue, insulin stimulates the processing of circulating lipoproteins to provide free fatty acids, facilitating triglyceride synthesis and storage by adipocytes; also directly inhibits the hydrolysis of triglycerides. In addition, insulin stimulates the cellular uptake of amino acids and increases cellular permeability to several ions, including potassium, magnesium, and phosphate. By activating sodium-potassium ATPases, insulin promotes the intracellular movement of potassium.

Insulins are categorized based on the onset, peak, and duration of effect (eg, rapid-, short-, intermediate-, and long-acting insulin).

Contraindications Hypersensitivity to regular insulin or any component of the formulation; during episodes of hypoglycemia

Warnings/Precautions Hypoglycemia is the most common adverse effect of insulin. The timing of hypoglycemia differs among various insulin formulations. Hypoglycemia may result from increased work or exercise without eating; use of long-acting insulin preparations (eg, insulin detemir, insulin glargine) may delay recovery from hypoglycemia. Profound and prolonged episodes of hypoglycemia may result in convulsions, unconsciousness, temporary or permanent brain damage or even death. Insulin requirements may be altered during illness, emotional disturbances or other stressors. Insulin may produce hypokalemia which, if left untreated, may result in respiratory paralysis, ventricular arrhythmia and even death. Use with caution in patients at risk for hypokalemia (eg, I.V. insulin use). Use with caution in renal or hepatic impairment. In the elderly, avoid use of sliding scale insulin in this population due to increased risk of hypoglycemia without benefits in management of hyperglycemia regardless of care setting (Beers Criteria).

Human insulin differs from animal-source insulin. Any change of insulin should be made cautiously; changing manufacturers, type, and/or method of manufacture may result in the need for a change of dosage. U-500 regular insulin is a concentrated insulin formulation which contains 500 units of insulin per mL; for SubQ administration only using a U-100 insulin syringe or tuberculin syringe; **not for I.V. administration**. To avoid dosing errors when using a U-100 insulin syringe, the prescribed dose should be written in actual insulin units and as unit markings on the U-100 insulin syringe (eg, 50 units [10 units on a U-100 insulin syringe]). To avoid dosing errors when using a tuberculin syringe, the prescribed dose should be written in actual insulin units and as a volume (eg, 50 units

[0.1 mL]). Mixing U-500 regular insulin with other insulin formulations is not recommended.

Regular insulin may be administered I.V. or I.M. in selected clinical situations; close monitoring of blood glucose and serum potassium, as well as medical supervision, is required.

The general objective of exogenous insulin therapy is to approximate the physiologic pattern of insulin secretion which is characterized by two distinct phases. Phase 1 insulin secretion suppresses hepatic glucose production and phase 2 insulin secretion occurs in response to carbohydrate ingestion; therefore, exogenous insulin therapy may consist of basal insulin (eg, intermediate- or long-acting insulin or via continuous subcutaneous insulin infusion [CSII]) and/or preprandial insulin (eg, short- or rapid-acting insulin) (see Related Information: Insulin Products). Patients with type 1 diabetes do not produce endogenous insulin; therefore, these patients require both basal and preprandial insulin administration. Patients with type 2 diabetes retain some beta-cell function in the early stages of their disease; however, as the disease progresses, phase 1 insulin secretion may become completely impaired and phase 2 insulin secretion becomes delayed and/or inadequate in response to meals. Therefore, patients with type 2 diabetes may be treated with oral antidiabetic agents, basal insulin, and/or preprandial insulin depending on the stage of disease and current glycemic control. Since treatment regimens often consist of multiple agents, dosage adjustments must address the specific phase of insulin release that is primarily contributing to the patient's impaired glycemic control. Diabetes self-management education (DSME) is essential to maximize the effectiveness of therapy. Treatment and monitoring regimens must be individualized.

Potentially significant drug-drug interactions may exist, requiring dose or frequency adjustment, additional monitoring, and/or selection of alternative therapy.

Drug Interactions

Avoid Concomitant Use There are no known interactions where it is recommended to avoid concomitant use.

Decreased Effect

The levels/effects of Insulin Regular may be decreased by: Corticosteroids (Orally Inhaled); Corticosteroids (Systemic); Loop Diuretics; Luteinizing Hormone-Releasing Hormone Analogs; Somatropin; Thiazide Diuretics

Increased Effect/Toxicity

Insulin Regular may increase the levels/effects of: Antidiabetic Agents (Thiazolidinedione); Hypoglycemic Agents; Quinolone Antibiotics

The levels/effects of Insulin Regular may be increased by: Beta-Blockers; Edetate CALCIUM Disodium; Edetate Disodium; Herbs

(Hypoglycemic Properties); MAO Inhibitors; Metreleptin; Pegvisomant; Salicylates; Selective Serotonin Reuptake Inhibitors

Nutritional/Ethanol Interactions

Ethanol: Use caution with ethanol; may increase risk of hypoglycemia.

Herb/Nutraceutical: Use caution with alfalfa, aloe, bilberry, bitter melon, burdock, celery, damiana, fenugreek, garcinia, garlic, ginger, ginseng (American), gymnema, marshmallow, stinging nettle; may increase risk of hypoglycemia.

Adverse Reactions Primarily symptoms of hypoglycemia

Cardiovascular: Pallor, palpitation, tachycardia

Central nervous system: Fatigue, headache, hypothermia, loss of consciousness, mental confusion

Dermatologic: Redness, urticaria

Endocrine & metabolic: Hypoglycemia, hypokalemia

Gastrointestinal: Hunger, nausea, numbness of mouth

Local: Atrophy or hypertrophy of SubQ fat tissue; edema, itching, pain or warmth at injection site; stinging

Neuromuscular & skeletal: Muscle weakness, paresthesia, tremor

Ocular: Transient presbyopia or blurred vision

Miscellaneous: Anaphylaxis, diaphoresis, local and/or systemic hypersensitivity reactions

Pharmacodynamics/Kinetics

Onset of Action SubQ: 0.5 hours; Peak effect: SubQ: 2.5-5 hours

Duration of Action SubQ:

U-100: 4-12 hours (may increase with dose)

U-500: Up to 24 hours

Available Dosage Forms

Solution, Injection:

HumuLIN R [OTC]: 100 units/mL (3 mL, 10 mL)

NovoLIN R [OTC]: 100 units/mL (10 mL)

NovoLIN R ReliOn [OTC]: 100 units/mL (10 mL)

Solution, Subcutaneous:

HumuLIN R U-500 (CONCENTRATED): 500 units/mL (20 mL)

General Dosage Range Dosage adjustment recommended in patients with renal impairment

I.V., SubQ: *Children and Adults:* Diabetes mellitus, type 1: Initial: 0.5-1 unit/kg/day in divided doses; Usual maintenance: 0.5-1.2 units/kg/day in divided doses. **Note:** Generally, 50% to 75% of the total daily dose (TDD) is given as an intermediate- or long-acting form of insulin (1-2 daily injections) and the remaining portion is then divided and administered before or at mealtime (depending on the formulation) as a rapid-acting or short-acting form of insulin.

Usual Infusion Concentrations: Pediatric I.V. infusion: 0.1 unit/mL, 0.5 unit/mL, **or** 1 unit/mL

Usual Infusion Concentrations: Adult I.V. infusion: 100 units in 100 mL (concentration: 1 unit/mL) of NS

Administration

I.M. Do not use if solution is viscous or cloudy; use only if clear and colorless. May be administered I.M. in selected clinical situations; close monitoring of blood glucose and serum potassium as well as medical supervision is required.

I.V. Do not use if solution is viscous or cloudy; use only if clear and colorless. May be administered I.V. with close monitoring of blood glucose and serum potassium; appropriate medical supervision is required. If possible, avoid I.V. bolus administration in pediatric patients with DKA; may increase risk of cerebral edema. **Do not administer mixtures of insulin formulations intravenously.** I.V. administration of U-500 regular insulin is not recommended.

I.V. infusions: To minimize insulin adsorption to I.V. tubing: Flush the I.V. tubing with a priming infusion of 20 mL from the insulin infusion, whenever a new IV tubing set is added to the insulin infusion container. (Jacobi, 2012; Thompson, 2012).

Note: Also refer to institution-specific protocols where appropriate.

If insulin is required prior to the availability of the insulin drip, regular insulin should be administered by I.V. push injection.

Because of insulin adsorption to I.V. tubing or infusion bags, the actual amount of insulin being administered via I.V. infusion could be substantially less than the apparent amount. Therefore, adjustment of the I.V. infusion rate should be based on effect and not solely on the apparent insulin dose. The apparent dose may be used as a starting point for determining the subsequent SubQ dosing regimen (Moghissi, 2009); however, the transition to SubQ administration requires continuous medical supervision, frequent monitoring of blood glucose, and careful adjustment of therapy. In addition, SubQ insulin should be given 1-4 hours prior to the discontinuation of I.V. insulin to prevent hyperglycemia (Moghissi, 2009).

Injectable Detail pH: 7-7.8

Subcutaneous Do not use if solution is viscous or cloudy; use only if clear and colorless. Regular insulin should be administered within 30-60 minutes before a meal. Cold injections should be avoided. SubQ administration is usually made into the thighs, arms, buttocks, or abdomen; rotate injection sites. When mixing regular insulin with other preparations of insulin, regular insulin should be drawn into syringe first. Regular insulin is not recommended for use in external SubQ insulin infusion pump.

Preparation for Administration

For SubQ administration:

Humulin® R: May be diluted with the universal diluent, Sterile Diluent for Humalog®, Humulin® N, Humulin® R, Humulin® 70/30, and Humulin®

R U-500, to a concentration of 10 units/mL (U-10) or 50 units/mL (U-50).

Novolin® R: Insulin Diluting Medium for Novo-Log® is **not** intended for use with Novolin® R or any insulin product other than insulin aspart.

For I.V. infusion:

Humulin® R: May be diluted in NS or D_5W to concentrations of 0.1-1 unit/mL.

Novolin® R: May be diluted in NS, D_5W, or $D_{10}W$ with 40 mEq/L potassium chloride at concentrations of 0.05-1 unit/mL.

Storage/Stability

Humulin® R, Humulin® R U-500: Store unopened vials in refrigerator between 2°C and 8°C (36°F to 46°F); do not freeze; keep away from heat and sunlight. Once punctured (in use), vials may be stored for up to 31 days in the refrigerator between 2°C and 8°C (36°F to 46°F) or at room temperature of ≤30°C (≤86°F).

Novolin® R: Store unopened vials in refrigerator between 2°C and 8°C (36°F to 46°F) until product expiration date or at room temperature ≤25°C (≤77°F) for up to 42 days; do not freeze; keep away from heat and sunlight. Once punctured (in use), store vials at room temperature ≤25°C (≤77°F) for up to 42 days (this includes any days stored at room temperature prior to opening vial); refrigeration of in-use vials is not recommended.

Canadian labeling (not in U.S. labeling): All products: Unopened vials, cartridges, and pens should be stored under refrigeration between 2°C and 8°C (36°F to 46°F) until the expiration date; do not freeze; keep away from heat and sunlight. Once punctured (in use), Humulin® vials, cartridges, and pens should be stored at room temperature <25°C (<77°F) for up to 4 weeks. Once punctured (in use), Novolin® ge vials, cartridges, and pens may be stored for up to 1 month at room temperature <25°C (<77°F) for vials or <30°C (<86°F) for pens/cartridges; do not refrigerate.

For SubQ administration:

Humulin® R: According to the manufacturer, diluted insulin should be stored at 30°C (86°F) and used within 14 days **or** at 5°C (41°F) and used within 28 days.

For I.V. infusion:

Humulin® R: Stable for 48 hours at room temperature or for 48 hours under refrigeration followed by 48 hours at room temperature.

Novolin® R: Stable for 24 hours at room temperature

Nursing Actions

Physical Assessment Monitor for hypoglycemia at regular intervals during therapy. Teach patient proper use, including appropriate injection technique and syringe/needle disposal, and monitoring requirements.

Patient Education

- Discuss specific use of drug and side effects with patient as it relates to treatment. (HCAHPS: During this hospital stay, were you given any medicine that you had not taken before? Before giving you any new medicine, how often did hospital staff tell you what the medicine was for? How often did hospital staff describe possible side effects in a way you could understand?)
- Patient may experience hypoglycemia, nausea, weight gain, or application site irritation. Have patient report immediately to prescriber rash, signs of infection, or severe hyperglycemia (HCAHPS).
- Educate patient about signs of a significant reaction (eg, wheezing; chest tightness; fever; itching; bad cough; blue skin color; seizures; or swelling of face, lips, tongue, or throat). **Note:** This is not a comprehensive list of all side effects. Patient should consult prescriber for additional questions.

Intended Use and Disclaimer: Should not be printed and given to patients. This information is intended to serve as a concise initial reference for healthcare professionals to use when discussing medications with a patient. You must ultimately rely on your own discretion, experience and judgment in diagnosing, treating and advising patients.

Dietary Considerations Individualized medical nutrition therapy (MNT) based on ADA recommendations is an integral part of therapy.

Related Information

Interferon Alfa-2b (in ter FEER on AL fa too bee)

Brand Names: U.S. Intron-A

Index Terms INF-alpha 2; Interferon Alpha-2b; rLFN-α2; α-2-interferon

Pharmacologic Category Antineoplastic Agent; Biological Response Modulator; Biological Response Modulator; Immunomodulator, Systemic; Interferon

Medication Safety Issues

Sound-alike/look-alike issues:

Interferon alfa-2b may be confused with interferon alfa-2a, interferon alfa-n3, pegylated interferon alfa-2b

Intron® A may be confused with PEG-Intron

International issues:

Interferon alfa-2b may be confused with interferon alpha multi-subtype which is available in international markets

Medication Guide Available Yes

Pregnancy Risk Factor C / X in combination with ribavirin

Lactation Enters breast milk/not recommended

Use

Patients ≥1 year of age: Chronic hepatitis B

Patients ≥3 years of age: Chronic hepatitis C (in combination with ribavirin)

Patients ≥18 years of age: Condyloma acuminata, chronic hepatitis B, chronic hepatitis C, hairy cell leukemia, malignant melanoma (high-risk of recurrence), AIDS-related Kaposi's sarcoma, follicular non-Hodgkin lymphoma

Unlabeled Use Treatment of cutaneous ulcerations of Behçet's disease, neuroendocrine tumors (including carcinoid syndrome and islet cell tumor), cutaneous T-cell lymphoma, desmoid tumor, hepatitis D, chronic myelogenous leukemia (CML), non-Hodgkin lymphomas (other than follicular lymphoma, see approved use), multiple myeloma, renal cell carcinoma, West Nile virus

Available Dosage Forms

Solution, Injection:

Intron-A: 6,000,000 units/mL (3.8 mL); 10,000,000 units/mL (3.2 mL)

Solution Reconstituted, Injection:

Intron-A: 10,000,000 units (1 ea); 18,000,000 units (1 ea); 50,000,000 units (1 ea)

General Dosage Range Dosage adjustment is recommended in patients who develop toxicities

I.M.:

Children 1-17 years: 3-5 million units/m^2 3 times weekly (maximum: 3 million units per dose)

Adults: Dosage varies greatly depending on indication

I.V.: *Adults:* 20 million units/m^2 for 5 consecutive days per week

Intralesional: *Adults:* 1 million units/lesion 3 times weekly, on alternate days (maximum: 5 lesions per treatment)

SubQ:

Children 1-17 years: Initial: 3 million units/m^2 3 times weekly for 1 week; Maintenance: 6 million units/m^2 3 times weekly (maximum: 10 million units 3 times weekly) **or** 3-5 million units/m^2 3 times weekly (maximum: 3 million units per dose)

Adults: Dosage varies greatly depending on indication

◀ **Administration**

I.M. Not all dosage forms are recommended for all administration routes; refer to manufacturer's labeling.

Administer dose in the evening (if possible) to enhance tolerability. Rotate injection sites. Some patients may be appropriate for self-administration with appropriate training. Allow to reach room temperature prior to injection. In hairy cell leukemia treatment, if platelets are <50,000/mm^3, do not administer intramuscularly (administer SubQ instead).

I.V. Not all dosage forms are recommended for all administration routes; refer to manufacturer's labeling.

Infuse over ~20 minutes. Administer dose in the evening (if possible) to enhance tolerability.

Injectable Detail pH: 6.9-7.5

Subcutaneous Not all dosage forms are recommended for all administration routes; refer to manufacturer's labeling.

SubQ: Suggested for those who are at risk for bleeding or are thrombocytopenic. Rotate SubQ injection site. Administer dose in the evening (if possible) to enhance tolerability. Patient should be well hydrated. Some patients may be appropriate for self-administration with appropriate training. Allow to reach room temperature prior to injection.

Other Not all dosage forms are recommended for all administration routes; refer to manufacturer's labeling.

Intralesional: Inject at an angle nearly parallel to the plane of the skin, directing the needle to center of the base of the wart to infiltrate the lesion core and cause a small wheal. Only infiltrate the keratinized layer; avoid administration which is too deep or shallow.

Nursing Actions

Physical Assessment Monitor for neuropsychiatric changes, especially depression, suicidal or homicidal ideation, psychosis, or mania; decreased pulmonary function; or ophthalmic changes. Evaluate immediately any reported changes in vision. Teach appropriate reconstitution, injection, and needle disposal.

Patient Education

• Discuss specific use of drug and side effects with patient as it relates to treatment. (HCAHPS: During this hospital stay, were you given any medicine that you had not taken before? Before giving you any new medicine, how often did hospital staff tell you what the medicine was for? How often did hospital staff describe possible side effects in a way you could understand?)

• Patient may experience flu-like syndrome, presyncope, fatigue, blurred vision, illogical thinking, headache, nausea, anemia, leukopenia, thrombocytopenia, depression, injection site irritation, xerostomia, diarrhea, loss of appetite, alopecia, or insomnia. Have patient report immediately to prescriber nervousness, emotional instability, anxiety, angina, tachycardia, dyspnea, severe dyspepsia, significant weight loss, ecchymosis, bleeding, severe asthenia, sudden vision changes, eye pain, eye irritation, or rash (HCAHPS).

• Educate patient about signs of a significant reaction (eg, wheezing; chest tightness; fever; itching; bad cough; blue skin color; seizures; or swelling of face, lips, tongue, or throat). **Note:** This is not a comprehensive list of all side effects. Patient should consult prescriber for additional questions.

Intended Use and Disclaimer: Should not be printed and given to patients. This information is intended to serve as a concise initial reference for healthcare professionals to use when discussing medications with a patient. You must ultimately rely on your own discretion, experience and judgment in diagnosing, treating and advising patients.

Interferon Alfacon-1

(in ter FEER on AL fa con one)

Brand Names: U.S. Infergen [DSC]

Pharmacologic Category Interferon

Medication Safety Issues

Sound-alike/look-alike issues:

Interferon alfacon-1 may be confused with interferon alfa-2a, interferon alfa-2b, interferon alfa-n3, peginterferon alfa-2b

International issues:

Interferon alfacon-1 may be confused with interferon alpha multi-subtype which is available in international markets

Medication Guide Available Yes

Pregnancy Risk Factor C

Lactation Excretion in breast milk unknown/use caution

Use Treatment of chronic hepatitis C virus (HCV) infection in patients ≥18 years of age with compensated liver disease and anti-HCV serum antibodies or HCV RNA; concurrent use with ribavirin in HCV-infected patients who have failed treatment with pegylated interferon/ribavirin (Bacon, 2009)

General Dosage Range Dosage adjustment recommended in patients who develop toxicities

SubQ: *Adults:* 9-15 mcg 3 times/week; may increase to 15 mcg 3 times/week

Administration

Other Interferon alfacon-1 is given by SubQ injection, 3 times/week, with at least 48 hours between doses. Allow to reach room temperature just prior to administration.

Nursing Actions

Physical Assessment Monitor for signs of depression and suicide ideation. Patient with pre-existing diabetes mellitus or hypertension should have an ophthalmic exam prior to beginning treatment. If self-administered, instruct patient in appropriate storage, injection technique, and syringe disposal.

Patient Education

- Discuss specific use of drug and side effects with patient as it relates to treatment. (HCAHPS: During this hospital stay, were you given any medicine that you had not taken before? Before giving you any new medicine, how often did hospital staff tell you what the medicine was for? How often did hospital staff describe possible side effects in a way you could understand?)
- Patient may experience flu-like syndrome, pre-syncope, fatigue, blurred vision, illogical thinking, headache, leukopenia, thrombocytopenia, dyspepsia, nausea, diarrhea, alopecia, or insomnia. Have patient report immediately to prescriber signs of infection, depression, nervousness, emotional instability, anxiety, angina, tachycardia, dyspnea, inability to eat, discolored urine, jaundice, severe asthenia, ecchymosis, bleeding, sudden vision changes, eye pain, eye irritation, or rash (HCAHPS).
- Educate patient about signs of a significant reaction (eg, wheezing; chest tightness; fever; itching; bad cough; blue skin color; seizures; or swelling of face, lips, tongue, or throat). **Note:** This is not a comprehensive list of all side effects. Patient should consult prescriber for additional questions.

Intended Use and Disclaimer: Should not be printed and given to patients. This information is intended to serve as a concise initial reference for healthcare professionals to use when discussing medications with a patient. You must ultimately rely on your own discretion, experience and judgment in diagnosing, treating and advising patients.

Interferon Beta-1a (in ter FEER on BAY ta won aye)

Brand Names: U.S. Avonex®; Avonex® Pen™; Rebif®; Rebif® Rebidose®; Rebif® Rebidose® Titration Pack; Rebif® Titration Pack

Index Terms rIFN beta-1a

Pharmacologic Category Interferon

Medication Safety Issues

Sound-alike/look-alike issues:

Avonex® may be confused with Avelox®

Medication Guide Available Yes

Pregnancy Risk Factor C

Lactation Enters breast milk/use caution

Breast-Feeding Considerations Small amounts of interferon beta-1a are excreted in breast milk. Milk samples were obtained from six lactating women (6-23 months postpartum) receiving Avonex® 30 mcg I.M. once weekly; sampling occurred at intervals for 72 hours after the dose. The highest reported concentration was 179 pg/mL and the relative infant dose was calculated to be <1% of the maternal dose. Adverse events were not observed in the nursing infants (Hale, 2012). The manufacturer recommends that caution be exercised when administering interferon beta-1a to nursing women.

Use Treatment of relapsing forms of multiple sclerosis (MS)

Canadian labeling: Additional uses (not in U.S. labeling): Avonex®: To decrease the number and volume of active brain lesions, decrease overall disease burden, and delay onset of clinically definite MS in patients who have experienced a single demyelinating event.

Mechanism of Action/Effect Mechanism in the treatment of MS is unknown; slows the accumulation of physical disability and decreases frequency of clinical MS exacerbations

Contraindications Hypersensitivity to natural or recombinant interferons, human albumin (only for albumin-containing formulations), or any other component of the formulation

Canadian labeling: Additional contraindications (not in U.S. labeling): Rebif®: Pregnancy; decompensated liver disease

Warnings/Precautions Interferons have been associated with severe psychiatric adverse events (psychosis, mania, depression, suicidal behavior/ideation) in patients with and without previous psychiatric symptoms, avoid use in severe psychiatric disorders and use caution in patients with a history of depression; patients exhibiting depressive symptoms should be closely monitored and discontinuation of therapy should be considered.

Autoimmune disorders including idiopathic thrombocytopenia, hyper- and hypothyroidism and rarely autoimmune hepatitis have been reported. Allergic reactions, including anaphylaxis, have been reported; some reactions may occur after prolonged use. Rare cases of severe hepatic injury, including cases of hepatic failure requiring transplantation, have been reported in patients receiving interferon beta-1a; risk may be increased by ethanol use or concurrent therapy with hepatotoxic drugs. Some reports indicate symptoms began after 1-6 months of treatment. Transaminase elevations may be asymptomatic. Use with caution in patients with active or a history of liver disease, alcohol abuse, or increased serum ALT (>2.5 times ULN) at baseline. Obtain liver function tests at 1-, 3-, and 6 months post therapy initiation, or as clinically necessary. Treatment should be suspended immediately if jaundice or symptoms of hepatic dysfunction occur. Consider dose reductions or temporary discontinuation if ALT >5 times ULN. Hematologic effects, including pancytopenia (rare), leukopenia, and thrombocytopenia, have been reported. Use with caution in patients with bone marrow suppression; monitor blood counts at 1-, 3-, and 6 months post therapy initiation, or as clinically necessary. Associated with a high incidence of flu-like adverse effects; use of analgesics and/or antipyretics on treatment days may be helpful. Use caution in patients with pre-existing cardiovascular disease, including angina, HF, and/or arrhythmia. Rare cases of new-onset cardiomyopathy and/or HF have been reported. Use caution in patients with seizure disorders. Thyroid abnormalities may develop with use; may worsen preexisting thyroid conditions. Monitor thyroid function tests every 6 months or as clinically necessary. Safety and efficacy in patients with chronic progressive MS have not been established. Albumin is a component of some formulations (contraindicated in albumin-sensitive patients); rare risk of CJD or viral transmission.

Drug Interactions

Avoid Concomitant Use There are no known interactions where it is recommended to avoid concomitant use.

Decreased Effect There are no known significant interactions involving a decrease in effect.

Increased Effect/Toxicity
Interferon Beta-1a may increase the levels/effects of: Theophylline Derivatives; Zidovudine

Adverse Reactions Note: Adverse reactions reported as a composite of both commercially-available products. Spectrum and incidence of reactions is generally similar between products, but consult individual product labels for specific incidence.

>10%:
Central nervous system: Headache (58% to 70%), fatigue (33% to 41%), fever (20% to 28%), pain (23%), chills (19%), depression (18% to 25%), dizziness (14%)
Gastrointestinal: Nausea (23%), abdominal pain (8% to 22%)
Genitourinary: Urinary tract infection (17%)
Hematologic: Leukopenia (28% to 36%)
Hepatic: ALT increased (20% to 27%), AST increased (10% to 17%)
Local: Injection site reaction (3% to 92%)
Neuromuscular & skeletal: Myalgia (25% to 29%), back pain (23% to 25%), weakness (24%), skeletal pain (10% to 15%), rigors (6% to 13%)
Ocular: Vision abnormal (7% to 13%)
Respiratory: Sinusitis (14%), upper respiratory tract infection (14%)
Miscellaneous: Flu-like syndrome (49% to 59%), neutralizing antibodies (significance not known; Avonex® 5%; Rebif® 24%), lymphadenopathy (11% to 12%)
1% to 10%:
Cardiovascular: Chest pain (5% to 6%), vasodilation (2%)

Central nervous system: Migraine (5%), somnolence (4% to 5%), malaise (4% to 5%), seizure (1% to 5%)
Dermatologic: Erythematous rash (5% to 7%), maculopapular rash (4% to 5%), alopecia (4%), urticaria
Endocrine & metabolic: Thyroid disorder (4% to 6%)
Gastrointestinal: Xerostomia (1% to 5%), toothache (3%)
Genitourinary: Micturition frequency (2% to 7%), urinary incontinence (2% to 4%)
Hematologic: Thrombocytopenia (2% to 8%), anemia (3% to 5%)
Hepatic: Bilirubinemia (2% to 3%)
Local: Injection site pain (8%), injection site bruising (6%), injection site necrosis (1% to 3%), injection site inflammation
Neuromuscular & skeletal: Arthralgia (9%), hypertonia (6% to 7%), coordination abnormal (4% to 5%)
Ocular: Eye disorder (4%), xerophthalmia (1% to 3%)
Respiratory: Bronchitis (8%)
Miscellaneous: Infection (7%)

Pharmacodynamics/Kinetics

Onset of Action Avonex®: 12 hours (based on biological response markers)

Duration of Action Avonex®: 4 days (based on biological response markers)

Available Dosage Forms

Injection, powder for reconstitution [preservative free]:
Avonex®: 33 mcg [contains albumin (human); provides 30 mcg/mL following reconstitution; supplied with diluent]

Injection, solution:
Avonex®, Avonex® Pen™: 30 mcg/0.5 mL (0.5 mL)

Injection, solution [preservative free]:
Rebif®: 22 mcg/0.5 mL (0.5 mL), 44 mcg/0.5 mL (0.5 mL)
Rebif® Rebidose®: 22 mcg/0.5 mL (0.5 mL), 44 mcg/0.5 mL (0.5 mL)

Injection, solution [preservative free, combination package]:
Rebif® Titration Pack: 8.8 mcg/0.2 mL (6s) and 22 mcg/0.5 mL (6s)
Rebif® Rebidose® Titration Pack: 8.8 mcg/0.2 mL (6s) and 22 mcg/0.5 mL (6s)

General Dosage Range Dosage adjustment recommended in patients who develop toxicities

I.M.: *Adults:* Initial: 30 mcg once weekly **or** 7.5 mcg (week 1) then titrate in increments of 7.5 mcg once weekly (weeks 2-4) to 30 mcg once weekly

SubQ: *Adults:* Initial: 4.4 or 8.8 mcg 3 times weekly for 2 weeks; Titration: 11 or 22 mcg 3 times weekly for 2 weeks; Maintenance: 22 or 44 mcg 3 times weekly

Administration

I.M. Avonex®: Must be administered by I.M. injection. Rotate injection site. Do not inject into area where skin is irritated, red, bruised, scarred, or infected. Two hours after injection, examine site for redness, swelling, or tenderness. Discard any unused portion.

Subcutaneous Rebif®, Rebif® Rebidose®: Administer SubQ at the same time of day on the same 3 days each week (ie, late afternoon/evening Mon, Wed, Fri; doses should be at least 48 hours apart); rotate injection site; do not inject into area where skin is sore, red, damaged, or infected. Discard any unused portion.

Preparation for Administration Avonex®: Reconstitute with 1.1 mL of diluent and swirl gently to dissolve. Do not shake. The reconstituted product contains no preservative and is for single-use only; discard unused portion.

Storage/Stability

Avonex®:

Prefilled syringe or pen: Store at 2°C to 8°C (36°F to 46°F); do not freeze. Protect from light. Allow to warm to room temperature prior to use (do not use external heat source). If refrigeration is not available, product may be stored at ≤25°C (77°F) for up to 7 days.

Vial: Store unreconstituted vial at 2°C to 8°C (36°F to 46°F). If refrigeration is not available, may be stored at 25°C (77°F) for up to 30 days; do not freeze. Protect from light. Following reconstitution, use immediately, but may be stored up to 6 hours at 2°C to 8°C (36°F to 46°F); do not freeze.

Rebif®, Rebif® Rebidose®: Store at 2°C to 8°C (36°F to 46°F); do not freeze. Protect from light. May also be stored ≤25°C (77°F) for up to 30 days if protected from heat and light.

Nursing Actions

Physical Assessment Monitor for signs of depression and suicide ideation. Instruct patient/caregiver on appropriate reconstitution, injection, and needle disposal.

Patient Education

- Discuss specific use of drug and side effects with patient as it relates to treatment. (HCAHPS: During this hospital stay, were you given any medicine that you had not taken before? Before giving you any new medicine, how often did hospital staff tell you what the medicine was for? How often did hospital staff describe possible side effects in a way you could understand?)
- Patient may experience flu-like syndrome, presyncope, fatigue, blurred vision, illogical thinking, nausea, dyspepsia, vision changes, leukopenia, or injection site irritation. Have patient report immediately to prescriber signs of infection, depression, nervousness, emotional instability, anxiety, angina, tachycardia, dyspnea, significant dizziness, considerable edema, inability to eat, discolored urine, jaundice, severe asthenia, ecchymosis, bleeding, pregnancy, or rash (HCAHPS).
- Educate patient about signs of a significant reaction (eg, wheezing; chest tightness; fever; itching; bad cough; blue skin color; seizures; or swelling of face, lips, tongue, or throat). **Note:** This is not a comprehensive list of all side effects. Patient should consult prescriber for additional questions.

Intended Use and Disclaimer: Should not be printed and given to patients. This information is intended to serve as a concise initial reference for healthcare professionals to use when discussing medications with a patient. You must ultimately rely on your own discretion, experience and judgment in diagnosing, treating and advising patients.

Interferon Beta-1b (in ter FEER on BAY ta won bee)

Brand Names: U.S. Betaseron; Extavia
Index Terms rIFN beta-1b
Pharmacologic Category Interferon
Medication Guide Available Yes
Pregnancy Risk Factor C
Lactation Excretion in breast milk unknown/not recommended
Breast-Feeding Considerations It is not known if interferon beta-1b is excreted in breast milk. Due to the potential for serious adverse reactions in the nursing infant, the decision to continue or discontinue breast-feeding during therapy should take into account the risk of exposure to the infant and the benefits of treatment to the mother.
Use Treatment of relapsing forms of multiple sclerosis (MS); treatment of first clinical episode with MRI features consistent with MS
Canadian labeling: Additional use (not in U.S. labeling): Treatment of secondary-progressive MS
Mechanism of Action/Effect Alters the expression and response to cell surface antigens and can enhance immune cell activities; mechanism in MS in unknown
Contraindications Hypersensitivity to natural or recombinant interferon beta, albumin human or any other component of the formulation
Canadian labeling: Additional contraindication (not in U.S. labeling): Pregnancy; decompensated liver disease
Warnings/Precautions Allergic reactions (eg, bronchospasm, dyspnea, skin rash, tongue edema, urticaria), including anaphylaxis (rare), have been reported with use; discontinue use if anaphylaxis occurs. Associated with a high incidence of flu-like adverse effects; use of analgesics and/or antipyretics on treatment days may be helpful. Improvement in symptoms occurs over time. Hepatotoxicity has been reported with beta interferons, including rare reports of hepatitis ▶

(autoimmune) and hepatic failure requiring transplant; use with caution in patients with concurrent exposure to other hepatotoxic drugs. Monitor liver function tests as clinically necessary. Consider discontinuation if serum transaminase levels increase significantly or are associated with clinical symptoms (eg, jaundice). Interferons have been associated with severe psychiatric adverse events (psychosis, mania, depression, suicidal behavior/ ideation) in patients with and without previous psychiatric symptoms; avoid use in severe psychiatric disorders and use caution in patients with a history of depression; patients exhibiting symptoms of depression should be closely monitored and discontinuation of therapy should be considered. Use with caution in patients with a history of seizure disorder.

Use with caution in patients with pre-existing cardiovascular disease. Rare cases of new-onset cardiomyopathy and/or HF have been reported. If HF worsens in the absence of another etiology, consider discontinuation of therapy. Use with caution in patients with hepatic impairment or in combination with alcohol. The Canadian labeling contraindicates use in patients with decompensated hepatic disease. Use with caution in patients with bone marrow suppression; may require increased monitoring. Leukopenia has also been observed; routine monitoring of complete blood counts with differentials is recommended. Dose reduction may be required. Thyroid abnormalities may develop with use; may worsen preexisting thyroid conditions. Monitor thyroid function tests every 6 months or as clinically necessary.

Severe injection site reactions (necrosis) may occur, which may or may not heal with continued therapy. Reactions generally arise within the first 4 months of therapy, but have occurred ≥1 year after initiation. Incidence of reactions tend to improve over time. Patient and/or caregiver competency in injection technique should be confirmed and periodically re-evaluated. Do not inject into affected area until completely healed; if multiple lesions occur, discontinue use until they are fully healed. Contains albumin, which may carry a remote risk of transmitting viral diseases.

Drug Interactions

Avoid Concomitant Use There are no known interactions where it is recommended to avoid concomitant use.

Decreased Effect There are no known significant interactions involving a decrease in effect.

Increased Effect/Toxicity

Interferon Beta-1b may increase the levels/effects of: Theophylline Derivatives; Zidovudine

Adverse Reactions Note: Flu-like syndrome (including at least two of the following - headache, fever, chills, malaise, diaphoresis, and myalgia) are reported in the majority of patients (60%) and decrease over time (average duration ~1 week).

>10%:

Cardiovascular: Peripheral edema (12% to 15%), chest pain (9% to 11%)

Central nervous system: Headache (50% to 57%), pain (42% to 51%), hypertonia (40% to 50%), myasthenia (46%), chills (21% to 25%), dizziness (24%), insomnia (21% to 24%), ataxia (17% to 21%)

Dermatologic: Skin rash (21% to 24%), dermatological disease (10% to 12%)

Gastrointestinal: Nausea (27%), constipation (20%), diarrhea (19%), abdominal pain (16% to 19%), dyspepsia (14%)

Genitourinary: Urinary urgency (11% to 13%), uterine hemorrhage (9% to 11%)

Hematologic & oncologic: Lymphocytopenia (86% to 88%), leukopenia (13% to 18%), neutropenia (13% to 14%)

Immunologic: Antibody development (≤45%; neutralizing; significance not known)

Local: Injection site reaction (78% to 85%, including inflammation [53%], pain [18%], tissue necrosis [4% to 5%], hypersensitivity reaction [4%], swelling [2% to 3%], residual mass [2%])

Neuromuscular & skeletal: Weakness (53% to 61%), arthralgia (31%), myalgia (23% to 27%)

Respiratory: Flu-like symptoms (decreases over treatment course; 57% to 60%)

Miscellaneous: Fever (31% to 36%)

1% to 10%:

Cardiovascular: Vasodilatation (8%), hypertension (6% to 7%), peripheral vascular disease (6%), palpitations (4%), tachycardia (4%)

Central nervous system: Anxiety (10%), malaise (6% to 8%), nervousness (7%)

Dermatologic: Diaphoresis (8%), alopecia (4%)

Endocrine & metabolic: Hypermenorrhea (8%), dysmenorrhea (7%), weight gain (7%)

Genitourinary: Impotence (8% to 9%), cystitis (8%), urinary frequency (7%), pelvic pain (6%), prostatic disease (3%)

Hematologic & oncologic: Lymphadenopathy (6% to 8%)

Hepatic: Increased serum ALT (>5x baseline: 10% to 12%), increased serum AST (>5x baseline: 3% to 4%)

Hypersensitivity: Hypersensitivity (3%)

Neuromuscular & skeletal: Leg cramps (4%)

Respiratory: Dyspnea (6% to 7%)

Available Dosage Forms

Kit, Subcutaneous:

Betaseron: 0.3 mg

Kit, Subcutaneous [preservative free]:

Extavia: 0.3 mg

General Dosage Range SubQ: *Adults:* 0.0625-0.25 mg every other day

Administration

Subcutaneous Withdraw dose of reconstituted solution from the vial into a sterile syringe fitted with a 27-gauge (Extavia) or 30-gauge (Betaseron) needle and inject the solution subcutaneously; sites for self-injection include outer surface of the arms, abdomen (**except** 2-inch area around the navel), hips, and thighs. Rotate SubQ injection site. Do not inject into area where skin is bruised, infected, or broken. Patient should be well hydrated. If a dose is missed, administer as soon as remembered; do not administer on 2 consecutive days. Time subsequent doses every 48 hours.

Preparation for Administration To reconstitute solution, inject 1.2 mL of diluent (provided); gently swirl to dissolve, do not shake. Reconstituted solution provides 0.25 mg/mL. Use product within 3 hours of reconstitution. Discard unused portion of vial. Foaming may occur if swirled or shaken too vigorously; allow vial to sit until foam settles.

Storage/Stability Store intact vials at 20°C to 25°C (68°F to 77°F); excursions permitted to 15°C to 30°C (59°F to 86°F) for ≤3 months. If not used immediately following reconstitution, refrigerate solution at 2°C to 8°C (35°F to 46°F) and use within 3 hours; do not freeze or shake solution. Discard unused portion of vial.

Nursing Actions

Physical Assessment Assess for psychiatric or suicide histories (eg, psychosis, mania, depression, suicide behavior/ideation). Monitor injection sites for signs of necrosis. Teach proper administration for SubQ injections and disposal of needles if appropriate. Emphasize the need for adequate hydration. Monitor for opportunistic infection.

Patient Education

- Discuss specific use of drug and side effects with patient as it relates to treatment. (HCAHPS: During this hospital stay, were you given any medicine that you had not taken before? Before giving you any new medicine, how often did hospital staff tell you what the medicine was for? How often did hospital staff describe possible side effects in a way you could understand?)
- Patient may experience injection site irritation, flu-like syndrome, constipation, dyspepsia, depression, or edema. Have patient report immediately to prescriber nervousness, emotional instability, anxiety, severe skin irritation, ecchymosis, bleeding, discolored urine, jaundice, severe asthenia, inability to eat, significant nausea, rash, or pregnancy (HCAHPS).
- Educate patient about signs of a significant reaction (eg, wheezing; chest tightness; fever; itching; bad cough; blue skin color; seizures; or swelling of face, lips, tongue, or throat). **Note:** This is not a comprehensive list of all side effects. Patient should consult prescriber for additional questions.

Intended Use and Disclaimer: Should not be printed and given to patients. This information is intended to serve as a concise initial reference for healthcare professionals to use when discussing medications with a patient. You must ultimately rely on your own discretion, experience and judgment in diagnosing, treating and advising patients.

Interferon Gamma-1b
(in ter FEER on GAM ah won bee)

Brand Names: U.S. Actimmune

Pharmacologic Category Interferon

Pregnancy Risk Factor C

Lactation Excretion in breast milk unknown/not recommended

Breast-Feeding Considerations Potential for serious adverse reactions. Because its use has not been evaluated during lactation, breast-feeding is not recommended

Use Reduce frequency and severity of serious infections associated with chronic granulomatous disease; delay time to disease progression in patients with severe, malignant osteopetrosis

Mechanism of Action/Effect Interferon gamma participates in immunoregulation. The exact mechanism of action for the treatment of chronic granulomatous disease or osteopetrosis has not been defined.

Contraindications Hypersensitivity to interferon gamma, *E. coli* derived proteins, or any component of the formulation

Warnings/Precautions Hypersensitivity reactions have been reported (rarely). Transient cutaneous rashes may occur. Dose-related bone marrow toxicity has been reported; use caution in patients with myelosuppression. May cause hepatotoxicity and the incidence may be increased in children <1 year of age. Doses >10 times the weekly recommended dose (used in studies for unlabeled indications) have been associated with a different pattern/frequency of adverse effects. Flu-like symptoms which may exacerbate pre-existing cardiovascular disorders (including ischemia, HF, or arrhythmias) and the development of neurologic disorders have been noted at the higher doses. Caution should also be used in patients with seizure disorders or compromised CNS function.

Drug Interactions

Avoid Concomitant Use There are no known interactions where it is recommended to avoid concomitant use.

Decreased Effect There are no known significant interactions involving a decrease in effect.

Increased Effect/Toxicity

Interferon Gamma-1b may increase the levels/effects of: Theophylline Derivatives; Zidovudine

Adverse Reactions Based on 50 mcg/m^2 dose administered 3 times weekly for chronic granulomatous disease

>10%:

Central nervous system: Fever (52%), headache (33%), chills (14%), fatigue (14%)

Dermatologic: Rash (17%)

Gastrointestinal: Diarrhea (14%), vomiting (13%)
Local: Injection site erythema or tenderness (14%)

1% to 10%:

Central nervous system: Depression (3%)

Gastrointestinal: Nausea (10%), abdominal pain (8%)

Neuromuscular & skeletal: Myalgia (6%), arthralgia (2%), back pain (2%)

Additional adverse reactions noted at doses >100 mcg/m^2 administered 3 times weekly: ALT increased, AST increased, autoantibodies increased, bronchospasm, chest discomfort, confusion, dermatomyositis exacerbation, disorientation, DVT, gait disturbance, GI bleeding, hallucinations, heart block, heart failure, hepatic insufficiency, hyperglycemia, hypertriglyceridemia, hyponatremia, hypotension, interstitial pneumonitis, lupus-like syndrome, MI, neutropenia, pancreatitis (may be fatal), Parkinsonian symptoms, PE, proteinuria, renal insufficiency (reversible), seizure, syncope, tachyarrhythmia, tachypnea, thrombocytopenia, TIA

Available Dosage Forms
Solution, Subcutaneous:
Actimmune: 2,000,000 units/0.5 mL (0.5 mL)

General Dosage Range Dosage adjustment recommended in patients who develop toxicities

SubQ: *Children and Adults:*
BSA ≤0.5 m^2: 1.5 mcg/kg/dose 3 times/week
BSA >0.5 m^2: 50 mcg/m^2 (1 million units/m^2) 3 times/week

Administration
Other Administer by SubQ injection into the right and left deltoid or anterior thigh.

Storage/Stability Store in refrigerator at 2°C to 8°C (36°F to 46°F); do not freeze. Do not shake. Discard if left unrefrigerated for >12 hours.

Nursing Actions
Physical Assessment Teach patient/caregiver appropriate reconstitution, injection, and needle disposal.

Patient Education
• Discuss specific use of drug and side effects with patient as it relates to treatment. (HCAHPS: During this hospital stay, were you given any medicine that you had not taken before? Before giving you any new medicine, how often did hospital staff tell you what the medicine was for? How often did hospital staff describe possible side effects in a way you could understand?)

• Patient may experience injection site irritation, flu-like syndrome, diarrhea, nausea, dyspepsia, asthenia, or depression. Have patient report immediately to prescriber nervousness, emotional instability, anxiety, ecchymosis, bleeding, discolored urine, jaundice, inability to eat, severe skin irritation, pregnancy, or rash (HCAHPS).

• Educate patient about signs of a significant reaction (eg, wheezing; chest tightness; fever;

itching; bad cough; blue skin color; seizures; or swelling of face, lips, tongue, or throat). **Note:** This is not a comprehensive list of all side effects. Patient should consult prescriber for additional questions.

Intended Use and Disclaimer: Should not be printed and given to patients. This information is intended to serve as a concise initial reference for healthcare professionals to use when discussing medications with a patient. You must ultimately rely on your own discretion, experience and judgment in diagnosing, treating and advising patients.

Ipilimumab (ip i LIM u mab)

Brand Names: U.S. Yervoy

Index Terms MDX-010; MDX-CTLA-4; MOAB-CTLA-4

Pharmacologic Category Antineoplastic Agent, Monoclonal Antibody

Medication Safety Issues
High alert medication:
This medication is in a class the Institute for Safe Medication Practices (ISMP) includes among its list of drug classes which have a heightened risk of causing significant patient harm when used in error.

Medication Guide Available Yes

Pregnancy Risk Factor C

Lactation Excretion in breast milk unknown/not recommended

Use Treatment of unresectable or metastatic melanoma

Available Dosage Forms
Solution, Intravenous [preservative free]:
Yervoy: 50 mg/10 mL (10 mL); 200 mg/40 mL (40 mL)

General Dosage Range Dosage adjustment recommended in patients who develop toxicities.
I.V.: *Adults:* 3 mg/kg every 3 weeks

Administration
I.V. Infuse over 90 minutes through a low protein-binding in-line filter. Flush with NS or D$_5$W at the end of infusion

Injectable Detail pH: 7 (solution in vial)

Nursing Actions
Patient Education
• Discuss specific use of drug and side effects with patient as it relates to treatment. (HCAHPS: During this hospital stay, were you given any medicine that you had not taken before? Before giving you any new medicine, how often did hospital staff tell you what the medicine was for? How often did hospital staff describe possible side effects in a way you could understand?)

• Patient may experience fatigue, diarrhea, nausea, loss of appetite, or rash. Have patient report immediately to prescriber signs of infection, dizziness or syncope, paresthesia, severe

headache, illogical thinking, intolerable dyspepsia, discolored urine, jaundice, inability to eat, ecchymosis, melena, significant mouth or skin irritation, or sudden vision changes (HCAHPS).
• Educate patient about signs of a significant reaction (eg, wheezing; chest tightness; fever; itching; bad cough; blue skin color; seizures; or swelling of face, lips, tongue, or throat). **Note:** This is not a comprehensive list of all side effects. Patient should consult prescriber for additional questions.

Intended Use and Disclaimer: Should not be printed and given to patients. This information is intended to serve as a concise initial reference for healthcare professionals to use when discussing medications with a patient. You must ultimately rely on your own discretion, experience and judgment in diagnosing, treating and advising patients.

Ipratropium (Oral Inhalation)
(i pra TROE pee um)

Brand Names: U.S. Atrovent HFA
Index Terms Ipratropium Bromide
Pharmacologic Category Anticholinergic Agent
Medication Safety Issues
Sound-alike/look-alike issues:
Atrovent® may be confused with Alupent, Serevent®
Ipratropium may be confused with tiotropium
Pregnancy Risk Factor B
Lactation Excretion in breast milk unknown/use caution
Breast-Feeding Considerations It is not known if ipratropium (oral inhalation) is excreted in breast milk. The manufacturer recommends that caution be exercised when administering ipratropium (oral inhalation) to nursing women.
Use Anticholinergic bronchodilator used in bronchospasm associated with COPD, bronchitis, and emphysema
Mechanism of Action/Effect Blocks the action of acetylcholine at parasympathetic sites in bronchial smooth muscle causing bronchodilation; local application to nasal mucosa inhibits serous and seromucous gland secretions.
Contraindications Hypersensitivity to ipratropium, atropine (and its derivatives), or any component of the formulation
Warnings/Precautions Immediate hypersensitivity reactions (urticaria, angioedema, rash, bronchospasm) have been reported. Rarely, paradoxical bronchospasm may occur with use of inhaled bronchodilating agents; this should be distinguished from inadequate response. Not indicated for the initial treatment of acute episodes of bronchospasm where rescue therapy is required for rapid response. Should only be used in acute exacerbations of asthma in conjunction with

short-acting beta-adrenergic agonists for acute episodes. Use with caution in patients with myasthenia gravis, narrow-angle glaucoma, benign prostatic hyperplasia (BPH), or bladder neck obstruction
Drug Interactions
Avoid Concomitant Use
Avoid concomitant use of Ipratropium (Oral Inhalation) with any of the following: Aclidinium; Anticholinergics; Potassium Chloride; Tiotropium; Umeclidinium
Decreased Effect
Ipratropium (Oral Inhalation) may decrease the levels/effects of: Acetylcholinesterase Inhibitors (Central); Secretin

The levels/effects of Ipratropium (Oral Inhalation) may be decreased by: Acetylcholinesterase Inhibitors (Central)
Increased Effect/Toxicity
Ipratropium (Oral Inhalation) may increase the levels/effects of: AbobotulinumtoxinA; Analgesics (Opioid); Anticholinergics; Cannabinoids; Mirabegron; OnabotulinumtoxinA; Potassium Chloride; RimabotulinumtoxinB; Thiazide Diuretics; Tiotropium; Topiramate

The levels/effects of Ipratropium (Oral Inhalation) may be increased by: Aclidinium; Pramlintide; Umeclidinium
Adverse Reactions
>10%: Respiratory: Bronchitis (10% to 23%), COPD exacerbation (8% to 23%), sinusitis (1% to 11%)
1% to 10%:
Central nervous system: Headache (6% to 7%), dizziness (3%)
Gastrointestinal: Dyspepsia (1% to 5%), nausea (4%), xerostomia (2% to 4%), taste perversion (1%)
Genitourinary: Urinary tract infection (2% to 10%)
Neuromuscular & skeletal: Back pain (2% to 7%)
Respiratory: Dyspnea (7% to 8%), cough (>3%), rhinitis (>3%), upper respiratory infection (>3%)
Miscellaneous: Flu-like syndrome (4% to 8%)
Pharmacodynamics/Kinetics
Onset of Action Bronchodilation: Within 15 minutes; Peak effect: 1-2 hours
Duration of Action 2-5 hours
Dosage Forms Considerations
Atrovent HFA 12.9 g canister contains 200 inhalations.
Available Dosage Forms
Aerosol Solution, Inhalation:
Atrovent HFA: 17 mcg/actuation (12.9 g)
Solution, Inhalation:
Generic: 0.02% (2.5 mL)
Solution, Inhalation [preservative free]:
Generic: 0.02% (2.5 mL)

General Dosage Range

Inhalation: *Children >12 years and Adults:* 2 inhalations 4 times/day (maximum: 12 inhalations/day)

Nebulization: *Children >12 years and Adults:* 500 mcg every 6-8 hours

Administration

Inhalation Atrovent® HFA: Prior to initial use, prime inhaler by releasing 2 test sprays into the air. If the inhaler has not been used for >3 days, reprime.

Storage/Stability

Aerosol: Store at controlled room temperature of 25°C (77°F). Do not store near heat or open flame.

Solution: Store at 15°C to 30°C (59°F to 86°F). Protect from light.

Nursing Actions

Physical Assessment Teach patient importance of proper administration.

Patient Education

- Discuss specific use of drug and side effects with patient as it relates to treatment. (HCAHPS: During this hospital stay, were you given any medicine that you had not taken before? Before giving you any new medicine, how often did hospital staff tell you what the medicine was for? How often did hospital staff describe possible side effects in a way you could understand?)
- Patient may experience headache, pharyngitis, rhinitis, or xerostomia. Have patient report immediately to prescriber dyspnea, sudden vision changes, eye pain, eye irritation, or rash (HCAHPS).
- Educate patient about signs of a significant reaction (eg, wheezing; chest tightness; fever; itching; bad cough; blue skin color; seizures; or swelling of face, lips, tongue, or throat). **Note:** This is not a comprehensive list of all side effects. Patient should consult prescriber for additional questions.

Intended Use and Disclaimer: Should not be printed and given to patients. This information is intended to serve as a concise initial reference for healthcare professionals to use when discussing medications with a patient. You must ultimately rely on your own discretion, experience and judgment in diagnosing, treating and advising patients.

Ipratropium (Nasal) (i pra TROE pee um)

Brand Names: U.S. Atrovent

Index Terms Ipratropium Bromide

Pharmacologic Category Anticholinergic Agent

Medication Safety Issues

Sound-alike/look-alike issues:

Atrovent® may be confused with Alupent, Serevent®

Ipratropium may be confused with tiotropium

Pregnancy Risk Factor B

Lactation Excretion in breast milk unknown/use caution

Use Symptomatic relief of rhinorrhea associated with the common cold and allergic and nonallergic rhinitis

Dosage Forms Considerations

Atrovent 0.03% (21 mcg/spray) nasal solution 30 mL bottles contain 345 sprays, and the 0.06% (42 mcg/spray) 15 mL bottles contain 165 sprays.

Available Dosage Forms

Solution, Nasal:

Atrovent: 0.03% (30 mL); 0.06% (15 mL)

Generic: 0.03% (30 mL); 0.06% (15 mL)

General Dosage Range Intranasal:

0.03% solution: *Children ≥6 years and Adults:* 2 sprays in each nostril 2-3 times/day

0.06% solution: *Children ≥5 years and Adults:* 2 sprays in each nostril 3-4 times/day

Administration

Inhalation Prior to initial use, prime inhaler by releasing 7 test sprays into the air. If the inhaler has not been used for >24 hours, reprime by releasing 2 test sprays into the air.

Nursing Actions

Physical Assessment Teach patient importance of proper administration.

Patient Education

- Discuss specific use of drug and side effects with patient as it relates to treatment. (HCAHPS: During this hospital stay, were you given any medicine that you had not taken before? Before giving you any new medicine, how often did hospital staff tell you what the medicine was for? How often did hospital staff describe possible side effects in a way you could understand?)
- Patient may experience xerostomia, headache, rhinitis, or epistaxis. Have patient report immediately to prescriber rash (HCAHPS).
- Educate patient about signs of a significant reaction (eg, wheezing; chest tightness; fever; itching; bad cough; blue skin color; seizures; or swelling of face, lips, tongue, or throat). **Note:** This is not a comprehensive list of all side effects. Patient should consult prescriber for additional questions.

Intended Use and Disclaimer: Should not be printed and given to patients. This information is intended to serve as a concise initial reference for healthcare professionals to use when discussing medications with a patient. You must ultimately rely on your own discretion, experience and judgment in diagnosing, treating and advising patients.

Ipratropium and Albuterol
(i pra TROE pee um & al BYOO ter ole)

Brand Names: U.S. Combivent® Respimat®; Combivent® [DSC]; DuoNeb®

Index Terms Albuterol and Ipratropium; Salbutamol and Ipratropium

Pharmacologic Category Anticholinergic Agent; Beta$_2$-Adrenergic Agonist

Medication Safety Issues

Sound-alike/look-alike issues:

Combivent® may be confused with Combivir®, Serevent®

DuoNeb® may be confused with DuoTrav™, Duovent® UDV

Pregnancy Risk Factor C

Use Treatment of COPD in those patients who are currently on a regular bronchodilator who continue to have bronchospasms and require a second bronchodilator

Available Dosage Forms

Solution, for nebulization: Ipratropium 0.5 mg and albuterol (base) 2.5 mg per 3 mL (30s, 60s)

DuoNeb®: Ipratropium 0.5 mg and albuterol (base) 2.5 mg per 3 mL (30s, 60s)

Solution, for oral inhalation [spray]:

Combivent® Respimat®: Ipratropium bromide 20 mcg and albuterol (base) 100 mcg per inhalation (4 g) [120 metered actuations]

General Dosage Range

Inhalation: *Adults:* 1 inhalation (Combivent® Respimat®) or 2 inhalations (Combivent®) 4 times daily (maximum: Combivent® Respimat®: 6 inhalations/24 hours; Combivent®: 12 inhalations/24 hours)

Nebulization: *Adults:* 3 mL every 6 hours (maximum: 3 mL every 4 hours)

Administration

Inhalation

Nebulization: Administer via jet nebulizer to an air compressor with an adequate air flow, equipped with a mouthpiece or face mask.

Metered-dose inhaler (MDI):

Combivent®: Shake canister vigorously for ≥10 seconds. Prior to first use (or if not used for >24 hours), a test spray of 3 sprays is recommended.

Combivent® Respimat®: Prior to first use (or if not used in >21 days), point towards ground and actuate until aerosol cloud is seen, then repeat 3 additional times before use. If not used for >3 days; actuate once before use.

Nursing Actions

Physical Assessment Monitor for FEV$_1$, peak flow, asthma symptoms, heart rate, blood pressure, and blood glucose. Monitor insulin and/or oral hypoglycemic therapy requirements in diabetics. Encourage patient to keep good records of home glucose monitoring, especially during initiation of drug therapy. Instruct patient to report if home glucose consistently high or if signs of hyperglycemia (eg, increased thirst, increased urination, sleepiness) occur.

Educate patients regarding importance of regular eye exams. Instruct patients to notify provider of change in vision or seeing rainbow-colored circles around lights. Educate male patients regarding possible urinary retention. Monitor urine output.

Patient Education

• Discuss specific use of drug and side effects with patient as it relates to treatment. (HCAHPS: During this hospital stay, were you given any medicine that you had not taken before? Before giving you any new medicine, how often did hospital staff tell you what the medicine was for? How often did hospital staff describe possible side effects in a way you could understand?)

• Patient may experience dyspepsia, xerostomia, rhinorrhea, tremors, or pharyngitis. Have patient report immediately to prescriber signs of hypokalemia, signs of hyperuricemia, angina, tachycardia, uncontrolled breathing attack, decreased peak flow measurement, severe anxiety, considerable dizziness, syncope, intolerable headache, vision changes, eye pain, eye irritation, paresthesia, dysuria, difficult urination, or edema (HCAHPS).

• Educate patient about signs of a significant reaction (eg, wheezing; chest tightness; fever; itching; bad cough; blue skin color; seizures; or swelling of face, lips, tongue, or throat). **Note:** This is not a comprehensive list of all side effects. Patient should consult prescriber for additional questions.

Intended Use and Disclaimer: Should not be printed and given to patients. This information is intended to serve as a concise initial reference for healthcare professionals to use when discussing medications with a patient. You must ultimately rely on your own discretion, experience and judgment in diagnosing, treating and advising patients.

Related Information

Albuterol *on page 51*

Ipratropium (Oral Inhalation) *on page 867*

Irbesartan (ir be SAR tan)

Brand Names: U.S. Avapro

Pharmacologic Category Angiotensin II Receptor Blocker; Antihypertensive

Medication Safety Issues

Sound-alike/look-alike issues:

Avapro may be confused with Anaprox

Pregnancy Risk Factor D

Lactation Excretion in breast milk unknown/not recommended

Breast-Feeding Considerations It is not known if irbesartan is excreted into breast milk. Due to the potential for serious adverse reactions in the nursing infant, the manufacturer recommends a decision be made whether to discontinue nursing or to discontinue the drug, taking into account the importance of treatment to the mother. Breast-fed infants of mothers taking medications for hypertension should be monitored for adverse effects (Chobanian, 2003).

Use Treatment of hypertension alone or in combination with other antihypertensives; treatment of diabetic nephropathy in patients with type 2 diabetes mellitus (noninsulin dependent, NIDDM) and hypertension

Unlabeled Use To slow the rate of progression of aortic-root dilation in pediatric patients with Marfan's syndrome

Mechanism of Action/Effect Irbesartan is an angiotensin receptor antagonist. Angiotensin II acts as a vasoconstrictor and stimulates the release of aldosterone, which results in reabsorption of sodium and water. These effects result in an elevation in blood pressure. Irbesartan blocks the AT1 angiotensin II receptor, thereby blocking the vasoconstriction and the aldosterone secreting effects of angiotensin II.

Contraindications Hypersensitivity to irbesartan or any component of the formulation; concomitant use with aliskiren in patients with diabetes mellitus *Canadian labeling:* Additional contraindications (not in U.S. labeling): Hypersensitivity to irbesartan or any component of the formulation; concomitant use with aliskiren in patients with moderate to severe renal impairment (GFR <60 mL/minute/ 1.73 m^2)

Warnings/Precautions [U.S. Boxed Warning]: Drugs that act on the renin-angiotensin system can cause injury and death to the developing fetus. Discontinue as soon as possible once pregnancy is detected. May cause hyperkalemia; avoid potassium supplementation unless specifically required by healthcare provider. May be associated with deterioration of renal function and/or increases in serum creatinine, particularly in patients with low renal blood flow (eg, renal artery stenosis, heart failure) whose glomerular filtration rate (GFR) is dependent on efferent arteriolar vasoconstriction by angiotensin II. Avoid use or use a much smaller dose in patients who are intravascularly volume-depleted; use caution in patients with unstented unilateral or bilateral renal artery stenosis. When unstented bilateral renal artery stenosis is present, use is generally avoided due to the elevated risk of deterioration in renal function unless possible benefits outweigh risks. AUCs of irbesartan (not the active metabolite) are about 50% greater in patients with CrCl <30 mL/minute and are doubled in hemodialysis patients.

Potentially significant drug interactions may exist, requiring dose or frequency adjustment, additional monitoring, and/or selection of alternative therapy.

Angioedema has been reported rarely with some angiotensin II receptor antagonists (ARBs) and may occur at any time during treatment (especially following first dose). It may involve the head and neck (potentially compromising airway) or the intestine (presenting with abdominal pain). Patients with idiopathic or hereditary angioedema or previous angioedema associated with ACE-inhibitor therapy may be at an increased risk. Prolonged frequent monitoring may be required, especially if tongue, glottis, or larynx are involved, as they are associated with airway obstruction. Patients with a history of airway surgery may have a higher risk of airway obstruction. Discontinue therapy immediately if angioedema occurs. Aggressive early management is critical. Intramuscular (I.M.) administration of epinephrine may be necessary. Do not readminister to patients who have had angioedema with ARBs.

Drug Interactions

Avoid Concomitant Use

Avoid concomitant use of Irbesartan with any of the following: Pimozide

Decreased Effect

The levels/effects of Irbesartan may be decreased by: Herbs (Hypertensive Properties); Methylphenidate; Nonsteroidal Anti-Inflammatory Agents; Rifamycin Derivatives; Yohimbine

Increased Effect/Toxicity

Irbesartan may increase the levels/effects of: ACE Inhibitors; Amifostine; Antihypertensives; ARIPiprazole; Bosentan; Carvedilol; CycloSPORINE (Systemic); CYP2C8 Substrates; CYP2C9 Substrates; Dofetilide; DULoxetine; Hypotensive Agents; Lithium; Lomitapide; Nonsteroidal Anti-Inflammatory Agents; Obinutuzumab; Pimozide; Potassium-Sparing Diuretics; RiTUXimab; Sodium Phosphates

The levels/effects of Irbesartan may be increased by: Alfuzosin; Aliskiren; Brimonidine (Topical); Canagliflozin; Diazoxide; Eplerenone; Fluconazole; Heparin; Heparin (Low Molecular Weight); Herbs (Hypotensive Properties); MAO Inhibitors; Pentoxifylline; Phosphodiesterase 5 Inhibitors; Potassium Salts; Prostacyclin Analogues; Tolvaptan; Trimethoprim

Nutritional/Ethanol Interactions Herb/Nutraceutical: Dong quai has estrogenic activity. Some herbal medications may worsen hypertension (eg, ephedra); garlic may have additional antihypertensive effects. Management: Avoid dong quai if using for hypertension. Avoid ephedra, yohimbe, ginseng, and garlic.

Adverse Reactions Unless otherwise indicated, percentage of incidence is reported for patients with hypertension.

>10%: Endocrine & metabolic: Hyperkalemia (19%, diabetic nephropathy; rarely seen in HTN)

1% to 10%:

Cardiovascular: Orthostatic hypotension (5%, diabetic nephropathy)

Central nervous system: Fatigue (4%), dizziness (10%, diabetic nephropathy)

Gastrointestinal: Diarrhea (3%), dyspepsia (2%)

Respiratory: Upper respiratory infection (9%), cough (2.8% versus 2.7% in placebo)

Pharmacodynamics/Kinetics
Onset of Action Peak levels in 1-2 hours
Duration of Action >24 hours
Available Dosage Forms
Tablet, Oral:
Avapro: 75 mg, 150 mg, 300 mg
Generic: 75 mg, 150 mg, 300 mg
General Dosage Range Oral:
Children 6-12 years: Initial: 75 mg once daily; Maintenance: 75-150 mg once daily
Children ≥13 years and Adults: Initial: 75-150 mg once daily; Maintenance: 75-300 mg once daily
Storage/Stability Store at room temperature of 15°C to 30°C (59°F to 86°F).
Nursing Actions
Physical Assessment Assess potential for interactions with other pharmacological agents or herbal products (risk of hyperkalemia or toxicity). Monitor for hypotension at regular intervals during therapy.
Patient Education
• Discuss specific use of drug and side effects with patient as it relates to treatment. (HCAHPS: During this hospital stay, were you given any medicine that you had not taken before? Before giving you any new medicine, how often did hospital staff tell you what the medicine was for? How often did hospital staff describe possible side effects in a way you could understand?)
• Patient may experience dizziness, hyperkalemia, dyspepsia, diarrhea, or worsening kidney function. Have patient report immediately to prescriber hyperhidrosis, vomiting, syncope, severe headache, rash, or pregnancy (HCAHPS).
• Educate patient about signs of a significant reaction (eg, wheezing; chest tightness; fever; itching; bad cough; blue skin color; seizures; or swelling of face, lips, tongue, or throat). **Note:** This is not a comprehensive list of all side effects. Patient should consult prescriber for additional questions,

Intended Use and Disclaimer: Should not be printed and given to patients. This information is intended to serve as a concise initial reference for healthcare professionals to use when discussing medications with a patient. You must ultimately rely on your own discretion, experience and judgment in diagnosing, treating and advising patients.
Dietary Considerations May be taken with or without food.

Irbesartan and Hydrochlorothiazide
(ir be SAR tan & hye droe klor oh THYE a zide)

Brand Names: U.S. Avalide
Index Terms Avapro® HCT; Hydrochlorothiazide and Irbesartan

Pharmacologic Category Angiotensin II Receptor Blocker; Antihypertensive; Diuretic, Thiazide
Medication Safety Issues
Sound-alike/look-alike issues:
Avalide may be confused with Avandia®
Pregnancy Risk Factor D
Use Combination therapy for the management of hypertension; may be used as initial therapy in patients likely to need multiple drugs to achieve blood pressure goals
Available Dosage Forms
Tablet, oral: 150/12.5: Irbesartan 150 mg and hydrochlorothiazide 12.5 mg; 300/12.5: Irbesartan 300 mg and hydrochlorothiazide 12.5 mg
Avalide: Irbesartan 150 mg and hydrochlorothiazide 12.5 mg; irbesartan 300 mg and hydrochlorothiazide 12.5 mg
General Dosage Range Oral: *Adults:* Irbesartan 150-300 mg and hydrochlorothiazide 12.5-25 mg once daily
Nursing Actions
Physical Assessment See individual agents.
Patient Education
• Discuss specific use of drug and side effects with patient as it relates to treatment. (HCAHPS: During this hospital stay, were you given any medicine that you had not taken before? Before giving you any new medicine, how often did hospital staff tell you what the medicine was for? How often did hospital staff describe possible side effects in a way you could understand?)
• Patient may experience dizziness, asthenia, or nausea. Have patient report immediately to prescriber signs of infection, signs of hyperglycemia, signs of renal impairment, paresthesia, angina, sexual dysfunction, strength differences from one side to another, akathisia, severe dyspepsia, dyspnea, significant weight gain, edema, ecchymosis, bleeding, jaundice, or vision changes (HCAHPS).
• Educate patient about signs of a significant reaction (eg, wheezing; chest tightness; fever; itching; bad cough; blue skin color; seizures; or swelling of face, lips, tongue, or throat). **Note:** This is not a comprehensive list of all side effects. Patient should consult prescriber for additional questions.

Intended Use and Disclaimer: Should not be printed and given to patients. This information is intended to serve as a concise initial reference for healthcare professionals to use when discussing medications with a patient. You must ultimately rely on your own discretion, experience and judgment in diagnosing, treating and advising patients.

Related Information
Hydrochlorothiazide *on page* 775
Irbesartan *on page* 869

Irinotecan (eye rye no TEE kan)

Brand Names: U.S. Camptosar

Index Terms Camptothecin-11; CPT-11; Irinotecan HCl; Irinotecan Hydrochloride

Pharmacologic Category Antineoplastic Agent, Camptothecin; Antineoplastic Agent, Topoisomerase I Inhibitor

Medication Safety Issues

Sound-alike/look-alike issues:

Irinotecan may be confused with topotecan

High alert medication:

This medication is in a class the Institute for Safe Medication Practices (ISMP) includes among its list of drug classes which have a heightened risk of causing significant patient harm when used in error.

Pregnancy Risk Factor D

Lactation Excretion in breast milk unknown/not recommended

Breast-Feeding Considerations Due to the potential for serious adverse reactions in the nursing infant, breast-feeding is not recommended.

Use Treatment of metastatic carcinoma of the colon or rectum

Unlabeled Use Treatment of cervical cancer (recurrent or metastatic), central nervous system tumors (recurrent glioblastoma), esophageal cancer, Ewing's sarcoma (recurrent or progressive), gastric cancer (metastatic or locally advanced), nonsmall cell lung cancer (advanced), ovarian cancer (recurrent), pancreatic cancer (advanced), small cell lung cancer (extensive stage)

Mechanism of Action/Effect Irinotecan and its active metabolite (SN-38) bind reversibly to topoisomerase I-DNA complex preventing religation of the cleaved DNA strand. This results in the accumulation of cleavable complexes and double-strand DNA breaks. As mammalian cells cannot efficiently repair these breaks, cell death consistent with S-phase cell cycle specificity occurs, leading to termination of cellular replication.

Contraindications Hypersensitivity to irinotecan or any component of the formulation

Warnings/Precautions Hazardous agent - use appropriate precautions for handling and disposal (NIOSH, 2012). Severe hypersensitivity reactions (including anaphylaxis) have occurred. For I.V. use only; monitor infusion site; may cause local tissue necrosis or thrombophlebitis if extravasation occurs (the manufacturer recommends flushing the site with sterile water and ice application).

[U.S. Boxed Warning]: Severe diarrhea may be dose-limiting and potentially fatal; early-onset and late-onset diarrhea may occur. Early diarrhea occurs during or within 24 hours of receiving irinotecan and is characterized by cholinergic symptoms (eg, increased salivation, rhinitis, miosis, diaphoresis, flushing, abdominal cramping, lacrimation); may be prevented or treated with atropine. Late diarrhea occurs more than 24 hours after treatment which may lead to dehydration, electrolyte imbalance, or sepsis; may be life-threatening and should be promptly treated with loperamide; dose reductions may be recommended for future doses within the current cycle. Antibiotics may be necessary if patient develops ileus, fever, or severe neutropenia. Patients with diarrhea should be carefully monitored and treated promptly; may require fluid and electrolyte therapy. Colitis, complicated by ulceration, bleeding, ileus, and infection has been reported; initiate antibiotics promptly in patients with ileus.

[U.S. Boxed Warning]: May cause severe myelosuppression. Deaths due to sepsis following severe neutropenia have been reported. Complications due to neutropenia should be promptly managed with antibiotics. Therapy should be temporarily discontinued if neutropenic fever occurs or if the absolute neutrophil count is <1000/mm^3. The dose of irinotecan should be reduced if there is a clinically significant decrease in the total WBC (<200/mm^3), neutrophil count (<1500/mm^3), hemoglobin (<8 g/dL), or platelet count (<100,000/mm^3). Routine administration of a colony-stimulating factor is generally not necessary, but may be considered for patients experiencing significant neutropenia. Fatal cases of interstitial pulmonary disease (IPD)-like events have been reported with single-agent and combination therapy. Promptly evaluate changes in baseline pulmonary symptoms or any new-onset pulmonary symptoms. Discontinue all chemotherapy if IPD is diagnosed.

Patients with even modest elevations in total serum bilirubin levels (1-2 mg/dL) have a significantly greater likelihood of experiencing first-course grade 3 or 4 neutropenia than those with bilirubin levels that were <1 mg/dL. Patients with abnormal glucuronidation of bilirubin, such as those with Gilbert's syndrome, may also be at greater risk of myelosuppression when receiving therapy with irinotecan. Use caution when treating patients with known hepatic dysfunction or hyperbilirubinemia; exposure to the active metabolite (SN-38) is increased; toxicities may be increased. Dosage adjustments should be considered.

Patients homozygous for the UGT1A1*28 allele are at increased risk of neutropenia; initial one-level dose reduction should be considered for both single-agent and combination regimens. Heterozygous carriers of the UGT1A1*28 allele may also be at increased risk; however, most patients have tolerated normal starting doses. Avoid vaccination with live vaccines during treatment (risk of infection may be increased due to immunosuppression). Although the response to vaccines may be diminished, inactivated vaccines may be administered during treatment.

Renal impairment and acute renal failure have been reported, possibly due to dehydration secondary to diarrhea. Use with caution in patients with renal impairment; not recommended in patients on dialysis. Patients with bowel obstruction should not be treated with irinotecan until resolution of obstruction. Use caution in patients who previously received pelvic/abdominal radiation, elderly patients with comorbid conditions, or baseline performance status of 2; close monitoring and dosage adjustments are recommended. Contains sorbitol; do not use in patients with hereditary fructose intolerance. Thromboembolic events have been reported. **[U.S. Boxed Warning]: Should be administered under the supervision of an experienced cancer chemotherapy physician.** Except as part of a clinical trial, use in combination with fluorouracil and leucovorin "Mayo Clinic" regimen is not recommended. Increased toxicity has also been noted in patients with a baseline performance status of 2 in other combination regimens containing irinotecan, leucovorin, and fluorouracil. High potential for CYP-mediated drug interactions; enzyme inducers may decrease exposure to irinotecan and SN-38 (active metabolite); enzyme inhibitors may increase exposure; for use in patients with CNS tumors (unlabeled use), selection of antiseizure medications which are not enzyme inducers is preferred.

Drug Interactions

Avoid Concomitant Use

Avoid concomitant use of Irinotecan with any of the following: Atazanavir; BCG; CloZAPine; Conivaptan; Fusidic Acid (Systemic); Grapefruit Juice; Natalizumab; Pimecrolimus; St Johns Wort; Tacrolimus (Topical); Tofacitinib; Vaccines (Live)

Decreased Effect

Irinotecan may decrease the levels/effects of: BCG; Coccidioidin Skin Test; Sipuleucel-T; Vaccines (Inactivated); Vaccines (Live)

The levels/effects of Irinotecan may be decreased by: Bosentan; CarBAMazepine; CYP3A4 Inducers (Strong); Dabrafenib; Deferasirox; Echinacea; Fosphenytoin; Mitotane; P-glycoprotein/ABCB1 Inducers; PHENobarbital; Phenytoin; St Johns Wort; Tocilizumab

Increased Effect/Toxicity

Irinotecan may increase the levels/effects of: CloZAPine; Leflunomide; Natalizumab; Tofacitinib; Vaccines (Live)

The levels/effects of Irinotecan may be increased by: Antifungal Agents (Azole Derivatives, Systemic); Atazanavir; Bevacizumab; Conivaptan; CYP2B6 Inhibitors (Moderate); CYP2B6 Inhibitors (Strong); CYP3A4 Inhibitors (Moderate); CYP3A4 Inhibitors (Strong); Dasatinib; Denosumab; Eltrombopag; Fusidic Acid (Systemic); Grapefruit Juice; Ivacaftor; Luliconazole; Mifepristone; P-glycoprotein/ABCB1 Inhibitors; Pimecrolimus; Quazepam; Regorafenib; Roflumilast; Simeprevir; SORAfenib; Stiripentol; Tacrolimus (Topical); Trastuzumab

Nutritional/Ethanol Interactions Herb/Nutraceutical: Avoid St John's wort (decreases the efficacy of irinotecan).

Adverse Reactions Frequency of adverse reactions reported for single-agent use of irinotecan only.

>10%:

Cardiovascular: Vasodilation (9% to 11%)

Central nervous system: Cholinergic toxicity (47% - includes rhinitis, increased salivation, miosis, lacrimation, diaphoresis, flushing and intestinal hyperperistalsis); fever (44% to 45%), pain (23% to 24%), dizziness (15% to 21%), insomnia (19%), headache (17%), chills (14%)

Dermatologic: Alopecia (46% to 72%), rash (13% to 14%)

Endocrine & metabolic: Dehydration (15%)

Gastrointestinal: Diarrhea, late (83% to 88%; grade 3/4: 14% to 31%), diarrhea, early (43% to 51%; grade 3/4: 7% to 22%), nausea (70% to 86%), abdominal pain (57% to 68%), vomiting (62% to 67%), cramps (57%), anorexia (44% to 55%), constipation (30% to 32%), mucositis (30%), weight loss (30%), flatulence (12%), stomatitis (12%)

Hematologic: Anemia (60% to 97%; grades 3/4: 5% to 7%), leukopenia (63% to 96%, grades 3/4: 14% to 28%), thrombocytopenia (96%, grades 3/4: 1% to 4%), neutropenia (30% to 96%; grades 3/4: 14% to 31%)

Hepatic: Bilirubin increased (84%), alkaline phosphatase increased (13%)

Neuromuscular & skeletal: Weakness (69% to 76%), back pain (14%)

Respiratory: Dyspnea (22%), cough (17% to 20%), rhinitis (16%)

Miscellaneous: Diaphoresis (16%), infection (14%)

1% to 10%:

Cardiovascular: Edema (10%), hypotension (6%), thromboembolic events (5%)

Central nervous system: Somnolence (9%), confusion (3%)

Gastrointestinal: Abdominal fullness (10%), dyspepsia (10%)

Hematologic: Neutropenic fever (grades 3/4: 2% to 6%), hemorrhage (grades 3/4: 1% to 5%), neutropenic infection (grades 3/4: 1% to 2%)

Hepatic: AST increased (10%), ascites and/or jaundice (grades 3/4: 9%)

Respiratory: Pneumonia (4%)

Note: In limited pediatric experience, dehydration (often associated with severe hypokalemia and hyponatremia) was among the most significant grade 3/4 adverse events, with a frequency up to 29%. In addition, grade 3/4 infection was reported in 24%.

Available Dosage Forms

Solution, Intravenous:

Camptosar: 40 mg/2 mL (2 mL); 100 mg/5 mL (5 mL); 300 mg/15 mL (15 mL)

Generic: 40 mg/2 mL (2 mL); 100 mg/5 mL (5 mL); 500 mg/25 mL (25 mL)

Solution, Intravenous [preservative free]:

Generic: 40 mg/2 mL (2 mL); 100 mg/5 mL (5 mL)

General Dosage Range Dosage adjustment recommended in patients with hepatic impairment or who develop toxicities

I.V.: *Adults:* Dosage varies greatly depending on indication

Administration

I.V. Administer by I.V. infusion, usually over 90 minutes. Premedication with dexamethasone and a 5-HT$_3$ blocker is recommended 30 minutes prior to administration; prochlorperazine may be considered for subsequent use (if needed). Consider atropine 0.25-1 mg I.V. or SubQ as premedication for or treatment of cholinergic symptoms (eg, increased salivation, rhinitis, miosis, diaphoresis, abdominal cramping) or early onset diarrhea.

The recommended regimen to manage late diarrhea is loperamide 4 mg orally at onset of late diarrhea, followed by 2 mg every 2 hours (or 4 mg every 4 hours at night) until 12 hours have passed without a bowel movement. If diarrhea recurs, then repeat administration. Loperamide should not be used for more than 48 consecutive hours.

Hazardous agent; use appropriate precautions for handling and disposal (NIOSH, 2012).

Injectable Detail pH: 3-3.8

Preparation for Administration Hazardous agent; use appropriate precautions for handling and disposal (NIOSH, 2012). Dilute in 250-500 mL D$_5$W (preferred) or NS to a final concentration of 0.12-2.8 mg/mL. Due to the relatively acidic pH, irinotecan appears to be more stable in D$_5$W than NS.

Storage/Stability Store intact vials at room temperature. Protect from light. Solutions diluted in NS may precipitate if refrigerated. Solutions diluted in D$_5$W are stable for 24 hours at room temperature or 48 hours under refrigeration at 2°C to 8°C, although the manufacturer recommends use within 24 hours if refrigerated, within 6 hours at room temperature, and/or within 12 hours at room temperature (including infusion time) only if prepared under strict aseptic conditions (eg, laminar flow hood). Do not freeze.

Nursing Actions

Physical Assessment Premedication with antiemetic may be ordered (emetic potential moderate). Monitor infusion site closely to prevent extravasation. Monitor for immediate or delayed diarrhea (can be fatal), neutropenia, sepsis, mucositis, and/or stomatitis.

Patient Education

• Discuss specific use of drug and side effects with patient as it relates to treatment. (HCAHPS: During this hospital stay, were you given any medicine that you had not taken before? Before giving you any new medicine, how often did hospital staff tell you what the medicine was for? How often did hospital staff describe possible side effects in a way you could understand?)

• Patient may experience anemia, leukopenia, thrombocytopenia, headache, nausea, diarrhea, alopecia, stomatitis, or fatigue. Have patient report immediately to prescriber signs of infection, dyspnea, dizziness or syncope, ecchymosis, melena, or rash (HCAHPS).

• Educate patient about signs of a significant reaction (eg, wheezing; chest tightness; fever; itching; bad cough; blue skin color; seizures; or swelling of face, lips, tongue, or throat). **Note:** This is not a comprehensive list of all side effects. Patient should consult prescriber for additional questions.

Intended Use and Disclaimer: Should not be printed and given to patients. This information is intended to serve as a concise initial reference for healthcare professionals to use when discussing medications with a patient. You must ultimately rely on your own discretion, experience and judgment in diagnosing, treating and advising patients.

Dietary Considerations Contains sorbitol; do not use in patients with hereditary fructose intolerance.

Related Information

Management of Drug Extravasations *on page 1700*

Iron Dextran Complex
(EYE ern DEKS tran KOM pleks)

Brand Names: U.S. Dexferrum; Infed

Index Terms High-Molecular-Weight Iron Dextran (DexFerrum); Imferon; Iron Dextran; Low-Molecular-Weight Iron Dextran (INFeD)

Pharmacologic Category Iron Salt

Medication Safety Issues

Sound-alike/look-alike issues:

Dexferrum may be confused with Desferal

Iron dextran complex may be confused with ferumoxytol

Pregnancy Risk Factor C

Lactation Enters breast milk/use caution

Use Iron deficiency: Treatment of iron deficiency in patients in whom oral administration is unsatisfactory or infeasible

Dosage Forms Considerations

Strength of iron dextran complex is expressed as elemental iron.

Available Dosage Forms
Solution, Injection:
Dexferrum: 50 mg/mL (1 mL, 2 mL)
Infed: 50 mg/mL (2 mL)
General Dosage Range Note: A 0.5 mL test dose (0.25 mL in infants) should be given prior to starting iron dextran therapy.
I.M., I.V.:
Children <5 kg and >4 months: Replacement iron (mg) = blood loss (mL) x Hct; **Note:** Total dose should be divided daily at not more than 25 mg/day
Children 5-15 kg and >4 months: Total Dose (mL) = 0.0442 (desired Hgb [usually 12 g/dL] - observed Hgb) x W (in kg) + (0.26 x W [in kg]) **or** replacement iron (mg) = blood loss (mL) x hematocrit; **Note:** Total dose should be divided daily at not more than 50 mg/day (5-10 kg) or 100 mg/day (10-15 kg)
Children >15 kg: Total Dose (mL) = 0.0442 (desired Hgb [usually 14.8 g/dL] - observed Hgb) x LBW + (0.26 x LBW) **or** replacement iron (mg) = blood loss (mL) x Hct; **Note:** Total dose should be divided daily at not more than 100 mg/day
Adults: Total Dose (mL) = 0.0442 (desired Hgb [usually 14.8 g/dL] - observed Hgb) x LBW + (0.26 x LBW) **or** replacement iron (mg) = blood loss (mL) x Hct; **Note:** Total dose should be divided daily at not more than 100 mg/day

Administration
I.M. Note: A test dose should be given on the first day of therapy; patient should be observed for 1 hour for hypersensitivity reaction, then the remainder of the day's dose (dose minus test dose) should be given. Resuscitation equipment, medication, and trained personnel should be available. An uneventful test dose does not ensure an anaphylactic-type reaction will not occur during administration of the therapeutic dose.

I.M. (INFeD): Use Z-track technique (displacement of the skin laterally prior to injection); injection should be deep into the upper outer quadrant of buttock; alternate buttocks with subsequent injections. Administer test dose at same recommended site using the same technique.

I.V. Test dose should be given gradually over at least 30 seconds (INFeD) or 5 minutes (Dexferrum), or over 1-2 minutes (INFeD) for cancer-/chemotherapy-associated anemia (Auerbach, 2004). Subsequent dose(s) may be administered by I.V. bolus undiluted at a rate not to exceed 50 mg/minute (maximum 100 mg). For total dose infusion in patients with cancer-/chemotherapy-associated anemia (unlabeled dose): 1 hour after the test dose, administer the balance of the dose diluted in 500 mL NS and infuse at 175 mL/hour (Auerbach, 2004) or administer over several hours (NCCN Anemia guidelines v.2.2104). Avoid dilutions with dextrose (increased incidence of local pain and phlebitis).
Injectable Detail pH: Undiluted: 4.5-7 (dexferrum); 5.2-6.5 (INFeD)

Nursing Actions
Physical Assessment Be alert to the potential for anaphylaxis. Resuscitation equipment and emergency medications should be available. Note that adverse response may occur some time (1-4 days) after administration. Monitor patient's tolerance of medication including evidence of symptoms such as arthralgias and myalgias.

Patient Education
• Discuss specific use of drug and side effects with patient as it relates to treatment. (HCAHPS: During this hospital stay, were you given any medicine that you had not taken before? Before giving you any new medicine, how often did hospital staff tell you what the medicine was for? How often did hospital staff describe possible side effects in a way you could understand?)
• Patient may experience injection site irritation, diarrhea, flushing, headache, dyspepsia, myalgia, nausea, or dysgeusia. Have patient report immediately to prescriber angina, severe dizziness, dyspnea, or rash (HCAHPS).
• Educate patient about signs of a significant reaction (eg, wheezing; chest tightness; fever; itching; bad cough; blue skin color; seizures; or swelling of face, lips, tongue, or throat). **Note:** This is not a comprehensive list of all side effects. Patient should consult prescriber for additional questions.

Intended Use and Disclaimer: Should not be printed and given to patients. This information is intended to serve as a concise initial reference for healthcare professionals to use when discussing medications with a patient. You must ultimately rely on your own discretion, experience and judgment in diagnosing, treating and advising patients.

Iron Sucrose (EYE ern SOO krose)

Brand Names: U.S. Venofer
Pharmacologic Category Iron Salt
Medication Safety Issues
Sound-alike/look-alike issues:
Iron sucrose may be confused with ferumoxytol
Pregnancy Risk Factor B
Lactation Excretion in breast milk unknown/use caution
Use Iron deficiency anemia: Treatment of iron-deficiency anemia in chronic kidney disease (CKD)
Unlabeled Use Chemotherapy-associated anemia
Dosage Forms Considerations
Strength of iron sucrose is expressed as elemental iron.

Available Dosage Forms

Solution, Intravenous [preservative free]:
Venofer: 20 mg/mL (2.5 mL, 5 mL, 10 mL)

General Dosage Range I.V.:

Children ≥2 years and Adolescents: Maintenance therapy: 0.5 mg/kg/dose (maximum: 100 mg) every 2 weeks for 6 doses **or** every 4 weeks for 3 doses

Adults: 100 mg during consecutive dialysis sessions for 10 doses (total cumulative dose: 1000 mg) **or** 200 mg on 5 different occasions within a 14-day period (total cumulative dose: 1000 mg) **or** two 300 mg infusions administered 14 days apart, followed by a single 400 mg infusion 14 days later (total cumulative dose: 1000 mg)

Administration

I.V. Administer intravenously as a slow I.V. injection (**not** for rapid I.V. injection) or as an I.V. infusion. Can be administered through dialysis line.

Children and Adolescents:

Slow I.V. injection: Administer undiluted over 5 minutes

Infusion: Infuse diluted solution over 5-60 minutes

Adults:

Slow I.V. injection: May administer doses ≤200 mg undiluted by slow I.V. injection over 2-5 minutes. When administering to hemodialysis-dependent patients, give iron sucrose early during the dialysis session.

Infusion: Infuse diluted doses ≤200 mg over at least 15 minutes; infuse diluted 300 mg dose over 1.5 hours; infuse diluted 400 mg dose over 2.5 hours; infuse diluted 500 mg dose over 3.5-4 hours (limited experience). When administering to hemodialysis-dependent patients, give iron sucrose early during the dialysis session.

Nursing Actions

Physical Assessment Facilities for cardiopulmonary resuscitation must be available during administration. Monitor vital signs, including blood pressure, closely during infusion. Hemodialysis patients are susceptible to hypotension related to total dose or rate of administration. Monitor for symptoms of an allergic reaction, including hives, itching, angioedema, and severe dizziness. Monitor patient for chest pain, dyspnea, or dysrhythmias. Monitor during and for 30 minutes after infusion is complete.

Patient Education

- Discuss specific use of drug and side effects with patient as it relates to treatment. (HCAHPS: During this hospital stay, were you given any medicine that you had not taken before? Before giving you any new medicine, how often did hospital staff tell you what the medicine was for? How often did hospital staff describe possible side effects in a way you could understand?)

- Patient may experience dizziness, dyspepsia, emesis, diarrhea, or headache. Have patient report immediately to prescriber angina or rash (HCAHPS).

- Educate patient about signs of a significant reaction (eg, wheezing; chest tightness; fever; itching; bad cough; blue skin color; seizures; or swelling of face, lips, tongue, or throat). **Note:** This is not a comprehensive list of all side effects. Patient should consult prescriber for additional questions.

Intended Use and Disclaimer: Should not be printed and given to patients. This information is intended to serve as a concise initial reference for healthcare professionals to use when discussing medications with a patient. You must ultimately rely on your own discretion, experience and judgment in diagnosing, treating and advising patients.

Isoniazid (eye soe NYE a zid)

Index Terms INH; Isonicotinic Acid Hydrazide

Pharmacologic Category Antitubercular Agent

Medication Safety Issues

International issues:

Hydra [Japan] may be confused with Hydrea brand name for hydroxyurea [U.S., Canada, and multiple international markets]

Pregnancy Risk Factor C

Lactation Enters breast milk/compatible

Breast-Feeding Considerations Small amounts of isoniazid are excreted in breast milk. However, women with tuberculosis should not be discouraged from breast-feeding. Pyridoxine supplementation is recommended for the mother and infant.

Use Treatment of susceptible tuberculosis infections; treatment of latent tuberculosis infection (LTBI)

Mechanism of Action/Effect Unknown, but may include the inhibition of mycolic acid synthesis resulting in disruption of the bacterial cell wall

Contraindications Hypersensitivity to isoniazid or any component of the formulation; acute liver disease; previous history of hepatic damage during isoniazid therapy; previous severe adverse reaction (drug fever, chills, arthritis) to isoniazid

Warnings/Precautions Use with caution in patients with severe renal impairment and liver disease. **[U.S. Boxed Warning]: Severe and sometimes fatal hepatitis may occur; usually occurs within the first 3 months of treatment, although may develop even after many months of treatment.** The risk of developing hepatitis is age-related, although isoniazid-induced hepatotoxicity has been reported in children; daily ethanol consumption may also increase the risk. Patients must report any prodromal symptoms of hepatitis, such as fatigue, weakness, malaise, anorexia, nausea, abdominal pain, jaundice, or vomiting.

Patients should be instructed to immediately discontinue therapy if any of these symptoms occur, even if a clinical evaluation has yet to be conducted. Treatment with isoniazid for latent tuberculosis infection should be deferred in patients with acute hepatic diseases. Periodic ophthalmic examinations are recommended even when usual symptoms do not occur. Pyridoxine (10-50 mg/day) is recommended in individuals at risk for development of peripheral neuropathies (eg, HIV infection, nutritional deficiency, diabetes, pregnancy). Children with low milk and low meat intake should receive concomitant pyridoxine therapy. Multidrug regimens should be utilized for the treatment of active tuberculosis to prevent the emergence of drug resistance.

Drug Interactions

Avoid Concomitant Use

Avoid concomitant use of Isoniazid with any of the following: Pimozide; Tegafur; Thioridazine

Decreased Effect

Isoniazid may decrease the levels/effects of: Clopidogrel; Codeine; Itraconazole; Ketoconazole (Systemic); Tamoxifen; Tegafur; TraMADol

The levels/effects of Isoniazid may be decreased by: Antacids; Corticosteroids (Systemic); Cyproterone

Increased Effect/Toxicity

Isoniazid may increase the levels/effects of: Acetaminophen; ARIPiprazole; Benzodiazepines (metabolized by oxidation); CarBAMazepine; Chlorzoxazone; Citalopram; CycloSERINE; CYP2A6 Substrates; CYP2C19 Substrates; CYP2D6 Substrates; CYP2E1 Substrates; Dofetilide; DOXOrubicin (Conventional); Fesoterodine; Fosphenytoin; Lomitapide; Metoprolol; Nebivolol; Phenytoin; Pimozide; Theophylline Derivatives; Thioridazine

The levels/effects of Isoniazid may be increased by: Disulfiram; Ethionamide; Propafenone; Rifamycin Derivatives

Nutritional/Ethanol Interactions

Ethanol: Ethanol increases the risk of hepatitis. Management: Avoid ethanol.

Food: Bioavailability is decreased if taken with food. Isoniazid may also decrease folic acid absorption and alters pyridoxine metabolism. Management: Take on an empty stomach 1 hour before or 2 hours after a meal; increase dietary intake of folate, niacin, and magnesium.

Tyramine-containing food: Isoniazid has weak monoamine oxidase inhibiting activity and may potentially inhibit tyramine metabolism. Several case reports of mild reactions (flushing, palpitations, headache, mild increase in blood pressure, diaphoresis) after ingestion of certain types of cheese or red wine, have been reported (Self, 1999; Toutoungi, 1985). Management: Manufacturer's labeling recommends avoiding tyramine-containing foods (eg, aged or matured cheese,

air-dried or cured meats including sausages and salamis; fava or broad bean pods, tap/draft beers, Marmite concentrate, sauerkraut, soy sauce, and other soybean condiments). However, the clinical relevance of the tyramine reaction for the vast majority of patients receiving isoniazid has been questioned due to isoniazid's weak MAO inhibition and the relatively few published case reports of the interaction. Although not fully investigated, it has been proposed that the reaction has a genetic component and may only be significant in poor or intermediate acetylators since isoniazid is primarily inactivated by acetylation (DiMartini, 1995; Toutoungi, 1985).

Histamine-containing food: Isoniazid may also inhibit diamine oxidase resulting in headache, sweating, palpitations, flushing, hypotension to histamine-containing foods (eg, skipjack, tuna, other tropical fish). Management: Manufacturer's labeling recommends avoiding histamine-containing foods.

Adverse Reactions Frequency not defined.

Cardiovascular: Hypertension, palpitation, tachycardia, vasculitis

Central nervous system: Depression, dizziness, encephalopathy, fever, lethargy, memory impairment, psychosis, seizure, slurred speech, toxic encephalopathy

Dermatologic: Flushing, rash (morbilliform, maculopapular, pruritic, or exfoliative)

Endocrine & metabolic: Gynecomastia, hyperglycemia, metabolic acidosis, pellagra, pyridoxine deficiency

Gastrointestinal: Anorexia, epigastric distress, nausea, stomach pain, vomiting

Hematologic: Agranulocytosis, anemia (sideroblastic, hemolytic, or aplastic), eosinophilia, thrombocytopenia

Hepatic: LFTs mildly increased (10% to 20%), hyperbilirubinemia, bilirubinuria, jaundice, hepatic dysfunction, hepatitis (may involve progressive liver damage; risk increases with age; 2.3% in patients >50 years)

Neuromuscular & skeletal: Arthralgia, hyperreflexia, paresthesia, peripheral neuropathy (dose-related incidence, 10% to 20% incidence with 10 mg/kg/day), weakness

Ocular: Blurred vision, loss of vision, optic neuritis and atrophy

Miscellaneous: Lupus-like syndrome, lymphadenopathy, rheumatic syndrome

Available Dosage Forms

Solution, Injection:
Generic: 100 mg/mL (10 mL)

Syrup, Oral:
Generic: 50 mg/5 mL (473 mL)

Tablet, Oral:
Generic: 100 mg, 300 mg

◄ **General Dosage Range Oral, I.M.:**
Children: 10-20 mg/kg/day once daily (maximum: 300 mg/day) **or** 20-40 mg/kg 2-3 times/week (maximum: 900 mg/dose)
Adults: 300 mg (5 mg/kg) once daily **or** 900 mg (15 mg/kg) 2-3 times/week

Administration

Oral Should be administered 1 hour before or 2 hours after meals on an empty stomach.

Storage/Stability
Tablet: Store at 20°C to 25°C (68°F to 77°F). Protect from light.
Oral solution: Store at 15°C to 30°C (59°F to 86°F). Protect from light.

Nursing Actions

Physical Assessment Monitor for liver damage, nausea, vomiting, peripheral neuropathy, and CNS changes at regular intervals during therapy. Teach patient importance of proper diet and ophthalmic examinations.

Patient Education

• Discuss specific use of drug and side effects with patient as it relates to treatment. (HCAHPS: During this hospital stay, were you given any medicine that you had not taken before? Before giving you any new medicine, how often did hospital staff tell you what the medicine was for? How often did hospital staff describe possible side effects in a way you could understand?)

• Patient may experience dyspepsia, nausea, or hepatic impairment. Have patient report immediately to prescriber inability to eat, discolored urine, jaundice, severe asthenia, paresthesia, sudden vision changes, eye pain, eye irritation, or rash (HCAHPS).

• Educate patient about signs of a significant reaction (eg, wheezing; chest tightness; fever; itching; bad cough; blue skin color; seizures; or swelling of face, lips, tongue, or throat). **Note:** This is not a comprehensive list of all side effects. Patient should consult prescriber for additional questions.

Intended Use and Disclaimer: Should not be printed and given to patients. This information is intended to serve as a concise initial reference for healthcare professionals to use when discussing medications with a patient. You must ultimately rely on your own discretion, experience and judgment in diagnosing, treating and advising patients.

Dietary Considerations Should be taken 1 hour before or 2 hours after meals on an empty stomach; increase dietary intake of folate, niacin, magnesium.

Isoproterenol (eye soe proe TER e nole)

Brand Names: U.S. Isuprel
Index Terms Isoproterenol Hydrochloride

Pharmacologic Category Beta$_1$- & Beta$_2$-Adrenergic Agonist Agent

Medication Safety Issues
Sound-alike/look-alike issues:
Isuprel® may be confused with Disophrol®, Isordil®

Pregnancy Risk Factor C

Lactation Excretion in breast milk unknown/use caution

Use Manufacturer's labeled indications (see **"Note"**): Mild or transient episodes of heart block that do not require electric shock or pacemaker therapy; serious episodes of heart block and Adams-Stokes attacks (except when caused by ventricular tachycardia or fibrillation); cardiac arrest until electric shock or pacemaker therapy is available; bronchospasm during anesthesia; adjunct to fluid and electrolyte replacement therapy and other drugs and procedures in the treatment of hypovolemic or septic shock and low cardiac output states (eg, decompensated heart failure, cardiogenic shock)

Note: The use of isoproterenol in advanced cardiac life support (ACLS) has largely been supplanted by the use of other adrenergic agents (eg, epinephrine and dopamine). The use of isoproterenol for bronchospasm during anesthesia and cardiogenic, hypovolemic, or septic shock is no longer recommended. See *Unlabeled Use* for more appropriate, yet unlabeled, uses.

Unlabeled Use Pharmacologic overdrive pacing for refractory torsade de pointes; pharmacologic provocation during tilt table testing for syncope; temporary control of bradycardia in denervated heart transplant patients unresponsive to atropine; ventricular arrhythmias due to AV nodal block; beta-blocker overdose; electrical storm associated with Brugada syndrome

Available Dosage Forms
Solution, Injection:
Isuprel: 0.2 mg/mL (1 mL, 5 mL)

General Dosage Range Continuous I.V. infusion:
Children: 0.05-2 mcg/**kg**/minute; titrate to patient response
Adults: 2-10 mcg/minute; titrate to patient response

Usual Infusion Concentrations: Pediatric I.V. infusion: 20 **mcg**/mL

Usual Infusion Concentrations: Adult I.V. infusion: 1 mg in 100 mL (10 **mcg**/mL), 1 mg in 500 mL (2 **mcg**/mL), **or** 4 mg in 250 mL (16 **mcg**/mL) of D$_5$W or NS

Administration
I.V. I.V. infusion administration requires the use of an infusion pump.

Injectable Detail pH: 2.5-4.5

Nursing Actions

Physical Assessment Monitor cardiac, respiratory, and hemodynamic status when used in acute or emergency situations.

Patient Education

- Discuss specific use of drug and side effects with patient as it relates to treatment. (HCAHPS: During this hospital stay, were you given any medicine that you had not taken before? Before giving you any new medicine, how often did hospital staff tell you what the medicine was for? How often did hospital staff describe possible side effects in a way you could understand?)
- Patient may experience headache, nervousness and anxiety, nausea, or injection site irritation. Have patient report immediately to prescriber dyspnea, angina, tachycardia, severe dizziness, paresthesia, or rash (HCAHPS).
- Educate patient about signs of a significant reaction (eg, wheezing; chest tightness; fever; itching; bad cough; blue skin color; seizures; or swelling of face, lips, tongue, or throat). **Note:** This is not a comprehensive list of all side effects. Patient should consult prescriber for additional questions.

Intended Use and Disclaimer: Should not be printed and given to patients. This information is intended to serve as a concise initial reference for healthcare professionals to use when discussing medications with a patient. You must ultimately rely on your own discretion, experience and judgment in diagnosing, treating and advising patients.

Isosorbide Dinitrate
(eye soe SOR bide dye NYE trate)

Brand Names: U.S. Dilatrate-SR; IsoDitrate ER; Isordil Titradose
Index Terms ISD; ISDN
Pharmacologic Category Antianginal Agent; Vasodilator
Medication Safety Issues
Sound-alike/look-alike issues:
  Isordil may be confused with Inderal, Isuprel, Plendil
Pregnancy Risk Factor C
Lactation Excretion in breast milk unknown/use caution
Breast-Feeding Considerations It is not known if isosorbide dinitrate is excreted in breast milk. The manufacturer recommends that caution be exercised when administering isosorbide dinitrate to nursing women.
Use Prevention and treatment of angina pectoris
  Note: Due to slower onset of action, not the drug of choice to abort an acute anginal episode.
Unlabeled Use Patients with heart failure with reduced ejection fraction (HFrEF) who do not tolerate an ACE inhibitor or an angiotensin receptor blocker (ARB) (in combination with hydralazine); African-American (self-identified) patients with HFrEF NYHA class III-IV remaining symptomatic despite optimal guideline-directed medical therapy (in combination with hydralazine); esophageal spastic disorders

Mechanism of Action/Effect Relaxes vascular smooth muscles, decreases arterial resistance and venous return which reduces cardiac oxygen demand. Additionally, coronary artery dilation improves collateral flow to ischemic regions.

Contraindications Hypersensitivity to isosorbide dinitrate or any component of the formulation; hypersensitivity to organic nitrates; concurrent use with phosphodiesterase-5 (PDE-5) inhibitors (sildenafil, tadalafil, or vardenafil)

Warnings/Precautions Severe hypotension can occur; paradoxical bradycardia and increased angina pectoris can accompany hypotension. Postural hypotension can also occur; ethanol may potentiate this effect. Use with caution in volume depletion and moderate hypotension, and use with extreme caution with inferior wall MI and suspected right ventricular infarctions. Avoid use in patients with hypertrophic cardiomyopathy (HCM) with outflow tract obstruction; nitrates may reduce preload, exacerbating obstruction and cause hypotension or syncope and/or worsening of heart failure (ACCF/AHA [Gersh, 2011]).

Use of isosorbide dinitrate sublingual tablets to treat acute angina attacks is recommended only in patients unresponsive to sublingual nitroglycerin; however, current clinical practice guidelines do not recommend use during an acute anginal episode. Avoid use of extended release formulations in acute MI or acute HF; cannot easily reverse effects if adverse events develop. Nitrates may precipitate or aggravate increased intracranial pressure and subsequently may worsen clinical outcomes in patients with neurologic injury (eg, intracranial hemorrhage, traumatic brain injury). Appropriate dosing intervals are needed to minimize tolerance development. Tolerance can only be overcome by short periods of nitrate absence from the body. Dose escalation does not overcome this effect. When used for HF in combination with hydralazine, tolerance is less of a concern (Gogia, 1995).

Avoid concurrent use with PDE-5 inhibitors (eg, sildenafil, tadalafil, vardenafil). When nitrate administration becomes medically necessary, may administer nitrates only if 24 hours have elapsed after use of sildenafil or vardenafil (48 hours after tadalafil use) (Trujillo, 2007).

Drug Interactions
Avoid Concomitant Use
  Avoid concomitant use of Isosorbide Dinitrate with any of the following: Conivaptan; Fusidic Acid (Systemic); Phosphodiesterase 5 Inhibitors; Riociguat

Decreased Effect
  The levels/effects of Isosorbide Dinitrate may be decreased by: Bosentan; CYP3A4 Inducers (Strong); Dabrafenib; Deferasirox; Herbs (CYP3A4 Inducers); Mitotane; Tocilizumab

Increased Effect/Toxicity

Isosorbide Dinitrate may increase the levels/ effects of: DULoxetine; Hypotensive Agents; Prilocaine; Riociguat; Rosiglitazone; Sodium Nitrite

The levels/effects of Isosorbide Dinitrate may be increased by: Conivaptan; CYP3A4 Inhibitors (Moderate); CYP3A4 Inhibitors (Strong); Dasatinib; Fusidic Acid (Systemic); Ivacaftor; Luliconazole; Mifepristone; Nitric Oxide; Phosphodiesterase 5 Inhibitors; Simeprevir; Stiripentol

Nutritional/Ethanol Interactions

Ethanol: Caution with ethanol (may increase risk of hypotension).

Herb/Nutraceutical: Avoid black cohosh, California poppy, coleus, golden seal, hawthorn, mistletoe, periwinkle, quinine, shepherd's purse (may cause hypotension).

Adverse Reactions Frequency not defined.

Cardiovascular: Crescendo angina (uncommon), hypotension, orthostatic hypotension, rebound hypertension (uncommon), syncope (uncommon)

Central nervous system: Headache (most common), lightheadedness (related to blood pressure changes)

Hematologic: Methemoglobinemia (rare, overdose)

Pharmacodynamics/Kinetics

Onset of Action Sublingual tablet: ~3 minutes; Oral tablet and capsule (includes extended-release formulations): ~1 hour

Duration of Action Sublingual tablet: 1-2 hours; Oral tablet and capsule (includes extended-release formulations): Up to 8 hours

Available Dosage Forms

Capsule Extended Release, Oral:
Dilatrate-SR: 40 mg

Tablet, Oral:
Isordil Titradose: 5 mg, 40 mg
Generic: 5 mg, 10 mg, 20 mg, 30 mg

Tablet Extended Release, Oral:
IsoDitrate ER: 40 mg
Generic: 40 mg

General Dosage Range

Oral:
Immediate release: *Adults:* 5-40 mg 2-3 times daily
Sustained release: *Adults:* 40-160 mg daily in divided doses
Sublingual: *Adults:* 2.5-5 mg every 5-10 minutes for maximum of 3 doses in 15-30 minutes **or** 2.5-5 mg 15 minutes prior to activities which may provoke an anginal episode

Administration

Oral May consider administration of first dose in physician office; observe for maximal cardiovascular dynamic effects and adverse effects (orthostatic hypotension, headache). Do not administer around the clock; allow nitrate-free interval ≥14 hours (immediate release products) and >18 hours (sustained release products). Do not crush sublingual tablets or extended release formulations.

Immediate release products: When prescribed twice daily, consider administering at 8 AM and 1 PM. For 3 times/day dosing, consider 8 AM, 1 PM, and 6 PM.

Sustained release products: Consider once daily in morning or twice-daily dosing at 8 AM and between 1-2 PM.

Nursing Actions

Physical Assessment Assess blood pressure and monitor for hypotension and tolerance at regular intervals during therapy. Teach patient importance of maintaining dosing schedule to provide drug-free period.

Patient Education

- Discuss specific use of drug and side effects with patient as it relates to treatment. (HCAHPS: During this hospital stay, were you given any medicine that you had not taken before? Before giving you any new medicine, how often did hospital staff tell you what the medicine was for? How often did hospital staff describe possible side effects in a way you could understand?)
- Patient may experience dizziness, flushing, or headache. Have patient report immediately to prescriber angina or rash (HCAHPS).
- Educate patient about signs of a significant reaction (eg, wheezing; chest tightness; fever; itching; bad cough; blue skin color; seizures; or swelling of face, lips, tongue, or throat). **Note:** This is not a comprehensive list of all side effects. Patient should consult prescriber for additional questions.

Intended Use and Disclaimer: Should not be printed and given to patients. This information is intended to serve as a concise initial reference for healthcare professionals to use when discussing medications with a patient. You must ultimately rely on your own discretion, experience and judgment in diagnosing, treating and advising patients.

Related Information

Oral Medications That Should Not Be Crushed or Altered *on page 1712*

Isosorbide Mononitrate
(eye soe SOR bide mon oh NYE trate)

Brand Names: U.S. Imdur

Index Terms ISMN

Pharmacologic Category Antianginal Agent; Vasodilator

Medication Safety Issues

Sound-alike/look-alike issues:

Imdur® may be confused with Imuran®, Inderal® LA, K-Dur®

Monoket® may be confused with Monopril®

Pregnancy Risk Factor B/C (manufacturer dependent)

Lactation Excretion in breast milk unknown/use caution

Use Prevention of angina pectoris

Available Dosage Forms

Tablet, Oral:

Generic: 10 mg, 20 mg

Tablet Extended Release 24 Hour, Oral:

Imdur: 30 mg, 60 mg, 120 mg

Generic: 30 mg, 60 mg, 120 mg

General Dosage Range Oral:

Extended release: *Adults:* Initial: 30-60 mg once daily; Maintenance: 30-240 mg once daily (maximum: 240 mg/day)

Regular release: *Adults:* 5-20 mg twice daily

Administration

Oral Do not administer around-the-clock. Immediate release tablet should be scheduled twice daily with doses 7 hours apart (8 AM and 3 PM); extended release tablet may be administered once daily in the morning upon rising with a half-glassful of fluid and should not be chewed or crushed.

Nursing Actions

Physical Assessment Tolerance to nitrates will develop and proper timing of doses is needed to minimize tolerance. Monitor for hypotension and GI disturbance when beginning therapy, when dose is adjusted, and at regular intervals during therapy. Teach patient importance of maintaining dosing schedule.

Patient Education

• Discuss specific use of drug and side effects with patient as it relates to treatment. (HCAHPS: During this hospital stay, were you given any medicine that you had not taken before? Before giving you any new medicine, how often did hospital staff tell you what the medicine was for? How often did hospital staff describe possible side effects in a way you could understand?)

• Patient may experience dizziness, flushing, or headache. Have patient report immediately to prescriber angina or rash (HCAHPS).

• Educate patient about signs of a significant reaction (eg, wheezing; chest tightness; fever; itching; bad cough; blue skin color; seizures; or swelling of face, lips, tongue, or throat). **Note:** This is not a comprehensive list of all side effects. Patient should consult prescriber for additional questions.

Intended Use and Disclaimer: Should not be printed and given to patients. This information is intended to serve as a concise initial reference for healthcare professionals to use when discussing medications with a patient. You must ultimately rely on your own discretion, experience and judgment in diagnosing, treating and advising patients.

Related Information

Oral Medications That Should Not Be Crushed or Altered *on page 1712*

Isotretinoin (eye soe TRET i noyn)

Brand Names: U.S. Absorica; Amnesteem; Claravis; Myorisan; Zenatane

Index Terms 13-*cis*-Retinoic Acid; 13-*cis*-Vitamin A Acid; 13-CRA; *Cis*-Retinoic Acid; Accutane; Isotretinoinum

Pharmacologic Category Acne Products; Antineoplastic Agent, Retinoic Acid Derivative; Retinoic Acid Derivative

Medication Safety Issues

Sound-alike/look-alike issues:

Accutane® may be confused with Accolate®, Accupril®

Claravis™ may be confused with Cleviprex®

ISOtretinoin may be confused with tretinoin

Other safety concerns:

Isotretinoin may be confused with tretinoin (which is also called all-*trans* retinoic acid, or ATRA); while both products may have uses in cancer treatment, they are **not** interchangeable.

Medication Guide Available Yes

Pregnancy Risk Factor X

Lactation Excretion in breast milk unknown/not recommended

Breast-Feeding Considerations It is not known if isotretinoin is excreted in breast milk. A case report describes a green discharge from the breast of a nonlactating woman which was determined to be iatrogenic galactorrhea due to isotretinoin (Larsen, 1985). Due to the potential for serious adverse reactions in the nursing infant, the manufacturer recommends a decision be made whether to discontinue nursing or to discontinue the drug, taking into account the importance of treatment to the mother.

Use Treatment of severe recalcitrant nodular acne unresponsive to conventional therapy

Unlabeled Use Management of moderate degrees of treatment-resistant acne, management of acne that produces physical or psychological scarring; treatment of cutaneous T-cell lymphomas (mycosis fungoides and Sézary syndrome); prevention of squamous cell skin cancers (in high-risk patients); treatment of high-risk neuroblastoma in children

Mechanism of Action/Effect Reduces sebaceous gland size and reduces sebum production in acne treatment; in neuroblastoma, decreases cell proliferation and induces differentiation

Contraindications Hypersensitivity to isotretinoin or any component of the formulation; sensitivity to parabens, vitamin A, or other retinoids; pregnant women or those who may become pregnant

Warnings/Precautions Hazardous agent - use appropriate precautions for handling and disposal (meets NIOSH, 2012 criteria). This medication ▶

should only be prescribed by prescribers competent in treating severe recalcitrant nodular acne and experienced with the use of systemic retinoids. Anaphylaxis and other types of allergic reactions, including cutaneous reactions and allergic vasculitis, have been reported. **[U.S. Boxed Warnings]: Birth defects (facial, eye, ear, skull, central nervous system, cardiovascular, thymus and parathyroid gland abnormalities) have been noted following isotretinoin exposure during pregnancy and the risk for severe birth defects is high, with any dose or even with short treatment duration. Low IQ scores have also been reported. The risk for spontaneous abortion and premature births is increased. Because of the high likelihood of teratogenic effects, all patients (male and female), prescribers, wholesalers, and dispensing pharmacists must register and be active in the iPLEDGE™ risk evaluation and mitigation strategy (REMS) program; do not prescribe isotretinoin for women who are or who are likely to become pregnant while using the drug. If pregnancy occurs during therapy, isotretinoin should be discontinued immediately and the patient referred to an obstetrician-gynecologist specializing in reproductive toxicity.** Women of childbearing potential must be capable of complying with effective contraceptive measures. Patients must select and commit to two forms of contraception. Therapy is begun after two negative pregnancy tests; effective contraception must be used for at least 1 month before beginning therapy, during therapy, and for 1 month after discontinuation of therapy. Prescriptions should be written for no more than a 30-day supply, and pregnancy testing and counseling should be repeated monthly.

May cause depression, psychosis, aggressive or violent behavior, and changes in mood; use with extreme caution in patients with psychiatric disorders. Rarely, suicidal thoughts and actions have been reported during isotretinoin usage. All patients should be observed closely for symptoms of depression or suicidal thoughts. Discontinuation of treatment alone may not be sufficient, further evaluation may be necessary. Cases of pseudotumor cerebri (benign intracranial hypertension) have been reported, some with concomitant use of tetracycline (avoid using together). Patients with papilledema, headache, nausea, vomiting, and visual disturbances should be referred to a neurologist and treatment with isotretinoin discontinued. Hearing impairment, which can continue after therapy is discontinued, may occur. Clinical hepatitis, elevated liver enzymes, inflammatory bowel disease, skeletal hyperostosis, premature epiphyseal closure, vision impairment, corneal opacities, decreased tolerance to contact lenses (due to dry eyes), and decreased night vision have also been reported with the use of isotretinoin. Rare postmarketing cases of severe skin reactions (eg,

Stevens-Johnson syndrome, erythema multiforme) have been reported with use.

Use with caution in patients with diabetes mellitus; impaired glucose control has been reported. Use caution in patients with hypertriglyceridemia; acute pancreatitis and fatal hemorrhagic pancreatitis (rare) have been reported. Bone mineral density may decrease; use caution in patients with a genetic predisposition to bone disorders (ie, osteoporosis, osteomalacia) and with disease states or concomitant medications that can induce bone disorders. Patients may be at risk when participating in activities with repetitive impact (such as sports). Patients should be instructed not to donate blood during therapy and for 1 month following discontinuation of therapy due to risk of donated blood being given to a pregnant female. Safety of long-term use is not established and is not recommended.

Absorica™: Absorption is ~83% greater than Accutane® when administered under fasting conditions; they are bioequivalent when taken with a high-fat meal. Absorica™ is **not** interchangeable with other generic isotretinoin products. Isotretinoin and tretinoin (which is also known as all-*trans* retinoic acid, or ATRA) may be confused, while both products may be used in cancer treatment, they are **not** interchangeable; verify product prior to dispensing and administration to prevent medication errors.

Drug Interactions

Avoid Concomitant Use

Avoid concomitant use of ISOtretinoin with any of the following: Multivitamins/Fluoride (with ADE); Multivitamins/Minerals (with ADEK, Folate, Iron); Multivitamins/Minerals (with AE, No Iron); Tetracycline Derivatives; Vitamin A

Decreased Effect

ISOtretinoin may decrease the levels/effects of: Contraceptives (Estrogens); Contraceptives (Progestins)

Increased Effect/Toxicity

ISOtretinoin may increase the levels/effects of: Mipomersen; Porfimer; Vitamin A

The levels/effects of ISOtretinoin may be increased by: Alcohol (Ethyl); Multivitamins/Fluoride (with ADE); Multivitamins/Minerals (with ADEK, Folate, Iron); Multivitamins/Minerals (with AE, No Iron); Tetracycline Derivatives

Nutritional/Ethanol Interactions

Ethanol: Avoid or limit ethanol (may increase triglyceride levels if taken in excess).

Food: Isotretinoin bioavailability increased if taken with food or milk.

Herb/Nutraceutical: Avoid dong quai, St John's wort (may also cause photosensitization and may decrease the effectiveness of oral contraceptives). Additional vitamin A supplements may lead to vitamin A toxicity (dry skin, irritation, arthralgias, myalgias, abdominal pain, hepatic changes); avoid use.

Adverse Reactions Frequency not always defined.

Cardiovascular: Chest pain, edema, flushing, palpitation, stroke, syncope, tachycardia, vascular thrombotic disease

Central nervous system: Aggressive behavior, depression, dizziness, drowsiness, emotional instability, fatigue, headache, insomnia, lethargy, malaise, nervousness, paresthesia, pseudotumor cerebri, psychosis, seizure, stroke, suicidal ideation, suicide attempts, suicide, violent behavior

Dermatologic: Abnormal wound healing acne fulminans, alopecia, bruising, cheilitis, cutaneous allergic reactions, dry nose, dry skin, eczema, eruptive xanthomas, facial erythema, fragility of skin, hair abnormalities, hirsutism, hyperpigmentation, hypopigmentation, increased sunburn susceptibility, nail dystrophy, paronychia, peeling of palms, peeling of soles, photoallergic reactions, photosensitizing reactions, pruritus, purpura, rash

Endocrine & metabolic: Triglycerides increased (25%), abnormal menses, blood glucose increased, cholesterol increased, HDL decreased, hyperuricemia

Gastrointestinal: Bleeding and inflammation of the gums, colitis, esophagitis, esophageal ulceration, inflammatory bowel disease, nausea, nonspecific gastrointestinal symptoms, pancreatitis, weight loss, xerostomia

Genitourinary: Nonspecific urogenital findings

Hematologic: Agranulocytosis (rare), anemia, neutropenia, pyogenic granuloma, thrombocytopenia

Hepatic: Alkaline phosphatase increased, ALT increased, AST increased, GGTP increased, hepatitis, LDH increased

Neuromuscular & skeletal: Back pain (29% in pediatric patients), arthralgia, arthritis, bone abnormalities, bone mineral density decreased, calcification of tendons and ligaments, CPK increased, myalgia, premature epiphyseal closure, skeletal hyperostosis, tendonitis, weakness

Ocular: Conjunctivitis (4%), blepharitis (1%), chalazion (1%), hordeolum (1%), cataracts, color vision disorder, corneal opacities, eyelid inflammation, keratitis, night vision decreased, optic neuritis, photophobia, visual disturbances

Otic: Hearing impairment, tinnitus

Renal: Glomerulonephritis, hematuria, proteinuria, pyuria, vasculitis

Respiratory: Bronchospasms, epistaxis, respiratory infection, voice alteration, Wegener's granulomatosis

Miscellaneous: Allergic reactions, anaphylactic reactions, disseminated herpes simplex, diaphoresis, infection, lymphadenopathy

Available Dosage Forms

Capsule, Oral:

Absorica: 10 mg, 20 mg, 30 mg, 40 mg

Amnesteem: 10 mg, 20 mg, 40 mg

Claravis: 10 mg, 20 mg, 30 mg, 40 mg

Myorisan: 10 mg, 20 mg, 40 mg

Zenatane: 10 mg, 20 mg, 40 mg

General Dosage Range Dosage adjustments recommended in patients with hepatic impairment

Oral:

Children 12-17 years: 0.5-1 mg/kg/day in 2 divided doses

Adults: 0.5-2 mg/kg/day in 2 divided doses

Administration

Oral Administer orally with a meal (except Absorica™ which may be taken without regard to meals). According to the manufacturers' labeling, capsules should be swallowed whole with a full glass of liquid. For patients unable to swallow capsule whole, an oral liquid may be prepared; may irritate esophagus if contents are removed from the capsule.

Hazardous agent; use appropriate precautions for handling and disposal (meets NIOSH, 2012 criteria).

Storage/Stability Store at room temperature of 59°F to 86°F (15°C to 30°C). Protect from light.

Nursing Actions

Physical Assessment Monitor patients with diabetes closely; monitor skin for unusual reactions. Observe for depression or suicide ideation.

Patient Education

• Discuss specific use of drug and side effects with patient as it relates to treatment. (HCAHPS: During this hospital stay, were you given any medicine that you had not taken before? Before giving you any new medicine, how often did hospital staff tell you what the medicine was for? How often did hospital staff describe possible side effects in a way you could understand?)

• Patient may experience depression, dyspepsia, nausea, xerostomia, stomatitis, rhinitis, skin irritation, eye irritation, vision changes, erythema, or osteopenia. Have patient report immediately to prescriber anger, significant dizziness, severe headache, considerable bloody stools, dysphagia, hearing impairment, polyuria, polydipsia, weight loss, inability to eat, severe asthenia, discolored urine, jaundice, rash, or pregnancy (HCAHPS).

• Educate patient about signs of a significant reaction (eg, wheezing; chest tightness; fever; itching; bad cough; blue skin color; seizures; or swelling of face, lips, tongue, or throat). **Note:** This is not a comprehensive list of all side effects. Patient should consult prescriber for additional questions.

Intended Use and Disclaimer: Should not be printed and given to patients. This information is intended to serve as a concise initial reference for healthcare professionals to use when discussing medications with a patient. You must ultimately rely on your own discretion, experience and

judgment in diagnosing, treating and advising patients.

Dietary Considerations Should be taken with food, except Absorbica™ which may be taken without regard to meals. Limit intake of vitamin A; avoid use of other vitamin A products. Some formulations may contain soybean oil.

Related Information

Oral Medications That Should Not Be Crushed or Altered *on page 1712*

Isradipine (iz RA di peen)

Pharmacologic Category Antihypertensive; Calcium Channel Blocker; Calcium Channel Blocker, Dihydropyridine

Pregnancy Risk Factor C

Lactation Excretion in breast milk unknown/not recommended

Use Management of hypertension (may be used alone or concurrently with thiazide-type diuretics).

Unlabeled Use Pediatric hypertension

Available Dosage Forms

Capsule, Oral:

Generic: 2.5 mg, 5 mg

General Dosage Range Dosage adjustment recommended in patients with hepatic or renal impairment

Oral: *Adults:* Initial: 2.5 mg twice daily; Usual range: 2.5-10 mg daily

Administration

Oral May be administered without regard to meals.

Nursing Actions

Physical Assessment Monitor for tachycardia, hypotension, edema, and dyspnea at regular intervals during therapy. When discontinuing, dose should be tapered slowly.

Patient Education

• Discuss specific use of drug and side effects with patient as it relates to treatment. (HCAHPS: During this hospital stay, were you given any medicine that you had not taken before? Before giving you any new medicine, how often did hospital staff tell you what the medicine was for? How often did hospital staff describe possible side effects in a way you could understand?)

• Patient may experience dizziness or headache. Have patient report immediately to prescriber tachycardia, dyspnea, or rash (HCAHPS).

• Educate patient about signs of a significant reaction (eg, wheezing; chest tightness; fever; itching; bad cough; blue skin color; seizures; or swelling of face, lips, tongue, or throat). **Note:** This is not a comprehensive list of all side effects. Patient should consult prescriber for additional questions.

Intended Use and Disclaimer: Should not be printed and given to patients. This information is intended to serve as a concise initial reference for healthcare professionals to use when discussing medications with a patient. You must ultimately rely on your own discretion, experience and judgment in diagnosing, treating and advising patients.

Itraconazole (i tra KOE na zole)

Brand Names: U.S. Onmel; Sporanox; Sporanox Pulsepak

Pharmacologic Category Antifungal Agent, Oral

Medication Safety Issues

Sound-alike/look-alike issues:

Itraconazole may be confused with fluconazole, voriconazole

Sporanox may be confused with Suprax, Topamax

Pregnancy Risk Factor C

Lactation Enters breast milk/not recommended

Breast-Feeding Considerations Itraconazole is excreted in breast milk. According to the manufacturer, the decision to continue or discontinue breast-feeding during therapy should take into account the risk of exposure to the infant and the benefits of treatment to the mother.

Use

Oral capsules: Treatment of susceptible fungal infections in immunocompromised and immunocompetent patients including blastomycosis and histoplasmosis; indicated for aspergillosis (in patients intolerant/refractory to amphotericin B), and onychomycosis of the toenail and fingernail (in nonimmunocompromised patients)

Oral solution: Treatment of oral and esophageal candidiasis

Oral tablets: Treatment of onychomycosis of the toenail (in nonimmunocompromised patients)

Canadian labeling: Oral capsules: Additional indications (not in U.S. labeling): Treatment of oral and esophageal candidiasis; treatment of cutaneous and lymphatic sporotrichosis, chromomycosis, or paracoccidioidomycosis in immunocompetent and immunosuppressed patients; treatment of onychomycosis in immunosuppressed patients; treatment of dermatomycoses due to tinea pedis, tinea cruris, tinea corporis and of pityriasis versicolor in immunocompetent and immunocompromised patients in whom oral therapy is appropriate

Mechanism of Action/Effect Interferes with cytochrome P450 activity, decreasing ergosterol synthesis (principal sterol in fungal cell membrane) and inhibiting cell membrane formation

Contraindications Hypersensitivity to itraconazole (use caution in patients with a history of hypersensitivity to other azoles), any component of the formulation; concurrent administration with cisapride, dofetilide, ergot derivatives, felodipine, levomethadyl, lovastatin, methadone, midazolam (oral), nisoldipine, pimozide, quinidine, simvastatin, or triazolam; treatment of onychomycosis (or other non-life-threatening indications) in patients with evidence of ventricular dysfunction, heart failure (HF) or a history of HF; treatment of onychomycosis in patients who are pregnant or intend on becoming pregnant

Canadian labeling: Oral capsule: Additional contraindications (not in U.S. labeling): Concurrent administration with eletriptan; treatment of dermatomycosis (tinea pedis, tinea cruris, tinea corporis) and of pityriasis versicolor in patients who are pregnant or intend on becoming pregnant

Warnings/Precautions [U.S. Boxed Warning]: Negative inotropic effects have been observed following intravenous administration. Discontinue or reassess use if signs or symptoms of HF (heart failure) occur during treatment. [U.S. Boxed Warning]: Use is contraindicated for treatment of onychomycosis in patients with ventricular dysfunction or a history of HF. Cases of HF, peripheral edema, and pulmonary edema have occurred in patients treated for onychomycosis. HF has been reported, particularly in patients receiving a total daily oral dose of 400 mg. Use with caution in patients with risk factors for HF (COPD, renal failure, edematous disorders, ischemic or valvular disease). Discontinue if signs or symptoms of HF or neuropathy occur during treatment. Due to potential toxicity, the manufacturer recommends confirmation of diagnosis testing of nail specimens prior to treatment of onychomycosis.

[U.S. Boxed Warning]: Serious cardiovascular adverse events including, QT prolongation, ventricular tachycardia, torsade de pointes, cardiac arrest and/or sudden death have been observed due to itraconazole-induced increased serum concentrations of the following: cisapride, dofetilide, ergot alkaloids (dihydroergotamine, ergonovine, ergotamine, methylergonovine), felodipine, levomethadyl, lovastatin, methadone, midazolam (oral), nisoldipine, pimozide, quinidine, simvastatin, or triazolam; concurrent use contraindicated. Other potentially significant interactions may exist, requiring dose or frequency adjustment, additional monitoring, and/or selection of alternative therapy.

Use with caution in patients with renal impairment. Rare cases of serious hepatotoxicity (including liver failure and death) have been reported (including some cases occurring within the first week of therapy); hepatotoxicity was reported in some patients without pre-existing liver disease or risk factors. Use with caution in patients with pre-existing hepatic impairment; monitor liver function closely. Not recommended for use in patients with active liver disease, elevated liver enzymes, or prior hepatotoxic reactions to other drugs unless the expected benefit exceeds the risk of hepatotoxicity. Discontinue treatment if signs or symptoms of hepatotoxicity develop. Transient or permanent

hearing loss has been reported. Quinidine (a contraindicated drug) was used concurrently in several of these cases. Hearing loss usually resolves after discontinuation, but may persist in some patients.

Large differences in itraconazole pharmacokinetic parameters have been observed in cystic fibrosis patients receiving the solution; if a patient with cystic fibrosis does not respond to therapy, alternate therapies should be considered. Due to differences in bioavailability, oral capsules and oral solution cannot be used interchangeably. Only the oral solution has proven efficacy for oral and esophageal candidiasis. Initiation of treatment with oral solution is not recommended in patients at immediate risk for systemic candidiasis (eg, patients with severe neutropenia).

Drug Interactions

Avoid Concomitant Use

Avoid concomitant use of Itraconazole with any of the following: Ado-Trastuzumab Emtansine; Alfuzosin; Aliskiren; ALPRAZolam; Apixaban; Avanafil; Axitinib; Bosutinib; Cabozantinib; Cisapride; Conivaptan; Crizotinib; CYP3A4 Inducers (Strong); Dihydroergotamine; Dofetilide; Dronedarone; Eletriptan; Eplerenone; Ergoloid Mesylates; Ergonovine; Ergotamine; Estazolam; Everolimus; Felodipine; Halofantrine; Ibrutinib; Imatinib; Ivabradine; Lapatinib; Lomitapide; Lovastatin; Lurasidone; Macitentan; Methadone; Methylergonovine; Midazolam; Nevirapine; Nilotinib; Nisoldipine; Pimozide; Pomalidomide; QuiNIDine; Ranolazine; Red Yeast Rice; Regorafenib; Rivaroxaban; Salmeterol; Silodosin; Simeprevir; Simvastatin; Tamsulosin; Ticagrelor; Tolvaptan; Topotecan; Toremifene; Triazolam; Ulipristal; Vemurafenib; VinCRIStine (Liposomal)

Decreased Effect

Itraconazole may decrease the levels/effects of: Amphotericin B; Ifosfamide; Prasugrel; Saccharomyces boulardii; Ticagrelor

The levels/effects of Itraconazole may be decreased by: Antacids; CYP3A4 Inducers (Strong); Dabrafenib; Deferasirox; Didanosine; Efavirenz; Etravirine; Fosphenytoin; Grapefruit Juice; H2-Antagonists; Herbs (CYP3A4 Inducers); Isoniazid; Nevirapine; Phenytoin; Proton Pump Inhibitors; Rifamycin Derivatives; Sucralfate; Tocilizumab

Increased Effect/Toxicity

Itraconazole may increase the levels/effects of: Ado-Trastuzumab Emtansine; Afatinib; Alfentanil; Alfuzosin; Aliskiren; Almotriptan; Alosetron; ALPRAZolam; Apixaban; ARIPiprazole; AtorvaSTATin; Avanafil; Axitinib; Bedaquiline; Benzodiazepines (metabolized by oxidation); Boceprevir; Bortezomib; Bosentan; Bosutinib; Brentuximab Vedotin; Brinzolamide; Budesonide (Nasal); Budesonide (Systemic, Oral Inhalation); BusPIRone; Busulfan; Cabozantinib; Calcium Channel Blockers; Cardiac Glycosides; Cilostazol;

Cisapride; Cobicistat; Colchicine; Conivaptan; Corticosteroids (Orally Inhaled); Corticosteroids (Systemic); Crizotinib; CycloSPORINE (Systemic); CYP3A4 Substrates; Dabigatran Etexilate; Darunavir; Dienogest; Dihydroergotamine; DOCEtaxel; Dofetilide; DOXOrubicin (Conventional); Dronedarone; Dutasteride; Eletriptan; Elvitegravir; Enzalutamide; Eplerenone; Ergoloid Mesylates; Ergonovine; Ergotamine; Estazolam; Etravirine; Everolimus; Felodipine; FentaNYL; Fesoterodine; Fexofenadine; Fluticasone (Nasal); Fluticasone (Oral Inhalation); Fosamprenavir; Fosphenytoin; GuanFACINE; Halofantrine; Highest Risk QTc-Prolonging Agents; Ibrutinib; Iloperidone; Imatinib; Indinavir; Irinotecan; Ivabradine; Ivacaftor; Ixabepilone; Lacosamide; Lapatinib; Levomilnacipran; Lomitapide; Losartan; Lovastatin; Lumefantrine; Lurasidone; Macitentan; Macrolide Antibiotics; Maraviroc; Methadone; Methylergonovine; MethylPREDNISolone; Midazolam; Mifepristone; Moderate Risk QTc-Prolonging Agents; Nilotinib; Nisoldipine; Ospemifene; OxyCODONE; Paliperidone; Paricalcitol; PAZOPanib; P-glycoprotein/ABCB1 Substrates; Phenytoin; Pimecrolimus; Pimozide; Pomalidomide; PONATinib; Pravastatin; Propafenone; Prucalopride; QUEtiapine; QuiNIDine; Ranolazine; Red Yeast Rice; Regorafenib; Repaglinide; Rifamycin Derivatives; Rilpivirine; Riociguat; Rivaroxaban; RomiDEPsin; Rosuvastatin; Ruxolitinib; Salmeterol; Saquinavir; Saxagliptin; Sildenafil; Silodosin; Simeprevir; Simvastatin; Sirolimus; Solifenacin; SORAfenib; SUNItinib; Tacrolimus (Systemic); Tacrolimus (Topical); Tadalafil; Tamsulosin; Telaprevir; Temsirolimus; Ticagrelor; Tofacitinib; Tolterodine; Tolvaptan; Topotecan; Toremifene; Triazolam; Ulipristal; Vardenafil; Vemurafenib; Vilazodone; VinBLAStine; VinCRIStine; VinCRIStine (Liposomal); Vinorelbine; Vitamin K Antagonists; Zolpidem; Zuclopenthixol

The levels/effects of Itraconazole may be increased by: Boceprevir; Cobicistat; Darunavir; Etravirine; Fosamprenavir; Grapefruit Juice; Indinavir; Lopinavir; Macrolide Antibiotics; Ritonavir; Saquinavir; Telaprevir; Tipranavir

Nutritional/Ethanol Interactions

Food:

Capsules: Absorption enhanced by food and possibly by gastric acidity. Cola drinks have been shown to increase the absorption of the capsules in patients with achlorhydria or those taking H_2-receptor antagonists or other gastric acid suppressors. Grapefruit/grapefruit juice may increase serum levels. Management: Take capsules immediately after meals. Avoid grapefruit juice.

Solution: Food decreases the bioavailability and increases the time to peak concentration. Management: Take solution on an empty stomach 1 hour before or 2 hours after meals.

Herb/Nutraceutical: St John's wort may decrease itraconazole levels.

Adverse Reactions

>10%: Gastrointestinal: Nausea (3% to 11%), diarrhea (3% to 11%)

1% to 10%:

Cardiovascular: Edema (4%), hypertension (3%), chest pain (3%)

Central nervous system: Headache (4% to 10%), fever (2% to 7%), dizziness (2% to 4%), anxiety (3%), depression (2% to 3%), fatigue (2% to 3%), pain (2% to 3%), malaise (1% to 3%), dreams abnormal (2%)

Dermatologic: Rash (3% to 9%), pruritus (≤5%)

Endocrine & metabolic: Hypertriglyceridemia (≤3%), hypokalemia (2%)

Gastrointestinal: Vomiting (5% to 7%), abdominal pain (2% to 6%), dyspepsia (≤4%), flatulence (≤4%), gingivitis (3%), stomatitis (ulcerative) (≤3%), constipation (2% to 3%), appetite increased (2%), gastritis (2%), gastroenteritis (2%)

Hepatic: LFTs abnormal (≤4%)

Neuromuscular & skeletal: Bursitis (3%), myalgia (≤3%), tremor (2%), weakness (≤2%)

Renal: Cystitis (3%), urinary tract infection (3%)

Respiratory: Rhinitis (5% to 9%), upper respiratory tract infection (8%), sinusitis (2% to 7%), cough (4%), dyspnea (2%), pharyngitis (≤2%), pneumonia (2%), sputum increased (2%)

Miscellaneous: Diaphoresis increased (3%), herpes zoster (2%)

Available Dosage Forms

Capsule, Oral:

Sporanox: 100 mg

Sporanox Pulsepak: 100 mg

Generic: 100 mg

Solution, Oral:

Sporanox: 10 mg/mL (150 mL)

Tablet, Oral:

Onmel: 200 mg

General Dosage Range Oral: *Adults:* 100-600 mg daily; doses >200 mg daily are given in 2-3 divided doses

Administration

Oral Doses >200 mg/day are given in 2 divided doses; do not administer with antacids. Capsule and oral solution formulations are not bioequivalent and thus are not interchangeable. Capsule and tablet absorption is best if taken with food, therefore, it is best to administer itraconazole after meals at the same time each day; solution should be taken on an empty stomach. When treating oropharyngeal and esophageal candidiasis, solution should be swished vigorously in mouth (10 mL at a time), then swallowed.

Storage/Stability

Capsule: Store at room temperature of 15°C to 25°C (59°F to 77°F). Protect from light and moisture.

Oral solution: Store at ≤25°C (77°F); do not freeze.

Tablet: Store at room temperature 15°C to 25°C (59°F to 77°F); excursions are permitted between 15°C and 30°C (59°F and 86°F). Protect from light and moisture.

Nursing Actions
Patient Education
- Discuss specific use of drug and side effects with patient as it relates to treatment. (HCAHPS: During this hospital stay, were you given any medicine that you had not taken before? Before giving you any new medicine, how often did hospital staff tell you what the medicine was for? How often did hospital staff describe possible side effects in a way you could understand?)
- Patient may experience headache, dyspepsia, nausea, diarrhea, flatulence, rhinorrhea, or parageusia. Have patient report immediately to prescriber signs of hypokalemia, signs of pancreatitis, paresthesia, hematuria, mastalgia, macromastia, urinary retention, oliguria, angina, tachycardia, sexual dysfunction, depression, dysphagia, severe dizziness, syncope, chills, pharyngitis, alopecia, arthralgia, tinnitus, tremors, insomnia, ecchymosis, hemorrhaging, xerostomia, xerophthalmia, vision changes, significant asthenia, hearing impairment, or signs of hepatic impairment (HCAHPS).
- Educate patient about signs of a significant reaction (eg, wheezing; chest tightness; fever; itching; bad cough; blue skin color; seizures; or swelling of face, lips, tongue, or throat). **Note:** This is not a comprehensive list of all side effects. Patient should consult prescriber for additional questions.

Intended Use and Disclaimer: Should not be printed and given to patients. This information is intended to serve as a concise initial reference for healthcare professionals to use when discussing medications with a patient. You must ultimately rely on your own discretion, experience and judgment in diagnosing, treating and advising patients.

Dietary Considerations
Capsule, tablet: Take with food.
Solution: Take without food, if possible.

Ivacaftor (eye va KAF tor)

Brand Names: U.S. Kalydeco
Index Terms VX-770
Pharmacologic Category Cystic Fibrosis Transmembrane Conductance Regulator Potentiator
Pregnancy Risk Factor B
Lactation Excretion unknown/use caution
Use Treatment of cystic fibrosis (CF) in patients who have one of the following mutations in the cystic fibrosis transmembrane conductance regulator (CFTR) gene: G551D, G1244E, G1349D, G178R, G551S, S1251N, S1255P, S549N, or S549R.

Note: Not effective in patients with CF who are homozygous for the F508del mutation in the CTFR gene

Available Dosage Forms
Tablet, Oral:
Kalydeco: 150 mg

General Dosage Range Dosage adjustment recommended in patients with hepatic impairment or on concomitant therapy.
Oral: *Children ≥6 years and Adults:* 150 mg every 12 hours

Administration
Oral Administer with high-fat-containing foods (eg, butter, cheese pizza, eggs, peanut butter).

Nursing Actions
Physical Assessment Monitor for liver function tests on a routine basis; educate patient about need to take with fatty foods. Assess pulmonary exam with use.

Patient Education
- Discuss specific use of drug and side effects with patient as it relates to treatment. (HCAHPS: During this hospital stay, were you given any medicine that you had not taken before? Before giving you any new medicine, how often did hospital staff tell you what the medicine was for? How often did hospital staff describe possible side effects in a way you could understand?)
- Patient may experience headache, dizziness, pharyngitis, rhinorrhea, diarrhea, dyspepsia, or nausea. Have patient report immediately to prescriber severe asthenia, discolored urine, jaundice, inability to eat, or rash (HCAHPS).
- Educate patient about signs of a significant reaction (eg, wheezing; chest tightness; fever; itching; bad cough; blue skin color; seizures; or swelling of face, lips, tongue, or throat). **Note:** This is not a comprehensive list of all side effects. Patient should consult prescriber for additional questions.

Intended Use and Disclaimer: Should not be printed and given to patients. This information is intended to serve as a concise initial reference for healthcare professionals to use when discussing medications with a patient. You must ultimately rely on your own discretion, experience and judgment in diagnosing, treating and advising patients.

Ketoconazole (Systemic)
(kee toe KOE na zole)

Index Terms Nizoral
Pharmacologic Category Antifungal Agent, Oral
Medication Safety Issues
Sound-alike/look-alike issues:
Nizoral may be confused with Nasarel, Neoral, Nitrol
Medication Guide Available Yes
Pregnancy Risk Factor C

Lactation Enters breast milk/not recommended

Use Fungal infections:

U.S. labeling: Systemic fungal infections: Treatment of susceptible fungal infections, including blastomycosis, histoplasmosis, paracoccidioidomycosis, coccidioidomycosis, and chromomycosis in patients who have failed or who are intolerant to other antifungal therapies

Canadian labeling: Treatment of serious or life-threatening systemic fungal infections (eg, systemic candidiasis, chronic mucocutaneous candidiasis, coccidioidomycosis, paracoccidioidomycosis, histoplasmosis, and chromomycosis) where alternate therapy is inappropriate or ineffective; may be considered for severe dermatophytoses unresponsive to other therapy

Unlabeled Use Treatment of advanced prostate cancer

Available Dosage Forms

Tablet, Oral:

Generic: 200 mg

General Dosage Range Oral:

Children ≥2 years: 3.3-6.6 mg/kg once daily

Adults: 200-400 mg once daily

Administration

Oral Administer oral tablets 2 hours prior to antacids to prevent decreased absorption due to the high pH of gastric contents. Patients with achlorhydria should administer with acidic liquid (eg, soda pop).

Nursing Actions

Physical Assessment Monitor liver function on a regular basis. Teach patient necessity of completing full therapy and importance of adequate hydration.

Patient Education

• Discuss specific use of drug and side effects with patient as it relates to treatment. (HCAHPS: During this hospital stay, were you given any medicine that you had not taken before? Before giving you any new medicine, how often did hospital staff tell you what the medicine was for? How often did hospital staff describe possible side effects in a way you could understand?)

• Patient may experience dyspepsia, diarrhea, or headache. Have patient report immediately to prescriber bloating, depression, suicidal ideation, tachycardia, arrhythmia, chills, pharyngitis, paresthesia, edema of extremities, abdominal edema, ecchymosis, hemorrhaging, vision changes, severe nausea, considerable asthenia, dizziness, angina, or syncope (HCAHPS).

• Educate patient about signs of a significant reaction (eg, wheezing; chest tightness; fever; itching; bad cough; blue skin color; seizures; or swelling of face, lips, tongue, or throat). **Note:** This is not a comprehensive list of all side effects. Patient should consult prescriber for additional questions.

Intended Use and Disclaimer: Should not be printed and given to patients. This information is intended to serve as a concise initial reference for healthcare professionals to use when discussing medications with a patient. You must ultimately rely on your own discretion, experience and judgment in diagnosing, treating and advising patients.

Ketoconazole (Topical) (kee toe KOE na zole)

Brand Names: U.S. Extina; Ketodan; Nizoral; Nizoral A-D [OTC]; Xolegel

Pharmacologic Category Antifungal Agent, Topical

Medication Safety Issues

Sound-alike/look-alike issues:

Nizoral® may be confused with Nasarel, Neoral®, Nitrol®

Pregnancy Risk Factor C

Lactation Excretion in breast milk unknown/use caution

Use

Cream: Treatment of tinea corporis, tinea cruris, tinea versicolor, cutaneous candidiasis, seborrheic dermatitis

Foam, gel: Treatment of seborrheic dermatitis

Shampoo: Treatment of dandruff, seborrheic dermatitis, tinea versicolor

Unlabeled Use Cream: Treatment of susceptible fungal infections in the oral cavity including candidiasis, oral thrush, and chronic mucocutaneous candidiasis

Available Dosage Forms

Cream, External:

Generic: 2% (15 g, 30 g, 60 g)

Foam, External:

Extina: 2% (50 g, 100 g)

Ketodan: 2% (100 g)

Gel, External:

Xolegel: 2% (45 g)

Kit, External:

Ketodan: 2%

Shampoo, External:

Nizoral: 2% (120 mL)

Nizoral A-D [OTC]: 1% (125 mL, 200 mL)

Generic: 2% (120 mL)

General Dosage Range Topical:

Cream: *Children ≥12 years and Adults:* Rub gently into the affected area 1-2 times daily

Foam: *Children ≥12 years and Adults:* Apply to affected area twice daily

Gel: *Children ≥12 years and Adults:* Apply gently to affected area once daily

Shampoo: *Children ≥12 years and Adults:* Apply up to twice weekly

Administration

Topical Cream, foam, gel, and shampoo are for external use only. Avoid exposure to flame or smoking immediately following application of gel or foam; do not apply directly to hands.

Nursing Actions

Physical Assessment Teach patient proper administration or application and necessity of completing full therapy.

Patient Education

- Discuss specific use of drug and side effects with patient as it relates to treatment. (HCAHPS: During this hospital stay, were you given any medicine that you had not taken before? Before giving you any new medicine, how often did hospital staff tell you what the medicine was for? How often did hospital staff describe possible side effects in a way you could understand?)
- Patient may experience scalp irritation, straight hair, alopecia, or skin irritation. Have patient report immediately to prescriber rash (HCAHPS).
- Educate patient about signs of a significant reaction (eg, wheezing; chest tightness; fever; itching; bad cough; blue skin color; seizures; or swelling of face, lips, tongue, or throat). **Note:** This is not a comprehensive list of all side effects. Patient should consult prescriber for additional questions.

Intended Use and Disclaimer: Should not be printed and given to patients. This information is intended to serve as a concise initial reference for healthcare professionals to use when discussing medications with a patient. You must ultimately rely on your own discretion, experience and judgment in diagnosing, treating and advising patients.

Ketoprofen (kee toe PROE fen)

Pharmacologic Category Nonsteroidal Anti-inflammatory Drug (NSAID), Oral

Medication Safety Issues

Sound-alike/look-alike issues:

Ketoprofen may be confused with ketotifen

BEERS Criteria medication:

This drug may be potentially inappropriate for use in geriatric patients (Quality of evidence - moderate; Strength of recommendation - strong).

Medication Guide Available Yes

Pregnancy Risk Factor C

Lactation Enters breast milk

Use Acute and long-term treatment of rheumatoid arthritis and osteoarthritis; primary dysmenorrhea; mild-to-moderate pain

Unlabeled Use Migraine prophylaxis

Available Dosage Forms

Capsule, Oral:

Generic: 50 mg, 75 mg

Capsule Extended Release 24 Hour, Oral:

Generic: 200 mg

General Dosage Range Dosage adjustment recommended in patients with hepatic and renal impairment

Oral:

Extended release: *Adults:* 200 mg once daily

Regular release: *Adults:* 25-50 mg 4 times/day or 75 mg 3 times/day (maximum: 300 mg/day)

Administration

Oral May take with food to reduce GI upset. Do not crush or break extended release capsules.

Nursing Actions

Physical Assessment Monitor blood pressure at the beginning of therapy and periodically during use. Monitor for GI effects, hepatotoxicity, and ototoxicity at beginning of therapy and periodically throughout therapy. Schedule ophthalmic evaluations for patients who develop eye complaints during long-term NSAID therapy.

Patient Education

- Discuss specific use of drug and side effects with patient as it relates to treatment. (HCAHPS: During this hospital stay, were you given any medicine that you had not taken before? Before giving you any new medicine, how often did hospital staff tell you what the medicine was for? How often did hospital staff describe possible side effects in a way you could understand?)
- Patient may experience headache, nausea, dyspepsia, pyrosis, constipation, or diarrhea. Have patient report immediately to prescriber angina, strength differences from one side to another, edema or pain of hands or feet, significant weight gain, melena, hematuria, ecchymosis, or rash (HCAHPS).
- Educate patient about signs of a significant reaction (eg, wheezing; chest tightness; fever; itching; bad cough; blue skin color; seizures; or swelling of face, lips, tongue, or throat). **Note:** This is not a comprehensive list of all side effects. Patient should consult prescriber for additional questions.

Intended Use and Disclaimer: Should not be printed and given to patients. This information is intended to serve as a concise initial reference for healthcare professionals to use when discussing medications with a patient. You must ultimately rely on your own discretion, experience and judgment in diagnosing, treating and advising patients.

Ketorolac (Systemic) (KEE toe role ak)

Index Terms Ketorolac Tromethamine; Toradol

Pharmacologic Category Nonsteroidal Anti-inflammatory Drug (NSAID), Oral; Nonsteroidal Anti-inflammatory Drug (NSAID), Parenteral

◀ **Medication Safety Issues**

Sound-alike/look-alike issues:

Ketorolac may be confused with Ketalar®

Toradol® may be confused with Foradil®, Inderal®, TEGretol®, traMADol, tromethamine

BEERS Criteria medication:

This drug may be potentially inappropriate for use in geriatric patients (Quality of evidence - high; Strength of recommendation - strong).

International issues:

Toradol [Canada and multiple international markets] may be confused with Theradol brand name for tramadol [Netherlands]

Medication Guide Available Yes

Pregnancy Risk Factor C

Lactation Enters breast milk/use caution

Breast-Feeding Considerations Low concentrations of ketorolac are found in breast milk (milk concentrations were <1% of the weight-adjusted maternal dose in one study [Wischnik, 1989]). The manufacturer recommends that caution be used if administered to nursing women.

Use Short-term (≤5 days) management of moderate-to-severe acute pain requiring analgesia at the opioid level

Mechanism of Action/Effect Reversibly inhibits cyclooxygenase-1 and 2 (COX-1 and 2) enzymes, which results in decreased formation of prostaglandin precursors; has antipyretic, analgesic, and anti-inflammatory properties

Contraindications Hypersensitivity to ketorolac, aspirin, other NSAIDs, or any component of the formulation; active or history of peptic ulcer disease; recent or history of GI bleeding or perforation; patients with advanced renal disease or risk of renal failure (due to volume depletion); prophylaxis before major surgery; suspected or confirmed cerebrovascular bleeding; hemorrhagic diathesis, incomplete hemostasis, or high risk of bleeding; concurrent use with ASA, other NSAIDs, probenecid or pentoxifylline; epidural or intrathecal administration; perioperative pain in the setting of coronary artery bypass graft (CABG) surgery; labor and delivery

Warnings/Precautions [U.S. Boxed Warning]: Inhibits platelet function; contraindicated in patients with cerebrovascular bleeding (suspected or confirmed), hemorrhagic diathesis, incomplete hemostasis and patients at high risk for bleeding. Effects on platelet adhesion and aggregation may prolong bleeding time. Anemia may occur; patients on long-term NSAID therapy should be monitored for anemia. Rarely, NSAID use has been associated with potentially severe blood dyscrasias (eg, agranulocytosis, thrombocytopenia, aplastic anemia).

[U.S. Boxed Warning]: NSAIDs are associated with an increased risk of adverse cardiovascular thrombotic events, including MI and stroke. Risk may be increased with duration of use or pre-existing cardiovascular risk factors or disease. Carefully evaluate individual cardiovascular risk profiles prior to prescribing. May cause new-onset hypertension or worsening of existing hypertension. Use caution with fluid retention. Avoid use in heart failure (ACCF/AHA [Yancy, 2013]). Concurrent use of aspirin has not been shown to consistently reduce thromboembolic events. **[U.S. Boxed Warning]: Use is contraindicated as prophylactic analgesic before any major surgery and is contraindicated for treatment of perioperative pain in the setting of coronary artery bypass graft (CABG) surgery.** Risk of MI and stroke may be increased with use following CABG surgery. Wound bleeding and postoperative hematomas have been associated with ketorolac use in the perioperative setting.

[U.S. Boxed Warning]: Ketorolac is contraindicated in patients with advanced renal impairment and in patients at risk for renal failure due to volume depletion. NSAID use may compromise existing renal function; dose-dependent decreases in prostaglandin synthesis may result from NSAID use, reducing renal blood flow which may cause renal decompensation. NSAID use may increase the risk for hyperkalemia. Patients with impaired renal function, dehydration, heart failure, liver dysfunction, those taking diuretics and ACE inhibitors, and the elderly are at greater risk of renal toxicity. Use with caution in patients with impaired renal function or history of kidney disease; dosage adjustment is required in patients with moderate elevation in serum creatinine. Monitor renal function closely. Acute renal failure, interstitial nephritis, and nephrotic syndrome have been reported with ketorolac use; papillary necrosis and renal injury have been reported with the use of NSAIDs. Use of NSAIDs can compromise existing renal function. Rehydrate patient before starting therapy.

[U.S. Boxed Warning]: NSAIDs may increase risk of gastrointestinal irritation, inflammation, ulceration, bleeding, and perforation. These events may occur at any time during therapy and without warning. Use is contraindicated in patients with active/history of peptic ulcer disease and recent/history of GI bleeding or perforation. Use caution with a history of inflammatory bowel disease, concurrent therapy with anticoagulants, and/or corticosteroids, smoking, use of alcohol, the elderly, or debilitated patients.

[U.S. Boxed Warning]: Ketorolac injection is contraindicated in patients with prior hypersensitivity reaction to aspirin or NSAIDs. NSAIDs may cause serious skin adverse events including exfoliative dermatitis, Stevens-Johnson syndrome (SJS), and toxic epidermal necrolysis (TEN); discontinue use at first sign of skin rash or hypersensitivity. Hypersensitivity or anaphylactoid reactions may occur, even without prior exposure;

patients with "aspirin triad" (bronchial asthma, aspirin intolerance, rhinitis) may be at increased risk. Do not use in patients who experience bronchospasm, asthma, rhinitis, or urticaria with NSAID or aspirin therapy. Use caution in other forms of asthma.

Use with caution in patients with hepatic impairment or a history of liver disease. Closely monitor patients with any abnormal LFT. Rarely, severe hepatic reactions (eg, fulminant hepatitis, hepatic necrosis, liver failure) have occurred with NSAID use; discontinue if signs or symptoms of liver disease develop, or if systemic manifestations occur.

[U.S. Boxed Warning]: Dosage adjustment is required for patients ≥65 years of age. Avoid use in older adults; use is associated with an increased risk of GI bleeding and peptic ulcer disease in older adults in high risk category (eg, >75 years or age or receiving concomitant oral/ parenteral corticosteroids, anticoagulants, or antiplatelet agents) (Beers Criteria). [U.S. Boxed Warning]: Dosage adjustment is required for patients weighing <50 kg (<110 pounds). [U.S. Boxed Warning]: Ketorolac is contraindicated during labor and delivery (may inhibit uterine contractions and adversely affect fetal circulation). [U.S. Boxed Warning]: Concurrent use of ketorolac with aspirin or other NSAIDs is contraindicated due to the increased risk of adverse reactions.

[U.S. Boxed Warning]: Contraindicated for epidural or intrathecal administration (formulation contains alcohol). [U.S. Boxed Warning]: Systemic ketorolac is indicated for short term (≤5 days) use in adults for treatment of moderately severe acute pain requiring opioid-level analgesia. Low doses of opioids may be needed for breakthrough pain. [U.S. Boxed Warning]: Oral therapy is only indicated for use as continuation treatment, following parenteral ketorolac and is not indicated for minor or chronic painful conditions. Do not exceed maximum daily recommended doses; does not improve efficacy but may increase the risk of serious adverse effects. The combined therapy duration (oral and parenteral) should not exceed 5 days. Use the lowest effective dose for the shortest duration of time, consistent with individual patient goals, to reduce risk of cardiovascular or GI adverse events. Alternate therapies should be considered for patients at high risk. [U.S. Boxed Warning]: Ketorolac is not indicated for use in children.

Potentially significant drug-drug interactions may exist, requiring dose or frequency adjustment, additional monitoring, and/or selection of alternative therapy.

NSAIDS may cause drowsiness, dizziness, blurred vision and other neurologic effects which may impair physical or mental abilities; patients must be cautioned about performing tasks which require mental alertness (eg, operating machinery or driving). Discontinue use with blurred or diminished vision and perform ophthalmologic exam.

Drug Interactions

Avoid Concomitant Use

Avoid concomitant use of Ketorolac (Systemic) with any of the following: Aspirin; Floctafenine; Ketorolac (Nasal); Nonsteroidal Anti-Inflammatory Agents; NSAID (COX-2 Inhibitor); Omacetaxine; Pentoxifylline; Probenecid; Urokinase

Decreased Effect

Ketorolac (Systemic) may decrease the levels/ effects of: ACE Inhibitors; Agents with Antiplatelet Properties; Aliskiren; Angiotensin II Receptor Blockers; Anticonvulsants; Aspirin; Beta-Blockers; Eplerenone; HydrALAZINE; Loop Diuretics; Potassium-Sparing Diuretics; Prostaglandins (Ophthalmic); Salicylates; Selective Serotonin Reuptake Inhibitors; Thiazide Diuretics

The levels/effects of Ketorolac (Systemic) may be decreased by: Bile Acid Sequestrants; Salicylates

Increased Effect/Toxicity

Ketorolac (Systemic) may increase the levels/ effects of: 5-ASA Derivatives; Agents with Antiplatelet Properties; Aliskiren; Aminoglycosides; Anticoagulants; Aspirin; Bisphosphonate Derivatives; Collagenase (Systemic); CycloSPORINE (Systemic); Dabigatran Etexilate; Deferasirox; Desmopressin; Digoxin; Eplerenone; Haloperidol; Ibritumomab; Lithium; Methotrexate; Neuromuscular-Blocking Agents (Nondepolarizing); Nonsteroidal Anti-Inflammatory Agents; NSAID (COX-2 Inhibitor); Omacetaxine; PEMEtrexed; Pentoxifylline; Porfimer; Potassium-Sparing Diuretics; PRALAtrexate; Quinolone Antibiotics; Rivaroxaban; Salicylates; Tenofovir; Thrombolytic Agents; Tositumomab and Iodine I 131 Tositumomab; Urokinase; Vancomycin; Vitamin K Antagonists

The levels/effects of Ketorolac (Systemic) may be increased by: ACE Inhibitors; Angiotensin II Receptor Blockers; Antidepressants (Tricyclic, Tertiary Amine); Corticosteroids (Systemic); CycloSPORINE (Systemic); Dasatinib; Floctafenine; Glucosamine; Herbs (Anticoagulant/Antiplatelet Properties); Ibrutinib; Ketorolac (Nasal); Multivitamins/Fluoride (with ADE); Multivitamins/ Minerals (with ADEK, Folate, Iron); Multivitamins/ Minerals (with AE, No Iron); Omega-3 Fatty Acids; Pentosan Polysulfate Sodium; Probenecid; Prostacyclin Analogues; Selective Serotonin Reuptake Inhibitors; Serotonin/Norepinephrine Reuptake Inhibitors; Sodium Phosphates; Tipranavir; Treprostinil; Vitamin E

Nutritional/Ethanol Interactions

Ethanol: Avoid ethanol (may enhance gastric mucosal irritation).

Food: Oral: High-fat meals may delay time to peak (by ~1 hour) and decrease peak concentrations.

Herb/Nutraceutical: Avoid alfalfa, anise, bilberry, bladderwrack, bromelain, cat's claw, celery, chamomile, coleus, cordyceps, dong quai, evening primrose, fenugreek, feverfew, garlic, ginger, ginkgo biloba, ginseng (American, Panax, Siberian), grapeseed, green tea, guggul, horse chestnut seed, horseradish, licorice, prickly ash, red clover, reishi, SAMe (S-adenosylmethionine), sweet clover, turmeric, and white willow (all have additional antiplatelet activity).

Adverse Reactions Frequencies noted for parenteral administration:

>10%:

Central nervous system: Headache (17%)

Gastrointestinal: Gastrointestinal pain (13%), dyspepsia (12%), nausea (12%)

>1% to 10%:

Cardiovascular: Edema (4%), hypertension

Central nervous system: Dizziness (7%), drowsiness (6%)

Dermatologic: Diaphoresis, pruritus, skin rash

Gastrointestinal: Diarrhea (7%), constipation, flatulence, gastrointestinal fullness, gastrointestinal hemorrhage, gastrointestinal perforation, gastrointestinal ulcer, heartburn, stomatitis, vomiting

Hematologic & oncologic: Anemia, prolonged bleeding time, purpura

Hepatic: Increased liver enzymes

Local: Pain at injection site (2%)

Otic: Tinnitus

Renal: Renal function abnormality

Pharmacodynamics/Kinetics

Onset of Action Analgesic: I.M., I.V.: ~30 minutes; Peak effect: Analgesic: ≤2-3 hours

Duration of Action Analgesic: 4-6 hours

Available Dosage Forms

Solution, Injection:

Generic: 15 mg/mL (1 mL); 30 mg/mL (1 mL); 60 mg/2 mL (2 mL); 300 mg/10 mL (10 mL)

Solution, Intramuscular:

Generic: 30 mg/mL (1 mL); 60 mg/2 mL (2 mL)

Tablet, Oral:

Generic: 10 mg

General Dosage Range Dosage adjustment recommended in patients with renal impairment

I.M.:

Adolescents ≥17 years and Adults <50 kg and Elderly ≥65 years: 30 mg as a single dose or 15 mg every 6 hours (maximum: 60 mg daily)

Adolescents ≥17 years and Adults ≥50 kg: 60 mg as a single dose or 30 mg every 6 hours (maximum: 120 mg daily)

I.V.:

Adolescents ≥17 years and Adults <50 kg and Elderly ≥65 years: 15 mg as a single dose or 15 mg every 6 hours (maximum: 60 mg daily)

Adolescents ≥17 years and Adults ≥50 kg: 30 mg as a single dose or 30 mg every 6 hours (maximum: 120 mg daily)

Oral:

Adolescents ≥17 years and Adults <50 kg and Elderly ≥65 years: 10 mg every 4-6 hours as needed (maximum: 40 mg daily)

Adolescents ≥17 years and Adults ≥50 kg: 20 mg, followed by 10 mg every 4-6 hours as needed (maximum: 40 mg daily)

Administration

I.M. Administer slowly and deeply into the muscle.

I.V. Administer I.V. bolus over a minimum of 15 seconds.

Injectable Detail pH: 6.9-7.9

Oral May take with food to reduce GI upset.

Storage/Stability

Injection: Store at room temperature of 15°C to 30°C (59°F to 86°F). Protect from light. Injection is clear and has a slight yellow color. Precipitation may occur at relatively low pH values.

Tablet: Store at room temperature of 15°C to 30°C (59°F to 86°F).

Nursing Actions

Physical Assessment Assess allergy history prior to treatment. I.V./I.M.: Monitor vital signs on a regular basis during infusion or following injection. Oral: Monitor blood pressure prior to treatment and periodically throughout.

Patient Education

• Discuss specific use of drug and side effects with patient as it relates to treatment. (HCAHPS: During this hospital stay, were you given any medicine that you had not taken before? Before giving you any new medicine, how often did hospital staff tell you what the medicine was for? How often did hospital staff describe possible side effects in a way you could understand?)

• Patient may experience headache, dyspepsia, nausea, or diarrhea. Have patient report immediately to prescriber angina, strength differences from one side to another, edema or pain of hands or feet, significant weight gain, melena, hematuria, ecchymosis, or rash (HCAHPS).

• Educate patient about signs of a significant reaction (eg, wheezing; chest tightness; fever; itching; bad cough; blue skin color; seizures; or swelling of face, lips, tongue, or throat). **Note:** This is not a comprehensive list of all side effects. Patient should consult prescriber for additional questions.

Intended Use and Disclaimer: Should not be printed and given to patients. This information is intended to serve as a concise initial reference for healthcare professionals to use when discussing medications with a patient. You must ultimately rely on your own discretion, experience and judgment in diagnosing, treating and advising patients.

Dietary Considerations Administer tablet with food or milk to decrease gastrointestinal distress.

Ketorolac (Nasal) (KEE toe role ak)

Brand Names: U.S. Sprix
Index Terms Ketorolac Tromethamine
Pharmacologic Category Nonsteroidal Antiinflammatory Drug (NSAID), Nasal
Medication Safety Issues
 Sound-alike/look-alike issues:
  Ketorolac may be confused with Ketalar®
 BEERS Criteria medication:
  This drug may be potentially inappropriate for use in geriatric patients (Quality of evidence - high; Strength of recommendation - strong).
Medication Guide Available Yes
Pregnancy Risk Factor C/D ≥30 weeks gestation
Lactation Enters breast milk/contraindicated (per manufacturer's labeling)
Use Short-term (≤5 days) management of moderate-to-moderately-severe acute pain requiring analgesia at the opioid level
Available Dosage Forms
 Solution, Nasal [preservative free]:
  Sprix: 15.75 mg/spray (1 ea)
General Dosage Range Dosage adjustment recommended in patients with renal impairment.
 Intranasal:
  Adults <65 years and ≥50 kg: one spray (15.75 mg) in each nostril (total dose: 31.5 mg) every 6-8 hours; maximum dose: 4 doses (126 mg)/day
  Adults <50 kg and/or Elderly ≥65 years: One spray (15.75 mg) in 1 nostril (total dose: 15.75 mg) every 6-8 hours; maximum dose: 4 doses (63 mg)/day
Administration
 Inhalation Each nasal spray contains medication for 1 day of therapy. Before first use of a nasal spray container, prime by pressing pump 5 times. There is no need to prime the pump again if more doses are administered during the next 24 hours using the same nasal container. Repeat priming each day prior to first use of each new nasal spray. Blow nose to clear nostrils. Sit up straight or stand; tilt head slightly forward. Insert tip of container into nostril, keeping bottle upright, and point container away from the center of nose. Spray once, pressing down evenly on both sides of container.

 Discard container within 24 hours of priming even if there is unused medication.
Nursing Actions
 Physical Assessment Monitor for pain effectiveness and bleeding (bruising, abdominal pain, dyspepsia). Make sure patient understands how to use nasal spray correctly.

Patient Education
- Discuss specific use of drug and side effects with patient as it relates to treatment. (HCAHPS: During this hospital stay, were you given any medicine that you had not taken before? Before giving you any new medicine, how often did hospital staff tell you what the medicine was for? How often did hospital staff describe possible side effects in a way you could understand?)
- Patient may experience rhinitis, lacrimation, dyspepsia, or diarrhea. Have patient report immediately to prescriber angina, strength differences from one side to another, severe nausea, considerable edema, significant weight gain, melena, hematuria, ecchymosis, or bleeding (HCAHPS).
- Educate patient about signs of a significant reaction (eg, wheezing; chest tightness; fever; itching; bad cough; blue skin color; seizures; or swelling of face, lips, tongue, or throat). **Note:** This is not a comprehensive list of all side effects. Patient should consult prescriber for additional questions.

Intended Use and Disclaimer: Should not be printed and given to patients. This information is intended to serve as a concise initial reference for healthcare professionals to use when discussing medications with a patient. You must ultimately rely on your own discretion, experience and judgment in diagnosing, treating and advising patients.

Ketorolac (Ophthalmic) (KEE toe role ak)

Brand Names: U.S. Acular; Acular LS; Acuvail
Index Terms Ketorolac Tromethamine
Pharmacologic Category Nonsteroidal Antiinflammatory Drug (NSAID), Ophthalmic
Medication Safety Issues
 Sound-alike/look-alike issues:
  Acular® may be confused with Acthar®, Ocular
  Ketorolac may be confused with Ketalar®
Pregnancy Risk Factor C
Lactation Use caution
Use Temporary relief of ocular itching due to seasonal allergic conjunctivitis; postoperative pain and/or inflammation following cataract extraction; reduction of ocular pain, burning, and stinging following corneal refractive surgery
Available Dosage Forms
 Solution, Ophthalmic:
  Acular: 0.5% (5 mL)
  Acular LS: 0.4% (5 mL)
  Generic: 0.4% (5 mL); 0.5% (3 mL, 5 mL, 10 mL)
 Solution, Ophthalmic [preservative free]:
  Acuvail: 0.45% (30 ea)
General Dosage Range Ophthalmic:
 Children ≥2 years, Adolescents, and Adults: Acular®: Instill 1 drop to affected eye(s) 4 times daily

Children ≥3 years, Adolescents, and Adults: Acular LS®: Instill 1 drop to affected eye(s) 4 times daily
Adults: Acuvail®: Instill 1 drop to affected eye(s) 2 times daily

Administration

Ophthalmic May contain benzalkonium chloride which may be absorbed by contact lenses; contact lenses should not be worn during treatment. May be administered with other ophthalmic medications including antibiotics, beta-blockers, carbonic anhydrase inhibitors, cycloplegics, and mydriatics; wait at least 5 minutes before administering other eye drops.

Nursing Actions

Patient Education

• Discuss specific use of drug and side effects with patient as it relates to treatment. (HCAHPS: During this hospital stay, were you given any medicine that you had not taken before? Before giving you any new medicine, how often did hospital staff tell you what the medicine was for? How often did hospital staff describe possible side effects in a way you could understand?)

• Patient may experience blurred vision. Have patient report immediately to prescriber vision changes, ophthalmalgia, severe eye irritation, or subconjunctival hemorrhage (HCAHPS).

• Educate patient about signs of a significant reaction (eg, wheezing; chest tightness; fever; itching; bad cough; blue skin color; seizures; or swelling of face, lips, tongue, or throat). **Note:** This is not a comprehensive list of all side effects. Patient should consult prescriber for additional questions.

Intended Use and Disclaimer: Should not be printed and given to patients. This information is intended to serve as a concise initial reference for healthcare professionals to use when discussing medications with a patient. You must ultimately rely on your own discretion, experience and judgment in diagnosing, treating and advising patients.

Ketotifen (Systemic) (kee toe TYE fen)

Index Terms Ketotifen Fumarate

Pharmacologic Category Histamine H₁ Antagonist; Histamine H₁ Antagonist, Second Generation; Mast Cell Stabilizer; Piperidine Derivative

Medication Safety Issues

Sound-alike/look-alike issues:

Ketotifen may be confused with ketoprofen

Zaditen® may be confused with Zaditor®

Lactation Enters breast milk/not recommended

Use Adjunctive therapy in the chronic treatment of pediatric patients ≥6 months of age with mild, atopic asthma

Mechanism of Action/Effect Relatively selective, noncompetitive H₁-receptor antagonist and mast cell stabilizer, inhibiting the release of mediators from cells involved in hypersensitivity reactions

Contraindications Hypersensitivity to ketotifen or any component of the formulation; use of ketotifen syrup in patients sensitive to benzoate compounds

Warnings/Precautions Indicated for prophylactic treatment; not effective for the prevention or treatment of acute asthma attacks. Therapy for acute symptoms of asthma (eg, corticosteroids, beta₂-agonists, xanthine derivatives) should be maintained and gradually reduced. Several weeks of oral ketotifen therapy may be needed to observe clinical response while maximum therapeutic response usually requires duration of therapy ≥10 weeks. Therapy should be maintained for at least 2-3 months to determine effectiveness. If therapy requires discontinuation, gradually reduce over 2-4 weeks. Oral dosage forms may cause sedation early in therapy. Sedative effects may be reduced by initiating therapy at one-half the recommended daily dose with gradual increase over 5 days to maintenance dose.

Caution patients about performing tasks which require mental alertness (eg, driving or operating machinery). Thrombocytopenia has occurred rarely when used concomitantly with oral antidiabetic agents. Use with caution in epileptic patients; may lower seizure threshold. Use caution in diabetics and individuals with benzoate allergies as the syrup preparation contains carbohydrates and benzoate compounds.

Adverse Reactions 1% to 10%:

Central nervous system: Sedation (8%; less than placebo), headache (1%), sleep disturbance (1%)

Dermatologic: Rash (4%), urticaria (1%)

Gastrointestinal: Weight gain (5%), abdominal pain (1%), appetite increased (1%)

Respiratory: Respiratory infection (4%), epistaxis (1%)

Miscellaneous: Flu (3%), puffy eyelid (1%)

Product Availability Not available in the U.S.

General Dosage Range Oral:

Children 6 months to 3 years: Initial: 0.05 mg/kg once daily or in 2 divided doses for 5 days; Maintenance: 0.05 mg/kg twice daily (maximum dose: 1 mg twice daily)

Children >3 years: Initial: 1 mg once daily or in 2 divided doses for 5 days; Maintenance: 1 mg twice daily

Administration

Oral Administer without regards to meals.

Storage/Stability

Syrup: Store at up to 25°C (up to 77°F).

Tablet: Store at up to 25°C (up to 77°F). Protect from moisture.

Nursing Actions

Patient Education

• Discuss specific use of drug and side effects with caregiver as it relates to treatment. (HCAHPS: During this hospital stay, were you given any medicine that you had not taken before? Before giving you any new medicine, how often did hospital staff tell you what the medicine was for? How often did hospital staff describe possible side effects in a way you could understand?)

• Patient may experience fatigue or weight gain. Have caregiver report immediately to prescriber rash (HCAHPS).

• Educate caregiver about signs of a significant reaction (eg, wheezing; chest tightness; fever; itching; bad cough; blue skin color; seizures; or swelling of face, lips, tongue, or throat). **Note:** This is not a comprehensive list of all side effects. Caregiver should consult prescriber for additional questions.

Intended Use and Disclaimer: Should not be printed and given to patients. This information is intended to serve as a concise initial reference for healthcare professionals to use when discussing medications with a patient. You must ultimately rely on your own discretion, experience and judgment in diagnosing, treating and advising patients.

Dietary Considerations May be taken without regard to meals. Syrup contains carbohydrate 4 g/5 mL.

Labetalol (la BET a lole)

Brand Names: U.S. Trandate

Index Terms Ibidomide Hydrochloride; Labetalol Hydrochloride

Pharmacologic Category Antihypertensive; Beta-Blocker With Alpha-Blocking Activity

Medication Safety Issues

Sound-alike/look-alike issues:

Labetalol may be confused with betaxolol, lamo-TRIgine, Lipitor®

Normodyne® may be confused with Norpramin®

Trandate® may be confused with traMADol, TRENtal®

High alert medication:

The Institute for Safe Medication Practices (ISMP) includes this medication among its list of drugs which have a heightened risk of causing significant patient harm when used in error.

Administration issues:

Significant differences exist between oral and I.V. dosing. Use caution when converting from one route of administration to another.

Pregnancy Risk Factor C

Lactation Enters breast milk/use caution

Breast-Feeding Considerations Low amounts of labetalol are found in breast milk and can be detected in the serum of nursing infants. The manufacturer recommends that caution be exercised when administering labetalol to nursing women.

Use Treatment of mild-to-severe hypertension; I.V. for severe hypertension (eg, hypertensive emergencies)

Unlabeled Use Pediatric hypertension; management of pre-eclampsia; severe hypertension in pregnancy; hypertension during acute ischemic stroke

Mechanism of Action/Effect Blocks alpha-, beta$_1$-, and beta$_2$-adrenergic receptor sites; elevated renins are reduced. The ratios of alpha- to beta-blockade differ depending on the route of administration: 1:3 (oral) and 1:7 (I.V.).

Contraindications Hypersensitivity to labetalol or any component of the formulation; severe bradycardia; heart block greater than first degree (except in patients with a functioning artificial pacemaker); cardiogenic shock; bronchial asthma; uncompensated cardiac failure; conditions associated with severe and prolonged hypotension

Warnings/Precautions Consider pre-existing conditions such as sick sinus syndrome before initiating. Symptomatic hypotension with or without syncope may occur with labetalol; close monitoring of patient is required especially with initial dosing and dosing increases; blood pressure must be lowered at a rate appropriate for the patient's clinical condition. Initiation with a low dose and gradual up-titration may help to decrease the occurrence of hypotension or syncope. Patients should be advised to avoid driving or other hazardous tasks during initiation of therapy due to the risk of syncope. Orthostatic hypotension may occur with I.V. administration; patient should remain supine during and for up to 3 hours after I.V. administration. Use with caution in impaired hepatic function; bioavailability is increased due to decreased first-pass metabolism. Severe hepatic injury including some fatalities have also been rarely reported with use: periodically monitor LFTs with prolonged use. Use with caution in patients with diabetes mellitus; may potentiate hypoglycemia and/or mask signs and symptoms. Bradycardia may be observed more frequently in elderly patients (>65 years of age); dosage reductions may be necessary. May also reduce release of insulin in response to hyperglycemia; dosage of antidiabetic agents may need to be adjusted. May mask signs of hyperthyroidism (eg, tachycardia); if hyperthyroidism is suspected, carefully manage and monitor; abrupt withdrawal may exacerbate symptoms of hyperthyroidism or precipitate thyroid storm. Elimination of labetalol is reduced in elderly patients; lower maintenance doses may be required.

Use only with extreme caution in compensated heart failure and monitor for a worsening of the condition. Beta-blocker therapy should not be withdrawn abruptly (particularly in patients with CAD), but gradually tapered to avoid acute tachycardia, hypertension, and/or ischemia. Chronic beta-blocker therapy should not be routinely withdrawn prior to major surgery. Use caution with concurrent use of digoxin, verapamil, or diltiazem; bradycardia or heart block can occur. Use with caution in patients receiving inhaled anesthetic agents known to depress myocardial contractility. Patients with bronchospastic disease should not receive beta-blockers; if used at all, should be used cautiously with close monitoring. Use with caution in patients with myasthenia gravis or psychiatric disease (may cause or exacerbate CNS depression). Can precipitate or aggravate symptoms of arterial insufficiency in patients with PVD and Raynaud's disease; use with caution and monitor for progression of arterial obstruction. If possible, obtain diagnostic tests for pheochromocytoma prior to use. May induce or exacerbate psoriasis. Labetalol has been shown to be effective in lowering blood pressure and relieving symptoms in patients with pheochromocytoma. However, some patients have experienced paradoxical hypertensive responses; use with caution in patients with pheochromocytoma. Additional alpha-blockade may be required during use of labetalol. Use caution with history of severe anaphylaxis to allergens; patients taking beta-blockers may become more sensitive to repeated challenges. Treatment of anaphylaxis (eg, epinephrine) in patients taking beta-blockers may be ineffective or promote undesirable effects.

Intraoperative floppy iris syndrome has been observed in cataract surgery patients who were on or were previously treated with alpha$_1$-blockers; causality has not been established and there appears to be no benefit in discontinuing alpha-blocker therapy prior to surgery. Instruct patients to inform ophthalmologist of labetalol use when considering eye surgery.

Drug Interactions

Avoid Concomitant Use
Avoid concomitant use of Labetalol with any of the following: Beta2-Agonists; Floctafenine; Methacholine

Decreased Effect
Labetalol may decrease the levels/effects of: Beta2-Agonists; Theophylline Derivatives

The levels/effects of Labetalol may be decreased by: Barbiturates; Herbs (Hypertensive Properties); Methylphenidate; Nonsteroidal Anti-Inflammatory Agents; Rifamycin Derivatives; Yohimbine

Increased Effect/Toxicity
Labetalol may increase the levels/effects of: Alpha-/Beta-Agonists (Direct-Acting); Alpha1-Blockers; Alpha2-Agonists; Amifostine; Antihypertensives; Antipsychotic Agents (Phenothiazines); Bupivacaine; Cardiac Glycosides; Cholinergic Agonists; DULoxetine; Ergot Derivatives; Fingolimod; Hypotensive Agents; Insulin; Lidocaine (Systemic); Lidocaine (Topical); Mepivacaine; Methacholine; Midodrine; Obinutuzumab; RiTUXimab; Sulfonylureas

The levels/effects of Labetalol may be increased by: Acetylcholinesterase Inhibitors; Alpha2-Agonists; Aminoquinolines (Antimalarial); Amiodarone; Anilidopiperidine Opioids; Antipsychotic Agents (Phenothiazines); Brimonidine (Topical); Calcium Channel Blockers (Dihydropyridine); Calcium Channel Blockers (Nondihydropyridine); Diazoxide; Dipyridamole; Disopyramide; Dronedarone; Floctafenine; Herbs (Hypotensive Properties); MAO Inhibitors; Pentoxifylline; Phosphodiesterase 5 Inhibitors; Propafenone; Prostacyclin Analogues; Regorafenib; Reserpine

Nutritional/Ethanol Interactions
Food: Labetalol serum concentrations may be increased if taken with food.

Herb/Nutraceutical: Avoid dong quai if using for hypertension (has estrogenic activity). Avoid ephedra, yohimbe, ginseng (may worsen hypertension). Avoid natural licorice (causes sodium and water retention and increases potassium loss). Avoid garlic (may have increased antihypertensive effect).

Adverse Reactions
>10%:
Cardiovascular: Orthostatic hypotension (I.V. use; ≤58%)
Central nervous system: Dizziness (1% to 20%), fatigue (1% to 11%)
Gastrointestinal: Nausea (≤19%)
1% to 10%:
Cardiovascular: Hypotension (1% to 5%), edema (≤2%), flushing (1%), ventricular arrhythmia (I.V. use; 1%)
Central nervous system: Somnolence (3%), headache (2%), vertigo (1% to 2%)
Dermatologic: Scalp tingling (≤7%), pruritus (1%), rash (1%)
Gastrointestinal: Dyspepsia (≤4%), vomiting (≤3%), taste disturbance (1%)
Genitourinary: Ejaculatory failure (≤5%), impotence (1% to 4%)
Hepatic: Transaminases increased (4%)
Neuromuscular & skeletal: Paresthesia (≤5%), weakness (1%)
Ocular: Vision abnormal (1%)
Renal: BUN increased (≤8%)
Respiratory: Nasal congestion (1% to 6%), dyspnea (2%)
Miscellaneous: Diaphoresis (≤4%)
Other adverse reactions noted with beta-adrenergic blocking agents include mental depression, catatonia, disorientation, short-term memory loss, emotional lability, clouded sensorium, intensification of pre-existing AV block, laryngospasm, respiratory distress, agranulocytosis, thrombocytopenic purpura, nonthrombocytopenic purpura, mesenteric artery thrombosis, and ischemic colitis.

Pharmacodynamics/Kinetics

Onset of Action Oral: 20 minutes to 2 hours; I.V.: 2-5 minutes; Peak effect: Oral: 1-4 hours; I.V.: 5-15 minutes

Duration of Action Blood pressure response: Oral: 8-12 hours (dose dependent)

I.V.: 2-18 hours (dose dependent; based on single and multiple sequential doses of 0.25-0.5 mg/kg with cumulative dosing up to 3.25 mg/kg)

Available Dosage Forms

Solution, Intravenous:

Generic: 5 mg/mL (4 mL, 20 mL, 40 mL)

Tablet, Oral:

Trandate: 100 mg, 200 mg, 300 mg

Generic: 100 mg, 200 mg, 300 mg

General Dosage Range

I.V.:

Children: 0.3-1 mg/kg/dose intermittently **or** 0.4-1 mg/kg/hour infusion (maximum: 3 mg/kg/hour)

Adults: Bolus: 20 mg, may give 40-80 mg at 10-minute intervals; Infusion: 2 mg/minute (maximum: 300 mg total cumulative dose)

Oral: *Adults:* Initial: 100 mg twice daily; Maintenance: 200-800 mg/day in 2 divided doses (maximum: 2.4 g/day)

Usual Infusion Concentrations: Pediatric I.V. infusion: 1 mg/mL

Usual Infusion Concentrations: Adult I.V. infusion: 500 mg in 250 mL (concentration: 2 mg/mL) of D_5W

Administration

I.V. Bolus dose may be administered I.V. push at a rate of 10 mg/minute; may follow with continuous I.V. infusion

Injectable Detail pH: 3-4

Storage/Stability

Tablets: Store at room temperature (refer to manufacturer's labeling for detailed storage requirements). Protect from light and excessive moisture.

Injectable: Store at room temperature (refer to manufacturer's labeling for detailed storage requirements); do not freeze. Protect from light. The solution is clear to slightly yellow.

Parenteral admixture: Stability of parenteral admixture at room temperature (25°C) and refrigeration temperature (4°C): 3 days.

Nursing Actions

Physical Assessment Monitor blood pressure and heart rate prior to and following first dose and with any change in dosage. Caution patients with diabetes to monitor glucose levels closely; beta-blockers may alter glucose tolerance. Monitor for CHF.

Patient Education

• Discuss specific use of drug and side effects with patient as it relates to treatment. (HCAHPS: During this hospital stay, were you given any medicine that you had not taken before? Before giving you any new medicine, how often did hospital staff tell you what the medicine was for? How often did hospital staff describe possible side effects in a way you could understand?)

• Patient may experience dizziness, nausea, asthenia, or impotence. Have patient report immediately to prescriber dyspnea, significant weight gain, or rash (HCAHPS).

• Educate patient about signs of a significant reaction (eg, wheezing; chest tightness; fever; itching; bad cough; blue skin color; seizures; or swelling of face, lips, tongue, or throat). **Note:** This is not a comprehensive list of all side effects. Patient should consult prescriber for additional questions.

Intended Use and Disclaimer: Should not be printed and given to patients. This information is intended to serve as a concise initial reference for healthcare professionals to use when discussing medications with a patient. You must ultimately rely on your own discretion, experience and judgment in diagnosing, treating and advising patients.

Lacosamide (la KOE sa mide)

Brand Names: U.S. Vimpat

Index Terms ADD 234037; Harkoseride; LCM; SPM 927

Pharmacologic Category Anticonvulsant, Miscellaneous

Medication Safety Issues

Sound-alike/look-alike issues:

Lacosamide may be confused with zonisamide

Vimpat may be confused with Vimovo

Medication Guide Available Yes

Pregnancy Risk Factor C

Lactation Excretion in breast milk unknown/not recommended

Breast-Feeding Considerations It is unknown if lacosamide is excreted in human milk. The manufacturer recommends a decision be made whether to discontinue nursing or to discontinue the drug, taking into account the importance of treatment to the mother.

Use Adjunctive therapy in the treatment of partial-onset seizures

Mechanism of Action/Effect Lacosamide stabilizes hyperexcitable neuronal membranes and inhibits repetitive neuronal firing to decrease epileptiform activity.

Contraindications

U.S. labeling: There are no contraindications listed in manufacturer's labeling.

Canadian labeling: Hypersensitivity to lacosamide or any component of the formulation; second- or third-degree atrioventricular (AV) block (current or history of).

Warnings/Precautions Antiepileptics are associated with an increased risk of suicidal behavior/thoughts with use (regardless of indication); ▶

patients should be monitored for signs/symptoms of depression, suicidal tendencies, and other unusual behavior changes during therapy and instructed to inform their healthcare provider immediately if symptoms occur. CNS effects may occur; patients should be cautioned about performing tasks which require alertness (eg, operating machinery or driving). Lacosamide may prolong PR interval; second degree and complete AV block has also been reported. Use caution in patients with conduction problems (eg, first/second degree atrioventricular block and sick sinus syndrome without pacemaker), sodium channelopathies (eg, Brugada Syndrome), myocardial ischemia, heart failure, structural heart disease, or if concurrent use with other drugs that prolong the PR interval; ECG is recommended prior to initiating therapy and when at steady state. Instruct patients to contact their healthcare provider if signs or symptoms of conduction problems occur (eg, low or irregular pulse, feeling of lightheadedness and fainting). During investigational trials, atrial fibrillation/flutter, or syncope occurred slightly more often in patients with diabetic neuropathy and/or cardiovascular disease. Use caution with renal or hepatic impairment and if these patients are taking strong inhibitors of CYP3A4 and CYP2C9; dosage adjustment may be necessary. Multiorgan hypersensitivity reactions can occur (rare); monitor patient and discontinue therapy if necessary. Withdraw therapy gradually (≥1 week) to minimize the potential of increased seizure frequency. Blurred vision and diplopia may occur during therapy. If visual disturbances persist, further assessment, including dose reduction and discontinuation should be considered. Monitor patients with known vision-related issues or ocular conditions. Effects with ethanol may be potentiated. Some products may contain phenylalanine.

Drug Interactions

Avoid Concomitant Use There are no known interactions where it is recommended to avoid concomitant use.

Decreased Effect

The levels/effects of Lacosamide may be decreased by: CarBAMazepine; Fosphenytoin; PHENobarbital; Phenytoin

Increased Effect/Toxicity

The levels/effects of Lacosamide may be increased by: CYP2C9 Inhibitors (Strong); CYP3A4 Inhibitors (Strong); Delavirdine; NiCARdipine

Nutritional/Ethanol Interactions Ethanol: Avoid ethanol (may increase CNS depression).

Adverse Reactions The majority of adverse events are dose-dependent.

>10%:
Central nervous system: Dizziness (16% to 53%), fatigue (7% to 15%), ataxia (4% to 15%), headache (11% to 14%)

Gastrointestinal: Nausea (7% to 17%), vomiting (6% to 16%)
Neuromuscular & skeletal: Tremor (6% to 12%)
Ophthalmic: Diplopia (6% to 16%), blurred vision (2% to 16%)

1% to 10%:
Cardiovascular: Syncope (adults 1%; dose-related: >400 mg/day)
Central nervous system: Drowsiness (8%), memory impairment (6%), equilibrium disturbance (1% to 6%), vertigo (3% to 5%), abnormal gait (2% to 4%), depression (2%)
Dermatologic: Pruritus (2% to 3%)
Gastrointestinal: Diarrhea (3% to 5%)
Hematologic & oncologic: Bruise (4%)
Hepatic: Increased serum ALT (1%)
Local: Pain at injection site (3%), local irritation (1%)
Neuromuscular & skeletal: Weakness (2% to 4%)
Ophthalmic: Nystagmus (5% to 10%)
Miscellaneous: Laceration (3%)

Controlled Substance C-V

Available Dosage Forms

Solution, Intravenous:
Vimpat: 200 mg/20 mL (20 mL)
Solution, Oral:
Vimpat: 10 mg/mL (200 mL, 465 mL)
Tablet, Oral:
Vimpat: 50 mg, 100 mg, 150 mg, 200 mg

General Dosage Range Dosage adjustment recommended in patients with hepatic or renal impairment

Oral: Adolescents ≥17 years and Adults: Initial: 50 mg twice daily; Maintenance dose: 200-400 mg daily in 2 divided doses

Administration

I.V. Administer over 30-60 minutes. Twice daily I.V. infusions have been used for up to 5 days. Can be administered without further dilution or may be mixed with compatible diluents (NS, LR, D$_5$W).

Injectable Detail pH: 3.5-5 (vial)

Oral Oral solution, tablets: May be administered with or without food. Oral solution should be administered with a calibrated measuring device (not a household teaspoon or tablespoon).

Preparation for Administration Injection: May be mixed with compatible diluents (NS, LR, D$_5$W) in glass or PVC.

Storage/Stability

Injection: Store at 20°C to 25°C (68°F to 77°F); excursions permitted between 15°C to 30°C (59°F to 86°F). Do not freeze. Stable when mixed with compatible diluents (NS, LR, D$_5$W) for at least 24 hours in glass or PVC at room temperature of 15°C to 30°C (59°F to 86°F). Discard any unused portion.

Oral solution, tablets: Store at 20°C to 25°C (68°F to 77°F); excursions permitted between 15°C to 30°C (59°F to 86°F). Do not freeze oral solution. Discard any unused portion of oral solution after 7 weeks.

Nursing Actions

Physical Assessment Taper dosage slowly when discontinuing. Do not discontinue abruptly. Monitor for depression. Be alert to suicide ideation. Teach patient safety and seizure precautions.

Patient Education

- Discuss specific use of drug and side effects with patient as it relates to treatment. (HCAHPS: During this hospital stay, were you given any medicine that you had not taken before? Before giving you any new medicine, how often did hospital staff tell you what the medicine was for? How often did hospital staff describe possible side effects in a way you could understand?)
- Patient may experience presyncope, fatigue, blurred vision, illogical thinking, headache, imbalance, dizziness, asthenia, or nausea. Have patient report immediately to prescriber depression, bradycardia, sudden vision changes, eye pain, eye irritation, or rash (HCAHPS).
- Educate patient about signs of a significant reaction (eg, wheezing; chest tightness; fever; itching; bad cough; blue skin color; seizures; or swelling of face, lips, tongue, or throat). **Note:** This is not a comprehensive list of all side effects. Patient should consult prescriber for additional questions.

Intended Use and Disclaimer: Should not be printed and given to patients. This information is intended to serve as a concise initial reference for healthcare professionals to use when discussing medications with a patient. You must ultimately rely on your own discretion, experience and judgment in diagnosing, treating and advising patients.

Dietary Considerations Some products may contain phenylalanine.

Lactulose (LAK tyoo lose)

Brand Names: U.S. Constulose; Enulose; Generlac; Kristalose

Pharmacologic Category Ammonium Detoxicant; Laxative, Osmotic

Medication Safety Issues

Sound-alike/look-alike issues:

Lactulose may be confused with lactose

Pregnancy Risk Factor B

Lactation Excretion in breast milk unknown/use caution

Use Prevention and treatment of portal-systemic encephalopathy (including hepatic precoma and coma); treatment of constipation

Available Dosage Forms

Packet, Oral:

Kristalose: 10 g (30 ea); 20 g (30 ea)

Solution, Oral:

Constulose: 10 g/15 mL (237 mL, 946 mL)

Enulose: 10 g/15 mL (473 mL)

Generlac: 10 g/15 mL (473 mL, 1892 mL)

Generic: 10 g/15 mL (15 mL, 30 mL, 236 mL, 237 mL, 473 mL, 500 mL, 946 mL, 1892 mL); 20 g/30 mL (30 mL)

General Dosage Range

Oral:

Infants: 1.7-6.7 g/day (2.5-10 mL/day) in divided doses

Older Children and Adolescents: 26.7-60 g/day (40-90 mL/day) in divided doses

Adults: PSE: 20-30 g (30-45 mL) every hour initially, then 3-4 times/day; Constipation: 10-40 g (15-60 mL) daily

Rectal: *Adults:* Constipation: 200 g (300 mL); may repeat every 4-6 hours

Administration

Oral

Oral solution: May mix with fruit juice, water, or milk.

Crystals for oral solution: Dissolve contents of packet in 120 mL water.

Other Rectal: Mix with water or normal saline; administer as retention enema using a rectal balloon catheter; retain for 30-60 minutes. Transition to oral lactulose when appropriate (able to take oral medication and no longer a risk for aspiration) prior to discontinuing rectal administration.

Nursing Actions

Physical Assessment Monitor therapeutic effectiveness (soft formed stools or resolution of CNS status in PSE). Monitor for CHF. Monitor frequency/consistency of stools. May need to adjust dose for severe diarrhea.

Patient Education

- Discuss specific use of drug and side effects with patient as it relates to treatment. (HCAHPS: During this hospital stay, were you given any medicine that you had not taken before? Before giving you any new medicine, how often did hospital staff tell you what the medicine was for? How often did hospital staff describe possible side effects in a way you could understand?)
- Patient may experience dyspepsia, pyrosis, or diarrhea. Have patient report immediately to prescriber severe dizziness or rash (HCAHPS).
- Educate patient about signs of a significant reaction (eg, wheezing; chest tightness; fever; itching; bad cough; blue skin color; seizures; or swelling of face, lips, tongue, or throat). **Note:** This is not a comprehensive list of all side effects. Patient should consult prescriber for additional questions.

Intended Use and Disclaimer: Should not be printed and given to patients. This information is intended to serve as a concise initial reference for healthcare professionals to use when discussing medications with a patient. You must ultimately rely on your own discretion, experience and

judgment in diagnosing, treating and advising patients.

LamiVUDine (la MI vyoo deen)

Brand Names: U.S. Epivir; Epivir HBV

Index Terms 3TC

Pharmacologic Category Antihepadnaviral, Reverse Transcriptase Inhibitor, Nucleoside (Anti-HBV); Antiretroviral, Reverse Transcriptase Inhibitor, Nucleoside (Anti-HIV)

Medication Safety Issues

Sound-alike/look-alike issues:

LamiVUDine may be confused with lamoTRIgine

Epivir may be confused with Combivir

Pregnancy Risk Factor C

Lactation Enters breast milk/contraindicated

Breast-Feeding Considerations Lamivudine is excreted into breast milk and can be detected in the serum of nursing infants.

Maternal or infant antiretroviral therapy does not completely eliminate the risk of postnatal HIV transmission. In addition, multiclass-resistant virus has been detected in breast-feeding infants despite maternal therapy. Therefore, in the United States, where formula is accessible, affordable, safe, and sustainable, and the risk of infant mortality due to diarrhea and respiratory infections is low, complete avoidance of breast-feeding by HIV-infected women is recommended to decrease potential transmission of HIV (DHHS [perinatal], 2012).

Use

Chronic hepatitis B (Epivir HBV): For the treatment of chronic hepatitis B associated with evidence of hepatitis B viral replication and active liver inflammation.

Limitations of use: Use only when an alternative antiviral agent with a higher genetic barrier to resistance is not available or appropriate; has not been evaluated in patients with HBV-HIV-1 coinfection, hepatitis C virus or hepatitis delta virus; has also not been evaluated in patients with chronic HBV infection with decompensated liver disease or in liver transplant recipients.

HIV infection (Epivir): In combination with other antiretroviral agents for the treatment of HIV

Unlabeled Use Postexposure prophylaxis for HIV exposure as part of a multidrug regimen

Mechanism of Action/Effect Lamivudine is a cytosine analog. In vitro, lamivudine is phosphorylated to its active 5'-triphosphate metabolite (L-TP), which inhibits HIV reverse transcription via viral DNA chain termination; L-TP also inhibits the RNA- and DNA-dependent DNA polymerase activities of reverse transcriptase. In hepatitis B, the monophosphate form is incorporated into viral DNA by hepatitis B virus polymerase, resulting in DNA chain termination.

Contraindications Clinically significant hypersensitivity (eg, anaphylaxis) to lamivudine or any component of the formulation

Warnings/Precautions Use caution with renal impairment; dosage reduction recommended. Use with extreme caution in children with history of pancreatitis or risk factors for development of pancreatitis. Pancreatitis has been reported, particularly in HIV-infected children with a history of nucleoside use. Do not use as monotherapy in treatment of HIV. Lamivudine combined with emtricitabine is not recommended as a dual-NRTI combination due to similar resistance patterns and negligible additive antiviral activity; lamivudine and tenofovir combination is preferred as the NRTIs in a fully suppressive antiretroviral regimen (DHHS, 2013). Treatment of HBV in patients with unrecognized/untreated HIV may lead to rapid HIV resistance. In addition, treatment of HIV in patients with unrecognized/untreated HBV may lead to rapid HBV resistance. Use with caution in combination with interferon alfa with or without ribavirin in HIV/HBV coinfected patients; monitor closely for hepatic decompensation, anemia, or neutropenia; dose reduction or discontinuation of interferon and/or ribavirin may be required if toxicity evident. In HIV/HBV coinfection, lamivudine and tenofovir are a preferred NRTI backbone in a fully suppressive antiretroviral regimen to provide activity against both HIV and HBV (DHHS, 2013). **[U.S. Boxed Warning]: Do not use Epivir HBV tablets or Epivir HBV oral solution for the treatment of HIV.**

[U.S. Boxed Warning]: Lactic acidosis and severe hepatomegaly with steatosis have been reported, including fatal cases. Use caution in hepatic impairment. Pregnancy, obesity, and/or prolonged therapy may increase the risk of lactic acidosis and liver damage.

Immune reconstitution syndrome may develop resulting in the occurrence of an inflammatory response to an indolent or residual opportunistic infection during initial HIV treatment or activation of autoimmune disorders (eg, Graves' disease, polymyositis, Guillain-Barré syndrome) later in therapy. May be associated with fat redistribution. Concomitant use of other lamivudine-containing products should be avoided.

[U.S. Boxed Warning]: Monitor patients closely for several months following discontinuation of therapy for chronic hepatitis B; clinical exacerbations may occur, including fatal cases. **Monitor hepatic function with clinical and laboratory follow up for at least several months after hepatitis B treatment discontinuation. Initiate antihepatitis B (HBV) medications if clinically appropriate. [U.S. Boxed Warning]: Risk of HIV-1 Resistance: HIV-1 resistance may emerge in chronic hepatitis B-infection patients with unrecognized or untreated HIV-1 infection.**

Counseling and (HIV) testing should be offered to all patients before beginning treatment with lamivudine for hepatitis B and then periodically during treatment. Lamivudine dosing for hepatitis B is subtherapeutic if used for HIV-1 infection treatment. Lamivudine monotherapy is not appropriate for HIV-1 infection treatment. Lamivudine resistant HIV-1 can develop rapidly and limit treatment options if used in unrecognized or untreated HIV-1 infection or if a patient becomes coinfected during HBV treatment. Lamivudine dosing for hepatitis B is also subtherapeutic if used for HIV-1/HBV coinfection treatment. If lamivudine is chosen as part of a HIV-1 treatment regimen in coinfected patients, the higher lamivudine dosage indicated for HIV-1 therapy should be used, with other drugs, in an appropriate combination regimen.

Not recommended as first-line therapy of chronic HBV due to high rate of resistance. Consider use only if other anti-HBV antiviral regimens with more favorable resistance patterns cannot be used. May be appropriate for short-term treatment of acute HBV (Lok, 2009). Potential compliance problems, frequency of administration, and adverse effects should be discussed with patients before initiating therapy to help prevent the emergence of resistance.

Drug Interactions

Avoid Concomitant Use

Avoid concomitant use of LamiVUDine with any of the following: Emtricitabine

Decreased Effect There are no known significant interactions involving a decrease in effect.

Increased Effect/Toxicity

LamiVUDine may increase the levels/effects of: Emtricitabine

The levels/effects of LamiVUDine may be increased by: Ganciclovir-Valganciclovir; Ribavirin; Trimethoprim

Nutritional/Ethanol Interactions Food: Food decreases the rate of absorption and C_{max}; however, there is no change in the systemic AUC. Therefore, may be taken with or without food.

Adverse Reactions Incidence data include patients on combination therapy with other antiretroviral agents.

>10%:
Central nervous system: Headache (21% to 35%), fatigue (24% to 27%), insomnia (11%)
Gastrointestinal: Nausea (15% to 33%), diarrhea (14% to 18%), pancreatitis (range: 0.3% to 18%; higher percentage in pediatric patients), abdominal pain (9% to 16%), vomiting (13% to 15%)
Hematologic: Neutropenia (7% to 15%)
Hepatic: Transaminases increased (2% to 11%)
Neuromuscular & skeletal: Myalgia (8% to 14%), neuropathy (12%), musculoskeletal pain (12%)
Respiratory: Nasal signs and symptoms (20%), cough (18%), sore throat (13%)

Miscellaneous: Infections (25%; includes ear, nose, and throat)
1% to 10%:
Central nervous system: Dizziness (10%), depression (9%), fever (7% to 10%), chills (7% to 10%)
Dermatologic: Rash (5% to 9%)
Gastrointestinal: Anorexia (10%), lipase increased (10%), abdominal cramps (6%), dyspepsia (5%), amylase increased (<1% to 4%), heartburn
Hematologic: Thrombocytopenia (1% to 4%), hemoglobinemia (2% to 3%)
Neuromuscular & skeletal: Creatine phosphokinase increased (9%), arthralgia (5% to 7%)

Available Dosage Forms

Solution, Oral:
Epivir: 10 mg/mL (240 mL)
Epivir HBV: 5 mg/mL (240 mL)
Tablet, Oral:
Epivir: 150 mg, 300 mg
Epivir HBV: 100 mg
Generic: 100 mg, 150 mg, 300 mg

General Dosage Range Dosage adjustment recommended in patients with renal impairment

Oral:
Infants 1-3 months: HIV (DHHS [pediatric], 2010): 4 mg/kg/dose twice daily
Children 3 months to 2 years: HIV: 4 mg/kg/dose twice daily (maximum: 150 mg twice daily)
Children 2-16 years and >16 years and <50 kg: Hepatitis B: 3 mg/kg/dose once daily (maximum: 100 mg/day); HIV: 4 mg/kg/dose twice daily (maximum: 150 mg twice daily)
Children >16 years and ≥50 kg: Hepatitis B: 3 mg/kg/dose once daily (maximum: 100 mg/day); HIV: 150 mg twice daily **or** 300 mg once daily
Adults <50 kg: Hepatitis B: 100 mg/day; HIV (DHHS [pediatric], 2010): 4 mg/kg/dose twice daily (maximum: 150 mg twice daily)
Adults ≥50 kg: Hepatitis B: 100 mg/day; HIV: 150 mg twice daily **or** 300 mg once daily

Administration

Oral May be administered without regard to meals. Adjust dosage in renal failure.

Storage/Stability

Oral solution:
Epivir: Store at 25°C (77°F) tightly closed.
Epivir HBV: Store at 20°C to 25°C (68°F to 77°F) tightly closed.
Tablet: Store at 25°C (77°F); excursions are permitted between 15°C and 30°C (59°F and 86°F).

Nursing Actions

Physical Assessment Monitor for headache, fatigue, and insomnia. Monitor patients closely for several months following discontinuation of therapy for chronic hepatitis B. Teach patient timing of multiple medications.

◀ **Patient Education**
- Discuss specific use of drug and side effects with patient as it relates to treatment. (HCAHPS: During this hospital stay, were you given any medicine that you had not taken before? Before giving you any new medicine, how often did hospital staff tell you what the medicine was for? How often did hospital staff describe possible side effects in a way you could understand?)
- Patient may experience headache, nausea, or diarrhea. Have patient report immediately to prescriber severe dyspepsia or rash (HCAHPS).
- Educate patient about signs of a significant reaction (eg, wheezing; chest tightness; fever; itching; bad cough; blue skin color; seizures; or swelling of face, lips, tongue, or throat). **Note:** This is not a comprehensive list of all side effects. Patient should consult prescriber for additional questions.

Intended Use and Disclaimer: Should not be printed and given to patients. This information is intended to serve as a concise initial reference for healthcare professionals to use when discussing medications with a patient. You must ultimately rely on your own discretion, experience and judgment in diagnosing, treating and advising patients.

Dietary Considerations May be taken without regard to meals. Some products may contain sucrose.

Lamivudine and Zidovudine
(la MI vyoo deen & zye DOE vyoo deen)

Brand Names: U.S. Combivir®
Index Terms AZT + 3TC (error-prone abbreviation); Zidovudine and Lamivudine
Pharmacologic Category Antiretroviral, Reverse Transcriptase Inhibitor, Nucleoside (Anti-HIV)
Medication Safety Issues
  Sound-alike/look-alike issues:
    Combivir® may be confused with Combivent®, Epivir®
  Other safety concerns:
    AZT is an error-prone abbreviation (mistaken as azaTHIOprine, aztreonam)
Pregnancy Risk Factor C
Lactation See individual agents.
Use Treatment of HIV infection when therapy is warranted based on clinical and/or immunological evidence of disease progression
Available Dosage Forms
  Tablet, oral: Lamivudine 150 mg and zidovudine 300 mg
  Combivir®: Lamivudine 150 mg and zidovudine 300 mg [scored]
General Dosage Range Oral: *Adolescents ≥30 kg and Adults:* 1 tablet (lamivudine 150 mg/zidovudine 300 mg) twice daily

Nursing Actions
Physical Assessment See individual agents.
Patient Education
- Discuss specific use of drug and side effects with patient as it relates to treatment. (HCAHPS: During this hospital stay, were you given any medicine that you had not taken before? Before giving you any new medicine, how often did hospital staff tell you what the medicine was for? How often did hospital staff describe possible side effects in a way you could understand?)
- Patient may experience headache, nausea, diarrhea, or pancreas irritation. Have patient report immediately to prescriber signs of infection, severe myalgia, back pain, or considerable asthenia (HCAHPS).
- Educate patient about signs of a significant reaction (eg, wheezing; chest tightness; fever; itching; bad cough; blue skin color; seizures; or swelling of face, lips, tongue, or throat). **Note:** This is not a comprehensive list of all side effects. Patient should consult prescriber for additional questions.

Intended Use and Disclaimer: Should not be printed and given to patients. This information is intended to serve as a concise initial reference for healthcare professionals to use when discussing medications with a patient. You must ultimately rely on your own discretion, experience and judgment in diagnosing, treating and advising patients.

Related Information
LamiVUDine *on page 900*
Zidovudine *on page 1630*

LamoTRIgine (la MOE tri jeen)

Brand Names: U.S. LaMICtal; LaMICtal ODT; LaMICtal Starter; LaMICtal XR
Index Terms BW-430C; LTG
Pharmacologic Category Anticonvulsant, Miscellaneous
Medication Safety Issues
  Sound-alike/look-alike issues:
    LamoTRIgine may be confused with labetalol, LamISIL®, lamiVUDine, levothyroxine, Lomotil®
    LaMICtal® may be confused with LamISIL®, Lomotil®
  Administration issues:
    Potential exists for medication errors to occur among different formulations of LaMICtal® (tablets, extended release tablets, orally disintegrating tablets, and chewable/dispersible tablets). Patients should be instructed to visually inspect tablets dispensed to verify receiving the correct medication and formulation. The medication

guide includes illustrations to aid in tablet verification.

International issues:

Lamictal [U.S., Canada, and multiple international markets] may be confused with Ludiomil brand name for maprotiline [multiple international markets]

Lamotrigine [U.S., Canada, and multiple international markets] may be confused with Ludiomil brand name for maprotiline [multiple international markets]

Medication Guide Available Yes

Pregnancy Risk Factor C

Lactation Enters breast milk/use caution

Breast-Feeding Considerations Lamotrigine is found in breast milk and may be as high as 50% of the maternal serum concentration. Adverse events observed in breast-feeding infants include apnea, drowsiness, and poor sucking. The manufacturer recommends that caution be used if administered to a breast-feeding woman and to monitor the nursing infant.

Use

U.S. labeling:

Immediate release: Adjunctive therapy in the treatment of generalized seizures of Lennox-Gastaut syndrome, primary generalized tonic-clonic seizures, and partial seizures; conversion to monotherapy in patients with partial seizures who are receiving treatment with a single antiepileptic drug (AED) (specifically carbamazepine, phenytoin, phenobarbital, primidone, or valproic acid); maintenance treatment of bipolar I disorder

Extended release: Adjunctive therapy for primary generalized tonic-clonic seizures and partial seizures (with or without secondary generalization); conversion to monotherapy in patients with partial seizures who are receiving treatment with a single antiepileptic drug AED

Canadian labeling: Immediate release: Adjunctive therapy for epilepsy uncontrolled by conventional therapy; monotherapy of epilepsy following withdrawal of concurrent antiepileptic agents; adjunctive therapy for Lennox-Gastaut syndrome

Mechanism of Action/Effect A triazine derivative which inhibits release of glutamate (an excitatory amino acid) and inhibits voltage-sensitive sodium channels, which stabilizes neuronal membranes. Lamotrigine has weak inhibitory effect on the 5-HT$_3$ receptor; *in vitro* inhibits dihydrofolate reductase.

Contraindications Hypersensitivity to lamotrigine or any component of the formulation

Warnings/Precautions [U.S. Boxed Warning]: Severe and potentially life-threatening skin rashes requiring hospitalization have been reported; incidence of serious rash is higher in pediatric patients than adults; risk may be increased by coadministration with valproic acid, higher than recommended starting doses, and exceeding recommended dose titration. The majority of cases occur in the first 8 weeks; however, isolated cases may occur after prolonged treatment or in patients without these risk factors. Discontinue at first sign of rash and do not reinitiate therapy unless rash is clearly not drug related. Rare cases of Stevens-Johnson syndrome, toxic epidermal necrolysis, and angioedema have been reported.

Antiepileptics are associated with an increased risk of suicidal behavior/thoughts with use (regardless of indication); patients should be monitored for signs/symptoms of depression, suicidal tendencies, and other unusual behavior changes during therapy and instructed to inform their healthcare provider immediately if symptoms occur.

A spectrum of hematologic effects have been reported with use (eg, neutropenia, leukopenia, thrombocytopenia, pancytopenia, anemias, and rarely, aplastic anemia and pure red cell aplasia); patients with a previous history of adverse hematologic reaction to any drug may be at increased risk. Early detection of hematologic change is important; advise patients of early signs and symptoms including fever, sore throat, mouth ulcers, infections, easy bruising, petechial or purpuric hemorrhage. May be associated with hypersensitivity syndrome (eg, anticonvulsant hypersensitivity syndrome). Multiorgan hypersensitivity reactions (drug reaction with eosinophilia and systemic symptoms [DRESS]) have been reported. Symptoms may include fever, rash, and/or lymphadenopathy; monitor for signs and symptoms of possible disparate manifestations associated with lymphatic, hepatic, renal, and/or hematologic organ systems. Evaluate patient with fever and lymphadenopathy, even if rash is not present; discontinuation and conversion to alternate therapy may be required. Increased risk of developing aseptic meningitis has been reported; symptoms (eg, headache, nuchal rigidity, fever, nausea/vomiting, rash, photophobia) have generally occurred within 1-45 days following therapy initiation. Use caution in patients with renal or hepatic impairment. Avoid abrupt cessation, taper over at least 2 weeks if possible.

May cause CNS depression, which may impair physical or mental abilities. Patients must be cautioned about performing tasks which require mental alertness (eg, operating machinery or driving). Effects with other sedative drugs or ethanol may be potentiated. Binds to melanin and may accumulate in the eye and other melanin-rich tissues; the clinical significance of this is not known. Safety and efficacy have not been established for use as initial monotherapy, conversion to monotherapy from antiepileptic drugs (AED) other than carbamazepine, phenytoin, phenobarbital, primidone or valproic acid or conversion to monotherapy from two or more AEDs. Patients treated for bipolar disorder should be monitored closely for clinical worsening or suicidality; prescriptions should be written for the smallest quantity consistent with good patient care. Hormonal contraceptives may cause a decrease in lamotrigine levels; dose adjustment of the lamotrigine maintenance dose may be required when initiating or discontinuing estrogen-containing oral contraceptives. Valproic acid may cause an increase in lamotrigine levels requiring dose adjustment. There is a potential for medication errors with similar-sounding medications and among different lamotrigine formulations; medication errors have occurred.

Drug Interactions

Avoid Concomitant Use

Avoid concomitant use of LamoTRIgine with any of the following: Azelastine (Nasal); Paraldehyde; Thalidomide

Decreased Effect

LamoTRIgine may decrease the levels/effects of: Contraceptives (Progestins)

The levels/effects of LamoTRIgine may be decreased by: Barbiturates; CarBAMazepine; Contraceptives (Estrogens); Ezogabine; Fosphenytoin; Ketorolac (Nasal); Ketorolac (Systemic); Mefloquine; Orlistat; Phenytoin; Primidone; Rifampin; Ritonavir

Increased Effect/Toxicity

LamoTRIgine may increase the levels/effects of: Alcohol (Ethyl); Azelastine (Nasal); Buprenorphine; CarBAMazepine; CNS Depressants; Desmopressin; Hydrocodone; MetFORMIN; Methotrimeprazine; Metyrosine; Mirtazapine; OLANZapine; Paraldehyde; Pramipexole; Procainamide; ROPINIRole; Rotigotine; Selective Serotonin Reuptake Inhibitors; Thalidomide; Zolpidem

The levels/effects of LamoTRIgine may be increased by: Brimonidine (Topical); Doxylamine; Droperidol; HydrOXYzine; Magnesium Sulfate; Methotrimeprazine; Perampanel; Sodium Oxybate; Tapentadol; Valproic Acid and Derivatives

Nutritional/Ethanol Interactions

Ethanol: May increase CNS depression; monitor for increased effects with coadministration. Caution patients about effects.

Food: Has no effect on absorption.

Herb/Nutraceutical: Avoid evening primrose (seizure threshold decreased).

Adverse Reactions Percentages reported in adults on monotherapy for epilepsy or bipolar disorder.

>10%: Gastrointestinal: Nausea (7% to 14%)

1% to 10%:

Cardiovascular: Chest pain (5%), peripheral edema (2% to 5%), edema (1% to 5%)

Central nervous system: Insomnia (5% to 10%), somnolence (9%), fatigue (8%), coordination impaired (7%), dizziness (7%), anxiety (5%), pain (5%), ataxia (2% to 5%), irritability (2% to 5%), suicidal ideation (2% to 5%), agitation (1% to 5%), amnesia (1% to 5%), depression (1% to

5%), dream abnormality (1% to 5%), emotional lability (1% to 5%), fever (1% to 5%), hypoesthesia (1% to 5%), migraine (1% to 5%), thought abnormality (1% to 5%), confusion (1%)

Dermatologic: Rash (nonserious: 7%), dermatitis (2% to 5%), dry skin (2% to 5%)

Endocrine & metabolic: Dysmenorrhea (5%), libido increased (2% to 5%)

Gastrointestinal: Vomiting (5% to 9%), dyspepsia (7%), abdominal pain (6%), xerostomia (2% to 6%), constipation (5%), weight loss (5%), anorexia (2% to 5%), peptic ulcer (2% to 5%), rectal hemorrhage (2% to 5%), flatulence (1% to 5%), weight gain (1% to 5%)

Genitourinary: Urinary frequency (1% to 5%)

Neuromuscular & skeletal: Back pain (8%), weakness (2% to 5%), arthralgia (1% to 5%), myalgia (1% 5%), neck pain (1% to 5%), paresthesia (1%)

Ocular: Nystagmus (2% to 5%), vision abnormal (2% to 5%), amblyopia (1%)

Respiratory: Rhinitis (7%), cough (5%), pharyngitis (5%), bronchitis (2% to 5%), dyspnea (2% to 5%), epistaxis (2% to 5%), sinusitis (1% to 5%)

Miscellaneous: Infection (5%), diaphoresis (2% to 5%), reflexes increased/decreased (2% to 5%), dyspraxia (1% to 5%)

Available Dosage Forms

Kit, Oral:

LaMICtal ODT: 50 mg (42s), 100 mg (14s), 25 mg (14s), 50 mg (14s) and 100 mg (7s), 25 mg (21s) and 50 mg (7s)

LaMICtal Starter: 25 mg (35s), 25 mg (84s) and 100 mg (14s), 25 mg (42s) and 100 mg (7s)

LaMICtal XR: 25 mg (21s) and 50 mg, (7s), 25 mg (14s), 50 mg (14s) and 100 mg (7s), 50 mg (14s), 100 mg (14s) and 200 mg (7s)

Tablet, Oral:

LaMICtal: 25 mg, 100 mg, 150 mg, 200 mg

Generic: 25 mg, 100 mg, 150 mg, 200 mg

Tablet Chewable, Oral:

LaMICtal: 2 mg, 5 mg, 25 mg

Generic: 5 mg, 25 mg

Tablet Dispersible, Oral:

LaMICtal ODT: 25 mg, 50 mg, 100 mg, 200 mg

Tablet Extended Release 24 Hour, Oral:

LaMICtal XR: 25 mg, 50 mg, 100 mg, 200 mg, 250 mg, 300 mg

Generic: 25 mg, 50 mg, 100 mg, 200 mg, 250 mg, 300 mg

General Dosage Range Dosage adjustment recommended in patients with hepatic or renal impairment or on concomitant therapy

Oral:

Immediate release formulation:

Children 2-12 years: Dosage varies greatly depending on indication

Children >12 years and Adults: Dosage varies greatly depending on indication

Extended release formulation: *Children ≥13 years and Adults:* Dosage varies greatly depending on indication

Administration

Oral Doses should be rounded down to the nearest whole tablet.

Lamictal® chewable/dispersible tablets: May be chewed, dispersed in water or diluted fruit juice, or swallowed whole. To disperse tablets, add to a small amount of liquid (just enough to cover tablet); let sit ~1 minute until dispersed; swirl solution and consume immediately. Do not administer partial amounts of liquid. If tablets are chewed, a small amount of water or diluted fruit juice should be used to aid in swallowing.

Lamictal® ODT™: Place tablets on tongue and move around in the mouth. Tablets will dissolve rapidly and can be swallowed with or without food or water.

Lamictal® XR™: Administer without regard to meals. Swallow whole; do not chew, crush, or cut.

Storage/Stability Store at 25°C (77°F); excursions permitted to 15°C to 30°C (59°F to 86°F). Protect from light.

Nursing Actions

Physical Assessment Monitor therapeutic response (seizure activity, type, duration) at beginning of therapy and periodically throughout. Report presence of skin rash immediately. Monitor for suicide ideation, depression, or unusual behavior changes. Taper dosage slowly when discontinuing. Observe and teach seizure/safety precautions.

Patient Education
• Discuss specific use of drug and side effects with patient as it relates to treatment. (HCAHPS: During this hospital stay, were you given any medicine that you had not taken before? Before giving you any new medicine, how often did hospital staff tell you what the medicine was for? How often did hospital staff describe possible side effects in a way you could understand?)
• Patient may experience presyncope, fatigue, blurred vision, illogical thinking, dizziness, imbalance, headache, or nausea. Have patient report immediately to prescriber depression, signs of infection, severe asthenia, significant myalgia, neck stiffness, sudden vision changes, discolored urine, jaundice, ecchymosis, bleeding, or rash (HCAHPS).
• Educate patient about signs of a significant reaction (eg, wheezing; chest tightness; fever; itching; bad cough; blue skin color; seizures; or swelling of face, lips, tongue, or throat). **Note:** This is not a comprehensive list of all side effects. Patient should consult prescriber for additional questions.

Intended Use and Disclaimer: Should not be printed and given to patients. This information is intended to serve as a concise initial reference for healthcare professionals to use when discussing medications with a patient. You must ultimately rely on your own discretion, experience and judgment in diagnosing, treating and advising patients.

Related Information
Oral Medications That Should Not Be Crushed or Altered *on page 1712*

Lansoprazole (lan SOE pra zole)

Brand Names: U.S. First-Lansoprazole; Heartburn Relief 24 Hour [OTC]; Prevacid; Prevacid 24HR [OTC]; Prevacid SoluTab

Pharmacologic Category Proton Pump Inhibitor; Substituted Benzimidazole

Medication Safety Issues
Sound-alike/look-alike issues:
Lansoprazole may be confused with aripiprazole, dexlansoprazole
Prevacid® may be confused with Pravachol®, Prevpac®, PriLOSEC®, Prinivil®

Medication Guide Available Yes
Pregnancy Risk Factor B
Lactation Excretion in breast milk unknown/not recommended

Breast-Feeding Considerations It is not known if lansoprazole is excreted into breast milk. Due to the potential for serious adverse reactions in the nursing infant, the manufacturer recommends a decision be made whether to discontinue nursing or to discontinue the drug, taking into account the importance of treatment to the mother.

Use Short-term (4 weeks) treatment of active duodenal ulcers; maintenance treatment of healed duodenal ulcers; as part of a multidrug regimen for *H. pylori* eradication to reduce the risk of duodenal ulcer recurrence; short-term (up to 8 weeks) treatment of active benign gastric ulcer; treatment of NSAID-associated gastric ulcer; to reduce the risk of NSAID-associated gastric ulcer in patients with a history of gastric ulcer who require an NSAID; short-term treatment of symptomatic GERD; short-term (up to 8 weeks) treatment for all grades of erosive esophagitis; to maintain healing of erosive esophagitis; long-term treatment of pathological hypersecretory conditions, including Zollinger-Ellison syndrome

OTC labeling: Relief of frequent heartburn (≥2 days/week)

Unlabeled Use Stress ulcer prophylaxis in the critically-ill

Mechanism of Action/Effect A proton pump inhibitor which decreases acid secretion in gastric parietal cells

Contraindications Hypersensitivity to lansoprazole or any component of the formulation

Warnings/Precautions Use of proton pump inhibitors (PPIs) may increase the risk of gastrointestinal infections (eg, *Salmonella, Campylobacter*). Relief of symptoms does not preclude the presence of a gastric malignancy. Atrophic gastritis (by biopsy) has been noted with long-term omeprazole therapy; this may also occur with lansoprazole. No reports of enterochromaffin-like (ECL) cell carcinoids, dysplasia, or neoplasia have occurred. Use of proton pump inhibitors (PPIs) may increase risk of CDAD, especially in hospitalized patients; consider CDAD diagnosis in patients with persistent diarrhea that does not improve. Use the lowest dose and shortest duration of PPI therapy appropriate for the condition being treated. Severe liver dysfunction may require dosage reductions. Decreased *H. pylori* eradication rates have been observed with short-term (≤7 days) combination therapy. The American College of Gastroenterology recommends 10-14 days of therapy (triple or quadruple) for eradication of *H. pylori* (Chey, 2007).

PPIs may diminish the therapeutic effect of clopidogrel thought to be due to reduced formation of the active metabolite of clopidogrel. The manufacturer of clopidogrel recommends either avoidance of both omeprazole (even when scheduled 12 hours apart) and esomeprazole or use of a PPI with comparatively less effect on the active metabolite of clopidogrel (eg, pantoprazole). Although lansoprazole exhibits the most potent CYP2C19 inhibition *in vitro* (Li, 2004; Ogilvie, 2011), an *in vivo* study of extensive CYP2C19 metabolizers showed less reduction of the active metabolite of clopidogrel by lansoprazole/dexlansoprazole compared to esomeprazole/omeprazole (Frelinger, 2012). The manufacturer of lansoprazole states that no dosage adjustment is necessary for clopidogrel when used concurrently. In contrast to these warnings, others have recommended the continued use of PPIs, regardless of the degree of inhibition, in patients with a history of GI bleeding or multiple risk factors for GI bleeding who are also receiving clopidogrel since no evidence has established clinically meaningful differences in outcome; however, a clinically-significant interaction cannot be excluded in those who are poor metabolizers of clopidogrel (Abraham, 2010; Levine, 2011). Additionally, concomitant use of lansoprazole with some drugs may require cautious use, may not be recommended, or may require dosage adjustments.

Increased incidence of osteoporosis-related bone fractures of the hip, spine, or wrist may occur with PPI therapy. Patients on high-dose or long-term therapy should be monitored. Use the lowest effective dose for the shortest duration of time, use vitamin D and calcium supplementation, and follow appropriate guidelines to reduce risk of fractures in patients at risk. Lansoprazole has been shown to be ineffective for the treatment of symptomatic GERD in children 1 month to <1 year.

Hypomagnesemia, reported rarely, usually with prolonged PPI use of >3 months (most cases >1 year of therapy); may be symptomatic or asymptomatic; severe cases may cause tetany, seizures, and cardiac arrhythmias. Consider obtaining serum magnesium concentrations prior to beginning long-term therapy, especially if taking concomitant digoxin, diuretics, or other drugs known to cause hypomagnesemia; and periodically thereafter. Hypomagnesemia may be corrected by magnesium supplementation, although discontinuation of lansoprazole may be necessary; magnesium levels typically return to normal within 1 week of stopping.

When used for self-medication, patients should be instructed not to use if they have difficulty swallowing, are vomiting blood, or have bloody or black stools. Prior to use, patients should contact healthcare provider if they have liver disease, heartburn for >3 months, heartburn with dizziness, lightheadedness, or sweating, MI symptoms, frequent chest pain, frequent wheezing (especially with heartburn), unexplained weight loss, nausea/vomiting, stomach pain, or are taking antifungals, atazanavir, digoxin, tacrolimus, theophylline, or warfarin. Patients should stop use and consult a healthcare provider if heartburn continues or worsens, or if they need to take for >14 days or more often than every 4 months. Patients should be informed that it may take 1-4 days for full effect to be seen; should not be used for immediate relief.

Drug Interactions

Avoid Concomitant Use

Avoid concomitant use of Lansoprazole with any of the following: Dasatinib; Delavirdine; Erlotinib; Nelfinavir; Pimozide; PONATinib; Rilpivirine; Risedronate

Decreased Effect

Lansoprazole may decrease the levels/effects of: Atazanavir; Bisphosphonate Derivatives; Bosutinib; Cefditoren; Clopidogrel; Dabigatran Etexilate; Dabrafenib; Dasatinib; Delavirdine; Erlotinib; Gefitinib; Indinavir; Iron Salts; Itraconazole; Ketoconazole (Systemic); Mesalamine; Multivitamins/Minerals (with ADEK, Folate, Iron); Mycophenolate; Nelfinavir; Nilotinib; PONATinib; Posaconazole; Rilpivirine; Riociguat; Risedronate; Vismodegib

The levels/effects of Lansoprazole may be decreased by: Bosentan; CYP2C19 Inducers (Strong); CYP3A4 Inducers (Strong); Dabrafenib; Deferasirox; Herbs (CYP3A4 Inducers); Mitotane; Tipranavir; Tocilizumab

Increased Effect/Toxicity

Lansoprazole may increase the levels/effects of: Amphetamine; ARIPiprazole; Dexmethylphenidate; Dextroamphetamine; Dofetilide; Imatinib; Lomitapide; Methotrexate; Methylphenidate; Pimozide; Raltegravir; Risedronate; Saquinavir; Tacrolimus (Systemic); Vitamin K Antagonists; Voriconazole

The levels/effects of Lansoprazole may be increased by: Fluconazole; Ketoconazole (Systemic); Voriconazole

Nutritional/Ethanol Interactions

Ethanol: Avoid ethanol (may cause gastric mucosal irritation).

Food: Lansoprazole serum concentrations may be decreased if taken with food.

Herb/Nutraceutical: Avoid St John's wort (may decrease the levels/effect of lansoprazole).

Adverse Reactions 1% to 10%:

Central nervous system: Headache (children 1-11 years 3%, 12-17 years 7%), dizziness (children 12-17 years 3%; adults <1%)

Gastrointestinal: Diarrhea (1% to 5%; 60 mg/day: 7%), abdominal pain (children 12-17 years 5%; adults 2%), constipation (children 1-11 years 5%; adults 1%), nausea (children 12-17 years 3%; adults 1%)

Pharmacodynamics/Kinetics

Onset of Action Gastric acid suppression: Oral: 1-3 hours

Duration of Action Gastric acid suppression: Oral: >1 day

Available Dosage Forms

Capsule Delayed Release, Oral:
Heartburn Relief 24 Hour [OTC]: 15 mg
Prevacid: 15 mg, 30 mg
Prevacid 24 HR [OTC]: 15 mg
Generic: 15 mg, 30 mg

Suspension, Oral:
First-Lansoprazole: 3 mg/mL (90 mL, 150 mL, 300 mL)

Tablet Dispersible, Oral:
Prevacid SoluTab: 15 mg, 30 mg

General Dosage Range Oral:

Children 1-11 years and ≤30 kg: 15 mg once daily (maximum: 30 mg twice daily)

Children 1-11 years and >30 kg: 30 mg once daily (maximum: 30 mg twice daily)

Children 12-17 years: 15-30 mg once daily

Adults: 15-180 mg/day in 1-2 divided doses

Administration

Oral

Administer before food; best if taken before breakfast. The intact granules should not be chewed or crushed; however, several options are available for those patients unable to swallow capsules:

Capsules may be opened and the intact granules sprinkled on 1 tablespoon of applesauce, Ensure® pudding, cottage cheese, yogurt, or strained pears. The granules should then be swallowed immediately.

Capsules may be opened and emptied into ~60 mL orange juice, apple juice, or tomato juice; mix and swallow immediately. Rinse the glass with additional juice and swallow to assure complete delivery of the dose.

Orally-disintegrating tablets: Should not be swallowed whole, broken, cut, or chewed. Place tablet on tongue; allow to dissolve (with or without water) until particles can be swallowed. Orally-disintegrating tablets may also be administered via an oral syringe: Place the 15 mg tablet in an oral syringe and draw up ~4 mL water, or place the 30 mg tablet in an oral syringe and draw up ~10 mL water. After tablet has dispersed, administer within 15 minutes. Refill the syringe with water (2 mL for the 15 mg tablet; 5 mL for the 30 mg tablet), shake gently, then administer any remaining contents.

Other Nasogastric tube administration:

Capsule: Capsule can be opened, the granules mixed (not crushed) with 40 mL of apple juice and then administered through the NG tube into the stomach, then flush tube with additional apple juice. Do not mix with other liquids. Thirty milligrams has also been suspended in 10 mL of 8.4% sodium bicarbonate solution (or apple juice) and administered via NG tube (Brophy, 2010).

Orally-disintegrating tablet: Nasogastric tube ≥8 French: Place a 15 mg tablet in a syringe and draw up ~4 mL water, or place the 30 mg tablet in a syringe and draw up ~10 mL water. After tablet has dispersed, administer within 15 minutes. Refill the syringe with ~5 mL water, shake gently, and then flush the nasogastric tube.

Storage/Stability Store at 25°C (77°F); excursions permitted to 15°C to 30°C (59°F to 86°F).

Nursing Actions

Physical Assessment Monitor effectiveness of ulcer symptom relief.

Patient Education

• Discuss specific use of drug and side effects with patient as it relates to treatment. (HCAHPS: During this hospital stay, were you given any medicine that you had not taken before? Before giving you any new medicine, how often did hospital staff tell you what the medicine was for? How often did hospital staff describe possible side effects in a way you could understand?)

• Patient may experience dizziness, headache, dyspepsia, constipation, or diarrhea. Have patient report immediately to prescriber syncope, tachycardia, osteodynia, myalgia, asthenia, ecchymosis, or rash (HCAHPS).

• Educate patient about signs of a significant reaction (eg, wheezing; chest tightness; fever; itching; bad cough; blue skin color; seizures; or swelling of face, lips, tongue, or throat). **Note:** This is not a comprehensive list of all side effects. Patient should consult prescriber for additional questions.

Intended Use and Disclaimer: Should not be printed and given to patients. This information is intended to serve as a concise initial reference for healthcare professionals to use when discussing medications with a patient. You must ultimately rely on your own discretion, experience and

judgment in diagnosing, treating and advising patients.

Dietary Considerations Should be taken before eating; best if taken before breakfast. Some products may contain phenylalanine.

Related Information

Oral Medications That Should Not Be Crushed or Altered *on page 1712*

Lansoprazole, Amoxicillin, and Clarithromycin

(lan SOE pra zole, a moks i SIL in, & kla RITH roe mye sin)

Brand Names: U.S. Prevpac®

Index Terms Amoxicillin, Clarithromycin, and Lansoprazole; Clarithromycin, Lansoprazole, and Amoxicillin; Lansoprazole, Amoxicillin, and Clarithromycin

Pharmacologic Category Antibiotic, Macrolide Combination; Antibiotic, Penicillin; Gastrointestinal Agent, Miscellaneous; Proton Pump Inhibitor; Substituted Benzimidazole

Medication Safety Issues

Sound-alike/look-alike issues:

Prevpac® may be confused with Prevacid®

Pregnancy Risk Factor C

Use Eradication of *H. pylori* to reduce the risk of recurrent duodenal ulcer

Available Dosage Forms

Combination package [each administration card contains]:

Prevpac®:

Capsule: Amoxicillin 500 mg (4 capsules/day)

Capsule, delayed release (Prevacid®): Lansoprazole 30 mg (2 capsules/day)

Tablet (Biaxin®): Clarithromycin 500 mg (2 tablets/day)

Generic:

Capsule: Amoxicillin 500 mg (4 capsules/day)

Capsule, delayed release: Lansoprazole 30 mg (2 capsules/day)

Tablet: Clarithromycin 500 mg (2 tablets/day)

General Dosage Range Oral: *Adults:* Lansoprazole 30 mg, amoxicillin 1 g, and clarithromycin 500 mg taken together twice daily

Nursing Actions

Physical Assessment See individual agents.

Patient Education

• Discuss specific use of drug and side effects with patient as it relates to treatment. (HCAHPS: During this hospital stay, were you given any medicine that you had not taken before? Before giving you any new medicine, how often did hospital staff tell you what the medicine was for? How often did hospital staff describe possible side effects in a way you could understand?)

• Patient may experience dyspepsia, abnormal taste, nausea, diarrhea, or vaginal yeast infection. Have patient report immediately to prescriber severe osteodynia (HCAHPS).

• Educate patient about signs of a significant reaction (eg, wheezing; chest tightness; fever; itching; bad cough; blue skin color; seizures; or swelling of face, lips, tongue, or throat). **Note:** This is not a comprehensive list of all side effects. Patient should consult prescriber for additional questions.

Intended Use and Disclaimer: Should not be printed and given to patients. This information is intended to serve as a concise initial reference for healthcare professionals to use when discussing medications with a patient. You must ultimately rely on your own discretion, experience and judgment in diagnosing, treating and advising patients.

Related Information

Amoxicillin *on page 92*

Clarithromycin *on page 335*

Lansoprazole *on page 905*

Lapatinib (la PA ti nib)

Brand Names: U.S. Tykerb

Index Terms GW572016; Lapatinib Ditosylate

Pharmacologic Category Antineoplastic Agent, Anti-HER2; Antineoplastic Agent, Epidermal Growth Factor Receptor (EGFR) Inhibitor; Antineoplastic Agent, Tyrosine Kinase Inhibitor

Medication Safety Issues

Sound-alike/look-alike issues:

Lapatinib may be confused with dasatinib, erlotinib, imatinib, regorafenib, SUNItinib, vandetanib

High alert medication:

This medication is in a class the Institute for Safe Medication Practices (ISMP) includes among its list of drug classes which have a heightened risk of causing significant patient harm when used in error.

Pregnancy Risk Factor D

Lactation Excretion in breast milk unknown/not recommended

Use

Breast cancer: Treatment of human epidermal growth receptor type 2 (HER2) overexpressing advanced or metastatic breast cancer (in combination with capecitabine) in patients who have received prior therapy (with an anthracycline, a taxane, and trastuzumab); HER2 overexpressing hormone receptor–positive metastatic breast cancer in postmenopausal women where hormone therapy is indicated (in combination with letrozole) Limitations of use: Patients should have disease progression on trastuzumab prior to initiation of treatment with lapatinib in combination with capecitabine.

Unlabeled Use Treatment (in combination with trastuzumab) of HER2 overexpressing metastatic breast cancer which had progressed on prior trastuzumab containing therapy; treatment of HER2

overexpressing metastatic breast cancer with brain metastases

Available Dosage Forms

Tablet, Oral:

Tykerb: 250 mg

General Dosage Range Dosage adjustment recommended in patients with hepatic impairment, on concomitant therapy, or who develop toxicities

Oral: *Adults:* 1250-1500 mg once daily

Administration

Oral Administer once daily, on an empty stomach, 1 hour before or 1 hour after a meal. Take full dose at the same time each day; dividing doses throughout the day is not recommended.

Hazardous agent; use appropriate precautions for handling and disposal (meets NIOSH, 2012 criteria).

Nursing Actions

Physical Assessment Check results of CBC, LFTs, electrolytes, and left ventricular ejection fraction at baseline and on a regular basis. Monitor and quantitate diarrhea, new pulmonary or cardiac symptoms regularly.

Patient Education

- Discuss specific use of drug and side effects with patient as it relates to treatment. (HCAHPS: During this hospital stay, were you given any medicine that you had not taken before? Before giving you any new medicine, how often did hospital staff tell you what the medicine was for? How often did hospital staff describe possible side effects in a way you could understand?)
- Patient may experience xeroderma, headache, alopecia, back pain, epistaxis, nail discoloration, stomatitis, lack of appetite, or insomnia. Have patient report immediately to prescriber signs of infection, dyspnea, signs of pulmonary disorder, excessive weight gain, edema of extremities, arrhythmia, angina, tachycardia, severe dizziness, syncope, considerable dyspepsia, significant nausea, diarrhea, dehydration, intolerable asthenia, ecchymosis, hemorrhaging, or eczema of hands or feet (HCAHPS).
- Educate patient about signs of a significant reaction (eg, wheezing; chest tightness; fever; itching; bad cough; blue skin color; seizures; or swelling of face, lips, tongue, or throat). **Note:** This is not a comprehensive list of all side effects. Patient should consult prescriber for additional questions.

Intended Use and Disclaimer: Should not be printed and given to patients. This information is intended to serve as a concise initial reference for healthcare professionals to use when discussing medications with a patient. You must ultimately rely on your own discretion, experience and judgment in diagnosing, treating and advising patients.

Latanoprost (la TA noe prost)

Brand Names: U.S. Xalatan

Pharmacologic Category Ophthalmic Agent, Antiglaucoma; Prostaglandin, Ophthalmic

Medication Safety Issues

Sound-alike/look-alike issues:

Latanoprost may be confused with Lantus®

Xalatan® may be confused with Lantus®, Travatan®, Xalacom™, Zarontin®

Pregnancy Risk Factor C

Lactation Excretion in breast milk unknown/use caution

Use Reduction of elevated intraocular pressure in patients with open-angle glaucoma or ocular hypertension

Available Dosage Forms

Solution, Ophthalmic:

Xalatan: 0.005% (2.5 mL)

Generic: 0.005% (2.5 mL)

General Dosage Range Ophthalmic: *Adults:* 1 drop (1.5 mcg) in the affected eye(s) once daily

Administration

Other If more than one topical ophthalmic drug is being used, administer the drugs at least 5 minutes apart. A delivery aid, Xal-Ease™, is available for administering Xalatan®.

Nursing Actions

Physical Assessment Monitor for blurred vision, burning and stinging, conjunctival hyperemia, foreign body sensation, itching, increased pigmentation of the iris, and punctate epithelial keratopathy.

Patient Education

- Discuss specific use of drug and side effects with patient as it relates to treatment. (HCAHPS: During this hospital stay, were you given any medicine that you had not taken before? Before giving you any new medicine, how often did hospital staff tell you what the medicine was for? How often did hospital staff describe possible side effects in a way you could understand?)
- Patient may experience light sensitivity, eye irritation, blurred vision, or change in eye color. Have patient report immediately to prescriber sudden vision changes, eye pain, or rash (HCAHPS).
- Educate patient about signs of a significant reaction (eg, wheezing; chest tightness; fever; itching; bad cough; blue skin color; seizures; or swelling of face, lips, tongue, or throat). **Note:** This is not a comprehensive list of all side effects. Patient should consult prescriber for additional questions.

Intended Use and Disclaimer: Should not be printed and given to patients. This information is intended to serve as a concise initial reference for healthcare professionals to use when discussing medications with a patient. You must ultimately

rely on your own discretion, experience and judgment in diagnosing, treating and advising patients.

Leflunomide (le FLOO noh mide)

Brand Names: U.S. Arava

Pharmacologic Category Antirheumatic, Disease Modifying

Medication Safety Issues

Sound-alike/look-alike issues:

Leflunomide may be confused with lenalidomide

Pregnancy Risk Factor X

Lactation Excretion in breast milk unknown/not recommended

Breast-Feeding Considerations It is not known whether leflunomide is secreted in human milk. Because the potential for serious adverse reactions exists in the nursing infant, a decision should be made whether to discontinue nursing or discontinue the drug, taking into account the importance of the drug to the mother.

Use Treatment of active rheumatoid arthritis; indicated to reduce signs and symptoms, and to inhibit structural damage and improve physical function

Unlabeled Use Treatment of cytomegalovirus (CMV) disease in transplant recipients resistant to standard antivirals; prevention of acute and chronic rejection in recipients of solid organ transplants

Mechanism of Action/Effect Leflunomide is an immunodulatory agent that inhibits pyrimidine synthesis, resulting in antiproliferative and anti-inflammatory effects. Leflunomide is a prodrug; the active metabolite is responsible for activity. For CMV, may interfere with virion assembly.

Contraindications Hypersensitivity to leflunomide or any component of the formulation; pregnancy

Warnings/Precautions Hazardous agent - use appropriate precautions for handling and disposal (NIOSH, 2012). **[U.S. Boxed Warning]: Use has been associated with rare reports of hepatotoxicity, hepatic failure, and death. Treatment should not be initiated in patients with preexisting acute or chronic liver disease or ALT >2 x ULN. Use caution in patients with concurrent exposure to potentially hepatotoxic drugs. Monitor ALT levels during therapy; discontinue if ALT >3 x ULN occurs and, if hepatotoxicity is likely leflunomide-induced, start drug elimination procedures** (eg, cholestyramine, activated charcoal).

Use has been associated (rarely) with interstitial lung disease; discontinue in patients who develop new onset or worsening of pulmonary symptoms. Drug elimination procedures should be considered (eg, cholestyramine, activated charcoal) if interstitial lung disease occurs; fatal outcomes have been reported. May increase susceptibility to infection, including opportunistic pathogens. Severe infections, sepsis, and fatalities have been reported.

Not recommended in patients with severe immunodeficiency, bone marrow dysplasia, or severe, uncontrolled infections. Caution should be exercised when considering the use in patients with a history of new/recurrent infections, with conditions that predispose them to infections, or with chronic, latent, or localized infections. Patients who develop a new infection while undergoing treatment should be monitored closely; consider discontinuation of therapy and drug elimination procedures if infection is serious.

Use may affect defenses against malignancies; impact on the development and course of malignancies is not fully defined. As compared to the general population, an increased risk of lymphoma has been noted in clinical trials; however, rheumatoid arthritis has been previously associated with an increased rate of lymphoma. Use with caution in patients with a prior history of significant hematologic abnormalities; avoid use with bone marrow dysplasia. Use has been associated with rare pancytopenia, agranulocytosis, and thrombocytopenia, generally when given concurrently or recently with methotrexate or other immunosuppressive agents. Monitoring of hematologic function is required; discontinue if evidence of bone marrow suppression and begin drug elimination procedures (eg, cholestyramine or activated charcoal). Rare cases of dermatologic reactions (including Stevens-Johnson syndrome and toxic epidermal necrolysis) have been reported; discontinue if evidence of severe dermatologic reaction occurs, and begin drug elimination procedures (eg, cholestyramine or activated charcoal). Cases of peripheral neuropathy have been reported; use with caution in patients >60 years of age, receiving concomitant neurotoxic medications, or patients with diabetes; discontinue if evidence of peripheral neuropathy occurs and begin drug elimination procedures (eg, cholestyramine, activated charcoal).

Safety has not been established in patients with latent tuberculosis infection. Patients should be screened for tuberculosis and if necessary, treated prior to initiating therapy. Use with caution in patients with renal impairment. **[U.S. Boxed Warning]: Women of childbearing potential should not receive therapy until pregnancy has been excluded,** they have been counseled concerning fetal risk and reliable contraceptive measures have been confirmed. Women of childbearing potential should also undergo drug elimination procedures (eg, cholestyramine, activated charcoal) following discontinuation of therapy. Patients should be brought up to date with all immunizations before initiating therapy. Live vaccines should not be given concurrently; there is no data available concerning secondary transmission of live vaccines in patients receiving therapy. Due to variations in clearance, it may take up to 2 years to reach low levels of leflunomide metabolite serum concentrations. A drug elimination procedure using cholestyramine or activated charcoal is recommended when a more rapid elimination is needed.

Drug Interactions

Avoid Concomitant Use

Avoid concomitant use of Leflunomide with any of the following: BCG; Natalizumab; Pimecrolimus; Tacrolimus (Topical); Teriflunomide; Tofacitinib

Decreased Effect

Leflunomide may decrease the levels/effects of: BCG; Coccidioidin Skin Test; Sipuleucel-T; Vaccines (Inactivated)

The levels/effects of Leflunomide may be decreased by: Bile Acid Sequestrants; Charcoal, Activated; Echinacea

Increased Effect/Toxicity

Leflunomide may increase the levels/effects of: Bosentan; Carvedilol; CYP2C9 Substrates; Natalizumab; Teriflunomide; Tofacitinib; TOLBUTamide; Vaccines (Live); Vitamin K Antagonists

The levels/effects of Leflunomide may be increased by: Denosumab; Immunosuppressants; Methotrexate; Pimecrolimus; Rifampin; Roflumilast; Tacrolimus (Topical); TOLBUTamide; Trastuzumab

Nutritional/Ethanol Interactions

Food: No interactions with food have been noted. Management: Maintain adequate hydration, unless instructed to restrict fluid intake.

Herb/Nutraceutical: Echinacea may diminish the therapeutic effect of leflunomide.

Adverse Reactions

>10%:

Gastrointestinal: Diarrhea (17%)

Respiratory: Respiratory tract infection (4% to 15%)

1% to 10%:

Cardiovascular: Hypertension (10%), chest pain (2%), edema (peripheral), palpitation, tachycardia, varicose vein, vasculitis, vasodilation

Central nervous system: Headache (7%), dizziness (4%), pain (2%), anxiety, depression, fever, insomnia, malaise, migraine, sleep disorder, vertigo

Dermatologic: Alopecia (10%), rash (10%), pruritus (4%), dry skin (2%), eczema (2%), acne, bruising, dermatitis, hair discoloration, hematoma, nail disorder, skin disorder/discoloration, skin ulcer, subcutaneous nodule

Endocrine & metabolic: Hypokalemia (1%), diabetes mellitus, hyperglycemia, hyperlipidemia, hyperthyroidism, menstrual disorder

Gastrointestinal: Nausea (9%), abdominal pain (5% to 6%), dyspepsia (5%), weight loss (4%), anorexia (3%), gastroenteritis (3%), mouth ulceration (3%), vomiting (3%), candidiasis (oral), colitis, constipation, esophagitis, flatulence, gastritis, gingivitis, melena, salivary gland enlarged, stomatitis, taste disturbance, xerostomia

Genitourinary: Urinary tract infection (5%), albuminuria, cystitis, dysuria, prostate disorder, urinary frequency, vaginal candidiasis

Hematologic: Anemia

Hepatic: Abnormal LFTs (5%), cholelithiasis

Local: Abscess

Neuromuscular & skeletal: Back pain (5%), joint disorder (4%), tenosynovitis (3%), weakness (3%), paresthesia (2%), synovitis (2%), arthralgia (1%), leg cramps (1%), arthrosis, bone necrosis, bone pain, bursitis, CPK increased, myalgia, neck pain, neuralgia, neuritis, pelvic pain, tendon rupture

Ocular: Blurred vision, cataract, conjunctivitis, eye disorder

Renal: Hematuria

Respiratory: Bronchitis (7%), cough (3%), pharyngitis (3%), pneumonia (2%), rhinitis (2%), sinusitis (2%), asthma, dyspnea, epistaxis

Miscellaneous: Accidental injury (5%), allergic reactions (2%), flu-like syndrome (2%), cyst, diaphoresis, hernia, herpes infection

Available Dosage Forms

Tablet, Oral:

Arava: 10 mg, 20 mg

Generic: 10 mg, 20 mg

General Dosage Range

Dosage adjustment recommended in patients who develop toxicities

Oral: *Adults:* Initial: 100 mg/day for 3 days; Maintenance range: 10-20 mg/day

Administration

Oral Administer without regard to meals.

Hazardous agent; use appropriate precautions for handling and disposal (NIOSH, 2012).

Storage/Stability Store at 25°C (77°F); excursions permitted to 15°C to 30°C (59°F to 86°F). Protect from light.

Nursing Actions

Physical Assessment Monitor for reduction of rheumatoid arthritis signs and symptoms and structural damage. Place and read PPD prior to initiating. Monitor for signs and symptoms of severe infection, hypertension, or hepatic dysfunction. Monitor for new onset or worsening of pulmonary symptoms.

Patient Education

• Discuss specific use of drug and side effects with patient as it relates to treatment. (HCAHPS: During this hospital stay, were you given any medicine that you had not taken before? Before giving you any new medicine, how often did hospital staff tell you what the medicine was for? How often did hospital staff describe possible side effects in a way you could understand?)

• Patient may experience lung infection, nausea, diarrhea, alopecia, or hepatic impairment. Have patient report immediately to prescriber signs of infection, dyspnea, severe dyspepsia, paresthesia, inability to eat, discolored urine, jaundice, considerable asthenia, rash, or pregnancy (HCAHPS).

• Educate patient about signs of a significant reaction (eg, wheezing; chest tightness; fever; itching; bad cough; blue skin color; seizures; or swelling of face, lips, tongue, or throat). **Note:** This is not a comprehensive list of all side effects. Patient should consult prescriber for additional questions.

Intended Use and Disclaimer: Should not be printed and given to patients. This information is intended to serve as a concise initial reference for healthcare professionals to use when discussing medications with a patient. You must ultimately rely on your own discretion, experience and judgment in diagnosing, treating and advising patients.

Dietary Considerations May be taken without regard to meals.

Related Information

Oral Medications That Should Not Be Crushed or Altered *on page 1712*

Lenalidomide (le na LID oh mide)

Brand Names: U.S. Revlimid

Index Terms CC-5013; IMid-1

Pharmacologic Category Angiogenesis Inhibitor; Antineoplastic Agent; Immunomodulator, Systemic

Medication Safety Issues

Sound-alike/look-alike issues:

Lenalidomide may be confused with leflunomide, pomalidomide, thalidomide

Revlimid may be confused with Thalomid

High alert medication:

This medication is in a class the Institute for Safe Medication Practices (ISMP) includes among its list of drug classes which have a heightened risk of causing significant patient harm when used in error.

International issues:

Revlimid may be confused with Revolade, a brand name for eltrombopag [Canada].

Medication Guide Available Yes

Pregnancy Risk Factor X

Lactation Excretion in breast milk unknown/not recommended

Use

Mantle cell lymphoma: Treatment of patients with mantle cell lymphoma that has relapsed or progressed after 2 prior therapies (one of which included bortezomib).

Multiple myeloma: Treatment of multiple myeloma (in combination with dexamethasone) in patients who have received at least one prior therapy

Myelodysplastic syndromes: Treatment of patients with transfusion-dependent anemia due to low- or intermediate-1-risk myelodysplastic syndromes (MDS) associated with a deletion 5q

(del 5q) cytogenetic abnormality with or without additional cytogenetic abnormalities

Unlabeled Use Treatment of non-Hodgkin lymphoma (diffuse large B-cell lymphoma); relapsed or refractory chronic lymphocytic leukemia (CLL); systemic light chain amyloidosis; lower-risk myelodysplastic syndrome (MDS) in transfusion-dependent patients without deletion 5q (del 5q); maintenance treatment for multiple myeloma (after response to primary treatment or following autologous stem cell transplant)

Available Dosage Forms

Capsule, Oral:

Revlimid: 2.5 mg, 5 mg, 10 mg, 15 mg, 20 mg, 25 mg

General Dosage Range Dosage adjustment recommended in patients with renal impairment or who develop toxicities

Oral: *Adults:* 10 once daily **or** 25 mg once daily for 21 of 28 days

Administration

Oral Administer at about the same time each day with water; administer with or without food. Swallow capsule whole; do not break, open, or chew.

Missed doses: May administer a missed dose if within 12 hours of usual dosing time. If greater than 12 hours, patient should skip dose for that day and resume usual dosing the following day. Patient should **not** take 2 doses to make up for a missed dose.

Hazardous agent; use appropriate precautions for handling and disposal (NIOSH, 2012).

Nursing Actions

Physical Assessment Verify that patient is not pregnant prior to initiating therapy. Instruct patient to use two reliable forms of contraception beginning 4 weeks prior to, during, and for 4 weeks after therapy and during therapy interruptions.

Monitor for signs of thromboembolism (shortness of breath, chest pain, or arm or leg swelling), deep vein thrombosis (swelling and tenderness of extremities), rash, angioedema, infection, or bleeding. Monitor for neutropenia and thrombocytopenia. Serious side effects also include fever, chills, unusual or abnormal bleeding.

Inform patient they will need to fill out forms and sign when picking up drug.

Patient Education

• Discuss specific use of drug and side effects with patient as it relates to treatment. (HCAHPS: During this hospital stay, were you given any medicine that you had not taken before? Before giving you any new medicine, how often did hospital staff tell you what the medicine was for? How often did hospital staff describe possible side effects in a way you could understand?)

• Patient may experience anemia, back pain, dyspepsia, blurred vision, diarrhea, headache, arthralgia, asthenia, rash, fatigue, dizziness, constipation, nausea, or edema. Have patient report immediately to prescriber signs of infection, angina, dyspnea, ecchymosis, bleeding, pregnancy, or severe skin irritation (HCAHPS).

• Educate patient about signs of a significant reaction (eg, wheezing; chest tightness; fever; itching; bad cough; blue skin color; seizures; or swelling of face, lips, tongue, or throat). **Note:** This is not a comprehensive list of all side effects. Patient should consult prescriber for additional questions.

Intended Use and Disclaimer: Should not be printed and given to patients. This information is intended to serve as a concise initial reference for healthcare professionals to use when discussing medications with a patient. You must ultimately rely on your own discretion, experience and judgment in diagnosing, treating and advising patients.

Related Information
Oral Medications That Should Not Be Crushed or Altered on page 1712

Lepirudin (leh puh ROO din)

Index Terms Lepirudin (rDNA); Recombinant Hirudin

Pharmacologic Category Anticoagulant; Anticoagulant, Direct Thrombin Inhibitor

Medication Safety Issues
High alert medication:
The Institute for Safe Medication Practices (ISMP) includes this medication among its list of drugs which have a heightened risk of causing significant patient harm when used in error.

Pregnancy Risk Factor B

Lactation Excretion unknown/not recommended

Breast-Feeding Considerations A case report describes lepirudin use in a breast-feeding woman, 7 weeks postpartum. The mother was using lepirudin 50 mg twice daily. Maternal serum concentrations were 0.73 mg/L and milk concentrations were below the limit of detection (0.1 mg/L) when measured 3 hours after administration (Lindhoff-Last, 2000).

Use Indicated for anticoagulation in patients with heparin-induced thrombocytopenia (HIT) and associated thromboembolic disease in order to prevent further thromboembolic complications

Mechanism of Action/Effect Lepirudin is a highly specific direct thrombin inhibitor. Each molecule is capable of binding one molecule of thrombin and inhibiting its thrombogenic activity.

Contraindications Hypersensitivity to hirudins or any component of the formulation

Warnings/Precautions Hemorrhagic events: Intracranial bleeding following concomitant thrombolytic therapy with rt-PA or streptokinase may be life threatening. For patients with an increased risk of bleeding, a careful assessment weighing the risk

of lepirudin administration versus its anticipated benefit has to be made by the treating physician. In particular, this includes the following conditions: Recent puncture of large vessels or organ biopsy; anomaly of vessels or organs; recent cerebrovascular accident, stroke, intracerebral surgery, or other neuroaxial procedures; severe uncontrolled hypertension; bacterial endocarditis; advanced renal impairment; hemorrhagic diathesis; recent major surgery; and recent major bleeding (eg, intracranial, gastrointestinal, intraocular, or pulmonary bleeding). With renal impairment, relative overdose might occur even with standard dosage regimen. The bolus dose and rate of infusion must be reduced in patients with known or suspected renal insufficiency.

Formation of antihirudin antibodies may increase the anticoagulant effect of lepirudin possibly due to delayed renal elimination of active lepirudin-antihirudin complexes. Therefore, strict monitoring of aPTT is necessary also during prolonged therapy. No evidence of neutralization of lepirudin or of allergic reactions associated with positive antibody test results was found. Allergic and hypersensitivity reactions, including anaphylaxis have been reported and may occur frequently in patients treated concomitantly with streptokinase; caution is warranted during re-exposure (anaphylaxis has been reported).

Serious liver injury (eg, liver cirrhosis) may enhance the anticoagulant effect of lepirudin due to coagulation defects secondary to reduced generation of vitamin K-dependent clotting factors.

Clinical trials have provided limited information to support any recommendations for re-exposure to lepirudin (anaphylaxis has been reported). Safety and efficacy have not been established in children.

Drug Interactions
Avoid Concomitant Use
Avoid concomitant use of Lepirudin with any of the following: Apixaban; Dabigatran Etexilate; Omacetaxine; Rivaroxaban; Urokinase

Decreased Effect
The levels/effects of Lepirudin may be decreased by: Estrogen Derivatives; Progestins

Increased Effect/Toxicity
Lepirudin may increase the levels/effects of: Anticoagulants; Collagenase (Systemic); Deferasirox; Ibritumomab; Omacetaxine; Rivaroxaban; Tositumomab and Iodine I 131 Tositumomab

The levels/effects of Lepirudin may be increased by: Agents with Antiplatelet Properties; Apixaban; Dabigatran Etexilate; Dasatinib; Herbs (Anticoagulant/Antiplatelet Properties); Ibrutinib; Nonsteroidal Anti-Inflammatory Agents; Omega-3 Fatty Acids; Pentosan Polysulfate Sodium; Prostacyclin Analogues; Salicylates; Sugammadex; Thrombolytic Agents; Tibolone; Tipranavir; Urokinase; Vitamin E

◄ **Nutritional/Ethanol Interactions** Herb/Nutraceutical: Avoid cat's claw, dong quai, evening primrose, feverfew, garlic, ginger, ginkgo, red clover, horse chestnut, green tea, ginseng (all have additional antiplatelet activity)

Adverse Reactions As with all anticoagulants, bleeding is the most common adverse event associated with lepirudin. Hemorrhage may occur at virtually any site. Risk is dependent on multiple variables.

HIT patients:
>10%: Hematologic: Anemia (12%), bleeding from puncture sites (11%), hematoma (11%)
1% to 10%:
Cardiovascular: Heart failure (3%), pericardial effusion (1%), ventricular fibrillation (1%)
Central nervous system: Fever (7%)
Dermatologic: Maculopapular rash (4%), eczema (3%)
Gastrointestinal: GI bleeding/rectal bleeding (5%)
Genitourinary: Vaginal bleeding (2%)
Hepatic: Transaminases increased (6%)
Renal: Hematuria (4%)
Respiratory: Epistaxis (4%)

Non-HIT populations (including those receiving thrombolytics and/or contrast media):
1% to 10%: Respiratory: Bronchospasm/stridor/dyspnea/cough

Product Availability Not available in the U.S.

General Dosage Range Dosage adjustment recommended in patients with renal impairment
I.V.: *Adults:* Bolus: 0.2-0.4 mg/kg; Infusion: 0.1-0.15 mg/kg/hour (maximum: 0.21 mg/kg/hour)

Administration
I.V. I.V. bolus: Inject slowly for continuous infusion; solutions with 0.2 or 0.4 mg/mL may be used.
Oral Administer **only** intravenously

Preparation for Administration
Intravenous bolus: Use a solution with a concentration of 5 mg/mL: Reconstitute one vial (50 mg) of lepirudin with 1 mL of sterile water for injection or 0.9% sodium chloride injection. The final concentration of 5 mg/mL is obtained by transferring the contents of the vial into a sterile, single-use syringe (of at least 10 mL capacity) and diluting the solution to a total volume of 10 mL using sterile water for injection, 0.9% sodium chloride, or 5% dextrose in water.

Intravenous infusion: For continuous intravenous infusion, solutions with concentrations of 0.2 or 0.4 mg/mL may be used. Reconstitute 2 vials (50 mg each) of lepirudin with 1 mL each using either sterile water for injection or 0.9% sodium chloride injection. The final concentration of 0.2 mg/mL or 0.4 mg/mL is obtained by transferring the contents of both vials into an infusion bag containing 500 mL or 250 mL of 0.9% sodium chloride injection or 5% dextrose injection.

Storage/Stability
Intact vials should be stored at 2°C to 25°C (36°F to 77°F). Manufacturer recommends using reconstituted solution immediately after preparation. Reconstituted solutions of lepirudin are stable for 24 hours at room temperature.

Nursing Actions
Physical Assessment Note Administration for infusion specifics. Bleeding precautions should be observed. Monitor for hypersensitivity reaction, bleeding, chest pain, and rash. Teach patient bleeding precautions.

Patient Education
• Discuss specific use of drug and side effects with patient as it relates to treatment. (HCAHPS: During this hospital stay, were you given any medicine that you had not taken before? Before giving you any new medicine, how often did hospital staff tell you what the medicine was for? How often did hospital staff describe possible side effects in a way you could understand?)
• Patient may experience bleeding problems. Have patient report immediately to prescriber severe dizziness, imbalance, illogical thinking, significant headache, ecchymosis, or rash (HCAHPS).
• Educate patient about signs of a significant reaction (eg, wheezing; chest tightness; fever; itching; bad cough; blue skin color; seizures; or swelling of face, lips, tongue, or throat). **Note:** This is not a comprehensive list of all side effects. Patient should consult prescriber for additional questions.

Intended Use and Disclaimer: Should not be printed and given to patients. This information is intended to serve as a concise initial reference for healthcare professionals to use when discussing medications with a patient. You must ultimately rely on your own discretion, experience and judgment in diagnosing, treating and advising patients.

Letrozole (LET roe zole)

Brand Names: U.S. Femara
Index Terms CGS-20267
Pharmacologic Category Antineoplastic Agent, Aromatase Inhibitor
Medication Safety Issues
Sound-alike/look-alike issues:
Femara may be confused with Famvir, femhrt, Provera
Letrozole may be confused with anastrozole
International issues:
Letaris, a formerly marketed Dutch brand name product for letrozole, may be confused with Letairis, a U.S. brand name for ambrisentan.
Pregnancy Risk Factor X
Lactation Excretion in breast milk unknown/not recommended

Breast-Feeding Considerations It is not known if letrozole is excreted in breast milk. Due to the potential for serious adverse reactions in the nursing infant, a decision should be made whether to discontinue nursing or to discontinue the drug, taking into account the importance of treatment to the mother.

Use For use in postmenopausal women in the adjuvant treatment of hormone receptor positive early breast cancer, extended adjuvant treatment of early breast cancer after 5 years of tamoxifen, advanced breast cancer with disease progression following antiestrogen therapy, hormone receptor positive or hormone receptor unknown, locally-advanced, or first-line (or second-line) treatment of advanced or metastatic breast cancer

Unlabeled Use Treatment of ovarian (epithelial) cancer, endometrial cancer

Mechanism of Action/Effect Nonsteroidal competitive inhibitor of the aromatase enzyme system, which catalyzes conversion of androgens to estrogens. Inhibition leads to a significant reduction in plasma estrogen levels. Does not affect synthesis of adrenal or thyroid hormones, aldosterone, or androgens.

Contraindications Use in women who are or may become pregnant

Canadian labeling: Additional contraindications (not in U.S. labeling): Hypersensitivity to letrozole, other aromatase inhibitors, or any component of the formulation; use in patients <18 years of age; breast-feeding

Warnings/Precautions Hazardous agent - use appropriate precautions for handling and disposal (NIOSH, 2012). Use caution with hepatic impairment; dose adjustment recommended in patients with cirrhosis or severe hepatic dysfunction. May cause dizziness, fatigue, and somnolence; patients should be cautioned before performing tasks which require mental alertness (eg, operating machinery or driving). May increase total serum cholesterol; in patients treated with adjuvant therapy and cholesterol levels within normal limits, an increase of >1.5 x ULN in total cholesterol has been demonstrated in 8.2% of letrozole-treated patients (25% requiring lipid-lowering medications) vs 3.2% of tamoxifen-treated patients (16% requiring medications); monitor cholesterol panel; may require antihyperlipidemics. May cause decreases in bone mineral density (BMD); a decrease in hip BMD by 3.8% from baseline in letrozole-treated patients vs 2% in placebo at 2 years has been demonstrated; however, there was no statistical difference in changes to the lumbar spine BMD scores; monitor BMD.

Drug Interactions

Avoid Concomitant Use

Avoid concomitant use of Letrozole with any of the following: Tegafur

Decreased Effect

Letrozole may decrease the levels/effects of: Cardiac Glycosides; Tegafur; Vitamin K Antagonists

The levels/effects of Letrozole may be decreased by: Tamoxifen

Increased Effect/Toxicity

Letrozole may increase the levels/effects of: CYP2A6 Substrates; Methadone; Vitamin K Antagonists

Adverse Reactions

>10%:
Cardiovascular: Edema (7% to 18%)
Central nervous system: Headache (4% to 20%), dizziness (3% to 14%), fatigue (8% to 13%)
Endocrine & metabolic: Hypercholesterolemia (3% to 52%), hot flashes (6% to 50%)
Gastrointestinal: Nausea (9% to 17%), weight gain (2% to 13%), constipation (2% to 11%)
Neuromuscular & skeletal: Weakness (4% to 34%), arthralgia (8% to 25%), arthritis (7% to 25%), bone pain (5% to 22%), back pain (5% to 18%), bone mineral density decreased/osteoporosis (5% to 15%), bone fracture (10% to 14%)
Respiratory: Dyspnea (6% to 18%), cough (6% to 13%)
Miscellaneous: Diaphoresis (≤24%), night sweats (15%)

1% to 10%:
Cardiovascular: Chest pain (6% to 8%), hypertension (5% to 8%), chest wall pain (6%), peripheral edema (5%); cerebrovascular accident including hemorrhagic stroke, thrombotic stroke (2% to 3%); thromboembolic event including venous thrombosis, thrombophlebitis, portal vein thrombosis, pulmonary embolism (2% to 3%); MI (1% to 2%), angina (1% to 2%), transient ischemic attack
Central nervous system: Insomnia (6% to 7%), pain (5%), anxiety (<5%), depression (<5%), vertigo (<5%), somnolence (3%)
Dermatologic: Rash (5%), alopecia (3% to 5%), pruritus (1%)
Endocrine & metabolic: Breast pain (2% to 7%), hypercalcemia (<5%)
Gastrointestinal: Diarrhea (5% to 8%), vomiting (3% to 7%), weight loss (6% to 7%), abdominal pain (6%), anorexia (1% to 5%), dyspepsia (3%)
Genitourinary: Urinary tract infection (6%), vaginal bleeding (5%), vaginal dryness (5%), vaginal hemorrhage (5%), vaginal irritation (5%)
Neuromuscular & skeletal: Limb pain (4% to 10%), myalgia (7% to 9%)
Ocular: Cataract (2%)
Renal: Renal disorder (5%)
Respiratory: Pleural effusion (<5%)
Miscellaneous: Infection (7%), influenza (6%), viral infection (6%), secondary malignancy (2% to 4%)

Available Dosage Forms
Tablet, Oral:
Femara: 2.5 mg
Generic: 2.5 mg
General Dosage Range Dosage adjustment recommended in patients with hepatic impairment
Oral: *Adults (postmenopausal females):* 2.5 mg once daily

Administration
Oral Administer with or without food.

Hazardous agent; use appropriate precautions for handling and disposal (NIOSH, 2012).
Storage/Stability Store at room temperature of 25°C (77°F); excursions permitted to 15°C to 30°C (59°F to 86°F).

Nursing Actions
Physical Assessment For use in postmenopausal women only. Monitor for hypertension, pain, gastrointestinal upset, hot flashes, and dyspnea on a regular basis.

Patient Education
• Discuss specific use of drug and side effects with patient as it relates to treatment. (HCAHPS: During this hospital stay, were you given any medicine that you had not taken before? Before giving you any new medicine, how often did hospital staff tell you what the medicine was for? How often did hospital staff describe possible side effects in a way you could understand?)
• Patient may experience dizziness, fatigue, flushing, headache, nausea, back pain, myalgia, edema, constipation, osteodynia, osteogenesis imperfecta, hyperlipidemia, or weight gain. Have patient report immediately to prescriber angina, tachycardia, syncope, dyspnea, strength differences from one side to another, significant weight loss, or rash (HCAHPS).
• Educate patient about signs of a significant reaction (eg, wheezing; chest tightness; fever; itching; bad cough; blue skin color; seizures; or swelling of face, lips, tongue, or throat). **Note:** This is not a comprehensive list of all side effects. Patient should consult prescriber for additional questions.

Intended Use and Disclaimer: Should not be printed and given to patients. This information is intended to serve as a concise initial reference for healthcare professionals to use when discussing medications with a patient. You must ultimately rely on your own discretion, experience and judgment in diagnosing, treating and advising patients.

Dietary Considerations May be taken without regard to meals. Calcium and vitamin D supplementation are recommended.

Leucovorin Calcium (loo koe VOR in KAL see um)

Index Terms 5-Formyl Tetrahydrofolate; Calcium Folinate; Calcium Leucovorin; Citrovorum Factor; Folinate Calcium; Folinic Acid (error prone synonym); Leucovorin
Pharmacologic Category Antidote; Chemotherapy Modulating Agent; Rescue Agent (Chemotherapy); Vitamin, Water Soluble
Medication Safety Issues
Sound-alike/look-alike issues:
Leucovorin may be confused with Leukeran®, Leukine®, LEVOleucovorin
Folinic acid may be confused with folic acid
Folinic acid is an error prone synonym and should not be used
Pregnancy Risk Factor C
Lactation Excretion in breast milk unknown/use caution
Breast-Feeding Considerations Leucovorin is a biologically active form of folic acid. Adequate amounts of folic acid are recommended in breast-feeding women. Refer to Folic Acid monograph.
Use Antidote for folic acid antagonists (methotrexate, trimethoprim, pyrimethamine) and rescue therapy following high-dose methotrexate; in combination with fluorouracil in the treatment of colon cancer; treatment of megaloblastic anemias when folate is deficient as in infancy, sprue, pregnancy, and nutritional deficiency when oral folate therapy is not possible
Unlabeled Use Adjunctive cofactor therapy in methanol toxicity; prevention of pyrimethamine hematologic toxicity in HIV-positive patients
Mechanism of Action/Effect A reduced form of folic acid, leucovorin supplies the necessary cofactor blocked by methotrexate. Leucovorin actively competes with methotrexate for transport sites, displaces methotrexate from intracellular binding sites, and restores active folate stores required for DNA/RNA synthesis. Stabilizes the binding of 5-dUMP and thymidylate synthetase, enhancing the activity of fluorouracil. When administered with pyrimethamine for the treatment of opportunistic infections, leucovorin reduces the risk for hematologic toxicity.

Methanol toxicity treatment: Formic acid (methanol's toxic metabolite) is normally metabolized to carbon dioxide and water by 10-formyltetrahydrofolate dehydrogenase after being bound to tetrahydrofolate. Administering a source of tetrahydrofolate may aid the body in eliminating formic acid.
Contraindications Pernicious anemia or vitamin B_{12}-deficient megaloblastic anemias
Warnings/Precautions When used for the treatment of accidental weak folic acid antagonist overdose, administer as soon as possible. When used for the treatment of a methotrexate overdose, administer as soon as possible. Do not wait for the results of a methotrexate level before initiating therapy. It is important to adjust the leucovorin dose once a methotrexate level is known. When used for methotrexate rescue therapy, methotrexate serum concentrations should be monitored to

determine dose and duration of leucovorin therapy. The dose may need to be increased or administration prolonged in situations where methotrexate excretion may be delayed (eg, ascites, pleural effusion, renal insufficiency, inadequate hydration); **never administer leucovorin intrathecally.** Combination of leucovorin and sulfamethoxazole-trimethoprim for the acute treatment of PCP in patients with HIV infection has been reported to cause increased rates of treatment failure. Leucovorin may increase the toxicity of 5-fluorouracil; dose of 5-fluorouracil may need decreased.

Powder for injection: When doses >10 mg/m² are required, reconstitute using sterile water for injection, not a solution containing benzyl alcohol.

Injection: Due to calcium content, do not administer I.V. solutions at a rate >160 mg/minute. Not intended for intrathecal use.

Drug Interactions
Avoid Concomitant Use
Avoid concomitant use of Leucovorin Calcium with any of the following: Raltitrexed; Trimethoprim
Decreased Effect
Leucovorin Calcium may decrease the levels/ effects of: Fosphenytoin; PHENobarbital; Phenytoin; Primidone; Raltitrexed; Trimethoprim

The levels/effects of Leucovorin Calcium may be decreased by: Glucarpidase
Increased Effect/Toxicity
Leucovorin Calcium may increase the levels/ effects of: Capecitabine; Fluorouracil (Systemic); Fluorouracil (Topical); Tegafur
Adverse Reactions Frequency not defined. Toxicities (especially gastrointestinal toxicity) of fluorouracil is higher when used in combination with leucovorin.
Dermatologic: Rash, pruritus, erythema, urticaria
Hematologic: Thrombocytosis
Respiratory: Wheezing
Miscellaneous: Allergic reactions, anaphylactoid reactions
Available Dosage Forms
Solution, Injection:
Generic: 300 mg/30 mL (30 mL)
Solution, Intravenous:
Generic: 10 mg/mL (50 mL)
Solution Reconstituted, Injection:
Generic: 50 mg (1 ea); 100 mg (1 ea); 200 mg (1 ea); 350 mg (1 ea); 500 mg (1 ea)
Solution Reconstituted, Injection [preservative free]:
Generic: 50 mg (1 ea); 100 mg (1 ea); 200 mg (1 ea); 350 mg (1 ea)
Tablet, Oral:
Generic: 5 mg, 10 mg, 15 mg, 25 mg
General Dosage Range
I.M.: *Children and Adults:* ≤1 mg/day [folate deficient megaloblastic anemia] **or** 15 mg (~10 mg/m²) every 6 hours for 10 doses [methotrexate rescue dose]
I.V.:
Children: 15 mg (~10 mg/m²) every 6 hours for 10 doses
Adults: Initial: 15 mg (~10 mg/m²) every 6 hours for 10 doses [methotrexate rescue dose] **or** 200 mg/m² **or** 20 mg/m² as a single dose [colorectal cancer]
Oral: *Children and Adults:* 5-15 mg/day [weak folic acid antagonist overdose] **or** 15 mg (~10 mg/m²) every 6 hours for 10 doses [methotrexate rescue dose]
Administration
I.V. Due to calcium content, do not administer I.V. solutions at a rate >160 mg/minute; not intended for intrathecal use.
Refer to individual protocols. Should be administered I.M., I.V. push, or I.V. infusion (15 minutes to 2 hours). Leucovorin should not be administered concurrently with methotrexate. It is commonly initiated 24 hours after the start of methotrexate. Toxicity to normal tissues may be irreversible if leucovorin is not initiated by ~40 hours after the start of methotrexate.
As a rescue after folate antagonists: Administer by I.V. bolus, I.M., or orally.
In combination with fluorouracil: Fluorouracil activity, the fluorouracil is usually given after, or at the midpoint, of the leucovorin infusion. Leucovorin is usually administered by I.V. bolus injection or short (10-120 minutes) I.V. infusion. Other administration schedules have been used; refer to individual protocols.
Injectable Detail pH: 8.1 (vials)
Oral Do not administer orally in the presence of nausea or vomiting. Doses >25 mg should be administered parenterally.
Preparation for Administration Powder for injection: Reconstitute with SWFI or BWFI; dilute in 100-1000 mL NS, D₅W for infusion. When doses >10 mg/m² are required, reconstitute using sterile water for injection, not a solution containing benzyl alcohol.
Storage/Stability
Powder for injection: Store at room temperature of 25°C (77°F). Protect from light. Solutions reconstituted with bacteriostatic water for injection U.S.P., must be used within 7 days. Solutions reconstituted with SWFI must be used immediately. Parenteral admixture is stable for 24 hours stored at room temperature (25°C) and for 4 days when stored under refrigeration (4°C).
Solution for injection: Prior to dilution, store vials under refrigeration at 2°C to 8°C (36°F to 46°F). Protect from light.
Tablet: Store at room temperature of 15°C to 30°C (59°F to 86°F).

Nursing Actions

Patient Education

- Discuss specific use of drug and side effects with patient as it relates to treatment. (HCAHPS: During this hospital stay, were you given any medicine that you had not taken before? Before giving you any new medicine, how often did hospital staff tell you what the medicine was for? How often did hospital staff describe possible side effects in a way you could understand?)
- Have patient report immediately to prescriber rash (HCAHPS).
- Educate patient about signs of a significant reaction (eg, wheezing; chest tightness; fever; itching; bad cough; blue skin color; seizures; or swelling of face, lips, tongue, or throat). **Note:** This is not a comprehensive list of all side effects. Patient should consult prescriber for additional questions.

Intended Use and Disclaimer: Should not be printed and given to patients. This information is intended to serve as a concise initial reference for healthcare professionals to use when discussing medications with a patient. You must ultimately rely on your own discretion, experience and judgment in diagnosing, treating and advising patients.

Dietary Considerations Solutions for injection contain calcium 0.004 mEq per leucovorin 1 mg

---

Leuprolide (loo PROE lide)

Brand Names: U.S. Eligard; Lupron Depot; Lupron Depot-Ped

Index Terms Abbott-43818; Leuprolide Acetate; Leuprorelin Acetate; TAP-144

Pharmacologic Category Antineoplastic Agent, Gonadotropin-Releasing Hormone Agonist; Gonadotropin Releasing Hormone Agonist

Medication Safety Issues

Sound-alike/look-alike issues:

Lupron Depot (1-month or 3-month formulation) may be confused with Lupron Depot-Ped (1-month or 3-month formulation)

Lupron Depot-Ped is available in two formulations, a 1-month formulation and a 3-month formulation. Both formulations offer an 11.25 mg strength which may further add confusion.

Pregnancy Risk Factor X

Lactation Excretion in breast milk unknown/contraindicated

Breast-Feeding Considerations It is not known if leuprolide is excreted into breast milk; use is contraindicated in nursing women.

Use Palliative treatment of advanced prostate cancer; management of endometriosis; treatment of anemia caused by uterine leiomyomata (fibroids); central precocious puberty

Unlabeled Use Treatment of breast cancer; infertility; treatment of paraphilia/hypersexuality

Mechanism of Action/Effect Leuprolide, is an agonist of luteinizing hormone-releasing hormone (LHRH). Acting as a potent inhibitor of gonadotropin secretion; continuous administration results in suppression of ovarian and testicular steroidogenesis due to decreased levels of LH and FSH with subsequent decrease in testosterone (male) and estrogen (female) levels. In males, testosterone levels are reduced to below castrate levels. Leuprolide may also have a direct inhibitory effect on the testes, and act by a different mechanism not directly related to reduction in serum testosterone.

Contraindications Hypersensitivity to leuprolide, GnRH, GnRH-agonist analogs, or any component of the formulation; undiagnosed abnormal vaginal bleeding; pregnancy; breast-feeding

Lupron Depot 22.5 mg, 30 mg, and 45 mg are also not indicated for use in women

Warnings/Precautions Hazardous agent - use appropriate precautions for handling and disposal (NIOSH, 2012). Transient increases in testosterone serum levels (~50% above baseline) occur at the start of treatment. Androgen-deprivation therapy (ADT) may increase the risk for cardiovascular disease (Levine, 2010); sudden cardiac death and stroke have been reported in men receiving GnRH agonists; long-term ADT may prolong the QT interval; consider the benefits of ADT versus the risk for QT prolongation in patients with a history of QT$_c$ prolongation, with medications known to prolong the QT interval, or with pre-existing cardiac disease. Tumor flare, bone pain, neuropathy, urinary tract obstruction, and spinal cord compression have been reported when used for prostate cancer; closely observe patients for weakness, paresthesias, hematuria, and urinary tract obstruction in first few weeks of therapy. Observe patients with metastatic vertebral lesions or urinary obstruction closely. Exacerbation of endometriosis or uterine leiomyomata may occur initially. Decreased bone density has been reported when used for ≥6 months; use caution in patients with additional risk factors for bone loss (eg, chronic alcohol use, corticosteroid therapy). In patients with prostate cancer, androgen deprivation therapy may increase the risk for cardiovascular disease, diabetes, insulin resistance, obesity, alterations in lipids, and fractures; monitor as clinically necessary. Use caution in patients with a history of psychiatric illness; alteration in mood, memory impairment, and depression have been associated with use. Rare cases of pituitary apoplexy (frequently secondary to pituitary adenoma) have been observed with GnRH agonist administration (onset from 1 hour to usually <2 weeks); may present as sudden headache, vomiting, visual or mental status changes, and infrequently cardiovascular collapse; immediate medical attention required. Convulsions have been observed in postmarketing reports; patients affected included both those with and without a history of cerebrovascular disorders, central nervous system anomalies or tumors, epilepsy, seizures, and those on concomitant medications which may lower the seizure threshold. If seizures occur, manage accordingly. Females treated for precocious puberty may experience menses or spotting during the first 2 months of treatment; notify healthcare provider if bleeding continues after the second month.

Some dosage forms may contain benzyl alcohol which has been associated with "gasping syndrome" in neonates; patients with benzyl alcohol allergy may demonstrate a hypersensitivity reaction (usually local) in the form of erythema and induration at the injection site. Vehicle used in depot injectable formulations (polylactide-co-glycolide microspheres) has rarely been associated with retinal artery occlusion in patients with abnormal arteriovenous anastomosis. Due to different release properties, combinations of dosage forms or fractions of dosage forms should not be interchanged.

Drug Interactions

Avoid Concomitant Use

Avoid concomitant use of Leuprolide with any of the following: Indium 111 Capromab Pendetide

Decreased Effect

Leuprolide may decrease the levels/effects of: Antidiabetic Agents; Indium 111 Capromab Pendetide

Increased Effect/Toxicity There are no known significant interactions involving an increase in effect.

Adverse Reactions

Children (percentages based on 1-month and 3-month pediatric formulations combined):
>10%: Local: Pain at injection site (≤20%)
2% to 10%:
Cardiovascular: Vasodilatation (2%)
Central nervous system: Emotional lability (5%), mood changes (5%), headache (3% to 5%), pain (3%)
Dermatologic: Acne vulgaris (3%), skin rash (3% including erythema multiforme), seborrhea (3%)
Endocrine & metabolic: Weight gain (≤7%)
Genitourinary: Vaginal hemorrhage (3%), vaginal discharge (3%), vaginitis (3%)
Local: Injection site reaction (≤9%)

Adults: Note: For prostate cancer treatment, an initial rise in serum testosterone concentrations may cause "tumor flare" or worsening of symptoms, including bone pain, neuropathy, hematuria, or ureteral or bladder outlet obstruction during the first 2 weeks. Similarly, an initial increase in estradiol levels, with a temporary worsening of symptoms, may occur in women treated with leuprolide.

Delayed release formulations:
>10%:
Cardiovascular: Edema (≤14%)
Central nervous system: Headache (≤65%), pain (<2% to 33%), depression (≤31%), insomnia (≤31%), fatigue (≤17%), dizziness (≤16%)
Dermatologic: Allergic skin reaction (≤12%)
Endocrine & metabolic: Hot flash (25% to 98%), weight changes (≤13%), hyperlipidemia (≤12%), libido decreased (≤11%)
Gastrointestinal: Nausea and vomiting (≤25%), change in bowel habits (≤14%)
Genitourinary: Vaginitis (11% to 28%), testicular atrophy (≤20%), genitourinary complaint (13% to 15%)
Local: Burning sensation at injection site burning (transient: ≤35%)
Neuromuscular & skeletal: Weakness (≤18%), arthropathy (≤12%)
Respiratory: Flu-like symptoms (≤12%)
1% to 10% (limited to important or life-threatening):
Cardiovascular: Angina pectoris (<5%), atrial fibrillation (<5%), bradycardia (<5%), cardiac arrhythmia (<5%), cardiac failure (<5%), deep thrombophlebitis (<5%), hyper-/hypotension (<5%), palpitation (<5%), syncope (<5%), tachycardia (<5%)
Central nervous system: Nervousness (≤8%), paresthesia (≤8%), anxiety (≤6%), confusion (<5%), delusions (<5%), dementia (<5%), neuropathy (<5%), paralysis (<5%), seizure (<5%), ostealgia (<2%)
Dermatologic: Acne vulgaris (≤10%), alopecia (≤5%), diaphoresis (≤5%), cellulitis (<5%), pruritus (≤3%), skin rash (≤2%)
Endocrine & metabolic: Dehydration (≤8%), gynecomastia (≤7%), decreased prostatic acid phosphatase (≥5%), decreased serum bicarbonate (≥5%), hypercholesterolemia (≥5%), hyperglycemia (≥5%), hyperphosphatemia (≥5%), hyperuricemia (≥5%), hypoalbuminemia (≥5%), hypocholesterolemia (≥5%), hypoproteinemia (≥5%), increased prostatic acid phosphatase (≥5%), menstrual disorder (≤2%), hirsutism (<2%)
Gastrointestinal: Anorexia (<5%), dysphagia (<5%), gastrointestinal hemorrhage (<5%), intestinal obstruction (<5%), gastric ulcer (<5%), constipation (≤3%), gastroenteritis (≤3%), diarrhea (≤2%)
Genitourinary: Mastalgia (≤6%), impotence (≤5%), balanitis (<5%), urinary incontinence (<5%), lactation (<5%), penile disease (<5%), testicular disease (<5%), urinary tract infection (<5%), nocturia (≤4%), testicular pain (≤4%), dysuria (≤2%), bladder spasm (<2%), erectile dysfunction (<2%), hematuria (<2%), urinary retention (<2%), urinary urgency (<2%)
Hematologic & oncologic: Eosinophilia (≥5%), leukopenia (≥5%), change in platelet count ▶

(increased; ≥5%), bruise (≤5%), lymphadenopathy (<5%), anemia

Hepatic: Abnormal hepatic function tests (≥5%), prolonged partial thromboplastin time (≥5%), prolonged prothrombin time (≥5%), hepatomegaly (<5%)

Hypersensitivity: Hypersensitivity reaction (<5%)

Infection: Infection (5%)

Local: Pain at injection site (2% to 5%), erythema at injection site (1% to 3%)

Neuromuscular & skeletal: Myalgia (≤8%), pathological fracture (<5%), arthralgia (≤1%)

Renal: Increased blood urea nitrogen (≥5%), increased serum creatinine (≥5%), decreased urine specific gravity (≥5%), increased urine specific gravity (≥5%), polyuria (2% to 4%)

Respiratory: Emphysema (<5%), epistaxis (<5%), hemoptysis (<5%), pleural effusion (<5%), pulmonary edema (<5%), dyspnea (≤2%), cough (≤1%)

Miscellaneous: Fever (<5%)

Immediate release formulation:

>10%:

Cardiovascular: ECG changes (19%), peripheral edema (12%)

Central nervous system: Pain (13%)

Endocrine & metabolic: Hot flash (55%)

1% to 10% (limited to important or life-threatening):

Cardiovascular: Hypertension (8%), heart murmur (3%), thrombophlebitis (2%), cardiac failure (1%), angina pectoris, cardiac arrhythmia, myocardial infarction, pulmonary embolism, syncope

Central nervous system: Headache (7%), insomnia (7%), dizziness (5%), ostealgia (5%), anxiety, depression, fatigue, fever, nervousness, peripheral neuropathy

Dermatologic: Dermatitis (5%), alopecia, hyperpigmentation, pruritus, skin lesion

Endocrine & metabolic: Decreased libido, diabetes mellitus, goiter, gynecomastia, hypercalcemia, hypoglycemia

Gastrointestinal: Constipation (7%), anorexia (6%), nausea and vomiting (5%), diarrhea, dysphagia, gastrointestinal hemorrhage, peptic ulcer, rectal polyps

Genitourinary: Decreased testicular size (7%), hematuria (6%), urinary frequency (6%), impotence (4%), urinary tract infection (3%), bladder spasm, dysuria, incontinence, mastalgia, testicular pain, urinary tract obstruction

Hematologic & oncologic: Anemia (5%), bruise

Infection: Infection

Local: Injection site reaction

Neuromuscular & skeletal: Weakness (10%)

Ophthalmic: Blurred vision

Renal: Increased blood urea nitrogen, increased serum creatinine

Respiratory: Dyspnea (2%), cough, pneumonia, pulmonary fibrosis

Miscellaneous: Fever, inflammation

Pharmacodynamics/Kinetics

Onset of Action Following transient increase, testosterone suppression occurs in ~2-4 weeks of continued therapy

Available Dosage Forms

Kit, Injection:

Generic: 1 mg/0.2 mL

Kit, Intramuscular:

Lupron Depot: 7.5 mg, 45 mg

Kit, Intramuscular [preservative free]:

Lupron Depot: 3.75 mg, 11.25 mg, 22.5 mg, 30 mg

Lupron Depot-Ped: 7.5 mg, 11.25 mg, 15 mg, 30 mg (Ped), 11.25 mg (Ped)

Kit, Subcutaneous:

Eligard: 7.5 mg, 22.5 mg, 30 mg, 45 mg

General Dosage Range I.M., SubQ: *Children and Adults:* Dosage varies greatly depending on indication

Administration

I.M. Lupron Depot, Lupron Depot-Ped: Administer as a single injection. Vary injection site periodically

Hazardous agent; use appropriate precautions for handling and disposal (NIOSH, 2012).

Subcutaneous

Eligard: Vary injection site; choose site with adequate subcutaneous tissue (eg, upper or mid-abdomen, upper buttocks); avoid areas that may be compressed or rubbed (eg, belt or waistband)

Leuprolide acetate 5 mg/mL solution: Vary injection site; if an alternate syringe from the syringe provided is required, insulin syringes should be used

Hazardous agent; use appropriate precautions for handling and disposal (NIOSH, 2012).

Preparation for Administration Hazardous agent; use appropriate precautions for handling and disposal (NIOSH, 2012).

Eligard: Packaged in two syringes; one contains the Atrigel polymer system and the second contains leuprolide acetate powder; follow package instructions for mixing

Lupron Depot, Lupron Depot-Ped: Reconstitute only with diluent provided

Storage/Stability

Eligard: Store at 2°C to 8°C (36°F to 46°C). Allow to reach room temperature prior to using; once mixed, must be administered within 30 minutes.

Lupron Depot, Lupron Depot-Ped: Store at room temperature of 25°C (77°F); excursions permitted to 15°C to 30°C (59°F to 86°F). Upon reconstitution, the suspension does not contain a preservative and should be used immediately; discard if not used within 2 hours.

Leuprolide acetate 5 mg/mL solution: Store at 20°C to 25°C (68°F to 77°F); excursions permitted to 15°C to 30°C (59°F to 86°F). Protect from light and store vial in carton until use. Do not freeze.

Nursing Actions

Physical Assessment Instruct patients with diabetes to monitor glucose levels closely; may impact effectiveness of antidiabetic agents. If self-administered, teach patient or caregiver proper storage, injection technique, and syringe/needle disposal. Wash hands before and after injection. Observe patients for weakness and paresthesias in the first few weeks of therapy. Monitor for symptoms of hypoglycemia.

Patient Education
- Discuss specific use of drug and side effects with patient as it relates to treatment. (HCAHPS: During this hospital stay, were you given any medicine that you had not taken before? Before giving you any new medicine, how often did hospital staff tell you what the medicine was for? How often did hospital staff describe possible side effects in a way you could understand?)
- Patient may experience flushing, osteodynia, hematuria, urinary retention, osteopenia, edema, headache, fatigue, nausea, depression, emotional instability, insomnia, short-term vaginal bleeding, or change in sex ability. Have patient report immediately to prescriber angina, illogical thinking, strength differences from one side to another, severe back pain, sudden vision changes, significant skin irritation, polydipsia, polyuria, weight loss, or rash (HCAHPS).
- Educate patient about signs of a significant reaction (eg, wheezing; chest tightness; fever; itching; bad cough; blue skin color; seizures; or swelling of face, lips, tongue, or throat). **Note:** This is not a comprehensive list of all side effects. Patient should consult prescriber for additional questions.

Intended Use and Disclaimer: Should not be printed and given to patients. This information is intended to serve as a concise initial reference for healthcare professionals to use when discussing medications with a patient. You must ultimately rely on your own discretion, experience and judgment in diagnosing, treating and advising patients.

Leuprolide and Norethindrone
(loo PROE lide & nor eth IN drone)

Brand Names: U.S. Lupaneta Pack

Index Terms Leuprolide Acetate and Norethindrone Acetate; Lupaneta Pack; Norethindrone and Leuprolide

Pharmacologic Category Gonadotropin Releasing Hormone Agonist; Progestin

Pregnancy Risk Factor X

Use Endometriosis: Management of initial and recurrent painful symptoms of endometriosis

Product Availability Lupaneta Pack: FDA approved December 2012: anticipated availability is fourth quarter of 2013. Refer to prescribing information for additional information.

Available Dosage Forms
Kit, Combination:
Lupaneta Pack: 1-month kit: leuprolide acetate 3.75 mg depot suspension for injection (1) and norethindrone acetate 5 mg oral tablets (30), 3-month kit: leuprolide acetate 11.25 mg depot suspension for injection (1) and norethindrone acetate 5 mg oral tablets (90)

General Dosage Range I.M./Oral: *Adults:*
Females:
1 month: Leuprolide 3.75 mg I.M. once every month and norethindrone 5 mg orally once daily (maximum initial therapy duration: 6 months; may repeat treatment once for a maximum cumulative therapy duration: 12 months)
3 month: Leuprolide 11.25 mg I.M. once every 3 months and norethindrone 5 mg orally once daily (maximum initial therapy duration: 6 months; may repeat treatment once for a maximum cumulative therapy duration: 12 months)

Administration
I.M. Injection: Leuprolide: Administer I.M. in the gluteal area, anterior thigh, or deltoid. Do not use if a blood vessel is accidently penetrated (will be able to see aspirated blood below the transparent luer lock).

Hazardous agent; use appropriate precautions for handling and disposal (NIOSH, 2012).

Oral Tablet: Norethindrone: Administer orally. Hazardous agent; use appropriate precautions for handling and disposal (NIOSH, 2012).

Nursing Actions
Physical Assessment Monitor for fatigue, hot flashes, memory impairment, decrease in sexual ability or desire, vaginal dryness, migraines, swelling of extremities, peripheral neuropathy, visual loss, proptosis, diplopia, injection site pain or bruising, or depression. Assess how patient is tolerating hot flashes. If patient is of childbearing age, ask about contraception methods and ensure patient is not pregnant.

Patient Education
- Discuss specific use of drug and side effects with patient as it relates to treatment. (HCAHPS: During this hospital stay, were you given any medicine that you had not taken before? Before giving you any new medicine, how often did hospital staff tell you what the medicine was for? How often did hospital staff describe possible side effects in a way you could understand?)
- Patient may experience acne vulgaris, hot flashes, asthenia, insomnia, constipation, diarrhea, or loss of libido. Have patient report immediately to prescriber signs of hepatic impairment, angina, tachycardia, depression, suicidal ideation, anxiety, emotional instability, illogical thinking, strength differences from one side to another, difficulty speaking, change in balance,

blurred vision, severe behavioral problems, significant headache, considerable nausea, edema of extremities, hemoptysis, intolerable dizziness, vision changes, blindness, exophthalmos, vaginitis, vaginal hemorrhaging, urinary retention, dysuria, dyspnea, significant weight gain, mastalgia, arrhythmia, hyperhidrosis, memory impairment, paresthesia, or osteopenia (HCAHPS).

- Educate patient about signs of a significant reaction (eg, wheezing; chest tightness; fever; itching; bad cough; blue skin color; seizures; or swelling or face, lips, tongue, or throat). **Note:** This is not a comprehensive list of all side effects. Patient should consult prescriber for additional questions.

Intended Use and Disclaimer: Should not be printed and given to patients. This information is intended to serve as a concise initial reference for healthcare professionals to use when discussing medications with a patient. You must ultimately rely on your own discretion, experience and judgment in diagnosing, treating and advising patients.

Related Information
Leuprolide on page 918
Norethindrone on page 1139

Levalbuterol (leve al BYOO ter ole)

Brand Names: U.S. Xopenex; Xopenex Concentrate; Xopenex HFA
Index Terms Levalbuterol Hydrochloride; Levalbuterol Tartrate; Levosalbutamol; R-albuterol
Pharmacologic Category Beta$_2$ Agonist
Medication Safety Issues
Sound-alike/look-alike issues:
Xopenex® may be confused with Xanax®
Pregnancy Risk Factor C
Lactation Excretion in breast milk unknown/use caution
Breast-Feeding Considerations It is not known whether levalbuterol is excreted in human milk. Although breast-feeding is not recommended by the manufacturer, the use of beta$_2$-receptor agonists are not considered a contraindication to breast-feeding (NAEPP, 2005).
Use Treatment or prevention of bronchospasm in children and adults with reversible obstructive airway disease
Mechanism of Action/Effect Relaxes bronchial smooth muscle by action on beta$_2$-receptors with little effect on heart rate
Contraindications Hypersensitivity to levalbuterol, albuterol, or any component of the formulation
Warnings/Precautions Optimize anti-inflammatory treatment before initiating maintenance treatment with levalbuterol. Do not use as a component of chronic therapy without an anti-inflammatory agent. Only the mildest form of asthma (Step 1

and/or exercise-induced) would not require concurrent use based upon asthma guidelines. Patient must be instructed to seek medical attention in cases where acute symptoms are not relieved or a previous level of response is diminished. The need to increase frequency of use may indicate deterioration of asthma, and treatment must not be delayed. A spacer device or valved holding chamber is recommended when using a metered-dose inhaler.

Use caution in patients with cardiovascular disease (arrhythmia or hypertension or HF), convulsive disorders, diabetes, glaucoma, hyperthyroidism, or hypokalemia. Beta-agonists may cause elevation in blood pressure, heart rate, and result in CNS stimulation/excitation. Beta$_2$-agonists may increase risk of arrhythmia, increase serum glucose, or decrease serum potassium.

Immediate hypersensitivity reactions (urticaria, angioedema, rash, bronchospasm) have been reported. Do not exceed recommended dose; serious adverse events including fatalities, have been associated with excessive use of inhaled sympathomimetics. Rarely, paradoxical bronchospasm may occur with use of inhaled bronchodilating agents; this should be distinguished from inadequate response. Use with caution during labor and delivery. Safety and efficacy have not been established in patients <4 years of age.

Drug Interactions
Avoid Concomitant Use
Avoid concomitant use of Levalbuterol with any of the following: Beta-Blockers (Nonselective); Iobenguane I 123
Decreased Effect
Levalbuterol may decrease the levels/effects of: Iobenguane I 123

The levels/effects of Levalbuterol may be decreased by: Beta-Blockers (Beta1 Selective); Beta-Blockers (Nonselective); Betahistine
Increased Effect/Toxicity
Levalbuterol may increase the levels/effects of: Atosiban; Loop Diuretics; Sympathomimetics; Thiazide Diuretics

The levels/effects of Levalbuterol may be increased by: AtoMOXetine; Cannabinoids; MAO Inhibitors; Tricyclic Antidepressants
Adverse Reactions
>10%:
Endocrine & metabolic: Serum glucose increased, serum potassium decreased
Neuromuscular & skeletal: Tremor (≤7%)
Respiratory: Rhinitis (3% to 11%)
Miscellaneous: Viral infection (7% to 12%)
>2% to 10%:
Central nervous system: Headache (8% to 12%), nervousness (3% to 10%), dizziness (1% to 3%), anxiety (≤3%), migraine (≤3%), weakness (3%)

Cardiovascular: Tachycardia (~3%)

Dermatologic: Rash (≤8%)

Gastrointestinal: Diarrhea (2% to 6%), dyspepsia (1% to 3%)

Neuromuscular & skeletal: Leg cramps (≤3%)

Respiratory: Asthma (9%), pharyngitis (3% to 10%), cough (1% to 4%), sinusitis (1% to 4%), nasal edema (1% to 3%)

Miscellaneous: Flu-like syndrome (1% to 4%), accidental injury (≤3%)

Note: Immediate hypersensitivity reactions have occurred (including angioedema, oropharyngeal edema, urticaria, and anaphylaxis).

Pharmacodynamics/Kinetics

Onset of Action Measured as a 15% increase in FEV_1:

Aerosol: 5.5-10.2 minutes; Peak effect: ~77 minutes

Nebulization: 10-17 minutes; Peak effect: 1.5 hours

Duration of Action Measured as a 15% increase in FEV_1:

Aerosol: 3-4 hours (up to 6 hours in some patients)

Nebulization: 5-6 hours (up to 8 hours in some patients)

Dosage Forms Considerations

Xopenex HFA 15 g canisters contain 200 inhalations.

Available Dosage Forms

Aerosol, Inhalation:

Xopenex HFA: 45 mcg/actuation (15 g)

Nebulization Solution, Inhalation:

Xopenex: 0.63 mg/3 mL (3 mL); 1.25 mg/3 mL (3 mL)

Generic: 0.63 mg/3 mL (3 mL)

Nebulization Solution, Inhalation [preservative free]:

Xopenex: 0.31 mg/3 mL (3 mL)

Xopenex Concentrate: 1.25 mg/0.5 mL (30 ea)

Generic: 0.31 mg/3 mL (3 mL); 0.63 mg/3 mL (3 mL); 1.25 mg/3 mL (3 mL); 1.25 mg/0.5 mL (1 ea, 30 ea)

General Dosage Range

Inhalation (metered-dose inhaler): *Children ≥4 years and Adults:* 1-2 puffs every 4-6 hours

Nebulization (solution):

Children ≤4 years: 0.31-1.25 mg every 4-6 hours as needed

Children 5-11 years: 0.31-0.63 mg 3 times/day

Children ≥12 years and Adults: 0.63-1.25 mg every 8 hours as needed

Elderly: Initial: 0.63 mg

Administration

Inhalation

Metered-dose inhaler: Shake well before use; prime with 4 test sprays prior to first use or if inhaler has not been used for more than 3 days. Clean actuator (mouthpiece) weekly. A spacer device or valved holding chamber is recommended when using a metered-dose inhaler.

Solution for nebulization: Safety and efficacy were established when administered with the following nebulizers: PARI LC Jet™, PARI LC Plus™, as well as the following compressors: PARI Master®, Dura-Neb® 2000, and Dura-Neb® 3000. Concentrated solution should be diluted prior to use. Blow-by administration is not recommended, use a mask device if patient unable to hold mouthpiece in mouth for administration.

Preparation for Administration Concentrated solution should be diluted with 2.5 mL NS prior to use.

Storage/Stability

Aerosol: Store at room temperature of 20°C to 25°C (68°F to 77°F); protect from freezing and direct sunlight. Store with mouthpiece down. Discard after 200 actuations.

Solution for nebulization: Store in protective foil pouch at room temperature of 20°C to 25°C (68°F to 77°F). Protect from light and excessive heat. Vials should be used within 2 weeks after opening protective pouch. Use within 1 week and protect from light if removed from pouch. Vials of concentrated solution should be used immediately after removing from protective pouch.

Nursing Actions

Physical Assessment Teach patient safe use of nebulizer.

Patient Education

- Discuss specific use of drug and side effects with patient as it relates to treatment. (HCAHPS: During this hospital stay, were you given any medicine that you had not taken before? Before giving you any new medicine, how often did hospital staff tell you what the medicine was for? How often did hospital staff describe possible side effects in a way you could understand?)

- Patient may experience headache, dizziness, xerostomia, rhinorrhea, nausea, tremors, or pharyngitis. Have patient report immediately to prescriber signs of hypokalemia, uncontrollable breathing attack, decreased peak flow measurement, angina, tachycardia, severe dizziness, syncope, significant anxiety, intolerable headache, or considerable dyspnea (HCAHPS).

- Educate patient about signs of a significant reaction (eg, wheezing; chest tightness; fever; itching; bad cough; blue skin color; seizures; or swelling of face, lips, tongue, or throat). **Note:** This is not a comprehensive list of all side effects. Patient should consult prescriber for additional questions.

Intended Use and Disclaimer: Should not be printed and given to patients. This information is intended to serve as a concise initial reference for healthcare professionals to use when discussing medications with a patient. You must ultimately rely on your own discretion, experience and judgment in diagnosing, treating and advising patients.

Levetiracetam (lee va tye RA se tam)

Brand Names: U.S. Keppra; Keppra XR

Pharmacologic Category Anticonvulsant, Miscellaneous

Medication Safety Issues

Sound-alike/look-alike issues:

Keppra may be confused with Keflex, Keppra XR

LevETIRAcetam may be confused with levOCARNitine, levofloxacin

Potential for dispensing errors between Keppra and Kaletra (lopinavir/ritonavir)

Medication Guide Available Yes

Pregnancy Risk Factor C

Lactation Enters breast milk/not recommended

Breast-Feeding Considerations Levetiracetam can be detected in breast milk. Using data from 11 women collected 4-23 days after delivery, the estimated exposure of levetiracetam to the breast-feeding infant would be ~2 mg/kg/day (relative infant dose 7.9% of the weight-adjusted maternal dose). Adverse events were not reported in the nursing infants (Tomson, 2007). Breast-feeding is not recommended by the manufacturer.

Use Adjunctive therapy in the treatment of partial onset, myoclonic, and/or primary generalized tonic-clonic seizures

Mechanism of Action/Effect The precise mechanism by which levetiracetam exerts its antiepileptic effect is unknown. However, several studies have suggested the mechanism may involve one or more central pharmacologic effects.

Contraindications There are no contraindications listed in the U.S. manufacturer's labeling.

Canadian labeling: Hypersensitivity to levetiracetam or any component of the formulation

Warnings/Precautions Antiepileptics are associated with an increased risk of suicidal behavior/thoughts with use (regardless of indication); patients should be monitored for signs/symptoms of depression, suicidal tendencies, and other unusual behavior changes during therapy and instructed to inform their healthcare provider immediately if symptoms occur.

Severe dermatologic reactions (toxic epidermal necrolysis and Stevens-Johnson syndrome) have been reported; onset usually within ~2 weeks of treatment initiation but may be delayed (>4 months); discontinue for any signs of a hypersensitivity reaction or unspecified rash.

Psychotic symptoms (psychosis, hallucinations) and behavioral symptoms (including aggression, anger, anxiety, depersonalization, depression, personality disorder) may occur; incidence may be increased in children. Dose reduction or discontinuation may be required. Levetiracetam should be withdrawn gradually, when possible, to minimize the potential of increased seizure frequency. Use caution with renal impairment; dosage adjustment

may be necessary. Impaired coordination, weakness, dizziness, and somnolence may occur, most commonly during the first month of therapy; use caution when driving or operating heavy machinery. Although rare, decreases in red blood cell counts, hemoglobin, hematocrit, white blood cell counts and neutrophils have been observed. Safety and efficacy of I.V. and extended release tablet formulations have not been established in children <16 years of age. Isolated elevations in diastolic blood pressure measurements have been reported in children <4 years of age; however, no observable differences were noted in mean diastolic measurements of children receiving levetiracetam vs placebo. Similar effects have not been observed in older children and adults.

Drug Interactions

Avoid Concomitant Use

Avoid concomitant use of LevETIRAcetam with any of the following: Azelastine (Nasal); Paraldehyde; Thalidomide

Decreased Effect

The levels/effects of LevETIRAcetam may be decreased by: Ketorolac (Nasal); Ketorolac (Systemic); Mefloquine; Orlistat

Increased Effect/Toxicity

LevETIRAcetam may increase the levels/effects of: Alcohol (Ethyl); Azelastine (Nasal); Buprenorphine; CNS Depressants; Hydrocodone; Methotrimeprazine; Metyrosine; Mirtazapine; Paraldehyde; Pramipexole; ROPINIRole; Rotigotine; Selective Serotonin Reuptake Inhibitors; Thalidomide; Zolpidem

The levels/effects of LevETIRAcetam may be increased by: Brimonidine (Topical); Doxylamine; Droperidol; HydrOXYzine; Magnesium Sulfate; Methotrimeprazine; Perampanel; Sodium Oxybate; Tapentadol

Nutritional/Ethanol Interactions

Ethanol: May increase CNS depression; monitor for increased effects with coadministration. Caution patients about effects.

Food: Food may delay, but does not affect the extent of absorption.

Adverse Reactions

>10%:

Cardiovascular: Increased blood pressure (diastolic; infants and children <4 years: 17%)

Central nervous system: Behavioral problems (including aggression, anger, apathy, depersonalization, hyperkinesias, neurosis: adults 5% to 13%; children 5% to 38%), drowsiness (2% to 23%), headache (14% to 19%), psychotic symptoms (infants and children <4 years: 17%; children 4-16 years: 2%; adults 1%), hostility (2% to 12%), irritability (2% to12%), fatigue (10% to 11%)

Gastrointestinal: Vomiting (children and adolescents 4-16 years: 15%), anorexia (3% to 13%)

Infection: Infection (2% to 13%)

Neuromuscular & skeletal: Weakness (9% to 15%)

Respiratory: Nasopharyngitis (7% to 15%), pharyngitis (6% to 14%), rhinitis (2% to 13%), cough (2% to 11%)

1% to 10%:

Cardiovascular: Facial edema (2%)

Central nervous system: Aggressive behavior (children and adolescents 4-16 years: 10%), nervousness (2% to 10%), dizziness (5% to 9%), personality disorder (8%), pain (6% to 7%), agitation (4% to 6%), emotional lability (2% to 6%), lethargy (children and adolescents 4-16 years: 6%), insomnia (children and adolescents 4-16 years: 5%), depression (2% to 5%), vertigo (3% to 5%), ataxia (3%), falling (children and adolescents 4-16 years: 3%), amnesia (2%), anxiety (2% to 3%), confusion (2%), paranoia (children and adolescents 4-16 years: 2%), paresthesia (2%), sedation (children 2%)

Dermatologic: Bruise (3% to 4%), pruritus (2%), skin discoloration (2%), skin rash (2%)

Endocrine & metabolic: Dehydration (2%)

Gastrointestinal: Upper abdominal pain (children and adolescents 4-16 years: 9%), decreased appetite (children and adolescents 4-16 years: 8%), diarrhea (6% to 8%), nausea (5%), gastroenteritis (2% to 4%), constipation (children and adolescents 4-16 years: 3%)

Genitourinary: Urine abnormality (2%)

Hematologic & oncologic: Eosinophilia (children and adolescents 4-16 years: 8%), decreased white blood cell count (3%)

Infection: Influenza (3% to 8%), viral infection (2%)

Neuromuscular & skeletal: Neck pain (2% to 8%), arthralgia (children and adolescents 4-16 years: 2%), hyperreflexia (2%), sprain (children and adolescents 4-16 years: 2%)

Ophthalmic: Conjunctivitis (2% to 3%), diplopia (2%), amblyopia (2%)

Otic: Otalgia (2%)

Renal: Albuminuria (4%)

Respiratory: Nasal congestion (children and adolescents 4-16 years: 9%), flu-like symptoms (3% to 8%), pharyngolaryngeal pain (children and adolescents 4-16 years: 7%), asthma (2%), sinusitis (2%)

Miscellaneous: Accidental injury (children and adolescents 4-16 years: 2% to 4%)

Pharmacodynamics/Kinetics

Onset of Action Peak effect: Oral: 1 hour

Available Dosage Forms

Solution, Intravenous:

Keppra: 500 mg/5 mL (5 mL)

Generic: 500 mg/100 mL (100 mL); 1000 mg/100 mL (100 mL); 1500 mg/100 mL (100 mL); 500 mg/5 mL (5 mL)

Solution, Intravenous [preservative free]:

Generic: 500 mg/5 mL (5 mL)

Solution, Oral:

Keppra: 100 mg/mL (473 mL)

Generic: 100 mg/mL (5 mL, 473 mL, 500 mL)

Tablet, Oral:

Keppra: 250 mg, 500 mg, 750 mg, 1000 mg

Generic: 250 mg, 500 mg, 750 mg, 1000 mg

Tablet Extended Release 24 Hour, Oral:

Keppra XR: 500 mg, 750 mg

Generic: 500 mg, 750 mg

General Dosage Range Dosage adjustment recommended in patients with renal impairment

Oral:

Immediate release:

Children 1 to <6 months: Initial: 7 mg/kg twice daily; Maintenance: 7-21 mg/kg/dose twice daily (maximum: 42 mg/kg/day)

Children 6 months to <4 years: Initial: 10 mg/kg twice daily; Maintenance: 10-25 mg/kg twice daily (maximum: 50 mg/kg/day)

Children 4 to <16 years: Initial: 10 mg/kg twice daily; Maintenance: 10-30 mg/kg twice daily (maximum: 60 mg/kg/day or 3000 mg/day)

Children ≥12 years: Initial: 500 mg twice daily; Maintenance: 500-1500 mg twice daily (maximum: 3000 mg/day)

Adults: Initial: 500 mg twice daily; Maintenance: 500-1500 mg twice daily (maximum: 3000 mg/day)

Extended release: *Children ≥16 years and Adults:* Initial: 1000 mg once daily; Maintenance: 1000-3000 mg once daily (maximum: 3000 mg/day)

I.V.: *Children ≥16 years and Adults:* Initial: 500 mg twice daily; Maintenance: 500-1500 mg twice daily (maximum: 3000 mg/day)

Administration

I.V. Infuse over 15 minutes

Injectable Detail pH: 5.5

Oral

May be administered without regard to meals.

Oral solution: Should be administered with a calibrated measuring device (not a household teaspoon or tablespoon)

Tablet (immediate release and extended release): Only administer as whole tablet; do not crush, break or chew.

Preparation for Administration Vials for injection: Must dilute dose in 100 mL of NS, LR, or D₅W.

Storage/Stability

Oral solution, tablets: Store at 25°C (77°F); excursions permitted to 15°C to 30°C (59°F to 86°F).

Premixed solution for infusion: Store at 20°C to 25°C (68°F to 77°F).

Vials for injection: Store at 25°C (77°F); excursions permitted to 15°C to 30°C (59°F to 86°F). Admixed solution is stable for 24 hours in PVC bags kept at room temperature.

Nursing Actions

Physical Assessment Monitor therapeutic response (seizure activity, force, type, duration) at beginning of therapy and periodically ▶

throughout. Monitor for CNS depression (somnolence and fatigue), behavioral abnormalities (psychosis, hallucinations, psychotic depression), and other behavioral symptoms (agitation, anger, aggression, irritability, hostility, anxiety, apathy, emotional lability, depersonalization, and depression). Taper dosage slowly when discontinuing. Observe and teach seizure/safety precautions.

Patient Education

- Discuss specific use of drug and side effects with patient as it relates to treatment. (HCAHPS: During this hospital stay, were you given any medicine that you had not taken before? Before giving you any new medicine, how often did hospital staff tell you what the medicine was for? How often did hospital staff describe possible side effects in a way you could understand?)
- Patient may experience presyncope, fatigue, blurred vision, illogical thinking, imbalance, headache, mood changes, rhinorrhea, pharyngitis, asthenia, nausea, or emotional instability. Have patient report immediately to prescriber signs of infection, depression, ecchymosis, bleeding, or rash (HCAHPS).
- Educate patient about signs of a significant reaction (eg, wheezing; chest tightness; fever; itching; bad cough; blue skin color; seizures; or swelling of face, lips, tongue, or throat). **Note:** This is not a comprehensive list of all side effects. Patient should consult prescriber for additional questions.

Intended Use and Disclaimer: Should not be printed and given to patients. This information is intended to serve as a concise initial reference for healthcare professionals to use when discussing medications with a patient. You must ultimately rely on your own discretion, experience and judgment in diagnosing, treating and advising patients.

Dietary Considerations May be taken without regard to meals.

Related Information
Oral Medications That Should Not Be Crushed or Altered *on page 1712*

Levocabastine (Nasal) (LEE voe kab as teen)

Index Terms Levocabastine Hydrochloride
Pharmacologic Category Histamine H_1 Antagonist; Histamine H_1 Antagonist, Second Generation; Piperidine Derivative
Medication Safety Issues
  Sound-alike/look-alike issues:
  Levocabastine may be confused with levobunolol, levOCARNitine
  Livostin® may be confused with lovastatin
  International issues:
  Livostin [Canada and multiple international markets] may be confused with Limoxin brand name for ambroxol [Indonesia] and amoxicillin

[Mexico]; Lovastin brand name for lovastatin [Malaysia, Poland, Singapore]
Use Symptomatic treatment of allergic rhinitis
Product Availability Not available in U.S.
General Dosage Range Intranasal: *Children ≥12 years and Adults ≤65 years:* 2 sprays in each nostril 2-4 times/day
Administration
  Other Intranasal: Shake bottle well before each use. Prior to initial use, bottle should be primed until a fine spray is delivered. Instruct patients to blow nose and clear nasal passages before administering spray and to inhale nasally while spraying.
Nursing Actions
Patient Education
- Discuss specific use of drug and side effects with patient as it relates to treatment. (HCAHPS: During this hospital stay, were you given any medicine that you had not taken before? Before giving you any new medicine, how often did hospital staff tell you what the medicine was for? How often did hospital staff describe possible side effects in a way you could understand?)
- Patient may experience xerostomia, presyncope, fatigue, blurred vision, illogical thinking, headache, or rhinitis. Have patient report immediately to prescriber severe dizziness, syncope, or rash (HCAHPS).
- Educate patient about signs of a significant reaction (eg, wheezing; chest tightness; fever; itching; bad cough; blue skin color; seizures; or swelling of face, lips, tongue, or throat). **Note:** This is not a comprehensive list of all side effects. Patient should consult prescriber for additional questions.

Intended Use and Disclaimer: Should not be printed and given to patients. This information is intended to serve as a concise initial reference for healthcare professionals to use when discussing medications with a patient. You must ultimately rely on your own discretion, experience and judgment in diagnosing, treating and advising patients.

Levocabastine (Ophthalmic)
(LEE voe kab as teen)

Index Terms Levocabastine Hydrochloride
Pharmacologic Category Histamine H_1 Antagonist; Histamine H_1 Antagonist, Second Generation; Piperidine Derivative
Medication Safety Issues
  Sound-alike/look-alike issues:
  Levocabastine may be confused with levobunolol, levOCARNitine
  Livostin® may be confused with lovastatin

International issues:
Livostin [Canada and multiple international markets] may be confused with Limoxin brand name for ambroxol [Indonesia] and amoxicillin [Mexico]; Lovastin brand name for lovastatin [Malaysia, Poland, Singapore]

Use Treatment of seasonal allergic conjunctivitis

Product Availability Not available in U.S.

General Dosage Range Ophthalmic: *Children ≥12 years and Adults ≤65 years:* Instill 1 drop in affected eye(s) 2-4 times/day

Administration
Other For topical ophthalmic use only. Shake bottle well. Wash hands prior to use. Avoid touching the dropper tip to surfaces to avoid contamination.

Nursing Actions
Patient Education
• Discuss specific use of drug and side effects with patient as it relates to treatment. (HCAHPS: During this hospital stay, were you given any medicine that you had not taken before? Before giving you any new medicine, how often did hospital staff tell you what the medicine was for? How often did hospital staff describe possible side effects in a way you could understand?)
• Patient may experience eye irritation. Have patient report immediately to prescriber sudden vision changes or rash (HCAHPS).
• Educate patient about signs of a significant reaction (eg, wheezing; chest tightness; fever; itching; bad cough; blue skin color; seizures; or swelling of face, lips, tongue, or throat). **Note:** This is not a comprehensive list of all side effects. Patient should consult prescriber for additional questions.

Intended Use and Disclaimer: Should not be printed and given to patients. This information is intended to serve as a concise initial reference for healthcare professionals to use when discussing medications with a patient. You must ultimately rely on your own discretion, experience and judgment in diagnosing, treating and advising patients.

Levocetirizine (LEE vo se TI ra zeen)

Brand Names: U.S. Xyzal

Index Terms Levocetirizine Dihydrochloride

Pharmacologic Category Histamine H₁ Antagonist; Histamine H₁ Antagonist, Second Generation; Piperazine Derivative

Medication Safety Issues
Sound-alike/look-alike issues:
Levocetirizine may be confused with cetirizine

Pregnancy Risk Factor B

Lactation Excretion in breast milk unknown/not recommended

Use Relief of symptoms of perennial and seasonal allergic rhinitis; treatment of skin manifestations (uncomplicated) of chronic idiopathic urticaria

Available Dosage Forms
Solution, Oral:
Xyzal: 2.5 mg/5 mL (148 mL)
Generic: 2.5 mg/5 mL (148 mL)
Tablet, Oral:
Xyzal: 5 mg
Generic: 5 mg

General Dosage Range Dosage adjustment recommended in patients with renal impairment
Oral:
Children 6 months to 5 years: 1.25 mg once daily
Children 6-11 years: 2.5 mg once daily
Children ≥12 years and Adults: 2.5-5 mg once daily

Administration
Oral Administer in the evening. May be administered without regard to meals.

Nursing Actions
Patient Education
• Discuss specific use of drug and side effects with patient as it relates to treatment. (HCAHPS: During this hospital stay, were you given any medicine that you had not taken before? Before giving you any new medicine, how often did hospital staff tell you what the medicine was for? How often did hospital staff describe possible side effects in a way you could understand?)
• Patient may experience presyncope, fatigue, blurred vision, illogical thinking, or xerostomia. Have patient report immediately to prescriber severe dizziness, syncope, urinary retention, or rash (HCAHPS).
• Educate patient about signs of a significant reaction (eg, wheezing; chest tightness; fever; itching; bad cough; blue skin color; seizures; or swelling of face, lips, tongue, or throat). **Note:** This is not a comprehensive list of all side effects. Patient should consult prescriber for additional questions.

Intended Use and Disclaimer: Should not be printed and given to patients. This information is intended to serve as a concise initial reference for healthcare professionals to use when discussing medications with a patient. You must ultimately rely on your own discretion, experience and judgment in diagnosing, treating and advising patients.

Levodopa, Carbidopa, and Entacapone
(lee voe DOE pa, kar bi DOE pa, & en TA ka pone)

Brand Names: U.S. Stalevo

Index Terms Carbidopa, Entacapone, and Levodopa; Carbidopa, Levodopa, and Entacapone; Entacapone, Carbidopa, and Levodopa

◀ **Pharmacologic Category** Anti-Parkinson's Agent, COMT Inhibitor; Anti-Parkinson's Agent, Decarboxylase Inhibitor; Anti-Parkinson's Agent, Dopamine Precursor

Medication Safety Issues

Administration issues:

Strengths listed in Stalevo brand names correspond to the **levodopa** component of the formulation only. All strengths of Stalevo contain a levodopa/carbidopa ratio of 4:1 plus entacapone 200 mg.

Pregnancy Risk Factor C

Use Parkinson disease: Treatment of idiopathic Parkinson disease.

Available Dosage Forms

Tablet:

Stalevo: 50: Levodopa 50 mg, carbidopa 12.5 mg, and entacapone 200 mg; 75: Levodopa 75 mg, carbidopa 18.75 mg, and entacapone 200 mg; 100: Levodopa 100 mg, carbidopa 25 mg, and entacapone 200 mg; 125: Levodopa 125 mg, carbidopa 31.25 mg, and entacapone 200 mg; 150: Levodopa 150 mg, carbidopa 37.5 mg, and entacapone 200 mg; 200: Levodopa 200 mg, carbidopa 50 mg, and entacapone 200 mg

Generic: Levodopa 50 mg, carbidopa 12.5 mg, and entacapone 200 mg; Levodopa 75 mg, carbidopa 18.75 mg, and entacapone 200 mg; Levodopa 100 mg, carbidopa 25 mg, and entacapone 200 mg; Levodopa 125 mg, carbidopa 31.25 mg, and entacapone 200 mg; Levodopa 150 mg, carbidopa 37.5 mg, and entacapone 200 mg; Levodopa 200 mg, carbidopa 50 mg, and entacapone 200 mg

General Dosage Range Oral: *Adults:* 1 tablet (50-200 mg levodopa/12.5-50 mg carbidopa/200 mg entacapone) at each dosing interval (maximum: 1600 mg/day entacapone or 300 mg/day carbidopa)

Administration

Oral Swallow tablet whole; do not crush, break, or chew. Only 1 tablet should be administered at each dosing interval. May be administered without regard to meals.

Nursing Actions

Physical Assessment See individual agents.

Patient Education

• Discuss specific use of drug and side effects with patient as it relates to treatment. (HCAHPS: During this hospital stay, were you given any medicine that you had not taken before? Before giving you any new medicine, how often did hospital staff tell you what the medicine was for? How often did hospital staff describe possible side effects in a way you could understand?)

• Patient may experience presyncope, fatigue, blurred vision, illogical thinking, dizziness, nausea, diarrhea, discolored bodily fluids, or hallucinations. Have patient report immediately to prescriber severe myalgia or significant asthenia (HCAHPS).

• Educate patient about signs of a significant reaction (eg, wheezing; chest tightness; fever; itching; bad cough; blue skin color; seizures; or swelling of face, lips, tongue, or throat). **Note:** This is not a comprehensive list of all side effects. Patient should consult prescriber for additional questions.

Intended Use and Disclaimer: Should not be printed and given to patients. This information is intended to serve as a concise initial reference for healthcare professionals to use when discussing medications with a patient. You must ultimately rely on your own discretion, experience and judgment in diagnosing, treating and advising patients.

Related Information

Entacapone *on page 535*

Levofloxacin (Systemic) (lee voe FLOKS a sin)

Brand Names: U.S. Levaquin

Pharmacologic Category Antibiotic, Fluoroquinolone; Antibiotic, Respiratory Fluoroquinolone

Medication Safety Issues

Sound-alike/look-alike issues:

Levaquin may be confused with Levoxyl, Levsin/SL, Lovenox

Levofloxacin may be confused with levETIRAcetam, levodopa, Levophed, levothyroxine

Medication Guide Available Yes

Pregnancy Risk Factor C

Lactation Enters breast milk/not recommended

Breast-Feeding Considerations Based on data from a case report, small amounts of levofloxacin are excreted in breast milk. Breast-feeding is not recommended by the manufacturer. Levofloxacin is the L-isomer of ofloxacin. Ofloxacin has also been shown to have minimal concentrations in human milk. Nondose-related effects could include modification of bowel flora.

Use Treatment of community-acquired pneumonia, including multidrug resistant strains of *S. pneumoniae* (MDRSP); nosocomial pneumonia; chronic bronchitis (acute bacterial exacerbation); acute bacterial rhinosinusitis (ABRS); prostatitis (chronic bacterial); urinary tract infection (uncomplicated or complicated); acute pyelonephritis; skin or skin structure infections (uncomplicated or complicated); reduce incidence or disease progression of inhalational anthrax (postexposure); prophylaxis and treatment of plague (pneumonic and septicemic) due to *Y. pestis*

Unlabeled Use Diverticulitis, enterocolitis (*Shigella* spp), epididymitis (nongonococcal), urethritis (nongonococcal), complicated intra-abdominal infections (in combination with metronidazole), Legionnaires' disease, peritonitis, PID (alternative therapy); traveler's diarrhea; oral phase treatment of prosthetic joint infection; surgical (preoperative) prophylaxis

Note: As of April 2007, the CDC no longer recommends the use of fluoroquinolones for the treatment of gonococcal disease due to increased prevalence of fluoroquinolone-resistant *Neisseria gonorrhoeae*.

Mechanism of Action/Effect Levofloxacin, a fluorinated quinolone, exerts a broad spectrum bactericidal effect. It inhibits DNA gyrase which is required for DNA replication and transcription, DNA repair, recombination, and transposition within the bacteria.

Contraindications Hypersensitivity to levofloxacin, any component of the formulation, or other quinolones

Canadian labeling: Additional contraindications (not in U.S. labeling): History of tendonitis or tendon rupture associated with use of any quinolone antimicrobial agent

Warnings/Precautions [U.S. Boxed Warning]: There have been reports of tendon inflammation and/or rupture with quinolone antibiotics; risk may be increased with concurrent corticosteroids, organ transplant recipients, and in patients >60 years of age. Rupture of the Achilles tendon sometimes requiring surgical repair has been reported most frequently; but other tendon sites (eg, rotator cuff, biceps) have also been reported. Strenuous physical activity, rheumatoid arthritis, and renal impairment may be an independent risk factor for tendonitis. Discontinue at first sign of tendon inflammation or pain. May occur even after discontinuation of therapy. Use with caution in patients with rheumatoid arthritis; may increase risk of tendon rupture. Safety of use in pediatric patients for >14 days of therapy has not been studied; increased incidence of musculoskeletal disorders (eg, arthralgia, tendon rupture) has been observed in children. CNS effects may occur (toxic psychoses, tremor, restlessness, anxiety, lightheadedness, paranoia, depression, nightmares, confusion, and very rarely hallucinations increased intracranial pressure (including pseudotumor cerebri, seizures, or toxic psychosis). Potential for seizures, although very rare, may be increased with concomitant NSAID therapy. Use with caution in individuals at risk of seizures, with known or suspected CNS disorders or renal dysfunction. Avoid excessive sunlight and take precautions to limit exposure (eg, loose fitting clothing, sunscreen); may cause moderate-to-severe phototoxicity reactions. Discontinue use if photosensitivity occurs.

Rare cases of torsade de pointes have been reported in patients receiving levofloxacin. Use caution in patients with known prolongation of QT interval, bradycardia, hypokalemia, hypomagnesemia, or in those receiving concurrent therapy with Class Ia or Class III antiarrhythmics.

Severe hypersensitivity reactions, including anaphylaxis, have occurred with quinolone therapy. Reactions may present as typical allergic symptoms after a single dose, or may manifest as severe idiosyncratic dermatologic, vascular, pulmonary, renal, hepatic, and/or hematologic events, usually after multiple doses. Prompt discontinuation of drug should occur if skin rash or other symptoms arise. Prolonged use may result in fungal or bacterial superinfection, including *C. difficile*-associated diarrhea (CDAD) and pseudomembranous colitis; CDAD has been observed >2 months postantibiotic treatment. Peripheral neuropathy has been reported (rare); may occur soon after initiation of therapy and may be irreversible; discontinue if symptoms of sensory or sensorimotor neuropathy occur. **[U.S. Boxed Warning]: Quinolones may exacerbate myasthenia gravis; avoid use (rare, potentially life-threatening weakness of respiratory muscles may occur).** Unrelated to hypersensitivity, severe hepatotoxicity (including acute hepatitis and fatalities) has been reported. Elderly patients may be at greater risk. Discontinue therapy immediately if signs and symptoms of hepatitis occur. Hemolytic reactions may (rarely) occur with quinolone use in patients with latent or actual G6PD deficiency.

Fluoroquinolones have been associated with the development of serious, and sometimes fatal, hypoglycemia, most often in elderly diabetics, but also in patients without diabetes. This occurred most frequently with gatifloxacin (no longer available systemically) but may occur at a lower frequency with other quinolones.

Drug Interactions

Avoid Concomitant Use

Avoid concomitant use of Levofloxacin (Systemic) with any of the following: BCG; Highest Risk QTc-Prolonging Agents; Ivabradine; Mifepristone; Strontium Ranelate

Decreased Effect

Levofloxacin (Systemic) may decrease the levels/effects of: BCG; Didanosine; Mycophenolate; Sodium Picosulfate; Sulfonylureas; Typhoid Vaccine

The levels/effects of Levofloxacin (Systemic) may be decreased by: Antacids; Calcium Salts; Didanosine; Iron Salts; Lanthanum; Magnesium Salts; Multivitamins/Minerals (with ADEK, Folate, Iron); Multivitamins/Minerals (with AE, No Iron); Quinapril; Sevelamer; Strontium Ranelate; Sucralfate; Zinc Salts

Increased Effect/Toxicity

Levofloxacin (Systemic) may increase the levels/effects of: Corticosteroids (Systemic); Highest Risk QTc-Prolonging Agents; Moderate Risk QTc-Prolonging Agents; Porfimer; Sulfonylureas; Tacrolimus (Systemic); Varenicline; Vitamin K Antagonists

◀ *The levels/effects of Levofloxacin (Systemic) may be increased by:* Insulin; Ivabradine; Mifepristone; Nonsteroidal Anti-Inflammatory Agents; Probenecid; QTc-Prolonging Agents (Indeterminate Risk and Risk Modifying)

Adverse Reactions 1% to 10%:
Cardiovascular: Chest pain (1%), edema (1%)
Central nervous system: Headache (6%), insomnia (4%), dizziness (3%)
Dermatologic: Rash (2%), pruritus (1%)
Gastrointestinal: Nausea (7%), diarrhea (5%), constipation (3%), abdominal pain (2%), dyspepsia (2%), vomiting (2%)
Genitourinary: Vaginitis (1%)
Local: Injection site reaction (1%)
Respiratory: Dyspnea (1%)
Miscellaneous: Moniliasis (1%)

Available Dosage Forms
Solution, Intravenous [preservative free]:
Levaquin: 250 mg/50 mL (50 mL); 500 mg/100 mL (100 mL); 750 mg/150 mL (150 mL)
Generic: 250 mg/50 mL (50 mL); 500 mg/100 mL (100 mL); 750 mg/150 mL (150 mL); 25 mg/mL (20 mL, 30 mL)
Solution, Oral:
Levaquin: 25 mg/mL (480 mL)
Generic: 25 mg/mL (10 mL, 20 mL, 100 mL, 200 mL, 480 mL)
Tablet, Oral:
Levaquin: 250 mg, 500 mg, 750 mg
Generic: 250 mg, 500 mg, 750 mg

General Dosage Range Dosage adjustment recommended in patients with renal impairment
Oral, I.V.:
Infants ≥6 months and Children ≤50 kg: 8 mg/kg every 12 hours (maximum: 250 mg/dose)
Children >50 kg: 500 mg once daily
Adults: 250-750 mg once daily

Administration
I.V. Infuse 250-500 mg I.V. solution over 60 minutes; infuse 750 mg I.V. solution over 90 minutes. Too rapid of infusion can lead to hypotension. Avoid administration through an intravenous line with a solution containing multivalent cations (eg, magnesium, calcium). Maintain adequate hydration of patient to prevent crystalluria or cylindruria.
Injectable Detail pH: 3.8-5.8
Oral Tablets may be administered without regard to meals. Oral solution should be administered 1 hour before or 2 hours after meals. Maintain adequate hydration of patient to prevent crystalluria.
Preparation for Administration Solution for injection: Single-use vials must be further diluted in compatible solution to a final concentration of 5 mg/mL prior to infusion.

Storage/Stability
Solution for injection:
Vial: Store at room temperature. Protect from light. Diluted solution (5 mg/mL) is stable for 72 hours when stored at room temperature; stable for 14 days when stored under refrigeration. When frozen, stable for 6 months; do not refreeze. Do not thaw in microwave or by bath immersion.
Premixed: Store at ≤25°C (77°F); do not freeze. Brief exposure to 40°C (104°F) does not affect product. Protect from light.
Tablet, oral solution: Store at 25°C (77°F); excursions permitted to 15°C to 30°C (59°F to 86°F).

Nursing Actions
Physical Assessment Results of culture and sensitivity tests and patient's allergy history should be assessed before initiating therapy. Monitor patient closely; if an allergic reaction occurs (itching, urticaria, dyspnea or facial edema, loss of consciousness, tingling, cardiovascular collapse), drug should be discontinued immediately and prescriber notified. Monitor for hypersensitivity reactions, opportunistic infection, tendon rupture, and persistent diarrhea (*C. difficile*-associated colitis can occur post-treatment).

Patient Education
• Discuss specific use of drug and side effects with patient as it relates to treatment. (HCAHPS: During this hospital stay, were you given any medicine that you had not taken before? Before giving you any new medicine, how often did hospital staff tell you what the medicine was for? How often did hospital staff describe possible side effects in a way you could understand?)
• Patient may experience dyspepsia, nausea, or diarrhea. Have patient report immediately to prescriber tachycardia, significant headache, illogical thinking, ankle pain, arthralgia, edema, severe asthenia, paresthesia, discolored urine, jaundice, inability to eat, sudden vision changes, tinnitus, or rash (HCAHPS).
• Educate patient about signs of a significant reaction (eg, wheezing; chest tightness; fever; itching; bad cough; blue skin color; seizures; or swelling of face, lips, tongue, or throat). **Note:** This is not a comprehensive list of all side effects. Patient should consult prescriber for additional questions.

Intended Use and Disclaimer: Should not be printed and given to patients. This information is intended to serve as a concise initial reference for healthcare professionals to use when discussing medications with a patient. You must ultimately rely on your own discretion, experience and judgment in diagnosing, treating and advising patients.

Dietary Considerations Tablets may be taken without regard to meals. Oral solution should be administered on an empty stomach (1 hour before or 2 hours after a meal). Take 2 hours before or 2 hours after multiple vitamins, antacids, or other products containing magnesium, aluminum, iron, or zinc.

LEVOleucovorin (lee voe loo koe VOR in)

Brand Names: U.S. Fusilev

Index Terms 6S-leucovorin; Calcium Levoleucovorin; L-leucovorin; Levo-folinic Acid; Levo-leucovorin; Levoleucovorin Calcium Pentahydrate; S-leucovorin

Pharmacologic Category Antidote; Chemotherapy Modulating Agent; Rescue Agent (Chemotherapy)

Medication Safety Issues

Sound-alike/look-alike issues:

LEVOleucovorin may be confused with leucovorin calcium, Leukeran®, Leukine®

Pregnancy Risk Factor C

Lactation Excretion in breast milk unknown/not recommended

Use Treatment of advanced, metastatic colorectal cancer (palliative) in combination with fluorouracil; rescue agent after high-dose methotrexate therapy in osteosarcoma; antidote for impaired methotrexate elimination and for inadvertent overdosage of folic acid antagonists

Available Dosage Forms

Solution Reconstituted, Intravenous:

Fusilev: 50 mg (1 ea)

General Dosage Range I.V.: *Children and Adults:* Dosing varies greatly depending on indication

Administration

I.V. For I.V. administration only; do not administer intrathecally. Administer by slow I.V. push or infusion over at least 3 minutes, not to exceed 160 mg/minute (due to calcium content).

For colorectal cancer: Levoleucovorin has also been administered (unlabeled administration rate) as I.V. infusion over 2 hours (Comella, 2000; Tournigand, 2006).

Other Do not administer intrathecally.

Nursing Actions

Physical Assessment Levoleucovorin is used in combination with the drug 5FU for the treatment of colorectal cancer. When it is given with 5FU, it is usually administered over 5 days. It is important to review the patient's medications and monitor if he or she takes sulfa medications, seizure medications (eg, phenytoin), or a multivitamin with folic acid.

Patient Education

• Discuss specific use of drug and side effects with patient as it relates to treatment. (HCAHPS: During this hospital stay, were you given any medicine that you had not taken before? Before giving you any new medicine, how often did hospital staff tell you what the medicine was

for? How often did hospital staff describe possible side effects in a way you could understand?)

• Patient may experience nausea, stomatitis, diarrhea, asthenia, alopecia, lack of appetite, or dyspepsia. Have patient report immediately to prescriber rash (HCAHPS).

• Educate patient about signs of a significant reaction (eg, wheezing; chest tightness; fever; itching; bad cough; blue skin color; seizures; or swelling of face, lips, tongue, or throat). **Note:** This is not a comprehensive list of all side effects. Patient should consult prescriber for additional questions.

Intended Use and Disclaimer: Should not be printed and given to patients. This information is intended to serve as a concise initial reference for healthcare professionals to use when discussing medications with a patient. You must ultimately rely on your own discretion, experience and judgment in diagnosing, treating and advising patients.

Levomilnacipran (lee voe mil NA si pran)

Brand Names: U.S. Fetzima; Fetzima Titration

Pharmacologic Category Antidepressant, Serotonin/Norepinephrine Reuptake Inhibitor

Medication Safety Issues

Sound-alike/look-alike issues:

Levomilnacipran may be confused with milnacipran

Medication Guide Available Yes

Pregnancy Risk Factor C

Lactation Excretion in breast milk unknown/not recommended

Breast-Feeding Considerations It is not known if levomilnacipran is excreted into breast milk. Due to the potential for serious adverse reactions in the nursing infant, the manufacturer recommends a decision be made whether to discontinue nursing or to discontinue the drug, taking into account the importance of treatment to the mother.

Use Major depressive disorder: Treatment of major depressive disorder (MDD)

Mechanism of Action/Effect Levomilnacipran, the more active enantiomer of milnacipran, is a potent inhibitor of norepinephrine and serotonin reuptake (Montgomery, 2013).

Contraindications Hypersensitivity to levomilnacipran, milnacipran, or any component of the formulation; use of MAO inhibitors intended to treat psychiatric disorders (concurrently or within 7 days of discontinuing levomilnacipran, or within 2 weeks of discontinuing the MAO inhibitor); initiation of levomilnacipran in a patient receiving linezolid or intravenous methylene blue; uncontrolled narrow-angle glaucoma

Warnings/Precautions [U.S. Boxed Warning]: Antidepressants increase the risk of suicidal thinking and behavior in children, adolescents, ▶

and young adults (18-24 years of age) with major depressive disorder (MDD) and other psychiatric disorders; consider risk prior to prescribing. Short-term studies did not show an increased risk in patients >24 years of age and showed a decreased risk in patients ≥65 years. Closely monitor for clinical worsening, suicidality, or unusual changes in behavior; the patient's family or caregiver should be instructed to closely observe the patient and communicate condition with healthcare provider. A medication guide should be dispensed with each prescription. **Levomilnacipran is not FDA approved for the treatment of major depressive disorder or for use in children.**

Suicide risks should be monitored in patients treated with SNRIs regardless of the indication. The possibility of a suicide attempt is inherent in major depression and may persist until remission occurs. Monitor for worsening of depression or suicidality, especially during initiation of therapy (generally first few months) or with dose increases or decreases. Use caution in high-risk patients. Worsening depression and severe abrupt suicidality that are not part of the presenting symptoms may require discontinuation or modification of drug therapy. The patient's family or caregiver should be alerted to monitor patients for the emergence of suicidality and associated behaviors (such as agitation, irritability, hostility, impulsivity, and hypomania) and call healthcare provider.

May precipitate a shift to mania or hypomania in patients with bipolar disorder. Monotherapy in patients with bipolar disorder should be avoided. Patients presenting with depressive symptoms should be screened for bipolar disorder. **Levomilnacipran is not FDA approved for the treatment of bipolar disorder.**

Potentially life-threatening serotonin syndrome (SS) has occurred with serotonergic agents (eg, SSRIs, SNRIs), particularly when used in combination with other serotonergic agents (eg, triptans, TCAs, fentanyl, lithium, tramadol, buspirone, St John's wort, tryptophan) or agents that impair metabolism of serotonin (eg, MAO inhibitors intended to treat psychiatric disorders, other MAO inhibitors [ie, linezolid and intravenous methylene blue]). Discontinue treatment (and any concomitant serotonergic agent) immediately if signs/symptoms arise. SSRIs and SNRIs have been associated with the development of SIADH; hyponatremia has been reported rarely (including severe cases with serum sodium <110 mmol/L). Age (the elderly), volume depletion and/or concurrent use of diuretics likely increases risk. Discontinue treatment in patients with symptomatic hyponatremia.

Potentially significant drug-drug interactions may exist, requiring dose or frequency adjustment, additional monitoring, and/or selection of alternative therapy. Concurrent use with MAO inhibitors is contraindicated. May cause sustained increase in blood pressure or heart rate. Control pre-existing hypertension and cardiovascular disease prior to initiation of levomilnacipran. Use caution in patients with renal impairment; dose reduction required in moderate or severe renal impairment. Use cautiously in patients with a history of seizures. May impair platelet aggregation, resulting in bleeding. May cause increased urinary hesitancy or retention. Use caution in patients with controlled narrow-angle glaucoma; use is contraindicated with uncontrolled narrow-angle glaucoma. Bone fractures have been associated with antidepressant treatment. Consider the possibility of a fragility fracture if an antidepressant-treated patient presents with unexplained bone pain, point tenderness, swelling, or bruising (Rabenda, 2013; Rizzoli, 2012). Use caution in elderly patients; may have a higher risk of SIADH or hyponatremia.

Abrupt discontinuation or interruption of antidepressant therapy has been associated with a discontinuation syndrome. Symptoms arising may vary with antidepressant however commonly include nausea, vomiting, diarrhea, headaches, light-headedness, dizziness, diminished appetite, sweating, chills, tremors, paresthesias, fatigue, somnolence, and sleep disturbances (eg, vivid dreams, insomnia). Greater risks for developing a discontinuation syndrome have been associated with antidepressants with shorter half-lives, longer durations of treatment, and abrupt discontinuation. For antidepressants of short or intermediate half-lives, symptoms may emerge within 2-5 days after treatment discontinuation and last 7-14 days (APA, 2010; Fava, 2006; Haddad, 2001; Shelton, 2001; Warner, 2006).

Drug Interactions

Avoid Concomitant Use

Avoid concomitant use of Levomilnacipran with any of the following: Fusidic Acid (Systemic); Iobenguane I 123; Linezolid; MAO Inhibitors; Methylene Blue; Urokinase

Decreased Effect

Levomilnacipran may decrease the levels/effects of: Alpha2-Agonists; Iobenguane I 123; Ioflupane I 123

The levels/effects of Levomilnacipran may be decreased by: Nonsteroidal Anti-Inflammatory Agents; Peginterferon Alfa-2b

Increased Effect/Toxicity

Levomilnacipran may increase the levels/effects of: Agents with Antiplatelet Properties; Alpha-/Beta-Agonists; Anticoagulants; Antipsychotics; Aspirin; Collagenase (Systemic); Dabigatran Etexilate; Ibritumomab; Methylene Blue; Metoclopramide; NSAID (Nonselective); Rivaroxaban; Salicylates; Serotonin Modulators; Thrombolytic Agents; Tositumomab and Iodine I 131 Tositumomab; Urokinase; Vitamin K Antagonists

The levels/effects of Levomilnacipran may be increased by: Alcohol (Ethyl); Antipsychotics; CYP3A4 Inhibitors (Moderate); CYP3A4 Inhibitors (Strong); Dasatinib; Fusidic Acid (Systemic); Glucosamine; Herbs (Anticoagulant/Antiplatelet Properties); Ibrutinib; Ivacaftor; Linezolid; Lulicaonazole; MAO Inhibitors; Mifepristone; Multivitamins/Fluoride (with ADE); Multivitamins/Minerals (with ADEK, Folate, Iron); Multivitamins/Minerals (with AE, No Iron); Nonsteroidal Anti-Inflammatory Agents; Omega-3 Fatty Acids; Pentosan Polysulfate Sodium; Pentoxifylline; Prostacyclin Analogues; Simeprevir; Tipranavir; Vitamin E

Nutritional/Ethanol Interactions

Ethanol: Ethanol may increase CNS depression and may accelerate drug release by interacting with extended-release properties. Management: Avoid ethanol.

Herb/Nutraceutical: Some herbal medications may increase risk of serotonin syndrome and/or excessive sedation. Management: Avoid valerian, St John's wort, SAMe, kava kava, and tryptophan.

Adverse Reactions

>10%:

Cardiovascular: Orthostatic hypotension (6% to 12%; dose related)

Gastrointestinal: Nausea (17%)

1% to 10%:

Cardiovascular: Increased heart rate (6%), tachycardia (6%), palpitations (5%), hypertension (3%), hypotension (3%), increased blood pressure (3%), angina pectoris (<2%), chest pain (<2%), supraventricular extrasystole (<2%), syncope (<2%), ventricular premature contractions (<2%)

Central nervous system: Ejaculatory disorder (5%), aggressive behavior (<2%), agitation (<2%), extrapyramidal reaction (<2%), migraine (<2%), outbursts of anger (<2%), panic attack (<2%), paresthesia (<2%), tension (<2%), yawning (<2%)

Dermatologic: Hyperhidrosis (9%), skin rash (2%), pruritus (<2%), urticaria (<2%), xeroderma (<2%)

Endocrine & metabolic: Hot flash (3%), hypercholesterolemia (<2%), increased thirst (<2%)

Gastrointestinal: Constipation (9%), vomiting (5%), decreased appetite (3%), abdominal pain (<2%), bruxism (<2%), flatulence (<2%)

Genitourinary: Erectile dysfunction (6% to 10%; dose related), urinary hesitancy (4% to 6%; dose related), testicular pain (4%), hematuria (<2%), pollakiuria (<2%), proteinuria (<2%)

Hepatic: Abnormal hepatic function tests (<2%)

Ophthalmic: Blurred vision (<2%), conjunctival hemorrhage (<2%), dry eye syndrome (<2%)

Available Dosage Forms

Capsule ER 24 Hour Therapy Pack, Oral:
Fetzima Titration: 20 & 40 mg (28 ea)

Capsule Extended Release 24 Hour, Oral:
Fetzima: 20 mg, 40 mg, 80 mg, 120 mg

General Dosage Range Dosage adjustment recommended in patients with renal impairment.

Oral: *Adults:* Initial: 20 mg once daily; Maintenance: 40-120 mg once daily; Maximum: 120 mg daily

Administration

Oral Administer with or without food at approximately the same time each day. Swallow whole, do not open, chew, or crush the capsule.

Storage/Stability Store at 25°C (77°F); excursions permitted between 15°C and 30°C (59°F and 86°F).

Nursing Actions

Patient Education

• Discuss specific use of drug and side effects with patient as it relates to treatment. (HCAHPS: During this hospital stay, were you given any medicine that you had not taken before? Before giving you any new medicine, how often did hospital staff tell you what the medicine was for? How often did hospital staff describe possible side effects in a way you could understand?)

• Patient may experience nausea, constipation, hyperhidrosis, or sexual dysfunction. Have patient report immediately to prescriber depression, suicidal ideation, nervousness, emotional instability, illogical thinking, anxiety, signs of hyponatremia, angina, significant change in balance, tachycardia, severe headache, considerable dizziness, ecchymosis asthenia, or dysuria (HCAHPS).

• Educate patient about signs of a significant reaction (eg, wheezing; chest tightness; fever; itching; bad cough; blue skin color; seizures; or swelling of face, lips, tongue, or throat). **Note:** This is not a comprehensive list of all side effects. Patient should consult prescriber for additional questions.

Intended Use and Disclaimer: Should not be printed and given to patients. This information is intended to serve as a concise initial reference for healthcare professionals to use when discussing medications with a patient. You must ultimately rely on your own discretion, experience and judgment in diagnosing, treating and advising patients.

Levonorgestrel (LEE voe nor jes trel)

Brand Names: U.S. Mirena; My Way [DSC]; Next Choice One Dose; Plan B; Plan B One-Step; Plan B One-Step [OTC]; Skyla

Index Terms LNg 20; Plan B

Pharmacologic Category Contraceptive; Progestin

Lactation Enters breast milk

Use

Intrauterine device (IUD): Prevention of pregnancy; treatment of heavy menstrual bleeding in women who also choose to use an IUD for contraception

Oral: Emergency contraception following unprotected intercourse or possible contraceptive failure

Available Dosage Forms

Intrauterine Device, Intrauterine:

Mirena: 20 mcg/24 hr

Skyla: 13.5 mg

Tablet, Oral:

Next Choice One Dose: 1.5 mg

Plan B: 0.75 mg

Plan B One-Step [OTC]: 1.5 mg, 1.5 mg

Generic: 0.75 mg, 1.5 mg

General Dosage Range

Intrauterine: *Adults:* Insert into uterine cavity, replace in 5 years (Mirena) **or** 3 years (Skyla)

Oral: *Adults:* 0.75 mg every 12 hours for 2 doses **or** 1.5 mg as a single dose

Administration

Oral Consider repeating the dose if vomiting occurs within 2 hours. If severe vomiting occurs, may consider administering the oral tablets vaginally (ACOG, 2010).

Hazardous agent; use appropriate precautions for handling and disposal (NIOSH, 2012).

Other Intrauterine device: Insert into the uterine cavity to the recommended depth with the provided insertion device; should not be forced into the uterus. Transvaginal ultrasound may be used to check proper placement. Remove if not positioned properly and insert a new IUD; do not reinsert removed IUD. Exclude perforation if exceptional pain or bleeding occurs after insertion.

Hazardous agent; use appropriate precautions for handling and disposal (NIOSH, 2012).

Intravaginal If severe vomiting occurs with oral tablets, may consider administering the oral tablets vaginally (ACOG, 2010). Hazardous agent; use appropriate precautions for handling and disposal (NIOSH, 2012).

Nursing Actions

Physical Assessment Pregnancy should be ruled out prior to insertion of levonorgestrel-coated IUD. Monitor for prolonged menstrual bleeding, amenorrhea, and irregularity of menses. Educate patient about need for annual medical exams.

If vomiting occurs within 2 hours of taking medication, patient may need another dose. If emergency contraception taken, next menstrual period can begin up to 1 week earlier or later than expected. If delay is longer than 1 week, contact prescriber because patient may be pregnant. Notify prescriber if patient experiences severe lower abdominal pain 3-5 weeks after taking.

Patient Education

- Discuss specific use of drug and side effects with patient as it relates to treatment. (HCAHPS: During this hospital stay, were you given any medicine that you had not taken before? Before giving you any new medicine, how often did hospital staff tell you what the medicine was for? How often did hospital staff describe possible side effects in a way you could understand?)
- Patient may experience weight gain, headache, nausea, acne, macromastia, vaginal yeast infection, menstrual irregularity, gallbladder disease, thrombosis, MI, application site pain, or hypertension. Have patient report immediately to prescriber severe dyspepsia, sudden vision changes, eye pain, eye irritation, mastalgia, pregnancy, emesis, dislodged device, painful intercourse, discolored urine, or jaundice (HCAHPS).
- Educate patient about signs of a significant reaction (eg, wheezing; chest tightness; fever; itching; bad cough; blue skin color; seizures; or swelling of face, lips, tongue, or throat). **Note:** This is not a comprehensive list of all side effects. Patient should consult prescriber for additional questions.

Intended Use and Disclaimer: Should not be printed and given to patients. This information is intended to serve as a concise initial reference for healthcare professionals to use when discussing medications with a patient. You must ultimately rely on your own discretion, experience and judgment in diagnosing, treating and advising patients.

Levorphanol (lee VOR fa nole)

Index Terms Levo-Dromoran; Levorphan Tartrate; Levorphanol Tartrate

Pharmacologic Category Analgesic, Opioid

Medication Safety Issues

High alert medication:

The Institute for Safe Medication Practices (ISMP) includes this medication among its list of drug classes which have a heightened risk of causing significant patient harm when used in error.

Pregnancy Risk Factor C

Lactation Excretion in breast milk unknown/not recommended

Use Relief of moderate-to-severe pain; preoperative sedation/analgesia; management of chronic pain (eg, cancer) requiring opioid therapy

Controlled Substance C-II

Available Dosage Forms

Tablet, Oral:

Generic: 2 mg

General Dosage Range Dosage adjustment recommended in patients with hepatic impairment

Oral: *Adults:* 2-4 mg every 6-8 hours as needed

Nursing Actions

Physical Assessment Monitor blood pressure, CNS and respiratory status, and degree of sedation at beginning of therapy and periodically thereafter. Assess patient's physical and/or psychological dependence. For inpatients, implement safety measures (eg, side rails up, call light within reach, instructions to call for assistance). Discontinue slowly after prolonged use.

Patient Education
- Discuss specific use of drug and side effects with patient as it relates to treatment. (HCAHPS: During this hospital stay, were you given any medicine that you had not taken before? Before giving you any new medicine, how often did hospital staff tell you what the medicine was for? How often did hospital staff describe possible side effects in a way you could understand?)
- Patient may experience fatigue, flushing, or nausea. Have patient report immediately to prescriber severe dizziness, syncope, illogical thinking, considerable constipation, significant asthenia, mood changes, difficult urination, tachycardia, bradycardia, or arrhythmia (HCAHPS).
- Educate patient about signs of a significant reaction (eg, wheezing; chest tightness; fever; itching; bad cough; blue skin color; seizures; or swelling of face, lips, tongue, or throat). **Note:** This is not a comprehensive list of all side effects. Patient should consult prescriber for additional questions.

Intended Use and Disclaimer: Should not be printed and given to patients. This information is intended to serve as a concise initial reference for healthcare professionals to use when discussing medications with a patient. You must ultimately rely on your own discretion, experience and judgment in diagnosing, treating and advising patients.

Levothyroxine (lee voe thye ROKS een)

Brand Names: U.S. Levothroid [DSC]; Levoxyl [DSC]; Synthroid; Tirosint; Unithroid; Unithroid Direct

Index Terms L-Thyroxine Sodium; Levothyroxine Sodium; T_4

Pharmacologic Category Thyroid Product

Medication Safety Issues

Sound-alike/look-alike issues:

Levothyroxine may be confused with lamoTRIgine, Lanoxin®, levofloxacin, liothyronine

Levoxyl® may be confused with Lanoxin®, Levaquin®, Luvox®

Synthroid® may be confused with Symmetrel®

Administration issues:

Significant differences exist between oral and I.V. dosing. Use caution when converting from one route of administration to another.

Other safety concerns:

To avoid errors due to misinterpretation of a decimal point, always express dosage in mcg (**not** mg).

Pregnancy Risk Factor A

Lactation Enters breast milk/use caution

Breast-Feeding Considerations Endogenous thyroid hormones are minimally found in breast milk. The amount of endogenous thyroxine found in breast milk does not influence infant plasma thyroid values. Levothyroxine was not found to cause adverse events to the infant or mother during breast-feeding. Adequate thyroid hormone concentrations are required to maintain normal lactation. Appropriate levothyroxine doses should be continued during breast-feeding.

Use Replacement or supplemental therapy in hypothyroidism; pituitary TSH suppression

Unlabeled Use Management of hemodynamically unstable potential organ donors increasing the quantity of organs available for transplantation

Mechanism of Action/Effect It is believed the thyroid hormone exerts its many metabolic effects through control of DNA transcription and protein synthesis

Contraindications Hypersensitivity to levothyroxine sodium or any component of the formulation; acute MI; thyrotoxicosis of any etiology; uncorrected adrenal insufficiency

Capsule: Additional contraindication: Inability to swallow capsules

Warnings/Precautions [U.S. Boxed Warning]: Thyroid supplements are ineffective and potentially toxic when used for the treatment of obesity or for weight reduction, especially in euthyroid patients. High doses may produce serious or even life-threatening toxic effects particularly when used with some anorectic drugs (eg, sympathomimetic amines). Routine use of T_4 for TSH suppression is not recommended in patients with benign thyroid nodules. In patients deemed appropriate candidates, treatment should never be fully suppressive (TSH <0.1 mIU/L). Use with caution and reduce dosage in patients with angina pectoris or other cardiovascular disease; decrease initial dose. Use cautiously in the elderly since they may be more likely to have compromised cardiovascular functions. Patients with adrenal insufficiency, myxedema, diabetes mellitus and insipidus may have symptoms exaggerated or aggravated. Chronic hypothyroidism predisposes patients to coronary artery disease. Long-term therapy can decrease bone mineral density. Levoxyl® may rapidly swell and disintegrate causing choking or gagging (should be administered with a ▶

full glass of water); use caution in patients with dysphagia or other swallowing disorders.

Drug Interactions

Avoid Concomitant Use

Avoid concomitant use of Levothyroxine with any of the following: Sodium Iodide I131; Sucroferric Oxyhydroxide

Decreased Effect

Levothyroxine may decrease the levels/effects of: Sodium Iodide I131; Theophylline Derivatives

The levels/effects of Levothyroxine may be decreased by: Aluminum Hydroxide; Bile Acid Sequestrants; Calcium Polystyrene Sulfonate; Calcium Salts; CarBAMazepine; Estrogen Derivatives; Fosphenytoin; Iron Salts; Lanthanum; Multivitamins/Minerals (with ADEK, Folate, Iron); Orlistat; Phenytoin; Raloxifene; Rifampin; Selective Serotonin Reuptake Inhibitors; Sevelamer; Sodium Polystyrene Sulfonate; Sucralfate; Sucroferric Oxyhydroxide

Increased Effect/Toxicity

Levothyroxine may increase the levels/effects of: Tricyclic Antidepressants; Vitamin K Antagonists

The levels/effects of Levothyroxine may be increased by: Piracetam

Nutritional/Ethanol Interactions Food: Taking levothyroxine with enteral nutrition may cause reduced bioavailability and may lower serum thyroxine levels leading to signs or symptoms of hypothyroidism. Soybean flour (infant formula), cottonseed meal, walnuts, and dietary fiber may decrease absorption of levothyroxine from the GI tract. Management: Take in the morning on an empty stomach at least 30 minutes before food. Consider an increase in dose if taken with enteral tube feed.

Adverse Reactions Frequency not defined.

Cardiovascular: Angina pectoris, cardiac arrest, cardiac arrhythmia, congestive heart failure, flushing, hypertension, increased pulse, myocardial infarction, palpitations, tachycardia

Central nervous system: Anxiety, choking sensation (Levoxyl), emotional lability, fatigue, headache, heat intolerance, hyperactivity, insomnia, irritability, myasthenia, nervousness, pseudotumor cerebri (children), seizure (rare)

Dermatologic: Alopecia, diaphoresis

Endocrine & metabolic: Menstrual disease, weight loss

Gastrointestinal: Abdominal cramps, diarrhea, dysphagia (Levoxyl), gag reflex (Levoxyl), increased appetite, vomiting

Genitourinary: Infertility

Hepatic: Increased liver enzymes

Hypersensitivity: Hypersensitivity (to inactive ingredients; symptoms include urticaria, pruritus, rash, flushing, angioedema, GI symptoms, fever, arthralgia, serum sickness, wheezing)

Neuromuscular & skeletal: Decreased bone mineral density, slipped capital femoral epiphysis (children), tremor

Respiratory: Dyspnea

Miscellaneous: Fever

Pharmacodynamics/Kinetics

Onset of Action Therapeutic: Oral: 3-5 days; I.V. 6-8 hours; Peak effect: I.V.: 24 hours

Available Dosage Forms

Capsule, Oral:

Tirosint: 13 mcg, 25 mcg, 50 mcg, 75 mcg, 88 mcg, 100 mcg, 112 mcg, 125 mcg, 137 mcg, 150 mcg

Solution Reconstituted, Intravenous [preservative free]:

Generic: 100 mcg (1 ea); 200 mcg (1 ea); 500 mcg (1 ea)

Tablet, Oral:

Synthroid: 25 mcg, 50 mcg, 75 mcg, 88 mcg, 100 mcg, 112 mcg, 125 mcg, 137 mcg, 150 mcg, 175 mcg, 200 mcg, 300 mcg

Unithroid: 25 mcg, 50 mcg, 75 mcg, 88 mcg, 100 mcg, 112 mcg, 125 mcg, 150 mcg, 175 mcg, 200 mcg, 300 mcg

Unithroid Direct: 25 mcg, 50 mcg, 75 mcg, 88 mcg, 100 mcg, 112 mcg, 125 mcg, 150 mcg, 175 mcg, 200 mcg, 300 mcg

Generic: 25 mcg, 50 mcg, 75 mcg, 88 mcg, 100 mcg, 112 mcg, 125 mcg, 137 mcg, 150 mcg, 175 mcg, 200 mcg, 300 mcg

General Dosage Range

I.M.: *Children and Adults:* 50% of oral dose

I.V.:

Children: 50% of oral dose

Adults: 50% of oral dose or 200-500 mcg, then 100-300 mcg the next day if needed

Oral:

Children 1-3 months: 10-15 mcg/kg/day

Children 3-6 months: 8-10 mcg/kg/day

Children 6-12 months: 6-8 mcg/kg/day

Children 1-5 years: 5-6 mcg/kg/day

Children 6-12 years: 4-5 mcg/kg/day

Children >12 years: 2-3 mcg/kg/day

Adults: Initial: 12.5-25 mcg/day **or** 1.7 mcg/kg/day (usual doses are ≤200 mcg/day)

*Elderly >50 years without cardiac disease **or** <50 years with cardiac disease:* Initial: 25-50 mcg/day

Elderly >50 years with cardiac disease: Initial: 12.5-25 mcg/day

Administration

I.V. Administer doses ≤100 mcg I.V. over 1 minute.

Oral Administer in the morning on an empty stomach, at least 30 minutes before food.

Capsule: Must be swallowed whole; do not cut, crush, or attempt to dissolve capsules in water to prepare a suspension.

Tablet: May be crushed and suspended in 5-10 mL of water; suspension should be used immediately. Levoxyl® should be administered with a full glass of water to prevent gagging (due to tablet swelling).

Other Nasogastric tube: Bioavailability of levothyroxine is reduced if administered with enteral tube feeds. Since holding feedings for at least 1 hour before and after levothyroxine administration may not completely resolve the interaction, an increase in dose (eg, additional 25 mcg) may be necessary (Dickerson, 2010).

Preparation for Administration Dilute vial for injection with 5 mL normal saline. Reconstituted concentrations for the 100 mcg, 200 mcg and 500 mcg vials are 20 mcg/mL, 40 mcg/mL, and 100 mcg/mL, respectively. Shake well and use immediately after reconstitution (manufacturer recommendation); discard any unused portions.

Storage/Stability Store capsules, tablets, and injection at room temperature; excursions permitted to 15°C to 30°C (59°F to 86°F). Protect from light and moisture.

Additional stability data:

Stability in polypropylene syringes (100 mcg/mL in NS) at 5°C ± 1°C is 7 days (Gupta, 2000).

Stability in latex-free, PVC minibags protected from light and stored at 15°C to 30°C (59°F to 86°F) was 12 hours for a 2 mcg/mL concentration or 18 hours for a 0.4 mcg/mL concentration in NS. May be exposed to light; however, stability time is significantly reduced, especially for the 2 mcg/mL concentration (Strong, 2010).

Nursing Actions

Physical Assessment Monitor for hyper-/hypothyroidism on a regular basis during therapy.

Patient Education

• Discuss specific use of drug and side effects with patient as it relates to treatment. (HCAHPS: During this hospital stay, were you given any medicine that you had not taken before? Before giving you any new medicine, how often did hospital staff tell you what the medicine was for? How often did hospital staff describe possible side effects in a way you could understand?)

• Patient may experience alopecia. Have patient report immediately to prescriber angina, tachycardia, arrhythmia, headache, dyspnea, change in appetite, excessive weight gain or loss, diarrhea, dyspepsia, nausea, behavioral changes, anxiety, tremors, insomnia, temperature sensitivity, hyperhidrosis, leg cramps, asthenia, or menstrual irregularities (HCAHPS).

• Educate patient about signs of a significant reaction (eg, wheezing; chest tightness; fever; itching; bad cough; blue skin color; seizures; or swelling of face, lips, tongue, or throat). **Note:** This is not a comprehensive list of all side effects. Patient should consult prescriber for additional questions.

Intended Use and Disclaimer: Should not be printed and given to patients. This information is intended to serve as a concise initial reference for healthcare professionals to use when discussing medications with a patient. You must ultimately rely on your own discretion, experience and judgment in diagnosing, treating and advising patients.

Dietary Considerations Should be taken on an empty stomach, at least 30 minutes before food.

Lidocaine (Systemic) (LYE doe kane)

Brand Names: U.S. Xylocaine; Xylocaine (Cardiac); Xylocaine-MPF

Index Terms Lidocaine Hydrochloride; Lignocaine Hydrochloride

Pharmacologic Category Antiarrhythmic Agent, Class Ib; Local Anesthetic

Medication Safety Issues

High alert medication:

The Institute for Safe Medication Practices (ISMP) includes this medication (epidural administration; I.V. formulation) among its list of drugs which have a heightened risk of causing significant patient harm when used in error.

International issues:

Lidosen [Italy] may be confused with Lincocin brand name for lincomycin [U.S., Canada, and multiple international markets]; Lodosyn brand name for carbidopa [U.S.]

Pregnancy Risk Factor B

Lactation Enters breast milk/use caution

Breast-Feeding Considerations Lidocaine is excreted into breast milk. The manufacturer recommends that caution be used when administered to a nursing woman. When administered by injection for dental or obstetric analgesia, small amounts are detected in breast milk; oral bioavailability to the nursing infant is expected to be low and the amount of lidocaine available to the nursing infant would not be expected to cause adverse events (Lebedevs, 1993; Ortega, 1999). Cumulative exposure from all routes of administration should be considered.

Use Local and regional anesthesia by infiltration, nerve block, epidural, or spinal techniques; acute treatment of ventricular arrhythmias from myocardial infarction or cardiac manipulation (eg, cardiac surgery)

Note: The routine prophylactic use of lidocaine to prevent arrhythmia associated with fibrinolytic administration or to suppress isolated ventricular premature beats, couplets, runs of accelerated idioventricular rhythm, and nonsustained VT is not recommended (Antman, 2004).

Unlabeled Use

ACLS guidelines: Hemodynamically stable monomorphic ventricular tachycardia (VT) (preserved ventricular function); polymorphic VT (preserved ventricular function); drug-induced monomorphic VT; when amiodarone is not available, pulseless VT or ventricular fibrillation (VF) (unresponsive to defibrillation, CPR, and vasopressor administration)

PALS guidelines: When amiodarone is not available, pulseless VT or VF (unresponsive to defibrillation, CPR, and epinephrine administration); consider in patients with cocaine overdose to prevent arrhythmias secondary to MI

I.V. infusion for chronic pain syndrome

Mechanism of Action/Effect Class Ib antiarrhythmic; suppresses automaticity of conduction tissue by increasing electrical stimulation threshold of ventricles, His-Purkinje system, and spontaneous depolarization of ventricles during diastole by direct action on tissues; blocks both initiation and conduction of nerve impulses by decreasing the neuronal membrane's permeability to sodium ions, which results in inhibition of depolarization with resultant blockade of conduction

Contraindications Hypersensitivity to lidocaine or any component of the formulation; hypersensitivity to another local anesthetic of the amide type; Adam-Stokes syndrome; Wolff-Parkinson-White syndrome; severe degrees of SA, AV, or intraventricular heart block (except in patients with a functioning artificial pacemaker); premixed injection may contain corn-derived dextrose and its use is contraindicated in patients with allergy to corn or corn-related products

Warnings/Precautions Use caution in patients with severe hepatic dysfunction or pseudocholinesterase deficiency; may have increased risk of lidocaine toxicity.

Intravenous: Constant ECG monitoring is necessary during I.V. administration. Use cautiously in hepatic impairment, HF, marked hypoxia, severe respiratory depression, hypovolemia, history of malignant hyperthermia, or shock. Increased ventricular rate may be seen when administered to a patient with atrial fibrillation. Correct electrolyte disturbances, especially hypokalemia or hypomagnesemia, prior to use and throughout therapy. Use is contraindicated in patients with Wolff-Parkinson-White syndrome and severe degrees of SA, AV, or intraventricular heart block (except in patients with a functioning artificial pacemaker). Correct any underlying causes of ventricular arrhythmias. Monitor closely for signs and symptoms of CNS toxicity. The elderly may be prone to increased CNS and cardiovascular side effects. Reduce dose in hepatic dysfunction and CHF.

Injectable anesthetic: Follow appropriate administration techniques so as not to administer any intravascularly. Continuous intra-articular infusion of local anesthetics after arthroscopic or other surgical procedures is **not** an approved use; chondrolysis (primarily in the shoulder joint) has occurred following infusion, with some cases requiring arthroplasty or shoulder replacement. Solutions containing antimicrobial preservatives should not be used for epidural or spinal anesthesia. Some solutions contain a bisulfite; avoid in patients who are allergic to bisulfite. Resuscitative equipment, medicine and oxygen should be available in case of emergency. Use products containing epinephrine cautiously in patients with significant vascular disease, compromised blood flow, or during or following general anesthesia (increased risk of arrhythmias). Adjust the dose for the elderly, pediatric, acutely ill, and debilitated patients.

Drug Interactions

Avoid Concomitant Use

Avoid concomitant use of Lidocaine (Systemic) with any of the following: Conivaptan; Fusidic Acid (Systemic); Saquinavir

Decreased Effect

Lidocaine (Systemic) may decrease the levels/ effects of: Technetium Tc 99m Tilmanocept

The levels/effects of Lidocaine (Systemic) may be decreased by: Bosentan; CYP1A2 Inducers (Strong); CYP3A4 Inducers (Strong); Cyproterone; Dabrafenib; Deferasirox; Etravirine; Herbs (CYP3A4 Inducers); Mitotane; Tocilizumab

Increased Effect/Toxicity

Lidocaine (Systemic) may increase the levels/ effects of: Prilocaine; Sodium Nitrite

The levels/effects of Lidocaine (Systemic) may be increased by: Abiraterone Acetate; Amiodarone; Beta-Blockers; Conivaptan; CYP1A2 Inhibitors (Moderate); CYP1A2 Inhibitors (Strong); CYP3A4 Inhibitors (Moderate); CYP3A4 Inhibitors (Strong); Dasatinib; Deferasirox; Disopyramide; Fusidic Acid (Systemic); Hyaluronidase; Ivacaftor; Luliconazole; Mifepristone; Nitric Oxide; Saquinavir; Simeprevir; Stiripentol; Telaprevir; Vemurafenib

Nutritional/Ethanol Interactions Herb/Nutraceutical: St John's wort may decrease lidocaine levels; avoid concurrent use.

Adverse Reactions Effects vary with route of administration. Many effects are dose related. Frequency not defined.

Cardiovascular: Arrhythmia, bradycardia, arterial spasms, cardiovascular collapse, defibrillator threshold increased, edema, flushing, heart block, hypotension, sinus node supression, vascular insufficiency (periarticular injections)

Central nervous system: Agitation, anxiety, apprehension, coma, confusion, disorientation, dizziness, drowsiness, euphoria, hallucinations, headache, hyperesthesia, hypoesthesia, lethargy, lightheadedness, nervousness, psychosis, seizure, slurred speech, somnolence, unconsciousness

Gastrointestinal: Metallic taste, nausea, vomiting

Local: Thrombophlebitis

Neuromuscular & skeletal: Paresthesia, transient radicular pain (subarachnoid administration; up to 1.9%), tremor, twitching, weakness

Otic: Tinnitus

Respiratory: Bronchospasm, dyspnea, respiratory depression or arrest

Miscellaneous: Allergic reactions, anaphylactic reaction, anaphylactoid reaction, sensitivity to temperature extremes

Following spinal anesthesia: Positional headache (3%), shivering (2%), double vision (<1%), cauda equina syndrome, hypotension, nausea, peripheral nerve symptoms, respiratory inadequacy

Pharmacodynamics/Kinetics

Onset of Action Single bolus dose: 45-90 seconds

Duration of Action 10-20 minutes

Available Dosage Forms

Solution, Injection:
Xylocaine: 0.5% (50 mL); 1% (20 mL, 50 mL); 2% (10 mL, 20 mL, 50 mL)
Xylocaine-MPF: 0.5% (50 mL); 1% (2 mL, 5 mL, 10 mL, 30 mL); 1.5% (10 mL, 20 mL); 2% (2 mL, 5 mL, 10 mL); 4% (5 mL)
Generic: 0.5% (50 mL); 1% (2 mL, 5 mL, 10 mL, 20 mL, 30 mL, 50 mL); 1.5% (20 mL); 2% (2 mL, 5 mL, 20 mL, 50 mL)

Solution, Injection [preservative free]:
Generic: 0.5% (50 mL); 1% (2 mL, 5 mL, 30 mL); 1.5% (20 mL); 2% (2 mL, 5 mL, 10 mL); 4% (5 mL)

Solution, Intravenous:
Xylocaine (Cardiac): 20 mg/mL (5 mL)
Generic: 10 mg/mL (5 mL); 20 mg/mL (5 mL); 0.4% [4 mg/mL] (250 mL, 500 mL); 0.8% [8 mg/mL] (250 mL); 2% (5 mL); 5% [50 mg/mL] (2 mL)

Solution, Intravenous [preservative free]:
Generic: 10 mg/mL (5 mL); 20 mg/mL (5 mL)

General Dosage Range Dosage adjustment recommended in patients with hepatic impairment.
I.V.:
Children: Loading dose: 1 mg/kg, may repeat 0.5-1 mg/kg; Infusion: 20-50 mcg/kg/minute
Adults: Bolus: 1-1.5 mg/kg, may repeat 0.5-0.75 mg/kg up to a total of 3 mg/kg; Infusion: 1-4 mg/minute
Local injection: Children and Adults: Maximum: 4.5 mg/kg/dose; do not repeat within 2 hours

Usual Infusion Concentrations: Pediatric Note: Premixed solutions available
I.V. infusion: 8000 mcg/mL

Usual Infusion Concentrations: Adult Note: Premixed solutions available
I.V. infusion: 1000 mg in 250 mL (concentration: 4 mg/mL) or 2000 mg in 250 mL (concentration: 8 mg/mL) of D_5W

Administration

I.V.
Bolus: According to the manufacturer, may administer at 25 to 50 mg/minute. In the setting of cardiac arrest (eg, ventricular fibrillation or pulseless ventricular tachycardia), may be infused rapidly into a peripheral vein (Dorian, 2002).

Continuous infusion: After initial bolus dosing, may administer as a continuous infusion; refer to indication-specific infusion rates in dosing for detailed recommendations. In the setting of cardiac arrest, infusion may be initiated once patient has return of spontaneous circulation resulting from lidocaine administration; however, there is no evidence to support subsequent continuous infusion to prevent recurrence (ACLS [Peberdy, 2010]). Local thrombophlebitis may occur in patients receiving prolonged I.V. infusions.

Injectable Detail pH: 5-7 (injection); 3.5-6 (premixed infusion solution in D_5W)

Endotracheal Endotracheal (unlabeled administration route): Dilute in NS or sterile water. Absorption is greater with sterile water and results in less impairment of PaO_2 (Hahnel, 1990). Stop compressions, spray drug quickly down tube. Flush with 5 mL of NS and follow immediately with several quick insufflations and continue chest compressions.

Intraosseous I.O. (unlabeled administration route): Intraosseous administration is a safe and effective alternative to venous access in children with cardiac arrest; the onset for most medications is similar to that of I.V. administration (PALS, 2010). In adults, I.O. administration is a reasonable alternative when quick I.V. access is not feasible (ACLS, 2010).

Preparation for Administration Local infiltration: Buffered lidocaine for injectable local anesthetic may be prepared: Add 2 mL of sodium bicarbonate 8.4% to 18 mL of lidocaine 1% (Christoph, 1988).

Storage/Stability Injection: Stable at room temperature. Stability of parenteral admixture at room temperature (25°C) is the expiration date on premixed bag; out of overwrap stability is 30 days.

Nursing Actions

Physical Assessment Dental/local anesthetic: Use caution to prevent gagging or choking. Avoid food or drink for 1 hour. **Antiarrhythmic: I.V.:** Monitor ECG, blood pressure, and respirations closely and continually. Keep patient supine to reduce hypotensive effects. Assess frequently for adverse reactions or signs of CNS toxicity (eg, drowsiness, lightheadedness, dizziness, tinnitus, blurred vision, vomiting, twitching, tremor, lethargy, coma, agitation, slurred speech, seizure, anxiety, euphoria, hallucinations, paresthesia, psychosis).

Patient Education

- Discuss specific use of drug and side effects with patient as it relates to treatment. (HCAHPS: During this hospital stay, were you given any medicine that you had not taken before? Before giving you any new medicine, how often did hospital staff tell you what the medicine was

for? How often did hospital staff describe possible side effects in a way you could understand?)
- Patient may experience injection site irritation, asthenia, dizziness, blurred vision, or paresthesia. Have patient report immediately to prescriber dyspnea, tachycardia, illogical thinking, nervousness and anxiety, or rash (HCAHPS).
- Educate patient about signs of a significant reaction (eg, wheezing; chest tightness; fever; itching; bad cough; blue skin color; seizures; or swelling of face, lips, tongue, or throat). **Note:** This is not a comprehensive list of all side effects. Patient should consult prescriber for additional questions.

Intended Use and Disclaimer: Should not be printed and given to patients. This information is intended to serve as a concise initial reference for healthcare professionals to use when discussing medications with a patient. You must ultimately rely on your own discretion, experience and judgment in diagnosing, treating and advising patients.

Dietary Considerations Premixed injection may contain corn-derived dextrose and its use is contraindicated in patients with allergy to corn-related products.

Related Information

Peak and Trough Guidelines *on page 1710*

Lidocaine (Topical) (LYE doe kane)

Brand Names: U.S. AneCream [OTC]; AneCream5 [OTC]; LC-4 Lidocaine [OTC]; LC-5 Lidocaine [OTC]; Lidoderm; LidoRx; LMX 4 Plus [OTC]; LMX 4 [OTC]; LMX 5 [OTC]; LTA 360 Kit; Predator [OTC]; RectiCare [OTC]; Tecnu First Aid [OTC]; Topicaine 5 [OTC]; Topicaine [OTC]; Xylocaine

Index Terms Lidocaine Hydrochloride; Lidocaine Patch; Lignocaine Hydrochloride; Viscous Lidocaine; Xylocaine Viscous

Pharmacologic Category Analgesic, Topical; Local Anesthetic

Pregnancy Risk Factor B

Lactation Enters breast milk/use caution

Use

Rectal: Temporary relief of pain and itching due to anorectal disorders

Topical: Local anesthetic for oral mucous membrane; use in laser/cosmetic surgeries; minor burns, cuts, and abrasions of the skin

Oral topical solution (2% viscous): Topical anesthesia of irritated or inflamed oral mucous membranes and pharyngeal tissue; reducing gagging during the taking of x-ray

Oral Topical solution (4%): Topical anesthesia of accessible mucous membranes of the oral and nasal cavities and proximal portions of the digestive tract.

Jelly: Prevention and control of pain in procedures involving the male and female urethra; for topical treatment of painful urethritis

Patch (Lidoderm): Relief of allodynia (painful hypersensitivity) and chronic pain in postherpetic neuralgia

Patch (LidoPatch): Temporary relief of localized pain

Available Dosage Forms

Cream, External:
AneCream [OTC]: 4% (5 g, 15 g, 30 g)
AneCream5 [OTC]: 5% (15 g, 30 g)
LC-4 Lidocaine [OTC]: 4% (45 g)
LC-5 Lidocaine [OTC]: 5% (45 g)
LMX 4 [OTC]: 4% (5 g, 15 g, 30 g)
LMX 5 [OTC]: 5% (15 g, 30 g)
Predator [OTC]: 4% (63 g)
RectiCare [OTC]: 5% (30 g)
Generic: 3% (28.3 g, 28.35 g, 85 g)

Gel, External:
LidoRx: 3% (10 mL, 30 mL)
Tecnu First Aid [OTC]: 0.2-2.5% (56.7 g)
Topicaine [OTC]: 4% (10 g, 30 g, 113 g)
Topicaine 5 [OTC]: 5% (10 g, 30 g, 113 g)
Generic: 2% (5 mL, 20 mL, 30 mL)

Gel, External [preservative free]:
Generic: 2% (5 mL, 10 mL)

Kit, External:
AneCream [OTC]: 4%
LMX 4 Plus [OTC]: 4%

Lotion, External:
Generic: 3% (177 mL)

Ointment, External:
Generic: 5% (30 g, 35.44 g, 50 g)

Patch, External:
Lidoderm: 5% (1 ea, 30 ea)
Generic: 5% (1 ea, 30 ea)

Solution, External:
Xylocaine: 4% (50 mL)
Generic: 4% (50 mL)

Solution, Mouth/Throat:
Generic: 2% (15 mL, 100 mL)

Solution, Mouth/Throat [preservative free]:
LTA 360 Kit: 4% (4 mL)
Generic: 4% (4 mL)

General Dosage Range Topical:

Cream: *Children, Adolescents, and Adults:* Dosage varies greatly depending on product

Gel, ointment, solution: *Adults:* Apply to affected area ≤4 times daily as needed (maximum: 4.5 mg/kg/dose; 300 mg per dose)

Jelly:
Children: Maximum: 4.5 mg/kg/dose
Adults: 3-30 mL (maximum: 30 mL [600 mg]/12-hour period)

Oral topical solution (2% viscous):
Infants and Children <3 years: 1.25 mL applied no more frequently than every 3 hours (maximum: 4 doses per 12-hour period)
Children ≥3 years and Adolescents: Should not exceed 4.5 mg/kg/dose (or 300 mg per dose);

swished in the mouth and spit out no more frequently than every 3 hours

Adults: 15 mL swished in the mouth and spit out or gargled no more frequently than every 3 hours (maximum: 4.5 mg/kg [or 300 mg per dose]; 8 doses per 24-hour period)

Patch: *Adults:*

Lidoderm: Apply up to 3 patches in a single application for up to 12 hours in any 24-hour period

LidoPatch: Apply 1 patch in a single application for up to 12 hours in any 24-hour period

Administration

Topical

Gel (Topicaine): Apply a moderately thick layer to affected area (~1/8 inch thick). Allow time for numbness to develop (~20-60 minutes after application). When used prior to laser surgery, avoid mucous membranes and remove prior to laser treatment.

Oral topical solution (2% viscous): Mouth irritation or inflammation: Have patient swish medication around mouth and then spit it out. In children <3 years, apply to affected area with cotton-tipped applicator. Do not eat for 60 minutes following use. For pharyngeal anesthesia, patient should gargle and may swallow medication. In children <3 years, apply to affected area with cotton-tipped applicator.

Patch:

Lidoderm: Apply to most painful area of skin immediately after removal from protective envelope. May be cut (with scissors, prior to removal of release liner) to appropriate size. Clothing may be worn over application area. After removal from skin, fold used patches so the adhesive side sticks to itself; avoid contact with eyes. Remove immediately if burning sensation occurs. Wash hands after application. Avoid exposing application site to external heat sources (eg, heating pad, electric blanket, heat lamp, hot tub).

LidoPatch: Remove protective film and apply to painful area. Avoid contact with eyes or mucous membranes. Wash hands after application. Avoid exposing application site to external heat sources (eg, heating pad, electric blanket, heat lamp, hot tub).

Nursing Actions

Patient Education

- Discuss specific use of drug and side effects with patient as it relates to treatment. (HCAHPS: During this hospital stay, were you given any medicine that you had not taken before? Before giving you any new medicine, how often did hospital staff tell you what the medicine was for? How often did hospital staff describe possible side effects in a way you could understand?)
- Patient may experience skin irritation. Have patient report immediately to prescriber severe

stomatitis, significant paresthesia, or rash (HCAHPS).

- Educate patient about signs of a significant reaction (eg, wheezing; chest tightness; fever; itching; bad cough; blue skin color; seizures; or swelling of face, lips, tongue, or throat). **Note:** This is not a comprehensive list of all side effects. Patient should consult prescriber for additional questions.

Intended Use and Disclaimer: Should not be printed and given to patients. This information is intended to serve as a concise initial reference for healthcare professionals to use when discussing medications with a patient. You must ultimately rely on your own discretion, experience and judgment in diagnosing, treating and advising patients.

Lidocaine and Epinephrine
(LYE doe kane & ep i NEF rin)

Brand Names: U.S. Lignospan® Forte; Lignospan® Standard; Xylocaine® MPF With Epinephrine; Xylocaine® With Epinephrine

Index Terms Epinephrine and Lidocaine

Pharmacologic Category Local Anesthetic

Pregnancy Risk Factor B

Lactation Lidocaine enters breast milk/use caution

Use Local infiltration anesthesia; AVS for nerve block

Available Dosage Forms

Injection, solution:

Generics:

0.5% / 1:200,000: Lidocaine hydrochloride 0.5% [5 mg/mL] and epinephrine 1:200,000 (50 mL)

1% / 1:100,000: Lidocaine hydrochloride 1% [10 mg/mL] and epinephrine 1:100,000 (20 mL, 30 mL, 50 mL)

2% / 1:100,000: Lidocaine hydrochloride 2% [20 mg/mL] and epinephrine 1:100,000 (30 mL, 50 mL)

Brands:

Xylocaine® with Epinephrine:

0.5% / 1:200,000: Lidocaine hydrochloride 0.5% [5 mg/mL] and epinephrine 1:200,000 (50 mL)

1% / 1:100,000: Lidocaine hydrochloride 1% [10 mg/mL] and epinephrine 1:100,000 (10 mL, 20 mL, 50 mL)

2% / 1:100,000: Lidocaine hydrochloride 2% [20 mg/mL] and epinephrine 1:100,000 (10 mL, 20 mL, 50 mL)

Injection, solution [preservative free]:

Generics:

1.5% / 1:200,000: Lidocaine hydrochloride 1.5% [15 mg/mL] and epinephrine 1:200,000 (5 mL, 30 mL)

2% / 1:200,000: Lidocaine hydrochloride 2% [20 mg/mL] and epinephrine 1:200,000 (20 mL)

◄ *Brands:*
Xylocaine®-MPF with Epinephrine:
1% / 1:200,000: Lidocaine hydrochloride 1% [10 mg/mL] and epinephrine 1:200,000 (5 mL, 10 mL, 30 mL)
1.5% / 1:200,000: Lidocaine hydrochloride 1.5% [15 mg/mL] and epinephrine 1:200,000 (5 mL, 10 mL, 30 mL)
2% / 1:200,000: Lidocaine hydrochloride 2% [20 mg/mL] and epinephrine 1:200,000 (5 mL, 10 mL, 20 mL)

Injection, solution [for dental use]:
Generics:
2% / 1:50,000: Lidocaine hydrochloride 2% [20 mg/mL] and epinephrine 1:50,000 (1.7 mL, 1.8 mL)
2% / 1:100,000: Lidocaine hydrochloride 2% [20 mg/mL] and epinephrine 1:100,000 (1.7 mL, 1.8 mL)
Brands:
Lignospan® Forte: 2% / 1:50,000: Lidocaine hydrochloride 2% [20 mg/mL] and epinephrine 1:50,000 (1.7 mL)
Lignospan® Standard: 2% / 1:100,000: Lidocaine hydrochloride 2% [20 mg/mL] and epinephrine 1:100,000 (1.7 mL)

General Dosage Range Conduction block or infiltration (dental):
Children <12 years: 20-30 mg (1-1.5 mL) of 2% lidocaine with epinephrine 1:100,000 (maximum: 4.5 mg/kg of lidocaine or 100-150 mg as a single dose)
Children ≥12 years and Adults: Do not exceed 7 mg/kg body weight up to a maximum range of 300 mg (usual dental practice) to 500 mg (approved product labeling) of lidocaine hydrochloride and 3 mcg (0.003 mg) of epinephrine/kg of body weight **or** 0.2 mg epinephrine per dental appointment.

Administration
Other Injection solution for infiltration: Before injecting, withdraw syringe plunger to ensure injection is not into vein or artery. Aspirate the syringe after tissue penetration and before injection to minimize chance of direct vascular injection.

Nursing Actions
Physical Assessment See individual agents.
Patient Education
• Discuss specific use of drug and side effects with patient as it relates to treatment. (HCAHPS: During this hospital stay, were you given any medicine that you had not taken before? Before giving you any new medicine, how often did hospital staff tell you what the medicine was for? How often did hospital staff describe possible side effects in a way you could understand?)
• Patient may experience injection site irritation. Have patient report immediately to prescriber significant change in balance, sudden vision changes, eye pain, eye irritation, paresthesia,

severe skin irritation, or illogical thinking (HCAHPS).
• Educate patient about signs of a significant reaction (eg, wheezing; chest tightness; fever; itching; bad cough; blue skin color; seizures; or swelling of face, lips, tongue, or throat). **Note:** This is not a comprehensive list of all side effects. Patient should consult prescriber for additional questions.

Intended Use and Disclaimer: Should not be printed and given to patients. This information is intended to serve as a concise initial reference for healthcare professionals to use when discussing medications with a patient. You must ultimately rely on your own discretion, experience and judgment in diagnosing, treating and advising patients.
Related Information
EPINEPHrine (Systemic, Oral Inhalation) *on page 538*
Lidocaine (Topical) *on page 940*

Linaclotide (lin AK loe tide)

Brand Names: U.S. Linzess
Index Terms Linaclotide Acetate
Pharmacologic Category Gastrointestinal Agent, Miscellaneous
Medication Guide Available Yes
Pregnancy Risk Factor C
Lactation Excretion in breast milk unknown/use caution
Breast-Feeding Considerations It is not known if linaclotide is excreted in breast milk; linaclotide and its metabolite are not measurable in plasma when used at recommended doses. The manufacturer recommends to use caution if administered to breast-feeding women.
Use Treatment of chronic idiopathic constipation (CIC); treatment of irritable bowel syndrome with constipation (IBS-C) in adults
Mechanism of Action/Effect Linaclotide increases intestinal fluid and reduces transit time; may decrease visceral pain.
Contraindications Use in pediatric patients ≤6 years of age; known or suspected mechanical gastrointestinal obstruction
Warnings/Precautions [U.S. Boxed Warning]: Use is contraindicated in pediatric patients ≤6 years of age. Use in pediatric patients 6-17 years of age should be avoided. Deaths were observed in young juvenile animals during non-clinical studies; deaths were not observed in older juvenile animals. There are not sufficient safety and efficacy data to support use in pediatric patients. May cause severe diarrhea; consider dose suspension if necessary. Patients should be instructed to discontinue use and contact their healthcare provider if severe diarrhea occurs.

Administration with a high-fat meal may worsen diarrhea.

Drug Interactions

Avoid Concomitant Use There are no known interactions where it is recommended to avoid concomitant use.

Decreased Effect There are no known significant interactions involving a decrease in effect.

Increased Effect/Toxicity There are no known significant interactions involving an increase in effect.

Adverse Reactions Adverse reactions reported with use in IBS-C and CIC.

>10%: Gastrointestinal: Diarrhea (16% to 20%; severe diarrhea: 2%)

1% to 10%:

Central nervous system: Headache (4%), fatigue (<2%)

Endocrine & metabolic: Dehydration (≤1%)

Gastrointestinal: Abdominal pain (7%), flatulence (4% to 6%), abdominal distension (2% to 3%), viral gastroenteritis (≤3%), dyspepsia (<2%), fecal incontinence (<2%), gastroesophageal reflux disease (<2%), vomiting (<2%)

Respiratory: Upper respiratory tract infection (5%), sinusitis (3%)

Available Dosage Forms

Capsule, Oral:

Linzess: 145 mcg, 290 mcg

General Dosage Range

Oral: *Adults:* 145 mcg or 290 mcg once daily

Administration

Oral Oral: Administer at least 30 minutes before breakfast on an empty stomach; loose stools and greater stool frequency may occur after administration with a high-fat breakfast. Swallow capsule whole; do not break or chew capsules.

Storage/Stability Store at 25°C (77°F) in tightly closed, original container with included desiccant packet; excursions permitted between 15°C and 30°C (59°F and 86°F). Do not repackage; protect from moisture.

Nursing Actions

Physical Assessment Monitor for efficacy. Educate patient about when to call if diarrhea occurs. Monitor volume status and frequency of bowel movements.

Patient Education

• Discuss specific use of drug and side effects with patient as it relates to treatment. (HCAHPS: During this hospital stay, were you given any medicine that you had not taken before? Before giving you any new medicine, how often did hospital staff tell you what the medicine was for? How often did hospital staff describe possible side effects in a way you could understand?)

• Patient may experience diarrhea, dyspepsia, gas, upper respiratory tract infection, and headache. Have patient report immediately to prescriber severe diarrhea or dizziness (HCAHPS).

• Educate patient about signs of a significant reaction (eg, wheezing; chest tightness; fever; itching; bad cough; blue skin color; seizures; or swelling of face, lips, tongue, or throat). **Note:** This is not a comprehensive list of all side effects. Patient should consult prescriber for additional questions.

Intended Use and Disclaimer: Should not be printed and given to patients. This information is intended to serve as a concise initial reference for healthcare professionals to use when discussing medications with a patient. You must ultimately rely on your own discretion, experience and judgment in diagnosing, treating and advising patients.

Dietary Considerations Take at least 30 minutes before breakfast on an empty stomach. Loose stools and greater stool frequency may occur after administration with a high-fat breakfast.

Related Information

Oral Medications That Should Not Be Crushed or Altered *on page 1712*

Linagliptin (lin a GLIP tin)

Brand Names: U.S. Tradjenta

Index Terms BI-1356; Trajenta

Pharmacologic Category Antidiabetic Agent, Dipeptidyl Peptidase IV (DPP-IV) Inhibitor

Medication Safety Issues

High alert medication:

The Institute for Safe Medication Practices (ISMP) includes this medication among its list of drug classes which have a heightened risk of causing significant patient harm when used in error.

Medication Guide Available Yes

Pregnancy Risk Factor B

Lactation Excretion in breast milk unknown/use caution

Breast-Feeding Considerations It is not known if linagliptin is excreted in breast milk. The manufacturer recommends that caution be used if administered to breast-feeding women.

Use Management of type 2 diabetes mellitus (non-insulin dependent, NIDDM) as an adjunct to diet and exercise as monotherapy or in combination with other antidiabetic agents

Mechanism of Action/Effect Linagliptin inhibits dipeptidyl peptidase IV (DPP-IV) enzyme resulting in increased insulin synthesis and release and decreased hepatic glucose production.

Contraindications Hypersensitivity to linagliptin or any component of the formulation

Canadian labeling: Additional contraindications: Use in type 1 diabetes mellitus or diabetic ketoacidosis

Warnings/Precautions Avoid use in type 1 diabetes mellitus (insulin dependent, IDDM) and ▶

diabetic ketoacidosis (DKA) due to lack of efficacy in these populations. Diabetes self-management education (DSME) is essential to maximize the effectiveness of therapy. Cases of acute pancreatitis, including fatalities, have been reported with use. Monitor for signs/symptoms of pancreatitis; discontinue use immediately if pancreatitis is suspected and initiate appropriate management. Use with caution in patients with a history of pancreatitis as it is not known if this population is at greater risk. Clinical trials included only a limited number of patients with heart failure (HF). No specific recommendations regarding this population are provided in the approved U.S. labeling (Canadian labeling recommends against use in this population). Potentially significant drug-drug interactions may exist, requiring dose or frequency adjustment, additional monitoring, and/or selection of alternative therapy.

Drug Interactions

Avoid Concomitant Use There are no known interactions where it is recommended to avoid concomitant use.

Decreased Effect

The levels/effects of Linagliptin may be decreased by: Bosentan; Corticosteroids (Orally Inhaled); Corticosteroids (Systemic); CYP3A4 Inducers (Strong); Dabrafenib; Deferasirox; Herbs (CYP3A4 Inducers); Loop Diuretics; Luteinizing Hormone-Releasing Hormone Analogs; P-glycoprotein/ABCB1 Inducers; Somatropin; Thiazide Diuretics; Tocilizumab

Increased Effect/Toxicity

Linagliptin may increase the levels/effects of: ACE Inhibitors; Hypoglycemic Agents

The levels/effects of Linagliptin may be increased by: Herbs (Hypoglycemic Properties); MAO Inhibitors; Pegvisomant; P-glycoprotein/ABCB1 Inhibitors; Ritonavir; Salicylates; Selective Serotonin Reuptake Inhibitors

Nutritional/Ethanol Interactions

Ethanol: Caution with ethanol (may cause hypoglycemia).

Herb/Nutraceutical: Herbs with hypoglycemic properties may enhance the hypoglycemic effect of linagliptin. This includes alfalfa, aloe, bilberry, bitter melon, burdock, celery, damiana, fenugreek, garcinia, garlic, ginger, ginseng (American), gymnema, marshmallow, stinging nettle.

Adverse Reactions

>10%: Endocrine & metabolic: Hypoglycemia (combined with metformin and/or sulfonylurea [15% to 23%]; monotherapy [<1% to 7%]; metformin [<1%], pioglitazone [<1%])

1% to 10%:

Central nervous system: Headache (6%)

Endocrine & metabolic: Hyperlipidemia (3%), hyperuricemia (3%), increased serum triglycerides (2% to 3%), weight gain (2%)

Gastrointestinal: Diarrhea (3%), constipation (2%)

Genitourinary: Urinary tract infection (3%)

Neuromuscular & skeletal: Arthralgia (6%), back pain (6%)

Respiratory: Nasopharyngitis (6% to 7%), cough (2%)

Available Dosage Forms

Tablet, Oral:

Tradjenta: 5 mg

General Dosage Range Oral: *Adults:* 5 mg once daily

Concomitant use with insulin and/or insulin secretagogues (eg, sulfonylureas): Reduced dose of insulin and/or insulin secretagogues may be needed.

Administration

Oral May be administered with or without food.

Storage/Stability Store at 25°C (77°F); excursions permitted between 15°C to 30°C (59°F to 86°F).

Nursing Actions

Patient Education

• Discuss specific use of drug and side effects with patient as it relates to treatment. (HCAHPS: During this hospital stay, were you given any medicine that you had not taken before? Before giving you any new medicine, how often did hospital staff tell you what the medicine was for? How often did hospital staff describe possible side effects in a way you could understand?)

• Patient may experience pharyngitis, rhinitis, rhinorrhea, or diarrhea. Have patient report immediately to prescriber signs of hypoglycemia or signs of pancreatitis (HCAHPS).

• Educate patient about signs of a significant reaction (eg, wheezing; chest tightness; fever; itching; bad cough; blue skin color; seizures; or swelling of face, lips, tongue, or throat). **Note:** This is not a comprehensive list of all side effects. Patient should consult prescriber for additional questions.

Intended Use and Disclaimer: Should not be printed and given to patients. This information is intended to serve as a concise initial reference for healthcare professionals to use when discussing medications with a patient. You must ultimately rely on your own discretion, experience and judgment in diagnosing, treating and advising patients.

Dietary Considerations May be taken without regard to food. Individualized medical nutrition therapy (MNT) based on ADA recommendations is an integral part of therapy.

Linagliptin and Metformin
(lin a GLIP tin & met FOR min)

Brand Names: U.S. Jentadueto

Index Terms Linagliptin and Metformin Hydrochloride; Metformin and Linagliptin; Metformin Hydrochloride and Linagliptin

Pharmacologic Category Antidiabetic Agent, Biguanide; Antidiabetic Agent, Dipeptidyl Peptidase IV (DPP-IV) Inhibitor

Medication Safety Issues

Sound-alike/look-alike issues:

Linagliptin and Metformin may be confused with Sitagliptin and Metformin

High alert medication:

The Institute for Safe Medication Practices (ISMP) includes this medication among its list of drug classes which have a heightened risk of causing significant patient harm when used in error.

Medication Guide Available Yes

Pregnancy Risk Factor B

Use Management of type 2 diabetes mellitus (non-insulin dependent, NIDDM) as an adjunct to diet and exercise in patients when treatment with both linagliptin and metformin is appropriate

Available Dosage Forms

Tablet, oral:

Jentadueto™ 2.5/500: Linagliptin 2.5 mg and metformin 500 mg

Jentadueto™ 2.5/850: Linagliptin 2.5 mg and metformin 850 mg

Jentadueto™ 2.5/1000: Linagliptin 2.5 mg and metformin 1000 mg

General Dosage Range Oral: *Adults:* Linagliptin 2.5 mg and metformin 500-1000 mg twice daily (maximum: 5 mg daily [linagliptin], 2000 mg daily [metformin])

Administration

Oral Administer with meals, at the same time each day.

Nursing Actions

Physical Assessment See individual agents.

Patient Education

• Discuss specific use of drug and side effects with patient as it relates to treatment. (HCAHPS: During this hospital stay, were you given any medicine that you had not taken before? Before giving you any new medicine, how often did hospital staff tell you what the medicine was for? How often did hospital staff describe possible side effects in a way you could understand?)

• Patient may experience dyspepsia, nausea, diarrhea, flatulence, asthenia, headache, pharyngitis, rhinitis, or rhinorrhea. Have patient report immediately to prescriber signs of hypoglycemia, signs of pancreatitis, or signs of lactic acidosis (HCAHPS).

• Educate patient about signs of a significant reaction (eg, wheezing; chest tightness; fever; itching; bad cough; blue skin color; seizures; or swelling of face, lips, tongue, or throat). **Note:** This is not a comprehensive list of all side effects. Patient should consult prescriber for additional questions.

Intended Use and Disclaimer: Should not be printed and given to patients. This information is intended to serve as a concise initial reference for healthcare professionals to use when discussing medications with a patient. You must ultimately rely on your own discretion, experience and judgment in diagnosing, treating and advising patients.

Related Information

Linagliptin *on page 943*

MetFORMIN *on page 1014*

Lindane (LIN dane)

Index Terms Benzene Hexachloride; Gamma Benzene Hexachloride; Hexachlorocyclohexane; Kwell

Pharmacologic Category Antiparasitic Agent, Topical; Pediculocide; Scabicidal Agent

Medication Guide Available Yes

Pregnancy Risk Factor C

Lactation Enters breast milk/not recommended

Use

Lotion: Treatment of *Sarcoptes scabiei* (scabies)

Shampoo: Treatment of *Pediculus capitis* (head lice) and *Phthirus pubis* (crab lice)

Note: Not recommended for first line-treatment; use should be reserved for patients who are intolerant to or have failed first-line agents.

Available Dosage Forms

Lotion, External:

Generic: 1% (60 mL)

Shampoo, External:

Generic: 1% (60 mL)

General Dosage Range Topical:

Lotion: *Infants, Children, Adolescents, and Adults* Apply a thin layer; bathe and remove drug after 8-12 hours (maximum: 60 mL). Do not retreat.

Shampoo: *Infants, Children, Adolescents, and Adults* Apply to dry hair (maximum: 60 mL). Do not retreat.

Administration

Topical Shake well prior to use. For topical use only; never administer orally. Caregivers should apply with gloves (avoid natural latex, may be permeable to lindane). Rinse off with warm (not hot) water.

Lotion: Apply to dry, cool skin; do not apply to face or eyes. Wait at least 1 hour after bathing or showering (wet or warm skin increases absorption). Skin should be clean and free of any other lotions, creams, or oil prior to lindane application. Do not use on open wounds or sores. Do not use occlusive dressings.

Shampoo: Apply to clean, dry hair. Wait at least 1 hour after washing hair before applying lindane shampoo. Hair should be washed with a shampoo not containing a conditioner; hair and skin of head and neck should be free of any lotions, oils, or creams prior to lindane application. Do not cover with shower cap or towel.

Hazardous agent; use appropriate precautions for handling and disposal (EPA, U-listed)

◀ ## Nursing Actions
Physical Assessment Assess head, hair, and skin surfaces for presence of lice and nits. Teach patient appropriate application.

Patient Education
- Discuss specific use of drug and side effects with patient as it relates to treatment. (HCAHPS: During this hospital stay, were you given any medicine that you had not taken before? Before giving you any new medicine, how often did hospital staff tell you what the medicine was for? How often did hospital staff describe possible side effects in a way you could understand?)
- Patient may experience xeroderma or headache. Have patient report immediately to prescriber severe dizziness, paresthesia, considerable skin irritation, or rash (HCAHPS).
- Educate patient about signs of a significant reaction (eg, wheezing; chest tightness; fever; itching; bad cough; blue skin color; seizures; or swelling of face, lips, tongue, or throat). **Note:** This is not a comprehensive list of all side effects. Patient should consult prescriber for additional questions.

Intended Use and Disclaimer: Should not be printed and given to patients. This information is intended to serve as a concise initial reference for healthcare professionals to use when discussing medications with a patient. You must ultimately rely on your own discretion, experience and judgment in diagnosing, treating and advising patients.

Linezolid (li NE zoh lid)

Brand Names: U.S. Zyvox
Pharmacologic Category Antibiotic, Oxazolidinone
Medication Safety Issues
Sound-alike/look-alike issues:
Zyvox may be confused with Zosyn, Zovirax
Pregnancy Risk Factor C
Lactation Excreted in breast milk/use caution
Breast-Feeding Considerations Linezolid is excreted into breast milk. The manufacturer advises caution if administering linezolid to a breast-feeding woman. Nondose-related effects could include modification of bowel flora.

Use Treatment of vancomycin-resistant *Enterococcus faecium* (VRE) infections, nosocomial pneumonia caused by *Staphylococcus aureus* (including MRSA) or *Streptococcus pneumoniae* (including multidrug-resistant strains [MDRSP]), complicated and uncomplicated skin and skin structure infections (including diabetic foot infections without concomitant osteomyelitis), and community-acquired pneumonia caused by susceptible gram-positive organisms

Unlabeled Use Treatment of prosthetic joint infection

Mechanism of Action/Effect Inhibits bacterial protein synthesis by binding to bacterial 23S ribosomal RNA of the 50S subunit. This prevents the formation of a functional 70S initiation complex that is essential for the bacterial translation process. Linezolid is bacteriostatic against enterococci and staphylococci and bactericidal against most strains of streptococci.

Contraindications Hypersensitivity to linezolid or any other component of the formulation; concurrent use or within 2 weeks of MAO inhibitors

Warnings/Precautions Myelosuppression has been reported and may be dependent on duration of therapy (generally >2 weeks of treatment); use with caution in patients with pre-existing myelosuppression, in patients receiving other drugs which may cause bone marrow suppression, or in chronic infection (previous or concurrent antibiotic therapy). Weekly CBC monitoring is recommended. Consider discontinuation in patients developing myelosuppression (or in whom myelosuppression worsens during treatment).

Lactic acidosis has been reported with use. Linezolid exhibits mild MAO inhibitor properties and has the potential to have the same interactions as other MAO inhibitors; use with caution and monitor closely in patients with uncontrolled hypertension, pheochromocytoma, carcinoid syndrome, or untreated hyperthyroidism; do not use in the absence of close monitoring. Hypoglycemic episodes have been reported; use with caution and closely monitor glucose in diabetic patients. Dose reductions/discontinuation of concurrent hypoglycemic agents or discontinuation of linezolid may be required. Symptoms of agitation, confusion, hallucinations, hyper-reflexia, myoclonus, shivering, and tachycardia may occur with concomitant proserotonergic drugs (eg, SSRIs/SNRIs, tricyclic antidepressants, triptans, meperidine, bupropion) or agents which reduce linezolid's metabolism; these medications should not be used concurrently unless patient is closely monitored for signs/symptoms of serotonin syndrome or neuroleptic malignant syndrome-like reactions. Patients maintained on proserotonergic drugs requiring urgent treatment with linezolid may receive linezolid if the other proserotonergic drug is discontinued promptly and the benefits of linezolid outweigh risks; monitor for 2 weeks (5 weeks for fluoxetine) after discontinuation of maintenance drug or 24 hours after last linezolid dose, whichever comes first. Unnecessary use may lead to the development of resistance to linezolid; consider alternatives before initiating outpatient treatment.

Peripheral and optic neuropathy (with vision loss) has been reported in adults and children and may occur primarily with extended courses of therapy >28 days; any symptoms of visual change or impairment warrant immediate ophthalmic evaluation and possible discontinuation of therapy.

Seizures have been reported; use with caution in patients with a history of seizures. Prolonged use may result in fungal or bacterial superinfection, including *C. difficile*-associated diarrhea (CDAD) and pseudomembranous colitis; CDAD has been observed >2 months postantibiotic treatment.

Due to inconsistent concentrations in the CSF, empiric use in pediatric patients with CNS infections is not recommended by the manufacturer; however, there are multiple case reports describing successful treatment of documented VRE and *Staphylococcus aureus* CNS and shunt infections in the literature. Linezolid should not be used in the empiric treatment of catheter-related bloodstream infection (CRBSI), but may be appropriate for targeted therapy (Mermel, 2009). Oral suspension contains phenylalanine.

Drug Interactions

Avoid Concomitant Use

Avoid concomitant use of Linezolid with any of the following: Anilidopiperidine Opioids; Apraclonidine; AtoMOXetine; Bezafibrate; Buprenorphine; BuPROPion; BusPIRone; CarBAMazepine; CloZAPine; Cyclobenzaprine; Cyproheptadine; Dexmethylphenidate; Dextromethorphan; Diethylpropion; Hydrocodone; HYDROmorphone; Isomethepene; Levonordefrin; MAO Inhibitors; Maprotiline; Meperidine; Methyldopa; Methylene Blue; Methylphenidate; Mirtazapine; Morphine (Liposomal); Morphine (Systemic); Nefazodone; Oxymorphone; Pizotifen; Selective Serotonin Reuptake Inhibitors; Serotonin 5-HT1D Receptor Agonists; Serotonin/Norepinephrine Reuptake Inhibitors; Tapentadol; Tetrabenazine; Tetrahydrozoline (Nasal); TraZODone; Tricyclic Antidepressants; Tryptophan

Decreased Effect

Linezolid may decrease the levels/effects of: Domperidone

The levels/effects of Linezolid may be decreased by: Cyproheptadine; Domperidone

Increased Effect/Toxicity

Linezolid may increase the levels/effects of: Antipsychotics; Apraclonidine; AtoMOXetine; Beta2-Agonists; Betahistine; Bezafibrate; Brimonidine (Ophthalmic); Brimonidine (Topical); BuPROPion; CloZAPine; Cyproheptadine; Dexmethylphenidate; Dextromethorphan; Diethylpropion; Domperidone; Doxapram; Doxylamine; EPINEPHrine (Nasal); Epinephrine (Racemic); EPINEPHrine (Systemic, Oral Inhalation); Hydrocodone; HYDROmorphone; Hypoglycemic Agents; Isometheptene; Levonordefrin; Lithium; Meperidine; Methadone; Methyldopa; Methylene Blue; Methylphenidate; Metoclopramide; Mirtazapine; Morphine (Liposomal); Morphine (Systemic); Nefazodone; Norepinephrine; OxyCODONE;

Pizotifen; Reserpine; Selective Serotonin Reuptake Inhibitors; Serotonin 5-HT1D Receptor Agonists; Serotonin Modulators; Serotonin/Norepinephrine Reuptake Inhibitors; Sympathomimetics; Tetrahydrozoline (Nasal); TraZODone; Tricyclic Antidepressants

The levels/effects of Linezolid may be increased by: Anilidopiperidine Opioids; Antipsychotics; Buprenorphine; BusPIRone; CarBAMazepine; COMT Inhibitors; Cyclobenzaprine; Levodopa; MAO Inhibitors; Maprotiline; Oxymorphone; Tapentadol; Tetrabenazine; TraMADol; Tryptophan

Nutritional/Ethanol Interactions

Ethanol: May cause additional CNS depressant effects and provide potential source of additional tyramine content. Management: Avoid ethanol.

Food: Concurrent ingestion of foods rich in tyramine may cause sudden and severe high blood pressure (hypertensive crisis). Food's freshness is also an important concern; improperly stored or spoiled food can create an environment where tyramine concentrations may increase. Management: Avoid tyramine-containing foods with MAOIs.

Herb/Nutraceutical: Ingestion of large quantities of supplements containing caffeine, tyrosine, tryptophan, or phenylalanine. May increase the risk of severe side effects (eg, hypertensive reactions, serotonin syndrome). Management: Avoid supplements containing caffeine, tyrosine, tryptophan, or phenylalanine.

Adverse Reactions

Percentages as reported in adults; frequency similar in pediatric patients unless otherwise noted.

>10%:

Central nervous system: Headache (<1% to 11%)

Gastrointestinal: Diarrhea (3% to 11%)

Hematologic & oncologic: Decreased hemoglobin (1% to 16%), thrombocytopenia (<1% to 13%), leukopenia (children 1% to 12%; adults <1% to 2%)

1% to 10%:

Central nervous system: Insomnia (3%), dizziness (≤3%), vertigo (children 1%)

Dermatologic: Skin rash (1% to 2%), pruritus (children 1%)

Endocrine & metabolic: Increased amylase (<1% to 2%), increased lactate dehydrogenase (<1% to 2%)

Gastrointestinal: Nausea (1% to 10%), vomiting (1% to 9%), increased serum lipase (3% to 4%), constipation (2%), dysgeusia (1% to 2%), loose stools (children 1% to 2%), oral candidiasis (1% to 2%), abdominal pain (≤2%), tongue discoloration (≤1%), pancreatitis

Genitourinary: Vulvovaginal candidiasis (1% to 2%)

Hematologic & oncologic: Neutropenia (children 1% to 6%; adults ≤1%), anemia (children ≤6%; adults ≤2%), eosinophilia (children ≤2%)

Hepatic: Increased serum ALT (≤10%), increased serum bilirubin (children ≤6%; adults ≤1%), increased serum AST (adults 2% to 5%), increased serum alkaline phosphatase (<1% to 4%), abnormal hepatic function tests (≤2%)

Infection: Fungal infection (≤1% to 2%)

Renal: Increased blood urea nitrogen (≤2%), increased serum creatinine (<1% to 2%)

Miscellaneous: Fever (2%)

Available Dosage Forms

Solution, Intravenous:

Zyvox: 2 mg/mL (100 mL, 300 mL)

Suspension Reconstituted, Oral:

Zyvox: 100 mg/5 mL (150 mL)

Tablet, Oral:

Zyvox: 600 mg

General Dosage Range

I.V.:

Children ≤11 years: 10 mg/kg (maximum dose: 600 mg) every 8 hours

Children ≥12 years and Adults: 600 mg every 12 hours

Oral:

Children <5 years: 10 mg/kg every 8 hours (maximum: 600 mg/dose)

Children 5-11 years: 10 mg/kg every 8-12 hours (maximum: 600 mg/dose)

Children ≥12 years and Adults: 400-600 mg every 12 hours

Administration

I.V. Administer intravenous infusion over 30-120 minutes. Do not mix or infuse with other medications. When the same intravenous line is used for sequential infusion of other medications, flush line with D₅W, NS, or LR before and after infusing linezolid. The yellow color of the injection may intensify over time without affecting potency.

Oral Oral suspension: Invert gently to mix prior to administration, do not shake. Administer without regard to meals.

Preparation for Administration Oral suspension: Reconstitute with 123 mL of distilled water (in 2 portions); shake vigorously. Concentration is 100 mg/5 mL. Prior to administration mix gently by inverting bottle; do not shake.

Storage/Stability

Infusion: Store at 25°C (77°F); excursions permitted to 15°C to 30°C (59°F to 86°F). Protect from light. Keep infusion bags in overwrap until ready for use. Protect infusion bags from freezing.

Oral suspension: Following reconstitution, store at 25°C (77°F); excursions permitted to 15°C to 30°C (59°F to 86°F). Use reconstituted suspension within 21 days. Protect from light.

Tablet: Store at 25°C (77°F); excursions permitted to 15°C to 30°C (59°F to 86°F). Protect from light; protect from moisture.

Nursing Actions

Physical Assessment Previous drug allergies should be assessed before administering first dose. Serotonergic agents may increase resistance to linezolid and increase risk of serotonin syndrome, hypertension with adrenergic agents, or myelosuppression with other drugs that may cause bone marrow suppression. Monitor for myelosuppression (anemia), lactic acidosis, or peripheral or optic neuropathy. Instruct patient to follow a tyramine-free diet.

Patient Education

• Discuss specific use of drug and side effects with patient as it relates to treatment. (HCAHPS: During this hospital stay, were you given any medicine that you had not taken before? Before giving you any new medicine, how often did hospital staff tell you what the medicine was for? How often did hospital staff describe possible side effects in a way you could understand?)

• Patient may experience anemia, headache, nausea, or diarrhea. Have patient report immediately to prescriber severe dizziness, dyspnea, illogical thinking, balance changes, signs of hypoglycemia, ecchymosis, bleeding, significant fatigue, sudden vision changes, or rash (HCAHPS).

• Educate patient about signs of a significant reaction (eg, wheezing; chest tightness; fever; itching; bad cough; blue skin color; seizures; or swelling of face, lips, tongue, or throat). **Note:** This is not a comprehensive list of all side effects. Patient should consult prescriber for additional questions.

Intended Use and Disclaimer: Should not be printed and given to patients. This information is intended to serve as a concise initial reference for healthcare professionals to use when discussing medications with a patient. You must ultimately rely on your own discretion, experience and judgment in diagnosing, treating and advising patients.

Dietary Considerations Take without regard to meals. Some products may contain sodium and/or phenylalanine. Avoid consuming large amounts of tyramine-containing foods/beverages. Some examples include aged or matured cheese, air-dried or cured meats (including sausages and salamis, fava or broad bean pods, tap/draft beers, Marmite concentrate, sauerkraut, soy sauce, and other soybean condiments.

Liraglutide (lir a GLOO tide)

Brand Names: U.S. Victoza

Index Terms NN2211

Pharmacologic Category Antidiabetic Agent, Glucagon-Like Peptide-1 (GLP-1) Receptor Agonist

Medication Safety Issues

Other safety concerns:

Cross-contamination may occur if pens are shared among multiple patients. Steps should be taken to prohibit sharing of pens.

Medication Guide Available Yes

Pregnancy Risk Factor C

Lactation Excretion in breast milk unknown/not recommended

Breast-Feeding Considerations It is not known if liraglutide is excreted into breast milk. Because tumors were observed in animal studies, the manufacturer recommends that a decision be made whether to discontinue nursing or to discontinue the drug, taking into account the importance of treatment to the mother.

Use Treatment of type 2 diabetes mellitus (non-insulin dependent, NIDDM) to improve glycemic control as an adjunct to diet and exercise

Mechanism of Action/Effect Liraglutide is a long acting analog of human glucagon-like peptide-1 (GLP-1) (an incretin hormone) which increases glucose-dependent insulin secretion, decreases inappropriate glucagon secretion, increases B-cell growth/replication, slows gastric emptying, and decreases food intake. Liraglutide administration results in decreases in hemoglobin A_{1c} by approximately 1%.

Contraindications Hypersensitivity to liraglutide or any component of the formulation; history of or family history of medullary thyroid carcinoma (MTC); patients with multiple endocrine neoplasia syndrome type 2 (MEN2)

Canadian labeling: Additional contraindications (not in U.S. labeling): Pregnancy; breast-feeding

Warnings/Precautions [U.S. Boxed Warning] Dose- and duration- dependent thyroid C-cell tumors have developed in animal studies with liraglutide therapy; relevance in humans unknown. Due to the finding in animal studies, patients were monitored with serum calcitonin or thyroid ultrasound during clinical trials; however, it is unknown if this is beneficial in decreasing the risk of thyroid tumors. Patients should be counseled on the risk and symptoms (eg, neck mass, dysphagia, dyspnea, persistent hoarseness) of thyroid tumors. Use is contraindicated in patients with or a family history of medullary thyroid cancer and in patients with multiple endocrine neoplasia syndrome type 2 (MEN2). During clinical studies, a few cases of thyroid C-cell hyperplasia were reported. Consultation with an endocrinologist is recommended in patients who develop elevated calcitonin concentrations.

Serious hypersensitivity reactions, including anaphylactic reactions and angioedema, have been reported with use; discontinue therapy in the event of a hypersensitivity reaction. Use with caution in patients with a history of angioedema to other GLP-1 receptor agonists (angioedema has been reported with other GLP-1 receptor agonists); potential for cross-sensitivity is unknown. Cases of acute and chronic pancreatitis (including one case of fatal necrotizing pancreatitis) have been reported although conclusive evidence to liraglutide therapy has not been established; monitor for signs and symptoms of pancreatitis (eg, persistent severe abdominal pain which may radiate to the back and which may or may not be accompanied by vomiting. If pancreatitis is suspected, discontinue use. Do not resume unless an alternative etiology of pancreatitis is confirmed. Use with caution in patients with a history of pancreatitis or consider antidiabetic therapies other than liraglutide. Use with caution in patients with cholelithiasis and/or alcohol abuse. Most common reactions are gastrointestinal related; these symptoms may be dose-related and may decrease in frequency/severity with gradual titration and continued use. Slows gastric emptying; has not been studied in patients with pre-existing gastroparesis. Use may be associated with weight loss (likely due to reduced intake) independent of the change in hemoglobin A_{1c}. Use with caution in patients with hepatic impairment. Use with caution in renal impairment, particularly during initiation of therapy and dose escalation; cases of acute renal failure and chronic renal failure exacerbation have been reported; some cases have been reported in patients with no known pre-existing renal disease.

Concomitant use of an insulin secretagogue (eg, sulfonylurea, meglitinide) or insulin may increase the risk of hypoglycemia; dosage reduction of secretagogues or insulin may be required. Concurrent use with prandial insulin therapy has not been evaluated. Due to its effects on gastric emptying, liraglutide may reduce the rate and extent of absorption of orally-administered drugs; use with caution in patients receiving medications with a narrow therapeutic window or require rapid absorption from the GI tract. Not recommended for first-line therapy; use as adjunct to diet and exercise. Do not use in patients with type 1 diabetes mellitus or for the treatment of diabetic ketoacidosis; not a substitute for insulin. Diabetes self-management education (DSME) is essential to maximize the effectiveness of therapy. According to the Centers for Disease Control and Prevention (CDC), pen-shaped injection devices should never be used for more than one person (even when the needle is changed) because of the risk of infection. The injection device should be clearly labeled with individual patient information to ensure that the correct pen is used (CDC, 2012).

Drug Interactions

Avoid Concomitant Use There are no known interactions where it is recommended to avoid concomitant use.

Decreased Effect

The levels/effects of Liraglutide may be decreased by: Corticosteroids (Orally Inhaled); Corticosteroids (Systemic); Luteinizing Hormone-Releasing Hormone Analogs; Somatropin; Thiazide Diuretics

Increased Effect/Toxicity

Liraglutide may increase the levels/effects of: Sulfonylureas

The levels/effects of Liraglutide may be increased by: Pegvisomant

Nutritional/Ethanol Interactions Ethanol: Ethanol may cause hypoglycemia. Management: Avoid ethanol.

Adverse Reactions Incidence reported in monotherapy trials unless otherwise specified.

>10%: Gastrointestinal: Nausea (28%), diarrhea (17%), vomiting (11%)

1% to 10%:

Central nervous system: Headache (9%)

Gastrointestinal: Constipation (10%), dyspepsia (combination trials: 9%)

Hepatic: Hyperbilirubinemia (monotherapy and combination trials: 4%)

Immunologic: Antibody development: Antiliraglutide antibodies (low titers [concentrations not requiring dilution of serum]; monotherapy and combination trials: 9%), cross-reacting antiliraglutide antibodies to native GLP-1 (monotherapy: 7%; combination trials: 5%)

Local: Injection site reactions (monotherapy and combination trials: 2% [includes rash, erythema])

Available Dosage Forms

Solution, Subcutaneous:

Victoza: 18 mg/3 mL (3 mL)

General Dosage Range SubQ: *Adults:* Initial: 0.6 mg once daily; maintenance: 1.2-1.8 mg/day

Administration

Other SubQ: Use only if clear, colorless, and free of particulate matter. Administer via injection in the upper arm, thigh, or abdomen. Administer without regard to meals or time of day. Change needle with each administration. Do not share pens between patients even if needle is changed. If using concomitantly with insulin, administer as separate injections (do **not** mix); may inject in the same body region as insulin, but not adjacent to one another.

Storage/Stability Prior to initial use, store under refrigeration at 2°C to 8°C (36°F to 46°F); after initial use, may be stored in refrigerator or at room temperature of 15°C to 30°C (59°F to 86°F). Do not freeze (discard if freezing occurs). Protect from heat and light. Pen should be discarded 30 days after initial use.

Nursing Actions

Physical Assessment Assess for use-related cautions (eg, renal or hepatic impairment, history of patient or familial medullary thyroid cancer, multiple endocrine neoplasia syndrome type 2 [MEN 2]). Teach patient diabetes self-management and proper injection techniques and syringe/needle disposal.

Patient Education

• Discuss specific use of drug and side effects with patient as it relates to treatment. (HCAHPS: During this hospital stay, were you given any medicine that you had not taken before? Before giving you any new medicine, how often did hospital staff tell you what the medicine was for? How often did hospital staff describe possible side effects in a way you could understand?)

• Patient may experience hypoglycemia, headache, nausea, diarrhea, or injection site irritation. Have patient report immediately to prescriber signs of infection, significant hyperglycemia, severe dyspepsia, dysphagia, lump on neck, or rash (HCAHPS).

• Educate patient about signs of a significant reaction (eg, wheezing; chest tightness; fever; itching; bad cough; blue skin color; seizures; or swelling of face, lips, tongue, or throat). **Note:** This is not a comprehensive list of all side effects. Patient should consult prescriber for additional questions.

Intended Use and Disclaimer: Should not be printed and given to patients. This information is intended to serve as a concise initial reference for healthcare professionals to use when discussing medications with a patient. You must ultimately rely on your own discretion, experience and judgment in diagnosing, treating and advising patients.

Dietary Considerations Individualized medical nutrition therapy (MNT) based on ADA recommendations is an integral part of therapy.

Lisdexamfetamine (lis dex am FET a meen)

Brand Names: U.S. Vyvanse

Index Terms Lisdexamfetamine Dimesylate; Lisdexamphetamine; NRP104

Pharmacologic Category Central Nervous System Stimulant

Medication Safety Issues

Sound-alike/look-alike issues:

Vyvanse may be confused with Visanne, ViVAXIM, Vytorin, Glucovance, Vivactil

Medication Guide Available Yes

Pregnancy Risk Factor C

Lactation Enters breast milk/not recommended

Breast-Feeding Considerations The majority of human data is based on illicit amphetamine/methamphetamine exposure and not from therapeutic maternal use (Golub, 2005). Amphetamines are excreted into breast milk and use may decrease milk production. Increased irritability, agitation, and crying have been reported in nursing infants (ACOG, 2011). According to the manufacturer, the decision to continue or discontinue breast-feeding during therapy should take into account the risk of exposure to the infant and the benefits of treatment to the mother.

Use Treatment of attention-deficit/hyperactivity disorder (ADHD)

Mechanism of Action/Effect Lisdexamfetamine dimesylate is a prodrug that is converted to the active component dextroamphetamine. Amphetamines release catecholamines from storage sites in the nerve terminals.

Contraindications

Hypersensitivity to amphetamine products or any component of the formulation; use during or within 14 days following MAO inhibitor therapy

Canadian labeling: Additional contraindications (not in U.S. labeling): Known hypersensitivity or idiosyncrasy to sympathomimetic amines; advanced arteriosclerosis; symptomatic cardiovascular disease; moderate-to-severe hypertension; hyperthyroidism; glaucoma; agitated states; history of drug abuse

Warnings/Precautions Sudden death, stroke, and myocardial infarction have been reported in adults receiving the recommended doses of CNS stimulants. In children and adolescents with pre-existing structural cardiac abnormalities or other serious heart problems, sudden death has been reported while receiving the recommended doses of CNS stimulants for ADHD. These products should be avoided in the patients with known serious structural cardiac abnormalities, cardiomyopathy, serious heart rhythm abnormalities, coronary artery disease (adults), or other serious cardiac problems that could increase the risk of sudden death that these conditions alone carry. Patients should be carefully evaluated for these cardiac disorders prior to initiation of therapy. Patients who develop chest pain, syncope, or arrhythmias during therapy should be evaluated promptly. CNS stimulants may increase heart rate (approximate mean increase: 3-6 bpm) and blood pressure (approximate mean increase: 2-4 mm Hg); monitor for adverse events related to tachycardia or hypertension. Stimulants are associated with peripheral vasculopathy, including Raynaud's phenomenon; signs/symptoms are usually mild and intermittent, and generally improve with dose reduction or discontinuation. Digital ulceration and/or soft tissue breakdown have been observed rarely; monitor for digital changes during therapy and seek further evaluation (eg, rheumatology) if necessary.

Use with caution in patients with psychiatric or seizure disorders. May exacerbate symptoms of behavior and thought disorder in psychotic patients. Stimulants may unmask tics in individuals with coexisting Tourette's syndrome. **[U.S. Boxed Warning]: CNS stimulants (including lisdexamfetamine) have a high potential for abuse and dependence; assess for abuse potential prior to use and monitor for signs of abuse and dependence during therapy.** Use with caution in patients with history of ethanol or drug abuse (Canadian labeling contraindicates use if history of drug abuse). Prescriptions should be written for the smallest quantity consistent with good patient care to minimize possibility of overdose. Abrupt discontinuation following high doses or for prolonged periods may result in symptoms for withdrawal (eg, depression, extreme fatigue). Recommended to be used as part of a comprehensive treatment program for attention deficit disorders. When used for extended periods, therapy should be periodically re-evaluated to determine if continued treatment is necessary; if possible, interrupt therapy to assess if behavioral symptoms recur.

Use with caution in the elderly due to CNS stimulant adverse effects. Appetite suppression may occur; monitor weight during therapy, particularly in children. Use of stimulants has been associated with slowing of growth rate; monitor growth rate during treatment. Treatment interruption may be necessary in patients who are not growing or gaining weight as expected. Potentially significant drug-drug interactions may exist, requiring dose or frequency adjustment, additional monitoring, and/or selection of alternative therapy.

Drug Interactions

Avoid Concomitant Use

Avoid concomitant use of Lisdexamfetamine with any of the following: Iobenguane I 123; MAO Inhibitors

Decreased Effect

Lisdexamfetamine may decrease the levels/effects of: Antihistamines; Ethosuximide; Iobenguane I 123; Ioflupane I 123; PHENobarbital; Phenytoin

The levels/effects of Lisdexamfetamine may be decreased by: Ammonium Chloride; Antipsychotics; Ascorbic Acid; Gastrointestinal Acidifying Agents; Lithium; Methenamine; Multivitamins/Fluoride (with ADE); Multivitamins/Minerals (with ADEK, Folate, Iron); Multivitamins/Minerals (with AE, No Iron); Urinary Acidifying Agents

Increased Effect/Toxicity

Lisdexamfetamine may increase the levels/effects of: Analgesics (Opioid); Sympathomimetics

The levels/effects of Lisdexamfetamine may be increased by: Alkalinizing Agents; Antacids; AtoMOXetine; Cannabinoids; Carbonic Anhydrase Inhibitors; MAO Inhibitors; Tricyclic Antidepressants

◀ **Nutritional/Ethanol Interactions**

Ethanol: Ethanol may increase CNS depression. Caffeine use may worsen problems with sleeping, headache, irritability, dizziness, nausea, vomiting, abdominal pain, and decreased appetite. Management: Avoid ethanol and caffeine.

Food: High-fat meal prolongs T_{max} by ~1 hour.

Adverse Reactions

>10%:

Central nervous system: Insomnia (13% to 27%)

Gastrointestinal: Decreased appetite (children and adolescents 34% to 39%; adults 27%), xerostomia (adults 26%; children and adolescents 4% to 5%), abdominal pain (children 12%)

1% to 10%:

Cardiovascular: Increased blood pressure (adults 3%), increased heart rate (adults 2%)

Central nervous system: Irritability (children 10%), anxiety (adults 6%), dizziness (children 5%), akathisia (adults 4%), agitation (adults 3%), emotional lability (children 3%), restlessness (adults 3%), drowsiness (children 2%), tics (children 2%)

Dermatologic: Hyperhidrosis (adults 3%), skin rash (children 3%)

Endocrine & metabolic: Weight loss (children and adolescents 9%; adults 3%)

Gastrointestinal: Vomiting (children 9%), diarrhea (adults 7%), nausea (6% to 7%), anorexia (adults 5%)

Genitourinary: Erectile dysfunction (adults 3%), decreased libido (adults <2%)

Neuromuscular & skeletal: Tremor (adults 2%)

Respiratory: Dyspnea (adults 2%)

Miscellaneous: Fever (children 2%)

Controlled Substance C-II

Available Dosage Forms

Capsule, Oral:

Vyvanse: 20 mg, 30 mg, 40 mg, 50 mg, 60 mg, 70 mg

General Dosage Range Oral: *Children ≥6 years, Adolescents, and Adults:* Initial: 30 mg once daily; Maintenance: Up to 70 mg once daily

Administration

Oral Administer in the morning without regard to meals; swallow capsule whole, do not chew; capsule may be opened and the entire contents dissolved in glass of water; stir until dispersed completely and consume the resulting solution immediately; do not store solution.

Storage/Stability Store at controlled room temperature of 25°C (77°F) excursions permitted to 15°C to 30°C (59°F to 86°F). Protect from light.

Nursing Actions

Physical Assessment Perform careful cardiovascular assessment prior to initiating therapy. Monitor weight, blood pressure, and vital signs at beginning of therapy and periodically throughout. Children should also have height measured often while taking this medication.

Patient Education

• Discuss specific use of drug and side effects with patient as it relates to treatment. (HCAHPS: During this hospital stay, were you given any medicine that you had not taken before? Before giving you any new medicine, how often did hospital staff tell you what the medicine was for? How often did hospital staff describe possible side effects in a way you could understand?)

• Patient may experience diarrhea, nausea, xerostomia, lack of appetite, weight loss, or insomnia. Have patient report immediately to prescriber depression, nervousness, emotional instability, anxiety, behavioral problems, severe headache, sudden vision changes, angina, tachycardia, or rash (HCAHPS).

• Educate patient about signs of a significant reaction (eg, wheezing; chest tightness; fever; itching; bad cough; blue skin color; seizures; or swelling of face, lips, tongue, or throat). **Note:** This is not a comprehensive list of all side effects. Patient should consult prescriber for additional questions.

Intended Use and Disclaimer: Should not be printed and given to patients. This information is intended to serve as a concise initial reference for healthcare professionals to use when discussing medications with a patient. You must ultimately rely on your own discretion, experience and judgment in diagnosing, treating and advising patients.

Lisinopril (lyse IN oh pril)

Brand Names: U.S. Prinivil; Zestril

Pharmacologic Category Angiotensin-Converting Enzyme (ACE) Inhibitor; Antihypertensive

Medication Safety Issues

Sound-alike/look-alike issues:

Lisinopril may be confused with fosinopril, Lioresal, Lipitor, RisperDAL

Prinivil® may be confused with Plendil, Pravachol, Prevacid, PriLOSEC, Proventil

Zestril® may be confused with Desyrel, Restoril, Vistaril, Zegerid, Zerit, Zetia, Zostrix, ZyPREXA

International issues:

Acepril [Malaysia] may be confused with Accupril which is a brand name for quinapril [U.S.]

Acepril: Brand name for lisinopril [Malaysia], but also the brand name for captopril [Great Britain]; enalapril [Hungary, Switzerland]

Pregnancy Risk Factor D

Lactation Excretion in breast milk unknown/not recommended

Breast-Feeding Considerations It is not known if lisinopril is excreted in breast milk. Breast-feeding is not recommended by the manufacturer.

Use Treatment of hypertension, either alone or in combination with other antihypertensive agents; adjunctive therapy in treatment of heart failure

(HF) (afterload reduction); treatment of acute myocardial infarction within 24 hours in hemodynamically-stable patients to improve survival; treatment of left ventricular dysfunction after myocardial infarction

Note: The ACCF/AHA 2013 heart failure guidelines recommend the use of ACE inhibitors, along with other guideline directed medical therapies, to prevent HF in patients with a reduced ejection fraction who have a history of MI (stage B HF), to prevent HF in any patient with a reduced ejection fraction (stage B HF), or to treat those with HF and reduced ejection fraction (stage C HFrEF) (Yancy, 2013).

Mechanism of Action/Effect Competitive inhibitor of angiotensin-converting enzyme (ACE); prevents conversion of angiotensin I to angiotensin II, a potent vasoconstrictor; results in lower levels of angiotensin II which causes an increase in plasma renin activity and a reduction in aldosterone secretion

Contraindications

Hypersensitivity to lisinopril or any component of the formulation; angioedema related to previous treatment with an ACE inhibitor; patients with idiopathic or hereditary angioedema; concomitant use with aliskiren in patients with diabetes mellitus

Canadian labeling: Additional contraindications (not in U.S. labeling): Concomitant use with aliskiren-containing drugs in patients with moderate-to-severe renal impairment (GFR <60 mL/minute/ 1.73 m^2)

Warnings/Precautions Anaphylactic reactions may occur rarely with ACE inhibitors. At any time during treatment (especially following first dose), angioedema may occur rarely with ACE inhibitors; it may involve the head and neck (potentially compromising airway) or the intestine (presenting with abdominal pain). African-Americans may be at an increased risk. Prolonged frequent monitoring may be required especially if tongue, glottis, or larynx are involved as they are associated with airway obstruction. Patients with a history of airway surgery may have a higher risk of airway obstruction. Aggressive early and appropriate management is critical. Use in patients with idiopathic or hereditary angioedema or previous angioedema associated with ACE inhibitor therapy is contraindicated. Severe anaphylactoid reactions may be seen during hemodialysis (eg, CVVHD) with high-flux dialysis membranes (eg, AN69), and rarely, during low density lipoprotein apheresis with dextran sulfate cellulose. Rare cases of anaphylactoid reactions have been reported in patients undergoing sensitization treatment with hymenoptera (bee, wasp) venom while receiving ACE inhibitors.

Symptomatic hypotension with or without syncope can occur with ACE inhibitors (usually with the first several doses); effects are most often observed in volume depleted patients; correct volume depletion prior to initiation; close monitoring of patient is required especially with initial dosing and dosing increases; blood pressure must be lowered at a rate appropriate for the patient's clinical condition. Initiation of therapy in patients with ischemic heart disease or cerebrovascular disease warrants close observation due to the potential consequences posed by falling blood pressure (eg, MI, stroke). Use with caution in hypertrophic cardiomyopathy with outflow tract obstruction, severe aortic stenosis, or before, during, or immediately after major surgery. **[U.S. Boxed Warning]: Drugs that act on the renin-angiotensin system can cause injury and death to the developing fetus. Discontinue as soon as possible once pregnancy is detected.**

Hyperkalemia may occur with ACE inhibitors; risk factors include renal dysfunction, diabetes mellitus, concomitant use of potassium-sparing diuretics, potassium supplements, and/or potassium-containing salts. Use cautiously, if at all, with these agents and monitor potassium closely. Cough may occur with ACE inhibitors. Other causes of cough should be considered (eg, pulmonary congestion in patients with heart failure) and excluded prior to discontinuation.

May be associated with deterioration of renal function and/or increases in serum creatinine, particularly in patients with low renal blood flow (eg, renal artery stenosis, heart failure) whose glomerular filtration rate (GFR) is dependent on efferent arteriolar vasoconstriction by angiotensin II; deterioration may result in oliguria, acute renal failure, and progressive azotemia. Small increases in serum creatinine may occur following initiation; consider discontinuation only in patients with progressive and/or significant deterioration in renal function. Use with caution in patients with unstented unilateral/bilateral renal artery stenosis. When unstented bilateral renal artery stenosis is present, use is generally avoided due to the elevated risk of deterioration in renal function unless possible benefits outweigh risks. Potentially significant drug-drug interactions may exist, requiring dose or frequency adjustment, additional monitoring, and/or selection of alternative therapy.

Rare toxicities associated with ACE inhibitors include cholestatic jaundice (which may progress to fulminant hepatic necrosis), agranulocytosis, neutropenia, or leukopenia with myeloid hypoplasia. Patients with collagen vascular diseases (especially with concomitant renal impairment) or renal impairment alone may be at increased risk for hematologic toxicity; periodically monitor CBC with differential in these patients. Safety and efficacy have not been established in children <6 years of age or children with a CrCl ≤30 mL/minute.

Drug Interactions

Avoid Concomitant Use There are no known interactions where it is recommended to avoid concomitant use.

Decreased Effect

The levels/effects of Lisinopril may be decreased by: Antacids; Aprotinin; Herbs (Hypertensive Properties); Icatibant; Lanthanum; Methylphenidate; Nonsteroidal Anti-Inflammatory Agents; Salicylates; Yohimbine

Increased Effect/Toxicity

Lisinopril may increase the levels/effects of: Allopurinol; Amifostine; Antihypertensives; AzaTHIOprine; CycloSPORINE (Systemic); DULoxetine; Ferric Gluconate; Gold Sodium Thiomalate; Hypotensive Agents; Iron Dextran Complex; Lithium; Nonsteroidal Anti-Inflammatory Agents; Obinutuzumab; RiTUXimab; Sodium Phosphates

The levels/effects of Lisinopril may be increased by: Alfuzosin; Aliskiren; Angiotensin II Receptor Blockers; Brimonidine (Topical); Canagliflozin; Diazoxide; DPP-IV Inhibitors; Eplerenone; Everolimus; Heparin; Heparin (Low Molecular Weight); Herbs (Hypotensive Properties); Loop Diuretics; MAO Inhibitors; Pentoxifylline; Phosphodiesterase 5 Inhibitors; Potassium Salts; Potassium-Sparing Diuretics; Prostacyclin Analogues; Sirolimus; Temsirolimus; Thiazide Diuretics; TiZANidine; Tolvaptan; Trimethoprim

Nutritional/Ethanol Interactions

Food: Potassium supplements and/or potassium-containing salts may cause or worsen hyperkalemia. Management: Consult prescriber before consuming a potassium-rich diet, potassium supplements, or salt substitutes.

Herb/Nutraceutical: Some herbal medications may worsen hypertension (eg, licorice); others may increase the antihypertensive effect of lisinopril (eg, shepherd's purse). Management: Avoid bayberry, blue cohosh, cayenne, ephedra, ginger, ginseng (American), kola, licorice, and yohimbe. Avoid black cohosh, California poppy, coleus, golden seal, hawthorn, mistletoe, periwinkle, quinine, and shepherd's purse.

Adverse Reactions Note: Frequency ranges include data from hypertension and heart failure trials. Higher rates of adverse reactions have generally been noted in patients with heart failure. However, the frequency of adverse effects associated with placebo is also increased in this population.

>10%:

Cardiovascular: Hypotension (1% to 11%)

Central nervous system: Dizziness (5% to 19%)

1% to 10%:

Cardiovascular: Syncope (5% to 7%), chest pain (3%), orthostatic effects (1%)

Central nervous system: Headache (4% to 6%), fatigue (3%)

Dermatologic: Skin rash (1% to 2%)

Endocrine & metabolic: Increased nonprotein nitrogen (7% to 9%), hyperkalemia (2% to 6%)

Gastrointestinal: Diarrhea (3% to 4%), abdominal pain (2%), nausea (2%), vomiting (1%)

Genitourinary: Impotence (1%)

Hematologic & oncologic: Decreased hemoglobin (small)

Infection: Common cold (1%)

Neuromuscular & skeletal: Weakness (1%)

Renal: Increased serum creatinine (7% to 10%; often transient), increased blood urea nitrogen (2%), renal insufficiency (in patients with bilateral renal artery stenosis or hypovolemia)

Respiratory: Cough (4% to 9%), upper respiratory tract infection (1% to 2%)

Pharmacodynamics/Kinetics

Onset of Action 1 hour; Peak effect: Hypotensive: Oral: ~6 hours

Duration of Action 24 hours

Available Dosage Forms

Tablet, Oral:

Prinivil: 5 mg, 10 mg, 20 mg

Zestril: 2.5 mg, 5 mg, 10 mg, 20 mg, 30 mg, 40 mg

Generic: 2.5 mg, 5 mg, 10 mg, 20 mg, 30 mg, 40 mg

General Dosage Range Dosage adjustment recommended in patients with renal impairment

Oral:

Children ≥6 years: Initial: 0.07 mg/kg once daily (up to 5 mg); Maintenance: Maximum: Doses >0.61 mg/kg or >40 mg have not been evaluated

Adults: Initial: 2.5-10 mg/day; Maintenance: 10-80 mg/day

Elderly: Initial: 2.5-5 mg/day (maximum: 40 mg/day)

Administration

Oral Watch for hypotensive effects within 1-3 hours of first dose or new higher dose.

Nursing Actions

Physical Assessment Assess potential for interactions with other pharmacological agents or herbal products that may impact fluid balance or cardiac status. Monitor for angioedema that may potentially affect airway or intestine, hypovolemia, postural hypotension, and anaphylactic reaction very closely following first dose, any increase in dose, and regularly during therapy.

Patient Education

• Discuss specific use of drug and side effects with patient as it relates to treatment. (HCAHPS: During this hospital stay, were you given any medicine that you had not taken before? Before giving you any new medicine, how often did hospital staff tell you what the medicine was for? How often did hospital staff describe possible side effects in a way you could understand?)

• Patient may experience dizziness, headache, or parageusia. Have patient report immediately to prescriber signs of infection, syncope, dyspnea, hyperhidrosis, diarrhea, significant weight gain, edema in legs or abdomen, discolored urine, jaundice, or rash (HCAHPS).

- Educate patient about signs of a significant reaction (eg, wheezing; chest tightness; fever; itching; bad cough; blue skin color; seizures; or swelling of face, lips, tongue, or throat). **Note:** This is not a comprehensive list of all side effects. Patient should consult prescriber for additional questions.

Intended Use and Disclaimer: Should not be printed and given to patients. This information is intended to serve as a concise initial reference for healthcare professionals to use when discussing medications with a patient. You must ultimately rely on your own discretion, experience and judgment in diagnosing, treating and advising patients.

Dietary Considerations Use potassium-containing salt substitutes cautiously in patients with diabetes, patients with renal dysfunction, or those maintained on potassium supplements or potassium-sparing diuretics.

Lisinopril and Hydrochlorothiazide
(lyse IN oh pril & hye droe klor oh THYE a zide)

Brand Names: U.S. Prinzide; Zestoretic
Index Terms Hydrochlorothiazide and Lisinopril
Pharmacologic Category Angiotensin-Converting Enzyme (ACE) Inhibitor; Antihypertensive; Diuretic, Thiazide
Pregnancy Risk Factor D
Use Treatment of hypertension
Available Dosage Forms
Tablet, oral: 10/12.5: Lisinopril 10 mg and hydrochlorothiazide 12.5 mg; 20/12.5: Lisinopril 20 mg and hydrochlorothiazide 12.5 mg; 20/25: Lisinopril 20 mg and hydrochlorothiazide 25 mg
Prinzide®:
10/12.5: Lisinopril 10 mg and hydrochlorothiazide 12.5 mg
Zestoretic®:
10/12.5: Lisinopril 10 mg and hydrochlorothiazide 12.5 mg
20/12.5: Lisinopril 20 mg and hydrochlorothiazide 12.5 mg
20/25: Lisinopril 20 mg and hydrochlorothiazide 25 mg
General Dosage Range Oral: *Adults:* Lisinopril 10-80 mg and hydrochlorothiazide 12.5-50 mg once daily
Nursing Actions
Physical Assessment See individual agents.
Patient Education
- Discuss specific use of drug and side effects with patient as it relates to treatment. (HCAHPS: During this hospital stay, were you given any medicine that you had not taken before? Before giving you any new medicine, how often did

hospital staff tell you what the medicine was for? How often did hospital staff describe possible side effects in a way you could understand?)
- Patient may experience dizziness or headache. Have patient report immediately to prescriber signs of infection, signs of hyperglycemia, signs of renal or hepatic impairment, angina, dyspnea, severe dyspepsia, bradycardia, arthralgia, akathisia, ecchymosis, bleeding, strength differences from one side to another, significant weight gain, paresthesia, dysuria, or vision changes (HCAHPS).
- Educate patient about signs of a significant reaction (eg, wheezing; chest tightness; fever; itching; bad cough; blue skin color; seizures; or swelling of face, lips, tongue, or throat). **Note:** This is not a comprehensive list of all side effects. Patient should consult prescriber for additional questions.

Intended Use and Disclaimer: Should not be printed and given to patients. This information is intended to serve as a concise initial reference for healthcare professionals to use when discussing medications with a patient. You must ultimately rely on your own discretion, experience and judgment in diagnosing, treating and advising patients.

Related Information
Hydrochlorothiazide *on page* 775
Lisinopril *on page* 952

Lithium (LITH ee um)

Brand Names: U.S. Lithobid
Index Terms Eskalith; Lithium Carbonate; Lithium Citrate
Pharmacologic Category Antimanic Agent
Medication Safety Issues
Sound-alike/look-alike issues:
Eskalith may be confused with Estratest
Lithium may be confused with lanthanum
Lithobid® may be confused with Levbid®, Lithostat®
Other safety concerns:
Do not confuse **mEq** (milliequivalent) with **mg** (milligram). **Note:** 300 mg lithium carbonate or citrate contain 8 mEq lithium. Dosage should be written in **mg** (milligrams) to avoid confusion.
Check prescriptions for unusually high volumes of the syrup for dosing errors.
Pregnancy Risk Factor D
Lactation Enters breast milk/not recommended
Breast-Feeding Considerations Lithium is excreted into breast milk and serum concentrations of nursing infants may be 10% to 50% of the maternal serum concentration (Grandjean, 2009). Hypotonia, hypothermia, cyanosis, electrocardiogram changes, and lethargy have been reported in nursing infants (ACOG, 2008). It is generally recommended that breast-feeding be avoided ▶

during maternal use of lithium; however, treatment may be continued in appropriately selected patients (Grandjean, 2009; Sharma, 2009; Viguera, 2007). The hydration status of the nursing infant and maternal serum concentrations of lithium should be monitored (ACOG, 2008). In addition, monitor the infant for lethargy, growth, and feeding problems; obtain infant serum concentrations only if clinical concerns arise (Bogen, 2012; Yonkers, 2011). Long-term effects on development and behavior have not been studied (ACOG, 2008; Grandjean, 2009).

Use Management of bipolar disorders; treatment of mania in individuals with bipolar disorder (maintenance treatment prevents or diminishes intensity of subsequent episodes)

Unlabeled Use Potential augmenting agent for antidepressants; aggression, post-traumatic stress disorder, conduct disorder in children

Mechanism of Action/Effect Stabilizes mood by actions on nerve cells of the central nervous system; involves serotonin, phosphatidylinositol cycle, and dopamine receptor sensitivity

Contraindications Hypersensitivity to lithium or any component of the formulation; avoid use in patients with severe cardiovascular or renal disease, or with severe debilitation, dehydration, or sodium depletion

Warnings/Precautions [U.S. Boxed Warning]: Lithium toxicity is closely related to serum levels and can occur at therapeutic doses; serum lithium determinations are required to monitor therapy. Use with caution in patients with thyroid disease, mild-moderate renal impairment, or mild-moderate cardiovascular disease. Use caution in patients receiving medications which alter sodium excretion (eg, diuretics, ACE inhibitors, NSAIDs), or in patients with significant fluid loss (protracted sweating, diarrhea, or prolonged fever); temporary reduction or cessation of therapy may be warranted. Some elderly patients may be extremely sensitive to the effects of lithium, see General Dosage Range. Chronic therapy results in diminished renal concentrating ability (nephrogenic DI); this is usually reversible when lithium is discontinued. Changes in renal function should be monitored, and re-evaluation of treatment may be necessary. Use caution in patients at risk of suicide (suicidal thoughts or behavior).

Use with caution in patients receiving neuroleptic medications - a syndrome resembling NMS has been associated with concurrent therapy. Lithium may impair the patient's alertness, affecting the ability to operate machinery or driving a vehicle. Neuromuscular-blocking agents should be administered with caution; the response may be prolonged.

Higher serum concentrations may be required and tolerated during an acute manic phase; however, the tolerance decreases when symptoms subside.

Normal fluid and salt intake must be maintained during therapy.

Drug Interactions

Avoid Concomitant Use There are no known interactions where it is recommended to avoid concomitant use.

Decreased Effect

Lithium may decrease the levels/effects of: Amphetamines; Antipsychotics; Desmopressin

The levels/effects of Lithium may be decreased by: Calcitonin; Calcium Polystyrene Sulfonate; Carbonic Anhydrase Inhibitors; Loop Diuretics; Sodium Bicarbonate; Sodium Chloride; Sodium Polystyrene Sulfonate; Theophylline Derivatives

Increased Effect/Toxicity

Lithium may increase the levels/effects of: Antipsychotics; Highest Risk QTc-Prolonging Agents; Metoclopramide; Moderate Risk QTc-Prolonging Agents; Neuromuscular-Blocking Agents; Selective Serotonin Reuptake Inhibitors; Serotonin Modulators; Tricyclic Antidepressants

The levels/effects of Lithium may be increased by: ACE Inhibitors; Angiotensin II Receptor Blockers; Antipsychotics; Calcium Channel Blockers (Nondihydropyridine); CarBAMazepine; Desmopressin; Eplerenone; Fosphenytoin; Loop Diuretics; MAO Inhibitors; Methyldopa; Mifepristone; Nonsteroidal Anti-Inflammatory Agents; Phenytoin; Potassium Iodide; Thiazide Diuretics; Topiramate

Nutritional/Ethanol Interactions Food: Limit caffeine.

Adverse Reactions Frequency not defined.

Cardiovascular: Cardiac arrhythmia, hypotension, sinus node dysfunction, flattened or inverted T waves (reversible), edema, bradycardia, syncope

Central nervous system: Blackout spells, coma, confusion, dizziness, dystonia, fatigue, headache, lethargy, pseudotumor cerebri, psychomotor retardation, restlessness, sedation, seizure, slowed intellectual functioning, slurred speech, stupor, tics, vertigo

Dermatologic: Dry or thinning of hair, folliculitis, alopecia, exacerbation of psoriasis, rash

Endocrine & metabolic: Euthyroid goiter and/or hypothyroidism, hyperthyroidism, hyperglycemia, diabetes insipidus

Gastrointestinal: Polydipsia, anorexia, nausea, vomiting, diarrhea, xerostomia, metallic taste, weight gain, salivary gland swelling, excessive salivation

Genitourinary: Incontinence, polyuria, glycosuria, oliguria, albuminuria

Hematologic: Leukocytosis

Neuromuscular & skeletal: Tremor, muscle hyperirritability, ataxia, choreoathetoid movements, hyperactive deep tendon reflexes, myasthenia gravis (rare)

Ocular: Nystagmus, blurred vision, transient scotoma

Miscellaneous: Coldness and painful discoloration of fingers and toes

Postmarketing and/or case reports: Drug-induced Brugada syndrome

Available Dosage Forms

Capsule, Oral:
Generic: 150 mg, 300 mg, 600 mg

Solution, Oral:
Generic: 8 mEq/5 mL (5 mL, 500 mL)

Tablet, Oral:
Generic: 300 mg

Tablet Extended Release, Oral:
Lithobid: 300 mg
Generic: 300 mg, 450 mg

General Dosage Range Dosage adjustment recommended in patients with renal impairment

Oral:
Immediate release:
Adults: 900-2400 mg/day in 3-4 divided doses
Elderly: Initial: 300 mg twice daily (maximum: >900-1200 mg/day)
Extended release: Adults: 900-1800 mg/day in 2 divided doses

Administration

Oral Administer with meals to decrease GI upset. Extended release tablets must be swallowed whole; do not crush or chew.

Nursing Actions

Physical Assessment Monitor cardiovascular status; assess for fluid retention. Educate patient about signs and symptoms of toxicity.

Patient Education
- Discuss specific use of drug and side effects with patient as it relates to treatment. (HCAHPS: During this hospital stay, were you given any medicine that you had not taken before? Before giving you any new medicine, how often did hospital staff tell you what the medicine was for? How often did hospital staff describe possible side effects in a way you could understand?)
- Patient may experience presyncope, fatigue, blurred vision, illogical thinking, tremors, headache, nausea, or polyuria. Have patient report immediately to prescriber severe dizziness, significant change in balance, hyperhidrosis, considerable asthenia, or rash (HCAHPS).
- Educate patient about signs of a significant reaction (eg, wheezing; chest tightness; fever; itching; bad cough; blue skin color; seizures; or swelling of face, lips, tongue, or throat). **Note:** This is not a comprehensive list of all side effects. Patient should consult prescriber for additional questions.

Intended Use and Disclaimer: Should not be printed and given to patients. This information is intended to serve as a concise initial reference for healthcare professionals to use when discussing medications with a patient. You must ultimately rely on your own discretion, experience and judgment in diagnosing, treating and advising patients.

Dietary Considerations May be taken with meals to avoid GI upset; maintain adequate fluid intake.

Related Information
Oral Medications That Should Not Be Crushed or Altered on page 1712
Peak and Trough Guidelines on page 1710

Lodoxamide (loe DOKS a mide)

Brand Names: U.S. Alomide
Index Terms Lodoxamide Tromethamine
Pharmacologic Category Mast Cell Stabilizer
Medication Safety Issues
International issues:
Thilomide [Greece, Turkey] may be confused with Thalomid brand name for thalidomide [U.S., Canada]

Pregnancy Risk Factor B
Lactation Excretion in breast milk unknown/use caution
Use Treatment of vernal keratoconjunctivitis, vernal conjunctivitis, and vernal keratitis

Available Dosage Forms
Solution, Ophthalmic:
Alomide: 0.1% (10 mL)

General Dosage Range Ophthalmic: Children >2 years and Adults: Instill 1-2 drops in eye(s) 4 times/day

Nursing Actions

Patient Education
- Discuss specific use of drug and side effects with patient as it relates to treatment. (HCAHPS: During this hospital stay, were you given any medicine that you had not taken before? Before giving you any new medicine, how often did hospital staff tell you what the medicine was for? How often did hospital staff describe possible side effects in a way you could understand?)
- Have patient report immediately to prescriber vision changes, ophthalmalgia, or severe eye irritation (HCAHPS).
- Educate patient about signs of a significant reaction (eg, wheezing; chest tightness; fever; itching; bad cough; blue skin color; seizures; or swelling of face, lips, tongue, or throat). **Note:** This is not a comprehensive list of all side effects. Patient should consult prescriber for additional questions.

Intended Use and Disclaimer: Should not be printed and given to patients. This information is intended to serve as a concise initial reference for healthcare professionals to use when discussing medications with a patient. You must ultimately rely on your own discretion, experience and judgment in diagnosing, treating and advising patients.

Lomitapide (loe MI ta pide)

Brand Names: U.S. Juxtapid
Index Terms AEGR-733; BMS 201038; Lomitapide Mesylate
Pharmacologic Category Antilipemic Agent, Microsomal Triglyceride Transfer Protein (MTP) Inhibitor
Medication Guide Available Yes
Pregnancy Risk Factor X
Lactation Excretion in breast milk unknown/not recommended
Breast-Feeding Considerations It is not known if lomitapide is excreted into breast milk. Due to the potential for serious adverse reactions in the nursing infant, a decision should be made whether to discontinue nursing or to discontinue the drug, taking into account the importance of treatment to the mother.
Use Homozygous familial hypercholesterolemia: Adjunct to a low-fat diet and other lipid-lowering treatments, including low-density lipoprotein (LDL) apheresis where available, to reduce LDL cholesterol, total cholesterol, apolipoprotein B (apo B), and non-high-density lipoprotein cholesterol (non-HDL-C) in patients with homozygous familial hypercholesterolemia.
Mechanism of Action/Effect Lomitapide directly binds to and inhibits microsomal triglyceride transfer protein (MTP) ultimately reducing plasma LDL-C concentrations.
Contraindications Pregnancy; coadministration with moderate or strong CYP3A4 inhibitors; moderate or severe hepatic impairment (Child-Pugh class B or C) and patients with active liver disease, including unexplained persistent elevations of serum transaminases.
Warnings/Precautions [U.S. Boxed Warning]: May cause transaminase elevations; elevations in ALT or AST ≥3 times upper limit of normal occurred during clinical trials (no clinically meaningful concomitant bilirubin, INR, or alkaline phosphatase elevation was observed). Lomitapide also increases hepatic fat, with or without concomitant transaminase elevations. Hepatic steatosis associated with lomitapide (reversible upon discontinuation) may be a risk factor for progressive liver disease including steatohepatitis and cirrhosis. Monitor hepatic function (ALT, AST, alkaline phosphatase and total bilirubin) prior to treatment; monitor ALT and AST regularly as recommended during treatment; dosage adjustment or discontinuation may be necessary; transaminases typically reduce within 1-4 weeks after discontinuation. Alcohol ingestion may increase the risk of hepatic steatosis; alcohol consumption should be limited to ≤1 drink/day. Use caution when administered concomitantly with other hepatotoxic medications (eg, acetaminophen (>4 g/day for ≥3 days/week),

amiodarone, isotretinoin, methotrexate, tetracyclines, and tamoxifen); may require more frequent monitoring of liver function tests. Concomitant administration with other LDL-lowering agents that also have the potential to increase hepatic fat is not recommended (has not been studied). Use with caution in patients with mild (Child-Pugh class A) hepatic impairment due to increased drug exposure; a reduced maximum dose is recommended. Use is contraindicated in patients with moderate to severe (Child-Pugh class B or C) impairment or active liver disease including unexplained persistent elevations of serum transaminases. Monitor liver function as recommended. Use with caution in patients with mild-to-severe renal impairment including end-stage renal disease (ESRD) not receiving dialysis (has not been evaluated); drug exposure may significantly increase. Use with caution in patients with ESRD receiving dialysis; a reduced maximum dose of 40 mg daily is recommended.

Significant gastrointestinal events (eg, diarrhea, nausea, dyspepsia, vomiting) occurred during treatment with lomitapide; absorption of other oral medications may be affected; adherence to a low-fat diet (<20% of energy from fat) and gradual titration of dosage will reduce the risk of gastrointestinal adverse events. Lomitapide may reduce the absorption of fat-soluble nutrients (eg, vitamin E, linoleic acid, alpha-linolenic acid, eicosapentaenoic acid, and docosahexaenoic acid); supplementation is recommended; patients with chronic bowel or pancreatic diseases predisposed to malabsorption are at increased risk for deficiency.

Potentially significant drug-drug interactions may exist, requiring dose or frequency adjustment, additional monitoring, and/or selection of alternative therapy. Contains lactose; avoid use in patients with hereditary galactose intolerance, Lapp lactase deficiency, or glucose-galactose malabsorption; may result in diarrhea and malabsorption. **[U.S. Boxed Warning]: Due to the risk for hepatotoxicity, access is restricted through a REMS program (Juxtapid™ REMS program).** Only certified healthcare providers and pharmacies may prescribe and dispense lomitapide.

Drug Interactions

Avoid Concomitant Use
Avoid concomitant use of Lomitapide with any of the following: Bosutinib; CYP3A4 Inhibitors (Moderate); CYP3A4 Inhibitors (Strong); Fusidic Acid (Systemic); Ibrutinib; Ivabradine; Lovastatin; PAZOPanib; Pimozide; Pomalidomide; Rivaroxaban; Silodosin; Simeprevir; Tolvaptan; Topotecan; Uliprstal; VinCRIStine (Liposomal)

Decreased Effect
Lomitapide may decrease the levels/effects of: Ifosfamide

The levels/effects of Lomitapide may be decreased by: Bile Acid Sequestrants; Bosentan; CYP3A4 Inducers (Strong); Dabrafenib; Deferasirox; Herbs (CYP3A4 Inducers); Mitotane; Tocilizumab

Increased Effect/Toxicity

Lomitapide may increase the levels/effects of: Afatinib; ARIPiprazole; Avanafil; Bosentan; Bosutinib; Budesonide (Systemic, Oral Inhalation); Colchicine; CYP3A4 Substrates; Dabigatran Etexilate; Dofetilide; DOXOrubicin (Conventional); Eplerenone; Everolimus; FentaNYL; Halofantrine; Ibrutinib; Imatinib; Ivabradine; Ivacaftor; Lovastatin; Lurasidone; OxyCODONE; PAZOPanib; P-glycoprotein/ABCB1 Substrates; Pimecrolimus; Pimozide; Pomalidomide; Propafenone; Prucalopride; Ranolazine; Rivaroxaban; Salmeterol; Saxagliptin; Silodosin; Simeprevir; Simvastatin; Tolvaptan; Topotecan; Ulipristal; Vilazodone; VinCRIStine (Liposomal); Warfarin; Zuclopenthixol

The levels/effects of Lomitapide may be increased by: Alcohol (Ethyl); CYP3A4 Inhibitors (Moderate); CYP3A4 Inhibitors (Strong); CYP3A4 Inhibitors (Weak); Dasatinib; Fusidic Acid (Systemic); Ivacaftor; Luliconazole; Mifepristone; Simeprevir

Nutritional/Ethanol Interactions

Ethanol: May increase the risk for hepatic steatosis. Management: Limit alcohol consumption to 1 drink per day.

Food:

Grapefruit juice may increase lomitapide plasma concentration. Management: Avoid grapefruit juice.

High-fat diet: Diets containing ≥20% of total calories from fat may increase the risk of gastrointestinal adverse reactions (eg, abdominal pain/discomfort, constipation, diarrhea, flatulence, and nausea/vomiting).

Herb/Nutraceutical: Absorption of fat-soluble nutrients may be reduced. Management: Take recommended daily supplements of vitamin E, alpha-linolenic acid (ALA), linoleic acid, eicosapentaenoic acid (EPA), and docosahexaenoic acid (DHA).

Adverse Reactions

>10%:

Cardiovascular: Chest pain (24%)

Central nervous system: Fatigue (17%)

Gastrointestinal: Diarrhea (79%; severe: 14%), nausea (65%), dyspepsia (38%), vomiting (34%; severe: 10%), abdominal pain (34%; severe: 7%), weight loss (24%), abdominal discomfort (21%; severe: 7%), abdominal distension (21%; severe: 7%), constipation (21%), flatulence (21%), gastroenteritis (14%)

Hepatic: Hepatic steatosis (increase in hepatic fat >5%: 78%; >20% fat increase: 13%), ALT increased (17%; severe: 10%), ALT and/or AST ≥3 times upper limit of normal (34%)

Neuromuscular & skeletal: Back pain (14%)

Respiratory: Nasopharyngitis (17%), pharyngolaryngeal pain (14%)

Miscellaneous: Influenza (21%)

1% to 10%:

Cardiovascular: Angina pectoris (10%), palpitation (10%)

Central nervous system: Dizziness (10%), fever (10%), headache (10%)

Gastrointestinal: Defecation urgency (10%), gastroesophageal reflux disease (10%), rectal tenesmus (10%)

Hepatic: Hepatotoxicity (severe: 10%)

Respiratory: Nasal congestion (10%)

Available Dosage Forms

Capsule, Oral:

Juxtapid: 5 mg, 10 mg, 20 mg

General Dosage Range
Dosage adjustment recommended in patients on concomitant therapy, with renal or hepatic impairment, or who develop toxicities.

Oral: *Adults:* 5-60 mg once daily

Administration

Oral Administer with a glass of water and without food; administer at least 2 hours after the evening meal since administration with food may increase risk of gastrointestinal adverse effects. Swallow capsules whole (do not open, crush, dissolve, or chew).

Storage/Stability Store at 20°C to 25°C (68°F to 77°F); excursions permitted between 15°C to 30°C (59°F to 86°F). Brief exposure up to 40°C (104°F) may be tolerated provided the mean temperature does not exceed 25°C (77°F); minimize this type of exposure. Protect from moisture.

Nursing Actions

Physical Assessment Monitor for GI tolerance; can cause nausea, vomiting, diarrhea, dyspepsia, and abdominal pain. Ensure proper administration to decrease GI distress. Monitor for hepatic tolerance as well, including obtaining liver function tests at specific intervals during treatment.

Patient Education

• Discuss specific use of drug and side effects with patient as it relates to treatment. (HCAHPS: During this hospital stay, were you given any medicine that you had not taken before? Before giving you any new medicine, how often did hospital staff tell you what the medicine was for? How often did hospital staff describe possible side effects in a way you could understand?)

• Patient may experience diarrhea, nausea, dyspepsia, asthenia, flatulence, pyrosis, weight loss, back pain, flu-like syndrome, or hepatic impairment. Have patient report immediately to prescriber angina, inability to eat, ecchymosis, bleeding, discolored urine, jaundice, significant myalgia, or pregnancy (HCAHPS).

- Educate patient about signs of a significant reaction (eg, wheezing; chest tightness; fever; itching; bad cough; blue skin color; seizures; or swelling of face, lips, tongue, or throat). **Note:** This is not a comprehensive list of all side effects. Patient should consult prescriber for additional questions.

Intended Use and Disclaimer: Should not be printed and given to patients. This information is intended to serve as a concise initial reference for healthcare professionals to use when discussing medications with a patient. You must ultimately rely on your own discretion, experience and judgment in diagnosing, treating and advising patients.

Related Information

Oral Medications That Should Not Be Crushed or Altered *on page 1712*

Loperamide (loe PER a mide)

Brand Names: U.S. Anti-Diarrheal [OTC]; Diamode [OTC]; Imodium A-D [OTC]; Loperamide A-D [OTC]

Index Terms Loperamide Hydrochloride

Pharmacologic Category Antidiarrheal

Medication Safety Issues

Sound-alike/look-alike issues:

Imodium® A-D may be confused with Indocin® Loperamide may be confused with furosemide, Lomotil®

International issues:

Indiaral [France] may be confused with Inderal and Inderal LA brand names for propranolol [U.S., Canada, and multiple international markets]

Lomotil: Brand name for loperamide [Mexico, Philippines], but also the brand name for diphenoxylate [U.S., Canada, and multiple international markets]

Lomotil [Mexico, Phillipines] may be confused with Ludiomil brand name for maprotiline [multiple international markets]

Pregnancy Risk Factor C

Lactation Enters breast milk/not recommended

Use Control and symptomatic relief of chronic diarrhea associated with inflammatory bowel disease and of acute nonspecific diarrhea; to reduce volume of ileostomy discharge

OTC labeling: Control of symptoms of diarrhea, including Traveler's diarrhea

Unlabeled Use Cancer treatment-induced diarrhea (eg, irinotecan induced); chronic diarrhea caused by bowel resection

Available Dosage Forms

Capsule, Oral:

Generic: 2 mg

Liquid, Oral:

Imodium A-D [OTC]: 1 mg/7.5 mL (30 mL, 120 mL, 240 mL, 360 mL)

Generic: 1 mg/5 mL (5 mL, 10 mL, 118 mL)

Suspension, Oral:

Generic: 1 mg/7.5 mL (120 mL)

Tablet, Oral:

Anti-Diarrheal [OTC]: 2 mg

Diamode [OTC]: 2 mg

Imodium A-D [OTC]: 2 mg

Loperamide A-D [OTC]: 2 mg

Tablet Chewable, Oral:

Imodium A-D [OTC]: 2 mg

General Dosage Range Oral:

Children 2-5 years (13-20 kg): Initial: 1 mg 3 times/day for first 24 hours; Maintenance: 0.1 mg/kg after each loose stool

Children 6-8 years (20-30 kg): Initial: 2 mg twice daily for first 24 hours; Maintenance: 0.1 mg/kg after each loose stool **or** 2 mg after first loose stool, followed by 1 mg after each subsequent stool (maximum: 4 mg/day)

Children 8-12 years (>30 kg): Initial: 2 mg 3 times/day for first 24 hours; Maintenance: 0.1 mg/kg after each loose stool

Children 9-11 years: 2 mg after first loose stool, followed by 1 mg after each subsequent stool (maximum: 6 mg/day)

Children ≥12 years: Initial: 4 mg after first loose stool, followed by 2 mg after each subsequent stool (maximum: 8 mg/day)

Adults: Initial: 4 mg followed by 2 mg after each loose stool (maximum: 8-16 mg/day) **or** 4-8 mg/day in divided doses

Nursing Actions

Physical Assessment Assess for cause of diarrhea before administering first dose.

Patient Education

- Discuss specific use of drug and side effects with patient as it relates to treatment. (HCAHPS: During this hospital stay, were you given any medicine that you had not taken before? Before giving you any new medicine, how often did hospital staff tell you what the medicine was for? How often did hospital staff describe possible side effects in a way you could understand?)

- Patient may experience presyncope, fatigue, blurred vision, illogical thinking, dyspepsia, nausea, or constipation. Have patient report immediately to prescriber severe dizziness, significant diarrhea, edema, melena, or rash (HCAHPS).

- Educate patient about signs of a significant reaction (eg, wheezing; chest tightness; fever; itching; bad cough; blue skin color; seizures; or swelling of face, lips, tongue, or throat). **Note:** This is not a comprehensive list of all side effects. Patient should consult prescriber for additional questions.

Intended Use and Disclaimer: Should not be printed and given to patients. This information is intended to serve as a concise initial reference for healthcare professionals to use when discussing medications with a patient. You must ultimately rely on your own discretion, experience and judgment in diagnosing, treating and advising patients.

Lopinavir and Ritonavir
(loe PIN a veer & ri TOE na vir)

Brand Names: U.S. Kaletra
Index Terms Ritonavir and Lopinavir
Pharmacologic Category Antiretroviral, Protease Inhibitor (Anti-HIV)
Medication Safety Issues
Sound-alike/look-alike issues:
Potential for dispensing errors between Kaletra® and Keppra® (levETIRAcetam)
Administration issues:
Children's doses are based on weight and calculated by milligrams of lopinavir. Care should be taken to accurately calculate the dose. The oral solution contains lopinavir 80 mg and ritonavir 20 mg per one mL. Children <12 years of age (and ≤40 kg) who are not taking certain concomitant antiretroviral medications will receive <5 mL of solution per dose.

Medication Guide Available Yes
Pregnancy Risk Factor C
Lactation Excretion in breast milk unknown/contraindicated
Use Treatment of HIV infection in combination with other antiretroviral agents
Available Dosage Forms
Solution, oral:
Kaletra: Lopinavir 80 mg and ritonavir 20 mg per mL
Tablet:
Kaletra:
Lopinavir 100 mg and ritonavir 25 mg
Lopinavir 200 mg and ritonavir 50 mg
General Dosage Range Dosage adjustment recommended in patients on concomitant therapy
Oral:
Children 14 days to 6 months: Lopinavir 16 mg/kg or 300 mg/m² twice daily
Children 6 months to 18 years and <15 kg: 12 mg lopinavir/kg twice daily (maximum dose: Lopinavir 400 mg/ritonavir 100 mg)
Children 6 months to 18 years and 15-40 kg: 10 mg lopinavir/kg twice daily (maximum dose: Lopinavir 400 mg/ritonavir 100 mg)
Children 6 months to 18 years and >40 kg: Lopinavir 400 mg/ritonavir 100 mg twice daily
Adults: Lopinavir 400 mg/ritonavir 100 mg twice daily **or** lopinavir 800 mg/ritonavir 200 mg once daily

Administration
Oral
Solution: Must be administered with food; if using didanosine, take didanosine 1 hour before or 2 hours after lopinavir/ritonavir. Administer using calibrated dosing syringe.
Tablet: May be taken with or without food. Swallow whole, do not break, crush, or chew. May be taken with didanosine when taken without food. Tablets are not recommended in patients <15 kg.
Nursing Actions
Physical Assessment If liquid dosing, flush feeding tube before and after administration. Monitor for signs of bleeding; serum lipase and amylase; lipid panel.
Patient Education
• Discuss specific use of drug and side effects with patient as it relates to treatment. (HCAHPS: During this hospital stay, were you given any medicine that you had not taken before? Before giving you any new medicine, how often did hospital staff tell you what the medicine was for? How often did hospital staff describe possible side effects in a way you could understand?)
• Patient may experience hyperlipidemia, hypertriglyceridemia, headache, nausea, dyspepsia, diarrhea, lipodystrophy, or asthenia. Have patient report immediately to prescriber tachycardia, severe dizziness, syncope, polydipsia, polyuria, weight loss, discolored urine, jaundice, inability to eat, or rash (HCAHPS).
• Educate patient about signs of a significant reaction (eg, wheezing; chest tightness; fever; itching; bad cough; blue skin color; seizures; or swelling of face, lips, tongue, or throat). **Note:** This is not a comprehensive list of all side effects. Patient should consult prescriber for additional questions.

Intended Use and Disclaimer: Should not be printed and given to patients. This information is intended to serve as a concise initial reference for healthcare professionals to use when discussing medications with a patient. You must ultimately rely on your own discretion, experience and judgment in diagnosing, treating and advising patients.
Related Information
Oral Medications That Should Not Be Crushed or Altered *on page 1712*
Ritonavir *on page 1366*

Loratadine (lor AT a deen)

Brand Names: U.S. Alavert [OTC]; Allergy Relief For Kids [OTC]; Allergy Relief [OTC]; Allergy [OTC]; Childrens Loratadine [OTC]; Claritin Reditabs [OTC]; Claritin [OTC]; Loradamed [OTC]; Loratadine Childrens [OTC]; Loratadine Hives Relief [OTC]; Triaminic Allerchews [OTC]

Index Terms Tavist ND

Pharmacologic Category Histamine H$_1$ Antagonist; Histamine H$_1$ Antagonist, Second Generation; Piperidine Derivative

Medication Safety Issues

Sound-alike/look-alike issues:

Claritin may be confused with clarithromycin

Claritin (loratadine) may be confused with Claritin Eye (ketotifen)

Lorcaserin hydrochloride may be confused with lorcaserin hydrochloride

BEERS Criteria medication:

This drug may be potentially inappropriate for use in geriatric patients (Quality of evidence - varies based on comorbidity; Strength of recommendation - varies based on comorbidity)

Use

Allergic rhinitis: Relief of nasal and non-nasal symptoms of seasonal allergic rhinitis

Urticaria: Treatment of itching due to hives (urticarial)

Available Dosage Forms

Capsule, Oral:

Claritin [OTC]: 10 mg

Solution, Oral:

Childrens Loratadine [OTC]: 5 mg/5 mL (120 mL)

Loratadine Childrens [OTC]: 5 mg/5 mL (120 mL)

Loratadine Hives Relief [OTC]: 5 mg/5 mL (120 mL)

Syrup, Oral:

Allergy Relief [OTC]: 5 mg/5 mL (236 mL)

Allergy Relief For Kids [OTC]: 5 mg/5 mL (120 mL)

Childrens Loratadine [OTC]: 5 mg/5 mL (120 mL)

Claritin [OTC]: 5 mg/5 mL (60 mL, 120 mL, 150 mL)

Loratadine Childrens [OTC]: 5 mg/5 mL (120 mL)

Tablet, Oral:

Alavert [OTC]: 10 mg

Allergy [OTC]: 10 mg

Allergy Relief [OTC]: 10 mg

Claritin [OTC]: 10 mg

Loradamed [OTC]: 10 mg

Generic: 10 mg

Tablet Chewable, Oral:

Claritin [OTC]: 5 mg

Tablet Dispersible, Oral:

Alavert [OTC]: 10 mg

Allergy [OTC]: 10 mg

Allergy Relief [OTC]: 10 mg

Claritin Reditabs [OTC]: 5 mg, 10 mg

Triaminic Allerchews [OTC]: 10 mg

General Dosage Range

Oral:

Children 2-5 years: 5 mg once daily

Children ≥6 years and Adults: 10 mg once daily

Administration

Oral May be administered without regard to meals.

Dispersible tablet: Place in month and allow to dissolve. Swallow with or without water.

Nursing Actions

Patient Education

• Discuss specific use of drug and side effects with patient as it relates to treatment. (HCAHPS: During this hospital stay, were you given any medicine that you had not taken before? Before giving you any new medicine, how often did hospital staff tell you what the medicine was for? How often did hospital staff describe possible side effects in a way you could understand?)

• Patient may experience presyncope, fatigue, blurred vision, illogical thinking, headache, or xerostomia. Have patient report immediately to prescriber severe dizziness, syncope, or rash (HCAHPS).

• Educate patient about signs of a significant reaction (eg, wheezing; chest tightness; fever; itching; bad cough; blue skin color; seizures; swelling of face, lips, tongue, or throat). **Note:** This is not a comprehensive list of all side effects. Patient should consult prescriber for additional questions.

Intended Use and Disclaimer: Should not be printed and given to patients. This information is intended to serve as a concise initial reference for healthcare professionals to use when discussing medications with a patient. You must ultimately rely on your own discretion, experience and judgment in diagnosing, treating and advising patients.

Loratadine and Pseudoephedrine
(lor AT a deen & soo doe e FED rin)

Brand Names: U.S. Alavert™ Allergy and Sinus [OTC]; Claritin-D® 12 Hour Allergy & Congestion [OTC]; Claritin-D® 24 Hour Allergy & Congestion [OTC]; Loratadine-D 12 Hour [OTC]

Index Terms Pseudoephedrine and Loratadine

Pharmacologic Category Alpha/Beta Agonist; Decongestant; Histamine H$_1$ Antagonist; Histamine H$_1$ Antagonist, Second Generation; Piperidine Derivative

Medication Safety Issues

Sound-alike/look-alike issues:

Claritin-D® may be confused with Claritin-D® 24

Claritin-D® 24 may be confused with Claritin-D®

Use Temporary relief of symptoms of seasonal allergic rhinitis, other upper respiratory allergies, or the common cold

Available Dosage Forms

Tablet, extended release: Loratadine 10 mg and pseudoephedrine 240 mg

Alavert™ Allergy and Sinus [OTC]: Loratadine 5 mg and pseudoephedrine 120 mg

Claritin-D® 12 Hour Allergy & Congestion [OTC]: Loratadine 5 mg and pseudoephedrine 120 mg

Claritin-D® 24 Hour Allergy & Congestion [OTC]: Loratadine 10 mg and pseudoephedrine 240 mg

Loratadine-D 12 Hour [OTC]: Loratadine 5 mg and pseudoephedrine sulfate 120 mg

General Dosage Range Dosage adjustment recommended in patients with renal impairment

Oral: *Children ≥12 years and Adults:* Alavert™ Allergy and Sinus, Claritin-D® 24-Hour: 1 tablet every 24 hours; Claritin-D® 12-Hour: 1 tablet every 12 hours

Nursing Actions

Physical Assessment See individual agents.

Patient Education

- Discuss specific use of drug and side effects with patient as it relates to treatment. (HCAHPS: During this hospital stay, were you given any medicine that you had not taken before? Before giving you any new medicine, how often did hospital staff tell you what the medicine was for? How often did hospital staff describe possible side effects in a way you could understand?)
- Patient may experience presyncope, fatigue, blurred vision, illogical thinking, headache, nervousness and anxiety, xerostomia, or insomnia. Have patient report immediately to prescriber angina, tachycardia, syncope, or considerable asthenia (HCAHPS).
- Educate patient about signs of a significant reaction (eg, wheezing; chest tightness; fever; itching; bad cough; blue skin color; seizures; or swelling of face, lips, tongue, or throat). **Note:** This is not a comprehensive list of all side effects. Patient should consult prescriber for additional questions.

Intended Use and Disclaimer: Should not be printed and given to patients. This information is intended to serve as a concise initial reference for healthcare professionals to use when discussing medications with a patient. You must ultimately rely on your own discretion, experience and judgment in diagnosing, treating and advising patients.

Related Information

Loratadine *on page 961*

Oral Medications That Should Not Be Crushed or Altered *on page 1712*

Pseudoephedrine *on page 1311*

LORazepam (lor A ze pam)

Brand Names: U.S. Ativan; LORazepam Intensol

Pharmacologic Category Benzodiazepine

Medication Safety Issues

Sound-alike/look-alike issues:

LORazepam may be confused with ALPRAZolam, clonazePAM, diazepam, KlonoPIN, Lovaza, temazepam, zolpidem

Ativan may be confused with Ambien, Atarax, Atgam, Avitene

BEERS Criteria medication:

This drug may be potentially inappropriate for use in geriatric patients (Quality of evidence - high; Strength of recommendation - strong).

Administration issues:

Injection dosage form contains propylene glycol. Monitor for toxicity when administering continuous lorazepam infusions.

Pregnancy Risk Factor D

Lactation Enters breast milk/not recommended

Breast-Feeding Considerations Lorazepam can be detected in breast milk. Drowsiness, lethargy, or weight loss in nursing infants have been observed in case reports following maternal use of some benzodiazepines (Iqbal, 2002). Breast-feeding is not recommended by the manufacturer.

Use

Anxiety (oral): Management of anxiety disorders, short-term (≤4 months) relief of anxiety symptoms, or anxiety associated with depressive symptoms, or anxiety/stress-associated insomnia

Anesthesia premedication (parenteral): Anesthesia premedication to relieve anxiety or to produce amnesia (diminish recall) or sedation

Status epilepticus (parenteral): Treatment of status epilepticus

Unlabeled Use Agitation in ICU patient (I.V.); alcohol withdrawal delirium; alcohol withdrawal syndrome; chemotherapy-associated nausea and vomiting (either as an adjunct to standard antiemetics or for breakthrough nausea/vomiting); partial complex seizures (refractory); psychogenic catatonia; rapid tranquilization of the agitated patient; status epilepticus (in pediatrics)

Mechanism of Action/Effect Binds to stereospecific benzodiazepine receptors on the postsynaptic GABA neuron at several sites within the central nervous system, including the limbic system, reticular formation. Enhancement of the inhibitory effect of GABA on neuronal excitability results by increased neuronal membrane permeability to chloride ions. This shift in chloride ions results in hyperpolarization (a less excitable state) and stabilization.

Contraindications Hypersensitivity to lorazepam, any component of the formulation, or other benzodiazepines (cross-sensitivity with other benzodiazepines may exist); acute narrow-angle glaucoma; sleep apnea (parenteral); intra-arterial injection of parenteral formulation; severe respiratory insufficiency (except during mechanical ventilation)

Warnings/Precautions Use with caution in elderly or debilitated patients, patients with hepatic disease (including alcoholics) or renal impairment. In older adults, benzodiazepines increase the risk of impaired cognition, delirium, falls, fractures, and motor vehicle accidents. Due to increased sensitivity in this age group, avoid use for treatment of insomnia, agitation, or delirium. (Beers Criteria). ▶

◀ Use with caution in patients with respiratory disease (COPD or sleep apnea) or limited pulmonary reserve, or impaired gag reflex. Initial doses in elderly or debilitated patients should be at the lower end of the dosing range. May worsen hepatic encephalopathy.

Causes CNS depression (dose-related) resulting in sedation, dizziness, confusion, or ataxia which may impair physical and mental capabilities. Patients must be cautioned about performing tasks which require mental alertness (eg, operating machinery or driving). Potentially significant drug-drug interactions may exist, requiring dose or frequency adjustment, additional monitoring, and/or selection of alternative therapy. Use with caution in patients receiving other CNS depressants or psychoactive agents. Effects with other sedative drugs or ethanol may be potentiated. Benzodiazepines have been associated with falls and traumatic injury and should be used with extreme caution in patients who are at risk of these events.

Lorazepam may cause anterograde amnesia. Paradoxical reactions, including hyperactive or aggressive behavior have been reported with benzodiazepines, particularly in adolescent/pediatric or psychiatric patients. Does not have analgesic, antidepressant, or antipsychotic properties.

Pre-existing depression may worsen or emerge during therapy. Not recommended for use in primary depressive or psychotic disorders. Should not be used in patients at risk for suicide without adequate antidepressant treatment. Risk of dependence increases in patients with a history of alcohol or drug abuse and those with significant personality disorders; use with caution in these patients. Tolerance, psychological and physical dependence may also occur with higher dosages and prolonged use. The risk of dependence is decreased with short-term treatment (2-4 weeks); evaluate the need for continued treatment prior to extending therapy duration. Benzodiazepines have been associated with dependence and acute withdrawal symptoms on discontinuation or reduction in dose. Acute withdrawal, including seizures, may be precipitated after administration of flumazenil to patients receiving long-term benzodiazepine therapy.

As a hypnotic agent, should be used only after evaluation of potential causes of sleep disturbance. Failure of sleep disturbance to resolve after 7-10 days may indicate psychiatric or medical illness. A worsening of insomnia or the emergence of new abnormalities of thought or behavior may represent unrecognized psychiatric or medical illness and requires immediate and careful evaluation.

Status epilepticus should not be treated with injectable benzodiazepines alone; requires close observation and management and possibly ventilatory support. When used as a component of preanesthesia, monitor for heavy sedation and airway obstruction; equipment necessary to maintain airway and ventilatory support should be available. Parenteral formulation of lorazepam contains polyethylene glycol which has resulted in toxicity during high-dose and/or longer-term infusions. Parenteral formulation also contains propylene glycol (PG) may be associated with dose-related toxicity and can occur ≥48 hours after initiation of lorazepam. Limited data suggest increased risk of PG accumulation at doses of ≥6 mg/hour for 48 hours or more (Nelson, 2008). Monitor for signs of toxicity which may include acute renal failure, lactic acidosis, and/or osmol gap. May consider using enteral delivery of lorazepam tablets to decrease the risk of PG toxicity (Lugo, 1999). Parenteral formulation also contains benzyl alcohol; avoid in neonates.

Drug Interactions

Avoid Concomitant Use
Avoid concomitant use of LORazepam with any of the following: Azelastine (Nasal); OLANZapine; Paraldehyde; Sodium Oxybate; Thalidomide

Decreased Effect
The levels/effects of LORazepam may be decreased by: Theophylline Derivatives; Yohimbine

Increased Effect/Toxicity
LORazepam may increase the levels/effects of: Alcohol (Ethyl); Azelastine (Nasal); Buprenorphine; CloZAPine; CNS Depressants; Fosphenytoin; Hydrocodone; Methotrimeprazine; Metyrosine; Mirtazapine; Paraldehyde; Phenytoin; Pramipexole; ROPINIRole; Rotigotine; Selective Serotonin Reuptake Inhibitors; Sodium Oxybate; Thalidomide; Zolpidem

The levels/effects of LORazepam may be increased by: Brimonidine (Topical); Doxylamine; Droperidol; HydrOXYzine; Loxapine; Magnesium Sulfate; Methotrimeprazine; OLANZapine; Perampanel; Probenecid; Tapentadol; Valproic Acid and Derivatives

Nutritional/Ethanol Interactions
Ethanol: May increase CNS depression; monitor for increased effects with coadministration. Caution patients about effects.

Herb/Nutraceutical: Avoid valerian, St John's wort, kava kava, gotu kola (may increase CNS depression).

Adverse Reactions Frequency not always defined.
Cardiovascular: Hypotension (≤2%)

Central nervous system: Sedation (≤16%), dizziness (≤7%), drowsiness (2% to 4%), unsteadiness (3%), headache (1%), coma (≤1%), stupor (≤1%), aggressive behavior, agitation, akathisia, amnesia, anxiety, central nervous system stimulation, disinhibition, disorientation, dysarthria, euphoria, excitement, extrapyramidal reaction, fatigue, hostility, hypothermia, irritability, mania, memory impairment, outbursts of anger, psychosis, seizures, sleep apnea (exacerbation), sleep disturbances, slurred speech, suicidal behavior, suicidal ideation, vertigo

Dermatologic: Alopecia, skin rash

Gastrointestinal: Changes in appetite, constipation

Endocrine & metabolic: Change in libido, hyponatremia, SIADH

Genitourinary: Impotence, orgasm disturbance

Hematologic & oncologic: Agranulocytosis, pancytopenia, thrombocytopenia

Hepatic: Increased serum alkaline phosphatase, increased serum bilirubin, increased serum transaminases, jaundice

Hypersensitivity: Anaphylaxis, anaphylactoid reaction, hypersensitivity reaction

Local: Pain at injection site (I.M.: 1% to 17%; I.V.: ≤2%), erythema at injection site (≤2%)

Neuromuscular & skeletal: Weakness (≤4%)

Ophthalmic: Visual disturbances (including diplopia and blurred vision)

Respiratory: Respiratory failure (1% to 2%), apnea (1%), hypoventilation (≤1%), exacerbation of obstructive pulmonary disease, nasal congestion, respiratory depression, worsening of sleep apnea

Pharmacodynamics/Kinetics

Onset of Action

Hypnosis: I.M.: 20-30 minutes

Sedation: I.V.: Within 2-3 minutes (Greenblatt, 1983)

Anticonvulsant: I.V.: Within 10 minutes; Oral: 30-60 minutes

Duration of Action Up to 8 hours

Controlled Substance C-IV

Available Dosage Forms

Concentrate, Oral:

LORazepam Intensol: 2 mg/mL (30 mL)

Generic: 2 mg/mL (30 mL)

Solution, Injection:

Ativan: 2 mg/mL (1 mL, 10 mL); 4 mg/mL (1 mL, 10 mL)

Generic: 2 mg/mL (1 mL, 10 mL); 4 mg/mL (1 mL, 10 mL)

Tablet, Oral:

Ativan: 0.5 mg, 1 mg, 2 mg

Generic: 0.5 mg, 1 mg, 2 mg

General Dosage Range Dosage adjustment recommended in patients on concomitant therapy.

I.M.: *Adults:* 0.5-1 mg every 30-60 minutes as needed **or** 0.05 mg/kg as a single dose (maximum dose: 4 mg)

I.V.: *Adults:* 0.044 mg/kg as a single dose (maximum dose: 4 mg) **or** 4 mg (may repeat)

Oral: *Adults:* 1-10 mg daily in 2-3 divided doses **or** 2-4 mg at bedtime

Administration

I.M. Should be administered (undiluted) deep into the muscle mass.

I.V.

I.V. injection: Dilute prior to use. Do not exceed 2 mg/minute or 0.05 mg/kg over 2-5 minutes.

Monitor I.V. site during administration. Avoid intra-arterial administration. Avoid extravasation.

Continuous I.V. infusion (unlabeled administration mode; Barr, 2013) solutions should have an in-line filter and the solution should be checked frequently for possible precipitation (Grillo, 1996).

Oral Lorazepam oral concentrate: Use only the provided calibrated dropper to withdraw the prescribed dose. Mix the dose with liquid (eg, water, juice, soda, soda-like beverage) or semisolid food (eg, applesauce, pudding), and stir for a few seconds to blend completely. The prepared mixture should be administered immediately.

Preparation for Administration

I.V. injection: Dilute I.V. dose prior to use with an equal volume of compatible diluent (D_5W, NS, SWFI).

Infusion: Use 2 mg/mL injectable vial to prepare; there may be decreased stability when using 4 mg/mL vial. Dilute to ≤1 mg/mL and mix in glass bottle. Precipitation may occur. Can also be administered undiluted via infusion.

I.M.: Administer undiluted.

Storage/Stability

Parenteral: Intact vials should be refrigerated (room temperature storage information may be available; contact product manufacturer to obtain current recommendations). Protect from light. Do not use discolored or precipitate-containing solutions. Parenteral admixture is stable at room temperature (25°C) for 24 hours.

Oral concentrate: Store at colder room temperature or refrigerate at 2°C to 8°C (36°F to 46°F). Discard open bottle after 90 days.

Tablet: Store at room temperature. Protect from light.

Nursing Actions

Physical Assessment Oral: Assess for history of addiction; long-term use can result in dependence, abuse, or tolerance; periodically evaluate need for continued use. For inpatient use, institute safety measures. Taper dosage slowly when discontinuing. **I.V./I.M.:** Monitor cardiac, respiratory, and CNS status and ability to void.

Patient Education

• Discuss specific use of drug and side effects with patient as it relates to treatment. (HCAHPS: During this hospital stay, were you given any medicine that you had not taken before? Before giving you any new medicine, how often did hospital staff tell you what the medicine was for? How often did hospital staff describe possible side effects in a way you could understand?)

• Patient may experience presyncope, fatigue, blurred vision, illogical thinking, xerostomia, or change in balance. Have patient report immediately to prescriber severe asthenia (HCAHPS).

• Educate patient about signs of a significant reaction (eg, wheezing; chest tightness; fever; itching; bad cough; blue skin color; seizures; or ▶

swelling of face, lips, tongue, or throat). **Note:** This is not a comprehensive list of all side effects. Patient should consult prescriber for additional questions.

Intended Use and Disclaimer: Should not be printed and given to patients. This information is intended to serve as a concise initial reference for healthcare professionals to use when discussing medications with a patient. You must ultimately rely on your own discretion, experience and judgment in diagnosing, treating and advising patients.

Lorcaserin (lor KA ser in)

Brand Names: U.S. Belviq
Index Terms Lorcaserin Hydrochloride
Pharmacologic Category Anorexiant; Serotonin 5-HT$_{2C}$ Receptor Agonist
Medication Safety Issues
Sound-alike/look-alike issues:
Lorcaserin hydrochloride may be confused with loratadine hydrochloride (Claritin®) and losartan (Cozaar®)
Lorcaserin may be confused with Lotensin®
Pregnancy Risk Factor X
Lactation Excretion in breast milk unknown/ not recommended
Breast-Feeding Considerations Lorcaserin may alter maternal serum prolactin concentrations. It is not known if lorcaserin is excreted into breast milk. According to the manufacturer, the decision to continue or discontinue breast-feeding during therapy should take into account the risk of exposure to the infant and the benefits of treatment to the mother. Weight-loss therapy is generally not recommended for lactating women. Weight-loss programs which include physical activity and nutrition components should be discussed at the 6-week postpartum visit (ADA, 2009; IOM, 2009).
Use Chronic weight management, as an adjunct to a reduced-calorie diet and increased physical activity, in patients with either an initial body mass index (BMI) of ≥30 kg/m^2 **or** an initial BMI of ≥27 kg/m^2 and at least one weight-related comorbid condition (eg, hypertension, dyslipidemia, type 2 diabetes)
Mechanism of Action/Effect Selective serotonin 5-HT$_{2C}$ receptor agonist that stimulates neurons in the hypothalamus leading to satiety and decreased food intake.
Contraindications Pregnancy
Warnings/Precautions Use may cause confusion, somnolence, fatigue, and cognitive impairment (difficulty with concentration/attention/memory); patients must be cautioned about performing tasks which require mental alertness (eg, operating machinery or driving). Agents affecting the CNS have been associated with depression and suicidal ideation; monitor patients closely

during use; discontinue for suicidal thoughts or behaviors. Priapism may occur with use; men with erections >4 hours should immediately discontinue lorcaserin and seek emergency medical attention to avoid irreversible damage to erectile tissue. Use with caution in men with conditions that increase the risk for priapism (eg, sickle cell anemia, multiple myeloma, leukemia) or men with anatomical penis deformities (eg, angulation, cavernosal fibrosis, Peyronie's disease). Rare WBC and RBC count decreases (including leukopenia, lymphopenia, neutropenia, anemia, decreases in hematocrit and hemoglobin) have been observed; consider monitoring CBC periodically during use. Increased prolactin levels may occur; obtain prolactin levels if signs or symptoms of hyperprolactinemia occur (eg, galactorrhea, gynecomastia).

Primary pulmonary hypertension (PPH) is a rare and frequently fatal pulmonary disease, which has been reported in patients receiving other centrally acting, serotonergic weight loss agents. Available data from clinical trials are inadequate to determine if lorcaserin increases the risk for pulmonary hypertension (due to the low incidence of PPH occurring in the general population); however, a theoretical risk cannot be excluded. Cardiac valvular disease has been associated with the use of agents exhibiting potent 5-HT$_{2B}$ agonist activity (eg, cabergoline, fenfluramine [not currently on the U.S. market], dexfenfluramine [not currently on the U.S. market]). Cardiac valvular disease is believed to result from activation of 5-HT$_{2B}$ receptors in interstitial cardiac cells. Lorcaserin has greater affinity for 5-HT$_{2C}$ receptors compared to 5-HT$_{2B}$ receptors (at therapeutic doses). However, a slight increase in incidence of regurgitant cardiac valve disease (mitral and/or aortic) has been observed with lorcaserin compared to placebo in some clinical trials (pooled RR: 1.16; 95% CI: 0.81-1.67). The incidence observed in both groups was low, making it difficult to ascertain the risk of valvular disease with lorcaserin therapy based on available data. Evaluate patients if signs/symptoms of valvular heart disease (eg, dyspnea, dependent edema, heart failure, new onset cardiac murmur) arise during therapy; consider discontinuing therapy if present. Use has not been studied in patients with hemodynamically-significant valvular heart disease. Do not use lorcaserin in combination with potent serotonergic and dopaminergic agents that are potent 5-HT$_{2B}$ receptor agonists (eg, cabergoline) due to the risk for cardiac valvulopathy.

Serotonin syndrome (SS)/neuroleptic malignant syndrome (NMS)-like reactions have occurred with serotonergic agents such as lorcaserin, particularly when used in combination with other serotonergic agents (eg, triptans, SNRIs, SSRIs, TCAs, bupropion, St John's wort, tryptophan), agents that impair metabolism of serotonin (eg, MAO inhibitors, dextromethorphan, tramadol, lithium), or antidopaminergic agents (eg, antipsychotics). Concurrent use with these agents should be avoided. If concomitant use cannot be avoided, coadminister with extreme caution, and closely monitor patients, particularly during treatment initiation. Discontinue treatment (and any concomitant serotonergic and/or antidopaminergic agents) immediately if signs/symptoms of SS or NMS-like reactions arise.

Use with caution in patients with bradycardia or heart block (second or third degree); bradycardia has been observed rarely with use. Use with caution in patients with heart failure (has not been studied). Effect of lorcaserin on cardiovascular morbidity and mortality has not been established. Use with caution in patients with type 2 diabetes mellitus; weight loss from therapy may result in decreased requirements of antidiabetic agents and an increased risk of hypoglycemia; monitor blood glucose. Use with caution in patients with severe hepatic impairment (not studied); lorcaserin undergoes extensive hepatic metabolism. Use is not recommended in patients with severe renal impairment or end stage renal disease. Use with caution in patients with moderate renal impairment. Serum concentrations and principal metabolite (M1 and M5) half-lives are increased in renal impairment.

In short-term studies, euphoria, hallucinations, and dissociation have been observed with lorcaserin at supratherapeutic doses. Data suggest lorcaserin may produce psychic dependence. Physical dependence or a withdrawal syndrome has not been observed. Pharmacotherapy for weight loss should be used in conjunction with a comprehensive weight management program including diet and exercise. Discontinue if significant weight loss has not occurred (ie, <5% within the first 12 weeks of treatment). Concomitant use of lorcaserin with other agents intended for weight loss (eg, phentermine, orlistat, OTC, or herbal preparations) has not been evaluated; safety and efficacy of coadministration with other weight loss agents are unknown.

Drug Interactions

Avoid Concomitant Use

Avoid concomitant use of Lorcaserin with any of the following: Ergot Derivatives; Thioridazine

Decreased Effect

Lorcaserin may decrease the levels/effects of: Codeine; Tamoxifen

Increased Effect/Toxicity

Lorcaserin may increase the levels/effects of: Antipsychotics; CYP2D6 Substrates; DOXOrubicin (Conventional); Ergot Derivatives; Fesoterodine; Metoclopramide; Metoprolol; Nebivolol; Phosphodiesterase 5 Inhibitors; Serotonin Modulators; Thioridazine

The levels/effects of Lorcaserin may be increased by: Antipsychotics; BuPROPion; Propafenone

Adverse Reactions

>10%:

Central nervous system: Headache (15% to 17%)

Endocrine & metabolic: Hypoglycemia (diabetic patients 29%; severe: 2%)

Hematologic: Lymphocytes decreased (12%)

Neuromuscular & skeletal: Back pain (6% to 12%)

Respiratory: Upper respiratory tract infection (14%), nasopharyngitis (11% to 13%)

1% to 10%:

Cardiovascular: Peripheral edema (5%), hypertension (5%), valvulopathy (at 1 year: 2.4%; placebo: 2.0%)

Central nervous system: Dizziness (7% to 9%), fatigue (7%), anxiety (4%), insomnia (4%), depression (2% to 3%; placebo: 2%), cognitive impairment (2%), psychiatric disorders (2%)

Dermatologic: Rash (2%)

Endocrine & metabolic: Diabetes mellitus exacerbation (3%), prolactin increased (<2 x ULN: 7%; 2 x ULN: 2%; 5 x ULN: <1%)

Gastrointestinal: Nausea (8% to 9%), diarrhea (7%), constipation (6%), xerostomia (5%), vomiting (4%), gastroenteritis (3%), toothache (3%), appetite decreased (2%)

Genitourinary: Urinary tract infection (7% to 9%)

Hematologic: Hemoglobin decreased (10%), neutrophils decreased (6%)

Neuromuscular & skeletal: Muscle spasms (5%), musculoskeletal pain (2%)

Ocular: Eye disorders (5%; diabetic patients 6%)

Respiratory: Cough (4% to 8%), oropharyngeal pain (4%), sinus congestion (3%)

Miscellaneous: Seasonal allergy (3%), stress (3%)

Controlled Substance C-IV

Available Dosage Forms

Tablet, Oral:

Belviq: 10 mg

General Dosage Range Oral: *Adults:* 10 mg twice daily (maximum: 10 mg twice daily)

Administration

Oral Administer orally with or without food.

Storage/Stability Store at 25°C (77°F); excursions permitted to 15°C to 30°C (59°F to 86°F).

Nursing Actions

Physical Assessment Monitor for efficacy (>5% weight loss). Educate patient on proper nutrition and importance of measuring weight and tracking progress. Monitor blood pressure and for signs of any valvular heart disease, such as dyspnea, dependent edema, heart failure, or new onset cardiac murmur. Educate males to seek emergency medical care for erections lasting >4 hours. Observe for signs of breast enlargement or drainage from breasts.

Observe for changes in mental status, such as depression, hallucinations, euphoria, or cognitive impairment (attention, memory). Counsel patient and caregiver to report mental status changes and thoughts of suicide.

Patient Education
- Discuss specific use of drug and side effects with patient as it relates to treatment. (HCAHPS: During this hospital stay, were you given any medicine that you had not taken before? Before giving you any new medicine, how often did hospital staff tell you what the medicine was for? How often did hospital staff describe possible side effects in a way you could understand?)
- Patient may experience headache, presyncope, dyspepsia, xerostomia, constipation, back pain, or hypoglycemia. Have patient report immediately to prescriber dyspnea, tachycardia, bradycardia, edema, depression, illogical thinking, significant imbalance, fasciculations, erection lasting >4 hours, severe emesis, considerable weight loss, asthenia, or rash (HCAHPS).
- Educate patient about signs of a significant reaction (eg, wheezing; chest tightness; fever; itching; bad cough; blue skin color; seizures; or swelling of face, lips, tongue, or throat). **Note:** This is not a comprehensive list of all side effects. Patient should consult prescriber for additional questions.

Intended Use and Disclaimer: Should not be printed and given to patients. This information is intended to serve as a concise initial reference for healthcare professionals to use when discussing medications with a patient. You must ultimately rely on your own discretion, experience and judgment in diagnosing, treating and advising patients.

Losartan (loe SAR tan)

Brand Names: U.S. Cozaar
Index Terms DuP 753; Losartan Potassium; MK594
Pharmacologic Category Angiotensin II Receptor Blocker; Antihypertensive
Medication Safety Issues
Sound-alike/look-alike issues:
Cozaar may be confused with Colace, Coreg, Hyzaar, Zocor
Losartan may be confused with locaserin, valsartan
Pregnancy Risk Factor D
Lactation Excretion in breast milk unknown/not recommended
Breast-Feeding Considerations It is not known if losartan is found in breast milk. Due to the potential for serious adverse reactions in the nursing infant, the manufacturer recommends a decision be made whether to discontinue nursing or to discontinue the drug, taking into account the importance of treatment to the mother.
Use Treatment of hypertension (HTN); treatment of diabetic nephropathy in patients with type 2

diabetes mellitus (noninsulin dependent, NIDDM) and a history of hypertension; stroke risk reduction in patients with HTN and left ventricular hypertrophy (LVH)
Unlabeled Use To slow the rate of progression of aortic-root dilation in pediatric patients with Marfan's syndrome; syndrome; heart failure (HF) patients intolerant of ACE inhibitors
Note: The ACCF/AHA 2013 heart failure guidelines recommend the use of ARBs (ie, candesartan, losartan, and valsartan) in patients with HF with reduced ejection fraction who cannot tolerate ACE inhibitors (due to cough) to reduce morbidity and mortality. They also suggest that ARBs are reasonable first-line alternatives to ACE inhibitors in patients already maintained on an ARB for other indications (ACCF/AHA [Yancy, 2013]).
Mechanism of Action/Effect As a selective and competitive, nonpeptide angiotensin II receptor antagonist, losartan blocks the vasoconstrictor and aldosterone-secreting effects of angiotensin II. Losartan increases urinary flow rate and in addition to being natriuretic and kaliuretic, increases excretion of chloride, magnesium, uric acid, calcium, and phosphate.
Contraindications
Hypersensitivity to losartan or any component of the formulation; concomitant use with aliskiren in patients with diabetes mellitus
Canadian labeling: Additional contraindications (not in U.S. labeling): Concomitant use with aliskiren in patients with moderate-to-severe renal impairment (GFR <60 mL/minute/1.73 m^2)
Warnings/Precautions [U.S. Boxed Warning]: Drugs that act on the renin-angiotensin system can cause injury and death to the developing fetus. Discontinue as soon as possible once pregnancy is detected. Avoid use or use a much smaller dose in patients who are volume-depleted; correct depletion first. Use with caution in patients with significant aortic/mitral stenosis. May cause hyperkalemia; avoid potassium supplementation unless specifically required by healthcare provider. May be associated with deterioration of renal function and/or increases in serum creatinine, particularly in patients with low renal blood flow (eg, renal artery stenosis, heart failure) whose glomerular filtration rate (GFR) is dependent on efferent arteriolar vasoconstriction by angiotensin II. Use caution in patients with unstented unilateral/bilateral renal artery stenosis. When unstented bilateral renal artery stenosis is present, use is generally avoided due to the elevated risk of deterioration in renal function unless possible benefits outweigh risks. Use with caution with pre-existing renal insufficiency. AUCs of losartan (not the active metabolite) are about 50% greater in patients with CrCl <30 mL/minute and are doubled in hemodialysis patients. Potentially significant drug interactions may exist, requiring dose or frequency

adjustment, additional monitoring, and/or selection of alternative therapy.

Angioedema has been reported rarely with some angiotensin II receptor antagonists (ARBs) and may occur at any time during treatment (especially following first dose). It may involve the head and neck (potentially compromising airway) or the intestine (presenting with abdominal pain). Patients with idiopathic or hereditary angioedema or previous angioedema associated with ACE-inhibitor therapy may be at an increased risk. Prolonged frequent monitoring may be required, especially if tongue, glottis, or larynx are involved, as they are associated with airway obstruction. Patients with a history of airway surgery may have a higher risk of airway obstruction. Discontinue therapy immediately if angioedema occurs. Aggressive early management is critical. Intramuscular (I.M.) administration of epinephrine may be necessary. Do not readminister to patients who have had angioedema with ARBs.

When used to reduce the risk of stroke in patients with HTN and LVH, may not be effective in African-American population. Use caution with hepatic dysfunction, dose adjustment may be needed.

Drug Interactions

Avoid Concomitant Use
Avoid concomitant use of Losartan with any of the following: Pimozide

Decreased Effect
The levels/effects of Losartan may be decreased by: Bosentan; CYP2C9 Inducers (Strong); CYP3A4 Inducers (Strong); Dabrafenib; Deferasirox; Herbs (CYP3A4 Inducers); Herbs (Hypertensive Properties); Methylphenidate; Mitotane; Nonsteroidal Anti-Inflammatory Agents; Peginterferon Alfa-2b; Rifamycin Derivatives; Tocilizumab; Yohimbine

Increased Effect/Toxicity
Losartan may increase the levels/effects of: ACE Inhibitors; Amifostine; Antihypertensives; ARIPiprazole; Bosentan; Carvedilol; CycloSPORINE (Systemic); CYP2C8 Substrates; CYP2C9 Substrates; Dofetilide; DULoxetine; Hypotensive Agents; Lithium; Lomitapide; Nonsteroidal Anti-Inflammatory Agents; Obinutuzumab; Pimozide; Potassium-Sparing Diuretics; RiTUXimab; Sodium Phosphates

The levels/effects of Losartan may be increased by: Alfuzosin; Aliskiren; Antifungal Agents (Azole Derivatives, Systemic); Brimonidine (Topical); Canagliflozin; CYP2C9 Inhibitors (Moderate); CYP2C9 Inhibitors (Strong); Diazoxide; Eplerenone; Fluconazole; Heparin; Heparin (Low Molecular Weight); Herbs (Hypotensive Properties); MAO Inhibitors; Mifepristone; Milk Thistle; Pentoxifylline; Phosphodiesterase 5 Inhibitors; Potassium Salts; Prostacyclin Analogues; Tolvaptan; Trimethoprim

Nutritional/Ethanol Interactions Herb/Nutraceutical: St John's wort may decrease levels of losartan. Some herbal medications may worsen hypertension (eg, licorice); others may increase the antihypertensive effect of losartan (eg, shepherd's purse). Some herbal medications may increase the hypoglycemic effects of losartan (eg, alfalfa). Management: Avoid St John's wort. Avoid bayberry, blue cohosh, ginseng (American), kola, licorice, and yohimbe. Avoid black cohosh, California poppy, coleus, golden seal, hawthorn, mistletoe, periwinkle, quinine, and shepherd's purse. Avoid alfalfa, aloe, bilberry, bitter melon, burdock, celery, damiana, fenugreek, garcinia, garlic, ginger, ginseng (American), gymnema, marshmallow, and stinging nettle.

Adverse Reactions Note: The incidence of some adverse reactions varied based on the underlying disease state. Notations are made, where applicable, for data derived from trials conducted in diabetic nephropathy and hypertensive patients, respectively.

>10%:
Cardiovascular: Chest pain (12% diabetic nephropathy)
Central nervous system: Fatigue (14% diabetic nephropathy)
Endocrine: Hypoglycemia (14% diabetic nephropathy)
Gastrointestinal: Diarrhea (2% hypertension to 15% diabetic nephropathy)
Genitourinary: Urinary tract infection (13% diabetic nephropathy)
Hematologic: Anemia (14% diabetic nephropathy)
Neuromuscular & skeletal: Weakness (14% diabetic nephropathy), back pain (2% hypertension to 12% diabetic nephropathy)
Respiratory: Cough (≤3% to 11%; similar to placebo; incidence higher in patients with previous cough related to ACE inhibitor therapy)

1% to 10%:
Cardiovascular: Hypotension (7% diabetic nephropathy), orthostatic hypotension (4% hypertension to 4% diabetic nephropathy), first-dose hypotension (dose related: <1% with 50 mg, 2% with 100 mg)
Central nervous system: Dizziness (4%), hypoesthesia (5% diabetic nephropathy), fever (4% diabetic nephropathy), insomnia (1%)
Dermatology: Cellulitis (7% diabetic nephropathy)
Endocrine: Hyperkalemia (<1% hypertension to 7% diabetic nephropathy)
Gastrointestinal: Gastritis (5% diabetic nephropathy), weight gain (4% diabetic nephropathy), dyspepsia (1% to 4%), abdominal pain (2%), nausea (2%)
Neuromuscular & skeletal: Muscular weakness (7% diabetic nephropathy), knee pain (5% diabetic nephropathy), leg pain (1% to 5%), muscle cramps (1%), myalgia (1%)

Respiratory: Bronchitis (10% diabetic nephropathy), upper respiratory infection (8%), nasal congestion (2%), sinusitis (1% hypertension to 6% diabetic nephropathy)

Miscellaneous: Infection (5% diabetic nephropathy), flu-like syndrome (10% diabetic nephropathy)

Pharmacodynamics/Kinetics
Onset of Action 6 hours
Available Dosage Forms
Tablet, Oral:
Cozaar: 25 mg, 50 mg, 100 mg
Generic: 25 mg, 50 mg, 100 mg

General Dosage Range Dosage adjustment recommended in patients with hepatic impairment
Oral:
Children 6-16 years: Initial: 0.7 mg/kg once daily (maximum: 50 mg/day); Maintenance: Maximum: ≤1.4 mg/kg; 100 mg
Adults: Initial: 25-50 mg once daily; Maintenance: 25-100 mg/day in 1-2 divided doses (maximum: 100 mg/day)

Administration
Oral May be administered without regard to meals.
Storage/Stability Store at 15°C to 30°C (59°F to 86°F). Protect from light.

Nursing Actions
Physical Assessment Monitor vital signs regularly during therapy. Caution patients with diabetes to monitor glucose levels closely; may alter glucose control. Monitor for symptomatic postural hypotension, especially during the first few weeks of therapy. Assess if patient orthostatic if complaining of dizziness. Instruct patient to get up slowly from a sitting or lying position, especially in the first few weeks of beginning therapy.

Patient Education
• Discuss specific use of drug and side effects with patient as it relates to treatment. (HCAHPS: During this hospital stay, were you given any medicine that you had not taken before? Before giving you any new medicine, how often did hospital staff tell you what the medicine was for? How often did hospital staff describe possible side effects in a way you could understand?)
• Patient may experience dizziness, hyperkalemia, diarrhea, or worsening kidney function. Have patient report immediately to prescriber syncope, severe headache, hyperhidrosis, vomiting, rash, or pregnancy (HCAHPS).
• Educate patient about signs of a significant reaction (eg, wheezing; chest tightness; fever; itching; bad cough; blue skin color; seizures; or swelling of face, lips, tongue, or throat). **Note:** This is not a comprehensive list of all side effects. Patients should consult prescriber for additional questions.

Intended Use and Disclaimer: Should not be printed and given to patients. This information is intended to serve as a concise initial reference for healthcare professionals to use when discussing medications with a patient. You must ultimately rely on your own discretion, experience and judgment in diagnosing, treating and advising patients.

Dietary Considerations May be taken without regard to meals. Some products may contain potassium.

Losartan and Hydrochlorothiazide
(loe SAR tan & hye droe klor oh THYE a zide)

Brand Names: U.S. Hyzaar®
Index Terms Hydrochlorothiazide and Losartan
Pharmacologic Category Angiotensin II Receptor Blocker; Antihypertensive; Diuretic, Thiazide
Medication Safety Issues
Sound-alike/look-alike issues:
Hyzaar may be confused with Cozaar
Pregnancy Risk Factor D
Use Treatment of hypertension; stroke risk reduction in patients with HTN and left ventricular hypertrophy (LVH)
Available Dosage Forms
Tablet, oral: 50/12.5: Losartan 50 mg and hydrochlorothiazide 12.5 mg; 100/12.5: Losartan 100 mg and hydrochlorothiazide 12.5 mg; 100/25: Losartan 100 mg and hydrochlorothiazide 25 mg
Hyzaar: 50/12.5: Losartan 50 mg and hydrochlorothiazide 12.5 mg; 100/12.5: Losartan 100 mg and hydrochlorothiazide 12.5 mg; 100/25: Losartan 100 mg and hydrochlorothiazide 25 mg
General Dosage Range Oral: *Adults:* Losartan 50-100 mg and hydrochlorothiazide 12.5-50 mg once daily
Nursing Actions
Physical Assessment See individual agents.
Patient Education
• Discuss specific use of drug and side effects with patient as it relates to treatment. (HCAHPS: During this hospital stay, were you given any medicine that you had not taken before? Before giving you any new medicine, how often did hospital staff tell you what the medicine was for? How often did hospital staff describe possible side effects in a way you could understand?)
• Patient may experience dizziness, back pain, diarrhea, or rhinitis. Have patient report immediately to prescriber signs of infection, signs of hyperglycemia, signs of renal impairment, severe headache, paresthesia, angina, discolored urine, jaundice, sexual dysfunction, bradycardia, strength differences from one side to another, akathisia, considerable dyspepsia, dyspnea, significant weight gain, edema, ecchymosis, bleeding, pallor, or vision changes (HCAHPS).
• Educate patient about signs of a significant reaction (eg, wheezing; chest tightness; fever; itching; bad cough; blue skin color; seizures; or

swelling of face, lips, tongue, or throat). **Note:** This is not a comprehensive list of all side effects. Patient should consult prescriber for additional questions.

Intended Use and Disclaimer: Should not be printed and given to patients. This information is intended to serve as a concise initial reference for healthcare professionals to use when discussing medications with a patient. You must ultimately rely on your own discretion, experience and judgment in diagnosing, treating and advising patients.

Related Information

Hydrochlorothiazide *on page 775*
Losartan *on page 968*

Loteprednol (loe te PRED nol)

Brand Names: U.S. Alrex; Lotemax
Index Terms Loteprednol Etabonate
Pharmacologic Category Corticosteroid, Ophthalmic
Pregnancy Risk Factor C
Lactation Excretion in breast milk unknown/use caution
Use

Alrex®: Temporary relief of signs and symptoms of seasonal allergic conjunctivitis

Lotemax®: Treatment of postoperative inflammation and pain following ocular surgery; treatment of inflammatory conditions (eg, steroid-responsive inflammatory conditions of the palpebral and bulbar conjunctiva, cornea, and anterior segment of the globe such as allergic conjunctivitis, acne rosacea, superficial punctate keratitis, herpes zoster keratitis, iritis, cyclitis, selected infective conjunctivitis, when the inherent hazard of steroid use is accepted to obtain an advisable diminution in edema and inflammation)

Available Dosage Forms

Gel, Ophthalmic:
Lotemax: 0.5% (5 g)
Ointment, Ophthalmic:
Lotemax: 0.5% (3.5 g)
Suspension, Ophthalmic:
Alrex: 0.2% (5 mL, 10 mL)
Lotemax: 0.5% (5 mL, 10 mL, 15 mL)

General Dosage Range Ophthalmic: *Adults:* Ointment: Apply ~1/2 inch ribbon into affected eye(s) 4 times daily; Gel: Instill 1-2 drops into affected eye(s) 4 times daily; Suspension: Instill 1-2 drops into affected eye(s) 4 times daily

Administration

Ophthalmic

Gel: While bottle is closed, invert and shake once to fill tip prior to instilling drops.
Suspension: Shake well before using.

Nursing Actions

Patient Education

- Discuss specific use of drug and side effects with patient as it relates to treatment. (HCAHPS: During this hospital stay, were you given any medicine that you had not taken before? Before giving you any new medicine, how often did hospital staff tell you what the medicine was for? How often did hospital staff describe possible side effects in a way you could understand?)
- Patient may experience additional eye pressure, headache, eye irritation, or blurred vision. Have patient report immediately to prescriber sudden vision changes, eye pain, or rash (HCAHPS).
- Educate patient about signs of a significant reaction (eg, wheezing; chest tightness; fever; itching; bad cough; blue skin color; seizures; or swelling of face, lips, tongue, or throat). **Note:** This is not a comprehensive list of all side effects. Patient should consult prescriber for additional questions.

Intended Use and Disclaimer: Should not be printed and given to patients. This information is intended to serve as a concise initial reference for healthcare professionals to use when discussing medications with a patient. You must ultimately rely on your own discretion, experience and judgment in diagnosing, treating and advising patients.

Loteprednol and Tobramycin
(loe te PRED nol & toe bra MYE sin)

Brand Names: U.S. Zylet®
Index Terms Loteprednol Etabonate and Tobramycin; Tobramycin and Loteprednol Etabonate
Pharmacologic Category Antibiotic/Corticosteroid, Ophthalmic
Pregnancy Risk Factor C
Lactation Excretion in breast milk unknown/use caution
Use Treatment of steroid-responsive ocular inflammatory conditions where either a superficial bacterial ocular infection or the risk of a superficial bacterial ocular infection exists

Available Dosage Forms

Suspension, ophthalmic [drops]:
Zylet®: Loteprednol 0.5% and tobramycin 0.3% (2.5 mL, 5 mL, 10 mL)

General Dosage Range Ophthalmic: *Children and Adults:* Instill 1-2 drops into the affected eye(s) every 4-6 hours

Administration

Other Contact lenses should not be worn during therapy. Shake well before using; Tilt head back, instill suspension in conjunctival sac and close eye(s). Do not touch dropper to eye. Apply light finger pressure on lacrimal sac for 1 minute following instillation.

Nursing Actions

Physical Assessment See individual agents.

Patient Education

- Discuss specific use of drug and side effects with patient as it relates to treatment. (HCAHPS: During this hospital stay, were you given any medicine that you had not taken before? Before giving you any new medicine, how often did hospital staff tell you what the medicine was for? How often did hospital staff describe possible side effects in a way you could understand?)
- Patient may experience eye irritation, blurred vision, or headache. Have patient report immediately to prescriber sudden vision changes or eye pain (HCAHPS).
- Educate patient about signs of a significant reaction (eg, wheezing; chest tightness; fever; itching; bad cough; blue skin color; seizures; or swelling of face, lips, tongue, or throat). **Note:** This is not a comprehensive list of all side effects. Patient should consult prescriber for additional questions.

Intended Use and Disclaimer: Should not be printed and given to patients. This information is intended to serve as a concise initial reference for healthcare professionals to use when discussing medications with a patient. You must ultimately rely on your own discretion, experience and judgment in diagnosing, treating and advising patients.

Related Information

Loteprednol on page 971

Lovastatin (LOE va sta tin)

Brand Names: U.S. Altoprev; Mevacor

Index Terms Mevinolin; Monacolin K

Pharmacologic Category Antilipemic Agent, HMG-CoA Reductase Inhibitor

Medication Safety Issues

Sound-alike/look-alike issues:

Lovastatin may be confused with atorvaSTATin, Leustatin, Livostin, Lotensin, nystatin, pitavastatin

Mevacor may be confused with Benicar, Lipitor

International issues:

Lovacol [Chile and Finland] may be confused with Levatol brand name for penbutolol [U.S.]

Lovastin [Malaysia, Poland, and Singapore] may be confused with Livostin brand name for levocabastine [multiple international markets]

Mevacor [U.S., Canada, and multiple international markets} may be confused with Mivacron brand name for mivacurium [multiple international markets]

Pregnancy Risk Factor X

Lactation Excretion in breast milk unknown/contraindicated

Use

Adjunct to dietary therapy to decrease elevated serum total and LDL-cholesterol concentrations in primary hypercholesterolemia

Primary prevention of coronary artery disease (patients without symptomatic disease with average to moderately elevated total and LDL-cholesterol and below average HDL-cholesterol); slow progression of coronary atherosclerosis in patients with coronary heart disease and reduce the risk of myocardial infarction, unstable angina, and coronary revascularization procedures.

Adjunct to dietary therapy in adolescent patients (10-17 years of age, females >1 year postmenarche) with heterozygous familial hypercholesterolemia having LDL >189 mg/dL, **or** LDL >160 mg/dL with positive family history of premature cardiovascular disease (CVD), **or** LDL >160 mg/dL with the presence of at least two other CVD risk factors

Primary and secondary prevention of atherosclerotic cardiovascular disease (ASCVD) according to the American College of Cardiology/American Heart Association: To reduce the risk of ASCVD in patients with clinical ASCVD (eg, coronary heart disease, stroke/TIA, or peripheral arterial disease presumed to be of atherosclerotic origin) who are greater than 75 years of age or not a candidate for high-intensity statin therapy; in patients without clinical ASCVD if LDL-C is 190 mg/dL or greater and not a candidate for high-intensity statin therapy; in patients without clinical ASCVD who have type 1 or type 2 diabetes and are between 40 and 75 years of age; in patients with an estimated 10-year ASCVD risk 7.5% or greater and who are between 40 and 75 years of age (Stone, 2013).

Available Dosage Forms

Tablet, Oral:

Mevacor: 20 mg, 40 mg

Generic: 10 mg, 20 mg, 40 mg

Tablet Extended Release 24 Hour, Oral:

Altoprev: 20 mg, 40 mg, 60 mg

General Dosage Range Dosage adjustment recommended in patients with renal impairment or on concomitant therapy

Oral:

Extended release: *Adults:* 20-60 mg once daily (maximum: 60 mg daily)

Immediate release:

Children 10-17 years: Initial: 10-20 mg once daily; Maintenance: 10-40 mg once daily (maximum: 40 mg daily)

Adults: Initial: 20 mg once daily; Maintenance: 20-80 mg once daily (maximum: 80 mg daily)

Administration

Oral Administer immediate release tablet with the evening meal. Administer extended release tablet at bedtime; do not crush or chew.

Nursing Actions

Physical Assessment Assess risk potential for interactions with other prescriptions or herbal products patient may be taking that may increase risk of myopathy or rhabdomyolysis. Monitor for signs/symptoms of myopathy (muscle pain, tenderness, or weakness). Teach proper diet and exercise program.

Patient Education

- Discuss specific use of drug and side effects with patient as it relates to treatment. (HCAHPS: During this hospital stay, were you given any medicine that you had not taken before? Before giving you any new medicine, how often did hospital staff tell you what the medicine was for? How often did hospital staff describe possible side effects in a way you could understand?)
- Patient may experience headache, dyspepsia, diarrhea, asthenia, or arthralgia. Have patient report immediately to prescriber flu-like syndrome, ecchymosis, bleeding, inability to eat, severe fatigue, discolored urine, jaundice, or rash (HCAHPS).
- Educate patient about signs of a significant reaction (eg, wheezing; chest tightness; fever; itching; bad cough; blue skin color; seizures; or swelling of face, lips, tongue, or throat). **Note:** This is not a comprehensive list of all side effects. Patient should consult prescriber for additional questions.

Intended Use and Disclaimer: Should not be printed and given to patients. This information is intended to serve as a concise initial reference for healthcare professionals to use when discussing medications with a patient. You must ultimately rely on your own discretion, experience and judgment in diagnosing, treating and advising patients.

Related Information

Oral Medications That Should Not Be Crushed or Altered *on page 1712*

Lubiprostone (loo bi PROS tone)

Brand Names: U.S. Amitiza
Index Terms RU 0211; SPI 0211
Pharmacologic Category Chloride Channel Activator; Gastrointestinal Agent, Miscellaneous
Pregnancy Risk Factor C
Lactation Excretion in breast milk unknown/use caution
Breast-Feeding Considerations It is not known if lubiprostone or its active metabolite are excreted into breast milk. The manufacturer recommends monitoring nursing infants for diarrhea.
Use Treatment of chronic idiopathic constipation; treatment of opioid-induced constipation with chronic non-cancer pain; treatment of irritable bowel syndrome with constipation in adult women
Mechanism of Action/Effect Activates chloride channel channels in the intestines to increase intestinal fluid and intestinal motility

Contraindications Known or suspected mechanical bowel obstruction
Warnings/Precautions Symptoms of mechanical gastrointestinal obstruction should be evaluated before prescribing this medicine; use is contraindicated in patients with bowel obstruction. Avoid use in patients with severe diarrhea. Nausea may occur; administer with food to reduce symptoms. Dyspnea, often described as chest tightness, has been observed with use; generally occurs following the first dose with an acute onset (within 30-60 minutes) and resolves within a few hours; however, has been frequently reported with subsequent dosing. Dose adjustment may be needed in patients with moderate-to-severe hepatic impairment (Child-Pugh class B or C). Not approved for use in males with irritable bowel syndrome with constipation. Diphenylheptane opioids (eg, methadone) may potentially decrease the efficacy of lubiprostone in a dose-dependent manner.

Drug Interactions

Avoid Concomitant Use There are no known interactions where it is recommended to avoid concomitant use.

Decreased Effect

The levels/effects of Lubiprostone may be decreased by: Methadone

Increased Effect/Toxicity There are no known significant interactions involving an increase in effect.

Adverse Reactions

>10%:
  Central nervous system: Headache (2% to 11%)
  Gastrointestinal: Nausea (8% to 29%; severe: 1% to 4%; dose related; male: 8%; elderly: 19%), diarrhea (7% to 12%; severe <1% to 2%)
1% to 10%:
  Cardiovascular: Edema (3%), peripheral edema (1% to 3%), chest discomfort (2%)
  Central nervous system: Dizziness (3%), fatigue (2%)
  Gastrointestinal: Abdominal pain (4% to 8%), flatulence (4% to 6%), abdominal distention (3% to 6%), abdominal distress (3%), loose stools (3%), vomiting (3%), dyspepsia (2%), xerostomia (1%)
  Respiratory: Dyspnea (<1% to 3%)

Available Dosage Forms

Capsule, Oral:
  Amitiza: 8 mcg, 24 mcg

General Dosage Range Dosage adjustment recommended in hepatic impairment and in patients who develop toxicities

Oral:
  Adults (females): 8 mcg twice daily **or** 24 mcg twice daily
  Adults (males): 24 mcg twice daily

Administration

Oral Administer with food and water. Swallow whole; do not break or chew.

◀ **Storage/Stability** Store at 25°C (77°F); excursions permitted to 15°C to 30°C (59°F to 86°F). Protect from light and extreme temperatures.

Nursing Actions

Patient Education

• Discuss specific use of drug and side effects with patient as it relates to treatment. (HCAHPS: During this hospital stay, were you given any medicine that you had not taken before? Before giving you any new medicine, how often did hospital staff tell you what the medicine was for? How often did hospital staff describe possible side effects in a way you could understand?)

• Patient may experience nausea, headache, dyspepsia, pyrosis, or diarrhea. Have patient report immediately to prescriber dyspnea, angina, or rash (HCAHPS).

• Educate patient about signs of a significant reaction (eg, wheezing; chest tightness; fever; itching; bad cough; blue skin color; seizures; or swelling of face, lips, tongue, or throat). **Note:** This is not a comprehensive list of all side effects. Patient should consult prescriber for additional questions.

Intended Use and Disclaimer: Should not be printed and given to patients. This information is intended to serve as a concise initial reference for healthcare professionals to use when discussing medications with a patient. You must ultimately rely on your own discretion, experience and judgment in diagnosing, treating and advising patients.

Dietary Considerations Take with food and water to decrease nausea.

Related Information

Oral Medications That Should Not Be Crushed or Altered on page 1712

Luliconazole (loo li KON a zole)

Brand Names: U.S. Luzu

Pharmacologic Category Antifungal Agent, Topical

Pregnancy Risk Factor C

Lactation Excretion in breast milk unknown/use caution

Use Fungal infections: Topical treatment of tinea pedis, tinea cruris, and tinea corporis caused by the organisms *Trichophyton rubrum* and *Epidermophyton floccosum*

Product Availability Luzu: FDA approved November 2013; anticipated availability is currently unknown.

Available Dosage Forms

Cream, External:
Luzu: 1% (60 g)

General Dosage Range Topical: *Adults:* Apply once daily.

Administration

Topical For topical use only. Not for ophthalmic, oral, or intravaginal use. Wash hands following application.

Tinea pedis: Apply a thin layer to affected area and ~1 inch of immediate surrounding area(s).

Tinea cruris or tinea corporis: Apply to the affected area and ~1 inch of the immediate surrounding area(s).

Nursing Actions

Patient Education

• Discuss specific use of drug and side effects with patient as it relates to treatment. (HCAHPS: During this hospital stay, were you given any medicine that you had not taken before? Before giving you any new medicine, how often did hospital staff tell you what the medicine was for? How often did hospital staff describe possible side effects in a way you could understand?)

• Have patient report immediately to prescriber severe skin irritation (HCAHPS).

• Educate patient about signs of a significant reaction (eg, wheezing; chest tightness; fever; itching; bad cough; blue skin color; seizures; or swelling of face, lips, tongue, or throat). **Note:** This is not a comprehensive list of all side effects. Patient should consult prescriber for additional questions.

Intended Use and Disclaimer: Should not be printed and given to patients. This information is intended to serve as a concise initial reference for healthcare professionals to use when discussing medications with a patient. You must ultimately rely on your own discretion, experience and judgment in diagnosing, treating and advising patients.

Lurasidone (loo RAS i done)

Brand Names: U.S. Latuda

Index Terms Lurasidone Hydrochloride; SM-13496

Pharmacologic Category Antipsychotic Agent, Atypical

Medication Safety Issues

Sound-alike/look-alike issues:

Latuda may be confused with Lantus

BEERS Criteria medication:

This drug may be potentially inappropriate for use in geriatric patients (Quality of evidence - moderate; Strength of recommendation - strong).

Pregnancy Risk Factor B

Lactation Excretion in breast milk unknown/not recommended

Breast-Feeding Considerations It is not known if lurasidone is excreted in breast milk. Due to the potential for serious adverse reactions in the nursing infant, the manufacturer recommends a decision be made whether to discontinue nursing or to discontinue the drug, taking into account the importance of the treatment to the mother.

Use Psychiatric issues:

U.S. labeling: Treatment of schizophrenia; monotherapy or adjunctive therapy of depressive episodes associated with bipolar I disorder

Canadian labeling: Treatment of schizophrenia

Mechanism of Action/Effect Atypical antipsychotic with high affinity for serotonin, dopamine, and moderate affinity for alpha$_2$-adrenergic receptors; no significant affinity for muscarinic or histamine receptors. Results in improvement of psychotic symptoms and reduction of extrapyramidal and antimuscarinic side effects as compared to typical antipsychotics.

Contraindications Hypersensitivity to lurasidone or any component of the formulation; concomitant use with strong CYP3A4 inhibitors (eg, ketoconazole) and inducers (eg, rifampin)

Warnings/Precautions [U.S. Boxed Warning]: Antidepressants increase the risk of suicidal thinking and behavior in children, adolescents, and young adults (18-24 years of age) with major depressive disorder and other psychiatric disorders; consider risk prior to prescribing. Lurasidone is not approved in the U.S. for use in children. Short-term studies did not show an increased risk in patients >24 years of age and showed a decreased risk in patients ≥65 years. **[U.S. Boxed Warning]: Closely monitor all patients for clinical worsening, suicidality, or unusual changes in behavior,** particularly during the initial 1-2 months of therapy or during periods of dosage adjustments (increases or decreases); the patient's family or caregiver should be instructed to closely observe the patient and communicate condition with healthcare provider. A medication guide concerning the use of antidepressants should be dispensed with each prescription.

The possibility of a suicide attempt is inherent in major depression and may persist until remission occurs. Patients treated with antidepressants (for any indication) should be observed for clinical worsening and suicidality, especially during the initial few months of a course of drug therapy, or at times of dose changes (increases or decreases). Worsening depression and severe abrupt suicidality that are not part of the presenting symptoms may require discontinuation or modification of drug therapy. Use caution in high-risk patients during initiation of therapy.

Prescriptions should be written for the smallest quantity consistent with good patient care. The patient's family or caregiver should be alerted to monitor patients for the emergence of suicidality and associated behaviors such as anxiety, agitation, panic attacks, insomnia, irritability, hostility, impulsivity, akathisia, hypomania, and mania; patients should be instructed to notify their healthcare provider if any of these symptoms or worsening depression or psychosis occur.

[U.S. Boxed Warning]: Elderly patients with dementia-related psychosis treated with antipsychotics are at an increased risk of death compared to placebo. Most deaths appeared to be either cardiovascular (eg, heart failure, sudden death) or infectious (eg, pneumonia) in nature. **Lurasidone is not approved for the treatment of dementia-related psychosis.** An increased incidence of cerebrovascular effects (eg, transient ischemic attack, stroke), including fatalities, has been reported in placebo-controlled trials of antipsychotics for the unapproved use in elderly patients with dementia-related psychosis.

Leukopenia, neutropenia, and agranulocytosis (sometimes fatal) have been reported in clinical trials and postmarketing reports with antipsychotic use; presence of risk factors (eg, pre-existing low WBC or history of drug-induced leuko-/neutropenia) should prompt periodic blood count assessment. Discontinue therapy at first signs of blood dyscrasias or if absolute neutrophil count <1000/mm^3.

Low to moderately sedating, use with caution in disorders where CNS depression is a feature; patients must be cautioned about performing tasks which require mental alertness (eg, operating machinery or driving). Use with caution in Parkinson's disease. Caution in patients with predisposition to seizures, including those with a history of seizures, head trauma, brain damage, alcoholism, or concurrent therapy with medications which may lower seizure threshold. Elderly patients may be at increased risk of seizures due to an increased prevalence of predisposing factors. Use with caution in renal or hepatic dysfunction; dose reduction recommended in moderate-to-severe impairment. Esophageal dysmotility and aspiration have been associated with antipsychotic use; use with caution in patients at risk of aspiration pneumonia (ie, Alzheimer's disease). Use is associated with increased prolactin levels; clinical significance of hyperprolactinemia in patients with breast cancer or other prolactin-dependent tumors is unknown. May alter temperature regulation.

Use with caution in patients with severe cardiac disease, hemodynamic instability, prior myocardial infarction or ischemic heart disease. May cause orthostatic hypotension; use with caution in patients at risk of this effect (eg, concurrent medication use which may predispose to hypotension/bradycardia or presence of hypovolemia) or in those who would not tolerate transient hypotensive episodes. Antipsychotics may alter cardiac conduction; life-threatening arrhythmias have occurred with therapeutic doses of antipsychotics. Relative to other antipsychotics, lurasidone has minimal effects on the QT$_c$ interval and therefore, risk for arrhythmias is low. However, Canadian labeling recommends avoiding use of lurasidone in patients with a history of cardiac arrhythmias, situations that ▶

may increase the risk of torsade de pointes and/or sudden death due to QT prolongation including bradycardia, congenital QT prolongation, electrolyte disturbances (ie, hypokalemia or hypomagnesemia), or in combination with other QT_c-prolonging agents. Increases in total cholesterol and triglyceride concentrations have been observed with atypical antipsychotic use; during clinical trials of lurasidone, there were no significant changes in total cholesterol or triglycerides observed. Potentially significant drug-drug interactions may exist, requiring dose or frequency adjustment, additional monitoring, and/or selection of alternative therapy. Consult drug interactions database for more detailed information.

May cause extrapyramidal symptoms (EPS), including pseudoparkinsonism, acute dystonic reactions, akathisia, and tardive dyskinesia (potentially irreversible). Risk of tardive dyskinesia may be increased in elderly patients, particularly elderly women. Risk of dystonia (and probably other EPS) may be greater with increased doses, use of conventional antipsychotics, males, and younger patients. Use may be associated with neuroleptic malignant syndrome (NMS); monitor for mental status changes, fever, muscle rigidity and/or autonomic instability (risk may be increased in patients with Parkinson's disease or Lewy body dementia). May cause hyperglycemia; in some cases may be extreme and associated with ketoacidosis, hyperosmolar coma, or death. Use with caution in patients with diabetes or other disorders of glucose regulation; monitor for worsening of glucose control. Significant weight gain has been observed with antipsychotic therapy; incidence varies with product. Monitor waist circumference and BMI.

Use in elderly patients with dementia is associated with an increased risk of mortality and cerebrovascular accidents; avoid antipsychotic use for behavioral problems associated with dementia unless alternative nonpharmacologic therapies have failed and patient may harm self or others. In addition, use may cause or exacerbate syndrome of inappropriate antidiuretic hormone secretion or hyponatremia; monitor sodium closely with initiation or dosage adjustments in older adults (Beers Criteria).

Drug Interactions

Avoid Concomitant Use

Avoid concomitant use of Lurasidone with any of the following: Amisulpride; Azelastine (Nasal); CYP3A4 Inducers (Strong); CYP3A4 Inhibitors (Strong); DOPamine; EPINEPHrine (Systemic, Oral Inhalation); Fusidic Acid (Systemic); Grapefruit Juice; Metoclopramide; Paraldehyde; Pimozide; St Johns Wort; Sulpiride; Thalidomide

Decreased Effect

Lurasidone may decrease the levels/effects of: Amphetamines; Anti-Parkinson's Agents (Dopamine Agonist); Quinagolide

The levels/effects of Lurasidone may be decreased by: Bosentan; CYP3A4 Inducers (Strong); Dabrafenib; Deferasirox; Lithium formulations; St Johns Wort; Tocilizumab

Increased Effect/Toxicity

Lurasidone may increase the levels/effects of: Alcohol (Ethyl); Amisulpride; ARIPiprazole; Azelastine (Nasal); Buprenorphine; CNS Depressants; Disopyramide; Dofetilide; Hydrocodone; Lomitapide; Methotrimeprazine; Methylphenidate; Paraldehyde; Pimozide; Procainamide; QuiNIDine; Serotonin Modulators; Sulpiride; Thalidomide; Zolpidem

The levels/effects of Lurasidone may be increased by: Acetylcholinesterase Inhibitors (Central); Brimonidine (Topical); CYP3A4 Inhibitors (Moderate); CYP3A4 Inhibitors (Strong); Dasatinib; DOPamine; Doxylamine; Droperidol; EPINEPHrine (Systemic, Oral Inhalation); Fusidic Acid (Systemic); Grapefruit Juice; HydrOXYzine; Ivacaftor; Lithium formulations; Luliconazole; Magnesium Sulfate; MAO Inhibitors; Methotrimeprazine; Methylphenidate; Metoclopramide; Metyrosine; Mifepristone; Perampanel; Serotonin Modulators; Simeprevir; Sodium Oxybate; Tetrabenazine

Nutritional/Ethanol Interactions

Ethanol: May increase CNS depression; monitor for increased effects with coadministration. Caution patients about effects.

Food: Administration with food (≥350 calories) increased C_{max} and AUC of lurasidone ~3 times and 2 times, respectively, compared to administration under fasting conditions. Lurasidone exposure was not affected by the fat content of the meal.

Adverse Reactions
Frequencies reported for schizophrenia unless otherwise noted.

10%:

Central nervous system: Drowsiness (dose-related: 8% to 27%; depressive episodes, monotherapy: 11%), extrapyramidal reaction (dose-related: 14% to 26%; depressive episodes, monotherapy: 7%), akathisia (dose-related: 6% to 22%; depressive episodes, monotherapy: 8% to 11%), parkinsonian-like syndrome (6% to 17%; depressive episodes, monotherapy: 8%)

Endocrine & metabolic: Increased serum triglycerides (10% to 14%), increased serum glucose (fasting, 10% to 14%), increased serum cholesterol (6% to 14%)

Gastrointestinal: Nausea (dose-related; 10%; depressive episodes, monotherapy: 14%)

1% to 10%:

Cardiovascular: Orthostatic hypotension (1% to 2%), tachycardia

Central nervous system: Insomnia (10%), agitation (5%; depressive episodes, monotherapy: 4%), anxiety (5%), dizziness (4%), dystonia

(≤7%; depressive episodes, monotherapy: ≤2%), restlessness (1% to 3%)

Dermatologic: Pruritus, skin rash

Endocrine & metabolic: Increased serum prolactin (≥5 x ULN: females: 8%; males: ≤2%), weight gain (≥7% increase in baseline body weight: 2% to 6%)

Gastrointestinal: Vomiting (8%; depressive episodes, monotherapy: 4%), dyspepsia (6%), xerostomia (depressive episodes, monotherapy: 5%), diarrhea (≥1%; depressive episodes, monotherapy: 4%), sialorrhea (2%), abdominal pain, decreased appetite

Genitourinary: Urinary tract infection (depressive episodes, monotherapy: 2%)

Infection: Influenza (depressive episodes, monotherapy: 2%)

Neuromuscular & skeletal: Back pain (3%; depressive episodes, monotherapy: 2%), increased creatine phosphokinase

Ophthalmic: Blurred vision

Renal: Increased serum creatinine (3% to 7%; depressive episodes, monotherapy: 2% to 4%)

Respiratory: Nasopharyngitis (depressive episodes, monotherapy: 4%)

Available Dosage Forms

Tablet, Oral:

Latuda: 20 mg, 40 mg, 60 mg, 80 mg, 120 mg

General Dosage Range Dosage adjustment recommended in patients with hepatic or renal impairment or on concomitant therapy.

Oral: *Adults:* Initial: 20-40 mg once daily (maximum: 120-160 mg daily)

Administration

Oral Administer with food (≥350 calories).

Storage/Stability Store at controlled room temperature of 25°C (77°F); excursions permitted to 15°C to 30°C (59°F to 86°F).

Nursing Actions

Physical Assessment Monitor weight prior to treatment and periodically throughout. Be alert to the potential for orthostatic hypotension. Taper dosage slowly when discontinuing.

Patient Education

• Discuss specific use of drug and side effects with patient as it relates to treatment. (HCAHPS: During this hospital stay, were you given any medicine that you had not taken before? Before giving you any new medicine, how often did hospital staff tell you what the medicine was for? How often did hospital staff describe possible side effects in a way you could understand?)

• Patient may experience presyncope, fatigue, blurred vision, illogical thinking, dizziness, nausea, weight gain, or hyperglycemia. Have patient report immediately to prescriber angina, significant change in balance, tremors, severe myalgia, polyuria, polydipsia, weight loss, significant asthenia, or rash (HCAHPS).

• Educate patient about signs of a significant reaction (eg, wheezing; chest tightness; fever;

itching; bad cough; blue skin color; seizures; or swelling of face, lips, tongue, or throat). **Note:** This is not a comprehensive list of all side effects. Patient should consult prescriber for additional questions.

Intended Use and Disclaimer: Should not be printed and given to patients. This information is intended to serve as a concise initial reference for healthcare professionals to use when discussing medications with a patient. You must ultimately rely on your own discretion, experience and judgment in diagnosing, treating and advising patients.

Dietary Considerations Should be taken with food (≥350 calories).

Lutropin Alfa (LOO troe pin AL fa)

Index Terms r-hLH; Recombinant Human Luteinizing Hormone

Pharmacologic Category Gonadotropin; Ovulation Stimulator

Pregnancy Risk Factor X

Lactation Excretion in breast milk unknown/use caution

Use Stimulation of follicular development in infertile hypogonadotropic hypogonadal (HH) women with profound luteinizing hormone (LH) deficiency (<1.2 units/L); to be used in combination with follitropin alfa

General Dosage Range SubQ: *Adults (females):* 75 units daily

Administration

Other SubQ: Administer on the stomach, a few inches above or below the navel. Do not shake solution; allow any bubbles to settle prior to administration.

Nursing Actions

Physical Assessment This medication should only be prescribed by a fertility specialist. For subcutaneous use only. Administer around navel area. Instruct patient in appropriate administration technique and disposal of used needles and syringes.

Patient Education

• Discuss specific use of drug and side effects with patient as it relates to treatment. (HCAHPS: During this hospital stay, were you given any medicine that you had not taken before? Before giving you any new medicine, how often did hospital staff tell you what the medicine was for? How often did hospital staff describe possible side effects in a way you could understand?)

• Patient may experience injection site irritation, ovarian cysts, nausea, or headache. Have patient report immediately to prescriber dyspnea, severe dyspepsia, significant weight gain, or rash (HCAHPS).

• Educate patient about signs of a significant reaction (eg, wheezing; chest tightness; fever;

itching; bad cough; blue skin color; seizures; or swelling of face, lips, tongue, or throat). **Note:** This is not a comprehensive list of all side effects. Patient should consult prescriber for additional questions.

Intended Use and Disclaimer: Should not be printed and given to patients. This information is intended to serve as a concise initial reference for healthcare professionals to use when discussing medications with a patient. You must ultimately rely on your own discretion, experience and judgment in diagnosing, treating and advising patients.

Macitentan (ma si TEN tan)

Brand Names: U.S. Opsumit
Index Terms ACT-064992
Pharmacologic Category Endothelin Receptor Antagonist; Vasodilator
Medication Guide Available Yes
Pregnancy Risk Factor X
Lactation Excretion in breast milk unknown/not recommended
Use Pulmonary arterial hypertension: Treatment of pulmonary arterial hypertension (PAH) (WHO Group I) to delay disease progression.
Available Dosage Forms
Tablet, Oral:
Opsumit: 10 mg
General Dosage Range Oral: *Adults:* 10 mg once daily
Administration
Oral Swallow tablet whole. Do not split, crush, or chew tablets. May be administered with or without food. Hazardous agent; use appropriate precautions for handling and disposal (NIOSH, 2012).
Nursing Actions
Patient Education
• Discuss specific use of drug and side effects with patient as it relates to treatment. (HCAHPS: During this hospital stay, were you given any medicine that you had not taken before? Before giving you any new medicine, how often did hospital staff tell you what the medicine was for? How often did hospital staff describe possible side effects in a way you could understand?)
• Patient may experience headache, rhinitis, pharyngitis, rhinorrhea, or flu-like symptoms. Have patient report immediately to prescriber signs of hepatic impairment, severe asthenia, dyspnea, considerable weight gain, edema of extremities, ecchymoses, hemorrhaging, dysuria, or difficult urination (HCAHPS).
• Educate patient about signs of a significant reaction (eg, wheezing; chest tightness; fever; itching; bad cough; blue skin color; seizures; or swelling of face, lips, tongue, or throat). **Note:** This is not a comprehensive list of all side effects. Patient should consult prescriber for additional questions.

Intended Use and Disclaimer: Should not be printed and given to patients. This information is intended to serve as a concise initial reference for healthcare professionals to use when discussing medications with a patient. You must ultimately rely on your own discretion, experience and judgment in diagnosing, treating and advising patients.

Magnesium Chloride (mag NEE zhum KLOR ide)

Brand Names: U.S. Chloromag; Mag-Delay [OTC]; Mag-SR Plus Calcium [OTC]; Mag-SR [OTC]; Slow Magnesium/Calcium [OTC]; Slow-Mag [OTC]
Pharmacologic Category Electrolyte Supplement, Oral; Electrolyte Supplement, Parenteral; Magnesium Salt
Pregnancy Risk Factor C
Lactation Enters breast milk
Use Correction or prevention of hypomagnesemia; dietary supplement
Dosage Forms Considerations
1 g magnesium chloride = elemental magnesium 120 mg = magnesium 9.85 mEq = magnesium 4.93 mmol
Elemental magnesium 64 mg = magnesium 5.26 mEq = magnesium 2.62 mmol
Available Dosage Forms
Solution, Injection:
Chloromag: 200 mg/mL (50 mL)
Generic: 200 mg/mL (50 mL)
Tablet Delayed Release, Oral:
Mag-SR Plus Calcium [OTC]: 64 mg
Slow Magnesium/Calcium [OTC]: 64 mg
Slow-Mag [OTC]: 71.5 mg
Tablet Extended Release, Oral:
Mag-Delay [OTC]: 535 mg
Mag-SR [OTC]: 535 mg
General Dosage Range
I.V.:
Children <50 kg: 0.3-0.5 mEq/kg/day
Children >50 kg: 10-30 mEq/day
Adults: 8-24 mEq/day added to TPN
Oral: RDA (elemental magnesium):
Children: 80-240 mg/day
Adults: 360-410 mg/day
Nursing Actions
Patient Education
• Discuss specific use of drug and side effects with patient as it relates to treatment. (HCAHPS: During this hospital stay, were you given any medicine that you had not taken before? Before giving you any new medicine, how often did hospital staff tell you what the medicine was for? How often did hospital staff describe possible side effects in a way you could understand?)

- Patient may experience diarrhea. Have patient report immediately to prescriber dyspnea, severe dizziness, significant flushing, considerable asthenia, illogical thinking, or rash (HCAHPS).
- Educate patient about signs of a significant reaction (eg, wheezing; chest tightness; fever; itching; bad cough; blue skin color; seizures; or swelling of face, lips, tongue, or throat). **Note:** This is not a comprehensive list of all side effects. Patient should consult prescriber for additional questions.

Intended Use and Disclaimer: Should not be printed and given to patients. This information is intended to serve as a concise initial reference for healthcare professionals to use when discussing medications with a patient. You must ultimately rely on your own discretion, experience and judgment in diagnosing, treating and advising patients.

Related Information

Oral Medications That Should Not Be Crushed or Altered *on page 1712*

Magnesium Gluconate
(mag NEE zhum GLOO koe nate)

Brand Names: U.S. Mag-G [OTC]; Magonate [OTC]

Pharmacologic Category Electrolyte Supplement, Oral; Magnesium Salt

Lactation Enters breast milk/compatible

Use Dietary supplement

Dosage Forms Considerations

1 g magnesium gluconate = elemental magnesium 54 mg = magnesium 4.5 mEq = magnesium 2.25 mmol

Available Dosage Forms

Liquid, Oral:

Magonate [OTC]: Magnesium carbonate equivalent to magnesium gluconate 1000 mg (54 mg elemental magnesium) per 5 mL (355 mL)

Tablet, Oral:

Mag-G [OTC]: 500 mg (27 mg elemental magnesium)

Magonate [OTC]: 500 mg (27 mg elemental magnesium)

Generic: Elemental magnesium 27.5 mg

Tablet, Oral [preservative free]:

Generic: 500 mg (27 mg elemental magnesium)

General Dosage Range Oral: RDA (elemental magnesium):

Children 1-13 years: 80-240 mg/day

Children ≥14 years and Adults: 310-420 mg/day

Administration

Oral Administer on an empty stomach

Nursing Actions

Patient Education

- Discuss specific use of drug and side effects with patient as it relates to treatment. (HCAHPS: During this hospital stay, were you given any medicine that you had not taken before? Before giving you any new medicine, how often did hospital staff tell you what the medicine was for? How often did hospital staff describe possible side effects in a way you could understand?)
- Patient may experience diarrhea. Have patient report immediately to prescriber dyspnea, illogical thinking, severe nausea, significant asthenia, or rash (HCAHPS).
- Educate patient about signs of a significant reaction (eg, wheezing; chest tightness; fever; itching; bad cough; blue skin color; seizures; or swelling of face, lips, tongue, or throat). **Note:** This is not a comprehensive list of all side effects. Patient should consult prescriber for additional questions.

Intended Use and Disclaimer: Should not be printed and given to patients. This information is intended to serve as a concise initial reference for healthcare professionals to use when discussing medications with a patient. You must ultimately rely on your own discretion, experience and judgment in diagnosing, treating and advising patients.

Magnesium Sulfate (mag NEE zhum SUL fate)

Brand Names: U.S. Epsom Salt [OTC]

Index Terms Epsom Salts; $MgSO_4$ (error-prone abbreviation)

Pharmacologic Category Anticonvulsant, Miscellaneous; Electrolyte Supplement, Parenteral; Magnesium Salt

Medication Safety Issues

Sound-alike/look-alike issues:

Magnesium sulfate may be confused with manganese sulfate, morphine sulfate

$MgSO_4$ is an error-prone abbreviation (mistaken as morphine sulfate)

High alert medication:

The Institute for Safe Medication Practices (ISMP) includes this medication (I.V. formulation) among its list of drugs which have a heightened risk of causing significant patient harm when used in error.

Pregnancy Risk Factor D

Lactation Enters breast milk/use caution

Use

Treatment and prevention of hypomagnesemia; prevention and treatment of seizures in severe pre-eclampsia or eclampsia, pediatric acute nephritis; torsade de pointes; treatment of cardiac arrhythmias (VT/VF) caused by hypomagnesemia

OTC labeling: Soaking aid for minor cuts and bruises; laxative for the relief of occasional constipation

Unlabeled Use Asthma exacerbation (life-threatening) unresponsive to 1 hour intensive conventional treatment

Dosage Forms Considerations

1 g of magnesium sulfate = elemental magnesium 98.6 mg = magnesium 8.12 mEq = magnesium 4.06 mmol

Magnesium sulfate 1% [10 mg/mL] in Dextrose 5% injection is equivalent to elemental magnesium 0.081 mEq/mL.

Magnesium sulfate 2% [20 mg/mL] in Dextrose 5% injection is equivalent to elemental magnesium 0.162 mEq/mL.

Magnesium sulfate 4% [40 mg/mL] in Water injection is equivalent to elemental magnesium 0.325 mEq/mL.

Magnesium sulfate 8% [80 mg/mL] in Water injection is equivalent to elemental magnesium 0.65 mEq/mL.

Magnesium sulfate 50% injection is equivalent to elemental magnesium 4 mEq/mL.

Available Dosage Forms

Capsule, Oral:
Generic: 70 mg

Granules, Oral:
Epsom Salt [OTC]: (454 g, 1810 g, 1816 g)

Solution, Injection:
Generic: 40 mg/mL (50 mL, 100 mL, 500 mL, 1000 mL); 80 mg/mL (50 mL); 50% (2 mL, 10 mL, 20 mL, 50 mL)

Solution, Intravenous:
Generic: 10 mg/mL (100 mL); 20 mg/mL (500 mL)

General Dosage Range

I.V.: *Children and Adults*: Dosage varies greatly depending on indication

Oral:
RDA (elemental magnesium):
Children 1-13 years: 80-240 mg daily
Children ≥14 years and Adults: 310-420 mg daily
Laxative:
Children 6-12 years: 1-2 teaspoons of granules dissolved in water once daily
Children >12 years, Adolescents, and Adults: 2-6 teaspoons of granules dissolved in water once daily

I.M.: *Adults*: Hypomagnesemia: 1-4 g daily in divided doses

Topical: *Adults*: Soaking aid: Dissolve 2 cupfuls of granules per gallon of warm water

Administration

I.M. Must be diluted prior to administration for children (Adults: 25% or 50% concentration; Children: ≤20% diluted solution)

I.V. Must be diluted to a ≤20% solution for I.V. infusion and may be administered I.V. push, IVPB, or continuous I.V. infusion. When giving I.V. push, must dilute first and should generally not be given any faster than 150 mg/minute; may administer over 1-2 minutes in patients with persistent pulseless VT or VF with known hypomagnesemia (Dager, 2006). ACLS guidelines recommend administration over 15 minutes in patients with torsade de pointes (ACLS, 2010). In patients not in cardiac arrest, hypotension and asystole may occur with rapid administration.

Maximal rate of infusion: Up to 50% of an I.V. dose may be eliminated in the urine, therefore, slower administration may improve retention. If severely symptomatic, may administer ≤4 g over 4-5 minutes. For doses <6 g, infuse over 8-12 hours and for larger doses infuse over 24 hours if patient asymptomatic (Kraft, 2005).

Oral When used as a laxative, the patient should drink a full 8 ounces of liquid following each dose. Lemon juice may be added to the initial solution to improve the taste.

Topical May dissolve granules to prepare a solution for use as a soaking aid or as a compress. To make a compress, use a towel to apply as a wet dressing.

Nursing Actions

Physical Assessment When administered parenterally, monitor serum magnesium concentration, respiratory rate, deep tendon reflex, and renal function.

Patient Education

• Discuss specific use of drug and side effects with patient as it relates to treatment. (HCAHPS: During this hospital stay, were you given any medicine that you had not taken before? Before giving you any new medicine, how often did hospital staff tell you what the medicine was for? How often did hospital staff describe possible side effects in a way you could understand?)

• Patient may experience hypotension, injection site irritation, or diarrhea. Have patient report immediately to prescriber angina, tachycardia, severe dizziness, significant asthenia, sudden vision changes, illogical thinking, considerable flushing, or rash (HCAHPS).

• Educate patient about signs of a significant reaction (eg, wheezing; chest tightness; fever; itching; bad cough; blue skin color; seizures; or swelling of face, lips, tongue, or throat). **Note:** This is not a comprehensive list of all side effects. Patient should consult prescriber for additional questions.

Intended Use and Disclaimer: Should not be printed and given to patients. This information is intended to serve as a concise initial reference for healthcare professionals to use when discussing medications with a patient. You must ultimately rely on your own discretion, experience and judgment in diagnosing, treating and advising patients.

Mannitol (MAN i tole)

Brand Names: U.S. Aridol; Osmitrol; Resectisol

Index Terms D-Mannitol

Pharmacologic Category Diagnostic Agent; Diuretic, Osmotic; Genitourinary Irrigant

Medication Safety Issues

Sound-alike/look-alike issues:

Osmitrol® may be confused with esmolol

Pregnancy Risk Factor C

Lactation Excretion in breast milk unknown/use caution

Use

Injection: Reduction of increased intracranial pressure associated with cerebral edema; reduction of increased intraocular pressure; promoting urinary excretion of toxic substances; genitourinary irrigant in transurethral prostatic resection or other transurethral surgical procedures

Note: Although FDA-labeled indications, the use of mannitol for the prevention of acute renal failure and/or promotion of diuresis is not routinely recommended (Kellum, 2008).

Genitourinary irrigation solution: Irrigation in transurethral prostatic resection or other transurethral surgical procedures

Powder for inhalation: Assessment of bronchial hyper-responsiveness

Unlabeled Use Improve renal transplant function

Available Dosage Forms

Kit, Inhalation:

Aridol:

Solution, Intravenous:

Osmitrol: 5% (1000 mL); 10% (500 mL); 15% (500 mL); 20% (250 mL, 500 mL)

Generic: 5% (1000 mL); 10% (1000 mL); 15% (500 mL); 20% (250 mL, 500 mL); 25% (50 mL)

Solution, Irrigation:

Resectisol: 5% (2000 mL)

General Dosage Range

Inhalation: *Children ≥6 years and Adults:* 0-635 mg administered in a stepwise fashion until a positive response or the full dose has been administered (whichever comes first)

I.V.: *Adults:* Reduction of intraocular pressure: 1.5-2 g/kg

Transurethral: *Adults:* Use 5% urogenital solution as required for irrigation

Administration

I.V. Concentration and rate of administration depends on indication/severity, or may be adjusted to urine flow. For cerebral edema or elevated ICP, administer over 30-60 minutes. Inspect for crystals prior to administration. If crystals present redissolve by warming solution. Use filter-type administration set for infusion solutions containing mannitol ≥20%. Do not administer with blood. Crenation and agglutination of red blood cells may occur if administered with whole blood.

Vesicant (at concentrations >5%); ensure proper catheter or needle position prior to and during I.V. infusion. Avoid extravasation of I.V. infusions.

Extravasation management: If extravasation occurs, stop infusion immediately and disconnect (leave needle/cannula in place); gently aspirate extravasated solution (do **NOT** flush the line); initiate hyaluronidase antidote; remove needle/cannula; apply dry cold compresses (Hurst, 2004); elevate extremity.

Hyaluronidase: ubQ: Administer multiple 0.5-1 mL injections of a 15 units/mL solution around the periphery of the extravasation (Kumar, 2003).

Injectable Detail pH: 4.5-7

Inhalation Inhalation (Aridol): Administer using supplied single patient use inhaler; do not puncture capsule more than once; do not swallow capsules. A nose clip may be used if preferred. The patient should exhale completely, followed by a controlled rapid deep inspiration from the device; hold breath for 5 seconds and exhale through the mouth. Measure FEV_1 in duplicate 60 seconds after inhalation; repeat process until positive response or full dose (635 mg) has been administered.

Other Irrigation: Administer using only the appropriate transurethral urologic instrumentation.

Nursing Actions

Physical Assessment Adequate renal function should be present prior to administration. Monitor infusion site closely for extravasation; this is a vesicant. Monitor renal and cardiovascular status during infusion. Monitor for circulatory overload, CHF, rash, and water intoxication.

Patient Education

• Discuss specific use of drug and side effects with patient as it relates to treatment. (HCAHPS: During this hospital stay, were you given any medicine that you had not taken before? Before giving you any new medicine, how often did hospital staff tell you what the medicine was for? How often did hospital staff describe possible side effects in a way you could understand?)

• Patient may experience hypokalemia, dizziness, headache, nausea, xerostomia, or dyspepsia. Have patient report immediately to prescriber dyspnea, angina, tachycardia, sudden vision changes, urinary retention, severe edema, or rash (HCAHPS).

• Educate patient about signs of a significant reaction (eg, wheezing; chest tightness; fever; itching; bad cough; blue skin color; seizures; or swelling of face, lips, tongue, or throat). **Note:** This is not a comprehensive list of all side effects. Patient should consult prescriber for additional questions.

Intended Use and Disclaimer: Should not be printed and given to patients. This information is intended to serve as a concise initial reference for ▶

healthcare professionals to use when discussing medications with a patient. You must ultimately rely on your own discretion, experience and judgment in diagnosing, treating and advising patients.

Related Information

Diagnostics and Surgical Aids *on page 1670*

Management of Drug Extravasations *on page 1700*

Maraviroc (mah RAV er rock)

Brand Names: U.S. Selzentry

Index Terms UK-427,857

Pharmacologic Category Antiretroviral, CCR5 Antagonist (Anti-HIV)

Medication Guide Available Yes

Pregnancy Risk Factor B

Lactation Excretion in breast milk unknown/contraindicated

Breast-Feeding Considerations It is not known if maraviroc is excreted into breast milk. Maternal or infant antiretroviral therapy does not completely eliminate the risk of postnatal HIV transmission. In addition, multiclass-resistant virus has been detected in breast-feeding infants despite maternal therapy. Therefore, in the United States, where formula is accessible, affordable, safe, and sustainable, and the risk of infant mortality due to diarrhea and respiratory infections is low, complete avoidance of breast-feeding by HIV-infected women is recommended to decrease potential transmission of HIV (DHHS [perinatal], 2012).

Use Treatment of CCR5-tropic HIV-1 infection, in combination with other antiretroviral agents

Mechanism of Action/Effect Inhibits CCR5-tropic HIV-1 virus from entering into CD4 cells

Contraindications Patients with severe renal impairment (CrCl <30 mL/minute) or end-stage renal disease (ESRD) who are taking potent CYP3A4 inhibitors or inducers

Canadian labeling: Additional contraindications (not in U.S. labeling): Hypersensitivity to maraviroc or any component of the formulation

Warnings/Precautions [U.S. Boxed Warning] Possible drug-induced hepatotoxicity with allergic type features has been reported; hepatotoxicity (usually after 1 month of treatment) may be preceded by allergic type reactions (eg, pruritic rash, eosinophilia, fever or increased IgE, excluding rash alone or Stevens-Johnson syndrome [DHHS, 2013]) and/or hepatic adverse events (transaminase increases or signs/symptoms of hepatitis); some cases have been life-threatening; immediately evaluate patients with signs and symptoms of allergic reaction or hepatitis. Use with caution in patients with preexisting hepatic dysfunction or coinfection with HBV or HCV, however symptoms have occurred in the absence of preexisting hepatic conditions. Monitor hepatic function at baseline and as clinically indicated during treatment. Consider discontinuation in any patient with possible hepatitis or with elevated transaminases combined with systemic allergic events.

Severe and life-threatening skin and hypersensitivity reactions, including Stevens-Johnson syndrome, toxic epidermal necrolysis and drug rash with eosinophilia with systemic symptoms (DRESS), have been reported with use, predominately in patients also receiving concomitant agents associated with these reactions. Rash and constitutional findings (eg, fever, muscle aches, conjunctivitis, oral lesions), with or without organ dysfunction, have also accompanied these reports. Discontinue maraviroc and any other suspected agent immediately if symptoms or signs of hypersensitivity occur. Monitor liver function tests and clinical status as appropriate.

Patients may develop immune reconstitution syndrome resulting in the occurrence of an inflammatory response to an indolent or residual opportunistic infection during initial HIV treatment or activation of autoimmune disorders (eg, Graves' disease, polymyositis, Guillain-Barré syndrome) later in therapy; further evaluation and treatment may be required. Monitor closely for signs/symptoms of developing infections; use associated with a small increase of certain upper respiratory tract infections and herpes virus infections during clinical trials. Use with caution in patients with cardiovascular disease or cardiac risk factors. During trials, a small increase in cardiovascular events (myocardial ischemia and/or infarction) occurred in treated patients compared to placebo, although a contributory relationship relative to therapy is unknown. Symptomatic postural hypotension has occurred; use caution in patients at risk for postural hypotension due to concomitant medication or history of condition. Adjust dose in patients with severe renal dysfunction if postural hypotension experienced.

Use caution in patients with mild-to-moderate hepatic impairment; maraviroc concentrations are increased; no dosage adjustment recommended. Maraviroc concentrations are further increased in patients with moderate hepatic impairment receiving concomitant strong CYP3A inhibitors; monitor closely for adverse events. Renal impairment may increase maraviroc concentrations. Use with caution in patients with mild-to-moderate renal impairment. Potentially significant interactions may exist, requiring dose or frequency adjustment, additional monitoring, and/or selection of alternative therapy. Prior to therapy, coreceptor tropism testing should be performed for presence of CCR5-tropic only virus HIV-1 infection. Therapy not recommended for use in patients with CXCR4- or dual/mixed tropic HIV-1 infection; efficacy not demonstrated in this population. In studies with treatment-naive patients, virologic failure and emergent lamivudine resistance was more common in maraviroc-treated patients compared to patients receiving efavirenz.

Drug Interactions

Avoid Concomitant Use

Avoid concomitant use of Maraviroc with any of the following: Fusidic Acid (Systemic); St Johns Wort

Decreased Effect

The levels/effects of Maraviroc may be decreased by: Bosentan; CYP3A4 Inducers (Strong); Dabrafenib; Deferasirox; St Johns Wort; Tocilizumab

Increased Effect/Toxicity

The levels/effects of Maraviroc may be increased by: CYP3A4 Inhibitors (Moderate); CYP3A4 Inhibitors (Strong); Dasatinib; Fusidic Acid (Systemic); Ivacaftor; Luliconazole; Mifepristone; Simeprevir

Nutritional/Ethanol Interactions Herb/Nutraceutical: St. John's wort may decrease maraviroc concentrations leading to loss of therapeutic efficacy and potentially increased risk of resistance; concomitant use not recommended.

Adverse Reactions

>10%:

Central nervous system: Fever (13%)

Dermatologic: Skin rash (11%)

Respiratory: Upper respiratory tract infection (23%), cough (14%)

2% to 10%:

Cardiovascular: Vascular hypertensive disorder (3%)

Central nervous system: Dizziness (9%; including postural dizziness), insomnia (8%), paresthesia (5%), anxiety (4%), impaired consciousness (4%), depression (4%), pain (4%), peripheral neuropathy (4%), sensory disturbance (4%), amnesia (3%)

Dermatologic: Folliculitis (4%), pruritus (4%), acne vulgaris (3%), skin neoplasm (benign; 3%), alopecia (2%), erythema (2%), tinea (4%)

Endocrine & metabolic: Lipodystrophy (4%)

Gastrointestinal: Decreased gastrointestinal motility (9%), change in appetite (8%), constipation (6%)

Genitourinary: Genitourinary complaint (urinary tract/bladder symptoms, 3% to 5%), warts (genital, 2%)

Hematologic & oncologic: Neutropenia (grades 3/4: 4%)

Hepatic: Increased serum AST (grades 3/4: 5%), increased serum ALT (grades 3/4: 3%), increased serum bilirubin (grades 3/4: 6%)

Infection: Herpes infection (8%), bacterial infection (3%), *Neisseria*, (3%),

Neuromuscular & skeletal: Arthralgia (7%), myalgia (3%)

Ophthalmic: Conjunctivitis (2%), eye infection (2%)

Otic: Otitis media (2%)

Respiratory: Bronchitis (7%), sinusitis (7%), paranasal sinus disease (3% to 6%), irregular breathing (4%), nasal congestion (4%), lower respiratory tract infection (3%)

Miscellaneous: Sweat gland disturbances (5%), flu-like symptoms (2%)

Available Dosage Forms

Tablet, Oral:

Selzentry: 150 mg, 300 mg

General Dosage Range Dosage adjustment recommended in patients with renal impairment or on concomitant therapy

Oral: *Children ≥16 years and Adults:* 300 mg twice daily

Administration

Oral Administer without regards to meals.

Storage/Stability Store at 25°C (77°F); excursions permitted to 15°C to 30°C (59°F to 86°F).

Nursing Actions

Physical Assessment Monitor for cardiotoxicity, hepatotoxicity, upper respiratory infections, hypotension, dizziness, insomnia, and rash. Teach patient proper timing of multiple medications.

Patient Education

- Discuss specific use of drug and side effects with patient as it relates to treatment. (HCAHPS: During this hospital stay, were you given any medicine that you had not taken before? Before giving you any new medicine, how often did hospital staff tell you what the medicine was for? How often did hospital staff describe possible side effects in a way you could understand?)
- Patient may experience dizziness, dyspepsia, myalgia, arthralgia, or hepatic impairment. Have patient report immediately to prescriber signs of infection, severe asthenia, discolored urine, jaundice, inability to eat, or rash (HCAHPS).
- Educate patient about signs of a significant reaction (eg, wheezing; chest tightness; fever; itching; bad cough; blue skin color; seizures; or swelling of face, lips, tongue, or throat). **Note:** This is not a comprehensive list of all side effects. Patient should consult prescriber for additional questions.

Intended Use and Disclaimer: Should not be printed and given to patients. This information is intended to serve as a concise initial reference for healthcare professionals to use when discussing medications with a patient. You must ultimately rely on your own discretion, experience and judgment in diagnosing, treating and advising patients.

Dietary Considerations May be taken without regards to meals.

Measles, Mumps, and Rubella Virus Vaccine (MEE zels, mumpz & roo BEL a VYE rus vak SEEN)

Brand Names: U.S. M-M-R II

Index Terms MMR; Mumps, Measles and Rubella Vaccines; Rubella, Measles and Mumps Vaccines

Pharmacologic Category Vaccine, Live (Viral)

Medication Safety Issues

Sound-alike/look-alike issues:

MMR (measles, mumps and rubella virus vaccine) may be confused with MMRV (measles, mumps, rubella, and varicella) vaccine

Pregnancy Risk Factor C

Lactation

Measles/mumps: Excretion in breast milk unknown/use caution

Rubella: Enters breast milk/use caution

Use Measles, mumps, and rubella prophylaxis

The Advisory Committee on Immunization Practices (ACIP) recommends routine vaccination for the following (CDC, 2013c):

- All children (first dose given at 12-15 months of age)
- Adults born 1957 or later (without evidence of immunity or documentation of vaccination). Vaccine may be given to adults born prior to 1957 if they do not have contraindications to the MMR vaccine.
- Adults at higher risk for exposure to and transmission of measles mumps and rubella should receive special consideration for vaccination, unless an acceptable evidence of immunity exists. This includes international travelers, persons attending colleges and other post high school education, persons working in healthcare facilities.

Available Dosage Forms

Injection, powder for reconstitution [preservative free]:

M-M-R® II: Measles virus ≥1000 $TCID_{50}$, mumps virus ≥20,000 $TCID_{50}$, and rubella virus ≥1000 $TCID_{50}$

General Dosage Range SubQ:

Children ≥12 months: 0.5 mL per dose for 2 doses

Adults: 0.5 mL per dose for 1 or 2 doses

Administration

I.M. Priorix (Canadian product, not available in the U.S.) may also be given by I.M. injection.

I.V. Not for I.V. administration.

Subcutaneous Administer SubQ in outer aspect of the upper arm in patients ≥12 months. **Not for I.V. administration.** The minimum interval between 2 doses of MMR vaccine is 28 days (CDC, 2013c).

Simultaneous administration of vaccines helps ensure the patients will be fully vaccinated by the appropriate age. Simultaneous administration of vaccines is defined as administering >1 vaccine on the same day at different anatomic sites. The use of licensed combination vaccines is generally preferred over separate injections of the equivalent components. Separate vaccines should not be combined in the same syringe unless indicated by product specific labeling. Separate needles and syringes should be used for each injection. The ACIP prefers each dose of a specific vaccine in a series come from the same manufacturer when possible. Adolescents and adults should be vaccinated while seated or lying down. In general, preterm infants should be vaccinated at the same chronological age as full-term infants (CDC, 2011).

Antipyretics have not been shown to prevent febrile seizures. Antipyretics may be used to treat fever or discomfort following vaccination (CDC, 2011). One study reported that routine prophylactic administration of acetaminophen to prevent fever prior to vaccination decreased the immune response of some vaccines; the clinical significance of this reduction in immune response has not been established (Prymula, 2009).

Nursing Actions

Physical Assessment U.S. federal law requires entry into the patient's medical record.

Patient Education

- Discuss specific use of vaccine and side effects with patient as it relates to treatment. (HCAHPS: During this hospital stay, were you given any medicine that you had not taken before? Before giving you any new medicine, how often did hospital staff tell you what the medicine was for? How often did hospital staff describe possible side effects in a way you could understand?)
- Patient may experience headache, nausea, diarrhea, or rhinitis. Have patient report immediately to prescriber severe asthenia or rash (HCAHPS).
- Educate patient about signs of a significant reaction (eg, wheezing; chest tightness; fever; itching; bad cough; blue skin color; seizures; or swelling of face, lips, tongue, or throat). **Note:** This is not a comprehensive list of all side effects. Patient should consult prescriber for additional questions.

Intended Use and Disclaimer: Should not be printed and given to patients. This information is intended to serve as a concise initial reference for healthcare professionals to use when discussing medications with a patient. You must ultimately rely on your own discretion, experience and judgment in diagnosing, treating and advising patients.

Related Information

Immunization Administration Recommendations *on page 1675*

Immunization Recommendations *on page 1680*

Measles, Mumps, Rubella, and Varicella Virus Vaccine

(MEE zels, mumpz, roo BEL a, & var i SEL a VYE rus vak SEEN)

Brand Names: U.S. ProQuad

Index Terms MMRV; Mumps, Rubella, Varicella, and Measles Vaccine; Rubella, Varicella, Measles, and Mumps Vaccine; Varicella, Measles, Mumps, and Rubella Vaccine

Pharmacologic Category Vaccine, Live (Viral)

Medication Safety Issues

Sound-alike/look-alike issues:

MMRV (measles, mumps, rubella, and varicella) vaccine may be confused with MMR (measles, mumps and rubella virus) vaccine.

Use

Measles, mumps, rubella, and varicella vaccination: To provide active immunization for the prevention of measles, mumps, rubella, and varicella in children 12 months to 12 years of age.

The Advisory Committee on Immunization Practices (ACIP) recommends routine vaccination against measles, mumps, rubella, and varicella in healthy children; the first dose should be given at 12-15 months of age and the second dose at 4-6 years of age. For children receiving their first dose at 12-47 months of age, either the MMRV combination vaccine or separate MMR and varicella vaccines can be used. (The ACIP prefers administration of separate MMR and varicella vaccines as the first dose in this age group unless the parent or caregiver expresses preference for the MMRV combination.) For children receiving the first dose at ≥48 months or their second dose at any age, use of MMRV is preferred. For children with a personal or family history of seizures, the ACIP recommends vaccination with separate MMR and varicella vaccines, as opposed to the MMRV combination vaccine (CDC, 2010).

Canadian labeling (not in U.S. labeling): MMRV combination vaccine is approved for use in healthy children 9 months to 6 years; may consider use in healthy children ≤12 years of age based upon prior experience with the separate component (live-attenuated MMR or live-attenuated varicella [OKA-strain]) vaccines.

Available Dosage Forms

Injection, powder for reconstitution [preservative free]:

ProQuad: Measles virus ≥3.00 $\log_{10}$ $TCID_{50}$, mumps virus ≥4.30 $\log_{10}$ $TCID_{50}$, rubella virus ≥3.00 $\log_{10}$ $TCID_{50}$, and varicella virus ≥3.99 $\log_{10}$ PFU

General Dosage Range SubQ: *Children 12 months to 12 years:* 1 dose (0.5 mL)

Administration

Subcutaneous Disinfectants (eg, alcohol) may inactivate the attenuated viruses in the vaccine. Allow disinfectant adequate time to evaporate from skin prior to administration.

U.S labeling: For SubQ injection only; inject in the outer aspect of the deltoid region of the upper arm or in the higher anterolateral area of the thigh. Administer immediately following reconstitution; discard reconstituted vaccine if not used within 30 minutes.

Canadian labeling: For SubQ or I.M. injection only; inject in the deltoid region of upper arm. Do not administer by I.M. injection in patients with bleeding disorders.

Note: The Canadian labeling states that Priorix-Tetra (MMRV) may be given simultaneously (at different injection sites) with the combination vaccine Infanrix-hexa (contains diphtheria-tetanus-acellular pertussis-hepatitis B-inactivated polio virus-*Haemophilus* influenzae type B [DTaP-HBV-IPV/Hib]) and with monovalent vaccines DTaP, Hib, IPV, HBV.

Simultaneous administration of vaccines helps ensure the patients will be fully vaccinated by the appropriate age. Simultaneous administration of vaccines is defined as administering >1 vaccine on the same day at different anatomic sites. The use of licensed combination vaccines is generally preferred over separate injections of the equivalent components. Separate vaccines should not be combined in the same syringe unless indicated by product specific labeling. Separate needles and syringes should be used for each injection. The ACIP prefers each dose of a specific vaccine in a series come from the same manufacturer when possible. Adolescents and adults should be vaccinated while seated or lying down. In general, preterm infants should be vaccinated at the same chronological age as full-term infants (CDC, 2011).

Antipyretics have not been shown to prevent febrile seizures. Antipyretics may be used to treat fever or discomfort following vaccination (CDC, 2011). One study reported that routine prophylactic administration of acetaminophen to prevent fever prior to vaccination decreased the immune response of some vaccines; the clinical significance of this reduction in immune response has not been established (Prymula, 2009).

Nursing Actions

Physical Assessment Assess hypersensitivity history and health status prior to administration. Treatment must be immediately available in event of anaphylactic or serious allergic reactions. U.S. federal law requires entry into the patient's medical record.

Patient Education

• Discuss specific use of vaccine and side effects with patient as it relates to treatment. (HCAHPS: During this hospital stay, were you given any medicine that you had not taken before? Before giving you any new medicine, how often did hospital staff tell you what the medicine was for? How often did hospital staff describe possible side effects in a way you could understand?)

• Patient may experience headache, nausea, diarrhea, or rhinitis. Have patient report immediately to prescriber severe asthenia or rash (HCAHPS).

• Educate patient about signs of a significant reaction (eg, wheezing; chest tightness; fever; itching; bad cough; blue skin color; seizures; or swelling of face, lips, tongue, or throat). **Note:** This is not a comprehensive list of all side

effects. Patient should consult prescriber for additional questions.

Intended Use and Disclaimer: Should not be printed and given to patients. This information is intended to serve as a concise initial reference for healthcare professionals to use when discussing medications with a patient. You must ultimately rely on your own discretion, experience and judgment in diagnosing, treating and advising patients.

Related Information
Immunization Administration Recommendations *on page 1675*
Immunization Recommendations *on page 1680*

Mebendazole (me BEN da zole)

Index Terms Vermox
Pharmacologic Category Anthelmintic
Medication Safety Issues
Sound-alike/look-alike issues:
Mebendazole may be confused with metroNIDA-ZOLE
Pregnancy Risk Factor C
Lactation Excretion in breast milk unknown/use caution
Use Treatment of *Ancylostoma duodenale* or *Necator amiericanus* (hookworms), *Ascaris lumbricoides* (roundworms), *Enterobius vermicularis* (pinworms), *Strongyloides stercoralis* (roundworm), *Taenia solium* (tapeworms), *Trichuris trichiura* (whipworms),
Unlabeled Use Treatment of *Ancylostoma caninum* (eosinophilic enterocolitis), *Capillaria philippinensis* (capillariasis), *Giardia duodenalis* (giardiasis), *Mansonella perstans* (filariasis), visceral larva migrans (toxocariasis)
General Dosage Range Oral: *Children ≥2 years; Adolescents, and Adults:* 100 mg as a single dose **or** twice daily
Administration
Oral Tablets may be chewed, swallowed whole, or crushed and mixed with food. Tablets may be administered with or without food.
Nursing Actions
Physical Assessment Since worm infestations are easily transmitted, all persons sharing same household should be treated. Teach transmission prevention.
Patient Education
• Discuss specific use of drug and side effects with patient as it relates to treatment. (HCAHPS: During this hospital stay, were you given any medicine that you had not taken before? Before giving you any new medicine, how often did hospital staff tell you what the medicine was for? How often did hospital staff describe possible side effects in a way you could understand?)
• Patient may experience headache, dyspepsia, nausea, or diarrhea. Have patient report immediately to prescriber asthenia or rash (HCAHPS).

• Educate patient about signs of a significant reaction (eg, wheezing; chest tightness; fever; itching; bad cough; blue skin color; seizures; or swelling of face, lips, tongue, or throat). **Note:** This is not a comprehensive list of all side effects. Patient should consult prescriber for additional questions.

Intended Use and Disclaimer: Should not be printed and given to patients. This information is intended to serve as a concise initial reference for healthcare professionals to use when discussing medications with a patient. You must ultimately rely on your own discretion, experience and judgment in diagnosing, treating and advising patients.

Meclizine (MEK li zeen)

Brand Names: U.S. Dramamine Less Drowsy [OTC]; Medi-Meclizine [OTC]; Travel Sickness [OTC]; UniVert; Vertin-32 [OTC]
Index Terms Antivert; Meclizine Hydrochloride; Meclozine Hydrochloride
Pharmacologic Category Antiemetic; Histamine H_1 Antagonist; Histamine H_1 Antagonist, First Generation; Piperazine Derivative
Medication Safety Issues
Sound-alike/look-alike issues:
Antivert® may be confused with Anzemet®, Axert®
BEERS Criteria medication:
This drug may be potentially inappropriate for use in geriatric patients (Quality of evidence - varies based on comorbidity; Strength of recommendation - varies based on comorbidity)
Pregnancy Risk Factor B
Lactation Excretion in breast milk unknown
Use Prevention and treatment of symptoms of motion sickness; management of vertigo with diseases affecting the vestibular system
Available Dosage Forms
Tablet, Oral:
Dramamine Less Drowsy [OTC]: 25 mg
Medi-Meclizine [OTC]: 25 mg
UniVert: 32 mg
Vertin-32 [OTC]: 32 mg
Generic: 12.5 mg, 25 mg
Tablet Chewable, Oral:
Travel Sickness [OTC]: 25 mg
Generic: 25 mg
General Dosage Range Oral: *Children ≥12 years and Adults:* 25-50 mg 1 hour before travel, may repeat every 24 hours if needed **or** 25-100 mg/day in divided doses
Nursing Actions
Physical Assessment Observe safety precautions (eg, bed rails up, call bell at hand).

Patient Education

- Discuss specific use of drug and side effects with patient as it relates to treatment. (HCAHPS: During this hospital stay, were you given any medicine that you had not taken before? Before giving you any new medicine, how often did hospital staff tell you what the medicine was for? How often did hospital staff describe possible side effects in a way you could understand?)
- Patient may experience presyncope, fatigue, blurred vision, illogical thinking, or xerostomia. Have patient report immediately to prescriber urinary retention, severe asthenia, or rash (HCAHPS).
- Educate patient about signs of a significant reaction (eg, wheezing; chest tightness; fever; itching; bad cough; blue skin color; seizures; or swelling of face, lips, tongue, or throat). **Note:** This is not a comprehensive list of all side effects. Patient should consult prescriber for additional questions.

Intended Use and Disclaimer: Should not be printed and given to patients. This information is intended to serve as a concise initial reference for healthcare professionals to use when discussing medications with a patient. You must ultimately rely on your own discretion, experience and judgment in diagnosing, treating and advising patients.

MedroxyPROGESTERone

(me DROKS ee proe JES te rone)

Brand Names: U.S. Depo-Provera; Depo-SubQ Provera 104; Provera

Index Terms Acetoxymethylprogesterone; Medroxyprogesterone Acetate; Methylacetoxyprogesterone; MPA

Pharmacologic Category Contraceptive; Progestin

Medication Safety Issues

Sound-alike/look-alike issues:

Depo-Provera® may be confused with depo-subQ provera 104™

MedroxyPROGESTERone may be confused with hydroxyprogesterone caproate, methylPREDNISolone, methylTESTOSTERone

Provera® may be confused with Covera®, Femara®, Parlodel®, Premarin®, Proscar®, PROzac®

Administration issues:

The injectable dosage form is available in different formulations. Carefully review prescriptions to assure the correct formulation and route of administration.

Pregnancy Risk Factor X

Lactation Enters breast milk

Breast-Feeding Considerations Medroxyprogesterone (MPA) is excreted into breast milk. Composition, quality, and quantity of breast milk are not affected; adverse developmental and behavioral effects have not been noted following exposure of infant to MPA while breast-feeding. The manufacturer does not recommend the use of MPA tablets in breast-feeding mothers; however, guidelines note that the injectable MPA contraceptives can be initiated immediately postpartum in women who are nursing (CDC, 2010; CDC, 2011; CDC, 2013).

Use Secondary amenorrhea or abnormal uterine bleeding due to hormonal imbalance; reduction of endometrial hyperplasia in nonhysterectomized postmenopausal women receiving conjugated estrogens; prevention of pregnancy; management of endometriosis-associated pain; adjunctive therapy and palliative treatment of recurrent and metastatic endometrial carcinoma

Unlabeled Use Treatment of low-grade endometrial stromal sarcoma; treatment of paraphilia/hypersexuality

Mechanism of Action/Effect Inhibits secretion of pituitary gonadotropins, which prevents follicular maturation and ovulation; causes endometrial thinning

Contraindications Hypersensitivity to medroxyprogesterone or any component of the formulation; history of or current thrombophlebitis or venous thromboembolic disorders (including DVT, PE); cerebral vascular disease; severe hepatic dysfunction or disease; carcinoma of the breast or other estrogen- or progesterone-dependent neoplasia; undiagnosed vaginal bleeding; missed abortion, diagnostic test for pregnancy, pregnancy

Warnings/Precautions Hazardous agent; use appropriate precautions for handling and disposal (NIOSH, 2012).

[U.S. Boxed Warning]: Prolonged use of medroxyprogesterone contraceptive injection may result in a loss of bone mineral density (BMD). It is not known if use during adolescence or early adulthood will decrease peak bone mass accretion or increase the risk for osteoporotic fractures later in life. Loss is related to the duration of use, may not be completely reversible on discontinuation of the drug, and incidence is not significantly different between the SubQ and I.M. dosage forms. The impact on peak bone mass in adolescents should be weighed against the potential for unintended pregnancies in treatment decision. Consider alternative contraceptive methods in patients at risk for osteoporosis (eg, metabolic bone disease, family history of osteoporosis, chronic use of medications associated with osteoporosis such as corticosteroids). **[U.S. Boxed Warning]: Long-term use (ie, >2 years) should be limited to situations where other birth control methods are inadequate.** Consider other methods of birth control in women with (or at risk for) osteoporosis. **[U.S. Boxed Warning]: Inform patients that injectable contraceptives do not protect against HIV infection**

▶

or other sexually-transmitted diseases. When used for contraception, the possibility of ectopic pregnancy should be considered in patients with abdominal pain. Anaphylaxis or anaphylactoid reactions have been reported with use of the injection; medication for the treatment of hypersensitivity reactions should be available for immediate use.

[U.S. Boxed Warning]: Estrogens with or without progestin should not be used to prevent cardiovascular disease. Using data from the Women's Health Initiative (WHI) studies, an increased risk of deep vein thrombosis (DVT) and stroke has been reported with CE and an increased risk of DVT, stroke, pulmonary emboli (PE) and myocardial infarction (MI) has been reported with CE with MPA in postmenopausal women. Additional risk factors include diabetes mellitus, hypercholesterolemia, hypertension, SLE, obesity, tobacco use, and/or history of venous thromboembolism (VTE). Risk factors should be managed appropriately; discontinue use if adverse cardiovascular events occur or are suspected. If thrombosis develops with contraceptive treatment, discontinue treatment (unless no other acceptable contraceptive alternative). Whenever possible, progestins in combination with estrogens should be discontinued at least 4-6 weeks prior to and for 2 weeks following elective surgery associated with an increased risk of thromboembolism or during periods of prolonged immobilization.

[U.S. Boxed Warning]: Estrogens with or without progestin should not be used to prevent dementia. In the Women's Health Initiative Memory Study (WHIMS), an increased incidence of dementia was observed in women ≥65 years of age taking CE alone or in combination with MPA.

[U.S. Boxed Warning]: Based on data from the Women's Health Initiative (WHI) studies, an increased risk of invasive breast cancer was observed in postmenopausal women using conjugated estrogens (CE) in combination with medroxyprogesterone acetate (MPA). This risk may be associated with duration of use and declines once combined therapy is discontinued (Chlebowski, 2009). The risk of invasive breast cancer was decreased in postmenopausal women with a hysterectomy using CE only, regardless of weight. However, the risk was not significantly decreased in women at high risk for breast cancer (family history of breast cancer, personal history of benign breast disease) (Anderson, 2012). An increase in abnormal mammogram findings has also been reported with estrogen alone or in combination with progestin therapy. Use is contraindicated in patients with known or suspected breast cancer.

MPA is used to reduce the risk of endometrial hyperplasia in nonhysterectomized postmenopausal women receiving conjugated estrogens. The use of unopposed estrogen in women with an intact uterus is associated with an increased risk of endometrial cancer. The addition of a progestin to estrogen therapy may decrease the risk of endometrial hyperplasia, a precursor to endometrial cancer. Adequate diagnostic measures, including endometrial sampling if indicated, should be performed to rule out malignancy in postmenopausal women with undiagnosed abnormal vaginal bleeding. Estrogens may exacerbate endometriosis. Malignant transformation of residual endometrial implants has been reported posthysterectomy with unopposed estrogen therapy. Consider adding a progestin in women with residual endometriosis posthysterectomy. Postmenopausal estrogen therapy and combined estrogen/progesterone therapy may increase the risk of ovarian cancer; however, the absolute risk to an individual woman is small. Although results from various studies are not consistent, risk does not appear to be significantly associated with the duration, route, or dose of therapy. In one study, the risk decreased after 2 years following discontinuation of therapy (Mørch, 2009). Although the risk of ovarian cancer is rare, women who are at an increased risk (eg, family history) should be counseled about the association (NAMS, 2012).

[U.S. Boxed Warning]: Estrogens with or without progestin should be used for the shortest duration possible at the lowest effective dose consistent with treatment goals. Before prescribing estrogen therapy to postmenopausal women, the risks and benefits must be weighed for each patient. Women should be informed of these risks and benefits, as well as possible effects of progestin when added to estrogen therapy. Patients should be reevaluated as clinically appropriate to determine if treatment is still necessary. Available data related to treatment risks are from Women's Health Initiative (WHI) studies, which evaluated oral CE 0.625 mg with or without MPA 2.5 mg relative to placebo in postmenopausal women. Other combinations and dosage forms of estrogens and progestins were not studied. Outcomes reported from clinical trials using CE with or without MPA should be assumed to be similar for other doses and other dosage forms of estrogens and progestins until comparable data becomes available.

Discontinue pending examination in cases of sudden partial or complete vision loss, sudden onset of proptosis, diplopia, or migraine; discontinue permanently if papilledema or retinal vascular lesions are observed on examination. Use with caution in patients with diseases that may be exacerbated by fluid retention (including asthma, epilepsy, migraine, cardiac, or renal dysfunction).

Contraceptive therapy with medroxyprogesterone commonly results in an average weight gain of ~2.5 kg after 1 year and ~3.7 kg after 2 years of treatment. Use caution with history of depression.

May have adverse effects on glucose tolerance; use caution in women with diabetes. MPA is extensively metabolized in the liver. Discontinue if jaundice develops or if acute or chronic hepatic disturbances occur. Use is contraindicated with severe hepatic disease. Unscheduled bleeding/spotting may occur. Presentation of irregular, unresolving vaginal bleeding following previously regular cycles warrants further evaluation including endometrial sampling, if indicated, to rule out malignancy. Not for use prior to menarche. The use of estrogens and/or progestins may change the results of some laboratory tests (eg, coagulation factors, lipids, glucose tolerance, binding proteins). The dose, route, and the specific estrogen/progestin influences these changes. In addition, personal risk factors (eg, cardiovascular disease, smoking, diabetes, age) also contribute to adverse events; use of specific products may be contraindicated in women with certain risk factors.

Drug Interactions

Avoid Concomitant Use

Avoid concomitant use of MedroxyPROGESTERone with any of the following: Axitinib; Griseofulvin; Indium 111 Capromab Pendetide; Simeprevir; Tranexamic Acid; Uliprista

Decreased Effect

MedroxyPROGESTERone may decrease the levels/effects of: Anticoagulants; ARIPiprazole; Axitinib; Ibrutinib; Indium 111 Capromab Pendetide; Saxagliptin; Simeprevir; Vitamin K Antagonists

The levels/effects of MedroxyPROGESTERone may be decreased by: Acitretin; Aminoglutethimide; Aprepitant; Artemether; Barbiturates; Bexarotene (Systemic); Bile Acid Sequestrants; Bosentan; CarBAMazepine; CloBAZam; CYP3A4 Inducers (Strong); Dabrafenib; Deferasirox; Eslicarbazepine; Felbamate; Fosaprepitant; Fosphenytoin; Griseofulvin; LamoTRIgine; Metreleptin; Mifepristone; Mitotane; Mycophenolate; Nelfinavir; Nevirapine; OXcarbazepine; Perampanel; Phenytoin; Primidone; Prucalopride; Retinoic Acid Derivatives; Rifamycin Derivatives; St Johns Wort; Sugammadex; Telaprevir; Tocilizumab; Topiramate; Uliprista

Increased Effect/Toxicity

MedroxyPROGESTERone may increase the levels/effects of: Benzodiazepines (metabolized by oxidation); Selegiline; Thalidomide; Tranexamic Acid; Voriconazole

The levels/effects of MedroxyPROGESTERone may be increased by: Atazanavir; Boceprevir; Cobicistat; Herbs (Progestogenic Properties); Metreleptin; Mifepristone; Voriconazole

Nutritional/Ethanol Interactions

Ethanol: Avoid ethanol (may increase risk of osteoporosis).

Food: Bioavailability of the oral tablet is increased when taken with food; half-life is unchanged.

Herb/Nutraceutical: St John's wort may diminish the therapeutic effect of progestin contraceptives (contraceptive failure is possible).

Adverse Reactions Adverse effects as reported with any dosage form; percent ranges presented are noted with the MPA I.M. contraceptive injection: >5%:

Central nervous system: Dizziness, headache, nervousness

Endocrine & metabolic: Libido decreased, menstrual irregularities (includes bleeding, amenorrhea, or both)

Gastrointestinal: Abdominal pain/discomfort, weight gain (>10 lbs at 24 months: 38%)

1% to 5%:

Cardiovascular: Edema

Central nervous system: Depression, fatigue, insomnia

Dermatologic: Acne, alopecia, rash

Endocrine & metabolic: Breast pain, hot flashes

Gastrointestinal: Bloating, nausea

Genitourinary: Dysmenorrhea, leukorrhea, vaginitis

Local: Injection site reaction (SubQ administration): Atrophy, induration, pain

Neuromuscular & skeletal: Arthralgia, backache, leg cramp, weakness

Available Dosage Forms

Suspension, Intramuscular:

Depo-Provera: 150 mg/mL (1 mL); 400 mg/mL (2.5 mL)

Generic: 150 mg/mL (1 mL)

Suspension, Subcutaneous:

Depo-SubQ Provera 104: 104 mg/0.65 mL (0.65 mL)

Tablet, Oral:

Provera: 2.5 mg, 5 mg, 10 mg

Generic: 2.5 mg, 5 mg, 10 mg

General Dosage Range Dosage adjustment recommended in patients with hepatic impairment.

I.M.:

Adolescents and Adults: Contraception: 150 mg every 3 months

Adults: Endometrial cancer: 400-1000 mg/week

Oral: *Adolescents and Adults:* 5-10 mg once daily

SubQ: *Adolescents and Adults:* 104 mg every 3 months (every 12-14 weeks)

Administration

I.M. Depo-Provera® Contraceptive: Administer first dose during the first 5 days of menstrual period, or within the first 5 days postpartum if not breastfeeding, or at the sixth week postpartum if breastfeeding exclusively. Shake vigorously prior to administration. Administer by deep I.M. injection in the gluteal or deltoid muscle. When switching from combined hormonal contraceptives ▸

(estrogen plus progestin), the first injection should be on the day after the last active tablet or (at the latest) the day after the final inactive tablet. When switching from other contraceptive methods, ensure continuous contraceptive coverage.

Hazardous agent; use appropriate precautions for handling and disposal (NIOSH, 2012).

Other SubQ: depo-subQ provera 104™: Administer first dose during the first 5 days of menstrual period, or at the sixth week postpartum if breastfeeding. Shake vigorously prior to administration. Administer by SubQ injection in the anterior thigh or abdomen; avoid boney areas and the umbilicus. Administer over 5-7 seconds. Do not rub the injection area. When switching from combined hormonal contraceptives (estrogen plus progestin), the first injection should be within 7 days after the last active pill, or removal of patch or ring. If switching from the I.M. to SubQ formulation, the next dose should be given within the prescribed dosing period for the I.M. injection to assure continuous coverage.

Hazardous agent; use appropriate precautions for handling and disposal (NIOSH, 2012).

Storage/Stability Store at controlled room temperature.

Nursing Actions

Physical Assessment Instruct patient on appropriate dose scheduling.

Patient Education
- Discuss specific use of drug and side effects with patient as it relates to treatment. (HCAHPS: During this hospital stay, were you given any medicine that you had not taken before? Before giving you any new medicine, how often did hospital staff tell you what the medicine was for? How often did hospital staff describe possible side effects in a way you could understand?)
- Patient may experience weight gain, osteopenia, headache, asthenia, dyspepsia, polyphagia, edema, or menstrual irregularity. Have patient report immediately to prescriber angina, dyspnea, or rash (HCAHPS).
- Educate patient about signs of a significant reaction (eg, wheezing; chest tightness; fever; itching; bad cough; blue skin color; seizures; or swelling of face, lips, tongue, or throat). **Note:** This is not a comprehensive list of all side effects. Patient should consult prescriber for additional questions.

Intended Use and Disclaimer: Should not be printed and given to patients. This information is intended to serve as a concise initial reference for healthcare professionals to use when discussing medications with a patient. You must ultimately rely on your own discretion, experience and judgment in diagnosing, treating and advising patients.

Dietary Considerations Ensure adequate calcium and vitamin D intake

Mefloquine (ME floe kwin)

Index Terms Mefloquine Hydrochloride
Pharmacologic Category Antimalarial Agent
Medication Safety Issues
International issues:
Lariam [multiple international markets] may be confused with Levaquin [Argentina, Brazil, Venezuela]
Medication Guide Available Yes
Pregnancy Risk Factor B
Lactation Enters breast milk/use caution
Use Treatment of mild-to-moderate acute malarial infections and prevention of malaria caused by *Plasmodium falciparum* (including chloroquine-resistant strains) or *P. vivax*

Note: Due to geographical resistance and cross-resistance, consult current CDC guidelines.
Unlabeled Use Treatment of uncomplicated, chloroquine-resistant *P. vivax* malaria
Available Dosage Forms
Tablet, Oral:
Generic: 250 mg
General Dosage Range Oral:
Children ≥6 months: Prophylaxis: 5 mg/kg/once weekly (maximum: 250 mg/dose); Treatment: 20-25 mg/kg/day in 2 divided doses (maximum: 1250 mg)
Adults: Prophylaxis: 250 mg once weekly; Treatment: 1250 mg (5 tablets) as a single dose
Administration
Oral Administer with food and with at least 8 oz of water. When used for malaria prophylaxis, dose should be taken once weekly on the same day each week. If vomiting occurs within 30 minutes after the dose, an additional full dose should be given; if it occurs within 30-60 minutes after dose, an additional half-dose should be given. Tablets may be crushed and suspended in a small amount of water, milk, or another beverage for persons unable to swallow tablets.
Nursing Actions
Physical Assessment Monitor for hypertension, cardiomyopathy, hyperglycemia, and hepatotoxicity on a regular basis throughout therapy. Monitor patient closely for any development of psychiatric symptoms (anxiety, paranoia, depression, hallucinations, and psychosis); may persist long after mefloquine has been discontinued. Advise patient about the importance of carrying medication guide and wallet provided when mefloquine is dispensed for malaria. Teach patient importance of adequate hydration.
Patient Education
- Discuss specific use of drug and side effects with patient as it relates to treatment. (HCAHPS: During this hospital stay, were you given any

medicine that you had not taken before? Before giving you any new medicine, how often did hospital staff tell you what the medicine was for? How often did hospital staff describe possible side effects in a way you could understand?)
- Patient may experience headache, presyncope, fatigue, blurred vision, illogical thinking, nausea, dizziness, hallucinations, insomnia, or nightmares. Have patient report immediately to prescriber depression, nervousness, emotional instability, anxiety, angina, tachycardia, dyspnea, flu-like syndrome, or rash (HCAHPS).
- Educate patient about signs of a significant reaction (eg, wheezing; chest tightness; fever; itching; bad cough; blue skin color; seizures; or swelling of face, lips, tongue, or throat). **Note:** This is not a comprehensive list of all side effects. Patient should consult prescriber for additional questions.

Intended Use and Disclaimer: Should not be printed and given to patients. This information is intended to serve as a concise initial reference for healthcare professionals to use when discussing medications with a patient. You must ultimately rely on your own discretion, experience and judgment in diagnosing, treating and advising patients.

Megestrol (me JES trole)

Brand Names: U.S. Megace ES; Megace Oral
Index Terms 5071-1DL(6); Megestrol Acetate
Pharmacologic Category Antineoplastic Agent, Hormone; Appetite Stimulant; Progestin
Medication Safety Issues
Sound-alike/look-alike issues:
  Megace® may be confused with Reglan®
  Megestrol may be confused with mesalamine
BEERS Criteria medication:
  This drug may be potentially inappropriate for use in geriatric patients (Quality of evidence - moderate; Strength of recommendation - strong).
Pregnancy Risk Factor D (tablet) / X (suspension)
Lactation Enters breast milk/not recommended
Use
Tablet: Palliative treatment of advanced breast and endometrial carcinoma
Suspension: Treatment of anorexia, cachexia, or unexplained significant weight loss in patients with AIDS
Available Dosage Forms
Suspension, Oral:
  Megace ES: 625 mg/5 mL (150 mL)
  Megace Oral: 40 mg/mL (240 mL)
  Generic: 40 mg/mL (10 mL, 240 mL, 480 mL); 400 mg/10 mL (10 mL)
Tablet, Oral:
  Generic: 20 mg, 40 mg

General Dosage Range Oral:
  Adults (females): Tablet: 40-320 mg/day in divided doses
  Adults (males/females): Suspension: 400-800 mg/day [Megace®] **or** 625 mg/day [Megace® ES]
Administration
Oral Megestrol acetate (Megace®) oral suspension is compatible with water, orange juice, apple juice, or Sustacal H.C. for immediate consumption. Shake suspension well before use.

Hazardous agent; use appropriate precautions for handling and disposal (NIOSH, 2012).
Nursing Actions
Physical Assessment Monitor for hypertension, CNS changes (confusion, insomnia), rash, changes in menses, gastrointestinal upset, jaundice, and thrombophlebitis regularly during therapy. Teach patient importance of adequate hydration.
Patient Education
- Discuss specific use of drug and side effects with patient as it relates to treatment. (HCAHPS: During this hospital stay, were you given any medicine that you had not taken before? Before giving you any new medicine, how often did hospital staff tell you what the medicine was for? How often did hospital staff describe possible side effects in a way you could understand?)
- Patient may experience emotional instability, nausea, hypertension, headache, increased appetite, weight gain, alopecia, impotence, or menstrual irregularities. Have patient report immediately to prescriber depression, illogical thinking, fatigue, tremors, tachycardia, dizziness, angina, dyspnea, edema or pain in leg or arm, polydipsia, polyuria, weight loss, or rash (HCAHPS).
- Educate patient about signs of a significant reaction (eg, wheezing; chest tightness; fever; itching; bad cough; blue skin color; seizures; or swelling of face, lips, tongue, or throat). **Note:** This is not a comprehensive list of all side effects. Patient should consult prescriber for additional questions.

Intended Use and Disclaimer: Should not be printed and given to patients. This information is intended to serve as a concise initial reference for healthcare professionals to use when discussing medications with a patient. You must ultimately rely on your own discretion, experience and judgment in diagnosing, treating and advising patients.

Meloxicam (mel OKS i kam)

Brand Names: U.S. Meloxicam Comfort Pac; Mobic
Pharmacologic Category Nonsteroidal Anti-inflammatory Drug (NSAID), Oral

◄ **Medication Safety Issues**

BEERS Criteria medication:
This drug may be potentially inappropriate for use in geriatric patients (Quality of evidence - moderate; Strength of recommendation - strong).

Medication Guide Available Yes

Pregnancy Risk Factor C / D ≥30 weeks gestation

Lactation Excretion in breast milk unknown/not recommended

Breast-Feeding Considerations It is not known whether meloxicam is excreted in human milk. Breast-feeding is not recommended by the manufacturer.

Use Relief of signs and symptoms of osteoarthritis, rheumatoid arthritis, and juvenile idiopathic arthritis (JIA)

Mechanism of Action/Effect Reversibly inhibits cyclooxygenase-1 and 2 (COX-1 and 2) enzymes, which results in decreased formation of prostaglandin precursors; has antipyretic, analgesic, and anti-inflammatory properties

Contraindications Hypersensitivity (eg, asthma, urticaria, allergic-type reactions) to meloxicam, aspirin, other NSAIDs, or any component of the formulation; perioperative pain in the setting of coronary artery bypass graft (CABG) surgery

Warnings/Precautions [U.S. Boxed Warning]: NSAIDs are associated with an increased risk of adverse cardiovascular thrombotic events, including MI and stroke. Risk may be increased with duration of use or pre-existing cardiovascular risk factors or disease. Carefully evaluate individual cardiovascular risk profiles prior to prescribing. May cause new-onset hypertension or worsening of existing hypertension. Use caution with fluid retention. Avoid use in heart failure (ACCF/AHA [Yancy, 2013]). Concurrent administration of ibuprofen, and potentially other nonselective NSAIDs, may interfere with aspirin's cardioprotective effect. **[U.S. Boxed Warning]: Use is contraindicated for treatment of perioperative pain in the setting of coronary artery bypass graft (CABG) surgery.** Risk of MI and stroke may be increased with use within the first 10-14 days following CABG surgery.

Platelet adhesion and aggregation may be decreased; may prolong bleeding time; patients with coagulation disorders or who are receiving anticoagulants should be monitored closely. Anemia may occur; patients on long-term NSAID therapy should be monitored for anemia. Rarely, NSAID use may cause severe blood dyscrasias (eg, agranulocytosis, aplastic anemia, thrombocytopenia).

NSAID use may compromise existing renal function; dose-dependent decreases in prostaglandin synthesis may result from NSAID use, reducing renal blood flow which may cause renal decompensation. NSAID use may increase the risk for hyperkalemia. Patients with impaired renal function, dehydration, heart failure, liver dysfunction, those taking diuretics, and ACE inhibitors, and the elderly are at greater risk of renal toxicity and hyperkalemia. Rehydrate patient before starting therapy; monitor renal function closely. Not recommended for use in patients with advanced renal disease. Long-term NSAID use may result in renal papillary necrosis.

[U.S. Boxed Warning]: NSAIDs may increase risk of gastrointestinal irritation, inflammation, ulceration, bleeding, and perforation. These events may occur at any time during therapy and without warning. Use caution with a history of GI disease (bleeding or ulcers), concurrent therapy with aspirin, anticoagulants and/or corticosteroids, smoking, use of alcohol, the elderly or debilitated patients. When used concomitantly with aspirin, a substantial increase in the risk of gastrointestinal complications (eg, ulcer) occurs; concomitant gastroprotective therapy (eg, proton pump inhibitors) is recommended (Bhatt, 2008).

Use the lowest effective dose for the shortest duration of time, consistent with individual patient goals, to reduce risk of cardiovascular or GI adverse events. Alternate therapies should be considered for patients at high risk.

NSAIDs may cause serious skin adverse events including exfoliative dermatitis, Stevens-Johnson syndrome (SJS) and toxic epidermal necrolysis (TEN); discontinue use at first sign of skin rash or hypersensitivity. Anaphylactoid reactions may occur, even without prior exposure; patients with "aspirin triad" (bronchial asthma, aspirin intolerance, rhinitis) may be at increased risk. Do not use in patients who experience bronchospasm, asthma, rhinitis, or urticaria with NSAID or aspirin therapy. Use caution in other forms of asthma.

Use with caution in patients with decreased hepatic function. Closely monitor patients with any abnormal LFT. Severe hepatic reactions (eg, fulminant hepatitis, liver failure) have occurred with NSAID use, rarely; discontinue if signs or symptoms of liver disease develop, or if systemic manifestations occur.

NSAIDS may cause drowsiness, dizziness, blurred vision and other neurologic effects which may impair physical or mental abilities; patients must be cautioned about performing tasks which require mental alertness (eg, operating machinery or driving). Discontinue use with blurred or diminished vision and perform ophthalmologic exam. Monitor vision with long-term therapy.

In the elderly, avoid chronic use (unless alternative agents ineffective and patient can receive concomitant gastroprotective agent); nonselective oral NSAID use is associated with an increased risk of GI bleeding and peptic ulcer disease in older adults in high risk category (eg, >75 years or age or receiving concomitant oral/parenteral corticosteroids, anticoagulants, or antiplatelet agents) (Beers Criteria).

Oral suspension formulation may contain sorbitol. Concomitant use with sodium polystyrene sulfonate (Kayexalate®) may cause intestinal necrosis (including fatal cases); combined use should be avoided. Withhold for at least 4-6 half-lives prior to surgical or dental procedures.

Drug Interactions

Avoid Concomitant Use

Avoid concomitant use of Meloxicam with any of the following: Calcium Polystyrene Sulfonate; Floctafenine; Ketorolac (Nasal); Ketorolac (Systemic); NSAID (COX-2 Inhibitor); Omacetaxine; Sodium Polystyrene Sulfonate; Urokinase

Decreased Effect

Meloxicam may decrease the levels/effects of: ACE Inhibitors; Agents with Antiplatelet Properties; Aliskiren; Angiotensin II Receptor Blockers; Beta-Blockers; Eplerenone; HydrALAZINE; Loop Diuretics; Potassium-Sparing Diuretics; Prostaglandins (Ophthalmic); Salicylates; Selective Serotonin Reuptake Inhibitors; Thiazide Diuretics

The levels/effects of Meloxicam may be decreased by: Bile Acid Sequestrants; Nonsteroidal Anti-Inflammatory Agents; Salicylates

Increased Effect/Toxicity

Meloxicam may increase the levels/effects of: 5-ASA Derivatives; Agents with Antiplatelet Properties; Aliskiren; Aminoglycosides; Anticoagulants; Bisphosphonate Derivatives; Calcium Polystyrene Sulfonate; Collagenase (Systemic); CycloSPORINE (Systemic); Dabigatran Etexilate; Deferasirox; Desmopressin; Digoxin; Eplerenone; Haloperidol; Ibritumomab; Lithium; Methotrexate; Nonsteroidal Anti-Inflammatory Agents; NSAID (COX-2 Inhibitor); Omacetaxine; PEMEtrexed; Porfimer; Potassium-Sparing Diuretics; PRALAtrexate; Quinolone Antibiotics; Rivaroxaban; Salicylates; Sodium Polystyrene Sulfonate; Tenofovir; Thrombolytic Agents; Tositumomab and Iodine I 131 Tositumomab; Urokinase; Vancomycin; Vitamin K Antagonists

The levels/effects of Meloxicam may be increased by: ACE Inhibitors; Angiotensin II Receptor Blockers; Antidepressants (Tricyclic, Tertiary Amine); Corticosteroids (Systemic); CycloSPORINE (Systemic); Dasatinib; Floctafenine; Glucosamine; Herbs (Anticoagulant/Antiplatelet Properties); Ibrutinib; Ketorolac (Nasal); Ketorolac (Systemic); Multivitamins/Fluoride (with ADE); Multivitamins/Minerals (with ADEK, Folate, Iron); Multivitamins/Minerals (with AE, No Iron); Nonsteroidal Anti-Inflammatory Agents; Omega-3 Fatty Acids; Pentosan Polysulfate Sodium; Pentoxifylline; Probenecid; Prostacyclin Analogues; Selective Serotonin Reuptake Inhibitors; Serotonin/Norepinephrine Reuptake Inhibitors; Sodium Phosphates; Tipranavir; Treprostinil; Vitamin E; Voriconazole

Nutritional/Ethanol Interactions

Ethanol: Avoid ethanol (may enhance gastric mucosal irritation).

Herb/Nutraceutical: Avoid alfalfa, anise, bilberry, bladderwrack, bromelain, cat's claw, celery, chamomile, coleus, cordyceps, dong quai, evening primrose, fenugreek, feverfew, garlic, ginger, ginkgo biloba, ginseng (American, Panax, Siberian), grapeseed, green tea, guggul, horse chestnut seed, horseradish, licorice, prickly ash, red clover, reishi, SAMe (S-adenosylmethionine), sweet clover, turmeric, white willow (all have additional antiplatelet activity).

Adverse Reactions Percentages reported in adult patients; abdominal pain, diarrhea, fever, headache, pyrexia, and vomiting were reported more commonly in pediatric patients

2% to 10%:

Cardiovascular: Edema (≤5%)

Central nervous system: Headache (2% to 8%), pain (1% to 5%), dizziness (≤4%), insomnia (≤4%)

Dermatologic: Pruritus (≤2%), rash (≤3%)

Gastrointestinal: Dyspepsia (4% to 10%), diarrhea (2% to 8%), nausea (2% to 7%), abdominal pain (2% to 5%), constipation (≤3%), flatulence (≤3%), vomiting (≤3%)

Genitourinary: Urinary tract infection (≤7%), micturition (≤2%)

Hematologic: Anemia (≤4%)

Neuromuscular & skeletal: Arthralgia (≤5%), back pain (≤3%)

Respiratory: Upper respiratory infection (≤8%), cough (≤2%), pharyngitis (≤3%)

Miscellaneous: Flu-like syndrome (2% to 6%), falls (≤3%)

Dosage Forms Considerations

Meloxicam Comfort Pac is a kit containing meloxicam oral tablets 15 mg, and Duraflex topical gel.

Available Dosage Forms

Kit, Combination:

Meloxicam Comfort Pac: 15 mg

Suspension, Oral:

Mobic: 7.5 mg/5 mL (100 mL)

Generic: 7.5 mg/5 mL (100 mL)

Tablet, Oral:

Mobic: 7.5 mg, 15 mg

Generic: 7.5 mg, 15 mg

General Dosage Range Oral:

Children ≥2 years: 0.125 mg/kg/day (maximum: 7.5 mg/day)

Adults: Initial: 7.5 mg once daily; Maintenance: 7.5-15 mg once daily (maximum: 15 mg/day)

Administration

Oral May be administered with or without meals; take with food or milk to minimize gastrointestinal irritation. Oral suspension: Shake gently prior to use.

Storage/Stability Store at 25°C (77°F). Protect tablets from moisture.

Nursing Actions

Physical Assessment Monitor blood pressure at the beginning of therapy and periodically during use. Monitor for gastrointestinal effects and oto-toxicity at beginning of therapy and periodically throughout.

Patient Education

• Discuss specific use of drug and side effects with patient as it relates to treatment. (HCAHPS: During this hospital stay, were you given any medicine that you had not taken before? Before giving you any new medicine, how often did hospital staff tell you what the medicine was for? How often did hospital staff describe possible side effects in a way you could understand?)

• Patient may experience headache, dyspepsia, nausea, or diarrhea. Have patient report immediately to prescriber angina, strength differences from one side to another, edema or pain of hands or feet, significant weight gain, melena, hematuria, ecchymosis, or rash (HCAHPS).

• Educate patient about signs of a significant reaction (eg, wheezing; chest tightness; fever; itching; bad cough; blue skin color; seizures; or swelling of face, lips, tongue, or throat). **Note:** This is not a comprehensive list of all side effects. Patient should consult prescriber for additional questions.

Intended Use and Disclaimer: Should not be printed and given to patients. This information is intended to serve as a concise initial reference for healthcare professionals to use when discussing medications with a patient. You must ultimately rely on your own discretion, experience and judgment in diagnosing, treating and advising patients.

Dietary Considerations Should be taken with food or milk to minimize gastrointestinal irritation.

Melphalan (MEL fa lan)

Brand Names: U.S. Alkeran

Index Terms L-PAM; L-Phenylalanine Mustard; L-Sarcolysin; Phenylalanine Mustard

Pharmacologic Category Antineoplastic Agent, Alkylating Agent; Antineoplastic Agent, Alkylating Agent (Nitrogen Mustard)

Medication Safety Issues

Sound-alike/look-alike issues:

Melphalan may be confused with Mephyton®, Myleran®

Alkeran® may be confused with Alferon®, Leukeran®, Myleran®

High alert medication:

This medication is in a class the Institute for Safe Medication Practices (ISMP) includes among its list of drug classes which have a heightened risk of causing significant patient harm when used in error.

Pregnancy Risk Factor D

Lactation Excretion in breast milk unknown/not recommended

Breast-Feeding Considerations According to the manufacturer, melphalan should not be administered if breast-feeding.

Use Palliative treatment of multiple myeloma and nonresectable epithelial ovarian carcinoma

Unlabeled Use Treatment of Hodgkin lymphoma, light chain amyloidosis; conditioning regimen for autologous hematopoietic stem cell transplantation in adults with hematologic disorders (eg, multiple myeloma) and autologous marrow or stem cell transplantation in pediatric neuroblastoma and Ewing's sarcoma

Mechanism of Action/Effect Alkylating agent which is a derivative of mechlorethamine that inhibits DNA and RNA synthesis via formation of carbonium ions; cross-links strands of DNA; acts on both resting and rapidly dividing tumor cells.

Contraindications Hypersensitivity to melphalan or any component of the formulation; patients whose disease was resistant to prior melphalan therapy

Warnings/Precautions Hazardous agent; use appropriate precautions for handling and disposal (NIOSH, 2012).

[U.S. Boxed Warning]: Bone marrow suppression is common; may be severe and result in infection or bleeding; has been demonstrated more with the I.V. formulation (compared to oral); myelosuppression is dose-related. Monitor blood counts; may require treatment delay or dose modification for thrombocytopenia or neutropenia. Use with caution in patients with prior bone marrow suppression, impaired renal function (consider dose reduction), or who have received prior (or concurrent) chemotherapy or irradiation. Myelotoxicity is generally reversible, although irreversible bone marrow failure has been reported. In patients who are candidates for autologous transplantation, avoid melphalan-containing regimens prior to transplant (due to the effects on stem cell reserve). Signs of infection, such as fever and WBC rise, may not occur; lethargy and confusion may be more prominent signs of infection.

[U.S. Boxed Warning]: Hypersensitivity reactions (including anaphylaxis) have occurred in ~2% of patients receiving I.V. melphalan, usually after multiple treatment cycles. Discontinue infusion and treat symptomatically. Hypersensitivity may also occur (rarely) with oral melphalan. Do not readminister (oral or I.V.) in patients who experience hypersensitivity to melphalan.

Gastrointestinal toxicities, including nausea, vomiting, diarrhea and mucositis, are common. When administering high-dose melphalan in autologous transplantation, cryotherapy is recommended to prevent mucositis (Keefe, 2007). Abnormal liver function tests may occur; hepatitis and jaundice have also been reported; hepatic sinusoidal obstruction syndrome (SOS; formerly called veno-occlusive disease) has been reported with I.V. melphalan. Pulmonary fibrosis (some fatal) and interstitial pneumonitis have been observed with treatment. Dosage reduction is recommended with I.V. melphalan in patients with renal impairment; reduced initial doses may also be recommended with oral melphalan. Closely monitor patients with azotemia.

[U.S. Boxed Warning]: Produces chromosomal changes and is leukemogenic and potentially mutagenic; secondary malignancies (including acute myeloid leukemia, myeloproliferative disease, and carcinoma) have been reported reported (some patients were receiving combination chemotherapy or radiation therapy); the risk is increased with increased treatment duration and cumulative doses. Suppresses ovarian function and produces amenorrhea; may also cause testicular suppression.

Extravasation may cause local tissue damage; administration by slow injection into a fast running I.V. solution into an injection port or via a central line is recommended; do not administer directly into a peripheral vein. **[U.S. Boxed Warning]: Should be administered under the supervision of an experienced cancer chemotherapy physician.** Avoid vaccination with live vaccines during treatment if immunocompromised. Toxicity may be increased in elderly; start with lowest recommended adult doses.

Drug Interactions
Avoid Concomitant Use
Avoid concomitant use of Melphalan with any of the following: BCG; CloZAPine; Nalidixic Acid; Natalizumab; Pimecrolimus; Tacrolimus (Topical); Tofacitinib; Vaccines (Live)

Decreased Effect
Melphalan may decrease the levels/effects of: BCG; Cardiac Glycosides; Coccidioidin Skin Test; Sipuleucel-T; Vaccines (Inactivated); Vaccines (Live); Vitamin K Antagonists

The levels/effects of Melphalan may be decreased by: Echinacea

Increased Effect/Toxicity
Melphalan may increase the levels/effects of: Carmustine; CloZAPine; CycloSPORINE (Systemic); Leflunomide; Natalizumab; Tofacitinib; Vaccines (Live); Vitamin K Antagonists

The levels/effects of Melphalan may be increased by: Denosumab; Nalidixic Acid; Pimecrolimus; Roflumilast; Tacrolimus (Topical); Trastuzumab

Nutritional/Ethanol Interactions
Ethanol: Avoid ethanol (due to GI irritation).
Food: Food interferes with oral absorption.

Adverse Reactions
>10%:
  Gastrointestinal: Nausea/vomiting, diarrhea, oral ulceration
  Hematologic: Myelosuppression, leukopenia (nadir: 14-21 days; recovery: 28-35 days), thrombocytopenia (nadir: 14-21 days; recovery: 28-35 days), anemia
  Miscellaneous: Secondary malignancy (<2% to 20%; cumulative dose and duration dependent, includes acute myeloid leukemia, myeloproliferative syndrome, carcinoma)
1% to 10%: Miscellaneous: Hypersensitivity (I.V.: 2%; includes bronchospasm, dyspnea, edema, hypotension, pruritus, rash, tachycardia, urticaria)

Available Dosage Forms
Solution Reconstituted, Intravenous:
  Alkeran: 50 mg (1 ea)
  Generic: 50 mg (1 ea)
Tablet, Oral:
  Alkeran: 2 mg

General Dosage Range Dosage adjustment recommended in patients with renal impairment or who develop toxicities
I.V.: *Adults:* 16 mg/m^2 administered at 2-week intervals for 4 doses, then repeat at 4-week intervals
Oral: *Adults:* Dosage varies greatly depending on indication

Administration
I.V. Due to limited stability, complete administration of I.V. dose should occur within 60 minutes of reconstitution. Infuse over 15-30 minutes. Extravasation may cause local tissue damage; administration by slow injection into a fast running I.V. solution into an injection port or via a central line is recommended; do not administer by direct injection into a peripheral vein.

Hazardous agent; use appropriate precautions for handling and disposal (NIOSH, 2012).
Injectable Detail pH: 6.5-7
Oral Administer on an empty stomach.

Hazardous agent; use appropriate precautions for handling and disposal (NIOSH, 2012).
Preparation for Administration Hazardous agent; use appropriate precautions for handling and disposal (NIOSH, 2012).
Injection: Stability is limited; must be prepared fresh. **The time between reconstitution/dilution and administration of parenteral melphalan must be kept to a minimum (manufacturer recommends <60 minutes) because reconstituted and diluted solutions are unstable.** Dissolve powder initially with 10 mL of supplied ▶

diluent to a concentration of 5 mg/mL; shake immediately and vigorously to dissolve. **Immediately** dilute dose in NS to a concentration of ≤0.45 mg/mL (manufacturer recommended concentration). Do not refrigerate solution; precipitation occurs. The manufacturer recommends administration within 60 minutes of reconstitution.

Storage/Stability

Tablet: Store in refrigerator at 2°C to 8°C (36°F to 46°F). Protect from light.

Injection: Store at room temperature of 15°C to 30°C (59°F to 86°F). Protect from light. Stability is limited; must be prepared fresh. A 5 mg/mL concentration is chemically and physically stable for ≤90 minutes when stored at room temperature, although the manufacturer recommends administration be completed within 60 minutes of reconstitution; **immediately** dilute dose in NS. Do not refrigerate solution; precipitation occurs.

Nursing Actions

Physical Assessment I.V.: Monitor infusion site carefully to prevent extravasation. Monitor for gastrointestinal upset, myelosuppression (leukopenia), diarrhea, and hypersensitivity reaction regularly during therapy.

Patient Education

• Discuss specific use of drug and side effects with patient as it relates to treatment. (HCAHPS: During this hospital stay, were you given any medicine that you had not taken before? Before giving you any new medicine, how often did hospital staff tell you what the medicine was for? How often did hospital staff describe possible side effects in a way you could understand?)

• Patient may experience nausea, anemia, leukopenia, thrombocytopenia, diarrhea, skin irritation, alopecia, menstrual irregularity, stomatitis, or discolored urine. Have patient report immediately to prescriber signs of infection, dyspnea, severe dyspepsia, ecchymosis, jaundice, asthenia, or rash (HCAHPS).

• Educate patient about signs of a significant reaction (eg, wheezing; chest tightness; fever; itching; bad cough; blue skin color; seizures; or swelling of face, lips, tongue, or throat). **Note:** This is not a comprehensive list of all side effects. Patient should consult prescriber for additional questions.

Intended Use and Disclaimer: Should not be printed and given to patients. This information is intended to serve as a concise initial reference for healthcare professionals to use when discussing medications with a patient. You must ultimately rely on your own discretion, experience and judgment in diagnosing, treating and advising patients.

Dietary Considerations Should be taken on an empty stomach (1 hour prior to or 2 hours after meals).

Related Information

Management of Drug Extravasations *on page 1700*

Memantine (me MAN teen)

Brand Names: U.S. Namenda; Namenda Titration Pak; Namenda XR; Namenda XR Titration Pack

Index Terms Memantine Hydrochloride

Pharmacologic Category N-Methyl-D-Aspartate Receptor Antagonist

Medication Safety Issues

Sound-alike/look-alike issues:

Memantine may be confused with mesalamine

Pregnancy Risk Factor B

Lactation Excretion in breast milk unknown/use caution

Breast-Feeding Considerations It is not known if memantine is excreted in breast milk. The manufacturer recommends that caution be exercised when administering memantine to nursing women.

Use Alzheimer disease: Treatment of moderate to severe dementia of the Alzheimer type.

Unlabeled Use Treatment of mild-to-moderate vascular dementia

Mechanism of Action/Effect Memantine is an uncompetitive antagonist of the N-methyl-D-aspartate (NMDA) type of glutamate receptors and reduces the decline in function in Alzheimer's disease; it has not been shown to prevent or slow neurodegeneration associated with this disease.

Contraindications Hypersensitivity to memantine or any component of the formulation

Warnings/Precautions Use with caution in patients with cardiovascular disease; an increased incidence of cardiac failure, angina, bradycardia, and hypertension (compared with placebo) was observed in clinical trials. Use caution with seizure disorders or severe hepatic impairment. Use with caution in severe renal impairment; dose adjustments may be required. Worsening of corneal condition has been observed in a clinical trial; periodic ophthalmic exams during use have been recommended (Canadian labeling). Clearance is significantly reduced by alkaline urine; use caution with medications, dietary changes, or patient conditions which may alter urine pH.

Drug Interactions

Avoid Concomitant Use There are no known interactions where it is recommended to avoid concomitant use.

Decreased Effect There are no known significant interactions involving a decrease in effect.

Increased Effect/Toxicity

Memantine may increase the levels/effects of: Trimethoprim

The levels/effects of Memantine may be increased by: Carbonic Anhydrase Inhibitors; Sodium Bicarbonate; Trimethoprim

Adverse Reactions Adverse reactions similar in immediate and extended release formulations except as noted.

1% to 10%:

Cardiovascular: Hypertension (4%), hypotension (extended release: 2%), cardiac failure, cerebrovascular accident, syncope, transient ischemic attacks

Central nervous system: Dizziness (5% to 7%), confusion (6%), headache (6%), anxiety (extended release: 4%), depression (extended release: 3%), hallucination (3%), pain (3%), drowsiness (3%), fatigue (2%), aggressive behavior (2%), ataxia, hypokinesia, vertigo

Dermatologic: Skin rash

Endocrine & metabolic: Weight gain (extended release: 3%), weight loss

Gastrointestinal: Constipation (3% to 5%), diarrhea (5%), vomiting (2% to 3%), abdominal pain (2%)

Genitourinary: Urinary incontinence (2%), urinary frequency

Hematologic & oncologic: Anemia

Hepatic: Increased serum alkaline phosphatase

Infection: Influenza (4%)

Neuromuscular & skeletal: Back pain (3%)

Ophthalmic: Cataract, conjunctivitis

Respiratory: Cough (4%), dyspnea (2%), pneumonia

Available Dosage Forms

Capsule Extended Release 24 Hour, Oral:

Namenda XR: 7 mg, 14 mg, 21 mg, 28 mg

Namenda XR Titration Pack: 7 mg (7s), 14 mg (7s), 21 mg (7s), and 28 mg (7s)

Solution, Oral:

Namenda: 10 mg/5 mL (360 mL)

Tablet, Oral:

Namenda: 5 mg, 10 mg

Namenda Titration Pak: 5 (28)-10 (21) mg

General Dosage Range Dosage adjustment recommended in patients with renal impairment

Oral: *Adults:* Immediate release: Initial: 5 mg once daily; Target: 20 mg daily in 2 divided doses; Extended release: Initial: 7 mg once daily; Target: 28 mg once daily

Administration

Oral Administer without regard to meals. Extended release capsules may be swallowed whole or entire contents of capsule may be sprinkled on applesauce and swallowed immediately; do not chew, crush, or divide.

Storage/Stability Store at 25°C (77°C); excursions permitted to 15°C to 30°C (59°F to 86°F).

Nursing Actions

Physical Assessment Monitor for hypertension, CNS changes, rash, and constipation on a regular basis throughout therapy.

Patient Education

• Discuss specific use of drug and side effects with patient as it relates to treatment. (HCAHPS: During this hospital stay, were you given any

medicine that you had not taken before? Before giving you any new medicine, how often did hospital staff tell you what the medicine was for? How often did hospital staff describe possible side effects in a way you could understand?)

• Patient may experience dizziness, headache, diarrhea, or constipation. Have patient report immediately to prescriber dyspnea, severe nausea, or rash (HCAHPS).

• Educate patient about signs of a significant reaction (eg, wheezing; chest tightness; fever; itching; bad cough; blue skin color; seizures; or swelling of face, lips, tongue, or throat). **Note:** This is not a comprehensive list of all side effects. Patient should consult prescriber for additional questions.

Intended Use and Disclaimer: Should not be printed and given to patients. This information is intended to serve as a concise initial reference for healthcare professionals to use when discussing medications with a patient. You must ultimately rely on your own discretion, experience and judgment in diagnosing, treating and advising patients.

Meningococcal Group C-CRM197 Conjugate Vaccine

(me NIN joe kok al groop see see ahr em wuhn nahyn tee sev uhn KON joo gate vak SEEN)

Index Terms MenC-CRM197; MenCC

Pharmacologic Category Vaccine

Lactation Excretion in breast milk unknown/use caution

Use To provide active immunization against invasive meningococcal disease caused by *N. meningitidis* serogroup C, in children ≥2 months and adults

The National Advisory Committee on Immunization (NACI) recommendations for persons considered at an increased risk for meningococcal disease:

Chemoprophylaxis and immunoprophylaxis: Selection of meningococcal vaccination to be based upon serogroup(s):

Individuals living in the same household or with close contact (eg, kissing, shared cigarettes, shared eating or drinking utensils) of infected patient

Employees and children of nursery schools or day care

Immunoprophylaxis: Selection of meningococcal vaccination to be based upon serogroup(s):

Adolescents and young adults

Laboratory workers routinely exposed to isolates of *N. meningitidis*

Military recruits

Persons traveling to or who reside in countries where *N. meningitidis* is hyperendemic or epidemic, particularly if contact with local population will be prolonged

Persons with terminal complement component deficiencies

Persons with anatomic or functional asplenia

Note: Use is also recommended during meningococcal outbreaks caused by serogroup C.

Chemoprophylaxis:

Healthcare workers with intensive unprotected contact with infected patients

Airline passengers sitting directly next to an infected patient for duration of at least 8 hours

See NACI guidelines for specific drug treatment at http://www.phac-aspc.gc.ca/naci-ccni

Product Availability Not available in U.S.

General Dosage Range I.M.:

Infants ≥2-12 months: 0.5 mL as a single dose for a total of 3 doses

Infants ≥4-11 months without prior vaccination: 0.5 mL as a single dose for a total of 2 doses

Children ≥1 year and Adults: 0.5 mL as a single dose

Administration

I.M. Administer by deep intramuscular injection only into the anterolateral thigh in infants and the deltoid area in older children, adolescents, and adults. Use separate injection sites if administering multiple vaccinations on the same day.

Acetaminophen may be used when needed to provide comfort; however, routine prophylactic administration of acetaminophen to prevent fever due to vaccine use is not recommended. There is evidence of a decreased immune response to some vaccines associated with acetaminophen administration; the clinical significance of this reduction in immune response has not been established.

I.V. Do not administer via I.V., SubQ, or I.D. routes.

Nursing Actions

Physical Assessment Use caution in immunocompromised patients, patients with bleeding disorders, or those taking anticoagulants. Anaphylactoid and/or hypersensitivity reactions may occur; treatment should be available for immediate use. All serious adverse reactions must be reported to the U.S. DHHS. U.S. federal law also requires entry into the patient's medical record.

Patient Education

• Discuss specific use of vaccine and side effects with patient as it relates to treatment. (HCAHPS: During this hospital stay, were you given any medicine that you had not taken before? Before giving you any new medicine, how often did hospital staff tell you what the medicine was for? How often did hospital staff describe possible side effects in a way you could understand?)

• Patient may experience headache, diarrhea, nausea, myalgia, asthenia, or injection site irritation. Have patient report immediately to prescriber rash (HCAHPS).

• Educate patient about signs of a significant reaction (eg, wheezing; chest tightness; fever; itching; bad cough; blue skin color; seizures; or swelling of face, lips, tongue, or throat). **Note:** This is not a comprehensive list of all side effects. Patient should consult prescriber for additional questions.

Intended Use and Disclaimer: Should not be printed and given to patients. This information is intended to serve as a concise initial reference for healthcare professionals to use when discussing medications with a patient. You must ultimately rely on your own discretion, experience and judgment in diagnosing, treating and advising patients.

Related Information

Immunization Administration Recommendations *on page 1675*

Immunization Recommendations *on page 1680*

Meningococcal (Groups A / C / Y and W-135) Diphtheria Conjugate Vaccine

(me NIN joe kok al groops aye, see, why & dubl yoo won thur tee fyve dif THEER ee a KON joo gate vak SEEN)

Brand Names: U.S. Menactra; Menveo

Index Terms MCV; MCV4; MenACWY; MenACWY-CRM (Menveo); MenACWY-D (Menactra); Meningococcal Conjugate Vaccine

Pharmacologic Category Vaccine, Inactivated (Bacterial)

Medication Safety Issues

Administration issue:

Menactra (MCV4) should be administered by intramuscular (I.M.) injection only. Inadvertent subcutaneous (SubQ) administration has been reported; possibly due to confusion of this product with Menomune (MPSV4), also a meningococcal polysaccharide vaccine, which is administered by the SubQ route.

Pregnancy Risk Factor B/C (manufacturer dependent)

Lactation Excretion in breast milk unknown/use caution

Use Provide active immunization of children and adults against invasive meningococcal disease caused by *N. meningitidis* serogroups A, C, Y, and W-135.

The Advisory Committee on Immunization Practices (ACIP) (CDC, 62[2], 2013):

ACIP recommends routine vaccination of the following:

- Children and adolescents 11-18 years of age
- Persons ≥2 months of age who are at increased risk of meningococcal disease
- Persons (in all recommended age groups) at increased risk who are part of outbreaks caused by vaccine preventable serogroups

Those at increased risk of meningococcal disease include the following:

- Persons ≥2 months of age with medical conditions such as anatomical or functional asplenia or persistent compliment component deficiencies (eg, C_5-C_9, properdin, factor H, or factor D)
- Persons ≥9 months of age that travel to or reside in countries where meningococcal disease is hyperendemic or epidemic, especially if contact with the local population will be prolonged
- Unvaccinated or incompletely vaccinated first year college students living in residence halls
- Military recruits
- Microbiologists with occupational exposure

The Canadian National Advisory Committee on Immunization (NACI): NACI recommends a routine vaccination at ~12 years of age but no booster unless at a continued high risk of exposure. Either quadrivalent vaccine may be used; NACI does not have a preference. NACI recommends use of Menveo (unlabeled use) for high risk persons 2 months to 2 years of age if vaccination with a quadrivalent vaccine is needed; may also be considered for use in persons ≥56 years of age (NACI, 39[1], 2013). Additional recommendations may be found at www.phac-aspc.gc.ca/publicat/ccdr-rmtc/13vol39/acs-dcc-1/index-eng.php

Available Dosage Forms

Injection, solution [preservative free]:

Menactra: 4 mcg each of polysaccharide antigen groups A, C, Y, and W-135 [bound to diphtheria toxoid 48 mcg] per 0.5 mL

Menveo: MenA oligosaccharide 10 mcg, MenC oligosaccharide 5 mcg, MenY oligosaccharide 5 mcg, and MenW-135 oligosaccharide 5 mcg [bound to CRM_{197} protein 32.7-64.1 mcg] per 0.5 mL

General Dosage Range I.M.:

Menactra:

Infants ≥9 months and Children <2 years: 0.5 mL/dose given as a 2-dose series, 3 months apart

Children ≥2 years, Adolescents, and Adults ≤55 years: 0.5 mL as a single dose

Menveo: Age at initial vaccination:

Infants ≥2 months to <7 months: 0.5 mL/dose given as a 4-dose series at 2, 4, 6, and 12 months of age

Infants ≥7 months and Children <2 years: 0.5 mL/dose given as a 2-dose series, with the second dose given during the second year of life and at least 3 months after the first dose

Children ≥2 to <6 years: 0.5 mL/dose given as a single dose; for children at continued high risk of meningococcal disease, may consider an additional dose given 2 months after the first dose

Children ≥6 years, Adolescents, and Adults ≤55 years: 0.5 mL/dose given as a single dose

Administration

I.M. Administer by I.M. route, preferably into the anterolateral aspect of the thigh (infants) or upper deltoid region (toddlers, adolescents, and adults). Do not administer via I.V., SubQ or I.D. route. For patients at risk of hemorrhage, the ACIP recommends "it should be administered intramuscularly if, in the opinion of a physician familiar with the patient's bleeding risk, the vaccine can be administered by this route with reasonable safety. If the patient receives antihemophilia or other similar therapy, intramuscular vaccination can be scheduled shortly after such therapy is administered. A fine needle (23 gauge or smaller) can be used for the vaccination and firm pressure applied to the site (without rubbing) for at least 2 minutes. The patient or family should be instructed concerning the risk of hematoma from the injection." Patients on anticoagulant therapy should be considered to have the same bleeding risks and treated as those with clotting factor disorders (CDC, 60[2], 2011).

For I.M. administration only. Based on limited data, inadvertent SubQ administration provides a lower serologic response, however, the response is still considered to be protective. If inadvertently administered by the SubQ route, revaccination is not necessary.

Simultaneous administration of vaccines helps ensure the patients will be fully vaccinated by the appropriate age. Simultaneous administration of vaccines is defined as administering >1 vaccine on the same day at different anatomic sites. Separate vaccines should not be combined in the same syringe unless indicated by product specific labeling. Separate needles and syringes should be used for each injection. The ACIP prefers each dose of a specific vaccine in a series come from the same manufacturer when possible. Adolescents and adults should be vaccinated while seated or lying down. In general, preterm infants should be vaccinated at the same chronological age as full-term infants (CDC, 60[2], 2011).

Antipyretics have not been shown to prevent febrile seizures. Antipyretics may be used to treat fever or discomfort following vaccination (CDC, 60[2], 2011). One study reported that routine prophylactic administration of acetaminophen to prevent fever prior to vaccination decreased the immune response of some vaccines; the clinical significance of this reduction in immune response has not been established (Prymula, 2009).

I.V. Do not administer via I.V., SubQ or I.D. route.

Other For I.M. administration only. Based on limited data, inadvertent SubQ administration provides a lower serologic response, however the response is still considered to be protective. If inadvertently administered by the SubQ route, revaccination is not necessary.

Nursing Actions

Physical Assessment Ensure appropriate aged patients have received proper vaccine regimen. May inquire about college patient is attending; may affect additional vaccine needs. U.S. federal law requires entry into the patient's medical record.

Instruct patient to report serious hypersensitivity reaction symptoms including respiratory distress, hypotension, urticaria, upper airway swelling or symptoms of swelling (eg, dizziness or trouble breathing). Other side effects include pain, redness, tenderness, or swelling at injection site along with headache or fever 1-2 days after injection.

Patient Education
- Discuss specific use of vaccine and side effects with patient as it relates to treatment. (HCAHPS: During this hospital stay, were you given any medicine that you had not taken before? Before giving you any new medicine, how often did hospital staff tell you what the medicine was for? How often did hospital staff describe possible side effects in a way you could understand?)
- Patient may experience pain, redness or swelling at injection site, headache, fatigue, nausea, emesis, diarrhea, or dyspepsia. Have patient report immediately to prescriber severe injection site reaction (HCAHPS).
- Educate patient about signs of a significant reaction (eg, wheezing; chest tightness; fever; itching; bad cough; blue skin color; seizures; or swelling of face, lips, tongue, or throat). **Note:** This is not a comprehensive list of all side effects. Patient should consult prescriber for additional questions.

Intended Use and Disclaimer: Should not be printed and given to patients. This information is intended to serve as a concise initial reference for healthcare professionals to use when discussing medications with a patient. You must ultimately rely on your own discretion, experience and judgment in diagnosing, treating and advising patients.

Related Information

Immunization Administration Recommendations *on page 1675*

Immunization Recommendations *on page 1680*

Meningococcal Polysaccharide (Groups C and Y) and *Haemophilus* b Tetanus Toxoid Conjugate Vaccine
(me NIN joe kok al pol i SAK a ride groops see & why & he MOF i lus bee TET a nus TOKS oyd KON joo gate vak SEEN)

Brand Names: U.S. Menhibrix

Index Terms Hib-MenCY-TT

Pharmacologic Category Vaccine, Inactivated (Bacterial)

Medication Safety Issues
Sound-alike/look-alike issues:
MenHibrix® (Meningococcal Polysaccharide (Groups C and Y) and *Haemophilus* b Tetanus Toxoid Conjugate Vaccine) may be confused with Hiberix® (*Haemophilus* b Conjugate Vaccine)

Pregnancy Risk Factor C

Use To provide active immunity to prevent invasive disease caused by meningococcal serogroups C and Y and *Haemophilus influenzae* type b

The Advisory Committee on Immunization Practices (ACIP) recommends vaccination only for infants 2-18 months of age who are at increased risk for meningococcal disease, including:
- Infants with persistent complement pathway deficiencies
- Infants with anatomic or functional asplenia, including sickle cell disease
- Infants in communities with serogroups C and Y meningococcal disease outbreaks

The ACIP does not recommend routine vaccination for infants not at increased risk for meningococcal disease. In addition, infants traveling to certain areas (eg, meningitis belt of sub-Saharan Africa) will require a meningococcal vaccine with serogroups A and W_{135}; vaccination with Hib-MenCY-TT will not be adequate (CDC, 2013).

Mechanism of Action/Effect Provides active immunity against disease caused by *Neisseria meningitidis* serogroups C and Y and *Haemophilus influenzae* type b

Contraindications Severe allergic reaction to any meningococcal, *H. influenza* type B, or tetanus toxoid-containing vaccine, or any component of the vaccine

Warnings/Precautions Use with caution in patients with a history of bleeding disorders (including thrombocytopenia) and/or patients on anticoagulant therapy; bleeding/hematoma may occur from I.M. administration. The decision to administer or delay vaccination because of current or recent febrile illness depends on the severity of symptoms and the etiology of the disease. Immunization should be delayed during the course of an acute febrile illness. Vaccination may not result in effective immunity in all patients. Response depends upon multiple factors (eg, type of vaccine, age of patient) and is improved by administering the vaccine at the recommended dose, route, and interval. Vaccines may not be effective if administered during periods of altered immune competence (CDC, 2011). Has not been evaluated for use in immunosuppressed children. In general, severely immunocompromised patients (eg, patients receiving chemo/radiation therapy or other immunosuppressive therapy [including high-dose corticosteroids]) may have a reduced response to vaccination. In general, inactivated vaccines should be administered ≥2 weeks prior to planned immunosuppression when feasible (Rubin, 2014). Syncope has been reported with use of injectable vaccines and may be accompanied by transient visual disturbances, weakness, or tonic-clonic movements. Procedures should be in place to avoid injuries from falling and to restore cerebral perfusion if syncope occurs. Use with caution in patients with history of GBS; carefully consider risks and benefits to vaccination in patients known to have experienced GBS within 6 weeks following previous influenza vaccination. Immediate treatment (including epinephrine 1:1000) for anaphylactoid and/or hypersensitivity reactions should be available during vaccine use. In order to maximize vaccination rates, the ACIP recommends simultaneous administration of all age-appropriate vaccines (live or inactivated) for which a person is eligible at a single clinic visit, unless contraindications exist. The use of combination vaccines is generally preferred over separate injections, taking into consideration provider assessment, patient preference, and adverse events. When using combination vaccines, the minimum age for administration is the oldest minimum age for any individual component; the minimum interval between dosing is the greatest minimum interval between any individual component. Not a substitute for routine tetanus immunization.

Drug Interactions

Avoid Concomitant Use There are no known interactions where it is recommended to avoid concomitant use.

Decreased Effect

The levels/effects of Meningococcal Polysaccharide (Groups C and Y) and Haemophilus b Tetanus Toxoid Conjugate Vaccine may be decreased by: Belimumab; Fingolimod; Immunosuppressants

Increased Effect/Toxicity There are no known significant interactions involving an increase in effect.

Adverse Reactions All serious adverse reactions must be reported to the U.S. Department of Health and Human Services (DHHS) Vaccine Adverse Event Reporting System (VAERS) 1-800-822-7967 or online at https://vaers.hhs. gov/esub/index. In Canada, adverse reactions may be reported to local provincial/territorial health agencies or to the Vaccine Safety Section at Public Health Agency of Canada (1-866-844-0018).

>10%:

Central nervous system: Irritability (62% to 71%), drowsiness (49% to 63%), fever ≥100.4°F/38°C (11% to 26%)

Gastrointestinal: Appetite decreased (30% to 34%)

Local: Injection site reactions: Pain (41% to 46%), redness (21% to 36%), swelling (15% to 25%)

Pharmacodynamics/Kinetics

Onset of Action Antibody response to the components of the vaccine occurs in ≥95% of children following the third dose and ≥98% following the fourth dose.

Available Dosage Forms

Solution Reconstituted, Intramuscular [preservative free]:

Menhibrix: 5 mcg each of polysaccharide antigen groups C and Y, and 2.5 mcg Haemophilus b capsular polysaccharide per 0.5 mL dose (1 ea)

General Dosage Range

I.M.: *Infants ≥6 weeks and Children ≤18 months:* 0.5 mL/dose given as a four-dose series at 2, 4, 6, and 12-15 months of age

Administration

I.M. Administer by I.M. injection in the anterolateral aspect of the thigh in children <1 year of age or the deltoid muscle in children >1 year of age. Do not administer I.V., SubQ, or intradermally.

Do not coadminister with other Hib-containing vaccines (CDC, 2013).

For patients at risk of hemorrhage following intramuscular injection, the ACIP recommends "it should be administered intramuscularly if, in the opinion of the physician familiar with the patient's bleeding risk, the vaccine can be administered by this route with reasonable safety. If the patient receives antihemophilia or other similar therapy, intramuscular vaccination can be scheduled shortly after such therapy is administered. A fine needle (23 gauge or smaller) can be used for the vaccination and firm pressure applied to the site (without rubbing) for at least 2 minutes. The patient should be instructed concerning the risk of hematoma from the injection." Patients on anticoagulant therapy should be considered to have the same bleeding risks and treated as those with clotting factor disorders (CDC, 2011).

Simultaneous administration of vaccines helps ensure the patients will be fully vaccinated by the appropriate age. Simultaneous administration of vaccines is defined as administering >1 vaccine on the same day at different anatomic sites. The use of licensed combination vaccines is generally preferred over separate injections of the equivalent components. Separate vaccines should not be combined in the same syringe unless indicated by product specific labeling. Separate needles and syringes should be used for each injection. The ACIP prefers each dose of a specific vaccine in a series come from the same manufacturer when possible. Adolescents and adults should be vaccinated while seated or lying down. In general, preterm infants should be vaccinated at the same chronological age as full-term infants (CDC, 2011).

Antipyretics have not been shown to prevent febrile seizures. Antipyretics may be used to treat fever or discomfort following vaccination (CDC, 2011). One study reported that routine prophylactic administration of acetaminophen to prevent fever prior to vaccination decreased the immune response of some vaccines; the clinical significance of this reduction in immune response has not been established (Prymula, 2009).

I.V. Do not administer via I.V., SubQ, or intradermally.

Preparation for Administration Reconstitute with provided diluent. Final solution should be clear and colorless. Use immediately after reconstitution.

Storage/Stability Prior to use, store lyophilized vaccine under refrigeration at 2°C to 8°C (36°F to 46°F). Protect from light. Diluent may be stored under refrigeration or at room temperature; do not freeze; discard if frozen.

Nursing Actions

Physical Assessment Ensure patient has received full vaccine series. Monitor for immediate anaphylactoid or hypersensitivity reaction and signs of bleeding at administration site for I.M. administration. Monitor for severe weakness or unusual feelings in arms and legs occurring 2-4 weeks after vaccinations. Monitor for fever. Record all side effects.

Patient Education

• Discuss specific use of vaccine and side effects with caregiver as it relates to treatment. (HCAHPS: During this hospital stay, were you given any medicine that you had not taken before? Before giving you any new medicine, how often did hospital staff tell you what the medicine was for? How often did hospital staff describe possible side effects in a way you could understand?)

• Patient may experience feelings of grouchiness, loss of appetite, fatigue, or irritation at injection site. Have caregiver report immediately to prescriber rash (HCAHPS).

• Educate caregiver about signs of a significant reaction (eg, wheezing; chest tightness; fever; itching; bad cough; blue skin color; seizures; or swelling of face, lips, tongue, or throat). **Note:** This is not a comprehensive list of all side effects. Caregiver should consult prescriber for additional questions.

Intended Use and Disclaimer: Should not be printed and given to patients. This information is intended to serve as a concise initial reference for healthcare professionals to use when discussing medications with a patient. You must ultimately rely on your own discretion, experience and judgment in diagnosing, treating and advising patients.

Related Information

Immunization Administration Recommendations *on page 1675*

Immunization Recommendations *on page 1680*

Meningococcal Polysaccharide Vaccine (Groups A / C / Y and W-135)

(me NIN joe kok al pol i SAK a ride vak SEEN groops aye, see, why & dubl yoo won thur tee fyve)

Brand Names: U.S. Menomune®-A/C/Y/W-135

Index Terms Meningococcal Polysaccharide Vaccine; MPSV; MPSV4

Pharmacologic Category Vaccine, Inactivated (Bacterial)

Medication Safety Issues

Administration issue:

Menomune® (MPSV4) should be administered by subcutaneous (SubQ) injection. Menactra® (MCV4), also a meningococcal polysaccharide vaccine, is to be administered by intramuscular (I.M.) injection only.

Pregnancy Risk Factor C

Lactation Excretion in breast milk unknown/use caution

Use Provide active immunity to meningococcal serogroups contained in the vaccine

The Advisory Committee on Immunization Practices (ACIP) recommends routine vaccination for persons at increased risk for meningococcal disease. Meningococcal quadrivalent conjugate vaccine (MenACWY) is preferred; meningococcal polysaccharide vaccine (MPSV4) is preferred in meningococcal vaccine-naive adults ≥56 years of age requiring only a single vaccination (CDC, 2013).

Those at increased risk of meningococcal disease include the following:

- Persons ≥2 months of age with medical conditions such as anatomical or functional asplenia or persistent compliment component deficiencies (eg, C_5-C_9, properdin, factor H, or factor D)

- Persons ≥9 months of age that travel to or reside in countries where meningococcal disease is hyperendemic or epidemic, especially if contact with the local population will be prolonged

- Unvaccinated or incompletely vaccinated first year college students living in residence halls

- Military recruits

- Microbiologists with occupational exposure

- Persons (in all recommended age groups) at risk who are part of outbreaks caused by vaccine preventable serogroups

Available Dosage Forms

Injection, powder for reconstitution [MPSV4]:

Menomune®-A/C/Y/W-135: 50 mcg each of polysaccharide antigen groups A, C, Y, and W-135 per 0.5 mL dose

General Dosage Range SubQ: *Children ≥2 years and Adults:* 0.5 mL as a single dose

Administration

Other Administer by SubQ injection to the deltoid region; do not administer intradermally, I.M., or I.V.

Simultaneous administration of vaccines helps ensure the patients will be fully vaccinated by the appropriate age. Simultaneous administration of vaccines is defined as administering ≥1 vaccine on the same day at different anatomic sites. Separate vaccines should not be combined in the same syringe unless indicated by product specific labeling. Separate needles and syringes should be used for each injection. The ACIP prefers each dose of a specific vaccine in a series come from the same manufacturer when possible. Adolescents and adults should be vaccinated while seated or lying down. In general, preterm infants should be vaccinated at the same chronological age as full-term infants (CDC, 2011).

Antipyretics have not been shown to prevent febrile seizures. Antipyretics may be used to treat fever or discomfort following vaccination (CDC, 2011). One study reported that routine prophylactic administration of acetaminophen to prevent fever prior to vaccination decreased the immune response of some vaccines; the clinical significance of this reduction in immune response has not been established (Prymula, 2009).

Nursing Actions

Physical Assessment Ensure that vaccine series is complete for full benefit.

U.S. federal law requires entry into the patient's medical record.

Instruct patient to report serious hypersensitivity reaction symptoms including respiratory distress, hypotension, urticaria, upper airway swelling or symptoms of swelling (eg, dizziness or trouble breathing). Other side effects include pain, redness, tenderness, or swelling at injection site along with headache or fever 1-2 days after injection.

Patient Education

• Discuss specific use of vaccine and side effects with patient as it relates to treatment. (HCAHPS: During this hospital stay, were you given any medicine that you had not taken before? Before giving you any new medicine, how often did hospital staff tell you what the medicine was for? How often did hospital staff describe possible side effects in a way you could understand?)

• Patient may experience pain, redness or swelling at injection site, headache, fatigue, nausea, emesis, diarrhea, or dyspepsia. Have patient report immediately to prescriber severe injection site reaction (HCAHPS).

• Educate patient about signs of a significant reaction (eg, wheezing; chest tightness; fever; itching; bad cough; blue skin color; seizures; or swelling of face, lips, tongue, or throat). **Note:** This is not a comprehensive list of all side effects. Patient should consult prescriber for additional questions.

Intended Use and Disclaimer: Should not be printed and given to patients. This information is intended to serve as a concise initial reference for healthcare professionals to use when discussing medications with a patient. You must ultimately rely on your own discretion, experience and judgment in diagnosing, treating and advising patients.

Related Information

Immunization Administration Recommendations *on page 1675*

Immunization Recommendations *on page 1680*

Menotropins (men oh TROE pins)

Brand Names: U.S. Menopur®; Repronex®

Index Terms hMG; Human Menopausal Gonadotropin

Pharmacologic Category Gonadotropin; Ovulation Stimulator

Medication Safety Issues

Sound-alike/look-alike issues:

Repronex® may be confused with Regranex®

Pregnancy Risk Factor X

Lactation Excretion in breast milk unknown/use caution

Breast-Feeding Considerations It is not known if menotropins is excreted in breast milk. The manufacturer recommends that caution be exercised when administering menotropins to nursing women.

Use Female:

In conjunction with hCG to induce ovulation and pregnancy in infertile females experiencing oligoanovulation or anovulation when the cause of anovulation is functional and not caused by primary ovarian failure (Repronex®)

Stimulation of multiple follicle development in ovulatory patients as part of an assisted reproductive technology (ART) (Menopur®, Repronex®)

Unlabeled Use Male: Stimulation of spermatogenesis in primary or secondary hypogonadotropic hypogonadism

Mechanism of Action/Effect Actions occur as a result of both follicle stimulating hormone (FSH) effects and luteinizing hormone (LH) effects; menotropins stimulate the development and maturation of the ovarian follicle (FSH), cause ovulation (LH), and stimulate the development of the corpus luteum (LH); in males it stimulates spermatogenesis (LH)

Contraindications Hypersensitivity to menotropins or any component of the formulation; primary ovarian failure as indicated by a high follicle-stimulating hormone (FSH) level; uncontrolled thyroid and adrenal dysfunction; abnormal bleeding of undetermined origin; intracranial lesion (ie, pituitary tumor); ovarian cyst or enlargement not due to polycystic ovary syndrome; infertility due to any cause other than anovulation (except candidates for *in vitro* fertilization); sex hormone-dependent tumors of the reproductive tract and accessory organs; pregnancy

Warnings/Precautions Hazardous agent; use appropriate precautions for handling and disposal (NIOSH, 2012). These medications should only be used by physicians who are thoroughly familiar with infertility problems and their management. Advise patient of frequency and potential hazards of multiple pregnancy. May cause ovarian hyperstimulation syndrome (OHSS); if severe, treatment should be discontinued and patient should be hospitalized (may become more severe if pregnancy occurs). Monitor for ovarian enlargement; to minimize the hazard of abnormal ovarian enlargement, use the lowest possible dose. Serious pulmonary conditions (atelectasis, acute respiratory distress syndrome) and arterial thromboembolism have been reported. Safety and efficacy have not been established in renal or hepatic impairment, or in pediatric and geriatric patients. Use may lead to multiple births.

Drug Interactions

Avoid Concomitant Use There are no known interactions where it is recommended to avoid concomitant use.

Decreased Effect There are no known significant interactions involving a decrease in effect.

Increased Effect/Toxicity There are no known significant interactions involving an increase in effect.

Adverse Reactions Adverse effects may vary according to specific product, route, and/or dosage.

>10%:

Central nervous system: Headache (up to 34%)

Gastrointestinal: Abdominal pain (up to 18%), nausea (up to 12%)

Genitourinary: OHSS (up to 13%, dose related)

Local: Injection site reaction (4% to 12%)

1% to 10%:

Cardiovascular: Flushing

Central nervous system: Dizziness, malaise, migraine

Endocrine & metabolic: Breast tenderness, hot flashes, menstrual irregularities

Gastrointestinal: Abdominal cramping, abdominal fullness, constipation, diarrhea, enlarged abdomen, vomiting

Genitourinary: Ectopic pregnancy, ovarian disease, vaginal hemorrhage

Local: Injection site edema/pain

Neuromuscular & skeletal: Back pain

Respiratory: Cough increased, respiratory disorder

Miscellaneous: Infection, flu-like syndrome

Frequency not defined:

Cardiovascular: Stroke, tachycardia, thrombosis (venous or arterial)

Dermatologic: Angioedema, rash, urticaria

Genitourinary: Adnexal torsion, hemoperitoneum, ovarian enlargement

Neuromuscular & skeletal: Limb necrosis

Respiratory: Acute respiratory distress syndrome, atelectasis, dyspnea, embolism, laryngeal edema, pulmonary infarction, tachypnea

Miscellaneous: Allergic reaction, anaphylaxis

Dosage Forms Considerations

75 units of menotropins represents 75 units each of FSH activity and LH activity

Available Dosage Forms

Injection, powder for reconstitution:

Menopur®, Repronex®: 75 units

General Dosage Range

I.M.: *Adults:* Repronex®: Initial: 150 units **or** 225 units daily (maximum: 450 units/day; 12 days of therapy)

SubQ: *Adults:* Menopur®: Initial: 225 units daily (maximum: 450 units/day; 20 days of therapy); Repronex®: Initial: 150 units **or** 225 units daily (maximum: 450 units/day; 12 days of therapy)

Administration

I.M. Repronex®: Administer deep in a large muscle.

Hazardous agent; use appropriate precautions for handling and disposal (NIOSH, 2012).

Other SubQ:

Menopur®: Administer to alternating sites of the abdomen. When administration to the lower abdomen is not possible, the injection may be given into the thigh.

Repronex®: Administer to alternating sites of the lower abdomen.

Hazardous agent; use appropriate precautions for handling and disposal (NIOSH, 2012).

Preparation for Administration Hazardous agent; use appropriate precautions for handling and disposal (NIOSH, 2012). After reconstitution inject immediately; discard any unused portion.

Storage/Stability Lyophilized powder may be refrigerated or stored at room temperature. Protect from light.

Nursing Actions

Physical Assessment Teach appropriate method for measuring basal body temperature to indicate ovulation. Stress importance of following prescriber's instructions for timing intercourse. If self-administered, teach appropriate injection technique and needle disposal.

Patient Education

• Discuss specific use of drug and side effects with patient as it relates to treatment. (HCAHPS: During this hospital stay, were you given any medicine that you had not taken before? Before giving you any new medicine, how often did hospital staff tell you what the medicine was

for? How often did hospital staff describe possible side effects in a way you could understand?)
- Patient may experience injection site irritation, ovarian cysts, nausea, dyspepsia, headache, macromastia, or ovarian hyperstimulation. Have patient report immediately to prescriber dyspnea, severe diarrhea, significant weight gain, considerable edema, or rash (HCAHPS).
- Educate patient about signs of a significant reaction (eg, wheezing; chest tightness; fever; itching; bad cough; blue skin color; seizures; or swelling of face, lips, tongue, or throat). **Note:** This is not a comprehensive list of all side effects. Patient should consult prescriber for additional questions.

Intended Use and Disclaimer: Should not be printed and given to patients. This information is intended to serve as a concise initial reference for healthcare professionals to use when discussing medications with a patient. You must ultimately rely on your own discretion, experience and judgment in diagnosing, treating and advising patients.

Meperidine (me PER i deen)

Brand Names: U.S. Demerol; Meperitab
Index Terms Isonipecaine Hydrochloride; Meperidine Hydrochloride; Pethidine Hydrochloride
Pharmacologic Category Analgesic, Opioid
Medication Safety Issues
 Sound-alike/look-alike issues:
  Meperidine may be confused with meprobamate
  Demerol® may be confused with Demulen®, Desyrel, Dilaudid®, Pamelor™
 High alert medication:
  The Institute for Safe Medication Practices (ISMP) includes this medication among its list of drug classes which have a heightened risk of causing significant patient harm when used in error.
 BEERS Criteria medication:
  This drug may be potentially inappropriate for use in geriatric patients (Quality of evidence - high; Strength of recommendation - strong).
 Other safety concerns:
  Avoid the use of meperidine for pain control, especially in elderly and renally-compromised patients because of the risk of neurotoxicity (American Pain Society, 2008; Institute for Safe Medication Practices [ISMP], 2007)
Pregnancy Risk Factor C
Lactation Enters breast milk/not recommended
Use Management of moderate-to-severe pain; adjunct to anesthesia and preoperative sedation
Unlabeled Use Reduce postoperative shivering; reduce rigors from amphotericin B (conventional)
Controlled Substance C-II

Available Dosage Forms
 Solution, Injection:
  Demerol: 25 mg/mL (1 mL); 25 mg/0.5 mL (0.5 mL); 50 mg/mL (1 mL, 30 mL); 75 mg/1.5 mL (1.5 mL); 100 mg/2 mL (2 mL); 75 mg/mL (1 mL); 100 mg/mL (1 mL, 20 mL)
  Generic: 10 mg/mL (30 mL); 25 mg/mL (1 mL); 50 mg/mL (1 mL); 100 mg/mL (1 mL)
 Solution, Oral:
  Generic: 50 mg/5 mL (500 mL)
 Tablet, Oral:
  Demerol: 50 mg, 100 mg
  Meperitab: 50 mg, 100 mg
  Generic: 50 mg, 100 mg
General Dosage Range Dosage adjustment recommended in patients with hepatic impairment
 I.M., SubQ:
  Children: 1.1-1.8 mg/kg/dose every 3-4 hours as needed (maximum: 50-150 mg/dose) **or** 1.1-2.2 mg/kg given 30-90 minutes before the beginning of anesthesia (maximum: 50-150 mg/dose)
  Adults: 50-150 mg every 3-4 hours as needed **or** 50-150 mg given 30-90 minutes before the beginning of anesthesia **or** 50-100 mg when pain becomes regular; may repeat at every 1-3 hours
  Elderly: Avoid use
 Oral:
  Children: 1.1-1.8 mg/kg/dose every 3-4 hours as needed (maximum: 50-150 mg/dose)
  Adults: Initial: 50-150 mg every 3-4 hours as needed
  Elderly: Avoid use
Administration
 I.V. Solution for injection: May be administered I.M., SubQ, or I.V.; I.V. push should be administered slowly using a diluted solution, use of a 10 mg/mL concentration has been recommended.
 Injectable Detail pH: 3.5-6
 Oral Oral solution: Administer solution in 1/2 glass of water; undiluted solution may exert topical anesthetic effect on mucous membranes
Nursing Actions
 Physical Assessment Monitor for effectiveness of pain relief. Monitor blood pressure, CNS and respiratory status, and degree of sedation at beginning of therapy and periodically thereafter. Assess patient's physical and/or psychological dependence. For inpatients, implement safety measures (eg, side rails up, call light within reach, instructions to call for assistance). Discontinue slowly after prolonged use.
Patient Education
- Discuss specific use of drug and side effects with patient as it relates to treatment. (HCAHPS: During this hospital stay, were you given any medicine that you had not taken before? Before giving you any new medicine, how often did hospital staff tell you what the medicine was

for? How often did hospital staff describe possible side effects in a way you could understand?)
• Patient may experience fatigue, flushing, lack of appetite, or hyperhidrosis. Have patient report immediately to prescriber severe dizziness, syncope, illogical thinking, considerable nausea, significant constipation, intolerable asthenia, angina, tachycardia, bradycardia, arrhythmia, difficult urination, hallucinations, mood changes, severe dyspepsia, dyspnea, considerable headache, tremors, difficulty with motor activity, or vision changes (HCAHPS).
• Educate patient about signs of a significant reaction (eg, wheezing; chest tightness; fever; itching; bad cough; blue skin color; seizures; or swelling of face, lips, tongue, or throat). **Note:** This is not a comprehensive list of all side effects. Patient should consult prescriber for additional questions.

Intended Use and Disclaimer: Should not be printed and given to patients. This information is intended to serve as a concise initial reference for healthcare professionals to use when discussing medications with a patient. You must ultimately rely on your own discretion, experience and judgment in diagnosing, treating and advising patients.

Mercaptopurine (mer kap toe PURE een)

Brand Names: U.S. Purinethol
Index Terms 6-Mercaptopurine (error-prone abbreviation); 6-MP (error-prone abbreviation)
Pharmacologic Category Antineoplastic Agent, Antimetabolite; Antineoplastic Agent, Antimetabolite (Purine Analog); Immunosuppressant Agent
Medication Safety Issues
Sound-alike/look-alike issues:
Mercaptopurine may be confused with methotrexate
Purinethol® may be confused with propylthiouracil
High alert medication:
This medication is in a class the Institute for Safe Medication Practices (ISMP) includes among its list of drug classes which have a heightened risk of causing significant patient harm when used in error.
Other safety concerns:
To avoid potentially serious dosage errors, the terms "6-mercaptopurine" or "6-MP" should be avoided; use of these terms has been associated with sixfold overdosages.
Azathioprine is metabolized to mercaptopurine; concurrent use of these commercially-available products has resulted in profound myelosuppression.
Pregnancy Risk Factor D
Lactation Excretion in breast milk unknown/not recommended

Breast-Feeding Considerations Mercaptopurine is the active metabolite of azathioprine. Following administration of azathioprine, mercaptopurine can be detected in breast milk (Gardiner, 2006). It is not known if/how much mercaptopurine is found in breast milk following oral administration. According to the manufacturer, the decision to discontinue mercaptopurine or discontinue breast-feeding during therapy should take into account the benefits of treatment to the mother.
Use Maintenance treatment component of acute lymphoblastic leukemia (ALL)
Unlabeled Use Steroid-sparing agent for corticosteroid-dependent Crohn's disease (CD) and ulcerative colitis (UC); maintenance of remission in CD; fistulizing Crohn's disease; maintenance treatment in acute promyelocytic leukemia (APL); treatment component for non Hodgkin lymphoma (NHL), treatment of autoimmune hepatitis
Mechanism of Action/Effect Purine antagonist which inhibits DNA and RNA synthesis
Contraindications Hypersensitivity to mercaptopurine or any component of the formulation; patients whose disease showed prior resistance to mercaptopurine
Warnings/Precautions Hazardous agent - use appropriate precautions for handling and disposal (NIOSH, 2012).

Hepatotoxicity has been reported, including jaundice, ascites, hepatic necrosis (may be fatal), intrahepatic cholestasis, parenchymal cell necrosis, and/or hepatic encephalopathy; may be due to direct hepatic cell damage or hypersensitivity. While hepatotoxicity or hepatic injury may occur at any dose, dosages >2.5 mg/kg/day are associated with a higher incidence. Signs of jaundice generally appear early in treatment, after ~1-2 months (range: 1 week to 8 years) and may resolve following discontinuation; recurrence with rechallenge has been noted. Monitor liver function tests (monitor more frequently if used in combination with other hepatotoxic drugs or in patients with pre-existing hepatic impairment. Consider a reduced dose in patients with hepatic impairment. Withhold treatment for clinical signs of jaundice (hepatomegaly, anorexia, tenderness), deterioration in liver function tests, toxic hepatitis, or biliary stasis until hepatotoxicity is ruled out.

Dose-related leukopenia, thrombocytopenia, and anemia are common; however, may be indicative of disease progression. Hematologic toxicity may be delayed. Bone marrow may appear hypoplastic (could also appear normal). Monitor for bleeding (due to thrombocytopenia) or infection (due to neutropenia). Patients with homozygous genetic defect of thiopurine methyltransferase (TPMT) are more sensitive to myelosuppressive effects; generally associated with rapid myelosuppression. Significant mercaptopurine dose reductions will be necessary (possibly with continued concomitant chemotherapy at normal doses). Patients who are heterozygous for TPMT defects will have intermediate activity; may have increased toxicity (primarily myelosuppression) although will generally tolerate normal mercaptopurine doses. Consider TPMT testing for severe toxicities/excessive myelosuppression. Patients on concurrent therapy with drugs which may inhibit TPMT (eg, olsalazine) or xanthine oxidase (eg, allopurinol) may be sensitive to myelosuppressive effects.

Immunosuppressive agents, including mercaptopurine, are associated with the development of lymphoma and other malignancies including hepatosplenic T-cell lymphoma (HSTCL). Because azathioprine is metabolized to mercaptopurine, concomitant use with azathioprine may result in profound myelosuppression and should be avoided. Mercaptopurine is immunosuppressive; the risk for infection is increased; common signs of infection, such as fever and leukocytosis may not occur; lethargy and confusion may be more prominent signs of infection. Immune response to vaccines may be diminished. Consider adjusting dosage in patients with renal impairment. Some renal adverse effects may be minimized with hydration and prophylactic antihyperuricemic therapy. To avoid potentially serious dosage errors, the terms "6-mercaptopurine" or "6-MP" should be avoided; use of these terms has been associated with sixfold overdosages.

Drug Interactions
Avoid Concomitant Use
Avoid concomitant use of Mercaptopurine with any of the following: AzaTHIOprine; BCG; CloZAPine; Febuxostat; Natalizumab; Pimecrolimus; Tacrolimus (Topical); Tofacitinib
Decreased Effect
Mercaptopurine may decrease the levels/effects of: BCG; Coccidioidin Skin Test; Sipuleucel-T; Vaccines (Inactivated); Vitamin K Antagonists

The levels/effects of Mercaptopurine may be decreased by: Echinacea
Increased Effect/Toxicity
Mercaptopurine may increase the levels/effects of: CloZAPine; Leflunomide; Natalizumab; Tofacitinib; Vaccines (Live); Vitamin K Antagonists

The levels/effects of Mercaptopurine may be increased by: 5-ASA Derivatives; Allopurinol; AzaTHIOprine; Denosumab; DOXOrubicin (Conventional); Febuxostat; Pimecrolimus; Roflumilast; Sulfamethoxazole; Tacrolimus (Topical); Trastuzumab; Trimethoprim

Nutritional/Ethanol Interactions Food: Absorption is variable with food. Management: Take on an empty stomach at the same time each day 1 hour before or 2 hours after a meal. Maintain adequate hydration, unless instructed to restrict fluid intake.

Adverse Reactions Frequency not defined.
Central nervous system: Drug fever

Dermatologic: Alopecia, hyperpigmentation, rash
Endocrine & metabolic: Hyperuricemia
Gastrointestinal: Anorexia, diarrhea, intestinal ulcers, mucositis/oral lesions (rare), nausea (minimal), pancreatitis, sprue-like symptoms, stomach pain, vomiting (minimal)
Genitourinary: Oligospermia
Hematologic: Myelosuppression (onset 7-10 days; nadir 14 days; recovery: 21 days); anemia, bleeding, granulocytopenia, leukopenia, marrow hypoplasia, thrombocytopenia
Hepatic: Hepatotoxicity, ascites, biliary stasis, hepatic damage/injury, hepatic encephalopathy, hepatic necrosis, hepatomegaly, intrahepatic cholestasis, jaundice, parenchymal cell necrosis, toxic hepatitis
Renal: Hyperuricosuria, renal toxicity
Miscellaneous: Hepatosplenic T cell lymphoma, immunosuppression, infection, secondary malignancy

Available Dosage Forms
Tablet, Oral:
Purinethol: 50 mg
Generic: 50 mg
General Dosage Range Dosage adjustment recommended in patients with hepatic or renal impairment or on concomitant therapy
Oral: *Children and Adults:* Maintenance: 1.5-2.5 mg/kg/day

Administration
Oral Preferably on an empty stomach (1 hour before or 2 hours after meals)

For the treatment of ALL in children (Schmiegelow, 1997): Administration in the evening has demonstration superior outcome; administration with food did not significantly affect outcome.

Hazardous agent; use appropriate precautions for handling and disposal (NIOSH, 2012).

Storage/Stability Store at room temperature of 15°C to 25°C (59°F to 77°F). Protect from moisture.

Nursing Actions
Physical Assessment Assess hepatic function; jaundice, ascites, and encephalopathy can occur some time following therapy. Monitor nutritional status and renal status. Monitor for dehydration, myelosuppression, anemia, and leukopenia on a regular basis. Teach patient importance of adequate hydration. Monitor for signs/symptoms of malignancy (eg, splenomegaly, hepatomegaly, abdominal pain, persistent fever, night sweats, weight loss).

Patient Education
• Discuss specific use of drug and side effects with patient as it relates to treatment. (HCAHPS: During this hospital stay, were you given any medicine that you had not taken before? Before giving you any new medicine, how often did hospital staff tell you what the medicine was for? How often did hospital staff describe possible side effects in a way you could understand?)

- Patient may experience diarrhea, loss of appetite, anemia, leukopenia, thrombocytopenia, change in skin color, or stomatitis. Have patient report immediately to prescriber signs of infection, dyspnea, angina, severe dyspepsia, significant nausea, fatigue, intolerable back pain, edema of hands or feet, ecchymosis, discolored urine, jaundice, nocturnal hyperhidrosis, significant weight gain or loss, or rash (HCAHPS).
- Educate patient about signs of a significant reaction (eg, wheezing; chest tightness; fever; itching; bad cough; blue skin color; seizures; or swelling of face, lips, tongue, or throat). **Note:** This is not a comprehensive list of all side effects. Patient should consult prescriber for additional questions.

Intended Use and Disclaimer: Should not be printed and given to patients. This information is intended to serve as a concise initial reference for healthcare professionals to use when discussing medications with a patient. You must ultimately rely on your own discretion, experience and judgment in diagnosing, treating and advising patients.

Dietary Considerations Should not be administered with meals.

Related Information
Oral Medications That Should Not Be Crushed or Altered *on page 1712*

Meropenem (mer oh PEN em)

Brand Names: U.S. Merrem
Pharmacologic Category Antibiotic, Carbapenem

Medication Safety Issues
Sound-alike/look-alike issues:
Meropenem may be confused with ertapenem, imipenem, metroNIDAZOLE

Pregnancy Risk Factor B

Lactation Excreted in breast milk/use caution

Breast-Feeding Considerations Small amounts of meropenem are excreted into breast milk (case report). The manufacturer recommends that caution be exercised when administering meropenem to breast-feeding women. Nondose-related effects could include modification of bowel flora.

Use
Treatment of intra-abdominal infections (complicated appendicitis and peritonitis); treatment of bacterial meningitis in pediatric patients ≥3 months of age caused by *S. pneumoniae*, *H. influenzae*, and *N. meningitidis*; treatment of complicated skin and skin structure infections caused by susceptible organisms
Canadian labeling: Additional indications (not in U.S. labeling): Treatment of lower respiratory tract infections (community-acquired and nosocomial pneumonias), complicated urinary tract infections, gynecologic infections (excluding chlamydia), and septicemia; treatment of bacterial meningitis in adults caused by *S. pneumoniae*, *H. influenzae*, and *N. meningitidis* (use in adult meningitis based on pediatric data)

Unlabeled Use *Burkholderia pseudomallei* (melioidosis), catheter-related blood stream infections; cystic fibrosis, pulmonary exacerbation; febrile neutropenia; pneumonia (hospital-acquired, healthcare-associated, or ventilator-associated); treatment of prosthetic joint infection

Mechanism of Action/Effect Inhibits cell wall synthesis in susceptible bacteria

Contraindications Hypersensitivity to meropenem, any component of the formulation, or other carbapenems (eg, doripenem, ertapenem, imipenem); patients who have experienced anaphylactic reactions to other beta-lactams

Warnings/Precautions Serious hypersensitivity reactions, including anaphylaxis, have been reported (some without a history of previous allergic reactions to beta-lactams). Carbapenems have been associated with CNS adverse effects, including confusional states and seizures (myoclonic); use caution with CNS disorders (eg, brain lesions and history of seizures) and adjust dose in renal impairment to avoid drug accumulation, which may increase seizure risk. Outpatient use may result in paresthesias, seizures, or headaches that can impair neuromotor function and alertness; patients should not operate machinery or drive until it is established that meropenem is well tolerated. Prolonged use may result in fungal or bacterial superinfection, including *C. difficile*-associated diarrhea (CDAD) and pseudomembranous colitis; CDAD has been observed >2 months postantibiotic treatment. Use with caution in patients with renal impairment; dosage adjustment required in patients with moderate-to-severe renal dysfunction. Thrombocytopenia has been reported in patients with renal dysfunction. Lower doses (based upon renal function) are often required in the elderly. May decrease divalproex sodium/valproic acid concentrations leading to breakthrough seizures; concomitant use not recommended. Alternative antimicrobial agents should be considered; if concurrent meropenem is necessary, consider additional antiseizure medication.

Drug Interactions

Avoid Concomitant Use
Avoid concomitant use of Meropenem with any of the following: BCG; Probenecid

Decreased Effect
Meropenem may decrease the levels/effects of: BCG; Sodium Picosulfate; Typhoid Vaccine; Valproic Acid and Derivatives

Increased Effect/Toxicity
The levels/effects of Meropenem may be increased by: Probenecid

Adverse Reactions 1% to 10%:
Central nervous system: Headache (2% to 8%), pain (≤5%)

Dermatologic: Rash (2% to 3%, includes diaper-area moniliasis in infants), pruritus (1%)

Endocrine & metabolic: Hypoglycemia

Gastrointestinal: Diarrhea (4% to 7%), nausea/vomiting (1% to 8%), constipation (1% to 7%), oral moniliasis (up to 2% in pediatric patients), glossitis (1%)

Hematologic: Anemia (≤6%)

Local: Inflammation at the injection site (2%), phlebitis/thrombophlebitis (1%), injection site reaction (1%)

Respiratory: Apnea (1%), pharyngitis, pneumonia

Miscellaneous: Sepsis (2%), shock (1%)

Available Dosage Forms

Solution Reconstituted, Intravenous:

Merrem: 500 mg (1 ea); 1 g (1 ea)

Generic: 500 mg (1 ea); 1 g (1 ea)

General Dosage Range Dosage adjustment recommended in patients with renal impairment

I.V.:

Children ≥3 months and <50 kg: 10-40 mg/kg every 8 hours (maximum: 2 **g** every 8 hours)

Children ≥50 kg and Adults: 500 mg to 2 **g** every 8 hours

Administration

I.V. Administer I.V. infusion over 15-30 minutes; I.V. bolus injection (5-20 mL) over 3-5 minutes

Extended infusion administration (unlabeled dosing): Administer over 3 hours (Crandon 2011; Dandekar, 2003). **Note:** Must consider meropenem's limited room temperature stability if using extended infusions

Injectable Detail pH: 7.3-8.3

Preparation for Administration Meropenem infusion vials may be reconstituted with SWFI. The 500 mg vials should be reconstituted with 10 mL, and 1 g vials with 20 mL. May be further diluted with compatible solutions for infusion. Consult detailed reference/product labeling for compatibility.

Storage/Stability Freshly prepared solutions should be used. However, constituted solutions maintain satisfactory potency under the conditions described below. Solutions should not be frozen.

Dry powder should be stored at controlled room temperature 20°C to 25°C (68°F to 77°F).

Injection reconstitution: Stability in vial when constituted (up to 50 mg/mL) with:

SWFI: Stable for up to 3 hours at up to 25°C (77°F) or for up to 13 hours at up to 5°C (41°F).

Infusion admixture (1-20 mg/mL): Solution is stable when diluted in NS for 1 hour at up to 25°C (77°F) or 15 hours at up to 5°C (41°F). Solutions constituted with dextrose injection 5% should be used immediately. **Note:** Meropenem stability (admixed with NS at a concentration of 20 mg/mL) at room temperature for >1 hour or under refrigeration for >15 hours is not supported by the manufacturer. Data exist supporting stability (admixed with NS at a concentration

of 20 mg/mL) at room temperature for ≤4 hours and under refrigeration ≤24 hours (Patel, 1997).

Nursing Actions

Physical Assessment Results of culture and sensitivity tests and patient's allergy history should be assessed prior to beginning treatment. Infusion site should be monitored closely to prevent phlebitis/thrombophlebitis. Teach patient importance of adequate hydration.

Patient Education

• Discuss specific use of drug and side effects with patient as it relates to treatment. (HCAHPS: During this hospital stay, were you given any medicine that you had not taken before? Before giving you any new medicine, how often did hospital staff tell you what the medicine was for? How often did hospital staff describe possible side effects in a way you could understand?)

• Patient may experience nausea, diarrhea, or vaginal yeast infection. Have patient report immediately to prescriber dizziness, syncope, or rash (HCAHPS).

• Educate patient about signs of a significant reaction (eg, wheezing; chest tightness; fever; itching; bad cough; blue skin color; seizures; or swelling of face, lips, tongue, or throat). **Note:** This is not a comprehensive list of all side effects. Patient should consult prescriber for additional questions.

Intended Use and Disclaimer: Should not be printed and given to patients. This information is intended to serve as a concise initial reference for healthcare professionals to use when discussing medications with a patient. You must ultimately rely on your own discretion, experience and judgment in diagnosing, treating and advising patients.

Dietary Considerations Some products may contain sodium.

Mesalamine (me SAL a meen)

Brand Names: U.S. Apriso; Asacol HD; Canasa; Delzicol; Lialda; Pentasa; Rowasa; SfRowasa

Index Terms 5-Aminosalicylic Acid; 5-ASA; Fisalamine; Mesalazine

Pharmacologic Category 5-Aminosalicylic Acid Derivative

Medication Safety Issues

Sound-alike/look-alike issues:

Mesalamine may be confused with mecamylamine, megestrol, memantine, metaxalone, methenamine

Apriso may be confused with Apri

Asacol may be confused with Ansaid, Os-Cal

Lialda may be confused with Aldara

Pentasa may be confused with Pancrease, Pangestyme

Pregnancy Risk Factor B/C (product specific)

Lactation Enters breast milk/use caution

◀ **Breast-Feeding Considerations** Low concentrations of the parent drug (undetectable to 0.11 mg/L) and higher concentrations of the N-acetyl metabolite of the parent drug (5-18 mg/L) have been detected in human breast milk following oral or rectal maternal doses of 500 mg to 3 g daily. Adverse effects (diarrhea) in a nursing infant have been reported while the mother received rectal administration of mesalamine within 12 hours after the first dose (Nelis, 1989). The manufacturer recommends that caution be used if administered to a nursing woman. Other sources consider use of mesalamine to be safe while breastfeeding (Habal, 2012; Mottet, 2009).

Use

U.S. labeling:

Oral:

Apriso: Maintenance of remission of ulcerative colitis

Asacol HD: Treatment of moderately-active ulcerative colitis

Delzicol, Lialda, Pentasa: Treatment and maintenance of remission of mildly- to moderately-active ulcerative colitis

Rectal: Treatment of active mild to moderate distal ulcerative colitis (suspension only), proctosigmoiditis (suspension only), or proctitis (suspension and suppository)

Canadian labeling:

Oral:

Asacol, Mezavant: Treatment and maintenance of remission of mildly- to moderately-active ulcerative colitis

Asacol 800: Treatment of moderately-active ulcerative colitis

Mesasal: Treatment and maintenance of remission of ulcerative colitis

Pentasa: Treatment and maintenance of remission of mildly- to moderately-active ulcerative colitis; treatment and maintenance of remission of mild to moderate Crohn's disease

Rectal: Treatment and maintenance of remission of distal ulcerative colitis (extending to splenic flexure) and as adjunctive therapy in more extensive disease (suspension only); treatment and maintenance of ulcerative proctitis (suppository only)

Mechanism of Action/Effect Mesalamine (5-aminosalicylic acid) is the active component of sulfasalazine; the specific mechanism of action of mesalamine is unknown; however, it is thought that it modulates local chemical mediators of the inflammatory response, especially leukotrienes, and is also postulated to be a free radical scavenger or an inhibitor of tumor necrosis factor (TNF); action appears topical rather than systemic

Contraindications

U.S. labeling: Hypersensitivity to mesalamine, aminosalicylates, salicylates, or any component of the formulation (including suppository vehicle of vegetable fatty acid esters)

Canadian labeling: Hypersensitivity to mesalamine, salicylates, or any component of the formulation; severe renal impairment (GFR <30 mL/minute/1.73 m^2); severe hepatic impairment

Additional contraindications per specific Canadian product labeling: Existing gastric or duodenal ulcer, urinary tract obstruction, use in children <2 years of age (Asacol, Asacol 800, Mesasal, Pentasa, Salofalk); hemorrhagic diathesis (Mesasal); patients unable to swallow intact tablet (Asacol, Asacol 800); renal parenchymal disease (Pentasa)

Warnings/Precautions May cause an acute intolerance syndrome (cramping, acute abdominal pain, bloody diarrhea; sometimes fever, headache, rash); discontinue if this occurs. Use caution in patients with active peptic ulcers. Patients with pyloric stenosis or other gastrointestinal obstructive disorders may have prolonged gastric retention of tablets, delaying the release of mesalamine in the colon. Pericarditis or myocarditis (mesalamine-induced cardiac hypersensitivity reactions) should be considered in patients with chest pain; use with caution in patients predisposed to these conditions. Pancreatitis should be considered in patients with new abdominal discomfort. Symptomatic worsening of colitis/IBD may occur following initiation of therapy. Oligospermia (rare, reversible) has been reported in males. Use caution in patients with sulfasalazine hypersensitivity. Use caution in patients with impaired hepatic function; hepatic failure has been reported. Canadian labeling contraindicates use in severe hepatic impairment. Renal disease (including minimal change nephropathy, acute/chronic interstitial nephritis, nephrotic syndrome, and rarely renal failure) has been reported; use caution with other medications converted to mesalamine. An evaluation of renal function is recommended prior to initiation of mesalamine products and periodically during treatment. Use caution in patients with renal impairment. Canadian labeling contraindicates use in severe renal impairment GFR <30 mL/minute/1.73 m^2; urinary tract obstruction and renal parenchymal disease are also included as contraindications in specific Canadian labels. Use caution with other medications converted to mesalamine. Post-marketing reports suggest an increased incidence of blood dyscrasias in patients >65 years of age. In addition, elderly may have difficulty administering and retaining rectal suppositories or may have decreased renal function; use with caution and monitor.

Apriso contains phenylalanine. The Asacol HD 800 mg tablet has not been shown to be bioequivalent to two Asacol 400 mg tablets [Canadian product] or two Delzicol 400 mg capsules. Canasa suppositories contain saturated vegetable fatty acid esters (contraindicated in patients with allergy to these components). Rowasa, Salofalk [Canadian product] and Pentasa [Canadian product] enema contain metabisulfite salts that may cause severe hypersensitivity reactions (ie, anaphylaxis) in patients with sulfite allergies.

Drug Interactions

Avoid Concomitant Use There are no known interactions where it is recommended to avoid concomitant use.

Decreased Effect

Mesalamine may decrease the levels/effects of: Cardiac Glycosides

The levels/effects of Mesalamine may be decreased by: Antacids; H2-Antagonists; Proton Pump Inhibitors

Increased Effect/Toxicity

Mesalamine may increase the levels/effects of: Heparin; Heparin (Low Molecular Weight); Thiopurine Analogs; Varicella Virus-Containing Vaccines

The levels/effects of Mesalamine may be increased by: Nonsteroidal Anti-Inflammatory Agents

Adverse Reactions Adverse effects vary depending upon dosage form. Incidence usually on lower end with enema and suppository dosage forms.

>10%:

Central nervous system: Headache (2% to 35%), pain (≤14%)

Gastrointestinal: Abdominal pain (1% to 18%), eructation (16%), nausea (3% to 13%)

Respiratory: Pharyngitis (11%)

1% to 10%:

Cardiovascular: Chest pain (3%), peripheral edema (3%), vasodilation (≥2%), hypertension (1%)

Central nervous system: Dizziness (2% to 8%), chills (3%), malaise (2% to 3%), fatigue (<3%), vertigo (<3%), anxiety (≥2%), migraine (≥2%), nervousness (≥2%), paresthesia (≥2%), insomnia (2%)

Dermatologic: Skin rash (1% to 6%), diaphoresis (3%), pruritus (1% to 3%), alopecia (<3%), acne vulgaris (1% to 2%)

Endocrine & metabolic: Increased serum triglycerides (<3%)

Gastrointestinal: Diarrhea (2% to 8%), dyspepsia (1% to 6%), flatulence (1% to 6%), constipation (5%), vomiting (1% to 5%), intolerance syndrome (3%), exacerbation of ulcerative colitis (1% to 3%), rectal hemorrhage (<3%), gastroenteritis (≥2%), gastrointestinal hemorrhage (≥2%), abnormal stools (≥2%), tenesmus (≥2%), rectal pain (1% to 2%), anorectal pain (on insertion of enema tip; 1%), hemorrhoids (1%), abdominal distention (≥1%)

Genitourinary: Polyuria (≥2%)

Hematologic & oncologic: Hematocrit/hemoglobin decreased (<3%)

Hepatic: Cholestatic hepatitis (<3%), increased serum transaminases (<3%), abnormal hepatic function tests (2%), increased serum ALT (1%)

Infection: Infection (≥2%)

Neuromuscular & skeletal: Back pain (1% to 7%), hypertonia (5%), arthralgia (≤5%), myalgia (3%), weakness (≥2%), arthritis (2%), musculoskeletal pain (leg/joint; 2%)

Ophthalmic: Visual disturbance (≥2%), conjunctivitis (2%)

Otic: Tinnitus (<3%), otalgia (≥2%)

Renal: Decreased creatinine clearance (<3%), hematuria (<3%)

Respiratory: Flu-like symptoms (1% to 5%), nasopharyngitis (1% to 4%), dyspnea (<3%), bronchitis (≥2%), sinusitis (≥2%), cough (≤2%)

Miscellaneous: Fever (1% to 6%)

Available Dosage Forms

Capsule Delayed Release, Oral:
Delzicol: 400 mg

Capsule Extended Release, Oral:
Pentasa: 250 mg, 500 mg

Capsule Extended Release 24 Hour, Oral:
Apriso: 0.375 g

Enema, Rectal:
SfRowasa: 4 g/60 mL (60 mL)
Generic: 4 g (60 mL)

Kit, Rectal:
Rowasa: 4 g
Generic: 4 g

Suppository, Rectal:
Canasa: 1000 mg (30 ea, 42 ea)

Tablet Delayed Release, Oral:
Asacol HD: 800 mg
Lialda: 1.2 g

General Dosage Range

Oral: *Adults:*

Capsule: Apriso: 1.5 g once daily; Delzicol: 800 mg 3 times daily or 1.6 g daily in 4 divided doses; Pentasa: 1 g 4 times daily

Tablet: Asacol HD: 1.6 g 3 times daily; Lialda: 2.4-4.8 g once daily

Rectal: *Adults:* Retention enema: 60 mL (4 g) at bedtime, retained overnight (~8 hours); Suppository: Insert 1000 mg at bedtime

Administration

Oral

Capsules:

Apriso: Administer with or without food; do not administer with antacids. The capsule should be swallowed whole per the manufacturer's labeling; however, opening the capsule and placing the contents (delayed release granules) on food with a pH <6 is not expected to affect the release of mesalamine once ingested (data on file, Salix Pharmaceuticals Medical Information). There is no safety/efficacy information regarding this practice. The contents of the capsules should not be chewed or crushed.

Delzicol: Administer 1 hour before or 2 hours after a meal. The capsule should be swallowed whole per the manufacturer's labeling; do not break, chew, or crush.

Pentasa: Administer with or without food. Although the manufacturer recommends swallowing the capsule whole, if a patient is unable to swallow the capsule, some clinicians support opening the capsules and placing the contents (controlled-release beads) on yogurt or peanut butter (Crohn's & Colitis Foundation of America). There are currently no published data evaluating the safety/efficacy of this practice. The contents of the capsules should not be chewed or crushed.

Tablets: Swallow whole; do not break, chew, or crush.

Asacol [Canadian product]: Do not break outer coating; administer with or without food.

Asacol HD, Asacol 800 [Canadian product]: Do not break outer coating; administer with or without food.

Lialda: Do not break outer coating; should be administered once daily with a meal

Mesasal [Canadian product]: Administer before meals.

Mezavant [Canadian product]: Do not break outer coating; should be administered once daily with a meal.

Pentasa [Canadian product]: Administer with meals.

Rectal

Rectal enema: Shake bottle well. Retain enemas for 8 hours or as long as practical.

Suppository: Remove foil wrapper; avoid excessive handling. Should be retained for at least 1-3 hours to achieve maximum benefit.

Storage/Stability

Capsule:

Apriso: Store at controlled room temperature of 20°C to 25°C (68°F to 77°F)

Delzicol: Store at controlled room temperature of 20°C to 25°C (68°F to 77°F); excursions permitted between 15°C and 30°C (59°F and 86°F).

Pentasa: Store at controlled room temperature of 15°C to 30°C (59°F to 86°F). Protect from light.

Enema: Store at controlled room temperature. Use promptly once foil wrap is removed. Contents may darken with time (do not use if dark brown).

Suppository: Store below 25°C (below 77°F). May store under refrigeration; do not freeze. Protect from direct heat, light, and humidity.

Tablet: Store at controlled room temperature:

Asacol HD: 20°C to 25°C (68°F to 77°F); excursions permitted between 15°C and 30°C (59°F and 86°F).

Asacol, Asacol 800 [Canadian products]: 15°C to 30°C (59°F to 86°F)

Lialda: 15°C to 30°C (59°F to 86°F)

Mezavant [Canadian product]: 15°C to 25°C (59°F to 77°F)

Nursing Actions

Physical Assessment Patient allergy history to salicylates should be assessed prior to beginning therapy. Monitor laboratory tests, therapeutic effectiveness, and adverse reactions (chest pain, CNS effects, gastrointestinal upset, exacerbation of colitis) on a regular basis throughout therapy. Teach patient proper use (according to formulation), possible side effects/appropriate interventions (eg, importance of adequate hydration), and adverse symptoms to report.

Patient Education

• Discuss specific use of drug and side effects with patient as it relates to treatment. (HCAHPS: During this hospital stay, were you given any medicine that you had not taken before? Before giving you any new medicine, how often did hospital staff tell you what the medicine was for? How often did hospital staff describe possible side effects in a way you could understand?)

• Patient may experience dyspepsia, nausea, constipation, headache, or pharyngitis. Have patient report immediately to prescriber dyspnea, angina, tablet shells in stool, or rash (HCAHPS).

• Educate patient about signs of a significant reaction (eg, wheezing; chest tightness; fever; itching; bad cough; blue skin color; seizures; or swelling of face, lips, tongue, or throat). **Note:** This is not a comprehensive list of all side effects. Patient should consult prescriber for additional questions.

Intended Use and Disclaimer: Should not be printed and given to patients. This information is intended to serve as a concise initial reference for healthcare professionals to use when discussing medications with a patient. You must ultimately rely on your own discretion, experience and judgment in diagnosing, treating and advising patients.

Dietary Considerations Some products may contain phenylalanine.

Apriso: Do not administer with antacids.

Canasa rectal suppository contains saturated vegetable fatty acid esters.

Related Information

Oral Medications That Should Not Be Crushed or Altered *on page 1712*

Mesna (MES na)

Brand Names: U.S. Mesnex

Index Terms Mercaptoethane Sulfonate; Sodium 2-Mercaptoethane Sulfonate

Pharmacologic Category Antidote; Chemoprotective Agent

Pregnancy Risk Factor B

Lactation Excretion in breast milk unknown/not recommended

Use Preventative agent to reduce the incidence of ifosfamide-induced hemorrhagic cystitis

Unlabeled Use Preventative agent to reduce the incidence of cyclophosphamide-induced hemorrhagic cystitis with high-dose cyclophosphamide

Available Dosage Forms
Solution, Intravenous:
Mesnex: 100 mg/mL (10 mL)
Generic: 100 mg/mL (10 mL)
Tablet, Oral:
Mesnex: 400 mg

General Dosage Range
I.V.: *Children and Adults:* 60% of the ifosfamide dose given in 3 divided doses
I.V., Oral: *Children and Adults:* 100% of the ifosfamide dose, given as 20% I.V., followed by 2 (40% each) doses orally

Administration
I.V. Administer by short (15-30 minutes) infusion or continuous infusion (maintain continuous infusion for 12-24 after completion of ifosfamide infusion) (Hensley, 2008)
Injectable Detail pH: 6.5-8.5
Oral Administer orally in tablet formulation or parenteral solution diluted in water, milk, juice, or carbonated beverages; patients who vomit within 2 hours after taking oral mesna should repeat the dose or receive I.V. mesna

Nursing Actions
Physical Assessment Assess frequently for hematuria/bladder hemorrhage. Hypersensitive reactions have been reported, ranging from mild hypersensitivity to systemic anaphylactic reactions. Monitor closely.

Patient Education
- Discuss specific use of drug and side effects with patient as it relates to treatment. (HCAHPS: During this hospital stay, were you given any medicine that you had not taken before? Before giving you any new medicine, how often did hospital staff tell you what the medicine was for? How often did hospital staff describe possible side effects in a way you could understand?)
- Patient may experience parageusia, diarrhea, nausea, dyspepsia, or injection site irritation. Have patient report immediately to prescriber hematuria, urinary retention, ecchymosis, bleeding, severe dizziness, or rash (HCAHPS).
- Educate patient about signs of a significant reaction (eg, wheezing; chest tightness; fever; itching; bad cough; blue skin color; seizures; or swelling of face, lips, tongue, or throat). **Note:** This is not a comprehensive list of all side effects. Patient should consult prescriber for additional questions.

Intended Use and Disclaimer: Should not be printed and given to patients. This information is intended to serve as a concise initial reference for healthcare professionals to use when discussing medications with a patient. You must ultimately rely on your own discretion, experience and judgment in diagnosing, treating and advising patients.

Metaxalone (me TAKS a lone)

Brand Names: U.S. Skelaxin
Pharmacologic Category Skeletal Muscle Relaxant
Medication Safety Issues
Sound-alike/look-alike issues:
Metaxalone may be confused with mesalamine, metolazone
Skelaxin® may be confused with Robaxin®
BEERS Criteria medication:
This drug may be potentially inappropriate for use in geriatric patients (Quality of evidence - moderate; Strength of recommendation - strong).
Lactation Excretion in breast milk unknown/not recommended
Breast-Feeding Considerations It is not known if metaxalone is excreted in breast milk. Breast-feeding is not recommended by the manufacturer.
Use Relief of discomfort associated with acute, painful musculoskeletal conditions
Mechanism of Action/Effect Precise mechanism has not been established; however, efficacy appears to result from disruption of the spasm-pain-spasm cycle, probably by a general CNS depressant mechanism. Does not have a direct effect on skeletal muscle.
Contraindications Hypersensitivity to metaxalone or any component of the formulation; significantly impaired hepatic or renal function, history of drug-induced hemolytic anemias or other anemias
Warnings/Precautions May cause CNS depression. CNS depressant effects may be augmented when used in conjunction with other depressants (eg, barbiturates, ethanol), when taken with food, or in the elderly. May impair mental and/or physical ability to perform hazardous tasks such as operating machinery or driving a motor vehicle. Use with caution in patients with impaired renal or hepatic function (contraindicated if significant impairment); routine monitoring of transaminases is recommended. An increase in bioavailability and half-life have been observed in female patients. Muscle relaxants are poorly tolerated by the elderly due to potent anticholinergic effects, sedation, and risk of fracture. Efficacy is questionable at dosages tolerated by elderly patients; avoid use (Beers Criteria). Safety and efficacy have not been established in children ≤12 years of age.
Drug Interactions
Avoid Concomitant Use
Avoid concomitant use of Metaxalone with any of the following: Azelastine (Nasal); Paraldehyde; Thalidomide
Decreased Effect
The levels/effects of Metaxalone may be decreased by: Peginterferon Alfa-2b
Increased Effect/Toxicity
Metaxalone may increase the levels/effects of: Alcohol (Ethyl); Azelastine (Nasal); ▶

Buprenorphine; CNS Depressants; Hydrocodone; Methotrimeprazine; Metyrosine; Mirtazapine; Paraldehyde; Pramipexole; ROPINIRole; Rotigotine; Selective Serotonin Reuptake Inhibitors; Thalidomide; Zolpidem

The levels/effects of Metaxalone may be increased by: Brimonidine (Topical); Doxylamine; Droperidol; HydrOXYzine; Magnesium Sulfate; Methotrimeprazine; Perampanel; Sodium Oxybate; Tapentadol

Nutritional/Ethanol Interactions

Ethanol: May increase CNS depression; monitor for increased effects with coadministration. Caution patients about effects.

Food: Bioavailability may be increased (may increase CNS depression).

Herb/Nutraceutical: Avoid valerian, St John's wort, kava kava, gotu kola (may increase CNS depression).

Adverse Reactions Frequency not defined.

Central nervous system: Dizziness, drowsiness, headache, irritability, nervousness

Dermatologic: Rash (with or without pruritus)

Gastrointestinal: Gastrointestinal upset, nausea, vomiting

Hematologic: Hemolytic anemia, leukopenia

Hepatic: Jaundice

Miscellaneous: Hypersensitivity (including rare anaphylactoid reactions)

Pharmacodynamics/Kinetics

Onset of Action ~1 hour

Duration of Action ~4-6 hours

Available Dosage Forms

Tablet, Oral:

Skelaxin: 800 mg

Generic: 800 mg

General Dosage Range Oral: *Children >12 years and Adults:* 800 mg 3-4 times/day

Administration

Oral May be administered with or without food. However, serum concentrations may be increased when administered with food; clinical significance has not been established. Patients should be monitored.

Storage/Stability Store at controlled room temperature of 15°C to 30°C (59°F to 86°F).

Nursing Actions

Patient Education

• Discuss specific use of drug and side effects with patient as it relates to treatment. (HCAHPS: During this hospital stay, were you given any medicine that you had not taken before? Before giving you any new medicine, how often did hospital staff tell you what the medicine was for? How often did hospital staff describe possible side effects in a way you could understand?)

• Patient may experience presyncope, fatigue, blurred vision, illogical thinking, dizziness, or nausea. Have patient report immediately to prescriber rash (HCAHPS).

• Educate patient about signs of a significant reaction (eg, wheezing; chest tightness; fever; itching; bad cough; blue skin color; seizures; or swelling of face, lips, tongue, or throat). **Note:** This is not a comprehensive list of all side effects. Patient should consult prescriber for additional questions.

Intended Use and Disclaimer: Should not be printed and given to patients. This information is intended to serve as a concise initial reference for healthcare professionals to use when discussing medications with a patient. You must ultimately rely on your own discretion, experience and judgment in diagnosing, treating and advising patients.

Dietary Considerations Administration with food may increase serum concentrations.

MetFORMIN (met FOR min)

Brand Names: U.S. Fortamet; Glucophage; Glucophage XR; Glumetza; Riomet

Index Terms Metformin Hydrochloride

Pharmacologic Category Antidiabetic Agent, Biguanide

Medication Safety Issues

Sound-alike/look-alike issues:

MetFORMIN may be confused with metroNIDAZOLE

Glucophage® may be confused with Glucotrol®, Glutofac®

High alert medication:

The Institute for Safe Medication Practices (ISMP) includes this medication among its list of drug classes which have a heightened risk of causing significant patient harm when used in error.

International issues:

Dianben [Spain] may be confused with Diovan brand name for valsartan [U.S., Canada, and multiple international markets]

Pregnancy Risk Factor B

Lactation Enters breast milk/not recommended

Breast-Feeding Considerations Low amounts of metformin (generally ≤1% of the weight-adjusted maternal dose) are excreted into breast milk. Because breast milk concentrations of metformin stay relatively constant, avoiding nursing around peak plasma concentrations in the mother would not be helpful in reducing metformin exposure to the infant (Briggs, 2005; Eyal, 2010; Gardiner, 2003; Hale, 2002). Growth and development were not affected in infants born to mothers with PCOS and who took metformin while breast-feeding (Glueck, 2006).

Breast-feeding is encouraged for all women, including those with diabetes; however, the safety of metformin during breast-feeding has not yet been established (Metzger, 2007). According to the manufacturer, due to the potential for hypoglycemia in the nursing infant, a decision should be made whether to discontinue nursing or to discontinue the drug, taking into account the importance of treatment to the mother.

Use Management of type 2 diabetes mellitus (non-insulin dependent, NIDDM) when hyperglycemia cannot be managed with diet and exercise alone.

Note: If not contraindicated and if tolerated, metformin is the preferred initial pharmacologic agent for type 2 diabetes management (ADA, 2013).

Unlabeled Use Gestational diabetes mellitus (GDM); polycystic ovary syndrome (PCOS); prevention of type 2 diabetes mellitus

Mechanism of Action/Effect Decreases hepatic glucose production, decreasing intestinal absorption of glucose and improves insulin sensitivity (increases peripheral glucose uptake and utilization)

Contraindications Note: Temporarily discontinue in patients undergoing radiologic studies in which intravascular iodinated contrast media are utilized.

U.S. labeling: Hypersensitivity to metformin or any component of the formulation; renal disease or renal dysfunction (serum creatinine ≥1.5 mg/dL in males or ≥1.4 mg/dL in females) or abnormal creatinine clearance from any cause, including shock, acute myocardial infarction, or septicemia; acute or chronic metabolic acidosis with or without coma (including diabetic ketoacidosis)

Canadian labeling: Hypersensitivity to metformin or any component of the formulation; renal function unknown, renal impairment, and serum creatinine levels above the upper limit of normal range; renal disease or renal dysfunction (serum creatinine ≥136 micromol/L in males or ≥124 micromol/L in females or abnormal creatinine clearance <60 mL/minute) which may result from conditions such as cardiovascular collapse (shock), acute myocardial infarction, and septicemia; unstable and/or insulin-dependent (Type I) diabetes mellitus; history of ketoacidosis with or without coma; history of lactic acidosis (regardless of precipitating factors); excessive alcohol intake (acute or chronic); severe hepatic dysfunction or clinical or laboratory evidence of hepatic disease; cardiovascular collapse and disease states associated with hypoxemia including cardiorespiratory insufficiency, which are often associated with hyperlactacidemia; stress conditions (eg, severe infection, trauma, surgery and postoperative recovery phase); severe dehydration; pregnancy; breast-feeding

Warnings/Precautions [U.S. Boxed Warning]: Lactic acidosis is a rare, but potentially severe consequence of therapy with metformin that requires urgent care and hospitalization. The risk is increased in patients with acute congestive heart failure, dehydration, excessive alcohol intake, hepatic or renal impairment, or sepsis. Symptoms may be nonspecific (eg, abdominal distress, malaise, myalgia, respiratory distress, somnolence); low pH, increased anion gap and elevated blood lactate may be observed. Discontinue immediately if acidosis is suspected. Lactic acidosis should be suspected in any patient with diabetes receiving metformin with evidence of acidosis but without evidence of ketoacidosis. Discontinue metformin in patients with conditions associated with dehydration, sepsis, or hypoxemia. The risk of accumulation and lactic acidosis increases with the degree of impairment of renal function. Use caution in patients with congestive heart failure requiring pharmacologic management, particularly in patients with unstable or acute CHF; risk of lactic acidosis may be increased secondary to hypoperfusion.

Metformin is substantially excreted by the kidney. The risk of accumulation and lactic acidosis increases with the degree of impairment of renal function. Patients with renal function below the limit of normal for their age should not receive metformin. Metformin should be withheld in patients with prerenal azotemia. In elderly patients, renal function should be monitored regularly; should not be initiated in patients ≥80 years of age unless normal renal function is confirmed. Use of concomitant medications that may affect renal function (ie, affect tubular secretion) may also affect metformin disposition. Therapy should be suspended for any surgical procedures (Canadian labeling recommends discontinuing use 48 hours prior to surgical procedures excluding minor procedures not associated with restricted food and fluid intake). Restart only after normal oral intake resumed and normal renal function is verified. Therapy should be temporarily discontinued prior to or at the time of intravascular administration of iodinated contrast media (potential for acute alteration in renal function). Metformin should be withheld for 48 hours after the radiologic study and restarted only after renal function has been confirmed as normal. It may be necessary to discontinue metformin and administer insulin if the patient is exposed to stress (fever, trauma, infection, surgery).

Avoid use in patients with impaired liver function. Patient must be instructed to avoid excessive acute or chronic ethanol use; ethanol may potentiate metformin's effect on lactate metabolism. Administration of oral antidiabetic drugs has been reported to be associated with increased cardiovascular mortality; metformin does not appear to share this risk. Insoluble tablet shell of Glumetza® 1000 mg extended release tablet may remain intact and be visible in the stool. Other extended released tablets (Fortamet®, Glucophage® XR, Glumetza® 500 mg) may appear in the stool as a soft mass resembling the tablet.

Drug Interactions

Avoid Concomitant Use There are no known interactions where it is recommended to avoid concomitant use.

Decreased Effect

MetFORMIN may decrease the levels/effects of: Trospium

The levels/effects of MetFORMIN may be decreased by: Corticosteroids (Orally Inhaled); Corticosteroids (Systemic); Luteinizing Hormone-Releasing Hormone Analogs; Somatropin; Thiazide Diuretics

Increased Effect/Toxicity

MetFORMIN may increase the levels/effects of: Dalfampridine; Dofetilide

The levels/effects of MetFORMIN may be increased by: Carbonic Anhydrase Inhibitors; Cephalexin; Cimetidine; Dalfampridine; Dolutegravir; Glycopyrrolate; Iodinated Contrast Agents; LamoTRIgine; Pegvisomant; Ranolazine; Topiramate; Trimethoprim

Nutritional/Ethanol Interactions

Ethanol: Avoid or limit ethanol (incidence of lactic acidosis may be increased; may cause hypoglycemia).

Food: Food decreases the extent and slightly delays the absorption. May decrease absorption of vitamin B_{12} and/or folic acid.

Herb/Nutraceutical: Caution with chromium, garlic, gymnema (may cause hypoglycemia).

Adverse Reactions

>10%:

Gastrointestinal: Diarrhea (IR tablet: 12% to 53%; ER tablet: 10% to 17%), nausea/vomiting (IR tablet: 7% to 26%; ER tablet: 7% to 9%), flatulence (12%)

Neuromuscular & skeletal: Weakness (9%)

1% to 10%:

Cardiovascular: Chest discomfort, flushing, palpitation

Central nervous system: Headache (6%), chills, dizziness, lightheadedness

Dermatologic: Rash

Endocrine & metabolic: Hypoglycemia

Gastrointestinal: Indigestion (7%), abdominal discomfort (6%), abdominal distention, abnormal stools, constipation, dyspepsia/ heartburn, taste disorder

Neuromuscular & skeletal: Myalgia

Respiratory: Dyspnea, upper respiratory tract infection

Miscellaneous: Decreased vitamin B_{12} levels (7%), increased diaphoresis, flu-like syndrome, nail disorder

Pharmacodynamics/Kinetics

Onset of Action Within days; maximum effects up to 2 weeks

Available Dosage Forms

Solution, Oral:

Riomet: 500 mg/5 mL (118 mL, 473 mL)

Tablet, Oral:

Glucophage: 500 mg, 850 mg, 1000 mg

Generic: 500 mg, 850 mg, 1000 mg

Tablet Extended Release 24 Hour, Oral:

Fortamet: 500 mg, 1000 mg

Glucophage XR: 500 mg, 750 mg

Glumetza: 500 mg, 1000 mg

Generic: 500 mg, 750 mg, 1000 mg

General Dosage Range Oral:

Extended release: *Adults:* Initial: 500 mg once daily; Maintenance: Up to 2000-2500 mg/day (varies by product) in 1-2 divided doses

Immediate release:

Children 10-16 years: Initial: 500 mg twice daily; Maintenance: Up to 2000 mg/day in divided doses

Children >16 years and Adults: Initial: 500 mg twice daily **or** 850 mg once daily; Maintenance: Up to 2000 mg daily in divided doses **or** 2550 mg daily in 3 divided doses

Administration

Oral Administer with a meal (to decrease GI upset).

Extended release: Swallow whole; do not crush, break, or chew. Administer once daily doses with the evening meal. Fortamet® should also be administered with a full glass of water.

Storage/Stability

Oral solution: Store at 15°C to 30°C (59°F to 86°F).

Tablets: Store at 20°C to 25°C (68°F to 77°F); excursion permitted to 15°C to 30°C (59°F to 86°F). Protect from light and moisture.

Nursing Actions

Physical Assessment Monitor for signs and symptoms of vitamin B_{12} and/or folic acid deficiency during therapy; supplementation may be required. Refer patient to diabetes educator for instruction if needed.

Patient Education

• Discuss specific use of drug and side effects with patient as it relates to treatment. (HCAHPS: During this hospital stay, were you given any medicine that you had not taken before? Before giving you any new medicine, how often did hospital staff tell you what the medicine was for? How often did hospital staff describe possible side effects in a way you could understand?)

• Patient may experience hypoglycemia, dyspepsia, nausea, diarrhea, lack of appetite, xerostomia, or signs of lactic acidosis. Have patient report immediately to prescriber hyperglycemia, severe dizziness, dyspnea, cold intolerance, significant weight loss, severe asthenia, or rash (HCAHPS).

• Educate patient about signs of a significant reaction (eg, wheezing; chest tightness; fever; itching; bad cough; blue skin color; seizures; or swelling of face, lips, tongue, or throat). **Note:** This is not a comprehensive list of all side effects. Patient should consult prescriber for additional questions.

Intended Use and Disclaimer: Should not be printed and given to patients. This information is intended to serve as a concise initial reference for healthcare professionals to use when discussing medications with a patient. You must ultimately rely on your own discretion, experience and judgment in diagnosing, treating and advising patients.

Dietary Considerations Drug may cause GI upset; take with food (to decrease GI upset). Take at the same time(s) each day. Dietary modification based on ADA recommendations is a part of therapy. Monitor for signs and symptoms of vitamin B_{12} and/or folic acid deficiency; supplementation may be required.

Related Information

Oral Medications That Should Not Be Crushed or Altered *on page 1712*

Methadone (METH a done)

Brand Names: U.S. Dolophine; Methadone HCl Intensol; Methadose; Methadose Sugar-Free

Index Terms Methadone Hydrochloride

Pharmacologic Category Analgesic, Opioid

Medication Safety Issues

Sound-alike/look-alike issues:

Methadone may be confused with dexmethylphenidate, Mephyton®, methylphenidate, Metadate CD®, Metadate® ER, metolazone, morphine

High alert medication:

The Institute for Safe Medication Practices (ISMP) includes this medication among its list of drug classes which have a heightened risk of causing significant patient harm when used in error.

Medication Guide Available Yes

Pregnancy Risk Factor C

Lactation Enters breast milk

Breast-Feeding Considerations Methadone is excreted into breast milk; the dose to a nursing infant has been calculated to be 2% to 3% of the maternal dose (following oral doses of 10-80 mg/day). Peak methadone levels appear in breast milk 4-5 hours after an oral dose. Methadone has been detected in the plasma of some breast-fed infants whose mothers are taking methadone. Sedation and respiratory depression have been reported in nursing infants. The manufacturer recommends that women monitor their nursing infants for sedation and that they should be instructed as to when to contact their healthcare provider for emergency care. In addition, the manufacturer recommends slowly weaning to prevent withdrawal symptoms in the nursing infant.

When methadone is used to treat opioid addiction in nursing women, guidelines do not contraindicate breast-feeding as long as the infant is tolerant to the dose and other contraindications do not exist (ACOG, 2012). If additional illicit substances are being abused, women treated with methadone should pump and discard breast milk until sobriety is established (ACOG, 2012; Dow, 2012).

Use Management of moderate-to-severe pain when a continuous, around-the-clock opioid analgesic is needed for an extended period of time; detoxification and maintenance treatment of opioid addiction through a certified program

Mechanism of Action/Effect Binds to opiate receptors in the CNS, causing inhibition of ascending pain pathways, altering the perception of and response to pain; produces generalized CNS depression. Methadone has also been shown to have weak N-methyl-D-aspartate (NMDA) receptor antagonism (Callahan, 2004).

Contraindications

Hypersensitivity to methadone or any component of the formulation; significant respiratory depression (in the absence of resuscitative equipment or in an unmonitored setting); acute or severe bronchial asthma (in the absence of resuscitative equipment or in an unmonitored setting) or hypercarbia; known or suspected paralytic ileus; concurrent use of selegiline (Ensam® product labeling)

Methadone is not to be used on an as-needed basis; it is not for pain that is mild or not expected to persist; it is not for acute pain or postoperative pain.

Canadian labeling: Additional contraindications (not in U.S. labeling): Diarrhea associated with pseudomembranous colitis or caused by poisoning until toxic material has been eliminated from the gastrointestinal tract

Warnings/Precautions The optimal analgesic dose varies widely among patients. Doses should be titrated to pain relief/prevention. Patients maintained on stable doses of methadone may need rescue doses of a immediate release analgesic in case of acute pain (eg, postoperative pain, physical trauma). Methadone is ineffective for the relief of anxiety.

[U.S. Boxed Warning]: QT_c interval prolongation and serious arrhythmias (eg, torsade de pointes) have occurred during treatment. Patients should be informed of the potential arrhythmia risk, evaluated for any history of structural heart disease, arrhythmia, syncope, and for existence of potential drug interactions including drugs that possess QT_c interval-prolonging properties, promote hypokalemia, hypomagnesemia, or hypocalcemia, or reduce elimination of methadone (eg, CYP3A4 inhibitors). Obtain baseline ECG for all patients and risk stratify according to QT_c interval; QT_c interval prolongation and torsade de pointes may be associated with doses >200 mg/day, but have also been observed with lower doses. Potentially significant drug-drug interactions may exist, requiring dose or frequency adjustment, additional monitoring, and/or selection of alternative therapy. May cause severe hypotension; use caution with severe volume depletion or other conditions which may compromise maintenance of normal blood pressure. Use caution with cardiovascular disease or patients predisposed to dysrhythmias.

[U.S. Boxed Warning]: Fatal respiratory depression may occur with the highest risk at initiation and with dose increases. Use caution in patients with respiratory disease or pre-existing respiratory conditions (eg, severe obesity, asthma, COPD, sleep apnea, CNS depression) and kyphoscoliosis or other skeletal disorder which may alter respiratory function. Because the respiratory effects last longer than the analgesic effects, slow titration is required. Use extreme caution during treatment initiation, dose titration and conversion from other opioid agonists. Incomplete cross tolerance may occur; patients tolerant to other mu opioid agonists may not be tolerant to methadone. Abrupt cessation may precipitate withdrawal symptoms. Gradually taper dose.

After chronic maternal exposure to opioids, neonatal withdrawal syndrome may occur in the newborn; monitor neonate closely. Signs and symptoms include irritability, hyperactivity and abnormal sleep pattern, high pitched cry, tremor, vomiting, diarrhea and failure to gain weight. Onset, duration and severity depend on the drug used, duration of use, maternal dose, and rate of drug elimination by the newborn. Opioid withdrawal syndrome in the neonate, unlike in adults, may be life-threatening and should be treated according to protocols developed by neonatology experts.

May cause CNS depression, which may impair physical or mental abilities. Patients must be cautioned about performing tasks which require mental alertness (eg, operating machinery or driving). Effects with other sedative drugs or ethanol may be potentiated. Use with caution in patients with depression or suicidal tendencies, or in patients with a history of drug or ethanol abuse. Tolerance or psychological and physical dependence may occur with prolonged use. **[U.S. Boxed Warning]: Monitor for signs of misuse, abuse and addiction during therapy.**

Avoid use of methadone in patients with CNS depression or coma as these patients are susceptible to intracranial effects of CO_2 retention. Use with caution in patients with head injury or increased intracranial pressure; reduced respiratory drive and resultant CO_2 retention may increase intracranial pressure. May obscure diagnosis or clinical course of patients with acute abdominal conditions. Avoid use in gastrointestinal obstruction.

Elderly may be more susceptible to adverse effects (eg, CNS, respiratory, gastrointestinal). Decrease initial dose and use caution in the elderly or debilitated; with hyper/hypothyroidism, morbid obesity, adrenal insufficiency, prostatic hyperplasia, or urethral stricture; or with severe renal or hepatic failure. Use with caution in patients with biliary tract dysfunction including acute pancreatitis; may cause constriction of sphincter of Oddi. **[U.S. Boxed Warning]: For oral administration only;** excipients to deter use by injection are contained in tablets.

[U.S. Boxed Warning]: When used for treatment of opioid addiction: May only be dispensed by certified opioid treatment programs. Exceptions include inpatient treatment of other conditions and emergency period (not >3 days) while definitive substance abuse treatment is being sought. **[U.S. Boxed Warning]: Accidental ingestion can result in fatal overdose, especially in children. [U.S. Boxed Warning]: Should only be prescribed by healthcare professionals who are knowledgeable in the use of potent opioids for chronic pain management.**

Drug Interactions

Avoid Concomitant Use

Avoid concomitant use of Methadone with any of the following: Alcohol (Ethyl); Azelastine (Nasal); Conivaptan; Fusidic Acid (Systemic); Highest Risk QTc-Prolonging Agents; Itraconazole; Ivabradine; Lopinavir; Mifepristone; Paraldehyde; Posaconazole; Thalidomide; Thioridazine

Decreased Effect

Methadone may decrease the levels/effects of: Codeine; Didanosine; Fosamprenavir; Lubiprostone; Pegvisomant; Tamoxifen; TraMADol

The levels/effects of Methadone may be decreased by: Ammonium Chloride; Boceprevir; Bosentan; CarBAMazepine; CYP3A4 Inducers (Strong); Dabrafenib; Darunavir; Deferasirox; Etravirine; Fosamprenavir; Fosphenytoin; Herbs (CYP3A4 Inducers); Lopinavir; Mitotane; Mixed Agonist / Antagonist Opioids; Nelfinavir; PHENobarbital; Phenytoin; Primidone; Reverse Transcriptase Inhibitors (Non-Nucleoside); Rifamycin Derivatives; Ritonavir; Saquinavir; Telaprevir; Tipranavir; Tocilizumab

Increased Effect/Toxicity

Methadone may increase the levels/effects of: Alvimopan; Azelastine (Nasal); CNS Depressants; CYP2D6 Substrates; Desmopressin; Diuretics; DOXOrubicin (Conventional); Fesoterodine; Highest Risk QTc-Prolonging Agents; Hydrocodone; Lomitapide; Lopinavir; Metoprolol; Metyrosine; Mirtazapine; Moderate Risk QTc-Prolonging Agents; Nebivolol; Paraldehyde; Pramipexole; ROPINIRole; Rotigotine; Saquinavir; Selective Serotonin Reuptake Inhibitors; Thalidomide; Thioridazine; Zidovudine; Zolpidem

The levels/effects of Methadone may be increased by: Alcohol (Ethyl); Amphetamines;

Anticholinergics; Antipsychotic Agents (Phenothiazines); Aromatase Inhibitors; Boceprevir; Brimonidine (Topical); Cannabinoids; Conivaptan; CYP2B6 Inhibitors (Moderate); CYP2B6 Inhibitors (Strong); CYP3A4 Inhibitors (Moderate); CYP3A4 Inhibitors (Strong); Dasatinib; Doxylamine; Fluconazole; Fusidic Acid (Systemic); HydrOXYzine; Interferons (Alfa); Itraconazole; Ivabradine; Ivacaftor; Ketoconazole (Systemic); Luliconazole; Magnesium Sulfate; MAO Inhibitors; Mifepristone; Perampanel; Posaconazole; QTc-Prolonging Agents (Indeterminate Risk and Risk Modifying); Quazepam; Selective Serotonin Reuptake Inhibitors; Simeprevir; Sodium Oxybate; Stiripentol; Succinylcholine; Tapentadol; Voriconazole

Nutritional/Ethanol Interactions

Ethanol: Ethanol may increase CNS depression. Management: Avoid ethanol.

Food: Grapefruit/grapefruit juice may increase levels of methadone. Management: Avoid concurrent use of grapefruit juice.

Herb/Nutraceutical: St John's wort may decrease methadone levels and increase CNS depression; valerian, kava kava, and gotu kola may increase CNS depression. Management: Avoid St John's wort, valerian, kava kava, and gotu kola.

Adverse Reactions Frequency not defined. During prolonged administration, adverse effects may decrease over several weeks; however, constipation and sweating may persist.

Cardiovascular: Arrhythmia, bigeminal rhythms, bradycardia, cardiac arrest, cardiomyopathy, ECG changes, edema, extrasystoles, faintness, flushing, heart failure, hypotension, palpitation, peripheral vasodilation, phlebitis, orthostatic hypotension, QT interval prolonged, shock, syncope, tachycardia, torsade de pointes, T-wave inversion, ventricular fibrillation, ventricular tachycardia

Central nervous system: Agitation, confusion, disorientation, dizziness, drowsiness, dysphoria, euphoria, hallucination, headache, insomnia, lightheadedness, sedation, seizure

Dermatologic: Hemorrhagic urticaria, pruritus, rash, urticaria

Endocrine & metabolic: Antidiuretic effect, amenorrhea, hypokalemia, hypomagnesemia, libido decreased

Gastrointestinal: Abdominal pain, anorexia, biliary tract spasm, constipation, glossitis, nausea, stomach cramps, vomiting, weight gain, xerostomia

Genitourinary: Impotence, urinary retention or hesitancy

Hematologic: Thrombocytopenia (reversible, reported in patients with chronic hepatitis)

Neuromuscular & skeletal: Weakness

Local: I.M./SubQ injection: Erythema, pain, swelling; I.V. injection: Hemorrhagic urticaria (rare), pruritus, urticaria, rash

Ocular: Miosis, visual disturbances

Respiratory: Pulmonary edema, respiratory depression, respiratory arrest

Miscellaneous: Death, diaphoresis, physical and psychological dependence

Pharmacodynamics/Kinetics

Onset of Action Oral: Analgesic: 0.5-1 hour; Parenteral: 10-20 minutes; Peak effect: Parenteral: 1-2 hours; Oral: Continuous dosing: 3-5 days

Duration of Action Analgesia: Oral: 4-8 hours (single-dose studies), increases to 22-48 hours with repeated doses; slow release from the liver and other tissues may prolong duration of action

Controlled Substance C-II

Available Dosage Forms

Concentrate, Oral:
Methadone HCl Intensol: 10 mg/mL (30 mL)
Methadose: 10 mg/mL (1000 mL)
Methadose Sugar-Free: 10 mg/mL (1000 mL)
Generic: 10 mg/mL (30 mL, 1000 mL)

Solution, Injection:
Generic: 10 mg/mL (20 mL)

Solution, Oral:
Generic: 5 mg/5 mL (500 mL); 10 mg/5 mL (500 mL)

Tablet, Oral:
Dolophine: 5 mg, 10 mg
Methadose: 10 mg
Generic: 5 mg, 10 mg

Tablet Soluble, Oral:
Methadose: 40 mg
Generic: 40 mg

General Dosage Range Dosage adjustment recommended in patients with renal impairment or who develop toxicities

I.M.:
Adults: Initial: 2.5 mg every 8-12 hours
Elderly: 2.5 mg every 8-12 hours

I.V., SubQ: *Adults:* Initial: 2.5 mg every 8-12 hours

Oral:
Adults: Detoxification: Initial: Up to 40 mg/day; Maintenance: 80-120 mg/day; Pain: 2.5-10 mg every 4-12 hours as needed
Elderly: 2.5 mg every 8-12 hours

Administration

I.M. Injectable solution can be administered I.M.

I.V. Injectable solution can be administered I.V.; rate of administration not defined.

Injectable Detail pH: 4.5-6.5

Oral Oral dose for detoxification and maintenance may be administered in fruit juice or water. Dispersible tablet should not be chewed or swallowed; add to liquid and allow to dissolve before administering. May rinse if residual remains.

Subcutaneous Injectable solution can be administered SubQ.

Storage/Stability

Injection: Store at controlled room temperature of 15°C to 30°C (59°F to 86°F). Protect from light.

Oral concentrate, oral solution, tablet: Store at controlled room temperature of 15°C to 30°C (59°F to 86°F).

Nursing Actions

Physical Assessment Monitor for effectiveness of pain relief. Monitor ECG, blood pressure, CNS and respiratory status, and degree of sedation at beginning of therapy and periodically thereafter. Assess patient's physical dependence and withdrawal symptoms, including diarrhea, runny nose, watery eyes, abdominal cramping, agitation, dilated pupils, yawning, goose bumps, nausea, and vomiting. For inpatients, implement safety measures (eg, side rails up, call light within reach, instructions to call for assistance) due to increased fall risk.

Patient Education

• Discuss specific use of drug and side effects with patient as it relates to treatment. (HCAHPS: During this hospital stay, were you given any medicine that you had not taken before? Before giving you any new medicine, how often did hospital staff tell you what the medicine was for? How often did hospital staff describe possible side effects in a way you could understand?)

• Patient may experience nausea, fatigue, or hyperidrosis. Have patient report immediately to prescriber signs of hypokalemia, severe dizziness, syncope, angina, tachycardia, bradycardia, illogical thinking, significant constipation, considerable asthenia, sexual dysfunction, hallucination, mood changes, intolerable dyspepsia, severe headache, dyspnea, excessive weight gain, edema of extremities, insomnia, difficult urination, ecchymosis, hemorrhaging, vision changes, menstrual irregularities, considerable injection site irritation (HCAHPS).

• Educate patient about signs of a significant reaction (eg, wheezing; chest tightness; fever; itching; bad cough; blue skin color; seizures; or swelling of face, lips, tongue, or throat). **Note:** This is not a comprehensive list of all side effects. Patient should consult prescriber for additional questions.

Intended Use and Disclaimer: Should not be printed and given to patients. This information is intended to serve as a concise initial reference for healthcare professionals to use when discussing medications with a patient. You must ultimately rely on your own discretion, experience and judgment in diagnosing, treating and advising patients.

Methamphetamine (meth am FET a meen)

Brand Names: U.S. Desoxyn
Index Terms Desoxyephedrine Hydrochloride; Methamphetamine Hydrochloride
Pharmacologic Category Anorexiant; Central Nervous System Stimulant; Sympathomimetic

Medication Safety Issues
  Sound-alike/look-alike issues:
    Desoxyn® may be confused with digoxin
Medication Guide Available Yes
Pregnancy Risk Factor C
Lactation Enters breast milk/not recommended
Use
  Attention deficit disorder with hyperactivity: For a stabilizing effect in children >6 years with a behavioral syndrome characterized by the following group of developmentally inappropriate symptoms: Moderate to severe distractibility, short attention span, hyperactivity, emotional lability, and impulsivity
  Exogenous obesity: Short-term (ie, a few weeks) adjunct in a regimen of weight reduction based on caloric restriction, for patients in whom obesity is refractory to alternative therapy (eg, repeated diets, group programs, other drugs)
Unlabeled Use Narcolepsy
Controlled Substance C-II
Available Dosage Forms
  Tablet, Oral:
    Desoxyn: 5 mg
    Generic: 5 mg
General Dosage Range Oral:
  Children ≥6 years: ADHD: Initial: 5 mg 1-2 times daily; Usual maintenance: 20-25 mg daily in 1 or 2 divided doses
  Children ≥12 years and Adults: Exogenous obesity: 5 mg before each meal
Administration
  Oral For obesity, administer 30 minutes before each meal. Late evening doses should be avoided due to potential for insomnia.
Nursing Actions
  Physical Assessment Monitor vital signs at beginning of therapy and periodically during therapy.
Patient Education
  • Discuss specific use of drug and side effects with patient as it relates to treatment. (HCAHPS: During this hospital stay, were you given any medicine that you had not taken before? Before giving you any new medicine, how often did hospital staff tell you what the medicine was for? How often did hospital staff describe possible side effects in a way you could understand?)
  • Patient may experience nervousness, anxiety, xerostomia, or insomnia. Have patient report immediately to prescriber angina, depression, emotional instability, behavioral problems, sudden vision changes, or rash (HCAHPS).
  • Educate patient about signs of a significant reaction (eg, wheezing; chest tightness; fever; itching; bad cough; blue skin color; seizures; or swelling of face, lips, tongue, or throat). **Note:** This is not a comprehensive list of all side effects. Patient should consult prescriber for additional questions.

Intended Use and Disclaimer: Should not be printed and given to patients. This information is intended to serve as a concise initial reference for healthcare professionals to use when discussing medications with a patient. You must ultimately rely on your own discretion, experience and judgment in diagnosing, treating and advising patients.

Methimazole (meth IM a zole)

Brand Names: U.S. Tapazole
Index Terms Thiamazole
Pharmacologic Category Antithyroid Agent; Thioamide
Medication Safety Issues
Sound-alike/look-alike issues:
Methimazole may be confused with metolazone
Pregnancy Risk Factor D
Lactation Enters breast milk
Use Treatment of hyperthyroidism (including preparation for radioactive iodine therapy or thyroidectomy)
Unlabeled Use
Treatment of Graves' disease
Available Dosage Forms
Tablet, Oral:
Tapazole: 5 mg, 10 mg
Generic: 5 mg, 10 mg
General Dosage Range Oral:
Children: Initial: 0.4 mg/kg/day in 3 divided doses; Maintenance: 0.2 mg/kg/day in 3 divided doses
Adults: Initial: 15-60 mg/day in 3 divided doses; Maintenance: 5-15 mg/day in 1-3 divided doses
Administration
Other Administer consistently in relation to meals every day. In thyrotoxic crisis, rectal administration has been described (Nabil, 1982).
Nursing Actions
Physical Assessment Monitor for improvement in hyperthyroid symptoms, rash, gastrointestinal upset, leucopenia, anemia, and arthralgia during therapy. Medication can lower blood counts leading to infections. Prolonged use may lead to hypothyroidism.
Patient Education
• Discuss specific use of drug and side effects with patient as it relates to treatment. (HCAHPS: During this hospital stay, were you given any medicine that you had not taken before? Before giving you any new medicine, how often did hospital staff tell you what the medicine was for? How often did hospital staff describe possible side effects in a way you could understand?)
• Patient may experience alopecia, nausea, changes in skin pigmentation, or parageusia. Have patient report immediately to prescriber signs of infection, arthralgia, myalgia, inability to eat, ecchymosis, bleeding, discolored urine, jaundice, severe asthenia, or rash (HCAHPS).

• Educate patient about signs of a significant reaction (eg, wheezing; chest tightness; fever; itching; bad cough; blue skin color; seizures; or swelling of face, lips, tongue, or throat). **Note:** This is not a comprehensive list of all side effects. Patient should consult prescriber for additional questions.

Intended Use and Disclaimer: Should not be printed and given to patients. This information is intended to serve as a concise initial reference for healthcare professionals to use when discussing medications with a patient. You must ultimately rely on your own discretion, experience and judgment in diagnosing, treating and advising patients.

Methocarbamol (meth oh KAR ba mole)

Brand Names: U.S. Robaxin; Robaxin-750
Pharmacologic Category Skeletal Muscle Relaxant
Medication Safety Issues
Sound-alike/look-alike issues:
Methocarbamol may be confused with mephobarbital
Robaxin® may be confused with ribavirin, Skelaxin®
BEERS Criteria medication:
This drug may be potentially inappropriate for use in geriatric patients (Quality of evidence - moderate; Strength of recommendation - strong).
International issues:
Robaxin [U.S., Canada, Great Britain, Greece, Spain] may be confused with Rubex brand name for ascorbic acid [Ireland]; doxorubicin [Brazil]
Pregnancy Risk Factor C
Lactation Excretion in breast milk unknown/use caution
Use Adjunctive treatment of muscle spasm associated with acute painful musculoskeletal conditions (eg, tetanus)
Available Dosage Forms
Solution, Injection:
Robaxin: 100 mg/mL (10 mL)
Tablet, Oral:
Robaxin: 500 mg
Robaxin-750: 750 mg
Generic: 500 mg, 750 mg
General Dosage Range
I.M.: *Adults:* 1 g every 8 hours (maximum dose: 3 g/day for 3 consecutive days)
I.V.:
Children: 15 mg/kg/dose **or** 500 mg/m^2/dose every 6 hours as needed (maximum dose: 1.8 g/m^2/day for 3 consecutive days)
Adults: 1-3 g every 6 hours **or** 1 g every 8 hours (maximum dose: 3 g/day for 3 consecutive days)
Oral: *Children ≥16 years and Adults:* Initial: 1.5 g 4 times/day for 2-3 days (maximum: 8 g/day); Maintenance: 4-4.5 g/day in 3-6 divided doses

Administration

I.M. Solution for injection: A maximum of 5 mL can be administered into each gluteal region.

I.V. Solution for injection: Maximum rate: 3 mL/minute; may be administered undiluted or diluted. Monitor closely for extravasation. Administer I.V. while in recumbent position. Maintain position for at least 10-15 minutes following infusion.

Oral Tablets may be crushed and mixed with food or liquid if needed.

Nursing Actions

Physical Assessment Assess allergies; packaging contains latex. Monitor I.V. site closely to prevent extravasation. Caution patient about sedation.

Patient Education

• Discuss specific use of drug and side effects with patient as it relates to treatment. (HCAHPS: During this hospital stay, were you given any medicine that you had not taken before? Before giving you any new medicine, how often did hospital staff tell you what the medicine was for? How often did hospital staff describe possible side effects in a way you could understand?)

• Patient may experience presyncope, fatigue, blurred vision, illogical thinking, dizziness, nausea, discolored urine, or parageusia. Have patient report immediately to prescriber rash (HCAHPS).

• Educate patient about signs of a significant reaction (eg, wheezing; chest tightness; fever; itching; bad cough; blue skin color; seizures; or swelling of face, lips, tongue, or throat). **Note:** This is not a comprehensive list of all side effects. Patient should consult prescriber for additional questions.

Intended Use and Disclaimer: Should not be printed and given to patients. This information is intended to serve as a concise initial reference for healthcare professionals to use when discussing medications with a patient. You must ultimately rely on your own discretion, experience and judgment in diagnosing, treating and advising patients.

Methotrexate (meth oh TREKS ate)

Brand Names: U.S. Otrexup; Rheumatrex; Trexall

Index Terms Amethopterin; Methotrexate Sodium; Methotrexatum; MTX (error-prone abbreviation)

Pharmacologic Category Antineoplastic Agent, Antimetabolite (Antifolate); Antirheumatic, Disease Modifying; Immunosuppressant Agent

Medication Safety Issues

Sound-alike/look-alike issues:

Methotrexate may be confused with mercaptopurine, methylPREDNISolone sodium succinate, metolazone, metroNIDAZOLE, mitoXANtrone, PRALAtrexate

High alert medication:

The Institute for Safe Medication Practices (ISMP) includes this medication among its list of drugs which have a heightened risk of causing significant patient harm when used in error.

Administration issues:

Errors have occurred (resulting in death) when methotrexate was administered as "daily" dose instead of "weekly" dose recommended for some indications.

Intrathecal medication safety: The American Society of Clinical Oncology (ASCO)/Oncology Nursing Society (ONS) chemotherapy administration safety standards (Jacobson, 2009) encourage the following safety measures for intrathecal chemotherapy:

• Intrathecal medication should not be prepared during the preparation of any other agents

• After preparation, keep in an isolated location or container clearly marked with a label identifying as "intrathecal" use only

• Delivery to the patient should only be with other medications also intended for administration into the central nervous system

Other safety concerns:

MTX is an error-prone abbreviation (mistaken as mitoxantrone or multivitamin)

International issues:

Trexall [U.S.] may be confused with Trexol brand name for tramadol [Mexico]; Truxal brand name for chlorprothixene [multiple international markets]

Pregnancy Risk Factor X (psoriasis, rheumatoid arthritis)

Lactation Enters breast milk/contraindicated

Breast-Feeding Considerations Low amounts of methotrexate are excreted into breast milk. Due to the potential for serious adverse reactions in a breast-feeding infant, use is contraindicated in nursing mothers.

Use

Oncology-related uses: Acute lymphoblastic leukemia (ALL) maintenance treatment, ALL meningeal leukemia (prophylaxis and treatment); treatment of trophoblastic neoplasms (gestational choriocarcinoma, chorioadenoma destruens and hydatidiform mole), breast cancer, head and neck cancer (epidermoid), cutaneous T-Cell lymphoma (advanced mycosis fungoides), lung cancer (squamous cell and small cell), advanced non-Hodgkin's lymphomas (NHL), osteosarcoma

Nononcology uses: Treatment of psoriasis (severe, recalcitrant, disabling), severe, active rheumatoid arthritis (RA), active polyarticular-course juvenile idiopathic arthritis (pJIA)

Unlabeled Use Treatment and maintenance of remission in Crohn disease; management of ectopic pregnancy; dermatomyositis/polymyositis;

treatment of bladder cancer, central nervous system tumors (including nonleukemic meningeal cancers), acute promyelocytic leukemia (maintenance treatment), soft tissue sarcoma (desmoid tumors); acute graft-versus-host disease (GVHD) prophylaxis; medical management of abortion; systemic lupus erythematosus; Takayasu arteritis

Mechanism of Action/Effect Methotrexate is a folate antimetabolite that inhibits DNA synthesis, repair, and cellular replication. Methotrexate irreversibly binds to and inhibits dihydrofolate reductase, inhibiting the formation of reduced folates, and thymidylate synthetase, resulting in inhibition of purine and thymidylic acid synthesis. Methotrexate is cell cycle specific for the S phase of the cycle.

The MOA in the treatment of rheumatoid arthritis is unknown, but may affect immune function. In psoriasis, methotrexate is thought to target rapidly proliferating epithelial cells in the skin.

In Crohn disease, it may have immune modulator and anti-inflammatory activity

Contraindications Known hypersensitivity to methotrexate or any component of the formulation; breast-feeding

Additional contraindications for patients with psoriasis or rheumatoid arthritis: Pregnancy, alcoholism, alcoholic liver disease or other chronic liver disease, immunodeficiency syndrome (overt or laboratory evidence); pre-existing blood dyscrasias (eg, bone marrow hypoplasia, leukopenia, thrombocytopenia, significant anemia)

Warnings/Precautions Hazardous agent - use appropriate precautions for handling and disposal (NIOSH, 2012).

[U.S. Boxed Warning]: Methotrexate has been associated with acute (elevated transaminases) and potentially fatal chronic (fibrosis, cirrhosis) hepatotoxicity. Risk is related to cumulative dose (≥1.5 g) and prolonged exposure. Monitor closely (with liver function tests, including serum albumin) for liver toxicities. Liver enzyme elevations may be noted, but may not be predictive of hepatic disease in long term treatment for psoriasis (but generally is predictive in rheumatoid arthritis [RA] treatment). With long-term use, liver biopsy may show histologic changes, fibrosis, or cirrhosis; periodic liver biopsy is recommended with long-term use for psoriasis patients with risk factors for hepatotoxicity and for persistent abnormal liver function tests in psoriasis patients without risk factors for hepatotoxicity and in RA patients; discontinue methotrexate with moderate-to-severe change in liver biopsy. Risk factors for hepatotoxicity include history of above moderate ethanol consumption, persistent abnormal liver chemistries, history of chronic liver disease (including hepatitis B or C), family history of inheritable liver disease, diabetes, obesity, hyperlipidemia, lack of folate

supplementation during methotrexate therapy, cumulative methotrexate dose exceeding 1.5 g, continuous daily methotrexate dosing and history of significant exposure to hepatotoxic drugs. Use caution with preexisting liver impairment; may require dosage reduction. Use caution when used with other hepatotoxic agents (azathioprine, retinoids, sulfasalazine). **[U.S. Boxed Warning]: Methotrexate elimination is reduced in patients with ascites and pleural effusions;** resulting in prolonged half-life and toxicity; may require dose reduction or discontinuation. Monitor closely for toxicity.

[U.S. Boxed Warning]: May cause renal damage leading to acute renal failure, especially with high-dose methotrexate; monitor renal function and methotrexate levels closely, maintain adequate hydration and urinary alkalinization. Use caution in osteosarcoma patients treated with high-dose methotrexate in combination with nephrotoxic chemotherapy (eg, cisplatin). **[U.S. Boxed Warning]: Methotrexate elimination is reduced in patients with renal impairment;** may require dose reduction or discontinuation; monitor closely for toxicity. **[U.S. Boxed Warning]: Tumor lysis syndrome may occur in patients with high tumor burden;** use appropriate prevention and treatment.

[U.S. Boxed Warning]: May cause potentially life-threatening pneumonitis (acute or chronic); may require treatment interruption; may be irreversible. Pulmonary symptoms may occur at any time during therapy and at any dosage; monitor closely for pulmonary symptoms, particularly dry, nonproductive cough. Other potential symptoms include fever, dyspnea, hypoxemia, or pulmonary infiltrate. **[U.S. Boxed Warning]: Methotrexate elimination is reduced in patients with pleural effusions;** may require dose reduction or discontinuation. Monitor closely for toxicity.

[U.S. Boxed Warning]: Bone marrow suppression may occur (sometimes fatal); aplastic anemia has been reported; anemia, pancytopenia, leukopenia, neutropenia, and/or thrombocytopenia may occur. Use caution in patients with pre-existing bone marrow suppression. Discontinue treatment (immediately) in RA or psoriasis if a significant decrease in hematologic components is noted. **[U.S. Boxed Warning]: Use of low-dose methotrexate has been associated with the development of malignant lymphomas;** may regress upon treatment discontinuation; treat lymphoma appropriately if regression is not induced by cessation of methotrexate. Discontinue methotrexate if lymphoma does not regress. Other secondary tumors have been reported.

[U.S. Boxed Warning]: Gastrointestinal toxicity may occur; diarrhea and ulcerative stomatitis may require treatment interruption; death from hemorrhagic enteritis or intestinal perforation has been reported. Use with caution in patients with peptic ulcer disease, ulcerative colitis. Doses ≥250 mg/m^2 (I.V.) are associated with moderate emetic potential; antiemetics are recommended to prevent nausea and vomiting.

May cause neurotoxicity including seizures (usually in pediatric ALL patients receiving intermediate-dose (1 g/m^2 methotrexate), leuko-encephalopathy (usually with concurrent cranial irradiation) and stroke-like encephalopathy (usually with high-dose regimens). Chemical arachnoiditis (headache, back pain, nuchal rigidity, fever) and myelopathy may result from intrathecal administration. Chronic leukoencephalopathy has been reported with high-dose and with intrathecal methotrexate; may be progressive and fatal. May cause dizziness and fatigue; may affect the ability to drive or operate heavy machinery.

[U.S. Boxed Warning]: Any dose level, route of administration, or duration of therapy may cause severe and potentially fatal dermatologic reactions, including toxic epidermal necrolysis, Stevens-Johnson syndrome, exfoliative dermatitis, skin necrosis, and erythema multiforme. Recovery has been reported with treatment discontinuation. Radiation dermatitis and sunburn may be precipitated by methotrexate administration. Psoriatic lesions may be worsened by concomitant exposure to ultraviolet radiation.

Potentially significant drug-drug interactions may exist, requiring dose or frequency adjustment, additional monitoring, and/or selection of alternative therapy. **[U.S. Boxed Warning]: Concomitant administration with NSAIDs may cause severe bone marrow suppression, aplastic anemia, and GI toxicity.** Do not administer NSAIDs prior to or during high-dose methotrexate therapy; may increase and prolong serum methotrexate levels. Doses used for psoriasis may still lead to unexpected toxicities; use caution when administering NSAIDs or salicylates with lower doses of methotrexate for RA. Methotrexate may increase the levels and effects of mercaptopurine; may require dosage adjustments. Vitamins containing folate may decrease response to systemic methotrexate; folate deficiency may increase methotrexate toxicity. Concomitant use of proton pump inhibitors with methotrexate (primarily high-dose methotrexate) may elevate and prolong serum methotrexate and metabolite (hydroxymethotrexate) levels; may lead to toxicities; use with caution. Immunization may be ineffective during methotrexate treatment. Immunization with live vaccines is not recommended; cases of disseminated vaccinia infections due to live vaccines have been reported. **[U.S. Boxed Warning]: Concomitant methotrexate administration with radiotherapy may increase the risk of soft tissue necrosis and osteonecrosis.**

[U.S. Boxed Warnings]: Should be administered under the supervision of a physician experienced in the use of antimetabolite therapy; serious and fatal toxicities have occurred at all dose levels. Immune suppression may lead to potentially fatal opportunistic infections, including *Pneumocystis jirovecii* pneumonia (PCP). Use methotrexate with extreme caution in patients with an active infection (contraindicated in patients with immunodeficiency syndrome). **[U.S. Boxed Warnings]: For rheumatoid arthritis and psoriasis, immunosuppressive therapy should only be used when disease is active, severe, recalcitrant, and disabling; and where less toxic, traditional therapy is ineffective. Methotrexate formulations and/or diluents containing preservatives should not be used for intrathecal or high-dose methotrexate therapy. May cause fetal death or congenital abnormalities; do not use for psoriasis or RA treatment in pregnant women.** May cause impairment of fertility, oligospermia, and menstrual dysfunction. Toxicity from methotrexate or any immunosuppressive is increased in the elderly. Methotrexate injection may contain benzyl alcohol and should not be used in neonates. Errors have occurred (some resulting in death) when methotrexate was administered as "daily" dose instead of a "weekly" dose intended for some indications.

When used for intrathecal administration, should not be prepared during the preparation of any other agents; after preparation, store intrathecal medications in an isolated location or container clearly marked with a label identifying as "intrathecal" use only; delivery of intrathecal medications to the patient should only be with other medications intended for administration into the central nervous system (Jacobson, 2009).

Drug Interactions

Avoid Concomitant Use

Avoid concomitant use of Methotrexate with any of the following: Acitretin; BCG; CloZAPine; Natalizumab; Pimecrolimus; Tacrolimus (Topical); Tofacitinib

Decreased Effect

Methotrexate may decrease the levels/effects of: BCG; Cardiac Glycosides; Coccidioidin Skin Test; Fosphenytoin-Phenytoin; Loop Diuretics; Saproterin; Sipuleucel-T; Vaccines (Inactivated); Vitamin K Antagonists

The levels/effects of Methotrexate may be decreased by: Bile Acid Sequestrants; Echinacea; P-glycoprotein/ABCB1 Inducers

Increased Effect/Toxicity

Methotrexate may increase the levels/effects of: CloZAPine; CycloSPORINE (Systemic); Leflunomide; Loop Diuretics; Natalizumab; Tegafur; Theophylline Derivatives; Tofacitinib; Vaccines (Live); Vitamin K Antagonists

The levels/effects of Methotrexate may be increased by: Acitretin; Alitretinoin (Systemic); Ciprofloxacin (Systemic); CycloSPORINE (Systemic); Denosumab; Eltrombopag; Loop Diuretics; Mipomersen; Nonsteroidal Anti-Inflammatory Agents; Penicillins; P-glycoprotein/ABCB1 Inhibitors; Pimecrolimus; Probenecid; Proton Pump Inhibitors; Roflumilast; Salicylates; SulfaSALAzine; Sulfonamide Derivatives; Tacrolimus (Topical); Trastuzumab; Trimethoprim

Nutritional/Ethanol Interactions

Ethanol: Ethanol may be associated with increased liver injury. Management: Avoid ethanol.

Food: Methotrexate peak serum levels may be decreased if taken with food. Milk-rich foods may decrease methotrexate absorption. Folate may decrease drug response.

Herb/Nutraceutical: Echinacea has immunostimulant properties. Management: Avoid echinacea.

Adverse Reactions Note: Adverse reactions vary by route and dosage. Hematologic and/or gastrointestinal toxicities may be common at dosages used in chemotherapy; these reactions are much less frequent when used at typical dosages for rheumatic diseases.

>10%:

Central nervous system (with intrathecal administration or very high-dose therapy):

Arachnoiditis: Acute reaction manifested as severe headache, nuchal rigidity, vomiting, and fever; may be alleviated by reducing the dose

Central nervous system toxicity (subacute): 10% of patients treated with 12-15 mg of intrathecal methotrexate may develop this in the second or third week of therapy; consists of motor paralysis of extremities, cranial nerve palsy, seizure, or coma. This has also been seen in pediatric cases receiving very high-dose I.V. methotrexate.

Demyelinating disease of the central nervous system: Seen months or years after receiving methotrexate; usually in association with cranial irradiation or other systemic chemotherapy

Dermatologic: Erythema

Endocrine & metabolic: Hyperuricemia

Gastrointestinal: Aphthous stomatitis, gingivitis, diarrhea, glossitis, intestinal perforation, mucositis (dose dependent; appears in 3-7 days after therapy, resolving within 2 weeks), nausea, vomiting

Genitourinary: Azotemia, oligospermia

Hematologic & oncologic: Bone marrow depression (nadir: 7-10 days), leukopenia, thrombocytopenia

Hepatic: Increased liver enzymes (chronic therapy)

Immunologic: Immunosuppression

Renal: Nephropathy, renal failure

Respiratory: Pharyngitis

1% to 10%:

Cardiovascular: Vasculitis

Central nervous system: Chills, dizziness, malaise

Dermatologic: Alopecia, burning sensation of skin (psoriasis), dermatitis, hyperpigmentation, hypopigmentation, pruritus, skin photosensitivity, skin rash

Endocrine & metabolic: Diabetes mellitus

Gastrointestinal: Periportal fibrosis (chronic therapy), stomatitis

Genitourinary: Cystitis

Hematologic & oncologic: Hemorrhage, pancytopenia

Hepatic: Cirrhosis (chronic therapy)

Infection: Infection

Neuromuscular & skeletal: Arthralgia

Ophthalmic: Blurred vision

Renal: Renal insufficiency: Manifested by an abrupt rise in serum creatinine and BUN and a fall in urine output; more common with high-dose methotrexate, and may be due to precipitation of the drug.

Respiratory: Pneumonitis: Associated with fever, cough, and interstitial pulmonary infiltrates; treatment is to withhold methotrexate during the acute reaction; interstitial pneumonitis has been reported to occur with an incidence of 1% in patients with RA (dose 7.5-15 mg/week)

Miscellaneous: Fever

Pharmacodynamics/Kinetics

Onset of Action Antirheumatic: 3-6 weeks; additional improvement may continue longer than 12 weeks

Available Dosage Forms

Solution, Injection:

Generic: 25 mg/mL (2 mL, 10 mL)

Solution, Injection [preservative free]:

Generic: 25 mg/mL (2 mL, 4 mL, 8 mL, 10 mL, 40 mL); 50 mg/2 mL (2 mL); 100 mg/4 mL (4 mL); 200 mg/8 mL (8 mL); 250 mg/10 mL (10 mL); 1 g/40 mL (40 mL)

Solution Auto-injector, Subcutaneous [preservative free]:

Otrexup: 10 mg/0.4 mL (0.4 mL); 15 mg/0.4 mL (0.4 mL); 20 mg/0.4 mL (0.4 mL); 25 mg/0.4 mL (0.4 mL)

Solution Reconstituted, Injection [preservative free]:

Generic: 1 g (1 ea)

Tablet, Oral:

Rheumatrex: 2.5 mg

Trexall: 5 mg, 7.5 mg, 10 mg, 15 mg

Generic: 2.5 mg

General Dosage Range Dosage adjustment recommended in patients with hepatic or renal impairment or who develop toxicities.

I.M., Oral, SubQ:
Children: 10-30 mg/m^2 once weekly
Adults: Dosage varies greatly depending on indication

I.V.: *Children and Adults:* Dosage varies greatly depending on indication

Intrathecal:
Children <1 year: 6 mg/dose
Children 1 year: 8 mg/dose
Children 2 years: 10 mg/dose
Children ≥3 years and Adults: 12 mg/dose

Administration

I.M. May be administered I.M. Hazardous agent; use appropriate precautions for handling and disposal (NIOSH, 2012).

I.V. May be administered I.V.; I.V. administration may be as slow push, short bolus infusion, or 24- to 42-hour continuous infusion

Specific dosing schemes vary, but high dose should be followed by leucovorin calcium to prevent toxicity; refer to Leucovorin Calcium monograph on page 916

Hazardous agent; use appropriate precautions for handling and disposal (NIOSH, 2012).

Oral Oral administration is often preferred when low doses are being administered. Hazardous agent; use appropriate precautions for handling and disposal (NIOSH, 2012).

Subcutaneous May be administered SubQ (depending on indication and product).

Otrexup is available in an autoinjector for once weekly subcutaneous use; patient may self-administer after appropriate training on preparation and administration, and with appropriate follow-up monitoring.

Hazardous agent; use appropriate precautions for handling and disposal (NIOSH, 2012).

Intrathecal May be administered intrathecally; must use preservative-free formulation for intrathecal administration. Hazardous agent; use appropriate precautions for handling and disposal (NIOSH, 2012).

Preparation for Administration Hazardous agent; use appropriate precautions for handling and disposal (NIOSH, 2012). **Use preservative-free preparations for intrathecal or high-dose methotrexate administration.**

I.V.: Dilute powder with D$_5$W or NS to a concentration of ≤25 mg/mL (20 mg and 50 mg vials) and 50 mg/mL (1 g vial). May further dilute in D$_5$W or NS.

Intrathecal: Prepare intrathecal solutions with preservative-free NS, lactated Ringer's, or Elliot's B solution to a final volume of up to 12 mL (volume generally based on institution or practitioner preference). Intrathecal methotrexate concentrations may be institution specific or based on practitioner preference, generally ranging from a final

concentration of 1 mg/mL (per prescribing information; Grossman, 1993; Lin, 2008) up to ~2-4 mg/mL (de Lemos, 2009; Glantz, 1999). For triple intrathecal therapy (methotrexate 12 mg/hydrocortisone 24 mg/cytarabine 36 mg), preparation to final volume of 12 mL is reported (Lin, 2008). Intrathecal medications should **NOT** be prepared during the preparation of any other agents.

Storage/Stability

Tablets: Store at room temperature of 20°C to 25°C (68°F to 77°F); excursions are permitted between 15°C and 30°C (59°F and 86°F). Protect from light.

Injection: Store intact vials and autoinjectors at room temperature 20°C to 25°C (68°F to 77°F); excursions may be permitted between 15°C and 30°C (59°F and 86°F). Protect from light.

I.V.: Solution diluted in D$_5$W or NS is stable for 24 hours at room temperature (21°C to 25°C). Reconstituted solutions with a preservative may be stored under refrigeration for up to 3 months, and up to 4 weeks at room temperature.

Intrathecal: Intrathecal dilutions are preservative-free and should be used as soon as possible after preparation. After preparation, store intrathecal medications (until use) in an isolated location or container clearly marked with a label identifying as "intrathecal" use only.

Nursing Actions

Physical Assessment Inform physician if patient has history of pericardial or pleural effusion, liver impairment, kidney disease, ulcerative colitis, or peptic ulcer disease. Monitor frequently for signs of pneumonitis such as dry, nonproductive cough; GI toxicities such as blood in stool or vomit, black, tarry stools, mucositis, or mouth ulcers; dermatological effects such as radiation recall and photosensitivity, and signs of renal failure such as decreased urine output, or dark, tea-colored urine. Instruct patient on importance of limited alcohol intake during treatment. Monitor for lethargy, decreased appetite, right upper quadrant pain, or yellowing of skin or eyes.

Patient Education
- Discuss specific use of drug and side effects with patient as it relates to treatment. (HCAHPS: During this hospital stay, were you given any medicine that you had not taken before? Before giving you any new medicine, how often did hospital staff tell you what the medicine was for? How often did hospital staff describe possible side effects in a way you could understand?)
- Patient may experience anemia, leukopenia, thrombocytopenia, nausea, loss of appetite, diarrhea, stomatitis, pharyngitis, headache, or alopecia. Have patient report immediately to prescriber signs of infection, angina, dyspnea, petechiae, severe dyspepsia, inability to eat, ecchymosis, discolored urine, jaundice, significant fatigue, pregnancy, or rash (HCAHPS).

- Educate patient about signs of a significant reaction (eg, wheezing; chest tightness; fever; itching; bad cough; blue skin color; seizures; or swelling of face, lips, tongue, or throat). **Note:** This is not a comprehensive list of all side effects. Patient should consult prescriber for additional questions.

Intended Use and Disclaimer: Should not be printed and given to patients. This information is intended to serve as a concise initial reference for healthcare professionals to use when discussing medications with a patient. You must ultimately rely on your own discretion, experience and judgment in diagnosing, treating and advising patients.
Dietary Considerations Some products may contain sodium.

Methoxsalen (Topical) (meth OKS a len)

Brand Names: U.S. Oxsoralen
Index Terms Methoxypsoralen
Pharmacologic Category Psoralen
Pregnancy Risk Factor C
Lactation Excretion in breast milk unknown/not recommended
Use Repigmentation of idiopathic vitiligo
Available Dosage Forms
  Lotion, External:
  Oxsoralen: 1% (29.57 mL)
General Dosage Range Topical: *Children ≥12 years and Adults:* Lotion is applied by healthcare provider prior to UVA light exposure, usually no more than once weekly
Administration
  Topical Hands and fingers of person applying the lotion should be protected to prevent possible photosensitization and/or burns.
Nursing Actions
  Physical Assessment This drug is administered in conjunction with ultraviolet light or ultraviolet radiation therapy. Teach patient sunlight precautions.
  Patient Education
  - Discuss specific use of drug and side effects with patient as it relates to treatment. (HCAHPS: During this hospital stay, were you given any medicine that you had not taken before? Before giving you any new medicine, how often did hospital staff tell you what the medicine was for? How often did hospital staff describe possible side effects in a way you could understand?)
  - Patient may experience erythema, or skin irritation. Have patient report immediately to prescriber rash (HCAHPS).
  - Educate patient about signs of a significant reaction (eg, wheezing; chest tightness; fever; itching; bad cough; blue skin color; seizures; or swelling of face, lips, tongue, or throat). **Note:** This is not a comprehensive list of all side

effects. Patient should consult prescriber for additional questions.

Intended Use and Disclaimer: Should not be printed and given to patients. This information is intended to serve as a concise initial reference for healthcare professionals to use when discussing medications with a patient. You must ultimately rely on your own discretion, experience and judgment in diagnosing, treating and advising patients.

Methyldopa (meth il DOE pa)

Index Terms Aldomet; Methyldopate Hydrochloride
Pharmacologic Category Alpha$_2$-Adrenergic Agonist; Antihypertensive
Medication Safety Issues
  Sound-alike/look-alike issues:
    Methyldopa may be confused with L-dopa, levodopa
  BEERS Criteria medication:
    This drug may be potentially inappropriate for use in geriatric patients (Quality of evidence - low; Strength of recommendation - strong).
Pregnancy Risk Factor B/C (injectable)
Lactation Enters breast milk/use caution
Use Management of moderate-to-severe hypertension
Available Dosage Forms
  Solution, Intravenous:
    Generic: 250 mg/5 mL (5 mL)
  Tablet, Oral:
    Generic: 250 mg, 500 mg
General Dosage Range Dosage adjustment recommended in patients with renal impairment
  I.V.:
    Children: 5-10 mg/kg/dose every 6-8 hours (maximum: 65 mg/kg/day; 3 g/day)
    Adults: 250-500 mg every 6-8 hours (maximum: 1 g every 6 hours)
  Oral:
    Children: Initial: 10 mg/kg/day in 2-4 divided doses; Maintenance: Up to 65 mg/kg/day (maximum: 3 g/day)
    Adults: Initial: 250 mg 2-3 times/day; Maintenance: 250-1000 mg/day in 2 divided doses (maximum: 3 g/day)
Administration
  I.V. Infuse over 30-60 minutes.
  Oral Administer new dosage increases in the evening to minimize sedation.
Nursing Actions
  Physical Assessment Monitor for hypotension, bradycardia, or CNS changes on a regular basis.
  Patient Education
  - Discuss specific use of drug and side effects with patient as it relates to treatment. (HCAHPS: During this hospital stay, were you given any medicine that you had not taken before? Before giving you any new medicine, how often did

hospital staff tell you what the medicine was for? How often did hospital staff describe possible side effects in a way you could understand?)

• Patient may experience presyncope, fatigue, blurred vision, illogical thinking, dizziness, headache, nervousness, anxiety, xerostomia, or impotence. Have patient report immediately to prescriber depression, severe edema, discolored urine, jaundice, significant asthenia, ecchymosis, bleeding, or rash (HCAHPS).

• Educate patient about signs of a significant reaction (eg, wheezing; chest tightness; fever; itching; bad cough; blue skin color; seizures; or swelling of face, lips, tongue, or throat). **Note:** This is not a comprehensive list of all side effects. Patient should consult prescriber for additional questions.

Intended Use and Disclaimer: Should not be printed and given to patients. This information is intended to serve as a concise initial reference for healthcare professionals to use when discussing medications with a patient. You must ultimately rely on your own discretion, experience and judgment in diagnosing, treating and advising patients.

Methylergonovine (meth il er goe NOE veen)

Index Terms Methylergometrine Maleate; Methylergonovine Maleate

Pharmacologic Category Ergot Derivative

Medication Safety Issues

Sound-alike/look-alike issues:

Methergine® may be confused with Brethine

Methylergonovine and terbutaline parenteral dosage forms look similar. Due to their contrasting indications, use care when administering these agents.

Administration issues:

Inadvertent administration of methylergonovine to newborns has been reported in place of routine medications (eg, vitamin K or hepatitis B vaccine); store methylergonovine injection separately from medications used for neonates.

Pregnancy Risk Factor C

Lactation Enters breast milk/not recommended

Use Management of uterine atony, hemorrhage and subinvolution of the uterus following delivery of the placenta; control of uterine hemorrhage following delivery of the anterior shoulder in the second stage of labor

Available Dosage Forms

Solution, Injection:

Generic: 0.2 mg/mL (1 mL)

Solution, Injection [preservative free]:

Generic: 0.2 mg/mL (1 mL)

Tablet, Oral:

Generic: 0.2 mg

General Dosage Range

I.M., I.V.: *Adults:* 0.2 mg after delivery; may repeat every 2-4 hours

Oral: *Adults:* 0.2 mg 3-4 times daily in the puerperium

Administration

I.M. May be administered intramuscularly. Hazardous agent; use appropriate precautions for handling and disposal (NIOSH, 2012).

I.V. Administer over ≥60 seconds. Should not be routinely administered I.V. because of possibility of inducing sudden hypertension and cerebrovascular accident. I.V. administration should only be considered during life-threatening situations. Hazardous agent; use appropriate precautions for handling and disposal (NIOSH, 2012).

Injectable Detail pH: 2.7-3.5

Oral Available in tablets for oral administration. Hazardous agent; use appropriate precautions for handling and disposal (NIOSH, 2012).

Nursing Actions

Physical Assessment Monitor blood pressure, CNS status, and vaginal bleeding on a regular basis. May cause nausea. Patient may require antiemetic.

Patient Education

• Discuss specific use of drug and side effects with patient as it relates to treatment. (HCAHPS: During this hospital stay, were you given any medicine that you had not taken before? Before giving you any new medicine, how often did hospital staff tell you what the medicine was for? How often did hospital staff describe possible side effects in a way you could understand?)

• Patient may experience hypertension, nausea, or headache. Have patient report immediately to prescriber angina, tachycardia, severe dizziness, dyspnea, or rash (HCAHPS).

• Educate patient about signs of a significant reaction (eg, wheezing; chest tightness; fever; itching; bad cough; blue skin color; seizures; or swelling of face, lips, tongue, or throat). **Note:** This is not a comprehensive list of all side effects. Patient should consult prescriber for additional questions.

Intended Use and Disclaimer: Should not be printed and given to patients. This information is intended to serve as a concise initial reference for healthcare professionals to use when discussing medications with a patient. You must ultimately rely on your own discretion, experience and judgment in diagnosing, treating and advising patients.

Methylnaltrexone (meth il nal TREKS one)

Brand Names: U.S. Relistor

Index Terms Methylnaltrexone Bromide; N-methylnaltrexone Bromide

Pharmacologic Category Gastrointestinal Agent, Miscellaneous; Opioid Antagonist, Peripherally-Acting

Medication Safety Issues
Sound-alike/look-alike issues:
Methylnaltrexone may be confused with naltrexone

Pregnancy Risk Factor B

Lactation Excretion in breast milk unknown/use caution

Breast-Feeding Considerations It is not known if methylnaltrexone is excreted in breast milk. The manufacturer recommends that caution be exercised when administering methylnaltrexone to nursing women.

Use Opioid-induced constipation: Treatment of opioid-induced constipation in patients with advanced illness (receiving palliative care) who have an inadequate response to conventional laxative regimens

Mechanism of Action/Effect Peripherally-acting mu-opioid receptor antagonist which decreases opioid-induced constipation without affecting opioid analgesic effects

Contraindications Known or suspected mechanical gastrointestinal obstruction.
Canadian labeling: Additional contraindications (not in U.S. labeling): Hypersensitivity to methylnaltrexone or any component of the formulation

Warnings/Precautions Discontinue treatment for severe or persistent diarrhea. Gastrointestinal perforation of the colon, duodenum, and stomach has been reported in patients with advanced illnesses associated with impaired structural integrity of the GI wall (eg, cancer, Ogilvie's syndrome, peptic ulcer). Use caution in patients with known or history of GI tract lesions; discontinue therapy if persistent, severe, or worsening abdominal symptoms occur. Use with caution in patients with renal impairment; dosage adjustment recommended for severe renal impairment (CrCl <30 mL/minute). Has not been studied in patients with end-stage renal impairment requiring dialysis. Discontinue methylnaltrexone if opioids are discontinued. Use beyond 4 months has not been studied.

Drug Interactions
Avoid Concomitant Use There are no known interactions where it is recommended to avoid concomitant use.
Decreased Effect
The levels/effects of Methylnaltrexone may be decreased by: Peginterferon Alfa-2b
Increased Effect/Toxicity There are no known significant interactions involving an increase in effect.

Adverse Reactions
>10%: Gastrointestinal: Abdominal pain (29%), flatulence (13%), nausea (12%)
1% to 10%:
Central nervous system: Dizziness (7%)

Dermatologic: Hyperhidrosis (7%)
Gastrointestinal: Diarrhea (6%)

Pharmacodynamics/Kinetics
Onset of Action Usually within 30-60 minutes (in responding patients)

Available Dosage Forms
Kit, Subcutaneous:
Relistor: 12 mg/0.6 mL
Solution, Subcutaneous:
Relistor: 8 mg/0.4 mL (0.4 mL); 12 mg/0.6 mL (0.6 mL)

General Dosage Range Dosage adjustment recommended in patients with renal impairment
SubQ:
Adults <38 kg and >114 kg: 0.15 mg/kg (round dose up to nearest 0.1 mL of volume) every other day as needed (maximum: 1 dose/24 hours)
Adults 38 to <62 kg: 8 mg every other day as needed (maximum: 1 dose/24 hours)
Adults 62-114 kg: 12 mg every other day as needed (maximum: 1 dose/24 hours)

Administration
Subcutaneous Administer subcutaneously into upper arm, abdomen, or thigh. Rotate injection site. Do not inject in tender, bruised, red, or hard areas.

Storage/Stability Store intact vials and prefilled syringes between 20°C and 25°C (68°F and 77°F); excursions are permitted between 15°C and 30°C (59°F and 86°F). Do not freeze. Protect from light. Solution withdrawn from the single use vial is stable in a syringe for 24 hours at room temperature.

Nursing Actions
Physical Assessment Contact prescriber if severe or persistent diarrhea occurs; may be discontinued. Must be discontinued if opioids are discontinued. Teach patient appropriate injection technique and syringe/needle disposal.

Patient Education
• Discuss specific use of drug and side effects with patient as it relates to treatment. HCAHPS: During this hospital stay, were you given any medicine that you had not taken before? Before giving you any new medicine, how often did hospital staff tell you what the medicine was for? How often did hospital staff describe possible side effects in a way you could understand?)
• Patient may experience dizziness, dyspepsia, nausea, or flatulence. Have patient report immediately to prescriber severe diarrhea or rash (HCAHPS).
• Educate patient about signs of a significant reaction (eg, wheezing; chest tightness; fever; itching; bad cough; blue skin color; seizures; or swelling of face, lips, tongue, or throat). **Note:** This is not a comprehensive list of all side effects. Patient should consult prescriber for additional questions.

◀ **Intended Use and Disclaimer:** Should not be printed and given to patients. This information is intended to serve as a concise initial reference for healthcare professionals to use when discussing medications with a patient. You must ultimately rely on your own discretion, experience and judgment in diagnosing, treating and advising patients.

Methylphenidate (meth il FEN i date)

Brand Names: U.S. Concerta; Daytrana; Metadate CD; Metadate ER; Methylin; Quillivant XR; Ritalin; Ritalin LA; Ritalin SR
Index Terms Methylphenidate Hydrochloride
Pharmacologic Category Central Nervous System Stimulant
Medication Safety Issues
Sound-alike/look-alike issues:
Metadate CD may be confused with Metadate ER
Metadate ER may be confused with methadone
Methylphenidate may be confused with methadone
Ritalin may be confused with Rifadin, ritodrine
Ritalin LA may be confused with Ritalin-SR
Medication Guide Available Yes
Pregnancy Risk Factor C
Lactation Enters breast milk/use caution
Breast-Feeding Considerations Methylphenidate excretion into breast milk has been noted in case reports. In both cases, the authors calculated the relative infant dose to be ≤0.2% of the weight adjusted maternal dose. Adverse events were not noted in either infant, however, both were older (6 months of age and 11 months of age) and exposure was limited (Hackett, 2006; Spigset, 2007). The manufacturer recommends that caution be used if administered to a nursing woman.
Use
U.S. labeling: Treatment of attention-deficit/hyperactivity disorder (ADHD); symptomatic management of narcolepsy (except Concerta, Daytrana, Metadate CD, Ritalin LA, and Quillivant XR)
Canadian labeling: Treatment of attention-deficit/hyperactivity disorder (ADHD); symptomatic management of narcolepsy (except Biphentin, Concerta)
Unlabeled Use Treatment of depression in medically-ill older adults or adult patients with terminal illness and/or receiving palliative care
Mechanism of Action/Effect Mild CNS stimulant; blocks the reuptake of norepinephrine and dopamine into presynaptic neurons; appears to stimulate the cerebral cortex and subcortical structures similar to amphetamines
Contraindications
U.S. labeling: Hypersensitivity to methylphenidate or any component of the formulation; marked anxiety, tension, and agitation; glaucoma; use during or within 14 days following MAO inhibitor

therapy; family history or diagnosis of Tourette's syndrome or tics
Additional contraindications: Metadate CD and Metadate ER: Severe hypertension, heart failure, arrhythmia, hyperthyroidism, recent MI or angina; concomitant use of halogenated anesthetics
Canadian labeling: Hypersensitivity to methylphenidate or any component of the formulation; marked anxiety, tension, and agitation; glaucoma; use during or within 14 days following MAO inhibitor therapy; family history or diagnosis of Tourette's syndrome or tics, thyrotoxicosis, advanced arteriosclerosis, symptomatic cardiovascular disease, or moderate-to-severe hypertension
Additional contraindications: Ritalin and Ritalin SR: Pheochromocytoma
Warnings/Precautions CNS stimulant use has been associated with serious cardiovascular events (eg, sudden death in children and adolescents; sudden death, stroke, and MI in adults) in patients with pre-existing structural cardiac abnormalities or other serious heart problems. These products should be avoided in patients with known serious structural cardiac abnormalities, cardiomyopathy, serious heart rhythm abnormalities, or other serious cardiac problems that could further increase their risk of sudden death. Patients should be carefully evaluated for cardiac disease prior to initiation of therapy. Use of stimulants can cause an increase in blood pressure (average 2-4 mm Hg) and increases in heart rate (average 3-6 bpm), although some patients may have larger than average increases. Use caution with hypertension, hyperthyroidism, or other cardiovascular conditions that might be exacerbated by increases in blood pressure or heart rate. Some products are contraindicated in patients with heart failure, arrhythmias, severe hypertension, hyperthyroidism, angina, or recent MI. Stimulants are associated with peripheral vasculopathy, including Raynaud's phenomenon; signs/symptoms are usually mild and intermittent, and generally improve with dose reduction or discontinuation. Digital ulceration and/or soft tissue breakdown have been observed rarely; monitor for digital changes during therapy and seek further evaluation (eg, rheumatology) if necessary. Prolonged and painful erections (priapism), sometimes requiring surgical intervention, have been reported with methylphenidate use in pediatric and adult patients. Priapism has been reported to develop after some time on the drug, often subsequent to an increase in dose and also during a period of drug withdrawal (drug holidays or discontinuation). Patients who develop abnormally sustained or frequent and painful erections should seek immediate medical attention.

Has demonstrated value as part of a comprehensive treatment program for ADHD. Use with caution in patients with bipolar disorder (may induce mixed/manic episode). May exacerbate symptoms of behavior and thought disorder in psychotic patients; new-onset psychosis or mania may occur with stimulant use; observe for symptoms of aggression and/or hostility. Use caution with seizure disorders (may reduce seizure threshold). Use caution in patients with history of ethanol or drug abuse. May exacerbate symptoms of behavior and thought disorder in psychotic patients. **[U.S. Boxed Warning]: Potential for drug dependency exists - avoid abrupt discontinuation in patients who have received for prolonged periods.** Visual disturbances have been reported (rare). Not labeled for use in children <6 years of age. Use of stimulants has been associated with suppression of growth in children; monitor growth rate during treatment.

Concerta should not be used in patients with esophageal motility disorders or pre-existing severe gastrointestinal narrowing (small bowel disease, short gut syndrome, history of peritonitis, cystic fibrosis, chronic intestinal pseudo-obstruction, Meckel's diverticulum). Concomitant use of Metadate CD and Metadate ER with halogenated anesthetics is contraindicated; may cause sudden elevations in blood pressure; if surgery is planned, do not administer Metadate CD or Metadate ER on the day of surgery. Transdermal system may cause allergic contact sensitization, characterized by intense local reactions (edema, papules) that may spread beyond the patch site; sensitization may subsequently manifest systemically with other routes of methylphenidate administration; monitor closely. Avoid exposure of application site to any direct external heat sources (eg, hair dryers, heating pads, electric blankets); may increase the rate and extent of absorption and risk of overdose. Efficacy of transdermal methylphenidate therapy for >7 weeks has not been established. Potentially significant interactions may exist, requiring dose or frequency adjustment, additional monitoring, and/or selection of alternative therapy. Consult drug interactions database for more detailed information. Biphentin [Canadian product] controlled release capsules are not interchangeable with other controlled release formulations. Some dosage forms may contain lactose or sucrose; use with caution in patients intolerant to either component (some manufacturer labels recommend avoiding use in such patients).

Drug Interactions

Avoid Concomitant Use

Avoid concomitant use of Methylphenidate with any of the following: Alcohol (Ethyl); Inhalational Anesthetics; Iobenguane I 123; MAO Inhibitors

Decreased Effect

Methylphenidate may decrease the levels/effects of: Antihypertensives; Iobenguane I 123; Ioflupane I 123

Increased Effect/Toxicity

Methylphenidate may increase the levels/effects of: Anti-Parkinson's Agents (Dopamine Agonist); Antipsychotics; CloNIDine; Fosphenytoin; Inhalational Anesthetics; PHENobarbital; Phenytoin; Primidone; Sympathomimetics; Tricyclic Antidepressants; Vitamin K Antagonists

The levels/effects of Methylphenidate may be increased by: Alcohol (Ethyl); Antacids; Antipsychotics; AtoMOXetine; Cannabinoids; H2-Antagonists; MAO Inhibitors; Proton Pump Inhibitors

Nutritional/Ethanol Interactions

Ethanol: Alcohol consumption increases the rate of methylphenidate release from Metadate CD and Ritalin LA (extended-release capsules), but not from Concerta (extended-release tablet); an *in vitro* study involving Metadate CD and Ritalin LA showed that an alcohol concentration of 40% resulted in 84% and 98% of the methylphenidate being released in the first hour, respectively. Alcohol may also exacerbate the CNS effects of psychoactive drugs, such as methylphenidate, regardless of dosage form. Management: Avoid consuming alcohol during therapy.

Food: Food may increase oral absorption of immediate release tablet/solution and chewable tablet. Management: Administer 30-45 minutes before meals.

Herb/Nutraceutical: Ephedra may cause hypertension or arrhythmias and yohimbe has CNS stimulatory activity. Management: Avoid ephedra and yohimbe.

Adverse Reactions

All dosage forms: Frequency not always defined.

Cardiovascular: Angina, cardiac arrhythmia, cerebral arteritis, cerebral hemorrhage, cerebral occlusion, cerebrovascular accidents, hyper-/hypotension, MI, murmur, palpitation, pulse increased/decreased, Raynaud's phenomenon, tachycardia, vasculitis

Central nervous system: Motion sickness (children 2%), tic (children 2%), aggression, agitation, anger, anxiety, confusional state, depression, dizziness, drowsiness, emotional lability, fatigue, fever, headache, hypervigilance, insomnia, irritability, lethargy, nervousness, neuroleptic malignant syndrome (NMS) (rare), restlessness, stroke, tension, Tourette's syndrome (rare), toxic psychosis, tremor, vertigo

Dermatologic: Excoriation (children 4%), alopecia, erythema multiforme, exfoliative dermatitis, hyperhidrosis, rash, urticaria

Endocrine & metabolic: Dysmenorrhea, growth retardation, libido decreased

Gastrointestinal: Abdominal pain, anorexia, appetite decreased, bruxism, constipation, diarrhea, dyspepsia, nausea, vomiting, weight loss, xerostomia

Genitourinary: Erectile dysfunction

Hematologic: Anemia, leukopenia, pancytopenia, thrombocytopenia, thrombocytopenic purpura

Hepatic: Bilirubin increased, hepatic coma, liver function tests abnormal, transaminases increased

Neuromuscular & skeletal: Arthralgia, dyskinesia, muscle tightness, paresthesia

Ocular: Eye pain (children 2%), blurred vision, dry eyes, mydriasis, visual accommodation disturbance

Renal: Necrotizing vasculitis

Respiratory: Cough increased, dyspnea, pharyngitis, pharyngolaryngeal pain, rhinitis, sinusitis, upper respiratory tract infection

Miscellaneous: Accidental injury, hypersensitivity reactions

Transdermal system: Frequency of adverse events as reported in trials of 7-week duration. Incidence of some events higher with extended use.

>10%:

Central nervous system: Headache (≤15%; longterm use in children: 28%), insomnia (6% to 13%; long-term use in children: 30%), irritability (7% to 11%)

Gastrointestinal: Appetite decreased (26%), nausea (10% to 12%)

Miscellaneous: Viral infection (long-term use in children: 28%)

1% to 10%:

Cardiovascular: Tachycardia (≤1%)

Central nervous system: Tic (7%), dizziness (adolescents 6%), emotional instability (6%)

Gastrointestinal: Vomiting (3% to 10%), weight loss (6% to 9%), abdominal pain (5% to 7%), anorexia (5%; long-term use in children: 46%)

Local: Application site reaction

Respiratory: Nasal congestion (6%) nasopharyngitis (5%)

Pharmacodynamics/Kinetics

Onset of Action Peak effect:

Immediate release tablet: Cerebral stimulation: ~2 hours

Controlled release capsule: Biphentin [Canadian product]: Initial: within 1 hour

Extended release capsule: Metadate CD, Ritalin LA: Biphasic; initial peak similar to immediate release product, followed by second rising portion (corresponding to extended release portion)

Extended release tablet: Concerta: Initial: 1-2 hours

Sustained release tablet: Ritalin-SR: 4-7 hours

Transdermal: ~2 hours; may be expedited by the application of external heat

Duration of Action Immediate release tablet: 3-6 hours; Sustained release tablet: Ritalin-SR: 8 hours; Extended release tablet: Metadate ER: 8 hours, Concerta: 12 hours; Controlled release

capsule: Biphentin [Canadian product]: ~10-12 hours

Controlled Substance C-II

Available Dosage Forms

Capsule Extended Release, Oral:

Metadate CD: 10 mg, 20 mg, 30 mg, 40 mg, 50 mg, 60 mg

Generic: 10 mg, 20 mg, 30 mg, 40 mg, 50 mg, 60 mg

Capsule Extended Release 24 Hour, Oral:

Ritalin LA: 10 mg, 20 mg, 30 mg, 40 mg

Generic: 20 mg, 30 mg, 40 mg

Patch, Transdermal:

Daytrana: 10 mg/9 hr (30 ea); 15 mg/9 hr (30 ea); 20 mg/9 hr (30 ea); 30 mg/9 hr (30 ea)

Solution, Oral:

Methylin: 5 mg/5 mL (500 mL); 10 mg/5 mL (500 mL)

Generic: 5 mg/5 mL (500 mL); 10 mg/5 mL (500 mL)

Suspension Reconstituted, Oral:

Quillivant XR: 25 mg/5 mL (60 mL, 120 mL, 150 mL, 180 mL)

Tablet, Oral:

Ritalin: 5 mg, 10 mg, 20 mg

Generic: 5 mg, 10 mg, 20 mg

Tablet Chewable, Oral:

Methylin: 2.5 mg, 5 mg, 10 mg

Tablet Extended Release, Oral:

Concerta: 18 mg, 27 mg, 36 mg, 54 mg

Metadate ER: 20 mg

Ritalin SR: 20 mg

Generic: 10 mg, 18 mg, 20 mg, 27 mg, 36 mg, 54 mg

General Dosage Range

Oral:

Immediate release: *Children ≥6 years, Adolescents, and Adults:* Initial: 5 mg twice daily; Maintenance: Increase by 5-10 mg daily at weekly intervals (maximum: 60 mg daily in 2-3 divided doses)

Extended and sustained release:

Children 6 to <13 years: Concerta: 18-54 mg once every morning (maximum: 54 mg daily); Metadate ER, Ritalin-SR: 20-60 mg daily (maximum: 60 mg daily); Metadate CD, Quillivant XR, Ritalin LA: Initial: 20 mg once daily (maximum: 60 mg daily)

Adolescents and Adults: Concerta: 18-72 mg once every morning (maximum: 72 mg daily); Metadate ER, Ritalin-SR: 20-60 mg daily (maximum: 60 mg daily); Metadate CD, Quillivant XR, Ritalin LA: Initial: 20 mg once daily (maximum: 60 mg daily)

Transdermal: *Children ≥6 and Adolescents <18 years:* Initial: 10 mg patch once daily; Maximum: 30 mg patch once daily

Administration

Oral

Controlled release capsule (Biphentin; Canadian product): Administer in the morning with breakfast. Swallow whole; do not crush or chew capsule. Alternatively, capsules may be opened and the contents sprinkled onto applesauce, ice cream, or yogurt, but the beads must not be crushed or chewed.

Immediate release (IR) tablet (Ritalin), IR solution (Methylin), chewable tablet (Methylin): Administer each dose 30-45 minutes before a meal. Ensure last daily dose is administered before 6 pm if difficulty sleeping occurs. Administer chewable tablet with at least 8 ounces of water or other fluid.

Extended release capsule (Metadate CD, Ritalin LA): Administer in the morning. May be taken with or without food. Alternatively, capsules may be opened and the contents sprinkled onto a small amount (equal to 1 tablespoon) of cold applesauce. Swallow applesauce without chewing. Do not crush or chew capsule contents.

Extended release suspension (Quillivant XR): Administer in the morning with or without food. Shake bottle ≥10 seconds prior to administration. Use the oral dosing dispenser provided; wash after each use.

Extended release tablet:

Metadate ER: May be taken with or without food. Swallow whole with water or other fluid; do not crush or chew tablet.

Concerta: Administer in the morning. May be taken with or without food, but must be taken with water or other fluid. Do not crush, chew, or divide tablet.

Sustained release tablet (Ritalin-SR): Administer 30-45 minutes before a meal. Swallow whole; do not crush or chew tablet.

Topical Transdermal (Daytrana): Apply to clean, dry, non-oily, intact skin to the hip area, avoiding the waistline; do not premedicate the patch site with hydrocortisone or other solutions, creams, ointments, or emollients. Apply at the same time each day to alternating hips. Press firmly for 30 seconds to ensure proper adherence. Avoid exposure of application site to external heat source, which may increase the amount of drug absorbed. If difficulty is experienced when separating the patch from the liner or if any medication (sticky substance) remains on the liner after separation; discard that patch and apply a new patch. Do not use a patch that has been damaged or torn. Do not cut patch. If patch should dislodge, may replace with new patch (to different site) but total wear time should not exceed 9 hours; do not reapply with dressings, tape, or common adhesives. Patch may be removed early if a shorter duration of effect is desired or if late day side effects occur. Wash hands with soap and water after handling. Avoid touching the sticky side of the patch. If patch removal is difficult, an oil-based product (eg, petroleum jelly, olive oil) may be applied to the patch edges to aid removal; never apply acetone-based products (eg, nail polish remover) to patch. Dispose of used patch by folding adhesive side onto itself, and discard in toilet or appropriate lidded container.

Preparation for Administration

Suspension: *Extended release (Quillivant XR):* Prior to dispensing, reconstitute with an appropriate amount of water (refer to bottle).

Storage/Stability

Capsule:

Extended release (Metadate CD, Ritalin LA): Store at 25°C (77°F); excursions permitted to 15°C to 30°C (59°F to 86°F). Protect from light.

Controlled release (Biphentin [Canadian product]): Store at 15°C to 30°C (59°F to 86°F).

Solution: *Immediate release (Methylin):* Store at 20°C to 25°C (68°F to 77°F).

Suspension: *Extended release (Quillivant XR):* Store at 25°C (77°F); excursions permitted to 15°C to 30°C (59°F to 86°F), before and after reconstitution. Reconstituted bottle must be used within 4 months.

Tablet:

Chewable (Methylin): Store at 20°C to 25°C (68°F to 77°F). Protect from light and moisture.

Extended release:

Metadate ER: Store at 20°C to 25°C (68°F to 77°F); excursions permitted to 15°C to 30°C (59°F to 86°F). Protect from light and moisture.

Concerta: Store at 25°C (77°F); excursions permitted to 15°C to 30°C (59°F to 86°F). Protect from humidity.

Immediate release (Ritalin): Store at 25°C (77°F); excursions permitted to 15°C to 30°C (59°F to 86°F). Protect from light and moisture.

Sustained release (Ritalin-SR): Store at 25°C (77°F); excursions permitted to 15°C to 30°C (59°F to 86°F). Protect from light and moisture.

Transdermal system: *Daytrana:* Store at 25°C (77°F); excursions permitted to 15°C to 30°C (59°F to 86°F). Keep patches stored in protective pouch. Once tray is opened, use patches within 2 months; once an individual patch has been removed from the pouch and the protective liner removed, use immediately. Do not refrigerate or freeze.

Nursing Actions

Physical Assessment Monitor height/weight routinely in all populations. Monitor vital signs; be aware of increased blood pressure and pulse. Monitor for changes in mood. Beware of requests for early refills or reports of lost prescription; may recommend random toxicology screening.

Patient Education

• Discuss specific use of drug and side effects with patient as it relates to treatment. HCAHPS: During this hospital stay, were you given any medicine that you had not taken before? Before giving you any new medicine, how often did hospital staff tell you what the medicine was for? How often did hospital staff describe possible side effects in a way you could understand?) ▶

- Patient may experience fatigue, xerostomia, weight loss, lack of appetite, insomnia, or dyspepsia. Have patient report immediately to prescriber severe skin irritation, arthralgia, skin or mouth discoloration, blurred vision, vision changes, tachycardia, bradycardia, arrhythmia, significant headache, considerable nausea, jaundice, chills, pharyngitis, tremors, difficulty with motor activity, hyperhidrosis, intolerable asthenia, extremity discoloration, paresthesia, wounds on extremities, signs of severe cardiac abnormalities, behavioral changes, mood changes, or depression (ie, suicidal ideation, anxiety, emotional instability, illogical thinking) (HCAHPS).
- Educate patient about signs of a significant reaction (eg, wheezing; chest tightness; fever; itching; bad cough; blue skin color; seizures; or swelling of face, lips, tongue, or throat). **Note:** This is not a comprehensive list of all side effects. Patient should consult prescriber for additional questions.

Intended Use and Disclaimer: Should not be printed and given to patients. This information is intended to serve as a concise initial reference for healthcare professionals to use when discussing medications with a patient. You must ultimately rely on your own discretion, experience and judgment in diagnosing, treating and advising patients.

Dietary Considerations Administer immediate release (IR) tablet (Ritalin), IR solution (Methylin), chewable tablet (Methylin), and sustained released tablet (Ritalin-SR) 30-45 minutes before meals. Some products may contain phenylalanine.

Related Information

Oral Medications That Should Not Be Crushed or Altered *on page 1712*

MethylPREDNISolone (meth il pred NIS oh lone)

Brand Names: U.S. A-Methapred; Depo-Medrol; Medrol; Medrol (Pak); Solu-MEDROL

Index Terms 6-α-Methylprednisolone; A-Methapred; Medrol Dose Pack; Methylprednisolone Acetate; Methylprednisolone Sodium Succinate; Solumedrol

Pharmacologic Category Corticosteroid, Systemic

Medication Safety Issues

Sound-alike/look-alike issues:

MethylPREDNISolone may be confused with medroxyPROGESTERone, methotrexate, methylTESTOSTERone, predniSONE

Depo-Medrol may be confused with Solu-Medrol

Medrol may be confused with Mebaral®

Solu-MEDROL may be confused with salmeterol, Solu-CORTEF

International issues:

Medrol [U.S., Canada, and multiple international markets] may be confused with Medral brand name for omeprazole [Mexico]

Pregnancy Risk Factor C

Lactation Enters breast milk/use caution

Breast-Feeding Considerations Corticosteroids are excreted in human milk. The manufacturer notes that when used systemically, maternal use of corticosteroids have the potential to cause adverse events in a nursing infant (eg, growth suppression, interfere with endogenous corticosteroid production) and therefore recommends a decision be made whether to discontinue nursing or to discontinue the drug, taking into account the importance of treatment to the mother. If there is concern about exposure to the infant, some guidelines recommend waiting 4 hours after the maternal dose of an oral systemic corticosteroid before breast-feeding in order to decrease potential exposure to the nursing infant (based on a study using prednisolone) (Bae, 2011; Leachman, 2006; Makol, 2011; Ost, 1985). Other guidelines note that maternal use of systemic corticosteroids is not a contraindication to breast-feeding (NAEPP, 2005).

Use Primarily as an anti-inflammatory or immunosuppressant agent in the treatment of a variety of diseases including those of hematologic, allergic, inflammatory, neoplastic, and autoimmune origin. Prevention and treatment of graft-versus-host disease following allogeneic bone marrow transplantation.

Unlabeled Use Acute spinal cord injury

Mechanism of Action/Effect In a tissue-specific manner, corticosteroids regulate gene expression subsequent to binding specific intracellular receptors and translocation into the nucleus. Corticosteroids exert a wide array of physiologic effects, including modulation of carbohydrate, protein, and lipid metabolism, and maintenance of fluid and electrolyte homeostasis. Moreover, cardiovascular, immunologic, musculoskeletal, endocrine, and neurologic physiology are influenced by corticosteroids.

Contraindications Hypersensitivity to methylprednisolone or any component of the formulation; systemic fungal infection (except intra-articular injection in localized joint conditions); administration of live virus vaccines. methylprednisolone formulations containing benzyl alcohol preservative are contraindicated in premature infants; I.M. administration in idiopathic thrombocytopenia purpura; intrathecal administration

Warnings/Precautions Use with caution in patients with thyroid disease, hepatic impairment, renal impairment, cardiovascular disease, diabetes, glaucoma, cataracts, myasthenia gravis, patients at risk for osteoporosis, patients at risk for seizures, or GI diseases (diverticulitis, peptic ulcer, ulcerative colitis) due to perforation risk. Not recommended for the treatment of optic neuritis; may increase frequency of new episodes. Use caution following acute MI (corticosteroids have been associated with myocardial rupture). Cardiomegaly and congestive heart failure have been reported following concurrent use of amphotericin B and hydrocortisone for the management of fungal infections.

Because of the risk of adverse effects, systemic corticosteroids should be used cautiously in the elderly in the smallest possible effective dose for the shortest duration. May affect growth velocity; growth should be routinely monitored in pediatric patients. Withdraw therapy with gradual tapering of dose.

May cause hypercorticism or suppression of hypothalamic-pituitary-adrenal (HPA) axis, particularly in younger children or in patients receiving high doses for prolonged periods. HPA axis suppression may lead to adrenal crisis. Withdrawal and discontinuation of a corticosteroid should be done slowly and carefully. Particular care is required when patients are transferred from systemic corticosteroids to inhaled products due to possible adrenal insufficiency or withdrawal from steroids, including an increase in allergic symptoms. Patients receiving >20 mg per day of prednisone (or equivalent) may be most susceptible. Fatalities have occurred due to adrenal insufficiency in asthmatic patients during and after transfer from systemic corticosteroids to aerosol steroids; aerosol steroids do not provide the systemic steroid needed to treat patients having trauma, surgery, or infections.

Acute myopathy has been reported with high dose corticosteroids, usually in patients with neuromuscular transmission disorders; may involve ocular and/or respiratory muscles; monitor creatine kinase; recovery may be delayed. Corticosteroid use may cause psychiatric disturbances, including depression, euphoria, insomnia, mood swings, and personality changes. Pre-existing psychiatric conditions may be exacerbated by corticosteroid use. Prolonged use of corticosteroids may also increase the incidence of secondary infection, cause activation of latent infections, mask acute infection (including fungal infections), prolong or exacerbate viral or parasitic infections, or limit response to vaccines. Exposure to chickenpox or measles should be avoided; corticosteroids should not be used to treat ocular herpes simplex. Corticosteroids should not be used for cerebral malaria or viral hepatitis. Close observation is required in patients with latent tuberculosis and/or TB reactivity; restrict use in active TB (only in conjunction with antituberculosis treatment). Amebiasis should be ruled out in any patient with recent travel to tropic climates or unexplained diarrhea prior to initiation of corticosteroids. Prolonged treatment with corticosteroids has been associated with the development of Kaposi's sarcoma (case reports); discontinuation may result in clinical improvement.

High-dose corticosteroids should not be used to manage acute head injury. Rare cases of anaphylactoid reactions have been observed in patients receiving corticosteroids. Avoid injection or leakage into the dermis; dermal and/or subdermal skin depression may occur at the site of injection. Avoid deltoid muscle injection; subcutaneous atrophy may occur. Some dosage forms contain benzyl alcohol which has been associated with "gasping syndrome" in neonates.

Drug Interactions

Avoid Concomitant Use

Avoid concomitant use of MethylPREDNISolone with any of the following: Aldesleukin; BCG; Indium 111 Capromab Pendetide; Mifepristone; Natalizumab; Pimecrolimus; Pimozide; Tacrolimus (Topical); Tofacitinib

Decreased Effect

MethylPREDNISolone may decrease the levels/effects of: Aldesleukin; Antidiabetic Agents; BCG; Calcitriol; Coccidioidin Skin Test; Corticorelin; CycloSPORINE (Systemic); Hyaluronidase; Indium 111 Capromab Pendetide; Isoniazid; Salicylates; Sipuleucel-T; Telaprevir; Urea Cycle Disorder Agents; Vaccines (Inactivated)

The levels/effects of MethylPREDNISolone may be decreased by: Aminoglutethimide; Antacids; Barbiturates; Bile Acid Sequestrants; CarBAMazepine; Echinacea; Fosphenytoin; Mifepristone; Mitotane; Phenytoin; Primidone; Rifamycin Derivatives

Increased Effect/Toxicity

MethylPREDNISolone may increase the levels/effects of: Acetylcholinesterase Inhibitors; Amphotericin B; ARIPiprazole; CycloSPORINE (Systemic); Deferasirox; Dofetilide; Leflunomide; Lomitapide; Loop Diuretics; Natalizumab; NSAID (COX-2 Inhibitor); NSAID (Nonselective); Pimozide; Thiazide Diuretics; Tofacitinib; Vaccines (Live); Warfarin

The levels/effects of MethylPREDNISolone may be increased by: Antifungal Agents (Azole Derivatives, Systemic); Aprepitant; Calcium Channel Blockers (Nondihydropyridine); CycloSPORINE (Systemic); CYP3A4 Inhibitors (Strong); Denosumab; Estrogen Derivatives; Fluconazole; Fosaprepitant; Indacaterol; Macrolide Antibiotics; Mifepristone; Neuromuscular-Blocking Agents (Nondepolarizing); Pimecrolimus; Quinolone Antibiotics; Roflumilast; Salicylates; Tacrolimus (Topical); Telaprevir; Trastuzumab

Nutritional/Ethanol Interactions

Ethanol: Ethanol may increase gastric mucosal irritation. Management: Avoid ethanol.

Food: Methylprednisolone interferes with calcium absorption. May cause GI upset. Management: Administer with food. Limit caffeine.

Herb/Nutraceutical: St John's wort may decrease methylprednisolone levels. Cat's claw and echinacea have immunostimulant properties. Management: Avoid St John's wort, cat's claw, and echinacea.

Adverse Reactions Frequency not defined.

Cardiovascular: Arrhythmias, bradycardia, cardiac arrest, cardiomegaly, circulatory collapse, congestive heart failure, edema, fat embolism, hypertension, hypertrophic cardiomyopathy in premature infants, myocardial rupture (post MI), syncope, tachycardia, thromboembolism, vasculitis

Central nervous system: Delirium, depression, emotional instability, euphoria, hallucinations, headache, intracranial pressure increased, insomnia, malaise, mood swings, nervousness, neuritis, personality changes, psychic disorders, pseudotumor cerebri (usually following discontinuation), seizure, vertigo

Dermatologic: Acne, allergic dermatitis, alopecia, dry scaly skin, ecchymoses, edema, erythema, hirsutism, hyper-/hypopigmentation, hypertrichosis, impaired wound healing, petechiae, rash, skin atrophy, sterile abscess, skin test reaction impaired, striae, urticaria

Endocrine & metabolic: Adrenal suppression, amenorrhea, carbohydrate intolerance increased, Cushing's syndrome, diabetes mellitus, fluid retention, glucose intolerance, growth suppression (children), hyperglycemia, hyperlipidemia, hypokalemia, hypokalemic alkalosis, menstrual irregularities, negative nitrogen balance, pituitary-adrenal axis suppression, protein catabolism, sodium and water retention

Gastrointestinal: Abdominal distention, appetite increased, bowel/bladder dysfunction (after intrathecal administration), gastrointestinal hemorrhage, gastrointestinal perforation, nausea, pancreatitis, peptic ulcer, perforation of the small and large intestine, ulcerative esophagitis, vomiting, weight gain

Hematologic: Leukocytosis (transient)

Hepatic: Hepatomegaly, transaminases increased

Local: Postinjection flare (intra-articular use), thrombophlebitis

Neuromuscular & skeletal: Arthralgia, arthropathy, aseptic necrosis (femoral and humoral heads), fractures, muscle mass loss, muscle weakness, myopathy (particularly in conjunction with neuromuscular disease or neuromuscular-blocking agents), neuropathy, osteoporosis, parasthesia, tendon rupture, vertebral compression fractures, weakness

Ocular: Cataracts, exophthalmoses, glaucoma, intraocular pressure increased

Renal: Glycosuria

Respiratory: Pulmonary edema

Miscellaneous: Abnormal fat disposition, anaphylactoid reaction, anaphylaxis, angioedema, avascular necrosis, diaphoresis, hiccups, hypersensitivity reactions, infections, secondary malignancy

Pharmacodynamics/Kinetics

Onset of Action Peak effect (route dependent): Oral: 1-2 hours; I.M.: 4-8 days; Intra-articular: 1 week; methylprednisolone sodium succinate is highly soluble and has a rapid effect by I.M. and I.V. routes

Duration of Action Route dependent: Oral: 30-36 hours; I.M.: 1-4 weeks; Intra-articular: 1-5 weeks; methylprednisolone acetate has a low solubility and has a sustained I.M. effect

Available Dosage Forms

Solution Reconstituted, Injection:
A-Methapred: 40 mg (1 ea); 125 mg (1 ea)
Solu-MEDROL: 500 mg (1 ea); 1000 mg (1 ea); 2 g (1 ea)
Generic: 40 mg (1 ea); 125 mg (1 ea); 500 mg (1 ea); 1000 mg (1 ea); 1 g (1 ea)

Solution Reconstituted, Injection [preservative free]:
Solu-MEDROL: 40 mg (1 ea); 125 mg (1 ea); 500 mg (1 ea); 1000 mg (1 ea)

Suspension, Injection:
Depo-Medrol: 20 mg/mL (5 mL); 40 mg/mL (1 mL, 5 mL, 10 mL); 80 mg/mL (1 mL, 5 mL)
Generic: 40 mg/mL (1 mL, 5 mL, 10 mL); 80 mg/mL (1 mL, 5 mL)

Tablet, Oral:
Medrol: 2 mg, 4 mg, 8 mg, 16 mg, 32 mg
Medrol (Pak): 4 mg
Generic: 4 mg, 8 mg, 16 mg, 32 mg

General Dosage Range

I.M.:
Acetate: *Adults:* 10-120 mg every 1-2 weeks
Sodium succinate:
Children: 0.5-1.7 mg/kg/day **or** 5-25 mg/m²/day divided every 6-12 hours; "Pulse" therapy: 15-30 mg/kg/dose given once daily for 3 days
Adults: 10-80 mg once daily

I.V. (sodium succinate): *Children and Adults:* Dosage varies greatly by indication

Intra-articular (acetate): *Adults:* Administer every 1-5 weeks
Large joints (eg, knee, ankle): 20-80 mg
Medium joints (eg, elbow, wrist): 10-40 mg
Small joints: 4-10 mg

Intralesional (acetate): *Adults:* 20-60 mg every 1-5 weeks

Oral:
Children: 0.5-1.7 mg/kg/day **or** 5-25 mg/m²/day divided every 6-12 hours; "Pulse" therapy: 15-30 mg/kg/dose once daily for 3 days
Adults: 2-60 mg/day in 1-4 divided doses

Administration

I.V. Only sodium succinate formulation may be given I.V. Acetate salt should not be given I.V.

Parenteral: Methylprednisolone sodium succinate may be administered I.M. or I.V.; I.V. administration may be IVP over one to several minutes or IVPB or continuous I.V. infusion. Avoid injection or leakage into the dermis; dermal and/or subdermal skin depression may occur at the site of injection.

I.V.: Succinate:
  Low dose: ≤1.8 mg/kg or ≤125 mg/dose: I.V. push over 3-15 minutes
  Moderate dose: ≥2 mg/kg or 250 mg/dose: I.V. over 15-30 minutes
  High dose: 15 mg/kg or ≥500 mg/dose: I.V. over ≥30 minutes
    Doses >15 mg/kg or ≥1 g: Administer over 1 hour
  Do **not** administer high-dose I.V. push; hypotension, cardiac arrhythmia, and sudden death have been reported in patients given high-dose methylprednisolone I.V. push (>0.5 g over <10 minutes). Intermittent infusion over 15-60 minutes; maximum concentration: I.V. push 125 mg/mL.

I.M.: Avoid injection into the deltoid muscle due to a high incidence of subcutaneous atrophy. Avoid injection or leakage into the dermis; dermal and/or subdermal skin depression may occur at the site of injection. Do not inject into areas that have evidence of acute local infection.

Injectable Detail pH: 7-8 (adjusted with sodium hydroxide)

Oral Administer with meals to decrease GI upset. Give daily dose in the morning to mimic normal peak blood levels.

Topical For external use only. Apply sparingly.

Preparation for Administration
Standard diluent (Solu-Medrol®): 40 mg/50 mL D₅W; 125 mg/50 mL D₅W.
Minimum volume (Solu-Medrol®): 50 mL D₅W.

Storage/Stability Intact vials of methylprednisolone sodium succinate should be stored at controlled room temperature of 20°C to 25°C (68°F to 77°F). Protect from light. Reconstituted solutions of methylprednisolone sodium succinate should be stored at room temperature of 20°C to 25°C (68°F to 77°F) and used within 48 hours. Stability of parenteral admixture at room temperature (25°C) and at refrigeration temperature (4°C) is 48 hours.

Nursing Actions

Physical Assessment Teach patients to report infection and adrenal suppression. Instruct patients with diabetes to monitor serum glucose levels closely; corticosteroids can alter glycemic response. Dose may need to be increased if patient is experiencing higher than normal levels of stress. When discontinuing, taper dose and frequency slowly.

Patient Education
• Discuss specific use of drug and side effects with patient as it relates to treatment. HCAHPS: During this hospital stay, were you given any medicine that you had not taken before? Before giving you any new medicine, how often did

hospital staff tell you what the medicine was for? How often did hospital staff describe possible side effects in a way you could understand?)
• Patient may experience nausea, insomnia, akathisia, or hyperhidrosis. Have patient report immediately to prescriber signs of infection, signs of hyperglycemia, signs of hypokalemia, signs of pancreatitis, severe asthenia, irritability, tremors, tachycardia, confusion, dizziness, dyspnea, excessive weight gain or loss, edema of extremities, skin changes, moon face, buffalo hump, significant headache, angina, menstrual irregularities, osteodynia, arthralgia, vision changes, mood changes, behavioral changes, depression, paresthesia, ecchymosis, hemorrhaging, intolerable dyspepsia, melena, hematemesis, injection site irritation, or blindness (HCAHPS).
• Educate patient about signs of a significant reaction (eg, wheezing; chest tightness; fever; itching; bad cough; blue skin color; seizures; or swelling of face, lips, tongue, or throat). **Note:** This is not a comprehensive list of all side effects. Patient should consult prescriber for additional questions.

Intended Use and Disclaimer: Should not be printed and given to patients. This information is intended to serve as a concise initial reference for healthcare professionals to use when discussing medications with a patient. You must ultimately rely on your own discretion, experience and judgment in diagnosing, treating and advising patients.

Dietary Considerations Take with meals to decrease GI upset; need diet rich in pyridoxine, vitamin C, vitamin D, folate, calcium, phosphorus, and protein.

MethylTESTOSTERone
(meth il tes TOS te rone)

Brand Names: U.S. Android; Methitest; Testred
Pharmacologic Category Androgen
Medication Safety Issues
  Sound-alike/look-alike issues:
  MethylTESTOSTERone may be confused with medroxyPROGESTERone, methylPREDNISolone
  BEERS Criteria medication:
  This drug may be potentially inappropriate for use in geriatric patients (Quality of evidence - moderate; Strength of recommendation - weak).

Pregnancy Risk Factor X
Lactation Excretion in breast milk unknown/not recommended
Use
Male: Hypogonadism; delayed puberty; impotence and climacteric symptoms
Female: Palliative treatment of metastatic breast cancer

▶

◀ **Unlabeled Use** Hypogonadism (male); delayed puberty (male)

Controlled Substance C-III

Available Dosage Forms

Capsule, Oral:
Android: 10 mg
Testred: 10 mg

Tablet, Oral:
Methitest: 10 mg

General Dosage Range

Oral:
Adults (females): 50-200 mg/day
Adults (males): 10-50 mg/day

Nursing Actions

Physical Assessment Assess potential for interactions with other pharmacological agents patient may be taking (eg, effects of hypoglycemic agents may be increased). Monitor for virilism (male and female), edema, CNS changes (anxiety, depression), acne, baldness, GI irritation, leukopenia, and hepatic dysfunction frequently during therapy. Caution patients with diabetes; effects of hypoglycemic agents may be increased.

Patient Education

- Discuss specific use of drug and side effects with patient as it relates to treatment. (HCAHPS: During this hospital stay, were you given any medicine that you had not taken before? Before giving you any new medicine, how often did hospital staff tell you what the medicine was for? How often did hospital staff describe possible side effects in a way you could understand?)
- Patient may experience acne, emotional instability, nausea, impotence, macromastia, or breast soreness. Have patient report immediately to prescriber significant weight gain, erection lasting >4 hours, severe edema, urinary retention, considerable nervousness and anxiety, asthenia, discolored urine, jaundice, dysphonia, hirsutism, menstrual changes, or rash (HCAHPS).
- Educate patient about signs of a significant reaction (eg, wheezing; chest tightness; fever; itching; bad cough; blue skin color; seizures; or swelling of face, lips, tongue, or throat). **Note:** This is not a comprehensive list of all side effects. Patient should consult prescriber for additional questions.

Intended Use and Disclaimer: Should not be printed and given to patients. This information is intended to serve as a concise initial reference for healthcare professionals to use when discussing medications with a patient. You must ultimately rely on your own discretion, experience and judgment in diagnosing, treating and advising patients.

Metoclopramide (met oh KLOE pra mide)

Brand Names: U.S. Metozolv ODT; Reglan

Pharmacologic Category Antiemetic; Gastrointestinal Agent, Prokinetic

Medication Safety Issues

Sound-alike/look-alike issues:
Metoclopramide may be confused with metolazone, metoprolol, metroNIDAZOLE
Reglan may be confused with Megace, Regonol, Renagel, Regitine

BEERS Criteria medication:
This drug may be potentially inappropriate for use in geriatric patients (Quality of evidence - moderate; Strength of recommendation - strong).

Medication Guide Available Yes

Pregnancy Risk Factor B

Lactation Enters breast milk/use caution

Breast-Feeding Considerations Metoclopramide enters breast milk. Information is available from studies conducted in mothers nursing preterm infants (n=14; delivered at 23-34 weeks gestation) or term infants (n=18) and taking metoclopramide 10 mg 3 times daily. The median concentration of metoclopramide in breast milk was ~45 ng/mL in the preterm infants and the mean concentration was ~48 ng/mL in the full term infants. The authors of both studies calculated the relative infant dose to be 3% to 5%, based on a therapeutic infant dose of 0.5 mg/kg/day. Metoclopramide was also detected in the serum of one nursing full term infant (Hansen, 2005; Kauppila, 1983). Metoclopramide may increase prolactin concentrations and cause galactorrhea and gynecomastia, but studies which evaluated its use to increase milk production for women who want to nurse have had mixed results. In addition, due to the potential for adverse events, nonpharmacologic measure should be considered prior to the use of medications as galactagogues (ABM, 2011). The manufacturer recommends that caution be used if administered to a nursing woman.

Use

Oral: Symptomatic treatment of diabetic gastroparesis; gastroesophageal reflux

I.V., I.M.: Symptomatic treatment of diabetic gastroparesis; postpyloric placement of enteral feeding tubes; prevention and/or treatment of nausea and vomiting associated with chemotherapy, or postsurgery; to stimulate gastric emptying and intestinal transit of barium during radiological examination of the stomach/small intestine

Unlabeled Use Management of gastroparesis (regardless of etiology)

Mechanism of Action/Effect Blocks dopamine receptors and (when given in higher doses) also blocks serotonin receptors in chemoreceptor trigger zone of the CNS; enhances the response to acetylcholine of tissue in upper GI tract causing enhanced motility and accelerated gastric emptying without stimulating gastric, biliary, or pancreatic secretions; increases lower esophageal sphincter tone

Contraindications Hypersensitivity to metoclopramide or any component of the formulation; GI obstruction, perforation or hemorrhage; pheochromocytoma; history of seizures or concomitant use of other agents likely to increase extrapyramidal reactions

Warnings/Precautions [U.S. Boxed Warning]: May cause tardive dyskinesia, which is often irreversible; duration of treatment and total cumulative dose are associated with an increased risk. Therapy durations >12 weeks should be avoided (except in rare cases following risk:benefit assessment). Risk appears to be increased in the elderly, women, and diabetics; however, it is not possible to predict which patients will develop tardive dyskinesia. Therapy should be discontinued in any patient if signs/symptoms of tardive dyskinesia appear.

May cause extrapyramidal symptoms, generally manifested as acute dystonic reactions within the initial 24-48 hours of use. Risk of these reactions is increased at higher doses, and in pediatric patients, and adults <30 years of age. Pseudoparkinsonism (eg, bradykinesia, tremor, rigidity) may also occur (usually within first 6 months of therapy) and is generally reversible following discontinuation. Use with caution or avoid in patients with Parkinson's disease. Avoid use in older adults (except for gastroparesis) due to risk of extrapyramidal effects, including tardive dyskinesia; risk potentially even greater in frail older adults (Beers Criteria). In addition, risk of tardive dyskinesia may be increased in older women. Neuroleptic malignant syndrome (NMS) has been reported (rarely) with metoclopramide.

May cause transient increase in serum aldosterone; use caution in patients who are at risk of fluid overload (HF, cirrhosis). Use caution in patients with hypertension or following surgical anastomosis/closure. Use caution with a history of mental illness; has been associated with depression. Abrupt discontinuation may (rarely) result in withdrawal symptoms (dizziness, headache, nervousness). Use caution and adjust dose in renal impairment. Patients with NADH-cytochrome b5 reductase deficiency are at increased risk of methemoglobinemia and/or sulfhemoglobinemia. Neonates may have an increased risk of methemoglobinemia due to decreased levels of NADH-cytochrome b5 reductase deficiency and prolonged clearance of metoclopramide.

Drug Interactions

Avoid Concomitant Use

Avoid concomitant use of Metoclopramide with any of the following: Antipsychotics; Droperidol; Promethazine; Tetrabenazine; Trimetazidine

Decreased Effect

Metoclopramide may decrease the levels/effects of: Anti-Parkinson's Agents (Dopamine Agonist); Atovaquone; Posaconazole; Quinagolide

The levels/effects of Metoclopramide may be decreased by: Peginterferon Alfa-2b

Increased Effect/Toxicity

Metoclopramide may increase the levels/effects of: Antipsychotics; CycloSPORINE (Systemic); Prilocaine; Promethazine; Selective Serotonin Reuptake Inhibitors; Sodium Nitrite; Tetrabenazine; Tricyclic Antidepressants; Trimetazidine; Venlafaxine

The levels/effects of Metoclopramide may be increased by: Droperidol; Metyrosine; Nitric Oxide; Serotonin Modulators

Nutritional/Ethanol Interactions Ethanol: Avoid ethanol (may increase CNS depression).

Adverse Reactions Frequency not always defined.

Cardiovascular: Atrioventricular block, bradycardia, congestive heart failure, flushing (following high I.V. doses), hypertension, hypotension, supraventricular tachycardia

Central nervous system: Drowsiness (~10% to 70%; dose related), dystonic reaction (<1% to 25%; dose and age related), lassitude (~10%), restlessness (~10%), fatigue (2% to 10%), headache (4% to 5%), dizziness (1% to 4%), somnolence (2% to 3%), akathisia, confusion, depression, drug-induced Parkinson's disease, hallucination (rare), insomnia, neuroleptic malignant syndrome (rare), seizure, suicidal ideation, tardive dyskinesia

Dermatologic: Skin rash, urticaria

Endocrine & metabolic: Amenorrhea, fluid retention, galactorrhea, gynecomastia, hyperprolactinemia, porphyria

Gastrointestinal: Nausea (4% to 6%), vomiting (1% to 2%), diarrhea

Genitourinary: Impotence, urinary frequency, urinary incontinence

Hematologic & oncologic: Agranulocytosis, leukopenia, methemoglobinemia, neutropenia, sulfhemoglobinemia

Hepatic: Hepatotoxicity (rare)

Hypersensitivity: Angioedema (rare), hypersensitivity reaction

Neuromuscular & skeletal: Laryngospasm (rare)

Ophthalmic: Visual disturbance

Respiratory: Bronchospasm, laryngeal edema (rare)

Pharmacodynamics/Kinetics

Onset of Action Oral: 30-60 minutes; I.V.: 1-3 minutes; I.M.: 10-15 minutes

Duration of Action Therapeutic: 1-2 hours, regardless of route

Available Dosage Forms

Solution, Injection:

Generic: 5 mg/mL (2 mL)

Solution, Injection [preservative free]:

Generic: 5 mg/mL (2 mL)

Solution, Oral:
Generic: 5 mg/5 mL (10 mL, 473 mL); 10 mg/10 mL (10 mL)
Tablet, Oral:
Reglan: 5 mg, 10 mg
Generic: 5 mg, 10 mg
Tablet Dispersible, Oral:
Metozolv ODT: 5 mg
General Dosage Range Dosage adjustment recommended in patients with renal impairment
I.M.: *Adults:* 10-20 mg as a single dose **or** 10 mg before each meal and at bedtime
I.V.:
Children <6 years: 0.1 mg/kg as a single dose
Children 6-14 years: 2.5-5 mg as a single dose
Children >14 years: 10 mg as a single dose
Adults: 10 mg before each meal and at bedtime **or** 1-2 mg/kg every 2-3 hours (maximum: 5 doses daily) **or** 10 mg as a single dose
Oral: *Adults:* 10-15 mg up to 4 times daily
Administration
I.M. May be administered I.M.
I.V. Injection solution may be given I.M., direct I.V. push, short infusion (15-30 minutes), or continuous infusion; lower doses (≤10 mg) of metoclopramide can be given I.V. push undiluted over 1-2 minutes; higher doses (>10 mg) to be diluted in 50 mL of compatible solution (preferably NS) and given IVPB over at least 15 minutes; continuous SubQ infusion and rectal administration have been reported. **Note:** Rapid I.V. administration may be associated with a transient (but intense) feeling of anxiety and restlessness, followed by drowsiness.
Injectable Detail pH: 3-6.5
Oral Orally-disintegrating tablets: Administer on an empty stomach at least 30 minutes prior to food. Do not remove from packaging until time of administration. If tablet breaks or crumbles while handling, discard and remove new tablet. Using dry hands, place tablet on tongue and allow to dissolve. Swallow with saliva.
Other Continuous SubQ infusion and rectal administration have been reported
Preparation for Administration Injection solution: Lower doses (≤10 mg): No dilution required; Higher doses (>10 mg): Dilute in 50 mL of compatible solution (preferably NS).
Storage/Stability
Injection solution: Store intact vial at controlled room temperature; injection is photosensitive and should be protected from light during storage; parenteral admixtures in D_5W or NS are stable for at least 24 hours and do not require light protection if used within 24 hours.
Tablet: Store at controlled room temperature of 20°C to 25°C (68°F to 77°F).
Nursing Actions
Physical Assessment Monitor vital signs during intravenous administration. Inpatients should use safety measures to prevent falls (eg, side rails up, call light within reach) and caution patient to call for assistance with ambulation. Monitor and report abnormal movements of the facial muscles, mouth, tongue, limbs, or pelvis. Report signs of restlessness or parkinsonism. Check for any sexual side effects such as missed menses, enlarged breasts or breast discharge, and sexual changes.
Patient Education
- Discuss specific use of drug and side effects with patient as it relates to treatment. (HCAHPS: During this hospital stay, were you given any medicine that you had not taken before? Before giving you any new medicine, how often did hospital staff tell you what the medicine was for? How often did hospital staff describe possible side effects in a way you could understand?)
- Patient may experience presyncope, fatigue, blurred vision, illogical thinking, headache, dyspepsia, diarrhea, anxiety, or insomnia. Have patient report immediately to prescriber tachycardia, severe dizziness, fasciculations, tremors, or rash (HCAHPS).
- Educate patient about signs of a significant reaction (eg, wheezing; chest tightness; fever; itching; bad cough; blue skin color; seizures; or swelling of face, lips, tongue, or throat). **Note:** This is not a comprehensive list of all side effects. Patient should consult prescriber for additional questions.

Intended Use and Disclaimer: Should not be printed and given to patients. This information is intended to serve as a concise initial reference for healthcare professionals to use when discussing medications with a patient. You must ultimately rely on your own discretion, experience and judgment in diagnosing, treating and advising patients.

Metolazone (me TOLE a zone)

Brand Names: U.S. Zaroxolyn
Pharmacologic Category Diuretic, Thiazide-Related
Medication Safety Issues
Sound-alike/look-alike issues:
Metolazone may be confused with metaxalone, methadone, methazolamide, methimazole, methotrexate, metoclopramide, metoprolol, minoxidil
Zaroxolyn may be confused with Zarontin
Pregnancy Risk Factor B
Lactation Enters breast milk/not recommended
Breast-Feeding Considerations It is not known if metolazone is excreted in breast milk. Due to the potential for serious adverse reactions in the nursing infant, a decision should be made whether to discontinue nursing or to discontinue the drug, taking into account the importance of treatment to the mother.

Use Management of mild-to-moderate hypertension; treatment of edema in heart failure and nephrotic syndrome, impaired renal function

Mechanism of Action/Effect Inhibits sodium reabsorption in the distal tubules causing increased excretion of sodium and water, as well as, potassium and hydrogen ions

Contraindications Hypersensitivity to metolazone, any component of the formulation, other thiazides, and sulfonamide derivatives; anuria; hepatic coma; pregnancy (expert analysis)

Warnings/Precautions Electrolyte disturbances (hypokalemia, hypochloremic alkalosis, hyponatremia) can occur. Large or prolonged fluid and electrolyte losses may occur with concomitant furosemide administration. Use with caution in severe hepatic dysfunction; hepatic encephalopathy can be caused by electrolyte disturbances. Gout can be precipitate in certain patients with a history of gout, a familial predisposition to gout, or chronic renal failure. Cautious use in patients with prediabetes or diabetes; may see a change in glucose control. Can cause SLE exacerbation or activation. Use caution in severe renal impairment. Use with caution in patients with moderate or high cholesterol concentrations. Photosensitization may occur.

Chemical similarities are present among sulfonamides, sulfonylureas, carbonic anhydrase inhibitors, thiazides, and loop diuretics (except ethacrynic acid). Use in patients with thiazide or sulfonamide allergy is specifically contraindicated in product labeling, however, a risk of cross-reaction exists in patients with allergy to any of these compounds; avoid use when previous reaction has been severe. Discontinue if signs of hypersensitivity are noted.

Drug Interactions

Avoid Concomitant Use

Avoid concomitant use of Metolazone with any of the following: Dofetilide

Decreased Effect

Metolazone may decrease the levels/effects of: Antidiabetic Agents

The levels/effects of Metolazone may be decreased by: Bile Acid Sequestrants; Herbs (Hypertensive Properties); Methylphenidate; Nonsteroidal Anti-Inflammatory Agents; Yohimbine

Increased Effect/Toxicity

Metolazone may increase the levels/effects of: ACE Inhibitors; Allopurinol; Amifostine; Antihypertensives; Calcium Salts; CarBAMazepine; Diazoxide; Dofetilide; DULoxetine; Hypotensive Agents; Ivabradine; Lithium; Multivitamins/Minerals (with ADEK, Folate, Iron); Multivitamins/Minerals (with AE, No Iron); Obinutuzumab; OXcarbazepine; Porfimer; RiTUXimab; Sodium Phosphates; Topiramate; Toremifene; Vitamin D Analogs

The levels/effects of Metolazone may be increased by: Alcohol (Ethyl); Alfuzosin; Analgesics (Opioid); Anticholinergic Agents; Barbiturates; Beta2-Agonists; Brimonidine (Topical); Corticosteroids (Orally Inhaled); Corticosteroids (Systemic); Herbs (Hypotensive Properties); Licorice; MAO Inhibitors; Multivitamins/Fluoride (with ADE); Pentoxifylline; Phosphodiesterase 5 Inhibitors; Prostacyclin Analogues; Selective Serotonin Reuptake Inhibitors

Nutritional/Ethanol Interactions

Ethanol: May potentiate hypotensive effect of metazolone.

Herb/Nutraceutical: Avoid herbs with *hypertensive* properties (bayberry, blue cohosh, cayenne, ephedra, ginger, ginseng [American], kola, licorice); may diminish the antihypertensive effect of metolazone. Avoid herbs with *hypotensive* properties (black cohosh, California poppy, coleus, golden seal, hawthorn, mistletoe, periwinkle, quinine, shepherd's purse); may enhance the hypotensive effect of metolazone.

Adverse Reactions Frequency not defined.

Cardiovascular: Chest pain/discomfort, necrotizing angiitis, orthostatic hypotension, palpitation, syncope, venous thrombosis, vertigo, volume depletion

Central nervous system: Chills, depression, dizziness, drowsiness, fatigue, headache, lightheadedness, restlessness

Dermatologic: Petechiae, photosensitivity, pruritus, purpura, rash, skin necrosis, Stevens-Johnson syndrome, toxic epidermal necrolysis, urticaria

Endocrine & metabolic: Gout attacks, hypercalcemia, hyperglycemia, hyperuricemia, hypochloremia, hypochloremic alkalosis, hypokalemia, hypomagnesemia, hyponatremia, hypophosphatemia

Gastrointestinal: Abdominal bloating, abdominal pain, anorexia, constipation, diarrhea, epigastric distress, nausea, pancreatitis, vomiting, xerostomia

Genitourinary: Impotence

Hematologic: Agranulocytosis, aplastic/hypoplastic anemia, hemoconcentration, leukopenia, thrombocytopenia

Hepatic: Cholestatic jaundice, hepatitis

Neuromuscular & skeletal: Joint pain, muscle cramps/spasm, neuropathy, paresthesia, weakness

Ocular: Blurred vision (transient)

Renal: BUN increased, glucosuria

Pharmacodynamics/Kinetics

Onset of Action Diuresis: ~60 minutes

Duration of Action ≥24 hours

Available Dosage Forms

Tablet, Oral:
Zaroxolyn: 2.5 mg, 5 mg
Generic: 2.5 mg, 5 mg, 10 mg

General Dosage Range Oral: *Adults:* 2.5-20 mg every 24 hours

◀ **Administration**

Oral May be taken with food or milk. Take early in day to avoid nocturia. Take the last dose of multiple doses no later than 6 PM unless instructed otherwise.

Nursing Actions

Physical Assessment Patient's renal status and allergy history (thiazides and sulfonamide derivatives) should be assessed prior to beginning therapy. Assess electrolytes and renal function. Monitor for hypersensitivity reactions, electrolyte imbalance, and hypotension.

Patient Education

• Discuss specific use of drug and side effects with patient as it relates to treatment. (HCAHPS: During this hospital stay, were you given any medicine that you had not taken before? Before giving you any new medicine, how often did hospital staff tell you what the medicine was for? How often did hospital staff describe possible side effects in a way you could understand?)

• Patient may experience hypokalemia, dizziness, nausea, xerostomia, or erythema. Have patient report immediately to prescriber rash (HCAHPS).

• Educate patient about signs of a significant reaction (eg, wheezing; chest tightness; fever; itching; bad cough; blue skin color; seizures; or swelling of face, lips, tongue, or throat). **Note:** This is not a comprehensive list of all side effects. Patient should consult prescriber for additional questions.

Intended Use and Disclaimer: Should not be printed and given to patients. This information is intended to serve as a concise initial reference for healthcare professionals to use when discussing medications with a patient. You must ultimately rely on your own discretion, experience and judgment in diagnosing, treating and advising patients.

Dietary Considerations Should be taken after breakfast; may require potassium supplementation

Metoprolol (me toe PROE lole)

Brand Names: U.S. Lopressor; Toprol XL

Index Terms Metoprolol Succinate; Metoprolol Tartrate

Pharmacologic Category Antianginal Agent; Antihypertensive; Beta-Blocker, Beta-1 Selective

Medication Safety Issues

Sound-alike/look-alike issues:

Lopressor may be confused with Lyrica

Metoprolol may be confused with metaproterenol, metoclopramide, metolazone, misoprostol

Metoprolol succinate may be confused with metoprolol tartrate

Toprol-XL may be confused with TEGretol, TEGretol-XR, Topamax

High alert medication:

The Institute for Safe Medication Practices (ISMP) includes this medication among its list of drugs which have a heightened risk of causing significant patient harm when used in error.

Administration issues:

Significant differences exist between oral and I.V. dosing. Use caution when converting from one route of administration to another.

Pregnancy Risk Factor C

Lactation Enters breast milk/use caution

Breast-Feeding Considerations Small amounts of metoprolol can be detected in breast milk. The manufacturer recommends that caution be exercised when administering metoprolol to nursing women.

Use Treatment of angina pectoris, hypertension, or hemodynamically-stable acute myocardial infarction

Extended release: Treatment of angina pectoris or hypertension; to reduce mortality/hospitalization in patients with heart failure (HF) (stable NYHA Class II or III) already receiving ACE inhibitors, diuretics, and/or digoxin

Note: The ACCF/AHA 2013 heart failure guidelines recommend the use of 1 of 3 beta blockers (ie, bisoprolol, carvedilol, or extended-release metoprolol succinate) for all patients with recent or remote history of MI or ACS and reduced ejection fraction (rEF) to reduce mortality, for all patients with rEF to prevent symptomatic HF (even if no history of MI), and for all patients with current or prior symptoms of HF with reduced ejection fraction (HFrEF), unless contraindicated, to reduce morbidity and mortality (ACCF/AHA [Yancy, 2013]).

Unlabeled Use Treatment of ventricular arrhythmias, atrial ectopy; migraine prophylaxis, essential tremor; prevention of reinfarction and sudden death after myocardial infarction; prevention and treatment of atrial fibrillation and atrial flutter; multifocal atrial tachycardia; symptomatic treatment of hypertrophic obstructive cardiomyopathy; management of thyrotoxicosis

Mechanism of Action/Effect Due to inhibition of beta$_1$-receptors, metoprolol reduces myocardial contractility, heart rate, and blood pressure.

Contraindications

Hypersensitivity to metoprolol, any component of the formulation, or other beta-blockers

Note: Additional contraindications are formulation and/or indication specific.

Immediate release tablets/injectable formulation:

Hypertension and angina: Sinus bradycardia; second- and third-degree heart block; cardiogenic shock; overt heart failure; sick sinus syndrome (except in patients with a functioning artificial pacemaker); severe peripheral arterial disease; pheochromocytoma (without alpha blockade)

Myocardial infarction: Severe sinus bradycardia (heart rate <45 beats/minute); significant first-degree heart block (P-R interval ≥0.24 seconds); second- and third-degree heart block; systolic blood pressure <100 mm Hg; moderate-to-severe cardiac failure

Extended release tablet: Severe bradycardia, second- and third degree heart block; cardiogenic shock; decompensated heart failure; sick sinus syndrome (except in patients with a functioning artificial pacemaker)

Warnings/Precautions [U.S. Boxed Warning]: Beta-blocker therapy should not be withdrawn abruptly (particularly in patients with CAD), but gradually tapered over 1-2 weeks to avoid acute tachycardia, hypertension, and/or ischemia. Consider pre-existing conditions such as sick sinus syndrome before initiating. Metoprolol commonly produces mild first-degree heart block (P-R interval >0.2-0.24 sec). May also produce severe first- (P-R interval ≥0.26 sec), second-, or third-degree heart block. Patients with acute MI (especially right ventricular MI) have a high risk of developing heart block of varying degrees. If severe heart block occurs, metoprolol should be discontinued and measures to increase heart rate should be employed. Symptomatic hypotension may occur with use. May precipitate or aggravate symptoms of arterial insufficiency in patients with PVD and Raynaud's disease; use with caution and monitor for progression of arterial obstruction. Potentially significant interactions may exist, requiring dose or frequency adjustment, additional monitoring, and/or selection of alternative therapy. Consult drug interactions database for more detailed information.

In general, beta-blockers should be avoided in patients with bronchospastic disease. Metoprolol, with B$_1$ selectivity, should be used cautiously in bronchospastic disease with close monitoring. Use cautiously in patients with diabetes because it can mask prominent hypoglycemic symptoms. May mask signs of hyperthyroidism (eg, tachycardia); if hyperthyroidism is suspected, carefully manage and monitor; abrupt withdrawal may exacerbate symptoms of hyperthyroidism or precipitate thyroid storm. Alterations in thyroid function tests may be observed. Use caution with hepatic dysfunction. Use with caution in patients with myasthenia gravis or psychiatric disease (may cause CNS depression). Although perioperative beta-blocker therapy is recommended prior to elective surgery in selected patients, use of high-dose extended release metoprolol in patients naïve to beta-blocker therapy undergoing noncardiac surgery has been associated with bradycardia, hypotension, stroke, and death. Chronic beta-blocker therapy should not be routinely withdrawn prior to major surgery. Use of beta-blockers may unmask

cardiac failure in patients without a history of dysfunction. Adequate alpha-blockade is required prior to use of any beta-blocker for patients with untreated pheochromocytoma. May induce or exacerbate psoriasis. Use caution with history of severe anaphylaxis to allergens; patients taking beta-blockers may become more sensitive to repeated allergen challenges. Treatment of anaphylaxis (eg, epinephrine) in patients taking beta-blockers may be ineffective or promote undesirable effects. Bradycardia may be observed more frequently in elderly patients (>65 years of age); dosage reductions may be necessary.

Extended release: Use with caution in patients with compensated heart failure; monitor for a worsening of heart failure.

Drug Interactions

Avoid Concomitant Use

Avoid concomitant use of Metoprolol with any of the following: Floctafenine; Methacholine

Decreased Effect

Metoprolol may decrease the levels/effects of: Beta2-Agonists; Theophylline Derivatives

The levels/effects of Metoprolol may be decreased by: Barbiturates; Herbs (Hypertensive Properties); Methylphenidate; Mirabegron; Nonsteroidal Anti-Inflammatory Agents; Peginterferon Alfa-2b; Rifamycin Derivatives; Yohimbine

Increased Effect/Toxicity

Metoprolol may increase the levels/effects of: Alpha-/Beta-Agonists (Direct-Acting); Alpha1-Blockers; Alpha2-Agonists; Amifostine; Antihypertensives; Antipsychotic Agents (Phenothiazines); ARIPiprazole; Bupivacaine; Cardiac Glycosides; Cholinergic Agonists; Ergot Derivatives; Fingolimod; Hypotensive Agents; Insulin; Lidocaine (Systemic); Lidocaine (Topical); Mepivacaine; Methacholine; Midodrine; Obinutuzumab; RiTUXimab; Sulfonylureas

The levels/effects of Metoprolol may be increased by: Acetylcholinesterase Inhibitors; Alpha2-Agonists; Aminoquinolines (Antimalarial); Amiodarone; Anilidopiperidine Opioids; Antipsychotic Agents (Phenothiazines); Brimonidine (Topical); Calcium Channel Blockers (Dihydropyridine); Calcium Channel Blockers (Nondihydropyridine); CYP2D6 Inhibitors; Darunavir; Diazoxide; Dipyridamole; Disopyramide; Dronedarone; Floctafenine; Herbs (Hypotensive Properties); MAO Inhibitors; Mirabegron; Pentoxifylline; Phosphodiesterase 5 Inhibitors; Propafenone; Prostacyclin Analogues; Regorafenib; Reserpine; Selective Serotonin Reuptake Inhibitors

Nutritional/Ethanol Interactions

Food: Food increases absorption. Metoprolol serum levels may be increased if taken with food. Management: Take immediate release tartrate tablets with food; succinate can be taken with or without food.

Herb/Nutraceutical: Some herbal medications may worsen hypertension (eg, licorice); others may increase the antihypertensive effect of metoprolol (eg, shepherd's purse). Management: Avoid bayberry, blue cohosh, cayenne, ephedra, ginger, ginseng (American), gotu kola, licorice, and yohimbe. Avoid black cohosh, California poppy, coleus, golden seal, hawthorn, mistletoe, periwinkle, quinine, and shepherd's purse.

Adverse Reactions Frequency may not be defined.

Cardiovascular: Hypotension (1% to 27%), bradycardia (2% to 16%), first-degree heart block (P-R interval ≥0.26 sec; 5%), arterial insufficiency (usually Raynaud type; 1%), chest pain (1%), CHF (1%), edema (peripheral; 1%), palpitation (1%), syncope (1%)

Central nervous system: Dizziness (2% to 10%), fatigue (1% to 10%), depression (5%), confusion, hallucinations, headache, insomnia, memory loss (short-term), nightmares, sleep disturbances, somnolence, vertigo

Dermatology: Pruritus (5%), rash (5%), photosensitivity, psoriasis exacerbated

Endocrine & metabolic: Libido decreased, Peyronie's disease (<1%), diabetes exacerbated

Gastrointestinal: Diarrhea (5%), constipation (1%), flatulence (1%), gastrointestinal pain (1%), heartburn (1%), nausea (1%), xerostomia (1%), vomiting

Hematologic: Claudication

Neuromuscular & skeletal: Musculoskeletal pain

Ocular: Blurred vision, visual disturbances

Otic: Tinnitus

Respiratory: Dyspnea (1% to 3%), bronchospasm (1%), wheezing (1%), rhinitis, shortness of breath

Miscellaneous: Cold extremities (1%)

Other events reported with beta-blockers: Catatonia, emotional lability, fever, hypersensitivity reactions, laryngospasm, nonthrombocytopenic purpura, respiratory distress, thrombocytopenic purpura

Pharmacodynamics/Kinetics

Onset of Action Peak effect: Oral: 1-2 hours (Regårdh, 1980); I.V.: 20 minutes (when infused over 10 minutes)

Duration of Action Oral: Immediate release: Variable (dose-related; 50% reduction in maximum heart rate after single doses of 20, 50, and 100 mg occurred at 3.3, 5, and 6.4 hours, respectively), Extended release: ~24 hours; I.V.: 5-8 hours

Available Dosage Forms

Solution, Intravenous:
Lopressor: 1 mg/mL (5 mL)
Generic: 1 mg/mL (5 mL); 5 mg/5 mL (5 mL)

Tablet, Oral:
Lopressor: 50 mg, 100 mg
Generic: 25 mg, 50 mg, 100 mg

Tablet Extended Release 24 Hour, Oral:
Toprol XL: 25 mg, 50 mg, 100 mg, 200 mg
Generic: 25 mg, 50 mg, 100 mg, 200 mg

General Dosage Range

I.V.: *Adults*: 1.25-5 mg every 6-12 hours (maximum: 15 mg every 3 hours) **or** 5 mg every 2 minutes for 3 doses (acute MI)

Oral:
Extended release:
Children ≥6 years: 1-2 mg/kg once daily (maximum: 2 mg/kg/day or 200 mg/day)
Adults: 12.5-200 mg/day (maximum: 400 mg/day)
Immediate release:
Children >1 year: 1-6 mg/kg/day divided twice daily (maximum: 200 mg/day)
Adults: 50-450 mg/day in 2-3 divided doses

Administration

I.V. I.V. dose is much smaller than oral dose. When administered acutely for cardiac treatment, monitor ECG and blood pressure; may administer by rapid infusion (I.V. push) over 1 minute. May also be administered by slow infusion (ie, 5-10 mg of metoprolol in 50 mL of fluid) over ~30-60 minutes during less urgent situations (eg, substitution for oral metoprolol).

Injectable Detail pH: 7.5

Oral Extended release tablets may be divided in half; do not crush or chew. Administer immediate release tablets with or immediately following food.

Storage/Stability

Injection: Store at 25°C (77°F); excursions permitted to 15°C to 30°C (59°F to 86°F). Protect from light and heat.

Tablet: Store at 25°C (77°F); excursions permitted to 15°C to 30°C (59°F to 86°F). Protect from moisture and heat.

Nursing Actions

Physical Assessment Monitor blood pressure and cardiac status. Monitor for fluid balance, heart failure symptoms, and postural hypotension. Taper dosage slowly when discontinuing. Report abdominal pain; unusual bleeding or bruising; or changes in color of urine or stool. Advise patients with diabetes to monitor glucose levels closely; beta-blockers may alter glucose tolerance.

Patient Education
- Discuss specific use of drug and side effects with patient as it relates to treatment. (HCAHPS: During this hospital stay, were you given any medicine that you had not taken before? Before giving you any new medicine, how often did hospital staff tell you what the medicine was for? How often did hospital staff describe possible side effects in a way you could understand?)
- Patient may experience presyncope, fatigue, blurred vision, illogical thinking, dizziness, impotence, asthenia, depression, diarrhea, or bradycardia. Have patient report immediately to prescriber nervousness, anxiety, emotional

instability, dyspnea, significant weight gain, pregnancy, or rash (HCAHPS).

• Educate patient about signs of a significant reaction (eg, wheezing; chest tightness; fever; itching; bad cough; blue skin color; seizures; or swelling of face, lips, tongue, or throat). **Note:** This is not a comprehensive list of all side effects. Patient should consult prescriber for additional questions.

Intended Use and Disclaimer: Should not be printed and given to patients. This information is intended to serve as a concise initial reference for healthcare professionals to use when discussing medications with a patient. You must ultimately rely on your own discretion, experience and judgment in diagnosing, treating and advising patients.

Dietary Considerations Immediate release tablets should be taken with food. Extended release tablets may be taken without regard to meals.

Related Information
Oral Medications That Should Not Be Crushed or Altered *on page 1712*

MetroNIDAZOLE (Systemic)
(met roe NYE da zole)

Brand Names: U.S. Flagyl; Flagyl ER; Metro
Index Terms Metronidazole Hydrochloride
Pharmacologic Category Amebicide; Antibiotic, Miscellaneous; Antiprotozoal, Nitroimidazole
Medication Safety Issues
Sound-alike/look-alike issues:
MetroNIDAZOLE may be confused with mebendazole, meropenem, metFORMIN, methotrexate, metoclopramide, miconazole

Pregnancy Risk Factor B
Lactation Enters breast milk/not recommended
Breast-Feeding Considerations Metronidazole and its active metabolite are measurable in the breast milk and infant plasma. Milk concentrations are similar to those in the maternal plasma and are highly variable. Peak concentrations of metronidazole in breast milk occur ~2-4 hours after the oral dose. In studies, the calculated relative infant doses have ranged from 0.13% to 36% of the weight-adjusted maternal dose. Use of metronidazole in a lactating patient is not recommended by the manufacturer. If metronidazole is given, breast-feeding should be withheld for 12-24 hours after the dose (CDC, 2010). Not recommended for treatment of *Clostridium difficile* infection in breast-feeding women (Surzwica, 2013).

Use
Oral: Treatment of susceptible anaerobic bacterial and protozoal infections in the following conditions: Amebiasis, symptomatic and asymptomatic trichomoniasis, skin and skin structure infections, bone and joint infections, CNS infections, endocarditis, gynecologic infections, intra-abdominal infections (as part of combination regimen), respiratory tract infections (lower), septicemia due to anaerobes (immediate-release only); bacterial vaginosis (extended-release only); treatment of *Clostridium difficile*-associated diarrhea (CDAD)
Injection: Treatment of susceptible anaerobic bacterial infections in the following conditions: Skin and skin structure infections, bone and joint infections, CNS infections, endocarditis, gynecologic infections, intra-abdominal infections (as part of combination regimen), respiratory tract infections (lower), septicemia; surgical (preoperative) prophylaxis (colorectal surgery); treatment of CDAD

Unlabeled Use Crohn's disease; urethritis
Mechanism of Action/Effect Inhibits DNA synthesis in susceptible organisms
Contraindications Hypersensitivity to metronidazole, nitroimidazole derivatives, or any component of the formulation; pregnancy (first trimester); use of disulfiram within the past 2 weeks; use of alcohol during therapy or within 3 days of therapy discontinuation

Warnings/Precautions [U.S. Boxed Warning]: Possibly carcinogenic based on animal data. Use with caution in patients with severe liver impairment and ESRD due to potential accumulation; reduce dosage in patients with severe liver impairment and consider dosage reduction in patients with severe renal impairment (CrCl <10 mL/minute) who are receiving prolonged therapy. Hemodialysis patients may need supplemental dosing. Use with caution in patients with blood dyscrasias, history of seizures, CHF or other sodium-retaining states.

Aseptic meningitis, encephalopathy, seizures, and neuropathies have been reported especially with increased doses and chronic treatment; monitor and consider discontinuation of therapy if symptoms occur. Prolonged use may result in fungal or bacterial superinfection, including *C. difficile*-associated diarrhea (CDAD) and pseudomembranous colitis; CDAD has been observed >2 months post-antibiotic treatment. The Infectious Disease Society of America (IDSA) recommends the use of oral metronidazole for initial treatment of mild-to-moderate *C. difficile* infection and the use of oral vancomycin for initial treatment of severe *C. difficile* infection with or without I.V. metronidazole depending on the presence of complications. May treat recurrent mild-to-moderate infection once with oral metronidazole; avoid use beyond first reoccurrence due to potential cumulative neurotoxicity (Cohen, 2010). The American College of Gastroenterology (ACG) recommends oral vancomycin and intravenous metronidazole for severe and complicated CDI (Surawicz, 2013). Candidiasis infection (known or unknown) maybe more prominent during metronidazole treatment, antifungal treatment required. If *H. pylori* is not eradicated in patients being treated with metronidazole in a ▶

regimen, it should be assumed that metronidazole-resistance has occurred and it should not again be used.

Disulfiram-like reactions to ethanol have been reported with oral metronidazole; avoid alcoholic beverages or products containing propylene glycol during and for at least 3 days after therapy. Use with caution in the elderly; dosage adjustment may be required based on renal and/or hepatic function.

Drug Interactions

Avoid Concomitant Use
Avoid concomitant use of MetroNIDAZOLE (Systemic) with any of the following: Alcohol (Ethyl); BCG; Carbocisteine; Disulfiram; Pimozide

Decreased Effect
MetroNIDAZOLE (Systemic) may decrease the levels/effects of: BCG; Mycophenolate; Sodium Picosulfate; Typhoid Vaccine

The levels/effects of MetroNIDAZOLE (Systemic) may be decreased by: Fosphenytoin; PHENobarbital; Phenytoin

Increased Effect/Toxicity
MetroNIDAZOLE (Systemic) may increase the levels/effects of: Alcohol (Ethyl); ARIPiprazole; Busulfan; Calcineurin Inhibitors; Carbocisteine; Dofetilide; Fluorouracil (Systemic); Fosphenytoin; Lomitapide; Phenytoin; Pimozide; Tegafur; Tipranavir; Vitamin K Antagonists

The levels/effects of MetroNIDAZOLE (Systemic) may be increased by: Disulfiram; Mebendazole

Nutritional/Ethanol Interactions
Ethanol: The manufacturer recommends to avoid all ethanol or any ethanol-containing drugs (may cause disulfiram-like reaction characterized by flushing, headache, nausea, vomiting, sweating, or tachycardia) during and for 3 days after therapy.

Food: Peak antibiotic serum concentration lowered and delayed, but total drug absorbed not affected.

Adverse Reactions Frequency not always defined.
Cardiovascular: Flattened T-wave on ECG, flushing, local thrombophlebitis (I.V.), syncope

Central nervous system: Headache (18%), metallic taste (9%), dizziness (4%), aseptic meningitis, ataxia, brain disease, confusion, depression, disulfiram-like reaction (with alcohol), dysarthria, dyspareunia, insomnia, irritability, peripheral neuropathy, seizure, vertigo

Dermatologic: Erythematous rash, pruritus, Stevens-Johnson syndrome, toxic epidermal necrolysis, urticaria

Gastrointestinal: Nausea (10% to ~12%), abdominal pain (4%), diarrhea (4%), xerostomia (2%), abdominal cramps, anorexia, constipation, epigastric distress, glossitis, hairy tongue, pancreatitis (rare), proctitis, stomatitis, vomiting

Genitourinary: Vaginitis (15%), genital pruritus (5%), dysmenorrhea (3%), urine abnormality (3%), urinary tract infection (2%), cystitis, dark urine (rare), decreased libido, dysuria, sensation of pelvic pressure, urinary incontinence, vaginal dryness, vulvovaginal candidiasis

Hematologic & oncologic: Neutropenia (reversible), thrombocytopenia (reversible, rare)

Immunologic: Serum sickness-like reaction (joint pains)

Infection: Bacterial infection (7%), candidiasis (3%)

Neuromuscular & skeletal: Weakness

Ophthalmic: Optic neuropathy

Renal: Polyuria

Respiratory: Flu-like symptoms (6%), upper respiratory tract infection (4%), pharyngitis (3%), nasal congestion, rhinitis, sinusitis

Miscellaneous: Fever, lesion (central nervous system, reversible)

Available Dosage Forms

Capsule, Oral:
Flagyl: 375 mg
Generic: 375 mg

Solution, Intravenous:
Metro: 500 mg (100 mL)
Generic: 500 mg (100 mL)

Solution, Intravenous [preservative free]:
Generic: 500 mg (100 mL)

Tablet, Oral:
Flagyl: 250 mg, 500 mg
Generic: 250 mg, 500 mg

Tablet Extended Release 24 Hour, Oral:
Flagyl ER: 750 mg

General Dosage Range
Dosage adjustment recommended in patients with hepatic or renal impairment

I.V.: *Adults:* 500 mg every 6-8 hours (maximum: 4 g/day)

Oral:
Extended release: *Adults:* 750 mg once daily
Regular release:
Infants and Children: 35-50 mg/kg/day divided every 8 hours
Adults: 250-750 mg every 6-12 hours (maximum: 4 g/day) **or** 2 g as a single dose

Administration
I.V. Infuse intravenously over 30-60 minutes. Avoid contact of drug solution with equipment containing aluminum.

Injectable Detail pH: 4.5-7 (ready to use)

Oral Immediate-release tablets and capsules may be administered with food to minimize stomach upset. Extended release tablets should be administered on an empty stomach (1 hour before or 2 hours after meals); do not split, crush, or chew.

Storage/Stability
Oral:
Extended-release: Store at 25°C (77°F); excursions are permitted to 15°C to 30°C (59°F to 86°F).
Immediate release: Store at 15°C to 25°C (59°F to 77°F). Protect the tablets from light.

Injection: Store at 25°C (77°F). Protect from light. Brief exposure up to 40°C does not adversely affect the product. Avoid excessive heat. Do not refrigerate. Do not remove unit from overwrap until ready for use. Discard unused solution.

Nursing Actions

Physical Assessment Monitor for CNS, neuromuscular, and dermatologic reactions. Assess patient for numbness or paresthesia of extremities, seizures, or other CNS abnormalities. Reenforce abstinence from alcohol during and immediately after therapy. Monitor for hypersensitivity reactions.

Patient Education
- Discuss specific use of drug and side effects with patient as it relates to treatment. (HCAHPS: During this hospital stay, were you given any medicine that you had not taken before? Before giving you any new medicine, how often did hospital staff tell you what the medicine was for? How often did hospital staff describe possible side effects in a way you could understand?)
- Patient may experience nausea, diarrhea, headache, lack of appetite, parageusia, or discolored urine. Have patient report immediately to prescriber severe dizziness, significant headache, difficulty speaking, paresthesia, or rash (HCAHPS).
- Educate patient about signs of a significant reaction (eg, wheezing; chest tightness; fever; itching; bad cough; blue skin color; seizures; or swelling of face, lips, tongue, or throat). **Note:** This is not a comprehensive list of all side effects. Patient should consult prescriber for additional questions.

Intended Use and Disclaimer: Should not be printed and given to patients. This information is intended to serve as a concise initial reference for healthcare professionals to use when discussing medications with a patient. You must ultimately rely on your own discretion, experience and judgment in diagnosing, treating and advising patients.

Dietary Considerations

Immediate-release tablets and capsules may be administered with food to minimize stomach upset. Extended release tablets should be taken on an empty stomach (1 hour before or 2 hours after meals).
Sodium: Injectable dosage form may contain sodium.
Alcohol: Use of alcohol is contraindicated during therapy and for 3 days after therapy discontinuation.

Related Information

Oral Medications That Should Not Be Crushed or Altered *on page 1712*

Miconazole (Oral) (mi KON a zole)

Brand Names: U.S. Oravig
Index Terms Miconazole Nitrate
Pharmacologic Category Antifungal Agent, Oral Nonabsorbed
Medication Safety Issues
Sound-alike/look-alike issues:
Miconazole may be confused with metroNIDAZOLE, Micronase, Micronor®
Pregnancy Risk Factor C
Lactation Excretion in breast milk unknown/use caution
Use Treatment of oropharyngeal candidiasis
Available Dosage Forms
Tablet, Buccal:
Oravig: 50 mg
General Dosage Range Buccal: *Children ≥16 years and Adults:* 50 mg (1 tablet) once daily
Administration
Oral Apply in the morning after brushing teeth. With dry hands, place either side of the tablet against the upper gum above the incisor tooth; hold with slight pressure over the upper lip for 30 seconds. Placing the rounded side of the tablet against the gum may be more comfortable. Alternate sides of the mouth with each application; do not crush, chew, or swallow. Avoid chewing gum while in place.

If the tablet does not adhere to the gum or falls off within 6 hours of application, the same tablet should be repositioned immediately. If the tablet does not adhere, use a new tablet. If the tablet is swallowed within 6 hours of application, the patient should drink a glass of water and apply a new tablet (only once). If the tablet falls off or is swallowed >6 hours after application, a new tablet should not be applied until the next regularly scheduled dose.

Nursing Actions

Patient Education
- Discuss specific use of drug and side effects with patient as it relates to treatment. (HCAHPS: During this hospital stay, were you given any medicine that you had not taken before? Before giving you any new medicine, how often did hospital staff tell you what the medicine was for? How often did hospital staff describe possible side effects in a way you could understand?)
- Patient may experience stomatitis, headache, nausea, diarrhea, or parageusia. Have patient report immediately to prescriber recurring yeast infection, severe dyspepsia, inability to eat, or rash (HCAHPS).
- Educate patient about signs of a significant reaction (eg, wheezing; chest tightness; fever; ▶

◄ itching; bad cough; blue skin color; seizures; or swelling of face, lips, tongue, or throat). **Note:** This is not a comprehensive list of all side effects. Patient should consult prescriber for additional questions.

Intended Use and Disclaimer: Should not be printed and given to patients. This information is intended to serve as a concise initial reference for healthcare professionals to use when discussing medications with a patient. You must ultimately rely on your own discretion, experience and judgment in diagnosing, treating and advising patients.

Related Information

Oral Medications That Should Not Be Crushed or Altered *on page 1712*

Miconazole (Topical) (mi KON a zole)

Brand Names: U.S. Aloe Vesta Antifungal [OTC]; Antifungal [OTC]; Azolen Tincture [OTC]; Baza Antifungal [OTC]; Carrington Antifungal [OTC]; Critic-Aid Clear AF [OTC]; Cruex Prescription Strength [OTC]; DermaFungal [OTC]; Desenex Jock Itch [OTC]; Desenex Spray [OTC]; Desenex [OTC]; Fungoid Tincture [OTC]; Lotrimin AF Deodorant Powder [OTC]; Lotrimin AF Jock Itch Powder [OTC]; Lotrimin AF Powder [OTC]; Lotrimin AF [OTC]; Micaderm [OTC]; Micatin [OTC]; Miconazole 3; Miconazole 3 Combo Pack [OTC]; Miconazole 7 [OTC]; Micro Guard [OTC]; Miranel AF [OTC]; Mitrazol [OTC]; Podactin [OTC]; Remedy Antifungal [OTC]; Secura Antifungal Extra Thick [OTC]; Secura Antifungal [OTC]; Soothe & Cool INZO Antifungal [OTC]; Triple Paste AF [OTC]; Vagistat-3 [OTC]; Zeasorb-AF [OTC]

Index Terms Miconazole Nitrate

Pharmacologic Category Antifungal Agent, Topical; Antifungal Agent, Vaginal

Medication Safety Issues

Sound-alike/look-alike issues:

Miconazole may be confused with metroNIDA-ZOLE, Micronase, Micronor®

Lotrimin® may be confused with Lotrisone®, Otrivin®

Micatin® may be confused with Miacalcin®

Lactation Excretion in breast milk unknown/use caution

Use Treatment of vulvovaginal candidiasis and a variety of skin and mucous membrane fungal infections

Available Dosage Forms

Aerosol, External:

Desenex Spray [OTC]: 2% (133 g)

Lotrimin AF [OTC]: 2% (150 g)

Aerosol Powder, External:

Cruex Prescription Strength [OTC]: 2% (85 g)

Desenex Jock Itch [OTC]: 2% (113 g)

Desenex Spray [OTC]: 2% (113 g)

Lotrimin AF Deodorant Powder [OTC]: 2% (133 g)

Lotrimin AF Jock Itch Powder [OTC]: 2% (133 g)

Lotrimin AF Powder [OTC]: 2% (133 g)

Cream, External:

Antifungal [OTC]: 2% (14 g, 28 g, 42.5 g, 113 g, 198 g)

Baza Antifungal [OTC]: 2% (4 g, 57 g, 142 g)

Carrington Antifungal [OTC]: 2% (141 g)

Micaderm [OTC]: 2% (30 g)

Micatin [OTC]: 2% (14 g)

Micro Guard [OTC]: 2% (57 g)

Podactin [OTC]: 2% (28.35 g)

Remedy Antifungal [OTC]: 2% (118 mL)

Secura Antifungal [OTC]: 2% (57 g)

Secura Antifungal Extra Thick [OTC]: 2% (92 g)

Soothe & Cool INZO Antifungal [OTC]: 2% (56.7 g, 141.7 g)

Generic: 2% (15 g, 28.4 g, 30 g)

Cream, Vaginal:

Miconazole 7 [OTC]: 2% (45 g)

Generic: 2% (45 g)

Kit, External:

Fungoid Tincture [OTC]: 2%

Kit, Vaginal:

Miconazole 3 Combo Pack [OTC]: Cream, topical: 2% (9 g) and Suppository, vaginal: 200 mg (3s)

Vagistat-3 [OTC]: Cream, topical: 2% (9 g) and Suppository, vaginal: 200 mg (3s)

Lotion, External:

Zeasorb-AF [OTC]: 2% (56 g)

Ointment, External:

Aloe Vesta Antifungal [OTC]: 2% (56 g, 141 g)

Critic-Aid Clear AF [OTC]: 2% (4 g, 57 g, 142 g)

DermaFungal [OTC]: 2% (113 g)

Triple Paste AF [OTC]: 2% (56.7 g)

Powder, External:

Desenex [OTC]: 2% (43 g, 85 g)

Lotrimin AF [OTC]: 2% (90 g)

Micro Guard [OTC]: 2% (85 g)

Mitrazol [OTC]: 2% (30 g)

Remedy Antifungal [OTC]: 2% (85 g)

Zeasorb-AF [OTC]: 2% (71 g)

Solution, External:

Azolen Tincture [OTC]: 2% (29.57 mL)

Fungoid Tincture [OTC]: 2% (29.57 mL)

Miranel AF [OTC]: 2% (28 g)

Suppository, Vaginal:

Miconazole 7 [OTC]: 100 mg (7 ea)

Miconazole 3: 200 mg (3 ea)

Generic: 100 mg (7 ea)

General Dosage Range

Intravaginal: *Children ≥12 years and Adults:* Insert 1 applicatorful or suppository (100 mg or 200 mg) once daily at bedtime **or** insert 1 suppository (1200 mg) as a single dose.

Topical: *Children and Adults:* Apply twice daily **or** dissolve 1 effervescent tablet in ~1 gallon of water and soak feet for 15-30 minutes

Nursing Actions

Physical Assessment Caution patients with diabetes to test serum glucose regularly; may inhibit the metabolism of oral sulfonylureas. Teach patient bleeding precautions.

Patient Education
- Discuss specific use of drug and side effects with patient as it relates to treatment. (HCAHPS: During this hospital stay, were you given any medicine that you had not taken before? Before giving you any new medicine, how often did hospital staff tell you what the medicine was for? How often did hospital staff describe possible side effects in a way you could understand?)
- Patient may experience dyspepsia or skin irritation. Have patient report immediately to prescriber reoccurring yeast infection or rash (HCAHPS).
- Educate patient about signs of a significant reaction (eg, wheezing; chest tightness; fever; itching; bad cough; blue skin color; seizures; or swelling of face, lips, tongue, or throat). **Note:** This is not a comprehensive list of all side effects. Patient should consult prescriber for additional questions.

Intended Use and Disclaimer: Should not be printed and given to patients. This information is intended to serve as a concise initial reference for healthcare professionals to use when discussing medications with a patient. You must ultimately rely on your own discretion, experience and judgment in diagnosing, treating and advising patients.

Midazolam (MID aye zoe lam)

Index Terms Midazolam Hydrochloride; Versed
Pharmacologic Category Benzodiazepine
Medication Safety Issues
　Sound-alike/look-alike issues:
　　Versed may be confused with VePesid, Vistaril®
　High alert medication:
　　The Institute for Safe Medication Practices (ISMP) includes this medication among its list of drugs which have a heightened risk of causing significant patient harm when used in error.

Pregnancy Risk Factor D
Lactation Enters breast milk/use caution
Breast-Feeding Considerations Midazolam and hydroxymidazolam can be detected in breast milk. Based on information from two women, 2-3 months postpartum, the half-life of midazolam in breast milk is ~1 hour. Milk concentrations were below the limit of detection (<5 nmol/L) 4 hours after a single maternal dose of midazolam 15 mg. Drowsiness, lethargy, or weight loss in nursing infants have been observed in case reports following maternal use of some benzodiazepines (Iqbal, 2002; Matheson, 1990). The manufacturer recommends that caution be exercised when administering midazolam to nursing women.

Use Preoperative sedation; moderate sedation prior to diagnostic or radiographic procedures; ICU sedation (continuous infusion); induction and maintenance of general anesthesia

Unlabeled Use Anxiety, status epilepticus, conscious sedation (intranasal route)

Mechanism of Action/Effect Binds to stereospecific benzodiazepine receptors on the postsynaptic GABA neuron at several sites within the central nervous system, including the limbic system, reticular formation. Enhancement of the inhibitory effect of GABA on neuronal excitability results by increased neuronal membrane permeability to chloride ions. This shift in chloride ions results in hyperpolarization (a less excitable state) and stabilization.

Contraindications Hypersensitivity to midazolam or any component of the formulation; intrathecal or epidural injection of parenteral forms containing preservatives (ie, benzyl alcohol); acute narrow-angle glaucoma; concurrent use of potent inhibitors of CYP3A4 (amprenavir, atazanavir, or ritonavir)

Per respective protease inhibitor manufacturer's labeling: Concurrent use of oral midazolam with amprenavir, atazanavir, darunavir, indinavir, lopinavir-ritonavir, nelfinavir, ritonavir, saquinavir, tipranavir and concurrent use of oral or injectable midazolam with fosamprenavir

Warnings/Precautions [U.S. Boxed Warning]: May cause severe respiratory depression, respiratory arrest, or apnea. Use with extreme caution, particularly in noncritical care settings. Appropriate resuscitative equipment and qualified personnel must be available for administration and monitoring. Initial dosing must be cautiously titrated and individualized, particularly in elderly or debilitated patients, patients with hepatic impairment (including alcoholics), or in renal impairment, particularly if other CNS depressants (including opioids) are used concurrently. **[U.S. Boxed Warning]: Initial doses in elderly or debilitated patients should be conservative; as little as 1 mg, but not to exceed 2.5 mg.** Use with caution in patients with respiratory disease or impaired gag reflex. Use during upper airway procedures may increase risk of hypoventilation. Prolonged responses have been noted following extended administration by continuous infusion (possibly due to metabolite accumulation) or in the presence of drugs which inhibit midazolam metabolism.

Causes CNS depression (dose-related) resulting in sedation, dizziness, confusion, or ataxia which may impair physical and mental capabilities. Patients must be cautioned about performing tasks which require mental alertness (eg, operating machinery or driving). A minimum of 1 day should elapse after midazolam administration before attempting these tasks. Use with caution in patients receiving other

CNS depressants or psychoactive agents. Effects with other sedative drugs or ethanol may be potentiated. Benzodiazepines have been associated with falls and traumatic injury and should be used with extreme caution in patients who are at risk of these events (especially the elderly).

Use with caution in patients receiving CYP3A4 inhibitors; may result in more intense and prolonged sedation; consider reducing midazolam dose and anticipate potential for prolongation and intensity of effect. The concurrent use of all protease inhibitors is contraindicated with oral midazolam per their respective manufacturer's labeling. The concurrent use of fosamprenavir is contraindicated with both oral and parenteral forms of midazolam.

May cause hypotension - hemodynamic events are more common in pediatric patients or patients with hemodynamic instability. Hypotension and/or respiratory depression may occur more frequently in patients who have received opioid analgesics. Use with caution in obese patients, chronic renal failure, and HF. Does not protect against increases in heart rate or blood pressure during intubation. Should not be used in shock, coma, or acute alcohol intoxication. **[U.S. Boxed Warning]: Do not administer by rapid I.V. injection in neonates; severe hypotension and seizures have been reported; risk may be increased with concomitant fentanyl use.**

Avoid intra-arterial administration or extravasation of parenteral formulation. Some parenteral dosage forms may contain benzyl alcohol which has been associated with "gasping syndrome" in neonates. Some formulations may contain cherry flavoring.

Midazolam causes anterograde amnesia. Paradoxical reactions, including hyperactive or aggressive behavior have been reported with benzodiazepines, particularly in adolescent/pediatric or psychiatric patients; may consider treatment with flumazenil (Massanari, 1997). Does not have analgesic, antidepressant, or antipsychotic properties.

Benzodiazepines have been associated with dependence and acute withdrawal symptoms on discontinuation or reduction in dose. Acute withdrawal, including seizures, may be precipitated after administration of flumazenil to patients receiving long-term benzodiazepine therapy.

Drug Interactions

Avoid Concomitant Use

Avoid concomitant use of Midazolam with any of the following: Azelastine (Nasal); Boceprevir; Cobicistat; Conivaptan; Efavirenz; Fusidic Acid (Systemic); Itraconazole; Ketoconazole (Systemic); OLANZapine; Paraldehyde; Pimozide; Protease Inhibitors; Sodium Oxybate; Telaprevir; Thalidomide

Decreased Effect

The levels/effects of Midazolam may be decreased by: Bosentan; CarBAMazepine; CYP3A4 Inducers (Strong); Dabrafenib; Deferasirox; Ginkgo Biloba; Herbs (CYP3A4 Inducers); Mitotane; Rifamycin Derivatives; Theophylline Derivatives; Tocilizumab; Yohimbine

Increased Effect/Toxicity

Midazolam may increase the levels/effects of: Alcohol (Ethyl); ARIPiprazole; Azelastine (Nasal); Buprenorphine; CloZAPine; CNS Depressants; Dofetilide; Fosphenytoin; Hydrocodone; Lomitapide; Methotrimeprazine; Metyrosine; Mirtazapine; Paraldehyde; Phenytoin; Pimozide; Pramipexole; Propofol; ROPINIRole; Rotigotine; Selective Serotonin Reuptake Inhibitors; Sodium Oxybate; Thalidomide; Zolpidem

The levels/effects of Midazolam may be increased by: Antifungal Agents (Azole Derivatives, Systemic); Aprepitant; AtorvaSTATin; Boceprevir; Brimonidine (Topical); Calcium Channel Blockers (Nondihydropyridine); Cimetidine; Cobicistat; Conivaptan; Contraceptives (Estrogens); Contraceptives (Progestins); CYP3A4 Inhibitors (Moderate); CYP3A4 Inhibitors (Strong); Dasatinib; Doxylamine; Droperidol; Efavirenz; Fosaprepitant; Fusidic Acid (Systemic); Grapefruit Juice; HydrOXYzine; Isoniazid; Itraconazole; Ivacaftor; Ketoconazole (Systemic); Luliconazole; Macrolide Antibiotics; Magnesium Sulfate; Methotrimeprazine; Mifepristone; OLANZapine; Perampanel; Propofol; Protease Inhibitors; Proton Pump Inhibitors; Selective Serotonin Reuptake Inhibitors; Simeprevir; Stiripentol; Tapentadol; Telaprevir

Nutritional/Ethanol Interactions

Ethanol: Ethanol may increase CNS depression. Management: Avoid ethanol.

Food: Grapefruit juice may increase serum concentrations of midazolam. Management: Avoid concurrent use of grapefruit juice with oral midazolam.

Herb/Nutraceutical: St John's wort may decrease midazolam levels and increase CNS depression; valerian, kava kava, and gotu kola may increase CNS depression. Management: Avoid concurrent use with St John's wort, valerian, kava kava, and gotu kola.

Adverse Reactions As reported in adults unless otherwise noted:

>10%: Respiratory: Decreased tidal volume and/or respiratory rate decrease, apnea (3% children)

1% to 10%:

Cardiovascular: Hypotension (3% children)

Central nervous system: Drowsiness (1%), oversedation, headache (1%), seizure-like activity (1% children)

Gastrointestinal: Nausea (3%), vomiting (3%)

Local: Pain and local reactions at injection site (4% I.M., 5% I.V.; severity less than diazepam)

Neuromuscular & skeletal: Myoclonic jerks (pre-term infants)

Ocular: Nystagmus (1% children)

Respiratory: Cough (1%)

Miscellaneous: Physical and psychological dependence with prolonged use, hiccups (4%, 1% children), paradoxical reaction (2% children)

Pharmacodynamics/Kinetics

Onset of Action I.M.: Sedation: ~15 minutes; I.V.: 3-5 minutes; Oral: 10-20 minutes; Intranasal: Children: 4-8 minutes (Lee-Kim, 2004); Peak effect: I.M.: 0.5-1 hour

Duration of Action I.M.: Up to 6 hours; Mean: 2 hours; Intranasal: Children: 18-41 minutes (Lee-Kim, 2004); I.V.: Single dose: <2 hours (dose-dependent) (Fragen, 1997); Cirrhosis: Up to 6 hours (MacGilcrhist, 1986)

Controlled Substance C-IV

Available Dosage Forms

Solution, Injection:
Generic: 2 mg/2 mL (2 mL); 5 mg/5 mL (5 mL); 10 mg/10 mL (10 mL); 5 mg/mL (1 mL, 2 mL, 5 mL, 10 mL); 10 mg/2 mL (2 mL); 25 mg/5 mL (5 mL); 50 mg/10 mL (10 mL)

Solution, Injection [preservative free]:
Generic: 2 mg/2 mL (2 mL); 5 mg/5 mL (5 mL); 5 mg/mL (1 mL); 10 mg/2 mL (2 mL)

Syrup, Oral:
Generic: 2 mg/mL (118 mL)

General Dosage Range

I.M.:
Children: 0.1-0.15 mg/kg 30-60 minutes prior to surgery/procedure (maximum: 10 mg total)
Adults: 0.07-0.08 mg/kg 30-60 minutes prior to surgery/procedure; Usual dose: 5 mg

I.V.:
Infants <6 months: 0.05-0.2 mg/kg loading dose followed by 0.4-6 mcg/kg/minute infusion
Infants 6 months to Children 5 years: Initial: 0.05-0.1 mg/kg once (maximum: 6 mg or 0.6 mg/kg total) **or** 0.05-0.2 mg/kg loading dose followed by 0.4-6 mcg/kg/minute infusion
Children 6-12 years: 0.025-0.05 mg/kg once (maximum: 10 mg or 0.4 mg/kg total) **or** 0.05-0.2 mg/kg loading dose followed by 0.4-6 mcg/kg/minute infusion
Children ≥12 years and Adults: Dosage varies greatly depending on indication

Oral:
Children <6 years: 0.25-0.5 mg/kg as single dose; may require as much as 1 mg/kg (maximum: 20 mg total)
Children 6-16 years: 0.25-0.5 mg/kg as a single dose (maximum: 20 mg total)

Usual Infusion Concentrations: Pediatric I.V. infusion: 0.5 mg/mL **or** 1 mg/mL

Usual Infusion Concentrations: Adult I.V. infusion: 100 mg in 100 mL (concentration: 1 mg/mL) of D_5W or NS

Administration

I.M. Give deep I.M. into large muscle.

I.V. Administer by slow I.V. injection over at least 2-5 minutes at a concentration of 1-5 mg/mL or by I.V. infusion. For induction of anesthesia, administer I.V. bolus over 5-30 seconds. Continuous infusions should be administered via an infusion pump.

Injectable Detail pH: 3 (adjusted)

Oral Do not mix with any liquid (such as grapefruit juice) prior to administration.

Other Intranasal: **Note:** Due to the low pH of the solution, burning upon administration is likely to occur. Use of an atomizer, such as the MAD 300 Mucosal Atomizer which attaches to a tuberculin syringe, can reduce irritation. If possible, based upon dose to be administered, use higher concentration injectable solution to minimize volume administered intranasal. Smaller volume will reduce irritation and swallowing of administered dose. The maximum recommended dose volume (of the 5 mg/mL concentration) per nare is 1 mL. Using the 5 mg/mL injectable solution, draw up desired dose with a 1-3 mL needleless syringe; may attach a nasal mucosal atomization device prior to delivering dose. Deliver half of the total dose volume into the first nare using the atomizer device or by dripping slowly into nostril, then deliver the other half of the dose into the second nare.

Storage/Stability The manufacturer states that midazolam, at a final concentration of 0.5 mg/mL, is stable for up to 24 hours when diluted with D_5W or NS. A final concentration of 1 mg/mL in NS has been documented to be stable for up to 10 days (McMullen, 1995). Admixtures do not require protection from light for short-term storage.

Nursing Actions

Physical Assessment I.V.: Monitor cardiac and respiratory status continuously. Monitor I.V. infusion site carefully for extravasation. For inpatient use, institute safety measures. I.V./I.M.: Monitor closely following administration. Provide bedrest and assistance with ambulation for several hours.

Patient Education
- Discuss specific use of drug and side effects with patient as it relates to treatment. (HCAHPS: During this hospital stay, were you given any medicine that you had not taken before? Before giving you any new medicine, how often did hospital staff tell you what the medicine was for? How often did hospital staff describe possible side effects in a way you could understand?)
- Patient may experience presyncope, fatigue, blurred vision, illogical thinking, xerostomia, or change in balance. Have patient report immediately to prescriber dyspnea or severe asthenia (HCAHPS).
- Educate patient about signs of a significant reaction (eg, wheezing; chest tightness; fever; itching; bad cough; blue skin color; seizures; or

swelling of face, lips, tongue, or throat). **Note:** This is not a comprehensive list of all side effects. Patient should consult prescriber for additional questions.

Intended Use and Disclaimer: Should not be printed and given to patients. This information is intended to serve as a concise initial reference for healthcare professionals to use when discussing medications with a patient. You must ultimately rely on your own discretion, experience and judgment in diagnosing, treating and advising patients.

Dietary Considerations Avoid grapefruit juice with oral syrup.

Midodrine (MI doe dreen)

Index Terms Midodrine Hydrochloride; ProAmatine
Pharmacologic Category Alpha$_1$ Agonist
Medication Safety Issues
   Sound-alike/look-alike issues:
   Midodrine may be confused with Midrin®, minoxidil
   ProAmatine may be confused with protamine
Pregnancy Risk Factor C
Lactation Excretion in breast milk is unknown/use caution
Use Orphan drug: Treatment of symptomatic orthostatic hypotension
Unlabeled Use Management of urinary incontinence; vasovagal syncope; prevention of dialysis-induced hypotension
Available Dosage Forms
   Tablet, Oral:
   Generic: 2.5 mg, 5 mg, 10 mg
General Dosage Range Dosage adjustment recommended in patients with renal impairment
   Oral: *Adults:* 10 mg 3 times/day (maximum: 40 mg/day)
Administration
   Oral Doses may be given in approximately 3- to 4-hour intervals (eg, shortly before or upon rising in the morning, at midday, in the late afternoon not later than 6 PM). Avoid dosing after the evening meal or within 4 hours of bedtime. Continue therapy only in patients who appear to attain symptomatic improvement during initial treatment. Standing systolic blood pressure may be elevated 15-30 mm Hg at 1 hour after a 10 mg dose. Some effect may persist for 2-3 hours.
Nursing Actions
   Physical Assessment Assess for reduction of hypotension and adverse reactions (eg, supine hypertension, urinary urgency/retention, rash) prior to treatment and periodically thereafter. Standing blood pressure may be elevated 1 hour after administration and remain slightly elevated 3-4 hours.

Patient Education
• Discuss specific use of drug and side effects with patient as it relates to treatment. (HCAHPS: During this hospital stay, were you given any medicine that you had not taken before? Before giving you any new medicine, how often did hospital staff tell you what the medicine was for? How often did hospital staff describe possible side effects in a way you could understand?)
• Patient may experience hypertension, headache, dyspepsia, or skin irritation. Have patient report immediately to prescriber angina, tachycardia, severe dizziness, sudden vision changes, tinnitus, urinary retention, paresthesia, or rash (HCAHPS).
• Educate patient about signs of a significant reaction (eg, wheezing; chest tightness; fever; itching; bad cough; blue skin color; seizures; or swelling of face, lips, tongue, or throat). **Note:** This is not a comprehensive list of all side effects. Patient should consult prescriber for additional questions.

Intended Use and Disclaimer: Should not be printed and given to patients. This information is intended to serve as a concise initial reference for healthcare professionals to use when discussing medications with a patient. You must ultimately rely on your own discretion, experience and judgment in diagnosing, treating and advising patients.

Mifepristone (mi FE pris tone)

Brand Names: U.S. Korlym; Mifeprex
Index Terms RU-38486; RU-486
Pharmacologic Category Abortifacient; Antineoplastic Agent, Hormone Antagonist; Antiprogestin; Cortisol Receptor Blocker
Medication Safety Issues
   Sound-alike/look-alike issues:
   Mifeprex® may be confused with Mirapex®
   Mifepristone may be confused with misoprostol
   High alert medication:
   The Institute for Safe Medication Practices (ISMP) includes this medication among its list of drug classes which have a heightened risk of causing significant patient harm when used in error.
Medication Guide Available Yes
Pregnancy Risk Factor X
Lactation Enters breast milk/not recommended
Use
   Korlym™: To control hyperglycemia occurring secondary to hypercortisolism in patients with endogenous Cushing's syndrome who have type 2 diabetes mellitus or glucose intolerance and who failed surgery or who are not surgical candidates
   Mifeprex®: Medical termination of intrauterine pregnancy, through day 49 of pregnancy. Patients

may need treatment with misoprostol and possibly surgery to complete therapy.

Unlabeled Use Treatment of unresectable meningioma; has been studied in the treatment of breast cancer and ovarian cancer; termination of pregnancy ≤63 days of pregnancy

Available Dosage Forms

Tablet, Oral:

Korlym: 300 mg

Mifeprex: 200 mg

General Dosage Range Dosage adjustment recommended in patients with hepatic or renal impairment or on concomitant therapy when treating hyperglycemia in patients with Cushing's syndrome.

Oral: *Adults:* Hyperglycemia in patients with Cushing's syndrome: 300-1200 mg once daily (maximum: 1200 mg once daily, not to exceed 20 mg/kg/day); Termination of pregnancy: Day 1: 600 mg (three 200 mg tablets) as a single dose

Administration

Oral

Hyperglycemia in patients with Cushing's syndrome: Administer as a single daily dose with a meal. Tablets should be swallowed whole, not crushed, split, or chewed.

Termination of pregnancy: To be taken as a single dose under physician supervision

Hazardous agent; use appropriate precautions for handling and disposal (NIOSH, 2012).

Nursing Actions

Physical Assessment

Korlym™: Monitor response of glucose; ensure the patient is not pregnant prior to initiating.

Mifeprex®: Monitor for excessive bleeding, successful termination of pregnancy. Monitor vital signs.

Patient Education

- Discuss specific use of drug and side effects with patient as it relates to treatment. (HCAHPS: During this hospital stay, were you given any medicine that you had not taken before? Before giving you any new medicine, how often did hospital staff tell you what the medicine was for? How often did hospital staff describe possible side effects in a way you could understand?)
- Patient may experience dizziness, headache, fatigue, dyspepsia, nausea, lack of appetite, diarrhea, vaginal bleeding, or hypoglycemia. Have patient report immediately to prescriber signs of infection, tachycardia, hypotension, menstrual irregularities, severe asthenia, or rash (HCAHPS).
- Educate patient about signs of a significant reaction (eg, wheezing; chest tightness; fever; itching; bad cough; blue skin color; seizures; or swelling of face, lips, tongue, or throat). **Note:** This is not a comprehensive list of all side effects. Patient should consult prescriber for additional questions.

Intended Use and Disclaimer: Should not be printed and given to patients. This information is intended to serve as a concise initial reference for healthcare professionals to use when discussing medications with a patient. You must ultimately rely on your own discretion, experience and judgment in diagnosing, treating and advising patients.

Miglitol (MIG li tol)

Brand Names: U.S. Glyset

Pharmacologic Category Antidiabetic Agent, Alpha-Glucosidase Inhibitor

Medication Safety Issues

Sound-alike/look-alike issues:

Glyset® may be confused with Cycloset®

Pregnancy Risk Factor B

Lactation Enters breast milk/not recommended

Use Type 2 diabetes mellitus (noninsulin-dependent, NIDDM):

Monotherapy as an adjunct to diet to improve glycemic control in patients with type 2 diabetes mellitus (noninsulin-dependent, NIDDM) whose hyperglycemia cannot be managed with diet alone

Combination therapy with a sulfonylurea when diet plus either miglitol or a sulfonylurea alone do not result in adequate glycemic control. The effect of miglitol to enhance glycemic control is additive to that of sulfonylureas when used in combination.

Available Dosage Forms

Tablet, Oral:

Glyset: 25 mg, 50 mg, 100 mg

General Dosage Range Oral: *Adults:* Initial: 25 mg 3 times daily; Maintenance: 25-100 mg 3 times daily (maximum: 300 mg daily)

Administration

Oral Administer at the start of each main meal.

Nursing Actions

Physical Assessment Teach patient importance of adequate diabetic control.

Patient Education

- Discuss specific use of drug and side effects with patient as it relates to treatment. (HCAHPS: During this hospital stay, were you given any medicine that you had not taken before? Before giving you any new medicine, how often did hospital staff tell you what the medicine was for? How often did hospital staff describe possible side effects in a way you could understand?)
- Patient may experience dyspepsia, flatulence, or diarrhea. Have patient report immediately to prescriber signs of infection, hyper-/hypoglycemia, or rash (HCAHPS).
- Educate patient about signs of a significant reaction (eg, wheezing; chest tightness; fever; itching; bad cough; blue skin color; seizures; or swelling of face, lips, tongue, or throat). **Note:** This is not a comprehensive list of all side

effects. Patient should consult prescriber for additional questions.

Intended Use and Disclaimer: Should not be printed and given to patients. This information is intended to serve as a concise initial reference for healthcare professionals to use when discussing medications with a patient. You must ultimately rely on your own discretion, experience and judgment in diagnosing, treating and advising patients.

Milnacipran (mil NAY ci pran)

Brand Names: U.S. Savella; Savella Titration Pack

Pharmacologic Category Antidepressant, Serotonin/Norepinephrine Reuptake Inhibitor

Medication Safety Issues

Sound-alike/look-alike issues:

Milnacipran may be confused with levomilnacipran

Savella® may be confused with cevimeline, sevelamer

Medication Guide Available Yes

Pregnancy Risk Factor C

Lactation Enters breast milk/use caution

Breast-Feeding Considerations Milnacipran is excreted into breast milk. The manufacturer recommends that caution be exercised when administering milnacipran to nursing women.

Use Management of fibromyalgia

Mechanism of Action/Effect Inhibits norepinephrine and serotonin reuptake; improves symptoms associated with fibromyalgia

Contraindications Use of MAOIs intended to treat psychiatric disorders (concurrently or within 5 days of discontinuing milnacipran, or within 2 weeks of discontinuing the MAOI); initiation of milnacipran in a patient receiving linezolid or methylene blue I.V.; uncontrolled narrow-angle glaucoma

Warnings/Precautions [U.S. Boxed Warning]: Milnacipran is a serotonin/norepinephrine reuptake inhibitor (SNRI) similar to SNRIs used to treat depression and other psychiatric disorders. Antidepressants increase the risk of suicidal thinking and behavior in children, adolescents, and young adults (18-24 years of age) with major depressive disorder (MDD) and other psychiatric disorders; consider risk prior to prescribing. Short-term studies did not show an increased risk in patients >24 years of age and showed a decreased risk in patients ≥65 years. Closely monitor for clinical worsening, suicidality, or unusual changes in behavior; the patient's family or caregiver should be instructed to closely observe the patient and communicate condition with healthcare provider. A medication guide concerning the use of antidepressants in children and teenagers should be dispensed with each prescription. **Milnacipran is not FDA approved for the treatment of major depressive disorder or for use in children.**

Suicide risks should be monitored in patients treated with SNRIs regardless of the indication. The possibility of a suicide attempt is inherent in major depression and may persist until remission occurs. Patients treated with antidepressants should be observed for clinical worsening and suicidality, especially during initial few months of a course of drug therapy, or at times of dose changes, either increases or decreases. Use caution in high-risk patients. Worsening depression and severe abrupt suicidality that are not part of the presenting symptoms may require discontinuation or modification of drug therapy. Prescriptions should be written for the smallest quantity consistent with good patient care. The patient's family or caregiver should be alerted to monitor patients for the emergence of suicidality and associated behaviors (such as anxiety, agitation, panic attacks, insomnia, irritability, hostility, impulsivity, akathisia, mania, and hypomania); patients should be instructed to notify their health care provider if any of these symptoms or worsening depression or psychosis occur.

Patients with major depressive disorder were excluded from clinical trials evaluating milnacipran for fibromyalgia; however, mania has been reported in patients with mood disorders taking similar medications. May worsen psychosis in some patients or precipitate a shift to mania or hypomania in patients with bipolar disorder. Patients presenting with depressive symptoms should be screened for bipolar disorder. Monotherapy in patients with bipolar disorder should be avoided. **Milnacipran is not FDA approved for the treatment of bipolar depression.**

Potentially life-threatening serotonin syndrome (SS) has occurred with serotonergic agents (eg, SSRIs, SNRIs), particularly when used in combination with other serotonergic agents (eg, triptans, TCAs, fentanyl, lithium, tramadol, buspirone, St John's wort, tryptophan) or agents that impair metabolism of serotonin (eg, MAO inhibitors intended to treat psychiatric disorders, other MAO inhibitors [ie, linezolid and intravenous methylene blue]). Monitor patients closely for signs of SS such as mental status changes (eg, agitation, hallucinations, delirium, coma); autonomic instability (eg, tachycardia, labile blood pressure, dizziness, diaphoresis, flushing, hyperthermia, incoordination); neuromuscular changes (eg, tremor, rigidity, myoclonus, hyperreflexia, incoordination); GI symptoms (eg, nausea, vomiting, diarrhea); and/or seizures. Discontinue treatment (and any concomitant serotonergic agent) immediately if signs/symptoms arise. Potential for severe reaction when used with MAO inhibitors; autonomic instability, coma, death, delirium, diaphoresis, hyperthermia, mental status changes/agitation, muscular rigidity, myoclonus, neuroleptic malignant syndrome features, and seizures may occur; concurrent use with MAO inhibitors is contraindicated. Do not use milnacipran in combination with an MAO inhibitor or within 14 days of discontinuing an MAO inhibitor; do not start an MAO inhibitor until ≥5 days after discontinuing milnacipran. Symptoms of serotonin syndrome may occur with concomitant proserotonergic drugs (ie, SSRIs/SNRIs or triptans), agents which reduce milnacipran's metabolism, or antidopaminergic agents (including antipsychotics). Concurrent use of serotonin precursors (eg, tryptophan) is not recommended.

May increase blood pressure and heart rate. Preexisting cardiovascular disease (including hypertension and tachyarrhythmias) should be treated prior to initiating therapy. Blood pressure and heart rate should be evaluated prior to initiating therapy and periodically thereafter; consider dose reduction or gradual discontinuation of therapy in individuals with sustained hypertension or tachycardia during therapy. Use with caution in patients with pre-existing hypertension, tachyarrhythmias (eg, atrial fibrillation), or other cardiovascular disease; and with concomitant medications known to increase blood pressure or heart rate. May impair platelet aggregation resulting in increased risk of bleeding events, particularly if used concomitantly with aspirin or NSAIDs due to ulcerogenic potential. Data are inconclusive regarding extent of bleeding risk of SNRIs in combination with warfarin or other anticoagulants. Bleeding related to SNRI use has been reported to range from relatively minor bruising and epistaxis to life-threatening hemorrhage. Avoid use in patients with substantial ethanol intake, evidence of chronic liver disease or hepatic impairment. Cases of increased liver enzymes and severe liver injury (including fulminant hepatitis) have been reported. Discontinue therapy with the presentation of jaundice or other signs of hepatic dysfunction and do not reinitiate therapy unless another source or cause is identified. Use caution in patients with a history of seizures. Use caution in patients with a history of dysuria, especially males with prostatic hypertrophy, prostatitis, or other lower urinary tract disorders. Use caution in patients with controlled narrow-angle glaucoma; use is contraindicated with uncontrolled narrow-angle glaucoma. SSRIs and SNRIs have been associated with the development of SIADH; hyponatremia has been reported rarely (including severe cases with serum sodium <110 mmol/L), predominately in the elderly. Volume depletion and/or concurrent use of diuretics likely increases risk. Bone fractures have been associated with antidepressant treatment. Use caution in elderly patients; may cause or exacerbate syndrome of inappropriate antidiuretic hormone secretion or hyponatremia. Consider the possibility of a fragility fracture if an antidepressant-treated patient presents with unexplained bone pain, point tenderness, swelling, or bruising (Rabenda, 2013; Rizzoli, 2012).

Abrupt discontinuation or interruption of antidepressant therapy has been associated with a discontinuation syndrome. Symptoms arising may vary with antidepressant however commonly include nausea, vomiting, diarrhea, headaches, light-headedness, dizziness, diminished appetite, sweating, chills, tremors, paresthesias, fatigue, somnolence, and sleep disturbances (eg, vivid dreams, insomnia). Greater risks for developing a discontinuation syndrome have been associated with antidepressants with shorter half-lives, longer durations of treatment, and abrupt discontinuation. For antidepressants of short or intermediate half-lives, symptoms may emerge within 2-5 days after treatment discontinuation and last 7-14 days (APA, 2010; Fava, 2006; Haddad, 2001; Shelton, 2001; Warner, 2006).

Drug Interactions

Avoid Concomitant Use

Avoid concomitant use of Milnacipran with any of the following: Iobenguane I 123; Linezolid; MAO Inhibitors; Methylene Blue; Urokinase

Decreased Effect

Milnacipran may decrease the levels/effects of: Alpha2-Agonists; Iobenguane I 123; Ioflupane I 123

The levels/effects of Milnacipran may be decreased by: Nonsteroidal Anti-Inflammatory Agents

Increased Effect/Toxicity

Milnacipran may increase the levels/effects of: Agents with Antiplatelet Properties; Alpha-/Beta-Agonists; Anticoagulants; Antipsychotics; Aspirin; Collagenase (Systemic); Dabigatran Etexilate; Digoxin; Ibritumomab; Methylene Blue; Metoclopramide; NSAID (Nonselective); Rivaroxaban; Salicylates; Serotonin Modulators; Thrombolytic Agents; Tositumomab and Iodine I 131 Tositumomab; Urokinase; Vitamin K Antagonists

The levels/effects of Milnacipran may be increased by: Alcohol (Ethyl); Antipsychotics; ClomiPRAMINE; Dasatinib; Glucosamine; Herbs (Anticoagulant/Antiplatelet Properties); Ibrutinib; Linezolid; MAO Inhibitors; Multivitamins/Fluoride (with ADE); Multivitamins/Minerals (with ADEK, Folate, Iron); Multivitamins/Minerals (with AE, No Iron); Nonsteroidal Anti-Inflammatory Agents; Omega-3 Fatty Acids; Pentosan Polysulfate Sodium; Pentoxifylline; Prostacyclin Analogues; Tipranavir; Vitamin E

Nutritional/Ethanol Interactions

Ethanol: Ethanol may increase CNS depression. Management: Avoid ethanol.

Herb/Nutraceutical: Some herbal medications may increase risk of serotonin syndrome and/or excessive sedation. Management: Avoid valerian, St John's wort, SAMe, kava kava, and tryptophan.

Adverse Reactions

>10%:

Central nervous system: Headache (18%), insomnia (12%)

Endocrine & metabolic: Hot flashes (12%)

Gastrointestinal: Nausea (37%), constipation (16%)

1% to 10%:

Cardiovascular: Palpitation (7%), heart rate increased (6%), hypertension (5%), blood pressure increased (3%), flushing (3%), tachycardia (2%), peripheral edema (≥1%)

Central nervous system: Dizziness (10%), migraine (5%), chills (2%), tremor (2%), depression (≥1%), fatigue (≥1%), fever (≥1%), irritability (≥1%), somnolence (≥1%)

Dermatologic: Hyperhidrosis (9%), rash (3%)

Endocrine & metabolic: Hypercholesterolemia (≥1%)

Gastrointestinal: Vomiting (7%), xerostomia (5%), abdominal pain (3%), appetite decreased (2%), abdominal distension (≥1%), abnormal taste (≥1%), diarrhea (≥1%), dyspepsia (≥1%), flatulence (≥1%), gastroesophageal reflux disease (≥1%), weight changes (≥1%)

Genitourinary: Dysuria (≥2%), ejaculation disorder/failure (≥2%), erectile dysfunction (≥2%), libido decreased (≥2%), prostatitis (≥2%), scrotal pain (≥2%), testicular pain (≥2%), testicular swelling (≥2%), urethral pain (≥2%), urinary hesitation (≥2%), urinary retention (≥2%), urine flow decreased (≥2%), cystitis (≥1%), urinary tract infection (≥1%)

Neuromuscular & skeletal: Falling (≥1%)

Ocular: Blurred vision (2%)

Respiratory: Dyspnea (2%)

Miscellaneous: Night sweats (≥1%)

Available Dosage Forms

Miscellaneous, Oral:

Savella Titration Pack: 12.5 mg (5s), 25 mg (8s), and 50 mg (42s)

Tablet, Oral:

Savella: 12.5 mg, 25 mg, 50 mg, 100 mg

General Dosage Range Dosage adjustment recommended in patients with renal impairment

Oral: *Adults:* 50 mg twice daily

Administration

Oral Administer with or without food; food may improve tolerability.

Storage/Stability Store at 25°C (77°F); excursions permitted between 15°C to 30°C (59°F to 86°F).

Nursing Actions

Physical Assessment Monitor blood pressure and heart rate prior to initiating therapy and periodically throughout. Monitor for signs and symptoms of suicide ideation (eg, anxiety, depression, behavior changes). Taper dosage when discontinuing.

Patient Education

• Discuss specific use of drug and side effects with patient as it relates to treatment. (HCAHPS: During this hospital stay, were you given any medicine that you had not taken before? Before giving you any new medicine, how often did hospital staff tell you what the medicine was for? How often did hospital staff describe possible side effects in a way you could understand?)

• Patient may experience dizziness, flushing, headache, nausea, constipation, or insomnia. Have patient report immediately to prescriber depression, dyspnea, angina, illogical thinking, significant change in balance, fasciculations, tremors, tachycardia, ecchymosis, bleeding, severe asthenia, or rash (HCAHPS).

• Educate patient about signs of a significant reaction (eg, wheezing; chest tightness; fever; itching; bad cough; blue skin color; seizures; or swelling of face, lips, tongue, or throat). **Note:** This is not a comprehensive list of all side effects. Patient should consult prescriber for additional questions.

Intended Use and Disclaimer: Should not be printed and given to patients. This information is intended to serve as a concise initial reference for healthcare professionals to use when discussing medications with a patient. You must ultimately rely on your own discretion, experience and judgment in diagnosing, treating and advising patients.

Milrinone (MIL ri none)

Index Terms Milrinone Lactate

Pharmacologic Category Inotrope; Phosphodiesterase-3 Enzyme Inhibitor

Medication Safety Issues

Sound-alike/look-alike issues:

Primacor may be confused with Primaxin

High alert medication:

The Institute for Safe Medication Practices (ISMP) includes this medication among its list of drugs which have a heightened risk of causing significant patient harm when used in error.

Pregnancy Risk Factor C

Lactation Excretion in breast milk unknown/use caution

Breast-Feeding Considerations It is not known if milrinone is excreted in breast milk. The manufacturer recommends that caution be exercised when administering milrinone to nursing women.

Use Short-term I.V. therapy of acutely-decompensated heart failure

American College of Cardiology/American Heart Association heart failure (HF) guideline recommendations (ACCF/AHA [Yancy, 2013]): To maintain systemic perfusion and preserve end-organ performance in patients with cardiogenic shock; bridge therapy in stage D HF unresponsive to guideline-directed medical therapy and device therapy in patients awaiting heart transplant or mechanical circulatory support; short-term management of hospitalized patients with severe systolic dysfunction presenting with low blood pressure and significantly depressed cardiac output; long-term management (palliative therapy) in select patients with stage D HF unresponsive to guideline-directed medical therapy and device therapy who are not candidates for heart transplant or mechanical circulatory support.

Unlabeled Use Inotropic therapy for patients unresponsive to other acute heart failure therapies (eg, dobutamine); outpatient inotropic therapy for heart transplant candidates; palliation of symptoms in end-stage heart failure patients who cannot otherwise be discharged from the hospital and are not transplant candidates

Mechanism of Action/Effect Phosphodiesterase inhibitor resulting in vasodilation

Contraindications Hypersensitivity to milrinone, inamrinone, or any component of the formulation; concurrent use of inamrinone

Warnings/Precautions Monitor closely for hypotension. Avoid in severe obstructive aortic or pulmonic valvular disease. Milrinone may aggravate outflow tract obstruction in hypertrophic subaortic stenosis. Supraventricular and ventricular arrhythmias have developed in high-risk patients. Ensure that ventricular rate controlled in atrial fibrillation/flutter prior to initiating milrinone. Not recommended for use in acute MI patients. Monitor and correct fluid and electrolyte problems. Adjust dose in renal dysfunction. Discontinue therapy if dose-related elevations in LFTs and clinical symptoms of hepatotoxicity occur. According to the ACCF/AHA 2013 heart failure guidelines, long-term use of intravenous inotropic therapy without a specific indication or for reasons other than palliation is potentially harmful.

Drug Interactions

Avoid Concomitant Use

Avoid concomitant use of Milrinone with any of the following: Riociguat

Decreased Effect There are no known significant interactions involving a decrease in effect.

Increased Effect/Toxicity

Milrinone may increase the levels/effects of: Riociguat

Adverse Reactions

>10%: Cardiovascular: Ventricular arrhythmia (ectopy 9%, NSVT 3%, sustained ventricular tachycardia 1%, ventricular fibrillation <1%)

1% to 10%:

Cardiovascular: Supraventricular arrhythmia (4%), hypotension (3%), angina/chest pain (1%)

Central nervous system: Headache (3%)

Pharmacodynamics/Kinetics

Onset of Action I.V.: 5-15 minutes

Available Dosage Forms

Solution, Intravenous:

Generic: 200 mcg/mL (100 mL, 200 mL); 10 mg/10 mL (10 mL); 20 mg/20 mL (20 mL); 50 mg/50 mL (50 mL)

Solution, Intravenous [preservative free]:

Generic: 200 mcg/mL (100 mL, 200 mL)

General Dosage Range Dosage adjustment recommended in patients with renal impairment

I.V.: *Adults:* Loading dose (optional): 50 mcg/kg; Maintenance: 0.125-0.75 mcg/kg/minute

Usual Infusion Concentrations: Pediatric Note: Premixed solutions available

I.V. infusion: 200 mcg/mL

Usual Infusion Concentrations: Adult Note: Premixed solutions available

I.V. infusion: 20 mg in 100 mL (total volume) (concentration: 200 mcg/mL) of D_5W

Administration

I.V. Infuse via infusion pump.

Injectable Detail Injectable solution and premixed solution: pH: 3.2-4

Preparation for Administration Standard dilution: For a final concentration of 0.2 mg/mL: Dilute Primacor® 1 mg/mL (20 mL) with 80 mL diluent (final volume: 100 mL) of ½NS, NS or D_5W. May also dilute 1 mg/mL (10 mL) with 40 mL diluent (final volume: 50 mL).

Storage/Stability Store at 15°C to 30°C (59°F to 86°F); avoid freezing. Stable at 0.2 mg/mL in ½NS, NS, or D_5W for 72 hours at room temperature in normal light.

Nursing Actions

Physical Assessment Monitor cardiac/hemodynamic status continuously during therapy and serum potassium at regular intervals. Monitor for fluid retention.

Patient Education

• Discuss specific use of drug and side effects with patient as it relates to treatment. (HCAHPS: During this hospital stay, were you given any medicine that you had not taken before? Before giving you any new medicine, how often did hospital staff tell you what the medicine was for? How often did hospital staff describe possible side effects in a way you could understand?)

• Patient may experience headache, hypotension, injection site irritation, or hepatic impairment. Have patient report immediately to prescriber angina, tachycardia, severe dizziness, ecchymosis, bleeding, or rash (HCAHPS).

• Educate patient about signs of a significant reaction (eg, wheezing; chest tightness; fever; itching; bad cough; blue skin color; seizures; or swelling of face, lips, tongue, or throat). **Note:** This is not a comprehensive list of all side effects. Patient should consult prescriber for additional questions.

Intended Use and Disclaimer: Should not be printed and given to patients. This information is intended to serve as a concise initial reference for healthcare professionals to use when discussing medications with a patient. You must ultimately rely on your own discretion, experience and

◀ judgment in diagnosing, treating and advising patients.

Minocycline (mi noe SYE kleen)

Brand Names: U.S. Dynacin [DSC]; Minocin; Solodyn

Index Terms Minocycline Hydrochloride; Ximino™

Pharmacologic Category Antibiotic, Tetracycline Derivative

Medication Safety Issues

Sound-alike/look-alike issues:

Dynacin® may be confused with Dyazide®, Dynapen

Minocin® may be confused with Indocin®, Lincocin®, Minizide®, niacin

Pregnancy Risk Factor D

Lactation Enters breast milk/not recommended

Breast-Feeding Considerations Minocycline is excreted in breast milk (Brogden, 1975). According to the manufacturer, the decision to continue or discontinue breast-feeding during therapy should take into account the risk of exposure to the infant and the benefits of treatment to the mother. Oral absorption is not affected by dairy products; therefore, oral absorption of minocycline by the breast-feeding infant would not be expected to be diminished by the calcium in the maternal milk. Non-dose-related effects could include modification of bowel flora. There have been case reports of black discoloration of breast milk in women taking minocycline (Basler, 1985; Hunt, 1996).

Use Treatment of susceptible bacterial infections of both gram-negative and gram-positive organisms; treatment of anthrax (inhalational, cutaneous, and gastrointestinal); moderate-to-severe acne; meningococcal (asymptomatic) carrier state; Rickettsial diseases (including Rocky Mountain spotted fever, Q fever); nongonococcal urethritis, gonorrhea; acute intestinal amebiasis; respiratory tract infection; skin/soft tissue infections; chlamydial infections

Extended release (Solodyn®): Only indicated for treatment of inflammatory lesions of non-nodular moderate-to-severe acne

Unlabeled Use Rheumatoid arthritis (patients with low disease activity of short duration); nocardiosis; alternative treatment for community-acquired MRSA infection; chronic oral antimicrobial suppression of prosthetic joint infection

Mechanism of Action/Effect Inhibits bacterial protein synthesis by binding with the 30S and possibly the 50S ribosomal subunit(s) of susceptible bacteria; cell wall synthesis is not affected

Rheumatoid arthritis: The mechanism of action of minocycline in rheumatoid arthritis is not completely understood. It is thought to have antimicrobial, anti-inflammatory, immunomodulatory, and chondroprotective effects. More specifically, it is thought to be a potent inhibitor of metalloproteinases, which are active in rheumatoid arthritis joint destruction.

Contraindications Hypersensitivity to minocycline, other tetracyclines, or any component of the formulation

Warnings/Precautions May be associated with increases in BUN secondary to antianabolic effects; use caution in patients with renal impairment (CrCl <80 mL/minute). Hepatotoxicity has been reported; use caution in patients with hepatic insufficiency. Autoimmune syndromes (eg, lupus-like, hepatitis, and vasculitis) have been reported; discontinue if symptoms occur. CNS effects (lightheadedness, vertigo) may occur; patients must be cautioned about performing tasks which require mental alertness (eg, operating machinery or driving). Pseudotumor cerebri has been (rarely) reported with tetracycline use; usually resolves with discontinuation. May cause photosensitivity; discontinue if skin erythema occurs. Prolonged use may result in fungal or bacterial superinfection, including *C. difficile*-associated diarrhea (CDAD) and pseudomembranous colitis; CDAD has been observed >2 months postantibiotic treatment. May cause tissue hyperpigmentation, enamel hypoplasia, or permanent tooth discoloration; use of tetracyclines should be avoided during tooth development (children <8 years of age) unless other drugs are not likely to be effective or are contraindicated. Do not use during pregnancy. In addition to affecting tooth development, tetracycline use has been associated with retardation of skeletal development and reduced bone growth. Rash, along with eosinophilia, fever, and organ failure (Drug Rash with Eosinophilia and Systemic Symptoms [DRESS] syndrome) has been reported; discontinue treatment immediately if DRESS syndrome is suspected.

Drug Interactions

Avoid Concomitant Use

Avoid concomitant use of Minocycline with any of the following: BCG; Retinoic Acid Derivatives; Strontium Ranelate

Decreased Effect

Minocycline may decrease the levels/effects of: Atazanavir; BCG; Penicillins; Sodium Picosulfate; Typhoid Vaccine

The levels/effects of Minocycline may be decreased by: Antacids; Bile Acid Sequestrants; Bismuth; Bismuth Subsalicylate; Calcium Salts; Iron Salts; Lanthanum; Magnesium Salts; Multivitamins/Minerals (with ADEK, Folate, Iron); Multivitamins/Minerals (with AE, No Iron); Quinapril; Strontium Ranelate; Sucralfate; Sucroferric Oxyhydroxide; Zinc Salts

Increased Effect/Toxicity

Minocycline may increase the levels/effects of: Mipomersen; Neuromuscular-Blocking Agents; Porfimer; Retinoic Acid Derivatives; Vitamin K Antagonists

Nutritional/Ethanol Interactions

Food: Minocycline serum concentrations are not significantly altered if taken with food or dairy products.

Herb/Nutraceutical: Avoid dong quai, St John's wort (may also cause photosensitization).

Adverse Reactions Frequency not defined.

Cardiovascular: Myocarditis, pericarditis, vasculitis

Central nervous system: Bulging fontanels, dizziness, fatigue, fever, headache, hypoesthesia, malaise, mood changes, paresthesia, pseudotumor cerebri, sedation, seizure, somnolence, vertigo

Dermatologic: Alopecia, angioedema, drug rash with eosinophilia and systemic symptoms (DRESS), erythema multiforme, erythema nodosum, erythematous rash, exfoliative dermatitis, hyperpigmentation of nails, maculopapular rash, photosensitivity, pigmentation of the skin and mucous membranes, pruritus, Stevens-Johnson syndrome, toxic epidermal necrolysis, urticaria

Endocrine & metabolic: Thyroid cancer, thyroid discoloration, thyroid dysfunction

Gastrointestinal: Anorexia, diarrhea, dyspepsia, dysphagia, enamel hypoplasia, enterocolitis, esophageal ulcerations, esophagitis, glossitis, inflammatory lesions (oral/anogenital), moniliasis, nausea, oral cavity discoloration, pancreatitis, pseudomembranous colitis, stomatitis, tooth discoloration, vomiting, xerostomia

Genitourinary: Balanitis, vulvovaginitis

Hematologic: Agranulocytosis, eosinophilia, hemolytic anemia, leukopenia, neutropenia, pancytopenia, thrombocytopenia

Hepatic: Autoimmune hepatitis, hepatic cholestasis, hepatic failure, hepatitis, hyperbilirubinemia, jaundice, liver enzyme increases

Local: Injection site reaction (I.V. administration)

Neuromuscular & skeletal: Arthralgia, arthritis, bone discoloration, joint stiffness, joint swelling, myalgia

Otic: Hearing loss, tinnitus

Renal: Acute renal failure, BUN increased, interstitial nephritis

Respiratory: Asthma, bronchospasm, cough, dyspnea, pneumonitis, pulmonary infiltrate (with eosinophilia)

Miscellaneous: Anaphylaxis, hypersensitivity, lupus erythematosus, lupus-like syndrome, serum sickness

Product Availability Ximino™ extended-release capsules: FDA approved July 2012; anticipated availability currently unknown. Consult prescribing information for additional information.

Available Dosage Forms

Capsule, Oral:
Minocin: 50 mg, 75 mg, 100 mg
Generic: 50 mg, 75 mg, 100 mg
Kit, Combination:
Minocin: 50 mg, 100 mg

Solution Reconstituted, Intravenous:
Minocin: 100 mg (1 ea)
Tablet, Oral:
Generic: 50 mg, 75 mg, 100 mg
Tablet Extended Release 24 Hour, Oral:
Solodyn: 55 mg, 65 mg, 80 mg, 105 mg, 115 mg
Generic: 45 mg, 90 mg, 135 mg

General Dosage Range Dosage adjustment recommended in patients with renal impairment

I.V.:
Children >8 years: 4 mg/kg initially, followed by 2 mg/kg/dose every 12 hours (maximum: 400 mg daily)
Adults: 200 mg initially, followed by 100 mg every 12 hours (maximum: 400 mg daily)

Oral:
Children >8 years: 4 mg/kg initially, followed by 2 mg/kg/dose every 12 hours
Children ≥12 years: Solodyn®: 45-135 mg once daily (weight-based)
Adults: 200 mg initially, followed by 100 mg every 12 hours **or** 50-100 mg twice daily (acne); Solodyn®: 45-135 mg once daily (weight-based)

Administration

I.V. I.V.: Infuse slowly; avoid rapid administration. The manufacturer's labeling does not provide a recommended administration rate. The injectable route should be used only if the oral route is not feasible or adequate. Prolonged intravenous therapy may be associated with thrombophlebitis.

Oral May be administered with or without food. Administer with adequate fluid to decrease the risk of esophageal irritation and ulceration. Swallow pellet-filled capsule and extended release tablet whole; do not chew, crush, or split.

Preparation for Administration Injection: Reconstitute with 5 mL of sterile water for injection, and further dilute in 500-1000 mL of NS, D_5W, D_5NS, Ringer's injection, or LR.

Storage/Stability

Capsule (including pellet-filled), tablet: Store at 20°C to 25°C (68°F to 77°F); protect from heat. Protect from light and moisture.

Extended release tablet: Store at 15°C to 30°C (59°F to 86°F); protect from heat. Protect from light and moisture.

Injection: Store vials at 20°C to 25°C (68°F to 77°F) prior to reconstitution. Reconstituted solution is stable at room temperature for 24 hours. Final dilutions should be administered immediately.

Nursing Actions

Physical Assessment Results of culture and sensitivity tests and allergy history should be assessed before beginning therapy. Teach patient importance of adequate hydration.

Patient Education

• Discuss specific use of drug and side effects with patient as it relates to treatment. (HCAHPS: During this hospital stay, were you given any medicine that you had not taken before? Before giving you any new medicine, how often did ▶

hospital staff tell you what the medicine was for? How often did hospital staff describe possible side effects in a way you could understand?)

- Patient may experience diarrhea, dizziness, fatigue, nausea, lack of appetite, or injection site irritation. Have patient report immediately to prescriber signs of hepatic impairment, signs of pancreatitis, vision changes, urinary retention, oliguria, chills, pharyngitis, hearing impairment, arthralgia, myalgia, severe headache, tinnitus, dyspnea, enlarged lymph nodes, dysphagia, ecchymosis, hemorrhaging, rectal irritation, significant asthenia, stomatitis, genital irritation, vaginal yeast infection, or signs of pseudomembranous colitis (HCAHPS).
- Educate patient about signs of a significant reaction (eg, wheezing; chest tightness; fever; itching; bad cough; blue skin color; seizures; or swelling of face, lips, tongue, or throat). **Note:** This is not a comprehensive list of all side effects. Patient should consult prescriber for additional questions.

Intended Use and Disclaimer: Should not be printed and given to patients. This information is intended to serve as a concise initial reference for healthcare professionals to use when discussing medications with a patient. You must ultimately rely on your own discretion, experience and judgment in diagnosing, treating and advising patients.

Dietary Considerations May be taken with or without food.

Related Information

Oral Medications That Should Not Be Crushed or Altered *on page 1712*

Mipomersen (mi poe MER sen)

Brand Names: U.S. Kynamro
Index Terms ISIS 301012; Mipomersen Sodium
Pharmacologic Category Antihyperlipidemic Agent, Apolipoprotein B Antisense Oligonucleotide
Medication Guide Available Yes
Pregnancy Risk Factor B
Lactation Excretion in breast milk unknown/not recommended
Breast-Feeding Considerations It is not known if mipomersen is excreted in breast milk. Breastfeeding is not recommended by the manufacturer.
Use Adjunct to dietary therapy and other lipid-lowering treatments to reduce low-density lipoprotein cholesterol (LDL-C), total cholesterol, apolipoprotein B, and non-high-density lipoprotein cholesterol (non-HDL-C) in patients with homozygous familial hypercholesterolemia (HoFH)
Mechanism of Action/Effect Mipomersen is an oligonucleotide inhibitor of apo B-100 synthesis. ApoB is the main component of LDL-C and very low density lipoprotein (VLDL), the precursor to LDL-C. Mipomersen binds to the messenger ribonucleic acid (mRNA) of apoB in a sequence-specific manner resulting in degradation or disruption of the mRNA thereby reducing formation of apoB.

Contraindications Hypersensitivity to mipomersen or any component of the formulation; moderate or severe hepatic impairment (Child-Pugh class B or C); active liver disease; unexplained persistent elevations of hepatic transaminases

Warnings/Precautions [U.S. Boxed Warning]: As seen in clinical trials, may cause hepatic transaminase elevation and increases in hepatic steatosis (with or without concomitant increases in transaminases) which may progress to steatohepatitis and cirrhosis; measure ALT, AST, alkaline phosphatase, and total bilirubin prior to initiation, then ALT and AST on a regular basis as recommended. Withhold dose of mipomersen if ALT or AST is ≥3 x ULN. Discontinue mipomersen if clinically significant hepatotoxicity occurs. Because mipomersen has a risk of hepatotoxicity, it is only available through a restricted program under a Risk Evaluation and Mitigation Strategy (REMS) program (Kynamro™ REMS). Alcohol consumption during treatment with mipomersen should be limited to ≤1 drink/day due to potential to increase levels of hepatic fat and induce or exacerbate liver injury. Use caution when used concomitantly with other medications known to cause hepatotoxicity (eg, isotretinoin, amiodarone, acetaminophen [>4 g/day for ≥3 days/week], methotrexate, tetracyclines, and tamoxifen); consider monitoring liver function tests more frequently. Concurrent use with LDL-C lowering medications that can also increase hepatic fat is not recommended. Use is contraindicated in patients with moderate or severe hepatic impairment or active liver disease including patients with unexplained persistent elevations of hepatic transaminases. If baseline liver function tests are abnormal, consider initiation after an appropriate work up and abnormalities are explained or resolved.

Within 2 days after an injection, influenza-like symptoms (eg, fever, chills, myalgia, arthralgia, malaise, or fatigue) have been reported in 30% of patients receiving mipomersen. Injection site reactions (eg, erythema, pain, tenderness, pruritus, and local swelling) were common in patients receiving mipomersen; minimize injection site reactions by using proper subcutaneous administration technique.

Safety and efficacy in patients with hepatic impairment have not been established; use is contraindicated in patients with moderate or severe hepatic impairment (Child-Pugh class B or C), active liver disease, or unexplained persistent elevations of hepatic transaminases. Safety and efficacy in patients with renal impairment including those who undergo hemodialysis have not been established; use is not recommended in patients with severe renal impairment, clinically significant proteinuria, or on hemodialysis.

In clinical trials, patients ≥65 years of age (n=59) experienced a higher incidence of hepatic steatosis, hypertension, and peripheral edema; use with caution in the elderly. Safety and efficacy of the treatment of hypercholesterolemia not due to homozygous familial hypercholesterolemia (HoFH) have not been established. The use of mipomersen as an adjunct to LDL-C apheresis is not recommended (use not established).

Drug Interactions

Avoid Concomitant Use There are no known interactions where it is recommended to avoid concomitant use.

Decreased Effect There are no known significant interactions involving a decrease in effect.

Increased Effect/Toxicity

Mipomersen may increase the levels/effects of: Methotrexate

The levels/effects of Mipomersen may be increased by: Acetaminophen; Alcohol (Ethyl); Amiodarone; ISOtretinoin; Tamoxifen; Tetracycline Derivatives

Nutritional/Ethanol Interactions Ethanol: Limit alcohol consumption during treatment with mipomersen to ≤1 drink/day due to potential for increased levels of hepatic fat and induced or exacerbated liver injury.

Adverse Reactions

>10%:
  Central nervous system: Fatigue (15%), headache (12%)
  Gastrointestinal: Nausea (14%)
  Hepatic: ALT increased (≥3 x ULN to <5 x ULN: 12%; ≥5 x ULN to <10 x ULN: 3%; ≥10 x ULN: 1%)
  Local: Injection site reactions: Erythema (59%), pain (56%), hematoma (32%), pruritus (29%), swelling (18%), discoloration (17%)
  Miscellaneous: Antibody formation (38% to 72%), flu-like syndrome (13% to 66%)
1% to 10%:
  Cardiovascular: Hypertension (7%), peripheral edema (5%), angina pectoris (4%), palpitations (3%)
  Central nervous system: Fever (8%), chills (6%), insomnia (3%)
  Gastrointestinal: Vomiting (4%), abdominal pain (3%)
  Hepatic: Hepatic steatosis (7%), AST increased (≥3 x ULN to <5 x ULN: 7%; ≥5 x ULN to <10 x ULN: 3%)
  Neuromuscular & skeletal: Limb pain (7%), musculoskeletal pain (4%)
  Renal: Proteinuria (9%)
  Miscellaneous: Neoplasms (4%, benign and malignant)

Available Dosage Forms

Solution, Subcutaneous [preservative free]:
  Kynamro: 200 mg/mL (1 mL)

General Dosage Range SubQ: *Adults:* 200 mg once weekly

Administration

Subcutaneous For subQ administration only. Do not administer I.M. or I.V. Remove from refrigerator, allow to reach room temperature (≥30 minutes prior to administration), and visually inspect prior to administration; do not administer if solution is cloudy or contains visible particulate matter (return to pharmacy). Administer first injection under the guidance/supervision of a qualified health care professional. Administer SubQ into the abdomen, thigh region, or outer area of upper arm; do not administer where there is active skin disease (eg, sunburns, skin rash, inflammation/infection) or into tattooed skin or scar. Administer on the same day every week. If dose is missed, administer at least 3 days before the next weekly dose.

Storage/Stability Store refrigerated solution at 2°C to 8°C (36°F to 46°F) or when refrigeration is not available, may store at ≤30°C (86°F) (away from heat sources) for up to 14 days. Protect from light. Keep in original container until time of use. For single use only; discard any unused drug after removal of dose.

Nursing Actions

Physical Assessment Monitor for signs and symptoms of liver injury (nausea, lethargy, jaundice, abdominal pain, fever, vomiting, or flu-like symptoms). Educate regarding importance of limiting alcohol intake to one drink per day. Monitor for drug-drug interactions with other hepatotoxic medications. Monitor for injection site reactions. Teach correct technique for subcutaneous injections.

Patient Education

• Discuss specific use of drug and side effects with patient as it relates to treatment. (HCAHPS: During this hospital stay, were you given any medicine that you had not taken before? Before giving you any new medicine, how often did hospital staff tell you what the medicine was for? How often did hospital staff describe possible side effects in a way you could understand?)
• Patient may experience nausea, headache, flu-like syndrome, injection site irritation, or hepatic impairment. Have patient report immediately to prescriber severe dyspepsia, considerable asthenia, inability to eat, discolored urine, jaundice, significant skin irritation, or rash (HCAHPS).
• Educate patient about signs of a significant reaction (eg, wheezing; chest tightness; fever; itching; bad cough; blue skin color; seizures; or swelling of face, lips, tongue, or throat). **Note:** This is not a comprehensive list of all side

effects. Patient should consult prescriber for additional questions.

Intended Use and Disclaimer: Should not be printed and given to patients. This information is intended to serve as a concise initial reference for healthcare professionals to use when discussing medications with a patient. You must ultimately rely on your own discretion, experience and judgment in diagnosing, treating and advising patients.

Dietary Considerations Limit alcohol consumption during treatment with mipomersen to ≤1 drink/day due to potential for increased levels of hepatic fat and induced or exacerbated liver injury.

Mirabegron (mir a BEG ron)

Brand Names: U.S. Myrbetriq
Index Terms YM-178
Pharmacologic Category Beta$_3$ Agonist
Pregnancy Risk Factor C
Lactation Excretion in breast milk unknown/not recommended
Breast-Feeding Considerations Excretion of mirabegron into breast milk is expected. According to the manufacturer, the decision to continue or discontinue breast-feeding during therapy should take into account the risk of exposure to the infant and the benefits of treatment to the mother.
Use Treatment of overactive bladder (OAB) with symptoms of urinary frequency, urgency, or urge incontinence
Mechanism of Action/Effect Increases bladder capacity by relaxing the smooth muscle of the bladder during the urine storage phase
Contraindications There are no contraindications listed in the manufacturer's U.S. product labeling.

Canadian labeling: Hypersensitivity to mirabegron or any component of the formulation; severe uncontrolled hypertension (systolic blood pressure ≥180 mm Hg and/or diastolic blood pressure ≥110 mm Hg); pregnancy

Warnings/Precautions Dose-related increases in blood pressure were observed in clinical trials (mean increase of ~0.5-1 mm Hg compared to placebo in overactive bladder patients treated with 50 mg); monitor blood pressure periodically during therapy. Not recommended for use in patients with severe uncontrolled hypertension (SBP ≥180 and/or DBP ≥110 mm Hg); if used in patients with controlled and less severe hypertension, use with caution and monitor blood pressure closely; exacerbation of pre-existing hypertension has been reported. Use with caution in patients with bladder outlet obstruction (BOO) or in patients taking concomitant antimuscarinic medications; the risk of urinary retention may be increased. Use with caution in patients with a history of QT interval prolongation or those receiving medications known to prolong the QT interval. In one thorough QT study,

supratherapeutic doses prolonged the QTc interval based on the individual subject-specific correction method (QTcI) in females but not in males (Malik, 2012). In general, mirabegron at the recommended dose has a low risk of QT interval prolongation (Sanford, 2013).

Mirabegron is a moderate CYP2D6 inhibitor; potentially significant drug-drug interactions may exist, requiring dose or frequency adjustment, additional monitoring, and/or selection of alternative therapy. Use with caution in patients with mild-to-moderate hepatic impairment; dosage adjustment is required in patients with moderate hepatic impairment. Use is not recommended in severe hepatic impairment. Use with caution in patients with renal impairment; dosage adjustment is required in patients with severe renal impairment. Use is not recommended in ESRD. Systemic exposure is increased in females compared to males; however, dosage adjustments are not necessary or recommended.

Drug Interactions
Avoid Concomitant Use
Avoid concomitant use of Mirabegron with any of the following: Pimozide; Thioridazine
Decreased Effect
Mirabegron may decrease the levels/effects of: Codeine; Metoprolol; Tamoxifen; TraMADol

The levels/effects of Mirabegron may be decreased by: Peginterferon Alfa-2b; Rifampin
Increased Effect/Toxicity
Mirabegron may increase the levels/effects of: ARIPiprazole; CYP2D6 Substrates; Desipramine; Digoxin; Dofetilide; DOXOrubicin (Conventional); Fesoterodine; Flecainide; Highest Risk QTc-Prolonging Agents; Lomitapide; Metoprolol; Moderate Risk QTc-Prolonging Agents; Nebivolol; Pimozide; Propafenone; Solifenacin; Thioridazine

The levels/effects of Mirabegron may be increased by: Anticholinergic Agents; Ketoconazole (Systemic); Mifepristone
Nutritional/Ethanol Interactions Food: Coadministration with a high-fat meal decreased C_{max} and AUC by 45% and 17%, respectively. Coadministration with a low-fat meal decreased C_{max} and AUC by 75% and 51%, respectively. However, safety and efficacy were unaffected by food intake, and mirabegron may be administered without regard to food.
Adverse Reactions
>10%: Cardiovascular: Hypertension (9% to 11%)
1% to 10%:
Cardiovascular: Tachycardia (2%)
Central nervous system: Headache (4%), dizziness (3%)
Gastrointestinal: Constipation (2% to 3%), xerostomia (3%), diarrhea (2%)
Genitourinary: Urinary tract infection (3% to 6%), cystitis (2%)

Neuromuscular & skeletal: Back pain (3%), arthralgia (2%)

Respiratory: Nasopharyngitis (4%), sinusitis (3%)

Miscellaneous: Flu-like syndrome (3%)

Pharmacodynamics/Kinetics

Onset of Action Efficacy is seen within 8 weeks; steady state achieved within 7 days

Available Dosage Forms

Tablet Extended Release 24 Hour, Oral:

Myrbetriq: 25 mg, 50 mg

General Dosage Range Dosage adjustment recommended in patients with renal and hepatic impairment

Oral: *Adults:* Initial: 25 mg once daily; Maintenance: 25-50 mg once daily

Administration

Oral Administer orally without regard to food. Swallow the tablet whole with water; do not chew, divide, or crush.

Storage/Stability Store at 25°C (77°F); excursions permitted to 15°C to 30°C (59°F to 86°F).

Nursing Actions

Physical Assessment Monitor blood pressure and heart rate. Monitor for improvement in underlying condition; assess for symptoms of urinary retention.

Patient Education

- Discuss specific use of drug and side effects with patient as it relates to treatment. (HCAHPS: During this hospital stay, were you given any medicine that you had not taken before? Before giving you any new medicine, how often did hospital staff tell you what the medicine was for? How often did hospital staff describe possible side effects in a way you could understand?)
- Patient may experience hypertension, headache, or rhinitis. Have patient report immediately to prescriber back pain, hematuria, severe dizziness, inability to urinate, or rash (HCAHPS).
- Educate patient about signs of a significant reaction (eg, wheezing; chest tightness; fever; itching; bad cough; blue skin color; seizures; or swelling of face, lips, tongue, or throat). **Note:** This is not a comprehensive list of all side effects. Patient should consult prescriber for additional questions.

Intended Use and Disclaimer: Should not be printed and given to patients. This information is intended to serve as a concise initial reference for healthcare professionals to use when discussing medications with a patient. You must ultimately rely on your own discretion, experience and judgment in diagnosing, treating and advising patients.

Related Information

Oral Medications That Should Not Be Crushed or Altered *on page 1712*

Mirtazapine (mir TAZ a peen)

Brand Names: U.S. Remeron; Remeron SolTab

Pharmacologic Category Antidepressant, Alpha-2 Antagonist

Medication Safety Issues

Sound-alike/look-alike issues:

Remeron® may be confused with Premarin®, ramelteon, Rozerem®, Zemuron®

BEERS Criteria medication:

This drug may be potentially inappropriate for use in geriatric patients (SIADH: Quality of evidence - moderate; Strength of recommendation - strong).

International issues:

Avanza [Australia] may be confused with Albenza brand name for albendazole [U.S.]; Avandia brand name for rosiglitazone [U.S., Canada, and multiple international markets]

Remeron [U.S., Canada, and multiple international markets] may be confused with Reneuron which is a brand name for fluoxetine [Spain]

Medication Guide Available Yes

Pregnancy Risk Factor C

Lactation Excreted in breast milk/use caution

Breast-Feeding Considerations Mirtazapine and its active metabolite are found in breast milk, with higher levels in the hindmilk than foremilk. Mirtazapine can also be detected in the serum of nursing infants; adverse events have generally not been observed, although possible sedation and weight gain was noted in one case report (Kristensen, 2007; Tonn, 2009). The manufacturer recommends that caution be used if administered to a breast-feeding woman.

Use Treatment of depression

Unlabeled Use Alzheimer's dementia-related depression; post-traumatic stress disorder (PTSD)

Mechanism of Action/Effect Mirtazapine is a tetracyclic antidepressant that works by its central presynaptic alpha$_2$-adrenergic antagonist effects, which results in increased release of norepinephrine and serotonin. It is also a potent antagonist of 5-HT$_2$ and 5-HT$_3$ serotonin receptors and H$_1$ histamine receptors and a moderate peripheral alpha$_1$-adrenergic and muscarinic antagonist; it does not inhibit the reuptake of norepinephrine or serotonin.

Contraindications Hypersensitivity to mirtazapine or any component of the formulation; use of MAO inhibitors intended to treat psychiatric disorders (concurrently or within 14 days of discontinuing either mirtazapine or the MAO inhibitor); initiation of mirtazapine in a patient receiving linezolid or intravenous methylene blue

◀ **Warnings/Precautions [U.S. Boxed Warning]: Antidepressants increase the risk of suicidal thinking and behavior in children, adolescents, and young adults (18-24 years of age) with major depressive disorder (MDD) and other psychiatric disorders;** consider risk prior to prescribing. Short-term studies did not show an increased risk in patients >24 years of age and showed a decreased risk in patients ≥65 years. Closely monitor for clinical worsening, suicidality, or unusual changes in behavior; the patient's family or caregiver should be instructed to closely observe the patient and communicate condition with healthcare provider. A medication guide should be dispensed with each prescription. **Mirtazapine is not FDA approved for use in children.**

The possibility of a suicide attempt is inherent in major depression and may persist until remission occurs. Monitor for worsening of depression or suicidality, especially during initiation of therapy (generally first 1-2 months) or with dose increases or decreases. Use caution in high-risk patients. Worsening depression and severe abrupt suicidality that are not part of the presenting symptoms may require discontinuation or modification of drug therapy. The patient's family or caregiver should be alerted to monitor patients for the emergence of suicidality and associated behaviors (such as agitation, irritability, hostility, impulsivity, and hypomania) and call healthcare provider.

May worsen psychosis in some patients or precipitate a shift to mania or hypomania in patients with bipolar disorder. Patients presenting with depressive symptoms should be screened for bipolar disorder. Monotherapy in patients with bipolar disorder should be avoided. **Mirtazapine is not FDA approved for the treatment of bipolar depression.**

Potentially life-threatening serotonin syndrome (SS) has occurred with serotonergic agents (eg, SSRIs, SNRIs), particularly when used in combination with other serotonergic agents (eg, triptans, TCAs, fentanyl, lithium, tramadol, buspirone, St John's wort, tryptophan) or agents that impair metabolism of serotonin (eg, MAO inhibitors intended to treat psychiatric disorders, other MAO inhibitors such as linezolid and intravenous methylene blue). Discontinue treatment (and any concomitant serotonergic agent) immediately if signs/symptoms arise. Discontinue immediately if signs and symptoms of neutropenia/agranulocytosis occur. May cause sedation, resulting in impaired performance of tasks requiring alertness (eg, operating machinery or driving). The degree of sedation is moderate-high relative to other antidepressants. Conversely, may increase psychomotor restlessness within first few weeks of therapy. The risks of orthostatic hypotension or anticholinergic effects are low relative to other antidepressants. The incidence of sexual dysfunction with mirtazapine

is generally lower than with selective serotonin reuptake inhibitors (SSRIs). May increase appetite and stimulate weight gain. In clinical trials, an increased incidence of weight gain in adults and children was observed with mirtazapine compared to placebo; up to 8% of patients discontinued therapy due to weight gain. May increase serum cholesterol and triglyceride levels. Potentially significant interactions may exist, requiring dose or frequency adjustment, additional monitoring, and/or selection of alternative therapy.

Use caution in patients with a previous seizure disorder or condition predisposing to seizures such as brain damage, alcoholism, or concurrent therapy with other drugs which lower the seizure threshold. Bone fractures have been associated with antidepressant treatment. Consider the possibility of a fragility fracture if an antidepressant-treated patient presents with unexplained bone pain, point tenderness, swelling, or bruising (Rabenda, 2013; Rizzoli, 2012). Use with caution in patients with hepatic or renal dysfunction. Use caution in elderly patients; may cause or exacerbate syndrome of inappropriate antidiuretic hormone secretion or hyponatremia; monitor sodium closely with initiation or dosage adjustments in older adults (Beers Criteria). Clinically significant transaminase elevations have been observed. Sol-Tab® formulation contains phenylalanine.

Abrupt discontinuation or interruption of antidepressant therapy has been associated with a discontinuation syndrome. Symptoms arising may vary with antidepressant however commonly include nausea, vomiting, diarrhea, headaches, lightheadedness, dizziness, diminished appetite, sweating, chills, tremors, paresthesias, fatigue, somnolence, and sleep disturbances (eg, vivid dreams, insomnia). Greater risks for developing a discontinuation syndrome have been associated with antidepressants with shorter half-lives, longer durations of treatment, and abrupt discontinuation. For antidepressants of short or intermediate half-lives, symptoms may emerge within 2-5 days after treatment discontinuation and last 7-14 days (APA, 2010; Fava, 2006; Haddad, 2001; Shelton, 2001; Warner, 2006).

Drug Interactions

Avoid Concomitant Use

Avoid concomitant use of Mirtazapine with any of the following: Alcohol (Ethyl); Azelastine (Nasal); Conivaptan; Fusidic Acid (Systemic); Linezolid; MAO Inhibitors; Methylene Blue; Paraldehyde; Thalidomide; Tryptophan

Decreased Effect

Mirtazapine may decrease the levels/effects of: Alpha2-Agonists

The levels/effects of Mirtazapine may be decreased by: Bosentan; CYP1A2 Inducers (Strong); CYP3A4 Inducers (Strong);

Cyproterone; Dabrafenib; Deferasirox; Mitotane; Peginterferon Alfa-2b; Tocilizumab

Increased Effect/Toxicity

Mirtazapine may increase the levels/effects of: Antipsychotics; Azelastine (Nasal); Buprenorphine; Dofetilide; Highest Risk QTc-Prolonging Agents; Hydrocodone; Lomitapide; Methylene Blue; Metoclopramide; Metyrosine; Moderate Risk QTc-Prolonging Agents; Paraldehyde; Pramipexole; ROPINIRole; Rotigotine; Serotonin Modulators; Thalidomide; Warfarin; Zolpidem

The levels/effects of Mirtazapine may be increased by: Abiraterone Acetate; Alcohol (Ethyl); Antipsychotics; Brimonidine (Topical); CNS Depressants; Conivaptan; CYP1A2 Inhibitors (Moderate); CYP1A2 Inhibitors (Strong); CYP2D6 Inhibitors (Moderate); CYP2D6 Inhibitors (Strong); CYP3A4 Inhibitors (Moderate); CYP3A4 Inhibitors (Strong); Darunavir; Dasatinib; Deferasirox; Doxylamine; Fusidic Acid (Systemic); HydrOXYzine; Ivacaftor; Linezolid; Luliconazole; Magnesium Sulfate; MAO Inhibitors; Mifepristone; Perampanel; Simeprevir; Sodium Oxybate; Stiripentol; Tryptophan; Vemurafenib

Nutritional/Ethanol Interactions

Ethanol: May increase CNS depression; monitor for increased effects with coadministration. Caution patients about effects.

Herb/Nutraceutical: Avoid St John's wort (may decrease mirtazapine levels). Avoid valerian, St John's wort, tryptophan, SAMe, kava kava (may increase CNS depression and/or increase the risk of serotonin syndrome).

Adverse Reactions

>10%:
Central nervous system: Somnolence (54%)
Endocrine & metabolic: Cholesterol increased
Gastrointestinal: Xerostomia (25%), appetite increased (17%), constipation (13%), weight gain (12%; weight gain of >7% reported in 8% of adults, ≤49% of pediatric patients)

1% to 10%:
Cardiovascular: Peripheral edema (2%), edema (1%), hypertension, vasodilatation
Central nervous system: Dizziness (7%), abnormal dreams (4%), abnormal thoughts (3%), confusion (2%), agitation, amnesia, anxiety, apathy, depression, hyper/hypokinesia, hypoesthesia, malaise, vertigo
Dermatologic: Pruritus, rash
Endocrine & metabolic: Triglycerides increased
Gastrointestinal: Abdominal pain, anorexia, vomiting
Genitourinary: Urinary frequency (2%), urinary tract infection
Hepatic: SGPT increased (≥3 times ULN: 2%)
Neuromuscular & skeletal: Weakness (8%), back pain (2%), myalgia (2%), tremor (2%), arthralgia, myasthenia, paresthesia, twitching

Respiratory: Dyspnea (1%), cough increased, sinusitis
Miscellaneous: Flu-like syndrome (5%), thirst

Available Dosage Forms

Tablet, Oral:
Remeron: 15 mg, 30 mg, 45 mg
Generic: 7.5 mg, 15 mg, 30 mg, 45 mg

Tablet Dispersible, Oral:
Remeron SolTab: 15 mg, 30 mg, 45 mg
Generic: 15 mg, 30 mg, 45 mg

General Dosage Range Oral: *Adults:* Initial: 15 mg nightly; Maintenance: 15-45 mg nightly

Administration

Oral

Orally disintegrating tablet: Administer without regard to meals. Open blister pack and place tablet on the tongue; tablet is formulated to dissolve on the tongue without water; do not split tablet.

Tablet: Administer without regard to meals. Canadian labeling does not recommend chewing tablet.

Storage/Stability

Orally disintegrating tablet: Store at controlled room temperature of 25°C (77°F); excursions permitted to 15°C to 30°C (59°F to 86°F). Protect from light and moisture. Use immediately upon opening tablet blister.

Tablet: Store at controlled room temperature of 25°C (77°F); excursions permitted to 15°C to 30°C (59°F to 86°F). Protect from light and moisture.

Nursing Actions

Physical Assessment Monitor therapeutic response (ie, mood, affect, mental status) at beginning of therapy and periodically throughout. Monitor for CNS depression/sedation. Monitor for clinical worsening and suicide ideation. Taper dosage slowly when discontinuing.

Patient Education

- Discuss specific use of drug and side effects with patient as it relates to treatment. (HCAHPS: During this hospital stay, were you given any medicine that you had not taken before? Before giving you any new medicine, how often did hospital staff tell you what the medicine was for? How often did hospital staff describe possible side effects in a way you could understand?)
- Patient may experience presyncope, fatigue, blurred vision, illogical thinking, dizziness, constipation, xerostomia, or weight gain. Have patient report immediately to prescriber signs of infection, tachycardia, severe nausea, significant change in balance, fasciculations, considerable asthenia, or rash (HCAHPS).
- Educate patient about signs of a significant reaction (eg, wheezing; chest tightness; fever; itching; bad cough; blue skin color; seizures; or swelling of face, lips, tongue, or throat). **Note:** This is not a comprehensive list of all side

effects. Patient should consult prescriber for additional questions.

Intended Use and Disclaimer: Should not be printed and given to patients. This information is intended to serve as a concise initial reference for healthcare professionals to use when discussing medications with a patient. You must ultimately rely on your own discretion, experience and judgment in diagnosing, treating and advising patients.

Dietary Considerations Some products may contain phenylalanine.

Misoprostol (mye soe PROST ole)

Brand Names: U.S. Cytotec
Pharmacologic Category Prostaglandin
Medication Safety Issues
Sound-alike/look-alike issues:
Cytotec® may be confused with Cytoxan
Misoprostol may be confused with metoprolol, mifepristone
Pregnancy Risk Factor X
Lactation Enters breast milk/use caution
Use
Prevention of NSAID-induced gastric ulcers
Medical termination of pregnancy of ≤49 days in conjunction with mifepristone (refer to Mifepristone monograph for details)
Unlabeled Use Cervical ripening and labor induction (except in women with prior cesarean delivery or major uterine surgery); prevention of postpartum hemorrhage; treatment of postpartum hemorrhage; treatment of incomplete or missed abortion in women <12 weeks gestation
Available Dosage Forms
Tablet, Oral:
Cytotec: 100 mcg, 200 mcg
Generic: 100 mcg, 200 mcg
General Dosage Range Oral: *Adults:* 100-200 mcg 4 times daily
Administration
Oral Incidence of diarrhea may be lessened by having patient take dose right after meals and avoiding magnesium-containing antacids. When used for the prevention of NSAID-induced ulcers, therapy is usually begun on the second or third day of the next normal menstrual period in women of childbearing potential.
Nursing Actions
Physical Assessment Teach appropriate diet and lifestyle if being used to prevent ulcers.
Patient Education
• Discuss specific use of drug and side effects with patient as it relates to treatment. (HCAHPS: During this hospital stay, were you given any medicine that you had not taken before? Before giving you any new medicine, how often did hospital staff tell you what the medicine was

for? How often did hospital staff describe possible side effects in a way you could understand?)
• Patient may experience headache, dyspepsia, nausea, or diarrhea. Have patient report immediately to prescriber asthenia or rash (HCAHPS).
• Educate patient about signs of a significant reaction (eg, wheezing; chest tightness; fever; itching; bad cough; blue skin color; seizures; or swelling of face, lips, tongue, or throat). **Note:** This is not a comprehensive list of all side effects. Patient should consult prescriber for additional questions.

Intended Use and Disclaimer: Should not be printed and given to patients. This information is intended to serve as a concise initial reference for healthcare professionals to use when discussing medications with a patient. You must ultimately rely on your own discretion, experience and judgment in diagnosing, treating and advising patients.

Mitotane (MYE toe tane)

Brand Names: U.S. Lysodren
Index Terms Chloditan; Chlodithane; Khloditan; Mytotan; o,p'-DDD; Ortho,para-DDD
Pharmacologic Category Antineoplastic Agent, Miscellaneous
Medication Safety Issues
Sound-alike/look-alike issues:
Mitotane may be confused with mitoMYcin, mitoXANtrone
High alert medication:
This medication is in a class the Institute for Safe Medication Practices (ISMP) includes among its list of drug classes which have a heightened risk of causing significant patient harm when used in error.
Pregnancy Risk Factor D
Lactation Enters breast milk/not recommended
Use Adrenocortical carcinoma: Treatment of inoperable adrenocortical carcinoma (both functional and non-functional types)
Unlabeled Use Treatment of Cushing syndrome
Available Dosage Forms
Tablet, Oral:
Lysodren: 500 mg
General Dosage Range Dosage adjustment recommended in patients who develop toxicities
Oral: *Adults:* Initial: 2-6 g daily in divided doses; Maintenance: 9-10 g daily in 3-4 divided doses (maximum: 18-19 g daily)
Administration
Oral Administer in 3-4 divided doses/day. Do not crush tablets. Mitotane is associated with a moderate emetic potential; antiemetics may be needed to prevent nausea and vomiting.

Hazardous agent; use appropriate precautions for handling and disposal (NIOSH, 2012). Wear impervious gloves when handling; avoid exposure to crushed or broken tablets.

Nursing Actions

Physical Assessment Evaluate for serious side effects such as abdominal pain, confusion, high fever, chills, or increased sweating. In addition, neurological deficits may occur with high doses taken more than 2 years. Patients should wear identification tag in case of emergency. Evaluate for depression or lethargy.

Patient Education
- Discuss specific use of drug and side effects with patient as it relates to treatment. (HCAHPS: During this hospital stay, were you given any medicine that you had not taken before? Before giving you any new medicine, how often did hospital staff tell you what the medicine was for? How often did hospital staff describe possible side effects in a way you could understand?)
- Patient may experience presyncope, fatigue, blurred vision, illogical thinking, dizziness, nausea, diarrhea, or loss of appetite. Have patient report immediately to prescriber signs of infection, syncope, or rash (HCAHPS).
- Educate patient about signs of a significant reaction (eg, wheezing; chest tightness; fever; itching; bad cough; blue skin color; seizures; or swelling of face, lips, tongue, or throat). **Note:** This is not a comprehensive list of all side effects. Patient should consult prescriber for additional questions.

Intended Use and Disclaimer: Should not be printed and given to patients. This information is intended to serve as a concise initial reference for healthcare professionals to use when discussing medications with a patient. You must ultimately rely on your own discretion, experience and judgment in diagnosing, treating and advising patients.

Related Information
Oral Medications That Should Not Be Crushed or Altered *on page 1712*

Mitoxantrone (mye toe ZAN trone)

Index Terms CL-232315; DHAD; DHAQ; Dihydroxyanthracenedione; Dihydroxyanthracenedione Dihydrochloride; Mitoxantrone Dihydrochloride; Mitoxantrone HCl; Mitoxantrone Hydrochloride; Mitozantrone; Novantrone

Pharmacologic Category Antineoplastic Agent, Anthracenedione; Antineoplastic Agent, Topoisomerase II Inhibitor

Medication Safety Issues

Sound-alike/look-alike issues:
MitoXANtrone may be confused with methotrexate, mitoMYcin, mitotane, Mutamycin®

High alert medication:
This medication is in a class the Institute for Safe Medication Practices (ISMP) includes among its list of drug classes which have a heightened risk of causing significant patient harm when used in error.

Medication Guide Available Yes

Pregnancy Risk Factor D

Lactation Enters breast milk/not recommended

Breast-Feeding Considerations Mitoxantrone is excreted in human milk and significant concentrations (18 ng/mL) have been reported for 28 days after the last administration. Because of the potential for serious adverse reactions in infants from mitoxantrone, breast-feeding should be discontinued before starting treatment.

Use Initial treatment of acute nonlymphocytic leukemias (ANLL [includes myelogenous, promyelocytic, monocytic and erythroid leukemias]); treatment of advanced hormone-refractory prostate cancer; secondary progressive or relapsing-remitting multiple sclerosis (MS)

Canadian labeling: Additional uses (not in U.S. labeling): Treatment of metastatic breast cancer, relapsed leukemia (adults), lymphoma, and hepatocellular carcinoma

Unlabeled Use Treatment of Hodgkin lymphoma (refractory), non-Hodgkin lymphomas (NHL), acute lymphocytic leukemia (ALL), relapsed acute myeloid leukemia (AML), breast cancer (metastatic), pediatric acute myelogenous leukemia (AML), pediatric acute promyelocytic leukemia (APL); part of a conditioning regimen for autologous hematopoietic stem cell transplantation (HSCT)

Mechanism of Action/Effect Related to the anthracyclines, mitoxantrone intercalates into DNA resulting in cross-links and strand breaks; also interferes with RNA and inhibits topoisomerase II; active throughout entire cell cycle (cell-cycle nonspecific)

Contraindications Hypersensitivity to mitoxantrone or any component of the formulation

Canadian labeling: Additional contraindications (not in U.S. labeling): Prior hypersensitivity to anthracyclines; prior substantial anthracycline exposure and abnormal cardiac function prior to initiation of mitoxantrone therapy; presence of severe myelosuppression due to prior chemo- and/or radiotherapy; severe hepatic impairment; intrathecal administration

Warnings/Precautions Hazardous agent - use appropriate precautions for handling and disposal (NIOSH, 2012).

[U.S. Boxed Warning]: Usually should not be administered if baseline neutrophil count <1500 cells/mm³ (except for treatment of ANLL). Monitor blood counts and monitor for infection due to neutropenia. Treatment may lead to severe myelosuppression; unless the expected benefit outweighs the risk, use is generally not recommended in patients with pre-existing myelosuppression from prior chemotherapy.

◄ **[U.S. Boxed Warning]: May cause myocardial toxicity and potentially-fatal heart failure (HF); risk increases with cumulative dosing. Effects may occur during therapy or may be delayed (months or years after completion of therapy).** Predisposing factors for mitoxantrone-induced cardiotoxicity include prior anthracycline or anthracenedione therapy, prior cardiovascular disease, concomitant use of cardiotoxic drugs, and mediastinal/pericardial irradiation, although may also occur in patients without risk factors. Prior to therapy initiation, evaluate all patients for cardiac-related signs/symptoms, including history, physical exam, and ECG; and evaluate baseline left ventricular ejection fraction (LVEF) with echocardiogram or multigated radionuclide angiography (MUGA) or MRI. Not recommended for use in MS patients when LVEF <50%, or baseline LVEF below the lower limit of normal (LLN). Evaluate for cardiac signs/symptoms (by history, physical exam, and ECG) and evaluate LVEF (using same method as baseline LVEF) in MS patients prior to each dose and if signs/symptoms of HF develop. Use in MS should be limited to a cumulative dose of ≤140 mg/m², and discontinued if LVEF falls below LLN or a significant decrease in LVEF is observed; decreases in LVEF and HF have been observed in patients with MS who have received cumulative doses <100 mg/m². Patients with MS should undergo annual LVEF evaluation following discontinuation of therapy to monitor for delayed cardiotoxicity.

[U.S. Boxed Warning]: For I.V. administration only, into a free-flowing I.V.; may cause severe local tissue damage if extravasation occurs; do not administer subcutaneously, intramuscularly, or intra-arterially. Do not administer intrathecally; may cause serious and permanent neurologic damage. Irritant with vesicant-like properties; extravasation resulting in burning, erythema, pain, swelling and skin discoloration (blue) has been reported; may result in tissue necrosis and require debridement for skin graft. Ensure proper needle or catheter placement prior to and during infusion. Avoid extravasation. May cause urine, saliva, tears, and sweat to turn blue-green for 24 hours postinfusion. Whites of eyes may have blue-green tinge. **[U.S. Boxed Warning]: Treatment with mitoxantrone increases the risk of developing secondary acute myelogenous leukemia (AML) in patients with cancer and in patients with MS;** acute promyelocytic leukemia (APL) has also been observed. Symptoms of acute leukemia include excessive bruising, bleeding and recurrent infections. The risk for secondary leukemia is increased in patients who are heavily pretreated, with higher doses, and with combination chemotherapy.

[U.S. Boxed Warning]: Should be administered under the supervision of a physician experienced in cancer chemotherapy agents. Dosage should be reduced in patients with impaired hepatobiliary function (clearance is reduced). Canadian labeling contraindicates use in severe hepatic impairment. Not for treatment of multiple sclerosis in patients with concurrent hepatic impairment. Not for treatment of primary progressive multiple sclerosis. Rapid lysis of tumor cells may lead to hyperuricemia.

Drug Interactions

Avoid Concomitant Use
Avoid concomitant use of MitoXANtrone with any of the following: BCG; CloZAPine; Natalizumab; Pimecrolimus; Pimozide; Tacrolimus (Topical); Tofacitinib; Vaccines (Live)

Decreased Effect
MitoXANtrone may decrease the levels/effects of: BCG; Coccidioidin Skin Test; Sipuleucel-T; Vaccines (Inactivated); Vaccines (Live)

The levels/effects of MitoXANtrone may be decreased by: Echinacea

Increased Effect/Toxicity
MitoXANtrone may increase the levels/effects of: ARIPiprazole; CloZAPine; Dofetilide; Leflunomide; Lomitapide; Natalizumab; Pimozide; Tofacitinib; Vaccines (Live)

The levels/effects of MitoXANtrone may be increased by: CycloSPORINE (Systemic); Denosumab; Pimecrolimus; Roflumilast; Tacrolimus (Topical); Trastuzumab

Nutritional/Ethanol Interactions Herb/Nutraceutical: Avoid echinacea (may diminish the immunosuppressant effect).

Adverse Reactions Includes events reported with any indication; incidence varies based on treatment, dose, and/or concomitant medications >10%:

Cardiovascular: Edema (10% to 30%), arrhythmia (3% to 18%), cardiac function changes (≤18%), ECG changes (≤11%)

Central nervous system: Fever (6% to 78%), pain (8% to 41%), fatigue (≤39%), headache (6% to 13%)

Dermatologic: Alopecia (20% to 61%), nail bed changes (≤11%), petechiae/bruising (6% to 11%)

Endocrine & metabolic: Menstrual disorder (26% to 61%), amenorrhea (28% to 53%), hyperglycemia (10% to 31%)

Gastrointestinal: Nausea (26% to 76%), vomiting (6% to 72%), diarrhea (14% to 47%), mucositis (10% to 29%; onset: ≤1 week), stomatitis (8% to 29%; onset: ≤1 week), anorexia (22% to 25%), weight gain/loss (13% to 17%), constipation (10% to 16%), GI bleeding (2% to 16%), abdominal pain (9% to 15%), dyspepsia (5% to 14%)

Genitourinary: Urinary tract infection (7% to 32%), abnormal urine (5% to 11%)

Hematologic: Neutropenia (79% to 100%; onset: ≤3 weeks; grade 4: 23% to 54%), leukopenia (9% to 100%), lymphopenia (72% to 95%), anemia/hemoglobin decreased (5% to 75%) thrombocytopenia (33% to 39%; grades 3/4: 3% to 4%), neutropenic fever (≤11%)

Hepatic: Alkaline phosphatase increased (≤37%), transaminases increased (5% to 20%), GGT increased (3% to 15%)

Neuromuscular & skeletal: Weakness (≤24%)

Renal: BUN increased (≤22%), creatinine increased (≤13%), hematuria (≤11%)

Respiratory: Upper respiratory tract infection (7% to 53%), pharyngitis (≤19%), dyspnea (6% to 18%), cough (5% to 13%)

Miscellaneous: Infection (4% to 60%), sepsis (ANLL 31% to 34%), fungal infection (9% to 15%)

1% to 10%:

Cardiovascular: CHF (≤5%), ischemia (≤5%), LVEF decreased (≤5%), hypertension (≤4%)

Central nervous system: Chills (≤5%), anxiety (5%), depression (5%), seizure (2% to 4%)

Dermatologic: Cutaneous mycosis (≤10%), skin infection (≤5%)

Endocrine & metabolic: Hypocalcemia (10%), hypokalemia (7% to 10%), hyponatremia (9%), menorrhagia (7%)

Gastrointestinal: Aphthosis (≤10%)

Genitourinary: Impotence (≤7%), sterility (≤5%)

Hematologic: Granulocytopenia (6%), hemorrhage (5% to 6%), secondary acute leukemias (≤3%; includes AML, APL)

Hepatic: Jaundice (3% to 7%)

Neuromuscular & skeletal: Back pain (6% to 8%), myalgia (≤5%), arthralgia (≤5%)

Ocular: Conjunctivitis (≤5%), blurred vision (≤3%)

Renal: Renal failure (≤8%), proteinuria (≤6%)

Respiratory: Rhinitis (10%), pneumonia (≤9%), sinusitis (≤6%)

Miscellaneous: Systemic infection (≤10%), diaphoresis (≤9%)

Available Dosage Forms

Concentrate, Intravenous:

Generic: 20 mg/10 mL (10 mL); 25 mg/12.5 mL (12.5 mL); 30 mg/15 mL (15 mL)

General Dosage Range I.V.: *Adults:* 12 mg/m^2/day once daily for 2-3 days **or** 12-14 mg/m^2 every 3 weeks **or** 12 mg/m^2 every 3 months (multiple sclerosis; maximum lifetime cumulative dose: 140 mg/m^2)

Administration

I.V. For I.V. administration only; do not administer intrathecally, subcutaneously, intramuscularly or intra-arterially. Must be diluted prior to use. Usually administered as a short I.V. infusion over 5-15 minutes; do not infuse over <3-5 minutes.

High doses for bone marrow transplant (unlabeled use) are usually given as 3 divided doses

over 1 hour each at 1-2 hour intervals on the same day (Oyan, 2006; Tarella, 2001).

Irritant with vesicant-like properties; ensure proper needle or catheter placement prior to and during infusion; avoid extravasation.

Extravasation management: If extravasation occurs, stop infusion immediately and disconnect (leave cannula/needle in place); gently aspirate extravasated solution (do **NOT** flush the line); remove needle/cannula; elevate extremity. Initiate antidote (dexrazoxane or dimethyl sulfate [DMSO]). Apply dry cold compresses for 20 minutes 4 times daily for 1-2 days (Perez Fidalgo, 2012); withhold cooling beginning 15 minutes before dexrazoxane infusion; continue withholding cooling until 15 minutes after infusion is completed. Topical DMSO should not be administered in combination with dexrazoxane; may lessen dexrazoxane efficacy.

Dexrazoxane: Adults: 1000 mg/m^2 (maximum dose: 2000 mg) I.V. (administer in a large vein remote from site of extravasation) over 1-2 hours days 1 and 2, then 500 mg/m^2 (maximum dose: 1000 mg) I.V. over 1-2 hours day 3; begin within 6 hours of extravasation. Day 2 and day 3 doses should be administered at approximately the same time (± 3 hours) as the dose on day 1 (Mouridsen, 2007; Perez Fidalgo, 2012). **Note:** Reduce dexrazoxane dose by 50% in patients with moderate to severe renal impairment (CrCl <40 mL/minute).

DMSO: Children and Adults: Apply topically to a region covering twice the affected area every 8 hours for 7 days; begin within 10 minutes of extravasation; do not cover with a dressing (Perez Fidalgo, 2012).

Hazardous agent; use appropriate precautions for handling and disposal (NIOSH, 2012).

Injectable Detail pH: 3-4.5 (concentrated solution in vial)

Preparation for Administration Hazardous agent; use appropriate precautions for handling and disposal (NIOSH, 2012). Dilute in at least 50 mL of NS or D$_5$W.

Storage/Stability Store intact vials at 15°C to 25°C (59°F to 77°F); do not freeze. Opened vials may be stored at room temperature for 7 days or under refrigeration for up to 14 days. Solutions diluted for administration are stable for 7 days at room temperature or under refrigeration, although the manufacturer recommends immediate use.

Nursing Actions

Physical Assessment Monitor infusion site closely to prevent extravasation, which may cause severe local tissue damage. Monitor for arrhythmia, hypersensitivity reactions, anemia, gastrointestinal upset, opportunistic infection, gout, and CHF (rales, dyspnea, edema) with each dose and throughout therapy. Caution patients with diabetes to monitor glucose levels closely; may cause hyperglycemia.

Patient Education

• Discuss specific use of drug and side effects with patient as it relates to treatment. (HCAHPS: During this hospital stay, were you given any medicine that you had not taken before? Before giving you any new medicine, how often did hospital staff tell you what the medicine was for? How often did hospital staff describe possible side effects in a way you could understand?)

• Patient may experience urine discoloration, dyspepsia, diarrhea, constipation, lack of appetite, headache, stomatitis, cheilitis, alopecia, back pain, or menstrual irregularities. Have patient report immediately to prescriber signs of infection, severe dizziness, syncope, considerable nausea, excessive weight loss, ecchymosis, hemorrhaging, significant asthenia, osteodynia, night sweats, or skin or nail discoloration (HCAHPS).

• Educate patient about signs of a significant reaction (eg, wheezing; chest tightness; fever; itching; bad cough; blue skin color; seizures; or swelling of face, lips, tongue, or throat). **Note:** This is not a comprehensive list of all side effects. Patient should consult prescriber for additional questions.

Intended Use and Disclaimer: Should not be printed and given to patients. This information is intended to serve as a concise initial reference for healthcare professionals to use when discussing medications with a patient. You must ultimately rely on your own discretion, experience and judgment in diagnosing, treating and advising patients.

Related Information

Management of Drug Extravasations *on page 1700*

Modafinil (moe DAF i nil)

Brand Names: U.S. Provigil

Pharmacologic Category Central Nervous System Stimulant

Medication Guide Available Yes

Pregnancy Risk Factor C

Lactation Excretion in breast milk unknown/use caution

Breast-Feeding Considerations It is not known if modafinil is excreted into breast milk. The manufacturer recommends caution be used if administered to nursing women.

Use Improve wakefulness in patients with excessive daytime sleepiness associated with narcolepsy and shift work sleep disorder (SWSD); adjunctive therapy for obstructive sleep apnea/hypopnea syndrome (OSAHS)

Unlabeled Use Attention-deficit/hyperactivity disorder (ADHD); treatment of fatigue in MS and other disorders

Mechanism of Action/Effect The exact mechanism of action is unclear, it does not appear to alter the release of dopamine or norepinephrine, it may exert its stimulant effects by decreasing GABA-mediated neurotransmission, although this theory has not yet been fully evaluated; several studies also suggest that an intact central alpha-adrenergic system is required for modafinil's activity; the drug increases high-frequency alpha waves while decreasing both delta and theta wave activity, and these effects are consistent with generalized increases in mental alertness

Contraindications Hypersensitivity to modafinil, armodafinil, or any component of the formulation

Canadian labeling: Additional contraindications (not in U.S. labeling): Patients in agitated states or with severe anxiety

Warnings/Precautions For use following complete evaluation of sleepiness and in conjunction with other standard treatments (eg, CPAP). The degree of sleepiness should be reassessed frequently; some patients may not return to a normal level of wakefulness. Use is not recommended with a history of angina, cardiac ischemia, recent history of myocardial infarction, left ventricular hypertrophy, or patients with mitral valve prolapse who have developed mitral valve prolapse syndrome with previous CNS stimulant use.

Serious and life-threatening rashes (including Stevens-Johnson syndrome and toxic epidermal necrolysis) have been reported with modafinil. Most cases have occurred within the first 5 weeks of therapy; however, rare cases have occurred after long-term use. No risk factors have been identified to predict occurrence or severity. Patients should be advised to discontinue at first sign of rash. The serious nature of these dermatologic adverse effects, as well as reports of psychiatric events, resulted in the FDA's Pediatric Advisory Committee unanimously recommending that a specific warning against the use of modafinil in children be added to the manufacturer's labeling. Modafinil is not FDA-approved for use in pediatrics for any indication.

In addition, rare cases of multiorgan hypersensitivity reactions in association with modafinil use, and lone cases of angioedema and anaphylactoid reactions with armodafinil, have been reported. Signs and symptoms are diverse, reflecting the involvement of specific organs. Patients typically present with fever and rash associated with organ-system dysfunction. Patients should be advised to report any signs and symptoms related to these effects; discontinuation of therapy is recommended.

Caution should be exercised when modafinil is given to patients with a history of psychosis; may impair the ability to engage in potentially hazardous activities. Stimulants may unmask tics in individuals with coexisting Tourette's syndrome. Use caution with renal or hepatic impairment (dosage adjustment in severe hepatic dysfunction is recommended).

Drug Interactions
Avoid Concomitant Use
Avoid concomitant use of Modafinil with any of the following: Axitinib; Bosutinib; Conivaptan; Fusidic Acid (Systemic); Iobenguane I 123; Pimozide; Simeprevir

Decreased Effect
Modafinil may decrease the levels/effects of: ARIPiprazole; Axitinib; Bosutinib; Clopidogrel; Contraceptives (Estrogens); CycloSPORINE (Systemic); Ibrutinib; Iobenguane I 123; Saxagliptin; Simeprevir

The levels/effects of Modafinil may be decreased by: Bosentan; CYP3A4 Inducers (Strong); Dabrafenib; Deferasirox; Herbs (CYP3A4 Inducers); Mitotane; Tocilizumab

Increased Effect/Toxicity
Modafinil may increase the levels/effects of: ARIPiprazole; Citalopram; CYP2C19 Substrates; Dofetilide; Lomitapide; Pimozide; Sympathomimetics

The levels/effects of Modafinil may be increased by: AtoMOXetine; Cannabinoids; Conivaptan; CYP3A4 Inhibitors (Moderate); CYP3A4 Inhibitors (Strong); Dasatinib; Fusidic Acid (Systemic); Ivacaftor; Linezolid; Luliconazole; Mifepristone; Simeprevir; Stiripentol

Nutritional/Ethanol Interactions
Ethanol: Avoid or limit ethanol.
Food: Delays absorption, but does not affect bioavailability.

Adverse Reactions
>10%:
Central nervous system: Headache (adults 34%; children 20%; dose related)
Gastrointestinal: Appetite decreased (children 16%), abdominal pain (children 12%), nausea (11%)
1% to 10%:
Cardiovascular: Chest pain (3%), hypertension (3%), palpitation (2%), tachycardia (2%), vasodilation (2%), edema (1%)
Central nervous system: Nervousness (7%), dizziness (5%), anxiety (5%; dose related), insomnia (5%), depression (2%), somnolence (2%), chills (1%), agitation (1%), confusion (1%), emotional lability (1%), vertigo (1%)
Dermatologic: Rash (1%; includes some severe cases requiring hospitalization)
Gastrointestinal: Diarrhea (6%), dyspepsia (5%), weight loss (children 5%), xerostomia (4%), anorexia (4%), constipation (2%), flatulence (1%), mouth ulceration (1%), taste perversion (1%)

Genitourinary: Abnormal urine (1%), hematuria (1%), pyuria (1%)
Hematologic: Eosinophilia (1%)
Hepatic: LFTs abnormal (2%)
Neuromuscular & skeletal: Back pain (6%), paresthesia (2%), dyskinesia (1%), hyperkinesia (1%), hypertonia (1%), neck rigidity (1%), tremor (1%)
Ocular: Amblyopia (1%), eye pain (1%), vision abnormal (1%)
Respiratory: Rhinitis (7%), pharyngitis (4%), lung disorder (2%), asthma (1%), epistaxis (1%)
Miscellaneous: Flu-like syndrome (4%), thirst (1%), diaphoresis (1%), herpes simplex infection (1%)

Controlled Substance C-IV
Available Dosage Forms
Tablet, Oral:
Provigil: 100 mg, 200 mg
Generic: 100 mg, 200 mg
General Dosage Range
Dosage adjustment recommended in patients with hepatic impairment.
Oral: *Adults:* 200 mg once daily (maximum: 400 mg daily)
Administration
Oral
U.S. labeling: For the treatment of narcolepsy and obstructive sleep apnea/hypopnea syndrome, administer dose in the morning. For the treatment of shift work sleep disorder, administer dose ~1 hour prior to start of work shift.
Canadian labeling: For the treatment of narcolepsy, administer in 2 divided doses with first dose given in the morning and the second dose given at noon (or no later than early afternoon) to avoid potential for insomnia. For treatment of obstructive sleep apnea, administer as a single dose in the morning. For the treatment of shift work sleep disorder, administer dose ~1 hour prior to start of work shift.
Storage/Stability
Provigil®: Store at 20°C to 25°C (68°F to 77°F).
Alertec® (Canadian availability; not available in U.S.): Store at 15°C to 30°C (59°F to 86°F).
Nursing Actions
Physical Assessment Perform careful cardiovascular assessment prior to initiating therapy.
Patient Education
• Discuss specific use of drug and side effects with patient as it relates to treatment. (HCAHPS: During this hospital stay, were you given any medicine that you had not taken before? Before giving you any new medicine, how often did hospital staff tell you what the medicine was for? How often did hospital staff describe possible side effects in a way you could understand?)
• Patient may experience akathisia, diarrhea, insomnia, back pain, dizziness, dyspepsia, or rhinitis. Have patient report immediately to prescriber signs of hepatic impairment, angina, tachycardia, depression (ie, suicidal ideation,

anxiety, emotional instability, illogical thinking), hallucinations, severe headache, arrhythmia, chills, pharyngitis, dyspnea, edema of extremities, ecchymosis, hemorrhaging, considerable asthenia, or Stevens-Johnson syndrome/toxic epidermal necrolysis (HCAHPS).

- Educate patient about signs of a significant reaction (eg, wheezing; chest tightness; fever; itching; bad cough; blue skin color; seizures; or swelling of face, lips, tongue, or throat). **Note:** This is not a comprehensive list of all side effects. Patient should consult prescriber for additional questions.

Intended Use and Disclaimer: Should not be printed and given to patients. This information is intended to serve as a concise initial reference for healthcare professionals to use when discussing medications with a patient. You must ultimately rely on your own discretion, experience and judgment in diagnosing, treating and advising patients.

Moexipril (mo EKS i pril)

Brand Names: U.S. Univasc
Index Terms Moexipril Hydrochloride
Pharmacologic Category Angiotensin-Converting Enzyme (ACE) Inhibitor; Antihypertensive
Medication Safety Issues
Sound-alike/look-alike issues:
Moexipril may be confused with Monopril
Pregnancy Risk Factor D
Lactation Excretion in breast milk unknown/use caution
Breast-Feeding Considerations It is not known if moexipril is excreted into breast milk. The manufacturer recommends that caution be exercised when administering moexipril to nursing women.
Use Treatment of hypertension, alone or in combination with thiazide diuretics
Mechanism of Action/Effect Competitive inhibitor of angiotensin-converting enzyme (ACE); prevents conversion of angiotensin I to angiotensin II, a potent vasoconstrictor; results in lower levels of angiotensin II which causes an increase in plasma renin activity and a reduction in aldosterone secretion
Contraindications Hypersensitivity to moexipril or any component of the formulation; angioedema related to previous treatment with an ACE inhibitor; concomitant use with aliskiren in patients with diabetes mellitus
Warnings/Precautions Anaphylactic reactions may occur rarely with ACE inhibitors. At any time during treatment (especially following first dose) angioedema may occur rarely with ACE inhibitors; it may involve the head and neck (potentially compromising airway) or the intestine (presenting with abdominal pain). African-Americans and patients with idiopathic or hereditary angioedema

may be at an increased risk. Prolonged frequent monitoring may be required especially if tongue, glottis, or larynx are involved as they are associated with airway obstruction. Patients with a history of airway surgery may have a higher risk of airway obstruction. Aggressive early and appropriate management is critical. Use in patients with previous angioedema associated with ACE inhibitor therapy is contraindicated. Severe anaphylactoid reactions may be seen during hemodialysis (eg, CVVHD) with high-flux dialysis membranes (eg, AN69), and rarely, during low density lipoprotein apheresis with dextran sulfate cellulose. Rare cases of anaphylactoid reactions have been reported in patients undergoing sensitization treatment with hymenoptera (bee, wasp) venom while receiving ACE inhibitors.

Symptomatic hypotension with or without syncope can occur with ACE inhibitors (usually with the first several doses); effects are most often observed in volume depleted patients; correct volume depletion prior to initiation; close monitoring of patient is required especially with initial dosing and dosing increases; blood pressure must be lowered at a rate appropriate for the patient's clinical condition. Initiation of therapy in patients with ischemic heart disease or cerebrovascular disease warrants close observation due to the potential consequences posed by falling blood pressure (eg, MI, stroke). Use with caution in hypertrophic cardiomyopathy with outflow tract obstruction, severe aortic stenosis, or before, during, or immediately after major surgery. **[U.S. Boxed Warning]: Drugs that act on the renin-angiotensin system can cause injury and death to the developing fetus. Discontinue as soon as possible once pregnancy is detected.**

Hyperkalemia may occur with ACE inhibitors; risk factors include renal dysfunction, diabetes mellitus, concomitant use of potassium-sparing diuretics, potassium supplements, and/or potassium-containing salts. Use cautiously, if at all, with these agents and monitor potassium closely. Cough may occur with ACE inhibitors. Other causes of cough should be considered (eg, pulmonary congestion in patients with heart failure) and excluded prior to discontinuation.

May be associated with deterioration of renal function and/or increases in serum creatinine, particularly in patients with low renal blood flow (eg, renal artery stenosis, heart failure) whose glomerular filtration rate (GFR) is dependent on efferent arteriolar vasoconstriction by angiotensin II; deterioration may result in oliguria, acute renal failure, and progressive azotemia. Small increases in serum creatinine may occur following initiation; consider discontinuation only in patients with progressive and/or significant deterioration in renal function. Use with caution in patients with unstented unilateral/bilateral renal artery stenosis. When unstented bilateral renal artery stenosis is present, use is generally avoided due to the elevated risk of deterioration in renal function unless possible benefits outweigh risks. Concomitant use of an angiotensin receptor blocker (ARB) or renin inhibitor (eg, aliskiren) is associated with an increased risk of hypotension, hyperkalemia, and renal dysfunction; concomitant use with aliskiren should be avoided in patients with GFR <60 mL/minute and is contraindicated in patients with diabetes mellitus (regardless of GFR).

Rare toxicities associated with ACE inhibitors include cholestatic jaundice (which may progress to fulminant hepatic necrosis), agranulocytosis, neutropenia, or leukopenia with myeloid hypoplasia. Patients with collagen vascular diseases (especially with concomitant renal impairment) or renal impairment alone may be at increased risk for hematologic toxicity; periodically monitor CBC with differential in these patients.

Drug Interactions

Avoid Concomitant Use There are no known interactions where it is recommended to avoid concomitant use.

Decreased Effect

The levels/effects of Moexipril may be decreased by: Antacids; Aprotinin; Herbs (Hypertensive Properties); Icatibant; Lanthanum; Methylphenidate; Nonsteroidal Anti-Inflammatory Agents; Salicylates; Yohimbine

Increased Effect/Toxicity

Moexipril may increase the levels/effects of: Allopurinol; Amifostine; Antihypertensives; AzaTHIOprine; CycloSPORINE (Systemic); DULoxetine; Ferric Gluconate; Gold Sodium Thiomalate; Highest Risk QTc-Prolonging Agents; Hypotensive Agents; Iron Dextran Complex; Lithium; Moderate Risk QTc-Prolonging Agents; Nonsteroidal Anti-Inflammatory Agents; Obinutuzumab; RiTUXimab; Sodium Phosphates

The levels/effects of Moexipril may be increased by: Alfuzosin; Aliskiren; Angiotensin II Receptor Blockers; Brimonidine (Topical); Canagliflozin; Diazoxide; DPP-IV Inhibitors; Eplerenone; Everolimus; Heparin; Heparin (Low Molecular Weight); Herbs (Hypotensive Properties); Loop Diuretics; MAO Inhibitors; Mifepristone; Pentoxifylline; Phosphodiesterase 5 Inhibitors; Potassium Salts; Potassium-Sparing Diuretics; Prostacyclin Analogues; Sirolimus; Temsirolimus; Thiazide Diuretics; TiZANidine; Tolvaptan; Trimethoprim

Nutritional/Ethanol Interactions

Food: Food may delay and reduce peak serum levels. Potassium supplements and/or potassium-containing salts may cause or worsen hyperkalemia. Management: Take on an empty stomach 1 hour before or 2 hours after a meal. Consult prescriber before consuming a potassium-rich diet, potassium supplements, or salt substitutes.

Herb/Nutraceutical: Some herbal medications may worsen hypertension (eg, licorice); others may increase the antihypertensive effect of moexipril (eg, shepherd's purse). Management: Avoid bayberry, blue cohosh, cayenne, ephedra, ginger, ginseng (American), kola, licorice, and yohimbe. Avoid black cohosh, California poppy, coleus, golden seal, hawthorn, mistletoe, periwinkle, quinine, and shepherd's purse.

Adverse Reactions 1% to 10%:

Cardiovascular: Hypotension, peripheral edema

Central nervous system: Headache, dizziness, fatigue

Dermatologic: Flushing, rash

Endocrine & metabolic: Hyperkalemia, hyponatremia

Gastrointestinal: Diarrhea, nausea, heartburn

Genitourinary: Polyuria

Neuromuscular & skeletal: Myalgia

Renal: Reversible increases in creatinine or BUN

Respiratory: Cough, pharyngitis, upper respiratory infection, sinusitis

Pharmacodynamics/Kinetics

Onset of Action Peak effect: 1-2 hours

Duration of Action >24 hours

Available Dosage Forms

Tablet, Oral:

Univasc: 7.5 mg, 15 mg

Generic: 7.5 mg, 15 mg

General Dosage Range Dosage adjustment recommended in patients with renal impairment

Oral: *Adults:* Initial: 3.75-7.5 mg once daily; Maintenance: 7.5-30 mg/day in 1 or 2 divided doses

Administration

Oral Administer on an empty stomach.

Nursing Actions

Physical Assessment Assess potential for interactions with other pharmacological agents or herbal products that may impact fluid balance or cardiac status. Patient should be monitored closely for anaphylactic reaction or angioedema which can occur at any time during treatment and may involve head and neck. Monitor blood pressure. Monitor for hypotension, rash, diarrhea, myalgia, and electrolyte imbalance regularly during therapy.

Patient Education

• Discuss specific use of drug and side effects with patient as it relates to treatment. (HCAHPS: During this hospital stay, were you given any medicine that you had not taken before? Before giving you any new medicine, how often did hospital staff tell you what the medicine was for? How often did hospital staff describe possible side effects in a way you could understand?)

• Patient may experience dizziness, headache, or parageusia. Have patient report immediately to prescriber signs of infection, syncope, dyspnea, hyperhidrosis, diarrhea, significant weight gain, edema in legs or abdomen, discolored urine, jaundice, or rash (HCAHPS).

- Educate patient about signs of a significant reaction (eg, wheezing; chest tightness; fever; itching; bad cough; blue skin color; seizures; or swelling of face, lips, tongue, or throat). **Note:** This is not a comprehensive list of all side effects. Patient should consult prescriber for additional questions.

Intended Use and Disclaimer: Should not be printed and given to patients. This information is intended to serve as a concise initial reference for healthcare professionals to use when discussing medications with a patient. You must ultimately rely on your own discretion, experience and judgment in diagnosing, treating and advising patients.

Dietary Considerations Take on an empty stomach.

Moexipril and Hydrochlorothiazide
(mo EKS i pril & hye droe klor oh THYE a zide)

Brand Names: U.S. Uniretic®
Index Terms Hydrochlorothiazide and Moexipril
Pharmacologic Category Angiotensin-Converting Enzyme (ACE) Inhibitor; Antihypertensive; Diuretic, Thiazide
Pregnancy Risk Factor D
Use Treatment of hypertension; not indicated for initial treatment of hypertension
Available Dosage Forms

Tablet, oral: 7.5/12.5: Moexipril 7.5 mg and hydrochlorothiazide 12.5; 15/12.5: Moexipril 15 mg and hydrochlorothiazide 12.5; 15/25: Moexipril 15 mg and hydrochlorothiazide 25

Uniretic®: 7.5/12.5: Moexipril 7.5 mg and hydrochlorothiazide 12.5 mg [scored]; 15/12.5: Moexipril 15 mg and hydrochlorothiazide 12.5 mg [scored]; 15/25: Moexipril 15 mg and hydrochlorothiazide 25 mg [scored]

General Dosage Range Oral: *Adults:* 7.5-30 mg of moexipril/day and ≤50 mg hydrochlorothiazide/day in a single or divided dose
Nursing Actions
Physical Assessment See individual agents.
Patient Education

- Discuss specific use of drug and side effects with patient as it relates to treatment. (HCAHPS: During this hospital stay, were you given any medicine that you had not taken before? Before giving you any new medicine, how often did hospital staff tell you what the medicine was for? How often did hospital staff describe possible side effects in a way you could understand?)
- Patient may experience dizziness, headache, diarrhea, dyspepsia, or asthenia. Have patient report immediately to prescriber signs of infection, signs of hyperglycemia, signs of renal or hepatic impairment, angina, urinary retention,

dysuria, bradycardia, paresthesia, strength differences from one side to another, akathisia, dyspnea, significant weight gain, edema, ecchymosis, bleeding, or vision changes (HCAHPS).

- Educate patient about signs of a significant reaction (eg, wheezing; chest tightness; fever; itching; bad cough; blue skin color; seizures; or swelling of face, lips, tongue, or throat). **Note:** This is not a comprehensive list of all side effects. Patient should consult prescriber for additional questions.

Intended Use and Disclaimer: Should not be printed and given to patients. This information is intended to serve as a concise initial reference for healthcare professionals to use when discussing medications with a patient. You must ultimately rely on your own discretion, experience and judgment in diagnosing, treating and advising patients.

Related Information
Hydrochlorothiazide *on page* 775
Moexipril *on page* 1072

Mometasone (Oral Inhalation)
(moe MET a sone)

Brand Names: U.S. Asmanex 120 Metered Doses; Asmanex 14 Metered Doses; Asmanex 30 Metered Doses; Asmanex 60 Metered Doses; Asmanex 7 Metered Doses
Index Terms Mometasone Furoate
Pharmacologic Category Corticosteroid, Inhalant (Oral)
Pregnancy Risk Factor C
Lactation Excretion in breast milk unknown/use caution
Breast-Feeding Considerations Systemic corticosteroids are excreted in human milk. It is not known if sufficient quantities of mometasone are absorbed following oral inhalation to produce detectable amounts in breast milk; however, oral absorption is limited (<1%). The manufacturer recommends that caution be exercised when administering mometasone to nursing women. The use of inhaled corticosteroids is not considered a contraindication to breast-feeding (NAEPP, 2005).
Use Maintenance treatment of asthma as prophylactic therapy
Mechanism of Action/Effect Blocks inflammation; reverses capillary permeability and release of inflammatory mediators (leukotrienes and prostaglandins); suppresses migration of polymorphonuclear leukocytes.
Contraindications Hypersensitivity to mometasone or any component of the formulation; hypersensitivity to milk proteins; primary treatment of status asthmaticus or acute bronchospasm

Canadian labeling: Additional contraindications (not in U.S. labeling): Untreated systemic fungal, bacterial, viral, or parasitic infections; active or quiet tuberculosis infection of the respiratory tract; ocular herpes simplex

Warnings/Precautions May cause hypercorticism or suppression of hypothalamic-pituitary-adrenal (HPA) axis, particularly in younger children or in patients receiving high doses for prolonged periods. HPA axis suppression may lead to adrenal crisis. Withdrawal and discontinuation of a corticosteroid should be done slowly and carefully. Particular care is required when patients are transferred from systemic corticosteroids to inhaled products due to possible adrenal insufficiency or withdrawal from steroids, including an increase in allergic symptoms. Patients receiving >20 mg per day of prednisone (or equivalent) may be most susceptible. Fatalities have occurred due to adrenal insufficiency in asthmatic patients during and after transfer from systemic corticosteroids to aerosol steroids; aerosol steroids do not provide the systemic steroid needed to treat patients having trauma, surgery, or infections. When transferring to oral inhaler, previously-suppressed allergic conditions (rhinitis, conjunctivitis, eczema) may be unmasked.

Bronchospasm may occur with wheezing after inhalation; if this occurs, stop steroid and treat with a fast-acting bronchodilator. Supplemental steroids (oral or parenteral) may be needed during stress or severe asthma attacks. Not to be used in status asthmaticus or for the relief of acute bronchospasm. Corticosteroid use may cause psychiatric disturbances, including depression, euphoria, insomnia, mood swings, and personality changes. Pre-existing psychiatric conditions may be exacerbated by corticosteroid use. Prolonged use of corticosteroids may also increase the incidence of secondary infection, mask acute infection (including fungal infections), prolong or exacerbate viral infections, or limit response to vaccines. Exposure to chickenpox should be avoided; corticosteroids should not be used to treat ocular herpes simplex. Corticosteroids should not be used for cerebral malaria or viral hepatitis. Close observation is required in patients with latent tuberculosis and/or TB reactivity; restrict use in active TB (only in conjunction with antituberculosis treatment). Canadian labeling contraindicates use in patients with untreated systemic fungal, bacterial, viral, or parasitic infections, active or quiet tuberculosis infection of the respiratory tract and ocular herpes simplex.

Prolonged treatment with corticosteroids has been associated with the development of Kaposi's sarcoma (case reports); if noted, discontinuation of therapy should be considered. Local oropharyngeal *Candida* infections have been reported; if occurs treat appropriately while continuing mometasone therapy. Patients should be instructed to rinse mouth after each use.

Reactions including, anaphylaxis, angioedema, pruritus, and rash have been reported; if these symptoms occur discontinue use. Use with caution in patients with thyroid disease, hepatic impairment, renal impairment, cardiovascular disease, diabetes, glaucoma, cataracts, myasthenia gravis, patients with or who are at risk for osteoporosis, patients at risk for seizures, or GI diseases (diverticulitis, peptic ulcer, ulcerative colitis) due to perforation risk. Use caution following acute MI (corticosteroids have been associated with myocardial rupture). Because of the risk of adverse effects, systemic corticosteroids should be used cautiously in the elderly in the smallest possible effective dose for the shortest duration.

Orally-inhaled corticosteroids may cause a reduction in growth velocity in pediatric patients (~1 centimeter per year [range: 0.3-1.8 cm per year] and related to dose and duration of exposure). To minimize the systemic effects of orally-inhaled corticosteroids, each patient should be titrated to the lowest effective dose. Growth should be routinely monitored in pediatric patients. Prior to use, the dose and duration of treatment should be based on the risk versus benefit for each individual patient. In general, use the smallest effective dose for the shortest duration of time to minimize adverse events. A gradual tapering of dose may be required prior to discontinuing therapy. There have been reports of systemic corticosteroid withdrawal symptoms (eg, joint/muscle pain, lassitude, depression) when withdrawing inhalation therapy. May contain lactose; very rare anaphylactic reactions have been reported in patients with severe milk protein allergy.

Drug Interactions

Avoid Concomitant Use

Avoid concomitant use of Mometasone (Oral Inhalation) with any of the following: Aldesleukin

Decreased Effect

Mometasone (Oral Inhalation) may decrease the levels/effects of: Aldesleukin; Antidiabetic Agents; Corticorelin; Hyaluronidase; Telaprevir

Increased Effect/Toxicity

Mometasone (Oral Inhalation) may increase the levels/effects of: Amphotericin B; Deferasirox; Loop Diuretics; Thiazide Diuretics

The levels/effects of Mometasone (Oral Inhalation) may be increased by: CYP3A4 Inhibitors (Strong); Telaprevir

Adverse Reactions

>10%:

Central nervous system: Headache (17% to 22%), fatigue (1% to 13%), depression (11%)

Neuromuscular & skeletal: Musculoskeletal pain (4% to 22%), arthralgia (13%)

Respiratory: Sinusitis (5% to 22%), rhinitis (4% to 20%), upper respiratory infection (8% to 15%), pharyngitis (8% to 13%)

Miscellaneous: Oral candidiasis (4% to 22%)

1% to 10%:
Central nervous system: Fever (children 7%), pain (1% to <3%)
Dermatologic: Bruising (children 2%)
Gastrointestinal: Abdominal pain (2% to 6%), dyspepsia (3% to 5%), nausea (1% to 3%), vomiting (1% to ≤3%), anorexia (1% to <3%), dry throat (1% to <3%), gastroenteritis (1% to <3%)
Genitourinary: Dysmenorrhea (4% to 9%), urinary tract infection (children 2%)
Neuromuscular & skeletal: Back pain (3% to 6%), myalgia (2% to 3%)
Ocular: Ocular pressure increased (3%), cataracts (1%)
Otic: Earache (1% to <3%)
Respiratory: Sinus congestion (9%), dysphonia (1% to <3%), epistaxis (1% to <3%), nasal irritation (1% to <3%)
Miscellaneous: Flu-like syndrome (1% to <3%), infection (1% to <3%)

Available Dosage Forms
Aerosol Powder Breath Activated, Inhalation:
Asmanex 120 Metered Doses: 220 mcg/INH (1 ea)
Asmanex 14 Metered Doses: 220 mcg/INH (1 ea)
Asmanex 30 Metered Doses: 110 mcg/INH (1 ea); 220 mcg/INH (1 ea)
Asmanex 60 Metered Doses: 220 mcg/INH (1 ea)
Asmanex 7 Metered Doses: 110 mcg/INH (1 ea)

General Dosage Range Inhalation:
Children 4-11 years: 110 mcg once daily (maximum: 110 mcg/day)
Children ≥12 years and Adults: 1-4 inhalations (220-880 mcg) in 1-2 divided doses (maximum: 880 mcg/day)

Administration
Inhalation Exhale fully prior to bringing the Twisthaler® up to the mouth. Place between lips and inhale quickly and deeply. Do not breathe out through the inhaler. Remove inhaler and hold breath for 10 seconds if possible. Rinse mouth after use.

Storage/Stability Store at 25°C (77°F); excursions permitted to 15°C to 30°C (59°F to 86°F). Discard when oral dose counter reads "00" (or 45 days [U.S. labeling] or 60 days [Canadian labeling] after opening the foil pouch).

Nursing Actions
Physical Assessment Long-term use: Assess for glaucoma and cataracts periodically. Monitor growth in pediatric patients.

Patient Education
• Discuss specific use of drug and side effects with patient as it relates to treatment. (HCAHPS: During this hospital stay, were you given any medicine that you had not taken before? Before giving you any new medicine, how often did hospital staff tell you what the medicine was for? How often did hospital staff describe possible side effects in a way you could understand?)

• Patient may experience headache, rhinitis, stomatitis, asthenia, myalgia, osteopenia, cataracts, or glaucoma. Have patient report immediately to prescriber signs of infection, irritability, tremors, tachycardia, confusion, dizziness, diaphoresis, dyspnea, or rash (HCAHPS).
• Educate patient about signs of a significant reaction (eg, wheezing; chest tightness; fever; itching; bad cough; blue skin color; seizures; or swelling of face, lips, tongue, or throat). **Note:** This is not a comprehensive list of all side effects. Patient should consult prescriber for additional questions.

Intended Use and Disclaimer: Should not be printed and given to patients. This information is intended to serve as a concise initial reference for healthcare professionals to use when discussing medications with a patient. You must ultimately rely on your own discretion, experience and judgment in diagnosing, treating and advising patients.

Dietary Considerations Asmanex® Twisthaler® contains lactose.

Mometasone (Nasal) (moe MET a sone)

Brand Names: U.S. Nasonex
Index Terms Mometasone Furoate
Pharmacologic Category Corticosteroid, Nasal
Pregnancy Risk Factor C
Lactation Excretion in breast milk unknown/use caution
Use Treatment of nasal symptoms of seasonal and perennial allergic rhinitis; prevention of nasal symptoms associated with seasonal allergic rhinitis; treatment of nasal polyps in adults
Canadian labeling: Additional use (not in U.S. labeling): Treatment of mild-to-moderate uncomplicated rhinosinusitis or as adjunctive treatment (with antimicrobials) in acute rhinosinusitis
Unlabeled Use Adjunct to antibiotics in empiric treatment of acute bacterial rhinosinusitis (ABRS) (Chow, 2012)
Dosage Forms Considerations
Nasonex 17 g bottles contain 120 sprays.
Available Dosage Forms
Suspension, Nasal:
Nasonex: 50 mcg/actuation (17 g)
General Dosage Range Intranasal:
Children 2-11 years: 1 spray (50 mcg) in each nostril once daily
Children ≥12 years and Adults: 2 sprays (100 mcg) in each nostril once or twice daily
Administration
Inhalation Shake well prior to use. Prior to first use, prime pump by actuating 10 times or until fine spray appears; may store for a maximum of 1 week (U.S. labeling recommendations) or 2 weeks (Canadian labeling recommendations) without repriming; if unused for greater than

recommended storage period, reprime by actuating 2 times or until fine spray appears. Spray should be administered once or twice daily, at a regular interval.

Nursing Actions

Physical Assessment Monitor growth with long-term use in pediatric patients.

Patient Education

- Discuss specific use of drug and side effects with patient as it relates to treatment. (HCAHPS: During this hospital stay, were you given any medicine that you had not taken before? Before giving you any new medicine, how often did hospital staff tell you what the medicine was for? How often did hospital staff describe possible side effects in a way you could understand?)
- Patient may experience headache, rhinitis, or epistaxis. Have patient report immediately to prescriber rash (HCAHPS).
- Educate patient about signs of a significant reaction (eg, wheezing; chest tightness; fever; itching; bad cough; blue skin color; seizures; or swelling of face, lips, tongue, or throat). **Note:** This is not a comprehensive list of all side effects. Patient should consult prescriber for additional questions.

Intended Use and Disclaimer: Should not be printed and given to patients. This information is intended to serve as a concise initial reference for healthcare professionals to use when discussing medications with a patient. You must ultimately rely on your own discretion, experience and judgment in diagnosing, treating and advising patients.

Mometasone (Topical) (moe MET a sone)

Brand Names: U.S. Elocon
Index Terms Mometasone Furoate
Pharmacologic Category Corticosteroid, Topical
Medication Safety Issues
  Sound-alike/look-alike issues:
  Elocon lotion may be confused with ophthalmic solutions. Manufacturer's labeling emphasizes the product is **NOT** for use in the eyes.
Pregnancy Risk Factor C
Lactation Enters breast milk/use caution
Use Relief of the inflammatory and pruritic manifestations of corticosteroid-responsive dermatoses (medium potency topical corticosteroid)
Available Dosage Forms
  Cream, External:
    Elocon: 0.1% (15 g, 45 g, 50 g)
    Generic: 0.1% (15 g, 45 g)
  Lotion, External:
    Elocon: 0.1% (30 mL, 60 mL)
  Ointment, External:
    Elocon: 0.1% (15 g, 45 g)
    Generic: 0.1% (15 g, 45 g)

Solution, External:
  Generic: 0.1% (30 mL, 60 mL)
General Dosage Range Topical:
  Cream, ointment: *Children ≥2 years, Adolescents, and Adults:* Apply a thin film to affected area once daily
  Lotion: *Children ≥12 years, Adolescents, and Adults:* Apply a few drops to affected area once daily
Administration
  Topical Apply sparingly; avoid eyes, face, underarms, and groin (including diaper area). Do not wrap or bandage affected area.
  Cream, ointment: Apply thin film to affected area.
  Lotion: Apply a few drops to affected area and massage lightly until medication disappears.
Nursing Actions
Patient Education

- Discuss specific use of drug and side effects with patient as it relates to treatment. (HCAHPS: During this hospital stay, were you given any medicine that you had not taken before? Before giving you any new medicine, how often did hospital staff tell you what the medicine was for? How often did hospital staff describe possible side effects in a way you could understand?)
- Have patient report immediately to prescriber signs of hyperglycemia, skin changes, or severe skin irritation (HCAHPS).
- Educate patient about signs of a significant reaction (eg, wheezing; chest tightness; fever; itching; bad cough; blue skin color; seizures; or swelling of face, lips, tongue, or throat). **Note:** This is not a comprehensive list of all side effects. Patient should consult prescriber for additional questions.

Intended Use and Disclaimer: Should not be printed and given to patients. This information is intended to serve as a concise initial reference for healthcare professionals to use when discussing medications with a patient. You must ultimately rely on your own discretion, experience and judgment in diagnosing, treating and advising patients.

Montelukast (mon te LOO kast)

Brand Names: U.S. Singulair
Index Terms Montelukast Sodium
Pharmacologic Category Leukotriene-Receptor Antagonist
Medication Safety Issues
  Sound-alike/look-alike issues:
  Singulair® may be confused with Oralair™, SINEquan®
Pregnancy Risk Factor B
Lactation Excretion in breast milk unknown/use caution
Breast-Feeding Considerations It is not known if montelukast is excreted into breast milk. The ▶

manufacturer recommends that caution be exercised when administering montelukast to nursing women.

Use Prophylaxis and chronic treatment of asthma; relief of symptoms of seasonal allergic rhinitis and perennial allergic rhinitis; prevention of exercise-induced bronchoconstriction

Unlabeled Use Urticaria (nonsteroidal anti-inflammatory drug–induced)

Mechanism of Action/Effect Montelukast is a selective leukotriene receptor antagonist which inhibits cysteinyl leukotriene. Leukotrienes are responsible for edema and smooth muscle contraction that is felt to be associated with the signs and symptoms of asthma. Cysteinyl leukotrienes are also released following allergen exposure leading to symptoms associated with allergic rhinitis.

Contraindications Hypersensitivity to montelukast or any component of the formulation

Warnings/Precautions Montelukast is not FDA approved for use in the reversal of bronchospasm in acute asthma attacks, including status asthmaticus; some studies, however, support its use as adjunctive therapy (Cylly, 2003; Ferreira, 2001; Harmancik, 2006). Appropriate rescue medication should be available. Montelukast treatment should continue during acute asthma exacerbation. When inhaled or systemic corticosteroid reduction is considered in patients initiating or receiving montelukast, appropriate clinical monitoring and a gradual dose reduction of the steroid are recommended.

Postmarketing reports of behavioral changes (eg, agitation, aggression, anxiety, attention deficit, depression, hallucinations, hostility, insomnia, irritability, restlessness, sleep disturbance, suicide ideation/behavior) have been noted in pediatric, adolescent, and adult patients. In a retrospective analysis performed by Merck, serious behavior-related events were rare (Philip, 2009a); assess patients for behavioral changes. Patients should be instructed to notify the prescriber if behavioral changes occur.

Potentially significant drug-drug interactions may exist, requiring dose or frequency adjustment, additional monitoring, and/or selection of alternative therapy. In rare cases, patients on therapy with montelukast may present with systemic eosinophilia, sometimes presenting with clinical features of vasculitis consistent with Churg-Strauss syndrome, a condition which is often treated with systemic corticosteroid therapy. Healthcare providers should be alert to eosinophilia, vasculitic rash, worsening pulmonary symptoms, cardiac complications, and/or neuropathy presenting in their patients. A causal association between montelukast and these underlying conditions has not been established. Montelukast will not interrupt bronchoconstrictor response to aspirin or other NSAIDs; aspirin sensitive asthmatics should

continue to avoid these agents. The chewable tablet contains phenylalanine.

Drug Interactions

Avoid Concomitant Use There are no known interactions where it is recommended to avoid concomitant use.

Decreased Effect

The levels/effects of Montelukast may be decreased by: Bosentan; CYP2C9 Inducers (Strong); CYP3A4 Inducers (Strong); Dabrafenib; Deferasirox; Herbs (CYP3A4 Inducers); Mitotane; Peginterferon Alfa-2b; Tocilizumab

Increased Effect/Toxicity

The levels/effects of Montelukast may be increased by: CYP2C9 Inhibitors (Moderate); CYP2C9 Inhibitors (Strong); Mifepristone

Nutritional/Ethanol Interactions Herb/Nutraceutical: St John's wort may decrease montelukast levels.

Adverse Reactions

Children ≥15 years and Adults:

>10%:

Central nervous system: Headache (18%)

1% to 10%:

Central nervous system: Dizziness (2%), fatigue (2%), fever (2%)

Dermatologic: Skin rash (2%)

Gastrointestinal: Dyspepsia (2%), gastroenteritis (2%), toothache (2%)

Hepatic: Increased serum AST (2%), increased serum ALT (≥1%)

Neuromuscular & skeletal: Weakness (2%)

Respiratory: Nasal congestion (2%), cough (≥1%), epistaxis (≥1%), sinusitis (≥1%), upper respiratory tract infection (≥1%)

Children 2 to ≤14 years: ≥2%:

Central nervous system: Fever, headache

Dermatologic: Dermatitis, eczema, skin rash, urticaria

Gastrointestinal: Abdominal pain, dyspepsia, gastroenteritis, nausea

Infection: Influenza, varicella, viral infection

Ophthalmic: Conjunctivitis

Otic: Otalgia, otitis

Respiratory: Laryngitis, pharyngitis, pneumonia, rhinorrhea, sinusitis, upper respiratory tract infection

Children 6 to 23 months: ≥2%:

Respiratory: Cough, otitis media, pharyngitis, rhinitis, tonsillitis, upper respiratory tract infection, wheezing

Pharmacodynamics/Kinetics

Duration of Action >24 hours

Available Dosage Forms

Packet, Oral:

Singulair: 4 mg (30 ea)

Generic: 4 mg (1 ea, 30 ea)

Tablet, Oral:

Singulair: 10 mg

Generic: 10 mg

Tablet Chewable, Oral:
Singulair: 4 mg, 5 mg
Generic: 4 mg, 5 mg

General Dosage Range Oral:
Children 6 months to <6 years: 4 mg once daily
Children ≥6 years and Adolescents <15 years:
5 mg once daily **or** 5 mg 2 hours prior to exercise
Children ≥15 years and Adults: 10 mg once daily
or 10 mg 2 hours prior to exercise

Administration

Oral When treating asthma, administer dose in the evening. Patients with allergic rhinitis may individualize administration time (morning or evening). Patients with **both** asthma and allergic rhinitis should take a single dose in the evening. May administer without regard to food or meals. Granules: May be administered directly in the mouth, dissolved in 5 mL of baby formula or breast milk, or mixed with a spoonful of applesauce, carrots, rice, or ice cream; do not add to any other liquids or foods. Administer within 15 minutes of opening packet.

Storage/Stability Store at room temperature of 25°C (77°F); excursions permitted to 15°C to 30°C (59°F to 86°F). Store in original package. Protect from moisture and light. Granules must be used within 15 minutes of opening packet.

Nursing Actions

Physical Assessment Educate patient about proper use of this medication in contrast to other asthma medications such as various inhalers. Monitor mental and mood status. Be alert to signs of depression, hallucinations, irritability, agitation, and suicide ideation. Some side effects may include include headache, sore throat, sinus infection, earache, runny nose, cough, gastric upset. Notify provider if patient develops a rash; worsening pulmonary symptoms including increased use of rescue inhalers; or has weakness, tingling, tremors, or shaking to extremities.

Patient Education

- Discuss specific use of drug and side effects with patient as it relates to treatment. (HCAHPS: During this hospital stay, were you given any medicine that you had not taken before? Before giving you any new medicine, how often did hospital staff tell you what the medicine was for? How often did hospital staff describe possible side effects in a way you could understand?)
- Patient may experience flu-like syndrome, nervousness and anxiety, dyspepsia, nausea, or rhinitis. Have patient report immediately to prescriber depression, emotional instability, illogical thinking, dyspnea, increased use of inhaler, paresthesia, discolored urine, jaundice, inability to eat, behavioral changes, or rash (HCAHPS).
- Educate patient about signs of a significant reaction (eg, wheezing; chest tightness; fever; itching; bad cough; blue skin color; seizures; or swelling of face, lips, tongue, or throat). **Note:** This is not a comprehensive list of all side effects. Patient should consult prescriber for additional questions.

Intended Use and Disclaimer: Should not be printed and given to patients. This information is intended to serve as a concise initial reference for healthcare professionals to use when discussing medications with a patient. You must ultimately rely on your own discretion, experience and judgment in diagnosing, treating and advising patients.

Dietary Considerations Some products may contain phenylalanine.

Morphine (Systemic) (MOR feen)

Brand Names: U.S. Astramorph; AVINza; Duramorph; Infumorph 200; Infumorph 500; Kadian; MS Contin

Index Terms MS (error-prone abbreviation and should not be used); MSO$_4$ (error-prone abbreviation and should not be used); Roxanol

Pharmacologic Category Analgesic, Opioid

Medication Safety Issues

Sound-alike/look-alike issues:
Morphine may be confused with HYDROmorphone, methadone
Morphine sulfate may be confused with magnesium sulfate
Kadian® may be confused with Kapidex [DSC]
MS Contin® may be confused with OxyCONTIN®
MSO$_4$ and MS are error-prone abbreviations (mistaken as magnesium sulfate)
AVINza® may be confused with Evista®, INVanz®
Roxanol may be confused with OxyFast®, Roxicet™, Roxicodone®

High alert medication:
The Institute for Safe Medication Practices (ISMP) includes this medication (I.V. formulation) among its list of drug classes which have a heightened risk of causing significant patient harm when used in error.

Other safety concerns:
Use care when prescribing and/or administering morphine solutions. These products are available in different concentrations. Always prescribe dosage in mg; **not** by volume (mL).
Use caution when selecting a morphine formulation for use in neurologic infusion pumps (eg, Medtronic delivery systems). The product should be appropriately labeled as "preservative-free" and suitable for intraspinal use via continuous infusion. In addition, the product should be formulated in a pH range that is compatible with the device operation specifications.
Significant differences exist between oral and I.V. dosing. Use caution when converting from one route of administration to another.

Medication Guide Available Yes

Pregnancy Risk Factor C

Lactation Enters breast milk

Breast-Feeding Considerations Morphine concentrates in breast milk, with a milk to plasma AUC ratio of 2.5:1. Detectable serum levels of morphine can be found in infants following morphine administration to nursing mothers.

Parenteral opioids used during labor have the potential to interfere with a newborn's natural reflex to nurse within the first few hours after birth. Morphine is recommended as an analgesic in nursing women due to the limited amounts found in breast milk and poor oral bioavailability in nursing infants. Nursing infants exposed to large doses of opioids should be monitored for apnea and sedation (Montgomery, 2012).

Treatment of the mother with single doses of morphine is not expected to cause detrimental effects in nursing infants. Breast-feeding following chronic use or in neonates with hepatic or renal dysfunction may lead to higher levels of morphine in the infant and a risk of adverse effects (Spigset, 2000).

The manufacturers of extended release products note that due to the potential for serious adverse reactions in the nursing infant, a decision should be made whether to discontinue nursing or to discontinue the drug, taking into account the importance of treatment to the mother.

Use Relief of moderate-to-severe acute and chronic pain; relief of pain of myocardial infarction; relief of dyspnea of acute left ventricular failure and pulmonary edema; preanesthetic medication

Infumorph: Used in continuous microinfusion devices for intrathecal or epidural administration in treatment of intractable chronic pain

Extended release products: Moderate-to-severe pain when continuous, around-the-clock opioid analgesia is needed for an extended period of time

Note: Opioid tolerance: Use of morphine sulfate extended release tablets/capsules ≥90 mg, and/or the oral solution 100 mg/5 mL (20 mg/mL) should be reserved for opioid-tolerant patients (ie, already taking at least 60 mg daily of oral morphine equivalent for at least 1 week).

Mechanism of Action/Effect Binds to opioid receptors in the CNS, causing inhibition of ascending pain pathways, altering the perception of and response to pain; produces generalized CNS depression

Contraindications Note: Some contraindications are product specific. For details, please see detailed product prescribing information.

Hypersensitivity to morphine sulfate or any component of the formulation; severe respiratory depression, acute or severe asthma (in an unmonitored setting or without resuscitative equipment); known or suspected paralytic ileus

Additional contraindication information (based on formulation):

Epidural/intrathecal:

Astramorph/PF™, Duramorph: Upper airway obstruction

Astramorph/PF™, Duramorph, Infumorph: Usual contraindications related to neuraxial analgesia apply (eg, presence of infection at infusion site, concomitant anticoagulant therapy, uncontrolled bleeding diathesis)

Extended release: GI obstruction

Immediate release tablets/solution: Hypercarbia

Injectable formulation: Heart failure due to chronic lung disease, cardiac arrhythmias; increased intracranial pressure, head injuries, brain tumors; acute alcoholism, deliriums tremens; seizure disorders; use during labor when a premature birth is anticipated

Suppository: Severe CNS depression; cardiac arrhythmias, heart failure due to chronic lung disease; increased intracranial or cerebrospinal pressure, head injuries, brain tumor; acute alcoholism, delirium tremens; seizure disorder; use after biliary tract surgery, suspected surgical abdomen, surgical anastomosis; concurrent use or within 2 weeks of MAO inhibitors

Warnings/Precautions An opioid-containing analgesic regimen should be tailored to each patient's needs and based upon the type of pain being treated (acute versus chronic), the route of administration, degree of tolerance for opioids (naive versus chronic user), age, weight, and medical condition. The optimal analgesic dose varies widely among patients. Doses should be titrated to pain relief/prevention. When used as an epidural injection, monitor for delayed sedation. **[U.S. Boxed Warning]: Healthcare provider should be alert to problems of abuse, misuse, and diversion. [U.S. Boxed Warning]: Extended release formulations, concentrated oral solution (100 mg/5 mL): Fatal overdose of morphine can result from accidental ingestion, especially in children.**

[U.S. Boxed Warning]: Fatal respiratory depression may occur. Greatest risk during initiation and dose increases. Use with caution in patients (particularly elderly, debilitated) with impaired respiratory function (especially hypoxia or hypercapnia), COPD, other obstructive pulmonary disease, decreased respiratory reserve, kyphoscoliosis or other skeletal disorder which may alter respiratory function. Infants <3 months of age are more susceptible to respiratory depression, use with caution and generally in reduced doses in this age group.

Use caution in morbid obesity, adrenal insufficiency, prostatic hyperplasia, thyroid dysfunction, urinary stricture, renal impairment, or severe hepatic dysfunction and in patients with hypersensitivity reactions to other phenanthrene derivative opioid agonists (codeine, hydrocodone, hydromorphone, levorphanol, oxycodone, oxymorphone). Avoid use in patients with CNS depression or coma as these patients are susceptible to intracranial effects of CO_2 retention. Use with caution in patients with biliary tract dysfunction including acute pancreatitis as may cause constriction of sphincter of Oddi. May obscure diagnosis or clinical course of patients with acute abdominal conditions. Some preparations contain sulfites which may cause allergic reactions.

May cause CNS depression, which may impair physical or mental abilities; patients must be cautioned about performing tasks which require mental alertness (eg, operating machinery or driving). Potentially significant drug interactions may exist, requiring dose or frequency adjustment, additional monitoring, and/or selection of alternative therapy. Effects may be potentiated when used with other sedative drugs. **[U.S. Boxed Warning]: Do not administer Avinza® with alcoholic beverages or ethanol-containing prescription or nonprescription products, which may disrupt extended-release characteristic of product.**

May cause hypotension; use with caution in patients with hypovolemia, cardiovascular disease (including acute MI), circulatory shock, or drugs which may exaggerate hypotensive effects (including phenothiazines or general anesthetics). May cause orthostatic hypotension and syncope in ambulatory patients. Use with extreme caution in patients with head injury, intracranial lesions, or elevated intracranial pressure; exaggerated elevation of ICP may occur if respiratory drive is depressed and CO_2 retention occurs. Use with caution in patients with seizure disorders, may exacerbate pre-existing seizures. Tolerance or drug dependence may result from extended use. Concurrent use of agonist/antagonist analgesics may precipitate withdrawal symptoms and/or reduced analgesic efficacy in patients following prolonged therapy with mu opioid agonists. Abrupt discontinuation following prolonged use may also lead to withdrawal symptoms. Gradually wean dose over a short period of time. Elderly may be particularly susceptible to adverse effects. Use epidural/intrathecal formulations with extreme caution in the elderly. After chronic maternal exposure to opioids, neonatal withdrawal syndrome may occur in the newborn; monitor neonate closely. Signs and symptoms include irritability, hyperactivity and abnormal sleep pattern, high pitched cry, tremor, vomiting, diarrhea and failure to gain weight. Onset, duration and severity depend on the drug used, duration of use, maternal dose, and rate of drug elimination by the newborn. Opioid withdrawal syndrome in the neonate, unlike in adults, may be life-threatening and should be treated according to protocols developed by neonatology experts.

[U.S. Boxed Warning]: Extended release dosage forms should not be crushed, dissolved, or chewed. Extended release products are not intended for "as needed (PRN)" use. Avinza® capsules contain fumaric acid; dangerous quantities of fumaric acid may be ingested when >1600 mg/day is used; serious renal toxicity may occur above the maximum dose. **Extended release products are not interchangeable;** when determining a generic equivalent or switching from one extended release product to another, review pharmacokinetic properties.

Highly concentrated oral solutions: **[U.S. Boxed Warning]: Check doses carefully when using highly concentrated oral solutions. The 100 mg/5 mL (20 mg/mL) concentration is indicated for use in opioid-tolerant patients only.**

Injections: Products are designed for administration by specific routes (ie, I.V., intrathecal, epidural). Use caution when prescribing, dispensing, or administering to use formulations only by intended route(s).

Astramorph/PF™, Duramorph, Infumorph: **[U.S. Boxed Warning]: Due to the risk of severe and/or sustained cardiopulmonary depressant effects, must be administered in a fully equipped room for resuscitation and staffed environment.** Naloxone injection should be immediately available. Patient should remain in this environment for at least 24 hours following the initial dose. **[U.S. Boxed Warning]: Accidental dermal exposure to Astramorph/PF™, Duramorph, Infumorph should be rinsed with water. Contaminated clothing should be removed.** For patients receiving Infumorph via microinfusion device, patient may be observed, as appropriate, for the first several days after catheter implantation. Thoracic epidural administration has been shown to dramatically increase the risk of early and late respiratory depression.

[U.S. Boxed Warning]: Improper or erroneous substitution of Infumorph for regular Duramorph is likely to result in serious overdosage, leading to seizures, respiratory depression and possibly a fatal outcome. Infumorph should only be used in microinfusion devices; not for I.V., I.M., or SubQ administration or for single-dose administration. Monitor closely, especially in the first 24 hours. Inflammatory masses (eg, granulomas), some resulting in severe neurologic impairment have occurred when receiving Infumorph via indwelling intrathecal catheter; monitor carefully for new neurologic signs/symptoms. **[U.S. Boxed Warning]: Intrathecal dosage is usually 1/10 (one-tenth) that of epidural dosage.**

Drug Interactions
Avoid Concomitant Use
Avoid concomitant use of Morphine (Systemic) with any of the following: Azelastine (Nasal); MAO Inhibitors; Paraldehyde; Thalidomide
Decreased Effect
Morphine (Systemic) may decrease the levels/ effects of: Clopidogrel; Pegvisomant

The levels/effects of Morphine (Systemic) may be decreased by: Ammonium Chloride; Mixed Agonist / Antagonist Opioids; Peginterferon Alfa-2b; P-glycoprotein/ABCB1 Inducers; Rifamycin Derivatives
Increased Effect/Toxicity
Morphine (Systemic) may increase the levels/ effects of: Alcohol (Ethyl); Alvimopan; Azelastine (Nasal); CNS Depressants; Desmopressin; Diuretics; Hydrocodone; Metyrosine; Mirtazapine; Paraldehyde; Pramipexole; ROPINIRole; Rotigotine; Selective Serotonin Reuptake Inhibitors; Thalidomide; Zolpidem

The levels/effects of Morphine (Systemic) may be increased by: Amphetamines; Anticholinergics; Antipsychotic Agents (Phenothiazines); Brimonidine (Topical); Cannabinoids; Doxylamine; Droperidol; HydrOXYzine; Magnesium Sulfate; MAO Inhibitors; Perampanel; P-glycoprotein/ABCB1 Inhibitors; Sodium Oxybate; Succinylcholine; Tapentadol

Nutritional/Ethanol Interactions
Ethanol: Alcoholic beverages or ethanol-containing products may disrupt extended release formulation resulting in rapid release of entire morphine dose. Ethanol may also increase CNS depression. Management: Avoid alcohol. **Do not administer Avinza® with alcoholic beverages or ethanol-containing prescription or nonprescription products.**

Food: Administration of oral morphine solution with food may increase bioavailability (ie, a report of 34% increase in morphine AUC when morphine oral solution followed a high-fat meal). The bioavailability of Avinza®, MS Contin®, or Kadian® does not appear to be affected by food. Management: Take consistently with or without meals.

Herb/Nutraceutical: Gotu kola, valerian, and kava kava may increase CNS depression. Management: Avoid gotu kola, valerian, and kava kava.

Adverse Reactions Note: Individual patient differences are unpredictable, and percentage may differ in acute pain (surgical) treatment. Reactions may be dose, formulation, and/or route dependent.

Frequency not defined:
Cardiovascular: Circulatory depression, flushing, shock
Central nervous system: Dysphonia, physical and psychological dependence, sedation
Endocrine & metabolic: Antidiuretic hormone release, hypogonadism

Neuromuscular & skeletal: Bone mineral density decreased
>10%:
Cardiovascular: Bradycardia, hypotension
Central nervous system: Drowsiness (9% to 48%; tolerance usually develops to drowsiness with regular dosing for 1-2 weeks), dizziness (6% to 20%), fever (<3% to >10%), confusion, headache (following epidural or intrathecal use)
Dermatologic: Pruritus (may be dose related)
Gastrointestinal: Xerostomia (78%), constipation (9% to 40%; tolerance develops very slowly if at all), nausea (7% to 28%; tolerance usually develops to nausea and vomiting with chronic use), vomiting
Genitourinary: Urinary retention (16%; may be prolonged, up to 20 hours, following epidural or intrathecal use)
Hematologic: Anemia (following intrathecal use)
Local: Pain at injection site
Neuromuscular & skeletal: Weakness
Respiratory: Oxygen saturation decreased
Miscellaneous: Histamine release
1% to 10%:
Cardiovascular: Atrial fibrillation (<3%), chest pain (<3%), edema, hypertension, palpitation, peripheral edema, syncope, tachycardia, vasodilation
Central nervous system: Amnesia, agitation, anxiety, apathy, apprehension, ataxia, chills, coma, delirium, depression, dream abnormalities, euphoria, false sense of well being, hallucination, hypoesthesia, insomnia, lethargy, malaise, nervousness, restlessness, seizure, slurred speech, somnolence, vertigo
Dermatologic: Dry skin, rash, urticaria
Endocrine & metabolic: Gynecomastia (<3%), hypokalemia, hyponatremia, libido decreased
Gastrointestinal: Abdominal distension, abdominal pain, anorexia, biliary colic, diarrhea, dyspepsia, dysphagia, flatulence, gastroenteritis, GERD, GI irritation, paralytic ileus, rectal disorder, taste perversion, weight loss
Genitourinary: Bladder spasm, dysuria, ejaculation abnormal, impotence, urination decreased
Hematologic: Leukopenia (<3%), thrombocytopenia (<3%), hematocrit decreased
Hepatic: Liver function tests increased
Neuromuscular & skeletal: Arthralgia, back pain, bone pain, foot drop, gait abnormalities, paresthesia, rigors, skeletal muscle rigidity, tremor
Ocular: Amblyopia, conjunctivitis, eye pain, vision problems/disturbance
Renal: Oliguria
Respiratory: Asthma, atelectasis, dyspnea, hiccups, hypercapnia, hypoxia, pulmonary edema (noncardiogenic), respiratory depression, rhinitis
Miscellaneous: Diaphoresis, flu-like syndrome, infection, thirst, voice alteration, withdrawal syndrome

Pharmacodynamics/Kinetics

Onset of Action Patient dependent; dosing must be individualized: Oral (immediate release): ~30 minutes; I.V.: 5-10 minutes

Duration of Action Patient dependent; dosing must be individualized: Pain relief:

Immediate release formulations: 4 hours

Extended release capsule and tablet: 8-24 hours (formulation dependent)

Controlled Substance C-II

Available Dosage Forms

Capsule Extended Release 24 Hour, Oral:

AVINza: 30 mg, 45 mg, 60 mg, 75 mg, 90 mg, 120 mg

Kadian: 10 mg, 20 mg, 30 mg, 40 mg, 50 mg, 60 mg, 70 mg, 80 mg, 100 mg, 130 mg, 150 mg, 200 mg

Generic: 10 mg, 20 mg, 30 mg, 45 mg, 50 mg, 60 mg, 75 mg, 80 mg, 90 mg, 100 mg, 120 mg

Device, Intramuscular:

Generic: 10 mg/0.7 mL (0.7 mL)

Solution, Injection:

Generic: 4 mg/mL (1 mL); 5 mg/mL (1 mL); 8 mg/mL (1 mL); 10 mg/mL (1 mL, 10 mL); 15 mg/mL (1 mL, 20 mL)

Solution, Injection [preservative free]:

Astramorph: 0.5 mg/mL (2 mL); 1 mg/mL (2 mL)

Duramorph: 0.5 mg/mL (10 mL); 1 mg/mL (10 mL)

Infumorph 200: 200 mg/20 mL (10 mL) (20 mL)

Infumorph 500: 500 mg/20 mL (25 mg/mL) (20 mL)

Generic: 0.5 mg/mL (10 mL); 1 mg/mL (10 mL)

Solution, Intravenous:

Generic: 1 mg/mL (10 mL, 30 mL, 250 mL); 25 mg/mL (4 mL, 10 mL); 50 mg/mL (20 mL, 50 mL)

Solution, Intravenous [preservative free]:

Generic: 1 mg/mL (30 mL); 2 mg/mL (1 mL); 4 mg/mL (1 mL); 150 mg/30 mL (30 mL); 8 mg/mL (1 mL); 10 mg/mL (1 mL); 15 mg/mL (1 mL); 25 mg/mL (10 mL)

Solution, Oral:

Generic: 10 mg/5 mL (5 mL, 100 mL, 500 mL); 20 mg/5 mL (5 mL, 100 mL, 500 mL); 20 mg/mL (15 mL, 30 mL, 120 mL, 240 mL); 100 mg/5 mL (30 mL, 120 mL)

Suppository, Rectal:

Generic: 5 mg (12 ea); 10 mg (12 ea); 20 mg (12 ea); 30 mg (12 ea)

Tablet, Oral:

Generic: 15 mg, 30 mg

Tablet Extended Release, Oral:

MS Contin: 15 mg, 30 mg, 60 mg, 100 mg, 200 mg

Generic: 15 mg, 30 mg, 60 mg, 100 mg, 200 mg

General Dosage Range Dosage adjustment recommended in patients with renal impairment

Epidural: *Adults:* 30-100 **mcg/kg** (2.5-3.75 mg; Astramorph/PF™, Duramorph) as a single dose **or** continuous infusion of 0.2-0.4 mg/hour **or** continuous microinfusion (Infumorph): Opioid-naive patients: 3.5-7.5 mg over 24 hours; Opioid-tolerant patients: 4.5-30 mg over 24 hours

I.M.:

Children >6 months and <50 kg: 0.1-0.2 mg/kg every 3-4 hours as needed

Adults: 5-15 mg every 4 hours as needed

I.T. (I.T. dose is usually 1/10 that of epidural dose):

Adults: Opioid-naive: 0.1-0.3 mg/dose as single dose (Astramorph/PF™, Duramorph) **or** as continuous microinfusion (Infumorph): Opioid-naive: 0.2-1 mg over 24 hours; Opioid-tolerant: 1-10 mg over 24 hours

I.V.:

Children >6 months and <50 kg: 0.05-0.3 mg/kg (maximum dose: 10 mg) every 3-4 hours as needed **or** 10-30 **mcg/kg/hour** as an initial continuous infusion

Adults: 2.5-5 mg every 3-4 hours **or** 0.8-10 mg/hour; Usual range: Up to 80 mg/hour

Adults (mechanically-ventilated): 2-4 mg every 1-2 hours **or** 4-8 mg every 3-4 hours **or** 2-30 mg/hour

Oral:

Extended release: *Adults:*

Capsules: Established daily dose on prompt-release formulations administered in 1-2 divided doses (every 12 hours)

Tablets: Established daily dose on prompt-release formulations administered in divided doses every 8-12 hours

Immediate release:

Children >6 months and <50 kg: 0.15-0.3 mg/kg every 3-4 hours as needed

Adults: 10-30 mg every 4 hours as needed; **Note:** Much higher doses may be necessary for chronic pain

PCA: *Adults:* Concentration: 1 mg/mL; Demand dose: 0.5-2.5 mg; Lockout interval: 5-10 minutes

Rectal: *Adults:* 10-20 mg every 3-4 hours

SubQ:

Adults: 5-15 mg every 3-4 hours as needed **or** 0.8-10 mg/hour (up to 80 mg/hour) as continuous infusion

Adults (mechanically-ventilated): 2-30 mg/hour

Usual Infusion Concentrations: Pediatric I.V. infusion: 0.1 mg/mL, 0.5 mg/mL, **or** 1 mg/mL

Usual Infusion Concentrations: Adult I.V. infusion: 1 mg/mL

Administration

I.V. When giving morphine I.V. push, it is best to first dilute with sterile water or NS for a final concentration of 1-2 mg/mL and then administer slowly over 4-5 minutes.

Injectable Detail pH: 2.5-6

Oral Do not crush, chew, or dissolve extended release drug product; swallow whole. Kadian® and Avinza® can be opened and sprinkled on applesauce and eaten immediately without chewing; do not crush, dissolve, or chew the beads as it can result in a rapid release of a potentially fatal dose of morphine. Ensure all pellets have been swallowed by rinsing mouth. Contents of Kadian® capsules may be opened and sprinkled over 10 mL water and flushed through prewetted 16F gastrostomy tube; do not administer Kadian® through gastric/nasogastric tubes.

Other Epidural: Use preservative-free solutions for epidural use. Infumorph may **only** be used as a continuous microinfusion via catheter.

Intrathecal Use preservative-free solutions for intrathecal use. Infumorph may **only** be used as a continuous microinfusion via catheter.

Storage/Stability

Capsule, extended release: Store at 25°C (77°F); excursions permitted to 15°C to 30°C (59°F to 86°F). Protect from light and moisture.

Injection: Store at controlled room temperature of 20°C to 25°C (68°F to 77°F); do not freeze. Protect from light. Degradation depends on pH and presence of oxygen; relatively stable in pH ≤4; darkening of solutions indicate degradation. Astramorph/PF™, Duramorph, Infumorph: Store in carton until use at controlled room temperature of 20°C to 25°C (68°F to 77°F); excursions permitted to 15°C to 30°C (59°F to 86°F); do not freeze; do not heat-sterilize. Contains no preservative or antioxidant. Protect from light.

Oral solution: Store at controlled room temperature of 15°C to 30°C (59°F to 86°F); do not freeze. Protect from moisture.

Suppositories: Store below controlled room temperature 25°C (77°F).

Tablet, extended release: Store at controlled room temperature of 25°C (77°F); excursions permitted to 15°C to 30°C (59°F to 86°F).

Tablet, immediate release: Store at controlled room temperature of 15°C to 30°C (59°F to 86°F). Protect from moisture.

Nursing Actions

Physical Assessment Monitor for effectiveness of pain relief. Monitor blood pressure, CNS and respiratory status, and degree of sedation at beginning of therapy and periodically thereafter. Assess patient's physical and/or psychological dependence. Observe for allergic reaction if patient has allergies to other opioids, such as methadone, codeine, hydrocodone, or dihydrocodeine. For inpatients, implement safety measures (eg, side rails up, call light within reach, instructions to call for assistance). Discontinue slowly after prolonged use. Educate ambulatory patients about use, risk of falls, and operating machinery including motor vehicles.

Patient Education

• Discuss specific use of drug and side effects with patient as it relates to treatment. (HCAHPS: During this hospital stay, were you given any medicine that you had not taken before? Before giving you any new medicine, how often did hospital staff tell you what the medicine was for? How often did hospital staff describe possible side effects in a way you could understand?)

• Patient may experience presyncope, fatigue, blurred vision, illogical thinking, dizziness, nausea, constipation, or xerostomia. Have patient report immediately to prescriber syncope, dyspnea, chronic pain, or severe asthenia (HCAHPS).

• Educate patient about signs of a significant reaction (eg, wheezing; chest tightness; fever; itching; bad cough; blue skin color; seizures; or swelling of face, lips, tongue, or throat). **Note:** This is not a comprehensive list of all side effects. Patient should consult prescriber for additional questions.

Intended Use and Disclaimer: Should not be printed and given to patients. This information is intended to serve as a concise initial reference for healthcare professionals to use when discussing medications with a patient. You must ultimately rely on your own discretion, experience and judgment in diagnosing, treating and advising patients.

Dietary Considerations Morphine may cause GI upset; take with food if GI upset occurs. Be consistent when taking morphine with or without meals.

Related Information

Oral Medications That Should Not Be Crushed or Altered *on page 1712*

Morphine and Naltrexone
(MOR feen & nal TREKS one)

Brand Names: U.S. Embeda™

Index Terms Morphine Sulfate and Naltrexone Hydrochloride; MS (error-prone abbreviation and should not be used); MSO$_4$ (error-prone abbreviation and should not be used); Naltrexone and Morphine

Pharmacologic Category Analgesic, Opioid; Opioid Antagonist

Medication Safety Issues

Sound-alike/look-alike issues:

Morphine may be confused with HYDROmorphone

Morphine sulfate may be confused with magnesium sulfate

Naltrexone may be confused with methylnaltrexone, naloxone

MSO$_4$ and MS are error-prone abbreviations (mistaken as magnesium sulfate)

High alert medication:

The Institute for Safe Medication Practices (ISMP) includes this medication among its list of drug classes which have a heightened risk of causing significant patient harm when used in error.

Medication Guide Available Yes

Pregnancy Risk Factor C

Lactation Enters breast milk/not recommended

Use Relief of moderate-to-severe pain when continual, around-the-clock therapy is needed for an extended period of time

Product Availability Embeda was voluntarily recalled from the market in March 2011 due to manufacturing issues resulting in stability requirements not being met during routine testing. As of November 2013, the FDA has approved a Prior Approval Supplement for Embeda, which included an update to the manufacturing process that addressed the stability requirement and allows for the product to return to the market; availability anticipated in the second quarter of 2014.

Controlled Substance C-II

Available Dosage Forms

Capsule, extended release, oral:

Embeda™ 20/0.8: Morphine 20 mg and naltrexone 0.8 mg

Embeda™ 30/1.2: Morphine 30 mg and naltrexone 1.2 mg

Embeda™ 50/2: Morphine 50 mg and naltrexone 2 mg

Embeda™ 80/3.2: Morphine 80 mg and naltrexone 3.2 mg

Embeda™ 100/4: Morphine 100 mg and naltrexone 4 mg

General Dosage Range Oral: *Adults:* Initial: 20 mg/0.8 mg once or twice daily; Maintenance: Adjust based on individual patient requirement

Administration

Oral Capsule should be swallowed whole. Contents of the capsule may be sprinkled on applesauce (do not divide in separate doses) and swallowed immediately. Rinse mouth to ensure all contents have been swallowed. Do not crush, chew, or dissolve pellets in the capsule prior to swallowing. Not for nasogastric/gastric tube administration. First dose may be taken at the same time as the last dose of immediate release opioid medication.

Nursing Actions

Physical Assessment See individual agents.

Patient Education

• Discuss specific use of drug and side effects with patient as it relates to treatment. (HCAHPS: During this hospital stay, were you given any medicine that you had not taken before? Before giving you any new medicine, how often did hospital staff tell you what the medicine was for? How often did hospital staff describe possible side effects in a way you could understand?)

• Patient may experience headache, fatigue, or xerostomia. Have patient report immediately to prescriber severe dizziness, syncope, signification nausea, or considerable constipation (HCAHPS).

• Educate patient about signs of a significant reaction (eg, wheezing; chest tightness; fever;

itching; bad cough; blue skin color; seizures; or swelling of face, lips, tongue, or throat). **Note:** This is not a comprehensive list of all side effects. Patient should consult prescriber for additional questions.

Intended Use and Disclaimer: Should not be printed and given to patients. This information is intended to serve as a concise initial reference for healthcare professionals to use when discussing medications with a patient. You must ultimately rely on your own discretion, experience and judgment in diagnosing, treating and advising patients.

Related Information

Morphine (Systemic) *on page 1079*

Naltrexone *on page 1100*

Moxifloxacin (Systemic) (moxs i FLOKS a sin)

Brand Names: U.S. Avelox; Avelox ABC Pack

Index Terms Moxifloxacin Hydrochloride

Pharmacologic Category Antibiotic, Fluoroquinolone; Antibiotic, Respiratory Fluoroquinolone

Medication Safety Issues

Sound-alike/look-alike issues:

Avelox may be confused with Avonex

Medication Guide Available Yes

Pregnancy Risk Factor C

Lactation Excretion in breast milk unknown/not recommended

Breast-Feeding Considerations It is not known if moxifloxacin is excreted into breast milk. Breast-feeding is not recommended by the manufacturer. Although there is no information on the use of moxifloxacin during breast-feeding, other quinolones are considered compatible. Nondose-related effects could include modification of bowel flora.

Use Treatment of mild-to-moderate community-acquired pneumonia, including multidrug-resistant *Streptococcus pneumoniae* (MDRSP); acute bacterial exacerbation of chronic bronchitis; acute bacterial rhinosinusitis (ABRS); complicated and uncomplicated skin and skin structure infections; complicated intra-abdominal infections

Unlabeled Use Treatment of *Legionella* pneumonia; treatment of mild-to-moderate community-acquired pneumonia (CAP), including multidrug-resistant *Streptococcus pneumoniae* (MDRSP) in adolescents with skeletal maturity; tuberculosis (second-line therapy); surgical (perioperative) prophylaxis

Mechanism of Action/Effect Moxifloxacin is a quinolone antibiotic with bactericidal activity against susceptible gram-negative and gram-positive microorganisms.

Contraindications Hypersensitivity to moxifloxacin, other quinolone antibiotics, or any component of the formulation

Warnings/Precautions [U.S. Boxed Warning]: There have been reports of tendon inflammation and/or rupture with quinolone antibiotics in all ages; risk may be increased with concurrent corticosteroids, solid organ transplant recipients, and in patients >60 years of age. Rupture of the Achilles tendon sometimes requiring surgical repair has been reported most frequently; but other tendon sites (eg, rotator cuff, biceps) have also been reported. Strenuous physical activity, rheumatoid arthritis, and renal impairment may be an independent risk factor for tendonitis. Inflammation and rupture may occur bilaterally. Cases have been reported within the first 48 hours, during, and up to several months after discontinuation of therapy. Discontinue at first sign of tendon inflammation or pain. Use with caution in patients with rheumatoid arthritis; may increase risk of tendon rupture. Use with caution in patients with a history of tendon disorders.

Use with caution in patients with significant bradycardia or acute myocardial ischemia. Moxifloxacin causes a concentration-dependent QT prolongation. Do not exceed recommended dose or infusion rate. Avoid use with uncorrected hypokalemia, with other drugs that prolong the QT interval or induce bradycardia, or with class Ia or III antiarrhythmic agents. CNS effects may occur (tremor, restlessness, confusion, and very rarely hallucinations, increased intracranial pressure [including pseudotumor cerebri] or seizures). Use with caution in patients with known or suspected CNS disorder. Potential for seizures, although very rare, may be increased with concomitant NSAID therapy. Use with caution in individuals at risk of seizures. Use with caution in patients with mild, moderate, or severe hepatic impairment or liver cirrhosis; may increase the risk of QT prolongation. Fulminant hepatitis potentially leading to liver failure (including fatalities) has been reported with use. Use with caution in diabetes; glucose regulation may be altered.

Fluoroquinolones have been associated with the development of serious, and sometimes fatal, hypoglycemia, most often in elderly diabetics, but also in patients without diabetes. This occurred most frequently with gatifloxacin (no longer available systemically) but may occur at a lower frequency with other quinolones.

Severe hypersensitivity reactions, including anaphylaxis, have occurred with quinolone therapy. Reactions may present as typical allergic symptoms after a single dose, or may manifest as severe idiosyncratic dermatologic, vascular, pulmonary, renal, hepatic, and/or hematologic events, usually after multiple doses. Prompt discontinuation of drug should occur if skin rash or other symptoms arise. Avoid excessive sunlight and take precautions to limit exposure (eg, loose fitting clothing, sunscreen); may cause moderate-to-severe phototoxicity reactions. Discontinue use if photosensitivity occurs. Prolonged use may result in fungal or bacterial superinfection, including *C. difficile*-associated diarrhea (CDAD) and pseudomembranous colitis; CDAD has been observed >2 months postantibiotic treatment.

[U.S. Boxed Warning]: Quinolones may exacerbate myasthenia gravis; avoid use (rare, potentially life-threatening weakness of respiratory muscles may occur). Peripheral neuropathy has been reported (rare); may occur soon after initiation of therapy and may be irreversible; discontinue if symptoms of sensory or sensorimotor neuropathy occur. Hemolytic reactions may (rarely) occur with quinolone use in patients with latent or actual G6PD deficiency. Adverse effects (eg, tendon rupture, QT changes) may be increased in the elderly. Some quinolones may exacerbate myasthenia gravis, use with caution (rare, potentially life-threatening weakness of respiratory muscles may occur). Safety and efficacy of systemically administered moxifloxacin (oral, intravenous) in patients <18 years of age have not been established.

Drug Interactions

Avoid Concomitant Use

Avoid concomitant use of Moxifloxacin (Systemic) with any of the following: BCG; Highest Risk QTc-Prolonging Agents; Ivabradine; Mifepristone; Strontium Ranelate

Decreased Effect

Moxifloxacin (Systemic) may decrease the levels/ effects of: BCG; Didanosine; Mycophenolate; Sodium Picosulfate; Sulfonylureas; Typhoid Vaccine

The levels/effects of Moxifloxacin (Systemic) may be decreased by: Antacids; Didanosine; Iron Salts; Lanthanum; Magnesium Salts; Multivitamins/Minerals (with ADEK, Folate, Iron); Multivitamins/Minerals (with AE, No Iron); Quinapril; Sevelamer; Strontium Ranelate; Sucralfate; Zinc Salts

Increased Effect/Toxicity

Moxifloxacin (Systemic) may increase the levels/ effects of: Corticosteroids (Systemic); Highest Risk QTc-Prolonging Agents; Moderate Risk QTc-Prolonging Agents; Porfimer; Sulfonylureas; Varenicline; Vitamin K Antagonists

The levels/effects of Moxifloxacin (Systemic) may be increased by: Insulin; Ivabradine; Mifepristone; Nonsteroidal Anti-Inflammatory Agents; Probenecid; QTc-Prolonging Agents (Indeterminate Risk and Risk Modifying)

Nutritional/Ethanol Interactions Food: Absorption is not affected by administration with a high-fat meal or yogurt.

Adverse Reactions

2% to 10%:

Central nervous system: Headache (≤4%), dizziness (3%), insomnia (2%)

Endocrine & metabolic: Chloride increased (≥2%), glucose decreased (≥2%), ionized calcium increased (≥2%)

Gastrointestinal: Nausea (7%), diarrhea (6%), amylase decreased (≥2%), constipation (2%), vomiting (2%), abdominal pain (1% to 2%)

Hematologic: Decreased serum levels of the following (≥2%): Basophils, eosinophils, hemoglobin, PT, RBC, neutrophils; increased serum levels of the following (≥2%): MCH, neutrophils, PT, WBC

Hepatic: Bilirubin decreased/increased (≥2%)

Renal: Albumin increased (≥2%)

Respiratory: PO_2 decreased (≥2%)

0.1% to <2%:

Cardiovascular: Angina, atrial fibrillation, bradycardia, cardiac arrest, edema, heart failure, hypertension, hypotension, palpitation, peripheral edema, QT_c prolongation, syncope, tachycardia

Central nervous system: Fever (1%), agitation, anxiety, chills, confusion, depression, disorientation, fatigue, hallucinations, hypoesthesia, lethargy, malaise, nervousness, pain, restlessness, somnolence, vertigo

Dermatologic: Allergic dermatitis, erythema, hyperhidrosis, pruritus, rash, urticaria

Endocrine & metabolic: Hypokalemia (1%), dehydration, hyperglycemia, hyperlipidemia, triglycerides increased, uric acid increased

Gastrointestinal: Dyspepsia (1%), abdominal discomfort, abdominal distension, amylase increased, anorexia, appetite decreased, flatulence, gastritis, gastroenteritis, gastroesophageal reflux disease, lactic dehydrogenase increased, lipase increased, taste perversion, xerostomia

Genitourinary: Dysuria, vaginitis, vulvovaginal candidiasis, vulvovaginal mycotic infection, vulvovaginal pruritus

Hematologic: Anemia (1%), eosinophilia, hematocrit decreased, leukocytosis, leukopenia, aPTT increased, thrombocythemia, thrombocytopenia

Hepatic: ALT increased (1%), AST increased, alkaline phosphatase increased, GGTP increased, liver function test abnormal

Local: Injection site extravasation, phlebitis

Neuromuscular & skeletal: Arthralgia, back pain, chest pain (noncardiac), facial pain, limb pain, muscle spasms, musculoskeletal pain, myalgia, paresthesia, tremor, weakness

Ocular: Blurred vision

Otic: Tinnitus

Renal: BUN increased, creatinine increased, renal failure

Respiratory: Asthma, bronchospasm, dyspnea, wheezing

Miscellaneous: Allergic reaction, candidiasis, fungal infection, night sweats, oral candidiasis

Available Dosage Forms

Solution, Intravenous [preservative free]:

Avelox: 400 mg/250 mL (250 mL)

Tablet, Oral:

Avelox: 400 mg

Avelox ABC Pack: 400 mg

Generic: 400 mg

General Dosage Range I.V., oral: *Adults:* 400 mg every 24 hours

Administration

I.V. Infuse over 60 minutes; do not infuse by rapid or bolus intravenous infusion

Storage/Stability Store at controlled room temperature of 25°C (77°F). Do not refrigerate infusion solution.

Nursing Actions

Physical Assessment Results of culture and sensitivity tests and patient's allergy history should be assessed before initiating therapy. Monitor patient closely; if an allergic reaction occurs (itching, urticaria, dyspnea or facial edema, loss of consciousness, tingling, cardiovascular collapse), drug should be discontinued immediately and prescriber notified. Monitor for hypersensitivity reactions, opportunistic infection, tendon rupture, and persistent diarrhea (*C. difficile*-associated colitis can occur post-treatment).

Patient Education

- Discuss specific use of drug and side effects with patient as it relates to treatment. (HCAHPS: During this hospital stay, were you given any medicine that you had not taken before? Before giving you any new medicine, how often did hospital staff tell you what the medicine was for? How often did hospital staff describe possible side effects in a way you could understand?)

- Patient may experience dizziness, nausea, diarrhea, dyspepsia, or headache. Have patient report immediately to prescriber tachycardia, ankle pain, severe asthenia, arthralgia, edema, paresthesia, or rash (HCAHPS).

- Educate patient about signs of a significant reaction (eg, wheezing; chest tightness; fever; itching; bad cough; blue skin color; seizures; or swelling of face, lips, tongue, or throat). **Note:** This is not a comprehensive list of all side effects. Patient should consult prescriber for additional questions.

Intended Use and Disclaimer: Should not be printed and given to patients. This information is intended to serve as a concise initial reference for healthcare professionals to use when discussing medications with a patient. You must ultimately rely on your own discretion, experience and judgment in diagnosing, treating and advising patients.

◀ **Dietary Considerations** May be taken without regard to meals. Take 4 hours before or 8 hours after multiple vitamins, antacids, or other products containing magnesium, aluminum, iron, or zinc. Avelox® I.V. infusion (premixed in sodium chloride 0.8%) contains sodium 34.2 mEq (~787 mg)/ 250 mL.

Moxifloxacin (Ophthalmic)
(moxs i FLOKS a sin)

Brand Names: U.S. Moxeza; Vigamox
Index Terms Moxifloxacin Hydrochloride
Pharmacologic Category Antibiotic, Fluoroquinolone; Antibiotic, Ophthalmic
Medication Safety Issues
International issues:
Vigamox [U.S., Canada, and multiple international markets] may be confused with Fisamox brand name for amoxicillin [Australia]
Pregnancy Risk Factor C
Lactation Use caution
Use Treatment of bacterial conjunctivitis caused by susceptible organisms
Available Dosage Forms
Solution, Ophthalmic:
Moxeza: 0.5% (3 mL)
Vigamox: 0.5% (3 mL)
General Dosage Range Ophthalmic:
Children ≥4 months and Adults: Moxeza™: Instill 1 drop into affected eye(s) 2 times/day
Children ≥1 year and Adults: Vigamox®: Instill 1 drop into affected eye(s) 3 times/day
Administration
Other For topical ophthalmic use only; avoid touching tip of applicator to eye or other surfaces.
Nursing Actions
Patient Education
• Discuss specific use of drug and side effects with patient as it relates to treatment. (HCAHPS: During this hospital stay, were you given any medicine that you had not taken before? Before giving you any new medicine, how often did hospital staff tell you what the medicine was for? How often did hospital staff describe possible side effects in a way you could understand?)
• Patient may experience short-term pain. Have patient report immediately to prescriber sudden vision changes, eye irritation, or rash (HCAHPS).
• Educate patient about signs of a significant reaction (eg, wheezing; chest tightness; fever; itching; bad cough; blue skin color; seizures; or swelling of face, lips, tongue, or throat). **Note:** This is not a comprehensive list of all side effects. Patient should consult prescriber for additional questions.

Intended Use and Disclaimer: Should not be printed and given to patients. This information is intended to serve as a concise initial reference for healthcare professionals to use when discussing medications with a patient. You must ultimately rely on your own discretion, experience and judgment in diagnosing, treating and advising patients.

Mycophenolate (mye koe FEN oh late)

Brand Names: U.S. CellCept; CellCept Intravenous; Myfortic
Index Terms MMF; MPA; Mycophenolate Mofetil; Mycophenolate Sodium; Mycophenolic Acid
Pharmacologic Category Immunosuppressant Agent
Medication Guide Available Yes
Pregnancy Risk Factor D
Lactation Excretion in breast milk unknown/not recommended
Breast-Feeding Considerations It is unknown if mycophenolate is excreted in human milk. Due to potentially serious adverse reactions, the decision to discontinue the drug or discontinue breast-feeding should be considered. Breast-feeding is not recommended during therapy or for 6 weeks after treatment is complete.
Use Prophylaxis of organ rejection concomitantly with cyclosporine and corticosteroids in patients receiving allogeneic renal (CellCept, Myfortic), cardiac (CellCept), or hepatic (CellCept) transplants
Unlabeled Use Treatment of rejection in liver transplant patients unable to tolerate tacrolimus or cyclosporine due to toxicity; treatment of recurrent or persistent rejection in heart transplant patients; treatment of moderate-severe psoriasis; treatment of lupus nephritis; treatment of myasthenia gravis; prevention of graft-versus-host disease (GVHD); treatment of refractory acute GVHD and chronic GVHD; treatment of refractory autoimmune hepatitis
Mechanism of Action/Effect Inhibition of purine synthesis of human lymphocytes and proliferation of human lymphocytes
Contraindications Hypersensitivity to mycophenolate mofetil, mycophenolic acid, mycophenolate sodium, or any component of the formulation
Cellcept: Intravenous formulation is also contraindicated in patients who are allergic to polysorbate 80
Warnings/Precautions Hazardous agent - use appropriate precautions for handling and disposal (NIOSH, 2012). **[U.S. Boxed Warning]: Risk for bacterial, viral, fungal, and protozoal infections, including opportunistic infections, is increased with immunosuppressant therapy;** infections may be serious and potentially fatal. Due to the risk of oversuppression of the immune system, which may increase susceptibility to infection, combination immunosuppressant therapy should be used with caution. Polyomavirus associated nephropathy (PVAN), JC virus-associated progressive multifocal leukoencephalopathy (PML),

cytomegalovirus (CMV) infections, reactivation of hepatitis B (HBV) or hepatitis C (HCV), have been reported with use. A reduction in immunosuppression should be considered for patients with new or reactivated viral infections; however, in transplant recipients, the risk that reduced immunosuppression presents to the functioning graft should also be considered. PVAN, primarily from activation of BK virus, may lead to the deterioration of renal function and/or renal graft loss. PML, a potentially fatal condition, commonly presents with hemiparesis, apathy, ataxia, cognitive deficiencies, confusion, and hemiparesis. Risk factors for development of PML include treatment with immunosuppressants and immune function impairment; consultation with a neurologist should be considered in any patient with neurological symptoms receiving immunosuppressants. Risk of CMV viremia or disease is increased in transplant recipients CMV seronegative at the time of transplant who receive a graft from a CMV seropositive donor. In patients infected with HBV or HCV, viral reactivation may occur; these patients should be monitored for signs of active HBV or HCV. **[U.S. Boxed Warning]: Risk of development of lymphoma and skin malignancy is increased.** The risk for malignancies is related to intensity/duration of therapy. Patients should be monitored appropriately, instructed to limit exposure to sunlight/UV light to decrease the risk of skin cancer, and given supportive treatment should these conditions occur. Post-transplant lymphoproliferative disorder related to EBV infection has been reported in immunosuppressed organ transplant patients; risk is highest in EBV seronegative patients (including many young children). Neutropenia (including severe neutropenia) may occur, requiring dose reduction or interruption of treatment (risk greater from day 31-180 post-transplant). Use may rarely be associated with gastric or duodenal ulcers, GI bleeding and/or perforation. Use caution in patients with active serious digestive system disease; patients with active peptic ulcers were not included in clinical studies. Use caution in renal impairment as toxicity may be increased; may require dosage adjustment in severe impairment.

[U.S. Boxed Warning]: Mycophenolate is associated with an increased risk of congenital malformations and first trimester pregnancy loss when used by pregnant women. Females of reproductive potential must be counseled about pregnancy prevention and planning. Alternative agents should be considered for women planning a pregnancy. Females of reproductive potential should have a negative pregnancy test with a sensitivity of ≥25 mIU/mL immediately before therapy and the test should be repeated 8-10 days later. Pregnancy tests should be repeated during routine follow-up visits. Acceptable forms of contraception should be used during treatment and for 6 weeks after therapy is discontinued. Females of childbearing potential should have a negative pregnancy test within 1 week prior to beginning therapy. Two reliable forms of contraception should be used beginning 4 weeks prior to, during, and for 6 weeks after therapy. Because mycophenolate mofetil has demonstrated teratogenic effects in rats and rabbits, tablets should not be crushed, and capsules should not be opened or crushed. Avoid inhalation or direct contact with skin or mucous membranes of the powder contained in the capsules and the powder for oral suspension. Caution should be exercised in the handling and preparation of solutions of intravenous mycophenolate. Avoid skin contact with the intravenous solution and reconstituted suspension. If such contact occurs, wash thoroughly with soap and water, rinse eyes with plain water.

Theoretically, use should be avoided in patients with the rare hereditary deficiency of hypoxanthine-guanine phosphoribosyltransferase (such as Lesch-Nyhan or Kelley-Seegmiller syndrome). Intravenous solutions should be given over at least 2 hours; never administer intravenous solution by rapid or bolus injection. Live attenuated vaccines should be avoided during use; vaccinations may be less effective during therapy. **[U.S. Boxed Warning]: Should be administered under the supervision of a physician experienced in immunosuppressive therapy.**

Note: CellCept and Myfortic dosage forms should not be used interchangeably due to differences in absorption. Some dosage forms may contain phenylalanine. The intravenous formulation contains polysorbate 80.

Drug Interactions
Avoid Concomitant Use
Avoid concomitant use of Mycophenolate with any of the following: BCG; Cholestyramine Resin; Natalizumab; Pimecrolimus; Rifamycin Derivatives; Tacrolimus (Topical); Tofacitinib; Vaccines (Live)

Decreased Effect
Mycophenolate may decrease the levels/effects of: BCG; Coccidioidin Skin Test; Contraceptives (Estrogens); Contraceptives (Progestins); Sipuleucel-T; Vaccines (Inactivated); Vaccines (Live)

The levels/effects of Mycophenolate may be decreased by: Antacids; Cholestyramine Resin; CycloSPORINE (Systemic); Echinacea; Magnesium Salts; MetroNIDAZOLE (Systemic); Penicillins; Proton Pump Inhibitors; Quinolone Antibiotics; Rifamycin Derivatives; Sevelamer

Increased Effect/Toxicity
Mycophenolate may increase the levels/effects of: Acyclovir-Valacyclovir; Ganciclovir-Valganciclovir; Leflunomide; Natalizumab; Tofacitinib; Vaccines (Live)

The levels/effects of Mycophenolate may be increased by: Acyclovir-Valacyclovir; Belatacept; Denosumab; Ganciclovir-Valganciclovir; Pimecrolimus; Probenecid; Roflumilast; Tacrolimus (Topical); Trastuzumab

Nutritional/Ethanol Interactions

Food: Food decreases C_{max} of MPA by 40% following CellCept administration and 33% following Myfortic use; the extent of absorption is not changed. Management: Take CellCept or Myfortic on an empty stomach to decrease variability; however, Cellcept may be taken with food if necessary in stable renal transplant patients.

Herb/Nutraceutical: Cat's claw and echinacea have immunostimulant properties. Management: Avoid cat's claw and echinacea.

Adverse Reactions Data for incidence >20% as reported in adults following oral dosing of CellCept alone in renal, cardiac, and hepatic allograft rejection studies. Profile in 3% to <20% range reflects use in combination with cyclosporine and corticosteroids. In general, lower doses used in renal rejection patients had less adverse effects than higher doses. Rates of adverse effects were similar for each indication, except for those unique to the specific organ involved. The type of adverse effects observed in pediatric patients was similar to those seen in adults, with the exception of abdominal pain, anemia, diarrhea, fever, hypertension, infection, pharyngitis, respiratory tract infection, sepsis, and vomiting; lymphoproliferative disorder was the only type of malignancy observed. Percentages of adverse reactions were similar in studies comparing CellCept to Myfortic in patients following renal transplant.

>20%:

Cardiovascular: Hypertension (28% to 78%), hypotension (33%), peripheral edema (27% to 64%), edema (27% to 28%), chest pain (26%), tachycardia (20% to 22%)

Central nervous system: Pain (31% to 76%), headache (16% to 54%), insomnia (41% to 52%), fever (21% to 52%), dizziness (29%), anxiety (28%)

Dermatologic: Rash (22%)

Endocrine & metabolic: Hyperglycemia (44% to 47%), hypercholesterolemia (41%), hypomagnesemia (39%), hypokalemia (32% to 37%), hypocalcemia (30%), hyperkalemia (22%)

Gastrointestinal: Abdominal pain (25% to 63%), nausea (20% to 55%), diarrhea (31% to 51%), constipation (19% to 41%), vomiting (33% to 34%), anorexia (25%), dyspepsia (22%)

Genitourinary: Urinary tract infection (37%)

Hematologic: Leukopenia (23% to 46%), anemia (26% to 43%; hypochromic 25%), leukocytosis (22% to 41%), thrombocytopenia (24% to 38%)

Hepatic: Liver function tests abnormal (25%), ascites (24%)

Neuromuscular & skeletal: Back pain (35% to 47%), weakness (35% to 43%), tremor (24% to 34%), paresthesia (21%)

Renal: Creatinine increased (39%), BUN increased (35%), kidney function abnormal (22% to 26%)

Respiratory: Dyspnea (31% to 37%), respiratory tract infection (22% to 37%), pleural effusion (34%), cough (31%), lung disorder (22% to 30%), sinusitis (26%)

Miscellaneous: Infection (18% to 27%), sepsis (27%), lactate dehydrogenase increased (23%), *Candida* (17% to 22%), herpes simplex (10% to 21%)

3% to <20%:

Cardiovascular: Angina, arrhythmia, arterial thrombosis, atrial fibrillation, atrial flutter, bradycardia, cardiac arrest, cardiac failure, CHF, extrasystole, facial edema, hyper-/hypovolemia, orthostatic hypotension, pallor, palpitation, pericardial effusion, peripheral vascular disorder, supraventricular extrasystoles, supraventricular tachycardia, syncope, thrombosis, vasodilation, vasospasm, venous pressure increased, ventricular extrasystole, ventricular tachycardia

Central nervous system: Agitation, chills with fever, confusion, delirium, depression, emotional lability, hallucinations, hypoesthesia, malaise, nervousness, psychosis, seizure, somnolence, thinking abnormal, vertigo

Dermatologic: Acne, alopecia, bruising, cellulitis, fungal dermatitis, hirsutism, petechia, pruritus, skin carcinoma, skin hypertrophy, skin ulcer, vesiculobullous rash

Endocrine & metabolic: Acidosis, alkalosis, Cushing's syndrome, dehydration, diabetes mellitus, gout, hypercalcemia, hyper-hypophosphatemia, hyperlipemia, hyperuricemia, hypochloremia, hypoglycemia, hyponatremia, hypoproteinemia, hypothyroidism, parathyroid disorder

Gastrointestinal: Abdomen enlarged, dysphagia, esophagitis, flatulence, gastritis, gastroenteritis, gastrointestinal hemorrhage, gastrointestinal moniliasis, gingivitis, gum hyperplasia, ileus, melena, mouth ulceration, oral moniliasis, stomach disorder, stomach ulcer, stomatitis, xerostomia, weight gain/loss

Genitourinary: Impotence, nocturia, pelvic pain, prostatic disorder, scrotal edema, urinary frequency, urinary incontinence, urinary retention, urinary tract disorder

Hematologic: Coagulation disorder, hemorrhage, neutropenia, pancytopenia, polycythemia, prothrombin time increased, thromboplastin time increased

Hepatic: Alkaline phosphatase increased, bilirubinemia, cholangitis, cholestatic jaundice, GGT increased, hepatitis, jaundice, liver damage, transaminases increased

Local: Abscess

Neuromuscular & skeletal: Arthralgia, hypertonia, joint disorder, leg cramps, myalgia, myasthenia, neck pain, neuropathy, osteoporosis

Ocular: Amblyopia, cataract, conjunctivitis, eye hemorrhage, lacrimation disorder, vision abnormal

Otic: Deafness, ear disorder, ear pain, tinnitus

Renal: Albuminuria, creatinine increased, dysuria, hematuria, hydronephrosis, oliguria, pyelonephritis, renal failure, renal tubular necrosis

Respiratory: Apnea, asthma, atelectasis, bronchitis, epistaxis, hemoptysis, hiccup, hyperventilation, hypoxia, respiratory acidosis, pharyngitis, pneumonia, pneumothorax, pulmonary edema, pulmonary hypertension, respiratory moniliasis, rhinitis, sputum increased, voice alteration

Miscellaneous: *Candida* (mucocutaneous 16% to 18%), CMV viremia/syndrome (12% to 14%), CMV tissue invasive disease (6% to 12%), herpes zoster cutaneous disease (4% to 10%), cyst, diaphoresis, flu-like syndrome, healing abnormal, hernia, ileus infection, neoplasm, peritonitis, thirst

Pharmacodynamics/Kinetics

Onset of Action Peak effect: Correlation of toxicity or efficacy is still being developed, however, one study indicated that 12-hour AUCs >40 mcg/mL/hour were correlated with efficacy and decreased episodes of rejection

Available Dosage Forms

Capsule, Oral:
CellCept: 250 mg
Generic: 250 mg

Solution Reconstituted, Intravenous:
CellCept Intravenous: 500 mg (1 ea)

Suspension Reconstituted, Oral:
CellCept: 200 mg/mL (160 mL)

Tablet, Oral:
CellCept: 500 mg
Generic: 500 mg

Tablet Delayed Release, Oral:
Myfortic: 180 mg, 360 mg
Generic: 180 mg, 360 mg

General Dosage Range Dosage adjustment recommended in patient with renal impairment and who develop toxicities

I.V.: CellCept: *Adults:* 1-1.5 g twice daily

Oral:
Cellcept:
Infants ≥3 months and Children (suspension): 600 mg/m²/dose twice daily (maximum: 1 g twice daily)
Children and Adolescents with BSA 1.25-1.5 m² (capsule): 750 mg twice daily
Children and Adolescents with BSA >1.5 m² (capsule or tablet): 1 g twice daily
Adults: 1-1.5 g twice daily
Myfortic:
Children ≥5 years and Adolescents with BSA 1.19-1.58 m²: 400 mg/m² twice daily **or** 540 mg twice daily (maximum: 1080 mg daily)

Children ≥5 years and Adolescents with BSA >1.58 m²: 400 mg/m² twice daily **or** 720 mg twice daily (maximum: 1440 mg daily)
Adults: 720 mg twice daily

Administration

I.V. Intravenous solutions should be given over at least 2 hours. Do not administer intravenous solution by rapid or bolus injection.

Hazardous agent; use appropriate precautions for handling and disposal (NIOSH, 2012).

Injectable Detail Reconstituted solution: pH 2.4-4.1

Oral Oral dosage formulations (tablet, capsule, suspension) should be administered on an empty stomach (1 hour before or 2 hours after meals) to avoid variability in MPA absorption. The oral solution may be administered via a nasogastric tube (minimum 8 French, 1.7 mm interior diameter); oral suspension should not be mixed with other medications. Delayed release tablets should not be crushed, cut, or chewed. Cellcept may be administered with food in stable renal transplant patients when necessary. If a dose is missed, administer as soon as it is remembered. If it is close to the next scheduled dose, skip the missed dose and resume at next regularly scheduled time; do not double a dose to make up for a missed dose.

Hazardous agent; use appropriate precautions for handling and disposal (NIOSH, 2012).

Preparation for Administration Hazardous agent; use appropriate precautions for handling and disposal (NIOSH, 2012).

Oral suspension: Should be constituted prior to dispensing to the patient and **not** mixed with any other medication. Add 47 mL of water to the bottle and shake well for ~1 minute. Add another 47 mL of water to the bottle and shake well for an additional minute. Final concentration is 200 mg/mL of mycophenolate mofetil.

I.V.: Reconstitute the contents of each vial with 14 mL of 5% dextrose injection; dilute the contents of a vial with 5% dextrose in water to a final concentration of 6 mg mycophenolate mofetil per mL.

Note: Vial is vacuum-sealed; if a lack of vacuum is noted during preparation, the vial should not be used.

Storage/Stability

Capsules: Store at 25°C (77°F); excursions permitted to 15°C to 30°C (59°F to 86°F).

Tablets: Store at 25°C (77°F); excursions permitted to 15°C to 30°C (59°F to 86°F). Protect from moisture and light.

Oral suspension: Store powder for oral suspension at 25°C (77°F); excursions permitted to 15°C to 30°C (59°F to 86°F). Once reconstituted, the oral solution may be stored at room temperature or under refrigeration. Do not freeze. The mixed suspension is stable for 60 days.

Injection: Store intact vials and diluted solutions at 25°C (77°F); excursions permitted to 15°C to 30°C (59°F to 86°F). Begin infusion within 4 hours of reconstitution.

Nursing Actions

Physical Assessment Monitor blood pressure periodically while receiving this medication. Assess for peripheral edema and other signs of fluid retention. Patients with diabetes should monitor glucose levels closely (this medication may alter glucose levels). Monitor for signs of opportunistic infection (eg, persistent fever, malaise, sore throat, unusual bleeding or bruising). Patient is at risk for lymphoproliferative disease and certain other malignancies; monitor closely.

Patient Education

- Discuss specific use of drug and side effects with patient as it relates to treatment. (HCAHPS: During this hospital stay, were you given any medicine that you had not taken before? Before giving you any new medicine, how often did hospital staff tell you what the medicine was for? How often did hospital staff describe possible side effects in a way you could understand?)
- Patient may experience hypertension, headache, nausea, anemia, leukopenia, thrombocytopenia, diarrhea, or edema. Have patient report immediately to prescriber signs of infection, dyspnea, tachycardia, significant change in balance, illogical thinking, ecchymosis, bleeding, severe skin irritation, considerable weight loss, significant asthenia, urinary retention, pregnancy, or rash (HCAHPS).
- Educate patient about signs of a significant reaction (eg, wheezing; chest tightness; fever; itching; bad cough; blue skin color; seizures; or swelling of face, lips, tongue, or throat). **Note:** This is not a comprehensive list of all side effects. Patient should consult prescriber for additional questions.

Intended Use and Disclaimer: Should not be printed and given to patients. This information is intended to serve as a concise initial reference for healthcare professionals to use when discussing medications with a patient. You must ultimately rely on your own discretion, experience and judgment in diagnosing, treating and advising patients.

Dietary Considerations Oral dosage formulations should be taken on an empty stomach to avoid variability in MPA absorption. However, in stable renal transplant patients, Cellcept may be administered with food if necessary. Some products may contain phenylalanine.

Related Information
Oral Medications That Should Not Be Crushed o Altered *on page 1712*

Nabilone (NA bi lone)

Brand Names: U.S. Cesamet
Pharmacologic Category Antiemetic
Pregnancy Risk Factor C
Lactation Excretion in breast milk unknown/no recommended
Use Treatment of refractory nausea and vomiting associated with cancer chemotherapy
Controlled Substance C-II
Available Dosage Forms
Capsule, Oral:
Cesamet: 1 mg
General Dosage Range Oral: *Adults:* 1-2 mg twice daily (maximum: 6 mg daily)
Administration
Oral Initial dose should be given 1-3 hours before chemotherapy.
Nursing Actions
Physical Assessment Monitor for CNS changes and psychotic reactions (can persist for 3 days following discontinuation); this medicine may have properties similar to marijuana and has the potential for abuse or dependence.

Patient Education

- Discuss specific use of drug and side effects with patient as it relates to treatment. (HCAHPS During this hospital stay, were you given any medicine that you had not taken before? Before giving you any new medicine, how often did hospital staff tell you what the medicine was for? How often did hospital staff describe possible side effects in a way you could understand?)
- Patient may experience presyncope, fatigue, blurred vision, illogical thinking, hypotension, dizziness, xerostomia, asthenia, imbalance, or headache. Have patient report immediately to prescriber depression, nervousness, emotional instability, anxiety, or rash (HCAHPS).
- Educate patient about signs of a significant reaction (eg, wheezing; chest tightness; fever; itching; bad cough; blue skin color; seizures; or swelling of face, lips, tongue, or throat). **Note:** This is not a comprehensive list of all side effects. Patient should consult prescriber for additional questions.

Intended Use and Disclaimer: Should not be printed and given to patients. This information is intended to serve as a concise initial reference for healthcare professionals to use when discussing medications with a patient. You must ultimately rely on your own discretion, experience and judgment in diagnosing, treating and advising patients.

Nabumetone (na BYOO me tone)

Index Terms Relafen

Pharmacologic Category Nonsteroidal Anti-inflammatory Drug (NSAID), Oral

Medication Safety Issues

BEERS Criteria medication:

This drug may be potentially inappropriate for use in geriatric patients (Quality of evidence - moderate; Strength of recommendation - strong).

Medication Guide Available Yes

Pregnancy Risk Factor C

Lactation Excretion in breast milk unknown/not recommended

Breast-Feeding Considerations It is not known if nabumetone or 6MNA are excreted into breast milk. Breast-feeding is not recommended by the manufacturer.

Use Management of osteoarthritis and rheumatoid arthritis

Unlabeled Use Moderate pain

Mechanism of Action/Effect Reversibly inhibits cyclooxygenase-1 and 2 (COX-1 and 2) enzymes, which results in decreased formation of prostaglandin precursors; has antipyretic, analgesic, and anti-inflammatory properties

Contraindications Hypersensitivity to nabumetone, aspirin, other NSAIDs, or any component of the formulation; perioperative pain in the setting of coronary artery bypass graft (CABG) surgery

Warnings/Precautions [U.S. Boxed Warning]: NSAIDs are associated with an increased risk of adverse cardiovascular thrombotic events, including MI and stroke. Risk may be increased with duration of use or pre-existing cardiovascular risk factors or disease. Carefully evaluate individual cardiovascular risk profiles prior to prescribing. May cause new-onset hypertension or worsening of existing hypertension. Use caution with fluid retention. Avoid use in heart failure (ACCF/AHA [Yancy, 2013]). Concurrent administration of ibuprofen, and potentially other nonselective NSAIDs, may interfere with aspirin's cardioprotective effect. **[U.S. Boxed Warning]: Use is contraindicated for treatment of perioperative pain in the setting of coronary artery bypass graft (CABG) surgery.** Risk of MI and stroke may be increased with use following CABG surgery.

Platelet adhesion and aggregation may be decreased; may prolong bleeding time; patients with coagulation disorders or who are receiving anticoagulants should be monitored closely. Anemia may occur; patients on long-term NSAID therapy should be monitored for anemia. Rarely, NSAID use may cause severe blood dyscrasias (eg, agranulocytosis, aplastic anemia, thrombocytopenia).

NSAID use may compromise existing renal function; dose-dependent decreases in prostaglandin synthesis may result from NSAID use, reducing renal blood flow which may cause renal decompensation. NSAID use may increase the risk for hyperkalemia. Patients with impaired renal function, dehydration, heart failure, liver dysfunction, those taking diuretics, and ACE inhibitors, and the elderly are at greater risk of renal toxicity and hyperkalemia. Rehydrate patient before starting therapy; monitor renal function closely. Not recommended for use in patients with advanced renal disease. Long-term NSAID use may result in renal papillary necrosis.

[U.S. Boxed Warning]: NSAIDs may increase risk of gastrointestinal irritation, inflammation, ulceration, bleeding, and perforation. These events may occur at any time during therapy and without warning. Use caution with a history of GI disease (bleeding or ulcers), concurrent therapy with aspirin, anticoagulants and/or corticosteroids, smoking, use of alcohol, the elderly or debilitated patients. When used concomitantly with aspirin, a substantial increase in the risk of gastrointestinal complications (eg, ulcer) occurs; concomitant gastroprotective therapy (eg, proton pump inhibitors) is recommended (Bhatt, 2008).

Use the lowest effective dose for the shortest duration of time, consistent with individual patient goals, to reduce risk of cardiovascular or GI adverse events. Alternate therapies should be considered for patients at high risk.

NSAIDs may cause serious skin adverse events including exfoliative dermatitis, Stevens-Johnson syndrome (SJS) and toxic epidermal necrolysis (TEN); discontinue use at first sign of skin rash or hypersensitivity. Anaphylactoid reactions may occur, even without prior exposure; patients with "aspirin triad" (bronchial asthma, aspirin intolerance, rhinitis) may be at increased risk. Do not use in patients who experience bronchospasm, asthma, rhinitis, or urticaria with NSAID or aspirin therapy. Use caution in other forms of asthma.

Use with caution in patients with decreased hepatic function. Closely monitor patients with any abnormal LFT. Severe hepatic reactions (eg, fulminant hepatitis, liver failure) have occurred with NSAID use, rarely; discontinue if signs or symptoms of liver disease develop, or if systemic manifestations occur.

NSAIDS may cause drowsiness, dizziness, blurred vision and other neurologic effects which may impair physical or mental abilities; patients must be cautioned about performing tasks which require mental alertness (eg, operating machinery or driving). Discontinue use with blurred or diminished vision and perform ophthalmologic exam. Monitor vision with long-term therapy.

In the elderly, avoid chronic use (unless alternative agents ineffective and patient can receive ▶

concomitant gastroprotective agent); nonselective oral NSAID use is associated with an increased risk of GI bleeding and peptic ulcer disease in older adults in high risk category (eg, >75 years or age or receiving concomitant oral/parenteral corticosteroids, anticoagulants, or antiplatelet agents) (Beers Criteria).

Withhold for at least 4-6 half-lives prior to surgical or dental procedures. May cause photosensitivity reactions.

Drug Interactions

Avoid Concomitant Use

Avoid concomitant use of Nabumetone with any of the following: Floctafenine; Ketorolac (Nasal); Ketorolac (Systemic); NSAID (COX-2 Inhibitor); Omacetaxine; Urokinase

Decreased Effect

Nabumetone may decrease the levels/effects of: ACE Inhibitors; Agents with Antiplatelet Properties; Aliskiren; Angiotensin II Receptor Blockers; Beta-Blockers; Eplerenone; HydrALAZINE; Loop Diuretics; Potassium-Sparing Diuretics; Prostaglandins (Ophthalmic); Salicylates; Selective Serotonin Reuptake Inhibitors; Thiazide Diuretics

The levels/effects of Nabumetone may be decreased by: Bile Acid Sequestrants; Nonsteroidal Anti-Inflammatory Agents; Salicylates

Increased Effect/Toxicity

Nabumetone may increase the levels/effects of: 5-ASA Derivatives; Agents with Antiplatelet Properties; Aliskiren; Aminoglycosides; Anticoagulants; Bisphosphonate Derivatives; Collagenase (Systemic); CycloSPORINE (Systemic); Dabigatran Etexilate; Deferasirox; Desmopressin; Digoxin; Eplerenone; Haloperidol; Ibritumomab; Lithium; Methotrexate; Nonsteroidal Anti-Inflammatory Agents; NSAID (COX-2 Inhibitor); Omacetaxine; PEMEtrexed; Porfimer; Potassium-Sparing Diuretics; PRALAtrexate; Quinolone Antibiotics; Rivaroxaban; Salicylates; Tenofovir; Thrombolytic Agents; Tositumomab and Iodine I 131 Tositumomab; Urokinase; Vancomycin; Vitamin K Antagonists

The levels/effects of Nabumetone may be increased by: ACE Inhibitors; Angiotensin II Receptor Blockers; Antidepressants (Tricyclic, Tertiary Amine); Corticosteroids (Systemic); CycloSPORINE (Systemic); Dasatinib; Floctafenine; Glucosamine; Herbs (Anticoagulant/Antiplatelet Properties); Ibrutinib; Ketorolac (Nasal); Ketorolac (Systemic); Multivitamins/Fluoride (with ADE); Multivitamins/Minerals (with ADEK, Folate, Iron); Multivitamins/Minerals (with AE, No Iron); Nonsteroidal Anti-Inflammatory Agents; Omega-3 Fatty Acids; Pentosan Polysulfate Sodium; Pentoxifylline; Probenecid; Prostacyclin Analogues; Selective Serotonin Reuptake Inhibitors; Serotonin/Norepinephrine Reuptake Inhibitors; Sodium Phosphates; Tipranavir; Treprostinil; Vitamin E

Nutritional/Ethanol Interactions

Ethanol: Avoid ethanol (may enhance gastric mucosal irritation).

Food: Nabumetone peak serum concentrations may be increased if taken with food or dairy products.

Herb/Nutraceutical: Avoid alfalfa, anise, bilberry, bladderwrack, bromelain, cat's claw, celery, chamomile, coleus, cordyceps, dong quai, evening primrose, fenugreek, feverfew, garlic, ginger, ginkgo biloba, ginseng (American, Panax, Siberian), grapeseed, green tea, guggul, horse chestnut seed, horseradish, licorice, prickly ash, red clover, reishi, SAMe (S-adenosylmethionine), sweet clover, turmeric, white willow (all have additional antiplatelet activity).

Adverse Reactions

>10%: Gastrointestinal: Diarrhea (14%), dyspepsia (13%), abdominal pain (12%)

1% to 10%:

Cardiovascular: Edema (3% to 9%)

Central nervous system: Dizziness (3% to 9%), headache (3% to 9%), fatigue (1% to 3%), insomnia (1% to 3%), nervousness (1% to 3%), somnolence (1% to 3%)

Dermatologic: Pruritus (3% to 9%), rash (3% to 9%)

Gastrointestinal: Constipation (3% to 9%), flatulence (3% to 9%), guaiac positive (3% to 9%), nausea (3% to 9%), gastritis (1% to 3%), stomatitis (1% to 3%), vomiting (1% to 3%), xerostomia (1% to 3%)

Otic: Tinnitus

Miscellaneous: Diaphoresis (1% to 3%)

Pharmacodynamics/Kinetics

Onset of Action Several days

Available Dosage Forms

Tablet, Oral:

Generic: 500 mg, 750 mg

General Dosage Range Dosage adjustment recommended in patients with renal impairment

Oral: *Adults:* 1000 mg/day in 1-2 divided doses (maximum: 2000 mg/day)

Nursing Actions

Physical Assessment Monitor blood pressure at the beginning of therapy and periodically during use. Monitor for GI effects, hepatotoxicity, and ototoxicity at beginning of therapy and periodically throughout. Schedule ophthalmic evaluations for patients who develop eye complaints during long-term NSAID therapy.

Patient Education

- Discuss specific use of drug and side effects with patient as it relates to treatment. (HCAHPS: During this hospital stay, were you given any medicine that you had not taken before? Before giving you any new medicine, how often did hospital staff tell you what the medicine was for? How often did hospital staff describe possible side effects in a way you could understand?)

- Patient may experience headache, dyspepsia, pyrosis, nausea, constipation, diarrhea, or edema. Have patient report immediately to prescriber angina, strength differences from one side to another, significant weight gain, melena, hematuria, ecchymosis, or rash (HCAHPS).
- Educate patient about signs of a significant reaction (eg, wheezing; chest tightness; fever; itching; bad cough; blue skin color; seizures; or swelling of face, lips, tongue, or throat). **Note:** This is not a comprehensive list of all side effects. Patient should consult prescriber for additional questions.

Intended Use and Disclaimer: Should not be printed and given to patients. This information is intended to serve as a concise initial reference for healthcare professionals to use when discussing medications with a patient. You must ultimately rely on your own discretion, experience and judgment in diagnosing, treating and advising patients.

Nadolol (NAY doe lol)

Brand Names: U.S. Corgard
Pharmacologic Category Antianginal Agent; Antihypertensive; Beta-Blocker, Nonselective
Medication Safety Issues
Sound-alike/look-alike issues:
Corgard® may be confused with Cognex®, Coreg®
International issues:
Nadolol may be confused with Mandol brand name for cefamandole [Belgium, Netherlands, New Zealand, Russia]
Pregnancy Risk Factor C
Lactation Enters breast milk/use caution consider risk:benefit
Use Treatment of hypertension and angina pectoris
Unlabeled Use Migraine headache prophylaxis; primary and secondary prophylaxis of variceal hemorrhage; management of thyrotoxicosis
Available Dosage Forms
Tablet, Oral:
Corgard: 20 mg, 40 mg, 80 mg
Generic: 20 mg, 40 mg, 80 mg
General Dosage Range Dosage adjustment recommended in patients with renal impairment
Oral:
Adults: Initial: 40 mg once daily; Maintenance: 40-320 mg once daily
Elderly: Initial: 20 mg once daily; Maintenance: 20-240 mg once daily
Administration
Oral May be administered without regard to meals.
Nursing Actions
Physical Assessment Assess blood pressure and heart rate prior to and following first dose, any change in dosage, and periodically thereafter. Monitor or advise patient to monitor weight, fluid

balance (I & O), and signs of CHF (edema, new cough or dyspnea, unresolved fatigue). Monitor serum glucose levels of patients with diabetes since beta-blockers may alter glucose tolerance.
Patient Education
- Discuss specific use of drug and side effects with patient as it relates to treatment. (HCAHPS: During this hospital stay, were you given any medicine that you had not taken before? Before giving you any new medicine, how often did hospital staff tell you what the medicine was for? How often did hospital staff describe possible side effects in a way you could understand?)
- Patient may experience presyncope, fatigue, blurred vision, illogical thinking, dizziness, or impotence. Have patient report immediately to prescriber dyspnea, significant weight gain, severe asthenia, or rash (HCAHPS).
- Educate patient about signs of a significant reaction (eg, wheezing; chest tightness; fever; itching; bad cough; blue skin color; seizures; or swelling of face, lips, tongue, or throat). **Note:** This is not a comprehensive list of all side effects. Patient should consult prescriber for additional questions.

Intended Use and Disclaimer: Should not be printed and given to patients. This information is intended to serve as a concise initial reference for healthcare professionals to use when discussing medications with a patient. You must ultimately rely on your own discretion, experience and judgment in diagnosing, treating and advising patients.

Nafarelin (naf a REL in)

Brand Names: U.S. Synarel
Index Terms Nafarelin Acetate
Pharmacologic Category Gonadotropin Releasing Hormone Agonist
Medication Safety Issues
Sound-alike/look-alike issues:
Nafarelin may be confused with Anafranil®, enalapril
Pregnancy Risk Factor X
Lactation Excretion in breast milk unknown/contraindicated
Use Treatment of endometriosis, including pain and reduction of lesions; treatment of central precocious puberty (CPP; gonadotropin-dependent precocious puberty) in children of both sexes
Available Dosage Forms
Solution, Nasal:
Synarel: 2 mg/mL (8 mL)
General Dosage Range Nasal:
Children: 2 sprays (400 mcg) into each nostril twice daily; may increase to 3 sprays (600 mcg) into alternating nostrils 3 times/day
Adults: 1 spray (200 mcg) in 1-2 nostrils twice daily

◄ **Administration**

Inhalation Nasal spray: Do not use topical nasal decongestant for at least 2 hours after nafarelin use. Allow ~30 seconds to elapse between sprays. Sneezing during or immediately after dosing should be avoided (may decrease drug absorption).

Hazardous agent; use appropriate precautions for handling and disposal (NIOSH, 2012).

Nursing Actions

Physical Assessment For treatment of precocious puberty. Teach patient or caregiver correct timing and administration of nasal spray.

Patient Education

- Discuss specific use of drug and side effects with patient as it relates to treatment. (HCAHPS: During this hospital stay, were you given any medicine that you had not taken before? Before giving you any new medicine, how often did hospital staff tell you what the medicine was for? How often did hospital staff describe possible side effects in a way you could understand?)
- Patient may experience headache, flushing, acne, vaginal irritation, rhinitis, osteopenia, emotional instability, changes in mood, impotence, or ovarian cysts. Have patient report immediately to prescriber angina, severe nausea, sudden vision changes, eye pain, eye irritation, illogical thinking, pregnancy, polyuria, polydipsia, weight loss, menstruation, or rash (HCAHPS).
- Educate patient about signs of a significant reaction (eg, wheezing; chest tightness; fever; itching; bad cough; blue skin color; seizures; or swelling of face, lips, tongue, or throat). **Note:** This is not a comprehensive list of all side effects. Patient should consult prescriber for additional questions.

Intended Use and Disclaimer: Should not be printed and given to patients. This information is intended to serve as a concise initial reference for healthcare professionals to use when discussing medications with a patient. You must ultimately rely on your own discretion, experience and judgment in diagnosing, treating and advising patients.

Nafcillin (naf SIL in)

Brand Names: U.S. Nallpen in Dextrose

Index Terms Ethoxynaphthamido Penicillin Sodium; Nafcillin Sodium; Nallpen; Sodium Nafcillin

Pharmacologic Category Antibiotic, Penicillin

Pregnancy Risk Factor B

Lactation Enters breast milk/use caution

Use Treatment of infections such as osteomyelitis, bacteremia, septicemia, endocarditis, and CNS infections caused by susceptible strains of *Staphylococcus* species

Available Dosage Forms

Solution, Intravenous:
Nallpen in Dextrose: 1 g/50 mL (50 mL); 2 g/100 mL (100 mL)

Solution Reconstituted, Injection:
Generic: 1 g (1 ea); 2 g (1 ea); 10 g (1 ea)

Solution Reconstituted, Injection [preservative free]:
Generic: 1 g (1 ea); 2 g (1 ea); 10 g (1 ea)

Solution Reconstituted, Intravenous:
Generic: 1 g (1 ea); 2 g (1 ea)

General Dosage Range I.M., I.V.: *Children and Adults:* Dosage varies greatly depending on indication

Administration

I.M. Administer as a deep intragluteal injection; rotate injection sites.

I.V.
Infuse over 30-60 minutes. Vesicant; ensure proper needle or catheter placement prior to and during I.V. infusion. Avoid extravasation.

Extravasation management: If extravasation occurs, stop infusion immediately and disconnect (leave needle/cannula in place); gently aspirate extravasated solution (do **NOT** flush the line); initiate hyaluronidase antidote; remove needle/cannula; apply dry cold compresses (Hurst, 2004); elevate extremity.

Hyaluronidase: Intradermal or SubQ: Inject a total of 1 mL (15 units/mL) as five separate 0.2 mL injections (using a 25-gauge needle) into area of extravasation at the leading edge in a clockwise manner (MacCara, 1983; Zenk, 1981a).

Injectable Detail
pH: 6-8.5 (solution in premixed bag for infusion)

Nursing Actions

Physical Assessment Assess results of culture and sensitivity tests and allergy history prior to starting therapy. Injection site must be monitored closely to prevent extravasation. Monitor for hypersensitivity and opportunistic infection (eg, fever, chills, unhealed sores, white plaques in mouth or vagina, purulent vaginal discharge).

Patient Education

- Discuss specific use of drug and side effects with patient as it relates to treatment. (HCAHPS: During this hospital stay, were you given any medicine that you had not taken before? Before giving you any new medicine, how often did hospital staff tell you what the medicine was for? How often did hospital staff describe possible side effects in a way you could understand?)
- Patient may experience nausea, diarrhea, or vaginal yeast infection. Have patient report immediately to prescriber ecchymosis, bleeding, or rash (HCAHPS).
- Educate patient about signs of a significant reaction (eg, wheezing; chest tightness; fever; itching; bad cough; blue skin color; seizures; or

swelling of face, lips, tongue, or throat). **Note:** This is not a comprehensive list of all side effects. Patient should consult prescriber for additional questions.

Intended Use and Disclaimer: Should not be printed and given to patients. This information is intended to serve as a concise initial reference for healthcare professionals to use when discussing medications with a patient. You must ultimately rely on your own discretion, experience and judgment in diagnosing, treating and advising patients.

Related Information

Management of Drug Extravasations *on page 1700*

Nalbuphine (NAL byoo feen)

Index Terms Nalbuphine Hydrochloride; Nubain
Pharmacologic Category Analgesic, Opioid; Analgesic, Opioid Partial Agonist
Medication Safety Issues
Sound-alike/look-alike issues:
Nalbuphine may be confused with naloxone
Nubain may be confused with Navane®, Nebcin
High alert medication:
The Institute for Safe Medication Practices (ISMP) includes this medication among its list of drug classes which have a heightened risk of causing significant patient harm when used in error.

Pregnancy Risk Factor C
Lactation Enters breast milk/use caution
Breast-Feeding Considerations Small amounts (<1% of maternal dose) of nalbuphine are excreted in breast milk. The manufacturer recommends that caution be exercised when administering nalbuphine to nursing women.

Parenteral opioids used during labor have the potential to interfere with a newborns natural reflex to nurse within the first few hours after birth. If nalbuphine is administered to a nursing woman, it is recommended to monitor both the mother and baby for psychotomimetic reactions. Nursing infants exposed to large doses of opioids should also be monitored for apnea and sedation (Montgomery, 2012).

Use Relief of moderate-to-severe pain; preoperative analgesia, postoperative and surgical anesthesia, and obstetrical analgesia during labor and delivery
Unlabeled Use Opioid-induced pruritus
Mechanism of Action/Effect Binds to opiate receptors in the CNS, causing inhibition of ascending pain pathways, altering the perception of and response to pain; produces generalized CNS depression
Contraindications Hypersensitivity to nalbuphine or any component of the formulation
Warnings/Precautions Use caution in CNS depression. Sedation and psychomotor impairment

are likely, and are additive with other CNS depressants or ethanol. May cause respiratory depression. Ambulatory patients must be cautioned about performing tasks which require mental alertness (eg, operating machinery or driving). Potentially significant drug interactions may exist, requiring dose or frequency adjustment, additional monitoring, and/or selection of alternative therapy. Effects may be potentiated when used with other sedative drugs or ethanol. Use with caution in patients with recent myocardial infarction, biliary tract impairment, pancreatitis, morbid obesity, thyroid dysfunction, head trauma, or increased intracranial pressure. Avoid use in patients with CNS depression or coma as these patients are susceptible to intracranial effects of CO_2 retention. Use caution in patients with prostatic hyperplasia and/or urinary stricture, adrenal insufficiency, decreased hepatic or renal function. Use with caution in patients with pre-existing respiratory compromise (hypoxia and/or hypercapnia), COPD or other obstructive pulmonary disease; critical respiratory depression may occur, even at therapeutic dosages. May cause hypotension; use with caution in patients with hypovolemia, cardiovascular disease (including acute MI), or drugs which may exaggerate hypotensive effects (including phenothiazines or general anesthetics). May obscure diagnosis or clinical course of patients with acute abdominal conditions. May result in tolerance and/or drug dependence with chronic use; use with caution in patients with a history of drug dependence. Abrupt discontinuation following prolonged use may lead to withdrawal symptoms. May precipitate withdrawal symptoms in patients following prolonged therapy with mu opioid agonists.

Use with caution in pregnancy (close neonatal monitoring required when used in labor and delivery). After chronic maternal exposure to opioids, neonatal withdrawal syndrome may occur in the newborn; monitor neonate closely. Signs and symptoms include irritability, hyperactivity and abnormal sleep pattern, high pitched cry, tremor, vomiting, diarrhea and failure to gain weight. Onset, duration and severity depend on the drug used, duration of use, maternal dose, and rate of drug elimination by the newborn. Opioid withdrawal syndrome in the neonate, unlike in adults, may be life-threatening and should be treated according to protocols developed by neonatology experts. Use with caution in the elderly and debilitated patients; may be more sensitive to adverse effects. Safety and efficacy in children have not been established.
Drug Interactions
Avoid Concomitant Use
Avoid concomitant use of Nalbuphine with any of the following: Azelastine (Nasal); Paraldehyde; Thalidomide

◀ **Decreased Effect**

Nalbuphine may decrease the levels/effects of:
Analgesics (Opioid); Pegvisomant

The levels/effects of Nalbuphine may be decreased by: Ammonium Chloride; Mixed Agonist / Antagonist Opioids

Increased Effect/Toxicity

Nalbuphine may increase the levels/effects of:
Alcohol (Ethyl); Alvimopan; Azelastine (Nasal); CNS Depressants; Desmopressin; Diuretics; Metyrosine; Mirtazapine; Paraldehyde; Pramipexole; ROPINIRole; Rotigotine; Selective Serotonin Reuptake Inhibitors; Thalidomide; Zolpidem

The levels/effects of Nalbuphine may be increased by: Amphetamines; Anticholinergics; Antipsychotic Agents (Phenothiazines); Brimonidine (Topical); Cannabinoids; Doxylamine; Droperidol; HydrOXYzine; Magnesium Sulfate; Perampanel; Sodium Oxybate; Succinylcholine

Nutritional/Ethanol Interactions

Ethanol: May increase CNS depression; monitor for increased effects with coadministration. Caution patients about effects.

Herb/Nutraceutical: Avoid valerian, St John's wort, kava kava, gotu kola (may increase CNS depression).

Adverse Reactions

>10%: Central nervous system: Sedation (36%)

1% to 10%:

Central nervous system: Dizziness (5%), headache (3%)

Gastrointestinal: Nausea/vomiting (6%), xerostomia (4%)

Miscellaneous: Clamminess (9%)

Pharmacodynamics/Kinetics

Onset of Action Peak effect: SubQ, I.M.: <15 minutes; I.V.: 2-3 minutes

Available Dosage Forms

Solution, Injection:

Generic: 10 mg/mL (1 mL, 10 mL); 20 mg/mL (1 mL, 10 mL)

General Dosage Range

I.M., SubQ: *Adults:* 10 mg/70 kg every 3-6 hours (maximum: 20 mg/dose; 160 mg/day)

I.V.: *Adults:* 10 mg/70 kg every 3-6 hours (maximum: 20 mg/dose; 160 mg/day) **or** 0.3-3 mg/kg over 10-15 minutes, then 0.25-0.5 mg/kg as required for anesthesia **or** 2.5-5 mg (1-2 doses)

Administration

Injectable Detail pH: 3.5-3.7 (adjusted)

Storage/Stability Store at room temperature of 15°C to 30°C (59°F to 86°F). Protect from light.

Nursing Actions

Physical Assessment Monitor for effectiveness of pain relief. Monitor blood pressure, CNS and respiratory status, and degree of sedation at beginning of therapy and periodically thereafter. For inpatients, implement safety measures (eg, side rails up, call light within reach, instructions to call for assistance). Assess patient's physical and/or psychological dependence. Discontinue slowly after prolonged use.

Patient Education

- Discuss specific use of drug and side effects with patient as it relates to treatment. (HCAHPS: During this hospital stay, were you given any medicine that you had not taken before? Before giving you any new medicine, how often did hospital staff tell you what the medicine was for? How often did hospital staff describe possible side effects in a way you could understand?)
- Patient may experience presyncope, fatigue, blurred vision, illogical thinking, dizziness, nausea, or constipation. Have patient report immediately to prescriber syncope, dyspnea, poor pain control, asthenia, or rash (HCAHPS).
- Educate patient about signs of a significant reaction (eg, wheezing; chest tightness; fever; itching; bad cough; blue skin color; seizures; or swelling of face, lips, tongue, or throat). **Note:** This is not a comprehensive list of all side effects. Patient should consult prescriber for additional questions.

Intended Use and Disclaimer: Should not be printed and given to patients. This information is intended to serve as a concise initial reference for healthcare professionals to use when discussing medications with a patient. You must ultimately rely on your own discretion, experience and judgment in diagnosing, treating and advising patients.

Naloxone (nal OKS one)

Index Terms *N*-allylnoroxymorphine Hydrochloride; Naloxone Hydrochloride; Narcan

Pharmacologic Category Antidote; Opioid Antagonist

Medication Safety Issues

Sound-alike/look-alike issues:

Naloxone may be confused with Lanoxin®, nalbuphine, naltrexone

Narcan may be confused with Marcaine®, Norcuron®

International issues:

Narcan [multiple international markets] may be confused with Marcen brand name for ketazolam [Spain]

Pregnancy Risk Factor C

Lactation Excretion in breast milk unknown/use caution

Breast-Feeding Considerations It is not known if naloxone is excreted into breast milk, however, systemic absorption following oral administration is low (Smith, 2012) and any exposure of naloxone to a nursing infant would therefore be limited. Since naloxone is used for opioid reversal, the opioid concentrations in the milk of a breast-feeding mother and potential transfer of the opioid to the infant should be considered.

Use Complete or partial reversal of opioid drug effects, including respiratory depression; management of known or suspected opioid overdose; diagnosis of suspected opioid dependence or acute opioid overdose

Unlabeled Use Opioid-induced pruritus

Mechanism of Action/Effect Pure opioid antagonist that competes and displaces opioids at opioid receptor sites

Contraindications Hypersensitivity to naloxone or any component of the formulation

Warnings/Precautions Due to an association between naloxone and acute pulmonary edema, use with caution in patients with cardiovascular disease or in patients receiving medications with potential adverse cardiovascular effects (eg, hypotension, pulmonary edema, or arrhythmias). Administration of naloxone causes the release of catecholamines; may precipitate acute withdrawal or unmask pain in those who regularly take opioids. Excessive dosages should be avoided after use of opioids in surgery. Abrupt postoperative reversal may result in nausea, vomiting, sweating, tachycardia, hypertension, seizures, and other cardiovascular events (including pulmonary edema and arrhythmias). May precipitate withdrawal symptoms in patients addicted to opioids, including pain, hypertension, sweating, agitation, irritability; in neonates, symptoms may include shrill cry, failure to feed; carefully titrate dose to reverse hypoventilation; do not fully awaken patient or reverse analgesic effect (postoperative patient). Use caution in patients with history of seizures; avoid use in treatment of meperidine-induced seizures. Recurrence of respiratory depression is possible if the opioid involved is long-acting; observe patients until there is no reasonable risk of recurrent respiratory depression.

To prevent overdose deaths, there are initiatives to dispense naloxone for self- or buddy-administration to patients at risk of opioid overdose (eg, recipients of high-dose opioids, suspected or confirmed history of illicit opioid use) and individuals likely to be present in an overdose situation (eg, family members of illicit drug users) (Albert, 2011; Bennett, 2011). Needleless administration via nebulization and the intranasal route by first responders and bystanders has also been described (Doe-Simkins, 2009; Weber, 2012). Needleless administration provides an alternative route of administration in patients with venous scarring due to illicit drug use (eg, heroin). There is a low incidence of death following naloxone reversal of opioid toxicity in patients who refuse transport to a healthcare facility (Wampler, 2011).

Drug Interactions

Avoid Concomitant Use There are no known interactions where it is recommended to avoid concomitant use.

Decreased Effect There are no known significant interactions involving a decrease in effect.

Increased Effect/Toxicity There are no known significant interactions involving an increase in effect.

Adverse Reactions Adverse reactions are related to reversing dependency and precipitating withdrawal. Withdrawal symptoms are the result of sympathetic excess. Adverse events occur secondarily to reversal (withdrawal) of opioid analgesia and sedation.

Cardiovascular: Cardiac arrest, fever, flushing, hypertension, hypotension, tachycardia, ventricular fibrillation ventricular tachycardia

Central nervous system: Agitation, coma, crying (excessive [neonates]), encephalopathy, hallucination, irritability, nervousness, restlessness, seizure (neonates), tremulousness

Gastrointestinal: Abdominal cramps, diarrhea, nausea, vomiting

Local: Injection site reaction

Neuromuscular & skeletal: Ache, hyperreflexia (neonates), paresthesia, piloerection, tremor, weakness

Respiratory: Dyspnea, hypoxia, pulmonary edema, respiratory depression, rhinorrhea, sneezing

Miscellaneous: Diaphoresis, hot flashes, shivering, yawning

Pharmacodynamics/Kinetics

Onset of Action Endotracheal, I.M., SubQ: 2-5 minutes; Inhalation via nebulization: ~5 minutes (Mycyk, 2003); Intranasal: ~8-13 minutes (Kelley, 2005; Robertson, 2009); I.V.: ~2 minutes

Duration of Action Depending on route of administration, ~30-120 minutes; I.V. has a shorter duration of action than I.M. administration; since naloxone's action is shorter than that of most opioids, repeated doses are usually needed

Available Dosage Forms

Solution, Injection:
Generic: 0.4 mg/mL (1 mL, 10 mL)
Solution, Injection [preservative free]:
Generic: 1 mg/mL (2 mL)

General Dosage Range I.M., I.V., SubQ: *Adults:* 0.1-2 mg every 2-3 minutes as needed (maximum: 10 mg)

Administration

I.M. May administer I.M. if unable to obtain I.V. access.

I.V.

I.V. push: Administer over 30 seconds as undiluted preparation **or** administer as diluted preparation slow I.V. push by diluting 0.4 mg (1 mL) ampul with 9 mL of normal saline for a total volume of 10 mL to achieve a concentration of 0.04 mg/mL (APS, 2008)

I.V. continuous infusion: Dilute to 4 **mcg**/mL in D₅W or normal saline

Subcutaneous May administer SubQ if unable to obtain I.V. access

Inhalation

Inhalation via nebulization (unlabeled route): Dilute 2 mg of naloxone with 3 mL of normal saline and administer via nebulizer face mask (Mycyk, 2003; Weber, 2012).

Intranasal (unlabeled route): Administer total dose equally divided into each nostril using a mucosal atomizer device (MAD) (Kelly, 2005; Robertson, 2009; Vanden Hoek, 2010).

Endotracheal Endotracheal (unlabeled route): There is only anecdotal support for this route of administration. May require a slightly higher dose than used in other routes. Dilute to 1-2 mL with normal saline; flush with 5 mL of saline and then administer 5 ventilations.

Preparation for Administration

I.V. push: Dilute naloxone 0.4 mg (1 mL ampul) with 9 mL of NS for a total volume of 10 mL to achieve a concentration of 0.04 mg/mL (APS, 2008)

I.V. infusion: Dilute naloxone 2 mg in 500 mL of NS or D₅W to make a final concentration of 4 **mcg**/mL; use within 24 hours

Inhalation via nebulization (unlabeled route): Dilute 2 mg of naloxone with 3 mL of normal saline (Mycyk, 2003; Weber, 2012)

Storage/Stability Store at 20°C to 25°C (68°F to 77°F). Protect from light.

Nursing Actions

Physical Assessment Assess patient for opioid dependency. Monitor vital signs and cardiorespiratory status continuously during infusion; maintain patent airway.

Patient Education

• Discuss specific use of drug and side effects with patient as it relates to treatment. (HCAHPS: During this hospital stay, were you given any medicine that you had not taken before? Before giving you any new medicine, how often did hospital staff tell you what the medicine was for? How often did hospital staff describe possible side effects in a way you could understand?)

• Patient may experience nausea or injection site irritation. Have patient report immediately to prescriber signs of depression (ie, suicidal ideation, anxiety, emotional instability, illogical thinking), severe dizziness, syncope, hyperhidrosis, akathisia, tremors, flushing, angina, tachycardia, or arrhythmia (HCAHPS).

• Educate patient about signs of a significant reaction (eg, wheezing; chest tightness; fever; itching; bad cough; blue skin color; seizures; or swelling of face, lips, tongue, or throat). **Note:** This is not a comprehensive list of all side effects. Patient should consult prescriber for additional questions.

Intended Use and Disclaimer: Should not be printed and given to patients. This information is intended to serve as a concise initial reference for healthcare professionals to use when discussing medications with a patient. You must ultimately rely on your own discretion, experience and judgment in diagnosing, treating and advising patients.

Naltrexone (nal TREKS one)

Brand Names: U.S. ReVia; Vivitrol
Index Terms Naltrexone Hydrochloride
Pharmacologic Category Antidote; Opioid Antagonist
Medication Safety Issues
Sound-alike/look-alike issues:
Naltrexone may be confused with methylnaltrexone, naloxone
ReVia may be confused with Revatio
Administration issues:
Vivitrol: For intramuscular (I.M.) gluteal injection only
Medication Guide Available Yes
Pregnancy Risk Factor C
Lactation Enters breast milk/not recommended
Breast-Feeding Considerations Naltrexone is excreted into breast milk. Due to the potential for serious adverse reactions in the nursing infant, the manufacturer recommends a decision be made whether to discontinue nursing or to discontinue the drug, taking into account the importance of treatment to the mother.
Use
Alcohol dependence: Treatment of alcohol dependence.
Opioid dependence: For the blockade of the effects of exogenously administered opioids.
Mechanism of Action/Effect Naltrexone (a pure opioid antagonist) is a cyclopropyl derivative of oxymorphone similar in structure to naloxone and nalorphine (a morphine derivative); it acts as a competitive antagonist at opioid receptor sites, showing the highest affinity for mu receptors.
Contraindications Hypersensitivity to naltrexone or any component of the formulation; opioid dependence or current use of opioid analgesics (including partial opioid agonists); acute opioid withdrawal; failure to pass naloxone challenge or positive urine screen for opioids
Warnings/Precautions Dose-related hepatocellular injury is possible; the margin of separation between the apparent safe and hepatotoxic doses appears to be ≤5-fold. Discontinue therapy if signs/symptoms of acute hepatitis develop. Clinicians should note that elevated transaminases may be a result of pre-existing alcoholic liver disease, hepatitis B and/or C infection, or concomitant use of other hepatotoxic drugs; abrupt opioid withdrawal may also lead to acute liver injury. Therapy may precipitate withdrawal symptoms in patients

addicted to opioids; patients should be opioid-free (including tramadol) for a minimum of 7-10 days; a naloxone challenge test may help to confirm patient is opioid-free prior to therapy if there is any suspicion since urinary opioid screen may not be sufficient proof. Patients transitioning from buprenorphine or methadone may be vulnerable to precipitation of withdrawal symptoms for as long as 2 weeks. Use of naltrexone does not eliminate or diminish withdrawal symptoms. Patients who had been treated with naltrexone may respond to lower opioid doses than previously used. This could result in potentially life-threatening opioid intoxication. Patients should be aware that they may be more sensitive to lower doses of opioids after naltrexone treatment is discontinued, after a missed dose, or near the end of the dosing interval. Warn patients that any attempt to overcome opioid blockade during naltrexone therapy, could potentially lead to fatal opioid overdose; the opioid competitive receptor blockade produced by naltrexone is potentially surmountable in the presence of large amounts of opioids. In naltrexone-treated patients requiring emergency pain management, consider alternatives to opioid therapy (eg, regional analgesia, nonopioid analgesics, general anesthesia). If opioid therapy is required for pain therapy, patients should be under the direct care of a trained anesthesia provider.

Suicidal thoughts, attempted suicide, and depression have been reported postmarketing; monitor closely. Hypersensitivity, including anaphylaxis, has been reported. Cases of eosinophilic pneumonia have been reported and should be considered in patients presenting with progressive hypoxia and dyspnea. Use with caution in patients with severe hepatic impairment (has not been studied; if coagulopathy presents, I.M. injection may cause hematoma formation). Use with caution in patients with moderate-to-severe renal impairment (has not been studied). Use I.M. injection with caution in patients with thrombocytopenia or any bleeding disorder (hemophilia and severe hepatic failure), and patients on anticoagulant therapy; bleeding/hematoma may occur from I.M. administration. Serious injection site reactions (eg, cellulitis, induration, hematoma, abscess, necrosis) have been reported with use, including severe cases requiring surgical debridement. Females appear to be at a higher risk. Patients should report any injection site pain, swelling, bruising, pruritus, or redness that does not improve (or worsens). For I.M. use only in the gluteal muscle; do **not** administer I.V., SubQ, or into fatty tissue; incorrect administration may increase the risk of injection site reactions. Vehicle used in the injectable naltrexone formulation (polylactide-co-glycolide microspheres) has rarely been associated with retinal artery occlusion in patients with abnormal arteriovenous anastomosis following injection of other drug products that also use the polylactide-co-glycolide microspheres vehicle.

Drug Interactions

Avoid Concomitant Use There are no known interactions where it is recommended to avoid concomitant use.

Decreased Effect There are no known significant interactions involving a decrease in effect.

Increased Effect/Toxicity There are no known significant interactions involving an increase in effect.

Adverse Reactions Combined reporting of adverse events from oral and injectable formulations:

>10%:
Cardiovascular: Syncope (13%)
Central nervous system: Headache (3% to 25%), insomnia (3% to 14%), dizziness (4% to 13%), anxiety (2% to 12%), decreased energy (>10%), nervousness (4% to >10%)
Gastrointestinal: Nausea (10% to 33%), vomiting (3% to 14%), appetite decreased (14%), diarrhea (13%), abdominal pain (11%), abdominal cramping
Hepatic: ALT increased (13%)
Local: Injection site reaction (≤69%; includes bruising, induration, nodules, pain, pruritus, swelling, tenderness)
Neuromuscular & skeletal: CPK increased (11% to 39%), arthralgia (12%), myalgia (>10%)
Respiratory: Pharyngitis (7% to 11%)

1% to 10%:
Cardiovascular: Hypertension (5%)
Central nervous system: Suicidal ideation (≤10%), depression (8%), somnolence (2% to 4%), fatigue (4%), chills, energy increased, feeling down, irritability
Dermatologic: Skin rash (6% to 10%)
Endocrine & metabolic: Increased thirst, polydipsia
Gastrointestinal: Dry mouth (5%), toothache (4%), constipation
Genitourinary: Delayed ejaculation (<10%), impotency (<10%)
Hepatic: AST increased (2% to 10%), GGT increased (7%)
Neuromuscular & skeletal: Muscle cramps (8%), back pain (6%)
Miscellaneous: Influenza (5%)

Pharmacodynamics/Kinetics

Duration of Action Oral: 50 mg: 24 hours; 100 mg: 48 hours; 150 mg: 72 hours; I.M.: 4 weeks

Available Dosage Forms

Suspension Reconstituted, Intramuscular:
Vivitrol: 380 mg (1 ea)

Tablet, Oral:
ReVia: 50 mg
Generic: 50 mg

General Dosage Range

I.M.: *Adults:* 380 mg once every 4 weeks
Oral: *Adults:* 25-50 mg once daily

◀ **Administration**

I.M. Vivitrol: Administer I.M. into the upper outer quadrant of the gluteal area; must inject dose using one of the provided needles for administration. Use either the 1.5-inch needle (for very lean patients) or the 2-inch needle (for patients with a larger amount of subcutaneous tissue overlying the gluteal muscle). Either needle may be used for patients with average body habitus. Avoid inadvertent injection into a blood vessel; do not administer I.V., SubQ, or into fatty tissue (the risk of serious injection site reaction is increased if given incorrectly as a SubQ injection or into fatty tissue instead of the gluteal muscle). Injection should alternate between the 2 buttocks. Do not substitute any components of the dose-pack.

Oral May be administered with or without food. Administration with food or after meals may minimize adverse gastrointestinal effects. Advise patient not to self-administer opioids while receiving naltrexone therapy.

Preparation for Administration Injection: Prior to reconstitution, allow drug vial and provided diluent to reach room temperature (~45 minutes). Using the provided 1-inch *preparation* needle, reconstitute with 3.4 mL of the diluent and allow to dissolve by vigorously shaking the vial for ~1 minute. Mixed suspension will be milky white, free of clumps, and will move freely down the walls of the vial. Immediately after suspension, withdraw 4.2 mL of the suspension using the same preparation needle.

Prior to administration, replace the preparation needle with the appropriate size provided *administration* needle (use the 2-inch needle with the needle protection device for patients with a larger amount of subcutaneous tissue overlying the gluteal muscle; for very lean patients, the 1.5-inch needle may be appropriate; either needle may be used for patients with average body habitus). Prior to injection, remove any air bubbles and push on the plunger until 4 mL of the suspension remains in the syringe. Following reconstitution of the suspension, administer immediately.

Storage/Stability

Injection: Store unopened kit at 2°C to 8°C (36°F to 46°F). Kit may be kept at room temperature of ≤25°C (77°F) for ≤7 days prior to use; do not freeze. Following reconstitution of the suspension, administer immediately.

Tablet: Store at 20°C to 25°C (68°F to 77°F).

Nursing Actions

Physical Assessment Do not use until patient has been opioid-free for 7-10 days. Assess carefully for several days following start of therapy for narcotic withdrawal symptoms or severe adverse reactions. Monitor injection site for reaction. Use non-narcotic analgesics for pain. Monitor for suicide ideation.

Patient Education

- Discuss specific use of drug and side effects with patient as it relates to treatment. (HCAHPS: During this hospital stay, were you given any medicine that you had not taken before? Before giving you any new medicine, how often did hospital staff tell you what the medicine was for? How often did hospital staff describe possible side effects in a way you could understand?)
- Patient may experience headache, dyspepsia, cramps, insomnia, nausea, fatigue, arthralgia, myalgia, lack of appetite, asthenia, xerostomia, or diarrhea. Have patient report immediately to prescriber signs of hepatic impairment, signs of depression (ie, suicidal ideation, anxiety, emotional instability, illogical thinking), severe dizziness, syncope, tachycardia, blurred vision, arrhythmia, hallucinations, dyspnea, significant injection site irritation (HCAHPS).
- Educate patient about signs of a significant reaction (eg, wheezing; chest tightness; fever; itching; bad cough; blue skin color; seizures; or swelling of face, lips, tongue, or throat). **Note:** This is not a comprehensive list of all side effects. Patient should consult prescriber for additional questions.

Intended Use and Disclaimer: Should not be printed and given to patients. This information is intended to serve as a concise initial reference for healthcare professionals to use when discussing medications with a patient. You must ultimately rely on your own discretion, experience and judgment in diagnosing, treating and advising patients.

Naproxen (na PROKS en)

Brand Names: U.S. Aleve [OTC]; All Day Pain Relief [OTC]; All Day Relief [OTC]; Anaprox; Anaprox DS; EC-Naprosyn; Flanax Pain Relief [OTC]; Mediproxen [OTC]; Naprelan; Naproderm [DSC]; Naprosyn; Naproxen Comfort Pac; Naproxen DR

Index Terms Naproxen Sodium

Pharmacologic Category Nonsteroidal Anti-inflammatory Drug (NSAID), Oral

Medication Safety Issues

Sound-alike/look-alike issues:

Naproxen may be confused with Natacyn®, Nebcin

Anaprox® may be confused with Anaspaz®, Avapro®

Naprelan® may be confused with Naprosyn®

Naprosyn® may be confused with Natacyn®, Nebcin

BEERS Criteria medication:

This drug may be potentially inappropriate for use in geriatric patients (Quality of evidence - moderate; Strength of recommendation - strong).

International issues:

Flogen [Mexico] may be confused with Flovent brand name for fluticasone [U.S., Canada]

Flogen [Mexico] may be confused with Floxin brand name for flunarizine [Thailand], norfloxacin [South Africa], ofloxacin [U.S., Canada], and perfloxacin [Philippines]

Medication Guide Available Yes

Pregnancy Risk Factor C

Lactation Enters breast milk/not recommended

Use

Acute gout/Ankylosing spondylitis/Bursitis/Juvenile arthritis/Juvenile rheumatoid arthritis/Osteoarthritis/Rheumatoid arthritis/Tendonitis (Rx products only): For the relief of the signs and symptoms of acute gout, ankylosing spondylitis, bursitis, juvenile arthritis (excluding ER tablets), juvenile rheumatoid arthritis (oral suspension only), osteoarthritis, rheumatoid arthritis, and tendonitis. Delayed-release naproxen is not recommended for initial treatment of acute pain.

Pain/Primary dysmenorrhea (Rx and OTC products): For the relief of mild-to-moderate pain and the treatment of primary dysmenorrhea. Delayed-release naproxen is not recommended for initial treatment of acute pain.

Unlabeled Use Migraine prophylaxis

Available Dosage Forms

Capsule, Oral:

Aleve [OTC]: 220 mg

Kit, Combination:

Naproxen Comfort Pac: 500 mg

Suspension, Oral:

Naprosyn: 125 mg/5 mL (480 mL)

Generic: 125 mg/5 mL (500 mL)

Tablet, Oral:

Aleve [OTC]: 220 mg

All Day Pain Relief [OTC]: 220 mg

All Day Relief [OTC]: 220 mg

Anaprox: 275 mg

Anaprox DS: 550 mg

Flanax Pain Relief [OTC]: 220 mg

Mediproxen [OTC]: 220 mg

Naprosyn: 250 mg, 375 mg, 500 mg

Generic: 220 mg, 250 mg, 275 mg, 375 mg, 500 mg, 550 mg

Tablet Delayed Release, Oral:

EC-Naprosyn: 375 mg, 500 mg

Naproxen DR: 375 mg, 500 mg

Tablet Extended Release 24 Hour, Oral:

Naprelan: 375 mg, 500 mg, 750 mg

General Dosage Range Oral:

Children >2-11 years: Naproxen base: 10 mg/kg/day in 2 divided doses (recommended maximum: 10 mg/kg/day; up to 15 mg/kg daily has been tolerated)

Children ≥12 years: Naproxen base: 10 mg/kg/day in 2 divided doses (maximum: 10 mg/kg/day) **or** 200 mg every 8-12 hours (maximum: 600 mg daily)

Adults: Naproxen base: Initial: 200-1500 mg as a single dose; Maintenance: 200-500 mg every 6-12 hours (maximum: 1500 mg daily)

Administration

Oral Administer with food, milk, or antacids to decrease GI adverse effects

Suspension: Shake suspension well before administration.

Tablet, delayed or extended release: Swallow tablet whole; do not break, crush, or chew.

Nursing Actions

Physical Assessment Monitor blood pressure at the beginning of therapy and periodically during use. Monitor for GI effects, hepatotoxicity, and ototoxicity at beginning of therapy and periodically throughout. Schedule ophthalmic evaluations for patients who develop eye complaints during long-term NSAID therapy.

Patient Education

- Discuss specific use of drug and side effects with patient as it relates to treatment. (HCAHPS: During this hospital stay, were you given any medicine that you had not taken before? Before giving you any new medicine, how often did hospital staff tell you what the medicine was for? How often did hospital staff describe possible side effects in a way you could understand?)
- Patient may experience headache, dyspepsia, pyrosis, nausea, or constipation. Have patient report immediately to prescriber angina, strength differences from one side to another, edema or pain of hands or feet, significant weight gain, melena, hematuria, ecchymosis, or rash (HCAHPS).
- Educate patient about signs of a significant reaction (eg, wheezing; chest tightness; fever; itching; bad cough; blue skin color; seizures; or swelling of face, lips, tongue, or throat). **Note:** This is not a comprehensive list of all side effects. Patient should consult prescriber for additional questions.

Intended Use and Disclaimer: Should not be printed and given to patients. This information is intended to serve as a concise initial reference for healthcare professionals to use when discussing medications with a patient. You must ultimately rely on your own discretion, experience and judgment in diagnosing, treating and advising patients.

◀ **Related Information**
Oral Medications That Should Not Be Crushed or Altered *on page 1712*

Naproxen and Esomeprazole
(na PROKS en & es oh ME pray zol)

Brand Names: U.S. Vimovo
Index Terms Esomeprazole and Naproxen
Pharmacologic Category Nonsteroidal Anti-inflammatory Drug (NSAID), Oral; Proton Pump Inhibitor; Substituted Benzimidazole
Medication Safety Issues
Sound-alike/look-alike issues:
Vimovo™ may be confused with Vimpat®
Medication Guide Available Yes
Pregnancy Risk Factor C/D ≥30 weeks gestation
Use Reduction of the risk of NSAID-associated gastric ulcers in patients at risk of developing gastric ulcers who require an NSAID for the treatment of rheumatoid arthritis, osteoarthritis, and ankylosing spondylitis
Available Dosage Forms
Tablet Delayed Release, Oral:
Vimovo: Naproxen [delayed release] 375 mg and esomeprazole [immediate release] 20 mg, Naproxen [delayed release] 500 mg and esomeprazole [immediate release] 20 mg
General Dosage Range Oral: *Adults:* 1 tablet (naproxen 375-500 mg/esomeprazole 20 mg) twice daily; Maximum dose of esomeprazole: 40 mg daily
Administration
Oral Administer dose at least 30 minutes prior to meals. Tablets should be swallowed whole; do not chew, crush, dissolve, or split tablet.
Nursing Actions
Physical Assessment See individual agents.
Patient Education
- Discuss specific use of drug and side effects with patient as it relates to treatment. (HCAHPS: During this hospital stay, were you given any medicine that you had not taken before? Before giving you any new medicine, how often did hospital staff tell you what the medicine was for? How often did hospital staff describe possible side effects in a way you could understand?)
- Patient may experience dyspepsia, pyrosis, headache, nausea, constipation, or diarrhea. Have patient report immediately to prescriber angina, tachycardia, strength differences from one side to another, significant weight gain, inability to eat, discolored urine, jaundice, severe asthenia, melena, hematuria, ecchymosis, bleeding, considerable edema, intolerable osteodynia, or significant myalgia (HCAHPS).
- Educate patient about signs of a significant reaction (eg, wheezing; chest tightness; fever; itching; bad cough; blue skin color; seizures; or swelling of face, lips, tongue, or throat). **Note:** This is not a comprehensive list of all side

effects. Patient should consult prescriber for additional questions.

Intended Use and Disclaimer: Should not be printed and given to patients. This information is intended to serve as a concise initial reference for healthcare professionals to use when discussing medications with a patient. You must ultimately rely on your own discretion, experience and judgment in diagnosing, treating and advising patients.
Related Information
Esomeprazole *on page 572*
Naproxen *on page 1102*
Oral Medications That Should Not Be Crushed or Altered *on page 1712*

Naratriptan (NAR a trip tan)

Brand Names: U.S. Amerge
Index Terms Naratriptan Hydrochloride
Pharmacologic Category Antimigraine Agent; Serotonin 5-HT$_{1B, 1D}$ Receptor Agonist
Medication Safety Issues
Sound-alike/look-alike issues:
Amerge may be confused with Altace, Amaryl
Pregnancy Risk Factor C
Lactation Excretion in breast milk unknown/use caution
Breast-Feeding Considerations It is not known if naratriptan is excreted in breast milk. Due to the potential for serious adverse reactions in the nursing infant, the manufacturer recommends a decision be made whether to discontinue nursing or to discontinue the drug, taking into account the importance of treatment to the mother.
Use Migraines: Acute treatment of migraine attacks with or without aura in adults.
Unlabeled Use Short-term prevention of menstrually associated migraines (MAMs)
Mechanism of Action/Effect Selective agonist for serotonin receptor in cranial arteries; causes vasoconstriction and relief of migraine
Contraindications
Ischemic coronary artery disease (CAD) (angina pectoris, history of myocardial infarction [MI], or documented silent ischemia); coronary artery vasospasm, including Prinzmetal's angina; Wolff-Parkinson-White syndrome or arrhythmias associated with other cardiac accessory conduction pathway disorders; history of stroke, transient ischemic attack (TIA), or history of hemiplegic or basilar migraine; peripheral vascular disease; ischemic bowel disease; uncontrolled hypertension; recent use (within 24 hours) of another 5-HT$_1$ agonist, ergotamine-containing medication, or ergot-type medication (eg, dihydroergotamine or methysergide); severe renal impairment (CrCl <15 mL/minute) or severe hepatic impairment; hypersensitivity to naratriptan or any component of the formulation

Canadian labeling: Additional contraindications (not in U.S. labeling): Cardiac arrhythmias (especially tachycardias); valvular heart disease, congenital heart disease, atherosclerotic disease; management of ophthalmoplegic migraine; Raynaud's syndrome

Documentation of allergenic cross-reactivity for triptans is limited. However, because of similarities in chemical structure and/or pharmacologic actions, the possibility of cross-sensitivity cannot be ruled out with certainty.

Warnings/Precautions Use only if there is a clear diagnosis of migraine. Use is contraindicated in patients with severe hepatic or renal impairment. Do not give to patients with risk factors for CAD until a cardiovascular evaluation has been performed; if evaluation is satisfactory, the healthcare provider should administer the first dose (consider ECG monitoring) and cardiovascular status should be periodically re-evaluated. Cardiac events (coronary artery vasospasm, transient ischemia, myocardial infarction, ventricular tachycardia/fibrillation, cardiac arrest, and death), cerebral/subarachnoid hemorrhage, stroke (some fatal), peripheral vascular ischemia, gastrointestinal vascular ischemia/infarction, splenic infarction, and Raynaud's syndrome have been reported with 5-HT$_1$ agonist administration. Partial vision loss and blindness (transient and permanent) have been reported with use of 5-HT$_1$ agonists; a causal relationship between these events and 5-HT$_1$ agonist administration has not been clearly determined. Patients who experience sensations of chest pain/pressure/tightness or symptoms suggestive of angina following dosing should be evaluated for coronary artery disease or Prinzmetal's angina before receiving additional doses; if dosing is resumed and similar symptoms recur, monitor with ECG. Significant elevation in blood pressure, including hypertensive crisis with acute impairment of organ systems, has been reported on rare occasions in patients with and without a history of hypertension; monitor blood pressure. Blood pressure increases may be more pronounced in the elderly. May cause CNS depression, such as dizziness, weakness, or drowsiness, which may impair physical or mental abilities; patients must be cautioned about performing tasks which require mental alertness (eg, operating machinery or driving). Only indicated for the acute treatment of migraine; not indicated for migraine prophylaxis, or for the treatment of cluster headache, hemiplegic or basilar migraine. Acute migraine agents (eg, triptans, opioids, ergotamine, or a combination of the agents) used for 10 or more days per month may lead to worsening of headaches (medication overuse headache); withdrawal treatment may be necessary in the setting of overuse. If a patient does not respond to the first dose, the diagnosis of migraine should be reconsidered; rule out underlying neurologic disease in patients with atypical headache and in patients with no prior history of migraine.

Potentially significant drug-drug interactions may exist, requiring dose or frequency adjustment, additional monitoring, and/or selection of alternative therapy. Symptoms of agitation, confusion, hallucinations, hyper-reflexia, myoclonus, shivering, and tachycardia may occur with concomitant proserotonergic drugs (ie, SSRIs/SNRIs or triptans) or agents which reduce naratriptan's metabolism. Concurrent use of serotonin precursors (eg, tryptophan) is not recommended. If concomitant administration with SSRIs is warranted, monitor closely, especially at initiation and with dose increases. Discontinue naratriptan if serotonin syndrome is suspected. Anaphylaxis, anaphylactoid, and hypersensitivity reactions (including angioedema) have occurred; may be life-threatening or fatal.

Drug Interactions

Avoid Concomitant Use

Avoid concomitant use of Naratriptan with any of the following: Ergot Derivatives

Decreased Effect There are no known significant interactions involving a decrease in effect.

Increased Effect/Toxicity

Naratriptan may increase the levels/effects of: Antipsychotics; Droxidopa; Ergot Derivatives; Metoclopramide; Serotonin Modulators

The levels/effects of Naratriptan may be increased by: Antipsychotics; Ergot Derivatives

Adverse Reactions 1% to 10%:

Central nervous system: Pain/pressure (2% to 4%), malaise/fatigue (2%), dizziness (1% to 2%), drowsiness (1% to 2%), vertigo (1%)

Gastrointestinal: Nausea (4% to 5%), hyposalivation (1%), vomiting (1%)

Neuromuscular & skeletal: Paresthesia (1% to 2%)

Ocular: Photophobia (1%)

Miscellaneous: Ear/nose/throat infection (1%), pressure/tightness/heaviness sensations (1%), warm/cold temperature sensations (1%)

Pharmacodynamics/Kinetics

Onset of Action ~1-2 hours (Bomhof, 1999; Tfelt-Hansen, 2000)

Available Dosage Forms

Tablet, Oral:

Amerge: 1 mg, 2.5 mg

Generic: 1 mg, 2.5 mg

General Dosage Range Dosage adjustment recommended in patients with hepatic or renal impairment

Oral: *Adults:* 1-2.5 mg, may repeat after 4 hours (maximum: 5 mg daily)

Administration

Oral Administer as soon as symptoms appear; may take with or without food. Do **not** crush or chew tablet; swallow whole with water.

Storage/Stability Store at 20°C to 25°C (68°F to 77°F).

Nursing Actions

Physical Assessment Assess potential for interactions with ergot-containing drugs and SSRIs patient may be taking. Monitor closely, especially after the first dose. Monitor for drowsiness, nausea/vomiting, paresthesias, hypertension, and cardiac events. Teach patient proper use (treatment of acute migraine).

Patient Education

- Discuss specific use of drug and side effects with patient as it relates to treatment. (HCAHPS: During this hospital stay, were you given any medicine that you had not taken before? Before giving you any new medicine, how often did hospital staff tell you what the medicine was for? How often did hospital staff describe possible side effects in a way you could understand?)
- Patient may experience fatigue, asthenia, or warmth sensation. Have patient report immediately to prescriber skin discoloration, paresthesia, constipation, considerable dyspepsia, melena, weight loss, leg cramps, leg pain, temperature sensitivity, paresthesia of feet, dyspnea, serotonin syndrome (ie, dizziness, severe headache, agitation, hallucinations, tachycardia, arrhythmia, flushing, tremors, hyperhidrosis, change in balance, illogical thinking, severe nausea, significant diarrhea), signs of severe cardiac abnormalities, strength differences from one side to another, difficulty speaking or thinking, or vision changes (HCAHPS).
- Educate patient about signs of a significant reaction (eg, wheezing; chest tightness; fever; itching; bad cough; blue skin color; seizures; or swelling of face, lips, tongue, or throat). **Note:** This is not a comprehensive list of all side effects. Patient should consult prescriber for additional questions.

Intended Use and Disclaimer: Should not be printed and given to patients. This information is intended to serve as a concise initial reference for healthcare professionals to use when discussing medications with a patient. You must ultimately rely on your own discretion, experience and judgment in diagnosing, treating and advising patients.

Natalizumab (na ta LIZ u mab)

Brand Names: U.S. Tysabri
Index Terms AN100226; Anti-4 Alpha Integrin; IgG4-Kappa Monoclonal Antibody
Pharmacologic Category Gastrointestinal Agent, Miscellaneous; Monoclonal Antibody, Selective Adhesion-Molecule Inhibitor
Medication Guide Available Yes
Pregnancy Risk Factor C
Lactation Enters breast milk

Use

Crohn disease: For inducing and maintaining clinical response and remission in adult patients with moderately to severely active Crohn disease with evidence of inflammation who have had an inadequate response to, or are unable to tolerate, conventional Crohn disease therapies and inhibitors of tumor necrosis factor-alpha (TNF-alpha).

Multiple sclerosis: As monotherapy for the treatment of patients with relapsing forms of multiple sclerosis (MS). Natalizumab increases the risk of PML. When initiating and continuing treatment with natalizumab, consider whether the expected benefit of natalizumab is sufficient to offset this risk.

Canada labeling: Treatment of relapsing forms of multiple sclerosis

Available Dosage Forms

Concentrate, Intravenous [preservative free]: Tysabri: 300 mg/15 mL (15 mL)
General Dosage Range I.V.: *Adults:* 300 mg every 4 weeks

Administration

I.V. Warm solution to room temperature prior to administration. Diluted solution should be infused over 1 hour; do not administer by I.V. bolus or push. Patients should be closely monitored for signs and symptoms of hypersensitivity during the infusion and for at least 1 hour after the infusion is complete. The infusion should be discontinued if a reaction occurs, and treatment of the reaction should be instituted. Following infusion, flush line with NS.

Injectable Detail pH: 6.1

Nursing Actions

Physical Assessment Monitor patient closely for infusion-related reactions (eg, urticaria, dizziness, fever, rash, rigors, pruritus, nausea, flushing, hypotension, dyspnea, chest pain) during and for 1 hour following infusion. If hypersensitivity reaction occurs, promptly discontinue infusion and notify prescriber. Monitor for hepatotoxicity; opportunistic infection (including herpes), nausea or vomiting, excessive fatigue, depression, anxiety, cognitive changes, suicidal ideation, vision changes, tremors, or rash.

Patient Education

- Discuss specific use of drug and side effects with patient as it relates to treatment. (HCAHPS: During this hospital stay, were you given any medicine that you had not taken before? Before giving you any new medicine, how often did hospital staff tell you what the medicine was for? How often did hospital staff describe possible side effects in a way you could understand?)
- Patient may experience depression, headache, nausea, diarrhea, dyspepsia, asthenia, fatigue, arthralgia, or hepatic impairment. Have patient report immediately to prescriber signs of infection, illogical thinking, sudden vision changes,

significant change in balance, discolored urine, jaundice, or rash (HCAHPS).

• Educate patient about signs of a significant reaction (eg, wheezing; chest tightness; fever; itching; bad cough; blue skin color; seizures; or swelling of face, lips, tongue, or throat). **Note:** This is not a comprehensive list of all side effects. Patient should consult prescriber for additional questions.

Intended Use and Disclaimer: Should not be printed and given to patients. This information is intended to serve as a concise initial reference for healthcare professionals to use when discussing medications with a patient. You must ultimately rely on your own discretion, experience and judgment in diagnosing, treating and advising patients.

Nateglinide (na te GLYE nide)

Brand Names: U.S. Starlix
Pharmacologic Category Antidiabetic Agent, Meglitinide Derivative
Medication Safety Issues
High alert medication:
The Institute for Safe Medication Practices (ISMP) includes this medication among its list of drug classes which have a heightened risk of causing significant patient harm when used in error.
Pregnancy Risk Factor C
Lactation Excretion in breast milk unknown/not recommended
Breast-Feeding Considerations It is not known if nateglinide is excreted in breast milk. Breast-feeding is not recommended by the manufacturer.
Use Type 2 diabetes mellitus: For the treatment of adults with type 2 diabetes mellitus as an adjunct to diet and exercise to improve glycemic control.
Mechanism of Action/Effect Nonsulfonylurea hypoglycemic agent which stimulates release from the pancreatic beta cells. Nateglinide-induced insulin release is glucose-dependent.
Contraindications Hypersensitivity to nateglinide or any component of the formulation; type 1 diabetes; diabetic ketoacidosis (this condition should be treated with insulin)
Warnings/Precautions Use with caution in patients with moderate-to-severe hepatic impairment. Use caution in severe renal dysfunction, elderly, malnourished, or patients with adrenal/pituitary dysfunction; may be more susceptible to glucose-lowering effects. All oral hypoglycemic agents are capable of producing hypoglycemia. Proper patient selection, dosage, and instructions to the patients are important to avoid hypoglycemic episodes. It may be necessary to discontinue nateglinide and administer insulin if the patient is exposed to stress (eg, fever, trauma, infection, surgery). Indicated for adjunctive therapy with

metformin; not to be used as a substitute for metformin monotherapy. Combination treatment with sulfonylureas is not recommended (no additional benefit). Patients not adequately controlled on oral agents which stimulate insulin release (eg, glyburide) should not be switched to nateglinide or have nateglinide added to therapy.
Drug Interactions
Avoid Concomitant Use
Avoid concomitant use of Nateglinide with any of the following: Conivaptan; Fusidic Acid (Systemic)
Decreased Effect
The levels/effects of Nateglinide may be decreased by: Bosentan; Corticosteroids (Orally Inhaled); Corticosteroids (Systemic); CYP2C9 Inducers (Strong); CYP3A4 Inducers (Strong); Dabrafenib; Deferasirox; Herbs (CYP3A4 Inducers); Loop Diuretics; Luteinizing Hormone-Releasing Hormone Analogs; Mitotane; Peginterferon Alfa-2b; Somatropin; Thiazide Diuretics; Tocilizumab
Increased Effect/Toxicity
Nateglinide may increase the levels/effects of: Hypoglycemic Agents

The levels/effects of Nateglinide may be increased by: Conivaptan; CYP2C9 Inhibitors (Moderate); CYP2C9 Inhibitors (Strong); CYP3A4 Inhibitors (Moderate); CYP3A4 Inhibitors (Strong); Dasatinib; Eltrombopag; Fusidic Acid (Systemic); Herbs (Hypoglycemic Properties); Ivacaftor; Luliconazole; MAO Inhibitors; Mifepristone; Pegvisomant; Salicylates; Selective Serotonin Reuptake Inhibitors; Simeprevir; Stiripentol
Nutritional/Ethanol Interactions
Ethanol: Ethanol may increase the risk of hypoglycemia. Management: Avoid ethanol.
Food: Rate of absorption is decreased and T_{max} is delayed when taken with food. Food does not affect AUC. Multiple peak plasma concentrations may be observed if fasting. Not affected by composition of meal.
Herb/Nutraceutical: Alfalfa, aloe, bilberry, bitter melon, burdock, celery, damiana, fenugreek, garcinia, garlic, ginger, ginseng (American), gymnema, marshmallow, and stinging nettle may enhance the hypoglycemic effects of antidiabetic agents. St. John's wort may decrease the levels/effect of nateglinide. Management: Avoid alfalfa, aloe, bilberry, bitter melon, burdock, celery, damiana, fenugreek, garcinia, garlic, ginger, ginseng (American), gymnema, marshmallow, and stinging nettle. Avoid St John's wort.
Adverse Reactions As reported with nateglinide monotherapy:
>10%: Respiratory: Upper respiratory infection (11%)

1% to 10%:
Central nervous system: Dizziness (4%)
Endocrine & metabolic: Hypoglycemia (2%), uric acid increased
Gastrointestinal: Diarrhea (3%), weight gain
Neuromuscular & skeletal: Back pain, (4%), arthropathy (3%)
Respiratory: Bronchitis (3%), cough (2%)
Miscellaneous: Flu-like syndrome (4%)

Pharmacodynamics/Kinetics
Onset of Action Insulin secretion: ~20 minutes; Peak effect: 1 hour
Duration of Action 4 hours
Available Dosage Forms
Tablet, Oral:
Starlix: 60 mg, 120 mg
Generic: 60 mg, 120 mg
General Dosage Range Oral: *Adults:* 60-120 mg 3 times daily

Administration
Oral Administer 1-30 minutes prior to meals. Scheduled dose should not be administered if a meal is missed to avoid hypoglycemia.
Storage/Stability Store at 25°C (77°F); excursions are permitted between 15°C and 30°C (59°F and 86°F).

Nursing Actions
Physical Assessment Teach patient importance of proper administration.
Patient Education
• Discuss specific use of drug and side effects with patient as it relates to treatment. (HCAHPS: During this hospital stay, were you given any medicine that you had not taken before? Before giving you any new medicine, how often did hospital staff tell you what the medicine was for? How often did hospital staff describe possible side effects in a way you could understand?)
• Have patient report immediately to prescriber signs of hypoglycemia (HCAHPS).
• Educate patient about signs of a significant reaction (eg, wheezing; chest tightness; fever; itching; bad cough; blue skin color; seizures; or swelling of face, lips, tongue, or throat). **Note:** This is not a comprehensive list of all side effects. Patient should consult prescriber for additional questions.

Intended Use and Disclaimer: Should not be printed and given to patients. This information is intended to serve as a concise initial reference for healthcare professionals to use when discussing medications with a patient. You must ultimately rely on your own discretion, experience and judgment in diagnosing, treating and advising patients.
Dietary Considerations Nateglinide should be taken 1-30 minutes prior to meals. Scheduled dose should not be taken if meal is missed to avoid hypoglycemia. Dietary modification based on ADA recommendations is a part of therapy.

Decreases blood glucose concentration. Hypoglycemia may occur. Must be able to recognize symptoms of hypoglycemia (sweating, dizziness, palpitations, increased appetite, trembling).

Nebivolol (ne BIV oh lole)

Brand Names: U.S. Bystolic
Index Terms Nebivolol Hydrochloride
Pharmacologic Category Antihypertensive; Beta-Blocker, Beta-1 Selective
Pregnancy Risk Factor C
Lactation Excretion in breast milk unknown/not recommended
Use Treatment of hypertension, alone or in combination with other agents
Unlabeled Use Heart failure
Available Dosage Forms
Tablet, Oral:
Bystolic: 2.5 mg, 5 mg, 10 mg, 20 mg
General Dosage Range Dosage adjustment recommended in patients with hepatic or renal impairment
Oral: *Adults:* Initial: 5 mg once daily; Maintenance: 5-40 mg once daily

Administration
Oral May be administered with or without food.
Nursing Actions
Physical Assessment Monitor therapeutic response, especially pulse rate and blood pressure, prior to initiation and periodically thereafter. Taper dosage slowly when discontinuing. Advise patients with diabetes to monitor glucose levels closely; beta-blockers may alter glucose tolerance.
Patient Education
• Discuss specific use of drug and side effects with patient as it relates to treatment. (HCAHPS: During this hospital stay, were you given any medicine that you had not taken before? Before giving you any new medicine, how often did hospital staff tell you what the medicine was for? How often did hospital staff describe possible side effects in a way you could understand?)
• Patient may experience dizziness, headache, bradycardia, or impotence. Have patient report immediately to prescriber depression, nervousness, emotional instability, anxiety, dyspnea, significant weight gain, severe asthenia, or rash (HCAHPS).
• Educate patient about signs of a significant reaction (eg, wheezing; chest tightness; fever; itching; bad cough; blue skin color; seizures; or swelling of face, lips, tongue, or throat). **Note:** This is not a comprehensive list of all side effects. Patient should consult prescriber for additional questions.

Intended Use and Disclaimer: Should not be printed and given to patients. This information is intended to serve as a concise initial reference for

healthcare professionals to use when discussing medications with a patient. You must ultimately rely on your own discretion, experience and judgment in diagnosing, treating and advising patients.

Nefazodone (nef AY zoe done)

Index Terms Nefazodone Hydrochloride; Serzone
Pharmacologic Category Antidepressant, Serotonin Reuptake Inhibitor/Antagonist
Medication Safety Issues
Sound-alike/look-alike issues:
Serzone® may be confused with selegiline, SEROquel®, sertraline
Medication Guide Available Yes
Pregnancy Risk Factor C
Lactation Enters breast milk/use caution
Use Treatment of depression
Unlabeled Use Post-traumatic stress disorder (PTSD)
Available Dosage Forms
Tablet, Oral:
Generic: 50 mg, 100 mg, 150 mg, 200 mg, 250 mg
General Dosage Range Oral:
Adults: Initial: 200 mg/day in 2 divided doses; Maintenance: 300-600 mg/day in 2 divided doses
Elderly: Initial: 50 mg twice daily; Maintenance: 200-400 mg/day in 2 divided doses
Administration
Oral Dosing after meals may decrease lightheadedness and postural hypotension, but may also decrease absorption and therefore effectiveness.
Nursing Actions
Physical Assessment Monitor therapeutic response (eg, mental status, mood). Monitor for clinical worsening and suicide ideation. Taper dosage slowly when discontinuing.
Patient Education
- Discuss specific use of drug and side effects with patient as it relates to treatment. (HCAHPS: During this hospital stay, were you given any medicine that you had not taken before? Before giving you any new medicine, how often did hospital staff tell you what the medicine was for? How often did hospital staff describe possible side effects in a way you could understand?)
- Patient may experience presyncope, fatigue, blurred vision, illogical thinking, dizziness, headache, nausea, constipation, or xerostomia. Have patient report immediately to prescriber discolored urine, jaundice, inability to eat, severe asthenia, or rash (HCAHPS).
- Educate patient about signs of a significant reaction (eg, wheezing; chest tightness; fever; itching; bad cough; blue skin color; seizures; or swelling of face, lips, tongue, or throat). **Note:** This is not a comprehensive list of all side effects. Patient should consult prescriber for additional questions.

Intended Use and Disclaimer: Should not be printed and given to patients. This information is intended to serve as a concise initial reference for healthcare professionals to use when discussing medications with a patient. You must ultimately rely on your own discretion, experience and judgment in diagnosing, treating and advising patients.

Nelfinavir (nel FIN a veer)

Brand Names: U.S. Viracept
Index Terms NFV
Pharmacologic Category Antiretroviral, Protease Inhibitor (Anti-HIV)
Medication Safety Issues
Sound-alike/look-alike issues:
Nelfinavir may be confused with nevirapine
Viracept may be confused with Viramune, Viramune XR
Pregnancy Risk Factor B
Lactation Excretion in breast milk unknown/contraindicated
Breast-Feeding Considerations Maternal or infant antiretroviral therapy does not completely eliminate the risk of postnatal HIV transmission. In addition, multiclass-resistant virus has been detected in breast-feeding infants despite maternal therapy. Therefore, in the United States, where formula is accessible, affordable, safe, and sustainable, and the risk of infant mortality due to diarrhea and respiratory infections is low, complete avoidance of breast-feeding by HIV-infected women is recommended to decrease potential transmission of HIV (DHHS [perinatal], 2012).
Use In combination with other antiretroviral therapy in the treatment of HIV infection
Mechanism of Action/Effect Blocks the site of HIV-1 protease activity, resulting in the formation of immature, noninfectious viral particles.
Contraindications Hypersensitivity to nelfinavir or any component of the formulation; concurrent therapy with alfuzosin, amiodarone, cisapride, dihydroergotamine, ergotamine, lovastatin, methylergonovine, midazolam (oral), pimozide, quinidine, rifampin, sildenafil (when used for pulmonary artery hypertension [eg, Revatio®]), simvastatin, St John's wort, triazolam
Warnings/Precautions High potential for drug interactions; concomitant use of nelfinavir with some drugs may require cautious use, may not be recommended, may require dosage adjustments, or may be contraindicated.

Use caution with hepatic impairment; use not recommended with moderate-to-severe impairment. Warn patients that redistribution of body fat can occur. New-onset diabetes mellitus, exacerbation of diabetes, and hyperglycemia have been ▶

reported in HIV-infected patients receiving protease inhibitors. Use with caution in patients with hemophilia A or B; increased bleeding during protease inhibitor therapy has been reported. Patients may develop immune reconstitution syndrome resulting in the occurrence of an inflammatory response to an indolent or residual opportunistic infection during initial HIV treatment or activation of autoimmune disorders (eg, Graves' disease, polymyositis, Guillain-Barré syndrome) later in therapy; further evaluation and treatment may be required.

Drug Interactions

Avoid Concomitant Use

Avoid concomitant use of Nelfinavir with any of the following: Ado-Trastuzumab Emtansine; Alfuzosin; Amiodarone; Apixaban; Avanafil; Axitinib; Bosutinib; Cabozantinib; Cisapride; Conivaptan; Crizotinib; Dronedarone; Eplerenone; Ergot Derivatives; Everolimus; Halofantrine; Ibrutinib; Imatinib; Ivabradine; Lapatinib; Lomitapide; Lovastatin; Lurasidone; Macitentan; Midazolam; Nilotinib; Nisoldipine; Pimozide; Pomalidomide; Proton Pump Inhibitors; QuiNIDine; Ranolazine; Red Yeast Rice; Regorafenib; Rifampin; Rivaroxaban; Salmeterol; Silodosin; Simeprevir; Simvastatin; St Johns Wort; Tamsulosin; Ticagrelor; Tolvaptan; Topotecan; Toremifene; Triazolam; Ulipristal; Vemurafenib; VinCRIStine (Liposomal)

Decreased Effect

Nelfinavir may decrease the levels/effects of: Abacavir; Boceprevir; Clarithromycin; Contraceptives (Estrogens); Contraceptives (Progestins); Delavirdine; Etravirine; Fosphenytoin; Ifosfamide; Lopinavir; Meperidine; Methadone; Phenytoin; Prasugrel; Pravastatin; Theophylline Derivatives; Ticagrelor; Valproic Acid and Derivatives; Warfarin; Zidovudine

The levels/effects of Nelfinavir may be decreased by: Antacids; Boceprevir; Bosentan; CarBAMazepine; CYP2C19 Inducers (Strong); CYP3A4 Inducers (Strong); Dabrafenib; Deferasirox; Fosphenytoin; Garlic; H2-Antagonists; Mitotane; Nevirapine; Peginterferon Alfa-2b; P-glycoprotein/ABCB1 Inducers; Phenytoin; Proton Pump Inhibitors; Rifabutin; Rifampin; St Johns Wort; Tocilizumab

Increased Effect/Toxicity

Nelfinavir may increase the levels/effects of: Ado-Trastuzumab Emtansine; Afatinib; Alfuzosin; Almotriptan; Alosetron; ALPRAZolam; Amiodarone; Apixaban; ARIPiprazole; AtorvaSTATin; Avanafil; Axitinib; Azithromycin (Systemic); Bedaquiline; Bortezomib; Bosentan; Bosutinib; Brentuximab Vedotin; Brinzolamide; Budesonide (Nasal); Budesonide (Systemic, Oral Inhalation); Cabozantinib; Calcium Channel Blockers (Dihydropyridine); Calcium Channel Blockers (Nondihydropyridine); CarBAMazepine; Cisapride; Clarithromycin; Colchicine; Conivaptan; Corticosteroids (Orally Inhaled); Crizotinib;

CycloSPORINE (Systemic); CYP3A4 Substrates; Dabigatran Etexilate; Dienogest; Digoxin; Dofetilide; DOXOrubicin (Conventional); Dronedarone; Dutasteride; Enfuvirtide; Enzalutamide; Eplerenone; Ergot Derivatives; Everolimus; FentaNYL; Fesoterodine; Fluticasone (Nasal); Fluticasone (Oral Inhalation); GuanFACINE; Halofantrine; Ibrutinib; Iloperidone; Imatinib; Ivabradine; Ivacaftor; Ixabepilone; Lacosamide; Lapatinib; Levomilnacipran; Lomitapide; Lovastatin; Lumefantrine; Lurasidone; Macitentan; Maraviroc; Meperidine; MethylPREDNISolone; Midazolam; Mifepristone; Nefazodone; Nilotinib; Nisoldipine; Ospemifene; OxyCODONE; Paricalcitol; PAZOPanib; P-glycoprotein/ABCB1 Substrates; Pimecrolimus; Pimozide; Pomalidomide; PONATinib; Propafenone; Protease Inhibitors; Prucalopride; QUEtiapine; QuiNIDine; Ranolazine; Red Yeast Rice; Regorafenib; Repaglinide; Rifabutin; Rilpivirine; Riociguat; Rivaroxaban; RomiDEPsin; Rosuvastatin; Ruxolitinib; Salmeterol; Saxagliptin; Sildenafil; Silodosin; Simeprevir; Simvastatin; Sirolimus; SORAfenib; Tacrolimus (Systemic); Tacrolimus (Topical); Tadalafil; Tamsulosin; Temsirolimus; Ticagrelor; Tofacitinib; Tolterodine; Tolvaptan; Topotecan; Toremifene; TraZODone; Triazolam; Tricyclic Antidepressants; Ulipristal; Vardenafil; Vemurafenib; Vilazodone; VinCRIStine (Liposomal); Warfarin; Zuclopenthixol

The levels/effects of Nelfinavir may be increased by: Clarithromycin; CycloSPORINE (Systemic); Delavirdine; Enfuvirtide; Etravirine; Lopinavir; P-glycoprotein/ABCB1 Inhibitors; Simeprevir; Voriconazole

Nutritional/Ethanol Interactions

Food: Nelfinavir taken with food increases plasma concentration time curve (AUC) by two- to threefold. Do not administer with acidic food or juice (orange juice, apple juice, or applesauce) since the combination may have a bitter taste.

Herb/Nutraceutical: St John's wort may decrease the levels/effects of protease inhibitors; concurrent use should probably be avoided.

Adverse Reactions Data presented on experience in adults, unless otherwise noted.

>10%: Gastrointestinal: Diarrhea (14% to 20%; children: 39% to 47%)

2% to 10%:

Dermatologic: Rash (1% to 3%)

Gastrointestinal: Nausea (3% to 7%), flatulence (1% to 5%)

Hematologic: Lymphocytes decreased (1% to 6%), neutrophils decreased (1% to 5%)

Available Dosage Forms

Tablet, Oral:

Viracept: 250 mg, 625 mg

General Dosage Range Oral:
Children 2-13 years: 45-55 mg/kg twice daily **or** 25-35 mg/kg 3 times daily (maximum: 2500 mg daily)
Adults: 750 mg 3 times daily **or** 1250 mg twice daily

Administration
Oral Tablets: Administer with a meal. If unable to swallow tablets, may dissolve tablets in a small amount of water; mix cloudy liquid well and consume immediately. Rinse glass with water to ensure receiving full dose.

Storage/Stability Store at room temperature of 15°C to 30°C (59°F to 86°F).

Nursing Actions
Physical Assessment Monitor for adherence to regimen. Monitor for gastrointestinal disturbance (nausea or diarrhea) that can lead to dehydration and weight loss. Caution patients to monitor glucose levels closely; may cause hyperglycemia or new-onset diabetes. Teach patient proper timing of multiple medications.

Patient Education
- Discuss specific use of drug and side effects with patient as it relates to treatment. (HCAHPS: During this hospital stay, were you given any medicine that you had not taken before? Before giving you any new medicine, how often did hospital staff tell you what the medicine was for? How often did hospital staff describe possible side effects in a way you could understand?)
- Patient may experience dyspepsia, nausea, or diarrhea. Have patient report immediately to prescriber rash (HCAHPS).
- Educate patient about signs of a significant reaction (eg, wheezing; chest tightness; fever; itching; bad cough; blue skin color; seizures; or swelling of face, lips, tongue, or throat). **Note:** This is not a comprehensive list of all side effects. Patient should consult prescriber for additional questions.

Intended Use and Disclaimer: Should not be printed and given to patients. This information is intended to serve as a concise initial reference for healthcare professionals to use when discussing medications with a patient. You must ultimately rely on your own discretion, experience and judgment in diagnosing, treating and advising patients.

Dietary Considerations Should be taken as scheduled with a meal.

Nepafenac (ne pa FEN ak)

Brand Names: U.S. Ilevro; Nevanac
Pharmacologic Category Nonsteroidal Anti-inflammatory Drug (NSAID), Ophthalmic
Pregnancy Risk Factor C
Lactation Excretion in breast milk unknown/use caution

Use Treatment of pain and inflammation associated with cataract surgery

Available Dosage Forms
Suspension, Ophthalmic:
Ilevro: 0.3% (1.7 mL)
Nevanac: 0.1% (3 mL)

General Dosage Range Ophthalmic: *Children ≥10 years, Adolescents, and Adults:*
Ilevro™: Instill 1 drop into affected eye(s) once daily
Nevanac®: Instill 1 drop into affected eye(s) 3 times/day

Administration
Ophthalmic For topical ophthalmic use only; shake well prior to use. Remove contact lenses prior to using solutions containing benzalkonium chloride. To avoid contamination, do not touch tip of container to any surface. May be administered with other eye drops; wait at least 5 minutes before administering other eye drops.

Nursing Actions
Patient Education
- Discuss specific use of drug and side effects with patient as it relates to treatment. (HCAHPS: During this hospital stay, were you given any medicine that you had not taken before? Before giving you any new medicine, how often did hospital staff tell you what the medicine was for? How often did hospital staff describe possible side effects in a way you could understand?)
- Have patient report immediately to prescriber vision changes, ophthalmalgia, or severe eye irritation (HCAHPS).
- Educate patient about signs of a significant reaction (eg, wheezing; chest tightness; fever; itching; bad cough; blue skin color; seizures; or swelling of face, lips, tongue, or throat). **Note:** This is not a comprehensive list of all side effects. Patient should consult prescriber for additional questions.

Intended Use and Disclaimer: Should not be printed and given to patients. This information is intended to serve as a concise initial reference for healthcare professionals to use when discussing medications with a patient. You must ultimately rely on your own discretion, experience and judgment in diagnosing, treating and advising patients.

Nesiritide (ni SIR i tide)

Brand Names: U.S. Natrecor
Index Terms B-type Natriuretic Peptide (Human); hBNP; Natriuretic Peptide
Pharmacologic Category Natriuretic Peptide, B-Type, Human

Medication Safety Issues

High alert medication:
The Institute for Safe Medication Practices (ISMP) includes this medication among its list of drugs which have a heightened risk of causing significant patient harm when used in error.

International issues:
Natrecor [U.S., Canada, Argentina, Venezuela] may be confused with Nitrocor brand name for nitroglycerin [Italy, Russia, Venezuela]

Pregnancy Risk Factor C

Lactation Excretion in breast milk unknown/use caution

Breast-Feeding Considerations It is not known if nesiritide is excreted in breast milk.

Use Treatment of acutely decompensated heart failure (HF) with dyspnea at rest or with minimal activity

Mechanism of Action/Effect Binds to cell surface receptors in vasculature, resulting in smooth muscle cell relaxation. Has been shown to produce dose-dependent reductions in pulmonary capillary wedge pressure (PCWP) and systemic arterial pressure providing symptomatic improvements (dyspnea decreased) for several days.

Contraindications Hypersensitivity to natriuretic peptide or any component of the formulation; cardiogenic shock (when used as primary therapy); hypotension (persistent systolic blood pressure <100 mm Hg) prior to therapy

Warnings/Precautions May cause hypotension; administer in clinical situations when blood pressure may be closely monitored. Effects may be additive with other agents capable of causing hypotension. Hypotensive effects may last for several hours.

Should not be used in patients with low cardiac filling pressures, or in patients with conditions which depend on venous return including significant valvular stenosis, restrictive or obstructive cardiomyopathy, constrictive pericarditis, and pericardial tamponade. May be associated with development of azotemia; use caution in patients with renal impairment or in patients where renal perfusion is dependent on renin-angiotensin-aldosterone system; avoid initiation at doses higher than recommended.

Monitor for allergic or anaphylactic reactions; use caution in patients with history of hypersensitivity to other recombinant peptides. Use caution with prolonged infusions; limited experience with infusions >96 hours.

Drug Interactions

Avoid Concomitant Use There are no known interactions where it is recommended to avoid concomitant use.

Decreased Effect There are no known significant interactions involving a decrease in effect.

Increased Effect/Toxicity
Nesiritide may increase the levels/effects of: DULoxetine; Hypotensive Agents

Nutritional/Ethanol Interactions Herb/Nutraceutical: Avoid bayberry, blue cohosh, cayenne, ephedra, ginger, ginseng (American), kola, and licorice (may increase blood pressure). Avoid black cohosh, California poppy, coleus, golden seal, hawthorn, mistletoe, periwinkle, quinine, and shepherd's purse (may enhance decreased blood pressure).

Adverse Reactions Note: Frequencies cited below were recorded in VMAC trial, unless otherwise noted, at dosages similar to approved labeling. Higher frequencies have been observed in trials using higher dosages of nesiritide. The percentages marked with an asterisk (*) indicate frequency less than or equal to placebo or other standard therapy.

>10%:
Cardiovascular: Hypotension (total: 11% [27% in ASCEND-HF trial]; symptomatic: 4% [7% in ASCEND-HF trial] at recommended dose, up to 17% at higher doses)
Renal: Increased serum creatinine (28% with >0.5 mg/dL increase over baseline)

1% to 10%:
Cardiovascular: Ventricular tachycardia (3%)*, ventricular extrasystoles (3%)*, angina (2%)*, bradycardia (1%), tachycardia, atrial fibrillation, AV node conduction abnormalities
Central nervous system: Headache (8%)*, dizziness (3%), insomnia (2%)*, anxiety (3%), confusion, fever, paresthesia, somnolence, tremor
Dermatologic: Pruritus, rash
Gastrointestinal: Nausea (4%)*, abdominal pain (1%)*, vomiting (1%)*
Hematologic: Anemia
Local: Injection site reaction, catheter pain
Neuromuscular & skeletal: Back pain (4%), leg cramps
Ocular: Amblyopia
Respiratory: Apnea, cough increased, hemoptysis
Miscellaneous: Diaphoresis

Pharmacodynamics/Kinetics

Onset of Action PCWP reduction: 15 minutes (60% of 3-hour effect achieved within this time period); Peak effect: Within 1 hour

Duration of Action >60 minutes (up to several hours) for systolic blood pressure; hemodynamic effects persist longer than serum half-life would predict

Available Dosage Forms

Solution Reconstituted, Intravenous:
Natrecor: 1.5 mg (1 ea)

General Dosage Range I.V.: *Adults:* Bolus: 2 mcg/kg; Infusion: Initial: 0.01 mcg/kg/minute (maximum: 0.03 mcg/kg/minute)

Usual Infusion Concentrations: Adult I.V. infusion: 1.5 mg in 250 mL (concentration: 6 **mcg**/mL) of D$_5$W or NS

Administration

I.V. Do not administer through a heparin-coated catheter (concurrent administration of heparin via a separate catheter is acceptable, per manufacturer).

Injectable Detail Prime I.V. tubing with 5 mL of infusion prior to connection with vascular access port and prior to administering bolus or starting the infusion. Withdraw bolus from the prepared infusion bag and administer over 60 seconds. Begin infusion immediately following administration of the bolus.

Preparation for Administration Reconstitute 1.5 mg vial with 5 mL of diluent removed from a prefilled 250 mL plastic I.V. bag (compatible with D$_5$W, D$_5$^{1}/$_2$NS, D$_5$^{1}/$_4$NS, NS). Do not shake vial to dissolve (roll gently). Withdraw entire contents of vial and add to 250 mL I.V. bag. Invert several times to mix. Resultant concentration of solution is ~6 mcg/mL.

Storage/Stability Vials may be stored below 25°C (77°F); do not freeze. Protect from light. Following reconstitution, vials are stable at 2°C to 25°C (36°F to 77°F) for up to 24 hours. Use reconstituted solution within 24 hours.

Nursing Actions

Physical Assessment Monitor blood pressure and cardiac function before, at frequent intervals during, and for 24 hours following infusion (hemodynamic monitoring with larger doses). Assess renal function and monitor for hypersensitivity reaction on a regular basis during therapy.

Patient Education

• Discuss specific use of drug and side effects with patient as it relates to treatment. (HCAHPS: During this hospital stay, were you given any medicine that you had not taken before? Before giving you any new medicine, how often did hospital staff tell you what the medicine was for? How often did hospital staff describe possible side effects in a way you could understand?)

• Patient may experience hypotension, renal impairment, headache, dyspepsia, nausea, or injection site irritation. Have patient report immediately to prescriber dyspnea, tachycardia, severe dizziness, or rash (HCAHPS).

• Educate patient about signs of a significant reaction (eg, wheezing; chest tightness; fever; itching; bad cough; blue skin color; seizures; or swelling of face, lips, tongue, or throat). **Note:** This is not a comprehensive list of all side effects. Patient should consult prescriber for additional questions.

Intended Use and Disclaimer: Should not be printed and given to patients. This information is intended to serve as a concise initial reference for healthcare professionals to use when discussing medications with a patient. You must ultimately rely on your own discretion, experience and judgment in diagnosing, treating and advising patients.

Nevirapine (ne VYE ra peen)

Brand Names: U.S. Viramune; Viramune XR

Index Terms NVP

Pharmacologic Category Antiretroviral, Reverse Transcriptase Inhibitor, Non-nucleoside (Anti-HIV)

Medication Safety Issues

Sound-alike/look-alike issues:

Nevirapine may be confused with nelfinavir

Viramune®, Viramune XR® may be confused with Viracept®

Medication Guide Available Yes

Pregnancy Risk Factor B

Lactation Enters breast milk/contraindicated

Breast-Feeding Considerations Although breast-feeding is not recommended, nevirapine is excreted into breast milk and measurable in the serum of nursing infants. Maternal or infant antiretroviral therapy does not completely eliminate the risk of postnatal HIV transmission. In addition, multiclass resistant virus has been detected in breast-feeding infants despite maternal therapy. Therefore, in the United States, where formula is accessible, affordable, safe, and sustainable, and the risk of infant mortality due to diarrhea and respiratory infections is low, complete avoidance of breast-feeding by HIV-infected women is recommended to decrease potential transmission of HIV (DHHS [perinatal], 2012).

Use In combination therapy with other antiretroviral agents for the treatment of HIV-1

Mechanism of Action/Effect Blocks the RNA-dependent DNA polymerase activity

Contraindications Moderate-to-severe hepatic impairment (Child-Pugh class B or C); use in occupational or nonoccupational postexposure prophylaxis (PEP) regimens

Canadian labeling: Additional contraindications (not in U.S. labeling): Clinically significant hypersensitivity to nevirapine or any component of the formulation; therapy rechallenge in patients with prior hypersensitivity reactions, severe rash, rash accompanied by constitutional symptoms, or clinical hepatitis due to nevirapine; severe hepatic dysfunction or AST or ALT >5 times ULN (pretreatment or during prior use of nevirapine); hereditary conditions of galactose intolerance (eg, galactosemia, Lapp lactase deficiency, glucose-galactose malabsorption); concomitant use of herbal products containing St John's wort

Warnings/Precautions [U.S. Boxed Warning]: Severe hepatotoxic reactions may occur (fulminant and cholestatic hepatitis, hepatic necrosis) and, in some cases, have resulted in hepatic failure and death. The greatest risk of ▶

these reactions is within the initial 6 weeks of treatment. Patients with a history of chronic hepatitis (B or C) or increased baseline transaminase levels may be at increased risk of hepatotoxic reactions. Female gender and patients with increased CD4$^+$-cell counts may be at substantially greater risk of hepatic events (often associated with rash). Therapy in antiretroviral naive patients should not be started with elevated CD4$^+$-cell counts unless the benefit of therapy outweighs the risk of serious hepatotoxicity (adult/postpubertal females: CD4$^+$-cell counts >250 cells/mm^3; adult males: CD4$^+$-cell counts >400 cells/mm^3). Use with caution in patients with pre-existing dysfunction; monitor closely for drug-induced hepatotoxicity. U.S. labeling contraindicates use in patients with moderate-to-severe impairment (Child-Pugh class B or C). Canadian labeling contraindicates use in severe impairment.

[U.S. Boxed Warning]: Severe life-threatening skin reactions (eg, Stevens-Johnson syndrome, toxic epidermal necrolysis, hypersensitivity reactions with rash and organ dysfunction), including fatal cases, have occurred. The greatest risk of these reactions is within the initial 6 weeks of treatment; intensive monitoring is required during the initial 18 weeks of therapy to detect potentially life-threatening dermatologic, hypersensitivity, and hepatic reactions. Risk is greatest in African-Americans, Asian, or Hispanic race/ethnicity or in females. A 14-day lead-in dosing period with immediate release formulation must be initiated to decrease the incidence of adverse effects. The lead-in dosing can be extended up to 28 days if necessary, but an alternative regimen is necessary if >28 days is required. If a severe dermatologic or hypersensitivity reaction occurs, or if signs and symptoms of hepatitis occur, nevirapine should be permanently discontinued. These events may include a severe rash, or a rash associated with fever, blisters, oral lesions, conjunctivitis, facial edema, muscle or joint aches, transaminase elevations, general malaise, hepatitis, eosinophilia, granulocytopenia, lymphadenopathy, or renal dysfunction. Coadministration of prednisone during the first 6 weeks of therapy increases incidence and severity of rash; concomitant prednisone is not recommended to prevent rash.

May cause redistribution of fat (eg, buffalo hump, peripheral wasting with increased abdominal girth, cushingoid appearance). Patients may develop immune reconstitution syndrome resulting in the occurrence of an inflammatory response to an indolent or residual opportunistic infection during initial HIV treatment or activation of autoimmune disorders (eg, Graves' disease, polymyositis, Guillain-Barré syndrome) later in therapy; further evaluation and treatment may be required. Rhabdomyolysis has been observed in conjunction with skin and/or hepatic adverse events during postmarketing surveillance. Termination of therapy is warranted with evidence of severe skin or liver toxicity.

Use with caution in patients taking strong CYP3A4 inhibitors, moderate or strong CYP3A4 inducers and major CYP3A4 substrates (see Drug Interactions); consider alternative agents that avoid or lessen the potential for CYP-mediated interactions. Concurrent use of St John's wort or efavirenz is not recommended; may decrease the therapeutic efficacy (St John's wort) or increase adverse effects (efavirenz). Canadian labeling contraindicates concurrent use with products containing St John's wort.

Nevirapine-based initial regimens should not be used in children <3 years of age if previously exposed to nevirapine during prevention of maternal-to-child transmission of HIV due to increased risk of resistance and treatment failure. Protease inhibitor-based initial regimens preferred in this population.

Due to rapid emergence of resistance, nevirapine should not be used as monotherapy or the only agent added to a failing regimen for the treatment of HIV. Consider alteration of antiretroviral therapies if disease progression occurs while patients are receiving nevirapine. Use care when timing discontinuation of regimens containing nevirapine; levels are sustained after levels of other medications decrease, leading to nevirapine resistance. Cross-resistance may be conferred to other nonnucleoside reverse transcriptase inhibitors (DHHS, 2012).

Drug Interactions

Avoid Concomitant Use

Avoid concomitant use of Nevirapine with any of the following: Abiraterone Acetate; Apixaban; Artemether; Atazanavir; Axitinib; Bedaquiline; Boceprevir; Bortezomib; Bosutinib; Cabozantinib; CarBAMazepine; CloZAPine; Crizotinib; Dienogest; Dolutegravir; Dronedarone; Efavirenz; Enzalutamide; Etravirine; Everolimus; Ibrutinib; Itraconazole; Ivacaftor; Ketoconazole (Systemic); Lapatinib; Lumefantrine; Lurasidone; Macitentan; Mifepristone; NIFEdipine; Nilotinib; Nisoldipine; PAZOPanib; Perampanel; Pimozide; Pomalidomide; PONATinib; Praziquantel; Ranolazine; Regorafenib; Rilpivirine; Rivaroxaban; Roflumilast; RomiDEPsin; Simeprevir; SORAfenib; St Johns Wort; Tasimelteon; Telaprevir; Ticagrelor; Tofacitinib; Tolvaptan; Toremifene; Uliprital; Vandetanib; Vemurafenib; VinCRIStine (Liposomal)

Decreased Effect

Nevirapine may decrease the levels/effects of: Abiraterone Acetate; Apixaban; ARIPiprazole; Artemether; Atazanavir; Axitinib; Bedaquiline; Boceprevir; Bortezomib; Bosutinib; Brentuximab Vedotin; Cabozantinib; CarBAMazepine;

Caspofungin; Clarithromycin; CloZAPine; Contraceptives (Estrogens); Contraceptives (Progestins); Crizotinib; CYP2B6 Substrates; CYP3A4 Substrates; Dasatinib; Dienogest; Dolutegravir; DOXOrubicin (Conventional); Dronedarone; Efavirenz; Enzalutamide; Etravirine; Everolimus; Exemestane; Fosamprenavir; Gefitinib; GuanFACINE; Ibrutinib; Imatinib; Indinavir; Itraconazole; Ivacaftor; Ixabepilone; Ketoconazole (Systemic); Lapatinib; Linagliptin; Lopinavir; Lumefantrine; Lurasidone; Macitentan; Maraviroc; Methadone; Mifepristone; Nelfinavir; NIFEdipine; Nilotinib; Nisoldipine; PAZOPanib; Perampanel; Pomalidomide; PONATinib; Praziquantel; QUEtiapine; Ranolazine; Regorafenib; Rifabutin; Rilpivirine; Rivaroxaban; Roflumilast; RomiDEPsin; Saquinavir; Saxagliptin; Simeprevir; SORAfenib; SUNItinib; Tadalafil; Tasimelteon; Telaprevir; Ticagrelor; Tofacitinib; Tolvaptan; Toremifene; Ulipristal; Vandetanib; Vemurafenib; Vilazodone; VinCRIStine (Liposomal); Voriconazole; Vortioxetine; Zuclopenthixol

The levels/effects of Nevirapine may be decreased by: Bosentan; CarBAMazepine; CYP3A4 Inducers (Strong); Dabrafenib; Deferasirox; Mitotane; Peginterferon Alfa-2b; Rifabutin; Rifampin; St Johns Wort; Tocilizumab

Increased Effect/Toxicity
Nevirapine may increase the levels/effects of: ARIPiprazole; Clarithromycin; Dofetilide; Efavirenz; Etravirine; Ifosfamide; Lomitapide; Pimozide; Rifabutin; Rilpivirine

The levels/effects of Nevirapine may be increased by: Atazanavir; Clarithromycin; Efavirenz; Fluconazole; Voriconazole

Nutritional/Ethanol Interactions Herb/Nutraceutical: Nevirapine serum concentration may be decreased by St John's wort; avoid concurrent use.

Adverse Reactions Note: Potentially life-threatening nevirapine-associated adverse effects may present with the following symptoms: Abrupt onset of flu-like symptoms, abdominal pain, jaundice, or fever with or without rash; may progress to hepatic failure with encephalopathy. Skin rash is present in ~50% of cases.
>10%:
Dermatologic: Rash (1% to 7%; grade 1/2: 13%; grade 3/4: 2%)
Endocrine & metabolic: Cholesterol increased (240-300 mg/dL: 18% to 19%; >300 mg/dL: 3% to 4%), LDL increased (160-190 mg/dL: 15%; >190 mg/dL: 5%)
Hematologic: Neutropenia (4% to 13%; grades 3/4: 1% to 2%)
Hepatic: ALT increased (2.6-5 x ULN: 10% to 13%; ≥5.1 x ULN: 6% to 7%), symptomatic hepatic events (including hepatitis and hepatic failure: 2% to 11%; risk higher in ARV-naive women with CD4 counts >250 cells/mm³ and

ARV-naive men with CD4 counts >400 cells/mm³)
1% to 10%:
Central nervous system: Fatigue (≤5%), headache (1% to 4%), fever (1% to 2%)
Gastrointestinal: Nausea (<1% to 9%), amylase increased (1.6-5 x ULN: 7% to 8%; ≥5.1 x ULN: <1%), abdominal pain (≤2%), diarrhea (≤2%)
Hepatic: AST increased (2.6-5 x ULN: 7% to 9%; ≥5.1 x ULN: 4% to 5%)
Neuromuscular & skeletal: Arthralgia (2%)

Available Dosage Forms
Suspension, Oral:
Viramune: 50 mg/5 mL (240 mL)
Generic: 50 mg/5 mL (240 mL)
Tablet, Oral:
Viramune: 200 mg
Generic: 200 mg
Tablet Extended Release 24 Hour, Oral:
Viramune XR: 100 mg, 400 mg

General Dosage Range Dosage adjustment recommended in patients who are receiving hemodialysis.
Oral, immediate release:
Infants and Children <8 years: Initial: 150-200 mg/m²/dose once daily (maximum: 200 mg daily); Maintenance: 150-200 mg/m²/dose twice daily (maximum: 400 mg daily).
Children ≥8 years: Initial: 120-150 mg/m²/dose once daily (maximum: 200 mg daily); Maintenance: 120-150 mg/m²/dose twice daily (maximum: 400 mg daily)
Adolescents and Adults: Initial: 200 mg once daily; Maintenance: 200 mg twice daily
Oral, extended release:
Children 6 to <18 years: Maintenance:
0.58 m² to 0.83 m²: 200 mg once daily
0.84 m² to 1.16 m²: 300 mg once daily
≥1.17 m²: 400 mg once daily (do not exceed 400 mg daily)
Adults: Maintenance: 400 mg once daily

Administration
Oral May be administered with or without food. May be administered with an antacid or didanosine. Shake suspension gently prior to administration; the use of an oral dosing syringe is recommended, especially if the dose is ≤5 mL; if using a dosing cup, after administration, rinse cup with water and also administer rinse. Extended release tablets must be swallowed whole and not crushed, chewed, or divided.

Storage/Stability Store at 25°C (77°F); excursion permitted to 15°C to 30°C (59°F to 86°F).

Nursing Actions
Physical Assessment Check results of LFTs during therapy. Monitor patient closely for any signs of hypersensitivity during 14 days of lead-in dosing. Monitor regularly and frequently during initial 18 weeks of therapy for symptoms of hypersensitivity/dermatologic reactions (which may include severe rash, rash with fever, blisters, oral ▶

lesions, conjunctivitis, facial edema, muscle or joint aches, general malaise, jaundice, hepatitis, or renal dysfunction). Assess adherence to therapy. Notify provider if patient's hepatic transaminases are elevated, if patient develops a rash, or if patient has signs or symptoms of hepatitis.

Patient Education

• Discuss specific use of drug and side effects with patient as it relates to treatment. (HCAHPS: During this hospital stay, were you given any medicine that you had not taken before? Before giving you any new medicine, how often did hospital staff tell you what the medicine was for? How often did hospital staff describe possible side effects in a way you could understand?)

• Patient may experience headache, nausea, diarrhea, asthenia, or dyspepsia. Have patient report immediately to prescriber inability to eat, severe mouth irritation, significant myalgia, discolored urine, jaundice, sudden vision changes, severe skin irritation, or rash (HCAHPS).

• Educate patient about signs of a significant reaction (eg, wheezing; chest tightness; fever; itching; bad cough; blue skin color; seizures; or swelling of face, lips, tongue, or throat). **Note:** This is not a comprehensive list of all side effects. Patient should consult prescriber for additional questions.

Intended Use and Disclaimer: Should not be printed and given to patients. This information is intended to serve as a concise initial reference for healthcare professionals to use when discussing medications with a patient. You must ultimately rely on your own discretion, experience and judgment in diagnosing, treating and advising patients.

Related Information

Oral Medications That Should Not Be Crushed or Altered *on page 1712*

Niacin (NYE a sin)

Brand Names: U.S. Niacin-50 [OTC]; Niacor; Niaspan; Slo-Niacin [OTC]

Index Terms Nicotinic Acid; Vitamin B_3

Pharmacologic Category Antilipemic Agent, Miscellaneous; Vitamin, Water Soluble

Medication Safety Issues

Sound-alike/look-alike issues:

Niacin may be confused with Minocin, niacinamide, Niaspan

Pregnancy Risk Factor C

Lactation Enters breast milk/consider risk:benefit

Breast-Feeding Considerations Niacin is excreted in human breast milk. When used as a dietary supplement, niacin requirements may be increased in nursing women compared to nonnursing women (IOM, 1998). Because lipid-lowering doses of niacin may cause serious adverse reactions in nursing infants, a decision should be made whether to discontinue nursing or discontinue the drug, taking into account the importance of the drug to the mother.

Use Treatment of dyslipidemias (Fredrickson types IIa and IIb or primary hypercholesterolemia) as mono- or adjunctive therapy; to lower the risk of recurrent MI in patients with a history of MI and hyperlipidemia; to slow progression or promote regression of coronary artery disease; treatment of hypertriglyceridemia in patients at risk of pancreatitis; dietary supplement

Unlabeled Use Treatment of pellagra

Mechanism of Action/Effect Component of two coenzymes which is necessary for tissue respiration, lipid metabolism, and glycogenolysis; inhibits the synthesis of very low density lipoproteins (VLDL) and low density lipoproteins (LDL); may also increase the rate of chylomicron triglyceride removal from plasma

Contraindications Hypersensitivity to niacin, niacinamide, or any component of the formulation; active hepatic disease or significant or unexplained persistent elevations in hepatic transaminases; active peptic ulcer; arterial hemorrhage

Warnings/Precautions Prior to initiation, secondary causes for hypercholesterolemia (eg, poorly controlled diabetes mellitus, hypothyroidism) should be excluded; management with diet and other nonpharmacologic measures (eg, exercise or weight reduction) should be attempted prior to initiation. Use has not been evaluated in Fredrickson type I or III dyslipidemias. Use with caution in patients with unstable angina or MI, renal disease, active gallbladder disease (can exacerbate), or with anticoagulants (may slightly increase prothrombin time). In patients with pre-existing coronary artery disease, the incidence of atrial fibrillation was observed more frequently in those receiving immediate release (crystalline) niacin as compared to placebo (Coronary Drug Project Research Group, 1975). Niacin should not be used if patient experiences new-onset atrial fibrillation during therapy (Stone, 2013). Use with caution in patients with diabetes (may interfere with glucose control); niacin should not be used if patient experiences persistent hyperglycemia during therapy (Stone, 2013). Use with caution in patients with gout; niacin should not be used if patient experiences acute gout during therapy (Stone, 2013).

Use with caution in patients with a past history of hepatic impairment and/or who consume substantial amounts of ethanol; contraindicated with active liver disease or unexplained persistent transaminase elevation. Niacin should not be used if hepatic transaminase elevations >2-3 times upper limit of normal occur during therapy (Stone, 2013). Rare cases of rhabdomyolysis have occurred during concomitant use with HMG-CoA reductase inhibitors. With concurrent use or if symptoms suggestive of myopathy occur, monitor creatine phosphokinase (CPK) and potassium; use with caution in patients with renal impairment, inadequately treated hypothyroidism, patients with diabetes or the elderly; risk for myopathy and rhabdomyolysis may be increased. May cause gastrointestinal distress, vomiting, diarrhea, or aggravate peptic ulcer. Use is contraindicated in patients with active peptic ulcer disease. Niacin should not be used if patient experiences unexplained abdominal pain or gastrointestinal symptoms or unexplained weight loss during therapy (Stone, 2013).

Immediate and extended or sustained release products are not interchangeable. Cases of severe hepatotoxicity have occurred when immediate release (crystalline) niacin products have been substituted with sustained-release (modified release, timed-release) niacin products at equivalent doses. Patients should be initiated with low doses (eg, 500 mg at bedtime) with titration to achieve desired response. Flushing and pruritus, common adverse effects of niacin, may be attenuated with a gradual increase in dose, and/or by taking aspirin (adults: 325 mg) or an NSAID 30 minutes before dosing (Stone, 2013). May also use other NSAIDs according to the manufacturer. Flushing associated with extended-release preparation is significantly reduced (Guyton, 2007). Compliance is enhanced with twice-daily dosing (extended-release product excluded). Niacin should not be used if patient experiences persistent severe cutaneous symptoms during therapy (Stone, 2013).

Drug Interactions

Avoid Concomitant Use There are no known interactions where it is recommended to avoid concomitant use.

Decreased Effect

The levels/effects of Niacin may be decreased by: Bile Acid Sequestrants

Increased Effect/Toxicity

Niacin may increase the levels/effects of: HMG-CoA Reductase Inhibitors

The levels/effects of Niacin may be increased by: Alcohol (Ethyl)

Nutritional/Ethanol Interactions Ethanol: Avoid heavy use; avoid use around niacin dose.

Adverse Reactions Frequency not defined.

Cardiovascular: Arrhythmias, atrial fibrillation, edema, flushing, hypotension, orthostasis, palpitation, syncope (rare), tachycardia

Central nervous system: Chills, dizziness, headache, insomnia, migraine, nervousness, pain

Dermatologic: Acanthosis nigricans, burning skin, dry skin, hyperpigmentation, maculopapular rash, pruritus, rash, skin discoloration, urticaria

Endocrine & metabolic: Glucose tolerance decreased, gout, phosphorous levels decreased, hyperuricemia

Gastrointestinal: Abdominal pain, amylase increased, diarrhea, dyspepsia, eructation, flatulence, nausea, peptic ulcers, vomiting

Hematologic: Platelet counts decreased

Hepatic: Hepatic necrosis (rare), hepatitis, jaundice, transaminases increased (dose-related), prothrombin time increased, total bilirubin increased

Neuromuscular & skeletal: CPK increased, leg cramps, myalgia, myasthenia, myopathy (with concurrent HMG-CoA reductase inhibitor), paresthesia, rhabdomyolysis (with concurrent HMG-CoA reductase inhibitor; rare), weakness

Ocular: Blurred vision, cystoid macular edema, toxic amblyopia

Respiratory: Cough, dyspnea

Miscellaneous: Diaphoresis, hypersensitivity reactions (rare; includes anaphylaxis, angioedema, laryngismus, vesiculobullous rash), LDH increased

Available Dosage Forms

Capsule Extended Release, Oral:
Generic: 250 mg, 500 mg

Capsule Extended Release, Oral [preservative free]:
Generic: 250 mg, 500 mg

Tablet, Oral:
Niacin-50 [OTC]: 50 mg
Niacor: 500 mg
Generic: 50 mg, 100 mg, 250 mg, 500 mg

Tablet, Oral [preservative free]:
Generic: 50 mg, 100 mg, 500 mg

Tablet Extended Release, Oral:
Niaspan: 500 mg, 750 mg, 1000 mg
Slo-Niacin [OTC]: 250 mg, 500 mg, 750 mg
Generic: 500 mg, 750 mg, 1000 mg

Tablet Extended Release, Oral [preservative free]:
Generic: 250 mg, 500 mg, 1000 mg

General Dosage Range Oral:
Extended release: *Adults:* 500 mg to 2 g once daily
Regular release: *Adults:* 100-250 mg daily in 1-2 divided doses **or** 1.5-6 g daily in 2-3 divided doses (maximum dose: 6 g daily in 3 divided doses)
Sustained release: *Adults:* Usual: 1-2 g daily

Administration

Oral Administer with food. To attenuate flushing symptoms, may premedicate with aspirin 325 mg administered 30 minutes before dose; avoid ingestion of hot liquids or alcohol concurrently with niacin (Stone, 2013). May also use other NSAIDs to prevent flushing according to the manufacturer.

Niaspan: Administer at bedtime. Tablet strengths are not interchangeable. When switching from immediate release tablet, initiate Niaspan at lower dose and titrate. If therapy is interrupted for an extended period, dose should be retitrated.

◄ Long-acting forms should not be crushed, broken, or chewed. Slo-Niacin may be broken along the score line. Do not substitute long-acting forms for immediate release ones.

Storage/Stability
Niaspan: Store at room temperature of 20°C to 25°C (68°F to 77°F).
Niacor: Store at controlled room temperature of 15°C to 30°C (59°F to 86°F).

Nursing Actions
Physical Assessment Monitor for signs/symptoms of myopathy (muscle weakness or pain, fatigue), nausea, vomiting, loss of appetite, decrease in urine output especially with dark urine, irregular heartbeat, or blurry vision. Monitor for flushing, which is a common side effect usually seen with initiation of medication and increase in dosage.

Patient Education
- Discuss specific use of drug and side effects with patient as it relates to treatment. (HCAHPS: During this hospital stay, were you given any medicine that you had not taken before? Before giving you any new medicine, how often did hospital staff tell you what the medicine was for? How often did hospital staff describe possible side effects in a way you could understand?)
- Patient may experience flushing or headache. Have patient report immediately to prescriber inability to eat, ecchymosis, bleeding, jaundice, or rash (HCAHPS).
- Educate patient about signs of a significant reaction (eg, wheezing; chest tightness; fever; itching; bad cough; blue skin color; seizures; or swelling of face, lips, tongue, or throat). **Note:** This is not a comprehensive list of all side effects. Patient should consult prescriber for additional questions.

Intended Use and Disclaimer: Should not be printed and given to patients. This information is intended to serve as a concise initial reference for healthcare professionals to use when discussing medications with a patient. You must ultimately rely on your own discretion, experience and judgment in diagnosing, treating and advising patients.

Dietary Considerations Should be taken with meal; low-fat meal if treating hyperlipidemia. Avoid hot drinks around the time of niacin dose.

Related Information
Oral Medications That Should Not Be Crushed or Altered *on page 1712*

Niacin and Simvastatin
(NYE a sin & sim va STAT in)

Brand Names: U.S. Simcor®
Index Terms Simvastatin and Niacin
Pharmacologic Category Antilipemic Agent, HMG-CoA Reductase Inhibitor; Antilipemic Agent, Miscellaneous

Pregnancy Risk Factor X
Use Reduce total cholesterol, LDL, Apo B, non-HDL, TG, and/or increase HDL in patients with primary hypercholesterolemia, mixed dyslipidemia, or hypertriglyceridemia in combination with standard cholesterol-lowering diet when simvastatin or niacin monotherapy is inadequate

Available Dosage Forms
Tablet, variable release, oral:
Simcor®: 500/20: Niacin 500 mg [extended release] and simvastatin 20 mg [immediate release]; 500/40: Niacin 500 mg [extended release] and simvastatin 40 mg [immediate release]; 750/20: Niacin 750 mg [extended release] and simvastatin 20 mg [immediate release]; 1000/20: Niacin 1000 mg [extended release] and simvastatin 20 mg [immediate release]; 1000/40: Niacin 1000 mg [extended release] and simvastatin 40 mg [immediate release]

General Dosage Range Oral: *Adults:* Niacin 500-2000 mg/simvastatin 20-40 mg once daily

Administration
Oral Tablets must be swallowed whole; do not crush or chew. Administer with a low-fat snack at bedtime.

Nursing Actions
Physical Assessment See individual agents.

Patient Education
- Discuss specific use of drug and side effects with patient as it relates to treatment. (HCAHPS: During this hospital stay, were you given any medicine that you had not taken before? Before giving you any new medicine, how often did hospital staff tell you what the medicine was for? How often did hospital staff describe possible side effects in a way you could understand?
- Patient may experience headache, dizziness, nausea, diarrhea, or back pain. Have patient report immediately to prescriber signs of hepatic impairment, signs of pancreatitis, melena, myalgia, arthralgia, paresthesia, illogical thinking, memory loss, depression, sexual dysfunction, vision changes, tachycardia, arrhythmia, ecchymosis, bleeding, considerable asthenia, dyspnea, hyperhidrosis, edema, urinary retention, pharyngitis, lack of appetite, emesis, or insomnia (HCAHPS).
- Educate patient about signs of a significant reaction (eg, wheezing; chest tightness; fever; itching; bad cough; blue skin color; seizures; or swelling of face, lips, tongue, or throat). **Note:** This is not a comprehensive list of all side effects. Patient should consult prescriber for additional questions.

Intended Use and Disclaimer: Should not be printed and given to patients. This information is intended to serve as a concise initial reference for healthcare professionals to use when discussing medications with a patient. You must ultimately

rely on your own discretion, experience and judgment in diagnosing, treating and advising patients.

Related Information

Niacin *on page 1116*

Simvastatin *on page 1414*

NiCARdipine (nye KAR de peen)

Brand Names: U.S. Cardene IV; Cardene SR

Index Terms Nicardipine Hydrochloride

Pharmacologic Category Antianginal Agent; Antihypertensive; Calcium Channel Blocker; Calcium Channel Blocker, Dihydropyridine

Medication Safety Issues

Sound-alike/look-alike issues:

NiCARdipine may be confused with niacinamide, NIFEdipine, niMODipine

Cardene may be confused with Cardizem, Cardura, codeine

Administration issues:

Significant differences exist between oral and I.V. dosing. Use caution when converting from one route of administration to another.

International issues:

Cardene [U.S., Great Britain, Netherlands] may be confused with Cardem brand name for celiprolol [Spain]; Cardin brand name for simvastatin [Poland]

Pregnancy Risk Factor C

Lactation Enters breast milk

Breast-Feeding Considerations Nicardipine is minimally excreted into breast milk. Per the manufacturer, the possibility of infant exposure should be considered. In one study, peak milk concentrations ranged from 1.9-18.8 mcg/mL following oral maternal doses of 40-150 mg/day. The estimated exposure to the breast-feeding infant was calculated to be 0.073% of the weight-adjusted maternal oral dose or 0.14% of the weight-adjusted maternal I.V. dose. Adverse events were not noted in the infants. Breast-fed infants of mothers taking medications for hypertension should be monitored for adverse effects (Chobanian, 2003).

Use Chronic stable angina (immediate-release product only); management of hypertension (immediate and sustained release products); parenteral only for short-term use when oral treatment is not feasible

Unlabeled Use Control of blood pressure in acute ischemic stroke and spontaneous intracranial hemorrhage, postoperative hypertension associated with carotid endarterectomy, perioperative hypertension, prevention of migraine headaches, subarachnoid hemorrhage associated cerebral vasospasm

Mechanism of Action/Effect Inhibits calcium ion from entering the "slow channels" or select voltage-sensitive areas of vascular smooth muscle and myocardium during depolarization, producing a relaxation of coronary vascular smooth muscle and coronary vasodilation; increases myocardial oxygen delivery in patients with vasospastic angina

Contraindications Hypersensitivity to nicardipine or any component of the formulation; advanced aortic stenosis

Warnings/Precautions Symptomatic hypotension with or without syncope can rarely occur; blood pressure must be lowered at a rate appropriate for the patient's clinical condition. Close monitoring of blood pressure and heart rate is required. Reflex tachycardia may occur resulting in angina and/or MI in patients with obstructive coronary disease especially in the absence of concurrent beta blockade. The most common side effect is peripheral edema (dose-dependent); occurs within 2-3 weeks of starting therapy. Use with caution in CAD (can cause increase in angina), aortic stenosis (may reduce coronary perfusion resulting in ischemia; use is contraindicated in patients with advanced aortic stenosis), and hypertrophic cardiomyopathy with outflow tract obstruction. The ACCF/AHA heart failure guidelines recommend to avoid use in patients with heart failure due to lack of benefit and/or worse outcomes with calcium channel blockers in general (Yancy, 2013). To minimize infusion site reactions, peripheral infusion sites (for I.V. therapy) should be changed every 12 hours; use of small peripheral veins should be avoided. Titrate I.V. dose cautiously in patients with renal or hepatic dysfunction. Use the I.V. form cautiously in patients with portal hypertension (can cause increase in hepatic pressure gradient). Initiate at the low end of the dosage range in the elderly.

Drug Interactions

Avoid Concomitant Use

Avoid concomitant use of NiCARdipine with any of the following: Ado-Trastuzumab Emtansine; Alfuzosin; Apixaban; Avanafil; Axitinib; Bosutinib; Cabozantinib; Conivaptan; Crizotinib; Dronedarone; Eplerenone; Everolimus; Fusidic Acid (Systemic); Halofantrine; Ibrutinib; Imatinib; Ivabradine; Lapatinib; Lomitapide; Lovastatin; Lurasidone; Macitentan; Nilotinib; Nisoldipine; Pimozide; Pomalidomide; Ranolazine; Red Yeast Rice; Regorafenib; Rivaroxaban; Salmeterol; Silodosin; Simeprevir; Simvastatin; Tamsulosin; Thioridazine; Ticagrelor; Tolvaptan; Topotecan; Toremifene; Ulipristal; Vemurafenib; VinCRIStine (Liposomal)

Decreased Effect

NiCARdipine may decrease the levels/effects of: Clopidogrel; Codeine; Ifosfamide; Prasugrel; QuiNIDine; Tamoxifen; Ticagrelor; TraMADol

The levels/effects of NiCARdipine may be decreased by: Barbiturates; Calcium Salts; CarBAMazepine; CYP3A4 Inducers (Strong); Dabrafenib; Deferasirox; Herbs (CYP3A4 Inducers); Herbs (Hypertensive Properties); Melatonin;

Methylphenidate; Mitotane; Nafcillin; Peginterferon Alfa-2b; P-glycoprotein/ABCB1 Inducers; Rifamycin Derivatives; Tocilizumab; Yohimbine

Increased Effect/Toxicity

NiCARdipine may increase the levels/effects of: Ado-Trastuzumab Emtansine; Afatinib; Alfuzosin; Almotriptan; Alosetron; Amifostine; Antihypertensives; Apixaban; ARIPiprazole; Atosiban; Avanafil; Axitinib; Bedaquiline; Beta-Blockers; Bortezomib; Bosentan; Bosutinib; Brentuximab Vedotin; Brinzolamide; Budesonide (Nasal); Budesonide (Systemic, Oral Inhalation); Cabozantinib; Calcium Channel Blockers (Nondihydropyridine); Carvedilol; Citalopram; Colchicine; Conivaptan; Corticosteroids (Orally Inhaled); Crizotinib; CYP2C19 Substrates; CYP2C9 Substrates; CYP2D6 Substrates; CYP3A4 Substrates; Dabigatran Etexilate; Diclofenac (Systemic); Dienogest; Dofetilide; DOXOrubicin (Conventional); Dronedarone; DULoxetine; Dutasteride; Enzalutamide; Eplerenone; Everolimus; FentaNYL; Fesoterodine; Fluticasone (Nasal); Fluticasone (Oral Inhalation); Fosphenytoin; GuanFACINE; Halofantrine; Highest Risk QTc-Prolonging Agents; Hypotensive Agents; Ibrutinib; Iloperidone; Imatinib; Ivabradine; Ivacaftor; Ixabepilone; Lacosamide; Lapatinib; Levomilnacipran; Lomitapide; Lovastatin; Lumefantrine; Lurasidone; Macitentan; Magnesium Salts; Maraviroc; MethylPREDNISolone; Metoprolol; Mifepristone; Moderate Risk QTc-Prolonging Agents; Neuromuscular-Blocking Agents (Nondepolarizing); Nilotinib; Nisoldipine; Nitroprusside; Obinutuzumab; Ospemifene; OxyCODONE; Paricalcitol; PAZOPanib; P-glycoprotein/ABCB1 Substrates; Phenytoin; Pimecrolimus; Pimozide; Pomalidomide; PONATinib; Propafenone; Propranolol; Prucalopride; QUEtiapine; QuiNIDine; Ranolazine; Red Yeast Rice; Regorafenib; Repaglinide; Rilpivirine; RiTUXimab; Rivaroxaban; RomiDEPsin; Ruxolitinib; Salmeterol; Saxagliptin; Sildenafil; Silodosin; Simeprevir; Simvastatin; SORAfenib; Tacrolimus (Systemic); Tadalafil; Tamsulosin; Thioridazine; Ticagrelor; Tofacitinib; Tolterodine; Tolvaptan; Topotecan; Toremifene; Ulipristal; Vardenafil; Vemurafenib; Vilazodone; VinCRIStine (Liposomal); Zuclopenthixol

The levels/effects of NiCARdipine may be increased by: Alpha1-Blockers; Antifungal Agents (Azole Derivatives, Systemic); Brimonidine (Topical); Calcium Channel Blockers (Nondihydropyridine); CycloSPORINE (Systemic); CYP3A4 Inhibitors (Moderate); CYP3A4 Inhibitors (Strong); Dasatinib; Diazoxide; Fluconazole; Fusidic Acid (Systemic); Grapefruit Juice; Herbs (Hypotensive Properties); Luliconazole; Macrolide Antibiotics; Magnesium Salts; MAO Inhibitors; Pentoxifylline; P-glycoprotein/ABCB1 Inhibitors; Prostacyclin Analogues; Protease Inhibitors; QuiNIDine; Stiripentol

Nutritional/Ethanol Interactions

Ethanol: Ethanol may increase CNS depression. Management: Avoid ethanol.

Food: Nicardipine average peak concentrations may be decreased if taken with food. Serum concentrations/toxicity of nicardipine may be increased by grapefruit juice. Management: Avoid grapefruit juice.

Herb/Nutraceutical: St John's wort may decrease levels. Some herbal medications may worsen hypertension (eg, licorice); others may increase the antihypertensive effect of nicardipine (eg, shepherd's purse). Management: Avoid St John's wort. Avoid bayberry, blue cohosh, cayenne, ephedra, ginger, ginseng (American), kola, licorice, and yohimbe. Avoid black cohosh, California poppy, coleus, golden seal, hawthorn, mistletoe, periwinkle, quinine, and shepherd's purse.

Adverse Reactions 1% to 10%:

Cardiovascular: Cardiovascular: Flushing (6% to 10%), peripheral edema (dose related; 6% to 8%), hypotension (I.V. 6%), increased angina (dose related; 6%), palpitation (3% to 4%), tachycardia (1% to 4%), vasodilation (1% to 5%), chest pain (I.V. 1%), ECG abnormal (I.V. 1%), extrasystoles (I.V. 1%), hemopericardium (I.V. 1%), hypertension (I.V. 1%), orthostasis (1%), supraventricular tachycardia (I.V. 1%), syncope (1%), ventricular extrasystoles (I.V. 1%), ventricular tachycardia (I.V. 1%)

Central nervous system: Headache (6% to 15%), dizziness (1% to 7%), hypoesthesia (1%), intracranial hemorrhage (1%) pain (1%), somnolence (1%)

Dermatologic: Rash (1%)

Endocrine & metabolic: Hypokalemia (I.V. 1%)

Gastrointestinal: Nausea (2% to 5%), vomiting (I.V. 5%), dyspepsia (oral 2%), abdominal pain (I.V. 1%), dry mouth (1%)

Genitourinary: Polyuria (1%)

Local: Injection site pain (I.V. 1%), injection site reaction (I.V. 1%)

Neuromuscular & skeletal: Weakness (1% to 6%), myalgia (1%), paresthesia (1%)

Renal: Hematuria (1%)

Respiratory: Dyspnea (1%)

Miscellaneous: Diaphoresis (1%)

Pharmacodynamics/Kinetics

Onset of Action Oral: 0.5-2 hours; I.V.: 10 minutes; Hypotension: ~20 minutes

Duration of Action I.V.: ≤8 hours; Oral: Immediate release capsules: ≤8 hours, Sustained release capsules: 8-12 hours

Available Dosage Forms

Capsule, Oral:
Generic: 20 mg, 30 mg

Capsule Extended Release 12 Hour, Oral:
Cardene SR: 30 mg, 60 mg

Solution, Intravenous:
Cardene IV: 20 mg (200 mL); 40 mg (200 mL); 2.5 mg/mL (10 mL)
Generic: 2.5 mg/mL (10 mL)
General Dosage Range Dosage adjustment recommended in patients with hepatic or renal impairment
I.V.: *Adults:* Initial: 5 mg/hour; Maintenance: 3-15 mg/hour
Oral:
Immediate release: *Adults:* Initial: 20 mg 3 times/day; Maintenance: 20-40 mg 3 times/day
Sustained release: *Adults:* Initial: 30 mg twice daily; Maintenance: Up to 60 mg twice daily
Usual Infusion Concentrations: Pediatric
Note: Premixed solutions available
I.V. infusion: 100 mcg/mL or 500 mcg/mL
Usual Infusion Concentrations: Adult Note: Premixed solutions available
I.V. infusion: 25 mg in 250 mL (total volume) (concentration: 0.1 mg/mL) **or** 25 mg in 50 mL (total volume) (concentration: 0.5 mg/mL) of D_5W or NS
Administration
I.V.
Vials must be diluted before use. Administer as a slow continuous infusion at a concentration of 0.1 mg/mL or 0.2 mg/mL. Peripheral venous irritation may be minimized by changing the site of infusion every 12 hours. Concentrations of 0.5 mg/mL may be administered via a central line only.
Premixed bags: No further dilution needed. For single use only, discard any unused portion. Use only if solution is clear; the manufacturer recommends not to admix or run in the same line as other medications.
Injectable Detail pH: Vial: 3.5; Premixed bag: 3.7-4.7
Oral The total daily dose of immediate-release product may not automatically be equivalent to the daily sustained-release dose; use caution in converting. Do not chew or crush the sustained release formulation, swallow whole. Do not open or cut capsules.
Preparation for Administration I.V.: Vial: Dilute 25 mg vial with 240 mL of compatible solution to provide a 250 mL total volume solution and a final concentration of 0.1 mg/mL.
Storage/Stability
I.V.:
Premixed bags: Store at controlled room temperature of 20°C to 25°C (68°F to 77°F). Protect from light and excessive heat. Do not freeze.
Vials: Store at controlled room temperature of 20°C to 25°C (68°F to 77°F). Protect from light. Diluted solution (0.1 mg/mL) is stable at room temperature for 24 hours in glass or PVC containers. Stability has also been demonstrated at room temperature at concentrations up to 0.5 mg/mL in PVC containers for 24 hours or

in glass containers for up to 7 days (Baaske, 1996).
Oral (Cardene®, Cardene SR®): Store at 15°C to 30°C (59°F to 86°F). Protect from light. Freezing does not affect stability.
Nursing Actions
Physical Assessment Infusion site must be monitored closely to prevent extravasation; peripheral infusion sites should be changed every 12 hours. Evaluate cardiac status and blood pressure and monitor for rash, hypotension, bradycardia, confusion, and nausea when starting, adjusting dose, or discontinuing. Teach patient orthostatic precautions.
Patient Education
• Discuss specific use of drug and side effects with patient as it relates to treatment. (HCAHPS: During this hospital stay, were you given any medicine that you had not taken before? Before giving you any new medicine, how often did hospital staff tell you what the medicine was for? How often did hospital staff describe possible side effects in a way you could understand?
• Patient may experience dizziness, flushing, edema, headache, or injection site irritation. Have patient report immediately to prescriber tachycardia, dyspnea, or rash (HCAHPS).
• Educate patient about signs of a significant reaction (eg, wheezing; chest tightness; fever; itching; bad cough; blue skin color; seizures; or swelling of face, lips, tongue, or throat). **Note:** This is not a comprehensive list of all side effects. Patient should consult prescriber for additional questions.

Intended Use and Disclaimer: Should not be printed and given to patients. This information is intended to serve as a concise initial reference for healthcare professionals to use when discussing medications with a patient. You must ultimately rely on your own discretion, experience and judgment in diagnosing, treating and advising patients.
Dietary Considerations Avoid grapefruit juice.
Related Information
Oral Medications That Should Not Be Crushed or Altered *on page 1712*

Nicotine (nik oh TEEN)

Brand Names: U.S. Nicoderm CQ [OTC]; Nicorelief [OTC]; NICOrelief [OTC] [DSC]; Nicorette Mini [OTC]; Nicorette Starter Kit [OTC]; Nicorette [OTC]; Nicotrol; Nicotrol NS; Thrive [OTC]
Index Terms Habitrol; Nicotine Patch
Pharmacologic Category Smoking Cessation Aid

Medication Safety Issues

Sound-alike/look-alike issues:
NicoDerm may be confused with Nitroderm
Nicorette may be confused with Nordette

Other safety concerns:
Transdermal patch may contain conducting metal (eg, aluminum); remove patch prior to MRI.

Pregnancy Risk Factor D (nasal)

Lactation Excretion in breast milk unknown/use caution

Use Smoking cessation: Treatment to aid smoking cessation for the relief of nicotine withdrawal symptoms (including nicotine craving)

Unlabeled Use Management of ulcerative colitis (transdermal)

Available Dosage Forms

Gum, Mouth/Throat:
Nicorelief [OTC]: 2 mg (50 ea, 110 ea); 4 mg (50 ea, 110 ea)
Nicorette [OTC]: 2 mg (20 ea, 40 ea, 100 ea, 110 ea, 160 ea, 170 ea, 190 ea, 200 ea); 4 mg (20 ea, 40 ea, 100 ea, 110 ea, 160 ea, 170 ea, 190 ea, 200 ea)
Nicorette Starter Kit [OTC]: 2 mg (100 ea, 110 ea); 4 mg (110 ea)
Thrive [OTC]: 2 mg (100 ea, 110 ea); 4 mg (100 ea, 110 ea)
Generic: 2 mg (20 ea, 40 ea, 50 ea, 100 ea, 110 ea); 4 mg (20 ea, 40 ea, 50 ea, 100 ea, 110 ea)

Inhaler, Inhalation:
Nicotrol: 10 mg (168 ea)

Kit, Transdermal:
Generic: 21 mg/24 hr; 14 mg/24 hr; 7 mg/24 hr

Lozenge, Mouth/Throat:
Nicorette [OTC]: 2 mg (72 ea, 81 ea, 108 ea, 168 ea); 4 mg (72 ea, 81 ea, 108 ea, 168 ea)
Nicorette Mini [OTC]: 2 mg (81 ea, 135 ea); 4 mg (81 ea, 135 ea)
Generic: 2 mg (72 ea); 4 mg (72 ea)

Patch 24 Hour, Transdermal:
Nicoderm CQ [OTC]: 7 mg/24 hr (14 ea); 14 mg/24 hr (14 ea, 21 ea); 21 mg/24 hr (7 ea, 14 ea, 21 ea)
Generic: 7 mg/24 hr (7 ea, 14 ea); 14 mg/24 hr (7 ea, 14 ea); 21 mg/24 hr (7 ea, 14 ea, 28 ea)

Solution, Nasal:
Nicotrol NS: 10 mg/mL (10 mL)

General Dosage Range Dosage adjustment recommended for transdermal route in patients on concomitant therapy

Inhalation:
Nasal: *Adults:* 1-2 sprays/hour (maximum: 10 sprays/hour; 80 sprays/day)
Oral: *Adults:* Usually 6 to 16 cartridges per day; best effect was achieved by frequent continuous puffing (20 minutes)

Oral: *Adults:* 2 mg or 4 mg every 1-2 hours (weeks 1-6); every 2-4 hours (weeks 7-9); and every 4-8 hours (weeks 10-12) (maximum: 24 pieces gum/day; 20 lozenges/day)

Transdermal:
Patients smoking >10 cigarettes/day: Begin with **step 1** (21 mg/day) for 6 weeks, followed by **step 2** (14 mg/day) for 2 weeks; finish with **step 3** (7 mg/day) for 2 weeks
Patients smoking ≤10 cigarettes/day: Begin with **step 2** (14 mg/day) for 6 weeks, followed by **step 3** (7 mg/day) for 2 weeks

Administration

Oral

Gum: Should be chewed slowly to avoid jaw ache and to maximize benefit. Chew slowly until it tingles, then park gum between cheek and gum until tingle is gone; repeat process until most of tingle is gone (~30 minutes).

Lozenge: Should not be chewed or swallowed; allow to dissolve slowly (~20-30 minutes)

Hazardous agent; use appropriate precautions for handling and disposal (EPA, P-listed).

Topical Apply new patch to nonhairy, clean, dry skin on the upper body or upper outer arm; each patch should be applied to a different site. Apply immediately after removing backing from patch; press onto skin for ~10 seconds. Patch may be worn for 16 or 24 hours. If cigarette cravings occur upon awakening, wear for 24 hours; if vivid dreams or other sleep disturbances occur, remove the patch at bedtime and apply a new patch in the morning. Do not cut patch; causes rapid evaporation, rendering the patch useless. Do not wear more than 1 patch at a time; do not leave patch on for more than 24 hours. Wash hands after applying or removing patch.

Hazardous agent; use appropriate precautions for handling and disposal (EPA, P-listed).

Inhalation

Nasal spray: Prime pump prior to first use (pump 6-8 times until fine spray appears) or if it has not been used for 24 hours (pump 1-2 times). Blow nose prior to use. Tilt head back slightly and insert tip of bottle into nostril. Breathe through mouth and spray once in each nostril. Do not sniff, swallow, or inhale through the nose during administration. After administration, wait 2-3 minutes before blowing nose.

Oral inhalant: Insert cartridge into inhaler and push hard until it pops into place. Replace mouthpiece and twist the top and bottom so that markings do not line up. Inhale deeply into the back of the throat or puff in short breaths. Nicotine in cartridge is used up after about 20 minutes of active puffing.

Hazardous agent; use appropriate precautions for handling and disposal (EPA, P-listed).

Nursing Actions

Physical Assessment Monitor cardiac status and vital signs prior to, when beginning, and periodically during therapy.

Patient Education

- Discuss specific use of drug and side effects with patient as it relates to treatment. (HCAHPS: During this hospital stay, were you given any medicine that you had not taken before? Before giving you any new medicine, how often did hospital staff tell you what the medicine was for? How often did hospital staff describe possible side effects in a way you could understand?
- Patient may experience hiccups, insomnia, nervousness and anxiety, headache, nausea, jaw ache, stomatitis, skin irritation, or rhinitis. Have patient report immediately to prescriber rash (HCAHPS).
- Educate patient about signs of a significant reaction (eg, wheezing; chest tightness; fever; itching; bad cough; blue skin color; seizures; or swelling of face, lips, tongue, or throat). **Note:** This is not a comprehensive list of all side effects. Patient should consult prescriber for additional questions.

Intended Use and Disclaimer: Should not be printed and given to patients. This information is intended to serve as a concise initial reference for healthcare professionals to use when discussing medications with a patient. You must ultimately rely on your own discretion, experience and judgment in diagnosing, treating and advising patients.

Related Information

Oral Medications That Should Not Be Crushed or Altered *on page 1712*

NIFEdipine (nye FED i peen)

Brand Names: U.S. Adalat CC; Afeditab CR; Nifediac CC; Nifedical XL; Procardia; Procardia XL

Pharmacologic Category Antianginal Agent; Antihypertensive; Calcium Channel Blocker; Calcium Channel Blocker, Dihydropyridine

Medication Safety Issues

Sound-alike/look-alike issues:

NIFEdipine may be confused with niCARdipine, niMODipine, nisoldipine

Procardia XL may be confused with Cartia XT

BEERS Criteria medication:

This drug may be potentially inappropriate for use in geriatric patients (Quality of evidence - high; Strength of recommendation - strong).

International issues:

Depin [India] may be confused with Depen brand name for penicillamine [U.S.]; Depon brand name for acetaminophen [Greece]; Dipen brand name for diltiazem [Greece]

Nipin [Italy and Singapore] may be confused with Nipent brand name for pentostatin [U.S., Canada, and multiple international markets]

Pregnancy Risk Factor C

Lactation Enters breast milk/not recommended

Use Management of chronic stable or vasospastic angina; treatment of hypertension (sustained release products only)

Unlabeled Use Management of pulmonary hypertension, preterm labor, and Raynaud's phenomenon; prevention and treatment of high altitude pulmonary edema

Available Dosage Forms

Capsule, Oral:

Procardia: 10 mg

Generic: 10 mg, 20 mg

Tablet Extended Release 24 Hour, Oral:

Adalat CC: 30 mg, 60 mg, 90 mg

Afeditab CR: 30 mg, 60 mg

Nifediac CC: 30 mg, 60 mg, 90 mg

Nifedical XL: 30 mg, 60 mg

Procardia XL: 30 mg, 60 mg, 90 mg

Generic: 30 mg, 60 mg, 90 mg

General Dosage Range Oral:

Immediate release: *Adults:* Initial: 10 mg 3-4 times/day (maximum: 180 mg/day)

Extended release: *Adults:* Initial: 30 mg once daily; Maintenance: 30-60 mg once daily (maximum: 120-180 mg/day)

Administration

Oral

Immediate release: In general, may be administered with or without food.

Extended release: Tablets should be swallowed whole; do not crush, split, or chew.

Adalat® CC, Afeditab® CR, Nifediac CC®: Administer on an empty stomach (per manufacturer). Other extended release products may not have this recommendation; consult product labeling.

Nursing Actions

Physical Assessment Monitor for hypotension, peripheral edema, and constipation when starting, adjusting dose, or discontinuing. Teach patient orthostatic precautions.

Patient Education

- Discuss specific use of drug and side effects with patient as it relates to treatment. (HCAHPS: During this hospital stay, were you given any medicine that you had not taken before? Before giving you any new medicine, how often did hospital staff tell you what the medicine was for? How often did hospital staff describe possible side effects in a way you could understand?
- Patient may experience tablet shell in stool, dizziness, flushing, headache, nausea, constipation, or edema. Have patient report immediately to prescriber tachycardia, dyspnea, severe asthenia, or rash (HCAHPS).
- Educate patient about signs of a significant reaction (eg, wheezing; chest tightness; fever; itching; bad cough; blue skin color; seizures; or swelling of face, lips, tongue, or throat). **Note:** This is not a comprehensive list of all side effects. Patient should consult prescriber for additional questions.

Intended Use and Disclaimer: Should not be printed and given to patients. This information is intended to serve as a concise initial reference for healthcare professionals to use when discussing medications with a patient. You must ultimately rely on your own discretion, experience and judgment in diagnosing, treating and advising patients.

Related Information

Oral Medications That Should Not Be Crushed or Altered *on page 1712*

Nilotinib (nye LOE ti nib)

Brand Names: U.S. Tasigna

Index Terms AMN107; Nilotinib Hydrochloride Monohydrate

Pharmacologic Category Antineoplastic Agent, BCR-ABL Tyrosine Kinase Inhibitor; Antineoplastic Agent, Tyrosine Kinase Inhibitor

Medication Safety Issues

Sound-alike/look-alike issues:

Nilotinib may be confused with bosutinib, dasatinib, imatinib, nilutamide, PONATinib, SUNItinib, vandetanib

High alert medication:

This medication is in a class the Institute for Safe Medication Practices (ISMP) includes among its list of drug classes which have a heightened risk of causing significant patient harm when used in error.

Medication Guide Available Yes

Pregnancy Risk Factor D

Lactation Excretion in breast milk unknown/not recommended

Breast-Feeding Considerations It is not known if nilotinib is excreted in breast milk. Due to the potential for serious adverse reactions in the nursing infant, the decision to discontinue breast-feeding during therapy or to discontinue nilotinib should take into account the benefits of treatment to the mother.

Use Chronic myeloid leukemia (CML): Treatment of newly-diagnosed Philadelphia chromosome-positive CML (Ph+ CML) in chronic phase; treatment of chronic and accelerated phase Ph+ CML refractory or intolerant to prior therapy (including imatinib)

Unlabeled Use Treatment of refractory gastrointestinal stromal tumor (GIST)

Mechanism of Action/Effect Selective tyrosine kinase inhibitor that inhibits leukemic cell proliferation.

Contraindications Use in patients with hypokalemia, hypomagnesemia, or long QT syndrome

Canadian labeling: Additional contraindication (not in U.S. labeling): Hypersensitivity to nilotinib or any component of the formulation

Warnings/Precautions Hazardous agent - use appropriate precautions for handling and disposal

(NIOSH, 2012). **[U.S. Boxed Warnings]: May prolong the QT interval; sudden deaths have been reported. Use in patients with hypokalemia, hypomagnesemia, or long QT syndrome is contraindicated. Correct hypomagnesemia and hypokalemia prior to initiating therapy; monitor electrolytes periodically. Monitor ECG and QT$_c$ (baseline, at 7 days, with dose change, and periodically). Avoid the use of QT-prolonging agents.** Avoid concurrent use with antiarrhythmics and other drugs which may prolong QT interval; may increase the risk of potentially-fatal arrhythmias. Sudden deaths appear to be related to dose-dependent ventricular repolarization abnormalities. Prolonged QT interval may result in torsade de pointes, which may cause syncope, seizure, and/or death. Patients with uncontrolled or significant cardiovascular disease were excluded from studies. **[U.S. Boxed Warning]: Administer on an empty stomach, at least 1 hour before and 2 hours after food;** administration with food may prolong the QT$_c$. Potentially significant drug-drug/drug-food interactions may exist, requiring dose or frequency adjustment, additional monitoring, and/or selection of alternative therapy. **[U.S. Boxed Warning]: Avoid concurrent use with strong CYP3A4 inhibitors** (including grapefruit juice); interrupt nilotinib treatment if a strong CYP3A4 inhibitor is required; if coadministration cannot be avoided, consider nilotinib dose reductions. CYP3A4 inducers (including St John's wort) should also be avoided. Nilotinib solubility is decreased at higher pH; concurrent use with proton pump inhibitors is not recommended. If necessary, H$_2$-receptor blockers may be administered ~10 hours before and 2 hours after a nilotonib dose. Antacids (eg, aluminum hydroxide, magnesium hydroxide, simethicone) may be administered ~2 hours before or 2 hours after nilotinib.

Atherosclerosis-related events such as peripheral arterial occlusive disease, femoral artery stenosis, coronary artery stenosis, carotid artery stenosis, and cerebrovascular accident have been reported. Use caution in patients with pre-existing risk factors, and monitor for new or worsening symptoms suggestive of atherosclerotic events.

Dosage reduction is recommended in patients with hepatic impairment, along with close monitoring of the QT interval. Nilotinib metabolism is primarily hepatic (exposure is increased in patients with hepatic impairment). May cause hepatotoxicity, including dose-limiting elevations in bilirubin, transaminases, and alkaline phosphatase; monitor liver function. UGT1A1 polymorphisms may be a risk factor for increased toxicity (eg, hyperbilirubinemia) (Shibata, 2013).

Reversible myelosuppression, including grades 3 and 4 thrombocytopenia, neutropenia, and anemia may occur; may require dose reductions and/or treatment delay; monitor blood counts. Use with caution in patients with a history of pancreatitis, may cause dose-limiting elevations of serum lipase and amylase; monitor. In patients with abdominal symptoms in conjunction with lipase increases, withhold treatment and consider diagnostics to exclude pancreatitis. Tumor lysis syndrome (TLS) has been reported in patients with resistant or intolerant CML; the majority of cases had malignant disease progression, high WBC counts, and/or dehydration; maintain adequate hydration and treat high uric acid levels prior to nilotinib. Consider alternative therapy or a dosage increase (with more frequent monitoring) in patients with total gastrectomy (nilotinib exposure is reduced). Capsules contain lactose; do not use with galactose intolerance, severe lactase deficiency, or glucose-galactose malabsorption syndromes.

Drug Interactions

Avoid Concomitant Use

Avoid concomitant use of Nilotinib with any of the following: BCG; Bosutinib; CloZAPine; CYP3A4 Inducers (Strong); CYP3A4 Inhibitors (Strong); Fusidic Acid (Systemic); Highest Risk QTc-Prolonging Agents; Ivabradine; Mifepristone; Moderate Risk QTc-Prolonging Agents; Natalizumab; Pimecrolimus; Pomalidomide; Silodosin; Tacrolimus (Topical); Thioridazine; Tofacitinib; Topotecan; Vaccines (Live); VinCRIStine (Liposomal)

Decreased Effect

Nilotinib may decrease the levels/effects of: BCG; Cardiac Glycosides; Coccidioidin Skin Test; Codeine; Sipuleucel-T; Tamoxifen; TraMADol; Vaccines (Inactivated); Vaccines (Live); Vitamin K Antagonists

The levels/effects of Nilotinib may be decreased by: Antacids; Bosentan; CYP3A4 Inducers (Strong); Dabrafenib; Deferasirox; Echinacea; H2-Antagonists; Herbs (CYP3A4 Inducers); Proton Pump Inhibitors; Tocilizumab

Increased Effect/Toxicity

Nilotinib may increase the levels/effects of: Afatinib; ARIPiprazole; Bosentan; Bosutinib; Carvedilol; CloZAPine; Colchicine; CYP2C8 Substrates; CYP2C9 Substrates; CYP2D6 Substrates; Dabigatran Etexilate; DOXOrubicin (Conventional); Everolimus; Fesoterodine; Highest Risk QTc-Prolonging Agents; Leflunomide; Lomitapide; Metoprolol; Natalizumab; Nebivolol; P-glycoprotein/ABCB1 Substrates; Pomalidomide; Prucalopride; Rivaroxaban; Silodosin; Thioridazine; Tofacitinib; Topotecan; Vaccines (Live); VinCRIStine (Liposomal); Vitamin K Antagonists

The levels/effects of Nilotinib may be increased by: CYP3A4 Inhibitors (Moderate); CYP3A4 Inhibitors (Strong); Dasatinib; Denosumab; Fusidic Acid (Systemic); Ivabradine; Ivacaftor; Luliconazole; Mifepristone; Moderate Risk QTc-Prolonging Agents; Pimecrolimus; QTc-Prolonging Agents (Indeterminate Risk and Risk Modifying); Roflumilast; Simeprevir; Tacrolimus (Topical); Trastuzumab

Nutritional/Ethanol Interactions

Food: Grapefruit juice may result in increased concentrations of nilotinib and potentiate QT prolongation. Management: Avoid grapefruit juice.

Herb/Nutraceutical: St John's wort may decrease nilotinib levels. Administration with grapefruit juice may result in increased concentrations of nilotinib and potentiate QT prolongation. Management: Avoid St John's wort and grapefruit juice.

Adverse Reactions

>10%:

Cardiovascular: Peripheral edema (8% to 15%), hypertension (10% to 11%)

Central nervous system: Headache (20% to 35%), fatigue (21% to 32%), fever (11% to 28%), insomnia (7% to 12%)

Dermatologic: Rash (29% to 38%), pruritus (20% to 32%), alopecia (11% to 13%)

Endocrine & metabolic: Hypophosphatemia (grades 3/4: 5% to 17%), hyperglycemia (grades 3/4: 6% to 12%)

Gastrointestinal: Nausea (20% to 37%), vomiting (11% to 29%), diarrhea (14% to 28%), constipation (17% to 26%), lipase increased (1% to ≥10%; grades 3/4: 7% to 18%), abdominal pain (12% to 17%), anorexia (12% to 15%)

Hematologic: Neutropenia (grades 3/4: 12% to 42%; median duration: 15 days), thrombocytopenia (grades 3/4: 10% to 42%; median duration: 22 days), anemia (grades 3/4: 4% to 27%)

Hepatic: Hyperbilirubinemia (≥10%; grades 3/4: 4% to 9%), ALT increased (≥10%; grades 3/4: 4%), AST increased (≥10%; grades 3/4: 1% to 3%)

Neuromuscular & skeletal: Arthralgia (16% to 26%), limb pain (11% to 20%), myalgia (14% to 19%), back pain (14% to 17%), weakness (11% to 16%), bone pain (14% to 15%), muscle spasm (11% to 15%), musculoskeletal pain (11% to 12%)

Respiratory: Cough (14% to 27%), nasopharyngitis (15% to 24%), dyspnea (9% to 15%), upper respiratory tract infection (≤15%), oropharyngeal pain (7% to 11%)

Miscellaneous: Night sweats (12% to 27%), flu-like syndrome (11%)

1% to 10%:

Cardiovascular: Arterial stenosis (5% to 6%), cerebrovascular accident (5% to 6%), peripheral arterial occlusive disease (5% to 6%), angina, arrhythmia (including AV block, atrial fibrillation, bradycardia, cardiac flutter, extrasystoles, and tachycardia), chest pain (including noncardiac), flushing, palpitation, QT interval prolonged

Central nervous system: Dizziness (10%), anxiety, depression, dysphonia, hypoesthesia, malaise, pain, vertigo

Dermatologic: Dry skin (>5% to <10%), acne, bruising, dermatitis (including allergic and ▶

acneiform), eczema, erythema, folliculitis, hyperhidrosis, skin papilloma, urticaria

Endocrine & metabolic: Hypokalemia (grades 3/4: ≤9%), hyponatremia (grades 3/4: ≤7%), hyperkalemia (grades 3/4: 2% to 6%), hypocalcemia (grades 3/4: ≤5%), albumin decreased (grades 3/4: ≤4%), diabetes mellitus, hypercalcemia, hypercholesterolemia, hyperlipidemia, hyperphosphatemia, hypomagnesemia

Gastrointestinal: Dyspepsia (4% to 10%), abdominal discomfort, abnormal taste, amylase increased, flatulence, pancreatitis, weight gain/loss

Genitourinary: Pollakiuria

Hematologic: Lymphopenia, neutropenic fever, pancytopenia

Hepatic: Alkaline phosphatase increased (grades 3/4: ≤1%), GGT increased

Neuromuscular & skeletal: Paresthesia, peripheral neuropathy

Ocular: Eyelid edema (1%), conjunctivitis, dry eye, eye hemorrhage, periorbital edema, pruritus

Respiratory: Pleural effusion (≤1%), dyspnea (exertional), epistaxis

Available Dosage Forms

Capsule, Oral:

Tasigna: 150 mg, 200 mg

General Dosage Range Dosage adjustment recommended in patients with hepatic impairment, on concomitant therapy, or who develop toxicities

Oral: *Adults:* 300-400 mg twice daily

Administration

Oral Administer twice daily doses ~12 hours apart. Administer on an empty stomach, at least 1 hour before or 2 hours after food. Capsules should be swallowed whole with water. If unable to swallow whole, may empty contents into 5 mL applesauce and administer within 15 minutes (do not save for later use).

Hazardous agent; use appropriate precautions for handling and disposal (NIOSH, 2012).

Storage/Stability Store at 25°C (77°F); excursions permitted to 15°C to 30°C (59°F to 86°F).

Nursing Actions

Physical Assessment Monitor for myelosuppression, cardiac changes, gastrointestinal disturbance, and hyperglycemia. Monitor pulmonary status.

Patient Education

• Discuss specific use of drug and side effects with patient as it relates to treatment. (HCAHPS: During this hospital stay, were you given any medicine that you had not taken before? Before giving you any new medicine, how often did hospital staff tell you what the medicine was for? How often did hospital staff describe possible side effects in a way you could understand?)

• Patient may experience anemia, leukopenia, thrombocytopenia, headache, nausea, loss of appetite, constipation, diarrhea, edema in arms or legs, hypertension, hyperglycemia, myalgia, alopecia, insomnia, rhinorrhea, fatigue, or skin irritation. Have patient report immediately to prescriber signs of infection, angina, tachycardia, syncope, dyspnea, severe dyspepsia, significant weight gain, ecchymosis, discolored urine, jaundice, sudden vision changes, or rash (HCAHPS).

• Educate patient about signs of a significant reaction (eg, wheezing; chest tightness; fever; itching; bad cough; blue skin color; seizures; or swelling of face, lips, tongue, or throat). **Note:** This is not a comprehensive list of all side effects. Patient should consult prescriber for additional questions.

Intended Use and Disclaimer: Should not be printed and given to patients. This information is intended to serve as a concise initial reference for healthcare professionals to use when discussing medications with a patient. You must ultimately rely on your own discretion, experience and judgment in diagnosing, treating and advising patients.

Dietary Considerations The bioavailability of nilotinib is increased with food. Take on an empty stomach, at least 1 hour before or 2 hours after food. Avoid grapefruit juice.

Related Information

Oral Medications That Should Not Be Crushed or Altered *on page 1712*

Nilutamide (ni LOO ta mide)

Brand Names: U.S. Nilandron

Index Terms RU-23908

Pharmacologic Category Antineoplastic Agent, Antiandrogen

Medication Safety Issues

Sound-alike/look-alike issues:

Nilutamide may be confused with nilotinib

Pregnancy Risk Factor C

Use Treatment of metastatic prostate cancer (in combination with surgical castration)

Available Dosage Forms

Tablet, Oral:

Nilandron: 150 mg

General Dosage Range Oral: *Adults:* Initial: 300 mg once daily; Maintenance: 150 mg once daily

Administration

Oral Administer without regard to meals.

Hazardous agent; use appropriate precautions for handling and disposal (NIOSH, 2012).

Nursing Actions

Physical Assessment Teach patient orthostatic precautions.

Patient Education

- Discuss specific use of drug and side effects with patient as it relates to treatment. (HCAHPS: During this hospital stay, were you given any medicine that you had not taken before? Before giving you any new medicine, how often did hospital staff tell you what the medicine was for? How often did hospital staff describe possible side effects in a way you could understand?)
- Patient may experience flushing, decreased night vision, nausea, macromastia, breast soreness, skin irritation, alopecia, or impotence. Have patient report immediately to prescriber signs of infection, dyspnea, angina, significant weight loss, severe edema, considerable dyspepsia, asthenia, discolored urine, jaundice, inability to eat, or rash (HCAHPS).
- Educate patient about signs of a significant reaction (eg, wheezing; chest tightness; fever; itching; bad cough; blue skin color; seizures; or swelling of face, lips, tongue, or throat). **Note:** This is not a comprehensive list of all side effects. Patient should consult prescriber for additional questions.

Intended Use and Disclaimer: Should not be printed and given to patients. This information is intended to serve as a concise initial reference for healthcare professionals to use when discussing medications with a patient. You must ultimately rely on your own discretion, experience and judgment in diagnosing, treating and advising patients.

NiMODipine (nye MOE di peen)

Brand Names: U.S. Nymalize
Pharmacologic Category Calcium Channel Blocker; Calcium Channel Blocker, Dihydropyridine
Medication Safety Issues
Sound-alike/look-alike issues:
NiMODipine may be confused with niCARdipine, NIFEdipine, nisoldipine
Administration issues:
For oral administration only. For patients unable to swallow a capsule, the drug should be dispensed in an oral syringe (preferably amber in color) labeled **"WARNING: For ORAL use only"** or **"Not for I.V. use."** Nimodipine has inadvertently been administered I.V. when withdrawn from capsules into a syringe for subsequent nasogastric tube administration. Severe cardiovascular adverse events, including fatalities, have resulted. Employ precautions against such an event.
Pregnancy Risk Factor C
Lactation Enters breast milk/not recommended
Breast-Feeding Considerations Nimodipine is excreted into breast milk; two case reports note concentrations to be <1% of the weight-adjusted maternal dose (Carcas, 1996; Tonks, 1995).

Breast-feeding is not recommended by the manufacturer.
Use Subarachnoid hemorrhage: For the improvement of neurological outcome by reducing the incidence and severity of ischemic deficits in adult patients with subarachnoid hemorrhage (SAH) from ruptured intracranial berry aneurysms regardless of their postictus neurological condition (ie, Hunt and Hess grades I to V)
Mechanism of Action/Effect Nimodipine shares the pharmacology of other calcium channel blockers; animal studies indicate that nimodipine has a greater effect on cerebral arterials than other arterials; inhibits calcium ion from entering the "slow channels" or select voltage sensitive areas of vascular smooth muscle and myocardium during depolarization
Contraindications There are no contraindications listed in the manufacturer's labeling.
Warnings/Precautions [U.S. Boxed Warning]: Nimodipine has inadvertently been administered I.V. when withdrawn from capsules into a syringe for subsequent nasogastric administration. Severe cardiovascular adverse events, including fatalities, have resulted; precautions (eg, adequate labeling, use of oral syringes) should be employed against such an event.

Increased angina and/or MI have occurred with initiation or dosage titration of calcium channel blockers. Reflex tachycardia may occur resulting in angina and/or MI in patients with obstructive coronary disease, especially in the absence of concurrent beta-blockade. Peripheral edema is a common adverse event; occurs within 2-3 weeks of starting therapy. Symptomatic hypotension with or without syncope can occur; blood pressure must be lowered at a rate appropriate for the patient's clinical condition. Monitor blood pressure closely during treatment. Use with caution in patients with cirrhosis due to the increased plasma concentrations of nimodipine and an increased risk of adverse reactions; a lower dose and close monitoring of blood pressure and heart rate is required. Intestinal pseudo-obstruction and ileus have been reported (rarely) during therapy.

Potentially significant drug-drug interactions may exist, requiring dose or frequency adjustment, additional monitoring, and/or selection of alternative therapy.
Drug Interactions
Avoid Concomitant Use
Avoid concomitant use of NiMODipine with any of the following: Conivaptan; Fusidic Acid (Systemic); Grapefruit Juice
Decreased Effect
NiMODipine may decrease the levels/effects of: Clopidogrel; QuiNIDine

The levels/effects of NiMODipine may be decreased by: Barbiturates; Bosentan; Calcium ▶

Salts; CarBAMazepine; CYP3A4 Inducers (Strong); Dabrafenib; Deferasirox; Herbs (CYP3A4 Inducers); Herbs (Hypertensive Properties); Melatonin; Methylphenidate; Mitotane; Nafcillin; Rifamycin Derivatives; Tocilizumab; Yohimbine

Increased Effect/Toxicity

NiMODipine may increase the levels/effects of: Amifostine; Antihypertensives; Atosiban; Beta-Blockers; Calcium Channel Blockers (Nondihydropyridine); DULoxetine; Fosphenytoin; Hypotensive Agents; Magnesium Salts; Neuromuscular-Blocking Agents (Nondepolarizing); Nitroprusside; Obinutuzumab; Phenytoin; QuiNIDine; RiTUXimab; Tacrolimus (Systemic)

The levels/effects of NiMODipine may be increased by: Alpha1-Blockers; Antifungal Agents (Azole Derivatives, Systemic); Brimonidine (Topical); Calcium Channel Blockers (Nondihydropyridine); Cimetidine; Conivaptan; CycloSPORINE (Systemic); CYP3A4 Inhibitors (Moderate); CYP3A4 Inhibitors (Strong); Dasatinib; Diazoxide; Fluconazole; FLUoxetine; Fusidic Acid (Systemic); Grapefruit Juice; Herbs (Hypotensive Properties); Ivacaftor; Luliconazole; Macrolide Antibiotics; Magnesium Salts; MAO Inhibitors; Mifepristone; Pentoxifylline; Phosphodiesterase 5 Inhibitors; Prostacyclin Analogues; Protease Inhibitors; QuiNIDine; Simeprevir; Stiripentol

Nutritional/Ethanol Interactions Food: Administration with a standard breakfast results in a 68% lower maximum plasma concentration and 38% lower bioavailability as compared to administration under fasted conditions. In addition, AUC and maximum plasma concentration were increased by an average of 51% and 24%, respectively, following administration of nimodipine with grapefruit juice (Fuhr, 1998). Management: Administer on an empty stomach, at least 1 hour before or 2 hours after meals. Avoid concurrent use of grapefruit juice and nimodipine.

Adverse Reactions

1% to 10%:

Cardiovascular: Decreased blood pressure (4% to 5%), bradycardia (1%)

Central nervous system: Headache (1%)

Gastrointestinal: Nausea (1%)

Available Dosage Forms

Capsule, Oral:

Generic: 30 mg

Solution, Oral:

Nymalize: 60 mg/20 mL (20 mL, 473 mL)

General Dosage Range Dosage adjustment recommended in patients with hepatic impairment

Oral: *Adults:* 60 mg every 4 hours

Administration

Oral For enteral administration ONLY. Life-threatening adverse events have occurred when administered parenterally. Administer on an empty stomach at least 1 hour before or 2 hours after meals.

Nasogastric (NG) or gastric tube administration:

Oral solution (Nymalzine): Administer using the supplied oral syringe labeled **"ORAL USE ONLY"**. Following administration, refill the oral syringe with 20 mL of NS and flush any remaining contents from NG or gastric tube into the stomach.

Capsules: If the capsules cannot be swallowed, the liquid may be removed by making a hole in each end of the capsule with an 18-gauge needle and extracting the contents into a syringe; transfer these contents into an oral syringe (amber-colored oral syringe preferred). It is strongly recommended that preparation be done in the pharmacy. Label oral syringe with **"WARNING: For ORAL use only"** or **"Not for I.V. use."** Follow with a flush of 30 mL NS.

Storage/Stability Store at 25°C (77°F); excursions are permitted to 15°C to 30°C (59°F to 86°F). Protect from capsules light and freezing. Protect solution from light and do not refrigerate.

Nursing Actions

Physical Assessment Measure vital signs and assess neurologic and cardiac status. Monitor for rash, hypotension, constipation, and peripheral edema when starting or adjusting dose and periodically during therapy.

Patient Education

• Discuss specific use of drug and side effects with patient as it relates to treatment. (HCAHPS: During this hospital stay, were you given any medicine that you had not taken before? Before giving you any new medicine, how often did hospital staff tell you what the medicine was for? How often did hospital staff describe possible side effects in a way you could understand?)

• Patient may experience dizziness or headache. Have patient report immediately to prescriber tachycardia, dyspnea, or rash (HCAHPS).

• Educate patient about signs of a significant reaction (eg, wheezing; chest tightness; fever; itching; bad cough; blue skin color; seizures; or swelling of face, lips, tongue, or throat). **Note:** This is not a comprehensive list of all side effects. Patient should consult prescriber for additional questions.

Intended Use and Disclaimer: Should not be printed and given to patients. This information is intended to serve as a concise initial reference for healthcare professionals to use when discussing medications with a patient. You must ultimately rely on your own discretion, experience and judgment in diagnosing, treating and advising patients.

Nisoldipine (nye SOL di peen)

Brand Names: U.S. Sular

Pharmacologic Category Antihypertensive; Calcium Channel Blocker; Calcium Channel Blocker, Dihydropyridine

Medication Safety Issues

Sound-alike/look-alike issues:

Nisoldipine may be confused with NIFEdipine, niMODipine

Pregnancy Risk Factor C

Lactation Excretion in breast milk unknown/not recommended

Breast-Feeding Considerations It is not known if nisoldipine is excreted into breast milk. The manufacturer recommends a decision be made whether to discontinue nursing or to discontinue the drug, taking into account the importance of treatment to the mother. Breast-fed infants of mothers taking medications for hypertension should be monitored for adverse effects (Chobanian, 2003).

Use Management of hypertension, alone or in combination with other antihypertensive agents

Mechanism of Action/Effect As a dihydropyridine calcium channel blocker, structurally similar to nifedipine, nisoldipine impedes the movement of calcium ions into vascular smooth muscle and cardiac muscle. Dihydropyridines are potent vasodilators and are not as likely to suppress cardiac contractility and slow cardiac conduction as other calcium antagonists such as verapamil and diltiazem; nisoldipine is 5-10 times as potent a vasodilator as nifedipine.

Contraindications Hypersensitivity to nisoldipine, any component of the formulation, or other dihydropyridine calcium channel blockers

Warnings/Precautions With initiation or dosage titration of dihydropyridine calcium channel blockers, reflex tachycardia may occur resulting in angina and/or MI in patients with obstructive coronary disease especially in the absence of concurrent beta-blockade. Use with caution in patients with severe aortic stenosis, and hypertrophic cardiomyopathy with outflow tract obstruction. The ACCF/AHA heart failure guidelines recommend to avoid use in patients with heart failure due to lack of benefit and/or worse outcomes with calcium channel blockers in general (Yancy, 2013). Use with caution in hepatic impairment; lower starting dose required. The most common side effect is peripheral edema; occurs within 2-3 weeks of starting therapy. Symptomatic hypotension with or without syncope can rarely occur; blood pressure must be lowered at a rate appropriate for the patient's clinical condition. Some dosage forms contain tartrazine, which may cause allergic reactions in certain individuals (eg, aspirin hypersensitivity). Use with caution in patients >65 years of age; lower starting dose recommended.

Drug Interactions

Avoid Concomitant Use

Avoid concomitant use of Nisoldipine with any of the following: CYP3A4 Inducers (Strong); CYP3A4 Inhibitors (Strong); Fusidic Acid (Systemic); Grapefruit Juice; Pimozide

Decreased Effect

Nisoldipine may decrease the levels/effects of: Clopidogrel

The levels/effects of Nisoldipine may be decreased by: Barbiturates; Bosentan; Calcium Salts; CarBAMazepine; CYP3A4 Inducers (Strong); Dabrafenib; Deferasirox; Herbs (CYP3A4 Inducers); Herbs (Hypertensive Properties); Melatonin; Methylphenidate; Nafcillin; Rifamycin Derivatives; Tocilizumab; Yohimbine

Increased Effect/Toxicity

Nisoldipine may increase the levels/effects of: Amifostine; Antihypertensives; ARIPiprazole; Atosiban; Beta-Blockers; Calcium Channel Blockers (Nondihydropyridine); Dofetilide; DULoxetine; Fosphenytoin; Hypotensive Agents; Lomitapide; Magnesium Salts; Neuromuscular-Blocking Agents (Nondepolarizing); Nitroprusside; Obinutuzumab; Phenytoin; Pimozide; RiTUXimab; Tacrolimus (Systemic)

The levels/effects of Nisoldipine may be increased by: Alpha1-Blockers; Antifungal Agents (Azole Derivatives, Systemic); Brimonidine (Topical); Calcium Channel Blockers (Nondihydropyridine); Cimetidine; CycloSPORINE (Systemic); CYP3A4 Inhibitors (Moderate); CYP3A4 Inhibitors (Strong); Dasatinib; Diazoxide; Fluconazole; Fusidic Acid (Systemic); Grapefruit Juice; Herbs (Hypotensive Properties); Ivacaftor; Luliconazole; Macrolide Antibiotics; Magnesium Salts; MAO Inhibitors; Mifepristone; Pentoxifylline; Phosphodiesterase 5 Inhibitors; Prostacyclin Analogues; Protease Inhibitors; Simeprevir

Nutritional/Ethanol Interactions

Food: Peak concentrations of nisoldipine may be significantly increased if taken with high-lipid foods; however, total exposure (AUC) may be reduced. Grapefruit juice has been shown to significantly increase the bioavailability of nisoldipine. Management: Take on an empty stomach 1 hour before or 2 hours after a meal. Avoid a high-fat diet. Avoid grapefruit products before and after dosing.

Herb/Nutraceutical: St John's wort may decrease nisoldipine levels. Some herbal medications may worsen hypertension (eg, licorice); others may increase the antihypertensive effect of nisoldipine (eg, shepherd's purse). Management: Avoid St John's wort. Avoid bayberry, blue cohosh, cayenne, ephedra, ginger, ginseng (American), kola, licorice, and yohimbe. Avoid black cohosh, California poppy, coleus, golden seal, hawthorn, mistletoe, periwinkle, quinine, and shepherd's purse.

Adverse Reactions

>10%:

Cardiovascular: Peripheral edema (dose related; 7% to 29%)

Central nervous system: Headache (22%)

1% to 10%:

Cardiovascular: Vasodilation (4%), palpitation (3%), angina exacerbation (2%), chest pain (2%)

Central nervous system: Dizziness (3% to 10%)

Dermatologic: Rash (2%)

Gastrointestinal: Nausea (2%)

Respiratory: Pharyngitis (5%), sinusitis (3%)

Pharmacodynamics/Kinetics

Duration of Action >24 hours

Available Dosage Forms

Tablet Extended Release 24 Hour, Oral:

Sular: 8.5 mg, 17 mg, 34 mg

Generic: 8.5 mg, 17 mg, 20 mg, 25.5 mg, 30 mg, 34 mg, 40 mg

General Dosage Range Dosage adjustment recommended in patients with hepatic impairment

Oral:

Adults:

Sular® (Geomatrix® delivery system): Initial: 17 mg once daily; Maintenance: 17-34 mg once daily (maximum: 34 mg/day)

Nisoldipine extended-release (original formulation): Initial: 20 mg once daily; Maintenance: 10-40 mg once daily (maximum: 60 mg/day)

Elderly: Sular® (Geomatrix® delivery system): Initial: 8.5 mg once daily; Nisoldipine extended-release (original formulation): Initial: 10 mg once daily

Administration

Oral Administer at the same time each day to ensure minimal fluctuation of serum levels. Avoid high-fat diet. Administer on an empty stomach (1 hour before or 2 hours after a meal). Swallow whole; do not crush, break, split, or chew.

Storage/Stability Store at controlled room temperature of 20°C to 25°C (68°F to 77°F). Protect from light; protect from moisture.

Nursing Actions

Physical Assessment Assess cardiac status and blood pressure. Monitor for chest pain, dyspnea, edema, rash, and constipation when starting or adjusting dose and periodically during therapy. Dose should be tapered gradually when discontinuing.

Patient Education

• Discuss specific use of drug and side effects with patient as it relates to treatment. (HCAHPS: During this hospital stay, were you given any medicine that you had not taken before? Before giving you any new medicine, how often did hospital staff tell you what the medicine was for? How often did hospital staff describe possible side effects in a way you could understand?)

• Patient may experience dizziness, headache, or edema. Have patient report immediately to prescriber tachycardia, dyspnea, or rash (HCAHPS).

• Educate patient about signs of a significant reaction (eg, wheezing; chest tightness; fever; itching; bad cough; blue skin color; seizures; or swelling of face, lips, tongue, or throat). **Note:** This is not a comprehensive list of all side effects. Patient should consult prescriber for additional questions.

Intended Use and Disclaimer: Should not be printed and given to patients. This information is intended to serve as a concise initial reference for healthcare professionals to use when discussing medications with a patient. You must ultimately rely on your own discretion, experience and judgment in diagnosing, treating and advising patients.

Dietary Considerations Take on an empty stomach (1 hour before or 2 hours after a meal). Avoid grapefruit juice before and after dosing. Avoid grapefuit juice; avoid high-fat diet.

Related Information

Oral Medications That Should Not Be Crushed or Altered *on page 1712*

Nitazoxanide (nye ta ZOX a nide)

Brand Names: U.S. Alinia

Index Terms NTZ

Pharmacologic Category Antiprotozoal

Pregnancy Risk Factor B

Lactation Excretion in breast milk unknown/use caution

Breast-Feeding Considerations It is not known if nitazoxanide is excreted in breast milk. The manufacturer recommends that caution be exercised when administering nitazoxanide to nursing women.

Use Treatment of diarrhea caused by *Cryptosporidium parvum* or *Giardia lamblia*

Unlabeled Use Alternative treatment for *Clostridium difficile*-associated diarrhea (CDAD)

Mechanism of Action/Effect Nitazoxanide is rapidly metabolized to the active metabolite tizoxanide *in vivo*. Nitazoxanide and its metabolite inhibit the growth of sporozoites and oocysts of *Cryptosporidium parvum* and trophozoites of *Giardia lamblia*.

Contraindications Hypersensitivity to nitazoxanide or any component of the formulation

Warnings/Precautions Use caution with renal or hepatic impairment. Safety and efficacy have not been established in patients with HIV infection or immunodeficiency. Oral suspension contains sucrose; use caution in patients with diabetes mellitus.

Drug Interactions

Avoid Concomitant Use There are no known interactions where it is recommended to avoid concomitant use.

Decreased Effect There are no known significant interactions involving a decrease in effect.

Increased Effect/Toxicity There are no known significant interactions involving an increase in effect.

Nutritional/Ethanol Interactions Food: Food increases AUC. Management: Take with food.

Adverse Reactions Rates of adverse effects were similar to those reported with placebo.

1% to 10%:
Central nervous system: Headache (1% to 3%)
Gastrointestinal: Abdominal pain (7% to 8%), diarrhea (2% to 4%), nausea (3%), vomiting (1%)

Available Dosage Forms
Suspension Reconstituted, Oral:
Alinia: 100 mg/5 mL (60 mL)
Tablet, Oral:
Alinia: 500 mg
General Dosage Range Oral:
Children 1-3 years: 100 mg every 12 hours (oral suspension)
Children 4-11 years: 200 mg every 12 hours (oral suspension)
Children ≥12 years and Adults: 500 mg every 12 hours (oral suspension or tablets)

Administration
Oral Administer with food. Shake suspension well prior to administration.

Preparation for Administration For preparation at time of dispensing, add 48 mL incrementally to 60 mL bottle; shake vigorously. Resulting suspension is 20 mg/mL (100 mg per 5 mL).

Storage/Stability
Suspension: Prior to and following reconstitution, store at 25°C (77°F); excursions permitted to 15°C to 30°C (59°F to 86°F). For preparation at time of dispensing, add 48 mL incrementally to 60 mL bottle; shake vigorously. Resulting suspension is 20 mg/mL (100 mg per 5 mL). Following reconstitution, discard unused portion of suspension after 7 days.
Tablet: Store at 25°C (77°F); excursions permitted to 15°C to 30°C (59°F to 86°F).

Nursing Actions
Patient Education
• Discuss specific use of drug and side effects with patient as it relates to treatment. (HCAHPS: During this hospital stay, were you given any medicine that you had not taken before? Before giving you any new medicine, how often did hospital staff tell you what the medicine was for? How often did hospital staff describe possible side effects in a way you could understand?)
• Patient may experience headache or dyspepsia. Have patient report immediately to prescriber severe nausea or rash (HCAHPS).
• Educate patient about signs of a significant reaction (eg, wheezing; chest tightness; fever; itching; bad cough; blue skin color; seizures; or

swelling of face, lips, tongue, or throat). **Note:** This is not a comprehensive list of all side effects. Patient should consult prescriber for additional questions.

Intended Use and Disclaimer: Should not be printed and given to patients. This information is intended to serve as a concise initial reference for healthcare professionals to use when discussing medications with a patient. You must ultimately rely on your own discretion, experience and judgment in diagnosing, treating and advising patients.

Dietary Considerations Should be taken with food.

Nitrofurantoin (nye troe fyoor AN toyn)

Brand Names: U.S. Furadantin; Macrobid; Macrodantin

Pharmacologic Category Antibiotic, Miscellaneous

Medication Safety Issues
Sound alike/look alike issues:
Macrobid may be confused with microK, Nitro-Bid
Nitrofurantoin may be confused with Neurontin®, nitroglycerin
BEERS Criteria medication:
This drug may be potentially inappropriate for use in geriatric patients (Quality of evidence - moderate; Strength of recommendation - strong).

Pregnancy Risk Factor B (contraindicated at term)

Lactation Enters breast milk/not recommended (infants <1 month)

Use
Urinary tract infections: For the treatment of urinary tract infections (UTIs) when caused by susceptible strains of *Escherichia coli*, enterococci, *Staphylococcus aureus*, and certain susceptible strains of *Klebsiella* and *Enterobacter* species.
Acute cystitis: Nitrofurantoin monohydrate/macrocrystals: Indicated only for the treatment of acute uncomplicated UTIs (acute cystitis) caused by susceptible strains of *E. coli* or *Staphylococcus saprophyticus* in patients ≥12 years of age.

Available Dosage Forms
Capsule, Oral:
Macrobid: 100 mg
Macrodantin: 25 mg, 50 mg, 100 mg
Generic: 50 mg, 100 mg
Suspension, Oral:
Furadantin: 25 mg/5 mL (230 mL)
Generic: 25 mg/5 mL (230 mL, 240 mL)
General Dosage Range Oral:
Children >1 month: Furadantin, Macrodantin: 5-7 mg/kg/day divided every 6 hours (maximum: 400 mg daily) **or** 1-2 mg/kg/day divided every 12-24 hours (maximum: 100 mg daily)
Children >12 years: Macrobid: 100 mg twice daily ▶

Adults: Furadantin, Macrodantin: 50-100 mg every 6 hours **or** once daily; Macrobid: 100 mg twice daily

Administration

Oral Administer with meals to improve absorption and decrease adverse effects; suspension may be mixed with water, milk, fruit juice, or infant formula. Shake suspension well before use.

Nursing Actions

Physical Assessment Monitor for any signs of allergy: Hives, swelling, difficulty breathing. Educate regarding change in urine color.

Patient Education

- Discuss specific use of drug and side effects with patient as it relates to treatment. (HCAHPS: During this hospital stay, were you given any medicine that you had not taken before? Before giving you any new medicine, how often did hospital staff tell you what the medicine was for? How often did hospital staff describe possible side effects in a way you could understand?)
- Patient may experience nausea, diarrhea, lack of appetite, flatulence, or urine discoloration. Have patient report immediately to prescriber signs of pancreatitis, vision changes, ophthalmalgia, involuntary eye movements, illogical thinking, severe headache, depression, skin or nail discoloration, significant asthenia, signs of pseudomembranous colitis, signs of pulmonary disorder, signs of hepatic impairment, or signs of severe neuropathy (HCAHPS).
- Educate patient about signs of a significant reaction (eg, wheezing; chest tightness; fever; itching; bad cough; blue skin color; seizures; or swelling of face, lips, tongue, or throat). **Note:** This is not a comprehensive list of all side effects. Patient should consult prescriber for additional questions.

Intended Use and Disclaimer: Should not be printed and given to patients. This information is intended to serve as a concise initial reference for healthcare professionals to use when discussing medications with a patient. You must ultimately rely on your own discretion, experience and judgment in diagnosing, treating and advising patients.

Nitroglycerin (nye troe GLI ser in)

Brand Names: U.S. Minitran; Nitro-Bid; Nitro-Dur; Nitro-Time; Nitrolingual; NitroMist; Nitrostat; Rectiv

Index Terms Glyceryl Trinitrate; Nitroglycerol; NTG; Tridil

Pharmacologic Category Antianginal Agent; Antidote, Extravasation; Vasodilator

Medication Safety Issues

Sound-alike/look-alike issues:

Nitroglycerin may be confused with nitrofurantoin, nitroprusside

Nitro-Bid may be confused with Macrobid

Nitroderm may be confused with NicoDerm

Nitrol may be confused with Nizoral

Nitrostat may be confused with Nilstat, nystatin

Other safety concerns:

Transdermal patch may contain conducting metal (eg, aluminum); remove patch prior to MRI.

International issues:

Nitrocor [Italy, Russia, and Venezuela] may be confused with Natrecor brand name for nesiritide [U.S., Canada, and multiple international markets]; Nutracort brand name for hydrocortisone in the [U.S. and multiple international markets]; Nitro-Dur [U.S., Canada, and multiple international markets]

Pregnancy Risk Factor C

Lactation Excretion in breast milk unknown/use caution

Breast-Feeding Considerations It is not known if nitroglycerin is excreted in breast milk. The manufacturer recommends that caution be exercised when administering nitroglycerin to nursing women. Information related to the use of nitroglycerin and breast-feeding is limited (Böttiger, 2010; O'Sullivan, 2011).

Use Treatment or prevention of angina pectoris

Intravenous (I.V.) administration: Treatment or prevention of angina pectoris; acute decompensated heart failure (especially when associated with acute myocardial infarction); perioperative hypertension (especially during cardiovascular surgery); induction of intraoperative hypotension

Intra-anal administration (Rectiv ointment): Treatment of moderate-to-severe pain associated with chronic anal fissure

Unlabeled Use Short-term management of pulmonary hypertension (I.V.); esophageal spastic disorders; uterine relaxation; treatment of sympathomimetic vasopressor extravasation injury (alternative to phentolamine)

Mechanism of Action/Effect Relaxes smooth muscle, producing a vasodilator effect on the peripheral veins and arteries with more prominent effects on the veins. Primarily reduces cardiac oxygen demand by decreasing preload (left ventricular end-diastolic pressure); may modestly reduce afterload; dilates coronary arteries and improves collateral flow to ischemic regions. For use in rectal fissures, intra-anal administration results in decreased sphincter tone and intra-anal pressure.

Contraindications Hypersensitivity to organic nitrates or any component of the formulation (includes adhesives for transdermal product); concurrent use with phosphodiesterase-5 (PDE-5) inhibitors (sildenafil, tadalafil, or vardenafil); increased intracranial pressure; severe anemia

Additional contraindications for I.V. product: Constrictive pericarditis; pericardial tamponade; restrictive cardiomyopathy

Note: According to the 2010 American Heart Association guidelines for the treatment of acute coronary syndromes, nitrates are considered contraindicated in the following conditions: Hypotension (SBP <90 mm Hg or ≥30 mm Hg below baseline), extreme bradycardia (<50 bpm), tachycardia in the absence of heart failure (>100 bpm), and right ventricular infarction (O'Connor, 2010).

Warnings/Precautions Severe hypotension can occur. Use with caution in volume depletion, moderate hypotension, and extreme caution with inferior wall MI and suspected right ventricular involvement. Use considered contraindicated in patients with severe hypotension (SBP <90 mm Hg or ≥30 mm Hg below baseline), extreme bradycardia (<50 bpm), and right ventricular MI (O'Connor, 2010). Avoid use in patients with hypertrophic cardiomyopathy (HCM) with outflow tract obstruction; nitrates may reduce preload, exacerbating obstruction and cause hypotension or syncope and/or worsening of heart failure (ACCF/AHA [Gersh, 2011]).

Paradoxical bradycardia and increased angina pectoris can accompany hypotension. Orthostatic hypotension can also occur. Ethanol can accentuate this. Tolerance does develop to nitrates and appropriate dosing is needed to minimize this (drug-free interval). Avoid use of long-acting agents in acute MI or acute HF; cannot easily reverse effects. Nitrates may aggravate angina caused by hypertrophic cardiomyopathy. Nitroglycerin may precipitate or aggravate increased intracranial pressure and subsequently may worsen clinical outcomes in patients with neurologic injury (eg, intracranial hemorrhage, traumatic brain injury). Nitroglycerin transdermal patches may contain conducting metal (eg, aluminum); remove patch prior to MRI. Potentially significant drug-drug interactions may exist, requiring dose or frequency adjustment, additional monitoring, and/or selection of alternative therapy. Avoid concurrent use with PDE-5 inhibitors (eg, sildenafil, tadalafil, vardenafil). When nitrate administration becomes medically necessary, may administer nitrates only if 24 hours have elapsed after use of sildenafil or vardenafil (48 hours after tadalafil use) (Trujillo, 2007).

Use caution when treating rectal anal fissures with nitroglycerin ointment formulation in patients with suspected or known significant cardiovascular disorders (eg, cardiomyopathies, heart failure, acute MI); intra-anal nitroglycerin administration may decrease systolic blood pressure and decrease arterial vascular resistance.

Drug Interactions

Avoid Concomitant Use

Avoid concomitant use of Nitroglycerin with any of the following: Ergot Derivatives; Phosphodiesterase 5 Inhibitors; Riociguat

Decreased Effect

Nitroglycerin may decrease the levels/effects of: Alteplase; Heparin

The levels/effects of Nitroglycerin may be decreased by: Ergot Derivatives

Increased Effect/Toxicity

Nitroglycerin may increase the levels/effects of: DULoxetine; Ergot Derivatives; Hypotensive Agents; Prilocaine; Riociguat; Rosiglitazone; Sodium Nitrite

The levels/effects of Nitroglycerin may be increased by: Alfuzosin; Nitric Oxide; Phosphodiesterase 5 Inhibitors

Nutritional/Ethanol Interactions

Ethanol: Avoid ethanol (may increase the hypotensive effects of nitroglycerin). Monitor.

Herb/Nutraceutical: Avoid bayberry, blue cohosh, cayenne, ephedra, ginger, ginseng (American), kola, licorice (may worsen hypertension). Avoid black cohosh, California poppy, coleus, golden seal, hawthorn, mistletoe, periwinkle, quinine, shepherd's purse (may cause hypotension).

Adverse Reactions Frequency not defined.

Cardiovascular: Bradycardia, flushing, hypotension, orthostatic hypotension, peripheral edema, syncope, tachycardia

Central nervous system: Headache (common), dizziness, lightheadedness

Gastrointestinal: Nausea, vomiting, xerostomia

Neuromuscular & skeletal: Paresthesia, weakness

Respiratory: Dyspnea, pharyngitis, rhinitis

Miscellaneous: Diaphoresis

Pharmacodynamics/Kinetics

Onset of Action Sublingual tablet: 1-3 minutes; Translingual spray: Similar to sublingual tablet; Extended release: ~60 minutes; Topical: 15-30 minutes; Transdermal: ~30 minutes; I.V.: Immediate

Peak effect: Sublingual tablet: 5 minutes; Translingual spray: 4-10 minutes; Extended release: 2.5-4 hours; Topical: ~60 minutes; Transdermal: 120 minutes; I.V.: Immediate

Duration of Action Sublingual tablet: At least 25 minutes; Translingual spray: Similar to sublingual tablet; Extended release: 4-8 hours (Gibbons, 2002); Topical: 7 hours; Transdermal: 10-12 hours; I.V.: 3-5 minutes

Available Dosage Forms

Aerosol Solution, Translingual:

NitroMist: 400 mcg/spray (4.1 g, 8.5 g)

Generic: 400 mcg/spray (4.1 g, 8.5 g)

Capsule Extended Release, Oral:

Nitro-Time: 2.5 mg, 6.5 mg, 9 mg

Generic: 2.5 mg, 6.5 mg, 9 mg

Ointment, Rectal:

Rectiv: 0.4% (30 g)

Ointment, Transdermal:

Nitro-Bid: 2% (1 g, 30 g, 60 g)

Patch 24 Hour, Transdermal:
Minitran: 0.1 mg/hr (30 ea); 0.2 mg/hr (30 ea); 0.4 mg/hr (30 ea); 0.6 mg/hr (30 ea)
Nitro-Dur: 0.1 mg/hr (30 ea, 100 ea); 0.2 mg/hr (30 ea, 100 ea); 0.3 mg/hr (30 ea, 100 ea); 0.4 mg/hr (30 ea, 100 ea); 0.6 mg/hr (30 ea, 100 ea); 0.8 mg/hr (30 ea, 100 ea)
Generic: 0.1 mg/hr (30 ea, 4350 ea); 0.2 mg/hr (30 ea, 4350 ea); 0.4 mg/hr (30 ea, 4350 ea); 0.6 mg/hr (30 ea, 4350 ea)

Solution, Intravenous:
Generic: 25 mg (250 mL); 50 mg (250 mL, 500 mL); 100 mg (250 mL); 200 mg (500 mL); 5 mg/mL (10 mL)

Solution, Translingual:
Nitrolingual: 0.4 mg/spray (4.9 g, 12 g)
Generic: 0.4 mg/spray (4.9 g, 12 g)

Tablet Sublingual, Sublingual:
Nitrostat: 0.3 mg, 0.4 mg, 0.6 mg

General Dosage Range

I.V.: *Adults:* Initial: 5 mcg/minute; Maintenance: 20-200 mcg/minute (maximum: 400 mcg/minute)
Intra-anal: *Adults:* 1 inch every 12 hours
Oral: *Adults:* 2.5-6.5 mg 3-4 times/day; Maintenance: Up to 26 mg 4 times/day
Sublingual: *Adults:* 0.3-0.6 mg every 5 minutes for maximum of 3 doses in 15 minutes **or** 5-10 minutes prior to activities which may provoke an attack
Topical: *Adults:*
Ointment: Apply 0.5" to 2" every 6 hours with a daily nitrate-free interval of ~10-12 hours
Patch: Initial: 0.2-0.4 mg/hour for 12-14 hours/day; Maintenance: 0.2-0.8 mg/hour for 12-14 hours
Translingual: *Adults:* 1-2 sprays under tongue every 3-5 minutes for maximum of 3 doses in 15 minutes **or** 5-10 minutes prior to activities which may provoke an attack

Usual Infusion Concentrations: Pediatric
Note: Premixed solutions available
I.V. infusion: 100 mcg/mL, 200 mcg/mL, or 400 mcg/mL

Usual Infusion Concentrations: Adult Note:
Premixed solutions available
I.V. infusion: 50 mg in 250 mL (concentration: 200 mcg/mL) **or** 100 mg in 250 mL (concentration: 400 mcg/mL) of D_5W

Administration
I.V. Prepare in glass bottles, EXCEL® or PAB® containers. Adsorption occurs to soft plastic (eg, PVC); use administration sets intended for nitroglycerin. Administer via infusion pump.
Injectable Detail Nitroglycerin can be absorbed by plastic (eg, PVC) tubing or containers. Infusion pump may not infuse accurately with different tubing. Be alert to potential for unregulated flow.

pH: 3-6.5

Oral
Oral (extended release capsule): Swallow whole. Do not chew, break, or crush. Take with a full glass of water.
Sublingual: Do not crush sublingual product (tablet). Place under tongue and allow to dissolve.
Translingual spray: Do not shake container. Prior to initial use, the pump must be primed by spraying 5 times (Nitrolingual®) or 10 times (Nitromist®) into the air. Priming sprays should be directed away from patient and others. Release spray onto or under tongue. Close mouth after administration. Do not rinse the mouth for at least 5-10 minutes. The end of the pump should be covered by the fluid in the bottle. If pump is unused for 6 weeks, a single priming spray (Nitrolingual®) or 2 priming sprays (Nitromist®) should be completed.

Topical
Topical ointment: Wash hands prior to and after use. Application site should be clean, dry, and hair-free. Apply to chest or back with the applicator or dose-measuring paper. Spread in a thin layer over a 2.25 x 3.5 inch area. Do not rub into skin. Tape applicator into place.
Drug extravasation management, (treatment), sympathomimetic vasopressors (alternative to phentolamine) (unlabeled use): Stop vesicant infusion immediately and disconnect I.V. line (leave needle/cannula in place); gently aspirate extravasated solution from the I.V. line (do **NOT** flush the line); remove needle/cannula; elevate extremity. Apply nitroglycerin ointment as a thin ribbon to the affected area (Wong, 1992). May also apply dry warm compresses (Hurst, 2004).
Topical patch, transdermal: Application site should be clean, dry and hair-free. Remove patch after 12-14 hours. Rotate patch sites.
Other Intra-anal ointment: Using a finger covering (eg, plastic wrap, surgical glove, finger cot), place finger beside 1 inch measuring guide on the box and squeeze ointment the length of the measuring line directly onto covered finger. Insert ointment into the anal canal using the covered finger up to first finger joint (do not insert further than the first finger joint) and apply ointment around the side of the anal canal. If intra-anal application is too painful, may apply the ointment to the outside of the anus. Wash hands following application.

Storage/Stability
I.V. solution: Doses should be made in glass bottles, EXCEL® or PAB® containers. Adsorption occurs to soft plastic (eg, PVC). Nitroglycerin diluted in D_5W or NS in glass containers is physically and chemically stable for 48 hours at room temperature and 7 days under refrigeration. In D_5W or NS in EXCEL®/PAB® containers it is physically and chemically stable for 24 hours at room temperature.

Store sublingual tablets, topical ointment, and rectal ointment in tightly closed containers at 20°C to 25°C (68°F to 77°F); slow release capsules at 20°C to 25°C (68°F to 77°F); translingual spray and transdermal patch at 15°C to 30°C (59°F to 86°F).

Nursing Actions

Physical Assessment Assess cardiac status and monitor for hypotension and GI disturbances. Teach patient importance of drug-free intervals.

Patient Education
- Discuss specific use of drug and side effects with patient as it relates to treatment. (HCAHPS: During this hospital stay, were you given any medicine that you had not taken before? Before giving you any new medicine, how often did hospital staff tell you what the medicine was for? How often did hospital staff describe possible side effects in a way you could understand?)
- Patient may experience dizziness, flushing, headache, or skin irritation. Have patient report immediately to prescriber angina, tachycardia, dyspnea, or rash (HCAHPS).
- Educate patient about signs of a significant reaction (eg, wheezing; chest tightness; fever; itching; bad cough; blue skin color; seizures; or swelling of face, lips, tongue, or throat). **Note:** This is not a comprehensive list of all side effects. Patient should consult prescriber for additional questions.

Intended Use and Disclaimer: Should not be printed and given to patients. This information is intended to serve as a concise initial reference for healthcare professionals to use when discussing medications with a patient. You must ultimately rely on your own discretion, experience and judgment in diagnosing, treating and advising patients.

Related Information

Management of Drug Extravasations *on page 1700*

Oral Medications That Should Not Be Crushed or Altered *on page 1712*

Nitroprusside (nye troe PRUS ide)

Brand Names: U.S. Nitropress

Index Terms Nitroprusside Sodium; Sodium Nitroferricyanide; Sodium Nitroprusside

Pharmacologic Category Antihypertensive; Vasodilator

Medication Safety Issues

Sound-alike/look-alike issues:

Nitroprusside may be confused with nitroglycerin

High alert medication:

The Institute for Safe Medication Practices (ISMP) includes this medication among its list of drugs which have a heightened risk of causing significant patient harm when used in error.

Pregnancy Risk Factor C

Lactation Excretion in breast milk unknown/not recommended

Breast-Feeding Considerations It is not known if nitroprusside is excreted in breast milk. Due to the potential for serious adverse reactions in the nursing infant, a decision should be made whether to discontinue nursing or to discontinue the drug, taking into account the importance of treatment to the mother.

Use Management of hypertensive crises; acute decompensated heart failure (HF); used for controlled hypotension to reduce bleeding during surgery

Unlabeled Use Management of hypertension during acute ischemic stroke

Mechanism of Action/Effect Causes peripheral vasodilation by direct action on venous and arteriolar smooth muscle, thus reducing peripheral resistance; will increase cardiac output by decreasing afterload; reduces aortal and left ventricular impedance

Contraindications Treatment of compensatory hypertension (aortic coarctation, arteriovenous shunting); to produce controlled hypotension during surgery in patients with known inadequate cerebral circulation or in moribund patients requiring emergency surgery; high output heart failure associated with reduced systemic vascular resistance (eg, septic shock); congenital optic atrophy or tobacco amblyopia

Warnings/Precautions [U.S. Boxed Warning] Excessive hypotension resulting in compromised perfusion of vital organs may occur; continuous blood pressure monitoring by experienced personnel is required. Except when used briefly or at low (<2 mcg/kg/minute) infusion rates, nitroprusside gives rise to large cyanide quantities. Do not use the maximum dose for more than 10 minutes; if blood pressure is not controlled by the maximum rate (ie, 10 mcg/kg/minute) after 10 minutes, discontinue infusion. Monitor for cyanide toxicity via acid-base balance and venous oxygen concentration; however, clinicians should note that these indicators may not always reliably indicate cyanide toxicity. Patients at risk of cyanide toxicity include those who are malnourished, have hepatic impairment, or those undergoing cardiopulmonary bypass, or therapeutic hypothermia (Rindone, 1992). Discontinue use of nitroprusside if signs and/or symptoms of cyanide toxicity (eg, metabolic acidosis, decreased oxygen saturation, bradycardia, confusion, convulsions) occur. Although not routinely done, sodium thiosulfate has been co-administered with nitroprusside using a 10:1 ratio of sodium thiosulfate to nitroprusside when higher doses of nitroprusside are used (eg, 4-10 mcg/kg/minute) for extended periods of time in order to prevent cyanide toxicity (Varon, 2008; Shulz, 2010); thiocyanate toxicity may still occur with this approach (Rindone, 1992). The use of ▶

◀ other agents (eg, clevidipine, labetalol, nicardipine) should be considered if blood pressure is not controlled with nitroprusside. Use the lowest end of the dosage range with renal impairment. Cyanide toxicity may occur in patients with decreased liver function. Thiocyanate toxicity occurs in patients with renal impairment or those on prolonged infusions.

When nitroprusside is used for controlled hypotension during surgery, correct pre-existing anemia and hypovolemia prior to use when possible. Use with extreme caution in patients with elevated intracranial pressure (head trauma, cerebral hemorrhage), severe renal impairment, hepatic failure, hypothyroidism. **[U.S. Boxed Warning]: Solution must be further diluted with 5% dextrose in water. Do not administer by direct injection.**

Drug Interactions

Avoid Concomitant Use There are no known interactions where it is recommended to avoid concomitant use.

Decreased Effect

The levels/effects of Nitroprusside may be decreased by: Herbs (Hypertensive Properties); Methylphenidate; Yohimbine

Increased Effect/Toxicity

Nitroprusside may increase the levels/effects of: Amifostine; Antihypertensives; DULoxetine; Hypotensive Agents; Obinutuzumab; Prilocaine; RiTUXimab; Sodium Nitrite

The levels/effects of Nitroprusside may be increased by: Alfuzosin; Brimonidine (Topical); Calcium Channel Blockers; Diazoxide; Herbs (Hypotensive Properties); MAO Inhibitors; Nitric Oxide; Pentoxifylline; Phosphodiesterase 5 Inhibitors; Prostacyclin Analogues

Adverse Reactions Frequency not defined.

Cardiovascular: Bradycardia, ECG changes, flushing, hypotension (excessive), palpitation, substernal distress, tachycardia

Central nervous system: Apprehension, dizziness, headache, intracranial pressure increased, restlessness

Dermatologic: Rash

Endocrine & metabolic: Metabolic acidosis (secondary to cyanide toxicity), hypothyroidism

Gastrointestinal: Abdominal pain, ileus, nausea, retching, vomiting

Hematologic: Methemoglobinemia, platelet aggregation decreased

Local: Injection site irritation

Neuromuscular & skeletal: Hyperreflexia (secondary to thiocyanate toxicity), muscle twitching

Ocular: Miosis (secondary to thiocyanate toxicity)

Otic: Tinnitus (secondary to thiocyanate toxicity)

Respiratory: Hyperoxemia (secondary to cyanide toxicity)

Miscellaneous: Cyanide toxicity, diaphoresis, thiocyanate toxicity

Pharmacodynamics/Kinetics

Onset of Action Hypotensive effect: <2 minutes

Duration of Action Hypotensive effect: 1-10 minutes

Available Dosage Forms

Solution, Intravenous:

Nitropress: 25 mg/mL (2 mL)

General Dosage Range I.V.: *Children and Adults:* Initial: 0.3 mcg/kg/minute; Usual dose: 3 mcg/kg/minute (maximum: 10 mcg/kg/minute)

Usual Infusion Concentrations: Pediatric I.V. infusion: 100 mcg/mL or 200 mcg/mL

Usual Infusion Concentrations: Adult I.V. infusion: 50 mg in 250 mL (concentration: 200 **mcg**/mL) or 100 mg in 250 mL (concentration: 400 **mcg**/mL) of D_5W

Administration

I.V. I.V. infusion only; infusion pump required; must be diluted prior to administration; not for direct injection. Due to potential for excessive hypotension, continuously monitor patient's blood pressure during therapy.

Injectable Detail pH: 3.5-6

Preparation for Administration

Prior to administration, nitroprusside sodium should be further diluted by diluting 50 mg in 250-1000 mL of D_5W (preferred), LR, or NS.

Use only clear solutions; solutions of nitroprusside exhibit a color described as brownish, brown, brownish-pink, light orange, and straw. Solutions are highly sensitive to light. Exposure to light causes decomposition, resulting in a highly colored solution of orange, dark brown or blue. **A blue color indicates almost complete decomposition.** Do not use discolored solutions (eg, blue, green, red) or solutions in which particulate matter is visible.

Prepared solutions should be wrapped with aluminum foil or other opaque material to protect from light (do as soon as possible).

Storage/Stability Store the intact vial at 20°C to 25°C (68°F to 77°F). Protect from light.

Stability of parenteral admixture at room temperature (25°C) and at refrigeration temperature (4°C) is 24 hours.

Nursing Actions

Physical Assessment Monitor infusion site closely to prevent extravasation. Monitor patient blood pressure continuously. Assess acid/base balance (metabolic acidosis is early sign of cyanide toxicity). Monitor for disorientation, hypoxia, and muscular twitching.

Patient Education

• Discuss specific use of drug and side effects with patient as it relates to treatment. (HCAHPS: During this hospital stay, were you given any medicine that you had not taken before? Before giving you any new medicine, how often did hospital staff tell you what the medicine was

for? How often did hospital staff describe possible side effects in a way you could understand?)
- Patient may experience flushing, headache, or injection site irritation. Have patient report immediately to prescriber dyspnea, tachycardia, severe dizziness, illogical thinking, tremors, fasciculations, fatigue, considerable nausea, or rash (HCAHPS).
- Educate patient about signs of a significant reaction (eg, wheezing; chest tightness; fever; itching; bad cough; blue skin color; seizures; or swelling of face, lips, tongue, or throat). **Note:** This is not a comprehensive list of all side effects. Patient should consult prescriber for additional questions.

Intended Use and Disclaimer: Should not be printed and given to patients. This information is intended to serve as a concise initial reference for healthcare professionals to use when discussing medications with a patient. You must ultimately rely on your own discretion, experience and judgment in diagnosing, treating and advising patients.

Nizatidine (ni ZA ti deen)

Brand Names: U.S. Axid; Axid AR [OTC]
Pharmacologic Category Histamine H₂ Antagonist
Medication Safety Issues
 Sound-alike/look-alike issues:
  Axid® may be confused with Ansaid®
 International issues:
  Tazac [Australia] may be confused with Tazact brand name for piperacillin/tazobactam [India]; Tiazac brand name for diltiazem [U.S., Canada]
Pregnancy Risk Factor B
Lactation Enters breast milk/consider risk:benefit
Use Treatment and maintenance of duodenal ulcer; treatment of benign gastric ulcer; treatment of gastroesophageal reflux disease (GERD)
Unlabeled Use Part of a multidrug regimen for *H. pylori* eradication to reduce the risk of duodenal ulcer recurrence
Available Dosage Forms
 Capsule, Oral:
  Axid: 300 mg
  Generic: 150 mg, 300 mg
 Solution, Oral:
  Axid: 15 mg/mL (480 mL)
  Generic: 15 mg/mL (473 mL, 480 mL)
 Tablet, Oral:
  Axid AR [OTC]: 75 mg
General Dosage Range Dosage adjustment recommended in patients with renal impairment
Oral:
 Children ≥12 years: 150 mg twice daily
 Adults: 300 mg/day in 1-2 divided doses **or** 75 mg twice daily (OTC dosing)

Nursing Actions
 Patient Education
- Discuss specific use of drug and side effects with patient as it relates to treatment. (HCAHPS: During this hospital stay, were you given any medicine that you had not taken before? Before giving you any new medicine, how often did hospital staff tell you what the medicine was for? How often did hospital staff describe possible side effects in a way you could understand?)
- Patient may experience dizziness, headache, constipation, or diarrhea. Have patient report immediately to prescriber angina, tachycardia, illogical thinking, ecchymosis, bleeding, or rash (HCAHPS).
- Educate patient about signs of a significant reaction (eg, wheezing; chest tightness; fever; itching; bad cough; blue skin color; seizures; or swelling of face, lips, tongue, or throat). **Note:** This is not a comprehensive list of all side effects. Patient should consult prescriber for additional questions.

Intended Use and Disclaimer: Should not be printed and given to patients. This information is intended to serve as a concise initial reference for healthcare professionals to use when discussing medications with a patient. You must ultimately rely on your own discretion, experience and judgment in diagnosing, treating and advising patients.

Norepinephrine (nor ep i NEF rin)

Brand Names: U.S. Levophed
Index Terms Levarterenol Bitartrate; Noradrenaline; Noradrenaline Acid Tartrate; Norepinephrine Bitartrate
Pharmacologic Category Alpha/Beta Agonist
Medication Safety Issues
 Sound-alike/look-alike issues:
  Levophed® may be confused with levofloxacin
 High alert medication:
  The Institute for Safe Medication Practices (ISMP) includes this medication among its list of drugs which have a heightened risk of causing significant patient harm when used in error.
Pregnancy Risk Factor C
Lactation Excretion in breast milk unknown/use caution
Breast-Feeding Considerations It is not known if norepinephrine is excreted in breast milk. The manufacturer recommends that caution be exercised when administering norepinephrine to nursing women.
Use Treatment of shock which persists after adequate fluid volume replacement; severe hypotension

Note: Recommended as the first-choice vasopressor for the treatment of sepsis and septic shock in adult patients (Dellinger, 2013)

◀ **Mechanism of Action/Effect** Stimulates $beta_1$-adrenergic receptors and alpha-adrenergic receptors causing increased contractility and heart rate as well as vasoconstriction, thereby increasing systemic blood pressure and coronary blood flow; clinically, alpha effects (vasoconstriction) are greater than beta effects (inotropic and chronotropic effects)

Contraindications Hypersensitivity to norepinephrine, bisulfites (contains metabisulfite), or any component of the formulation; hypotension from hypovolemia except as an emergency measure to maintain coronary and cerebral perfusion until volume could be replaced; mesenteric or peripheral vascular thrombosis unless it is a life-saving procedure; during anesthesia with cyclopropane (not available in U.S.) or halothane (not available in U.S.) anesthesia (risk of ventricular arrhythmias)

Warnings/Precautions Assure adequate circulatory volume to minimize need for vasoconstrictors. Avoid hypertension; monitor blood pressure closely and adjust infusion rate. Use with extreme caution in patients taking MAO-Inhibitors. Vesicant; ensure proper needle or catheter placement prior to and during infusion. Avoid extravasation; infuse into a large vein if possible. Avoid infusion into leg veins. Montior I.V. site closely. **[U.S. Boxed Warning]: If extravasation occurs, infiltrate the area with diluted phentolamine (5-10 mg in 10-15 mL of saline) with a fine hypodermic needle. Phentolamine should be administered as soon as possible after extravasation is noted to prevent sloughing/necrosis**. Product may contain sodium metabisulfite.

Drug Interactions

Avoid Concomitant Use

Avoid concomitant use of Norepinephrine with any of the following: Ergot Derivatives; Inhalational Anesthetics; Iobenguane I 123

Decreased Effect

Norepinephrine may decrease the levels/effects of: Benzylpenicilloyl Polylysine; Iobenguane I 123; Ioflupane I 123

The levels/effects of Norepinephrine may be decreased by: Alpha1-Blockers; Spironolactone

Increased Effect/Toxicity

Norepinephrine may increase the levels/effects of: Droxidopa; Sympathomimetics

The levels/effects of Norepinephrine may be increased by: Antacids; AtoMOXetine; Beta-Blockers; Cannabinoids; Carbonic Anhydrase Inhibitors; COMT Inhibitors; Ergot Derivatives; Hyaluronidase; Inhalational Anesthetics; MAO Inhibitors; Serotonin/Norepinephrine Reuptake Inhibitors; Tricyclic Antidepressants

Adverse Reactions Frequency not defined.

Cardiovascular: Arrhythmias, bradycardia, peripheral (digital) ischemia

Central nervous system: Anxiety, headache (transient)

Local: Skin necrosis (with extravasation)

Respiratory: Dyspnea, respiratory difficulty

Pharmacodynamics/Kinetics

Onset of Action I.V.: Very rapid-acting

Duration of Action Vasopressor: 1-2 minutes

Available Dosage Forms

Solution, Injection:

Levophed: 1 mg/mL (4 mL)

Generic: 1 mg/mL (4 mL)

Solution, Injection [preservative free]:

Generic: 1 mg/mL (4 mL)

General Dosage Range I.V.:

Children: Initial: 0.05-0.1 mcg/kg/minute; Maintenance: Titrate to desired effect (maximum: 2 mcg/kg/minute)

Adults: Initial: 8-12 mcg/minute; Maintenance: Titrate to desired effect (usual maintenance range: 2-4 mcg/minute)

Usual Infusion Concentrations: Pediatric I.V. infusion: 8 mcg/mL or 16 mcg/mL

Usual Infusion Concentrations: Adult I.V. infusion: 4 mg in 250 mL (concentration: 16 mcg/mL) or 8 mg in 250 mL (concentration: 32 mcg/mL) of D_5W or NS

Administration

I.V. Administer as a continuous infusion with the use of an infusion pump. Dilute prior to use. Administration via central line recommended (may cause severe ischemic necrosis if extravasated). Do not administer sodium bicarbonate (or any alkaline solution) through an I.V. line containing norepinephrine; inactivation of norepinephrine may occur.

Vesicant; ensure proper needle or catheter placement prior to and during infusion; avoid extravasation.

Extravasation management: If extravasation occurs, stop infusion immediately and disconnect (leave cannula/needle in place); gently aspirate extravasated solution (do **NOT** flush the line); remove needle/cannula; elevate extremity. Initiate phentolamine (or alternative) antidote. Apply dry warm compresses (Hurst, 2004).

Phentolamine: Dilute 5-10 mg in 10-15 mL NS and administer into extravasation site as soon as possible after extravasation (Peberdy, 2010) or dilute 5-10 mg in 10 mL NS and administer into extravasation area (within 12 hours of extravasation).

Alternatives to phentolamine (due to shortage):

Nitroglycerin topical 2% ointment (based on limited case reports in neonates/infants): Apply 4 mm/kg as a thin ribbon to the affected areas; may repeat after 8 hours if needed (Wong, 1992) or apply a 1-inch strip on the affected site (Denkler, 1989).

Terbutaline (based on limited case reports): Infiltrate extravasation area using a solution of terbutaline 1 mg diluted to 10 mL in NS (large extravasation site; administration volume varied from 3-10 mL) **or** 1 mg diluted in 1 mL NS (small/distal extravasation site; administration volume varied from 0.5-1 mL) (Stier, 1999).

Preparation for Administration Dilute with D_5W, D_5NS, or NS; dilution in NS is not recommended by the manufacturer; however, stability in NS has been demonstrated (Tremblay, 2008).

Storage/Stability Readily oxidized. Protect from light. Do not use if brown coloration. Stability of parenteral admixture at room temperature (25°C) is 24 hours.

Nursing Actions

Physical Assessment Monitor blood pressure and cardiac status, CNS status, skin temperature, and color during and following infusion. Monitor fluid status (I & O). Assess infusion site frequently for extravasation. Blanching along vein pathway is a preliminary sign of extravasation.

Patient Education

• Discuss specific use of drug and side effects with patient as it relates to treatment. (HCAHPS: During this hospital stay, were you given any medicine that you had not taken before? Before giving you any new medicine, how often did hospital staff tell you what the medicine was for? How often did hospital staff describe possible side effects in a way you could understand?)

• Patient may experience dizziness, nausea, nervousness, anxiety, or application site irritation. Have patient report immediately to prescriber rash (HCAHPS).

• Educate patient about signs of a significant reaction (eg, wheezing; chest tightness; fever; itching; bad cough; blue skin color; seizures; or swelling of face, lips, tongue, or throat). **Note:** This is not a comprehensive list of all side effects. Patient should consult prescriber for additional questions.

Intended Use and Disclaimer: Should not be printed and given to patients. This information is intended to serve as a concise initial reference for healthcare professionals to use when discussing medications with a patient. You must ultimately rely on your own discretion, experience and judgment in diagnosing, treating and advising patients.

Related Information

Management of Drug Extravasations *on page 1700*

Norethindrone (nor ETH in drone)

Brand Names: U.S. Aygestin; Camila; Errin; Heather; Jencycla; Jolivette; Lyza; Nor-QD; Nora-BE; Ortho Micronor

Index Terms Norethindrone Acetate; Norethisterone

Pharmacologic Category Contraceptive; Progestin

Medication Safety Issues

Sound-alike/look-alike issues:

Micronor® may be confused with miconazole, Micronase

Pregnancy Risk Factor X

Lactation Enters breast milk/use caution

Use Treatment of amenorrhea; abnormal uterine bleeding; endometriosis; prevention of pregnancy

Available Dosage Forms

Tablet, Oral:

Aygestin: 5 mg

Camila: 0.35 mg

Errin: 0.35 mg

Heather: 0.35 mg

Jencycla: 0.35 mg

Jolivette: 0.35 mg

Lyza: 0.35 mg

Nor-QD: 0.35 mg

Nora-BE: 0.35 mg

Ortho Micronor: 0.35 mg

Generic: 0.35 mg, 5 mg

General Dosage Range Oral:

Norethindrone: *Children (postmenarche) and Adults:* 0.35 mg every day

Norethindrone acetate: *Adolescents and Adults:* 2.5-15 mg once daily for 5-14 days of menstrual cycle

Administration

Oral Administer at the same time each day. When used for the prevention of pregnancy, a back up method of contraception should be used for 48 hours if dose is missed or taken ≥3 hours late.

Hazardous agent; use appropriate precautions for handling and disposal (NIOSH, 2012).

Nursing Actions

Physical Assessment Teach appropriate administration schedule. Schedule physical exam with reference to the breasts and pelvis, including a Papanicolaou smear. Exam may be deferred if appropriate; pregnancy should be ruled out prior to use. Monitor patient closely for loss of vision, sudden onset of proptosis, diplopia, migraine, blood pressure, signs and symptoms of thromboembolic disorders, signs or symptoms of depression, glycemic control in diabetics, and lipid profiles in patients being treated for hyperlipidemias. Adequate diagnostic measures, including endometrial sampling, if indicated, should be performed to rule out malignancy in all cases of undiagnosed abnormal vaginal bleeding. Emphasize need for regular breast self-exam and necessity of annual physical check-up with long-term use.

Patient Education

• Discuss specific use of drug and side effects with patient as it relates to treatment. (HCAHPS: During this hospital stay, were you given any medicine that you had not taken before? Before

giving you any new medicine, how often did hospital staff tell you what the medicine was for? How often did hospital staff describe possible side effects in a way you could understand?)

• Patient may experience headache, nausea, dizziness, mastalgia, or menstrual irregularity. Have patient report immediately to prescriber depression, nervousness, emotional instability, anxiety, angina, dyspnea, edema, or rash (HCAHPS).

• Educate patient about signs of a significant reaction (eg, wheezing; chest tightness; fever; itching; bad cough; blue skin color; seizures; or swelling of face, lips, tongue, or throat). **Note:** This is not a comprehensive list of all side effects. Patient should consult prescriber for additional questions.

Intended Use and Disclaimer: Should not be printed and given to patients. This information is intended to serve as a concise initial reference for healthcare professionals to use when discussing medications with a patient. You must ultimately rely on your own discretion, experience and judgment in diagnosing, treating and advising patients.

Norethindrone and Mestranol
(nor eth IN drone & MES tra nole)

Brand Names: U.S. Necon® 1/50; Norinyl® 1+50
Index Terms Mestranol and Norethindrone; Ortho Novum 1/50
Pharmacologic Category Contraceptive; Estrogen and Progestin Combination
Medication Safety Issues
Sound-alike/look-alike issues:
Norinyl® may be confused with Nardil®
Pregnancy Risk Factor X
Lactation Enters breast milk/not recommended
Use Prevention of pregnancy
Unlabeled Use Treatment of hypermenorrhea (menorrhagia); pain associated with endometriosis; dysmenorrhea; dysfunctional uterine bleeding; treatment of polycystic ovary syndrome (PCOS) in women with menstrual irregularities and hirsutism/acne
Available Dosage Forms
Tablet, monophasic formulations:
Necon® 1/50: Norethindrone 1 mg and mestranol 0.05 mg [21 light blue tablets and 7 white inactive tablets] (28s)
Norinyl® 1+50: Norethindrone 1 mg and mestranol 0.05 mg [21 white tablets and 7 orange inactive tablets] (28s)
General Dosage Range Oral:
21-tablet package: *Children (menarche) and Adults:* 1 tablet daily for 21 days, followed by 7 days off
28-tablet package: *Children (menarche) and Adults:* 1 tablet daily

Administration
Oral Administer at the same time each day. Administer at bedtime to minimize occurrence of adverse effects. Hazardous agent; use appropriate precautions for handling and disposal (NIOSH, 2012).
Nursing Actions
Physical Assessment See individual agents.
Patient Education
• Discuss specific use of drug and side effects with patient as it relates to treatment. (HCAHPS: During this hospital stay, were you given any medicine that you had not taken before? Before giving you any new medicine, how often did hospital staff tell you what the medicine was for? How often did hospital staff describe possible side effects in a way you could understand?)

• Patient may experience weight gain, headache, dyspepsia, nausea, macromastia, vaginal yeast infection, or menstrual irregularity. Have patient report immediately to prescriber angina, dyspnea, edema, sudden vision changes, eye pain, eye irritation, contact lens discomfort, mastalgia, or pregnancy (HCAHPS).

• Educate patient about signs of a significant reaction (eg, wheezing; chest tightness; fever; itching; bad cough; blue skin color; seizures; or swelling of face, lips, tongue, or throat). **Note:** This is not a comprehensive list of all side effects. Patient should consult prescriber for additional questions.

Intended Use and Disclaimer: Should not be printed and given to patients. This information is intended to serve as a concise initial reference for healthcare professionals to use when discussing medications with a patient. You must ultimately rely on your own discretion, experience and judgment in diagnosing, treating and advising patients.

Related Information
Norethindrone *on page 1139*

Nortriptyline (nor TRIP ti leen)

Brand Names: U.S. Pamelor
Index Terms Nortriptyline Hydrochloride
Pharmacologic Category Antidepressant, Tricyclic (Secondary Amine)
Medication Safety Issues
Sound-alike/look-alike issues:
Aventyl® HCl may be confused with Bentyl®
Nortriptyline may be confused with amitriptyline, desipramine, Norpramin®
Pamelor™ may be confused with Demerol®, Tambocor™

BEERS Criteria medication:
This drug may be potentially inappropriate for use in geriatric patients (SIADH: Quality of evidence - moderate; Strength of recommendation - strong).

Medication Guide Available Yes

Lactation Enters breast milk

Use Treatment of symptoms of depression

Unlabeled Use Chronic pain (including neuropathic pain), myofascial pain, burning mouth sydrome, anxiety disorders, attention-deficit/hyperactivity disorder (ADHD); enuresis; adjunctive therapy for smoking cessation

Available Dosage Forms

Capsule, Oral:
Pamelor: 10 mg, 25 mg, 50 mg, 75 mg
Generic: 10 mg, 25 mg, 50 mg, 75 mg

Solution, Oral:
Generic: 10 mg/5 mL (473 mL)

General Dosage Range Oral:
Adults: 25 mg 3-4 times/day (maximum: 150 mg/day)
Elderly: Initial: 10-25 mg once daily; Maintenance: 75 mg/day in 1-2 divided doses

Nursing Actions

Physical Assessment Assess for suicidal tendencies before beginning therapy. Assess therapeutic response (mental status, mood, affect). Monitor for suicide ideation at beginning of therapy and periodically throughout. Dosage should be tapered slowly when discontinuing. Caution patients with diabetes to monitor glucose levels closely; may increase or decrease serum glucose levels.

Patient Education

- Discuss specific use of drug and side effects with patient as it relates to treatment. (HCAHPS: During this hospital stay, were you given any medicine that you had not taken before? Before giving you any new medicine, how often did hospital staff tell you what the medicine was for? How often did hospital staff describe possible side effects in a way you could understand?)
- Patient may experience presyncope, fatigue, blurred vision, illogical thinking, dizziness, constipation, or xerostomia. Have patient report immediately to prescriber urinary retention, severe asthenia, or rash (HCAHPS).
- Educate patient about signs of a significant reaction (eg, wheezing; chest tightness; fever; itching; bad cough; blue skin color; seizures; or swelling of face, lips, tongue, or throat). **Note:** This is not a comprehensive list of all side effects. Patient should consult prescriber for additional questions.

Intended Use and Disclaimer: Should not be printed and given to patients. This information is intended to serve as a concise initial reference for healthcare professionals to use when discussing medications with a patient. You must ultimately rely on your own discretion, experience and judgment in diagnosing, treating and advising patients.

Related Information
Peak and Trough Guidelines *on page 1710*

Nystatin (Oral) (nye STAT in)

Brand Names: U.S. Bio-Statin

Pharmacologic Category Antifungal Agent, Oral Nonabsorbed

Medication Safety Issues

Sound-alike/look-alike issues:
Nystatin may be confused with HMG-CoA reductase inhibitors (also known as "statins"; eg, atorvaSTATin, fluvastatin, lovastatin, pitavastatin, pravastatin, rosuvastatin, simvastatin), Nitrostat®

Pregnancy Risk Factor C

Lactation Excretion in breast milk unknown/use caution

Use Treatment of susceptible cutaneous, mucocutaneous, and oral cavity fungal infections normally caused by the *Candida* species

Available Dosage Forms

Capsule, Oral [preservative free]:
Bio-Statin: 500,000 units, 1,000,000 units

Powder, Oral:
Bio-Statin: (1 ea)
Generic: (1 ea)

Suspension, Mouth/Throat:
Generic: 100,000 units/mL (5 mL, 60 mL, 473 mL, 480 mL)

Tablet, Oral:
Generic: 500,000 units

General Dosage Range Oral:
Premature infants: 100,000 units 4 times/day
Infants: 200,000 units 4 times/day
Children: 400,000-600,000 units 4 times/day
Adults: 400,000-1,000,000 units/day in 3-4 divided doses

Administration

Oral Suspension: Shake well before using. Should be swished about the mouth and retained in the mouth for as long as possible (several minutes) before swallowing. For neonates and infants, paint nystatin suspension into recesses of the mouth.

Nursing Actions

Patient Education

- Discuss specific use of drug and side effects with patient as it relates to treatment. (HCAHPS: During this hospital stay, were you given any medicine that you had not taken before? Before giving you any new medicine, how often did hospital staff tell you what the medicine was for? How often did hospital staff describe possible side effects in a way you could understand?)
- Patient may experience dyspepsia or nausea. Have patient report immediately to prescriber reoccurring yeast infection, dysphagia, or rash (HCAHPS).

• Educate patient about signs of a significant reaction (eg, wheezing; chest tightness; fever; itching; bad cough; blue skin color; seizures; or swelling of face, lips, tongue, or throat). **Note:** This is not a comprehensive list of all side effects. Patient should consult prescriber for additional questions.

Intended Use and Disclaimer: Should not be printed and given to patients. This information is intended to serve as a concise initial reference for healthcare professionals to use when discussing medications with a patient. You must ultimately rely on your own discretion, experience and judgment in diagnosing, treating and advising patients.

Nystatin (Topical) (nye STAT in)

Brand Names: U.S. Nyamyc; Nystop; Pedi-Dri; Pediaderm AF Complete

Pharmacologic Category Antifungal Agent, Topical

Medication Safety Issues

Sound-alike/look-alike issues:
Nystatin may be confused with HMG-CoA reductase inhibitors (also known as "statins"; eg, atorvaSTATin, fluvastatin, lovastatin, pitavastatin, pravastatin, rosuvastatin, simvastatin), Nitrostat

Pregnancy Risk Factor C

Lactation Excretion in breast milk unknown/not recommended

Use Treatment of susceptible cutaneous and mucocutaneous fungal infections normally caused by the *Candida* species

Available Dosage Forms

Cream, External:
Generic: 100,000 units/g (15 g, 30 g)

Kit, External:
Pediaderm AF Complete: 100,000 units/g

Ointment, External:
Generic: 100,000 units/g (15 g, 30 g)

Powder, External:
Nyamyc: 100,000 units/g (15 g, 30 g, 60 g)
Nystop: 100,000 units/g (15 g, 30 g, 60 g)
Pedi-Dri: 100,000 units/g (56.7 g)
Generic: 100,000 units/g (15 g, 30 g, 60 g)

General Dosage Range
Topical: *Children and Adults:* Apply 2-3 times/day to affected areas

Nursing Actions

Physical Assessment Determine that cause of infection is fungal. Avoid skin contact when applying.

Patient Education
• Discuss specific use of drug and side effects with patient as it relates to treatment. (HCAHPS: During this hospital stay, were you given any medicine that you had not taken before? Before giving you any new medicine, how often did

hospital staff tell you what the medicine was for? How often did hospital staff describe possible side effects in a way you could understand?)
• Have patient report immediately to prescriber severe skin irritation (HCAHPS).
• Educate patient about signs of a significant reaction (eg, wheezing; chest tightness; fever; itching; bad cough; blue skin color; seizures; or swelling of face, lips, tongue, or throat). **Note:** This is not a comprehensive list of all side effects. Patient should consult prescriber for additional questions.

Intended Use and Disclaimer: Should not be printed and given to patients. This information is intended to serve as a concise initial reference for healthcare professionals to use when discussing medications with a patient. You must ultimately rely on your own discretion, experience and judgment in diagnosing, treating and advising patients.

Nystatin and Triamcinolone
(nye STAT in & trye am SIN oh lone)

Index Terms Triamcinolone and Nystatin

Pharmacologic Category Antifungal Agent, Topical; Corticosteroid, Topical

Pregnancy Risk Factor C

Lactation Excretion in breast milk unknown/use caution

Use Treatment of cutaneous candidiasis

Available Dosage Forms

Cream: Nystatin 100,000 units and triamcinolone 0.1% (15 g, 30 g, 60 g)

Ointment: Nystatin 100,000 units and triamcinolone 0.1% (15 g, 30 g, 60 g)

General Dosage Range Topical: *Children and Adults:* Apply sparingly to affected area(s) twice daily

Administration

Topical External use only; do not use on open or weeping wounds; do not use with occlusive dressings.

Nursing Actions

Physical Assessment See individual agents.

Patient Education
• Discuss specific use of drug and side effects with patient as it relates to treatment. (HCAHPS: During this hospital stay, were you given any medicine that you had not taken before? Before giving you any new medicine, how often did hospital staff tell you what the medicine was for? How often did hospital staff describe possible side effects in a way you could understand?)
• Patient may experience skin irritation. Have patient report immediately to prescriber reoccurring yeast infection (HCAHPS).
• Educate patient about signs of a significant reaction (eg, wheezing; chest tightness; fever; itching; bad cough; blue skin color; seizures; or

swelling of face, lips, tongue, or throat). **Note:** This is not a comprehensive list of all side effects. Patient should consult prescriber for additional questions.

Intended Use and Disclaimer: Should not be printed and given to patients. This information is intended to serve as a concise initial reference for healthcare professionals to use when discussing medications with a patient. You must ultimately rely on your own discretion, experience and judgment in diagnosing, treating and advising patients.

Related Information

Nystatin (Topical) *on page 1142*
Triamcinolone (Topical) *on page 1565*

Octreotide (ok TREE oh tide)

Brand Names: U.S. SandoSTATIN; SandoSTATIN LAR Depot
Index Terms Longastatin; Octreotide Acetate
Pharmacologic Category Antidiarrheal; Antidote; Somatostatin Analog
Medication Safety Issues
Sound-alike/look-alike issues:
Octreotide may be confused with pasireotide
SandoSTATIN may be confused with SandIM-MUNE, SandoSTATIN LAR, sargramostim, simvastatin
Pregnancy Risk Factor B
Lactation Excreted in breast milk/use caution
Use Control of symptoms (diarrhea and flushing) in patients with metastatic carcinoid tumors; treatment of watery diarrhea associated with vasoactive intestinal peptide-secreting tumors (VIPomas); treatment of acromegaly
Unlabeled Use Treatment of AIDS-associated diarrhea (including *Cryptosporidiosis*), chemotherapy-induced diarrhea, graft-versus-host disease (GVHD) associated diarrhea, postgastrectomy dumping syndrome; control of bleeding of esophageal varices; second-line treatment for thymic malignancies; Cushing's syndrome (ectopic); insulinomas; small bowel fistulas; islet cell tumors; Zollinger-Ellison syndrome; congenital hyperinsulinism; hypothalamic obesity; treatment of hypoglycemia secondary to sulfonylurea poisoning; treatment of malignant bowel obstruction
Available Dosage Forms
Kit, Intramuscular:
SandoSTATIN LAR Depot: 10 mg, 20 mg, 30 mg
Solution, Injection:
SandoSTATIN: 50 mcg/mL (1 mL); 100 mcg/mL (1 mL); 200 mcg/mL (5 mL); 500 mcg/mL (1 mL); 1000 mcg/mL (5 mL)
Generic: 50 mcg/mL (1 mL); 100 mcg/mL (1 mL); 200 mcg/mL (5 mL); 1000 mcg/5 mL (5 mL); 500 mcg/mL (1 mL); 1000 mcg/mL (5 mL)
Solution, Injection [preservative free]:
Generic: 100 mcg/mL (1 mL); 500 mcg/mL (1 mL)

General Dosage Range Dosage adjustment recommended in patients with hepatic or renal impairment
I.M.: *Adults:* Depot: 20 mg every 4 weeks (maximum: 40 mg every 2 weeks)
I.V., SubQ: *Adults:* 50-1500 mcg/day in 2-4 divided doses
Usual Infusion Concentrations: Adult I.V. infusion: 500 mcg in 250 mL (concentration: 2 **mcg/mL**) of D₅W or NS

Administration
I.M. Depot formulation: Administer I.M. intragluteal (avoid deltoid administration); alternate gluteal injection sites to avoid irritation. **Do not** administer Sandostatin LAR® intravenously or subcutaneously; must be administered immediately after mixing.
I.V. Regular injection only (not suspension): I.V. administration may be I.V. push (undiluted over 3 minutes), intermittent I.V. infusion (over 15-30 minutes), or continuous I.V. infusion (unlabeled route).
Injectable Detail Do not use if solution contains particles or is discolored.

pH: Solution: ~4.2
Other SubQ: Use the concentration with smallest volume to deliver dose to reduce injection site pain. Rotate injection site; may bring to room temperature prior to injection.

Nursing Actions
Physical Assessment May effect response to insulin or sulfonylureas and/or response to cardiovascular medications. Monitor for hyperglycemia, hypothyroidism, bradycardia, chest pain, GI disturbances, CNS changes, and dyspnea. Caution patients with diabetes to monitor serum glucose closely; may affect response to insulin or sulfonylureas. Teach patient appropriate injection technique and syringe/needle disposal.

Patient Education
• Discuss specific use of drug and side effects with patient as it relates to treatment. (HCAHPS: During this hospital stay, were you given any medicine that you had not taken before? Before giving you any new medicine, how often did hospital staff tell you what the medicine was for? How often did hospital staff describe possible side effects in a way you could understand?)
• Patient may experience flatulence, flu-like syndrome, constipation, dizziness, or injection site irritation. Have patient report immediately to prescriber signs of hyperglycemia, signs of hypothyroidism, signs of cholelithiasis, angina, severe nausea, considerable diarrhea, significant dyspepsia, bradycardia, arrhythmia, bloating, abdominal edema, jaundice, intolerable asthenia, severe headache, or signs of hypoglycemia (HCAHPS).

◀ • Educate patient about signs of a significant reaction (eg, wheezing; chest tightness; fever; itching; bad cough; blue skin color; seizures; or swelling of face, lips, tongue, or throat). **Note:** This is not a comprehensive list of all side effects. Patient should consult prescriber for additional questions.

Intended Use and Disclaimer: Should not be printed and given to patients. This information is intended to serve as a concise initial reference for healthcare professionals to use when discussing medications with a patient. You must ultimately rely on your own discretion, experience and judgment in diagnosing, treating and advising patients.

Ofatumumab (oh fa TOOM yoo mab)

Brand Names: U.S. Arzerra
Index Terms HuMax-CD20
Pharmacologic Category Antineoplastic Agent, Anti-CD20; Antineoplastic Agent, Monoclonal Antibody
Medication Safety Issues
Sound-alike/look-alike issues:
Ofatumumab may be confused with obinutuzumab, omalizumab
High alert medication:
This medication is in a class the Institute for Safe Medication Practices (ISMP) includes among its list of drug classes which have a heightened risk of causing significant patient harm when used in error.
Pregnancy Risk Factor C
Lactation Excretion in breast milk unknown/use caution
Use Chronic lymphocytic leukemia: Treatment of refractory chronic lymphocytic leukemia (CLL)
Available Dosage Forms
Concentrate, Intravenous [preservative free]:
Arzerra: 100 mg/5 mL (5 mL); 1000 mg/50 mL (50 mL)
General Dosage Range Dosage adjustment recommended in patients who develop toxicities
I.V.: *Adults:* 300 mg week 1, followed 1 week later by 2000 mg once weekly for 7 doses (doses 2-8), followed 4 weeks later by 2000 mg once every 4 weeks for 4 doses (doses 9-12; for a total of 12 doses)
Administration
I.V. Do not administer I.V. push or as a bolus. Premedicate with acetaminophen, an antihistamine and a corticosteroid 30-120 minutes prior to administration. Administer with an in-line filter (supplied). Do not mix with or infuse with other medications. Flush line before and after infusion with NS. Begin infusion within 12 hours of preparation. The final concentration of dose 1 is 0.3 mg/mL and final concentration of doses 2-12 is 2 mg/mL.

Premedication: Premedicate with oral acetaminophen (1000 mg), an oral or I.V. antihistamine (eg, cetirizine 10 mg orally or equivalent), and an I.V. corticosteroid. Full dose corticosteroid is recommended for doses 1, 2, and 9; in the absence of infusion reaction ≥grade 3, may gradually reduce corticosteroid dose for doses 3-8; administer full or half corticosteroid dose with doses 10-12 if ≥grade 3 did not occur with dose 9.
Doses 1 and 2: Initiate infusion at 12 mL/hour for 30 minutes, if tolerated (no infusion reaction) increase to 25 mL/hour for 30 minutes, if tolerated, increase to 50 mL/hour for 30 minutes, if tolerated, increase to 100 mL/hour for 30 minutes, if tolerated, increase to 200 mL/hour for duration of infusion.
Doses 3-12: Initiate infusion at 25 mL/hour for 30 minutes, if tolerated (no infusion reaction) increase to 50 mL/hour for 30 minutes, if tolerated, increase to 100 mL/hour for 30 minutes, if tolerated, increase to 200 mL/hour for 30 minutes, if tolerated, increase to 400 mL/hour for remainder of infusion.
Injectable Detail pH: 6.5
Nursing Actions
Physical Assessment Premedication may be ordered. Monitor patient very closely for infusion reactions; emergency medical equipment and medications for hypersensitivity reactions should be available. Instruct patient to report signs of HSR including shortness of breath, chills, chest pain, or other abnormal symptoms during infusion. Patient should have hepatitis B screening prior to first dose as drug may cause reactivation of hepatitis B virus. Instruct patients to have follow-up and check labs frequently throughout treatment. Inform about safety and bleeding precautions with thrombocytopenia, and infection precautions with low white blood cells. Rare cases of PML have occurred; patients should report any vision changes, memory loss, difficulty speaking, or new onset of clumsiness.
Patient Education
• Discuss specific use of drug and side effects with patient as it relates to treatment. (HCAHPS: During this hospital stay, were you given any medicine that you had not taken before? Before giving you any new medicine, how often did hospital staff tell you what the medicine was for? How often did hospital staff describe possible side effects in a way you could understand?)
• Patient may experience anemia, leukopenia, fatigue, nausea, diarrhea, chills, hives, or angina. Have patient report immediately to prescriber signs of infection, illogical thinking, dizziness or syncope, change in balance, dyspnea, difficulty speaking, severe dyspepsia, jaundice, ecchymosis, or rash (HCAHPS).
• Educate patient about signs of a significant reaction (eg, wheezing; chest tightness; fever;

itching; bad cough; blue skin color; seizures; or swelling of face, lips, tongue, or throat). **Note:** This is not a comprehensive list of all side effects. Patient should consult prescriber for additional questions.

Intended Use and Disclaimer: Should not be printed and given to patients. This information is intended to serve as a concise initial reference for healthcare professionals to use when discussing medications with a patient. You must ultimately rely on your own discretion, experience and judgment in diagnosing, treating and advising patients.

Ofloxacin (Ophthalmic) (oh FLOKS a sin)

Brand Names: U.S. Ocuflox
Pharmacologic Category Antibiotic, Fluoroquinolone; Antibiotic, Ophthalmic
Medication Safety Issues
  Sound-alike/look-alike issues:
  Ocuflox® may be confused with Occlusal™-HP, Ocufen®
Pregnancy Risk Factor C
Lactation Enters breast milk/not recommended
Use Treatment of superficial ocular infections involving the conjunctiva or cornea due to strains of susceptible organisms
Available Dosage Forms
  Solution, Ophthalmic:
  Ocuflox: 0.3% (5 mL)
  Generic: 0.3% (5 mL, 10 mL)
General Dosage Range Ophthalmic: *Children >1 year and Adults:* Initial: 1-2 drops every 30 minutes to 4 hours; Maintenance: 1-2 drops every 4-6 hours
Administration
  Other For ophthalmic use only; avoid touching tip of applicator to eye or other surfaces.
Nursing Actions
  Physical Assessment Instruct patient to report allergic reaction and tendon pain.
Patient Education
  • Discuss specific use of drug and side effects with patient as it relates to treatment. (HCAHPS: During this hospital stay, were you given any medicine that you had not taken before? Before giving you any new medicine, how often did hospital staff tell you what the medicine was for? How often did hospital staff describe possible side effects in a way you could understand?)
  • Patient may experience dizziness or eye irritation. Have patient report immediately to prescriber ankle pain, arthralgia, edema, sudden vision changes, or rash (HCAHPS).
  • Educate patient about signs of a significant reaction (eg, wheezing; chest tightness; fever; itching; bad cough; blue skin color; seizures; or swelling of face, lips, tongue, or throat). **Note:** This is not a comprehensive list of all side

effects. Patient should consult prescriber for additional questions.

Intended Use and Disclaimer: Should not be printed and given to patients. This information is intended to serve as a concise initial reference for healthcare professionals to use when discussing medications with a patient. You must ultimately rely on your own discretion, experience and judgment in diagnosing, treating and advising patients.

Ofloxacin (Otic) (oh FLOKS a sin)

Index Terms Floxin Otic Singles
Pharmacologic Category Antibiotic, Fluoroquinolone; Antibiotic, Otic
Medication Safety Issues
  Sound-alike/look-alike issues:
  Floxin may be confused with Flexeril®
  International issues:
  Floxin: Brand name for ofloxacin [U.S., Canada], but also the brand name for flunarizine [Thailand], norfloxacin [South Africa], and perfloxacin [Philippines]
  Floxin [U.S., Canada] may be confused with Flexin brand name for diclofenac [Argentina], cyclobenzaprine [Chile], and orphenadrine [Israel]; Flogen brand name for naproxen [Mexico]
Pregnancy Risk Factor C
Lactation Enters breast milk/not recommended
Use Otitis externa, chronic suppurative otitis media, acute otitis media
Available Dosage Forms
  Solution, Otic:
  Generic: 0.3% (5 mL, 10 mL)
General Dosage Range
  Otic:
  Children <6 months: Dosage not established
  Children ≥6 months to 12 years: 5 drops daily
  Children >12 years: 10 drops once or twice daily
  Adults: 10 drops once or twice daily
Administration
  Other Prior to use, warm solution by holding container in hands for 1-2 minutes. Patient should lie down with affected ear upward and medication instilled. Pump tragus 4 times to ensure penetration of medication. Patient should remain in this position for 5 minutes.
Nursing Actions
  Patient Education
  • Discuss specific use of drug and side effects with patient as it relates to treatment. (HCAHPS: During this hospital stay, were you given any medicine that you had not taken before? Before giving you any new medicine, how often did hospital staff tell you what the medicine was for? How often did hospital staff describe possible side effects in a way you could understand?)

- Patient may experience dizziness, skin irritation, or otalgia. Have patient report immediately to prescriber severe ear pain, ankle pain, arthralgia, edema, or rash (HCAHPS).
- Educate patient about signs of a significant reaction (eg, wheezing; chest tightness; fever; itching; bad cough; blue skin color; seizures; or swelling of face, lips, tongue, or throat). **Note:** This is not a comprehensive list of all side effects. Patient should consult prescriber for additional questions.

Intended Use and Disclaimer: Should not be printed and given to patients. This information is intended to serve as a concise initial reference for healthcare professionals to use when discussing medications with a patient. You must ultimately rely on your own discretion, experience and judgment in diagnosing, treating and advising patients.

OLANZapine (oh LAN za peen)

Brand Names: U.S. ZyPREXA; ZyPREXA Relprevv; ZyPREXA Zydis

Index Terms LY170053; Olanzapine Pamoate; Zyprexa Zydis

Pharmacologic Category Antimanic Agent; Antipsychotic Agent, Atypical

Medication Safety Issues

Sound-alike/look-alike issues:

OLANZapine may be confused with olsalazine, QUEtiapine

ZyPREXA may be confused with CeleXA, Reprexain, Zestril, ZyrTEC

ZyPREXA Zydis may be confused with Zelapar, zolpidem

ZyPREXA Relprevv may be confused with ZyPREXA IntraMuscular

BEERS Criteria medication:

This drug may be potentially inappropriate for use in geriatric patients (Quality of evidence - moderate; Strength of recommendation - strong).

Medication Guide Available Yes

Pregnancy Risk Factor C

Lactation Enters breast milk/not recommended

Breast-Feeding Considerations Olanzapine is excreted into breast milk. At steady-state concentrations, it is estimated that a breast-fed infant may be exposed to ~2% of the maternal dose. In one study, the median time to peak milk concentration was ~5 hours after the maternal dose and serum concentrations in the nursing infants were low (<5 ng/mL; n=5) (Gardiner, 2003). An increased risk of adverse events in nursing infants has not been reported (Gardiner, 2003; Gilad, 2011). Breast-feeding is not recommended by the manufacturer.

Use

Oral: Treatment of the manifestations of schizophrenia; treatment of acute or mixed mania episodes associated with bipolar I disorder (as monotherapy or in combination with lithium or valproate); maintenance treatment of bipolar disorder; in combination with fluoxetine for treatment-resistant or bipolar I depression

I.M., extended-release (Zyprexa Relprevv): Treatment of schizophrenia

I.M., short-acting (Zyprexa IntraMuscular): Treatment of acute agitation associated with schizophrenia and bipolar I mania

Unlabeled Use Treatment of psychosis/schizophrenia in children; chronic pain; prevention of chemotherapy-associated delayed nausea or vomiting; psychosis/agitation related to Alzheimer's dementia; acute treatment of delirium

Mechanism of Action/Effect The efficacy of olanzapine in schizophrenia and bipolar disorder is thought to be mediated through combined antagonism of dopamine and serotonin type 2 receptor sites.

Contraindications There are no contraindications listed in the manufacturer's labeling.

Canadian labeling: Hypersensitivity to olanzapine or any component of the formulation

Warnings/Precautions [U.S. Boxed Warning]: Elderly patients with dementia-related psychosis treated with antipsychotics are at an increased risk of death compared to placebo. Most deaths appeared to be either cardiovascular (eg, heart failure, sudden death) or infectious (eg, pneumonia) in nature. In addition, an increased incidence of cerebrovascular effects (eg, transient ischemic attack, stroke) has been reported in studies of placebo-controlled trials of olanzapine in elderly patients with dementia-related psychosis. Olanzapine is not approved for the treatment of dementia-related psychosis.

Moderate to highly sedating, use with caution in disorders where CNS depression is a feature; patients must be cautioned about performing tasks which require mental alertness (eg, operating machinery or driving). Use caution in patients with cardiac disease. Use with caution in Parkinson's disease, predisposition to seizures, or severe hepatic or renal disease. Life-threatening arrhythmias have occurred with therapeutic doses of some neuroleptics. May induce orthostatic hypotension; use caution with history of cardiovascular disease, hemodynamic instability, prior myocardial infarction, or ischemic heart disease. Increases in cholesterol and triglycerides have been noted. Use with caution in patients with pre-existing abnormal lipid profile. Esophageal dysmotility and aspiration have been associated with antipsychotic use; use with caution in patients at risk of aspiration pneumonia. May increase prolactin levels; clinical significance of hyperprolactinemia in patients with breast cancer or other prolactin-dependent tumors is unknown. Significant weight gain (>7% of baseline weight) may occur; monitor waist circumference and BMI. Impaired core body temperature regulation may occur; caution with strenuous exercise, heat exposure, dehydration, and concomitant medication possessing anticholinergic effects.

Leukopenia, neutropenia, and agranulocytosis (sometimes fatal) have been reported in clinical trials and postmarketing reports with antipsychotic use; presence of risk factors (eg, pre-existing low WBC or history of drug-induced leuko-/neutropenia) should prompt periodic blood count assessment. Discontinue therapy at first signs of blood dyscrasias or if absolute neutrophil count <1000/mm^3.

May cause anticholinergic effects; use with caution in patients with decreased gastrointestinal motility, urinary retention, BPH, xerostomia, or narrow-angle glaucoma. Relative to other neuroleptics, olanzapine has a moderate potency of cholinergic blockade. May cause extrapyramidal symptoms (EPS), although risk of these reactions is lower relative to other neuroleptics. Risk of dystonia (and probably other EPS) may be greater with increased doses, use of conventional antipsychotics, males, and younger patients. May be associated with neuroleptic malignant syndrome (NMS). May cause extreme and life-threatening hyperglycemia; use with caution in patients with diabetes or other disorders of glucose regulation; monitor. Olanzapine levels may be lower in patients who smoke; the manufacturer does not require dosage adjustments, although dosage adjustments may be considered. Use in adolescent patients ≥13 years of age may result in increased weight gain and sedation, as well as greater increases in LDL cholesterol, total cholesterol, triglycerides, prolactin, and liver transaminase levels when compared to adults. Adolescent patients should be maintained on the lowest dose necessary.

Use in elderly patients with dementia is associated with an increased risk of mortality and cerebrovascular accidents; avoid antipsychotic use for behavioral problems associated with dementia unless alternative nonpharmacologic therapies have failed and patient may harm self or others. In addition, use may cause or exacerbate syndrome of inappropriate antidiuretic hormone secretion or hyponatremia; monitor sodium closely with initiation or dosage adjustments in older adults. May also be inappropriate in older adults depending on comorbidities (eg, dementia, delirium) due to its potent anticholinergic effects (Beers Criteria).

The possibility of a suicide attempt is inherent in psychotic illness or bipolar disorder; use caution in high-risk patients during initiation of therapy. Prescriptions should be written for the smallest quantity consistent with good patient care.

There are two Zyprexa formulations for intramuscular injection: Zyprexa Relprevv is an extended-release formulation and Zyprexa Intramuscular is short-acting:

Extended-release I.M. injection (Zyprexa Relprevv): Monitor for post injection delirium/ sedation syndrome; patients should be continuously watched (≥3 hours) for symptoms of olanzapine overdose. Only available through a restricted drug distribution program.

Short-acting I.M. injection (Zyprexa IntraMuscular): Patients should remain recumbent if drowsy/dizzy until hypotension, bradycardia, and/or hypoventilation have been ruled out. Concurrent use of I.M./I.V. benzodiazepines is not recommended (fatalities have been reported, though causality not determined).

Drug Interactions
Avoid Concomitant Use
Avoid concomitant use of OLANZapine with any of the following: Aclidinium; Amisulpride; Azelastine (Nasal); Benzodiazepines; Ipratropium (Oral Inhalation); Metoclopramide; Paraldehyde; Pimozide; Sulpiride; Thalidomide; Tiotropium; Umeclidinium

Decreased Effect
OLANZapine may decrease the levels/effects of: Amphetamines; Anti-Parkinson's Agents (Dopamine Agonist); Quinagolide

The levels/effects of OLANZapine may be decreased by: CYP1A2 Inducers (Strong); Cyproterone; Lithium formulations; Peginterferon Alfa-2b; Valproic Acid and Derivatives

Increased Effect/Toxicity
OLANZapine may increase the levels/effects of: Alcohol (Ethyl); Amisulpride; Analgesics (Opioid); Anticholinergics; ARIPiprazole; Azelastine (Nasal); Benzodiazepines; Buprenorphine; CNS Depressants; Dofetilide; Highest Risk QTc-Prolonging Agents; Hydrocodone; Lomitapide; Methotrimeprazine; Methylphenidate; Moderate Risk QTc-Prolonging Agents; Paraldehyde; Pimozide; Serotonin Modulators; Sulpiride; Thalidomide; Tiotropium; Zolpidem

The levels/effects of OLANZapine may be increased by: Abiraterone Acetate; Acetylcholinesterase Inhibitors (Central); Aclidinium; Brimonidine (Topical); CYP1A2 Inhibitors (Moderate); CYP1A2 Inhibitors (Strong); Deferasirox; Doxylamine; Droperidol; FluvoxaMINE; HydrOXYzine; Ipratropium (Oral Inhalation); LamoTRIgine; Lithium formulations; Magnesium Sulfate; Methotrimeprazine; Methylphenidate; Metoclopramide; Metyrosine; Mifepristone; Perampanel; Pramlintide; Serotonin Modulators; Sodium Oxybate; Tetrabenazine; Umeclidinium; Vemurafenib

Nutritional/Ethanol Interactions
Ethanol: May increase CNS depression; monitor for increased effects with coadministration. Caution patients about effects.

Herb/Nutraceutical: Avoid dong quai, St John's wort (may also cause photosensitization). Avoid kava kava, gotu kola, valerian, St John's wort (may increase CNS depression).

Adverse Reactions

Oral: Unless otherwise noted, adverse events are reported for placebo-controlled trials in adult patients on monotherapy:

>10%:

Central nervous system: Somnolence (dose dependent; 20% to 39%; adolescents 39% to 48%), extrapyramidal symptoms (dose dependent; ≤32%), dizziness (11% to 18%), headache (adolescents 17%), fatigue (adolescents 3% to 14%), insomnia (12%)

Endocrine & metabolic: Prolactin increased (30%; adolescents 47%)

Gastrointestinal: Weight gain (5% to 6%, has been reported as high as 40%; adolescents 29% to 31%), appetite increased (3% to 6%; adolescents 17% to 29%), xerostomia (dose dependent; 3% to 22%), constipation (9% to 11%), dyspepsia (7% to 11%)

Hepatic: ALT increased ≥3 x ULN (adolescents 12%; adults 5%)

Neuromuscular & skeletal: Weakness (dose dependent; 8% to 20%)

Miscellaneous: Accidental injury (12%)

1% to 10%:

Cardiovascular: Chest pain, hypertension, orthostatic hypotension, peripheral edema, tachycardia

Central nervous system: Fever, personality changes, restlessness (adolescents)

Dermatologic: Bruising

Endocrine & metabolic: Breast-related events ([adolescents] discharge, enlargement, galactorrhea, gynecomastia, lactation disorder); menstrual-related events (amenorrhea, hypomenorrhea, menstruation delayed, oligomenorrhea); sexual function-related events (anorgasmia, ejaculation delayed, erectile dysfunction, changes in libido, abnormal orgasm, sexual dysfunction)

Gastrointestinal: Abdominal pain (adolescents), diarrhea (adolescents), flatulence, nausea (dose dependent), vomiting

Genitourinary: Incontinence, UTI

Hepatic: Hepatic enzymes increased

Neuromuscular & skeletal: Abnormal gait, akathisia, articulation impairment, back pain, falling, hypertonia, joint/extremity pain, muscle stiffness (adolescents), tremor (dose dependent)

Ocular: Amblyopia

Respiratory: Cough, epistaxis (adolescents), pharyngitis, respiratory tract infection (adolescents), rhinitis, sinusitis (adolescents)

Injection: Unless otherwise noted, adverse events are reported for placebo-controlled trials in adult patients on extended-release I.M. injection

(Zyprexa Relprevv). Also refer to adverse reactions noted with oral therapy.

>10%: Central nervous system: Headache (13% to 18%), sedation (8% to 13%)

1% to 10%:

Cardiovascular: Hypertension, hypotension (short-acting), orthostatic hypotension (short-acting), QT prolongation

Central nervous system: Abnormal dreams, abnormal thinking, auditory hallucination, dizziness, dysarthria, extrapyramidal symptoms, fatigue, fever, pain, restlessness, somnolence

Dermatologic: Acne

Gastrointestinal: Abdominal pain, appetite increased, diarrhea, flatulence, nausea, vomiting, weight gain, xerostomia

Genitourinary: Vaginal discharge

Hepatic: Liver enzymes increased

Local: Injection site pain

Neuromuscular & skeletal: Arthralgia, back pain, muscle spasms, stiffness, tremor, weakness (short-acting)

Otic: Ear pain

Respiratory: Cough, nasal congestion, nasopharyngitis, pharyngolaryngeal pain, sneezing, upper respiratory tract infection

Miscellaneous: Toothache, tooth infection, viral infection

<1%, postmarketing, and/or case reports (limited to important or life-threatening): CPK increased, post-injection delirium/sedation syndrome, syncope (short-acting)

Available Dosage Forms

Solution Reconstituted, Intramuscular:
ZyPREXA: 10 mg (1 ea)
Generic: 10 mg (1 ea)

Suspension Reconstituted, Intramuscular:
ZyPREXA Relprevv: 210 mg (1 ea); 300 mg (1 ea); 405 mg (1 ea)

Tablet, Oral:
ZyPREXA: 2.5 mg, 5 mg, 7.5 mg, 10 mg, 15 mg, 20 mg
Generic: 2.5 mg, 5 mg, 7.5 mg, 10 mg, 15 mg, 20 mg

Tablet Dispersible, Oral:
ZyPREXA Zydis: 5 mg, 10 mg, 15 mg, 20 mg
Generic: 5 mg, 10 mg, 15 mg, 20 mg

General Dosage Range

I.M.: *Adults:*

Extended release: 150-300 mg every 2 weeks **or** 300-405 mg every 4 weeks (maximum: 300 mg every 2 weeks; 405 mg every 4 weeks)

Short-acting: Initial: 10 mg/dose; 2-4 hours between doses (maximum: 30 mg daily)

Oral:

Children and Adolescents 10-17 years (in combination with fluoxetine): Initial 2.5 mg once daily; dosing range: 2.5-12 mg daily

Adolescents ≥13 years: Initial: 2.5-5 mg once daily; dosing range: 2.5-20 mg daily

Adults: Initial: 5-15 mg once daily; Maintenance: 5-20 mg once daily

Elderly: Initial: 2.5-5 mg daily

Administration

I.M.

Short-acting I.M. injection: **For I.M. administration only**; do not administer injection intravenously or subcutaneously; inject slowly, deep into muscle. If dizziness and/or drowsiness are noted, patient should remain recumbent until examination indicates postural hypotension and/or bradycardia are not a problem.

Extended-release I.M. injection: **For I.M. gluteal injection only**; do not administer I.V. or subcutaneously. After needle insertion into muscle, aspirate to verify that no blood appears. Do not massage injection site. Use diluent, syringes, and needles provided in convenience kit; obtain a new kit if aspiration of blood occurs.

Oral

Tablet: May be administered without regard to meals.

Orally-disintegrating tablet: Remove from foil blister by peeling back (do not push tablet through the foil). Place tablet in mouth immediately upon removal. Tablet dissolves rapidly in saliva and may be swallowed with or without liquid. May be administered with or without food/meals.

Preparation for Administration

Injection, extended-release: Dilute as directed to final concentration of 150 mg/mL. Shake vigorously to mix; will form yellow, opaque suspension. Following reconstitution, suspension may be stored at room temperature and used within 24 hours. Shake vigorously to resuspend prior to administration. Use immediately once suspension is in syringe. Suspension may be irritating to skin; wear gloves during reconstitution.

Injection, short-acting: Reconstitute 10 mg vial with 2.1 mL SWFI. Resulting solution is ~5 mg/mL. Use immediately (within 1 hour) following reconstitution. Discard any unused portion.

Storage/Stability

Injection, extended-release: Store at 20°C to 25°C (68°F to 77°F); excursions permitted to 15°C to 30°C (59°F to 86°F).

Injection, short-acting: Store at 20°C to 25°C (68°F to 77°F); excursions permitted to 15°C to 30°C (59°F to 86°F); do not freeze. Protect from light.

Tablet and orally-disintegrating tablet: Store at 20°C to 25°C (68°F to 77°F); excursions permitted to 15°C to 30°C (59°F to 86°F). Protect from light and moisture.

Nursing Actions

Physical Assessment Initiate at lower doses. Taper dosage slowly when discontinuing. Instruct patients with diabetes to monitor blood glucose levels closely; may cause hyperglycemia. Assess for extrapyramidal symptoms, suicide ideation, sedation, CNS changes, and neuroleptic malignant syndrome prior to treatment and periodically throughout. Monitor weight prior to initiating therapy and at least monthly. If Zyprexa® Relprevv™ is administered, monitor closely for at least 3 hours for symptoms of oversedation and/or delirium.

Patient Education

• Discuss specific use of drug and side effects with patient as it relates to treatment. (HCAHPS: During this hospital stay, were you given any medicine that you had not taken before? Before giving you any new medicine, how often did hospital staff tell you what the medicine was for? How often did hospital staff describe possible side effects in a way you could understand?)

• Patient may experience presyncope, fatigue, blurred vision, illogical thinking, dizziness, nervousness and anxiety, hyperlipidemia, hostility, constipation, xerostomia, weight gain, hyperglycemia, or insomnia. Have patient report immediately to prescriber depression, emotional instability, significant change in balance, tremors, anhidrosis, dysphagia, severe asthenia, polyuria, polydipsia, weight loss, pregnancy, or rash (HCAHPS).

• Educate patient about signs of a significant reaction (eg, wheezing; chest tightness; fever; itching; bad cough; blue skin color; seizures; or swelling of face, lips, tongue, or throat). **Note:** This is not a comprehensive list of all side effects. Patient should consult prescriber for additional questions.

Intended Use and Disclaimer: Should not be printed and given to patients. This information is intended to serve as a concise initial reference for healthcare professionals to use when discussing medications with a patient. You must ultimately rely on your own discretion, experience and judgment in diagnosing, treating and advising patients.

Dietary Considerations Tablets may be taken without regard to meals. Some products may contain phenylalanine.

Olanzapine and Fluoxetine
(oh LAN za peen & floo OKS e teen)

Brand Names: U.S. Symbyax

Index Terms Fluoxetine and Olanzapine; Olanzapine and Fluoxetine Hydrochloride

Pharmacologic Category Antidepressant, Selective Serotonin Reuptake Inhibitor; Antipsychotic Agent, Atypical

Medication Safety Issues

Sound-alike/look-alike issues:

Symbyax may be confused with Cymbalta

BEERS Criteria medication:

This drug may be potentially inappropriate for use in geriatric patients (Quality of evidence - moderate; Strength of recommendation - strong).

Medication Guide Available Yes

Pregnancy Risk Factor C

Use Treatment of depressive episodes associated with bipolar I disorder; treatment-resistant depression (unresponsive to 2 trials of different antidepressants in the current episode)

Available Dosage Forms

Capsule, oral: 3/25: Olanzapine 3 mg and fluoxetine 25 mg; 6/25: Olanzapine 6 mg and fluoxetine 25 mg; 6/50: Olanzapine 6 mg and fluoxetine 50 mg; 12/25: Olanzapine 12 mg and fluoxetine 25 mg; 12/50: Olanzapine 12 mg and fluoxetine 50 mg

Symbyax:

3/25: Olanzapine 3 mg and fluoxetine 25 mg
6/25: Olanzapine 6 mg and fluoxetine 25 mg
6/50: Olanzapine 6 mg and fluoxetine 50 mg
12/25: Olanzapine 12 mg and fluoxetine 25 mg
12/50: Olanzapine 12 mg and fluoxetine 50 mg

General Dosage Range Dosage adjustment recommended in patients with hepatic impairment

Oral:

Children and Adolescents 10-17 years: Initial: Olanzapine 3mg and fluoxetine 25 mg once daily; Maintenance: Olanzapine 6-12 mg and fluoxetine 25-50 mg once daily

Adults: Initial: Olanzapine 6 mg and fluoxetine 25 mg once daily; Maintenance: Olanzapine 6-12 mg and fluoxetine 25-50 mg once daily

Elderly >65 years: Initial: Olanzapine 3-6 mg and fluoxetine 25 mg once daily

Administration

Oral Capsules should be taken once daily in the evening. May be taken without regard to meals.

Nursing Actions

Physical Assessment See individual agents.

Patient Education

- Discuss specific use of drug and side effects with patient as it relates to treatment. (HCAHPS: During this hospital stay, were you given any medicine that you had not taken before? Before giving you any new medicine, how often did hospital staff tell you what the medicine was for? How often did hospital staff describe possible side effects in a way you could understand?)
- Patient may experience hyperglycemia, presyncope, fatigue, blurred vision, illogical thinking, dizziness, diarrhea, xerostomia, or weight gain. Have patient report immediately to prescriber fasciculations, diaphoresis, myalgia, significant change in balance, tremors, considerable nervousness and anxiety, severe asthenia, polyuria, polydipsia, weight loss, tachycardia, intolerable nausea, ecchymosis, or bleeding (HCAHPS).
- Educate patient about signs of a significant reaction (eg, wheezing; chest tightness; fever; itching; bad cough; blue skin color; seizures; or swelling of face, lips, tongue, or throat). **Note:** This is not a comprehensive list of all side effects. Patient should consult prescriber for additional questions.

Intended Use and Disclaimer: Should not be printed and given to patients. This information is intended to serve as a concise initial reference for healthcare professionals to use when discussing medications with a patient. You must ultimately rely on your own discretion, experience and judgment in diagnosing, treating and advising patients.

Related Information

FLUoxetine *on page 679*
OLANZapine *on page 1146*

Olmesartan (ole me SAR tan)

Brand Names: U.S. Benicar

Index Terms Olmesartan Medoxomil

Pharmacologic Category Angiotensin II Receptor Blocker; Antihypertensive

Medication Safety Issues

Sound-alike/look-alike issues:
Benicar may be confused with Mevacor

Pregnancy Risk Factor D

Lactation Excretion in breast milk unknown/not recommended

Breast-Feeding Considerations It is not known if olmesartan is excreted into breast milk. Due to the potential for serious adverse reactions in the nursing infant, the manufacturer recommends a decision be made whether to discontinue nursing or to discontinue the drug, taking into account the importance of treatment to the mother. Breast-fed infants of mothers taking medications for hypertension should be monitored for adverse effects (Chobanian, 2003).

Use Treatment of hypertension with or without concurrent use of other antihypertensive agents

Mechanism of Action/Effect As a selective and competitive, nonpeptide angiotensin II receptor antagonist, olmesartan blocks the vasoconstrictor and aldosterone-secreting effects of angiotensin II. Olmesartan increases urinary flow rate and in addition to being natriuretic and kaliuretic, increases excretion of chloride, magnesium, uric acid, calcium, and phosphate.

Contraindications Concomitant use with aliskiren in patients with diabetes mellitus

Canadian labeling: Additional contraindications (not in U.S. labeling): Hypersensitivity to olmesartan or any component of the formulation; concomitant use with aliskiren in patients with moderate to severe renal impairment (GFR <60 mL/minute/1.73 m²)

Warnings/Precautions [U.S. Boxed Warning]: Drugs that act on the renin-angiotensin system can cause injury and death to the developing fetus. Discontinue as soon as possible once pregnancy is detected. May cause hyperkalemia; avoid potassium supplementation unless specifically required by healthcare provider. Avoid use or use a smaller dose in patients who are volume depleted; correct depletion first. May be associated with deterioration of renal function and/or increases in serum creatinine, particularly in patients with low renal blood flow (eg, renal artery stenosis, heart failure) whose glomerular filtration rate (GFR) is dependent on efferent arteriolar vasoconstriction by angiotensin II. Use with caution in unstented unilateral/bilateral renal artery stenosis. When unstented bilateral renal artery stenosis is present, use is generally avoided due to the elevated risk of deterioration in renal function unless possible benefits outweigh risks. Use with caution with pre-existing renal insufficiency; significant aortic/mitral stenosis. Potentially significant drug-drug interactions may exist, requiring dose or frequency adjustment, additional monitoring, and/or selection of alternative therapy.

Symptoms of sprue-like enteropathy (ie, severe, chronic diarrhea with significant weight loss) has been reported; may develop years after treatment initiation with villous atrophy commonly found on intestinal biopsy. Once other etiologies have been excluded, discontinue treatment and consider other antihypertensive treatment. Clinical and histologic improvement was noted after treatment was discontinued in a case series of 22 patients (Rubio-Tapia, 2012).

Angioedema has been reported rarely with some angiotensin II receptor antagonists (ARBs) and may occur at any time during treatment (especially following first dose). It may involve the head and neck (potentially compromising airway) or the intestine (presenting with abdominal pain). Patients with idiopathic or hereditary angioedema or previous angioedema associated with ACE-inhibitor therapy may be at an increased risk. Prolonged frequent monitoring may be required, especially if tongue, glottis, or larynx are involved, as they are associated with airway obstruction. Patients with a history of airway surgery may have a higher risk of airway obstruction. Discontinue therapy immediately if angioedema occurs. Aggressive early management is critical. Intramuscular (I.M.) administration of epinephrine may be necessary. Do not readminister to patients who have had angioedema with ARBs.

Drug Interactions

Avoid Concomitant Use There are no known interactions where it is recommended to avoid concomitant use.

Decreased Effect

The levels/effects of Olmesartan may be decreased by: Colesevelam; Herbs (Hypertensive Properties); Methylphenidate; Nonsteroidal Anti-Inflammatory Agents; Yohimbine

Increased Effect/Toxicity

Olmesartan may increase the levels/effects of: ACE Inhibitors; Amifostine; Antihypertensives;

CycloSPORINE (Systemic); DULoxetine; Hypotensive Agents; Lithium; Nonsteroidal Anti-Inflammatory Agents; Obinutuzumab; Potassium-Sparing Diuretics; RiTUXimab; Sodium Phosphates

The levels/effects of Olmesartan may be increased by: Alfuzosin; Aliskiren; Brimonidine (Topical); Canagliflozin; Diazoxide; Eltrombopag; Eplerenone; Heparin; Heparin (Low Molecular Weight); Herbs (Hypotensive Properties); MAO Inhibitors; Pentoxifylline; Phosphodiesterase 5 Inhibitors; Potassium Salts; Prostacyclin Analogues; Tolvaptan; Trimethoprim

Nutritional/Ethanol Interactions

Food: Does not affect olmesartan bioavailability. Potassium supplements and/or potassium-containing salts may cause or worsen hyperkalemia. Management: Consult prescriber before consuming a potassium-rich diet, potassium supplements, or salt substitutes.

Herb/Nutraceutical: Some herbal medications may worsen hypertension (eg, licorice); others may increase the antihypertensive effect of olmesartan (eg, shepherd's purse). Management: Avoid bayberry, blue cohosh, cayenne, ephedra, ginger, ginseng (American), kola, licorice, and yohimbe. Avoid black cohosh, California poppy, coleus, golden seal, hawthorn, mistletoe, periwinkle, quinine, and shepherd's purse.

Adverse Reactions 1% to 10%:

Central nervous system: Dizziness (3%), headache

Endocrine & metabolic: Hyperglycemia, hypertriglyceridemia

Gastrointestinal: Diarrhea

Neuromuscular & skeletal: Back pain, CPK increased

Renal: Hematuria

Respiratory: Bronchitis, pharyngitis, rhinitis, sinusitis

Miscellaneous: Flu-like syndrome

Available Dosage Forms

Tablet, Oral:

Benicar: 5 mg, 20 mg, 40 mg

General Dosage Range Oral:

Children 6-16 years:

20 kg to <35 kg: Initial: 10 mg once daily (maximum: 20 mg once daily)

≥35 kg: Initial: 20 mg once daily (maximum: 40 mg once daily)

Adolescents >16 years and Adults: Initial: 20 mg once daily; Maintenance: 20-40 mg once daily

Elderly: Initial: 5-20 mg once daily

Administration

Oral May be administered with or without food.

Storage/Stability Store at 20°C to 25°C (68°F to 77°F).

◄ **Nursing Actions**

Physical Assessment Monitor blood pressure. Monitor for tachycardia, hypotension, diarrhea, and bronchitis on a regular basis throughout therapy. Instruct patients with diabetes to monitor glucose levels closely (may cause hyperglycemia).

Patient Education

• Discuss specific use of drug and side effects with patient as it relates to treatment. (HCAHPS: During this hospital stay, were you given any medicine that you had not taken before? Before giving you any new medicine, how often did hospital staff tell you what the medicine was for? How often did hospital staff describe possible side effects in a way you could understand?)

• Patient may experience dizziness, diarrhea, hyperkalemia, or worsening kidney function. Have patient report immediately to prescriber syncope, severe headache, hyperhidrosis, vomiting, rash, or pregnancy (HCAHPS).

• Educate patient about signs of a significant reaction (eg, wheezing; chest tightness; fever; itching; bad cough; blue skin color; seizures; or swelling of face, lips, tongue, or throat). **Note:** This is not a comprehensive list of all side effects. Patients should consult prescriber for additional questions.

Intended Use and Disclaimer: Should not be printed and given to patients. This information is intended to serve as a concise initial reference for healthcare professionals to use when discussing medications with a patient. You must ultimately rely on your own discretion, experience and judgment in diagnosing, treating and advising patients.

Dietary Considerations May be taken with or without food.

Olmesartan, Amlodipine, and Hydrochlorothiazide

(ole me SAR tan, am LOE di peen, & hye droe klor oh THYE a zide)

Brand Names: U.S. Tribenzor™

Index Terms Amlodipine Besylate, Olmesartan Medoxomil, and Hydrochlorothiazide; Amlodipine, Hydrochlorothiazide, and Olmesartan; Hydrochlorothiazide, Olmesartan, and Amlodipine; Olmesartan, Hydrochlorothiazide, and Amlodipine

Pharmacologic Category Angiotensin II Receptor Blocker; Antianginal Agent; Antihypertensive; Calcium Channel Blocker; Calcium Channel Blocker, Dihydropyridine; Diuretic, Thiazide

Pregnancy Risk Factor D

Use Treatment of hypertension (not for initial therapy)

Available Dosage Forms

Tablet, oral:

Tribenzor™: Olmesartan medoxomil 40 mg, amlodipine 5 mg, and hydrochlorothiazide

25 mg, olmesartan medoxomil 40 mg, amlodipine 10 mg, and hydrochlorothiazide 25 mg, olmesartan medoxomil 20 mg, amlodipine 5 mg, and hydrochlorothiazide 12.5 mg, olmesartan medoxomil 40 mg, amlodipine 5 mg, and hydrochlorothiazide 12.5 mg, olmesartan medoxomil 40 mg, amlodipine 10 mg, and hydrochlorothiazide 12.5 mg

General Dosage Range Oral: *Adults:* Amlodipine 5-10 mg and olmesartan 20-40 mg and hydrochlorothiazide 12.5-25 mg once daily (maximum 10 mg/day [amlodipine]; 25 mg/day [hydrochlorothiazide]; 40 mg/day [olmesartan])

Administration

Oral Administer with or without food.

Nursing Actions

Physical Assessment See individual agents.

Patient Education

• Discuss specific use of drug and side effects with patient as it relates to treatment. (HCAHPS: During this hospital stay, were you given any medicine that you had not taken before? Before giving you any new medicine, how often did hospital staff tell you what the medicine was for? How often did hospital staff describe possible side effects in a way you could understand?)

• Patient may experience dizziness, headache, dyspepsia, pharyngitis, rhinitis, rhinorrhea, or asthenia. Have patient report immediately to prescriber signs of infection, signs of hyperglycemia, signs of renal or hepatic impairment, paresthesia, dysuria, bradycardia, arthralgia, dyspnea, significant weight gain, edema, angina, changes to teeth or gums, ecchymosis, bleeding, akathisia, or vision changes (HCAHPS).

• Educate patient about signs of a significant reaction (eg, wheezing; chest tightness; fever; itching; bad cough; blue skin color; seizures; or swelling of face, lips, tongue, or throat). **Note:** This is not a comprehensive list of all side effects. Patient should consult prescriber for additional questions.

Intended Use and Disclaimer: Should not be printed and given to patients. This information is intended to serve as a concise initial reference for healthcare professionals to use when discussing medications with a patient. You must ultimately rely on your own discretion, experience and judgment in diagnosing, treating and advising patients.

Related Information

AmLODIPine *on page 87*
Hydrochlorothiazide *on page 775*
Olmesartan *on page 1150*

Olmesartan and Hydrochlorothiazide

(ole me SAR tan & hye droe klor oh THYE a zide)

Brand Names: U.S. Benicar HCT

Index Terms Hydrochlorothiazide and Olmesartan Medoxomil; Olmesartan Medoxomil and Hydrochlorothiazide

Pharmacologic Category Angiotensin II Receptor Blocker; Diuretic, Thiazide

Pregnancy Risk Factor D

Use Treatment of hypertension (not recommended for initial treatment)

Available Dosage Forms

Tablet:

Benicar HCT®: 20/12.5: Olmesartan 20 mg and hydrochlorothiazide 12.5 mg; 40/12.5: Olmesartan 40 mg and hydrochlorothiazide 12.5 mg; 40/25: Olmesartan 40 mg and hydrochlorothiazide 25 mg

General Dosage Range Oral: *Adults:* Olmesartan 20-40 mg and hydrochlorothiazide 12.5-25 mg once daily (maximum: 25 mg/day [hydrochlorothiazide]; 40 mg/day [olmesartan])

Administration

Oral May be administered with or without food. Take early in day to avoid nocturia.

Nursing Actions

Physical Assessment See individual agents.

Patient Education

• Discuss specific use of drug and side effects with patient as it relates to treatment. (HCAHPS: During this hospital stay, were you given any medicine that you had not taken before? Before giving you any new medicine, how often did hospital staff tell you what the medicine was for? How often did hospital staff describe possible side effects in a way you could understand?)

• Patient may experience dizziness or dyspepsia. Have patient report immediately to prescriber signs of infection, signs of hyperglycemia, signs of renal impairment, angina, sexual dysfunction, akathisia, dyspnea, significant weight gain, edema, ecchymosis, bleeding, jaundice, or vision changes (HCAHPS).

• Educate patient about signs of a significant reaction (eg, wheezing; chest tightness; fever; itching; bad cough; blue skin color; seizures; or swelling of face, lips, tongue, or throat). **Note:** This is not a comprehensive list of all side effects. Patient should consult prescriber for additional questions.

Intended Use and Disclaimer: Should not be printed and given to patients. This information is intended to serve as a concise initial reference for healthcare professionals to use when discussing medications with a patient. You must ultimately rely on your own discretion, experience and judgment in diagnosing, treating and advising patients.

Related Information

Hydrochlorothiazide *on page 775*
Olmesartan *on page 1150*

Olopatadine (Nasal) (oh la PAT a deen)

Brand Names: U.S. Patanase

Index Terms Olopatadine Hydrochloride

Pharmacologic Category Histamine H_1 Antagonist; Histamine H_1 Antagonist, Second Generation; Piperidine Derivative

Pregnancy Risk Factor C

Lactation Excretion in breast milk unknown/use caution

Use Treatment of the symptoms of seasonal allergic rhinitis

Dosage Forms Considerations

Patanase 30.5 g bottles contain 240 sprays.

Available Dosage Forms

Solution, Nasal:

Patanase: 0.6% (30.5 g)

General Dosage Range Intranasal:

Children 6-11 years: 1 spray into each nostril twice daily

Children ≥12 years, Adolescents, and Adults: 2 sprays into each nostril twice daily

Administration

Inhalation For intranasal use only. Before initial use of the nasal spray, the delivery system should be primed with 5 sprays or until a fine mist appears. If 7 or more days have elapsed since last use, the delivery system should be reprimed with 2 sprays or until a fine mist appears. Blow nose to clear nostrils. Keep head tilted downward when spraying. Insert applicator into nostril, keeping bottle upright, and close off the other nostril. Breathe in through nose. While inhaling, press pump to release spray. Alternate sprays between nostrils. After each use, wipe the spray tip with a clean tissue or cloth.

Nursing Actions

Physical Assessment Assess nasal mucosa periodically for ulceration.

Patient Education

• Discuss specific use of drug and side effects with patient as it relates to treatment. (HCAHPS: During this hospital stay, were you given any medicine that you had not taken before? Before giving you any new medicine, how often did hospital staff tell you what the medicine was for? How often did hospital staff describe possible side effects in a way you could understand?)

• Patient may experience presyncope, fatigue, blurred vision, illogical thinking, headache, or

parageusia. Have patient report immediately to prescriber rash (HCAHPS).
• Educate patient about signs of a significant reaction (eg, wheezing; chest tightness; fever; itching; bad cough; blue skin color; seizures; or swelling of face, lips, tongue, or throat). **Note:** This is not a comprehensive list of all side effects. Patient should consult prescriber for additional questions.

Intended Use and Disclaimer: Should not be printed and given to patients. This information is intended to serve as a concise initial reference for healthcare professionals to use when discussing medications with a patient. You must ultimately rely on your own discretion, experience and judgment in diagnosing, treating and advising patients.

Olopatadine (Ophthalmic) (oh la PAT a deen)

Brand Names: U.S. Pataday; Patanol
Index Terms Olopatadine Hydrochloride
Pharmacologic Category Histamine H$_1$ Antagonist; Histamine H$_1$ Antagonist, Second Generation; Piperidine Derivative
Medication Safety Issues
Sound-alike/look-alike issues:
Patanol® may be confused with Platinol
International issues:
Patanol [U.S., Canada, and multiple international markets] may be confused with Bétanol brand name for metipranolol [Monaco]
Pregnancy Risk Factor C
Lactation Excretion in breast milk unknown/use caution
Use Treatment of the signs and symptoms of allergic conjunctivitis
Available Dosage Forms
Solution, Ophthalmic:
Pataday: 0.2% (2.5 mL)
Patanol: 0.1% (5 mL)
General Dosage Range Ophthalmic:
Children ≥3 years, Adolescents, and Adults: Patanol®: Instill 1 drop into each affected eye twice daily
Children ≥2 years, Adolescents, and Adults: Pataday™: Instill 1 drop into each affected eye once daily
Administration
Other For topical ophthalmic use only. Wash hands prior to use. Do not touch tip of container to eye. After instilling drops, wait at least 10 minutes before inserting contact lenses. Do not insert contacts if eyes are red.
Nursing Actions
Patient Education
• Discuss specific use of drug and side effects with patient as it relates to treatment. (HCAHPS: During this hospital stay, were you given any medicine that you had not taken before? Before

giving you any new medicine, how often did hospital staff tell you what the medicine was for? How often did hospital staff describe possible side effects in a way you could understand?)
• Patient may experience headache. Have patient report immediately to prescriber vision changes, ophthalmalgia, or severe eye irritation (HCAHPS).
• Educate patient about signs of a significant reaction (eg, wheezing; chest tightness; fever; itching; bad cough; blue skin color; seizures; or swelling of face, lips, tongue, or throat). **Note:** This is not a comprehensive list of all side effects. Patient should consult prescriber for additional questions.

Intended Use and Disclaimer: Should not be printed and given to patients. This information is intended to serve as a concise initial reference for healthcare professionals to use when discussing medications with a patient. You must ultimately rely on your own discretion, experience and judgment in diagnosing, treating and advising patients.

Olsalazine (ole SAL a zeen)

Brand Names: U.S. Dipentum
Index Terms Olsalazine Sodium
Pharmacologic Category 5-Aminosalicylic Acid Derivative
Medication Safety Issues
Sound-alike/look-alike issues:
Olsalazine may be confused with OLANZapine
Dipentum® may be confused with Dilantin®
Pregnancy Risk Factor C
Lactation Enters breast milk/not recommended
Use Maintenance of remission of ulcerative colitis in patients intolerant to sulfasalazine
Available Dosage Forms
Capsule, Oral:
Dipentum: 250 mg
General Dosage Range Oral: *Adults:* 1 g/day in 2 divided doses
Administration
Oral Administer with food in evenly divided doses.
Nursing Actions
Physical Assessment Assess allergy history before initiating therapy (salicylates, sulfasalazine, or mesalamine). Monitor for reduction of clinical signs of ulcerative colitis. Monitor for diarrhea.
Patient Education
• Discuss specific use of drug and side effects with patient as it relates to treatment. (HCAHPS: During this hospital stay, were you given any medicine that you had not taken before? Before giving you any new medicine, how often did hospital staff tell you what the medicine was for? How often did hospital staff describe possible side effects in a way you could understand?)

- Patient may experience dyspepsia, nausea, or diarrhea. Have patient report immediately to prescriber bloody stools or rash (HCAHPS).
- Educate patient about signs of a significant reaction (eg, wheezing; chest tightness; fever; itching; bad cough; blue skin color; seizures; or swelling of face, lips, tongue, or throat). **Note:** This is not a comprehensive list of all side effects. Patient should consult prescriber for additional questions.

Intended Use and Disclaimer: Should not be printed and given to patients. This information is intended to serve as a concise initial reference for healthcare professionals to use when discussing medications with a patient. You must ultimately rely on your own discretion, experience and judgment in diagnosing, treating and advising patients.

Omacetaxine (oh ma se TAX een)

Brand Names: U.S. Synribo
Index Terms CGX-625; HHT; Homoharringtonine; Omacetaxine Mepesuccinate
Pharmacologic Category Antineoplastic Agent, Cephalotaxine; Antineoplastic Agent, Protein Synthesis Inhibitor
Medication Safety Issues
High alert medication:
  This medication is in a class the Institute for Safe Medical Practices (ISMP) includes among its list of drug classes which have a heightened risk of causing significant patient harm when used in error.
Pregnancy Risk Factor D
Lactation Excretion in breast milk unknown/not recommended
Use Treatment of chronic or accelerated phase chronic myelogenous leukemia (CML) in patients resistant and/or intolerant to ≥2 tyrosine kinase inhibitors
Available Dosage Forms
Solution Reconstituted, Subcutaneous [preservative free]:
  Synribo: 3.5 mg (1 ea)
General Dosage Range SubQ: *Adults:* Induction: 1.25 mg/m^2 twice daily for 14 days of a 28-day treatment cycle; Maintenance: 1.25 mg/m^2 twice daily for 7 consecutive days of a 28-day treatment cycle
Administration
Subcutaneous Administer subcutaneously.

  Hazardous agent: Use appropriate precautions for handling and disposal (meets NIOSH, 2012 criteria).
Nursing Actions
Physical Assessment Assess for signs and symptoms of bleeding such as bleeding gums, black tarry stools, or blood in the urine. Monitor blood glucose levels and assess for signs of

hyperglycemia. Older patients >65 years may not tolerate effects on bone marrow as well as younger patients.
Patient Education
- Discuss specific use of drug and side effects with patient as it relates to treatment. (HCAHPS: During this hospital stay, were you given any medicine that you had not taken before? Before giving you any new medicine, how often did hospital staff tell you what the medicine was for? How often did hospital staff describe possible side effects in a way you could understand?)
- Patient may experience headache, lack of appetite, myalgia, arthralgia, back pain, alopecia, or insomnia. Have patient report immediately to prescriber signs of infection, signs of hemorrhaging, strength differences from one side to another, difficulty speaking or thinking, change in balance, blurred vision, signs of hyperglycemia, severe asthenia, considerable nausea, significant diarrhea, intolerable dyspepsia, severe constipation, edema of extremities, or significant injection site irritation (HCAHPS).
- Educate patient about signs of a significant reaction (eg, wheezing; chest tightness; fever; itching; bad cough; blue skin color; seizures; or swelling of face, lips, tongue, or throat). **Note:** This is not a comprehensive list of all side effects. Patient should consult prescriber for additional questions.

Intended Use and Disclaimer: Should not be printed and given to patients. This information is intended to serve as a concise initial reference for healthcare professionals to use when discussing medications with a patient. You must ultimately rely on your own discretion, experience and judgment in diagnosing, treating and advising patients.

Omalizumab (oh mah lye ZOO mab)

Brand Names: U.S. Xolair
Index Terms rhuMAb-E25
Pharmacologic Category Monoclonal Antibody, Anti-Asthmatic
Medication Safety Issues
Sound-alike/look-alike issues:
  Omalizumab may be confused with obinutuzumab, ofatumumab
Medication Guide Available Yes
Pregnancy Risk Factor B
Lactation Excretion in breast milk unknown/use caution
Breast-Feeding Considerations It is not known if omalizumab is excreted in breast milk; however, IgG is excreted in human milk and excretion of omalizumab is expected. Effects to nursing infant are not known; use with caution.

Use Treatment of moderate-to-severe, persistent allergic asthma in patients with a positive skin test or *in vitro* reactivity to a perennial aeroallergen and not adequately controlled with inhaled corticosteroids

Mechanism of Action/Effect Blocks the binding of IgE to mast cells and basophils, decreasing the allergic response, corticosteroid usage, and asthma exacerbations.

Contraindications Severe hypersensitivity to omalizumab or any component of the formulation

Warnings/Precautions [U.S. Boxed Warning]: Anaphylaxis, including delayed-onset anaphylaxis, has been reported following administration; anaphylaxis may present as bronchospasm, hypotension, syncope, urticaria, and/ or angioedema of the throat or tongue. Anaphylaxis has occurred after the first dose and in some cases >1 year after initiation of regular treatment. Due to the risk, patients should be observed closely for an appropriate time period after administration and should receive treatment only under direct medical supervision. Healthcare providers should be prepared to administer appropriate therapy for managing potentially life-threatening anaphylaxis. Patients should be instructed on identifying signs/symptoms of anaphylaxis and to seek immediate care if they arise. In postmarketing reports, anaphylaxis usually occurred with the first or second dose and with a time to onset of ≤60 minutes; however, reactions have been reported with subsequent doses (after 39 doses) and with a time to onset of up to 4 days after administration. Discontinue therapy following any severe reaction.

In rare cases, patients may present with systemic eosinophilia, sometimes presenting with clinical features of vasculitis consistent with Churg-Strauss syndrome, a condition which is often treated with systemic corticosteroid therapy. Healthcare providers should be alert to eosinophilia, vasculitic rash, worsening pulmonary symptoms, cardiac complications, and/or neuropathy presenting in their patients. A causal association between omalizumab and these underlying conditions has not been established. Reports of a constellation of symptoms including fever, arthritis or arthralgia, rash, and lymphadenopathy have been reported with postmarketing use (symptoms resemble those seen in patients experiencing serum sickness, although circulating immune complexes or a skin biopsy consistent with a Type III hypersensitivity reaction were not been observed with these cases). Onset of symptoms generally occurred 1-5 days following the first or subsequent doses. Discontinue therapy in any patient reporting this constellation of signs/symptoms. Malignant neoplasms have been reported rarely with use in short-term studies; impact of long-term use is not known. Use caution with and monitor patients at

high risk for parasitic (helminth) infections (risk of infection may be increased).

Therapy has not been shown to alleviate acute asthma exacerbations; do not use to treat acute bronchospasm or status asthmaticus. Dosing is based on body weight and pretreatment total IgE serum levels. IgE levels remain elevated up to 1 year following treatment, therefore, levels taken during treatment cannot and should not be used as a dosage guide. Gradually taper systemic or inhaled corticosteroid therapy; do not discontinue corticosteroids abruptly following initiation of omalizumab therapy.

Drug Interactions

Avoid Concomitant Use

Avoid concomitant use of Omalizumab with any of the following: BCG; Natalizumab; Pimecrolimus; Tacrolimus (Topical); Tofacitinib; Vaccines (Live)

Decreased Effect

Omalizumab may decrease the levels/effects of: BCG; Coccidioidin Skin Test; Sipuleucel-T; Vaccines (Inactivated); Vaccines (Live)

The levels/effects of Omalizumab may be decreased by: Echinacea

Increased Effect/Toxicity

Omalizumab may increase the levels/effects of: Leflunomide; Natalizumab; Tofacitinib; Vaccines (Live)

The levels/effects of Omalizumab may be increased by: Denosumab; Pimecrolimus; Roflumilast; Tacrolimus (Topical); Trastuzumab

Adverse Reactions

>10%: Local: Injection site reaction (45%; placebo 43%; severe 12%). Most reactions occurred within 1 hour, lasted <8 days, and decreased in frequency with additional dosing.

1% to 10%:

Central nervous system: Pain (7%), dizziness (3%), fatigue (3%)

Dermatologic: Dermatitis (2%), pruritus (2%)

Neuromuscular & skeletal: Arthralgia (8%), leg pain (4%), arm pain (2%), bone fracture (2%)

Otic: Otalgia (2%)

Available Dosage Forms

Solution Reconstituted, Subcutaneous [preservative free]:

Xolair: 150 mg (1 ea)

General Dosage Range SubQ:

Pretreatment serum IgE ≥30-100 units/mL:

Children ≥12 years and Adults 30-90 kg: 150 mg every 4 weeks

Children ≥12 years and Adults >90-150 kg: 300 mg every 4 weeks

Pretreatment serum IgE >100-200 units/mL:

Children ≥12 years and Adults 30-90 kg: 300 mg every 4 weeks

Children ≥12 years and Adults >90-150 kg: 225 mg every 2 weeks

Pretreatment serum IgE >200-300 units/mL:
Children ≥12 years and Adults 30-60 kg: 300 mg every 4 weeks
Children ≥12 years and Adults >60-90 kg: 225 mg every 2 weeks
Children ≥12 years and Adults >90-150 kg: 300 mg every 2 weeks

Pretreatment serum IgE >300-400 units/mL:
Children ≥12 years and Adults 30-70 kg: 225 mg every 2 weeks
Children ≥12 years and Adults >70-90 kg: 300 mg every 2 weeks
Children ≥12 years and Adults >90 kg: Do not administer dose

Pretreatment serum IgE >400-500 units/mL:
Children ≥12 years and Adults 30-70 kg: 300 mg every 2 weeks
Children ≥12 years and Adults >70-90 kg: 375 mg every 2 weeks
Children ≥12 years and Adults >90 kg: Do not administer dose

Pretreatment serum IgE >500-600 units/mL:
Children ≥12 years and Adults 30-60 kg: 300 mg every 2 weeks
Children ≥12 years and Adults >60-70 kg: 375 mg every 2 weeks
Children ≥12 years and Adults >70 kg: Do not administer dose

Pretreatment serum IgE >600-700 units/mL:
Children ≥12 years and Adults 30-60 kg: 375 mg every 2 weeks
Children ≥12 years and Adults >60 kg: Do not administer dose

Administration

Subcutaneous Doses >150 mg should be divided over more than one injection site (eg, 225 mg or 300 mg administered as two injections, 375 mg administered as three injections). Injections may take 5-10 seconds to administer (solution is slightly viscous). Administer only under direct medical supervision and observe patient for a minimum of 2 hours following administration of any dose given.

Preparation for Administration Reconstitute using SWFI, USP only; add SWFI 1.4 mL to upright vial using a 1-inch, 18-gauge needle on a 3 mL syringe and swirl gently for ~1 minute to evenly wet the powder; do not shake. Then gently swirl the upright vial for 5-10 seconds approximately every 5 minutes until dissolved; generally takes 15-20 minutes to dissolve completely. If it takes >20 minutes to dissolve completely, continue to swirl the upright vial for 5-10 seconds every 5 minutes until no gel-like particles are visible in the solution; do not use if contents are not completely dissolved after 40 minutes. Resulting solution is 150 mg/1.2 mL. Invert the vial for 15 seconds so the solution drains toward the stopper. Remove all of the solution by inserting a new 3 mL syringe with a 1-inch, 18-gauge needle into the inverted vial. Replace the 18-gauge needle with a 25-gauge needle for subcutaneous injection, and expel any air, bubbles, or excess solution to obtain the 1.2 mL dose.

Storage/Stability Prior to reconstitution, store under refrigeration at 2°C to 8°C (36°F to 46°F); product may be shipped at room temperature. Following reconstitution, protect from direct sunlight. May be stored for up to 8 hours if refrigerated or 4 hours if stored at room temperature.

Nursing Actions

Physical Assessment For SubQ use only. Evaluate pulmonary function tests at baseline and as necessary with treatment. Anaphylactic reactions have been reported within 2-24 hours of initial dose; monitor patient for a minimum of 2 hours following injection; appropriate equipment and medications for the treatment of hypersensitivity reactions should be available. Monitor for hypersensitivity reaction, infection, dermatitis, and arthralgia at beginning of and periodically during therapy. Educate patient about signs and symptoms of hypersensitivity and when to call doctor.

Patient Education
- Discuss specific use of drug and side effects with patient as it relates to treatment. (HCAHPS: During this hospital stay, were you given any medicine that you had not taken before? Before giving you any new medicine, how often did hospital staff tell you what the medicine was for? How often did hospital staff describe possible side effects in a way you could understand?)
- Patient may experience dizziness, headache, myalgia, otalgia, or injection site irritation. Have patient report immediately to prescriber signs of infection, angina, tachycardia, strength differences from one side to another, significant weight gain or loss, edema, decreased peak flow measurement, or rash (HCAHPS).
- Educate patient about signs of a significant reaction (eg, wheezing; chest tightness; fever; itching; bad cough; blue skin color; seizures; or swelling of face, lips, tongue, or throat). **Note:** This is not a comprehensive list of all side effects. Patient should consult prescriber for additional questions.

Intended Use and Disclaimer: Should not be printed and given to patients. This information is intended to serve as a concise initial reference for healthcare professionals to use when discussing medications with a patient. You must ultimately rely on your own discretion, experience and judgment in diagnosing, treating and advising patients.

Omega-3-Acid Ethyl Esters
(oh MEG a three AS id ETH il ES ters)

Brand Names: U.S. Lovaza

Index Terms Docosahexaenoic Acid; Eicosapentaenoic Acid; Ethyl Esters of Omega-3 Fatty Acids; Fish Oil; Omega 3; P-OM3

◄ **Pharmacologic Category** Antilipemic Agent, Omega-3 Fatty Acids

Medication Safety Issues

Sound-alike/look-alike issues:

Lovaza may be confused with LORazepam

International issues:

Omacor [multiple international markets] may be confused with Amicar brand name for aminocaproic acid [U.S.]

Other safety concerns:

The Institute for Safe Medication Practices (ISMP) reported a case of a foam plastic cup dissolving after contact with the liquid contents from a Lovaza capsule. ISMP is requesting the manufacturer to add warnings to its labeling and that healthcare providers add Lovaza to their list of medications to not crush.

Pregnancy Risk Factor C

Lactation Enters breast milk/use caution

Use Lovaza: Adjunct to diet therapy in the treatment of hypertriglyceridemia (≥500 mg/dL)

Note: The Endocrine Society recommends that omega-3 fatty acids such as Lovaza may be considered for triglyceride levels >1000 mg/dL and may be used alone or in combination with HMG-CoA reductase inhibitors (Berglund, 2012). A number of OTC formulations containing omega-3 fatty acids are marketed as nutritional supplements; these do not have FDA-approved indications and may not contain the same amounts of the active ingredient.

Unlabeled Use Lovaza: Treatment of IgA nephropathy

Available Dosage Forms

Capsule, liquid gel, oral:

Lovaza: 1 g

General Dosage Range Oral: *Adults:* 4 g/day in 1-2 divided doses

Administration

Oral May be administered with or without food. Administer whole, do not break, crush, dissolve, or chew.

Nursing Actions

Physical Assessment Do not use if allergic to fish. Encourage diet and exercise along with use of this medication.

Patient Education

• Discuss specific use of drug and side effects with patient as it relates to treatment. (HCAHPS: During this hospital stay, were you given any medicine that you had not taken before? Before giving you any new medicine, how often did hospital staff tell you what the medicine was for? How often did hospital staff describe possible side effects in a way you could understand?)

• Patient may experience flatulence, xerostomia, or nausea. Have patient report immediately to prescriber tachycardia, severe diarrhea, ecchymosis, bleeding, significant dyspepsia, dyspnea,

considerable weight gain, discolored urine, jaundice, inability to eat, or rash (HCAHPS).

• Educate patient about signs of a significant reaction (eg, wheezing; chest tightness; fever; itching; bad cough; blue skin color; seizures; or swelling of face, lips, tongue, or throat). **Note:** This is not a comprehensive list of all side effects. Patient should consult prescriber for additional questions.

Intended Use and Disclaimer: Should not be printed and given to patients. This information is intended to serve as a concise initial reference for healthcare professionals to use when discussing medications with a patient. You must ultimately rely on your own discretion, experience and judgment in diagnosing, treating and advising patients.

Related Information

Oral Medications That Should Not Be Crushed or Altered *on page 1712*

Omeprazole (oh MEP ra zole)

Brand Names: U.S. First-Omeprazole; Omeprazole+Syrspend SF Alka; PriLOSEC; PriLOSEC OTC [OTC]

Index Terms Omeprazole Magnesium

Pharmacologic Category Proton Pump Inhibitor; Substituted Benzimidazole

Medication Safety Issues

Sound-alike/look-alike issues:

Omeprazole may be confused with aripiprazole, esomeprazole, fomepizole

PriLOSEC® may be confused with Plendil®, Prevacid®, predniSONE, prilocaine, Prinivil®, Proventil®, PROzac®

International issues:

Losec [multiple international markets] may be confused with Lasix brand name for furosemide [U.S., Canada, and multiple international markets]

Medral [Mexico] may be confused with Medrol brand name for methylprednisolone [U.S., Canada, and multiple international markets]

Norpramin: Brand name for omeprazole [Spain], but also the brand name for desipramine [U.S., Canada] and enalapril/hydrochlorothiazide [Portugal]

Medication Guide Available Yes

Pregnancy Risk Factor C

Lactation Enters breast milk/use caution

Breast-Feeding Considerations Omeprazole is excreted into breast milk. Milk concentrations of omeprazole were studied in a breast-feeding woman at 3 weeks postpartum. The mother had taken omeprazole 20 mg daily starting her 29th week of gestation and continued after delivery. Following administration of omeprazole 20 mg, peak concentrations in the maternal serum occurred 240 minutes after the dose and peak concentrations in the breast milk were 180 minutes after the dose. The concentrations of omeprazole detected in the breast milk were <7% of the highest maternal serum concentration (Marshall, 1998). The manufacturer recommends caution be used if administered to a nursing woman. The acidic content of the nursing infants' stomach may potentially inactivate any ingested omeprazole (Marshall, 1998).

Use Short-term (4-8 weeks) treatment of active duodenal ulcer disease or active benign gastric ulcer; treatment of heartburn and other symptoms associated with gastroesophageal reflux disease (GERD); short-term (4-8 weeks) treatment of endoscopically-diagnosed erosive esophagitis; maintenance healing of erosive esophagitis; long-term treatment of pathological hypersecretory conditions (eg, Zollinger-Ellison syndrome); as part of a multidrug regimen for *H. pylori* eradication to reduce the risk of duodenal ulcer recurrence

OTC labeling: Short-term treatment of frequent, uncomplicated heartburn occurring ≥2 days/week

Unlabeled Use Healing NSAID-induced ulcers; prevention of NSAID-induced ulcer; stress ulcer prophylaxis in the critically-ill

Mechanism of Action/Effect Proton pump inhibitor; suppresses gastric basal and stimulated acid secretion by inhibiting the parietal cell H+/K+ ATP pump

Contraindications Hypersensitivity to omeprazole, other substituted benzimidazole proton pump inhibitors, or any component of the formulation

Warnings/Precautions Use of proton pump inhibitors (PPIs) may increase the risk of gastrointestinal infections (eg, *Salmonella, Campylobacter*). Relief of symptoms does not preclude the presence of a gastric malignancy. Atrophic gastritis (by biopsy) has been noted with long-term omeprazole therapy. In long-term (2-year) studies in rats, omeprazole produced a dose-related increase in gastric carcinoid tumors. While available endoscopic evaluations and histologic examinations of biopsy specimens from human stomachs have not detected a risk from short-term exposure to omeprazole, further human data on the effect of sustained hypochlorhydria and hypergastrinemia are needed to rule out the possibility of an increased risk for the development of tumors in humans receiving long-term therapy. Use of PPIs may increase risk of *Clostridium difficile*-associated diarrhea (CDAD), especially in hospitalized patients; consider CDAD diagnosis in patients with persistent diarrhea that does not improve. Use the lowest dose and shortest duration of PPI therapy appropriate for the condition being treated.

PPIs may diminish the therapeutic effect of clopidogrel, thought to be due to reduced formation of the active metabolite of clopidogrel. The manufacturer of clopidogrel recommends either avoidance both omeprazole (even when scheduled 12 hours

apart) and esomeprazole or use of a PPI with comparatively less effect on the active metabolite of clopidogrel (eg, pantoprazole). In contrast to these warnings, others have recommended the continued use of PPIs, regardless of the degree of inhibition, in patients with a history of GI bleeding or multiple risk factors for GI bleeding who are also receiving clopidogrel since no evidence has established clinically meaningful differences in outcome; however, a clinically-significant interaction cannot be excluded in those who are poor metabolizers of clopidogrel (Abraham, 2010; Levine, 2011). Additionally, concomitant use of omeprazole with some drugs may require cautious use, may not be recommended, or may require dosage adjustments.

Increased incidence of osteoporosis-related bone fractures of the hip, spine, or wrist may occur with PPI therapy. Patients on high-dose (multiple daily doses) or long-term (≥1 year) therapy should be monitored. Use the lowest effective dose for the shortest duration of time, use vitamin D and calcium supplementation, and follow appropriate guidelines to reduce risk of fractures in patients at risk.

Hypomagnesemia, reported rarely, usually with prolonged PPI use of >3 months (most cases >1 year of therapy); may be symptomatic or asymptomatic; severe cases may cause tetany, seizures, and cardiac arrhythmias. Consider obtaining serum magnesium concentrations prior to beginning long-term therapy, especially if taking concomitant digoxin, diuretics, or other drugs known to cause hypomagnesemia; and periodically thereafter. Hypomagnesemia may be corrected by magnesium supplementation, although discontinuation of omeprazole may be necessary; magnesium levels typically return to normal within 1 week of stopping. Serum chromogranin A levels may be increased if assessed while patient on omeprazole; may lead to diagnostic errors related to neuroendocrine tumors.

Decreased *H. pylori* eradication rates have been observed with short-term (≤7 days) combination therapy. The American College of Gastroenterology recommends 10-14 days of therapy (triple or quadruple) for eradication of *H. pylori* (Chey, 2007). Bioavailability may be increased in Asian populations and patients with hepatic dysfunction; consider dosage reductions, especially for maintenance healing of erosive esophagitis. Bioavailability may be increased in the elderly. When used for self-medication (OTC), do not use for >14 days.

Drug Interactions

Avoid Concomitant Use

Avoid concomitant use of Omeprazole with any of the following: Clopidogrel; Dasatinib; Delavirdine; Erlotinib; Nelfinavir; Pimozide; PONATinib; Rifampin; Rilpivirine; Risedronate; St Johns Wort

Decreased Effect

Omeprazole may decrease the levels/effects of: Atazanavir; Bisphosphonate Derivatives; Bosutinib; Cefditoren; Clopidogrel; CloZAPine; Dabigatran Etexilate; Dabrafenib; Dasatinib; Delavirdine; Erlotinib; Gefitinib; Indinavir; Iron Salts; Itraconazole; Ketoconazole (Systemic); Mesalamine; Multivitamins/Minerals (with ADEK, Folate, Iron); Mycophenolate; Nelfinavir; Nilotinib; PONATinib; Posaconazole; Rilpivirine; Riociguat; Risedronate; Vismodegib

The levels/effects of Omeprazole may be decreased by: CYP2C19 Inducers (Strong); Dabrafenib; Fosphenytoin; Peginterferon Alfa-2b; Phenytoin; Rifampin; St Johns Wort; Tipranavir

Increased Effect/Toxicity

Omeprazole may increase the levels/effects of: Amphetamine; ARIPiprazole; Benzodiazepines (metabolized by oxidation); Bosentan; Carvedilol; Cilostazol; Citalopram; CloZAPine; CycloSPORINE (Systemic); CYP2C19 Substrates; CYP2C9 Substrates; Dexmethylphenidate; Dextroamphetamine; Dofetilide; Escitalopram; Fosphenytoin; Lomitapide; Methotrexate; Methylphenidate; Phenytoin; Pimozide; Raltegravir; Risedronate; Saquinavir; Tacrolimus (Systemic); Vitamin K Antagonists; Voriconazole

The levels/effects of Omeprazole may be increased by: Fluconazole; Ketoconazole (Systemic); Voriconazole

Nutritional/Ethanol Interactions

Ethanol: Avoid ethanol (may cause gastric mucosal irritation).

Food: Food delays absorption.

Herb/Nutraceutical: Avoid use of St John's wort (may decrease efficacy of omeprazole).

Adverse Reactions 1% to 10%:

Central nervous system: Headache (7%), dizziness (2%)

Dermatologic: Rash (2%)

Gastrointestinal: Abdominal pain (5%), diarrhea (4%), nausea (4%), vomiting (3%), flatulence (3%), acid regurgitation (2%), constipation (2%)

Neuromuscular & skeletal: Back pain (1%), weakness (1%)

Respiratory: Upper respiratory infection (2%), cough (1%)

Pharmacodynamics/Kinetics

Onset of Action Antisecretory: ~1 hour; Peak effect: Within 2 hours

Duration of Action Up to 72 hours; 50% of maximum effect at 24 hours; after stopping treatment, secretory activity gradually returns over 3-5 days

Available Dosage Forms

Capsule Delayed Release, Oral:

PriLOSEC: 10 mg, 20 mg, 40 mg

Generic: 10 mg, 20 mg, 40 mg, 20 mg

Packet, Oral:

PriLOSEC: 2.5 mg (30 ea); 10 mg (30 ea)

Suspension, Oral:

First-Omeprazole: 2 mg/mL (90 mL, 150 mL, 300 mL)

Omeprazole+Syrspend SF Alka: 2 mg/mL (100 mL)

Tablet Delayed Release, Oral:

PriLOSEC OTC [OTC]: 20 mg

Generic: 20 mg

General Dosage Range Oral:

Children 1-16 years and 5 kg to <10 kg: 5 mg once daily

Children 1-16 years and 10 kg to <20 kg: 10 mg once daily

Children 1-16 years and ≥20 kg: 20 mg once daily

Adults: 20-40 mg daily (may be given in 2 divided doses); doses up to 360 mg daily [pathological hypersecretory syndrome]

Administration

Oral Best if administered before breakfast.

Capsule: Should be swallowed whole; do not chew or crush. Delayed release capsule may be opened and contents added to 1 tablespoon of applesauce (use immediately after adding to applesauce); mixture should not be chewed or warmed.

Oral suspension: Following reconstitution, the suspension should be left to thicken for 2-3 minutes and administered within 30 minutes. If any material remains after administration, add more water, stir, and administer immediately.

Tablet: Should be swallowed whole; do not crush or chew.

Other Nasogastric/orogastric (NG/OG) tube administration:

Oral suspension (using packets): After removing a catheter-tip syringe plunger, add 5 mL of water to the syringe and the contents of a 2.5 mg packet (or 15 mL of water for the 10 mg packet). Immediately shake syringe and leave to thicken for 2-3 minutes; shake syringe again and within 30 minutes administer via NG or gastric tube (French size 6 or larger). Refill syringe with an equal amount of water, shake, and flush remaining contents through NG or gastric tube

Oral suspension (using capsules): The manufacturer of Prilosec® does not give recommendations for extemporaneous preparation of omeprazole capsules for NG/OG administration. Consider using the packets for oral suspension. If packets are unavailable, methods of preparation of capsules for NG/OG administration have been described (Balaban, 1997; Phillips, 1996). An extemporaneously prepared suspension with extended stability may also be used (DiGiacinto, 2000; Quercia, 1997; Sharma, 1999).

Preparation for Administration Granules for oral suspension: For oral administration, empty the contents of the 2.5 mg packet into 5 mL of water (10 mg packet into 15 mL of water); stir. For NG administration, add 5 mL of water into a catheter-tipped syringe, and then add the contents of a

2.5 mg packet (15 mL water for the 10 mg packet); shake. **Note:** Regardless of the route of administration, the suspension should be left to thicken for 2-3 minutes prior to administration.

Storage/Stability
Capsules, tablets: Store at 15°C to 30°C (59°F to 86°F). Protect from light and moisture.

Granules for oral suspension: Store at 25°C (77°F); excursions permitted to 15°C to 30°C (59°F to 86°F).

Nursing Actions
Physical Assessment Optimize prevention of fractures in patients with osteoporosis.

Patient Education
- Discuss specific use of drug and side effects with patient as it relates to treatment. (HCAHPS: During this hospital stay, were you given any medicine that you had not taken before? Before giving you any new medicine, how often did hospital staff tell you what the medicine was for? How often did hospital staff describe possible side effects in a way you could understand?)
- Patient may experience headache, dyspepsia, nausea, or diarrhea. Have patient report immediately to prescriber severe dizziness, syncope, tachycardia, ecchymosis, osteodynia, myalgia, asthenia, or rash (HCAHPS).
- Educate patient about signs of a significant reaction (eg, wheezing; chest tightness; fever; itching; bad cough; blue skin color; seizures; or swelling of face, lips, tongue, or throat). **Note:** This is not a comprehensive list of all side effects. Patient should consult prescriber for additional questions.

Intended Use and Disclaimer: Should not be printed and given to patients. This information is intended to serve as a concise initial reference for healthcare professionals to use when discussing medications with a patient. You must ultimately rely on your own discretion, experience and judgment in diagnosing, treating and advising patients.

Dietary Considerations Should be taken on an empty stomach; best if taken before breakfast.

Related Information
Oral Medications That Should Not Be Crushed or Altered *on page 1712*

Omeprazole and Sodium Bicarbonate
(oh MEP ra zole & SOW dee um bye KAR bun ate)

Brand Names: U.S. Zegerid OTC™ [OTC]; Zegerid®

Index Terms Sodium Bicarbonate and Omeprazole

Pharmacologic Category Proton Pump Inhibitor; Substituted Benzimidazole

Medication Safety Issues
Sound-alike/look-alike issues:
Zegerid® may be confused with Zestril®

Medication Guide Available Yes
Pregnancy Risk Factor C
Use Short-term (4-8 weeks) treatment of active duodenal ulcer or active benign gastric ulcer; treatment of heartburn and other symptoms associated with gastroesophageal reflux disease (GERD); short-term (4-8 weeks) treatment of endoscopically-diagnosed erosive esophagitis; maintenance healing of erosive esophagitis; reduction of risk of upper gastrointestinal bleeding in critically-ill patients

OTC labeling: Short-term (2 weeks) treatment of frequent (2 days/week), uncomplicated heartburn

Available Dosage Forms
Capsule, oral: Omeprazole 20 mg [immediate release] and sodium bicarbonate 1100 mg; omeprazole 40 mg [immediate release] and sodium bicarbonate 1100 mg
Zegerid®: Omeprazole 20 mg [immediate release] and sodium bicarbonate 1100 mg
Zegerid®: Omeprazole 40 mg [immediate release] and sodium bicarbonate 1100 mg
Zegerid OTC™ [OTC]: Omeprazole 20 mg [immediate release] and sodium bicarbonate 1100 mg

Powder for suspension, oral:
Zegerid®: Omeprazole 20 mg and sodium bicarbonate 1680 mg per packet
Zegerid®: Omeprazole 40 mg and sodium bicarbonate 1680 mg per packet

General Dosage Range Oral: *Adults:* 20-40 mg/day in 1-2 divided doses

Administration
Oral Note: Both strengths of Zegerid® capsule and powder for oral suspension have identical sodium bicarbonate content, respectively. Do not substitute two 20 mg capsules/packets for one 40 mg dose.

Capsule: Should be swallowed whole with water (do not use other liquids); do not chew or crush. Capsules should **not** be opened, sprinkled on food, or administered via NG. Best if taken at least 1 hour before breakfast.

Powder for oral suspension: Administer 1 hour before a meal. Mix with 15-30 mL of water; stir well and drink immediately. Rinse cup with water and drink. Do not use other liquids or sprinkle on food.

Other Nasogastric/orogastric tube: Powder for oral suspension: Mix well with 20 mL of water (do not use other liquids) and administer immediately; flush tube with an additional 20 mL of water. Suspend enteral feeding for 3 hours before and 1 hour after administering.

Nursing Actions
Physical Assessment See individual agents.
Patient Education
- Discuss specific use of drug and side effects with patient as it relates to treatment. (HCAHPS: During this hospital stay, were you given any

medicine that you had not taken before? Before giving you any new medicine, how often did hospital staff tell you what the medicine was for? How often did hospital staff describe possible side effects in a way you could understand?)

- Patient may experience signs of hypokalemia, headache, or diarrhea. Have patient report immediately to prescriber severe dizziness, tachycardia, considerable dyspepsia, significant edema, ecchymosis, bleeding, intolerable osteodynia, or severe myalgia (HCAHPS).
- Educate patient about signs of a significant reaction (eg, wheezing; chest tightness; fever; itching; bad cough; blue skin color; seizures; or swelling of face, lips, tongue, or throat). **Note:** This is not a comprehensive list of all side effects. Patient should consult prescriber for additional questions.

Intended Use and Disclaimer: Should not be printed and given to patients. This information is intended to serve as a concise initial reference for healthcare professionals to use when discussing medications with a patient. You must ultimately rely on your own discretion, experience and judgment in diagnosing, treating and advising patients.

Related Information

Omeprazole *on page 1158*

Oral Medications That Should Not Be Crushed or Altered *on page 1712*

Sodium Bicarbonate *on page 1424*

Ondansetron (on DAN se tron)

Brand Names: U.S. Zofran; Zofran ODT; Zuplenz

Index Terms GR38032R; Ondansetron Hydrochloride; Zuplenz®

Pharmacologic Category Antiemetic; Selective 5-HT$_3$ Receptor Antagonist

Medication Safety Issues

Sound-alike/look-alike issues:

Ondansetron may be confused with dolasetron, granisetron, palonosetron

Zofran® may be confused with Zantac®, Zosyn®

Pregnancy Risk Factor B

Lactation Excretion in breast milk unknown/use caution

Breast-Feeding Considerations It is not known if ondansetron is excreted into breast milk. The manufacturer recommends caution be used if administered to nursing women.

Use

I.V.: Prevention of nausea and vomiting associated with initial and repeat courses of emetogenic cancer chemotherapy (including high-dose cisplatin); prevention of postoperative nausea and/or vomiting (PONV); treatment of PONV if no prophylactic dose of ondansetron received

Oral: Prevention of nausea and vomiting associated with highly emetogenic cancer chemotherapy (including high-dose cisplatin); prevention of nausea and vomiting associated with initial and repeat courses of moderately emetogenic cancer chemotherapy; prevention of nausea and vomiting associated with radiotherapy (either total body irradiation, single high-dose fraction to the abdomen, or daily fractions to the abdomen); prevention of PONV

Unlabeled Use Hyperemesis gravidarum (severe or refractory); breakthrough treatment of nausea and vomiting associated with chemotherapy

Mechanism of Action/Effect Selective 5-HT$_3$ receptor antagonist, blocking serotonin, both peripherally on vagal nerve terminals and centrally in the chemoreceptor trigger zone

Contraindications Hypersensitivity to ondansetron or any component of the formulation; concomitant use of apomorphine

Warnings/Precautions Ondansetron should be used on a scheduled basis, not on an "as needed" (PRN) basis, since data support the use of this drug only in the prevention of nausea and vomiting (due to antineoplastic therapy) and not in the rescue of nausea and vomiting. Ondansetron should only be used in the first 24-48 hours of chemotherapy. Data do not support any increased efficacy of ondansetron in delayed nausea and vomiting. Does not stimulate gastric or intestinal peristalsis; may mask progressive ileus and/or gastric distension. Use with caution in patients allergic to other 5-HT$_3$ receptor antagonists; cross-reactivity has been reported.

Dose-dependent QT interval prolongation occurs with ondansetron use. Cases of torsade de pointes have also been reported to the manufacturer. Selective 5-HT$_3$ antagonists, including ondansetron, have been associated with a number of dose-dependent increases in ECG intervals (eg, PR, QRS duration, QT/QT$_c$, JT), usually occurring 1-2 hours after I.V. administration. Single doses >16 mg ondansetron I.V. are no longer recommended due to the potential for an increased risk of QT prolongation. In most patients, these changes are not clinically relevant; however, when used in conjunction with other agents that prolong these intervals or in those at risk for QT prolongation, arrhythmia may occur. When used with agents that prolong the QT interval (eg, Class I and III antiarrhythmics) or in patients with cardiovascular disease, clinically relevant QT interval prolongation may occur resulting in torsade de pointes. Avoid ondansetron use in patients with congenital long QT syndrome. Use caution and monitor ECG in patients with other risk factors for QT prolongation (eg, medications known to prolong QT interval, electrolyte abnormalities [hypokalemia or hypomagnesemia], heart failure, bradyarrhythmias, and cumulative high-dose anthracycline therapy). I.V. formulations of 5-HT$_3$ antagonists have more association with ECG interval changes, compared to oral formulations. Dose limitations are recommended for patients with severe hepatic impairment (Child-Pugh class C); use with caution in mild-moderate hepatic impairment; clearance is decreased and half-life increased in hepatic impairment.

Orally-disintegrating tablets contain phenylalanine.

Drug Interactions

Avoid Concomitant Use

Avoid concomitant use of Ondansetron with any of the following: Apomorphine; Highest Risk QTc-Prolonging Agents; Ivabradine; Mifepristone

Decreased Effect

Ondansetron may decrease the levels/effects of: Tapentadol; TraMADol

The levels/effects of Ondansetron may be decreased by: Bosentan; CYP3A4 Inducers (Strong); Dabrafenib; Deferasirox; Herbs (CYP3A4 Inducers); Mitotane; Peginterferon Alfa-2b; P-glycoprotein/ABCB1 Inducers; Rifamycin Derivatives; Tocilizumab

Increased Effect/Toxicity

Ondansetron may increase the levels/effects of: Apomorphine; ARIPiprazole; Highest Risk QTc-Prolonging Agents; Moderate Risk QTc-Prolonging Agents

The levels/effects of Ondansetron may be increased by: Ivabradine; Mifepristone; P-glycoprotein/ABCB1 Inhibitors; QTc-Prolonging Agents (Indeterminate Risk and Risk Modifying)

Nutritional/Ethanol Interactions

Food: Tablet: Food slightly increases the extent of absorption.

Herb/Nutraceutical: St John's wort may decrease ondansetron levels.

Adverse Reactions Note: Percentages reported in adult patients.

>10%:

Central nervous system: Headache (9% to 27%), malaise/fatigue (9% to 13%)

Gastrointestinal: Constipation (6% to 11%)

1% to 10%:

Central nervous system: Drowsiness (8%), dizziness (7%), anxiety (6%), paresthesia (2%), sensation of cold (2%)

Dermatologic: Pruritus (2% to 5%), skin rash (1%)

Gastrointestinal: Diarrhea (2% to 7%)

Genitourinary: Gynecologic disease (7%), urinary retention (5%)

Hepatic: Increased serum ALT (>2 times ULN: 1% to 5%), increased serum AST (>2 times ULN: 1% to 5%)

Local: Injection site reaction (4%; pain, redness, burning)

Respiratory: Hypoxia (9%)

Miscellaneous: Fever (2% to 8%)

Pharmacodynamics/Kinetics

Onset of Action ~30 minutes

Available Dosage Forms

Film, Oral:

Zuplenz: 4 mg (1 ea, 10 ea); 8 mg (1 ea, 10 ea)

Solution, Injection:

Zofran: 40 mg/20 mL (20 mL)

Generic: 4 mg/2 mL (2 mL); 40 mg/20 mL (20 mL)

Solution, Injection [preservative free]:

Generic: 4 mg/2 mL (2 mL)

Solution, Oral:

Zofran: 4 mg/5 mL (50 mL)

Generic: 4 mg/5 mL (50 mL)

Tablet, Oral:

Zofran: 4 mg, 8 mg

Generic: 4 mg, 8 mg, 24 mg

Tablet Dispersible, Oral:

Zofran ODT: 4 mg, 8 mg

Generic: 4 mg, 8 mg

General Dosage Range Dosage adjustment recommended in patients with hepatic impairment

I.M.: *Adults:* 4 mg as a single dose

I.V.:

Infants 1-6 months: 0.1 mg/kg as a single dose

Children 6 months to 12 years and ≤40 kg: 0.1 mg/kg as a single dose **or** 0.15 mg/kg/dose (maximum: 16 mg/dose) for 3 doses

Children 6 months to 12 years and >40 kg and Children >12 years to 18 years: 4 mg as a single dose **or** 0.15 mg/kg/dose (maximum: 16 mg/dose) for 3 doses

Adults: 0.15 mg/kg/dose (maximum: 16 mg/dose) for 3 doses **or** 4 mg as a single dose

Oral:

Children 4-11 years: 4 mg every 4 hours for 3 doses (day 1), then 4 mg every 8 hours for 1-2 days

Children ≥12 years and Adults: 16 mg or 24 mg as a single dose **or** 8 mg every 8-12 hours

Administration

I.M. Should be given undiluted.

I.V.

IVPB: Infuse diluted solution over 15-30 minutes; 24-hour continuous infusions have been reported, but are rarely used.

Chemotherapy-induced nausea and vomiting: Give first dose 30 minutes prior to beginning chemotherapy.

I.V. push: Prevention of postoperative nausea and vomiting: Single doses may be administered I.V. injection over 2-5 minutes as undiluted solution.

Injectable Detail pH: 3-4

Oral Oral dosage forms should be given 30 minutes prior to chemotherapy; 1-2 hours before radiotherapy; 1 hour prior to the induction of anesthesia

Orally-disintegrating tablets: Do not remove from blister until needed. Peel backing off the blister, do not push tablet through. Using dry hands, place tablet on tongue and allow to dissolve. Swallow with saliva.

Oral soluble film: Do not remove from pouch until immediately before use. Using dry hands, place ▶

film on top of tongue and allow to dissolve (4-20 seconds). Swallow with or without liquid. If using more than one film, each film should be allowed to dissolve completely before administering the next film.

Preparation for Administration Prior to I.V. infusion, dilute in 50 mL D₅W or NS.

Storage/Stability

Oral soluble film: Store between 20°C and 25°C (68°F and 77°F). Store pouches in cartons; keep film in individual pouch until ready to use.

Oral solution: Store between 15°C and 30°C (59°F and 86°F). Protect from light.

Tablet: Store between 2°C and 30°C (36°F and 86°F).

Vial: Store between 2°C and 30°C (36°F and 86°F). Protect from light. Stable when mixed in D₅W or NS for 48 hours at room temperature.

Nursing Actions

Physical Assessment Allergy history to selective 5-HT₃ receptor antagonists should be assessed prior to administering. Assess other drugs patient may be taking that may prolong QT interval. I.V.: Follow infusion specifics. Oral and I.V. doses have different schedules and should not be administered on "PRN" basis.

Patient Education

• Discuss specific use of drug and side effects with patient as it relates to treatment. (HCAHPS: During this hospital stay, were you given any medicine that you had not taken before? Before giving you any new medicine, how often did hospital staff tell you what the medicine was for? How often did hospital staff describe possible side effects in a way you could understand?)

• Patient may experience headache, asthenia, constipation, dizziness, presyncope, fatigue, blurred vision, or illogical thinking. Have patient report immediately to prescriber tachycardia or rash (HCAHPS).

• Educate patient about signs of a significant reaction (eg, wheezing; chest tightness; fever; itching; bad cough; blue skin color; seizures; or swelling of face, lips, tongue, or throat). **Note:** This is not a comprehensive list of all side effects. Patient should consult prescriber for additional questions.

Intended Use and Disclaimer: Should not be printed and given to patients. This information is intended to serve as a concise initial reference for healthcare professionals to use when discussing medications with a patient. You must ultimately rely on your own discretion, experience and judgment in diagnosing, treating and advising patients.

Dietary Considerations Take without regard to meals. Some products may contain phenylalanine.

Opium Tincture (OH pee um TING chur)

Index Terms Deodorized Tincture of Opium (error-prone synonym); DTO (error-prone abbreviation); Opium Tincture, Deodorized; Tincture of Opium

Pharmacologic Category Analgesic, Opioid, Antidiarrheal

Medication Safety Issues

Sound-alike/look-alike issues:

Opium tincture may be confused with camphorated tincture of opium (paregoric)

High alert medication:

The Institute for Safe Medication Practices (ISMP) includes this medication among its list of drugs which have a heightened risk of causing significant patient harm when used in error.

Administration issues:

Use care when prescribing opium tincture; opium tincture is 25 times more concentrated than paregoric, each undiluted mL of opium tincture contains the equivalent of morphine 10 mg/mL.

If opium tincture is used in neonates, a 25-fold dilution should be prepared (final concentration 0.4 mg/mL morphine). Of note, paregoric (which contains the equivalent of morphine 0.4 mg/mL) is **not** recommended for use in neonates due to the high alcohol content (~45%) and the presence of other additives; as an alternative to the use of diluted opium tincture or paregoric, ISMP recommends using a diluted preservative free injectable morphine solution orally.

Although historically opium tincture is dosed as mL/kg, the preferred dosing units are **mg**/kg (Levine, 2001). ISMP suggests hospitals evaluate the need for this product at their institution.

Other safety concerns:

DTO is an error-prone abbreviation and should never be used as an abbreviation for opium tincture (also known as *Deodorized* Tincture of Opium) due to potential for being mistaken as *Diluted* Tincture of Opium

Pregnancy Risk Factor C

Lactation Enters breast milk/use caution

Use Treatment of diarrhea in adults

Controlled Substance C-II

Available Dosage Forms

Tincture, Oral:

Generic: 10 mg/mL (1%) (118 mL, 473 mL)

General Dosage Range

Oral: Opium tincture contains morphine 10 mg/mL. Use caution in ordering, dispensing, and/or administering. The following doses are expressed in **mg** (milligram) dosing units of morphine.

Adults: Usual: 6 **mg** of undiluted opium tincture (10 mg/mL) 4 times daily

Administration

Oral May administer with food to decrease GI upset.

Nursing Actions

Physical Assessment If being used to control diarrhea, monitor stools. Monitor for effectiveness. Monitor blood pressure, CNS and respiratory status, and degree of sedation at beginning of therapy and periodically thereafter. Assess patient's physical and/or psychological dependence. For inpatients, implement safety measures (eg, side rails up, call light within reach, instructions to call for assistance). Discontinue slowly after prolonged use.

Patient Education

- Discuss specific use of drug and side effects with patient as it relates to treatment. (HCAHPS: During this hospital stay, were you given any medicine that you had not taken before? Before giving you any new medicine, how often did hospital staff tell you what the medicine was for? How often did hospital staff describe possible side effects in a way you could understand?)
- Patient may experience nausea. Have patient report immediately to prescriber severe dizziness, syncope, illogical thinking, considerable constipation, difficult urination, tachycardia, bradycardia, dyspnea, or vision changes (HCAHPS).
- Educate patient about signs of a significant reaction (eg, wheezing; chest tightness; fever; itching; bad cough; blue skin color; seizures; or swelling of face, lips, tongue, or throat). **Note:** This is not a comprehensive list of all side effects. Patient should consult prescriber for additional questions.

Intended Use and Disclaimer: Should not be printed and given to patients. This information is intended to serve as a concise initial reference for healthcare professionals to use when discussing medications with a patient. You must ultimately rely on your own discretion, experience and judgment in diagnosing, treating and advising patients.

Orlistat (OR li stat)

Brand Names: U.S. Alli [OTC]; Xenical
Pharmacologic Category Lipase Inhibitor
Medication Safety Issues
  Sound-alike/look-alike issues:
  Xenical may be confused with Xeloda®
Pregnancy Risk Factor X
Lactation Excretion in breast milk unknown/use caution
Breast-Feeding Considerations Weight-loss therapy is generally not recommended for lactating women. Weight-loss programs which include physical activity and nutrition components should be discussed at the 6-week postpartum visit (ADA, 2009; IOM, 2009).
Use Management of obesity, including weight loss and weight management, when used in conjunction with a reduced-calorie and low-fat diet; reduce the risk of weight regain after prior weight loss; indicated for obese patients with an initial body mass index (BMI) ≥ 30 kg/m^2 or ≥ 27 kg/m^2 in the presence of other risk factors (eg, diabetes, dyslipidemia, hypertension)

Mechanism of Action/Effect Inhibits gastric and pancreatic lipases, thus inhibiting the absorption of dietary fats (by 30% at doses of 120 mg 3 times/day)

Contraindications Hypersensitivity to orlistat or any component of the formulation; chronic malabsorption syndrome or cholestasis; pregnancy

Warnings/Precautions Prior to use other causes for obesity (eg, hypothyroidism) should be ruled out. Cases of severe liver injury (some fatal) with hepatocellular necrosis or acute hepatic failure have been reported (rare); liver transplantation has been required in some patients. Patients should be instructed to report any symptoms of hepatic dysfunction (eg, anorexia, pruritus, jaundice, dark urine, light colored stools, right upper quadrant pain); discontinue orlistat and obtain liver function test immediately if symptoms occur. Advise patients to adhere to dietary guidelines; if taken with a diet high in fat (>30% total daily calories from fat) gastrointestinal adverse events may increase. Distribute daily fat intake over 3 main meals. If taken with any 1 meal very high in fat, the possibility of gastrointestinal effects increases. Counsel patients to take a multivitamin supplement that contains fat-soluble vitamins ≥ 2 hours before or after orlistat administration to ensure adequate nutrition; orlistat has been shown to reduce the absorption of some fat-soluble vitamins and beta-carotene. Increased levels of urinary oxalate following treatment may occur in some patients; monitor renal function in patients at risk for renal failure; use with caution in patients with a history of hyperoxaluria or calcium oxalate nephrolithiasis. Orlistat may decrease cyclosporine plasma concentrations; administer cyclosporine ≥ 3 hours before or after orlistat and monitor frequently. The potential exists for misuse in inappropriate patient populations (eg, patients with anorexia nervosa or bulimia) similar to any weight loss agent. In general, substantial weight loss may increase the risk of cholelithiasis.

Self-medication (OTC use): Prior to use, patients should contact their healthcare provider if they have ever had kidney stones, gall bladder disease, or pancreatitis. Patients taking medications for diabetes or thyroid disease, anticoagulants, or other weight-loss products should consult their healthcare provider or pharmacist. Patients who have had an organ transplant should not use orlistat. If severe and/or continuous abdominal pain, itching, yellowing of the eyes or skin, dark urine, or loss of appetite occurs, use should be discontinued and healthcare provider consulted.

Drug Interactions

Avoid Concomitant Use There are no known interactions where it is recommended to avoid concomitant use.

Decreased Effect

Orlistat may decrease the levels/effects of: Amiodarone; Anticonvulsants; CycloSPORINE (Systemic); Levothyroxine; Multivitamins/Fluoride (with ADE); Multivitamins/Minerals (with ADEK, Folate, Iron); Multivitamins/Minerals (with AE, No Iron); Paricalcitol; Propafenone; Vitamin D Analogs; Vitamins (Fat Soluble)

Increased Effect/Toxicity

Orlistat may increase the levels/effects of: Warfarin

Nutritional/Ethanol Interactions Fat-soluble vitamins: Absorption of vitamins A, D, E, and K may be decreased by orlistat. A multivitamin containing the fat-soluble vitamins (A, D, E, and K) should be administered once daily at least 2 hours before or after orlistat.

Adverse Reactions Note: The frequency of most adverse reactions (especially gastrointestinal effects) decreases over time.

>10%:
Central nervous system: Headache (≤31%)
Gastrointestinal: Oily spotting (4% to 27%), abdominal pain/discomfort (≤26%), flatus with discharge (2% to 24%), fecal urgency (3% to 22%), fatty/oily stool (6% to 20%), oily evacuation (2% to 12%), defecation increased (3% to 11%)
Neuromuscular & skeletal: Back pain (≤14%)
Respiratory: Upper respiratory infection (26% to 38%)
Miscellaneous: Influenza (≤40%)
1% to 10%:
Cardiovascular: Pedal edema (≤3%)
Central nervous system: Fatigue (3% to 7%), anxiety (3% to 5%), sleep disorder (≤4%)
Dermatologic: Dry skin (≤2%)
Endocrine & metabolic: Menstrual irregularities (≤10%)
Gastrointestinal: Nausea (4% to 8%), fecal incontinence (2% to 8%), infectious diarrhea (≤5%), rectal pain/discomfort (3% to 5%), tooth disorder (3% to 4%), gingival disorder (2% to 4%)
Genitourinary: Urinary tract infection (6% to 8%), vaginitis (3% to 4%)
Neuromuscular & skeletal: Myalgia (≤4%)
Otic: Otitis (3% to 4%)
Respiratory: Lower respiratory infection (≤8%)

Pharmacodynamics/Kinetics

Onset of Action 24-48 hours
Duration of Action 48-72 hours

Available Dosage Forms

Capsule, Oral:
Alli [OTC]: 60 mg
Xenical: 120 mg

General Dosage Range Oral:

Children ≥12 years and Adults: Xenical®: 120 mg 3 times/day
Adults: Alli™ (OTC labeling): 60 mg 3 times/day

Administration

Oral Administer during or up to 1 hour after each main meal containing fat.

Storage/Stability Store at 25°C (77°F); excursions permitted to 15°C to 30°C (59°F to 86°F).

Nursing Actions

Patient Education

• Discuss specific use of drug and side effects with patient as it relates to treatment. (HCAHPS: During this hospital stay, were you given any medicine that you had not taken before? Before giving you any new medicine, how often did hospital staff tell you what the medicine was for? How often did hospital staff describe possible side effects in a way you could understand?)

• Patient may experience headache, back pain, dyspepsia, or flatulence. Have patient report immediately to prescriber severe nausea, significant weight loss, inability to eat, considerable asthenia, discolored urine, jaundice, hematuria, or rash (HCAHPS).

• Educate patient about signs of a significant reaction (eg, wheezing; chest tightness; fever; itching; bad cough; blue skin color; seizures; or swelling of face, lips, tongue, or throat). **Note:** This is not a comprehensive list of all side effects. Patient should consult prescriber for additional questions.

Intended Use and Disclaimer: Should not be printed and given to patients. This information is intended to serve as a concise initial reference for healthcare professionals to use when discussing medications with a patient. You must ultimately rely on your own discretion, experience and judgment in diagnosing, treating and advising patients.

Dietary Considerations Multivitamin supplements that contain fat-soluble vitamins should be taken once daily at least 2 hours before or after the administration of orlistat (ie, bedtime). Gastrointestinal effects of orlistat may increase if taken with any one meal very high in fat. Distribute daily intake of carbohydrates, fat (~30% of daily calories), and protein over three main meals.

Orphenadrine (or FEN a dreen)

Brand Names: U.S. Norflex
Index Terms Orphenadrine Citrate
Pharmacologic Category Skeletal Muscle Relaxant

Medication Safety Issues

Sound-alike/look-alike issues:
Norflex™ may be confused with norfloxacin, Noroxin®

BEERS Criteria medication:
This drug may be potentially inappropriate for use in geriatric patients (Quality of evidence - moderate; Strength of recommendation - strong).

International issues:
Flexin: Brand name for orphenadrine [Israel] but is also the brand name for cyclobenzaprine [Chile] and diclofenac [Argentina]

Flexin [Israel] may be confused with Floxin which is a brand name for flunarizine [Thailand], norfloxacin [South Africa], ofloxacin [U.S., Canada], and perfloxacin [Philippines]

Pregnancy Risk Factor C

Use Treatment of muscle spasm associated with acute painful musculoskeletal conditions

Available Dosage Forms

Solution, Injection:
Norflex: 30 mg/mL (2 mL)
Generic: 30 mg/mL (2 mL)

Solution, Injection [preservative free]:
Generic: 30 mg/mL (2 mL)

Tablet Extended Release 12 Hour, Oral:
Generic: 100 mg

General Dosage Range

I.M., I.V.: *Adults:* 60 mg every 12 hours
Oral: *Adults:* 100 mg twice daily

Administration

Oral Do not crush sustained release drug product.

Nursing Actions

Physical Assessment Do not discontinue abruptly if patient using chronically; taper dosage slowly.

Patient Education
• Discuss specific use of drug and side effects with patient as it relates to treatment. (HCAHPS: During this hospital stay, were you given any medicine that you had not taken before? Before giving you any new medicine, how often did hospital staff tell you what the medicine was for? How often did hospital staff describe possible side effects in a way you could understand?)
• Patient may experience presyncope, fatigue, blurred vision, illogical thinking, dizziness, or nausea. Have patient report immediately to prescriber rash (HCAHPS).
• Educate patient about signs of a significant reaction (eg, wheezing; chest tightness; fever; itching; bad cough; blue skin color; seizures; or swelling of face, lips, tongue, or throat). **Note:** This is not a comprehensive list of all side effects. Patient should consult prescriber for additional questions.

Intended Use and Disclaimer: Should not be printed and given to patients. This information is intended to serve as a concise initial reference for healthcare professionals to use when discussing medications with a patient. You must ultimately rely on your own discretion, experience and judgment in diagnosing, treating and advising patients.

Related Information

Oral Medications That Should Not Be Crushed or Altered *on page 1712*

Oseltamivir (oh sel TAM i vir)

Brand Names: U.S. Tamiflu
Pharmacologic Category Antiviral Agent; Neuraminidase Inhibitor

Medication Safety Issues

Sound-alike/look-alike issues:
Tamiflu may be confused with Tambocor, Thera-Flu

Other safety concerns:
Oseltamivir (Tamiflu) oral suspension is available in a 6 mg/mL concentration and is packaged with an oral syringe calibrated in **milliliters** up to a total of 10 mL. **Instructions to the patient should be provided based on these units of measure (ie, mL). When providing oseltamivir suspension for children <1 year of age, use a lower calibrated (ie, <10 mL) oral syringe to ensure accurate dosing.**

When commercially-prepared oseltamivir oral suspension is not available, an extemporaneously prepared suspension may be compounded to provide a 6 mg/mL concentration.

Pregnancy Risk Factor C

Lactation Enters breast milk/not recommended

Breast-Feeding Considerations Small amounts of oseltamivir and oseltamivir carboxylate have been detected in breast milk. Breast-feeding is not recommended by the manufacturer. According to the CDC, breast-feeding while taking oseltamivir can be continued. The CDC recommends that women infected with the influenza virus follow general precautions (eg, frequent hand washing) to decrease viral transmission to the child. Mothers with influenza-like illnesses at delivery should consider avoiding close contact with the infant until they have received 48 hours of antiviral medication, fever has resolved, and cough and secretions can be controlled. These measures may help decrease (but not eliminate) the risk of transmitting influenza to the newborn. During this time, breast milk can be expressed and bottle-fed to the infant by another person who is well. Protective measures, such as wearing a face mask, changing into a clean gown or clothing, and strict hand hygiene should be continued by the mother for ≥7 days after the onset of symptoms or until symptom-free for 24 hours. Infant care should be performed by a non-infected person when possible (consult current CDC guidelines). Influenza may cause serious illness in postpartum women and prompt evaluation for febrile respiratory illnesses is recommended.

Use

Prophylaxis of influenza: Prophylaxis of influenza (A or B) infection in children ≥1 year of age and adults.

Treatment of influenza: Treatment of uncomplicated acute illness due to influenza (A or B) infection in children ≥2 weeks of age and adults who have been symptomatic for no more than 2 days.

The Advisory Committee on Immunization Practices (ACIP) recommends that **treatment** be considered for the following:

- Persons with severe, complicated or progressive illness
- Hospitalized persons
- Persons at higher risk for influenza complications:
  - Children <2 years of age (highest risk in children <6 months of age)
  - Adults ≥65 years of age
  - Persons with chronic disorders of the pulmonary (including asthma) or cardiovascular systems (except hypertension)
  - Persons with chronic metabolic diseases (including diabetes mellitus), hepatic disease, renal dysfunction, hematologic disorders (including sickle cell disease), or immunosuppression (including immunosuppression caused by medications or HIV)
  - Persons with neurologic/neuromuscular conditions (including conditions such as spinal cord injuries, seizure disorders, cerebral palsy, stroke, mental retardation, moderate to severe developmental delay, or muscular dystrophy) which may compromise respiratory function, the handling of respiratory secretions, or that can increase the risk of aspiration
  - Pregnant or postpartum women (≤2 weeks after delivery)
  - Persons <19 years of age on long-term aspirin therapy
  - American Indians and Alaskan Natives
  - Persons who are morbidly obese (BMI ≥40)
  - Residents of nursing homes or other chronic care facilities
- Use may also be considered for previously healthy, nonhigh-risk outpatients with confirmed or suspected influenza based on clinical judgment when treatment can be started within 48 hours of illness onset.

The ACIP recommends that **prophylaxis** be considered for the following:

- Postexposure prophylaxis may be considered for family or close contacts of suspected or confirmed cases, who are at higher risk of influenza complications, and who have not been vaccinated against the circulating strain at the time of the exposure.
- Postexposure prophylaxis may be considered for unvaccinated healthcare workers who had occupational exposure without protective equipment.
- Pre-exposure prophylaxis should only be used for persons at very high risk of influenza complications who cannot be otherwise protected at times of high risk for exposure.
- Prophylaxis should also be administered to all eligible residents of institutions that house patients at high risk when needed to control outbreaks.

The ACIP recommends that treatment and prophylaxis be given to children <1 year of age when indicated.

Mechanism of Action/Effect Thought to inhibit influenza virus by altering virus particle aggregation and release

Contraindications Hypersensitivity to oseltamivir or any component of the formulation

Warnings/Precautions Oseltamivir is not a substitute for the influenza virus vaccine. It has not been shown to prevent primary or concomitant bacterial infections that may occur with influenza virus. Use caution with renal impairment; dosage adjustment is required for creatinine clearance <30 mL/minute. Safety and efficacy for use in patients with chronic cardiac and/or kidney disease, severe hepatic impairment, or for treatment or prophylaxis in immunocompromised patients have not been established. Rare but severe hypersensitivity reactions, including anaphylaxis and severe dermatologic reactions (eg, Stevens-Johnson syndrome, erythema multiforme), have been associated with use. Discontinue use immediately if hypersensitivity occurs or is suspected and treat appropriately. Rare occurrences of neuropsychiatric events (including confusion, delirium, hallucinations, and/or self-injury) have been reported from postmarketing surveillance (primarily in pediatric patients); direct causation is difficult to establish (influenza infection may also be associated with behavioral and neurologic changes). Monitor closely for signs of any unusual behavior.

Antiviral treatment should begin within 48 hours of symptom onset. However, the CDC recommends that treatment may still be beneficial and should be started in hospitalized patients with severe, complicated or progressive illness if >48 hours. Treatment should not be delayed while awaiting results of laboratory tests for influenza. Nonhospitalized persons who are not at high risk for developing severe or complicated illness and who have a mild disease are not likely to benefit if treatment is started >48 hours after symptom onset. Nonhospitalized persons who are already beginning to recover do not need treatment. Oral suspension contains sorbitol (delivers ~2 g sorbitol per 75 mg dose); use with caution in patients with hereditary fructose intolerance.

Drug Interactions

Avoid Concomitant Use There are no known interactions where it is recommended to avoid concomitant use.

Decreased Effect

Oseltamivir may decrease the levels/effects of: Influenza Virus Vaccine (Live/Attenuated)

Increased Effect/Toxicity

The levels/effects of Oseltamivir may be increased by: Probenecid

Adverse Reactions

>10%: Gastrointestinal: Vomiting (2% to 15%)

1% to 10%:

Gastrointestinal: Nausea (4% to 10%), abdominal pain (2% to 5%), diarrhea (1% to 3%)

Ocular: Conjunctivitis (1%)

Respiratory: Epistaxis (1%)

Available Dosage Forms

Capsule, Oral:

Tamiflu: 30 mg, 45 mg, 75 mg

Suspension Reconstituted, Oral:

Tamiflu: 6 mg/mL (60 mL)

General Dosage Range Dosage adjustment recommended in patients with renal impairment

Oral:

Infants ≥2 weeks: 3 mg/kg/dose twice daily

Children 1-12 years and ≤15 kg: 30 mg once or twice daily

Children 1-12 years and >15 to ≤23 kg: 45 mg once or twice daily

Children 1-12 years and >23 to ≤40 kg: 60 mg once or twice daily

Children 1-12 years and >40 kg, Adolescents, and Adults: 75 mg once or twice daily

Administration

Oral May be administered without regard to meals; take with food to improve tolerance. Capsules may be opened and mixed with sweetened liquid (eg, chocolate syrup, corn syrup, caramel topping, light brown sugar dissolved in water). Administer oral suspension using the supplied oral syringe (exception: for children <1 year, a smaller volume [ie, <10 mL] oral syringe should be used in place of the supplied oral syringe to ensure accurate dosing); shake well before each use. If oral suspension is not available and/or appropriate strength of capsules are not available to mix with sweetened liquids, an extemporaneous preparation may be prepared.

Other Mechanically ventilated critically ill patients: May administer via naso- or orogastric (NG/OG) tube. For a 150 mg dose, dissolve powder from two 75 mg capsules in 20 mL of sterile water and inject down the NG/OG tube; follow with a 10 mL sterile water flush (Taylor, 2008).

Preparation for Administration Oral suspension: Reconstitute with 55 mL of water to a final concentration of 6 mg/mL (to make 60 mL total suspension).

Storage/Stability

Capsules: Store at 25°C (77°F); excursions permitted to 15°C to 30°C (59°F to 86°F).

Oral suspension: Store powder for suspension at 25°C (77°F); excursions permitted to 15°C to 30°C (59°F to 86°F). Once reconstituted, store suspension under refrigeration at 2°C to 8°C (36°F to 46°F) or at room temperature; do not freeze. Use within 10 days of preparation if stored at room temperature or within 17 days of preparation if stored under refrigeration.

Nursing Actions

Physical Assessment Assess effectiveness of therapy as there can be resistance. Children <1 year old require a specific dosing device as the one that comes with the medicine may not be accurate with small doses. Be sure to educate caregivers about this.

Monitor for nausea and vomiting or neuropsychiatric events (these may rarely occur). Severe allergic reactions are not common but can occur.

Patient Education

- Discuss specific use of drug and side effects with patient as it relates to treatment. (HCAHPS: During this hospital stay, were you given any medicine that you had not taken before? Before giving you any new medicine, how often did hospital staff tell you what the medicine was for? How often did hospital staff describe possible side effects in a way you could understand?)
- Patient may experience dizziness, dyspepsia, nausea, diarrhea, headache, or fatigue. Have patient report immediately to prescriber illogical thinking, behavioral problems, or rash (HCAHPS).
- Educate patient about signs of a significant reaction (eg, wheezing; chest tightness; fever; itching; bad cough; blue skin color; seizures; or swelling of face, lips, tongue, or throat). **Note:** This is not a comprehensive list of all side effects. Patient should consult prescriber for additional questions.

Intended Use and Disclaimer: Should not be printed and given to patients. This information is intended to serve as a concise initial reference for healthcare professionals to use when discussing medications with a patient. You must ultimately rely on your own discretion, experience and judgment in diagnosing, treating and advising patients.

Dietary Considerations Take without regard to meals; take with food to improve tolerance.

Ospemifene (os PEM i feen)

Brand Names: U.S. Osphena

Index Terms FC1271a

Pharmacologic Category Selective Estrogen Receptor Modulator (SERM)

Medication Safety Issues
Sound-alike/look-alike issues:
Ospemifene may be confused with raloxifene, toremifene

Pregnancy Risk Factor X

Lactation Excretion in breast milk unknown

Breast-Feeding Considerations It is not known if ospemifene is excreted into breast milk.

Use Treatment of moderate-to-severe dyspareunia due to vulvar and vaginal atrophy (VVA) of menopause

Mechanism of Action/Effect Ospemifene improves vaginal changes associated with the decrease in natural estrogen production associated with menopause and significantly decreases vaginal dryness and pain associated with sexual activity.

Contraindications Undiagnosed abnormal vaginal bleeding; DVT or PE (current or history of); active or history of arterial thromboembolic disease (eg, stroke, MI); estrogen-dependent tumor (known or suspected); women who are or may become pregnant

Warnings/Precautions [U.S. Boxed Warning]: The use of unopposed estrogen in women with an intact uterus is associated with an increased risk of endometrial cancer. The addition of a progestin to estrogen therapy may decrease the risk of endometrial hyperplasia, a precursor to endometrial cancer. Adequate diagnostic measures, including endometrial sampling if indicated, should be performed to rule out malignancy in postmenopausal women with undiagnosed abnormal vaginal bleeding. Ospemifene is an estrogen agonist/antagonist with agonistic effects on the endometrium. For women with an intact uterus using an estrogen without a progestin, the risk of endometrial cancer is dependent upon dose and duration of therapy. Endometrial cancer was not reported in clinical studies of ospemifene (duration ≤52 weeks) and the use of progestins was not evaluated. Ospemifene was not studied in women with breast cancer. Use is not currently recommended in women with carcinoma of the breast (known, suspected or history of) and use is contraindicated with an estrogen-dependent tumor.

[U.S. Boxed Warning]: Using data from the Women's Health Initiative (WHI) studies, an increased risk of deep vein thrombosis (DVT) and stroke has been reported with oral conjugated estrogens. The following were reported with ospemifene in clinical trials lasting ≤15 months duration: thromboembolic stroke 0.72/1000 women (placebo 1.04/1000 women); hemorrhagic stroke 1.45/1000 women (placebo 0/1000 women); DVT 1.45/1000 women (placebo 1.04/1000 women). Risk factors for cardiovascular disorders, arterial vascular disorders and /or venous thromboembolism (VTE) should be

managed appropriately. Risk factors include diabetes mellitus, hypercholesterolemia, hypertension, SLE, obesity, tobacco use, and/or history of VTE. Discontinue immediately if a VTE, thromboembolic or hemorrhagic stroke occur or are suspected.

[U.S. Boxed Warning]: Ospemifene should be used for the shortest duration possible consistent with treatment goals and risks for the individual woman.

Ospemifene has not been studied in patients with severe hepatic impairment; use is not recommended. Potentially significant interactions may exist, requiring dose or frequency adjustment, additional monitoring, and/or selection of alternative therapy. Consult drug interactions database for more detailed information. Whenever possible, discontinue at least 4-6 weeks prior to elective surgery associated with an increased risk of thromboembolism or during periods of prolonged immobilization.

Hazardous agent: Use appropriate precautions for handling and disposal (meets NIOSH, 2012 criteria).

Drug Interactions
Avoid Concomitant Use
Avoid concomitant use of Ospemifene with any of the following: Estrogen Derivatives; Fluconazole; Pimozide; Selective Estrogen Receptor Modulators

Decreased Effect
The levels/effects of Ospemifene may be decreased by: Bosentan; CYP2C9 Inducers (Strong); CYP3A4 Inducers (Strong); Dabrafenib; Deferasirox; Estrogen Derivatives; Herbs (CYP3A4 Inducers); Mitotane; Peginterferon Alfa-2b; Selective Estrogen Receptor Modulators; Tocilizumab

Increased Effect/Toxicity
Ospemifene may increase the levels/effects of: ARIPiprazole; Dofetilide; Lomitapide; Pimozide

The levels/effects of Ospemifene may be increased by: CYP2C9 Inhibitors (Strong); CYP3A4 Inhibitors (Strong); Estrogen Derivatives; Fluconazole; Selective Estrogen Receptor Modulators

Adverse Reactions 1% to 10%:
Dermatologic: Hyperhidrosis (2%)
Endocrine & metabolic: Hot flashes (8%)
Genitourinary: Vaginal discharge (4%), genital discharge (1%)
Neuromuscular & skeletal: Muscle spasm (3%)

Pharmacodynamics/Kinetics
Onset of Action A significant decrease in vaginal dryness and dyspareunia were observed after 12 weeks of therapy (Bachmann, 2010).

Available Dosage Forms
Tablet, Oral:
Osphena: 60 mg

General Dosage Range Oral: *Adults (postmenopausal females):* 60 mg once daily

Administration

Oral Administer with food.

Hazardous agent: Use appropriate precautions for handling and disposal (meets NIOSH, 2012 criteria).

Storage/Stability Store at controlled room temperature of 20°C to 25°C (68°F to 77°F); excursions permitted to 15°C to 30°C (59°F to 86°F).

Nursing Actions

Physical Assessment Assess efficacy of treatment. Assess for signs of a stroke: Facial or arm drooping and slurred speech; unilateral weakness. Assess for signs of DVT: Pain, tenderness in calf, redness, difficulty with ambulation. Monitor for signs of PE or cardiac event: Sudden onset of shortness of breath and chest pain. Educate patient about need to stop therapy prior to surgery or at times of immobility to reduce risk of blood clots.

Patient Education

- Discuss specific use of drug and side effects with patient as it relates to treatment. (HCAHPS: During this hospital stay, were you given any medicine that you had not taken before? Before giving you any new medicine, how often did hospital staff tell you what the medicine was for? How often did hospital staff describe possible side effects in a way you could understand?)
- Patient may experience hot flashes, vaginal discharge, fasciculations, or hyperhidrosis. Have patient report immediately to prescriber angina, dyspnea, strength differences from one side to another, significant asthenia, severe headache, edema, or considerable vaginal bleeding (HCAHPS).
- Educate patient about signs of a significant reaction (eg, wheezing; chest tightness; fever; itching; bad cough; blue skin color; seizures; or swelling of face, lips, tongue, or throat). **Note:** This is not a comprehensive list of all side effects. Patient should consult prescriber for additional questions.

Intended Use and Disclaimer: Should not be printed and given to patients. This information is intended to serve as a concise initial reference for healthcare professionals to use when discussing medications with a patient. You must ultimately rely on your own discretion, experience and judgment in diagnosing, treating and advising patients.

Oxaliplatin (ox AL i pla tin)

Brand Names: U.S. Eloxatin

Index Terms Diaminocyclohexane Oxalatoplatinum; L-OHP; Oxalatoplatin; Oxalatoplatinum

Pharmacologic Category Antineoplastic Agent, Alkylating Agent; Antineoplastic Agent, Platinum Analog

Medication Safety Issues

Sound-alike/look-alike issues:

Oxaliplatin may be confused with Aloxi®, carboplatin, cisplatin

High alert medication:

This medication is in a class the Institute for Safe Medication Practices (ISMP) includes among its list of drug classes which have a heightened risk of causing significant patient harm when used in error.

Pregnancy Risk Factor D

Lactation Excretion in breast milk unknown/not recommended

Breast-Feeding Considerations It is not known if oxaliplatin is excreted in breast milk. Due to the potential for serious adverse reactions in the nursing infant, the decision to discontinue breast-feeding or to discontinue oxaliplatin should take into account the benefits of treatment to the mother.

Use Treatment of stage III colon cancer (adjuvant) after complete resection of primary tumor; treatment of advanced colorectal cancer

Unlabeled Use Treatment of esophageal cancer, gastric cancer, hepatobiliary cancer (advanced), non-Hodgkin's lymphoma (refractory), ovarian cancer (advanced, platinum-pretreated), pancreatic cancer (advanced), testicular cancer (refractory)

Mechanism of Action/Effect Oxaliplatin, a platinum derivative, is an alkylating agent. Following intracellular hydrolysis, the platinum compound binds to DNA forming cross-links which inhibit DNA replication and transcription, resulting in cell death. Cytotoxicity is cell-cycle nonspecific.

Contraindications Hypersensitivity to oxaliplatin, other platinum-containing compounds, or any component of the formulation

Canadian labeling: Additional contraindications (not in U.S. labeling): Pregnancy, breast-feeding; severe renal impairment (CrCl <30 mL/minute)

Warnings/Precautions Hazardous agent - use appropriate precautions for handling and disposal (NIOSH, 2012). **[U.S. Boxed Warning]: Anaphylactic/anaphylactoid reactions have been reported with oxaliplatin (may occur within minutes of administration); symptoms may be managed with epinephrine, corticosteroids, antihistamines,** and discontinuation; oxygen and bronchodilators have also been used (Kim, 2009). Grade 3 or 4 hypersensitivity has been observed. Allergic reactions are similar to reactions reported with other platinum analogs, and may occur with any cycle. Reactions typically occur after multiple cycles; in retrospective reviews, reaction occurred at a median of 7-9 cycles, with an onset of 5-70 minutes (Kim, 2009; Polyzos, 2009). Symptoms may include bronchospasm (rare), erythema, hypotension (rare), pruritus, rash, and/or urticaria;

previously-untreated patients have also experienced flushing, diaphoresis, diarrhea, shortness of breath, chest pain, hypotension, syncope, and disorientation. According to the manufacturer, rechallenge is contraindicated (deaths due to anaphylaxis have been associated with platinum derivatives). In patients rechallenged after mild hypersensitivity, reaction recurred at a higher level of severity; for patients with severe hypersensitivity, rechallenge (with 2-3 days of antihistamine and corticosteroid premedication, and prolongation of infusion time) allowed for 2-4 additional oxaliplatin cycles; however, rechallenge was not feasible in nearly two-thirds of patients due to the severity of the initial reaction (Polyzos, 2009).

Two different types of peripheral sensory neuropathy may occur: First, an acute (within hours to 1-2 days), reversible (resolves within 14 days), with primarily peripheral symptoms that are often exacerbated by cold (may include pharyngolaryngeal dysesthesia); commonly recur with subsequent doses; avoid mucositis prophylaxis with ice chips during oxaliplatin infusion. Secondly, a more persistent (>14 days) presentation that often interferes with daily activities (eg, writing, buttoning, swallowing), these symptoms may improve in some patients upon discontinuing treatment. In a retrospective evaluation of patients treated with oxaliplatin for colorectal cancer, the incidence of peripheral sensory neuropathy was similar between diabetic and nondiabetic patients (Ramanathan, 2010). Several retrospective studies (as well as a small, underpowered randomized trial) have suggested calcium and magnesium infusions before and after oxaliplatin administration may reduce incidence of cumulative sensory neuropathy; however, a recent abstract of an ongoing randomized, placebo-controlled, double-blind study in patients with colorectal cancer suggests there is no benefit of calcium and magnesium in preventing sensory neuropathy or in decreasing oxaliplatin discontinuation rates (Loprinzi, 2013).

Oxaliplatin is associated with a moderate emetic potential; antiemetics are recommended to prevent nausea and vomiting. Cases of reversible posterior leukoencephalopathy syndrome (RPLS) have been reported. Signs/symptoms include headache, mental status changes, seizure, blurred vision, blindness and/or other vision changes; may be associated with hypertension; diagnosis is confirmed with brain imaging. May cause pulmonary fibrosis; withhold treatment for unexplained pulmonary symptoms (eg, crackles, dyspnea, nonproductive cough, pulmonary infiltrates) until interstitial lung disease or pulmonary fibrosis are excluded. Hepatotoxicity (including rare cases of hepatitis and hepatic failure) has been reported. Liver biopsy has revealed peliosis, nodular regenerative hyperplasia, sinusoidal alterations, perisinusoidal fibrosis, and veno-occlusive lesions; the presence of hepatic vascular disorders (including veno-occlusive disease) should be considered, especially in individuals developing portal hypertension or who present with increased liver function tests. Use caution with renal dysfunction; increased toxicity may occur; reduce initial dose in severe impairment. Potentially significant drug-drug interactions may exist, requiring dose or frequency adjustment, additional monitoring, and/or selection of alternative therapy. Elderly patients are more sensitive to some adverse events including diarrhea, dehydration, hypokalemia, leukopenia, fatigue and syncope. Oxaliplatin is an irritant with vesicant-like properties; ensure proper needle or catheter placement prior to and during infusion; avoid extravasation.

Drug Interactions
Avoid Concomitant Use
Avoid concomitant use of Oxaliplatin with any of the following: BCG; CloZAPine; Natalizumab; Pimecrolimus; Tacrolimus (Topical); Tofacitinib; Vaccines (Live)
Decreased Effect
Oxaliplatin may decrease the levels/effects of: BCG; Cardiac Glycosides; Coccidioidin Skin Test; Fosphenytoin-Phenytoin; Sipuleucel-T; Vaccines (Inactivated); Vaccines (Live); Vitamin K Antagonists

The levels/effects of Oxaliplatin may be decreased by: Echinacea
Increased Effect/Toxicity
Oxaliplatin may increase the levels/effects of: CloZAPine; Leflunomide; Natalizumab; Taxane Derivatives; Tofacitinib; Topotecan; Vaccines (Live); Vitamin K Antagonists

The levels/effects of Oxaliplatin may be increased by: Denosumab; Pimecrolimus; Roflumilast; Tacrolimus (Topical); Trastuzumab
Adverse Reactions Percentages reported with monotherapy.
>10%:
Central nervous system: Peripheral neuropathy (may be dose limiting; 76% to 92%; acute 65%; grades 3/4: 5%; persistent 43%; grades 3/4: 3%), fatigue (61%), pain (14%), headache (13%), insomnia (11%)
Gastrointestinal: Nausea (64%), diarrhea (46%), vomiting (37%), abdominal pain (31%), constipation (31%), anorexia (20%), stomatitis (14%)
Hematologic & oncologic: Anemia (64%; grades 3/4: 1%), thrombocytopenia (30%; grades 3/4: 3%), leukopenia (13%)
Hepatic: Increased serum AST (54%; grades 3/4: 4%), increased serum ALT (36%; grades 3/4: 1%), increased serum bilirubin (13%; grades 3/4: 5%)
Neuromuscular & skeletal: Back pain (11%)
Respiratory: Dyspnea (13%), cough (11%)
Miscellaneous: Fever (25%)

1% to 10%:

Cardiovascular: Edema (10%), chest pain (5%), peripheral edema (5%), flushing (3%), thromboembolism (2%)

Central nervous system: Rigors (9%), dizziness (7%)

Dermatologic: Skin rash (5%), alopecia (3%), palmar-plantar erythrodysesthesia (1%)

Endocrine & metabolic: Dehydration (5%), hypokalemia (3%)

Gastrointestinal: Dyspepsia (7%), dysgeusia (5%), flatulence (3%), hiccups (2%), mucositis (2%), gastroesophageal reflux disease (1%), dysphagia (acute 1% to 2%)

Genitourinary: Dysuria (1%)

Hematologic & oncologic: Neutropenia (7%)

Hypersensitivity: Hypersensitivity reaction (3%; includes urticaria, pruritus, facial flushing, shortness of breath, bronchospasm, diaphoresis, hypotension, syncope: grades 3/4: 2% to 3%)

Local: Injection site reaction (9%; redness/swelling/pain)

Neuromuscular & skeletal: Arthralgia (7%)

Ocular: Abnormal lacrimation (1%)

Renal: Increased serum creatinine (5% to 10%)

Respiratory: Upper respiratory tract infection (7%), rhinitis (6%), epistaxis (2%), pharyngitis (2%), pharyngolaryngeal dysesthesia (grades 3/4: 1% to 2%)

Available Dosage Forms

Solution, Intravenous [preservative free]:

Eloxatin: 50 mg/10 mL (10 mL); 100 mg/20 mL (20 mL); 200 mg/40 mL (40 mL)

Generic: 50 mg/10 mL (10 mL); 100 mg/20 mL (20 mL)

Solution Reconstituted, Intravenous [preservative free]:

Generic: 50 mg (1 ea); 100 mg (1 ea)

General Dosage Range Dosage adjustment recommended in patients with renal impairment or who develop toxicities

I.V.: *Adults:* 85 mg/m^2 every 2 weeks

Administration

I.V. Administer as I.V. infusion over 2 hours; extend infusion time to 6 hours for acute toxicities. Flush infusion line with D$_5$W prior to administration of any concomitant medication. Patients should receive an antiemetic premedication regimen. Avoid mucositis prophylaxis with ice chips during oxaliplatin infusion (may exacerbate acute neurological symptoms). Do not use needles or administration sets containing aluminum.

Oxaliplatin is associated with a moderate emetic potential; antiemetics are recommended to prevent nausea and vomiting.

Irritant with vesicant-like properties; ensure proper needle or catheter placement prior to and during infusion. Avoid extravasation; monitor I.V. site for redness, swelling, or pain.

Extravasation management: If extravasation occurs, stop infusion immediately and disconnect (leave cannula/needle in place); gently aspirate extravasated solution (do **NOT** flush the line); remove needle/cannula; elevate extremity. Information conflicts regarding use of warm or cold compresses. Cold compresses could potentially precipitate or exacerbate peripheral neuropathy (de Lemos, 2005).

Hazardous agent; use appropriate precautions for handling and disposal (NIOSH, 2012).

Preparation for Administration

Hazardous agent; use appropriate precautions for handling and disposal (NIOSH, 2012).

Do not prepare using a chloride-containing solution such as NaCl due to rapid conversion to monochloroplatinum, dichloroplatinum, and diaquoplatinum; all highly reactive in sodium chloride (Takimoto, 2007). Do not use needles or administration sets containing aluminum during preparation.

Aqueous solution: Dilution with D$_5$W (250 or 500 mL) is required prior to administration.

Lyophilized powder: Use only SWFI or D$_5$W to reconstitute powder. To obtain final concentration of 5 mg/mL add 10 mL of diluent to 50 mg vial or 20 mL diluent to 100 mg vial. Gently swirl vial to dissolve powder. Dilution with D$_5$W (250 or 500 mL) is required prior to administration. Discard unused portion of vial.

Storage/Stability Store intact vials at room temperature of 25°C (77°F); excursions permitted to 15°C to 30°C (59°F to 86°F); do not freeze. Protect concentrated solution from light (store in original outer carton). According to the manufacturer, solutions diluted for infusion are stable up to 6 hours at room temperature of 20°C to 25°C (68°F to 77°F) or up to 24 hours under refrigeration at 2°C to 8°C (36°F to 46°F). Oxaliplatin solution diluted with D$_5$W to a final concentration of 0.7 mg/mL (polyolefin container) has been shown to retain >90% of the original concentration for up to 30 days when stored at room temperature or refrigerated; artificial light did not affect the concentration (Andre, 2007). As this study did not examine sterility, refrigeration would be preferred to limit microbial growth. Solutions diluted for infusion do not require protection from light.

Nursing Actions

Physical Assessment Patient must be observed closely for anaphylactic-like reactions (can occur within minutes of administration; appropriate medications for the treatment of hypersensitivity reactions should be available). Monitor for pulmonary and hepatic toxicity, neuropathy (acute or persistent), GI disturbance, anemia, chest pain, and thromboembolism during and between each infusion.

▶

Patient Education

- Discuss specific use of drug and side effects with patient as it relates to treatment. (HCAHPS: During this hospital stay, were you given any medicine that you had not taken before? Before giving you any new medicine, how often did hospital staff tell you what the medicine was for? How often did hospital staff describe possible side effects in a way you could understand?)
- Patient may experience paresthesia, dysphagia, nausea, diarrhea, headache, stomatitis, constipation, dyspepsia, anemia, leukopenia, thrombocytopenia, asthenia, or hypertension. Have patient report immediately to prescriber signs of infection, dyspnea, abnormal gait, dizziness or syncope, illogical thinking, sudden vision changes, ecchymosis, discolored urine, jaundice, inability to eat, or rash (HCAHPS).
- Educate patient about signs of a significant reaction (eg, wheezing; chest tightness; fever; itching; bad cough; blue skin color; seizures; or swelling of face, lips, tongue, or throat). **Note:** This is not a comprehensive list of all side effects. Patient should consult prescriber for additional questions.

Intended Use and Disclaimer: Should not be printed and given to patients. This information is intended to serve as a concise initial reference for healthcare professionals to use when discussing medications with a patient. You must ultimately rely on your own discretion, experience and judgment in diagnosing, treating and advising patients.

Related Information

Management of Drug Extravasations *on page 1700*

Oxaprozin (oks a PROE zin)

Brand Names: U.S. Daypro

Pharmacologic Category Nonsteroidal Anti-inflammatory Drug (NSAID), Oral

Medication Safety Issues

Sound-alike/look-alike issues:

Oxaprozin may be confused with oxazepam

BEERS Criteria medication:

This drug may be potentially inappropriate for use in geriatric patients (Quality of evidence - moderate; Strength of recommendation - strong).

Medication Guide Available Yes

Pregnancy Risk Factor C

Lactation Excretion in breast milk unknown/not recommended

Use Management of signs and symptoms of osteoarthritis, rheumatoid arthritis, and juvenile idiopathic arthritis (JIA)

Available Dosage Forms

Tablet, Oral:

Daypro: 600 mg

Generic: 600 mg

General Dosage Range Dosage adjustment recommended in patients with renal impairment

Oral:

Children 6-16 years and 22-31 kg: 600 mg once daily

Children 6-16 years and 32-54 kg: 900 mg once daily

Children 6-16 years and ≥55 kg: 1200 mg once daily

Adults: 600-1800 mg once daily (maximum: 1200 mg daily [<50 kg]; 1800 mg daily or 26 mg/kg/day (whichever lower) [>50 kg])

Nursing Actions

Physical Assessment Monitor blood pressure at the beginning of therapy and periodically during use. Monitor for GI effects, hepatotoxicity, and ototoxicity at beginning of therapy and periodically throughout. Schedule ophthalmic evaluations for patients who develop eye complaints during long-term NSAID therapy.

Patient Education

- Discuss specific use of drug and side effects with patient as it relates to treatment. (HCAHPS: During this hospital stay, were you given any medicine that you had not taken before? Before giving you any new medicine, how often did hospital staff tell you what the medicine was for? How often did hospital staff describe possible side effects in a way you could understand?)
- Patient may experience headache, dyspepsia, pyrosis, nausea, constipation, or diarrhea. Have patient report immediately to prescriber angina, strength differences from one side to another, edema or pain of hands or feet, significant weight gain, melena, hematuria, ecchymosis, or rash (HCAHPS).
- Educate patient about signs of a significant reaction (eg, wheezing; chest tightness; fever; itching; bad cough; blue skin color; seizures; or swelling of face, lips, tongue, or throat). **Note:** This is not a comprehensive list of all side effects. Patient should consult prescriber for additional questions.

Intended Use and Disclaimer: Should not be printed and given to patients. This information is intended to serve as a concise initial reference for healthcare professionals to use when discussing medications with a patient. You must ultimately rely on your own discretion, experience and judgment in diagnosing, treating and advising patients.

Oxazepam (oks A ze pam)

Index Terms Serax

Pharmacologic Category Benzodiazepine

Medication Safety Issues

Sound-alike/look-alike issues:

Oxazepam may be confused with oxcarbazepine, oxaprozin, quazepam

Serax may be confused with Eurax®, Urex, Zyr-TEC®

BEERS Criteria medication:

This drug may be potentially inappropriate for use in geriatric patients (Quality of evidence - high; Strength of recommendation - strong).

International issues:

Murelax [Australia] may be confused with MiraLax brand name for polyethylene glycol 3350 [U.S.]

Use Management of anxiety disorders, including anxiety associated with depression; management of ethanol withdrawal

Controlled Substance C-IV

Available Dosage Forms

Capsule, Oral:

Generic: 10 mg, 15 mg, 30 mg

General Dosage Range Oral:

Children >12 years, Adolescents, and Adults: 10-30 mg 3-4 times daily

Elderly: Initial: 10 mg 3 times daily; Maintenance: 10-15 mg 3-4 times daily

Administration

Oral Administer orally in divided doses.

Nursing Actions

Physical Assessment Assess for history of addiction; long-term use can result in dependence, abuse, or tolerance; periodically evaluate need for continued use. For inpatient use, institute safety measures to prevent falls. Monitor for oversedation, dizziness, confusion, or ataxia which may impair physical and mental capabilities.

Patient Education

- Discuss specific use of drug and side effects with patient as it relates to treatment. (HCAHPS: During this hospital stay, were you given any medicine that you had not taken before? Before giving you any new medicine, how often did hospital staff tell you what the medicine was for? How often did hospital staff describe possible side effects in a way you could understand?)
- Patient may experience presyncope, fatigue, blurred vision, illogical thinking, xerostomia, or change in balance. Have patient report immediately to prescriber rash (HCAHPS)
- Educate patient about signs of a significant reaction (eg, wheezing; chest tightness; fever; itching; bad cough; blue skin color; seizures; or swelling of face, lips, tongue, or throat). **Note:** This is not a comprehensive list of all side effects. Patient should consult prescriber for additional questions.

Intended Use and Disclaimer: Should not be printed and given to patients. This information is intended to serve as a concise initial reference for healthcare professionals to use when discussing medications with a patient. You must ultimately rely on your own discretion, experience and judgment in diagnosing, treating and advising patients.

OXcarbazepine (ox car BAZ e peen)

Brand Names: U.S. Oxtellar XR; Trileptal

Index Terms GP 47680; OCBZ

Pharmacologic Category Anticonvulsant, Miscellaneous

Medication Safety Issues

Sound-alike/look-alike issues:

OXcarbazepine may be confused with carBAMazepine, oxazepam

Trileptal® may be confused with TriLipix®

Medication Guide Available Yes

Pregnancy Risk Factor C

Lactation Enters breast milk/not recommended

Breast-Feeding Considerations Oxcarbazepine and the active 10-hydroxy metabolite (MHD) are found in breast milk (small amounts). According to the manufacturer, the decision to continue or discontinue breast-feeding during therapy should take into account the risk of exposure to the infant and the benefits of treatment to the mother.

Use

Oxtellar XR™: Adjunctive therapy in the treatment of partial seizures in patients with epilepsy

Trileptal®: Monotherapy or adjunctive therapy in the treatment of partial seizures in patients with epilepsy

Unlabeled Use Bipolar disorder; treatment of neuropathic pain

Mechanism of Action/Effect Precise mechanism of action has not been determined. Believed to prevent the spread of seizures by decreasing propagation of synaptic impulses.

Contraindications Hypersensitivity to oxcarbazepine or any component of the formulation

Warnings/Precautions Hazardous agent - use appropriate precautions for handling and disposal (NIOSH, 2012). Antiepileptics are associated with an increased risk of suicidal behavior/thoughts with use (regardless of indication); patients should be monitored for signs/symptoms of depression, suicidal tendencies, and other unusual behavior changes during therapy and instructed to inform their healthcare provider immediately if symptoms occur.

Clinically-significant hyponatremia (serum sodium <125 mmol/L) may develop during oxcarbazepine use. Rare cases of anaphylaxis and angioedema have been reported, even after initial dosing; permanently discontinue should symptoms occur. Use caution in patients with previous hypersensitivity to carbamazepine (cross-sensitivity occurs in 25% to 30% of patients). Potentially serious, sometimes fatal, dermatologic reactions (eg, Stevens-Johnson, toxic epidermal necrolysis) and multiorgan hypersensitivity reactions have been reported in adults and children; monitor for signs and symptoms of skin reactions and possible disparate manifestations associated with lymphatic, hepatic, renal, and/or hematologic organ systems; discontinuation and conversion to alternate therapy may be required. As with all antiepileptic drugs, oxcarbazepine should be withdrawn gradually to minimize the potential of increased seizure frequency. Use of oxcarbazepine has been associated with CNS-related adverse events, most significant of these were cognitive symptoms including psychomotor slowing, difficulty with concentration, speech or language problems, somnolence or fatigue, and coordination abnormalities, including ataxia and gait disturbances. Effects with other sedative drugs or ethanol may be potentiated. Single-dose studies show that half-life of the primary active metabolite is prolonged three- to fourfold and AUC is doubled in patients with CrCl <30 mL/minute; dose adjustment required in these patients. May reduce the efficacy of oral contraceptives (nonhormonal contraceptive measures are recommended). Agranulocytosis, leukopenia, and pancytopenia have been reported with use (rare). Discontinuation and conversion to alternate therapy may be required.

Drug Interactions

Avoid Concomitant Use

Avoid concomitant use of OXcarbazepine with any of the following: Abiraterone Acetate; Apixaban; Artemether; Axitinib; Bedaquiline; Boceprevir; Bortezomib; Bosutinib; Cabozantinib; CloZAPine; Crizotinib; Dienogest; Dolutegravir; Dronedarone; Enzalutamide; Everolimus; Ibrutinib; Itraconazole; Ivacaftor; Lapatinib; Lumefantrine; Lurasidone; Macitentan; Mifepristone; NIFEdipine; Nilotinib; Nisoldipine; PAZOPanib; Pomalidomide; PONATinib; Praziquantel; Ranolazine; Regorafenib; Rilpivirine; Rivaroxaban; Roflumilast; RomiDEPsin; Selegiline; Simeprevir; Sofosbuvir; SORAfenib; Tasimelteon; Telaprevir; Ticagrelor; Tofacitinib; Tolvaptan; Toremifene; Ulipristal; Vandetanib; Vemurafenib; VinCRIStine (Liposomal)

Decreased Effect

OXcarbazepine may decrease the levels/effects of: Abiraterone Acetate; Apixaban; ARIPiprazole; Artemether; Axitinib; Bedaquiline; Boceprevir; Bortezomib; Bosutinib; Brentuximab Vedotin; Cabozantinib; Clarithromycin; CloZAPine; Cobicistat; Contraceptives (Estrogens); Contraceptives (Progestins); Crizotinib; CYP3A4 Substrates; Dasatinib; Dienogest; Dolutegravir; DOXOrubicin (Conventional); Dronedarone; Elvitegravir; Enzalutamide; Everolimus; Exemestane; Gefitinib; GuanFACINE; Ibrutinib; Imatinib; Itraconazole; Ivacaftor; Ixabepilone; Lapatinib; Linagliptin; Lumefantrine; Lurasidone; Macitentan; Maraviroc; Mifepristone; NIFEdipine; Nilotinib; Nisoldipine; PAZOPanib; Perampanel; Pomalidomide; PONATinib; Praziquantel; QUEtiapine; Ranolazine; Regorafenib; Rilpivirine; Rivaroxaban; Roflumilast; RomiDEPsin; Saxagliptin; Simeprevir; Sofosbuvir; SORAfenib; SUNItinib; Tadalafil; Tasimelteon; Telaprevir; Ticagrelor; Tofacitinib; Tolvaptan; Toremifene; Ulipristal; Vandetanib; Vemurafenib; Vilazodone; VinCRIStine (Liposomal); Vortioxetine; Zuclopenthixol

The levels/effects of OXcarbazepine may be decreased by: CarBAMazepine; Fosphenytoin-Phenytoin; Ketorolac (Nasal); Ketorolac (Systemic); Mefloquine; Orlistat; PHENobarbital; Valproic Acid and Derivatives

Increased Effect/Toxicity

OXcarbazepine may increase the levels/effects of: Clarithromycin; Fosphenytoin-Phenytoin; Ifosfamide; PHENobarbital; Selegiline

The levels/effects of OXcarbazepine may be increased by: Clarithromycin; Perampanel; Thiazide Diuretics

Nutritional/Ethanol Interactions

Ethanol: Avoid ethanol (may increase CNS depression).

Herb/Nutraceutical: St John's wort may decrease oxcarbazepine levels. Avoid evening primrose (seizure threshold decreased). Avoid valerian, St John's wort, kava kava, gotu kola.

Adverse Reactions Incidence in children was similar.

>10%:
Central nervous system: Dizziness (22% to 49%), drowsiness (20% to 36%), headache (13% to 32%), ataxia (1% to 31%), fatigue (12% to 15%), vertigo (6% to 15%)
Gastrointestinal: Vomiting (7% to 36%), nausea (15% to 29%), abdominal pain (10% to 13%)
Neuromuscular & skeletal: Abnormal gait (5% to 17%), tremor (3% to 16%)
Ophthalmic: Diplopia (14% to 40%), nystagmus (7% to 26%), visual disturbance (4% to 14%)
1% to 10%:
Cardiovascular: Hypotension (≤2%), lower extremity edema (1% to 2%)
Central nervous system: Nervousness (2% to 5%), amnesia (4%), abnormality in thinking (≤4%), insomnia (2% to 4%), fever (3%), dysmetria (1% to 3%), speech disorder (1% to 3%), feeling abnormal (≤2%), abnormal electroencephalogram (≤2%), agitation (1% to 2%), confusion (1% to 2%)
Dermatologic: Skin rash (4%), acne vulgaris (1% to 2%)
Endocrine & metabolic: Hyponatremia (1% to 3%)
Gastrointestinal: Diarrhea (5% to 7%), dyspepsia (5% to 6%), constipation (2% to 6%), dysgeusia (5%), xerostomia (3%), gastritis (1% to 2%), weight gain (1% to 2%)
Genitourinary: Urinary frequency (2%)
Neuromuscular & skeletal: Weakness (3% to 6%), back pain (4%), falling (4%), sprain (≤2%), myasthenia (1% to 2%)

Ophthalmic: Accommodation disturbance (≤2%)
Respiratory: Upper respiratory tract infection (7%), rhinitis (2% to 5%), pulmonary infection (4%), epistaxis (4%), sinusitis (4%)

Available Dosage Forms

Suspension, Oral:
Trileptal: 300 mg/5 mL (250 mL)
Generic: 300 mg/5 mL (250 mL)

Tablet, Oral:
Trileptal: 150 mg, 300 mg, 600 mg
Generic: 150 mg, 300 mg, 600 mg

Tablet Extended Release 24 Hour, Oral:
Oxtellar XR: 150 mg, 300 mg, 600 mg

General Dosage Range Dosage adjustment recommended in patients with renal impairment

Oral:
Children 2-3 years and <20 kg: Immediate release (Trileptal®): Initial: 8-20 mg/kg/day (maximum: 600 mg daily) in 2 divided doses; Maintenance: Maximum of 60 mg/kg/day in 2 divided doses

Children 2-3 years and ≥20 kg: Immediate release (Trileptal®): Initial: 8-10 mg/kg/day (maximum: 600 mg daily) in 2 divided doses; Maintenance: Maximum of 60 mg/kg/day in 2 divided doses

Children 4-16 years: Immediate release (Trileptal®): Initial: 8-10 mg/kg/day (maximum: 600 mg daily) in 2 divided doses; Maintenance: Dependent on patient weight and indication

Children 6-17 years and ≤29 kg: Extended release (Oxtellar XR™): Initial: 8-10 mg/kg once daily (maximum: 600 mg daily in the first week); Maintenance: Up to 900 mg once daily

Children 6-17 years and ≥29.1-39 kg: Extended release (Oxtellar XR™): Initial: 8-10 mg/kg once daily (maximum: 600 mg daily in the first week); Maintenance: Up to 1200 mg once daily

Children 6-17 years and >39 kg: Extended release (Oxtellar XR™): Initial: 8-10 mg/kg once daily (maximum: 600 mg daily in the first week); Maintenance: Up to 1800 mg once daily

Children >16 years and Adults: Immediate release (Trileptal®): Initial: 600 mg daily in 2 divided doses; Maintenance: 1200-2400 mg daily in 2 divided doses (maximum: 2400 mg daily)

Children >17 years and Adults: Extended release (Oxtellar XR™): Initial: 600 mg once daily; Maintenance: 1200-2400 mg once daily (maximum: 2400 mg daily)

Administration

Oral

Immediate release: Administer twice daily without regard to meals.
Suspension: Prior to using for the first time, firmly insert the plastic adapter provided with the bottle. Cover adapter with child-resistant cap when not in use. Shake bottle for at least 10 seconds, remove child-resistant cap, and insert the oral dosing syringe provided to withdraw appropriate dose. Dose may be taken directly from oral syringe or may be mixed in a small glass of water immediately prior to swallowing. Rinse syringe with warm water after use and allow to dry thoroughly. Discard any unused portion after 7 weeks of first opening bottle.

Extended release: Administer once daily on an empty stomach at least 1 hour before or 2 hours after food. Swallow whole; do not cut, crush, or chew the tablets.

Hazardous agent; use appropriate precautions for handling and disposal (NIOSH, 2012).

Storage/Stability Store tablets and suspension at 25°C (77°F); excursions permitted to 15°C to 30°C (59°F to 86°F). Use suspension within 7 weeks of first opening container.

Nursing Actions

Physical Assessment Obtain allergy history (cross-sensitivity to carbamazepine). Monitor effectiveness. Assess GI tolerance. Monitor for sedation, dizziness, CNS changes, mood or cognitive changes, visual changes, and skin reactions. Be alert for emergence of depression, including suicidal ideation. Dosage should be tapered when discontinuing to reduce risk of increased seizures. If being used to prevent seizures, teach patient safety and seizure precautions to caregivers/family in the event of a seizure.

Patient Education

- Discuss specific use of drug and side effects with patient as it relates to treatment. (HCAHPS: During this hospital stay, were you given any medicine that you had not taken before? Before giving you any new medicine, how often did hospital staff tell you what the medicine was for? How often did hospital staff describe possible side effects in a way you could understand?)

- Patient may experience presyncope, fatigue, blurred vision, illogical thinking, dizziness, imbalance, headache, or nausea. Have patient report immediately to prescriber depression, nervousness, emotional instability, anxiety, sudden vision changes, eye pain, eye irritation, severe asthenia, jaundice, ecchymosis, or bleeding (HCAHPS).

- Educate patient about signs of a significant reaction (eg, wheezing; chest tightness; fever; itching; bad cough; blue skin color; seizures; or swelling of face, lips, tongue, or throat). **Note:** This is not a comprehensive list of all side effects. Patient should consult prescriber for additional questions.

Intended Use and Disclaimer: Should not be printed and given to patients. This information is intended to serve as a concise initial reference for healthcare professionals to use when discussing medications with a patient. You must ultimately rely on your own discretion, experience and judgment in diagnosing, treating and advising patients.

Related Information
Oral Medications That Should Not Be Crushed or Altered *on page 1712*

Oxybutynin (oks i BYOO ti nin)

Brand Names: U.S. Ditropan XL; Gelnique; Oxytrol; Oxytrol For Women [OTC]

Index Terms Ditropan; Oxybutynin Chloride

Pharmacologic Category Antispasmodic Agent, Urinary

Medication Safety Issues

Sound-alike/look-alike issues:

Oxybutynin may be confused with OxyCONTIN

Ditropan may be confused with Detrol, diazepam, Diprivan, dithranol

BEERS Criteria medication:

This drug may be potentially inappropriate for use in geriatric patients (Quality of evidence - varies based on comorbidity; Strength of recommendation - varies based on comorbidity)

Other safety concerns:

Transdermal patch may contain conducting metal (eg, aluminum); remove patch prior to MRI.

Pregnancy Risk Factor B

Lactation Excretion in breast milk unknown/use caution

Breast-Feeding Considerations It is not known if oxybutynin is excreted into breast milk. The manufacturer recommends that caution be used if administered to a nursing woman. Suppression of lactation has been reported.

Use Treatment of symptoms associated with overactive uninhibited neurogenic or reflex neurogenic bladder (eg, urgency, frequency, leakage, urge incontinence, dysuria); treatment of symptoms associated with detrusor overactivity due to a neurological condition (eg, spina bifida) (extended release tablet only)

Mechanism of Action/Effect Direct antispasmodic effect on smooth muscle, also inhibits the action of acetylcholine on smooth muscle (exhibits $1/5$ the anticholinergic activity of atropine, but has 4-10 times the antispasmodic activity); does not block effects at skeletal muscle or at autonomic ganglia; increases bladder capacity, decreases uninhibited contractions, and delays desire to void, therefore, decreases urgency and frequency

Contraindications Hypersensitivity to oxybutynin or any component of the formulation; patients with or at risk for uncontrolled narrow-angle glaucoma, urinary retention, gastric retention or conditions with severely decreased GI motility

OTC labeling: When used for self-medication, do not use if you have pain or burning when urinating, blood in urine, unexplained lower back or side pain, cloudy or foul-smelling urine; in males; age <18 years; only experience accidental urine loss when cough, sneeze, or laugh; diagnosis of urinary or gastric retention; glaucoma; hypersensitivity to oxybutynin.

Warnings/Precautions Cases of angioedema involving the face, lips, tongue, and/or larynx have been reported with oral oxybutynin; some cases have occurred after a single dose. Discontinue immediately if tongue, hypopharynx, or larynx is involved; promptly initiate appropriate management. Use with caution in patients with bladder outflow obstruction (may increase the risk of urinary retention), treated angle-closure glaucoma (use is contraindicated in uncontrolled narrow-angle glaucoma), hyperthyroidism, coronary artery disease, heart failure, hypertension, cardiac arrhythmias, hepatic or renal impairment, prostatic hyperplasia (may cause urinary retention), hiatal hernia, myasthenia gravis, dementia. Use with caution in patients with decreased GI motility or gastrointestinal obstructive disorders (eg, ulcerative colitis, intestinal atony, pyloric stenosis); may increase the risk of gastric retention. In patients with ulcerative colitis, use may decrease gastric motility to the point of increasing the risk of paralytic ileus or toxic megacolon. Use with caution in patients with gastroesophageal reflux or with medications that may exacerbate esophagitis (eg, bisphosphonates). May increase the risk of heat prostration. Anticholinergics may cause agitation, confusion, drowsiness, dizziness, hallucinations, headache, and/or blurred vision, which may impair physical or mental abilities; patients must be cautioned about performing tasks which require mental alertness (eg, operating machinery or driving). Dose reduction or discontinuation should be considered if CNS effects occur.

Potentially significant drug-drug interactions may exist, requiring dose or frequency adjustment, additional monitoring, and/or selection of alternative therapy. This medication is associated with potent anticholinergic properties which may be inappropriate in older adults depending on comorbidities (eg, dementia, delirium) (Beers Criteria).

The extended release formulation consists of drug within a nondeformable matrix; following drug release/absorption, the matrix/shell is expelled in the stool. The use of nondeformable products in patients with known stricture/narrowing of the GI tract has been associated with symptoms of obstruction. Transdermal patch may contain conducting metal (eg, aluminum); remove patch prior to MRI. When using the topical gel, cover treatment area with clothing after gel has dried to minimize transferring medication to others. Discontinue gel if skin irritation occurs. Gel contains ethanol; do not expose to open flame or smoking until gel has dried.

When used for self-medication (OTC), other causes of frequent urination (UTI, diabetes, early pregnancy, other serious conditions) may need to be considered prior to use. Patients should contact a health care provider if symptoms do not improve within 2 weeks of initial use or for new or worsening symptoms.

Drug Interactions

Avoid Concomitant Use

Avoid concomitant use of Oxybutynin with any of the following: Aclidinium; Ipratropium (Oral Inhalation); Pimozide; Potassium Chloride; Tiotropium; Umeclidinium

Decreased Effect

Oxybutynin may decrease the levels/effects of: Acetylcholinesterase Inhibitors (Central); Secretin

The levels/effects of Oxybutynin may be decreased by: Acetylcholinesterase Inhibitors (Central)

Increased Effect/Toxicity

Oxybutynin may increase the levels/effects of: AbobotulinumtoxinA; Analgesics (Opioid); Anticholinergics; ARIPiprazole; Cannabinoids; Dofetilide; Lomitapide; Mirabegron; OnabotulinumtoxinA; Pimozide; Potassium Chloride; RimabotulinumtoxinB; Thiazide Diuretics; Tiotropium; Topiramate

The levels/effects of Oxybutynin may be increased by: Aclidinium; Ipratropium (Oral Inhalation); Pramlintide; Umeclidinium

Nutritional/Ethanol Interactions Ethanol: Use ethanol with caution (may increase CNS depression and toxicity). Watch for sedation.

Adverse Reactions

Oral:

>10%:

Central nervous system: Dizziness (4% to 17%), drowsiness (2% to 14%)

Gastrointestinal: Xerostomia (29% to 71%; dose related), constipation (7% to 15%), nausea (2% to 12%)

1% to 10%:

Cardiovascular: Cardiac arrhythmia (sinus; 1% to <5%), chest pain (1% to <5%), decreased blood pressure (1% to <5%), edema (1% to <5%), flushing (1% to <5%), hypertension (1% to <5%), palpitations (1% to <5%), peripheral edema (1% to <5%)

Central nervous system: Headache (6% to 10%), nervousness (1% to 7%), pain (1% to 7%), insomnia (1% to 6%), confusion (1% to <5%), depression (1% to <5%), fatigue (1% to <5%)

Dermatologic: Pruritus (1% to <5%), xeroderma (1% to <5%)

Endocrine & metabolic: Fluid retention (1% to <5%), hyperglycemia (1% to <5%)

Gastrointestinal: Diarrhea (1% to 9%), dyspepsia (5% to 7%), abdominal pain (1% to <5%), dry throat (1% to <5%), dysphagia (1% to <5%), eructation (1% to <5%), flatulence (1% to <5%), gastroesophageal reflux disease (1% to <5%), unpleasant taste (1% to <5%), vomiting (1% to <5%)

Genitourinary: Urinary hesitancy (1% to 9%), urinary tract infection (5% to 7%), urinary retention (1% to 6%), cystitis (1% to <5%), dysuria (1% to <5%), pollakiuria (1% to <5%)

Infection: Fungal infection (1% to <5%)

Neuromuscular & skeletal: Weakness (1% to 7%), arthralgia (1% to <5%), back pain (1% to <5%), flank pain (1% to <5%), limb pain (1% to <5%)

Ophthalmic: Blurred vision (1% to 10%), xerophthalmia (3% to 6%), eye irritation (1% to <5%), keratoconjunctivitis sicca (1% to <5%)

Respiratory: Asthma (1% to <5%), bronchitis (1% to <5%), cough (1% to <5%), dry throat (1% to <5%), hoarseness (1% to <5%), nasal congestion (1% to <5%), dry nose (1% to <5%), nasopharyngitis (1% to <5%), pharyngolaryngeal pain (1% to <5%), sinus congestion (1% to <5%), upper respiratory tract infection (1% to <5%)

Miscellaneous: Increased thirst (1% to <5%)

Topical gel:

>10%:

Gastrointestinal: Xerostomia (2% to 12%)

Local: Application site reaction (4% to 14%; includes erythema [4%], pruritus [3%], dermatitis [2%], anesthesia, irritation, pain, papules, rash [3%])

1% to 10%:

Central nervous system: Dizziness (2% to 3%), fatigue (2%), headache (2%)

Dermatologic: Pruritus (1%)

Gastrointestinal: Gastroenteritis (2%), constipation (1%)

Genitourinary: Urinary tract infection (5% to 7%)

Ophthalmic: Conjunctivitis (4%), blurred vision (<2%), xerophthalmia (<2%)

Respiratory: Nasopharyngitis (3% to 5%), upper respiratory tract infection (5%)

Transdermal:

>10%: Local: Pruritus (14% to 17%)

1% to 10%:

Gastrointestinal: Xerostomia (4% to 10%), constipation (3%), diarrhea (3%)

Genitourinary: Dysuria (2%)

Local: Erythema (6% to 8%), localized vesiculation (3%), macular eruption (3%), skin rash (3%)

Ophthalmic: Visual disturbance (3%)

Pharmacodynamics/Kinetics

Onset of Action Oral: Immediate release: 30-60 minutes; Peak effect: 3-6 hours

Duration of Action Oral: Immediate release: 6-10 hours; Extended release: Up to 24 hours

Available Dosage Forms

Gel, Transdermal:

Gelnique: 10% (1 g); 3% (92 g)

Patch Biweekly, Transdermal:

Oxytrol: 3.9 mg/24 hr (1 ea, 2 ea, 4 ea, 8 ea)

Oxytrol For Women [OTC]: 3.9 mg/24 hr (8 ea); 3.9 mg/24hr (4 ea)

Syrup, Oral:
Generic: 5 mg/5 mL (5 mL, 473 mL)
Tablet, Oral:
Generic: 5 mg
Tablet Extended Release 24 Hour, Oral:
Ditropan XL: 5 mg, 10 mg, 15 mg
Generic: 5 mg, 10 mg, 15 mg
General Dosage Range
Oral:
Extended release:
Children ≥6 years: 5 mg once daily (maximum: 20 mg daily)
Adults: Initial: 5-10 mg once daily; Maintenance: 5-30 mg once daily (maximum: 30 mg daily)
Immediate release:
Children ≥5 years: 5 mg 2-3 times daily (maximum: 15 mg daily)
Adults: 5 mg 2-4 times daily(maximum: 20 mg daily)
Elderly: 2.5 mg 2-3 times daily
Topical gel: *Adults:* Genlique 3%: Apply 3 pumps (84 mg) once daily; Genlique 10%: Apply contents of 1 sachet (100 mg/g) once daily
Transdermal: *Adults:* Apply one 3.9 mg/day patch twice weekly
Administration
Oral Administer without regard to meals. Extended release tablets must be swallowed whole with liquid; do not crush, divide, or chew; take at approximately the same time each day.

Topical Topical gel: For topical use only. Apply to clean, dry, intact skin on abdomen, thighs, or upper arms/shoulders. Wash hands after use. Cover treated area with clothing after gel has dried to prevent transfer of medication to others. Do not bathe, shower, or swim until 1 hour after gel applied. Do not apply to recently shaved skin.
Genlique 3%: Prior to initial use, press pump 4 times to prime pump; discard any gel dispensed from pump during priming. Rotate application sites to avoid skin irritation.
Genlique 10%: Rotate site; do not apply to same site on consecutive days.

Other Transdermal: Apply to clean, dry skin on abdomen, hip, or buttock. Select a new site for each new system (avoid reapplication to same site within 7 days). Wear patch under clothing; do not expose to sunlight.
Storage/Stability
Immediate release tablet and syrup: Store at 20°C to 25°C (68°F to 77°F). Protect from light.
Extended release tablet: Store at 25°C (77°F); excursions permitted to 15°C to 30°C (59°F to 86°F). Protect from moisture and humidity.
Topical gel (pump or sachets): Store at 25°C (77°F); excursions permitted to 15°C to 30°C (59°F to 86°F). Protect from moisture and humidity. Keep gel away from open flame. Do not store sachets outside the sealed pouch; apply immediately after removal from the protective pouch. Discard used sachets such that accidental application or ingestion by children, pets, or others is avoided.

Transdermal patch: Store at 20°C to 25°C (68°F to 77°F). Protect from moisture and humidity. Do not store outside the sealed pouch; apply immediately after removal from the protective pouch. Discard used patches such that accidental application or ingestion by children, pets, or others is avoided.
Nursing Actions
Physical Assessment Assess voiding pattern, incontinent episodes, frequency, urgency, distention, and urinary retention prior to beginning therapy and periodically throughout.
Patient Education
- Discuss specific use of drug and side effects with patient as it relates to treatment. (HCAHPS: During this hospital stay, were you given any medicine that you had not taken before? Before giving you any new medicine, how often did hospital staff tell you what the medicine was for? How often did hospital staff describe possible side effects in a way you could understand?)
- Patient may experience tablet shell in stool, presyncope, fatigue, blurred vision, illogical thinking, headache, nausea, constipation, xerostomia, or skin irritation. Have patient report immediately to prescriber nervousness and anxiety, severe flushing, or rash (HCAHPS).
- Educate patient about signs of a significant reaction (eg, wheezing; chest tightness; fever; itching; bad cough; blue skin color; seizures; or swelling of face, lips, tongue, or throat). **Note:** This is not a comprehensive list of all side effects. Patient should consult prescriber for additional questions.

Intended Use and Disclaimer: Should not be printed and given to patients. This information is intended to serve as a concise initial reference for healthcare professionals to use when discussing medications with a patient. You must ultimately rely on your own discretion, experience and judgment in diagnosing, treating and advising patients.

Dietary Considerations Food causes a slight delay in the absorption of the oral solution and bioavailability is increased by ~25%. Absorption of the extended release tablet is not affected by food. May be taken without regard to meals.
Related Information
Oral Medications That Should Not Be Crushed or Altered *on page 1712*

OxyCODONE (oks i KOE done)

Brand Names: U.S. Oxecta; OxyCONTIN; Roxicodone
Index Terms Dihydrohydroxycodeinone; Oxecta; Oxycodone Hydrochloride
Pharmacologic Category Analgesic, Opioid

Medication Safety Issues
Sound-alike/look-alike issues:

OxyCODONE may be confused with HYDRO-codone, OxyCONTIN, oxymorphone

OxyCONTIN may be confused with MS Contin, oxybutynin

OxyFast may be confused with Roxanol

Roxicodone may be confused with Roxanol

High alert medication:

The Institute for Safe Medication Practices (ISMP) includes this medication among its list of drug classes which have a heightened risk of causing significant patient harm when used in error.

Medication Guide Available Yes

Pregnancy Risk Factor B

Lactation Enters breast milk/not recommended

Breast-Feeding Considerations Oxycodone is excreted into breast milk. Breast-feeding is not recommended by the manufacturer. Sedation and/or respiratory depression may occur in the infant; symptoms of opioid withdrawal may occur following the cessation of breast-feeding. Nursing infants exposed to large doses of opioids should be monitored for apnea and sedation. Use caution in a woman who may be an ultrarapid metabolizer; oxycodone is a substrate for CYP2D6 and their nursing infants may be at higher risk for adverse events (Montgomery, 2012).

Use Management of moderate-to-severe pain, normally used in combination with nonopioid analgesics

OxyContin is indicated for around-the-clock management of moderate-to-severe pain when a continuous analgesic is needed for an extended period of time.

Mechanism of Action/Effect Binds to opiate receptors in the CNS, causing inhibition of ascending pain pathways, altering the perception of and response to pain; produces generalized CNS depression

Contraindications Hypersensitivity to oxycodone or any component of the formulation; significant respiratory depression; hypercarbia; acute or severe bronchial asthma; paralytic ileus (known or suspected); GI obstruction

Warnings/Precautions May cause CNS depression, which may impair physical or mental abilities; patients must be cautioned about performing tasks which require mental alertness (eg, operating machinery or driving). Potentially significant drug interactions may exist, requiring dose or frequency adjustment, additional monitoring, and/or selection of alternative therapy. Effects may be potentiated when used with other sedative drugs or ethanol. Use with caution in patients with hypersensitivity reactions to other phenanthrene derivative opioid agonists (morphine, hydrocodone, hydromorphone, levorphanol, oxymorphone), respiratory diseases including asthma, emphysema, or COPD.

Use with caution in pancreatitis or biliary tract disease, acute alcoholism (including delirium tremens), morbid obesity, adrenocortical insufficiency, history of seizure disorders, kyphoscoliosis (or other skeletal disorder which may alter respiratory function), hypothyroidism (including myxedema), prostatic hyperplasia, urethral stricture, and toxic psychosis. May obscure diagnosis or clinical course of patients with acute abdominal conditions. Avoid use in patients with CNS depression/coma as these patients are susceptible to intracranial effects of CO_2 retention.

Use with caution in the elderly, debilitated, or cachectic patients, and hepatic or renal dysfunction. Hemodynamic effects (hypotension, orthostasis) may be exaggerated in patients with hypovolemia, concurrent vasodilating drugs, or in patients with head injury. Monitor for symptoms of hypotension following initiation or dose titration. Respiratory depressant effects and capacity to elevate CSF pressure may be exaggerated in presence of head injury, other intracranial lesion, or pre-existing intracranial pressure.

Concomitant use with CYP3A4 inhibitors may result in increased effects and potentially fatal respiratory depression. Concurrent use of agonist/antagonist analgesics may precipitate withdrawal symptoms and/or reduced analgesic efficacy in patients following prolonged therapy with mu opioid agonists. Abrupt discontinuation following prolonged use may also lead to withdrawal symptoms. Healthcare provider should be alert to problems of abuse, misuse, and diversion; abuse of products by crushing, chewing, snorting, or injecting may result in severe overdose, adverse effects, or death.

After chronic maternal exposure to opioids, neonatal withdrawal syndrome may occur in the newborn; monitor neonate closely. Signs and symptoms include irritability, hyperactivity and abnormal sleep pattern, high pitched cry, tremor, vomiting, diarrhea and failure to gain weight. Onset, duration and severity depend on the drug used, duration of use, maternal dose, and rate of drug elimination by the newborn. Opioid withdrawal syndrome in the neonate, unlike in adults, may be life-threatening and should be treated according to protocols developed by neonatology experts.

Controlled-release tablets: OxyContin is not intended for use as an "as needed" analgesic or for the treatment of mild pain, acute pain, or postoperative pain requiring short-term analgesia (should be used postoperatively only if the patient has received it prior to surgery or if severe, persistent pain is anticipated). **[U.S. Boxed Warning]: May cause potentially life-threatening respiratory depression even with therapeutic use. Ensure proper dosing and titration; monitor for respiratory depression especially within** the first 24-72 hours of initiation or dose escalation. Oxycodone controlled-release tablets should only be prescribed by healthcare professionals familiar with the use of potent opioids for chronic pain. Do NOT crush, break, chew or dissolve controlled-release tablets (may result in a potentially fatal overdose); 60 mg and 80 mg strengths, a single dose >40 mg, or a total dose of >80 mg/day are for use only in opioid-tolerant patients. Tablets may be difficult to swallow and could become lodged in throat; patients with swallowing difficulties may be at increased risk. Cases of intestinal obstruction or diverticulitis exacerbation have also been reported, including cases requiring medical intervention to remove the tablet; patients with an underlying GI disease (eg, esophageal cancer, colon cancer) may be at increased risk. **[U.S. Boxed Warning]: Accidental exposure may result in fatal overdose of oxycodone, especially in children. [U.S. Boxed Warning]: Healthcare provider should be alert to problems of abuse, misuse, and diversion. Tolerance or drug dependence may result from extended use. Patients should be assessed for risk of abuse or addiction prior to therapy and all patients should be monitored for signs of misuse, abuse, and addiction. Risk of opioid abuse is increased in patients with a history or family history of alcohol or drug abuse or mental illness.**

Oral solutions: **[U.S. Boxed Warning]: Highly concentrated oral solution (20 mg/mL) should only be used in opioid tolerant patients (taking ≥30 mg/day of oxycodone or equivalent for ≥1 week). [U.S. Boxed Warning]: Orders for oxycodone oral solutions (20 mg/mL or 5 mg/5 mL) should be clearly written to include the intended dose (in mg vs mL) and the intended product concentration to be dispensed to avoid potential dosing errors. Products should be stored out of reach of children; seek immediate medical care in the event of accidental ingestion.**

Drug Interactions

Avoid Concomitant Use
Avoid concomitant use of OxyCODONE with any of the following: Azelastine (Nasal); Fusidic Acid (Systemic); Paraldehyde; Thalidomide

Decreased Effect
OxyCODONE may decrease the levels/effects of: Pegvisomant

The levels/effects of OxyCODONE may be decreased by: Ammonium Chloride; Bosentan; CYP3A4 Inducers (Strong); Dabrafenib; Deferasirox; Mitotane; Mixed Agonist / Antagonist Opioids; Rifampin; St Johns Wort; Tocilizumab

Increased Effect/Toxicity
OxyCODONE may increase the levels/effects of: Alcohol (Ethyl); Alvimopan; Azelastine (Nasal); CNS Depressants; Desmopressin; Diuretics; Hydrocodone; Metyrosine; Mirtazapine; Paraldehyde; Pramipexole; ROPINIRole; Rotigotine; Selective Serotonin Reuptake Inhibitors; Thalidomide; Zolpidem

The levels/effects of OxyCODONE may be increased by: Amphetamines; Anticholinergics; Antipsychotic Agents (Phenothiazines); Brimonidine (Topical); Cannabinoids; CYP3A4 Inhibitors (Moderate); CYP3A4 Inhibitors (Strong); Dasatinib; Doxylamine; Droperidol; Fusidic Acid (Systemic); HydrOXYzine; Ivacaftor; Luliconazole; Magnesium Sulfate; MAO Inhibitors; Mifepristone; Perampanel; Simeprevir; Sodium Oxybate; Succinylcholine; Tapentadol; Voriconazole

Nutritional/Ethanol Interactions
Ethanol: May increase CNS depression; monitor for increased effects with coadministration. Caution patients about effects.

Herb/Nutraceutical: Avoid valerian, St John's wort, kava kava, gotu kola (may increase CNS depression).

Adverse Reactions Note: Percentages as reported with OxyContin
>10%:
Central nervous system: Somnolence (23%), dizziness (13%)

Dermatologic: Pruritus (13%)

Gastrointestinal: Constipation (23%), nausea (23%), vomiting (12%)

1% to 10%:
Cardiovascular: Orthostatic hypotension (1% to 5%)

Central nervous system: Headache (7%), abnormal dreams (1% to 5%), anxiety (1% to 5%), chills (1% to 5%), confusion (1% to 5%), dysphoria (1% to 5%), euphoria (1% to 5%), fever (1% to 5%), insomnia (1% to 5%), nervousness (1% to 5%), thought abnormalities (1% to 5%)

Dermatologic: Rash (1% to 5%)

Gastrointestinal: Xerostomia (6%), abdominal pain (1% to 5%), anorexia (1% to 5%), diarrhea (1% to 5%), dyspepsia (1% to 5%), gastritis (1% to 5%)

Neuromuscular & skeletal: Weakness (6%), twitching (1% to 5%)

Respiratory: Dyspnea (1% to 5%), hiccups (1% to 5%)

Miscellaneous: Diaphoresis (5%)

Pharmacodynamics/Kinetics
Onset of Action Pain relief: Immediate release: 10-15 minutes; Peak effect: Immediate release: 0.5-1 hour

Duration of Action Immediate release: 3-6 hours; Controlled release: ≤12 hours

Controlled Substance C-II

Available Dosage Forms

Capsule, Oral:

Generic: 5 mg

Concentrate, Oral:

Generic: 20 mg/mL (30 mL)

Solution, Oral:

Generic: 5 mg/5 mL (5 mL, 15 mL, 500 mL)

Tablet, Oral:

Roxicodone: 5 mg, 15 mg, 30 mg

Generic: 5 mg, 10 mg, 15 mg, 20 mg, 30 mg

Tablet Abuse-Deterrent, Oral:

Oxecta: 5 mg, 7.5 mg

Tablet ER 12 Hour Abuse-Deterrent, Oral:

OxyCONTIN: 10 mg, 15 mg, 20 mg, 30 mg, 40 mg, 60 mg, 80 mg

General Dosage Range Dosage adjustment recommended in patients with renal or hepatic impairment, or on concomitant therapy

Oral:

Controlled release: *Adults:* 10-160 mg every 12 hours

Immediate release: *Adults:* 5-20 mg every 4-6 hours as needed

Administration

Oral

Controlled release: Swallow tablet whole. Do not moisten, dissolve, cut, crush, break, or chew controlled release tablets. Controlled release tablets are not indicated for rectal administration; increased risk of adverse events due to better rectal absorption. Controlled release tablets should be administered one at a time and each followed with water immediately after placing in the mouth.

Immediate release (Oxecta): Must be swallowed whole with enough water to ensure complete swallowing immediately after placing in the mouth. The tablet should not be wet prior to placing in the mouth. Do not crush, chew, or dissolve the tablets. Do not administer via feeding tubes (eg, gastric, NG) due to potential for obstruction. The formulation uses technology designed to discourage common methods of tampering to prevent misuse/abuse.

Appropriate laxatives should be administered to avoid the constipating side effects associated with use. Antiemetics may be needed for persistent nausea.

Storage/Stability Store at 25°C (77°F); excursions permitted between 15°C to 30°C (59°F to 86°F). Protect from light.

Nursing Actions

Physical Assessment Monitor for effectiveness of pain relief. Monitor blood pressure, CNS and respiratory status, and degree of sedation at beginning of therapy and periodically thereafter. Assess patient's physical and/or psychological dependence. For inpatients, implement safety measures (eg, side rails up, call light within reach, instructions to call for assistance). Discontinue slowly after prolonged use.

Patient Education

- Discuss specific use of drug and side effects with patient as it relates to treatment. (HCAHPS: During this hospital stay, were you given any medicine that you had not taken before? Before giving you any new medicine, how often did hospital staff tell you what the medicine was for? How often did hospital staff describe possible side effects in a way you could understand?)
- Patient may experience nausea, fatigue, headache, insomnia, or xerostomia. Have patient report immediately to prescriber severe dizziness, syncope, illogical thinking, considerable constipation, significant dyspepsia, intolerable asthenia, dyspnea, difficult urination, tachycardia, bradycardia, arrhythmia, tremors, vision changes, angina, hallucinations, mood changes, memory loss, difficulty speaking, abnormal gait, or edema of extremities (HCAHPS).
- Educate patient about signs of a significant reaction (eg, wheezing; chest tightness; fever; itching; bad cough; blue skin color; seizures; or swelling of face, lips, tongue, or throat). **Note:** This is not a comprehensive list of all side effects. Patient should consult prescriber for additional questions.

Intended Use and Disclaimer: Should not be printed and given to patients. This information is intended to serve as a concise initial reference for healthcare professionals to use when discussing medications with a patient. You must ultimately rely on your own discretion, experience and judgment in diagnosing, treating and advising patients.

Dietary Considerations Instruct patient to avoid high-fat meals when taking some products (food has no effect on the reformulated OxyContin).

Related Information

Oral Medications That Should Not Be Crushed or Altered *on page 1712*

Oxycodone and Acetaminophen
(oks i KOE done & a seet a MIN oh fen)

Brand Names: U.S. Endocet; Magnacet [DSC]; Percocet; Primlev; Roxicet; Roxicet 5/500

Index Terms Acetaminophen and Oxycodone; Tylox; Xartemis XR

Pharmacologic Category Analgesic Combination (Opioid)

Medication Safety Issues

Sound-alike/look-alike issues:

Oxycodone and Acetaminophen may be confused with Hydrocodone and Acetaminophen

Endocet may be confused with Indocid

Percocet may be confused with Fioricet, Percodan

Roxicet may be confused with Roxanol

◀ Tylox may be confused with Trimox, Tylenol, Xanax

High alert medication:
The Institute for Safe Medication Practices (ISMP) includes this medication among its list of drug classes which have a heightened risk of causing significant patient harm when used in error.

Other safety concerns:
Duplicate therapy issues: This product contains acetaminophen, which may be a component of other combination products. Do not exceed the maximum recommended daily dose of acetaminophen.

Medication Guide Available Yes

Pregnancy Risk Factor C

Use Moderate to moderately severe pain: Management of moderate to moderately-severe pain

Product Availability Xartemis XR: FDA approved March 2014; anticipated availability is currently unknown. Xartemis XR is an extended-release oral formulation of oxycodone and acetaminophen with immediate-release and extended-release components. Refer to the prescribing information for additional information.

Controlled Substance C-II

Available Dosage Forms
Caplet, oral: Oxycodone 5 mg and acetaminophen 500 mg
Roxicet 5/500: Oxycodone 5 mg and acetaminophen 500 mg
Capsule, oral: Oxycodone 5 mg and acetaminophen 500 mg
Solution, oral: Oxycodone 5 mg and acetaminophen 325 mg per 5 mL
Roxicet: Oxycodone 5 mg and acetaminophen 325 mg per 5 mL
Tablet, oral: 2.5/325: Oxycodone hydrochloride 2.5 mg and acetaminophen 325 mg; 5/325: Oxycodone hydrochloride 5 mg and acetaminophen 325 mg; 7.5/325: Oxycodone hydrochloride 7.5 mg and acetaminophen 325 mg; 7.5/500: Oxycodone hydrochloride 7.5 mg and acetaminophen 500 mg; 10/325: Oxycodone hydrochloride 10 mg and acetaminophen 325 mg; 10/650: Oxycodone hydrochloride 10 mg and acetaminophen 650 mg
Endocet 5/325 [scored]: Oxycodone 5 mg and acetaminophen 325 mg
Endocet 7.5/325: Oxycodone 7.5 mg and acetaminophen 325 mg
Endocet 10/325: Oxycodone 10 mg and acetaminophen 325 mg
Percocet 2.5/325: Oxycodone 2.5 mg and acetaminophen 325 mg
Percocet 5/325 [scored]: Oxycodone 5 mg and acetaminophen 325 mg
Percocet 7.5/325: Oxycodone 7.5 mg and acetaminophen 325 mg
Percocet 7.5/500: Oxycodone 7.5 mg and acetaminophen 500 mg
Percocet 10/325: Oxycodone 10 mg and acetaminophen 325 mg
Percocet 10/650: Oxycodone 10 mg and acetaminophen 650 mg
Primlev 5/300: Oxycodone 5 mg and acetaminophen 300 mg
Primlev 7.5/300: Oxycodone 7.5 mg and acetaminophen 300 mg
Primlev 10/300: Oxycodone 10 mg and acetaminophen 300 mg
Roxicet [scored]: Oxycodone 5 mg and acetaminophen 325 mg

General Dosage Range
Oral: *Adults:*
Acetaminophen: 325-650 mg every 4-6 hours (maximum: 4 g daily)
Oxycodone: 2.5-10 mg/dose every 6 hours as needed (do not exceed acetaminophen maximum of 4 g daily)

Nursing Actions
Physical Assessment See individual agents.

Patient Education
• Discuss specific use of drug and side effects with patient as it relates to treatment. (HCAHPS: During this hospital stay, were you given any medicine that you had not taken before? Before giving you any new medicine, how often did hospital staff tell you what the medicine was for? How often did hospital staff describe possible side effects in a way you could understand?)
• Patient may experience fatigue, flushing, or nausea. Have patient report immediately to prescriber signs of hepatic impairment, severe dizziness, syncope, dyspnea, illogical thinking, considerable constipation, significant asthenia, paresthesia, urinary retention, oliguria, tachycardia, bradycardia, arrhythmia, chills, pharyngitis, hallucinations, mood changes, hearing impairment, intolerable headache, back pain, dyspepsia, tremors, ecchymosis, hemorrhaging, vision changes, or Stevens-Johnson syndrome/toxic epidermal necrolysis (HCAHPS).
• Educate patient about signs of a significant reaction (eg, wheezing; chest tightness; fever; itching; bad cough; blue skin color; seizures; or swelling of face, lips, tongue, or throat). **Note:** This is not a comprehensive list of all side effects. Patient should consult prescriber for additional questions.

Intended Use and Disclaimer: Should not be printed and given to patients. This information is intended to serve as a concise initial reference for healthcare professionals to use when discussing medications with a patient. You must ultimately rely on your own discretion, experience and judgment in diagnosing, treating and advising patients.

Related Information
Acetaminophen *on page 31*
OxyCODONE *on page 1180*

Oxycodone and Ibuprofen
(oks i KOE done & eye byoo PROE fen)

Index Terms Ibuprofen and Oxycodone
Pharmacologic Category Analgesic Combination (Opioid); Nonsteroidal Anti-inflammatory Drug (NSAID), Oral
Medication Safety Issues
High alert medication:
The Institute for Safe Medication Practices (ISMP) includes this medication among its list of drug classes which have a heightened risk of causing significant patient harm when used in error.
Medication Guide Available Yes
Pregnancy Risk Factor C/D ≥30 weeks gestation
Lactation Enters breast milk/not recommended
Use Short-term (≤7 days) management of acute, moderate-to-severe pain
Controlled Substance C-II
Available Dosage Forms
Tablet: Oxycodone 5 mg and ibuprofen 400 mg
General Dosage Range Oral: *Adults:* 1 tablet as needed (maximum: 4 tablets/day; 7 days)
Administration
Oral Administer without regard to meals.
Nursing Actions
Physical Assessment See individual agents.
Patient Education
• Discuss specific use of drug and side effects with patient as it relates to treatment. (HCAHPS: During this hospital stay, were you given any medicine that you had not taken before? Before giving you any new medicine, how often did hospital staff tell you what the medicine was for? How often did hospital staff describe possible side effects in a way you could understand?)
• Patient may experience fatigue or headache. Have patient report immediately to prescriber severe dizziness, syncope, angina, tachycardia, strength differences from one side to another, difficulty speaking or thinking, change in balance, blurred vision, dyspnea, significant nausea, considerable dyspepsia, excessive weight gain, edema of extremities, melena, intolerable constipation, ecchymosis, hemorrhaging, severe asthenia, jaundice, arrhythmia, flu-like syndrome, urinary retention, oliguria, mood changes, neck rigidity, or hematemesis (HCAHPS).
• Educate patient about signs of a significant reaction (eg, wheezing; chest tightness; fever; itching; bad cough; blue skin color; seizures; or swelling of face, lips, tongue, or throat). **Note:** This is not a comprehensive list of all side effects. Patient should consult prescriber for additional questions.

Intended Use and Disclaimer: Should not be printed and given to patients. This information is intended to serve as a concise initial reference for healthcare professionals to use when discussing medications with a patient. You must ultimately rely on your own discretion, experience and judgment in diagnosing, treating and advising patients.
Related Information
Ibuprofen *on page 798*
OxyCODONE *on page 1180*

Oxycodone and Naloxone
(oks i KOE done & nal OKS one)

Index Terms Naloxone and Oxycodone; Oxycodone Hydrochloride and Naloxone Hydrochloride
Pharmacologic Category Analgesic, Opioid; Opioid Antagonist
Medication Safety Issues
Sound-alike/look-alike issues:
Targin® may be confused with Talwin®
High alert medication:
The Institute for Safe Medication Practices (ISMP) includes this medication among its list of drug classes which have a heightened risk of causing significant patient harm when used in error.
Use Treatment of moderate-to-severe pain in patients requiring around-the-clock opioid analgesia; combined with an opioid antagonist for the relief of opioid-induced constipation
Product Availability Not available in the U.S.
Controlled Substance CDSA I
General Dosage Range Dosage adjustment required in renal and hepatic impairment.
Oral: *Adults:* Dosing is individualized and may vary based on prior exposure to opioids and/or tolerance to the respiratory depressant effects of oxycodone. Maximum single dose: Oxycodone 40 mg/naloxone 20 mg; maximum daily dose: Oxycodone 80 mg/naloxone 40 mg
Administration
Oral Swallow tablet whole with 4-6 ounces of water. Do not moisten, dissolve, cut, crush, break, or chew tablets. Tablets are not indicated for rectal administration; increased risk of adverse events due to enhanced rectal absorption. Controlled release tablets should be administered 1 at a time and each followed with water immediately after placing in the mouth. May be administered without regard to meals. Missed doses should be taken at the next regularly scheduled time.
Nursing Actions
Patient Education
• Discuss specific use of drug and side effects with patient as it relates to treatment. (HCAHPS: During this hospital stay, were you given any medicine that you had not taken before? Before giving you any new medicine, how often did hospital staff tell you what the medicine was ▶

for? How often did hospital staff describe possible side effects in a way you could understand?)
- Patient may experience fatigue, dizziness, nausea, diarrhea, constipation, headache, or hyperhidrosis. Have patient report immediately to prescriber dyspnea, illogical thinking, or poor pain control (HCAHPS).
- Educate patient about signs of a significant reaction (eg, wheezing; chest tightness; fever; itching; bad cough; blue skin color; seizures; or swelling of face, lips, tongue, or throat). **Note:** This is not a comprehensive list of all side effects. Patient should consult prescriber for additional questions.

Intended Use and Disclaimer: Should not be printed and given to patients. This information is intended to serve as a concise initial reference for healthcare professionals to use when discussing medications with a patient. You must ultimately rely on your own discretion, experience and judgment in diagnosing, treating and advising patients.

Related Information
Naloxone *on page 1098*
OxyCODONE *on page 1180*

Oxymorphone (oks i MOR fone)

Brand Names: U.S. Opana; Opana ER
Index Terms Oxymorphone Hydrochloride
Pharmacologic Category Analgesic, Opioid
Medication Safety Issues
Sound-alike/look-alike issues:
Oxymorphone may be confused with oxycodone, oxymetholone
High alert medication:
The Institute for Safe Medication Practices (ISMP) includes this medication among its list of drug classes which have a heightened risk of causing significant patient harm when used in error.
Medication Guide Available Yes
Pregnancy Risk Factor C
Lactation Excretion in breast milk unknown/use caution
Breast-Feeding Considerations Some opioids can be found in breast milk. Withdrawal symptoms may be observed in breast-feeding infants when opioid analgesics are discontinued. The manufacturer recommends that caution be used if administered to a nursing woman. Nursing infants exposed to large doses of opioids should be monitored for apnea and sedation (Montgomery, 2012).
Use
Parenteral: Management of moderate-to-severe acute pain; analgesia during labor; preoperative medication; anesthesia support; relief of anxiety in patients with dyspnea associated with pulmonary edema secondary to acute left ventricular failure

Oral, regular release: Management of moderate-to-severe acute pain
Oral, extended release: Management of moderate-to-severe pain in patients requiring around-the-clock opioid treatment for an extended period of time
Mechanism of Action/Effect Oxymorphone hydrochloride is a potent opioid analgesic with uses similar to those of morphine. The drug is a semisynthetic derivative of morphine (phenanthrene derivative) and is closely related to hydromorphone chemically (Dilaudid®).
Contraindications Hypersensitivity to oxymorphone, other morphine analogs (phenanthrene derivatives), or any component of the formulation; paralytic ileus (known or suspected); moderate-to-severe hepatic impairment; severe respiratory depression (unless using immediate release or parenteral formulation in monitored setting with resuscitative equipment); acute/severe bronchial asthma; hypercarbia
Note: Parenteral formulation is also contraindicated in the treatment of upper airway obstruction and pulmonary edema due to a chemical respiratory irritant.
Warnings/Precautions An opioid-containing analgesic regimen should be tailored to each patient's needs and based upon the type of pain being treated (acute versus chronic), the route of administration, degree of tolerance for opioids (naive versus chronic user), age, weight, and patient comorbidities. The optimal analgesic dose varies widely among patients. Doses should be titrated to pain relief/prevention.

May cause CNS depression, which may impair physical or mental abilities; patients must be cautioned about performing tasks which require mental alertness (eg, operating machinery or driving). Potentially significant drug interactions may exist, requiring dose or frequency adjustment, additional monitoring, and/or selection of alternative therapy. Effects may be potentiated when used with other sedative drugs or ethanol. Use not recommended within 14 days of MAO inhibitors. Due to structural similarities, hypersensitivity to other phenanthrene-derivative opioid agonists (codeine, hydrocodone, hydromorphone, levorphanol, morphine) may result in similar hypersensitivity reaction if oxymorphone is used; therefore, the use of oxymorphone is contraindicated in patients with previous hypersensitivity to other phenanthrene derivatives. May cause respiratory depression. Use extreme caution in patients with COPD or other chronic respiratory conditions characterized by hypoxia, hypercapnia, or diminished respiratory reserve (myxedema, cor pulmonale, kyphoscoliosis, obstructive sleep apnea, severe obesity). Use with caution in patients (particularly elderly or debilitated) with impaired respiratory function, adrenal disease, morbid obesity, seizure disorders, toxic psychosis, thyroid dysfunction, prostatic hyperplasia, or renal impairment. Use caution in mild hepatic dysfunction; use is contraindicated in moderate-to-severe hepatic impairment. Avoid use in patients with CNS depression or coma as these patients are susceptible to intracranial effects of CO_2 retention. Use only with extreme caution (if at all) in patients with head injury or increased intracranial pressure (ICP); potential to elevate ICP and/or blunt papillary response may be greatly exaggerated in these patients. Use with caution in patients with biliary tract dysfunction including acute pancreatitis; may cause constriction of sphincter of Oddi. May obscure diagnosis or clinical course of patients with acute abdominal conditions.

Oxymorphone shares the toxic potential of opioid agonists and usual precautions of opioid agonist therapy should be observed; may cause hypotension in patients with acute myocardial infarction, volume depletion, or concurrent drug therapy which may exaggerate vasodilation. The elderly may be particularly susceptible to adverse effects of opioids.

[U.S. Boxed Warning]: Healthcare provider should be alert to problems of abuse, misuse, and diversion. Tolerance or drug dependence may result from extended use. Use caution in patients with a history of drug dependence or abuse. Abrupt discontinuation may precipitate withdrawal syndrome. After chronic maternal exposure to opioids, neonatal withdrawal syndrome may occur in the newborn; monitor neonate closely. Signs and symptoms include irritability, hyperactivity and abnormal sleep pattern, high pitched cry, tremor, vomiting, diarrhea and failure to gain weight. Onset, duration and severity depend on the drug used, duration of use, maternal dose, and rate of drug elimination by the newborn. Opioid withdrawal syndrome in the neonate, unlike in adults, may be life-threatening and should be treated according to protocols developed by neonatology experts.

Extended release formulation:

[U.S. Boxed Warnings]: Opana® ER is an extended release oral formulation of oxymorphone and is not suitable for use as an "as needed" analgesic. Tablets should not be broken, chewed, dissolved, or crushed; tablets should be swallowed whole. Opana® ER is intended for use in long-term, continuous management of moderate-to-severe chronic pain. It is not indicated for use in the immediate postoperative period (12-24 hours). Cases of thrombotic thrombocytopenic purpura (TTP) resulting in kidney failure (requiring dialysis) and death have been reported as a result of misuse by drug abusers injecting the extended-release tablets intravenously; tablets are intended for oral administration only. **[U.S. Boxed Warning]: The coingestion of**

ethanol or ethanol-containing medications with Opana® ER may result in accelerated release of drug from the dosage form, abruptly increasing plasma levels, which may have fatal consequences.

Drug Interactions

Avoid Concomitant Use

Avoid concomitant use of Oxymorphone with any of the following: Azelastine (Nasal); MAO Inhibitors; Paraldehyde; Thalidomide

Decreased Effect

Oxymorphone may decrease the levels/effects of: Pegvisomant

The levels/effects of Oxymorphone may be decreased by: Ammonium Chloride; Mixed Agonist / Antagonist Opioids

Increased Effect/Toxicity

Oxymorphone may increase the levels/effects of: Alcohol (Ethyl); Alvimopan; Azelastine (Nasal); CNS Depressants; Desmopressin; Diuretics; Hydrocodone; MAO Inhibitors; Metyrosine; Mirtazapine; Paraldehyde; Pramipexole; ROPINIRole; Rotigotine; Selective Serotonin Reuptake Inhibitors; Thalidomide; Zolpidem

The levels/effects of Oxymorphone may be increased by: Amphetamines; Anticholinergics; Antipsychotic Agents (Phenothiazines); Brimonidine (Topical); Cannabinoids; Doxylamine; Droperidol; HydrOXYzine; Magnesium Sulfate; Perampanel; Sodium Oxybate; Succinylcholine; Tapentadol

Nutritional/Ethanol Interactions

Ethanol: Ethanol ingestion with extended-release tablets is specifically contraindicated due to possible accelerated release and potentially fatal overdose. Ethanol may also increase CNS depression; monitor for increased effects with coadministration. Caution patients about effects.

Food: When taken orally with a high-fat meal, peak concentration is 38% to 50% greater. Both immediate-release and extended-release tablets should be taken 1 hour before or 2 hours after eating.

Herb/Nutraceutical: Avoid valerian, St John's wort, kava kava, gotu kola (may increase CNS depression).

Adverse Reactions Incidence usually on higher end with extended release (ER) tablet.

>10%:

Central nervous system: Somnolence (9% to 19%), dizziness (7% to 18%), fever (1% to 14%), headache (7% to 12%)

Dermatologic: Pruritus (8% to 15%)

Gastrointestinal: Nausea (19% to 33%), constipation (4% to 28%), vomiting (9% to 16%)

1% to 10%:

Cardiovascular: Hypotension (<10%), tachycardia (<10%), edema (<10%), flushing (<10%), hypertension (<10%)

Central nervous system: Anxiety (1% to <10%), sedation (1% to <10%), depression (<10%), disorientation (<10%), lethargy (<10%), nervousness (<10%), restlessness (<10%), fatigue (≤4%), insomnia (≤4%), confusion (3%)

Endocrine & metabolic: Dehydration (<10%)

Gastrointestinal: Abdominal distension (<10%), flatulence (1% to <10%), xerostomia (1% to <10%), dyspepsia (<10%), weight loss (<10%), diarrhea (≤4%), abdominal pain (≤3%), appetite decreased (≤3%)

Neuromuscular & skeletal: Weakness (<10%)

Ocular: Blurred vision (<10%)

Respiratory: Hypoxia (<10%), dyspnea (<10%)

Miscellaneous: Diaphoresis (1% to <10%)

Pharmacodynamics/Kinetics

Onset of Action Parenteral: 5-10 minutes

Duration of Action Analgesic: Parenteral: 3-6 hours

Controlled Substance C-II

Available Dosage Forms

Solution, Injection:

Opana: 1 mg/mL (1 mL)

Tablet, Oral:

Opana: 5 mg, 10 mg

Generic: 5 mg, 10 mg

Tablet ER 12 Hour Abuse-Deterrent, Oral:

Opana ER: 5 mg, 7.5 mg, 10 mg, 15 mg, 20 mg, 30 mg, 40 mg

Tablet Extended Release 12 Hour, Oral:

Generic: 5 mg, 7.5 mg, 10 mg, 15 mg, 20 mg, 30 mg, 40 mg

General Dosage Range Dosage adjustment recommended in patients with hepatic or renal impairment

I.M., SubQ: *Adults:* Initial: 0.5 mg; Maintenance: 1-1.5 mg every 4-6 hours as needed

I.V.: *Adults:* Initial: 0.5 mg

Oral:

Extended release: *Adults (opioid-naive):* Initial: 5 mg every 12 hours; Maintenance: Titrate upward with 5-10 mg every 12 hours at 3-7 day intervals until desired response

Immediate release: *Adults (opioid-naive):* Initial: 5-10 mg every 4-6 hours; Maintenance: Titrate upward to desired response

Administration

Injectable Detail pH: 2.7-4.5

Oral Administer immediate release and extended release tablets 1 hour before or 2 hours after eating. Opana® ER tablet should be swallowed whole; do not break, crush, dissolve, or chew.

Storage/Stability Injection solution, tablet: Store at 25°C (77°F); excursions permitted to 15°C to 30°C (59°F to 86°F). Protect injection from light.

Nursing Actions

Physical Assessment If used to control diarrhea, monitor stools. Monitor for effectiveness of pain relief. Monitor blood pressure, CNS and respiratory status, and degree of sedation at beginning of therapy and periodically thereafter. Assess patient's physical and/or psychological dependence. For inpatients, implement safety measures (eg, side rails up, call light within reach, instructions to call for assistance). Discontinue slowly after prolonged use.

Patient Education

• Discuss specific use of drug and side effects with patient as it relates to treatment. (HCAHPS: During this hospital stay, were you given any medicine that you had not taken before? Before giving you any new medicine, how often did hospital staff tell you what the medicine was for? How often did hospital staff describe possible side effects in a way you could understand?)

• Patient may experience fatigue, xerostomia, flatulence, hyperhidrosis, asthenia, or tablet shell in stool. Have patient report immediately to prescriber severe dizziness, dyspnea, illogical thinking, significant nausea, considerable constipation, angina, tachycardia, bradycardia, arrhythmia, hallucinations, mood changes, intolerable dyspepsia, severe headache, difficult urination, edema, vision changes, or memory loss (HCAHPS).

• Educate patient about signs of a significant reaction (eg, wheezing; chest tightness; fever; itching; bad cough; blue skin color; seizures; or swelling of face, lips, tongue, or throat). **Note:** This is not a comprehensive list of all side effects. Patient should consult prescriber for additional questions.

Intended Use and Disclaimer: Should not be printed and given to patients. This information is intended to serve as a concise initial reference for healthcare professionals to use when discussing medications with a patient. You must ultimately rely on your own discretion, experience and judgment in diagnosing, treating and advising patients.

Dietary Considerations Immediate release and extended release tablets should be taken 1 hour before or 2 hours after eating.

Related Information

Oral Medications That Should Not Be Crushed or Altered *on page 1712*

Oxytocin (oks i TOE sin)

Brand Names: U.S. Pitocin

Index Terms Pit

Pharmacologic Category Oxytocic Agent

Medication Safety Issues

High alert medication:

The Institute for Safe Medication Practices (ISMP) includes this medication among its list of drugs which have a heightened risk of causing significant patient harm when used in error.

Pregnancy Risk Factor C (manufacturer specific)

Lactation Excretion in breast milk unknown/use caution

Breast-Feeding Considerations Endogenous levels of oxytocin naturally increase during breast-feeding.

Use Induction of labor in patients with a medical indication; stimulation or reinforcement of labor; adjunctive therapy in management of abortion; to produce uterine contractions during the third stage of labor; control of postpartum bleeding

Mechanism of Action/Effect Oxytocin stimulates uterine contraction by activating G-protein-coupled receptors that trigger increases in intracellular calcium levels in uterine myofibrils. Oxytocin also increases local prostaglandin production, further stimulating uterine contraction.

Contraindications Hypersensitivity to oxytocin or any component of the formulation; significant cephalopelvic disproportion; unfavorable fetal positions; fetal distress when delivery is not imminent; hypertonic or hyperactive uterus; contraindicated vaginal delivery (invasive cervical cancer, active genital herpes, prolapse of the cord, cord presentation, total placenta previa, or vasa previa); obstetrical emergencies where surgical intervention is favored; where adequate uterine activity fails to achieve satisfactory progress

Warnings/Precautions Hazardous agent - use appropriate precautions for handling and disposal (NIOSH, 2012). **[U.S. Boxed Warning]: To be used for medical rather than elective induction of labor.** Medical indications for labor induction may include Rh problems, maternal diabetes, preeclampsia at or near term, when delivery is in the best interest of mother or fetus, or premature rupture of membranes when delivery is indicated. Use is generally not recommended in the following conditions: Fetal distress, hydramnios, partial placenta previa, prematurity, borderline cephalopelvic disproportion, or conditions where there is a predisposition for uterine rupture. May produce antidiuretic effect (ie, water intoxication). Severe water intoxication with convulsions, coma, and death is associated with a slow oxytocin infusion over 24 hours. High doses or hypersensitivity to oxytocin may cause uterine hypertonicity, spasm, tetanic contraction, or rupture of the uterus. Intravenous preparations should be administered by adequately trained individuals familiar with its use and able to identify complications.

Drug Interactions

Avoid Concomitant Use
Avoid concomitant use of Oxytocin with any of the following: Carboprost Tromethamine

Decreased Effect There are no known significant interactions involving a decrease in effect.

Increased Effect/Toxicity
Oxytocin may increase the levels/effects of: Highest Risk QTc-Prolonging Agents; Moderate Risk QTc-Prolonging Agents

The levels/effects of Oxytocin may be increased by: Carboprost Tromethamine; Dinoprostone; Mifepristone; Misoprostol

Adverse Reactions Frequency not defined.
Fetus or neonate:
Cardiovascular: Arrhythmias (including premature ventricular contractions), bradycardia
Central nervous system: Brain or CNS damage (permanent), neonatal seizure
Hepatic: Neonatal jaundice
Ocular: Neonatal retinal hemorrhage
Miscellaneous: Fetal death, low Apgar score (5 minute)
Mother:
Cardiovascular: Arrhythmias (including premature ventricular contractions), hypertensive episodes
Gastrointestinal: Nausea, vomiting
Genitourinary: Pelvic hematoma, postpartum hemorrhage, uterine hypertonicity, tetanic contraction of the uterus, uterine rupture, uterine spasm
Hematologic: Afibrinogenemia (fatal)
Miscellaneous: Anaphylactic reaction, subarachnoid hemorrhage; severe water intoxication with convulsions, coma, and death is associated with a slow oxytocin infusion over 24 hours

Pharmacodynamics/Kinetics
Onset of Action Uterine contractions: I.M.: 3-5 minutes; I.V.: ~1 minute
Duration of Action I.M.: 2-3 hour; I.V.: 1 hour

Available Dosage Forms
Solution, Injection:
Pitocin: 10 units/mL (1 mL, 10 mL, 50 mL)
Generic: 10 units/mL (1 mL, 10 mL, 30 mL)

General Dosage Range
I.M.: *Adults:* Total dose of 10 units after delivery of the placenta
I.V.: *Adults:* Dosage varies greatly depending on indication

Administration
I.V. An infusion pump is required for administration.
Hazardous agent; use appropriate precautions for handling and disposal (NIOSH, 2012).

Preparation for Administration Hazardous agent; use appropriate precautions for handling and disposal (NIOSH, 2012).
I.V.:
Induction or stimulation of labor: Add oxytocin 10 units to NS or LR 1000 mL to yield a solution containing oxytocin 10 milliunits/mL. Rotate solution to mix.
Postpartum uterine bleeding: Add oxytocin 10-40 units to running I.V. infusion; maximum: 40 units/1000 mL.
Adjunctive management of abortion: Add oxytocin 10 units to 500 mL of a physiologic saline solution or D5W.

Storage/Stability Store at 20°C to 25°C (68°F to 77°F); excursions permitted to 15°C to 30°C (59°F to 86°F); do not freeze.

◀ **Nursing Actions**

Physical Assessment Monitor blood pressure, fluid intake and output, and labor closely if using oxytocin for induction; fetal monitoring is strongly recommended.

Patient Education

- Discuss specific use of drug and side effects with patient as it relates to treatment. (HCAHPS: During this hospital stay, were you given any medicine that you had not taken before? Before giving you any new medicine, how often did hospital staff tell you what the medicine was for? How often did hospital staff describe possible side effects in a way you could understand?)
- Patient may experience injection site irritation or nausea. Have patient report immediately to prescriber heavy bleeding, tachycardia, severe headache, significant dyspepsia, or rash (HCAHPS).
- Educate patient about signs of a significant reaction (eg, wheezing; chest tightness; fever; itching; bad cough; blue skin color; seizures; or swelling of face, lips, tongue, or throat). **Note:** This is not a comprehensive list of all side effects. Patient should consult prescriber for additional questions.

Intended Use and Disclaimer: Should not be printed and given to patients. This information is intended to serve as a concise initial reference for healthcare professionals to use when discussing medications with a patient. You must ultimately rely on your own discretion, experience and judgment in diagnosing, treating and advising patients.

Paclitaxel (pac li TAKS el)

Index Terms Conventional Paclitaxel; Paclitaxel (Conventional); Taxol

Pharmacologic Category Antineoplastic Agent, Antimicrotubular; Antineoplastic Agent, Taxane Derivative

Medication Safety Issues

Sound-alike/look-alike issues:

PACLitaxel may be confused with cabazitaxel, DOCEtaxel, PARoxetine, Paxil®

PACLitaxel (conventional) may be confused with PACLitaxel (protein-bound)

Taxol® may be confused with Abraxane®, Paxil®, Taxotere®

High alert medication:

This medication is in a class the Institute for Safe Medication Practices (ISMP) includes among its list of drug classes which have a heightened risk of causing significant patient harm when used in error.

Pregnancy Risk Factor D

Lactation Enters breast milk/not recommended

Use Treatment of breast, nonsmall cell lung, and ovarian cancers; treatment of AIDS-related Kaposi's sarcoma (KS)

Unlabeled Use Treatment of bladder, cervical, small cell lung, and head and neck cancers; treatment of (unknown primary) adenocarcinoma

Available Dosage Forms

Concentrate, Intravenous:

Generic: 100 mg/16.7 mL (16.7 mL); 30 mg/5 mL (5 mL); 150 mg/25 mL (25 mL); 300 mg/50 mL (50 mL)

Concentrate, Intravenous [preservative free]:

Generic: 100 mg/16.7 mL (16.7 mL); 30 mg/5 mL (5 mL); 300 mg/50 mL (50 mL)

General Dosage Range Dosage adjustment recommended in patients with hepatic impairment or who develop toxicities

I.V.: *Adults:* Dosage varies greatly depending on indication

Administration

I.V. IInfuse over 1-96 hours. When administered as a part of a combination chemotherapy regimen, sequence of administration may vary by regimen; refer to specific protocol for sequence recommendation.

Premedication with dexamethasone (20 mg orally or I.V. at 12 and 6 hours **or** 14 and 7 hours before the dose; reduce to 10 mg with advanced HIV disease), diphenhydramine (50 mg I.V. 30-60 minutes prior to the dose), and cimetidine 300 mg, famotidine 20 mg, or ranitidine 50 mg (I.V. 30-60 minutes prior to the dose) is recommended.

Administer I.V. infusion over 1-24 hours; infuse through a 0.22 micron in-line filter and nonsorbing administration set.

Irritant with vesicant-like properties; avoid extravasation. Ensure proper needle or catheter position prior to administration.

Extravasation management: If extravasation occurs, stop infusion immediately and disconnect (leave cannula/needle in place); gently aspirate extravasated solution (do **NOT** flush the line); remove needle/cannula; initiate antidote (hyaluronidase); remove needle/cannula; elevate extremity. Information conflicts regarding the use of warm or cold compresses (Perez Fidalgo, 2012; Polovich, 2009).

Hyaluronidase: If needle/cannula still in place: Administer 1-6 mL (150 units/mL) into existing I.V. line; usual dose is 1 mL for each 1 mL of extravasated drug; if needle/cannula has been removed, inject subcutaneously in a clockwise manner around area of extravasation; may repeat several times over the next 3-4 hours (Ener, 2004).

Hazardous agent; use appropriate precautions for handling and disposal (NIOSH, 2012).

Injectable Detail pH: 4.4-5.6

Other Intraperitoneal: 1- to 2-hour infusion

Hazardous agent; use appropriate precautions for handling and disposal (NIOSH, 2012).

Nursing Actions

Physical Assessment Monitor infusion site closely to avoid extravasation. Monitor for hypersensitivity reaction, cardiovascular abnormalities, sensory neuropathy, myelosuppression, and GI irritation prior to, during, and between each infusion.

Patient Education

- Discuss specific use of drug and side effects with patient as it relates to treatment. (HCAHPS: During this hospital stay, were you given any medicine that you had not taken before? Before giving you any new medicine, how often did hospital staff tell you what the medicine was for? How often did hospital staff describe possible side effects in a way you could understand?)
- Patient may experience chills, hives, angina, anemia, leukopenia, thrombocytopenia, fatigue, nausea, diarrhea, stomatitis, alopecia, flushing, edema, paresthesia, myalgia, arthralgia, or infertility. Have patient report immediately to prescriber signs of infection, dyspnea, severe dyspepsia, ecchymosis, inability to eat, discolored urine, jaundice, or rash (HCAHPS).
- Educate patient about signs of a significant reaction (eg, wheezing; chest tightness; fever; itching; bad cough; blue skin color; seizures; or swelling of face, lips, tongue, or throat). **Note:** This is not a comprehensive list of all side effects. Patient should consult prescriber for additional questions.

Intended Use and Disclaimer: Should not be printed and given to patients. This information is intended to serve as a concise initial reference for healthcare professionals to use when discussing medications with a patient. You must ultimately rely on your own discretion, experience and judgment in diagnosing, treating and advising patients.

Related Information

Management of Drug Extravasations *on page 1700*

Paclitaxel (Protein Bound)
(pac li TAKS el PROE teen bownd)

Brand Names: U.S. Abraxane

Index Terms ABI-007; Albumin-Bound Paclitaxel; Albumin-Stabilized Nanoparticle Paclitaxel; nab-Paclitaxel; Nanoparticle Albumin-Bound Paclitaxel; Paclitaxel (Nanoparticle Albumin Bound); Paclitaxel, Albumin-Bound; Protein-Bound Paclitaxel

Pharmacologic Category Antineoplastic Agent, Antimicrotubular; Antineoplastic Agent, Taxane Derivative

Medication Safety Issues

Sound-alike/look-alike issues:

PACLitaxel (protein bound) may be confused with PACLitaxel (conventional)

Abraxane may be confused with Paxil, Taxol, Taxotere

High alert medication:

This medication is in a class the Institute for Safe Medication Practices (ISMP) includes among its list of drug classes which have a heightened risk of causing significant patient harm when used in error.

Pregnancy Risk Factor D

Lactation Enters breast milk/not recommended

Use

Breast cancer: Treatment of refractory (metastatic) or relapsed (within 6 months of adjuvant therapy) breast cancer after failure of combination chemotherapy (including anthracycline-based therapy unless clinically contraindicated)

Nonsmall cell lung cancer (NSCLC): First-line treatment of locally advanced or metastatic NSCLC (in combination with carboplatin) in patients ineligible for curative surgery or radiation therapy

Pancreatic cancer: First-line treatment of patients with metastatic adenocarcinoma of the pancreas (in combination with gemcitabine)

Unlabeled Use Treatment of recurrent or persistent ovarian, fallopian tube, or primary peritoneal cancers

Available Dosage Forms

Suspension Reconstituted, Intravenous:

Abraxane: 100 mg (1 ea)

General Dosage Range Dosage adjustment recommended in patients with hepatic impairment or who develop toxicities

I.V.: *Adults:* Dosage varies greatly depending on indication.

Administration

I.V. Administer over 30 minutes (breast cancer and NSCLC) or over 30-40 minutes (pancreatic cancer); limiting the infusion rate to 30 minutes reduces the risk for infusion-related reaction; do not use an in-line filter. Monitor infusion site; avoid extravasation. When given on a weekly (unlabeled) schedule, infusions were administered over ~30 minutes (Gradishar, 2009; Rizvi, 2008). When administered as part of a combination chemotherapy regimen, sequence of administration may vary by regimen; refer to specific protocol for sequence of administration. According to the manufacturer, paclitaxel (protein bound should be given first, followed immediately by carboplatin (NSCLC) or gemcitabine (pancreatic cancer).

Hazardous agent; use appropriate precautions for handling and disposal (NIOSH, 2012). ▶

◀ Nursing Actions

Physical Assessment Monitor for hypersensitivity reactions. Paclitaxel (protein bound) is not interchangeable with paclitaxel. Monitor for cardiovascular abnormalities, sensory neuropathy (numbness, tingling, burning pain), myelosuppression (anemia, opportunistic infection), and GI irritation (nausea, vomiting, mucositis, stomatitis) prior to, during, and between each infusion. Notify physician with any symptoms of fever, chills, cough, sore throat, or painful urination. Serious side effects, which require immediate attention, include jaw, left arm, or chest pain; coughing up blood; weakness on one side of the body; slurred speech; confusion; or severe headache. Educate patients about avoidance of certain vaccines (live vaccines) during treatment. Educate patient to use reliable forms of birth control while receiving this drug.

Patient Education
• Discuss specific use of drug and side effects with patient as it relates to treatment. (HCAHPS: During this hospital stay, were you given any medicine that you had not taken before? Before giving you any new medicine, how often did hospital staff tell you what the medicine was for? How often did hospital staff describe possible side effects in a way you could understand?)
• Patient may experience anemia, leukopenia, tachycardia, fatigue, stomatitis, edema, alopecia, nausea, diarrhea, paresthesia, myalgia, or arthralgia. Have patient report immediately to prescriber signs of infection, dyspnea, severe dyspepsia, angina, ecchymosis, bleeding, inability to eat, discolored urine, jaundice, or severe asthenia (HCAHPS).
• Educate patient about signs of a significant reaction (eg, wheezing; chest tightness; fever; itching; bad cough; blue skin color; seizures; or swelling of face, lips, tongue, or throat). **Note:** This is not a comprehensive list of all side effects. Patient should consult prescriber for additional questions.

Intended Use and Disclaimer: Should not be printed and given to patients. This information is intended to serve as a concise initial reference for healthcare professionals to use when discussing medications with a patient. You must ultimately rely on your own discretion, experience and judgment in diagnosing, treating and advising patients.

Related Information
Management of Drug Extravasations *on page 1700*

Paliperidone (pal ee PER i done)

Brand Names: U.S. Invega; Invega Sustenna
Index Terms 9-hydroxy-risperidone; 9-OH-risperidone; Paliperidone Palmitate

Pharmacologic Category Antipsychotic Agent, Atypical
Medication Safety Issues
BEERS Criteria medication:
This drug may be potentially inappropriate for use in geriatric patients (Quality of evidence - moderate; Strength of recommendation - strong).
Pregnancy Risk Factor C
Lactation Enters breast milk/not recommended
Breast-Feeding Considerations Paliperidone is excreted into breast milk. According to the manufacturer, the decision to continue or discontinue breast-feeding during therapy should take into account the risk of exposure to the infant and the benefits of treatment to the mother.
Use
Oral: Treatment of schizophrenia; acute treatment of schizoaffective disorder (monotherapy or adjunctive therapy to mood stabilizers and/or antidepressants)
Injection: Treatment of schizophrenia
Unlabeled Use Psychosis/agitation related to Alzheimer's dementia
Mechanism of Action/Effect Paliperidone is the primary active metabolite of risperidone. Mixed central serotonergic and dopaminergic antagonism is thought to improve negative symptoms of psychoses and reduce the incidence of extrapyramidal side effects.
Contraindications Hypersensitivity to paliperidone, risperidone, or any component of the formulation
Warnings/Precautions [U.S. Boxed Warning]: Elderly patients with dementia-related psychosis treated with antipsychotics are at an increased risk of death compared to placebo. Most deaths appeared to be either cardiovascular (eg, heart failure, sudden death) or infectious (eg, pneumonia) in nature. In addition, an increased incidence of cerebrovascular adverse effects (eg, transient ischemic attack, cerebrovascular accidents) has been reported in studies of placebo-controlled trials of risperidone (paliperidone is the primary active metabolite of risperidone) in elderly patients with dementia-related psychosis. Paliperidone is not approved for the treatment of dementia-related psychosis. In addition, patients with Lewy body dementia (LBD) may be more sensitive to CNS-related and extrapyramidal effects.

Compared with risperidone, paliperidone is low to moderately sedating; use with caution in disorders where CNS depression is a feature. Use caution in patients with predisposition to seizures. Use with caution in mild renal dysfunction; dose reduction recommended. Not recommended in patients with moderate-to-severe impairment. Esophageal dysmotility and aspiration have been associated with antipsychotic use; use with caution in patients at risk of aspiration pneumonia (eg, Alzheimer's disease).

Leukopenia, neutropenia, and agranulocytosis (sometimes fatal) have been reported in clinical trials and postmarketing reports with antipsychotic use; presence of risk factors (eg, pre-existing low WBC or history of drug-induced leuko-/neutropenia) should prompt periodic blood count assessment. Discontinue therapy at first signs of blood dyscrasias or if absolute neutrophil count <1000/mm^3.

Paliperidone is associated with increased prolactin levels; clinical significance of hyperprolactinemia in patients with breast cancer or other prolactin-dependent tumors is unknown. May alter temperature regulation. May mask toxicity of other drugs or conditions (eg, intestinal obstruction, Reye's syndrome, brain tumor) due to antiemetic effects. Priapism has been reported rarely with use.

May cause orthostasis and syncope. Use with caution in patients with cardiovascular diseases (eg, heart failure, history of myocardial infarction or ischemia, cerebrovascular disease, conduction abnormalities). Use caution in patients receiving medications for hypertension (orthostatic effects may be exacerbated) or in patients with hypovolemia or dehydration. May alter cardiac conduction; life-threatening arrhythmias have occurred with therapeutic doses of neuroleptics. Avoid use in combination with QT$_c$-prolonging drugs. Avoid use in patients with congenital long QT syndrome and in patients with history of cardiac arrhythmia.

May cause extrapyramidal symptoms (EPS), including pseudoparkinsonism, acute dystonic reactions, akathisia, and tardive dyskinesia (risk of these reactions is low relative to other neuroleptics, and is dose dependent). Risk of dystonia (and probably other EPS) may be greater with increased doses, use of conventional antipsychotics, males, and younger patients. Risk of neuroleptic malignant syndrome (NMS) may be increased in patients with Parkinson's disease or Lewy body dementia; monitor for symptoms of confusion, obtundation, postural instability and extrapyramidal symptoms. May cause hyperglycemia; in some cases may be extreme and associated with ketoacidosis, hyperosmolar coma, or death. Use with caution in patients with diabetes (or risk factors) or other disorders of glucose regulation; monitor for worsening of glucose control. Significant weight gain has been observed with antipsychotic therapy; incidence varies with product. Monitor waist circumference and BMI. May cause lipid abnormalities (LDL and triglycerides increased; HDL decreased). Few case reports describe intraoperative floppy iris syndrome (IFIS) in patients receiving risperidone and undergoing cataract surgery (Ford, 2011). IFIS has not been reported with paliperidone but caution is advised since it is the active metabolite of risperidone. Prior to cataract surgery, evaluate for prior or current paliperidone or risperidone use. The benefits or risks of interrupting paliperidone or risperidone prior to surgery have not been established; clinicians are advised to proceed with surgery cautiously.

The possibility of a suicide attempt is inherent in psychotic illness or bipolar disorder; use caution in high-risk patients during initiation of therapy. Prescriptions should be written for the smallest quantity consistent with good patient care.

Use in elderly patients with dementia is associated with an increased risk of mortality and cerebrovascular accidents; avoid antipsychotic use for behavioral problems associated with dementia unless alternative nonpharmacologic therapies have failed and patient may harm self or others. In addition, use may cause or exacerbate syndrome of inappropriate antidiuretic hormone secretion or hyponatremia; monitor sodium closely with initiation or dosage adjustments in older adults (Beers Criteria).

The tablet formulation consists of drug within a nonabsorbable shell that is expelled and may be visible in the stool. Use is not recommended in patients with pre-existing severe gastrointestinal narrowing disorders. Patients with upper GI tract alterations in transit time may have increased or decreased bioavailability of paliperidone. Do not use in patients unable to swallow the tablet whole.

Drug Interactions

Avoid Concomitant Use

Avoid concomitant use of Paliperidone with any of the following: Amisulpride; Azelastine (Nasal); Highest Risk QTc-Prolonging Agents; Ivabradine; Metoclopramide; Mifepristone; Moderate Risk QTc-Prolonging Agents; Paraldehyde; Sulpiride; Thalidomide

Decreased Effect

Paliperidone may decrease the levels/effects of: Amphetamines; Anti-Parkinson's Agents (Dopamine Agonist); Quinagolide

The levels/effects of Paliperidone may be decreased by: CarBAMazepine; Lithium formulations; P-glycoprotein/ABCB1 Inducers

Increased Effect/Toxicity

Paliperidone may increase the levels/effects of: Alcohol (Ethyl); Amisulpride; Azelastine (Nasal); Buprenorphine; CNS Depressants; Highest Risk QTc-Prolonging Agents; Hydrocodone; Methotrimeprazine; Methylphenidate; Paraldehyde; Serotonin Modulators; Sulpiride; Thalidomide; Zolpidem

The levels/effects of Paliperidone may be increased by: Acetylcholinesterase Inhibitors (Central); Brimonidine (Topical); Doxylamine; HydrOXYzine; Itraconazole; Ivabradine; Lithium formulations; Magnesium Sulfate; Methotrimeprazine; Methylphenidate; Metoclopramide; Metyrosine; Mifepristone; Moderate Risk QTc-Prolonging Agents; Perampanel; P-glycoprotein/ABCB1

Inhibitors; QTc-Prolonging Agents (Indeterminate Risk and Risk Modifying); RisperiDONE; Serotonin Modulators; Sodium Oxybate; Tetrabenazine; Valproic Acid and Derivatives

Nutritional/Ethanol Interactions
Ethanol: May increase CNS depression; monitor for increased effects with coadministration. Caution patients about effects.

Herb/Nutraceutical: Paliperidone may increase the serotonergic effect of St John's wort; use caution and monitor for serotonin toxicity or NMS during concomitant use. St John's wort is also a strong CYP3A4 inducer; dose of paliperidone may need to be increased when St John's wort is coadministered and decreased when St. John's wort is discontinued.

Adverse Reactions Unless otherwise noted, frequency of adverse effects is reported for the oral/I.M. formulation in adults.

>10%:
Cardiovascular: Tachycardia (1% to 14%)
Central nervous system: EPS (≤26%; dose dependent), insomnia (10% to 15%), headache (6% to 15%), parkinsonism (3% to 14%; dose dependent), somnolence (adolescents 9% to 26%; adults 1% to 12%; dose dependent)
Neuromuscular & skeletal: Tremor (2% to 12%)

3% to 10%:
Cardiovascular: Orthostatic hypotension (1% to 4%; dose dependent), bundle branch block (≤3%)
Central nervous system: Agitation (4% to 10%), akathisia (adolescents 4% to 17%; adults 1% to 10%; dose dependent), anxiety (adolescents ≤9%; adults 3% to 8%), dizziness (1% to 6%), dystonia (1% to 5%; dose dependent), dysarthria (1% to 4%; dose dependent), fatigue (adolescents ≤4%), sleep disorder (≤3%), lethargy (adolescents ≤3%)
Endocrine & metabolic: Amenorrhea (adolescents ≤6%), galactorrhea (adolescents ≤4%), gynecomastia (adolescents ≤3%)
Gastrointestinal: Weight gain (1% to 9%; dose dependent), nausea (2% to 8%), dyspepsia (5% to 6%), vomiting (adolescents ≤11%; adults 2% to 5%), constipation (1% to 5%), salivation increased (adolescents ≤6%; adults ≤4%; dose dependent), appetite increased (2% to 3%), toothache (1% to 3%), abdominal pain (≤3%), diarrhea (≤3%), xerostomia (≤3%); tongue swelling (adolescents ≤3%), tongue paralysis (adolescents ≤3%)
Local: I.M. formulation: Injection site reaction (≤10%)
Neuromuscular & skeletal: Hyperkinesia (2% to 10% dose dependent), dyskinesia (1% to 9%), weakness (≤4%), myalgia (≤4% dose dependent), back pain (1% to 3%), extremity pain (≤3%)
Ocular: Blurred vision (adolescents ≤3%)
Respiratory: Nasopharyngitis (≤5%; dose dependent), upper respiratory tract infection (1% to 4%), cough (≤3%; dose dependent), rhinitis (1% to 3%; dose dependent)

Available Dosage Forms
Suspension, Intramuscular:
Invega Sustenna: 39 mg/0.25 mL (0.25 mL); 78 mg/0.5 mL (0.5 mL); 117 mg/0.75 mL (0.75 mL); 156 mg/mL (1 mL); 234 mg/1.5 mL (1.5 mL)

Tablet Extended Release 24 Hour, Oral:
Invega: 1.5 mg, 3 mg, 6 mg, 9 mg

General Dosage Range Dosage adjustment recommended in patients with renal impairment
I.M.: *Adults:* Initial: 234 mg, then 156 mg 1 week later; Maintenance: 39-234 mg monthly
Oral: *Adolescents 12-17 years and Adults:* 3-12 mg once daily (maximum: 12 mg daily)

Administration
I.M. Invega® Sustenna™ should be administered by I.M. route only as a single injection (do not divide); do not administer I.V. or subcutaneously. Avoid inadvertent injection into vasculature. Prior to injection, shake syringe for at least 10 seconds to ensure a homogenous suspension. The 2 initial injections should be administered in the deltoid muscle using a 1½ inch, 22-gauge needle for patients ≥90 kg, and a 1 inch, 23-gauge needle for patients <90 kg. The 2 initial deltoid intramuscular injections help attain therapeutic concentrations rapidly. Alternate deltoid injections (right and left deltoid muscle). The second dose may be administered 4 days before or after the weekly time point (Canadian labeling suggests the second dose may be administered 2 days before or after the weekly time point). Monthly maintenance doses can be administered in either the deltoid or gluteal muscle. Administer injections in the gluteal muscle using a 1½ inch, 22-gauge needle in the upper-outer quadrant of the gluteal area. Alternate gluteal injections (right and left gluteal muscle). The monthly maintenance dose may be administered 7 days before or after the monthly time point.
I.V. Do not administer I.V. or SubQ.
Oral Administer in the morning without regard to meals. Extended release tablets should be swallowed whole with liquids; do not crush, chew, or divide.

Storage/Stability Store at controlled room temperature of ≤25°C (77°F); excursions permitted to 15°C to 30°C (59°F to 86°F). Protect tablets from moisture.

Nursing Actions
Physical Assessment Educate patient about increased risk for weight gain; monitor weight and BMI regularly. Educate regarding healthy food choices and exercise. Monitor lab work, particularly in those with existing diabetes. Educate about possible orthostasis and the need to keep well-hydrated and make position changes slowly if dizziness occurs. Monitor for development of EPS anytime during treatment. Ongoing

monitoring of mental status and response to medication is important.

Patient Education
- Discuss specific use of drug and side effects with patient as it relates to treatment. (HCAHPS: During this hospital stay, were you given any medicine that you had not taken before? Before giving you any new medicine, how often did hospital staff tell you what the medicine was for? How often did hospital staff describe possible side effects in a way you could understand?)
- Patient may experience tablet shell in stool, presyncope, asthenia, blurred vision, illogical thinking, dizziness, hyperglycemia, headache, weight gain, nervousness, anxiety, insomnia, or application site irritation. Have patient report immediately to prescriber angina, tachycardia, significant change in balance, tremors, polyuria, polydipsia, weight loss, erection lasting >4 hours, pregnancy, or rash (HCAHPS).
- Educate patient about signs of a significant reaction (eg, wheezing; chest tightness; fever; itching; bad cough; blue skin color; seizures; or swelling of face, lips, tongue, or throat). **Note:** This is not a comprehensive list of all side effects. Patient should consult prescriber for additional questions.

Intended Use and Disclaimer: Should not be printed and given to patients. This information is intended to serve as a concise initial reference for healthcare professionals to use when discussing medications with a patient. You must ultimately rely on your own discretion, experience and judgment in diagnosing, treating and advising patients.

Dietary Considerations May be taken without regard to meals.

Related Information
Oral Medications That Should Not Be Crushed or Altered on page 1712

Palonosetron (pal oh NOE se tron)

Brand Names: U.S. Aloxi

Index Terms Palonosetron Hydrochloride; RS-25259; RS-25259-197

Pharmacologic Category Antiemetic; Selective 5-HT$_3$ Receptor Antagonist

Medication Safety Issues
Sound-alike/look-alike issues:
Aloxi® may be confused with Eloxatin®, oxaliplatin
Palonosetron may be confused with dolasetron, granisetron, ondansetron

Pregnancy Risk Factor B

Lactation Excretion in breast milk unknown/not recommended

Breast-Feeding Considerations The extent to which palonosetron is excreted in breast milk, if at all, is unknown. Due to the potential for adverse effects in the nursing infant, breast-feeding is not recommended.

Use Prevention of chemotherapy-associated nausea and vomiting; indicated for prevention of acute (highly-emetogenic therapy) as well as acute and delayed (moderately-emetogenic therapy) nausea and vomiting; prevention of postoperative nausea and vomiting (PONV)

Mechanism of Action/Effect Selective 5-HT$_3$ receptor antagonist, blocking serotonin, both on vagal nerve terminals in the periphery and centrally in the chemoreceptor trigger zone

Contraindications Hypersensitivity to palonosetron or any component of the formulation

Warnings/Precautions Hypersensitivity has been observed rarely with I.V. palonosetron. Use caution in patients allergic to other 5-HT$_3$ receptor antagonists; cross-reactivity is possible. Some selective 5-HT$_3$ receptor antagonists have been associated with dose-dependent increases in ECG intervals (eg, PR, QRS duration, QT/QT$_c$, JT), usually occurring 1-2 hours after I.V. administration. In general, these changes are not clinically relevant, however, when these agents are used in conjunction with other agents that prolong these intervals, arrhythmia may occur. When used with agents that prolong the QT interval (eg, Class I and III antiarrhythmics), clinically relevant QT interval prolongation could result in torsade de pointes. A number of trials have shown that 5-HT$_3$ antagonists produce QT interval prolongation to variable degrees. Use with caution in patients at risk of QT prolongation and/or ventricular arrhythmia. Reduction in heart rate may also occur with the 5-HT$_3$ antagonists. Use with caution in patients with congenital long QT syndrome or other risk factors for QT prolongation (eg, medications known to prolong QT interval, electrolyte abnormalities, and cumulative high dose anthracycline therapy).

Not intended for treatment of nausea and vomiting or for chronic continuous therapy. **For chemotherapy, should be used on a scheduled basis, not on an "as needed" (PRN) basis,** since data support the use of this drug only in the prevention of nausea and vomiting (due to antineoplastic therapy) and not in the rescue of nausea and vomiting. For PONV, may use for low expectation of PONV if it is essential to avoid nausea and vomiting in the postoperative period; use is not recommended if there is little expectation of nausea and vomiting.

Drug Interactions
Avoid Concomitant Use
Avoid concomitant use of Palonosetron with any of the following: Apomorphine

Decreased Effect
Palonosetron may decrease the levels/effects of: Tapentadol; TraMADol

The levels/effects of Palonosetron may be decreased by: Peginterferon Alfa-2b

Increased Effect/Toxicity

Palonosetron may increase the levels/effects of:
Apomorphine

Adverse Reactions Adverse events may vary according to indication.

1% to 10%:

Cardiovascular: QT prolongation (chemotherapy-associated <1%; PONV 1% to 5%), bradycardia (chemotherapy-associated 1%; PONV 4%), hypotension (≤1%), sinus bradycardia (≤1%), tachycardia (nonsustained) (≤1%)

Central nervous system: Headache (chemotherapy-associated 5% to 9%; PONV 3%), anxiety (1%), dizziness (≤1%)

Dermatologic: Pruritus (≤1%)

Endocrine & metabolic: Hyperkalemia (1%)

Gastrointestinal: Constipation (2% to 5%), diarrhea (≤1%), flatulence (≤1%)

Genitourinary: Urinary retention (≤1%)

Hepatic: ALT increased (≤1%; transient), AST increased (≤1%; transient)

Neuromuscular & skeletal: Weakness (1%)

Available Dosage Forms

Solution, Intravenous:

Aloxi: 0.25 mg/5 mL (5 mL)

General Dosage Range I.V.: *Adults:* 0.25 mg or 0.075 mg as a single dose

Administration

I.V. Flush I.V. line with NS prior to and following administration.

Chemotherapy-associated nausea and vomiting: Infuse over 30 seconds, 30 minutes prior to the start of chemotherapy

PONV: Infuse over 10 seconds immediately prior to anesthesia induction

Injectable Detail pH: 4.5-5.5

Storage/Stability Store intact vials at room temperature of 20°C to 25°C (68°F to 77°F); excursions permitted to 15°C to 30°C (59°F to 86°F); do not freeze. Protect from light. Solutions of 5 mcg/mL and 30 mcg/mL in NS, D_5W, $D_5^{1/2}NS$, and D_5LR injection are stable for 48 hours at room temperature and 14 days under refrigeration (Trissel, 2004).

Nursing Actions

Physical Assessment Allergy history to selective 5-HT$_3$ receptor antagonists should be assessed prior to administering. Assess other drugs patient may be taking that may prolong QT interval. To be used on a scheduled basis for prevention of nausea and vomiting associated with cancer chemotherapy and postoperative nausea and vomiting; not recommended for treatment of existing chemotherapy-induced emesis. I.V.: Follow infusion specifics.

Patient Education

• Discuss specific use of drug and side effects with patient as it relates to treatment. (HCAHPS: During this hospital stay, were you given any medicine that you had not taken before? Before giving you any new medicine, how often did hospital staff tell you what the medicine was for? How often did hospital staff describe possible side effects in a way you could understand?)

• Patient may experience headache, constipation, or injection site irritation. Have patient report immediately to prescriber illogical thinking, tachycardia, severe asthenia, or rash (HCAHPS).

• Educate patient about signs of a significant reaction (eg, wheezing; chest tightness; fever; itching; bad cough; blue skin color; seizures; or swelling of face, lips, tongue, or throat). **Note:** This is not a comprehensive list of all side effects. Patient should consult prescriber for additional questions.

Intended Use and Disclaimer: Should not be printed and given to patients. This information is intended to serve as a concise initial reference for healthcare professionals to use when discussing medications with a patient. You must ultimately rely on your own discretion, experience and judgment in diagnosing, treating and advising patients.

Pamidronate (pa mi DROE nate)

Index Terms Pamidronate Disodium

Pharmacologic Category Bisphosphonate Derivative

Medication Safety Issues

Sound-alike/look-alike issues:

Aredia® may be confused with Adriamycin®

Pamidronate may be confused with papaverine

Pregnancy Risk Factor D

Lactation Excretion in breast milk unknown/not recommended

Breast-Feeding Considerations It is not known if pamidronate is excreted into breast milk. Pamidronate was not detected in the milk of a nursing woman receiving pamidronate 30 mg I.V. monthly (therapy started ~6 months postpartum). Following the first infusion, milk was pumped and collected for 0-24 hours and 25-48 hours, and each day pooled for analysis. Pamidronate readings were below the limit of quantification (<0.4 micromole/L). During therapy, breast milk was pumped and discarded for the first 48 hours following each infusion prior to resuming nursing. The infant was breast-fed >80% of the time; adverse events were not observed in the nursing infant (Simonoski, 2000). Monitoring the serum calcium concentrations of nursing infants is recommended (Stathopoulos, 2011). Due to the potential for serious adverse reactions in the nursing infant, the manufacturer recommends a decision be made whether to discontinue nursing or to discontinue the drug, taking into account the importance of treatment to the mother.

Use Treatment of moderate or severe hypercalcemia associated with malignancy (in conjunction with adequate hydration) with or without bone metastases; treatment of osteolytic bone lesions associated with multiple myeloma or metastatic breast cancer; moderate-to-severe Paget's disease of bone

Unlabeled Use Treatment of osteogenesis imperfecta; treatment of symptomatic bone metastases of thyroid cancer; prevention of bone loss associated with androgen deprivation treatment in prostate cancer

Mechanism of Action/Effect Nitrogen-containing bisphosphonate; inhibits bone resorption and decreases mineralization by disrupting osteoclast activity (Gralow, 2009; Rogers, 2011)

Contraindications Hypersensitivity to pamidronate, other bisphosphonates, or any component of the formulation

Warnings/Precautions Hazardous agent - use appropriate precautions for handling and disposal (meets NIOSH, 2012 criteria). Osteonecrosis of the jaw (ONJ) has been reported in patients receiving bisphosphonates. Risk factors include invasive dental procedures (eg, tooth extraction, dental implants, boney surgery); a diagnosis of cancer, with concomitant chemotherapy, radiotherapy, or corticosteroids; poor oral hygiene, ill-fitting dentures; and comorbid disorders (anemia, coagulopathy, infection, pre-existing dental disease). Most reported cases occurred after I.V. bisphosphonate therapy; however, cases have been reported following oral therapy. A dental exam and preventative dentistry should be performed prior to placing patients with risk factors on chronic bisphosphonate therapy. There is no evidence that discontinuing therapy reduces the risk of developing ONJ (Assael, 2009). The benefit/risk must be assessed by the treating physician and/or dentist/surgeon prior to any invasive dental procedure. Patients developing ONJ while on bisphosphonates should receive care by an oral surgeon.

Atypical femur fractures (after minimal or no trauma) have been reported. The fractures include subtrochanteric femur (bone just below the hip joint) and diaphyseal femur (long segment of the thigh bone). Some patients experience prodromal pain weeks or months before the fracture occurs. It is unclear if bisphosphonate therapy is the cause for these fractures. Patients receiving long-term (>3-5 years) bisphosphonate therapy may be at an increased risk. Consider discontinuing pamidronate in patients with a suspected femoral shaft fracture. Patients who present with thigh or groin pain in the absence of trauma should be evaluated. Infrequently, severe (and occasionally debilitating) musculoskeletal (bone, joint, and/or muscle) pain have been reported during bisphosphonate treatment. The onset of pain ranged from a single day to several months. Consider discontinuing therapy in patients who experience severe symptoms; symptoms usually resolve upon discontinuation.

Some patients experienced recurrence when rechallenged with same drug or another bisphosphonate; avoid use in patients with a history of these symptoms in association with bisphosphonate therapy.

Initial or single doses have been associated with renal deterioration, progressing to renal failure and dialysis. Withhold pamidronate treatment (until renal function returns to baseline) in patients with evidence of renal deterioration. Glomerulosclerosis (focal segmental) with or without nephrotic syndrome has also been reported. Longer infusion times (>2 hours) may reduce the risk for renal toxicity, especially in patients with pre-existing renal insufficiency. Single pamidronate doses should not exceed 90 mg. Patients with serum creatinine >3 mg/dL were not studied in clinical trials; limited data are available in patients with CrCl <30 mL/minute. Evaluate serum creatinine prior to each treatment. For the treatment of bone metastases, use is not recommended in patients with severe renal impairment; for renal impairment in indications other than bone metastases, use clinical judgment to determine if benefits outweigh potential risks.

Use has been associated with asymptomatic electrolyte abnormalities (including hypophosphatemia, hypokalemia, hypomagnesemia, and hypocalcemia). Rare cases of symptomatic hypocalcemia, including tetany have been reported. Patients with a history of thyroid surgery may have relative hypoparathyroidism; predisposing them to pamidronate-related hypocalcemia. Patients with pre-existing anemia, leukopenia, or thrombocytopenia should be closely monitored during the first 2 weeks of treatment.

Multiple myeloma: According to the American Society of Clinical Oncology (ASCO) guidelines for bisphosphonates in multiple myeloma, treatment with pamidronate is not recommended for asymptomatic (smoldering) or indolent myeloma or with solitary plasmacytoma (Kyle, 2007). The National Comprehensive Cancer Network® (NCCN) multiple myeloma guidelines (v.2.2013) recommend bisphosphonates for all patients receiving treatment for symptomatic disease; the use of bisphosphonates in stage 1 or smoldering disease may be considered, although preferably as part of a clinical trial. Patients with Bence-Jones proteinuria and dehydration should be adequately hydrated prior to therapy.

Hypercalcemia of malignancy (HCM): Adequate hydration is required during treatment (urine output ~2 L/day); avoid overhydration, especially in patients with heart failure.

Drug Interactions

Avoid Concomitant Use There are no known interactions where it is recommended to avoid concomitant use.

Decreased Effect

The levels/effects of Pamidronate may be decreased by: Proton Pump Inhibitors

Increased Effect/Toxicity

Pamidronate may increase the levels/effects of: Deferasirox; Phosphate Supplements

The levels/effects of Pamidronate may be increased by: Aminoglycosides; Nonsteroidal Anti-Inflammatory Agents; Systemic Angiogenesis Inhibitors; Thalidomide

Adverse Reactions Note: Actual percentages may vary by indication; treatment for multiple myeloma is associated with higher percentage.

>10%:

Central nervous system: Fever (18% to 39%; transient), fatigue (≤37%), headache (≤26%), insomnia (≤22%)

Endocrine & metabolic: Hypophosphatemia (≤18%), hypokalemia (4% to 18%), hypomagnesemia (4% to 12%), hypocalcemia (≤12%)

Gastrointestinal: Nausea (≤54%), vomiting (≤36%), anorexia (≤26%), abdominal pain (≤23%), dyspepsia (≤23%)

Genitourinary: Urinary tract infection (≤19%)

Hematologic: Anemia (≤43%), granulocytopenia (≤20%)

Local: Infusion site reaction (≤18%; includes induration, pain, redness and swelling)

Neuromuscular & skeletal: Myalgia (≤26%), weakness (≤22%), arthralgia (≤14%), osteonecrosis of the jaw (cancer patients: 1% to 11%)

Renal: Serum creatinine increased (≤19%)

Respiratory: Dyspnea (≤30%), cough (≤26%), upper respiratory tract infection (≤24%), sinusitis (≤16%), pleural effusion (≤11%)

1% to 10%:

Cardiovascular: Atrial fibrillation (≤6%), hypertension (≤6%), syncope (≤6%), tachycardia (≤6%), atrial flutter (≤1%), cardiac failure (≤1%), edema (≤1%)

Central nervous system: Somnolence (≤6%), psychosis (≤4%), seizure (≤2%)

Endocrine & metabolic: Hypothyroidism (≤6%)

Gastrointestinal: Constipation (≤6%), gastrointestinal hemorrhage (≤6%), diarrhea (≤1%), stomatitis (≤1%)

Hematologic: Leukopenia (≤4%), neutropenia (≤1%), thrombocytopenia (≤1%)

Neuromuscular & skeletal: Back pain, bone pain

Renal: Uremia (≤4%)

Respiratory: Rales (≤6%), rhinitis (≤6%)

Miscellaneous: Moniliasis (≤6%)

Pharmacodynamics/Kinetics

Onset of Action

Hypercalcemia of malignancy (HCM): ≤24 hours for decrease in albumin-corrected serum calcium; maximum effect: ≤7 days

Paget's disease: ~1 month for ≥50% decrease in serum alkaline phosphatase

Duration of Action HCM: 7-14 days; Paget's disease: 1-372 days

Available Dosage Forms

Solution, Intravenous:

Generic: 30 mg/10 mL (10 mL); 90 mg/10 mL (10 mL)

Solution, Intravenous [preservative free]:

Generic: 30 mg/10 mL (10 mL); 6 mg/mL (10 mL); 90 mg/10 mL (10 mL)

Solution Reconstituted, Intravenous:

Generic: 30 mg (1 ea); 90 mg (1 ea)

General Dosage Range Dosage adjustment recommended in patients with renal impairment

I.V.: *Adults:* 60-90 mg as a single dose, may repeat every 3-4 weeks **or** 30 mg daily for 3 consecutive days

Administration

I.V. Infusion rate varies by indication. Longer infusion times (>2 hours) may reduce the risk for renal toxicity, especially in patients with pre-existing renal insufficiency. The manufacturer recommends infusing over 2-24 hours for hypercalcemia of malignancy; over 2 hours for osteolytic bone lesions with metastatic breast cancer; and over 4 hours for Paget's disease and for osteolytic bone lesions with multiple myeloma. The ASCO guidelines for bisphosphonate use in multiple myeloma recommend infusing pamidronate over at least 2 hours; if therapy is withheld due to renal toxicity, infuse over at least 4 hours upon reintroduction of treatment after renal recovery (Kyle, 2007).

Hazardous agent; use appropriate precautions for handling and disposal (meets NIOSH, 2012 criteria).

Injectable Detail pH: 6-7.4 (reconstituted solution)

Preparation for Administration Hazardous agent; use appropriate precautions for handling and disposal (meets NIOSH, 2012 criteria).

Powder for injection: Reconstitute by adding 10 mL of SWFI to each vial of lyophilized pamidronate disodium powder, the resulting solution will be 30 mg/10 mL or 90 mg/10 mL.

Pamidronate may be further diluted in 250-1000 mL of 0.45% or 0.9% sodium chloride or 5% dextrose. (The manufacturer recommends dilution in 1000 mL for hypercalcemia of malignancy, 500 mL for Paget's disease and bone metastases of myeloma, and 250 mL for bone metastases of breast cancer.)

Storage/Stability

Powder for reconstitution: Store at or below 30°C (86°F). The reconstituted solution is stable for 24 hours stored under refrigeration at 2°C to 8°C (36°F to 46°F).

Solution for injection: Store at 20°C to 25°C (68°F to 77°F).

Pamidronate solution for infusion is stable at room temperature for up to 24 hours.

Nursing Actions

Physical Assessment Educate patient about the importance of dental care and regular dental exams. Check results of laboratory monitoring (serum creatinine, calcium, phosphate, magnesium, potassium, and CBC with differential).

Patient Education
- Discuss specific use of drug and side effects with patient as it relates to treatment. (HCAHPS: During this hospital stay, were you given any medicine that you had not taken before? Before giving you any new medicine, how often did hospital staff tell you what the medicine was for? How often did hospital staff describe possible side effects in a way you could understand?)
- Patient may experience nausea, injection site irritation, lack of appetite, headache, insomnia, rhinorrhea, anemia, hypophosphatemia, asthenia, arthralgia, myalgia, or osteodynia. Have patient report immediately to prescriber signs of infection; angina; urinary retention; severe jaw, groin, or thigh pain; or rash (HCAHPS).
- Educate patient about signs of a significant reaction (eg, wheezing; chest tightness; fever; itching; bad cough; blue skin color; seizures; or swelling of face, lips, tongue, or throat). **Note:** This is not a comprehensive list of all side effects. Patient should consult prescriber for additional questions.

Intended Use and Disclaimer: Should not be printed and given to patients. This information is intended to serve as a concise initial reference for healthcare professionals to use when discussing medications with a patient. You must ultimately rely on your own discretion, experience and judgment in diagnosing, treating and advising patients.

Dietary Considerations Multiple myeloma or metastatic bone lesions from solid tumors or Paget's disease: Take adequate daily calcium and vitamin D supplement (if patient is not hypercalcemic).

Pancrelipase (pan kre LYE pase)

Brand Names: U.S. Creon; Pancreaze; Pancrelipase (Lip-Prot-Amyl); Pertzye; Ultresa; Viokace; Zenpep

Index Terms Amylase, Lipase, and Protease; Lipancreatin; Lipase, Protease, and Amylase; Pancreatic Enzymes; Protease, Lipase, and Amylase

Pharmacologic Category Enzyme

Medication Safety Issues

Sound-alike/look-alike issues:

Pancrelipase may be confused with pancreatin

Medication Guide Available Yes

Pregnancy Risk Factor C

Lactation Excretion in breast milk unknown/use caution

Use Treatment of exocrine pancreatic insufficiency (EPI) due to conditions such as cystic fibrosis (Creon, Pancreaze, Pertzye, Ultresa, Zenpep); chronic pancreatitis (Creon, Viokace); or pancreatectomy (Creon, Viokace)

Note: Viokace must be administered with a proton pump inhibitor (PPI) since it is not enteric coated.

Available Dosage Forms

Capsule, delayed release, bicarbonate buffered enteric coated microspheres, oral [porcine derived]:

Pertzye: Lipase 8,000 USP units, protease 28,750 USP units, and amylase 30,250 USP units

Pertzye: Lipase 16,000 USP units, protease 57,500 USP units, and amylase 60,500 USP units

Capsule, delayed release, enteric coated beads, oral [porcine derived]:

Pancrelipase (Lip-Prot-Amyl): Lipase 5000 USP units, protease 17,000 USP units, and amylase 27,000 USP units

Zenpep: Lipase 3000 USP units, protease 10,000 USP units, and amylase 16,000 USP units

Zenpep: Lipase 5000 USP units, protease 17,000 USP units, and amylase 27,000 USP units

Zenpep: Lipase 10,000 USP units, protease 34,000 USP units, and amylase 55,000 USP units

Zenpep: Lipase 15,000 USP units, protease 51,000 USP units, and amylase 82,000 USP units

Zenpep: Lipase 20,000 USP units, protease 68,000 USP units, and amylase 109,000 USP units

Zenpep: Lipase 25,000 USP units, protease 85,000 USP units, and amylase 136,000 USP units

Capsule, delayed release, enteric coated microspheres, oral [porcine derived]:

Creon: Lipase 3000 USP units, protease 9500 USP units, and amylase 15,000 USP units

Creon: Lipase 6000 USP units, protease 19,000 USP units, and amylase 30,000 USP units

Creon: Lipase 12,000 USP units, protease 38,000 USP units, and amylase 60,000 USP units

Creon: Lipase 24,000 USP units, protease 76,000 USP units, and amylase 120,000 USP units

Creon: Lipase 36,000 USP units, protease 114,000 USP units, and amylase 180,000 USP units

Capsule, delayed release, enteric coated microtablets, oral [porcine derived]:

Pancreaze: Lipase 4200 USP units, protease 10,000 USP units, and amylase 17,500 USP units

Pancreaze: Lipase 10,500 USP units, protease 25,000 USP units, and amylase 43,750 USP units

Pancreaze: Lipase 16,800 USP units, protease 40,000 USP units, and amylase 70,000 USP units

Pancreaze: Lipase 21,000 USP units, protease 37,000 USP units, and amylase 61,000 USP units

Capsule, delayed release, enteric coated mini-tablets, oral [porcine derived]:

Ultresa: Lipase 13,800 USP units, protease 27,600 USP units, and amylase 27,600 USP units

Ultresa: Lipase 20,700 USP units, protease 41,400 USP units, and amylase 41,400 USP units

Ultresa: Lipase 23,000 USP units, protease 46,000 USP units, and amylase 46,000 USP units

Tablet, oral [porcine derived]:

Viokace: Lipase 10,440 USP units, protease 39,150 USP units, and amylase 39,150 USP units

Viokace: Lipase 20,880 USP units, protease 78,300 USP units, and amylase 78,300 USP units

General Dosage Range Oral:

Infants ≤1 year: Lipase 2000-4000 units per 120 mL of formula or per breast-feeding

Children >1 and <4 years: Lipase 1000-2500 units/kg/meal; Maximum: Lipase ≤2500 units/kg/**meal or** lipase ≤10,000 units/kg/**day or** lipase <4000 units/g of fat daily

Children ≥4 years, Adolescents, and Adults: Lipase 500-2500 units/kg/meal **or** lipase 72,000 units/meal (while consuming ≥100 g of fat per day); Maximum: Lipase ≤2500 units/kg/**meal or** lipase ≤10,000 units/kg/**day or** lipase <4000 units/g of fat daily

Administration

Oral Administer with meals or snacks and swallow whole with a generous amount of liquid. Do not crush or chew; retention in the mouth before swallowing may cause mucosal irritation and stomatitis.

Capsules, delayed release: If necessary, capsules may also be opened and contents added to a small amount of an acidic food (pH ≤4.5), such as applesauce. The food should be at room temperature and swallowed immediately after mixing. The contents of the capsule should not be crushed or chewed. Follow with water or juice to ensure complete ingestion and that no medication remains in the mouth.

When administering to infants <1 year of age, do not mix with breast milk or infant formula. Open capsule and place the contents directly into the mouth or mix with a small amount of acidic soft food (pH ≤4.5), such as applesauce or other acidic commercially prepared baby food (pears or bananas) at room temperature. Administer immediately after mixing (or within 15 minutes of mixing using Pancreaze). Follow with infant formula or breast milk to ensure complete ingestion and that no medication remains in the mouth.

Tablets: Viokace: Tablets are not enteric coated and should be taken with a proton pump inhibitor.

Other Administration via gastrostomy (G) tube: An *in vitro* study demonstrated that Creon delayed-release capsules sprinkled onto a small amount of baby food (pH <4.5; applesauce or bananas manufactured by both Gerber and Beech-Nut) stirred gently and after 15 minutes was administered through the following G-tubes without significant loss of lipase activity: Kimberly-Clark MIC Bolus size 18 Fr, Kimberly-Clark MIC-KEY size 16 Fr, Bard Tri-Funnel size 18 Fr, and Bard Button size 18 Fr (Shlieout, 2011).

Nursing Actions

Physical Assessment Dosing and administration depend on purpose for use and formulation (available products are not interchangeable).

Patient Education

• Discuss specific use of drug and side effects with patient as it relates to treatment. (HCAHPS: During this hospital stay, were you given any medicine that you had not taken before? Before giving you any new medicine, how often did hospital staff tell you what the medicine was for? How often did hospital staff describe possible side effects in a way you could understand?)

• Patient may experience dizziness, dyspepsia, headache, flatulence, nausea, or diarrhea. Have patient report immediately to prescriber dyspnea, severe constipation, significant arthralgia, or rash (HCAHPS).

• Educate patient about signs of a significant reaction (eg, wheezing; chest tightness; fever; itching; bad cough; blue skin color; seizures; or swelling of face, lips, tongue, or throat). **Note:** This is not a comprehensive list of all side effects. Patient should consult prescriber for additional questions.

Intended Use and Disclaimer: Should not be printed and given to patients. This information is intended to serve as a concise initial reference for healthcare professionals to use when discussing medications with a patient. You must ultimately rely on your own discretion, experience and judgment in diagnosing, treating and advising patients.

Related Information

Oral Medications That Should Not Be Crushed or Altered *on page 1712*

Pancuronium (pan kyoo ROE nee um)

Index Terms Pancuronium Bromide; Pavulon [DSC]

Pharmacologic Category Neuromuscular Blocker Agent, Nondepolarizing

Medication Safety Issues

High alert medication:

The Institute for Safe Medication Practices (ISMP) includes this medication among its list of drugs which have a heightened risk of causing significant patient harm when used in error.

Other safety concerns:

United States Pharmacopeia (USP) 2006: The Interdisciplinary Safe Medication Use Expert Committee of the USP has recommended the following:

- Hospitals, clinics, and other practice sites should institute special safeguards in the storage, labeling, and use of these agents and should include these safeguards in staff orientation and competency training.
- Healthcare professionals should be on high alert (especially vigilant) whenever a neuromuscular-blocking agent (NMBA) is stocked, ordered, prepared, or administered.

Pregnancy Risk Factor C

Use Facilitation of endotracheal intubation and relaxation of skeletal muscles during surgery; facilitation of mechanical ventilation in ICU patients; does not relieve pain or produce sedation

Available Dosage Forms

Solution, Intravenous:

Generic: 1 mg/mL (10 mL); 2 mg/mL (2 mL, 5 mL)

General Dosage Range Dosage adjustment recommended in patients with renal impairment

I.V.: *Children >1 month and Adults:*

ICU paralysis: 0.06-0.1 mg/kg bolus followed by 1-2 **mcg**/kg/**minute** infusion **or** 0.1-0.2 mg/kg every 1-3 hours

Surgery: Intubation: Initial: 0.06-1 mg/kg **or** 0.05 mg/kg after succinylcholine; Maintenance: 0.01 mg/kg administered 60-100 minutes after initial dose and then every 25-60 minutes

Administration

I.V. May be administered undiluted by rapid I.V. injection.

Injectable Detail pH: 4 (adjusted)

Nursing Actions

Physical Assessment Ventilatory support must be instituted and maintained until adequate respiratory muscle function and/or airway protection are assured. This drug is not an anesthetic or analgesic; pain must be treated with other agents. Continuous monitoring of vital signs, cardiac status, respiratory status, and degree of neuromuscular block (objective assessment with peripheral external nerve stimulator) is mandatory until full muscle tone has returned. It may take longer for return of muscle tone in obese or elderly patients or patients with renal or hepatic disease, myasthenia gravis, myopathy, other neuromuscular disease, dehydration, electrolyte imbalance, or severe acid/base imbalance.

Long-term use: Monitor level of neuromuscular blockade, skeletal muscle movement, and

respiratory effort. Reposition patient and provide appropriate skin care, mouth care, and care of patient's eyes every 2-3 hours while sedated. Provide appropriate emotional and sensory support (auditory and environmental).

Patient Education

- Discuss specific use of drug and side effects with patient as it relates to treatment. (HCAHPS: During this hospital stay, were you given any medicine that you had not taken before? Before giving you any new medicine, how often did hospital staff tell you what the medicine was for? How often did hospital staff describe possible side effects in a way you could understand?)
- Patient may experience dizziness or flushing. Have patient report immediately to prescriber tachycardia or rash (HCAHPS).
- Educate patient about signs of a significant reaction (eg, wheezing; chest tightness; fever; itching; bad cough; blue skin color; seizures; or swelling of face, lips, tongue, or throat). **Note:** This is not a comprehensive list of all side effects. Patient should consult prescriber for additional questions.

Intended Use and Disclaimer: Should not be printed and given to patients. This information is intended to serve as a concise initial reference for healthcare professionals to use when discussing medications with a patient. You must ultimately rely on your own discretion, experience and judgment in diagnosing, treating and advising patients.

Panitumumab (pan i TOOM yoo mab)

Brand Names: U.S. Vectibix

Index Terms ABX-EGF; MOAB ABX-EGF; Monoclonal Antibody ABX-EGF; rHuMAb-EGFr

Pharmacologic Category Antineoplastic Agent, Epidermal Growth Factor Receptor (EGFR) Inhibitor; Antineoplastic Agent, Monoclonal Antibody

Medication Safety Issues

Sound-alike/look-alike issues:

Panitumumab may be confused with pertuzumab

Pregnancy Risk Factor C

Lactation Excretion in breast milk unknown/not recommended

Use

Colorectal cancer: As a single agent for the treatment of EGFR-expressing metastatic colorectal carcinoma (mCRC) with disease progression on or following fluoropyrimidine-, oxaliplatin-, and irinotecan-containing chemotherapy regimens.

Limitations of use: Panitumumab is not indicated for the treatment of patients with *KRAS* mutation-positive mCRC or for whom *KRAS* mCRC status is unknown. Retrospective subset analyses of mCRC trials have not shown a treatment benefit for panitumumab in patients whose tumors had *KRAS* mutations in codon 12 or 13. Panitumumab in combination with oxaliplatin-based chemotherapy is not indicated for the treatment of patients with *RAS* (*KRAS* or *NRAS*) mutation-positive mCRC or for whom *RAS* status is unknown.

Unlabeled Use Treatment of metastatic colorectal cancer (KRAS wild-type) in combination with other chemotherapy agents

Available Dosage Forms

Solution, Intravenous [preservative free]:

Vectibix: 100 mg/5 mL (5 mL); 400 mg/20 mL (20 mL)

General Dosage Range Dosage adjustment recommended in patients who develop toxicities

I.V.: *Adults:* 6 mg/kg every 14 days

Administration

I.V. Doses ≤1000 mg, infuse over 1 hour; doses >1000 mg, infuse over 90 minutes (via infusion pump); do not administer I.V. push or as a bolus. Administer through a low protein-binding 0.2 or 0.22 micrometer in-line filter. Flush line with NS before and after infusion. Reduce infusion rate by 50% for mild-to-moderate infusion reactions (grades 1 and 2); stop infusion for severe infusion reactions (grades 3 and 4) and consider permanent discontinuation.

Injectable Detail pH: 5.6-6 (liquid for intravenous injection)

Nursing Actions

Physical Assessment Monitor patient closely during and following infusion for infusion reaction; appropriate medical support for the management of infusion reactions should be readily available. Infusion reactions may include dyspnea, shortness of breath, wheezing, chest tightness, or bronchospasm. Other reactions include hives, itching, and rash; nausea/vomiting; and dizziness. Monitor for severe skin reactions which include blistering, peeling, or burning, peripheral edema, and gastrointestinal upset (pain, nausea, diarrhea, constipation, vomiting) at each infusion and throughout therapy. Instruct patient to use appropriate sunscreen and protective clothing.

Patient Education

• Discuss specific use of drug and side effects with patient as it relates to treatment. (HCAHPS: During this hospital stay, were you given any medicine that you had not taken before? Before giving you any new medicine, how often did hospital staff tell you what the medicine was for? How often did hospital staff describe possible side effects in a way you could understand?)

• Patient may experience eye or skin irritation, rash, fatigue, dyspepsia, nausea, constipation, diarrhea, edema in arms or legs, chills, hives, or angina. Have patient report immediately to prescriber signs of infection, dyspnea, infusion reaction, sudden vision changes, or urinary retention (HCAHPS).

• Educate patient about signs of a significant reaction (eg, wheezing; chest tightness; fever; itching; bad cough; blue skin color; seizures; or swelling of face, lips, tongue, or throat). **Note:** This is not a comprehensive list of all side effects. Patient should consult prescriber for additional questions.

Intended Use and Disclaimer: Should not be printed and given to patients. This information is intended to serve as a concise initial reference for healthcare professionals to use when discussing medications with a patient. You must ultimately rely on your own discretion, experience and judgment in diagnosing, treating and advising patients.

Pantoprazole (pan TOE pra zole)

Brand Names: U.S. Protonix

Index Terms Pantoprazole Magnesium; Pantoprazole Sodium

Pharmacologic Category Proton Pump Inhibitor; Substituted Benzimidazole

Medication Safety Issues

Sound-alike/look-alike issues:

Pantoprazole may be confused with ARIPiprazole

Protonix may be confused with Lotronex, Lovenox, protamine

Administration issues:

Vials containing Protonix I.V. for injection are not recommended for use with spiked I.V. system adaptors. Nurses and pharmacists have reported breakage of the glass vials during attempts to connect spiked I.V. system adaptors, which may potentially result in injury to healthcare professionals.

International issues:

Protonix [U.S., Canada] may be confused with Pretanix brand name for indapamide [Hungary]

Medication Guide Available Yes

Pregnancy Risk Factor B

Lactation Enters breast milk/not recommended

Breast-Feeding Considerations Pantoprazole is excreted into breast milk. The excretion of pantoprazole into breast milk was studied in a nursing woman, 10 months postpartum. Following a single dose of pantoprazole 40 mg, maternal milk and serum samples were obtained over 24 hours. Peak concentrations appeared in both the plasma and milk 2 hours after the dose. Pantoprazole concentrations in breast milk were below the limits of detection during most of the study period. Based on this single dose study, the authors calculated the expected exposure to a nursing infant to be 0.14% of the weight-adjusted maternal dose (Plante, 2004). Due to the potential for serious adverse reactions in the nursing infant, the manufacturer recommends a decision be made whether to discontinue nursing or to discontinue the drug, taking into account the importance of treatment to the mother; however, the acidic content of the nursing infants' stomach may potentially inactivate any ingested pantoprazole (Plante, 2004).

Use

Oral: Short-term (up to 8 weeks) treatment and maintenance of healing of erosive esophagitis associated with GERD; reduction in relapse rates of daytime and nighttime heartburn symptoms in GERD; hypersecretory disorders associated with Zollinger-Ellison syndrome or other GI hypersecretory disorders

I.V.: Short-term treatment (7-10 days) of patients with gastroesophageal reflux disease (GERD) and a history of erosive esophagitis; hypersecretory disorders associated with Zollinger-Ellison syndrome or other GI hypersecretory disorders

Canadian labeling: Additional use (not in U.S. labeling): Oral: Peptic ulcer disease (eg, duodenal or gastric ulcer); adjunct treatment with antibiotics for *Helicobacter pylori* eradication; prevention of GI lesions in patients receiving prolonged NSAID therapy

Unlabeled Use Peptic ulcer disease, active ulcer bleeding (parenteral formulation); adjunct treatment with antibiotics for *Helicobacter pylori* eradication; stress ulcer prophylaxis in the critically-ill (parenteral formulation)

Mechanism of Action/Effect Suppresses gastric acid secretion by inhibiting the parietal cell H^+/K^+ ATP pump

Contraindications Hypersensitivity to pantoprazole, substituted benzimidazole proton pump inhibitors, or any component of the formulation

Warnings/Precautions Use of proton pump inhibitors (PPIs) may increase the risk of gastrointestinal infections (eg, *Salmonella, Campylobacter*). Relief of symptoms does not preclude the presence of a gastric malignancy. Long-term pantoprazole therapy (especially in patients who were *H. pylori* positive) has caused biopsy-proven atrophic gastritis. Benign and malignant neoplasia has been observed in long-term rodent studies; while not reported in humans, the relevance of these findings in regards to tumorigenicity in humans is not known. Use of PPIs may increase risk of *Clostridium difficile*-associated diarrhea (CDAD), especially in hospitalized patients; consider CDAD diagnosis in patients with persistent diarrhea that does not improve. Use the lowest dose and shortest duration of PPI therapy appropriate for the condition being treated. Prolonged treatment (typically >3 years) may lead to vitamin B_{12} malabsorption and subsequent deficiency. Intravenous preparation contains edetate sodium (EDTA); use caution in patients who are at risk for zinc deficiency if other EDTA-containing solutions are coadministered. Decreased *H. pylori* eradication rates have been observed with short-term (≤7 days) combination therapy. The American College of Gastroenterology recommends 10-14 days of therapy (triple or quadruple) for eradication of *H. pylori* (Chey, 2007).

PPIs may diminish the therapeutic effect of clopidogrel, thought to be due to reduced formation of the active metabolite of clopidogrel. The manufacturer of clopidogrel recommends either avoidance of both omeprazole (even when scheduled 12 hours apart) and esomeprazole or use of a PPI with comparatively less effect on the active metabolite of clopidogrel. Of the PPIs, pantoprazole has the lowest degree of CYP2C19 inhibition *in vitro* (Li, 2004) and has been shown to have less effect on conversion of clopidogrel to its active metabolite compared to omeprazole (Angiolillo, 2011). In contrast to these warnings, others have recommended the continued use of PPIs, regardless of the degree of inhibition, in patients with a history of GI bleeding or multiple risk factors for GI bleeding who are also receiving clopidogrel since no evidence has established clinically meaningful differences in outcome; however, a clinically-significant interaction cannot be excluded in those who are poor metabolizers of clopidogrel (Abraham, 2010; Levine, 2011). Concomitant use of pantoprazole with some drugs may require cautious use, may not be recommended, or may require dosage adjustments.

Increased incidence of osteoporosis-related bone fractures of the hip, spine, or wrist may occur with PPI therapy. Patients on high-dose or long-term therapy (≥1 year) should be monitored. Use the lowest effective dose for the shortest duration of time, use vitamin D and calcium supplementation, and follow appropriate guidelines to reduce risk of fractures in patients at risk. Thrombophlebitis and hypersensitivity reactions including anaphylaxis, Stevens-Johnson syndrome, and toxic epidermal necrolysis have been reported with IV administration.

Hypomagnesemia, reported rarely, usually with prolonged PPI use of >3 months (most cases >1 year of therapy); may be symptomatic or asymptomatic; severe cases may cause tetany, seizures, and cardiac arrhythmias. Consider obtaining serum magnesium concentrations prior to beginning long-term therapy, especially if taking concomitant digoxin, diuretics, or other drugs known to cause hypomagnesemia; and periodically thereafter. Hypomagnesemia may be corrected by magnesium supplementation, although discontinuation of pantoprazole may be necessary; magnesium levels typically return to normal within 2 weeks of stopping.

Drug Interactions

Avoid Concomitant Use

Avoid concomitant use of Pantoprazole with any of the following: Dasatinib; Delavirdine; Erlotinib; Nelfinavir; PAZOPanib; PONATinib; Rilpivirine; Risedronate

Decreased Effect

Pantoprazole may decrease the levels/effects of: Atazanavir; Bisphosphonate Derivatives; ▶

Bosutinib; Cefditoren; Clopidogrel; Dabigatran Etexilate; Dabrafenib; Dasatinib; Delavirdine; Erlotinib; Gefitinib; Indinavir; Iron Salts; Itraconazole; Ketoconazole (Systemic); Mesalamine; Multivitamins/Minerals (with ADEK, Folate, Iron); Mycophenolate; Nelfinavir; Nilotinib; PONATinib; Posaconazole; Rilpivirine; Riociguat; Risedronate; Vismodegib

The levels/effects of Pantoprazole may be decreased by: CYP2C19 Inducers (Strong); Dabrafenib; Peginterferon Alfa-2b; Tipranavir

Increased Effect/Toxicity

Pantoprazole may increase the levels/effects of: Amphetamine; Dexmethylphenidate; Dextroamphetamine; Methotrexate; Methylphenidate; PAZOPanib; Raltegravir; Risedronate; Saquinavir; Topotecan; Voriconazole

The levels/effects of Pantoprazole may be increased by: Fluconazole; Ketoconazole (Systemic); Voriconazole

Nutritional/Ethanol Interactions

Ethanol: Avoid ethanol (may cause gastric mucosal irritation).

Herb/Nutraceutical: Prolonged treatment (typically >3 years) may lead to vitamin B_{12} malabsorption and subsequent deficiency.

Adverse Reactions

>10%: Central nervous system: Headache (adults 12%; children >4%)

1% to 10%:

Cardiovascular: Facial edema (≤4%), generalized edema (≤2%)

Central nervous system: Dizziness (≤4%), vertigo (≤4%), depression (≤2%), fever (adults ≤2%; children >4%)

Dermatologic: Rash (adults ≤2%; children >4%), urticaria (≤4%), photosensitivity (≤2%), pruritus (≤2%)

Endocrine & metabolic: Triglycerides increased (≤4%)

Gastrointestinal: Diarrhea (≤9%), abdominal pain (children >4%), vomiting (≥4%), constipation (≤4%), flatulence (children ≤4%), nausea (children ≤4%), xerostomia (≤2%)

Hematologic: Leukopenia (≤2%), thrombocytopenia (≤2%)

Hepatic: Liver function tests abnormal (≤4%), hepatitis (≤2%)

Local: Injection site reaction (thrombophlebitis ≤2%)

Neuromuscular & skeletal: Arthralgia (≤4%), myalgia (≤4%), CPK increased (≤4%)

Ocular: Blurred vision (≤2%)

Respiratory: Upper respiratory tract infection (children >4%)

Miscellaneous: Allergic reaction (≤4%)

Available Dosage Forms

Packet, Oral:

Protonix: 40 mg (1 ea, 30 ea)

Solution Reconstituted, Intravenous:

Protonix: 40 mg (1 ea)

Generic: 40 mg (1 ea)

Tablet Delayed Release, Oral:

Protonix: 20 mg, 40 mg

Generic: 20 mg, 40 mg

General Dosage Range

I.V.: *Adults:* Erosive gastritis: 40 mg once daily; Hypersecretory disorders: 160-240 mg daily in divided doses

Oral:

Children ≥5 years: ≥15 to <40 kg: 20 mg once daily; ≥40 kg: 40 mg once daily

Adults: 20-40 mg once or twice daily (maximum: 240 mg daily normally reserved for treatment of hypersecretory conditions)

Usual Infusion Concentrations: Adult I.V. infusion: 80 mg in 100 mL (concentration: 0.8 mg/mL) of D_5W or NS

Administration

I.V. Flush I.V. line before and after administration. In-line filter not required.

2-minute infusion: The volume of reconstituted solution (4 mg/mL) to be injected may be administered intravenously over at least 2 minutes.

15-minute infusion: Infuse over 15 minutes at a rate not to exceed 7 mL/minute (3 mg/minute).

Oral

Tablet: Should be swallowed whole, do not crush or chew. Best if taken before breakfast.

Delayed-release oral suspension: Should only be administered in apple juice or applesauce and taken ~30 minutes before a meal. Do not administer with any other liquid (eg, water) or foods.

Oral administration in **applesauce**: Sprinkle intact granules on 1 tablespoon of applesauce and swallow within 10 minutes of preparation.

Oral administration in **apple juice**: Empty intact granules into 5 mL of apple juice, stir for 5 seconds, and swallow immediately after preparation. Rinse container once or twice with apple juice and swallow immediately.

Nasogastric tube administration: Separate the plunger from the barrel of a 60 mL catheter tip syringe and connect to a ≥16 French nasogastric tube. Holding the syringe attached to the tubing as high as possible, empty the contents of the packet into barrel of the syringe, add 10 mL of apple juice and gently tap/shake the barrel of the syringe to help empty the syringe. Add an additional 10 mL of apple juice and gently tap/shake the barrel to help rinse. Repeat rinse with at least 2-10 mL aliquots of apple juice. No granules should remain in the syringe.

Preparation for Administration

Reconstitute with 10 mL NS (final concentration 4 mg/mL). When administering by I.V. infusion, reconstituted solution may be added to 100 mL D_5W, NS, or LR.

Storage/Stability

Oral: Store tablet and oral suspension at controlled room temperature of 20°C to 25°C (68°F to 77°F); excursions permitted to 15°C to 30°C (59°F to 86°F).

I.V.: Prior to reconstitution, store at controlled room temperature of 20°C to 25°C (68°F to 77°F); excursions permitted to 15°C to 30°C (59°F to 86°F). Do not freeze. Protect from light prior to reconstitution; upon reconstitution, protection from light is not required. Per manufacturer's labeling, reconstituted solution is stable at room temperature for 6 hours; further diluted (admixed) solution should be stored at room temperature and used within 24 hours from the time of initial reconstitution. However, studies have shown that reconstituted solution (4 mg/mL) in polypropylene syringes is stable up to 96 hours at room temperature (Johnson, 2005). Upon further dilution, the admixed solution should be used within 96 hours from the time of initial reconstitution. The preparation should be stored at 3°C to 5°C (37°F to 41°F) if it is stored beyond 48 hours to minimize discoloration.

Nursing Actions

Physical Assessment Monitor for rebleeding.

Patient Education

- Discuss specific use of drug and side effects with patient as it relates to treatment. (HCAHPS: During this hospital stay, were you given any medicine that you had not taken before? Before giving you any new medicine, how often did hospital staff tell you what the medicine was for? How often did hospital staff describe possible side effects in a way you could understand?)
- Patient may experience headache or diarrhea. Have patient report immediately to prescriber severe dizziness, syncope, tachycardia, dyspepsia, osteodynia, myalgia, asthenia, ecchymosis, or rash (HCAHPS).
- Educate patient about signs of a significant reaction (eg, wheezing; chest tightness; fever; itching; bad cough; blue skin color; seizures; or swelling of face, lips, tongue, or throat). **Note:** This is not a comprehensive list of all side effects. Patient should consult prescriber for additional questions.

Intended Use and Disclaimer: Should not be printed and given to patients. This information is intended to serve as a concise initial reference for healthcare professionals to use when discussing medications with a patient. You must ultimately rely on your own discretion, experience and judgment in diagnosing, treating and advising patients.

Dietary Considerations

Oral: May be taken with or without food; best if taken before breakfast.

I.V.: Due to EDTA in preparation, zinc supplementation may be needed in patients prone to zinc deficiency.

Related Information

Oral Medications That Should Not Be Crushed or Altered *on page 1712*

Papillomavirus (Types 6, 11, 16, 18) Vaccine (Human, Recombinant)
(pap ih LO ma VYE rus typs six e LEV en SIX teen AYE teen vak SEEN YU man ree KOM be nant)

Brand Names: U.S. Gardasil

Index Terms HPV Vaccine (Quadrivalent); HPV4; Human Papillomavirus Vaccine (Quadrivalent); Papillomavirus Vaccine, Recombinant; Quadrivalent Human Papillomavirus Vaccine

Pharmacologic Category Vaccine, Inactivated (Viral)

Medication Safety Issues

Sound-alike/look-alike issues:

Papillomavirus vaccine types 6, 11, 16, 18 (Gardasil) may be confused with Papillomavirus vaccine types 16, 18 (Cervarix)

Pregnancy Risk Factor B

Lactation Excretion in breast milk unknown/use caution

Use

U.S. labeling:

Females 9 to 26 years of age:

For the prevention of the following diseases: cervical, vulvar, vaginal, and anal cancer caused by HPV types 16 and 18; genital warts (condyloma acuminatum) caused by HPV types 6 and 11;

For the prevention of the following precancerous or dysplastic lesions caused by HPV types 6, 11, 16, and 18: cervical intraepithelial neoplasia (CIN) grade 2/3 and cervical adenocarcinoma in situ; CIN grade 1; vulvar intraepithelial neoplasia grade 2 and 3; vaginal intraepithelial neoplasia grade 2 and 3; and anal intraepithelial neoplasia grades 1, 2, and 3.

Males 9 through 26 years of age:

For the prevention of the following diseases: anal cancer caused by HPV types 16 and 18; genital warts (condyloma acuminata) caused by HPV types 6 and 11;

For the prevention of anal intraepithelial neoplasia grades 1, 2, and 3 caused by HPV types 6, 11, 16, and 18.

Limitations of use: Does not provide protection against vaccine HPV types to which a person has already been previously exposed, or HPV types not contained in the vaccine; does not prevent CIN grade 2/3 or worse in women >26 years of age. Not intended for the treatment of active external genital lesions or cervical, vulvar, vaginal, and anal cancers.

PAPILLOMAVIRUS (TYPES 6, 11, 16, 18) VACCINE (HUMAN, RECOMBINANT)

◀ *Canadian labeling:*
Females ≥9 years and ≤26 years of age: Prevention of anal cancer caused by HPV types 16 and 18; anal intraepithelial neoplasia caused by HPV types 6, 11, 16, and 18

Females ≥9 years and ≤45 years of age: Prevention of cervical, vulvar, and vaginal cancer caused by HPV types 16 and 18; genital warts caused by HPV types 6 and 11; cervical adenocarcinoma *in situ*, vulvar, vaginal, or cervical intraepithelial neoplasia caused by HPV types 6, 11, 16, and 18

Males ≥9 years and ≤26 years of age: Prevention of anal cancer caused by HPV types 16 and 18; anal intraepithelial neoplasia caused by HPV types 6, 11, 16, and 18; genital warts caused by HPV types 6 and 11

The Advisory Committee on Immunization Practices (ACIP) recommends routine vaccination for females and males 11-12 years of age; catch-up vaccination is recommended for females 13-26 years of age and males 13-21 years of age. Males 22-26 years may also be vaccinated. The ACIP also recommends routine vaccination for men who have sex with men (MSM) through 26 years of age (CDC, 2007; CDC, 59[20], 2010; CDC, 60[50], 2011). Vaccination is also recommended for immunocompromised persons or MSM through 26 years of age who were not previously vaccinated when they were younger. Although not specifically recommended for their profession, health care providers within the recommended age groups should also receive the HPV vaccine (CDC, 2013a).

Available Dosage Forms

Injection, suspension [preservative free]:
Gardasil: HPV 6 L1 protein 20 mcg, HPV 11 L1 protein 40 mcg, HPV 16 L1 protein 40 mcg, and HPV 18 L1 protein 20 mcg per 0.5 mL (0.5 mL)

General Dosage Range I.M.: *Children ≥9 years, Adolescents, and Adults ≤26 years:* 0.5 mL initial dose, followed by 0.5 mL 2 and 6 months later

Administration

I.M. Shake suspension well before use. Inject the entire dose I.M. into the deltoid region of the upper arm or higher anterolateral thigh area. Observe for syncope for 15 minutes following administration. If the vaccine series is interrupted and only one dose was given, administer the second dose as soon as possible (CDC, 2007). Minimum interval between first and second doses is 4 weeks; the minimum interval between first and third doses is 24 weeks (CDC, 59[20], 2010; CDC, 2013a). Inadequate doses or doses received following a shorter than recommended dosing interval should be repeated (CDC, 2007). The HPV vaccine series should be completed with the same product whenever possible (CDC, 59[20], 2010).

For patients at risk of hemorrhage following intramuscular injection, the ACIP recommends "it should be administered intramuscularly if, in the opinion of the physician familiar with the patient's bleeding risk, the vaccine can be administered by this route with reasonable safety. If the patient receives antihemophilia or other similar therapy, intramuscular vaccination can be scheduled shortly after such therapy is administered. A fine needle (23 gauge or smaller) can be used for the vaccination and firm pressure applied to the site (without rubbing) for at least 2 minutes. The patient should be instructed concerning the risk of hematoma from the injection." Patients on anticoagulant therapy should be considered to have the same bleeding risks and treated as those with clotting factor disorders (CDC 60[2], 2011).

Simultaneous administration of vaccines helps ensure the patients will be fully vaccinated by the appropriate age. Simultaneous administration of vaccines is defined as administering >1 vaccine on the same day at different anatomic sites. Separate vaccines should not be combined in the same syringe unless indicated by product specific labeling. Separate needles and syringes should be used for each injection. The ACIP prefers each dose of a specific vaccine in a series come from the same manufacturer when possible. Adolescents and adults should be vaccinated while seated or lying down. In general, preterm infants should be vaccinated at the same chronological age as full-term infants (CDC 60[2], 2011).

Antipyretics have not been shown to prevent febrile seizures. Antipyretics may be used to treat fever or discomfort following vaccination (CDC 60 [2], 2011). One study reported that routine prophylactic administration of acetaminophen to prevent fever prior to vaccination decreased the immune response of some vaccines; the clinical significance of this reduction in immune response has not been established (Prymula, 2009).

Nursing Actions

Physical Assessment Observe patient for 15 minutes after administration for syncope. Treatment for anaphylactic/anaphylactoid reaction should be available during vaccine use; if there is a hypersensitivity response after receiving a dose of Gardasil, patient should not receive further doses. All patients should be informed that the vaccine is not a treatment for active disease and is not a substitute for regular, routine cervical screening. All serious adverse reactions must be reported to the U.S. DHHS. U.S. federal law also requires entry into the patient's medical record. Monitor for less-severe side effects: Headaches, nausea, injection site reactions, dizziness, and low-grade fever.

Patient Education

- Discuss specific use of vaccine and side effects with patient as it relates to treatment. (HCAHPS: During this hospital stay, were you given any medicine that you had not taken before? Before giving you any new medicine, how often did hospital staff tell you what the medicine was for? How often did hospital staff describe possible side effects in a way you could understand?)
- Patient may experience pain, redness or swelling at injection site, headache, fatigue, nausea, emesis, diarrhea, or dyspepsia. Have patient report immediately to prescriber severe injection site reaction (HCAHPS).
- Educate patient about signs of a significant reaction (eg, wheezing; chest tightness; fever; itching; bad cough; blue skin color; seizures; or swelling of face, lips, tongue, or throat). **Note:** This is not a comprehensive list of all side effects. Patient should consult prescriber for additional questions.

Intended Use and Disclaimer: Should not be printed and given to patients. This information is intended to serve as a concise initial reference for healthcare professionals to use when discussing medications with a patient. You must ultimately rely on your own discretion, experience and judgment in diagnosing, treating and advising patients.

Related Information

Immunization Administration Recommendations *on page 1675*

Immunization Recommendations *on page 1680*

Papillomavirus (Types 16, 18) Vaccine (Human, Recombinant)

(pap ih LO ma VYE rus typs SIX teen AYE teen vak SEEN YU man ree KOM be nant)

Brand Names: U.S. Cervarix®

Index Terms Bivalent Human Papillomavirus Vaccine; GSK-580299; HPV 16/18 L1 VLP/AS04 VAC; HPV Vaccine (Bivalent); HPV2; Human Papillomavirus Vaccine (Bivalent); Papillomavirus Vaccine, Recombinant

Pharmacologic Category Vaccine, Inactivated (Viral)

Medication Safety Issues

Sound-alike/look-alike issues:

Papillomavirus vaccine types 16, 18 (Cervarix®) may be confused with Papillomavirus vaccine types 6, 11, 16, 18 (Gardasil®)

Cervarix® may be confused with Cerebyx®, CeleBREX®

Pregnancy Risk Factor B

Lactation Excretion in breast milk unknown/use caution

Use

U.S. labeling: Females 9 through 25 years of age: Prevention of cervical cancer, cervical adenocarcinoma *in situ*, and cervical intraepithelial neoplasia caused by human papillomavirus (HPV) types 16, 18

The Advisory Committee on Immunization Practices (ACIP) recommends routine vaccination for females 11-12 years of age; catch-up vaccination is recommended for females 13-25 years of age (CDC, 59[20], 2010). Vaccination is also recommended for immunocompromised females through 26 years of age who were not previously vaccinated when they were younger. Although not specifically recommended for their profession, female health care providers within the recommended age groups should also receive the HPV vaccine (CDC, 2013).

Canadian labeling: Females 9 through 45 years of age: Prevention of cervical cancer, cervical adenocarcinoma *in situ*, and cervical intraepithelial neoplasia caused by human papillomavirus (HPV) types 16, 18

The National Advisory Committee on Immunization (NACI) recommends routine vaccination for females between 9 and 26 years of age. It should not be administered in females <9 years but may be administered to females >26 years (CCDR, 2012).

Available Dosage Forms

Injection, suspension [preservative free]:

Cervarix®: HPV 16 L1 protein 20 mcg and HPV 18 L1 protein 20 mcg per 0.5 mL (0.5 mL)

General Dosage Range I.M.: *Children ≥9 years, Adolescents, and Adults ≤25 years: Females:* 0.5 mL initial dose, followed by 0.5 mL 1 and 6 months later

Administration

I.M. Shake well prior to use. Do not use if discolored or if containing particulate matter, or if vial or syringe is cracked. Inject I.M. into the deltoid region of the upper arm. Do not administer I.V., SubQ, or intradermally.

For patients at risk of hemorrhage following intramuscular injection, the ACIP recommends "it should be administered intramuscularly if, in the opinion of the physician familiar with the patient's bleeding risk, the vaccine can be administered by this route with reasonable safety. If the patient receives antihemophilia or other similar therapy, intramuscular vaccination can be scheduled shortly after such therapy is administered. A fine needle (23 gauge or smaller) can be used for the vaccination and firm pressure applied to the site (without rubbing) for at least 2 minutes. The patient should be instructed concerning the risk of hematoma from the injection." Patients on anticoagulant therapy should be considered to have the same bleeding risks and treated as those with clotting factor disorders (CDC, 2011).

Simultaneous administration of vaccines helps ensure the patients will be fully vaccinated by ▶

the appropriate age. Simultaneous administration of vaccines is defined as administering >1 vaccine on the same day at different anatomic sites. Separate vaccines should not be combined in the same syringe unless indicated by product specific labeling. Separate needles and syringes should be used for each injection. The ACIP prefers each dose of a specific vaccine in a series come from the same manufacturer when possible. Adolescents and adults should be vaccinated while seated or lying down. In general, preterm infants should be vaccinated at the same chronological age as full-term infants (CDC, 2011).

Antipyretics have not been shown to prevent febrile seizures. Antipyretics may be used to treat fever or discomfort following vaccination (CDC, 2011). One study reported that routine prophylactic administration of acetaminophen to prevent fever prior to vaccination decreased the immune response of some vaccines; the clinical significance of this reduction in immune response has not been established (Prymula, 2009).

Nursing Actions

Physical Assessment Have emergency treatment for anaphylactoid or hypersensitivity reaction available. Syncope following administration may occur. If latex sensitive, be advised that packaging may contain latex. Emphasize necessity to complete all 3 doses for maximum efficacy. All serious adverse reactions must be reported to the U.S. DHHS. U.S. federal law also requires entry into the patient's medical record.

Patient Education

- Discuss specific use of vaccine and side effects with patient as it relates to treatment. (HCAHPS: During this hospital stay, were you given any medicine that you had not taken before? Before giving you any new medicine, how often did hospital staff tell you what the medicine was for? How often did hospital staff describe possible side effects in a way you could understand?)
- Patient may experience pain, redness or swelling at injection site, headache, fatigue, nausea, emesis, diarrhea, or dyspepsia. Have patient report immediately to prescriber severe injection site reaction (HCAHPS).
- Educate patient about signs of a significant reaction (eg, wheezing; chest tightness; fever; itching; bad cough; blue skin color; seizures; or swelling of face, lips, tongue, or throat). **Note:** This is not a comprehensive list of all side effects. Patient should consult prescriber for additional questions.

Intended Use and Disclaimer: Should not be printed and given to patients. This information is intended to serve as a concise initial reference for healthcare professionals to use when discussing medications with a patient. You must ultimately rely on your own discretion, experience and judgment in diagnosing, treating and advising patients.

Related Information

Immunization Administration Recommendations *on page 1675*

Immunization Recommendations *on page 1680*

Paregoric (par e GOR ik)

Index Terms Camphorated Tincture of Opium (error-prone synonym)

Pharmacologic Category Analgesic, Opioid

Medication Safety Issues

Sound-alike/look-alike issues:

Camphorated tincture of opium is an error-prone synonym (mistaken as opium tincture)

Paregoric may be confused with Percogesic®

High alert medication:

The Institute for Safe Medication Practices (ISMP) includes this medication among its list of drug classes which have a heightened risk of causing significant patient harm when used in error.

Administration issues:

Use care when prescribing opium products; paregoric contains the equivalent of morphine 0.4 mg/mL; opium tincture contains the equivalent of morphine 10 mg/mL

Pregnancy Risk Factor C

Lactation Enters breast milk/use caution

Use Treatment of diarrhea

Controlled Substance C-III

Available Dosage Forms

Tincture, Oral:

Generic: 2 mg/5 mL (473 mL)

General Dosage Range Oral:

Children: 0.25-0.5 mL/kg 1-4 times daily

Adults: 5-10 mL 1-4 times daily

Nursing Actions

Physical Assessment If used to control diarrhea, monitor stools. Monitor for excessive sedation, respiratory depression, or hypotension. For inpatients, implement safety measures (eg, side rails up, call light within reach, patient instructions to call for assistance). Assess patient's physical and/or psychological dependence. Discontinue slowly after prolonged use

Patient Education

- Discuss specific use of drug and side effects with patient as it relates to treatment. (HCAHPS: During this hospital stay, were you given any medicine that you had not taken before? Before giving you any new medicine, how often did hospital staff tell you what the medicine was for? How often did hospital staff describe possible side effects in a way you could understand?)
- Patient may experience fatigue or nausea. Have patient report immediately to prescriber severe dizziness, syncope, dyspnea, illogical thinking, tachycardia, arrhythmia, mood changes,

considerable constipation, or vision changes (HCAHPS).
- Educate patient about signs of a significant reaction (eg, wheezing; chest tightness; fever; itching; bad cough; blue skin color; seizures; or swelling of face, lips, tongue, or throat). **Note:** This is not a comprehensive list of all side effects. Patient should consult prescriber for additional questions.

Intended Use and Disclaimer: Should not be printed and given to patients. This information is intended to serve as a concise initial reference for healthcare professionals to use when discussing medications with a patient. You must ultimately rely on your own discretion, experience and judgment in diagnosing, treating and advising patients.

Paricalcitol (pah ri KAL si tole)

Brand Names: U.S. Zemplar
Pharmacologic Category Vitamin D Analog
Medication Safety Issues
Sound alike/look alike issues:
Paricalcitol may be confused with calcitriol
Zemplar may be confused with zaleplon, Zelapar, zolpidem, ZyPREXA Zydis
Pregnancy Risk Factor C
Lactation Excretion in breast milk unknown/not recommended
Use
I.V.: Prevention and treatment of secondary hyperparathyroidism associated with stage 5 chronic kidney disease (CKD)
Oral: Prevention and treatment of secondary hyperparathyroidism associated with stage 3 and 4 CKD and stage 5 CKD patients on hemodialysis or peritoneal dialysis
Available Dosage Forms
Capsule, Oral:
Zemplar: 1 mcg, 2 mcg, 4 mcg
Generic: 1 mcg, 2 mcg, 4 mcg
Solution, Intravenous:
Zemplar: 2 mcg/mL (1 mL); 5 mcg/mL (1 mL, 2 mL)
General Dosage Range Dosage adjustment recommended in patients with renal impairment
I.V.: *Children ≥5 years and Adults:* 0.04-0.24 mcg/kg (2.8-16.8 mcg) every other day during dialysis
Oral: *Adults:* 1-2 mcg/day **or** 2-4 mcg 3 times/week
Administration
I.V. Administered as a bolus dose at anytime during dialysis. Doses should not be administered more often than every other day.
Oral May be administered with or without food. With the 3 times/week dosing schedule, doses should not be given more frequently than every other day.

Nursing Actions
Physical Assessment Instruct patient on dietary requirements.
Patient Education
- Discuss specific use of drug and side effects with patient as it relates to treatment. (HCAHPS: During this hospital stay, were you given any medicine that you had not taken before? Before giving you any new medicine, how often did hospital staff tell you what the medicine was for? How often did hospital staff describe possible side effects in a way you could understand?)
- Patient may experience dizziness, hypercalcemia, nausea, or diarrhea. Have patient report immediately to prescriber illogical thinking, severe constipation, inability to eat, significant weight loss, severe asthenia, or rash (HCAHPS).
- Educate patient about signs of a significant reaction (eg, wheezing; chest tightness; fever; itching; bad cough; blue skin color; seizures; or swelling of face, lips, tongue, or throat). **Note:** This is not a comprehensive list of all side effects. Patient should consult prescriber for additional questions.

Intended Use and Disclaimer: Should not be printed and given to patients. This information is intended to serve as a concise initial reference for healthcare professionals to use when discussing medications with a patient. You must ultimately rely on your own discretion, experience and judgment in diagnosing, treating and advising patients.

PARoxetine (pa ROKS e teen)

Brand Names: U.S. Brisdelle; Paxil; Paxil CR; Pexeva
Index Terms Brisdelle; Paroxetine Hydrochloride; Paroxetine Mesylate
Pharmacologic Category Antidepressant, Selective Serotonin Reuptake Inhibitor
Medication Safety Issues
Sound-alike/look-alike issues:
PARoxetine may be confused with FLUoxetine, PACLitaxel, piroxicam, pyridoxine, vortioxetine
Paxil may be confused with Doxil, PACLitaxel, Plavix, PROzac, Taxol
BEERS Criteria medication:
This drug may be potentially inappropriate for use in geriatric patients (SIADH: Quality of evidence - moderate; Strength of recommendation - strong).
Medication Guide Available Yes
Pregnancy Risk Factor D//X (product specific)
Lactation Enters breast milk/use caution
Breast-Feeding Considerations Paroxetine is excreted in breast milk and concentrations in the hindmilk are higher than in foremilk. Paroxetine has not been detected in the serum of nursing infants.

Adverse reactions have been reported in nursing infants exposed to some SSRIs. The manufacturer recommends that caution be exercised when administering paroxetine to nursing women. Maternal use of an SSRI during pregnancy may cause delayed milk secretion. The American Academy of Breastfeeding Medicine suggests that paroxetine may be considered for the treatment of postpartum depression in appropriately selected women who are nursing. Mothers should be monitored for changes in symptoms and infants should be monitored for growth. The long-term effects on development and behavior have not been studied.

Use

Generalized anxiety disorder (immediate release): For the treatment of generalized anxiety disorder (GAD)

Major depressive disorder (immediate and controlled release): For the treatment of major depressive disorder (MDD)

Obsessive-compulsive disorder (immediate release): For the treatment of obsessions and compulsions in patients with obsessive-compulsive disorder (OCD)

Panic disorder (immediate and controlled release): For the treatment of panic disorder, with or without agoraphobia

Post-traumatic stress disorder (immediate release): For the treatment of post-traumatic stress disorder (PTSD)

Premenstrual dysphoric disorder (controlled release): For the treatment of premenstrual dysphoric disorder (PMDD)

Social anxiety disorder (immediate and controlled release): For the treatment of social anxiety disorder, also known as social phobia

Vasomotor symptoms of menopause (Brisdelle only): For the treatment of moderate to severe vasomotor symptoms associated with menopause

Unlabeled Use May be useful in eating disorders, impulse control disorders; treatment of obsessive-compulsive disorder (OCD) in children

Mechanism of Action/Effect Paroxetine is a selective serotonin reuptake inhibitor, chemically unrelated to tricyclic, tetracyclic, or other antidepressants; presumably, the inhibition of serotonin reuptake from brain synapse stimulated serotonin activity in the brain

Contraindications Concurrent use with or within 14 days of MAOIs intended to treat psychiatric disorders; initiation in patients being treated with linezolid or methylene blue I.V.; concomitant use with pimozide or thioridazine; hypersensitivity to paroxetine or any of its inactive ingredients; pregnancy (Brisdelle only).

Warnings/Precautions Hazardous agent - use appropriate precautions for handling and disposal (NIOSH, 2012). **[U.S. Boxed Warning]: Antidepressants increase the risk of suicidal thinking and behavior in children, adolescents, and young adults (18-24 years of age) with major depressive disorder (MDD) and other psychiatric disorders;** consider risk prior to prescribing. Short-term studies did not show an increased risk in patients >24 years of age and showed a decreased risk in patients ≥65 years. Closely monitor patients for clinical worsening, suicidality, or unusual changes in behavior, particularly during the initial 1-2 months of therapy or during periods of dosage adjustments (increases or decreases); the patient's family or caregiver should be instructed to closely observe the patient and communicate condition with healthcare provider. A medication guide concerning the use of antidepressants should be dispensed with each prescription. **Paroxetine is not FDA approved for use in children.**

The possibility of a suicide attempt is inherent in major depression and may persist until remission occurs. Patients treated with antidepressants (for any indication) should be observed for clinical worsening and suicidality, especially during the initial few months of a course of drug therapy, or at times of dose changes, either increases or decreases. Use caution in high-risk patients. Worsening depression and severe abrupt suicidality that are not part of the presenting symptoms may require discontinuation or modification of drug therapy. The patient's family or caregiver should be alerted to monitor patients for the emergence of suicidality and associated behaviors (such as agitation, irritability, hostility, impulsivity, and hypomania) and call healthcare provider.

May worsen psychosis in some patients or precipitate a shift to mania or hypomania in patients with bipolar disorder. Patients presenting with depressive symptoms should be screened for bipolar disorder. Monotherapy in patients with bipolar disorder should be avoided. **Paroxetine is not FDA approved for the treatment of bipolar depression.**

Potentially life-threatening serotonin syndrome (SS) has occurred with serotonergic agents (eg, SSRIs, SNRIs), particularly when used in combination with other serotonergic agents (eg, triptans, TCAs, fentanyl, lithium, tramadol, buspirone, St John's wort, tryptophan) or agents that impair metabolism of serotonin (eg, MAO inhibitors intended to treat psychiatric disorders, other MAO inhibitors [ie, linezolid and intravenous methylene blue]). Discontinue treatment (and any concomitant serotonergic agent) immediately if signs/symptoms arise.

Paroxetine may increase the risks associated with electroconvulsive therapy. Has a low potential to impair cognitive or motor performance - use caution when operating hazardous machinery or driving. Symptoms of agitation and/or restlessness may occur during initial few weeks of therapy.

Low potential for sedation or anticholinergic effects relative to cyclic antidepressants. Bone fractures have been associated with SSRI treatment. Consider the possibility of a fragility fracture if an SSRI-treated patient presents with unexplained bone pain, point tenderness, swelling, or bruising.

Use caution in elderly patients; may cause or exacerbate syndrome of inappropriate antidiuretic hormone secretion or hyponatremia; monitor sodium closely with initiation or dosage adjustments in older adults. Medication associated with potent anticholinergic properties which may be inappropriate in older adults depending on comorbidities (eg, dementia, delirium) (Beers Criteria).

Use caution in patients with a previous seizure disorder or condition predisposing to seizures such as brain damage, alcoholism, or concurrent therapy with other drugs which lower the seizure threshold. Use with caution in patients with hepatic dysfunction. May cause SIADH; volume depletion and/or diuretics may increase risk. Potentially significant drug-drug interactions may exist, requiring dose or frequency adjustment, additional monitoring, and/or selection of alternative therapy. Use with caution in patients with renal insufficiency or other concurrent illness (due to limited experience); dose reduction recommended with severe renal impairment. May cause or exacerbate sexual dysfunction. Use caution in patients with narrow-angle glaucoma. Avoid use in the first trimester of pregnancy. Menopausal vasomotor symptoms do not occur during pregnancy; therefore, the use of paroxetine for the treatment of menopausal vasomotor symptoms is contraindicated in pregnant women.

Brisdelle contains a lower dose than what is required for the treatment of psychiatric conditions. Patients who require paroxetine for the treatment of psychiatric conditions should discontinue Brisdelle and begin treatment with a paroxetine-containing medication which provides an adequate dosage.

Abrupt discontinuation or interruption of antidepressant therapy has been associated with a discontinuation syndrome. Symptoms arising may vary with antidepressant however commonly include nausea, vomiting, diarrhea, headaches, lightheadedness, dizziness, diminished appetite, sweating, chills, tremors, paresthesias, fatigue, somnolence, and sleep disturbances (eg, vivid dreams, insomnia). Greater risks for developing a discontinuation syndrome have been associated with antidepressants with shorter half-lives, longer durations of treatment, and abrupt discontinuation. For antidepressants of short or intermediate half-lives, symptoms may emerge within 2-5 days after treatment discontinuation and last 7-14 days (APA, 2010; Fava, 2006; Haddod, 2001; Shelton, 2001; Warner, 2006).

Drug Interactions

Avoid Concomitant Use

Avoid concomitant use of PARoxetine with any of the following: Dosulepin; Iobenguane I 123; Linezolid; MAO Inhibitors; Methylene Blue; Pimozide; Tamoxifen; Thioridazine; Tryptophan; Urokinase

Decreased Effect

PARoxetine may decrease the levels/effects of: Aprepitant; Codeine; Fosaprepitant; Iloperidone; Iobenguane I 123; Ioflupane I 123; Tamoxifen; Thyroid Products; TraMADol

The levels/effects of PARoxetine may be decreased by: Aprepitant; CarBAMazepine; Cyproheptadine; Darunavir; Fosamprenavir; Fosaprepitant; NSAID (COX-2 Inhibitor); NSAID (Nonselective); Peginterferon Alfa-2b

Increased Effect/Toxicity

PARoxetine may increase the levels/effects of: Agents with Antiplatelet Properties; Anticoagulants; Antidepressants (Serotonin Reuptake Inhibitor/Antagonist); Antipsychotics; ARIPiprazole; Asenapine; Aspirin; AtoMOXetine; Beta-Blockers; BusPIRone; CarBAMazepine; CloZAPine; Collagenase (Systemic); CYP2B6 Substrates; CYP2D6 Substrates; Dabigatran Etexilate; Desmopressin; Dextromethorphan; Dofetilide; Dosulepin; DOXOrubicin (Conventional); DULoxetine; Fesoterodine; Galantamine; Highest Risk QTc-Prolonging Agents; Hypoglycemic Agents; Ibritumomab; Iloperidone; Lomitapide; Methadone; Methylene Blue; Metoclopramide; Metoprolol; Mexiletine; Moderate Risk QTc-Prolonging Agents; Nebivolol; NSAID (COX-2 Inhibitor); NSAID (Nonselective); Pimozide; Propafenone; RisperiDONE; Rivaroxaban; Salicylates; Serotonin Modulators; Tetrabenazine; Thiazide Diuretics; Thioridazine; Thrombolytic Agents; Tositumomab and Iodine I 131 Tositumomab; TraMADol; Tricyclic Antidepressants; Urokinase; Vitamin K Antagonists; Vortioxetine

The levels/effects of PARoxetine may be increased by: Abiraterone Acetate; Alcohol (Ethyl); Analgesics (Opioid); ARIPiprazole; Asenapine; BuPROPion; BusPIRone; Cimetidine; CNS Depressants; Cobicistat; CYP2D6 Inhibitors (Moderate); CYP2D6 Inhibitors (Strong); Dasatinib; DULoxetine; Glucosamine; Herbs (Anticoagulant/Antiplatelet Properties); Ibrutinib; Linezolid; Lithium; MAO Inhibitors; Metoclopramide; Metyrosine; Mifepristone; Multivitamins/Fluoride (with ADE); Multivitamins/Minerals (with ADEK, Folate, Iron); Multivitamins/Minerals (with AE, No Iron); Omega-3 Fatty Acids; Pentosan Polysulfate Sodium; Pentoxifylline; Pravastatin; Prostacyclin Analogues; Tipranavir; TraMADol; Tryptophan; Vitamin E

Nutritional/Ethanol Interactions

Ethanol: May increase CNS depression; monitor for increased effects with coadministration. Caution patients about effects.

Food: Peak concentration is increased, but bioavailability is not significantly altered by food.

Herb/Nutraceutical: Avoid valerian, St John's wort, tryptophan, SAMe, kava kava.

Adverse Reactions Frequency varies by dose and indication. Adverse reactions reported as a composite of all indications.

>10%:

Central nervous system: Drowsiness (15% to 24%), insomnia (11% to 24%), headache (6% to 18%), dizziness (6% to 14%)

Dermatologic: Diaphoresis (5% to 14%)

Endocrine & metabolic: Decreased libido (3% to 15%)

Gastrointestinal: Nausea (19% to 26%), xerostomia (9% to 18%), constipation (5% to 16%), diarrhea (9% to 12%)

Genitourinary: Ejaculatory disorder (13% to 28%)

Neuromuscular & skeletal: Weakness (12% to 22%), tremor (4% to 11%)

1% to 10%:

Cardiovascular: Vasodilatation (2% to 4%), chest pain (3%), palpitations (2% to 3%), hypertension (≥1%), tachycardia (≥1%)

Central nervous system: Nervousness (4% to 9%), anxiety (5%), fatigue (5%), agitation (3% to 5%), paresthesia (4%), abnormal dreams (3% to 4%), lack of concentration (3% to 4%), yawning (2% to 4%), depersonalization (≤3%), myoclonus (2% to 3%), amnesia (2%), chills (2%), emotional lability (≥1%), vertigo (≥1%), confusion (1%), myasthenia (1%)

Dermatologic: Skin rash (2% to 3%), pruritus (≥1%)

Endocrine & metabolic: Orgasm disturbance (2% to 9%), dysmenorrhea (5%), weight gain (≥1%)

Gastrointestinal: Decreased appetite (5% to 9%), dyspepsia (2% to 5%), flatulence (4%), abdominal pain (4%), nausea and vomiting (4%), increased appetite (2% to 4%), vomiting (2% to 3%), dysgeusia (2%)

Genitourinary: Male genital disease (10%), female genital tract disease (2% to 9%), impotence (2% to 9%), urinary frequency (2% to 3%), urinary tract infection (2%)

Infection: Infection (5% to 6%)

Neuromuscular & skeletal: Myalgia (2% to 4%), back pain (3%), myopathy (2%), arthralgia (≥1%)

Ophthalmic: Blurred vision (4%), visual disturbance (2% to 4%)

Otic: Tinnitus (≥1%)

Respiratory: Dyspnea (≤7%), pharyngitis (4%), sinusitis (≤4%), rhinitis (3%)

Pharmacodynamics/Kinetics

Onset of Action Depression: The onset of action is within a week, however, individual response varies greatly and full response may not be seen until 8-12 weeks after initiation of treatment.

Available Dosage Forms

Capsule, Oral:

Brisdelle: 7.5 mg

Suspension, Oral:

Paxil: 10 mg/5 mL (250 mL)

Tablet, Oral:

Paxil: 10 mg, 20 mg, 30 mg, 40 mg

Pexeva: 10 mg, 20 mg, 30 mg, 40 mg

Generic: 10 mg, 20 mg, 30 mg, 40 mg

Tablet Extended Release 24 Hour, Oral:

Paxil CR: 12.5 mg, 25 mg, 37.5 mg

Generic: 12.5 mg, 25 mg, 37.5 mg

General Dosage Range

Oral:

Capsules: *Adults:* 7.5 mg once daily at bedtime; no dosage adjustment is necessary in patients with hepatic or renal impairment.

Tablets: Dosage adjustment recommended in patients with hepatic or renal impairment

Controlled release:

Adults: Initial: 12.5-25 mg once daily; Maintenance: 12.5-75 mg once daily (maximum: 75 mg/day)

Elderly: Initial: 12.5 mg once daily; Maintenance: 12.5-50 mg/day (maximum: 50 mg/day)

Immediate release:

Adults: Initial: 10-20 mg once daily: Maintenance: 10-60 mg once daily (maximum: 60 mg/day)

Elderly: Initial: 10 mg once daily; Maintenance: 10-40 mg once daily (maximum: 40 mg/day)

Suspension: Dosage adjustment recommended in patients with hepatic or renal impairment

Adults: Initial: 10-20 mg once daily: Maintenance: 10-60 mg once daily (maximum: 60 mg/day)

Elderly: Initial: 10 mg once daily; Maintenance: 10-40 mg once daily (maximum: 40 mg/day)

Administration

Oral May be administered without regard to meals. Paxil, Paxil CR, and Pexeva should preferentially be administered in the morning; whereas Brisdelle is recommended to be administered at bedtime. Do not crush, break, or chew controlled-release tablets.

Hazardous agent; use appropriate precautions for handling and disposal (NIOSH, 2012).

Storage/Stability

Capsules: Store between 20°C and 25°C (68°F and 77°F); excursions permitted between 15°C and 30°C (59°F and 86°F). Protect from light and humidity.

Tablets: Store immediate-release tablets between 15°C and 30°C (59°F and 86°F) and controlled-release tablets at or below 25°C (77°F).

Suspension: Store at or below 25°C (77°F).

Nursing Actions

Physical Assessment Evaluate mental status, particularly mood and thought content for suicidal ideations. Provide patients with local and national suicide prevention crisis phone numbers when using antidepressant therapy. Educate patients about possible side effects: Dry mouth, constipation, sedation, weight gain, urinary retention, sexual dysfunction.

Patient Education
- Discuss specific use of drug and side effects with patient as it relates to treatment. (HCAHPS: During this hospital stay, were you given any medicine that you had not taken before? Before giving you any new medicine, how often did hospital staff tell you what the medicine was for? How often did hospital staff describe possible side effects in a way you could understand?)
- Patient may experience presyncope, fatigue, blurred vision, illogical thinking, nervousness or excitability, headache, nausea, diarrhea, xerostomia, change in sex ability, or insomnia. Have patient report immediately to prescriber change in balance, agitation, fasciculations, muscle stiffness, tachycardia, ecchymosis, or rash (HCAHPS).
- Educate patient about signs of a significant reaction (eg, wheezing; chest tightness; fever; itching; bad cough; blue skin color; seizures; or swelling of face, lips, tongue, or throat). **Note:** This is not a comprehensive list of all side effects. Patient should consult prescriber for additional questions.

Intended Use and Disclaimer: Should not be printed and given to patients. This information is intended to serve as a concise initial reference for healthcare professionals to use when discussing medications with a patient. You must ultimately rely on your own discretion, experience and judgment in diagnosing, treating and advising patients.

Dietary Considerations May be taken without regard to meals.

Related Information
Oral Medications That Should Not Be Crushed or Altered *on page 1712*

Pasireotide (pas i REE oh tide)

Brand Names: U.S. Signifor
Index Terms Pasireotide Diaspartate; SOM230
Pharmacologic Category Somatostatin Analog
Medication Safety Issues
　Sound-alike/look-alike issues:
　　Pasireotide may be confused with lanreotide, octreotide
Medication Guide Available Yes
Pregnancy Risk Factor C
Lactation Excretion in breast milk unknown/use caution

Use Treatment of Cushing's disease in patients for whom pituitary surgery is not an option or has not been curative

Available Dosage Forms
Solution, Subcutaneous:
　Signifor: 0.3 mg/mL (1 mL); 0.6 mg/mL (1 mL); 0.9 mg/mL (1 mL)
General Dosage Range Dosage adjustment recommended in patients with hepatic impairment.
SubQ: *Adults:* Initial: 0.6 mg or 0.9 mg twice daily; titrate based on response and tolerability. Recommended dosage range: 0.3-0.9 mg twice daily.

Administration

Subcutaneous Administer by subcutaneous injection into the top of the thigh or abdomen (excluding the navel and waistline). Do not inject into inflamed or irritated skin. Alternate the injection site. Do not use if vial contains particulates or solution is discolored.

Nursing Actions

Physical Assessment Monitor for weakness, fatigue, nausea/vomiting, and hyperglycemia. Look at patient's glucose chart. Check vital signs. Check to see if any signs of gallstones. Educate patient about monitoring glucose at home and keeping a chart of the results. Educate patient about signs and symptoms of hyperglycemia or gallstones. Have patient call prescriber if symptoms occur or if blood sugar tests increase.

Patient Education
- Discuss specific use of drug and side effects with patient as it relates to treatment. (HCAHPS: During this hospital stay, were you given any medicine that you had not taken before? Before giving you any new medicine, how often did hospital staff tell you what the medicine was for? How often did hospital staff describe possible side effects in a way you could understand?)
- Patient may experience dyspepsia, headache, asthenia, nausea, diarrhea, hyper-/hypoglycemia, alopecia, short-term pain, bradycardia, or gallstones. Have patient report immediately to prescriber severe dizziness or inability to eat (HCAHPS).
- Educate patient about signs of a significant reaction (eg, wheezing; chest tightness; fever; itching; bad cough; blue skin color; seizures; or swelling of face, lips, tongue, or throat). **Note:** This is not a comprehensive list of all side effects. Patient should consult prescriber for additional questions.

Intended Use and Disclaimer: Should not be printed and given to patients. This information is intended to serve as a concise initial reference for healthcare professionals to use when discussing medications with a patient. You must ultimately rely on your own discretion, experience and judgment in diagnosing, treating and advising patients.

PAZOPanib (paz OH pa nib)

Brand Names: U.S. Votrient

Index Terms GW786034; Pazopanib Hydrochloride

Pharmacologic Category Antineoplastic Agent, Tyrosine Kinase Inhibitor; Antineoplastic Agent, Vascular Endothelial Growth Factor (VEGF) Inhibitor

Medication Safety Issues

Sound-alike/look-alike issues:

PAZOPanib may be confused with axitinib, pegaptanib, PONATinib, regorafenib, SUNItinib, vandetanib

Votrient may be confused with vorinostat

High alert medication:

This medication is in a class the Institute for Safe Medication Practices (ISMP) includes among its list of drug classes which have a heightened risk of causing significant patient harm when used in error.

Medication Guide Available Yes

Pregnancy Risk Factor D

Lactation Excretion in breast milk unknown/not recommended

Use

Renal cell cancer (RCC): Treatment of advanced RCC

Soft tissue sarcoma (STS): Treatment of advanced STS (in patients previously treated with chemotherapy)

Note: Efficacy for adipocytic STS or gastrointestinal stromal tumor (GIST) has not been demonstrated

Unlabeled Use Treatment of advanced, differentiated thyroid cancer

Available Dosage Forms

Tablet, Oral:

Votrient: 200 mg

General Dosage Range Dosage adjustment recommended in patients with hepatic impairment, on concomitant therapy, or who develop toxicities

Oral: *Adults:* 800 mg once daily

Administration

Oral Administer on an empty stomach, 1 hour before or 2 hours after a meal. Do not crush tablet (rate of absorption may be increased; may affect systemic exposure).

Hazardous agent; use appropriate precautions for handling and disposal (NIOSH, 2012).

Nursing Actions

Physical Assessment Monitor for hypertension, gastrointestinal perforation, diarrhea, hyper-/hypoglycemia, and cardiac changes; dose adjustments may be necessary.

Patient Education

• Discuss specific use of drug and side effects with patient as it relates to treatment. (HCAHPS: During this hospital stay, were you given any medicine that you had not taken before? Before giving you any new medicine, how often did hospital staff tell you what the medicine was for? How often did hospital staff describe possible side effects in a way you could understand?)

• Patient may experience headache, diarrhea, lack of appetite, dysgeusia, stomatitis, hair discoloration, alopecia, myalgia, weight loss, insomnia, or nail changes. Have patient report immediately to prescriber signs of infection, signs of hemorrhaging, angina, arrhythmia, tachycardia, severe dizziness, syncope, edema of extremities, illogical thinking, blindness, significant dyspepsia, considerable nausea, intolerable asthenia, urinary retention, oliguria, eczema of hands or feet, abdominal edema, signs of severe cardiac abnormalities, or signs of thrombotic thrombocytopenic purpura/hemolytic uremic syndrome (TTP/HUS) (HCAHPS).

• Educate patient about signs of a significant reaction (eg, wheezing; chest tightness; fever; itching; bad cough; blue skin color; seizures; or swelling of face, lips, tongue, or throat). **Note:** This is not a comprehensive list of all side effects. Patient should consult prescriber for additional questions.

Intended Use and Disclaimer: Should not be printed and given to patients. This information is intended to serve as a concise initial reference for healthcare professionals to use when discussing medications with a patient. You must ultimately rely on your own discretion, experience and judgment in diagnosing, treating and advising patients.

Related Information

Oral Medications That Should Not Be Crushed or Altered *on page 1712*

Pegaspargase (peg AS par jase)

Brand Names: U.S. Oncaspar

Index Terms L-asparaginase with Polyethylene Glycol; PEG-ASP; PEG-asparaginase; PEG-L-asparaginase; PEGLA; Polyethylene Glycol-L-asparaginase

Pharmacologic Category Antineoplastic Agent, Enzyme; Antineoplastic Agent, Miscellaneous

Medication Safety Issues

Sound-alike/look-alike issues:

Oncaspar® may be confused with Elspar®

Pegaspargase may be confused with asparaginase, peginesatide

High alert medication:

The Institute for Safe Medication Practices (ISMP) includes this medication among its list of drugs which have a heightened risk of causing significant patient harm when used in error.

Pregnancy Risk Factor C

Lactation Excretion in breast milk unknown/not recommended

Breast-Feeding Considerations Due to the potential for serious adverse reactions in the nursing infant, breast-feeding is not recommended.

Use Treatment of acute lymphocytic leukemia (ALL); treatment of ALL with previous hypersensitivity to native L-asparaginase

Mechanism of Action/Effect Pegaspargase is a modified version of asparaginase. Leukemic cells, especially lymphoblasts, require exogenous asparagine; normal cells can synthesize asparagine. Asparaginase contains L-asparaginase amidohydrolase type EC-2 which inhibits protein synthesis by deaminating asparagine to aspartic acid and ammonia in the plasma and extracellular fluid and therefore deprives tumor cells of the amino acid for protein synthesis. Asparaginase is cycle-specific for the G_1 phase of the cell cycle.

Contraindications History of serious allergic reactions to pegaspargase; history of any of the following with prior L-asparaginase treatment: pancreatitis, serious hemorrhagic events, serious thrombosis

Warnings/Precautions Hazardous agent - use appropriate precautions for handling and disposal (NIOSH, 2012). Serious allergic reactions may occur; discontinue in patients with serious allergic reaction. Observe patients for at least 1 hour after administration; immediate treatment for hypersensitivity reactions should be available during administration. Pegaspargase is indicated for use in patients who have had hypersensitivity reactions to native L-asparaginase; however, in one study, 32% of patients with a history of allergic reaction to E. coli asparaginase products also experienced allergic reaction to pegaspargase.

Serious thrombotic events, including sagittal sinus thrombosis may occur; discontinue with serious thrombotic event. Pancreatitis may occur; promptly evaluate patients with abdominal pain; discontinue if pancreatitis occurs during treatment. May cause glucose intolerance; irreversible in some cases; use with caution in patients with hyperglycemia, or diabetes. Coagulopathy has been reported; monitor coagulation parameters; severe or symptomatic coagulopathy may require treatment with fresh-frozen plasma; use with caution in patients with underlying coagulopathy. Reversible hepatotoxicity (hyperbilirubinemia and liver enzyme elevation) may occur; use with caution in patients with hepatic dysfunction or concomitant hepatotoxic medications. Use cautiously in patients with previous hematologic complications from asparaginase.

Drug Interactions

Avoid Concomitant Use

Avoid concomitant use of Pegaspargase with any of the following: BCG; Natalizumab; Pimecrolimus; Tacrolimus (Topical); Tofacitinib; Vaccines (Live)

Decreased Effect

Pegaspargase may decrease the levels/effects of: BCG; Coccidioidin Skin Test; Sipuleucel-T; Vaccines (Inactivated); Vaccines (Live)

The levels/effects of Pegaspargase may be decreased by: Echinacea; Pegloticase

Increased Effect/Toxicity

Pegaspargase may increase the levels/effects of: Leflunomide; Natalizumab; Tofacitinib; Vaccines (Live)

The levels/effects of Pegaspargase may be increased by: Denosumab; Pimecrolimus; Roflumilast; Tacrolimus (Topical); Trastuzumab

Adverse Reactions

>5%:

Cardiovascular: Edema

Central nervous system: Fever, malaise

Dermatologic: Rash

Gastrointestinal: Nausea, vomiting

Hematologic: Coagulopathy (7%; grades 3/4: 2%)

Hepatic: Transaminases increased (11%; grades 3/4: 3%)

Miscellaneous: Allergic reactions (including bronchospasm, chills, dyspnea, edema, erythema, hypotension, rash, swelling, urticaria; no prior asparaginase hypersensitivity: 1% to 10%; grades 3/4: 2%; prior asparaginase hypersensitivity: 32%; grades 3/4: 8%)

1% to 5%:

Cardiovascular: Hypotension, peripheral edema, tachycardia, thrombosis (4%)

Central nervous system: Chills, CNS thrombosis (2% to 4%; grades 3/4: 3%), CNS hemorrhage (2%), headache, seizure

Dermatologic: Lip edema, urticaria

Endocrine & metabolic: Hyperglycemia (3% to 5%; grades 3/4: ≤5%), hyperuricemia, hypoglycemia, hypoproteinemia

Gastrointestinal: Abdominal pain, anorexia, diarrhea, pancreatitis (1% to 2%; grades 3/4: 2%)

Hematologic: Anticoagulant effect decreased, disseminated intravascular coagulation (DIC), fibrinogen decreased, hemolytic anemia, leukopenia, pancytopenia, thrombocytopenia, thromboplastin increased, myelosuppression

Hepatic: Liver function tests abnormal (grades 3/4: 5%), hyperbilirubinemia (grades 3/4: 2%), jaundice

Local: Injection site hypersensitivity, pain or reaction

Neuromuscular & skeletal: Arthralgia, limb pain, myalgia, paresthesia

Respiratory: Dyspnea

Miscellaneous: Anaphylactic reactions, night sweats

Pharmacodynamics/Kinetics

Onset of Action Asparagine depletion: I.M.: Within 4 days

Duration of Action Asparagine depletion: I.M.: ~21 days; I.V. (in asparaginase naive adults): 2-4 weeks

Available Dosage Forms

Solution, Injection [preservative free]:
Oncaspar: 750 units/mL (5 mL)

General Dosage Range I.M., I.V.: *Children and Adults:* 2500 units/m² every 14 days

Administration

I.M. Must only be administered as a deep intramuscular injection into a large muscle. Do not exceed 2 mL per injection site; use multiple injection sites for I.M. injection volume >2 mL.

Hazardous agent; use appropriate precautions for handling and disposal (NIOSH, 2012).

I.V. Administer over 1-2 hours through a running I.V. infusion line; **do not administer I.V. push.**

Hazardous agent; use appropriate precautions for handling and disposal (NIOSH, 2012).

Injectable Detail Have available appropriate agents for maintenance of an adequate airway and treatment of a hypersensitivity reaction (antihistamine, epinephrine, oxygen, I.V. corticosteroids). Be prepared to treat anaphylaxis at each administration.

pH: 7.3

Preparation for Administration Hazardous agent; use appropriate precautions for handling and disposal (NIOSH, 2012).

I.V.: Dilute in 100 mL NS or D$_5$W.

Storage/Stability Refrigerate unused vials at 2°C to 8°C (36°F to 46°F); do not freeze. Do not shake; protect from light. Discard vial if previously frozen, stored at room temperature for >48 hours, excessively shaken/agitated, or if cloudy, discolored, or if precipitate is present. If not used immediately, solutions for infusion should be refrigerated at 2°C to 8°C (36°F to 46°F) and used within 48 hours (including administration time).

Nursing Actions

Physical Assessment Monitor patient during and for at least 1 hour following administration; treatment for anaphylactic reactions should be available. Monitor for GI disturbance, thrombotic events, pancreatitis, depression of clotting factors, glucose intolerance, and hypotension.

Patient Education

• Discuss specific use of drug and side effects with patient as it relates to treatment. (HCAHPS: During this hospital stay, were you given any medicine that you had not taken before? Before giving you any new medicine, how often did hospital staff tell you what the medicine was for? How often did hospital staff describe possible side effects in a way you could understand?)

• Patient may experience nausea. Have patient report immediately to prescriber signs of pancreatitis, signs of hyperglycemia, signs of hepatic impairment, strength differences from one side to another, difficulty speaking or thinking, change in balance, blurred vision, angina, edema of extremities, hemoptysis, dyspnea, severe headache, ecchymosis, hemorrhaging, hallucinations, vision changes, illogical thinking, urinary retention, or oliguria (HCAHPS).

• Educate patient about signs of a significant reaction (eg, wheezing; chest tightness; fever; itching; bad cough; blue skin color; seizures; or swelling of face, lips, tongue, or throat). **Note:** This is not a comprehensive list of all side effects. Patient should consult prescriber for additional questions.

Intended Use and Disclaimer: Should not be printed and given to patients. This information is intended to serve as a concise initial reference for healthcare professionals to use when discussing medications with a patient. You must ultimately rely on your own discretion, experience and judgment in diagnosing, treating and advising patients.

Peginterferon Alfa-2a
(peg in ter FEER on AL fa too aye)

Brand Names: U.S. Pegasys; Pegasys ProClick

Index Terms Interferon Alfa-2a (PEG Conjugate); PEG-IFN Alfa-2a; Pegylated Interferon Alfa-2a

Pharmacologic Category Interferon

Medication Guide Available Yes

Pregnancy Risk Factor C / X in combination with ribavirin

Lactation Excretion in breast milk unknown/not recommended

Breast-Feeding Considerations Breast milk samples obtained from a lactating mother prior to and after administration of interferon alfa-2b showed that interferon alfa is present in breast milk and administration of the medication did not significantly affect endogenous levels. Breast-feeding is not linked to the spread of hepatitis C virus; however, if nipples are cracked or bleeding, breast-feeding is not recommended. Mothers coinfected with HIV are discouraged from breast-feeding to decrease potential transmission of HIV.

Use

Chronic hepatitis B: Treatment of adults with hepatitis B e antigen (HBeAg)-positive and HBeAG-negative chronic hepatitis B virus (HBV) infection who have compensated liver disease and evidence of viral replication and liver inflammation

Chronic hepatitis C:
Treatment of patients with chronic hepatitis C virus (HCV) infection who have compensated liver disease and have not been previously

treated with interferon alfa, alone or in combination with ribavirin (monotherapy with peginterferon alfa-2a is not recommended for treatment of chronic hepatitis C infection unless a patient has a contraindication to or significant intolerance of ribavirin). Efficacy was demonstrated in patients with compensated liver disease and histological evidence of cirrhosis (Child-Pugh class A), and adult patients with clinically stable HIV disease (CD4 count >100 cells/mm^3).

Combination with ribavirin and an HCV NS3/4A protease inhibitor is indicated in adults with HCV genotype 1.

Combination with ribavirin is indicated in patients with HCV genotypes other than 1, children ≥5 years of age and adolescents, or patients with HCV genotype 1 where use of an HCV NS3/4A protease inhibitor is not warranted based on tolerability, contraindications or other clinical factors.

Mechanism of Action/Effect Alpha interferons are a family of proteins, produced by nucleated cells that have antiviral, antiproliferative, and immune-regulating activity. There are 16 known subtypes of alpha interferons. Interferons interact with cells through high affinity cell surface receptors. Following activation, multiple effects can be detected including induction of gene transcription. Interferons inhibit cellular growth, alter the state of cellular differentiation, interfere with oncogene expression, alter cell surface antigen expression, increase phagocytic activity of macrophages, and augment cytotoxicity of lymphocytes for target cells.

Contraindications Hypersensitivity to polyethylene glycol (PEG), interferon alfa, or any component of the formulation; autoimmune hepatitis; decompensated liver disease in cirrhotic patients (Child-Pugh score >6); decompensated liver disease (Child-Pugh score ≥6, class B and C) in CHC coinfected with HIV; neonates and infants

Warnings/Precautions [U.S. Boxed Warning]: May cause or exacerbate life-threatening neuropsychiatric disorders; monitor closely; discontinue treatment with worsening or persistently severe signs/symptoms of neuropsychiatric disorders. In most cases these effects were reversible following discontinuation, but not all cases. Neuropsychiatric adverse effects include depression, suicidal ideation, suicide attempt, homicidal ideation, drug overdose, and relapse of drug addiction, and may occur in patients with or without a prior history of psychiatric disorder. Avoid use in severe psychiatric disorders; use with extreme caution in patients with a history of depression. Patients who experience dizziness, confusion, somnolence or fatigue should use caution when performing tasks which require mental alertness (eg, operating machinery or driving).

[U.S. Boxed Warning]: May cause or exacerbate autoimmune disorders; monitor closely; discontinue treatment in patients with worsening or persistently severe signs/symptoms of autoimmune disease. Thyroiditis, thrombotic thrombocytopenic purpura, immune thrombocytopenia (ITP), rheumatoid arthritis, interstitial nephritis, systemic lupus erythematosus, and psoriasis have been reported with interferon therapy; use with caution in patients with autoimmune disorders.

[U.S. Boxed Warning]: May cause or aggravate infectious disorders; monitor closely; discontinue treatment in patients with worsening or persistently severe signs/symptoms of infectious disorders. Serious and severe infections (bacterial, viral, and fungal) have been reported with treatment. Interferon therapy is commonly associated with flu-like symptoms, including fever; however, rule out other causes/infection with persistent or high fever.

[U.S. Boxed Warning]: May cause or aggravate ischemic disorders and hemorrhagic cerebrovascular events; monitor closely; discontinue treatment in patients with worsening or persistent ischemia. Has been reported in patients without risk factors for stroke.

[U.S. Boxed Warning]: Combination treatment with ribavirin may cause birth defects and/or fetal mortality (avoid pregnancy in females and female partners of male patients); hemolytic anemia (which may worsen cardiac disease), genotoxicity, mutagenicity, and may possibly be carcinogenic.

May cause myelosuppression (including neutropenia, thrombocytopenia, lymphopenia, aplastic anemia). Use caution with baseline neutrophil count <1500/mm^3, platelet count <90,000/mm^3 or hemoglobin <10 g/dL. Discontinue therapy (at least temporarily) if ANC <500/mm^3 or platelet count <25,000/mm^3.

Hepatic decompensation and death have been associated with the use of alpha interferons including Pegasys®, in cirrhotic chronic hepatitis C patients; patients coinfected with HIV and receiving highly active antiretroviral therapy have shown an increased risk. Monitor hepatic function closely during use; discontinue if decompensation occurs (Child-Pugh score >6) in monoinfected patients and (Child-Pugh score ≥6, class B and C) in patients coinfected with HIV. In hepatitis B patients, flares (transient and potentially severe increases in serum ALT) may occur during or after treatment; more frequent monitoring of LFTs and a dose reduction are recommended. Discontinue if ALT elevation continues despite dose reduction or if increased bilirubin or hepatic decompensation occur.

Gastrointestinal hemorrhage, ulcerative and hemorrhagic/ischemic colitis have been observed with interferon alfa treatment; may be severe and/or life-threatening; discontinue if symptoms of colitis (eg, abdominal pain, bloody diarrhea, and/or fever) develop. Colitis generally resolves within 1-3 weeks of discontinuation. Discontinue therapy if known or suspected pancreatitis develops.

Use with caution in patients with diabetes mellitus; hyper- or hypoglycemia have been reported which may require adjustments in medications. Use with caution in patients with pre-existing thyroid disease; thyroid disorders (hyper- or hypothyroidism) or exacerbations have been reported. Use with caution in patients with prior cardiovascular disease; hypertension, arrhythmia, chest pain, and MI have been observed with treatment.

Severe acute hypersensitivity reactions (including anaphylaxis) have occurred rarely; prompt discontinuation is advised. Serious cutaneous reactions, including vesiculobullous eruptions, Stevens-Johnson syndrome and exfoliative dermatitis, have been reported (rarely) with use, with or without ribavirin therapy; discontinue with signs or symptoms of severe skin reactions.

Discontinue if new or worsening ophthalmologic disorders occur including decreased vision, retinal hemorrhages, retinal detachment (serous), cotton wool spots, and retinal artery or vein obstruction; if any ocular symptoms occur during use, a complete eye exam should be performed promptly. Prior to use, all patients should have a visual exam and patients with pre-existing disorders (eg, diabetic or hypertensive retinopathy) should have exams periodically during therapy.

May cause or aggravate dyspnea, pulmonary infiltrates, pneumonia, bronchiolitis obliterans, interstitial pneumonia, and sarcoidosis, resulting in potentially fatal respiratory failure; may recur upon rechallenge with interferons. Discontinue with unexplained pulmonary infiltrates or evidence of impaired pulmonary function. Use caution in patients with a history of pulmonary disease. Use with caution in patients with renal dysfunction (CrCl <30 mL/minute); monitor for signs/symptoms of toxicity (dosage adjustment required if toxicity occurs).

Safety and efficacy have not been established in patients who have failed other alpha interferon therapy, have received liver or other organ transplants, have been coinfected with HBV **and** HCV or HIV, have been coinfected with HCV **and** HBV or HIV with a CD4+ cell count <100 cells/mm³, or been treated for >48 weeks.

Due to differences in dosage, patients should not change brands of interferon without the concurrence of their healthcare provider.

Delay in weight and height increases have been noted in children treated with interferon alfa and concomitant ribavirin for 48 weeks. At two-year follow up after treatment, most children had returned to their baseline growth curve percentiles. Use with caution in the elderly; certain adverse effects (eg, neuropsychiatric, cardiac, flu-like reactions) may be more severe. Pretreatment hematological and biochemical tests are recommended for all patients; pregnancy screening (if woman of childbearing age) and ECG (if preexisting cardiac abnormalities) are also recommended.

Drug Interactions

Avoid Concomitant Use

Avoid concomitant use of Peginterferon Alfa-2a with any of the following: CloZAPine; Telbivudine

Decreased Effect

The levels/effects of Peginterferon Alfa-2a may be decreased by: Pegloticase

Increased Effect/Toxicity

Peginterferon Alfa-2a may increase the levels/ effects of: Aldesleukin; CloZAPine; Methadone; Ribavirin; Telbivudine; Theophylline Derivatives; Zidovudine

Nutritional/Ethanol Interactions Ethanol: Avoid use in patients with hepatitis C virus.

Adverse Reactions Note: Percentages are reported for peginterferon alfa-2a in chronic hepatitis C (CHC) patients. Other percentages indicated as "with ribavirin" or "in HIV/CHC" are those which significantly exceed incidence reported for peginterferon monotherapy in CHC patients.

>10%:

Central nervous system: Headache (54%), fatigue (56%), fever (37%; 41% with ribavirin; 54% in hepatitis B), insomnia (19%; 30% with ribavirin), depression (18%), dizziness (16%), irritability/anxiety/nervousness (19%; 33% with ribavirin), pain (11%)

Dermatologic: Alopecia (23%; 28% with ribavirin), pruritus (12%; 19% with ribavirin), dermatitis (16% with ribavirin)

Endocrine & metabolic: Growth suppression (children) percentile decrease (≥15 percentiles), weight (43%), height (25%)

Gastrointestinal: Nausea/vomiting (24%), anorexia (17%; 24% with ribavirin), diarrhea (16%), weight loss (16% in HIV/CHC), abdominal pain (15%)

Hematologic: Neutropenia (21%; 27% with ribavirin; 40% in HIV/CHC), lymphopenia (14% with ribavirin), anemia (11% with ribavirin; 14% in HIV/CHC)

Hepatic: ALT increases 5-10 x ULN during treatment (25% to 27% in hepatitis B); ALT increases >10 x ULN during treatment (12% to 18% in hepatitis B); ALT increases 5-10 x ULN after treatment (13% to 16% in hepatitis B); ALT increases >10 x ULN after treatment (7% to 12% in hepatitis B)

Local: Injection site reaction (22%)

Neuromuscular & skeletal: Weakness (56%; 65% with ribavirin), myalgia (37%), rigors (35%; 25% to 27% in hepatitis B), arthralgia (28%)

Respiratory: Dyspnea (13% with ribavirin)

1% to 10%:

Central nervous system: Concentration impaired (8%), memory impaired (5%), mood alteration (3%; 9% in HIV/CHC)

Dermatologic: Dermatitis (8%), rash (5%), dry skin (4%; 10% with ribavirin), eczema (1%; 5% with ribavirin)

Endocrine & metabolic: Hypothyroidism (3% to 4%), hyperthyroidism (≤1%)

Gastrointestinal: Xerostomia (6%), dyspepsia (<1%; 6% with ribavirin), weight loss (4%; 10% with ribavirin)

Hematologic: Thrombocytopenia (5%; 8% in HIV/CHC), lymphopenia (3%), anemia (2%)

Hepatic: Hepatic decompensation (2% in CHC/HIV)

Neuromuscular & skeletal: Back pain (9%)

Ocular: Blurred vision (4%)

Respiratory: Cough (4%; 10% with ribavirin), dyspnea (4%), exertional dyspnea (4% with ribavirin)

Miscellaneous: Diaphoresis (6%), bacterial infection (3%; 5% in HIV/CHC)

Available Dosage Forms

Kit, Subcutaneous [preservative free]:

Pegasys: 180 mcg/0.5 mL

Solution, Subcutaneous [preservative free]:

Pegasys: 180 mcg/mL (1 mL); 180 mcg/0.5 mL (0.5 mL)

Pegasys ProClick: 135 mcg/0.5 mL (0.5 mL); 180 mcg/0.5 mL (0.5 mL)

General Dosage Range Dosage adjustment recommended in patients with hepatic or renal impairment or who develop toxicities

SubQ:

Children ≥5 years: 180 mcg/1.73 m^2 x BSA once weekly (maximum dose: 180 mcg)

Adults: 180 mcg once weekly

Administration

Subcutaneous Administer in the abdomen or thigh. Rotate injection site. Do not use if solution contains particulate matter or is discolored. Discard unused solution. Administration should be done on the same day and at approximately the same time each week.

Storage/Stability Store in refrigerator at 2°C to 8°C (36°F to 46°F). Do not freeze or shake. Protect from light. The following stability information has also been reported:

Intact vial: May be stored at room temperature for up to 14 days (Cohen, 2007).

Prefilled syringe: May be stored at room temperature for up to 6 days (Cohen, 2007).

Nursing Actions

Physical Assessment Monitor for autoimmune disorders, psychiatric symptoms (eg, depression, irritability, anxiety, insomnia), LFTs, hypo-/hyperthyroidism, ischemic disorders, and signs/symptoms of toxicity. Remind patient to get baseline eye exam. Teach patient appropriate injection technique and syringe/needle disposal. In children, assess height and weight.

Patient Education

• Discuss specific use of drug and side effects with patient as it relates to treatment. (HCAHPS: During this hospital stay, were you given any medicine that you had not taken before? Before giving you any new medicine, how often did hospital staff tell you what the medicine was for? How often did hospital staff describe possible side effects in a way you could understand?)

• Patient may experience anemia, leukopenia, thrombocytopenia, flu-like syndrome, presyncope, asthenia, blurred vision, illogical thinking, headache, dyspepsia, emesis, diarrhea, lack of appetite, hair loss, insomnia, or application site irritation. Have patient report immediately to prescriber angina, tachycardia, dyspnea, alteration in muscle strength, trouble speaking or thinking, change in balance, blurred vision, ecchymosis, hematuria, discolored skin or eyes, polyuria, significant weight loss, or rash (HCAHPS).

• Educate patient about signs of a significant reaction (eg, wheezing; chest tightness; fever; itching; bad cough; blue skin color; seizures; or swelling of face, lips, tongue, or throat). **Note:** This is not a comprehensive list of all side effects. Patient should consult prescriber for additional questions.

Intended Use and Disclaimer: Should not be printed and given to patients. This information is intended to serve as a concise initial reference for healthcare professionals to use when discussing medications with a patient. You must ultimately rely on your own discretion, experience and judgment in diagnosing, treating and advising patients.

Dietary Considerations Avoid ethanol use in patients with hepatitis C virus.

Peginterferon Alfa-2b
(peg in ter FEER on AL fa too bee)

Brand Names: U.S. Peg-Intron; Peg-Intron Redipen; Peg-Intron Redipen Pak 4; Sylatron

Index Terms Interferon Alfa-2b (PEG Conjugate); PEG-IFN Alfa-2b; Pegylated Interferon Alfa-2b; Polyethylene Glycol Interferon Alfa-2b

Pharmacologic Category Antineoplastic Agent, Biological Response Modulator; Biological Response Modulator; Immunomodulator, Systemic; Interferon

Medication Safety Issues
Sound-alike/look-alike issues:
Peginterferon alfa-2b may be confused with interferon alfa-2a, interferon alfa-2b, interferon alfa-n3, peginterferon alfa-2a

PegIntron may be confused with Intron A, Pegasys

International issues:
Peginterferon alfa-2b may be confused with interferon alpha multi-subtype which is available in international markets

Medication Guide Available Yes

Pregnancy Risk Factor C / X in combination with ribavirin

Lactation Excretion in breast milk unknown/not recommended

Use
PegIntron: Treatment of chronic hepatitis C (CHC; in combination with ribavirin) in patients who have compensated liver disease; treatment of chronic hepatitis C (as monotherapy) in adult patients with compensated liver disease who have never received alfa interferons and are intolerant to ribavirin or have contraindications to ribavirin. **Note:** Combination therapy with ribavirin provides better response rates than peginterferon monotherapy

Sylatron: Adjuvant treatment of melanoma (with microscopic or gross nodal involvement within 84 days of definitive surgical resection, including complete lymphadenectomy)

Available Dosage Forms
Kit, Subcutaneous:
Peg-Intron: 50 mcg/0.5 mL, 80 mcg/0.5 mL, 120 mcg/0.5 mL, 150 mcg/0.5 mL
Peg-Intron Redipen: 50 mcg/0.5 mL, 80 mcg/0.5 mL, 120 mcg/0.5 mL, 150 mcg/0.5 mL
Sylatron: 296 mcg, 444 mcg, 888 mcg, 4 X 296 mcg, 4 X 444 mcg, 4 X 888 mcg
Kit, Subcutaneous [preservative free]:
Peg-Intron Redipen Pak 4: 50 mcg/0.5 mL, 80 mcg/0.5 mL, 120 mcg/0.5 mL, 150 mcg/0.5 mL

General Dosage Range Dosage adjustment recommended in patients with renal impairment or who develop toxicities
SubQ: Melanoma:
Adults: Initial: 6 mcg/kg/week; Maintenance: 3 mcg/kg/week
SubQ: Chronic hepatitis C:
Children ≥3 years: 60 mcg/m²/week (in combination with ribavirin)
Adults: Peginterferon monotherapy (based on average weekly dose of 1 mcg/kg):
Adults ≤45 kg: 40 mcg once weekly
Adults 46-56 kg: 50 mcg once weekly
Adults 57-72 kg: 64 mcg once weekly
Adults 73-88 kg: 80 mcg once weekly
Adults 89-106 kg: 96 mcg once weekly
Adults 107-136 kg: 120 mcg once weekly
Adults 137-160 kg: 150 mcg once weekly

Adults: Combination therapy with ribavirin (based on average weekly dose of 1.5 mcg/kg):
Adults <40 kg: 50 mcg once weekly (with ribavirin 800 mg/day)
Adults 40-50 kg: 64 mcg once weekly (with ribavirin 800 mg/day)
Adults 51-60 kg: 80 mcg once weekly (with ribavirin 800 mg/day)
Adults 61-65 kg: 96 mcg once weekly (with ribavirin 800 mg/day)
Adults 66-75 kg: 96 mcg once weekly (with ribavirin 1000 mg/day)
Adults 76-80 kg: 120 mcg once weekly (with ribavirin 1000 mg/day)
Adults 81-85 kg: 120 mcg once weekly (with ribavirin 1200 mg/day)
Adults 86-105 kg: 150 mcg once weekly (with ribavirin 1200 mg/day)
Adults >105 kg: 1.5 mcg/kg once weekly (with ribavirin 1400 mg/day)

Administration
Subcutaneous For SubQ administration; rotate injection site; thigh, outer surface of upper arm, and abdomen are preferred injection sites; do not inject near navel or waistline; patients who are thin should only use thigh or upper arm. Do not inject into bruised, infected, irritated, red, or scarred skin. The weekly dose may be administered at bedtime to reduce flu-like symptoms. For the treatment of CHC, the administration volume depends on the patient's weight and the peginterferon concentration used.

Nursing Actions
Physical Assessment Evaluate for changes in mental status, depression, and other psychiatric symptoms before and during therapy. Monitor vital signs. Report any new or worsening vision problems, excessive diarrhea, mental status changes, signs of infection, diabetes, or jaundice. Teach patient appropriate injection technique, medication storage, and syringe/needle disposal.

Patient Education
• Discuss specific use of drug and side effects with patient as it relates to treatment. (HCAHPS: During this hospital stay, were you given any medicine that you had not taken before? Before giving you any new medicine, how often did hospital staff tell you what the medicine was for? How often did hospital staff describe possible side effects in a way you could understand?)
• Patient may experience presyncope, asthenia, blurred vision, illogical thinking, headache, dyspepsia, emesis, diarrhea, lack of appetite, skin irritation, alopecia, insomnia, anemia, leukopenia, or thrombocytopenia. Have patient report immediately to prescriber angina, dyspnea, ecchymosis, sudden change in eyesight, discolored urine, jaundice, significant weight gain or loss, polyuria, cold intolerance, or rash (HCAHPS).

- Educate patient about signs of a significant reaction (eg, wheezing; chest tightness; fever; itching; bad cough; blue skin color; seizures; or swelling of face, lips, tongue, or throat). **Note:** This is not a comprehensive list of all side effects. Patient should consult prescriber for additional questions.

Intended Use and Disclaimer: Should not be printed and given to patients. This information is intended to serve as a concise initial reference for healthcare professionals to use when discussing medications with a patient. You must ultimately rely on your own discretion, experience and judgment in diagnosing, treating and advising patients.

Pegloticase (peg LOE ti kase)

Brand Names: U.S. Krystexxa

Index Terms PEG-Uricase; Pegylated Urate Oxidase; Polyethylene Glycol-Conjugated Uricase; Recombinant Urate Oxidase, Pegylated; Urate Oxidase, Pegylated

Pharmacologic Category Enzyme; Enzyme, Urate-Oxidase (Recombinant)

Medication Guide Available Yes

Pregnancy Risk Factor C

Lactation Excretion in breast milk unknown/not recommended

Breast-Feeding Considerations Due to the potential for serious adverse reactions in the nursing infant, breast-feeding is not recommended.

Use Treatment of chronic gout refractory to conventional therapy

Mechanism of Action/Effect Converts uric acid to allantoin (an inactive and water soluble metabolite of uric acid) which lowers serum uric acid concentrations; it does not inhibit the formation of uric acid

Contraindications Glucose-6-phosphate dehydrogenase (G6PD) deficiency

Warnings/Precautions [U.S. Boxed Warning]: Anaphylaxis and infusion reactions have been reported during and after administration; patients should be closely monitored during infusion and for an appropriate period of time after the infusion. Therapy should be administered in a healthcare facility by skilled medical personnel prepared for the immediate treatment of anaphylaxis. All patients should be premedicated with antihistamines and corticosteroids. Anaphylaxis may occur at any time during treatment (including the initial dose). **Reactions generally occur within 2 hours of administration; however, delayed hypersensitivity reactions have also been reported.** Infusion reactions are varied; symptoms range from chest pain, pruritus/urticaria, or dyspnea to a clinical presentation of anaphylaxis (eg, hemodynamic instability, perioral or lingual edema). If a less

severe (nonanaphylactic) infusion reaction occurs, the infusion may be slowed, or stopped and restarted at a slower rate, at the physician's discretion. **Risk of an infusion reaction is increased in patients whose uric acid is >6 mg/dL; therefore, monitor serum uric acid concentrations prior to infusion and consider discontinuing treatment if concentrations exceed 6 mg/dL, particularly in the event of 2 consecutive concentrations >6 mg/dL.** Concurrent use with oral antihyperuricemic agents may delay interpretations of ineffective pegloticase treatment (ie, serum uric acid >6 mg/dL) and ultimately increase risk for anaphylactoid and/or infusion reactions. Discontinue use of oral antihyperuricemic agents prior to and do not initiate during the course of pegloticase therapy.

Therapy with antihyperuricemic agents commonly results in gout flare, particularly upon initiation due to rapid lowering of urate concentrations; gout flare-ups during treatment do not warrant discontinuation of therapy. Gout flare prophylaxis is recommended, using nonsteroidal anti-inflammatory agents (NSAID) or colchicines, unless contraindicated, beginning ≥1 week before initiation of pegloticase and continuing for at least 6 months. Exacerbation of heart failure has been observed in clinical trials; use caution in patients with preexisting heart failure. Due to the risk for hemolysis and methemoglobinemia, pegloticase is contraindicated in patients with G6PD deficiency. Patients at higher risk for G6PD deficiency (eg, African, Mediterranean) should be screened prior to therapy. Therapy is not appropriate for the treatment of asymptomatic hyperuricemia. Potential for immunogenicity exists with the use of therapeutic proteins. Antipegloticase antibodies and antiPEG antibodies commonly occurred during clinical trials in pegloticase-treated patients. High antipegloticase antibody titers were associated with failure to maintain uric acid normalization and were also associated with a higher incidence of infusion reactions. Due to potential for immunogenicity, closely monitor patients who reinitiate therapy after discontinuing treatment for >4 weeks; patients may be at increased risk for anaphylaxis and infusion reactions.

Drug Interactions

Avoid Concomitant Use

Avoid concomitant use of Pegloticase with any of the following: Allopurinol; Febuxostat; Probenecid

Decreased Effect

Pegloticase may decrease the levels/effects of: Certolizumab Pegol; Pegademase Bovine; Pegaptanib; Pegaspargase; Pegfilgrastim; Peginterferon Alfa-2a; Peginterferon Alfa-2b; Pegvisomant

Increased Effect/Toxicity

The levels/effects of Pegloticase may be increased by: Allopurinol; Febuxostat; Probenecid

Adverse Reactions

>10%:

Dermatologic: Bruising (11%), urticaria (11%)

Gastrointestinal: Nausea (12%)

Miscellaneous: Antibody formation (antipegloti-case antibodies: 92%; antiPEG antibodies: 42%), gout flare (74% within the first 3 months), infusion reactions (26%)

1% to 10%:

Cardiovascular: Chest pain (6% to 10%)

Dermatologic: Erythema (10%), pruritus (10%)

Gastrointestinal: Constipation (6%), vomiting (5%)

Respiratory: Dyspnea (7%), nasopharyngitis (7%)

Miscellaneous: Anaphylaxis (≤7%)

Frequency not defined: Anemia, diarrhea, headache, muscle spasms, nephrolithiasis

Pharmacodynamics/Kinetics

Onset of Action ~24 hours following the first dose, serum uric acid concentrations decreased

Duration of Action >300 hours (12.5 days)

Available Dosage Forms

Solution, Intravenous:

Krystexxa: 8 mg/mL (1 mL)

General Dosage Range I.V.: *Adults:* 8 mg every 2 weeks

Administration

I.V. Administer diluted solution by I.V. infusion over ≥120 minutes via gravity feed or an infusion pump or syringe-type pump. Do **not** administer by I.V. push or bolus. Administer in a healthcare setting by healthcare providers prepared to manage potential anaphylaxis. Monitor closely for infusion reactions during infusion and for an appropriate period of time after the infusion (anaphylaxis has been reported within 2 hours of the infusion). In the event or a less severe infusion reaction, infusion may be slowed, or stopped and restarted at a slower rate, based on the discretion of the physician.

Preparation for Administration To prepare solution for administration, withdraw 1 mL (8 mg) and add to a 250 mL bag of NS or 1/2NS; invert bag several times to mix thoroughly (do **not** shake). Do not use vial if particulate matter is present or if solution is discolored (solution should be a clear and colorless). After withdrawal, discard any unused portion of the product remaining in the vial.

Storage/Stability Prior to use, vials must be stored in the carton to protect from light and kept under refrigeration between 2°C to 8°C (36°F to 46°F) at all times. Do **not** shake or freeze.

Diluted solution may be stored up to 4 hours at 2°C to 8°C (36°F to 46°F). Diluted solution is also stable for 4 hours at room temperature of 20°C to 25°C (68°F to 77°F); however, refrigeration is preferred. The diluted solution should be protected from light, not frozen, and used within 4 hours of dilution. Prior to administration, allow the diluted solution to reach room temperature; do not warm to room temperature using any form of artificial heating such as a microwave or warm water bath.

Nursing Actions

Patient Education

• Discuss specific use of drug and side effects with patient as it relates to treatment. (HCAHPS: During this hospital stay, were you given any medicine that you had not taken before? Before giving you any new medicine, how often did hospital staff tell you what the medicine was for? How often did hospital staff describe possible side effects in a way you could understand?)

• Patient may experience nausea, myalgia, or ecchymosis. Have patient report immediately to prescriber angina, severe dizziness, dyspnea, significant constipation, bleeding, or rash (HCAHPS).

• Educate patient about signs of a significant reaction (eg, wheezing; chest tightness; fever; itching; bad cough; blue skin color; seizures; or swelling of face, lips, tongue, or throat). **Note:** This is not a comprehensive list of all side effects. Patient should consult prescriber for additional questions.

Intended Use and Disclaimer: Should not be printed and given to patients. This information is intended to serve as a concise initial reference for healthcare professionals to use when discussing medications with a patient. You must ultimately rely on your own discretion, experience and judgment in diagnosing, treating and advising patients.

Pegvisomant (peg VI soe mant)

Brand Names: U.S. Somavert

Index Terms B2036-PEG

Pharmacologic Category Growth Hormone Receptor Antagonist

Medication Safety Issues

Sound-alike/look-alike issues:

Pegvisomant may be confused with peginesatide

Pregnancy Risk Factor C

Lactation Excretion in breast milk unknown/use caution

Use Acromegaly: Treatment of acromegaly in patients who have had an inadequate response to surgery or radiation therapy, or for whom these therapies are not appropriate.

Available Dosage Forms

Solution Reconstituted, Subcutaneous:

Somavert: 10 mg (1 ea); 15 mg (1 ea); 20 mg (1 ea)

General Dosage Range SubQ: *Adults:* Initial loading dose: 40 mg; Maintenance: 10-30 mg/day (maximum: 30 mg/day)

Administration

Other For SubQ administration only; to minimize the risk for lipohypertrophy, rotate injection site daily; if 2 injections are required, select a different injection site for second injection; may administer in upper arm, thigh, abdomen, or buttocks; do not rub injection site. Do not use on area of skin with rash, lumps, bruising or on broken skin. The manufacturer recommends the initial dose be administered under the supervision of prescribing healthcare provider.

Nursing Actions

Physical Assessment First dose should be administered under supervision of prescriber. Teach patient proper storage, reconstitution, injection technique, site rotation, and disposal of syringes/needles.

Patient Education

• Discuss specific use of drug and side effects with patient as it relates to treatment. (HCAHPS: During this hospital stay, were you given any medicine that you had not taken before? Before giving you any new medicine, how often did hospital staff tell you what the medicine was for? How often did hospital staff describe possible side effects in a way you could understand?)

• Patient may experience hypertension, nausea, diarrhea, flu-like syndrome, injection site irritation, or hepatic impairment. Have patient report immediately to prescriber severe dizziness, significant change in balance, discolored urine, jaundice, considerable asthenia, inability to eat, severe skin irritation, or rash (HCAHPS).

• Educate patient about signs of a significant reaction (eg, wheezing; chest tightness; fever; itching; bad cough; blue skin color; seizures; or swelling of face, lips, tongue, or throat). **Note:** This is not a comprehensive list of all side effects. Patient should consult prescriber for additional questions.

Intended Use and Disclaimer: Should not be printed and given to patients. This information is intended to serve as a concise initial reference for healthcare professionals to use when discussing medications with a patient. You must ultimately rely on your own discretion, experience and judgment in diagnosing, treating and advising patients.

Pemetrexed (pem e TREKS ed)

Brand Names: U.S. Alimta

Index Terms LY231514; Pemetrexed Disodium

Pharmacologic Category Antineoplastic Agent, Antimetabolite; Antineoplastic Agent, Antimetabolite (Antifolate)

Medication Safety Issues

Sound-alike/look-alike issues:

PEMEtrexed may be confused with methotrexate, PRALAtrexate

High alert medication:

This medication is in a class the Institute for Safe Medication Practices (ISMP) includes among its list of drug classes which have a heightened risk of causing significant patient harm when used in error.

Pregnancy Risk Factor D

Lactation Excretion in breast milk unknown/not recommended

Breast-Feeding Considerations According to the manufacturer, the decision to continue or discontinue breast-feeding during therapy should take into account the risk of exposure to the infant and the benefits of treatment to the mother.

Use Treatment of unresectable malignant pleural mesothelioma (in combination with cisplatin); treatment of locally advanced or metastatic **non**squamous nonsmall cell lung cancer (NSCLC; as initial treatment in combination with cisplatin, as single-agent maintenance treatment after 4 cycles of initial platinum-based double therapy, and single-agent treatment after prior chemotherapy)

Note: Not indicated for the treatment of **squamous** cell NSCLC

Unlabeled Use Treatment of bladder cancer (metastatic), cervical cancer (recurrent or metastatic), ovarian cancer (recurrent or persistent), thymic malignancies; treatment of malignant pleural mesothelioma (either as a single agent or in combination with carboplatin)

Mechanism of Action/Effect Disrupts folate-dependent metabolic processes essential for cell replication.

Contraindications Severe hypersensitivity to pemetrexed or any component of the formulation

Canadian labeling (additional contraindications; not in U.S. labeling): Concomitant yellow fever vaccine

Warnings/Precautions Hazardous agent - use appropriate precautions for handling and disposal (NIOSH, 2012). Hypersensitivity (including anaphylaxis) has been reported with use. May cause bone marrow suppression (anemia, neutropenia, thrombocytopenia and/or pancytopenia); frequent laboratory monitoring is necessary (myelosuppression is often dose-limiting). Dose reductions in subsequent cycles may be required. Prophylactic folic acid and vitamin B_{12} supplements are necessary to reduce hematologic and gastrointestinal toxicity and infection; initiate supplementation 1 week before the first dose of pemetrexed. Pretreatment with dexamethasone is necessary to reduce the incidence and severity of cutaneous reactions. Rarely, Stevens-Johnson syndrome and toxic epidermal necrolysis have been reported. Although the effect of third space fluid is not fully defined, studies have determined pemetrexed concentrations in patients with mild-to-moderate ascites/pleural effusions were similar to concentrations in trials of patients without third space fluid accumulation. Drainage of fluid from ascites/effusions may be considered, but is not likely necessary. Use caution with hepatic dysfunction not due to metastases; may require dose adjustment. Interstitial pneumonitis with respiratory insufficiency has been

▶

observed with use; interrupt therapy and evaluate promptly with progressive dyspnea and cough.

The manufacturer does not recommend use in patients with CrCl <45 mL/minute. Decreased renal function results in increased toxicity. Use caution in patients receiving concurrent nephrotoxins; may result in delayed pemetrexed clearance. NSAIDs may reduce the clearance of pemetrexed. In patients with CrCl 45-79 mL/minute, interruption of NSAID therapy may be necessary prior to, during, and immediately after pemetrexed therapy. Not indicated for use in patients with squamous cell NSCLC.

Drug Interactions
Avoid Concomitant Use
Avoid concomitant use of PEMEtrexed with any of the following: BCG; CloZAPine; Natalizumab; Pimecrolimus; Tacrolimus (Topical); Tofacitinib; Vaccines (Live)

Decreased Effect
PEMEtrexed may decrease the levels/effects of: BCG; Coccidioidin Skin Test; Sipuleucel-T; Vaccines (Inactivated); Vaccines (Live)

The levels/effects of PEMEtrexed may be decreased by: Echinacea

Increased Effect/Toxicity
PEMEtrexed may increase the levels/effects of: CloZAPine; Leflunomide; Natalizumab; Tofacitinib; Vaccines (Live)

The levels/effects of PEMEtrexed may be increased by: Denosumab; NSAID (Nonselective); Pimecrolimus; Roflumilast; Tacrolimus (Topical); Trastuzumab

Nutritional/Ethanol Interactions Lower ANC nadirs occur in patients with elevated baseline cystathionine or homocysteine concentrations. Levels of these substances can be reduced by folic acid and vitamin B_{12} supplementation.

Adverse Reactions
>10%:
Central nervous system: Fatigue (18% to 34%; dose-limiting)
Dermatologic: Rash/desquamation (10% to 14%)
Gastrointestinal: Nausea (12% to 31%), anorexia (19% to 22%), vomiting (6% to 16%), stomatitis (5% to 15%), diarrhea (5% to 13%)
Hematologic: Anemia (15% to 19%; grades 3/4: 3% to 5%), leukopenia (6% to 12%; grades 3/4: 2% to 4%), neutropenia (6% to 11%; grades 3/4: 3% to 5%; dose-limiting; nadir: 8-10 days; recovery: 4-8 days after nadir)
Respiratory: Pharyngitis (15%)
Central nervous system: Fatigue (25% to 34%; dose-limiting)
Dermatologic: Rash/desquamation (10% to 14%)
Gastrointestinal: Nausea (19% to 31%), anorexia (19% to 22%), vomiting (9% to 16%), stomatitis (7% to 15%), diarrhea (5% to 13%)

Hematologic: Anemia (15% to 19%; grades 3/4: 3% to 4%), leukopenia (6% to 12%; grades 3/4: 2% to 4%), neutropenia (6% to 11%; grades 3/4: 3% to 5%; dose-limiting; nadir: 8-10 days; recovery: 4-8 days after nadir)
Respiratory: Pharyngitis (15%)
1% to 10%:
Cardiovascular: Edema (1% to 5%)
Central nervous system: Fever (1% to 8%)
Dermatologic: Pruritus (1% to 7%), alopecia (1% to 6%), erythema multiforme (≤5%)
Gastrointestinal: Constipation (1% to 6%), weight loss (1%), abdominal pain (≤5%)
Hematologic: Thrombocytopenia (1% to 8%; grades 3/4: 2%; dose-limiting), febrile neutropenia (grades 3/4: 2%)
Hepatic: ALT increased (8% to 10%; grades 3/4: ≤2%), AST increased (7% to 8%; grades 3/4: ≤1%)
Neuromuscular & skeletal: Sensory neuropathy (≤9%), motor neuropathy (≤5%)
Ocular: Conjunctivitis (≤5%), lacrimation increased (≤5%)
Renal: Creatinine increased/creatinine clearance decreased (1% to 5%)
Miscellaneous: Allergic reaction/hypersensitivity (≤5%), infection (≤5%), sepsis (1%)

Available Dosage Forms
Solution Reconstituted, Intravenous:
Alimta: 100 mg (1 ea); 500 mg (1 ea)

General Dosage Range Dosage adjustment recommended in patients with hepatic impairment, on concomitant therapy, or who develop toxicities
I.V.: *Adults:* 500 mg/m^2 on day 1 of each 21-day cycle

Administration
I.V. Infuse over 10 minutes.

Hazardous agent; use appropriate precautions for handling and disposal (NIOSH, 2012).
Injectable Detail pH: 6.6-7.8
Preparation for Administration Hazardous agent; use appropriate precautions for handling and disposal (NIOSH, 2012). Reconstitute with NS (preservative free); add 4.2 mL to the 100 mg vial and 20 mL to the 500 mg vial, resulting in a 25 mg/mL concentration. Gently swirl. Solution may be colorless to green-yellow. Further dilute in 100 mL NS for infusion; may also dilute in D_5W (Zhang, 2006), although the manufacturer recommends NS.

Storage/Stability Store intact vials at room temperature of 25°C (77°F); excursions permitted to 15°C to 30°C (59°F to 86°F). Reconstituted solution in NS and infusion solutions (in D_5W or NS) are stable for 24 hours when refrigerated at 2°C to 8°C (36°F to 46°F). Concentrations at 25 mg/mL are stable in polypropylene syringes for 2 days at room temperature (23°C) (Zhang, 2005).

Nursing Actions

Physical Assessment Pre- and post-treatment medication may be prescribed (eg, oral folic acid and vitamin B_{12} 1 week [injection] before first dose). Corticosteroids may be ordered to reduce cutaneous reactions. Monitor for CNS changes, GI upset (nausea, vomiting, diarrhea, constipation), anemia, neuropathy, rash, and infection.

Patient Education
- Discuss specific use of drug and side effects with patient as it relates to treatment. (HCAHPS: During this hospital stay, were you given any medicine that you had not taken before? Before giving you any new medicine, how often did hospital staff tell you what the medicine was for? How often did hospital staff describe possible side effects in a way you could understand?)
- Patient may experience anemia, leukopenia, thrombocytopenia, fatigue, nausea, diarrhea, loss of appetite, stomatitis, pharyngitis, edema, or skin irritation. Have patient report immediately to prescriber signs of infection, angina, dyspnea, ecchymosis, rash, or pregnancy (HCAHPS).
- Educate patient about signs of a significant reaction (eg, wheezing; chest tightness; fever; itching; bad cough; blue skin color; seizures; or swelling of face, lips, tongue, or throat). **Note:** This is not a comprehensive list of all side effects. Patient should consult prescriber for additional questions.

Intended Use and Disclaimer: Should not be printed and given to patients. This information is intended to serve as a concise initial reference for healthcare professionals to use when discussing medications with a patient. You must ultimately rely on your own discretion, experience and judgment in diagnosing, treating and advising patients.

Dietary Considerations Initiate folic acid supplementation 1 week before first dose of pemetrexed, continue for full course of therapy, and for 21 days after last dose. Institute vitamin B_{12} 1 week before the first dose; administer every 9 weeks thereafter.

Penicillin G Benzathine
(pen i SIL in jee BENZ a theen)

Brand Names: U.S. Bicillin L-A
Index Terms Benzathine Benzylpenicillin; Benzathine Penicillin G; Benzylpenicillin Benzathine
Pharmacologic Category Antibiotic, Penicillin
Medication Safety Issues
Sound-alike/look-alike issues:
Penicillin may be confused with penicillamine
Bicillin® may be confused with Wycillin®
Administration issues:
Penicillin G benzathine may only be administered by deep intramuscular injection; intravenous administration of penicillin G benzathine has been associated with cardiopulmonary arrest and death.

Other safety concerns:
Bicillin® C-R (penicillin G benzathine and penicillin G procaine) may be confused with Bicillin® L-A (penicillin G benzathine). Penicillin G benzathine is the only product currently approved for the treatment of syphilis. Administration of penicillin G benzathine and penicillin G procaine combination instead of Bicillin® L-A may result in inadequate treatment response.

Pregnancy Risk Factor B
Lactation Enters breast milk/use caution
Use Active against some gram-positive organisms, few gram-negative organisms such as *Neisseria gonorrhoeae*, and some anaerobes and spirochetes; used in the treatment of syphilis; used only for the treatment of mild to moderately-severe upper respiratory tract infections caused by organisms susceptible to low concentrations of penicillin G or for prophylaxis of infections caused by these organisms; primary and secondary prevention of rheumatic fever
Available Dosage Forms
Suspension, Intramuscular:
Bicillin L-A: 600,000 units/mL (1 mL); 1,200,000 units/2 mL (2 mL); 2,400,000 units/4 mL (4 mL)
General Dosage Range I.M.:
Children ≤27 kg: 600,000 units/dose
Children >27 kg: 1.2 million units/dose
Adults: 1.2-2.4 million units as a single dose
Administration
I.M. Warm to room temperature before administration to lessen the pain associated with injection. Administer by deep I.M. injection in the upper outer quadrant of the buttock; in children <2 years of age, I.M. injections should be made into the midlateral muscle of the thigh, not the gluteal region. Do not inject near an artery or a nerve; permanent neurological damage or gangrene may result. When doses are repeated, rotate the injection site. **Do not administer I.V., intra-arterially, or SubQ.**
Nursing Actions
Physical Assessment Results of culture and sensitivity tests and patient's allergy history should be assessed prior to starting therapy. Monitor for hypersensitivity reactions and opportunistic infection.
Patient Education
- Discuss specific use of drug and side effects with patient as it relates to treatment. (HCAHPS: During this hospital stay, were you given any medicine that you had not taken before? Before giving you any new medicine, how often did hospital staff tell you what the medicine was for? How often did hospital staff describe possible side effects in a way you could understand?)
- Patient may experience nausea, diarrhea, or vaginal yeast infection. Have patient report

immediately to prescriber ecchymosis, bleeding, or rash (HCAHPS).

- Educate patient about signs of a significant reaction (eg, wheezing; chest tightness; fever; itching; bad cough; blue skin color; seizures; or swelling of face, lips, tongue, or throat). **Note:** This is not a comprehensive list of all side effects. Patient should consult prescriber for additional questions.

Intended Use and Disclaimer: Should not be printed and given to patients. This information is intended to serve as a concise initial reference for healthcare professionals to use when discussing medications with a patient. You must ultimately rely on your own discretion, experience and judgment in diagnosing, treating and advising patients.

Penicillin G (Parenteral/Aqueous)
(pen i SIL in jee, pa REN ter al, AYE kwee us)

Brand Names: U.S. Pfizerpen-G

Index Terms Benzylpenicillin Potassium; Benzylpenicillin Sodium; Crystalline Penicillin; Penicillin G Potassium; Penicillin G Sodium

Pharmacologic Category Antibiotic, Penicillin

Medication Safety Issues
Sound-alike/look-alike issues:
Penicillin may be confused with penicillamine

Pregnancy Risk Factor B

Lactation Enters breast milk/use caution

Breast-Feeding Considerations Very small amounts of penicillin G transfer into breast milk. Peak milk concentrations occur at approximately 1 hour after an IM dose and are higher if multiple doses are given. The manufacturer recommends that caution be exercised when administering penicillin to nursing women. Nondose-related effects could include modification of bowel flora and allergic sensitization.

Use Treatment of infections (including sepsis, pneumonia, pericarditis, endocarditis, meningitis, anthrax) caused by susceptible organisms; active against some gram-positive organisms, generally not *Staphylococcus aureus*; some gram-negative organisms such as *Neisseria gonorrhoeae*, and some anaerobes and spirochetes

Mechanism of Action/Effect Interferes with bacterial cell wall synthesis during active multiplication, causing cell wall death and resultant bactericidal activity against susceptible bacteria

Contraindications Hypersensitivity to penicillin or any component of the formulation

Warnings/Precautions Avoid intra-arterial administration or injection into or near major peripheral nerves or blood vessels since such injections may cause severe and/or permanent neurovascular damage; use with caution in patients with renal impairment (dosage reduction required), concomitant renal and hepatic impairment (further dosage

adjustment may be required), pre-existing seizure disorders, or with a history of hypersensitivity to cephalosporins. Prolonged use may result in fungal or bacterial superinfection, including *C. difficile*-associated diarrhea (CDAD) and pseudomembranous colitis; CDAD has been observed >2 months postantibiotic treatment. Serious and occasionally severe or fatal hypersensitivity (anaphylactoid) reactions have been reported in patients on penicillin therapy, especially with a history of beta-lactam hypersensitivity, history of sensitivity to multiple allergens, or previous IgE-mediated reactions (eg, anaphylaxis, angioedema, urticaria). Use with caution in asthmatic patients. Extended duration of therapy or use associated with high serum concentrations may be associated with an increased risk for some adverse reactions. Neonates may have decreased renal clearance of penicillin and require frequent dosage adjustments depending on age. Product contains sodium and potassium; high doses of I.V. therapy may alter serum levels.

Drug Interactions
Avoid Concomitant Use
Avoid concomitant use of Penicillin G (Parenteral/Aqueous) with any of the following: BCG

Decreased Effect
Penicillin G (Parenteral/Aqueous) may decrease the levels/effects of: BCG; Mycophenolate; Sodium Picosulfate; Typhoid Vaccine

The levels/effects of Penicillin G (Parenteral/Aqueous) may be decreased by: Tetracycline Derivatives

Increased Effect/Toxicity
Penicillin G (Parenteral/Aqueous) may increase the levels/effects of: Methotrexate; Vitamin K Antagonists

The levels/effects of Penicillin G (Parenteral/Aqueous) may be increased by: Probenecid

Adverse Reactions Frequency not defined.

Cardiovascular: Localized phlebitis, local thrombophlebitis

Central nervous system: Coma (high doses), hyperreflexia (high doses), myoclonus (high doses), seizure (high doses)

Dermatologic: Contact dermatitis, skin rash

Endocrine & metabolic: Electrolyte disturbance (high doses)

Gastrointestinal: Pseudomembranous colitis

Hematologic & oncologic: Neutropenia, positive direct Coombs test (rare, high doses)

Hypersensitivity: Anaphylaxis, hypersensitivity reaction (immediate and delayed), serum sickness

Immunologic: Jarisch-Herxheimer reaction

Local: Injection site reaction

Renal: Acute interstitial nephritis (high doses), renal tubular disease (high doses)

Available Dosage Forms

Solution, Intravenous:

Generic: 20,000 units/mL (50 mL); 40,000 units/ mL (50 mL); 60,000 units/mL (50 mL)

Solution Reconstituted, Injection:

Pfizerpen-G: 5,000,000 units (1 ea); 20,000,000 units (1 ea)

Generic: 5,000,000 units (1 ea); 20,000,000 units (1 ea)

Solution Reconstituted, Injection [preservative free]:

Generic: 20,000,000 units (1 ea)

General Dosage Range Dosage adjustment recommended in patients with renal impairment

I.M., I.V.:

Infants ≥1 month and Children: 100,000-400,000 units/kg/day in divided doses every 4-6 hours (maximum: 24 million units/day)

Adults: 2-30 million units/day in divided doses every 4-6 hours

Administration

I.M. Administer I.M. by deep injection in the upper outer quadrant of the buttock. Administer injection around-the-clock to promote less variation in peak and trough levels. **Note:** The 20 million unit dosage form may be administered by continuous I.V. infusion only.

I.V. Usually administered by intermittent infusion. In some centers, large doses may be administered by continuous I.V. infusion. **Note:** The 20 million unit dosage form may be administered by continuous I.V. infusion only.

Intermittent I.V.: May be dissolved in small amounts of SWFI, NS, D_5W and administered peripherally as a 50,000-100,000 unit/mL solution. In fluid-restricted patients, 146,000 units/ mL in SW results in a maximum recommended osmolality for peripheral infusion. Infuse over 15-30 minutes.

Continuous I.V. infusion: Determine the volume of fluid and rate of its administration required by the patient in a 24-hour period. Add the appropriate daily dosage of penicillin to this fluid. For example, if the daily dose is 10 million units and 2 L of fluid/day is required, add 5 million units to 1 L and adjust the rate of flow so the liter will be infused over 12 hours (83 mL/hour). Repeat steps (5 million units/L at 83 mL/hour) for the remaining 12 hours.

Injectable Detail pH: 6-7.5

Preparation for Administration

Intermittent I.V.: 5 million unit vial: Add 8.2 mL for a final concentration of 500,000 units/mL; add 3.2 mL for a final concentration of 1,000,000 units/ mL. Dilute further to 50,000-145,000 units/mL prior to infusion.

Continuous I.V. infusion: 20 million unit vial: Add 11.5 mL for a final concentration of 1,000,000 units/mL. Dilute further in 1-2 L of infusion solution and administer over a 24-hour period.

Storage/Stability

Penicillin G potassium powder for injection should be stored below 86°F (30°C). Following reconstitution, solution may be stored for up to 7 days under refrigeration. Premixed bags for infusion should be stored in the freezer (-20°C or -4°F); frozen bags may be thawed at room temperature or in refrigerator. Once thawed, solution is stable for 14 days if stored in refrigerator or for 24 hours when stored at room temperature. Do not refreeze once thawed.

Penicillin G sodium powder for injection should be stored at controlled room temperature. Reconstituted solution may be stored under refrigeration for up to 3 days.

Nursing Actions

Physical Assessment Results of culture and sensitivity tests and patient's allergy history should be assessed prior to starting therapy. Avoid intravascular or intra-arterial administration or injection into or near major peripheral nerves or blood vessels; may cause severe and/or permanent neurovascular damage. Monitor for hypersensitivity reactions, opportunistic infection (fever, chills, unhealed sores, white plaques in mouth or vagina, purulent vaginal discharge), CNS changes, and thrombophlebitis.

Patient Education

• Discuss specific use of drug and side effects with patient as it relates to treatment. (HCAHPS: During this hospital stay, were you given any medicine that you had not taken before? Before giving you any new medicine, how often did hospital staff tell you what the medicine was for? How often did hospital staff describe possible side effects in a way you could understand?)

• Patient may experience nausea, diarrhea, or vaginal yeast infection. Have patient report immediately to prescriber ecchymosis, bleeding, or rash (HCAHPS).

• Educate patient about signs of a significant reaction (eg, wheezing; chest tightness; fever; itching; bad cough; blue skin color; seizures; or swelling of face, lips, tongue, or throat). **Note:** This is not a comprehensive list of all side effects. Patient should consult prescriber for additional questions.

Intended Use and Disclaimer: Should not be printed and given to patients. This information is intended to serve as a concise initial reference for healthcare professionals to use when discussing medications with a patient. You must ultimately rely on your own discretion, experience and judgment in diagnosing, treating and advising patients.

Dietary Considerations Some products may contain potassium and/or sodium.

Penicillin G Procaine
(pen i SIL in jee PROE kane)

Index Terms APPG; Aqueous Procaine Penicillin G; Procaine Benzylpenicillin; Procaine Penicillin G; Wycillin

Pharmacologic Category Antibiotic, Penicillin

Medication Safety Issues
Sound-alike/look-alike issues:
Penicillin G procaine may be confused with penicillin V potassium
Wycillin® may be confused with Bicillin®

Pregnancy Risk Factor B

Lactation Enters breast milk/use caution

Use Treatment of moderately-severe infections due to *Treponema pallidum* and other penicillin G-sensitive microorganisms that are susceptible to low, but prolonged serum penicillin concentrations; anthrax due to *Bacillus anthracis* (postexposure) to reduce the incidence or progression of disease following exposure to aerolized *Bacillus anthracis*

Available Dosage Forms
Suspension, Intramuscular:
Generic: 600,000 units/mL (1 mL, 2 mL)

General Dosage Range Dosage adjustment recommended in patients with renal impairment
I.M.:
Children: 25,000-50,000 units/kg/day in divided doses 1-2 times/day (maximum: 4.8 million units/day)
Adults: 0.6-4.8 million units/day in divided doses every 12-24 hours

Administration
I.M. Procaine suspension is for deep I.M. injection only. Rotate the injection site. Do not inject in gluteal muscle in children <2 years of age. Avoid I.V., intravascular, or intra-arterial administration of penicillin G procaine since severe and/or permanent neurovascular damage may occur.

Nursing Actions
Physical Assessment Results of culture and sensitivity tests and patient's allergy history should be assessed prior to starting therapy. Avoid intravascular or intra-arterial administration or injection into or near major peripheral nerves or blood vessels; may cause severe and/or permanent neurovascular damage. Monitor for hypersensitivity reactions, opportunistic infection (fever, chills, unhealed sores, white plaques in mouth or vagina, purulent vaginal discharge), CNS changes, and thrombophlebitis.

Patient Education
• Discuss specific use of drug and side effects with patient as it relates to treatment. (HCAHPS: During this hospital stay, were you given any medicine that you had not taken before? Before giving you any new medicine, how often did hospital staff tell you what the medicine was for? How often did hospital staff describe possible side effects in a way you could understand?)

• Patient may experience nausea, diarrhea, short-term pain, or vaginal yeast infection. Have patient report immediately to prescriber ecchymosis, bleeding, or rash (HCAHPS).
• Educate patient about signs of a significant reaction (eg, wheezing; chest tightness; fever; itching; bad cough; blue skin color; seizures; or swelling of face, lips, tongue, or throat). **Note:** This is not a comprehensive list of all side effects. Patient should consult prescriber for additional questions.

Intended Use and Disclaimer: Should not be printed and given to patients. This information is intended to serve as a concise initial reference for healthcare professionals to use when discussing medications with a patient. You must ultimately rely on your own discretion, experience and judgment in diagnosing, treating and advising patients.

Penicillin V Potassium
(pen i SIL in vee poe TASS ee um)

Index Terms Pen VK; Phenoxymethyl Penicillin

Pharmacologic Category Antibiotic, Penicillin

Medication Safety Issues
Sound-alike/look-alike issues:
Penicillin V procaine may be confused with penicillin G potassium

Lactation Enters breast milk

Breast-Feeding Considerations Penicillin V is excreted into breast milk (low concentrations) and may be detected in the urine of some breast-feeding infants. Loose stools and rash have been reported in nursing infants.

Use Treatment of infections caused by susceptible organisms involving the respiratory tract, otitis media, sinusitis, skin, and soft tissues; prophylaxis in rheumatic fever

Unlabeled Use Chronic antimicrobial suppression of prosthetic joint infection; community-acquired cutaneous anthrax; cutaneous erysipeloid; group A streptococcal chronic carrier eradication; pneumococcal prophylaxis in patients with sickle cell disease or asplenia

Mechanism of Action/Effect Inhibits bacterial cell wall synthesis by binding to one or more of the penicillin-binding proteins (PBPs); which in turn inhibits the final transpeptidation step of peptidoglycan synthesis in bacterial cell walls, thus inhibiting cell wall biosynthesis. Bacteria eventually lyse due to ongoing activity of cell wall autolytic enzymes (autolysins and murein hydrolases) while cell wall assembly is arrested.

Contraindications Hypersensitivity to penicillin or any component of the formulation

Warnings/Precautions Use with caution in patients with severe renal impairment or history of seizures. Serious and occasionally severe or fatal hypersensitivity (anaphylactoid) reactions have been reported in patients on penicillin therapy, especially with a history of beta-lactam hypersensitivity, history of sensitivity to multiple allergens, or previous IgE-mediated reactions (eg, anaphylaxis, angioedema, urticaria). Use with caution in asthmatic patients. Extended duration of therapy or use associated with high serum concentrations may be associated with an increased risk for some adverse reactions. Prolonged use may result in fungal or bacterial superinfection, including *C. difficile*-associated diarrhea (CDAD) and pseudomembranous colitis; CDAD has been observed >2 months post-antibiotic treatment.

Drug Interactions

Avoid Concomitant Use

Avoid concomitant use of Penicillin V Potassium with any of the following: BCG

Decreased Effect

Penicillin V Potassium may decrease the levels/effects of: BCG; Mycophenolate; Sodium Picosulfate; Typhoid Vaccine

The levels/effects of Penicillin V Potassium may be decreased by: Tetracycline Derivatives

Increased Effect/Toxicity

Penicillin V Potassium may increase the levels/effects of: Methotrexate; Vitamin K Antagonists

The levels/effects of Penicillin V Potassium may be increased by: Probenecid

Nutritional/Ethanol Interactions Food:
Decreases drug absorption rate; decreases drug serum concentration. Management: Take on an empty stomach 1 hour before or 2 hours after meals around-the-clock to promote less variation in peak and trough serum levels.

Adverse Reactions >10%: Gastrointestinal: Mild diarrhea, vomiting, nausea, oral candidiasis

Available Dosage Forms

Solution Reconstituted, Oral:
Generic: 125 mg/5 mL (100 mL, 200 mL); 250 mg/5 mL (100 mL, 200 mL)

Tablet, Oral:
Generic: 250 mg, 500 mg

General Dosage Range Oral:

Children <12 years: 25-50 mg/kg/day divided every 6-8 hours (maximum: 3000 mg daily)

Children ≥12 years and Adults: 125-500 mg every 6-8 hours

Administration

Injectable Detail pH: 6-8.5 (reconstituted solution)

Oral Administer around-the-clock to promote less variation in peak and trough serum levels. Take on an empty stomach 1 hour before or 2 hours after meals, to enhance absorption, take until gone, do not skip doses.

Storage/Stability Refrigerate suspension after reconstitution; discard after 14 days.

Nursing Actions

Physical Assessment Results of culture and sensitivity tests and patient's allergy history should be assessed prior to starting therapy. Monitor for hypersensitivity reactions and opportunistic infection (fever, chills, unhealed sores, white plaques in mouth or vagina, purulent vaginal discharge, fatigue).

Patient Education

- Discuss specific use of drug and side effects with patient as it relates to treatment. (HCAHPS: During this hospital stay, were you given any medicine that you had not taken before? Before giving you any new medicine, how often did hospital staff tell you what the medicine was for? How often did hospital staff describe possible side effects in a way you could understand?)

- Patient may experience nausea, diarrhea, or vaginal yeast infection. Have patient report immediately to prescriber ecchymosis, bleeding, or rash (HCAHPS).

- Educate patient about signs of a significant reaction (eg, wheezing; chest tightness; fever; itching; bad cough; blue skin color; seizures; or swelling of face, lips, tongue, or throat). **Note:** This is not a comprehensive list of all side effects. Patient should consult prescriber for additional questions.

Intended Use and Disclaimer: Should not be printed and given to patients. This information is intended to serve as a concise initial reference for healthcare professionals to use when discussing medications with a patient. You must ultimately rely on your own discretion, experience and judgment in diagnosing, treating and advising patients.

Dietary Considerations Take on an empty stomach 1 hour before or 2 hours after meals.

Pentamidine (pen TAM i deen)

Brand Names: U.S. Nebupent; Pentam

Index Terms Pentamidine Isethionate

Pharmacologic Category Antifungal Agent; Antiprotozoal

Pregnancy Risk Factor C

Lactation Excretion in breast milk unknown/not recommended

Use

I.M., I.V.: Treatment of pneumonia caused by *Pneumocystis jirovecii* pneumonia (PCP)

Inhalation: Prevention of PCP in high-risk, HIV-infected patients either with a history of PCP or with a CD4+ count ≤200/mm^3

Unlabeled Use Prevention of PCP in nonHIV-infected patients; treatment of African trypanosomiasis, cutaneous leishmaniasis, and amebic meningoencephalitis

Available Dosage Forms

Solution Reconstituted, Inhalation:
Nebupent: 300 mg (1 ea)

Solution Reconstituted, Injection:
Pentam: 300 mg (1 ea)

General Dosage Range Dosage adjustment recommended in patients with renal impairment

I.M.: *Children >4 months and Adults:* 4 mg/kg once daily for 14-21 days

I.V.: *Children >4 months and Adults:* 4 mg/kg once daily for 14-21 days

Inhalation: *Children >16 years and Adults:* 300 mg/dose every 4 weeks

Administration

I.M. Administer deep I.M. Do not use NS as a diluent.

Hazardous agent; use appropriate precautions for handling and disposal (NIOSH, 2012).

I.V.

Do not use NS as an initial diluent. Infuse slowly over 60-120 minutes.

Irritant with vesicant-like properties; ensure proper needle or catheter placement prior to and during infusion. Avoid extravasation.

Extravasation management: If extravasation occurs, stop infusion immediately and disconnect (leave cannula/needle in place); gently aspirate extravasated solution (do **NOT** flush the line); remove needle/cannula; elevate extremity. Apply dry warm compresses (Reynolds, 2014).

Hazardous agent; use appropriate precautions for handling and disposal (NIOSH, 2012).

Inhalation Deliver via Respirgard® II nebulizer until nebulizer is emptied (30-45 minutes). Administer at a flow rate of 5-7 L/minute from a 40-50 pound-per-square inch (PSI) oxygen or air source. A 40-50 PSI air compressor can be used alternatively, with a set flow rate at 5-7 L/minute or a set pressure of 22-25 PSI. Air compressors <20 PSI should not be used. Use appropriate precautions to minimize exposure to healthcare personnel; refer to individual institutional policy.

Hazardous agent; use appropriate precautions for handling and disposal (NIOSH, 2012).

Nursing Actions

Physical Assessment I.V., I.M.: Patients should be lying down. Blood pressure, cardiac status, and respiratory function should be monitored closely during administration and several times thereafter until blood pressure is stable. Monitor for hypotension, rash, confusion, hallucinations, hypoglycemia, dyspnea, and cough. If self-administered, teach patient proper use of nebulizer.

Patient Education

• Discuss specific use of drug and side effects with patient as it relates to treatment. (HCAHPS: During this hospital stay, were you given any medicine that you had not taken before? Before giving you any new medicine, how often did hospital staff tell you what the medicine was for? How often did hospital staff describe possible side effects in a way you could understand?)

• Patient may experience dizziness, parageusia, asthenia, lack of appetite, injection site irritation, nausea, hypoglycemia, anemia, or thrombocytopenia. Have patient report immediately to prescriber signs of infection, angina, tachycardia, illogical thinking, severe hypertension, significant diarrhea, ecchymosis, bleeding, or rash (HCAHPS).

• Educate patient about signs of a significant reaction (eg, wheezing; chest tightness; fever; itching; bad cough; blue skin color; seizures; or swelling of face, lips, tongue, or throat). **Note:** This is not a comprehensive list of all side effects. Patient should consult prescriber for additional questions.

Intended Use and Disclaimer: Should not be printed and given to patients. This information is intended to serve as a concise initial reference for healthcare professionals to use when discussing medications with a patient. You must ultimately rely on your own discretion, experience and judgment in diagnosing, treating and advising patients.

Related Information

Management of Drug Extravasations *on page 1700*

Pentazocine and Naloxone
(pen TAZ oh seen & nal OKS one)

Index Terms Naloxone Hydrochloride and Pentazocine; Pentazocine Hydrochloride and Naloxone Hydrochloride; Talwin NX

Pharmacologic Category Analgesic, Opioid; Analgesic, Opioid Partial Agonist

Medication Safety Issues

High alert medication:

The Institute for Safe Medication Practices (ISMP) includes this medication among its list of drug classes which have a heightened risk of causing significant patient harm when used in error.

Pregnancy Risk Factor C

Lactation Pentazocine enters breast milk/use caution

Use Relief of moderate-to-severe pain; indicated for oral use only

Controlled Substance C-IV

Available Dosage Forms

Tablet, oral: Pentazocine 50 mg and naloxone 0.5 mg

General Dosage Range Dosage adjustment recommended in patients with renal impairment

Oral: *Children ≥12 years and Adults:* Based upon pentazocine: 50-100 mg every 3-4 hours (maximum: 600 mg/day)

Nursing Actions

Physical Assessment See individual agents.

Patient Education

- Discuss specific use of drug and side effects with patient as it relates to treatment. (HCAHPS: During this hospital stay, were you given any medicine that you had not taken before? Before giving you any new medicine, how often did hospital staff tell you what the medicine was for? How often did hospital staff describe possible side effects in a way you could understand?)
- Patient may experience presyncope, fatigue, blurred vision, illogical thinking, dizziness, nausea, or constipation. Have patient report immediately to prescriber dyspnea, poor pain control, or severe asthenia (HCAHPS).
- Educate patient about signs of a significant reaction (eg, wheezing; chest tightness; fever; itching; bad cough; blue skin color; seizures; or swelling of face, lips, tongue, or throat). **Note:** This is not a comprehensive list of all side effects. Patient should consult prescriber for additional questions.

Intended Use and Disclaimer: Should not be printed and given to patients. This information is intended to serve as a concise initial reference for healthcare professionals to use when discussing medications with a patient. You must ultimately rely on your own discretion, experience and judgment in diagnosing, treating and advising patients.

Related Information

Naloxone *on page 1098*

Pentosan Polysulfate Sodium
(PEN toe san pol i SUL fate SOW dee um)

Brand Names: U.S. Elmiron
Index Terms PPS
Pharmacologic Category Analgesic, Urinary
Medication Safety Issues
  Sound-alike/look-alike issues:
  Pentosan may be confused with pentostatin
  Elmiron® may be confused with Imuran®
Pregnancy Risk Factor B
Lactation Excretion in breast milk unknown/use caution
Use Relief of bladder pain or discomfort due to interstitial cystitis
Available Dosage Forms
  Capsule, Oral:
  Elmiron: 100 mg
General Dosage Range Oral: *Children ≥16 years and Adults:* 100 mg 3 times/day
Administration
  Oral Should be administered with water 1 hour before or 2 hours after meals.
Nursing Actions
  Patient Education
  - Discuss specific use of drug and side effects with patient as it relates to treatment. (HCAHPS: During this hospital stay, were you given any

medicine that you had not taken before? Before giving you any new medicine, how often did hospital staff tell you what the medicine was for? How often did hospital staff describe possible side effects in a way you could understand?)
- Patient may experience nausea, diarrhea, headache, or alopecia. Have patient report immediately to prescriber ecchymosis, bleeding, or rash (HCAHPS).
- Educate patient about signs of a significant reaction (eg, wheezing; chest tightness; fever; itching; bad cough; blue skin color; seizures; or swelling of face, lips, tongue, or throat). **Note:** This is not a comprehensive list of all side effects. Patient should consult prescriber for additional questions.

Intended Use and Disclaimer: Should not be printed and given to patients. This information is intended to serve as a concise initial reference for healthcare professionals to use when discussing medications with a patient. You must ultimately rely on your own discretion, experience and judgment in diagnosing, treating and advising patients.

Pentoxifylline (pen toks IF i lin)

Brand Names: U.S. TRENtal [DSC]
Index Terms Oxpentifylline
Pharmacologic Category Blood Viscosity Reducer Agent
Medication Safety Issues
  Sound-alike/look-alike issues:
  Pentoxifylline may be confused with tamoxifen
  TRENtal® may be confused with Bentyl®, TEGretol®, Trandate®
Pregnancy Risk Factor C
Lactation Enters breast milk/not recommended
Use Treatment of intermittent claudication on the basis of chronic occlusive arterial disease of the limbs; may improve function and symptoms, but not intended to replace more definitive therapy

Note: The American College of Chest Physicians (ACCP) discourages the use of pentoxifylline for the treatment of intermittent claudication refractory to exercise therapy (and smoking cessation) (Guyatt, 2012).

Unlabeled Use Severe alcoholic hepatitis; venous leg ulcers (with compression therapy)
Available Dosage Forms
  Tablet Extended Release, Oral:
  Generic: 400 mg
General Dosage Range Dosage adjustment recommended in patients with renal impairment
Oral: *Adults:* 400 mg 2-3 times/day
Administration
  Oral Tablets should be swallowed whole; do not chew, break, or crush. May be administered with food.

Nursing Actions

Physical Assessment For claudication: Monitor ability to increase walking distance without discomfort.

For liver disease: Monitor improvement of liver disease.

Tell prescriber if patient has renal dysfunction; dose adjustment may be required.

Patient Education

- Discuss specific use of drug and side effects with patient as it relates to treatment. (HCAHPS: During this hospital stay, were you given any medicine that you had not taken before? Before giving you any new medicine, how often did hospital staff tell you what the medicine was for? How often did hospital staff describe possible side effects in a way you could understand?)
- Patient may experience presyncope, fatigue, blurred vision, illogical thinking, dyspepsia, or nausea. Have patient report immediately to prescriber angina, tachycardia, severe dizziness, paresthesia, significant headache, ecchymosis, bleeding, or rash (HCAHPS).
- Educate patient about signs of a significant reaction (eg, wheezing; chest tightness; fever; itching; bad cough; blue skin color; seizures; or swelling of face, lips, tongue, or throat). **Note:** This is not a comprehensive list of all side effects. Patient should consult prescriber for additional questions.

Intended Use and Disclaimer: Should not be printed and given to patients. This information is intended to serve as a concise initial reference for healthcare professionals to use when discussing medications with a patient. You must ultimately rely on your own discretion, experience and judgment in diagnosing, treating and advising patients.

Related Information

Oral Medications That Should Not Be Crushed or Altered *on page 1712*

Perampanel (per AM pa nel)

Brand Names: U.S. Fycompa

Pharmacologic Category AMPA Glutamate Receptor Antagonist; Anticonvulsant, Miscellaneous

Medication Guide Available Yes

Pregnancy Risk Factor C

Lactation Excretion in breast milk unknown/use caution

Breast-Feeding Considerations It is not known if perampanel is excreted in breast milk. The manufacturer recommends that caution be exercised when administering perampanel to nursing women.

Use Adjunctive therapy in the treatment of partial-onset seizures (with or without generalized seizures)

Mechanism of Action/Effect Perampanel is a noncompetitive antagonist of the ionotropic alpha-amino-3-hydroxy-5-methyl-4-isoxazolepropionic acid (AMPA) glutamate receptor on postsynaptic neurons.

Contraindications There are no contraindications listed in manufacturer's labeling.

Warnings/Precautions [U.S. Boxed Warning]: Dose-related serious and/or life-threatening neuropsychiatric events (including aggression, anger, homicidal thoughts, hostility, and irritability) have been reported most often occurring in first 6 weeks of therapy in patients with or without pre-existing psychiatric disease; monitor patients closely especially during dosage adjustments and when receiving higher doses. Adjust dose or immediately discontinue use if severe or worsening symptoms occur. Inform patients and caregivers to contact their healthcare provider immediately if they experience any atypical behavioral and/or mood changes. Pooled analysis of trials involving various antiepileptics (regardless of indication) showed an increased risk of suicidal thoughts/behavior (incidence rate: 0.43% treated patients compared to 0.24% of patients receiving placebo); risk observed as early as 1 week after initiation and continued through duration of trials (most trials ≤24 weeks). Monitor all patients for notable changes in behavior that might indicate suicidal thoughts or depression; notify healthcare provider immediately if symptoms occur. Dizziness, fatigue (including lethargy and weakness), gait disturbances (including abnormal coordination, ataxia, and balance disorder), and somnolence may occur during therapy; patients should be cautioned about performing tasks which require alertness (eg, operating machinery or driving). Concomitant use with CNS depressant (including alcohol) may increase the risk of CNS depression. Use caution if a CNS depressant must be used concurrently with perampanel. Not recommended for use in patients with severe hepatic impairment, renal impairment, or on hemodialysis; dosage adjustment recommended for mild-to-moderate hepatic impairment. Use with extreme caution in patients who are at risk of falls; perampanel has been associated with falls and traumatic injury. Anticonvulsants should not be discontinued abruptly because of the possibility of increasing seizure frequency; therapy should be withdrawn gradually (≥1 week) to minimize the potential of increased seizure frequency, unless safety concerns require a more rapid withdrawal.

Drug Interactions

Avoid Concomitant Use

Avoid concomitant use of Perampanel with any of the following: Alcohol (Ethyl); Axitinib; Azelastine (Nasal); CYP3A4 Inducers (Strong); Paraldehyde; Simeprevir; St Johns Wort; Thalidomide

Decreased Effect

Perampanel may decrease the levels/effects of: ARIPiprazole; Axitinib; Contraceptives (Progestins); Ibrutinib; Saxagliptin; Simeprevir

The levels/effects of Perampanel may be decreased by: Bosentan; CarBAMazepine; CYP3A4 Inducers (Strong); Dabrafenib; Deferasirox; Fosphenytoin; Ketorolac (Nasal); Ketorolac (Systemic); Mefloquine; Orlistat; OXcarbazepine; Phenytoin; St Johns Wort; Tocilizumab

Increased Effect/Toxicity

Perampanel may increase the levels/effects of: Alcohol (Ethyl); Azelastine (Nasal); Buprenorphine; CNS Depressants; Hydrocodone; Methotrimeprazine; Metyrosine; Mirtazapine; OXcarbazepine; Paraldehyde; Pramipexole; ROPINIRole; Rotigotine; Selective Serotonin Reuptake Inhibitors; Thalidomide; Zolpidem

The levels/effects of Perampanel may be increased by: Brimonidine (Topical); Doxylamine; Droperidol; HydrOXYzine; Magnesium Sulfate; Methotrimeprazine; Sodium Oxybate; Tapentadol

Nutritional/Ethanol Interactions

Ethanol: Avoid ethanol (may increase CNS depression).

Herb/Nutraceutical: St John's wort may decrease perampanel levels. Avoid valerian, St John's wort, kava kava, gotu kola (may increase CNS depression).

Adverse Reactions

>10%: Central nervous system: Dizziness (16% to 43%), somnolence (9% to 18%), headache (13%), fatigue (8% to 12%), irritability (4% to 12%)

1% to 10%:

Cardiovascular: Peripheral edema (2%)

Central nervous system: Ataxia (1% to 8%), vertigo (3% to 5%), balance impaired (≤5%), gait disturbance (4%), anxiety (2% to 4%), aggression (2% to 3%), hypersomnia (1% to 3%), anger (≤3%), hypoesthesia (≤3%), confusion (2%), coordination impaired (≤2%), euphoria (≤2%), memory impaired (≤2%), mood changes (1% to 2%)

Dermatologic: Bruising (≤2%), skin laceration (≤2%)

Endocrine & metabolic: Hyponatremia (≤2%)

Gastrointestinal: Weight gain (4% to 9%), nausea (6% to 8%), vomiting (4%), constipation (3%)

Neuromuscular & skeletal: Falling (5% to 10%), back pain (5%), dysarthria (1% to 4%), myalgia (3%), arthralgia (≤3%), limb pain (≤3%), limb injury (2%), musculoskeletal pain (2%), weakness (2%), paresthesia (≤2%)

Ocular: Blurred vision (3% to 4%), diplopia (3%)

Respiratory: Cough (4%), upper respiratory tract infection (4%), oropharyngeal pain (2%)

Miscellaneous: Head injury (3%)

Controlled Substance C-III

Available Dosage Forms

Tablet, Oral:

Fycompa: 2 mg, 4 mg, 6 mg, 8 mg, 10 mg, 12 mg

General Dosage Range Dosage adjustment recommended in patients with hepatic impairment and on concomitant therapy.

Oral: *Children ≥12 years, Adolescents, and Adults:* Initial: 2 mg once daily at bedtime; maintenance dose: 8-12 mg once daily

Administration

Oral

Administer at bedtime. May be administered without regard to meals.

Storage/Stability Store at 25°C (77°F); excursions permitted between 15°C to 30°C (59°F to 86°F).

Nursing Actions

Physical Assessment Monitor hepatic and renal lab tests. Monitor patient for signs of serious neuropsychiatric events, including somnolence, aggression, anger, homicidal thoughts, hostility, and irritability. Monitor for seizure control. Provide safe environment for patient. Warn patient of increased risk of falls.

Patient Education

- Discuss specific use of drug and side effects with patient as it relates to treatment. (HCAHPS: During this hospital stay, were you given any medicine that you had not taken before? Before giving you any new medicine, how often did hospital staff tell you what the medicine was for? How often did hospital staff describe possible side effects in a way you could understand?)
- Patient may experience presyncope, asthenia, blurred vision, illogical thinking, dizziness, mood changes, headache, change in balance, dyspepsia, emesis, or weight gain. Have patient report immediately to prescriber tachycardia, lack of appetite, pregnancy, or rash (HCAHPS).
- Educate patient about signs of a significant reaction (eg, wheezing; chest tightness; fever; itching; bad cough; blue skin color; seizures; or swelling of face, lips, tongue, or throat). **Note:** This is not a comprehensive list of all side effects. Patient should consult prescriber for additional questions.

Intended Use and Disclaimer: Should not be printed and given to patients. This information is intended to serve as a concise initial reference for healthcare professionals to use when discussing medications with a patient. You must ultimately rely on your own discretion, experience and judgment in diagnosing, treating and advising patients.

Dietary Considerations May be taken without regard to meals.

Perindopril (per IN doe pril)

Brand Names: U.S. Aceon

Index Terms Perindopril Erbumine
Pharmacologic Category Angiotensin-Converting Enzyme (ACE) Inhibitor; Antihypertensive
Pregnancy Risk Factor D
Lactation Excretion in breast milk unknown/use caution
Use Treatment of hypertension; reduction of cardiovascular mortality or nonfatal myocardial infarction in patients with stable coronary artery disease
Canadian labeling: Additional use (unlabeled use in U.S.): Treatment of mild-moderate (NYHA I-III) heart failure (HF)

Note: The ACCF/AHA 2013 heart failure guidelines recommend the use of ACE inhibitors, along with other guideline-directed medical therapies, to prevent HF in patients with a reduced ejection fraction who have a history of MI (stage B HF), to prevent HF in any patient with a reduced ejection fraction (stage B HF), or to treat those with HF and reduced ejection fraction (stage C HFrEF) (ACCF/AHA [Yancy, 2013])
Unlabeled Use To delay the progression of nephropathy and reduce risks of cardiovascular events in hypertensive patients with type 1 or 2 diabetes mellitus
Available Dosage Forms
Tablet, Oral:
Aceon: 4 mg, 8 mg
Generic: 2 mg, 4 mg, 8 mg
General Dosage Range Dosage adjustment recommended in patients with renal impairment
Oral: *Adults:* Initial: 2-4 mg once daily; Maintenance: 4-8 mg/day in 1-2 divided doses (maximum: 16 mg/day)
Administration
Oral Administer prior to a meal.
Nursing Actions
Physical Assessment Monitor first dose carefully (hypotension can occur, especially with first dose; angioedema can occur at any time during treatment, especially following first dose). Monitor BP (standing and sitting), cardiac status, and fluid balance at beginning of therapy, when adjusting dose, and periodically throughout.
Patient Education
• Discuss specific use of drug and side effects with patient as it relates to treatment. (HCAHPS: During this hospital stay, were you given any medicine that you had not taken before? Before giving you any new medicine, how often did hospital staff tell you what the medicine was for? How often did hospital staff describe possible side effects in a way you could understand?)
• Patient may experience dizziness, headache, or diarrhea. Have patient report immediately to prescriber signs of infection, syncope, dyspnea, hyperhidrosis, significant weight gain, edema in legs or abdomen, discolored urine, jaundice, rash, or pregnancy (HCAHPS).

• Educate patient about signs of a significant reaction (eg, wheezing; chest tightness; fever; itching; bad cough; blue skin color; seizures; or swelling of face, lips, tongue, or throat). **Note:** This is not a comprehensive list of all side effects. Patient should consult prescriber for additional questions.

Intended Use and Disclaimer: Should not be printed and given to patients. This information is intended to serve as a concise initial reference for healthcare professionals to use when discussing medications with a patient. You must ultimately rely on your own discretion, experience and judgment in diagnosing, treating and advising patients.

Perphenazine (per FEN a zeen)

Index Terms Trilafon
Pharmacologic Category Antiemetic; Antipsychotic Agent, Typical, Phenothiazine
Medication Safety Issues
Sound-alike/look-alike issues:
Trilafon may be confused with Tri-Levlen®
BEERS Criteria medication:
This drug may be potentially inappropriate for use in geriatric patients (Quality of evidence - moderate; Strength of recommendation - strong).
Use Treatment of schizophrenia; severe nausea and vomiting
Unlabeled Use Psychosis; psychosis/agitation related to Alzheimer's dementia (risks vs benefits)
Available Dosage Forms
Tablet, Oral:
Generic: 2 mg, 4 mg, 8 mg, 16 mg
General Dosage Range Oral: *Adults:* 4-16 mg 2-4 times/day (maximum: 64 mg/day)
Administration
Oral May be administered without regard to meals.
Nursing Actions
Physical Assessment Monitor blood pressure and therapeutic response (mental status, mood, affect) at beginning of therapy and periodically throughout. Monitor for orthostatic hypotension, anticholinergic response, extrapyramidal symptoms, and pigmentary retinopathy.
Patient Education
• Discuss specific use of drug and side effects with patient as it relates to treatment. (HCAHPS: During this hospital stay, were you given any medicine that you had not taken before? Before giving you any new medicine, how often did hospital staff tell you what the medicine was for? How often did hospital staff describe possible side effects in a way you could understand?)
• Patient may experience presyncope, fatigue, blurred vision, illogical thinking, dizziness, nervousness and anxiety, constipation, xerostomia, weight gain, or impotence. Have patient report immediately to prescriber imbalance, tremors,

urinary retention, severe asthenia, pregnancy, or rash (HCAHPS).

- Educate patient about signs of a significant reaction (eg, wheezing; chest tightness; fever; itching; bad cough; blue skin color; seizures; or swelling of face, lips, tongue, or throat). **Note:** This is not a comprehensive list of all side effects. Patient should consult prescriber for additional questions.

Intended Use and Disclaimer: Should not be printed and given to patients. This information is intended to serve as a concise initial reference for healthcare professionals to use when discussing medications with a patient. You must ultimately rely on your own discretion, experience and judgment in diagnosing, treating and advising patients.

Pertuzumab (per TU zoo mab)

Brand Names: U.S. Perjeta

Index Terms 2C4 Antibody; MOAB 2C4; Monoclonal Antibody 2C4; Omnitarg; rhuMAb-2C4

Pharmacologic Category Antineoplastic Agent, Anti-HER2; Antineoplastic Agent, Monoclonal Antibody

Medication Safety Issues

Sound-alike/look-alike issues:

Pertuzumab may be confused with ado-trastuzumab emtansine, panitumumab, trastuzumab

High alert medication:

This medication is in a class the Institute for Safe Medication Practices (ISMP) includes among its list of drug classes which have a heightened risk of causing significant patient harm when used in error.

Pregnancy Risk Factor D

Lactation Excretion in breast milk unknown/not recommended

Use

Breast cancer, metastatic: Treatment of human epidermal growth factor receptor 2 (HER2)-positive metastatic breast cancer (in combination with trastuzumab and docetaxel) in patients who have not received prior anti-HER2 therapy or chemotherapy to treat metastatic disease

Breast cancer, neoadjuvant treatment: Neoadjuvant treatment of locally advanced, inflammatory, or early stage HER2-positive, breast cancer (either greater than 2 cm in diameter or node positive) in combination with trastuzumab and docetaxel (as part of a complete treatment regimen for early breast cancer).

Available Dosage Forms

Solution, Intravenous [preservative free]:

Perjeta: 420 mg/14 mL (14 mL)

General Dosage Range I.V.: *Adults:* Initial: 840 mg; Maintenance: 420 mg every 3 weeks

Administration

I.V. For I.V. infusion only, as a short infusion; infuse initial dose (840 mg) over 60 minutes; infuse maintenance dose (420 mg) over 30-60 minutes. Do not administer I.V. push or as a rapid bolus. Do not mix with other medications. For pertuzumab, trastuzumab, and docetaxel combination regimens, pertuzumab and trastuzumab may be administered in any order; however, docetaxel should be given after pertuzumab and trastuzumab. Observe patients for 30-60 minutes after each pertuzumab infusion and before subsequent infusions of trastuzumab or docetaxel.

Hazardous agent; use appropriate precautions for handling and disposal (meets NIOSH, 2012 criteria).

Injectable Detail pH: 6 (in vial)

Nursing Actions

Physical Assessment Monitor for infusion reactions. Have appropriate infusion reaction medications at bedside. Educate patients about need for heart function monitoring. Instruct patients to monitor weight daily and report >2 lb. weight gain in a day, swelling of lower extremities, or shortness of breath. In female patients of reproductive years, discuss effective birth control methods. Educate patient about watching for signs and symptoms of infection.

Patient Education

- Discuss specific use of drug and side effects with patient as it relates to treatment. (HCAHPS: During this hospital stay, were you given any medicine that you had not taken before? Before giving you any new medicine, how often did hospital staff tell you what the medicine was for? How often did hospital staff describe possible side effects in a way you could understand?)
- Patient may experience anemia, leukopenia, fatigue, dizziness, headache, diarrhea, nausea, mouth irritation or sores, myalgia, loss of appetite, parageusia, rash, or xeroderma. Have patient report immediately to prescriber signs of infection, dyspnea, angina, tachycardia, syncope, significant weight gain, ecchymosis, or pregnancy (HCAHPS).
- Educate patient about signs of a significant reaction (eg, wheezing; chest tightness; fever; itching; bad cough; blue skin color; seizures; or swelling of face, lips, tongue, or throat). **Note:** This is not a comprehensive list of all side effects. Patient should consult prescriber for additional questions.

Intended Use and Disclaimer: Should not be printed and given to patients. This information is intended to serve as a concise initial reference for healthcare professionals to use when discussing medications with a patient. You must ultimately rely on your own discretion, experience and judgment in diagnosing, treating and advising patients.

Phenazopyridine (fen az oh PEER i deen)

Brand Names: U.S. Azo-Gesic [OTC]; Baridium [OTC]; Pyridium; Urinary Pain Relief [OTC]
Index Terms Phenazopyridine Hydrochloride; Phenylazo Diamino Pyridine Hydrochloride
Pharmacologic Category Analgesic, Urinary
Medication Safety Issues
Sound-alike/look-alike issues:
Phenazopyridine may be confused with phenoxybenzamine
Pyridium® may be confused with Dyrenium®, Perdiem®, pyridoxine, pyrithione
Pregnancy Risk Factor B
Lactation Excretion in breast milk unknown
Use Symptomatic relief of urinary burning, itching, frequency, and urgency in association with urinary tract infection or following urologic procedures
Available Dosage Forms
Tablet, Oral:
Azo-Gesic [OTC]: 95 mg
Baridium [OTC]: 97.2 mg
Pyridium: 100 mg, 200 mg
Urinary Pain Relief [OTC]: 95 mg
Generic: 95 mg, 100 mg, 200 mg
General Dosage Range Dosage adjustment recommended in patients with renal impairment
Oral:
Children: 12 mg/kg/day in 3 divided doses
Adults: 100-200 mg 3 times/day
Administration
Oral Administer after meals.
Nursing Actions
Physical Assessment Instruct patients with diabetes to use serum glucose monitoring (phenazopyridine may interfere with certain urine testing reagents).
Patient Education
• Discuss specific use of drug and side effects with patient as it relates to treatment. (HCAHPS: During this hospital stay, were you given any medicine that you had not taken before? Before giving you any new medicine, how often did hospital staff tell you what the medicine was for? How often did hospital staff describe possible side effects in a way you could understand?)
• Patient may experience headache or dyspepsia. Have patient report immediately to prescriber severe nausea, inability to eat, discolored urine, jaundice, significant asthenia, or rash (HCAHPS).
• Educate patient about signs of a significant reaction (eg, wheezing; chest tightness; fever; itching; bad cough; blue skin color; seizures; or swelling of face, lips, tongue, or throat). **Note:** This is not a comprehensive list of all side effects. Patient should consult prescriber for additional questions.

Intended Use and Disclaimer: Should not be printed and given to patients. This information is intended to serve as a concise initial reference for healthcare professionals to use when discussing medications with a patient. You must ultimately rely on your own discretion, experience and judgment in diagnosing, treating and advising patients.

Phenelzine (FEN el zeen)

Brand Names: U.S. Nardil
Index Terms Phenelzine Sulfate
Pharmacologic Category Antidepressant, Monoamine Oxidase Inhibitor
Medication Safety Issues
Sound-alike/look-alike issues:
Phenelzine may be confused with phenytoin
Nardil® may be confused with Norinyl®
Medication Guide Available Yes
Pregnancy Risk Factor C
Lactation Excretion in breast milk unknown/not recommended
Use Symptomatic treatment of atypical, nonendogenous, or neurotic depression
Available Dosage Forms
Tablet, Oral:
Nardil: 15 mg
Generic: 15 mg
General Dosage Range Oral: *Adults:* Initial: 45 mg/day in 3 divided doses; Maintenance: 15-90 mg/day in 1-3 divided doses
Nursing Actions
Physical Assessment Monitor blood pressure, mental status, mood, affect, and suicide ideation. Observe for clinical worsening, suicidality, and unusual behavior changes, especially during the initial few months of therapy or during dosage changes. Patients with diabetes should monitor serum glucose closely (phenelzine may lower glucose level). Instruct patient to follow a tyramine-free diet.
Patient Education
• Discuss specific use of drug and side effects with patient as it relates to treatment. (HCAHPS: During this hospital stay, were you given any medicine that you had not taken before? Before giving you any new medicine, how often did hospital staff tell you what the medicine was for? How often did hospital staff describe possible side effects in a way you could understand?)
• Patient may experience presyncope, fatigue, blurred vision, illogical thinking, dizziness, headache, constipation, or insomnia. Have patient report immediately to prescriber angina, tachycardia, nervousness, tremors, fasciculations, severe nausea, or rash (HCAHPS).
• Educate patient about signs of a significant reaction (eg, wheezing; chest tightness; fever; itching; bad cough; blue skin color; seizures; or

swelling of face, lips, tongue, or throat). **Note:** This is not a comprehensive list of all side effects. Patient should consult prescriber for additional questions.

Intended Use and Disclaimer: Should not be printed and given to patients. This information is intended to serve as a concise initial reference for healthcare professionals to use when discussing medications with a patient. You must ultimately rely on your own discretion, experience and judgment in diagnosing, treating and advising patients.

PHENobarbital (fee noe BAR bi tal)

Brand Names: U.S. Luminal

Index Terms Luminal Sodium; Phenobarbital Sodium; Phenobarbitone; Phenylethylmalonylurea

Pharmacologic Category Anticonvulsant, Barbiturate; Barbiturate

Medication Safety Issues

Sound-alike/look-alike issues:

PHENobarbital may be confused with PENTobarbital, Phenergan®, phenytoin

BEERS Criteria medication:

This drug may be potentially inappropriate for use in geriatric patients (Quality of evidence - high; Strength of recommendation - strong).

Pregnancy Risk Factor B/D (manufacturer dependent)

Lactation Enters breast milk/use caution

Use Management of generalized tonic-clonic (grand mal), status epilepticus, and partial seizures; sedative/hypnotic

Note: Use to treat insomnia is not recommended (Schutte-Rodin, 2008)

Unlabeled Use Prevention and treatment of neonatal hyperbilirubinemia and lowering of bilirubin in chronic cholestasis; neonatal seizures

Controlled Substance C-IV

Available Dosage Forms

Elixir, Oral:

Generic: 20 mg/5 mL (473 mL)

Solution, Injection:

Luminal: 130 mg/mL (1 mL)

Generic: 65 mg/mL (1 mL); 130 mg/mL (1 mL)

Solution, Oral:

Generic: 20 mg/5 mL (473 mL)

Tablet, Oral:

Generic: 15 mg, 16.2 mg, 30 mg, 32.4 mg, 60 mg, 64.8 mg, 97.2 mg, 100 mg

General Dosage Range Dosage adjustment recommended in patients with renal impairment

I.M.:

Children: 3-5 mg/kg at bedtime or 1-3 mg/kg 1-1.5 hours before procedure

Adults: Dosage varies greatly depending on indication

I.V.:

Infants: Loading dose: 10-20 mg/kg in a single or divided dose; Maintenance: 5-8 mg/kg/day in 1-2 divided doses

Children: Loading dose: 15-20 mg/kg in a single or divided dose; Maintenance: Dosage varies greatly depending on indication

Adults: Loading dose: 10-20 mg/kg; may repeat dose in 20-minute intervals as needed (maximum total dose: 30 mg/kg); Maintenance: Dosage varies greatly depending on indication

Oral:

Infants: 5-8 mg/kg/day in 1-2 divided doses

Children and Adults: Dosage varies greatly depending on indication

Administration

I.M. Inject deep into muscle. Do not exceed 5 mL per injection site due to potential for tissue irritation.

I.V. Avoid rapid I.V. administration >60 mg/minute in adults and >30 mg/minute in children. Avoid extravasation. Intra-arterial injection is contraindicated. Avoid subcutaneous administration.

Injectable Detail Parenteral solutions are highly alkaline.

pH: 9.2-10.2

Nursing Actions

Physical Assessment Assess for history of addiction or suicide ideation; long-term use can result in dependence, abuse, or tolerance. **I.V.:** Keep patient under observation (vital signs, neurologic, cardiac, and respiratory status); use safety precautions.

Patient Education

- Discuss specific use of drug and side effects with patient as it relates to treatment. (HCAHPS: During this hospital stay, were you given any medicine that you had not taken before? Before giving you any new medicine, how often did hospital staff tell you what the medicine was for? How often did hospital staff describe possible side effects in a way you could understand?)
- Patient may experience presyncope, fatigue, blurred vision, illogical thinking, or dizziness. Have patient report immediately to prescriber dyspnea, imbalance, nervousness, anxiety, severe asthenia, or rash (HCAHPS).
- Educate patient about signs of a significant reaction (eg, wheezing; chest tightness; fever; itching; bad cough; blue skin color; seizures; or swelling of face, lips, tongue, or throat). **Note:** This is not a comprehensive list of all side effects. Patient should consult prescriber for additional questions.

Intended Use and Disclaimer: Should not be printed and given to patients. This information is intended to serve as a concise initial reference for healthcare professionals to use when discussing medications with a patient. You must ultimately rely on your own discretion, experience and

judgment in diagnosing, treating and advising patients.

Related Information
Peak and Trough Guidelines *on page 1710*

Phentermine and Topiramate
(FEN ter meen & toe PYRE a mate)

Brand Names: U.S. Qsymia™
Index Terms Qnexa; Topiramate and Phentermine
Pharmacologic Category Anorexiant; Anticonvulsant, Miscellaneous; Sympathomimetic
Medication Guide Available Yes
Pregnancy Risk Factor X
Lactation Excreted in breast milk/not recommended
Use Chronic weight management, as an adjunct to a reduced-calorie diet and increased physical activity, in patients with either an initial body mass index (BMI) of ≥30 kg/m^2 **or** an initial BMI of ≥27 kg/m^2 and at least one weight-related comorbid condition (eg, hypertension, dyslipidemia, type 2 diabetes)
Controlled Substance C-IV
Available Dosage Forms
Capsule, extended release, oral:
Qsymia™: 3.75/23: Phentermine 3.75 mg [immediate release] and topiramate 23 mg [extended release]
Qsymia™: 7.5/46: Phentermine 7.5 mg [immediate release] and topiramate 46 mg [extended release]
Qsymia™: 11.25/69: Phentermine 11.25 mg [immediate release] and topiramate 69 mg [extended release]
Qsymia™: 15/92: Phentermine 15 mg [immediate release] and topiramate 92 mg [extended release]
General Dosage Range Dosage adjustment recommended in patients with renal impairment or hepatic impairment.
Oral: *Adults:* Phentermine 3.75-15 mg/topiramate 23-92 mg once daily.
Administration
Oral Administer in the morning without regard to meals; avoid late evening administration (potential for insomnia).
Nursing Actions
Patient Education
• Discuss specific use of drug and side effects with patient as it relates to treatment. (HCAHPS: During this hospital stay, were you given any medicine that you had not taken before? Before giving you any new medicine, how often did hospital staff tell you what the medicine was for? How often did hospital staff describe possible side effects in a way you could understand?)
• Patient may experience dizziness, headache, constipation, xerostomia, insomnia, or paresthesia. Have patient report immediately to prescriber depression, nervousness, emotional

instability, illogical thinking, anxiety, angina, sudden vision changes, back pain, dyspepsia, hematuria, anhidrosis, pregnancy, or rash (HCAHPS).
• Educate patient about signs of a significant reaction (eg, wheezing; chest tightness; fever; itching; bad cough; blue skin color; seizures; or swelling of face, lips, tongue, or throat). **Note:** This is not a comprehensive list of all side effects. Patient should consult prescriber for additional questions.

Intended Use and Disclaimer: Should not be printed and given to patients. This information is intended to serve as a concise initial reference for healthcare professionals to use when discussing medications with a patient. You must ultimately rely on your own discretion, experience and judgment in diagnosing, treating and advising patients.
Related Information
Topiramate *on page 1541*

Phentolamine (fen TOLE a meen)

Brand Names: U.S. OraVerse
Index Terms Phentolamine Mesylate; Regitine [DSC]
Pharmacologic Category Alpha$_1$ Blocker; Antidote, Extravasation; Antihypertensive
Medication Safety Issues
Sound-alike/look-alike issues:
Phentolamine may be confused with phentermine, Ventolin
Regitine may be confused with Reglan
Pregnancy Risk Factor C
Lactation Excretion in breast milk unknown/use caution
Use Diagnosis of pheochromocytoma via the phentolamine-blocking test (see **"Note"**); prevention and management of hypertensive episodes associated with pheochromocytoma resulting from stress or manipulation during the perioperative period; prevention and treatment of dermal necrosis/sloughing after extravasation of norepinephrine

OraVerse™: Reversal of soft tissue anesthesia and the associated functional deficits resulting from a local dental anesthetic containing a vasoconstrictor

Note: The phentolamine-blocking test for the diagnosis of pheochromocytoma has largely been supplanted by the measurement of catecholamine concentrations and catecholamine metabolites (eg, metanephrine) in the plasma and urine; reserve phentolamine for cases when additional confirmation is necessary to determine diagnosis.
Unlabeled Use Management of extravasations of sympathomimetic vasopressors (in addition to norepinephrine) including dopamine, epinephrine and phenylephrine; treatment of hypertensive crisis

Available Dosage Forms

Solution, Injection:

Generic: 5 mg/mL (1 mL)

Solution Reconstituted, Injection:

Generic: 5 mg (1 ea)

General Dosage Range

Local infiltration: *Children and Adults:* Infiltrate extravasation site with 5-10 mg as soon as possible, within 12 hours of extravasation

I.M.:

Children: 3 mg as a single dose **or** 1 mg given 1-2 hours before procedure; repeat if needed

Adults: 5 mg as a single dose **or** 1-2 hours before procedure; repeat if needed

I.V.:

Children: 1 mg as a single dose **or** 1 mg given 1-2 hours before procedure (may repeat if needed) with 1 mg repeated as needed during procedure

Adults: 5 mg as a single dose **or** 5 mg 1-2 hours before procedure (may repeat if needed) with 5 mg repeated as needed during procedure

Submucosal injection:

Children 15-30 kg and <12 years: 0.2 mg (maximum)

Children >30 kg and <12 years: 0.4 mg (maximum)

Children >30 kg and ≥12 years and Adults: 0.2 mg to 0.8 mg (depending on number of cartridges of anesthesia)

Administration

I.M.

Pheochromocytoma diagnosis: Patient should be supine throughout test, preferable in a quiet, dark room. Blood pressure should be monitored every 10 minutes for at least 30 minutes, delay phentolamine administration until after blood pressure is stable (at an untreated, hypertensive level). A drop in blood pressure >35 mm Hg (systolic) and >25 mm Hg (diastolic) is considered a positive response. If blood pressure is elevated, unchanged, or decrease is <35 mm Hg (systolic) and <25 mm Hg (diastolic), then response is negative. Confirm positive response with other diagnostic measure. Negative responses do not exclude a pheochromocytoma diagnosis, particularly in patients with paroxysmal hypertension where an incidence of false negatives is high.

I.M.: After I.M. injection, monitor blood pressure every 5 minutes for 35-40 minutes. Blood pressure drops to above parameters within 20 minutes are considered positive.

Pheochromocytoma-associated hypertensive episode: Administer 1-2 hours prior to surgery and repeat during surgery (I.V.) if necessary.

I.V.

Pheochromocytoma diagnosis: Patient should be supine throughout test, preferable in a quiet, dark room. Blood pressure should be monitored every 10 minutes for at least 30 minutes, delay phentolamine administration until after blood pressure is stable (at an untreated, hypertensive level). A drop in blood pressure >35 mm Hg (systolic) and >25 mm Hg (diastolic) is considered a positive response. If blood pressure is elevated, unchanged, or decrease is <35 mm Hg (systolic) and <25 mm Hg (diastolic), then response is negative. Confirm positive response with other diagnostic measure. Negative responses do not exclude a pheochromocytoma diagnosis, particularly in patients with paroxysmal hypertension where an incidence of false negatives is high.

I.V.: Inject rapidly (after venous response to venipuncture has subsided); then monitor blood pressure immediately after injection, every 30 seconds for 3 minutes, then every minute for 7 minutes. Maximum response is generally achieved within 2 minutes; duration may last 15-30 minutes (although return to prior blood pressure may be sooner).

Pheochromocytoma-associated hypertensive episode: Administer 1-2 hours prior to surgery and repeat during surgery (I.V.) if necessary.

Hypertensive crisis (unlabeled use): Administer as an I.V. bolus (Chobanian, 2003).

Injectable Detail pH: 4.5-6.5

Other

Extravasation management (treatment), sympathomimetic vasopressors: Stop vesicant infusion immediately and disconnect I.V. line (leave needle/cannula in place); gently aspirate extravasated solution from the I.V. line (do **NOT** flush the line); remove needle/cannula; elevate extremity. Inject phentolamine 5-10 mg/10 mL saline into extravasation site (as soon as possible but within 12 hours of extravasation). AHA recommends diluting 5-10 mg in 10-15 mL saline and administering into the site (Peberdy, 2010).

Reversal of oral soft tissue (lip, tongue) anesthesia (OraVerse™): Submucosal oral injection: Use the same location and dental technique employed for administration of the local anesthetic.

Nursing Actions

Physical Assessment When used to prevent tissue necrosis after extravasation, monitor effectiveness of treatment closely. Utilize other local supportive therapies to help with extravasation. For other uses, avoid sudden position changes to prevent orthostatic variations.

Patient Education

• Discuss specific use of drug and side effects with patient as it relates to treatment. (HCAHPS: During this hospital stay, were you given any medicine that you had not taken before? Before giving you any new medicine, how often did hospital staff tell you what the medicine was for? How often did hospital staff describe possible side effects in a way you could understand?)

• Patient may experience dizziness, headache, nausea, or impotence. Have patient report immediately to prescriber angina, tachycardia, or rash (HCAHPS).

• Educate patient about signs of a significant reaction (eg, wheezing; chest tightness; fever; itching; bad cough; blue skin color; seizures; or swelling of face, lips, tongue, or throat). **Note:** This is not a comprehensive list of all side effects. Patient should consult prescriber for additional questions.

Intended Use and Disclaimer: Should not be printed and given to patients. This information is intended to serve as a concise initial reference for healthcare professionals to use when discussing medications with a patient. You must ultimately rely on your own discretion, experience and judgment in diagnosing, treating and advising patients.

Related Information

Management of Drug Extravasations *on page 1700*

Phenylephrine (Systemic) (fen il EF rin)

Brand Names: U.S. Little Colds Decongestant [OTC]; Medi-Phenyl [OTC]; Nasal Decongestant PE Max St [OTC]; Nasal Decongestant [OTC]; Neo-Synephrine [DSC]; Non-Pseudo Sinus Decongestant [OTC]; Sudafed PE Childrens [OTC]; Sudafed PE Maximum Strength [OTC]; Sudogest PE [OTC]

Index Terms Phenylephrine Hydrochloride

Pharmacologic Category Alpha-Adrenergic Agonist

Medication Safety Issues

Sound-alike/look-alike issues:

Sudafed PE® may be confused with Sudafed®

High alert medication:

The Institute for Safe Medication Practices (ISMP) includes this medication among its list of drugs which have a heightened risk of causing significant patient harm when used in error.

Pregnancy Risk Factor C

Lactation Excretion in breast milk unknown/use caution

Breast-Feeding Considerations It is not known if phenylephrine is excreted into breast milk. The manufacturer recommends that caution be exercised when administering phenylephrine to nursing women.

Use Treatment of hypotension, vascular failure in shock (see **"Note"**); as a vasoconstrictor in regional analgesia; supraventricular tachycardia (see **"Note"**); as a decongestant [OTC]

Note: Not recommended for routine use in the treatment of septic shock or supraventricular tachycardias.

Mechanism of Action/Effect Potent, direct-acting alpha-adrenergic agonist with virtually no beta-adrenergic activity; produces systemic arterial vasoconstriction

Contraindications Hypersensitivity to phenylephrine or any component of the formulation

Injection: Severe hypertension; ventricular tachycardia

Oral: Use with or within 14 days of MAO inhibitor therapy

Warnings/Precautions Some products contain sulfites which may cause allergic reactions in susceptible individuals. Use with extreme caution in patients taking MAO inhibitors.

Intravenous: Use with caution in the elderly, patients with hyperthyroidism, bradycardia, partial heart block, myocardial disease, or severe CAD. Avoid or use with extreme caution in patients with heart failure or cardiogenic shock; increased systemic vascular resistance may significantly reduce cardiac output. Assure adequate circulatory volume to minimize need for vasoconstrictors. Avoid use in patients with hypertension (contraindicated in severe hypertension); monitor blood pressure closely and adjust infusion rate. Vesicant; ensure proper needle or catheter placement prior to and during infusion; avoid extravasation. **[U.S. Boxed Warning]: Should be administered by adequately trained individuals familiar with its use.**

Oral: When used for self-medication (OTC), use caution with asthma, bowel obstruction/narrowing, hyperthyroidism, diabetes mellitus, cardiovascular disease, ischemic heart disease, hypertension, increased intraocular pressure, prostatic hyperplasia or in the elderly. Notify healthcare provider if symptoms do not improve within 7 days or are accompanied by fever. Discontinue and contact healthcare provider if nervousness, dizziness, or sleeplessness occur.

Drug Interactions

Avoid Concomitant Use

Avoid concomitant use of Phenylephrine (Systemic) with any of the following: Ergot Derivatives; Hyaluronidase; Iobenguane I 123; MAO Inhibitors

Decreased Effect

Phenylephrine (Systemic) may decrease the levels/effects of: Benzylpenicilloyl Polylysine; FentaNYL; Iobenguane I 123

The levels/effects of Phenylephrine (Systemic) may be decreased by: Alpha1-Blockers

Increased Effect/Toxicity

Phenylephrine (Systemic) may increase the levels/effects of: Sympathomimetics

The levels/effects of Phenylephrine (Systemic) may be increased by: AtoMOXetine; Cannabinoids; Ergot Derivatives; Hyaluronidase; Linezolid; MAO Inhibitors; Tricyclic Antidepressants

Nutritional/Ethanol Interactions Herb/Nutraceutical: Avoid ephedra, yohimbe (may cause CNS stimulation).

Adverse Reactions Frequency not defined.

Injection:

Cardiovascular: Arrhythmia (rare), decreased cardiac output, hypertension, pallor, precordial pain or discomfort, reflex bradycardia, severe peripheral and visceral vasoconstriction

Central nervous system: Anxiety, dizziness, excitability, giddiness, headache, insomnia, nervousness, restlessness

Endocrine & metabolic: Metabolic acidosis

Gastrointestinal: Gastric irritation, nausea

Local: I.V.: Extravasation which may lead to necrosis and sloughing of surrounding tissue, blanching of skin

Neuromuscular & skeletal: Paresthesia, pilomotor response, tremor, weakness

Renal: Decreased renal perfusion, reduced urine output

Respiratory: Respiratory distress

Miscellaneous: Hypersensitivity reactions (including rash, urticaria, leukopenia, agranulocytosis, thrombocytopenia)

Oral: Central nervous system: Anxiety, dizziness, excitability, giddiness, headache, insomnia, nervousness, restlessness

Pharmacodynamics/Kinetics

Onset of Action

Blood pressure increase/vasoconstriction: I.M., SubQ: 10-15 minutes; I.V.: Immediate

Nasal decongestant: Oral: 15-30 minutes (Kollar, 2007)

Duration of Action

Blood pressure increase/vasoconstriction: I.M.: 1-2 hours; I.V.: ~15-20 minutes; SubQ: 50 minutes

Nasal decongestant: Oral: ≤4 hours (Kollar, 2007)

Available Dosage Forms

Liquid, Oral:

Little Colds Decongestant [OTC]: 2.5 mg/mL (30 mL)

Solution, Injection:

Generic: 10 mg/mL (1 mL, 5 mL, 10 mL)

Solution, Oral:

Sudafed PE Childrens [OTC]: 2.5 mg/5 mL (118 mL)

Tablet, Oral:

Medi-Phenyl [OTC]: 5 mg

Nasal Decongestant [OTC]: 10 mg

Nasal Decongestant PE Max St [OTC]: 10 mg

Non-Pseudo Sinus Decongestant [OTC]: 10 mg

Sudafed PE Maximum Strength [OTC]: 10 mg

Sudogest PE [OTC]: 10 mg

General Dosage Range

I.V.:

Children: Bolus: 5-20 mcg/kg/dose every 10-15 minutes as needed; Infusion: 0.1-0.5 mcg/kg/minute

Adults: Bolus: 100-500 mcg/dose every 10-15 minutes as needed (maximum: 500 mcg); Infusion: Initial: 100-180 mcg/minute

Oral:

Children 4 to <6 years: 2.5 mg every 4 hours as needed (maximum: 15 mg/24 hours)

Children 6 to <12 years: 5 mg every 4 hours as needed (maximum: 30 mg/24 hours)

Children ≥12 years and Adults: 10 mg every 4 hours as needed (maximum: 60 mg/24 hours)

Usual Infusion Concentrations: Pediatric I.V. infusion: 20 **mcg**/mL, 40 **mcg**/mL, or 60 **mcg**/mL

Usual Infusion Concentrations: Adult I.V. infusion: 10 mg in 500 mL (concentration: 20 **mcg**/mL) of D$_5$W or NS, 50 mg in 500 mL (concentration: 100 **mcg**/mL) of NS, **or** 100 mg in 500 mL (concentration: 200 **mcg**/mL) of NS

Other institutions may use concentrations of 40 **mcg**/mL **or** 160 **mcg**/mL; however, stability information is not available for these concentrations.

Administration

I.V. Administer by slow injection or as a continuous infusion (after diluting); when administering as a continuous infusion, central line administration is preferred. I.V. infusions require an infusion pump.

Vesicant; ensure proper needle or catheter placement prior to and during infusion; avoid extravasation.

Extravasation management: If extravasation occurs, stop infusion immediately and disconnect (leave cannula/needle in place); gently aspirate extravasated solution (do **NOT** flush the line); remove needle/cannula; elevate extremity. Initiate phentolamine (or alternative antidote). Apply dry warm compresses (Hurst, 2004).

Phentolamine: Dilute 5-10 mg in 10-15 mL NS and administer into extravasation site as soon as possible after extravasation (Peberdy, 2010).

Alternatives to phentolamine (due to shortage):

Nitroglycerin topical 2% ointment (based on limited case reports in neonates/infants): Apply 4 mm/kg as a thin ribbon to the affected areas; may repeat after 8 hours if needed (Wong, 1992) **or** apply a 1-inch strip on the affected site (Denkler, 1989).

Terbutaline (based on limited case reports): Infiltrate extravasation area using a solution of terbutaline 1 mg diluted to 10 mL in NS (large extravasation site; administration volume varied from 3-10 mL) **or** 1 mg diluted in 1 mL NS (small/distal extravasation site; administration volume varied from 0.5-1 mL) (Stier, 1999).

Injectable Detail pH: 3-6.5 (10 mg/mL solution in vial)

◄ **Preparation for Administration** Solution for injection:

I.V. infusion: May dilute 10 mg in 500 mL NS or D$_5$W. May also dilute 50 mg in 500 mL NS or 100 mg in 500 mL NS; both concentrations are stable for at least 14 days at room temperature of 25°C (77°F) (Gupta, 2004). Dilution of 1250 mg in 500 mL NS retained potency for at least 24 hours at 22°C (Weber, 1970).

I.V. injection: May dilute with SWFI to a concentration of 1 mg/mL.

Stability in syringes (Kiser, 2007): Concentration of 0.1 mg/mL in NS (polypropylene syringes) is stable for at least 30 days at -20°C (-4°F), 3°C to 5°C (37°F to 41°F), or 23°C to 25°C (73.4°F to 77°F).

Storage/Stability

Solution for injection: Store vials at controlled room temperature of 15°C to 25°C (59°F to 77°F). Protect from light. Do not use solution if brown or contains a precipitate.

Oral: Store at controlled room temperature of 15°C to 25°C (59°F to 77°F). Protect from light.

Nursing Actions

Physical Assessment Parenteral: Monitor arterial blood gases, vital signs, and adverse reactions; monitor infusion site frequently for patency. If extravasation should occur, implement extravasation management immediately; can cause tissue sloughing.

Patient Education

• Discuss specific use of drug and side effects with patient as it relates to treatment. (HCAHPS: During this hospital stay, were you given any medicine that you had not taken before? Before giving you any new medicine, how often did hospital staff tell you what the medicine was for? How often did hospital staff describe possible side effects in a way you could understand?)

• Patient may experience hypertension, nervousness, anxiety, xerostomia, or inability to sleep. Have patient report immediately to prescriber angina, tachycardia, severe headache, or rash (HCAHPS).

• Educate patient about signs of a significant reaction (eg, wheezing; chest tightness; fever; itching; bad cough; blue skin color; seizures; or swelling of face, lips, tongue, or throat). **Note:** This is not a comprehensive list of all side effects. Patient should consult prescriber for additional questions.

Intended Use and Disclaimer: Should not be printed and given to patients. This information is intended to serve as a concise initial reference for healthcare professionals to use when discussing medications with a patient. You must ultimately rely on your own discretion, experience and judgment in diagnosing, treating and advising patients.

Dietary Considerations Some products may contain phenylalanine and/or sodium.

Related Information

Management of Drug Extravasations *on page 1700*

Phenylephrine (Nasal) (fen il EF rin)

Brand Names: U.S. 4-Way Fast Acting [OTC]; 4-Way Menthol [OTC]; Afrin Childrens [OTC]; Nasal Four [OTC]; Neo-Synephrine [OTC]; Rhinall [OTC]

Index Terms Phenylephrine Hydrochloride

Pharmacologic Category Alpha-Adrenergic Agonist; Decongestant

Medication Safety Issues

Sound-alike/look-alike issues:

Neo-Synephrine® (phenylephrine, nasal) may be confused with Neo-Synephrine® (oxymetazoline)

Use For OTC use as symptomatic relief of nasal and nasopharyngeal mucosal congestion

Available Dosage Forms

Solution, Nasal:

4-Way Fast Acting [OTC]: 1% (14.8 mL, 29.6 mL)

4-Way Menthol [OTC]: 1% (14.8 mL, 29.6 mL)

Afrin Childrens [OTC]: 0.25% (15 mL)

Nasal Four [OTC]: 1% (29.6 mL)

Neo-Synephrine [OTC]: 0.25% (15 mL); 0.5% (15 mL); 1% (15 mL)

Rhinall [OTC]: 0.25% (30 mL, 40 mL)

General Dosage Range Intranasal:

Children 2-6 years: 0.125% solution: Instill 1 drop in each nostril every 2-4 hours as needed for ≤3 days

Children 6-12 years: 0.25% solution: Instill 2-3 sprays in each nostril every 4 hours as needed for ≤3 days

Children >12 years: 0.25% to 0.5% solution: Instill 2-3 sprays or 2-3 drops in each nostril every 4 hours as needed for ≤3 days

Adults: 0.25% to 1% solution: Instill 2-3 sprays or 2-3 drops in each nostril every 4 hours as needed for ≤3 days

Nursing Actions

Physical Assessment Ensure patient is not using chronically; may cause rebound congestion when discontinued.

Patient Education

• Discuss specific use of drug and side effects with patient as it relates to treatment. (HCAHPS: During this hospital stay, were you given any medicine that you had not taken before? Before giving you any new medicine, how often did hospital staff tell you what the medicine was for? How often did hospital staff describe possible side effects in a way you could understand?)

• Patient may experience rhinitis. Have patient report immediately to prescriber severe headache or rash (HCAHPS).

- Educate patient about signs of a significant reaction (eg; wheezing; chest tightness; fever; itching; bad cough; blue skin color; seizures; or swelling of face, lips, tongue, or throat). **Note:** This is not a comprehensive list of all side effects. Patient should consult prescriber for additional questions.

Intended Use and Disclaimer: Should not be printed and given to patients. This information is intended to serve as a concise initial reference for healthcare professionals to use when discussing medications with a patient. You must ultimately rely on your own discretion, experience and judgment in diagnosing, treating and advising patients.

Phenylephrine (Ophthalmic) (fen il EF rin)

Brand Names: U.S. Altafrin; Mydfrin; Neofrin; Refresh Redness Relief
Index Terms Phenylephrine Hydrochloride
Pharmacologic Category Alpha-Adrenergic Agonist; Ophthalmic Agent, Antiglaucoma; Ophthalmic Agent, Mydriatic
Medication Safety Issues
Sound-alike/look-alike issues:
Mydfrin® may be confused with Midrin®
Pregnancy Risk Factor C
Lactation Excretion in breast milk unknown/use caution
Use Used as a mydriatic in ophthalmic procedures and treatment of wide-angle glaucoma; OTC use as symptomatic relief of redness of the eye due to irritation
Available Dosage Forms
Solution, Ophthalmic:
Altafrin: 2.5% (15 mL); 10% (5 mL)
Mydfrin: 2.5% (3 mL, 5 mL)
Neofrin: 2.5% (15 mL); 10% (5 mL)
Generic: 2.5% (2 mL, 3 mL, 5 mL, 15 mL); 10% (5 mL)
Solution, Ophthalmic [preservative free]:
Generic: 2.5% (1 ea)
General Dosage Range Ophthalmic:
Infants <1 year: Instill 1 drop of 2.5% solution 15-30 minutes before procedures
Children ≥1 year and Adults: Instill 1 drop of 2.5% or 10% solution; may repeat in 10-60 minutes as needed **or** 1-2 drops of 0.12% solution up to 4 times/day [OTC dosing] (maximum: 72 hours)
Nursing Actions
Physical Assessment Systemic absorption from ophthalmic instillation is minimal, so there are no specific monitoring recommendations to identify adverse events.
Patient Education
- Discuss specific use of drug and side effects with patient as it relates to treatment. (HCAHPS: During this hospital stay, were you given any medicine that you had not taken before? Before giving you any new medicine, how often did hospital staff tell you what the medicine was for? How often did hospital staff describe possible side effects in a way you could understand?)
- Patient may experience eye irritation. Have patient report immediately to prescriber severe headache, sudden vision changes, eye pain, or rash (HCAHPS).
- Educate patient about signs of a significant reaction (eg, wheezing; chest tightness; fever; itching; bad cough; blue skin color; seizures; or swelling of face, lips, tongue, or throat). **Note:** This is not a comprehensive list of all side effects. Patient should consult prescriber for additional questions.

Intended Use and Disclaimer: Should not be printed and given to patients. This information is intended to serve as a concise initial reference for healthcare professionals to use when discussing medications with a patient. You must ultimately rely on your own discretion, experience and judgment in diagnosing, treating and advising patients.

Phenytoin (FEN i toyn)

Brand Names: U.S. Dilantin; Dilantin Infatabs; Phenytek; Phenytoin Infatabs
Index Terms Diphenylhydantoin; DPH; Phenytoin Sodium; Phenytoin Sodium, Extended; Phenytoin Sodium, Prompt
Pharmacologic Category Anticonvulsant, Hydantoin
Medication Safety Issues
Sound-alike/look-alike issues:
Phenytoin may be confused with phenelzine, phentermine, PHENobarbital
Dilantin may be confused with Dilaudid, diltiazem, Dipentum
High alert medication:
The Institute for Safe Medication Practices (ISMP) includes this medication (I.V. formulation) among its list of drug classes which have a heightened risk of causing significant patient harm when used in error.
International issues:
Dilantin [U.S., Canada, and multiple international markets] may be confused with Dolantine brand name for pethidine [Belgium]
Medication Guide Available Yes
Pregnancy Risk Factor D
Lactation Enters breast milk/not recommended
Breast-Feeding Considerations Phenytoin is excreted in breast milk; however, the amount to which the infant is exposed is considered small. The manufacturers of phenytoin do not recommend breast-feeding during therapy.
Use Management of generalized tonic-clonic (grand mal), complex partial seizures; prevention of seizures following neurosurgery

Unlabeled Use Prevention of early (within 1 week) post-traumatic seizures (PTS) following traumatic brain injury

Mechanism of Action/Effect Stabilizes neuronal membranes and decreases seizure activity by increasing efflux or decreasing influx of sodium ions across cell membranes in the motor cortex during generation of nerve impulses; prolongs effective refractory period and suppresses ventricular pacemaker automaticity, shortens action potential in the heart

Contraindications Hypersensitivity to phenytoin, other hydantoins, or any component of the formulation; concurrent use of delavirdine (due to loss of virologic response and possible resistance to delavirdine or other non-nucleoside reverse transcriptase inhibitors [NNRTIs])

I.V.: Sinus bradycardia, sinoatrial block, second- and third-degree heart block, Adams-Stokes syndrome

Warnings/Precautions Antiepileptics are associated with an increased risk of suicidal behavior/ thoughts with use (regardless of indication); patients should be monitored for signs/symptoms of depression, suicidal tendencies, and other unusual behavior changes during therapy and instructed to inform their healthcare provider immediately if symptoms occur.

[U.S. Boxed Warning]: Phenytoin must be administered slowly. Intravenous administration should not exceed 50 mg/minute in adult patients. In pediatric patients, intravenous administration rate should not exceed 1-3 mg/kg/minute or 50 mg/minute whichever is slower. Hypotension and severe cardiac arrhythmias (eg, heart block, ventricular tachycardia, ventricular fibrillation) may occur with rapid administration; adverse cardiac events have been reported at or below the recommended infusion rate. Cardiac monitoring is necessary during and after administration of intravenous phenytoin; reduction in rate of administration or discontinuation of infusion may be necessary. For nonemergency use, intravenous phenytoin should be administered more slowly; the use of oral phenytoin should be used whenever possible. Vesicant (intravenous administration); ensure proper catheter or needle position prior to and during infusion; avoid extravasation; I.V. form may cause soft tissue irritation and inflammation, and skin necrosis at I.V. site; avoid I.V. administration in small veins. The "purple glove syndrome" (ie, discoloration with edema and pain of distal limb) may occur following peripheral I.V. administration of phenytoin; may or may not be associated with drug extravasation; symptoms may resolve spontaneously; however, skin necrosis and limb ischemia may occur; interventions such as fasciotomies, skin grafts, and amputation (rare) may be required. May increase frequency of petit mal seizures; use with caution in patients with porphyria; discontinue if rash or lymphadenopathy occurs; a spectrum of hematologic effects have been reported with use (eg, agranulocytosis, neutropenia, leukopenia, thrombocytopenia, pancytopenia, and anemias); use with caution in patients with hepatic dysfunction, hypothyroidism, or underlying cardiac disease; I.V. use is contraindicated in patients with sinus bradycardia, sinoatrial block, or second- and third-degree heart block; use with caution in elderly or debilitated patients, or in any condition associated with low serum albumin levels, which will increase the free fraction of phenytoin in the serum and, therefore, the pharmacologic response. Sedation, confusional states, or cerebellar dysfunction (loss of motor coordination) may occur at higher total serum concentrations, or at lower total serum concentrations when the free fraction of phenytoin is increased. Effects with other sedative drugs or ethanol may be potentiated. Abrupt withdrawal may precipitate status epilepticus. Severe reactions, including toxic epidermal necrolysis and Stevens-Johnson syndromes, although rarely reported, have resulted in fatalities; drug should be discontinued if there are any signs of rash and evaluate for signs and symptoms of drug reaction with eosinophilia and systemic symptoms (DRESS). Patients of Asian descent with the variant *HLA-B*1502* may be at an increased risk of developing Stevens-Johnson syndrome and/or toxic epidermal necrolysis. Chronic use of phenytoin has been associated with decreased bone mineral density (osteopenia, osteoporosis, and osteomalacia) and bone fractures. Chronic use may result in decreased vitamin D concentrations due to hepatic enzyme induction and may lead to hypocalcemia and hypophosphatemia; monitor as appropriate and consider implementing vitamin D and calcium supplementation.

Drug Interactions

Avoid Concomitant Use

Avoid concomitant use of Phenytoin with any of the following: Abiraterone Acetate; Apixaban; Artemether; Axitinib; Azelastine (Nasal); Bedaquiline; Boceprevir; Bortezomib; Bosutinib; Cabozantinib; CloZAPine; Crizotinib; Dabigatran Etexilate; Darunavir; Delavirdine; Dienogest; Dolutegravir; Dronedarone; Enzalutamide; Etravirine; Everolimus; Ibrutinib; Itraconazole; Ivacaftor; Lapatinib; Lumefantrine; Lurasidone; Macitentan; Mifepristone; NIFEdipine; Nilotinib; Nisoldipine; Paraldehyde; PAZOPanib; Pomalidomide; PONATinib; Praziquantel; Ranolazine; Regorafenib; Rilpivirine; Rivaroxaban; Roflumilast; RomiDEPsin; Simeprevir; Sofosbuvir; SORAfenib; Stiripentol; Tasimelteon; Telaprevir; Thalidomide; Ticagrelor; Tofacitinib; Tolvaptan; Toremifene; Ulipristal; Vandetanib; Vemurafenib; VinCRIStine (Liposomal)

Decreased Effect

Phenytoin may decrease the levels/effects of: Abiraterone Acetate; Acetaminophen; Afatinib; Albendazole; Amiodarone; Antifungal Agents (Azole Derivatives, Systemic); Apixaban; ARIPiprazole; Artemether; Axitinib; Bedaquiline; Boceprevir; Bortezomib; Bosutinib; Brentuximab Vedotin; Busulfan; Cabozantinib; Canagliflozin; CarBAMazepine; Caspofungin; Chloramphenicol; Clarithromycin; CloZAPine; Cobicistat; Contraceptives (Estrogens); Contraceptives (Progestins); Crizotinib; CycloSPORINE (Systemic); CYP2B6 Substrates; CYP2C19 Substrates; CYP2C8 Substrates; CYP2C9 Substrates; CYP3A4 Substrates; Dabigatran Etexilate; Darunavir; Dasatinib; Deferasirox; Delavirdine; Diclofenac (Systemic); Dienogest; Disopyramide; Dolutegravir; DOXOrubicin (Conventional); Doxycycline; Dronedarone; Efavirenz; Elvitegravir; Enzalutamide; Eslicarbazepine; Ethosuximide; Etoposide; Etoposide Phosphate; Etravirine; Everolimus; Exemestane; Ezogabine; Felbamate; Flunarizine; Gefitinib; GuanFACINE; HMG-CoA Reductase Inhibitors; Ibrutinib; Imatinib; Irinotecan; Itraconazole; Ivacaftor; Ixabepilone; Lacosamide; LamoTRIgine; Lapatinib; Levodopa; Linagliptin; Loop Diuretics; Lopinavir; Lumefantrine; Lurasidone; Macitentan; Maraviroc; Mebendazole; Meperidine; Methadone; MethylPREDNISolone; MetroNIDAZOLE (Systemic); Metyrapone; Mexiletine; Mifepristone; Nelfinavir; Neuromuscular-Blocking Agents (Nondepolarizing); NIFEdipine; Nilotinib; Nisoldipine; Omeprazole; OXcarbazepine; PAZOPanib; Perampanel; P-glycoprotein/ABCB1 Substrates; Pomalidomide; PONATinib; Praziquantel; PredmisoLONE (Systemic); PredniSONE; Primidone; QUEtiapine; QuiNIDine; QuiNINE; Ranolazine; Regorafenib; Rilpivirine; Ritonavir; Rivaroxaban; Roflumilast; RomiDEPsin; Rufinamide; Saxagliptin; Sertraline; Simeprevir; Sirolimus; Sofosbuvir; SORAfenib; SUNItinib; Tacrolimus (Systemic); Tadalafil; Tasimelteon; Telaprevir; Temsirolimus; Teniposide; Theophylline Derivatives; Thyroid Products; Ticagrelor; Tipranavir; Tofacitinib; Tolvaptan; Topiramate; Topotecan; Toremifene; TraZODone; Treprostinil; Trimethoprim; Ulipristal; Valproic Acid and Derivatives; Vandetanib; Vemurafenib; Vilazodone; VinCRIStine; VinCRIStine (Liposomal); Vortioxetine; Zonisamide; Zuclopenthixol

The levels/effects of Phenytoin may be decreased by: Alcohol (Ethyl); Amphetamines; Antacids; Bleomycin; CarBAMazepine; Ciprofloxacin (Systemic); Colesevelam; CYP2C19 Inducers (Strong); CYP2C9 Inducers (Strong); Dabrafenib; Diazoxide; Enzalutamide; Folic Acid; Fosamprenavir; Ketorolac (Nasal); Ketorolac (Systemic); Leucovorin Calcium-Levoleucovorin; Levomefolate; Lopinavir; Mefloquine; Methotrexate; Methylfolate; Multivitamins/Minerals (with ADEK, Folate, Iron); Nelfinavir; Orlistat; Peginterferon Alfa-2b; PHENobarbital; Platinum Derivatives; Pyridoxine; Rifampin; Ritonavir; Stiripentol; Theophylline Derivatives; Tipranavir; Valproic Acid and Derivatives; Vigabatrin; VinCRIStine

Increased Effect/Toxicity

Phenytoin may increase the levels/effects of: Azelastine (Nasal); Buprenorphine; Clarithromycin; CNS Depressants; Fosamprenavir; Hydrocodone; Ifosfamide; Lithium; Methotrimeprazine; Metyrosine; Mirtazapine; Neuromuscular-Blocking Agents (Nondepolarizing); Paraldehyde; PHENobarbital; Pramipexole; Prilocaine; ROPINIRole; Rotigotine; Selective Serotonin Reuptake Inhibitors; Sodium Nitrite; Thalidomide; Vitamin K Antagonists; Zolpidem

The levels/effects of Phenytoin may be increased by: Alcohol (Ethyl); Allopurinol; Amiodarone; Antifungal Agents (Azole Derivatives, Systemic); Benzodiazepines; Brimonidine (Topical); Calcium Channel Blockers; Capecitabine; CarBAMazepine; Carbonic Anhydrase Inhibitors; CeFAZolin; Chloramphenicol; Cimetidine; Clarithromycin; Cosyntropin; CYP2C19 Inhibitors (Moderate); CYP2C19 Inhibitors (Strong); CYP2C9 Inhibitors (Moderate); CYP2C9 Inhibitors (Strong); Delavirdine; Dexmethylphenidate; Disulfiram; Doxylamine; Droperidol; Efavirenz; Eslicarbazepine; Ethosuximide; Felbamate; Floxuridine; Fluconazole; Fluorouracil (Systemic); Fluorouracil (Topical); FLUoxetine; FluvoxaMINE; Halothane; HydrOXYzine; Isoniazid; Luliconazole; Magnesium Sulfate; Methotrimeprazine; Methylphenidate; MetroNIDAZOLE (Systemic); Nitric Oxide; Omeprazole; OXcarbazepine; Rufinamide; Sertraline; Sodium Oxybate; Tacrolimus (Systemic); Tapentadol; Tegafur; Telaprevir; Ticlopidine; Topiramate; TraZODone; Trimethoprim; Vitamin K Antagonists

Nutritional/Ethanol Interactions

Ethanol:

Acute use: Ethanol inhibits metabolism of phenytoin and may also increase CNS depression. Management: Avoid or limit ethanol. Caution patients about effects.

Chronic use: Ethanol stimulates metabolism of phenytoin. Management: Avoid or limit ethanol.

Food: Phenytoin serum concentrations may be altered if taken with food. If taken with enteral nutrition, phenytoin serum concentrations may be decreased. Tube feedings decrease bioavailability. Phenytoin may decrease calcium, folic acid, and vitamin D levels. Supplementing folic acid may lower the seizure threshold. Management: Hold tube feedings 1-2 hours before and 1-2 hours after phenytoin administration. Do not supplement folic acid. Consider vitamin D supplementation. Take preferably on an empty stomach.

Herb/Nutraceutical: Evening primrose may decrease the seizure threshold; other herbal medications may increase CNS depression. Management: Avoid evening primrose, valerian, St John's wort, kava kava, and gotu kola.

Adverse Reactions I.V. effects: Hypotension, bradycardia, cardiac arrhythmia, cardiovascular collapse (especially with rapid I.V. use), venous irritation and pain, thrombophlebitis

Effects not related to plasma phenytoin concentrations: Hypertrichosis, gingival hypertrophy, thickening of facial features, carbohydrate intolerance, folic acid deficiency, peripheral neuropathy, vitamin D deficiency, osteomalacia, systemic lupus erythematosus

Concentration-related effects: Nystagmus, blurred vision, diplopia, ataxia, slurred speech, dizziness, drowsiness, lethargy, coma, rash, fever, nausea, vomiting, gum tenderness, confusion, mood changes, folic acid depletion, osteomalacia, hyperglycemia

Related to elevated concentrations:
>20 mcg/mL: Far lateral nystagmus
>30 mcg/mL: 45° lateral gaze nystagmus and ataxia
>40 mcg/mL: Decreased mentation
>100 mcg/mL: Death

Cardiovascular: Bradycardia, cardiac arrhythmia, cardiovascular collapse, hypotension

Central nervous system: Dizziness, drowsiness, headache, insomnia, psychiatric changes, slurred speech, vertigo

Dermatologic: Rash

Gastrointestinal: Constipation, enlargement of lips, gingival hyperplasia, hepatic injury, nausea, taste disturbance, vomiting

Genitourinary: Peyronie's disease

Hematologic: Agranulocytosis, granulocytopenia, leukopenia, pancytopenia, thrombocytopenia

Hepatic: Acute hepatic failure, hepatitis, toxic hepatitis

Local: I.V. administration: Inflammation, irritation, necrosis, sloughing, tenderness, thrombophlebitis

Neuromuscular & skeletal: Paresthesia, peripheral neuropathy, tremor

Ocular: Blurred vision, diplopia, nystagmus

Rarely seen effects: Anaphylaxis, blood dyscrasias, coarsening of facial features, DRESS, dyskinesias, hepatitis, Hodgkin lymphoma, hypertrichosis, immunoglobulin abnormalities, lymphadenopathy, lymphoma, macrocytosis, megaloblastic anemia, periarteritis nodosa, pseudolymphoma, SLE-like syndrome, Stevens-Johnson syndrome, toxic epidermal necrolysis, venous irritation and pain

Pharmacodynamics/Kinetics

Onset of Action I.V.: ~0.5-1 hour

Available Dosage Forms

Capsule, Oral:
Dilantin: 30 mg, 100 mg
Phenytek: 200 mg, 300 mg
Generic: 100 mg, 200 mg, 300 mg

Solution, Injection:
Generic: 50 mg/mL (2 mL, 5 mL)

Suspension, Oral:
Dilantin: 125 mg/5 mL (237 mL)
Generic: 125 mg/5 mL (4 mL, 237 mL)

Tablet Chewable, Oral:
Dilantin Infatabs: 50 mg
Phenytoin Infatabs: 50 mg
Generic: 50 mg

General Dosage Range

I.V.:
Infants and Children: Loading dose: 15-20 mg/kg; Maintenance: 4-8 mg/kg/day in 2-3 divided doses

Adolescents and Adults: Loading dose: 10-20 mg/kg; Maintenance: 300-400 mg daily in 3 or 4 divided doses

Oral:
Children: Loading dose: 15-20 mg/kg in divided doses; Maintenance: 4-8 mg/kg/day in divided doses

Adolescents and Adults: Loading dose: 15-20 mg/kg in 3 divided doses every 2-4 hours; Maintenance: 300 mg daily in 1-3 divided doses or 5-6 mg/kg/day in 1-3 divided doses (range: 300-600 mg daily)

Administration

I.V. Fosphenytoin may be considered for loading in patients who are in status epilepticus, hemodynamically unstable, or develop hypotension/bradycardia with I.V. administration of phenytoin. Although, phenytoin may be administered by direct I.V. injection, it is preferable that phenytoin be administered via infusion pump either undiluted or diluted in normal saline as an I.V. piggyback (IVPB) to prevent exceeding the maximum infusion rate (monitor closely for extravasation during infusion). The maximum rate of I.V. administration is 50 mg/minute in adults. Highly sensitive patients (eg, elderly, patients with pre-existing cardiovascular conditions) should receive phenytoin more slowly (eg, 20 mg/minute) (Meek, 1999). In neonates, the manufacturer recommends a maximum rate of 1-3 mg/kg/minute; however, a lower maximum rate of 0.5-1 mg/kg/minute is used clinically (Sankar, 2010; Shields, 1989). An in-line 0.22-0.55 micron filter is recommended for IVPB solutions due to the potential for precipitation of the solution. Avoid extravasation. Following I.V. administration, NS should be injected through the same needle or I.V. catheter to prevent irritation.

Vesicant; ensure proper needle or catheter placement prior to and during I.V. infusion. Avoid extravasation.

Extravasation management: If extravasation occurs, stop infusion immediately and disconnect (leave needle/cannula in place); gently aspirate extravasated solution (do **NOT** flush the line); remove needle/cannula; elevate extremity. There is conflicting information regarding an antidote; some sources recommend not to use an antidote (Montgomery, 1999 [pediatric reference]), while other sources recommend hyaluronidase.

Hyaluronidase (if appropriate): SubQ: Administer four separate 0.2 mL injections of a 15 units/mL solution (using a 25-gauge needle) into area of extravasation (Sokol, 1998)

Injectable Detail pH: 12 (undiluted)

Oral Suspension: Shake well prior to use. Absorption is impaired when phenytoin suspension is given concurrently to patients who are receiving continuous nasogastric feedings. A method to resolve this interaction is to divide the daily dose of phenytoin and withhold the administration of nutritional supplements for 1-2 hours before and after each phenytoin dose.

Subcutaneous SubQ administration is not recommended because of the possibility of local tissue damage (due to high pH).

Other Avoid I.M. administration due to severe risk of local tissue destruction and necrosis; use **fos**phenytoin if I.M. administration necessary (Boucher, 1996; Meek, 1999). The manufacturer's labeling includes I.M. administration; however, in general the I.M. route should be avoided and should **NOT** be used for status epilepticus.

Preparation for Administration I.V.: May be further diluted in NS to a final concentration ≥5 mg/mL; infusion must be completed within 4 hours after preparation. Do not refrigerate.

Storage/Stability

Capsule, tablet: Store at 20°C to 25°C (68°F to 77°F). Protect capsules from light. Protect capsules and tablets from moisture.

Oral suspension: Store at room temperature of 20°C to 25°C (68°F to 77°F); do not freeze. Protect from light.

Solution for injection: Store at room temperature of 15°C to 30°C (59°F to 86°F). Use only clear solutions free of precipitate and haziness; slightly yellow solutions may be used. Precipitation may occur if solution is refrigerated and may dissolve at room temperature.

Nursing Actions

Physical Assessment When oral phenytoin is discontinued, dose should be tapered gradually; abrupt discontinuance can cause status epilepticus. I.V.: Monitor blood pressure. Monitor infusion site closely to prevent extravasation. Monitor patient closely for adverse results (eg, cardiorespiratory, CNS status, suicide ideation).

Patient Education

- Discuss specific use of drug and side effects with patient as it relates to treatment. (HCAHPS: During this hospital stay, were you given any medicine that you had not taken before? Before giving you any new medicine, how often did hospital staff tell you what the medicine was for? How often did hospital staff describe possible side effects in a way you could understand?)

- Patient may experience presyncope, fatigue, blurred vision, illogical thinking, dizziness, nausea, or constipation. Have patient report immediately to prescriber depression, imbalance, severe asthenia, significant skin irritation, stomatitis, discolored urine, jaundice, ecchymosis, bleeding, or rash (HCAHPS).

- Educate patient about signs of a significant reaction (eg, wheezing; chest tightness; fever; itching; bad cough; blue skin color; seizures; or swelling of face, lips, tongue, or throat). **Note:** This is not a comprehensive list of all side effects. Patient should consult prescriber for additional questions.

Intended Use and Disclaimer: Should not be printed and given to patients. This information is intended to serve as a concise initial reference for healthcare professionals to use when discussing medications with a patient. You must ultimately rely on your own discretion, experience and judgment in diagnosing, treating and advising patients.

Dietary Considerations

Folic acid: Phenytoin may decrease mucosal uptake of folic acid; to avoid folic acid deficiency and megaloblastic anemia, some clinicians recommend giving patients on anticonvulsants prophylactic doses of folic acid and cyanocobalamin. Folic acid 0.5 mg/day has been shown to reduce the incidence of phenytoin-induced gingival overgrowth in children (Arya, 2011). However, folate supplementation may increase seizures in some patients (dose dependent). Discuss with healthcare provider prior to using any supplements.

Calcium: Hypocalcemia has been reported in patients taking prolonged high-dose therapy with an anticonvulsant. Some clinicians have given an additional 4000 units/week of vitamin D (especially in those receiving poor nutrition and getting no sun exposure) to prevent hypocalcemia.

Vitamin D: Phenytoin interferes with vitamin D metabolism and osteomalacia may result; may need to supplement with vitamin D

Tube feedings: Tube feedings decrease phenytoin absorption. To avoid decreased serum levels with continuous NG feeds, hold feedings for 1-2 hours prior to and 1-2 hours after phenytoin administration, if possible. There is a variety of opinions on how to administer phenytoin with enteral feedings. Be **consistent** throughout therapy.

Injection may contain sodium.

Related Information

Management of Drug Extravasations *on page 1700*

Peak and Trough Guidelines *on page 1710*

Phytonadione (fye toe na DYE one)

Brand Names: U.S. Mephyton®

Index Terms Methylphytyl Napthoquinone; Phyllo-quinone; Phytomenadione; Vitamin K; Vitamin K_1

Pharmacologic Category Vitamin, Fat Soluble

Medication Safety Issues

Sound-alike/look-alike issues:
Mephyton® may be confused with melphalan, methadone

Pregnancy Risk Factor C

Lactation Enters breast milk/use caution

Breast-Feeding Considerations Small amounts of dietary vitamin K can be detected in breast milk and the dietary requirements of vitamin K are the same in nursing and non-nursing women (IOM, 2000). Information following the use of phytonadione has not been located. The manufacturer recommends caution be used if phytonadione is administered to a nursing woman.

Use Prevention and treatment of hypoprothrombinemia caused by vitamin K antagonist (VKA)-induced (eg, warfarin-induced) or other drug-induced vitamin K deficiency, altered activity, or altered metabolism; hypoprothrombinemia caused by malabsorption or inability to synthesize vitamin K; prophylaxis and treatment of hemorrhagic disease of the newborn

Unlabeled Use Treatment of hypoprothrombinemia caused by long-acting anticoagulant rodenticides (LAARs)

Mechanism of Action/Effect Promotes liver synthesis of clotting factors (II, VII, IX, X); however, the exact mechanism as to this stimulation is unknown. Menadiol is a water soluble form of vitamin K; phytonadione has a more rapid and prolonged effect than menadione; menadiol sodium diphosphate (K_4) is half as potent as menadione (K_3).

Contraindications Hypersensitivity to phytonadione or any component of the formulation

Warnings/Precautions [U.S. Boxed Warning]: Severe reactions resembling hypersensitivity reactions (eg, anaphylaxis) have occurred rarely during or immediately after I.V. administration (even with proper dilution and rate of administration); some patients had no previous exposure to phytonadione. Anaphylactoid reactions typically occurred when patients received large I.V. doses administered rapidly with formulations containing polyethoxylated castor oil; proper dosing, dilution, and administration will minimize risk (Ageno, 2012; Riegert-Johnson, 2002). Limit I.V. administration to situations where an alternative route of administration is not feasible and the benefit of therapy outweighs the risk of hypersensitivity reactions. Allergic reactions have also occurred with I.M. and SubQ injections, albeit less frequently. In obstructive jaundice or with biliary fistulas concurrent administration of bile salts is necessary. Manufacturers recommend the SubQ route over other parenteral routes. SubQ is less predictable when compared to the oral route. The American College of Chest Physicians recommends the I.V. route in patients with major bleeding secondary to warfarin. The I.V. route should be restricted to emergency situations where oral phytonadione cannot be used. Efficacy is delayed regardless of route of administration; patient management may require other treatments in the interim. In patients receiving a therapeutic vitamin K antagonist (VKA) (eg, warfarin), administer a dose of phytonadione that will quickly lower the INR into a safe range without causing resistance to warfarin. High phytonadione doses may lead to warfarin resistance for at least one week. Patients with LAAR-induced coagulopathy require much larger doses and longer treatment durations (up to months) after exposure compared to that needed to reverse VKA-induced coagulopathy. Use caution in newborns especially premature infants; hemolysis, jaundice and hyperbilirubinemia have been reported with larger than recommended doses. Some dosage forms contain benzyl alcohol which has been associated with "gasping syndrome" in premature infants. In liver disease, if initial doses do not reverse coagulopathy then higher doses are unlikely to have any effect. Ineffective in hereditary hypoprothrombinemia. Injectable products may contain aluminum; may result in toxic levels following prolonged administration. Product may contain polysorbate 80. Some dosage forms contain Cremophor® EL which has been associated with anaphylactoid reactions; use these formulations with caution.

Drug Interactions

Avoid Concomitant Use There are no known interactions where it is recommended to avoid concomitant use.

Decreased Effect

Phytonadione may decrease the levels/effects of: Vitamin K Antagonists

The levels/effects of Phytonadione may be decreased by: Mineral Oil; Orlistat

Increased Effect/Toxicity There are no known significant interactions involving an increase in effect.

Adverse Reactions Frequency not defined.

Cardiovascular: Cyanosis, flushing, hyper-/hypotension

Central nervous system: Dizziness

Dermatologic: Erythematous skin eruptions, pruritus, scleroderma-like lesions

Endocrine & metabolic: Hyperbilirubinemia (newborn; greater than recommended doses)

Gastrointestinal: Abnormal taste

Local: Injection site reactions

Respiratory: Dyspnea

Miscellaneous: Diaphoresis, hypersensitivity reactions, nonimmunologic anaphylaxis (formerly known as anaphylactoid reaction), sweating

Pharmacodynamics/Kinetics

Onset of Action

Onset of action: Increased coagulation factors: Oral: 6-10 hours; I.V.: 1-2 hours

Peak effect: INR values return to normal: Oral: 24-48 hours; I.V.: 12-14 hours

Available Dosage Forms

Injection, aqueous colloidal: 1 mg/0.5 mL (0.5 mL); 10 mg/mL (1 mL)

Injection, aqueous colloidal [preservative free]: 1 mg/0.5 mL (0.5 mL)

Tablet, oral: 100 mcg

Mephyton®: 5 mg

General Dosage Range

I.M.:

Newborns: Prophylaxis: 0.5-1 mg within 1 hour of birth; Treatment: 1 mg/dose/day

Adults: Initial: 2.5-25 mg/dose (maximum: 50 mg)

I.V.: *Adults:* Initial: 2.5-25 mg/dose (maximum: 50 mg)

Oral: *Adults:* Initial: 2.5-25 mg/dose (maximum: 50 mg)

SubQ:

Newborns: 1 mg/dose/day

Adults: Initial: 2.5-25 mg/dose (maximum: 50 mg)

Administration

I.V. Infuse slowly; rate of infusion should not exceed 1 mg/minute (3 mg/m^2/minute in children and infants). Alternatively, dilute dose in a minimum of 50 mL of compatible solution and administer using an infusion pump over at least 20 minutes (Ageno, 2012). The injectable route should be used only if the oral route is not feasible or there is a greater urgency to reverse anticoagulation.

Injectable Detail pH: 3.5-7

Oral The parenteral formulation may also be used for small oral doses (eg, 1 mg) or situations in which tablets cannot be swallowed (Crowther, 2000; O'Connor, 1986).

Preparation for Administration Dilute injection solution in preservative-free NS, D$_5$W, or D$_5$NS. To reduce the incidence of anaphylactoid reaction upon I.V. administration, dilute dose in a minimum of 50 mL of compatible solution and administer using an infusion pump over at least 20 minutes (Ageno, 2012).

Storage/Stability

Injection: Store at 15°C to 30°C (59°F to 86°F). Protect from light. **Note:** Store Hospira product at 20°C to 25°C (68°F to 77°F).

Oral: Store tablets at 15°C to 30°C (59°F to 86°F). Protect from light.

Nursing Actions

Physical Assessment Note dosing specifics according to use. Monitor degree of bleeding.

Patient Education

• Discuss specific use of drug and side effects with patient as it relates to treatment. (HCAHPS: During this hospital stay, were you given any medicine that you had not taken before? Before giving you any new medicine, how often did hospital staff tell you what the medicine was for? How often did hospital staff describe possible side effects in a way you could understand?)

• Patient may experience injection site pain or irritation, dysgeusia, or flushing. Have patient report immediately to prescriber tachycardia, arrhythmia, severe dizziness, syncope, dyspnea, hyperhydrosis, or skin or nail discoloration (HCAHPS).

• Educate patient about signs of a significant reaction (eg, wheezing; chest tightness; fever; itching; bad cough; blue skin color; seizures; or swelling of face, lips, tongue, or throat). **Note:** This is not a comprehensive list of all side effects. Patient should consult prescriber for additional questions.

Intended Use and Disclaimer: Should not be printed and given to patients. This information is intended to serve as a concise initial reference for healthcare professionals to use when discussing medications with a patient. You must ultimately rely on your own discretion, experience and judgment in diagnosing, treating and advising patients.

Pimozide (PI moe zide)

Brand Names: U.S. Orap

Pharmacologic Category Antipsychotic Agent, Typical

Medication Safety Issues

BEERS Criteria medication:

This drug may be potentially inappropriate for use in geriatric patients (Quality of evidence - moderate; Strength of recommendation - strong).

Pregnancy Risk Factor C

Lactation Excretion in breast milk unknown/not recommended

Use Suppression of severe motor and phonic tics in patients with Tourette's disorder who have failed to respond satisfactorily to standard treatment

Unlabeled Use Psychosis; reported use in individuals with delusions focused on physical symptoms (ie, preoccupation with parasitic infestation); Huntington's chorea

Available Dosage Forms

Tablet, Oral:

Orap: 1 mg, 2 mg

General Dosage Range Dosage adjustment recommended in patients who develop toxicities or those with a CYP2D6 poor metabolizer status.

Oral:

Children 2-12 years: Initial: 0.05 mg/kg once daily (preferably bedtime); Maintenance: 2-4 mg once daily (maximum: 10 mg/day [0.2 mg/kg/day])

Children >12 years and Adults: Initial: 1-2 mg in divided doses (maximum: 10 mg/day [0.2 mg/kg/day])

Nursing Actions

Physical Assessment Review ophthalmic exam and monitor blood pressure at beginning of therapy and periodically throughout. Monitor for endocrine changes, extrapyramidal symptoms, and neuroleptic malignant syndrome. Conduct ECG at baseline and periodically during therapy (especially during dosage adjustment).

Patient Education

- Discuss specific use of drug and side effects with patient as it relates to treatment. (HCAHPS: During this hospital stay, were you given any medicine that you had not taken before? Before giving you any new medicine, how often did hospital staff tell you what the medicine was for? How often did hospital staff describe possible side effects in a way you could understand?)
- Patient may experience presyncope, fatigue, blurred vision, illogical thinking, dizziness, nervousness and anxiety, constipation, xerostomia, weight gain, or impotence. Have patient report immediately to prescriber tachycardia, significant change in balance, tremors, urinary retention, severe asthenia, pregnancy, or rash (HCAHPS).
- Educate patient about signs of a significant reaction (eg, wheezing; chest tightness; fever; itching; bad cough; blue skin color; seizures; or swelling of face, lips, tongue, or throat). **Note:** This is not a comprehensive list of all side effects. Patient should consult prescriber for additional questions.

Intended Use and Disclaimer: Should not be printed and given to patients. This information is intended to serve as a concise initial reference for healthcare professionals to use when discussing medications with a patient. You must ultimately rely on your own discretion, experience and judgment in diagnosing, treating and advising patients.

Pindolol (PIN doe lole)

Pharmacologic Category Antihypertensive; Beta-Blocker With Intrinsic Sympathomimetic Activity

Medication Safety Issues

Sound-alike/look-alike issues:

Pindolol may be confused with Parlodel, Plendil
Visken may be confused with Visine, Viskazide

Pregnancy Risk Factor B

Lactation Enters breast milk/not recommended

Use

U.S. labeling: Treatment of hypertension, alone or in combination with other agents

Canadian labeling: Treatment of hypertension, alone or in combination with other agents; prophylaxis of angina pectoris

Unlabeled Use Potential augmenting agent for antidepressants; ventricular arrhythmias/tachycardia, antipsychotic-induced akathisia, situational anxiety; aggressive behavior associated with dementia

Available Dosage Forms

Tablet, Oral:

Generic: 5 mg, 10 mg

General Dosage Range Dosage adjustment recommended in patients with hepatic impairment

Oral:

Adults: Initial: 5 mg twice daily; Maintenance: 10-40 mg twice daily (maximum: 60 mg daily)

Elderly: Initial: 5 mg once daily

Administration

Oral May be administered without regard to meals.

Nursing Actions

Patient Education

- Discuss specific use of drug and side effects with patient as it relates to treatment. (HCAHPS: During this hospital stay, were you given any medicine that you had not taken before? Before giving you any new medicine, how often did hospital staff tell you what the medicine was for? How often did hospital staff describe possible side effects in a way you could understand?)
- Patient may experience presyncope, fatigue, blurred vision, illogical thinking, dizziness, insomnia, or impotence. Have patient report immediately to prescriber dyspnea, severe asthenia, or rash (HCAHPS).
- Educate patient about signs of a significant reaction (eg, wheezing; chest tightness; fever; itching; bad cough; blue skin color; seizures; or swelling of face, lips, tongue, or throat). **Note:** This is not a comprehensive list of all side effects. Patient should consult prescriber for additional questions.

Intended Use and Disclaimer: Should not be printed and given to patients. This information is intended to serve as a concise initial reference for healthcare professionals to use when discussing medications with a patient. You must ultimately rely on your own discretion, experience and judgment in diagnosing, treating and advising patients.

Pioglitazone (pye oh GLI ta zone)

Brand Names: U.S. Actos

Pharmacologic Category Antidiabetic Agent, Thiazolidinedione

Medication Safety Issues

Sound-alike/look-alike issues:

Actos® may be confused with Actidose®, Actonel®

High alert medication:

The Institute for Safe Medication Practices (ISMP) includes this medication among its list of drug classes which have a heightened risk of causing significant patient harm when used in error.

International issues:

Tiazac: Brand name for pioglitazone [Chile], but also the brand name for diltiazem [U.S, Canada]

Medication Guide Available Yes

Pregnancy Risk Factor C

Lactation Excretion in breast milk unknown/not recommended

Use Type 2 diabetes mellitus (noninsulin dependent, NIDDM), monotherapy or combination therapy: Adjunct to diet and exercise, to improve glycemic control

Available Dosage Forms

Tablet, Oral:

Actos: 15 mg, 30 mg, 45 mg

Generic: 15 mg, 30 mg, 45 mg

General Dosage Range Dosage adjustment recommended in patients on concomitant therapy.

Oral: *Adults:* Initial: 15-30 mg once daily; Maintenance: 15-45 mg once daily (maximum: 45 mg/day)

Administration

Oral May be administered without regard to meals.

Nursing Actions

Physical Assessment Monitor for signs of heart failure (weight gain, edema, dyspnea). Teach risks of hyperglycemia. Refer patient to a diabetic educator, if available.

Patient Education

• Discuss specific use of drug and side effects with patient as it relates to treatment. (HCAHPS: During this hospital stay, were you given any medicine that you had not taken before? Before giving you any new medicine, how often did hospital staff tell you what the medicine was for? How often did hospital staff describe possible side effects in a way you could understand?)

• Patient may experience headache, rhinitis, pharyngitis, myalgia, or flatulence. Have patient report immediately to prescriber strength differences from one side to another, difficulty speaking or thinking, change in balance, blurred vision, osteodynia, severe asthenia, angina, vision changes, dysuria, hematuria, polyuria, signs of hypoglycemia, or signs of hepatic impairment (HCAHPS).

• Educate patient about signs of a significant reaction (eg, wheezing; chest tightness; fever; itching; bad cough; blue skin color; seizures; or swelling of face, lips, tongue, or throat). **Note:** This is not a comprehensive list of all side effects. Patient should consult prescriber for additional questions.

Intended Use and Disclaimer: Should not be printed and given to patients. This information is intended to serve as a concise initial reference for healthcare professionals to use when discussing medications with a patient. You must ultimately rely on your own discretion, experience and judgment in diagnosing, treating and advising patients.

Pioglitazone and Glimepiride

(pye oh GLI ta zone & GLYE me pye ride)

Brand Names: U.S. Duetact™

Index Terms Glimepiride and Pioglitazone; Glimepiride and Pioglitazone Hydrochloride

Pharmacologic Category Antidiabetic Agent, Sulfonylurea; Antidiabetic Agent, Thiazolidinedione; Hypoglycemic Agent, Oral

Medication Safety Issues

High alert medication:

The Institute for Safe Medication Practices (ISMP) includes this medication among its list of drugs which have a heightened risk of causing significant patient harm when used in error.

Medication Guide Available Yes

Pregnancy Risk Factor C

Use Management of type 2 diabetes mellitus (noninsulin dependent, NIDDM) as an adjunct to diet and exercise in patients already treated with a thiazolidinedione and a sulfonylurea or who have inadequate control on either agent alone

Available Dosage Forms

Tablet: 30/2: Pioglitazone 30 mg and glimepiride 2 mg; 30/4: Pioglitazone 30 mg and glimepiride 4 mg

Duetact™: 30 mg/2 mg: Pioglitazone 30 mg and glimepiride 2 mg; 30 mg/4 mg: Pioglitazone 30 mg and glimepiride 4 mg

General Dosage Range Dosage adjustment recommended in patients with renal impairment

Oral:

Adults:

Patients inadequately controlled on **glimepiride** alone: Initial dose: Pioglitazone 30 mg and glimepiride 2-4 mg once daily (maximum: 45 mg/day [pioglitazone]; 8 mg/day [glimepiride])

Patients inadequately controlled on **pioglitazone** alone: Initial dose: Pioglitazone 30 mg and glimepiride 2 mg once daily (maximum: 45 mg/day [pioglitazone]; 8 mg/day [glimepiride])

Elderly: Initial: Glimepiride 1 mg/day prior to initiating Duetact™

Administration

Oral Administer once daily with the first main meal of the day. To avoid hypoglycemia, patients without oral intake may need to have the dose held.

Nursing Actions

Physical Assessment Monitor for weight gain of >5 lbs in 1 week, difficulty breathing, increased edema, or jaundice. Instruct patient about diabetic care. Monitor insulin and/or oral hypoglycemic therapy requirements. Encourage patient to keep good records of home glucose monitoring, especially during initiation of drug therapy. Instruct patient to report if home glucose consistently high/low.

Patient Education

- Discuss specific use of drug and side effects with patient as it relates to treatment. (HCAHPS: During this hospital stay, were you given any medicine that you had not taken before? Before giving you any new medicine, how often did hospital staff tell you what the medicine was for? How often did hospital staff describe possible side effects in a way you could understand?)
- Patient may experience headache, diarrhea, rhinitis, pharyngitis, or dyspepsia. Have patient report immediately to prescriber signs of hepatic impairment, strength differences from one side to another, difficulty speaking or thinking, change in balance, blurred vision, vision changes, severe asthenia, dysuria, hematuria, polyuria, ecchymosis, hemorrhaging, osteodynia, or signs of hypoglycemia (HCAHPS).
- Educate patient about signs of a significant reaction (eg, wheezing; chest tightness; fever; itching; bad cough; blue skin color; seizures; or swelling of face, lips, tongue, or throat). **Note:** This is not a comprehensive list of all side effects. Patient should consult prescriber for additional questions.

Intended Use and Disclaimer: Should not be printed and given to patients. This information is intended to serve as a concise initial reference for healthcare professionals to use when discussing medications with a patient. You must ultimately rely on your own discretion, experience and judgment in diagnosing, treating and advising patients.

Related Information

Glimepiride *on page 740*
Pioglitazone *on page 1250*

Pioglitazone and Metformin
(pye oh GLI ta zone & met FOR min)

Brand Names: U.S. Actoplus Met®; Actoplus Met® XR

Index Terms Metformin Hydrochloride and Pioglitazone Hydrochloride

Pharmacologic Category Antidiabetic Agent, Biguanide; Antidiabetic Agent, Thiazolidinedione

Medication Safety Issues
High alert medication:
The Institute for Safe Medication Practices (ISMP) includes this medication among its list of drug classes which have a heightened risk of causing significant patient harm when used in error.

Medication Guide Available Yes

Pregnancy Risk Factor C

Breast-Feeding Considerations Metformin is excreted into breast milk; excretion of pioglitazone is not known. Due to the potential for serious adverse reactions in the nursing infant, the manufacturer recommends a decision be made whether to discontinue nursing or to discontinue the drug, taking into account the importance of treatment to the mother. See individual agents.

Use Management of type 2 diabetes mellitus (noninsulin dependent, NIDDM) in patients already receiving a thiazolidinedione and metformin or who have inadequate control on either agent

Mechanism of Action/Effect

Pioglitazone is a thiazolidinedione antidiabetic agent that lowers blood glucose by improving target cell response to insulin, without increasing pancreatic insulin secretion. It has a mechanism of action that is dependent on the presence of insulin for activity.

Metformin decreases hepatic glucose production, decreasing intestinal absorption of glucose, and improves insulin sensitivity (increases peripheral glucose uptake and utilization).

Contraindications Hypersensitivity to pioglitazone, metformin, or any component of the formulation; NYHA Class III/IV heart failure (initiation of therapy); renal disease or renal dysfunction (serum creatinine ≥1.5 mg/dL [males] or ≥1.4 mg/dL [females], or abnormal creatinine clearance which may also result from conditions such as cardiovascular collapse, acute myocardial infarction, and septicemia); acute or chronic metabolic acidosis with or without coma (including diabetic ketoacidosis)

Note: Temporarily discontinue in patients undergoing radiologic studies in which intravascular iodinated contrast media are utilized.

Warnings/Precautions [U.S. Boxed Warning]: Lactic acidosis is a rare, but potentially severe consequence of therapy with metformin that requires urgent care and hospitalization. The risk is increased in patients with acute congestive heart failure, dehydration, excessive alcohol intake, hepatic or renal impairment, or sepsis. Symptoms may be nonspecific (eg, abdominal distress, malaise, myalgia, respiratory distress, somnolence); low pH, increased anion gap and elevated blood lactate may be observed. Discontinue immediately if acidosis is suspected. Lactic acidosis should be suspected in any patient with diabetes receiving metformin with evidence of acidosis but without evidence of ketoacidosis. Discontinue metformin in patients with conditions associated with dehydration, sepsis, or hypoxemia. Use caution in patients with heart failure requiring pharmacologic management, particularly in patients with unstable or acute CHF; risk of lactic acidosis may be increased secondary to hypoperfusion.

Metformin is substantially excreted by the kidney. The risk of accumulation and lactic acidosis increases with the degree of impairment of renal function. Patients with renal function below the limit of normal for their age should not receive metformin. In elderly patients, renal function should be monitored regularly; should not be used in any patient ≥80 years of age unless normal renal function is confirmed. Use of concomitant medications that may affect renal function (ie, affect tubular secretion) may also affect metformin disposition. Therapy should be suspended for any surgical procedures requiring food or fluid restriction (resume only after normal intake resumed and normal renal function is verified). Metformin therapy should be temporarily discontinued prior to or at the time of intravascular administration of iodinated contrast media (potential for acute alteration in renal function). Metformin should be withheld for 48 hours after the radiologic study and restarted only after renal function has been confirmed as normal.

[U.S. Boxed Warning]: Thiazolidinediones, including pioglitazone, may cause or exacerbate heart failure; closely monitor for signs and symptoms of heart failure (eg, rapid weight gain, dyspnea, edema), particularly after initiation or dose increases; if heart failure develops, treat accordingly and consider dose reduction or discontinuation. Not recommended for use in any patient with symptomatic heart failure; initiation of therapy is contraindicated in patients with NYHA class III or IV heart failure. If used in patients with NYHA class I or II (systolic) heart failure, initiate at lowest dosage and monitor closely. In addition, metformin should be used with caution in patients with heart failure requiring pharmacologic management, particularly in unstable or acute heart failure due to risk of lactic acidosis secondary to hypoperfusion. Dose reduction or discontinuation is recommended if heart failure suspected. Dose-related edema and weight gain observed with pioglitazone use; use with caution in patients with edema; monitor for signs/symptoms of heart failure.

Avoid metformin use in patients with impaired liver function due to potential for lactic acidosis. Hepatic failure, including fatalities, has been reported with pioglitazone. Monitor for signs/symptoms of liver injury closely during therapy; discontinuation of therapy may be necessary. Due to the possible risk of drug-induced liver injury with pioglitazone use, serum liver tests (ALT, AST, alkaline phosphatase, and total bilirubin) should be obtained prior to initiation in all patients. In patients with abnormal hepatic tests, therapy should be initiated with caution. During therapy, if signs/symptoms of liver injury (eg, fatigue, anorexia, jaundice, dark urine, right upper abdominal discomfort) arise, interrupt therapy, obtain liver tests immediately, and evaluate alternative etiologies. Routine periodic monitoring of serum liver tests during therapy is not necessary unless patient has liver disease or signs/symptoms of liver injury arise during use. Idiosyncratic hepatotoxicity has been reported with another thiazolidinedione agent (troglitazone);

avoid use in patients who previously experienced jaundice during troglitazone therapy. Instruct patients to avoid excessive acute or chronic ethanol use; ethanol may potentiate metformin's effect on lactate metabolism.

Mechanism of pioglitazone requires the presence of insulin; therefore, use in type 1 diabetes (insulin dependent, IDDM) or diabetic ketoacidosis is not recommended. It may be necessary to discontinue metformin and administer insulin if the patient is exposed to stress (fever, trauma, infection, surgery). Increased incidence of bone fractures in females treated with pioglitazone; majority of fractures occurred in the lower limb and distal upper limb. Consider risk of fracture prior to initiation and during use. Clinical trial data suggest an increased risk of bladder cancer in patients exposed to pioglitazone; risk may be increased with duration of use. Avoid use in patients with active bladder cancer and consider risks vs benefits prior to initiating therapy in patients with a history of bladder cancer.

Pioglitazone may decrease hemoglobin/hematocrit; effects may be related to increased plasma volume. Metformin may impair vitamin B_{12} absorption; monitor for anemia. Use pioglitazone with caution in premenopausal, anovulatory women; may result in a resumption of ovulation, increasing the risk of pregnancy. Macular edema has been reported with thiazolidinedione use, including pioglitazone. Patients should be seen by an ophthalmologist if any visual symptoms arise during therapy and all diabetic patients should have regular eye exams. The risk of hypoglycemia is increased when pioglitazone is combined with insulin or other diabetic medications; dosage adjustment of concomitant hypoglycemic agents may be necessary. Concomitant administration of pioglitazone with a strong CYP2C8 inhibitor increases pioglitazone exposure 3-fold; dosage adjustments are recommended if coadministered with a strong CYP2C8 inhibitor (eg, gemfibrozil).

Drug Interactions

Avoid Concomitant Use

Avoid concomitant use of Pioglitazone and Metformin with any of the following: Axitinib; Simeprevir

Decreased Effect

Pioglitazone and Metformin may decrease the levels/effects of: ARIPiprazole; Axitinib; Ibrutinib; Saxagliptin; Simeprevir; Trospium

The levels/effects of Pioglitazone and Metformin may be decreased by: Corticosteroids (Orally Inhaled); Corticosteroids (Systemic); CYP2C8 Inducers (Strong); Dabrafenib; Loop Diuretics; Luteinizing Hormone-Releasing Hormone Analogs; Rifampin; Somatropin; Thiazide Diuretics

Increased Effect/Toxicity

Pioglitazone and Metformin may increase the levels/effects of: CYP2C8 Substrates; Dalfampridine; Dofetilide; Hypoglycemic Agents

The levels/effects of Pioglitazone and Metformin may be increased by: Carbonic Anhydrase Inhibitors; Cephalexin; Cimetidine; CYP2C8 Inhibitors (Moderate); CYP2C8 Inhibitors (Strong); Dalfampridine; Deferasirox; Dolutegravir; Gemfibrozil; Glycopyrrolate; Herbs (Hypoglycemic Properties); Insulin; Iodinated Contrast Agents; LamoTRIgine; MAO Inhibitors; Mifepristone; Pegvisomant; Pregabalin; Ranolazine; Salicylates; Selective Serotonin Reuptake Inhibitors; Topiramate; Trimethoprim

Nutritional/Ethanol Interactions See individual agents.

Adverse Reactions Also see individual agents. Percentages of adverse effects as reported with the combination product.

>10%:
　Cardiovascular: Edema (lower limb, 3% to 11%)
　Respiratory: Upper respiratory infection (12% to 16%)

1% to 10%:
　Central nervous system: Headache (2% to 6%), dizziness (5%)
　Endocrine & metabolic: Weight gain (3% to 7%)
　Gastrointestinal: Diarrhea (5% to 6%), nausea (4% to 6%)
　Genitourinary: Urinary tract infection (5% to 6%)
　Hematologic: Anemia (≤2%)
　Respiratory: Sinusitis (4% to 5%)

Available Dosage Forms

Tablet, oral: 15/500: Pioglitazone 15 mg and metformin hydrochloride 500 mg; 15/850: Pioglitazone 15 mg and metformin hydrochloride 850 mg

Actoplus Met®: 15/500: Pioglitazone 15 mg and metformin 500 mg; 15/850: Pioglitazone 15 mg and metformin 850 mg

Tablet, variable release, oral:

Actoplus Met® XR: 15/1000: Pioglitazone 15 mg and metformin 1000 mg; 30/1000: Pioglitazone 30 mg and metformin 1000 mg

General Dosage Range Dosage adjustment recommended in patients on concomitant therapy.

Oral: *Adults:*

Immediate release tablet: Pioglitazone 15-45 mg/day and metformin 500-2550 mg/day (maximum: 45 mg/day [pioglitazone]; 2550 mg/day [metformin])

Variable release tablet: Pioglitazone 15-45 mg/day and metformin 1000-2000 mg/day (maximum: 45 mg/day [pioglitazone]; 2000 mg/day [metformin])

Administration

Oral

Immediate release formulation: Administer with meals.

Variable release formulation: Administer with the evening meal. Tablets should be swallowed whole; do not crush, split, or chew. Inactive tablet ingredients may be eliminated in the feces as a soft mass that resembles the original tablet.

Storage/Stability Store at 25°C (77°F); excursions permitted to 15°C to 30°C (59°F to 86°F). Protect from moisture and humidity

Nursing Actions

Physical Assessment See individual agents.

Patient Education

- Discuss specific use of drug and side effects with patient as it relates to treatment. (HCAHPS: During this hospital stay, were you given any medicine that you had not taken before? Before giving you any new medicine, how often did hospital staff tell you what the medicine was for? How often did hospital staff describe possible side effects in a way you could understand?)

- Patient may experience nausea, diarrhea, flatulence, headache, rhinitis, or pharyngitis. Have patient report immediately to prescriber signs of hepatic impairment, strength differences from one side to another, difficulty speaking or thinking, change in balance, blurred vision, osteodynia, severe asthenia, vision changes, dysuria, hematuria, polyuria, signs of hypoglycemia, or signs of lactic acidosis (HCAHPS).

- Educate patient about signs of a significant reaction (eg, wheezing; chest tightness; fever; itching; bad cough; blue skin color; seizures; or swelling of face, lips, tongue, or throat). **Note:** This is not a comprehensive list of all side effects. Patient should consult prescriber for additional questions.

Intended Use and Disclaimer: Should not be printed and given to patients. This information is intended to serve as a concise initial reference for healthcare professionals to use when discussing medications with a patient. You must ultimately rely on your own discretion, experience and judgment in diagnosing, treating and advising patients.

Dietary Considerations Immediate release tablets should be administered with meals. Variable release tablets should be administered with the evening meal. Avoid ethanol. Dietary modification based on ADA recommendations is a part of therapy. Monitor for signs and symptoms of vitamin B_{12} and/or folic acid deficiency; supplementation may be required.

Related Information

MetFORMIN *on page 1014*

Oral Medications That Should Not Be Crushed or Altered *on page 1712*

Pioglitazone *on page 1250*

Piperacillin and Tazobactam
(pi PER a sil in & ta zoe BAK tam)

Brand Names: U.S. Zosyn

Index Terms Piperacillin and Tazobactam Sodium; Piperacillin Sodium and Tazobactam Sodium; Tazobactam and Piperacillin

Pharmacologic Category Antibiotic, Penicillin

Medication Safety Issues

Sound-alike/look-alike issues:

Zosyn may be confused with Zofran, Zyvox

International issues:

Tazact [India] may be confused with Tazac brand name for nizatidine [Australia]; Tiazac brand name for diltiazem [U.S., Canada]

Pregnancy Risk Factor B

Breast-Feeding Considerations Low concentrations of piperacillin are excreted in breast milk; information for tazobactam is not available. The manufacturer recommends that caution be used when administering piperacillin/tazobactam to nursing women. Nondose-related effects could include modification of bowel flora.

Use

Moderate to severe bacterial infections: For the treatment of patients with moderate to severe infections caused by susceptible isolates of the designated bacteria in the following conditions.

Community-acquired pneumonia: Treatment of moderate severity community-acquired pneumonia (CAP) caused by beta-lactamase-producing strains of *Haemophilus influenzae*. IDSA/ATS guidelines only recommend piperacillin/tazobactam for CAP caused by *P. aeruginosa* or due to aspiration (Mandell, 2007).

Intra-abdominal infections: Treatment of appendicitis complicated by rupture or abscess and peritonitis caused by beta-lactamase-producing strains of *Escherichia coli*, *Bacteroides fragilis*, *Bacteroides ovatus*, *Bacteroides thetaiotaomicron*, or *Bacteroides vulgatus*.

Nosocomial pneumonia: Treatment of moderate to severe nosocomial pneumonia caused by beta-lactamase-producing strains of *Staphylococcus aureus* and by piperacillin/tazobactam-susceptible *Acinetobacter baumanii*, *H. influenzae*, *Klebsiella pneumoniae*, and *Pseudomonas aeruginosa* (nosocomial pneumonia caused by *P. aeruginosa* should be treated in combination with an aminoglycoside).

Pelvic infections: Treatment of postpartum endometriosis or pelvic inflammatory disease caused by beta-lactamase-producing strains of *E. coli*.

Skin and skin structure infections: Treatment of skin and skin structure infections, including cellulitis, cutaneous abscesses, and ischemic/diabetic foot infections caused by beta-lactamase-producing strains of *S. aureus*.

Unlabeled Use Treatment of moderate-to-severe infections caused by susceptible organisms, including urinary tract infections, bone and joint infections, septicemia, endocarditis, and cystic fibrosis exacerbations; surgical (perioperative) prophylaxis

Mechanism of Action/Effect Piperacillin interferes with bacterial cell wall synthesis during active multiplication, causing cell wall death and resultant bactericidal activity against susceptible bacteria. Piperacillin exhibits time-dependent killing. Tazobactam prevents degradation of piperacillin by binding to the active side on beta-lactamase; tazobactam inhibits many beta-lactamases, including staphylococcal penicillinase and Richmond-Sykes types 2, 3, 4, and 5, including extended spectrum enzymes; it has only limited activity against class 1 beta-lactamases other than class 1C types.

Contraindications Hypersensitivity to penicillins, cephalosporins, beta-lactamase inhibitors, or any component of the formulation

Warnings/Precautions Serious and occasionally severe or fatal hypersensitivity (anaphylactic/anaphylactoid) reactions have been reported in patients on penicillin therapy, especially with a history of beta-lactam hypersensitivity, history of sensitivity to multiple allergens, or previous IgE-mediated reactions (eg, anaphylaxis, angioedema, urticaria). Serious skin reactions, including toxic epidermal necrolysis (TEN) and Stevens-Johnson syndrome (SJS), have been reported. If a skin rash develops, monitor closely. Discontinue if lesions progress.

Bleeding disorders have been observed, particularly in patients with renal impairment; discontinue if thrombocytopenia or bleeding occurs. Leukopenia/neutropenia may occur; appears to be reversible and most frequently associated with prolonged administration. Assess hematologic parameters periodically, especially with prolonged (≥21 days) use.

Assess electrolytes periodically in patients with low potassium reserves, especially those receiving cytotoxic therapy or diuretics. Due to sodium load and to the adverse effects of high serum concentrations of penicillins, dosage modification is required in patients with impaired or underdeveloped renal function; use with caution in patients with seizures or in patients with history of beta-lactam allergy; associated with an increased incidence of rash and fever in cystic fibrosis patients. Use may result in fungal or bacterial superinfection, including *C. difficile*-associated diarrhea (CDAD) and pseudomembranous colitis; CDAD has been observed >2 months postantibiotic treatment.

Potentially significant drug-drug interactions may exist, requiring dose or frequency adjustment, additional monitoring, and/or selection of alternative therapy.

Drug Interactions

Avoid Concomitant Use

Avoid concomitant use of Piperacillin and Tazobactam with any of the following: BCG

◀ **Decreased Effect**

Piperacillin and Tazobactam may decrease the levels/effects of: Aminoglycosides; BCG; Mycophenolate; Sodium Picosulfate; Typhoid Vaccine

The levels/effects of Piperacillin and Tazobactam may be decreased by: Tetracycline Derivatives

Increased Effect/Toxicity

Piperacillin and Tazobactam may increase the levels/effects of: Floxacillin; Methotrexate; Vecuronium; Vitamin K Antagonists

The levels/effects of Piperacillin and Tazobactam may be increased by: Probenecid

Adverse Reactions

>10%: Gastrointestinal: Diarrhea (7% to 11%)

1% to 10%:

Cardiovascular: Hypertension (2%), chest pain (1%), edema (1%), phlebitis (1%)

Central nervous system: Headache (8%), insomnia (7%), agitation (2%), pain (2%), anxiety (1% to 2%), dizziness (1% to 2%)

Dermatologic: Skin rash (4%), pruritus (3%)

Gastrointestinal: Constipation (1% to 8%), nausea (7%), oral candidiasis (4%), vomiting (3% to 4%), dyspepsia (3%), change in stool (2%), abdominal pain (1% to 2%)

Hepatic: Increased serum AST (1%)

Infection: Abscess (2%), candidiasis (2%), infection (2%), sepsis (2%)

Local: Local irritation (3%)

Respiratory: Pharyngitis (2%), dyspnea (1%), rhinitis (1%)

Miscellaneous: Fever (2% to 5%)

Available Dosage Forms 8:1 ratio of piperacillin sodium/tazobactam sodium

Infusion [premixed iso-osmotic solution, frozen]: Zosyn®:

2.25 g: Piperacillin 2 g and tazobactam 0.25 g (50 mL)

3.375 g: Piperacillin 3 g and tazobactam 0.375 g (50 mL)

4.5 g: Piperacillin 4 g and tazobactam 0.5 g (100 mL)

Injection, powder for reconstitution: 2.25 g: Piperacillin 2 g and tazobactam 0.25 g; 3.375 g: Piperacillin 3 g and tazobactam 0.375 g; 4.5 g: Piperacillin 4 g and tazobactam 0.5 g; 40.5 g: Piperacillin 36 g and tazobactam 4.5 g

Zosyn®:

2.25 g: Piperacillin 2 g and tazobactam 0.25 g

3.375 g: Piperacillin 3 g and tazobactam 0.375 g

4.5 g: Piperacillin 4 g and tazobactam 0.5 g

40.5 g: Piperacillin 36 g and tazobactam 4.5 g

General Dosage Range Dosage adjustment recommended in patients with renal impairment.

I.V.:

Children 2-8 months: 80 mg/kg every 8 hours

Children ≥9 months and ≤40 kg: 100 mg/kg every 8 hours

Children >40 kg, Adolescents, and Adults: 3.375 g every 6 hours **or** 4.5 g every 6 hours (maximum: 18 g daily)

Administration

I.V. Administer by I.V. infusion over 30 minutes. For extended infusion administration (unlabeled dosing), administer over 3-4 hours (Kim 2007; Shea, 2009).

Some penicillins (eg, carbenicillin, ticarcillin, and piperacillin) have been shown to inactivate aminoglycosides *in vitro*. This has been observed to a greater extent with tobramycin and gentamicin, while amikacin has shown greater stability against inactivation. Concurrent use of these agents may pose a risk of reduced antibacterial efficacy *in vivo*, particularly in the setting of profound renal impairment. However, definitive clinical evidence is lacking. If combination penicillin/aminoglycoside therapy is desired in a patient with renal dysfunction, separation of doses (if feasible), and routine monitoring of aminoglycoside levels, CBC, and clinical response should be considered. **Note:** Reformulated Zosyn® containing EDTA has been shown to be compatible *in vitro* for Y-site infusion with amikacin and gentamicin diluted in NS or D_5W (applies **only** to specific concentrations and varies by product; consult manufacturer's labeling). Reformulated Zosyn® containing EDTA is **not** compatible with tobramycin.

Preparation for Administration Reconstitute single-dose vials with 5 mL of diluent per 1 g of piperacillin and then further dilute to a volume of 50-150 mL. Reconstitute pharmacy bulk vials with 152 mL of diluent to yield a concentration of piperacillin 200 mg/mL and tazobactam 25 mg/mL; transfer reconstituted solution and further dilute to a volume of 50-150 mL for administration.

Storage/Stability

Vials: Store at 20°C to 25°C (68°F to 77°F) prior to reconstitution. Use single-dose or bulk vials immediately after reconstitution. Discard any unused portion after 24 hours if stored at 20°C to 25°C (68°F to 77°F) or after 48 hours if stored refrigerated (2°C to 8°C [36°F to 46°F]). Do not freeze vials after reconstitution. Stability in I.V. bags has been demonstrated for up to 24 hours at room temperature and up to 1 week at refrigerated temperature. Stability in an ambulatory I.V. infusion pump has been demonstrated for a period of 12 hours at room temperature.

Galaxy containers: Store at or below -20°C (-4°F). The thawed solution is stable for 14 days under refrigeration (2°C to 8°C [36°F to 46°F]) or 24 hours at 20°C to 25°C (68°F to 77°F). Do not refreeze.

Nursing Actions

Physical Assessment Assess results of culture and sensitivity tests and patient's allergy history prior to starting therapy. Use with caution in presence of renal impairment. Monitor for hypersensitivity reactions and opportunistic infection (eg, fever, chills, unhealed sores, white plaques in mouth or vagina, purulent vaginal discharge, fatigue).

Patient Education
- Discuss specific use of drug and side effects with patient as it relates to treatment. (HCAHPS: During this hospital stay, were you given any medicine that you had not taken before? Before giving you any new medicine, how often did hospital staff tell you what the medicine was for? How often did hospital staff describe possible side effects in a way you could understand?)
- Patient may experience nausea, diarrhea, headache, or vaginal yeast infection. Have patient report immediately to prescriber ecchymosis, bleeding, or rash (HCAHPS).
- Educate patient about signs of a significant reaction (eg, wheezing; chest tightness; fever; itching; bad cough; blue skin color; seizures; or swelling of face, lips, tongue, or throat). **Note:** This is not a comprehensive list of all side effects. Patient should consult prescriber for additional questions.

Intended Use and Disclaimer: Should not be printed and given to patients. This information is intended to serve as a concise initial reference for healthcare professionals to use when discussing medications with a patient. You must ultimately rely on your own discretion, experience and judgment in diagnosing, treating and advising patients.

Dietary Considerations Some products may contain sodium.

Piroxicam (peer OKS i kam)

Brand Names: U.S. Feldene
Pharmacologic Category Nonsteroidal Anti-inflammatory Drug (NSAID), Oral
Medication Safety Issues
Sound-alike/look-alike issues:
Feldene may be confused with FLUoxetine
Piroxicam may be confused with PARoxetine
BEERS Criteria medication:
This drug may be potentially inappropriate for use in geriatric patients (Quality of evidence - moderate; Strength of recommendation - strong).
International issues:
Flogene [Brazil] may be confused with Flogen brand name for naproxen [Mexico]; Florone brand name for diflorasone [Germany, Greece]; Flovent brand name for fluticasone [U.S., Canada]

Medication Guide Available Yes
Pregnancy Risk Factor C
Lactation Enters breast milk/not recommended
Use Symptomatic treatment of acute and chronic rheumatoid arthritis and osteoarthritis

Canadian labeling: Additional use (not in U.S. labeling): Symptomatic treatment of ankylosing spondylitis
Available Dosage Forms
Capsule, Oral:
Feldene: 10 mg, 20 mg
Generic: 10 mg, 20 mg
General Dosage Range Oral: *Adults:* 10-20 mg daily in 1-2 divided doses (maximum: 20 mg daily)
Administration
Oral May administer with food or milk to decrease GI upset.
Rectal Rectal suppository [Canadian product]: Remove plastic wrapping covering suppository prior to inserting suppository into rectum.
Nursing Actions
Physical Assessment Monitor blood pressure at the beginning of therapy and periodically during use. Monitor for GI effects, hepatotoxicity, and ototoxicity at beginning of therapy and periodically throughout. Schedule ophthalmic evaluations for patients who develop eye complaints during long-term NSAID therapy.
Patient Education
- Discuss specific use of drug and side effects with patient as it relates to treatment. (HCAHPS: During this hospital stay, were you given any medicine that you had not taken before? Before giving you any new medicine, how often did hospital staff tell you what the medicine was for? How often did hospital staff describe possible side effects in a way you could understand?)
- Patient may experience dizziness, dyspepsia, pyrosis, or nausea. Have patient report immediately to prescriber syncope, angina, strength differences from one side to another, edema or pain of hands or feet, significant weight gain, melena, hematuria, ecchymosis, or rash (HCAHPS).
- Educate patient about signs of a significant reaction (eg, wheezing; chest tightness; fever; itching; bad cough; blue skin color; seizures; or swelling of face, lips, tongue, or throat). **Note:** This is not a comprehensive list of all side effects. Patient should consult prescriber for additional questions.

Intended Use and Disclaimer: Should not be printed and given to patients. This information is intended to serve as a concise initial reference for healthcare professionals to use when discussing medications with a patient. You must ultimately rely on your own discretion, experience and judgment in diagnosing, treating and advising patients.

Related Information
Oral Medications That Should Not Be Crushed or Altered *on page 1712*

Pitavastatin (pi TA va sta tin)

Brand Names: U.S. Livalo
Index Terms Pitavastatin Calcium
Pharmacologic Category Antilipemic Agent, HMG-CoA Reductase Inhibitor
Medication Safety Issues
Sound-alike/look-alike issues:
Pitavastatin may be confused with atorvaSTATin, fluvastatin, lovastatin, nystatin, pravastatin, rosuvastatin, simvastatin
Pregnancy Risk Factor X
Lactation Excretion in breast milk unknown/contraindicated
Breast-Feeding Considerations It is not known if pitavastatin is excreted into breast milk. Due to the potential for serious adverse reactions in a nursing infant, use while breast-feeding is contraindicated by the manufacturer.
Use Adjunct to dietary therapy to reduce elevations in total cholesterol (TC), LDL-C, apolipoprotein B (Apo B), and triglycerides (TG), and to increase low HDL-C in patients with primary hyperlipidemia and mixed dyslipidemia
Unlabeled Use
Primary and secondary prevention of atherosclerotic cardiovascular disease (ASCVD) according to the American College of Cardiology/American Heart Association: To reduce the risk of ASCVD in patients with clinical ASCVD (eg, coronary heart disease, stroke/TIA, or peripheral arterial disease presumed to be of atherosclerotic origin) who are greater than 75 years of age or not a candidate for high-intensity statin therapy; in patients without clinical ASCVD if LDL-C is 190 mg/dL or greater and not a candidate for high-intensity statin therapy; in patients without clinical ASCVD who have type 1 or type 2 diabetes and are between 40 and 75 years of age; in patients with an estimated 10-year ASCVD risk 7.5% or greater and who are between 40 and 75 years of age (Stone, 2013).
Mechanism of Action/Effect Inhibitor of 3-hydroxy-3-methylglutaryl coenzyme A (HMG-CoA) reductase, the rate-limiting enzyme in cholesterol synthesis (reduces the production of mevalonic acid from HMG-CoA); this then results in a compensatory increase in the expression of LDL receptors on hepatocyte membranes and a stimulation of LDL catabolism
Contraindications Hypersensitivity to pitavastatin or any component of the formulation; active liver disease including unexplained persistent elevations of hepatic transaminases; concurrent use with cyclosporine; pregnancy; breast-feeding
Warnings/Precautions Secondary causes of hyperlipidemia should be ruled out prior to therapy.

Pitavastatin has not been studied when the primary lipid abnormality is chylomicron elevation (Fredrickson types I and V) or in familial dysbetalipoproteinemia (Fredrickson type III). May cause hepatic dysfunction; in all patients, liver function must be monitored prior to initiation of therapy; repeat LFTs if clinically indicated thereafter; routine periodic monitoring of liver enzymes is not necessary. Use with caution in patients who consume large amounts of ethanol or have a history of liver disease; use is contraindicated in patients with active liver disease or unexplained persistent elevations of serum transaminases. If serious hepatotoxicity with clinical symptoms and/or hyperbilirubinemia or jaundice occurs during treatment, interrupt therapy. If an alternate etiology is not identified, do not restart pitavastatin.

Myopathy and rhabdomyolysis with acute renal failure have occurred with use. Risk is dose related and is increased with concurrent use of lipid-lowering agents which may cause rhabdomyolysis (fibric acid derivatives or niacin at doses ≥1 g/day) or during concurrent use with erythromycin or protease inhibitors. Use caution in patients with renal impairment, inadequately treated hypothyroidism, and those taking other drugs associated with myopathy (eg, colchicine); these patients are predisposed to myopathy. Monitor closely if used with other drugs associated with myopathy. Weigh the risk versus benefit when combining any of these drugs with pitavastatin. Immune-mediated necrotizing myopathy (IMNM), an autoimmune-mediated myopathy, has been reported (rarely) with HMG-CoA reductase inhibitor therapy. IMNM presents as proximal muscle weakness with elevated CPK levels, which persists despite discontinuation of HMG-CoA reductase inhibitor therapy; additionally, muscle biopsy may show necrotizing myopathy with limited inflammation; immunosuppressive therapy (eg, corticosteroids, azathioprine) may be used for treatment. The manufacturer recommends temporary discontinuation for elective major surgery, acute medical or surgical conditions, or in any patient experiencing an acute or serious condition predisposing to renal failure (eg, sepsis, hypotension, trauma, uncontrolled seizures). However, based upon current evidence, HMG-CoA reductase inhibitor therapy should be continued in the perioperative period unless risk outweighs cardioprotective benefit. Patients should be instructed to report unexplained muscle pain, tenderness, weakness, or brown urine. Concurrent use with cyclosporine is contraindicated. Ensure patient is on the lowest effective pitavastatin dose. Use with caution in elderly patients, as these patients are predisposed to myopathy. Increases in Hb A_{1c} and fasting blood glucose have been reported with HMG-CoA reductase inhibitors; however, the benefits of statin therapy far outweigh the risk of dysglycemia.

Drug Interactions

Avoid Concomitant Use

Avoid concomitant use of Pitavastatin with any of the following: CycloSPORINE (Systemic); Fusidic Acid (Systemic); Gemfibrozil; Red Yeast Rice

Decreased Effect

Pitavastatin may decrease the levels/effects of: Lanthanum

The levels/effects of Pitavastatin may be decreased by: Antacids; Bosentan

Increased Effect/Toxicity

Pitavastatin may increase the levels/effects of: DAPTOmycin; PAZOPanib; Trabectedin; Vitamin K Antagonists

The levels/effects of Pitavastatin may be increased by: Atazanavir; Bezafibrate; Boceprevir; Clarithromycin; Colchicine; CycloSPORINE (Systemic); Danazol; Eltrombopag; Erythromycin (Systemic); Fenofibrate and Derivatives; Fusidic Acid (Systemic); Gemfibrozil; Niacin; Niacinamide; Raltegravir; Red Yeast Rice; Rifamycin Derivatives; Sildenafil; Simeprevir; Telaprevir; Telithromycin

Nutritional/Ethanol Interactions

Ethanol: Avoid excessive ethanol consumption (due to potential hepatic effects).

Food: Red yeast rice contains an estimated 2.4 mg lovastatin per 600 mg rice.

Adverse Reactions

2% to 10%:

Gastrointestinal: Constipation (2% to 4%), diarrhea (2% to 3%)

Neuromuscular & skeletal: Back pain (1% to 4%), myalgia (2% to 3%), pain in extremities (1% to 2%)

Additional class-related events or case reports (not necessarily reported with pitavastatin therapy): Cataracts, cirrhosis, dermatomyositis, eosinophilia, extraocular muscle movement impaired, fulminant hepatic necrosis, gynecomastia, hypersensitivity syndrome (symptoms may include anaphylaxis, angioedema, arthralgia, erythema multiforme, eosinophilia, hemolytic anemia, immune-mediated necrotizing myopathy (IMNM), interstitial lung disease, lupus syndrome, photosensitivity, polymyalgia rheumatica, positive ANA, purpura, Stevens-Johnson syndrome, toxic epidermal necrolysis, urticaria, vasculitis), ophthalmoplegia, peripheral nerve palsy, rhabdomyolysis, renal failure (secondary to rhabdomyolysis), thyroid dysfunction, tremor, vertigo

Available Dosage Forms

Tablet, Oral:

Livalo: 1 mg, 2 mg, 4 mg

General Dosage Range Dosage adjustment recommended in patients with renal impairment or on concomitant therapy

Oral: *Adults:* Initial: 2 mg once daily; Maintenance: 2-4 mg once daily (maximum: 4 mg/day)

Administration

Oral May be administered with or without food; may take without regard to time of day.

Storage/Stability Store at controlled room temperature of 15°C to 30°C (59°F to 86°F). Protect from light.

Nursing Actions

Physical Assessment Monitor for signs and symptoms of myopathy (muscle pain and weakness, fatigue). Assess risk potential for interactions with other prescriptions or herbal products patient may be taking that may increase risk of myopathy or rhabdomyolysis. Teach proper diet and exercise regimen.

Patient Education

• Discuss specific use of drug and side effects with patient as it relates to treatment. (HCAHPS: During this hospital stay, were you given any medicine that you had not taken before? Before giving you any new medicine, how often did hospital staff tell you what the medicine was for? How often did hospital staff describe possible side effects in a way you could understand?)

• Patient may experience back pain, constipation, diarrhea, asthenia, or arthralgia. Have patient report immediately to prescriber flu-like syndrome, ecchymosis, bleeding, discolored urine, jaundice, or rash (HCAHPS).

• Educate patient about signs of a significant reaction (eg, wheezing; chest tightness; fever; itching; bad cough; blue skin color; seizures; or swelling of face, lips, tongue, or throat). **Note:** This is not a comprehensive list of all side effects. Patient should consult prescriber for additional questions.

Intended Use and Disclaimer: Should not be printed and given to patients. This information is intended to serve as a concise initial reference for healthcare professionals to use when discussing medications with a patient. You must ultimately rely on your own discretion, experience and judgment in diagnosing, treating and advising patients.

Dietary Considerations May be taken with or without food; may take without regard to time of day. Red yeast rice contains an estimated 2.4 mg lovastatin per 600 mg rice.

Plerixafor (pler IX a fore)

Brand Names: U.S. Mozobil

Index Terms AMD3100; LM3100

Pharmacologic Category Hematopoietic Agent; Hematopoietic Stem Cell Mobilizer

Pregnancy Risk Factor D

Lactation Excretion in breast milk unknown/not recommended

Use Peripheral stem cell mobilization: Mobilization of hematopoietic stem cells (HSC) for collection and subsequent autologous transplantation (in combination with filgrastim) in patients with non-Hodgkin lymphoma (NHL) and multiple myeloma (MM)

Available Dosage Forms

Solution, Subcutaneous [preservative free]:
Mozobil: 24 mg/1.2 mL (1.2 mL)

General Dosage Range Dosage adjustment recommended in patients with renal impairment

SubQ: *Adults:* 0.24 mg/kg/day (maximum dose: 40 mg daily)

Administration

Injectable Detail pH: 6-7.5 (solution in vial)

Subcutaneous Administer subcutaneously, ~11 hours prior to initiation of apheresis. In some clinical trials, plerixafor administration began in the evening prior to apheresis; filgrastim was begun on day 1, plerixafor initiated in the evening on day 4 and apheresis in the morning on day 5; with filgrastim, plerixafor, and apheresis then continued daily until sufficient cell collection for autologous transplant (DiPersio, 2009a; DiPersio, 2009b).

Hazardous agent; use appropriate precautions for handling and disposal (NIOSH, 2012).

Nursing Actions

Physical Assessment Teach patient appropriate injection techniques and syringe/needle disposal.

Patient Education

• Discuss specific use of drug and side effects with patient as it relates to treatment. (HCAHPS: During this hospital stay, were you given any medicine that you had not taken before? Before giving you any new medicine, how often did hospital staff tell you what the medicine was for? How often did hospital staff describe possible side effects in a way you could understand?)

• Patient may experience dizziness, asthenia, headache, short-term pain, nausea, diarrhea, or arthralgia. Have patient report immediately to prescriber dyspnea, severe shoulder pain, ecchymosis, bleeding, or rash (HCAHPS).

• Educate patient about signs of a significant reaction (eg, wheezing; chest tightness; fever; itching; bad cough; blue skin color; seizures; or swelling of face, lips, tongue, or throat). **Note:** This is not a comprehensive list of all side effects. Patient should consult prescriber for additional questions.

Intended Use and Disclaimer: Should not be printed and given to patients. This information is intended to serve as a concise initial reference for healthcare professionals to use when discussing medications with a patient. You must ultimately rely on your own discretion, experience and judgment in diagnosing, treating and advising patients.

Pneumococcal Conjugate Vaccine (10-Valent)
(noo moe KOK al KON ju gate vak SEEN, ten vay lent)

Index Terms 10-Valent Pneumococcal Nontypeable *Haemophilus influenzae* Protein D Conjugate Vaccine; PHiD-CV; Pneumococcal Conjugate Vaccine (Nontypeable *Haemophilus influenzae* [NTHi] Protein D, Diphtheria or Tetanus Toxoid Conjugates) Adsorbed

Pharmacologic Category Vaccine, Inactivated (Bacterial)

Medication Safety Issues
Sound-alike/look-alike issues:
Synflorix™ may be confused with Synagis®

Breast-Feeding Considerations Inactivated vaccines do not affect the safety of breast-feeding for the mother or the infant. Breast-feeding infants should be vaccinated according to the recommended schedules (CDC, 2011).

Use Immunization of infants and children against *Streptococcus pneumoniae* infection and invasive diseases caused by serotypes included in the vaccine

Mechanism of Action/Effect Promotes active immunization against invasive disease caused by *S. pneumoniae* capsular serotypes 1, 4, 5, 6B, 7F, 9V, 14, 18C, 19F, and 23F, all which are individually conjugated to a carrier protein (protein D, tetanus toxoid, or diphtheria toxoid); the aluminum salt, a mineral adjuvant, enhances the antibody response.

Contraindications Hypersensitivity to any component of the vaccine

Warnings/Precautions Immediate treatment (including epinephrine 1:1000) for anaphylactoid and/or hypersensitivity reactions should be available during vaccine use. Packaging may contain natural latex rubber. Apnea has been reported following I.M. vaccine administration in premature infants; consider risk versus benefit in infants born prematurely. Infants born ≤28 weeks gestation, particularly those with a prior history of respiratory immaturity, may require respiratory function monitoring for 2-3 days after administration. Syncope has been reported with use of injectable vaccines and may be accompanied by transient visual disturbances, weakness, or tonic-clonic movements. Procedures should be in place to avoid injuries from falling and to restore cerebral perfusion if syncope occurs.

Not to be used to treat pneumococcal infections. Safety and efficacy in children at increased risk for pneumococcal infection (eg, sickle cell disease, splenic dysfunction, HIV infection, malignancy, nephrotic syndrome) has not been established. Use with caution in severely immunocompromised patients (eg, HIV, patients receiving chemo/radiation therapy, or other immunosuppressive therapy including high-dose corticosteroids); may have a reduced response to vaccination. In general, inactivated vaccines should be administered ≥2 weeks prior to planned immunosuppression when feasible (Rubin, 2014). Use with caution in patients with a history of bleeding disorders (including thrombocytopenia) and/or patients on anticoagulant therapy; bleeding/hematoma may occur from I.M. administration.

Antibody response is provided only against pneumococcal serotypes included in the vaccine. Antibody response may also be observed to diphtheria toxoid, tetanus toxoid, and protein D (derived from nontypeable *Haemophilus influenzae*); however, recommended routine administration schedules for diphtheria, tetanus or *H. influenzae* type b vaccines should still be followed. In order to maximize vaccination rates, the Canadian National Advisory Committee on Immunization (NACI) recommends simultaneous administration of all age-appropriate vaccines (live or inactivated) for which a person is eligible at a single clinic visit, unless contraindications exist. The decision to administer or delay vaccination because of current or recent febrile illness depends on the severity of symptoms and the etiology of the disease. Immunization should be delayed during the course of an acute severe febrile illness; may administer to patients with mild acute illness. Vaccination may not result in effective immunity in all patients. Response depends upon multiple factors (eg, type of vaccine, age of patient) and may be improved by administering the vaccine at the recommended dose, route, and interval. Vaccines may not be effective if administered during periods of altered immune competence (CDC, 2011).

Administration of acetaminophen prior to or immediately following vaccination may reduce incidence and severity of vaccine related fever, although it has been reported that routine prophylactic administration of acetaminophen to prevent fever prior to vaccination, decreased the immune response of some vaccines; the clinical significance of this reduction in immune response has not been established (Prymula, 2009).

Drug Interactions

Avoid Concomitant Use There are no known interactions where it is recommended to avoid concomitant use.

Decreased Effect

The levels/effects of Pneumococcal Conjugate Vaccine (10-Valent) may be decreased by: Belimumab; Fingolimod; Immunosuppressants

Increased Effect/Toxicity There are no known significant interactions involving an increase in effect.

Adverse Reactions In Canada, adverse reactions may be reported to local provincial/territorial health agencies or to the Vaccine Safety Section at Public Health Agency of Canada (1-866-844-0018).

Frequency not always defined:
>10%:
  Central nervous system: Irritability (51% to 66%), drowsiness (33% to 58%), fever (≥38°C rectally ages <2 years: 26% to 37%)
  Gastrointestinal: Loss of appetite (17% to 31%)
  Local: Injection site reactions: Pain (23% to 57%), redness (38% to 53%), swelling (28% to 37%)
1% to 10%:
  Central nervous system: Fever (>39°C rectally age <2 years: 2% to 3%; ≥38°C rectally age 2-5 years)
  Local: Injection site induration

Product Availability Not available in the U.S.

General Dosage Range I.M.:

Infants 6 weeks to 6 months: 0.5 mL dose at 2, 4 and 6 months (minimum interval of 1 month between each of the first 3 doses), followed by booster dose of 0.5 mL administered at 12-15 months (minimum interval of 6 months between doses 3 and 4) **or** 0.5 mL dose at 2 and 4 months (minimum interval of 2 months between doses 1 and 2), followed by an additional 0.5 mL dose at 11-12 months (minimum interval of 6 months between doses 2 and 3)

Infants 7-11 months (previously unvaccinated): 0.5 mL for 2 doses administered at least 1 month apart, followed by a third dose administered after 1 year of age (minimum interval of 2 months between doses 2 and 3)

Children 12 months to <6 years (previously unvaccinated): 0.5 mL for a total of 2 doses administered at least 2 months apart

Administration

I.M. Shake well before use. Administer by I.M. injection only, preferably into the anterolateral aspect of the thigh in infants and into the deltoid in children. Do not administer intravenously or intradermally. Subcutaneous administration has not been studied.

Rule out bleeding disorders in patients <2 years of age prior to immunization. NACI recommends that patients with bleeding disorders receive all routine recommended vaccinations according to schedule. Bleeding disorders should be corrected prior to immunization (when possible) or immunization should be scheduled shortly after antihemophilia or other similar therapy. In patients with bleeding disorder that cannot be corrected, I.M. gluteal injections should be avoided (if possible). When immunizing patients with bleeding disorders, a fine-gauge needle of the appropriate length can be used for the vaccination and firm pressure applied to the site (without rubbing) for at least 5 minutes. The patient should be instructed concerning the risk of hematoma from the injection. Patients on anticoagulant therapy (eg, aspirin, warfarin, heparin) may be immunized via intramuscular injection without discontinuation of their anticoagulant therapy (NACI, 2006).

Simultaneous administration of vaccines helps ensure the patients will be fully vaccinated by the appropriate age. Simultaneous administration of vaccines is defined as administering >1 vaccine on the same day at different anatomic sites. Separate vaccines should not be combined in the same syringe unless indicated by product specific labeling.

I.V. Do **not** administer intravenously.

Storage/Stability Store at 2°C to 8°C (36°F to 46°F) and in original packaging to protect from light. Do not freeze; discard the vaccine if frozen or exposed to temperatures >37°C (>99°F). Vaccine should be administered upon removal from refrigeration; however, the manufacturer's labeling states the vaccine may be administered if left outside of refrigeration for ≤3 days at 8°C to 25°C (46°F to 77°F) or if left outside of refrigeration for ≤1 day at 25°C to 37°C (77°F to 99°F).

Nursing Actions

Patient Education

- Discuss specific use of vaccine and side effects with caregiver as it relates to treatment. (HCAHPS: During this hospital stay, were you given any medicine that you had not taken before? Before giving you any new medicine, how often did hospital staff tell you what the medicine was for? How often did hospital staff describe possible side effects in a way you could understand?)
- Patient may experience asthenia, mood changes, loss of appetite, or redness or swelling at injection site. Have caregiver report immediately to prescriber severe injection site reaction (HCAHPS).
- Educate caregiver about signs of a significant reaction (eg, wheezing; chest tightness; fever; itching; bad cough; blue skin color; seizures; or swelling of face, lips, tongue, or throat). **Note:** This is not a comprehensive list of all side effects. Caregiver should consult prescriber for additional questions.

Intended Use and Disclaimer: Should not be printed and given to patients. This information is intended to serve as a concise initial reference for healthcare professionals to use when discussing medications with a patient. You must ultimately rely on your own discretion, experience and judgment in diagnosing, treating and advising patients.

Related Information

Immunization Administration Recommendations *on page 1675*

Immunization Recommendations *on page 1680*

Pneumococcal Conjugate Vaccine (13-Valent)

(noo moe KOK al KON ju gate vak SEEN, thur TEEN vay lent)

Brand Names: U.S. Prevnar 13

Index Terms PCV13; Pneumococcal 13-Valent Conjugate Vaccine

Pharmacologic Category Vaccine, Inactivated (Bacterial)

Medication Safety Issues

Sound-alike/look-alike issues:

Pneumococcal 13-Valent Conjugate Vaccine (Prevnar 13) may be confused with Pneumococcal 7-Valent Conjugate Vaccine (Prevnar) or with Pneumococcal 23-Valent Polysaccharide Vaccine (Pneumovax 23)

Pregnancy Risk Factor B

Lactation Excretion in breast milk unknown/use caution

Use

U.S. labeling:

Immunization of children 6 weeks through 17 years of age against *Streptococcus pneumoniae* infection caused by serotypes included in the vaccine

Immunization of children 6 weeks through 5 years of age against otitis media caused by *Streptococcus pneumoniae* serotypes 4, 6B, 9V, 14, 18C, 19F, and 23F

Immunization of adults ≥50 years against pneumococcal pneumonia and invasive disease caused by *Streptococcus pneumoniae* serotypes included in the vaccine

Canadian labeling:

Immunization of children 6 weeks through 17 years of age against *Streptococcus pneumoniae* infection caused by serotypes included in the vaccine

Immunization of adults ≥50 years against pneumococcal pneumonia and invasive disease caused by *Streptococcus pneumoniae* serotypes included in the vaccine

The Advisory Committee on Immunization Practices (ACIP) recommends routine vaccination for the following (CDC 59[RR-11], 2010):

All children age 2-59 months

Children 60-71 months with underlying medical conditions including:

Immunocompetent children with chronic heart disease (particularly cyanotic congenital heart disease and heart failure), chronic lung disease (including asthma if treated with high dose corticosteroids), diabetes, cerebrospinal fluid leaks, or cochlear implants

Children with functional or anatomic asplenia, including sickle cell disease or other hemoglobinopathies, congenital or acquired asplenia, or splenic dysfunction.

Children with immunocompromising conditions including congenital immunodeficiency (includes B or T cell deficiency, compliment deficiencies and phagocytic disorders; excludes chronic granulomatous disease), HIV infection, chronic renal failure, nephrotic syndrome, leukemia, lymphoma, Hodgkin disease, generalized malignancies, solid organ transplant, or other diseases requiring immunosuppressive drugs (including long term systemic corticosteroids and radiation therapy)

Children who received ≥1 dose of PCV7

Note: Routine use is not recommended for healthy children ≥5 years of age.

Children ≥6 years and Adolescents ≤18 years of age (CDC, 2013c), and Adults ≥19 years of age (CDC, 2012): The ACIP also recommends routine vaccination for persons with the following underlying medical conditions:

Immunocompetent persons with cerebrospinal fluid leaks or cochlear implants

Persons with functional or anatomic asplenia, including sickle cell disease or other hemoglobinopathies, congenital or acquired asplenia

Persons with immunocompromising conditions including congenital or acquired immunodeficiency (includes B or T cell deficiency, compliment deficiencies and phagocytic disorders; excludes chronic granulomatous disease), HIV infection, chronic renal failure, nephrotic syndrome, leukemia, lymphoma, Hodgkin disease, generalized malignancies, solid organ transplant, multiple myeloma, or other diseases requiring immunosuppressive drugs (including long term systemic corticosteroids and radiation therapy)

Available Dosage Forms

Injection, suspension:

Prevnar 13: 2 mcg of each capsular saccharide for serotypes 1, 3, 4, 5, 6A, 7F, 9V, 14, 18C, 19A, 19F, and 23F, and 4 mcg of serotype 6B [bound to diphtheria CRM_{197} protein ~34 mcg] per 0.5 mL (0.5 mL)

General Dosage Range I.M.:

Infants 2-6 months: 0.5 mL at approximately 2-month intervals for 3 consecutive doses, followed by a fourth dose of 0.5 mL at 12-15 months of age

Infants 7-11 months (previously unvaccinated): 0.5 mL for a total of 3 doses, 2 doses at least 4 weeks apart, followed by a third dose at 12-15 months (at least 2 months after second dose)

Children 12-23 months (previously unvaccinated) and Children 24-71 months (previously unvaccinated) with underlying conditions: 0.5 mL for a total of 2 doses, separated by at least 8 weeks

Healthy Children 24-59 months (previously unvaccinated) and Children 6-18 years at high risk for invasive pneumococcal disease: 0.5 mL as a single dose

Children 14-71 months (previously completing vaccination with PCV7): 0.5 mL supplemental dose

Children 6 through 17 years: 0.5 mL as a single dose

Adults ≥50 years: 0.5 mL as a single dose

Administration

I.M. Shake well prior to use. Do not use if a homogenous white suspension does not form. Administer I.M. (deltoid muscle for toddlers, young children, and adults or lateral midthigh in infants). Do not inject I.V. or SubQ; avoid intradermal route. Concurrent administration of PCV13 and PPV23 has not been studied and is not recommended (CDC, 2010).

For patients at risk of hemorrhage following intramuscular injection, the ACIP recommends "it should be administered intramuscularly if, in the opinion of the physician familiar with the patient's bleeding risk, the vaccine can be administered by this route with reasonable safety. If the patient receives antihemophilia or other similar therapy, intramuscular vaccination can be scheduled shortly after such therapy is administered. A fine needle (23 gauge or smaller) can be used for the vaccination and firm pressure applied to the site (without rubbing) for at least 2 minutes. The patient should be instructed concerning the risk of hematoma from the injection." Patients on anticoagulant therapy should be considered to have the same bleeding risks and treated as those with clotting factor disorders (CDC, 2011).

Antipyretics have not been shown to prevent febrile seizures. Antipyretics may be used to treat fever or discomfort following vaccination (CDC, 2011). One study reported that routine prophylactic administration of acetaminophen to prevent fever prior to vaccination decreased the immune response of some vaccines; the clinical significance of this reduction in immune response has not been established (Prymula, 2009).

Simultaneous administration of vaccines helps ensure the patients will be fully vaccinated by the appropriate age. Simultaneous administration of vaccines is defined as administering >1 vaccine on the same day at different anatomic sites. Separate vaccines should not be combined in the same syringe unless indicated by product specific labeling. Separate needles and syringes should be used for each injection. The ACIP prefers each dose of a specific vaccine in a series come from the same manufacturer when possible. Adolescents and adults should be vaccinated while seated or lying down. In general, preterm infants should be vaccinated at the same chronological age as full-term infants (CDC, 2011).

Nursing Actions

Physical Assessment Screen for chronic illnesses, asplenia, HIV, and sickle cell disease before administering this vaccine. Hold pressure (without rubbing) on puncture site for 2-5 minutes for patients with history of bleeding disorder. Observe for hematoma formation or other signs of bleeding. Monitor for signs of hypersensitivity reactions or vasovagal responses.

Patient Education

• Discuss specific use of vaccine and side effects with patient as it relates to treatment. (HCAHPS: During this hospital stay, were you given any medicine that you had not taken before? Before giving you any new medicine, how often did hospital staff tell you what the medicine was for? How often did hospital staff describe possible side effects in a way you could understand?)

• Patient may experience pain, redness, or swelling at injection site; headache; fatigue; nausea; emesis; diarrhea; or dyspepsia. Have patient report immediately to prescriber severe injection site reaction (HCAHPS).

• Educate patient about signs of a significant reaction (eg, wheezing; chest tightness; fever; itching; bad cough; blue skin color; seizures; or swelling of face, lips, tongue, or throat). **Note:** This is not a comprehensive list of all side effects. Patient should consult prescriber for additional questions.

Intended Use and Disclaimer: Should not be printed and given to patients. This information is intended to serve as a concise initial reference for healthcare professionals to use when discussing medications with a patient. You must ultimately rely on your own discretion, experience and judgment in diagnosing, treating and advising patients.

Related Information

Immunization Administration Recommendations *on page 1675*

Immunization Recommendations *on page 1680*

Pneumococcal Polysaccharide Vaccine (Polyvalent)
(noo moe KOK al pol i SAK a ride vak SEEN, pol i VAY lent)

Brand Names: U.S. Pneumovax® 23

Index Terms 23-Valent Pneumococcal Polysaccharide Vaccine; 23PS; PPSV; PPSV23; PPV23

Pharmacologic Category Vaccine, Inactivated (Bacterial)

Medication Safety Issues

Sound-alike/look-alike issues:

Pneumococcal 23-Valent Polysaccharide Vaccine (Pneumovax® 23) may be confused with Pneumococcal 7-Valent Conjugate Vaccine (Prevnar®) or with Pneumococcal 13-Valent Conjugate Vaccine (Prevnar 13®)

Pregnancy Risk Factor C

Lactation Excretion in breast milk unknown/use caution

Use Immunization against pneumococcal disease caused by serotypes included in the vaccine. Routine vaccination is recommended for persons ≥50 years of age and persons ≥2 years in certain situations.

The Advisory Committee on Immunization Practices (ACIP) recommends routine vaccination for patients with the following underlying medical conditions (CDC, 59[34], 2010; CDC, 59[11], 2010; CDC, 2012):

Children ≥2 years of age and adults 19-64 years with functional or anatomic asplenia, including sickle cell disease or other hemoglobinopathies, congenital or acquired asplenia, splenic dysfunction, or splenectomy

Immunocompetent children ≥2 years of age with chronic heart disease (particularly cyanotic congenital heart disease and heart failure), chronic lung disease (including asthma if treated with high dose corticosteroids), diabetes, cerebrospinal fluid leaks, or cochlear implants

Immunocompetent adults 19-64 years with chronic heart disease (including heart failure and cardiomyopathies; excluding hypertension), chronic lung disease (including COPD, emphysema, and asthma), diabetes, cerebrospinal fluid leaks, cochlear implants, alcoholism, chronic liver disease, cirrhosis, and cigarette smokers

Immunocompromised children ≥2 years of age and adults 19-64 years with congenital or acquired immunodeficiency (includes B or T cell deficiency, compliment deficiencies and phagocytic disorders; excludes chronic granulomatous disease), HIV infection, chronic renal failure, nephrotic syndrome, leukemia, lymphoma, Hodgkin disease, generalized malignancies, solid organ transplant, multiple myeloma, or other diseases requiring immunosuppressive drugs (including long-term systemic corticosteroids and radiation therapy)

All adults ≥65 years of age

Available Dosage Forms

Injection, solution:

Pneumovax® 23: 25 mcg each of 23 capsular polysaccharide isolates/0.5 mL (0.5 mL, 2.5 mL)

General Dosage Range I.M., SubQ: *Children ≥2 years and Adults:* 0.5 mL

Administration

I.M. Do not inject I.V.; avoid intradermal administration (may cause severe local reactions); administer SubQ or I.M. (deltoid muscle or lateral midthigh)

For patients at risk of hemorrhage following intramuscular injection, the ACIP recommends "it should be administered intramuscularly if, in the opinion of the physician familiar with the patient's bleeding risk, the vaccine can be administered by this route with reasonable safety. If the patient receives antihemophilia or other similar therapy, intramuscular vaccination can be scheduled shortly after such therapy is administered. A fine needle (23 gauge or smaller) can be used for the vaccination and firm pressure applied to the site (without rubbing) for at least 2 minutes. The patient should be instructed concerning the risk of hematoma from the injection." Patients on anticoagulant therapy should be considered to have the same bleeding risks and treated as those with clotting factor disorders (CDC, 2011).

Antipyretics have not been shown to prevent febrile seizures. Antipyretics may be used to treat fever or discomfort following vaccination (CDC, 2011). One study reported that routine prophylactic administration of acetaminophen to prevent fever prior to vaccination decreased the immune response of some vaccines; the clinical significance of this reduction in immune response has not been established (Prymula, 2009).

Simultaneous administration of vaccines helps ensure the patients will be fully vaccinated by the appropriate age. Simultaneous administration of vaccines is defined as administering >1 vaccine on the same day at different anatomic sites. Separate vaccines should not be combined in the same syringe unless indicated by product specific labeling. Separate needles and syringes should be used for each injection. The ACIP prefers each dose of a specific vaccine in a series come from the same manufacturer when possible. Adolescents and adults should be vaccinated while seated or lying down. In general, preterm infants should be vaccinated at the same chronological age as full-term infants (CDC, 2011).

Subcutaneous Do not inject I.V., avoid intradermal administration (may cause severe local reactions); administer SubQ or I.M. (deltoid muscle or lateral midthigh).

Nursing Actions

Physical Assessment Screen for current health status prior to administering vaccine. Monitor for signs of hypersensitivity reactions, behavior changes, localized reactions, and vasovagal reactions.

Patient Education
- Discuss specific use of vaccine and side effects with patient as it relates to treatment. (HCAHPS: During this hospital stay, were you given any medicine that you had not taken before? Before giving you any new medicine, how often did hospital staff tell you what the medicine was for? How often did hospital staff describe possible side effects in a way you could understand?)
- Patient may experience pain, redness, or swelling at injection site; headache; fatigue; nausea; emesis; diarrhea; or dyspepsia. Have patient report immediately to prescriber severe injection site reaction (HCAHPS).
- Educate patient about signs of a significant reaction (eg, wheezing; chest tightness; fever; itching; bad cough; blue skin color; seizures; or swelling of face, lips, tongue, or throat). **Note:** This is not a comprehensive list of all side effects. Patient should consult prescriber for additional questions.

Intended Use and Disclaimer: Should not be printed and given to patients. This information is intended to serve as a concise initial reference for healthcare professionals to use when discussing medications with a patient. You must ultimately rely on your own discretion, experience and judgment in diagnosing, treating and advising patients.

Related Information

Immunization Administration Recommendations *on page 1675*

Immunization Recommendations *on page 1680*

Poliovirus Vaccine (Inactivated)
(POE lee oh VYE rus vak SEEN, in ak ti VAY ted)

Brand Names: U.S. IPOL®

Index Terms Enhanced-Potency Inactivated Poliovirus Vaccine; IPV; Polio Vaccine; Salk Vaccine

Pharmacologic Category Vaccine, Inactivated (Viral)

Medication Safety Issues

Administration issues:

Poliovirus vaccine (inactivated) may be confused with tuberculin products. Medication errors have occurred when poliovirus vaccine (IPV) has been inadvertently administered instead of tuberculin skin tests (PPD). These products are refrigerated and often stored in close proximity to each other.

Pregnancy Risk Factor C

Lactation Excretion into breast milk unknown/use caution

Use Active immunization against poliomyelitis caused by poliovirus types 1, 2, and 3. **Note:** Combination products containing polio vaccine are also available and may be preferred in certain age groups if recipients are likely to be susceptible to the agents contained within each vaccine.

The Advisory Committee on Immunization Practices (ACIP) recommends routine vaccination for the following:
- All children (first dose given at 2 months of age)

Routine immunization of adults in the United States is generally not recommended. Adults with previous wild poliovirus disease, who have never been immunized, or those who are incompletely immunized may receive inactivated poliovirus vaccine if they fall into one of the following categories:
- Travelers to regions or countries where poliomyelitis is endemic or epidemic
- Healthcare workers in close contact with patients who may be excreting poliovirus
- Laboratory workers handling specimens that may contain poliovirus
- Members of communities or specific population groups with diseases caused by wild poliovirus

- Incompletely vaccinated or unvaccinated adults in a household or with other close contact with children receiving oral poliovirus (may be at increased risk of vaccine associated paralytic poliomyelitis)

Available Dosage Forms

Injection, suspension:

IPOL®: Type 1 poliovirus 40 D-antigen units, type 2 poliovirus 8 D-antigen units, and type 3 poliovirus 32 D-antigen units per 0.5 mL (0.5 mL, 5 mL)

General Dosage Range I.M., SubQ:

Children: Primary immunization: Administer three 0.5 mL doses at 2, 4, and 6-18 months of age; do not administer more frequently than 4 weeks apart (preferably given more than 8 weeks apart). Booster dose: 0.5 mL at 4-6 years of age; Minimum interval between booster and previous dose is 6 months.

Adults (previously unvaccinated): Two 0.5 mL doses administered at 1- to 2-month intervals followed by a third dose 6-12 months later.

Administration

I.M. Administer to midlateral aspect of the thigh in infants and small children. Administer in the deltoid area to adults or older children.

I.V. Do not administer I.V.

Subcutaneous SubQ: Administer to midlateral aspect of the thigh in infants and small children. Administer in the deltoid area to adults or older children.

Other Simultaneous administration of vaccines helps ensure the patients will be fully vaccinated by the appropriate age. Simultaneous administration of vaccines is defined as administering >1 vaccine on the same day at different anatomic sites. The use of licensed combination vaccines is generally preferred over separate injections of the equivalent components. Separate vaccines should not be combined in the same syringe unless indicated by product specific labeling. Separate needles and syringes should be used for each injection. The ACIP prefers each dose of a specific vaccine in a series come from the same manufacturer when possible. Adolescents and adults should be vaccinated while seated or lying down. In general, preterm infants should be vaccinated at the same chronological age as full-term infants (CDC, 2011).

Antipyretics have not been shown to prevent febrile seizures. Antipyretics may be used to treat fever or discomfort following vaccination (CDC, 2011). One study reported that routine prophylactic administration of acetaminophen to prevent fever prior to vaccination decreased the immune response of some vaccines; the clinical significance of this reduction in immune response has not been established (Prymula, 2009).

Nursing Actions

Physical Assessment All serious adverse reactions must be reported to the U.S. DHHS. U.S. federal law also requires entry into the patient's medical record.

Patient Education

- Discuss specific use of vaccine and side effects with patient as it relates to treatment. (HCAHPS: During this hospital stay, were you given any medicine that you had not taken before? Before giving you any new medicine, how often did hospital staff tell you what the medicine was for? How often did hospital staff describe possible side effects in a way you could understand?)
- Patient may experience pain, redness or swelling at injection site, headache, fatigue, nausea, emesis, diarrhea, or dyspepsia. Have patient report immediately to prescriber severe injection site reaction (HCAHPS).
- Educate patient about signs of a significant reaction (eg, wheezing; chest tightness; fever; itching; bad cough; blue skin color; seizures; or swelling of face, lips, tongue, or throat). **Note:** This is not a comprehensive list of all side effects. Patient should consult prescriber for additional questions.

Intended Use and Disclaimer: Should not be printed and given to patients. This information is intended to serve as a concise initial reference for healthcare professionals to use when discussing medications with a patient. You must ultimately rely on your own discretion, experience and judgment in diagnosing, treating and advising patients.

Related Information

Immunization Administration Recommendations *on page 1675*

Immunization Recommendations *on page 1680*

Polyethylene Glycol-Electrolyte Solution

(pol i ETH i leen GLY kol ee LEK troe lite soe LOO shun)

Brand Names: U.S. Colyte; GaviLyte-C; GaviLyte-G; GaviLyte-N; GoLYTELY; MoviPrep; NuLYTELY; TriLyte

Index Terms Electrolyte Lavage Solution

Pharmacologic Category Laxative, Osmotic

Medication Safety Issues

Sound-alike/look-alike issues:

GoLYTELY may be confused with NuLYTELY

TriLyte may be confused with TriLipix

Medication Guide Available Yes

Pregnancy Risk Factor C

Lactation Excretion in breast milk unknown/use caution

Use Bowel cleansing prior to colonoscopy or barium enema X-ray examination

Unlabeled Use Whole bowel irrigation (WBI) in the following toxic ingestions: Packets of illicit drugs (body packers, body stuffers), potentially toxic sustained-release or enteric-coated agents, substantial amounts of iron (AACT, 2004)

Available Dosage Forms

Powder, for solution, oral: PEG 3350 240 g, sodium sulfate 22.72 g, sodium bicarbonate 6.72 g, sodium chloride 5.84 g, and potassium 2.98 g (4000 mL); PEG 3350 236 g, sodium sulfate 22.74 g, sodium bicarbonate 6.74 g, sodium chloride 5.86 g, and potassium chloride 2.97 g (4000 mL); PEG 3350 240 g, sodium bicarbonate 5.72 g, sodium chloride 11.2 g, and potassium chloride 1.48 g (4000 mL)

Colyte: PEG 3350 227.1 g, sodium sulfate 21.5 g, sodium bicarbonate 6.36 g, sodium chloride 5.53 g, and potassium chloride 2.82 g (3785 mL)

Colyte: PEG 3350 240 g, sodium sulfate 22.72 g, sodium bicarbonate 6.72 g, sodium chloride 5.84 g, and potassium 2.98 g (4000 mL)

GaviLyte-C: PEG 3350 240 g, sodium sulfate 22.72 g, sodium bicarbonate 6.72 g, sodium chloride 5.84 g, and potassium chloride 2.98 g (4000 mL)

GaviLyte-G: PEG 3350 236 g, sodium sulfate 22.74 g, sodium bicarbonate 6.74 g, sodium chloride 5.86 g, and potassium chloride 2.97 g (4000 mL)

GaviLyte-N: PEG 3350 420 g, sodium bicarbonate 5.72 g, sodium chloride 11.2 g, and potassium chloride 1.48 g (4000 mL)

GoLYTELY: PEG 3350 227.1 g, sodium sulfate 21.5 g, sodium bicarbonate 6.36 g, sodium chloride 5.53 g, and potassium 2.82 g per packet (1s)

GoLYTELY: PEG 3350 236 g, sodium sulfate 22.74 g, sodium bicarbonate 6.74 g, sodium chloride 5.86 g, and potassium 2.97 g (4000 mL)

MoviPrep: Pouch A: PEG 3350 100g, sodium sulfate 7.5 g, sodium chloride 2.69 g, potassium chloride 1.015 g; Pouch B: Ascorbic acid 4.7 g, sodium ascorbate 5.9 g

NuLYTELY: PEG 3350 420 g, sodium bicarbonate 5.72 g, sodium chloride 11.2 g, and potassium 1.48 g

TriLyte: PEG 3350 420 g, sodium bicarbonate 5.72 g, sodium chloride 11.2 g, and potassium 1.48 g

General Dosage Range

Nasogastric:

Infants ≥6 months, Children, and Adolescents (GaviLyte-N, NuLYTELY, TriLyte): 25 mL/kg/hour until the rectal effluent is clear (maximum total dose: 4 L)

Adults (CoLyte, GaviLyte-C, GaviLyte-G, GaviLyte-N, GoLYTELY, NuLYTELY, TriLyte): 20-30 mL/minute (1.2-1.8 L/hour) until 4 L are administered or the rectal effluent is clear

Oral:

Infants ≥6 months, Children, and Adolescents (GaviLyte-N, NuLYTELY, TriLyte): 25 mL/kg/hour until the rectal effluent is clear (maximum total dose: 4 L)

Adults: CoLyte, GaviLyte-C, GaviLyte-G, GaviLyte-N, GoLYTELY, NuLYTELY, TriLyte: 240 mL (8 oz) every 10 minutes, until 4 L are consumed or the rectal effluent is clear; MoviPrep: 240 mL (8 oz) every 15 minutes until 1 L consumed; repeat 1 time

Administration

Oral

Oral: Rapid drinking of each portion is preferred to drinking small amounts continuously. No additional ingredients or flavors (other than the flavor packets provided) should be added to the polyethylene glycol-electrolyte solution. Chilling the solution may improve palatability; administration of a chilled solution is **not** recommended in infants. Oral medications should not be administered within 1 hour of start of therapy.

Nasogastric administration: CoLyte, GaviLyte-C, GaviLyte-G, GaviLyte-N, GoLYTELY, NuLYTELY, TriLyte: The solution may be administered via nasogastric tube for bowel cleansing and whole bowel irrigation (preferred route; unlabeled use) in patients who are unwilling or unable to drink the solution.

Nursing Actions

Patient Education

- Discuss specific use of drug and side effects with patient as it relates to treatment. (HCAHPS: During this hospital stay, were you given any medicine that you had not taken before? Before giving you any new medicine, how often did hospital staff tell you what the medicine was for? How often did hospital staff describe possible side effects in a way you could understand?)
- Patient may experience anal irritation, dyspepsia, bloating, nausea, or asthenia. Have patient report immediately to prescriber inability to drink solution, severe dizziness, significant headache, urinary retention, or rash (HCAHPS).
- Educate patient about signs of a significant reaction (eg, wheezing; chest tightness; fever; itching; bad cough; blue skin color; seizures; or swelling of face, lips, tongue, or throat). **Note:** This is not a comprehensive list of all side effects. Patient should consult prescriber for additional questions.

Intended Use and Disclaimer: Should not be printed and given to patients. This information is intended to serve as a concise initial reference for healthcare professionals to use when discussing medications with a patient. You must ultimately rely on your own discretion, experience and judgment in diagnosing, treating and advising patients.

Polyethylene Glycol-Electrolyte Solution and Bisacodyl

(pol i ETH i leen GLY kol ee LEK troe lite soe LOO shun & bis a KOE dil)

Brand Names: U.S. HalfLytely® and Bisacodyl

Index Terms Bisacodyl and Polyethylene Glycol-Electrolyte Solution; Electrolyte Lavage Solution

Pharmacologic Category Laxative, Bowel Evacuant; Laxative, Stimulant

Medication Guide Available Yes

Pregnancy Risk Factor C

Lactation Excretion in breast milk unknown/use caution

Use Bowel cleansing prior to colonoscopy

Available Dosage Forms

Kit [each kit contains]:

HalfLytely® and Bisacodyl:

Powder for solution, oral (HalfLytely®): PEG 3350 210 g, sodium bicarbonate 2.86 g, sodium chloride 5.6 g, potassium chloride 0.74 g (2000 mL) [contains 4 flavor packs (each 1 g) cherry, lemon-lime, orange, pineapple flavors]

Tablet, delayed release (Bisacodyl): 5 mg (1s)

General Dosage Range Oral: *Adults:* 5 mg of bisacodyl as a single dose, after bowel movement or 6 hours (whichever occurs first) initiate 8 ounces of polyethylene glycol-electrolyte solution every 10 minutes until 2 L are consumed

Administration

Oral Administer bisacodyl tablet with water; do not chew or crush tablet. Do not take antacids within 1 hour of taking bisacodyl. Rapidly drinking the polyethylene glycol-electrolyte solution is preferred to drinking small amount continuously. If severe bloating, distention, or abdominal pain occurs, administration should be slowed or temporarily discontinued until symptoms resolve.

Nursing Actions

Patient Education

- Discuss specific use of drug and side effects with patient as it relates to treatment. (HCAHPS: During this hospital stay, were you given any medicine that you had not taken before? Before giving you any new medicine, how often did hospital staff tell you what the medicine was for? How often did hospital staff describe possible side effects in a way you could understand?)
- Patient may experience abdominal discomfort, dyspepsia, or nausea. Have patient report immediately to prescriber severe dizziness, significant headache, or urinary retention (HCAHPS).
- Educate patient about signs of a significant reaction (eg, wheezing; chest tightness; fever; itching; bad cough; blue skin color; seizures; or swelling of face, lips, tongue, or throat). **Note:** This is not a comprehensive list of all side effects. Patient should consult prescriber for additional questions.

Intended Use and Disclaimer: Should not be printed and given to patients. This information is intended to serve as a concise initial reference for healthcare professionals to use when discussing medications with a patient. You must ultimately rely on your own discretion, experience and judgment in diagnosing, treating and advising patients.

Pomalidomide (poe ma LID oh mide)

Brand Names: U.S. Pomalyst

Index Terms CC-4047

Pharmacologic Category Angiogenesis Inhibitor; Antineoplastic Agent; Immunomodulator, Systemic

Medication Safety Issues

Sound-alike/look-alike issues:

Pomalidomide may be confused with lenalidomide, thalidomide

High alert medication:

This medication is in a class the Institute for Safe Medication Practices (ISMP) includes among its list of drug classes which have a heightened risk of causing significant patient harm when used in error.

Medication Guide Available Yes

Pregnancy Risk Factor X

Lactation Excretion in breast milk unknown/not recommended

Use Treatment of multiple myeloma in patients who have received at least two prior therapies (including lenalidomide and bortezomib) and have continued disease progression on or within 60 days of completion of the last therapy

Available Dosage Forms

Capsule, Oral:

Pomalyst: 1 mg, 2 mg, 3 mg, 4 mg

General Dosage Range Dosage adjustment recommended in patients who develop toxicities.

Oral: *Adults:* 4 mg once daily on days 1-21 of 28-day cycles

Administration

Oral U.S. labeling recommends administering on an empty stomach with water (at least 2 hours before or 2 hours after a meal). Canadian labeling recommends administering without regard to meals. Should be swallowed whole; do not break, chew, or open the capsules. May administer a missed dose if within 12 hours of usual dosing time. If >12 hours, skip the dose for that day and resume usual dosing the following day. Do not take 2 doses to make up for a skipped dose.

Hazardous agent; use appropriate precautions for handling and disposal (meets NIOSH, 2012 criteria).

Nursing Actions

Physical Assessment Ensure that females of childbearing age are preventing pregnancy, as are men who are having sexual contact with women of childbearing age. Appropriate birth control must be used even for a time after therapy is completed. Use with caution with cardiac history, heart failure, and past MI. Check CBC with differential results to evaluate for severe myelosuppression. Increased risk of infection due to neutropenia. Evaluate for peripheral neuropathy. Evaluate for increased bilirubin and transaminases. Monitor for lower extremity swelling, redness, or pain or shortness of breath. Increased risk for blood clots with drug.

Patient Education

- Discuss specific use of drug and side effects with patient as it relates to treatment. (HCAHPS: During this hospital stay, were you given any medicine that you had not taken before? Before giving you any new medicine, how often did hospital staff tell you what the medicine was for? How often did hospital staff describe possible side effects in a way you could understand?)
- Patient may experience anemia, leukopenia, thrombocytopenia, presyncope, fatigue, blurred vision, illogical thinking, asthenia, constipation, diarrhea, nausea, back pain, edema, or thrombosis. Have patient report immediately to prescriber signs of infection, dyspnea, angina, paresthesia, ecchymosis, bleeding, thrombosis, or pregnancy (HCAHPS).
- Educate patient about signs of a significant reaction (eg, wheezing; chest tightness; fever; itching; bad cough; blue skin color; seizures; or swelling of face, lips, tongue, or throat). **Note:** This is not a comprehensive list of all side effects. Patient should consult prescriber for additional questions.

Intended Use and Disclaimer: Should not be printed and given to patients. This information is intended to serve as a concise initial reference for healthcare professionals to use when discussing medications with a patient. You must ultimately rely on your own discretion, experience and judgment in diagnosing, treating and advising patients.

Related Information

Oral Medications That Should Not Be Crushed or Altered *on page 1712*

PONATinib (poe NA ti nib)

Brand Names: U.S. Iclusig
Index Terms AP24534; Ponatinib Hydrochloride
Pharmacologic Category Antineoplastic Agent, BCR-ABL Tyrosine Kinase Inhibitor; Antineoplastic Agent, Tyrosine Kinase Inhibitor

Medication Safety Issues

Sound-alike/look-alike issues:
PONATinib may be confused with axitinib, bosutinib, cabozantinib, crizotinib, dasatinib, imatinib, nilotinib, PAZOPanib, pegaptanib, regorafenib, ruxolitinib, vemurafenib

High alert medication:
This medication is in a class the Institute for Safe Medical Practices (ISMP) includes among its list of drug classes which have a heightened risk of causing significant patient harm when used in error.

Medication Guide Available Yes
Pregnancy Risk Factor D
Lactation Excretion in breast milk unknown/not recommended

Use

Acute lymphoblastic leukemia: Treatment of Philadelphia chromosome-positive acute lymphoblastic leukemia (Ph+ ALL) for whom no other tyrosine kinase inhibitor therapy is indicated or who are T315I positive

Chronic myeloid leukemia: Treatment of chronic myeloid leukemia (CML) in chronic, accelerated, or blast phase for whom no other tyrosine kinase inhibitor therapy is indicated or who are T315I positive

Available Dosage Forms

Tablet, Oral:
Iclusig: 15 mg, 45 mg

General Dosage Range Dosage adjustment recommended in patients on concomitant therapy or who develop toxicities.
Oral: *Adults:* 45 mg once daily

Administration

Oral Administer with or without food. Swallow tablets whole (do not crush or dissolve).

Hazardous agent; use appropriate precautions for handling and disposal (meets NIOSH, 2012 criteria).

Nursing Actions

Physical Assessment Monitor vital signs; signs/symptoms such as new cough; shortness of breath; edema; radiating chest pain to neck, jaw, or arms; stroke symptoms, fever, sore throat, chills; unusual bleeding or bruising; black, tarry, or bright red blood in stool; yellow skin or eyes, itching, or pain in right upper quadrant of abdomen. Instruct patients to get immediate help for symptoms of stroke, chest pain, severe headache, shortness of breath, or irregular heart rate, fever, chills, bleeding, or abdominal pain. Monitor labs including metabolic panel, uric acid, LFTs, and CBC with differential. Assess older patients closely as they may not tolerate treatment as well.

Patient Education

- Discuss specific use of drug and side effects with patient as it relates to treatment. (HCAHPS: During this hospital stay, were you given any medicine that you had not taken before? Before

giving you any new medicine, how often did hospital staff tell you what the medicine was for? How often did hospital staff describe possible side effects in a way you could understand?)

• Patient may experience anemia, leukopenia, thrombocytopenia, headache, asthenia, arthralgia, nausea, constipation, rash, xeroderma, dyspepsia, or hypertension. Have patient report immediately to prescriber dyspnea, angina, tachycardia, severe dizziness, edema, inability to eat, significant weight gain, ecchymosis, bleeding, discolored urine, jaundice, urinary retention, poor healing, or rash (HCAHPS).

• Educate patient about signs of a significant reaction (eg, wheezing; chest tightness; fever; itching; bad cough; blue skin color; seizures; or swelling of face, lips, tongue, or throat). **Note:** This is not a comprehensive list of all side effects. Patient should consult prescriber for additional questions.

Intended Use and Disclaimer: Should not be printed and given to patients. This information is intended to serve as a concise initial reference for healthcare professionals to use when discussing medications with a patient. You must ultimately rely on your own discretion, experience and judgment in diagnosing, treating and advising patients.

Related Information
Oral Medications That Should Not Be Crushed or Altered *on page 1712*

Posaconazole (poe sa KON a zole)

Brand Names: U.S. Noxafil
Index Terms SCH 56592
Pharmacologic Category Antifungal Agent, Oral
Medication Safety Issues
Sound-alike/look-alike issues:
Noxafil may be confused with minoxidil
International issues:
Noxafil [U.S. and multiple international markets] may be confused with Noxidil brand name for minoxidil [Thailand]
Pregnancy Risk Factor C
Lactation Excretion in breast milk unknown/not recommended
Breast-Feeding Considerations Excretion in breast milk has not been investigated; use only if the benefit to the mother justifies potential risk to the fetus.
Use
U.S. labeling:
Invasive *Aspergillus* and *Candida* infections: Suspension and delayed release tablets: Prophylaxis of invasive *Aspergillus* and *Candida* infections in severely-immunocompromised patients (eg, hematopoietic stem cell transplant [HSCT] recipients with graft-versus-host disease [GVHD] or those with prolonged neutropenia

secondary to chemotherapy for hematologic malignancies)
Oropharyngeal candidiasis: Suspension: Treatment of oropharyngeal candidiasis (including patients refractory to itraconazole and/or fluconazole)
Canadian labeling:
Invasive *Aspergillus* and *Candida* infections: Prophylaxis of invasive *Aspergillus* and *Candida* infections in severely-immunocompromised patients (eg, hematopoietic stem cell transplant [HSCT] recipients with graft-versus-host disease [GVHD] or those with prolonged neutropenia); treatment of invasive aspergillosis in patients refractory to or intolerant of itraconazole or amphotericin B; treatment of oropharyngeal candidiasis
Unlabeled Use Salvage therapy of refractory or relapsed invasive fungal infections; mucormycosis; pulmonary infection (nonimmunosuppressed)
Mechanism of Action/Effect Interferes with fungal cytochrome P450 (latosterol-14α-demethylase) activity, decreasing ergosterol synthesis (principal sterol in fungal cell membrane) and inhibiting fungal cell membrane formation.
Contraindications Coadministration with sirolimus, ergot alkaloids (eg, ergotamine, dihydroergotamine), HMG-CoA reductase inhibitors that are primarily metabolized through CYP3A4 (eg, atorvastatin, lovastatin, simvastatin), or CYP3A4 substrates that prolong the QT interval (eg, pimozide, quinidine); hypersensitivity to posaconazole, other azole antifungal agents, or any component of the formulation.
Warnings/Precautions Hepatic dysfunction has occurred, ranging from mild/moderate increases of ALT, AST, alkaline phosphatase, total bilirubin, and/or clinical hepatitis to severe reactions (cholestasis, hepatic failure including death). Consider discontinuation of therapy in patients who develop clinical evidence of liver disease that may be secondary to posaconazole. Elevations in liver function tests have been generally reversible after posaconazole has been discontinued; some cases resolved without drug interruption. More severe reactions have been observed in patients with underlying serious medical conditions (eg, hematologic malignancy) and primarily with suspension total daily doses of 800 mg. Monitor liver function tests at baseline and periodically during therapy. If increases occur, monitor for severe hepatic injury development. Use caution in patients with an increased risk of arrhythmia (long QT syndrome, concurrent QT$_c$-prolonging drugs, drugs metabolized through CYP3A4, hypokalemia). Correct electrolyte abnormalities (eg, potassium, magnesium, and calcium) before initiating therapy. Concurrent use with cyclosporine or tacrolimus may significantly increase cyclosporine/tacrolimus concentrations and may result in rare serious adverse events (eg, nephrotoxicity, leukoencephalopathy, and

death); dose reduction and close monitoring are recommended with initiation of posaconazole therapy. Concurrent use with midazolam may increase midazolam concentrations and potentiate midazolam-related adverse effects. Potentially significant drug-drug interactions may exist, requiring dose or frequency adjustment, additional monitoring, and/or selection of alternative therapy.

U.S. labeling contraindicates use in patients with hypersensitivity to other azole antifungal agents; Canadian labeling does not contraindicate use, but recommends using caution in hypersensitivity with other azole antifungal agents; cross-reaction may occur, but has not been established. Consider alternative therapy or closely monitor for breakthrough fungal infections in patients receiving drugs that decrease absorption or increase the metabolism of posaconazole or in any patient unable to eat or tolerate an oral liquid nutritional supplement. Use caution in severe renal impairment; monitor for breakthrough fungal infections. Patients weighing ≥120 kg may have lower plasma drug exposure; monitor closely for breakthrough fungal infections.

Drug Interactions
Avoid Concomitant Use
Avoid concomitant use of Posaconazole with any of the following: Ado-Trastuzumab Emtansine; Alfuzosin; Apixaban; AtorvaSTATin; Avanafil; Axitinib; Bosutinib; Cabozantinib; Cisapride; Conivaptan; Crizotinib; Dihydroergotamine; Dofetilide; Dronedarone; Efavirenz; Eletriptan; Eplerenone; Ergoloid Mesylates; Ergonovine; Ergotamine; Everolimus; Halofantrine; Ibrutinib; Imatinib; Ivabradine; Lapatinib; Lomitapide; Lovastatin; Lurasidone; Macitentan; Methadone; Methylergonovine; Nilotinib; Nisoldipine; Pimozide; Pomalidomide; QuiNIDine; Ranolazine; Red Yeast Rice; Regorafenib; Rivaroxaban; Salmeterol; Silodosin; Simeprevir; Simvastatin; Sirolimus; Tamsulosin; Ticagrelor; Tolvaptan; Toremifene; Ulipristal; Vemurafenib; VinCRIStine (Liposomal)

Decreased Effect
Posaconazole may decrease the levels/effects of: Amphotericin B; Ifosfamide; Prasugrel; Saccharomyces boulardii; Ticagrelor

The levels/effects of Posaconazole may be decreased by: Didanosine; Efavirenz; Etravirine; Fosamprenavir; Fosphenytoin; H2-Antagonists; Metoclopramide; Phenytoin; Proton Pump Inhibitors; Rifamycin Derivatives; Sucralfate

Increased Effect/Toxicity
Posaconazole may increase the levels/effects of: Ado-Trastuzumab Emtansine; Alfentanil; Alfuzosin; Almotriptan; Alosetron; Antineoplastic Agents (Vinca Alkaloids); Apixaban; ARIPiprazole; Atazanavir; AtorvaSTATin; Avanafil; Axitinib; Bedaquiline; Benzodiazepines (metabolized by oxidation); Boceprevir; Bortezomib; Bosentan; Bosutinib; Brentuximab Vedotin; Brinzolamide; Budesonide (Nasal); Budesonide (Systemic, Oral Inhalation); BusPIRone; Busulfan; Cabozantinib; Calcium Channel Blockers; Cilostazol; Cisapride; Colchicine; Conivaptan; Corticosteroids (Orally Inhaled); Corticosteroids (Systemic); Crizotinib; CycloSPORINE (Systemic); CYP3A4 Substrates; Dienogest; Digoxin; Dihydroergotamine; DOCEtaxel; Dofetilide; DOXOrubicin (Conventional); Dronedarone; Dutasteride; Eletriptan; Enzalutamide; Eplerenone; Ergoloid Mesylates; Ergonovine; Ergotamine; Etravirine; Everolimus; FentaNYL; Fesoterodine; Fluticasone (Nasal); Fluticasone (Oral Inhalation); Fosamprenavir; Fosphenytoin; GlipiZIDE; GuanFACINE; Halofantrine; Highest Risk QTc-Prolonging Agents; Ibrutinib; Iloperidone; Imatinib; Irinotecan; Ivabradine; Ivacaftor; Ixabepilone; Lacosamide; Lapatinib; Levomilnacipran; Lomitapide; Losartan; Lovastatin; Lumefantrine; Lurasidone; Macitentan; Macrolide Antibiotics; Maraviroc; Methadone; Methylergonovine; MethylPREDNISolone; Mifepristone; Moderate Risk QTc-Prolonging Agents; Nilotinib; Nisoldipine; Ospemifene; OxyCODONE; Paricalcitol; PAZOPanib; Phenytoin; Pimecrolimus; Pimozide; Pomalidomide; PONATinib; Propafenone; QUEtiapine; QuiNIDine; Ranolazine; Red Yeast Rice; Regorafenib; Repaglinide; Rifamycin Derivatives; Rilpivirine; Ritonavir; Rivaroxaban; RomiDEPsin; Ruxolitinib; Salmeterol; Saxagliptin; Sildenafil; Silodosin; Simeprevir; Simvastatin; Sirolimus; Solifenacin; SORAfenib; SUNItinib; Tacrolimus (Systemic); Tacrolimus (Topical); Tadalafil; Tamsulosin; Telaprevir; Temsirolimus; Ticagrelor; Tofacitinib; Tolterodine; Tolvaptan; Toremifene; Uliprisal; Vardenafil; Vemurafenib; Vilazodone; VinCRIStine (Liposomal); Vitamin K Antagonists; Zolpidem; Zuclopenthixol

The levels/effects of Posaconazole may be increased by: Boceprevir; Etravirine; Macrolide Antibiotics; Telaprevir

Nutritional/Ethanol Interactions Food: Bioavailability increased ~3 times when posaconazole is administered with a nonfat meal or an oral liquid nutritional supplement; increased ~4 times when administered with a high-fat meal. Management: Suspension must be administered with or within 20 minutes of a full meal or an oral liquid nutritional supplement, or may be administered with an acidic carbonated beverage (eg, ginger ale). Take tablet with food. Consider alternative antifungal therapy in patients with inadequate oral intake or severe diarrhea/vomiting.

Adverse Reactions Note: Percentages reflect data from use in comparator trials with multiple concomitant conditions and medications; some adverse reactions may be due to underlying condition(s).

>10%:

Cardiovascular: Hypertension (11% to 18%), peripheral edema (16%), edema (9% to 15%), hypotension (14%), tachycardia (12%)

Central nervous system: Headache (8% to 28%), rigors (≤20%), fatigue (3% to 17%), insomnia (1% to 17%), dizziness (11%), pain (1% to 11%)

Dermatologic: Skin rash (16%), pruritus (11%)

Endocrine & metabolic: Hypokalemia (≤30%), hypomagnesemia (10% to 18%), weight loss (1% to 14%), hyperglycemia (11%), dehydration (1% to 11%)

Gastrointestinal: Diarrhea (10% to 42%), nausea (2% to 38%), vomiting (7% to 29%), abdominal pain (5% to 27%), constipation (10% to 21%), anorexia (2% to 19%), mucositis (17%), oral candidiasis (1% to 12%)

Hematologic & oncologic: Thrombocytopenia (14% to 29%), anemia (2% to 25%), neutropenia (4% to 23%), febrile neutropenia (20%), petechia (11%)

Hepatic: Increased serum ALT (6% to 17%)

Infection: Bacteremia (18%), herpes simplex infection (3% to 15%), cytomegalovirus disease (14%)

Neuromuscular & skeletal: Musculoskeletal pain (16%), weakness (2% to 13%), arthralgia (11%)

Respiratory: Cough (3% to 25%), dyspnea (1% to 20%), epistaxis (14%), stomatitis (14%), pharyngitis (12%)

Miscellaneous: Fever (6% to 45%)

1% to 10%:

Central nervous system: Chills (10%), anxiety (9%)

Dermatologic: Diaphoresis (2% to 10%)

Endocrine & metabolic: Hypocalcemia (9%)

Gastrointestinal: Dyspepsia (10%)

Genitourinary: Vaginal hemorrhage (10%)

Hepatic: Hyperbilirubinemia (7% to 10%), increased serum AST (3% to 4%), increased serum alkaline phosphatase (1% to 3%)

Neuromuscular & skeletal: Back pain (10%)

Respiratory: Pneumonia (3% to 10%), upper respiratory tract infection (7%)

Product Availability Noxafil injection: FDA approved March 2014; availability anticipated in April 2014.

Available Dosage Forms

Suspension, Oral:
Noxafil: 40 mg/mL (105 mL)

Tablet Delayed Release, Oral:
Noxafil: 100 mg

General Dosage Range Oral: *Children ≥13 years, Adolescents, and Adults:* 100-800 mg daily

Administration

Oral

Suspension: Shake well before use. Must be administered during or within 20 minutes following a full meal or an oral liquid nutritional supplement; alternatively, posaconazole may be administered with an acidic carbonated beverage (eg, ginger ale). In patients able to swallow, administer oral suspension using dosing spoon provided by the manufacturer; spoon should be rinsed clean with water after each use and before storage.

Tablets (delayed release): Swallow tablets whole; do not divide, crush, or chew. Administer with food.

Consider alternative antifungal therapy in patients with inadequate oral intake or severe diarrhea/vomiting; if alternative therapy is not an option, closely monitoring for breakthrough fungal infections. Adequate posaconazole absorption from GI tract and subsequent plasma concentrations are dependent on food for efficacy. Lower average plasma concentrations have been associated with an increased risk of treatment failure.

Storage/Stability Suspension: Store at 25°C (77°F); excursions are permitted between 15°C and 30°C (59°F and 86°F). Do not freeze.

Tablets: Store between 20°C and 25°C (68°F and 77°F); excursions are permitted between 15°C and 30°C (59°F and 86°F).

Nursing Actions

Physical Assessment Monitor for gastrointestinal disturbance, vision changes, hepatic toxicity (increased liver enzymes, jaundice), and CNS changes on a regular basis during therapy.

Patient Education

- Discuss specific use of drug and side effects with patient as it relates to treatment. (HCAHPS: During this hospital stay, were you given any medicine that you had not taken before? Before giving you any new medicine, how often did hospital staff tell you what the medicine was for? How often did hospital staff describe possible side effects in a way you could understand?)

- Patient may experience constipation, arthralgia, back pain, or insomnia. Have patient report immediately to prescriber signs of hepatic impairment, signs of hypokalemia, severe edema, angina, tachycardia, significant dizziness, syncope, intolerable dyspepsia, considerable diarrhea, severe nausea, dyspnea, excessive weight gain, edema of extremities, paresthesia, urinary retention, oliguria, chills, pharyngitis, stomatitis, significant headache, tremors, ecchymosis, hemorrhaging, vaginal hemorrhaging, or considerable asthenia (HCAHPS).

- Educate patient about signs of a significant reaction (eg, wheezing; chest tightness; fever; itching; bad cough; blue skin color; seizures; or swelling of face, lips, tongue, or throat). **Note:** This is not a comprehensive list of all side effects. Patient should consult prescriber for additional questions.

Intended Use and Disclaimer: Should not be printed and given to patients. This information is intended to serve as a concise initial reference for

healthcare professionals to use when discussing medications with a patient. You must ultimately rely on your own discretion, experience and judgment in diagnosing, treating and advising patients.

Dietary Considerations

Tablets (delayed release): Take with food.

Suspension: Give during or within 20 minutes following a full meal or liquid nutritional supplement; alternatively, posaconazole may be administered with an acidic carbonated beverage (eg, ginger ale).

Consider alternative antifungal therapy in patients with inadequate oral intake or severe diarrhea/ vomiting; if alternative therapy is not an option, closely monitoring for breakthrough fungal infections.

Adequate posaconazole absorption from GI tract and subsequent plasma concentrations are dependent on food for efficacy. Lower average plasma concentrations have been associated with an increased risk of treatment failure.

Potassium Bicarbonate
(poe TASS ee um bye KAR bun ate)

Brand Names: U.S. K-Bicarb [OTC]; K-Effervescent; K-Prime; K-Vescent

Pharmacologic Category Electrolyte Supplement, Oral

Pregnancy Risk Factor C

Use Potassium deficiency, hypokalemia

Available Dosage Forms

Capsule, Oral:
K-Bicarb [OTC]: 99 mg

Tablet Effervescent, Oral:
K-Effervescent: 25 mEq
K-Prime: 25 mEq
K-Vescent: 25 mEq
Generic: 25 mEq

General Dosage Range Oral:
Children: 1-4 mEq/kg/day
Adults: 25 mEq 2-4 times/day

Nursing Actions

Patient Education

- Discuss specific use of drug and side effects with patient as it relates to treatment. (HCAHPS: During this hospital stay, were you given any medicine that you had not taken before? Before giving you any new medicine, how often did hospital staff tell you what the medicine was for? How often did hospital staff describe possible side effects in a way you could understand?)
- Patient may experience dyspepsia, nausea, diarrhea, and flatulence. Have patient report immediately to prescriber tachycardia, severe dizziness, asthenia, paresthesia, ecchymosis, bleeding, or rash (HCAHPS).
- Educate patient about signs of a significant reaction (eg, wheezing; chest tightness; fever; itching; bad cough; blue skin color; seizures; or

swelling of face, lips, tongue, or throat). **Note:** This is not a comprehensive list of all side effects. Patient should consult prescriber for additional questions.

Intended Use and Disclaimer: Should not be printed and given to patients. This information is intended to serve as a concise initial reference for healthcare professionals to use when discussing medications with a patient. You must ultimately rely on your own discretion, experience and judgment in diagnosing, treating and advising patients.

Potassium Bicarbonate and Potassium Chloride
(poe TASS ee um bye KAR bun ate & poe TASS ee um KLOR ide)

Index Terms K-Lyte/Cl; Potassium Bicarbonate and Potassium Chloride (Effervescent)

Pharmacologic Category Electrolyte Supplement, Oral

Pregnancy Risk Factor C

Lactation Not recommended

Use Treatment or prevention of hypokalemia

Available Dosage Forms

Tablet for solution, oral [effervescent]: Potassium chloride 25 mEq

General Dosage Range

Oral:
Children: 1-4 mEq/kg/day in divided doses
Adults: Prevention: 16-24 mEq/day in 2-4 divided doses; Treatment: 40-100 mEq/day in 2-4 divided doses

Administration

Oral Administer with meals; solution should be sipped slowly, over 5-10 minutes

Nursing Actions

Physical Assessment See individual agents.

Patient Education

- Discuss specific use of drug and side effects with patient as it relates to treatment. (HCAHPS: During this hospital stay, were you given any medicine that you had not taken before? Before giving you any new medicine, how often did hospital staff tell you what the medicine was for? How often did hospital staff describe possible side effects in a way you could understand?)
- Patient may experience dyspepsia, nausea, diarrhea, or flatulence. Have patient report immediately to prescriber tachycardia, severe dizziness, paresthesia, ecchymosis, or bleeding (HCAHPS).
- Educate patient about signs of a significant reaction (eg, wheezing; chest tightness; fever; itching; bad cough; blue skin color; seizures; or swelling of face, lips, tongue, or throat). **Note:** This is not a comprehensive list of all side effects. Patient should consult prescriber for additional questions.

Intended Use and Disclaimer: Should not be printed and given to patients. This information is intended to serve as a concise initial reference for healthcare professionals to use when discussing medications with a patient. You must ultimately rely on your own discretion, experience and judgment in diagnosing, treating and advising patients.

Related Information

Oral Medications That Should Not Be Crushed or Altered *on page 1712*

Potassium Bicarbonate *on page 1273*

Potassium Chloride *on page 1274*

Potassium Bicarbonate and Potassium Citrate

(poe TASS ee um bye KAR bun ate & poe TASS ee um SIT rate)

Brand Names: U.S. Effer-K®; Klor-Con®/EF

Index Terms Potassium Bicarbonate and Potassium Citrate (Effervescent)

Pharmacologic Category Electrolyte Supplement, Oral

Medication Safety Issues

Sound-alike/look-alike issues:

Klor-Con® may be confused with Klaron®

Pregnancy Risk Factor C

Lactation Not recommended

Use Treatment or prevention of hypokalemia, particularly when it is necessary to avoid chloride or the acid/base status requires bicarbonate

Available Dosage Forms

Tablet for solution, oral [effervescent]:

Effer-K®: Potassium 10 mEq; potassium 20 mEq; potassium 25 mEq

Klor-Con®/EF: Potassium 25 mEq

General Dosage Range

Oral: *Adults:* Prevention: 10-80 mEq/day in 1-4 divided doses; Treatment: 40-100 mEq/day in 2-4 divided doses

Administration

Oral Dissolve tablet completely in 3-4 ounces of cold water or juice. May further dilute if GI adverse effects occur.

Nursing Actions

Physical Assessment See individual agents.

Patient Education

• Discuss specific use of drug and side effects with patient as it relates to treatment. (HCAHPS: During this hospital stay, were you given any medicine that you had not taken before? Before giving you any new medicine, how often did hospital staff tell you what the medicine was for? How often did hospital staff describe possible side effects in a way you could understand?)

• Patient may experience dyspepsia, nausea, or diarrhea. Have patient report immediately to prescriber tachycardia, severe dizziness, paresthesia, ecchymosis, or bleeding (HCAHPS).

• Educate patient about signs of a significant reaction (eg, wheezing; chest tightness; fever; itching; bad cough; blue skin color; seizures; or swelling of face, lips, tongue, or throat). **Note:** This is not a comprehensive list of all side effects. Patient should consult prescriber for additional questions.

Intended Use and Disclaimer: Should not be printed and given to patients. This information is intended to serve as a concise initial reference for healthcare professionals to use when discussing medications with a patient. You must ultimately rely on your own discretion, experience and judgment in diagnosing, treating and advising patients.

Related Information

Oral Medications That Should Not Be Crushed or Altered *on page 1712*

Potassium Bicarbonate *on page 1273*

Potassium Citrate *on page 1276*

Potassium Chloride (poe TASS ee um KLOR ide)

Brand Names: U.S. K-Lor; K-Tabs; K-Vescent; Klor-Con; Klor-Con 10; Klor-Con M10; Klor-Con M15; Klor-Con M20; Micro-K

Index Terms KCl; Kdur

Pharmacologic Category Electrolyte Supplement, Oral; Electrolyte Supplement, Parenteral

Medication Safety Issues

Sound-alike/look-alike issues:

Kaon-Cl-10 may be confused with kaolin

KCl may be confused with HCl

Klor-Con may be confused with Klaron®

microK may be confused with Macrobid®, Micronase

High alert medication:

The Institute for Safe Medication Practices (ISMP) includes this medication (I.V. formulation) among its list of drugs which have a heightened risk of causing significant patient harm when used in error.

Other safety concerns:

Per JCAHO recommendations, concentrated electrolyte solutions should not be available in patient care areas.

Consider special storage requirements for intravenous potassium salts; I.V. potassium salts have been administered IVP in error, leading to fatal outcomes.

Pregnancy Risk Factor C

Lactation Enters breast milk/not recommended

Breast-Feeding Considerations Potassium is excreted into breast milk (IOM, 2004). The normal content of potassium in human milk is ~13 mEq/L. Supplementation (that does not cause maternal hyperkalemia) would not be expected to affect normal concentrations.

Use Treatment or prevention of hypokalemia

Contraindications Hypersensitivity to any component of the formulation; hyperkalemia. In addition, solid oral dosage forms are contraindicated in patients in whom there is a structural, pathological, and/or pharmacologic cause for delay or arrest in passage through the GI tract.

Warnings/Precautions Close monitoring of serum potassium concentrations is needed to avoid hyperkalemia. Use with caution in patients with renal impairment, cardiac disease, acid/base disorders, or potassium-altering conditions/disorders. Use with caution in digitalized patients or patients receiving concomitant medications or therapies that increase potassium (eg, ACEI, potassium-sparing diuretics, potassium containing salt substitutes). Do **NOT** administer undiluted or I.V. push; inappropriate parenteral administration may be fatal. Always administer potassium further diluted; refer to appropriate dilution and administration rate recommendations. Vesicant/irritant (at concentrations >0.1 mEq/mL); ensure proper catheter or needle position prior to and during infusion; avoid extravasation. Pain and phlebitis may occur during parenteral infusion requiring a decrease in infusion rate or potassium concentration. Avoid administering potassium diluted in dextrose solutions during initial therapy; potential for transient decreases in serum potassium due to intracellular shift of potassium from dextrose-stimulated insulin release. May cause GI upset (eg, nausea, vomiting, diarrhea, abdominal pain, discomfort) and lead to GI ulceration, bleeding, perforation, and/or obstruction. Oral liquid preparations (not solid) should be used in patients with esophageal compression or delayed gastric emptying.

Drug Interactions

Avoid Concomitant Use

Avoid concomitant use of Potassium Chloride with any of the following: Anticholinergic Agents; Glycopyrrolate

Decreased Effect There are no known significant interactions involving a decrease in effect.

Increased Effect/Toxicity

Potassium Chloride may increase the levels/effects of: ACE Inhibitors; Angiotensin II Receptor Blockers; Potassium-Sparing Diuretics

The levels/effects of Potassium Chloride may be increased by: Anticholinergic Agents; Eplerenone; Glycopyrrolate; Heparin; Heparin (Low Molecular Weight)

Adverse Reactions Frequency not defined.
Dermatologic: Rash
Endocrine & metabolic: Hyperkalemia
Gastrointestinal: Abdominal pain/discomfort, diarrhea, flatulence, GI bleeding (oral), GI obstruction (oral), GI perforation (oral), nausea, vomiting

Dosage Forms Considerations
750 mg potassium chloride = elemental potassium
390 mg = potassium 10 mEq = potassium 10 mmol

Available Dosage Forms
Capsule Extended Release, Oral:
Micro-K: 8 mEq, 10 mEq
Generic: 8 mEq, 10 mEq
Liquid, Oral:
Generic: 20 mEq/15 mL (10%) (473 mL); 40 mEq/15 mL (20%) (473 mL)
Packet, Oral:
K-Lor: 20 mEq (30 ea, 100 ea)
K-Vescent: 20 mEq (100 ea)
Klor-Con: 20 mEq (1 ea, 30 ea, 100 ea); 25 mEq (30 ea, 100 ea)
Generic: 20 mEq (30 ea, 100 ea)
Solution, Intravenous:
Generic: 5 mEq (250 mL); 10 mEq (500 mL, 1000 mL); 20 mEq (1000 mL); 30 mEq (1000 mL); 40 mEq (1000 mL); 0.4 mEq/mL (50 mL); 10 mEq/100 mL (100 mL); 10 mEq/50 mL (50 mL); 20 mEq/100 mL (100 mL); 20 mEq/50 mL (50 mL); 40 mEq/100 mL (100 mL); 2 mEq/mL (5 mL, 10 mL, 15 mL, 20 mL, 30 mL, 250 mL); 20 mEq/L (1000 mL); 40 mEq/L (1000 mL)
Solution, Oral:
Generic: 20 mEq/15 mL (10%) (15 mL, 30 mL, 473 mL)
Tablet Extended Release, Oral:
K-Tabs: 10 mEq
Klor-Con: 8 mEq
Klor-Con 10: 10 mEq
Klor-Con M10: 10 mEq
Klor-Con M15: 15 mEq
Klor-Con M20: 20 mEq
Generic: 8 mEq, 10 mEq, 20 mEq

General Dosage Range
I.V.:
Children: Initial: 0.5-1 mEq/kg/dose (maximum dose: 40 mEq); repeat as needed based on lab values
Adults: Intermittent infusion: ≤10 mEq/hour; repeat as needed based on lab values (maximum: 200 mEq/day)
Oral:
Children: 1-2 mEq/kg/day in 1-2 divided doses or as needed based on lab values
Adults: Initial: 6-10 mEq/dose (maximum: 40 mEq/dose); Maintenance: 40-100 mEq/day in divided doses or as needed based on lab values

Administration
I.V. Potassium must be diluted prior to parenteral administration. Do not administer I.V. push. In general, the dose, concentration of infusion and rate of administration may be dependent on patient condition and specific institution policy. Some clinicians recommend that the maximum concentration for peripheral infusion is 10 mEq/100 mL and maximum rate of administration for peripheral infusion is 10 mEq/hour. ECG monitoring is recommended for peripheral or central infusions >10 mEq/hour in adults. Concentrations and rates of infusion may be greater with central line administration. Some clinicians recommend ▶

that the maximum concentration for central infusion is 20-40 mEq/100 mL and maximum rate of administration for central infusion is 40 mEq/hour.

Vesicant/irritant (at concentrations >0.1 mEq/mL); ensure proper needle or catheter placement prior to and during I.V. infusion. Avoid extravasation.

Extravasation management: If extravasation occurs, stop infusion immediately and disconnect (leave needle/cannula in place); gently aspirate extravasated solution (do **NOT** flush the line); initiate hyaluronidase antidote; remove needle/cannula; apply dry cold compresses (Hurst, 2004); elevate extremity.

Hyaluronidase: Intradermal or SubQ: Inject a total of 1 mL (15 units/mL) as five separate 0.2 mL injections (using a 25-gauge needle) into area of extravasation at the leading edge in a clockwise manner (MacCara, 1983; Zenk, 1981).

Oral Oral dosage forms should be taken with meals and a full glass of water or other liquid to minimize the risk of GI irritation. Prescribing information for the various oral preparations recommend that no more than 20 mEq or 25 mEq should be given as single dose.

Capsule: MicroK®: Swallow whole, do not chew. Capsules may also be opened and contents sprinkled on a spoonful of applesauce or pudding and should be swallowed immediately without chewing.

Powder: Klor-Con®: Dissolve one packet in 4-5 ounces of water or other beverage prior to administration.

Tablet:

K-Tab®, Kaon-Cl®, Klor-Con®: Swallow tablets whole; do not crush, chew, or suck on tablet.

Klor-Con® M: Swallow tablets whole; do not crush, chew, or suck on tablet. Tablet may also be broken in half and each half swallowed separately; the whole tablet may be dissolved in ~4 ounces of water (allow ~2 minutes to dissolve, stir well and drink immediately)

Preparation for Administration Parenteral: Potassium must be diluted prior to parenteral administration. The concentration of infusion may be dependent on patient condition and specific institution policy. Some clinicians recommend that the maximum concentration for peripheral infusion is 10 mEq/100 mL and 20-40 mEq/100 mL for central infusions.

Storage/Stability

Capsule: MicroK®: Store between 20°C to 25°C (68°F to 77°F).

Powder for oral solution: Klor-Con®: Store at room temperature of 15°C to 30°C (59°F to 86°F).

Solution for injection: Store at room temperature; do not freeze. Use only clear solutions. Use admixtures within 24 hours.

Tablet: K-Tab®: Store below 30°C (86°F).

Nursing Actions

Physical Assessment Monitor infusion site closely.

Patient Education

• Discuss specific use of drug and side effects with patient as it relates to treatment. (HCAHPS: During this hospital stay, were you given any medicine that you had not taken before? Before giving you any new medicine, how often did hospital staff tell you what the medicine was for? How often did hospital staff describe possible side effects in a way you could understand?)

• Patient may experience dyspepsia, nausea, or diarrhea. Have patient report immediately to prescriber tachycardia, severe dizziness, asthenia, paresthesia, melena, ecchymosis, bleeding, or rash (HCAHPS).

• Educate patient about signs of a significant reaction (eg, wheezing; chest tightness; fever; itching; bad cough; blue skin color; seizures; or swelling of face, lips, tongue, or throat). **Note:** This is not a comprehensive list of all side effects. Patient should consult prescriber for additional questions.

Intended Use and Disclaimer: Should not be printed and given to patients. This information is intended to serve as a concise initial reference for healthcare professionals to use when discussing medications with a patient. You must ultimately rely on your own discretion, experience and judgment in diagnosing, treating and advising patients.

Dietary Considerations Administer with plenty of fluid to decrease stomach irritation and discomfort. Some dietary sources of potassium include leafy green vegetables (eg, spinach, cabbage), tomatoes, cucumbers, zucchini, fruits (eg, apples, oranges, and bananas), root vegetables (eg, carrots, radishes), beans, and peas.

Related Information

Management of Drug Extravasations *on page 1700*

Oral Medications That Should Not Be Crushed or Altered *on page 1712*

Potassium Citrate (poe TASS ee um SIT rate)

Brand Names: U.S. Urocit-K 10; Urocit-K 15; Urocit-K 5

Pharmacologic Category Alkalinizing Agent, Oral

Medication Safety Issues

Sound-alike/look-alike issues:

Urocit®-K may be confused with Urised

Pregnancy Risk Factor C

Lactation Excreted in breast milk/not recommended

Use Prevention of uric acid nephrolithiasis; prevention of calcium renal stones in patients with hypocitraturia; urinary alkalinizer when sodium citrate is contraindicated

Available Dosage Forms

Tablet Extended Release, Oral:

Urocit-K 5: 5 mEq (540 mg)

Urocit-K 10: 10 mEq (1080 mg)

Urocit-K 15: 15 mEq (1620 mg)

Generic: 10 mEq (1080 mg), 15 mEq (1620 mg), 5 mEq (540 mg)

General Dosage Range Oral: *Adults:*

Immediate release: 10-20 mEq 3 times/day or 15 mEq 4 times/day (maximum: 100 mEq/day)

Extended release: 15-30 mEq 2 times/day or 10-20 mEq 3 times/day (maximum: 100 mEq/day)

Administration

Oral Administer with meals or bedtime snack (or within 30 minutes after). Swallow tablets whole with a full glass of water.

Nursing Actions

Physical Assessment Assess kidney function prior to treatment. Monitor cardiac status and serum potassium prior to treatment and at regular intervals.

Patient Education

• Discuss specific use of drug and side effects with patient as it relates to treatment. (HCAHPS: During this hospital stay, were you given any medicine that you had not taken before? Before giving you any new medicine, how often did hospital staff tell you what the medicine was for? How often did hospital staff describe possible side effects in a way you could understand?)

• Patient may experience hyperkalemia, nausea, diarrhea, or dyspepsia. Have patient report immediately to prescriber severe dizziness, paresthesia, illogical thinking, significant asthenia, or rash (HCAHPS).

• Educate patient about signs of a significant reaction (eg, wheezing; chest tightness; fever; itching; bad cough; blue skin color; seizures; or swelling of face, lips, tongue, or throat). **Note:** This is not a comprehensive list of all side effects. Patient should consult prescriber for additional questions.

Intended Use and Disclaimer: Should not be printed and given to patients. This information is intended to serve as a concise initial reference for healthcare professionals to use when discussing medications with a patient. You must ultimately rely on your own discretion, experience and judgment in diagnosing, treating and advising patients.

Related Information

Oral Medications That Should Not Be Crushed or Altered *on page 1712*

Potassium Iodide (poe TASS ee um EYE oh dide)

Brand Names: U.S. SSKI; ThyroShield [OTC]

Index Terms KI; Saturated Potassium Iodide Solution; Saturated Solution of Potassium Iodide

Pharmacologic Category Antidote; Antithyroid Agent; Expectorant

Medication Safety Issues

Sound-alike/look-alike issues:

Potassium iodide products, including saturated solution of potassium iodide (SSKI®) may be confused with potassium iodide and iodine (Strong Iodide Solution or Lugol's solution)

Other safety concerns:

Dosage volume: Dosing errors have been reported during the prescribing, dispensing, and administration of potassium iodide-containing solutions (eg, Lugol's, SSKI). Errors have occurred when **mL** doses were administered, when only **drops** were indicated for the dose. Carefully review dosage and administration information; appropriate oral dosage is most commonly expressed as drops to provide doses less than 1 mL. Dispensing unit doses is also highly recommended; pharmacists should never dispense quantities that could be lethal if consumed as a single dose. (ISMP, 2011).

Pregnancy Risk Factor D

Lactation Enters breast milk/use caution

Use Expectorant for the symptomatic treatment of chronic pulmonary diseases complicated by mucous; block thyroidal uptake of radioactive isotopes of iodine in a nuclear radiation emergency

Unlabeled Use Lymphocutaneous and cutaneous sporotrichosis; reduce thyroid vascularity prior to thyroidectomy; management of thyrotoxic crisis; block thyroidal uptake of radioactive isotopes of iodine after therapeutic or diagnostic exposure to radioactive iodine

Available Dosage Forms

Solution, Oral:

SSKI: 1 g/mL (30 mL, 237 mL)

ThyroShield [OTC]: 65 mg/mL (30 mL)

General Dosage Range Oral:

Infants <1 month: iOSAT™, ThyroSafe®, ThyroShield®: 16.25 mg once daily

Infants 1-12 months and Children 1-3 years: iOSAT™, ThyroSafe®, ThyroShield®: 32.5 mg once daily

Children 3-12 years and Children 12-18 years weighing <68 kg: iOSAT™, ThyroSafe®, ThyroShield®: 65 mg once daily

Children 12-18 years weighing ≥68 kg and Adults: iOSAT™, ThyroSafe®, ThyroShield®: 130 mg once daily

Adults: SSKI®: 300-600 mg 3-4 times daily

Administration

Oral

SSKI®: Dilute in a glassful of water, fruit juice, or milk. Take with food or milk to decrease gastric irritation.

iOSAT™, Thyrosafe®, Thyroshield®: Take as soon as possible after instructed to do so by public officials. Take every 24 hours; do not take more than 1 dose in 24 hours. Tablets may be crushed and mixed with water, low fat milk (white or chocolate), orange juice, soda (flat), raspberry syrup, or infant formula.

Nursing Actions

Physical Assessment Monitor patient for skin rash, swelling of the salivary glands. Patient may complain of a metallic taste; burning in the mouth and throat; or sore teeth and gums. Monitor for allergic reactions, which include fever; joint pain; edema; difficulty breathing, speaking, or swallowing; wheezing or shortness of breath.

Patient Education

- Discuss specific use of drug and side effects with patient as it relates to treatment. (HCAHPS: During this hospital stay, were you given any medicine that you had not taken before? Before giving you any new medicine, how often did hospital staff tell you what the medicine was for? How often did hospital staff describe possible side effects in a way you could understand?)
- Patient may experience rash, parageusia, nausea, or asthenia. Have patient report immediately to prescriber tachycardia, flu-like syndrome, severe dyspepsia, ecchymosis, bleeding, significant edema, or paresthesia (HCAHPS).
- Educate patient about signs of a significant reaction (eg, wheezing; chest tightness; fever; itching; bad cough; blue skin color; seizures; or swelling of face, lips, tongue, or throat). **Note:** This is not a comprehensive list of all side effects. Patient should consult prescriber for additional questions.

Intended Use and Disclaimer: Should not be printed and given to patients. This information is intended to serve as a concise initial reference for healthcare professionals to use when discussing medications with a patient. You must ultimately rely on your own discretion, experience and judgment in diagnosing, treating and advising patients.

Potassium Iodide and Iodine
(poe TASS ee um EYE oh dide & EYE oh dine)

Index Terms Iodine and Potassium Iodide; Lugol's Solution; Strong Iodine Solution

Pharmacologic Category Antithyroid Agent

Medication Safety Issues

Sound-alike/look-alike issues:

Potassium iodide and iodine (Strong Iodide Solution or Lugol's solution) may be confused with potassium iodide products, including saturated solution of potassium iodide (SSKI®)

Other safety concerns:

Dosage volume: Dosing errors have been reported during the prescribing, dispensing, and administration of potassium iodide-containing solutions (eg, Lugol's, SSKI). Errors have

occurred when **mL** doses were administered, when only **drops** were indicated for the dose. Carefully review dosage and administration information; appropriate oral dosage is most commonly expressed as drops to provide doses less than 1 mL. Dispensing unit doses is also highly recommended; pharmacists should never dispense quantities that could be lethal if consumed as a single dose. (ISMP, 2011).

Pregnancy Risk Factor D (potassium iodide)

Lactation Enters breast milk/use caution

Use Topical antiseptic

Unlabeled Use Reduce thyroid vascularity prior to thyroidectomy and management of thyrotoxic crisis; block thyroidal uptake of radioactive isotopes of iodine in a radiation emergency or after therapeutic/diagnostic use of radioactive iodine

Available Dosage Forms

Solution, oral: Potassium iodide 100 mg/mL and iodine 50 mg/mL (473 mL)

Solution, topical: Potassium iodide 100 mg/mL and iodine 50 mg/mL (8 mL)

General Dosage Range Topical: *Adults:* Apply directly to area(s) requiring antiseptic

Administration

Oral Has been used orally (unlabeled route)

Topical Apply topically directly to area(s) requiring antiseptic.

Nursing Actions

Patient Education

- Discuss specific use of drug and side effects with patient as it relates to treatment. (HCAHPS: During this hospital stay, were you given any medicine that you had not taken before? Before giving you any new medicine, how often did hospital staff tell you what the medicine was for? How often did hospital staff describe possible side effects in a way you could understand?)
- Patient may experience rash, abnormal taste, nausea, or asthenia. Have patient report immediately to prescriber tachycardia, flu-like symptoms, severe dyspepsia, ecchymosis, bleeding, considerable edema, or paresthesia (HCAHPS).
- Educate patient about signs of a significant reaction (eg, wheezing; chest tightness; fever; itching; bad cough; blue skin color; seizures; or swelling of face, lips, tongue, or throat). **Note:** This is not a comprehensive list of all side effects. Patient should consult prescriber for additional questions.

Intended Use and Disclaimer: Should not be printed and given to patients. This information is intended to serve as a concise initial reference for healthcare professionals to use when discussing medications with a patient. You must ultimately rely on your own discretion, experience and judgment in diagnosing, treating and advising patients.

Related Information

Potassium Iodide *on page 1277*

Potassium Phosphate
(poe TASS ee um FOS fate)

Brand Names: U.S. Neutra-Phos®-K [OTC] [DSC]

Index Terms Phosphate, Potassium

Pharmacologic Category Electrolyte Supplement, Parenteral

Medication Safety Issues

High alert medication:

The Institute for Safe Medication Practices (ISMP) includes this medication (I.V. formulation) among its list of drugs which have a heightened risk of causing significant patient harm when used in error.

Other safety concerns:

Per JCAHO recommendations, concentrated electrolyte solutions should not be available in patient care areas.

Consider special storage requirements for intravenous potassium salts; I.V. potassium salts have been administered IVP in error, leading to fatal outcomes.

Safe Prescribing: Because inorganic phosphate exists as monobasic and dibasic anions, with the mixture of valences dependent on pH, ordering by mEq amounts is unreliable and may lead to large dosing errors. In addition, I.V. phosphate is available in the sodium and potassium salt; therefore, the content of these cations must be considered when ordering phosphate. The most reliable method of ordering I.V. phosphate is by millimoles, then specifying the potassium or sodium salt. For example, an order for 15 mmol of phosphate as potassium phosphate in one liter of normal saline.

Pregnancy Risk Factor C

Breast-Feeding Considerations Phosphorus, sodium, and potassium are normal constituents of human milk.

Use Treatment and prevention of hypophosphatemia; **Note:** The concomitant amount of potassium must be calculated into the total electrolyte content. For each 1 mmol of phosphate, ~1.5 mEq of potassium will be administered. Therefore, if ordering 30 mmol of potassium phosphate, the patient will receive ~45 mEq of potassium.

Mechanism of Action/Effect

Phosphorus in the form of organic and inorganic phosphate has a variety of important biochemical functions in the body and is involved in many significant metabolic and enzymatic reactions in almost all organs and tissues. It exerts a modifying influence on the steady state of calcium levels, a buffering effect on acid-base equilibrium and a primary role in the renal excretion of hydrogen ion.

Potassium is the major cation of intracellular fluid and is essential for the conduction of nerve impulses in heart, brain, and skeletal muscle; contraction of cardiac, skeletal and smooth muscles; maintenance of normal renal function, acid-base balance, carbohydrate metabolism, and gastric secretion.

Contraindications Hyperphosphatemia, hyperkalemia, hypocalcemia

Warnings/Precautions Close monitoring of serum potassium concentrations is needed to avoid hyperkalemia. Use with caution in patients with renal insufficiency, cardiac disease, metabolic alkalosis. Use with caution in digitalized patients and patients receiving concomitant potassium-altering therapies. Parenteral potassium may cause pain and phlebitis, requiring a decrease in infusion rate or potassium concentration. Solutions for injection may contain aluminum; toxic levels may occur following prolonged administration in premature neonates or patients with renal impairment.

Drug Interactions

Avoid Concomitant Use There are no known interactions where it is recommended to avoid concomitant use.

Decreased Effect

The levels/effects of Potassium Phosphate may be decreased by: Antacids; Calcium Salts; Iron Salts; Magnesium Salts; Multivitamins/Minerals (with ADEK, Folate, Iron); Sucralfate

Increased Effect/Toxicity

Potassium Phosphate may increase the levels/effects of: ACE Inhibitors; Angiotensin II Receptor Blockers; Potassium-Sparing Diuretics

The levels/effects of Potassium Phosphate may be increased by: Bisphosphonate Derivatives; Eplerenone; Heparin; Heparin (Low Molecular Weight)

Nutritional/Ethanol Interactions Food: Avoid administering with oxalate (berries, nuts, chocolate, beans, celery, tomato) or phytate-containing foods (bran, whole wheat).

Adverse Reactions Frequency not defined.

Cardiovascular: Arrhythmia, bradycardia, chest pain, ECG changes, edema, heart block, hypotension

Central nervous system: Listlessness, mental confusion, tetany (with large doses of phosphate)

Endocrine & metabolic: Hyperkalemia

Gastrointestinal: Diarrhea, nausea, stomach pain, vomiting

Genitourinary: Urine output decreased

Local: Phlebitis

Neuromuscular & skeletal: Paralysis, paresthesia, weakness

Renal: Acute renal failure

Respiratory: Dyspnea

Dosage Forms Considerations

Potassium 4.4 mEq is equivalent to potassium 170 mg

Phosphorous 3 mmol is equivalent to phosphorus 93 mg

Available Dosage Forms

Injection, solution: Potassium 4.4 mEq and phosphorus 3 mmol per mL (5 mL, 15 mL, 50 mL)

General Dosage Range

I.V.:

Children: 0.08-1 mmol phosphate/kg **or** Parenteral nutrition Infusion: 0.5-2 mmol/kg/24 hours

Adults: 0.08-1 mmol phosphate/kg **or** Parenteral nutrition: Infusion: 20-40 mmol/24 hours

Administration

I.V. Injection must be diluted in appropriate I.V. solution and volume prior to administration. In general, the dose, concentration of infusion, and rate of administration may be dependent on patient condition and specific institution policy. Must consider administration precautions for phosphate and potassium when prescribing. **Note:** Due to the potential presence of translucent visible particles, American Regent, Inc recommends the use of a 0.22 micron in-line filter for I.V. administration (1.2 micron filter if admixture contains lipids) (Important Drug Administration Information, American Regent, 2013); a similar recommendation has not been noted by other manufacturers.

For adult patients with severe symptomatic hypophosphatemia (ie, <1.5 mg/dL), may administer at rates up to 15 mmol phosphate/hour (this rate will deliver potassium at 22.5 mEq/hour) (Charron, 2003; Rosen, 1995). Potassium infusion rates >10 mEq/hour should be administered via central line (minimizes burning and phlebitis). ECG monitoring is recommended for potassium infusions >10 mEq/hour in adults or >0.5 mEq/kg/hour in children. In patients with renal dysfunction and/or less severe hypophosphatemia, slower administration rates (eg, over 4-6 hours) or oral repletion is recommended.

Preparation for Administration In general, the dose, concentration of infusion, and rate of administration may be dependent on patient condition and specific institution policy. Intermittent infusion doses of potassium phosphate are typically prepared in 100-250 mL of NS or D$_5$W (usual phosphate concentration range: 0.15-0.6 mmol/mL) (Charron, 2003; Rosen, 1995). Suggested maximum concentrations:

Central line administration: 26.8 mmoL potassium phosphate/100 mL (40 mEq potassium/100 mL)

Peripheral line administration: 6.7 mmoL potassium phosphate/100 mL (10 mEq potassium/100 mL)

Observe the vial for the presence of translucent visible particles. Do not use vial if particles are present. Dilute in a compatible I.V. fluid. **Note:** Due to the potential presence of particulates, American Regent, Inc recommends the use of a 5 micron filter when preparing I.V. sodium phosphate-containing solutions (Important Drug Administration Information, American Regent, 2013); a similar recommendation has not been noted by other manufacturers.

Storage/Stability Store intact vials at 20°C to 25°C (68°F to 77°F); excursions permitted between 15°C and 30°C (59°F and 86°F).

Nursing Actions

Patient Education

- Discuss specific use of drug and side effects with patient as it relates to treatment. (HCAHPS: During this hospital stay, were you given any medicine that you had not taken before? Before giving you any new medicine, how often did hospital staff tell you what the medicine was for? How often did hospital staff describe possible side effects in a way you could understand?)
- Patient may experience dyspepsia, nausea, or diarrhea. Have patient report immediately to prescriber tachycardia, severe dizziness, asthenia, paresthesia, melena, ecchymosis, bleeding, or rash (HCAHPS).
- Educate patient about signs of a significant reaction (eg, wheezing; chest tightness; fever; itching; bad cough; blue skin color; seizures; or swelling of face, lips, tongue, or throat). **Note:** This is not a comprehensive list of all side effects. Patient should consult prescriber for additional questions.

Intended Use and Disclaimer: Should not be printed and given to patients. This information is intended to serve as a concise initial reference for healthcare professionals to use when discussing medications with a patient. You must ultimately rely on your own discretion, experience and judgment in diagnosing, treating and advising patients.

Potassium Phosphate and Sodium Phosphate

(poe TASS ee um FOS fate & SOW dee um FOS fate)

Brand Names: U.S. K-Phos® Neutral; K-Phos® No. 2; Phos-NaK; Phospha 250™ Neutral

Index Terms Neutra-Phos; Sodium Phosphate and Potassium Phosphate

Pharmacologic Category Electrolyte Supplement, Oral

Medication Safety Issues

Sound-alike/look-alike issues:

K-Phos® Neutral may be confused with Neutra-Phos-K®

Pregnancy Risk Factor C

Lactation Excretion in breast milk unknown/use caution

Use Phosphorus supplement; to increase urinary phosphate and pyrophosphate; to acidify the urine to lower calcium concentrations; to increase the antibacterial activity of methenamine; reduce odor and rash caused by ammonia in urine

Available Dosage Forms

Powder for solution, oral:

Phos-NaK: Dibasic potassium phosphate, monobasic potassium phosphate, dibasic sodium phosphate, and monobasic sodium phosphate per packet (100s)

Tablet, oral:

K-Phos® Neutral: Monobasic potassium phosphate 155 mg, dibasic sodium phosphate 852 mg, and monobasic sodium phosphate 130 mg

K-Phos® No. 2: Potassium phosphate 305 mg and sodium phosphate 700 mg

Phospha 250™ Neutral: Monobasic potassium phosphate 155 mg, dibasic sodium phosphate 852 mg, and monobasic sodium phosphate 130 mg

General Dosage Range Oral:

Children ≥4 years and Adolescents: 250 mg elemental phosphorus 4 times daily

Adults: 250-500 mg elemental phosphorus 4 times daily; may be increased to 250 mg elemental phosphorus every 2 hours (maximum daily dose: 2000 mg elemental phosphorus)

Administration

Oral Administer with a full glass of water at mealtime and at bedtime; administration with food may reduce risk of diarrhea.

Oral powder: Phos-NaK: Following dilution of powder with water or juice, solution may be chilled to increase palatability.

Nursing Actions

Patient Education

• Discuss specific use of drug and side effects with patient as it relates to treatment. (HCAHPS: During this hospital stay, were you given any medicine that you had not taken before? Before giving you any new medicine, how often did hospital staff tell you what the medicine was for? How often did hospital staff describe possible side effects in a way you could understand?)

• Patient may experience dyspepsia, nausea, or diarrhea. Have patient report immediately to prescriber tachycardia, severe dizziness, paresthesia, melena, ecchymosis, or bleeding (HCAHPS).

• Educate patient about signs of a significant reaction (eg, wheezing; chest tightness; fever; itching; bad cough; blue skin color; seizures; or swelling of face, lips, tongue, or throat). **Note:** This is not a comprehensive list of all side effects. Patient should consult prescriber for additional questions.

Intended Use and Disclaimer: Should not be printed and given to patients. This information is intended to serve as a concise initial reference for healthcare professionals to use when discussing medications with a patient. You must ultimately rely on your own discretion, experience and judgment in diagnosing, treating and advising patients.

Related Information

Potassium Phosphate *on page 1279*

Pralatrexate (pral a TREX ate)

Brand Names: U.S. Folotyn

Index Terms PDX

Pharmacologic Category Antineoplastic Agent, Antimetabolite; Antineoplastic Agent, Antimetabolite (Antifolate)

Medication Safety Issues

Sound-alike/look-alike issues:

PRALAtrexate may be confused with methotrexate, PEMEtrexed, raltitrexed

Folotyn® may be confused with Focalin®

High alert medication:

This medication is in a class the Institute for Safe Medication Practices (ISMP) includes among its list of drug classes which have a heightened risk of causing significant patient harm when used in error.

Pregnancy Risk Factor D

Lactation Excretion in breast milk unknown/not recommended

Use Treatment of relapsed or refractory peripheral T-cell lymphoma (PTCL)

Unlabeled Use Treatment of relapsed or refractory cutaneous T-cell lymphomas (mycosis fungoides [MF] and Sézary syndrome [SS])

Available Dosage Forms

Solution, Intravenous [preservative free]:

Folotyn: 20 mg/mL (1 mL); 40 mg/2 mL (2 mL)

General Dosage Range Dosage adjustment recommended in patients with renal impairment, hepatic impairment, or who develop toxicities.

I.V.: *Adults:* 30 mg/m^2 once weekly for 6 weeks of a 7-week treatment cycle

Administration

I.V. Administer I.V. push (undiluted) over 3-5 minutes into the line of a free-flowing normal saline I.V.

Hazardous agent; use appropriate precautions for handling and disposal (NIOSH, 2012).

Injectable Detail pH: 7.5-8.5

Nursing Actions

Physical Assessment Drugs with significant renal clearance may affect the levels/effects of pralatrexate. Monitor for mucositis, gastrointestinal disturbance, and renal or hepatic impairment.

Patient Education

• Discuss specific use of drug and side effects with patient as it relates to treatment. (HCAHPS: During this hospital stay, were you given any medicine that you had not taken before? Before giving you any new medicine, how often did hospital staff tell you what the medicine was for? How often did hospital staff describe possible side effects in a way you could understand?) ▶

• Patient may experience anemia, leukopenia, thrombocytopenia, fatigue, nausea, mouth irritation or sores, pharyngitis, epistaxis, edema, constipation, diarrhea, or back pain. Have patient report immediately to prescriber signs of infection, angina, dyspnea, ecchymosis, inability to eat, discolored urine, jaundice, severe skin irritation, rash, or pregnancy (HCAHPS).

• Educate patient about signs of a significant reaction (eg, wheezing; chest tightness; fever; itching; bad cough; blue skin color; seizures; or swelling of face, lips, tongue, or throat). **Note:** This is not a comprehensive list of all side effects. Patient should consult prescriber for additional questions.

Intended Use and Disclaimer: Should not be printed and given to patients. This information is intended to serve as a concise initial reference for healthcare professionals to use when discussing medications with a patient. You must ultimately rely on your own discretion, experience and judgment in diagnosing, treating and advising patients.

Pramipexole (pra mi PEKS ole)

Brand Names: U.S. Mirapex; Mirapex ER
Index Terms Pramipexole Dihydrochloride Monohydrate
Pharmacologic Category Anti-Parkinson's Agent, Dopamine Agonist
Medication Safety Issues
Sound-alike/look-alike issues:
Mirapex® may be confused with Hiprex®, Mifeprex®, MiraLax®
Pregnancy Risk Factor C
Lactation Excretion in breast milk unknown/not recommended
Breast-Feeding Considerations It is not known if pramipexole is excreted into breast milk; however, pramipexole inhibits prolactin secretion in humans and may potentially inhibit lactation. Due to the potential for serious adverse reactions in the nursing infant, the manufacturer recommends a decision be made whether to discontinue nursing or to discontinue the drug, taking into account the importance of treatment to the mother.
Use
Immediate release: Treatment of the signs and symptoms of idiopathic Parkinson's disease; treatment of moderate-to-severe primary Restless Legs Syndrome (RLS)
Extended release: Treatment of the signs and symptoms of idiopathic Parkinson's disease
Unlabeled Use Treatment of depression in bipolar disorder; treatment of fibromyalgia
Mechanism of Action/Effect Pramipexole is a nonergot dopamine agonist with specificity for the D_2 subfamily dopamine receptor, and has also been shown to bind to D_3 and D_4 receptors. By

binding to these receptors, it is thought that pramipexole can stimulate dopamine activity on the nerves of the striatum and substantia nigra.
Contraindications There are no contraindications listed in the manufacturer's labeling.
Warnings/Precautions Caution should be taken in patients with renal insufficiency; dose adjustment may be necessary. May cause or exacerbate dyskinesias; use caution in patients with pre-existing dyskinesias. May cause orthostatic hypotension; Parkinson's disease patients appear to have an impaired capacity to respond to a postural challenge. Use with caution in patients at risk of hypotension or where transient hypotensive episodes would be poorly tolerated. Parkinson's patients being treated with dopaminergic agonists ordinarily require careful monitoring for signs and symptoms of postural hypotension, especially during dose escalation. May cause hallucinations.

Dopamine agonists have been associated with compulsive behaviors and/or loss of impulse control, which has manifested as pathological gambling, libido increases (hypersexuality), and/or binge eating. Causality has not been established, and controversy exists as to whether this phenomenon is related to the underlying disease, prior behaviors/addictions and/or drug therapy. Dose reduction or discontinuation of therapy has been reported to reverse these behaviors in some, but not all cases. Risk for melanoma development is increased in Parkinson's disease patients; drug causation or factors contributing to risk have not been established. Patients should be monitored closely and periodic skin examinations should be performed.

Taper gradually when discontinuing therapy in Parkinson's disease; dopaminergic agents have been associated with a syndrome resembling neuroleptic malignant syndrome on abrupt withdrawal or significant dosage reduction after long-term use. Ergot-derived dopamine agonists have been associated with fibrotic complications (eg, retroperitoneal fibrosis, pleural thickening, and pulmonary infiltrates). Although pramipexole is not an ergot, there have been postmarketing reports of possible fibrotic complications (peritoneal, pleural, pulmonary) with pramipexole; monitor closely for signs and symptoms of fibrosis.

Pramipexole has been associated with somnolence, particularly at higher dosages (>1.5 mg/day). In addition, patients have been reported to fall asleep during activities of daily living, including driving, while taking this medication. Whether these patients exhibited somnolence prior to these events is not clear. Patients should be advised of this issue and factors which may increase risk (sleep disorders, other sedating medications, or concomitant medications which increase pramipexole concentrations) and instructed to report daytime somnolence or sleepiness to the prescriber. Patients should use caution in performing activities which require alertness (driving or operating machinery), and to avoid other medications which may cause CNS depression, including ethanol. Use caution in the elderly as they may be more sensitive to these adverse drug reactions.

Pathologic degenerative changes were observed in the retinas of albino rats during studies with this agent, but were not observed in the retinas of albino mice or in other species. The significance of these data for humans remains uncertain. Augmentation (earlier onset of symptoms in the evening/afternoon, increase and/or spread of symptoms to other extremities) or rebound (shifting of symptoms to early morning hours) may occur in some RLS patients.

Drug Interactions

Avoid Concomitant Use

Avoid concomitant use of Pramipexole with any of the following: Amisulpride; Sulpiride

Decreased Effect

Pramipexole may decrease the levels/effects of: Amisulpride; Antipsychotics (Typical); Sulpiride

The levels/effects of Pramipexole may be decreased by: Amisulpride; Antipsychotics (Atypical); Antipsychotics (Typical); Metoclopramide; Sulpiride

Increased Effect/Toxicity

Pramipexole may increase the levels/effects of: BuPROPion

The levels/effects of Pramipexole may be increased by: Alcohol (Ethyl); Cimetidine; CNS Depressants; MAO Inhibitors; Methylphenidate

Nutritional/Ethanol Interactions

Ethanol: May increase CNS depression; monitor for increased effects with coadministration. Caution patients about effects.

Food: Food intake does not affect the extent of drug absorption although the time to maximal plasma concentration is delayed when taken with a meal.

Herb/Nutraceutical: Avoid valerian, St John's wort, SAMe, kava kava (may increase risk of serotonin syndrome and/or excessive sedation).

Adverse Reactions

Parkinson's disease: Actual frequency may be dependent on dose and/or formulation:

>10%:

Cardiovascular: Orthostatic hypotension (dose related; ≤53%)

Central nervous system: Somnolence (dose related; 9% to 36%), extrapyramidal syndrome (28%), insomnia (4% to 27%), dizziness (2% to 26%), hallucinations (5% to 17%), abnormal dreams (11%), headache (4% to 7%)

Gastrointestinal: Nausea (dose related; 11% to 28%), constipation (dose related; 6% to 14%)

Neuromuscular & skeletal: Dyskinesia (17% to 47%), weakness (1% to 14%)

Miscellaneous: Accidental injury (17%)

1% to 10%:

Cardiovascular: Edema (2% to 8%), chest pain (3%)

Central nervous system: Confusion (4% to 10%), dystonia (2% to 8%), fatigue (6%), amnesia (dose related; 4% to 6%), sudden onset of sleep (3% to 6%), vertigo (2% to 4%), hypesthesia (3%), abnormal thinking (2% to 3%), akathisia (2% to 3%), malaise (2% to 3%), paranoia (2%), sleep disorder (1% to 3%), depression (≤2%), delusions (1%), fever (1%), myoclonus (1%)

Endocrine & metabolic: Libido decreased (1%)

Gastrointestinal: Xerostomia (4% to 7%), anorexia (1% to 5%), vomiting (4%), abdominal discomfort/pain (1% to 4%), dyspepsia (3%), appetite increased (2% to 3%), dysphagia (2%), weight loss (2%), salivary hypersecretion (≤2%), diarrhea (1% to 2%)

Genitourinary: Urinary frequency (6%), urinary tract infection (4%), impotence (2%), urinary incontinence (2%)

Neuromuscular & skeletal: Gait abnormalities (7%), hypertonia (7%), muscle spasm (3% to 5%), falls (4%), arthritis (3%), tremor (3%), back pain (2% to 3%), bursitis (2%), muscle twitching (2%), balance abnormalities (≤2%), CPK increased (1%), myasthenia (1%)

Ocular: Accommodation abnormalities (4%), vision abnormalities (3%), diplopia (1%)

Respiratory: Dyspnea (4%), cough (3%), rhinitis (3%), pneumonia (2%)

Restless legs syndrome: Actual frequency may be dependent on dose:

>10%:

Central nervous system: Headache (16%), insomnia (9% to 13%)

Gastrointestinal: Nausea (11% to 27%)

1% to 10%:

Central nervous system: Fatigue (3% to 9%), abnormal dreams (1% to 8%), somnolence (6%)

Gastrointestinal: Diarrhea (1% to 7%), constipation (4%), xerostomia (3%)

Neuromuscular & skeletal: Limb pain (3% to 7%)

Respiratory: Nasal congestion (≤6%)

Miscellaneous: Influenza (1% to 7%)

Available Dosage Forms

Tablet, Oral:

Mirapex: 0.125 mg, 0.25 mg, 0.5 mg, 0.75 mg, 1 mg, 1.5 mg

Generic: 0.125 mg, 0.25 mg, 0.5 mg, 0.75 mg, 1 mg, 1.5 mg

Tablet Extended Release 24 Hour, Oral:

Mirapex ER: 0.375 mg, 0.75 mg, 1.5 mg, 2.25 mg, 3 mg, 3.75 mg, 4.5 mg

General Dosage Range Dosage adjustment recommended in patients with renal impairment

Oral: Immediate release: *Adults:* Initial: 0.125 mg 3 times daily **or** 0.125 mg once daily before bedtime; Maintenance: 0.5-1.5 mg 3 times daily **or** 0.125-0.5 mg once daily before bedtime

Oral: Extended release: *Adults:* 0.375-4.5 mg once daily

Administration

Oral Doses should be titrated gradually in all patients to avoid the onset of intolerable side effects. The dosage should be increased to achieve a maximum therapeutic effect, balanced against the side effects of dyskinesia, hallucinations, somnolence, and dry mouth. May be administered with or without food; may be administered with food to decrease nausea. Extended release tablets should be swallowed whole and not chewed, crushed, or divided.

Storage/Stability Store at 25°C (77°F); excursions permitted to 15°C to 30°C (59°F to 86°F). Protect from light and high humidity.

Nursing Actions

Physical Assessment Monitor blood pressure when patient lying down and standing; orthostasis can be a problem. Assess degree of somnolence.

Monitor for sleep disorders, hallucinations, and falls. Monitor for symptoms of dyskinesia, dizziness, confusion, weight loss, joint pain, frequent urination, swelling of extremities, chest pain, shortness of breath, dark-colored urine, and muscle stiffness. Educate patient about getting up slowly to prevent dizziness and falls.

Patient Education
- Discuss specific use of drug and side effects with patient as it relates to treatment. (HCAHPS: During this hospital stay, were you given any medicine that you had not taken before? Before giving you any new medicine, how often did hospital staff tell you what the medicine was for? How often did hospital staff describe possible side effects in a way you could understand?)
- Patient may experience presyncope, fatigue, blurred vision, illogical thinking, dizziness, headache, hallucinations, nausea, constipation, or insomnia. Have patient report immediately to prescriber narcolepsy, uncontrollable compulsions, significant change in balance, or severe asthenia (HCAHPS).
- Educate patient about signs of a significant reaction (eg, wheezing; chest tightness; fever; itching; bad cough; blue skin color; seizures; or swelling of face, lips, tongue, or throat). **Note:** This is not a comprehensive list of all side effects. Patient should consult prescriber for additional questions.

Intended Use and Disclaimer: Should not be printed and given to patients. This information is intended to serve as a concise initial reference for healthcare professionals to use when discussing medications with a patient. You must ultimately rely on your own discretion, experience and judgment in diagnosing, treating and advising patients.

Dietary Considerations May be taken with or without food. May be taken with food to decrease nausea.

Pramlintide (PRAM lin tide)

Brand Names: U.S. SymlinPen 120; SymlinPen 60

Index Terms Pramlintide Acetate

Pharmacologic Category Amylinomimetic; Antidiabetic Agent

Medication Safety Issues

High alert medication:

The Institute for Safe Medication Practices (ISMP) includes this medication among its list of drug classes which have a heightened risk of causing significant patient harm when used in error.

Medication Guide Available Yes

Pregnancy Risk Factor C

Lactation Excretion in breast milk unknown/not recommended

Breast-Feeding Considerations It is not known if pramlintide is present in breast milk. The manufacturer recommends that pramlintide be used in nursing women only when the potential benefit to the mother outweighs the possible risk to the infant.

Use

Adjunctive treatment with mealtime insulin in type 1 diabetes mellitus (insulin dependent, IDDM) patients who have failed to achieve desired glucose control despite optimal insulin therapy

Adjunctive treatment with mealtime insulin in type 2 diabetes mellitus (noninsulin dependent, NIDDM) patients who have failed to achieve desired glucose control despite optimal insulin therapy, with or without concurrent sulfonylurea and/or metformin

Mechanism of Action/Effect Human amylin analog which, in conjunction with insulin, reduces postprandial glucose

Contraindications Hypersensitivity to pramlintide or any component of the formulation; confirmed diagnosis of gastroparesis; hypoglycemia unawareness

Warnings/Precautions [U.S. Boxed Warning]: Coadministration with insulin may induce severe hypoglycemia (usually within 3 hours following administration); coadministration with insulin therapy is an approved indication but does require an initial dosage reduction of insulin and frequent pre and post blood glucose monitoring to reduce risk of severe hypoglycemia. Concurrent use of other glucose-lowering agents may increase risk of hypoglycemia. Avoid use in patients with poor compliance with their insulin regimen and/or blood glucose monitoring. Do not use in patients with HbA_{1c} levels >9% or recent, recurrent episodes of hypoglycemia; obtain detailed history of glucose control (eg, HbA$_{1c}$, incidence of hypoglycemia, glucose monitoring, and medication compliance) and body weight before initiating therapy. Use caution in patients with visual or dexterity impairment. Use caution when driving or operating heavy machinery until effects on blood sugar are known. Use caution with certain antihypertensive agents (eg, beta-adrenergic blockers) which may mask signs/symptoms of hypoglycemia. Avoid use in patients with conditions or concurrent medications likely to impair gastric motility (eg, anticholinergics); do not use in patients requiring medication(s) to stimulate gastric emptying. According to the Centers for Disease Control and Prevention (CDC), pen-shaped injection devices should never be used for more than one person (even when the needle is changed) because of the risk of infection. The injection device should be clearly labeled with individual patient information to ensure that the correct pen is used (CDC, 2012).

Drug Interactions

Avoid Concomitant Use There are no known interactions where it is recommended to avoid concomitant use.

Decreased Effect There are no known significant interactions involving a decrease in effect.

Increased Effect/Toxicity
Pramlintide may increase the levels/effects of: Anticholinergics

Nutritional/Ethanol Interactions

Ethanol: Use caution with ethanol (may increase hypoglycemia).

Herb/Nutraceutical: Use caution with garlic, chromium, gymnema (may increase hypoglycemia).

Adverse Reactions

>10%:

Central nervous system: Headache (5% to 13%)

Gastrointestinal: Nausea (28% to 48%), vomiting (7% to 11%), anorexia (≤17%)

Endocrine & metabolic: Severe hypoglycemia (type 1 diabetes ≤17%)

Miscellaneous: Inflicted injury (8% to 14%)

1% to 10%:

Central nervous system: Fatigue (3% to 7%), dizziness (2% to 6%)

Endocrine & metabolic: Severe hypoglycemia (type 2 diabetes ≤8%)

Gastrointestinal: Abdominal pain (2% to 8%)

Respiratory: Pharyngitis (3% to 5%), cough (2% to 6%)

Neuromuscular & skeletal: Arthralgia (2% to 7%)

Miscellaneous: Allergic reaction (≤6%)

Pharmacodynamics/Kinetics

Duration of Action 3 hours

Available Dosage Forms

Solution, Subcutaneous:

SymlinPen 60: 1500 mcg/1.5 mL (1.5 mL)

SymlinPen 120: 2700 mcg/2.7 mL (2.7 mL)

General Dosage Range SubQ: *Adults:*

Type 1 diabetes mellitus (insulin dependent, IDDM): Initial: 15 mcg immediately prior to meals; Target dose: 30-60 mcg prior to meals

Type 2 diabetes mellitus (noninsulin dependent, NIDDM): Initial: 60 mcg immediately prior to meals; after 3-7 days increase to 120 mcg prior to meals

Administration

Subcutaneous Do not mix with insulins; administer subcutaneously into abdominal or thigh areas at sites distinct from concomitant insulin injections (do not administer into arm due to variable absorption); rotate injection sites frequently. Allow solution to reach room temperature before administering; may reduce injection site reactions. For oral medications in which a rapid onset of action is desired, administer 1 hour before, or 2 hours after pramlintide, if possible. Do not transfer drug from the pen injector to a syringe; dosing errors could occur.

Storage/Stability Store at 2°C to 8°C (36°F to 46°F); do not freeze. After initial use, may be kept refrigerated or at room temperature ≤30°C (≤86°F); discard after 30 days. Protect from light.

Nursing Actions

Physical Assessment Monitor for hypoglycemia. Teach patient appropriate injection techniques and syringe/needle disposal.

Patient Education

• Discuss specific use of drug and side effects with patient as it relates to treatment. (HCAHPS: During this hospital stay, were you given any medicine that you had not taken before? Before giving you any new medicine, how often did hospital staff tell you what the medicine was for? How often did hospital staff describe possible side effects in a way you could understand?)

• Patient may experience hypoglycemia, headache, nausea, weight loss, lack of appetite, or application site irritation. Have patient report immediately to prescriber signs of infection or rash (HCAHPS).

• Educate patient about signs of a significant reaction (eg, wheezing; chest tightness; fever; itching; bad cough; blue skin color; seizures; or swelling of face, lips, tongue, or throat). **Note:** This is not a comprehensive list of all side effects. Patient should consult prescriber for additional questions.

Intended Use and Disclaimer: Should not be printed and given to patients. This information is intended to serve as a concise initial reference for healthcare professionals to use when discussing medications with a patient. You must ultimately rely on your own discretion, experience and judgment in diagnosing, treating and advising patients.

▶

Dietary Considerations Dietary modification based on ADA recommendations is a part of therapy; pramlintide to be administered prior to major meals consisting of ≥250 Kcal or ≥30 g carbohydrates

---

Prasugrel (PRA soo grel)

Brand Names: U.S. Effient
Index Terms CS-747; LY-640315; Prasugrel Hydrochloride
Pharmacologic Category Antiplatelet Agent; Antiplatelet Agent, Thienopyridine
Medication Safety Issues
Sound-alike/look-alike issues:
Prasugrel may be confused with pravastatin, propranolol
BEERS Criteria medication:
This drug may be potentially inappropriate for use in geriatric patients (Quality of evidence - moderate; Strength of recommendation - weak).
Medication Guide Available Yes
Pregnancy Risk Factor B
Lactation Excretion in breast milk unknown/use caution
Breast-Feeding Considerations It is not known if prasugrel is excreted into breast milk. According to the manufacturer, use in nursing women only if the potential benefit to the mother is greater than the possible risk to the infant.
Use Acute coronary syndrome to be managed with percutaneous coronary intervention (PCI): To reduce the rate of thrombotic cardiovascular events (including stent thrombosis) in patients who are to be managed with PCI for unstable angina (UA), non-ST-segment elevation MI (NSTEMI), or ST-elevation MI (STEMI).
Unlabeled Use Initial treatment of UA/NSTEMI in patients undergoing PCI with allergy or major gastrointestinal intolerance to aspirin (**Note:** Dual antiplatelet therapy with another P2Y12 receptor inhibitor is not recommended in this situation [Jneid, 2012].)
Mechanism of Action/Effect Irreversibly blocks platelet activation and aggregation
Contraindications Active pathological bleeding such as peptic ulcer or intracranial hemorrhage; prior TIA or stroke; hypersensitivity (eg, anaphylaxis) to prasugrel or any component of the formulation.
Warnings/Precautions [U.S. Boxed Warning]: May cause significant or fatal bleeding. Use is contraindicated in patients with active pathological bleeding or history of TIA or stroke. Use with caution in patients who may be at risk of increased bleeding, including patients with active PUD, recent or recurrent GI bleeding, severe hepatic impairment, end-stage renal disease (ESRD), trauma, or surgery. Additional risk factors include body weight <60 kg, CABG or other surgical

procedure, concomitant use of medications that increase risk of bleeding.

[U.S. Boxed Warning]: In patients ≥75 years, use is generally not recommended due to increased risk of fatal and intracranial bleeding and uncertain benefit; use may be considered in high-risk situations (eg, patients with diabetes or history of MI). Risk of bleeding is increased in older adults (Beers Criteria). **[U.S. Boxed Warning]: Do not initiate therapy in patients likely to undergo urgent CABG surgery; when possible, discontinue ≥7 days prior to any surgery; increased risk of bleeding.** The American College of Chest Physicians (ACCP) recommends discontinuing prasugrel 5 days before surgery (Guyatt, 2012). When urgent CABG is necessary, the ACCF/AHA CABG guidelines suggest that it may be reasonable to perform surgery within 7 days of discontinuing prasugrel (Hillis, 2011).

Hypersensitivity, including angioedema, has been reported, including in patients with a previous history of thienopyridine hypersensitivity. Because of structural similarities, cross-reactivity is possible among the thienopyridines (clopidogrel, prasugrel, and ticlopidine); use with caution or avoid in patients with previous history of thienopyridine hypersensitivity. Use of prasugrel is contraindicated in patients with hypersensitivity (eg, anaphylaxis) to prasugrel. If necessary, discontinue therapy for active bleeding, elective surgery, stroke, or TIA; reinitiate therapy as soon as possible unless patient suffers stroke or TIA where subsequent use is contraindicated. If possible, manage bleeding without discontinuing prasugrel. Potentially significant drug-drug interactions may exist, requiring dose or frequency adjustment, additional monitoring, and/or selection of alternative therapy. Use caution in concurrent treatment with mediations that increase the risk of bleeding (eg, oral anticoagulants, NSAIDs, or fibrinolytics; bleeding risk is increased. Use with caution in patients with severe hepatic impairment or end-stage renal disease (patients are generally are at higher risk of bleeding). Cases of thrombotic thrombocytopenic purpura (TTP) (usually occurring within the first 2 weeks of therapy), resulting in some fatalities, have been reported with prasugrel; urgent plasmapheresis is required. In patients <60 kg, risk of bleeding increased; consider lower maintenance dose.

Drug Interactions
Avoid Concomitant Use
Avoid concomitant use of Prasugrel with any of the following: Urokinase
Decreased Effect
The levels/effects of Prasugrel may be decreased by: CYP3A4 Inhibitors (Strong); Nonsteroidal Anti-Inflammatory Agents; Ranitidine; Rifampin

Increased Effect/Toxicity

Prasugrel may increase the levels/effects of: Agents with Antiplatelet Properties; Anticoagulants; Collagenase (Systemic); Dabigatran Etexilate; Ibritumomab; Rivaroxaban; Salicylates; Thrombolytic Agents; Tositumomab and Iodine I 131 Tositumomab; Urokinase

The levels/effects of Prasugrel may be increased by: Dasatinib; Glucosamine; Herbs (Anticoagulant/Antiplatelet Properties); Ibrutinib; Multivitamins/Fluoride (with ADE); Multivitamins/Minerals (with ADEK, Folate, Iron); Multivitamins/Minerals (with AE, No Iron); Nonsteroidal Anti-Inflammatory Agents; Omega-3 Fatty Acids; Pentosan Polysulfate Sodium; Pentoxifylline; Prostacyclin Analogues; Tipranavir; Vitamin E

Adverse Reactions As with all drugs which may affect hemostasis, bleeding is associated with prasugrel. Hemorrhage may occur at virtually any site. Risk is dependent on multiple variables, including patient susceptibility and concurrent use of multiple agents which alter hemostasis.

2% to 10%:

Cardiovascular: Hypertension (8%), hypotension (4%), atrial fibrillation (3%), bradycardia (3%), noncardiac chest pain (3%), peripheral edema (3%)

Central nervous system: Headache (6%), dizziness (4%), fatigue (4%), fever (3%), extremity pain (3%)

Dermatologic: Rash (3%)

Endocrine & metabolic: Hypercholesterolemia/hyperlipidemia (7%)

Gastrointestinal: Nausea (5%), diarrhea (2%), gastrointestinal hemorrhage (2%)

Hematologic: Leukopenia (3%), anemia (2%)

Neuromuscular & skeletal: Back pain (5%)

Respiratory: Epistaxis (6%), dyspnea (5%), cough (4%)

Pharmacodynamics/Kinetics

Onset of Action Inhibition of platelet aggregation (IPA): Dose dependent: 60 mg loading dose: <30 minutes; median time to reach ≥20% IPA: 30 minutes (Brandt, 2007)

Peak effect: Time to maximal IPA: Dose-dependent: **Note:** Degree of IPA based on adenosine diphosphate (ADP) concentration used during light aggregometry: 60 mg loading dose: Occurs ~4 hours post administration; Mean IPA (ADP 5 micromol/L): ~84.1%; Mean IPA (ADP 20 micromole/L): ~78.8% (Brandt, 2007)

Duration of Action Duration of effect: Platelet aggregation gradually returns to baseline values over 5-9 days after discontinuation; reflective of new platelet production

Available Dosage Forms

Tablet, Oral:

Effient: 5 mg, 10 mg

General Dosage Range Oral: *Adults:* Loading dose: 60 mg; Maintenance dose: 10 mg once daily (in combination with aspirin 75-325 mg/day)

Administration

Oral Administer without regard to meals. Per the prescribing information, do not break the tablet. According to the manufacturer, however, chewing, breaking, or crushing the tablet is not expected to alter the stability or potency of prasugrel if administered immediately (not evaluated). Therefore, if it becomes necessary, tablets may be chewed and swallowed (bitter to taste) or crushed and mixed in food or liquid (eg, applesauce, juice, or water) and immediately administered by mouth or gastric tube. **Note:** Administration via an enteral tube that bypasses the acidic environment of the stomach may result in reduced bioavailability of prasugrel (data on file, Daiichi Sankyo-Lilly, 2012).

Storage/Stability Store at 25°C (77°F); excursions are permitted between 15°C and 30°C (59°F and 86°F).

Nursing Actions

Physical Assessment Monitor for signs and symptoms of bleeding. Educate patient regarding bleeding precautions like use of electric razor. Hold pressure on cuts for 5 minutes or until bleeding stops. Educate patient about sharing medication history with doctors, dentists, and surgeons.

Patient Education

• Discuss specific use of drug and side effects with patient as it relates to treatment. (HCAHPS: During this hospital stay, were you given any medicine that you had not taken before? Before giving you any new medicine, how often did hospital staff tell you what the medicine was for? How often did hospital staff describe possible side effects in a way you could understand?)

• Patient may experience dizziness, nausea, or headache. Have patient report immediately to prescriber angina, strength differences from one side to another, difficulty speaking or thinking, change in balance, blurred vision, dyspnea, illogical thinking, melena, hematuria, ecchymosis, bleeding, petechiae, jaundice, significant asthenia, sudden vision changes, or rash (HCAHPS).

• Educate patient about signs of a significant reaction (eg, wheezing; chest tightness; fever; itching; bad cough; blue skin color; seizures; or swelling of face, lips, tongue, or throat). **Note:** This is not a comprehensive list of all side effects. Patient should consult prescriber for additional questions.

Intended Use and Disclaimer: Should not be printed and given to patients. This information is intended to serve as a concise initial reference for healthcare professionals to use when discussing medications with a patient. You must ultimately

rely on your own discretion, experience and judgment in diagnosing, treating and advising patients.

Pravastatin (prav a STAT in)

Brand Names: U.S. Pravachol
Index Terms Pravastatin Sodium
Pharmacologic Category Antilipemic Agent, HMG-CoA Reductase Inhibitor
Medication Safety Issues
Sound-alike/look-alike issues:
Pravachol may be confused with atorvaSTATin, Prevacid, Prinivil, propranolol
Pravastatin may be confused with nystatin, pitavastatin, prasugrel
Pregnancy Risk Factor X
Lactation Enters breast milk/contraindicated
Breast-Feeding Considerations A small amount of pravastatin is excreted into breast milk. Data is available from eight lactating females administered pravastatin 20 mg twice daily for 2.5 days. After the fifth dose, maximum maternal serum concentrations were ~40 ng/mL (pravastatin) and ~26 ng/mL (metabolite) and maximum milk concentrations were ~3.9 ng/mL (pravastatin) and ~2.1 ng/mL (metabolite). Maximum milk concentrations were detected ~3 hours after the dose (Pan, 1988). Due to the potential for serious adverse reactions in a nursing infant, use while breast-feeding is contraindicated by the manufacturer.
Use Use with dietary therapy for the following:
Primary prevention of coronary events: In hypercholesterolemic patients without established coronary heart disease to reduce cardiovascular morbidity (myocardial infarction, coronary revascularization procedures) and mortality.
Secondary prevention of cardiovascular events in patients with established coronary heart disease: To slow the progression of coronary atherosclerosis; to reduce cardiovascular morbidity (myocardial infarction, coronary vascular procedures) and to reduce mortality; to reduce the risk of stroke and transient ischemic attacks
Primary and secondary prevention of atherosclerotic cardiovascular disease (ASCVD) according to the American College of Cardiology/American Heart Association: To reduce the risk of ASCVD in patients with clinical ASCVD (eg, coronary heart disease, stroke/TIA, or peripheral arterial disease presumed to be of atherosclerotic origin) who are greater than 75 years of age or not a candidate for high-intensity statin therapy; in patients without clinical ASCVD if LDL-C is 190 mg/dL or greater and not a candidate for high-intensity statin therapy; in patients without clinical ASCVD who have type 1 or type 2 diabetes and are between 40 and 75 years of age; in patients with an estimated 10-year ASCVD risk 7.5% or greater and who are between 40 and 75 years of age.

Hyperlipidemias: Reduce elevations in total cholesterol, LDL-C, apolipoprotein B, and triglycerides (elevations of 1 or more components are present in Fredrickson type IIa, IIb, III, and IV hyperlipidemias)
Heterozygous familial hypercholesterolemia (HeFH): In pediatric patients, 8-18 years of age, with HeFH having LDL-C ≥190 mg/dL or LDL ≥160 mg/dL with positive family history of premature cardiovascular disease (CVD) or 2 or more CVD risk factors in the pediatric patient
Mechanism of Action/Effect Pravastatin is a competitive inhibitor of 3-hydroxy-3-methylglutaryl coenzyme A (HMG-CoA) reductase, which is the rate-limiting enzyme involved in *de novo* cholesterol synthesis.
Contraindications Hypersensitivity to pravastatin or any component of the formulation; active liver disease; unexplained persistent elevations of serum transaminases; pregnancy; breast-feeding
Warnings/Precautions Secondary causes of hyperlipidemia should be ruled out prior to therapy. Liver function must be monitored by periodic laboratory assessment. Rhabdomyolysis with acute renal failure has occurred. Risk may be increased with concurrent use of other drugs which may cause rhabdomyolysis (including colchicine, gemfibrozil, fibric acid derivatives, or niacin at doses ≥1 g/day). Discontinue in any patient in which CPK levels are markedly elevated (>10 times ULN) or if myopathy is suspected/diagnosed. Immune-mediated necrotizing myopathy (IMNM), an autoimmune-mediated myopathy, has been reported (rarely) with HMG-CoA reductase inhibitor therapy. IMNM presents as proximal muscle weakness with elevated CPK levels, which persists despite discontinuation of HMG-CoA reductase inhibitor therapy; additionally, muscle biopsy may show necrotizing myopathy with limited inflammation; immunosuppressive therapy (eg, corticosteroids, azathioprine) may be used for treatment. The manufacturer recommends temporary discontinuation for elective major surgery, acute medical or surgical conditions, or in any patient experiencing an acute or serious condition predisposing to renal failure (eg, sepsis, hypotension, trauma, uncontrolled seizures). However, based upon current evidence, HMG-CoA reductase inhibitor therapy should be continued in the perioperative period unless risk outweighs cardioprotective benefit. Use with caution in patients with advanced age, these patients are predisposed to myopathy. Use caution in patients with previous liver disease or heavy ethanol use. If serious hepatotoxicity with clinical symptoms and/or hyperbilirubinemia or jaundice occurs during treatment, interrupt therapy. If an alternate etiology is not identified, do not restart pravastatin. Liver enzyme tests should be obtained at baseline and as clinically indicated; routine periodic monitoring of liver enzymes is not necessary. Increases in Hb A_{1c} and fasting blood

glucose have been reported with HMG-CoA reductase inhibitors; however, the benefits of statin therapy far outweigh the risk of dysglycemia. Treatment in patients <8 years of age is not recommended.

Drug Interactions

Avoid Concomitant Use

Avoid concomitant use of Pravastatin with any of the following: Fusidic Acid (Systemic); Gemfibrozil; Pimozide; Red Yeast Rice

Decreased Effect

Pravastatin may decrease the levels/effects of: Lanthanum

The levels/effects of Pravastatin may be decreased by: Antacids; Bile Acid Sequestrants; Efavirenz; Fosphenytoin; Nelfinavir; P-glycoprotein/ABCB1 Inducers; Phenytoin; Rifamycin Derivatives; Saquinavir

Increased Effect/Toxicity

Pravastatin may increase the levels/effects of: ARIPiprazole; CycloSPORINE (Systemic); DAPTOmycin; Dofetilide; Lomitapide; PARoxetine; PAZOPanib; Pimozide; Trabectedin; Vitamin K Antagonists

The levels/effects of Pravastatin may be increased by: Bezafibrate; Boceprevir; Clarithromycin; Colchicine; CycloSPORINE (Systemic); Darunavir; Eltrombopag; Erythromycin (Systemic); Fenofibrate and Derivatives; Fusidic Acid (Systemic); Gemfibrozil; Itraconazole; Niacin; Niacinamide; P-glycoprotein/ABCB1 Inhibitors; Raltegravir; Red Yeast Rice; Simeprevir; Telaprevir; Telithromycin

Nutritional/Ethanol Interactions

Ethanol: Consumption of large amounts of ethanol may increase the risk of liver damage with HMG-CoA reductase inhibitors.

Food: Red yeast rice contains an estimated 2.4 mg lovastatin per 600 mg rice.

Herb/Nutraceutical: St John's wort may decrease pravastatin levels.

Adverse Reactions As reported in short-term trials; safety and tolerability with long-term use were similar to placebo

1% to 10%:

Cardiovascular: Chest pain (4%)

Central nervous system: Headache (2% to 6%), fatigue (4%), dizziness (1% to 3%)

Dermatologic: Rash (4%)

Gastrointestinal: Nausea/vomiting (7%), diarrhea (6%), heartburn (3%)

Hepatic: Transaminases increased (>3x normal on two occasions: 1%)

Neuromuscular & skeletal: Myalgia (2%)

Respiratory: Cough (3%)

Miscellaneous: Influenza (2%)

Additional class-related events or case reports (not necessarily reported with pravastatin therapy): Angioedema, blood glucose increased, cataracts, depression, diabetes mellitus (new onset), dyspnea, eosinophilia, erectile dysfunction, facial paresis, glycosylated hemoglobin (Hb A_{1c}) increased, hypersensitivity reaction, immune-mediated necrotizing myopathy (IMNM), impaired extraocular muscle movement, impotence, interstitial lung disease, leukopenia, malaise, memory loss, ophthalmoplegia, paresthesia, peripheral neuropathy, photosensitivity, psychic disturbance, skin discoloration, thrombocytopenia, thyroid dysfunction, toxic epidermal necrolysis, transaminases increased, vomiting

Pharmacodynamics/Kinetics

Onset of Action Several days; Peak effect: 4 weeks

Available Dosage Forms

Tablet, Oral:

Pravachol: 20 mg, 40 mg, 80 mg

Generic: 10 mg, 20 mg, 40 mg, 80 mg

General Dosage Range Dosage adjustment recommended in patients with hepatic or renal impairment or on concomitant therapy

Oral:

Children 8-13 years: 20 mg once daily

Children 14-18 years: 40 mg once daily

Adults: Initial: 10-40 mg once daily; Maintenance: 10-80 mg once daily (maximum: 80 mg/day)

Administration

Oral May be administered without regard to meals.

Storage/Stability Store at 25°C (77°F); excursions permitted to 15°C to 30°C (59°F to 86°F). Protect from moisture and light.

Nursing Actions

Physical Assessment Monitor for signs and symptoms of myopathy (muscle pain and weakness, fatigue). Assess risk potential for interactions with other prescriptions or herbal products patient may be taking that may increase risk of myopathy or rhabdomyolysis. Teach proper diet and exercise regimen.

Patient Education

• Discuss specific use of drug and side effects with patient as it relates to treatment. (HCAHPS: During this hospital stay, were you given any medicine that you had not taken before? Before giving you any new medicine, how often did hospital staff tell you what the medicine was for? How often did hospital staff describe possible side effects in a way you could understand?)

• Patient may experience headache, dyspepsia, asthenia, arthralgia, dizziness, or diarrhea. Have patient report immediately to prescriber flu-like syndrome, ecchymosis, bleeding, discolored urine, jaundice, or rash (HCAHPS).

• Educate patient about signs of a significant reaction (eg, wheezing; chest tightness; fever; itching; bad cough; blue skin color; seizures; or swelling of face, lips, tongue, or throat). **Note:** This is not a comprehensive list of all side effects. Patient should consult prescriber for additional questions.

Intended Use and Disclaimer: Should not be printed and given to patients. This information is intended to serve as a concise initial reference for healthcare professionals to use when discussing medications with a patient. You must ultimately rely on your own discretion, experience and judgment in diagnosing, treating and advising patients.

Dietary Considerations May be taken without regard to meals. Before initiation of therapy, patients should be placed on a standard cholesterol-lowering diet for 6 weeks and the diet should be continued during drug therapy. Red yeast rice contains an estimated 2.4 mg lovastatin per 600 mg rice.

PrednisoLONE (Systemic)
(pred NISS oh lone)

Brand Names: U.S. Flo-Pred; Millipred; Millipred DP; Millipred DP 12-Day; Orapred; Orapred ODT; Pediapred; Prelone; Veripred 20

Index Terms Prednisolone Sodium Phosphate

Pharmacologic Category Corticosteroid, Systemic

Medication Safety Issues
Sound-alike/look-alike issues:
PrednisoLONE may be confused with predniSONE
Pediapred may be confused with Pediazole
Prelone may be confused with PROzac

Pregnancy Risk Factor C/D (manufacturer specific)

Lactation Enters breast milk/use caution

Breast-Feeding Considerations Prednisolone is excreted into breast milk. In one study (n=6), milk concentrations were 5% to 25% of the maternal serum concentration with peak concentrations occurring ~1 hour after the maternal dose. The milk/plasma ratio was found to be 0.2 with doses ≥30 mg/day and 0.1 with doses <30 mg/day. Following a maternal dose of prednisolone 80 mg/day, it was calculated that a breast-feeding infant would ingest <0.1% of the maternal dose (Ost, 1985). One manufacturer notes that when used systemically, maternal use of corticosteroids have the potential to cause adverse events in a nursing infant (eg, growth suppression, interfere with endogenous corticosteroid production) and therefore caution should be used when administered to nursing women. In order to decrease potential exposure to a nursing infant, one manufacturer recommends administering the dose after nursing, at the time of day with the longest interval between feeds. Other sources recommend waiting 4 hours after the maternal dose before breast-feeding (Bae, 2012; Leachman, 2006; Makol, 2011; Ost, 1985). Other guidelines note that maternal use of systemic corticosteroids is not a contraindication to breast-feeding (NAEPP, 2005).

Use Treatment of endocrine disorders, rheumatic disorders, collagen diseases, allergic states, respiratory diseases, hematologic disorders, neoplastic diseases, edematous states, and gastrointestinal diseases; resolution of acute exacerbations of multiple sclerosis; management of fulminating or disseminated tuberculosis and trichinosis; acute or chronic solid organ rejection

Unlabeled Use Severe alcoholic hepatitis; Bell's palsy; acute exacerbations of chronic obstructive pulmonary disease (COPD)

Mechanism of Action/Effect Decreases inflammation by suppression of migration of polymorphonuclear leukocytes and reversal of increased capillary permeability; suppresses the immune system by reducing activity and volume of the lymphatic system

Contraindications Hypersensitivity to prednisolone or any component of the formulation; acute superficial herpes simplex keratitis; live or attenuated virus vaccines (with immunosuppressive doses of corticosteroids); systemic fungal infections; varicella

Warnings/Precautions May cause hypercorticism or suppression of hypothalamic-pituitary-adrenal (HPA) axis, particularly in younger children or in patients receiving high doses for prolonged periods. HPA axis suppression may lead to adrenal crisis. Withdrawal and discontinuation of a corticosteroid should be done slowly and carefully. Particular care is required when patients are transferred from systemic corticosteroids to inhaled products due to possible adrenal insufficiency or withdrawal from steroids, including an increase in allergic symptoms. Patients receiving >20 mg per day of prednisone (or equivalent) may be most susceptible. Fatalities have occurred due to adrenal insufficiency in asthmatic patients during and after transfer from systemic corticosteroids to aerosol steroids; aerosol steroids do **not** provide the systemic steroid needed to treat patients having trauma, surgery, or infections.

Acute myopathy has been reported with high dose corticosteroids, usually in patients with neuromuscular transmission disorders; may involve ocular and/or respiratory muscles; monitor creatine kinase; recovery may be delayed. Corticosteroid use may cause psychiatric disturbances, including depression, euphoria, insomnia, mood swings, and personality changes. Pre-existing psychiatric conditions may be exacerbated by corticosteroid use. Prolonged use of corticosteroids may also increase the incidence of secondary infection, mask acute infection (including fungal infections), prolong or exacerbate viral infections, or limit response to vaccines. Exposure to chickenpox should be avoided; corticosteroids should not be used to treat ocular herpes simplex. Corticosteroids should not be used for cerebral malaria or viral hepatitis. Close observation is required in patients with latent tuberculosis and/or TB reactivity; restrict use in active TB (only in conjunction with antituberculosis treatment). Prolonged use of corticosteroids may result in glaucoma; cataract formation may occur. Prolonged treatment with corticosteroids has been associated with the development of Kaposi's sarcoma (case reports); if noted, discontinuation of therapy should be considered.

Use with caution in patients with thyroid disease, hepatic impairment, renal impairment, cardiovascular disease, diabetes, glaucoma, cataracts, myasthenia gravis, patients at risk for osteoporosis, patients at risk for seizures, or GI diseases (diverticulitis, peptic ulcer, ulcerative colitis) due to perforation risk. Use caution following acute MI (corticosteroids have been associated with myocardial rupture). Because of the risk of adverse effects, systemic corticosteroids should be used cautiously in the elderly in the smallest possible effective dose for the shortest duration. Withdraw therapy with gradual tapering of dose. May affect growth velocity; growth should be routinely monitored in pediatric patients. Potentially significant drug-drug interactions may exist, requiring dose or frequency adjustment, additional monitoring, and/or selection of alternative therapy.

Drug Interactions
Avoid Concomitant Use
Avoid concomitant use of PrednisoLONE (Systemic) with any of the following: Aldesleukin; BCG; Indium 111 Capromab Pendetide; Mifepristone; Natalizumab; Pimecrolimus; Pimozide; Tacrolimus (Topical); Tofacitinib

Decreased Effect
PrednisoLONE (Systemic) may decrease the levels/effects of: Aldesleukin; Antidiabetic Agents; BCG; Calcitriol; Coccidioidin Skin Test; Corticorelin; CycloSPORINE (Systemic); Hyaluronidase; Indium 111 Capromab Pendetide; Isoniazid; Salicylates; Sipuleucel-T; Telaprevir; Urea Cycle Disorder Agents; Vaccines (Inactivated)

The levels/effects of PrednisoLONE (Systemic) may be decreased by: Aminoglutethimide; Antacids; Barbiturates; Bile Acid Sequestrants; Echinacea; Fosphenytoin; Mifepristone; Mitotane; Phenytoin; Primidone; Rifamycin Derivatives

Increased Effect/Toxicity
PrednisoLONE (Systemic) may increase the levels/effects of: Acetylcholinesterase Inhibitors; Amphotericin B; ARIPiprazole; CycloSPORINE (Systemic); Deferasirox; Dofetilide; Leflunomide; Lomitapide; Loop Diuretics; Natalizumab; NSAID (COX-2 Inhibitor); NSAID (Nonselective); Pimozide; Thiazide Diuretics; Tofacitinib; Vaccines (Live); Warfarin

The levels/effects of PrednisoLONE (Systemic) may be increased by: Antifungal Agents (Azole Derivatives, Systemic); Aprepitant; Boceprevir; Calcium Channel Blockers (Nondihydropyridine); CycloSPORINE (Systemic); Denosumab; Estrogen Derivatives; Fluconazole; Fosaprepitant; Indacaterol; Macrolide Antibiotics; Mifepristone; Neuromuscular-Blocking Agents (Nondepolarizing); Pimecrolimus; Quinolone Antibiotics; Ritonavir; Roflumilast; Salicylates; Tacrolimus (Topical); Telaprevir; Trastuzumab

Nutritional/Ethanol Interactions
Ethanol: Avoid ethanol (may increase gastric mucosal irritation).
Food: Prednisolone interferes with calcium absorption. Limit caffeine.
Herb/Nutraceutical: St John's wort may decrease prednisolone levels. Avoid cat's claw, echinacea (have immunostimulant properties).

Adverse Reactions Frequency not defined.
Cardiovascular: Cardiomyopathy, CHF, edema, facial edema, hypertension
Central nervous system: Headache, insomnia, malaise, nervousness, pseudotumor cerebri, psychic disorders, seizure, vertigo
Dermatologic: Bruising, facial erythema, hirsutism, petechiae, skin test reaction suppression, thin fragile skin, urticaria
Endocrine & metabolic: Carbohydrate tolerance decreased, Cushing's syndrome, diabetes mellitus, growth suppression, hyperglycemia, hypernatremia, hypokalemia, hypokalemic alkalosis, menstrual irregularities, negative nitrogen balance, pituitary adrenal axis suppression
Gastrointestinal: Abdominal distention, increased appetite, indigestion, nausea, pancreatitis, peptic ulcer, ulcerative esophagitis, weight gain
Hepatic: LFTs increased (usually reversible)
Neuromuscular & skeletal: Arthralgia, aseptic necrosis (humeral/femoral heads), fractures, muscle mass decreased, muscle weakness, osteoporosis, steroid myopathy, tendon rupture, weakness
Ocular: Cataracts, exophthalmus, eyelid edema, glaucoma, intraocular pressure increased, irritation
Respiratory: Epistaxis
Miscellaneous: Diaphoresis increased, impaired wound healing

Pharmacodynamics/Kinetics
Duration of Action 18-36 hours
Available Dosage Forms
Solution, Oral:
  Millipred: 10 mg/5 mL (237 mL)
  Orapred: 15 mg/5 mL (20 mL, 237 mL)
  Pediapred: 5 mg/5 mL (120 mL)
  Veripred 20: 20 mg/5 mL (237 mL)
  Generic: 15 mg/5 mL (237 mL, 240 mL, 480 mL); 25 mg/5 mL (237 mL); 5 mg/5 mL (120 mL)
Suspension, Oral:
  Flo-Pred: 15 mg/5 mL (30 mL)
Syrup, Oral:
  Prelone: 15 mg/5 mL (240 mL)
  Generic: 15 mg/5 mL (240 mL, 480 mL)

Tablet, Oral:
Millipred: 5 mg
Millipred DP: 5 mg
Millipred DP 12-Day: 5 mg
Tablet Dispersible, Oral:
Orapred ODT: 10 mg, 15 mg, 30 mg
General Dosage Range Oral:
Children: Dosage varies greatly depending on indication
Adults: 5-60 mg daily **or** 200 mg daily for 1 week followed by 80 mg every other day for 1 month
Administration
Oral Administer oral formulation with food or milk to decrease GI effects.
Flo-Pred: Administer using the provided calibrated syringe (supplied by manufacturer) to accurately measure the dose. Syringe should be washed prior to next use.
Orapred ODT: Do not break or use partial tablet. Remove tablet from blister pack just prior to use. May swallow whole or allow to dissolve on tongue.
Storage/Stability
Flo-Pred™: Store at 20°C to 25°C (68°F to 77°F). Flo-Pred™ should be dispensed in the original container (to avoid loss of formulation during transfer).
Millipred™: Store at 20°C to 25°C (68°F to 77°F).
Orapred ODT®: Store at 20°C to 25°C (68°F to 77°F) in blister pack. Protect from moisture.
Orapred®, Veripred™ 20: 2°C to 8°C (36°F to 46°F).
Pediapred®: 4°C to 25°C (39°F to 77°F); may be refrigerated.
Nursing Actions
Physical Assessment Teach patients to report infection and adrenal suppression. Instruct patients with diabetes to monitor serum glucose levels closely; corticosteroids can alter glycemic response. Dose may need to be increased if patient is experiencing higher than normal levels of stress. When discontinuing, taper dose and frequency slowly.
Patient Education
• Discuss specific use of drug and side effects with patient as it relates to treatment. (HCAHPS: During this hospital stay, were you given any medicine that you had not taken before? Before giving you any new medicine, how often did hospital staff tell you what the medicine was for? How often did hospital staff describe possible side effects in a way you could understand?)
• Patient may experience nausea, insomnia, akathisia, or hyperhidrosis. Have patient report immediately to prescriber signs of infection, signs of hyperglycemia, signs of hypokalemia, signs of pancreatitis, severe asthenia, irritability, tremors, tachycardia, confusion, dizziness, dyspnea, excessive weight gain, edema of extremities, skin changes, moon face, buffalo hump, significant headache, bradycardia,

arrhythmia, angina, menstrual irregularities, arthralgia, myalgia, vision changes, mood changes, behavioral changes, depression, paresthesia, ecchymosis, hemorrhaging, intolerable dyspepsia, melena, or hematemesis (HCAHPS).
• Educate patient about signs of a significant reaction (eg, wheezing; chest tightness; fever; itching; bad cough; blue skin color; seizures; or swelling of face, lips, tongue, or throat). **Note:** This is not a comprehensive list of all side effects. Patient should consult prescriber for additional questions.

Intended Use and Disclaimer: Should not be printed and given to patients. This information is intended to serve as a concise initial reference for healthcare professionals to use when discussing medications with a patient. You must ultimately rely on your own discretion, experience and judgment in diagnosing, treating and advising patients.

Dietary Considerations Should be taken after meals or with food or milk to decrease GI effects; increase dietary intake of pyridoxine, vitamin C, vitamin D, folate, calcium, and phosphorus.

PrednisoLONE (Ophthalmic)
(pred NISS oh lone)

Brand Names: U.S. Omnipred; Pred Forte; Pred Mild
Index Terms Econopred; Prednisolone Acetate, Ophthalmic; Prednisolone Sodium Phosphate, Ophthalmic
Pharmacologic Category Corticosteroid, Ophthalmic
Medication Safety Issues
Sound-alike/look-alike issues:
PrednisoLONE may be confused with predniSONE

Pregnancy Risk Factor C
Use Treatment of palpebral and bulbar conjunctivitis; corneal injury from chemical, radiation, thermal burns, or foreign body penetration; steroid-responsive inflammatory ophthalmic diseases
Available Dosage Forms
Solution, Ophthalmic:
Generic: 1% (10 mL)
Suspension, Ophthalmic:
Omnipred: 1% (5 mL, 10 mL)
Pred Forte: 1% (1 mL, 5 mL, 10 mL, 15 mL)
Pred Mild: 0.12% (5 mL, 10 mL)
Generic: 1% (5 mL, 10 mL, 15 mL)
General Dosage Range Ophthalmic: *Children and Adults:* Initial: Instill 1-2 drops into conjunctival sac every hour during day, every 2 hours at night; Maintenance: 1 drop every 4 hours

Nursing Actions

Patient Education

- Discuss specific use of drug and side effects with patient as it relates to treatment. (HCAHPS: During this hospital stay, were you given any medicine that you had not taken before? Before giving you any new medicine, how often did hospital staff tell you what the medicine was for? How often did hospital staff describe possible side effects in a way you could understand?)
- Patient may experience short-term pain, cataracts, or glaucoma. Have patient report immediately to prescriber sudden vision changes, eye pain, eye irritation, or rash (HCAHPS).
- Educate patient about signs of a significant reaction (eg, wheezing; chest tightness; fever; itching; bad cough; blue skin color; seizures; or swelling of face, lips, tongue, or throat). **Note:** This is not a comprehensive list of all side effects. Patient should consult prescriber for additional questions.

Intended Use and Disclaimer: Should not be printed and given to patients. This information is intended to serve as a concise initial reference for healthcare professionals to use when discussing medications with a patient. You must ultimately rely on your own discretion, experience and judgment in diagnosing, treating and advising patients.

PredniSONE (PRED ni sone)

Brand Names: U.S. PredniSONE Intensol; Rayos
Index Terms Deltacortisone; Deltadehydrocortisone
Pharmacologic Category Corticosteroid, Systemic
Medication Safety Issues
Sound-alike/look-alike issues:
PredniSONE may be confused with methylPREDNISolone, Pramosone, prazosin, predniso-LONE, PriLOSEC, primidone, promethazine
Pregnancy Risk Factor C
Lactation Enters breast milk/Not recommended
Breast-Feeding Considerations Prednisone and its metabolite, prednisolone, are found in low concentrations in breast milk. Following a maternal dose of 10 mg (n=1), milk concentrations were measured ~2 hours after the maternal dose (prednisone 0.0016 mcg/mL; prednisolone 0.0267 mcg/mL) (Katz, 1975). In a study which included six mother/infant pairs, adverse events were not observed in nursing infants (maternal prednisone dose not provided) (Ito, 1993).

The manufacturer notes that when used systemically, maternal use of corticosteroids have the potential to cause adverse events in a nursing infant (eg, growth suppression, interfere with endogenous corticosteroid production) and therefore, a decision should be made whether to discontinue nursing or to discontinue the drug, taking into account the importance of treatment to the mother. If there is concern about exposure to the infant, some guidelines recommend waiting 4 hours after the maternal dose of an oral systemic corticosteroid before breast-feeding in order to decrease potential exposure to the nursing infant (based on a study using prednisolone) (Bae, 2011; Leachman, 2006; Makol, 2011; Ost, 1985). Other guidelines note that maternal use of prednisone is not a contraindication to breast-feeding (NAEPP, 2005).

Use Treatment of a variety of diseases, including:
Allergic conditions: Atopic dermatitis, drug hypersensitivity reactions, allergic rhinitis, serum sickness, adjunctive treatment of anaphylaxis
Dermatologic diseases: Bullous dermatitis herpetiformis, contact dermatitis, exfoliative erythroderma, mycosis fungoides, pemphigus, severe erythema multiforme (Stevens-Johnson syndrome), severe seborrheic dermatitis (immediate release only)
Endocrine conditions: Congenital adrenal hyperplasia, hypercalcemia of malignancy, nonsuppurative thyroiditis, adrenocortical insufficiency
Gastrointestinal diseases: Crohn's disease, ulcerative colitis
Hematologic diseases: Acquired (autoimmune) hemolytic anemia, Diamond-Blackfan anemia, immune thrombocytopenia (ITP), pure red cell aplasia, secondary thrombocytopenia
Infectious diseases: Trichinosis with neurologic or myocardial involvement, tuberculosis meningitis with subarachnoid block or impending block
Neoplastic conditions: Acute leukemia, aggressive lymphomas
Nervous system conditions (delayed release only): Acute exacerbations of multiple sclerosis, cerebral edema associated with primary or metastatic brain tumor, craniotomy or head injury
Ophthalmic conditions:
Immediate release only: Allergic conjunctivitis, keratitis, allergic corneal marginal ulcers, herpes zoster ophthalmicus, iritis and iridocyclitis, chorioretinitis, anterior segment inflammation, diffuse posterior uveitis and choroiditis, optic neuritis
Delayed release only: Uveitis, and ocular inflammatory conditions
Organ transplantation-related conditions (delayed release only): Solid organ rejection
Pulmonary diseases: Aspiration pneumonitis, asthma, pulmonary tuberculosis, symptomatic sarcoidosis
Immediate release only: Loeffler's syndrome not manageable by other means, berylliosis
Delayed release only: Acute exacerbations of chronic obstructive pulmonary disease (COPD), allergic bronchopulmonary aspergillosis, hypersensitivity pneumonitis, idiopathic bronchiolitis

obliterans with organizing pneumonia, idiopathic eosinophilic pneumonias, idiopathic pulmonary fibrosis, *Pneumocystis jiroveci* (formerly *carinii*) pneumonia (PCP)

Renal conditions: Nephrotic syndrome (idiopathic or related to lupus erythematosus), without uremia

Rheumatologic conditions, short-term therapy: Psoriatic arthritis, rheumatoid and juvenile arthritis, ankylosing spondylitis, acute gouty arthritis, systemic lupus erythematosus, dermatomyositis/polymyositis

Immediate release only: Bursitis, tenosynovitis, posttraumatic osteoarthritis, synovitis of osteoarthritis, epicondolyitis acute rheumatic carditis

Delayed release only: Polymyalgia rheumatica, relapsing polychondritis, Sjogren's syndrome, vasculitis

Rheumatologic conditions, maintenance therapy: Rheumatoid and juvenile arthritis, systemic lupus erythematosus, dermatomyositis/polymyositis

Immediate release only: Acute rheumatic carditis

Delayed release only: Ankylosing spondylitis, polymyalgia rheumatic, psoriatic arthritis, relapsing polychondritis, Sjogren's syndrome, vasculitis

Unlabeled Use Autoimmune hepatitis; Bell's palsy, adjunctive therapy for pain management in immunocompetent patients with herpes zoster; Takayasu arteritis; giant cell arteritis; Grave's ophthalmopathy prophylaxis; subacute thyroiditis; thyrotoxicosis (type II amiodarone-induced); acute exacerbation of chronic obstructive pulmonary disease (COPD) (immediate release products)

Mechanism of Action/Effect Decreases inflammation by suppression of migration of polymorphonuclear leukocytes and reversal of increased capillary permeability; suppresses the immune system by reducing activity and volume of the lymphatic system; suppresses adrenal function at high doses

Contraindications Hypersensitivity to any component of the formulation; systemic fungal infections; administration of live or live attenuated vaccines with immunosuppressive doses of prednisone

Warnings/Precautions May cause hypercorticism or suppression of hypothalamic-pituitary-adrenal (HPA) axis, particularly in younger children or in patients receiving high doses for prolonged periods. HPA axis suppression may lead to adrenal crisis. Withdrawal and discontinuation of a corticosteroid should be done slowly and carefully. Particular care is required when patients are transferred from systemic corticosteroids to inhaled products due to possible adrenal insufficiency or withdrawal from steroids, including an increase in allergic symptoms. Patients receiving >20 mg per day of prednisone (or equivalent) may be most susceptible. Fatalities have occurred due to adrenal insufficiency in asthmatic patients during and after transfer from systemic corticosteroids to aerosol steroids; aerosol steroids do **not** provide the systemic steroid needed to treat patients having trauma, surgery, or infections.

Acute myopathy has been reported with high dose corticosteroids, usually in patients with neuromuscular transmission disorders; may involve ocular and/or respiratory muscles; monitor creatine kinase; recovery may be delayed. Prolonged use of corticosteroids may increase the incidence of secondary infection, mask acute infection (including fungal infections), prolong or exacerbate viral infections, or limit response to vaccines. Exposure to chickenpox should be avoided. Corticosteroids should not be used to treat ocular herpes simplex or cerebral malaria. Close observation is required in patients with latent tuberculosis and/or TB reactivity; restrict use in active TB (only in conjunction with antituberculosis treatment). Prolonged treatment with corticosteroids has been associated with the development of Kaposi's sarcoma (case reports); if noted, discontinuation of therapy should be considered. Prolonged use may cause posterior subcapsular cataracts, glaucoma (with possible nerve damage) and may increase the risk for ocular infections. Corticosteroid use may cause psychiatric disturbances, including depression, euphoria, insomnia, mood swings, and personality changes. Pre-existing psychiatric conditions may be exacerbated by corticosteroid use.

Use with caution in patients with HF, diabetes, GI diseases (diverticulitis, peptic ulcer, ulcerative colitis; due to risk of perforation), hepatic impairment, myasthenia gravis, MI, patients with or who are at risk for osteoporosis, seizure disorders or thyroid disease. May affect growth velocity; growth should be routinely monitored in pediatric patients.

Prior to use, the dose and duration of treatment should be based on the risk versus benefit for each individual patient. In general, use the smallest effective dose for the shortest duration of time to minimize adverse events. A gradual tapering of dose may be required prior to discontinuing therapy. Potentially significant drug-drug interactions may exist, requiring dose or frequency adjustment, additional monitoring, and/or selection of alternative therapy.

Drug Interactions

Avoid Concomitant Use

Avoid concomitant use of PredniSONE with any of the following: Aldesleukin; Axitinib; BCG; Indium 111 Capromab Pendetide; Mifepristone; Natalizumab; Pimecrolimus; Simeprevir; Tacrolimus (Topical); Tofacitinib

Decreased Effect

PredniSONE may decrease the levels/effects of: Aldesleukin; Antidiabetic Agents; ARIPiprazole; Axitinib; BCG; Calcitriol; Coccidioidin Skin Test; Corticorelin; CycloSPORINE (Systemic); Hyaluronidase; Ibrutinib; Indium 111 Capromab Pendetide; Isoniazid; Salicylates; Simeprevir;

Sipuleucel-T; Telaprevir; Urea Cycle Disorder Agents; Vaccines (Inactivated)

The levels/effects of PredniSONE may be decreased by: Aminoglutethimide; Antacids; Barbiturates; Bile Acid Sequestrants; Echinacea; Fosphenytoin; Mifepristone; Mitotane; Phenytoin; Primidone; Rifamycin Derivatives; Somatropin; Tesamorelin

Increased Effect/Toxicity

PredniSONE may increase the levels/effects of: Acetylcholinesterase Inhibitors; Amphotericin B; CycloSPORINE (Systemic); Deferasirox; Leflunomide; Loop Diuretics; Natalizumab; NSAID (COX-2 Inhibitor); NSAID (Nonselective); Thiazide Diuretics; Tofacitinib; Vaccines (Live); Warfarin

The levels/effects of PredniSONE may be increased by: Antifungal Agents (Azole Derivatives, Systemic); Aprepitant; Boceprevir; Calcium Channel Blockers (Nondihydropyridine); CycloSPORINE (Systemic); Denosumab; Estrogen Derivatives; Fluconazole; Fosaprepitant; Indacaterol; Macrolide Antibiotics; Mifepristone; Neuromuscular-Blocking Agents (Nondepolarizing); Pimecrolimus; Quinolone Antibiotics; Ritonavir; Roflumilast; Salicylates; Tacrolimus (Topical); Telaprevir; Trastuzumab

Nutritional/Ethanol Interactions

Ethanol: Avoid ethanol (may increase gastric mucosal irritation)

Food: Prednisone interferes with calcium absorption. Limit caffeine.

Herb/Nutraceutical: St John's wort may decrease prednisone levels. Avoid cat's claw, echinacea (have immunostimulant properties).

Adverse Reactions Frequency not defined.

Cardiovascular: Congestive heart failure (in susceptible patients), hypertension

Central nervous system: Emotional instability, headache, intracranial pressure increased (with papilledema), psychic derangements (including euphoria, insomnia, mood swings, personality changes, severe depression), seizure, vertigo

Dermatologic: Bruising, facial erythema, petechiae, thin fragile skin, urticaria, wound healing impaired

Endocrine & metabolic: Adrenocortical and pituitary unresponsiveness (in times of stress), carbohydrate intolerance, Cushing's syndrome, diabetes mellitus, fluid retention, growth suppression (in children), hypokalemic alkalosis, hypothyroidism enhanced, menstrual irregularities, negative nitrogen balance due to protein catabolism, potassium loss, sodium retention

Gastrointestinal: Abdominal distension, pancreatitis, peptic ulcer (with possible perforation and hemorrhage), ulcerative esophagitis

Hepatic: ALT increased, AST increased, alkaline phosphatase increased

Neuromuscular & skeletal: Aseptic necrosis of femoral and humeral heads, muscle mass loss, muscle weakness, osteoporosis, pathologic fracture of long bones, steroid myopathy, tendon rupture (particularly Achilles tendon), vertebral compression fractures

Ocular: Exophthalmos, glaucoma, intraocular pressure increased, posterior subcapsular cataracts

Miscellaneous: Allergic reactions, anaphylactic reactions, diaphoresis, hypersensitivity reactions, infections, Kaposi's sarcoma

Available Dosage Forms

Concentrate, Oral:
PredniSONE Intensol: 5 mg/mL (30 mL)

Solution, Oral:
Generic: 5 mg/5 mL (5 mL, 120 mL, 500 mL)

Tablet, Oral:
Generic: 1 mg, 2.5 mg, 5 mg, 10 mg, 20 mg, 50 mg

Tablet Delayed Release, Oral:
Rayos: 1 mg, 2 mg, 5 mg

General Dosage Range Oral: *Children and Adults:* Initial: 5-60 mg daily

Administration

Oral Administer with food to decrease GI upset. Delayed release tablet (Rayos®) should be swallowed whole; do not crush or chew.

Nursing Actions

Physical Assessment Teach patient to report opportunistic infection and adrenal suppression. Instruct patients with diabetes to monitor serum glucose levels closely; corticosteroids can alter glucose tolerance. Monitor growth with long-term use in pediatric patients. Dose may need to be increased if patient is experiencing higher than normal levels of stress. When discontinuing, taper dose and frequency slowly.

Patient Education
• Discuss specific use of drug and side effects with patient as it relates to treatment. (HCAHPS: During this hospital stay, were you given any medicine that you had not taken before? Before giving you any new medicine, how often did hospital staff tell you what the medicine was for? How often did hospital staff describe possible side effects in a way you could understand?)
• Patient may experience nausea, insomnia, akathisia, or hyperhidrosis. Have patient report immediately to prescriber signs of infection, signs of hyperglycemia, signs of hypokalemia, signs of pancreatitis, severe asthenia, irritability, tremors, tachycardia, confusion, dizziness, dyspnea, excessive weight gain, edema of extremities, skin changes, moon face, buffalo hump, significant headache, bradycardia, arrhythmia, angina, menstrual irregularities, arthralgia, myalgia, vision changes, mood changes, behavioral changes, depression, paresthesia, considerable dyspepsia, ecchymosis, hemorrhaging, melena, or hematemesis (HCAHPS).
• Educate patient about signs of a significant reaction (eg, wheezing; chest tightness; fever; itching; bad cough; blue skin color; seizures; or

1295

swelling of face, lips, tongue, or throat). **Note:** This is not a comprehensive list of all side effects. Patient should consult prescriber for additional questions.

Intended Use and Disclaimer: Should not be printed and given to patients. This information is intended to serve as a concise initial reference for healthcare professionals to use when discussing medications with a patient. You must ultimately rely on your own discretion, experience and judgment in diagnosing, treating and advising patients.

Dietary Considerations Should be taken after meals or with food or milk; may require increased dietary intake of pyridoxine, vitamin C, vitamin D, folate, calcium, and phosphorus; may require decreased dietary intake of sodium

---

Pregabalin (pre GAB a lin)

Brand Names: U.S. Lyrica
Index Terms CI-1008; S-(+)-3-isobutylgaba
Pharmacologic Category Analgesic, Miscellaneous; Anticonvulsant, Miscellaneous
Medication Safety Issues
Sound-alike/look-alike issues:
Lyrica® may be confused with Lopressor®
Other safety concerns:
Pregabalin (Lyrica®) oral solution (20 mg/mL): Prescriptions should be written in terms of mg. The pharmacist will calculate the appropriate dose in mL for dispensing.
Medication Guide Available Yes
Pregnancy Risk Factor C
Lactation Excretion in breast milk unknown/not recommended
Breast-Feeding Considerations It is not known if pregabalin is excreted in breast milk. Due to the potential for serious adverse reactions in the nursing infant, a decision should be made whether to discontinue nursing or to discontinue the drug, taking into account the importance of treatment to the mother.
Use Management of neuropathic pain associated with diabetic peripheral neuropathy or with spinal cord injury; management of postherpetic neuralgia; adjunctive therapy for partial-onset seizure disorder; management of fibromyalgia
Mechanism of Action/Effect Decreases symptoms of painful peripheral neuropathies and, as adjunctive therapy in partial seizures, decreases the frequency of seizures
Contraindications Hypersensitivity to pregabalin or any component of the formulation
Warnings/Precautions Antiepileptics are associated with an increased risk of suicidal behavior/thoughts with use (regardless of indication); patients should be monitored for signs/symptoms of depression, suicidal tendencies, and other unusual behavior changes during therapy and

instructed to inform their healthcare provider immediately if symptoms occur.

Angioedema has been reported; may be life threatening; use with caution in patients with a history of angioedema episodes. Concurrent use with other drugs known to cause angioedema (eg, ACE inhibitors) may increase risk. Hypersensitivity reactions, including skin redness, blistering, hives, rash, dyspnea, and wheezing have been reported; discontinue treatment of hypersensitivity occurs. Dizziness and somnolence are commonly reported; effects generally occur shortly after initiation and occur more frequently at higher doses. Patients must be cautioned about performing tasks which require mental alertness (eg, operating machinery or driving). Visual disturbances (blurred vision, decreased acuity and visual field changes) have been associated with pregabalin therapy; patients should be instructed to notify their physician if these effects are noted.

Pregabalin has been associated with increases in CPK and rare cases of rhabdomyolysis. Patients should be instructed to notify their prescriber if unexplained muscle pain, tenderness, or weakness, particularly if fever and/or malaise are associated with these symptoms. Use may cause peripheral edema or weight gain; use with caution in patients with heart failure (NYHA Class III or IV) due to limited data in this patient population. In addition, effect on weight gain/edema may be additive with the thiazolidinedione class of antidiabetic agents; use caution when coadministering these agents, particularly in patients with prior cardiovascular disease. May decrease platelet count or prolong PR interval.

Has been noted to be tumorigenic (increased incidence of hemangiosarcoma) in animal studies; significance of these findings in humans is unknown. Pregabalin has been associated with discontinuation symptoms following abrupt cessation, and increases in seizure frequency (when used as an antiepileptic) may occur. Should not be discontinued abruptly; dosage tapering over at least 1 week is recommended. Use caution in renal impairment; dosage adjustment required.
Drug Interactions
Avoid Concomitant Use
Avoid concomitant use of Pregabalin with any of the following: Azelastine (Nasal); Paraldehyde; Thalidomide
Decreased Effect
The levels/effects of Pregabalin may be decreased by: Ketorolac (Nasal); Ketorolac (Systemic); Mefloquine; Orlistat
Increased Effect/Toxicity
Pregabalin may increase the levels/effects of: Alcohol (Ethyl); Antidiabetic Agents (Thiazolidinedione); Azelastine (Nasal); Buprenorphine; CNS Depressants; Hydrocodone; Methotrimeprazine;

Metyrosine; Mirtazapine; Paraldehyde; Pramipexole; ROPINIRole; Rotigotine; Selective Serotonin Reuptake Inhibitors; Thalidomide; Zolpidem

The levels/effects of Pregabalin may be increased by: Brimonidine (Topical); Doxylamine; Droperidol; HydrOXYzine; Magnesium Sulfate; Methotrimeprazine; Perampanel; Sodium Oxybate; Tapentadol

Nutritional/Ethanol Interactions

Ethanol: May increase CNS depression; monitor for increased effects with coadministration. Caution patients about effects.

Herb/Nutraceutical: Avoid valerian, St John's wort, kava kava, gotu kola (may increase CNS depression).

Adverse Reactions Note: Frequency of adverse effects may be influenced by dose or concurrent therapy. In add-on trials in epilepsy, frequency of CNS and visual adverse effects were higher than those reported in pain management trials. Range noted below is inclusive of all trials.

>10%:

Cardiovascular: Peripheral edema (≤16%)

Central nervous system: Dizziness (8% to 45%), somnolence (4% to 36%), ataxia (1% to 20%), headache (5% to 14%), fatigue (5% to 11%)

Gastrointestinal: Weight gain (≤16%), xerostomia (1% to 15%)

Neuromuscular & skeletal: Tremor (≤11%)

Ocular: Blurred vision (1% to 12%), diplopia (≤12%)

Miscellaneous: Infection (3% to 14%), accidental injury (2% to 11%)

1% to 10%:

Cardiovascular: Edema (≤8%), chest pain (1% to 4%), hypertension (2%), hypotension (2%)

Central nervous system: Neuropathy (2% to 9%), thinking abnormal (≤9%), confusion (≤7%), euphoria (≤7%), speech disorder (≤7%), attention disturbance (4% to 6%), amnesia (≤6%), incoordination (≤6%), pain (2% to 5%), insomnia (4%), memory impaired (1% to 4%), vertigo (1% to 4%), hypoesthesia (2% to 3%), feeling abnormal (1% to 3%), anxiety (2%), lethargy (1% to 2%), drunk feeling (1% to 2%), disorientation (≤2%), depersonalization (≥1%), fever (≥1%), hypertonia (≥1%), sedation (≥1%), stupor (≥1%), nervousness (≤1%)

Dermatologic: Decubitus ulcer (3%), facial edema (≤3%), bruising (≥1%), pruritus (≥1%)

Endocrine & metabolic: Fluid retention (2% to 3%), hypoglycemia (1% to 3%), libido decreased (≥1%)

Gastrointestinal: Constipation (≤10%), appetite increased (2% to 7%), nausea (5%), flatulence (≤3%), vomiting (1% to 3%), abdominal distension (2%), abdominal pain (≥1%), gastroenteritis (≥1%)

Genitourinary: Incontinence (≤3%), anorgasmia (≥1%), impotence (≥1%), urinary frequency (≥1%)

Hematologic: Thrombocytopenia (≥1%)

Neuromuscular & skeletal: Balance disorder (2% to 9%), abnormal gait (≤8%), weakness (2% to 7%), arthralgia (3% to 6%), twitching (≤5%), muscle spasm (2% to 4%), back pain (≤4%), myoclonus (≤4%), CPK increased (3%), neck pain (3%), pain in extremity (3%), joint swelling (2%), paresthesia (2%), leg cramps (≥1%), myalgia (≥1%), myasthenia (1%)

Ocular: Visual abnormalities (≤5%), eye disorder (≤2%), conjunctivitis (≥1%), nystagmus (≥1%)

Otic: Otitis media (≥1%), tinnitus (≥1%)

Respiratory: Nasopharyngitis (8%), sinusitis (4% to 7%), pharyngolaryngeal pain (1% to 3%), bronchitis (≤3%), dyspnea (≤3%)

Miscellaneous: Flu-like syndrome (1% to 2%), allergic reaction (≥1%)

Pharmacodynamics/Kinetics

Onset of Action Pain management: Effects may be noted as early as the first week of therapy

Controlled Substance C-V

Available Dosage Forms

Capsule, Oral:

Lyrica: 25 mg, 50 mg, 75 mg, 100 mg, 150 mg, 200 mg, 225 mg, 300 mg

Solution, Oral:

Lyrica: 20 mg/mL (473 mL)

General Dosage Range Dosage adjustment recommended in patients with renal impairment

Oral: *Adults:* Initial: 150 mg daily in 2-3 divided doses; Maintenance: 150-600 mg daily in 2-3 divided doses (maximum: 600 mg daily)

Administration

Oral May be administered with or without food.

Storage/Stability Store at 25°C (77°F); excursions permitted to15°C to 30°C (59°F to 86°F).

Nursing Actions

Physical Assessment Monitor weight. Assess for signs of fluid retention. Taper dosage over at least one week when discontinuing.

Patient Education

• Discuss specific use of drug and side effects with patient as it relates to treatment. (HCAHPS: During this hospital stay, were you given any medicine that you had not taken before? Before giving you any new medicine, how often did hospital staff tell you what the medicine was for? How often did hospital staff describe possible side effects in a way you could understand?)

• Patient may experience presyncope, fatigue, blurred vision, illogical thinking, vertigo, change in balance, weight gain, myalgia, headache, shakiness, xerostomia, emotional ups and downs, or nausea. Have patient report immediately to prescriber depression, thoughts of suicide, anxiety, flu-like symptoms, severe vertigo or syncope, significant asthenia, edema of legs or belly, vision changes, severe myalgia, significant skin irritation, or rash (HCAHPS).

- Educate patient about signs of a significant reaction (eg, wheezing; chest tightness; fever; itching; bad cough; blue skin color; seizures; or swelling of face, lips, tongue, or throat). **Note:** This is not a comprehensive list of all side effects. Patient should consult prescriber for additional questions.

Intended Use and Disclaimer: Should not be printed and given to patients. This information is intended to serve as a concise initial reference for healthcare professionals to use when discussing medications with a patient. You must ultimately rely on your own discretion, experience and judgment in diagnosing, treating and advising patients.

Dietary Considerations May be taken with or without food.

Primidone (PRI mi done)

Brand Names: U.S. Mysoline

Index Terms Desoxyphenobarbital; Primaclone

Pharmacologic Category Anticonvulsant, Miscellaneous; Barbiturate

Medication Safety Issues

Sound-alike/look-alike issues:

Primidone may be confused with predniSONE, primaquine, pyridoxine

Medication Guide Available Yes

Lactation Enters breast milk/not recommended

Use Management of grand mal, psychomotor, and focal seizures

Unlabeled Use Benign familial tremor (essential tremor)

Available Dosage Forms

Tablet, Oral:

Mysoline: 50 mg, 250 mg

Generic: 50 mg, 250 mg

General Dosage Range Dosage adjustment recommended in patients with renal impairment

Oral:

Children <8 years: Initial: 50 mg once daily at bedtime; Maintenance: 375-750 mg/day (10-25 mg/kg/day) in 3-4 divided doses

Children ≥8 years and Adults: Initial: 100-125 mg/day at bedtime; Maintenance: 750-1500 mg/day in 3-4 divided doses (maximum: 2 g/day)

Nursing Actions

Physical Assessment Monitor for signs and symptoms of depression or suicide ideation. Monitor therapeutic response (seizure activity, force, type, duration) at beginning of therapy and periodically throughout. Teach patient safety and seizure precautions.

Patient Education

- Discuss specific use of drug and side effects with patient as it relates to treatment. (HCAHPS: During this hospital stay, were you given any medicine that you had not taken before? Before giving you any new medicine, how often did hospital staff tell you what the medicine was for? How often did hospital staff describe possible side effects in a way you could understand?)
- Patient may experience presyncope, fatigue, blurred vision, illogical thinking, dizziness, or nausea. Have patient report immediately to prescriber depression, dyspnea, imbalance, severe asthenia, ecchymosis, or bleeding (HCAHPS).
- Educate patient about signs of a significant reaction (eg, wheezing; chest tightness; fever; itching; bad cough; blue skin color; seizures; or swelling of face, lips, tongue, or throat). **Note:** This is not a comprehensive list of all side effects. Patient should consult prescriber for additional questions.

Intended Use and Disclaimer: Should not be printed and given to patients. This information is intended to serve as a concise initial reference for healthcare professionals to use when discussing medications with a patient. You must ultimately rely on your own discretion, experience and judgment in diagnosing, treating and advising patients.

Related Information

Peak and Trough Guidelines on page 1710

Probenecid (proe BEN e sid)

Index Terms Benemid [DSC]

Pharmacologic Category Uricosuric Agent

Medication Safety Issues

Sound-alike/look-alike issues:

Probenecid may be confused with Procanbid

Lactation Based on a single case report, very small amounts of probenecid have been detected in breast milk (Ilett, 2006).

Use Treatment of hyperuricemia associated with gout or gouty arthritis; prolongation and elevation of beta-lactam plasma levels (eg, uncomplicated gonococcal infection)

Unlabeled Use Prolongation and elevation of beta-lactam plasma levels (eg, neurosyphilis, pelvic inflammatory disease)

Available Dosage Forms

Tablet, Oral:

Generic: 500 mg

General Dosage Range Avoid use if CrCl <30 mL/minute.

Oral:

Children 2-14 years: Prolong penicillin serum levels: Initial: 25 mg/kg then 40 mg/kg/day given 4 times/day (maximum: 500 mg/dose)

Children >50 kg and Adults:

Gonorrhea, PID: 1 g as a single dose

Gout: Initial: 250 mg twice daily (maximum: 2 g/day)

Neurosyphilis: 500 mg 4 times/day for 10-14 days

Prolong PCN levels: 500 mg 4 times/day

Administration

Oral Administer with food or antacids to minimize GI effects.

Nursing Actions

Physical Assessment Monitor frequency and severity of gouty attacks.

Patient Education

- Discuss specific use of drug and side effects with patient as it relates to treatment. (HCAHPS: During this hospital stay, were you given any medicine that you had not taken before? Before giving you any new medicine, how often did hospital staff tell you what the medicine was for? How often did hospital staff describe possible side effects in a way you could understand?)
- Patient may experience dizziness, headache, flushing, nausea, or lack of appetite. Have patient report immediately to prescriber signs of infection, dyspepsia, back pain, hematuria, ecchymosis, bleeding, severe asthenia, or rash (HCAHPS).
- Educate patient about signs of a significant reaction (eg, wheezing; chest tightness; fever; itching; bad cough; blue skin color; seizures; or swelling of face, lips, tongue, or throat). **Note:** This is not a comprehensive list of all side effects. Patient should consult prescriber for additional questions.

Intended Use and Disclaimer: Should not be printed and given to patients. This information is intended to serve as a concise initial reference for healthcare professionals to use when discussing medications with a patient. You must ultimately rely on your own discretion, experience and judgment in diagnosing, treating and advising patients.

Procainamide (pro KANE a mide)

Index Terms PCA (error-prone abbreviation); Procainamide Hydrochloride; Procaine Amide Hydrochloride; Procanbid; Pronestyl

Pharmacologic Category Antiarrhythmic Agent, Class Ia

Medication Safety Issues

Sound-alike/look-alike issues:

Procanbid may be confused with probenecid, Procan SR®

Pronestyl may be confused with Ponstel®

High alert medication:

The Institute for Safe Medication Practices (ISMP) includes this medication among its list of drugs which have a heightened risk of causing significant patient harm when used in error.

BEERS Criteria medication:

This drug may be potentially inappropriate for use in geriatric patients (Quality of evidence - high; Strength of recommendation - strong).

Administration issues:

Procainamide hydrochloride is available in 10 mL vials of 100 mg/mL and in 2 mL vials with 500 mg/mL. Note that **BOTH** vials contain 1 gram of drug; confusing the strengths can lead to massive overdoses or underdoses.

Other safety concerns:

PCA is an error-prone abbreviation (mistaken as patient controlled analgesia)

Pregnancy Risk Factor C

Lactation Enters breast milk/not recommended

Use

Intravenous: Treatment of life-threatening ventricular arrhythmias

Oral (Canadian labeling; not available in U.S.): Treatment of supraventricular arrhythmias. **Note:** In the treatment of atrial fibrillation, use only when preferred treatment is ineffective or cannot be used. Use in paroxysmal atrial tachycardia when reflex stimulation or other measures are ineffective.

Unlabeled Use

Paroxysmal supraventricular tachycardia (PSVT); prevent recurrence of ventricular tachycardia; symptomatic premature ventricular contractions

ACLS guidelines: I.V.: Treatment of the following arrhythmias in patients with preserved left ventricular function: Stable monomorphic VT; pre-excited atrial fibrillation; stable wide complex regular tachycardia (likely VT)

PALS guidelines: I.V.: Tachycardia with pulses and poor perfusion (probable SVT [unresponsive to vagal maneuvers and adenosine or synchronized cardioversion]; probable VT [unresponsive to synchronized cardioversion or adenosine])

Available Dosage Forms

Solution, Injection:

Generic: 100 mg/mL (10 mL); 500 mg/mL (2 mL)

General Dosage Range Dosage adjustment recommended in patients with hepatic or renal impairment

I.M.:

Children: 20-30 mg/kg/day divided every 4-6 hours (maximum: 4 g/day)

Adults: 50 mg/kg/day divided every 3-6 hours **or** 0.5-1 g every 4-8 hours

I.V.:

Children: Loading dose: 3-6 mg/kg/dose over 5 minutes (maximum: 100 mg/dose), may repeat every 5-10 minutes to maximum of 15 mg/kg/load; Infusion: 20-80 mcg/kg/minute (maximum: 2 g/day)

Adults: Loading dose: 15-18 mg/kg administered as slow infusion over 25-30 minutes **or** 100 mg/dose at a rate not to exceed 50 mg/minute repeated every 5 minutes as needed (maximum total dose: 1 g); Infusion: 1-4 mg/minute

Usual Infusion Concentrations: Adult I.V. infusion: 1000 mg in 500 mL (concentration: 2 mg/mL), 1000 mg in 250 mL (concentration: 4 mg/mL), **or** 2000 mg in 250 mL (concentration: 8 mg/mL) of D$_5$W or NS

Administration

I.V. Must dilute prior to I.V. administration. Dilute loading dose to a maximum concentration of 20 mg/mL; administer loading dose at a maximum rate of 50 mg/minute

Injectable Detail pH: 4-6

Oral Do **not** crush or chew sustained release drug products (not available in the U.S.).

Nursing Actions

Physical Assessment I.V. requires use of infusion pump and continuous cardiac and hemodynamic monitoring. Monitor cardiac status at beginning of therapy, when titrating dosage, and on a regular basis. Monitor QT$_c$, QRS, and PR intervals.

Patient Education

- Discuss specific use of drug and side effects with patient as it relates to treatment. (HCAHPS: During this hospital stay, were you given any medicine that you had not taken before? Before giving you any new medicine, how often did hospital staff tell you what the medicine was for? How often did hospital staff describe possible side effects in a way you could understand?)
- Patient may experience hypotension or lupus-like disease. Have patient report immediately to prescriber tachycardia, severe asthenia, significant dyspepsia, considerable nausea, inability to eat, arthralgia, edema, or rash (HCAHPS).
- Educate patient about signs of a significant reaction (eg, wheezing; chest tightness; fever; itching; bad cough; blue skin color; seizures; or swelling of face, lips, tongue, or throat). **Note:** This is not a comprehensive list of all side effects. Patient should consult prescriber for additional questions.

Intended Use and Disclaimer: Should not be printed and given to patients. This information is intended to serve as a concise initial reference for healthcare professionals to use when discussing medications with a patient. You must ultimately rely on your own discretion, experience and judgment in diagnosing, treating and advising patients.

Procarbazine (proe KAR ba zeen)

Brand Names: U.S. Matulane

Index Terms Benzmethyzin; Ibenzmethyzin; N-Methylhydrazine; PCB; PCZ; Procarbazine Hydrochloride

Pharmacologic Category Antineoplastic Agent, Alkylating Agent

Medication Safety Issues

Sound-alike/look-alike issues:
Procarbazine may be confused with dacarbazine

High alert medication:
This medication is in a class the Institute for Safe Medication Practices (ISMP) includes among its list of drug classes which have a heightened risk of causing significant patient harm when used in error.

Pregnancy Risk Factor D

Lactation Excretion in breast milk unknown/not recommended

Breast-Feeding Considerations It is not known if procarbazine is excreted in breast milk. Due to the potential for serious adverse reactions in the nursing infant, nursing is not recommended during treatment with procarbazine.

Use Treatment of Hodgkin lymphoma

Unlabeled Use Treatment of CNS tumors (anaplastic oligodendroglioma/oligoastrocytoma), non-Hodgkin lymphomas, and primary CNS lymphomas

Mechanism of Action/Effect Inhibits DNA, RNA, and protein synthesis by inhibiting transmethylation of methionine into transfer RNA; may also damage DNA directly through alkylation.

Contraindications Hypersensitivity to procarbazine or any component of the formulation; inadequate bone marrow reserve

Warnings/Precautions Hazardous agent - use appropriate precautions for handling and disposal (NIOSH, 2012). Hematologic toxicity (leukopenia and thrombocytopenia) may occur 2-8 weeks after treatment initiation. Allow ≥1 month interval between radiation therapy or myelosuppressive chemotherapy and initiation of procarbazine treatment. Withhold treatment for leukopenia (WBC <4000/mm^3) or thrombocytopenia (platelets <100,000/mm^3). Monitor for infections due to neutropenia. May cause hemolysis and/or presence of Heinz inclusion bodies in erythrocytes. Procarbazine is associated with a high emetic potential; antiemetics are recommended to prevent nausea and vomiting. May cause diarrhea and stomatitis; withhold treatment for diarrhea or stomatitis. Withhold treatment for CNS toxicity, hemorrhage, or hypersensitivity. Azoospermia and infertility have been reported with procarbazine when used in combination with other chemotherapy agents. Possibly carcinogenic; acute myeloid leukemia and lung cancer have been reported following use.

Use with caution in patients with hepatic or renal impairment. Potentially significant drug-drug interactions may exist, requiring dose or frequency adjustment, additional monitoring, and/or selection of alternative therapy. Possesses MAO inhibitor activity and has potential for severe drug and food interactions; follow MAOI diet (avoid tyramine-containing foods). Avoid ethanol consumption, may cause disulfiram-like reaction. **[U.S. Boxed Warning]: Should be administered under the supervision of an experienced cancer chemotherapy physician.**

Drug Interactions

Avoid Concomitant Use

Avoid concomitant use of Procarbazine with any of the following: Alpha-/Beta-Agonists (Indirect-Acting); Alpha1-Agonists; Amphetamines; Anilidopiperidine Opioids; Antidepressants (Serotonin Reuptake Inhibitor/Antagonist); Apraclonidine; AtoMOXetine; BCG; Bezafibrate; Buprenorphine; BuPROPion; BusPIRone; CarBAMazepine; CloZAPine; Cyclobenzaprine; Cyproheptadine; Dexmethylphenidate; Dextromethorphan; Diethylpropion; Hydrocodone; HYDROmorphone; Isometheptene; Levonordefrin; Linezolid; Maprotiline; Meperidine; Methyldopa; Methylene Blue; Methylphenidate; Mirtazapine; Morphine (Liposomal); Morphine (Systemic); Natalizumab; Oxymorphone; Pimecrolimus; Pizotifen; Selective Serotonin Reuptake Inhibitors; Serotonin 5-HT1D Receptor Agonists; Serotonin/Norepinephrine Reuptake Inhibitors; Tacrolimus (Topical); Tapentadol; Tetrabenazine; Tetrahydrozoline (Nasal); Tofacitinib; Tricyclic Antidepressants; Tryptophan; Vaccines (Live)

Decreased Effect

Procarbazine may decrease the levels/effects of: BCG; Cardiac Glycosides; Coccidioidin Skin Test; Domperidone; Sipuleucel-T; Vaccines (Inactivated); Vaccines (Live); Vitamin K Antagonists

The levels/effects of Procarbazine may be decreased by: Cyproheptadine; Domperidone; Echinacea

Increased Effect/Toxicity

Procarbazine may increase the levels/effects of: Alpha-/Beta-Agonists (Indirect-Acting); Alpha1-Agonists; Amphetamines; Antidepressants (Serotonin Reuptake Inhibitor/Antagonist); Antihypertensives; Antipsychotics; Apraclonidine; AtoMOXetine; Beta2-Agonists; Betahistine; Bezafibrate; Brimonidine (Ophthalmic); Brimonidine (Topical); BuPROPion; Carbocisteine; CloZAPine; Cyproheptadine; Dexmethylphenidate; Dextromethorphan; Diethylpropion; Domperidone; Doxapram; Doxylamine; EPINEPHrine (Nasal); Epinephrine (Racemic); EPINEPHrine (Systemic, Oral Inhalation); Hydrocodone; HYDROmorphone; Hypoglycemic Agents; Isometheptene; Leflunomide; Levonordefrin; Linezolid; Lithium; Meperidine; Methadone; Methyldopa; Methylene Blue; Methylphenidate; Metoclopramide; Mirtazapine; Morphine (Liposomal); Morphine (Systemic); Natalizumab; Norepinephrine; Orthostatic Hypotension Producing Agents; OxyCODONE;

Pizotifen; Reserpine; Selective Serotonin Reuptake Inhibitors; Serotonin 5-HT1D Receptor Agonists; Serotonin Modulators; Serotonin/Norepinephrine Reuptake Inhibitors; Tetrahydrozoline (Nasal); Tofacitinib; Tricyclic Antidepressants; Vaccines (Live); Vitamin K Antagonists

The levels/effects of Procarbazine may be increased by: Altretamine; Anilidopiperidine Opioids; Antipsychotics; Buprenorphine; BusPIRone; CarBAMazepine; COMT Inhibitors; Cyclobenzaprine; Denosumab; Levodopa; MAO Inhibitors; Maprotiline; Oxymorphone; Pimecrolimus; Roflumilast; Tacrolimus (Topical); Tapentadol; Tetrabenazine; TraMADol; Trastuzumab; Tryptophan

Nutritional/Ethanol Interactions

Ethanol: Ethanol may enhance the adverse/toxic effects of procarbazine or cause a disulfiram reaction. Management: Avoid ethanol.

Food: Concurrent ingestion of foods rich in tyramine may cause sudden and severe high blood pressure (hypertensive crisis or serotonin syndrome). Management: Avoid tyramine-containing foods (aged or matured cheese, air-dried or cured meats including sausages and salamis; fava or broad bean pods, tap/draft beers, Marmite concentrate, sauerkraut, soy sauce, and other soybean condiments). Food's freshness is also an important concern; improperly stored or spoiled food can create an environment in which tyramine concentrations may increase.

Herb/Nutraceutical: Supplements containing caffeine, tyrosine, tryptophan, or phenylalanine may increase the risk of severe side effects (eg, hypertensive reactions, serotonin syndrome). Echinacea may diminish the therapeutic effect of immunosuppressants. Management: Avoid supplements containing caffeine, tyrosine, tryptophan, or phenylalanine. Consider avoiding echinacea.

Adverse Reactions Frequency not always defined.

Cardiovascular: Edema, flushing, hypotension, syncope, tachycardia

Central nervous system: Apprehension, ataxia, chills, coma, confusion, depression, dizziness, drowsiness, falling, fatigue, hallucination, headache, hyporeflexia, insomnia, lethargy, nervousness, neuropathy, nightmares, pain, paresthesia, seizure, slurred speech, unsteadiness

Dermatologic: Alopecia, dermatitis, diaphoresis, hyperpigmentation, pruritus, skin rash, urticaria

Endocrine & metabolic: Gynecomastia (in prepubertal and early pubertal males)

Gastrointestinal: Nausea and vomiting (60% to 90%; increasing the dose in a stepwise fashion over several days may minimize), abdominal pain, anorexia, constipation, diarrhea, dysphagia, hematemesis, melena, stomatitis, xerostomia

Genitourinary: Reduced fertility (>10%), azoospermia (reported with combination chemotherapy), hematuria, nocturia

Hematologic & oncologic: Malignant neoplasm (2% to 15%; secondary; nonlymphoid; reported with combination therapy), anemia, bone marrow depression, eosinophilia, hemolysis (in patients with G6PD deficiency), hemolytic anemia, pancytopenia, petechia, purpura, thrombocytopenia

Hepatic: Hepatic insufficiency, jaundice

Hypersensitivity: Hypersensitivity reaction

Infection: Herpes virus infection, increased susceptibility to infection

Neuromuscular & skeletal: Arthralgia, foot-drop, myalgia, tremor, weakness

Ophthalmic: Accommodation disturbance, diplopia, nystagmus, papilledema, photophobia, retinal hemorrhage

Otic: Hearing loss

Renal: Polyuria

Respiratory: Cough, epistaxis, hemoptysis, hoarseness, pleural effusion, pneumonitis, pulmonary toxicity (<1%)

Miscellaneous: Fever

Available Dosage Forms

Capsule, Oral:

Matulane: 50 mg

General Dosage Range Dosage adjustment recommended in patients who develop toxicities and those with hepatic impairment.

Oral: *Children and Adults:* Dosage varies greatly depending on indication

Administration

Oral May be given as a single daily dose or in 2-3 divided doses. Procarbazine is associated with a high emetic potential; antiemetics are recommended to prevent nausea and vomiting.

Hazardous agent; use appropriate precautions for handling and disposal (NIOSH, 2012).

Storage/Stability Protect from light.

Nursing Actions

Physical Assessment Use of CNS depressants increases risk of adverse reactions. Emetic potential is high; antiemetic is generally required. Monitor for neurotoxicity, nausea and vomiting, pneumonitis, arthralgia, and paresthesia. Instruct patient about dietary and alcohol cautions (procarbazine has some MAO inhibitory effects; can result in life-threatening hypertension with ingestion of tyramine-containing food; alcohol may cause disulfiram-like reaction).

Patient Education

• Discuss specific use of drug and side effects with patient as it relates to treatment. (HCAHPS: During this hospital stay, were you given any medicine that you had not taken before? Before giving you any new medicine, how often did hospital staff tell you what the medicine was for? How often did hospital staff describe possible side effects in a way you could understand?)

• Patient may experience presyncope, fatigue, blurred vision, illogical thinking, nausea, alopecia, or infertility. Have patient report immediately to prescriber dyspnea, diarrhea, ecchymosis, stomatitis, or rash (HCAHPS).

• Educate patient about signs of a significant reaction (eg, wheezing; chest tightness; fever; itching; bad cough; blue skin color; seizures; or swelling of face, lips, tongue, or throat). **Note:** This is not a comprehensive list of all side effects. Patient should consult prescriber for additional questions.

Intended Use and Disclaimer: Should not be printed and given to patients. This information is intended to serve as a concise initial reference for healthcare professionals to use when discussing medications with a patient. You must ultimately rely on your own discretion, experience and judgment in diagnosing, treating and advising patients.

Dietary Considerations Avoid tyramine-containing foods/beverages. Some examples include aged or matured cheese, air-dried or cured meats (including sausages and salamis), fava or broad bean pods, tap/draft beers, Marmite concentrate, sauerkraut, soy sauce and other soybean condiments.

Related Information

Oral Medications That Should Not Be Crushed or Altered *on page 1712*

Prochlorperazine (proe klor PER a zeen)

Brand Names: U.S. Compazine; Compro

Index Terms Chlormeprazine; Prochlorperazine Edisylate; Prochlorperazine Maleate; Prochlorperazine Mesylate

Pharmacologic Category Antiemetic; Antipsychotic Agent, Typical, Phenothiazine

Medication Safety Issues

Sound-alike/look-alike issues:

Prochlorperazine may be confused with chlorproMAZINE

Compazine may be confused with Copaxone, Coumadin

BEERS Criteria medication:

This drug may be potentially inappropriate for use in geriatric patients (Quality of evidence - varies based on comorbidity; Strength of recommendation - varies based on comorbidity)

Other safety concerns:

CPZ (occasional abbreviation for Compazine) is an error-prone abbreviation (mistaken as chlorpromazine)

Lactation Excretion in breast milk unknown

Use Management of nausea and vomiting; psychotic disorders, including schizophrenia and anxiety; nonpsychotic anxiety

Unlabeled Use Behavioral syndromes in dementia; psychosis/agitation related to Alzheimer's dementia

Available Dosage Forms

Solution, Injection:

Generic: 5 mg/mL (2 mL, 10 mL)

Suppository, Rectal:

Compazine: 25 mg (12 ea)

Compro: 25 mg (12 ea)

Generic: 25 mg (12 ea, 1000 ea)

Tablet, Oral:

Compazine: 5 mg, 10 mg

Generic: 5 mg, 10 mg

General Dosage Range

I.M. (as edisylate):

Children ≥2 years and ≥9 kg: 0.13 mg/kg/dose; change to oral as soon as possible

Adults:

Antiemetic: 5-10 mg every 3-4 hours **or** 5-10 mg as a single dose with surgery, may repeat (maximum: 40 mg/day)

Antipsychotic: Initial: 10-20 mg every 2-4 hours to gain control (more than 3-4 doses are rarely needed); Maintenance: 10-20 mg every 4-6 hours

I.V. (as edisylate): *Adults*: 2.5-10 mg every 3-4 hours as needed (maximum: 40 mg/day) **or** 5-10 mg as a single dose with surgery, may repeat

Oral, rectal:

Children ≥2 years and ≥9 kg: Antiemetic:

9-13 kg: 2.5 mg 1-2 times/day as needed (maximum: 7.5 mg/day)

>13-18 kg: 2.5 mg 2-3 times/day as needed (maximum: 10 mg/day)

>18-39 kg: 2.5 mg 3 times/day or 5 mg 2 times/day as needed (maximum: 15 mg/day)

Children 2-12 years: Antipsychotic: Initial: 2.5 mg 2-3 times/day; Maintenance: Increase as needed to maximum of 20 mg/day for 2-5 years and 25 mg/day for 6-12 years

Adults:

Antiemetic: 5-10 mg 3-4 times/day (maximum: 40 mg/day)

Antipsychotic: Initial: 5-10 mg 3-4 times/day; Maintenance: Up to 150 mg/day

Nonpsychotic anxiety: 15-20 mg/day in divided doses; do not give doses >20 mg/day or for longer than 12 weeks

Administration

I.M. Inject by deep I.M. into outer quadrant of buttocks.

I.V. May be administered by slow I.V. push at a rate not exceeding 5 mg/minute or I.V. infusion. Do not administer as a bolus injection. To reduce the risk of hypotension, patients receiving I.V. prochlorperazine must remain lying down and be observed for at least 30 minutes following administration. Avoid skin contact with injection solution, contact dermatitis has occurred.

Injectable Detail Do not dilute with any diluent containing parabens as a preservative.

pH: 4.2-6.2

Oral Administer tablet without regard to meals.

Nursing Actions

Physical Assessment For I.V., continuously monitor blood pressure and heart rate during administration. Monitor blood pressure and heart rate, fluid balance (I & O ratio), and for dehydration. Monitor for seizures, especially with known seizure disorder. Monitor for excessive sedation, neuromuscular malignant syndrome, autonomic instability (eg, anticholinergic effects, such as flushing, excessive sweating, constipation, urinary retention), and extrapyramidal symptoms (eg, tardive dyskinesia, akathisia, pseudoparkinsonism).

Patient Education

• Discuss specific use of drug and side effects with patient as it relates to treatment. (HCAHPS: During this hospital stay, were you given any medicine that you had not taken before? Before giving you any new medicine, how often did hospital staff tell you what the medicine was for? How often did hospital staff describe possible side effects in a way you could understand?)

• Patient may experience presyncope, fatigue, blurred vision, illogical thinking, dizziness, nervousness and anxiety, constipation, xerostomia, weight gain, or impotence. Have patient report immediately to prescriber imbalance, tremors, urinary retention, severe asthenia, pregnancy, or rash (HCAHPS).

• Educate patient about signs of a significant reaction (eg, wheezing; chest tightness; fever; itching; bad cough; blue skin color; seizures; or swelling of face, lips, tongue, or throat). **Note:** This is not a comprehensive list of all side effects. Patient should consult prescriber for additional questions.

Intended Use and Disclaimer: Should not be printed and given to patients. This information is intended to serve as a concise initial reference for healthcare professionals to use when discussing medications with a patient. You must ultimately rely on your own discretion, experience and judgment in diagnosing, treating and advising patients.

Progesterone (proe JES ter one)

Brand Names: U.S. Crinone; Endometrin; First-Progesterone VGS 100; First-Progesterone VGS 200; First-Progesterone VGS 25; First-Progesterone VGS 400; First-Progesterone VGS 50; Prometrium

Index Terms Pregnenedione; Progestin

Pharmacologic Category Progestin

Pregnancy Risk Factor B (Prometrium®; none established for vaginal gel, vaginal tablet, or injection

Lactation Enters breast milk/use caution

Use

Oral: Prevention of endometrial hyperplasia in non-hysterectomized, postmenopausal women who are receiving conjugated estrogen tablets; secondary amenorrhea

I.M.: Amenorrhea; abnormal uterine bleeding due to hormonal imbalance

Intravaginal gel: Part of assisted reproductive technology (ART) for infertile women with progesterone deficiency; secondary amenorrhea

Vaginal tablet: Part of ART for infertile women with progesterone deficiency

Unlabeled Use Reduce the risk of recurrent spontaneous preterm birth in appropriately selected women

Available Dosage Forms

Capsule, Oral:

Prometrium: 100 mg, 200 mg

Generic: 100 mg, 200 mg

Gel, Vaginal:

Crinone: 4% (1.125 g); 8% (1.125 g)

Insert, Vaginal:

Endometrin: 100 mg (21 ea)

Oil, Intramuscular:

Generic: 50 mg/mL (10 mL)

Suppository, Vaginal:

First-Progesterone VGS 25: 25 mg (30 ea)

First-Progesterone VGS 50: 50 mg (30 ea)

First-Progesterone VGS 100: 100 mg (30 ea)

First-Progesterone VGS 200: 200 mg (30 ea)

First-Progesterone VGS 400: 400 mg (30 ea)

General Dosage Range

I.M.: *Adults (females):* 5-10 mg/day for 6 doses

Intravaginal: *Adults (females):*

ART: 90 mg (8% gel) once or twice daily or 100 mg (vaginal tablet) 2-3 times/day

Secondary amenorrhea: 45 mg (4% gel) every other day, may increase to 90 mg (8% gel) every other day if needed (maximum: 6 doses)

Oral: *Adults (females):*

Amenorrhea: 400 mg once daily in the evening for 10 days

Endometrial hyperplasia prevention: 200 mg once daily in the evening for 12 days sequentially per 28-day cycle

Administration

I.M. Administer deep I.M. only

Hazardous agent; use appropriate precautions for handling and disposal (NIOSH, 2012).

Oral Oral capsule: For patients who experience difficulty swallowing the capsules, taking with a full glass of water in the standing position may be beneficial.

Hazardous agent; use appropriate precautions for handling and disposal (NIOSH, 2012).

Other

Vaginal gel: (A small amount of gel will remain in the applicator following insertion): Administer into the vagina directly from sealed applicator. Remove applicator from wrapper; holding applicator by thickest end, shake down to move contents to thin end; while holding applicator by flat section of thick end, twist off tab; gently insert into vagina and squeeze thick end of applicator.

For use at altitudes above 2500 feet: Remove applicator from wrapper; hold applicator on both sides of bubble in the thick end; using a lancet, make a single puncture in the bubble to relieve air pressure; holding applicator by thickest end, shake down to move contents to thin end; while holding applicator by flat section of thick end, twist off tab; gently insert into vagina and squeeze thick end of applicator.

Vaginal tablet: Insert tablet in vagina using disposable applicator provided.

Hazardous agent; use appropriate precautions for handling and disposal (NIOSH, 2012).

Nursing Actions

Physical Assessment Assess blood pressure, mammogram, and results of Pap smears and pregnancy tests before beginning treatment and at least annually. Teach patient importance of annual physicals, Pap smears, and vision assessment.

Patient Education

• Discuss specific use of drug and side effects with patient as it relates to treatment. (HCAHPS: During this hospital stay, were you given any medicine that you had not taken before? Before giving you any new medicine, how often did hospital staff tell you what the medicine was for? How often did hospital staff describe possible side effects in a way you could understand?)

• Patient may experience dizziness, headache, dyspepsia, nausea, macromastia, mastalgia, myalgia, or arthralgia. Have patient report immediately to prescriber depression, nervousness, emotional instability, illogical thinking, anxiety, angina, dyspnea, edema, sudden vision changes, eye pain, eye irritation, rash, or menstrual irregularities (HCAHPS).

• Educate patient about signs of a significant reaction (eg, wheezing; chest tightness; fever; itching; bad cough; blue skin color; seizures; or swelling of face, lips, tongue, or throat). **Note:** This is not a comprehensive list of all side effects. Patient should consult prescriber for additional questions.

Intended Use and Disclaimer: Should not be printed and given to patients. This information is intended to serve as a concise initial reference for healthcare professionals to use when discussing medications with a patient. You must ultimately rely on your own discretion, experience and

judgment in diagnosing, treating and advising patients.

Related Information

Herbal and Nutritional Products *on page 1672*

Promethazine (proe METH a zeen)

Brand Names: U.S. Phenadoz; Phenergan; Promethegan

Index Terms Promethazine Hydrochloride

Pharmacologic Category Antiemetic; Histamine H_1 Antagonist; Histamine H_1 Antagonist, First Generation; Phenothiazine Derivative

Medication Safety Issues

Sound-alike/look-alike issues:

Promethazine may be confused with chlorproMA-ZINE, predniSONE

Phenergan® may be confused with PHENobarbital, Phrenilin®, Theragran

High alert medication:

The Institute for Safe Medication Practices (ISMP) includes this medication (I.V. formulation) among its list of drugs which have a heightened risk of causing significant patient harm when used in error.

BEERS Criteria medication:

This drug may be potentially inappropriate for use in geriatric patients (Quality of evidence - high; Strength of recommendation - strong).

Administration issues:

To prevent or minimize tissue damage during I.V. administration, the Institute for Safe Medication Practices (ISMP) has the following recommendations:

- Limit concentration available to the 25 mg/mL product
- Consider limiting initial doses to 6.25-12.5 mg
- Further dilute the 25 mg/mL strength into 10-20 mL NS
- Administer through a large bore vein (not hand or wrist)
- Administer via running I.V. line at port farthest from patient's vein
- Consider administering over 10-15 minutes
- Instruct patients to report immediately signs of pain or burning

International issues:

Sominex: Brand name for promethazine in Great Britain, but also is a brand name for diphenhydrAMINE in the U.S.

Pregnancy Risk Factor C

Lactation Excretion in breast milk unknown/not recommended

Use Symptomatic treatment of various allergic conditions; antiemetic; motion sickness; sedative; adjunct to postoperative analgesia and anesthesia

Unlabeled Use Treatment of nausea and vomiting of pregnancy (NVP)

Available Dosage Forms

Solution, Injection:

Phenergan: 25 mg/mL (1 mL); 50 mg/mL (1 mL)

Generic: 25 mg/mL (1 mL); 50 mg/mL (1 mL)

Solution, Oral:

Generic: 6.25 mg/5 mL (118 mL, 473 mL)

Suppository, Rectal:

Phenadoz: 12.5 mg (12 ea); 25 mg (12 ea)

Promethegan: 12.5 mg (12 ea); 25 mg (12 ea, 1000 ea); 50 mg (12 ea)

Generic: 12.5 mg (1 ea, 12 ea); 25 mg (1 ea, 12 ea)

Syrup, Oral:

Generic: 6.25 mg/5 mL (118 mL, 473 mL)

Tablet, Oral:

Generic: 12.5 mg, 25 mg, 50 mg

General Dosage Range

I.M., I.V.:

Children ≥2 years: 0.25-1 mg/kg 4-6 times/day as needed (maximum: 25 mg/dose; sedation: 50 mg/dose)

Adults: 12.5-75 mg/dose as a single dose **or** 12.5-50 mg every 4-6 hours as needed

Oral, rectal:

Children ≥2 years:

Allergic reactions: 0.1 mg/kg every 6 hours (maximum: 12.5 mg) during the day and 0.5 mg/kg (maximum: 25 mg/dose) at bedtime as needed

Antiemetic: 0.25-1 mg/kg 4-6 times/day as needed (maximum: 25 mg/dose)

Motion sickness: 0.5 mg/kg 30 minutes to 1 hour before departure, then every 12 hours as needed (maximum: 25 mg twice daily)

Sedation: 12.5-25 mg as single dose (maximum: 25 mg/dose)

Adults: 6.25-25 mg every 4-8 hours as needed **or** 12.5-50 mg as a single dose **or** 25 mg 30-60 minutes before departure, then every 12 hours as needed

Administration

I.M. Preferred route of administration; administer into deep muscle

I.V. I.V. administration is **not** the preferred route; severe tissue damage may occur. Solution for injection should be administered in a maximum concentration of 25 mg/mL (more dilute solutions are recommended). Administer via running I.V. line at port farthest from patient's vein, or through a large bore vein (not hand or wrist). Consider administering over 10-15 minutes (maximum: 25 mg/minute).

Vesicant; ensure proper needle or catheter placement prior to and during infusion; avoid extravasation. Discontinue immediately if burning or pain occurs with administration; evaluate for inadvertent arterial injection or extravasation.

Extravasation management: If extravasation occurs, stop infusion immediately and disconnect (leave cannula/needle in place); gently aspirate extravasated solution (do **NOT** flush the line); remove needle/cannula; elevate extremity. Apply dry cold compresses (Hurst, 2004).

Injectable Detail Rapid I.V. administration may produce a transient fall in blood pressure.

pH: 4-5.5

Subcutaneous Not for SubQ administration.

Nursing Actions

Physical Assessment I.M. is the preferred route of administration. I.V.: Infusion site must be monitored closely; severe tissue damage may result. Do not give SubQ or intra-arterially; necrotic lesions may occur. Monitor for sedation, bradycardia, akathisia, delirium, extrapyramidal symptoms, dermatitis, gastrointestinal upset, urinary retention, blurred vision, and respiratory depression. May be sedating and impair physical or mental abilities; use and teach sedation safety measures (eg, side rails up, call light within reach).

Patient Education

- Discuss specific use of drug and side effects with patient as it relates to treatment. (HCAHPS: During this hospital stay, were you given any medicine that you had not taken before? Before giving you any new medicine, how often did hospital staff tell you what the medicine was for? How often did hospital staff describe possible side effects in a way you could understand?)
- Patient may experience presyncope, fatigue, blurred vision, illogical thinking, dizziness, constipation, or xerostomia. Have patient report immediately to prescriber dyspnea, tachycardia, injection site pain, tremors, severe asthenia, urinary retention, or rash (HCAHPS).
- Educate patient about signs of a significant reaction (eg, wheezing; chest tightness; fever; itching; bad cough; blue skin color; seizures; or swelling of face, lips, tongue, or throat). **Note:** This is not a comprehensive list of all side effects. Patient should consult prescriber for additional questions.

Intended Use and Disclaimer: Should not be printed and given to patients. This information is intended to serve as a concise initial reference for healthcare professionals to use when discussing medications with a patient. You must ultimately rely on your own discretion, experience and judgment in diagnosing, treating and advising patients.

Related Information

Management of Drug Extravasations *on page 1700*

Propafenone (pro PAF en one)

Brand Names: U.S. Rythmol; Rythmol SR

Index Terms Propafenone Hydrochloride

Pharmacologic Category Antiarrhythmic Agent, Class Ic

Medication Safety Issues

BEERS Criteria medication:

This drug may be potentially inappropriate for use in geriatric patients (Quality of evidence - high; Strength of recommendation - strong).

Pregnancy Risk Factor C

Lactation Enters breast milk/not recommended

Use Treatment of life-threatening ventricular arrhythmias; treatment of paroxysmal atrial fibrillation/flutter (PAF) or paroxysmal supraventricular tachycardia (PSVT) in patients with disabling symptoms and without structural heart disease

Extended release capsule: Prolong the time to recurrence of symptomatic atrial fibrillation in patients without structural heart disease

Unlabeled Use Cardioversion of recent-onset atrial fibrillation (single dose); supraventricular tachycardia in patients with Wolff-Parkinson-White syndrome

Available Dosage Forms

Capsule Extended Release 12 Hour, Oral:
Rythmol SR: 225 mg, 325 mg, 425 mg
Generic: 225 mg, 325 mg, 425 mg

Tablet, Oral:
Rythmol: 150 mg, 225 mg
Generic: 150 mg, 225 mg, 300 mg

General Dosage Range Dosage adjustment recommended in patients with hepatic impairment

Oral:

Extended release: *Adults:* Initial: 225 mg every 12 hours; Maintenance: 225-425 mg every 12 hours

Immediate release: *Adults:* Initial: 150 mg every 8 hours; Maintenance: 150-300 mg every 8 hours

Administration

Oral Capsules should be swallowed whole; do not crush or chew; may be taken without regard to meals.

Nursing Actions

Physical Assessment Correct electrolyte abnormalities prior to and throughout use. May cause new or worsened arrhythmias.

Patient Education

- Discuss specific use of drug and side effects with patient as it relates to treatment. (HCAHPS: During this hospital stay, were you given any medicine that you had not taken before? Before giving you any new medicine, how often did hospital staff tell you what the medicine was for? How often did hospital staff describe possible side effects in a way you could understand?)
- Patient may experience presyncope, fatigue, blurred vision, illogical thinking, headache, or nausea. Have patient report immediately to prescriber signs of infection, angina, tachycardia, dyspnea, severe dizziness, edema, significant weight gain, or rash (HCAHPS).
- Educate patient about signs of a significant reaction (eg, wheezing; chest tightness; fever; itching; bad cough; blue skin color; seizures; or

swelling of face, lips, tongue, or throat). **Note:** This is not a comprehensive list of all side effects. Patient should consult prescriber for additional questions.

Intended Use and Disclaimer: Should not be printed and given to patients. This information is intended to serve as a concise initial reference for healthcare professionals to use when discussing medications with a patient. You must ultimately rely on your own discretion, experience and judgment in diagnosing, treating and advising patients.

Related Information

Oral Medications That Should Not Be Crushed or Altered *on page 1712*

Propranolol (proe PRAN oh lole)

Brand Names: U.S. Inderal LA; Inderal XL; Inno-Pran XL

Index Terms Propranolol Hydrochloride

Pharmacologic Category Antianginal Agent; Antiarrhythmic Agent, Class II; Antihypertensive; Beta-Adrenergic Blocker, Nonselective

Medication Safety Issues

Sound-alike/look-alike issues:

Propranolol may be confused with prasugrel, Pravachol, Propulsid

Inderal may be confused with Adderall, Enduron, Imdur, Imuran, Inderide, Isordil, Toradol

High alert medication:

The Institute for Safe Medication Practices (ISMP) includes this medication among its list of drugs which have a heightened risk of causing significant patient harm when used in error.

Administration issues:

Significant differences exist between oral and I.V. dosing. Use caution when converting from one route of administration to another.

International issues:

Inderal [Canada and multiple international markets] and Inderal LA [U.S.] may be confused with Indiaral brand name for loperamide [France]

Pregnancy Risk Factor C

Lactation Enters breast milk/use caution

Use Management of hypertension; angina pectoris; pheochromocytoma; essential tremor; supraventricular arrhythmias (such as atrial fibrillation and flutter, AV nodal re-entrant tachycardias), ventricular tachycardias (catecholamine-induced arrhythmias, digoxin toxicity); prevention of myocardial infarction; migraine headache prophylaxis; symptomatic treatment of hypertrophic subaortic stenosis (hypertrophic obstructive cardiomyopathy)

Unlabeled Use Tremor due to Parkinson's disease; aggressive behavior (not recommended for dementia-associated aggression), anxiety, schizophrenia; antipsychotic-induced akathisia; primary and secondary prophylaxis of variceal

hemorrhage; acute panic; thyrotoxicosis; tetralogy of Fallot (TOF) hypercyanotic spells

Available Dosage Forms

Capsule Extended Release 24 Hour, Oral:

Inderal LA: 60 mg, 80 mg, 120 mg, 160 mg

Inderal XL: 80 mg, 120 mg

InnoPran XL: 80 mg, 120 mg

Generic: 60 mg, 80 mg, 120 mg, 160 mg

Solution, Intravenous:

Generic: 1 mg/mL (1 mL)

Solution, Oral:

Generic: 20 mg/5 mL (500 mL); 40 mg/5 mL (500 mL)

Tablet, Oral:

Generic: 10 mg, 20 mg, 40 mg, 60 mg, 80 mg

General Dosage Range

I.V.: *Adults:* 1-3 mg, repeat every 2-5 minutes up to a total of 5 mg **or** 0.1 mg/kg divided into 3 equal doses given at 2- to 3-minute intervals; may repeat total dose in 2 minutes if needed

Oral:

Extended release: *Adults:* Initial: 80 mg once daily; Maintenance: 60-320 mg once daily (maximum: 640 mg/day)

Regular release: *Adults:* 30-320 mg/day in 2-4 divided doses (maximum: 640 mg/day)

Administration

I.V. I.V. dose is much smaller than oral dose. When administered acutely for cardiac treatment, monitor ECG and blood pressure. May administer by rapid infusion (I.V. push) at a rate of 1 mg/minute or by slow infusion over ~30 minutes. Necessary monitoring for surgical patients who are unable to take oral beta-blockers (prolonged ileus) has not been defined. Some institutions require monitoring of baseline and postinfusion heart rate and blood pressure when a patient's response to beta-blockade has not been characterized (ie, the patient's initial dose or following a change in dose). Consult individual institutional policies and procedures.

Injectable Detail pH: 2.8-3.5

Oral Do not crush long-acting forms.

Nursing Actions

Physical Assessment I.V. infusion usually requires hemodynamic monitoring; consult institution protocols. When discontinuing, drug must be tapered gradually over 2 weeks to avoid acute tachycardia, hypertension, and/or ischemia. Caution patients with diabetes to monitor blood glucose levels closely; beta-blockers can mask hypoglycemic symptoms.

Patient Education

• Discuss specific use of drug and side effects with patient as it relates to treatment. (HCAHPS: During this hospital stay, were you given any medicine that you had not taken before? Before giving you any new medicine, how often did hospital staff tell you what the medicine was for? How often did hospital staff describe possible side effects in a way you could understand?)

• Patient may experience presyncope, fatigue, blurred vision, illogical thinking, dizziness, or impotence. Have patient report immediately to prescriber dyspnea, significant weight gain, asthenia, severe skin irritation, or rash (HCAHPS).

• Educate patient about signs of a significant reaction (eg, wheezing; chest tightness; fever; itching; bad cough; blue skin color; seizures; or swelling of face, lips, tongue, or throat). **Note:** This is not a comprehensive list of all side effects. Patient should consult prescriber for additional questions.

Intended Use and Disclaimer: Should not be printed and given to patients. This information is intended to serve as a concise initial reference for healthcare professionals to use when discussing medications with a patient. You must ultimately rely on your own discretion, experience and judgment in diagnosing, treating and advising patients.

Related Information
Oral Medications That Should Not Be Crushed or Altered *on page 1712*

Propranolol and Hydrochlorothiazide
(proe PRAN oh lole & hye droe klor oh THYE a zide)

Index Terms Hydrochlorothiazide and Propranolol; Inderide

Pharmacologic Category Antihypertensive; Beta-Blocker, Nonselective; Diuretic, Thiazide

Medication Safety Issues
Sound-alike/look-alike issues:
Inderide may be confused with Inderal®

Pregnancy Risk Factor C

Use Management of hypertension

Available Dosage Forms
Tablet: Propranolol 40 mg and hydrochlorothiazide 25 mg; propranolol 80 mg and hydrochlorothiazide 25 mg

General Dosage Range Oral: *Adults:* Propranolol 80-160 mg/day and hydrochlorothiazide 12.5-50 mg/day in 2 divided doses

Nursing Actions
Physical Assessment See individual agents.

Patient Education
• Discuss specific use of drug and side effects with patient as it relates to treatment. (HCAHPS: During this hospital stay, were you given any medicine that you had not taken before? Before giving you any new medicine, how often did hospital staff tell you what the medicine was for? How often did hospital staff describe possible side effects in a way you could understand?)

• Patient may experience signs of hypokalemia, presyncope, fatigue, blurred vision, illogical thinking, dizziness, nausea, sexual dysfunction, or xerostomia. Have patient report immediately

to prescriber dyspnea, severe asthenia, urinary retention, significant skin irritation, sudden vision changes, eye pain, or eye irritation (HCAHPS).

• Educate patient about signs of a significant reaction (eg, wheezing; chest tightness; fever; itching; bad cough; blue skin color; seizures; swelling of face, lips, tongue, or throat). **Note:** This is not a comprehensive list of all side effects. Patient should consult prescriber for additional questions.

Intended Use and Disclaimer: Should not be printed and given to patients. This information is intended to serve as a concise initial reference for healthcare professionals to use when discussing medications with a patient. You must ultimately rely on your own discretion, experience and judgment in diagnosing, treating and advising patients.

Related Information
Hydrochlorothiazide *on page 775*
Propranolol *on page 1307*

Propylthiouracil (proe pil thye oh YOOR a sil)

Index Terms PTU (error-prone abbreviation)

Pharmacologic Category Antithyroid Agent; Thioamide

Medication Safety Issues
Sound-alike/look-alike issues:
Propylthiouracil may be confused with Purinethol®
PTU is an error-prone abbreviation (mistaken as mercaptopurine [Purinethol®; 6-MP])

Medication Guide Available Yes

Pregnancy Risk Factor D

Lactation Enters breast milk

Use Adjunctive therapy in patients intolerant of methimazole to ameliorate hyperthyroidism symptoms in preparation for surgical treatment or radioactive iodine therapy; treatment of hyperthyroidism in patients intolerant of methimazole and not candidates for surgical/radiotherapy

Unlabeled Use Management of Graves' disease, thyrotoxic crisis, or thyroid storm

Available Dosage Forms
Tablet, Oral:
Generic: 50 mg

General Dosage Range Oral:
Children 6-10 years: 50-150 mg/day
Children >10 years: 150-300 mg/day
Adults: Initial: 300-900 mg/day in 3 divided doses; Maintenance: 100-150 mg/day

Administration
Oral Administer at the same time in relation to meals each day, either always with meals or always between meals.

Nursing Actions
Physical Assessment Monitor for rash, goiter, nausea, vomiting, leucopenia, agranulocytosis,

anemia, jaundice, arthralgia, and CNS stimulation or depression.

Patient Education
- Discuss specific use of drug and side effects with patient as it relates to treatment. (HCAHPS: During this hospital stay, were you given any medicine that you had not taken before? Before giving you any new medicine, how often did hospital staff tell you what the medicine was for? How often did hospital staff describe possible side effects in a way you could understand?)
- Patient may experience headache, nausea, dyspepsia, or hepatic impairment. Have patient report immediately to prescriber inability to eat, ecchymosis, bleeding, discolored urine, jaundice, severe asthenia, or rash (HCAHPS).
- Educate patient about signs of a significant reaction (eg, wheezing; chest tightness; fever; itching; bad cough; blue skin color; seizures; or swelling of face, lips, tongue, or throat). **Note:** This is not a comprehensive list of all side effects. Patient should consult prescriber for additional questions.

Intended Use and Disclaimer: Should not be printed and given to patients. This information is intended to serve as a concise initial reference for healthcare professionals to use when discussing medications with a patient. You must ultimately rely on your own discretion, experience and judgment in diagnosing, treating and advising patients.

Protamine (PROE ta meen)

Index Terms Protamine Sulfate
Pharmacologic Category Antidote
Medication Safety Issues
Sound-alike/look-alike issues:
Protamine may be confused with ProAmatine, Protonix®, Protopam®
Pregnancy Risk Factor C
Lactation Excretion in breast milk unknown/use caution
Use Treatment of heparin overdosage; neutralize heparin during surgery or dialysis procedures
Unlabeled Use Treatment of low molecular weight heparin (LMWH) overdose
Available Dosage Forms
Solution, Intravenous:
Generic: 10 mg/mL (5 mL, 25 mL)
Solution, Intravenous [preservative free]:
Generic: 10 mg/mL (5 mL, 25 mL)
General Dosage Range I.V.: *Children and Adults:* 1 mg of protamine neutralizes ~100 units of heparin (maximum dose: 50 mg)
Administration
I.V. For I.V. use only. Administer slow IVP (50 mg over 10 minutes). Rapid I.V. infusion causes hypotension. Inject without further dilution over

1-3 minutes; maximum of 50 mg in any 10-minute period.
Injectable Detail pH: 6-7
Nursing Actions
Physical Assessment Monitor closely for hemodynamic changes. Monitor infusion rate. Slowing infusion rate may improve hypotension.
Patient Education
- Discuss specific use of drug and side effects with patient as it relates to treatment. (HCAHPS: During this hospital stay, were you given any medicine that you had not taken before? Before giving you any new medicine, how often did hospital staff tell you what the medicine was for? How often did hospital staff describe possible side effects in a way you could understand?)
- Patient may experience nausea or hypoglycemia. Have patient report immediately to prescriber dyspnea, severe dizziness, ecchymosis, bleeding, or rash (HCAHPS).
- Educate patient about signs of a significant reaction (eg, wheezing; chest tightness; fever; itching; bad cough; blue skin color; seizures; or swelling of face, lips, tongue, or throat). **Note:** This is not a comprehensive list of all side effects. Patient should consult prescriber for additional questions.

Intended Use and Disclaimer: Should not be printed and given to patients. This information is intended to serve as a concise initial reference for healthcare professionals to use when discussing medications with a patient. You must ultimately rely on your own discretion, experience and judgment in diagnosing, treating and advising patients.

Prucalopride (proo KAL oh pride)

Index Terms Prucalopride Succinate; R093877; R108512
Pharmacologic Category Serotonin 5-HT$_4$ Receptor Agonist
Medication Safety Issues
Sound-alike/look-alike issues:
Resotran™ may be confused with Restoril™
Lactation Enters breast milk/not recommended
Breast-Feeding Considerations Prucalopride is excreted into breast milk. Breast-feeding is not recommended by the manufacturer.
Use Treatment of chronic idiopathic constipation in adult females with inadequate response to laxatives
Unlabeled Use Opioid-induced constipation in chronic pain (noncancer) patients
Mechanism of Action/Effect Prucalopride is a selective, high-affinity 5-HT$_4$ receptor agonist whose action at the receptor site leads to neurotransmitter release and stimulation of the peristaltic reflex, intestinal secretions and gastrointestinal motility.

◀ **Contraindications** Hypersensitivity to prucalopride or any component of the formulation; renal impairment requiring dialysis; intestinal perforation or obstruction due to structural or functional disorder of the gut wall, obstructive ileus, severe inflammatory conditions of the GI tract (eg, Crohn's disease, ulcerative colitis, toxic megacolon).

Warnings/Precautions Use with caution in patients with a history of arrhythmias, ischemic cardiovascular disease, pre-excitation syndromes (eg, Wolff-Parkinson-White syndrome), or A-V nodal rhythm disorders. Slight increases in heart rate and shortened PR intervals were observed in healthy subjects during clinical trials; treatment-related effects on QRS duration or QTc interval were not observed. Palpitations have also been observed; monitoring of cardiovascular status is recommended. Instruct patients to report severe or persistent palpitations.

Use with caution in renal impairment; manufacturer's labeling recommends a dose reduction in severe impairment; contraindicated in patients requiring dialysis. Use with caution in patients with severe and unstable concomitant disease (eg, cancer, AIDS, psychiatric, hepatic, pulmonary, insulin-dependent diabetes mellitus); has not been studied. Patients with severe or persistent diarrhea should discontinue therapy and consult healthcare provider. Ischemic colitis has not observed during clinical trials but is a potential concern with treatment; instruct patients with onset of severe or worsening GI symptoms, bloody diarrhea or rectal bleeding to discontinue treatment and consult healthcare provider.

Dizziness and fatigue have been observed with initiation of therapy (generally the first day of therapy); caution patients in regards to operating dangerous machinery or driving. May contain lactose; do not use in patients with galactose intolerance, Lapp lactase deficiency, or glucose-galactose malabsorption syndromes. Use with caution in the elderly (limited data); dose reductions may be necessary. Efficacy not established in males. Women of childbearing potential should use effective contraceptive methods during treatment. An additional method of contraception is recommended in patients receiving oral contraceptives who experience severe diarrhea (potential decreased efficacy of the oral contraceptive). Cases of unintended pregnancies have been reported with prucalopride. Use is not recommended in children <18 years of age.

Drug Interactions

Avoid Concomitant Use There are no known interactions where it is recommended to avoid concomitant use.

Decreased Effect

Prucalopride may decrease the levels/effects of: Contraceptives (Estrogens); Contraceptives (Progestins)

Increased Effect/Toxicity

The levels/effects of Prucalopride may be increased by: P-glycoprotein/ABCB1 Inhibitors

Adverse Reactions

>10%:

Central nervous system: Headache (22%)

Gastrointestinal: Nausea (17%), abdominal pain (12%), diarrhea (12%)

1% to 10%:

Cardiovascular: Palpitation (1%; similar to placebo)

Central nervous system: Dizziness (4%), fatigue (3%), fever (1%), malaise (1%)

Genitourinary: Pollakiuria (1%)

Gastrointestinal: Upper abdominal pain (5%), flatulence (5%), vomiting (5%), dyspepsia (3%), bowel sounds abnormal (2%), anorexia (1%), gastroenteritis (1%)

Neuromuscular & skeletal: Muscle spasms (2%)

Product Availability Not available in U.S.

General Dosage Range Dosage adjustment recommended in patients with renal impairment.

Oral:

Adults (females ≥18 years): 2 mg once daily

Elderly (females >65 years): Initial: 1 mg once daily; maintenance: 1-2 mg once daily

Administration

Oral May administer without regard to meals. If a dose is missed, do not double to make up for a missed dose.

Storage/Stability Store at 15°C to 30°C (59°F to 86°F). Store in original container to protect from moisture.

Nursing Actions

Physical Assessment Monitor for cardiac event, clinically significant diarrhea, and ischemic colitis (rectal bleeding, bloody diarrhea, abdominal pain) frequently when beginning therapy and at regular intervals during treatment.

Patient Education

• Discuss specific use of drug and side effects with patient as it relates to treatment. (HCAHPS: During this hospital stay, were you given any medicine that you had not taken before? Before giving you any new medicine, how often did hospital staff tell you what the medicine was for? How often did hospital staff describe possible side effects in a way you could understand?)

• Patient may experience headache, nausea, diarrhea, or dyspepsia. Have patient report immediately to prescriber melena or rash (HCAHPS).

• Educate patient about signs of a significant reaction (eg, wheezing; chest tightness; fever; itching; bad cough; blue skin color; seizures; or swelling of face, lips, tongue, or throat). **Note:** This is not a comprehensive list of all side effects. Patient should consult prescriber for additional questions.

Pseudoephedrine (soo doe e FED rin)

Brand Names: U.S. Childrens Silfedrine [OTC]; Decongestant 12Hour Max St [OTC]; Decongestant [OTC]; ElixSure Congestion [OTC]; Genaphed [OTC]; Nasal Decongestant [OTC]; Nexafed [OTC]; Psudatabs [OTC]; Simply Stuffy [OTC]; Sudafed 12 Hour [OTC]; Sudafed 24 Hour [OTC]; Sudafed Childrens [OTC]; Sudafed [OTC]; Sudanyl [OTC]; SudoGest 12 Hour [OTC]; SudoGest [OTC]; Suphedrine [OTC]; Zephrex-D [OTC]

Index Terms d-Isoephedrine Hydrochloride; Pseudoephedrine Hydrochloride; Pseudoephedrine Sulfate; Sudafed

Pharmacologic Category Alpha/Beta Agonist; Decongestant

Medication Safety Issues

Sound-alike/look-alike issues:

Sudafed® may be confused with sotalol, Sudafed PE®, Sufenta®

Lactation Enters breast milk

Use Temporary symptomatic relief of nasal congestion due to common cold, upper respiratory allergies, and sinusitis; also promotes nasal or sinus drainage

Available Dosage Forms

Gel, Oral:

ElixSure Congestion [OTC]: 15 mg/5 mL (120 mL)

Liquid, Oral:

Childrens Silfedrine [OTC]: 15 mg/5 mL (118 mL, 237 mL)

Nasal Decongestant [OTC]: 30 mg/5 mL (118 mL)

Sudafed Childrens [OTC]: 15 mg/5 mL (118 mL)

Syrup, Oral:

Nasal Decongestant [OTC]: 30 mg/5 mL (473 mL)

Tablet, Oral:

Decongestant [OTC]: 30 mg

Genaphed [OTC]: 30 mg

Nasal Decongestant [OTC]: 30 mg

Psudatabs [OTC]: 30 mg

Simply Stuffy [OTC]: 30 mg

Sudafed [OTC]: 30 mg

Sudanyl [OTC]: 30 mg

SudoGest [OTC]: 30 mg, 60 mg

Suphedrine [OTC]: 30 mg

Generic: 30 mg, 60 mg

Tablet Abuse-Deterrent, Oral:

Nexafed [OTC]: 30 mg

Zephrex-D [OTC]: 30 mg

Tablet Extended Release 12 Hour, Oral:

Decongestant 12Hour Max St [OTC]: 120 mg

Sudafed 12 Hour [OTC]: 120 mg

SudoGest 12 Hour [OTC]: 120 mg

Generic: 120 mg

Tablet Extended Release 24 Hour, Oral:

Sudafed 24 Hour [OTC]: 240 mg

General Dosage Range Oral:

Immediate release:

Children 4-5 years: 15 mg every 4-6 hours (maximum: 60 mg/day)

Children 6-12 years: 30 mg every 4-6 hours (maximum: 120 mg/day)

Adults: 60 mg every 4-6 hours (maximum: 240 mg/day)

Extended release: *Adults:* 120 mg every 12 hours or 240 mg every 24 hours (maximum: 240 mg/day)

Administration

Oral Do not crush extended release drug product, swallow whole. May administer with or without food. Sudafed® 24 Hour tablet may not completely dissolve and appear in stool

Nursing Actions

Physical Assessment Monitor relief of congestion. Monitor for cardiac and CNS changes prior to treatment and throughout.

Patient Education

• Discuss specific use of drug and side effects with patient as it relates to treatment. (HCAHPS: During this hospital stay, were you given any medicine that you had not taken before? Before giving you any new medicine, how often did hospital staff tell you what the medicine was for? How often did hospital staff describe possible side effects in a way you could understand?)

• Patient may experience hypertension, nervousness, anxiety, headache, or insomnia. Have patient report immediately to prescriber angina, tachycardia, or rash (HCAHPS).

• Educate patient about signs of a significant reaction (eg, wheezing; chest tightness; fever; itching; bad cough; blue skin color; seizures; or swelling of face, lips, tongue, or throat). **Note:** This is not a comprehensive list of all side effects. Patient should consult prescriber for additional questions.

◄ **Related Information**
Oral Medications That Should Not Be Crushed or Altered *on page 1712*

Pyrazinamide (peer a ZIN a mide)

Index Terms Pyrazinoic Acid Amide
Pharmacologic Category Antitubercular Agent
Pregnancy Risk Factor C
Lactation Enters breast milk/use caution
Use Adjunctive treatment of tuberculosis in combination with other antituberculosis agents
Available Dosage Forms
Tablet, Oral:
Generic: 500 mg
General Dosage Range Dosage adjustment recommended in patients with renal impairment
Oral:
Children: 15-30 mg/kg once daily (maximum: 2 g/day) **or** 50 mg/kg/dose twice weekly (maximum: 2 g/dose)
Adults 40-55 kg: 1000 mg once daily **or** 2000 mg twice weekly **or** 1500 mg 3 times/week
Adults 56-75 kg: 1500 mg once daily **or** 3000 mg twice weekly **or** 2500 mg 3 times/week
Adults 76-90 kg: 2000 mg once daily (maximum dose regardless of weight) **or** 4000 mg twice weekly (maximum dose regardless of weight) **or** 3000 mg 3 times/week (maximum dose regardless of weight)
Nursing Actions
Physical Assessment Assess patient history for use cautions and evaluate any history of alcohol intake prior to beginning treatment. Monitor chest x-ray regularly.
Patient Education
• Discuss specific use of drug and side effects with patient as it relates to treatment. (HCAHPS: During this hospital stay, were you given any medicine that you had not taken before? Before giving you any new medicine, how often did hospital staff tell you what the medicine was for? How often did hospital staff describe possible side effects in a way you could understand?)
• Patient may experience nausea, asthenia, or hepatic impairment. Have patient report immediately to prescriber inability to eat, discolored urine, jaundice, severe arthralgia, or rash (HCAHPS).
• Educate patient about signs of a significant reaction (eg, wheezing; chest tightness; fever; itching; bad cough; blue skin color; seizures; or swelling of face, lips, tongue, or throat). **Note:** This is not a comprehensive list of all side effects. Patient should consult prescriber for additional questions.

Intended Use and Disclaimer: Should not be printed and given to patients. This information is intended to serve as a concise initial reference for healthcare professionals to use when discussing medications with a patient. You must ultimately rely on your own discretion, experience and judgment in diagnosing, treating and advising patients.

Pyrethrins and Piperonyl Butoxide
(pye RE thrins & pi PER oh nil byo TOKS ide)

Brand Names: U.S. A-200® Lice Treatment Kit [OTC]; A-200® Maximum Strength [OTC]; Licide® [OTC]; Pronto® Complete Lice Removal System [OTC]; Pronto® Plus Lice Killing Mousse Plus Vitamin E [OTC]; Pronto® Plus Lice Killing Mousse Shampoo Plus Natural Extracts and Oils [OTC]; Pronto® Plus Warm Oil Treatment and Conditioner [OTC]; RID® Maximum Strength [OTC]
Index Terms Piperonyl Butoxide and Pyrethrins
Pharmacologic Category Antiparasitic Agent, Topical; Pediculocide; Shampoo, Pediculocide
Pregnancy Risk Factor C
Use Treatment of *Pediculus humanus* infestations (head lice, body lice, pubic lice, and their eggs)
Available Dosage Forms
Kit:
A-200® Lice Treatment Kit [OTC]:
Shampoo: Pyrethrins 0.33% and piperonyl butoxide 4% (120 mL)
Solution: Permethrin 0.5% (180 mL)
Pronto® Complete Lice Removal System [OTC]:
Shampoo: Pyrethrins 0.33% and piperonyl butoxide 4% (60 mL)
Solution, topical: Benzalkonium chloride 0.1% (60 mL)
Oil, topical:
Pronto® Plus Warm Oil Treatment and Conditioner [OTC]: Pyrethrins 0.33% and piperonyl butoxide 4% (36 mL)
Shampoo:
A-200® Maximum Strength [OTC]: Pyrethrins 0.33% and piperonyl butoxide 4% (60 mL, 120 mL)
Licide® [OTC], Pronto® Plus Lice Killing Mousse Shampoo Plus Vitamin E [OTC]: Pyrethrins 0.33% and piperonyl butoxide 4% (120 mL)
Pronto® Plus Lice Killing Mousse Shampoo Plus Natural Extracts and Oils [OTC]: Pyrethrins 0.33% and piperonyl butoxide 4% (60 mL)
Pronto® Plus Lice Killing Mousse Shampoo Plus Vitamin E [OTC]: Pyrethrins 0.33% and piperonyl butoxide 4% (120 mL)
RID® Maximum Strength [OTC]: Pyrethrins 0.33% and piperonyl butoxide 4% (60 mL, 120 mL, 180 mL, 240 mL)
General Dosage Range Topical: *Children and Adults:* Apply to infested area, keep on for 10 minutes, wash, and rinse; may repeat once in a 24-hour period and then again in 7-10 days
Administration
Topical For external use only. Avoid touching eyes, mouth, or other mucous membranes.

Nursing Actions
Patient Education

- Discuss specific use of drug and side effects with patient as it relates to treatment. (HCAHPS: During this hospital stay, were you given any medicine that you had not taken before? Before giving you any new medicine, how often did hospital staff tell you what the medicine was for? How often did hospital staff describe possible side effects in a way you could understand?)
- Patient may experience scalp irritation, skin irritation, or short-term pain. Have patient report immediately to prescriber dyspnea or rash (HCAHPS).
- Educate patient about signs of a significant reaction (eg, wheezing; chest tightness; fever; itching; bad cough; blue skin color; seizures; or swelling of face, lips, tongue, or throat). **Note:** This is not a comprehensive list of all side effects. Patient should consult prescriber for additional questions.

Intended Use and Disclaimer: Should not be printed and given to patients. This information is intended to serve as a concise initial reference for healthcare professionals to use when discussing medications with a patient. You must ultimately rely on your own discretion, experience and judgment in diagnosing, treating and advising patients.

Pyridostigmine (peer id oh STIG meen)

Brand Names: U.S. Mestinon; Regonol
Index Terms Pyridostigmine Bromide
Pharmacologic Category Acetylcholinesterase Inhibitor
Medication Safety Issues
Sound-alike/look-alike issues:
 Pyridostigmine may be confused with physostigmine
 Regonol® may be confused with Reglan®, Renagel®
Pregnancy Risk Factor B
Lactation Enters breast milk/compatible
Use Symptomatic treatment of myasthenia gravis; antagonism of nondepolarizing neuromuscular blockers
Military use: Pretreatment for Soman nerve gas exposure
Available Dosage Forms
Solution, Injection:
 Regonol: 5 mg/mL (2 mL)
Syrup, Oral:
 Mestinon: 60 mg/5 mL (473 mL)
Tablet, Oral:
 Mestinon: 60 mg
 Generic: 60 mg
Tablet Extended Release, Oral:
 Mestinon: 180 mg

General Dosage Range
I.M.:
 Children: 0.05-0.15 mg/kg/dose
 Adults: ~1/30th of oral dose
I.V.:
 Children: 0.05-0.25 mg/kg/dose
 Adults: IVP: ~1/30th of oral dose **or** 0.1-0.25 mg/kg/dose (usual: 10-20 mg); Infusion: 2 mg/hour with gradual titration in increments of 0.5-1 mg/hour (maximum: 4 mg/hour)
Oral:
 Immediate release:
  Children: 7 mg/kg/day divided into 5-6 doses
  Adults: 60-1500 mg/day in 5-6 divided doses (usual: 600 mg/day)
 Sustained release: *Adults:* 180-540 mg once or twice daily (doses separated by at least 6 hours)
Administration
Injectable Detail pH: 5
Oral Do **not** crush sustained release tablet.
Nursing Actions
Physical Assessment When used to reverse neuromuscular block (anesthesia or excessive acetylcholine), monitor patient safety until full return of neuromuscular functioning. Assess bladder and sphincter adequacy prior to treatment. Monitor for cholinergic crisis: DUMBELS - **d**iarrhea, **u**rination, **m**iosis, **b**ronchospasm/bradycardia, **e**xcitability, **l**acrimation, and **s**alivation/ excessive sweating.
Patient Education

- Discuss specific use of drug and side effects with patient as it relates to treatment. (HCAHPS: During this hospital stay, were you given any medicine that you had not taken before? Before giving you any new medicine, how often did hospital staff tell you what the medicine was for? How often did hospital staff describe possible side effects in a way you could understand?)
- Patient may experience nausea, dyspepsia, or diarrhea. Have patient report immediately to prescriber significant change in balance or rash (HCAHPS).
- Educate patient about signs of a significant reaction (eg, wheezing; chest tightness; fever; itching; bad cough; blue skin color; seizures; or swelling of face, lips, tongue, or throat). **Note:** This is not a comprehensive list of all side effects. Patient should consult prescriber for additional questions.

Intended Use and Disclaimer: Should not be printed and given to patients. This information is intended to serve as a concise initial reference for healthcare professionals to use when discussing medications with a patient. You must ultimately rely on your own discretion, experience and judgment in diagnosing, treating and advising patients.

Related Information

Oral Medications That Should Not Be Crushed or Altered *on page 1712*

Pyridoxine (peer i DOKS een)

Brand Names: U.S. Neuro-K-250 T.D. [OTC]; Neuro-K-250 Vitamin B6 [OTC]; Neuro-K-50 [OTC]; Neuro-K-500 [OTC]; Pyri 500 [OTC]

Index Terms B6; B_6; Pyridoxine Hydrochloride; Vitamin B_6

Pharmacologic Category Vitamin, Water Soluble

Medication Safety Issues

Sound-alike/look-alike issues:

Pyridoxine may be confused with paroxetine, pralidoxime, Pyridium®

International issues:

Doxal [Brazil] may be confused with Doxil brand name for DOXOrubicin [U.S.]

Doxal: Brand name for pyridoxine/thiamine combination [Brazil], but also the brand name for doxepin [Finland]

Pregnancy Risk Factor A

Lactation Enters breast milk/compatible

Use Prevention and treatment of vitamin B_6 deficiency

Unlabeled Use Treatment and prophylaxis of neurological toxicities (ie, seizures, coma) associated with isoniazid and Gyromitrin-containing mushroom (false morel) overdose/toxicity; nausea and vomiting of pregnancy; prevention of peripheral neuropathy associated with isoniazid therapy for *Mycobacterium tuberculosis*

Available Dosage Forms

Capsule, Oral:

Neuro-K-250 T.D. [OTC]: 250 mg

Solution, Injection:

Generic: 100 mg/mL (1 mL)

Tablet, Oral:

Neuro-K-50 [OTC]: 50 mg

Neuro-K-500 [OTC]: 500 mg

Neuro-K-250 Vitamin B6 [OTC]: 250 mg

Pyri 500 [OTC]: 500 mg

Generic: 25 mg, 50 mg, 100 mg, 250 mg

Tablet, Oral [preservative free]:

Generic: 25 mg, 50 mg, 100 mg

Tablet Extended Release, Oral:

Generic: 200 mg

General Dosage Range

I.M., I.V.: *Adults:* 10-20 mg/day

Oral:

Infants 1-6 months: Adequate intake: 0.1 mg/day

Infants 7-12 months: Adequate intake: 0.3 mg/day

Children 1-3 years: RDA: 0.5 mg

Children 4-8 years: RDA: 0.6 mg

Children 9-13 years: RDA: 1 mg

Children 14-18 years: RDA: 1.2 mg (females); 1.3 mg (males)

Adults 19-50 years: RDA: 1.3 mg

Adults ≥51 years: RDA: 1.5 mg (females); 1.7 mg (males)

Pregnancy: RDA: 1.9 mg

Lactation: RDA: 2 mg

Administration

I.M. Burning may occur at the injection site after I.M. or SubQ administration.

I.V. Seizures have occurred following I.V. administration of very large doses.

Isoniazid toxicity (unlabeled use): Initial doses should be administered at a rate of 0.5-1 g/minute. If the parenteral formulation is not available, anecdotal reports suggest that pyridoxine tablets may be crushed and made into a slurry and given at the same dose orally or via nasogastric (NG) tube (Boyer, 2006). Oral administration is not recommended for acutely poisoned patients with seizure activity.

Injectable Detail pH: 2-3.8

Nursing Actions

Physical Assessment Provide patient appropriate dietary instructions.

Patient Education

- Discuss specific use of drug and side effects with patient as it relates to treatment. (HCAHPS: During this hospital stay, were you given any medicine that you had not taken before? Before giving you any new medicine, how often did hospital staff tell you what the medicine was for? How often did hospital staff describe possible side effects in a way you could understand?)

- Patient may experience headache, nausea, peripheral neuropathy, injection site irritation, or short-term pain. Have patient report immediately to prescriber paresthesia or rash (HCAHPS).

- Educate patient about signs of a significant reaction (eg, wheezing; chest tightness; fever; itching; bad cough; blue skin color; seizures; or swelling of face, lips, tongue, or throat). **Note:** This is not a comprehensive list of all side effects. Patient should consult prescriber for additional questions.

Intended Use and Disclaimer: Should not be printed and given to patients. This information is intended to serve as a concise initial reference for healthcare professionals to use when discussing medications with a patient. You must ultimately rely on your own discretion, experience and judgment in diagnosing, treating and advising patients.

QUEtiapine (kwe TYE a peen)

Brand Names: U.S. SEROquel; SEROquel XR

Index Terms Quetiapine Fumarate

Pharmacologic Category Antipsychotic Agent, Atypical

Medication Safety Issues
Sound-alike/look-alike issues:

QUEtiapine may be confused with OLANZapine

SEROquel may be confused with Serzone, SINE-quan

BEERS Criteria medication:

This drug may be potentially inappropriate for use in geriatric patients (Quality of evidence - moderate; Strength of recommendation - strong).

Medication Guide Available Yes

Pregnancy Risk Factor C

Lactation Enters breast milk/not recommended

Breast-Feeding Considerations Quetiapine is excreted into breast milk. Based on information from 8 mother-infant pairs, concentrations of quetiapine in breast milk have been reported from undetectable to 170 mcg/L. The estimated exposure to the breast-feeding infant would be up to 0.1 mg/kg/day (relative infant dose up to 0.43% based on a weight adjusted maternal dose of 400 mg/day). Due to the potential for serious adverse reactions in the nursing infant, the manufacturer recommends a decision be made whether to discontinue nursing or to discontinue the drug, taking into account the importance of treatment to the mother.

Use
Bipolar disorder: Acute treatment of manic (both immediate release and extended release [ER]) or mixed (ER only) episodes associated with bipolar I disorder, both as monotherapy and as an adjunct to lithium or divalproex; maintenance treatment of bipolar I disorder, as an adjunct to lithium or divalproex; acute treatment of depressive episodes associated with bipolar disorder

Major depressive disorder (ER only): Adjunctive therapy to antidepressants for the treatment of major depressive disorder.

Schizophrenia: Treatment of schizophrenia.

Unlabeled Use Delirium in the critically-ill patient; psychosis/agitation related to Alzheimer's dementia; augmentation in treatment-resistant obsessive compulsive disorder

Mechanism of Action/Effect Quetiapine is a dibenzothiazepine atypical antipsychotic. It has been proposed that this drug's antipsychotic activity is mediated through a combination of dopamine type 2 and serotonin type 2 antagonism.

Antagonism at receptors other than dopamine and 5-HT$_2$ with similar receptor affinities may explain some of the other effects of quetiapine. The drug's antagonism of histamine H$_1$-receptors may explain the somnolence observed. The drug's antagonism of adrenergic alpha$_1$-receptors may explain the orthostatic hypotension observed.

Contraindications Hypersensitivity to quetiapine or any component of the formulation

Warnings/Precautions [U.S. Boxed Warning]: Antidepressants increase the risk of suicidal thinking and behavior in children, adolescents, and young adults (18-24 years of age) with major depressive disorder (MDD) and other psychiatric disorders; consider risk prior to prescribing. Short-term studies did not show an increased risk in patients >24 years of age and showed a decreased risk in patients ≥65 years. Closely monitor all patients for clinical worsening, suicidality, or unusual changes in behavior; particularly during the initial 1-2 months of therapy or during periods of dosage adjustments (increased or decreases); the patient's family or caregiver should be instructed to closely observe the patient and communicate condition with healthcare provider. A medication guide concerning the use of antidepressants should be dispensed with each prescription. **Quetiapine is not approved in the U.S. for use in children <10 years of age.**

May precipitate a shift to mania or hypomania in patients with bipolar disorder. Patients presenting with depressive symptoms should be screened for bipolar disorder; the screening should include a detailed psychiatric history covering a family history of suicide, bipolar disorder, and depression. Quetiapine is approved in the U.S. for the treatment of bipolar depression. Pharmacologic treatment for pediatric bipolar I disorder or schizophrenia should be initiated only after thorough diagnostic evaluation and a careful consideration of potential risks vs benefits. If a pharmacologic agent is initiated, it should be a component of a total treatment program including psychological, educational and social interventions. Increased blood pressure (including hypertensive crisis) has been reported in children and adolescents; monitor blood pressure at baseline and periodically during use.

Leukopenia, neutropenia, and agranulocytosis (sometimes fatal) have been reported with antipsychotic use; presence of risk factors (eg, pre-existing low WBC or history of drug-induced leuko-/neutropenia) should prompt periodic blood count assessment. Discontinue therapy at first signs of blood dyscrasias or if absolute neutrophil count <1000/mm^3.

May cause orthostatic hypotension; use with caution in patients at risk of this effect or in those who would not tolerate transient hypotensive episodes (cerebrovascular disease, cardiovascular disease, dehydration, hypovolemia, or concurrent medication use which may predispose to hypotension/bradycardia) especially during the initial dose titration period. Use has been associated with QT prolongation; postmarketing reports have occurred in patients with concomitant illness, quetiapine overdose, or who were receiving concomitant therapy known to increase QT interval or cause electrolyte imbalance. Avoid use in patients at increased risk of torsade de pointes/sudden death (eg, hypokalemia, hypomagnesemia, history of cardiac arrhythmias, congenital prolongation of

QT interval, concomitant medications with QT$_c$ interval-prolonging properties). Use with caution in patients at increased risk of QT prolongation (eg, cardiovascular disease, heart failure, cardiac hypertrophy, elderly, family history of QT prolongation). May cause hyperglycemia; in some cases may be extreme and associated with ketoacidosis, hyperosmolar coma, or death. All patients should be monitored for symptoms of hyperglycemia (eg, polydipsia, polyuria, polyphagia, weakness) and undergo a fasting blood glucose test if symptoms develop during treatment. Patients with risk factors for diabetes (eg, obesity or family history) should have a baseline fasting blood sugar (FBS) and periodically during treatment. Use with caution in patients with pre-existing abnormal lipid profile. Significant weight gain has been observed with antipsychotic therapy; incidence varies with product. Monitor waist circumference and BMI.

[U.S. Boxed Warning]: Elderly patients with dementia-related psychosis treated with antipsychotics are at an increased risk of death compared to placebo. Most deaths appeared to be either cardiovascular (eg, heart failure, sudden death) or infectious (eg, pneumonia) in nature. Quetiapine is not approved for the treatment of dementia-related psychosis. Avoid antipsychotic use for behavioral problems associated with dementia unless alternative nonpharmacologic therapies have failed and patient may harm self or others. In addition, use may cause or exacerbate syndrome of inappropriate antidiuretic hormone secretion or hyponatremia; monitor sodium closely with initiation or dosage adjustments in older adults (Beers Criteria).

May cause dose-related decreases in thyroid levels, including cases requiring thyroid replacement therapy. Measure both TSH and free T$_4$, along with clinical assessment, at baseline and follow-up to determine thyroid status; measurement of TSH alone may not be accurate (exact mechanism of quetiapine's effect on the thyroid axis is unknown). Due to anticholinergic effects, use with caution in patients with decreased gastrointestinal motility, urinary retention, BPH, xerostomia, visual problems, and narrow-angle glaucoma. Relative to other antipsychotics, quetiapine has a moderate potency of cholinergic blockade. May cause extrapyramidal symptoms (EPS) and/or tardive dyskinesia. Risk of dystonia (and probably other EPS) may be greater with increased doses, use of conventional antipsychotics, males, and younger patients. Impaired core body temperature regulation may occur; caution with strenuous exercise, heat exposure, dehydration, and concomitant medication possessing anticholinergic effects. Use may be associated with neuroleptic malignant syndrome (NMS); monitor for mental status changes, fever, muscle rigidity and/or autonomic instability. Rare cases have been reported with quetiapine.

Esophageal dysmotility and aspiration have been associated with antipsychotic use; use with caution in patients at risk of aspiration pneumonia (eg, Alzheimer disease). Development of cataracts has been observed in animal studies; lens changes have been observed in humans during long-term treatment. Lens examination, such as a slit-lamp exam, on initiation of therapy and every 6 months thereafter is recommended by manufacturer. Use caution with Parkinson disease, history of seizures, and renal impairment. Use caution with hepatic impairment; may cause elevations of liver enzymes. May cause CNS depression, which may impair physical or mental abilities; patients must be cautioned about performing tasks that require mental alertness (eg, operating machinery or driving). Anaphylactic reactions have been reported with use. May increase prolactin levels; clinical significance of hyperprolactinemia in patients with breast cancer or other prolactin-dependent tumors is unknown. Potentially significant drug-drug interactions may exist, requiring dose or frequency adjustment, additional monitoring, and/or selection of alternative therapy. May cause withdrawal symptoms (rare) with abrupt cessation; gradually taper dose during discontinuation.

Drug Interactions

Avoid Concomitant Use

Avoid concomitant use of QUEtiapine with any of the following: Aclidinium; Amisulpride; Azelastine (Nasal); Fusidic Acid (Systemic); Highest Risk QTc-Prolonging Agents; Ipratropium (Oral Inhalation); Ivabradine; Metoclopramide; Mifepristone; Moderate Risk QTc-Prolonging Agents; Paraldehyde; Sulpiride; Thalidomide; Tiotropium; Umeclidinium

Decreased Effect

QUEtiapine may decrease the levels/effects of: Amphetamines; Anti-Parkinson's Agents (Dopamine Agonist); Quinagolide

The levels/effects of QUEtiapine may be decreased by: Bosentan; CYP3A4 Inducers (Strong); Dabrafenib; Deferasirox; Lithium formulations; Peginterferon Alfa-2b; St Johns Wort; Tocilizumab

Increased Effect/Toxicity

QUEtiapine may increase the levels/effects of: Alcohol (Ethyl); Amisulpride; Analgesics (Opioid); Anticholinergics; Azelastine (Nasal); Buprenorphine; CNS Depressants; Highest Risk QTc-Prolonging Agents; Hydrocodone; Hypotensive Agents; Methotrimeprazine; Methylphenidate; Paraldehyde; Serotonin Modulators; St Johns Wort; Sulpiride; Thalidomide; Tiotropium; Zolpidem

The levels/effects of QUEtiapine may be increased by: Acetylcholinesterase Inhibitors (Central); Aclidinium; Brimonidine (Topical); CYP3A4 Inhibitors (Moderate); CYP3A4

Inhibitors (Strong); Dasatinib; Doxylamine; Fusidic Acid (Systemic); HydrOXYzine; Ipratropium (Oral Inhalation); Ivabradine; Ivacaftor; Lithium formulations; Luliconazole; Magnesium Sulfate; Methotrimeprazine; Methylphenidate; Metoclopramide; Metyrosine; Mifepristone; Moderate Risk QTc-Prolonging Agents; Perampanel; Pramlintide; QTc-Prolonging Agents (Indeterminate Risk and Risk Modifying); Serotonin Modulators; Simeprevir; Sodium Oxybate; Tetrabenazine; Umeclidinium

Nutritional/Ethanol Interactions

Ethanol: Concomitant use with ethanol may increase CNS depression. Management: Advise patient that ethanol may enhance CNS depression; monitor for increased effects.

Food: In healthy volunteers, administration of quetiapine (immediate release) with food resulted in an increase in the peak serum concentration and AUC by 25% and 15%, respectively, compared to the fasting state. Administration of the extended release formulation with a high-fat meal (~800-1000 calories) resulted in an increase in peak serum concentration by 44% to 52% and AUC by 20% to 22% for the 50 mg and 300 mg tablets; administration with a light meal (≤300 calories) had no significant effect on the C_{max} or AUC. Management: Administer without food or with a light meal (≤300 calories).

Herb/Nutraceutical: Some herbal medications should be avoided due to the risk of CNS depression with concomitant use. St John's wort may decrease quetiapine levels. Management: Avoid valerian, St John's wort, kava kava, gotu kola.

Adverse Reactions Actual frequency may be dependent upon dose and/or indication. Unless otherwise noted, frequency of adverse effects is reported for adult patients; spectrum and incidence of adverse effects similar in children (with significant exceptions noted).

>10%:

Cardiovascular: Hypertension (diastolic; children and adolescents 41%), systolic hypertension (children and adolescents 15%), tachycardia (1% to 11%)

Central nervous system: Drowsiness (18% to 57%), headache (7% to 21%), agitation (5% to 20%), dizziness (1% to 19%), fatigue (3% to 14%), extrapyramidal reaction (1% to 13%)

Endocrine & metabolic: Weight gain (dose related; 3% to 23%), increased serum triglycerides (≥200 mg/dL, 8% to 22%), decreased HDL cholesterol (≤40 mg/dL, 6% to 19%), total cholesterol (≥240 mg/dL, 7% to 18%), increased LDL cholesterol (≥160 mg/dL, 4% to 17%), hyperglycemia (≥200 mg/dL post glucose challenge or fasting glucose ≥126 mg/dL, 2% to 12%)

Gastrointestinal: Xerostomia (9% to 44%; children and adolescents 4% to 10%), increased appetite (2% to 12%), constipation (2% to 11%)

1% to 10%:

Cardiovascular: Orthostatic hypotension (2% to 7%; children and adolescents <1%), syncope (<5%), palpitations (4%), peripheral edema (4%), increased heart rate (2% to 4%), hypotension (3%), hypertension (1% to 2%)

Central nervous system: Insomnia (9%), akathisia (≤8%), pain (1% to 7%), dystonia (≤6%), dysarthria (1% to 5%), irritability (1% to 5%), lethargy (1% to 5%), drooling (<5%), tardive dyskinesia (<5%), hypertonia (4%), twitching (4%), anxiety (2% to 4%), ataxia (2% to 4%), drug-induced Parkinson's disease (≤4%), abnormal dreams (2% to 3%), aggressive behavior (children and adolescents 1% to 3%), depression (1% to 3%), hypersomnia (1% to 3%), paresthesia (≤3%), abnormality in thinking (2%), decreased mental acuity (2%), disorientation (2%), hypoesthesia (2%), lack of concentration (2%), migraine (2%), restless leg syndrome (2%), vertigo (2%), confusion (1% to 2%), restlessness (1% to 2%), falling (≤2%), chills (1%)

Dermatologic: Skin rash (4%), acne vulgaris (children and adolescents 2% to 3%), diaphoresis (2%), hyperhidrosis (2%), pallor (children and adolescents 1% to 2%)

Endocrine & metabolic: Hyperprolactinemia (4%), decreased libido (≤2%), hypothyroidism (≤2%), increased thirst (children and adolescents ≤2%), increased gamma-glutamyl transferase (1%)

Gastrointestinal: Nausea (5% to 10%), vomiting (1% to 8%), dyspepsia (dose related; 2% to 7%), abdominal pain (1% to 7%), gastroenteritis (2% to 4%), toothache (2% to 3%), periodontal abscess (adolescents 1% to 3%), decreased appetite (2%), dysphagia (2%), flatulence (2%), gastroesophageal reflux disease (2%), anorexia (≥1%), unpleasant taste (1%), abdominal distension (≤1%)

Genitourinary: Pollakiuria (2%), urinary tract infection (2%), impotence (1%), lactation (female 1%)

Hematologic & oncologic: Neutropenia (≤2%), leukopenia (≥1%), hemorrhage (1%), lymphadenopathy (1%)

Hepatic: Increased serum transaminases (1% to 6%)

Hypersensitivity: Seasonal allergy (2%)

Neuromuscular & skeletal: Weakness (1% to 10%), tremor (2% to 8%), back pain (1% to 5%), dyskinesia (≤4%), arthralgia (1% to 4%), muscle rigidity (≤3%), muscle spasm (1% to 3%), stiffness (children and adolescents 1% to 3%), limb pain (2%), myalgia (2%), neck pain (2%), neck stiffness (1%)

Ophthalmic: Blurred vision (1% to 4%), amblyopia (2% to 3%)

Otic: Otalgia (≤2%)

Respiratory: Pharyngitis (4% to 6%), nasal congestion (3% to 6%), rhinitis (3% to 4%), cough (3%), upper respiratory tract infection (2% to 3%), epistaxis (adolescents ≤3%), sinus congestion (≤3%), sinus headache (2%), sinusitis (2%), flu-like symptoms (1% to 2%), dyspnea (≥1%), dry throat (1%)

Miscellaneous: Fever (1% to 4%)

Available Dosage Forms

Tablet, Oral:

SEROquel: 25 mg, 50 mg, 100 mg, 200 mg, 300 mg, 400 mg

Generic: 25 mg, 50 mg, 100 mg, 200 mg, 300 mg, 400 mg

Tablet Extended Release 24 Hour, Oral:

SEROquel XR: 50 mg, 150 mg, 200 mg, 300 mg, 400 mg

General Dosage Range Dosage adjustment recommended in patients with hepatic impairment and during concomitant therapy with CYP3A4 inhibitors and CYP3A4 inducers.

Oral:

Immediate release:

Children ≥10 to ≤12 years: Initial: 25 mg twice daily; Usual dosage range: 400-600 mg daily in 2-3 divided doses; maximum: 600 mg daily

Adolescents ≥13 to ≤17 years: Initial: 25 mg twice daily; Usual dosage range: 400-800 mg daily in 2-3 divided doses; maximum: 800 mg daily

Adults: Initial: 25-50 mg twice daily **or** 50 mg once daily; Usual dosage range: 150-800 mg daily in 2-3 divided doses

Elderly: Initial: 50 mg daily

Extended release:

Children ≥10 to ≤12 years: Initial: 50 mg once daily; Usual dosage range: 400-600 mg once daily; maximum: 600 mg once daily

Adolescents ≥13 to ≤17 years: Initial: 50 mg once daily; Usual dosage range: 400-800 mg once daily; maximum: 800 mg once daily

Adults: Initial: 50-300 mg once daily; Usual dosage range: 150-800 mg daily

Elderly: Initial: 50 mg once daily

Administration

Oral

Immediate release tablet: Administer with or without food.

Extended release tablet: Administer without food or with a light meal (≤300 calories), preferably in the evening. Swallow tablet whole; do not break, crush, or chew.

Other Nasogastric/enteral tube (unlabeled route): Hold tube feeds for 30 minutes before administration; flush with 25 mL of sterile water. Crush dose using immediate-release formulation, mix in 10 mL water and administer via NG/enteral tube; follow with a 50 mL flush of sterile water (Devlin, 2010).

Storage/Stability Store at 25°C (77°F); excursions permitted between 15°C and 30°C (59°F and 86°F).

Nursing Actions

Physical Assessment Monitor CNS responses, orthostatic hypotension, and seizure threshold. Assess mental status for depression and suicide ideation and observe for abnormal involuntary movements. Evaluate for cataracts before initiating treatment and every 6 months during chronic treatment. Monitor weight prior to initiating therapy and at least monthly.

Patient Education

• Discuss specific use of drug and side effects with patient as it relates to treatment. (HCAHPS: During this hospital stay, were you given any medicine that you had not taken before? Before giving you any new medicine, how often did hospital staff tell you what the medicine was for? How often did hospital staff describe possible side effects in a way you could understand?)

• Patient may experience presyncope, fatigue, blurred vision, illogical thinking, dizziness, headache, hypertension, hyperlipidemia, hypertriglyceridemia, nervousness and anxiety, constipation, xerostomia, weight gain, or hyperglycemia. Have patient report immediately to prescriber angina, significant change in balance, tremors, severe asthenia, polyuria, polydipsia, weight loss, menstrual irregularities, pregnancy, or rash (HCAHPS).

• Educate patient about signs of a significant reaction (eg, wheezing; chest tightness; fever; itching; bad cough; blue skin color; seizures; or swelling of face, lips, tongue, or throat). **Note:** This is not a comprehensive list of all side effects. Patient should consult prescriber for additional questions.

Intended Use and Disclaimer: Should not be printed and given to patients. This information is intended to serve as a concise initial reference for healthcare professionals to use when discussing medications with a patient. You must ultimately rely on your own discretion, experience and judgment in diagnosing, treating and advising patients.

Dietary Considerations Administer extended release tablet without food or with a light meal (≤300 calories).

Related Information

Oral Medications That Should Not Be Crushed or Altered *on page 1712*

Quinapril (KWIN a pril)

Brand Names: U.S. Accupril

Index Terms Quinapril Hydrochloride

Pharmacologic Category Angiotensin-Converting Enzyme (ACE) Inhibitor; Antihypertensive

Medication Safety Issues

Sound-alike/look-alike issues:
Accupril may be confused with Accolate, Accutane, AcipHex, Monopril

International issues:
Accupril [U.S., Canada] may be confused with Acepril which is a brand name for captopril [Great Britain]; enalapril [Hungary, Switzerland]; lisinopril [Malaysia]

Pregnancy Risk Factor D

Lactation Enters breast milk/use caution

Breast-Feeding Considerations Quinapril is excreted in breast milk. The manufacturer recommends that caution be exercised when administering quinapril to nursing women. The Canadian labeling contraindicates use in nursing women.

Use

Hypertension: Treatment of hypertension

Heart failure: Adjunctive treatment of heart failure (HF)

Note: The ACCF/AHA 2013 heart failure guidelines recommend the use of ACE inhibitors, along with other guideline directed medical therapies, to prevent HF in patients with a reduced ejection fraction who have a history of MI (stage B HF), to prevent HF in any patient with a reduced ejection fraction (stage B HF), or to treat those with HF and reduced ejection fraction (stage C HFrEF). (ACCF/AHA [Yancy, 2013])

Unlabeled Use Treatment of left ventricular dysfunction after myocardial infarction; pediatric hypertension; to delay the progression of nephropathy and reduce risks of cardiovascular events in hypertensive patients with type 1 or 2 diabetes mellitus

Mechanism of Action/Effect Competitive inhibitor of angiotensin-converting enzyme (ACE); prevents conversion of angiotensin I to angiotensin II, a potent vasoconstrictor; results in lower levels of angiotensin II which causes an increase in plasma renin activity and a reduction in aldosterone secretion

Contraindications

Hypersensitivity to quinapril or any component of the formulation; angioedema related to previous treatment with an ACE inhibitor; concomitant use with aliskiren in patients with diabetes mellitus.

Documentation of allergenic cross-reactivity for ACE inhibitors is limited. However, because of similarities in chemical structure and/or pharmacologic actions, the possibility of cross-sensitivity cannot be ruled out with certainty.

Canadian labeling: Additional contraindications (not in U.S. labeling): Women who are pregnant, intend to become pregnant, or of childbearing potential and not using adequate contraception; breast-feeding; concomitant use with aliskiren in patients with moderate-to-severe renal impairment (GFR <60 mL/minute/1.73 m^2)

Warnings/Precautions Anaphylactic reactions may occur rarely with ACE inhibitors. At any time during treatment (especially following first dose) angioedema may occur rarely with ACE inhibitors; it may involve the head and neck (potentially compromising airway) or the intestine (presenting with abdominal pain). African-Americans and patients with idiopathic or hereditary angioedema may be at an increased risk. Prolonged frequent monitoring may be required especially if tongue, glottis, or larynx are involved as they are associated with airway obstruction. Patients with a history of airway surgery may have a higher risk of airway obstruction. Aggressive early and appropriate management is critical. Use in patients with previous angioedema associated with ACE inhibitor therapy is contraindicated. Severe anaphylactoid reactions may be seen during hemodialysis (eg, CVVHD) with high-flux dialysis membranes (eg, AN69), and rarely, during low density lipoprotein apheresis with dextran sulfate cellulose. Rare cases of anaphylactoid reactions have been reported in patients undergoing sensitization treatment with hymenoptera (bee, wasp) venom while receiving ACE inhibitors. Formulation may contain lactose.

Symptomatic hypotension with or without syncope can occur with ACE inhibitors (usually with the first several doses); effects are most often observed in volume-depleted patients; close monitoring of patient is required especially with initial dosing and dosing increases; blood pressure must be lowered at a rate appropriate for the patient's clinical condition. Initiation of therapy in patients with ischemic heart disease or cerebrovascular disease warrants close observation due to the potential consequences posed by falling blood pressure (eg, MI, stroke). Use with caution in hypertrophic cardiomyopathy with outflow tract obstruction, severe aortic stenosis, or before, during, or immediately after major surgery. **[U.S. Boxed Warning]: Drugs that act on the renin-angiotensin system can cause injury and death to the developing fetus. Discontinue as soon as possible once pregnancy is detected.**

Hyperkalemia may occur with ACE inhibitors; risk factors include renal dysfunction, diabetes mellitus, concomitant use of potassium-sparing diuretics, potassium supplements, and/or potassium-containing salts. Use cautiously, if at all, with these agents and monitor potassium closely. Cough may occur with ACE inhibitors. Other causes of cough should be considered (eg, pulmonary congestion in patients with heart failure) and excluded prior to discontinuation.

May be associated with deterioration of renal function and/or increases in serum creatinine, particularly in patients with low renal blood flow (eg, renal artery stenosis, heart failure) whose glomerular filtration rate (GFR) is dependent on efferent arteriolar vasoconstriction by angiotensin II; deterioration may result in oliguria, acute renal failure, and progressive azotemia. Small increases in serum creatinine may occur following initiation; consider discontinuation only in patients with progressive and/or significant deterioration in renal function. Use with caution in patients with unstented unilateral/bilateral renal artery stenosis. When unstented bilateral renal artery stenosis is present, use is generally avoided due to the elevated risk of deterioration in renal function unless possible benefits outweigh risks. Potentially significant drug-drug interactions may exist, requiring dose or frequency adjustment, additional monitoring, and/or selection of alternative therapy.

Rare toxicities associated with ACE inhibitors include cholestatic jaundice (which may progress to fulminant hepatic necrosis), agranulocytosis, neutropenia, or leukopenia with myeloid hypoplasia. Patients with collagen vascular diseases (especially with concomitant renal impairment) or renal impairment alone may be at increased risk for hematologic toxicity; periodically monitor CBC with differential in these patients.

Drug Interactions

Avoid Concomitant Use There are no known interactions where it is recommended to avoid concomitant use.

Decreased Effect

Quinapril may decrease the levels/effects of: Quinolone Antibiotics; Tetracycline Derivatives

The levels/effects of Quinapril may be decreased by: Antacids; Aprotinin; Herbs (Hypertensive Properties); Icatibant; Lanthanum; Methylphenidate; Nonsteroidal Anti-Inflammatory Agents; Salicylates; Yohimbine

Increased Effect/Toxicity

Quinapril may increase the levels/effects of: Allopurinol; Amifostine; Antihypertensives; AzaTHIOprine; CycloSPORINE (Systemic); DULoxetine; Ferric Gluconate; Gold Sodium Thiomalate; Hypotensive Agents; Iron Dextran Complex; Lithium; Nonsteroidal Anti-Inflammatory Agents; Obinutuzumab; RiTUXimab; Sodium Phosphates

The levels/effects of Quinapril may be increased by: Alfuzosin; Aliskiren; Angiotensin II Receptor Blockers; Brimonidine (Topical); Canagliflozin; Diazoxide; DPP-IV Inhibitors; Eplerenone; Everolimus; Heparin; Heparin (Low Molecular Weight); Herbs (Hypotensive Properties); Loop Diuretics; MAO Inhibitors; Pentoxifylline; Phosphodiesterase 5 Inhibitors; Potassium Salts; Potassium-Sparing Diuretics; Prostacyclin Analogues; Sirolimus; Temsirolimus; Thiazide Diuretics; TiZANidine; Tolvaptan; Trimethoprim

Nutritional/Ethanol Interactions

Food: Potassium supplements and/or potassium-containing salts may cause or worsen hyperkalemia. Management: Consult prescriber before consuming a potassium-rich diet, potassium supplements, or salt substitutes.

Herb/Nutraceutical: Some herbal medications may worsen hypertension (eg, licorice); others may increase the antihypertensive effects of quinapril (eg, shepherd's purse). Management: Avoid bayberry, blue cohosh, cayenne, ephedra, ginger, ginseng (American), kola, licorice, and yohimbe. Avoid black cohosh, California poppy, coleus, golden seal, hawthorn, mistletoe, periwinkle, quinine, and shepherd's purse.

Adverse Reactions Note: Frequency ranges include data from hypertension and heart failure trials. Higher rates of adverse reactions have generally been noted in patients with CHF. However, the frequency of adverse effects associated with placebo is also increased in this population.

1% to 10%:
Cardiovascular: Hypotension (3%), chest pain (2%), first-dose hypotension (up to 3%)
Central nervous system: Dizziness (4% to 8%), headache (2% to 6%), fatigue (3%)
Dermatologic: Rash (1%)
Endocrine & metabolic: Hyperkalemia (2%)
Gastrointestinal: Vomiting/nausea (1% to 2%), diarrhea (2%)
Neuromuscular & skeletal: Myalgias (2% to 5%), back pain (1%)
Renal: BUN/serum creatinine increased (2%, transient elevations may occur with a higher frequency), worsening of renal function (in patients with bilateral renal artery stenosis or hypovolemia)
Respiratory: Upper respiratory symptoms, cough (2% to 4%; up to 13% in some studies), dyspnea (2%)

Pharmacodynamics/Kinetics
Onset of Action 1 hour
Duration of Action 24 hours

Available Dosage Forms
Tablet, Oral:
Accupril: 5 mg, 10 mg, 20 mg, 40 mg
Generic: 5 mg, 10 mg, 20 mg, 40 mg

General Dosage Range Dosage adjustment recommended in patients with renal impairment
Oral:
Adults: Initial: 5-20 mg daily in 1-2 divided doses; Maintenance: 10-80 mg daily in 1-2 divided doses
Elderly: Initial: 10 mg daily

Administration
Oral Administer without regard to meals.
Storage/Stability Store at 15°C to 30°C (59°F to 86°F). Protect from light.

Nursing Actions
Physical Assessment Assess potential for interactions with other pharmacological agents or herbal products that may impact fluid balance or cardiac status. Monitor blood pressure carefully (hypotension or angioedema can occur at any time during treatment, especially following first dose). Monitor cardiac status and blood pressure.

Monitor for hypovolemia, angioedema, and postural hypotension on a regular basis during therapy.

Patient Education
• Discuss specific use of drug and side effects with patient as it relates to treatment. (HCAHPS: During this hospital stay, were you given any medicine that you had not taken before? Before giving you any new medicine, how often did hospital staff tell you what the medicine was for? How often did hospital staff describe possible side effects in a way you could understand?)
• Patient may experience dizziness, headache, or myalgia. Have patient report immediately to prescriber signs of infection, syncope, dyspnea, hyperhidrosis, diarrhea, significant weight gain, edema in legs or abdomen, discolored urine, jaundice, or rash (HCAHPS).
• Educate patient about signs of a significant reaction (eg, wheezing; chest tightness; fever; itching; bad cough; blue skin color; seizures; or swelling of face, lips, tongue, or throat). **Note:** This is not a comprehensive list of all side effects. Patient should consult prescriber for additional questions.

Intended Use and Disclaimer: Should not be printed and given to patients. This information is intended to serve as a concise initial reference for healthcare professionals to use when discussing medications with a patient. You must ultimately rely on your own discretion, experience and judgment in diagnosing, treating and advising patients.

Quinapril and Hydrochlorothiazide
(KWIN a pril & hye droe klor oh THYE a zide)

Brand Names: U.S. Accuretic®
Index Terms Hydrochlorothiazide and Quinapril; Quinaretic
Pharmacologic Category Angiotensin-Converting Enzyme (ACE) Inhibitor; Antihypertensive; Diuretic, Thiazide
Pregnancy Risk Factor D
Use Hypertension: Treatment of hypertension (not for initial therapy)
Available Dosage Forms
Tablet, oral: 10/12.5: Quinapril 10 mg and hydrochlorothiazide 12.5 mg; 20/12.5: Quinapril 20 mg and hydrochlorothiazide 12.5 mg; 20/25: Quinapril 20 mg and hydrochlorothiazide 25 mg
Accuretic®: 10/12.5: Quinapril 10 mg and hydrochlorothiazide 12.5 mg; 20/12.5: Quinapril 20 mg and hydrochlorothiazide 12.5 mg; 20/25: Quinapril 20 mg and hydrochlorothiazide 25 mg
General Dosage Range Oral: *Adults:* Initial: 10-20 mg quinapril and 12.5 mg hydrochlorothiazide once daily; Maintenance: 5-40 mg quinapril and 6.25-25 mg hydrochlorothiazide once daily
Nursing Actions
Physical Assessment See individual agents.

Patient Education
• Discuss specific use of drug and side effects with patient as it relates to treatment. (HCAHPS: During this hospital stay, were you given any medicine that you had not taken before? Before giving you any new medicine, how often did hospital staff tell you what the medicine was for? How often did hospital staff describe possible side effects in a way you could understand?)
• Patient may experience dizziness, headache, diarrhea, asthenia, or dyspepsia. Have patient report immediately to prescriber signs of infection, signs of hyperglycemia, signs of hepatic or renal impairment, angina, bradycardia, akathisia, dyspnea, dysarthria, ecchymosis, bleeding, arthralgia, significant weight gain, or vision changes (HCAHPS).
• Educate patient about signs of a significant reaction (eg, wheezing; chest tightness; fever; itching; bad cough; blue skin color; seizures; or swelling of face, lips, tongue, or throat). **Note:** This is not a comprehensive list of all side effects. Patient should consult prescriber for additional questions.

Intended Use and Disclaimer: Should not be printed and given to patients. This information is intended to serve as a concise initial reference for healthcare professionals to use when discussing medications with a patient. You must ultimately rely on your own discretion, experience and judgment in diagnosing, treating and advising patients.

Related Information
Hydrochlorothiazide *on page* 775
Quinapril *on page* 1318

QuiNIDine (KWIN i deen)

Index Terms Quinidine Gluconate; Quinidine Polygalacturonate; Quinidine Sulfate
Pharmacologic Category Antiarrhythmic Agent, Class Ia; Antimalarial Agent
Medication Safety Issues
Sound-alike/look-alike issues:
QuiNIDine may be confused with cloNIDine, quiNINE
High alert medication:
The Institute for Safe Medication Practices (ISMP) includes this medication (I.V. formulation) among its list of drug classes which have a heightened risk of causing significant patient harm when used in error.
BEERS Criteria medication:
This drug may be potentially inappropriate for use in geriatric patients (Quality of evidence - high; Strength of recommendation - strong).
Pregnancy Risk Factor C
Lactation Enters breast milk/not recommended

Use

Quinidine gluconate and sulfate salts: Conversion and prevention of relapse into atrial fibrillation and/or flutter; suppression of ventricular arrhythmias. **Note:** Due to proarrhythmic effects, use should be reserved for life-threatening arrhythmias. Moreover, the use of quinidine has largely been replaced by more effective/safer antiarrhythmic agents and/or nonpharmacologic therapies (eg, radiofrequency ablation).

Quinidine gluconate (I.V. formulation): Conversion of atrial fibrillation/flutter and ventricular tachycardia. **Note:** The use of I.V. quinidine gluconate for these indications has been replaced by more effective/safer antiarrhythmic agents (eg, amiodarone and procainamide).

Quinidine gluconate (I.V. formulation) and quinidine sulfate: Treatment of malaria (*Plasmodium falciparum*)

Unlabeled Use Paroxysmal supraventricular tachycardia, paroxysmal AV junctional rhythm, and symptomatic atrial or ventricular premature contractions; short QT syndrome; Brugada syndrome

Available Dosage Forms

Solution, Injection:
Generic: 80 mg/mL (10 mL)
Tablet, Oral:
Generic: 200 mg, 300 mg
Tablet Extended Release, Oral:
Generic: 300 mg, 324 mg

General Dosage Range Dosages expressed in terms of the salt. Dosage adjustment recommended in patients with renal impairment.

I.V.: Quinidine gluconate: *Children and Adults:* 10 mg/kg bolus followed by 0.02 mg/kg/minute **or** 24 mg/kg bolus followed by 12 mg/kg every 8 hours

Oral:
Immediate release: Quinidine sulfate: *Adults:* Initial: 200-400 mg/dose every 6 hours
Extended release:
Quinidine gluconate: *Adults:* Initial: 324 mg every 8-12 hours
Quinidine sulfate: *Adults:* Initial: 300 mg every 8-12 hours

Usual Infusion Concentrations: Adult I.V. infusion: Quinidine gluconate: 800 mg in 50 mL (concentration: 16 mg/mL) of D_5W

Administration

I.V. Minimize use of PVC tubing to enhance bioavailability; shorter tubing lengths are recommended by the manufacturer

Injectable Detail pH: 5.5-7 (injection)

Oral Do not crush, chew, or break sustained release dosage forms. Give around-the-clock to promote less variation in peak and trough serum levels. Some preparations of quinidine gluconate extended release tablets may be split in half to facilitate dosage titration; tablets are not scored.

Nursing Actions

Physical Assessment I.V. requires use of infusion pump and continuous cardiac and hemodynamic monitoring. Monitor cardiac status at beginning of therapy, when titrating dosage, and on a regular basis. Quinidine has a low toxic:therapeutic ratio and overdose may easily produce severe and life-threatening reactions.

Patient Education

- Discuss specific use of drug and side effects with patient as it relates to treatment. (HCAHPS: During this hospital stay, were you given any medicine that you had not taken before? Before giving you any new medicine, how often did hospital staff tell you what the medicine was for? How often did hospital staff describe possible side effects in a way you could understand?)
- Patient may experience dizziness, nausea, diarrhea, dyspepsia, or parageusia. Have patient report immediately to prescriber tachycardia, severe asthenia, inability to eat, ecchymosis, bleeding, discolored urine, jaundice, or rash (HCAHPS).
- Educate patient about signs of a significant reaction (eg, wheezing; chest tightness; fever; itching; bad cough; blue skin color; seizures; or swelling of face, lips, tongue, or throat). **Note:** This is not a comprehensive list of all side effects. Patient should consult prescriber for additional questions.

Intended Use and Disclaimer: Should not be printed and given to patients. This information is intended to serve as a concise initial reference for healthcare professionals to use when discussing medications with a patient. You must ultimately rely on your own discretion, experience and judgment in diagnosing, treating and advising patients.

Related Information

Oral Medications That Should Not Be Crushed or Altered *on page 1712*

QuiNINE (KWYE nine)

Brand Names: U.S. Qualaquin

Index Terms Quinine Sulfate

Pharmacologic Category Antimalarial Agent

Medication Safety Issues

Sound-alike/look-alike issues:
QuiNINE may be confused with quiNIDine

Medication Guide Available Yes

Pregnancy Risk Factor C

Lactation Enters breast milk/use caution

Use In conjunction with other antimalarial agents, treatment of uncomplicated chloroquine-resistant *P. falciparum* malaria

Unlabeled Use Treatment of *Babesia microti* infection in conjunction with clindamycin; treatment of uncomplicated chloroquine-resistant *P. vivax*

malaria (in conjunction with other antimalarial agents)

Available Dosage Forms

Capsule, Oral:

Qualaquin: 324 mg

Generic: 324 mg

General Dosage Range Dosage adjustment recommended in patients with renal impairment

Oral:

Children: 30 mg/kg/day divided every 8 hours

Adults: 648 mg every 8 hours

Administration

Oral Avoid use of aluminum- or magnesium-containing antacids because of drug absorption problems. Swallow dose whole to avoid bitter taste. May be administered with food.

Nursing Actions

Physical Assessment Allergy history should be assessed prior to beginning therapy.

Patient Education

- Discuss specific use of drug and side effects with patient as it relates to treatment. (HCAHPS: During this hospital stay, were you given any medicine that you had not taken before? Before giving you any new medicine, how often did hospital staff tell you what the medicine was for? How often did hospital staff describe possible side effects in a way you could understand?)
- Patient may experience hypoglycemia, dyspepsia, nausea, diarrhea, headache, or flushing. Have patient report immediately to prescriber dyspnea, tachycardia, hearing impairment, signs of hypotension, severe dizziness, tinnitus, petechiae, ecchymosis, bleeding, sudden vision changes, or rash (HCAHPS).
- Educate patient about signs of a significant reaction (eg, wheezing; chest tightness; fever; itching; bad cough; blue skin color; seizures; or swelling of face, lips, tongue, or throat). **Note:** This is not a comprehensive list of all side effects. Patient should consult prescriber for additional questions.

Intended Use and Disclaimer: Should not be printed and given to patients. This information is intended to serve as a concise initial reference for healthcare professionals to use when discussing medications with a patient. You must ultimately rely on your own discretion, experience and judgment in diagnosing, treating and advising patients.

Quinupristin and Dalfopristin
(kwi NYOO pris tin & dal FOE pris tin)

Brand Names: U.S. Synercid®

Index Terms Dalfopristin and Quinupristin; RP-59500

Pharmacologic Category Antibiotic, Streptogramin

Pregnancy Risk Factor B

Lactation Excretion in breast milk unknown/use caution

Use Treatment of complicated skin and skin structure infections caused by methicillin-susceptible *Staphylococcus aureus* or *Streptococcus pyogenes*

Unlabeled Use Treatment of persistent MRSA bacteremia associated with vancomycin failure

Available Dosage Forms

Injection, powder for reconstitution:

Synercid®: 500 mg: Quinupristin 150 mg and dalfopristin 350 mg

General Dosage Range I.V.: *Children ≥12 years and Adults:* 7.5 mg/kg every 12 hours

Administration

I.V. Line should be flushed with 5% dextrose in water prior to and following administration. Infusion should be completed over 60 minutes (toxicity may be increased with shorter infusion). If severe venous irritation occurs following peripheral administration, quinupristin/dalfopristin may be further diluted (to 500 mL or 750 mL), infusion site changed, or infused by a peripherally-inserted central catheter (PICC) or a central venous catheter.

Nursing Actions

Physical Assessment Infusion site must be closely monitored. Monitor for arthralgia, headache, rash, hyperglycemia, opportunistic infection (fever, chills, sore throat, burning urination, fatigue), pseudomembranous colitis, hyperbilirubinemia, dyspnea, and ataxia.

Patient Education

- Discuss specific use of drug and side effects with patient as it relates to treatment. (HCAHPS: During this hospital stay, were you given any medicine that you had not taken before? Before giving you any new medicine, how often did hospital staff tell you what the medicine was for? How often did hospital staff describe possible side effects in a way you could understand?)
- Patient may experience injection site irritation, headache, nausea, diarrhea, arthralgia, or myalgia. Have patient report immediately to prescriber discolored urine, jaundice, severe fatigue, ecchymosis, bleeding, or rash (HCAHPS).
- Educate patient about signs of a significant reaction (eg, wheezing; chest tightness; fever; itching; bad cough; blue skin color; seizures; or swelling of face, lips, tongue, or throat). **Note:** This is not a comprehensive list of all side effects. Patient should consult prescriber for additional questions.

Intended Use and Disclaimer: Should not be printed and given to patients. This information is intended to serve as a concise initial reference for healthcare professionals to use when discussing medications with a patient. You must ultimately rely on your own discretion, experience and

judgment in diagnosing, treating and advising patients.

Rabeprazole (ra BEP ra zole)

Brand Names: U.S. Aciphex; AcipHex Sprinkle
Index Terms Pariprazole
Pharmacologic Category Proton Pump Inhibitor; Substituted Benzimidazole
Medication Safety Issues
Sound-alike/look-alike issues:
AcipHex may be confused with Acephen, Accupril, Aricept, pHisoHex
RABEprazole may be confused with ARIPiprazole, donepezil, lansoprazole, omeprazole, raloxifene
Medication Guide Available Yes
Pregnancy Risk Factor B
Lactation Excretion in breast milk unknown/use caution
Breast-Feeding Considerations It is not known if rabeprazole is excreted into breast milk. The manufacturer recommends that caution be exercised when administering rabeprazole to nursing women.
Use
Duodenal ulcers: Short-term (4 weeks or fewer) treatment in the healing and symptomatic relief of duodenal ulcers in adults.
Gastroesophageal reflux disease:
Erosive or ulcerative: Short-term (4 to 8 weeks) treatment in the healing and symptomatic relief of erosive or ulcerative gastroesophageal reflux disease (GERD) in adults; for maintaining healing and reduction in relapse rates of heartburn symptoms in adults with erosive or ulcerative GERD.
Symptomatic: Treatment of symptomatic GERD in adults and pediatric patients 1 year and older.
Helicobacter pylori eradication: In combination with amoxicillin and clarithromycin as a 3-drug regimen for the treatment of adults with *H. pylori* infection and duodenal ulcer disease (active or history of within the past 5 years) to eradicate *H. pylori*.
Pathological hypersecretory conditions: Long-term treatment of pathological hypersecretory conditions, including Zollinger-Ellison syndrome in adults.

Canadian labeling: Additional uses (not in U.S. labeling): Treatment of nonerosive reflux disease (NERD); treatment of gastric ulcers
Unlabeled Use Maintenance of healing and prevention of relapse for duodenal ulcer; treatment and prevention of NSAID-induced ulcer
Mechanism of Action/Effect Prevents gastric acid secretion
Contraindications Hypersensitivity to rabeprazole, substituted benzimidazoles, or any component of the formulation

Warnings/Precautions Use of proton pump inhibitors (PPIs) may increase the risk of gastrointestinal infections (eg, *Salmonella, Campylobacter*). Use caution in severe hepatic impairment. Relief of symptoms with rabeprazole does not preclude the presence of a gastric malignancy. Use of PPIs may increase risk of *Clostridium difficile*-associated diarrhea (CDAD), especially in hospitalized patients; consider CDAD diagnosis in patients with persistent diarrhea that does not improve. Use the lowest dose and shortest duration of PPI therapy appropriate for the condition being treated. Decreased *H. pylori* eradication rates have been observed with short-term (≤7 days) combination therapy. The American College of Gastroenterology recommends 10-14 days of therapy (triple or quadruple) for eradication of *H. pylori* (Chey, 2007).

PPIs may diminish the therapeutic effect of clopidogrel, thought to be due to reduced formation of the active metabolite of clopidogrel. The manufacturer of clopidogrel recommends either avoidance of both omeprazole (even when scheduled 12 hours apart) and esomeprazole or use of a PPI with comparatively less effect on the active metabolite of clopidogrel. Avoidance of rabeprazole appears prudent due to potent *in vitro* CYP2C19 inhibition (Li, 2004) and lack of sufficient comparative *in vivo* studies with other PPIs. In contrast to these warnings, others have recommended the continued use of PPIs, regardless of the degree of inhibition, in patients with a history of GI bleeding or multiple risk factors for GI bleeding who are also receiving clopidogrel since no evidence has established clinically meaningful differences in outcome; however, a clinically-significant interaction cannot be excluded in those who are poor metabolizers of clopidogrel (Abraham, 2010; Levine, 2011). Potentially significant drug-drug interactions may exist, requiring dose or frequency adjustment, additional monitoring, and/or selection of alternative therapy.

Increased incidence of osteoporosis-related bone fractures of the hip, spine, or wrist may occur with PPI therapy. Patients on high-dose (multiple daily doses) or long-term therapy (≥1 year) should be monitored. Use the lowest effective dose for the shortest duration of time, use vitamin D and calcium supplementation, and follow appropriate guidelines to reduce risk of fractures in patients at risk.

Hypomagnesemia, reported rarely, usually with prolonged PPI use of >3 months (most cases >1 year of therapy); may be symptomatic or asymptomatic; severe cases may cause tetany, seizures, and cardiac arrhythmias. Consider obtaining serum magnesium concentrations prior to beginning long-term therapy, especially if taking concomitant digoxin, diuretics, or other drugs known to cause hypomagnesemia; and periodically thereafter. Hypomagnesemia may be corrected by magnesium supplementation, although discontinuation of rabeprazole may be necessary; magnesium levels typically return to normal within 1 week of stopping.

Drug Interactions

Avoid Concomitant Use

Avoid concomitant use of RABEprazole with any of the following: Dasatinib; Delavirdine; Erlotinib; Nelfinavir; Pimozide; PONATinib; Rilpivirine; Risedronate

Decreased Effect

RABEprazole may decrease the levels/effects of: Atazanavir; Bisphosphonate Derivatives; Bosutinib; Cefditoren; Clopidogrel; Dabigatran Etexilate; Dabrafenib; Dasatinib; Delavirdine; Erlotinib; Gefitinib; Indinavir; Iron Salts; Itraconazole; Ketoconazole (Systemic); Mesalamine; Multivitamins/Minerals (with ADEK, Folate, Iron); Mycophenolate; Nelfinavir; Nilotinib; PONATinib; Posaconazole; Rilpivirine; Riociguat; Risedronate; Vismodegib

The levels/effects of RABEprazole may be decreased by: Bosentan; CYP2C19 Inducers (Strong); CYP3A4 Inducers (Strong); Dabrafenib; Deferasirox; Herbs (CYP3A4 Inducers); Mitotane; Tipranavir; Tocilizumab

Increased Effect/Toxicity

RABEprazole may increase the levels/effects of: Amphetamine; ARIPiprazole; CYP2C8 Substrates; Dexmethylphenidate; Dextroamphetamine; Dofetilide; Lomitapide; Methotrexate; Methylphenidate; Pimozide; Raltegravir; Risedronate; Saquinavir; Tacrolimus (Systemic); Voriconazole

The levels/effects of RABEprazole may be increased by: Fluconazole; Ketoconazole (Systemic); Voriconazole

Nutritional/Ethanol Interactions

Ethanol: Ethanol may cause gastric mucosal irritation. Management: Avoid concomitant administration of ethanol.

Food: High-fat meals may delay absorption of tablets, but C_{max} and AUC are not altered. Administration of capsule granules (sprinkled on applesauce) with a high-fat meal resulted in a decrease in C_{max} and AUC by 55% and 35%, respectively. Management: Tablets may be administered with or without food; capsules should be administered before a meal.

Herb/Nutraceutical: St John's wort may increase the metabolism and thus decrease the levels/effects of rabeprazole. Management: Avoid concomitant administration of St. John's wort.

Adverse Reactions Frequency not always defined.

1% to 10%:

Cardiovascular: Peripheral edema

Central nervous system: Headache (2% to 10%), pain (3%), dizziness

Gastrointestinal: Diarrhea (2% to 5%), nausea (2% to 5%), abdominal pain (4%), vomiting (4%), flatulence (3%), constipation (2%), xerostomia

Hepatic: Hepatic encephalopathy, hepatic enzymes increased, hepatitis

Neuromuscular & skeletal: Arthralgia, myalgia

Respiratory: Pharyngitis (3%)

Miscellaneous: Infection (2%)

Pharmacodynamics/Kinetics

Onset of Action Within 1 hour

Duration of Action 24 hours

Available Dosage Forms

Capsule Sprinkle, Oral:

AcipHex Sprinkle: 5 mg, 10 mg

Tablet Delayed Release, Oral:

Aciphex: 20 mg

Generic: 20 mg

General Dosage Range Oral:

Children 1-11 years: 5 to 10 mg once daily

Children ≥12 years and Adolescents: 20 mg once daily

Adults: 10-20 mg once to twice daily **or** 60 mg once daily

Administration

Oral May be administered with an antacid.

Capsules: Administer 30 minutes before a meal. Open capsule and sprinkle contents on a small amount of soft food (eg, applesauce, fruit or vegetable based baby food, yogurt) or empty contents into a small amount of liquid (eg, infant formula, apple juice, pediatric electrolyte solution); food or liquid should be at or below room temperature. Do not chew or crush granules; administer whole dose within 15 minutes of preparation (do not store for future use).

Tablets: May be administered with or without food. However, when used for the healing of duodenal ulcers, administration after breakfast is recommended. When used for the eradication of *H. pylori*, administration with the morning and evening meals is recommended. Swallow tablets whole; do not crush, split, or chew.

Storage/Stability Store at 25°C (77°F); excursions are permitted between 15°C and 30°C (59°F and 86°F). Protect from moisture.

Nursing Actions

Physical Assessment Assess those medications requiring acid environment for absorption. Monitor reduction in symptoms.

Patient Education

- Discuss specific use of drug and side effects with patient as it relates to treatment. (HCAHPS: During this hospital stay, were you given any medicine that you had not taken before? Before giving you any new medicine, how often did hospital staff tell you what the medicine was for? How often did hospital staff describe possible side effects in a way you could understand?)
- Patient may experience headache, diarrhea, or flatulence. Have patient report immediately to prescriber severe dizziness, syncope,

tachycardia, dyspepsia, osteodynia, myalgia, asthenia, ecchymosis, or rash (HCAHPS).
- Educate patient about signs of a significant reaction (eg, wheezing; chest tightness; fever; itching; bad cough; blue skin color; seizures; or swelling of face, lips, tongue, or throat). **Note:** This is not a comprehensive list of all side effects. Patient should consult prescriber for additional questions.

Intended Use and Disclaimer: Should not be printed and given to patients. This information is intended to serve as a concise initial reference for healthcare professionals to use when discussing medications with a patient. You must ultimately rely on your own discretion, experience and judgment in diagnosing, treating and advising patients.

Dietary Considerations
Capsules: Take 30 minutes before a meal.
Tablets: May be taken with or without food. However, when used for the healing of duodenal ulcers, it is best if taken after breakfast. When used for the eradication of *Helicobacter pylori*, take with the morning and evening meals.

Related Information
Oral Medications That Should Not Be Crushed or Altered *on page 1712*

Rabies Vaccine (RAY beez vak SEEN)

Brand Names: U.S. Imovax Rabies; RabAvert
Index Terms HDCV; Human Diploid Cell Cultures Rabies Vaccine; PCEC; Purified Chick Embryo Cell
Pharmacologic Category Vaccine, Inactivated (Viral)
Pregnancy Risk Factor C
Lactation Excretion in breast milk unknown
Use Pre-exposure and postexposure vaccination against rabies

The Advisory Committee on Immunization Practices (ACIP) recommends a primary course of prophylactic immunization (pre-exposure vaccination) for the following:
- Persons with continuous risk of infection, including rabies research laboratory and biologics production workers
- Persons with frequent risk of infection in areas where rabies is enzootic, including rabies diagnostic laboratory workers, cavers, veterinarians and their staff, and animal control and wildlife workers; persons who frequently handle bats
- Persons with infrequent risk of infection, including veterinarians and animal control staff with terrestrial animals in areas where rabies infection is rare, veterinary students, and travelers visiting areas where rabies is enzootic and immediate access to medical care and biologicals is limited

The ACIP recommends the use of postexposure vaccination for a particular person be assessed by the severity and likelihood versus the actual risk of acquiring rabies. Consideration should include the type of exposure, epidemiology of rabies in the area, species of the animal, circumstances of the incident, and the availability of the exposing animal for observation or rabies testing. Postexposure vaccination is used in both previously vaccinated and previously unvaccinated individuals.

Available Dosage Forms
Injectable, Intramuscular [preservative free]:
Imovax Rabies: 2.5 units/mL (1 ea)
Suspension Reconstituted, Intramuscular:
RabAvert: (1 ea)
General Dosage Range I.M.: *Children and Adults:* 1 mL

Administration
I.M. For I.M. administration only; this rabies vaccine product must not be administered intradermally; in adults and children, administer I.M. injections in the deltoid muscle, not the gluteal; for younger children, use the outer aspect of the thigh. Postexposure prophylaxis should begin with immediate cleansing of wounds with soap and water; if available, a virucidal agent (eg, povidone-iodine solution) should be used to irrigate the wounds.

For patients at risk of hemorrhage following intramuscular injection, the ACIP recommends "it should be administered intramuscularly if, in the opinion of the physician familiar with the patient's bleeding risk, the vaccine can be administered by this route with reasonable safety. If the patient receives antihemophilia or other similar therapy, intramuscular vaccination can be scheduled shortly after such therapy is administered. A fine needle (23 gauge or smaller) can be used for the vaccination and firm pressure applied to the site (without rubbing) for at least 2 minutes. The patient should be instructed concerning the risk of hematoma from the injection." Patients on anticoagulant therapy should be considered to have the same bleeding risks and treated as those with clotting factor disorders (CDC, 2011).

Simultaneous administration of vaccines helps ensure the patients will be fully vaccinated by the appropriate age. Simultaneous administration of vaccines is defined as administering >1 vaccine on the same day at different anatomic sites. The use of licensed combination vaccines is generally preferred over separate injections of the equivalent components. Separate vaccines should not be combined in the same syringe unless indicated by product specific labeling. Separate needles and syringes should be used for each injection. The ACIP prefers each dose of a specific vaccine in a series come from the same manufacturer when possible. Adolescents and adults should be vaccinated while seated or lying down. In general, preterm infants should be vaccinated at the same chronological age as full-term infants (CDC, 2011).

Antipyretics have not been shown to prevent febrile seizures. Antipyretics may be used to treat fever or discomfort following vaccination (CDC, 2011). One study reported that routine prophylactic administration of acetaminophen to prevent fever prior to vaccination decreased the immune response of some vaccines; the clinical significance of this reduction in immune response has not been established (Prymula, 2009).

Nursing Actions

Physical Assessment All serious adverse reactions must be reported to the U.S. DHHS. U.S. federal law also requires entry into the patient's medical record.

Patient Education

• Discuss specific use of vaccine and side effects with patient as it relates to treatment. (HCAHPS: During this hospital stay, were you given any medicine that you had not taken before? Before giving you any new medicine, how often did hospital staff tell you what the medicine was for? How often did hospital staff describe possible side effects in a way you could understand?)

• Patient may experience pain, redness or swelling at injection site, headache, fatigue, nausea, emesis, diarrhea, or dyspepsia. Have patient report immediately to prescriber severe injection site reaction (HCAHPS).

• Educate patient about signs of a significant reaction (eg, wheezing; chest tightness; fever; itching; bad cough; blue skin color; seizures; or swelling of face, lips, tongue, or throat). **Note:** This is not a comprehensive list of all side effects. Patient should consult prescriber for additional questions.

Intended Use and Disclaimer: Should not be printed and given to patients. This information is intended to serve as a concise initial reference for healthcare professionals to use when discussing medications with a patient. You must ultimately rely on your own discretion, experience and judgment in diagnosing, treating and advising patients.

Related Information

Immunization Administration Recommendations *on page 1675*

Immunization Recommendations *on page 1680*

Raloxifene (ral OKS i feen)

Brand Names: U.S. Evista

Index Terms Keoxifene Hydrochloride; Raloxifene Hydrochloride

Pharmacologic Category Selective Estrogen Receptor Modulator (SERM)

Medication Safety Issues

Sound-alike/look-alike issues:

Evista® may be confused with AVINza®, Eovist®

Raloxifene may be confused with ospemifene, toremifene

Medication Guide Available Yes

Pregnancy Risk Factor X

Lactation Excretion in breast milk unknown/contraindicated

Breast-Feeding Considerations It is not known if raloxifene is excreted into breast milk. Breast-feeding is contraindicated by the manufacturer.

Use Prevention and treatment of osteoporosis in postmenopausal women; risk reduction for invasive breast cancer in postmenopausal women with osteoporosis and in postmenopausal women with high risk for invasive breast cancer

Mechanism of Action/Effect A selective estrogen receptor modulator (SERM), meaning that it affects some of the same receptors that estrogen does, but not all, and in some instances, it antagonizes or blocks estrogen; it acts like estrogen to prevent bone loss and has the potential to block some estrogen effects in the breast uterine cancer tissues. Raloxifene decreases bone resorption, increasing bone mineral density and decreasing fracture incidence.

Contraindications History of or current venous thromboembolic disorders (including DVT, PE, and retinal vein thrombosis); pregnancy or women who could become pregnant; breast-feeding

Warnings/Precautions Hazardous agent - use appropriate precautions for handling and disposal (NIOSH, 2012). **[U.S. Boxed Warning]: May increase the risk for DVT or PE; use contraindicated in patients with history of or current venous thromboembolic disorders.** Use with caution in patients at high risk for venous thromboembolism; the risk for DVT and PE are higher in the first 4 months of treatment. Discontinue at least 72 hours prior to and during prolonged immobilization (postoperative recovery or prolonged bedrest). **[U.S. Boxed Warning]: The risk of death due to stroke may be increased in women with coronary heart disease or in women at risk for coronary events;** use with caution in patients with cardiovascular disease. Not be used for the prevention of cardiovascular disease. Use caution with moderate-to-severe renal dysfunction, hepatic impairment, unexplained uterine bleeding, and in women with a history of elevated triglycerides in response to treatment with oral estrogens (or estrogen/progestin). Safety with concomitant estrogen therapy has not been established. Safety and efficacy in premenopausal women or men have not been established. Not indicated for treatment of invasive breast cancer, to reduce the risk of recurrence of invasive breast cancer or to reduce the risk of noninvasive breast cancer. The efficacy (for breast cancer risk reduction) in women with inherited BRCA1 and BRCA1 mutations has not been established.

Drug Interactions

Avoid Concomitant Use

Avoid concomitant use of Raloxifene with any of the following: Ospemifene

Decreased Effect

Raloxifene may decrease the levels/effects of: Levothyroxine; Ospemifene

The levels/effects of Raloxifene may be decreased by: Bile Acid Sequestrants

Increased Effect/Toxicity

Raloxifene may increase the levels/effects of: Ospemifene

Nutritional/Ethanol Interactions Ethanol: Avoid ethanol (may increase risk of osteoporosis).

Adverse Reactions Note: Raloxifene has been associated with increased risk of thromboembolism (DVT, PE) and superficial thrombophlebitis; risk is similar to reported risk of HRT

>10%:

Cardiovascular: Peripheral edema (3% to 14%)

Endocrine & metabolic: Hot flashes (8% to 29%)

Neuromuscular & skeletal: Arthralgia (11% to 16%), leg cramps/muscle spasm (6% to 12%)

Miscellaneous: Flu syndrome (14% to 15%), infection (11%)

1% to 10%:

Cardiovascular: Chest pain (3%), venous thromboembolism (1% to 2%)

Central nervous system: Insomnia (6%)

Dermatologic: Rash (6%)

Endocrine & metabolic: Breast pain (4%)

Gastrointestinal: Weight gain (9%), abdominal pain (7%), vomiting (5%), flatulence (2% to 3%), cholelithiasis (≤3%), gastroenteritis (≤3%)

Genitourinary: Vaginal bleeding (6%), leukorrhea (3%), urinary tract disorder (3%), uterine disorder (3%), vaginal hemorrhage (3%), endometrial disorder (≤3%)

Neuromuscular & skeletal: Myalgia (8%), tendon disorder (4%)

Respiratory: Bronchitis (10%), sinusitis (10%), pharyngitis (8%), pneumonia (3%), laryngitis (≤2%)

Miscellaneous: Diaphoresis (3%)

Pharmacodynamics/Kinetics

Onset of Action 8 weeks

Available Dosage Forms

Tablet, Oral:

Evista: 60 mg

General Dosage Range Oral: *Adults (females):* 60 mg/day

Administration

Oral May be administered without regard to meals

Hazardous agent; use appropriate precautions for handling and disposal (NIOSH, 2012).

Storage/Stability Store at controlled room temperature of 20°C to 25°C (68°F to 77°F); excursions permitted to 15°C to 30°C (59°F to 86°F).

Nursing Actions

Physical Assessment Evaluate lipid profile and BMD. Monitor for DVT, PE, chest pain, migraine, and rash on a regular basis during therapy.

Patient Education

- Discuss specific use of drug and side effects with patient as it relates to treatment. (HCAHPS: During this hospital stay, were you given any medicine that you had not taken before? Before giving you any new medicine, how often did hospital staff tell you what the medicine was for? How often did hospital staff describe possible side effects in a way you could understand?)
- Patient may experience edema, hot flashes, headache, nausea, diarrhea, arthralgia, leg cramps, or insomnia. Have patient report immediately to prescriber depression, nervousness, emotional instability, illogical thinking, anxiety, angina, dyspnea, significant weight gain, sudden vision changes, eye pain, eye irritation, mastalgia, severe vaginal bleeding, or rash (HCAHPS).
- Educate patient about signs of a significant reaction (eg, wheezing; chest tightness; fever; itching; bad cough; blue skin color; seizures; or swelling of face, lips, tongue, or throat). **Note:** This is not a comprehensive list of all side effects. Patient should consult prescriber for additional questions.

Intended Use and Disclaimer: Should not be printed and given to patients. This information is intended to serve as a concise initial reference for healthcare professionals to use when discussing medications with a patient. You must ultimately rely on your own discretion, experience and judgment in diagnosing, treating and advising patients.

Dietary Considerations May be taken without regard to meals. Osteoporosis prevention or treatment: Ensure adequate calcium and vitamin D intake; if dietary intake is inadequate, dietary supplementation is recommended. Women and men should consume:

Calcium: 1000 mg/day (men: 50-70 years) **or** 1200 mg/day (women ≥51 years and men ≥71 years) (IOM, 2011; NOF, 2013)

Vitamin D: 800-1000 IU/day (men and women ≥50 years) (NOF, 2013). Recommended Dietary Allowance (RDA): 600 IU/day (men and women ≤70 years) **or** 800 IU/day (men and women ≥71 years) (IOM, 2011).

Related Information

Oral Medications That Should Not Be Crushed or Altered *on page 1712*

Raltegravir (ral TEG ra vir)

Brand Names: U.S. Isentress

Index Terms MK-0518; RAL

Pharmacologic Category Antiretroviral, Integrase Inhibitor (Anti-HIV)

Pregnancy Risk Factor C

Lactation Excretion in breast milk unknown/contraindicated

Breast-Feeding Considerations Maternal or infant antiretroviral therapy does not completely eliminate the risk of postnatal HIV transmission. In addition, multiclass-resistant virus has been detected in breast-feeding infants despite maternal therapy. Therefore, in the United States, where formula is accessible, affordable, safe, and sustainable, and the risk of infant mortality due to diarrhea and respiratory infections is low, complete avoidance of breast-feeding by HIV-infected women is recommended to decrease potential transmission of HIV (DHHS [perinatal], 2012).

Use HIV-1 infection: Treatment of HIV-1 infection in combination with other antiretroviral agents

Unlabeled Use Postexposure prophylaxis for occupational exposure to HIV

Mechanism of Action/Effect Inhibits the integration of viral DNA into host DNA, thereby blocking subsequent viral replication.

Contraindications There are no contraindications listed in the manufacturer's labeling.

Canadian labeling: Hypersensitivity to raltegravir or any other component of the formulation

Warnings/Precautions Patients may develop immune reconstitution syndrome resulting in the occurrence of an inflammatory response to an indolent or residual opportunistic infection during initial HIV treatment or activation of autoimmune disorders (eg, Graves' disease, polymyositis, Guillain-Barré syndrome) later in therapy; further evaluation and treatment may be required. Severe, life-threatening or fatal cases of Stevens-Johnson syndrome and toxic epidermal necrolysis have been reported. Hypersensitivity reactions (rash [may occur with fever, fatigue, malaise, conjunctivitis, or other constitutional symptoms], organ dysfunction and/or hepatic failure) have also been reported. Discontinue immediately if a severe skin reaction or hypersensitivity symptoms develop. Monitor liver transaminases and start supportive therapy. Myopathy and rhabdomyolysis have been reported; use caution in patients with risk factors for CK elevations and/or skeletal muscle abnormalities. Potentially significant drug-drug interactions may exist, requiring dose or frequency adjustment, additional monitoring, and/or selection of alternative therapy. Avoid use as a boosted PI replacement in antiretroviral experienced patients with documented resistance to nucleoside reverse transcriptase inhibitors. Chewable tablet contains phenylalanine.

Drug Interactions

Avoid Concomitant Use

Avoid concomitant use of Raltegravir with any of the following: Aluminum Hydroxide; Magnesium Salts

Decreased Effect

Raltegravir may decrease the levels/effects of: Fosamprenavir

The levels/effects of Raltegravir may be decreased by: Aluminum Hydroxide; Efavirenz; Fosamprenavir; Magnesium Salts; Rifabutin; Rifampin; Tipranavir

Increased Effect/Toxicity

Raltegravir may increase the levels/effects of: Fibric Acid Derivatives; HMG-CoA Reductase Inhibitors; Zidovudine

The levels/effects of Raltegravir may be increased by: Proton Pump Inhibitors

Nutritional/Ethanol Interactions

Food: Variable absorption depending upon meal type (low- vs high-fat meal) and dosage form; raltegravir was administered without regard to meals in clinical trials.

Herb/Nutraceutical: Avoid St John's wort (may decrease the levels/effects of raltegravir).

Adverse Reactions

>10%:

Hepatic: Increased serum ALT (1% to 11%; incidence higher with hepatitis B and/or C coinfection)

2% to 10%:

Central nervous system: Insomnia (4%), headache (2% to 4%), dizziness (2%), fatigue (2%)

Endocrine & metabolic: Increased serum glucose (126 to 250 mg/dL: 7% to 10%; 251 to 500 mg/dL: 2% to 3%)

Gastrointestinal: Increased serum lipase (2% to 5%), increased serum amylase (2% to 4%), nausea (3%)

Hematologic: Abnormal absolute neutrophil count (2% to 3%), thrombocytopenia (1% to 3%)

Hepatic: Increased serum AST (1% to 9%; incidence higher with hepatitis B and/or C coinfection), hyperbilirubinemia (<1% to 6%), increased serum alkaline phosphatase (<1% to 2%)

Neuromuscular & skeletal: Increased creatine phosphokinase (10 to 19.9 x ULN: 4%; ≥20 x ULN: 3%)

Product Availability Isentress (100 mg single use packets for oral suspension): FDA approved December 2013; anticipated availability is the third quarter of 2014.

Available Dosage Forms

Tablet, Oral:

Isentress: 400 mg

Tablet Chewable, Oral:

Isentress: 25 mg, 100 mg

General Dosage Range Dosage adjustment recommended in patients on concomitant therapy

◄ **Oral:**

Children 2 to <6 years: Chewable tablet: Weight-based dosing: 75-300 mg twice daily
Children 6 to <12 years: Chewable tablet: Weight-based dosing: 75-300 mg twice daily; if ≥25 kg, refer to weight-based dosing or adult dosing
Adolescents ≥12 years and Adults: Film-coated tablet: 400 mg twice daily

Administration

Oral May be administered without regard to meals.

Storage/Stability

Chewable tablet: Store in the original package with the bottle tightly closed, at room temperature of 20°C to 25°C (68°F to 77°F); excursions permitted to 15°C to 30°C (59°F to 86°F). Keep the desiccant in the bottle to protect from moisture.

Film-coated tablet: Store at room temperature of 20°C to 25°C (68°F to 77°F); excursions permitted to 15°C to 30°C (59°F to 86°F).

Nursing Actions

Physical Assessment Monitor for muscle pain and tenderness, changes in cholesterol, and signs and symptoms of depression.

Patient Education

- Discuss specific use of drug and side effects with patient as it relates to treatment. (HCAHPS: During this hospital stay, were you given any medicine that you had not taken before? Before giving you any new medicine, how often did hospital staff tell you what the medicine was for? How often did hospital staff describe possible side effects in a way you could understand?)
- Patient may experience insomnia, headache, dizziness, or dyspepsia. Have patient report immediately to prescriber signs of hepatic impairment, signs of renal impairment, myalgia, arthralgia, severe asthenia, ecchymosis, hemorrhaging, depression, or signs of Stevens-Johnson syndrome/toxic epidermal necrolysis (HCAHPS).
- Educate patient about signs of a significant reaction (eg, wheezing; chest tightness; fever; itching; bad cough; blue skin color; seizures; or swelling of face, lips, tongue, or throat). **Note:** This is not a comprehensive list of all side effects. Patient should consult prescriber for additional questions.

Intended Use and Disclaimer: Should not be printed and given to patients. This information is intended to serve as a concise initial reference for healthcare professionals to use when discussing medications with a patient. You must ultimately rely on your own discretion, experience and judgment in diagnosing, treating and advising patients.

Dietary Considerations May be taken without regard to meals. Some products may contain phenylalanine.

Ramelteon (ra MEL tee on)

Brand Names: U.S. Rozerem

Index Terms TAK-375

Pharmacologic Category Hypnotic, Miscellaneous; Melatonin Receptor Agonist

Medication Safety Issues

Sound-alike/look-alike issues:

Ramelteon may be confused with Remeron
Rozerem may be confused with Razadyne, Remeron

Medication Guide Available Yes

Pregnancy Risk Factor C

Lactation Excretion in breast milk unknown/use caution

Breast-Feeding Considerations It is not known if ramelteon is excreted in breast milk. The manufacturer recommends that caution be exercised when administering ramelteon to nursing women.

Use Treatment of insomnia characterized by difficulty with sleep onset

Mechanism of Action/Effect Activates melatonin receptors within an area of the CNS controlling circadian rhythms and sleep-wake cycle.

Contraindications History of angioedema with previous ramelteon therapy (do not rechallenge); concurrent use with fluvoxamine

Warnings/Precautions Symptomatic treatment of insomnia should be initiated only after careful evaluation of potential causes of sleep disturbance. Failure of sleep disturbance to resolve after a reasonable period of treatment may indicate psychiatric and/or medical illness. Because of the rapid onset of action, administer immediately prior to bedtime or after the patient has gone to bed and is having difficulty falling asleep. Hypnotics/sedatives have been associated with abnormal thinking and behavior changes including decreased inhibition, aggression, bizarre behavior, agitation, hallucinations, and depersonalization. These changes may occur unpredictably and may indicate previously unrecognized psychiatric disorders; evaluate appropriately. Postmarketing studies have indicated that the use of hypnotic/sedative agents (including ramelteon) for sleep has been associated with hypersensitivity reactions including anaphylaxis as well as angioedema. Do not rechallenge patients who have developed angioedema with ramelteon therapy. An increased risk for hazardous sleep-related activities such as sleep-driving; cooking and eating food, and making phone calls while asleep have also been noted. Use caution with pre-existing depression or other psychiatric conditions. Caution when using with other CNS depressants; avoid engaging in hazardous activities or activities requiring mental alertness. Not recommended for use in patients with severe sleep apnea or COPD. Use caution with moderate hepatic impairment; not recommended in patients with severe impairment. May cause disturbances of hormonal regulation. Use caution when administered concomitantly with strong CYP1A2 inhibitors.

Drug Interactions

Avoid Concomitant Use

Avoid concomitant use of Ramelteon with any of the following: Azelastine (Nasal); FluvoxaMINE; Paraldehyde; Sodium Oxybate; Thalidomide

Decreased Effect

The levels/effects of Ramelteon may be decreased by: Rifamycin Derivatives

Increased Effect/Toxicity

Ramelteon may increase the levels/effects of: Alcohol (Ethyl); Azelastine (Nasal); Buprenorphine; CNS Depressants; Hydrocodone; Methotrimeprazine; Metyrosine; Mirtazapine; Paraldehyde; Pramipexole; ROPINIRole; Rotigotine; Selective Serotonin Reuptake Inhibitors; Sodium Oxybate; Thalidomide; Zolpidem

The levels/effects of Ramelteon may be increased by: Abiraterone Acetate; Brimonidine (Topical); CYP1A2 Inhibitors (Moderate); CYP1A2 Inhibitors (Strong); Deferasirox; Doxylamine; Droperidol; Fluconazole; FluvoxaMINE; HydrOXYzine; Ketoconazole (Systemic); Magnesium Sulfate; Methotrimeprazine; Perampanel; Tapentadol; Vemurafenib

Nutritional/Ethanol Interactions

Ethanol: May increase CNS depression. Management: Avoid or limit ethanol.

Food: Taking with high-fat meal delays T_{max} and increases AUC (~31%). Management: Do not take with a high-fat meal.

Herb/Nutraceutical: Some herbal medications may increase CNS depression. Management: Avoid valerian, St John's wort, kava kava, and gotu kola.

Adverse Reactions 1% to 10%:

Central nervous system: Dizziness (4% to 5%), somnolence (3% to 5%), fatigue (3% to 4%), insomnia worsened (3%), depression (2%)

Endocrine & metabolic: Serum cortisol decreased (1%)

Gastrointestinal: Nausea (3%), taste perversion (2%)

Neuromuscular & skeletal: Myalgia (2%), arthralgia (2%)

Respiratory: Upper respiratory infection (3%)

Miscellaneous: Influenza (1%)

Pharmacodynamics/Kinetics

Onset of Action 30 minutes

Available Dosage Forms

Tablet, Oral:

Rozerem: 8 mg

General Dosage Range Oral: *Adults:* 8 mg at bedtime

Administration

Oral Do not administer with a high-fat meal. Swallow tablet whole; do not break.

Storage/Stability Store at 25°C (77°F); excursions permitted to 15°C to 30°C (59°F to 86°F). Protect from moisture.

Nursing Actions

Physical Assessment Monitor for CNS changes, abnormal thinking, and behavior changes.

Patient Education

• Discuss specific use of drug and side effects with patient as it relates to treatment. (HCAHPS: During this hospital stay, were you given any medicine that you had not taken before? Before giving you any new medicine, how often did hospital staff tell you what the medicine was for? How often did hospital staff describe possible side effects in a way you could understand?)

• Patient may experience dizziness, asthenia, menstrual irregularity, or impotence. Have patient report immediately to prescriber depression, nervousness, emotional instability, illogical thinking, anxiety, memory loss, or rash (HCAHPS).

• Educate patient about signs of a significant reaction (eg, wheezing; chest tightness; fever; itching; bad cough; blue skin color; seizures; or swelling of face, lips, tongue, or throat). **Note:** This is not a comprehensive list of all side effects. Patient should consult prescriber for additional questions.

Intended Use and Disclaimer: Should not be printed and given to patients. This information is intended to serve as a concise initial reference for healthcare professionals to use when discussing medications with a patient. You must ultimately rely on your own discretion, experience and judgment in diagnosing, treating and advising patients.

Dietary Considerations Do not take with high-fat meal.

Ramipril (RA mi pril)

Brand Names: U.S. Altace

Pharmacologic Category Angiotensin-Converting Enzyme (ACE) Inhibitor; Antihypertensive

Medication Safety Issues

Sound-alike/look-alike issues:

Ramipril may be confused with enalapril, Monopril, Amaryl

Altace may be confused with Altace HCT, alteplase, Amaryl, Amerge, Artane

Pregnancy Risk Factor D

Lactation Excretion in breast milk unknown/not recommended

Breast-Feeding Considerations Ramipril and its metabolites were not detected in breast milk following a single oral dose of 10 mg. It is not known if multiple doses will produce detectable levels. Breast-feeding is not recommended by the manufacturer.

Use

Heart failure post-myocardial infarction: Treatment of heart failure (HF) after myocardial infarction (MI)

Note: The ACCF/AHA 2013 heart failure guidelines recommend the use of ACE inhibitors, along with other guideline-directed medical therapies, to prevent HF in patients with a reduced ejection fraction who have a history of MI (stage B HF), to prevent HF in any patient with a reduced ejection fraction (stage B HF), or to treat those with HF and reduced ejection fraction (stage C HFrEF) (Yancy, 2013)

Hypertension: Treatment of hypertension, alone or in combination with thiazide diuretics

Reduction in risk of MI, stroke, and death from cardiovascular causes: To reduce the risk of MI, stroke, and death in patients ≥55 years of age at high risk of developing major cardiovascular events

Unlabeled Use Treatment of heart failure; to delay the progression of nephropathy and reduce risks of cardiovascular events in hypertensive patients with type 1 or 2 diabetes mellitus

Mechanism of Action/Effect Ramipril is an ACE inhibitor which prevents the formation of angiotensin II from angiotensin I and exhibits pharmacologic effects that are similar to captopril. Ramipril must undergo conversion in the liver to its biologically active metabolite, ramiprilat. The pharmacodynamic effects of ramipril result from the high-affinity, competitive, reversible binding of ramiprilat to angiotensin-converting enzyme thus preventing the formation of the potent vasoconstrictor angiotensin II.

Contraindications Hypersensitivity to ramipril or any component of the formulation; prior hypersensitivity (including angioedema) to ACE inhibitors; concomitant use with aliskiren in patients with diabetes mellitus

Warnings/Precautions Anaphylactic reactions may occur rarely with ACE inhibitors. At any time during treatment (especially following first dose) angioedema may occur rarely with ACE inhibitors; it may involve the head and neck (potentially compromising airway) or the intestine (presenting with abdominal pain). African-Americans and patients with idiopathic or hereditary angioedema may be at an increased risk. Prolonged frequent monitoring may be required especially if tongue, glottis, or larynx are involved as they are associated with airway obstruction. Patients with a history of airway surgery may have a higher risk of airway obstruction. Aggressive early and appropriate management is critical. Use in patients with previous angioedema associated with ACE inhibitor therapy is contraindicated. Severe anaphylactoid reactions may be seen during hemodialysis (eg, CVVHD) with high-flux dialysis membranes (eg, AN69), and rarely, during low density lipoprotein apheresis with dextran sulfate cellulose. Rare cases of anaphylactoid reactions have been reported in patients undergoing sensitization treatment with hymenoptera (bee, wasp) venom while receiving ACE inhibitors.

Symptomatic hypotension with or without syncope can occur with ACE inhibitors (usually with the first several doses); effects are most often observed in volume-depleted patients; close monitoring of patient is required especially with initial dosing and dosing increases; blood pressure must be lowered at a rate appropriate for the patient's clinical condition. Initiation of therapy in patients with ischemic heart disease or cerebrovascular disease warrants close observation due to the potential consequences posed by falling blood pressure (eg, MI, stroke). Use with caution in hypertrophic cardiomyopathy with outflow tract obstruction, severe aortic stenosis, or before, during, or immediately after major surgery. **[U.S. Boxed Warning]: Drugs that act on the renin-angiotensin system can cause injury and death to the developing fetus. Discontinue as soon as possible once pregnancy is detected.**

Hyperkalemia may occur with ACE inhibitors; risk factors include renal dysfunction, diabetes mellitus, concomitant use of potassium-sparing diuretics, potassium supplements, and/or potassium containing salts. Use cautiously, if at all, with these agents and monitor potassium closely. Cough may occur with ACE inhibitors. Other causes of cough should be considered (eg, pulmonary congestion in patients with heart failure) and excluded prior to discontinuation.

May be associated with deterioration of renal function and/or increases in serum creatinine, particularly in patients with low renal blood flow (eg, renal artery stenosis, heart failure) whose glomerular filtration rate (GFR) is dependent on efferent arteriolar vasoconstriction by angiotensin II; deterioration may result in oliguria, acute renal failure, and progressive azotemia. Small increases in serum creatinine may occur following initiation; consider discontinuation only in patients with progressive and/or significant deterioration in renal function. Use with caution in patients with unstented unilateral/bilateral renal artery stenosis. When unstented bilateral renal artery stenosis is present, use is generally avoided due to the elevated risk of deterioration in renal function unless possible benefits outweigh risks. Potentially significant drug-drug interactions may exist, requiring dose or frequency adjustment, additional monitoring, and/or selection of alternative therapy.

Rare toxicities associated with ACE inhibitors include cholestatic jaundice (which may progress to fulminant hepatic necrosis), agranulocytosis, neutropenia, or leukopenia with myeloid hypoplasia. Patients with collagen vascular diseases (especially with concomitant renal impairment) or renal impairment alone may be at increased risk for hematologic toxicity; periodically monitor CBC with differential in these patients.

Drug Interactions

Avoid Concomitant Use

Avoid concomitant use of Ramipril with any of the following: Telmisartan

Decreased Effect

The levels/effects of Ramipril may be decreased by: Aprotinin; Herbs (Hypertensive Properties); Icatibant; Lanthanum; Methylphenidate; Nonsteroidal Anti-Inflammatory Agents; Salicylates; Yohimbine

Increased Effect/Toxicity

Ramipril may increase the levels/effects of: Allopurinol; Amifostine; Antihypertensives; AzaTHIOprine; CycloSPORINE (Systemic); DULoxetine; Ferric Gluconate; Gold Sodium Thiomalate; Hypotensive Agents; Iron Dextran Complex; Lithium; Nonsteroidal Anti-Inflammatory Agents; Obinutuzumab; RiTUXimab; Sodium Phosphates

The levels/effects of Ramipril may be increased by: Alfuzosin; Aliskiren; Angiotensin II Receptor Blockers; Brimonidine (Topical); Canagliflozin; Diazoxide; DPP-IV Inhibitors; Eplerenone; Everolimus; Heparin; Heparin (Low Molecular Weight); Herbs (Hypotensive Properties); Loop Diuretics; MAO Inhibitors; Pentoxifylline; Phosphodiesterase 5 Inhibitors; Potassium Salts; Potassium-Sparing Diuretics; Prostacyclin Analogues; Sirolimus; Telmisartan; Temsirolimus; Thiazide Diuretics; TiZANidine; Tolvaptan; Trimethoprim

Nutritional/Ethanol Interactions

Food: Potassium supplements and/or potassium-containing salts may cause or worsen hyperkalemia. Management: Advise patient to consult prescriber before consuming a potassium-rich diet, potassium supplements, or salt substitutes.

Herb/Nutraceutical: Bayberry, blue cohosh, cayenne, ephedra, ginger, ginseng (American), kola, licorice (may worsen hypertension). Black cohosh, California poppy, coleus, golden seal, hawthorn, mistletoe, periwinkle, quinine, shepherd's purse (may have increased antihypertensive effect). Management: Advise patients to consult prescriber before taking herbs with hyper/hypotensive properties during therapy.

Adverse Reactions Note: Frequency ranges include data from hypertension and heart failure trials. Higher rates of adverse reactions have generally been noted in patients with CHF. However, the frequency of adverse effects associated with placebo is also increased in this population.

>10%: Respiratory: Cough increased (7% to 12%)
1% to 10%:
Cardiovascular: Hypotension (11%), angina (up to 3%), orthostatic hypotension (2%), syncope (up to 2%)

Central nervous system: Headache (1% to 5%), dizziness (2% to 4%), fatigue (2%), vertigo (up to 2%)
Endocrine & metabolic: Hyperkalemia (1% to 10%)
Gastrointestinal: Nausea/vomiting (1% to 2%)
Neuromuscular & skeletal: Chest pain (noncardiac) (1%)
Renal: Renal dysfunction (1%), serum creatinine increased (1% to 2%), BUN increased (<1% to 3%); transient increases of creatinine and/or BUN may occur more frequently
Respiratory: Cough (estimated 1% to 10%)
Worsening of renal function may occur in patients with bilateral renal artery stenosis or in hypovolemia. In addition, a syndrome which may include fever, myalgia, arthralgia, interstitial nephritis, vasculitis, rash, eosinophilia and positive ANA, and elevated ESR has been reported with ACE inhibitors. Risk of pancreatitis and agranulocytosis may be increased in patients with collagen vascular disease or renal impairment.

Pharmacodynamics/Kinetics

Onset of Action 1-2 hours
Duration of Action 24 hours

Available Dosage Forms

Capsule, Oral:
Altace: 1.25 mg, 2.5 mg, 5 mg, 10 mg
Generic: 1.25 mg, 2.5 mg, 5 mg, 10 mg

General Dosage Range Dosage adjustment recommended in patients with renal impairment
Oral: *Adults:* 2.5-20 mg daily

Administration

Oral Swallow capsule whole; may open the capsule and the mix contents with 120 mL of water, apple juice, or applesauce.

Storage/Stability Store at 15°C to 30°C (59°F to 86°F). Ramipril mixed with applesauce, apple juice, or water may be stored at room temperature for up to 24 hours or for up to 48 hours under refrigeration.

Nursing Actions

Physical Assessment Assess potential for interactions with other pharmacological agents or herbal products that may impact fluid balance or cardiac status. Monitor first dose carefully (hypotension or angioedema can occur at any time during treatment, especially following first dose). Monitor blood pressure and cardiac status. Monitor for cough, renal dysfunction, nausea/vomiting, hypovolemia, angioedema, and postural hypotension on a regular basis during therapy.

Patient Education
• Discuss specific use of drug and side effects with patient as it relates to treatment. (HCAHPS: During this hospital stay, were you given any medicine that you had not taken before? Before giving you any new medicine, how often did hospital staff tell you what the medicine was for? How often did hospital staff describe possible side effects in a way you could understand?)

• Patient may experience dizziness, headache, or parageusia. Have patient report immediately to prescriber signs of infection, syncope, dyspnea, hyperhidrosis, diarrhea, significant weight gain, edema in legs or abdomen, discolored urine, jaundice, or rash (HCAHPS).

• Educate patient about signs of a significant reaction (eg, wheezing; chest tightness; fever; itching; bad cough; blue skin color; seizures; or swelling of face, lips, tongue, or throat). **Note:** This is not a comprehensive list of all side effects. Patient should consult prescriber for additional questions.

Intended Use and Disclaimer: Should not be printed and given to patients. This information is intended to serve as a concise initial reference for healthcare professionals to use when discussing medications with a patient. You must ultimately rely on your own discretion, experience and judgment in diagnosing, treating and advising patients.

Ranitidine (ra NI ti deen)

Brand Names: U.S. Acid Reducer Maximum Strength [OTC] [DSC]; Acid Reducer [OTC]; Ranitidine Acid Reducer [OTC]; Zantac; Zantac 150 Maximum Strength [OTC]; Zantac 75 [OTC]; Zantac in NaCl [DSC]

Index Terms Ranitidine Hydrochloride

Pharmacologic Category Histamine H_2 Antagonist

Medication Safety Issues
Sound-alike/look-alike issues:
Ranitidine may be confused with amantadine, rimantadine
Zantac may be confused with Xanax, Zarontin, Zofran, ZyrTEC

Pregnancy Risk Factor B

Lactation Enters breast milk/use caution

Breast-Feeding Considerations Ranitidine is excreted into breast milk. The manufacturer recommends that caution be exercised when administering ranitidine to nursing women. Peak milk concentrations of ranitidine occur ~5.5 hours after the dose (case report).

Use
Zantac: Short-term and maintenance therapy of duodenal ulcer, gastric ulcer, gastroesophageal reflux disease (GERD), active benign ulcer, erosive esophagitis, and pathological hypersecretory conditions; as part of a multidrug regimen for *H. pylori* eradication to reduce the risk of duodenal ulcer recurrence
Zantac 75 [OTC]: Relief of heartburn, acid indigestion, and sour stomach

Unlabeled Use Recurrent postoperative ulcer, upper GI bleeding, prevention of acid-aspiration pneumonitis during surgery, and prevention of stress-induced ulcers

Mechanism of Action/Effect Competitive inhibition of histamine at H_2-receptors, gastric acid secretion, gastric volume and hydrogen ion concentration are reduced

Contraindications Hypersensitivity to ranitidine or any component of the formulation

Warnings/Precautions Ranitidine has been associated with confusional states (rare). Use with caution in patients with hepatic impairment; use with caution in renal impairment, dosage modification required. Avoid use in patients with history of acute porphyria (may precipitate attacks); long-term therapy may be associated with vitamin B_{12} deficiency. Symptoms of GI distress may be associated with a variety of conditions; symptomatic response to H_2 antagonists does not rule out the potential for significant pathology (eg, malignancy).

Drug Interactions
Avoid Concomitant Use
Avoid concomitant use of Ranitidine with any of the following: Dasatinib; Delavirdine; PONATinib; Risedronate

Decreased Effect
Ranitidine may decrease the levels/effects of: Atazanavir; Bosutinib; Cefditoren; Cefpodoxime; Cefuroxime; Dabrafenib; Dasatinib; Delavirdine; Erlotinib; Fosamprenavir; Gefitinib; Indinavir; Iron Salts; Itraconazole; Ketoconazole (Systemic); Mesalamine; Multivitamins/Minerals (with ADEK, Folate, Iron); Nelfinavir; Nilotinib; PONATinib; Posaconazole; Prasugrel; Rilpivirine; Vismodegib

The levels/effects of Ranitidine may be decreased by: Peginterferon Alfa-2b; P-glycoprotein/ABCB1 Inducers

Increased Effect/Toxicity
Ranitidine may increase the levels/effects of: ARIPiprazole; Dexmethylphenidate; Methylphenidate; Procainamide; Risedronate; Saquinavir; Sulfonylureas; Varenicline; Warfarin

The levels/effects of Ranitidine may be increased by: P-glycoprotein/ABCB1 Inhibitors

Nutritional/Ethanol Interactions
Ethanol: Avoid ethanol (may cause gastric mucosal irritation).
Food: Does not interfere with absorption of ranitidine.

Adverse Reactions Frequency not defined.
Cardiovascular: Asystole, atrioventricular block, bradycardia (with rapid I.V. administration), premature ventricular beats, tachycardia, vasculitis
Central nervous system: Agitation, dizziness, depression, hallucinations, headache, insomnia, malaise, mental confusion, somnolence, vertigo
Dermatologic: Alopecia, erythema multiforme, rash
Endocrine & metabolic: Prolactin levels increased
Gastrointestinal: Abdominal discomfort/pain, constipation, diarrhea, nausea, necrotizing enterocolitis (VLBW neonates; Guillet, 2006), pancreatitis, vomiting

Hematologic: Acquired immune hemolytic anemia, acute porphyritic attack, agranulocytosis, aplastic anemia, granulocytopenia, leukopenia, pancytopenia, thrombocytopenia

Hepatic: Cholestatic hepatitis, hepatic failure, hepatitis, jaundice

Local: Transient pain, burning or itching at the injection site

Neuromuscular & skeletal: Arthralgia, involuntary motor disturbance, myalgia

Ocular: Blurred vision

Renal: Acute interstitial nephritis, serum creatinine increased

Respiratory: Pneumonia (causal relationship not established)

Miscellaneous: Anaphylaxis, angioneurotic edema, hypersensitivity reactions (eg, bronchospasm, fever, eosinophilia)

Available Dosage Forms

Capsule, Oral:
Generic: 150 mg, 300 mg

Solution, Injection:
Zantac: 50 mg/2 mL (2 mL); 150 mg/6 mL (6 mL); 1000 mg/40 mL (40 mL)
Generic: 50 mg/2 mL (2 mL); 150 mg/6 mL (6 mL); 1000 mg/40 mL (40 mL)

Syrup, Oral:
Generic: 15 mg/mL (10 mL, 473 mL, 474 mL, 480 mL); 75 mg/5 mL (473 mL, 480 mL); 150 mg/10 mL (10 mL)

Tablet, Oral:
Acid Reducer [OTC]: 75 mg
Ranitidine Acid Reducer [OTC]: 75 mg
Zantac 75 [OTC]: 75 mg
Zantac: 150 mg, 300 mg
Zantac 150 Maximum Strength [OTC]: 150 mg
Generic: 75 mg, 150 mg, 300 mg

General Dosage Range Dosage adjustment recommended in patients with renal impairment

I.M.: *Children >16 years and Adults:* 50 mg every 6-8 hours

I.V.:
Children 1 month to 16 years: 2-4 mg/kg/day divided every 6-8 hours (maximum: 200 mg/day)
Children >16 years and Adults: 50 mg every 6-8 hours **or** Infusion: 6.25 mg/hour **or** 1-2.5 mg/kg/hour

Oral:
Children 1 month to 11 years: 2-4 mg/kg/dose once or twice daily **or** 5-10 mg/kg/day in 2 divided doses (maximum: 300 mg/day)
Children ≥12 to 16 years: 2-4 mg/kg once or twice daily **or** 5-10 mg/kg/day in 2 divided doses (maximum: 300 mg/day); OTC dosing: 75 mg 30-60 minutes before eating or drinking (maximum: 150 mg/day)
Children >16 years and Adults: 150 mg 1-4 times/day **or** 300 mg once daily; OTC dosing: 75 mg 30-60 minutes before eating or drinking (maximum: 150 mg/day)

Usual Infusion Concentrations: Pediatric
Note: Premixed solutions available
I.V. infusion: 0.5 mg/mL
Usual Infusion Concentrations: Adult Note:
Premixed solutions available
I.V. infusion: 50 mg in 50 mL (concentration: 1 mg/mL) **or** 500 mg in 250 mL (concentration: 2 mg/mL) of D_5W or NS

Administration
I.M. No dilution is needed.
I.V. I.V. must be diluted; may be administered I.V. push, intermittent I.V. infusion, or continuous I.V. infusion

I.V. push: Manufacturer recommends a maximum rate of administration of 10 mg/minute (or over 5 minutes); however, may also be administered at a maximum rate of 25 mg/minute (or over 2 minutes) if necessary (Coursin, 1988; Goelzer, 1988; Smith, 1987).

Intermittent I.V. infusion: Administer over 15-20 minutes

Continuous I.V. infusion: Titrate dosage based on gastric pH.

Injectable Detail pH: 6.7-7.3

Preparation for Administration Vials can be mixed with NS or D_5W.
Intermittent bolus injection, continuous infusion: Dilute to maximum of 2.5 mg/mL.
Intermittent infusion: Dilute to maximum of 0.5 mg/mL.

Storage/Stability
Injection: Vials: Store between 4°C to 25°C (39°F to 77°F); excursion permitted to 30°C (86°F). Protect from light. Solution is a clear, colorless to yellow solution; slight darkening does not affect potency. Vials mixed with NS or D_5W are stable for 48 hours at room temperature.
Premixed bag: Store between 2°C to 25°C (36°F to 77°F). Protect from light.
Syrup: Store between 4°C to 25°C (39°F to 77°F). Protect from light.
Tablets: Store in dry place, between 15°C to 30°C (59°F to 86°F). Protect from light.

Nursing Actions
Physical Assessment Monitor for CNS changes (depression, hallucinations, confusion, malaise), rash, and GI disturbance.

Patient Education
- Discuss specific use of drug and side effects with patient as it relates to treatment. (HCAHPS: During this hospital stay, were you given any medicine that you had not taken before? Before giving you any new medicine, how often did hospital staff tell you what the medicine was for? How often did hospital staff describe possible side effects in a way you could understand?)
- Patient may experience nausea, constipation, diarrhea, or injection site irritation. Have patient report immediately to prescriber severe dizziness, syncope, illogical thinking, angina, tachycardia, arrhythmia, significant headache, urinary

retention, ecchymosis, hemorrhaging, or signs of hepatic impairment (HCAHPS).
- Educate patient about signs of a significant reaction (eg, wheezing; chest tightness; fever; itching; bad cough; blue skin color; seizures; or swelling of face, lips, tongue, or throat). **Note:** This is not a comprehensive list of all side effects. Patient should consult prescriber for additional questions.

Intended Use and Disclaimer: Should not be printed and given to patients. This information is intended to serve as a concise initial reference for healthcare professionals to use when discussing medications with a patient. You must ultimately rely on your own discretion, experience and judgment in diagnosing, treating and advising patients.

Dietary Considerations Some products may contain phenylalanine and/or sodium. Oral dosage forms may be taken with or without food.

Ranolazine (ra NOE la zeen)

Brand Names: U.S. Ranexa

Pharmacologic Category Antianginal Agent; Cardiovascular Agent, Miscellaneous

Medication Safety Issues
Sound-alike/look-alike issues:
Ranexa may be confused with CeleXA

Pregnancy Risk Factor C

Lactation Excretion in breast milk unknown/not recommended

Breast-Feeding Considerations It is not known if ranolazine is excreted into breast milk. Due to the potential for serious adverse reactions in the nursing infant, the manufacturer recommends a decision be made whether to discontinue nursing or to discontinue the drug, taking into account the importance of treatment to the mother.

Use Chronic angina: Treatment of chronic angina **Note:** According to the 2012 ACCF/AHA/ACP/AATS/PCNA/SCAI/STS guidelines for patients with stable ischemic heart disease, ranolazine may be useful when prescribed as a substitute for beta blockers for relief of symptoms if initial treatment with beta blockers leads to unacceptable side effects, is less effective, or if initial treatment with beta blockers is contraindicated. May also be used in combination with beta blockers, for relief of symptoms when initial treatment with beta blockers is not successful (Fihn, 2012).

Mechanism of Action/Effect May increase myocardial relaxation during myocardial ischemia and improve energy supply during ischemia.

Contraindications Hepatic cirrhosis; concurrent strong CYP3A inhibitors; concurrent CYP3A inducers

Warnings/Precautions Ranolazine has been shown to prolong QT interval in a dose/plasma concentration-related manner. Cirrhotic patients with mild to moderate hepatic impairment demonstrated a 3-fold increase in QT prolongation. The incidence of symptomatic arrhythmias was similar to placebo in one trial (Morrow, 2007). Risk versus benefit should be assessed in patient maintained on a higher dose (>2000 mg/day) or exposure, concurrent use of other QT-prolonging drugs, potassium-channel variants known to cause QT prolongation, family history of or congenital long QT syndrome, or known acquired QT interval prolongation. Use is contraindicated in patients with hepatic cirrhosis. Ranolazine plasma levels increase in patients with mild and moderate hepatic impairment. Acute renal failure has been observed in some patients with severe renal impairment (CrCl <30 mL/minute); if acute renal failure develops (marked increase in serum creatinine associated with increased BUN), discontinue ranolazine and manage appropriately. Monitor renal function periodically in patients with moderate to severe renal impairment; particularly for increases in serum creatinine accompanied but increased BUN. In a renal impairment study, patients with severe impairment exhibited an initial elevation in diastolic blood pressure (~12-17 mm Hg at day 3), however this diminished to ~4 mm Hg increase by day 5 (Jerling, 2005); consider monitoring blood pressure in patients with renal dysfunction. Ranolazine has not been evaluated in patients requiring dialysis.

Ranolazine will not relieve acute angina episode and has not demonstrated benefit in acute coronary syndrome. Although ranolazine produces small reductions in hemoglobin A_{1c}, it is not a treatment for diabetes. Potentially significant drug-drug interactions may exist, requiring dose or frequency adjustment, additional monitoring, and/or selection of alternative therapy. Use is contraindicated with inducers and strong inhibitors of CYP3A. Use with caution in patients ≥75 years of age; they may experience more adverse events (including serious adverse events) and drug discontinuations due to adverse events.

Drug Interactions

Avoid Concomitant Use
Avoid concomitant use of Ranolazine with any of the following: Antifungal Agents (Azole Derivatives, Systemic); Bosutinib; CYP3A4 Inducers (Strong); CYP3A4 Inhibitors (Strong); Fusidic Acid (Systemic); Highest Risk QTc-Prolonging Agents; Ivabradine; Mifepristone; Pomalidomide; Rifampin; Silodosin; St Johns Wort; Topotecan; VinCRIStine (Liposomal)

Decreased Effect
The levels/effects of Ranolazine may be decreased by: Bosentan; CYP3A4 Inducers (Strong); Dabrafenib; Deferasirox; Peginterferon Alfa-2b; P-glycoprotein/ABCB1 Inducers; Rifampin; St Johns Wort; Tocilizumab

Increased Effect/Toxicity

Ranolazine may increase the levels/effects of: Afatinib; ARIPiprazole; AtorvaSTATin; Bosutinib; Colchicine; Dabigatran Etexilate; Digoxin; DOXOrubicin (Conventional); Everolimus; Highest Risk QTc-Prolonging Agents; Lomitapide; Lovastatin; MetFORMIN; Moderate Risk QTc-Prolonging Agents; P-glycoprotein/ABCB1 Substrates; Pomalidomide; Prucalopride; Rivaroxaban; Silodosin; Simvastatin; Tacrolimus (Systemic); Topotecan; VinCRIStine (Liposomal)

The levels/effects of Ranolazine may be increased by: Antifungal Agents (Azole Derivatives, Systemic); Calcium Channel Blockers (Nondihydropyridine); CYP3A4 Inhibitors (Moderate); CYP3A4 Inhibitors (Strong); Dasatinib; Fusidic Acid (Systemic); Ivabradine; Ivacaftor; Luliconazole; Mifepristone; P-glycoprotein/ABCB1 Inhibitors; QTc-Prolonging Agents (Indeterminate Risk and Risk Modifying); Simeprevir

Nutritional/Ethanol Interactions

Food: Grapefruit, grapefruit juice, or grapefruit-containing products may increase the serum concentration of ranolazine. Management: Avoid grapefruit-containing products or dose adjustment of ranolazine may be required.

Herb/Nutraceutical: St John's wort may decrease the serum concentration of ranolazine. Management: Avoid St John's wort.

Adverse Reactions >0.5% to 10%:

Cardiovascular: Bradycardia (≤4%), hypotension (≤4%), orthostatic hypotension (≤4%), palpitation (≤4%), peripheral edema (≤4%), QTc prolongation (>500 msec: ≤1%)

Central nervous system: Headache (≤6%), dizziness (1% to 6%), confusion (≤4%), vasovagal attacks (≤4%), vertigo (≤4%)

Dermatologic: Hyperhidrosis (≤4%)

Gastrointestinal: Constipation (≤9%), abdominal pain (≤4%), anorexia (≤4%), dyspepsia (≤4%), nausea (≤4%; dose related), vomiting (≤4%), xerostomia (≤4%)

Neuromuscular: Weakness (≤4%)

Ocular: Blurred vision (≤4%)

Otic: Tinnitus (≤4%)

Renal: Hematuria (≤4%)

Respiratory: Dyspnea (≤4%)

Available Dosage Forms

Tablet Extended Release 12 Hour, Oral:

Ranexa: 500 mg, 1000 mg

General Dosage Range Dosage adjustment recommended in patients on concomitant therapy

Oral: *Adults:* Initial: 500 mg twice daily; Maintenance: 500-1000 mg twice daily (maximum: 2000 mg daily)

Administration

Oral Administer with or without meals. Swallow tablet whole; do not crush, break, or chew.

Storage/Stability Store at 25°C (77°F); excursions permitted to 15°C to 30°C (59°F to 86°F).

Nursing Actions

Physical Assessment Check QTc if ECG obtained. Stress that this medication is not intended to treat an acute angina episode. Instruct patient in appropriate measures to take if an acute episode of angina occurs.

Patient Education

• Discuss specific use of drug and side effects with patient as it relates to treatment. (HCAHPS: During this hospital stay, were you given any medicine that you had not taken before? Before giving you any new medicine, how often did hospital staff tell you what the medicine was for? How often did hospital staff describe possible side effects in a way you could understand?)

• Patient may experience dizziness, headache, nausea, or constipation. Have patient report immediately to prescriber tachycardia, dyspnea, or rash (HCAHPS).

• Educate patient about signs of a significant reaction (eg, wheezing; chest tightness; fever; itching; bad cough; blue skin color; seizures; or swelling of face, lips, tongue, or throat). **Note:** This is not a comprehensive list of all side effects. Patient should consult prescriber for additional questions.

Intended Use and Disclaimer: Should not be printed and given to patients. This information is intended to serve as a concise initial reference for healthcare professionals to use when discussing medications with a patient. You must ultimately rely on your own discretion, experience and judgment in diagnosing, treating and advising patients.

Dietary Considerations Limit the use of grapefruit juice; the ranolazine dose should not exceed 500 mg twice daily when taken with grapefruit juice or grapefruit-containing products.

Related Information

Oral Medications That Should Not Be Crushed or Altered *on page 1712*

Rasagiline (ra SA ji leen)

Brand Names: U.S. Azilect

Index Terms AGN 1135; Rasagiline Mesylate; TVP-1012

Pharmacologic Category Anti-Parkinson's Agent, MAO Type B Inhibitor

Medication Safety Issues

Sound-alike/look-alike issues:

Azilect® may be confused with Aricept®

Pregnancy Risk Factor C

Lactation Excretion in breast milk unknown/use caution

Breast-Feeding Considerations Animal studies have shown rasagiline is capable of inhibiting prolactin secretion.

Use Treatment of idiopathic Parkinson's disease (initial monotherapy or as adjunct to levodopa)

Mechanism of Action/Effect Rasagiline selectively inhibits MAO-B which enhances brain dopamine levels, thus reducing symptomatic motor deficits.

Contraindications Concomitant use of cyclobenzaprine, dextromethorphan, methadone, propoxyphene, St John's wort, or tramadol; concomitant use of meperidine or an MAO inhibitor (including selective MAO-B inhibitors) within 14 days of rasagiline

Warnings/Precautions Hazardous agent - use appropriate precautions for handling and disposal (NIOSH, 2012).

Cardiovascular system: May cause orthostatic hypotension, particularly in combination with levodopa; use with caution in patients with hypotension or patients who would not tolerate transient hypotensive episodes (cardiovascular or cerebrovascular disease); orthostasis is usually most problematic during first 2 months of therapy and tends to abate thereafter. Due to the potential for hemodynamic instability, patients should not undergo elective surgery requiring general anesthesia and should avoid local anesthesia containing sympathomimetic vasoconstrictors within 14 days of discontinuing rasagiline. If surgery is required, benzodiazepines, mivacurium, fentanyl, morphine or codeine may be used cautiously. In patients taking recommended doses of rasagiline, dietary restriction of most tyramine-containing products is not necessary; however, certain foods (eg, aged cheeses) may contain high amounts (>150 mg) of tyramine and could lead to hypertensive crisis. Avoid concomitant use with foods high in tyramine.

Central nervous system: Serotonin syndrome (SS)/neuroleptic malignant syndrome (NMS)-like reactions may occur rarely, particularly when used at doses exceeding recommendations or when used in combination with an antidepressant (eg, SSRI, SNRI, TCA). May cause hallucinations; signs of severe CNS toxicity (some fatal), including hyperpyrexia, hyperthermia, rigidity, altered mental status, seizure and coma have been reported with selective and nonselective MAO inhibitor use in combination with antidepressants. Do not use within 5 weeks of fluoxetine discontinuation; do not initiate tricyclic, SSRI, or SNRI therapy within 2 weeks of discontinuing rasagiline. Addition to levodopa therapy may result in exacerbation of dyskinesias, requiring a reduction in levodopa dosage.

Dermatologic: Risk of melanoma may be increased with rasagiline, although increased risk has been associated with Parkinson's disease itself; patients should have regular and frequent skin examinations.

Organ dysfunction: Use caution in mild hepatic impairment; dose reduction recommended. Do not use with moderate-to-severe hepatic impairment.

Drug Interactions

Avoid Concomitant Use

Avoid concomitant use of Rasagiline with any of the following: Alpha-/Beta-Agonists (Indirect-Acting); Alpha1-Agonists; Amphetamines; Anilidopiperidine Opioids; Antidepressants (Serotonin Reuptake Inhibitor/Antagonist); Apraclonidine; AtoMOXetine; Bezafibrate; Buprenorphine; BuPROPion; BusPIRone; CarBAMazepine; Cyclobenzaprine; Cyproheptadine; Dexmethylphenidate; Dextromethorphan; Diethylpropion; Hydrocodone; HYDROmorphone; IsomethepTene; Levonordefrin; Linezolid; Maprotiline; Meperidine; Methyldopa; Methylene Blue; Methylphenidate; Mirtazapine; Morphine (Liposomal); Morphine (Systemic); Oxymorphone; Pizotifen; Selective Serotonin Reuptake Inhibitors; Serotonin 5-HT1D Receptor Agonists; Serotonin/Norepinephrine Reuptake Inhibitors; Tapentadol; Tetrabenazine; Tetrahydrozoline (Nasal); Tricyclic Antidepressants; Tryptophan

Decreased Effect

Rasagiline may decrease the levels/effects of: Domperidone

The levels/effects of Rasagiline may be decreased by: CYP1A2 Inducers (Strong); Cyproheptadine; Cyproterone; Domperidone

Increased Effect/Toxicity

Rasagiline may increase the levels/effects of: Alpha-/Beta-Agonists (Indirect-Acting); Alpha1-Agonists; Amphetamines; Antidepressants (Serotonin Reuptake Inhibitor/Antagonist); Antihypertensives; Antipsychotics; Apraclonidine; AtoMOXetine; Beta2-Agonists; Betahistine; Bezafibrate; Brimonidine (Ophthalmic); Brimonidine (Topical); BuPROPion; Cyproheptadine; Dexmethylphenidate; Dextromethorphan; Diethylpropion; Domperidone; Doxapram; Doxylamine; EPINEPHrine (Nasal); Epinephrine (Racemic); EPINEPHrine (Systemic, Oral Inhalation); Hydrocodone; HYDROmorphone; Hypoglycemic Agents; IsomethepTene; Levonordefrin; Linezolid; Lithium; Meperidine; Methadone; Methyldopa; Methylene Blue; Methylphenidate; Metoclopramide; Mirtazapine; Morphine (Liposomal); Morphine (Systemic); Norepinephrine; Orthostatic Hypotension Producing Agents; OxyCODONE; Pizotifen; Reserpine; Selective Serotonin Reuptake Inhibitors; Serotonin 5-HT1D Receptor Agonists; Serotonin Modulators; Serotonin/Norepinephrine Reuptake Inhibitors; Tetrahydrozoline (Nasal); Tricyclic Antidepressants

The levels/effects of Rasagiline may be increased by: Abiraterone Acetate; Altretamine; Anilidopiperidine Opioids; Antipsychotics; Buprenorphine; BusPIRone; CarBAMazepine; COMT Inhibitors; Cyclobenzaprine; CYP1A2 Inhibitors (Moderate);

CYP1A2 Inhibitors (Strong); Deferasirox; Levodopa; MAO Inhibitors; Maprotiline; Oxymorphone; Tapentadol; Tetrabenazine; TraMADol; Tryptophan; Vemurafenib

Nutritional/Ethanol Interactions

Ethanol: Management: Avoid ethanol.

Food: Concurrent ingestion of foods rich in tyramine may cause sudden and severe high blood pressure (hypertensive crisis). Management: Avoid foods containing high amounts (>150 mg) of tyramine (aged or matured cheese, air-dried or cured meats including sausages and salamis; fava or broad bean pods, tap/draft beers, Marmite concentrate, sauerkraut, soy sauce, and other soybean condiments. Food's freshness is also an important concern; improperly stored or spoiled food can create an environment in which tyramine concentrations may increase. Avoid these foods during and for 2 weeks after discontinuation of medication.

Herb/Nutraceutical: Some herbal medications may cause excessive sedation; others may increase the risk of serotonin syndrome or hypertensive reactions. Management: Avoid valerian, St John's wort, SAMe, and kava kava; avoid supplements containing caffeine, tyrosine, tryptophan, or phenylalanine.

Adverse Reactions Unless otherwise noted, the following adverse reactions are as reported for monotherapy. Spectrum of adverse events was generally similar with adjunctive (levodopa) therapy, though the incidence tended to be higher.

>10%:

Cardiovascular: Orthostatic hypotension (6% to 13% adjunct therapy, dose dependent)

Central nervous system: Dyskinesia (18% adjunct therapy), headache (14%)

Gastrointestinal: Nausea (10% to 12% adjunct therapy)

1% to 10%:

Cardiovascular: Angina, bundle branch block, chest pain, syncope

Central nervous system: Depression (5%), hallucinations (4% to 5% adjunct therapy), fever (3%), malaise (2%), vertigo (2%), anxiety, dizziness

Dermatologic: Bruising (2%), alopecia, skin carcinoma, vesiculobullous rash

Endocrine & metabolic: Impotence, libido decreased

Gastrointestinal: Constipation (4% to 9% adjunct therapy), weight loss (2% to 9% adjunct therapy; dose dependent), dyspepsia (7%), xerostomia (2% to 6% adjunct therapy; dose dependent), gastroenteritis (3%), anorexia, diarrhea, gastrointestinal hemorrhage, vomiting

Genitourinary: Hematuria, urinary incontinence

Hematologic: Leukopenia

Hepatic: Liver function tests increased

Neuromuscular & skeletal: Arthralgia (7%), neck pain (2%), arthritis (2%), paresthesia (2%), abnormal gait, hyperkinesias, hypertonia, neuropathy, tremor, weakness

Ocular: Conjunctivitis (3%)

Renal: Albuminuria

Respiratory: Rhinitis (3%), asthma, cough increased

Miscellaneous: Fall (5%), flu-like syndrome (5%), allergic reaction

Pharmacodynamics/Kinetics

Onset of Action Therapeutic: Within 1 hour

Duration of Action ~1 week (irreversible inhibition); may require ~14-40 days for complete restoration of (brain) MAO-B activity

Available Dosage Forms

Tablet, Oral:

Azilect: 0.5 mg, 1 mg

General Dosage Range Dosage adjustment recommended in patients with hepatic impairment or on concomitant therapy

Oral: *Adults:* 0.5-1 mg once daily

Administration

Oral Administer without regard to meals.

Hazardous agent; use appropriate precautions for handling and disposal (NIOSH, 2012).

Storage/Stability Store at 25°C (77°F); excursions permitted to 15°C to 30°C (59°F to 86°F).

Nursing Actions

Physical Assessment Monitor blood pressure. Be alert to suicide ideation. Patient should be cautioned against eating foods high in tyramine.

Patient Education

• Discuss specific use of drug and side effects with patient as it relates to treatment. (HCAHPS: During this hospital stay, were you given any medicine that you had not taken before? Before giving you any new medicine, how often did hospital staff tell you what the medicine was for? How often did hospital staff describe possible side effects in a way you could understand?)

• Patient may experience flu-like syndrome, constipation, fatigue, xerostomia, lack of appetite, dyspepsia, weight loss, nightmares, or arthralgia. Have patient report immediately to prescriber difficulty with motor activity, fasciculations, dysphagia, difficulty speaking, tremors, bradykinesia, rigidity, syncope, uncontrollable urges, skin growths, mole changes, angina, behavioral changes, mood changes, dyspnea, paresthesia, or serotonin syndrome (ie, dizziness, severe headache, agitation, hallucinations, tachycardia, arrhythmia, flushing, tremors, hyperhidrosis, change in balance, illogical thinking, severe nausea, significant diarrhea) (HCAHPS).

• Educate patient about signs of a significant reaction (eg, wheezing; chest tightness; fever; itching; bad cough; blue skin color; seizures; or swelling of face, lips, tongue, or throat). **Note:** This is not a comprehensive list of all side

effects. Patient should consult prescriber for additional questions.

Intended Use and Disclaimer: Should not be printed and given to patients. This information is intended to serve as a concise initial reference for healthcare professionals to use when discussing medications with a patient. You must ultimately rely on your own discretion, experience and judgment in diagnosing, treating and advising patients.

Dietary Considerations May be taken without regard to meals. Avoid products containing high amounts of tyramine (>150 mg), such as aged cheeses (eg, Stilton cheese). Restriction of tyramine-containing products with lower amounts (<150 mg) of tyramine is not necessary in patients taking recommended doses. Some examples of tyramine-containing products include aged or matured cheese, air-dried or cured meats (including sausages and salamis), fava or broad bean pods, tap/draft beers, Marmite concentrate, sauerkraut, soy sauce and other soybean condiments. Food's freshness is also an important concern; improperly stored or spoiled food can create an environment where tyramine concentrations may increase.

Rasburicase (ras BYOOR i kayse)

Brand Names: U.S. Elitek

Index Terms Recombinant Urate Oxidase; Urate Oxidase

Pharmacologic Category Enzyme; Enzyme, Urate-Oxidase (Recombinant)

Pregnancy Risk Factor C

Lactation Excretion in breast milk unknown/not recommended

Use Initial management of uric acid levels in patients with leukemia, lymphoma, and solid tumor malignancies receiving chemotherapy expected to result in tumor lysis and elevation of plasma uric acid

Available Dosage Forms

Solution Reconstituted, Intravenous:
Elitek: 1.5 mg (1 ea); 7.5 mg (1 ea)

General Dosage Range I.V.: *Children and Adults:* 0.2 mg/kg once daily

Administration

I.V. I.V. infusion over 30 minutes; do **not** administer as a bolus infusion. Do **not** filter during infusion. If not possible to administer through a separate line, I.V. line should be flushed with at least 15 mL saline prior to and following rasburicase infusion. The optimal timing of rasburicase administration (with respect to chemotherapy administration) is not specified in the manufacturer's labeling. In some studies, chemotherapy was administered 4-24 hours after the first rasburicase dose (Cortes, 2010; Kikuchi, 2009; Vadhan-Raj,

2012); however, rasburicase generally may be administered irrespective of chemotherapy timing.

Nursing Actions

Physical Assessment Monitor patient closely for hypersensitivity reaction.

Patient Education

• Discuss specific use of drug and side effects with patient as it relates to treatment. (HCAHPS: During this hospital stay, were you given any medicine that you had not taken before? Before giving you any new medicine, how often did hospital staff tell you what the medicine was for? How often did hospital staff describe possible side effects in a way you could understand?)

• Patient may experience headache, edema, nausea, constipation, diarrhea, dyspepsia, pharyngitis, or stomatitis. Have patient report immediately to prescriber angina, dyspnea, or rash (HCAHPS).

• Educate patient about signs of a significant reaction (eg, wheezing; chest tightness; fever; itching; bad cough; blue skin color; seizures; or swelling of face, lips, tongue, or throat). **Note:** This is not a comprehensive list of all side effects. Patient should consult prescriber for additional questions.

Intended Use and Disclaimer: Should not be printed and given to patients. This information is intended to serve as a concise initial reference for healthcare professionals to use when discussing medications with a patient. You must ultimately rely on your own discretion, experience and judgment in diagnosing, treating and advising patients.

Raxibacumab (rax i BAK ue mab)

Index Terms ABthrax

Pharmacologic Category Antidote; Monoclonal Antibody

Pregnancy Risk Factor B

Lactation Excretion in breast milk unknown

Use Treatment of inhalational anthrax following exposure to *Bacillus anthracis* in combination with appropriate antimicrobial therapy; prophylaxis of inhalational anthrax when alternative therapies are unavailable or not appropriate

Available Dosage Forms Injection, solution: 50 mg/mL (34 mL)

General Dosage Range I.V.:
Children and Adolescents:
≤15 kg: 80 mg/kg
>15 kg to 50 kg: 60 mg/kg
>50 kg: 40 mg/kg
Adults: 40 mg/kg

Administration

I.V. Premedicate with diphenhydramine ≤1 hour prior to raxibacumab infusion. Administer over 2 hours and 15 minutes; administration rate should be slower over the first 20 minutes to monitor for adverse reactions; slow or interrupt infusion if adverse reactions (including infusion-related reactions) occur. Administer as follows:

Body weight: ≤1 kg: Infuse at 0.5 mL/hour for 20 minutes; increase rate to 3.5 mL/hour for the remaining infusion

Body weight 1.1 to 2 kg: Infuse at 1 mL/hour for 20 minutes; increase rate to 7 mL/hour for the remaining infusion

Body weight 2.1 to 3 kg: Infuse at 1.2 mL/hour for 20 minutes; increase rate to 10 mL/hour for the remaining infusion

Body weight 3.1 to 4.9 kg: Infuse at 1.5 mL/hour for 20 minutes; increase rate to 12 mL/hour for the remaining infusion

Body weight 5 to 10 kg: Infuse at 3 mL/hour for 20 minutes; increase rate to 25 mL/hour for the remaining infusion

Body weight 11 to 30 kg: Infuse at 6 mL/hour for 20 minutes; increase rate to 50 mL/hour for the remaining infusion

Body weight ≥31 kg: Infuse at 15 mL/hour for 20 minutes; increase rate to 125 mL/hour for the remaining infusion

Injectable Detail pH: 6.5 (vial)

Nursing Actions

Physical Assessment Patient must be monitored closely for infusion-related reactions, including rash, urticaria, pain in the arms and legs, and pruritus. Administer diphenhydramine within 1 hour prior to the raxibacumab infusion to reduce the risk of infusion-related reactions; administer diphenhydramine via the oral or I.V. route depending on the proximity to the start of the raxibacumab infusion. The infusion rate should be slower over the first 20 minutes to monitor for adverse reactions; slow or interrupt the infusion if adverse reactions (including infusion-related reactions) occur. Instruct patient to continue taking oral antibiotics.

Patient Education

- Discuss specific use of drug and side effects with patient as it relates to treatment. (HCAHPS: During this hospital stay, were you given any medicine that you had not taken before? Before giving you any new medicine, how often did hospital staff tell you what the medicine was for? How often did hospital staff describe possible side effects in a way you could understand?)
- Patient may experience asthenia or limb pain. Have patient report immediately to prescriber signs of infection (HCAHPS).

- Educate patient about signs of a significant reaction (eg, wheezing; chest tightness; fever; itching; bad cough; blue skin color; seizures; or swelling of face, lips, tongue, or throat). **Note:** This is not a comprehensive list of all side effects. Patient should consult prescriber for additional questions.

Intended Use and Disclaimer: Should not be printed and given to patients. This information is intended to serve as a concise initial reference for healthcare professionals to use when discussing medications with a patient. You must ultimately rely on your own discretion, experience and judgment in diagnosing, treating and advising patients.

Regorafenib (re goe RAF e nib)

Brand Names: U.S. Stivarga

Index Terms BAY 73-4506

Pharmacologic Category Antineoplastic Agent, Tyrosine Kinase Inhibitor; Antineoplastic Agent, Vascular Endothelial Growth Factor (VEGF) Inhibitor

Medication Safety Issues

Sound-alike/look-alike issues:

Regorafenib may be confused with axitinib, crizotinib, dasatinib, erlotinib, imatinib, lapatinib, nilotinib, PAZOPanib, PONATinib, ruxolitinib, sorafenib, sunitinib, vemurafenib

High alert medication:

This medication is in a class the Institute for Safe Medication Practices (ISMP) includes among its list of drug classes which have a heightened risk of causing significant patient harm when used in error.

Pregnancy Risk Factor D

Lactation Excretion in breast milk unknown/not recommended

Use

Gastrointestinal stromal tumors: Treatment of locally-advanced, unresectable, or metastatic gastrointestinal stromal tumor (GIST) in patients previously treated with imatinib and sunitinib

Metastatic colorectal cancer: Treatment of metastatic colorectal cancer in patients previously treated with fluoropyrimidine-, oxaliplatin-, and irinotecan-based chemotherapy, anti-VEGF therapy, or anti-EGFR therapy (if *KRAS* wild type)

Available Dosage Forms

Tablet, Oral:

Stivarga: 40 mg

General Dosage Range Dosage adjustment recommended in patients who develop toxicities

Oral: *Adults:* 160 mg once daily

◀ **Administration**

Oral Take at the same time each day with a low-fat (<30% fat) breakfast; swallow tablets whole.

Hazardous agent; use appropriate precautions for handling and disposal (meets NIOSH, 2012 criteria).

Nursing Actions

Physical Assessment Monitor blood pressure, especially during the first 6 weeks of therapy. Watch for new or acute heart ischemia or infarction; dermatological toxicity (any rash), especially symptoms of hand-foot syndrome. Monitor for signs of severe bleeding, severe pain, swelling, or high fevers; signs/symptoms of gastrointestinal perforation; hepatic dysfunction (eg, jaundice, dark urine); impaired wound healing especially after surgery. Educate patients to tell all doctors and dentists about poor wound healing. Evaluate signs/symptoms of RPLS; severe headaches, seizure, confusion, or change in vision. Check results of CBC with differential and serum electrolytes.

Patient Education

- Discuss specific use of drug and side effects with patient as it relates to treatment. (HCAHPS: During this hospital stay, were you given any medicine that you had not taken before? Before giving you any new medicine, how often did hospital staff tell you what the medicine was for? How often did hospital staff describe possible side effects in a way you could understand?)
- Patient may experience anemia, leukopenia, thrombocytopenia, diarrhea, asthenia, hypertension, pain, headache, weight loss, lack of appetite, skin irritation of palms and soles, stomatitis, dysphonia, or rash. Have patient report immediately to prescriber signs of infection, illogical thinking, sudden vision changes, severe dizziness, tachycardia, angina, dyspnea, significant nausea, ecchymosis, bleeding, considerable weight gain, wounds not healing, discolored urine, or jaundice (HCAHPS).
- Educate patient about signs of a significant reaction (eg, wheezing; chest tightness; fever; itching; bad cough; blue skin color; seizures; or swelling of face, lips, tongue, or throat). **Note:** This is not a comprehensive list of all side effects. Patient should consult prescriber for additional questions.

Intended Use and Disclaimer: Should not be printed and given to patients. This information is intended to serve as a concise initial reference for healthcare professionals to use when discussing medications with a patient. You must ultimately rely on your own discretion, experience and judgment in diagnosing, treating and advising patients.

Related Information

Oral Medications That Should Not Be Crushed or Altered *on page 1712*

Repaglinide (re PAG li nide)

Brand Names: U.S. Prandin

Pharmacologic Category Antidiabetic Agent, Meglitinide Derivative

Medication Safety Issues

Sound-alike/look-alike issues:

Prandin® may be confused with Avandia®

High alert medication:

The Institute for Safe Medication Practices (ISMP) includes this medication among its list of drug classes which have a heightened risk of causing significant patient harm when used in error.

Pregnancy Risk Factor C

Lactation Excretion in breast milk unknown/not recommended

Breast-Feeding Considerations It is not known if repaglinide is excreted in breast milk. Breast-feeding is not recommended by the manufacturer.

Use Management of type 2 diabetes mellitus (non-insulin dependent, NIDDM) as an adjunct to diet and exercise; may be used in combination with metformin or thiazolidinediones

Mechanism of Action/Effect Nonsulfonylurea hypoglycemic agent of the meglitinide class (the nonsulfonylurea moiety of glyburide) used in the management of type 2 diabetes mellitus; stimulates insulin release from the pancreatic beta cells. Repaglinide-induced insulin release is glucose-dependent.

Contraindications Hypersensitivity to repaglinide or any component of the formulation; diabetic ketoacidosis, with or without coma; type 1 diabetes (insulin dependent, IDDM); concurrent gemfibrozil therapy

Warnings/Precautions Use with caution in patients with hepatic impairment. Use caution in severe renal dysfunction, elderly, malnourished, or patients with adrenal/pituitary dysfunction; may be more susceptible to glucose-lowering effects. May cause hypoglycemia; appropriate patient selection, dosage, and patient education are important to avoid hypoglycemic episodes. It may be necessary to discontinue repaglinide and administer insulin if the patient is exposed to stress (fever, trauma, infection, surgery). Theoretically, repaglinide may increase cardiovascular events as observed in some studies using sulfonylureas, but there are no long-term studies assessing this concern. Not indicated for use in combination with NPH insulin as there have been case reports of myocardial ischemia; further evaluation required to assess the safety of this combination.

Drug Interactions
Avoid Concomitant Use
Avoid concomitant use of Repaglinide with any of the following: Gemfibrozil
Decreased Effect
The levels/effects of Repaglinide may be decreased by: Bosentan; Corticosteroids (Orally Inhaled); Corticosteroids (Systemic); CYP2C8 Inducers (Strong); CYP3A4 Inducers (Strong); Dabrafenib; Herbs (CYP3A4 Inducers); Loop Diuretics; Luteinizing Hormone-Releasing Hormone Analogs; Mitotane; Rifampin; Somatropin; Thiazide Diuretics; Tocilizumab
Increased Effect/Toxicity
Repaglinide may increase the levels/effects of: Hypoglycemic Agents

The levels/effects of Repaglinide may be increased by: CycloSPORINE (Systemic); CYP2C8 Inhibitors (Moderate); CYP2C8 Inhibitors (Strong); CYP3A4 Inhibitors (Strong); Deferasirox; Eltrombopag; Gemfibrozil; Herbs (Hypoglycemic Properties); Macrolide Antibiotics; MAO Inhibitors; Mifepristone; Pegvisomant; Salicylates; Selective Serotonin Reuptake Inhibitors; Telaprevir; Teriflunomide; Trimethoprim
Nutritional/Ethanol Interactions
Ethanol: Ethanol may increase risk of hypoglycemia. Management: Avoid ethanol.

Food: When given with food, the AUC of repaglinide is decreased. Taking medication without eating may cause hypoglycemia. Management: Administer 15-30 minutes prior to a meal. If a meal is skipped, skip dose for that meal.

Herb/Nutraceutical: St John's wort may decrease the levels/effect of repaglinide. Other herbal medications may enhance the hypoglycemic effects of repaglinide. Management: Avoid St John's wort, alfalfa, aloe, bilberry, bitter melon, burdock, celery, damiana, fenugreek, garcinia, garlic, ginger, ginseng (American), gymnema, marshmallow, and stinging nettle.
Adverse Reactions
>10%:
Central nervous system: Headache (9% to 11%)
Endocrine & metabolic: Hypoglycemia (16% to 31%)
Respiratory: Upper respiratory tract infection (10% to 16%)
1% to 10%:
Cardiovascular: Ischemia (4%), chest pain (2% to 3%)
Gastrointestinal: Diarrhea (4% to 5%), constipation (2% to 3%)
Genitourinary: Urinary tract infection (2% to 3%)
Neuromuscular & skeletal: Back pain (5% to 6%), arthralgia (3% to 6%)
Respiratory: Sinusitis (3% to 6%), bronchitis (2% to 6%)
Miscellaneous: Allergy (1% to 2%)

Pharmacodynamics/Kinetics
Onset of Action Single dose: Increased insulin levels: ~15-60 minutes
Duration of Action 4-6 hours
Available Dosage Forms
Tablet, Oral:
Prandin: 0.5 mg, 1 mg, 2 mg
Generic: 0.5 mg, 1 mg, 2 mg
General Dosage Range Dosage adjustment recommended in patients with renal impairment
Oral: *Adults:* Initial: 0.5-2 mg before each meal; Maintenance: 0.5-4 mg before each meal (maximum: 16 mg/day)
Administration
Oral Administer 15 minutes before meals; however, time may vary from immediately preceding a meal to as long as 30 minutes before a meal. If the patient misses a meal or is unable to take anything by mouth, repaglinide should not be administered to avoid hypoglycemia. Patients consuming extra meals should be instructed to add a dose for the extra meal.
Storage/Stability Do not store above 25°C (77°F). Protect from moisture.
Nursing Actions
Physical Assessment Instruct patient to treat signs of hypoglycemia and report them to health care provider.
Patient Education
- Discuss specific use of drug and side effects with patient as it relates to treatment. (HCAHPS: During this hospital stay, were you given any medicine that you had not taken before? Before giving you any new medicine, how often did hospital staff tell you what the medicine was for? How often did hospital staff describe possible side effects in a way you could understand?)
- Patient may experience headache, rhinorrhea, rhinitis, diarrhea, or arthralgia. Have patient report immediately to prescriber ecchymosis, hemorrhaging, angina, chills, pharyngitis, or signs of hypoglycemia (HCAHPS).
- Educate patient about signs of a significant reaction (eg, wheezing; chest tightness; fever; itching; bad cough; blue skin color; seizures; or swelling of face, lips, tongue, or throat). **Note:** This is not a comprehensive list of all side effects. Patient should consult prescriber for additional questions.

Intended Use and Disclaimer: Should not be printed and given to patients. This information is intended to serve as a concise initial reference for healthcare professionals to use when discussing medications with a patient. You must ultimately rely on your own discretion, experience and judgment in diagnosing, treating and advising patients.

◀ **Dietary Considerations** Take repaglinide 15-30 minutes before meals. Individualized medical nutrition therapy (MNT) based on ADA recommendations is an integral part of therapy. May cause hypoglycemia. Must be able to recognize symptoms of hypoglycemia (palpitations, tachycardia, sweaty palms, diaphoresis, lightheadedness).

Repaglinide and Metformin
(re PAG li nide & met FOR min)

Brand Names: U.S. PrandiMet®

Index Terms Metformin and Repaglinide; Repaglinide and Metformin Hydrochloride

Pharmacologic Category Antidiabetic Agent, Biguanide; Antidiabetic Agent, Meglitinide Derivative; Hypoglycemic Agent, Oral

Medication Safety Issues

Sound-alike/look-alike issues:

PrandiMet® may be confused with Avandamet®, Prandin®

High alert medication:

The Institute for Safe Medication Practices (ISMP) includes this medication among its list of drug classes which have a heightened risk of causing significant patient harm when used in error.

Pregnancy Risk Factor C

Use Management of type 2 diabetes mellitus (non-insulin dependent, NIDDM), as an adjunct to diet and exercise, in patients currently receiving or not adequately controlled on metformin and/or a meglitinide

Available Dosage Forms

Tablet:

PrandiMet®: 1/500: Repaglinide 1 mg and metformin hydrochloride 500 mg; 2/500: Repaglinide 2 mg and metformin hydrochloride 500 mg

General Dosage Range Oral: *Adults:* Repaglinide 1-2 mg and metformin 500 mg 2-3 times daily with meals (maximum single dose: 4 mg/dose [repaglinide], 1000 mg/dose [metformin]; maximum daily dose: 10 mg/day [repaglinide], 2500 mg/day [metformin])

Administration

Oral Administer 15-30 minutes before meals to avoid risk of hypoglycemia/GI upset; if a meal skipped or patient is unable to take anything by mouth, do not administer dose.

Nursing Actions

Physical Assessment See individual agents.

Patient Education

• Discuss specific use of drug and side effects with patient as it relates to treatment. (HCAHPS: During this hospital stay, were you given any medicine that you had not taken before? Before giving you any new medicine, how often did hospital staff tell you what the medicine was for? How often did hospital staff describe possible side effects in a way you could understand?)

• Patient may experience headache, flatulence, nausea, diarrhea, rhinitis, or rhinorrhea. Have patient report immediately to prescriber ecchymosis, hemorrhaging, angina, chills, pharyngitis, signs of hypoglycemia, or signs of lactic acidosis (HCAHPS).

• Educate patient about signs of a significant reaction (eg, wheezing; chest tightness; fever; itching; bad cough; blue skin color; seizures; or swelling of face, lips, tongue, or throat). **Note:** This is not a comprehensive list of all side effects. Patient should consult prescriber for additional questions.

Intended Use and Disclaimer: Should not be printed and given to patients. This information is intended to serve as a concise initial reference for healthcare professionals to use when discussing medications with a patient. You must ultimately rely on your own discretion, experience and judgment in diagnosing, treating and advising patients.

Related Information

MetFORMIN *on page 1014*
Repaglinide *on page 1342*

Reteplase (RE ta plase)

Brand Names: U.S. Retavase; Retavase Half-Kit

Index Terms r-PA; Recombinant Plasminogen Activator

Pharmacologic Category Thrombolytic Agent

Medication Safety Issues

High alert medication:

The Institute for Safe Medication Practices (ISMP) includes this medication (I.V.) among its list of drugs which have a heightened risk of causing significant patient harm when used in error.

Pregnancy Risk Factor C

Lactation Excretion in breast milk unknown/use caution

Breast-Feeding Considerations It is not known if reteplase is excreted in breast milk. The manufacturer recommends that caution be exercised when administering reteplase to nursing women.

Use Management of ST-elevation myocardial infarction (STEMI) for the improvement of ventricular function, the reduction of the incidence of CHF, and the reduction of mortality following STEMI

Recommended criteria for treatment of STEMI (ACCF/AHA; O'Gara, 2013): Ischemic symptoms within 12 hours of treatment or evidence of ongoing ischemia 12-24 hours after symptom onset with a large area of myocardium at risk or hemodynamic instability.

STEMI ECG definition: New ST-segment elevation at the J point in at least 2 contiguous leads of ≥2 mm (0.2 mV) in men or ≥1.5 mm (0.15 mV) in women in leads V_2-V_3 and/or of ≥1 mm (0.1 mV) in other contiguous precordial leads or limb leads on ECG. New or presumably new left bundle branch block (LBBB) may interfere with ST-elevation analysis and should not be considered diagnostic in isolation.

At non-PCI-capable hospitals, the ACCF/AHA recommends thrombolytic therapy administration when the anticipated first medical contact (FMC)-to-device time at a PCI-capable hospital is >120 minutes due to unavoidable delays.

Mechanism of Action/Effect Reteplase initiates local fibrinolysis by binding to fibrin in a thrombus (clot) and converting entrapped plasminogen to plasmin. Dissolution of thrombus occluding a coronary artery restores perfusion to ischemic myocardium. Reteplase is manufactured by recombinant DNA technology using *E. coli.*

Contraindications Active internal bleeding; history of cerebrovascular accident; recent (ie, within 2 months) intracranial or intraspinal surgery or trauma; intracranial neoplasm, arteriovenous malformations, or aneurysm; known bleeding diathesis; severe uncontrolled hypertension

Additional contraindications (ACCF/AHA; O'Gara, 2013): Ischemic stroke within 3 months; prior intracranial hemorrhage; active bleeding (excluding menses); suspected aortic dissection; significant closed head or facial trauma within 3 months

Warnings/Precautions Use with caution in patients receiving oral anticoagulants; increased risk of bleeding. Adjunctive use of parenteral anticoagulants (eg, enoxaparin, heparin, or fondaparinux) is recommended to improve vessel patency and prevent reocclusion (ACCF/AHA; O'Gara, 2013); however, these may also contribute to bleeding; monitor for bleeding. I.M. injections and nonessential handling of the patient should be avoided. Venipunctures should be performed carefully and only when necessary. If arterial puncture is necessary, use an upper extremity vessel that can be manually compressed. If serious bleeding occurs then the infusion of reteplase and heparin should be stopped.

For the following conditions the risk of bleeding is higher with use of reteplase and should be weighed against the benefits of therapy: recent major surgery (eg, CABG, obstetrical delivery, organ biopsy), recent puncture of noncompressible vessels, cerebrovascular disease, recent gastrointestinal or genitourinary bleeding, recent trauma including CPR, hypertension (systolic BP >180 mm Hg and/or diastolic BP >110 mm Hg), high likelihood of left heart thrombus (eg, mitral stenosis with atrial fibrillation), acute pericarditis, subacute bacterial endocarditis, hemostatic defects including ones caused by severe renal or hepatic dysfunction, significant hepatic or renal dysfunction, diabetic hemorrhagic retinopathy or other hemorrhagic ophthalmic conditions, septic thrombophlebitis or occluded AV cannula at seriously infected site, advanced age (eg, >75 years), patients receiving oral anticoagulants, any other condition in which bleeding constitutes a significant hazard or would be particularly difficult to manage because of location.

Coronary thrombolysis may result in reperfusion arrhythmias. Follow standard MI management. Rare anaphylactic reactions can occur.

Drug Interactions

Avoid Concomitant Use There are no known interactions where it is recommended to avoid concomitant use.

Decreased Effect

The levels/effects of Reteplase may be decreased by: Aprotinin

Increased Effect/Toxicity

Reteplase may increase the levels/effects of: Anticoagulants; Dabigatran Etexilate

The levels/effects of Reteplase may be increased by: Agents with Antiplatelet Properties; Herbs (Anticoagulant/Antiplatelet Properties); Salicylates

Adverse Reactions Bleeding is the most frequent adverse effect associated with reteplase. Heparin and aspirin have been administered concurrently with reteplase in clinical trials. The incidence of adverse events is a reflection of these combined therapies, and is comparable to comparison thrombolytics.

>10%: Local: Injection site bleeding (5% to 49%)

1% to 10%:

Gastrointestinal: Bleeding (2% to 9%)

Genitourinary: Bleeding (1% to 10%)

Hematologic: Anemia (1% to 3%)

Other adverse effects noted are frequently associated with MI (and therefore may or may not be attributable to Retavase®) and include arrhythmia, AV block, cardiac arrest, cardiogenic shock, embolism, heart failure, hypotension, myocardial rupture, mitral regurgitation, pericardial effusion, pericarditis, pulmonary edema, recurrent ischemia, reinfarction, tamponade, thrombosis

Pharmacodynamics/Kinetics

Onset of Action Thrombolysis: 30-90 minutes

Available Dosage Forms

Kit, Intravenous [preservative free]:

Retavase: 10.4 units

Retavase Half-Kit: 10.4 units

General Dosage Range I.V.: *Adults:* 10 units; repeat after 30 minutes

Administration

I.V. Reconstituted dose should be administered I.V. over 2 minutes; no other medication should be added to the injection.

Preparation for Administration Reteplase should be reconstituted using the diluent, syringe, needle, and dispensing pin provided with each kit. Do not shake while reconstituting; swirl gently. Once reconstituted, use within 4 hours.

Storage/Stability Dosage kits should be stored at 2°C to 25°C (36°F to 77°F) and remain sealed until use in order to protect from light.

Nursing Actions

Physical Assessment Use caution when there is significant risk of bleeding. Monitor patient closely for bleeding during and following treatment. Monitor infusion site, neurological status (eg, intracranial hemorrhage), vital signs, and ECG. Maintain bleeding precautions; avoid I.M. injections, venipunctures (unless absolutely necessary), and nonessential handling of the patient. If arterial puncture is necessary, use an upper extremity vessel that can be manually compressed.

Patient Education

• Discuss specific use of drug and side effects with patient as it relates to treatment. (HCAHPS: During this hospital stay, were you given any medicine that you had not taken before? Before giving you any new medicine, how often did hospital staff tell you what the medicine was for? How often did hospital staff describe possible side effects in a way you could understand?)

• Patient may experience severe bleeding. Have patient report immediately to prescriber angina, illogical thinking, severe headache, significant back pain, considerable dyspepsia, ecchymosis, severe asthenia, or rash (HCAHPS).

• Educate patient about signs of a significant reaction (eg, wheezing; chest tightness; fever; itching; bad cough; blue skin color; seizures; or swelling of face, lips, tongue, or throat). **Note:** This is not a comprehensive list of all side effects. Patient should consult prescriber for additional questions.

Intended Use and Disclaimer: Should not be printed and given to patients. This information is intended to serve as a concise initial reference for healthcare professionals to use when discussing medications with a patient. You must ultimately rely on your own discretion, experience and judgment in diagnosing, treating and advising patients.

Rh$_o$(D) Immune Globulin
(ar aych oh (dee) i MYUN GLOB yoo lin)

Brand Names: U.S. HyperRHO S/D; MICRho-GAM Ultra-Filtered Plus; RhoGAM Ultra-Filtered Plus; Rhophylac; WinRho SDF

Index Terms Anti-D Immunoglobulin; RhIG; Rho (D) Immune Globulin (Human); RholGIV; RholVIM

Pharmacologic Category Blood Product Derivative; Immune Globulin

Pregnancy Risk Factor C

Use

Suppression of Rh isoimmunization: Use in the following situations when an Rh$_o$(D)-negative individual is exposed to Rh$_o$(D)-positive blood: During delivery of an Rh$_o$(D)-positive infant; abortion;

amniocentesis; chorionic villus sampling; ruptured tubal pregnancy; abdominal trauma; hydatidiform mole; transplacental hemorrhage. Used when the mother is Rh$_o$(D)-negative, the father of the child is either Rh$_o$(D)-positive or Rh$_o$(D)-unknown, or the baby is either Rh$_o$(D)-positive or Rh$_o$(D)-unknown.

Transfusion: Suppression of Rh isoimmunization in Rh$_o$(D)-negative individuals transfused with Rh$_o$(D) antigen-positive RBCs or blood components containing Rh$_o$(D) antigen-positive RBCs

Treatment of immune thrombocytopenia (ITP): Used intravenously in the following nonsplenectomized Rh$_o$(D)-positive individuals: Children with acute or chronic ITP, adults with chronic ITP, and children and adults with ITP secondary to HIV infection

Available Dosage Forms

Injectable, Intramuscular [preservative free]:
HyperRHO S/D: 50 mcg (1 ea); 300 mcg (1 ea)
MICRhoGAM Ultra-Filtered Plus: 50 mcg (1 ea)
RhoGAM Ultra-Filtered Plus: 300 mcg (1 ea)

Solution, Injection:
WinRho SDF: 2500 units/2.2 mL (2.2 mL); 5000 units/4.4 mL (4.4 mL); 1500 units/1.3 mL (1.3 mL); 15,000 units/13 mL (13 mL)

Solution, Injection [preservative free]:
Rhophylac: 1500 units/2 mL (2 mL)
WinRho SDF: 2500 units/2.2 mL (2.2 mL); 5000 units/4.4 mL (4.4 mL); 1500 units/1.3 mL (1.3 mL); 15,000 units/13 mL (13 mL)

General Dosage Range I.M., I.V.: *Children and Adults:* Dosage varies greatly depending on indication

Administration

I.M. Administer into the deltoid muscle of the upper arm or anterolateral aspect of the upper thigh. Avoid gluteal region due to risk of sciatic nerve injury. If large doses (>5 mL) are needed, administration in divided doses at different sites is recommended. **Note:** Do not administer I.M. Rh$_o$(D) immune globulin for ITP.

I.V.

WinRho® SDF: Infuse over at least 3-5 minutes; do not administer with other medications

Rhophylac®: ITP: Infuse at 2 mL per 15-60 seconds

Injectable Detail Note: If preparing dose using liquid formulation, withdraw the entire contents of the vial to ensure accurate calculation of the dosage requirement.

Nursing Actions

Physical Assessment Monitor blood pressure; may cause hyper-/hypotension. Be alert to the possibility of anaphylaxis. Assess for signs and symptoms of intravascular hemolysis (IVH) in patients with ITP, anemia, renal insufficiency, back pain, shaking, chills, discolored urine, or hematuria; observe patient for side effects for 8 hours following administration.

Patient Education

- Discuss specific use of vaccine and side effects with patient as it relates to treatment. (HCAHPS: During this hospital stay, were you given any medicine that you had not taken before? Before giving you any new medicine, how often did hospital staff tell you what the medicine was for? How often did hospital staff describe possible side effects in a way you could understand?)
- Patient may experience headache or injection site irritation. Have patient report immediately to prescriber dyspnea, severe back pain, significant edema, discolored urine, or rash (HCAHPS).
- Educate patient about signs of a significant reaction (eg, wheezing; chest tightness; fever; itching; bad cough; blue skin color; seizures; or swelling of face, lips, tongue, or throat). **Note:** This is not a comprehensive list of all side effects. Patient should consult prescriber for additional questions.

Intended Use and Disclaimer: Should not be printed and given to patients. This information is intended to serve as a concise initial reference for healthcare professionals to use when discussing medications with a patient. You must ultimately rely on your own discretion, experience and judgment in diagnosing, treating and advising patients.

Ribavirin (rye ba VYE rin)

Brand Names: U.S. Copegus; Moderiba; Rebetol; Ribasphere; Ribasphere RibaPak; Virazole
Index Terms RTCA; Tribavirin
Pharmacologic Category Antihepaciviral, Nucleoside (Anti-HCV)
Medication Safety Issues
Sound-alike/look-alike issues:
Ribavirin may be confused with riboflavin, rifampin, Robaxin
Medication Guide Available Yes
Pregnancy Risk Factor X
Lactation Excretion in breast milk unknown/not recommended
Breast-Feeding Considerations It is not known if ribavirin is excreted in breast milk. Due to the potential for serious adverse reactions in the nursing infant, a decision should be made whether to discontinue nursing or to discontinue the drug, taking into account the importance of treatment to the mother.
Use
Inhalation: Treatment of hospitalized infants and young children with respiratory syncytial virus (RSV) infections; specially indicated for treatment of severe lower respiratory tract RSV infections in patients with an underlying compromising condition (prematurity, cardiopulmonary disease, or immunosuppression)

Oral capsule: In combination with interferon alfa 2b (pegylated or nonpegylated) injection for the treatment of chronic hepatitis C in interferon alfa-naive or experienced-patients with compensated liver disease. Patients likely to fail retreatment after a prior failed course include previous nonresponders, those who received previous pegylated interferon treatment, patients who have significant bridging fibrosis or cirrhosis, or those with genotype 1 infection.

Oral solution: In combination with interferon alfa-2b (pegylated or nonpegylated) injection for the treatment of chronic hepatitis C in interferon alfa-naive or experienced patients ≥3 years of age with compensated liver disease. Patients likely to fail retreatment after a prior failed course include previous nonresponders, those who received previous pegylated interferon treatment, patients who have significant bridging fibrosis or cirrhosis, or those with genotype 1 infection.

Oral tablet: In combination with peginterferon alfa-2a for the treatment of adults (Copegus, Moderiba, Ribasphere) and patients ≥5 years of age (Copegus only) with chronic HCV infection who have compensated liver disease and have not previously been treated with interferon alpha, and in adult chronic hepatitis C patients coinfected with HIV

Unlabeled Use
Inhalation: Treatment for RSV in adult hematopoietic stem cell or heart/lung transplant recipients
Used in other viral infections including influenza A and B and adenovirus
Mechanism of Action/Effect Inhibits viral protein synthesis
Contraindications
Inhalation: Hypersensitivity to ribavirin or any component of the formulation; women who are pregnant or may become pregnant
Oral formulations: Hypersensitivity to ribavirin or any component of the formulation; women who are pregnant or may become pregnant; males whose female partners are pregnant; patients with hemoglobinopathies (eg, thalassemia major, sickle cell anemia); patients with autoimmune hepatitis; concomitant use with didanosine
Ribasphere capsules and Rebetol capsules/solution: Additional contraindications: Patients with a CrCl <50 mL/minute
Oral combination therapy with alfa interferons: Autoimmune hepatitis, hepatic decompensation (Child-Pugh score >6; class B and C) in cirrhotic chronic hepatitis C monoinfected patients prior to treatment, hepatic decompensation (Child-Pugh score ≥6) in cirrhotic chronic hepatitis C patients coinfected with HIV prior to treatment. Also refer to individual monographs for Interferon Alfa-2b (Intron A), Peginterferon Alfa-2b, and Peginterferon Alfa-2a (Pegasys) for additional contraindication information.

Warnings/Precautions Hazardous agent - use appropriate precautions for handling and disposal (NIOSH, 2012).

Oral: **[U.S. Boxed Warning]: Significant teratogenic effects have been observed in all animal studies.** A negative pregnancy test is required before initiation and monthly thereafter. Avoid pregnancy in female patients and female partners of male patients, during therapy, and for at least 6 months after treatment; two forms of contraception should be used. Safety and efficacy have not been established in patients who have received organ transplants, or been coinfected with hepatitis B or HIV (ribavirin tablets may be used in adult HIV-coinfected patients unless CD4+ cell count is <100 cells/microliter and HIV-1 RNA <5000 cells/mm^3). Hemoglobin at initiation must be ≥12 g/dL (women) or ≥13 g/dL (men) in CHC monoinfected patients and ≥11 g/dL (women) or ≥12 g/dL (men) in CHC and HIV coinfected patients. Oral ribavirin should not be used for adenovirus, RSV, influenza or parainfluenza infections; ribavirin inhalation is approved for severe RSV infection in children.

[U.S. Boxed Warning]: Monotherapy not effective for chronic hepatitis C infection. Severe psychiatric events have occurred including depression and suicidal behavior during combination therapy. Avoid use in patients with a psychiatric history; discontinue if severe psychiatric symptoms occur. Acute hypersensitivity reactions (eg, anaphylaxis, angioedema, bronchoconstriction, and urticaria) have been observed (rarely) with ribavirin and alfa interferon combination therapy. Severe cutaneous reactions, including Stevens-Johnson syndrome and exfoliative dermatitis have been reported (rarely) with ribavirin and alfa interferon combination therapy; discontinue with signs or symptoms of severe skin reactions. Use with caution in patients with renal impairment; dosage adjustment or discontinuation may be required. Elderly patients are more susceptible to adverse effects; use caution.

[U.S. Boxed Warning]: Hemolytic anemia is the primary clinical toxicity of oral therapy; anemia associated with ribavirin may worsen underlying cardiac disease and lead to fatal and nonfatal myocardial infarctions. Avoid use in patients with significant/unstable cardiac disease. Anemia usually occurs within 1-2 weeks of therapy initiation; observed in ~10% to 13% of patients when alfa interferons were combined with ribavirin. Assess cardiac function before initiation of therapy. If patient has underlying cardiac disease, assess electrocardiogram prior to and periodically during treatment. If any deterioration in cardiovascular status occurs, discontinue therapy. Use caution in patients with baseline risk of severe anemia. Assess hemoglobin and hematocrit at baseline and, at minimum, weeks 2 and 4 of therapy since initial drop may be significant.

Patients with renal dysfunction and/or those >50 years of age should be carefully assessed for development of anemia. Pancytopenia and bone marrow suppression have been reported with the combination of ribavirin, interferon, and azathioprine. Use caution in pulmonary disease; pulmonary symptoms have been associated with administration. Discontinue therapy if evidence of hepatic decompensation is observed. Use caution in patients with sarcoidosis (exacerbation reported). Dental and periodontal disorders have been reported with ribavirin and interferon therapy; patients should be instructed to brush teeth twice daily and have regular dental exams. Serious ophthalmologic disorders have occurred with combination therapy. All patients require an eye exam at baseline; those with pre-existing ophthalmologic disorders (eg, diabetic or hypertensive retinopathy) require periodic follow up. Delay in weight and height increases have been noted in children treated with combination therapy for CHC. In clinical studies, decreases were noted in weight and height for age z-scores and normative growth curve percentiles. Following treatment, rebound growth and weight gain occurred in most patients; however, a small percentage did not. Long-term data indicate that combination therapy may inhibit growth resulting in reduced adult height. Growth should be closely monitored in pediatric patients during therapy and post-treatment for growth catch-up.

Inhalation: **[U.S. Boxed Warning]: Use with caution in patients requiring assisted ventilation because precipitation of the drug in the respiratory equipment may interfere with safe and effective patient ventilation; sudden deterioration of respiratory function has been observed;** monitor carefully in patients with COPD and asthma for deterioration of respiratory function. Ribavirin is potentially mutagenic, tumor-promoting, and gonadotoxic. Although anemia has not been reported with inhalation therapy, consider monitoring for anemia 1-2 weeks post-treatment. Pregnant health care workers may consider unnecessary occupational exposure; ribavirin has been detected in healthcare workers' urine. Health care professionals or family members who are pregnant (or may become pregnant) should be counseled about potential risks of exposure and counseled about risk reduction strategies. Hazardous agent - use appropriate precautions for handling and disposal.

Drug Interactions

Avoid Concomitant Use

Avoid concomitant use of Ribavirin with any of the following: Didanosine

Decreased Effect

Ribavirin may decrease the levels/effects of: Influenza Virus Vaccine (Live/Attenuated)

Increased Effect/Toxicity
Ribavirin may increase the levels/effects of: Aza-THIOprine; Didanosine; Reverse Transcriptase Inhibitors (Nucleoside)

The levels/effects of Ribavirin may be increased by: Interferons (Alfa); Zidovudine

Nutritional/Ethanol Interactions Food: Oral: High-fat meal increases the AUC and C_{max}. Management: Capsule (in combination with peginterferon alfa-2b) and tablet should be administered with food. Other dosage forms and combinations should be taken consistently in regards to food.

Adverse Reactions

Inhalation:

1% to 10%:

Central nervous system: Fatigue, headache, insomnia

Gastrointestinal: Nausea, anorexia

Hematologic: Anemia

Oral (all adverse reactions are documented while receiving combination therapy with alfa interferons; percentages as reported in adults unless noted, most common pediatric adverse reactions were similar to adults); asterisked (*) percentages are those similar to interferon therapy alone:

>10%:

Central nervous system: Fatigue (60% to 70% [30% in pediatric patients])*, headache (43% to 66%)*, fever (32% to 55%)*, insomnia (26% to 41% [9% in pediatric patients]), depression (20% to 36%)*, irritability (23% to 33%), dizziness (14% to 26%), impaired concentration (10% to 21%)*, emotional lability (7% to 12%)*, anxiety (11%)

Dermatologic: Alopecia (27% to 36% [17% in pediatric patients]), pruritus (13% to 29% [11% in pediatric patients]), rash (5% to 28%), dry skin (10% to 24%), dermatitis (≤16%)

Endocrine and metabolic: Growth suppression (pediatric) percentile decrease (≥15 percentiles: weight 43%; height 25%), hyperuricemia (33% to 38%)

Gastrointestinal: Nausea (25% to 47% [18% in pediatric patients]), anorexia (21% to 32%), weight decrease (10% to 29%), vomiting (9% to 25%)*, diarrhea (10% to 22%), dyspepsia (6% to 16%), abdominal pain (8% to 13% [21% in pediatric patients]), xerostomia (≤12%), RUQ pain (≤12%)

Hematologic: Leukopenia (6% to 45%), neutropenia (8% to 42%; grade 4: 2% to 11%; 40% with HIV coinfection), hemoglobin decreased (11% to 35%), anemia (11% to 17%), thrombocytopenia (<1% to 15%), lymphopenia (12% to 14%), hemolytic anemia (10% to 13%)

Hepatic: Bilirubin increase (10% to 32%)

Local: Injection site reaction (36% to 58%), inflammation at injection site (18% to 25%)

Neuromuscular & skeletal: Decreased linear skeletal growth (including lagging weight gain; 70% in pediatric patients), myalgia (40% to 64% [17% in pediatric patients])*, rigors (25% to 48%), arthralgia (21% to 34%)*, musculoskeletal pain (19% to 28% [35% in pediatric patients])

Respiratory: Upper respiratory tract infection (60% in pediatric patients), dyspnea (13% to 26%), cough (7% to 23%), pharyngitis (≤13%), sinusitis (≤12%)*

Miscellaneous: Flu-like syndrome (13% to 18% [up to 91% in pediatric patients])*, viral infection (≤12%), diaphoresis (≤11%)

1% to 10%:

Cardiovascular: Chest pain (5% to 9%)*, flushing (≤4%)

Central nervous system: Mood alteration (≤6%; 9% with HIV coinfection), agitation (5% to 8%), nervousness (6%)*, memory impairment (≤6%), malaise (≤6%), suicidal ideation (adolescents: 2%; adults: 1%)

Dermatologic: Eczema (4% to 5%)

Endocrine & metabolic: Menstrual disorder (≤7%), hypothyroidism (≤5%)

Gastrointestinal: Taste perversion (4% to 9%), constipation (5%)

Hepatic: Hepatomegaly (4%), transaminases increased (1% to 3%), hepatic decompensation (2% with HIV coinfection)

Neuromuscular & skeletal: Weakness (9% to 10%), back pain (5%)

Ocular: Blurred vision (≤6%), conjunctivitis (≤5%)

Respiratory: Rhinitis (≤8%), exertional dyspnea (≤7%)

Miscellaneous: Fungal infection (≤6%), bacterial infection (3% to 5%)

Note: Incidence of headache, fever, suicidal ideation, and vomiting are higher in children.

Available Dosage Forms

Capsule, oral: 200 mg

Rebetol: 200 mg

Ribasphere: 200 mg

Powder for solution, for nebulization:

Virazole: 6 g

Solution, oral:

Rebetol: 40 mg/mL (100 mL)

Tablet, oral: 200 mg

Copegus: 200 mg

Ribasphere: 200 mg, 400 mg, 600 mg

Tablet, oral [dose-pack]:

Ribasphere RibaPak 600: 200 mg AM dose, 400 mg PM dose (14s, 56s)

Ribasphere RibaPak 800: 400 mg AM dose, 400 mg PM dose (14s, 56s)

Ribasphere RibaPak 1000: 600 mg AM dose, 400 mg PM dose (14s, 56s)

Ribasphere RibaPak 1200: 600 mg AM dose, 600 mg PM dose (14s, 56s)

General Dosage Range Dosage adjustment recommended in patients with renal impairment and in patients who develop toxicities.

Inhalation: *Children:* 20 mg/mL (6 **g** in 300 mL) solution; continuous: 12-18 hours daily

Oral capsules:

Children 47-59 kg: 800 mg daily

Children 60-73 kg: 1000 mg daily

Children >73 kg: 1200 mg daily

Adults: 800-1400 mg daily

Oral solution:

Children <47 kg: 15 mg/kg/day in 2 divided doses

Adults: 800-1400 mg daily

Oral tablet (Copegus):

Children 23-33 kg: 400 mg daily

Children 34-46 kg: 600 mg daily

Children 47-59 kg: 800 mg daily

Children 60-74 kg: 1000 mg daily

Children ≥75 kg: 1200 mg daily

Adults: 800-1200 mg daily

Oral tablet (Moderiba, Ribasphere): *Adults:* 800-1200 mg daily

Administration

Oral Capsule: Administer with food. Capsule should not be opened, crushed, chewed, or broken.

Solution: Administer with food. Use oral solution for children <47 kg, or those who cannot swallow capsules.

Tablet: Administer with food.

Hazardous agent; use appropriate precautions for handling and disposal (NIOSH, 2012).

Inhalation Ribavirin should be administered in well-ventilated rooms (at least 6 air changes/hour). In mechanically-ventilated patients, ribavirin can potentially be deposited in the ventilator delivery system depending on temperature, humidity, and electrostatic forces; this deposition can lead to malfunction or obstruction of the expiratory valve, resulting in inadvertently high positive end-expiratory pressures. The use of one-way valves in the inspiratory lines, a breathing circuit filter in the expiratory line, and frequent monitoring and filter replacement have been effective in preventing these problems. Solutions in SPAG-2 unit should be discarded at least every 24 hours and when the liquid level is low before adding newly reconstituted solution. Should not be mixed with other aerosolized medication.

Hazardous agent; use appropriate precautions for handling and disposal (NIOSH, 2012).

Preparation for Administration Hazardous agent; use appropriate precautions for handling and disposal (NIOSH, 2012).

Inhalation: Do not use any water containing an antimicrobial agent to reconstitute drug. Reconstituted solution is stable for 24 hours at room temperature.

Storage/Stability

Inhalation: Store vials in a dry place at 15°C to 30°C (59°F to 86°F).

Oral: Store at controlled room temperature of 25°C (77°F); excursions permitted between 15°C and 30°C (59°F and 86°F). Keep bottle tightly closed. Solution may also be refrigerated at 2°C to 8°C (36°F to 46°F).

Nursing Actions

Physical Assessment Note specific cautions for healthcare professionals' exposure risks with inhalation formulation. Monitor weight on a regular basis throughout therapy. Monitor for headache; fatigue; irritability; impaired concentration; nausea, vomiting, or anorexia; anemia; or deterioration of hepatic, respiratory, or cardiac status on a regular basis.

Patient Education

• Discuss specific use of vaccine and side effects with patient as it relates to treatment. (HCAHPS: During this hospital stay, were you given any medicine that you had not taken before? Before giving you any new medicine, how often did hospital staff tell you what the medicine was for? How often did hospital staff describe possible side effects in a way you could understand?)

• Patient may experience anemia, leukopenia, thrombocytopenia, presyncope, fatigue, blurred vision, illogical thinking, headache, dyspepsia, insomnia, nausea, diarrhea, xerostomia, loss of appetite, alopecia, or skin irritation. Have patient report immediately to prescriber angina, tachycardia, dizziness or syncope, dyspnea, significant weight gain or loss, inability to eat, pregnancy, or rash (HCAHPS).

• Educate patient about signs of a significant reaction (eg, wheezing; chest tightness; fever; itching; bad cough; blue skin color; seizures; or swelling of face, lips, tongue, or throat). **Note:** This is not a comprehensive list of all side effects. Patient should consult prescriber for additional questions.

Intended Use and Disclaimer: Should not be printed and given to patients. This information is intended to serve as a concise initial reference for healthcare professionals to use when discussing medications with a patient. You must ultimately rely on your own discretion, experience and judgment in diagnosing, treating and advising patients.

Dietary Considerations Capsules, solution, and tablets should be taken with food.

Rifabutin (rif a BYOO tin)

Brand Names: U.S. Mycobutin

Index Terms Ansamycin

Pharmacologic Category Antibiotic, Miscellaneous; Antitubercular Agent

Medication Safety Issues
Sound-alike/look-alike issues:
Rifabutin may be confused with rifampin

Pregnancy Risk Factor B

Lactation Excretion in breast milk unknown/not recommended

Breast-Feeding Considerations In the United States, where formula is accessible, affordable, safe, and sustainable, and the risk of infant mortality due to diarrhea and respiratory infections is low, complete avoidance of breast-feeding by HIV-infected women is recommended to decrease potential transmission of HIV (DHHS [perinatal], 2011).

Use Prevention of disseminated *Mycobacterium avium* complex (MAC) in patients with advanced HIV infection

Unlabeled Use Utilized in multidrug regimens for treatment of MAC; alternative to rifampin as prophylaxis for latent tuberculosis infection (LTBI) or part of multidrug regimen for treatment active tuberculosis infection

Mechanism of Action/Effect Inhibits DNA-dependent RNA polymerase at the beta subunit which prevents chain initiation

Contraindications Hypersensitivity to rifabutin, any other rifamycins, or any component of the formulation

Warnings/Precautions Rifabutin must not be administered for MAC prophylaxis to patients with active tuberculosis since its use may lead to the development of tuberculosis that is resistant to both rifabutin and rifampin. May be associated with neutropenia and/or thrombocytopenia (rarely). Dosage reduction recommended in severe impairment (CrCl <30 mL/minute). Prolonged use may result in fungal or bacterial superinfection, including *C. difficile*-associated diarrhea (CDAD) and pseudomembranous colitis; CDAD has been observed >2 months postantibiotic treatment. May cause brown/orange discoloration of urine, feces, saliva, sweat, tears, and skin. Remove soft contact lenses during therapy since permanent staining may occur.

Drug Interactions
Avoid Concomitant Use
Avoid concomitant use of Rifabutin with any of the following: Abiraterone Acetate; Apixaban; Artemether; Atovaquone; Axitinib; BCG; Bedaquiline; Boceprevir; Bortezomib; Bosutinib; Cabozantinib; CloZAPine; Cobicistat; Crizotinib; Dienogest; Dronedarone; Elvitegravir; Enzalutamide; Everolimus; Ibrutinib; Itraconazole; Ivacaftor; Lapatinib; Lumefantrine; Lurasidone; Macitentan; Mifepristone; Mycophenolate; NIFEdipine; Nilotinib; Nisoldipine; PAZOPanib; Perampanel; Pomalidomide; PONATinib; Praziquantel; Ranolazine; Regorafenib; Rilpivirine; Rivaroxaban; Roflumilast; RomiDEPsin; Simeprevir; Sofosbuvir; SORAfenib; Tasimelteon; Telaprevir; Ticagrelor; Tofacitinib; Tolvaptan; Toremifene; Ulipristal;

Vandetanib; Vemurafenib; VinCRIStine (Liposomal); Voriconazole

Decreased Effect
Rifabutin may decrease the levels/effects of: Abiraterone Acetate; Alfentanil; Angiotensin II Receptor Blockers; Antiemetics (5HT3 Antagonists); Antifungal Agents (Azole Derivatives, Systemic); Apixaban; ARIPiprazole; Artemether; Atovaquone; Axitinib; Barbiturates; BCG; Bedaquiline; Benzodiazepines (metabolized by oxidation); Boceprevir; Bortezomib; Bosutinib; Brentuximab Vedotin; BusPIRone; Cabozantinib; Calcium Channel Blockers; Clarithromycin; CloZAPine; Cobicistat; Contraceptives (Estrogens); Contraceptives (Progestins); Corticosteroids (Systemic); Crizotinib; CycloSPORINE (Systemic); CYP3A4 Substrates; Dapsone (Systemic); Dasatinib; Delavirdine; Dienogest; DOXOrubicin (Conventional); Dronedarone; Efavirenz; Elvitegravir; Enzalutamide; Etravirine; Everolimus; Exemestane; FentaNYL; Gefitinib; GuanFACINE; HMG-CoA Reductase Inhibitors; Ibrutinib; Imatinib; Indinavir; Itraconazole; Ivacaftor; Ixabepilone; Lapatinib; Linagliptin; Lumefantrine; Lurasidone; Macitentan; Maraviroc; Mifepristone; Morphine (Systemic); Mycophenolate; Nelfinavir; Nevirapine; NIFEdipine; Nilotinib; Nisoldipine; PAZOPanib; Perampanel; Pomalidomide; PONATinib; Praziquantel; Propafenone; QUEtiapine; QuiNIDine; Raltegravir; Ramelteon; Ranolazine; Regorafenib; Rilpivirine; Rivaroxaban; Roflumilast; RomiDEPsin; Saxagliptin; Simeprevir; Sodium Picosulfate; Sofosbuvir; SORAfenib; SUNItinib; Tacrolimus (Systemic); Tadalafil; Tamoxifen; Tasimelteon; Telaprevir; Temsirolimus; Ticagrelor; Tofacitinib; Tolvaptan; Toremifene; Typhoid Vaccine; Ulipristal; Vandetanib; Vemurafenib; Vilazodone; VinCRIStine (Liposomal); Vitamin K Antagonists; Voriconazole; Vortioxetine; Zaleplon; Zolpidem; Zuclopenthixol

The levels/effects of Rifabutin may be decreased by: Bosentan; CYP3A4 Inducers (Strong); Dabrafenib; Deferasirox; Efavirenz; Herbs (CYP3A4 Inducers); Mitotane; Nevirapine; Tocilizumab

Increased Effect/Toxicity
Rifabutin may increase the levels/effects of: Clarithromycin; Clopidogrel; Darunavir; Fosamprenavir; Ifosfamide; Isoniazid; Lopinavir; Pitavastatin

The levels/effects of Rifabutin may be increased by: Antifungal Agents (Azole Derivatives, Systemic); Atazanavir; Boceprevir; Clarithromycin; Darunavir; Delavirdine; Fosamprenavir; Indinavir; Lopinavir; Macrolide Antibiotics; Nelfinavir; Nevirapine; Ritonavir; Saquinavir; Telaprevir; Tipranavir; Voriconazole

Nutritional/Ethanol Interactions Food: High-fat meal may decrease the rate but not the extent of absorption.

◄ **Adverse Reactions**
>10%:
Dermatologic: Rash (11%)
Genitourinary: Discoloration of urine (30%)
Hematologic: Neutropenia (25%), leukopenia (17%)
1% to 10%:
Central nervous system: Headache (3%), fever (2%)
Gastrointestinal: Nausea (3% to 6%), abdominal pain (4%), dyspepsia (3%), eructation (3%), taste perversion (3%), vomiting (3%), flatulence (2%)
Hematologic: Thrombocytopenia (5%)
Hepatic: ALT increased (7% to 9%; incidence less than placebo), AST increased (7% to 9%; incidence less than placebo)
Neuromuscular & skeletal: Myalgia (2%)

Available Dosage Forms
Capsule, Oral:
Mycobutin: 150 mg

General Dosage Range Dosage adjustment recommended in patients with renal impairment or on concomitant therapy
Oral:
Children <6 years: 5 mg/kg once daily
Children ≥6 years and Adults: 300 mg once daily

Administration
Oral May be taken with meals to minimize nausea or vomiting.

Storage/Stability Store at 25°C (77°F); excursions permitted to 15°C to 30°C (59°F to 86°F).

Nursing Actions
Physical Assessment Monitor for anemia, neutropenia, GI disturbance, and rash.

Patient Education
• Discuss specific use of drug and side effects with patient as it relates to treatment. (HCAHPS: During this hospital stay, were you given any medicine that you had not taken before? Before giving you any new medicine, how often did hospital staff tell you what the medicine was for? How often did hospital staff describe possible side effects in a way you could understand?)
• Patient may experience leukopenia, thrombocytopenia, orange-colored body fluids, discolored contact lenses, dyspepsia, diarrhea, dizziness, or flu-like syndrome. Have patient report immediately to prescriber severe nausea, inability to eat, discolored urine, jaundice, significant fatigue, or rash (HCAHPS).
• Educate patient about signs of a significant reaction (eg, wheezing; chest tightness; fever; itching; bad cough; blue skin color; seizures; or swelling of face, lips, tongue, or throat). **Note:** This is not a comprehensive list of all side effects. Patient should consult prescriber for additional questions.

Intended Use and Disclaimer: Should not be printed and given to patients. This information is intended to serve as a concise initial reference for healthcare professionals to use when discussing medications with a patient. You must ultimately rely on your own discretion, experience and judgment in diagnosing, treating and advising patients.

Dietary Considerations May be taken with meals.

Rifampin (rif AM pin)

Brand Names: U.S. Rifadin
Index Terms Rifampicin
Pharmacologic Category Antibiotic, Miscellaneous; Antitubercular Agent
Medication Safety Issues
Sound-alike/look-alike issues:
Rifadin® may be confused with Rifater®, Ritalin®
Rifampin may be confused with ribavirin, rifabutin, Rifamate®, rifapentine, rifaximin

Pregnancy Risk Factor C
Lactation Enters breast milk/not recommended
Breast-Feeding Considerations The manufacturer does not recommend breast-feeding due to tumorigenicity observed in animal studies; however, the CDC does not consider rifampin a contraindication to breast-feeding.

Use Management of active tuberculosis in combination with other agents; elimination of meningococci from the nasopharynx in asymptomatic carriers

Unlabeled Use Prophylaxis of *Haemophilus influenzae* type b infection; *Legionella* pneumonia; used in combination with other anti-infectives in the treatment of staphylococcal infections; treatment of *M. leprae* infections; used in combination with penicillin for the treatment of chronic carriers of pharyngeal group A streptococci

Mechanism of Action/Effect Inhibits bacterial RNA synthesis by binding to the beta subunit of DNA-dependent RNA polymerase, blocking RNA transcription

Contraindications Hypersensitivity to rifampin, any rifamycins, or any component of the formulation; concurrent use of amprenavir, saquinavir/ritonavir (possibly other protease inhibitors)

Warnings/Precautions Use with caution and modify dosage in patients with liver impairment; observe for hyperbilirubinemia; discontinue therapy if this in conjunction with clinical symptoms or any signs of significant hepatocellular damage develop. Use with caution in patients receiving concurrent medications associated with hepatotoxicity. Use with caution in patients with a history of alcoholism (even if ethanol consumption is discontinued during therapy). Since rifampin since rifampin has enzyme-inducing properties, porphyria exacerbation is possible; use with caution in patients with porphyria; do not use for meningococcal disease, only for short-term treatment of asymptomatic carrier states

Regimens of >600 mg once or twice weekly have been associated with a high incidence of adverse reactions including a flu-like syndrome, hypersensitivity, thrombocytopenia, leukopenia, and anemia. Urine, feces, saliva, sweat, tears, and CSF may be discolored to red/orange; remove soft contact lenses during therapy since permanent staining may occur. Do not administer I.V. form via I.M. or SubQ routes; restart infusion at another site if extravasation occurs. Prolonged use may result in fungal or bacterial superinfection, including *C. difficile*-associated diarrhea (CDAD) and pseudomembranous colitis; CDAD has been observed >2 months postantibiotic treatment. Monitor for compliance in patients on intermittent therapy.

Drug Interactions
Avoid Concomitant Use
Avoid concomitant use of Rifampin with any of the following: Abiraterone Acetate; Apixaban; Artemether; Atazanavir; Atovaquone; Axitinib; BCG; Bedaquiline; Boceprevir; Bortezomib; Bosutinib; Cabozantinib; CloZAPine; Cobicistat; Crizotinib; Dabigatran Etexilate; Darunavir; Dienogest; Dronedarone; Elvitegravir; Enzalutamide; Esomeprazole; Etravirine; Everolimus; Fosamprenavir; Ibrutinib; Indinavir; Itraconazole; Ivacaftor; Lapatinib; Lopinavir; Lumefantrine; Lurasidone; Macitentan; Mifepristone; Mycophenolate; Nelfinavir; NIFEdipine; Nilotinib; Nisoldipine; Omeprazole; PAZOPanib; Perampanel; Pirfenidone; Pomalidomide; PONATinib; Praziquantel; QuiNINE; Ranolazine; Regorafenib; Rilpivirine; Ritonavir; Rivaroxaban; Roflumilast; RomiDEPsin; Saquinavir; Simeprevir; Sofosbuvir; SORAfenib; Tasimelteon; Telaprevir; Ticagrelor; Tipranavir; Tofacitinib; Tolvaptan; Toremifene; Ulipristal; Vandetanib; Vemurafenib; VinCRIStine (Liposomal); Voriconazole

Decreased Effect
Rifampin may decrease the levels/effects of: Abiraterone Acetate; Afatinib; Alfentanil; Amiodarone; Angiotensin II Receptor Blockers; Antidiabetic Agents (Thiazolidinedione); Antiemetics (5HT3 Antagonists); Antifungal Agents (Azole Derivatives, Systemic); Apixaban; Aprepitant; ARIPiprazole; Artemether; Atazanavir; Atovaquone; Axitinib; Barbiturates; Bazedoxifene; BCG; Bedaquiline; Bendamustine; Benzodiazepines (metabolized by oxidation); Beta-Blockers; Boceprevir; Bortezomib; Bosentan; Bosutinib; Brentuximab Vedotin; BusPIRone; Cabozantinib; Calcium Channel Blockers; Canagliflozin; Caspofungin; Chloramphenicol; Citalopram; Clarithromycin; CloZAPine; Cobicistat; Contraceptives (Estrogens); Contraceptives (Progestins); Corticosteroids (Systemic); Crizotinib; CycloSPORINE (Systemic); CYP1A2 Substrates; CYP2A6 Substrates; CYP2B6 Substrates; CYP2C19 Substrates; CYP2C8 Substrates; CYP2C9 Substrates; CYP3A4 Substrates; Dabigatran Etexilate; Dapsone (Systemic); Darunavir;

Dasatinib; Deferasirox; Delavirdine; Diclofenac (Systemic); Dienogest; Disopyramide; Dolutegravir; DOXOrubicin (Conventional); Doxycycline; Dronedarone; Efavirenz; Elvitegravir; Enzalutamide; Erlotinib; Esomeprazole; Etravirine; Everolimus; Exemestane; FentaNYL; Fexofenadine; Fosamprenavir; Fosaprepitant; Fosphenytoin; Gefitinib; GuanFACINE; HMG-CoA Reductase Inhibitors; Ibrutinib; Imatinib; Indinavir; Itraconazole; Ivacaftor; Ixabepilone; LamoTRIgine; Lapatinib; Linagliptin; Lopinavir; Lumefantrine; Lurasidone; Macitentan; Maraviroc; Methadone; Mifepristone; Mirabegron; Morphine (Systemic); Mycophenolate; Nelfinavir; Nevirapine; NIFEdipine; Nilotinib; Nisoldipine; Omeprazole; OxyCODONE; PAZOPanib; Perampanel; P-glycoprotein/ABCB1 Substrates; Phenytoin; Pirfenidone; Pomalidomide; PONATinib; Prasugrel; Praziquantel; Propafenone; QUEtiapine; QuiNIDine; QuiNINE; Raltegravir; Ramelteon; Ranolazine; Regorafenib; Repaglinide; Rilpivirine; Ritonavir; Rivaroxaban; Roflumilast; Saquinavir; Saxagliptin; Simeprevir; Sirolimus; Sodium Picosulfate; Sofosbuvir; SORAfenib; Sulfonylureas; SUNItinib; Tacrolimus (Systemic); Tadalafil; Tamoxifen; Tasimelteon; Telaprevir; Temsirolimus; Terbinafine (Systemic); Thyroid Products; Ticagrelor; Tipranavir; Tofacitinib; Tolvaptan; Toremifene; Treprostinil; Typhoid Vaccine; Ulipristal; Valproic Acid and Derivatives; Vandetanib; Vemurafenib; Vilazodone; VinCRIStine (Liposomal); Vitamin K Antagonists; Voriconazole; Vortioxetine; Zaleplon; Zidovudine; Zolpidem; Zuclopenthixol

The levels/effects of Rifampin may be decreased by: P-glycoprotein/ABCB1 Inducers

Increased Effect/Toxicity
Rifampin may increase the levels/effects of: Bosentan; Clarithromycin; Clopidogrel; Fexofenadine; Ifosfamide; Isoniazid; Leflunomide; Lopinavir; Pitavastatin; Propofol; RomiDEPsin; Saquinavir

The levels/effects of Rifampin may be increased by: Antifungal Agents (Azole Derivatives, Systemic); Clarithromycin; Delavirdine; Eltrombopag; Macrolide Antibiotics; P-glycoprotein/ABCB1 Inhibitors; Pyrazinamide; Voriconazole

Nutritional/Ethanol Interactions
Ethanol: Avoid ethanol (may increase risk of hepatotoxicity).

Food: Food decreases the extent of absorption; rifampin concentrations may be decreased if taken with food.

Herb/Nutraceutical: St John's wort may decrease rifampin levels.

Adverse Reactions
1% to 10%:
Dermatologic: Rash (1% to 5%)
Gastrointestinal (1% to 2%): Anorexia, cramps, diarrhea, epigastric distress, flatulence,

heartburn, nausea, pseudomembranous colitis, pancreatitis, vomiting

Hepatic: LFTs increased (up to 14%)

Frequency not defined:

Cardiovascular: Edema, flushing

Central nervous system: Ataxia, behavioral changes, concentration impaired, confusion, dizziness, drowsiness, fatigue, fever, headache, numbness, psychosis

Dermatologic: Pemphigoid reaction, pruritus, urticaria

Endocrine & metabolic: Adrenal insufficiency, menstrual disorders

Hematologic: Agranulocytosis (rare), DIC, eosinophilia, hemoglobin decreased, hemolysis, hemolytic anemia, leukopenia, thrombocytopenia (especially with high-dose therapy)

Hepatic: Hepatitis (rare), jaundice

Neuromuscular & skeletal: Myalgia, osteomalacia, weakness

Ocular: Exudative conjunctivitis, visual changes

Renal: Acute renal failure, BUN increased, hemoglobinuria, hematuria, interstitial nephritis, uric acid increased

Miscellaneous: Flu-like syndrome

Pharmacodynamics/Kinetics

Duration of Action ≤24 hours

Available Dosage Forms

Capsule, Oral:

Rifadin: 150 mg, 300 mg

Generic: 150 mg, 300 mg

Solution Reconstituted, Intravenous:

Rifadin: 600 mg (1 ea)

Generic: 600 mg (1 ea)

General Dosage Range I.V., Oral:

Children <12 years: 10-20 mg/kg/day in 1-2 divided doses or 10-20 mg/kg twice weekly (maximum: 600 mg/day)

Children ≥12 years and Adults: 10 mg/kg/day or 10 mg/kg 2-3 times/week or 600 mg every 12-24 hours

Administration

I.M. Do not administer I.M. or SubQ

I.V. Administer I.V. preparation by slow I.V. infusion over 30 minutes to 3 hours at a final concentration not to exceed 6 mg/mL.

Injectable Detail Avoid extravasation.

pH: 7.8-8.8

Oral Administer on an empty stomach with a glass of water (ie, 1 hour prior to, or 2 hours after meals or antacids) to increase total absorption (food may delay and reduce the amount of rifampin absorbed). The compounded oral suspension must be shaken well before using. May mix contents of capsule with applesauce or jelly.

Preparation for Administration Reconstitute vial with 10 mL SWFI. Prior to injection, dilute in appropriate volume of a compatible solution (eg, 100 mL D_5W).

Storage/Stability Store capsules and intact vials at 25°C (77°F); excursions permitted to 15°C to 30°C (59°F to 86°F); avoid excessive heat (>40°C [104°F]). Protect the intact vials from light. Reconstituted vials are stable for 24 hours at room temperature.

Stability of parenteral admixture at room temperature (25°C [77°F]) is 4 hours for D_5W and 24 hours for NS.

Nursing Actions

Physical Assessment Concurrent use with rifampin may decrease levels/effects of multiple other drugs. Infusion site must be monitored to prevent extravasation. Monitor chest x-ray. Monitor for hypersensitivity reactions, hepatotoxicity, CNS changes, hematologic changes, visual disturbances, and gastrointestinal upset on a regular basis during therapy. Monitor patient compliance with treatment regimen.

Patient Education

- Discuss specific use of drug and side effects with patient as it relates to treatment. (HCAHPS: During this hospital stay, were you given any medicine that you had not taken before? Before giving you any new medicine, how often did hospital staff tell you what the medicine was for? How often did hospital staff describe possible side effects in a way you could understand?)
- Patient may experience orange-colored body fluids, discolored contact lenses, dyspepsia, diarrhea, dizziness, or flu-like syndrome. Have patient report immediately to prescriber severe nausea, inability to eat, discolored urine, jaundice, significant fatigue, or rash (HCAHPS).
- Educate patient about signs of a significant reaction (eg, wheezing; chest tightness; fever; itching; bad cough; blue skin color; seizures; or swelling of face, lips, tongue, or throat). **Note:** This is not a comprehensive list of all side effects. Patient should consult prescriber for additional questions.

Intended Use and Disclaimer: Should not be printed and given to patients. This information is intended to serve as a concise initial reference for healthcare professionals to use when discussing medications with a patient. You must ultimately rely on your own discretion, experience and judgment in diagnosing, treating and advising patients.

Dietary Considerations Rifampin should be taken on an empty stomach.

Rifampin and Isoniazid
(rif AM pin & eye soe NYE a zid)

Brand Names: U.S. IsonaRif; Rifamate

Index Terms Isoniazid and Rifampin

Pharmacologic Category Antibiotic, Miscellaneous

Medication Safety Issues

Sound-alike/look-alike issues:
Rifamate may be confused with rifampin

Pregnancy Risk Factor C

Lactation Enters breast milk/compatible

Use Management of active tuberculosis; see individual agents for additional information

Available Dosage Forms

Capsule, oral:
IsonaRif™, Rifamate®: Rifampin 300 mg and isoniazid 150 mg

General Dosage Range Oral: *Adults:* 2 capsules (rifampin 300 mg/isoniazid 150 mg/capsule) once daily

Nursing Actions

Physical Assessment See individual agents.

Patient Education

- Discuss specific use of drug and side effects with patient as it relates to treatment. (HCAHPS: During this hospital stay, were you given any medicine that you had not taken before? Before giving you any new medicine, how often did hospital staff tell you what the medicine was for? How often did hospital staff describe possible side effects in a way you could understand?)

- Patient may experience discolored body fluids, change in color of contact lenses, dyspepsia, nausea, diarrhea, dizziness, or hepatic impairment. Have patient report immediately to prescriber inability to eat, discolored urine, jaundice, severe asthenia, sudden vision changes, eye pain, eye irritation, or paresthesia (HCAHPS).

- Educate patient about signs of a significant reaction (eg, wheezing; chest tightness; fever; itching; bad cough; blue skin color; seizures; or swelling of face, lips, tongue, or throat). **Note:** This is not a comprehensive list of all side effects. Patient should consult prescriber for additional questions.

Intended Use and Disclaimer: Should not be printed and given to patients. This information is intended to serve as a concise initial reference for healthcare professionals to use when discussing medications with a patient. You must ultimately rely on your own discretion, experience and judgment in diagnosing, treating and advising patients.

Related Information

Isoniazid *on page 876*
Rifampin *on page 1352*

Rilonacept (ri LON a sept)

Brand Names: U.S. Arcalyst
Pharmacologic Category Interleukin-1 Inhibitor
Pregnancy Risk Factor C
Lactation Excretion in breast milk unknown/use caution
Use Treatment of cryopyrin-associated periodic syndromes (CAPS) including familial cold autoinflammatory syndrome (FCAS) and Muckle-Wells syndrome (MWS)

Available Dosage Forms

Solution Reconstituted, Subcutaneous [preservative free]:
Arcalyst: 220 mg (1 ea)

General Dosage Range SubQ:
Children ≥12 years: Loading dose 4.4 mg/kg (maximum dose: 320 mg); Maintenance dose: 2.2 mg/kg once weekly (maximum dose: 160 mg)
Adults: Loading dose: 320 mg; Maintenance dose: 160 mg once weekly

Administration

Other SubQ: Rotate injection sites (thigh, abdomen, upper arm); injections should never be made at sites that are bruised, red, tender, or hard. If 2 injections are necessary to complete a dose, administer at different injection sites. Discard any unused portion.

Nursing Actions

Physical Assessment Evaluate for signs and symptoms of infection. This drug should not be used when active or chronic infections are present. Immunization should be given prior to initiating therapy. Teach patient appropriate injection techniques and syringe/needle disposal.

Patient Education

- Discuss specific use of drug and side effects with patient as it relates to treatment. (HCAHPS: During this hospital stay, were you given any medicine that you had not taken before? Before giving you any new medicine, how often did hospital staff tell you what the medicine was for? How often did hospital staff describe possible side effects in a way you could understand?)

- Patient may experience injection site irritation or hyperlipidemia. Have patient report immediately to prescriber signs of infection, severe skin irritation, or rash (HCAHPS).

- Educate patient about signs of a significant reaction (eg, wheezing; chest tightness; fever; itching; bad cough; blue skin color; seizures; or swelling of face, lips, tongue, or throat). **Note:** This is not a comprehensive list of all side effects. Patient should consult prescriber for additional questions.

Intended Use and Disclaimer: Should not be printed and given to patients. This information is intended to serve as a concise initial reference for healthcare professionals to use when discussing medications with a patient. You must ultimately rely on your own discretion, experience and judgment in diagnosing, treating and advising patients.

Rilpivirine (ril pi VIR een)

Brand Names: U.S. Edurant
Index Terms TMC278

Pharmacologic Category Antiretroviral, Reverse Transcriptase Inhibitor, Non-nucleoside (Anti-HIV)

Pregnancy Risk Factor B

Lactation Excretion in breast milk unknown/contra-indicated

Breast-Feeding Considerations Maternal or infant antiretroviral therapy does not completely eliminate the risk of postnatal HIV transmission. In addition, multiclass-resistant virus has been detected in breast-feeding infants despite maternal therapy. Therefore, in the United States, where formula is accessible, affordable, safe, and sustainable, and the risk of infant mortality due to diarrhea and respiratory infections is low, complete avoidance of breast-feeding by HIV-infected women is recommended to decrease potential transmission of HIV (DHHS [perinatal], 2012).

Use Treatment of HIV-1 infections in treatment-naive patients with HIV-1 RNA ≤100,000 copies/mL in combination with at least 2 other antiretroviral agents

Mechanism of Action/Effect As a non-nucleoside reverse transcriptase inhibitor, rilpivirine has activity against HIV-1 by binding to reverse transcriptase. It consequently blocks the RNA-dependent and DNA-dependent DNA polymerase activities, including HIV-1 replication. It does not require intracellular phosphorylation for antiviral activity.

Contraindications Concurrent use of carbamazepine, dexamethasone (>1 dose), oxcarbazepine, phenobarbital, phenytoin, proton pump inhibitors (PPIs), rifabutin, rifampin, rifapentine, or St John's wort

Warnings/Precautions Use in treatment-naive patients with HIV-1 RNA ≤100,000 copies/mL; not for use in treatment-experienced patients. May cause depressive disorders (depression, depressed mood, dysphoria, mood changes, negative thoughts, suicide attempts, or suicidal ideation); monitor for changes and need for intervention. Causes hepatotoxicity; patients with significant transaminase elevations or hepatitis B or C prior to treatment may be at greater risk; has occurred in a few patients with no prior hepatic disease or risk factors. Baseline and periodic laboratory LFT evaluation during therapy is recommended. May cause redistribution of fat (eg, buffalo hump, peripheral wasting with increased abdominal girth, cushingoid appearance). Patients may develop immune reconstitution syndrome resulting in the occurrence of an inflammatory response to an indolent or residual opportunistic infection during initial HIV treatment or activation of autoimmune disorders (eg, Graves' disease, polymyositis, Guillain-Barré syndrome) later in therapy; further evaluation and treatment may be required.

Potentially significant interactions may exist, requiring dose or frequency adjustment, additional monitoring, and/or selection of alternative therapy.

Doses >25 mg daily (ie, 75 mg daily, 300 mg daily) have been associated with QT$_c$ prolongation; use caution when coadministering with a drug with a known risk of torsade de pointes (DHHS, 2013).

Drug Interactions

Avoid Concomitant Use

Avoid concomitant use of Rilpivirine with any of the following: CarBAMazepine; Dexamethasone (Systemic); Etravirine; Fosphenytoin; OXcarbazepine; PHENobarbital; Phenytoin; Primidone; Proton Pump Inhibitors; Reverse Transcriptase Inhibitors (Non-Nucleoside); Rifamycin Derivatives; St Johns Wort

Decreased Effect

Rilpivirine may decrease the levels/effects of: CarBAMazepine; Didanosine; Etravirine; Ketoconazole (Systemic); Methadone

The levels/effects of Rilpivirine may be decreased by: Antacids; Bosentan; CarBAMazepine; CYP3A4 Inducers (Strong); Dabrafenib; Deferasirox; Dexamethasone (Systemic); Didanosine; Fosphenytoin; H2-Antagonists; Mitotane; OXcarbazepine; PHENobarbital; Phenytoin; Primidone; Proton Pump Inhibitors; Reverse Transcriptase Inhibitors (Non-Nucleoside); Rifamycin Derivatives; St Johns Wort; Tocilizumab

Increased Effect/Toxicity

Rilpivirine may increase the levels/effects of: Etravirine; Highest Risk QTc-Prolonging Agents; Moderate Risk QTc-Prolonging Agents

The levels/effects of Rilpivirine may be increased by: Boceprevir; CYP3A4 Inhibitors (Strong); Darunavir; Ketoconazole (Systemic); Lopinavir; Macrolide Antibiotics; Mifepristone; Reverse Transcriptase Inhibitors (Non-Nucleoside); Simeprevir

Nutritional/Ethanol Interactions

Food: Absorption increased by ~40% when taken with a normal- to high-calorie meal. Management: Administer with a normal- to high-calorie meal. Administration with a protein supplement drink alone does not increase absorption.

Herb/Nutraceutical: St John's wort may decrease the levels/effects of rilpivirine. Management: Avoid St John's wort; concurrent use is contraindicated.

Adverse Reactions

>10%:

Endocrine & metabolic: Cholesterol increased (7% to 17%; grade 3: <1%), LDL increased (5% to 14%; grade 3: 1%)

Hepatic: ALT increased (5% to 18%; grade 3/4: 1%), AST increased (4% to 16%; grade 3/4: 1% to 2%)

2% to 10%:

Central nervous system: Depressive disorders (depression, depressed mood, dysphoria, mood changes, negative thoughts, suicide attempts, suicidal ideation) (4% to 9%; grades 3/4: 1%), headache (3%), insomnia (3%), abnormal dreams (2%), fatigue (2%)

Dermatologic: Rash (3%)

Endocrine & metabolic: Triglycerides increased (2%; grade 3/4: ≤1%)

Gastrointestinal: Abdominal pain (2%)

Hepatic: Total bilirubin increased (3% to 5%; grade 3/4: ≤1%)

Renal: Creatinine increased (1% to 6%; grade 3/4: ≤1%)

Available Dosage Forms

Tablet, Oral:
Edurant: 25 mg

General Dosage Range Oral: *Adults:* 25 mg once daily

Administration

Oral Administer with a normal- to high-calorie meal. Taking with a protein supplement drink alone does not increase absorption.

Storage/Stability Store at 25°C (77°F); excursions permitted to 15°C to 30°C (59°F to 86°F). Keep in original container; protect from light.

Nursing Actions

Physical Assessment This is not a cure for HIV. Monitor closely for mood changes, depression, or suicide tendencies, as this requires immediate medical attention. Review patient's medications, as proton pump inhibitors or H$_2$ blockers reduce the absorption of the drug, resulting in decreased effectiveness. Rilpivirine should be used with caution in liver impairment. Patients with an impaired immune system (eg, HIV patients) need to be monitored for symptoms of infection, which may include fever, chills, cough, wheezing, and shortness of breath.

Patient Education

- Discuss specific use of drug and side effects with patient as it relates to treatment. (HCAHPS: During this hospital stay, were you given any medicine that you had not taken before? Before giving you any new medicine, how often did hospital staff tell you what the medicine was for? How often did hospital staff describe possible side effects in a way you could understand?)
- Patient may experience headache, mood changes, or insomnia. Have patient report immediately to prescriber depression, severe dyspepsia, inability to eat, asthenia, discolored urine, jaundice, or rash (HCAHPS).
- Educate patient about signs of a significant reaction (eg, wheezing; chest tightness; fever; itching; bad cough; blue skin color; seizures; or swelling of face, lips, tongue, or throat). **Note:** This is not a comprehensive list of all side effects. Patient should consult prescriber for additional questions.

Intended Use and Disclaimer: Should not be printed and given to patients. This information is intended to serve as a concise initial reference for healthcare professionals to use when discussing medications with a patient. You must ultimately rely on your own discretion, experience and judgment in diagnosing, treating and advising patients.

Dietary Considerations Take with a normal- to high-calorie meal. Taking with a protein supplement drink alone does not increase absorption.

Riluzole (RIL yoo zole)

Brand Names: U.S. Rilutek

Index Terms 2-Amino-6-Trifluoromethoxy-benzothiazole; RP-54274

Pharmacologic Category Glutamate Inhibitor

Pregnancy Risk Factor C

Lactation Excretion in breast milk unknown/not recommended

Breast-Feeding Considerations It is not known if riluzole is excreted in breast milk. Breast-feeding is not recommended by the manufacturer.

Use Treatment of amyotrophic lateral sclerosis (ALS); riluzole can extend survival or time to tracheostomy

Mechanism of Action/Effect Mechanism of action is not known. Pharmacologic properties include inhibitory effect on glutamate release, inactivation of voltage-dependent sodium channels; and ability to interfere with intracellular events that follow transmitter binding at excitatory amino acid receptors

Contraindications Severe hypersensitivity reactions to riluzole or any component of the formulation

Warnings/Precautions Among 4000 patients given riluzole for ALS, there were 3 cases of marked neutropenia (ANC <500/mm^3), all seen within the first 2 months of treatment. Interstitial lung disease (primarily hypersensitivity pneumonitis) has occurred, requires prompt evaluation and possible discontinuation. Use with caution in patients with concomitant renal insufficiency. Use with caution in patients with current evidence or history of abnormal liver function; do not administer if baseline liver function tests are elevated. May cause elevations in transaminases (usually transient). May cause elevations in transaminases (usually transient) within first 3 months of therapy; discontinue if ALT levels are ≥5 times upper limit of normal or if jaundice develops. The elderly or female patients may have decreased clearance of riluzole; use with caution. May cause dizziness or somnolence; caution should be used performing tasks which require alertness (operating machinery or driving).

Drug Interactions

Avoid Concomitant Use There are no known interactions where it is recommended to avoid concomitant use.

Decreased Effect

The levels/effects of Riluzole may be decreased by: CYP1A2 Inducers (Strong); Cyproterone

Increased Effect/Toxicity There are no known significant interactions involving an increase in effect.

Nutritional/Ethanol Interactions

Ethanol: Avoid ethanol (due to CNS depression and possible risk of liver toxicity).

Food: A high-fat meal decreases absorption of riluzole (decreasing AUC by 20% and peak blood levels by 45%). Charbroiled food may increase riluzole elimination.

Adverse Reactions

>10%:

Gastrointestinal: Nausea (16%)

Neuromuscular & skeletal: Weakness (19%)

1% to 10%:

Cardiovascular: Hypertension (5%), peripheral edema (3%), tachycardia (3%)

Central nervous system: Dizziness (4%), somnolence (2%), vertigo (2%), malaise (1%)

Dermatologic: Pruritus (4%), eczema (2%), exfoliative dermatitis (1%)

Gastrointestinal: Abdominal pain (5%), vomiting (4%), flatulence (3%), oral moniliasis (1%), stomatitis (1%), tooth caries (1%)

Genitourinary: Urinary tract infection (3%), dysuria (1%)

Hepatic: Liver function tests increased (8% >3 x ULN; 2% >5 x ULN)

Neuromuscular & skeletal: Arthralgia (4%), paresthesia (circumoral; 2%), tremor (1%)

Respiratory: Lung function decreased (10%), cough increased (3%)

Available Dosage Forms

Tablet, Oral:

Rilutek: 50 mg

Generic: 50 mg

General Dosage Range Oral: *Adults:* 50 mg every 12 hours

Administration

Oral Administer at the same time each day, at least 1 hour before or 2 hours after a meal.

Storage/Stability Store at 20°C to 25°C (68°F to 77°F). Protect from bright light.

Nursing Actions

Patient Education

• Discuss specific use of drug and side effects with patient as it relates to treatment. (HCAHPS: During this hospital stay, were you given any medicine that you had not taken before? Before giving you any new medicine, how often did hospital staff tell you what the medicine was for? How often did hospital staff describe possible side effects in a way you could understand?)

• Patient may experience dizziness, nausea, asthenia, or dyspepsia. Have patient report immediately to prescriber signs of infection, dyspnea, inability to eat, severe headache, jaundice, or rash (HCAHPS).

• Educate patient about signs of a significant reaction (eg, wheezing; chest tightness; fever; itching; bad cough; blue skin color; seizures; or swelling of face, lips, tongue, or throat). **Note:** This is not a comprehensive list of all side effects. Patient should consult prescriber for additional questions.

Intended Use and Disclaimer: Should not be printed and given to patients. This information is intended to serve as a concise initial reference for healthcare professionals to use when discussing medications with a patient. You must ultimately rely on your own discretion, experience and judgment in diagnosing, treating and advising patients.

Dietary Considerations Take at least 1 hour before or 2 hours after a meal.

Rimantadine (ri MAN ta deen)

Brand Names: U.S. Flumadine

Index Terms Rimantadine Hydrochloride

Pharmacologic Category Antiviral Agent; Antiviral Agent, Adamantane

Medication Safety Issues

Sound-alike/look-alike issues:

Rimantadine may be confused with amantadine, ranitidine, Rimactane

Flumadine® may be confused with fludarabine, flunisolide, flutamide

Pregnancy Risk Factor C

Lactation Excretion in breast milk unknown/ not recommended

Breast-Feeding Considerations Do not use in nursing mothers due to potential adverse effect in infants. The CDC recommends that women infected with the influenza virus follow general precautions (eg, frequent hand washing) to decrease viral transmission to the child. Mothers with influenza-like illnesses at delivery should consider avoiding close contact with the infant until they have received 48 hours of antiviral medication, fever has resolved, and cough and secretions can be controlled. These measures may help decrease (but not eliminate) the risk of transmitting influenza to the newborn during breast-feeding. During this time, breast milk can be expressed and bottle-fed to the infant by another person who is not infected. Protective measures, such as wearing a face mask, changing into a clean gown or clothing, and strict hand hygiene should be continued by the mother for ≥7 days after the onset of symptoms or until symptom-free for 24 hours. Infant care should be performed by a noninfected person when possible (consult current CDC guidelines).

Use Prophylaxis (adults and children >1 year of age) and treatment (adults) of influenza A viral infection (per manufacturer's labeling; also refer to current ACIP guidelines for recommendations during current flu season)

Note: In certain circumstances, the ACIP recommends use of rimantadine in combination with oseltamivir for the treatment or prophylaxis of influenza A infection when resistance to oseltamivir is suspected.

Mechanism of Action/Effect Exerts its inhibitory effect on three antigenic subtypes of influenza A virus (H1N1, H2N2, H3N2) early in the viral replicative cycle, possibly inhibiting the uncoating process; it has no activity against influenza B virus and is two- to eightfold more active than amantadine

Contraindications Hypersensitivity to drugs of the adamantine class, including rimantadine and amantadine, or any component of the formulation

Warnings/Precautions Use with caution in patients with renal and hepatic dysfunction; avoid use, if possible, in patients with uncontrolled psychosis or severe psychoneurosis. An increase in seizure incidence may occur in patients with seizure disorders; discontinue drug if seizures occur; resistance may develop during treatment; viruses exhibit cross-resistance between amantadine and rimantadine. Due to increased resistance, the ACIP has recommended that rimantadine and amantadine no longer be used for the treatment or prophylaxis of influenza A in the United States until susceptibility has been re-established; consult current guidelines. Rimantadine is not effective in the prevention or treatment of influenza B virus infections. The elderly are at higher risk for CNS (eg, dizziness, headache, weakness) and gastrointestinal (eg, nausea/vomiting, abdominal pain) adverse events; dosage adjustment is recommended in elderly patients >65 years of age.

Drug Interactions

Avoid Concomitant Use There are no known interactions where it is recommended to avoid concomitant use.

Decreased Effect

Rimantadine may decrease the levels/effects of: Influenza Virus Vaccine (Live/Attenuated)

Increased Effect/Toxicity

The levels/effects of Rimantadine may be increased by: MAO Inhibitors

Nutritional/Ethanol Interactions Food: Food does not affect rate or extent of absorption

Adverse Reactions 1% to 10%:

Central nervous system: Insomnia (2% to 3%), concentration impaired (≤2%), dizziness (1% to 2%), nervousness (1% to 2%), fatigue (1%), headache (1%)

Gastrointestinal: Nausea (3%), anorexia (2%), vomiting (2%), xerostomia (2%), abdominal pain (1%)

Neuromuscular & skeletal: Weakness (1%)

Pharmacodynamics/Kinetics

Onset of Action Antiviral activity: No data exist establishing a correlation between plasma concentration and antiviral effect

Available Dosage Forms

Tablet, Oral:
Flumadine: 100 mg
Generic: 100 mg

General Dosage Range Dosage adjustment recommended in patients with hepatic or renal impairment

Oral:

Children 1-9 years: 5 mg/kg/day in 1-2 divided doses (maximum: 150 mg/day)

Children ≥10 years and <40 kg: 5 mg/kg/day in 2 divided doses

Children ≥10 years and Adults: 100 mg twice daily

Elderly: 100 mg daily

Administration

Oral Initiation of rimantadine within 48 hours of the onset of influenza A illness halves the duration of illness and significantly reduces the duration of viral shedding and increased peripheral airways resistance. Continue therapy for 5-7 days after symptoms begin; discontinue as soon as clinically warranted to reduce the emergence of antiviral drug resistant viruses

Storage/Stability Store at 25°C (77°F); excursions permitted to 15°C to 30°C (59°F to 86°F).

Nursing Actions

Physical Assessment Recommendations for antiviral susceptibility and effectiveness may change. Validate with the CDC recommendations for use prior to prescribing. Monitor for hypotension, CNS changes (confusion, anxiety, agitation), gastrointestinal upset, and anticholinergic effects (dry mouth, urinary retention, mydriases).

Patient Education

• Discuss specific use of drug and side effects with patient as it relates to treatment. (HCAHPS: During this hospital stay, were you given any medicine that you had not taken before? Before giving you any new medicine, how often did hospital staff tell you what the medicine was for? How often did hospital staff describe possible side effects in a way you could understand?)

• Patient may experience nausea, dizziness, or insomnia. Have patient report immediately to prescriber change in balance, illogical thinking, or rash (HCAHPS).

• Educate patient about signs of a significant reaction (eg, wheezing; chest tightness; fever; itching; bad cough; blue skin color; seizures; or swelling of face, lips, tongue, or throat). **Note:** This is not a comprehensive list of all side effects. Patient should consult prescriber for additional questions.

Intended Use and Disclaimer: Should not be printed and given to patients. This information is

intended to serve as a concise initial reference for healthcare professionals to use when discussing medications with a patient. You must ultimately rely on your own discretion, experience and judgment in diagnosing, treating and advising patients.

Riociguat (rye oh SIG ue at)

Brand Names: U.S. Adempas
Index Terms Adempas; BAY 63-2521
Pharmacologic Category Soluble Guanylate Cyclase (sGC) Stimulator
Pregnancy Risk Factor X
Lactation Excretion unknown/not recommended
Use
Chronic thromboembolic pulmonary hypertension: Treatment of adults with persistent/recurrent chronic thromboembolic pulmonary hypertension (CTEPH) (WHO group 4) after surgical treatment or inoperable CTEPH to improve exercise capacity and WHO functional class
Pulmonary arterial hypertension: Treatment of adults with pulmonary artery hypertension (PAH) (WHO group 1) to improve exercise capacity, improve WHO functional class and to delay clinical worsening
Available Dosage Forms
Tablet, Oral:
Adempas: 0.5 mg, 1 mg, 1.5 mg, 2 mg, 2.5 mg
General Dosage Range Dosage adjustment recommended in patients on concomitant therapy, smokers, and in patients who develop toxicities.
Oral: *Adults:* 0.5-1 mg 3 times daily; maximum dose: 2.5 mg 3 times daily.
Administration
Oral Administer with or without food.
Nursing Actions
Physical Assessment Monitor for signs/symptoms of hypotension, bleeding, and pulmonary edema. Screen for smoking. Dose adjustment may be required with smoking or smoking cessation. Advise patient that if a dose is missed, take the next regularly scheduled dose. If treatment is interrupted for ≥3 days, retitration is required.
Patient Education
• Discuss specific use of drug and side effects with patient as it relates to treatment. (HCAHPS: During this hospital stay, were you given any medicine that you had not taken before? Before giving you any new medicine, how often did hospital staff tell you what the medicine was for? How often did hospital staff describe possible side effects in a way you could understand?)
• Patient may experience headache, nausea, pyrosis, dizziness, diarrhea, or constipation. Have patient report immediately to prescriber signs of hemorrhaging, arrhythmia, dysphagia, abdominal or extremity edema, angina, pallor, or severe asthenia (HCAHPS).

• Educate patient about signs of a significant reaction (eg, wheezing; chest tightness; fever; itching; bad cough; blue skin color; seizures; or swelling of face, lips, tongue, or throat). **Note:** This is not a comprehensive list of all side effects. Patient should consult prescriber for additional questions.

Intended Use and Disclaimer: Should not be printed and given to patients. This information is intended to serve as a concise initial reference for healthcare professionals to use when discussing medications with a patient. You must ultimately rely on your own discretion, experience and judgment in diagnosing, treating and advising patients.

Risedronate (ris ED roe nate)

Brand Names: U.S. Actonel; Atelvia
Index Terms Risedronate Sodium
Pharmacologic Category Bisphosphonate Derivative
Medication Safety Issues
Sound-alike/look-alike issues:
Actonel® may be confused with Actos®
Risedronate may be confused with alendronate
Medication Guide Available Yes
Pregnancy Risk Factor C
Lactation Excretion in breast milk unknown/not recommended
Breast-Feeding Considerations It is not known if risedronate is excreted into breast milk. Due to the potential for serious adverse reactions in the nursing infant, the manufacturer recommends a decision be made whether to discontinue nursing or to discontinue the drug, taking into account the importance of treatment to the mother.
Use
Actonel®: Treatment of Paget's disease of the bone; treatment and prevention of glucocorticoid-induced osteoporosis; treatment and prevention of osteoporosis in postmenopausal women; treatment of osteoporosis in men
Atelvia™: Treatment of osteoporosis in postmenopausal women
Mechanism of Action/Effect A bisphosphonate which inhibits bone resorption via actions on osteoclasts or on osteoclast precursors; decreases the rate of bone resorption, leading to an indirect increase in bone mineral density. In Paget's disease, characterized by disordered resorption and formation of bone, inhibition of resorption leads to an indirect decrease in bone formation; but the newly-formed bone has a more normal architecture.
Contraindications Hypersensitivity to risedronate, bisphosphonates, or any component of the formulation; hypocalcemia; inability to stand or sit upright for at least 30 minutes; abnormalities of the

esophagus (eg, stricture, achalasia) which delay esophageal emptying

Warnings/Precautions Bisphosphonates may cause upper gastrointestinal disorders such as dysphagia, esophagitis, esophageal ulcer, and gastric ulcer; risk increases in patients unable to comply with dosing instructions. Use with caution in patients with dysphagia, esophageal disease, gastritis, duodenitis, or ulcers (may worsen underlying condition). Discontinue if new or worsening symptoms occur. Use caution in patients with renal impairment (not recommended in patients with a CrCl <30 mL/minute). Hypocalcemia must be corrected before therapy initiation with risedronate. Ensure adequate calcium and vitamin D intake, especially for patients with Paget's disease in whom the pretreatment rate of bone turnover may be greatly elevated.

Bisphosphonate therapy has been associated with osteonecrosis, primarily of the jaw. Risk factors for osteonecrosis of the jaw (ONJ) include invasive dental procedures (eg, tooth extraction, dental implants, boney surgery); a diagnosis of cancer, with concomitant chemotherapy or corticosteroids; poor oral hygiene, ill-fitting dentures; and comorbid disorders (anemia, coagulopathy, infection, preexisting dental disease); risk may increase with duration of bisphosphonate use. Most reported cases occurred after I.V. bisphosphonate therapy; however, cases have been reported following oral therapy. A dental exam and preventative dentistry should be performed prior to placing patients with risk factors on chronic bisphosphonate therapy. The manufacturer's labeling states that discontinuing bisphosphonates in patients requiring invasive dental procedures may reduce the risk of ONJ. However, other experts suggest that there is no evidence that discontinuing therapy reduces the risk of developing ONJ (Assael, 2009). The benefit/risk must be assessed by the treating physician and/or dentist/surgeon prior to any invasive dental procedure. Patients developing ONJ while on bisphosphonates should receive care by an oral surgeon.

Atypical femur fractures have been reported in patients receiving bisphosphonates for treatment/prevention of osteoporosis. The fractures include subtrochanteric femur (bone just below the hip joint) and diaphyseal femur (long segment of the thigh bone). Some patients experience prodromal pain weeks or months before the fracture occurs. It is unclear if bisphosphonate therapy is the cause for these fractures, although the majority of cases have been reported in patients taking bisphosphonates. Patients receiving long-term (>3-5 years) therapy may be at an increased risk. Discontinue bisphosphonate therapy in patients who develop a femoral shaft fracture.

Infrequently, severe (and occasionally debilitating) bone, joint, and/or muscle pain have been reported

during bisphosphonate treatment. The onset of pain ranged from a single day to several months. Consider discontinuing therapy in patients who experience severe symptoms; symptoms usually resolve upon discontinuation. Some patients experienced recurrence when rechallenged with same drug or another bisphosphonate; avoid use in patients with a history of these symptoms in association with bisphosphonate therapy.

In the management of osteoporosis, re-evaluate the need for continued therapy periodically; the optimal duration of treatment has not yet been determined. Consider discontinuing after 3-5 years of use in patients at low-risk for fracture; following discontinuation, re-evaluate fracture risk periodically. When using for glucocorticoid-induced osteoporosis, evaluate sex steroid hormonal status prior to treatment initiation; consider appropriate hormone replacement if necessary. Not approved for use in pediatric patients with osteogenesis imperfecta due to lack of efficacy in reducing the risk of fracture. Potentially significant drug-drug interactions may exist, requiring dose or frequency adjustment, additional monitoring, and/or selection of alternative therapy.

Drug Interactions

Avoid Concomitant Use

Avoid concomitant use of Risedronate with any of the following: H2-Antagonists; Proton Pump Inhibitors

Decreased Effect

The levels/effects of Risedronate may be decreased by: Antacids; Calcium Salts; Iron Salts; Magnesium Salts; Multivitamins/Minerals (with ADEK, Folate, Iron); Multivitamins/Minerals (with AE, No Iron); Proton Pump Inhibitors; Sucroferric Oxyhydroxide

Increased Effect/Toxicity

Risedronate may increase the levels/effects of: Deferasirox; Phosphate Supplements

The levels/effects of Risedronate may be increased by: Aminoglycosides; H2-Antagonists; Nonsteroidal Anti-Inflammatory Agents; Proton Pump Inhibitors; Systemic Angiogenesis Inhibitors

Nutritional/Ethanol Interactions

Ethanol: Avoid ethanol (may increase risk of osteoporosis).

Food: Food reduces absorption (similar to other bisphosphonates); mean oral bioavailability is decreased when given with food.

Adverse Reactions Frequency may vary with product, dose, and indication.

>10%:

Cardiovascular: Hypertension (11%)

Central nervous system: Headache (3% to 18%)

Dermatologic: Skin rash (8% to 12%)

Endocrine & metabolic: Increased parathyroid hormone (transient; <30%)

Gastrointestinal: Diarrhea (5% to 20%), nausea (4% to 13%), constipation (3% to 13%), abdominal pain (2% to 12%), dyspepsia (4% to 11%)

Genitourinary: Urinary tract infection (11%)

Infection: Increased susceptibility to infection (≤31%)

Neuromuscular & skeletal: Arthralgia (7% to 33%), back pain (6% to 28%)

1% to 10%:

Cardiovascular: Peripheral edema (8%), chest pain (5% to 7%), cardiac arrhythmia (2%)

Central nervous system: Depression (7%), dizziness (3% to 7%)

Endocrine & metabolic: Hypocalcemia (≤5%), hypophosphatemia (<3%)

Gastrointestinal: Vomiting (2% to 5%), gastritis (3%), duodenitis (≤1%), glossitis (≤1%)

Genitourinary: Benign prostatic hyperplasia (5%), nephrolithiasis (3%)

Immunologic: Acute phase reaction (≤8%; includes fever, influenza-like illness)

Neuromuscular & skeletal: Myalgia (2% to 7%), neck pain (5%), muscle spasm (1% to 2%)

Ophthalmic: Cataract (7%)

Respiratory: Flu-like symptoms (10%), bronchitis (3% to 10%), pharyngitis (6%), rhinitis (6%), dyspnea (4%)

Pharmacodynamics/Kinetics

Onset of Action May require weeks

Available Dosage Forms

Tablet, Oral:

Actonel: 5 mg, 30 mg, 35 mg, 150 mg

Tablet Delayed Release, Oral:

Atelvia: 35 mg

General Dosage Range Oral: *Adults:* 5 mg or 30 mg once daily **or** 35 mg once weekly **or** 150 mg once a month

Administration

Oral Note: Avoid administration of oral calcium supplements, antacids, magnesium supplements/laxatives, and iron preparations within 30 minutes of risedronate administration.

Immediate release tablet: Risedronate immediate release tablets must be taken on an empty stomach with a full glass (6-8 oz) of **plain water** (not mineral water) at least 30 minutes before any food, drink, or other medications orally to avoid interference with absorption. Patient must remain sitting upright or standing for at least 30 minutes after taking (to reduce esophageal irritation). Tablet should be swallowed whole; do not crush or chew.

Delayed release tablet: Risedronate delayed release tablets must be taken with at least 4 oz of **plain water** (not mineral water) immediately **after** breakfast. Patient must remain sitting upright or standing for at least 30 minutes after taking (to reduce esophageal irritation). Tablet should be swallowed whole; do not cut, split, crush, or chew.

Storage/Stability Store at room temperature of 20°C to 25°C (68°F to 77°F).

Nursing Actions

Physical Assessment Teach patient specific administration directions. Instruct patient in lifestyle and dietary changes that may help decrease risk of worsening osteoporosis. Educate patient about importance of routine dental exams and follow up to prevent osteonecrosis of the jaw.

Patient Education

• Discuss specific use of drug and side effects with patient as it relates to treatment. (HCAHPS: During this hospital stay, were you given any medicine that you had not taken before? Before giving you any new medicine, how often did hospital staff tell you what the medicine was for? How often did hospital staff describe possible side effects in a way you could understand?)

• Patient may experience headache, nausea, constipation, diarrhea, hypertension, dyspepsia, arthralgia, myalgia, or osteopenia. Have patient report immediately to prescriber angina; dysphagia; severe jaw, groin, or thigh pain; paresthesia; fasciculations; or rash (HCAHPS).

• Educate patient about signs of a significant reaction (eg, wheezing; chest tightness; fever; itching; bad cough; blue skin color; seizures; or swelling of face, lips, tongue, or throat). **Note:** This is not a comprehensive list of all side effects. Patient should consult prescriber for additional questions.

Intended Use and Disclaimer: Should not be printed and given to patients. This information is intended to serve as a concise initial reference for healthcare professionals to use when discussing medications with a patient. You must ultimately rely on your own discretion, experience and judgment in diagnosing, treating and advising patients.

Dietary Considerations Ensure adequate calcium and vitamin D intake; if dietary intake is inadequate, dietary supplementation is recommended. Women and men should consume:

Calcium: 1000 mg/day (men: 50-70 years) **or** 1200 mg/day (women ≥51 years and men ≥71 years) (IOM, 2011; NOF, 2013)

Vitamin D: 800-1000 IU/day (men and women ≥50 years) (NOF, 2013). Recommended Dietary Allowance (RDA): 600 IU/day (men and women ≤70 years) **or** 800 IU/day (men and women ≥71 years) (IOM, 2011).

Take immediate release tablet with at least 6 oz of **plain water** (not mineral water) ≥30 minutes before the first food or drink of the day other than water. Take delayed release tablet with at least 4 ounces of **plain water** immediately **after** breakfast.

Related Information
Oral Medications That Should Not Be Crushed or Altered *on page 1712*

Risperidone (ris PER i done)

Brand Names: U.S. RisperDAL; RisperDAL Consta; RisperDAL M-TAB; RisperiDONE M-TAB

Index Terms Risperdal M-Tab

Pharmacologic Category Antimanic Agent; Antipsychotic Agent, Atypical

Medication Safety Issues

Sound-alike/look-alike issues:

RisperiDONE may be confused with reserpine, rOPINIRole

RisperDAL may be confused with lisinopril, reserpine, Restoril

BEERS Criteria medication:

This drug may be potentially inappropriate for use in geriatric patients (Quality of evidence - moderate; Strength of recommendation - strong).

Pregnancy Risk Factor C

Lactation Enters breast milk/not recommended

Breast-Feeding Considerations Risperidone and its metabolite are excreted in breast milk. Due to the potential for serious adverse reactions in the nursing infant, the manufacturer recommends a decision be made whether to discontinue nursing or to discontinue the drug, taking into account the importance of treatment to the mother. It is also recommended that women using Risperdal Consta not breast-feed during therapy or for 12 weeks after the last injection.

Use

Oral: Treatment of schizophrenia; treatment of acute mania or mixed episodes associated with bipolar I disorder (as monotherapy in children or adults, or in combination with lithium or valproate in adults); treatment of irritability/aggression associated with autistic disorder

Injection: Treatment of schizophrenia; maintenance treatment of bipolar I disorder in adults as monotherapy or in combination with lithium or valproate

Unlabeled Use Treatment of Tourette's syndrome; psychosis/agitation related to Alzheimer's dementia; post-traumatic stress disorder (PTSD)

Mechanism of Action/Effect Risperidone is a benzisoxazole atypical antipsychotic with affinity for dopamine and serotonin. Results in improvement of psychotic symptoms and reduction of extrapyramidal side effects.

Contraindications Hypersensitivity to risperidone or any component of the formulation

Warnings/Precautions Hazardous agent - use appropriate precautions for handling and disposal (NIOSH, 2012). **[U.S. Boxed Warning]: Elderly patients with dementia-related psychosis treated with antipsychotics are at an increased risk of death compared to placebo.** Most deaths appeared to be either cardiovascular (eg, heart failure, sudden death) or infectious (eg, pneumonia) in nature. In addition, an increased incidence of cerebrovascular effects (eg, transient ischemic attack, cerebrovascular accidents) has been reported in studies of placebo-controlled trials of risperidone in elderly patients with dementia-related psychosis. Risperidone is not approved for the treatment of dementia-related psychosis.

Leukopenia, neutropenia, and agranulocytosis (sometimes fatal) have been reported in clinical trials and postmarketing reports with antipsychotic use; presence of risk factors (eg, pre-existing low WBC or history of drug-induced leuko-/neutropenia) should prompt periodic blood count assessment. Discontinue therapy at first signs of blood dyscrasias or if absolute neutrophil count <1000/mm^3.

Low to moderately sedating, use with caution in disorders where CNS depression is a feature. Use with caution in Parkinson's disease. Caution in patients with predisposition to seizures. Use with caution in renal or hepatic dysfunction; dose reduction recommended. Esophageal dysmotility and aspiration have been associated with antipsychotic use; use with caution in patients at risk of aspiration pneumonia (ie, Alzheimer's disease). Risperidone is associated with greater increases in prolactin levels as compared to other antipsychotic agents; clinical significance of hyperprolactinemia in patients with breast cancer or other prolactin-dependent tumors is unknown. May alter temperature regulation. May mask toxicity of other drugs or conditions (eg, intestinal obstruction, Reyes syndrome, brain tumor) due to antiemetic effects. Neutropenia has been reported with antipsychotic use, including fatal cases of agranulocytosis. Pre-existing myelosuppression (disease or drug-induced) increases risk and these patients should have frequent CBC monitoring; decreased blood counts in absence of other causative factors should prompt discontinuation of therapy.

Use with caution in patients with cardiovascular diseases (eg, heart failure, history of myocardial infarction or ischemia, cerebrovascular disease, conduction abnormalities). May cause orthostatic hypotension; use with caution in patients at risk of this effect (eg, concurrent medication use which may predispose to hypotension/bradycardia or presence of hypovolemia) or in those who would not tolerate transient hypotensive episodes. May alter cardiac conduction (low risk relative to other neuroleptics); life-threatening arrhythmias have occurred with therapeutic doses of neuroleptics.

May cause anticholinergic effects (confusion, agitation, constipation, xerostomia, blurred vision, urinary retention); therefore, they should be used with caution in patients with decreased gastrointestinal motility, urinary retention, BPH, xerostomia, or visual problems (including narrow-angle glaucoma). Relative to other neuroleptics, risperidone has a low potency of cholinergic blockade. Few case reports describe intraoperative floppy iris syndrome (IFIS) in patients receiving risperidone and undergoing cataract surgery (Ford, 2011). Prior to cataract surgery, evaluate for prior or current risperidone use. The benefits or risks of interrupting risperidone prior to surgery have not been established; clinicians are advised to proceed with surgery cautiously.

May cause extrapyramidal symptoms (EPS), including pseudoparkinsonism, acute dystonic reactions, akathisia, and tardive dyskinesia (risk of these reactions is low relative to other neuroleptics, and is dose dependent). Risk of dystonia (and probably other EPS) may be greater with increased doses, use of conventional antipsychotics, males, and younger patients. Risk of neuroleptic malignant syndrome (NMS) may be increased in patients with Parkinson's disease or Lewy body dementia; monitor for symptoms of confusion, obtundation, postural instability and extrapyramidal symptoms. May cause hyperglycemia; in some cases may be extreme and associated with ketoacidosis, hyperosmolar coma, or death. Use with caution in patients with diabetes or other disorders of glucose regulation; monitor for worsening of glucose control. Dyslipidemia has been reported with atypical antipsychotics; risk profile may differ between agents. Discrepant results have been reported in clinical trials, regarding lipid changes associated with risperidone (American Diabetes Association, 2004). Significant weight gain has been observed with antipsychotic therapy; incidence varies with product. Monitor waist circumference and BMI. Rare cases of priapism have been reported.

Use in elderly patients with dementia is associated with an increased risk of mortality and cerebrovascular accidents; avoid antipsychotic use for behavioral problems associated with dementia unless alternative nonpharmacologic therapies have failed and patient may harm self or others. In addition, use may cause or exacerbate syndrome of inappropriate antidiuretic hormone secretion or hyponatremia; monitor sodium closely with initiation or dosage adjustments in older adults (Beers Criteria).

The possibility of a suicide attempt is inherent in psychotic illness or bipolar disorder; use caution in high-risk patients during initiation of therapy. Prescriptions should be written for the smallest quantity consistent with good patient care. Long-term effects on growth or sexual maturation have not been evaluated. Vehicle used in injectable (polylactide-co-glycolide microspheres) has rarely been associated with retinal artery occlusion in patients with abnormal arteriovenous anastomosis.

Drug Interactions
Avoid Concomitant Use
Avoid concomitant use of RisperiDONE with any of the following: Aclidinium; Amisulpride; Azelastine (Nasal); Ipratropium (Oral Inhalation); Metoclopramide; Paraldehyde; Pimozide; Sulpiride; Thalidomide; Tiotropium; Umeclidinium

Decreased Effect
RisperiDONE may decrease the levels/effects of: Amphetamines; Anti-Parkinson's Agents (Dopamine Agonist); Quinagolide

The levels/effects of RisperiDONE may be decreased by: CarBAMazepine; Lithium formulations; Peginterferon Alfa-2b; P-glycoprotein/ABCB1 Inducers

Increased Effect/Toxicity
RisperiDONE may increase the levels/effects of: Alcohol (Ethyl); Amisulpride; Analgesics (Opioid); Anticholinergics; ARIPiprazole; Azelastine (Nasal); Buprenorphine; CNS Depressants; Dofetilide; Highest Risk QTc-Prolonging Agents; Hydrocodone; Lomitapide; Methotrimeprazine; Methylphenidate; Moderate Risk QTc-Prolonging Agents; Paliperidone; Paraldehyde; Pimozide; Serotonin Modulators; Sulpiride; Thalidomide; Tiotropium; Zolpidem

The levels/effects of RisperiDONE may be increased by: Abiraterone Acetate; Acetylcholinesterase Inhibitors (Central); Aclidinium; Brimonidine (Topical); CYP2D6 Inhibitors (Moderate); CYP2D6 Inhibitors (Strong); Darunavir; Doxylamine; Droperidol; HydrOXYzine; Ipratropium (Oral Inhalation); Lithium formulations; Loop Diuretics; Magnesium Sulfate; Methotrimeprazine; Methylphenidate; Metoclopramide; Metyrosine; Mifepristone; Perampanel; P-glycoprotein/ABCB1 Inhibitors; Pramlintide; Selective Serotonin Reuptake Inhibitors; Serotonin Modulators; Sodium Oxybate; Tetrabenazine; Umeclidinium; Valproic Acid and Derivatives; Verapamil

Nutritional/Ethanol Interactions
Ethanol: Ethanol may increase CNS depression. Management: Limit or avoid ethanol.

Food: Oral solution is not compatible with beverages containing tannin or pectinate (cola or tea). Management: Administer oral solution with water, coffee, orange juice, or low-fat milk.

Herb/Nutraceutical: Some herbal medications may increase CNS depression. Management: Avoid kava kava, gotu kola, valerian, and St John's wort.

Adverse Reactions
>10%:
Central nervous system: Sedation (children 12% to 63%; adults 5% to 11%), parkinsonism (children: 28% to 62%; adults 8% to 25%), somnolence (adults 5% to 41%; children 4% to 11%), insomnia (≤32%), fatigue (children 18% to 31%; adults 1% to 9%), headache (12% to 21%), anxiety (≤8% to 16%), dizziness (3% to 16%),

fever (children 16%; adults 1% to 2%), akathisia (5% to 11%)

Gastrointestinal: Appetite increased (children 4% to 44%; adults 4%), weight gain (≥7% kg increase from baseline: children 8% to 33%; adults 4% to 21%), vomiting (children 10% to 20%; adults <4%), constipation (5% to 17%), nausea (5% to 16%), abdominal pain (children 6% to 16%; adults <4%), drooling (children 12%; adults <4%)

Genitourinary: Urinary incontinence (children 5% to 22%; adults <4%), enuresis (children 16%; adults <1%)

Neuromuscular & skeletal: Tremor (adults ≤24%; children ≤11%)

Respiratory: Nasopharyngitis (children 19%; adults ≤4%), cough (children ≤17%; adults ≤4%), rhinorrhea (children 12%; adults <4%)

1% to 10%:

Cardiovascular: Atrioventricular block first degree (<4%), bradycardia (<4%), bundle branch block (<4%), chest pain (<4%), ECG changes (<4%), facial edema (<4%), hypotension (<4%), orthostatic hypotension (<4%), palpitation (<4%), QT prolongation (<4%), tachycardia (adults <4%; children <1%), hypertension (≤3%), peripheral edema (≤3%), syncope (1% to 2%)

Central nervous system: Gait disturbance (4%), pain (1% to 4%), attention span decreased (≤4%), agitation (<4%), akinesia (<4%), coordination impaired (<4%), depression (<4%), malaise (<4%), nervousness (<4%), postural dizziness (<4%), seizure (<4%), sleep disturbances (<4%), sluggishness (<4%), vertigo (<4%), lethargy (2%), hypoesthesia (≤2%)

Dermatologic: Rash (<4% to 8%), eczema (<4%), pruritus (<4%), dry skin (≤3%), acne (<1% to 2%)

Endocrine & metabolic: Menorrhea (≤4%), breast discomfort (<4%), ejaculation disorder/delayed (<4%), erectile dysfunction (<4%), galactorrhea (<4%), gynecomastia (<4%), hyperglycemia (<4%), hyperprolactinemia (<4%), libido decreased (<4%), menstrual irregularities (<4%), sexual dysfunction (<4%)

Gastrointestinal: Dyspepsia (3% to 10%), xerostomia (≤7% to 10%), salivation increased (1% to 10%), diarrhea (<4% to 8%), appetite decreased (≤6%), anorexia (<1% to <4%), weight loss (≤4%), gastritis (<4%), gastroenteritis (<4%), toothache (≤3%)

Genitourinary: Cystitis (<4%), glucosuria (<4%), urinary tract infection (<4%)

Hematologic: Anemia (<4%), neutropenia (<4%)

Hepatic: ALT increased (<4%), AST increased (<4%), GGT increased (<4%)

Local: Abscess (<4%); injection site induration, pain, reaction, swelling (<4%)

Neuromuscular & skeletal: Dystonia (2% to 6%), limb pain (2% to 6%), dyskinesia (adults ≤6%; children <1%), arthralgia (2% to 4%), back pain (≤4%), buttock pain (<4%), dysarthria (<4%), hypokinesia (<4%), musculoskeletal chest pain (<4%), myalgia (<4%), neck pain (<4%), paresthesia (<4%), posture abnormal (<4%), tardive dyskinesia (<4%), weakness (<4%), creatine phosphokinase increased (≤2%)

Ocular: Blurred vision (2% to 7%), conjunctivitis (<4%), visual acuity reduced (<4%)

Otic: Earache (≤4%), otitis media (<4%)

Respiratory: Nasal congestion (≤6% to 10%), pharyngolaryngeal pain (3% to 10%), rhinitis (<4% to 9%), respiratory infection (≤6% to 8%), bronchitis (<4%), dyspnea (<4%), pharyngitis (<4%), pneumonia (<4%), sinusitis (<4%), epistaxis (≤2%)

Miscellaneous: Thirst (children ≤7%; adults <1%), flu-like syndrome (<4%), hypersensitivity (<4%), infection (<4%), viral infection (<4%)

Available Dosage Forms

Solution, Oral:
RisperDAL: 1 mg/mL (30 mL)
Generic: 1 mg/mL (30 mL)

Suspension Reconstituted, Intramuscular:
RisperDAL Consta: 12.5 mg (1 ea); 25 mg (1 ea); 37.5 mg (1 ea); 50 mg (1 ea)

Tablet, Oral:
RisperDAL: 0.25 mg, 0.5 mg, 1 mg, 2 mg, 3 mg, 4 mg
Generic: 0.25 mg, 0.5 mg, 1 mg, 2 mg, 3 mg, 4 mg

Tablet Dispersible, Oral:
RisperDAL M-TAB: 0.5 mg, 1 mg, 2 mg, 3 mg, 4 mg
RisperiDONE M-TAB: 0.5 mg, 1 mg, 2 mg, 3 mg, 4 mg
Generic: 0.25 mg, 0.5 mg, 1 mg, 2 mg, 3 mg, 4 mg

General Dosage Range Dosage adjustment recommended in patients with hepatic or renal impairment

I.M.:
Adults: 25 mg every 2 weeks (range: 12.5-50 mg every 2 weeks; maximum: 50 mg every 2 weeks)
Elderly: 12.5-25 mg every 2 weeks

Oral:
Children ≥5 years: Autism: Initial: 0.25 mg daily (<20 kg) or 0.5 mg daily (≥20 kg); Maximum dose: 1 mg daily (<20 kg) or 2.5 mg daily (≥20 kg) (3 mg daily in children >45 kg); Recommended target dose: 0.5 mg daily (<20 kg) or 1 mg daily (≥20 kg); dosing range 0.5-3 mg
Children 10-17 years: Bipolar disorder: Initial: 0.5 mg once daily; Recommended target dose: 1-2.5 mg daily; dosing range 1-6 mg daily
Children: 13-17 years: Schizophrenia: Initial: 0.5 mg once daily; Recommended target dose: 3 mg daily; dosing range 1-6 mg daily
Adults: Initial: 2-3 mg daily in 1-2 divided doses; Maintenance: 1-8 mg daily in 1-2 divided doses
Elderly: Initial: 0.5 mg twice daily

Administration

I.M. Risperdal® Consta® should be administered I.M. into either the deltoid muscle or the upper outer quadrant of the gluteal area. Avoid inadvertent injection into vasculature. Injection should alternate between the two arms or buttocks. Do not combine two different dosage strengths into one single administration. Do not substitute any components of the dose-pack; administer with needle provided (1-inch needle for deltoid administration or 2-inch needle for gluteal administration).

Hazardous agent; use appropriate precautions for handling and disposal (NIOSH, 2012).

Oral

Oral: May be administered without regard to meals.

Oral solution can be administered directly from the provided pipette or may be mixed with water, coffee, orange juice, or low-fat milk, but is **not compatible** with cola or tea.

In children or adolescents experiencing somnolence, half the daily dose may be administered twice daily **or** the once-daily dose may be administered at bedtime.

Risperdal® M-Tab® should not be removed from blister pack until administered. Do not push tablet through foil (tablet may become damaged); peel back foil to expose tablet. Using dry hands, place immediately on tongue. Tablet will dissolve within seconds, and may be swallowed with or without liquid. Do not split or chew.

Hazardous agent; use appropriate precautions for handling and disposal (NIOSH, 2012).

Preparation for Administration Hazardous agent; use appropriate precautions for handling and disposal (NIOSH, 2012). Risperdal® Consta®: Bring to room temperature prior to reconstitution. Reconstitute with provided diluent only. Shake vigorously to mix; will form thick, milky suspension. Following reconstitution, store at room temperature and use within 6 hours. Suspension settles in ~2 minutes; shake vigorously to resuspend prior to administration.

Storage/Stability

Injection: Risperdal® Consta®: Store in refrigerator at 2°C to 8°C (36°F to 46°F) and protect from light. May be stored at room temperature of 25°C (77°F) for up to 7 days prior to administration. Following reconstitution, store at room temperature and use within 6 hours. Suspension settles in ~2 minutes; shake vigorously to resuspend prior to administration.

Oral solution, tablet: Store at 15°C to 25°C (59°F to 77°F). Protect from light and moisture. Keep orally-disintegrating tablets sealed in foil pouch until ready to use. Do not freeze solution.

Nursing Actions

Physical Assessment Review ophthalmic exam and monitor mental status, mood, affect, CNS responses, anticholinergic and extrapyramidal symptoms, and orthostatic hypotension prior to treatment and periodically throughout. Monitor weight prior to initiating therapy and at least monthly. Be alert to the possibility of suicide ideation.

Patient Education

• Discuss specific use of drug and side effects with patient as it relates to treatment. (HCAHPS: During this hospital stay, were you given any medicine that you had not taken before? Before giving you any new medicine, how often did hospital staff tell you what the medicine was for? How often did hospital staff describe possible side effects in a way you could understand?)

• Patient may experience presyncope, fatigue, blurred vision, illogical thinking, dizziness, hyperglycemia, weight gain, impotence, hypersalivation, or insomnia. Have patient report immediately to prescriber significant change in balance, tremors, polyuria, polydipsia, weight loss, nervousness and anxiety, severe asthenia, pregnancy, or rash (HCAHPS).

• Educate patient about signs of a significant reaction (eg, wheezing; chest tightness; fever; itching; bad cough; blue skin color; seizures; or swelling of face, lips, tongue, or throat). **Note:** This is not a comprehensive list of all side effects. Patient should consult prescriber for additional questions.

Intended Use and Disclaimer: Should not be printed and given to patients. This information is intended to serve as a concise initial reference for healthcare professionals to use when discussing medications with a patient. You must ultimately rely on your own discretion, experience and judgment in diagnosing, treating and advising patients.

Dietary Considerations May be taken without regard to meals. Some products may contain phenylalanine.

Related Information

Oral Medications That Should Not Be Crushed or Altered *on page 1712*

Ritonavir (ri TOE na veer)

Brand Names: U.S. Norvir

Pharmacologic Category Antiretroviral, Protease Inhibitor (Anti-HIV)

Medication Safety Issues

Sound-alike/look-alike issues:

Ritonavir may be confused with Retrovir®

Norvir® may be confused with Norvasc®

Pregnancy Risk Factor B

Lactation Excretion in breast milk unknown/not recommended

Breast-Feeding Considerations Maternal or infant antiretroviral therapy does not completely eliminate the risk of postnatal HIV transmission.

In addition, multiclass-resistant virus has been detected in breast-feeding infants despite maternal therapy. Therefore, in the United States, where formula is accessible, affordable, safe, and sustainable, and the risk of infant mortality due to diarrhea and respiratory infections is low, complete avoidance of breast-feeding by HIV-infected women is recommended to decrease potential transmission of HIV (DHHS [perinatal], 2012).

Use Treatment of HIV infection; should always be used as part of a multidrug regimen

Unlabeled Use Used as a pharmacokinetic "booster" for other protease inhibitors

Mechanism of Action/Effect Blocks the site of HIV-1 protease activity, resulting in the formation of immature, noninfectious viral particles.

Contraindications Hypersensitivity to ritonavir or any component of the formulation; concurrent alfuzosin, amiodarone, cisapride, dihydroergotamine, ergonovine, ergotamine, flecainide, lovastatin, methylergonovine, midazolam (oral), pimozide, propafenone, quinidine, sildenafil (when used for the treatment of pulmonary arterial hypertension [eg, Revatio®]), simvastatin, St John's wort, triazolam, and voriconazole (when ritonavir ≥800 mg/day)

Canadian labeling: Additional contraindications (not in U.S. labeling): Concurrent use with rivaroxaban, voriconazole (regardless of ritonavir dose), salmeterol, vardenafil, bepridil, astemizole, or terfenadine

Warnings/Precautions [U.S. Boxed Warning]: Ritonavir may interact with many medications, including antiarrhythmics, ergot alkaloids, and sedatives/hypnotics, resulting in potentially serious and/or life-threatening adverse events. Some interactions may require dose or frequency adjustment, additional monitoring, and/or selection of alternative therapy. Pancreatitis has been observed (including fatalities); use with caution in patients with increased triglycerides; monitor serum lipase and amylase and for gastrointestinal symptoms. Increases in total cholesterol and triglycerides have been reported; screening should be done prior to therapy and periodically throughout treatment. Temporary or permanent discontinuation may be clinically indicated.

Protease inhibitors have been associated with a variety of hypersensitivity events (some severe), including rash, anaphylaxis (rare), angioedema, bronchospasm, erythema multiforme, toxic epidermal necrolysis, and/or Stevens-Johnson syndrome (rare). It is generally recommended to discontinue treatment if severe rash or moderate symptoms accompanied by other systemic symptoms occur. Use with caution in patients with cardiomyopathy, ischemic heart disease, pre-existing conduction abnormalities, or structural heart disease; may be at increased risk of conduction abnormalities (eg, second- or third-degree AV block). Ritonavir has

been associated with AV block due to prolongation of PR interval; use caution with drugs that prolong the PR interval. Use with caution in patients with hemophilia A or B; increased bleeding during protease inhibitor therapy has been reported and additional Factor VIII may be needed. Changes in glucose tolerance, hyperglycemia, exacerbation of diabetes, DKA, and new-onset diabetes mellitus have been reported in patients receiving protease inhibitors. May be associated with fat redistribution (buffalo hump, increased abdominal girth, breast engorgement, facial atrophy, and dyslipidemia). Immune reconstitution syndrome may develop resulting in the occurrence of an inflammatory response to an indolent or residual opportunistic infection during initial HIV treatment or activation of autoimmune disorders (eg, Graves' disease, polymyositis, Guillain-Barré syndrome) later in therapy; further evaluation and treatment may be required. May cause hepatitis or exacerbate pre-existing hepatic dysfunction (including fatalities); use with caution in patients with hepatitis B or C, cirrhosis, or those with high baseline transaminases; consider increased monitoring of transaminases in these patients. Norvir® tablets are **not** bioequivalent to Norvir® capsules. Gastrointestinal side effects (eg, nausea, vomiting, abdominal pain, diarrhea) or paresthesias may be more common when patients are switching from the capsule to the tablet formulation due to a higher C_{max} (26% increase) observed with the tablet formulation compared to the capsule. These side effects should decrease as therapy is continued.

Oral solution contains ethanol and propylene glycol; healthcare providers should pay special attention to accurate calculation, measurement, and administration of dose; ethanol competitively inhibits propylene glycol metabolism; preterm infants may be at increased risk of toxicity due to decreased ability to metabolize propylene glycol. Postmarketing adverse reactions (cardiac toxicity, lactic acidosis, renal failure, CNS depression, respiratory complications, acute renal failure including fatalities) have been reported in preterm neonates receiving ritonavir-containing solutions. Do not use in neonates with a postmenstrual age (first day of mother's last menstrual period to birth plus elapsed time after birth) <44 weeks, unless benefit outweighs risk and neonate is closely monitored (serum creatinine and osmolality, CNS depression, renal toxicity, lactic acidosis, cardiac conduction abnormalities, hemolysis).

Drug Interactions

Avoid Concomitant Use

Avoid concomitant use of Ritonavir with any of the following: Ado-Trastuzumab Emtansine; Alfuzosin; Amiodarone; Apixaban; Atovaquone; Avanafil; Axitinib; Bosutinib; Cabozantinib; Cisapride; Conivaptan; Crizotinib; Disulfiram; Dronedarone; Eplerenone; Ergot Derivatives; Etravirine;

Everolimus; Flecainide; Fluticasone (Nasal); Fusidic Acid (Systemic); Halofantrine; Ibrutinib; Imatinib; Ivabradine; Lapatinib; Lomitapide; Lovastatin; Lurasidone; Macitentan; Midazolam; Nilotinib; Nisoldipine; Pimozide; Pomalidomide; Propafenone; QuiNIDine; QuiNINE; Ranolazine; Red Yeast Rice; Regorafenib; Rifampin; Rivaroxaban; Salmeterol; Silodosin; Simeprevir; Simvastatin; St Johns Wort; Tamoxifen; Tamsulosin; Thioridazine; Ticagrelor; Tolvaptan; Topotecan; Toremifene; Triazolam; Ulipristal; Vemurafenib; VinCRIStine (Liposomal); Voriconazole

Decreased Effect

Ritonavir may decrease the levels/effects of: Abacavir; Atovaquone; Boceprevir; BuPROPion; Canagliflozin; Clarithromycin; Codeine; Contraceptives (Estrogens); Deferasirox; Delavirdine; Etravirine; Fosphenytoin; Ifosfamide; Iloperidone; LamoTRIgine; Meperidine; Methadone; Phenytoin; Prasugrel; Proguanil; QuiNINE; Tamoxifen; Telaprevir; Theophylline Derivatives; Ticagrelor; TraMADol; Valproic Acid and Derivatives; Voriconazole; Warfarin; Zidovudine

The levels/effects of Ritonavir may be decreased by: Antacids; Boceprevir; CarBAMazepine; CYP3A4 Inducers (Strong); Dabrafenib; Fosphenytoin; Garlic; Mitotane; Peginterferon Alfa-2b; P-glycoprotein/ABCB1 Inducers; Phenytoin; Rifampin; St Johns Wort; Tocilizumab

Increased Effect/Toxicity

Ritonavir may increase the levels/effects of: Ado-Trastuzumab Emtansine; Afatinib; Alfuzosin; Almotriptan; Alosetron; ALPRAZolam; Amiodarone; Apixaban; ARIPiprazole; AtoMOXetine; AtorvaSTATin; Avanafil; Axitinib; Bedaquiline; Bortezomib; Bosentan; Bosutinib; Brentuximab Vedotin; Brinzolamide; Budesonide (Nasal); Budesonide (Systemic, Oral Inhalation); Cabozantinib; Calcium Channel Blockers (Dihydropyridine); Calcium Channel Blockers (Nondihydropyridine); CarBAMazepine; Cisapride; Clarithromycin; Clorazepate; Colchicine; Conivaptan; Corticosteroids (Orally Inhaled); Crizotinib; CycloSPORINE (Systemic); CYP2C8 Substrates; CYP2D6 Substrates; CYP3A4 Substrates; Dabigatran Etexilate; Diazepam; Dienogest; Digoxin; Dofetilide; DOXOrubicin (Conventional); Dronabinol; Dronedarone; Dutasteride; Efavirenz; Enfuvirtide; Enzalutamide; Eplerenone; Ergot Derivatives; Estazolam; Everolimus; FentaNYL; Fesoterodine; Flecainide; Flurazepam; Fluticasone (Nasal); Fluticasone (Oral Inhalation); Fusidic Acid (Systemic); GuanFACINE; Halofantrine; Highest Risk QTc-Prolonging Agents; Ibrutinib; Iloperidone; Imatinib; Itraconazole; Ivabradine; Ivacaftor; Ixabepilone; Ketoconazole (Systemic); Lacosamide; Lapatinib; Levomilnacipran; Linagliptin; Lomitapide; Lovastatin; Lumefantrine; Lurasidone; Macitentan; Maraviroc; Meperidine; MethylPREDNISolone;

Metoprolol; Midazolam; Mifepristone; Moderate Risk QTc-Prolonging Agents; Nebivolol; Nefazodone; Nilotinib; Nisoldipine; Ospemifene; OxyCODONE; Paricalcitol; PAZOPanib; P-glycoprotein/ABCB1 Substrates; Pimecrolimus; Pimozide; Pioglitazone; Pomalidomide; PONATinib; PredniSOLONE (Systemic); PredniSONE; Propafenone; Protease Inhibitors; Prucalopride; QUEtiapine; QuiNIDine; QuiNINE; Ranolazine; Red Yeast Rice; Regorafenib; Repaglinide; Rifabutin; Rilpivirine; Riociguat; Rivaroxaban; RomiDEPsin; Rosuvastatin; Ruxolitinib; Salmeterol; Saxagliptin; Sildenafil; Silodosin; Simeprevir; Simvastatin; SORAfenib; Tacrolimus (Systemic); Tacrolimus (Topical); Tadalafil; Tamsulosin; Telaprevir; Temsirolimus; Tetrabenazine; Thioridazine; Ticagrelor; Tofacitinib; Tolterodine; Tolvaptan; Topotecan; Toremifene; Treprostinil; Triamcinolone (Systemic); Triazolam; Tricyclic Antidepressants; Ulipristal; Vardenafil; Vemurafenib; Vilazodone; VinBLAStine; VinCRIStine; VinCRIStine (Liposomal); Vortioxetine; Zuclopenthixol

The levels/effects of Ritonavir may be increased by: ARIPiprazole; Clarithromycin; CycloSPORINE (Systemic); Delavirdine; Disulfiram; Efavirenz; Enfuvirtide; Fusidic Acid (Systemic); MetroNIDAZOLE (Topical); P-glycoprotein/ABCB1 Inhibitors; Posaconazole; QuiNINE; Simeprevir

Nutritional/Ethanol Interactions

Food: Food enhances absorption. Management: Manufacturer recommends taking with food. Maintain adequate hydration, unless instructed to restrict fluid intake.

Herb/Nutraceutical: St John's wort may decrease ritonavir serum levels. Garlic may decrease the serum concentration of ritonavir. Management: Avoid St John's wort; concurrent use is contraindicated. Garlic supplementation is not recommended.

Adverse Reactions Percentages as reported for combined experiences in both treatment-naive and experienced adults:

>10%:

Endocrine & metabolic: Hypercholesterolemia (>240 mg/dL: 37% to 45%), increased serum triglycerides (>800 mg/dL: 17% to 34%; >1500 mg/dL: 1% to 13%)

Gastrointestinal: Nausea (26% to 30%), diarrhea (15% to 23%), vomiting (14% to 17%), dysgeusia (7% to 11%)

Hepatic: Increased gamma-glutamyl transferase (5% to 20%)

Neuromuscular & skeletal: Weakness (10% to 15%), increased creatine phosphokinase (9% to 12%)

2% to 10%:

Cardiovascular: Vasodilatation (2%), syncope (1% to 2%)

Central nervous system: Headache (6% to 7%), paresthesia (3% to 7%), dizziness (3% to 4%), insomnia (2% to 3%), drowsiness (2% to 3%), depression (2%), anxiety (≤2%), malaise (1% to 2%)

Dermatologic: Skin rash (≤4%), diaphoresis (2% to 3%)

Genitourinary: Uricosuria (≤4%)

Gastrointestinal: Abdominal pain (6% to 8%), anorexia (2% to 8%), dyspepsia (≤6%), throat irritation (local, 2% to 3%), flatulence (1% to 2%)

Hepatic: Increased serum transaminases (6% to 10%)

Neuromuscular & skeletal: Arthralgia (≤2%), myalgia (2%)

Respiratory: Pharyngitis (≤1% to 3%)

Miscellaneous: Fever (1% to 5%)

Available Dosage Forms

Capsule, Oral:
Norvir: 100 mg

Solution, Oral:
Norvir: 80 mg/mL (240 mL)

Tablet, Oral:
Norvir: 100 mg

General Dosage Range Dosage adjustment recommended in patients on concurrent therapy

Oral:

Infants >1 month and Children: Initial: 250 mg/m^2 twice daily; Maintenance: 350-400 mg/m^2 twice daily (maximum dose: 1200 mg daily)

Adolescents and Adults: 300-600 mg twice daily (maximum: 1200 mg daily)

Administration

Oral Administer all formulations with food, per the manufacturer. DHHS guidelines recommend administering the tablets with food and administering capsules or oral solution with food, if possible, to improve tolerability (DHHS, 2013). Liquid formulations usually have an unpleasant taste. Consider mixing it with chocolate milk or a liquid nutritional supplement and taking within 60 minutes. Whenever possible, administer oral solution with calibrated dosing syringe. Shake solution well before use. Tablets should be swallowed whole; do not chew, break, or crush.

Storage/Stability

Capsule: Store under refrigeration at 2°C to 8°C (36°F to 46°F); may be left out at room temperature of <25°C (<77°F) if used within 30 days. Protect from light. Avoid exposure to excessive heat.

Solution: Store at room temperature at 20°C to 25°C (68°F to 77°F); do not refrigerate. Avoid exposure to excessive heat. Keep cap tightly closed.

Tablet: Store at ≤30 (86°F); exposure to temperatures ≤50°C (122°F) permitted for ≤7 days. Exposure to high humidity outside of the original container (or a USP equivalent container) for >2 weeks is not recommended.

Nursing Actions

Physical Assessment Monitor for adherence to regimen. Help patient figure out best way to administer medication. Monitor for gastrointestinal disturbance (nausea, vomiting, diarrhea) that can lead to dehydration and weight loss, hyperlipidemia and redistribution of body fat, rash, CNS effects (malaise, insomnia, abnormal thinking), and electrolyte imbalance. Teach patient proper timing of multiple medications and drugs that should not be used concurrently. Instruct patient on glucose testing (protease inhibitors may cause hyperglycemia; exacerbation or new-onset diabetes).

Patient Education

- Discuss specific use of drug and side effects with patient as it relates to treatment. (HCAHPS: During this hospital stay, were you given any medicine that you had not taken before? Before giving you any new medicine, how often did hospital staff tell you what the medicine was for? How often did hospital staff describe possible side effects in a way you could understand?)

- Patient may experience hyperlipidemia, presyncope, fatigue, blurred vision, illogical thinking, dizziness, nausea, diarrhea, loss of appetite, parageusia, lipodystrophy, headache, dyspepsia, or asthenia. Have patient report immediately to prescriber tachycardia, syncope, polydipsia, polyuria, weight loss, discolored urine, jaundice, paresthesia, or rash (HCAHPS).

- Educate patient about signs of a significant reaction (eg, wheezing; chest tightness; fever; itching; bad cough; blue skin color; seizures; or swelling of face, lips, tongue, or throat). **Note:** This is not a comprehensive list of all side effects. Patient should consult prescriber for additional questions.

Intended Use and Disclaimer: Should not be printed and given to patients. This information is intended to serve as a concise initial reference for healthcare professionals to use when discussing medications with a patient. You must ultimately rely on your own discretion, experience and judgment in diagnosing, treating and advising patients.

Dietary Considerations The manufacturer recommends taking with food. Oral solution contains 43% ethanol by volume.

Related Information

Oral Medications That Should Not Be Crushed or Altered *on page 1712*

RITUXimab (ri TUK si mab)

Brand Names: U.S. Rituxan

Index Terms Anti-CD20 Monoclonal Antibody; C2B8 Monoclonal Antibody; IDEC-C2B8

Pharmacologic Category Antineoplastic Agent, Anti-CD20; Antineoplastic Agent, Monoclonal Antibody; Antirheumatic Miscellaneous; Immunosuppressant Agent; Monoclonal Antibody

◀ **Medication Safety Issues**

Sound-alike/look-alike issues:

Rituxan may be confused with Remicade

RiTUXimab may be confused with brentuximab, bevacizumab, inFLIXimab, ruxolitinib

High alert medication:

The medication is in a class the Institute for Safe Medication Practices (ISMP) includes among its list of drug classes which have a heightened risk of causing significant patient harm when used in error.

Administration issues:

The rituximab dose for rheumatoid arthritis is a flat dose (1000 mg) and is not based on body surface area (BSA).

Medication Guide Available Yes

Pregnancy Risk Factor C

Lactation Excretion in breast milk unknown/not recommended

Breast-Feeding Considerations It is not known if rituximab is excreted in human milk. However, human IgG is excreted in breast milk, and therefore, rituximab may also be excreted in milk. Although rituximab would not be expected to enter the circulation of a nursing infant in significant amounts, the decision to discontinue rituximab or discontinue breast-feeding should take into account the benefits of treatment to the mother.

Use

Treatment of CD20-positive non-Hodgkin lymphomas (NHL):

Relapsed or refractory, low-grade or follicular B-cell NHL (as a single agent)

Follicular B-cell NHL, previously untreated (in combination with first-line chemotherapy, and as single-agent maintenance therapy if response to first-line rituximab with chemotherapy)

Nonprogressing, low-grade B-cell NHL (as a single agent after first-line CVP treatment)

Diffuse large B-cell NHL, previously untreated (in combination with CHOP chemotherapy [or other anthracycline-based regimen])

Treatment of CD20-positive chronic lymphocytic leukemia (CLL) (in combination with fludarabine and cyclophosphamide)

Treatment of moderately- to severely-active rheumatoid arthritis (in combination with methotrexate) in adult patients with inadequate response to one or more TNF antagonists

Treatment of granulomatosis with polyangiitis (GPA; Wegener's granulomatosis) (in combination with glucocorticoids)

Treatment of microscopic polyangiitis (MPA) (in combination with glucocorticoids)

Unlabeled Use Treatment of Burkitt's lymphoma, central nervous system lymphoma, Hodgkin's lymphoma (lymphocyte predominant); mucosal associated lymphoid tissue (MALT) lymphoma (gastric and nongastric), splenic marginal zone lymphoma;

Waldenström's macroglobulinemia (WM); post-transplant lymphoproliferative disorder (PTLD); autoimmune hemolytic anemia (AIHA) in children; chronic immune thrombocytopenia (ITP); refractory pemphigus vulgaris; treatment of steroid-refractory chronic graft-versus-host disease (GVHD); refractory lupus nephritis; relapsed/refractory thrombotic thrombocytopenic purpura-hemolytic uremic syndrome (TTP-HUS), resistant idiopathic membranous nephropathy (IMN), refractory nephrotic syndrome (children)

Mechanism of Action/Effect Binds to the CD20 antigen on B-lymphocytes and recruits immune effector functions to mediate B-cell lysis *in vitro*. The antibody induces cell death in the DHL-4 human B-cell lymphoma line. B-cells are believed to play a role in the development and progression of rheumatoid arthritis. Signs and symptoms of RA are reduced by targeting B-cells and the progression of structural damage is delayed.

Contraindications There are no contraindications listed in the FDA-approved manufacturer's labeling.

Canadian labeling (not in U.S. labeling): Type 1 hypersensitivity or anaphylactic reaction to murine proteins, Chinese Hamster Ovary (CHO) cell proteins, or any component of the formulation; patients who have or have had progressive multifocal leukoencephalopathy (PML)

Warnings/Precautions [U.S. Boxed Warning]: Severe (occasionally fatal) infusion-related reactions have been reported, usually with the first infusion; fatalities have been reported within 24 hours of infusion; monitor closely during infusion; discontinue for severe reactions and provide medical intervention for grades 3 or 4 infusion reactions. Reactions usually occur within 30-120 minutes and may include hypotension, angioedema, bronchospasm, hypoxia, urticaria, and in more severe cases pulmonary infiltrates, acute respiratory distress syndrome, myocardial infarction, ventricular fibrillation, cardiogenic shock and/or anaphylaxis. Risk factors associated with fatal outcomes include chronic lymphocytic leukemia, female gender, mantle cell lymphoma, or pulmonary infiltrates. Closely monitor patients with a history of prior cardiopulmonary reactions or with pre-existing cardiac or pulmonary conditions and patients with high numbers of circulating malignant cells (>25,000/mm^3). Prior to infusion, premedicate patients with acetaminophen and an antihistamine (and methylprednisolone for patients with RA). Discontinue infusion for severe reactions; treatment is symptomatic. Medications for the treatment of hypersensitivity reactions (eg, bronchodilators, epinephrine, antihistamines, corticosteroids) should be available for immediate use. Discontinue infusion for serious or life-threatening cardiac arrhythmias. Perform cardiac monitoring during and after the infusion in patients who develop clinically significant arrhythmias or who have a history of arrhythmia or angina. Mild-to-moderate infusion-related reactions (eg, chills, fever, rigors) occur frequently and are typically managed through slowing or interrupting the infusion. Infusion may be resumed at a 50% infusion rate reduction upon resolution of symptoms. Due to the potential for hypotension, consider withholding antihypertensives 12 hours prior to treatment.

[U.S. Boxed Warning]: Hepatitis B virus (HBV) reactivation may occur with use and may result in fulminant hepatitis, hepatic failure, and death. Screen all patients for HBV infection by measuring hepatitis B surface antigen (HBsAG) and hepatitis B core antibody (anti-HBc) prior to therapy initiation; monitor patients for clinical and laboratory signs of hepatitis or HBV during and for several months after treatment. Discontinue rituximab (and concomitant medications) if viral hepatitis develops and initiate appropriate antiviral therapy. Reactivation has occurred in patients who are HBsAg positive as well as in those who are HBsAg negative but are anti-HBc positive; HBV reactivation has also been observed in patients who had previously resolved HBV infection. HBV reactivation has been reported up to 24 months after therapy discontinuation. Use cautiously in patients who show evidence of prior HBV infection (eg, HBsAg positive [regardless of antibody status] or HBsAG negative but anti-HBc positive); consult with appropriate clinicians regarding monitoring and consideration of antiviral therapy before and/or during rituximab treatment. The safety of resuming rituximab treatment following HBV reactivation is not known; discuss reinitiation of therapy in patients with resolved HBV reactivation with physicians experienced in HBV management.

[U.S. Boxed Warning]: Progressive multifocal leukoencephalopathy (PML) due to JC virus infection has been reported with rituximab use; may be fatal. Cases were reported in patients with hematologic malignancies receiving rituximab either with combination chemotherapy, or with hematopoietic stem cell transplant. Cases were also reported in patients receiving rituximab for autoimmune diseases who had received prior or concurrent immunosuppressant therapy. Onset may be delayed, although most cases were diagnosed within 12 months of the last rituximab dose. A retrospective analysis of patients (n=57) diagnosed with PML following rituximab therapy, found a median of 16 months (following rituximab initiation), 5.5 months (following last rituximab dose), and 6 rituximab doses preceded PML diagnosis. Clinical findings included confusion/disorientation, motor weakness/hemiparesis, altered vision/speech, and poor motor coordination with symptoms progressing over weeks to months (Carson, 2009). Promptly evaluate any patient presenting with neurological changes; consider neurology consultation, brain MRI and lumbar puncture for suspected PML. Discontinue rituximab in patients who develop PML; consider reduction/discontinuation of concurrent chemotherapy or immunosuppressants. Avoid use if severe active infection is present. Serious and potentially fatal bacterial, fungal, and either new or reactivated viral infections may occur during treatment and after completing rituximab. Infections have been observed in patients with prolonged hypogammaglobulinemia, defined as hypogammaglobulinemia >11 months after rituximab exposure; monitor immunoglobulin levels as necessary. Associated new or reactivated viral infections have included cytomegalovirus, herpes simplex virus, parvovirus B19, varicella zoster virus, West Nile virus, and hepatitis B and C. Discontinue rituximab in patients who develop other serious infections and initiate appropriate anti-infective treatment.

Tumor lysis syndrome leading to acute renal failure requiring dialysis (some fatal) may occur 12-24 hours following the first dose when used as a single agent in the treatment of NHL. Hyperkalemia, hypocalcemia, hyperuricemia, and/or hyperphosphatemia may occur. Administer prophylaxis (antihyperuricemic therapy, hydration) in patients at high risk (high numbers of circulating malignant cells ≥25,000/mm^3 or high tumor burden). May cause fatal renal toxicity in patients with hematologic malignancies. Patients who received combination therapy with cisplatin and rituximab for NHL experienced renal toxicity during clinical trials; this combination is not an approved treatment regimen. Monitor for signs of renal failure; discontinue rituximab with increasing serum creatinine or oliguria. Correct electrolyte abnormalities; monitor hydration status.

[U.S. Boxed Warning]: Severe and sometimes fatal mucocutaneous reactions (lichenoid dermatitis, paraneoplastic pemphigus, Stevens-Johnson syndrome, toxic epidermal necrolysis and vesiculobullous dermatitis) have been reported; onset has been variable but has occurred as early as the first day of exposure. Discontinue in patients experiencing severe mucocutaneous skin reactions; the safety of re-exposure following mucocutaneous reactions has not been evaluated. Use caution with pre-existing cardiac or pulmonary disease, or prior cardiopulmonary events. Rheumatoid arthritis patients are at increased risk for cardiovascular events; monitor closely during and after each infusion. Elderly patients are at higher risk for cardiac (supraventricular arrhythmia) and pulmonary adverse events (pneumonia, pneumonitis). Abdominal pain, bowel obstruction, and perforation (rarely fatal) have been reported with an average onset of symptoms of ~6 days (range: 1-77 days); complaints of abdominal pain or repeated vomiting should be evaluated, especially if early in the treatment course. Live vaccines should not be given concurrently with rituximab; there is no data available concerning secondary transmission of live vaccines with or following rituximab treatment. RA patients should be brought up to date with nonlive immunizations (following current guidelines) at least 4 weeks before initiating therapy; evaluate risks of therapy delay versus benefit (of nonlive vaccines) for NHL patients. Safety and efficacy of rituximab in combination with biologic agents or disease-modifying antirheumatic drugs (DMARDs) other than methotrexate have not been established. Rituximab is not recommended for use in RA patients who have not had prior inadequate response to TNF antagonists. Safety and efficacy of retreatment for RA have not been established. The safety of concomitant immunosuppressants other than corticosteroids has not been evaluated in patients with granulomatosis with polyangiitis (GPA; Wegener's granulomatosis) or microscopic polyangiitis (MPA) after rituximab-induced B-cell depletion. There are only limited data on subsequent courses of rituximab for GPA or MPA; safety and efficacy of retreatment have not been established.

Drug Interactions

Avoid Concomitant Use

Avoid concomitant use of RiTUXimab with any of the following: Abatacept; BCG; Belimumab; Certolizumab Pegol; CloZAPine; Natalizumab; Pimecrolimus; Tacrolimus (Topical); Tofacitinib; Vaccines (Live)

Decreased Effect

RiTUXimab may decrease the levels/effects of: BCG; Coccidioidin Skin Test; Sipuleucel-T; Vaccines (Inactivated); Vaccines (Live)

The levels/effects of RiTUXimab may be decreased by: Echinacea

Increased Effect/Toxicity

RiTUXimab may increase the levels/effects of: Abatacept; Belimumab; Certolizumab Pegol; CloZAPine; Leflunomide; Natalizumab; Tofacitinib; Vaccines (Live)

The levels/effects of RiTUXimab may be increased by: Abciximab; Antihypertensives; Denosumab; Pimecrolimus; Roflumilast; Tacrolimus (Topical); Trastuzumab

Nutritional/Ethanol Interactions Herb/Nutraceutical: Avoid echinacea (may diminish the therapeutic effect of immunosuppressants). Avoid hypoglycemic herbs, including alfalfa, aloe, bilberry, bitter melon, burdock, celery, damiana, fenugreek, garcinia, garlic, ginger, ginseng (American), gymnema, marshmallow, and stinging nettle (may enhance the hypoglycemic effect of rituximab).

Adverse Reactions Note: Patients treated with rituximab for rheumatoid arthritis (RA) may experience fewer adverse reactions.

>10%:

Cardiovascular: Peripheral edema (8% to 16%), hypertension (6% to 12%)

Central nervous system: Fever (5% to 53%), fatigue (13% to 39%), chills (3% to 33%), headache (17% to 19%), insomnia (≤14%), pain (12%)

Dermatologic: Rash (10% to 17%; grades 3/4: 1%), pruritus (5% to 17%), angioedema (11%; grades 3/4: 1%)

Gastrointestinal: Nausea (8% to 23%), diarrhea (10% to 17%), abdominal pain (2% to 14%), weight gain (11%)

Hematologic: Cytopenias (grades 3/4: ≤48%; may be prolonged), lymphopenia (48%; grades 3/4: 40%; median duration 14 days), anemia (8% to 35%; grades 3/4: 3%), leukopenia (NHL: 14%; grades 3/4: 4%; CLL: grades 3/4: 23%; GPA/MPA: 10%), neutropenia (NHL: 14%; grades 3/4: 4% to 6%; median duration 13 days; CLL: grades 3/4: 30% to 49%), neutropenic fever (CLL: grades 3/4: 9% to 15%), thrombocytopenia (12%; grades 3/4: 2% to 11%)

Hepatic: ALT increased (≤13%)

Neuromuscular & skeletal: Neuropathy (≤30%), weakness (2% to 26%), muscle spasm (≤17%), arthralgia (6% to 13%)

Respiratory: Cough (13%), rhinitis (3% to 12%), epistaxis (≤11%)

Miscellaneous: Infusion-related reactions (lymphoma: first dose 77%; decreases with subsequent infusions; may include angioedema, bronchospasm, chills, dizziness, fever, headache, hyper-/hypotension, myalgia, nausea, pruritus, rash, rigors, urticaria, and vomiting; reactions reported are lower [first infusion: 32%] in RA; CLL: 59%; grades 3/4: 7% to 9%; GPA/MPA: 12%); infection (19% to 62%; grades 3/4: 4%; bacterial: 19%; viral 10%; fungal: 1%), human antichimeric antibody (HACA) positive (1% to 23%), night sweats (15%)

1% to 10%:

Cardiovascular: Hypotension (10%; grades 3/4: 2%), flushing (5%)

Central nervous system: Dizziness (10%), anxiety (2% to 5%), migraine (RA: 2%)

Dermatologic: Urticaria (2% to 8%)

Endocrine & metabolic: Hyperglycemia (9%)

Gastrointestinal: Vomiting (10%), dyspepsia (RA: 3%)

Neuromuscular & skeletal: Back pain (10%), myalgia (10%), paresthesia (2%)

Respiratory: Dyspnea (≤10%), throat irritation (2% to 9%), bronchospasm (8%), dyspnea (7%), upper respiratory tract infection (RA: 7%), sinusitis (6%)

Miscellaneous: LDH increased (7%)

Pharmacodynamics/Kinetics

Duration of Action Detectable in serum 3-6 months after completion of treatment; B-cell recovery begins ~6 months following completion of treatment; median B-cell levels return to normal by 12 months following completion of treatment

Available Dosage Forms

Concentrate, Intravenous [preservative free]:
Rituxan: 10 mg/mL (10 mL, 50 mL)

General Dosage Range I.V.: *Adults:* Dosage varies greatly depending on indication

Administration

I.V. Do **not** administer I.V. push or bolus. If a reaction occurs, slow or stop the infusion. If the reaction abates, restart infusion at 50% of the previous rate. Discontinue infusion in the event of serious or life-threatening cardiac arrhythmias.

I.V.: Initial infusion: Start rate of 50 mg/hour; if there is no reaction, increase the rate by 50 mg/hour increments every 30 minutes, to a maximum rate of 400 mg/hour.

Subsequent infusions:

Standard infusion rate: If patient tolerated initial infusion, start at 100 mg/hour; if there is no reaction, increase the rate by 100 mg/hour increments every 30 minutes, to a maximum rate of 400 mg/hour.

Accelerated infusion rate (90 minutes): For patients with previously untreated follicular NHL and diffuse large B-cell NHL who are receiving a corticosteroid as part of their combination chemotherapy regimen, have a circulating lymphocyte count <5000/mm^3, or have no significant cardiovascular disease. After tolerance has been established (no grade 3 or 4 infusion-related event) at the recommended infusion rate in cycle 1, a rapid infusion rate may be used beginning with cycle 2. The daily corticosteroid, acetaminophen, and diphenhydramine are administered prior to treatment, then the rituximab dose is administered over 90 minutes, with 20% of the dose administered over the first 30 minutes and the remaining 80% is given over 60 minutes (Sehn, 2007). If the 90-minute infusion in cycle 2 is tolerated, the same rate may be used for the remainder of the treatment regimen (through cycles 6 or 8).

Injectable Detail pH: 6.5

Preparation for Administration Withdraw necessary amount of rituximab and dilute to a final concentration of 1-4 mg/mL with 0.9% sodium chloride or 5% dextrose in water. Gently invert the bag to mix the solution. Do not shake.

Storage/Stability Store intact vials refrigerated at 2°C to 8°C (36°F to 46°F); do not freeze. Do not shake. Protect vials from direct sunlight. Solutions for infusion are stable at 2°C to 8°C (36°F to 46°F) for 24 hours and at room temperature for an additional 24 hours.

Nursing Actions

Physical Assessment Premedication may be ordered. Monitor patient closely for chills, fever, rigors, dizziness, angioedema, respiratory distress, myalgia, nausea, pruritus, rash, and vomiting during and following each infusion.

Emergency equipment and medications (epinephrine, antihistamines, corticosteroids) should be immediately available during infusion. In the event of severe infusion reaction, infusion should be stopped and prescriber notified immediately. Monitor patient closely for abdominal pain (bowel obstruction and perforation), hyper-/hypotension, CNS changes, hyper-/hypoglycemia, and rash after each dose and following discontinuation of therapy. Bowel obstruction and perforation can occur early in therapy; acute tumor lysis syndrome leading to acute renal failure can occur 12-24 hours after first dose; severe mucocutaneous reactions can occur from 1-13 weeks following treatment; and new or reactivated serious viral infection may occur up to one year following discontinuation of therapy.

Patient Education

• Discuss specific use of drug and side effects with patient as it relates to treatment. (HCAHPS: During this hospital stay, were you given any medicine that you had not taken before? Before giving you any new medicine, how often did hospital staff tell you what the medicine was for? How often did hospital staff describe possible side effects in a way you could understand?)

• Patient may experience flu-like syndrome, hypotension, fatigue, dizziness, headache, nausea, dyspepsia, diarrhea, rhinorrhea, edema in arms or legs, leukopenia, thrombocytopenia, or hypertension. Have patient report immediately to prescriber signs of infection, angina, tachycardia, sudden vision changes, illogical thinking, syncope, change in balance, strength differences from one side to another, difficulty walking or speaking, dyspnea, jaundice, ecchymosis, severe mouth or skin irritation, or rash (HCAHPS).

• Educate patient about signs of a significant reaction (eg, wheezing; chest tightness; fever; itching; bad cough; blue skin color; seizures; or swelling of face, lips, tongue, or throat). **Note:** This is not a comprehensive list of all side effects. Patient should consult prescriber for additional questions.

Intended Use and Disclaimer: Should not be printed and given to patients. This information is intended to serve as a concise initial reference for healthcare professionals to use when discussing medications with a patient. You must ultimately rely on your own discretion, experience and judgment in diagnosing, treating and advising patients.

Rivaroxaban (riv a ROX a ban)

Brand Names: U.S. Xarelto
Index Terms BAY 59-7939
Pharmacologic Category Anticoagulant; Anticoagulant, Factor Xa Inhibitor

◀ **Medication Safety Issues**
  High alert medication:
    This medication is in a class the Institute for Safe
    Medication Practices (ISMP) includes among its
    list of drug classes which have a heightened risk
    of causing significant patient harm when used in
    error.
Medication Guide Available Yes
Pregnancy Risk Factor C
Lactation Excretion in breast milk unknown/not
recommended
Breast-Feeding Considerations It is not known if
rivaroxaban is excreted into breast milk. Due to the
potential for serious adverse reactions in the nursing infant, the decision to discontinue rivaroxaban
or to discontinue breast-feeding during therapy
should take into account the benefits of treatment
to the mother; use of alternative anticoagulants is
preferred (Guyatt, 2012). Use in breast-feeding
mothers is contraindicated in the Canadian labeling.
Use
  Deep vein thrombosis prophylaxis: Postopera-
    tive thrombophylaxis of deep vein thrombosis
    (DVT) which may lead to pulmonary embolism
    in patients undergoing knee or hip replacement
    surgery.
  Deep vein thrombosis treatment: Treatment
    of DVT.
  Nonvalvular atrial fibrillation: Prevention of
    stroke and systemic embolism in patients with
    nonvalvular atrial fibrillation.
  Pulmonary embolism treatment: Treatment of
    pulmonary embolism.
  **Reduction in the risk of recurrence of deep vein
    thrombosis and pulmonary embolism:** Reduc-
    tion in the risk of recurrence of DVT and pulmo-
    nary embolism following initial 6 months of
    treatment for DVT and/or pulmonary embolism.
Mechanism of Action/Effect
Inhibits platelet activation and fibrin clot formation
via direct and selective inhibition of factor Xa (FXa)
Contraindications Severe hypersensitivity to
rivaroxaban or any component of the formulation;
active pathological bleeding

Canadian labeling: Additional contraindications
(not in U.S. labeling): Hepatic disease (including
Child-Pugh classes B and C) associated with
coagulopathy and clinically relevant bleeding risk;
clinically significant active bleeding, including hemorrhagic manifestations and bleeding diathesis;
lesions at increased risk of clinically significant
bleeding (eg, hemorrhagic or ischemic cerebral
infarction) within previous 6 months; spontaneous
hemostasis impairment; concomitant systemic
treatment with strong CYP3A4 and P-glycoprotein
(P-gp) inhibitors; pregnancy; lactation
Warnings/Precautions Most common complication is bleeding; major hemorrhages (eg, intracranial, GI, retinal, epidural hematoma, adrenal

bleeding) have been reported. Certain patients
are at increased risk of bleeding; risk factors
include bacterial endocarditis, congenital or
acquired bleeding disorders, thrombocytopenia,
recent puncture of large vessels or organ biopsy,
stroke, intracerebral surgery, or other neuraxial
procedure, severe uncontrolled hypertension, renal
impairment, recent major surgery, recent major
bleeding (intracranial, GI, intraocular, or pulmonary), concomitant use of drugs that affect hemostasis, and advanced age. Monitor for signs and
symptoms of bleeding. Prompt clinical evaluation is
warranted with any unexplained decrease in hemoglobin or blood pressure. **Note:** No specific antidote exists for rivaroxaban reversal; not dialyzable
due to high plasma protein binding. Protamine
sulfate and vitamin K are not expected to affect
the anticoagulant activity of rivaroxaban. The use
of activated prothrombin complex concentrate
(aPCC) or recombinant factor VIIa has not been
evaluated. The use of a four-factor PCC (Cofact,
not available in the U.S.) in healthy subjects has
been shown to reverse the anticoagulant effect (ie,
normalize the prothrombin time) of rivaroxaban
(Eerenberg, 2011).

**[U.S. Boxed Warning]: Spinal or epidural hem-
atomas may occur with neuraxial anesthesia
(epidural or spinal anesthesia) or spinal puncture in patients who are anticoagulated; may
result in long-term or permanent paralysis. The
risk of spinal/epidural hematoma is increased
with the use of indwelling epidural catheters,
concomitant administration of other drugs that
affect hemostasis (eg, NSAIDS, platelet inhibitors, other anticoagulants), in patients with a
history of traumatic or repeated epidural or
spinal punctures, or a history of spinal deformity or spinal surgery. Monitor for signs of neurologic impairment (eg, numbness/weakness of
legs, bowel/bladder dysfunction); prompt diagnosis and treatment are necessary. In patients
who are anticoagulated or pharmacologic
thromboprophylaxis is anticipated, assess
risks versus benefits prior to neuraxial interventions.** In patients who receive both rivaroxaban
and neuraxial anesthesia, avoid removal of epidural catheter for at least 18 hours following last
rivaroxaban dose; avoid rivaroxaban administration for at least 6 hours following epidural catheter
removal; if traumatic puncture occurs, avoid rivaroxaban administration for at least 24 hours.

**[U.S. Boxed Warning]: As with any oral anti-
coagulant in the absence of adequate alternative anticoagulation, an increased risk of
thrombotic events (including stroke) may occur
with premature discontinuation of rivaroxaban.
Consider the addition of alternative anticoagulant therapy when discontinuing rivaroxaban
for reasons other than pathological bleeding
or completion of a course of therapy.** An

increased rate of stroke was observed during the transition from rivaroxaban to warfarin in clinical trials in atrial fibrillation patients. In a post-hoc analysis of the ROCKET AF trial, patients who temporarily (>3 days) or permanently discontinued anticoagulation, the risk of stroke or non-CNS embolism was similar with rivaroxaban as compared to warfarin (Patel, 2013).

Avoid use in patients with moderate-to-severe hepatic impairment (Child-Pugh classes B and C) or in patients with any hepatic disease associated with coagulopathy; use in this patient population is contraindicated in the Canadian labeling. Use with caution in patients with moderate renal impairment (CrCl 30-49 mL/minute) when used for postoperative thromboprophylaxis including patients receiving concomitant drug therapy that may increase rivaroxaban systemic exposure and those with deteriorating renal function. Monitor for any signs or symptoms of blood loss. Avoid use in severe renal impairment (DVT/PE, postoperative thromboprophylaxis: CrCl <30 mL/minute; nonvalvular atrial fibrillation: CrCl <15 mL/minute) since rivaroxaban exposure is expected to increase; discontinue use in patients who develop acute renal failure. Use with caution in the elderly. Elderly patients exhibit higher rivaroxaban concentrations compared to younger patients due primarily to reduced clearance. Overall, efficacy of rivaroxaban in the elderly (age ≥65 years) was similar to that of patients <65 years of age. Both thrombotic and bleeding events were higher in the elderly; however, the risk to benefit profile was favorable among all age groups.

Potentially significant drug-drug interactions may exist, requiring dose or frequency adjustment, additional monitoring, and/or selection of alternative therapy. In patients with renal impairment, concomitant use of rivaroxaban with combined P-gp and weak or moderate CYP3A4 inhibitors should only occur if the potential benefit outweighs the risk of bleeding. Formulation contains lactose; use is not recommended in patients with lactose or galactose intolerance (eg, Lapp lactase deficiency, glucose-galactose malabsorption).

Discontinue rivaroxaban at least 24 hours prior to surgery/invasive procedures; reinitiate when adequate hemostasis has been achieved unless oral therapy cannot be administered then consider administration of a parenteral anticoagulant. Safety and efficacy have not been established in patients with prosthetic heart valves or significant rheumatic heart disease (eg, mitral stenosis); use is not recommended. Non-valvular atrial fibrillation is defined as atrial fibrillation that occurs in the absence of rheumatic mitral valve disease, mitral valve repair, or prosthetic heart valve (Fuster, 2011). Rivaroxaban is **not** recommended as an alternative to unfractionated heparin in the treatment of acute pulmonary embolism in hemodynamically unstable patients or patients requiring thrombolysis or pulmonary embolectomy.

Drug Interactions
Avoid Concomitant Use
Avoid concomitant use of Rivaroxaban with any of the following: Anticoagulants; Apixaban; CYP3A4 Inducers (Strong); CYP3A4 Inhibitors (Moderate); CYP3A4 Inhibitors (Strong); Dabigatran Etexilate; Omacetaxine; St Johns Wort; Urokinase

Decreased Effect
The levels/effects of Rivaroxaban may be decreased by: Bosentan; CYP3A4 Inducers (Strong); Dabrafenib; Deferasirox; Estrogen Derivatives; P-glycoprotein/ABCB1 Inducers; Progestins; St Johns Wort; Tocilizumab

Increased Effect/Toxicity
Rivaroxaban may increase the levels/effects of: Collagenase (Systemic); Deferasirox; Ibritumomab; Omacetaxine; Tositumomab and Iodine I 131 Tositumomab

The levels/effects of Rivaroxaban may be increased by: Agents with Antiplatelet Properties; Anticoagulants; Apixaban; Azithromycin (Systemic); Clarithromycin; CYP3A4 Inhibitors (Moderate); CYP3A4 Inhibitors (Strong); Dabigatran Etexilate; Dasatinib; Erythromycin (Systemic); Fusidic Acid (Systemic); Herbs (Anticoagulant/Antiplatelet Properties); Ibrutinib; Ivacaftor; Luliconazole; Mifepristone; Nonsteroidal Anti-Inflammatory Agents; Omega-3 Fatty Acids; Pentosan Polysulfate Sodium; P-glycoprotein/ABCB1 Inhibitors; Prostacyclin Analogues; Salicylates; Simeprevir; Sugammadex; Thrombolytic Agents; Tibolone; Tipranavir; Urokinase; Verapamil; Vitamin E

Nutritional/Ethanol Interactions
Food: Grapefruit juice may increase levels/effects of rivaroxaban; use caution.

Herb/Nutraceutical: Avoid concomitant use of St John's wort if possible (may decrease levels/effects of rivaroxaban; use with caution and consider dosage adjustment of rivaroxaban if concomitant use cannot be avoided).

Adverse Reactions 1% to 10%:
Cardiovascular: Peripheral edema (≤6%)

Central nervous system: Dizziness (≤6%), headache (3% to 5%), pyrexia (1% to 3%), fatigue (≤3%), syncope (≤2%)

Dermatologic: Bruising (3%), pruritus (≤2%), rash (2%), blister (1%)

Gastrointestinal: Diarrhea (≤5%), constipation (≤3%), abdominal pain (≤2%), nausea (1% to 3%), dyspepsia (≤2%), vomiting (≤2%), oropharyngeal pain (≤1%), toothache (≤1%)

Genitourinary: Hematuria (≤4%), urinary tract infection (≤1%)

Hematologic: Bleeding (atrial fibrillation: 21% [major: 6%]; DVT prophylaxis: 5% to 6% [major: <1%]; DVT treatment: 6% to 10% [major: 1%]), hematoma (≤3%), anemia (1% to 3%)

Local: Wound secretion (≤3%)

Neuromuscular & skeletal: Extremity pain (≤5%), back pain (≤4%), osteoarthritis (≤2%), muscle spasm (1%)

Respiratory: Epistaxis (4% to 10%), hemoptysis (≤1%), sinusitis (≤1%)

Available Dosage Forms

Tablet, Oral:

Xarelto: 10 mg, 15 mg, 20 mg

General Dosage Range Dosage adjustment recommended in patients with renal impairment.

Oral: *Adults:* 10-20 mg once daily or an initial dose of 15 mg twice daily followed by 20 mg once daily

Administration

Oral Administer doses ≥15 mg/day with food; dose of 10 mg/day may be administered without regard to meals. For nonvalvular atrial fibrillation, administer with the evening meal. For patients who cannot swallow whole tablets, the manufacturer's labeling states the 15 mg and 20 mg tablets may be crushed and mixed with applesauce immediately prior to use (**Note:** the manufacturer's labeling does not specify the 10 mg tablets can be crushed although the 10 mg, 15 mg, and 20 mg tablets are all biconvex film-coated tablets); immediately follow administration with food.

Missed doses: Patients receiving 15 mg twice daily dosing who miss a dose should take a dose immediately to ensure 30 mg of rivaroxaban is administered per day (two 15 mg tablets may be taken together); resume therapy the following day as previously taken. Patients receiving once-daily dosing who miss a dose should take a dose as soon as possible on the same day; resume therapy the following day as previously taken.

Other For nasogastric/gastric feeding tube administration, the manufacturer's labeling states the 15 mg and 20 mg tablets may be crushed and mixed in 50 mL of water (**Note:** The manufacturer's labeling does not specify the 10 mg tablets can be crushed although the 10 mg, 15 mg, and 20 mg tablets are all biconvex film-coated tablets); administer the suspension within 4 hours of preparation and follow administration immediately with enteral feeding. Avoid administration distal to the stomach; a decrease in the AUC and C_{max} (29% and 56%, respectively) was observed when rivaroxaban was delivered to the proximal small intestine; further decreases may be seen with delivery to the distal small intestine or ascending colon.

Storage/Stability Store at 25°C (77°F); excursions permitted to 15°C to 30°C (59°F to 86°F).

Nursing Actions

Physical Assessment After neuraxial anesthesia, monitor for development of hematoma at site of catheter. Monitor for unusual bleeding and for neurological compromise in the setting of epidural or spinal hematoma. Educate patient about signs and symptoms of bleeding and who to contact in the event of bleeding. Advise patient to tell all doctors and dentists about use of an anticoagulant.

Patient Education

• Discuss specific use of drug and side effects with patient as it relates to treatment. (HCAHPS: During this hospital stay, were you given any medicine that you had not taken before? Before giving you any new medicine, how often did hospital staff tell you what the medicine was for? How often did hospital staff describe possible side effects in a way you could understand?)

• Patient may experience bleeding problems, headache, nausea, or dizziness. Have patient report immediately to prescriber paresthesia, illogical thinking, or ecchymosis (HCAHPS).

• Educate patient about signs of a significant reaction (eg, wheezing; chest tightness; fever; itching; bad cough; blue skin color; seizures; or swelling of face, lips, tongue, or throat). **Note:** This is not a comprehensive list of all side effects. Patient should consult prescriber for additional questions.

Intended Use and Disclaimer: Should not be printed and given to patients. This information is intended to serve as a concise initial reference for healthcare professionals to use when discussing medications with a patient. You must ultimately rely on your own discretion, experience, and judgment in diagnosing, treating and advising patients.

Rivastigmine (ri va STIG meen)

Brand Names: U.S. Exelon

Index Terms ENA 713; Rivastigmine Tartrate; SDZ ENA 713

Pharmacologic Category Acetylcholinesterase Inhibitor (Central)

Pregnancy Risk Factor B

Lactation Excretion in breast milk unknown/not recommended

Breast-Feeding Considerations It is not known if rivastigmine is excreted in breast milk. Rivastigmine is not indicated in nursing mothers.

Use Dementia associated with Alzheimer's or Parkinson's disease:

U.S. labeling: Treatment of mild, moderate, or severe dementia associated with Alzheimer's disease; treatment of mild-to-moderate dementia associated with Parkinson's disease

Canadian labeling: Treatment of mild-to-moderate dementia associated with Alzheimer's disease; treatment of mild-to-moderate dementia associated with Parkinson's disease

Unlabeled Use Treatment of dementia with Lewy bodies

Mechanism of Action/Effect Rivastigmine increases acetylcholine in the central nervous system through reversible inhibition of its hydrolysis by cholinesterase

Contraindications Hypersensitivity to rivastigmine, other carbamate derivatives (eg, neostigmine, pyridostigmine, physostigmine), or any component of the formulation; history of application site reactions with rivastigmine patch

Canadian labeling: Additional contraindications (not in U.S. labeling): Severe hepatic impairment

Warnings/Precautions Significant nausea/vomiting/diarrhea or anorexia/weight loss/decreased appetite are associated with use; occurs more frequently in women and during the titration phase. The incidence and severity of these reactions are dose-related. Monitor weight during therapy. Therapy should be initiated at lowest dose and titrated; if treatment is interrupted for >3 days, reinstate at the lowest daily dose. May have vagotonic effects which may cause bradycardia and/or heart block with or without a history of cardiac disease. Alzheimer's treatment guidelines consider bradycardia to be a relative contraindication for use of centrally-active cholinesterase inhibitors. Postmarketing cases of overdose (including fatalities) have been reported in association with medication errors/improper use of rivastigmine transdermal patches. No more than 1 patch should be applied daily and existing patch must be removed prior to applying new patch.

Use of patch may result in allergic contact dermatitis; discontinue therapy if an intense local reaction occurs (eg, increasing erythema, edema, papules, vesicles) and if symptoms do not improve after 48 hours of patch removal. If therapy is still required, oral rivastigmine may be used following negative allergy testing; some patients may not be able to take rivastigmine in any form. Postmarketing reports of disseminated hypersensitivity skin reactions have occurred with use of oral or transdermal products; discontinue use of all rivastigmine therapy in these cases.

Use caution in patients with a history of peptic ulcer disease or concurrent NSAID use; may increase gastric acid secretion. Monitor for active or occult bleeding. Use caution in patients with sick-sinus syndrome, bradycardia or supraventricular conduction conditions, urinary obstruction, seizure disorders, or pulmonary conditions such as asthma or COPD. May exacerbate or induce extrapyramidal symptoms; worsening of symptoms (eg, tremor) in patients with Parkinson's disease has been observed. May cause CNS depression, which may impair physical or mental abilities; patients must be cautioned about performing tasks which require mental alertness (eg, operating machinery or driving). Systemic exposure may be increased in patients <50 kg and decreased in patients >100 kg. Consider dose reduction if toxicities develop in patients <50 kg (oral and transdermal). Consider a dose increase in patients >100 kg (transdermal).

Potentially significant drug-drug interactions may exist, requiring dose or frequency adjustment, additional monitoring, and/or selection of alternative therapy.

Drug Interactions

Avoid Concomitant Use There are no known interactions where it is recommended to avoid concomitant use.

Decreased Effect

Rivastigmine may decrease the levels/effects of: Anticholinergics; Neuromuscular-Blocking Agents (Nondepolarizing)

The levels/effects of Rivastigmine may be decreased by: Anticholinergics; Dipyridamole

Increased Effect/Toxicity

Rivastigmine may increase the levels/effects of: Antipsychotics; Beta-Blockers; Cholinergic Agonists; Succinylcholine

The levels/effects of Rivastigmine may be increased by: Corticosteroids (Systemic)

Nutritional/Ethanol Interactions

Smoking: Nicotine increases the clearance of rivastigmine by 23%.

Ethanol: Avoid ethanol (due to risk of sedation; may increase GI irritation).

Food: Food delays absorption by 90 minutes, lowers C_{max} by 30% and increases AUC by 30%.

Herb/Nutraceutical: Avoid ginkgo biloba (may increase cholinergic effects).

Adverse Reactions Note: Many concentration-related effects are reported at a lower frequency by transdermal route.

>10%:

Central nervous system: Dizziness (1% to 21%), headache (3% to 17%), agitation (3% to 14%), falling (6% to 12%)

Dermatologic: Application site reactions (including erythema, irritation, pruritus, and rash <1% to 13%)

Gastrointestinal: Nausea (3% to 47%), vomiting (3% to 31%), weight loss (3% to 26%), diarrhea (<1% to 19%), anorexia (3% to 17%), abdominal pain (1% to 13%)

Neuromuscular & skeletal: Tremor (1% to 23%)

1% to 10%:

Cardiovascular: Syncope (3%), hypertension (3%)

Central nervous system: Fatigue (1% to 9%), insomnia (1% to 9%), confusion (8%), depression (4% to 6%), somnolence (4% to 6%), malaise (5%), anxiety (2% to 5%), hallucinations (2% to 5%), psychomotor hyperactivity (3%), aggressiveness (2% to 3%), parkinsonism symptoms worsening (2% to 3%), cogwheel rigidity (1% to 3%), restlessness (1% to 3%), vertigo (≤2%), paranoia (>1%)

Gastrointestinal: Dyspepsia (9%), appetite decreased (1% to 9%), constipation (5%), flatulence (4%), upper abdominal pain (1% to 4%), eructation (2%), dehydration (1% to 2%), sialorrhea (1% to 2%)

Genitourinary: Urinary tract infection (1% to 10%), urinary incontinence (2% to 3%)

Neuromuscular & skeletal: Weakness (2% to 6%), bradykinesia (3% to 4%), hypokinesia (1% to 4%), dyskinesia (1% to 3%), back pain (>1%)

Respiratory: Rhinitis (4%)

Miscellaneous: Accidental trauma (10%), diaphoresis (2% to 4%), flu-like syndrome (3%)

Pharmacodynamics/Kinetics

Duration of Action Anticholinesterase activity (CSF): ~10 hours (6 mg oral dose)

Available Dosage Forms

Capsule, Oral:

Exelon: 1.5 mg, 3 mg, 4.5 mg, 6 mg

Generic: 1.5 mg, 3 mg, 4.5 mg, 6 mg

Patch 24 Hour, Transdermal:

Exelon: 4.6 mg/24 hr (1 ea, 30 ea); 9.5 mg/24 hr (1 ea, 30 ea); 13.3 mg/24 hr (1 ea, 30 ea)

Solution, Oral:

Exelon: 2 mg/mL (120 mL)

General Dosage Range Dosage adjustment recommended (transdermal patch) in patients with hepatic impairment or who develop toxicities.

Oral: *Adults:* Initial: 1.5 mg twice daily; Maintenance: 1.5-6 mg twice daily (maximum: 12 mg daily)

Transdermal patch: *Adults:* Initial: 4.6 mg/24 hours; Maintenance: (9.5-13.3) mg/24 hours (maximum dose: 13.3 mg/24 hours)

Administration

Oral Administer with meals (breakfast and dinner). Capsule should be swallowed whole. Liquid form, which is available for patients who cannot swallow capsules, can be swallowed directly from syringe or mixed with water, soda, or cold fruit juice. Stir well and drink within 4 hours of mixing.

Topical Transdermal patch: Apply transdermal patch to upper or lower back (alternatively, may apply to upper arm or chest). Do not use patch if the pouch seal is broken or if the patch is cut, altered, or damaged. Avoid reapplication to same spot of skin for 14 days (eg, may rotate sections of back). Apply to clean, dry, and hairless skin. Patch should be pressed down firmly by applying pressure with the hand over the entire patch for at least 30 seconds, making sure edges stick well. Do not apply to red, irritated, or broken skin. Avoid areas of recent application of lotion or powder. After removal, fold patch to press adhesive surfaces together, place in previously saved pouch, and discard. Avoid eye contact; wash hands after handling patch. Remove old patch and replace with a new patch every 24 hours (at the same time each day). If a dose is missed or if the patch falls off, apply a new patch immediately and replace the following day at the usual application time. Avoid exposing the patch to external sources of heat (eg, sauna, excessive light) for prolonged periods of time. No more than 1 patch

should be applied daily and existing patch must be removed prior to applying new patch.

Storage/Stability

Oral: Store at 25°C (77°F); excursions permitted between 15°C and 30°C (59°F to 86°F); do not freeze. Store solution in an upright position. Stable at room temperature for up to 4 hours when solution is mixed with cold fruit juice or soda.

Transdermal patch: Store at 25°C (77°F); excursions permitted between 15°C and 30°C (59°F to 86°F). Patches should be kept in sealed pouch until use.

Nursing Actions

Physical Assessment Assess bladder and sphincter adequacy prior to treatment. Monitor weight and vital signs regularly. Educate patient and family about concerning side effects: Falls, fainting, urinary problems, incontinence, loss of appetite, vomiting, bloody stools, weight loss, behavioral changes, aggression, increased confusion. Assess cognitive function at periodic intervals.

Patient Education

• Discuss specific use of drug and side effects with patient as it relates to treatment. (HCAHPS: During this hospital stay, were you given any medicine that you had not taken before? Before giving you any new medicine, how often did hospital staff tell you what the medicine was for? How often did hospital staff describe possible side effects in a way you could understand?)

• Patient may experience dizziness, headache, dyspepsia, nausea, lack of appetite, or diarrhea. Have patient report immediately to prescriber depression, mood changes, dyspnea, significant weight loss, or rash (HCAHPS).

• Educate patient about signs of a significant reaction (eg, wheezing; chest tightness; fever; itching; bad cough; blue skin color; seizures; or swelling of face, lips, tongue, or throat). **Note:** This is not a comprehensive list of all side effects. Patient should consult prescriber for additional questions.

Intended Use and Disclaimer: Should not be printed and given to patients. This information is intended to serve as a concise initial reference for healthcare professionals to use when discussing medications with a patient. You must ultimately rely on your own discretion, experience and judgment in diagnosing, treating and advising patients.

Rizatriptan (rye za TRIP tan)

Brand Names: U.S. Maxalt; Maxalt-MLT

Index Terms MK462

Pharmacologic Category Antimigraine Agent; Serotonin 5-HT$_{1B, 1D}$ Receptor Agonist

Pregnancy Risk Factor C

Lactation Excretion in breast milk unknown/use caution

Breast-Feeding Considerations It is not known if rizatriptan is excreted in breast milk. The manufacturer recommends that caution be exercised when administering rizatriptan to nursing women.

Use Acute treatment of migraine with or without aura

Mechanism of Action/Effect Selective agonist for serotonin receptor in cranial arteries; causes vasoconstriction and relief of migraine

Contraindications Hypersensitivity to rizatriptan or any component of the formulation; documented ischemic heart disease or other significant cardiovascular disease; coronary artery vasospasm (including Prinzmetal's angina); history of stroke or transient ischemic attack; peripheral vascular disease; ischemic bowel disease; uncontrolled hypertension; basilar or hemiplegic migraine; during or within 2 weeks of MAO inhibitors; during or within 24 hours of treatment with another 5-HT$_1$ agonist, or an ergot-containing or ergot-type medication (eg, methysergide, dihydroergotamine)

Warnings/Precautions Only indicated for treatment of acute migraine; not for the prevention of migraines or the treatment of cluster headache. If a patient does not respond to the first dose, the diagnosis of migraine should be reconsidered. Coronary artery vasospasm, transient ischemia, myocardial infarction, ventricular tachycardia/fibrillation, cardiac arrest, and death have been reported with 5-HT$_1$ agonist administration. Patients who experience sensations of chest pain/pressure/tightness or symptoms suggestive of angina following dosing should be evaluated for coronary artery disease or Prinzmetal's angina before receiving additional doses; if dosing is resumed and similar symptoms recur, monitor with ECG. Should not be given to patients who have risk factors for CAD (eg, hypertension, hypercholesterolemia, smoker, obesity, diabetes, strong family history of CAD, menopause, male >40 years of age) without adequate cardiac evaluation. Patients with suspected CAD should have cardiovascular evaluation to rule out CAD before considering use; if cardiovascular evaluation is "satisfactory," first dose should be given in the healthcare provider's office (consider ECG monitoring). Periodic evaluation of cardiovascular status should be done in all patients. Significant elevation in blood pressure, including hypertensive crisis, has also been reported on rare occasions in patients with and without a history of hypertension. Cerebral/subarachnoid hemorrhage, stroke, peripheral vascular ischemia, gastrointestinal ischemia/infarction, splenic infarction and Raynaud's syndrome have been reported with 5-HT$_1$ agonist administration. Use is contraindicated in patients with a history of stroke or transient ischemic attack. Rarely, partial vision loss and blindness (transient and permanent) have been reported with 5-HT$_1$ agonists.

Use with caution in elderly or patients with hepatic or renal impairment (including dialysis patients). Symptoms of agitation, confusion, hallucinations, hyper-reflexia, myoclonus, shivering, and tachycardia may occur with concomitant proserotonergic drugs (eg, SSRIs/SNRIs or triptans) or agents which reduce rizatriptan's metabolism. Concurrent use of serotonin precursors (eg, tryptophan) is not recommended. If concomitant administration with SSRIs is warranted, monitor closely, especially at initiation and with dose increases. Overuse of medications for acute migraine, including 5-HT$_1$ agonists, may lead to headache exacerbation. Maxalt-MLT® tablets contain phenylalanine.

Drug Interactions

Avoid Concomitant Use

Avoid concomitant use of Rizatriptan with any of the following: Ergot Derivatives; MAO Inhibitors

Decreased Effect There are no known significant interactions involving a decrease in effect.

Increased Effect/Toxicity

Rizatriptan may increase the levels/effects of: Antipsychotics; Droxidopa; Ergot Derivatives; Metoclopramide; Serotonin Modulators

The levels/effects of Rizatriptan may be increased by: Antipsychotics; Ergot Derivatives; MAO Inhibitors; Propranolol

Nutritional/Ethanol Interactions Food: Food delays absorption.

Adverse Reactions 1% to 10%:

Cardiovascular: Chest pain (<2% to 3%), flushing (>1%), palpitation (>1%)

Central nervous system: Dizziness (4% to 9%), somnolence (4% to 8%), fatigue (adults 4% to 7%; children >1%), pain (3%), headache (≤2%), euphoria (>1%), hypoesthesia (>1%)

Dermatologic: Skin flushing

Gastrointestinal: Nausea (4% to 6%), xerostomia (3%), abdominal discomfort (children >1%), diarrhea (>1%), vomiting (>1%)

Neuromuscular & skeletal: Weakness (4% to 7%), paresthesia (3% to 4%); neck, throat, and jaw pain/tightness/pressure (≤2%), tremor (>1%)

Respiratory: Dyspnea (>1%)

Miscellaneous: Feeling of heaviness (<1% to 2%)

Pharmacodynamics/Kinetics

Onset of Action Most patients have response to treatment within 2 hours

Available Dosage Forms

Tablet, Oral:

Maxalt: 5 mg, 10 mg

Generic: 5 mg, 10 mg

Tablet Dispersible, Oral:

Maxalt-MLT: 5 mg, 10 mg

Generic: 5 mg, 10 mg

General Dosage Range Oral:
Children 6-17 years: <40 kg: 5 mg as a single dose; ≥40 kg: 10 mg as a single dose
Adults: 5-10 mg once, repeat if needed (maximum: 30 mg/day)

Administration
Oral May be administered with or without food. For orally-disintegrating tablets (Maxalt-MLT®), patient should be instructed to place tablet on tongue and allow to dissolve. Dissolved tablet will be swallowed with saliva.

Storage/Stability Store at room temperature of 15°C to 30°C (59°F to 86°F); orally disintegrating tablets should be stored in blister pack until administration.

Nursing Actions
Physical Assessment For use only with clear diagnosis of migraine. Presence of or risk for coronary disease should be assessed prior to beginning therapy. Monitor for hypertension, cardiac events, drowsiness, nausea/vomiting, chest pain, and palpitations. Teach patient proper use (treatment of acute migraine).

Patient Education
- Discuss specific use of drug and side effects with patient as it relates to treatment. (HCAHPS: During this hospital stay, were you given any medicine that you had not taken before? Before giving you any new medicine, how often did hospital staff tell you what the medicine was for? How often did hospital staff describe possible side effects in a way you could understand?)
- Patient may experience fatigue, head heaviness or pressure, paresthesia, or asthenia. Have patient report immediately to prescriber vision changes, blindness, constipation, considerable dyspepsia, melena, weight loss, leg cramps, leg pain, temperature sensitivity, paresthesia of feet, dyspnea, mood changes, skin discoloration, serotonin syndrome (ie, dizziness, severe headache, agitation, hallucinations, tachycardia, arrhythmia, flushing, tremors, hyperhidrosis, change in balance, illogical thinking, severe nausea, significant diarrhea), signs of severe cardiac abnormalities, strength differences from one side to another, or difficulty speaking or thinking (HCAHPS).
- Educate patient about signs of a significant reaction (eg, wheezing; chest tightness; fever; itching; bad cough; blue skin color; seizures; or swelling of face, lips, tongue, or throat). **Note:** This is not a comprehensive list of all side effects. Patient should consult prescriber for additional questions.

Intended Use and Disclaimer: Should not be printed and given to patients. This information is intended to serve as a concise initial reference for healthcare professionals to use when discussing medications with a patient. You must ultimately rely on your own discretion, experience and judgment in diagnosing, treating and advising patients.

Dietary Considerations Some products may contain phenylalanine.

Roflumilast (roe FLUE mi last)

Brand Names: U.S. Daliresp
Pharmacologic Category Phosphodiesterase-4 Enzyme Inhibitor
Medication Guide Available Yes
Pregnancy Risk Factor C
Breast-Feeding Considerations Roflumilast and/or its metabolites are excreted into the breast milk of lactating rats. Excretion into human breast milk is likely. Avoid use while breast-feeding.
Use Adjunct to bronchodilator therapy in the maintenance treatment of severe chronic obstructive pulmonary disease (COPD) associated with chronic bronchitis
Mechanism of Action/Effect Roflumilast and its active metabolite selectively inhibit phosphodiesterase-4 (PDE4) leading to an accumulation of cyclic AMP (cAMP) within inflammatory and structural cells important in the development of COPD. Inflammation, pulmonary remodeling, and mucociliary malfunction are decreased.
Contraindications Moderate or severe hepatic impairment (Child-Pugh class B or C)

Canadian labeling: Additional contraindication (not in U.S. labeling): Hypersensitivity to roflumilast or any component of the formulation

Warnings/Precautions Not indicated for relieving acute bronchospasms or for use as monotherapy of COPD; use only as adjunctive therapy to bronchodilator therapy. Neuropsychiatric effects (eg, anxiety, depression) have been reported with use; rarely, suicidal behavior/ ideation and completed suicide were reported. Avoid use in patients with a history of depression with suicidal behavior/ideations; instruct patients/caregivers to report psychiatric symptoms and consider discontinuation of therapy in such patients. Systemic exposure may be increased in patients with mild hepatic impairment; use in moderate-to-severe impairment is contraindicated.

May cause weight loss and/or diarrhea (sometimes severe); weight loss usually observed within 6 months of initiating therapy and diarrhea within 4 weeks. Instruct patients to monitor weight regularly. Avoid initiation of therapy or discontinue therapy with unexplained/pronounced weight loss.

Drug Interactions
Avoid Concomitant Use
Avoid concomitant use of Roflumilast with any of the following: CYP3A4 Inducers (Strong); Rifampin

Decreased Effect

The levels/effects of Roflumilast may be decreased by: Bosentan; CYP3A4 Inducers (Strong); Dabrafenib; Deferasirox; Herbs (CYP3A4 Inducers); Rifampin

Increased Effect/Toxicity

Roflumilast may increase the levels/effects of: Immunosuppressants

The levels/effects of Roflumilast may be increased by: Cimetidine; Ciprofloxacin (Systemic); FluvoxaMINE

Adverse Reactions

2% to 10%:

Central nervous system: Headache (4%), dizziness (2%), insomnia (2%)

Endocrine & metabolic: Weight loss (5% to 10% of body weight: 8% to 20%; >10% loss: 7%)

Gastrointestinal: Diarrhea (10%), nausea (5%), decreased appetite (2%)

Infection: Influenza (3%)

Neuromuscular & skeletal: Back pain (3%)

Available Dosage Forms

Tablet, Oral:

Daliresp: 500 mcg

General Dosage Range Oral: *Adults:* 500 mcg once daily

Administration

Oral Administer without regard to meals.

Storage/Stability Store at 20°C to 25°C (68°F to 77°F), excursions permitted from 15°C to 30°C (59°F to 86°F).

Nursing Actions

Physical Assessment This drug reduces inflammation in the lungs, which helps to slow progression of COPD. It is not a bronchodilator and therefore is not to be used for treatment of acute bronchospasms. This drug can cause depression, thoughts of suicide, or mood swings. Instruct patient and family to be aware of behavior or mood changes. If patient has moderate-to-severe liver damage, roflumilast is not indicated. Monitor patient's weight, as rapid weight loss is a serious side effect.

Patient Education

• Discuss specific use of drug and side effects with patient as it relates to treatment. (HCAHPS: During this hospital stay, were you given any medicine that you had not taken before? Before giving you any new medicine, how often did hospital staff tell you what the medicine was for? How often did hospital staff describe possible side effects in a way you could understand?)

• Patient may experience dizziness, dyspepsia, nausea, diarrhea, weight loss, headache, or insomnia. Have patient report immediately to prescriber uncontrollable breaking attack, tachycardia, depression, nervousness, emotional instability, illogical thinking, anxiety, or rash (HCAHPS).

• Educate patient about signs of a significant reaction (eg, wheezing; chest tightness; fever; itching; bad cough; blue skin color; seizures; or swelling of face, lips, tongue, or throat). **Note:** This is not a comprehensive list of all side effects. Patient should consult prescriber for additional questions.

Intended Use and Disclaimer: Should not be printed and given to patients. This information is intended to serve as a concise initial reference for healthcare professionals to use when discussing medications with a patient. You must ultimately rely on your own discretion, experience and judgment in diagnosing, treating and advising patients.

Dietary Considerations May be given with or without food.

Ropinirole (roe PIN i role)

Brand Names: U.S. Requip; Requip XL

Index Terms Ropinirole Hydrochloride

Pharmacologic Category Anti-Parkinson's Agent, Dopamine Agonist

Medication Safety Issues

Sound-alike/look-alike issues:

Requip® may be confused with Reglan®

ROPINIRole may be confused with RisperDAL®, risperiDONE, ropivacaine

Pregnancy Risk Factor C

Lactation Excretion in breast milk unknown/not recommended

Breast-Feeding Considerations It is not known if ropinirole is excreted into breast milk. Ropinirole inhibits prolactin secretion in humans and may potentially inhibit lactation. Due to the potential for serious adverse reactions, the manufacturer recommends that a decision be made whether to discontinue nursing or discontinue the drug, taking into account the importance of the drug to the mother.

Use Treatment of idiopathic Parkinson's disease; in patients with early Parkinson's disease who were not receiving concomitant levodopa therapy as well as in patients with advanced disease on concomitant levodopa; treatment of moderate-to-severe primary Restless Legs Syndrome (RLS)

Contraindications Hypersensitivity to ropinirole or any component of the formulation

Warnings/Precautions Syncope, sometimes associated with bradycardia, was observed in association with ropinirole in both early Parkinson's disease (without levodopa) patients and advanced Parkinson's disease (with levodopa) patients. Dopamine agonists appear to impair the systemic regulation of blood pressure resulting in postural hypotension, especially during dose escalation. Parkinson's disease patients appear to have an impaired capacity to respond to a postural challenge; use with caution in patients at risk of hypotension (ie, those receiving antihypertensive or antiarrhythmic drugs) or where transient hypotensive episodes would be poorly tolerated (cardiovascular disease or cerebrovascular disease). Parkinson's patients being treated with dopaminergic agonists ordinarily require careful monitoring for signs and symptoms of postural hypotension, especially during dose escalation, and should be informed of this risk.

May cause hallucinations (dose dependent); risk may be increased in the elderly. Use with caution in patients with pre-existing dyskinesia, hepatic or severe renal dysfunction (use in patients with severe renal impairment and who are not undergoing regular hemodialysis is not recommended in the Canadian labeling). Avoid use in patients with a major psychotic disorder; may exacerbate psychosis.

Patients treated with ropinirole have reported falling asleep while engaging in activities of daily living; this has been reported to occur without significant warning signs. Monitor for daytime somnolence or pre-existing sleep disorder; caution with concomitant sedating medication; discontinue if significant daytime sleepiness or episodes of falling asleep occur. Patients must be cautioned about performing tasks which require mental alertness (eg, operating machinery or driving). Use with caution in patients receiving other CNS depressants or psychoactive agents. Effects with other sedative drugs or ethanol may be potentiated.

Dopamine agonists have been associated with compulsive behaviors and/or loss of impulse control, which has manifested as pathological gambling, libido increases (hypersexuality), and/or binge eating. Causality has not been established, and controversy exists as to whether this phenomenon is related to the underlying disease, prior behaviors/addictions and/or drug therapy. Dose reduction or discontinuation of therapy has been reported to reverse these behaviors in some, but not all cases. Risk for melanoma development is increased in Parkinson's disease patients; drug causation or factors contributing to risk have not been established. Patients should be monitored closely and periodic skin examinations should be performed.

Some patients treated for RLS may experience worsening of symptoms in the early morning hours (rebound) or an increase and/or spread of daytime symptoms (augmentation); clinical management of these phenomena has not been evaluated in controlled clinical trials. Pathologic degenerative changes were observed in the retinas of albino rats during studies with this agent, but were not observed in the retinas of albino mice or in other species. The significance of these data for humans remains uncertain.

Other dopaminergic agents have been associated with a syndrome resembling neuroleptic malignant syndrome on withdrawal or significant dosage reduction after long-term use. Risk of fibrotic complications (eg, pleural effusion/fibrosis, interstitial lung disease) and melanoma has been reported in patients receiving ropinirole; drug causation has not been established.

Drug Interactions
Avoid Concomitant Use
Avoid concomitant use of ROPINIRole with any of the following: Amisulpride; Sulpiride

Decreased Effect
ROPINIRole may decrease the levels/effects of: Amisulpride; Antipsychotics (Typical); Sulpiride

The levels/effects of ROPINIRole may be decreased by: Amisulpride; Antipsychotics (Atypical); Antipsychotics (Typical); CYP1A2 Inducers (Strong); Cyproterone; Metoclopramide; Sulpiride

Increased Effect/Toxicity
ROPINIRole may increase the levels/effects of: BuPROPion

The levels/effects of ROPINIRole may be increased by: Abiraterone Acetate; Alcohol (Ethyl); Ciprofloxacin (Systemic); CNS Depressants; CYP1A2 Inhibitors (Moderate); CYP1A2 Inhibitors (Strong); Deferasirox; Estrogen Derivatives; MAO Inhibitors; Methylphenidate; Vemurafenib

Nutritional/Ethanol Interactions
Ethanol: Avoid ethanol (may increase CNS depression).

Herb/Nutraceutical: Avoid kava kava, gotu kola, valerian, St John's wort (may increase CNS depression).

Adverse Reactions
Data inclusive of trials in early Parkinson's disease (without levodopa) and Restless Legs Syndrome:

>10%:

Cardiovascular: Syncope (1% to 12%)

Central nervous system: Somnolence (11% to 40%), dizziness (6% to 40%), fatigue (8% to 11%)

Gastrointestinal: Nausea (immediate release: 40% to 60%; extended release: 19%), vomiting (11% to 12%)

Miscellaneous: Viral infection (11%)

1% to 10%:

Cardiovascular: Dependent/leg edema (2% to 7%), orthostasis (1% to 6%), hypertension (5%), chest pain (4%), flushing (3%), palpitation (3%), peripheral ischemia (2% to 3%), atrial fibrillation (2%), extrasystoles (2%), hypotension (2%), tachycardia (2%)

Central nervous system: Pain (3% to 8%), headache (extended release: 6%), confusion (5%), hallucinations (up to 5%; dose related), hypoesthesia (4%), amnesia (3%), malaise (3%), yawning (3%), concentration impaired (2%), vertigo (2%)

Dermatologic: Hyperhidrosis (3%)

Gastrointestinal: Dyspepsia (4% to 10%), abdominal pain (3% to 7%), constipation (≥5%), xerostomia (3% to 5%), diarrhea (5%), anorexia (4%), flatulence (3%)

Genitourinary: Urinary tract infection (5%), impotence (3%)

Hepatic: Alkaline phosphatase increased (3%)

Neuromuscular & skeletal: Weakness (6%), arthralgia (4%), muscle cramps (3%), paresthesia (3%), hyperkinesia (2%)

Ocular: Abnormal vision (6%), xerophthalmia (2%)

Respiratory: Pharyngitis (6% to 9%), rhinitis (4%), sinusitis (4%), bronchitis (3%), dyspnea (3%), influenza (3%), cough (3%), nasal congestion (2%)

Miscellaneous: Diaphoresis increased (3% to 6%)

Advanced Parkinson's disease (with levodopa):
>10%:

Central nervous system: Dizziness (immediate release: 26%; extended-release: 8%), somnolence (immediate release: 20%, extended release: 7%), headache (17%)

Gastrointestinal: Nausea (immediate release: 30%; extended-release: 11%)

Neuromuscular & skeletal: Dyskinesias (immediate release: 34%; extended-release: 13%; dose related)

1% to 10%:

Cardiovascular: Hypotension (2% to 5%; including orthostatic), peripheral edema (4%), syncope (3%), hypertension (3%; dose related)

Central nervous system: Hallucinations (7% to 10%; dose related), confusion (9%), anxiety (2% to 6%), amnesia (5%), nervousness (5%), pain (5%), vertigo (4%), abnormal dreaming (3%), paresis (3%), aggravated parkinsonism, insomnia

Gastrointestinal: Abdominal pain (6% to 9%), vomiting (7%), constipation (4% to 6%), diarrhea (3% to 5%), xerostomia (2% to 5%), dysphagia (2%), flatulence (2%), salivation increased (2%), weight loss (2%)

Genitourinary: Urinary tract infection (6%), pyuria (2%), urinary incontinence (2%)

Hematologic: Anemia (2%)

Neuromuscular & skeletal: Falls (2% to 10%; dose related), arthralgia (7%), tremor (6%), hypokinesia (5%), paresthesia (5%), arthritis (3%), back pain (3%)

Ocular: Diplopia (2%)

Respiratory: Upper respiratory tract infection (9%), dyspnea (3%)

Miscellaneous: Injury, diaphoresis increased (7%), viral infection, increased drug level (7%)

Other adverse effects (all phase 2/3 trials for Parkinson's disease and Restless Leg Syndrome): ≥1%: Asthma, BUN increased, depression, gastroenteritis, gastrointestinal reflux, irritability, migraine, muscle spasm, myalgia, neck pain, neuralgia, osteoarthritis, pharyngolaryngeal pain, rash, rigors, sleep disorder, tendonitis

Available Dosage Forms

Tablet, Oral:

Requip: 0.25 mg, 0.5 mg, 1 mg, 2 mg, 3 mg, 4 mg, 5 mg

Generic: 0.25 mg, 0.5 mg, 1 mg, 2 mg, 3 mg, 4 mg, 5 mg

Tablet Extended Release 24 Hour, Oral:

Requip XL: 2 mg, 4 mg, 6 mg, 8 mg, 12 mg

Generic: 2 mg, 4 mg, 6 mg, 8 mg, 12 mg

General Dosage Range Oral: *Adults:*

Parkinson's:

Immediate release: Initial: 0.25 mg 3 times/day; Maintenance: 0.75-24 mg/day in 3 divided doses

Extended release: Initial: 2 mg once daily; Maintenance: 2-24 mg once daily (maximum: 24 mg/day)

Restless legs: Immediate release: Initial: 0.25 mg prior to bedtime; Maintenance: 0.25-4 mg prior to bedtime

Administration

Oral May be administered without regard to meals; taking with food may reduce nausea. Swallow extended-release tablet whole; do not crush, split, or chew.

Storage/Stability Store at controlled room temperature of 20°C to 25°C (68°F to 77°F). Protect from light.

Nursing Actions

Physical Assessment Monitor blood pressure periodically. Monitor for CNS depression/somnolence.

Patient Education

- Discuss specific use of drug and side effects with patient as it relates to treatment. (HCAHPS: During this hospital stay, were you given any medicine that you had not taken before? Before giving you any new medicine, how often did hospital staff tell you what the medicine was for? How often did hospital staff describe possible side effects in a way you could understand?)

- Patient may experience presyncope, fatigue, blurred vision, illogical thinking, dizziness, or nausea. Have patient report immediately to prescriber narcolepsy, severe diarrhea, significant asthenia, or rash (HCAHPS).

- Educate patient about signs of a significant reaction (eg, wheezing; chest tightness; fever; itching; bad cough; blue skin color; seizures; or swelling of face, lips, tongue, or throat). **Note:** This is not a comprehensive list of all side effects. Patient should consult prescriber for additional questions.

Intended Use and Disclaimer: Should not be printed and given to patients. This information is intended to serve as a concise initial reference for healthcare professionals to use when discussing medications with a patient. You must ultimately rely on your own discretion, experience and judgment in diagnosing, treating and advising patients.

Dietary Considerations May be taken without regard to meals; taking with food may reduce nausea.

Related Information

Oral Medications That Should Not Be Crushed or Altered *on page 1712*

Rosiglitazone (roh si GLI ta zone)

Brand Names: U.S. Avandia

Pharmacologic Category Antidiabetic Agent, Thiazolidinedione

Medication Safety Issues

Sound-alike/look-alike issues:

Avandia® may be confused with Avalide®, Coumadin®, Prandin®

High alert medication:

The Institute for Safe Medication Practices (ISMP) includes this medication among its list of drug classes which have a heightened risk of causing significant patient harm when used in error.

International issues:

Avandia [U.S., Canada, and multiple international markets] may be confused with Avanza brand name for mirtazapine [Australia]

Medication Guide Available Yes

Pregnancy Risk Factor C

Lactation Excretion in breast milk unknown/not recommended

Breast-Feeding Considerations It is not known if rosiglitazone is excreted in breast milk. Although breast-feeding is encouraged for all women, including those with diabetes, the safety of rosiglitazone during breast-feeding has not yet been established (Metzger, 2007). Breast-feeding is not recommended by the manufacturer.

Use Type 2 diabetes: Adjunct to diet and exercise to improve glycemic control in adults with type 2 diabetes mellitus (noninsulin dependent, NIDDM); may be used as monotherapy or in combination with metformin or a sulfonylurea.

Mechanism of Action/Effect Thiazolidinedione antidiabetic agent that lowers blood glucose by improving target cell response to insulin, without increasing pancreatic insulin secretion. It has a mechanism of action that is dependent on the presence of insulin for activity.

Contraindications

U.S. labeling: NYHA Class III/IV heart failure (initiation of therapy)

Canadian labeling: Hypersensitivity to rosiglitazone or any component of the formulation; any stage of heart failure (eg, NYHA Class I, II, III, IV); serious hepatic impairment; pregnancy

Warnings/Precautions [U.S. Boxed Warning]: Thiazolidinediones, including rosiglitazone, may cause or exacerbate congestive heart failure; closely monitor for signs/symptoms of congestive heart failure (eg, rapid weight gain, dyspnea, edema), particularly after initiation or dose increases. If heart failure develops, treat accordingly and consider dose reduction or discontinuation. Not recommended for use in any patient with symptomatic heart failure. In the U.S., initiation of therapy is contraindicated in patients with NYHA class III or IV heart failure; in Canada use is contraindicated in patients with any stage of heart failure (NYHA class I, II, III, IV). Use with caution in patients with edema; may increase plasma volume and/or cause fluid retention, leading to heart failure. Monitor for signs/symptoms of heart failure. Dose-related weight gain observed with use; mechanism unknown but likely associated with fluid retention and fat accumulation. Use may also be associated with an increased risk of angina and MI. Use caution in patients at risk for cardiovascular events and monitor closely. Discontinue if any deterioration in cardiac status occurs.

[U.S. Boxed Warning]: Due to cardiovascular risks, rosiglitazone-containing medications are only available through the Avandia-Rosiglitazone Medicines Access Program™. Patients and prescribers must be registered and meet conditions of the program. Call 1-800-282-6342 or visit www.avandia.com for more information.

Should not be used in diabetic ketoacidosis. Mechanism requires the presence of insulin; therefore, use in type 1 diabetes (insulin dependent, IDDM) is not recommended. It may be necessary to discontinue therapy and administer insulin if the patient is exposed to stress (fever, trauma, infection, surgery). Do not initiate in patients with stable ischemic heart disease due to an increased risk of cardiovascular complications (Fihn, 2012).

Potentially significant drug-drug interactions may exist, requiring dose or frequency adjustment, additional monitoring, and/or selection of alternative therapy.

Use with caution in patients with elevated transaminases (AST or ALT); do not initiate in patients with active liver disease or ALT >2.5 times ULN at baseline; evaluate patients with ALT ≤2.5 times ULN at baseline or during therapy for cause of enzyme elevation; during therapy, if ALT >3 times ULN, reevaluate levels promptly and discontinue if elevation persists or if jaundice occurs at any time during use. Idiosyncratic hepatotoxicity has been reported with another thiazolidinedione agent (troglitazone); avoid use in patients who previously experienced jaundice during troglitazone therapy. Monitoring should include periodic determinations of liver function. Increased incidence of bone fractures in females treated with rosiglitazone observed during analysis of long-term trial; majority of fractures occurred in the upper arm, hand, and foot (differing from the hip or spine fractures usually associated with postmenopausal osteoporosis). May decrease hemoglobin/hematocrit and/or WBC count (slight); effects may be related to increased plasma volume and/or dose related; use with caution in patients with anemia; may reduce hemoglobin and hematocrit.

Rosiglitazone has been associated with new onset and/or worsening of macular edema in patients with diabetes. Rosiglitazone should be used with caution in patients with a pre-existing macular edema or diabetic retinopathy. Discontinuation of rosiglitazone should be considered in any patient who reports visual deterioration. In addition, ophthalmological consultation should be initiated in these patients. Use with caution in premenopausal, anovulatory women; may result in resumption of ovulation, increasing the risk of pregnancy.

Additional Canadian warnings (not included in U.S. labeling): If glycemic control is inadequate, rosiglitazone may be added to metformin or a sulfonylurea (if metformin use is contraindicated or not tolerated); use of triple therapy (rosiglitazone in combination with both metformin and a sulfonylurea) is not indicated due to increased risks of heart failure and fluid retention.

Drug Interactions
Avoid Concomitant Use There are no known interactions where it is recommended to avoid concomitant use.

Decreased Effect
The levels/effects of Rosiglitazone may be decreased by: Cholestyramine Resin; Corticosteroids (Orally Inhaled); Corticosteroids (Systemic); CYP2C8 Inducers (Strong); Dabrafenib; Loop Diuretics; Luteinizing Hormone-Releasing Hormone Analogs; Rifampin; Somatropin; Thiazide Diuretics

Increased Effect/Toxicity
Rosiglitazone may increase the levels/effects of: CYP2C8 Substrates; Hypoglycemic Agents

The levels/effects of Rosiglitazone may be increased by: CYP2C8 Inhibitors (Moderate); CYP2C8 Inhibitors (Strong); Deferasirox; Gemfibrozil; Herbs (Hypoglycemic Properties); Insulin; MAO Inhibitors; Mifepristone; Pegvisomant; Pregabalin; Salicylates; Selective Serotonin Reuptake Inhibitors; Trimethoprim; Vasodilators (Organic Nitrates)

Nutritional/Ethanol Interactions
Ethanol: Ethanol may cause hypoglycemia. Management: Avoid ethanol during therapy.

Herb/Nutraceutical: Concurrent use of some herbal products may enhance hypoglycemic effects. Management: Avoid alfalfa, aloe, bilberry, bitter melon, burdock, celery, damiana, fenugreek, garcinia, garlic, ginger, ginseng (American), gymnema, marshmallow, stinging nettle.

Adverse Reactions Note: The rate of certain adverse reactions (eg, anemia, edema, hypoglycemia) may be higher with some combination therapies.

>10%: Endocrine & metabolic: HDL-cholesterol increased, LDL-cholesterol increased, total cholesterol increased, weight gain

1% to 10%:
Cardiovascular: Edema (5%), hypertension (4%); heart failure/CHF (up to 2% to 3% in patients receiving insulin; incidence likely higher in patients with pre-existing HF; myocardial ischemia (3%; incidence likely higher in patients with preexisting CAD)
Central nervous system: Headache (6%)
Endocrine & metabolic: Hypoglycemia (1% to 3%; combination therapy with insulin: 12% to 14%)
Gastrointestinal: Diarrhea (3%)
Hematologic: Anemia (2%)
Neuromuscular & skeletal: Fractures (up to 9%; incidence greater in females; usually upper arm, hand, or foot), arthralgia (5%), back pain (4% to 5%)
Respiratory: Upper respiratory tract infection (4% to 10%), nasopharyngitis (6%)
Miscellaneous: Injury (8%)

Pharmacodynamics/Kinetics
Onset of Action Delayed; Maximum effect: Up to 12 weeks

Available Dosage Forms
Tablet, Oral:
Avandia: 2 mg, 4 mg, 8 mg

General Dosage Range Oral: *Adults:* Initial: 4 mg daily in 1-2 divided doses; Maintenance: 4-8 mg daily in 1-2 divided doses; Maximum dose: 8 mg daily

Administration
Oral May be administered without regard to meals.

Storage/Stability Store at 25°C (77°F); excursions are permitted between 15°C and 30°C (59°F and 86°F). Protect from light.

Nursing Actions
Physical Assessment Monitor laboratory results closely. Assess for signs of fluid retention and heart failure. Monitor weight. Monitor response to therapy closely until response is stable. Advise women using oral contraceptives about need for alternative method of contraception. Teach risks of hyperglycemia, its symptoms, treatment, and predisposing conditions. Refer patient to a diabetic educator, if possible.

Patient Education

- Discuss specific use of drug and side effects with patient as it relates to treatment. (HCAHPS: During this hospital stay, were you given any medicine that you had not taken before? Before giving you any new medicine, how often did hospital staff tell you what the medicine was for? How often did hospital staff describe possible side effects in a way you could understand?)
- Patient may experience headache, rhinitis, or pharyngitis. Have patient report immediately to prescriber signs of hepatic impairment, strength differences from one side to another, difficulty speaking or thinking, change in balance, blurred vision, osteodynia, vision changes, severe asthenia, or signs of hypoglycemia (HCAHPS).
- Educate patient about signs of a significant reaction (eg, wheezing; chest tightness; fever; itching; bad cough; blue skin color; seizures; or swelling of face, lips, tongue, or throat). **Note:** This is not a comprehensive list of all side effects. Patient should consult prescriber for additional questions.

Intended Use and Disclaimer: Should not be printed and given to patients. This information is intended to serve as a concise initial reference for healthcare professionals to use when discussing medications with a patient. You must ultimately rely on your own discretion, experience and judgment in diagnosing, treating and advising patients.

Dietary Considerations Management of type 2 diabetes mellitus (noninsulin dependent, NIDDM) should include diet control.

Rosiglitazone and Glimepiride
(roh si GLI ta zone & GLYE me pye ride)

Brand Names: U.S. Avandaryl

Index Terms Glimepiride and Rosiglitazone Maleate

Pharmacologic Category Antidiabetic Agent, Sulfonylurea; Antidiabetic Agent, Thiazolidinedione

Medication Safety Issues
High alert medication:

The Institute for Safe Medication Practices (ISMP) includes this medication among its list of drugs which have a heightened risk of causing significant patient harm when used in error.

Medication Guide Available Yes

Pregnancy Risk Factor C

Use Type 2 diabetes: Adjunct to diet and exercise to improve glycemic control in adults with type 2 diabetes mellitus (noninsulin dependent, NIDDM) and in whom dual rosiglitazone/glimepiride therapy is appropriate

Available Dosage Forms
Tablet:

Avandaryl®: 4 mg/1 mg: Rosiglitazone 4 mg and glimepiride 1 mg; 4 mg/2 mg: Rosiglitazone 4 mg and glimepiride 2 mg; 4 mg/4 mg: Rosiglitazone 4 mg and glimepiride 4 mg; 8 mg/2 mg: Rosiglitazone 8 mg and glimepiride 2 mg; 8 mg/4 mg: Rosiglitazone 8 mg and glimepiride 4 mg

General Dosage Range Dosage adjustment recommended in patients with hepatic or renal impairment

Oral:

Adults: Initial: Rosiglitazone 4 mg and glimepiride 1-2 mg once daily; Maintenance: Rosiglitazone 4-8 mg and glimepiride 1-4 mg once daily

Elderly: Initial: Rosiglitazone 4 mg and glimepiride 1 mg once daily

Administration
Oral Should be administered with the first meal of the day.

Nursing Actions
Physical Assessment See individual agents.

Patient Education

- Discuss specific use of drug and side effects with patient as it relates to treatment. (HCAHPS: During this hospital stay, were you given any medicine that you had not taken before? Before giving you any new medicine, how often did hospital staff tell you what the medicine was for? How often did hospital staff describe possible side effects in a way you could understand?)
- Patient may experience headache, rhinitis, or pharyngitis. Have patient report immediately to prescriber signs of hepatic impairment, strength differences from one side to another, difficulty speaking or thinking, change in balance, blurred vision, osteodynia, ecchymosis, hemorrhaging, vision changes, severe asthenia, or signs of hypoglycemia (HCAHPS).
- Educate patient about signs of a significant reaction (eg, wheezing; chest tightness; fever; itching; bad cough; blue skin color; seizures; or swelling of face, lips, tongue, or throat). **Note:** This is not a comprehensive list of all side effects. Patient should consult prescriber for additional questions.

Intended Use and Disclaimer: Should not be printed and given to patients. This information is intended to serve as a concise initial reference for healthcare professionals to use when discussing medications with a patient. You must ultimately rely on your own discretion, experience and judgment in diagnosing, treating and advising patients.

Related Information
Glimepiride *on page 740*
Rosiglitazone *on page 1384*

Rosiglitazone and Metformin
(roh si GLI ta zone & met FOR min)

Brand Names: U.S. Avandamet
Index Terms Metformin and Rosiglitazone; Metformin Hydrochloride and Rosiglitazone Maleate; Rosiglitazone Maleate and Metformin Hydrochloride
Pharmacologic Category Antidiabetic Agent, Biguanide; Antidiabetic Agent, Thiazolidinedione
Medication Safety Issues
Sound-alike/look-alike issues:
Avandamet® may be confused with Anzemet®
High alert medication:
The Institute for Safe Medication Practices (ISMP) includes this medication among its list of drug classes which have a heightened risk of causing significant patient harm when used in error.
Medication Guide Available Yes
Pregnancy Risk Factor C
Use Type 2 diabetes: As an adjunct to diet and exercise to improve glycemic control in adults with type 2 diabetes mellitus (noninsulin dependent, NIDDM) when treatment with both rosiglitazone and metformin is appropriate.
Available Dosage Forms
Tablet, Oral:
Avandamet: 2/500: Rosiglitazone 2 mg and metformin 500 mg; 4/500: Rosiglitazone 4 mg and metformin 500 mg; 2/1000: Rosiglitazone 2 mg and metformin 1000 mg; 4/1000: Rosiglitazone 4 mg and metformin 1000 mg
General Dosage Range Oral: *Adults:* Initial: Rosiglitazone 2 mg and metformin 500 mg once or twice daily; titrate gradually (maximum: rosiglitazone 8 mg daily; metformin 2000 mg daily)
Administration
Oral Administer with meals, generally in divided doses. Patients who are NPO may need to have their dose held to avoid hypoglycemia.
Nursing Actions
Physical Assessment See individual agents.
Patient Education
• Discuss specific use of drug and side effects with patient as it relates to treatment. (HCAHPS: During this hospital stay, were you given any medicine that you had not taken before? Before giving you any new medicine, how often did hospital staff tell you what the medicine was for? How often did hospital staff describe possible side effects in a way you could understand?)
• Patient may experience dyspepsia, diarrhea, flatulence, headache, rhinitis, pharyngitis, arthralgia, or dizziness. Have patient report immediately to prescriber signs of hepatic impairment, strength differences from one side

to another, difficulty speaking or thinking, change in balance, blurred vision, osteodynia, vision changes, severe asthenia, signs of hypoglycemia, or signs of lactic acidosis (HCAHPS).
• Educate patient about signs of a significant reaction (eg, wheezing; chest tightness; fever; itching; bad cough; blue skin color; seizures; or swelling of face, lips, tongue, or throat). **Note:** This is not a comprehensive list of all side effects. Patient should consult prescriber for additional questions.

Intended Use and Disclaimer: Should not be printed and given to patients. This information is intended to serve as a concise initial reference for healthcare professionals to use when discussing medications with a patient. You must ultimately rely on your own discretion, experience and judgment in diagnosing, treating and advising patients.
Related Information
MetFORMIN *on page 1014*
Rosiglitazone *on page 1384*

Rosuvastatin (roe soo va STAT in)

Brand Names: U.S. Crestor
Index Terms Rosuvastatin Calcium
Pharmacologic Category Antilipemic Agent, HMG-CoA Reductase Inhibitor
Medication Safety Issues
Sound-alike/look-alike issues:
Rosuvastatin may be confused with atorvaSTA-Tin, nystatin, pitavastatin
Pregnancy Risk Factor X
Lactation Excretion in breast milk unknown/contraindicated
Breast-Feeding Considerations It is not known if rosuvastatin is excreted into breast milk. Due to the potential for serious adverse reactions in a nursing infant, use while breast-feeding is contraindicated by the manufacturer.
Use
Heterozygous familial hypercholesterolemia in children: Adjunct to diet to reduce total cholesterol, low-density lipoprotein cholesterol (LDL-C), and apolipoprotein B (apo B) levels in adolescent males and females who are at least 1 year postmenarche and are 10-17 years of age with heterozygous familial hypercholesteremia if after an adequate trial of diet therapy the following findings are present: LDL-C more than 190 mg/dL or more than 160 mg/dL and there is a positive family history of premature cardiovascular (CV) disease or 2 or more other CV disease risk factors.
Homozygous familial hypercholesterolemia: To reduce LDL-C, total cholesterol, and apo B in adults with homozygous familial hypercholesterolemia as an adjunct to other lipid-lowering

treatments (eg, LDL apheresis) or alone if such treatments are unavailable.

Hyperlipidemia and mixed dyslipidemia: Adjunctive therapy to diet to reduce elevated total cholesterol, LDL-C, apo B, non–high-density lipoprotein cholesterol (non-HDL-C), and triglyceride levels, and to increase HDL-C in patients with primary hyperlipidemia or mixed dyslipidemia.

Hypertriglyceridemia: Adjunct to diet for the treatment of adults with hypertriglyceridemia.

Primary dysbetalipoproteinemia (type III hyperlipoproteinemia): Adjunct to diet for the treatment of patients with primary dysbetalipoproteinemia (type III hyperlipoproteinemia).

Prevention of cardiovascular disease:

Primary prevention: To reduce the risk of stroke, myocardial infarction, or arterial revascularization procedures in patients without clinically evident coronary heart disease or lipid abnormalities but with all of the following: 1) an increased risk of cardiovascular disease based on age ≥50 years old in men and ≥60 years old in women, 2) hsCRP ≥2 mg/L, and 3) the presence of at least one additional cardiovascular disease risk factor such as hypertension, low HDL-C, smoking, or a family history of premature coronary heart disease.

Secondary prevention: Adjunctive therapy to diet to slow the progression of atherosclerosis in adults as part of a treatment strategy to lower total cholesterol and LDL-C to target levels.

Primary and secondary prevention of atherosclerotic cardiovascular disease (ASCVD) according to the American College of Cardiology/American Heart Association: To reduce the risk of ASCVD in patients with clinical ASCVD (eg, coronary heart disease, stroke/TIA, or peripheral arterial disease presumed to be of atherosclerotic origin) who are less than 75 years of age; in patients without clinical ASCVD if LDL-C is 190 mg/dL or greater; in patients without clinical ASCVD who have type 1 or type 2 diabetes and are between 40 and 75 years of age with an estimated 10-year ASCVD risk 7.5% or greater; in patients with an estimated 10-year ASCVD risk 7.5% or greater and who are between 40 and 75 years of age. (Stone, 2013).

Mechanism of Action/Effect Inhibitor of 3-hydroxy-3-methylglutaryl coenzyme A (HMG-CoA) reductase, the rate limiting enzyme in cholesterol synthesis (reduces the production of mevalonic acid from HMG-CoA); lowers TC, LDL-C, TG and improves HDL:LDL ratio

Contraindications Known hypersensitivity to any component of the formulation; active liver disease or unexplained persistent elevations of serum transaminases; pregnancy; breast-feeding.

Canadian labeling: Additional contraindications (not in U.S. labeling): Concomitant administration of cyclosporine; use of 40 mg dose in Asian patients, patients with predisposing risk factors for myopathy/rhabdomyolysis (eg, hereditary muscle disorders, history of myotoxicity with other HMG-CoA reductase inhibitors, concomitant use with fibrates or niacin, severe hepatic impairment, severe renal impairment [CrCl <30 mL/minute/1.73 m^2], hypothyroidism, alcohol abuse)

Warnings/Precautions Secondary causes of hyperlipidemia should be ruled out prior to therapy. Rosuvastatin has not been studied when the primary lipid abnormality is chylomicron elevation (Fredrickson types I and V). Postmarketing reports of fatal and nonfatal hepatic failure are rare. If serious hepatotoxicity with clinical symptoms and/or hyperbilirubinemia or jaundice occurs during treatment, interrupt therapy. If an alternate etiology is not identified, do not restart rosuvastatin. Liver enzyme tests should be obtained at baseline and as clinically indicated; routine periodic monitoring of liver enzymes is not necessary. Use with caution in patients who consume large amounts of ethanol or have a history of liver disease; use is contraindicated with active liver disease or unexplained transaminase elevations. Hematuria (microscopic) and proteinuria have been observed; more commonly reported in patients receiving rosuvastatin 40 mg daily, but typically transient and not associated with a decrease in renal function. Consider dosage reduction if unexplained hematuria and proteinuria persists. HMG-CoA reductase inhibitors may cause rhabdomyolysis with acute renal failure and/or myopathy. Discontinue in any patient in which CPK levels are markedly elevated (>10 times ULN) or if myopathy is suspected/diagnosed. This risk is dose-related and is increased with concurrent use of other lipid-lowering medications (fibric acid derivatives or niacin doses ≥1 g/day), other interacting drugs, drugs associated with myopathy (eg, colchicine), age ≥65 years, female gender, certain subgroups of Asian ancestry, uncontrolled hypothyroidism, and renal dysfunction. Dose reductions may be necessary. Immune-mediated necrotizing myopathy (IMNM), an autoimmune-mediated myopathy, has been reported (rarely) with HMG-CoA reductase inhibitor therapy. IMNM presents as proximal muscle weakness with elevated CPK levels, which persists despite discontinuation of HMG-CoA reductase inhibitor therapy; additionally, muscle biopsy may show necrotizing myopathy with limited inflammation; immunosuppressive therapy (eg, corticosteroids, azathioprine) may be used for treatment.

The manufacturer recommends temporary discontinuation for elective major surgery, acute medical or surgical conditions, or in any patient experiencing an acute or serious condition predisposing to renal failure (eg, sepsis, dehydration, electrolyte disorders, hypotension, trauma, uncontrolled seizures). However, based upon current evidence, HMG-CoA reductase inhibitor therapy should be continued in the perioperative period unless risk outweighs cardioprotective benefit. Patients should be instructed to report unexplained muscle pain, tenderness, weakness, or dark urine; in Canada, concomitant use with cyclosporine or niacin is contraindicated, and rosuvastatin at a dose of 40 mg/day in Asian patients is contraindicated. Small increases in Hb A_{1c} (mean: ~0.1%) and fasting blood glucose have been reported with rosuvastatin; however, the benefits of statin therapy far outweigh the risk of dysglycemia.

Potentially significant interactions may exist, requiring dose or frequency adjustment, additional monitoring, and/or selection of alternative therapy. Consult drug interactions database for more detailed information. Dosage adjustment required in patients with a CrCl <30 mL/minute/1.73 m² and not receiving hemodialysis (contraindicated in the Canadian labeling). Use with caution in elderly patients as they are more predisposed to myopathy.

Drug Interactions

Avoid Concomitant Use

Avoid concomitant use of Rosuvastatin with any of the following: Fusidic Acid (Systemic); Gemfibrozil; Red Yeast Rice

Decreased Effect

Rosuvastatin may decrease the levels/effects of: Lanthanum

The levels/effects of Rosuvastatin may be decreased by: Antacids; Eslicarbazepine

Increased Effect/Toxicity

Rosuvastatin may increase the levels/effects of: DAPTOmycin; PAZOPanib; Trabectedin; Vitamin K Antagonists

The levels/effects of Rosuvastatin may be increased by: Amiodarone; Bezafibrate; Boceprevir; Colchicine; CycloSPORINE (Systemic); Dronedarone; Eltrombopag; Fenofibrate and Derivatives; Fusidic Acid (Systemic); Gemfibrozil; Itraconazole; Niacin; Niacinamide; Protease Inhibitors; Raltegravir; Red Yeast Rice; Simeprevir; Telaprevir

Nutritional/Ethanol Interactions

Ethanol: Avoid excessive ethanol consumption (due to potential hepatic effects).

Food: Red yeast rice contains an estimated 2.4 mg lovastatin per 600 mg rice.

Adverse Reactions

>10%: Neuromuscular & skeletal: Myalgia (3% to 13%)

2% to 10%:

Central nervous system: Headache (6%), dizziness (4%)

Endocrine & metabolic: Diabetes mellitus (3%)

Gastrointestinal: Nausea (3%), abdominal pain (2%), constipation (2%)

Hepatic: Increased serum ALT (2%; >3 times ULN)

Neuromuscular & skeletal: Arthralgia (4% to 10%), increased creatine phosphokinase (3%; >10 x ULN: Children 3%), weakness (3%)

Pharmacodynamics/Kinetics

Onset of Action Within 1 week; maximal at 4 weeks

Available Dosage Forms

Tablet, Oral:

Crestor: 5 mg, 10 mg, 20 mg, 40 mg

General Dosage Range Dosage adjustment recommended in patients with severe renal impairment, on concomitant drug therapy, or who develop toxicities

Oral:

Children and Adolescents 10-17 years (females >1 year postmenarche): Initial: 5-20 mg once daily (maximum: 20 mg daily)

Adults: Initial: 5-20 mg once daily; Maintenance: 5-40 mg once daily (maximum: 40 mg daily)

Administration

Oral May be administered with or without food. May be taken at any time of the day.

Storage/Stability Store between 20°C and 25°C (68°F to 77°F). Protect from moisture.

Nursing Actions

Physical Assessment Monitor for signs and symptoms of myopathy (muscle tenderness, pain, or weakness). Assess risk potential for interactions with other prescriptions or herbal products patient may be taking that may increase risk of myopathy or rhabdomyolysis. Assess cholesterol profile prior to treatment and at regular intervals. Assess LFT prior to initiating therapy and recheck when clinically indicated. Teach proper diet and exercise regimen.

Patient Education

- Discuss specific use of drug and side effects with patient as it relates to treatment. (HCAHPS: During this hospital stay, were you given any medicine that you had not taken before? Before giving you any new medicine, how often did hospital staff tell you what the medicine was for? How often did hospital staff describe possible side effects in a way you could understand?)
- Patient may experience headache, diarrhea, dyspepsia, asthenia, or arthralgia. Have patient report immediately to prescriber flu-like syndrome, ecchymosis, bleeding, discolored urine, jaundice, or rash (HCAHPS).
- Educate patient about signs of a significant reaction (eg, wheezing; chest tightness; fever; itching; bad cough; blue skin color; seizures; or swelling of face, lips, tongue, or throat). **Note:** This is not a comprehensive list of all side effects. Patient should consult prescriber for additional questions.

Intended Use and Disclaimer: Should not be printed and given to patients. This information is intended to serve as a concise initial reference for healthcare professionals to use when discussing

medications with a patient. You must ultimately rely on your own discretion, experience and judgment in diagnosing, treating and advising patients.

Dietary Considerations Red yeast rice contains an estimated 2.4 mg lovastatin per 600 mg rice.

Rotavirus Vaccine (ROE ta vye rus vak SEEN)

Brand Names: U.S. Rotarix; RotaTeq

Index Terms Human Rotavirus Vaccine, Attenuated (HRV); Pentavalent Human-Bovine Reassortant Rotavirus Vaccine (PRV); Rotavirus Vaccine, Pentavalent; RV1 (Rotarix); RV5 (RotaTeq)

Pharmacologic Category Vaccine, Live (Viral)

Pregnancy Risk Factor C

Use Prevention of rotavirus gastroenteritis in infants and children

The Advisory Committee on Immunization Practices (ACIP) recommends routine vaccination of all infants (CDC, 2009).

Available Dosage Forms

Powder, for suspension, oral [preservative free; human derived]:

Rotarix: G1P[8] ≥10^6 CCID$_{50}$ per 1 mL

Solution, oral [preservative free]:

RotaTeq: G1 ≥2.2 x 10^6 infectious units, G2 ≥2.8 x 10^6 infectious units, G3 ≥2.2 x 10^6 infectious units, G4 ≥2 x 10^6 infectious units, and P1A [8] ≥2.3 x 10^6 infectious units per 2 mL (2 mL)

General Dosage Range Oral:

Infants 6-24 weeks: Rotarix: A total of two 1 mL doses administered at 2 and 4 months of age

Infants 6-32 weeks: RotaTeq: A total of three 2 mL doses given at 2, 4, and 6 months of age

Administration

Oral

Rotarix: Using oral applicator, administer contents into infant's inner cheek. Dispose of applicator and vaccine vial in biologic waste container.

RotaTeq: Gently squeeze dose from ready-to-use dosing tube into infant's inner cheek. After use, dispose of the empty tube and cap in a biologic waste container.

Note: A single dose of the rotavirus vaccine should not be readministered to an infant who regurgitates, spits out, or vomits the vaccine during administration. Any remaining dose(s) should be administered on schedule (CDC, 2009).

Simultaneous administration of vaccines helps ensure the patients will be fully vaccinated by the appropriate age. Simultaneous administration of vaccines is defined as administering >1 vaccine on the same day at different anatomic sites. Separate vaccines should not be combined in the same syringe unless indicated by product specific labeling. The ACIP prefers each dose of a specific vaccine in a series come from the same manufacturer when possible. In general, preterm

infants should be vaccinated at the same chronological age as full-term infants (CDC, 2011).

Antipyretics have not been shown to prevent febrile seizures. Antipyretics may be used to treat fever or discomfort following vaccination (CDC, 2011). One study reported that routine prophylactic administration of acetaminophen to prevent fever prior to vaccination decreased the immune response of some vaccines; the clinical significance of this reduction in immune response has not been established (Prymula, 2009).

Nursing Actions

Physical Assessment Have treatment for anaphylactoid or hypersensitivity reaction available. If latex sensitive, be advised that packaging may contain latex. Consider deferring administration in patients with moderate or severe acute illness (with or without fever); may administer to patients with mild acute illness (with or without fever). U.S. federal law requires entry into the patient's medical record.

Patient Education

• Discuss specific use of vaccine and side effects with caregiver as it relates to treatment. (HCAHPS: During this hospital stay, were you given any medicine that you had not taken before? Before giving you any new medicine, how often did hospital staff tell you what the medicine was for? How often did hospital staff describe possible side effects in a way you could understand?)

• Patient may experience headache, nausea, diarrhea, or rhinitis. Have caregiver report immediately to prescriber severe asthenia or rash (HCAHPS).

• Educate caregiver about signs of a significant reaction (eg, wheezing; chest tightness; fever; itching; bad cough; blue skin color; seizures; or swelling of face, lips, tongue, or throat). **Note:** This is not a comprehensive list of all side effects. Caregiver should consult prescriber for additional questions.

Intended Use and Disclaimer: Should not be printed and given to patients. This information is intended to serve as a concise initial reference for healthcare professionals to use when discussing medications with a patient. You must ultimately rely on your own discretion, experience and judgment in diagnosing, treating and advising patients.

Related Information

Immunization Administration Recommendations *on page 1675*

Immunization Recommendations *on page 1680*

Rotigotine (roe TIG oh teen)

Brand Names: U.S. Neupro

Index Terms N-0923

Pharmacologic Category Anti-Parkinson's Agent, Dopamine Agonist

Medication Safety Issues

Sound-alike/look-alike issues:

Neupro may be confused with Neupogen

Transdermal patch contains metal (eg, aluminum); remove patch prior to MRI or cardioversion

Pregnancy Risk Factor C

Lactation Excretion in breast milk unknown/use caution

Breast-Feeding Considerations Prolactin secretion is decreased and lactation may be inhibited. The Canadian labeling recommends discontinuing breast-feeding in women who require therapy.

Use Treatment of the signs and symptoms of idiopathic Parkinson's disease (early-stage to advanced-stage disease); treatment of moderate-to-severe primary restless legs syndrome (RLS)

Mechanism of Action/Effect Rotigotine is a non-ergot dopamine agonist with specificity for D_3-, D_2-, and D_1-dopamine receptors. Although the precise mechanism of action of rotigotine is unknown, it is believed to be due to stimulation of postsynaptic dopamine D_2-type auto receptors within the substantia nigra in the brain, leading to improved dopaminergic transmission in the motor areas of the basal ganglia, notably the caudate nucleus/putamen regions.

Contraindications Hypersensitivity to rotigotine or any component of the formulation

Warnings/Precautions Use is commonly associated with somnolence. In addition, falling asleep during activities of daily living, including while driving, has also been reported and may occur without significant warning signs. Monitor for daytime somnolence or pre-existing sleep disorder. Patients must be cautioned about performing tasks which require mental alertness (eg, operating machinery or driving). Use with caution in patients receiving other CNS depressants or psychoactive agents; discontinue if significant daytime sleepiness or episodes of falling asleep occur. Effects with other sedative drugs or ethanol may be potentiated.

Dopamine agonists may cause orthostatic hypotension and syncope; Parkinson's disease patients appear to have an impaired capacity to respond to a postural challenge. Use with caution in patients at risk of hypotension (such as those receiving antihypertensive drugs) or where transient hypotensive episodes would be poorly tolerated (cardiovascular disease or cerebrovascular disease). Parkinson's and restless legs syndrome (RLS) patients being treated with dopaminergic agonists ordinarily require careful monitoring for signs and symptoms of postural hypotension, especially during dose escalation, and should be informed of this risk. Weight gain and fluid retention have been reported, primarily associated with development of peripheral edema in Parkinson's disease patients; use caution in patients with heart failure or renal insufficiency. Therapy has also been associated with increases in blood pressure (may be significant), and increased heart rate; use caution in pre-existing cardiovascular disease.

Dopamine agonists have been associated with compulsive behaviors and/or loss of impulse control, which has manifested as pathological gambling, libido increases (hypersexuality), and/or binge eating. Causality has not been established, and controversy exists as to whether this phenomenon is related to the underlying disease, prior behaviors/addictions and/or drug therapy. Dose reduction or discontinuation of therapy has been reported to reverse these behaviors in some, but not all cases.

In RLS patents, augmentation (earlier onset of symptoms each day and/or an overall increase in symptom severity) or rebound (considered to be an end of dose effect) may occur.

Use with caution in patients with pre-existing dyskinesia; therapy may exacerbate. Therapy may also cause hallucinations (dose-related) and other psychotic like behaviors (eg, agitation, delirium, delusions, aggression); in general, avoid use in patients with pre-existing major psychotic disorders. Risk for melanoma development is increased in Parkinson's disease patients; drug causation or factors contributing to risk have not been established. Patients receiving therapy for any indication should be monitored closely and periodic skin examinations should be performed. Other dopaminergic agents have been associated with a syndrome resembling neuroleptic malignant syndrome on withdrawal and/or significant dosage reduction. Taper treatment when discontinuing therapy; do not stop abruptly. Rare cases of pleural effusion, pleural thickening, pulmonary infiltrates, retroperitoneal fibrosis, pericarditis and/or cardiac valvulopathy have been reported in patients treated with ergot-derived dopamine agonists, generally with prolonged use. The potential of rotigotine, a non-ergot-derived dopamine agonist, to cause similar fibrotic complications is unknown.

Patch contains aluminum; remove patch prior to magnetic resonance imaging or cardioversion to avoid skin burns. Patch also contains sodium metabisulfite which may cause allergic reaction in susceptible individuals. Dose-dependent application site reactions, potentially severe, have been observed; daily rotation of application sites has been shown to decrease incidence of reactions. If a generalized (nonapplication site) skin reaction occurs; discontinue therapy. Avoid exposure of application site to any direct external heat sources (eg, hair dryers, heating pads, electric blankets, saunas, hot tubs, direct sunlight); heat exposure has not been studied with the rotigotine patch, but an increase in the rate and extent of absorption has been observed with other transdermal products.

Drug Interactions

Avoid Concomitant Use

Avoid concomitant use of Rotigotine with any of the following: Amisulpride

Decreased Effect

Rotigotine may decrease the levels/effects of: Amisulpride; Antipsychotics (Typical)

The levels/effects of Rotigotine may be decreased by: Amisulpride; Antipsychotics (Atypical); Antipsychotics (Typical); Metoclopramide

Increased Effect/Toxicity

Rotigotine may increase the levels/effects of: BuPROPion

The levels/effects of Rotigotine may be increased by: Alcohol (Ethyl); CNS Depressants; MAO Inhibitors; Methylphenidate

Nutritional/Ethanol Interactions Ethanol: Ethanol may increase CNS depression. Management: Avoid concurrent use of ethanol.

Adverse Reactions

>10%:

Cardiovascular: Peripheral edema (dose related; 2% to 14%)

Central nervous system: Somnolence (dose related; 5% to 32%), dizziness (5% to 23%), headache (8% to 18%), fatigue (6% to 18%), orthostatic hypotension (1% to 18%), sleep disorder (disturbance in initiating/maintaining sleep; dose related; 2% to 14%), hallucinations (dose related; 7% to 14%), insomnia (5% to 11%)

Dermatologic: Application site reactions (dose related; 27% to 46%), hyperhidrosis (dose related; 1% to 11%)

Gastrointestinal: Nausea (dose related; 15% to 48%), vomiting (dose related; 2% to 20%)

Neuromuscular & skeletal: Dyskinesia (dose related; 14% to 17%), arthralgia (8% to 11%)

1% to 10%:

Cardiovascular: Hypertension (dose related; 1% to 5%), T-wave abnormalities on ECG (≤3%), syncope

Central nervous system: Abnormal dreams (dose related; 1% to 7%), nightmare (dose related; 3% to 5%), depression (≤5%), vertigo (1% to 4%), early morning awakening (dose related; ≤3%), balance disorder (2% to 3%), lethargy (1% to 2%), postural dizziness (1% to 2%), sleep attacks (dose related; ≤2%)

Dermatologic: Pruritus (3% to 7%), erythema (dose related; ≤6%), pruritic rash (dose related; ≤3%)

Endocrine & metabolic: Hot flash (≤3%), serum ferritin decreased (dose related; 1% to 2%); serum glucose decreased

Gastrointestinal: Constipation (2% to 9%), weight gain (2% to 9%), diarrhea (5% to 7%), anorexia (≤8%), xerostomia (dose related; 3% to 7%), appetite decreased (≤3%), dyspepsia (dose related; ≤3%), weight loss (dose related; ≤3%)

Genitourinary: Erectile dysfunction (dose related; ≤3%), urinary WBC positive (≤3%)

Hematologic: Contusion (dose related; ≤4%), hemoglobin decreased, hematocrit decreased

Neuromuscular & skeletal: Paresthesia (dose related 5% to 6%), tremor (3% to 4%), weakness (3% to 4%), muscle spasms (dose related; 1% to 4%), musculoskeletal pain (2%)

Ocular: Vision changes

Otic: Tinnitus (≤3%)

Renal: BUN increased

Respiratory: Nasopharyngitis (7% to 10%), upper respiratory tract infection (≤5%), cough (3%), nasal congestion (3%), sinus congestion (2% to 3%), sinusitis (dose related; ≤3%), pharyngolaryngeal pain (≤2%)

Miscellaneous: Hiccups (dose related; 2% to 3%)

Available Dosage Forms

Patch 24 Hour, Transdermal:

Neupro: 1 mg/24 hr (30 ea); 2 mg/24 hr (30 ea); 3 mg/24 hr (30 ea); 4 mg/24 hr (30 ea); 6 mg/24 hr (30 ea); 8 mg/24 hr (30 ea)

General Dosage Range

Transdermal: *Adults:* 1-4 mg/24 hours; Maintenance (usual): 1-8 mg/24 hours (maximum: varies by indication)

Administration

Topical Transdermal patch: Apply patch to clean, dry, hairless area of intact healthy skin on the front of the abdomen, thigh, hip, flank, shoulder, or upper arm at approximately the same time daily. Remove from pouch immediately before use and press patch firmly in place on skin for 30 seconds. Application sites should be rotated on a daily basis. Do not apply to same application site more than once every 14 days or apply patch to oily, irritated or damaged skin. Avoid exposing patch to external heat sources (eg, heating pad, electric blanket, heat lamp, hot tub, direct sunlight). If applied to hairy area, shave ≥3 days prior to applying patch. If patch falls off, immediately apply a new one to a new site.

Storage/Stability Store at 20°C to 25°C (68°F to 77°F). Store in original pouch until application.

Nursing Actions

Physical Assessment Assess other prescription and OTC medications patient may be taking to avoid duplications and interactions. Monitor therapeutic response and adverse reactions at the beginning and periodically throughout therapy. Taper dosage slowly when discontinuing. Do not discontinue abruptly. Assess knowledge/teach patient appropriate use, side effects, and symptoms to report.

Patient Education

• Discuss specific use of drug and side effects with patient as it relates to treatment. (HCAHPS: During this hospital stay, were you given any medicine that you had not taken before? Before giving you any new medicine, how often did hospital staff tell you what the medicine was

for? How often did hospital staff describe possible side effects in a way you could understand?)
• Patient may experience presyncope, fatigue, blurred vision, illogical thinking, dizziness, nausea, hypertension, weight gain, or skin irritation. Have patient report immediately to prescriber narcolepsy, uncontrollable compulsions, severe asthenia, edema, or rash (HCAHPS).
• Educate patient about signs of a significant reaction (eg, wheezing; chest tightness; fever; itching; bad cough; blue skin color; seizures; or swelling of face, lips, tongue, or throat). **Note:** This is not a comprehensive list of all side effects. Patient should consult prescriber for additional questions.

Intended Use and Disclaimer: Should not be printed and given to patients. This information is intended to serve as a concise initial reference for healthcare professionals to use when discussing medications with a patient. You must ultimately rely on your own discretion, experience and judgment in diagnosing, treating and advising patients.

Rufinamide (roo FIN a mide)

Brand Names: U.S. Banzel
Index Terms CGP 33101; E 2080; RUF 331; Xilep
Pharmacologic Category Anticonvulsant, Triazole Derivative
Medication Guide Available Yes
Pregnancy Risk Factor C
Lactation Excretion in breast milk unknown/not recommended
Use Adjunctive therapy in the treatment of generalized seizures of Lennox-Gastaut syndrome
Available Dosage Forms
Suspension, Oral:
Banzel: 40 mg/mL (460 mL)
Tablet, Oral:
Banzel: 200 mg, 400 mg
General Dosage Range Oral:
Children ≥4 years: Initial: 10 mg/kg/day in 2 equally divided doses (maximum: 45 mg/kg/day or 3200 mg/day)
Adults: Initial: 400-800 mg/day in 2 equally divided doses (maximum: 3200 mg/day)
Administration
Oral Administer with food. Tablets may be swallowed whole, split in half, or crushed. Oral suspension should be administered using the provided adapter and oral syringe; shake well before every administration.
Nursing Actions
Physical Assessment Monitor for signs and symptoms of suicide ideation (eg, anxiety, depression, unusual mood or behavior changes).

Patient Education
• Discuss specific use of drug and side effects with patient as it relates to treatment. (HCAHPS: During this hospital stay, were you given any medicine that you had not taken before? Before giving you any new medicine, how often did hospital staff tell you what the medicine was for? How often did hospital staff describe possible side effects in a way you could understand?)
• Patient may experience presyncope, fatigue, blurred vision, illogical thinking, dizziness, headache, or nausea. Have patient report immediately to prescriber depression, nervousness, emotional instability, anxiety, severe asthenia, or rash (HCAHPS).
• Educate patient about signs of a significant reaction (eg, wheezing; chest tightness; fever; itching; bad cough; blue skin color; seizures; or swelling of face, lips, tongue, or throat). **Note:** This is not a comprehensive list of all side effects. Patient should consult prescriber for additional questions.

Intended Use and Disclaimer: Should not be printed and given to patients. This information is intended to serve as a concise initial reference for healthcare professionals to use when discussing medications with a patient. You must ultimately rely on your own discretion, experience and judgment in diagnosing, treating and advising patients.

Ruxolitinib (rux oh LI ti nib)

Brand Names: U.S. Jakafi
Index Terms INCB 18424; INCB018424; INCB424; Ruxolitinib Phosphate
Pharmacologic Category Antineoplastic Agent, Janus Associated Kinase Inhibitor; Antineoplastic Agent, Tyrosine Kinase Inhibitor; Janus Associated Kinase Inhibitor
Medication Safety Issues
Sound-alike/look-alike issues:
Ruxolitinib may be confused with PONATinib, riTUXimab
Pregnancy Risk Factor C
Lactation Excretion in breast milk unknown/ not recommended
Use Treatment of intermediate or high-risk myelofibrosis, including primary myelofibrosis, post-polycythemia vera (post-PV) myelofibrosis and post-essential thrombocythemia (post-ET) myelofibrosis
Available Dosage Forms
Tablet, Oral:
Jakafi: 5 mg, 10 mg, 15 mg, 20 mg, 25 mg
General Dosage Range Dosage adjustment recommended in patients with hepatic impairment, renal impairment, on concomitant strong CYP3A4 inhibitor therapy, or who develop toxicities.
Oral: *Adults:* 15-20 mg twice daily; maximum dose: 25 mg twice daily

◀ **Administration**

Oral May be administered orally with or without food. If a dose is missed, return to the usual dosing schedule and do **not** administer an additional dose.

If unable to ingest tablets, may administer through a nasogastric (NG) tube (≥8 Fr): Suspend 1 tablet in ~40 mL water and stir for ~10 minutes and administer (within 6 hours after dispersion) with appropriate syringe; rinse NG tube with ~75 mL water (effect of enteral tube feeding on ruxolitinib exposure has not been evaluated)

Hazardous agent; use appropriate precautions for handling and disposal (meets NIOSH, 2012 criteria).

Nursing Actions

Physical Assessment Monitor vital signs throughout therapy. Assess for viral, fungal, or bacterial infections. Ongoing infections should be resolved prior to therapy. Instruct patient to report shortness of breath, painful skin rash, or blisters. Canadian labeling recommends obtaining an ECG at baseline and then periodically during therapy; check ECG results. Monitor CBC with differential throughout therapy.

Patient Education

• Discuss specific use of drug and side effects with patient as it relates to treatment. (HCAHPS: During this hospital stay, were you given any medicine that you had not taken before? Before giving you any new medicine, how often did hospital staff tell you what the medicine was for? How often did hospital staff describe possible side effects in a way you could understand?)

• Patient may experience dizziness, headache, weight gain, or flatulence. Have patient report immediately to prescriber signs of infection, nausea, dyspnea, asthenia, ecchymosis, hemorrhaging, or signs of multifocal leukoencephalopathy (PML) (HCAHPS).

• Educate patient about signs of a significant reaction (eg, wheezing; chest tightness; fever; itching; bad cough; blue skin color; seizures; or swelling of face, lips, tongue, or throat). **Note:** This is not a comprehensive list of all side effects. Patient should consult prescriber for additional questions.

Intended Use and Disclaimer: Should not be printed and given to patients. This information is intended to serve as a concise initial reference for healthcare professionals to use when discussing medications with a patient. You must ultimately rely on your own discretion, experience and judgment in diagnosing, treating and advising patients.

Salmeterol (sal ME te role)

Brand Names: U.S. Serevent Diskus

Index Terms Salmeterol Xinafoate

Pharmacologic Category Beta₂ Agonist; Beta₂-Adrenergic Agonist, Long-Acting

Medication Safety Issues
Sound-alike/look-alike issues:
Salmeterol may be confused with Salbutamol, Solu-Medrol®
Serevent® may be confused with Atrovent®, Combivent®, sertraline, Sinemet®, Spiriva®, Zoloft®

Medication Guide Available Yes

Pregnancy Risk Factor C

Lactation Excretion unknown/use caution

Breast-Feeding Considerations It is not known if salmeterol is excreted into breast milk. According to the manufacturer, the decision to continue or discontinue breast-feeding during therapy should take into account the risk of exposure to the infant and the benefits of treatment to the mother. The use of beta₂-receptor agonists are not considered a contraindication to breast-feeding (NAEPP, 2005).

Use Maintenance treatment of asthma and prevention of bronchospasm (as concomitant therapy) in patients with reversible obstructive airway disease, including patients with symptoms of nocturnal asthma; prevention of exercise-induced bronchospasm (monotherapy may be indicated in patients without persistent asthma); maintenance treatment of bronchospasm associated with COPD

Mechanism of Action/Effect Relaxes bronchial smooth muscle by selective action on beta₂-receptors with little effect on heart rate; salmeterol acts locally in the lung.

Contraindications Hypersensitivity to salmeterol or any component of the formulation (milk proteins); monotherapy in the treatment of asthma (ie, use without a concomitant long-term asthma control medication, such as an inhaled corticosteroid); status asthmaticus or other acute episodes of asthma or COPD

Warnings/Precautions Asthma treatment: **[U.S. Boxed Warning]: Long-acting beta₂-agonists (LABAs) increase the risk of asthma-related deaths. Salmeterol should only be used in asthma patients as adjuvant therapy in patients who are currently receiving but are not adequately controlled on a long-term asthma control medication (ie, an inhaled corticosteroid).** Monotherapy with an LABA is contraindicated in the treatment of asthma. In a large, randomized, placebo-controlled U.S. clinical trial (SMART, 2006), salmeterol was associated with an increase in asthma-related deaths (when added to usual asthma therapy); risk is considered a class effect among all LABAs. Data are not available to determine if the addition of an inhaled corticosteroid lessens this increased risk of death associated with LABA use. Assess patients at regular intervals once asthma control is maintained on combination therapy to determine if step-down therapy is appropriate and the LABA can be discontinued (without loss of asthma control), and the patient can be maintained on an inhaled corticosteroid. LABAs are not appropriate in patients whose asthma is adequately controlled on low- or medium-dose inhaled corticosteroids. Do **not** use for acute bronchospasm. Short-acting beta₂-agonist (eg, albuterol) should be used for acute symptoms and symptoms occurring between treatments. Do **not** initiate in patients with significantly worsening or acutely deteriorating asthma; reports of severe (sometimes fatal) respiratory events have been reported when salmeterol has been initiated in this situation. Corticosteroids should not be stopped or reduced when salmeterol is initiated. During initiation, watch for signs of worsening asthma. Patients must be instructed to use short-acting beta₂-agonists (eg, albuterol) for acute asthmatic or COPD symptoms and to seek medical attention in cases where acute symptoms are not relieved or a previous level of response is diminished. The need to increase frequency of use of short-acting beta₂-agonist may indicate deterioration of asthma, and treatment must not be delayed. Because LABAs may disguise poorly controlled persistent asthma, frequent or chronic use of LABAs for exercise-induced bronchospasm is discouraged by the NIH Asthma Guidelines (NIH, 2007). Salmeterol should not be used more than twice daily; do not use with other long-acting beta₂-agonists. **[U.S. Boxed Warning]: LABAs may increase the risk of asthma-related hospitalization in pediatric and adolescent patients.** In general, a combination product containing a LABA and an inhaled corticosteroid is preferred in patients <18 years of age to ensure compliance.

COPD treatment: Appropriate use: Do **not** use for acute episodes of COPD. Do **not** initiate in patients with significantly worsening or acutely deteriorating COPD. Data are not available to determine if LABA use increases the risk of death in patients with COPD.

Concurrent diseases: Use caution in patients with cardiovascular disease (eg, arrhythmia, hypertension, or HF), seizure disorders, diabetes, hyperthyroidism, hepatic impairment, or hypokalemia. Beta-agonists may cause elevation in blood pressure, heart rate, CNS stimulation/excitation, increased risk of arrhythmia, increase serum glucose, or decrease serum potassium.

Adverse events: Immediate hypersensitivity reactions (urticaria, angioedema, rash, bronchospasm) have been reported. There have been reports of laryngeal spasm, irritation, swelling (stridor, choking) with use. Salmeterol should not be used more than twice daily; do not exceed recommended dose; do not use with other long-acting beta₂-agonists; serious adverse events have been associated with excessive use of inhaled sympathomimetics. Rarely, paradoxical bronchospasm may occur with use of inhaled bronchodilating agents; this should be distinguished from inadequate response. Use with strong CYP3A4 inhibitors (see Drug Interactions) is not recommended due to potential for an increased risk of cardiovascular events. Powder for oral inhalation contains lactose; very rare anaphylactic reactions have been reported in patients with severe milk protein allergy.

Drug Interactions

Avoid Concomitant Use

Avoid concomitant use of Salmeterol with any of the following: Beta-Blockers (Nonselective); Cobicistat; CYP3A4 Inhibitors (Strong); Fusidic Acid (Systemic); Iobenguane I 123; Long-Acting Beta2-Agonists; Telaprevir

Decreased Effect

Salmeterol may decrease the levels/effects of: Iobenguane I 123

The levels/effects of Salmeterol may be decreased by: Beta-Blockers (Beta1 Selective); Beta-Blockers (Nonselective); Betahistine

Increased Effect/Toxicity

Salmeterol may increase the levels/effects of: Atosiban; Highest Risk QTc-Prolonging Agents; Long-Acting Beta2-Agonists; Loop Diuretics; Moderate Risk QTc-Prolonging Agents; Sympathomimetics; Thiazide Diuretics

The levels/effects of Salmeterol may be increased by: AtoMOXetine; Cannabinoids; Cobicistat; CYP3A4 Inhibitors (Moderate); CYP3A4 Inhibitors (Strong); Dasatinib; Fusidic Acid (Systemic); Ivacaftor; Luliconazole; MAO Inhibitors; Mifepristone; Simeprevir; Telaprevir; Tricyclic Antidepressants

Adverse Reactions

>10%:

Central nervous system: Headache (13% to 17%)

Neuromuscular & skeletal: Pain (1% to 12%)

1% to 10%:

Cardiovascular: Hypertension (4%), edema (1% to 3%), pallor

Central nervous system: Dizziness (4%), sleep disturbance (1% to 3%), fever (1% to 3%), anxiety (1% to 3%), migraine (1% to 3%)

Dermatologic: Rash (1% to 4%), contact dermatitis (1% to 3%), eczema (1% to 3%), urticaria (3%), photodermatitis (1% to 2%)

Endocrine & metabolic: Hyperglycemia (1% to 3%)

Gastrointestinal: Throat irritation (7%), nausea (1% to 3%), dyspepsia (1% to 3%), dental pain (1% to 3%), gastrointestinal infection (1% to 3%), oropharyngeal candidiasis (1% to 3%), xerostomia (1% to 3%)

Hepatic: Liver enzymes increased

Neuromuscular & skeletal: Muscular cramps/spasm (3%), articular rheumatism (1% to 3%), arthralgia (1% to 3%), joint pain (1% to 3%), muscular stiffness (1% to 3%), paresthesia (1% to 3%), rigidity (1% to 3%)

Ocular: Keratitis/conjunctivitis (1% to 3%)

Respiratory: Nasal congestion (4% to 9%), tracheitis/bronchitis (7%), pharyngitis (≤6%), cough (5%), influenza (5%), viral respiratory tract infection (5%), sinusitis (4% to 5%), rhinitis (4% to 5%), asthma (3% to 4%)

Pharmacodynamics/Kinetics

Onset of Action Asthma: 30-48 minutes, COPD: 2 hours; Peak effect: Asthma: 3 hours, COPD: 2-5 hours

Duration of Action 12 hours

Available Dosage Forms

Aerosol Powder Breath Activated, Inhalation: Serevent Diskus: 50 mcg/dose (28 ea, 60 ea)

General Dosage Range Inhalation: *Children ≥4 years and Adults:* 1 inhalation (50 mcg) twice daily

Administration

Inhalation Not to be used for the relief of acute attacks. Not for use with a spacer device. Administer with Diskus® in a level, horizontal position. Do not wash mouthpiece; Diskus® should be kept dry. Discard device 6 weeks after removal from foil pouch or when the dose counter reads "0" (whichever comes first).

Storage/Stability Inhalation powder (Serevent® Diskus®): Store at controlled room temperature 20°C to 25°C (68°F to 77°F) in a dry place away from direct heat or sunlight. Stable for 6 weeks after removal from foil pouch.

Nursing Actions

Physical Assessment Not for use to relieve acute asthmatic attacks. Monitor for increased use of short-acting beta$_2$-agonist inhalers; may be marker of a deteriorating asthma condition. For inpatient care, monitor vital signs and lung sounds prior to and periodically during therapy.

Patient Education

• Discuss specific use of drug and side effects with patient as it relates to treatment. (HCAHPS: During this hospital stay, were you given any medicine that you had not taken before? Before giving you any new medicine, how often did hospital staff tell you what the medicine was for? How often did hospital staff describe possible side effects in a way you could understand?)

• Patient may experience headache, nervousness and anxiety, myalgia, xerostomia, or pharyngitis. Have patient report immediately to prescriber uncontrollable breathing attack, decreased peak flow measurement, frequent use of inhaler, angina, tachycardia, dyspnea, or rash (HCAHPS).

• Educate patient about signs of a significant reaction (eg, wheezing; chest tightness; fever; itching; bad cough; blue skin color; seizures; or swelling of face, lips, tongue, or throat). **Note:** This is not a comprehensive list of all side effects. Patient should consult prescriber for additional questions.

Intended Use and Disclaimer: Should not be printed and given to patients. This information is intended to serve as a concise initial reference for healthcare professionals to use when discussing medications with a patient. You must ultimately rely on your own discretion, experience and judgment in diagnosing, treating and advising patients.

Dietary Considerations Some products may contain lactose; very rare anaphylactic reactions have been reported in patients with severe milk protein allergy.

Saquinavir (sa KWIN a veer)

Brand Names: U.S. Invirase

Index Terms Saquinavir Mesylate; SQV

Pharmacologic Category Antiretroviral, Protease Inhibitor (Anti-HIV)

Medication Safety Issues

Sound-alike/look-alike issues:

Saquinavir may be confused with SINEquan®

Medication Guide Available Yes

Pregnancy Risk Factor B

Lactation Excretion in breast milk unknown/contraindicated

Breast-Feeding Considerations Maternal or infant antiretroviral therapy does not completely eliminate the risk of postnatal HIV transmission. In addition, multiclass-resistant virus has been detected in breast-feeding infants despite maternal therapy. Therefore, in the United States, where formula is accessible, affordable, safe, and sustainable, and the risk of infant mortality due to diarrhea and respiratory infections is low, complete avoidance of breast-feeding by HIV-infected women is recommended to decrease potential transmission of HIV (DHHS [perinatal], 2012).

Use Treatment of HIV infection; used in combination with ritonavir and other antiretroviral agents

Mechanism of Action/Effect Blocks the site of HIV-1 protease activity, resulting in the formation of immature, noninfectious viral particles.

Contraindications Hypersensitivity to saquinavir or any component of the formulation; congenital or acquired QT prolongation, refractory hypokalemia or hypomagnesemia, concomitant use of other medications that both increase saquinavir plasma concentrations and prolong the QT interval; complete AV block (without implanted ventricular pacemaker) or patients at high risk of complete AV block; severe hepatic impairment; coadministration of saquinavir/ritonavir with alfuzosin, amiodarone, bepridil, cisapride, dofetilide, ergot derivatives, flecainide, lidocaine (systemic), lovastatin, midazolam (oral), pimozide, propafenone, quinidine, rifampin, sildenafil (when used for pulmonary artery hypertension [eg, Revatio®]), simvastatin, trazodone, or triazolam

Canadian labeling: Additional contraindications (not in U.S. labeling): Concurrent use with procainamide, sotalol, astemizole, or terfenadine

Warnings/Precautions Use caution in patients with hepatic insufficiency. May exacerbate pre-existing hepatic dysfunction; use with caution in patients with hepatitis B or C and in cirrhosis. May be associated with fat redistribution (buffalo hump, increased abdominal girth, breast engorgement, facial atrophy). Use caution in hemophilia. May increase cholesterol and/or triglycerides. Changes in glucose tolerance, hyperglycemia, exacerbation of diabetes, DKA, and new-onset diabetes mellitus have been reported in patients receiving protease inhibitors.

Altered cardiac conduction: Saquinavir/ritonavir prolongs the QT interval, potentially leading to torsade de pointes, and prolongs the PR interval, potentially leading to heart block. Second- or third-degree AV block has been reported (rare). An ECG should be performed for all patients prior to starting saquinavir/ritonavir therapy; do not initiate therapy in patients with a baseline QT interval >450 msec or diagnosed with long QT syndrome. If baseline QT interval <450 msec, may initiate therapy but a subsequent ECG is recommended after ~3-4 days of therapy. If subsequent QT interval is >480 msec or is prolonged over baseline by >20 msec, therapy should be discontinued. Patients who may be at increased risk for QT- or PR-interval prolongation include those with heart failure, bradyarrhythmias, hepatic impairment, electrolyte abnormalities, ischemic heart disease, cardiomyopathy, structural heart disease, or those with pre-existing cardiac conduction abnormalities; ECG monitoring is recommended for these patients.

Must be used in combination with ritonavir. Continued administration after loss of viral suppression efficacy may increase the likelihood of cross-resistance to other protease inhibitors. Promptly discontinue therapy if viral suppression response is lost. High potential for drug interactions; concomitant use of saquinavir with some drugs may require cautious use, may not be recommended, may require dosage adjustments, or may be contraindicated. Consult drug interactions database for more detailed information. Patients may develop immune reconstitution syndrome resulting in the occurrence of an inflammatory response to an indolent or residual opportunistic infection during initial HIV treatment or activation of autoimmune disorders (eg, Graves' disease, polymyositis, Guillain-Barré syndrome) later in therapy; further evaluation and treatment may be required. Formulation contains lactose; Canadian product labeling recommends against use in patients with galactose intolerance, Lapp lactase deficiency or glucose-galactose malabsorption.

Drug Interactions

Avoid Concomitant Use

Avoid concomitant use of Saquinavir with any of the following: Ado-Trastuzumab Emtansine; Alfuzosin; Amiodarone; Apixaban; Avanafil; Axitinib; Bepridil [Off Market]; Bosutinib; Cabozantinib; Cisapride; Conivaptan; Crizotinib; Darunavir; Dofetilide; Dronedarone; Eplerenone; Ergot Derivatives; Everolimus; Flecainide; Fusidic Acid (Systemic); Halofantrine; Highest Risk QTc-Prolonging Agents; Ibrutinib; Imatinib; Ivabradine; Lapatinib; Lidocaine (Systemic); Lomitapide; Lovastatin; Lurasidone; Macitentan; Midazolam; Mifepristone; Nilotinib; Nisoldipine; Pimozide; Pomalidomide; Propafenone; QuiNIDine; Ranolazine; Red Yeast Rice; Regorafenib; Rifampin; Rivaroxaban; Salmeterol; Silodosin; Simeprevir; Simvastatin; St Johns Wort; Tamsulosin; Ticagrelor; Tolvaptan; Topotecan; Toremifene; TraZODone; Triazolam; Ulipristal; Vemurafenib; VinCRIStine (Liposomal)

Decreased Effect

Saquinavir may decrease the levels/effects of: Abacavir; Boceprevir; Clarithromycin; Contraceptives (Estrogens); Darunavir; Delavirdine; Etravirine; Ifosfamide; Meperidine; Methadone; Prasugrel; Pravastatin; Theophylline Derivatives; Ticagrelor; Valproic Acid and Derivatives; Zidovudine

The levels/effects of Saquinavir may be decreased by: Antacids; Boceprevir; Bosentan; CarBAMazepine; CYP3A4 Inducers (Strong); Dabrafenib; Deferasirox; Efavirenz; Garlic; Mitotane; Nevirapine; Peginterferon Alfa-2b; P-glycoprotein/ABCB1 Inducers; Rifampin; St Johns Wort; Tocilizumab

Increased Effect/Toxicity

Saquinavir may increase the levels/effects of: Ado-Trastuzumab Emtansine; Afatinib; Alfuzosin; Almotriptan; Alosetron; ALPRAZolam; Amiodarone; Apixaban; ARIPiprazole; AtorvaSTATin; Avanafil; Axitinib; Bedaquiline; Bepridil [Off Market]; Bortezomib; Bosentan; Bosutinib; Brentuximab Vedotin; Brinzolamide; Budesonide (Nasal); Budesonide (Systemic, Oral Inhalation); Cabozantinib; Calcium Channel Blockers (Dihydropyridine); Calcium Channel Blockers (Nondihydropyridine); CarBAMazepine; Cisapride; Clarithromycin; Clorazepate; Colchicine; Conivaptan; Corticosteroids (Orally Inhaled); Crizotinib; CycloSPORINE (Systemic); CYP3A4 Substrates; Dabigatran Etexilate; Diazepam; Dienogest; Digoxin; Dofetilide; DOXOrubicin (Conventional); Dronedarone; Dutasteride; Efavirenz; Enfuvirtide; Enzalutamide; Eplerenone; Ergot Derivatives; Everolimus; FentaNYL; Fesoterodine; Flecainide; Flurazepam; Fluticasone (Nasal); Fluticasone (Oral Inhalation); Fusidic Acid (Systemic); GuanFACINE; Halofantrine; Highest Risk QTc-Prolonging Agents; Ibrutinib; ▶

Iloperidone; Imatinib; Itraconazole; Ivabradine; Ivacaftor; Ixabepilone; Ketoconazole (Systemic); Lacosamide; Lapatinib; Levomilnacipran; Lidocaine (Systemic); Lomitapide; Lovastatin; Lumefantrine; Lurasidone; Macitentan; Maraviroc; Meperidine; MethylPREDNISolone; Midazolam; Mifepristone; Moderate Risk QTc-Prolonging Agents; Nefazodone; Nilotinib; Nisoldipine; Ospemifene; OxyCODONE; Paricalcitol; PAZOPanib; P-glycoprotein/ABCB1 Substrates; Pimecrolimus; Pimozide; Pomalidomide; PONATinib; Propafenone; Protease Inhibitors; Prucalopride; QUEtiapine; QuiNIDine; Ranolazine; Red Yeast Rice; Regorafenib; Repaglinide; Rifabutin; Rilpivirine; Riociguat; Rivaroxaban; RomiDEPsin; Rosuvastatin; Ruxolitinib; Salmeterol; Saxagliptin; Sildenafil; Silodosin; Simeprevir; Simvastatin; SORAfenib; Tacrolimus (Systemic); Tacrolimus (Topical); Tadalafil; Tamsulosin; Temsirolimus; Ticagrelor; Tofacitinib; Tolterodine; Tolvaptan; Topotecan; Toremifene; TraZODone; Triazolam; Tricyclic Antidepressants; Ulipristal; Vardenafil; Vemurafenib; Vilazodone; VinCRIStine (Liposomal); Warfarin; Zuclopenthixol

The levels/effects of Saquinavir may be increased by: Bepridil [Off Market]; Clarithromycin; CycloSPORINE (Systemic); Delavirdine; Enfuvirtide; Etravirine; Fusidic Acid (Systemic); H2-Antagonists; Itraconazole; Ivabradine; Ketoconazole (Systemic); Methadone; Mifepristone; P-glycoprotein/ABCB1 Inhibitors; Proton Pump Inhibitors; QTc-Prolonging Agents (Indeterminate Risk and Risk Modifying); Rifampin; Simeprevir

Nutritional/Ethanol Interactions

Food: A high-fat meal maximizes bioavailability. Saquinavir levels may increase if taken with grapefruit juice. Management: Administer within 2 hours of a full meal.

Herb/Nutraceutical: Saquinavir serum concentrations may be decreased by St John's wort and garlic capsules. Management: Avoid St John's wort. Avoid garlic supplementation.

Adverse Reactions

Incidence data shown for saquinavir soft gel capsule formulation (no longer available) in combination with ritonavir.

10%: Gastrointestinal: Nausea (11%)

1% to 10%:

Cardiovascular: Chest pain

Central nervous system: Fatigue (6%), fever (3%), anxiety, depression, headache, insomnia, pain

Dermatologic: Pruritus (3%), rash (3%), dry lips/skin (2%), eczema (2%), verruca

Endocrine & metabolic: Lipodystrophy (5%), hyperglycemia (3%), hypoglycemia, hyperkalemia, libido disorder, serum amylase increased

Gastrointestinal: Diarrhea (8%), vomiting (7%), abdominal pain (6%), constipation (2%), abdominal discomfort, appetite decreased,

buccal mucosa ulceration, dyspepsia, flatulence, taste alteration

Hepatic: AST increased, ALT increased, bilirubin increased

Neuromuscular & skeletal: Back pain (2%), CPK increased, paresthesia, weakness

Renal: Creatinine kinase increased

Respiratory: Pneumonia (5%), bronchitis (3%), sinusitis (3%)

Miscellaneous: Influenza (3%)

Incidence not currently defined (limited to significant reactions; reported for hard or soft gel capsule with/without ritonavir)

Cardiovascular: Cyanosis, heart valve disorder (including murmur), hyper-/hypotension, peripheral vasoconstriction, prolonged QT interval, prolonged PR interval, syncope, thrombophlebitis

Central nervous system: Agitation, amnesia, ataxia, confusion, hallucination, hyper-/hyporeflexia, myelopolyradiculoneuritis, neuropathies, poliomyelitis, progressive multifocal encephalopathy, psychosis, seizures, somnolence, speech disorder, suicide attempt

Dermatologic: Alopecia, bullous eruption, dermatitis, erythema, maculopapular rash, photosensitivity, Stevens-Johnson syndrome, skin ulceration, urticaria

Endocrine & metabolic: Dehydration, diabetes, electrolyte changes, TSH increased

Gastrointestinal: Ascites, colic, dysphagia, esophagitis, bloody stools, gastritis, intestinal obstruction, hemorrhage (rectal), pancreatitis, stomatitis

Genitourinary: impotence, prostate enlarged, hematuria, UTI

Hematologic; Acute myeloblastic leukemia, anemia (including hemolytic), leukopenia, neutropenia, pancytopenia, splenomegaly, thrombocytopenia

Hepatic: Alkaline phosphatase increased, GGT increased, hepatitis, hepatomegaly, hepatosplenomegaly, jaundice, liver disease exacerbation

Neuromuscular & skeletal: Arthritis, LDH increased

Ocular: Blepharitis, visual disturbance

Otic: Otitis, hearing decreased, tinnitus

Renal: Nephrolithiasis, renal calculus

Respiratory: Dyspnea, hemoptysis, pharyngitis, upper respiratory tract infection

Miscellaneous: Immune reconstitution syndrome, infections (bacterial, fungal, viral)

Available Dosage Forms

Capsule, Oral:

Invirase: 200 mg

Tablet, Oral:

Invirase: 500 mg

General Dosage Range Dosage adjustment recommended in patients on concomitant therapy

Oral: *Children >16 years and Adults:* 1000 mg twice daily

Administration

Oral Administer saquinavir and ritonavir at the same time and within 2 hours after a full meal.

Patients unable to swallow capsules may open capsules and mix contents with 15 mL of syrup (or sorbitol if diabetic or glucose intolerant) or with 3 teaspoons of jam. Mixture should be stirred for 30-60 seconds and then administered entirely. Suspension should be at room temperature prior to administration.

Storage/Stability Invirase®: Store at 25°C (77°F); excursions permitted to 15°C to 30°C (59°F to 86°F).

Nursing Actions

Physical Assessment Monitor for adherence to regimen. Monitor for gastrointestinal disturbance (nausea, vomiting, diarrhea) that can lead to dehydration and weight loss, hyperlipidemia, and redistribution of body fat, rash, CNS effects (malaise, insomnia, abnormal thinking), and electrolyte imbalance at regular intervals during therapy. Teach patient proper timing of multiple medications. Instruct patient on glucose testing (protease inhibitors may cause hyperglycemia, exacerbation or new-onset diabetes).

Patient Education
- Discuss specific use of drug and side effects with patient as it relates to treatment. (HCAHPS: During this hospital stay, were you given any medicine that you had not taken before? Before giving you any new medicine, how often did hospital staff tell you what the medicine was for? How often did hospital staff describe possible side effects in a way you could understand?)
- Patient may experience headache, dyspepsia, pyrosis, nausea, diarrhea, lipodystrophy, or diabetes. Have patient report immediately to prescriber severe dizziness, syncope, tachycardia, bradycardia, discolored urine, jaundice, inability to eat, asthenia, polydipsia, polyuria, weight loss, or rash (HCAHPS).
- Educate patient about signs of a significant reaction (eg, wheezing; chest tightness; fever; itching; bad cough; blue skin color; seizures; or swelling of face, lips, tongue, or throat). **Note:** This is not a comprehensive list of all side effects. Patient should consult prescriber for additional questions.

Intended Use and Disclaimer: Should not be printed and given to patients. This information is intended to serve as a concise initial reference for healthcare professionals to use when discussing medications with a patient. You must ultimately rely on your own discretion, experience and judgment in diagnosing, treating and advising patients.

Dietary Considerations Take within 2 hours of a meal. Invirase® capsules and tablets contain lactose (not expected to induce symptoms of intolerance).

Sargramostim (sar GRAM oh stim)

Brand Names: U.S. Leukine

Index Terms GM-CSF; GMCSF; Granulocyte-Macrophage Colony Stimulating Factor; Prokine; Recombinant Granulocyte-Macrophage Colony Stimulating Factor; rhuGM-CSF

Pharmacologic Category Colony Stimulating Factor; Hematopoietic Agent

Medication Safety Issues
Sound-alike/look-alike issues:
Leukine may be confused with Leukeran, leucovorin

Pregnancy Risk Factor C

Lactation Excretion in breast milk unknown/not recommended

Breast-Feeding Considerations It is not known if sargramostim is excreted in breast milk. Breast-feeding is not recommended by the manufacturer.

Use
Acute myelogenous leukemia (AML): To shorten time to neutrophil recovery and to reduce the incidence of severe and life-threatening infections and infections resulting in death following induction chemotherapy in older adults (≥55 years of age)

Bone marrow transplant (allogeneic or autologous): For graft failure or engraftment delay

Myeloid reconstitution after allogeneic bone marrow transplantation: To accelerate myeloid recovery

Myeloid reconstitution after autologous bone marrow transplantation: To accelerate myeloid recovery following transplantation in non-Hodgkin lymphoma (NHL), acute lymphoblastic leukemia (ALL), Hodgkin lymphoma

Peripheral stem cell transplantation: Mobilization of hematopoietic progenitor cells for leukapheresis and myeloid reconstitution following autologous peripheral stem cell transplantation

Unlabeled Use
Primary prophylaxis of neutropenia in patients receiving chemotherapy (outside transplant and AML) or who are at high risk for neutropenic fever

Treatment of radiation-induced myelosuppression of the bone marrow

Mechanism of Action/Effect Stimulates proliferation, differentiation and functional activity of neutrophils, eosinophils, monocytes, and macrophages.

Contraindications Hypersensitivity to sargramostim, yeast-derived products, or any component of the formulation; concurrent (24 hours preceding/following) use with myelosuppressive chemotherapy or radiation therapy; patients with excessive (≥10%) leukemic myeloid blasts in bone marrow or peripheral blood

Warnings/Precautions Simultaneous administration or administration 24 hours preceding/following cytotoxic chemotherapy or radiotherapy is ▶

contraindicated due to the sensitivity of rapidly dividing hematopoietic progenitor cells. If there is a rapid increase in blood counts (ANC >20,000/mm³, WBC >50,000/mm³, or platelets >500,000/mm³), decrease the dose by 50% or discontinue therapy. Excessive blood counts should fall to normal within 3-7 days after the discontinuation of therapy. Monitor CBC with differential twice weekly during treatment. Limited response to sargramostim may be seen in patients who have received bone marrow purged by chemical agents which do not preserve an adequate number of responsive hematopoietic progenitors (eg, <1.2 x 10⁴/kg progenitors). In patients receiving autologous bone marrow transplant, response to sargramostim may be limited if extensive radiotherapy to the abdomen or chest or multiple myelotoxic agents were administered prior to transplantation. May potentially act as a growth factor for any tumor type, particularly myeloid malignancies; caution should be exercised when using in any malignancy with myeloid characteristics. Tumors of nonhematopoietic origin may have surface receptors for sargramostim. Discontinue use if disease progression occurs during treatment.

Anaphylaxis or other serious allergic reactions have been reported; discontinue immediately and initiate appropriate therapy if a serious allergic or anaphylactic reaction occurs. A "first-dose effect", characterized by respiratory distress, hypoxia, flushing, hypotension, syncope, and/or tachycardia, may occur (rarely) with the first dose of a cycle and resolve with appropriate symptomatic treatment; symptoms do not usually occur with subsequent doses within that cycle. Dyspnea may occur; monitor respiratory symptoms during and following I.V. infusion. Decrease infusion rate by 50% if dyspnea occurs; discontinue the infusion if dyspnea persists despite reduction in the rate of administration. Subsequent doses may be administered at the standard rate with careful monitoring. Use with caution in patients with hypoxia or preexisting pulmonary disease. Edema, capillary leak syndrome, pleural and/or pericardial effusion have been reported; fluid retention has been shown to be reversible with dosage reduction or discontinuation of sargramostim with or without concomitant use of diuretics. Use with caution in patients with pre-existing fluid retention, pulmonary infiltrates, or congestive heart failure; may exacerbate fluid retention.

Use with caution in patients with pre-existing cardiac disease. Reversible transient supraventricular arrhythmias have been reported, especially in patients with a history of arrhythmias. Use with caution in patients with hepatic impairment (hyperbilirubinemia and elevated transaminases have been observed) or renal impairment (serum creatinine elevations have been observed). Monitor hepatic and renal function at least every other week in patients with history of impairment. Solution contains benzyl alcohol; do not use in premature infants or neonates.

Drug Interactions

Avoid Concomitant Use There are no known interactions where it is recommended to avoid concomitant use.

Decreased Effect There are no known significant interactions involving a decrease in effect.

Increased Effect/Toxicity

Sargramostim may increase the levels/effects of: Bleomycin

Adverse Reactions

>10%:

Cardiovascular: Hypertension (34%), edema (13% to 25%), pericardial effusion (4% to 25%), thrombosis (19%), chest pain (15%), peripheral edema (11%), tachycardia (11%)

Central nervous system: Malaise (57%), headache (26%), chills (25%), anxiety (11%), insomnia (11%)

Dermatologic: Skin rash (44% to 77%), pruritus (23%)

Endocrine & metabolic: Weight loss (37%), hyperglycemia (25%), hypercholesterolemia (17%), hypomagnesemia (15%)

Gastrointestinal: Diarrhea (81% to 89%), nausea (58% to 70%), vomiting (46% to 70%), gastric ulcer (50%), abdominal pain (38%), anorexia (13%), hematemesis (13%), dysphagia (11%), gastrointestinal hemorrhage (11%)

Hepatic: Hyperbilirubinemia (30%)

Neuromuscular & skeletal: Weakness (66%), ostealgia (21%), arthralgia (11% to 21%), myalgia (18%)

Ophthalmic: Retinal hemorrhage (11%)

Renal: Increased blood urea nitrogen (23%), increased serum creatinine (15%)

Respiratory: Pharyngitis (23%), epistaxis (17%), dyspnea (15%)

Miscellaneous: Fever (81%)

1% to 10%:

Immunologic: Antibody development (2%)

Respiratory: Pleural effusion (1%)

Pharmacodynamics/Kinetics

Onset of Action Increase in WBC: 7-14 days

Duration of Action WBCs return to baseline within 1 week of discontinuing drug

Available Dosage Forms

Solution Reconstituted, Intravenous [preservative free]:

Leukine: 250 mcg (1 ea)

General Dosage Range

I.V.: *Adults:* Infusion: 250 mcg/m² once daily (maximum: 500 mcg/m²/day)

SubQ: *Adults:* 250 mcg/m² once daily

Administration

I.V. I.V.: Infuse over 2 hours, 4 hours or 24 hours (indication specific). An in-line membrane filter should **NOT** be used for intravenous administration. When administering GM-CSF subcutaneously, rotate injection sites.

Injectable Detail pH: 6.7-7.7 (injection solution); 7.1-7.7 (reconstituted solution)

Subcutaneous Administer undiluted; rotate injection sites, avoiding navel/waistline.

Preparation for Administration

Powder for injection: May be reconstituted with 1 mL of preservative free SWFI or bacteriostatic water for injection. Direct the diluent toward the side of the vial and gently swirl to reconstitute; do not shake. Do not mix the contents of vials which have been reconstituted with different diluents.

SubQ: May be administered without further dilution.

I.V.: Further dilution with NS is required. If the final sargramostim concentration is <10 mcg/mL, 1 mg of human albumin per 1 mL of NS should be added (eg, add 1 mL of 5% human albumin per 50 mL of NS).

Storage/Stability Store intact vials at 2°C to 8°C (36°F to 46°F); do not freeze. Do not shake.

Solution for injection: May be stored for up to 20 days at 2°C to 8°C (36°F to 46°F) once the vial has been entered. Discard remaining solution after 20 days.

Powder for injection: Preparations made with SWFI should be administered as soon as possible, and discarded within 6 hours of reconstitution. Solutions reconstituted with bacteriostatic water may be stored for up to 20 days at 2°C to 8°C (36°F to 46°F); do not freeze.

Nursing Actions

Physical Assessment Patient must be monitored closely during and following infusion for respiratory symptoms and "first-dose effect" (hypotension, tachycardia, flushing, and syncope with the first dose of a cycle). Monitor for respiratory symptoms, fluid balance (I and O), rash, hypotension, tachycardia, GI disturbance (diarrhea, stomatitis, mucositis), myalgia, and bone pain.

Patient Education

• Discuss specific use of drug and side effects with patient as it relates to treatment. (HCAHPS: During this hospital stay, were you given any medicine that you had not taken before? Before giving you any new medicine, how often did hospital staff tell you what the medicine was for? How often did hospital staff describe possible side effects in a way you could understand?)

• Patient may experience injection site irritation, headache, insomnia, edema, osteodynia, myalgia, arthralgia, asthenia, hypertension, diarrhea, hypotension, tachycardia, or flushing. Have patient report immediately to prescriber dyspnea, severe dizziness, edema, significant weight gain, or rash (HCAHPS).

• Educate patient about signs of a significant reaction (eg, wheezing; chest tightness; fever; itching; bad cough; blue skin color; seizures; or

swelling of face, lips, tongue, or throat). **Note:** This is not a comprehensive list of all side effects. Patient should consult prescriber for additional questions.

Intended Use and Disclaimer: Should not be printed and given to patients. This information is intended to serve as a concise initial reference for healthcare professionals to use when discussing medications with a patient. You must ultimately rely on your own discretion, experience and judgment in diagnosing, treating and advising patients.

Saxagliptin and Metformin
(sax a GLIP tin & met FOR min)

Brand Names: U.S. Kombiglyze™ XR

Index Terms Metformin and Saxagliptin; Metformin Hydrochloride and Saxagliptin; Saxagliptin and Metformin Hydrochloride

Pharmacologic Category Antidiabetic Agent, Biguanide; Antidiabetic Agent, Dipeptidyl Peptidase IV (DPP-IV) Inhibitor

Medication Safety Issues

Sound-alike/look-alike issues:

Saxagliptin and Metformin may be confused with sitaGLIPtin and Metformin

Kombiglyze™ XR (U.S. brand name for **extended release** saxagliptin/metformin combination) may be confused with Komboglyze™ (Canadian brand name for **immediate release** saxagliptin/metformin combination)

High alert medication:

The Institute for Safe Medication Practices (ISMP) includes this medication among its list of drug classes which have a heightened risk of causing significant patient harm when used in error.

Medication Guide Available Yes

Pregnancy Risk Factor B

Use Management of type 2 diabetes mellitus (non-insulin dependent, NIDDM) as an adjunct to diet and exercise when treatment with both saxagliptin and metformin is appropriate

Available Dosage Forms

Tablet, variable release, oral:

Kombiglyze™ XR 2.5/1000: Saxagliptin 2.5 mg [immediate release] and metformin hydrochloride 1000 mg [extended release]; 5/500: Saxagliptin 5 mg [immediate release] and metformin hydrochloride 500 mg [extended release]; 5/1000: Saxagliptin 5 mg [immediate release] and metformin hydrochloride 1000 mg [extended release]

General Dosage Range Dosage adjustment recommended in patients on concomitant therapy

Oral: *Adults:* Saxagliptin 2.5-5 mg and metformin 500-2000 mg once daily (maximum: 5 mg daily [saxagliptin], 2000 mg daily [metformin])

Administration

Oral Administer once daily with the evening meal. Swallow whole; do not crush, cut, or chew tablets.

Komboglyze™ (Canadian availability; immediate release formulation not available in U.S.): Administer twice daily with meals (eg, breakfast and dinner).

Nursing Actions

Physical Assessment See individual agents.

Patient Education
- Discuss specific use of drug and side effects with patient as it relates to treatment. (HCAHPS: During this hospital stay, were you given any medicine that you had not taken before? Before giving you any new medicine, how often did hospital staff tell you what the medicine was for? How often did hospital staff describe possible side effects in a way you could understand?)
- Patient may experience nausea, diarrhea, flatulence, asthenia, headache, rhinitis, or rhinorrhea. Have patient report immediately to prescriber angina, chills, pharyngitis, dysuria, difficult urination, foul-smelling urine, signs of hypoglycemia, signs of pancreatitis, or signs of lactic acidosis (HCAHPS).
- Educate patient about signs of a significant reaction (eg, wheezing; chest tightness; fever; itching; bad cough; blue skin color; seizures; or swelling of face, lips, tongue, or throat). **Note:** This is not a comprehensive list of all side effects. Patient should consult prescriber for additional questions.

Intended Use and Disclaimer: Should not be printed and given to patients. This information is intended to serve as a concise initial reference for healthcare professionals to use when discussing medications with a patient. You must ultimately rely on your own discretion, experience and judgment in diagnosing, treating and advising patients.

Related Information

MetFORMIN *on page 1014*

Oral Medications That Should Not Be Crushed or Altered *on page 1712*

Scopolamine (Systemic) (skoe POL a meen)

Brand Names: U.S. Transderm-Scop

Index Terms Hyoscine Butylbromide; Scopolamine Base; Scopolamine Butylbromide; Scopolamine Hydrobromide

Pharmacologic Category Anticholinergic Agent

Medication Safety Issues

BEERS Criteria medication:
This drug may be potentially inappropriate for use in geriatric patients (Quality of evidence - moderate; Strength of recommendation - strong).

Other safety concerns:
Transdermal patch may contain conducting metal (eg, aluminum); remove patch prior to MRI.

Pregnancy Risk Factor C

Lactation Enters breast milk/use caution

Use

Scopolamine base: Transdermal: Prevention of nausea/vomiting associated with motion sickness and recovery from anesthesia and surgery

Scopolamine hydrobromide: Injection: Preoperative medication to produce amnesia, sedation, tranquilization, antiemetic effects, and decrease salivary and respiratory secretions

Scopolamine butylbromide [not available in the U.S.]: Oral/injection: Treatment of smooth muscle spasm of the genitourinary or gastrointestinal tract; injection may also be used prior to radiological/diagnostic procedures to prevent spasm

Unlabeled Use Scopolamine base: Transdermal: Breakthrough treatment of nausea and vomiting associated with chemotherapy

Available Dosage Forms

Patch 72 Hour, Transdermal:
Transderm-Scop: 1.5 mg (1 ea, 4 ea, 10 ea, 24 ea)

Solution, Injection:
Generic: 0.4 mg/mL (1 mL)

General Dosage Range

I.M., I.V., SubQ:
Children 6 months to 3 years: 0.1-0.15 mg
Children 3-6 years: 0.2-0.3 mg
Adults: 0.3-0.65 mg (single dose) **or** 0.6 mg 3-4 times/day

Transdermal: *Adults:* Apply 1 patch every 3 days as needed

Administration

I.M. Butylbromide: Intramuscular injections should be administered 10-15 minutes prior to radiological/diagnostic procedures.

I.V.
Butylbromide: No dilution is necessary prior to injection; inject at a rate of 1 mL/minute
Hydrobromide: Dilute with an equal volume of sterile water and administer by direct I.V.; inject over 2-3 minutes

Injectable Detail Hydrobromide: pH: 3.5-6.5

Oral Tablet should be swallowed whole and taken with a full glass of water.

Topical Transdermal: Apply to hairless area of skin behind the ear. Wash hands before and after applying the disc to avoid drug contact with eyes. Do not use any patch that has been damaged, cut, or manipulated in any way. Topical patch is programmed to deliver 1 mg over 3 days. Once applied, do not remove the patch for 3 full days (motion sickness). When used postoperatively for nausea/vomiting, the patch should be removed 24 hours after surgery. If patch becomes displaced, discard and apply a new patch.

Other Butylbromide or hydrobromide: May administer by subcutaneous injection.

Nursing Actions

Physical Assessment When used preoperatively, safety precautions should be observed and patient should be advised about blurred vision.

Patient Education

- Discuss specific use of drug and side effects with patient as it relates to treatment. (HCAHPS: During this hospital stay, were you given any medicine that you had not taken before? Before giving you any new medicine, how often did hospital staff tell you what the medicine was for? How often did hospital staff describe possible side effects in a way you could understand?)
- Patient may experience presyncope, fatigue, blurred vision, illogical thinking, constipation, or xerostomia. Have patient report immediately to prescriber severe dizziness, urinary retention, or rash (HCAHPS).
- Educate patient about signs of a significant reaction (eg, wheezing; chest tightness; fever; itching; bad cough; blue skin color; seizures; or swelling of face, lips, tongue, or throat). **Note:** This is not a comprehensive list of all side effects. Patient should consult prescriber for additional questions.

Intended Use and Disclaimer: Should not be printed and given to patients. This information is intended to serve as a concise initial reference for healthcare professionals to use when discussing medications with a patient. You must ultimately rely on your own discretion, experience and judgment in diagnosing, treating and advising patients.

Selegiline (se LE ji leen)

Brand Names: U.S. Eldepryl; Emsam; Zelapar
Index Terms Deprenyl; L-Deprenyl; Selegiline Hydrochloride
Pharmacologic Category Anti-Parkinson's Agent, MAO Type B Inhibitor; Antidepressant, Monoamine Oxidase Inhibitor
Medication Safety Issues
Sound-alike/look-alike issues:
Selegiline may be confused with Salagen, sertraline, Serzone, Stelazine
Eldepryl may be confused with Elavil, enalapril
Zelapar may be confused with zaleplon, Zemplar, zolpidem, ZyPREXA Zydis
Medication Guide Available Yes
Pregnancy Risk Factor C
Lactation Excretion in breast milk unknown/not recommended
Breast-Feeding Considerations It is not known if selegiline is excreted in breast milk. The manufacturer recommends discontinuing all unessential drugs in nursing women.
Use Adjunct in the management of parkinsonian patients in which levodopa/carbidopa therapy is

deteriorating (oral products); treatment of major depressive disorder (transdermal product)
Unlabeled Use Early Parkinson's disease; attention-deficit/hyperactivity disorder (ADHD)
Mechanism of Action/Effect At lower oral doses (capsule/tablet ≤10 mg/day; orally disintegrating tablet <2.5 mg/day), selegiline is a selective monoamine oxidase (MAO) type B inhibitor, which increases dopaminergic synaptic activity thus reducing symptoms of Parkinsonism. At higher oral doses or administered transdermally in recommended doses, selegiline nonselectively inhibits both MAO-B and MAO-A which blocks catabolism of other centrally-active biogenic amine neurotransmitters leading to improved mood
Contraindications Hypersensitivity to selegiline or any component of the formulation; concomitant use of meperidine
Orally disintegrating tablet: Additional contraindications: Concomitant use of dextromethorphan, methadone, propoxyphene, tramadol, oral selegiline, other MAO inhibitors
Transdermal: Additional contraindications: Pheochromocytoma; concomitant use of bupropion, selective or dual serotonin reuptake inhibitors (including SSRIs and SNRIs), tricyclic antidepressants, tramadol, propoxyphene, methadone, dextromethorphan, St. John's wort, mirtazapine, cyclobenzaprine, oral selegiline and other MAO inhibitors; carbamazepine, and oxcarbazepine; elective surgery requiring general anesthesia (selegiline should be discontinued at least 10 days prior to elective surgery); local anesthesia containing sympathomimetic vasoconstrictors; sympathomimetics (and related compounds); foods high in tyramine content; supplements containing tyrosine, phenylalanine, tryptophan, or caffeine
Warnings/Precautions
Oral: MAO-B selective inhibition should not pose a problem with tyramine-containing products as long as the typical oral doses are employed, however, rare reactions have been reported. Increased risk of nonselective MAO inhibition occurs with oral capsule/tablet doses >10 mg/day or orally disintegrating tablet doses >2.5 mg/day. Use of oral selegiline with tricyclic antidepressants and SSRIs has also been associated with rare reactions and should generally be avoided. Addition to levodopa therapy may result in exacerbation of levodopa adverse effects, requiring a reduction in levodopa dosage. Dopaminergic agents used for Parkinson's disease or restless legs syndrome have been associated with compulsive behaviors and/or loss of impulse control, which has manifested as pathological gambling, libido increases (hypersexuality), and/or binge eating. Causality has not been established, and controversy exists as to whether this phenomenon is related to the underlying disease, prior behaviors/addictions and/or drug therapy. Dose reduction or discontinuation of therapy has ▶

been reported to reverse these behaviors in some, but not all cases. Use caution in patients with hepatic or renal impairment. Incidence of orthostatic hypotension may be increased in older adults and when titrating to the 2.5 mg dosage in patients taking the orally disintegrating tablet. Risk for melanoma development is increased in Parkinson's disease patients; drug causation or factors contributing to risk have not been established. Patients should be monitored closely and periodic skin examinations should be performed. Orally disintegrating tablet may cause oral mucosa edema, irritation, pain, ulceration and/or swallowing pain. Do not use orally disintegrating tablet concurrently with other selegiline products; wait at least 14 days from discontinuation before initiating treatment with another selegiline dosage form. Some products may contain phenylalanine.

Transdermal: Nonselective MAO inhibition occurs with transdermal delivery and is necessary for antidepressant efficacy. Hypertensive crisis as a result of ingesting tyramine-rich foods is always a concern with nonselective MAO inhibition. Although transdermal delivery minimizes inhibition of MAO-A in the gut, there is limited data with higher transdermal doses; dietary modifications are recommended with doses >6 mg/24 hours.

Transdermal patch: May cause orthostatic hypotension; use with caution in patients at risk of this effect or in those who would not tolerate transient hypotensive episodes (cerebrovascular disease, cardiovascular disease, hypovolemia, or concurrent medication use which may predispose to hypotension/bradycardia). May contain conducting metal (eg, aluminum); remove patch prior to MRI. Avoid exposure of application site and surrounding area to direct external heat sources.

Transdermal: **[U.S. Boxed Warning]: Antidepressants increase the risk of suicidal thinking and behavior in children, adolescents, and young adults (18-24 years of age) with major depressive disorder (MDD) and other psychiatric disorders;** consider risk prior to prescribing. Short-term studies did not show an increased risk in patients >24 years of age and showed a decreased risk in patients ≥65 years. Closely monitor patients for worsening of depression, suicidality and/or associated behaviors, particularly during the initial 1-2 months of therapy or during periods of dosage adjustments (increases or decreases); the patient's family or caregiver should be instructed to closely observe the patient and communicate condition with healthcare provider. A medication guide concerning the use of antidepressants should be dispensed with each prescription. **Transdermal selegiline is not FDA approved for use in children <12 years of age.**

Transdermal: The possibility of a suicide attempt is inherit in major depression and may persist until remission occurs. Patients treated with antidepressants (for any indication) should be observed for clinical worsening and suicidality, especially during the initial few months of a course of drug therapy, or at times of dose changes, either increases or decreases. Use caution in high-risk patients. Worsening depression and severe abrupt suicidality that are not part of the presenting symptoms may require discontinuation or modification of drug therapy. Use caution in high-risk patients during initiation of therapy. The patient's family or caregiver should be alerted to monitor patients for the emergence of suicidality and associated behaviors (such as agitation, irritability, hostility, and hypomania) and call healthcare provider.

Transdermal selegiline may worsen psychosis in some patients or precipitate a shift to mania or hypomania in patients with bipolar disorder. Monotherapy in patients with bipolar disorder should be avoided. Patients presenting with depressive symptoms should be screened for bipolar disorder. **Selegiline is not FDA approved for the treatment of bipolar depression.**

Abrupt discontinuation or interruption of antidepressant therapy has been associated with a discontinuation syndrome. Symptoms arising may vary with antidepressant however commonly include nausea, vomiting, diarrhea, headaches, lightheadedness, dizziness, diminished appetite, sweating, chills, tremors, paresthesias, fatigue, somnolence, and sleep disturbances (eg, vivid dreams, insomnia). Greater risks for developing a discontinuation syndrome have been associated with antidepressants with shorter half-lives, longer durations of treatment, and abrupt discontinuation. More severe symptoms have also been associated with MAO inhibitors. For antidepressants of short or intermediate half-lives, symptoms may emerge within 2-5 days after treatment discontinuation and last 7-14 days (APA, 2010; Fava, 2006; Haddad, 2001; Shelton, 2001; Warner, 2006).

Drug Interactions

Avoid Concomitant Use

Avoid concomitant use of Selegiline with any of the following: Alpha-/Beta-Agonists (Indirect-Acting); Alpha1-Agonists; Amphetamines; Anilidopiperidine Opioids; Antidepressants (Serotonin Reuptake Inhibitor/Antagonist); Apraclonidine; AtoMOXetine; Bezafibrate; Buprenorphine; BuPROPion; BusPIRone; CarBAMazepine; Cyclobenzaprine; Cyproheptadine; Dexmethylphenidate; Dextromethorphan; Diethylpropion; Hydrocodone; HYDROmorphone; Isomethepene; Levonordefrin; Linezolid; Maprotiline; Meperidine; Methyldopa; Methylene Blue; Methylphenidate; Mirtazapine; Morphine (Liposomal); Morphine (Systemic); OXcarbazepine; Oxymorphone; Pizotifen; Selective Serotonin Reuptake Inhibitors; Serotonin 5-HT1D Receptor Agonists; Serotonin/Norepinephrine Reuptake Inhibitors;

Tapentadol; Tetrabenazine; Tetrahydrozoline (Nasal); Tricyclic Antidepressants; Tryptophan

Decreased Effect

Selegiline may decrease the levels/effects of: Domperidone; Ioflupane I 123

The levels/effects of Selegiline may be decreased by: CYP2B6 Inducers (Strong); Cyproheptadine; Dabrafenib; Domperidone; Peginterferon Alfa-2b

Increased Effect/Toxicity

Selegiline may increase the levels/effects of: Alpha-/Beta-Agonists (Indirect-Acting); Alpha1-Agonists; Amphetamines; Antidepressants (Serotonin Reuptake Inhibitor/Antagonist); Antihypertensives; Antipsychotics; Apraclonidine; AtoMOXetine; Beta2-Agonists; Betahistine; Bezafibrate; Brimonidine (Ophthalmic); Brimonidine (Topical); BuPROPion; Cyproheptadine; Dexmethylphenidate; Dextromethorphan; Diethylpropion; Dofetilide; Domperidone; Doxapram; Doxylamine; EPINEPHrine (Nasal); Epinephrine (Racemic); EPINEPHrine (Systemic, Oral Inhalation); Hydrocodone; HYDROmorphone; Hypoglycemic Agents; Isometheptene; Levonordefrin; Linezolid; Lithium; Lomitapide; Meperidine; Methadone; Methyldopa; Methylene Blue; Methylphenidate; Metoclopramide; Mirtazapine; Morphine (Liposomal); Morphine (Systemic); Norepinephrine; Orthostatic Hypotension Producing Agents; OxyCODONE; Pizotifen; Reserpine; Selective Serotonin Reuptake Inhibitors; Serotonin 5-HT1D Receptor Agonists; Serotonin Modulators; Serotonin/Norepinephrine Reuptake Inhibitors; Tetrahydrozoline (Nasal); Tricyclic Antidepressants

The levels/effects of Selegiline may be increased by: Altretamine; Anilidopiperidine Opioids; Antipsychotics; Buprenorphine; BusPIRone; CarBAMazepine; COMT Inhibitors; Contraceptives (Estrogens); Contraceptives (Progestins); Cyclobenzaprine; CYP2B6 Inhibitors (Moderate); CYP2B6 Inhibitors (Strong); Levodopa; MAO Inhibitors; Maprotiline; OXcarbazepine; Oxymorphone; Quazepam; Tapentadol; Tetrabenazine; TraMADol; Tryptophan

Nutritional/Ethanol Interactions

Ethanol: Ethanol may enhance the adverse/toxic effects of selegiline. Beverages containing tyramine (eg, hearty red wine and beer) may increase toxic effects. Management: Avoid ethanol and beverages containing tyramine.

Food: Concurrent ingestion of foods rich in tyramine, dopamine, tyrosine, phenylalanine, tryptophan, or caffeine may cause sudden and severe high blood pressure (hypertensive crisis or serotonin syndrome). Management: Avoid tyramine-containing foods (aged or matured cheese, air-dried or cured meats including sausages and salamis; fava or broad bean pods, tap/draft beers, Marmite concentrate, sauerkraut, soy sauce, and other soybean condiments. Food's freshness is also an important concern; improperly stored or spoiled food can create an environment in which tyramine concentrations may increase. Avoid foods containing dopamine, tyrosine, phenylalanine, tryptophan, or caffeine.

Herb/Nutraceutical: Kava kava, valerian, St John's wort, and SAMe may increase risk of serotonin syndrome and/or excessive sedation. Supplements containing caffeine, tyrosine, tryptophan, or phenylalanine may increase the risk of severe side effects like hypertensive reactions or serotonin syndrome. Management: Avoid kava kava, valerian, St John's wort, SAMe, and supplements containing caffeine, tyrosine, tryptophan, or phenylalanine.

Adverse Reactions Unless otherwise noted, the percentage of adverse events is reported for the transdermal patch (**Note:** ODT = orally disintegrating tablet, Oral = capsule/tablet)

>10%:

Central nervous system: Headache (18%; ODT 7%; oral 4%), insomnia (12%; ODT 7%), dizziness (oral 14%; ODT 11%)

Gastrointestinal: Nausea (oral 20%; ODT 11%)

Local: Application site reaction (24%)

1% to 10%:

Cardiovascular: Hypotension (including postural 3% to 10%), palpitation (oral 2%), chest pain (≥1%; ODT 2%), hypertension (≥1%; ODT 3%), peripheral edema (≥1%)

Central nervous system: Pain (ODT 8%; oral 2%), hallucinations (oral 6%; ODT 4%), confusion (oral 6%; ODT 4%), vivid dreams (oral 4%), ataxia (ODT 3%), somnolence (ODT 3%), lethargy (oral 2%), agitation (≥1%), amnesia (≥1%), paresthesia (≥1%), thinking abnormal (≥1%), depression (<1%; ODT 2%)

Dermatologic: Rash (4%), bruising (≥1%; ODT 2%), pruritus (≥1%), acne (≥1%)

Endocrine & metabolic: Weight loss (5%; oral 2%), hypokalemia (ODT 2%), sexual side effects (≤1%)

Gastrointestinal: Diarrhea (9%; ODT 2%; oral 2%), xerostomia (8%; oral 6%; ODT 4%), stomatitis (ODT 5%), abdominal pain (oral 8%), dyspepsia (4%; ODT 5%), dysphagia (ODT 2%), dental caries (ODT 2%), constipation (≥1%; ODT 4%), flatulence (≥1%; ODT 2%), anorexia (≥1%), gastroenteritis (≥1%), taste perversion (≥1%; ODT 2%), vomiting (≥1%; ODT 3%)

Genitourinary: Urinary retention (oral 2%), dysmenorrhea (≥1%), metrorrhagia (≥1%), UTI (≥1%), urinary frequency (≥1%)

Neuromuscular & skeletal: Dyskinesia (ODT 6%), back pain (ODT 5%; oral 2%), ataxia (<1%; ODT 3%), leg cramps (ODT 3%; oral 2%), myalgia (≥1%; ODT 3%), neck pain (≥1%), tremor (<1%; ODT 3%)

Otic: Tinnitus (≥1%)

Respiratory: Rhinitis (ODT 7%), pharyngitis (3%; ODT 4%), sinusitis (3%), cough (≥1%), bronchitis (≥1%), dyspnea (<1%; ODT 3%)

Miscellaneous: Diaphoresis (≥1%)

Pharmacodynamics/Kinetics

Onset of Action Therapeutic: Oral: Within 1 hour

Duration of Action Oral: 24-72 hours

Available Dosage Forms

Capsule, Oral:

Eldepryl: 5 mg

Generic: 5 mg

Patch 24 Hour, Transdermal:

Emsam: 6 mg/24 hr (30 ea); 9 mg/24 hr (30 ea); 12 mg/24 hr (30 ea)

Tablet, Oral:

Generic: 5 mg

Tablet Dispersible, Oral:

Zelapar: 1.25 mg

General Dosage Range

Oral:

Capsule/Tablet: *Adults:* 5 mg twice daily

Disintegrating tablet: *Adults:* Initial: 1.25 mg daily; Maintenance: 1.25-2.5 mg daily (maximum: 2.5 mg daily)

Transdermal:

Adults: Initial: 6 mg once daily; Maintenance: 6-12 mg once daily (maximum: 12 mg/day)

Elderly: 6 mg once daily

Administration

Oral Orally disintegrating tablet (Zelapar®): Take in morning before breakfast; place on top of tongue and allow to dissolve. Avoid food or liquid 5 minutes before and after administration.

Topical Transdermal (Emsam®): Apply to clean, dry, intact skin to the upper torso (below the neck and above the waist), upper thigh, or outer surface of the upper arm. Avoid exposure of application site to external heat source, which may increase the amount of drug absorbed. Apply at the same time each day and rotate application sites. Wash hands with soap and water after handling. Avoid touching the sticky side of the patch.

Storage/Stability

Capsule, tablet, transdermal: Store at 20°C to 25°C (68°F to 77°F). Store patch in sealed pouch and apply immediately after removal.

Orally disintegrating tablet: Store at controlled room temperature 25°C (77°F); excursions permitted to 15°C to 30°C (59°F to 86°F). Use within 3 months of opening pouch and immediately after opening individual blister.

Nursing Actions

Physical Assessment Monitor therapeutic response (eg, mental status, involuntary movements) at beginning of therapy and periodically throughout. Monitor blood pressure. Be alert to suicide ideation. Patient should be cautioned against eating foods high in tyramine. Discontinue transdermal product at least 10 days prior to elective surgery. Taper dose when discontinuing.

Patient Education

• Discuss specific use of drug and side effects with patient as it relates to treatment. (HCAHPS: During this hospital stay, were you given any medicine that you had not taken before? Before giving you any new medicine, how often did hospital staff tell you what the medicine was for? How often did hospital staff describe possible side effects in a way you could understand?)

• Patient may experience presyncope, fatigue, blurred vision, illogical thinking, dizziness, headache, nausea, insomnia, or skin irritation. Have patient report immediately to prescriber tachycardia, significant change in balance, uncontrollable compulsions, nervousness and anxiety, severe flushing, or rash (HCAHPS).

• Educate patient about signs of a significant reaction (eg, wheezing; chest tightness; fever; itching; bad cough; blue skin color; seizures; or swelling of face, lips, tongue, or throat). **Note:** This is not a comprehensive list of all side effects. Patient should consult prescriber for additional questions.

Intended Use and Disclaimer: Should not be printed and given to patients. This information is intended to serve as a concise initial reference for healthcare professionals to use when discussing medications with a patient. You must ultimately rely on your own discretion, experience and judgment in diagnosing, treating and advising patients.

Dietary Considerations Avoid or limit tyramine-containing foods/beverages (product and/or dose-dependent). Some examples include aged or matured cheese, air-dried or cured meats (including sausages and salamis), fava or broad bean pods, tap/draft beers, Marmite concentrate, sauerkraut, soy sauce and other soybean condiments. Food's freshness is also an important concern; improperly stored or spoiled food can create an environment where tyramine concentrations may increase.

Emsam®: 9 mg/24 hours or 12 mg/24 hours: Avoid tyramine-rich foods or beverages beginning the first day of treatment or for 2 weeks after discontinuation or dose reduction to 6 mg/24 hours. Zelapar®: Do not take with food or liquid. Some products may contain phenylalanine.

Sertraline (SER tra leen)

Brand Names: U.S. Zoloft

Index Terms Sertraline Hydrochloride

Pharmacologic Category Antidepressant, Selective Serotonin Reuptake Inhibitor

Medication Safety Issues

Sound-alike/look-alike issues:

Sertraline may be confused with cetirizine, selegiline, Serevent, Soriatane

Zoloft may be confused with Zocor

BEERS Criteria medication:

This drug may be potentially inappropriate for use in geriatric patients (Quality of evidence - moderate; Strength of recommendation - strong).

Medication Guide Available Yes

Pregnancy Risk Factor C

Lactation Enters breast milk/use caution

Breast-Feeding Considerations Sertraline and desmethylsertraline are excreted in breast milk. Adverse events have been reported in nursing infants exposed to some SSRIs. The American Academy of Breastfeeding Medicine suggests that sertraline may be considered for the treatment of postpartum depression in appropriately selected women who are nursing. Infants exposed to sertraline while breast-feeding generally receive a low relative dose and serum concentrations are not detectable in most infants. Sertraline concentrations in the hindmilk are higher than in foremilk. If the benefits of the mother receiving the sertraline and breast-feeding outweigh the risks, the mother may consider pumping and discarding breast milk with the feeding 7-9 hours after the daily dose to decrease sertraline exposure to the infant. The long-term effects on development and behavior have not been studied. The manufacturer recommends that caution be exercised when administering sertraline to nursing women. Maternal use of an SSRI during pregnancy may cause delayed milk secretion.

Use

Major depressive disorder: Treatment of major depressive disorder (MDD) in adults.

Obsessive-compulsive disorder: Treatment of obsessions and compulsions in patients with obsessive-compulsive disorder (OCD).

Panic disorder: Treatment of panic disorder in adults with or without agoraphobia.

Post-traumatic stress disorder: Treatment of post-traumatic stress disorder (PTSD) in adults.

Premenstrual dysphoric disorder: Treatment of premenstrual dysphoric disorder (PMDD) in adults.

Social anxiety disorder: Treatment of social anxiety disorder (social phobia) in adults.

Unlabeled Use Binge-eating disorder; bulimia nervosa; generalized anxiety disorder (GAD)

Mechanism of Action/Effect Antidepressant with selective inhibitory effects on presynaptic serotonin (5-HT) reuptake and only very weak effects on norepinephrine and dopamine neuronal uptake

Contraindications

Use of MAOIs intended to treat psychiatric disorders (concurrently or within 14 days of stopping an MAOI or sertraline); concurrent use with pimozide; initiation in patients treated with linezolid or methylene blue IV; hypersensitivity to sertraline or any component of the formulation; concurrent use with disulfiram (oral concentrate only).

Documentation of allergenic cross-reactivity for SSRIs is limited. However, because of similarities in chemical structure and/or pharmacologic actions, the possibility of cross-sensitivity cannot be ruled out with certainty.

Warnings/Precautions [U.S. Boxed Warning]: Antidepressants increase the risk of suicidal thinking and behavior in children, adolescents, and young adults (18-24 years of age) with major depressive disorder (MDD) and other psychiatric disorders; consider risk prior to prescribing. Short-term studies did not show an increased risk in patients >24 years of age and showed a decreased risk in patients ≥65 years. Closely monitor patients for clinical worsening, suicidality, or unusual changes in behavior, particularly during the initial 1-2 months of therapy or during periods of dosage adjustments (increases or decreases); the patient's family or caregiver should be instructed to closely observe the patient and communicate condition with healthcare provider. A medication guide concerning the use of antidepressants should be dispensed with each prescription. **Sertraline is not FDA approved for use in children with major depressive disorder (MDD). However, it is approved for the treatment of obsessive-compulsive disorder (OCD) in children ≥6 years of age.**

The possibility of a suicide attempt is inherent in major depression and may persist until remission occurs. Use caution in high-risk patients. Worsening depression and severe abrupt suicidality that are not part of the presenting symptoms may require discontinuation or modification of drug therapy. The patient's family or caregiver should be alerted to monitor patients for the emergence of suicidality and associated behaviors (such as agitation, irritability, hostility, impulsivity, and hypomania) and call healthcare provider.

May precipitate a mixed/manic episode in patients at risk for bipolar disorder. Use with caution in patients with a family history of bipolar disorder, mania, or hypomania. Patients presenting with depressive symptoms should be screened for bipolar disorder. **Sertraline is not FDA approved for the treatment of bipolar depression.**

Potentially life-threatening serotonin syndrome (SS) has occurred with serotonergic agents (eg, SSRIs, SNRIs), particularly when used in combination with other serotonergic agents (eg, triptans, TCAs, fentanyl, lithium, tramadol, buspirone, St John's wort, tryptophan) or agents that impair metabolism of serotonin (eg, MAO inhibitors intended to treat psychiatric disorders, other MAO inhibitors [ie, linezolid and intravenous methylene blue]). Discontinue treatment (and any concomitant serotonergic agent) immediately if signs/symptoms arise. Has a very low potential to impair cognitive or motor performance. However, caution patients regarding activities requiring alertness until response to sertraline is known. Does not appear to potentiate the effects of alcohol, however, ethanol use is not advised.

Use with caution in patients with risk factors for QTc prolongation; cases of QTc prolongation and torsade de pointes have been reported. Use caution in patients with a previous seizure disorder or condition predisposing to seizures such as brain damage, alcoholism, or concurrent therapy with other drugs which lower the seizure threshold. May increase the risks associated with electroconvulsive therapy. Use with caution in patients with narrow-angle glaucoma or a history of glaucoma; may cause mydriasis, which can exacerbate symptoms. Use with caution in patients with hepatic dysfunction and in elderly patients. May cause hyponatremia/SIADH (elderly at increased risk); volume depletion (diuretics may increase risk). Use caution in elderly patients; may cause or exacerbate syndrome of inappropriate antidiuretic hormone secretion or hyponatremia; monitor sodium closely with initiation or dosage adjustments in older adults (Beers Criteria). Sertraline acts as a mild uricosuric; use with caution in patients at risk of uric acid nephropathy. Use with caution in patients where weight loss is undesirable. May cause or exacerbate sexual dysfunction. Potentially significant drug-drug interactions may exist, requiring dose or frequency adjustment, additional monitoring, and/or selection of alternative therapy.

Use oral concentrate formulation with caution in patients with latex sensitivity; dropper dispenser contains dry natural rubber. Monitor growth in pediatric patients. Given their lower body weight, lower doses are advisable in pediatric patients in order to avoid excessive plasma levels, despite slightly greater metabolism efficiency than adults.

Abrupt discontinuation or interruption of antidepressant therapy has been associated with a discontinuation syndrome. Symptoms arising may vary with antidepressant however commonly include nausea, vomiting, diarrhea, headaches, lightheadedness, dizziness, diminished appetite, sweating, chills, tremors, paresthesias, fatigue, somnolence, and sleep disturbances (eg, vivid dreams, insomnia). Greater risks for developing a discontinuation syndrome have been associated with antidepressants with shorter half-lives, longer durations of treatment, and abrupt discontinuation. For antidepressants of short or intermediate half-lives, symptoms may emerge within 2-5 days after treatment discontinuation and last 7-14 days (APA, 2010; Fava, 2006; Haddad, 2001; Shelton, 2001; Warner, 2006).

Drug Interactions

Avoid Concomitant Use

Avoid concomitant use of Sertraline with any of the following: Disulfiram; Dosulepin; Iobenguane I 123; Linezolid; MAO Inhibitors; Methylene Blue; Pimozide; Thioridazine; Tryptophan; Urokinase

Decreased Effect

Sertraline may decrease the levels/effects of: Clopidogrel; Iobenguane I 123; Ioflupane I 123; Tamoxifen; Thyroid Products

The levels/effects of Sertraline may be decreased by: CarBAMazepine; Cyproheptadine; Darunavir; Efavirenz; Fosphenytoin; NSAID (COX-2 Inhibitor); NSAID (Nonselective); Peginterferon Alfa-2b; Phenytoin

Increased Effect/Toxicity

Sertraline may increase the levels/effects of: Agents with Antiplatelet Properties; Anticoagulants; Antidepressants (Serotonin Reuptake Inhibitor/Antagonist); Antipsychotics; ARIPiprazole; Aspirin; Beta-Blockers; BusPIRone; CarBAMazepine; CloZAPine; Collagenase (Systemic); CYP2B6 Substrates; CYP2C19 Substrates; CYP2D6 Substrates; Dabigatran Etexilate; Desmopressin; Dextromethorphan; Dofetilide; Dosulepin; DOXOrubicin (Conventional); Fesoterodine; Fosphenytoin; Galantamine; Highest Risk QTc-Prolonging Agents; Hypoglycemic Agents; Ibritumomab; Lomitapide; Methadone; Methylene Blue; Metoclopramide; Metoprolol; Moderate Risk QTc-Prolonging Agents; NSAID (COX-2 Inhibitor); NSAID (Nonselective); Phenytoin; Pimozide; Propafenone; RisperiDONE; Rivaroxaban; Salicylates; Serotonin Modulators; Thiazide Diuretics; Thioridazine; Thrombolytic Agents; Tositumomab and Iodine I 131 Tositumomab; TraMADol; Tricyclic Antidepressants; Urokinase; Vitamin K Antagonists

The levels/effects of Sertraline may be increased by: Alcohol (Ethyl); Analgesics (Opioid); Antipsychotics; BusPIRone; Cimetidine; CNS Depressants; Cobicistat; Dasatinib; Disulfiram; Glucosamine; Grapefruit Juice; Herbs (Anticoagulant/Antiplatelet Properties); Ibrutinib; Linezolid; Lithium; Macrolide Antibiotics; MAO Inhibitors; Metoclopramide; Metyrosine; Mifepristone; Multivitamins/Fluoride (with ADE); Multivitamins/Minerals (with ADEK, Folate, Iron); Multivitamins/Minerals (with AE, No Iron); Omega-3 Fatty Acids; Pentosan Polysulfate Sodium; Pentoxifylline; Prostacyclin Analogues; Tipranavir; TraMADol; Tryptophan; Vitamin E

Nutritional/Ethanol Interactions

Ethanol: Concurrent use with ethanol may increase CNS depression. Management: Monitor for increased effects with coadministration. Caution patients about effects.

Food: Sertraline average peak serum levels may be increased if taken with food.

Herb/Nutraceutical: Concurrent use with some herbal medications may increase the risk of serotonin syndrome and/or CNS depression. Management: Avoid valerian, St John's wort, tryptophan, kava kava, gotu kola.

Adverse Reactions

>10%:

Central nervous system: Dizziness, fatigue, headache, insomnia, somnolence

Endocrine & metabolic: Libido decreased

Gastrointestinal: Anorexia, diarrhea, nausea, xerostomia

Genitourinary: Ejaculatory disturbances

Neuromuscular & skeletal: Tremors

Miscellaneous: Diaphoresis

1% to 10%:

Cardiovascular: Chest pain, palpitation

Central nervous system: Agitation, anxiety, hypoesthesia, malaise, nervousness, pain

Dermatologic: Rash

Endocrine & metabolic: Impotence

Gastrointestinal: Appetite increased, constipation, dyspepsia, flatulence, vomiting, weight gain

Neuromuscular & skeletal: Back pain, hypertonia, myalgia, paresthesia, weakness

Ocular: Visual difficulty, abnormal vision

Otic: Tinnitus

Respiratory: Rhinitis

Miscellaneous: Yawning

Pediatric patients: Additional adverse reactions reported in pediatric patients (frequency >2%): Aggressiveness, epistaxis, hyperkinesia, purpura, sinusitis, urinary incontinence

Pharmacodynamics/Kinetics

Onset of Action Depression: The onset of action is within a week, however, individual response varies greatly and full response may not be seen until 8-12 weeks after initiation of treatment.

Available Dosage Forms

Concentrate, Oral:

Zoloft: 20 mg/mL (60 mL)

Generic: 20 mg/mL (60 mL)

Tablet, Oral:

Zoloft: 25 mg, 50 mg, 100 mg

Generic: 25 mg, 50 mg, 100 mg

General Dosage Range Dosage adjustment recommended in patients with hepatic impairment

Oral:

Children 6-12 years: Initial: 25 mg once daily; Maintenance: 25-200 mg once daily (maximum: 200 mg daily)

Children 13-17 years: Initial: 50 mg once daily; Maintenance: 25-200 mg once daily (maximum: 200 mg daily)

Adults: Initial: 25-50 mg once daily; Maintenance: 50-200 mg once daily (maximum: 200 mg daily)

Administration

Oral Administer once daily either in the morning or evening; if somnolence is noted, administer at bedtime.

Oral concentrate: Must be diluted immediately before use. **Note:** Use with caution in patients with latex sensitivity; dropper dispenser contains dry natural rubber.

Preparation for Administration Oral concentrate: Must be diluted before use. **Immediately before administration**, use the dropper provided to measure the required amount of concentrate; mix with 4 ounces (1/2 cup) of water, ginger ale, lemon/lime soda, lemonade, or orange juice only. Do not mix with any other liquids than these. The dose should be taken immediately after mixing; do not mix in advance. A slight haze may appear after mixing; this is normal.

Storage/Stability Store at 25°C (77°F); excursions are permitted between 15°C and 30°C (59°F and 86°F).

Nursing Actions

Physical Assessment Assess mental status for worsening of depression, suicide ideation, anxiety, social functioning, mania, or panic attack (especially during initiation of therapy and when dosage is changed). Pediatric patients: Monitor growth pattern.

Patient Education

• Discuss specific use of drug and side effects with patient as it relates to treatment. (HCAHPS: During this hospital stay, were you given any medicine that you had not taken before? Before giving you any new medicine, how often did hospital staff tell you what the medicine was for? How often did hospital staff describe possible side effects in a way you could understand?)

• Patient may experience fatigue, asthenia, dyspepsia, xerostomia, constipation, sexual dysfunction, insomnia, or lack of appetite. Have patient report immediately to prescriber signs of hyponatremia, signs of depression (ie, suicidal ideation, anxiety, emotional instability, illogical thinking), signs of hemorrhaging, behavioral changes, angina, vision changes, incontinence, excessive weight gain or loss, menstrual irregularities, serotonin syndrome (ie, dizziness, severe headache, agitation, hallucinations, tachycardia, arrhythmia, flushing, tremors, hyperhidrosis, change in balance, severe nausea, significant diarrhea), or priapism (HCAHPS).

• Educate patient about signs of a significant reaction (eg, wheezing; chest tightness; fever; itching; bad cough; blue skin color; seizures; or swelling of face, lips, tongue, or throat). **Note:** This is not a comprehensive list of all side effects. Patient should consult prescriber for additional questions.

Intended Use and Disclaimer: Should not be printed and given to patients. This information is intended to serve as a concise initial reference for healthcare professionals to use when discussing medications with a patient. You must ultimately

◀ rely on your own discretion, experience and judgment in diagnosing, treating and advising patients.

Sevelamer (se VEL a mer)

Brand Names: U.S. Renagel; Renvela
Index Terms Sevelamer Carbonate; Sevelamer Hydrochloride
Pharmacologic Category Phosphate Binder
Medication Safety Issues
Sound-alike/look-alike issues:
Renagel® may be confused with Reglan®, Regonol®, Renvela®
Renvela® may be confused with Reglan®, Regonol®, Renagel®
Sevelamer may be confused with Savella®
International issues:
Renagel [U.S., Canada, and multiple international markets] may be confused with Remegel brand name for aluminium hydroxide and magnesium carbonate [Netherlands] and for calcium carbonate [Hungary, Great Britain and Ireland] and with Remegel Wind Relief brand name for calcium carbonate and simethicone [Great Britain]
Pregnancy Risk Factor C
Use Reduction or control of serum phosphorous in patients with chronic kidney disease on hemodialysis
Available Dosage Forms
Packet, Oral:
Renvela: 0.8 g (1 ea, 90 ea); 2.4 g (1 ea, 90 ea)
Tablet, Oral:
Renagel: 400 mg, 800 mg
Renvela: 800 mg
General Dosage Range Oral: *Adults:* Initial: 800-1600 mg 3 times/day; Maintenance: Up to 2400-14,000 mg/day in 3 divided doses
Administration
Oral Must be administered with meals.
Powder for oral suspension: Stir vigorously to suspend mixture just prior to drinking; powder does not dissolve. Drink within 30 minutes of preparing and resuspend just prior to drinking.
Tablets: Swallow whole; do not crush, chew, or break.
Nursing Actions
Physical Assessment Monitor blood pressure; may cause high blood pressure.
Patient Education
• Discuss specific use of drug and side effects with patient as it relates to treatment. (HCAHPS: During this hospital stay, were you given any medicine that you had not taken before? Before giving you any new medicine, how often did hospital staff tell you what the medicine was for? How often did hospital staff describe possible side effects in a way you could understand?)
• Patient may experience dyspepsia, nausea, diarrhea, flatulence, or constipation. Have patient report immediately to prescriber rash (HCAHPS).
• Educate patient about signs of a significant reaction (eg, wheezing; chest tightness; fever; itching; bad cough; blue skin color; seizures; or swelling of face, lips, tongue, or throat). **Note:** This is not a comprehensive list of all side effects. Patient should consult prescriber for additional questions.

Intended Use and Disclaimer: Should not be printed and given to patients. This information is intended to serve as a concise initial reference for healthcare professionals to use when discussing medications with a patient. You must ultimately rely on your own discretion, experience and judgment in diagnosing, treating and advising patients.
Related Information
Oral Medications That Should Not Be Crushed or Altered *on page 1712*

Sildenafil (sil DEN a fil)

Brand Names: U.S. Revatio; Viagra
Index Terms Sildenafil Citrate; UK92480
Pharmacologic Category Phosphodiesterase-5 Enzyme Inhibitor
Medication Safety Issues
Sound-alike/look-alike issues:
Revatio may be confused with ReVia, Revonto
Sildenafil may be confused with silodosin, tadalafil, vardenafil
Viagra may be confused with Allegra, Vaniqa
Pregnancy Risk Factor B
Lactation Excretion in breast milk unknown/use caution
Breast-Feeding Considerations It is not known if sildenafil is excreted in breast milk. The manufacturer recommends that caution be exercised when administering sildenafil to nursing women.
Use
Revatio: Treatment of pulmonary arterial hypertension (PAH) (WHO Group I) in adults to improve exercise ability and delay clinical worsening.
Viagra: Treatment of erectile dysfunction (ED)
Unlabeled Use Pulmonary hypertension (WHO Group II, III, and IV); persistent pulmonary hypertension after recent left ventricular assist device placement
Mechanism of Action/Effect Sildenafil enhances the effect of nitric oxide by inhibiting phosphodiesterase type 5 (PDE-5), resulting in smooth muscle relaxation. In erectile dysfunction, smooth muscle relaxation results in the inflow of blood into the corpus cavernosum with sexual stimulation. In pulmonary hypertension, smooth muscle relaxation results in pulmonary vasculature; vasodilation reducing pulmonary pressure.
Contraindications Hypersensitivity to sildenafil or any component of the formulation; concurrent use

(regularly/intermittently) of organic nitrates in any form (eg, nitroglycerin, isosorbide dinitrate); concurrent use with a protease inhibitor regimen when sildenafil is used for pulmonary artery hypertension (eg, Revatio)

Warnings/Precautions Decreases in blood pressure may occur due to vasodilator effects; use with caution in patients with left ventricular outflow obstruction (aortic stenosis or hypertrophic obstructive cardiomyopathy), those on antihypertensive therapy, with resting hypotension (BP <90/50 mm Hg), fluid depletion, or autonomic dysfunction; may be more sensitive to hypotensive actions. Patients should be hemodynamically stable prior to initiating therapy at the lowest possible dose. Avoid or limit concurrent substantial alcohol consumption as this may increase the risk of symptomatic hypotension. Use with caution in patients with uncontrolled hypertension (>170/110 mm Hg); life-threatening arrhythmias, stroke or MI within the last 6 months; cardiac failure or coronary artery disease causing unstable angina; safety and efficacy have not been studied in these patients. There is a degree of cardiac risk associated with sexual activity; therefore, physicians should consider the cardiovascular status of their patients prior to initiating any treatment for erectile dysfunction. If pulmonary edema occurs when treating pulmonary arterial hypertension (PAH), consider the possibility of pulmonary veno-occlusive disease (PVOD); continued use is not recommended in patient with PVOD.

Sildenafil should be used with caution in patients with anatomical deformation of the penis (angulation, cavernosal fibrosis, or Peyronie's disease) and in patients who have conditions which may predispose them to priapism (sickle cell anemia, multiple myeloma, leukemia). All patients should be instructed to seek medical attention if erection persists >4 hours.

Vision loss may occur and be a sign of nonarteritic anterior ischemic optic neuropathy (NAION). Risk may be increased with history of vision loss. Other risk factors for NAION include low cup-to-disc ratio ("crowded disc"), coronary artery disease, diabetes, hypertension, hyperlipidemia, smoking, and age >50 years. May cause dose-related impairment of color discrimination. Use caution in patients with retinitis pigmentosa; a minority have genetic disorders of retinal phosphodiesterases (no safety information available). Sudden decrease or loss of hearing has been reported; hearing changes may be accompanied by tinnitus and dizziness. A direct relationship between therapy and vision or hearing loss has not been determined.

The potential underlying causes of erectile dysfunction should be evaluated prior to treatment. The safety and efficacy of sildenafil with other treatments for erectile dysfunction have not been

established; use is not recommended. Adding sildenafil to bosentan therapy does not result in any beneficial effect on PAH exercise capacity. Potentially significant drug-drug interactions may exist, requiring dose or frequency adjustment, additional monitoring, and/or selection of alternative therapy. Use with caution in patients taking strong CYP3A4 inhibitors or alpha-blockers. Concomitant use with all forms of nitrates is contraindicated. If nitrate administration is medically necessary, it is not known when nitrates can be safely administered following the use of sildenafil (per manufacturer); the ACC/AHA 2007 guidelines supports administration of nitrates only if 24 hours have elapsed.

Avoid abrupt discontinuation, especially if used as monotherapy in PAH as exacerbation may occur. Use caution in patients with bleeding disorders or with active peptic ulcer disease; safety and efficacy have not been established. Efficacy has not been established for treatment of pulmonary hypertension associated with sickle cell disease. Use with caution in the elderly, or patients with renal or hepatic dysfunction; dose adjustment may be needed. Use of Revatio, especially chronic use, is not recommended in children. After 2 years of treatment, increased mortality seen in long-term (median treatment exposure: 3.8 years) study at higher doses (20-80 mg [depending upon weight] 3 times/day) (Barst, 2012a; Barst, 2012b).

Drug Interactions

Avoid Concomitant Use

Avoid concomitant use of Sildenafil with any of the following: Alprostadil; Amyl Nitrite; Boceprevir; Cobicistat; Fusidic Acid (Systemic); Phosphodiesterase 5 Inhibitors; Pimozide; Riociguat; Telaprevir; Vasodilators (Organic Nitrates)

Decreased Effect

The levels/effects of Sildenafil may be decreased by: Bosentan; CYP3A4 Inducers (Strong); Dabrafenib; Deferasirox; Etravirine; Herbs (CYP3A4 Inducers); Mitotane; Peginterferon Alfa-2b; Tocilizumab

Increased Effect/Toxicity

Sildenafil may increase the levels/effects of: Alpha1-Blockers; Alprostadil; Amyl Nitrite; Antihypertensives; ARIPiprazole; Bosentan; Dofetilide; HMG-CoA Reductase Inhibitors; Lomitapide; Phosphodiesterase 5 Inhibitors; Pimozide; Riociguat; Vasodilators (Organic Nitrates)

The levels/effects of Sildenafil may be increased by: Alcohol (Ethyl); Boceprevir; Cobicistat; CYP3A4 Inhibitors (Moderate); CYP3A4 Inhibitors (Strong); Dasatinib; Erythromycin (Systemic); Fluconazole; Fusidic Acid (Systemic); Itraconazole; Ivacaftor; Ketoconazole (Systemic); Lorcaserin; Luliconazole; Mifepristone; Posaconazole; Protease Inhibitors; Sapropterin; Simeprevir; Telaprevir; Voriconazole

Nutritional/Ethanol Interactions Ethanol: Substantial consumption of ethanol may increase the risk of hypotension and orthostasis. Lower ethanol consumption has not been associated with significant changes in blood pressure or increase in orthostatic symptoms. Management: Avoid or limit ethanol consumption.

Food: Avoid grapefruit juice.

Herb/Nutraceutical: St John's wort may decrease sildenafil levels. Management: Avoid St John's wort.

Adverse Reactions Based upon normal doses for either indication or route. (Adverse effects such as flushing, diarrhea, myalgia, and visual disturbances may be increased with adult doses >100 mg/24 hours.)

>10%:

Central nervous system: Headache (16% to 46%)

Gastrointestinal: Dyspepsia (7% to 17%; dose related)

2% to 10%:

Cardiovascular: Flushing (10%)

Central nervous system: Insomnia (≤7%), pyrexia (6%), dizziness (2%)

Dermatologic: Erythema (6%), rash (2%)

Gastrointestinal: Diarrhea (3% to 9%), gastritis (≤3%)

Genitourinary: Urinary tract infection (3%)

Hepatic: LFTs increased

Neuromuscular & skeletal: Myalgia (≤7%), paresthesia (≤3%)

Ocular: Abnormal vision (color changes, blurred vision, or increased sensitivity to light 3% to 11%; dose related)

Respiratory: Epistaxis (9% to 13%), dyspnea exacerbated (≤7%), nasal congestion (4%), rhinitis (4%), sinusitis (3%)

Pharmacodynamics/Kinetics

Onset of Action ~60 minutes

Duration of Action 2-4 hours

Product Availability Revatio oral suspension is not currently available in the U.S. Launch date for U.S. availability is unknown.

Available Dosage Forms

Solution, Intravenous:

Revatio: 10 mg/12.5 mL (12.5 mL)

Tablet, Oral:

Revatio: 20 mg

Viagra: 25 mg, 50 mg, 100 mg

Generic: 20 mg

General Dosage Range Dosage adjustment recommended in patients with hepatic or renal impairment or on concomitant therapy

I.V.: *Adults:* Revatio: 2.5 mg or 10 mg 3 times daily

Oral:

Adults: Revatio: 5 mg or 20 mg 3 times daily; Viagra: 25-100 mg once daily

Elderly: Viagra: Initial: 25 mg

Administration

I.V. Revatio: Administer injection as an I.V. bolus.

Oral

Revatio: Administer tablets without regard to meals at least 4-6 hours apart.

Viagra: Administer orally 30 minutes to 4 hours before sexual activity.

Storage/Stability Store at 20°C to 25°C (68°F to 77°F); excursions are permitted between 15°C and 30°C (59°F and 86°F).

Nursing Actions

Patient Education

• Discuss specific use of drug and side effects with patient as it relates to treatment. (HCAHPS: During this hospital stay, were you given any medicine that you had not taken before? Before giving you any new medicine, how often did hospital staff tell you what the medicine was for? How often did hospital staff describe possible side effects in a way you could understand?)

• Patient may experience flushing, hypotension, headache, dyspepsia, pyrosis, rhinitis, or vision changes. Have patient report immediately to prescriber erection lasting >4 hours, dyspnea, angina, tachycardia, severe dizziness, hearing impairment, or rash (HCAHPS).

• Educate patient about signs of a significant reaction (eg, wheezing; chest tightness; fever; itching; bad cough; blue skin color; seizures; or swelling of face, lips, tongue, or throat). **Note:** This is not a comprehensive list of all side effects. Patient should consult prescriber for additional questions.

Intended Use and Disclaimer: Should not be printed and given to patients. This information is intended to serve as a concise initial reference for healthcare professionals to use when discussing medications with a patient. You must ultimately rely on your own discretion, experience and judgment in diagnosing, treating and advising patients.

Dietary Considerations Avoid grapefruit juice.

Silodosin (SI lo doe sin)

Brand Names: U.S. Rapaflo

Index Terms KMD 3213

Pharmacologic Category Alpha$_1$ Blocker

Medication Safety Issues

Sound-alike/look-alike issues:

Rapaflo® may be confused with Rapamune®

Silodosin may be confused with sildenafil

Pregnancy Risk Factor B

Use Treatment of signs and symptoms of benign prostatic hyperplasia (BPH)

Mechanism of Action/Effect Selectively antagonizes alpha$_{1A}$-adrenoreceptors in the prostate (and bladder) which mediate the dynamic component of urine flow obstruction by regulating smooth muscle tone of the bladder neck and prostate. When given to patients with BPH, blockade of alpha-receptors leads to relaxation of these muscles, resulting in an improvement in urine flow rate and symptoms. Alpha-blockade does not influence the static component of urinary obstruction, which is related to tissue proliferation.

Contraindications

U.S. labeling: Hypersensitivity to silodosin or any component of the formulation, concurrent use with strong CYP3A4 inhibitors (eg, clarithromycin, itraconazole, ketoconazole, ritonavir); severe renal impairment (CrCl <30 mL/minute); severe hepatic impairment (Child-Pugh class C)

Canadian labeling: Additional contraindications (not in U.S. labeling): Concurrent use with other alpha-blockers (eg, prazosin, terazosin, doxazosin)

Warnings/Precautions Not intended for use as an antihypertensive drug. May cause significant orthostatic hypotension with or without syncope, especially with first dose; anticipate a similar effect if therapy is interrupted for a few days, if dosage is rapidly increased, or if another antihypertensive drug (particularly vasodilators) or a PDE-5 inhibitor (eg, sildenafil, tadalafil, vardenafil) is introduced although coadministration of sildenafil or tadalafil with silodosin was not associated with a clinically significant risk of orthostatic hypotension in one clinical trial (MacDiarmid, 2010). "First-dose" orthostatic hypotension may occur 4-8 hours after dosing; may be dose related. Patients should be cautioned about performing hazardous tasks, driving, or operating heavy machinery when starting new therapy or adjusting dosage upward. Rule out prostatic carcinoma before beginning therapy with silodosin. Intraoperative floppy iris syndrome has been observed in cataract surgery patients who were on or were previously treated with alpha$_1$-blockers; causality has not been established and there appears to be no benefit in discontinuing alpha-blocker therapy prior to surgery. Use with caution in patients with mild-to-moderate hepatic impairment; contraindicated with severe impairment; not studied. Use with caution in patients with moderate renal impairment; dosage adjustment recommended. Contraindicated in patients with severe impairment (CrCl <30 mL/minute). Use with caution in the elderly; risk of orthostatic hypotension increases with increasing age. Patients ≥65 years of age experienced an incidence of up to 5% in clinical trials. Not indicated for use in women or children.

Drug Interactions

Avoid Concomitant Use

Avoid concomitant use of Silodosin with any of the following: Alpha1-Blockers; CYP3A4 Inhibitors (Strong); Fusidic Acid (Systemic); P-glycoprotein/ABCB1 Inhibitors

Decreased Effect

Silodosin may decrease the levels/effects of: Alpha-/Beta-Agonists; Alpha1-Agonists

The levels/effects of Silodosin may be decreased by: Bosentan; CYP3A4 Inducers (Strong); Dabrafenib; Deferasirox; Herbs (CYP3A4 Inducers); Mitotane; P-glycoprotein/ABCB1 Inducers; Tocilizumab

Increased Effect/Toxicity

Silodosin may increase the levels/effects of: Alpha1-Blockers; Calcium Channel Blockers

The levels/effects of Silodosin may be increased by: Beta-Blockers; CYP3A4 Inhibitors (Moderate); CYP3A4 Inhibitors (Strong); Dasatinib; Fusidic Acid (Systemic); Ivacaftor; Luliconazole; MAO Inhibitors; Mifepristone; P-glycoprotein/ABCB1 Inhibitors; Phosphodiesterase 5 Inhibitors; Simeprevir

Nutritional/Ethanol Interactions

Food: AUC decrease by 4% to 49% and C_{max} decreased by ~18% to 43% with moderate calorie/fat meal. Management: Take once daily with a meal.

Herb/Nutraceutical: St John's wort may decrease the levels/effects of silodosin; other herbal medications may have hypotensive properties. There is limited data regarding use with saw palmetto. Management: Avoid St John's wort, black cohosh, California poppy, coleus, golden seal, hawthorn, mistletoe, periwinkle, quinine, and shepherd's purse. Avoid saw palmetto.

Adverse Reactions

>10%: Genitourinary: Retrograde ejaculation (28%)

1% to 10%:

Cardiovascular: Orthostatic hypotension (3%; increased in elderly ≥65 years up to 5%)

Central nervous system: Dizziness (3%), headache (2%), insomnia (1% to 2%)

Gastrointestinal: Diarrhea (3%), abdominal pain (1% to 2%)

Genitourinary: Prostate specific antigen increased (1% to 2%)

Neuromuscular & skeletal: Weakness (1% to 2%)

Respiratory: Nasal congestion (2%), rhinorrhea (1% to 2%), sinusitis (1% to 2%)

Available Dosage Forms

Capsule, Oral:

Rapaflo: 4 mg, 8 mg

General Dosage Range Dosage adjustment recommended in patients with renal impairment

Oral: Adults: Males: 8 mg once daily

Administration

Oral Administer with a meal. Capsules may be opened and the powder sprinkled onto a tablespoon of applesauce (not hot). The applesauce should be swallowed within 5 minutes without chewing and followed with 8 oz of cool water. Subdividing the capsule contents is not recommended. Do not store for future use.

Storage/Stability Store at room temperature of 25°C (77°F); excursions permitted to 15°C to 30°C (59°F to 86°F). Protect from light. Protect from moisture.

Nursing Actions

Physical Assessment Assess potential for inter-actions or toxicity with other antihypertensives or drugs that may increase hypotensive effect. Mon-itor symptomatic relief of BPH regularly. Monitor for orthostatic hypotension and syncope when beginning therapy, if therapy is interrupted, or if dose is increased (dose may need to be adjusted). When discontinuing, dose should be tapered and blood pressure monitored closely.

Patient Education

• Discuss specific use of drug and side effects with patient as it relates to treatment. (HCAHPS: During this hospital stay, were you given any medicine that you had not taken before? Before giving you any new medicine, how often did hospital staff tell you what the medicine was for? How often did hospital staff describe possi-ble side effects in a way you could understand?)

• Patient may experience dizziness, headache, diarrhea, or impotence. Have patient report immediately to prescriber angina, discolored urine, jaundice, or rash (HCAHPS).

• Educate patient about signs of a significant reaction (eg, wheezing; chest tightness; fever; itching; bad cough; blue skin color; seizures; or swelling of face, lips, tongue, or throat). **Note:** This is not a comprehensive list of all side effects. Patient should consult prescriber for additional questions.

Intended Use and Disclaimer: Should not be printed and given to patients. This information is intended to serve as a concise initial reference for healthcare professionals to use when discussing medications with a patient. You must ultimately rely on your own discretion, experience and judg-ment in diagnosing, treating and advising patients.

Dietary Considerations Take with a meal.

Simeprevir (sim E pre vir)

Brand Names: U.S. Olysio
Index Terms TMC435
Pharmacologic Category Antihepaciviral, Pro-tease Inhibitor (Anti-HCV)
Pregnancy Risk Factor X
Lactation Excretion in breast milk unknown/not recommended
Use Chronic hepatitis C: Treatment of genotype 1 chronic hepatitis C (in combination with peginter-feron alfa and ribavirin) in patients with compen-sated liver disease (including cirrhosis)
Available Dosage Forms
Capsule, Oral:
Olysio: 150 mg
General Dosage Range
Oral: Adults: 150 mg once daily

Administration

Oral Administer with food. Administer concurrently with peginterferon alfa and ribavirin. Maintain adequate fluid intake/hydration. Swallow capsu-les whole; do not chew, crush, break, cut, or dissolve the capsule.

Nursing Actions

Physical Assessment Monitor patient for rash, especially during the first 4 weeks of treatment. Patients should be taught to protect skin from sun exposure; monitor for burning, erythema, exuda-tion, edema, and blistering. Monitor for irritation of the eyes. This medication will cause fetal toxicity. Monitor results of pregnancy testing.

Patient Education

• Discuss specific use of drug and side effects with patient as it relates to treatment. (HCAHPS: During this hospital stay, were you given any medicine that you had not taken before? Before giving you any new medicine, how often did hospital staff tell you what the medicine was for? How often did hospital staff describe possi-ble side effects in a way you could understand?)

• Patient may experience dyspepsia or myalgia. Have patient report immediately to prescriber dyspnea, severe skin irritation, stomatitis, or eye irritation (HCAHPS).

• Educate patient about signs of a significant reaction (eg, wheezing; chest tightness; fever; itching; bad cough; blue skin color; seizures; or swelling of face, lips, tongue, or throat). **Note:** This is not a comprehensive list of all side effects. Patient should consult prescriber for additional questions.

Intended Use and Disclaimer: Should not be printed and given to patients. This information is intended to serve as a concise initial reference for healthcare professionals to use when discussing medications with a patient. You must ultimately rely on your own discretion, experience and judg-ment in diagnosing, treating and advising patients.

Simvastatin (sim va STAT in)

Brand Names: U.S. Zocor
Pharmacologic Category Antilipemic Agent, HMG-CoA Reductase Inhibitor
Medication Safety Issues
Sound-alike/look-alike issues:
Simvastatin may be confused with atorvaSTATin, nystatin, pitavastatin
Zocor may be confused with Cozaar, Lipitor, Zoloft, ZyrTEC
International issues:
Cardin [Poland] may be confused with Cardem brand name for celiprolol [Spain]; Cardene brand name for nicardipine [U.S., Great Britain, Netherlands]
Pregnancy Risk Factor X

Lactation Excretion in breast milk unknown/contraindicated

Breast-Feeding Considerations It is not known if simvastatin is excreted into breast milk. Due to the potential for serious adverse reactions in a nursing infant, breast-feeding is contraindicated by the manufacturer.

Use Used with dietary therapy for the following:

Secondary prevention of cardiovascular events in hypercholesterolemic patients with established coronary heart disease (CHD) or at high risk for CHD: To reduce cardiovascular morbidity (myocardial infarction, coronary/noncoronary revascularization procedures) and mortality; to reduce the risk of stroke

Hyperlipidemias: To reduce elevations in total cholesterol (total-C), LDL-C, apolipoprotein B, triglycerides, and VLDL-C, and to increase HDL-C in patients with primary hypercholesterolemia (elevations of 1 or more components are present in Fredrickson type IIa, IIb, III, and IV hyperlipidemias); treatment of homozygous familial hypercholesterolemia

Heterozygous familial hypercholesterolemia (HeFH): In adolescent patients (10-17 years of age, females >1 year postmenarche) with HeFH having LDL-C ≥190 mg/dL **or** LDL-C ≥160 mg/dL with positive family history of premature cardiovascular disease (CVD), or 2 or more CVD risk factors in the adolescent patient

Primary and secondary prevention of atherosclerotic cardiovascular disease (ASCVD) according to the American College of Cardiology/American Heart Association: To reduce the risk of ASCVD in patients with clinical ASCVD (eg, coronary heart disease, stroke/TIA, or peripheral arterial disease presumed to be of atherosclerotic origin) who are greater than 75 years of age or not a candidate for high-intensity statin therapy; in patients without clinical ASCVD if LDL-C is 190 mg/dL or greater and not a candidate for high-intensity statin therapy; in patients without clinical ASCVD who have type 1 or type 2 diabetes and are between 40 and 75 years of age; in patients with an estimated 10-year ASCVD risk 7.5% or greater and who are between 40 and 75 years of age (Stone, 2013).

Mechanism of Action/Effect Simvastatin is a derivative of lovastatin that acts by competitively inhibiting 3-hydroxy-3-methylglutaryl-coenzyme A (HMG-CoA) reductase, the enzyme that catalyzes the rate-limiting step in cholesterol biosynthesis; lowers total and LDL-cholesterol with increase in HDL

Contraindications Hypersensitivity to simvastatin or any component of the formulation; active liver disease; unexplained persistent elevations of serum transaminases; concomitant use of strong CYP3A4 inhibitors (eg, clarithromycin, erythromycin, itraconazole, ketoconazole, nefazodone, posaconazole, voriconazole, protease inhibitors [including boceprevir and telaprevir], telithromycin,

cobicistat-containing products), cyclosporine, danazol, and gemfibrozil; pregnancy; breast-feeding

Warnings/Precautions Secondary causes of hyperlipidemia should be ruled out prior to therapy. Liver enzyme tests should be obtained at baseline and as clinically indicated; routine periodic monitoring of liver enzymes is not necessary. Use with caution in patients who consume large amounts of ethanol or have a history of liver disease; use is contraindicated with active liver disease and with unexplained transaminase elevations. Rhabdomyolysis with acute renal failure has occurred. Risk of rhabdomyolysis is dose-related and increased with high doses (80 mg), concurrent use of lipid-lowering agents which may also cause rhabdomyolysis (other fibrates or niacin doses ≥1 g/day), or moderate-to-strong CYP3A4 inhibitors (eg, amiodarone, grapefruit juice in large quantities, or verapamil), age ≥65 years, female gender, uncontrolled hypothyroidism, and renal dysfunction. In Chinese patients, do not use high-dose simvastatin (80 mg) if concurrently taking niacin ≥1 g/day; may increase risk of myopathy. Immune-mediated necrotizing myopathy (IMNM), an autoimmune-mediated myopathy, has been reported (rarely) with HMG-CoA reductase inhibitor therapy. IMNM presents as proximal muscle weakness with elevated CPK levels, which persists despite discontinuation of HMG-CoA reductase inhibitor therapy; additionally, muscle biopsy may show necrotizing myopathy with limited inflammation; immunosuppressive therapy (eg, corticosteroids, azathioprine) may be used for treatment. Concomitant use of simvastatin with some drugs may require cautious use, may not be recommended, may require dosage adjustments, or may be contraindicated. If concurrent use of a contraindicated interacting medication is unavoidable, treatment with simvastatin should be suspended during use or consider the use of an alternative HMG-CoA reductase inhibitor void of CYP3A4 metabolism. Monitor closely if used with other drugs associated with myopathy (eg, colchicine). Increases in Hb A_{1c} and fasting blood glucose have been reported with HMG-CoA reductase inhibitors; however, the benefits of statin therapy far outweigh the risk of dysglycemia. The manufacturer recommends temporary discontinuation for elective major surgery, acute medical or surgical conditions, or in any patient experiencing an acute or serious condition predisposing to renal failure (eg, sepsis, hypotension, trauma, uncontrolled seizures). However, based upon current evidence, HMG-CoA reductase inhibitor therapy should be continued in the perioperative period unless risk outweighs cardioprotective benefit. Use with caution in patients with severe renal impairment; initial dosage adjustment is necessary; monitor closely.

◀ **Drug Interactions**

Avoid Concomitant Use

Avoid concomitant use of Simvastatin with any of the following: Boceprevir; Clarithromycin; Cyclo-SPORINE (Systemic); CYP3A4 Inhibitors (Strong); Erythromycin (Systemic); Fusidic Acid (Systemic); Gemfibrozil; Mifepristone; Protease Inhibitors; Red Yeast Rice; Telaprevir; Telithromycin

Decreased Effect

Simvastatin may decrease the levels/effects of: Lanthanum

The levels/effects of Simvastatin may be decreased by: Antacids; Bosentan; CYP3A4 Inducers (Strong); Dabrafenib; Deferasirox; Efavirenz; Eslicarbazepine; Etravirine; Fosphenytoin; Mitotane; Phenytoin; Rifamycin Derivatives; St Johns Wort; Tocilizumab

Increased Effect/Toxicity

Simvastatin may increase the levels/effects of: ARIPiprazole; DAPTOmycin; Diltiazem; PAZOPanib; Trabectedin; Vitamin K Antagonists

The levels/effects of Simvastatin may be increased by: Amiodarone; AmLODIPine; Azithromycin (Systemic); Bezafibrate; Boceprevir; Clarithromycin; Colchicine; CycloSPORINE (Systemic); CYP3A4 Inhibitors (Moderate); CYP3A4 Inhibitors (Strong); Cyproterone; Danazol; Dasatinib; Diltiazem; Dronedarone; Eltrombopag; Erythromycin (Systemic); Fenofibrate and Derivatives; Fluconazole; Fusidic Acid (Systemic); Gemfibrozil; Grapefruit Juice; Green Tea; Imatinib; Ivacaftor; Lomitapide; Luliconazole; Mifepristone; Niacin; Niacinamide; Protease Inhibitors; QuiNINE; Raltegravir; Ranolazine; Red Yeast Rice; Sildenafil; Simeprevir; Telaprevir; Telithromycin; Ticagrelor; Verapamil

Nutritional/Ethanol Interactions

Ethanol: Excessive ethanol consumption has the potential to cause hepatic effects. Management: Avoid or limit ethanol consumption.

Food: Simvastatin serum concentration may be increased when taken with grapefruit juice. Red yeast rice contains an estimated 2.4 mg lovastatin per 600 mg rice. Management: Avoid concurrent intake of large quantities of grapefruit juice (>1 quart/day).

Herb/Nutraceutical: St John's wort may decrease simvastatin levels. Management: Avoid St John's wort.

Adverse Reactions

1% to 10%:

Cardiovascular: Atrial fibrillation (6%; placebo 5%), edema (3%; placebo 2%)

Central nervous system: Headache (3% to 7%), vertigo (5%)

Dermatologic: Eczema (5%)

Gastrointestinal: Abdominal pain (7%), constipation (2% to 7%), gastritis (5%), nausea (5%)

Hepatic: Transaminases increased (>3 x ULN; 1%)

Neuromuscular & skeletal: CPK increased (>3 x normal; 5%), myalgia (4%)

Respiratory: Upper respiratory infections (9%), bronchitis (7%)

Additional class-related events or case reports (not necessarily reported with simvastatin therapy): Alteration in taste, anorexia, anxiety, bilirubin increased, cataracts, cholestatic jaundice, cirrhosis, decreased libido, depression, erectile dysfunction/impotence, facial paresis, fatty liver, fulminant hepatic necrosis, gynecomastia, hepatoma, hyperbilirubinemia, immune-mediated necrotizing myopathy (IMNM), impaired extraocular muscle movement, increased CPK (>10 x normal), interstitial lung disease, ophthalmoplegia, peripheral nerve palsy, psychic disturbance, renal failure (secondary to rhabdomyolysis), thyroid dysfunction, tremor, vertigo

Pharmacodynamics/Kinetics

Onset of Action >3 days; Peak effect: 2 weeks

Available Dosage Forms

Tablet, Oral:

Zocor: 5 mg, 10 mg, 20 mg, 40 mg, 80 mg

Generic: 5 mg, 10 mg, 20 mg, 40 mg, 80 mg

General Dosage Range Dosage adjustment recommended in patients with renal impairment or on concomitant therapy

Oral:

Children 10-17 years (females >1 year postmenarche): Initial: 10 mg once daily; Maintenance: 10-40 mg once daily (maximum: 40 mg/day)

Adults: Initial: 10-20 mg once daily; Maintenance: 5-40 mg once daily (maximum: 40 mg daily [80 mg daily may be used in patients taking this dose ≥12 months with no evidence of myopathy])

Administration

Oral May be administered without regard to meals. Administer in the evening for maximal efficacy.

Storage/Stability Tablets should be stored in tightly-closed containers at temperatures between 5°C to 30°C (41°F to 86°F).

Nursing Actions

Physical Assessment Monitor for signs and symptoms of myopathy (muscle tenderness, pain, or weakness). Assess risk potential for interactions with other prescriptions or herbal products patient may be taking that may increase risk of myopathy or rhabdomyolysis. Assess cholesterol profile prior to treatment and at regular intervals. Assess LFT prior to initiating therapy and recheck when clinically indicated. Teach proper diet and exercise regimen.

Patient Education

• Discuss specific use of drug and side effects with patient as it relates to treatment. (HCAHPS: During this hospital stay, were you given any medicine that you had not taken before? Before

giving you any new medicine, how often did hospital staff tell you what the medicine was for? How often did hospital staff describe possible side effects in a way you could understand?)
- Patient may experience headache, dyspepsia, constipation, diarrhea, asthenia, or arthralgia. Have patient report immediately to prescriber flu-like syndrome, ecchymosis, bleeding, discolored urine, jaundice, inability to eat, severe fatigue, or rash (HCAHPS).
- Educate patient about signs of a significant reaction (eg, wheezing; chest tightness; fever; itching; bad cough; blue skin color; seizures; or swelling of face, lips, tongue, or throat). **Note:** This is not a comprehensive list of all side effects. Patient should consult prescriber for additional questions.

Intended Use and Disclaimer: Should not be printed and given to patients. This information is intended to serve as a concise initial reference for healthcare professionals to use when discussing medications with a patient. You must ultimately rely on your own discretion, experience and judgment in diagnosing, treating and advising patients.

Dietary Considerations May be taken without regard to meals. Red yeast rice contains an estimated 2.4 mg lovastatin per 600 mg rice.

Sinecatechins (sin e KAT e kins)

Brand Names: U.S. Veregen
Index Terms Catechins; Green Tea Extract; Kunecatechins; Polyphenols; Polyphenon E
Pharmacologic Category Immunomodulator, Topical; Topical Skin Product
Pregnancy Risk Factor C
Lactation Excretion in breast milk unknown
Use Treatment of external genital and perianal warts secondary to condylomata acuminata
Available Dosage Forms
Ointment, External:
Veregen: 15% (15 g, 30 g)
General Dosage Range Topical: *Adults:* Apply a thin layer (~0.5 cm strand) 3 times/day
Administration
Topical Wash hands before and after application; apply with fingers, leaving a thin layer of ointment; do not wash ointment off affected area after application. Discontinue treatment if the severity of local skin reactions becomes unacceptable. Do not apply internally; do not apply to open wounds; do not apply occlusive dressing. Sexual contact should be avoided while ointment is on skin. For females requiring tampon use during treatment, tampon should be inserted prior to application of ointment to prevent accidental application of ointment into the vagina. May stain clothing or bedding.

Nursing Actions
Patient Education
- Discuss specific use of drug and side effects with patient as it relates to treatment. (HCAHPS: During this hospital stay, were you given any medicine that you had not taken before? Before giving you any new medicine, how often did hospital staff tell you what the medicine was for? How often did hospital staff describe possible side effects in a way you could understand?)
- Have patient report immediately to prescriber severe skin irritation or pain, blisters, hemorrhaging, dysuria, difficult urination, or groin or pelvic pain (HCAHPS).
- Educate patient about signs of a significant reaction (eg, wheezing; chest tightness; fever; itching; bad cough; blue skin color; seizures; or swelling of face, lips, tongue, or throat). **Note:** This is not a comprehensive list of all side effects. Patient should consult prescriber for additional questions.

Intended Use and Disclaimer: Should not be printed and given to patients. This information is intended to serve as a concise initial reference for healthcare professionals to use when discussing medications with a patient. You must ultimately rely on your own discretion, experience and judgment in diagnosing, treating and advising patients.

Sirolimus (sir OH li mus)

Brand Names: U.S. Rapamune
Index Terms Rapamycin
Pharmacologic Category Immunosuppressant Agent; mTOR Kinase Inhibitor
Medication Safety Issues
Sound-alike/look-alike issues:
Rapamune® may be confused with Rapaflo®
Sirolimus may be confused with everolimus, pimecrolimus, tacrolimus, temsirolimus
Medication Guide Available Yes
Pregnancy Risk Factor C
Lactation Excretion in breast milk unknown/not recommended
Breast-Feeding Considerations It is not known if sirolimus is excreted in breast milk. Due to the potential for adverse reactions in the breast-fed infant, including possible immunosuppression, breast-feeding is not recommended.
Use Prophylaxis of organ rejection in patients receiving renal transplants
Unlabeled Use Prophylaxis of organ rejection and allograft vasculopathy in heart transplant recipients; prevention acute graft-versus-host disease (GVHD) in allogeneic stem cell transplantation; treatment of refractory acute or chronic GVHD; treatment of chordoma, renal angiomyolipoma, or lymphangioleiomyomatosis

◄ **Mechanism of Action/Effect** Sirolimus inhibits T-lymphocyte activation and proliferation in response to antigenic and cytokine stimulation and inhibits antibody production (mechanism differs from other immunosuppressants) to inhibit acute rejection of allografts and prolongs graft survival. Sirolimus binds to FKBP-12, an intracellular protein, to form an immunosuppressive complex which inhibits the regulatory kinase, mTOR (mammalian target of rapamycin), which suppresses cytokine mediated T-cell proliferation, halting progression from the G1 to the S phase of the cell cycle.

Contraindications Hypersensitivity to sirolimus or any component of the formulation

Warnings/Precautions Hazardous agent - use appropriate precautions for handling and disposal (NIOSH, 2012). **[U.S. Boxed Warning]: Immunosuppressive agents, including sirolimus, increase the risk of infection and may be associated with the development of lymphoma.** Immune suppression may also increase the risk of opportunistic infections (including activation of latent viral infections including BK virus-associated nephropathy), fatal infections, and sepsis. Prophylactic treatment for *Pneumocystis jirovecii* pneumonia (PCP) should be administered for 1 year post-transplant; prophylaxis for cytomegalovirus (CMV) should be taken for 3 months post-transplant in patients at risk for CMV. Progressive multifocal leukoencephalopathy (PML), an opportunistic CNS infection caused by reactivation of the JC virus, has been reported in patients receiving immunosuppressive therapy, including sirolimus. Clinical findings of PML include apathy, ataxia, cognitive deficiency, confusion, and hemiparesis; promptly evaluate any patient presenting with neurological changes; consider decreasing the degree of immunosuppression with consideration to the risk of organ rejection in transplant patients.

[U.S. Boxed Warning]: Sirolimus is not recommended for use in liver or lung transplantation. Bronchial anastomotic dehiscence cases have been reported in lung transplant patients when sirolimus was used as part of an immunosuppressive regimen; most of these reactions were fatal. Studies indicate an association with an increased risk of hepatic artery thrombosis (HAT), graft failure, and increased mortality (with evidence of infection) in liver transplant patients when sirolimus is used in combination with cyclosporine and/or tacrolimus. Most cases of HAT occurred within 30 days of transplant.

In renal transplant patients, *de novo* use without cyclosporine has been associated with higher rates of acute rejection. Sirolimus should be used in combination with cyclosporine (and corticosteroids) initially. Cyclosporine may be withdrawn in low-to-moderate immunologic risk patients after 2-4 months, in conjunction with an increase in sirolimus dosage. In high immunologic risk patients, use in combination with cyclosporine and corticosteroids is recommended for the first year. Safety and efficacy of combination therapy with cyclosporine in high immunologic risk patients has not been studied beyond 12 months of treatment; adjustment of immunosuppressive therapy beyond 12 months should be considered based on clinical judgement. Monitor renal function closely when combined with cyclosporine; consider dosage adjustment or discontinue in patients with increasing serum creatinine.

May increase serum creatinine and decrease GFR. Use caution when used concurrently with medications which may alter renal function. May delay recovery of renal function in patients with delayed allograft function. Increased urinary protein excretion has been observed when converting renal transplant patients from calcineurin inhibitors to sirolimus during maintenance therapy. A higher level of proteinuria prior to sirolimus conversion correlates with a higher degree of proteinuria after conversion. In some patients, proteinuria may reach nephrotic levels; nephrotic syndrome (new onset) has been reported. Increased risk of BK viral-associated nephropathy which may impair renal function and cause graft loss; consider decreasing immunosuppressive burden if evidence of deteriorating renal function.

Use caution with hepatic impairment; a reduction in the maintenance dose is recommended. Has been associated with an increased risk of fluid accumulation and lymphocele; peripheral edema, lymphedema, ascites, and pleural and pericardial effusions (including significant effusions and tamponade) were reported; use with caution in patients in whom fluid accumulation may be poorly tolerated, such as in cardiovascular disease (heart failure or hypertension) and pulmonary disease. Cases of interstitial lung disease (eg, pneumonitis, bronchiolitis obliterans organizing pneumonia [BOOP], pulmonary fibrosis) have been observed; risk may be increased with higher trough levels. Potentially significant drug-drug interactions may exist, requiring dose or frequency adjustment, additional monitoring, and/or selection of alternative therapy. Concurrent use with a calcineurin inhibitor (cyclosporine, tacrolimus) may increase the risk of calcineurin inhibitor-induced hemolytic uremic syndrome/thrombotic thrombocytopenic purpura/thrombotic microangiopathy (HUS/TTP/TMA).

Hypersensitivity reactions, including anaphylactic/anaphylactoid reactions, angioedema, exfoliative dermatitis, and hypersensitivity vasculitis have been reported. Concurrent use with other drugs known to cause angioedema (eg, ACE inhibitors) may increase risk. Immunosuppressant therapy is associated with an increased risk of skin cancer; limit sun and ultraviolet light exposure; use appropriate sun protection. May increase serum lipids (cholesterol and triglycerides); use with caution in patients with hyperlipidemia; monitor cholesterol/lipids; if hyperlipidemia occurs, follow current guidelines for management (diet, exercise, lipid lowering agents); antihyperlipidemic therapy may not be effective in normalizing levels. May be associated with wound dehiscence and impaired healing; use caution in the perioperative period. Patients with a body mass index (BMI) >30 kg/m^2 are at increased risk for abnormal wound healing.

Sirolimus tablets and oral solution are not bioequivalent, due to differences in absorption. Clinical equivalence was seen using 2 mg tablet and 2 mg solution. It is not known if higher doses are also clinically equivalent. Monitor sirolimus levels if changes in dosage forms are made. **[U.S. Boxed Warning]: Should only be used by physicians experienced in immunosuppressive therapy and management of transplant patients. Adequate laboratory and supportive medical resources must be readily available.** Sirolimus concentrations are dependent on the assay method (eg, chromatographic and immunoassay) used; assay methods are not interchangeable. Variations in methods to determine sirolimus whole blood concentrations, as well as interlaboratory variations, may result in improper dosage adjustments, which may lead to subtherapeutic or toxic levels. Determine the assay method used to assure consistency (or accommodations if changes occur), and for monitoring purposes, be aware of alterations to assay method or reference range. The manufacturer recommends high performance liquid chromatography (HPLC) as the reference standard to determine sirolimus trough concentrations.

Drug Interactions

Avoid Concomitant Use

Avoid concomitant use of Sirolimus with any of the following: BCG; CloZAPine; Conivaptan; Crizotinib; Enzalutamide; Fusidic Acid (Systemic); Mifepristone; Natalizumab; Pimecrolimus; Pimozide; Posaconazole; Tacrolimus (Systemic); Tacrolimus (Topical); Tofacitinib; Vaccines (Live); Voriconazole

Decreased Effect

Sirolimus may decrease the levels/effects of: BCG; Coccidioidin Skin Test; Sipuleucel-T; Tacrolimus (Systemic); Vaccines (Inactivated); Vaccines (Live)

The levels/effects of Sirolimus may be decreased by: Bosentan; CYP3A4 Inducers (Strong); Dabrafenib; Deferasirox; Echinacea; Efavirenz; Enzalutamide; Fosphenytoin; Herbs (CYP3A4 Inducers); Mitotane; P-glycoprotein/ABCB1 Inducers; Phenytoin; Rifampin; Tocilizumab

Increased Effect/Toxicity

Sirolimus may increase the levels/effects of: ACE Inhibitors; ARIPiprazole; CloZAPine; CycloSPORINE (Systemic); Dofetilide; Leflunomide; Lomitapide; Natalizumab; Pimozide; Tacrolimus (Systemic); Tacrolimus (Topical); Tofacitinib; Vaccines (Live)

The levels/effects of Sirolimus may be increased by: Boceprevir; Conivaptan; Crizotinib; CycloSPORINE (Systemic); CYP3A4 Inhibitors (Moderate); CYP3A4 Inhibitors (Strong); Dasatinib; Denosumab; Fluconazole; Fusidic Acid (Systemic); Itraconazole; Ivacaftor; Ketoconazole (Systemic); Luliconazole; Macrolide Antibiotics; Mifepristone; Nelfinavir; P-glycoprotein/ABCB1 Inhibitors; Pimecrolimus; Posaconazole; Roflumilast; Stiripentol; Tacrolimus (Systemic); Tacrolimus (Topical); Telaprevir; Trastuzumab; Voriconazole

Nutritional/Ethanol Interactions

Food: Grapefruit juice may decrease clearance of sirolimus. Ingestion with high-fat meals decreases peak concentrations but increases AUC by 23% to 35%. Management: Avoid grapefruit juice. Take consistently (either with or without food) to minimize variability.

Herb/Nutraceutical: St John's wort may decrease sirolimus levels. Some herbal medications have immunostimulant properties (eg, echinacea). Herbs with hypoglycemic properties may increase the risk of sirolimus-induced hypoglycemia (eg, alfalfa). Management: Avoid St John's wort, cat's claw, and echinacea. Avoid alfalfa, aloe, bilberry, bitter melon, burdock, celery, damiana, fenugreek, garcinia, garlic, ginger, ginseng (American), gymnema, marshmallow, and stinging nettle.

Adverse Reactions Incidence of many adverse effects is dose related.

>20%:

Cardiovascular: Peripheral edema (54% to 58%), hypertension (45% to 49%), edema (18% to 20%)

Central nervous system: Headache (34%), pain (20% to 33%), insomnia (13% to 22%)

Dermatologic: Acne (22%)

Endocrine & metabolic: Hypertriglyceridemia (45% to 57%), hypercholesterolemia (43% to 46%)

Gastrointestinal: Constipation (36% to 38%), abdominal pain (29% to 36%), diarrhea (25% to 36%), nausea (25% to 31%)

Genitourinary: Urinary tract infection (26% to 33%)

Hematologic: Anemia (23% to 33%), thrombocytopenia (14% to 30%)

Neuromuscular & skeletal: Arthralgia (25% to 31%)

Renal: Serum creatinine increased (39% to 40%)

3% to 20%:

Cardiovascular: Atrial fibrillation, CHF, DVT, facial edema, hypervolemia, hypotension, orthostatic hypotension, palpitation, peripheral vascular disorder, syncope, tachycardia, thrombosis, vasodilation

Central nervous system: Anxiety, chills, confusion, depression, dizziness, emotional lability, hypoesthesia, malaise, neuropathy, somnolence

Dermatologic: Rash (10% to 20%), skin carcinoma (up to 3%; includes basal cell carcinoma, squamous cell carcinoma, melanoma), cellulitis, dermal ulcer, dermatitis (fungal), ecchymosis, hirsutism, pruritus, skin hypertrophy, wound healing abnormal

Endocrine & metabolic: Acidosis, Cushing's syndrome, dehydration, diabetes mellitus, glycosuria, hypercalcemia, hyperglycemia, hyperphosphatemia, hypocalcemia, hypoglycemia, hypokalemia, hypomagnesemia, hyponatremia

Gastrointestinal: Abdomen enlarged, anorexia, dysphagia, eructation, esophagitis, flatulence, gastritis, gastroenteritis, gingival hyperplasia, gingivitis, ileus, mouth ulceration, oral moniliasis, stomatitis, weight loss

Genitourinary: Amenorrhea, hypermenorrhea, impotence, menstrual disease, ovarian cyst, pelvic pain, scrotal edema, testis disorder

Hematologic: Hemolytic-uremic syndrome, hemorrhage, leukopenia, leukocytosis, polycythemia, TTP

Hepatic: Abnormal liver function tests, alkaline phosphatase increased, LDH increased

Local: Thrombophlebitis

Neuromuscular & skeletal: Arthrosis, bone necrosis, CPK increased, hyper-/hypotonia, leg cramps, myalgia, osteoporosis, paresthesia, tetany

Ocular: Abnormal vision, cataract, conjunctivitis

Otic: Ear pain, otitis media, tinnitus

Renal: Albuminuria, bladder pain, BUN increased, dysuria, hematuria, hydronephrosis, kidney pain, nephropathy (toxic), nocturia, oliguria, pyelonephritis, pyuria, tubular necrosis, urinary frequency, urinary incontinence, urinary retention

Respiratory: Asthma, atelectasis, bronchitis, cough, epistaxis, hypoxia, lung edema, pleural effusion, pneumonia, pulmonary embolism, rhinitis, sinusitis

Miscellaneous: Lymphoproliferative disease/lymphoma (1% to 3%), abscess, diaphoresis, flu-like syndrome, hernia, herpesvirus infection, infection (including opportunistic), lymphadenopathy, lymphocele, peritonitis, sepsis

Available Dosage Forms

Solution, Oral:

Rapamune: 1 mg/mL (60 mL)

Tablet, Oral:

Rapamune: 0.5 mg, 1 mg, 2 mg

Generic: 0.5 mg

General Dosage Range Dosage adjustment recommended in patients with hepatic impairment

Oral:

Adolescents ≥13 years and Adults <40 kg: Low-to-moderate immunologic risk: Loading dose: 3 mg/m^2 on day 1; Maintenance: 1 mg/m^2/day

Adolescents ≥13 years and Adults ≥40 kg: Low-to-moderate immunologic risk: Loading dose: 6 mg on day 1; Maintenance: 2 mg/day (maximum: 40 mg/day)

Adults: High risk: Loading dose: Up to 15 mg on day 1; Maintenance: 5 mg/day (maximum: 40 mg/day)

Administration

Oral Initial dose should be administered as soon as possible after transplant. Sirolimus should be taken 4 hours after oral cyclosporine (Neoral® or Gengraf®). Should be administered consistently (either with or without food).

Solution: Mix (by stirring vigorously) with at least 2 ounces of water or orange juice. No other liquids should be used for dilution. Patient should drink diluted solution immediately. The cup should then be refilled with an additional 4 ounces of water or orange juice, stirred vigorously, and the patient should drink the contents at once.

Tablet: Do not crush, split, or chew.

Hazardous agent; use appropriate precautions for handling and disposal (NIOSH, 2012).

Storage/Stability

Oral solution: Store under refrigeration, 2°C to 8°C (36°F to 46°F). Protect from light. A slight haze may develop in refrigerated solutions, but the quality of the product is not affected. After opening, solution should be used in 1 month. If necessary, may be stored at temperatures up to 25°C (77°F) for ≤15 days after opening. Product may be stored in amber syringe for a maximum of 24 hours (at room temperature or refrigerated). Discard syringe after single use. Solution should be used immediately following dilution.

Tablet: Store at room temperature of 20°C to 25°C (68°F to 77°F). Protect from light.

Nursing Actions

Physical Assessment Monitor blood pressure, weight, and renal function. Assess for signs of fluid retention and infection. Monitor lab work and report abnormalities to prescriber. Educate patient about need for adherence to medication and regular follow-up with doctor. Review potential for greater cancer risk and how frequent skin checks and follow-up are important.

Patient Education

• Discuss specific use of drug and side effects with patient as it relates to treatment. (HCAHPS: During this hospital stay, were you given any medicine that you had not taken before? Before giving you any new medicine, how often did hospital staff tell you what the medicine was for? How often did hospital staff describe possible side effects in a way you could understand?)

- Patient may experience hypertension, hyperlipidemia, anemia, thrombocytopenia, asthenia, headache, dyspepsia, constipation, diarrhea, nausea, arthralgia, edema, acne, or renal impairment. Have patient report immediately to prescriber signs of infection, dyspnea, wound that will not heal, urinary retention, ecchymosis, bleeding, or rash (HCAHPS).
- Educate patient about signs of a significant reaction (eg, wheezing; chest tightness; fever; itching; bad cough; blue skin color; seizures; or swelling of face, lips, tongue, or throat). **Note:** This is not a comprehensive list of all side effects. Patient should consult prescriber for additional questions.

Intended Use and Disclaimer: Should not be printed and given to patients. This information is intended to serve as a concise initial reference for healthcare professionals to use when discussing medications with a patient. You must ultimately rely on your own discretion, experience and judgment in diagnosing, treating and advising patients.

Dietary Considerations Take consistently (either with or without food) to minimize variability of absorption.

Related Information
Oral Medications That Should Not Be Crushed or Altered *on page 1712*

SitaGLIPtin (sit a GLIP tin)

Brand Names: U.S. Januvia
Index Terms MK-0431; Sitagliptin Phosphate
Pharmacologic Category Antidiabetic Agent, Dipeptidyl Peptidase IV (DPP-IV) Inhibitor
Medication Safety Issues
Sound-alike/look-alike issues:
Januvia® may be confused with Enjuvia™, Janumet®, Jantoven®
SitaGLIPtin may be confused with saxagliptin, SUMAtriptan
High alert medication:
The Institute for Safe Medication Practices (ISMP) includes this medication among its list of drug classes which have a heightened risk of causing significant patient harm when used in error.

Medication Guide Available Yes
Pregnancy Risk Factor B
Lactation Excretion in breast milk unknown/use caution

Breast-Feeding Considerations It is not known if sitagliptin is excreted in breast milk. The manufacturer recommends that caution be used if administered to breast-feeding women.

Use Management of type 2 diabetes mellitus (noninsulin dependent, NIDDM) as an adjunct to diet and exercise as monotherapy or in combination therapy with other antidiabetic agents

Mechanism of Action/Effect Sitagliptin inhibits dipeptidyl peptidase IV (DPP-IV) enzyme resulting in prolonged active incretin levels. Incretin hormones (eg, glucagon-like peptide-1 [GLP-1] and glucose-dependent insulinotropic polypeptide [GIP]) regulate glucose homeostasis by increasing insulin synthesis and release from pancreatic beta cells and decreasing glucagon secretion from pancreatic alpha cells. Decreased glucagon secretion results in decreased hepatic glucose production. Under normal physiologic circumstances, incretin hormones are released by the intestine throughout the day and levels are increased in response to a meal; incretin hormones are rapidly inactivated by the DPP-IV enzyme.

Contraindications Serious hypersensitivity (eg, anaphylaxis, angioedema) to sitagliptin or any component of the formulation

Warnings/Precautions Avoid use in type 1 diabetes mellitus (insulin dependent, IDDM) and diabetic ketoacidosis (DKA) due to lack of efficacy in these populations. Use caution when used in conjunction with insulin or insulin secretagogues; risk of hypoglycemia is increased. Monitor blood glucose closely; dosage adjustments of insulin or insulin secretagogues may be necessary. Use with caution in patients with moderate-to-severe renal dysfunction and end-stage renal disease (ESRD) requiring hemodialysis or peritoneal dialysis; dosing adjustment required. Safety and efficacy have not been established in severe hepatic dysfunction.

Rare hypersensitivity reactions, including anaphylaxis, angioedema, and/or severe dermatologic reactions (such as Stevens-Johnson syndrome), have been reported in postmarketing surveillance; discontinue if signs/symptoms of hypersensitivity reactions occur. Use with caution if patient has experienced angioedema with other DPP-IV inhibitor use. Cases of acute pancreatitis (including hemorrhagic and necrotizing with some fatalities) have been reported with use; monitor for signs/symptoms of pancreatitis. Discontinue use immediately if pancreatitis is suspected and initiate appropriate management. Use with caution in patients with a history of pancreatitis (not known if this population is at greater risk).

Clinical trials included only a limited number of patients with heart failure (HF). No specific recommendations regarding this population are provided in the approved U.S. labeling (Canadian labeling recommends against use in this population). Diabetes self-management education (DSME) is essential to maximize the effectiveness of therapy.

Drug Interactions
Avoid Concomitant Use There are no known interactions where it is recommended to avoid concomitant use.
Decreased Effect
The levels/effects of SitaGLIPtin may be decreased by: Corticosteroids (Orally Inhaled); ▶

Corticosteroids (Systemic); Loop Diuretics; Luteinizing Hormone-Releasing Hormone Analogs; P-glycoprotein/ABCB1 Inducers; Somatropin; Thiazide Diuretics

Increased Effect/Toxicity

SitaGLIPtin may increase the levels/effects of: ACE Inhibitors; Digoxin; Hypoglycemic Agents

The levels/effects of SitaGLIPtin may be increased by: Herbs (Hypoglycemic Properties); MAO Inhibitors; Pegvisomant; P-glycoprotein/ABCB1 Inhibitors; Salicylates; Selective Serotonin Reuptake Inhibitors

Adverse Reactions As reported with monotherapy: 1% to 10%:
Cardiovascular: Peripheral edema (2%)
Endocrine & metabolic: Hypoglycemia (1%)
Gastrointestinal: Diarrhea (4%), constipation (3%), nausea (2%)
Neuromuscular & skeletal: Osteoarthritis (1%)
Respiratory: Nasopharyngitis (5%), pharyngitis (1%), upper respiratory tract infection (viral; 1%)

Available Dosage Forms
Tablet, Oral:
Januvia: 25 mg, 50 mg, 100 mg

General Dosage Range Dosage adjustment recommended in patients with renal impairment
Oral: *Adults:* 100 mg once daily

Administration

Oral May be administered with or without food.

Storage/Stability Store at 20°C to 25°C (68°F to 77°F); excursions permitted to 15°C to 30°C (59°F to 86°F).

Nursing Actions

Physical Assessment With insulin or sulfonylureas, the risk of hypoglycemia may be increased and dosage adjustments may be necessary. Monitor renal function prior to treatment and throughout. Monitor for hypersensitivity reactions and development of pancreatitis. Refer patient to diabetic educator for diabetic education if necessary.

Patient Education
- Discuss specific use of drug and side effects with patient as it relates to treatment. (HCAHPS: During this hospital stay, were you given any medicine that you had not taken before? Before giving you any new medicine, how often did hospital staff tell you what the medicine was for? How often did hospital staff describe possible side effects in a way you could understand?)
- Patient may experience headache, pharyngitis, rhinitis, rhinorrhea, or diarrhea. Have patient report immediately to prescriber urinary retention, oliguria, signs of hypoglycemia, or signs of pancreatitis (HCAHPS).
- Educate patient about signs of a significant reaction (eg, wheezing; chest tightness; fever; itching; bad cough; blue skin color; seizures; or swelling of face, lips, tongue, or throat). **Note:** This is not a comprehensive list of all side

effects. Patient should consult prescriber for additional questions.

Intended Use and Disclaimer: Should not be printed and given to patients. This information is intended to serve as a concise initial reference for healthcare professionals to use when discussing medications with a patient. You must ultimately rely on your own discretion, experience and judgment in diagnosing, treating and advising patients.

Dietary Considerations May be taken with or without food. Individualized medical nutrition therapy (MNT) based on ADA recommendations is an integral part of therapy.

Related Information

Oral Medications That Should Not Be Crushed or Altered *on page 1712*

Sitagliptin and Metformin
(sit a GLIP tin & met FOR min)

Brand Names: U.S. Janumet; Janumet XR

Index Terms Metformin and Sitagliptin; Sitagliptin Phosphate and Metformin Hydrochloride

Pharmacologic Category Antidiabetic Agent, Biguanide; Antidiabetic Agent, Dipeptidyl Peptidase IV (DPP-IV) Inhibitor; Hypoglycemic Agent, Oral

Medication Safety Issues
Sound-alike/look-alike issues:
Janumet may be confused with Jantoven, Januvia
Sitagliptin and Metformin may be confused with Linagliptin and Metformin
Sitagliptin and Metformin may be confused with Saxagliptin and Metformin

High alert medication:
The Institute for Safe Medication Practices (ISMP) includes this medication among its list of drug classes which have a heightened risk of causing significant patient harm when used in error.

Medication Guide Available Yes

Pregnancy Risk Factor B

Use Type 2 diabetes mellitus: As an adjunct to diet and exercise to improve glycemic control in adults with type 2 diabetes mellitus when treatment with both sitagliptin and metformin is appropriate

Available Dosage Forms
Tablet, oral:
Janumet: 50/500: Sitagliptin 50 mg and metformin 500 mg; 50/1000: Sitagliptin 50 mg and metformin 1000 mg
Tablet, extended release, oral:
Janumet XR: 50/500: Sitagliptin 50 mg and metformin 500 mg
Janumet XR: 50/1000: Sitagliptin 50 mg and metformin 1000 mg
Janumet XR: 100/1000: Sitagliptin 100 mg and metformin 1000 mg

General Dosage Range Oral: *Adults:*

Immediate release: Sitagliptin 50 mg and metformin 500-1000 mg twice daily (maximum: 100 mg daily [sitagliptin], 2000 mg daily [metformin])

Extended release: Sitagliptin 100 mg and metformin 1000-2000 mg once daily (maximum: 100 mg daily [sitagliptin], 2000 mg daily [metformin])

Administration

Oral Administer with meals, at the same time each day (evening meal preferable for extended release tablets). Swallow extended release tablets whole; do not split, crush, or chew; do not split or divide regular release tablets.

Nursing Actions

Physical Assessment See individual agents.

Patient Education

- Discuss specific use of drug and side effects with patient as it relates to treatment. (HCAHPS: During this hospital stay, were you given any medicine that you had not taken before? Before giving you any new medicine, how often did hospital staff tell you what the medicine was for? How often did hospital staff describe possible side effects in a way you could understand?)
- Patient may experience dyspepsia, nausea, diarrhea, flatulence, asthenia, headache, rhinitis, or rhinorrhea. Have patient report immediately to prescriber signs of angina, chills, pharyngitis, urinary retention, oliguria, signs of hypoglycemia, signs of pancreatitis, or signs of lactic acidosis (HCAHPS).
- Educate patient about signs of a significant reaction (eg, wheezing; chest tightness; fever; itching; bad cough; blue skin color; seizures; or swelling of face, lips, tongue, or throat). **Note:** This is not a comprehensive list of all side effects. Patient should consult prescriber for additional questions.

Intended Use and Disclaimer: Should not be printed and given to patients. This information is intended to serve as a concise initial reference for healthcare professionals to use when discussing medications with a patient. You must ultimately rely on your own discretion, experience and judgment in diagnosing, treating and advising patients.

Related Information

MetFORMIN *on page 1014*

Oral Medications That Should Not Be Crushed or Altered *on page 1712*

SitaGLIPtin *on page 1421*

Sitagliptin and Simvastatin
(sit a GLIP tin & sim va STAT in)

Brand Names: U.S. Juvisync™ [DSC]

Index Terms Simvastatin and Sitagliptin; Sitagliptin Phosphate and Simvastatin

Pharmacologic Category Antidiabetic Agent, Dipeptidyl Peptidase IV (DPP-IV) Inhibitor; Antilipemic Agent, HMG-CoA Reductase Inhibitor

Medication Safety Issues

High alert medication:

The Institute for Safe Medication Practices (ISMP) includes this medication among its list of drug classes which have a heightened risk of causing significant patient harm when used in error.

Medication Guide Available Yes

Pregnancy Risk Factor X

Use For use when treatment with both sitagliptin and simvastatin is appropriate:

Sitagliptin: Management of type 2 diabetes mellitus (noninsulin dependent, NIDDM) as an adjunct to diet and exercise as monotherapy or in combination therapy with other antidiabetic agents

Simvastatin: Used with dietary therapy for the following:

Secondary prevention of cardiovascular events in hypercholesterolemic patients with established coronary heart disease (CHD) or at high risk for CHD: To reduce cardiovascular morbidity (myocardial infarction, coronary/noncoronary revascularization procedures) and mortality; to reduce the risk of stroke

Hyperlipidemias: To reduce elevations in total cholesterol (total-C), LDL-C, apolipoprotein B, triglycerides, and VLDL-C, and to increase HDL-C in patients with primary hypercholesterolemia (elevations of 1 or more components are present in Fredrickson type IIa, IIb, III, and IV hyperlipidemias); treatment of homozygous familial hypercholesterolemia

General Dosage Range Dosage adjustment recommended in patients on concomitant therapy or with renal impairment.

Oral: *Adults:* Initial: Sitagliptin 100 mg and simvastatin 40 mg once daily

Administration

Oral Administer in the evening. Do not split or divide tablet.

Nursing Actions

Physical Assessment See individual agents.

Patient Education

- Discuss specific use of drug and side effects with patient as it relates to treatment. (HCAHPS: During this hospital stay, were you given any medicine that you had not taken before? Before giving you any new medicine, how often did hospital staff tell you what the medicine was for? How often did hospital staff describe possible side effects in a way you could understand?)
- Patient may experience headache, rhinitis, dyspepsia, or constipation. Have patient report immediately to prescriber signs of hepatic impairment, urinary retention, oliguria, myalgia, arthralgia, ecchymosis, hemorrhaging, paresthesia, dizziness, illogical thinking, memory loss,

▶

depression, sexual dysfunction, tachycardia, arrhythmia, chills, pharyngitis, dyspnea, insomnia, severe asthenia, signs of hypoglycemia, signs of pancreatitis, or Stevens-Johnson syndrome/toxic epidermal necrolysis (HCAHPS).

• Educate patient about signs of a significant reaction (eg, wheezing; chest tightness; fever; itching; bad cough; blue skin color; seizures; or swelling of face, lips, tongue, or throat). **Note:** This is not a comprehensive list of all side effects. Patient should consult prescriber for additional questions.

Intended Use and Disclaimer: Should not be printed and given to patients. This information is intended to serve as a concise initial reference for healthcare professionals to use when discussing medications with a patient. You must ultimately rely on your own discretion, experience and judgment in diagnosing, treating and advising patients.

Related Information
Simvastatin on page 1414
SitaGLIPtin on page 1421

Sodium Bicarbonate
(SOW dee um bye KAR bun ate)

Brand Names: U.S. Neut
Index Terms Baking Soda; NaHCO$_3$; Sodium Acid Carbonate; Sodium Hydrogen Carbonate
Pharmacologic Category Alkalinizing Agent; Antacid; Electrolyte Supplement, Oral; Electrolyte Supplement, Parenteral
Pregnancy Risk Factor C
Lactation Enters breast milk
Breast-Feeding Considerations Sodium is found in breast milk (IOM, 2004).
Use
Management of metabolic acidosis; gastric hyperacidity; as an alkalinization agent for the urine; treatment of hyperkalemia; management of overdose of certain drugs, including tricyclic antidepressants and aspirin
Neutralizing additive (dental use): Improves onset of analgesia and reduces injection site pain by adjusting lidocaine with epinephrine solution to a more physiologic pH.
Unlabeled Use Prevention of contrast-induced nephropathy (CIN)
Mechanism of Action/Effect
Dissociates to provide bicarbonate ion which neutralizes hydrogen ion concentration and raises blood and urinary pH
Neutralizing additive (dental use): Increases pH of lidocaine and epinephrine solution to improve tolerability and increase tissue uptake
Contraindications
Alkalosis, hypernatremia, severe pulmonary edema, hypocalcemia, unknown abdominal pain

Neutralizing additive (dental use): Not for use as a systemic alkalizer
Warnings/Precautions Rapid administration in neonates and children <2 years of age has led to hypernatremia, decreased CSF pressure and intracranial hemorrhage. **Use of I.V. NaHCO$_3$ should be reserved for documented metabolic acidosis and for hyperkalemia-induced cardiac arrest.** Routine use in cardiac arrest is not recommended. Vesicant (at concentrations ≥8.4%); ensure proper catheter or needle position prior to and during infusion; avoid extravasation (tissue necrosis may occur due to hypertonicity). May cause sodium retention especially if renal function is impaired; not to be used in treatment of peptic ulcer; use with caution in patients with HF, edema, cirrhosis, or renal failure. Not the antacid of choice for the elderly because of sodium content and potential for systemic alkalosis.
Drug Interactions
Avoid Concomitant Use
Avoid concomitant use of Sodium Bicarbonate with any of the following: PONATinib
Decreased Effect
Sodium Bicarbonate may decrease the levels/effects of: ACE Inhibitors; Anticonvulsants (Hydantoin); Antipsychotic Agents (Phenothiazines); Atazanavir; Bisacodyl; Bosutinib; Cefditoren; Cefpodoxime; Cefuroxime; Chloroquine; Corticosteroids (Oral); Dabigatran Etexilate; Dabrafenib; Dasatinib; Delavirdine; Elvitegravir; Erlotinib; Flecainide; Gabapentin; HMG-CoA Reductase Inhibitors; Hyoscyamine; Iron Salts; Isoniazid; Itraconazole; Ketoconazole (Systemic); Lithium; Mesalamine; Methenamine; Multivitamins/Minerals (with ADEK, Folate, Iron); Nilotinib; PenicillAMINE; Phosphate Supplements; PONATinib; Potassium Acid Phosphate; Protease Inhibitors; Rilpivirine; Riociguat; Sulpiride; Tetracycline Derivatives; Trientine; Vismodegib
Increased Effect/Toxicity
Sodium Bicarbonate may increase the levels/effects of: Alpha-/Beta-Agonists; Amphetamines; Calcium Polystyrene Sulfonate; Dexmethylphenidate; Flecainide; Memantine; Methylphenidate; QuiNIDine; QuiNINE

The levels/effects of Sodium Bicarbonate may be increased by: AcetaZOLAMIDE
Nutritional/Ethanol Interactions Herb/Nutraceutical: Concurrent doses with iron may decrease iron absorption.
Adverse Reactions Frequency not defined.
Cardiovascular: Cerebral hemorrhage, CHF (aggravated), edema
Central nervous system: Tetany
Gastrointestinal: Belching, flatulence (with oral), gastric distension
Endocrine & metabolic: Hypernatremia, hyperosmolality, hypocalcemia, hypokalemia, increased affinity of hemoglobin for oxygen-reduced pH in

myocardial tissue necrosis when extravasated, intracranial acidosis, metabolic alkalosis, milk-alkali syndrome (especially with renal dysfunction)

Respiratory: Pulmonary edema

Pharmacodynamics/Kinetics

Onset of Action Oral: Rapid; I.V.: 15 minutes

Duration of Action Oral: 8-10 minutes; I.V.: 1-2 hours

Dosage Forms Considerations

Sodium bicarbonate solution 4.2% [42 mg/mL] provides 0.5 mEq/mL each of sodium and bicarbonate

Sodium bicarbonate solution 7.5% [75 mg/mL] provides 0.9 mEq/mL each of sodium and bicarbonate

Sodium bicarbonate solution 8.4% [84 mg/mL] provides 1 mEq/mL each of sodium and bicarbonate

Available Dosage Forms

Powder, Oral:

Generic: (1 g, 120 g, 454 g, 500 g, 1000 g, 2270 g, 2500 g, 12000 g, 45000 g)

Solution, Intravenous:

Neut: 4% (5 mL)

Generic: 4.2% (5 mL, 10 mL); 7.5% (50 mL); 8.4% (10 mL, 50 mL)

Tablet, Oral:

Generic: 325 mg, 650 mg

General Dosage Range

I.V.: *Children and Adults*: Dosage varies greatly depending on indication

Oral:

Children: 1-10 mEq/kg/day as a single dose **or** divided every 4-6 hours

Adults <60 years: 0.5-200 mEq/kg/day in 4-5 divided doses **or** 325 mg to 2 g 1-4 times/day (maximum: 16 g [200 mEq] day)

Adults ≥60 years: 0.5-100 mEq/kg/day in 4-6 divided doses **or** 325 mg to 2 g 1-4 times/day (maximum: 8 g [100 mEq] day)

Administration

I.V. For I.V. administration to infants, use the 0.5 mEq/mL solution or dilute the 1 mEq/mL solution 1:1 with **sterile water**; for direct I.V. infusion in emergencies, administer slowly (maximum rate in infants: 10 mEq/minute); for infusion, dilute to a maximum concentration of 0.5 mEq/mL in dextrose solution and infuse over 2 hours (maximum rate of administration: 1 mEq/kg/hour).

Vesicant (at concentrations ≥8.4%); ensure proper needle or catheter placement prior to and during I.V. infusion. Avoid extravasation.

Extravasation management: If extravasation occurs, stop infusion immediately and disconnect (leave needle/cannula in place); gently aspirate extravasated solution (do NOT flush the line); initiate hyaluronidase antidote; remove needle/cannula; apply dry cold compresses (Hurst, 2004); elevate extremity.

Hyaluronidase: SubQ: Inject four to five separate 0.2 mL injections of 15 units/mL around area of extravasation (Hurst, 2004).

Injectable Detail pH: 7-8.5

Oral Oral product should be administered 1-3 hours after meals.

Other Infiltration: Neutralizing additive (dental use): Add specified volume of 8.4% sodium bicarbonate directly with lidocaine and epinephrine injection and mix; use immediately after mixing.

Preparation for Administration

Prevention of contrast-induced nephropathy (unlabeled use): Remove 154 mL from 1000 mL bag of D_5W; replace with 154 mL of 8.4% sodium bicarbonate; resultant concentration is 154 mEq/L (Merten, 2004); more practically, institutions may remove 150 mL from 1000 mL bag of D_5W and replace with 150 mL of 8.4% sodium bicarbonate; resultant concentration is 150 mEq/L

Neutralizing additive (dental use): Add specified volume of 8.4% sodium bicarbonate directly with lidocaine and epinephrine injection and mix; use immediately after mixing.

Storage/Stability

Store injection at room temperature. Protect from heat and from freezing. Use only clear solutions.

Neutralizing additive (dental use): Store at 20°C to 25°C (68°F to 77°F).

Nursing Actions

Physical Assessment I.V.: Monitor cardiac status, arterial blood gases, and electrolytes. Monitor for CHF. Monitor infusion site for patency (if extravasation occurs, elevate extravasation site and apply warm compresses).

Patient Education

- Discuss specific use of drug and side effects with patient as it relates to treatment. (HCAHPS: During this hospital stay, were you given any medicine that you had not taken before? Before giving you any new medicine, how often did hospital staff tell you what the medicine was for? How often did hospital staff describe possible side effects in a way you could understand?)

- Patient may experience dyspepsia, bloating, flatulence, polydipsia, or hypokalemia. Have patient report immediately to prescriber dyspnea, illogical thinking, severe edema, or rash (HCAHPS).

- Educate patient about signs of a significant reaction (eg, wheezing; chest tightness; fever; itching; bad cough; blue skin color; seizures; or swelling of face, lips, tongue, or throat). **Note:** This is not a comprehensive list of all side effects. Patient should consult prescriber for additional questions.

Intended Use and Disclaimer: Should not be printed and given to patients. This information is intended to serve as a concise initial reference for healthcare professionals to use when discussing medications with a patient. You must ultimately ▶

rely on your own discretion, experience and judgment in diagnosing, treating and advising patients.

Dietary Considerations Some products may contain sodium. Oral product should be taken 1-3 hours after meals.

Related Information
Management of Drug Extravasations *on page 1700*

Sodium Citrate and Citric Acid
(SOW dee um SIT rate & SI trik AS id)

Brand Names: U.S. Cytra-2; Oracit®; Shohl's Solution (Modified)

Index Terms Bicitra; Citric Acid and Sodium Citrate; Modified Shohl's Solution

Pharmacologic Category Alkalinizing Agent, Oral

Medication Safety Issues
Sound-alike/look-alike issues:
Bicitra may be confused with Polycitra

Pregnancy Risk Factor Not established

Lactation Excretion in breast milk unknown/compatible

Use Treatment of metabolic acidosis; alkalinizing agent in conditions where long-term maintenance of an alkaline urine is desirable

Dosage Forms Considerations
Each mL provides 1 mEq sodium, and is equivalent to 1 mEq bicarbonate

Available Dosage Forms
Solution, oral:
Generic: Sodium citrate 500 mg and citric acid 334 mg per 5 mL
Cytra-2: Sodium citrate 500 mg and citric acid 334 mg per 5 mL
Oracit®: Sodium citrate 490 mg and citric acid 640 mg per 5 mL
Shohl's Solution (Modified): Sodium citrate 500 mg and citric acid 300 mg er 5 mL

General Dosage Range Oral:
Infants and Children: 2-3 mEq/kg/day in 3-4 divided doses **or** 5-15 mL after meals and at bedtime
Adults: 10-30 mL after meals and at bedtime

Administration
Oral Administer after meals. Dilute with 30-90 mL of water to enhance taste. Chilling solution prior to dosing helps to enhance palatability.

Nursing Actions
Physical Assessment Assess kidney function prior to treatment. Monitor cardiac status and serum potassium prior to treatment and at regular intervals.

Patient Education
• Discuss specific use of drug and side effects with patient as it relates to treatment. (HCAHPS: During this hospital stay, were you given any medicine that you had not taken before? Before giving you any new medicine, how often did hospital staff tell you what the medicine was

for? How often did hospital staff describe possible side effects in a way you could understand?)
• Patient may experience hyperkalemia or diarrhea. Have patient report immediately to prescriber rash (HCAHPS).
• Educate patient about signs of a significant reaction (eg, wheezing; chest tightness; fever; itching; bad cough; blue skin color; seizures; or swelling of face, lips, tongue, or throat). **Note:** This is not a comprehensive list of all side effects. Patient should consult prescriber for additional questions.

Intended Use and Disclaimer: Should not be printed and given to patients. This information is intended to serve as a concise initial reference for healthcare professionals to use when discussing medications with a patient. You must ultimately rely on your own discretion, experience and judgment in diagnosing, treating and advising patients.

Sodium Picosulfate, Magnesium Oxide, and Citric Acid
(SOW dee um pye ko SUL fate mag NEE zhum OKS ide & SI trik AS id)

Brand Names: U.S. Prepopik™

Index Terms Citric Acid, Sodium Picosulfate, and Magnesium Oxide; DA-1773; Magnesium Oxide, Sodium Picosulfate, and Citric Acid; Prepopik™; Sodium Picosulphate, Magnesium Oxide, and Citric Acid

Pharmacologic Category Laxative, Osmotic; Laxative, Stimulant

Medication Guide Available Yes

Pregnancy Risk Factor B

Lactation Excretion in breast milk unknown/use caution

Breast-Feeding Considerations Lactating women (n=8) were administered sodium picosulfate 10 mg as an oral solution once daily for 8 days. The active metabolite, BPHM, was detected in plasma and urine, but below the limit of detection in breast milk (<1 ng/mL) (Friedrich, 2011). Also refer to individual monographs.

Use Bowel cleansing prior to colonoscopy
Canadian labeling: Additional uses (not in U.S. labeling): Bowel cleansing prior to x-ray examination, endoscopy, or surgery

Mechanism of Action/Effect Stimulates colonic peristalsis and induces catharsis

Contraindications Hypersensitivity to sodium picosulfate, magnesium oxide, anhydrous citric acid, or any component of the formulation; GI obstruction or ileus; bowel perforation; gastric retention; toxic colitis; toxic megacolon; severe renal impairment (CrCl <30 mL/minute).
Canadian labeling: Additional contraindications (not in U.S. labeling): Congestive heart failure;

GI ulceration; nausea; vomiting; acute surgical abdominal conditions (eg, acute appendicitis)

Warnings/Precautions Serious arrhythmias have occurred rarely with the use of ionic osmotic laxative products; use caution in patients at increased risk for arrhythmias (eg, recent MI, unstable angina, cardiomyopathy, history of prolonged QT, HF, uncontrolled arrhythmias); consider baseline and post-colonoscopy ECGs in patients at increased risk for arrhythmias. Administration may cause fluid and electrolyte disturbances, particularly in patients at increased risk (eg, renal impairment, concomitant mediations that alter electrolyte balance). Any pre-existing electrolyte abnormalities should be corrected prior to use and patients should be adequately hydrated before, during, and after use. Consider evaluating for and treating post-colonoscopy electrolyte abnormalities in patients who develop significant vomiting, dehydration, or orthostatic hypotension. Seizures associated with electrolyte abnormalities (eg, hyponatremia, hypokalemia) and low serum osmolality have occurred; use with caution in patients with underlying electrolyte disturbances and in patients at increased risk for seizures (eg, concomitant medications that lower seizure threshold, withdrawal from alcohol or benzodiazepines). Osmotic laxatives may produce colonic mucosal aphthous ulcerations, including cases of ischemic colitis. Use caution when interpreting colonoscopy results in patients with inflammatory bowel disease.

Use with caution in patients with renal impairment and/or in patients taking medications that may adversely affect renal function (eg, diuretics, NSAIDs, ACE inhibitors); adequate hydration is particularly important in these patients. Patients with impaired renal function who develop severe vomiting should be closely monitored including measurement of electrolytes. Use with caution in patients with severe ulcerative colitis. Observe unconscious or semiconscious patients with impaired gag reflex or those who are otherwise prone to regurgitation or aspiration during administration of this product.

Patients with symptoms of bowel obstruction/perforation (nausea, vomiting, abdominal pain or distension) should be evaluated prior to use of this product. Each packet must be diluted with water prior to use, because inadvertent administration of undiluted solution may increase the risk of nausea, vomiting, and fluid/electrolyte abnormalities.

Oral medications administered ≤1 hour prior to the start of the bowel preparation regimen may not be absorbed. Chlorpromazine, digoxin, fluoroquinolones, iron, penicillamine, and tetracycline should be administered at least 2 hours before and 6 hours after administration of magnesium oxide to avoid chelation with magnesium. Sodium picosulfate requires the presence of colonic bacteria for the conversion to an active metabolite; prior or concomitant administration of antibiotics may reduce the efficacy of sodium picosulfate.

Drug Interactions

Avoid Concomitant Use

Avoid concomitant use of Sodium Picosulfate, Magnesium Oxide, and Citric Acid with any of the following: Calcium Polystyrene Sulfonate; Raltegravir; Sodium Polystyrene Sulfonate

Decreased Effect

Sodium Picosulfate, Magnesium Oxide, and Citric Acid may decrease the levels/effects of: Bisphosphonate Derivatives; Deferiprone; Dolutegravir; Eltrombopag; Gabapentin; Multivitamins/Fluoride (with ADE); Mycophenolate; Phosphate Supplements; Quinolone Antibiotics; Raltegravir; Tetracycline Derivatives; Trientine

The levels/effects of Sodium Picosulfate, Magnesium Oxide, and Citric Acid may be decreased by: Antibiotics; Trientine

Increased Effect/Toxicity

Sodium Picosulfate, Magnesium Oxide, and Citric Acid may increase the levels/effects of: Aluminum Hydroxide; Calcium Channel Blockers; Calcium Polystyrene Sulfonate; Neuromuscular-Blocking Agents; Sodium Polystyrene Sulfonate

The levels/effects of Sodium Picosulfate, Magnesium Oxide, and Citric Acid may be increased by: Alfacalcidol; Calcitriol; Calcium Channel Blockers

Adverse Reactions

>10%:
  Endocrine & metabolic: Hypermagnesemia (9% to 12%)
  Renal: GFR decreased (≤48 hours after colonoscopy: 10% to 29%)
1% to 10%:
  Central nervous system: Headache (2% to 3%)
  Endocrine & metabolic: Hypokalemia (5% to 7%), hypochloremia (1% to 4%), hyponatremia (1% to 4%)
  Gastrointestinal: Nausea (3%), vomiting (1%)
  Renal: Serum creatinine increased (<1% to 5%)

Available Dosage Forms

Powder for solution, oral:
  Prepopik™: Sodium picosulfate 10 mg, magnesium oxide 3.5 g, and citric acid 12 g per packet (2s)

General Dosage Range Oral: *Adults:* Two 150 mL (5 oz) doses

Administration

Oral

Prepopik™: Following the first dose, administer five 8-ounce clear liquid drinks (eg, water, clear broth, apple juice, white cranberry juice, white grape juice, ginger ale, plain gelatin [not purple or red], frozen juice bars [not purple or red]) within 5 hours. Following the second dose, administer three 8-ounce clear liquid drinks within 5 hours of administration. Clear liquids may be consumed up until 2 hours prior to the colonoscopy. In patients who develop bloating, distension, or abdominal pain, temporarily discontinue administration or increase the dosing interval until symptoms improve.

Purg-Odan™ (Canadian availability): Drink ~250 mL (8 oz) of clear liquids every hour while the effects of the bowel preparation regimen are apparent. Clear liquids may be consumed up until 2 hours prior to the procedure.

Pico-Salax® (Canadian availability):

At least 3 days prior to the procedure: Avoid eating seeds, nuts, fresh fruits and vegetables, and multigrain bread.

Day prior to the procedure: Consume clear liquids only (eg, water, clear power drinks, apple juice, white [not red] cranberry juice, white [not purple] grape juice, ginger ale, broth, tea [without milk, cream, or soy]), and no solid food. Patients with diabetes may drink a fiber-free supplement.

Following each dose: Adults should drink 1.5-2 L of clear fluids up until 2 hours prior to the procedure; children should drink one 8-ounce drink every hour while awake and up until 2 hours prior to the procedure.

Preparation for Administration Reconstitute immediately prior to each administration; do not prepare the solution in advance. To reconstitute, fill the supplied dosing cup with 5 ounces of cold water (up to the lower line) and add the contents of one packet to the cup; stir for 2-3 minutes.

Storage/Stability Store at 25°C (77°F); excursions permitted to15°C to 30°C (59°F to 86°F). Use the reconstituted solution immediately.

Nursing Actions

Physical Assessment Monitor patients prone to regurgitation or aspiration during administration. "Split dose" administration method preferred. Educate patient about proper use and function of bowel cleansing.

Reconstitute with cold water right before use, do not prepare solution in advance. Not for direct ingestion; must be dissolved and taken with additional water. Separate dosing of patient's usual medications from the administration of this one by 1 hour.

Monitor for severe bloating, distention, or abdominal pain. If present, delay the second dose until symptoms resolve. Specific patient groups may be sensitive to fluid shifts (older adults, patients taking routine medications that cause fluid shifts, patients with underling heart disease). Monitor them closely and educate them about rehydration.

Patient Education

• Discuss specific use of drug and side effects with patient as it relates to treatment. (HCAHPS: During this hospital stay, were you given any medicine that you had not taken before? Before giving you any new medicine, how often did hospital staff tell you what the medicine was

for? How often did hospital staff describe possible side effects in a way you could understand?)

• Patient may experience headache, hypokalemia, hypochloremia, hyponatremia, nausea, or emesis. Have patient report immediately to prescriber hypermagnesemia, or GFR decrease (HCAHPS).

• Educate patient about signs of a significant reaction (eg, wheezing; chest tightness; fever; itching; bad cough; blue skin color; seizures; or swelling of face, lips, tongue, or throat). **Note:** This is not a comprehensive list of all side effects. Patient should consult prescriber for additional questions.

Intended Use and Disclaimer: Should not be printed and given to patients. This information is intended to serve as a concise initial reference for healthcare professionals to use when discussing medications with a patient. You must ultimately rely on your own discretion, experience and judgment in diagnosing, treating and advising patients.

Sodium Polystyrene Sulfonate
(SOW dee um pol ee STYE reen SUL fon ate)

Brand Names: U.S. Kalexate; Kayexalate; Kionex; SPS

Pharmacologic Category Antidote

Medication Safety Issues

Sound-alike/look-alike issues:

Kayexalate® may be confused with Kaopectate® Sodium polystyrene sulfonate may be confused with calcium polystyrene sulfonate

Administration issues:

Always prescribe either one-time doses or as a specific number of doses (eg, 15 g q6h x 2 doses). Scheduled doses with no dosage limit could be given for days leading to dangerous hypokalemia.

International issues:

Kionex [U.S.] may be confused with Kinex brand name for biperiden [Mexico]

Pregnancy Risk Factor C

Lactation Excretion in breast milk unknown/use caution

Breast-Feeding Considerations It is not known if sodium polystyrene sulfonate is excreted in breast milk. The manufacturer recommends that caution be exercised when administering sodium polystyrene sulfonate to nursing women.

Use Treatment of hyperkalemia

Mechanism of Action/Effect Removes potassium by exchanging sodium ions for potassium ions in the intestine (especially the large intestine) before the resin is passed from the body

Contraindications Hypersensitivity to sodium polystyrene sulfonate or any component of the formulation; hypokalemia; obstructive bowel disease; neonates with reduced gut motility (postoperatively or drug-induced); oral administration in neonates

Additional contraindications: Sodium polystyrene sulfonate suspension (**with** sorbitol): Rectal administration in neonates (particularly in premature infants); any postoperative patient until normal bowel function resumes

Warnings/Precautions Intestinal necrosis (including fatalities) and other serious gastrointestinal events (eg, bleeding, ischemic colitis, perforation) have been reported, especially when administered with sorbitol. Increased risk may be associated with a history of intestinal disease or surgery, hypovolemia, prematurity, and renal insufficiency or failure; use with sorbitol is not recommended. Avoid use in any postoperative patient until normal bowel function resumes or in patients at risk for constipation or impaction; discontinue use if constipation occurs. Oral or rectal administration of sorbitol-containing sodium polystyrene sulfonate suspensions is contraindicated in neonates (particularly with prematurity). Use with caution in patients with severe HF, hypertension, or edema; sodium load may exacerbate condition. Effective lowering of serum potassium from sodium polystyrene sulfonate may take hours to days after administration; consider alternative measures (eg, dialysis) or concomitant therapy (eg, I.V. sodium bicarbonate) in situations where rapid correction of severe hyperkalemia is required. Severe hypokalemia may occur; frequent monitoring of serum potassium is recommended within each 24-hour period; ECG monitoring may be appropriate in select patients. In addition to serum potassium-lowering effects, cation-exchange resins may also affect other cation concentrations possibly resulting in decreased serum magnesium and calcium. Large oral doses may cause fecal impaction (especially in elderly).

Concomitant administration of oral sodium polystyrene sulfonate with nonabsorbable cation-donating antacids or laxatives (eg, magnesium hydroxide) may result in systemic alkalosis and may diminish ability to reduce serum potassium concentrations; use with such agents is not recommended. In addition, intestinal obstruction has been reported with concomitant administration of aluminum hydroxide due to concretion formation. Enema will reduce the serum potassium faster than oral administration, but the oral route will result in a greater reduction over several hours. Oral administration in neonates and use in neonates with reduced gut motility (postoperatively or drug-induced) is contraindicated. Oral or rectal administration of sorbitol-containing sodium polystyrene sulfonate suspensions in neonates (particularly with prematurity) is also contraindicated due to propylene glycol content and risk of intestinal necrosis and digestive hemorrhage. Use sodium polystyrene sulfonate (**without** sorbitol) with caution in premature or low-birth-weight infants. Use with caution in children when administering

rectally; excessive dosage or inadequate dilution may result in fecal impaction.

Drug Interactions

Avoid Concomitant Use

Avoid concomitant use of Sodium Polystyrene Sulfonate with any of the following: Laxatives; Meloxicam; Sorbitol

Decreased Effect

Sodium Polystyrene Sulfonate may decrease the levels/effects of: Lithium; Thyroid Products

Increased Effect/Toxicity

Sodium Polystyrene Sulfonate may increase the levels/effects of: Aluminum Hydroxide; Digoxin

The levels/effects of Sodium Polystyrene Sulfonate may be increased by: Antacids; Laxatives; Meloxicam; Sorbitol

Nutritional/Ethanol Interactions Food: Some liquids may contain potassium: Management: Do not mix in orange juice or in any fruit juice known to contain potassium.

Adverse Reactions Frequency not defined.

Endocrine & metabolic: Hypernatremia, hypocalcemia, hypokalemia, hypomagnesemia, sodium retention

Gastrointestinal: Anorexia, constipation, diarrhea, fecal impaction, intestinal necrosis (rare), intestinal obstruction (due to concretions in association with aluminum hydroxide), nausea, vomiting

Pharmacodynamics/Kinetics

Onset of Action 2-24 hours

Available Dosage Forms

Powder, Oral:

Kalexate: (454 g)

Kayexalate: (453.6 g)

Kionex: (454 g)

Generic: (453.6 g, 454 g)

Suspension, Oral:

Kionex: 15 g/60 mL (60 mL, 473 mL)

SPS: 15 g/60 mL (60 mL, 120 mL, 473 mL)

Generic: 15 g/60 mL (60 mL, 480 mL, 500 mL)

Suspension, Rectal:

Generic: 30 g/120 mL (120 mL); 50 g/200 mL (200 mL)

General Dosage Range

Oral:

Children: 1 g/kg/dose every 6 hours

Adults: 15 g 1-4 times/day

Rectal:

Children: 1 g/kg/dose every 2-6 hours

Adults: 30-50 g every 6 hours

Administration

Oral Shake suspension well prior to administration. Administer orally (or via NG tube) as a suspension. **Do not mix in orange juice.** Chilling the oral mixture will increase palatability.

Powder for suspension: For each 1 g of the powdered resin, add 3-4 mL of water or syrup (amount of fluid usually ranges from 20-100 mL)

Other Rectal: Enema route is less effective than oral administration. Administer cleansing enema ▶

first. Each dose of the powder for suspension should be suspended in 100 mL of aqueous vehicle and administered as a warm emulsion (body temperature). The commercially available suspension should also be warmed to body temperature. During administration, the solution should be agitated gently. Retain enema in colon for at least 30-60 minutes and for several hours, if possible. Once retention time is complete, irrigate colon with a nonsodium-containing solution to remove resin.

Storage/Stability Store at 25°C (77°F); excursions permitted to 15°C to 30°C (59°F to 86°F). Store repackaged product in refrigerator and use within 14 days. Freshly prepared suspensions should be used within 24 hours. Do not heat resin suspension.

Nursing Actions

Physical Assessment Monitor ECG until potassium levels are normal. Monitor bowel function; can cause constipation and/or fecal impaction.

Patient Education

- Discuss specific use of drug and side effects with patient as it relates to treatment. (HCAHPS: During this hospital stay, were you given any medicine that you had not taken before? Before giving you any new medicine, how often did hospital staff tell you what the medicine was for? How often did hospital staff describe possible side effects in a way you could understand?)
- Patient may experience nausea, constipation, lack of appetite, or hypokalemia. Have patient report immediately to prescriber severe dyspepsia, melena, or rash (HCAHPS).
- Educate patient about signs of a significant reaction (eg, wheezing; chest tightness; fever; itching; bad cough; blue skin color; seizures; or swelling of face, lips, tongue, or throat). **Note:** This is not a comprehensive list of all side effects. Patient should consult prescriber for additional questions.

Intended Use and Disclaimer: Should not be printed and given to patients. This information is intended to serve as a concise initial reference for healthcare professionals to use when discussing medications with a patient. You must ultimately rely on your own discretion, experience and judgment in diagnosing, treating and advising patients.

Dietary Considerations Do **not** mix in orange juice or in any fruit juice known to contain potassium. Some products may contain sodium.

Sofosbuvir (soe FOS bue vir)

Brand Names: U.S. Sovaldi
Index Terms Sovaldi
Pharmacologic Category Antihepaciviral, Polymerase Inhibitor (Anti-HCV)

Pregnancy Risk Factor B (sofosbuvir)/X (in combination with ritonavir or peginterferon alfa/ribavirin)

Lactation Excretion in breast milk unknown/not recommended.

Breast-Feeding Considerations

It is not known if sofosbuvir is excreted into breast milk. Due to the potential for serious adverse reactions in the nursing infant, the manufacturer recommends a decision be made whether to discontinue nursing or to discontinue the drug, taking into account the importance of treatment to the mother. Breast-feeding is not linked to the spread of hepatitis C virus; however, if nipples are cracked or bleeding, breast-feeding is not recommended (Workowski, 2010). Mothers coinfected with HIV are discouraged from breast-feeding to decrease potential transmission of HIV (DHHS [perinatal], 2012). Also refer to the Peginterferon Alfa and Ribavirin monographs for additional information.

Use Chronic hepatitis C: Treatment of genotype 1, 2, 3, or 4 chronic hepatitis C (CHC) (in combination with ribavirin or with peginterferon alfa and ribavirin), including patients with hepatocellular carcinoma meeting Milan criteria (awaiting liver transplantation) and those with HCV/HIV-1 coinfection

Mechanism of Action/Effect Sofosbuvir, a direct-acting antiviral agents against the hepatitis C virus, is a prodrug converted to its pharmacologically active form (GS-461203) via intracellular metabolism. It inhibits HCV NS5B RNA-dependent RNA polymerase, essential for viral replication, and acts as a chain terminator.

Contraindications All contraindications also applicable to ribavirin and peginterferon alfa including pregnancy and use by male partners of pregnant women.

Also refer to Peginterferon Alfa and Ribavirin monographs for individual product contraindications.

Warnings/Precautions Avoid pregnancy in females and female partners of male patients during therapy and for at least 6 months following treatment since used in combination with ribavirin for all indications; two nonhormonal forms of effective contraception must be used. Combination therapy with ribavirin is contraindicated in pregnancy; ribavirin may cause birth defects and/or death of the exposed fetus. Do not use as monotherapy; use only in combination with ribavirin (with or without peginterferon alfa depending upon the clinical indication). Potentially significant drug-drug interactions may exist, requiring dose or frequency adjustment, additional monitoring, and/or selection of alternative therapy, including use with potent P-gp inhibitors (eg, rifampin, St John's wort).

Drug Interactions

Avoid Concomitant Use

Avoid concomitant use of Sofosbuvir with any of the following: OXcarbazepine; P-glycoprotein/ABCB1 Inducers; Rifabutin; Rifapentine

Decreased Effect

The levels/effects of Sofosbuvir may be decreased by: OXcarbazepine; P-glycoprotein/ABCB1 Inducers; Rifabutin; Rifapentine

Increased Effect/Toxicity

The levels/effects of Sofosbuvir may be increased by: P-glycoprotein/ABCB1 Inhibitors

Adverse Reactions

>10%:

Central nervous system: Fatigue (30% to 59%), headache (24% to 36%), insomnia (15% to 25%), chills (2% to 17%), irritability (10% to 13%)

Dermatologic: Pruritus (11% to 27%), skin rash (8% to 18%)

Gastrointestinal: Nausea (22% to 34%), decreased appetite (18%), diarrhea (9% to 12%)

Hematologic & oncologic: Decreased hemoglobin (<10 g/dL: 6% to 23%; <8.5 g/dL: ≤2%), anemia (6% to 21%), neutropenia (<1% [interferon-free regimen] to 17% [interferon-containing regimen]), decreased neutrophils (≥0.5 to <0.75 times 10^9/L: <1% [interferon-free regimen] to 15%; <0.5 times 10^9/L: ≤5%)

Neuromuscular & skeletal: Weakness (5% to 21%), myalgia (6% to 14%)

Respiratory: Flu-like symptoms (6% to 16%)

Miscellaneous: Fever (4% to 18%)

1% to 10%:

Gastrointestinal: Increased serum lipase (>3 times ULN: ≤2%)

Hematologic & oncologic: Thrombocytopenia (≤1%)

Hepatic: Increased serum bilirubin (>2.5 times ULN: 3%)

Renal: Increased creatine kinase (≥10 times ULN: 1% to 2%)

Available Dosage Forms

Tablet, Oral:

Sovaldi: 400 mg

Administration

Oral Administer with or without food.

Storage/Stability
Store at room temperature below 30°C (86°F). Dispense only in original container.

Nursing Actions

Physical Assessment Monitor hematocrit and hemoglobin levels. Assess skin for rash. Monitor patient for nausea, itching, anorexia, and diarrhea.

Patient Education

• Discuss specific use of drug and side effects with patient as it relates to treatment. (HCAHPS: During this hospital stay, were you given any medicine that you had not taken before? Before giving you any new medicine, how often did hospital staff tell you what the medicine was for? How often did hospital staff describe possible side effects in a way you could understand?)

• Patient may experience headache, dyspepsia, or insomnia. Have patient report immediately to prescriber depression, suicidal ideation, anxiety, emotional instability, illogical thinking, dyspnea, severe asthenia, or pallor (HCAHPS).

• Educate patient about signs of a significant reaction (eg, wheezing; chest tightness; fever; itching; bad cough; blue skin color; seizures; or swelling of face, lips, tongue, or throat). **Note:** This is not a comprehensive list of all side effects. Patient should consult prescriber for additional questions.

Intended Use and Disclaimer: Should not be printed and given to patients. This information is intended to serve as a concise initial reference for healthcare professionals to use when discussing medications with a patient. You must ultimately rely on your own discretion, experience and judgment in diagnosing, treating and advising patients.

Solifenacin (sol i FEN a sin)

Brand Names: U.S. VESIcare

Index Terms Solifenacin Succinate; YM905

Pharmacologic Category Anticholinergic Agent

Medication Safety Issues

BEERS Criteria medication:

This drug may be potentially inappropriate for use in geriatric patients (Quality of evidence - varies based on comorbidity; Strength of recommendation - varies based on comorbidity)

Pregnancy Risk Factor C

Lactation Excretion in breast milk unknown/not recommended

Breast-Feeding Considerations It is not known if solifenacin is excreted in breast milk. The manufacturer recommends a decision be made whether to discontinue nursing or to discontinue the drug.

Use Treatment of overactive bladder with symptoms of urinary frequency, urgency, or urge incontinence

Mechanism of Action/Effect Inhibits muscarinic receptors resulting in decreased urinary bladder contraction, increased residual urine volume, and decreased detrusor muscle pressure.

Contraindications Hypersensitivity to solifenacin or any component of the formulation; urinary retention; gastric retention; uncontrolled narrow-angle glaucoma.

Warnings/Precautions Cases of angioedema involving the face, lips, tongue, and/or larynx have been reported during treatment; some cases have occurred after the first dose. Immediately discontinue if tongue, hypopharynx, or larynx is involved. Anaphylactic reactions have been reported rarely with solifenacin; immediately discontinue therapy if ▶

anaphylactic reaction develops. Do not use in patients with a known or suspected hypersensitivity. Central nervous system effects have been reported (eg, headache, confusion, hallucinations, somnolence); monitor, particularly at treatment initiation or dose increase, reduce dose or discontinue if necessary. May cause drowsiness and/or blurred vision, which may impair physical or mental abilities; patients must be cautioned about performing tasks which require mental alertness (eg, operating machinery or driving). Heat prostration may occur in the presence of increased environmental temperature; use caution in hot weather and/or exercise. Use with caution in patients with bladder outflow obstruction, gastrointestinal obstructive disorders, and decreased gastrointestinal motility. Use with caution in patients with a known history of QT prolongation or other risk factors for QT prolongation (eg, concomitant use of medications known to prolong QT interval and/or electrolyte abnormalities); the risk for QT prolongation is dose-related. Use with caution in patients with controlled (treated) narrow-angle glaucoma; use is contraindicated with uncontrolled narrow-angle glaucoma. Dosage adjustment is required for patients with severe renal impairment (CrCl <30 mL/minute) or moderate (Child-Pugh class B) hepatic impairment; use is not recommended with severe hepatic impairment (Child-Pugh class C). Patients on potent CYP3A4 inhibitors require the lower dose of solifenacin. This medication is associated with potent anticholinergic properties which may be inappropriate in older adults depending on comorbidities (eg, dementia, delirium) (Beers Criteria).

Drug Interactions

Avoid Concomitant Use

Avoid concomitant use of Solifenacin with any of the following: Aclidinium; Conivaptan; Fusidic Acid (Systemic); Ipratropium (Oral Inhalation); Potassium Chloride; Tiotropium; Umeclidinium

Decreased Effect

Solifenacin may decrease the levels/effects of: Acetylcholinesterase Inhibitors (Central); Secretin

The levels/effects of Solifenacin may be decreased by: Acetylcholinesterase Inhibitors (Central); Bosentan; CYP3A4 Inducers (Strong); Dabrafenib; Deferasirox; Herbs (CYP3A4 Inducers); Mitotane; Tocilizumab

Increased Effect/Toxicity

Solifenacin may increase the levels/effects of: AbobotulinumtoxinA; Analgesics (Opioid); Anticholinergics; Cannabinoids; Highest Risk QTc-Prolonging Agents; Moderate Risk QTc-Prolonging Agents; OnabotulinumtoxinA; Potassium Chloride; RimabotulinumtoxinB; Thiazide Diuretics; Tiotropium; Topiramate

The levels/effects of Solifenacin may be increased by: Aclidinium; Antifungal Agents (Azole Derivatives, Systemic); Conivaptan; CYP3A4 Inhibitors (Moderate); CYP3A4 Inhibitors (Strong); Dasatinib; Fusidic Acid (Systemic); Ipratropium (Oral Inhalation); Ivacaftor; Luliconazole; Mifepristone; Mirabegron; Pramlintide; Simeprevir; Stiripentol; Umeclidinium

Nutritional/Ethanol Interactions

Food: Grapefruit juice may increase the serum level effects of solifenacin.

Herb/Nutraceutical: St John's wort (*Hypericum*) may decrease the levels/effects of solifenacin.

Adverse Reactions

>10%: Gastrointestinal: Xerostomia (11% to 28%; dose-related), constipation (5% to 13%; dose-related)

1% to 10%:

Cardiovascular: Edema (≤1%), hypertension (≤1%)

Central nervous system: Fatigue (1% to 2%), depression (≤1%)

Gastrointestinal: Dyspepsia (1% to 4%), nausea (2% to 3%), upper abdominal pain (1% to 2%)

Genitourinary: Urinary tract infection (3% to 5%), urinary retention (≤1%)

Ocular: Blurred vision (4% to 5%), dry eye syndrome (≤2%)

Respiratory: Cough (≤1%)

Miscellaneous: Influenza (≤2%)

Available Dosage Forms

Tablet, Oral:

VESIcare: 5 mg, 10 mg

General Dosage Range
Dosage adjustment recommended in patients with hepatic or renal impairment and on concomitant therapy

Oral: *Adults:* 5-10 mg/day

Administration

Oral Swallow tablet whole; administer with liquids; may be administered without regard to meals.

Storage/Stability
Store at controlled room temperature of 25°C (77°F); excursions permitted to 15°C to 30°C (59°F to 86°F).

Nursing Actions

Physical Assessment Monitor urination pattern.

Patient Education

- Discuss specific use of drug and side effects with patient as it relates to treatment. (HCAHPS: During this hospital stay, were you given any medicine that you had not taken before? Before giving you any new medicine, how often did hospital staff tell you what the medicine was for? How often did hospital staff describe possible side effects in a way you could understand?)
- Patient may experience headache, dyspepsia, pyrosis, blurred vision, constipation, or xerostomia. Have patient report immediately to prescriber severe dizziness, dyspnea, illogical thinking, urinary retention, or rash (HCAHPS).
- Educate patient about signs of a significant reaction (eg, wheezing; chest tightness; fever; itching; bad cough; blue skin color; seizures; or swelling of face, lips, tongue, or throat). **Note:** This is not a comprehensive list of all side

effects. Patient should consult prescriber for additional questions.

Intended Use and Disclaimer: Should not be printed and given to patients. This information is intended to serve as a concise initial reference for healthcare professionals to use when discussing medications with a patient. You must ultimately rely on your own discretion, experience and judgment in diagnosing, treating and advising patients.

Dietary Considerations May be taken without regard to meals.

Related Information

Oral Medications That Should Not Be Crushed or Altered *on page 1712*

Somatropin (soe ma TROE pin)

Brand Names: U.S. Genotropin; Genotropin Mini-Quick; Humatrope; Norditropin FlexPro; Norditropin NordiFlex Pen; Nutropin AQ NuSpin 10; Nutropin AQ NuSpin 20; Nutropin AQ NuSpin 5; Nutropin AQ Pen; Nutropin [DSC]; Omnitrope; Saizen; Saizen Click.Easy; Serostim; Tev-Tropin; Zorbtive

Index Terms Growth Hormone, Human; hGH; Human Growth Hormone

Pharmacologic Category Growth Hormone

Medication Safety Issues

Sound-alike/look-alike issues:

Humatrope may be confused with homatropine

Somatrem may be confused with somatropin

Somatropin may be confused with homatropine, sumatriptan

BEERS Criteria medication:

This drug may be potentially inappropriate for use in geriatric patients (Quality of evidence - high; Strength of recommendation - strong).

Pregnancy Risk Factor B/C (depending upon manufacturer)

Lactation Excretion in breast milk unknown/use caution

Breast-Feeding Considerations It is not known if somatropin is excreted in breast milk. The manufacturer recommends that caution be exercised when administering somatropin to nursing women.

Use

Children:

Treatment of growth failure due to inadequate endogenous growth hormone secretion (Genotropin, Humatrope, Norditropin, Nutropin, Nutropin AQ, Omnitrope, Saizen, Tev-Tropin)

Treatment of short stature associated with Turner syndrome (Genotropin, Humatrope, Norditropin, Nutropin, Nutropin AQ, Omnitrope)

Treatment of Prader-Willi syndrome (Genotropin, Omnitrope)

Treatment of growth failure associated with chronic renal insufficiency (CRI) up until the time of renal transplantation (Nutropin, Nutropin AQ)

Treatment of growth failure in children born small for gestational age who fail to manifest catch-up growth by 2 years of age (Genotropin, Omnitrope) or by 2-4 years of age (Humatrope, Norditropin)

Treatment of idiopathic short stature (nongrowth hormone-deficient short stature) defined by height standard deviation score (SDS) ≤-2.25 and growth rate not likely to attain normal adult height (Genotropin, Humatrope, Nutropin, Nutropin AQ, Omnitrope)

Treatment of short stature or growth failure associated with short stature homeobox gene (SHOX) deficiency (Humatrope)

Treatment of short stature associated with Noonan syndrome (Norditropin)

Adults:

HIV patients with wasting or cachexia with concomitant antiviral therapy (Serostim)

Replacement of endogenous growth hormone in patients with adult growth hormone deficiency who meet both of the following criteria (Genotropin, Humatrope, Norditropin, Nutropin, Nutropin AQ, Omnitrope, Saizen):

Biochemical diagnosis of adult growth hormone deficiency by means of a subnormal response to a standard growth hormone stimulation test (peak growth hormone ≤5 mcg/L). Confirmatory testing may not be required in patients with congenital/genetic growth hormone deficiency or multiple pituitary hormone deficiencies due to organic diseases.

and

Adult-onset: Patients who have adult growth hormone deficiency whether alone or with multiple hormone deficiencies (hypopituitarism) as a result of pituitary disease, hypothalamic disease, surgery, radiation therapy, or trauma

or

Childhood-onset: Patients who were growth hormone deficient during childhood, confirmed as an adult before replacement therapy is initiated

Treatment of short-bowel syndrome (Zorbtive)

Unlabeled Use Pediatric HIV patients with wasting/cachexia (Serostim); HIV-associated adipose redistribution syndrome (HARS) (Serostim)

Mechanism of Action/Effect Human growth hormone assists in growth of linear bone, skeletal muscle, and organs; stimulates erythropoietin which increases red blood cell mass; exerts both insulin-like and diabetogenic effects; enhances transmucosal transport of water, electrolytes, and nutrients across the gut

Contraindications Hypersensitivity to growth hormone or any component of the formulation; growth promotion in pediatric patients with closed epiphyses; progression or recurrence of any underlying intracranial lesion or actively growing intracranial tumor; acute critical illness due to complications following open heart or abdominal surgery; multiple accidental trauma or acute respiratory failure;

evidence of active malignancy; active proliferative or severe nonproliferative diabetic retinopathy; use in patients with Prader-Willi syndrome **without** growth hormone deficiency (except Genotropin) or in patients with Prader-Willi syndrome **with** growth hormone deficiency who are severely obese, have a history of upper airway obstruction or sleep apnea, or have severe respiratory impairment

Warnings/Precautions Initiation of somatropin is contraindicated with acute critical illness due to complications following open heart or abdominal surgery, multiple accidental trauma, or acute respiratory failure; mortality may be increased. The safety of continuing somatropin in patients who develop these illnesses during therapy has not been established; use with caution. Use in contraindicated with active malignancy; monitor patients with pre-existing tumors or growth failure secondary to an intracranial lesion for recurrence or progression of underlying disease; discontinue therapy with evidence of recurrence. An increased risk of second neoplasm has been reported in childhood cancer survivors treated with somatropin; the most common second neoplasms were meningiomas in patients treated with radiation to the head for their first neoplasm. Monitor patients for any malignant transformation of skin lesions.

Somatropin may decrease insulin sensitivity; use with caution in patients with diabetes or with risk factors for impaired glucose tolerance. Adjustment of antidiabetic medications may be necessary. Pancreatitis has been rarely reported; incidence in children (especially girls) with Turner syndrome may be greater than adults. Monitor for hypersensitivity reactions. Patients with hypoadrenalism may require increased dosages of glucocorticoids (especially cortisone acetate and prednisone) due to somatropin-mediated inhibition of 11 beta-hydroxysteroid dehydrogenase type 1; undiagnosed central hypoadrenalism may be unmasked. Excessive glucocorticoid therapy may inhibit the growth promoting effects of somatropin in children; monitor and adjust glucocorticoids carefully. Untreated/undiagnosed hypothyroidism may decrease response to therapy; monitor thyroid function test periodically and initiate/adjust thyroid replacement therapy as needed. Closely monitor other hormonal replacement treatments in patients with hypopituitarism. Obese patients may experience an increased incidence of adverse events when using a weight-based dosing regimen. Intracranial hypertension (IH) with headache, nausea, papilledema, visual changes, and/or vomiting has been reported with somatropin; funduscopic examination prior to initiation of therapy and periodically thereafter is recommended. Treatment should be discontinued in patients who develop papilledema; resuming treatment at a lower dose may be considered once IH-associated signs and symptoms have resolved. Patients with Turner syndrome, chronic renal failure and Prader-Willi syndrome may be at increased risk for IH. Progression of scoliosis may occur in children experiencing rapid growth. Patients with growth hormone deficiency may develop slipped capital epiphyses more frequently, evaluate any child with new onset of a limp or with complaints of hip or knee pain. Patients with Turner syndrome are at increased risk for otitis media and other ear/hearing disorders, cardiovascular disorders (including stroke, aortic aneurysm, hypertension), and thyroid disease, monitor carefully. Fluid retention may occur frequently in adults during use; manifestations of fluid retention (eg, edema, arthralgia, myalgia, nerve compression syndromes/paresthesias) are generally transient and dose dependent. Products may contain benzyl alcohol or m-cresol. When administering to newborns, reconstitute with sterile water or saline for injection. Not for I.V. injection. According to the Centers for Disease Control and Prevention (CDC), pen-shaped injection devices should never be used for more than one person (even when the needle is changed) because of the risk of infection. The injection device should be clearly labeled with individual patient information to ensure that the correct pen is used (CDC, 2012).

Fatalities have been reported in pediatric patients with Prader-Willi syndrome following the use of growth hormone. The reported fatalities occurred in patients with one or more risk factors, including severe obesity, sleep apnea, respiratory impairment, or unidentified respiratory infection; male patients with one or more of these factors may be at greater risk. Treatment interruption is recommended in patients who show signs of upper airway obstruction, including the onset of, or increased, snoring. In addition, evaluation of and/or monitoring for sleep apnea and respiratory infections are recommended.

Patients with HIV infection should be maintained on antiretroviral therapy to prevent the potential increase in viral replication.

Avoid use in the elderly, except as hormone replacement following pituitary gland removal; use results in minimal effect on body composition and is associated with edema, arthralgia, carpal tunnel syndrome, gynecomastia, and impaired fasting glucose (Beers Criteria). Elderly may be more sensitive to the actions of somatropin; consider lower starting doses.

Safety and efficacy have not been established for the treatment of Noonan syndrome in children with significant cardiac disease. Children with epiphyseal closure who are treated for adult GHD need reassessment of therapy and dose. Administration site rotation is necessary to prevent tissue atrophy.

Drug Interactions

Avoid Concomitant Use There are no known interactions where it is recommended to avoid concomitant use.

Decreased Effect

Somatropin may decrease the levels/effects of: Antidiabetic Agents; Cortisone; PredniSONE

The levels/effects of Somatropin may be decreased by: Estrogen Derivatives

Increased Effect/Toxicity There are no known significant interactions involving an increase in effect.

Adverse Reactions

Growth hormone deficiency: Adverse reactions reported with growth hormone deficiency vary greatly by age. Generally, percentages are less in pediatric patients than adults, and many of the reactions reported in adults are dose related. Percentages reported also vary by product. Below is a listing by age group; events reported more commonly overall are noted with an asterisk (*).

Children: Antibodies development, arthralgia, benign intracranial hypertension, edema, eosinophilia, glycosuria, Hb A_{1c} increased, headache, hematoma, hematuria, hyperglycemia (mild), hypertriglyceridemia, hypoglycemia, hypothyroidism, injection site reaction, intracranial tumor, leg pain, lipoatrophy, leukemia, meningioma, muscle pain, papilledema, pseudotumor cerebri, psoriasis exacerbation, rash, scoliosis progression, seizure, slipped capital femoral epiphysis, weakness

Adults: Acne, ALT increased, AST increased, arthralgia*, back pain, bronchitis, carpal tunnel syndrome, chest pain, cough, depression, diabetes mellitus (type 2), diaphoresis, dizziness, edema*, fatigue, flu-like syndrome*, gastritis, glucose intolerance, glucosuria, headache*, hyperglycemia (mild), hypertension, hypoesthesia, hypothyroidism, infection, insomnia, insulin resistance, joint disorder, leg edema, muscle pain, myalgia*, nausea, pain in extremities, paresthesia*, peripheral edema*, pharyngitis, retinopathy, rhinitis, skeletal pain*, stiffness in extremities, surgical procedure, upper respiratory tract infection, weakness

Additional/postmarketing reactions observed with growth hormone deficiency: Gynecomastia, increased growth of pre-existing nevi, pancreatitis

HARS: Serostim®: Limited to >10%: Edema (peripheral) (19% to 45%), arthralgia (28% to 37%), pain (extremity) (5% to 19%), hypoesthesia (9% to 15%), headache (4% to 14%), blood glucose increased (4% to 14%), paresthesia (11% to 13%), myalgia (3% to 13%)

Idiopathic short stature: Percentages reported using Humatrope® versus placebo: Myalgia (24%), scoliosis (19%), otitis media (16%), arthralgia (11%), arthrosis (11%), hyperlipidemia

(8%), gynecomastia (5%), hip pain (3%), hypertension (3%). Additional adverse reactions listed as reported using other products from ISS NCGS Cohort (frequencies <1%): Aggressiveness, benign intracranial hypertension, diabetes, edema, hair loss, headache, injection site reaction

Prader-Willi syndrome: Genotropin® (frequency not defined): Aggressiveness, arthralgia, edema, hair loss, headache, benign intracranial hypertension, myalgia; fatalities associated with use in this population have been reported

Turner syndrome: Percentages reported using Humatrope® compared to untreated patients. Additional adverse reactions reported from other products, frequency not specified: Surgical procedures (45%), otitis media (43%), ear disorders (18%), joint pain, respiratory illness, urinary tract infection

HIV patients with wasting or cachexia: Serostim® (limited to ≥5%): Musculoskeletal disorders (arthralgia, arthrosis, myalgia: 78%), peripheral edema (26%), headache (13%), nausea (9%), paresthesia (8%), edema (6%), gynecomastia (6%), hypoesthesia (5%)

Short-bowel syndrome: Zorbtive® (limited to >10%): Peripheral edema (69% to 81%), facial edema (44% to 50%), arthralgia (31% to 44%), nausea (13% to 31%), injection site pain (up to 31%), flatulence (25%), injection site reaction (19% to 25%), abdominal pain (13% to 25%), vomiting (19%), pain (6% to 19%), chest pain (up to 19%), dehydration (up to 19%), infection (up to 19%), rhinitis (up to 19%), hearing symptoms (13%), dizziness (6% to 13%), rash (6% to 13%), diaphoresis (up to 13%), generalized edema (up to 13%), malaise (up to 13%), moniliasis (up to 13%), myalgia (up to 13%)

SHOX deficiency: Humatrope®: Arthralgia (11%), gynecomastia (8%), excessive cutaneous nevi (7%), scoliosis (4%)

Small for gestational age: Genotropin®, Humatrope® (frequency not defined): Mild, transient hyperglycemia; benign intracranial hypertension (rare); central precocious puberty; jaw prominence (rare); aggravation of pre-existing scoliosis (rare); injection site reactions; progression of pigmented nevi; carpal tunnel syndrome (rare) diabetes mellitus (rare); otitis media; headache; slipped capital femoral epiphysis

Pharmacodynamics/Kinetics

Duration of Action Maintains supraphysiologic levels for 18-20 hours

Available Dosage Forms

Solution, Subcutaneous:

Norditropin FlexPro: 5 mg/1.5 mL (1.5 mL); 10 mg/1.5 mL (1.5 mL); 15 mg/1.5 mL (1.5 mL)

Norditropin NordiFlex Pen: 30 mg/3 mL (3 mL)

Nutropin AQ NuSpin 5: 5 mg/2 mL (2 mL)

Nutropin AQ NuSpin 10: 10 mg/2 mL (2 mL)

Nutropin AQ NuSpin 20: 20 mg/2 mL (2 mL)

Nutropin AQ Pen: 10 mg/2 mL (2 mL); 20 mg/2 mL (2 mL)
Omnitrope: 5 mg/1.5 mL (1.5 mL); 10 mg/1.5 mL (1.5 mL)

Solution Reconstituted, Injection:
Humatrope: 5 mg (1 ea); 6 mg (1 ea); 12 mg (1 ea); 24 mg (1 ea)
Saizen: 5 mg (1 ea); 8.8 mg (1 ea)
Saizen Click.Easy: 8.8 mg (1 ea)

Solution Reconstituted, Subcutaneous:
Genotropin: 5 mg (1 ea); 12 mg (1 ea)
Omnitrope: 5.8 mg (1 ea)
Serostim: 4 mg (1 ea); 5 mg (1 ea); 6 mg (1 ea)
Tev-Tropin: 5 mg (1 ea)
Zorbtive: 8.8 mg (1 ea)

Solution Reconstituted, Subcutaneous [preservative free]:
Genotropin MiniQuick: 0.2 mg (1 ea); 0.4 mg (1 ea); 0.6 mg (1 ea); 0.8 mg (1 ea); 1 mg (1 ea); 1.2 mg (1 ea); 1.4 mg (1 ea); 1.6 mg (1 ea); 1.8 mg (1 ea); 2 mg (1 ea)

General Dosage Range I.M., SubQ: *Children and Adults:* Dosage varies greatly depending on indication

Administration

I.M. Not all products are approved for I.M. administration. Rotate administration sites to avoid tissue atrophy.

Other Do not shake; administer SubQ or I.M. (not all products are approved for I.M. administration). Rotate administration sites to avoid tissue atrophy. When administering to newborns, do not reconstitute with a diluent that contains benzyl alcohol; sterile water for injection may be used as an alternative. Norditropin cartridge must be administered using the corresponding color-coded NordiPen injection pen. Solution in the Omnitrope cartridges must be administered using the Omnitrope pen; when installing a new cartridge, prime pen prior to first use. When administering Tev-Tropin, SubQ injections of solutions >1 mL not recommended.

Preparation for Administration

Genotropin: Reconstitute with diluent provided.
Genotropin MiniQuick: Reconstitute with diluent provided. Consult the instructions provided with the reconstitution device.
Humatrope:
Cartridge: Consult HumatroPen User Guide for complete instructions for reconstitution. **Dilute with solution provided with cartridges ONLY; do not use diluent provided with vials.**
Vial: 5 mg: Reconstitute with 1.5-5 mL diluent provided. Swirl gently; do not shake.
Nutropin: Vial:
5 mg: Reconstitute with 1-5 mL bacteriostatic water for injection. Swirl gently, do not shake.
10 mg: Reconstitute with 1-10 mL bacteriostatic water for injection. Swirl gently, do not shake.
Omnitrope powder: Reconstitute with provided diluent. Swirl gently; do not shake.

Saizen: Vial:
5 mg: Reconstitute with 1-3 mL bacteriostatic water for injection or sterile water for injection. Gently swirl; do not shake.
8.8 mg: Reconstitute with 2-3 mL bacteriostatic water for injection or sterile water for injection. Gently swirl; do not shake.
Serostim: Vial: Reconstitute with 0.5-1 mL sterile water for injection.
Tev-Tropin: Reconstitute with 1-5 mL of diluent provided. Gently swirl; do not shake. May use preservative-free NS for use in newborns.
Zorbtive: 8.8 mg vial: Reconstitute with 1-2 mL bacteriostatic water for injection. Swirl gently.

Storage/Stability

Genotropin: Store at 2°C to 8°C (36°F to 46°F); do not freeze. Protect from light. Following reconstitution of 5.8 mg and 13.8 mg cartridge, store under refrigeration and use within 28 days.
Genotropin Miniquick: Store in refrigerator prior to dispensing, but may be stored ≤25°C (77°F) for up to 3 months after dispensing. Once reconstituted, solution must be refrigerated and used within 24 hours. Discard unused portion.
Humatrope:
Vial: Before and after reconstitution, store at 2°C to 8°C (36°F to 46°F); do not freeze. When reconstituted with provided diluent or bacteriostatic water for injection, use within 14 days. When reconstituted with sterile water for injection, use within 24 hours and discard unused portion.
Cartridge: Before and after reconstitution, store at 2°C to 8°C (36°F to 46°F); do not freeze. Following reconstitution with provided diluent, stable for 28 days under refrigeration.
Norditropin: Store at 2°C to 8°C (36°F to 46°F); do not freeze. Avoid direct light. When refrigerated, prefilled pen must be used within 4 weeks after initial injection. Orange and blue prefilled pens may also be stored up to 3 weeks at ≤25°C (77°F).
Nutropin: Before and after reconstitution, store at 2°C to 8°C (36°F to 46°F); do not freeze.
Nutropin vial: Use reconstituted vials within 14 days. When reconstituted with sterile water for injection, use immediately and discard unused portion.
Nutropin AQ formulations: Use within 28 days following initial use.
Omnitrope:
Powder for injection: Prior to reconstitution, store under refrigeration at 2°C to 8°C (36°F to 46°F); do not freeze. Protect from light. Reconstitute with provided diluent. Swirl gently; do not shake. Following reconstitution with the provided diluents, the 5.8 mg vial may be stored under refrigeration for up to 3 weeks. Store vial in carton to protect from light.
Solution: Prior to use, store under refrigeration at 2°C to 8°C (36°F to 46°F). Once the cartridge is

loaded into the pen delivery system, store under refrigeration for up to 28 days after first use.

Saizen: Prior to reconstitution, store at room temperature 15°C to 30°C (59°F to 86°F). Following reconstitution with bacteriostatic water for injection, reconstituted solution should be refrigerated and used within 14 days. When reconstituted with sterile water for injection, use immediately and discard unused portion. The Saizen easy click cartridge, when reconstituted with the provided bacteriostatic water, should be stored under refrigeration and used within 21 days.

Serostim: Prior to reconstitution, store at room temperature 15°C to 30°C (59°F to 86°F). When reconstituted with sterile water for injection, use immediately and discard unused portion.

Tev-Tropin: Prior to reconstitution, store at 2°C to 8°C (36°F to 46°F). Following reconstitution with bacteriostatic NS, solution should be refrigerated and used within 14 days. Some cloudiness may occur; do not use if cloudiness persists after warming to room temperature.

Zorbtive: Store unopened vials and diluent at room temperature of 15°C to 30°C (59°F to 86°F). Store reconstituted vial under refrigeration at 2°C to 8°C (36°F to 46°F) for up to 14 days; do not freeze.

Nursing Actions

Physical Assessment Instruct patients with diabetes to monitor glucose levels closely. Encourage funduscopic examinations at initiation of therapy and periodically during treatment. Instruct patient in proper use if self-administered (storage, reconstitution, injection techniques, and syringe/needle disposal). Pediatrics: Monitor growth curve; annually determine bone age.

Patient Education
- Discuss specific use of drug and side effects with patient as it relates to treatment. (HCAHPS: During this hospital stay, were you given any medicine that you had not taken before? Before giving you any new medicine, how often did hospital staff tell you what the medicine was for? How often did hospital staff describe possible side effects in a way you could understand?)
- Patient may experience headache, edema, osteopenia, myalgia, arthralgia, dyspepsia, nausea, injection site irritation, or pancreas irritation. Have patient report immediately to prescriber sudden vision changes, polyuria, polydipsia, weight loss, paresthesia, or rash (HCAHPS).
- Educate patient about signs of a significant reaction (eg, wheezing; chest tightness; fever; itching; bad cough; blue skin color; seizures; or swelling of face, lips, tongue, or throat). **Note:** This is not a comprehensive list of all side effects. Patient should consult prescriber for additional questions.

Intended Use and Disclaimer: Should not be printed and given to patients. This information is intended to serve as a concise initial reference for healthcare professionals to use when discussing medications with a patient. You must ultimately rely on your own discretion, experience and judgment in diagnosing, treating and advising patients.

Dietary Considerations

Prader-Willi syndrome: All patients should have effective weight control (use is contraindicated in severely-obese patients).

Short-bowel syndrome: Intravenous parenteral nutrition requirements may need reassessment as gastrointestinal absorption improves.

Sorafenib (sor AF e nib)

Brand Names: U.S. NexAVAR

Index Terms BAY 43-9006; Sorafenib Tosylate

Pharmacologic Category Antineoplastic Agent, Tyrosine Kinase Inhibitor; Antineoplastic Agent, Vascular Endothelial Growth Factor (VEGF) Inhibitor

Medication Safety Issues

Sound-alike/look-alike issues:

NexAVAR may be confused with NexIUM

SORAfenib may be confused with axitinib, gefitinib, imatinib, regorafenib, SUNItinib, vandetanib, vemurafenib

High alert medication:

This medication is in a class the Institute for Safe Medication Practices (ISMP) includes among its list of drug classes which have a heightened risk of causing significant patient harm when used in error.

Pregnancy Risk Factor D

Lactation Excretion in breast milk unknown/not recommended

Breast-Feeding Considerations It is not known if sorafenib is excreted in human milk. Due to the potential for serious adverse reactions in the nursing infant, the decision to discontinue sorafenib or to discontinue breast-feeding during therapy should take into account the benefits of treatment to the mother.

Use

Hepatocellular cancer: Treatment of unresectable hepatocellular cancer (HCC)

Renal cell cancer, advanced: Treatment of advanced renal cell cancer (RCC)

Thyroid cancer, differentiated: Treatment of locally recurrent or metastatic, progressive, differentiated thyroid cancer (refractory to radioactive iodine treatment)

Unlabeled Use Treatment of recurrent or metastatic angiosarcoma, resistant gastrointestinal stromal tumor (GIST)

Mechanism of Action/Effect Prevents tumor growth by inhibiting both tumor cell proliferation and tumor angiogenesis through kinase inhibition

Contraindications Known severe hypersensitivity to sorafenib or any component of the formulation;

use in combination with carboplatin and paclitaxel in patients with squamous cell lung cancer

Warnings/Precautions Hazardous agent - use appropriate precautions for handling and disposal (NIOSH, 2012). May cause hypertension (generally mild-to-moderate), especially in the first 6 weeks of treatment; monitor; use caution in patients with underlying or poorly-controlled hypertension; consider discontinuing (temporary or permanent) in patients who develop severe or persistent hypertension while on appropriate antihypertensive therapy. May cause cardiac ischemia or infarction; consider discontinuing (temporarily or permanently) in patients who develop these conditions; use in patients with unstable coronary artery disease or recent myocardial infarction has not been studied. QT prolongation has been observed; may increase the risk for ventricular arrhythmia. Avoid use in patients with congenital long QT syndrome; monitor electrolytes and ECG in patients with heart failure, bradyarrhythmias, and concurrent medications known to prolong the QT interval; correct electrolyte (calcium, magnesium, potassium) imbalances; interrupt treatment for QTc interval >500 msec or for ≥60 msec increase from baseline.

Serious bleeding events may occur (consider permanently discontinuing if serious); monitor PT/INR in patients on warfarin therapy. Thyroid cancer patients with tracheal, bronchial, and esophageal infiltration should be treated with local therapy prior to administering sorafenib due to the potential bleeding risk. May complicate wound healing; temporarily withhold treatment for patients undergoing major surgical procedures (the appropriate timing for reinitiation after surgical procedures has not been determined). Gastrointestinal perforation has been reported (rare); monitor patients for signs/symptoms (abdominal pain, constipation, or vomiting); discontinue treatment if gastrointestinal perforation occurs. Potentially significant drug-drug interactions may exist, requiring dose or frequency adjustment, additional monitoring, and/or selection of alternative therapy. Avoid concurrent use with strong CYP3A4 inducers (eg, carbamazepine, dexamethasone, phenobarbital, phenytoin, rifampin, St John's wort); may decrease sorafenib levels/effects. Use caution when administering sorafenib with compounds that are metabolized predominantly via UGT1A1 (eg, irinotecan). Use in combination with carboplatin and paclitaxel in patients with squamous cell lung cancer is contraindicated.

Hand-foot skin reaction and rash (generally grades 1 or 2) are the most common drug-related adverse events, and typically appear within the first 6 weeks of treatment; usually managed with topical treatment, treatment delays, and/or dose reductions. Consider permanently discontinuing with severe or persistent dermatological toxicities. The risk for hand-foot syndrome increased with cumulative doses of sorafenib (Azad, 2009). The incidence of hand-foot syndrome is also increased in patients treated with sorafenib plus bevacizumab in comparison to those treated with sorafenib monotherapy (Azad, 2009). Severe dermatologic toxicities, including Stevens-Johnson syndrome (SJS) and toxic epidermal necrolysis (TEN) have been reported; may be life-threatening; discontinue sorafenib for suspected SJS or TEN.

Sorafenib impairs exogenous thyroid suppression; TSH level elevations were commonly observed in the thyroid cancer study; monitor TSH levels monthly and as clinically necessary, and adjust thyroid replacement as needed. Sorafenib levels in patients with mild-to-moderate hepatic impairment (Child-Pugh classes A and B) were similar to levels observed in patients without hepatic impairment; has not been studied in patients with severe hepatic impairment. In a small study of Asian patients with advanced HCC, sorafenib demonstrated efficacy with adequate tolerability in a hepatitis B-endemic area (Yau, 2009). There have been reports of sorafenib-induced hepatitis (including hepatic failure and death) which is characterized by hepatocellular liver damage and transaminase increases (significant); increased bilirubin and INR may also occur. Monitor hepatic function regularly; discontinue sorafenib for unexplained significant transaminase increases.

Drug Interactions

Avoid Concomitant Use

Avoid concomitant use of SORAfenib with any of the following: BCG; CARBOplatin; CloZAPine; CYP3A4 Inducers (Strong); Highest Risk QTc-Prolonging Agents; Ivabradine; Mifepristone; Natalizumab; PACLitaxel; Pimecrolimus; St Johns Wort; Tacrolimus (Topical); Tofacitinib; Vaccines (Live)

Decreased Effect

SORAfenib may decrease the levels/effects of: BCG; Cardiac Glycosides; Coccidioidin Skin Test; Dacarbazine; Fluorouracil (Systemic); Fluorouracil (Topical); Sipuleucel-T; Vaccines (Inactivated); Vaccines (Live); Vitamin K Antagonists

The levels/effects of SORAfenib may be decreased by: CYP3A4 Inducers (Strong); Echinacea; Neomycin; St Johns Wort

Increased Effect/Toxicity

SORAfenib may increase the levels/effects of: Acetaminophen; Bisphosphonate Derivatives; Bosentan; CARBOplatin; Carvedilol; CloZAPine; CYP2B6 Substrates; CYP2C9 Substrates; DOCEtaxel; DOXOrubicin (Conventional); Fluorouracil (Systemic); Fluorouracil (Topical); Highest Risk QTc-Prolonging Agents; Irinotecan; Leflunomide; Moderate Risk QTc-Prolonging Agents; Natalizumab; PACLitaxel; Tofacitinib; Vaccines (Live); Vitamin K Antagonists; Warfarin

The levels/effects of SORAfenib may be increased by: Acetaminophen; Bevacizumab; CYP3A4 Inhibitors (Strong); Denosumab; Ivabradine; Mifepristone; Pimecrolimus; QTc-Prolonging Agents (Indeterminate Risk and Risk Modifying); Roflumilast; Tacrolimus (Topical); Trastuzumab

Nutritional/Ethanol Interactions

Food: Bioavailability is decreased 29% with a high-fat meal (bioavailability is similar to fasting state when administered with a moderate-fat meal). Management: Administer on an empty stomach 1 hour before or 2 hours after eating.

Herb/Nutraceutical: St John's wort may decrease the levels/effects of sorafenib. Management: Avoid St John's wort.

Adverse Reactions

>10%:

Cardiovascular: Hypertension (9% to 41%; grade 3: 3% to 4%; grade 4: <1%; grades 3/4: 10%, onset: ~3 weeks)

Central nervous system: Fatigue (37% to 46%), headache (≤10% to 17%), mouth pain (14%), voice disorder (13%), sensory neuropathy (≤13%), pain (11%)

Dermatologic: Hand-foot syndrome (21% to 69%; grade 3: 6% to 8%; grades 3/4: 19%), alopecia (14% to 67%), rash/desquamation (19% to 40%), pruritus (14% to 20%), grade 3: ≤1%; grades 3/4: 5%), dry skin (10% to 13%), erythema (≥10%)

Endocrine & metabolic: Hypoalbuminemia (≤59%), hypophosphatemia (35% to 45%; grade 3: 11% to 13%; grade 4: <1%), increased thyroid stimulating hormone (>0.5 mU/L: 41%; due to impairment of exogenous thyroid suppression), hypocalcemia (12% to 36%)

Gastrointestinal: Diarrhea (43% to 68%; grade 3: 2% to 10%; grade 4: <1%), weight loss (10% to 49%), lipase increased (40% to 41% [usually transient]), amylase increased (30% to 34% [usually transient]), abdominal pain (11% to 31%), decreased appetite (30%), anorexia (16% to 29%), stomatitis (24%), nausea (21% to 24%), constipation (14% to 16%), vomiting (11% to 16%)

Hematologic: Lymphopenia (23% to 47%; grades 3/4: ≤13%), thrombocytopenia (12% to 46%; grades 3/4: 1% to 4%), INR increased (≤42%), neutropenia (≤18%; grades 3/4: ≤5%), hemorrhage (15% to 17%; grade 3: 2%), leukopenia

Hepatic: Increased serum ALT (59%; grades 3/4: 4%), increased serum AST (54%; grades 3/4: 2%), liver dysfunction (≤11%; grade 3: 2%; grade 4: 1%)

Infection: Infection

Neuromuscular & skeletal: Limb pain (15%), weakness (12%), muscle pain

Respiratory: Dyspnea (≤14%), cough (≤13%)

Miscellaneous: Fever (11%)

1% to 10%:

Cardiovascular: Cardiac ischemia/infarction (≤3%), heart failure (2%, congestive), flushing

Central nervous system: Depression

Dermatologic: Hyperkeratosis (7%), acne, exfoliative dermatitis, folliculitis

Endocrine & metabolic: Hypokalemia (5% to 10%), hyponatremia, hypothyroidism

Gastrointestinal: Dysgeusia (6%), dyspepsia, dysphagia, gastroesophageal reflux disease, glossodynia, mucositis, xerostomia

Genitourinary: Erectile dysfunction

Hematologic: Squamous cell carcinoma of skin (3%; grades 3/4: 3%), anemia

Hepatic: Transaminases increased (transient)

Neuromuscular & skeletal: Muscle spasm (10%), joint pain (≤10%), myalgia

Renal: Proteinuria, renal failure

Respiratory: Epistaxis (7%), hoarseness, rhinorrhea

Miscellaneous: Flu-like syndrome

Available Dosage Forms

Tablet, Oral:

NexAVAR: 200 mg

General Dosage Range Dosage adjustments recommended in patients with hepatic or renal impairment, or who develop toxicities

Oral: *Adults:* 400 mg twice daily

Administration

Oral Administer on an empty stomach (1 hour before or 2 hours after eating).

Hazardous agent; use appropriate precautions for handling and disposal (NIOSH, 2012).

Storage/Stability Store at 25°C (77°F); excursions are permitted between 15°C and 30°C (59°F and 86°F). Protect from moisture.

Nursing Actions

Physical Assessment Monitor for gastrointestinal perforation including black tarry stool, blood in vomit, or bloody diarrhea. Serious side effects include fever, low blood counts, fatigue, rash, or dose-reducing hand-foot syndrome. Monitor for symptoms of hypothyroidism, which include fatigue, weight gain, dry skin/hair, constipation, bradycardia, hypothermia. Monitor CBC, metabolic panel, and TSH. Educate patient about vaccine use while on this medication.

Patient Education

- Discuss specific use of drug and side effects with patient as it relates to treatment. (HCAHPS: During this hospital stay, were you given any medicine that you had not taken before? Before giving you any new medicine, how often did hospital staff tell you what the medicine was for? How often did hospital staff describe possible side effects in a way you could understand?)
- Patient may experience constipation, xeroderma, alopecia, lack of appetite, weight loss, arthralgia, or myalgia. Have patient report immediately to prescriber signs of infection, signs of

hemorrhaging, dyspnea, vision changes, syncope, angina, significant dyspepsia, edema of extremities, painful extremities, significant asthenia, paresthesia, eczema of hands or feet, serotonin syndrome (ie, dizziness, severe headache, agitation, hallucinations, tachycardia, arrhythmia, flushing, tremors, hyperhidrosis, change in balance, illogical thinking, severe nausea, significant diarrhea), or signs of hepatic impairment (HCAHPS).

- Educate patient about signs of a significant reaction (eg, wheezing; chest tightness; fever; itching; bad cough; blue skin color; seizures; or swelling of face, lips, tongue, or throat). **Note:** This is not a comprehensive list of all side effects. Patient should consult prescriber for additional questions.

Intended Use and Disclaimer: Should not be printed and given to patients. This information is intended to serve as a concise initial reference for healthcare professionals to use when discussing medications with a patient. You must ultimately rely on your own discretion, experience and judgment in diagnosing, treating and advising patients.

Dietary Considerations Take without food (1 hour before or 2 hours after eating).

Sorbitol (SOR bi tole)

Brand Names: U.S. Ora-Sweet SF [OTC]
Pharmacologic Category Genitourinary Irrigant; Laxative, Osmotic
Pregnancy Risk Factor C
Lactation Use caution
Use Genitourinary irrigant in transurethral prostatic resection or other transurethral resection or other transurethral surgical procedures; diuretic; humectant; sweetening agent; hyperosmotic laxative; facilitate the passage of sodium polystyrene sulfonate through the intestinal tract
Available Dosage Forms
Solution, Irrigation:
Generic: 3% (3000 mL); 3.3% (2000 mL, 4000 mL)
Solution, Oral:
Generic: 70% (30 mL, 473 mL, 474 mL, 480 mL, 3840 mL)
Syrup, Oral:
Ora-Sweet SF [OTC]: (473 mL)
General Dosage Range
Oral:
Children 2-11 years: 2 mL/kg (70% solution) as a single dose
Children ≥12 years and Adults: 30-150 mL (70% solution) as a single dose
Rectal:
Children 2-11 years: 30-60 mL (25% to 30% solution) as a single dose

Children ≥12 years and Adults: 120 mL (25% to 30% solution) as a single dose
Topical: Adults: 3% to 3.3% as a transurethral irrigation
Nursing Actions
Physical Assessment When used as cathartic, determine cause of constipation before use.
Patient Education
- Discuss specific use of drug and side effects with patient as it relates to treatment. (HCAHPS: During this hospital stay, were you given any medicine that you had not taken before? Before giving you any new medicine, how often did hospital staff tell you what the medicine was for? How often did hospital staff describe possible side effects in a way you could understand?)
- Patient may experience dyspepsia, pyrosis, abdominal cramps, flatulence, or rectal irritation. Have patient report immediately to prescriber severe diarrhea, significant dyspepsia, nausea, dizziness, edema, weight gain, or asthenia (HCAHPS).
- Educate patient about signs of a significant reaction (eg, wheezing; chest tightness; fever; itching; bad cough; blue skin color; seizures; or swelling of face, lips, tongue, or throat). **Note:** This is not a comprehensive list of all side effects. Patient should consult prescriber for additional questions.

Intended Use and Disclaimer: Should not be printed and given to patients. This information is intended to serve as a concise initial reference for healthcare professionals to use when discussing medications with a patient. You must ultimately rely on your own discretion, experience and judgment in diagnosing, treating and advising patients.

Sotalol (SOE ta lole)

Brand Names: U.S. Betapace; Betapace AF; Sorine
Index Terms Sotalol Hydrochloride
Pharmacologic Category Antiarrhythmic Agent, Class II; Antiarrhythmic Agent, Class III; Beta-Adrenergic Blocker, Nonselective
Medication Safety Issues
Sound-alike/look-alike issues:
Sotalol may be confused with Stadol, Sudafed®
Betapace® may be confused with Betapace AF®
High alert medication:
The Institute for Safe Medication Practices (ISMP) includes this medication (I.V. formulation) among its list of drugs which have a heightened risk of causing significant patient harm when used in error.
BEERS Criteria medication:
This drug may be potentially inappropriate for use in geriatric patients (Quality of evidence - high; Strength of recommendation - strong).

Pregnancy Risk Factor B

Lactation Enters breast milk/consider risk:benefit

Breast-Feeding Considerations Sotalol is excreted into breast milk in concentrations higher than those found in the maternal serum. Although adverse events in nursing infants have not been observed in case reports, close monitoring for bradycardia, hypotension, respiratory distress, and hypoglycemia is advised. According to the manufacturer, the decision to continue or discontinue breast-feeding during therapy should take into account the risk of exposure to the infant and the benefits of treatment to the mother.

Use Treatment of documented ventricular arrhythmias (ie, sustained ventricular tachycardia), that in the judgment of the physician are life-threatening; maintenance of normal sinus rhythm in patients with symptomatic atrial fibrillation and atrial flutter who are currently in sinus rhythm. Manufacturer states substitutions should not be made for Betapace AF® since Betapace AF® is distributed with a patient package insert specific for atrial fibrillation/flutter.

Injection: Substitution for oral sotalol in those who are unable to take sotalol orally

Unlabeled Use Fetal tachycardia; alternative antiarrhythmic for the treatment of atrial fibrillation in patients with hypertrophic cardiomyopathy (HCM)

Mechanism of Action/Effect

Beta-blocker which contains both beta-adrenoreceptor-blocking (Vaughan Williams Class II) and cardiac action potential duration prolongation (Vaughan Williams Class III) properties

Class II effects: Increased sinus cycle length, slowed heart rate, decreased AV nodal conduction, and increased AV nodal refractoriness

Class III effects: Prolongation of the atrial and ventricular monophasic action potentials, and effective refractory prolongation of atrial muscle, ventricular muscle, and atrioventricular accessory pathways in both the antegrade and retrograde directions

Contraindications Hypersensitivity to sotalol or any component of the formulation; bronchial asthma; sinus bradycardia; second- or third-degree AV block (unless a functioning pacemaker is present); congenital or acquired long QT syndromes; cardiogenic shock; uncontrolled heart failure

Additional contraindications: Betapace AF® and the injectable formulation: Baseline QT_c interval >450 msec; bronchospastic conditions; CrCl <40 mL/minute; serum potassium <4 mEq/L; sick sinus syndrome

Warnings/Precautions [U.S. Boxed Warning] Manufacturer recommends initiation (or reinitiation) and doses increased in a hospital setting with continuous monitoring and staff familiar with the recognition and treatment of life-threatening arrhythmias. Some experts will initiate therapy on an outpatient basis in a patient without heart disease or bradycardia, who has a baseline uncorrected QT interval <450 msec, and normal serum potassium and magnesium levels; close ECG monitoring during this time is necessary. ACC/AHA guidelines for management of atrial fibrillation also recommend that for outpatient initiation the patient not have risk factors predisposing to drug-induced ventricular proarrhythmia (Fuster, 2006). Dosage should be adjusted gradually with 3 days between dosing increments to achieve steady-state concentrations, and to allow time to monitor QT intervals. **[U.S. Boxed Warning]: Adjust dosing interval based on creatinine clearance to decrease risk of proarrhythmia; QT interval prolongation is directly related to sotalol concentration.** Creatinine clearance must be calculated with dose initiation and dose increases. Use cautiously in the renally-impaired (dosage adjustment required). Betapace AF® and the injectable formulation are contraindicated in patients with CrCl <40 mL/minute.

[U.S. Boxed Warning]: Sotalol injection: Sotalol can cause life-threatening ventricular tachycardia associated with QT-interval prolongation (ie, torsade de pointes). Do not initiate if baseline QT_c interval is >450 msec. If QT_c exceeds 500 msec during therapy, reduce the dose, prolong the infusion duration, or discontinue use. If while on oral sotalol therapy baseline QT_c interval is >500 msec, use I.V. sotalol with particular caution; serious consideration should be given to reducing the dose or discontinuing I.V. sotalol when QT_c exceeds 520 msec. QT_c prolongation is directly related to the concentration of sotalol; reduced creatinine clearance, female gender, and large doses increase the risk of QT_c prolongation and subsequent torsade de pointes. Monitor and adjust dose to prevent QT_c prolongation. Concurrent use with other QT_c-prolonging drugs (including Class I and Class III antiarrhythmics) and use within 3 months of discontinuing amiodarone is generally not recommended. To reduce the chance of excessive QT_c-prolongation, withhold QT_c-prolonging drugs for at least 3 half-lives (or 3 months for amiodarone) before initiating sotalol.

Correct electrolyte imbalances before initiating (especially hypokalemia and hypomagnesemia). Consider pre-existing conditions such as sick sinus syndrome before initiating. Conduction abnormalities can occur particularly sinus bradycardia. Use cautiously within the first 2 weeks post-MI especially in patients with markedly impaired ventricular function (experience limited). Administer cautiously in compensated heart failure and monitor for a worsening of the condition. May precipitate or aggravate symptoms of arterial insufficiency in patients with PVD and Raynaud's disease; use with caution and monitor for progression of arterial obstruction. Bradycardia may be observed more ▶

frequently in elderly patients (>65 years of age); dosage reductions may be necessary. In the treatment of atrial fibrillation, avoid antiarrhythmics as first-line treatment. In older adults, data suggests rate control may provide more benefits than risks compared to rhythm control for most patients (Beers Criteria). Beta-blocker therapy should not be withdrawn abruptly (particularly in patients with CAD), but gradually tapered to avoid acute tachycardia, hypertension, and/or ischemia. Chronic beta-blocker therapy should not be routinely withdrawn prior to major surgery. Use caution with concurrent use of digoxin, verapamil, or diltiazem; bradycardia or heart block can occur. Use with caution in patients receiving inhaled anesthetic agents known to depress myocardial contractility. Use cautiously in diabetics because it can mask prominent hypoglycemic symptoms. Use with caution in patients with bronchospastic disease, myasthenia gravis or psychiatric disease. Adequate alpha-blockade is required prior to use of any beta-blocker for patients with untreated pheochromocytoma. May mask signs of hyperthyroidism (eg, tachycardia); if hyperthyroidism is suspected, carefully manage and monitor; abrupt withdrawal may exacerbate symptoms of hyperthyroidism or precipitate thyroid storm. Use caution with history of severe anaphylaxis to allergens; patients taking beta-blockers may become more sensitive to repeated challenges. Treatment of anaphylaxis (eg, epinephrine) in patients taking beta-blockers may be ineffective or promote undesirable effects.

[U.S. Boxed Warning]: Betapace® should not be substituted for Betapace® AF; Betapace® AF is distributed with an educational insert specifically for patients with atrial fibrillation/flutter.

Drug Interactions

Avoid Concomitant Use

Avoid concomitant use of Sotalol with any of the following: Beta2-Agonists; Fingolimod; Floctafenine; Highest Risk QTc-Prolonging Agents; Ivabradine; Methacholine; Mifepristone; Moderate Risk QTc-Prolonging Agents; Propafenone

Decreased Effect

Sotalol may decrease the levels/effects of: Beta2-Agonists; Theophylline Derivatives

The levels/effects of Sotalol may be decreased by: Barbiturates; Herbs (Hypertensive Properties); Methylphenidate; Nonsteroidal Anti-Inflammatory Agents; Rifamycin Derivatives; Yohimbine

Increased Effect/Toxicity

Sotalol may increase the levels/effects of: Alpha-/Beta-Agonists (Direct-Acting); Alpha1-Blockers; Alpha2-Agonists; Amifostine; Antihypertensives; Antipsychotic Agents (Phenothiazines); Bupivacaine; Cardiac Glycosides; Cholinergic Agonists; DULoxetine; Ergot Derivatives; Fingolimod; Highest Risk QTc-Prolonging Agents; Hypotensive Agents; Insulin; Lidocaine (Systemic); Lidocaine (Topical); Mepivacaine; Methacholine; Midodrine; Obinutuzumab; RiTUXimab; Sulfonylureas

The levels/effects of Sotalol may be increased by: Acetylcholinesterase Inhibitors; Alpha2-Agonists; Aminoquinolines (Antimalarial); Amiodarone; Anilidopiperidine Opioids; Antipsychotic Agents (Phenothiazines); Brimonidine (Topical); Calcium Channel Blockers (Dihydropyridine); Calcium Channel Blockers (Nondihydropyridine); Diazoxide; Dipyridamole; Disopyramide; Dronedarone; Fingolimod; Floctafenine; Herbs (Hypotensive Properties); Ivabradine; Lidocaine (Topical); MAO Inhibitors; Mifepristone; Moderate Risk QTc-Prolonging Agents; Pentoxifylline; Phosphodiesterase 5 Inhibitors; Propafenone; Prostacyclin Analogues; QTc-Prolonging Agents (Indeterminate Risk and Risk Modifying); Regorafenib; Reserpine

Nutritional/Ethanol Interactions

Food: Sotalol peak serum concentrations may be decreased if taken with food.

Herb/Nutraceutical: Avoid ephedra (may worsen arrhythmia).

Adverse Reactions Note: No clinical experience with I.V. sotalol; however, since exposure is similar between I.V. and oral sotalol, adverse reactions are expected to be similar.

>10%:

Cardiovascular: Bradycardia (13% to 16%), chest pain (3% to 16%), palpitation (14%)

Central nervous system: Fatigue (20%), dizziness (20%), lightheadedness (12%)

Neuromuscular & skeletal: Weakness (13%)

Respiratory: Dyspnea (21%)

1% to 10%:

Cardiovascular: Edema (8%), abnormal ECG (7%), hypotension (6%), proarrhythmia (5%), syncope (5%), CHF (5%), torsade de pointes (dose related; 1% to 4%), peripheral vascular disorders (3%), ventricular tachycardia worsened (1%), QT_c interval prolongation (dose related)

Central nervous system: Headache (8%), sleep problems (8%), mental confusion (6%), anxiety (4%), depression (4%)

Dermatologic: Itching/rash (5%)

Endocrine & metabolic: Sexual ability decreased (3%)

Gastrointestinal: Nausea/vomiting (10%), diarrhea (7%), stomach discomfort (3% to 6%), flatulence (2%)

Genitourinary: Impotence (2%)

Hematologic: Bleeding (2%)

Neuromuscular & skeletal: Extremity pain (7%), paresthesia (4%), back pain (3%)

Ocular: Visual problems (5%)

Respiratory: Upper respiratory problems (5% to 8%), asthma (2%)

Pharmacodynamics/Kinetics

Onset of Action Oral: Rapid, 1-2 hours; when administered I.V. for ongoing VT over 5 minutes, onset of action is ~5-10 minutes (Ho, 1994)

Duration of Action 8-16 hours

Available Dosage Forms

Tablet, Oral:

Betapace: 80 mg, 120 mg, 160 mg

Betapace AF: 80 mg, 120 mg, 160 mg

Sorine: 80 mg, 120 mg, 160 mg, 240 mg

Generic: 80 mg, 120 mg, 160 mg, 240 mg

General Dosage Range Dosage adjustment recommended in patients with renal impairment or who develop toxicities

I.V.: *Adults:* Initial: 75 mg twice daily; Maintenance: 75-150 mg twice daily (maximum: 300 mg/day)

Oral:

Children ≤2 years: Dosage should be adjusted (decreased) by plotting of the child's age on a logarithmic scale; **Note:** Refer to manufacturer's package labeling

Children >2 years: Initial: 90 mg/m^2/day in 3 divided doses; Maintenance: 90-180 mg/m^2/day in 3 divided doses (maximum: 180 mg/m^2/day)

Adults: Initial: 80 mg twice daily; Maintenance: 240-320 mg/day in 2-3 divided doses (maximum: 320 mg/day)

Administration

I.V.

Substitution for oral: Administer over 5 hours.

Hemodynamically stable monomorphic VT: Administer I.V. push over 5 minutes; use with caution due to increased risk of adverse events (eg, bradycardia, hypotension, torsade de pointes) (ACLS, 2010)

Oral Administer without regard to meals.

Storage/Stability Store at 25°C (77°F); excursions permitted to 15°C to 30°C (59°F to 86°F). To prepare sotalol infusion, see manufacturer's prescribing information.

Nursing Actions

Physical Assessment Monitor laboratory tests, blood pressure, and heart rate prior to and following first dose and with any change in dosage. Monitor cardiac and pulmonary status. Advise patients with diabetes to monitor glucose levels closely; beta-blockers may alter glucose tolerance. Should not be stopped abruptly; dose should be tapered gradually when discontinuing. Teach patient hypotension precautions.

Patient Education

• Discuss specific use of drug and side effects with patient as it relates to treatment. (HCAHPS: During this hospital stay, were you given any medicine that you had not taken before? Before giving you any new medicine, how often did hospital staff tell you what the medicine was for? How often did hospital staff describe possible side effects in a way you could understand?)

• Patient may experience presyncope, fatigue, blurred vision, illogical thinking, bradycardia, dizziness, asthenia, or impotence. Have patient report immediately to prescriber angina, tachycardia, dyspnea, significant weight gain, or rash (HCAHPS).

• Educate patient about signs of a significant reaction (eg, wheezing; chest tightness; fever; itching; bad cough; blue skin color; seizures; or swelling of face, lips, tongue, or throat). **Note:** This is not a comprehensive list of all side effects. Patient should consult prescriber for additional questions.

Intended Use and Disclaimer: Should not be printed and given to patients. This information is intended to serve as a concise initial reference for healthcare professionals to use when discussing medications with a patient. You must ultimately rely on your own discretion, experience and judgment in diagnosing, treating and advising patients.

Dietary Considerations May be taken without regard to meals.

Spinosad (SPIN oh sad)

Brand Names: U.S. Natroba

Index Terms NatrOVA

Pharmacologic Category Antiparasitic Agent, Topical; Pediculocide

Pregnancy Risk Factor B

Lactation Use caution

Use Topical treatment of head lice (*Pediculosis capitis*) infestation in adults and children ≥4 years of age

Unlabeled Use Topical treatment of head lice (*Pediculosis capitis*) infestation in children ≥6 months and <4 years of age

Available Dosage Forms

Suspension, External:

Natroba: 0.9% (120 mL)

Generic: 0.9% (120 mL)

General Dosage Range Topical: *Children ≥4 years old and Adults:* Apply sufficient amount to cover dry scalp and hair; may repeat in 7 days

Administration

Topical Topical suspension. For external use only. Shake bottle well. Apply to dry scalp and rub gently until the scalp is thoroughly moistened, then apply to dry hair; completely covering scalp and hair. Leave on for 10 minutes (start timing treatment after the scalp and hair have been completely covered). The hair should then be rinsed thoroughly with warm water. Shampoo may be used immediately after the product is completely rinsed off. If live lice are seen 7 days after the first treatment, repeat with second application. Avoid contact with the eyes. Nit combing is not required, although a fine-tooth comb may be used to remove treated lice and nits.

Spinosad should be a portion of a whole lice removal program, which should include washing or dry cleaning all clothing, hats, bedding and towels recently worn or used by the patient and washing combs, brushes, and hair accessories in hot water.

Nursing Actions

Patient Education

- Discuss specific use of drug and side effects with patient as it relates to treatment. (HCAHPS: During this hospital stay, were you given any medicine that you had not taken before? Before giving you any new medicine, how often did hospital staff tell you what the medicine was for? How often did hospital staff describe possible side effects in a way you could understand?)
- Patient may experience scalp irritation or skin irritation. Have patient report immediately to prescriber rash (HCAHPS).
- Educate patient about signs of a significant reaction (eg, wheezing; chest tightness; fever; itching; bad cough; blue skin color; seizures; or swelling of face, lips, tongue, or throat). **Note:** This is not a comprehensive list of all side effects. Patient should consult prescriber for additional questions.

Intended Use and Disclaimer: Should not be printed and given to patients. This information is intended to serve as a concise initial reference for healthcare professionals to use when discussing medications with a patient. You must ultimately rely on your own discretion, experience and judgment in diagnosing, treating and advising patients.

Spironolactone (speer on oh LAK tone)

Brand Names: U.S. Aldactone

Pharmacologic Category Antihypertensive; Diuretic, Potassium-Sparing; Selective Aldosterone Blocker

Medication Safety Issues

Sound-alike/look-alike issues:

Aldactone may be confused with Aldactazide

BEERS Criteria medication:

This drug may be potentially inappropriate for use in geriatric patients (Quality of evidence - moderate; Strength of recommendation - strong).

International issues:

Aldactone: Brand name for spironolactone [U.S., Canada, multiple international markets], but also the brand name for potassium canrenoate [Austria, Czech Republic, Germany, Hungary, Poland]

Pregnancy Risk Factor C

Lactation Enters breast milk/not recommended

Breast-Feeding Considerations The active metabolite of spironolactone (canrenone) has been found in breast milk. Information is available from a case report following maternal use of

spironolactone 25 mg twice daily throughout pregnancy, then 4 times daily after delivery. Milk and maternal serum samples were obtained 17 days after birth. Two hours after the maternal dose, canrenone concentrations were ~144 ng/mL (serum) and ~104 ng/mL (milk). When measured 14.5 hours after the dose, canrenone concentrations were ~92 ng/mL (serum) and ~47 ng/mL (milk). The authors calculated the estimated maximum amount of canrenone to the nursing infant to be ~0.2% of the maternal dose (Phelps, 1977). Effects to humans are not known; however, this metabolite was found to be carcinogenic in rats. Diuretics have the potential to decrease milk volume and suppress lactation. Breast-fed infants of mothers taking medications for hypertension should be monitored for adverse effects (Chobanian, 2003). According to the manufacturer, the decision to continue or discontinue breast-feeding during therapy should take into account the risk of exposure to the infant and the benefits of treatment to the mother; if use of spironolactone is essential, an alternative method of feeding should be used.

Use Management of edema associated with excessive aldosterone excretion or with congestive heart failure (HF) unresponsive to other therapies; hypertension; primary hyperaldosteronism (establishing diagnosis, short-term preoperative treatment, and long-term maintenance therapy in selected patients); hypokalemia; cirrhosis of liver accompanied by edema or ascites; nephrotic syndrome; severe HF (NYHA class III-IV) to increase survival and reduce hospitalization when added to standard therapy

Note: The ACCF/AHA 2013 heart failure guidelines recommend the use of aldosterone antagonists, along with other guideline-directed medical therapies, to reduce morbidity and mortality in patients with HF (NYHA class III-IV) with LVEF ≤35% (Yancy, 2013).

Unlabeled Use Female acne (adjunctive therapy); hirsutism; hypertension (pediatric); diuretic (pediatric)

The ACCF/AHA 2013 Heart failure (HF) guidelines recommend the use of aldosterone antagonists, along with other guideline-directed medical therapies, to reduce morbidity and mortality in patients with HF (NYHA class II) with LVEF ≤35% who have a history of prior cardiovascular hospitalization or elevated plasma natriuretic peptide levels and those patients with a LVEF ≤40% following acute MI who develop symptoms of HF or have a history of diabetes mellitus (ACCF/AHA [Yancy, 2013]).

Mechanism of Action/Effect Competes with aldosterone for receptor sites in the distal renal tubules, increasing sodium chloride and water excretion while conserving potassium and hydrogen ions; may block the effect of aldosterone on arteriolar smooth muscle as well

Contraindications Anuria; acute renal insufficiency; significant impairment of renal excretory function; hyperkalemia; Addison's disease or other conditions associated with hyperkalemia; concomitant use with eplerenone

Canadian labeling: Additional contraindications (not in U.S. labeling): Hypersensitivity to spironolactone or any component of the formulation; concomitant use with heparin or low molecular weight heparin

Warnings/Precautions [U.S. Boxed Warning]: Shown to be a tumorigen in chronic toxicity animal studies. Avoid unnecessary use.

Monitor closely for hyperkalemia; increases in serum potassium are dose related and rates of hyperkalemia also increase with declining renal function. The concurrent use of larger doses of ACE inhibitors (eg, ≥ lisinopril 10 mg daily) also increases the risk of hyperkalemia (ACCF/AHA [Yancy, 2013]). Dose reduction or interruption of therapy may be necessary with development of hyperkalemia. Use is contraindicated in patients with hyperkalemia or conditions associated with hyperkalemia (eg, Addison's disease). Risk of hyperkalemia is increased with declining renal function. Use with caution in patients with mild renal impairment; contraindicated with anuria, acute renal insufficiency, or significant impairment of renal excretory function. Avoid potassium supplements, potassium-containing salt substitutes, a diet rich in potassium, or other drugs that can cause hyperkalemia. Potentially significant drug-drug interactions may exist, requiring dose or frequency adjustment, additional monitoring, and/or selection of alternative therapy. Somnolence and dizziness have been reported with use; advise patients to use caution when driving or operating machinery until response to initial treatment has been determined. Excess amounts can lead to profound diuresis with fluid and electrolyte loss; close medical supervision and dose evaluation are required. Watch for and correct electrolyte disturbances; adjust dose to avoid dehydration. In cirrhosis, avoid electrolyte and acid/base imbalances that might lead to hepatic encephalopathy. Gynecomastia is related to dose and duration of therapy; typically is reversible following discontinuation of therapy but may persist (rare). Discontinue use prior to adrenal vein catheterization. When evaluating a heart failure patient for spironolactone treatment, eGFR should be >30 mL/minute/1.73 m^2 or creatinine should be ≤2.5 mg/dL (men) or ≤2 mg/dL (women) with no recent worsening and potassium <5 mEq/L with no history of severe hyperkalemia (ACCF/AHA [Yancy, 2013]). Serum potassium levels require close monitoring and management if elevated. The manufacturer recommends to discontinue or interrupt therapy if serum potassium >5 mEq/L or serum creatinine >4 mg/dL. The ACCF/AHA recommends considering discontinuation upon the development of serum potassium >5.5 mEq/L or worsening renal function with careful evaluation of the entire medical regimen. Avoid routine triple therapy with the combined use of an ACE inhibitor, ARB, and spironolactone. Instruct patients with heart failure to discontinue use during an episode of diarrhea or dehydration or when loop diuretic therapy is interrupted (ACCF/AHA [Yancy, 2013]).

In the elderly, avoid use of doses >25 mg/day in patients with heart failure or with reduced renal function (eg, CrCl <30 mL/minute or eGFR ≤30 mL/minute/1.73 m^2 [Yancy, 2013]); risk of hyperkalemia is increased for heart failure patients receiving >25 mg/day, particularly if taking concomitant medications such as NSAIDS, ACE inhibitor, angiotensin receptor blocker, or potassium supplements (Beers Criteria).

Drug Interactions

Avoid Concomitant Use

Avoid concomitant use of Spironolactone with any of the following: AMILoride; CycloSPORINE (Systemic); Tacrolimus (Systemic); Triamterene

Decreased Effect

Spironolactone may decrease the levels/effects of: Abiraterone Acetate; Alpha-/Beta-Agonists; Cardiac Glycosides; Mitotane; QuiNIDine

The levels/effects of Spironolactone may be decreased by: Herbs (Hypertensive Properties); Methylphenidate; Nonsteroidal Anti-Inflammatory Agents; Yohimbine

Increased Effect/Toxicity

Spironolactone may increase the levels/effects of: ACE Inhibitors; Amifostine; Ammonium Chloride; Antihypertensives; Cardiac Glycosides; Cyclo-SPORINE (Systemic); Digoxin; DULoxetine; Hypotensive Agents; Neuromuscular-Blocking Agents (Nondepolarizing); Obinutuzumab; RiTUXimab; Sodium Phosphates; Tacrolimus (Systemic)

The levels/effects of Spironolactone may be increased by: Alfuzosin; AMILoride; Analgesics (Opioid); Angiotensin II Receptor Blockers; AtorvaSTATin; Brimonidine (Topical); Canagliflozin; Cholestyramine Resin; Diazoxide; Drospirenone; Eplerenone; Heparin; Heparin (Low Molecular Weight); Herbs (Hypotensive Properties); MAO Inhibitors; Nitrofurantoin; Nonsteroidal Anti-Inflammatory Agents; Pentoxifylline; Phosphodiesterase 5 Inhibitors; Potassium Salts; Prostacyclin Analogues; Tolvaptan; Triamterene; Trimethoprim

Nutritional/Ethanol Interactions

Ethanol: Increases risk of orthostasis.

Food: Food increases absorption.

Herb/Nutraceutical: Avoid natural licorice (due to mineralocorticoid activity)

◄ **Adverse Reactions** Frequency not defined.
Cardiovascular: Vasculitis
Central nervous system: Ataxia, confusion, drowsiness, headache, lethargy
Dermatologic: Erythematous maculopapular rash, Stevens-Johnson syndrome, toxic epidermal necrolysis, urticaria
Endocrine & metabolic: Amenorrhea, gynecomastia, hyperkalemia
Gastrointestinal: Abdominal cramps, diarrhea, gastritis, gastrointestinal hemorrhage, gastrointestinal ulcer, nausea, vomiting
Genitourinary: Impotence, irregular menses, postmenopausal bleeding
Hematologic & oncologic: Agranulocytosis, malignant neoplasm of breast
Hepatic: Hepatotoxicity
Hypersensitivity: Anaphylaxis
Immunologic: DRESS syndrome
Renal: Increased blood urea nitrogen, renal failure, renal insufficiency
Miscellaneous: Fever

Pharmacodynamics/Kinetics
Duration of Action 2-3 days

Available Dosage Forms
Tablet, Oral:
Aldactone: 25 mg, 50 mg, 100 mg
Generic: 25 mg, 50 mg, 100 mg

General Dosage Range Dosage adjustment recommended in patients with renal impairment
Oral:
Adults: 12.5-400 mg daily in 1-2 divided doses

Storage/Stability Store below 25°C (77°F).

Nursing Actions
Physical Assessment Diuretic effect may be delayed 2-3 days. Monitor serum electrolytes on a regular basis during therapy. Assess fluid status and monitor for CNS changes (drowsiness, headache, confusion), rash, gynecomastia, and hyperkalemia during therapy.

Patient Education
• Discuss specific use of drug and side effects with patient as it relates to treatment. (HCAHPS: During this hospital stay, were you given any medicine that you had not taken before? Before giving you any new medicine, how often did hospital staff tell you what the medicine was for? How often did hospital staff describe possible side effects in a way you could understand?)
• Patient may experience hyperkalemia, dizziness, nausea, or impotence. Have patient report immediately to prescriber severe diarrhea, menstrual irregularity, macromastia (males), or rash (HCAHPS).
• Educate patient about signs of a significant reaction (eg, wheezing; chest tightness; fever; itching; bad cough; blue skin color; seizures; or swelling of face, lips, tongue, or throat). **Note:** This is not a comprehensive list of all side effects. Patient should consult prescriber for additional questions.

Intended Use and Disclaimer: Should not be printed and given to patients. This information is intended to serve as a concise initial reference for healthcare professionals to use when discussing medications with a patient. You must ultimately rely on your own discretion, experience and judgment in diagnosing, treating and advising patients.

Dietary Considerations Should be taken with food to decrease gastrointestinal irritation and to increase absorption. Excessive potassium intake (eg, salt substitutes, low-salt foods, bananas, nuts) should be avoided.

Stavudine (STAV yoo deen)

Brand Names: U.S. Zerit
Index Terms d4T
Pharmacologic Category Antiretroviral, Reverse Transcriptase Inhibitor, Nucleoside (Anti-HIV)
Medication Safety Issues
Sound-alike/look-alike issues:
Zerit® may be confused with Zestril®, Ziac®, ZyrTEC®
Medication Guide Available Yes
Pregnancy Risk Factor C
Lactation Excretion in breast milk unknown/contraindicated
Breast-Feeding Considerations Maternal or infant antiretroviral therapy does not completely eliminate the risk of postnatal HIV transmission. In addition, multiclass-resistant virus has been detected in breast-feeding infants despite maternal therapy. Therefore, in the United States, where formula is accessible, affordable, safe, and sustainable, and the risk of infant mortality due to diarrhea and respiratory infections is low, complete avoidance of breast-feeding by HIV-infected women is recommended to decrease potential transmission of HIV (DHHS [perinatal], 2012).
Use Treatment of HIV infection in combination with other antiretroviral agents
Mechanism of Action/Effect Inhibits reverse transcriptase of the human immunodeficiency virus (HIV)
Contraindications Hypersensitivity to stavudine or any component of the formulation
Warnings/Precautions Use with caution in patients who demonstrate previous hypersensitivity to zidovudine, didanosine, zalcitabine, pre-existing bone marrow suppression, renal insufficiency (dosage adjustment recommended), hepatic impairment, or peripheral neuropathy. Peripheral neuropathy may be a treatment-limiting side effect; consider permanent discontinuation. Zidovudine should not be used in combination with stavudine. **[U.S. Boxed Warning]: Lactic acidosis and severe hepatomegaly with steatosis have been reported with stavudine use, including fatal cases;** combination therapy with didanosine may

increase risk; use with caution in patients with risk factors for liver disease (although acidosis has occurred in patients without known risk factors, risk may be increased with female gender, obesity, pregnancy, or prolonged exposure). Suspend treatment in any patient who develops clinical or laboratory findings suggestive of lactic acidosis or hepatotoxicity. Mortality of 50% associated in some case series, notably with serum lactate >10 mmol/L (DHHS, 2012). Severe motor weakness (resembling Guillain-Barré syndrome) has been reported (including fatal cases, usually in association with lactic acidosis); manufacturer recommends discontinuation if motor weakness develops (with or without lactic acidosis). May cause redistribution of fat (eg, buffalo hump, peripheral wasting with increased abdominal girth, cushingoid appearance). Patients may develop immune reconstitution syndrome resulting in the occurrence of an inflammatory response to an indolent or residual opportunistic infection during initial HIV treatment or activation of autoimmune disorders (eg, Graves' disease, polymyositis, Guillain-Barré syndrome) later in therapy; further evaluation and treatment may be required. **[U.S. Boxed Warning]: Pancreatitis (including some fatal cases) has occurred during combination therapy with didanosine.** Suspend stavudine and didanosine combination therapy, and any other agents toxic to the pancreas, in patients with suspected pancreatitis. If pancreatitis diagnosis confirmed, use extreme caution if reinitiating stavudine; monitor closely and do not use didanosine in regimen. Use with caution in combination with interferon alfa with or without ribavirin in HIV/HBV coinfected patients; monitor closely for hepatic decompensation, anemia, or neutropenia; dose reduction or discontinuation of interferon and/or ribavirin may be required if toxicity evident. Combination therapy with didanosine or hydroxyurea may increase risk of hepatotoxicity, pancreatitis, or severe peripheral neuropathy; avoid stavudine or hydroxyurea combination.

Drug Interactions

Avoid Concomitant Use
Avoid concomitant use of Stavudine with any of the following: Hydroxyurea; Zidovudine

Decreased Effect
The levels/effects of Stavudine may be decreased by: DOXOrubicin (Conventional); DOXOrubicin (Liposomal); Zidovudine

Increased Effect/Toxicity
Stavudine may increase the levels/effects of: Didanosine; Hydroxyurea

The levels/effects of Stavudine may be increased by: Hydroxyurea; Ribavirin

Adverse Reactions Adverse reactions reported below represent experience with combination therapy with other nucleoside analogues and protease inhibitors.

>10%:
  Central nervous system: Headache (25% to 46%)
  Dermatologic: Rash (18% to 30%)
  Gastrointestinal: Nausea (43% to 53%; less than comparator group), vomiting (18% to 30%; less than comparator group), diarrhea (34% to 45%)
  Hepatic: Hyperbilirubinemia (65% to 68%; grade 3/4: 7% to 16%), AST increased (42% to 53%; grade 3/4: 5% to 7%), ALT increased (40% to 50%; grade 3/4: 6% to 8%), GGT increased (15% to 28%; grade 3/4: 2% to 5%)
  Neuromuscular & skeletal: Peripheral neuropathy (8% to 21%)
  Miscellaneous: Amylase increased (21% to 31%; grade 3/4: 4% to 8%), lipase increased (~27%; grade 3/4: 5% to 6%)

Available Dosage Forms
  Capsule, Oral:
    Zerit: 15 mg, 20 mg, 30 mg, 40 mg
    Generic: 15 mg, 20 mg, 30 mg, 40 mg
  Solution Reconstituted, Oral:
    Zerit: 1 mg/mL (200 mL)
    Generic: 1 mg/mL (200 mL)

General Dosage Range Dosage adjustment recommended in patients with renal impairment.
  Oral:
    Newborns (Birth to 13 days): 0.5 mg/kg every 12 hours
    Children ≥14 days and <30 kg: 1 mg/kg every 12 hours
    Children and Adults 30-59 kg: 30 mg every 12 hours
    Children and Adults ≥60 kg: 40 mg every 12 hours

Administration
Oral May be administered without regard to meals. Oral solution should be shaken vigorously prior to use.

Preparation for Administration Reconstitute powder for oral suspension with 202 mL of purified water as specified on the bottle. Shake vigorously until suspended. Final suspension will be 1 mg/mL (200 mL).

Storage/Stability Capsules and powder for reconstitution may be stored at controlled room temperature of 25°C (77°F). Reconstituted oral solution should be stored in refrigerator at 2°C to 8°C (36°F to 46°F) and is stable for 30 days.

Nursing Actions
Physical Assessment Allergy history should be assessed prior to beginning treatment. Monitor patient closely for peripheral neuropathy, lactic acidosis, hepatomegaly, and motor weakness; may require suspension of therapy. Teach patient proper timing of multiple medications.

Patient Education
 • Discuss specific use of drug and side effects with patient as it relates to treatment. (HCAHPS: During this hospital stay, were you given any medicine that you had not taken before? Before giving you any new medicine, how often did ▶

hospital staff tell you what the medicine was for? How often did hospital staff describe possible side effects in a way you could understand?)
- Patient may experience headache, nausea, diarrhea, lipodystrophy, or nerve problems. Have patient report immediately to prescriber dyspnea, paresthesia, severe dyspepsia, significant weight loss, jaundice, inability to eat, asthenia, considerable myalgia, sensation of cold, ecchymosis, or rash (HCAHPS).
- Educate patient about signs of a significant reaction (eg, wheezing; chest tightness; fever; itching; bad cough; blue skin color; seizures; or swelling of face, lips, tongue, or throat). **Note:** This is not a comprehensive list of all side effects. Patient should consult prescriber for additional questions.

Intended Use and Disclaimer: Should not be printed and given to patients. This information is intended to serve as a concise initial reference for healthcare professionals to use when discussing medications with a patient. You must ultimately rely on your own discretion, experience and judgment in diagnosing, treating and advising patients.

Dietary Considerations May be taken without regard to meals. Some products may contain sucrose.

Stiripentol (stir i PEN tol)

Index Terms BCX 2600; Estiripentol
Pharmacologic Category Anticonvulsant, Miscellaneous
Medication Safety Issues
Other safety concerns:
ALERT: Canadian Boxed Warning: The Health Canada-approved labeling includes a boxed warning. For verbatim wording of the boxed warning, consult the product labeling or www.-healthcanada.com.
Lactation Excretion in breast milk unknown/not recommended.
Use Dravet syndrome: Adjunctive treatment of refractory generalized tonic-clonic seizures in conjunction with clobazam and valproic acid in patients with severe myoclonic epilepsy in infancy (SMEI, Dravet syndrome) and whose seizures are not adequately controlled with clobazam and valproic acid alone.
Product Availability Not available in the U.S.
General Dosage Range Oral: *Children ≥3 years, Adolescents, and Adults:* Titrate dose upward over 3 days to 50 mg/kg daily given in 2 or 3 divided doses (maximum daily dose: 50 mg/kg)
Administration
Oral Administer in 2 or 3 divided doses daily with a meal. Capsule should be swallowed whole with a glass of water. Do not crush, chew, or open capsule. Powder for suspension should be mixed with a glass of water and consumed immediately.
Nursing Actions
Patient Education
- Discuss specific use of drug and side effects with patient as it relates to treatment. (HCAHPS: During this hospital stay, were you given any medicine that you had not taken before? Before giving you any new medicine, how often did hospital staff tell you what the medicine was for? How often did hospital staff describe possible side effects in a way you could understand?)
- Patient may experience back pain, sialorrhea, fatigue, skin irritation, lack of appetite, dyspepsia, nausea, insomnia, or weight gain or loss. Have patient report immediately to prescriber sings of hepatic impairment, illogical thinking, chills, pharyngitis, flu-like symptoms, hallucinations, nightmares, severe dizziness, tremors, rigidity, difficulty speaking, inability to focus, ecchymosis, hemorrhaging, or asthenia (HCAHPS).
- Educate patient about signs of a significant reaction (eg, wheezing; chest tightness; fever; itching; bad cough; blue skin color; seizures; or swelling of face, lips, tongue, or throat). **Note:** This is not a comprehensive list of all side effects. Patient should consult prescriber for additional questions.

Intended Use and Disclaimer: Should not be printed and given to patients. This information is intended to serve as a concise initial reference for healthcare professionals to use when discussing medications with a patient. You must ultimately rely on your own discretion, experience and judgment in diagnosing, treating and advising patients.

Streptozocin (strep toe ZOE sin)

Brand Names: U.S. Zanosar
Index Terms Streptozotocin
Pharmacologic Category Antineoplastic Agent, Alkylating Agent; Antineoplastic Agent, Alkylating Agent (Nitrosourea)
Medication Safety Issues
Sound-alike/look-alike issues:
Streptozocin may be confused with streptomycin
High alert medication:
This medication is in a class the Institute for Safe Medication Practices (ISMP) includes among its list of drug classes which have a heightened risk of causing significant patient harm when used in error.
Pregnancy Risk Factor D
Lactation Excretion in breast milk unknown/not recommended
Use Treatment of metastatic islet cell carcinoma of the pancreas (symptomatic or progressive disease)

Unlabeled Use Treatment of metastatic adrenal carcinoma

Available Dosage Forms

Solution Reconstituted, Intravenous:

Zanosar: 1 g (1 ea)

General Dosage Range Dosage adjustment recommended in patients with renal impairment or who develop toxicities.

I.V.: *Adults:* 500 mg/m² for 5 consecutive days every 6 weeks **or** 1000-1500 mg/m² once weekly (maximum dose: 1500 mg/m²)

Administration

I.V. Administer as either a rapid I.V. injection **or** as short or prolonged infusion.

Irritant with vesicant-like properties; ensure proper needle or catheter placement prior to and during infusion; avoid extravasation.

Extravasation management: If extravasation occurs, stop infusion immediately and disconnect (leave cannula/needle in place); gently aspirate extravasated solution (do **NOT** flush the line); remove needle/cannula; elevate extremity.

Hazardous agent; use appropriate precautions for handling and disposal (NIOSH, 2012).

Injectable Detail pH: 3.5-4.5 (reconstituted solution in vial)

Nursing Actions

Physical Assessment Antiemetic should be administered prior to therapy (emetic potential 100%). Infusion site should be monitored closely to prevent extravasation. Monitor for nephrotoxicity (I & O, edema, hematuria, BUN), hepatotoxicity (jaundice, fatigue, LFTs), hypoglycemia, and diarrhea (dehydration) on a regular basis. Caution patients with diabetes to monitor glucose levels closely (may precipitate hypoglycemia).

Patient Education

• Discuss specific use of drug and side effects with patient as it relates to treatment. (HCAHPS: During this hospital stay, were you given any medicine that you had not taken before? Before giving you any new medicine, how often did hospital staff tell you what the medicine was for? How often did hospital staff describe possible side effects in a way you could understand?)

• Patient may experience hypoglycemia, nausea, diarrhea, application site irritation, or renal impairment. Have patient report immediately to prescriber signs of infection, dyspnea, ecchymosis, severe dyspepsia, discolored urine, jaundice, or rash (HCAHPS).

• Educate patient about signs of a significant reaction (eg, wheezing; chest tightness; fever; itching; bad cough; blue skin color; seizures; or swelling of face, lips, tongue, or throat). **Note:** This is not a comprehensive list of all side effects. Patient should consult prescriber for additional questions.

Intended Use and Disclaimer: Should not be printed and given to patients. This information is intended to serve as a concise initial reference for healthcare professionals to use when discussing medications with a patient. You must ultimately rely on your own discretion, experience and judgment in diagnosing, treating and advising patients.

Related Information

Management of Drug Extravasations *on page 1700*

Succinylcholine (suks in il KOE leen)

Brand Names: U.S. Anectine; Quelicin; Quelicin-1000

Index Terms Succinylcholine Chloride; Suxamethonium Chloride

Pharmacologic Category Neuromuscular Blocker Agent, Depolarizing

Medication Safety Issues

High alert medication:

The Institute for Safe Medication Practices (ISMP) includes this medication among its list of drugs which have a heightened risk of causing significant patient harm when used in error.

Other safety concerns:

United States Pharmacopeia (USP) 2006: The Interdisciplinary Safe Medication Use Expert Committee of the USP has recommended the following:

- Hospitals, clinics, and other practice sites should institute special safeguards in the storage, labeling, and use of these agents and should include these safeguards in staff orientation and competency training.

- Healthcare professionals should be on high alert (especially vigilant) whenever a neuromuscular-blocking agent (NMBA) is stocked, ordered, prepared, or administered.

International issues:

Quelicin [U.S., Brazil, Canada, Indonesia] may be confused with Keflin brand name for cefalotin [Argentina, Brazil, Mexico, Netherlands, Norway]

Pregnancy Risk Factor C

Lactation Excretion in breast milk unknown/use caution

Use To facilitate both rapid sequence and routine endotracheal intubation and to relax skeletal muscles during surgery

Note: Does not relieve pain or produce sedation

Unlabeled Use To reduce the intensity of muscle contractions of electroconvulsive therapy (ECT)

Available Dosage Forms

Solution, Injection:

Anectine: 20 mg/mL (10 mL)

Quelicin: 20 mg/mL (10 mL)

Quelicin-1000: 100 mg/mL (10 mL)

General Dosage Range Dosage adjustment recommended in patients with renal or hepatic impairment

I.M.: *Children and Adults:* Up to 3-4 mg/kg (maximum: 150 mg total dose)

I.V.:

Smaller Children: Intermittent: Initial: 2 mg/kg/ dose; Maintenance: 0.3-0.6 mg/kg/dose every 5-10 minutes as needed

Older Children and Adolescents: Intermittent: Initial: 1 mg/kg/dose; Maintenance: 0.3-0.6 mg/kg every 5-10 minutes as needed

Adults: Intubation: 0.6 mg/kg (range: 0.3-1.1 mg/kg); Rapid sequence intubation: 1-1.5 mg/kg

Administration

I.M. I.M. injections should be made deeply, preferably high into deltoid muscle. Use only when I.V. access is not available.

I.V. May be given by rapid I.V. injection without further dilution.

Injectable Detail pH: 3-4.5

Nursing Actions

Physical Assessment Ventilatory support must be instituted and maintained until adequate respiratory muscle function and/or airway protection are assured. This drug is not an anesthetic or analgesic; pain must be treated with appropriate analgesic agents. Continuous monitoring of vital signs, cardiac status, respiratory status, and degree of neuromuscular block (objective assessment with external nerve stimulator) is mandatory during infusion and until full muscle tone has returned. Safety precautions regarding ventilation must be maintained until full muscle tone has returned.

Patient Education

• Discuss specific use of drug and side effects with patient as it relates to treatment. (HCAHPS: During this hospital stay, were you given any medicine that you had not taken before? Before giving you any new medicine, how often did hospital staff tell you what the medicine was for? How often did hospital staff describe possible side effects in a way you could understand?)

• Patient may experience dizziness, additional eye pressure, or myalgia. Have patient report immediately to prescriber tachycardia or rash (HCAHPS).

• Educate patient about signs of a significant reaction (eg, wheezing; chest tightness; fever; itching; bad cough; blue skin color; seizures; or swelling of face, lips, tongue, or throat). **Note:** This is not a comprehensive list of all side effects. Patient should consult prescriber for additional questions.

Intended Use and Disclaimer: Should not be printed and given to patients. This information is intended to serve as a concise initial reference for healthcare professionals to use when discussing medications with a patient. You must ultimately rely on your own discretion, experience and judgment in diagnosing, treating and advising patients.

Sucralfate (soo KRAL fate)

Brand Names: U.S. Carafate

Index Terms Aluminum Sucrose Sulfate, Basic

Pharmacologic Category Gastrointestinal Agent, Miscellaneous

Medication Safety Issues

Sound-alike/look-alike issues:

Sucralfate may be confused with salsalate

Carafate® may be confused with Cafergot®

Administration issues:

For oral administration only. Fatal pulmonary or cerebral embolism has been reported following inadvertent I.V. administration of sucralfate.

Pregnancy Risk Factor B

Lactation Excretion in breast milk unknown/use caution

Use Short-term (≤8 weeks) management of duodenal ulcers; maintenance therapy for duodenal ulcers

Available Dosage Forms

Suspension, Oral:

Carafate: 1 g/10 mL (420 mL)

Tablet, Oral:

Carafate: 1 g

Generic: 1 g

General Dosage Range Oral: *Adults:* 1 g 2-4 times/day

Administration

Oral Administer with water on an empty stomach. To reduce the potential of adversely affecting the absorption of other drugs, administer other drugs 2 hours prior to sucralfate.

Nursing Actions

Physical Assessment Teach patient proper timing of other medications. May cause constipation.

Patient Education

• Discuss specific use of drug and side effects with patient as it relates to treatment. (HCAHPS: During this hospital stay, were you given any medicine that you had not taken before? Before giving you any new medicine, how often did hospital staff tell you what the medicine was for? How often did hospital staff describe possible side effects in a way you could understand?)

• Patient may experience constipation. Have patient report immediately to prescriber signs of hyperglycemia, ecchymosis, or hemorrhaging (HCAHPS).

• Educate patient about signs of a significant reaction (eg, wheezing; chest tightness; fever; itching; bad cough; blue skin color; seizures; or swelling of face, lips, tongue, or throat). **Note:** This is not a comprehensive list of all side effects. Patient should consult prescriber for additional questions.

Sucroferric Oxyhydroxide
(soo kroe FER ik ox ee hye DROX ide)

Brand Names: U.S. Velphoro
Index Terms PA21; Polynuclear Iron (III)-Oxyhydroxide (pn-FeOOH)
Pharmacologic Category Phosphate Binder
Medication Safety Issues
Sound-alike/look-alike issues:
Sucroferric oxyhydroxide may be confused with iron sucrose (Venofer). sucrose
Medication Guide Available false
Pregnancy Risk Factor B
Lactation Excretion in breast milk unknown
Use Control of serum phosphorus: For the control of serum phosphorus levels in patients with chronic kidney disease (CKD) receiving dialysis
Available Dosage Forms
Tablet Chewable, Oral:
Velphoro: 500 mg
General Dosage Range Oral: *Adults:* Initial: 500 mg iron 3 times daily (1.5 g iron daily); usual maintenance: 1.5-2 g iron daily
Administration
Oral Tablets must be chewed; do not swallow whole. Tablets may be crushed to aid with chewing and swallowing. Must administer with meals. The total daily dose should be divided across the meals of the day.
Nursing Actions
Physical Assessment Monitor serum phosphorus levels, iron levels, and serum hepcidin. Can cause diarrhea and discoloration of feces. Monitor for nausea.
Patient Education
• Discuss specific use of drug and side effects with patient as it relates to treatment. (HCAHPS: During this hospital stay, were you given any medicine that you had not taken before? Before giving you any new medicine, how often did hospital staff tell you what the medicine was for? How often did hospital staff describe possible side effects in a way you could understand?)
• Patient may experience melena. Have patient report immediately to prescriber severe nausea, considerable dyspepsia, or significant diarrhea (HCAHPS).
• Educate patient about signs of a significant reaction (eg, wheezing; chest tightness; fever; itching; bad cough; blue skin color; seizures; or swelling of face, lips, tongue, or throat). **Note:** This is not a comprehensive list of all side effects. Patient should consult prescriber for additional questions.

SulfADIAZINE (sul fa DYE a zeen)

Pharmacologic Category Antibiotic, Sulfonamide Derivative
Medication Safety Issues
Sound-alike/look-alike issues:
SulfADIAZINE may be confused with sulfaSALAzine, sulfiSOXAZOLE
Pregnancy Risk Factor C
Lactation Enters breast milk/contraindicated
Use Treatment of the following conditions (per product labeling): Chancroid, trachoma, inclusion conjunctivitis, nocardiosis, urinary tract infections, toxoplasmosis encephalitis, malaria, meningococcal meningitis, acute otitis media, rheumatic fever (prophylaxis), meningitis (adjunctive)

Refer to current guidelines for appropriate use.
Available Dosage Forms
Tablet, Oral:
Generic: 500 mg
General Dosage Range Oral:
Children >2 months: Initial: 75 mg/kg; Maintenance: 150 mg/kg/day (maximum: 6 g/24 hours)
Children <30 kg and Adults <30 kg: 0.5 g/day (rheumatic fever prophylaxis)
Children ≥30 kg and Adults ≥30 kg: 1 g/day (rheumatic fever prophylaxis)
Adults: 2-4 g/day in divided doses
Administration
Oral Administer with at least 8 ounces of water and around-the-clock to promote less variation in peak and trough serum levels. Oral sodium bicarbonate may be used to alkalinize the urine of patients unable to maintain adequate fluid intake (in order to prevent crystalluria, azotemia, oliguria) (Lerner, 1996).
Nursing Actions
Physical Assessment Allergy history should be assessed prior to starting therapy (sulfonamides). Monitor for rash, photosensitivity, gastrointestinal disturbance (nausea, vomiting, anorexia), anemia, jaundice, and hematuria. Have patient call prescriber immediately if any signs of rash.
Patient Education
• Discuss specific use of drug and side effects with patient as it relates to treatment. (HCAHPS: During this hospital stay, were you given any medicine that you had not taken before? Before giving you any new medicine, how often did

hospital staff tell you what the medicine was for? How often did hospital staff describe possible side effects in a way you could understand?)
- Patient may experience headache, nausea, diarrhea, or inability to eat. Have patient report immediately to prescriber severe fatigue, significant skin irritation, considerable dyspepsia, discolored urine, jaundice, ecchymosis, bleeding, or rash (HCAHPS).
- Educate patient about signs of a significant reaction (eg, wheezing; chest tightness; fever; itching; bad cough; blue skin color; seizures; or swelling of face, lips, tongue, or throat). **Note:** This is not a comprehensive list of all side effects. Patient should consult prescriber for additional questions.

Intended Use and Disclaimer: Should not be printed and given to patients. This information is intended to serve as a concise initial reference for healthcare professionals to use when discussing medications with a patient. You must ultimately rely on your own discretion, experience and judgment in diagnosing, treating and advising patients.

Sulfamethoxazole and Trimethoprim
(sul fa meth OKS a zole & trye METH oh prim)

Brand Names: U.S. Bactrim; Bactrim DS; Septra DS; Sulfatrim
Index Terms Co-Trimoxazole; Septra; SMX-TMP; SMZ-TMP; Sulfatrim; TMP-SMX; TMP-SMZ; Trimethoprim and Sulfamethoxazole
Pharmacologic Category Antibiotic, Miscellaneous; Antibiotic, Sulfonamide Derivative
Medication Safety Issues
Sound-alike/look-alike issues:
Bactrim may be confused with bacitracin, Bactine, Bactroban
Co-trimoxazole may be confused with clotrimazole
Septra may be confused with Ceptaz, Sectral
Septra DS may be confused with Semprex-D
Pregnancy Risk Factor D
Lactation Enters breast milk/use caution
Use
Oral: Treatment of urinary tract infections due to *E. coli*, *Klebsiella* and *Enterobacter* sp, *M. morganii*, *P. mirabilis* and *P. vulgaris*; acute otitis media; acute exacerbations of chronic bronchitis due to susceptible strains of *H. influenzae* or *S. pneumoniae*; treatment and prophylaxis of *Pneumocystis jirovecii* pneumonia (PCP); traveler's diarrhea due to enterotoxigenic *E. coli*; treatment of enteritis caused by *Shigella flexneri* or *Shigella sonnei*
I.V.: Treatment of *Pneumocystis jirovecii* pneumonia (PCP); treatment of enteritis caused by *Shigella flexneri* or *Shigella sonnei*; treatment of severe or complicated urinary tract infections due to *E. coli*, *Klebsiella* and *Enterobacter* spp, *M. morganii*, *P. mirabilis*, and *P. vulgaris*

Unlabeled Use Cholera and *Salmonella*-type infections and nocardiosis; chronic prostatitis; as prophylaxis in neutropenic patients with *P. jirovecii* infections, in leukemia patients, and in patients following renal transplantation, to decrease incidence of PCP; treatment of *Cyclospora* infection, typhoid fever, *Nocardia asteroides* infection; prophylaxis against urinary tract infection; alternative treatment for MRSA infections; oral phase treatment of prosthetic joint infection; chronic antimicrobial suppression of prosthetic joint infection, treatment of Q fever (*Coxiella burnetii*)
Available Dosage Forms The 5:1 ratio (SMX: TMP) remains constant in all dosage forms.
Injection, solution: Sulfamethoxazole 80 mg and trimethoprim 16 mg per mL (5 mL, 10 mL, 30 mL)
Suspension, oral: Sulfamethoxazole 200 mg and trimethoprim 40 mg per 5 mL
Sulfatrim: Sulfamethoxazole 200 mg and trimethoprim 40 mg per 5 mL
Tablet, oral: Sulfamethoxazole 400 mg and trimethoprim 80 mg
Bactrim: Sulfamethoxazole 400 mg and trimethoprim 80 mg
Tablet, double-strength, oral: Sulfamethoxazole 800 mg and trimethoprim 160 mg
Bactrim DS, Septra DS: Sulfamethoxazole 800 mg and trimethoprim 160 mg
General Dosage Range Dosage adjustment recommended in patients with renal impairment
I.V.: *Children >2 months and Adults:* 8-20 mg TMP/kg/day divided every 6-12 hours
Oral:
Children >2 months: 6-20 mg TMP/kg/day divided every 6-12 hours **or** 150 mg TMP/m^2/day in divided doses every 12-24 hours for 3-7 days/week (maximum: sulfamethoxazole 1600 mg/day; trimethoprim 320 mg/day)
Adults: 1 or 2 double-strength tablets (sulfamethoxazole 800-1600 mg; trimethoprim 160-320 mg) every 12-24 hours **or** 15-20 mg TMP/kg/day in 3-4 divided doses
Administration
I.V. Infuse diluted solution I.V. over 60-90 minutes; not for I.M. injection.
Injectable Detail pH: 10
Oral Administer without regard to meals. Administer with at least 8 ounces of water.
Nursing Actions
Physical Assessment Perform culture and sensitivity tests prior to initiating therapy.
Patient Education
- Discuss specific use of drug and side effects with patient as it relates to treatment. (HCAHPS: During this hospital stay, were you given any medicine that you had not taken before? Before giving you any new medicine, how often did hospital staff tell you what the medicine was for? How often did hospital staff describe possible side effects in a way you could understand?)

- Patient may experience nausea, diarrhea, or lack of appetite. Have patient report immediately to prescriber discolored urine, jaundice, or rash (HCAHPS).
- Educate patient about signs of a significant reaction (eg, wheezing; chest tightness; fever; itching; bad cough; blue skin color; seizures; or swelling of face, lips, tongue, or throat). **Note:** This is not a comprehensive list of all side effects. Patient should consult prescriber for additional questions.

Intended Use and Disclaimer: Should not be printed and given to patients. This information is intended to serve as a concise initial reference for healthcare professionals to use when discussing medications with a patient. You must ultimately rely on your own discretion, experience and judgment in diagnosing, treating and advising patients.

Related Information
Trimethoprim *on page 1567*

Sulfasalazine (sul fa SAL a zeen)

Brand Names: U.S. Azulfidine; Azulfidine EN-tabs; Sulfazine; Sulfazine EC
Index Terms Salicylazosulfapyridine
Pharmacologic Category 5-Aminosalicylic Acid Derivative
Medication Safety Issues
 Sound-alike/look-alike issues:
  SulfaSALAzine may be confused with salsalate, sulfADIAZINE, sulfiSOXAZOLE
  Azulfidine may be confused with Augmentin®, azaTHIOprine
Pregnancy Risk Factor B
Lactation Enters breast milk/use caution
Use
 U.S. labeling: Treatment of mild-to-moderate ulcerative colitis or as adjunctive therapy in severe ulcerative colitis; enteric coated tablets are also used for rheumatoid arthritis (including juvenile idiopathic arthritis [JIA]) in patients who inadequately respond to analgesics and NSAIDs
 Canadian labeling: Adjunctive therapy in severe ulcerative colitis, distal ulcerative colitis or proctitis, and Crohn's disease; enteric coated tablets are also used for rheumatoid arthritis unsuccessfully treated with first-line therapy
Unlabeled Use Ankylosing spondylitis, Crohn's disease, psoriasis, psoriatic arthritis
Available Dosage Forms
 Tablet, Oral:
  Azulfidine: 500 mg
  Sulfazine: 500 mg
  Generic: 500 mg
 Tablet Delayed Release, Oral:
  Azulfidine EN-tabs: 500 mg
  Sulfazine EC: 500 mg
  Generic: 500 mg

General Dosage Range Oral:
 Delayed release:
  Children ≥6 years: Initial: 1/4 to 1/3 of expected maintenance dose; Maintenance: 30-50 mg/kg/day in 2 divided doses (maximum: 2 g daily)
  Adults: Initial: 0.5-1 g daily; Maintenance: 2 g/day in 2 divided doses (maximum: 3 g daily)
 Immediate release:
  Children ≥6 years: Initial: 40-60 mg/kg/day in 3-6 divided doses; Maintenance: 30 mg/kg/day in 4 divided doses
  Adults: Initial: 3-4 g daily in evenly divided doses at ≤8-hour intervals; Maintenance: 2 g daily in divided doses at ≤8-hour intervals
Administration
 Oral Tablets should be administered in evenly divided doses, preferably after meals. Enteric coated tablets should be swallowed whole.
Nursing Actions
 Physical Assessment Allergy history should be assessed prior to starting therapy (sulfa drugs, salicylates). Monitor for photosensitivity, gastrointestinal disturbance [nausea, vomiting, anorexia], anemia, jaundice, or hematuria. Caution patients with diabetes to monitor glucose levels closely; may cause altered effect of oral hypoglycemic agents.
 Patient Education
- Discuss specific use of drug and side effects with patient as it relates to treatment. (HCAHPS: During this hospital stay, were you given any medicine that you had not taken before? Before giving you any new medicine, how often did hospital staff tell you what the medicine was for? How often did hospital staff describe possible side effects in a way you could understand?)
- Patient may experience headache, dyspepsia, pyrosis, or nausea. Have patient report immediately to prescriber severe fatigue, tablet shell in stool, bloody stools, significant skin irritation, jaundice, inability to eat, or rash (HCAHPS).
- Educate patient about signs of a significant reaction (eg, wheezing; chest tightness; fever; itching; bad cough; blue skin color; seizures; or swelling of face, lips, tongue, or throat). **Note:** This is not a comprehensive list of all side effects. Patient should consult prescriber for additional questions.

Intended Use and Disclaimer: Should not be printed and given to patients. This information is intended to serve as a concise initial reference for healthcare professionals to use when discussing medications with a patient. You must ultimately rely on your own discretion, experience and judgment in diagnosing, treating and advising patients.

Related Information
Oral Medications That Should Not Be Crushed or
Altered *on page 1712*

Sulindac (SUL in dak)

Index Terms Clinoril
Pharmacologic Category Nonsteroidal Anti-
inflammatory Drug (NSAID), Oral
Medication Safety Issues
Sound-alike/look-alike issues:
Clinoril may be confused with Cleocin, Clozaril
BEERS Criteria medication:
This drug may be potentially inappropriate for use
in geriatric patients (Quality of evidence - mod-
erate; Strength of recommendation - strong).
Medication Guide Available Yes
Pregnancy Risk Factor C
Lactation Excretion in breast milk unknown/not
recommended
Breast-Feeding Considerations It is not known if
sulindac is excreted into breast milk. Breast-feeding is not recommended by the manufacturer.
Use Management of inflammatory diseases including osteoarthritis, rheumatoid arthritis, acute gouty
arthritis, ankylosing spondylitis, acute painful
shoulder (bursitis/tendonitis)
Unlabeled Use Management of preterm labor
Mechanism of Action/Effect Reversibly inhibits
cyclooxygenase-1 and 2 (COX-1 and 2) enzymes,
which results in decreased formation of prostaglandin precursors; has antipyretic, analgesic, and anti-
inflammatory properties
Contraindications Hypersensitivity or allergic-
type reactions to sulindac, aspirin, other NSAIDs,
or any component of the formulation; perioperative
pain in the setting of coronary artery bypass graft
(CABG) surgery
Warnings/Precautions [U.S. Boxed Warning]:
NSAIDs are associated with an increased risk
of adverse cardiovascular thrombotic events,
including MI and stroke. Use caution with fluid
retention. Avoid use in heart failure (ACCF/AHA
[Yancy, 2013]). Concurrent administration of ibuprofen, and potentially other nonselective NSAIDs,
may interfere with aspirin's cardioprotective effect.
May cause new-onset hypertension or worsening
of existing hypertension. NSAID use may compromise existing renal function; dose-dependent
decreases in prostaglandin synthesis may result
from NSAID use, reducing renal blood flow which
may cause renal decompensation. NSAID use may
increase the risk for hyperkalemia. Patients with
impaired renal function, dehydration, heart failure,
liver dysfunction, those taking diuretics, and ACE
inhibitors, and the elderly are at greater risk of renal
toxicity and hyperkalemia. Rehydrate patient
before starting therapy; monitor renal function
closely. Not recommended for use in patients with
advanced renal disease. Long-term NSAID use

may result in renal papillary necrosis. Use caution
in patients with renal lithiasis; sulindac metabolites
have been reported as components of renal
stones. Maintain adequate hydration in patients
with a history of renal stones. Use with caution in
patients with decreased hepatic function. May
require dosage adjustment in hepatic dysfunction;
sulfide and sulfone metabolites may accumulate.
The elderly are at increased risk for adverse
effects. **[U.S. Boxed Warning]: Use is contra-**
indicated for treatment of perioperative pain in
the setting of coronary artery bypass graft
(CABG) surgery. Risk of MI and stroke may be
increased with use following CABG surgery.

[U.S. Boxed Warning]: NSAIDs may increase
risk of gastrointestinal irritation, inflammation,
ulceration, bleeding, and perforation. Use the
lowest effective dose for the shortest duration of
time, consistent with individual patient goals, to
reduce risk of cardiovascular or GI adverse events.
When used concomitantly with aspirin, a substantial increase in the risk of gastrointestinal complications (eg, ulcer) occurs; concomitant
gastroprotective therapy (eg, proton pump inhibitors) is recommended (Bhatt, 2008). Pancreatitis
has been reported; discontinue with suspected
pancreatitis.

Avoid chronic use in the elderly (unless alternative
agents ineffective and patient can receive concomitant gastroprotective agent); nonselective oral
NSAID use is associated with an increased risk
of GI bleeding and peptic ulcer disease in older
adults in high risk category (eg, >75 years or age or
receiving concomitant oral/parenteral corticosteroids, anticoagulants, or antiplatelet agents) (Beers
Criteria).

NSAIDS may cause drowsiness, dizziness, blurred
vision and other neurologic effects which may
impair physical or mental abilities; patients must
be cautioned about performing tasks which require
mental alertness (eg, operating machinery or driving). Discontinue use with blurred or diminished
vision and perform ophthalmologic exam. Monitor
vision with long-term therapy.

Platelet adhesion and aggregation may be
decreased, may prolong bleeding time; patients
with coagulation disorders or who are receiving
anticoagulants should be monitored closely. Anemia may occur; patients on long-term NSAID therapy should be monitored for anemia. Rarely,
NSAID use may cause severe blood dyscrasias
(eg, agranulocytosis, aplastic anemia, thrombocytopenia). NSAIDs may cause serious skin adverse
events including exfoliative dermatitis, Stevens-
Johnson syndrome (SJS) and toxic epidermal necrolysis (TEN); discontinue use at first sign of skin
rash or hypersensitivity. Anaphylactoid reactions
may occur. Do not use in patients who experience
bronchospasm, asthma, rhinitis, or urticaria with

NSAID or aspirin therapy. Use caution in other forms of asthma. May increase the risk of aseptic meningitis, especially in patients with systemic lupus erythematosus (SLE) and mixed connective tissue disorders.

Withhold for at least 4-6 half-lives prior to surgical or dental procedures.

Drug Interactions

Avoid Concomitant Use

Avoid concomitant use of Sulindac with any of the following: Floctafenine; Ketorolac (Nasal); Ketorolac (Systemic); NSAID (COX-2 Inhibitor); Omacetaxine; Urokinase

Decreased Effect

Sulindac may decrease the levels/effects of: ACE Inhibitors; Agents with Antiplatelet Properties; Aliskiren; Angiotensin II Receptor Blockers; Beta-Blockers; Eplerenone; HydrALAZINE; Loop Diuretics; Potassium-Sparing Diuretics; Prostaglandins (Ophthalmic); Salicylates; Selective Serotonin Reuptake Inhibitors; Thiazide Diuretics

The levels/effects of Sulindac may be decreased by: Bile Acid Sequestrants; Nonsteroidal Anti-Inflammatory Agents; Salicylates

Increased Effect/Toxicity

Sulindac may increase the levels/effects of: 5-ASA Derivatives; Agents with Antiplatelet Properties; Aliskiren; Aminoglycosides; Anticoagulants; Bisphosphonate Derivatives; Collagenase (Systemic); CycloSPORINE (Systemic); Dabigatran Etexilate; Deferasirox; Desmopressin; Digoxin; Eplerenone; Haloperidol; Ibritumomab; Methotrexate; Nonsteroidal Anti-Inflammatory Agents; NSAID (COX-2 Inhibitor); Omacetaxine; PEMEtrexed; Porfimer; Potassium-Sparing Diuretics; PRALAtrexate; Quinolone Antibiotics; Rivaroxaban; Salicylates; Tenofovir; Thrombolytic Agents; Tositumomab and Iodine I 131 Tositumomab; Urokinase; Vancomycin; Vitamin K Antagonists

The levels/effects of Sulindac may be increased by: ACE Inhibitors; Angiotensin II Receptor Blockers; Antidepressants (Tricyclic, Tertiary Amine); Corticosteroids (Systemic); CycloSPORINE (Systemic); Dasatinib; Dimethyl Sulfoxide; Floctafenine; Glucosamine; Herbs (Anticoagulant/Antiplatelet Properties); Ibrutinib; Ketorolac (Nasal); Ketorolac (Systemic); Multivitamins/Fluoride (with ADE); Multivitamins/Minerals (with ADEK, Folate, Iron); Multivitamins/Minerals (with AE, No Iron); Nonsteroidal Anti-Inflammatory Agents; Omega-3 Fatty Acids; Pentosan Polysulfate Sodium; Pentoxifylline; Probenecid; Prostacyclin Analogues; Selective Serotonin Reuptake Inhibitors; Serotonin/Norepinephrine Reuptake Inhibitors; Sodium Phosphates; Tipranavir; Treprostinil; Vitamin E

Nutritional/Ethanol Interactions

Ethanol: Avoid ethanol (may enhance gastric mucosal irritation).

Herb/Nutraceutical: Avoid alfalfa, anise, bilberry, bladderwrack, bromelain, cat's claw, celery, chamomile, coleus, cordyceps, dong quai, evening primrose, fenugreek, feverfew, garlic, ginger, ginkgo biloba, ginseng (American, Panax, Siberian), grapeseed, green tea, guggul, horse chestnut seed, horseradish, licorice, prickly ash, red clover, reishi, SAMe (S-adenosylmethionine), sweet clover, turmeric, white willow (all have additional antiplatelet activity).

Adverse Reactions 1% to 10%:

Cardiovascular: Edema (1% to 3%)

Central nervous system: Dizziness (3% to 9%), headache (3% to 9%), nervousness (1% to 3%)

Dermatologic: Rash (3% to 9%), pruritus (1% to 3%)

Gastrointestinal: GI pain (10%), constipation (3% to 9%), diarrhea (3% to 9%), dyspepsia (3% to 9%), nausea (3% to 9%), abdominal cramps (1% to 3%), anorexia (1% to 3%), flatulence (1% to 3%), vomiting (1% to 3%)

Otic: Tinnitus (1% to 3%)

Available Dosage Forms

Tablet, Oral:

Generic: 150 mg, 200 mg

General Dosage Range Dosage adjustment recommended in patients with hepatic impairment

Oral: *Adults:* 150-200 mg twice daily (maximum: 400 mg/day)

Administration

Oral Should be administered with food or milk.

Storage/Stability Store at room temperature of 15°C to 30°C (59°F to 86°F).

Nursing Actions

Physical Assessment Monitor blood pressure at the beginning of therapy and periodically during use. Monitor for adverse GI and respiratory response, hepatotoxicity, and ototoxicity at beginning of therapy and periodically throughout. Schedule ophthalmic evaluations for patients who develop eye complaints during long-term NSAID therapy.

Patient Education

• Discuss specific use of drug and side effects with patient as it relates to treatment. (HCAHPS: During this hospital stay, were you given any medicine that you had not taken before? Before giving you any new medicine, how often did hospital staff tell you what the medicine was for? How often did hospital staff describe possible side effects in a way you could understand?)

• Patient may experience headache, dyspepsia, nausea, constipation, or diarrhea. Have patient report immediately to prescriber angina, dyspnea, strength differences from one side to another, edema or pain of hands or feet, significant weight gain, melena, hematuria, ecchymosis, discolored urine, jaundice, or rash (HCAHPS).

• Educate patient about signs of a significant reaction (eg, wheezing; chest tightness; fever; ▶

itching; bad cough; blue skin color; seizures; or swelling of face, lips, tongue, or throat). **Note:** This is not a comprehensive list of all side effects. Patient should consult prescriber for additional questions.

Intended Use and Disclaimer: Should not be printed and given to patients. This information is intended to serve as a concise initial reference for healthcare professionals to use when discussing medications with a patient. You must ultimately rely on your own discretion, experience and judgment in diagnosing, treating and advising patients.

Dietary Considerations Drug may cause GI upset, bleeding, ulceration, perforation; take with food or milk to minimize GI upset.

SUMAtriptan (soo ma TRIP tan)

Brand Names: U.S. Alsuma; Imitrex; Imitrex STATdose Refill; Imitrex STATdose System; Sumavel DosePro

Index Terms Sumatriptan Succinate

Pharmacologic Category Antimigraine Agent; Serotonin 5-HT$_{1B, 1D}$ Receptor Agonist

Medication Safety Issues

Sound-alike/look-alike issues:

SUMAtriptan may be confused with saxagliptin, sitaGLIPtin, somatropin, ZOLMitriptan

Pregnancy Risk Factor C

Lactation Enters breast milk/not recommended

Breast-Feeding Considerations The excretion of sumatriptan into breast milk was studied in five lactating women, 10-28 weeks postpartum (mean: 22.2 weeks). Sumatriptan 6 mg SubQ was administered and maternal milk and blood samples were collected over 8 hours after the dose. Sumatriptan was detected in breast milk. Maximum concentrations in the maternal blood (mean: 80.2 mcg/L; 0.25 hours after the dose) and milk (mean: 87.2 mcg/L; 2.5 hours after the dose) were similar. However, the amount of sumatriptan an infant would be exposed to following breast-feeding is considered to be small (although the mean milk-to-plasma ratio is ~4.9, weight-adjusted doses estimates suggest breast-fed infants receive 3.5% of a maternal dose). Expressing and discarding the milk for 8-12 hours after a single dose is suggested to reduce the amount present even further (Wojnar-Horton, 1996). Breast-feeding is not recommended by some manufacturers; however, according to other sources if treatment is needed, breast-feeding does not need to be discontinued (Jürgens, 2009; MacGregor, 2012).

Use

Intranasal, Oral, SubQ, Transdermal: Acute treatment of migraine with or without aura

SubQ: Acute treatment of cluster headache episodes

Mechanism of Action/Effect Selective agonist for serotonin receptor in cranial arteries; causes vasoconstriction and relief of migraine

Contraindications Hypersensitivity to sumatriptan or any component of the formulation, including allergic contact dermatitis to the transdermal patch; patients with ischemic heart disease or signs or symptoms of ischemic heart disease (including Prinzmetal's angina, angina pectoris, myocardial infarction, silent myocardial ischemia); cerebrovascular syndromes (including strokes, transient ischemic attacks); peripheral vascular disease (including ischemic bowel disease); uncontrolled hypertension; use within 24 hours of ergotamine derivatives; use within 24 hours of another 5-HT$_1$ agonist; concurrent administration or within 2 weeks of discontinuing an MAO type A inhibitors (oral, transdermal, and nasal sumatriptan only; see Warnings/Precautions); management of hemiplegic or basilar migraine; Wolff-Parkinson-White syndrome or arrhythmias associated with other cardiac accessory conduction pathway disorders (injectable Imitrex and transdermal only); severe hepatic impairment (oral, transdermal, and nasal sumatriptan, and injectable Imitrex only); not for I.V. administration

Warnings/Precautions Sumatriptan is only indicated for the acute treatment of migraine or cluster headache (product dependent); not indicated for migraine prophylaxis, or for the treatment of hemiplegic or basilar migraine. Acute migraine agents (eg, triptans, opioids, ergotamine, or a combination of the agents) used for 10 or more days per month may lead to worsening of headaches (medication overuse headache); withdrawal treatment may be necessary in the setting of overuse. May cause CNS depression, such as dizziness, weakness, or drowsiness, which may impair physical or mental abilities; patients must be cautioned about performing tasks which require mental alertness (eg, operating machinery or driving). If a patient does not respond to the first dose, the diagnosis of migraine or cluster headache should be reconsidered; rule out underlying neurologic disease in patients with atypical headache and in patients with no prior history of migraine or cluster headache. Cardiac events (coronary artery vasospasm, transient ischemia, myocardial infarction, ventricular tachycardia/fibrillation, cardiac arrest and death), cerebral/subarachnoid hemorrhage, and stroke have been reported with 5-HT$_1$ agonist administration. Patients who experience sensations of chest pain/pressure/tightness or symptoms suggestive of angina following dosing should be evaluated for coronary artery disease or Prinzmetal's angina before receiving additional doses; if dosing is resumed and similar symptoms recur, monitor with ECG. Do not give to patients with risk factors for CAD until a cardiovascular evaluation has been performed; if evaluation is satisfactory, the healthcare provider should administer the first dose (consider ECG monitoring) and cardiovascular status should be periodically evaluated.

Significant elevation in blood pressure, including hypertensive crisis, has also been reported on rare occasions in patients with and without a history of hypertension; use is contraindicated in patients with uncontrolled hypertension. Vasospasm-related reactions have been reported other than coronary artery vasospasm. Peripheral vascular ischemia, colonic ischemia with abdominal pain and bloody diarrhea, splenic infarction, and Raynaud syndrome have occurred. Transient and permanent blindness and significant partial vision loss have been very rarely reported. Use with caution in patients with a history of seizure disorder or in patients with a lowered seizure threshold. Use the oral formulation with caution (and with dosage limitations) in patients with hepatic impairment where treatment is necessary and advisable. Presystemic clearance of orally administered sumatriptan is reduced in hepatic impairment, leading to increased plasma concentrations; dosage reduction of the oral product is recommended. Non-oral routes of administration (nasal, subcutaneous formulations) do not undergo similar hepatic first-pass metabolism and are not expected to result in significantly altered pharmacokinetics in patients with hepatic impairment. Use of the oral, nasal, transdermal, or Imitrex injectable is contraindicated in severe hepatic impairment. Allergic contact dermatitis may occur with use of transdermal patch; erythematous plaque and/or erythemato-vesicular or erythemato-bullous eruptions may develop. Erythema alone is common and not by itself an indication of sensitization. Discontinue use if allergic contact dermatitis is suspected. Patients sensitized from use of transdermal system may develop systemic sensitization or other systemic reactions if sumatriptan-containing products are taken by other routes (oral, subcutaneous); if treatment with sumatriptan by other routes is required, first dose should be taken under close medical supervision. Do not apply transdermal patch in areas near or over electrically-active implantable or body-worn medical devices (eg, implantable cardiac pacemaker, body-worn insulin pump, implantable deep brain stimulator);patch contains metal parts and must be removed before magnetic resonance imaging (MRI) procedures.

Potentially significant drug-drug interactions may exist, requiring dose or frequency adjustment, additional monitoring, and/or selection of alternative therapy. Serotonin syndrome may occur with triptans, particularly when used concomitantly with other serotonergic drugs; symptoms (eg, mental status changes, tachycardia, hyperthermia, nausea, vomiting, diarrhea, hyperreflexia, incoordination) typically occur minutes to hours after initiation/dose increase of a serotonergic drug. Discontinue use if serotonin syndrome is suspected. Not recommended for use in elderly patients; older adults are at a higher risk for coronary artery disease and may be more likely to have reduced hepatic function.

Drug Interactions

Avoid Concomitant Use

Avoid concomitant use of SUMAtriptan with any of the following: Ergot Derivatives; MAO Inhibitors

Decreased Effect There are no known significant interactions involving a decrease in effect.

Increased Effect/Toxicity

SUMAtriptan may increase the levels/effects of: Antipsychotics; Droxidopa; Ergot Derivatives; Metoclopramide; Serotonin Modulators

The levels/effects of SUMAtriptan may be increased by: Antipsychotics; Ergot Derivatives; MAO Inhibitors

Adverse Reactions

Injection:

>10%:

Central nervous system: Paresthesia (5% to 14%), dizziness (12%), localized warm feeling (11%)

Local: Injection site reaction (≤86%; includes bleeding, bruising, swelling, and erythema)

1% to 10%:

Cardiovascular: Flushing (7%), chest discomfort (2% to 5%)

Central nervous system: Burning sensation (7%), feeling of heaviness (7%), pressure sensation (7%), feeling of tightness (5%), drowsiness (3%), feeling strange (2%), headache (2%), tight feeling in head (2%), anxiety (1%), cold sensation (1%), malaise (1%)

Dermatologic: Diaphoresis (2%)

Gastrointestinal: Nausea and vomiting (4%), sore throat (3%), abdominal distress (1%), dysphagia (1%)

Neuromuscular & skeletal: Neck pain (5%), numbness (5%), weakness (5%), jaw pain (2%), myalgia (2%), muscle cramps (1%)

Ophthalmic: Visual disturbance (1%)

Respiratory: Nasal signs and symptoms (2%), bronchospasm (1%)

Nasal spray:

>10%: Gastrointestinal: Unpleasant taste (13% to 24%), nausea (11% to 13%), vomiting (11% to 13%)

1% to 10%:

Central nervous system: Dizziness (1% to 2%)

Gastrointestinal: Sore throat (1% to 2%)

Respiratory: Nasal signs and symptoms (2% to 4%)

Tablet:

1% to 10%:

Cardiovascular: Hot and cold flashes (2% to 3%, placebo 2%), chest pain (1% to 2%), palpitations (1%), syncope (1%)

Central nervous system: Paresthesia (3% to 5%), sensation of pressure (neck/throat/jaw: 2% to 3%; nonspecified: 1% to 3%, placebo 2%), burning sensation (1%), dizziness (>1%), drowsiness (>1%), malaise (2% to 3%), headache (>1%), pain (nonspecified; 1% to 2%, placebo 1%), vertigo (<1% to 2%), migraine (>1%), sleepiness (>1%), hyperacusis (1%), numbness (1%)

Gastrointestinal: Diarrhea (1%), nausea (>1%), vomiting (>1%), reduced salivation (>1%)

Genitourinary: Hematuria (1%)

Hematologic & oncologic: Hemolytic anemia (1%), hemorrhage (ear: 1%; nose/throat: 1%)

Hypersensitivity: Hypersensitivity reaction (1%)

Neuromuscular & skeletal: Myalgia (1%)

Otic: Hearing loss (1%), tinnitus (1%)

Respiratory: Allergic rhinitis (1%), dyspnea (1%), rhinitis (1%), sinusitis (1%), upper respiratory tract inflammation (1%)

Transdermal system:

>10%: Local: Localized pain (26%)

1% to 10%:

Central nervous system: Localized warm feeling (6%), feeling abnormal (paresthesia, warm/cold sensation: 2%), sensation of pressure (chest/neck/throat/jaw: 2%)

Dermatologic: Skin discoloration (application site: 3% to 5%), allergic contact dermatitis (4%), skin vesicle (application site: 3%)

Hematologic & oncologic: Bruise (application site: 1% to 2%)

Local: Localized pruritus (8%), localized irritation (4%)

<1%: Skin erosion (application site)

Pharmacodynamics/Kinetics

Onset of Action Oral: ~30 minutes; Nasal: ~15-30 minutes; SubQ: ~10 minutes

Product Availability Zecuity (transdermal system): FDA approved January 2013; anticipated availability is currently unknown. Refer to prescribing information for additional information.

Available Dosage Forms

Device, Subcutaneous:

Sumavel DosePro: 6 mg/0.5 mL (0.5 mL)

Solution, Nasal:

Imitrex: 5 mg/actuation (1 ea); 20 mg/actuation (1 ea)

Generic: 5 mg/actuation (1 ea); 20 mg/actuation (1 ea)

Solution, Subcutaneous:

Alsuma: 6 mg/0.5 mL (0.5 mL)

Imitrex: 6 mg/0.5 mL (0.5 mL)

Imitrex STATdose Refill: 4 mg/0.5 mL (0.5 mL); 6 mg/0.5 mL (0.5 mL)

Imitrex STATdose System: 4 mg/0.5 mL (0.5 mL); 6 mg/0.5 mL (0.5 mL)

Generic: 4 mg/0.5 mL (0.5 mL); 6 mg/0.5 mL (0.5 mL)

Solution, Subcutaneous [preservative free]:

Generic: 6 mg/0.5 mL (0.5 mL)

Tablet, Oral:

Imitrex: 25 mg, 50 mg, 100 mg

Generic: 25 mg, 50 mg, 100 mg

General Dosage Range Dosage adjustment recommended for oral route in patients with hepatic impairment

Intranasal: *Adults:* 5-20 mg in one nostril as a single dose (may divide dose into both nostrils); may repeat after 2 hours (maximum: 40 mg/day)

Oral: *Adults:* 25-100 mg as a single dose; may repeat after 2 hours (maximum: 200 mg/day)

SubQ: *Adults:* Initial: Up to 6 mg; may repeat if needed ≥1 hour after initial dose (maximum: Two 6 mg injections per 24-hour period)

Transdermal: *Adults:* Initial: Apply one patch (provides 6.5 mg per 4 hours) a second patch may be applied no sooner than 2 hours after activation of the first patch (maximum: 2 patches per 24-hour period)

Administration

Oral Should be administered as soon as symptoms appear.

Topical Transdermal patch: Should be administered as soon as symptoms appear.

Apply patch to dry intact, non-irritated skin on the upper arm or thigh on a site that is relatively hair free and without scars, tattoos, abrasions, or other skin conditions (ie, generalized skin irritation, eczema, psoriasis, melanoma, contact dermatitis); secure with medical tape if needed. Do not apply to a previous application site until the site remains erythema free for at least 3 days. After application, the activation button must be pushed, and the red light emitting diode (LED) will turn on; the system will stop operating when dosing is completed and the LED will turn off, signaling that the patch can be removed; if the LED turns off before 4 hours, dosing has stopped and the patch can be removed. If headache relief is incomplete, a second patch can be applied to a different site, if >2 hours have elapsed since the first patch was applied. After use, fold the patch so the adhesive side sticks to itself and discard away from children and pets. The patch contains lithium-manganese dioxide batteries; dispose in accordance with state and local regulations.

Subcutaneous Should be administered as soon as symptoms appear.

Not for I.M. or I.V. use. Needle penetrates 1/4 inch of skin; use in areas of the body with adequate skin and subcutaneous thickness. Alsuma is a prefilled single-use autoinjector device.

Needleless administration (Sumavel DosePro): Administer to the abdomen (>2 inches from the navel) or thigh; not for I.M. or I.V. administration. Do not administer to other areas of the body (eg, arm). Device is for single use only, discard after use; do not use if the tip of the device is tilted or broken.

Inhalation Nasal spray: Should be administered as soon as symptoms appear.

Each nasal spray unit is preloaded with 1 dose; **do not** test the spray unit before use; remove unit from plastic pack when ready to use; while sitting down, gently blow nose to clear nasal passages; keep head upright and close one nostril gently with index finger; hold container with other hand, with thumb supporting bottom and index and middle fingers on either side of nozzle; insert nozzle into nostril about 1/2 inch; close mouth; take a breath through nose while releasing spray into nostril by pressing firmly on blue plunger; remove nozzle from nostril; keep head level for 10-20 seconds and gently breathe in through nose and out through mouth; **do not breathe deeply**.

Storage/Stability

Alsuma: Store at 25°C (77°F); excursions permitted between 15°C and 30°C (59°F and 86°F); do not refrigerate. Protect from light.

Imitrex injectable, tablet, nasal spray: Store at 2°C to 30°C (36°F to 86°F). Protect from light.

Sumavel DosePro: Store at 20°C to 25°C (68°F to 77°F); excursions permitted between 15°C and 30°C (59°F and 86°F); do not freeze.

Zecuity: Store at 20°C to 25°C (68°F to 77°F); excursions permitted between 15°C and 30°C (59°F and 86°F); do not refrigerate or freeze.

Nursing Actions

Physical Assessment For use only with a clear diagnosis of acute migraine or cluster headaches (not for prophylaxis). Cardiovascular status should be evaluated prior to initiating medication and periodically thereafter. Evaluate carefully for use-related cautions (eg, history of, current, or risk factors for coronary heart disease; hepatic impairment; or seizure history). Monitor for hypertension, cardiac event, cerebrovascular event, dizziness, tingling, drowsiness, myalgia, vision alternation, nausea, and vomiting. With SubQ, teach patient appropriate injection technique and syringe/needle disposal.

Patient Education

• Discuss specific use of drug and side effects with patient as it relates to treatment. (HCAHPS: During this hospital stay, were you given any medicine that you had not taken before? Before giving you any new medicine, how often did hospital staff tell you what the medicine was for? How often did hospital staff describe possible side effects in a way you could understand?)

• Patient may experience flushing, head heaviness or pressure, asthenia, fatigue, parageusia, rhinitis, pharyngitis, warmth sensation, or injection site irritation. Have patient report immediately to prescriber blindness, paresthesia, skin discoloration, constipation, considerable dyspepsia, melena, weight loss, leg cramps, leg pain, temperature sensitivity, paresthesia of feet, dyspnea, hearing impairment, serotonin syndrome (ie, dizziness, severe headache, agitation, hallucinations, tachycardia, arrhythmia, flushing, tremors, hyperhidrosis, change in balance, illogical thinking, severe nausea, significant diarrhea), signs of severe cardiac abnormalities, strength differences from one side to another, difficulty speaking or thinking, or vision changes (HCAHPS).

• Educate patient about signs of a significant reaction (eg, wheezing; chest tightness; fever; itching; bad cough; blue skin color; seizures; or swelling of face, lips, tongue, or throat). **Note:** This is not a comprehensive list of all side effects. Patient should consult prescriber for additional questions.

Intended Use and Disclaimer: Should not be printed and given to patients. This information is intended to serve as a concise initial reference for healthcare professionals to use when discussing medications with a patient. You must ultimately rely on your own discretion, experience and judgment in diagnosing, treating and advising patients.

Sumatriptan and Naproxen
(soo ma TRIP tan & na PROKS en)

Brand Names: U.S. Treximet®

Index Terms Naproxen and Sumatriptan; Naproxen Sodium and Sumatriptan; Naproxen Sodium and Sumatriptan Succinate; Sumatriptan Succinate and Naproxen; Sumatriptan Succinate and Naproxen Sodium

Pharmacologic Category Antimigraine Agent; Nonsteroidal Anti-inflammatory Drug (NSAID), Oral; Serotonin 5-HT$_{1B, 1D}$ Receptor Agonist

Medication Safety Issues

Sound-alike/look-alike issues:

Naproxen may be confused with Natacyn, Nebcin, neomycin, niacin

SUMAtriptan may be confused with somatropin, ZOLMitriptan

Treximet may be confused with Trexall

Medication Guide Available Yes

Pregnancy Risk Factor C

Use Acute treatment of migraine with or without aura

Available Dosage Forms

Tablet, oral:

Treximet® 85/500: Sumatriptan 85 mg and naproxen sodium 500 mg

General Dosage Range Oral: *Adults:* 1 tablet (sumatriptan 85 mg and naproxen 500 mg); may repeat in 2 hours if needed (maximum: 2 tablets/24 hours)

Administration

Oral May be administered with or without food. Swallow tablet whole; tablet should not be divided, crushed, or chewed.

Nursing Actions

Physical Assessment See individual agents.

Patient Education

- Discuss specific use of drug and side effects with patient as it relates to treatment. (HCAHPS: During this hospital stay, were you given any medicine that you had not taken before? Before giving you any new medicine, how often did hospital staff tell you what the medicine was for? How often did hospital staff describe possible side effects in a way you could understand?)
- Patient may experience dizziness, nausea, or xerostomia. Have patient report immediately to prescriber angina, tachycardia, illogical thinking, strength differences from one side to another, severe headache, considerable dyspepsia, fasciculations, diaphoresis, myalgia, intolerable edema, significant weight gain, melena, hematuria, ecchymosis, bleeding, sudden vision changes, eye pain, or eye irritation (HCAHPS).
- Educate patient about signs of a significant reaction (eg, wheezing; chest tightness; fever; itching; bad cough; blue skin color; seizures; or swelling of face, lips, tongue, or throat). **Note:** This is not a comprehensive list of all side effects. Patient should consult prescriber for additional questions.

Intended Use and Disclaimer: Should not be printed and given to patients. This information is intended to serve as a concise initial reference for healthcare professionals to use when discussing medications with a patient. You must ultimately rely on your own discretion, experience and judgment in diagnosing, treating and advising patients.

Related Information

Naproxen *on page 1102*
Oral Medications That Should Not Be Crushed or Altered *on page 1712*
SUMAtriptan *on page 1456*

Tacrolimus (Systemic) (ta KROE li mus)

Brand Names: U.S. Astagraf XL; Hecoria; Prograf
Index Terms FK506
Pharmacologic Category Calcineurin Inhibitor; Immunosuppressant Agent
Medication Safety Issues
Sound-alike/look-alike issues:
Prograf may be confused with Gengraf, PROzac
Tacrolimus may be confused with everolimus, pimecrolimus, sirolimus, temsirolimus

Other safety concerns:
The immediate release (Hecoria, Prograf) and extended release (Astagraf XL, Advagraf [Canadian product]) oral formulations are not interchangeable and are not substitutable.

Medication Guide Available Yes
Pregnancy Risk Factor C
Lactation Enters breast milk/not recommended

Breast-Feeding Considerations Tacrolimus is excreted into breast milk; concentrations are variable and lower than that of the maternal serum. The low bioavailability of tacrolimus following oral absorption may also decrease the amount of exposure to a nursing infant (Bramham, 2013; French, 2003; Gardiner, 2006). In one study, tacrolimus serum concentrations in the infants did not differ between those who were bottle fed or breast-fed (all infants were exposed to tacrolimus throughout pregnancy) (Bramham, 2013). Available information suggests that tacrolimus exposure to the nursing infant is ≤0.5% of the weight-adjusted maternal dose (Bramham, 2013; French, 2003; Gardiner, 2006). The manufacturer recommends that nursing be discontinued, taking into consideration the importance of the drug to the mother.

Use Organ rejection prophylaxis:

U.S. labeling:
Astagraf XL: Prevention of organ rejection in kidney transplant recipients
Hecoria: Prevention of organ rejection in heart, kidney, and liver transplant recipients
Prograf: Prevention of organ rejection in heart, kidney, and liver transplant recipients

Canadian labeling:
Advagraf: Prevention of organ rejection in kidney transplant recipients
Prograf: Prevention of organ rejection in heart, kidney, or liver transplant recipients; treatment of refractory rejection in kidney or liver transplant recipients; treatment of active rheumatoid arthritis in adult patients nonresponsive to disease-modifying antirheumatic drug (DMARD) therapy or when DMARD therapy is inappropriate

Unlabeled Use Prevention of organ rejection in lung, small bowel transplant recipients; prevention and treatment of graft-versus-host disease (GVHD) in allogeneic hematopoietic stem cell transplantation

Mechanism of Action/Effect Suppresses cellular immunity (inhibits T-lymphocyte activation)

Contraindications Hypersensitivity to tacrolimus or any component of the formulation

Warnings/Precautions Hazardous agent: Use appropriate precautions for handling and disposal (NIOSH, 2012). **[U.S. Boxed Warning]: Risk of developing infections (including bacterial, viral [including CMV], fungal, and protozoal infections [including opportunistic infections]) is increased.** Latent viral infections may be activated, including BK virus (associated with polyoma virus-associated nephropathy [PVAN]) and JC virus (associated with progressive multifocal leukoencephalopathy [PML]); may result in serious adverse effects. Immunosuppression increases the risk for CMV viremia and/or CMV disease; the risk of CMV disease is increased for patients who are CMV-seronegative prior to transplant and receive a graft from a CMV-seropositive donor. Consider reduction in immunosuppression if

PVAN, PML, CMV viremia and/or CMV disease occurs. **[U.S. Boxed Warning]: Immunosuppressive therapy may result in the development of lymphoma and other malignancies (predominantly skin malignancies).** The risk for new-onset diabetes and insulin-dependent post-transplant diabetes mellitus (PTDM) is increased with tacrolimus use after transplantation, including in patients without pretransplant history of diabetes mellitus; insulin dependence may be reversible; monitor blood glucose frequently; risk is increased in African-American and Hispanic kidney transplant patients. Nephrotoxicity (acute or chronic) has been reported, especially with higher doses; to avoid excess nephrotoxicity do not administer simultaneously with other nephrotoxic drugs (eg, sirolimus, cyclosporine). Neurotoxicity may occur especially when used in high doses; tremor headache, coma and delirium have been reported and are associated with serum concentrations. Seizures may also occur. Posterior reversible encephalopathy syndrome (PRES) has been reported; symptoms (altered mental status, headache, hypertension, seizures, and visual disturbances) are reversible with dose reduction or discontinuation of therapy; stabilize blood pressure and reduce dose with suspected or confirmed PRES diagnosis.

Pure red cell aplasia (PRCA) has been reported in patients receiving tacrolimus. Use with caution in patients with risk factors for PRCA including parvovirus B19 infection, underlying disease, or use of concomitant medications associated with PRCA (eg, mycophenolate). Discontinuation of therapy should be considered with diagnosis of PRCA. Monitoring of serum concentrations (trough for oral therapy) is essential to prevent organ rejection and reduce drug-related toxicity. Use caution in renal or hepatic dysfunction, dosing adjustments may be required. Delay initiation of therapy in kidney transplant patients if postoperative oliguria occurs; begin therapy no sooner than 6 hours and within 24 hours post-transplant, but may be delayed until renal function has recovered. Mild-to-severe hyperkalemia may occur; monitor serum potassium levels. Hypertension may commonly occur; antihypertensive treatment may be necessary; avoid use of potassium-sparing diuretics due to risk of hyperkalemia; concurrent use of calcium channel blockers may require tacrolimus dosage adjustment. Gastrointestinal perforation may occur; all reported cases were considered to be a complication of transplant surgery or accompanied by infection, diverticulum, or malignant neoplasm. Myocardial hypertrophy has been reported (rare). Prolongation of the QT/QTc and torsade de pointes may occur; avoid use in patients with congenital long QT syndrome. Consider obtaining electrocardiograms and monitoring electrolytes (magnesium, potassium, calcium) periodically during treatment in patients with congestive heart failure, bradyarrhythmias, those taking certain antiarrhythmic medications or other medicinal products that lead to QT prolongation, and those with electrolyte disturbances such as hypokalemia, hypocalcemia, or hypomagnesemia. Potentially significant drug-drug/drug-food interactions may exist, requiring dose or frequency adjustment, additional monitoring, and/or selection of alternative therapy. In liver transplantation, the tacrolimus dose and target range should be reduced to minimize the risk of nephrotoxicity when used in combination with everolimus. Extended release tacrolimus in combination with sirolimus is not recommended in renal transplant patients; the safety and efficacy of immediate release tacrolimus in combination with sirolimus has not been established in this patient population. Concomitant use was associated with increased mortality, graft loss, and hepatic artery thrombosis in liver transplant patients, as well as increased risk of renal impairment, wound healing complications, and PTDM in heart transplant recipients.

Immediate release and extended release capsules are NOT interchangeable or substitutable. The extended release formulation is a once daily preparation; and immediate release is intended for twice daily administration. Serious adverse events, including organ rejection may occur if inadvertently substituted. **[U.S. Boxed Warning]: Extended release tacrolimus was associated with increased mortality in female liver transplant recipients; the use of extended release tacrolimus is not recommended in liver transplantation.** Mortality at 12 months was 18% in females who received extended release tacrolimus compared to 8% for females who received regular release tacrolimus. Each mL of injection contains polyoxyl 60 hydrogenated castor oil (HCO-60) (200 mg) and dehydrated alcohol USP 80% v/v. Anaphylaxis has been reported with the injection, use should be reserved for those patients not able to take oral medications. Patients should not be immunized with live vaccines during or shortly after treatment and should avoid close contact with recently vaccinated (live vaccine) individuals. Oral formulations contain lactose; the Canadian labeling does not recommend use of these products in patients who may be lactose intolerant (eg, Lapp lactase deficiency, glucose-galactose malabsorption, galactose intolerance). **[U.S. Boxed Warning]: Should be administered under the supervision of a physician experienced in immunosuppressive therapy and organ transplantation in a facility appropriate for monitoring and managing therapy.**

Drug Interactions

Avoid Concomitant Use

Avoid concomitant use of Tacrolimus (Systemic) with any of the following: BCG; Bosutinib; CloZAPine; Conivaptan; Crizotinib; CycloSPORINE ▶

(Systemic); Enzalutamide; Eplerenone; Fusidic Acid (Systemic); Grapefruit Juice; Mifepristone; Natalizumab; PAZOPanib; Pimecrolimus; Pimozide; Pomalidomide; Potassium-Sparing Diuretics; Silodosin; Sirolimus; Tacrolimus (Topical); Temsirolimus; Tofacitinib; Topotecan; Vaccines (Live); VinCRIStine (Liposomal)

Decreased Effect

Tacrolimus (Systemic) may decrease the levels/effects of: BCG; Coccidioidin Skin Test; Sipuleucel-T; Vaccines (Inactivated); Vaccines (Live)

The levels/effects of Tacrolimus (Systemic) may be decreased by: Bosentan; Caspofungin; Cinacalcet; CYP3A4 Inducers (Strong); Dabrafenib; Deferasirox; Echinacea; Efavirenz; Enzalutamide; Fosphenytoin; Mitotane; P-glycoprotein/ABCB1 Inducers; Phenytoin; Rifamycin Derivatives; Sirolimus; St Johns Wort; Temsirolimus; Tocilizumab

Increased Effect/Toxicity

Tacrolimus (Systemic) may increase the levels/effects of: Afatinib; ARIPiprazole; Bosutinib; CloZAPine; Colchicine; CycloSPORINE (Systemic); Dabigatran Etexilate; Dofetilide; DOXOrubicin (Conventional); Everolimus; Fenofibrate and Derivatives; Fosphenytoin; Highest Risk QTc-Prolonging Agents; Leflunomide; Lomitapide; Moderate Risk QTc-Prolonging Agents; Natalizumab; PAZOPanib; P-glycoprotein/ABCB1 Substrates; Phenytoin; Pimozide; Pomalidomide; Prucalopride; Rivaroxaban; Silodosin; Sirolimus; Temsirolimus; Tofacitinib; Topotecan; Vaccines (Live); VinCRIStine (Liposomal)

The levels/effects of Tacrolimus (Systemic) may be increased by: Antidepressants (Serotonin Reuptake Inhibitor/Antagonist); Boceprevir; Calcium Channel Blockers (Dihydropyridine); Calcium Channel Blockers (Nondihydropyridine); Chloramphenicol; Clotrimazole (Oral); Conivaptan; Crizotinib; CycloSPORINE (Systemic); CYP3A4 Inhibitors (Moderate); CYP3A4 Inhibitors (Strong); Danazol; Dasatinib; Denosumab; Eplerenone; Ertapenem; Fluconazole; Fusidic Acid (Systemic); Grapefruit Juice; Itraconazole; Ivacaftor; Ketoconazole (Systemic); Levofloxacin (Systemic); Luliconazole; Macrolide Antibiotics; MetroNIDAZOLE (Systemic); Mifepristone; P-glycoprotein/ABCB1 Inhibitors; Pimecrolimus; Posaconazole; Potassium-Sparing Diuretics; Protease Inhibitors; Proton Pump Inhibitors; Ranolazine; Roflumilast; Sirolimus; Stiripentol; Tacrolimus (Topical); Telaprevir; Temsirolimus; Trastuzumab; Voriconazole

Nutritional/Ethanol Interactions

Ethanol: Alcohol may increase the rate of release of extended-release tacrolimus and adversely affect tacrolimus safety and/or efficacy. Management: Avoid alcohol.

Food: Food decreases rate and extent of absorption. High-fat meals have most pronounced effect (37% and 25% decrease in AUC, respectively,

and 77% and 25% decrease in C_{max}, respectively, for immediately release and extended release formulations). Grapefruit juice, a CYP3A4 inhibitor, may increase serum level and/or toxicity of tacrolimus. Management: Administer with or without food (immediate release), but be consistent. Administer extended release on an empty stomach. Avoid concurrent use of grapefruit juice.

Herb/Nutraceutical: St John's wort may reduce tacrolimus serum concentrations. Management: Avoid St John's wort.

Adverse Reactions As reported for kidney, liver, and heart transplantation:

≥15%:

Cardiovascular: Hypertension (13% to 89%), peripheral edema (11% to 36%), chest pain (19%), edema (<15% to 18%), pericardial effusion (heart transplant 15%; Astagraf XL <15%)

Central nervous system: Headache (10% to 64%), insomnia (9% to 64%), pain (24% to 63%), paresthesia (<15% to 40%), dizziness (<15% to 19%), fatigue (2% to 16%)

Dermatologic: Pruritus (<15% to 36%), skin rash (10% to 24%)

Endocrine & metabolic: Diabetes mellitus (posttransplant; kidney transplant 20% to 75%; heart transplant 13% to 22%; liver transplant 11% to 18%), hyperglycemia (16% to 70%), hypertriglyceridemia (65%), hypoglycemia (<15% to 61%), hypercholesterolemia (<15% to 57%), hypophosphatemia (5% to 49%), hypomagnesemia (3% to 48%), hyperkalemia (13% to 45%), hyperlipidemia (7% to 34%), hypokalemia (13% to 29%)

Gastrointestinal: Diarrhea (25% to 72%), abdominal pain (29% to 59%; Astagraf XL <15%), nausea (13% to 46%), constipation (14% to 40%), anorexia (7% to 34%), vomiting (13% to 29%), dyspepsia (18% to 28%; Astagraf XL <15%)

Genitourinary: Urinary tract infection (1% to 34%), oliguria (<15% to 19%)

Hematologic & oncologic: Anemia (5% to 50%; hemoglobin <10 g/dL 65%), leukopenia (11% to 48%), leukocytosis (8% to 32%), thrombocytopenia (14% to 24%)

Hepatic: Abnormal hepatic function tests (6% to 36%), ascites (7% to 27%)

Infection: Infection (15% to 45%), bacterial infection (8% to 41%), cytomegalovirus disease (heart transplant 32%; kidney transplant 6% to 12%), serious infection (19% to 24%)

Local: Postoperative wound complication (kidney transplant 28%)

Neuromuscular & skeletal: Tremor (15% to 56%; heart transplant 15%), weakness (11% to 52%), back pain (17% to 30%), arthralgia (25%; Astagraf XL <15%)

Renal: Renal function abnormality (36% to 56%), increased serum creatinine (16% to 45%), increased blood urea nitrogen (12% to 30%)

Respiratory: Pleural effusion (30% to 36%), respiratory tract infection (22% to 34%), dyspnea (5% to 29%), atelectasis (5% to 28%), cough (<15% to 18%), bronchitis (17%)

Miscellaneous: Fever (19% to 48%), postoperative pain (kidney transplant 29%), graft complications (kidney transplant 14% to 24%)

<15%:

Cardiovascular: Angina pectoris, atrial fibrillation, atrial flutter, bradycardia, cardiac arrest, cardiac arrhythmia, cardiac failure, cardiorespiratory arrest, cerebral infarction, cerebral ischemia, decreased heart rate, deep vein thrombophlebitis, deep vein thrombosis, ECG abnormality (QRS or ST segment or T wave), flushing, hemorrhagic stroke, hypertrophic cardiomyopathy, hypotension, ischemic heart disease, myocardial infarction, orthostatic hypotension, peripheral vascular disease, phlebitis, syncope, tachycardia, thrombosis, vasodilatation, ventricular premature contractions

Central nervous system: Abnormal dreams, abnormality in thinking, agitation, amnesia, anxiety, aphasia, ataxia, brain disease, carpal tunnel syndrome, chills, confusion, convulsions, depression, drowsiness, emotional lability, excessive crying, falling, flaccid paralysis, hallucination, hypertonia, hypoesthesia, mental status changes, mood elevation, myasthenia, myoclonus, nervousness, neurotoxicity, nightmares, paresis, peripheral neuropathy, psychosis, seizure, vertigo, voice disorder, writing difficulty

Dermatologic: Acne vulgaris, alopecia, bruise, cellulitis, condyloma acuminatum, dermal ulcer, dermatitis (including fungal), dermatological reaction, diaphoresis, exfoliative dermatitis, hypotrichosis, skin discoloration, skin photosensitivity

Endocrine & metabolic: Acidosis, albuminuria, alkalosis, anasarca, Cushing's syndrome, decreased serum bicarbonate, decreased serum iron, dehydration, gout, hirsutism, hypercalcemia, hyperphosphatemia, hyperuricemia, hypervolemia, hypocalcemia, hyponatremia, increased gamma-glutamyl transferase, increased lactate dehydrogenase, weight changes

Gastrointestinal: Gastroenteritis (2% to 7%), aphthous stomatitis, cholangitis, colitis, delayed gastric emptying, duodenitis, dysphagia, enlargement of abdomen, esophagitis (including ulcerative), flatulence, gastric ulcer, gastritis, gastroesophageal reflux disease, gastrointestinal hemorrhage, gastrointestinal perforation, hernia, hiccups, increased appetite, intestinal obstruction, oral candidiasis, pancreatic disease (pseudocyst), pancreatitis (including hemorrhagic and necrotizing), peritonitis, rectal disease, stomach cramps, stomatitis

Genitourinary: Anuria, bladder spasm, cystitis, dysuria, hematuria, nocturia, proteinuria, toxic nephrosis, urinary frequency, urinary incontinence, urinary retention, urinary urgency, vaginitis

Hematologic & oncologic: Blood coagulation disorder, decreased prothrombin time, hemolytic anemia, hemorrhage, hypochromic anemia, hypoproteinemia, increased hematocrit, increased INR, Kaposi's sarcoma, malignant neoplasm of bladder, malignant neoplasm of thyroid (papillary), neutropenia, pancytopenia, polycythemia, skin neoplasm

Hepatic: Cholestatic jaundice, hepatic injury, hepatitis (including acute, chronic, and granulomatous), hyperbilirubinemia, increased liver enzymes, increased serum alkaline phosphatase, jaundice

Hypersensitivity: Hypersensitivity reaction

Infection: Polyoma virus infection (≤5%), abscess, Epstein Barr virus infection, herpes simplex infection, sepsis, tinea versicolor

Local: Localized phlebitis

Neuromuscular & skeletal: Arthropathy, leg cramps, muscle spasm, muscle weakness of the extremities, myalgia, neuropathy (including compression), osteopenia, osteoporosis

Ophthalmic: Amblyopia, blurred vision, conjunctivitis, visual disturbance

Otic: Hearing loss, otalgia, otitis externa, otitis media, tinnitus

Renal: Acute renal failure, hydronephrosis, renal disease (BK nephropathy), renal tubular necrosis

Respiratory: Allergic rhinitis, asthma, emphysema, flu-like symptoms, pharyngitis, pneumonia, pneumothorax, pulmonary disease, pulmonary edema, pulmonary infiltrates, respiratory depression, respiratory failure, rhinitis, sinusitis

Miscellaneous: Wound healing impairment

Available Dosage Forms

Capsule, Oral:

Hecoria: 0.5 mg, 1 mg, 5 mg

Prograf: 0.5 mg, 1 mg, 5 mg

Generic: 0.5 mg, 1 mg, 5 mg

Capsule Extended Release 24 Hour, Oral:

Astagraf XL: 0.5 mg, 1 mg, 5 mg

Solution, Intravenous:

Prograf: 5 mg/mL (1 mL)

General Dosage Range

I.V.:

Children: 0.03-0.05 mg/kg/day as a continuous infusion

Adults: 0.01-0.05 mg/kg/day as a continuous infusion

Oral: Immediate release:

Children: 0.15-0.2 mg/kg/day in divided doses every 12 hours (titrate to target trough)

Adults: 0.075-0.2 mg/kg/day in divided doses every 12 hours (titrate to target trough)

◄ **Oral:** Extended release: *Adults:* 0.1 mg/kg as a single dose **or** 0.15-0.2 mg/kg once daily (titrate to target trough)

Administration

I.V. If I.V. administration is necessary, administer by continuous infusion only. Do not use PVC tubing when administering diluted solutions. Tacrolimus is usually intended to be administered as a continuous infusion over 24 hours. Do not mix with solutions with a pH ≥9 (eg, acyclovir or ganciclovir) due to chemical degradation of tacrolimus (use different ports in multilumen lines). Do not alter dose with concurrent T-tube clamping. Adsorption of the drug to PVC tubing may become clinically significant with low concentrations.

Hazardous agent - use appropriate precautions for handling and disposal (NIOSH, 2012).

Oral

Immediate release: Administer with or without food; be consistent with timing and composition of meals if GI intolerance occurs and administration with food becomes necessary (per manufacturer). If dosed once daily, administer in the morning. If dosed twice daily, doses should be 12 hours apart. If the morning and evening doses differ, the larger dose (differences are never >0.5-1 mg) should be given in the morning. If dosed 3 times daily, separate doses by 8 hours.

Combination therapy with everolimus for liver transplantation: Administer tacrolimus at the same time as everolimus.

Extended release: Administer on an empty stomach at least 1 hour before or 2 hours after a meal. Swallow whole, do not chew, crush, or divide. Take once daily in the morning at a consistent time each day. Missed doses may be taken up to 14 hours after scheduled time; if >14 hours, resume at next regularly scheduled time; do not double a dose to make up for a missed dose.

Hazardous agent - use appropriate precautions for handling and disposal (NIOSH, 2012).

Preparation for Administration Hazardous agent - use appropriate precautions for handling and disposal (NIOSH, 2012).

Injection: Dilute with 5% dextrose injection or 0.9% sodium chloride injection to a final concentration between 0.004 mg/mL and 0.02 mg/mL.

Storage/Stability

Injection: Prior to dilution, store at 5°C to 25°C (41°F to 77°F). Following dilution, stable for 24 hours in D_5W or NS in glass or polyethylene containers.

Capsules:

Astagraf XL, Prograf: Store at 25°C (77°F); excursions permitted between 15°C and 30°C (59°F and 86°F).

Hecoria: Store at 20°C to 25°C (68°F to 77°F).

Nursing Actions

Physical Assessment Monitor blood pressure frequently; can cause hypertension. Teach patient how to monitor blood glucose levels. Have patient bring glucose diary to clinic. Monitor for signs of opportunistic infection (eg, persistent fever, malaise, sore throat, unusual bleeding, or bruising). Monitor for signs and symptoms to neurotoxicity including headache, altered mental status, seizure, visual disturbance, delirium, and coma. Check lab and ECG results.

Patient Education

• Discuss specific use of drug and side effects with patient as it relates to treatment. (HCAHPS: During this hospital stay, were you given any medicine that you had not taken before? Before giving you any new medicine, how often did hospital staff tell you what the medicine was for? How often did hospital staff describe possible side effects in a way you could understand?)

• Patient may experience hypertension, renal impairment, dizziness, headache, nausea, diarrhea, insomnia, or erythema. Have patient report immediately to prescriber signs of infection, ecchymosis, bleeding, polyuria, polydipsia, weight loss, urinary retention, severe edema, or rash (HCAHPS).

• Educate patient about signs of a significant reaction (eg, wheezing; chest tightness; fever; itching; bad cough; blue skin color; seizures; or swelling of face, lips, tongue, or throat). **Note:** This is not a comprehensive list of all side effects. Patient should consult prescriber for additional questions.

Intended Use and Disclaimer: Should not be printed and given to patients. This information is intended to serve as a concise initial reference for healthcare professionals to use when discussing medications with a patient. You must ultimately rely on your own discretion, experience and judgment in diagnosing, treating and advising patients.

Dietary Considerations Capsule: Administer immediate release with or without food; be consistent with timing and composition of meals, food decreases bioavailability. Administer extended release on an empty stomach 1 hour before or 2 hours after a meal. Avoid grapefruit juice. Avoid alcohol.

Related Information

Oral Medications That Should Not Be Crushed or Altered *on page 1712*

Tacrolimus (Topical) (ta KROE li mus)

Brand Names: U.S. Protopic

Pharmacologic Category Calcineurin Inhibitor; Immunosuppressant Agent; Topical Skin Product

Medication Safety Issues
Sound-alike/look-alike issues:
Tacrolimus may be confused with everolimus, pimecrolimus, sirolimus, temsirolimus
Medication Guide Available Yes
Pregnancy Risk Factor C
Lactation Enters breast milk/not recommended
Use Moderate-to-severe atopic dermatitis in immunocompetent patients not responsive to conventional therapy or when conventional therapy is not appropriate
Canadian labeling: Additional use (not in U.S. labeling): Maintenance therapy to prevent flares and extend flare-free intervals in patients with moderate-to-severe atopic dermatitis who are responsive to initial therapy and experiencing ≥5 flares per year

Available Dosage Forms
Ointment, External:
Protopic: 0.03% (30 g, 60 g, 100 g); 0.1% (30 g, 60 g, 100 g)

General Dosage Range Topical:
Children ≥2-15 years: Apply thin layer of 0.03% to affected area twice daily
Children >15 years and Adults: Apply thin layer of 0.03% or 0.1% to affected area twice daily

Administration
Topical Do not use with occlusive dressings. Burning at the application site is most common in first few days; improves as atopic dermatitis improves. Limit application to involved areas. Continue as long as signs and symptoms persist; discontinue if resolution occurs; re-evaluate if symptoms persist >6 weeks.

Hazardous agent; use appropriate precautions for handling and disposal (NIOSH, 2012).

Nursing Actions
Physical Assessment Monitor for signs of opportunistic infection.
Patient Education
• Discuss specific use of drug and side effects with patient as it relates to treatment. (HCAHPS: During this hospital stay, were you given any medicine that you had not taken before? Before giving you any new medicine, how often did hospital staff tell you what the medicine was for? How often did hospital staff describe possible side effects in a way you could understand?)
• Patient may experience flu-like syndrome, headache, or skin irritation. Have patient report immediately to prescriber signs of infection or rash (HCAHPS).
• Educate patient about signs of a significant reaction (eg, wheezing; chest tightness; fever; itching; bad cough; blue skin color; seizures; or swelling of face, lips, tongue, or throat). **Note:** This is not a comprehensive list of all side effects. Patient should consult prescriber for additional questions.

Intended Use and Disclaimer: Should not be printed and given to patients. This information is intended to serve as a concise initial reference for healthcare professionals to use when discussing medications with a patient. You must ultimately rely on your own discretion, experience and judgment in diagnosing, treating and advising patients.

Tadalafil (tah DA la fil)

Brand Names: U.S. Adcirca; Cialis
Index Terms GF196960
Pharmacologic Category Phosphodiesterase-5 Enzyme Inhibitor
Medication Safety Issues
Sound-alike/look-alike issues:
Tadalafil may be confused with sildenafil, vardenafil
Adcirca may be confused with Advair Diskus, Advair HFA, Advicor
Pregnancy Risk Factor B
Lactation Excretion in breast milk unknown/use caution
Breast-Feeding Considerations It is not known if tadalafil is excreted in breast milk. The manufacturer recommends that caution be exercised when administering tadalafil to nursing women.
Use
Benign prostatic hyperplasia (Cialis only): For the treatment of the signs and symptoms of benign prostatic hyperplasia (BPH).
Erectile dysfunction (Cialis only): For the treatment of erectile dysfunction.
Erectile dysfunction and benign prostatic hyperplasia (Cialis only): For the treatment of erectile dysfunction and the signs and symptoms of BPH.
Pulmonary arterial hypertension (Adcirca only): Pulmonary arterial hypertension (Adcirca only): Studies establishing effectiveness included predominately patients with New York Heart Association (NYHA) functional class II to III symptoms and etiologies of idiopathic or heritable pulmonary arterial hypertension (61%) or pulmonary arterial hypertension associated with connective tissue diseases (23%).
Mechanism of Action/Effect
BPH: Exact mechanism unknown; effects likely due to PDE-5 mediated reduction and/or relaxation of prostate and bladder tissues, nerves and muscles
Erectile dysfunction: Tadalafil enhances the effect of nitric oxide (NO) by inhibiting phosphodiesterase type 5 (PDE-5), which is responsible for degradation of cGMP in the corpus cavernosum; when sexual stimulation causes local release of NO, inhibition of PDE-5 by tadalafil causes increased levels of cGMP in the corpus cavernosum, resulting in smooth muscle relaxation and inflow of blood to the corpus cavernosum. At ▶

recommended doses, it has no effect in the absence of sexual stimulation.

PAH: Inhibits phosphodiesterase type 5 (PDE-5) in smooth muscle of pulmonary vasculature where PDE-5 is responsible for the degradation of cyclic guanosine monophosphate (cGMP). Increased cGMP concentration results in pulmonary vasculature relaxation; vasodilation in the pulmonary bed and the systemic circulation (to a lesser degree) may occur.

Contraindications Known serious hypersensitivity to tadalafil or any component of the formulation; concurrent use (regularly/intermittently) of organic nitrates in any form (eg, nitroglycerin, isosorbide dinitrate)

Warnings/Precautions There is a degree of cardiac risk associated with sexual activity; therefore, physicians should consider the cardiovascular status of their patients prior to initiation. Use is not recommended in patients with hypotension (<90/50 mm Hg), uncontrolled hypertension (>170/100 mm Hg), NYHA class II-IV heart failure within the last 6 months, uncontrolled arrhythmias, stroke within the last 6 months, MI within the last 3 months, unstable angina or angina during sexual intercourse; safety and efficacy have not been evaluated in these patients. Safety and efficacy in PAH have not been evaluated in patients with clinically significant aortic and/or mitral valve disease, life-threatening arrhythmias, hypotension (<90/50 mm Hg), uncontrolled hypertension, significant left ventricular dysfunction, pericardial constriction, restrictive or congestive cardiomyopathy, symptomatic coronary artery disease. Use caution in patients with left ventricular outflow obstruction (eg, aortic stenosis, hypertrophic obstructive cardiomyopathy); may be more sensitive to vasodilator effects.

Patients experiencing anginal chest pain after tadalafil administration should seek immediate medical attention. Concomitant use (regularly/intermittently) with all forms of nitrates is contraindicated. When used for BPH, erectile dysfunction, or PAH and nitrate administration is medically necessary following use, at least 48 hours should elapse after the tadalafil dose and nitrate administration. When used for PAH, per the manufacturer, nitrate may be administered within 48 hours of tadalafil. For both situations, administration of nitrates should only be done under close medical supervision with hemodynamic monitoring.

Concurrent use with alpha-adrenergic antagonist therapy may cause symptomatic hypotension; patients should be hemodynamically stable prior to initiating tadalafil therapy at the lowest possible dose. Avoid or limit concurrent substantial alcohol consumption as this may increase the risk of symptomatic hypotension. When used for BPH or erectile dysfunction, use caution in patients receiving strong CYP3A4 inhibitors. When used for PAH, avoid use in patients taking strong CYP3A4 inducers/inhibitors. Use in patients receiving or about to receive ritonavir requires dosage adjustment or interruption of therapy, respectively. Canadian labeling does not recommend use of tadalafil in patients with PAH who are also receiving protease inhibitors.

Pulmonary vasodilators may exacerbate the cardiovascular status in patients with pulmonary veno-occlusive disease (PVOD); use is not recommended. In patients with unrecognized PVOD, signs of pulmonary edema should prompt investigation into this diagnosis. Use with caution in patients with mild-to-moderate hepatic impairment; dosage adjustment/limitation is needed. Use is not recommended in patients with severe hepatic impairment or cirrhosis. Use with caution in patients with renal impairment; dosage adjustment/limitation is needed. Safety and efficacy with other tadalafil brands or other PDE-5 inhibitors (ie, sildenafil and vardenafil) have not been established. Patients should be informed not to take with other tadalafil brands or other PDE-5 inhibitors. Use caution in patients with bleeding disorders or peptic ulcer disease due to effect on platelets (bleeding).

When used to treat BPH or erectile dysfunction, potential underlying causes of BPH or erectile dysfunction should be evaluated prior to treatment. Use with caution in patients with anatomical deformation of the penis (angulation, cavernosal fibrosis, or Peyronie's disease), or who have conditions which may predispose them to priapism (sickle cell anemia, multiple myeloma, leukemia). Instruct patients to seek immediate medical attention if erection persists >4 hours. Safety and efficacy with other tadalafil brands or other PDE-5 inhibitors (ie, sildenafil and vardenafil) have not been established. Patients should be informed not to take with other tadalafil brands or other PDE-5 inhibitors. The safety and efficacy of tadalafil with other treatments for erectile dysfunction have not been studied and are, therefore, not recommended as combination therapy.

Rare cases of nonarteritic anterior ischemic optic neuropathy (NAION) have been reported; risk may be increased with history of vision loss or NAION in one eye. Other risk factors for NAION include heart disease, diabetes, hypertension, smoking, age >50 years, or history of certain eye problems. Sudden decrease or loss of hearing has been reported rarely; hearing changes may be accompanied by tinnitus and dizziness. A direct relationship between therapy and vision or hearing loss has not been determined. Instruct patients to seek medical assistance for sudden loss of vision in one or both eyes, sudden decrease in hearing, or sudden loss of hearing.

Patients with genetic retinal disorders (eg, retinitis pigmentosa) were not evaluated in clinical trials; use is not recommended. Use with caution in the elderly.

Drug Interactions

Avoid Concomitant Use

Avoid concomitant use of Tadalafil with any of the following: Alprostadil; Amyl Nitrite; Fusidic Acid (Systemic); Phosphodiesterase 5 Inhibitors; Riociguat; Vasodilators (Organic Nitrates)

Decreased Effect

The levels/effects of Tadalafil may be decreased by: Bosentan; CYP3A4 Inducers (Strong); Etravirine

Increased Effect/Toxicity

Tadalafil may increase the levels/effects of: Alpha1-Blockers; Alprostadil; Amyl Nitrite; Antihypertensives; Bosentan; Phosphodiesterase 5 Inhibitors; Riociguat; Vasodilators (Organic Nitrates)

The levels/effects of Tadalafil may be increased by: Alcohol (Ethyl); Boceprevir; Cobicistat; CYP3A4 Inhibitors (Moderate); CYP3A4 Inhibitors (Strong); Dasatinib; Fluconazole; Fusidic Acid (Systemic); Itraconazole; Ivacaftor; Ketoconazole (Systemic); Lorcaserin; Luliconazole; Mifepristone; Posaconazole; Ritonavir; Sapropterin; Simeprevir; Telaprevir; Voriconazole

Nutritional/Ethanol Interactions Ethanol: Substantial consumption of ethanol may increase the risk of hypotension and orthostasis. Lower ethanol consumption has not been associated with significant changes in blood pressure or increase in orthostatic symptoms. Management: Avoid or limit ethanol consumption.

Food: Rate and extent of absorption are not affected by food. Grapefruit juice may increase serum levels/toxicity of tadalafil. Management: Use of grapefruit juice should be limited or avoided.

Herb/Nutraceutical: St John's wort may decrease the levels/effectiveness of tadalafil. Management: Avoid or use caution with concomitant use.

Adverse Reactions Based upon usual doses for either indication. For erectile dysfunction, similar adverse events are reported with once-daily versus intermittent dosing, but are generally lower than with doses used intermittently.

>10%:
Cardiovascular: Flushing (1% to 13%; dose related)
Central nervous system: Headache (3% to 42%; dose related)
Gastrointestinal: Dyspepsia (1% to 13%), nausea (10% to 11%)
Neuromuscular & skeletal: Myalgia (1% to 14%; dose related), back pain (2% to 12%), extremity pain (1% to 11%)
Respiratory: Respiratory tract infection (3% to 13%), nasopharyngitis (2% to 13%)

2% to 10%:
Cardiovascular: Hypertension (1% to 3%)
Gastrointestinal: Gastroenteritis (viral; 3% to 5%), GERD (1% to 3%), abdominal pain (1% to 2%), diarrhea (1% to 2%)
Genitourinary: Urinary tract infection (≤2%)
Respiratory: Nasal congestion (≤9%), cough (2% to 4%), bronchitis (≤2%)
Miscellaneous: Flu-like syndrome (2% to 5%)

Pharmacodynamics/Kinetics

Onset of Action Within 1 hour
Peak effect: Pulmonary artery vasodilation: 75-90 minutes (Ghofrani, 2004)

Duration of Action Erectile dysfunction: Up to 36 hours

Available Dosage Forms

Tablet, Oral:
Adcirca: 20 mg
Cialis: 2.5 mg, 5 mg, 10 mg, 20 mg

General Dosage Range Dosage adjustment recommended in patient with hepatic or renal impairment or on concomitant therapy

Oral: *Adults:* Benign prostatic hyperplasia: 5 mg once daily; Erectile dysfunction: As-needed dosing: 5-20 mg prior to anticipated sexual activity as a single dose (maximum: 1 dose/day); Once-daily dosing: 2.5-5 mg once daily; Pulmonary arterial hypertension: 40 mg once daily

Administration

Oral May be administered with or without food.
Adcirca®: Administer daily dose all at once; dividing doses throughout the day is not advised.
Cialis®: When used on an as-needed basis, should be taken at least 30 minutes prior to sexual activity. When used on a once-daily basis, should be taken at the same time each day, without regard to timing of sexual activity.

Storage/Stability Store at 25°C (77°F); excursions permitted to 15°C to 30°C (59°F to 86°F).

Nursing Actions

Physical Assessment Monitor for postural hypotension.

Patient Education
• Discuss specific use of drug and side effects with patient as it relates to treatment. (HCAHPS: During this hospital stay, were you given any medicine that you had not taken before? Before giving you any new medicine, how often did hospital staff tell you what the medicine was for? How often did hospital staff describe possible side effects in a way you could understand?)
• Patient may experience flushing, headache, dyspepsia, pyrosis, back pain, rhinitis, or vision changes. Have patient report immediately to prescriber erection lasting >4 hours, angina, tachycardia, severe dizziness, hearing impairment, or rash (HCAHPS).

• Educate patient about signs of a significant reaction (eg, wheezing; chest tightness; fever; itching; bad cough; blue skin color; seizures; or swelling of face, lips, tongue, or throat). **Note:** This is not a comprehensive list of all side effects. Patient should consult prescriber for additional questions.

Intended Use and Disclaimer: Should not be printed and given to patients. This information is intended to serve as a concise initial reference for healthcare professionals to use when discussing medications with a patient. You must ultimately rely on your own discretion, experience and judgment in diagnosing, treating and advising patients.

Dietary Considerations May be taken with or without food.

Tafluprost (TA floo prost)

Brand Names: U.S. Zioptan
Pharmacologic Category Ophthalmic Agent, Antiglaucoma; Prostaglandin, Ophthalmic
Pregnancy Risk Factor C
Lactation Excretion in breast milk unknown/use caution
Use Reduction of intraocular pressure (IOP) in patients with open-angle glaucoma or ocular hypertension
Available Dosage Forms
Solution, Ophthalmic [preservative free]:
Zioptan: 0.0015% (30 ea, 90 ea)
General Dosage Range Ophthalmic: *Adults:* One drop in the affected eye(s) once daily
Administration
Other For ophthalmic use only. Wash hands before use. Avoid touching the tip of the single-use container to eye or other surfaces. Each single-use container has adequate solution to treat both eyes (if applicable); discard immediately after use. If more than one topical ophthalmic drug is being used, administer the drugs at least 5 minutes apart.
Nursing Actions
Physical Assessment Monitor for blurred vision, burning and stinging, conjunctival hyperemia, foreign body sensation, itching, increased pigmentation of the iris, and punctate epithelial keratopathy.
Patient Education
• Discuss specific use of drug and side effects with patient as it relates to treatment. (HCAHPS: During this hospital stay, were you given any medicine that you had not taken before? Before giving you any new medicine, how often did hospital staff tell you what the medicine was for? How often did hospital staff describe possible side effects in a way you could understand?)
• Patient may experience eye irritation, blurred vision, or change in eye color. Have patient

report immediately to prescriber sudden vision changes, eye pain, or rash (HCAHPS).
• Educate patient about signs of a significant reaction (eg, wheezing; chest tightness; fever; itching; bad cough; blue skin color; seizures; or swelling of face, lips, tongue, or throat). **Note:** This is not a comprehensive list of all side effects. Patient should consult prescriber for additional questions.

Intended Use and Disclaimer: Should not be printed and given to patients. This information is intended to serve as a concise initial reference for healthcare professionals to use when discussing medications with a patient. You must ultimately rely on your own discretion, experience and judgment in diagnosing, treating and advising patients.

Tamoxifen (ta MOKS i fen)

Brand Names: U.S. Soltamox
Index Terms ICI-46474; Nolvadex; Tamoxifen Citras; Tamoxifen Citrate
Pharmacologic Category Antineoplastic Agent, Estrogen Receptor Antagonist; Selective Estrogen Receptor Modulator (SERM)
Medication Safety Issues
Sound-alike/look-alike issues:
Tamoxifen may be confused with pentoxifylline, Tambocor™, tamsulosin, temazepam
Medication Guide Available Yes
Pregnancy Risk Factor D
Lactation Excretion in breast milk unknown/not recommended
Breast-Feeding Considerations It is not known if tamoxifen is excreted in breast milk, however, it has been shown to inhibit lactation. Due to the potential for adverse reactions, women taking tamoxifen should not breast-feed.
Use Treatment of metastatic (female and male) breast cancer; adjuvant treatment of breast cancer after primary treatment with surgery and radiation; reduce risk of invasive breast cancer in women with ductal carcinoma *in situ* (DCIS) after surgery and radiation; reduce the incidence of breast cancer in women at high risk
Unlabeled Use Treatment of mastalgia, gynecomastia, ovarian cancer, endometrial cancer, and desmoid tumors; risk reduction in women with Paget's disease of the breast (with ER-positive DCIS or without associated cancer); induction of ovulation; treatment of precocious puberty in females, secondary to McCune-Albright syndrome
Mechanism of Action/Effect Competitively binds to estrogen receptors on tumors and other tissue targets, producing a nuclear complex that decreases DNA synthesis and inhibits estrogen effects; nonsteroidal agent with potent antiestrogenic properties which compete with estrogen for binding sites in breast and other tissues; cells

accumulate in the G_0 and G_1 phases; therefore, tamoxifen is cytostatic rather than cytocidal.

Contraindications Hypersensitivity to tamoxifen or any component of the formulation; concurrent warfarin therapy or history of deep vein thrombosis or pulmonary embolism (when tamoxifen is used for breast cancer risk reduction in women at high risk for breast cancer or with ductal carcinoma *in situ* [DCIS])

Warnings/Precautions Hazardous agent - use appropriate precautions for handling and disposal (NIOSH, 2012). **[U.S. Boxed Warning]: Serious and life-threatening events (some fatal), including stroke, pulmonary emboli, and uterine or endometrial malignancies, have occurred at an incidence greater than placebo during use for breast cancer risk reduction in women at high-risk for breast cancer and in women with ductal carcinoma *in situ* (DCIS). In women already diagnosed with breast cancer, the benefits of tamoxifen treatment outweigh risks; evaluate risks versus benefits (and discuss with patients) when used for breast cancer risk reduction.** An increased incidence of thromboembolic events, including DVT and pulmonary embolism, has been associated with use for breast cancer; risk is increased with concomitant chemotherapy; use with caution in individuals with a history of thromboembolic events. Thrombocytopenia and/or leukopenia may occur; neutropenia and pancytopenia have been reported rarely. Although the relationship to tamoxifen therapy is uncertain, rare hemorrhagic episodes have occurred in patients with significant thrombocytopenia. Use with caution in patients with hyperlipidemias; infrequent postmarketing cases of hyperlipidemias have been reported. Decreased visual acuity, retinal vein thrombosis, retinopathy, corneal changes, color perception changes, and increased incidence of cataracts (and the need for cataract surgery), have been reported. Hypercalcemia has occurred in some patients with bone metastasis, usually within a few weeks of therapy initiation; institute appropriate hypercalcemia management; discontinue if severe. Local disease flare and increased bone and tumor pain may occur in patients with metastatic breast cancer; may be associated with (good) tumor response.

Potentially significant drug-drug interactions may exist, requiring dose or frequency adjustment, additional monitoring, and/or selection of alternative therapy. Decreased efficacy and an increased risk of breast cancer recurrence has been reported with concurrent moderate or strong CYP2D6 inhibitors (Aubert, 2009; Dezentje, 2009). Concomitant use with select SSRIs may result in decreased tamoxifen efficacy. Strong CYP2D6 inhibitors (eg, fluoxetine, paroxetine) and moderate CYP2D6 inhibitors (eg, sertraline) are reported to interfere with transformation to the active metabolite

endoxifen; when possible, select alternative medications with minimal or no impact on endoxifen levels (NCCN Breast Cancer Risk Reduction Guidelines v.1.2013; Sideras, 2010). Weak CYP2D6 inhibitors (eg, venlafaxine, citalopram) have minimal effect on the conversion to endoxifen (Jin, 2005; NCCN Breast Cancer Risk Reduction Guidelines v.1.2013); escitalopram is also a weak CYP2D6 inhibitor. In a retrospective analysis of breast cancer patients taking tamoxifen and SSRIs, concomitant use of paroxetine and tamoxifen was associated with an increased risk of death due to breast cancer (Kelly, 2010). Lower plasma concentrations of endoxifen have been observed in patients associated with reduced CYP2D6 activity (Jin, 2005; Schroth, 2009) and may be associated with reduced efficacy, although data is conflicting. Routine CYP2D6 testing is not recommended at this time in order to determine optimal endocrine therapy (NCCN Breast Cancer Guidelines v.2.2013; Visvanathan, 2009).

Tamoxifen use may be associated with changes in bone mineral density (BMD) and the effects may be dependent upon menstrual status. In postmenopausal women, tamoxifen use is associated with a protective effect on bone mineral density (BMD), preventing loss of BMD which lasts over the 5-year treatment period. In premenopausal women, a decline (from baseline) in BMD mineral density has been observed in women who continued to menstruate; may be associated with an increased risk of fractures. Liver abnormalities such as cholestasis, fatty liver, hepatitis, and hepatic necrosis have occurred. Hepatocellular carcinomas have been reported in some studies; relationship to treatment is unclear. Tamoxifen is associated with an increased incidence of uterine or endometrial cancers. Endometrial hyperplasia, polyps, endometriosis, uterine fibroids, and ovarian cysts have occurred. Monitor and promptly evaluate any report of abnormal vaginal bleeding. Amenorrhea and menstrual irregularities have been reported with tamoxifen use.

Drug Interactions

Avoid Concomitant Use

Avoid concomitant use of Tamoxifen with any of the following: Bosutinib; Conivaptan; CYP2D6 Inhibitors (Strong); Fusidic Acid (Systemic); Ospemifene; PAZOPanib; Pimozide; Pomalidomide; Silodosin; Topotecan; VinCRIStine (Liposomal); Vitamin K Antagonists

Decreased Effect

Tamoxifen may decrease the levels/effects of: Anastrozole; Letrozole; Ospemifene

The levels/effects of Tamoxifen may be decreased by: Aminoglutethimide; Bexarotene (Systemic); Bosentan; CYP2C9 Inducers (Strong); CYP2D6 Inhibitors (Moderate); CYP2D6 Inhibitors (Strong); CYP3A4 Inducers (Strong); Dabrafenib; Deferasirox; Herbs (CYP3A4

Inducers); Mitotane; Peginterferon Alfa-2b; Rifamycin Derivatives; Tocilizumab

Increased Effect/Toxicity

Tamoxifen may increase the levels/effects of: Afatinib; ARIPiprazole; Bosutinib; Colchicine; CYP2C8 Substrates; Dabigatran Etexilate; Dofetilide; DOXOrubicin (Conventional); Everolimus; Highest Risk QTc-Prolonging Agents; Lomitapide; Mipomersen; Moderate Risk QTc-Prolonging Agents; Ospemifene; PAZOPanib; P-glycoprotein/ABCB1 Substrates; Pimozide; Pomalidomide; Prucalopride; Rivaroxaban; Silodosin; Topotecan; VinCRIStine (Liposomal); Vitamin K Antagonists

The levels/effects of Tamoxifen may be increased by: Abiraterone Acetate; Conivaptan; CYP2C9 Inhibitors (Moderate); CYP2C9 Inhibitors (Strong); CYP3A4 Inhibitors (Moderate); CYP3A4 Inhibitors (Strong); Darunavir; Dasatinib; Fusidic Acid (Systemic); Ivacaftor; Luliconazole; Mifepristone; Simeprevir

Nutritional/Ethanol Interactions

Food: Grapefruit juice may decrease the metabolism of tamoxifen. Management: Avoid grapefruit juice.

Herb/Nutraceutical: Black cohosh and dong quai have estrogenic properties. St John's wort may decrease levels/effects of tamoxifen. Management: Avoid black cohosh and dong quai in estrogen-dependent tumors. Avoid St John's wort.

Adverse Reactions

>10%:

Cardiovascular: Vasodilation (41%), flushing (33%), hypertension (11%), peripheral edema (11%)

Central nervous system: Mood changes (12% to 18%), pain (3% to 16%), depression (2% to 12%)

Dermatologic: Skin changes (6% to 19%), rash (13%)

Endocrine & metabolic: Hot flashes (3% to 80%), fluid retention (32%), altered menses (13% to 25%), amenorrhea (16%)

Gastrointestinal: Nausea (5% to 26%), weight loss (23%), vomiting (12%)

Genitourinary: Vaginal discharge (13% to 55%), vaginal bleeding (2% to 23%)

Neuromuscular & skeletal: Weakness (18%), arthritis (14%), arthralgia (11%)

Respiratory: Pharyngitis (14%)

Miscellaneous: Lymphedema (11%)

1% to 10%:

Cardiovascular: Chest pain (5%), venous thrombotic events (5%), edema (4%), cardiovascular ischemia (3%), angina (2%), deep venous thrombus (≤2%), MI (1%)

Central nervous system: Insomnia (9%), dizziness (8%), headache (8%), anxiety (6%), fatigue (4%)

Dermatologic: Alopecia (≤5%)

Endocrine & metabolic: Oligomenorrhea (9%), breast pain (6%), menstrual disorder (6%), breast neoplasm (5%), hypercholesterolemia (4%)

Gastrointestinal: Abdominal pain (9%), weight gain (9%), constipation (4% to 8%), diarrhea (7%), dyspepsia (6%), throat irritation (oral solution 5%), abdominal cramps (1%), anorexia (1%)

Genitourinary: Urinary tract infection (10%), leukorrhea (9%), vaginal hemorrhage (6%), vaginitis (5%), vulvovaginitis (5%), ovarian cyst (3%)

Hematologic: Thrombocytopenia (≤10%), anemia (5%)

Hepatic: AST increased (5%), serum bilirubin increased (2%)

Neuromuscular & skeletal: Back pain (10%), bone pain (6% to 10%), osteoporosis (7%), fracture (7%), arthrosis (5%), joint disorder (5%), myalgia (5%), paresthesia (5%), musculoskeletal pain (3%)

Ocular: Cataract (7%)

Renal: Serum creatinine increased (≤2%)

Respiratory: Cough (4% to 9%), dyspnea (8%), bronchitis (5%), sinusitis (5%)

Miscellaneous: Infection/sepsis (≤9%), diaphoresis (6%), flu-like syndrome (6%), cyst (5%), neoplasm (5%), allergic reaction (3%)

Available Dosage Forms

Solution, Oral:

Soltamox: 10 mg/5 mL (150 mL)

Tablet, Oral:

Generic: 10 mg, 20 mg

General Dosage Range Oral: *Adults:* 20-40 mg daily

Administration

Oral Administer tablets or oral solution with or without food. Use supplied dosing cup for oral solution.

Hazardous agent; use appropriate precautions for handling and disposal (NIOSH, 2012).

Storage/Stability

Oral solution: Store at ≤25°C (77°F); do not freeze or refrigerate. Protect from light. Discard opened bottle after 3 months.

Tablets: Store at 20°C to 25°C (68°F to 77°F). Protect from light.

Nursing Actions

Physical Assessment Evaluate for use-related precautions prior to beginning therapy. Monitor for thromboembolism, flushing, fluid retention, hot flashes, vaginal bleeding or discharge, constipation, rash, or mood changes. Teach patient importance of periodic ophthalmic evaluations and annual gynecological exams and mammograms with long-term use.

Patient Education

• Discuss specific use of drug and side effects with patient as it relates to treatment. (HCAHPS: During this hospital stay, were you given any

medicine that you had not taken before? Before giving you any new medicine, how often did hospital staff tell you what the medicine was for? How often did hospital staff describe possible side effects in a way you could understand?)

- Patient may experience flushing, menstrual irregularities, nausea, change in sex ability, vaginal discharge, mood changes, weight loss, or fatigue. Have patient report immediately to prescriber angina, dyspnea, edema in leg or arm, severe lower belly pain, paresthesia, strength differences from one side to another, sudden vision changes, discolored urine, jaundice, inability to eat, or rash (HCAHPS).
- Educate patient about signs of a significant reaction (eg, wheezing; chest tightness; fever; itching; bad cough; blue skin color; seizures; or swelling of face, lips, tongue, or throat). **Note:** This is not a comprehensive list of all side effects. Patient should consult prescriber for additional questions.

Intended Use and Disclaimer: Should not be printed and given to patients. This information is intended to serve as a concise initial reference for healthcare professionals to use when discussing medications with a patient. You must ultimately rely on your own discretion, experience and judgment in diagnosing, treating and advising patients.

Dietary Considerations Tablets and oral solution may be taken with or without food. Avoid grapefruit and grapefruit juice.

Related Information
Oral Medications That Should Not Be Crushed or Altered *on page 1712*

Tamsulosin (tam SOO loe sin)

Brand Names: U.S. Flomax
Index Terms Tamsulosin Hydrochloride
Pharmacologic Category Alpha$_1$ Blocker
Medication Safety Issues
Sound-alike/look-alike issues:
Flomax® may be confused with Flonase®, Flovent®, Foltx®, Fosamax®
Tamsulosin may be confused with tacrolimus, tamoxifen, terazosin

International issues:
Flomax [U.S., Canada, and multiple international markets] may be confused with Flomox brand name for cefcapene [Japan]; Volmax brand name for salbutamol [multiple international markets]
Flomax: Brand name for tamsulosin [U.S., Canada, and multiple international markets], but also the brand name for morniflumate [Italy]

Pregnancy Risk Factor B
Use Treatment of signs and symptoms of benign prostatic hyperplasia (BPH)

Unlabeled Use Symptomatic treatment of bladder outlet obstruction or dysfunction; facilitation of expulsion of ureteral stones

Mechanism of Action/Effect Antagonizes alpha$_{1A}$-adrenoreceptors in the prostate which mediate the dynamic component of urine flow obstruction by regulating smooth muscle tone of the bladder neck and prostate. When given to patients with BPH, blockade of alpha-receptors leads to relaxation of these muscles, resulting in an improvement in urine flow rate and symptoms. Alpha-blockade does not influence the static component of urinary obstruction, which is related to tissue proliferation.

Contraindications Hypersensitivity to tamsulosin or any component of the formulation

Warnings/Precautions Not intended for use as an antihypertensive drug. May cause significant orthostatic hypotension and syncope, especially with first dose; anticipate a similar effect if therapy is interrupted for a few days, if dosage is rapidly increased, or if another antihypertensive drug (particularly vasodilators) or a PDE-5 inhibitor (eg, sildenafil, tadalafil, vardenafil) is introduced. "First-dose" orthostatic hypotension may occur 4-8 hours after dosing; may be dose related. Patients should be cautioned about performing hazardous tasks when starting new therapy or adjusting dosage upward. Discontinue if symptoms of angina occur or worsen. Rule out prostatic carcinoma before beginning therapy with tamsulosin. Intraoperative floppy iris syndrome (IFIS) has been observed in cataract surgery patients who were on or were previously treated with alpha$_1$-blockers, particularly with tamsulosin use (Abdel-Aziz, 2009); in some cases, patients had discontinued the alpha1-blocker 5 weeks to 9 months prior to the surgery. The benefit of discontinuing alpha-blocker therapy prior to cataract surgery has not been established. IFIS may increase the risk of ocular complications during and after surgery. May require modifications to surgical technique; instruct patients to inform ophthalmologist of current or previous alpha$_1$-blocker use when considering eye surgery. Initiation of tamsulosin therapy in patients with planned cataract surgery is not recommended. Priapism has been associated with use (rarely). Rarely, patients with a sulfa allergy have also developed an allergic reaction to tamsulosin; avoid use when previous reaction has been severe.

Drug Interactions
Avoid Concomitant Use
Avoid concomitant use of Tamsulosin with any of the following: Alpha1-Blockers; CYP3A4 Inhibitors (Strong); Fusidic Acid (Systemic)
Decreased Effect
Tamsulosin may decrease the levels/effects of: Alpha-/Beta-Agonists; Alpha1-Agonists

The levels/effects of Tamsulosin may be decreased by: Bosentan; CYP3A4 Inducers (Strong); Dabrafenib; Deferasirox; Herbs (CYP3A4 Inducers); Mitotane; Peginterferon Alfa-2b; Tocilizumab

Increased Effect/Toxicity

Tamsulosin may increase the levels/effects of: Alpha1-Blockers; Calcium Channel Blockers

The levels/effects of Tamsulosin may be increased by: Beta-Blockers; CYP3A4 Inhibitors (Moderate); CYP3A4 Inhibitors (Strong); Dasatinib; Fusidic Acid (Systemic); Ivacaftor; Luliconazole; MAO Inhibitors; Mifepristone; Phosphodiesterase 5 Inhibitors; Simeprevir

Nutritional/Ethanol Interactions

Food: Fasting increases bioavailability by 30% and peak concentration 40% to 70%. Management: Administer 30 minutes after the same meal each day.

Herb/Nutraceutical: St John's wort may decrease the levels/effects of tamsulosin. Some herbal medications have hypotensive properties or may increase the hypotensive effect of tamsulosin. Limited information is available regarding combination with saw palmetto. Management: Avoid St John's wort, black cohosh, California poppy, coleus, golden seal, hawthorn, mistletoe, periwinkle, quinine, and shepherd's purse. Avoid saw palmetto.

Adverse Reactions

>10%:

Cardiovascular: Orthostatic hypotension (6% to 19%)

Central nervous system: Headache (19% to 21%), dizziness (15% to 17%)

Genitourinary: Abnormal ejaculation (8% to 18%)

Respiratory: Rhinitis (13% to 18%)

Miscellaneous: Infection (9% to 11%)

1% to 10%:

Cardiovascular: Chest pain (4%)

Central nervous system: Somnolence (3% to 4%), insomnia (1% to 2%), vertigo (≤1%)

Endocrine & metabolic: Libido decreased (1% to 2%)

Gastrointestinal: Diarrhea (4% to 6%), nausea (3% to 4%), gum pain, toothache

Neuromuscular & skeletal: Weakness (8% to 9%), back pain (7% to 8%)

Ocular: Blurred vision (≤2%)

Respiratory: Pharyngitis (5% to 6%), cough (3% to 5%), sinusitis (2% to 4%)

Available Dosage Forms

Capsule, Oral:

Flomax: 0.4 mg

Generic: 0.4 mg

General Dosage Range Oral: *Adults:* Initial: 0.4 mg once daily; Maintenance: 0.4-0.8 mg once daily

Administration

Oral Administer 30 minutes after the same meal each day. Capsules should be swallowed whole; do not crush, chew, or open.

Storage/Stability Store at room temperature of 25°C (77°F); excursions permitted to 15°C to 30°C (59°F to 86°F).

Nursing Actions

Physical Assessment Assess blood pressure and monitor for hypotension, dizziness, somnolence, and impotence at beginning of therapy and on a regular basis.

Patient Education

• Discuss specific use of drug and side effects with patient as it relates to treatment. (HCAHPS: During this hospital stay, were you given any medicine that you had not taken before? Before giving you any new medicine, how often did hospital staff tell you what the medicine was for? How often did hospital staff describe possible side effects in a way you could understand?)

• Patient may experience dizziness, headache, rhinitis, or impotence. Have patient report immediately to prescriber erection lasting >4 hours or rash (HCAHPS).

• Educate patient about signs of a significant reaction (eg, wheezing; chest tightness; fever; itching; bad cough; blue skin color; seizures; or swelling of face, lips, tongue, or throat). **Note:** This is not a comprehensive list of all side effects. Patient should consult prescriber for additional questions.

Intended Use and Disclaimer: Should not be printed and given to patients. This information is intended to serve as a concise initial reference for healthcare professionals to use when discussing medications with a patient. You must ultimately rely on your own discretion, experience and judgment in diagnosing, treating and advising patients.

Dietary Considerations Take once daily, 30 minutes after the same meal each day.

Related Information

Oral Medications That Should Not Be Crushed or Altered *on page 1712*

Tapentadol (ta PEN ta dol)

Brand Names: U.S. Nucynta; Nucynta ER

Index Terms CG5503; Tapentadol Hydrochloride

Pharmacologic Category Analgesic, Opioid

Medication Safety Issues

Sound-alike/look-alike issues:

Tapentadol may be confused with traMADol

High alert medication:

The Institute for Safe Medication Practices (ISMP) includes this medication among its list of drug classes which have a heightened risk of causing significant patient harm when used in error.

Medication Guide Available Yes

Pregnancy Risk Factor C

Lactation Excretion in breast milk unknown/not recommended

Breast-Feeding Considerations Limited information is available on the excretion of tapentadol in human milk; however, data suggests it may be excreted in human milk. The possibility of sedation or respiratory depression in the nursing infant should be considered; withdrawal may occur when maternal therapy is stopped. Due to the potential for serious adverse reactions in the nursing infant, the U.S. manufacturer recommends a decision be made whether to discontinue nursing or to discontinue the drug, taking into account the importance of treatment to the mother. Use while breast-feeding is contraindicated in the Canadian labeling.

Use

Immediate release formulation: Relief of moderate-to-severe acute pain

Long acting formulation: Relief of moderate-to-severe chronic pain or neuropathic pain associated with diabetic peripheral neuropathy (DPN) when continuous, around-the-clock analgesia is necessary for an extended period of time

Mechanism of Action/Effect Binds to μ-opiate receptors in the CNS causing inhibition of ascending pain pathways, altering the perception of and response to pain; also inhibits the reuptake of norepinephrine, which also modifies the ascending pain pathway

Contraindications Hypersensitivity to tapentadol or any component of the formulation; significant respiratory depression; acute or severe asthma or hypercapnia in unmonitored settings or in absence of resuscitative equipment or ventilatory support; known or suspected paralytic ileus; use with or within 14 days of MAO inhibitors

Canadian labeling: Additional contraindications (not in U.S. labeling): Hypersensitivity to opioids; acute respiratory depression, cor pulmonale; gastrointestinal obstruction or any disease/condition that affects bowel transit (eg, ileus of any type, strictures); severe renal impairment (CrCl <30 mL/minute); severe hepatic impairment (Child-Pugh class C); mild, intermittent, or short-duration pain that can be managed with alternative pain medication; management of perioperative pain (controlled release tablets); acute alcoholism, delirium tremens, and seizure disorders; severe CNS depression, increased cerebrospinal or intracranial pressure or head injury; pregnancy; breast-feeding; use during labor/delivery

Warnings/Precautions Use with caution in patients with respiratory disease or respiratory compromise (eg, asthma, chronic obstructive pulmonary disease [COPD], cor pulmonale, sleep apnea, severe obesity, kyphoscoliosis, hypoxia, hypercapnia); critical respiratory depression may occur, even at therapeutic dosages. Use with caution in debilitated or cachectic patients; there is a greater potential for critical respiratory depression, even at therapeutic dosages. Use with extreme caution in patients with head injury, intracranial lesions, or elevated intracranial pressure (ICP); exaggerated elevation of ICP may occur. Use caution in patients with a history of seizures or conditions predisposing patients to seizures; patients with a history of seizures were excluded in clinical trials of tapentadol. Tramadol, an analgesic with similar pharmacologic properties to tapentadol, has been associated with seizures, particularly in patients with predisposing factors. May cause severe hypotension; use with caution in patients with risk factors (eg, hypovolemia, concomitant use of other hypotensive agents). Avoid use in patients with circulatory shock.

Opioids may obscure diagnosis or clinical course of patients with acute abdominal conditions. May cause CNS depression, which may impair physical or mental abilities; patients must be cautioned about performing tasks which require mental alertness (eg, operating machinery or driving). Effects may be potentiated when used with other sedative drugs or ethanol. Potentially significant drug-drug interactions may exist, requiring dose or frequency adjustment, additional monitoring, and/or selection of alternative therapy.

Use with caution in patients with adrenal insufficiency (including Addison's disease), patients with biliary tract dysfunction or acute pancreatitis (opioids may cause spasm of the sphincter of Oddi), patients with CNS depression (avoid use in patients with impaired consciousness or coma as these patients are susceptible to intracranial effects of CO_2 retention), patients with hypothyroidism, prostatic hyperplasia and/or urinary stricture. Use opioids with caution in the elderly; consider decreasing initial dose. May have a greater potential for critical respiratory depression. Serum concentrations are increased in hepatic impairment; use with caution in patients with moderate hepatic impairment (dosage adjustment required). Not recommended for use in severe hepatic impairment (not studied). Use with caution in patients with mild-to-moderate renal impairment; no dosage adjustments recommended. Not recommended for use in severe renal impairment (not studied).

Prolonged use increases risk of abuse, addiction, and withdrawal symptoms. An opioid-containing regimen should be tailored to each patient's needs with respect to degree of tolerance for opioids (naïve versus chronic user), age, weight, and medical condition. Abrupt discontinuation may lead to withdrawal symptoms. Symptoms may be decreased by tapering prior to discontinuation. Mixed agonist/antagonist opioids may diminish the analgesic effect of tapentadol or precipitate withdrawal symptoms. Abuse of products by ▶

crushing, chewing, snorting, or injecting may result in severe overdose, adverse effects, or death.

After chronic maternal exposure to opioids, neonatal withdrawal syndrome may occur in the newborn; monitor neonate closely. Signs and symptoms include irritability, hyperactivity and abnormal sleep pattern, high pitched cry, tremor, vomiting, diarrhea and failure to gain weight. Onset, duration and severity depend on the drug used, duration of use, maternal dose, and rate of drug elimination by the newborn. Opioid withdrawal syndrome in the neonate, unlike in adults, may be life-threatening and should be treated according to protocols developed by neonatology experts.

Extended release tablets:
[U.S. Boxed Warning]: Respiratory depression, possibly fatal, may occur. Proper dosing, titration, and monitoring are essential. Extended release tablets must be swallowed whole and should NOT be split, crushed, broken, chewed, or dissolved in order to avoid rapid release and potential for fatal dose. Risk for respiratory depression is greatest during the initiation of therapy or with dose increases. Use is contraindicated in patients with significant respiratory depression or conditions that may increase that risk.

[U.S. Boxed Warning]: Accidental exposure, especially in children, may lead to fatal overdose. Not intended for use as an as-needed analgesic; **not** intended for the management of acute or postoperative pain; approved for the treatment of chronic pain only (not an as-needed basis).

[U.S. Boxed Warning]: Use of alcohol may increase tapentadol systemic exposure which may lead to possible fatal overdose. Avoid alcohol or alcohol containing medications during therapy.

[U.S. Boxed Warning]: Healthcare provider should be alert to problems of abuse, misuse, and diversion. Potential for abuse may be increased in patients with a history of or family history of substance abuse or mental illness. Use with caution in patients with a history of drug abuse or acute alcoholism. Tolerance, psychological and physical dependence may occur with prolonged use.

Drug Interactions
Avoid Concomitant Use
Avoid concomitant use of Tapentadol with any of the following: Alcohol (Ethyl); Azelastine (Nasal); MAO Inhibitors; Paraldehyde; Thalidomide

Decreased Effect
Tapentadol may decrease the levels/effects of: Pegvisomant

The levels/effects of Tapentadol may be decreased by: Ammonium Chloride; Antiemetics (5HT3 Antagonists); Mixed Agonist / Antagonist Opioids; Peginterferon Alfa-2b

Increased Effect/Toxicity
Tapentadol may increase the levels/effects of: Alvimopan; Antipsychotics; Azelastine (Nasal); CNS Depressants; Desmopressin; Diuretics; Hydrocodone; MAO Inhibitors; Metoclopramide; Metyrosine; Paraldehyde; Pramipexole; ROPINIRole; Rotigotine; Selective Serotonin Reuptake Inhibitors; Serotonin Modulators; Thalidomide; Zolpidem

The levels/effects of Tapentadol may be increased by: Alcohol (Ethyl); Amphetamines; Anticholinergics; Antipsychotic Agents (Phenothiazines); Antipsychotics; Brimonidine (Topical); Cannabinoids; Doxylamine; HydrOXYzine; Magnesium Sulfate; Perampanel; Sodium Oxybate; Succinylcholine

Nutritional/Ethanol Interactions
Ethanol: Concomitant use with alcohol may increase CNS depression and can increase the bioavailability of extended release tablets. Management: Avoid use of alcohol during therapy.

Food: When administered after a high fat/calorie meal, the AUC and C_{max} increased by 25% and 16%, respectively; may administer without regard to meals.

Herb/Nutraceutical: Avoid St John's wort (may increase CNS depression and risk of serotonin syndrome).

Adverse Reactions
Immediate release:
>10%:
Central nervous system: Dizziness (24%), somnolence (15%)
Gastrointestinal: Nausea (30%), vomiting (18%)
1% to 10%:
Central nervous system: Fatigue (3%), insomnia (2%), anxiety (1%), confusion (1%), dreams abnormal (1%), lethargy (1%)
Dermatologic: Pruritus (3% to 5%), hyperhidrosis (3%), rash (1%)
Endocrine & metabolic: Hot flushes (1%)
Gastrointestinal: Constipation (8%), xerostomia (4%), appetite decreased (2%), dyspepsia (2%)
Genitourinary: Urinary tract infection (1%)
Neuromuscular & skeletal: Arthralgia (1%), tremor (1%)
Respiratory: Nasopharyngitis (1%), upper respiratory tract infection (1%)

Extended release:
>10%:
Central nervous system: Dizziness (17% to 18%), headache (10% to 15%), somnolence (12% to 14%)
Gastrointestinal: Nausea (21% to 27%), constipation (13% to 17%), vomiting (8% to 12%)
1% to 10%:
Cardiovascular: Hypotension (1%)
Central nervous system: Fatigue (9%), anxiety (2% to 5%), insomnia (4%), irritability (2%), lethargy (2%), abnormal dreams (1% to 2%),

vertigo (1% to 2%), attention disturbances (1%), chills (1%), depression/depressed mood (1%), hypoesthesia (1%), nervousness (1%), sedation (1%), withdrawal syndrome (1%)

Dermatologic: Pruritus (1% to 8%), hyperhidrosis (3% to 5%), rash (1%)

Endocrine & metabolic: Hot flushes (2% to 3%)

Gastrointestinal: Diarrhea (7%), xerostomia (7%), appetite decreased (2% to 6%), dyspepsia (1% to 3%), abdominal discomfort (1%)

Genitourinary: Erectile dysfunction (1%)

Neuromuscular & skeletal: Tremor (1% to 3%), weakness (2%)

Ocular: Vision blurred (1%)

Respiratory: Dyspnea (1%)

Product Availability Nucynta Oral Solution: FDA approved October 2012; anticipated availability currently unknown. Refer to prescribing information for additional information.

Controlled Substance C-II

Available Dosage Forms

Tablet, Oral:

Nucynta: 50 mg, 75 mg, 100 mg

Tablet Extended Release 12 Hour, Oral:

Nucynta ER: 50 mg, 100 mg, 150 mg, 200 mg, 250 mg

General Dosage Range Dosage adjustment recommended in patients with hepatic impairment

Oral:

Immediate release: *Adults:* 50-100 mg every 4-6 hours as needed (maximum: 700 mg/day on day 1; 600 mg/day subsequent days)

Extended release: *Adults:* 50-250 mg twice daily (maximum: 500 mg/day)

Administration

Oral Administer orally with or without food. Long acting formulations must be swallowed whole and should **not** be split, crushed, broken, chewed, or dissolved; patients should be instructed to swallow 1 tablet at a time, immediately after placing in mouth. The Canadian product labeling recommends that immediate release tablets be swallowed whole.

Storage/Stability Store at room temperature up to 25°C (77°F); excursions permitted to 15°C to 30°C (59°F to 86°F). Protect from moisture.

Nursing Actions

Physical Assessment Monitor respiratory and CNS status. Assess patient's physical and/or psychological dependence. For inpatients, implement safety measures (eg, side rails up, call light within reach, instructions to call for assistance). Discontinue slowly after prolonged use. If case of overdose, call Poison Help at 1-800-222-1222.

Patient Education

• Discuss specific use of drug and side effects with patient as it relates to treatment. (HCAHPS: During this hospital stay, were you given any medicine that you had not taken before? Before giving you any new medicine, how often did hospital staff tell you what the medicine was

for? How often did hospital staff describe possible side effects in a way you could understand?)

• Patient may experience vertigo, presyncope, fatigue, blurred vision, illogical thinking, headache, pruritus, nausea, or constipation. Have patient report immediately to prescriber syncope, dyspnea, significant change in balance, agitation, fasciculations, hyperhidrosis, muscle stiffness, poor pain control, asthenia, or rash (HCAHPS).

• Educate patient about signs of a significant reaction (eg, wheezing; chest tightness; fever; itching; bad cough; blue skin color; seizures; or swelling of face, lips, tongue, or throat). **Note:** This is not a comprehensive list of all side effects. Patient should consult prescriber for additional questions.

Intended Use and Disclaimer: Should not be printed and given to patients. This information is intended to serve as a concise initial reference for healthcare professionals to use when discussing medications with a patient. You must ultimately rely on your own discretion, experience and judgment in diagnosing, treating and advising patients.

Dietary Considerations May be taken without regard to meals.

Related Information

Oral Medications That Should Not Be Crushed or Altered *on page 1712*

Tazarotene (taz AR oh teen)

Brand Names: U.S. Avage; Fabior; Tazorac

Pharmacologic Category Acne Products; Keratolytic Agent; Topical Skin Product, Acne

Pregnancy Risk Factor X

Lactation Excretion in breast milk unknown/not recommended

Use Topical treatment of facial acne vulgaris; topical treatment of stable plaque psoriasis; mitigation (palliation) of facial skin wrinkling, facial mottled hyper-/hypopigmentation, and benign facial lentigines

Available Dosage Forms

Cream, External:

Avage: 0.1% (30 g)

Tazorac: 0.05% (30 g, 60 g); 0.1% (30 g, 60 g)

Foam, External:

Fabior: 0.1% (50 g, 100 g)

Gel, External:

Tazorac: 0.05% (30 g, 100 g); 0.1% (30 g, 100 g)

General Dosage Range Topical: *Children ≥12 years, Adolescents, and Adults:* Apply a pea-sized amount or thin film **or** 2 mg/cm² once daily

Administration

Topical Do not apply to eczematous or sunburned skin; avoid eyes and mouth.

Acne: Apply in evening after gently cleansing and drying face; apply enough to cover entire affected area.

Foam: Dispense a small amount of foam into palm of the hand. Use fingertips to lightly cover the entire affected area of the face and/or upper trunk with a thin layer; massage into skin until foam disappears. Wash hands after use. Moisturizer may be used if necessary.

Palliation of fine facial wrinkles, facial mottled hyper-/hypopigmentation, benign facial lentigines: Apply to clean dry face at bedtime; lightly cover entire face including eyelids if desired. Emollients or moisturizers may be applied before or after; if applied before tazarotene, ensure cream or lotion has absorbed into the skin and has dried completely.

Psoriasis: Apply in evening. If a bath or shower is taken prior to application, dry the skin before applying. If emollients are used, apply them at least 1 hour prior to application. Unaffected skin may be more susceptible to irritation, avoid application to these areas.

Nursing Actions

Physical Assessment Assess for accumulated photosensitivity.

Patient Education
- Discuss specific use of drug and side effects with patient as it relates to treatment. (HCAHPS: During this hospital stay, were you given any medicine that you had not taken before? Before giving you any new medicine, how often did hospital staff tell you what the medicine was for? How often did hospital staff describe possible side effects in a way you could understand?)
- Patient may experience application site pain, skin irritation, or xeroderma. Have patient report immediately to prescriber pregnancy or rash (HCAHPS).
- Educate patient about signs of a significant reaction (eg, wheezing; chest tightness; fever; itching; bad cough; blue skin color; seizures; or swelling of face, lips, tongue, or throat). **Note:** This is not a comprehensive list of all side effects. Patient should consult prescriber for additional questions.

Intended Use and Disclaimer: Should not be printed and given to patients. This information is intended to serve as a concise initial reference for healthcare professionals to use when discussing medications with a patient. You must ultimately rely on your own discretion, experience and judgment in diagnosing, treating and advising patients.

Teduglutide (te due GLOO tide)

Brand Names: U.S. Gattex
Index Terms ALX-0600; Teduglutide Recombinant; Teduglutide [rDNA origin]

Pharmacologic Category Glucagon-Like Peptide-2 (GLP-2) Analog
Medication Guide Available Yes
Pregnancy Risk Factor B
Lactation Excretion in breast milk unknown/not recommended
Use Treatment of short bowel syndrome (SBS) in patients requiring parenteral nutrition support
Available Dosage Forms
Kit, Subcutaneous [preservative free]:
Gattex: 5 mg
General Dosage Range Dosage adjustment recommended in patients with renal impairment.
SubQ: *Adults:* 0.05 mg/kg once daily
Administration
Subcutaneous Rotate injection site between thighs, upper arms, and quadrants of the abdomen. Do not administer I.M. or I.V.
Nursing Actions
Physical Assessment Monitor for efficacy; assess frequency and consistency of bowel movements. Also monitor for other abdominal symptoms, injection site redness, nausea, headaches, stoma site (if patient has one), and fluid overload. Educate patient about need for colonoscopy follow-up.
Patient Education
- Discuss specific use of drug and side effects with patient as it relates to treatment. (HCAHPS: During this hospital stay, were you given any medicine that you had not taken before? Before giving you any new medicine, how often did hospital staff tell you what the medicine was for? How often did hospital staff describe possible side effects in a way you could understand?)
- Patient may experience edema, flatulence, nausea, dyspepsia, headache, or injection site irritation. Have patient report immediately to prescriber angina, significant weight gain, or severe constipation (HCAHPS).
- Educate patient about signs of a significant reaction (eg, wheezing; chest tightness; fever; itching; bad cough; blue skin color; seizures; or swelling of face, lips, tongue, or throat). **Note:** This is not a comprehensive list of all side effects. Patient should consult prescriber for additional questions.

Intended Use and Disclaimer: Should not be printed and given to patients. This information is intended to serve as a concise initial reference for healthcare professionals to use when discussing medications with a patient. You must ultimately rely on your own discretion, experience and judgment in diagnosing, treating and advising patients.

Tegaserod (teg a SER od)

Brand Names: U.S. Zelnorm®
Index Terms HTF919; Tegaserod Maleate

Pharmacologic Category Serotonin 5-HT$_4$ Receptor Agonist

Pregnancy Risk Factor B

Lactation Excretion in breast milk unknown/not recommended

Use Emergency treatment of irritable bowel syndrome with constipation (IBS-C) and chronic idiopathic constipation (CIC) in women (<55 years of age) in which no alternative therapy exists

Available Dosage Forms

Tablet, oral:
Zelnorm®: 2 mg, 6 mg

General Dosage Range Oral: *Adults (females <55 years of age):* 6 mg twice daily

Administration

Oral Administer 30 minutes before meals.

Nursing Actions

Physical Assessment For emergency use only under FDA emergency investigational new drug process. Monitor for cardiac event, clinically-significant diarrhea (hypovolemia, hypotension, syncope), and ischemic colitis (rectal bleeding, bloody diarrhea, abdominal pain) frequently when beginning therapy and at regular intervals during treatment.

Patient Education

• Discuss specific use of drug and side effects with patient as it relates to treatment. (HCAHPS: During this hospital stay, were you given any medicine that you had not taken before? Before giving you any new medicine, how often did hospital staff tell you what the medicine was for? How often did hospital staff describe possible side effects in a way you could understand?)
• Patient may experience headache, diarrhea, gas, or back pain. Have patient report immediately to prescriber severe diarrhea, dizziness, new or worsening dyspepsia, chest pain, or signs or symptoms of a stroke (HCAHPS).
• Educate patient about signs of a significant reaction (eg, wheezing; chest tightness; fever; itching; bad cough; blue skin color; seizures; or swelling of face, lips, tongue, or throat). **Note:** This is not a comprehensive list of all side effects. Patient should consult prescriber for additional questions.

Intended Use and Disclaimer: Should not be printed and given to patients. This information is intended to serve as a concise initial reference for healthcare professionals to use when discussing medications with a patient. You must ultimately rely on your own discretion, experience and judgment in diagnosing, treating and advising patients.

Telaprevir (tel A pre vir)

Brand Names: U.S. Incivek

Index Terms LY570310; MP-424; MP424; VRT111950; VX-950; VX950

Pharmacologic Category Antihepaciviral, Protease Inhibitor (Anti-HCV)

Medication Guide Available Yes

Pregnancy Risk Factor B / X (in combination with ribavirin)

Lactation Excretion in breast milk unknown/not recommended

Breast-Feeding Considerations It is not known if telaprevir or ribavirin are excreted into breast milk. The manufacturer recommends that breast-feeding be discontinued prior to the initiation of treatment.

Use Chronic hepatitis C: Treatment of genotype 1 chronic hepatitis C (in combination with peginterferon alfa and ribavirin) in adult patients with compensated liver disease (including cirrhosis) who are treatment naive or who have received previous interferon-based treatment, including null or partial responders, and treatment relapsers.

Mechanism of Action/Effect Inhibits viral protein synthesis; direct-acting antiviral against the hepatitis C virus

Contraindications

Combination treatment with ribavirin: Pregnancy; male partners of pregnant women

Coadministration with alfuzosin, cisapride, ergot derivatives (eg, dihydroergotamine, ergonovine, ergotamine, methylergonovine), lovastatin, midazolam [oral], pimozide, sildenafil/tadalafil [when used for treatment of pulmonary arterial hypertension], simvastatin, triazolam), rifampin, St John's wort, carbamazepine, phenobarbital, phenytoin

Canadian labeling: Additional contraindications (not in U.S. labeling): Hypersensitivity to telaprevir or any component of the formulation; coadministration with amiodarone, atorvastatin, eletriptan, flecainide, propafenone, quinidine, terfenadine, vardenafil

Also refer to Peginterferon Alfa and Ribavirin monographs for individual product contraindications.

Warnings/Precautions [U.S. Boxed Warning] Serious skin reactions (some fatal) including Stevens-Johnson syndrome (SJS), drug reaction with eosinophilia and systemic symptoms (DRESS), and toxic epidermal necrolysis (TEN), have been reported with telaprevir combination therapy. Fatal cases have been reported in patients with progressive rash and systemic symptoms who received ongoing therapy after diagnoses of serious skin reactions. Discontinue Telaprevir, Peginterferon Alfa, and Ribavirin immediately for serious skin reactions (including rash with systemic symptoms or a progressive severe rash) and refer for immediate medical care. Rash has been typically observed within first 4 weeks of therapy initiation but may occur at any time. Severe rashes (other than DRESS, SJS) are generalized, bullous, vesicular or ulcerative; may also have an eczematous appearance. Discontinue telaprevir (may continue peginterferon alfa and ribavirin) for severe rash or for mild-to-moderate rash that progresses; if no improvement in rash within 1 week of stopping telaprevir, interruption or discontinuation of peginterferon alfa and/or ribavirin should be considered (or sooner if clinically indicated). May use oral antihistamines/topical corticosteroids for rash treatment; do not use systemic corticosteroids. Do not restart telaprevir if discontinued due to any skin reaction.

Prerenal azotemia (with or without acute renal failure) and uric acid nephropathy have been reported. Assess serum electrolytes, creatinine, and uric acid pretreatment, at weeks 2, 4, 8, and 12, and when clinically indicated. Maintain adequate hydration. Anemia has been reported with peginterferon alfa and ribavirin; addition of telaprevir is associated with further hemoglobin decreases. Low hemoglobin levels were measured during the first 4 weeks of treatment, and the lowest at the end of telaprevir treatment (week 12). Dose modifications of ribavirin were needed more often in patients also taking telaprevir. Assess hematologic parameters (CBC with differential and platelet count) pretreatment, at weeks 2, 4, 8, and 12, and when clinically indicated. May require ribavirin dose reduction, interruption or discontinuation of treatment; if ribavirin dose reductions are inadequate, may consider discontinuing telaprevir. Do not reduce telaprevir dose. If ribavirin is discontinued, telaprevir must also be discontinued. Do not restart telaprevir if ribavirin therapy is reinitiated.

Avoid pregnancy in female patients and female partners of male patients, during therapy, and for at least 6 months after treatment; two forms of nonhormonal contraception should be used. Hormonal contraceptives may not be effective in patients taking telaprevir or for two weeks after discontinuing therapy. Safety and efficacy have not been established in patients who have uncompensated cirrhosis, received liver transplants, or who have failed to respond to other NS3/4A inhibitors (including repeated courses of telaprevir). Monotherapy is not effective for chronic hepatitis C infection. Not recommended in moderate or severe hepatic impairment (Child-Pugh class B or C) or decompensated hepatic disease. Potentially significant drug-drug interactions may exist, requiring dose or frequency adjustments, additional monitoring, and/or selection of alternative therapy.

Drug Interactions
Avoid Concomitant Use
Avoid concomitant use of Telaprevir with any of the following: Ado-Trastuzumab Emtansine; Alfuzosin; Apixaban; AtorvaSTATin; Avanafil; Axitinib; Bosutinib; Cabozantinib; CarBAMazepine; Cisapride; Conivaptan; Crizotinib; CYP3A4 Inducers (Strong); Darunavir; Dihydroergotamine; Dronedarone; Eplerenone; Ergoloid Mesylates; Ergonovine; Ergotamine; Everolimus; Fosamprenavir; Fosphenytoin; Fusidic Acid (Systemic); Halofantrine; Ibrutinib; Imatinib; Ivabradine; Lapatinib; Lomitapide; Lopinavir; Lovastatin; Lurasidone; Macitentan; Methylergonovine; Midazolam; Nilotinib; Nisoldipine; PHENobarbital; Phenytoin; Pimozide; Pomalidomide; Ranolazine; Red Yeast Rice; Regorafenib; Rifabutin; Rifampin; Rivaroxaban; Salmeterol; Sildenafil; Silodosin; Simeprevir; Simvastatin; St Johns Wort; Tamsulosin; Ticagrelor; Tolvaptan; Topotecan; Toremifene; Triazolam; Ulipristal; Vemurafenib; VinCRIStine (Liposomal)

Decreased Effect
Telaprevir may decrease the levels/effects of: Contraceptives (Estrogens); Contraceptives (Progestins); Darunavir; Efavirenz; Escitalopram; Fosamprenavir; Ifosfamide; Methadone; Prasugrel; Ticagrelor; Voriconazole; Warfarin; Zolpidem

The levels/effects of Telaprevir may be decreased by: Atazanavir; Bosentan; CarBAMazepine; Corticosteroids; Corticosteroids (Systemic); CYP3A4 Inducers (Strong); Dabrafenib; Darunavir; Deferasirox; Efavirenz; Etravirine; Fosamprenavir; Fosphenytoin; Lopinavir; P-glycoprotein/ABCB1 Inducers; PHENobarbital; Phenytoin; Rifabutin; Rifampin; Ritonavir; St Johns Wort; Tocilizumab

Increased Effect/Toxicity
Telaprevir may increase the levels/effects of: Ado-Trastuzumab Emtansine; Afatinib; Alfuzosin; Almotriptan; Alosetron; ALPRAZolam; Amiodarone; Apixaban; ARIPiprazole; Atazanavir; AtorvaSTATin; Avanafil; Axitinib; Bedaquiline; Bepridil [Off Market]; Bortezomib; Bosentan; Bosutinib; Brentuximab Vedotin; Brinzolamide; Budesonide (Nasal); Budesonide (Systemic, Oral Inhalation); Cabozantinib; CarBAMazepine; Cisapride; Clarithromycin; Colchicine; Conivaptan; Corticosteroids; Corticosteroids (Orally Inhaled); Corticosteroids (Systemic); Crizotinib; CycloSPORINE (Systemic); CYP3A4 Substrates; Dabigatran Etexilate; Dienogest; Digoxin; Dihydroergotamine; Dofetilide; DOXOrubicin (Conventional); Dronedarone; Dutasteride; Enzalutamide; Eplerenone; Ergoloid Mesylates; Ergonovine; Ergotamine; Erythromycin (Systemic); Everolimus; FentaNYL; Fesoterodine; Flecainide; Fluticasone (Nasal); Fluticasone (Oral Inhalation); Fluvastatin; Fosphenytoin; GuanFACINE; Halofantrine; Ibrutinib; Iloperidone; Imatinib; Itraconazole; Ivabradine; Ivacaftor; Ixabepilone; Ketoconazole (Systemic); Lacosamide; Lapatinib; Levomilnacipran; Lidocaine (Systemic); Lomitapide; Lovastatin; Lumefantrine; Lurasidone; Macitentan; Maraviroc; Methylergonovine; MethylPREDNISolone; Midazolam; Mifepristone; Nilotinib; Nisoldipine; Ospemifene; OxyCODONE; Paricalcitol; PAZOPanib; P-glycoprotein/ABCB1 Substrates; Phenytoin; Pimecrolimus; Pimozide;

Pitavastatin; Pomalidomide; PONATinib; Posaconazole; Pravastatin; Propafenone; Prucalopride; QUEtiapine; QuiNIDine; Ranolazine; Red Yeast Rice; Regorafenib; Repaglinide; Rifabutin; Rilpivirine; Rivaroxaban; RomiDEPsin; Rosuvastatin; Ruxolitinib; Salmeterol; Saxagliptin; Sildenafil; Silodosin; Simeprevir; Simvastatin; Sirolimus; SORAfenib; Tacrolimus (Systemic); Tadalafil; Tamsulosin; Telithromycin; Tenofovir; Ticagrelor; Tofacitinib; Tolterodine; Tolvaptan; Topotecan; Toremifene; TraZODone; Triazolam; Ulipristal; Vardenafil; Vemurafenib; Vilazodone; VinCRIStine (Liposomal); Voriconazole; Warfarin; Zuclopenthixol

The levels/effects of Telaprevir may be increased by: Clarithromycin; CYP3A4 Inhibitors (Moderate); CYP3A4 Inhibitors (Strong); Dasatinib; Erythromycin (Systemic); Fusidic Acid (Systemic); Itraconazole; Ketoconazole (Systemic); Luliconazole; P-glycoprotein/ABCB1 Inhibitors; Posaconazole; Ritonavir; Stiripentol; Telithromycin; Voriconazole

Adverse Reactions
>10%:
Central nervous system: Fatigue (56%)
Dermatologic: Rash (56%), pruritus (47%)
Endocrine and Metabolic: Hyperuricemia (<12.1 mg/dL: 66%; ≥12.1 mg/dL: 7%)
Gastrointestinal: Nausea (39%), diarrhea (26%), vomiting (13%), hemorrhoids (12%), anorectal discomfort (11%)
Hematologic: Anemia (36%), lymphopenia (15%)
Hepatic: Hyperbilirubinemia (<2.6 x ULN: 37%; ≥2.6 x ULN: 4%)
1% to 10%:
Gastrointestinal: Abnormal taste (10%), anal pruritus (6%)
Hematologic: Thrombocytopenia (3%)

Available Dosage Forms
Tablet, Oral:
Incivek: 375 mg
General Dosage Range Oral: Adults: 1125 mg twice daily
Administration
Oral Administer with a meal (not low fat) within 30 minutes prior to each dose. Doses should be taken approximately every 10-14 hours. Administer concurrently with peginterferon alfa and ribavirin. Maintain adequate fluid intake/hydration. Patients should be instructed to swallow INCIVEK tablets whole (eg, patients should not chew, crush, break, cut, or dissolve the tablets). If a dose is missed within 6 hours of the time it is usually taken, take as soon as possible. If more than 6 hours have passed since the dose is usually taken, the missed dose should not be taken and the patient should resume the usual schedule.
Storage/Stability Store at 25°C (77°F); excursions permitted to 15°C to 30°C (59°F to 86°F).

Nursing Actions
Physical Assessment This drug is typically not indicated for use alone; it must be taken along with peginterferon alfa-2a and ribavirin. These drugs are known to cause birth defects so there must be a negative pregnancy test prior to treatment and two forms of birth control must be used for 6 months after treatment. Do not use with moderate-to-severe liver damage. Instruct patient that medication must be taken with food. There is no renal impairment with this drug, so monitoring renal function is not necessary.
Patient Education
• Discuss specific use of drug and side effects with patient as it relates to treatment. (HCAHPS: During this hospital stay, were you given any medicine that you had not taken before? Before giving you any new medicine, how often did hospital staff tell you what the medicine was for? How often did hospital staff describe possible side effects in a way you could understand?)
• Patient may experience fatigue, anemia, parageusia, nausea, or diarrhea. Have patient report immediately to prescriber dizziness or syncope, dyspnea, ecchymosis, melena, stomatitis, severe skin irritation, or rash (HCAHPS).
• Educate patient about signs of a significant reaction (eg, wheezing; chest tightness; fever; itching; bad cough; blue skin color; seizures; or swelling of face, lips, tongue, or throat). **Note:** This is not a comprehensive list of all side effects. Patient should consult prescriber for additional questions.

Intended Use and Disclaimer: Should not be printed and given to patients. This information is intended to serve as a concise initial reference for healthcare professionals to use when discussing medications with a patient. You must ultimately rely on your own discretion, experience and judgment in diagnosing, treating and advising patients.
Dietary Considerations Take with a meal (not low fat).

Telbivudine (tel BI vyoo deen)

Brand Names: U.S. Tyzeka
Index Terms L-Deoxythymidine; LdT
Pharmacologic Category Antihepadnaviral, Reverse Transcriptase Inhibitor, Nucleoside (Anti-HBV)
Medication Guide Available Yes
Pregnancy Risk Factor B
Lactation Excretion in breast milk unknown/not recommended
Breast-Feeding Considerations It is not known if telbivudine is excreted in breast milk. Breast-feeding is not recommended by the manufacturer.

Use Treatment of chronic hepatitis B with evidence of viral replication and either persistent transaminase elevations or histologically-active disease

Mechanism of Action/Effect Telbivudine, a synthetic thymidine nucleoside analogue (L-enantiomer of thymidine), is intracellularly phosphorylated to the active triphosphate form, which competes with the natural substrate, thymidine 5'-triphosphate, to inhibit hepatitis B viral DNA polymerase; enzyme inhibition blocks reverse transcriptase activity thereby reducing viral DNA replication.

Contraindications Concurrent use with peginterferon alfa-2a

Canadian labeling: Additional contraindications (not in U.S. labeling): Hypersensitivity to telbivudine or any component of the formulation

Warnings/Precautions [U.S. Boxed Warnings]: Cases of lactic acidosis and severe hepatomegaly with steatosis, some fatal, have been reported with the use of nucleoside analogues. Severe, acute exacerbation of hepatitis B may occur upon discontinuation. Monitor liver function several months after stopping treatment; reinitiation of antihepatitis B therapy may be required. Myopathy (eg, unexplained muscle aches and/or muscle weakness in conjunction with increases serum creatine kinase) has been reported with telbivudine initiation after several weeks to months; therapy should be interrupted if myopathy suspected and discontinued if diagnosed. Patients taking concomitant medications associated with myopathy should be monitored closely. Peripheral neuropathy may occur alone or in combination with pegylated interferon alfa-2a (concurrent use is contraindicated) or possibly other interferons. Symptoms have been observed within 3 months after initiation of therapy. Interrupt treatment for suspected peripheral neuropathy and discontinue if confirmed; symptoms may be reversible with discontinuation. Use caution in patients with renal impairment or patients receiving concomitant therapy which may reduce renal function; dosage adjustment required (CrCl <50 mL/minute). Monitor renal function before and during treatment in liver transplant patients receiving concurrent therapy of cyclosporine or tacrolimus; telbivudine may need to be adjusted. Safety and efficacy have not been established in liver transplant patients, Black/African-American patients, or Hispanic patients.

Not recommended as first-line therapy of chronic HBV due to high rate of resistance; use may be appropriate in short-term treatment of acute HBV (Lok, 2009). Cross-resistance among other antivirals for hepatitis B may occur; use caution in patients failing previous therapy with lamivudine. Telbivudine does not exhibit any clinically-relevant activity against human immunodeficiency virus (HIV type 1). Safety and efficacy have not been studied in patients coinfected with HIV, hepatitis C virus (HCV), or hepatitis D virus (HDV).

Drug Interactions

Avoid Concomitant Use

Avoid concomitant use of Telbivudine with any of the following: Interferon Alfa-2b; Peginterferon Alfa-2a; Peginterferon Alfa-2b

Decreased Effect There are no known significant interactions involving a decrease in effect.

Increased Effect/Toxicity

The levels/effects of Telbivudine may be increased by: Interferon Alfa-2b; Peginterferon Alfa-2a; Peginterferon Alfa-2b

Nutritional/Ethanol Interactions

Ethanol: Should be avoided in hepatitis B infection due to potential hepatic toxicity.

Food: Does not have a significant effect on telbivudine absorption.

Adverse Reactions

>10%:

Central nervous system: Fatigue (13%)

Neuromuscular & skeletal: Increased creatine phosphokinase (79%; grades 3/4: 16%, most asymptomatic and transient)

1% to 10%:

Central nervous system: Headache (10%), dizziness (4%), fever (4%), insomnia (3%)

Dermatologic: Skin rash (4%), pruritus (2%)

Endocrine & metabolic: Increased serum lipase (grades 3/4: 2%)

Gastrointestinal: Diarrhea (6%), abdominal pain (3% to 6%), nausea (5%), abdominal distension (3%), dyspepsia (3%)

Hematologic & oncologic: Neutropenia (grades 3/4: 2%)

Hepatic: Increased serum ALT (grades 3/4: 5% to 7%), increased serum AST (grades 3/4: 6%)

Infection: Exacerbation of hepatitis B (2%)

Neuromuscular & skeletal: Arthralgia (4%), back pain (4%), myalgia (3%)

Respiratory: Cough (6%), pharyngolaryngeal pain (5%)

Available Dosage Forms

Tablet, Oral:

Tyzeka: 600 mg

General Dosage Range Dosage adjustment recommended in patients with renal impairment

Oral: *Children ≥16 years and Adults:* 600 mg once daily

Administration

Oral May be administered without regard to food.

Storage/Stability Store at 25°C (77°F); excursions permitted to 15°C to 30°C (59°F to 86°F).

Nursing Actions

Physical Assessment Monitor for peripheral neuropathy or myopathy (may be necessary to discontinue drug), gastrointestinal effects (pain or vomiting), or upper respiratory infection. Monitor closely for several months following discontinuation for possible clinical exacerbations.

Patient Education

- Discuss specific use of drug and side effects with patient as it relates to treatment. (HCAHPS: During this hospital stay, were you given any medicine that you had not taken before? Before giving you any new medicine, how often did hospital staff tell you what the medicine was for? How often did hospital staff describe possible side effects in a way you could understand?)
- Patient may experience dyspepsia, headache, asthenia, or diarrhea. Have patient report immediately to prescriber signs of hepatic impairment, signs of lactic acidosis, paresthesia, change in balance, abnormal gait, urinary retention, oliguria, chills, pharyngitis, abdominal edema, or myalgia (HCAHPS).
- Educate patient about signs of a significant reaction (eg, wheezing; chest tightness; fever; itching; bad cough; blue skin color; seizures; or swelling of face, lips, tongue, or throat). **Note:** This is not a comprehensive list of all side effects. Patient should consult prescriber for additional questions.

Intended Use and Disclaimer: Should not be printed and given to patients. This information is intended to serve as a concise initial reference for healthcare professionals to use when discussing medications with a patient. You must ultimately rely on your own discretion, experience and judgment in diagnosing, treating and advising patients.

Dietary Considerations May be taken without regard to food.

Telithromycin (tel ith roe MYE sin)

Brand Names: U.S. Ketek
Index Terms HMR 3647
Pharmacologic Category Antibiotic, Ketolide
Medication Safety Issues
Sound-alike/look-alike issues:
Telithromycin may be confused with telavancin
Medication Guide Available Yes
Pregnancy Risk Factor C
Lactation Excretion in breast milk unknown/use caution
Breast-Feeding Considerations It is not known if telithromycin is excreted in breast milk. The manufacturer recommends caution if using telithromycin in a breast-feeding woman.
Use Treatment of community-acquired pneumonia (mild-to-moderate) caused by susceptible strains of *Streptococcus pneumoniae* (including multidrug-resistant isolates), *Haemophilus influenzae*, *Chlamydophila pneumoniae*, *Moraxella catarrhalis*, and *Mycoplasma pneumoniae*
Mechanism of Action/Effect Inhibits bacterial protein synthesis by binding to two sites on the 50S ribosomal subunit.

Contraindications Hypersensitivity to telithromycin, macrolide antibiotics, or any component of the formulation; myasthenia gravis; history of hepatitis and/or jaundice associated with telithromycin or other macrolide antibiotic use; concurrent use of colchicine (if patient has concomitant renal or hepatic impairment), cisapride, pimozide, lovastatin, or simvastatin

Warnings/Precautions Acute hepatic failure and severe liver injury, including hepatitis and hepatic necrosis (leading to some fatalities) have been reported, in some cases after only a few doses; if signs/symptoms of hepatitis or liver damage occur, discontinue therapy and initiate liver function tests. **[U.S. Boxed Warning]: Life-threatening (including fatal) respiratory failure has occurred in patients with myasthenia gravis;** use in these patients is contraindicated. May prolong QT$_c$ interval, leading to a risk of ventricular arrhythmias; closely-related antibiotics have been associated with malignant ventricular arrhythmias and torsade de pointes. Avoid in patients with prolongation of QT$_c$ interval due to congenital causes, history of long QT syndrome, uncorrected electrolyte disturbances (hypokalemia or hypomagnesemia), significant bradycardia (<50 bpm), or concurrent therapy with QT$_c$-prolonging drugs (eg, class Ia and class III antiarrhythmics). Avoid use in patients with a prior history of confirmed cardiogenic syncope or ventricular arrhythmias while receiving macrolide antibiotics or other QT$_c$-prolonging drugs. May cause severe visual disturbances (eg, changes in accommodation ability, diplopia, blurred vision). May cause loss of consciousness (possibly vagal-related); caution patients that these events may interfere with ability to operate machinery or drive, and to use caution until effects are known. Use caution in renal impairment; severe impairment (CrCl <30 mL/minute) requires dosage adjustment. Pseudomembranous colitis has been reported. Safety and efficacy not established in pediatric patients <13 years of age per Canadian approved labeling and <18 years of age per U.S. approved labeling.

Drug Interactions
Avoid Concomitant Use
Avoid concomitant use of Telithromycin with any of the following: Ado-Trastuzumab Emtansine; Alfuzosin; Apixaban; Avanafil; Axitinib; BCG; Bosutinib; Cabozantinib; Cisapride; Conivaptan; Crizotinib; Disopyramide; Dronedarone; Eplerenone; Everolimus; Fusidic Acid (Systemic); Halofantrine; Highest Risk QTc-Prolonging Agents; Ibrutinib; Imatinib; Ivabradine; Lapatinib; Lomitapide; Lovastatin; Lurasidone; Macitentan; Mifepristone; Nilotinib; Nisoldipine; Pimozide; Pomalidomide; QuiNIDine; QuiNINE; Ranolazine; Red Yeast Rice; Regorafenib; Rivaroxaban; Salmeterol; Silodosin; Simeprevir; Simvastatin; Tamsulosin; Terfenadine; Ticagrelor; Tolvaptan;

Toremifene; Ulipristal; Vemurafenib; VinCRIStine (Liposomal)

Decreased Effect

Telithromycin may decrease the levels/effects of: BCG; Clopidogrel; Ifosfamide; Prasugrel; Sodium Picosulfate; Ticagrelor; Typhoid Vaccine

The levels/effects of Telithromycin may be decreased by: CYP3A4 Inducers (Strong); Dabrafenib; Deferasirox; Etravirine; Herbs (CYP3A4 Inducers); Mitotane; Tocilizumab

Increased Effect/Toxicity

Telithromycin may increase the levels/effects of: Ado-Trastuzumab Emtansine; Alfentanil; Alfuzosin; Almotriptan; Alosetron; ALPRAZolam; Antifungal Agents (Azole Derivatives, Systemic); Antineoplastic Agents (Vinca Alkaloids); Apixaban; ARIPiprazole; AtorvaSTATin; Avanafil; Axitinib; Bedaquiline; Bortezomib; Bosentan; Bosutinib; Brentuximab Vedotin; Brinzolamide; Budesonide (Nasal); Budesonide (Systemic, Oral Inhalation); BusPIRone; Cabozantinib; Calcium Channel Blockers; CarBAMazepine; Cardiac Glycosides; Cilostazol; Cisapride; CloZAPine; Cobicistat; Colchicine; Conivaptan; Corticosteroids (Orally Inhaled); Corticosteroids (Systemic); Crizotinib; CycloSPORINE (Systemic); CYP3A4 Substrates; Dienogest; Disopyramide; Dofetilide; DOXOrubicin (Conventional); Dronedarone; Dutasteride; Eletriptan; Enzalutamide; Eplerenone; Ergot Derivatives; Estazolam; Everolimus; FentaNYL; Fesoterodine; Fluticasone (Nasal); Fluticasone (Oral Inhalation); GuanFACINE; Halofantrine; Highest Risk QTc-Prolonging Agents; Ibrutinib; Iloperidone; Imatinib; Ivabradine; Ivacaftor; Ixabepilone; Lacosamide; Lapatinib; Levomilnacipran; Lomitapide; Lovastatin; Lumefantrine; Lurasidone; Macitentan; Maraviroc; MethylPREDNISolone; Midazolam; Mifepristone; Moderate Risk QTc-Prolonging Agents; Nilotinib; Nisoldipine; Ospemifene; OxyCODONE; Paricalcitol; PAZOPanib; Pimecrolimus; Pimozide; Pitavastatin; Pomalidomide; PONATinib; Pravastatin; Propafenone; QUEtiapine; QuiNIDine; QuiNINE; Ranolazine; Red Yeast Rice; Regorafenib; Repaglinide; Rifamycin Derivatives; Rilpivirine; Rivaroxaban; RomiDEPsin; Ruxolitinib; Salmeterol; Saxagliptin; Selective Serotonin Reuptake Inhibitors; Sildenafil; Silodosin; Simeprevir; Simvastatin; Sirolimus; SORAfenib; Tacrolimus (Systemic); Tacrolimus (Topical); Tadalafil; Tamsulosin; Telaprevir; Temsirolimus; Terfenadine; Ticagrelor; Tofacitinib; Tolterodine; Tolvaptan; Toremifene; Triazolam; Ulipristal; Vardenafil; Vemurafenib; Verapamil; Vilazodone; VinCRIStine (Liposomal); Vitamin K Antagonists; Zopiclone; Zuclopenthixol

The levels/effects of Telithromycin may be increased by: Antifungal Agents (Azole Derivatives, Systemic); Cobicistat; CYP3A4 Inhibitors (Moderate); CYP3A4 Inhibitors (Strong); Dasatinib; Fusidic Acid (Systemic); Ivabradine; Luliconazole; Mifepristone; QTc-Prolonging Agents (Indeterminate Risk and Risk Modifying); Stiripentol; Telaprevir

Nutritional/Ethanol Interactions Herb/Nutraceutical: St John's wort: May decrease the levels/effects of telithromycin.

Adverse Reactions

>10%: Gastrointestinal: Diarrhea (10% to 11%)

2% to 10%:

Central nervous system: Headache (2% to 6%), dizziness (3% to 4%)

Gastrointestinal: Nausea (7% to 8%), vomiting (2% to 3%), loose stools (2%), dysgeusia (2%)

≥0.2% to <2%:

Central nervous system: Fatigue, insomnia, somnolence, vertigo

Dermatologic: Rash

Gastrointestinal: Abdominal distension, abdominal pain, anorexia, constipation, dyspepsia, flatulence, gastritis, gastroenteritis, GI upset, glossitis, stomatitis, watery stools, xerostomia

Genitourinary: Vaginal candidiasis

Hematologic: Platelets increased

Hepatic: Transaminases increased

Ocular: Blurred vision, accommodation delayed, diplopia

Miscellaneous: Candidiasis, diaphoresis increased

Available Dosage Forms

Tablet, Oral:

Ketek: 300 mg, 400 mg

General Dosage Range Dosage adjustment recommended in patients with renal impairment

Oral: *Adults:* 800 mg once daily

Administration

Oral May be administered with or without food.

Storage/Stability Store at 15°C to 30°C (59°F to 86°F).

Nursing Actions

Physical Assessment Culture and sensitivity report and previous allergy history should be assessed prior to therapy. Monitor LFTs. Monitor for jaundice, gastrointestinal disturbance (nausea, vomiting, diarrhea), CNS (vertigo, insomnia), rash, opportunistic infection, QT prolongation, and arrhythmias. Teach patient to report any signs of jaundice or hepatic impairment.

Patient Education

• Discuss specific use of drug and side effects with patient as it relates to treatment. (HCAHPS: During this hospital stay, were you given any medicine that you had not taken before? Before giving you any new medicine, how often did hospital staff tell you what the medicine was for? How often did hospital staff describe possible side effects in a way you could understand?)

• Patient may experience dizziness, headache, nausea, diarrhea, increased/decreased appetite, vaginal yeast infection, or parageusia. Have patient report immediately to prescriber tachycardia, discolored urine, jaundice, ecchymosis,

inability to eat, severe fatigue, bleeding, sudden vision changes, significant dyspepsia, or rash (HCAHPS).
- Educate patient about signs of a significant reaction (eg, wheezing; chest tightness; fever; itching; bad cough; blue skin color; seizures; or swelling of face, lips, tongue, or throat). **Note:** This is not a comprehensive list of all side effects. Patient should consult prescriber for additional questions.

Intended Use and Disclaimer: Should not be printed and given to patients. This information is intended to serve as a concise initial reference for healthcare professionals to use when discussing medications with a patient. You must ultimately rely on your own discretion, experience and judgment in diagnosing, treating and advising patients.

Dietary Considerations May be taken with or without food.

Related Information
Oral Medications That Should Not Be Crushed or Altered *on page 1712*

Telmisartan (tel mi SAR tan)

Brand Names: U.S. Micardis
Pharmacologic Category Angiotensin II Receptor Blocker; Antihypertensive
Pregnancy Risk Factor D
Lactation Excretion in breast milk unknown/not recommended
Breast-Feeding Considerations It is not known if telmisartan is excreted in breast milk. Due to the potential for serious adverse reactions in the nursing infant, a decision should be made whether to discontinue nursing or to discontinue the drug, taking into account the importance of treatment to the mother. The Canadian labeling contraindicates use in nursing women. Breast-fed infants of mothers taking medications for hypertension should be monitored for adverse effects (Chobanian, 2003).

Use
Cardiovascular risk reduction: Cardiovascular risk reduction in patients ≥55 years of age unable to take ACE inhibitors and who are at high risk of major cardiovascular events (eg, MI, stroke, death)
Hypertension: For the treatment of hypertension, alone or in combination with other antihypertensive agents
Mechanism of Action/Effect Telmisartan, a nonpeptide angiotensin receptor antagonist, binds to the AT1 angiotensin II receptor thereby blocking the vasoconstriction and the aldosterone secreting effects of angiotensin II.
Contraindications Known hypersensitivity (eg, anaphylaxis, angioedema) to telmisartan or any component of the formulation; concurrent use of aliskiren in patients with diabetes

Canadian labeling: Additional contraindications: Concomitant use with aliskiren in patients with moderate-to-severe renal impairment (GFR <60 mL/min/1.73m^2); pregnancy; breast-feeding; fructose intolerance
Warnings/Precautions [U.S. Boxed Warning]: Drugs that act on the renin-angiotensin system can cause injury and death to the developing fetus. Discontinue as soon as possible once pregnancy is detected. May cause hyperkalemia; avoid potassium supplementation unless specifically required by healthcare provider. Avoid use or use a smaller dose in patients who are volume depleted; correct depletion first. May be associated with deterioration of renal function and/or increases in serum creatinine, particularly in patients with low renal blood flow (eg, renal artery stenosis, heart failure) whose glomerular filtration rate (GFR) is dependent on efferent arteriolar vasoconstriction by angiotensin II. Use with caution in unstented unilateral/bilateral renal artery stenosis. When unstented bilateral renal artery stenosis is present, use is generally avoided due to the elevated risk of deterioration in renal function unless possible benefits outweigh risks. Use with caution with preexisting renal insufficiency; significant aortic/mitral stenosis. Potentially significant drug-drug interactions may exist, requiring dose or frequency adjustment, additional monitoring, and/or selection of alternative therapy. Use with caution in patients who have biliary obstructive disorders or hepatic dysfunction. Product contains sorbitol. The Canadian labeling contraindicates use in fructose intolerant patients.

Angioedema has been reported rarely with some angiotensin II receptor antagonists (ARBs) and may occur at any time during treatment (especially following first dose). It may involve the head and neck (potentially compromising airway) or the intestine (presenting with abdominal pain). Patients with idiopathic or hereditary angioedema or previous angioedema associated with ACE-inhibitor therapy may be at an increased risk. Prolonged frequent monitoring may be required, especially if tongue, glottis, or larynx are involved, as they are associated with airway obstruction. Patients with a history of airway surgery may have a higher risk of airway obstruction. Discontinue therapy immediately if angioedema occurs. Aggressive early management is critical. Intramuscular (I.M.) administration of epinephrine may be necessary. Do not readminister to patients who have had angioedema with ARBs.
Drug Interactions
Avoid Concomitant Use
Avoid concomitant use of Telmisartan with any of the following: Ramipril

Decreased Effect

The levels/effects of Telmisartan may be decreased by: Herbs (Hypertensive Properties); Methylphenidate; Nonsteroidal Anti-Inflammatory Agents; Yohimbine

Increased Effect/Toxicity

Telmisartan may increase the levels/effects of: ACE Inhibitors; Amifostine; Antihypertensives; Cardiac Glycosides; CycloSPORINE (Systemic); DULoxetine; Hypotensive Agents; Lithium; Nonsteroidal Anti-Inflammatory Agents; Obinutuzumab; Potassium-Sparing Diuretics; Ramipril; RiTUXimab; Sodium Phosphates

The levels/effects of Telmisartan may be increased by: Alfuzosin; Aliskiren; Brimonidine (Topical); Canagliflozin; Diazoxide; Eplerenone; Heparin; Heparin (Low Molecular Weight); Herbs (Hypotensive Properties); MAO Inhibitors; Pentoxifylline; Phosphodiesterase 5 Inhibitors; Potassium Salts; Prostacyclin Analogues; Tolvaptan; Trimethoprim

Nutritional/Ethanol Interactions Herb/Nutraceutical: Some herbal medications may have hypertensive or hypotensive properties; others may increase or decrease the antihypertensive effect of telmisartan. Management: Avoid bayberry, blue cohosh, cayenne, ephedra, ginger, ginseng (American), kola, licorice, and yohimbe. Avoid black cohosh, California poppy, coleus, golden seal, hawthorn, mistletoe, periwinkle, quinine, and shepherd's purse.

Adverse Reactions May be associated with worsening of renal function in patients dependent on renin-angiotensin-aldosterone system.

1% to 10%:
Cardiovascular: Intermittent claudication (7%; placebo 6%), chest pain (≥1%), hypertension (≥1%), peripheral edema (≥1%)
Central nervous system: Dizziness (≥1%), fatigue (≥1%), headache (≥1%), pain (≥1%)
Dermatologic: Skin ulcer (3%; placebo 2%)
Gastrointestinal: Diarrhea (3%), abdominal pain (≥1%), dyspepsia (≥1%), nausea (≥1%)
Genitourinary: Urinary tract infection (≥1%)
Neuromuscular & skeletal: Back pain (3%), myalgia (≥1%)
Respiratory: Upper respiratory infection (7%), sinusitis (3%), cough (≥1%), pharyngitis (1%)

Pharmacodynamics/Kinetics

Onset of Action 1-2 hours; Peak effect: 0.5-1 hours

Duration of Action Up to 24 hours

Available Dosage Forms

Tablet, Oral:
Micardis: 20 mg, 40 mg, 80 mg
Generic: 20 mg, 40 mg, 80 mg

General Dosage Range Oral: *Adults:* Initial: 40-80 mg once daily; Maintenance: 20-80 mg daily once daily

Administration

Oral May be administered without regard to meals.

Storage/Stability Store at 25°C (77°F); excursions are permitted between 15°C and 30°C (59°F and 86°F). Tablets should not be removed from blisters until immediately before administration.

Nursing Actions

Physical Assessment Assess potential for interactions with other pharmacological agents and herbal products (eg, increased risk of hyperkalemia or increased hypotensive effects). Monitor for hypotension, diarrhea, URI, and cough on a regular basis during therapy. Teach patient need for regular blood pressure monitoring.

Patient Education

- Discuss specific use of drug and side effects with patient as it relates to treatment. (HCAHPS: During this hospital stay, were you given any medicine that you had not taken before? Before giving you any new medicine, how often did hospital staff tell you what the medicine was for? How often did hospital staff describe possible side effects in a way you could understand?)
- Patient may experience dizziness, dyspepsia, hyperkalemia, or worsening kidney function. Have patient report immediately to prescriber syncope, severe headache, hyperhidrosis, vomiting, rash, or pregnancy (HCAHPS).
- Educate patient about signs of a significant reaction (eg, wheezing; chest tightness; fever; itching; bad cough; blue skin color; seizures; or swelling of face, lips, tongue, or throat). **Note:** This is not a comprehensive list of all side effects. Patient should consult prescriber for additional questions.

Intended Use and Disclaimer: Should not be printed and given to patients. This information is intended to serve as a concise initial reference for healthcare professionals to use when discussing medications with a patient. You must ultimately rely on your own discretion, experience and judgment in diagnosing, treating and advising patients.

Dietary Considerations May be taken without regard to meals. Product contains sorbitol.

Telmisartan and Amlodipine
(tel mi SAR tan & am LOE di peen)

Brand Names: U.S. Twynsta

Index Terms Amlodipine and Telmisartan; Amlodipine Besylate and Telmisartan

Pharmacologic Category Angiotensin II Receptor Blocker; Antianginal Agent; Antihypertensive; Calcium Channel Blocker; Calcium Channel Blocker, Dihydropyridine

Pregnancy Risk Factor D

Use Hypertension:

U.S. labeling: Treatment of hypertension, including initial treatment in patients who will require multiple antihypertensives for adequate control

Canadian labeling: Treatment of mild-to-moderate hypertension in patients whom combination therapy is appropriate; not indicated for initial therapy

Available Dosage Forms

Tablet, oral:

Twynsta® 40/5: Telmisartan 40 mg and amlodipine 5 mg; Twynsta® 40/10: telmisartan 40 mg and amlodipine 10 mg; Twynsta® 80/5: telmisartan 80 mg and amlodipine 5 mg; Twynsta® 80/10: telmisartan 80 mg and amlodipine10 mg

General Dosage Range Oral: *Adults:* Amlodipine 5-10 mg and telmisartan 40-80 mg once daily (maximum: 10 mg/day [amlodipine]; 80 mg/day [telmisartan])

Administration

Oral May be administered without regard to meals.

Nursing Actions

Physical Assessment See individual agents.

Patient Education

- Discuss specific use of drug and side effects with patient as it relates to treatment. (HCAHPS: During this hospital stay, were you given any medicine that you had not taken before? Before giving you any new medicine, how often did hospital staff tell you what the medicine was for? How often did hospital staff describe possible side effects in a way you could understand?)
- Patient may experience dizziness, dyspepsia, diarrhea, fatigue, flushing, headache, back pain, nausea, or asthenia. Have patient report immediately to prescriber signs of infection, signs of hepatic impairment, urinary retention, angina, tachycardia, bradycardia, arrhythmia, mood changes, myalgia, dyspnea, significant weight gain, edema, or hyperhidrosis (HCAHPS).
- Educate patient about signs of a significant reaction (eg, wheezing; chest tightness; fever; itching; bad cough; blue skin color; seizures; or swelling of face, lips, tongue, or throat). **Note:** This is not a comprehensive list of all side effects. Patient should consult prescriber for additional questions.

Intended Use and Disclaimer: Should not be printed and given to patients. This information is intended to serve as a concise initial reference for healthcare professionals to use when discussing medications with a patient. You must ultimately rely on your own discretion, experience and judgment in diagnosing, treating and advising patients.

Related Information

AmLODIPine *on page 87*
Telmisartan *on page 1483*

Telmisartan and Hydrochlorothiazide

(tel mi SAR tan & hye droe klor oh THYE a zide)

Brand Names: U.S. Micardis HCT

Index Terms Hydrochlorothiazide and Telmisartan

Pharmacologic Category Angiotensin II Receptor Blocker; Antihypertensive; Diuretic, Thiazide

Pregnancy Risk Factor D

Use Hypertension: Treatment of hypertension; **Note:** A fixed-dose combination product should not be used for initial therapy

Available Dosage Forms

Tablet, oral:

Micardis® HCT: 40/12.5: Telmisartan 40 mg and hydrochlorothiazide 12.5 mg; 80/12.5: Telmisartan 80 mg and hydrochlorothiazide 12.5 mg; 80/25: Telmisartan 80 mg and hydrochlorothiazide 25 mg

General Dosage Range Dosage adjustment recommended in patients with hepatic impairment.

Oral: *Adults:* Initial: Telmisartan 80 mg and hydrochlorothiazide 12.5-25 mg once daily; Maintenance: Telmisartan 80-160 mg and hydrochlorothiazide 12.5-25 mg once daily

Administration

Oral May be administered without regard to meals.

Nursing Actions

Physical Assessment See individual agents.

Patient Education

- Discuss specific use of drug and side effects with patient as it relates to treatment. (HCAHPS: During this hospital stay, were you given any medicine that you had not taken before? Before giving you any new medicine, how often did hospital staff tell you what the medicine was for? How often did hospital staff describe possible side effects in a way you could understand?)
- Patient may experience dizziness, diarrhea, dyspepsia, or asthenia. Have patient report immediately to prescriber signs of infection, signs of hyperglycemia, signs of renal impairment, angina, sexual dysfunction, urinary retention, dysuria, hyperhidrosis, akathisia, dyspnea, significant weight gain, edema, ecchymosis, bleeding, jaundice, or vision changes (HCAHPS).
- Educate patient about signs of a significant reaction (eg, wheezing; chest tightness; fever; itching; bad cough; blue skin color; seizures; or swelling of face, lips, tongue, or throat). **Note:** This is not a comprehensive list of all side effects. Patient should consult prescriber for additional questions.

Intended Use and Disclaimer: Should not be printed and given to patients. This information is

intended to serve as a concise initial reference for healthcare professionals to use when discussing medications with a patient. You must ultimately rely on your own discretion, experience and judgment in diagnosing, treating and advising patients.

Related Information

Hydrochlorothiazide *on page 775*

Telmisartan *on page 1483*

Temazepam (te MAZ e pam)

Brand Names: U.S. Restoril

Pharmacologic Category Benzodiazepine

Medication Safety Issues

Sound-alike/look-alike issues:

Temazepam may be confused with flurazepam, LORazepam, tamoxifen

Restoril may be confused with Resotran, Risper-DAL, Vistaril, Zestril

BEERS Criteria medication:

This drug may be potentially inappropriate for use in geriatric patients (Quality of evidence - high; Strength of recommendation - strong).

Medication Guide Available Yes

Pregnancy Risk Factor X

Lactation Enters breast milk/use caution

Use Insomnia: Short-term treatment of insomnia

Controlled Substance C-IV

Available Dosage Forms

Capsule, Oral:

Restoril: 7.5 mg, 15 mg, 22.5 mg, 30 mg

Generic: 7.5 mg, 15 mg, 22.5 mg, 30 mg

General Dosage Range Oral:

Adults: 7.5-30 mg at bedtime

Elderly: Initial: 7.5 mg at bedtime

Nursing Actions

Physical Assessment Assess for history of addiction, dependence, or abuse. Educate patients about fall risks. For inpatient use, institute safety measures (side rails, night light, call bell, assistance with ambulation) to prevent falls. For outpatients, monitor for CNS depression at beginning of therapy and periodically throughout.

Patient Education

• Discuss specific use of drug and side effects with patient as it relates to treatment. (HCAHPS: During this hospital stay, were you given any medicine that you had not taken before? Before giving you any new medicine, how often did hospital staff tell you what the medicine was for? How often did hospital staff describe possible side effects in a way you could understand?)

• Patient may experience presyncope, fatigue, blurred vision, illogical thinking, xerostomia, or change in balance. Have patient report immediately to prescriber memory loss or rash (HCAHPS).

• Educate patient about signs of a significant reaction (eg, wheezing; chest tightness; fever; itching; bad cough; blue skin color; seizures; or swelling of face, lips, tongue, or throat). **Note:** This is not a comprehensive list of all side effects. Patient should consult prescriber for additional questions.

Intended Use and Disclaimer: Should not be printed and given to patients. This information is intended to serve as a concise initial reference for healthcare professionals to use when discussing medications with a patient. You must ultimately rely on your own discretion, experience and judgment in diagnosing, treating and advising patients.

Temozolomide (te moe ZOE loe mide)

Brand Names: U.S. Temodar

Index Terms SCH 52365; TMZ

Pharmacologic Category Antineoplastic Agent, Alkylating Agent (Triazene)

Medication Safety Issues

Sound-alike/look-alike issues:

Temodar may be confused with Tambocor

Temozolomide may be confused with temsirolimus

High alert medication:

This medication is in a class the Institute for Safe Medication Practices (ISMP) includes among its list of drug classes which have a heightened risk of causing significant patient harm when used in error.

Pregnancy Risk Factor D

Lactation Excretion in breast milk unknown/not recommended

Use

Anaplastic astrocytoma: Treatment of refractory anaplastic astrocytoma (refractory to a regimen containing a nitrosourea and procarbazine)

Glioblastoma multiforme: Treatment of newly-diagnosed glioblastoma multiforme (initially in combination with radiotherapy, then as maintenance treatment)

Canadian labeling: Treatment of newly-diagnosed glioblastoma multiforme (initially in combination with radiotherapy, then as maintenance treatment), treatment of recurrent or progressive glioblastoma multiforme or anaplastic astrocytoma

Unlabeled Use Treatment of recurrent glioblastoma multiforme, low-grade astrocytoma, low-grade oligodendroglioma, anaplastic oligodendroglioma, metastatic CNS lesions, refractory primary CNS lymphoma, advanced or metastatic melanoma, advanced cutaneous T-cell lymphomas (mycosis fungoides [MF] and Sézary syndrome [SS]), advanced neuroendocrine tumors (carcinoid or islet cell), Ewing's sarcoma (recurrent or progressive), soft tissue sarcomas (extremity/retroperitoneal/intra-abdominal or hemangiopericytoma/solitary fibrous tumor), treatment of pediatric neuroblastoma

Available Dosage Forms

Capsule, Oral:

Temodar: 5 mg, 20 mg, 100 mg, 140 mg, 180 mg, 250 mg

Generic: 5 mg, 20 mg, 100 mg, 140 mg, 180 mg, 250 mg

Solution Reconstituted, Intravenous:

Temodar: 100 mg (1 ea)

General Dosage Range Dosage adjustment recommended in patients who develop toxicities.

I.V., Oral: *Adults:* Dosage varies greatly depending on indication

Administration

I.V. Infuse over 90 minutes. Flush line before and after administration. May be administered through the same I.V. line as sodium chloride 0.9%; do not administer other medications through the same I.V. line.

Note: Temozolomide is associated with a moderate emetic potential; antiemetics are recommended to prevent nausea and vomiting.

Hazardous agent; use appropriate precautions for handling and disposal (NIOSH, 2012).

Oral Swallow capsules whole with a glass of water. Absorption is affected by food; therefore, administer consistently either with food or without food (was administered in studies under fasting and nonfasting conditions). May administer on an empty stomach or at bedtime to reduce nausea and vomiting. Do not repeat dose if vomiting occurs after dose is administered; wait until the next scheduled dose. Do not open or chew capsules; avoid contact with skin or mucous membranes if capsules are accidentally opened or damaged.

Note: Temozolomide is associated with a moderate emetic potential; antiemetics are recommended to prevent nausea and vomiting.

Hazardous agent; use appropriate precautions for handling and disposal (NIOSH, 2012).

Nursing Actions

Physical Assessment Monitor for convulsions, fatigue, impaired coordination, ataxia, gastrointestinal disturbance (nausea, vomiting, constipation), myelosuppression, rash, opportunistic infection, vision disturbance, and cough on a regular basis.

Patient Education

• Discuss specific use of drug and side effects with patient as it relates to treatment. (HCAHPS: During this hospital stay, were you given any medicine that you had not taken before? Before giving you any new medicine, how often did hospital staff tell you what the medicine was for? How often did hospital staff describe possible side effects in a way you could understand?)

• Patient may experience headache, nausea, constipation, diarrhea, edema in arms or legs, alopecia, asthenia, loss of appetite, leukopenia,

thrombocytopenia, or application site irritation. Have patient report immediately to prescriber ecchymosis or rash (HCAHPS).

• Educate patient about signs of a significant reaction (eg, wheezing; chest tightness; fever; itching; bad cough; blue skin color; seizures; or swelling of face, lips, tongue, or throat). **Note:** This is not a comprehensive list of all side effects. Patient should consult prescriber for additional questions.

Intended Use and Disclaimer: Should not be printed and given to patients. This information is intended to serve as a concise initial reference for healthcare professionals to use when discussing medications with a patient. You must ultimately rely on your own discretion, experience and judgment in diagnosing, treating and advising patients.

Related Information

Oral Medications That Should Not Be Crushed or Altered *on page 1712*

Temsirolimus (tem sir OH li mus)

Brand Names: U.S. Torisel

Index Terms CCI-779

Pharmacologic Category Antineoplastic Agent, mTOR Kinase Inhibitor

Medication Safety Issues

Sound-alike/look-alike issues:

Temsirolimus may be confused with everolimus, sirolimus, tacrolimus, temozolomide, tesamorelin

High alert medication:

This medication is in a class the Institute for Safe Medication Practices (ISMP) includes among its list of drug classes which have a heightened risk of causing significant patient harm when used in error.

Administration issues:

Temsirolimus requires a two-step dilution process prior to administration. The medication is supplied in a vial containing a total amount of 30 mg in a total volume of 1.2 mL (25 mg/mL). The vial must initially be diluted to 10 mg/mL (with provided 1.8 mL of diluent), then the intended dose should be withdrawn from the 10 mg/mL diluted vial (ie, 2.5 mL for a 25 mg dose) and further diluted for infusion in 250 mL sodium chloride 0.9%. Errors have occurred due to improper preparation.

Temsirolimus, for the treatment of advanced renal cell cancer, is a flat dose (25 mg if no dosage reductions) and is not based on body surface area (BSA).

Pregnancy Risk Factor D

Lactation Excretion in breast milk unknown/not recommended

Use Treatment of advanced renal cell cancer (RCC)

Available Dosage Forms
Solution, Intravenous:
Torisel: 25 mg/mL (1 mL)

General Dosage Range Dosage adjustment recommended in patients with hepatic impairment, on concomitant therapy, or who develop toxicities
I.V.: *Adults:* 25 mg once weekly

Administration
I.V. Infuse over 30-60 minutes via an infusion pump (preferred). Use polyethylene-lined non-DEHP administration tubing. Administer through an inline polyethersulfone filter ≤5 micron; if set does not contain an inline filter, a polyethersulfone end filter (0.2-5 micron) should be added (do not use both an inline and an end filter). Premedicate with an H_1 antagonist (eg, diphenhydramine 25-50 mg I.V.) ~30 minutes prior to infusion. Monitor during infusion; interrupt infusion for hypersensitivity/infusion reaction; monitor for 30-60 minutes; may reinitiate at a reduced infusion rate (over 60 minutes) with discretion, 30 minutes after administration of a histamine H_1 antagonist and/or a histamine H_2 antagonist (eg, famotidine or ranitidine). Administration should be completed within 6 hours of admixture.

Hazardous agent; use appropriate precautions for handling and disposal (NIOSH, 2012).

Nursing Actions
Physical Assessment Administer premedication as ordered prior to infusion. Monitor patient closely for anaphylaxis, dyspnea, flushing, and chest pain during and following each infusion; medication/equipment for treating reactions should be readily available. Monitor for altered glucose control (hyper-/hypoglycemia), opportunistic infection, interstitial lung disease (dyspnea, cough, hypoxia, fever, worsening respiratory condition), bowel perforation (abdominal pain, blood in stool), and renal failure at each infusion and throughout therapy; notify prescriber of serious adverse reactions.

Patient Education
- Discuss specific use of drug and side effects with patient as it relates to treatment. (HCAHPS: During this hospital stay, were you given any medicine that you had not taken before? Before giving you any new medicine, how often did hospital staff tell you what the medicine was for? How often did hospital staff describe possible side effects in a way you could understand?)
- Patient may experience anemia, leukopenia, thrombocytopenia, hyperlipidemia, hyperglycemia, edema, nausea, stomatitis, constipation, diarrhea, insomnia, xeroderma, asthenia, or loss of appetite. Have patient report immediately to prescriber signs of infection, dyspnea, severe dyspepsia, melena, polydipsia, polyuria, weight loss, ecchymosis, wound that will not heal, or rash (HCAHPS).

- Educate patient about signs of a significant reaction (eg, wheezing; chest tightness; fever; itching; bad cough; blue skin color; seizures; or swelling of face, lips, tongue, or throat). **Note:** This is not a comprehensive list of all side effects. Patient should consult prescriber for additional questions.

Intended Use and Disclaimer: Should not be printed and given to patients. This information is intended to serve as a concise initial reference for healthcare professionals to use when discussing medications with a patient. You must ultimately rely on your own discretion, experience and judgment in diagnosing, treating and advising patients.

Tenecteplase (ten EK te plase)

Brand Names: U.S. TNKase
Pharmacologic Category Thrombolytic Agent
Medication Safety Issues
Sound-alike/look-alike issues:
TNKase® may be confused with Activase®, t-PA
TNK (occasional abbreviation for TNKase®) is an error-prone abbreviation (mistaken as TPA)
High alert medication:
The Institute for Safe Medication Practices (ISMP) includes this medication (I.V.) among its list of drugs which have a heightened risk of causing significant patient harm when used in error.
Pregnancy Risk Factor C
Lactation Excretion in breast milk unknown/use caution
Breast-Feeding Considerations It is not known if tenecteplase is excreted in breast milk. The manufacturer recommends that caution be exercised when administering tenecteplase to nursing women.
Use Management of ST-elevation myocardial infarction (STEMI) for the lysis of thrombi in the coronary vasculature to restore perfusion and reduce mortality.
Recommended criteria for treatment of STEMI (ACCF/AHA; O'Gara, 2013): Ischemic symptoms within 12 hours of treatment or evidence of ongoing ischemia 12-24 hours after symptom onset with a large area of myocardium at risk or hemodynamic instability.
STEMI ECG definition: New ST-segment elevation at the J point in at least 2 contiguous leads of ≥2 mm (0.2 mV) in men or ≥1.5 mm (0.15 mV) in women in leads V_2-V_3 and/or of ≥1 mm (0.1 mV) in other contiguous precordial leads or limb leads on ECG. New or presumably new left bundle branch block (LBBB) may interfere with ST-elevation analysis and should not be considered diagnostic in isolation.

At non-PCI-capable hospitals, the ACCF/AHA recommends thrombolytic therapy administration when the anticipated first medical contact (FMC)-to-device time at a PCI-capable hospital is >120 minutes due to unavoidable delays.

Mechanism of Action/Effect Promotes initiation of fibrinolysis by binding to fibrin and converting plasminogen to plasmin.

Contraindications Active internal bleeding; history of cerebrovascular accident; recent (ie, within 2 months) intracranial/intraspinal surgery or trauma; intracranial neoplasm; arteriovenous malformation or aneurysm; bleeding diathesis; severe uncontrolled hypertension

Additional contraindications (ACCF/AHA; O'Gara, 2013): Ischemic stroke within 3 months; prior intracranial hemorrhage; active bleeding (excluding menses); suspected aortic dissection; significant closed head or facial trauma within 3 months

Warnings/Precautions Use with caution in patients receiving oral anticoagulants; increased risk of bleeding. Adjunctive use of parenteral anticoagulants (eg, enoxaparin, heparin, or fondaparinux) is recommended to improve vessel patency and prevent reocclusion and may also contribute to bleeding; monitor for bleeding (ACCF/AHA; O'Gara, 2013). Stop antiplatelet agents and heparin if serious bleeding occurs. Avoid I.M. injections and nonessential handling of the patient for a few hours after administration. Monitor for bleeding complications. Venipunctures should be performed carefully and only when necessary. If arterial puncture is necessary, then use an upper extremity that can be easily compressed manually. For the following conditions, the risk of bleeding is higher with use of tenecteplase and the use of tenecteplase should be weighed against the benefits: Recent major surgery, cerebrovascular disease, recent GI or GU bleed, recent trauma, uncontrolled hypertension (systolic BP >180 mm Hg and/or diastolic BP >110 mm Hg), suspected left heart thrombus, acute pericarditis, subacute bacterial endocarditis, hemostatic defects, severe hepatic dysfunction, hemorrhagic diabetic retinopathy or other hemorrhagic ophthalmic conditions, pregnancy, septic thrombophlebitis or occluded arteriovenous cannula at seriously infected site, advanced age, anticoagulants, recent administration of GP IIb/IIIa inhibitors. Use with caution in patients with advanced age; increased risk of bleeding. Mortality and rate of intracranial hemorrhage increases with increasing age >65 years of age; the risks and benefits of use should be weighed carefully in the elderly. Coronary thrombolysis may result in reperfusion arrhythmias. Caution with readministration of tenecteplase.

Drug Interactions

Avoid Concomitant Use There are no known interactions where it is recommended to avoid concomitant use.

Decreased Effect
The levels/effects of Tenecteplase may be decreased by: Aprotinin

Increased Effect/Toxicity
Tenecteplase may increase the levels/effects of: Anticoagulants; Dabigatran Etexilate

The levels/effects of Tenecteplase may be increased by: Agents with Antiplatelet Properties; Herbs (Anticoagulant/Antiplatelet Properties); Salicylates

Adverse Reactions As with all drugs which may affect hemostasis, bleeding is the major adverse effect associated with tenecteplase. Hemorrhage may occur at virtually any site. Risk is dependent on multiple variables, including the dosage administered, concurrent use of multiple agents which alter hemostasis, and patient predisposition. Rapid lysis of coronary artery thrombi by thrombolytic agents may be associated with reperfusion-related arterial and/or ventricular arrhythmia. The incidence of stroke and bleeding increase in patients >65 years.

>10%:
Hematologic: Bleeding (22% minor: ASSENT-2 trial)
Local: Hematoma (12% minor)
1% to 10%:
Central nervous system: Stroke (2%)
Gastrointestinal: Epistaxis (2% minor), GI hemorrhage (1% major, 2% minor)
Genitourinary: GU bleeding (4% minor)
Hematologic: Bleeding (5% major: ASSENT-2 trial)
Local: Bleeding at catheter puncture site (4% minor), hematoma (2% major)
Respiratory: Pharyngeal bleeding (3% minor)
Additional cardiovascular events associated with use in MI: Arrhythmia, AV block, cardiac arrest, cardiac tamponade, cardiogenic shock, embolism, electromechanical dissociation, fever, heart failure, hypotension, mitral regurgitation, myocardial reinfarction, myocardial rupture, nausea, pericardial effusion, pericarditis, pulmonary edema, recurrent myocardial ischemia, thrombosis, vomiting

Available Dosage Forms
Kit, Intravenous:
TNKase: 50 mg
General Dosage Range I.V.:
Adults <60 kg: 30 mg as a single dose
Adults ≥60 to <70 kg: 35 mg as a single dose
Adults ≥70 to <80 kg: 40 mg as a single dose
Adults ≥80 to <90 kg: 45 mg as a single dose
Adults ≥90 kg: 50 mg as a single dose
Administration
I.V. Tenecteplase is **incompatible** with dextrose solutions. Dextrose-containing lines must be flushed with a saline solution before and after administration. Administer as a single I.V. bolus ▶

over 5 seconds. Avoid I.M. injections and nonessential handling of patient.

Preparation for Administration Tenecteplase should be reconstituted using the supplied 10 mL syringe with TwinPak™ Dual Cannula Device and 10 mL sterile water for injection. Do not shake when reconstituting. Slight foaming is normal and will dissipate if left standing for several minutes. The reconstituted solution is 5 mg/mL. Any unused solution should be discarded. If reconstituted and not used immediately, store in refrigerator and use within 8 hours.

Storage/Stability Store under refrigeration of 2°C to 8°C (36°F to 46°F) or at room temperature; do not exceed 30°C (86°F). If reconstituted and not used immediately, store in refrigerator and use within 8 hours.

Nursing Actions

Physical Assessment Monitor patient closely for bleeding during and following treatment. Monitor infusion site, neurological status (eg, intracranial hemorrhage), vital signs, and ECG (reperfusion arrhythmias). Arrhythmias may occur; antiarrhythmic drugs should be immediately available. Maintain bedrest and bleeding precautions. Avoid I.M. injections, venipuncture (unless absolutely necessary), and nonessential handling of the patient. If arterial puncture is necessary, an upper extremity vessel that can be manually compressed should be used.

Patient Education

• Discuss specific use of drug and side effects with patient as it relates to treatment. (HCAHPS: During this hospital stay, were you given any medicine that you had not taken before? Before giving you any new medicine, how often did hospital staff tell you what the medicine was for? How often did hospital staff describe possible side effects in a way you could understand?)

• Patient may experience severe bleeding. Have patient report immediately to prescriber angina, illogical thinking, severe headache, significant back pain, considerable dyspepsia, ecchymosis, severe asthenia, or rash (HCAHPS).

• Educate patient about signs of a significant reaction (eg, wheezing; chest tightness; fever; itching; bad cough; blue skin color; seizures; or swelling of face, lips, tongue, or throat). **Note:** This is not a comprehensive list of all side effects. Patient should consult prescriber for additional questions.

Intended Use and Disclaimer: Should not be printed and given to patients. This information is intended to serve as a concise initial reference for healthcare professionals to use when discussing medications with a patient. You must ultimately rely on your own discretion, experience and judgment in diagnosing, treating and advising patients.

Tenofovir (ten OF oh vir)

Brand Names: U.S. Viread

Index Terms PMPA; TDF; Tenofovir Disoproxil Fumarate

Pharmacologic Category Antihepadnaviral, Reverse Transcriptase Inhibitor, Nucleotide (Anti-HBV); Antiretroviral, Reverse Transcriptase Inhibitor, Nucleotide (Anti-HIV)

Pregnancy Risk Factor B

Lactation Enters breast milk/contraindicated

Breast-Feeding Considerations Maternal or infant antiretroviral therapy does not completely eliminate the risk of postnatal HIV transmission. In addition, multiclass-resistant virus has been detected in breast-feeding infants despite maternal therapy. Therefore, in the United States, where formula is accessible, affordable, safe, and sustainable, and the risk of infant mortality due to diarrhea and respiratory infections is low, complete avoidance of breast-feeding by HIV-infected women is recommended to decrease potential transmission of HIV (DHHS [perinatal], 2012).

Use

U.S. labeling:

Chronic hepatitis B: Treatment of chronic hepatitis B virus (HBV) in patients ≥12 years of age

HIV infection: In combination with other antiretroviral agents for the treatment of HIV-1 infection in adults and pediatric patients ≥2 years of age

Canadian labeling: Management of HIV infections in combination with at least two other antiretroviral agents in patients ≥12 years of age; treatment of chronic hepatitis B virus (HBV) in patients with compensated or decompensated liver disease in patients ≥18 years of age

Mechanism of Action/Effect Tenofovir blocks replication of HIV virus by inhibiting the reverse transcriptase enzyme. It is chemically similar to adenosine 5'-monophosphate (a nucleotide), which is required to form DNA. Tenofovir inhibits replication of HBV by inhibiting HBV polymerase.

Contraindications

U.S. labeling: There are no contraindications listed in the manufacturer's labeling.

Canadian labeling: Hypersensitivity to tenofovir or any component of the formulation; concurrent use with fixed-dose combination products that contain tenofovir (Truvada, Atripla, Complera, or Stribild); concurrent use with adefovir (Hepsera)

Warnings/Precautions [U.S Boxed Warning]: Lactic acidosis and severe hepatomegaly with steatosis have been reported with tenofovir and other nucleoside analogues, including fatal cases; use with caution in patients with risk factors for liver disease (risk may be increased in obese patients or prolonged exposure) and suspend treatment in any patient who develops clinical or laboratory findings suggestive of lactic acidosis (transaminase elevation may/may not accompany hepatomegaly and steatosis). May cause redistribution of fat (eg, buffalo hump, peripheral wasting with increased abdominal girth, cushingoid appearance). Immune reconstitution syndrome may develop resulting in the occurrence of an inflammatory response to an indolent or residual opportunistic infection during initial HIV treatment or activation of autoimmune disorders (eg, Graves' disease, polymyositis, Guillain-Barré syndrome) later in therapy; further evaluation and treatment may be required. Use caution in hepatic impairment; limited data supporting treatment of chronic hepatitis B in patients with decompensated liver disease; observe for increased adverse reactions, including renal dysfunction.

In clinical trials, use has been associated with decreases in bone mineral density in HIV-1 infected adults and increases in bone metabolism markers. Serum parathyroid hormone and 1,25 vitamin D levels were also higher. Decreases in bone mineral density have also been observed in clinical trials of HIV-1 infected pediatric patients. Observations in chronic hepatitis B infected pediatric patients (aged 12-18 years) were similar. Consider monitoring of bone density in adult and pediatric patients with a history of pathologic fractures or with other risk factors for bone loss or osteoporosis. Consider calcium and vitamin D supplementation for all patients; effect of supplementation has not been studied but may be beneficial. Long-term bone health and fracture risk unknown. Skeletal growth (height) appears to be unaffected in tenofovir-treated children and adolescents.

May cause osteomalacia with proximal renal tubulopathy. Bone pain, extremity pain, fractures, arthralgias, weakness and muscle pain have been reported. In patients at risk for renal dysfunction, persistent or worsening bone or muscle symptoms should be evaluated for hypophosphatemia and osteomalacia.

Do not use as monotherapy in treatment of HIV. Clinical trials in HIV-infected patients whose regimens contained only three nucleoside reverse transcriptase inhibitors (NRTI) show less efficacy, early virologic failure and high rates of resistance substitutions. Use three NRTI regimens with caution and monitor response carefully. Triple drug regimens with two NRTIs in combination with a non-nucleoside reverse transcriptase inhibitor or a HIV-1 protease inhibitor are usually more effective. Treatment of HIV in patients with unrecognized/untreated hepatitis B virus (HBV) may lead to rapid HBV resistance. Patients should be tested for presence of chronic hepatitis B infection prior to initiation of therapy. In patients coinfected with HIV and HBV, an appropriate antiretroviral combination should be selected due to HIV resistance potential;

these patients should receive tenofovir dosed for HIV therapy.

Tenofovir is predominately eliminated renally; use caution in renal impairment. May cause acute renal failure or Fanconi syndrome; use caution with other nephrotoxic agents (including high dose or multiple NSAID use or those which compete for active tubular secretion). Acute renal failure has occurred in HIV-infected patients with risk factors for renal impairment who were on a stable tenofovir regimen to which a high dose or multiple NSAID therapy was added. Consider alternatives to NSAIDS in patients taking tenofovir and at risk for renal impairment. Calculate creatinine clearance prior to initiation of therapy and monitor renal function (including recalculation of creatinine clearance and serum phosphorus) during therapy. Dosage adjustment required in patients with CrCl <50 mL/minute. Use caution in patients with low body weight, or concurrent medications which increase tenofovir levels. Use caution in the elderly; dosage adjustment based on renal function may be required.

[U.S. Boxed Warning]: If treating HBV, acute exacerbation of hepatitis B may occur upon discontinuation. Monitor liver function closely for several months after discontinuing treatment; reinitiation of antihepatitis B therapy may be required. Treatment of HBV in patients with unrecognized/untreated HIV may lead to HIV resistance; patients should be tested for presence of HIV infection prior to initiating therapy. Do not use as monotherapy in treatment of HIV. Treatment of HIV in patients with unrecognized/untreated HBV may lead to rapid HBV resistance. Patients should be tested for presence of chronic hepatitis B prior to initiation of therapy. Potentially significant drug-drug interactions may exist, requiring dose or frequency adjustment, additional monitoring, and/or selection of alternative therapy. Do not use concurrently with adefovir or tenofovir combination products.

Drug Interactions

Avoid Concomitant Use

Avoid concomitant use of Tenofovir with any of the following: Adefovir; Dabigatran Etexilate; Didanosine; Pomalidomide; VinCRIStine (Liposomal)

Decreased Effect

Tenofovir may decrease the levels/effects of: Afatinib; Atazanavir; Dabigatran Etexilate; Didanosine; DOXOrubicin (Conventional); Linagliptin; P-glycoprotein/ABCB1 Substrates; Pomalidomide; Simeprevir; Tipranavir; VinCRIStine (Liposomal)

The levels/effects of Tenofovir may be decreased by: Adefovir; Tipranavir

Increased Effect/Toxicity

Tenofovir may increase the levels/effects of: Adefovir; Aminoglycosides; Darunavir; Didanosine; Ganciclovir-Valganciclovir

The levels/effects of Tenofovir may be increased by: Acyclovir-Valacyclovir; Adefovir; Aminoglycosides; Atazanavir; Cidofovir; Darunavir; Diclofenac (Systemic); Ganciclovir-Valganciclovir; Lopinavir; Nonsteroidal Anti-Inflammatory Agents; Simeprevir; Telaprevir

Nutritional/Ethanol Interactions Food: Fatty meals may increase the bioavailability of tenofovir. Tenofovir may be taken with or without food.

Adverse Reactions Includes data from both treatment-naive and treatment-experienced HIV patients and in chronic hepatitis B.

>10%:
Central nervous system: Insomnia (3% to 18%), headache (5% to 14%), pain (12% to 13%), dizziness (8% to 13%), depression (4% to 11%)
Dermatologic: Skin rash (includes maculopapular, pustular, or vesiculobullous rash; pruritus; or urticaria: 5% to 18%), pruritus (16%)
Endocrine & metabolic: Hypercholesterolemia (19% to 22%), increased serum triglycerides (1% to 4%)
Gastrointestinal: Abdominal pain (4% to 22%), nausea (8% to 20%), diarrhea (9% to 16%), vomiting (2% to 13%)
Neuromuscular & skeletal: Decreased bone mineral density (28%; ≥5% at spine or ≥7% at hip), increased creatine phosphokinase (2% to 12%), weakness (6% to 11%)
Miscellaneous: Fever (4% to 11%)
1% to 10%:
Cardiovascular: Chest pain (3%)
Central nervous system: Fatigue (9%), anxiety (6%), peripheral neuropathy (1% to 5%)
Dermatologic: Diaphoresis (3%)
Endocrine & metabolic: Weight loss (2% to 4%), glycosuria (grades 3/4: ≤3%), hyperglycemia (grades 3/4: 2% to 3%), lipodystrophy (1%)
Gastrointestinal: Increased serum amylase (grades 3/4: 4% to 9%), anorexia (3% to 4%), dyspepsia (3% to 4%), flatulence (3% to 4%)
Genitourinary: Hematuria (≤ grades 3/4: 3% to 7%)
Hematologic & oncologic: Neutropenia (3%)
Hepatic: Increased serum ALT (2% to 10%), increased serum AST (3% to 5%), increased serum transaminases (2% to 5%), increased serum alkaline phosphatase (1%)
Neuromuscular & skeletal: Back pain (4% to 9%), arthralgia (5%), myalgia (4%)
Renal: Increased serum creatinine (9%), renal failure (7%)
Respiratory: Sinusitis (8%), upper respiratory tract infection (8%), nasopharyngitis (5%), pneumonia (2% to 5%)

Available Dosage Forms
Powder, Oral:
Viread: 40 mg/g (60 g)
Tablet, Oral:
Viread: 150 mg, 200 mg, 250 mg, 300 mg

General Dosage Range Dosage adjustment recommended in patients with renal impairment
Oral:
Children 2 to <12 years: 8 mg/kg once daily (maximum: 300 mg once daily)
Children ≥12 years (and ≥35 kg), Adolescents, and Adults: 300 mg once daily

Administration
Oral Tablets may be administered without regard to meals. Powder should be mixed with 2-4 ounces of soft food (applesauce, baby food, yogurt) and swallowed immediately (avoids bitter taste); do not mix in liquid (powder may float on top of the liquid even after stirring). Measure powder using only the supplied dosing scoop.

Storage/Stability Store at 25°C (77°F); excursions are permitted between 15°C and 30°C (59°F and 86°F). Dispense only in original container.

Nursing Actions
Physical Assessment Allergy history should be assessed prior to beginning treatment. Monitor for lactic acidosis, elevated transaminases, osteomalacia, depression, increased triglyceride level, nausea, vomiting, diarrhea, neutropenia, myalgia, and peripheral neuropathy on a regular basis. With long-term use or use in children, assess bone strength. Observe for weakness; dark yellow or brown urine; unusual bleeding or bruising; flu-like symptoms; and jaundice.

Patient Education
• Discuss specific use of drug and side effects with patient as it relates to treatment. (HCAHPS: During this hospital stay, were you given any medicine that you had not taken before? Before giving you any new medicine, how often did hospital staff tell you what the medicine was for? How often did hospital staff describe possible side effects in a way you could understand?)
• Patient may experience headache, nausea, diarrhea, asthenia, or osteopenia. Have patient report immediately to prescriber signs of infection, dyspnea, severe dizziness or syncope, tachycardia, significant dyspepsia, inability to eat, severe myalgia, discolored urine, jaundice, or cold intolerance (HCAHPS).
• Educate patient about signs of a significant reaction (eg, wheezing; chest tightness; fever; itching; bad cough; blue skin color; seizures; or swelling of face, lips, tongue, or throat). **Note:** This is not a comprehensive list of all side effects. Patient should consult prescriber for additional questions.

Intended Use and Disclaimer: Should not be printed and given to patients. This information is intended to serve as a concise initial reference for healthcare professionals to use when discussing medications with a patient. You must ultimately rely on your own discretion, experience and judgment in diagnosing, treating and advising patients.

Dietary Considerations Consider calcium and vitamin D supplementation.

Terazosin (ter AY zoe sin)

Index Terms Hytrin
Pharmacologic Category Alpha₁ Blocker; Antihypertensive
Medication Safety Issues
  BEERS Criteria medication:
    This drug may be potentially inappropriate for use in geriatric patients (Quality of evidence - moderate; Strength of recommendation - strong).
Pregnancy Risk Factor C
Lactation Excretion in breast milk unknown/use caution
Use Management of mild-to-moderate hypertension; alone or in combination with other agents such as diuretics or beta-blockers; benign prostate hyperplasia (BPH)
Unlabeled Use Pediatric hypertension
Available Dosage Forms
  Capsule, Oral:
    Generic: 1 mg, 2 mg, 5 mg, 10 mg
General Dosage Range Dosage adjustment recommended in patients on concomitant therapy
  Oral: *Adults:* Initial: 1 mg at bedtime; Maintenance: 1-20 mg once daily (maximum: 20 mg/day)
Administration
  Oral Administered without regard to meals at the same time each day.
Nursing Actions
  Physical Assessment Monitor blood pressure and for hypotension, dizziness, somnolence, and impotence at beginning of therapy and on a regular basis. When discontinuing, dose should be tapered and blood pressure monitored closely.
  Patient Education
    • Discuss specific use of drug and side effects with patient as it relates to treatment. (HCAHPS: During this hospital stay, were you given any medicine that you had not taken before? Before giving you any new medicine, how often did hospital staff tell you what the medicine was for? How often did hospital staff describe possible side effects in a way you could understand?)
    • Patient may experience dizziness, rhinitis, asthenia, or impotence. Have patient report immediately to prescriber angina, erection lasting >4 hours, or rash (HCAHPS).
    • Educate patient about signs of a significant reaction (eg, wheezing; chest tightness; fever; itching; bad cough; blue skin color; seizures; or swelling of face, lips, tongue, or throat). **Note:** This is not a comprehensive list of all side effects. Patient should consult prescriber for additional questions.

  Intended Use and Disclaimer: Should not be printed and given to patients. This information is intended to serve as a concise initial reference for healthcare professionals to use when discussing medications with a patient. You must ultimately rely on your own discretion, experience and judgment in diagnosing, treating and advising patients.

Terbinafine (Systemic) (TER bin a feen)

Brand Names: U.S. LamISIL; Terbinex
Index Terms Terbinafine Hydrochloride
Pharmacologic Category Antifungal Agent, Oral
Medication Safety Issues
  Sound-alike/look-alike issues:
    Terbinafine may be confused with terbutaline
    LamISIL may be confused with LaMICtal, Lomotil
Pregnancy Risk Factor B
Lactation Enters breast milk/not recommended
Breast-Feeding Considerations Terbinafine is excreted in breast milk; the milk/plasma ratio is 7:1. Breast-feeding is not recommended by the manufacturer.
Use
  Onychomycosis (tablets only): Treatment of onychomycosis of the toenail or fingernail caused by dermatophytes (tinea unguium).
  Tinea capitis (granules only): Treatment of tinea capitis in patients 4 years and older.
  Canadian labeling: Additional use (not in U.S. labeling): Severe tineal skin infections (tinea cruris and tinea pedis) unresponsive to topical therapy
Unlabeled Use Sporotrichosis: Treatment of sporotrichosis (lymphocutaneous and cutaneous)
Mechanism of Action/Effect Synthetic allylamine derivative which inhibits squalene epoxidase, a key enzyme in sterol biosynthesis in fungi. This results in a deficiency of ergosterol within the fungal cell wall and results in fungal cell death.
Contraindications Hypersensitivity to terbinafine or any component of the formulation
Warnings/Precautions Due to potential toxicity, confirmation of diagnostic testing of nail or skin specimens prior to treatment of onychomycosis or dermatomycosis is recommended. Use caution in patients sensitive to allylamine antifungals (eg, naftifine, butenafine); cross sensitivity to terbinafine may exist. Transient decreases in absolute lymphocyte counts were observed in clinical trials; severe neutropenia (reversible upon discontinuation) has also been reported. Monitor CBC in patients with pre-existing immunosuppression if therapy is to continue >6 weeks and discontinue therapy if ANC ≤1000/mm³.

Serious skin and hypersensitivity reactions (eg, Stevens-Johnson syndrome, toxic epidermal necrolysis, erythema multiforme, exfoliative dermatitis, bullous dermatitis, drug reaction with eosinophilia and systemic symptoms [DRESS] syndrome) have occurred. If progressive skin rash or signs and symptoms of a hypersensitivity reaction occur, ▶

discontinue treatment. Cases of hepatic failure, some leading to liver transplant or death, have been reported; not recommended for use in patients with active or chronic liver disease. If clinical evidence of liver injury develops (eg, nausea, anorexia, fatigue, vomiting, right upper abdominal pain, jaundice, dark urine, pale stools), assess hepatic function immediately; discontinue therapy in cases of elevated liver function tests. Use with caution in patients with renal dysfunction (CrCl ≤50 mL/minute) (per Canadian labeling, not recommended for use); clearance is reduced by ~50%.

Disturbances of taste and/or smell may occur; resolution may be delayed (eg, >1 year) following discontinuation of therapy or in some cases, disturbance may be permanent. Discontinue therapy in patients with symptoms of taste or smell disturbance.

Drug Interactions

Avoid Concomitant Use

Avoid concomitant use of Terbinafine (Systemic) with any of the following: Axitinib; Pimozide; Simeprevir; Tamoxifen; Thioridazine

Decreased Effect

Terbinafine (Systemic) may decrease the levels/effects of: Axitinib; Codeine; Ibrutinib; Iloperidone; Saccharomyces boulardii; Saxagliptin; Simeprevir; Tamoxifen; TraMADol

The levels/effects of Terbinafine (Systemic) may be decreased by: Rifampin

Increased Effect/Toxicity

Terbinafine (Systemic) may increase the levels/effects of: ARIPiprazole; AtoMOXetine; CYP2D6 Substrates; DOXOrubicin (Conventional); Fesoterodine; Iloperidone; Metoprolol; Nebivolol; Pimozide; Propafenone; Tetrabenazine; Thioridazine; Tricyclic Antidepressants; Vortioxetine

Adverse Reactions Adverse events listed for tablets unless otherwise specified. Granules were studied in patients 4-12 years of age.

>10%: Central nervous system: Headache (13%; granules 7%)

1% to 10%:
Dermatologic: Skin rash (6%; granules 2%), pruritus (3%; granules 1%), urticaria (1%)
Gastrointestinal: Diarrhea (6%; granules 3%), vomiting (<1%; granules 5%), dyspepsia (4%), dysgeusia (may be severe and result in weight loss and depression; 3%), nausea (3%; granules 2%), abdominal pain (2%; granules 2% to 4%), flatulence (2%), sore throat (granules 2%), toothache (granules 1%)
Hepatic: Liver enzyme disorder (3%)
Infection: Influenza (granules 2%)
Ophthalmic: Visual disturbance (1%)
Respiratory: Nasopharyngitis (granules 10%), cough (granules 6%), upper respiratory tract infection (granules 5%), nasal congestion (granules 2%), rhinorrhea (granules 2%)
Miscellaneous: Fever (granules 7%)

Available Dosage Forms

Cream, External:
LamISIL AT [OTC]: 1% (12 g)

Kit, Combination:
Terbinex: 250 mg & 1%

Packet, Oral:
LamISIL: 125 mg (1 ea, 14 ea); 187.5 mg (1 ea, 14 ea)

Tablet, Oral:
LamISIL: 250 mg
Generic: 250 mg

General Dosage Range

Oral granules: *Children ≥4 years, Adolescents, and Adults:*
<25 kg: 125 mg once daily for 6 weeks
25-35 kg: 187.5 mg once daily for 6 weeks
>35 kg: 250 mg once daily for 6 weeks

Oral tablet: *Adults:* 250 mg once daily for 6-12 weeks

Administration

Oral Administer tablets without regard to meals. Administer granules with food; sprinkle granules on a spoonful of pudding or other soft, nonacidic food (eg, mashed potatoes); swallow entire spoonful without chewing; do not mix granules with applesauce or other fruit-based foods.

Storage/Stability

Granules: Store at 25°C (77°F); excursions permitted between 15°C to 30°C (59°F to 86°F).
Tablet: Store below 25°C (77°F). Protect from light.

Nursing Actions

Physical Assessment Use with caution in presence of hepatic or renal impairment.

Patient Education

- Discuss specific use of drug and side effects with patient as it relates to treatment. (HCAHPS: During this hospital stay, were you given any medicine that you had not taken before? Before giving you any new medicine, how often did hospital staff tell you what the medicine was for? How often did hospital staff describe possible side effects in a way you could understand?)
- Patient may experience headache, dyspepsia, nausea, diarrhea, or parageusia. Have patient report immediately to prescriber inability to eat, significant weight gain, discolored urine, jaundice, severe asthenia, sudden vision changes, eye pain, eye irritation, or rash (HCAHPS).
- Educate patient about signs of a significant reaction (eg, wheezing; chest tightness; fever; itching; bad cough; blue skin color; seizures; or swelling of face, lips, tongue, or throat). **Note:** This is not a comprehensive list of all side effects. Patient should consult prescriber for additional questions.

Intended Use and Disclaimer: Should not be printed and given to patients. This information is intended to serve as a concise initial reference for healthcare professionals to use when discussing

medications with a patient. You must ultimately rely on your own discretion, experience and judgment in diagnosing, treating and advising patients.

Terbutaline (ter BYOO ta leen)

Index Terms Brethaire; Brethine; Bricanyl; Terbutaline Sulfate

Pharmacologic Category Antidote, Extravasation; Beta$_2$ Agonist

Medication Safety Issues

Sound-alike/look-alike issues:

Brethine may be confused with Methergine®

Terbutaline may be confused with terbinafine, TOLBUTamide

Terbutaline and methylergonovine parenteral dosage forms look similar. Due to their contrasting indications, use care when administering these agents.

Pregnancy Risk Factor C

Lactation Enters breast milk/not recommended

Use Bronchodilator in reversible airway obstruction and bronchial asthma

Unlabeled Use Injection: Tocolytic agent (short-term [≤72 hours]) prevention or management of preterm labor; management of extravasation of sympathomimetic vasoconstrictors (based on limited case reports)

Available Dosage Forms

Solution, Injection:

Generic: 1 mg/mL (1 mL)

Tablet, Oral:

Generic: 2.5 mg, 5 mg

General Dosage Range Dosage adjustment recommended in patients with renal impairment

Oral:

Children 12-15 years: 2.5 mg every 6 hours 3 times/day (maximum: 7.5 mg/day)

Children >15 years and Adults: 2.5-5 mg every 6 hours 3 times/day (maximum: 15 mg/day)

SubQ:

Children <12 years: 0.005-0.01 mg/kg/dose to a maximum of 0.4 mg/dose; may repeat in 15-20 minutes

Children ≥12 years and Adults: 0.25 mg/dose; may repeat in 15-30 minutes (maximum: 0.5 mg/4-hour period)

Administration

I.V. Use infusion pump.

Injectable Detail pH: 4 (solution in vial)

Oral Administer around-the-clock to promote less variation in peak and trough serum levels.

Subcutaneous Extravasation management, sympathomimetic vasopressors (unlabeled use): Stop vesicant infusion immediately and disconnect I.V. line (leave needle/cannula in place); gently aspirate extravasated solution from the I.V. line (do **NOT** flush the line); remove needle/cannula; elevate extremity. Infiltrate extravasation area with terbutaline solution 1 mg diluted with 9 mL (large extravasation site) **or** 1 mg diluted with 1 mL (small/distal extravasation site) of 0.9% sodium chloride into extravasation site (Stier, 1999).

Inhalation Bricanyl® Turbuhaler® (Canadian availability): After removing lid, patient should hold inhaler upright and turn blue grip as far as it will go in one direction then turn it back to original position. Clicking sound indicates that inhaler is ready for use. Patient should exhale fully but not into the inhaler and then place mouthpiece gently between teeth, close lips around inhaler and inhale deeply. Inhaler should be removed from mouth prior to exhaling. Instruct patients to rinse mouth with water after each inhalation as some medication may stick to the inside of the mouth and throat. If inhaler is dropped or shaken, or if patient exhales into the inhaler after a dose is loaded, the dose will be lost and a new dose should be loaded and inhaled. Outside of mouthpiece should be cleaned once weekly with a dry tissue. Instruct patient to keep inhaler dry. First appearance of red mark in dose indicator (window underneath mouthpiece) indicates that 20 doses remain. When red mark reaches bottom of dose indicator no doses remain and Turbuhaler should be discarded.

Nursing Actions

Physical Assessment Respiratory use: Monitor for cardiac and CNS changes at beginning of therapy and periodically throughout. For inpatient care, monitor vital signs and lung sounds prior to and periodically during therapy. **Preterm labor use: Inpatient:** Monitor maternal vital signs; respiratory, fluid, cardiac, and electrolyte status; frequency, duration, and intensity of contractions; and fetal heart rate. Subcutaneous administration only; not intravenous administration. Monitor for common side effects: Nervousness, drowsiness, headache, palpitations, tachycardia, nausea, and tremors.

Patient Education

- Discuss specific use of drug and side effects with patient as it relates to treatment. (HCAHPS: During this hospital stay, were you given any medicine that you had not taken before? Before giving you any new medicine, how often did hospital staff tell you what the medicine was for? How often did hospital staff describe possible side effects in a way you could understand?)

- Patient may experience nervousness and anxiety, headache, nausea, xerostomia, insomnia, hypotension, flushing, hypokalemia, or hyperglycemia. Have patient report immediately to prescriber uncontrollable breathing attack, angina, tachycardia, decreased peak flow measurement, dyspnea, or rash (HCAHPS).

• Educate patient about signs of a significant reaction (eg, wheezing; chest tightness; fever; itching; bad cough; blue skin color; seizures; or swelling of face, lips, tongue, or throat). **Note:** This is not a comprehensive list of all side effects. Patient should consult prescriber for additional questions.

Intended Use and Disclaimer: Should not be printed and given to patients. This information is intended to serve as a concise initial reference for healthcare professionals to use when discussing medications with a patient. You must ultimately rely on your own discretion, experience and judgment in diagnosing, treating and advising patients.

Related Information
Management of Drug Extravasations *on page 1700*

Terconazole (ter KONE a zole)

Brand Names: U.S. Terazol 3; Terazol 7; Zazole
Index Terms Triaconazole
Pharmacologic Category Antifungal Agent, Vaginal
Medication Safety Issues
Sound-alike/look-alike issues:
Terconazole may be confused with tioconazole
International issues:
Terazol [U.S., Canada] may be confused with Theradol brand name for tramadol [Netherlands]
Pregnancy Risk Factor C
Lactation Excretion in breast milk unknown/not recommended
Use Candidiasis: For the local treatment of vulvovaginal candidiasis (moniliasis). As terconazole is effective only for vulvovaginitis caused by the genus *Candida*, the diagnosis should be confirmed by KOH smears or cultures.
Available Dosage Forms
Cream, Vaginal:
Terazol 7: 0.4% (45 g)
Terazol 3: 0.8% (20 g)
Zazole: 0.4% (45 g); 0.8% (20 g)
Generic: 0.4% (45 g); 0.8% (20 g)
Suppository, Vaginal:
Terazol 3: 80 mg (3 ea)
Zazole: 80 mg (3 ea)
Generic: 80 mg (3 ea)
General Dosage Range Intravaginal: *Adults, females:* Insert 1 applicatorful or suppository at bedtime
Administration
Intravaginal
Vaginal cream: Use applicator provided by manufacturer. Insertion should be as far as possible into the vagina without causing discomfort. Wash applicator after each use; allow to dry thoroughly before putting back together.

Vaginal suppository: Remove foil package prior to use. Insertion should be as far as possible into the vagina without causing discomfort. If the provided applicator is used for insertion, wash and dry thoroughly prior to additional use.
Nursing Actions
Patient Education
• Discuss specific use of drug and side effects with patient as it relates to treatment. (HCAHPS: During this hospital stay, were you given any medicine that you had not taken before? Before giving you any new medicine, how often did hospital staff tell you what the medicine was for? How often did hospital staff describe possible side effects in a way you could understand?)
• Patient may experience headache or dyspepsia. Have patient report immediately to prescriber reoccurring yeast infection or rash (HCAHPS).
• Educate patient about signs of a significant reaction (eg, wheezing; chest tightness; fever; itching; bad cough; blue skin color; seizures; or swelling of face, lips, tongue, or throat). **Note:** This is not a comprehensive list of all side effects. Patient should consult prescriber for additional questions.

Intended Use and Disclaimer: Should not be printed and given to patients. This information is intended to serve as a concise initial reference for healthcare professionals to use when discussing medications with a patient. You must ultimately rely on your own discretion, experience and judgment in diagnosing, treating and advising patients.

Teriflunomide (ter i FLOO noh mide)

Brand Names: U.S. Aubagio
Index Terms A771726; HMR1726
Pharmacologic Category Pyrimidine Synthesis Inhibitor
Medication Guide Available Yes
Pregnancy Risk Factor X
Lactation Excretion in breast milk unknown/not recommended
Breast-Feeding Considerations It is not known whether teriflunomide is secreted in human milk. Because the potential for serious adverse reactions exists in the nursing infant, a decision should be made whether to discontinue nursing or discontinue the drug, taking into account the importance of the drug to the mother.
Use Multiple sclerosis: Treatment of relapsing forms of multiple sclerosis
Mechanism of Action/Effect Teriflunomide is an immunomodulatory agent that inhibits pyrimidine synthesis, resulting in antiproliferative and anti-inflammatory effects.

Contraindications

Severe hepatic impairment; concomitant use with leflunomide; women of childbearing age who will not use contraception reliably; pregnancy

Canadian labeling: Additional contraindications (not in U.S. labeling): Hypersensitivity to teriflunomide, leflunomide or any component of the formulation; immunodeficiency states (eg, AIDS); impaired bone marrow function or significant anemias, leucopenia, neutropenia, or thrombocytopenia; serious active infections

Warnings/Precautions Hazardous agent; use appropriate precautions for handling and disposal (meets NIOSH, 2012 criteria). **[U.S. Boxed Warning]: Use of leflunomide has been associated with rare reports of hepatotoxicity, hepatic failure, and death, therefore, a similar risk is expected with teriflunomide. Treatment should not be initiated in patients with pre-existing acute or chronic liver disease or ALT >2 x ULN; use is contraindicated in patients with severe impairment. Use caution in patients with concurrent exposure to potentially hepatotoxic drugs. Monitor ALT levels at least monthly for first 6 months during therapy; discontinue if ALT >3 x ULN occurs and, if hepatotoxicity is likely teriflunomide-induced, start drug elimination procedures** (eg, cholestyramine, activated charcoal) and monitor liver function tests weekly until normalized.

Use of leflunomide has been associated (rarely) with interstitial lung disease; discontinue in patients who develop new onset or worsening of pulmonary symptoms. Drug elimination procedures should be considered (eg, cholestyramine, activated charcoal) if evidence of interstitial lung disease; fatal outcomes have been reported. May increase susceptibility to infection, including opportunistic pathogens. Severe infections, sepsis, and fatalities have been reported with leflunomide. One case of fatal sepsis has been reported with teriflunomide. Not recommended in patients with severe immunodeficiency, bone marrow dysplasia, or severe, uncontrolled infections. Caution should be exercised when considering the use in patients with a history of new/recurrent infections, with conditions that predispose them to infections, or with chronic, latent, or localized infections. Patients who develop a new infection while undergoing treatment should be monitored closely; consider discontinuation of therapy and drug elimination procedures if infection is serious.

Use may affect defenses against malignancies; impact on the development and course of malignancies is not fully defined. As compared to the general population, an increased risk of lymphoma has been noted in clinical trials with use of some immunosuppressive medications. Use with caution in patients with a prior history of significant hematologic abnormalities; avoid use with bone marrow

dysplasia. Neutropenia, leukopenia, and thrombocytopenia have been reported in clinical trials. Use of leflunomide has been associated with rare pancytopenia, agranulocytosis, and thrombocytopenia, therefore, a similar risk may be expected with teriflunomide. Monitoring of hematologic function is required; discontinue if evidence of bone marrow suppression and begin drug elimination procedures (eg, cholestyramine, activated charcoal). If coadministered with other potential immunosuppressive agents or switching from teriflunomide to another known immunosuppressant, increased monitoring for hematological adverse effects is necessary. Rare cases of dermatologic reactions (including Stevens-Johnson syndrome and toxic epidermal necrolysis) have been reported with leflunomide, therefore patients taking teriflunomide may also be at risk; discontinue if evidence of severe dermatologic reaction occurs, and begin drug elimination procedures (eg, cholestyramine or activated charcoal). Cases of peripheral neuropathy have been reported; use with caution in patients >60 years of age, receiving concomitant neurotoxic medications, or patients with diabetes; discontinue if evidence of peripheral neuropathy occurs and begin drug elimination procedures (eg, cholestyramine, activated charcoal).

Transient acute renal failure, most likely due to acute uric acid nephropathy has been reported. Increased serum creatinine typically occurred 12 weeks to 2 years after the first dose; serum creatinine usually normalized with continued use. Severe hyperkalemia (>7.0 mmol/L) has been reported. Monitor levels in patients with symptoms or acute renal failure. Increases in blood pressure have been reported; monitor at initiation of therapy and periodically thereafter.

Safety has not been established in patients with latent tuberculosis infection. Patients should be screened for tuberculosis and if necessary, treated prior to initiating therapy. Potentially significant drug-drug interactions may exist, requiring dose or frequency adjustment, additional monitoring, and/or selection of alternative therapy. Patients should be brought up to date with all immunizations before initiating therapy. Live vaccines should not be given concurrently; there is no data available concerning secondary transmission of live vaccines in patients receiving therapy. Due to variations in clearance, it may take up to 2 years to reach low levels of teriflunomide metabolite serum concentrations. A drug elimination procedure using cholestyramine or activated charcoal is recommended when a more rapid elimination is needed. If a response to teriflunomide had already been observed, the use of a rapid elimination procedure may result in the return of disease activity. **[U.S. Boxed Warning]: Based on animal data, teriflunomide may cause major birth defects if used in pregnant women. Teriflunomide is** ▶

contraindicated in pregnant women or women of childbearing potential who are not using reliable contraception. Pregnancy must be avoided during therapy or prior to completing the accelerated elimination treatment protocol.

Drug Interactions

Avoid Concomitant Use

Avoid concomitant use of Teriflunomide with any of the following: BCG; Leflunomide; Natalizumab; Pimecrolimus; Tacrolimus (Topical); Tofacitinib; Vaccines (Live)

Decreased Effect

Teriflunomide may decrease the levels/effects of: BCG; Caffeine; Coccidioidin Skin Test; Sipuleucel-T; Vaccines (Inactivated); Vaccines (Live); Warfarin

The levels/effects of Teriflunomide may be decreased by: Bile Acid Sequestrants; Charcoal, Activated; Echinacea

Increased Effect/Toxicity

Teriflunomide may increase the levels/effects of: CYP2C8 Substrates; Natalizumab; Repaglinide; Tofacitinib; Vaccines (Live)

The levels/effects of Teriflunomide may be increased by: Denosumab; Leflunomide; Pimecrolimus; Roflumilast; Tacrolimus (Topical); Trastuzumab

Adverse Reactions

>10%:
Central nervous system: Headache (19% to 22%)
Dermatologic: Alopecia (10% to 13%)
Endocrine & metabolic: Hypophosphatemia (5% to 18%)
Gastrointestinal: Diarrhea (15% to 18%), nausea (9% to 14%)
Hematologic: Neutropenia (2% to 15%)
Hepatic: ALT increased (12% to 14%)
Miscellaneous: Influenza (12%)

1% to 10%:
Cardiovascular: Hypertension (4%), palpitation (2% to 3%)
Central nervous system: Anxiety (3% to 4%)
Dermatologic: Pruritus (3% to 4%), acne (3%), burning sensation (2% to 3%)
Endocrine & metabolic: Hyperkalemia (1%)
Gastrointestinal: Abdominal pain (5% to 6%), toothache (4%), viral gastroenteritis (2% to 4%), weight loss (2% to 3%), abdominal distension (1% to 2%)
Genitourinary: Cystitis (2% to 4%)
Hematologic: Thrombocytopenia (10%), lymphocytopenia (7% to 10%), leukopenia (1% to 2%)
Hepatic: GGT increased (3% to 5%), AST increased (2% to 3%)
Neuromuscular & skeletal: Paresthesia (9% to 10%), musculoskeletal pain (4% to 5%), myalgia (3% to 4%), sciatica (3%), carpal tunnel syndrome (1% to 3%), peripheral neuropathy (1% to 2%)
Ocular: Blurred vision (3%), conjunctivitis (3%)

Renal: Renal failure (transient, 1%)
Respiratory: Upper respiratory tract infection (9%), bronchitis (8%), sinusitis (6%)
Miscellaneous: Herpes simplex (4%), seasonal allergy (2% to 3%)

Available Dosage Forms

Tablet, Oral:
Aubagio: 7 mg, 14 mg

General Dosage Range Oral: *Adults:* 7 mg or 14 mg once daily

Administration

Oral Administer without regard to meals.

Hazardous agent; use appropriate precautions for handling and disposal (meets NIOSH, 2012 criteria).

Storage/Stability Store at 20°C to 25°C (68°F to 77°F); excursions permitted to 15°C to 30°C (59°F to 86°F).

Nursing Actions

Physical Assessment Monitor CBC, liver function, and kidney function. Observe for hair loss, headache, diarrhea, nausea, low white blood cell count, or liver dysfunction. Monitor blood pressure and manage as needed during treatment. Instruct men and women of childbearing age about the need for birth control while taking this drug and for a period of time after discontinuation.

Patient Education
• Discuss specific use of drug and side effects with patient as it relates to treatment. (HCAHPS: During this hospital stay, were you given any medicine that you had not taken before? Before giving you any new medicine, how often did hospital staff tell you what the medicine was for? How often did hospital staff describe possible side effects in a way you could understand?)
• Patient may experience headache, dyspepsia, emesis, diarrhea, hair loss, or harm to liver. Have patient report immediately to prescriber dyspnea; paresthesia; inability to eat; change in color of urine, skin, or eyes; considerable asthenia; significant skin irritation; pregnancy; or rash (HCAHPS).
• Educate patient about signs of a significant reaction (eg, wheezing; chest tightness; fever; itching; bad cough; blue skin color; seizures; or swelling of face, lips, tongue, or throat). **Note:** This is not a comprehensive list of all side effects. Patient should consult prescriber for additional questions.

Intended Use and Disclaimer: Should not be printed and given to patients. This information is intended to serve as a concise initial reference for healthcare professionals to use when discussing medications with a patient. You must ultimately rely on your own discretion, experience and judgment in diagnosing, treating and advising patients.

Dietary Considerations May be taken with or without food.

Teriparatide (ter i PAR a tide)

Brand Names: U.S. Forteo

Index Terms Parathyroid Hormone (1-34); Recombinant Human Parathyroid Hormone (1-34); rhPTH(1-34)

Pharmacologic Category Parathyroid Hormone Analog

Medication Safety Issues

Sound-alike/look-alike issues:

Forteo® may be confused with Forfivo™ XL

Medication Guide Available Yes

Pregnancy Risk Factor C

Lactation Excretion in breast milk unknown/not recommended

Breast-Feeding Considerations Indicated for use in postmenopausal women. Studies have not been conducted to determine excretion in breast milk. Not recommended for use in breast-feeding women.

Use Treatment of osteoporosis in postmenopausal women at high risk of fracture; treatment of primary or hypogonadal osteoporosis in men at high risk of fracture; treatment of glucocorticoid-induced osteoporosis in men and women at high risk for fracture

Mechanism of Action/Effect An analog of parathyroid hormone, teriparatide stimulates osteoblast function, increases gastrointestinal calcium absorption, and increases renal tubular reabsorption of calcium. Treatment with teriparatide increases bone mineral density, bone mass, and strength. In postmenopausal women, it has been shown to decrease osteoporosis-related fractures.

Contraindications Hypersensitivity to teriparatide or any component of the formulation

Canadian labeling: Additional contraindications (not in U.S. labeling): Pre-existing hypercalcemia; severe renal impairment; metabolic bone diseases other than primary osteoporosis (including hyperparathyroidism and Paget's disease of the bone); unexplained elevations of alkaline phosphatase; prior external beam or implant radiation therapy involving the skeleton; bone metastases or history of skeletal malignancies; pregnancy; breast-feeding mothers; pediatric patients or young adults with open epiphysis

Warnings/Precautions [U.S. Boxed Warning]: In animal studies, teriparatide has been associated with an increase in osteosarcoma; risk was dependent on both dose and duration. Avoid use in patients with an increased risk of osteosarcoma (including Paget's disease, prior radiation, unexplained elevation of alkaline phosphatase, or in patients with open epiphyses). Do not use in patients with a history of skeletal metastases, hyperparathyroidism, or pre-existing hypercalcemia. Not for use in patients with metabolic bone disease other than osteoporosis. Use caution in patients with active or recent urolithiasis. Use caution in patients at risk of orthostasis (including concurrent antihypertensive therapy), or in patients who may not tolerate transient hypotension (cardiovascular or cerebrovascular disease). Use caution in patients with cardiac, renal or hepatic impairment (limited data available concerning safety and efficacy). Use in severe renal impairment is contraindicated in the Canadian labeling. Use of teriparatide for longer than 2 years is not recommended. Not approved for use in pediatric patients.

Drug Interactions

Avoid Concomitant Use There are no known interactions where it is recommended to avoid concomitant use.

Decreased Effect There are no known significant interactions involving a decrease in effect.

Increased Effect/Toxicity There are no known significant interactions involving an increase in effect.

Nutritional/Ethanol Interactions

Ethanol: Excessive intake may increase risk of osteoporosis.

Herb/Nutraceutical: Ensure adequate calcium and vitamin D intake.

Adverse Reactions

>10%: Endocrine & metabolic: Hypercalcemia (transient increases noted 4-6 hours postdose [women 11%; men 6%])

1% to 10%:

Cardiovascular: Orthostatic hypotension (5%; transient), chest pain (3%), syncope (3%)

Central nervous system: Dizziness (8%), insomnia (4% to 5%), anxiety (≤4%), depression (4%), vertigo (4%)

Dermatologic: Rash (5%)

Endocrine & metabolic: Hyperuricemia (3%)

Gastrointestinal: Nausea (9% to 14%), gastritis (≤7%), dyspepsia (5%), vomiting (3%)

Neuromuscular & skeletal: Arthralgia (10%), weakness (9%), leg cramps (3%)

Respiratory: Rhinitis (10%), pharyngitis (6%), dyspnea (4% to 6%), pneumonia (4% to 6%)

Miscellaneous: Antibodies to teriparatide (3% of women in long-term treatment; hypersensitivity reactions or decreased efficacy were not associated in preclinical trials), herpes zoster (≤3%)

Available Dosage Forms

Solution, Subcutaneous:

Forteo: 600 mcg/2.4 mL (2.4 mL)

General Dosage Range

SubQ: *Adults:* 20 mcg once daily

Administration

Other Administer by subcutaneous injection into the thigh or abdominal wall. Initial administration should occur under circumstances in which the patient may sit or lie down, in the event of orthostasis. **Note:** The 3 mL prefilled pen (Canadian availability; not available in U.S.) must be primed prior to each dose.

Storage/Stability Store at 2°C to 8°C (36°F to 46°F); do not freeze. Protect from light. Discard ▶

pen 28 days after first injection. Do not use if solution is cloudy, colored, or contains solid particles.

Nursing Actions

Physical Assessment Initial administration should occur where patient may sit or lie down, in the event of orthostasis. Monitor for chest pain, hypotension, nausea, vomiting, arthralgia, leg cramps, and dyspnea. Teach patient proper administration and disposal and proper diet with adequate calcium and vitamin D.

Patient Education

- Discuss specific use of drug and side effects with patient as it relates to treatment. (HCAHPS: During this hospital stay, were you given any medicine that you had not taken before? Before giving you any new medicine, how often did hospital staff tell you what the medicine was for? How often did hospital staff describe possible side effects in a way you could understand?)
- Patient may experience asthenia, dizziness, headache, leg cramps, myalgia, nausea, or rhinitis. Have patient report immediately to prescriber angina or rash (HCAHPS).
- Educate patient about signs of a significant reaction (eg, wheezing; chest tightness; fever; itching; bad cough; blue skin color; seizures; or swelling of face, lips, tongue, or throat). **Note:** This is not a comprehensive list of all side effects. Patient should consult prescriber for additional questions.

Intended Use and Disclaimer: Should not be printed and given to patients. This information is intended to serve as a concise initial reference for healthcare professionals to use when discussing medications with a patient. You must ultimately rely on your own discretion, experience and judgment in diagnosing, treating and advising patients.

Dietary Considerations Ensure adequate calcium and vitamin D intake; if dietary intake is inadequate, dietary supplementation is recommended. Women and men should consume:

Calcium: 1000 mg/day (men: 50-70 years) **or** 1200 mg/day (women ≥51 years and men ≥71 years) (IOM, 2011; NOF, 2013)

Vitamin D: 800-1000 IU/day (men and women ≥50 years) (NOF, 2013). Recommended Dietary Allowance (RDA): 600 IU/day (men and women ≤70 years) **or** 800 IU/day (men and women ≥71 years) (IOM, 2011).

Tesamorelin (tes a moe REL in)

Brand Names: U.S. Egrifta
Index Terms Tesamorelin Acetate; TH9507
Pharmacologic Category Growth Hormone Releasing Factor

Medication Safety Issues
Sound-alike/look-alike issues:
Tesamorelin may be confused with temsirolimus
Pregnancy Risk Factor X
Lactation Excretion in breast milk unknown/not recommended
Use Lipodystrophy in HIV-infected patients: For the reduction of excess abdominal fat in HIV-infected patients with lipodystrophy
Available Dosage Forms
Solution Reconstituted, Subcutaneous [preservative free]:
Egrifta: 2 mg (1 ea)
General Dosage Range SubQ: *Adults:* 2 mg once daily

Administration

Subcutaneous The abdomen is the preferred site of administration; rotate site within the abdomen. Avoid injection into scar tissue, bruises, or the navel.

Nursing Actions

Patient Education

- Discuss specific use of drug and side effects with patient as it relates to treatment. (HCAHPS: During this hospital stay, were you given any medicine that you had not taken before? Before giving you any new medicine, how often did hospital staff tell you what the medicine was for? How often did hospital staff describe possible side effects in a way you could understand?)
- Patient may experience edema, injection site irritation, hyperglycemia, nausea, arthralgia, or asthenia. Have patient report immediately to prescriber tachycardia, severe dizziness, dyspnea, significant edema, polyuria, polydipsia, weight loss, paresthesia, severe skin irritation, or rash (HCAHPS).
- Educate patient about signs of a significant reaction (eg, wheezing; chest tightness; fever; itching; bad cough; blue skin color; seizures; or swelling of face, lips, tongue, or throat). **Note:** This is not a comprehensive list of all side effects. Patient should consult prescriber for additional questions.

Intended Use and Disclaimer: Should not be printed and given to patients. This information is intended to serve as a concise initial reference for healthcare professionals to use when discussing medications with a patient. You must ultimately rely on your own discretion, experience and judgment in diagnosing, treating and advising patients.

Testosterone (tes TOS ter one)

Brand Names: U.S. Androderm; AndroGel; AndroGel Pump; Axiron; Depo-Testosterone; First-Testosterone; First-Testosterone MC; Fortesta; Striant; Testim; Testopel

Index Terms AVEED; Testosterone Cypionate; Testosterone Enanthate; Testosterone Undecanoate

Pharmacologic Category Androgen

Medication Safety Issues

Sound-alike/look-alike issues:

Testosterone may be confused with testolactone

Testoderm may be confused with Estraderm

AndroGel 1% may be confused with AndroGel 1.62%

Bio-T-Gel may be confused with T-Gel

BEERS Criteria medication:

This drug may be potentially inappropriate for use in geriatric patients (Quality of evidence - moderate; Strength of recommendation - weak).

Other safety concerns:

Transdermal patch may contain conducting metal (eg, aluminum); remove patch prior to MRI.

Medication Guide Available Yes

Pregnancy Risk Factor X

Lactation Enters breast milk/contraindicated

Breast-Feeding Considerations High levels of endogenous maternal testosterone, such as those caused by certain ovarian cysts, suppress milk production. Maternal serum testosterone levels generally fall following pregnancy and return to normal once breast-feeding is stopped. The amount of testosterone present in breast milk or the effect to the nursing infant following maternal supplementation is not known. Some products are contraindicated while breast-feeding. Females who are nursing should avoid skin-to-skin contact to areas where testosterone has been applied topically on another person.

Use

Injection: Androgen replacement therapy in the treatment of delayed male puberty; male hypogonadism (primary or hypogonadotropic); inoperable metastatic female breast cancer (enanthate only)

Pellet: Androgen replacement therapy in the treatment of delayed male puberty; male hypogonadism (primary or hypogonadotropic)

Buccal system, topical gel, topical solution, transdermal system: Male hypogonadism (primary or hypogonadotropic)

Capsule (not available in U.S.): Conditions associated with a deficiency or absence of endogenous testosterone

Mechanism of Action/Effect Principal endogenous androgen responsible for promoting the growth and development of the male sex organs and maintaining secondary sex characteristics in androgen-deficient males

Contraindications Hypersensitivity to testosterone or any component of the formulation; males with known or suspected carcinoma of the breast or prostate; women who are breast-feeding, pregnant, or who may become pregnant (**Note:** Striant® is contraindicated in all women.)

Depo-Testosterone: Also contraindicated in serious hepatic, renal, or cardiac disease

Warnings/Precautions Hazardous agent; use appropriate precautions for handling and disposal (NIOSH, 2012).

When used to treat delayed male puberty, perform radiographic examination of the hand and wrist every 6 months to determine the rate of bone maturation. May cause hypercalcemia in patients with prolonged immobilization or cancer. May accelerate bone maturation without producing compensating gain in linear growth. Has both androgenic and anabolic activity, the anabolic action may enhance hypoglycemia. May alter serum lipid profile; use caution with history of MI or coronary artery disease. Use caution in elderly patients or patients with other demographic factors which may increase the risk of prostatic carcinoma; careful monitoring is required. Discontinue therapy if urethral obstruction develops in patients with BPH (use lower dose if restarted). Withhold therapy pending urological evaluation in patients with palpable prostate nodule or induration, PSA >4 ng/mL, or PSA >3 ng/mL in men at high risk of prostate cancer (Bhasin, 2010). Use with caution in patients with conditions influenced by edema (eg, cardiovascular disease, migraine, seizure disorder, renal or hepatic impairment) or medications that enhance edema formation (eg, corticosteroids); testosterone may cause fluid retention. May cause gynecomastia. Large doses may suppress spermatogenesis. During treatment for metastatic breast cancer, women should be monitored for signs of virilization; discontinue if mild virilization is present to prevent irreversible symptoms.

May be inappropriate in the elderly due to potential risk of cardiac problems and contraindication for use in men with prostate cancer; in general, avoid use in older adults except in the setting of moderate-to-severe hypogonadism (Beers Criteria). In addition, elderly patients may be at greater risk for prostatic hyperplasia, prostate cancer, fluid retention, and transaminase elevations.

Prolonged use of high doses of oral androgens has been associated with serious hepatic effects (peliosis hepatis, hepatic neoplasms, cholestatic hepatitis, jaundice). Prolonged use of intramuscular testosterone enanthate has been associated with multiple hepatic adenomas. May potentiate sleep apnea in some male patients (obesity or chronic lung disease). May increase hematocrit requiring dose adjustment or discontinuation; discontinue therapy if hematocrit exceeds 54%; may reinitiate at lower dose (Bhasin, 2010).

[U.S. Boxed Warning]: Virilization in children has been reported following contact with unwashed or unclothed application sites of men using topical testosterone. Patients should strictly adhere to instructions for use

in order to prevent secondary exposure. Virilization of female sexual partners has also been reported with male use of topical testosterone. Symptoms of virilization generally regress following removal of exposure; however, in some children, enlarged genitalia and bone age did not fully return to age appropriate normal. Signs of inappropriate virilization in women or children following secondary exposure to topical testosterone should be brought to the attention of a healthcare provider. Topical testosterone products (gels and solution) may have different doses, strengths, or application instructions that may result in different systemic exposure; these products are not interchangeable. Transdermal patch may contain conducting metal (eg, aluminum); remove patch prior to MRI. Gels, solution, transdermal, and buccal system have not been evaluated in males <18 years of age; safety and efficacy of injection have not been established in males <12 years of age. Some testosterone products may be chemically synthesized from soy. Some products may contain benzyl alcohol. Use of Axiron® in males with BMI >35 kg/m^2 has not been established.

Drug Interactions

Avoid Concomitant Use

Avoid concomitant use of Testosterone with any of the following: Dehydroepiandrosterone

Decreased Effect There are no known significant interactions involving a decrease in effect.

Increased Effect/Toxicity

Testosterone may increase the levels/effects of: CycloSPORINE (Systemic); Vitamin K Antagonists

The levels/effects of Testosterone may be increased by: Dehydroepiandrosterone

Nutritional/Ethanol Interactions Herb/Nutraceutical: St John's wort may decrease testosterone levels.

Adverse Reactions Frequency not always defined.

Cardiovascular: Deep venous thrombosis, edema, hypertension, vasodilation

Central nervous system: Blood pressure increased (1%), headache (1%), insomnia (≤1%), mood swings (≤1%), abnormal dreams, aggressive behavior, anger, amnesia, anxiety, blood pressure decreased, chills, depression, dizziness, emotional lability, excitation, fatigue, hostility, malaise, memory loss, nervousness, seizure, sleep apnea, sleeplessness, suicidal ideation

Dermatologic: Acne, alopecia, contact dermatitis, dry skin, erythema, folliculitis, hair discoloration, hirsutism (increase in pubic hair growth), pruritus, rash, seborrhea

Endocrine & metabolic: Gynecomastia (≤1%), hot flashes (≤1%), breast pain/soreness, gonadotropin secretion decreased, growth acceleration, hypercalcemia, hyperchloremia, hypercholesterolemia, hyper-/hypoglycemia, hyper-/hypokalemia, hyperlipidemia, hypernatremia, inorganic phosphate retention, libido changes, menstrual problems (including amenorrhea), virilism, water retention

Gastrointestinal: Taste disorder (1%), appetite increased, diarrhea, gastroesophageal reflux, GI bleeding, GI irritation, nausea, vomiting, weight gain

Following buccal administration (most common): Bitter taste, gum edema, gum or mouth irritation, gum pain, gum tenderness, taste perversion

Genitourinary: Penile erections (≤1%; spontaneous), bladder irritability, impotence, oligospermia, priapism, prostatic carcinoma, prostatic hyperplasia, prostatitis, PSA increased, testicular atrophy, urinary tract infection, urination impaired

Hepatic: Bilirubin increased, cholestatic hepatitis, cholestatic jaundice, hepatic dysfunction, hepatic necrosis, hepatocellular neoplasms, liver function test changes, peliosis hepatis

Hematologic: Hematocrit/hemoglobin increased (1% to 3%), anemia, bleeding, leukopenia, polycythemia, suppression of clotting factors

Local: Application site reaction (gel, solution), injection site inflammation/pain

Transdermal system: Pruritus at application site (17% to 37%), burn-like blisters under system (12%), erythema at application site (≤7%), vesicles at application site (6%), allergic contact dermatitis to system (4%), burning at application site (3%), induration at application site (3%), exfoliation at application site (<3%)

Neuromuscular & skeletal: Back pain, hemarthrosis, hyperkinesias, paresthesia, weakness

Ocular: Lacrimation increased

Renal: Creatinine increased, hematuria, polyuria

Respiratory: Dyspnea, nasopharyngitis

Miscellaneous: Smell disorder (≤1%), anaphylactoid reactions, diaphoresis, hypersensitivity reactions

Pharmacodynamics/Kinetics

Duration of Action Route and ester dependent; I.M.: Cypionate and enanthate esters have longest duration, ≤2-4 weeks; gel: 24-48 hours

Product Availability AVEED (testosterone undecanoate) injection: FDA approved March 2014; availability anticipated in March 2014

Controlled Substance C-III

Available Dosage Forms

Cream, Transdermal:
First-Testosterone MC: 2% (60 g)

Gel, Transdermal:
AndroGel: 25 mg/2.5 g (2.5 g); 50 mg/5 g (5 g); 40.5 mg/2.5 g (1.62%) (2.5 g); 20.25 mg/1.25 g (1.62%) (1.25 g)
AndroGel Pump: 12.5 mg/acutation (1%) (75 g); 20.25 mg/acutation (1.62%) (75 g)
Fortesta: 10 mg/actuation (2%) (60 g)
Testim: 50 mg/5 g (5 g)

Miscellaneous, Buccal:
Striant: 30 mg (60 ea)

Oil, Intramuscular:
Depo-Testosterone: 100 mg/mL (10 mL); 200 mg/mL (1 mL, 10 mL)
Generic: 100 mg/mL (10 mL); 200 mg/mL (1 mL, 5 mL, 10 mL)

Ointment, Transdermal:
First-Testosterone: 2% (60 g)

Patch 24 Hour, Transdermal:
Androderm: 2 mg/24 hr (1 ea, 60 ea); 4 mg/24 hr (1 ea, 30 ea)

Pellet, Implant:
Testopel: 75 mg (10 ea, 100 ea)

Solution, Transdermal:
Axiron: 30 mg/actuation (90 mL)

General Dosage Range

Buccal: *Adults (males):* 30 mg every 12 hours

I.M.: *Adolescents and Adults (males):* 50-400 mg every 2-4 weeks

SubQ: *Adolescents and Adults (males):* 150-450 mg every 3-6 months

Topical: *Adults (males):* AndroGel® 1%: Apply 50-100 mg daily; AndroGel® 1.62%: Apply 20.25-81 mg daily; Axiron®: Apply 30-120 mg daily; Fortesta™: Apply 10-70 mg daily; Testim®: Apply 50-100 mg daily

Transdermal: *Adults (males):* Androderm®: Apply 2-7.5 mg daily

Administration

I.M. Warm injection to room temperature and shaking vial will help redissolve crystals that have formed after storage. Administer by deep I.M. injection into the gluteal muscle.

Hazardous agent; use appropriate precautions for handling and disposal (NIOSH, 2012).

Oral

Oral, buccal application (Striant®): One mucoadhesive for buccal application (buccal system) should be applied to a comfortable area above the incisor tooth. Place the flat side of the system on your fingertip. Gently push the curved side against your upper gum. Rotate to alternate sides of mouth with each application. Hold buccal system firmly in place for 30 seconds to ensure adhesion. The buccal system should adhere to gum for 12 hours. If the buccal system falls out, replace with a new system. If the system falls out within 4 hours of next dose, the new buccal system should remain in place until the time of the following scheduled dose. System will soften and mold to shape of gum as it absorbs moisture from mouth. Do not chew or swallow the buccal system. The buccal system will not dissolve; gently remove by sliding downwards from gum; avoid scratching gum.

Oral, capsule (Andriol®; not available in the U.S.): Should be administered with meals. Should be swallowed whole; do not crush or chew.

Hazardous agent; use appropriate precautions for handling and disposal (NIOSH, 2012).

Topical

Topical gel and solution: Apply to clean, dry, intact skin. Application sites should be allowed to dry for a few minutes prior to dressing. Hands should be washed with soap and water after application. **Do not apply testosterone gel or solution to the genitals.** Alcohol-based gels and solutions are flammable; avoid fire, flames, or smoking until dry. Testosterone may be transferred to another person following skin-to-skin contact with the application site. Strict adherence to application instructions is needed in order to decrease secondary exposure. Thoroughly wash hands after application and cover application site with clothing (ie, shirt) once gel or solution has dried, or clean application site thoroughly with soap and water prior to contact in order to minimize transfer. In addition to skin-to-skin contact, secondary exposure has also been reported following exposure to secondary items (eg, towel, shirt, sheets). If secondary exposure occurs, the other person should thoroughly wash the skin with soap and water as soon as possible.

AndroGel® 1%, AndroGel® 1.62%, Testim®: Apply (preferably in the morning) to the shoulder and upper arms. AndroGel® 1% may also be applied to the abdomen; do not apply AndroGel® 1.62% or Testim® to the abdomen. Area of application should be limited to what will be covered by a short sleeve t-shirt. Apply at the same time each day. Upon opening the packet(s), the entire contents should be squeezed into the palm of the hand and immediately applied to the application site(s). Alternatively, a portion may be squeezed onto palm of hand and applied, repeating the process at the same or other site until entire packet has been applied. Application site(s) should not be washed for ≥2 hours following application of AndroGel® 1.62% or Testim®, or >5 hours for AndroGel® 1%.

AndroGel® 1% multidose pump: Prime pump 3 times (and discard this portion of product) prior to initial use. Each actuation delivers 12.5 mg of testosterone (4 actuations = 50 mg; 6 actuations = 75 mg; 8 actuations = 100 mg); each actuation may be applied individually or all at the same time. Application site should not be washed for >5 hours following application.

AndroGel® 1.62% multidose pump: Prime pump 3 times (and discard this portion of product) prior to initial use. Each actuation delivers 20.25 mg of testosterone (2 actuations = 40.5 mg; 3 actuations = 60.75 mg; 4 actuations = 81 mg); each actuation may be applied individually or all at the same time. Avoid washing the site or swimming for ≥2 hours following application.

Axiron®: Apply using the applicator to the axilla at the same time each morning. Do not apply to other parts of the body (eg, abdomen, genitals, shoulders, upper arms). Avoid washing the site or swimming for 2 hours after application. Prior to first use, prime the applicator pump by depressing it 3 times (discard this portion of the product). After priming, position the nozzle over the applicator cup and depress pump fully one time; ensure liquid enters cup. Each pump actuation delivers testosterone 30 mg. No more than 30 mg (one pump) should be added to the cup at one time. The total dose should be divided between axilla (example, 30 mg/day: apply to one axilla only; 60 mg/day: apply 30 mg to each axilla; 90 mg/day: apply 30 mg to each axilla, allow to dry, then apply an additional 30 mg to one axilla; etc). To apply dose, keep applicator upright and wipe into the axilla; if solution runs or drips, use cup to wipe. Do not rub into skin with fingers or hand. If more than one 30 mg dose is needed, repeat process. Apply roll-on or stick antiperspirants or deodorants prior to testosterone. Once application site is dry, cover with clothing. After use, rinse applicator under running water and pat dry with a tissue. The application site and dose of this product are not interchangeable with other topical testosterone products.

Fortesta™: Apply to skin of front and inner thighs. Do not apply to other parts of the body. Use one finger to rub gel evenly onto skin of each thigh. Avoid showering, washing the site, or swimming for 2 hours after application. Prior to first dose, prime the pump by holding canister upright and fully depressing the pump 8 times (discard this portion of the product). Each pump actuation delivers testosterone 10 mg. The total dose should be divided between thighs (example, 10 mg/day: apply 10 mg to one thigh only; 20 mg/day: apply 10 mg to each thigh; 30 mg/day: apply 20 mg to one thigh and 10 mg to the other thigh; etc). Once application site is dry, cover with clothing. The application site and dose of this product are not interchangeable with other topical testosterone products.

Transdermal patch (Androderm®): Apply patch to clean, dry area of skin on the back, abdomen, upper arms, or thigh. Do not apply to bony areas or parts of the body that are subject to prolonged pressure while sleeping or sitting. **Do not apply to the scrotum.** Avoid showering, washing the site, or swimming for 3 hours after application. Following patch removal, mild skin irritation may be treated with OTC hydrocortisone cream. A small amount of triamcinolone acetonide 0.1% cream may be applied under the system to decrease irritation; do not use ointment. Patch should be applied nightly. Rotate administration sites, allowing 7 days between applying to the same site.

Hazardous agent; use appropriate precautions for handling and disposal (NIOSH, 2012).

Other Subcutaneous implant (Testopel®): Using strict sterile technique, must be surgically implanted.

Hazardous agent; use appropriate precautions for handling and disposal (NIOSH, 2012).

Storage/Stability

Androderm: Store at room temperature. Do not store outside of pouch. Excessive heat may cause system to burst.

AndroGel 1%, AndroGel 1.62%, Axiron, Delatestryl, Striant, Testim: Store at room temperature.

Depo-Testosterone: Store at room temperature. Protect from light.

Fortesta: Store at room temperature; do not freeze

Testopel: Store in a cool location.

Nursing Actions

Physical Assessment Instruct patients to apply to clean, dry skin and that area should be covered with clothing to prevent transmission.

Patient Education

- Discuss specific use of drug and side effects with patient as it relates to treatment. (HCAHPS: During this hospital stay, were you given any medicine that you had not taken before? Before giving you any new medicine, how often did hospital staff tell you what the medicine was for? How often did hospital staff describe possible side effects in a way you could understand?)
- Patient may experience macromastia, headache, emotional instability, flushing, or nausea. Have patient report immediately to prescriber inability to eat, erection lasting >4 hours, severe edema, urinary retention, considerable nervousness and anxiety, acne, enlarged sex organs, changes in body hair, jaundice, or rash (HCAHPS).
- Educate patient about signs of a significant reaction (eg, wheezing; chest tightness; fever; itching; bad cough; blue skin color; seizures; or swelling of face, lips, tongue, or throat). **Note:** This is not a comprehensive list of all side effects. Patient should consult prescriber for additional questions.

Intended Use and Disclaimer: Should not be printed and given to patients. This information is intended to serve as a concise initial reference for healthcare professionals to use when discussing medications with a patient. You must ultimately rely on your own discretion, experience and judgment in diagnosing, treating and advising patients.

Dietary Considerations Testosterone USP may be synthesized from soy. Food and beverages have not been found to interfere with buccal system; ensure system is in place following eating, drinking, or brushing teeth.

Tetrabenazine (tet ra BEN a zeen)

Brand Names: U.S. Xenazine
Pharmacologic Category Central Monoamine-Depleting Agent
Medication Guide Available Yes
Pregnancy Risk Factor C
Lactation Excretion in breast milk unknown/not recommended
Use Treatment of chorea associated with Huntington's disease
Canadian labeling: Treatment of hyperkinetic movement disorders, including Huntington's chorea, hemiballismus, senile chorea, Tourette syndrome, and tardive dyskinesia
Available Dosage Forms
Tablet, Oral:
Xenazine: 12.5 mg, 25 mg
General Dosage Range Dosage adjustment recommended in patients on concomitant therapy or who develop toxicities
Oral: *Adults:* 12.5 mg once daily; Maintenance: 25-100 mg/day in 2-3 divided doses
Administration
Oral May administer without regard to meals.
Nursing Actions
Physical Assessment Monitor psychiatric status and for CNS changes at beginning of therapy, with any dose change, and at frequent intervals during therapy.
Patient Education
- Discuss specific use of drug and side effects with patient as it relates to treatment. (HCAHPS: During this hospital stay, were you given any medicine that you had not taken before? Before giving you any new medicine, how often did hospital staff tell you what the medicine was for? How often did hospital staff describe possible side effects in a way you could understand?)
- Patient may experience presyncope, fatigue, blurred vision, illogical thinking, dizziness, bradykinesia, depression, nervousness and anxiety, hypotension, nausea, or insomnia. Have patient report immediately to prescriber emotional instability, dysphagia, tremors, missed dosage of >5 days, or rash (HCAHPS).
- Educate patient about signs of a significant reaction (eg, wheezing; chest tightness; fever; itching; bad cough; blue skin color; seizures; or swelling of face, lips, tongue, or throat). **Note:** This is not a comprehensive list of all side effects. Patient should consult prescriber for additional questions.

Intended Use and Disclaimer: Should not be printed and given to patients. This information is intended to serve as a concise initial reference for healthcare professionals to use when discussing medications with a patient. You must ultimately rely on your own discretion, experience and judgment in diagnosing, treating and advising patients.

Tetracycline (tet ra SYE kleen)

Index Terms Achromycin; TCN; Tetracycline Hydrochloride
Pharmacologic Category Antibiotic, Tetracycline Derivative
Medication Safety Issues
Sound-alike/look-alike issues:
Tetracycline may be confused with tetradecyl sulfate
Achromycin may be confused with actinomycin, Adriamycin
Pregnancy Risk Factor D
Lactation Enters breast milk/not recommended
Use Treatment of susceptible bacterial infections of both gram-positive and gram-negative organisms; also infections due to *Mycoplasma, Chlamydia,* and *Rickettsia*; indicated for acne, exacerbations of chronic bronchitis, and treatment of gonorrhea and syphilis in patients who are allergic to penicillin; as part of a multidrug regimen for *H. pylori* eradication to reduce the risk of duodenal ulcer recurrence
Unlabeled Use Treatment of periodontitis associated with presence of *Actinobacillus actinomycetemcomitans* (AA)
Available Dosage Forms
Capsule, Oral:
Generic: 250 mg, 500 mg
General Dosage Range Dosage adjustment recommended in patients with renal impairment
Oral:
Children >8 years: 25-50 mg/kg/day divided every 6 hours
Adults: 250-500 mg 2-4 times/day
Administration
Oral Oral should be given on an empty stomach (ie, 1 hour prior to, or 2 hours after meals) to increase total absorption. Administer at least 1-2 hours prior to, or 4 hours after antacid because aluminum and magnesium cations may chelate with tetracycline and reduce its total absorption. Administer around-the-clock to promote less variation in peak and trough serum levels.

Hazardous agent; use appropriate precautions for handling and disposal (NIOSH, 2012).
Nursing Actions
Physical Assessment Results of culture and sensitivity tests and patient's allergy history should be assessed prior to beginning therapy. Monitor for nausea, diarrhea, pericarditis, photosensitivity, rash, opportunistic infection, and hypersensitivity.
Patient Education
- Discuss specific use of drug and side effects with patient as it relates to treatment. (HCAHPS: During this hospital stay, were you given any ▶

medicine that you had not taken before? Before giving you any new medicine, how often did hospital staff tell you what the medicine was for? How often did hospital staff describe possible side effects in a way you could understand?)

• Patient may experience dyspepsia, lack of appetite, nausea, diarrhea, or vaginal yeast infection. Have patient report immediately to prescriber severe headache or rash (HCAHPS).

• Educate patient about signs of a significant reaction (eg, wheezing; chest tightness; fever; itching; bad cough; blue skin color; seizures; or swelling of face, lips, tongue, or throat). **Note:** This is not a comprehensive list of all side effects. Patient should consult prescriber for additional questions.

Intended Use and Disclaimer: Should not be printed and given to patients. This information is intended to serve as a concise initial reference for healthcare professionals to use when discussing medications with a patient. You must ultimately rely on your own discretion, experience and judgment in diagnosing, treating and advising patients.

Related Information

Oral Medications That Should Not Be Crushed or Altered *on page 1712*

Thalidomide (tha LI doe mide)

Brand Names: U.S. Thalomid
Pharmacologic Category Angiogenesis Inhibitor; Antineoplastic Agent; Immunomodulator, Systemic
Medication Safety Issues
Sound-alike/look-alike issues:
Thalidomide may be confused with flutamide, lenalidomide, pomalidomide
Thalomid may be confused with Revlimid, thiamine
High alert medication:
This medication is in a class the Institute for Safe Medication Practices (ISMP) includes among its list of drug classes that have a heightened risk of causing significant patient harm when used in error.
International issues:
Thalomid [U.S., Canada] may be confused with Thilomide brand name for Iodoxamide [Greece, Turkey]
Medication Guide Available Yes
Pregnancy Risk Factor X
Lactation Excretion in breast milk unknown/not recommended
Use
Erythema nodosum leprosum: Acute treatment of cutaneous manifestations of moderate to severe erythema nodosum leprosum; maintenance treatment for prevention and suppression of cutaneous manifestations of erythema nodosum leprosum recurrence

Multiple myeloma: Treatment of newly-diagnosed multiple myeloma (in combination with dexamethasone)
Unlabeled Use Treatment of chronic graft-versus-host disease (GVHD) in hematopoietic stem cell transplantation; AIDS-related aphthous stomatitis; Waldenström's macroglobulinemia; maintenance therapy of multiple myeloma (following autologous stem cell transplant); salvage therapy for multiple myeloma; systemic light chain amyloidosis
Available Dosage Forms
Capsule, Oral:
Thalomid: 50 mg, 100 mg, 150 mg, 200 mg
General Dosage Range Dosage adjustment recommended in patients who develop toxicities
Oral: *Children ≥12 years and Adults:* Initial: 100-300 mg once daily (maximum: 400 mg daily)
Administration
Oral Do not open or crush capsules. Avoid extensive handling of capsules; capsules should remain in blister pack until ingestion. If exposed to the powder content from broken capsules or body fluids from patients receiving thalidomide, the exposed area should be washed with soap and water.

U.S. labeling: Administer orally with water, preferably at bedtime once daily, at least 1 hour after the evening meal. Doses >400 mg/day may be given in divided doses at least 1 hour after meals. For missed doses, if <12 hours patient may receive dose; if >12 hours wait till next dose due.

Canadian labeling: Administer orally as a single dose at the same time each day; may be taken without regard to meals. May be administered at bedtime to decrease somnolence. Capsules should be swallowed whole, preferably with water.

Hazardous agent; use appropriate precautions for handling and disposal (NIOSH, 2012). Wear gloves to prevent cutaneous exposure.
Nursing Actions
Physical Assessment Patient must be capable of complying with STEPS® program. Instruct patient on risks of pregnancy, appropriate contraceptive measures, and necessity for frequent pregnancy testing (schedule pregnancy testing at time of dispensing and give patient schedule in writing). Monitor for signs of fluid retention, weight gain, and hypotension. Monitor closely for signs of neuropathy (ie, numbness, tingling, and pain in extremities), CNS depression, and altered blood counts.

Patient Education
• Discuss specific use of drug and side effects with patient as it relates to treatment. (HCAHPS: During this hospital stay, were you given any medicine that you had not taken before? Before giving you any new medicine, how often did hospital staff tell you what the medicine was

for? How often did hospital staff describe possible side effects in a way you could understand?)
- Patient may experience presyncope, dizziness, asthenia, fatigue, constipation, headache, anemia, hypocalcemia, edema, rash, nausea, or lack of appetite. Have patient report immediately to prescriber dyspnea, angina, paresthesia, blood clot, or pregnancy (HCAHPS).
- Educate patient about signs of a significant reaction (eg, wheezing; chest tightness; fever; itching; bad cough; blue skin color; seizures; or swelling of face, lips, tongue, or throat). **Note:** This is not a comprehensive list of all side effects. Patient should consult prescriber for additional questions.

Intended Use and Disclaimer: Should not be printed and given to patients. This information is intended to serve as a concise initial reference for healthcare professionals to use when discussing medications with a patient. You must ultimately rely on your own discretion, experience and judgment in diagnosing, treating and advising patients.

Related Information
Oral Medications That Should Not Be Crushed or Altered *on page 1712*

Theophylline (thee OFF i lin)

Brand Names: U.S. Elixophyllin; Theo-24; Theochron
Index Terms Theophylline Anhydrous
Pharmacologic Category Phosphodiesterase Enzyme Inhibitor, Nonselective
Pregnancy Risk Factor C
Lactation Enters breast milk/compatible
Use Treatment of symptoms and reversible airway obstruction due to chronic asthma, or other chronic lung diseases

Note: The Global Initiative for Asthma Guidelines (2009) and the National Heart, Lung and Blood Institute Guidelines (2007) do not recommend oral theophylline as a long-term control medication for asthma in children ≤5 years of age; use has been shown to be effective as an add-on (but not preferred) agent in older children and adults with severe asthma treated with inhaled or oral glucocorticoids. The guidelines do not recommend theophylline for the treatment of exacerbations of asthma.

The Global Initiative for Chronic Obstructive Lung Disease Guidelines (2013) suggest that while higher doses of slow release formulations of theophylline have been proven to be effective for use in COPD, it is not a preferred agent due to its potential for toxicity.

Available Dosage Forms
Capsule Extended Release 24 Hour, Oral:
Theo-24: 100 mg, 200 mg, 300 mg, 400 mg

Elixir, Oral:
Elixophyllin: 80 mg/15 mL (473 mL)
Solution, Intravenous:
Generic: 400 mg (250 mL, 500 mL); 800 mg (500 mL)
Solution, Oral:
Generic: 80 mg/15 mL (473 mL)
Tablet Extended Release 12 Hour, Oral:
Theochron: 100 mg, 200 mg, 300 mg
Generic: 100 mg, 200 mg, 300 mg, 450 mg
Tablet Extended Release 24 Hour, Oral:
Generic: 400 mg, 600 mg

General Dosage Range
I.V.:
Infants 6-52 weeks: mg/kg/hour = (0.008) (age in weeks) + 0.21
Children 1-9 years: 0.8 mg/kg/hour
Children 9-12 years and Adolescents 12-16 years (cigarette or marijuana smokers): 0.7 mg/kg/hour
Adolescents 12-16 years (nonsmokers): 0.5 mg/kg/hour; maximum: 900 mg/day unless serum levels indicate need for larger dose
Adults 16-60 years (otherwise healthy, nonsmokers): 0.4 mg/kg/hour; maximum: 900 mg/day unless serum levels indicate need for larger dose
Adults >60 years: 0.3 mg/kg/hour; maximum: 400 mg/day unless serum levels indicate need for larger dose

Oral solution:
Full-term Infants and Infants <26 weeks: Total daily dose (mg) = [(0.2 x age in weeks) +5] x (weight in kg); divide dose into 3 equal amounts and administer at 8-hour intervals
Full-term Infants and Infants ≥26 weeks and <52 weeks: Total daily dose (mg) = [(0.2 x age in weeks) +5] x (weight in kg); divide dose into 4 equal amounts and administer at 6-hour intervals
Children ≥1 year and <45 kg: Initial: 10-14 mg/kg/day in divided doses (maximum dose: 300 mg/day); titrate to maintenance dose: 20 mg/kg/day in divided doses every 4-6 hours (maximum dose: 600 mg/day)
Children >45 kg and Adults: Initial: 300 mg/day in divided doses; titrate to maintenance dose: 600 mg/day in divided doses every 6-8 hours

Oral extended release formulations:
Children ≥1 year and <45 kg: Initial: 10-14 mg/kg once daily (maximum dose: 300 mg/day); titrate to maintenance dose: 20 mg/kg once daily (maximum dose: 600 mg/day)
Children >45 kg and Adults: 300-600 mg once daily

Administration
I.V. Administer loading dose over 30 minutes; follow with a continuous infusion as appropriate.
Injectable Detail pH: 4.3

Oral Long-acting preparations should be taken with a full glass of water, swallowed whole, or cut in half if scored. Do **not** crush. Extended release capsule forms may be opened and the contents sprinkled on soft foods; do **not** chew beads.

Nursing Actions

Physical Assessment Evaluate effectiveness of therapy (prevention of bronchospasm). Monitor for cardiac and CNS changes at beginning of therapy and periodically throughout.

Patient Education
- Discuss specific use of drug and side effects with patient as it relates to treatment. (HCAHPS: During this hospital stay, were you given any medicine that you had not taken before? Before giving you any new medicine, how often did hospital staff tell you what the medicine was for? How often did hospital staff describe possible side effects in a way you could understand?)
- Patient may experience nervousness and anxiety or nausea. Have patient report immediately to prescriber tachycardia, severe dizziness, decreased peak flow measurement, or rash (HCAHPS).
- Educate patient about signs of a significant reaction (eg, wheezing; chest tightness; fever; itching; bad cough; blue skin color; seizures; or swelling of face, lips, tongue, or throat). **Note:** This is not a comprehensive list of all side effects. Patient should consult prescriber for additional questions.

Intended Use and Disclaimer: Should not be printed and given to patients. This information is intended to serve as a concise initial reference for healthcare professionals to use when discussing medications with a patient. You must ultimately rely on your own discretion, experience and judgment in diagnosing, treating and advising patients.

Related Information

Oral Medications That Should Not Be Crushed or Altered *on page 1712*

Peak and Trough Guidelines *on page 1710*

Thiamine (THYE a min)

Index Terms Aneurine Hydrochloride; Thiamin; Thiamine Hydrochloride; Thiaminium Chloride Hydrochloride; Vitamin B_1

Pharmacologic Category Vitamin, Water Soluble

Medication Safety Issues

Sound-alike/look-alike issues:
Thiamine may be confused with Tenormin, Thalomid, Thorazine

International issues:
Doxal [Brazil] may be confused with Doxil brand name for doxorubicin [U.S.]

Doxal: Brand name for pyridoxine/thiamine [Brazil], but also the brand name for doxepin [Finland]

Pregnancy Risk Factor A

Lactation Enters breast milk/use caution

Use Treatment of thiamine deficiency including beriberi, Wernicke's encephalopathy, Korsakoff's syndrome, neuritis associated with pregnancy, or in alcoholic patients; dietary supplement

Available Dosage Forms

Capsule, Oral:
Generic: 50 mg

Solution, Injection:
Generic: 100 mg/mL (2 mL)

Tablet, Oral:
Generic: 50 mg, 100 mg, 250 mg

Tablet, Oral [preservative free]:
Generic: 100 mg

General Dosage Range

I.M., I.V.:
Children: 10-25 mg/dose daily (thiamine deficiency)
Adults: 5-30 mg/dose 3 times/day (thiamine deficiency) **or** 50-250 mg/day (Wernicke's encephalopathy)

Oral:
Infants: 0.2-0.3 mg/day (adequate intake)
Children: 0.5-1.4 mg/day (recommended daily intake) **or** 5-50 mg/day (thiamine deficiency)
Adults: 1.1-1.4 mg/day (recommended daily intake) **or** 5-30 mg/day in 1-3 divided doses (thiamine deficiency)

Administration

I.M. Parenteral form may be administered I.M.

I.V. Parenteral form may be administered by I.V. injection. Various rates of administration have been reported (eg, 100 mg over 5 minutes). An extended infusion time is preferred for doses ≥100 mg. Local injection reactions may be minimized by slow administration (~30 minutes) into larger, more proximal veins. Thiamine should be administered prior to parenteral glucose solutions to prevent precipitation of acute symptoms of thiamine deficiency in the poorly nourished.

Injectable Detail pH: 2.5-4.5

Nursing Actions

Physical Assessment If self-administered, teach patient appropriate injection technique and needle disposal. Provide patient appropriate dietary instruction. Be alert to the potential for hypersensitivity reaction, especially if given I.V.

Patient Education
- Discuss specific use of drug and side effects with patient as it relates to treatment. (HCAHPS: During this hospital stay, were you given any medicine that you had not taken before? Before giving you any new medicine, how often did hospital staff tell you what the medicine was for? How often did hospital staff describe possible side effects in a way you could understand?)

• Patient may experience nausea or injection site irritation. Have patient report immediately to prescriber rash (HCAHPS).

• Educate patient about signs of a significant reaction (eg, wheezing; chest tightness; fever; itching; bad cough; blue skin color; seizures; or swelling of face, lips, tongue, or throat). **Note:** This is not a comprehensive list of all side effects. Patient should consult prescriber for additional questions.

Intended Use and Disclaimer: Should not be printed and given to patients. This information is intended to serve as a concise initial reference for healthcare professionals to use when discussing medications with a patient. You must ultimately rely on your own discretion, experience and judgment in diagnosing, treating and advising patients.

Thioguanine (thye oh GWAH neen)

Brand Names: U.S. Tabloid
Index Terms 2-Amino-6-Mercaptopurine; 6-TG (error-prone abbreviation); 6-Thioguanine (error-prone abbreviation); TG; Tioguanine
Pharmacologic Category Antineoplastic Agent, Antimetabolite; Antineoplastic Agent, Antimetabolite (Purine Analog)
Medication Safety Issues
Sound-alike/look-alike issues:
Thioguanine may be confused with thiotepa
High alert medication:
This medication is in a class the Institute for Safe Medication Practices (ISMP) includes among its list of drug classes which have a heightened risk of causing significant patient harm when used in error.
Other safety concerns:
6-thioguanine and 6-TG are error-prone abbreviations (associated with sixfold overdoses of thioguanine)
International issues:
Lanvis [Canada and multiple international markets] may be confused with Lantus brand name for insulin glargine [U.S., Canada, and multiple international markets]
Pregnancy Risk Factor D
Lactation Excretion in breast milk unknown/not recommended
Use Treatment of acute myelogenous (nonlymphocytic) leukemia (AML)
Unlabeled Use Treatment of pediatric acute lymphoblastic leukemia (ALL)
Available Dosage Forms
Tablet, Oral:
Tabloid: 40 mg

Administration
Oral For oral use; total daily dose can be given at one time.

Hazardous agent; use appropriate precautions for handling and disposal (NIOSH, 2012).
Nursing Actions
Physical Assessment Monitor for myelosuppression, nausea, vomiting, anorexia, malaise, and hepatotoxicity weekly when beginning therapy, then monthly. Teach patient necessity for contraception and importance of adequate hydration.
Patient Education
• Discuss specific use of drug and side effects with patient as it relates to treatment. (HCAHPS: During this hospital stay, were you given any medicine that you had not taken before? Before giving you any new medicine, how often did hospital staff tell you what the medicine was for? How often did hospital staff describe possible side effects in a way you could understand?)
• Patient may experience nausea, stomatitis, anemia, leukopenia, or thrombocytopenia. Have patient report immediately to prescriber signs of infection, severe diarrhea, ecchymosis, fatigue, severe dyspepsia, significant edema, considerable weight gain, discolored urine, jaundice, inability to eat, or rash (HCAHPS).
• Educate patient about signs of a significant reaction (eg, wheezing; chest tightness; fever; itching; bad cough; blue skin color; seizures; or swelling of face, lips, tongue, or throat). **Note:** This is not a comprehensive list of all side effects. Patient should consult prescriber for additional questions.

Intended Use and Disclaimer: Should not be printed and given to patients. This information is intended to serve as a concise initial reference for healthcare professionals to use when discussing medications with a patient. You must ultimately rely on your own discretion, experience and judgment in diagnosing, treating and advising patients.
Related Information
Oral Medications That Should Not Be Crushed or Altered *on page 1712*

Thioridazine (thye oh RID a zeen)

Index Terms Mellaril; Thioridazine Hydrochloride
Pharmacologic Category Antipsychotic Agent, Typical, Phenothiazine

◀ **Medication Safety Issues**
Sound-alike/look-alike issues:
Thioridazine may be confused with thiothixene, Thorazine
Mellaril may be confused with Elavil, Mebaral®
BEERS Criteria medication:
This drug may be potentially inappropriate for use in geriatric patients (Quality of evidence - moderate; Strength of recommendation - strong).

Use Management of schizophrenic patients who fail to respond adequately to treatment with other antipsychotic drugs, either because of insufficient effectiveness or the inability to achieve an effective dose due to intolerable adverse effects from those medications

Unlabeled Use Behavior problems (children); severe psychoses (children); schizophrenia/psychoses (children); depressive disorders/dementia (children and adults); behavioral symptoms associated with dementia (elderly); psychosis/agitation related to Alzheimer's dementia

Available Dosage Forms
Tablet, Oral:
Generic: 10 mg, 25 mg, 50 mg, 100 mg
General Dosage Range Oral:
Children >2-12 years: 0.5-3 mg/kg/day in 2-3 divided doses **or** 10-25 mg 2-3 times/day (maximum: 3 mg/kg/day)
Children >12 years and Adults: Initial: 50-100 mg 3 times/day; Maintenance: 150-800 mg/day in 2-4 divided doses (maximum: 800 mg/day) **or** Initial: 25 mg 3 times/day; Maintenance: 20-200 mg/day
Elderly: Initial: 10-25 mg 1-2 times/day; Maintenance: 10-400 mg/day in 1-2 divided doses (maximum: 400 mg/day)

Administration
Oral Do not take antacid within 2 hours of taking drug.

Nursing Actions
Physical Assessment Monitor for excess sedation, extrapyramidal symptoms, tardive dyskinesia, and CNS changes. Monitor level of sedation.
Patient Education
• Discuss specific use of drug and side effects with patient as it relates to treatment. (HCAHPS: During this hospital stay, were you given any medicine that you had not taken before? Before giving you any new medicine, how often did hospital staff tell you what the medicine was for? How often did hospital staff describe possible side effects in a way you could understand?)
• Patient may experience presyncope, fatigue, blurred vision, illogical thinking, dizziness, nervousness and anxiety, constipation, xerostomia, weight gain, or impotence. Have patient report immediately to prescriber tachycardia, significant change in balance, tremors, urinary retention, severe asthenia, or rash (HCAHPS).
• Educate patient about signs of a significant reaction (eg, wheezing; chest tightness; fever; itching; bad cough; blue skin color; seizures; or

swelling of face, lips, tongue, or throat). **Note:** This is not a comprehensive list of all side effects. Patient should consult prescriber for additional questions.

Intended Use and Disclaimer: Should not be printed and given to patients. This information is intended to serve as a concise initial reference for healthcare professionals to use when discussing medications with a patient. You must ultimately rely on your own discretion, experience and judgment in diagnosing, treating and advising patients.

Thiotepa (thye oh TEP a)

Index Terms TESPA; Thiophosphoramide; Thioplex; Triethylenethiophosphoramide; TSPA
Pharmacologic Category Antineoplastic Agent, Alkylating Agent
Medication Safety Issues
Sound-alike/look-alike issues:
Thiotepa may be confused with thioguanine
High alert medication:
This medication is in a class the Institute for Safe Medication Practices (ISMP) includes among its list of drug classes which have a heightened risk of causing significant patient harm when used in error.
Administration issues:
Intrathecal medication safety: The American Society of Clinical Oncology (ASCO)/Oncology Nursing Society (ONS) chemotherapy administration safety standards (Jacobson, 2009) encourage the following safety measures for intrathecal chemotherapy:
• Intrathecal medication should not be prepared during the preparation of any other agents
• After preparation, keep in an isolated location or container clearly marked with a label identifying as "intrathecal" use only
• Delivery to the patient should only be with other medications intended for administration into the central nervous system

Pregnancy Risk Factor D
Lactation Excretion in breast milk unknown/not recommended
Use Treatment of superficial papillary bladder cancer; palliative treatment of adenocarcinoma of breast or ovary; controlling intracavitary effusions caused by metastatic tumors
Unlabeled Use Intrathecal treatment of leptomeningeal metastases
Available Dosage Forms
Solution Reconstituted, Injection:
Generic: 15 mg (1 ea)
General Dosage Range Dosage adjustment recommended in patients who develop toxicities
I.V.: *Adults:* 0.3-0.4 mg/kg every 1-4 weeks
Intracavitary: *Adults:* 0.6-0.8 mg/kg

Intravesical: *Adults:* 60 mg retained for 2 hours once weekly for 4 weeks

Administration

I.V. Administer as a rapid injection. Infusion times may be longer for high-dose (unlabeled use) treatment; refer to specific protocols.

Hazardous agent; use appropriate precautions for handling and disposal (NIOSH, 2012).

Injectable Detail pH: 5.5-7.5

Other Intravesical instillation: Instill directly into the bladder and retain for 2 hours; patient should be repositioned every 15-30 minutes for maximal exposure.

Hazardous agent; use appropriate precautions for handling and disposal (NIOSH, 2012).

Nursing Actions

Physical Assessment Monitor laboratory tests regularly during treatment and for at least 3 weeks following treatment. Monitor for myelosuppression, leukopenia, dysuria, bleeding, and infection. Teach patient importance of adequate hydration.

Patient Education

- Discuss specific use of drug and side effects with patient as it relates to treatment. (HCAHPS: During this hospital stay, were you given any medicine that you had not taken before? Before giving you any new medicine, how often did hospital staff tell you what the medicine was for? How often did hospital staff describe possible side effects in a way you could understand?)
- Patient may experience anemia, leukopenia, thrombocytopenia, headache, nausea, alopecia, skin irritation, or infertility. Have patient report immediately to prescriber dyspnea, asthenia, severe dyspepsia, significant weight loss, ecchymosis, or rash (HCAHPS).
- Educate patient about signs of a significant reaction (eg, wheezing; chest tightness; fever; itching; bad cough; blue skin color; seizures; or swelling of face, lips, tongue, or throat). **Note:** This is not a comprehensive list of all side effects. Patient should consult prescriber for additional questions.

Intended Use and Disclaimer: Should not be printed and given to patients. This information is intended to serve as a concise initial reference for healthcare professionals to use when discussing medications with a patient. You must ultimately rely on your own discretion, experience and judgment in diagnosing, treating and advising patients.

Related Information

Management of Drug Extravasations *on page 1700*

Thiothixene (thye oh THIKS een)

Index Terms Navane; Tiotixene

Pharmacologic Category Antipsychotic Agent, Typical

Medication Safety Issues

Sound-alike/look-alike issues:

Thiothixene may be confused with FLUoxetine, thioridazine

Navane may be confused with Norvasc, Nubain

BEERS Criteria medication:

This drug may be potentially inappropriate for use in geriatric patients (Quality of evidence - moderate; Strength of recommendation - strong).

Use Schizophrenia: For the management of schizophrenia

Unlabeled Use Schizophrenia (children); psychosis/agitation related to Alzheimer dementia

Available Dosage Forms

Capsule, Oral:

Generic: 1 mg, 2 mg, 5 mg, 10 mg

General Dosage Range Oral: *Adults:* Initial: 6-10 mg daily in 2-3 divided doses; Maintenance: 15-30 mg/day in 2-3 divided doses (maximum: 60 mg daily)

Nursing Actions

Physical Assessment Monitor vital signs for orthostatic hypotension; monitor for other side effects including constipation, dry mouth, urinary retention, extrapyramidal side effects, sedation.

Patient Education

- Discuss specific use of drug and side effects with patient as it relates to treatment. (HCAHPS: During this hospital stay, were you given any medicine that you had not taken before? Before giving you any new medicine, how often did hospital staff tell you what the medicine was for? How often did hospital staff describe possible side effects in a way you could understand?)
- Patient may experience presyncope, fatigue, blurred vision, illogical thinking, dizziness, nervousness and anxiety, constipation, xerostomia, weight gain, or impotence. Have patient report immediately to prescriber significant change in balance, tremors, urinary retention, severe asthenia, pregnancy, or rash (HCAHPS).
- Educate patient about signs of a significant reaction (eg, wheezing; chest tightness; fever; itching; bad cough; blue skin color; seizures; or swelling of face, lips, tongue, or throat). **Note:** This is not a comprehensive list of all side effects. Patient should consult prescriber for additional questions.

Intended Use and Disclaimer: Should not be printed and given to patients. This information is intended to serve as a concise initial reference for healthcare professionals to use when discussing medications with a patient. You must ultimately rely on your own discretion, experience and judgment in diagnosing, treating and advising patients.

Thyroid, Desiccated (THYE roid DES i kay tid)

Brand Names: U.S. Armour Thyroid; Nature-Thyroid; NP Thyroid; Westhroid; Westhroid-P [DSC]; WP Thyroid

Index Terms Desiccated Thyroid; Levothyroxine and Liothyronine; Tetraiodothyronine and Triiodothyronine; Thyroid Extract; Thyroid USP

Pharmacologic Category Thyroid Product

Medication Safety Issues

BEERS Criteria medication:

This drug may be potentially inappropriate for use in geriatric patients (Quality of evidence - low; Strength of recommendation - strong).

Pregnancy Risk Factor A

Lactation Enters breast milk/use caution

Use Replacement or supplemental therapy in hypothyroidism; pituitary TSH suppressants (thyroid nodules, thyroiditis, multinodular goiter, thyroid cancer)

Available Dosage Forms

Tablet, Oral:

Armour Thyroid: 15 mg, 30 mg, 60 mg, 90 mg, 120 mg, 180 mg, 240 mg, 300 mg

Nature-Thyroid: 16.25 mg, 32.5 mg, 48.75 mg, 65 mg, 81.25 mg, 97.5 mg, 113.75 mg, 130 mg, 146.25 mg, 162.5 mg, 195 mg, 260 mg, 325 mg

NP Thyroid: 30 mg, 60 mg, 90 mg

Westhroid: 16.25 mg, 32.5 mg, 48.75 mg, 65 mg, 81.25 mg, 97.5 mg, 113.75 mg, 130 mg, 146.25 mg, 162.5 mg, 195 mg, 260 mg, 325 mg

WP Thyroid: 16.25 mg, 32.5 mg, 48.75 mg, 65 mg, 97.5 mg, 130 mg

General Dosage Range Oral:

Children 0-6 months: 15-30 mg/day or 4.8-6 mg/kg/day

Children 6-12 months: 30-45 mg/day or 3.6-4.8 mg/kg/day

Children 1-5 years: 45-60 mg/day or 3-3.6 mg/kg/day

Children 6-12 years: 60-90 mg/day or 2.4-3 mg/kg/day

Children >12 years: >90 mg/day or 1.2-1.8 mg/kg/day

Adults: Initial: 15-30 mg/day; Maintenance: 60-120 mg/day

Administration

Oral Administer on an empty stomach. Take in the morning before breakfast.

Nursing Actions

Physical Assessment Ineffective for weight reduction. Monitor for hyperthyroidism (weight loss, nervousness, sweating, tachycardia, insomnia, heat intolerance, palpitations, vomiting, psychosis, fever, seizures, angina, arrhythmias). Caution patients with diabetes to monitor glucose levels closely (may increase need for oral hypoglycemics or insulin).

Patient Education

- Discuss specific use of drug and side effects with patient as it relates to treatment. (HCAHPS: During this hospital stay, were you given any medicine that you had not taken before? Before giving you any new medicine, how often did hospital staff tell you what the medicine was for? How often did hospital staff describe possible side effects in a way you could understand?)
- Patient may experience polyphagia, loss of appetite, weight gain or loss, nervousness and anxiety, tremors, temperature sensitivity, hyperhidrosis, headache, nausea, diarrhea, mood changes, leg cramps, or insomnia. Have patient report immediately to prescriber angina, tachycardia, dyspnea, or rash (HCAHPS).
- Educate patient about signs of a significant reaction (eg, wheezing; chest tightness; fever; itching; bad cough; blue skin color; seizures; or swelling of face, lips, tongue, or throat). **Note:** This is not a comprehensive list of all side effects. Patient should consult prescriber for additional questions.

Intended Use and Disclaimer: Should not be printed and given to patients. This information is intended to serve as a concise initial reference for healthcare professionals to use when discussing medications with a patient. You must ultimately rely on your own discretion, experience and judgment in diagnosing, treating and advising patients.

TiaGABine (tye AG a been)

Brand Names: U.S. Gabitril

Index Terms Tiagabine Hydrochloride

Pharmacologic Category Anticonvulsant, Miscellaneous

Medication Safety Issues

Sound-alike/look-alike issues:

TiaGABine may be confused with tiZANidine

Medication Guide Available Yes

Pregnancy Risk Factor C

Lactation Enters breast milk/not recommended

Breast-Feeding Considerations Levels of excretion of tiagabine and/or its metabolites in human milk have not been determined and effects on the nursing infant are unknown. According to the manufacturer, the decision to continue or discontinue breast-feeding during therapy should take into account the risk of exposure to the infant and the benefits of treatment to the mother.

Use Adjunctive therapy in adults and children ≥12 years of age in the treatment of partial seizures

Mechanism of Action/Effect The exact mechanism by which tiagabine exerts antiseizure activity is not definitively known; however, *in vitro* experiments demonstrate that it enhances the activity of gamma aminobutyric acid (GABA), the major neuroinhibitory transmitter in the nervous system; it is thought that binding to the GABA uptake carrier inhibits the uptake of GABA into presynaptic neurons, allowing an increased amount of GABA to be available to postsynaptic neurons; based on *in vitro* studies, tiagabine does not inhibit the uptake of dopamine, norepinephrine, serotonin, glutamate, or choline

Contraindications Hypersensitivity to tiagabine or any component of the formulation

Warnings/Precautions Antiepileptics are associated with an increased risk of suicidal behavior/ thoughts with use (regardless of indication); patients should be monitored for signs/symptoms of depression, suicidal tendencies, and other unusual behavior changes during therapy and instructed to inform their healthcare provider immediately if symptoms occur. New-onset seizures and status epilepticus have been associated with tiagabine use when taken for unlabeled indications. Often these seizures have occurred shortly after the initiation of treatment or shortly after a dosage increase. Seizures have also occurred with very low doses or after several months of therapy. In most cases, patients were using concomitant medications (eg, antidepressants, antipsychotics, stimulants, opioids). In these instances, the discontinuation of tiagabine, followed by an evaluation for an underlying seizure disorder, is suggested. Use for unapproved indications, however, has not been proven to be safe or effective and is not recommended. When tiagabine is used as an adjunct in partial seizures (an FDA-approved indication), it should not be abruptly discontinued because of the possibility of increasing seizure frequency, unless safety concerns require a more rapid withdrawal. Rarely, nonconvulsive status epilepticus has been reported following abrupt discontinuation or dosage reduction.

Use with caution in patients with hepatic impairment. Experience in patients not receiving enzyme-inducing drugs has been limited; caution should be used in treating any patient who is not receiving one of these medications (decreased dose and slower titration may be required). Weakness, sedation, and confusion may occur with tiagabine use. Patients must be cautioned about performing tasks which require mental alertness (eg, operating machinery or driving). Effects with other sedative drugs or ethanol may be potentiated. May cause serious rash, including Stevens-Johnson syndrome.

Drug Interactions

Avoid Concomitant Use
Avoid concomitant use of TiaGABine with any of the following: Azelastine (Nasal); Conivaptan; Fusidic Acid (Systemic); Paraldehyde; Thalidomide

Decreased Effect
The levels/effects of TiaGABine may be decreased by: Bosentan; CYP3A4 Inducers (Strong); Dabrafenib; Deferasirox; Herbs (CYP3A4 Inducers); Ketorolac (Nasal); Ketorolac (Systemic); Mefloquine; Mitotane; Orlistat; Tocilizumab

Increased Effect/Toxicity
TiaGABine may increase the levels/effects of: Alcohol (Ethyl); Azelastine (Nasal); Buprenorphine; CNS Depressants; Hydrocodone; Methotrimeprazine; Metyrosine; Mirtazapine; Paraldehyde; Pramipexole; ROPINIRole; Rotigotine; Selective Serotonin Reuptake Inhibitors; Thalidomide; Zolpidem

The levels/effects of TiaGABine may be increased by: Brimonidine (Topical); Conivaptan; CYP3A4 Inhibitors (Moderate); CYP3A4 Inhibitors (Strong); Dasatinib; Doxylamine; Droperidol; Fusidic Acid (Systemic); HydrOXYzine; Ivacaftor; Luliconazole; Magnesium Sulfate; Methotrimeprazine; Mifepristone; Perampanel; Simeprevir; Sodium Oxybate; Stiripentol; Tapentadol

Nutritional/Ethanol Interactions
Ethanol: May increase CNS depression; monitor for increased effects with coadministration. Caution patients about effects.

Food: Food reduces the rate but not the extent of absorption.

Herb/Nutraceutical: St John's wort may decrease tiagabine levels. Avoid valerian, St John's wort, kava kava, gotu kola (may increase CNS depression).

Adverse Reactions
>10%:
Central nervous system: Concentration decreased, dizziness, nervousness, somnolence
Gastrointestinal: Nausea
Neuromuscular & skeletal: Weakness, tremor
1% to 10%:
Cardiovascular: Chest pain, edema, hypertension, palpitation, peripheral edema, syncope, tachycardia, vasodilation
Central nervous system: Agitation, ataxia, chills, confusion, difficulty with memory, confusion, depersonalization, depression, euphoria, hallucination, hostility, insomnia, malaise, migraine, paranoid reaction, personality disorder, speech disorder
Dermatologic: Alopecia, bruising, dry skin, pruritus, rash
Gastrointestinal: Abdominal pain, diarrhea, gingivitis, increased appetite, mouth ulceration, stomatitis, vomiting, weight gain/loss
Neuromuscular & skeletal: Abnormal gait, arthralgia, dysarthria, hyper-/hypokinesia, hyper-/hypotonia, myasthenia, myalgia, myoclonus, neck pain, paresthesia, reflexes decreased, stupor, twitching, vertigo
Ocular: Abnormal vision, amblyopia, nystagmus
Otic: Ear pain, hearing impairment, otitis media, tinnitus

Respiratory: Bronchitis, cough, dyspnea, epistaxis, pneumonia

Miscellaneous: Allergic reaction, cyst, diaphoresis, flu-like syndrome, lymphadenopathy

Available Dosage Forms

Tablet, Oral:

Gabitril: 2 mg, 4 mg, 12 mg, 16 mg

Generic: 2 mg, 4 mg

General Dosage Range Dosage adjustment recommended in patients on concomitant therapy

Oral:

Children 12-18 years: Initial: 4 mg once daily; Maintenance: 8-32 mg/day in 2-4 divided doses

Adults: Initial: 4 mg once daily; Maintenance: 8-56 mg/day in 2-4 divided doses

Nursing Actions

Physical Assessment Monitor therapeutic response (seizure activity, type, duration) at beginning of therapy and throughout. Use and teach seizure/safety precautions.

Patient Education

• Discuss specific use of drug and side effects with patient as it relates to treatment. (HCAHPS: During this hospital stay, were you given any medicine that you had not taken before? Before giving you any new medicine, how often did hospital staff tell you what the medicine was for? How often did hospital staff describe possible side effects in a way you could understand?)

• Patient may experience presyncope, fatigue, blurred vision, illogical thinking, dizziness, nausea, diarrhea, xerostomia, increased appetite, tremors, nervousness, or anxiety. Have patient report immediately to prescriber depression, imbalance, sudden vision changes, eye pain, eye irritation, severe asthenia, or rash (HCAHPS).

• Educate patient about signs of a significant reaction (eg, wheezing; chest tightness; fever; itching; bad cough; blue skin color; seizures; or swelling of face, lips, tongue, or throat). **Note:** This is not a comprehensive list of all side effects. Patient should consult prescriber for additional questions.

Intended Use and Disclaimer: Should not be printed and given to patients. This information is intended to serve as a concise initial reference for healthcare professionals to use when discussing medications with a patient. You must ultimately rely on your own discretion, experience and judgment in diagnosing, treating and advising patients.

Dietary Considerations Take with food.

Ticagrelor (tye KA grel or)

Brand Names: U.S. Brilinta

Index Terms AZD6140

Pharmacologic Category Antiplatelet Agent; Antiplatelet Agent, Cyclopentyltriazolopyrimidine

Medication Guide Available Yes

Pregnancy Risk Factor C

Breast-Feeding Considerations Excretion into breast milk is unknown; use is not recommended.

Use Used in conjunction with aspirin for secondary prevention of thrombotic events in patients with unstable angina (UA), non-ST-elevation myocardial infarction (NSTEMI), or ST-elevation myocardial infarction (STEMI) managed medically or with percutaneous coronary intervention (PCI) and/or coronary artery bypass graft (CABG)

Unlabeled Use In patients with allergy or major gastrointestinal intolerance to aspirin, initial treatment of UA/NSTEMI; **Note:** Dual antiplatelet therapy with another $P2Y_{12}$ receptor inhibitor is not recommended in this situation (Jneid, 2012).

Mechanism of Action/Effect Reversibly and noncompetitively blocks ADP-mediated platelet aggregation; recovery of platelet function is likely to depend on serum concentrations of ticagrelor and its active metabolite.

Contraindications Hypersensitivity (eg, angioedema) to ticagrelor or any component of the formulation; active pathological bleeding (eg, peptic ulcer or intracranial hemorrhage); history of intracranial hemorrhage; severe hepatic impairment

Canadian labeling: Additional contraindications (not in U.S. labeling): Moderate hepatic impairment; concomitant use of strong CYP3A4 inhibitors (eg, ketoconazole, clarithromycin, ritonavir, atazanavir, nefazodone)

Warnings/Precautions [U.S. Boxed Warning]: Ticagrelor increases the risk of bleeding including significant and sometimes fatal bleeding. Use is contraindicated in patients with active pathological bleeding and presence or history of intracranial hemorrhage. Additional risk factors for bleeding include propensity to bleed (eg, recent trauma or surgery, recent or recurrent GI bleeding, active PUD, moderate-to-severe hepatic impairment), CABG or other surgical procedure, concomitant use of medications that increase risk of bleeding (eg, warfarin, NSAIDs), and advanced age. Bleeding should be suspected if patient becomes hypotensive after undergoing recent coronary angiography, PCI, CABG, or other surgical procedure even if overt signs of bleeding do not exist. **Where possible, manage bleeding without discontinuing ticagrelor as the risk of cardiovascular events is increased upon discontinuation.** If discontinuation of ticagrelor is necessary, resume as soon as possible after the bleeding source is identified and controlled. Hemostatic benefits of platelet transfusions are not known; may inhibit transfused platelets. Premature discontinuation of therapy may increase the risk of cardiac events (eg, stent thrombosis with subsequent fatal or nonfatal MI). Duration of therapy, in general, is determined by the type of stent placed (bare metal or drug eluting) and whether an ACS event was ongoing at the time of placement. Use with caution in patients who are at an increased risk of bradycardia (eg, second- or third-degree AV block, sick sinus syndrome) or taking other bradycardic-inducing agents (eg, beta blockers, nondihydropyridine calcium channel blockers). Ventricular pauses ≥3 seconds were noted more frequently with ticagrelor than with clopidogrel in a substudy of the Platelet Inhibition and Patient Outcomes (PLATO) trial. Dyspnea (often mild-to-moderate and transient) was observed more frequently in patients receiving ticagrelor than clopidogrel during clinical trials. Ticagrelor-related dyspnea does not require specific treatment nor does it warrant therapy interruption; however, therapy should be discontinued in patients unable to tolerate ticagrelor-related dyspnea.

[U.S. Boxed Warning]: Maintenance doses of aspirin greater than 100 mg/day reduce the efficacy of ticagrelor and should be avoided. Use of higher maintenance doses of aspirin (ie, >100 mg/day) was associated with relatively unfavorable outcomes for ticagrelor versus clopidogrel in the PLATO trial (Gaglia, 2011; Wallentin, 2009). Canadian labeling recommends a maximum maintenance aspirin dose of 150 mg/day.

[U.S. Boxed Warning]: Avoid initiation of ticagrelor when urgent CABG surgery is planned; when possible discontinue use at least 5 days before any surgery. Discontinue 5 days before elective surgery (except in patients with cardiac stents that have not completed their full course of dual antiplatelet therapy; patient-specific situations need to be discussed with cardiologist). When urgent CABG is necessary, the ACCF/AHA CABG guidelines recommend discontinuation for at least 24 hours prior to surgery (Hillis, 2011).

Use is contraindicated in patients with severe hepatic impairment (Canadian labeling also contraindicates use in moderate-to-severe hepatic impairment). Use with caution in patients with renal impairment, a history of hyperuricemia or gouty arthritis. Canadian labeling does not recommend use in patients with uric acid nephropathy. Avoid concomitant use with strong CYP3A4 inhibitors (eg, ketoconazole, ritonavir, nefazodone) or strong CYP3A4 inducers (eg, rifampin, carbamazepine, dexamethasone, phenobarbital, phenytoin). Canadian labeling contraindicates use with strong CYP3A4 inhibitors.

Drug Interactions

Avoid Concomitant Use

Avoid concomitant use of Ticagrelor with any of the following: CYP3A4 Inducers (Strong); CYP3A4 Inhibitors (Strong); Urokinase

Decreased Effect

The levels/effects of Ticagrelor may be decreased by: Aspirin; Bosentan; CYP3A4 Inducers (Strong); CYP3A4 Inhibitors (Strong); Dabrafenib;

Deferasirox; Herbs (CYP3A4 Inducers); Nonsteroidal Anti-Inflammatory Agents; Tocilizumab

Increased Effect/Toxicity

Ticagrelor may increase the levels/effects of: Agents with Antiplatelet Properties; Anticoagulants; ARIPiprazole; Bosentan; Carvedilol; Collagenase (Systemic); CycloSPORINE (Systemic); CYP2C9 Substrates; Dabigatran Etexilate; Digoxin; Ibritumomab; Lovastatin; Rivaroxaban; Salicylates; Simvastatin; Thrombolytic Agents; Tositumomab and Iodine I 131 Tositumomab; Urokinase

The levels/effects of Ticagrelor may be increased by: Aspirin; CycloSPORINE (Systemic); CYP3A4 Inhibitors (Strong); Dasatinib; Glucosamine; Grapefruit Juice; Herbs (Anticoagulant/Antiplatelet Properties); Ibrutinib; Multivitamins/Fluoride (with ADE); Multivitamins/Minerals (with ADEK, Folate, Iron); Multivitamins/Minerals (with AE, No Iron); Nonsteroidal Anti-Inflammatory Agents; Omega-3 Fatty Acids; Pentosan Polysulfate Sodium; Pentoxifylline; Prostacyclin Analogues; Tipranavir; Vitamin E

Adverse Reactions Note: As with all drugs which may affect hemostasis, bleeding is associated with ticagrelor. Hemorrhage may occur at virtually any site. Risk is dependent on multiple variables, including the concurrent use of multiple agents which alter hemostasis and patient susceptibility. Frequencies as reported in PLATO trial versus clopidogrel:

>10%: Respiratory: Dyspnea (≤14%)

1% to 10%:

Cardiovascular: Ventricular pauses (6%; 2% after 1 month of therapy), atrial fibrillation (4%), hypertension (4%), angina (3%), hypotension (3%), bradycardia (1% to 3%), cardiac failure (2%), peripheral edema (2%), ventricular tachycardia (2%), palpitation (1%), syncope (1%), ventricular extrasystoles (1%), ventricular fibrillation (1%)

Central nervous system: Headache (7%), dizziness (5%), fatigue (3%), fever (3%), anxiety (2%), insomnia (2%), vertigo (2%), depression (1%)

Dermatologic: Bruising (2% to 4%), rash (2%), pruritus (1%), subcutaneous or dermal bleeding

Endocrine & metabolic: Hypokalemia (2%), diabetes mellitus (1%), dyslipidemia (1%), hypercholesterolemia (1%)

Gastrointestinal: Diarrhea (4%), nausea (4%), vomiting (3%), abdominal pain (2%), constipation (2%), dyspepsia (2%), GI hemorrhage

Genitourinary: Urinary tract infection (2%), urinary tract bleeding

Hematologic: Major bleeding (12%; composite of major fatal/life threatening and other major bleeding events), minor bleeding (~5%), anemia (2%), hematoma (2%), postprocedural hemorrhage (2%)

Local: Puncture site hematoma (2%)

Neuromuscular & skeletal: Back pain (4%), non-cardiac chest pain (4%), extremity pain (2%), arthralgia (2%), musculoskeletal pain (2%), weakness (2%), myalgia (1%)

Renal: Creatinine increased (7%; mechanism undetermined), hematuria (2%), renal failure (1%)

Respiratory: Epistaxis (6%), cough (5%), nasopharyngitis (2%), bronchitis (1%), pneumonia (1%)

Pharmacodynamics/Kinetics

Onset of Action Inhibition of platelet aggregation (IPA): 180 mg loading dose: ~41% within 30 minutes (similar to clopidogrel 600 mg at 8 hours); Peak effect: Time to maximal IPA: 180 mg loading dose: IPA ~88% at 2 hours post administration

Duration of Action IPA: 180 mg loading dose: 87% to 89% maintained from 2-8 hours; 24 hours after the last maintenance dose, IPA is 58% (similar to maintenance clopidogrel)

Time after discontinuation when IPA is 30%: ~56 hours; IPA 10%: ~110 hours (Gurbel, 2009). Mean IPA observed with ticagrelor at 3 days post-discontinuation was comparable to that observed with clopidogrel at 5 days post discontinuation.

Available Dosage Forms

Tablet, Oral:

Brilinta: 90 mg

General Dosage Range Oral: *Adults:* Loading dose: 180 mg; Maintenance: 90 mg twice daily

Administration

Oral May be administered without regard to meals. Missed doses should be taken at their next regularly scheduled time. For patients unable to swallow whole, tablets may be crushed to create a suspension for oral or NG use (data on file, AstraZeneca).

Storage/Stability Store at 25°C (77°F); excursions permitted to 15°C to 30°C (59°F to 86°F).

Nursing Actions

Physical Assessment Not to be used in patients with significant active bleeding. Drug should be held prior to surgery except with stent patients; discuss with cardiologist. Shortness of breath can occur early in therapy; treatment is not required but healthcare provider needs to be notified to ensure that there is not another cause of symptom. Other serious side effects include allergic reactions and bleeding.

Patient Education

• Discuss specific use of drug and side effects with patient as it relates to treatment. (HCAHPS: During this hospital stay, were you given any medicine that you had not taken before? Before giving you any new medicine, how often did hospital staff tell you what the medicine was for? How often did hospital staff describe possible side effects in a way you could understand?)

• Patient may experience headache, dizziness, dyspepsia, nausea, asthenia, constipation, or diarrhea. Have patient report immediately to prescriber angina, changes in strength, difficulty speaking, change in balance, blurred vision, dyspnea, illogical thinking, sudden vision changes, ecchymosis, bleeding, arthralgia, edema, or rash (HCAHPS).

• Educate patient about signs of a significant reaction (eg, wheezing; chest tightness; fever; itching; bad cough; blue skin color; seizures; or swelling of face, lips, tongue, or throat). **Note:** This is not a comprehensive list of all side effects. Patient should consult prescriber for additional questions.

Intended Use and Disclaimer: Should not be printed and given to patients. This information is intended to serve as a concise initial reference for healthcare professionals to use when discussing medications with a patient. You must ultimately rely on your own discretion, experience and judgment in diagnosing, treating and advising patients.

Dietary Considerations May be taken without regard to meals.

Ticarcillin and Clavulanate Potassium

(tye kar SIL in & klav yoo LAN ate poe TASS ee um)

Brand Names: U.S. Timentin

Index Terms Ticarcillin and Clavulanic Acid

Pharmacologic Category Antibiotic, Penicillin

Pregnancy Risk Factor B

Lactation Enters breast milk/use caution

Use

Bone and joint infections: Treatment of bone and joint infections caused by beta-lactamase-producing isolates of *Staphylococcus aureus*.

Endometritis: Treatment of endometritis caused by beta-lactamase-producing isolates of *Prevotella melaninogenicus*, *Enterobacter* species (including *E. cloacae*), *Klebsiella pneumoniae*, *Escherichia coli*, *S. aureus*, or *Staphylococcus epidermidis*.

Lower respiratory tract infections: Treatment of lower respiratory tract infections caused by beta-lactamase-producing isolates of *S. aureus*, *Haemophilus influenzae*, or *Klebsiella* species.

Peritonitis: Treatment of peritonitis caused by beta-lactamase-producing isolates of *E. coli*, *K. pneumonia*, or *Bacteroides fragilis* group.

Septicemia: Treatment of septicemia (including bacteremia) caused by beta-lactamase-producing isolates of *Klebsiella* species, *E. coli*, *S. aureus*, or *Pseudomonas aeruginosa* (or other *Pseudomonas* species).

Skin and skin structure infections: Treatment of skin and skin structure infections caused by beta-lactamase-producing isolates of *S. aureus*, *Klebsiella* species, or *E. coli*.

Urinary tract infections: Treatment of complicated and uncomplicated urinary tract infections caused by beta-lactamase-producing isolates of *E. coli*, *Klebsiella* species, *P. aeruginosa* (and other *Pseudomonas* species), *Citrobacter* species, *Enterobacter cloacae*, *Serratia marcescens*, or *S. aureus*.

Unlabeled Use Treatment of complicated intra-abdominal infections (Solomkin 2010), cystic fibrosis exacerbations (Zobell, 2013)

Available Dosage Forms

Infusion [premixed, frozen]:
Timentin®: Ticarcillin 3 g and clavulanic acid 0.1 g (100 mL)

Injection, powder for reconstitution:
Timentin®: Ticarcillin 3 g and clavulanic acid 0.1 g (3.1 g, 31 g)

General Dosage Range Dosage adjustment recommended in patients with hepatic or renal impairment

I.V.: *Infants ≥3 months, Children, Adolescents, and Adults:*
<60 kg: 200-300 mg ticarcillin/kg/day in divided doses every 4-6 hours (maximum: 18 g daily)
≥60 kg: 3.1 g every 4-6 hours

Administration

I.V. Infuse over 30 minutes.
Some penicillins (eg, carbenicillin, ticarcillin, and piperacillin) have been shown to inactivate aminoglycosides *in vitro*. This has been observed to a greater extent with tobramycin and gentamicin, while amikacin has shown greater stability against inactivation. Concurrent use of these agents may pose a risk of reduced antibacterial efficacy *in vivo*, particularly in the setting of profound renal impairment. However, definitive clinical evidence is lacking. If combination penicillin/aminoglycoside therapy is desired in a patient with renal dysfunction, separation of doses (if feasible), and routine monitoring of aminoglycoside levels, CBC, and clinical response should be considered.

Injectable Detail pH: 5.5-7.5

Nursing Actions

Patient Education
- Discuss specific use of drug and side effects with patient as it relates to treatment. (HCAHPS: During this hospital stay, were you given any medicine that you had not taken before? Before giving you any new medicine, how often did hospital staff tell you what the medicine was for? How often did hospital staff describe possible side effects in a way you could understand?)
- Patient may experience nausea, diarrhea, headache, or vaginal yeast infection. Have patient report immediately to prescriber ecchymosis, bleeding, or rash (HCAHPS).

- Educate patient about signs of a significant reaction (eg, wheezing; chest tightness; fever; itching; bad cough; blue skin color; seizures; or swelling of face, lips, tongue, or throat). **Note:** This is not a comprehensive list of all side effects. Patient should consult prescriber for additional questions.

Intended Use and Disclaimer: Should not be printed and given to patients. This information is intended to serve as a concise initial reference for healthcare professionals to use when discussing medications with a patient. You must ultimately rely on your own discretion, experience and judgment in diagnosing, treating and advising patients.

Tigecycline (tye ge SYE kleen)

Brand Names: U.S. Tygacil
Index Terms GAR-936
Pharmacologic Category Antibiotic, Glycylcycline
Pregnancy Risk Factor D
Lactation Excretion in breast milk unknown/use caution

Use

Community-acquired bacterial pneumonia: Treatment of community-acquired pneumonia in patients 18 years and older caused by *Streptococcus pneumoniae* (penicillin-susceptible isolates), including cases with concurrent bacteremia, *Haemophilus influenzae* (beta-lactamase negative isolates), and *Legionella pneumophila*.

Complicated intra-abdominal infections: Treatment of complicated intra-abdominal infections in patients 18 years and older caused by *Citrobacter freundii*, *Enterobacter cloacae*, *Escherichia coli*, *Klebsiella oxytoca*, *Klebsiella pneumoniae*, *Enterococcus faecalis* (vancomycin-susceptible isolates), *Staphylococcus aureus* (methicillin-susceptible and methicillin-resistant isolates), *Streptococcus anginosus* group (includes *S. anginosus*, *Streptococcus intermedius*, and *Streptococcus constellatus*), *Bacteroides fragilis*, *Bacteroides thetaiotaomicron*, *Bacteroides uniformis*, *Bacteroides vulgatus*, *Clostridium perfringens*, and *Peptostreptococcus micros*.

Complicated skin and skin structure infections: Treatment of skin and skin structure infections in patients 18 years and older caused by *E. coli*, *E. faecalis* (vancomycin-susceptible isolates), *S. aureus* (methicillin-susceptible and methicillin-resistant isolates), *Streptococcus agalactiae*, *S. anginosus* group (includes *S. anginosus*, *S. intermedius*, and *S. constellatus*), *Streptococcus pyogenes*, *E. cloacae*, *K. pneumoniae*, and *B. fragilis*.

Available Dosage Forms

Solution Reconstituted, Intravenous:
Tygacil: 50 mg (1 ea)

General Dosage Range Dosage adjustment recommended in patients with hepatic impairment
I.V.: *Adults:* Initial: 100 mg as a single dose; Maintenance: 50 mg every 12 hours
Administration
I.V. Infuse over 30-60 minutes through dedicated line or via Y-site
Nursing Actions
Physical Assessment Culture and sensitivity tests should be assessed prior to beginning therapy. May cause life-threatening anaphylaxis/anaphylactoid reactions. Monitor for nausea, vomiting, diarrhea, headache, rash, anemia, dyspnea, and opportunistic infection.
Patient Education
- Discuss specific use of drug and side effects with patient as it relates to treatment. (HCAHPS: During this hospital stay, were you given any medicine that you had not taken before? Before giving you any new medicine, how often did hospital staff tell you what the medicine was for? How often did hospital staff describe possible side effects in a way you could understand?)
- Patient may experience nausea, diarrhea, or injection site irritation. Have patient report immediately to prescriber severe skin irritation or rash (HCAHPS).
- Educate patient about signs of a significant reaction (eg, wheezing; chest tightness; fever; itching; bad cough; blue skin color; seizures; or swelling of face, lips, tongue, or throat). **Note:** This is not a comprehensive list of all side effects. Patient should consult prescriber for additional questions.

Intended Use and Disclaimer: Should not be printed and given to patients. This information is intended to serve as a concise initial reference for healthcare professionals to use when discussing medications with a patient. You must ultimately rely on your own discretion, experience and judgment in diagnosing, treating and advising patients.

Tiludronate (tye LOO droe nate)

Brand Names: U.S. Skelid
Index Terms Tiludronate Disodium
Pharmacologic Category Bisphosphonate Derivative
Pregnancy Risk Factor C
Lactation Excretion in breast milk unknown/use caution
Use Treatment of Paget's disease of the bone (osteitis deformans) in patients who have a level of serum alkaline phosphatase (SAP) at least twice the upper limit of normal, or who are symptomatic, or who are at risk for future complications of their disease

Available Dosage Forms
Tablet, Oral:
Skelid: 200 mg
General Dosage Range Oral: *Adults:* 400 mg once daily
Administration
Oral Administer as a single oral dose, take with 6-8 oz of plain water. Should not be taken with beverages containing minerals (eg, mineral water), food, or with other medications (may reduce absorption). Do not take within 2 hours of food. Take calcium or mineral supplements at least 2 hours before or after tiludronate. Take aluminum- or magnesium-containing antacids at least 2 hours after taking tiludronate. Patients should be instructed to stay upright (not to lie down) for at least 30 minutes and until after first food of the day (to reduce esophageal irritation).
Nursing Actions
Physical Assessment Monitor blood pressure at the beginning of therapy and periodically during use. Patients at risk for osteonecrosis of the jaw (eg, chemotherapy, corticosteroids, poor oral hygiene) should have dental exams; necessary preventive dentistry should be done before beginning bisphosphonate therapy. Teach patient appropriate administration of medication (eg, timing with food, supplements, and other medications). Instruct patient in lifestyle and dietary changes.
Patient Education
- Discuss specific use of drug and side effects with patient as it relates to treatment. (HCAHPS: During this hospital stay, were you given any medicine that you had not taken before? Before giving you any new medicine, how often did hospital staff tell you what the medicine was for? How often did hospital staff describe possible side effects in a way you could understand?)
- Patient may experience nausea, diarrhea, arthralgia, myalgia, or osteopenia. Have patient report immediately to prescriber angina; dysphagia; significant dyspepsia, severe jaw, groin, or thigh pain; or rash (HCAHPS).
- Educate patient about signs of a significant reaction (eg, wheezing; chest tightness; fever; itching; bad cough; blue skin color; seizures; or swelling of face, lips, tongue, or throat). **Note:** This is not a comprehensive list of all side effects. Patient should consult prescriber for additional questions.

Intended Use and Disclaimer: Should not be printed and given to patients. This information is intended to serve as a concise initial reference for healthcare professionals to use when discussing medications with a patient. You must ultimately rely on your own discretion, experience and judgment in diagnosing, treating and advising patients.

Timolol (Ophthalmic) (TIM oh lol)

Brand Names: U.S. Betimol; Istalol; Timoptic; Timoptic Ocudose; Timoptic-XE
Index Terms Timolol Hemihydrate; Timolol Maleate
Pharmacologic Category Beta-Blocker, Nonselective; Ophthalmic Agent, Antiglaucoma
Medication Safety Issues
Sound-alike/look-alike issues:
Timolol may be confused with atenolol, Tylenol®
Timoptic® may be confused with Betoptic S®, Talacen, Viroptic®
Other safety concerns:
Bottle cap color change: Timoptic®: Both the 0.25% and 0.5% strengths are now packaged in bottles with yellow caps; previously, the color of the cap on the product corresponded to different strengths.
International issues:
Betimol [U.S.] may be confused with Betanol brand name for metipranolol [Monaco]
Pregnancy Risk Factor C
Lactation Enters breast milk/consider risk:benefit
Use Treatment of elevated intraocular pressure such as glaucoma or ocular hypertension
Available Dosage Forms
Gel Forming Solution, Ophthalmic:
Timoptic-XE: 0.25% (5 mL); 0.5% (5 mL)
Generic: 0.25% (5 mL); 0.5% (5 mL)
Solution, Ophthalmic:
Betimol: 0.25% (5 mL); 0.5% (5 mL, 10 mL, 15 mL)
Istalol: 0.5% (2.5 mL, 5 mL)
Timoptic: 0.25% (5 mL); 0.5% (5 mL, 10 mL)
Generic: 0.25% (5 mL, 10 mL, 15 mL); 0.5% (5 mL, 10 mL, 15 mL)
Solution, Ophthalmic [preservative free]:
Timoptic Ocudose: 0.25% (60 ea); 0.5% (60 ea)
General Dosage Range Ophthalmic:
Gel-forming solution: *Children and Adults:* Instill 1 drop (0.25% or 0.5%) once daily
Solution: *Children and Adults:* Initial: Instill 1 drop (0.25%) twice daily; Maintenance: Instill 1 drop (0.25% or 0.5%) 1-2 times daily (maximum: 2 drops/day [0.5%])
Administration
Ophthalmic Ophthalmic: Administer other topically-applied ophthalmic medications at least 10 minutes before Timoptic-XE®; wash hands before use; invert closed bottle and shake once before use; remove cap carefully so that tip does not touch anything; hold bottle between thumb and index finger; use index finger of other hand to pull down the lower eyelid to form a pocket for the eye drop and tilt head back; place the dispenser tip close to the eye and gently squeeze the bottle to administer 1 drop; remove pressure after a single drop has been released; **do not allow the dispenser tip to touch the eye**; replace cap and store bottle in an upright position in a clean area;

do **not** enlarge hole of dispenser; do **not** wash tip with water, soap, or any other cleaner. Some solutions contain benzalkonium chloride; wait at least 10 minutes after instilling solution before inserting soft contact lenses.
Nursing Actions
Patient Education
• Discuss specific use of drug and side effects with patient as it relates to treatment. (HCAHPS: During this hospital stay, were you given any medicine that you had not taken before? Before giving you any new medicine, how often did hospital staff tell you what the medicine was for? How often did hospital staff describe possible side effects in a way you could understand?)
• Patient may experience eye irritation. Have patient report immediately to prescriber sudden vision changes, eye pain, or rash (HCAHPS).
• Educate patient about signs of a significant reaction (eg, wheezing; chest tightness; fever; itching; bad cough; blue skin color; seizures; or swelling of face, lips, tongue, or throat). **Note:** This is not a comprehensive list of all side effects. Patient should consult prescriber for additional questions.

Intended Use and Disclaimer: Should not be printed and given to patients. This information is intended to serve as a concise initial reference for healthcare professionals to use when discussing medications with a patient. You must ultimately rely on your own discretion, experience and judgment in diagnosing, treating and advising patients.

Tinidazole (tye NI da zole)

Brand Names: U.S. Tindamax
Pharmacologic Category Amebicide; Antibiotic, Miscellaneous; Antiprotozoal, Nitroimidazole
Pregnancy Risk Factor C
Lactation Enters breast milk/contraindicated
Breast-Feeding Considerations Tinidazole is excreted into breast milk in concentrations similar to those in the maternal serum and can be detected for up to 72 hours after administration. Tinidazole is contraindicated in nursing mothers unless breast-feeding is interrupted during therapy and for 3 days after the last dose.
Use Treatment of trichomoniasis caused by *T. vaginalis*; treatment of giardiasis caused by *G. duodenalis* (*G. lamblia*); treatment of intestinal amebiasis and amebic liver abscess caused by *E. histolytica*; treatment of bacterial vaginosis caused by *Bacteroides* spp, *Gardnerella vaginalis*, and *Prevotella* spp in nonpregnant females
Mechanism of Action/Effect After diffusing into the organism, it is proposed that tinidazole causes cytotoxicity by damaging DNA and preventing further DNA synthesis.

◄ **Contraindications** Hypersensitivity to tinidazole, nitroimidazole derivatives (including metronidazole), or any component of the formulation; pregnancy (1st trimester); breast-feeding

Warnings/Precautions Use caution with CNS diseases; seizures and peripheral neuropathy have been reported with tinidazole and other nitroimidazole derivatives. **[U.S. Boxed Warning]: Carcinogenicity has been observed with another nitroimidazole derivative (metronidazole) in animal studies;** use should be reserved for approved indications only. Use caution with current or history of blood dyscrasias or hepatic impairment. When used for amebiasis, not indicated for the treatment of asymptomatic cyst passage. Prolonged use may result in fungal or bacterial superinfection, including *C. difficile*-associated diarrhea (CDAD), pseudomembranous colitis, and/or vaginal candidiasis. CDAD has been observed >2 months postantibiotic treatment. Safety and efficacy have not been established in children ≤3 years of age.

Drug Interactions

Avoid Concomitant Use

Avoid concomitant use of Tinidazole with any of the following: Alcohol (Ethyl); Disulfiram

Decreased Effect There are no known significant interactions involving a decrease in effect.

Increased Effect/Toxicity

Tinidazole may increase the levels/effects of: Alcohol (Ethyl); Disulfiram

Nutritional/Ethanol Interactions

Ethanol: The manufacturer recommends to avoid all ethanol or any ethanol-containing drugs (may cause disulfiram-like reaction characterized by flushing, headache, nausea, vomiting, sweating or tachycardia) during and for at least 3 days after completion of treatment.

Food: Peak antibiotic serum concentration lowered and delayed, but total drug absorbed not affected.

Adverse Reactions

1% to 10%:

Central nervous system: Fatigue/malaise (1% to 2%), dizziness (≤1%), headache (≤1%)

Endocrine & metabolic: Menorrhagia (>2%)

Gastrointestinal: Metallic/bitter taste (4% to 6%), nausea (3% to 5%), anorexia (2% to 3%), appetite decreased (>2%), flatulence (>2%), dyspepsia/cramps/epigastric discomfort (1% to 2%), vomiting (1% to 2%), constipation (≤1%)

Genitourinary: *Candida* vaginitis (5%), painful urination (>2%), pelvic pain (>2%), urine abnormality (>2%), vaginal odor (>2%), vulvovaginal discomfort (>2%)

Neuromuscular & skeletal: Weakness (1% to 2%)

Renal: Urinary tract infection (>2%)

Respiratory: Upper respiratory tract infection (>2%)

Frequency not defined:

Cardiovascular: Flushing, palpitation

Central nervous system: Ataxia, coma (rare), confusion (rare), depression (rare), drowsiness, fever, giddiness, insomnia, seizure, vertigo

Dermatologic: Angioedema, pruritus, rash, urticaria

Gastrointestinal: Abdominal pain, diarrhea, furry tongue (rare), oral candidiasis, salivation, stomatitis, thirst, tongue discoloration, xerostomia

Genitourinary: Urine darkened, vaginal discharge increased

Hematologic: Leukopenia (transient), neutropenia (transient), thrombocytopenia (reversible; rare)

Hepatic: Transaminases increased

Neuromuscular & skeletal: Arthralgia, arthritis, myalgia, peripheral neuropathy (transient, includes numbness and paresthesia)

Respiratory: Bronchospasm (rare), dyspnea (rare), pharyngitis (rare)

Miscellaneous: Burning sensation, *Candida* overgrowth, diaphoresis

Available Dosage Forms

Tablet, Oral:

Tindamax: 250 mg, 500 mg

Generic: 250 mg, 500 mg

General Dosage Range Oral:

Children >3 years: 50 mg/kg/day (maximum: 2 g/day)

Adults: 1-2 g/day

Administration

Oral Administer with food.

Storage/Stability Store at controlled room temperature of 15°C to 30°C (59°F to 86°F). Protect from light.

Nursing Actions

Patient Education

• Discuss specific use of drug and side effects with patient as it relates to treatment. (HCAHPS: During this hospital stay, were you given any medicine that you had not taken before? Before giving you any new medicine, how often did hospital staff tell you what the medicine was for? How often did hospital staff describe possible side effects in a way you could understand?)

• Patient may experience nausea, parageusia, asthenia, or vaginal yeast infection. Have patient report immediately to prescriber severe diarrhea, paresthesia, or rash (HCAHPS).

• Educate patient about signs of a significant reaction (eg, wheezing; chest tightness; fever; itching; bad cough; blue skin color; seizures; or swelling of face, lips, tongue, or throat). **Note:** This is not a comprehensive list of all side effects. Patient should consult prescriber for additional questions.

Intended Use and Disclaimer: Should not be printed and given to patients. This information is intended to serve as a concise initial reference for healthcare professionals to use when discussing

medications with a patient. You must ultimately rely on your own discretion, experience and judgment in diagnosing, treating and advising patients.

Dietary Considerations Take with food. The manufacturer recommends that ethanol be avoided during treatment and for 3 days after therapy is complete.

Tinzaparin (tin ZA pa rin)

Index Terms Tinzaparin Sodium
Pharmacologic Category Anticoagulant; Anticoagulant, Low Molecular Weight Heparin
Medication Safety Issues
High alert medication:
The Institute for Safe Medication Practices (ISMP) includes this medication among its list of drug classes which have a heightened risk of causing significant patient harm when used in error.

Lactation Excretion in breast milk unknown/use caution

Breast-Feeding Considerations Small amounts of LMWH have been detected in breast milk; however, because it has a low oral bioavailability, it is unlikely to cause adverse events in a nursing infant. Use of LMWH may be continued in breast-feeding women (Guyatt, 2012).

Use Treatment of deep vein thrombosis (DVT) and/or pulmonary embolism (PE) (except in patients with severe hemodynamic instability); prevention of venous thromboembolism (VTE) following orthopedic surgery or following general surgery in patients at high risk of VTE; prevention of clotting in indwelling intravenous lines and extracorporeal circuit during hemodialysis (in patients without high bleeding risk)

Mechanism of Action/Effect Tinzaparin is a low molecular weight heparin that binds antithrombin III, enhancing the inhibition of several clotting factors, particularly factor Xa. Low molecular weight heparins have a small effect on the activated partial thromboplastin time.

Contraindications Hypersensitivity to tinzaparin sodium, heparin or other low molecular weight heparins (LMWH), or any component of the formulation; active bleeding; history of confirmed or suspected immunologically mediated heparin-induced thrombocytopenia (HIT) or positive *in vitro* platelet-aggregation test in the presence of tinzaparin; acute or subacute endocarditis; generalized hemorrhage tendency and other conditions involving increased risks of hemorrhage (eg, severe hepatic insufficiency, imminent abortion); hemophilia or major blood clotting disorders; acute cerebral insult or hemorrhagic cerebrovascular accidents without systemic emboli; uncontrolled severe hypertension; diabetic or hemorrhagic retinopathy; injury or surgery involving the brain, spinal cord, eyes or ears; spinal/epidural

anesthesia in patients requiring treatment dosages of tinzaparin; use of multidose vials containing benzyl alcohol in children <2 years of age, premature infants, and neonates

Note: Use of tinzaparin in patients with current HIT or HIT with thrombosis is **not** recommended and considered contraindicated due to high cross-reactivity to heparin-platelet factor-4 antibody (Guyatt [ACCP], 2012; Warkentin, 1999).

Warnings/Precautions Spinal or epidural hematomas, including subsequent paralysis, may occur with recent or anticipated neuraxial anesthesia (epidural or spinal) or spinal puncture in patients anticoagulated with low molecular weight heparin (LMWH) or heparinoids. Consider risk versus benefit prior to spinal procedures; risk is increased by the use of concomitant agents which may alter hemostasis, the use of indwelling epidural catheters for analgesia, a history of spinal deformity or spinal surgery, as well as traumatic or repeated epidural or spinal punctures. Avoid invasive spinal procedures for 12 hours following tinzaparin administration and withhold the next tinzaparin dose for at least 2 hours after the spinal procedure. Patient should be observed closely for signs and symptoms of neurological impairment. Not to be used interchangeably (unit for unit) with heparin or any other LMWHs.

Monitor patient closely for signs or symptoms of bleeding. Certain patients are at increased risk of bleeding. Risk factors include bacterial endocarditis; congenital or acquired bleeding disorders; active ulcerative or angiodysplastic GI diseases; severe uncontrolled hypertension; history of hemorrhagic stroke; use shortly after brain, spinal, or ophthalmologic surgery; those concomitantly treated with drugs that increase bleeding risk (eg, antiplatelet agents, anticoagulants); recent GI bleeding; thrombocytopenia or platelet defects; severe liver disease; hypertensive or diabetic retinopathy; or in patients undergoing invasive procedures. Withhold or discontinue for minor bleeding. Protamine infusion may be necessary for serious bleeding. Cases of thrombocytopenia including thrombocytopenia with thrombosis have occurred. Use with caution in patients with history of thrombocytopenia (drug-induced or congenital) or platelet defects; monitor platelet count closely. Use is contraindicated in patients with history of confirmed or suspected heparin-induced thrombocytopenia (HIT) or positive *in vitro* test for antiplatelet antibodies in the presence of tinzaparin. Discontinue therapy and consider alternative treatment if platelets are <100,000/mm^3 and/or thrombosis develops. Asymptomatic thrombocytosis has been observed with use, particularly in patients undergoing orthopedic surgery or with concurrent inflammatory process; discontinue use with increased platelet counts and evaluate the risks/necessity of further therapy. Prosthetic valve thrombosis has ▶

been reported in patients receiving thromboprophylaxis therapy with LMWHs. Pregnant women may be at increased risk.

Use with caution in hepatic impairment; associated with transient, dose-dependent increases in AST/ALT which typically resolve within 2-4 weeks of therapy discontinuation. Use with caution in patients with renal insufficiency. Reduced tinzaparin clearance has been observed in patients with moderate-to-severe renal impairment; Consider dosage reduction in patients with CrCl <30 mL/minute. Use with caution in the elderly (delayed elimination may occur). Use is not recommended in patients >70 years of age with renal impairment. An increase in all-cause mortality has been observed in patients ≥70 years (mean age: >82 years) with CrCl ≤60 mL/minute treated with tinzaparin compared to unfractionated heparin for acute DVT (Leizorovicz, 2011).

Heparin can cause hyperkalemia by suppressing aldosterone production; similar reactions could occur with LMWHs. Monitor for hyperkalemia which most commonly occurs in patients with risk factors for the development of hyperkalemia (eg, renal dysfunction, concomitant use of potassium-sparing diuretics or potassium supplements, hematoma in body tissues). For subcutaneous use only; do not administer intramuscularly or intravenously. Use with caution in patients <45 kg or >120 kg; limited experience in these patients. Individualized clinical and laboratory monitoring are recommended. Derived from porcine intestinal mucosa. Some dosage forms may contain benzyl alcohol or sodium metabisulfite.

Drug Interactions

Avoid Concomitant Use

Avoid concomitant use of Tinzaparin with any of the following: Apixaban; Dabigatran Etexilate; Omacetaxine; Rivaroxaban; Urokinase

Decreased Effect

The levels/effects of Tinzaparin may be decreased by: Estrogen Derivatives; Progestins

Increased Effect/Toxicity

Tinzaparin may increase the levels/effects of: ACE Inhibitors; Aliskiren; Angiotensin II Receptor Blockers; Anticoagulants; Canagliflozin; Collagenase (Systemic); Deferasirox; Eplerenone; Ibritumomab; Omacetaxine; Palifermin; Potassium Salts; Potassium-Sparing Diuretics; Rivaroxaban; Tositumomab and Iodine I 131 Tositumomab

The levels/effects of Tinzaparin may be increased by: 5-ASA Derivatives; Agents with Antiplatelet Properties; Apixaban; Dabigatran Etexilate; Dasatinib; Herbs (Anticoagulant/Antiplatelet Properties); Ibrutinib; Nonsteroidal Anti-Inflammatory Agents; Omega-3 Fatty Acids; Pentosan Polysulfate Sodium; Pentoxifylline; Prostacyclin Analogues; Salicylates; Sugammadex; Thrombolytic

Agents; Tibolone; Tipranavir; Urokinase; Vitamin E

Adverse Reactions
As with all anticoagulants, bleeding is the major adverse effect of tinzaparin. Hemorrhage may occur at virtually any site. Risk is dependent on multiple variables. **Note:** Incidence not always reported.

>10%:
Hepatic: ALT increased (≤13%)
Local: Injection site hematoma
1% to 10%:
Cardiovascular: Chest pain (2%), angina pectoris (≥1%), arrhythmia (≥1%), coronary thrombosis/MI (≥1%), dependent edema (≥1%), thromboembolism (≥1%)
Central nervous system: Fever (2%), headache (2%), pain (2%)
Dermatologic: Bullous eruption (≥1%), erythematous rash (≥1%), maculopapular rash (≥1%), skin necrosis (≥1%)
Gastrointestinal: Nausea (2%), abdominal pain (1%), constipation (1%), diarrhea (1%), vomiting (1%)
Genitourinary: Urinary tract infection (4%)
Hematologic: Bleeding events (major events including intracranial, retroperitoneal, or bleeding into a major prosthetic joint: ≤3%; hemorrhage site not specified (2%); other bleeding events reported at an incidence of ≥1% include anorectal bleeding, GI hemorrhage, hemarthrosis, hematemesis, hematuria, hemopericardium, injection site bleeding, melena, purpura, intra-abdominal bleeding, vaginal bleeding, wound hemorrhage), granulocytopenia (≥1%), thrombocytopenia (≥1%)
Hepatic: AST increased (9%)
Local: Injection site cellulitis (≥1%)
Neuromuscular & skeletal: Back pain (2%)
Respiratory: Epistaxis (2%), dyspnea (1%)
Miscellaneous: Allergic reaction (≥1%), neoplasm (≥1%)

Pharmacodynamics/Kinetics

Onset of Action 2-3 hours

Duration of Action Detectable anti-Xa activity persists for 24 hours

General Dosage Range Dosage adjustment recommended in renal impairment and extended (>4 hours) hemodialysis sessions.

I.V. or added to hemodialysis circuit: *Adults:* 2250-4500 anti-Xa units

SubQ: *Adults:* 50 anti-Xa units/kg or 3500 anti-Xa units/kg preoperatively; 75-3500 anti-Xa units/kg once daily (maximum: 18,000 anti-Xa units daily)

Administration

Other Patient should be lying down or sitting. Administer by deep SubQ injection into the lower abdomen, outer thigh, lower back, or upper arm. Injection site should be varied daily. To minimize bruising, do not rub the injection site. In hemodialysis patients, may be administered I.V. (patients with high or low hemorrhage risk) or added to the dialyzer circuit (patients with low hemorrhage risk).

Storage/Stability Store at 15°C to 25°C (59°F to 77°F).

Nursing Actions

Physical Assessment Monitor for bleeding, rash, and confusion on a regular basis throughout therapy. Observe and teach bleeding precautions. If self-administered, teach patient appropriate injection technique and syringe/needle disposal.

Patient Education
• Discuss specific use of drug and side effects with patient as it relates to treatment. (HCAHPS: During this hospital stay, were you given any medicine that you had not taken before? Before giving you any new medicine, how often did hospital staff tell you what the medicine was for? How often did hospital staff describe possible side effects in a way you could understand?)
• Patient may experience bleeding problems. Have patient report immediately to prescriber severe dizziness, edema, illogical thinking, significant headache, asthenia, paresthesia, ecchymosis, bleeding, or rash (HCAHPS).
• Educate patient about signs of a significant reaction (eg, wheezing; chest tightness; fever; itching; bad cough; blue skin color; seizures; or swelling of face, lips, tongue, or throat). **Note:** This is not a comprehensive list of all side effects. Patient should consult prescriber for additional questions.

Intended Use and Disclaimer: Should not be printed and given to patients. This information is intended to serve as a concise initial reference for healthcare professionals to use when discussing medications with a patient. You must ultimately rely on your own discretion, experience and judgment in diagnosing, treating and advising patients.

Tioconazole (tye oh KONE a zole)

Brand Names: U.S. Vagistat-1 [OTC]
Pharmacologic Category Antifungal Agent, Vaginal
Medication Safety Issues
Sound-alike/look-alike issues:
Tioconazole may be confused with terconazole
Use Local treatment of vulvovaginal candidiasis
Available Dosage Forms
Ointment, Vaginal:
Vagistat-1 [OTC]: 6.5% (4.6 g)
General Dosage Range Intravaginal: *Adults:* Insert 1 applicatorful prior to bedtime, as a single dose
Nursing Actions
Patient Education
• Discuss specific use of drug and side effects with patient as it relates to treatment. (HCAHPS: During this hospital stay, were you given any

medicine that you had not taken before? Before giving you any new medicine, how often did hospital staff tell you what the medicine was for? How often did hospital staff describe possible side effects in a way you could understand?)
• Patient may experience dyspepsia. Have patient report immediately to prescriber reoccurring yeast infection or rash (HCAHPS).
• Educate patient about signs of a significant reaction (eg, wheezing; chest tightness; fever; itching; bad cough; blue skin color; seizures; or swelling of face, lips, tongue, or throat). **Note:** This is not a comprehensive list of all side effects. Patient should consult prescriber for additional questions.

Intended Use and Disclaimer: Should not be printed and given to patients. This information is intended to serve as a concise initial reference for healthcare professionals to use when discussing medications with a patient. You must ultimately rely on your own discretion, experience and judgment in diagnosing, treating and advising patients.

Tiotropium (ty oh TRO pee um)

Brand Names: U.S. Spiriva HandiHaler
Index Terms Tiotropium Bromide Monohydrate
Pharmacologic Category Anticholinergic Agent; Anticholinergic Agent, Long-Acting
Medication Safety Issues
Sound-alike/look-alike issues:
Spiriva® may be confused with Inspra™, Serevent®
Tiotropium may be confused with ipratropium
Administration issues:
Spiriva® capsules for inhalation are for administration via HandiHaler® device and are **not** for oral use
Pregnancy Risk Factor C
Lactation Excretion in breast milk unknown/use caution
Breast-Feeding Considerations It is not known if tiotropium is excreted in breast milk. The manufacturer recommends that caution be exercised when administering tiotropium to nursing women.
Use Maintenance treatment of bronchospasm associated with COPD (including bronchitis and emphysema); reduction of COPD exacerbations
Mechanism of Action/Effect Blocks the action of acetylcholine at parasympathetic sites in bronchial smooth muscle causing bronchodilation
Contraindications Hypersensitivity to tiotropium or ipratropium, or any component of the formulation (contains lactose)
Warnings/Precautions Rarely, paradoxical bronchospasm may occur with use of inhaled bronchodilating agents; discontinue use and consider other therapy if bronchospasm occurs.

Not indicated for the initial (rescue) treatment of acute episodes of bronchospasm. Use with caution in patients with myasthenia gravis, narrow-angle glaucoma, prostatic hyperplasia, moderate-severe renal impairment (CrCl ≤50 mL/minute), or bladder neck obstruction; avoid inadvertent instillation of powder into the eyes. Immediate hypersensitivity reactions may occur; discontinue immediately if signs/symptoms occur. Use with caution in patients with a history of hypersensitivity to atropine.

The contents of Spiriva® capsules are for inhalation only via the HandiHaler® device. There have been reports of incorrect administration (swallowing of the capsules). Capsule for oral inhalation contains lactose; use with caution in patients with severe milk protein allergy.

Drug Interactions

Avoid Concomitant Use
Avoid concomitant use of Tiotropium with any of the following: Aclidinium; Anticholinergics; Ipratropium (Oral Inhalation); Potassium Chloride; Umeclidinium

Decreased Effect
Tiotropium may decrease the levels/effects of: Acetylcholinesterase Inhibitors (Central); Secretin

The levels/effects of Tiotropium may be decreased by: Acetylcholinesterase Inhibitors (Central); Peginterferon Alfa-2b

Increased Effect/Toxicity
Tiotropium may increase the levels/effects of: AbobotulinumtoxinA; Analgesics (Opioid); Anticholinergics; Cannabinoids; Mirabegron; OnabotulinumtoxinA; Potassium Chloride; RimabotulinumtoxinB; Thiazide Diuretics; Topiramate

The levels/effects of Tiotropium may be increased by: Aclidinium; Anticholinergics; Ipratropium (Oral Inhalation); Pramlintide; Umeclidinium

Adverse Reactions
>10%:
Gastrointestinal: Xerostomia (5% to 16%)
Respiratory: Upper respiratory tract infection (41%), pharyngitis (9% to 13%), sinusitis (7% to 11%)
1% to 10%:
Cardiovascular: Chest pain (1% to 7%), edema (dependent, 5%)
Central nervous system: Headache (6%), insomnia (4%), depression (1% to 4%), dysphonia (1% to 3%)
Dermatologic: Rash (4%)
Endocrine & metabolic: Hypercholesterolemia (1% to 3%), hyperglycemia (1% to 3%)
Gastrointestinal: Dyspepsia (6%), abdominal pain (5%), constipation (4% to 5%), vomiting (4%), gastroesophageal reflux (1% to 3%), stomatitis (including ulcerative; 1% to 3%)
Genitourinary: Urinary tract infection (7%)

Neuromuscular & skeletal: Arthralgia (4%), myalgia (4%), arthritis (≥3%), leg pain (1% to 3%), paresthesia (1% to 3%), skeletal pain (1% to 3%)
Ocular: Cataract (1% to 3%)
Respiratory: Rhinitis (6%), epistaxis (4%), cough (≥3%), laryngitis (1% to 3%)
Miscellaneous: Infection (4%), moniliasis (4%), flu-like syndrome (≥3%), allergic reaction (1% to 3%), herpes zoster (1% to 3%)

Available Dosage Forms
Capsule, Inhalation:
Spiriva HandiHaler: 18 mcg
General Dosage Range Inhalation: *Adults:* Contents of 1 capsule (18 mcg) once daily

Administration
Oral For oral inhalation only. Capsule should not be swallowed.

Inhalation Administer once daily at the same time each day. Remove capsule from foil blister immediately before use. Capsule should not be swallowed. Place capsule in the capsule-chamber in the base of the HandiHaler® Inhaler. Must only use the HandiHaler® Inhaler. Close mouthpiece until a click is heard, leaving dustcap open. Exhale fully. Do not exhale into inhaler. Tilt head slightly back and inhale (rapidly, steadily and deeply); the capsule vibration may be heard within the device. Hold breath as long as possible. If any powder remains in capsule, exhale and inhale again. Repeat until capsule is empty. Throw away empty capsule; do not leave in inhaler. Do not use a spacer with the HandiHaler® Inhaler. Do not use HandiHaler® device for other medications. Always keep capsules and inhaler dry.

Delivery of dose: Instruct patient to place mouthpiece gently between teeth, closing lips around inhaler. Instruct patient to inhale deeply and hold breath for 5-10 seconds. The amount of drug delivered is small, and the individual will not sense the medication as it is inhaled. Remove mouthpiece prior to exhalation. Patient should not breathe out through the mouthpiece.

Storage/Stability Store at 25°C (77°F); excursions permitted to 15°C to 30°C (59°F to 86°F). Avoid excessive temperatures and moisture. Do not store capsules in HandiHaler® device. Capsules should be stored in the blister pack and only removed immediately before use. Once protective foil is peeled back and/or removed the capsule should be used immediately; if capsule is not used immediately it should be discarded.

Nursing Actions
Physical Assessment Monitor pulmonary tests prior to and periodically during therapy.

Patient Education
• Discuss specific use of drug and side effects with patient as it relates to treatment. (HCAHPS: During this hospital stay, were you given any

medicine that you had not taken before? Before giving you any new medicine, how often did hospital staff tell you what the medicine was for? How often did hospital staff describe possible side effects in a way you could understand?)
- Patient may experience constipation, xerostomia, or pharyngitis. Have patient report immediately to prescriber dyspnea, rhinitis, sudden vision changes, decreased peak flow rate, increased inhaler use, or rash (HCAHPS).
- Educate patient about signs of a significant reaction (eg, wheezing; chest tightness; fever; itching; bad cough; blue skin color; seizures; or swelling of face, lips, tongue, or throat). **Note:** This is not a comprehensive list of all side effects. Patient should consult prescriber for additional questions.

Intended Use and Disclaimer: Should not be printed and given to patients. This information is intended to serve as a concise initial reference for healthcare professionals to use when discussing medications with a patient. You must ultimately rely on your own discretion, experience and judgment in diagnosing, treating and advising patients.

Tipranavir (tip RA na veer)

Brand Names: U.S. Aptivus
Index Terms PNU-140690E; TPV
Pharmacologic Category Antiretroviral, Protease Inhibitor (Anti-HIV)
Pregnancy Risk Factor C
Lactation Excretion in breast milk unknown/contraindicated
Breast-Feeding Considerations Maternal or infant antiretroviral therapy does not completely eliminate the risk of postnatal HIV transmission. In addition, multiclass-resistant virus has been detected in breast-feeding infants despite maternal therapy. Therefore, in the United States, where formula is accessible, affordable, safe, and sustainable, and the risk of infant mortality due to diarrhea and respiratory infections is low, complete avoidance of breast-feeding by HIV-infected women is recommended to decrease potential transmission of HIV (DHHS [perinatal], 2012).
Use Treatment of HIV-1 infections in combination with ritonavir and other antiretroviral agents; limited to highly treatment-experienced or multiprotease inhibitor-resistant patients.
Mechanism of Action/Effect Blocks the site of HIV-1 protease activity, resulting in the formation of immature, noninfectious viral particles.
Contraindications Concurrent therapy of tipranavir/ritonavir with alfuzosin, amiodarone, bepridil, cisapride, ergot derivatives (eg, dihydroergotamine, ergonovine, ergotamine, methylergonovine), flecainide, lovastatin, midazolam (oral), pimozide, propafenone, quinidine, rifampin, sildenafil (for pulmonary arterial hypertension [eg, Revatio®]), simvastatin, St John's wort, and triazolam; moderate-to-severe hepatic impairment (Child-Pugh class B or C)

Warnings/Precautions [U.S. Boxed Warning]: In combination with ritonavir, may cause hepatitis (including fatalities) and/or exacerbate preexisting hepatic dysfunction (causal relationship not established); patients with chronic hepatitis B or C are at increased risk. Monitor patients closely; discontinue use if signs or symptoms of toxicity occur or if asymptomatic AST/ALT elevations >10 times upper limit of normal or AST/ALT elevations >5-10 times upper limit of normal concurrently with total bilirubin >2.5 times the upper limit of normal occur. Use with caution in patients with mild hepatic impairment; contraindicated in moderate-to-severe impairment. May be associated with fat redistribution (buffalo hump, increased abdominal girth, breast engorgement, facial atrophy). Use caution in hemophilia. May increase cholesterol and/or triglycerides; hypertriglyceridemia may increase risk of pancreatitis. May cause hyperglycemia. Use with caution in patients with sulfonamide allergy. Protease inhibitors have been associated with a variety of hypersensitivity events (some severe), including rash, anaphylaxis (rare), angioedema, bronchospasm, erythema multiforme, and/or Stevens-Johnson syndrome (rare). It is generally recommended to discontinue treatment if severe rash or moderate symptoms accompanied by other systemic symptoms occur. Patients may develop immune reconstitution syndrome resulting in the occurrence of an inflammatory response to an indolent or residual opportunistic infection during initial HIV treatment or activation of autoimmune disorders (eg, Graves' disease, polymyositis, Guillain-Barré syndrome) later in therapy; further evaluation and treatment may be required.

[U.S. Boxed Warning]: Tipranavir in combination with ritonavir has been associated with rare reports of fatal and nonfatal intracranial hemorrhage; causal relationship not established. Events often occurred in patients with medical conditions (eg, CNS lesions, head trauma, recent neurosurgery, coagulopathy, alcohol abuse) or concurrent therapy which may have influenced these events. Tipranavir may inhibit platelet aggregation. Use with caution in patients who may be at risk for increased bleeding (trauma, surgery or other medical conditions) or in patients receiving concurrent medications which may increase the risk of bleeding, including antiplatelet agents and anticoagulants.

High potential for drug interactions; concomitant use of tipranavir with some drugs may require cautious use, may not be recommended, may require dosage adjustments, or may be contraindicated.

◄ **Drug Interactions**

Avoid Concomitant Use

Avoid concomitant use of Tipranavir with any of the following: Alfuzosin; Amiodarone; AtorvaSTA-Tin; Bepridil [Off Market]; Cisapride; Dabigatran Etexilate; Ergot Derivatives; Etravirine; Flecainide; Ketoconazole (Systemic); Lovastatin; Midazolam; Pimozide; Pomalidomide; Propafenone; QuiNIDine; Rifampin; Simeprevir; Simvastatin; Sofosbuvir; St Johns Wort; Tamoxifen; Thioridazine; Triazolam; VinCRIStine (Liposomal)

Decreased Effect

Tipranavir may decrease the levels/effects of: Abacavir; Afatinib; Boceprevir; Clarithromycin; Codeine; Contraceptives (Estrogens); Dabigatran Etexilate; Delavirdine; Didanosine; Dolutegravir; Estrogen Derivatives; Etravirine; Fosphenytoin; Iloperidone; Linagliptin; Meperidine; Methadone; P-glycoprotein/ABCB1 Substrates; PHENobarbital; Phenytoin; Pomalidomide; Proton Pump Inhibitors; Raltegravir; Sofosbuvir; Tamoxifen; Tenofovir; Theophylline Derivatives; TraMADol; Valproic Acid and Derivatives; VinCRIStine (Liposomal); Zidovudine

The levels/effects of Tipranavir may be decreased by: Antacids; Boceprevir; Bosentan; CarBAMazepine; CYP3A4 Inducers (Strong); Dabrafenib; Deferasirox; Fosphenytoin; Garlic; Mitotane; PHENobarbital; Phenytoin; Rifampin; St Johns Wort; Tenofovir; Tocilizumab

Increased Effect/Toxicity

Tipranavir may increase the levels/effects of: Agents with Antiplatelet Properties; Alfuzosin; ALPRAZolam; Amiodarone; Anticoagulants; ARIPiprazole; AtoMOXetine; AtorvaSTATin; Bepridil [Off Market]; Bosentan; Calcium Channel Blockers (Dihydropyridine); Calcium Channel Blockers (Nondihydropyridine); CarBAMazepine; Cisapride; Clarithromycin; CycloSPORINE (Systemic); CYP2D6 Substrates; Digoxin; DOXOrubicin (Conventional); Enfuvirtide; Ergot Derivatives; Fesoterodine; Flecainide; Iloperidone; Itraconazole; Ketoconazole (Systemic); Lovastatin; Meperidine; Metoprolol; Midazolam; Nebivolol; Nefazodone; Pimozide; Propafenone; Protease Inhibitors; QuiNIDine; Rifabutin; Riociguat; Rosuvastatin; Sildenafil; Simeprevir; Simvastatin; Tacrolimus (Systemic); Tacrolimus (Topical); Temsirolimus; Tetrabenazine; Thioridazine; TraZODone; Triazolam; Tricyclic Antidepressants; Vardenafil; Vitamin E; Vortioxetine

The levels/effects of Tipranavir may be increased by: Clarithromycin; CycloSPORINE (Systemic); Delavirdine; Disulfiram; Enfuvirtide; Estrogen Derivatives; Fluconazole; MetroNIDAZOLE (Systemic); MetroNIDAZOLE (Topical); Simeprevir

Nutritional/Ethanol Interactions

Ethanol: Capsules contain dehydrated alcohol 7% w/w (0.1 g per capsule)

Herb/Nutraceutical: St John's wort may decrease the levels/effects of tipranavir/ritonavir. Vitamin E (high dose) may increase the risk of bleeding. Garlic may decrease the serum concentration of tipranavir. Management: Avoid St John's wort; concurrent use is contraindicated. Avoid vitamin E supplementation. Garlic supplementation is not recommended.

Adverse Reactions

>10%:

Dermatologic: Rash (children 21%; adults 3% to 10%)

Endocrine & metabolic: Hypertriglyceridemia (>400 mg/dL: 61%), hypercholesterolemia (>300 mg/dL: 22%)

Gastrointestinal: Diarrhea (15%)

Hepatic: Transaminases increased (>2.5 x ULN: 26% to 32%; grade 3/4: 10% to 20%)

Neuromuscular & skeletal: CPK increased (grade 3/4: children 11%)

2% to 10%:

Central nervous system: Fever (6% to 8%), fatigue (6%), headache (5%)

Endocrine & metabolic: Dehydration (2%)

Gastrointestinal: Nausea (5% to 9%), amylase increased (grade 3: 6% to 8%), vomiting (6%), abdominal pain (4%), diarrhea (children 4%), weight loss (3%)

Hematologic: Bleeding (children 8%), WBC decreased (grades 3: 5%), anemia (3%), neutropenia (2%)

Hepatic: ALT increased (2%, grades 3/4: 10%), AST increased (grades 3/4: 6%), GGT increased (2%)

Neuromuscular & skeletal: Myalgia (2%)

Respiratory: Cough (children 6%), dyspnea (2%), epistaxis (children 4%)

Available Dosage Forms

Capsule, Oral:

Aptivus: 250 mg

Solution, Oral:

Aptivus: 100 mg/mL (95 mL)

General Dosage Range Dosage adjustment recommended in patients on concomitant therapy

Oral:

Children ≥2 years: 12-14 mg/kg or 290-375 mg/m² (maximum: 500 mg/dose) twice daily

Adults: 500 mg twice daily

Administration

Oral Coadministration with ritonavir is required. Administer with ritonavir capsules or solution without regard to meals; administer with ritonavir tablets with meals.

Storage/Stability

Capsule: Prior to opening bottle, store under refrigeration at 2°C to 8°C (36°F to 46°F). After bottle is opened, may be stored at controlled room temperature of 25°C (77°F) for up to 60 days.

Oral solution: Store at 15°C to 30°C (59°F to 86°F). After bottle is open, use within 60 days. Do not refrigerate or freeze oral solution.

Nursing Actions

Physical Assessment Monitor for adherence to regimen. Monitor for gastrointestinal disturbance (nausea, vomiting, diarrhea) that can lead to dehydration and weight loss, hyperlipidemia, redistribution of body fat, and rash. Caution patients to monitor glucose levels closely; may alter effects of hypoglycemic agents or cause hyperglycemia. Teach patient proper timing of multiple medications. Instruct patient on glucose testing.

Patient Education

• Discuss specific use of drug and side effects with patient as it relates to treatment. (HCAHPS: During this hospital stay, were you given any medicine that you had not taken before? Before giving you any new medicine, how often did hospital staff tell you what the medicine was for? How often did hospital staff describe possible side effects in a way you could understand?)

• Patient may experience hyperlipidemia, hypertriglyceridemia, headache, nausea, diarrhea, lipodystrophy, or asthenia. Have patient report immediately to prescriber severe dyspepsia, ecchymosis, illogical thinking, discolored urine, jaundice, inability to eat, or rash (HCAHPS).

• Educate patient about signs of a significant reaction (eg, wheezing; chest tightness; fever; itching; bad cough; blue skin color; seizures; or swelling of face, lips, tongue, or throat). **Note:** This is not a comprehensive list of all side effects. Patient should consult prescriber for additional questions.

Intended Use and Disclaimer: Should not be printed and given to patients. This information is intended to serve as a concise initial reference for healthcare professionals to use when discussing medications with a patient. You must ultimately rely on your own discretion, experience and judgment in diagnosing, treating and advising patients.

Dietary Considerations Capsule contains dehydrated ethanol. Oral solution formulation contains vitamin E; additional vitamin E supplements should be avoided.

Related Information
Oral Medications That Should Not Be Crushed or Altered *on page 1712*

Tirofiban (tye roe FYE ban)

Brand Names: U.S. Aggrastat
Index Terms MK383; Tirofiban Hydrochloride
Pharmacologic Category Antiplatelet Agent, Glycoprotein IIb/IIIa Inhibitor

Medication Safety Issues
Sound-alike/look-alike issues:
Aggrastat may be confused with Aggrenox, argatroban

High alert medication:
The Institute for Safe Medication Practices (ISMP) includes this medication among its list of drugs which have a heightened risk of causing significant patient harm when used in error.

Pregnancy Risk Factor B

Lactation Excretion in breast milk unknown/not recommended

Breast-Feeding Considerations It is not known if tirofiban is excreted in breast milk. Due to the potential for serious adverse reactions in the nursing infant, a decision should be made whether to discontinue nursing or to discontinue the drug, taking into account the importance of treatment to the mother.

Use Unstable angina/non-ST-elevation myocardial infarction: To decrease the rate of thrombotic cardiovascular events (combined end point of death, MI, or refractory ischemia/repeat cardiac procedure) in patients with non-ST-elevation acute coronary syndrome (unstable angina/non-ST-elevation myocardial infarction [UA/NSTEMI]).

Unlabeled Use To support PCI (administered at the time of PCI) for ST-elevation myocardial infarction (STEMI), UA/NSTEMI, and stable ischemic heart disease (ie, elective PCI)

Mechanism of Action/Effect A reversible antagonist of fibrinogen binding to the glycoprotein (GP) IIb/IIIa receptor, the major platelet surface receptor involved in platelet aggregation. Platelet aggregation inhibition is reversible following cessation of the infusion.

Contraindications Severe hypersensitivity reaction (ie, anaphylactic reaction) to tirofiban or any component of the formulation; history of thrombocytopenia following prior exposure to tirofiban; active internal bleeding or a history of bleeding diathesis, major surgical procedure, or severe physical trauma within the previous month

Warnings/Precautions Bleeding is the most common complication encountered during this therapy; most major bleeding occurs at the arterial access site for cardiac catheterization. Caution in patients with platelets <150,000/mm^3; patients with hemorrhagic retinopathy; chronic dialysis patients; when used in combination with other drugs impacting on coagulation. Percutaneous coronary intervention (unlabeled use): Prior to pulling the sheath, ACT should be <180 seconds or aPTT <50 seconds (Levine, 2011). Use standard compression techniques after sheath removal. Watch the site closely afterwards for further bleeding. Sheath hemostasis should be achieved at least 4 hours before hospital discharge. Other trauma and vascular punctures should be minimized. Avoid obtaining vascular access through a noncompressible site (eg, subclavian or jugular vein).

Profound thrombocytopenia has been reported with use of tirofiban. If during therapy platelet count decreases to <90,000/mm^3, monitor platelet counts to exclude pseudothrombocytopenia. If thrombocytopenia is confirmed, discontinue tirofiban and heparin if administered concurrently. Previous exposure to a glycoprotein IIb/IIIa inhibitor may increase the risk of thrombocytopenia. Use is contraindicated in patients with a history of thrombocytopenia following exposure to tirofiban.

Discontinue at least 2-4 hours prior to coronary artery bypass graft surgery (Anderson, 2013; Hillis, 2011). Dosage reduction of the maintenance infusion rate is necessary in patients with CrCl ≤60 mL/minute.

Drug Interactions

Avoid Concomitant Use
Avoid concomitant use of Tirofiban with any of the following: Urokinase

Decreased Effect
The levels/effects of Tirofiban may be decreased by: Nonsteroidal Anti-Inflammatory Agents

Increased Effect/Toxicity
Tirofiban may increase the levels/effects of: Agents with Antiplatelet Properties; Anticoagulants; Collagenase (Systemic); Dabigatran Etexilate; Ibritumomab; Rivaroxaban; Salicylates; Thrombolytic Agents; Tositumomab and Iodine I 131 Tositumomab; Urokinase

The levels/effects of Tirofiban may be increased by: Dasatinib; Glucosamine; Herbs (Anticoagulant/Antiplatelet Properties); Ibrutinib; Multivitamins/Fluoride (with ADE); Multivitamins/Minerals (with ADEK, Folate, Iron); Multivitamins/Minerals (with AE, No Iron); Nonsteroidal Anti-Inflammatory Agents; Omega-3 Fatty Acids; Pentosan Polysulfate Sodium; Pentoxifylline; Prostacyclin Analogues; Tipranavir; Vitamin E

Adverse Reactions
Bleeding is the major drug-related adverse effect. Patients received background treatment with aspirin and heparin. Adverse reactions reported are derived from both the high-dose bolus regimen **and** the dosing regimen used in studies that established the effectiveness of tirofiban.

>10%: Hematologic & oncologic: Minor hemorrhage (TIMI criteria minor bleeding; 10.5% to 12%; transfusion required: 4% to 4.3%)

1% to 10%:
Cardiovascular: Coronary artery dissection (5%), bradycardia (4%), edema (2%)
Central nervous system: Dizziness (3%), vasovagal reaction (2%), fever (>1%), headache (>1%)
Gastrointestinal: Nausea (>1%)
Genitourinary: Pelvic pain (6%)
Hematologic & oncologic: Major hemorrhage (TIMI criteria major bleeding; 1.4% to 2.2%; including hematoma [femoral]: 2%; [Valgimigli,

2005], intracranial bleeding, GI bleeding, retroperitoneal bleeding [Aydin, 2003], GU bleeding, myocardial rupture [left ventricular free wall; Valgimigli, 2005], pulmonary alveolar hemorrhage [Guo, 2012], spinal-epidural hematoma), thrombocytopenia: <90,000/mm^3 (1.5% to 1.9%), <50,000/mm^3 (0.3% to 0.5%)
Neuromuscular & skeletal: Leg pain (3%)
Miscellaneous: Diaphoresis (2%)

Pharmacodynamics/Kinetics
Onset of Action >90% inhibition of platelet aggregation (reversible after discontinuation) seen within 10 minutes

Available Dosage Forms
Solution, Intravenous:
Aggrastat: 50 mcg/mL (100 mL, 250 mL)

General Dosage Range Dosage adjustment recommended in patients with renal impairment
I.V.: *Adults:* Loading dose: 25 mcg/kg over 3 minutes; Maintenance infusion: 0.15 mcg/kg/minute continued for up to 18 hours

Administration
I.V. Infuse loading dose over 3 minutes, followed by continuous infusion. May be administered through the same catheter as heparin.

Storage/Stability Store at 25°C (77°F); excursions are permitted between 15°C and 30°C (59°F and 86°F); do not freeze. Protect from light during storage.

Nursing Actions
Physical Assessment Monitor vital signs prior to, during, and after therapy. Assess infusion insertion site during and after therapy (every 15 minutes or as institutional policy). Monitor closely for unusual or excessive bleeding (eg, CNS changes; blood in urine, stool, or vomitus; unusual bruising or bleeding). Monitor platelet counts.

Patient Education
• Discuss specific use of drug and side effects with patient as it relates to treatment. (HCAHPS: During this hospital stay, were you given any medicine that you had not taken before? Before giving you any new medicine, how often did hospital staff tell you what the medicine was for? How often did hospital staff describe possible side effects in a way you could understand?)
• Patient may experience bleeding problems, dizziness, or injection site irritation. Have patient report immediately to prescriber imbalance, illogical thinking, severe headache, ecchymosis, bleeding, or rash (HCAHPS).
• Educate patient about signs of a significant reaction (eg, wheezing; chest tightness; fever; itching; bad cough; blue skin color; seizures; or swelling of face, lips, tongue, or throat). **Note:** This is not a comprehensive list of all side effects. Patient should consult prescriber for additional questions.

TiZANidine (tye ZAN i deen)

Brand Names: U.S. Zanaflex
Index Terms Sirdalud
Pharmacologic Category Alpha$_2$-Adrenergic Agonist
Medication Safety Issues
Sound-alike/look-alike issues:
TiZANidine may be confused with tiaGABine
Zanaflex may be confused with Xiaflex
BEERS Criteria medication:
This drug may be potentially inappropriate for use in geriatric patients (Quality of evidence - varies based on comorbidity; Strength of recommendation - varies based on comorbidity)
Other safety concerns:
Zanaflex capsules and Zanaflex tablets (or generic tizanidine tablets) are not interchangeable in the fed state
Pregnancy Risk Factor C
Lactation Excretion in breast milk unknown
Breast-Feeding Considerations Excretion in breast milk is unknown, but expected due to lipid solubility.
Use Muscle spasticity: Management of spasticity; reserve treatment with tizanidine for daily activities and times when relief of spasticity is most important.
Unlabeled Use Tension headaches, acute low back pain
Mechanism of Action/Effect Acts within CNS at the level of the spinal cord to reduce excitation of motor neurons, resulting in muscle relaxation
Contraindications Concomitant therapy with ciprofloxacin or fluvoxamine (potent CYP1A2 inhibitors)
Warnings/Precautions Significant hypotension, syncope, and sedation may occur; use caution in patients at risk for severe hypotensive effects (eg, patients taking concurrent medications which may predispose to hypotension) or sedative effects (patients must be cautioned about performing tasks which require mental alertness [eg, operating machinery or driving]). Potentially significant drug-drug interactions may exist, requiring dose or frequency adjustment, additional monitoring, and/or selection of alternative therapy. Use caution in any patient with renal impairment. Clearance decreased significantly in patients with severe impairment (CrCl <25 mL/minute); dose reductions recommended. Use not recommended in patients with hepatic impairment; potential for hepatotoxicity likely due to extensive hepatic metabolism. Monitor aminotransferases prior to and during use or if hepatic injury is suspected.

May be inappropriate in older adults depending on comorbidities (eg, dementia, delirium) due to its potent anticholinergic effects (Beers Criteria). Use with caution; clearance decreased fourfold in the elderly; may increase risk of adverse effects and/or duration of effects. Elderly with severe renal impairment (CrCl <25 mL/minute) may have clearance reduced by >50% compared to healthy elderly subjects.

Use has been associated with visual hallucinations or delusions; use caution in patients with psychiatric disorders. Consider discontinuation of therapy if hallucinations occur. Withdrawal resulting in rebound hypertension, tachycardia, and hypertonia may occur upon discontinuation; doses should be decreased slowly, particularly in patients taking concomitant narcotics or receiving high doses (20 to 28 mg daily) for prolonged periods (≥9 weeks). Food alters absorption profile relative to administration under fasting conditions. In addition, bioequivalence between capsules and tablets is altered by food; capsules and tablets are bioequivalent under fasting conditions, but not under nonfasting conditions.

Drug Interactions
Avoid Concomitant Use
Avoid concomitant use of TiZANidine with any of the following: Azelastine (Nasal); Ciprofloxacin (Systemic); FluvoxaMINE; Iobenguane I 123; Paraldehyde; Thalidomide
Decreased Effect
TiZANidine may decrease the levels/effects of: Iobenguane I 123

The levels/effects of TiZANidine may be decreased by: Antidepressants (Alpha2-Antagonist); Serotonin/Norepinephrine Reuptake Inhibitors; Tricyclic Antidepressants
Increased Effect/Toxicity
TiZANidine may increase the levels/effects of: ACE Inhibitors; Alcohol (Ethyl); Azelastine (Nasal); Beta-Blockers; Buprenorphine; CNS Depressants; Highest Risk QTc-Prolonging Agents; Hydrocodone; Hypotensive Agents; Lisinopril; Methotrimeprazine; Metyrosine; Moderate Risk QTc-Prolonging Agents; Paraldehyde; Pramipexole; ROPINIRole; Rotigotine; Selective Serotonin Reuptake Inhibitors; Thalidomide; Zolpidem

The levels/effects of TiZANidine may be increased by: Abiraterone Acetate; Beta-Blockers; Brimonidine (Topical); Ciprofloxacin (Systemic); Contraceptives (Estrogens); CYP1A2 Inhibitors (Moderate); CYP1A2 Inhibitors (Strong); Deferasirox; Doxylamine; Droperidol; FluvoxaMINE; HydrOXYzine; Magnesium Sulfate; MAO Inhibitors; Methotrimeprazine;

◄ Mifepristone; Perampanel; Sodium Oxybate; Tapentadol; Vemurafenib

Nutritional/Ethanol Interactions

Ethanol: May increase CNS depression; monitor for increased effects with coadministration. Caution patients about effects.

Food: The tablet and capsule dosage forms are not bioequivalent when administered with food. Food increases both the time to peak concentration and the extent of absorption for both the tablet and capsule. However, maximal concentrations of tizanidine achieved when administered with food were increased by 30% for the tablet, but decreased by 20% for the capsule. Under fed conditions, the capsule is approximately 80% bioavailable relative to the tablet.

Herb/Nutraceutical: Avoid valerian, St John's wort, kava kava, gotu kola (may increase CNS depression). Avoid black cohosh, California poppy, coleus, golden seal, hawthorn, mistletoe, periwinkle, quinine, shepherd's purse (may increase hypotensive effects).

Adverse Reactions Frequency percentages below reported during multiple-dose studies, unless specified otherwise.

>10%:

Cardiovascular: Hypotension (16% to 33%)

Central nervous system: Somnolence (48%), dizziness (16%)

Gastrointestinal: Xerostomia (49%)

Neuromuscular & skeletal: Weakness (41%)

1% to 10%:

Cardiovascular: Bradycardia (2% to 10%)

Central nervous system: Nervousness (3%), speech disorder (3%), visual hallucinations/delusions (3%), anxiety (1%), depression (1%), fever (1%)

Dermatologic: Rash (1%), skin ulcer (1%)

Gastrointestinal: Constipation (4%), vomiting (3%), abdominal pain (1%), diarrhea (1%), dyspepsia (1%)

Genitourinary: UTI (10%), urinary frequency (3%)

Hepatic: Liver enzymes increased (3% to 5%)

Neuromuscular & skeletal: Dyskinesia (3%), back pain (1%), myasthenia (1%), paresthesia (1%)

Ocular: Blurred vision (3%)

Respiratory: Pharyngitis (3%), rhinitis (3%)

Miscellaneous: Infection (6%), flu-like syndrome (3%), diaphoresis (1%)

Pharmacodynamics/Kinetics

Onset of Action Single dose (8 mg): Peak effect: 1-2 hours

Duration of Action Single dose (8 mg): 3-6 hours

Available Dosage Forms

Capsule, Oral:

Zanaflex: 2 mg, 4 mg, 6 mg

Generic: 2 mg, 4 mg, 6 mg

Tablet, Oral:

Zanaflex: 4 mg

Generic: 2 mg, 4 mg

General Dosage Range Oral: *Adults:* Initial: 2 mg up to 3 times daily (at 6- to 8-hour intervals); maximum: 36 mg daily

Administration

Oral Capsules may be opened and contents sprinkled on food; however, extent of absorption is increased up to 20% relative to administration of the capsule under fasted conditions.

Storage/Stability Store at 25°C (77°F); excursions are permitted between 15°C and 30°C (59°F and 86°F).

Nursing Actions

Physical Assessment May cause hypotension; monitor blood pressure periodically. Do not discontinue medication abruptly; can cause hypertension and tachycardia.

Patient Education

• Discuss specific use of drug and side effects with patient as it relates to treatment. (HCAHPS: During this hospital stay, were you given any medicine that you had not taken before? Before giving you any new medicine, how often did hospital staff tell you what the medicine was for? How often did hospital staff describe possible side effects in a way you could understand?)

• Patient may experience presyncope, fatigue, blurred vision, illogical thinking, dizziness, or xerostomia. Have patient report immediately to prescriber severe dyspepsia, significant nausea, inability to eat, discolored urine, jaundice, considerable asthenia, or rash (HCAHPS).

• Educate patient about signs of a significant reaction (eg, wheezing; chest tightness; fever; itching; bad cough; blue skin color; seizures; or swelling of face, lips, tongue, or throat). **Note:** This is not a comprehensive list of all side effects. Patient should consult prescriber for additional questions.

Intended Use and Disclaimer: Should not be printed and given to patients. This information is intended to serve as a concise initial reference for healthcare professionals to use when discussing medications with a patient. You must ultimately rely on your own discretion, experience and judgment in diagnosing, treating and advising patients.

Dietary Considerations Administration with food compared to administration in the fasting state results in clinically-significant differences in absorption and other pharmacokinetic parameters. Patients should be consistent and should not switch administration of the tablets or the capsules between the fasting and nonfasting state. In addition, switching between the capsules and the tablets in the fed state will also result in significant differences. Opening capsule contents to sprinkle on applesauce compared to swallowing intact capsules whole will also result in significant absorption differences. Patients should be consistent with regards to administration.

Tobramycin (Systemic, Oral Inhalation) (toe bra MYE sin)

Brand Names: U.S. Bethkis; Tobi; Tobi Podhaler
Index Terms Tobramycin Sulfate
Pharmacologic Category Antibiotic, Aminoglycoside
Medication Safety Issues
Sound-alike/look-alike issues:
Tobramycin may be confused with Trobicin, vancomycin
International issues:
Nebcin [Multiple international markets] may be confused with Naprosyn brand name for naproxen [U.S., Canada, and multiple international markets]; Nubain brand name for nalbuphine [Multiple international markets]
High alert medication:
The Institute for Safe Medication Practices (ISMP) includes this medication (intrathecal administration) among its list of drug classes which have a heightened risk of causing significant patient harm when used in error.
Pregnancy Risk Factor D
Lactation Enters breast milk/not recommended
Breast-Feeding Considerations Tobramycin is excreted into breast milk and breast-feeding is not recommended by the manufacturer; however, tobramycin is not well absorbed when taken orally. This limited oral absorption may minimize exposure to the nursing infant. Nondose-related effects could include modification of bowel flora.
Use Treatment of documented or suspected infections caused by susceptible gram-negative bacilli, including *Pseudomonas aeruginosa*. Tobramycin solution for inhalation and powder for inhalation are indicated for the management of cystic fibrosis patients with *Pseudomonas aeruginosa*.
Mechanism of Action/Effect Interferes with bacterial protein synthesis, resulting in a defective bacteriocidal cell membrane
Contraindications Hypersensitivity to tobramycin, other aminoglycosides, or any component of the formulation
Warnings/Precautions [U.S. Boxed Warning]: Aminoglycosides may cause neurotoxicity and/or nephrotoxicity; usual risk factors include pre-existing renal impairment, concomitant neuro-/nephrotoxic medications, advanced age, and dehydration. Ototoxicity may be directly proportional to the amount of drug given and the duration of treatment; tinnitus or vertigo are indications of vestibular injury and impending hearing loss; renal damage is usually reversible. Tinnitus and/or hearing loss have also been reported with powder for oral inhalation use. May cause neuromuscular blockade and respiratory paralysis, especially when given soon after anesthesia or muscle relaxants. **[U.S. Boxed Warnings]: Aminoglycosides** may cause fetal harm if administered to a pregnant woman.

Not intended for long-term therapy due to toxic hazards associated with extended administration; use caution in pre-existing renal insufficiency, vestibular or cochlear impairment, myasthenia gravis, Parkinson's disease, hypocalcemia, and conditions which depress neuromuscular transmission. Dosage modification required in patients with impaired renal function during systemic therapy. Prolonged use may result in fungal or bacterial superinfection, including *C. difficile*-associated diarrhea (CDAD) and pseudomembranous colitis; CDAD has been observed >2 months postantibiotic treatment. Solution may contain sodium metabisulfate; use caution in patients with sulfite allergy. Solution for injection may contain sodium metabisulfate; use caution in patients with sulfite allergy. Bronchospasm may occur with tobramycin solution for inhalation; bronchospasm or wheezing should be treated appropriately if either arise. Safety and efficacy of the solution for inhalation have not been demonstrated in patients with FEV_1 <40% or >80% predicted (Bethkis, TOBI), or FEV_1 <25% or >80% predicted (TOBI Podhaler), in patients colonized with *Burkholderia cepacia*, or in patients ≤6 years of age. With powder for inhalation, consider baseline audiogram in patients at increased risk of auditory dysfunction. If any patient experiences tinnitus or hearing loss during treatment, audiological assessment should be performed. Serum tobramycin concentrations do not need to be monitored; one hour after powder inhalation, serum concentrations of 1-2 mcg/mL have been observed. If ototoxicity or nephrotoxicity occur, discontinue therapy until serum concentrations fall below 2 mcg/mL.

Potentially significant drug-drug interactions may exist, requiring dose or frequency adjustment, additional monitoring, and/or selection of alternative therapy.
Drug Interactions
Avoid Concomitant Use
Avoid concomitant use of Tobramycin (Systemic, Oral Inhalation) with any of the following: BCG; Gallium Nitrate
Decreased Effect
Tobramycin (Systemic, Oral Inhalation) may decrease the levels/effects of: BCG; Sodium Picosulfate; Typhoid Vaccine

The levels/effects of Tobramycin (Systemic, Oral Inhalation) may be decreased by: Penicillins
Increased Effect/Toxicity
Tobramycin (Systemic, Oral Inhalation) may increase the levels/effects of: AbobotulinumtoxinA; Bisphosphonate Derivatives; CARBOplatin; Colistimethate; CycloSPORINE (Systemic); Gallium Nitrate; Neuromuscular-Blocking Agents;

OnabotulinumtoxinA; RimabotulinumtoxinB; Tenofovir

The levels/effects of Tobramycin (Systemic, Oral Inhalation) may be increased by: Amphotericin B; Capreomycin; Cephalosporins (2nd Generation); Cephalosporins (3rd Generation); Cephalosporins (4th Generation); CISplatin; Loop Diuretics; Nonsteroidal Anti-Inflammatory Agents; Tenofovir; Vancomycin

Adverse Reactions

Injection: Frequency not defined:

Central nervous system: Confusion, disorientation, dizziness, headache, lethargy, vertigo

Dermatologic: Exfoliative dermatitis, pruritus, skin rash, urticaria

Endocrine & metabolic: Decreased serum calcium, decreased serum magnesium, decreased serum potassium and/or decreased serum sodium, increased lactate dehydrogenase

Gastrointestinal: Diarrhea, nausea, vomiting

Genitourinary: Casts in urine, oliguria, proteinuria

Hematologic & oncologic: Anemia, eosinophilia, granulocytopenia, leukocytosis, leukopenia, thrombocytopenia

Hepatic: Increased serum ALT, increased serum AST, increased serum bilirubin

Local: Pain at injection site

Miscellaneous: Fever

Otic: Auditory ototoxicity, hearing loss, tinnitus, vestibular ototoxicity

Renal: Increased blood urea nitrogen, increased serum creatinine

Inhalation

>10%:

Central nervous system: Voice disorder (powder 14%, solution 4%), headache (11% to 12%)

Miscellaneous: Fever (12% to 16%)

Respiratory: Cough (powder 10% to 48%, solution 31%), pulmonary disease (30% to 34%), reduced forced expiratory volume (solution 1% to 31%, powder 4%), discoloration of sputum (solution 21%), productive cough (18% to 20%), rales (solution 6% to 19%, powder 7%), dyspnea (12% to 16%), respiratory depression (2% to 16%), oropharyngeal pain (11% to 14%), hemoptysis (12% to 13%), pharyngolaryngeal pain (powder 11%, solution 3%)

1% to 10%:

Cardiovascular: Chest discomfort (3% to 7%)

Central nervous system: Malaise (6%)

Dermatologic: Skin rash (2%)

Endocrine: Increased serum glucose (powder 3%, solution <1%)

Gastrointestinal: Nausea (8% to 10%), dysgeusia (powder 4% to 7%, solution <1%), vomiting (6%), diarrhea (2% to 4%), xerostomia (powder 2%)

Hematologic & oncologic: Increased erythrocyte sedimentation rate (solution 8%), eosinophilia

(solution 2%), increased serum immunoglobulins (solution 2%)

Neuromuscular & skeletal: Musculoskeletal chest pain (<1% to 5%)

Otic: Hypoacusis (powder 10%), tinnitus (2% to 3%)

Respiratory: Upper respiratory tract infection (7% to 9%), nasal congestion (1% to 8%), wheezing (5% to 7%), throat irritation (2% to 5%), bronchospasm (≤1% to 5%), bronchitis (solution 3%), epistaxis (2% to 3%), rhinitis (solution 2%), tonsillitis (solution 2%)

Available Dosage Forms

Capsule, Inhalation:

Tobi Podhaler: 28 mg

Nebulization Solution, Inhalation [preservative free]:

Bethkis: 300 mg/4 mL (4 mL)

Tobi: 300 mg/5 mL (5 mL)

Generic: 300 mg/5 mL (5 mL)

Solution, Injection:

Generic: 10 mg/mL (2 mL); 80 mg/2 mL (2 mL); 1.2 g/30 mL (30 mL); 2 g/50 mL (50 mL)

Solution, Intravenous:

Generic: 80 mg (100 mL)

Solution Reconstituted, Injection:

Generic: 1.2 g (1 ea)

Solution Reconstituted, Injection [preservative free]:

Generic: 1.2 g (1 ea)

General Dosage Range Dosage adjustment recommended for the I.M. and I.V. routes in patients with renal impairment

I.M.:

Infants and Children <5 years: 2.5 mg/kg every 8 hours

Children ≥5 years: 2-3.3 mg/kg every 6-8 hours

Adults: 1-2.5 mg/kg every 8-12 hours (1 mg/kg used for synergy) **or** 4-7 mg/kg/day as a single daily dose

Elderly: 1.5-5 mg/kg/day in 1-2 divided doses

I.V.:

Infants and Children <5 years: 2.5 mg/kg every 8 hours

Children ≥5 years: 2-3.3 mg/kg every 6-8 hours

Adults: 1-2.5 mg/kg every 8-12 hours (1 mg/kg/dose used for synergy) **or** 4-7 mg/kg/day as a single daily dose

Elderly: 1.5-5 mg/kg/day in 1-2 divided doses **or** 5-7 mg/kg given every 24, 36, or 48 hours based on CrCl

Inhalation: *Children ≥6 years and Adults:* Bethkis, TOBI: 300 mg every 12 hours; TOBI Podhaler: 112 mg every 12 hours

Administration

I.V. Infuse over 30-60 minutes.

Some penicillins (eg, carbenicillin, ticarcillin, and piperacillin) have been shown to inactivate aminoglycosides *in vitro*. This has been observed to a greater extent with tobramycin and gentamicin, while amikacin has shown greater stability against inactivation. Concurrent use of these agents may pose a risk of reduced antibacterial efficacy *in vivo*, particularly in the setting of profound renal impairment. However, definitive clinical evidence is lacking. If combination penicillin/aminoglycoside therapy is desired in a patient with renal dysfunction, separation of doses (if feasible), and routine monitoring of aminoglycoside levels, CBC, and clinical response should be considered.

Injectable Detail pH: 3-6.5 (injection, adjusted); 6-8 (reconstituted solution from powder)

Inhalation

Bethkis, TOBI: To be inhaled over ~15 minutes using a handheld reusable nebulizer (PARI-LC PLUS) with a PARI Vios air compressor (Bethkis) or a DeVilbiss Pulmo-Aide air compressor (TOBI). If multiple different nebulizer treatments are required, administer bronchodilator first, followed by chest physiotherapy, any other nebulized medications, and then TOBI or Bethkis last. Do not mix with other nebulizer medications.

TOBI Podhaler: Capsules should be administered by oral inhalation via Podhaler device following manufacturer recommendations for use and handling. Capsules should be removed from the blister packaging immediately prior to use and should not be swallowed. Patients requiring bronchodilator therapy should administer the bronchodilator 15-90 minutes prior to TOBI Podhaler. The sequence of chest physiotherapy and additional inhaled therapies is at the discretion of the healthcare provider; however, TOBI Podhaler should always be administered last. The Canadian labeling recommends that patients requiring bronchodilator therapy should administer the bronchodilator 15-90 minutes prior to administering TOBI Podhaler.

Preparation for Administration Solution for injection: Dilute in 50-100 mL NS or D_5W for I.V. infusion.

Storage/Stability

Injection: Stable at room temperature both as the clear, colorless solution and as the dry powder. Reconstituted solutions remain stable for 24 hours at room temperature and 96 hours when refrigerated.

Powder, for inhalation (TOBI Podhaler): Store in original package at 25°C (77°F); excursions permitted to 15°C to 30°C (59°F to 86°F). Protect from moisture.

Solution, for inhalation (Bethkis, TOBI): Store under refrigeration at 2°C to 8°C (36°F to 46°F). May be stored in foil pouch (opened or unopened) at room temperature of 25°C (77°F) for up to 28 days. The colorless to pale yellow solution may darken over time if not stored under refrigeration; however, the color change does not affect product quality. Do not use if solution is cloudy, contains particles, or has been stored at room temperature for >28 days.

Nursing Actions

Physical Assessment Assess patient's hearing level before, during, and following therapy; report changes to prescriber immediately. Monitor for neurotoxicity (vertigo, ataxia) and opportunistic infection (fever, mouth and vaginal sores or plaques) at beginning of therapy and throughout.

Patient Education

• Discuss specific use of drug and side effects with patient as it relates to treatment. (HCAHPS: During this hospital stay, were you given any medicine that you had not taken before? Before giving you any new medicine, how often did hospital staff tell you what the medicine was for? How often did hospital staff describe possible side effects in a way you could understand?)

• Patient may experience parageusia, decreased renal function, or hearing impairment. Have patient report immediately to prescriber significant change in balance, asthenia, severe nervousness and anxiety, considerable nausea, significant diarrhea, urinary retention, or rash (HCAHPS).

• Educate patient about signs of a significant reaction (eg, wheezing; chest tightness; fever; itching; bad cough; blue skin color; seizures; or swelling of face, lips, tongue, or throat). **Note:** This is not a comprehensive list of all side effects. Patient should consult prescriber for additional questions.

Intended Use and Disclaimer: Should not be printed and given to patients. This information is intended to serve as a concise initial reference for healthcare professionals to use when discussing medications with a patient. You must ultimately rely on your own discretion, experience and judgment in diagnosing, treating and advising patients.

Dietary Considerations May require supplementation of calcium, magnesium, potassium.

Related Information

Peak and Trough Guidelines *on page 1710*

Tofacitinib (toe fa SYE ti nib)

Brand Names: U.S. Xeljanz

Index Terms CP-690, 550; Tofacitinib Citrate

Pharmacologic Category Antirheumatic Miscellaneous; Antirheumatic, Disease Modifying; Janus Associated Kinase Inhibitor

Medication Guide Available Yes

Pregnancy Risk Factor C

Lactation Excretion in breast milk unknown/not recommended

Breast-Feeding Considerations It is not known if tofacitinib is excreted into breast milk. Due to the potential for adverse reactions in a nursing infant, the decision to continue or discontinue breast-feeding during therapy should take into account ▶

the risk of exposure to the infant and the benefits of treatment to the mother.

Use Treatment of moderately- to severely-active rheumatoid arthritis (as monotherapy or in combination with methotrexate or other nonbiologic disease-modifying antirheumatic drugs [DMARDs]) in patients who have had an inadequate response to, or are intolerant of, methotrexate

Mechanism of Action/Effect Tofacitinib inhibits Janus kinase (JAK) enzymes, which are intracellular enzymes involved in stimulating hematopoiesis and immune cell function through extracellular cytokine or growth factor signaling. Inhibition of JAKs inhibits cytokine- or growth factor-mediated gene expression and intracellular activity of immune cells, reduces circulating CD16/56+ natural killer cells, serum IgG, IgM, IgA, and C-reactive protein, and increases B cells.

Contraindications There are no contraindications listed in the manufacturer's labeling.

Warnings/Precautions [U.S. Boxed Warning]: Patients receiving tofacitinib are at increased risk for serious infections, which may result in hospitalization and/or fatality; infections often developed in patients receiving concomitant immunosuppressive agents (eg, methotrexate or corticosteroids) and may present as disseminated disease. Active tuberculosis (disseminated or extrapulmonary), invasive fungal (including cryptococcosis and pneumocystosis) and bacterial, viral or other opportunistic infections (including esophageal candidiasis, multidermatomal herpes zoster, cytomegalovirus, and BK virus) have been reported in patients receiving tofacitinib. Reactivation of viral infections (eg, herpes zoster) was observed in clinical trials; the incidence of chronic viral hepatitis reactivation is unknown. Use with caution in patients that have been exposed to tuberculosis, with a history of serious or opportunistic infection, taking concomitant immunosuppressants, with comorbid conditions that predispose them to infections (eg, diabetes), or in patients who live in or travel to/from areas of endemic mycoses (ie, blastomycosis, coccidioidomycosis, histoplasmosis). Consider risks versus benefits prior to use in patients with a history of chronic or recurrent infection; do not initiate tofacitinib in patients with active infections, including localized infections. Monitor closely for signs/symptoms of infection during therapy; interrupt therapy if serious infections or sepsis develop. Use with caution in elderly patients; general incidence of infection is higher in elderly.

[U.S. Boxed Warning]: Tuberculosis (disseminated or extrapulmonary) has been reported in patients receiving tofacitinib. Patients should be evaluated for tuberculosis risk factors and active or latent infection (with a tuberculin skin test) before and during therapy. Treatment of latent tuberculosis should be initiated before use. Patients with initial negative tuberculin skin tests should receive continued monitoring for tuberculosis throughout treatment; active tuberculosis has developed in this population during treatment with tofacitinib. Use with caution in patients who have resided in regions where tuberculosis is endemic. Consider antituberculosis therapy if an adequate course of treatment cannot be confirmed in patients with a history of latent or active tuberculosis or for patients with risk factors despite negative skin test.

[U.S. Boxed Warning]: Lymphoma and other malignancies have been reported in patients receiving tofacitinib; Epstein Barr Virus-associated post-transplant lymphoproliferative disorder has been observed at an increased rate in renal transplant patients receiving tofacitinib and concomitant immunosuppressive medications. The most common types of malignancy observed were lung, breast, gastric, colorectal, renal cell, prostate, lymphoma, and malignant melanoma. Consider risks versus benefits prior to use in patients with a known malignancy (other than successfully treated nonmelanoma skin cancers [NMSC]) or when continuing tofacitinib in patients who develop a new malignancy.

Lymphocytopenia (after an initial lymphocytosis), neutropenia (<2000 cells/mm^3), and anemia have been observed with tofacitinib therapy. Lymphocyte counts <500 cells/mm^3 were associated with increased incidence of treated and serious infections; avoid tofacitinib initiation in patients with lymphocytes <500 cells/mm^3 at baseline. Avoid use in patients with ANC <1000 cells/mm^3 at baseline; interrupt therapy if ANC is persistently between 500-1000 cells/mm^3 or if ANC <500 cells/mm^3 during treatment. Consider resuming tofacitinib when ANC ≥1000 cells/mm^3. Avoid use in patients with hemoglobin <9 g/dL; interrupt therapy if hemoglobin decreases >2 g/dL or if hemoglobin <8 g/dL. Monitor lymphocyte counts at baseline and every 3 months thereafter; ANC, platelet counts, and hemoglobin should be assessed at baseline, after 4-8 weeks of therapy, and every 3 months thereafter.

Use with caution in patients at increased risk for gastrointestinal perforation (eg, history of diverticulitis); perforations have been reported in clinical trials. Promptly evaluate new-onset abdominal symptoms in patients taking tofacitinib. Increases in lipid parameters (eg, total cholesterol, LDL, and HDL cholesterol) were observed in patients receiving tofacitinib; maximum lipid increases were typically seen within 6 weeks of initiation. Assess lipids 4-8 weeks after tofacitinib initiation and manage lipid abnormalities accordingly. Increased incidence of liver enzyme elevation was observed in patients taking tofacitinib compared to placebo. Routine liver function test monitoring is recommended; interrupt therapy if drug-induced liver injury is suspected.

Immunization status should be current before initiating therapy. Live vaccines should not be given concomitantly with tofacitinib; no data are available concerning vaccination response or secondary transmission of infection by live vaccines in patients receiving therapy.

Tofacitinib should not be administered in combination with strong immunosuppressive medications (eg, azathioprine, tacrolimus, cyclosporine) due to the risk of additive immunosuppression; such combinations have not been studied in rheumatoid arthritis. Tofacitinib should not be administered in combination with biologic DMARDs.

Use is not recommended in patients with severe hepatic impairment; dosage reduction required in patients with moderate hepatic impairment. Dosage reduction required in patients with moderate or severe renal impairment.

Drug Interactions
Avoid Concomitant Use
Avoid concomitant use of Tofacitinib with any of the following: Abatacept; Anakinra; Anti-TNF Agents; BCG; CloZAPine; CYP3A4 Inducers (Strong); Fusidic Acid (Systemic); Immunosuppressants; Natalizumab; Pimecrolimus; RiTUXimab; Tacrolimus (Topical); Tocilizumab; Vaccines (Live)

Decreased Effect
Tofacitinib may decrease the levels/effects of: BCG; Coccidioidin Skin Test; Sipuleucel-T; Vaccines (Inactivated); Vaccines (Live)

The levels/effects of Tofacitinib may be decreased by: Bosentan; CYP3A4 Inducers (Strong); Dabrafenib; Deferasirox; Echinacea; Herbs (CYP3A4 Inducers)

Increased Effect/Toxicity
Tofacitinib may increase the levels/effects of: CloZAPine; Leflunomide; Natalizumab; Vaccines (Live)

The levels/effects of Tofacitinib may be increased by: Abatacept; Anakinra; Anti-TNF Agents; CYP3A4 Inhibitors (Moderate); CYP3A4 Inhibitors (Strong); Denosumab; Fluconazole; Fusidic Acid (Systemic); Ivacaftor; Luliconazole; Mifepristone; Pimecrolimus; RiTUXimab; Roflumilast; Simeprevir; Sitaxentan; Tacrolimus (Topical); Tocilizumab; Trastuzumab

Adverse Reactions
Percentages noted include the highest frequency regardless of dosage. Frequencies may vary for specific doses; consult prescribing information.
>10%: Miscellaneous: Infections (20%)
1% to 10%:
Cardiovascular: Hypertension (2%)
Central nervous system: Headache (4%)
Gastrointestinal: Diarrhea (4%)

Genitourinary: Urinary tract infection (2%)
Hepatic: ALT increased (>3 x upper limit of normal; 1%)
Renal: Serum creatinine increased (<2%)
Respiratory: Upper respiratory tract infections (5%), nasopharyngitis (4%)
Miscellaneous: Serious infections (2%)
<1%: Abdominal pain, anemia, arthralgia, cough, dehydration, dyspepsia, dyspnea, erythema, fatigue, gastritis, hepatic steatosis, insomnia, joint swelling, lymphocytopenia, malignancies, musculoskeletal pain, nausea, neutropenia, paresthesia, peripheral edema, pruritus, pyrexia, rash, sinus congestion, tendonitis, tuberculosis, vomiting
Postmarketing and/or case reports: Drug-induced liver injury

Available Dosage Forms
Tablet, Oral:
Xeljanz: 5 mg
General Dosage Range Dosage adjustment recommended in patients with renal impairment, hepatic impairment, on concomitant therapy, and who develop toxicities.
Oral: *Adults:* 5 mg twice daily

Administration
Oral May be taken without regard to food.

Storage/Stability Store between 20°C and 25°C (68°F to 77°F).

Nursing Actions
Physical Assessment Monitor for signs and symptoms of infection. Monitor blood pressure as hypertension can occur. Monitor for fever, sweating, chills, cough, shortness of breath, hemoptysis, burning with urination, diarrhea, and unexplained weight loss. Do not give live vaccines while the patient is receiving this medication. Rarely, gastrointestinal perforations may occur; observe for abdominal pain, severe nausea and vomiting, and blood in the stool.

Patient Education
• Discuss specific use of drug and side effects with patient as it relates to treatment. (HCAHPS: During this hospital stay, were you given any medicine that you had not taken before? Before giving you any new medicine, how often did hospital staff tell you what the medicine was for? How often did hospital staff describe possible side effects in a way you could understand?)
• Patient may experience headache, diarrhea, rhinorrhea, or pharyngitis. Have patient report immediately to prescriber signs of infection, dyspnea, ecchymosis, bleeding, severe asthenia, inability to eat, significant dyspepsia, discolored urine, or jaundice (HCAHPS).
• Educate patient about signs of a significant reaction (eg, wheezing; chest tightness; fever; itching; bad cough; blue skin color; seizures; or swelling of face, lips, tongue, or throat). **Note:** This is not a comprehensive list of all side effects. Patient should consult prescriber for additional questions.

Intended Use and Disclaimer: Should not be printed and given to patients. This information is intended to serve as a concise initial reference for healthcare professionals to use when discussing medications with a patient. You must ultimately rely on your own discretion, experience and judgment in diagnosing, treating and advising patients.

Tolcapone (TOLE ka pone)

Brand Names: U.S. Tasmar
Pharmacologic Category Anti-Parkinson's Agent, COMT Inhibitor
Medication Safety Issues
Sound-alike/look-alike issues:
Tolcapone may be confused with TOLAZamide, TOLBUTamide, tolmetin, tolterodine
International issues:
Tolcapone may be confused with Tolcamin, international brand name for ifosfamide.
Tasmar may be confused with Tasmen, international brand name for acetaminophen.
Pregnancy Risk Factor C
Lactation Excretion in breast milk unknown/use caution
Breast-Feeding Considerations It is not known if tolcapone is excreted in breast milk. The manufacturer recommends that caution be exercised when administering tolcapone to nursing women.
Use Adjunct to levodopa and carbidopa for the treatment of signs and symptoms of idiopathic Parkinson's disease in patients with motor fluctuations not responsive to other therapies
Mechanism of Action/Effect Tolcapone is a selective and reversible inhibitor of catechol-o-methyltransferase (COMT) which leads to more sustained blood levels of levodopa.
Contraindications Hypersensitivity to tolcapone or any component of the formulation; patients with liver disease or a history of tolcapone-induced hepatocellular injury; history of nontraumatic rhabdomyolysis or hyperpyrexia and confusion potentially related to medication
Warnings/Precautions [U.S. Boxed Warning]: Due to reports of fatal liver injury associated with use of this drug, the manufacturer is advising that tolcapone be reserved for patients who are experiencing inadequate symptom control or who are not appropriate candidates for other available treatments. Patients must provide written consent acknowledging the risks of hepatic injury. Close monitoring for potential hepatotoxicity is required during use. Do not initiate in patients with clinical evidence of liver disease or with two transaminases values greater than the upper limit of normal. Discontinue if signs and/or symptoms of hepatic injury are noted (eg, anorexia, jaundice, lethargy, transaminases >2 times upper limit of normal) or if clinical improvement is not evident after 3 weeks of therapy.

Tolcapone should not be reinitiated in patients who discontinued therapy due to evidence of liver injury; may be at increased risk for liver injury. Use with caution in patients with pre-existing dyskinesias; exacerbation of pre-existing dyskinesia has been reported. Levodopa dosage reduction may be required, particularly in patients with levodopa dosages >600 mg daily or with moderate-to-severe dyskinesia prior to initiation.

May cause orthostatic hypotension and syncope; Parkinson's disease patients appear to have an impaired capacity to respond to a postural challenge; use with caution in patients at risk of hypotension (such as those receiving antihypertensive drugs) or where transient hypotensive episodes would be poorly tolerated (cardiovascular disease or cerebrovascular disease). Parkinson's patients being treated with dopaminergic agonists ordinarily require careful monitoring for signs and symptoms of postural hypotension, especially during dose escalation, and should be informed of this risk. Patients have reported falling asleep while engaging in activities of daily living; this has been reported to occur without significant warning signs. Monitor for daytime somnolence or pre-existing sleep disorder. Use caution with other CNS depressants, sedating agents, psychoactive drugs or ethanol. Patients must be cautioned about performing tasks which require mental alertness (eg, operating machinery or driving). Discontinuation of treatment may be required in patients experiencing significant drowsiness. May cause hallucinations (onset within 2 weeks), which may improve with reduction in levodopa therapy; incidence may be increased in patients >75 years of age. Abnormal thinking and behavior changes have been reported and may include paranoid ideation, delusions, confusion, psychotic-like behavior, disorientation, aggressive behavior, agitation, and delirium. Avoid use in patients with a major psychotic disorder; may exacerbate psychosis. Use with caution in patients with lower gastrointestinal disease or an increased risk of dehydration; tolcapone has been associated with delayed development of diarrhea (onset after 2-12 weeks).

Potentially significant interactions may exist, requiring dose or frequency adjustment, additional monitoring, and/or selection of alternative therapy. Concomitant use of tolcapone and nonselective MAO inhibitors should be avoided. Selegiline is a selective MAO type B inhibitor (when given orally at ≤10 mg/day) and can be taken with tolcapone. Dopaminergic agents used for Parkinson's disease or restless legs syndrome have been associated with compulsive behaviors and/or loss of impulse control, which has manifested as pathological gambling, libido increases (hypersexuality), and/or binge eating. Causality has not been established, and controversy exists as to whether this phenomenon is related to the underlying disease, prior behaviors/addictions and/or drug therapy. Dose reduction or discontinuation of therapy has been reported to reverse these behaviors in some, but not all cases. Severe rhabdomyolysis has been reported with use. Risk for melanoma development is increased in Parkinson's disease patients; drug causation or factors contributing to risk have not been established. Patients should be monitored closely and periodic skin examinations should be performed. Dopaminergic agents from the ergot class have also been associated with fibrotic complications, such as retroperitoneal fibrosis, pulmonary infiltrates or effusion and pleural thickening. It is unknown whether nonergot, pro-dopaminergic agents like tolcapone confer this risk. Use caution in patients with severe renal impairment. Dopaminergic agents have been associated with a syndrome resembling neuroleptic malignant syndrome upon withdrawal or abrupt dosage reduction; patients should be monitored closely if therapy is discontinued.

Drug Interactions

Avoid Concomitant Use

Avoid concomitant use of Tolcapone with any of the following: Azelastine (Nasal); Paraldehyde; Thalidomide

Decreased Effect There are no known significant interactions involving a decrease in effect.

Increased Effect/Toxicity

Tolcapone may increase the levels/effects of: Alcohol (Ethyl); Azelastine (Nasal); Buprenorphine; CNS Depressants; COMT Substrates; Hydrocodone; MAO Inhibitors; Methotrimeprazine; Metyrosine; Mirtazapine; Paraldehyde; Pramipexole; ROPINIRole; Rotigotine; Selective Serotonin Reuptake Inhibitors; Thalidomide; Zolpidem

The levels/effects of Tolcapone may be increased by: Brimonidine (Topical); Doxylamine; Droperidol; HydrOXYzine; Magnesium Sulfate; MAO Inhibitors; Methotrimeprazine; Perampanel; Sodium Oxybate; Tapentadol

Nutritional/Ethanol Interactions

Ethanol: May increase CNS depression; monitor for increased effects with coadministration. Caution patients about effects.

Food: Tolcapone, taken with food within 1 hour before or 2 hours after the dose, decreases bioavailability by 10% to 20%.

Avoid valerian, St John's wort, kava kava, gotu kola (may increase CNS depression).

Adverse Reactions

>10%:

Cardiovascular: Orthostatic hypotension (17%)

Central nervous system: Somnolence (14% to 32%), sleep disorder (24% to 25%), hallucinations (8% to 24%), excessive dreaming (16% to 21%), dizziness (6% to 13%), headache (10% to 11%), confusion (10% to 11%)

Gastrointestinal: Nausea (28% to 50%), diarrhea (16% to 34%; approximately 3% to 4% severe), anorexia (19% to 23%)

Neuromuscular & skeletal: Dyskinesia (42% to 51%), dystonia (19% to 22%), muscle cramps (17% to 18%)

1% to 10%:

Cardiovascular: Syncope (4% to 5%), chest pain (1% to 3%), hypotension (2%), palpitation (1% to 3%)

Central nervous system: Fatigue (3% to 7%), loss of balance (2% to 3%), agitation (1%), euphoria (1%), hyperactivity (1%), malaise (1%), panic reaction (1%), irritability (1%), mental deficiency (1%), fever (1%), depression, hypoesthesia, tremor, speech disorder, vertigo, emotional lability, hyperkinesia

Dermatologic: Alopecia (1%), bleeding (1%), tumor (1%), rash

Gastrointestinal: Vomiting (8% to 10%), constipation (6% to 8%), xerostomia (5% to 6%), abdominal pain (5% to 6%), dyspepsia (3% to 4%), flatulence (2% to 4%)

Genitourinary: UTI (5%), hematuria (4% to 5%), urine discoloration (2% to 3%), urination disorder (1% to 2%), uterine tumor (1%), incontinence, impotence

Hepatic: Transaminases increased (1% to 3%; 3 times ULN, usually with first 6 months of therapy)

Neuromuscular & skeletal: Paresthesia (1% to 3%), hyper-/hypokinesia (1% to 3%), arthritis (1% to 2%), neck pain (2%), stiffness (2%), myalgia, rhabdomyolysis

Ocular: Cataract (1%), eye inflammation (1%)

Otic: Tinnitus

Respiratory: Upper respiratory infection (5% to 7%), dyspnea (3%), sinus congestion (1% to 2%), bronchitis, pharyngitis

Miscellaneous: Diaphoresis (4% to 7%), influenza (3% to 4%), burning (1% to 2%), flank pain, injury, infection

Available Dosage Forms

Tablet, Oral:

Tasmar: 100 mg

General Dosage Range Oral: *Adults:* Initial: 100 mg 3 times daily; Maintenance: 100-200 mg 3 times daily

Administration

Oral May be administered without regard to meals. In clinical studies, the first dose of the day was administered with carbidopa/levodopa, and the subsequent doses were administered 6 hours and 12 hours later.

Storage/Stability Store at 20°C to 25°C (68°F to 77°F).

Nursing Actions

Physical Assessment May exacerbate the adverse effects of levodopa, including levodopa toxicity. Assess therapeutic response (eg, mental status and involuntary movements). Monitor for CNS depression. Monitor blood pressure.

Patient Education
- Discuss specific use of drug and side effects with patient as it relates to treatment. (HCAHPS: During this hospital stay, were you given any medicine that you had not taken before? Before giving you any new medicine, how often did hospital staff tell you what the medicine was for? How often did hospital staff describe possible side effects in a way you could understand?)
- Patient may experience presyncope, fatigue, blurred vision, illogical thinking, dizziness, bradykinesia, nausea, or diarrhea. Have patient report immediately to prescriber severe dyspepsia, inability to eat, discolored urine, jaundice, significant asthenia, or rash (HCAHPS).
- Educate patient about signs of a significant reaction (eg, wheezing; chest tightness; fever; itching; bad cough; blue skin color; seizures; or swelling of face, lips, tongue, or throat). **Note:** This is not a comprehensive list of all side effects. Patient should consult prescriber for additional questions.

Intended Use and Disclaimer: Should not be printed and given to patients. This information is intended to serve as a concise initial reference for healthcare professionals to use when discussing medications with a patient. You must ultimately rely on your own discretion, experience and judgment in diagnosing, treating and advising patients.

Dietary Considerations May be taken without regard to meals.

Tolterodine (tole TER oh deen)

Brand Names: U.S. Detrol; Detrol LA
Index Terms Tolterodine Tartrate
Pharmacologic Category Anticholinergic Agent
Medication Safety Issues
 Sound-alike/look-alike issues:
  Tolterodine may be confused with fesoterodine, tolcapone
  Detrol® may be confused with Ditropan
 BEERS Criteria medication:
  This drug may be potentially inappropriate for use in geriatric patients (Quality of evidence - varies based on comorbidity; Strength of recommendation - varies based on comorbidity)
Pregnancy Risk Factor C
Lactation Excretion in breast milk unknown/not recommended
Breast-Feeding Considerations It is not known if tolterodine is excreted in breast milk. Due to the potential for serious adverse reactions in the nursing infant, a decision should be made whether to discontinue nursing or to discontinue the drug, taking into account the importance of treatment to the mother.

Use Treatment of patients with an overactive bladder with symptoms of urinary frequency, urgency, or urge incontinence

Mechanism of Action/Effect Antagonizes muscarinic receptors of the urinary bladder resulting in decreased bladder pressure and contraction.

Contraindications Hypersensitivity to tolterodine or fesoterodine (both are metabolized to 5-hydroxymethyl tolterodine) or any component of the formulation; urinary retention; gastric retention; uncontrolled narrow-angle glaucoma

Warnings/Precautions Cases of angioedema have been reported; some cases have occurred after a single dose. Discontinue immediately if angioedema and associated difficulty breathing, airway obstruction, or hypotension develop. May cause drowsiness, dizziness, and/or blurred vision, which may impair physical or mental abilities; patients must be cautioned about performing tasks which require mental alertness (eg, operating machinery or driving). Consider dose reduction or discontinuation if CNS effects occur. Use with caution in patients with bladder flow obstruction, may increase the risk of urinary retention. Use with caution in patients with gastrointestinal obstructive disorders (ie, pyloric stenosis), may increase the risk of gastric retention. Use with caution in patients with myasthenia gravis and controlled (treated) narrow-angle glaucoma; metabolized in the liver and excreted in the urine and feces, dosage adjustment is required for patients with renal or hepatic impairment. Tolterodine has been associated with QT$_c$ prolongation at high (supratherapeutic) doses. The manufacturer recommends caution in patients with congenital prolonged QT or in patients receiving concurrent therapy with QT$_c$-prolonging drugs (class Ia or III antiarrhythmics). However, the mean change in QT$_c$ even at supratherapeutic dosages was less than 15 msec. Individuals who are CYP2D6 poor metabolizers or in the presence of inhibitors of CYP2D6 and CYP3A4 may be more likely to exhibit prolongation. Dosage adjustment is recommended in patients receiving CYP3A4 inhibitors (a lower dose of tolterodine is recommended). This medication is associated with potent anticholinergic properties which may be inappropriate in older adults depending on comorbidities (eg, dementia, delirium) (Beers Criteria).

Drug Interactions
 Avoid Concomitant Use
  Avoid concomitant use of Tolterodine with any of the following: Aclidinium; Fusidic Acid (Systemic); Ipratropium (Oral Inhalation); Potassium Chloride; Tiotropium; Umeclidinium
 Decreased Effect
  Tolterodine may decrease the levels/effects of: Acetylcholinesterase Inhibitors (Central); Secretin

  The levels/effects of Tolterodine may be decreased by: Acetylcholinesterase Inhibitors (Central); Bosentan; CYP3A4 Inducers (Strong);

Dabrafenib; Deferasirox; Herbs (CYP3A4 Inducers); Mitotane; Peginterferon Alfa-2b; Tocilizumab

Increased Effect/Toxicity

Tolterodine may increase the levels/effects of: AbobotulinumtoxinA; Analgesics (Opioid); Anticholinergics; Cannabinoids; Highest Risk QTc-Prolonging Agents; Mirabegron; Moderate Risk QTc-Prolonging Agents; OnabotulinumtoxinA; Potassium Chloride; RimabotulinumtoxinB; Thiazide Diuretics; Tiotropium; Topiramate; Warfarin

The levels/effects of Tolterodine may be increased by: Abiraterone Acetate; Aclidinium; Antifungal Agents (Azole Derivatives, Systemic); CYP2D6 Inhibitors (Moderate); CYP2D6 Inhibitors (Strong); CYP3A4 Inhibitors (Moderate); CYP3A4 Inhibitors (Strong); Dasatinib; Fluconazole; Fusidic Acid (Systemic); Ipratropium (Oral Inhalation); Ivacaftor; Luliconazole; Mifepristone; Pramlintide; Simeprevir; Umeclidinium; VinBLAStine

Nutritional/Ethanol Interactions

Food: Increases bioavailability (~53% increase) of tolterodine tablets (dose adjustment not necessary); does not affect the pharmacokinetics of tolterodine extended release capsules. As a CYP3A4 inhibitor, grapefruit juice may increase the serum level and/or toxicity of tolterodine, but unlikely secondary to high oral bioavailability.

Herb/Nutraceutical: St John's wort (*Hypericum*) appears to induce CYP3A enzymes.

Adverse Reactions As reported with immediate release tablet, unless otherwise specified

>10%: Gastrointestinal: Dry mouth (35%; extended release capsules 23%)

1% to 10%:

Cardiovascular: Chest pain (2%)

Central nervous system: Headache (7%; extended release capsules 6%), dizziness (5%; extended release capsules 2%), fatigue (4%; extended release capsules 2%), somnolence (3%; extended release capsules 3%), anxiety (extended release capsules 1%)

Dermatologic: Dry skin (1%)

Gastrointestinal: Constipation (7%; extended release capsules 6%), abdominal pain (5%; extended release capsules 4%), diarrhea (4%), dyspepsia (4%; extended release capsules 3%), weight gain (1%)

Genitourinary: Dysuria (2%; extended release capsules 1%)

Neuromuscular & skeletal: Arthralgia (2%)

Ocular: Dry eyes (3%; extended release capsules 3%), abnormal vision (2%; extended release capsules 1%)

Respiratory: Bronchitis (2%), sinusitis (extended release capsules 2%)

Miscellaneous: Flu-like syndrome (3%), infection (1%)

Available Dosage Forms

Capsule Extended Release 24 Hour, Oral:

Detrol LA: 2 mg, 4 mg

Generic: 2 mg, 4 mg

Tablet, Oral:

Detrol: 1 mg, 2 mg

Generic: 1 mg, 2 mg

General Dosage Range Dosage adjustment recommended in patients with hepatic or renal impairment and on concomitant therapy

Oral: *Adults:* Extended release capsule: 2-4 mg once daily; Immediate release tablet: 1-2 mg twice daily

Administration

Oral Extended release capsule: Swallow whole; do not crush, chew, or open

Storage/Stability Store at 25°C (77°F); excursions permitted to 15°C to 30°C (59°F to 86°F). Protect from light.

Nursing Actions

Patient Education

- Discuss specific use of drug and side effects with patient as it relates to treatment. (HCAHPS: During this hospital stay, were you given any medicine that you had not taken before? Before giving you any new medicine, how often did hospital staff tell you what the medicine was for? How often did hospital staff describe possible side effects in a way you could understand?)

- Patient may experience dizziness, headache, dyspepsia, constipation, presyncope, fatigue, blurred vision, illogical thinking, or xerostomia. Have patient report immediately to prescriber dyspnea, urinary retention, or rash (HCAHPS).

- Educate patient about signs of a significant reaction (eg, wheezing; chest tightness; fever; itching; bad cough; blue skin color; seizures; or swelling of face, lips, tongue, or throat). **Note:** This is not a comprehensive list of all side effects. Patient should consult prescriber for additional questions.

Intended Use and Disclaimer: Should not be printed and given to patients. This information is intended to serve as a concise initial reference for healthcare professionals to use when discussing medications with a patient. You must ultimately rely on your own discretion, experience and judgment in diagnosing, treating and advising patients.

Related Information

Oral Medications That Should Not Be Crushed or Altered *on page 1712*

Tolvaptan (tol VAP tan)

Brand Names: U.S. Samsca

Index Terms OPC-41061

Pharmacologic Category Vasopressin Antagonist

Medication Guide Available Yes

◄ **Pregnancy Risk Factor** C

Lactation Excretion in breast milk unknown/not recommended

Breast-Feeding Considerations It is not known if tolvaptan is excreted in breast milk. Due to the potential for serious adverse reactions in the nursing infant, a decision should be made whether to discontinue nursing or to discontinue the drug, taking into account the importance of treatment to the mother.

Use Treatment of clinically significant hypervolemic or euvolemic hyponatremia associated with heart failure or SIADH with either a serum sodium <125 mEq/L or less marked hyponatremia that is symptomatic and resistant to fluid restriction

Mechanism of Action/Effect Tolvaptan blocks the antidiuretic action of arginine vasopressin in the kidney, leading to the excretion of free water without loss of serum sodium.

Contraindications Hypersensitivity (eg, anaphylactic shock, generalized rash) to tolvaptan or any component of the formulation; hypovolemic hyponatremia; urgent need to raise serum sodium acutely; use in patients unable to sense or appropriately respond to thirst; anuria; concurrent use with strong CYP3A inhibitors (eg, ketoconazole, itraconazole, ritonavir, indinavir, nelfinavir, saquinavir, nefazodone, telithromycin, clarithromycin)

Canadian labeling: Additional contraindications (not in U.S. labeling): Hypersensitivity to tolvaptan or any component of the formulation

Warnings/Precautions [U.S. Boxed Warning]: Tolvaptan should be initiated and reinitiated in patients only in a hospital where serum sodium can be closely monitored. Too rapid correction of hyponatremia (ie, >12 mEq/L/24 hours) can cause osmotic demyelination resulting in dysarthria, mutism, dysphagia, lethargy, affective changes, spastic quadriparesis, seizures, coma, and death. In susceptible patients (including those with severe malnutrition, or alcoholism), slower rates of correction may be advisable. Patients with SIADH or very low baseline serum sodium concentrations may be at greater risk of overly-rapid correction.

Tolvaptan may increase the risk of serious hepatotoxicity, including fatal hepatotoxicity. Cases usually occurred after 3 months of therapy although some cases occurred prior to 3 months. Therefore, treatment should be limited to 30 days. If hepatotoxicity is suspected, discontinue use. Avoid use in patients with liver disease, including those with cirrhosis, since the ability to recover from further liver injury may be impaired. In addition, patients with cirrhosis have a higher risk of gastrointestinal bleeding.

Interrupt or discontinue therapy in patients who develop medically significant signs or symptoms of hypovolemia. Patients should ingest fluids in response to thirst. Reductions in extracellular fluid volumes may cause hyperkalemia. Patients with a pretreatment serum potassium >5 mEq/L should be monitored after initiation of therapy.

Use in patients with creatinine clearance <10 mL/minute has not been studied; use is contraindicated in patients who are anuric. Use with hypertonic saline is not recommended. Potentially significant drug-drug interactions may exist, requiring dose or frequency adjustment, additional monitoring, and/or selection of alternative therapy.

Monitor closely for rate of serum sodium increase and neurological status; rapid serum sodium correction (>12 mEq/L/24 hours) can lead to permanent neurological damage. Discontinue use if rate of serum sodium increase is undesirable; fluid restriction during the first 24 hours of sodium correction can increase the risk of overly-rapid correction and should generally be avoided; not intended for urgent correction of serum sodium to prevent or treat serious neurologic symptoms; it has not been demonstrated that raising serum sodium with tolvaptan provides a symptomatic benefit.

Drug Interactions

Avoid Concomitant Use

Avoid concomitant use of Tolvaptan with any of the following: CYP3A4 Inducers (Strong); CYP3A4 Inhibitors (Moderate); CYP3A4 Inhibitors (Strong); Fusidic Acid (Systemic); Pimozide; Sodium Chloride

Decreased Effect

The levels/effects of Tolvaptan may be decreased by: Bosentan; CYP3A4 Inducers (Strong); Dabrafenib; Deferasirox; Herbs (CYP3A4 Inducers); P-glycoprotein/ABCB1 Inducers; Tocilizumab

Increased Effect/Toxicity

Tolvaptan may increase the levels/effects of: ACE Inhibitors; Angiotensin II Receptor Blockers; ARIPiprazole; Digoxin; Dofetilide; Lomitapide; Pimozide; Potassium-Sparing Diuretics

The levels/effects of Tolvaptan may be increased by: CYP3A4 Inhibitors (Moderate); CYP3A4 Inhibitors (Strong); Dasatinib; Fusidic Acid (Systemic); Ivacaftor; Luliconazole; Mifepristone; P-glycoprotein/ABCB1 Inhibitors; Simeprevir; Sodium Chloride

Nutritional/Ethanol Interactions

Food: Tolvaptan exposure may be doubled when taken with grapefruit juice. Management: Avoid grapefruit juice.

Herb/Nutraceutical: St John's wort may decrease tolvaptan serum concentrations. Management: Avoid St John's wort.

Adverse Reactions
>10%:
Gastrointestinal: Nausea (21%), xerostomia (7% to 13%)
Renal: Pollakiuria (4% to 11%), polyuria (4% to 11%)
Miscellaneous: Thirst (12% to 16%)
2% to 10%:
Central nervous system: Fever (4%)
Endocrine & metabolic: Hyperglycemia (6%), hypernatremia (<2%)
Gastrointestinal: GI bleeding (cirrhosis patients 10%), constipation (7%), anorexia (4%), hepatotoxicity (≤4%)
Neuromuscular & skeletal: Weakness (9%)

Pharmacodynamics/Kinetics
Onset of Action 2-4 hour; Peak effect: 4-8 hours
Duration of Action 60% peak serum sodium elevation is retained at 24 hours; urinary excretion of free water is no longer elevated

Available Dosage Forms
Tablet, Oral:
Samsca: 15 mg, 30 mg
General Dosage Range Oral: *Adults:* 15-60 mg once daily

Administration
Oral Treatment should be initiated or reinitiated in a hospital. May be administered without regards to meals.
Other Nasogastric (NG) tube: Administration via NG tube resulted in an ~25% reduction in AUC and a modest reduction in C_{max} in one study; 24-hour urine output was reduced by only 2.8%. Therefore, until further studies are done to determine a bioequivalent dose when administering via NG tube, NG tube administration of a crushed 15 mg tablet appears to be a viable alternative method of administration (McNeely, 2012).

Storage/Stability Store at 25°C (77°F); excursions permitted between 15°C and 30°C (59°F and 86°F).

Nursing Actions
Physical Assessment Monitor neurologic status. Teach patient about directions for fluid intake.

Patient Education
• Discuss specific use of drug and side effects with patient as it relates to treatment. (HCAHPS: During this hospital stay, were you given any medicine that you had not taken before? Before giving you any new medicine, how often did hospital staff tell you what the medicine was for? How often did hospital staff describe possible side effects in a way you could understand?)
• Patient may experience polydipsia, nausea, constipation, xerostomia, signs of hyperglycemia, or mood changes. Have patient report immediately to prescriber severe dizziness, significant diarrhea, considerable asthenia, illogical thinking, dysphasia, difficulty speaking, dyspraxia, ecchymosis, bleeding, urinary retention, severe dyspepsia, discolored urine, jaundice, inability to eat, or rash (HCAHPS).
• Educate patient about signs of a significant reaction (eg, wheezing; chest tightness; fever; itching; bad cough; blue skin color; seizures; or swelling of face, lips, tongue, or throat). **Note:** This is not a comprehensive list of all side effects. Patient should consult prescriber for additional questions.

Intended Use and Disclaimer: Should not be printed and given to patients. This information is intended to serve as a concise initial reference for healthcare professionals to use when discussing medications with a patient. You must ultimately rely on your own discretion, experience and judgment in diagnosing, treating and advising patients.

Dietary Considerations May be taken without regards to meals. Avoid grapefruit juice.

Topiramate (toe PYRE a mate)

Brand Names: U.S. Topamax; Topamax Sprinkle; Topiragen; Trokendi XR
Index Terms Qudexy XR
Pharmacologic Category Anticonvulsant, Miscellaneous

Medication Safety Issues
Sound-alike/look-alike issues:
Topamax may be confused with Sporanox, TEGretol, TEGretol-XR, Toprol-XL

Medication Guide Available Yes
Pregnancy Risk Factor D
Lactation Enters breast milk/use caution

Breast-Feeding Considerations Topiramate is excreted into breast milk. Based on information from five nursing infants, infant plasma concentrations of topiramate have been reported as 10% to 20% of the maternal plasma concentration. The manufacturer recommends that caution be used if administered to a nursing woman.

Use
Epilepsy:
Monotherapy: As initial monotherapy in patients 2 years and older (immediate release) or 10 years and older (extended release [ER]) with partial-onset or primary generalized tonic-clonic seizures
Adjunctive therapy: As adjunctive therapy in patients 2 years and older (immediate release) or 6 years and older (ER) with partial-onset seizures, primary generalized tonic-clonic seizures, or seizures associated with Lennox-Gastaut syndrome
Migraine (immediate release only): For the prophylaxis of migraine headache in adults
Unlabeled Use Diabetic neuropathy, infantile spasms, neuropathic pain; prophylaxis of cluster headache

Mechanism of Action/Effect Anticonvulsant activity may be due to a combination of potential mechanisms: Blocks neuronal voltage-dependent sodium channels, enhances GABA(A) activity, antagonizes AMPA/kainate glutamate receptors, and weakly inhibits carbonic anhydrase.

Contraindications

Extended release: Recent alcohol use (ie, within 6 hours prior to and 6 hours after administration); patients with metabolic acidosis who are taking concomitant metformin

Immediate release: There are no contraindications listed in the manufacturer's labeling.

Canadian labeling (not in U.S. labeling): Hypersensitivity to topiramate or any component of the formulation or container; pregnancy and women in childbearing years not using effective contraception (migraine prophylaxis only)

Warnings/Precautions Antiepileptics are associated with an increased risk of suicidal behavior/thoughts with use (regardless of indication); patients should be monitored for signs/symptoms of depression, suicidal tendencies, and other unusual behavior changes during therapy and instructed to inform their healthcare provider immediately if symptoms occur. Use with caution in patients with hepatic, respiratory, or renal impairment. Topiramate may decrease serum bicarbonate concentrations (up to 67% of patients); treatment-emergent metabolic acidosis is less common. Risk may be increased in patients with a predisposing condition (organ dysfunction, diarrhea, ketogenic diet, status epilepticus, or concurrent treatment with other drugs which may cause acidosis). Metabolic acidosis may occur at dosages as low as 50 mg/day. Monitor serum bicarbonate as well as potential complications of chronic acidosis (nephrolithiasis, osteomalacia, and reduced growth rates and/or weight in children). Kidney stones have been reported in both children and adults; the risk of kidney stones is about 2-4 times that of the untreated population; the risk of this event may be reduced by increasing fluid intake.

Cognitive dysfunction, psychiatric disturbances (depression or mood disorders), and sedation (somnolence or fatigue) may occur with topiramate use; incidence may be related to rapid titration and higher doses. Patients must be cautioned about performing tasks which require mental alertness (eg, operating machinery or driving). Topiramate may also cause paresthesia, dizziness, and ataxia. Topiramate has been associated with acute myopia and secondary angle-closure glaucoma in adults and children, typically within 1 month of initiation; discontinue in patients with acute onset of decreased visual acuity or ocular pain. Visual field defects have also been reported independent of increased intraocular pressure; generally reversible upon discontinuation. Consider discontinuation if visual problems occur at any time during treatment. Hyperammonemia with or without encephalopathy may occur with or without concomitant valproate administration; valproic acid dose-dependency was observed in limited pediatric studies; use with caution in patients with inborn errors of metabolism or decreased hepatic mitochondrial activity. Hypothermia (core body temperature <35°C [95°F]) has been reported with concomitant use of topiramate and valproic acid; may occur with or without associated hyperammonemia and may develop after topiramate initiation or dosage increase; discontinuation of topiramate or valproic acid may be necessary. Topiramate may be associated (rarely) with severe oligohydrosis and hyperthermia, most frequently in children; use caution and monitor closely during strenuous exercise, during exposure to high environmental temperature, or in patients receiving receiving other carbonic anhydrase inhibitors and drugs with anticholinergic activity. Potentially significant interactions may exist, requiring dose or frequency adjustment, additional monitoring, and/or selection of alternative therapy. Consult drug interactions database for more detailed information.

Avoid abrupt withdrawal of topiramate therapy; it should be withdrawn/tapered slowly to minimize the potential of increased seizure frequency. Doses were also gradually withdrawn in migraine prophylaxis studies.

Drug Interactions

Avoid Concomitant Use

Avoid concomitant use of Topiramate with any of the following: Alcohol (Ethyl); Axitinib; Azelastine (Nasal); Carbonic Anhydrase Inhibitors; Paraldehyde; Simeprevir; Thalidomide

Decreased Effect

Topiramate may decrease the levels/effects of: ARIPiprazole; Axitinib; Contraceptives (Estrogens); Contraceptives (Progestins); Ibrutinib; Methenamine; Primidone; Saxagliptin; Simeprevir

The levels/effects of Topiramate may be decreased by: CarBAMazepine; Fosphenytoin; Ketorolac (Nasal); Ketorolac (Systemic); Mefloquine; Orlistat; Phenytoin

Increased Effect/Toxicity

Topiramate may increase the levels/effects of: Alpha-/Beta-Agonists; Amphetamines; Anticonvulsants (Barbiturate); Anticonvulsants (Hydantoin); Azelastine (Nasal); Buprenorphine; Carbonic Anhydrase Inhibitors; CNS Depressants; Flecainide; Fosphenytoin; Hydrocodone; Lithium; Memantine; MetFORMIN; Methotrimeprazine; Metyrosine; Mirtazapine; Paraldehyde; Phenytoin; Pramipexole; Primidone; QuiNIDine; ROPINIRole; Rotigotine; Selective Serotonin Reuptake Inhibitors; Thalidomide; Valproic Acid and Derivatives; Zolpidem

The levels/effects of Topiramate may be increased by: Alcohol (Ethyl); Anticholinergic Agents; Brimonidine (Topical); Doxylamine; Droperidol; HydrOXYzine; Loop Diuretics; Magnesium Sulfate; Methotrimeprazine; Perampanel; Salicylates; Sodium Oxybate; Tapentadol; Thiazide Diuretics

Nutritional/Ethanol Interactions

Ethanol: May increase CNS depression; monitor for increased effects with coadministration. Caution patients about effects.

Food: Ketogenic diet may increase the possibility of acidosis and/or kidney stones.

Herb/Nutraceutical: Avoid evening primrose (seizure threshold decreased).

Adverse Reactions Adverse events are reported for placebo-controlled trials of adjunctive therapy in adult and pediatric patients. Unless otherwise noted, the percentages refer to incidence in epilepsy trials. **Note:** A wide range of dosages were studied; incidence of adverse events was frequently lower in the pediatric population studied.

>10%:

Central nervous system: Paresthesia (migraine trial: 35% to 51%; epilepsy trials: 1% to 11%), drowsiness (15% to 29%), dizziness (4% to 25%; dose dependent), nervousness (9% to 18%), fatigue (9% to 16%; dose dependent), ataxia (4% to 16%), psychomotor retardation (3% to 13%; dose dependent), impaired speech (2% to 13%), memory impairment (2% to 12%), abnormal behavior (children 11%), confusion (4% to 11%)

Endocrine & metabolic: Decreased serum bicarbonate (dose related: 7% to 67%; marked reductions [to <17 mEq/L] 1% to 11%)

Gastrointestinal: Anorexia (4% to 24%; dose dependent), nausea (6% to 10%; migraine trial: 9% to 14%)

Ophthalmic: Visual disturbance (2% to 13%)

Renal: Increased serum creatinine (children and adolescents 12-16 years 18%; with 100 mg dose)

Respiratory: Upper respiratory infection (migraine trial: 12% to 14%)

Miscellaneous: Accidental injury (14%)

1% to 10%:

Cardiovascular: Chest pain (2% to 4%), edema (2%), hypertension (1% to 2%), bradycardia (1%), pallor (1%), syncope (1%)

Central nervous system: Lack of concentration (5% to 10%), depression (5% to 9%; dose dependent), aggressive behavior (2% to 9%), insomnia (4% to 8%), mood disorder (≤6%), ataxia (4%), agitation (3%), cognitive dysfunction (3%), emotional lability (3%), anxiety (2% to 3%; dose dependent), hypoesthesia (2%; migraine trial: 6% to 8%), stupor (2%), vertigo (2%), fever (migraine trial: 1% to 2%), apathy (1%), hallucination (1%), hyporeflexia (2%),

neurosis (1%), psychosis (1%), rigors (1%), seizure (1%), suicide attempt (1%)

Dermatologic: Pruritus (migraine trial: 2% to 4%), dermatological reaction (2% to 3%), alopecia (2%), dermatitis (2%), hypertrichosis (2%), erythematous rash (1% to 2%), body odor (1%), diaphoresis (1%), eczema (1%), seborrhea (1%), skin discoloration (1%)

Endocrine & metabolic: Decreased serum phosphate (6%), mastalgia (4%), amenorrhea (2%), hypermenorrhea (2%), increased thirst (2%), hot flash (1% to 2%), menstrual disease (1% to 2%), decreased libido (<1% to 2%), hypoglycemia (1%), weight gain (1%), metabolic acidosis (hyperchloremia, nonanion gap)

Gastrointestinal: Weight loss (4% to 9%), dyspepsia (2% to 7%), abdominal pain (5% to 6%), sialorrhea (6%), constipation (4% to 5%), gastroenteritis (2% to 3%), vomiting (migraine trial: 1% to 3%), diarrhea (2%; migraine trial: 9% to 11%), dysgeusia (2%; migraine trial: 8% to 15%), xerostomia (2%), loss of sense of taste (migraine trial: ≤2%), appetite increased (1%), dysphagia (1%), fecal incontinence (1%), flatulence (1%), gastroesophageal reflux disease (1%), gingival hyperplasia (1%), gingivitis (1%), glossitis (1%)

Genitourinary: Urinary incontinence (2% to 4%), premature ejaculation (migraine trial: ≤3%), cystitis (2%), hematuria (2%), leukorrhea (2%), prostatic disease (2%), urinary tract infection (2%), impotence (1%), nocturia (1%), urine abnormality (1%)

Hematologic & oncologic: Purpura (8%), leukopenia (2%), anemia (1%), hematoma (1%), prolonged prothrombin time (1%), thrombocytopenia (1%)

Hepatic: Increased serum alkaline phosphatase (3%)

Hypersensitivity: Hypersensitivity reaction (2%)

Infection: Viral infection (2% to 7%: migraine trial: 3% to 4%), infection (2%), candidiasis (1%)

Neuromuscular & skeletal: Tremor (3% to 9%), abnormal gait (3% to 8%), arthralgia (migraine trial: 1% to 7%), weakness (6%), hyperkinesia (5%), back pain (1% to 5%), muscle spasm (2%; migraine trial: 2% to 4%), leg cramps (2%), leg pain (2%), myalgia (2%), musculoskeletal pain (1%)

Ophthalmic: Nystagmus (10%), diplopia (1% to 10%), eye disease (2%), abnormal lacrimation (1%), conjunctivitis (1%), myopia (1%)

Otic: Auditory impairment (2%), tinnitus (2%), otitis media (migraine trial: 1% to 2%)

Renal: Nephrolithiasis (1% to 7%; migraine trial ≤2%)

Respiratory: Rhinitis (4% to 7%), pharyngitis (6%), sinusitis (5%; migraine trial: 6% to 10%), pneumonia (5%), cough (migraine trial: 2% to 4%), epistaxis (2% to 4%), bronchitis (migraine trial: 3%), flu-like symptoms (3%), dyspnea (migraine trial: 1% to 3%)

Product Availability Qudexy XR: FDA approved March 2014; availability anticipated in the second quarter of 2014.

Available Dosage Forms

Capsule Extended Release 24 Hour, Oral:
Trokendi XR: 25 mg, 50 mg, 100 mg, 200 mg

Capsule Sprinkle, Oral:
Topamax Sprinkle: 15 mg, 25 mg
Generic: 15 mg, 25 mg

Tablet, Oral:
Topamax: 25 mg, 50 mg, 100 mg, 200 mg
Topiragen: 25 mg, 50 mg, 100 mg, 200 mg
Generic: 25 mg, 50 mg, 100 mg, 200 mg

General Dosage Range Dosage adjustment recommended in patients with renal impairment

Oral:

Immediate release:
Children 2-9 years: Initial: 25 mg once daily **or** 1-3 mg/kg/day; Maintenance: 150-400 mg/day in 2 divided doses **or** 5-9 mg/kg/day in 2 divided doses

Children 10-16 years: Initial: 25 mg once or twice daily **or** 1-3 mg/kg/day; Maintenance: 5-9 mg/kg/day in 2 divided doses **or** 25-200 mg twice daily

Children ≥17 years: Initial: 25 mg once or twice daily; Maintenance: 100-200 mg twice daily

Adults: Initial: 25-50 mg/day in 1-2 divided doses; Maintenance: 50-200 mg twice daily

Extended release:
Children 6-9 years: Initial: 25 mg once daily **or** 1-3 mg/kg/day; maintenance: 5-9 mg/kg/day

Children 10-16 years: Initial: 25-50 mg once daily **or** 1-3 mg/kg/day; maintenance: 5-9 mg/kg/day in 2 divided doses **or** 400 mg once daily

Adults: Initial: 25-50 mg/day once daily; Maintenance: 200-400 mg once daily

Administration

Oral Administer without regard to meals. Administer the immediate release formulation in divided doses; do not break the tablets. Swallow the extended release (ER) capsules whole; do not sprinkle on food, chew, or crush. Avoid alcohol use with topiramate ER within 6 hours prior to and 6 hours after administration.

Sprinkle capsules may be swallowed whole or opened to sprinkle the entire contents on a small amount (~1 teaspoon) of soft food; swallow immediately and do not chew. Do not store mixture for future use.

Storage/Stability

Extended release capsules: Store at 25°C (77°F); excursions permitted at 15°C to 30°C (59°F to 86°F). Protect from moisture. Protect from light.

Sprinkle capsules: Store at or below 25°C (77°F). Protect from moisture.

Tablets: Store at 15°C to 30°C (59°F to 86°F). Protect from moisture.

Nursing Actions

Physical Assessment Monitor therapeutic response (seizure activity, force, type, duration) at beginning of therapy and throughout. Use and teach seizure/safety precautions. May cause weight loss; monitor weight periodically.

Patient Education

- Discuss specific use of drug and side effects with patient as it relates to treatment. (HCAHPS: During this hospital stay, were you given any medicine that you had not taken before? Before giving you any new medicine, how often did hospital staff tell you what the medicine was for? How often did hospital staff describe possible side effects in a way you could understand?)

- Patient may experience nausea, dysgeusia, lack of appetite, diarrhea, anxiety, fatigue, headache, xerostomia, or alopecia. Have patient report immediately to prescriber signs of hyperuricemia, signs of infection, illogical thinking, inability to focus, change in balance, severe dizziness, inability to eat, back pain, abdominal pain, hematuria, difficult urination, anhidrosis, paresthesia, significant weight loss, osteodynia, angina, memory impairment, myalgia, asthenia, tinnitus, difficulty speaking, tremors, difficulty walking, ecchymosis, hemorrhaging, or involuntary eye movements (HCAHPS).

- Educate patient about signs of a significant reaction (eg, wheezing; chest tightness; fever; itching; bad cough; blue skin color; seizures; or swelling of face, lips, tongue, or throat). **Note:** This is not a comprehensive list of all side effects. Patient should consult prescriber for additional questions.

Intended Use and Disclaimer: Should not be printed and given to patients. This information is intended to serve as a concise initial reference for healthcare professionals to use when discussing medications with a patient. You must ultimately rely on your own discretion, experience and judgment in diagnosing, treating and advising patients.

Related Information

Oral Medications That Should Not Be Crushed or Altered *on page 1712*

Topotecan (toe poe TEE kan)

Brand Names: U.S. Hycamtin

Index Terms Hycamptamine; SKF 104864; SKF 104864-A; Topotecan Hydrochloride

Pharmacologic Category Antineoplastic Agent, Camptothecin; Antineoplastic Agent, Topoisomerase I Inhibitor

Medication Safety Issues

Sound-alike/look-alike issues:

Hycamtin may be confused with Mycamine

Topotecan may be confused with irinotecan

High alert medication:

This medication is in a class the Institute for Safe Medication Practices (ISMP) includes among its list of drug classes which have a heightened risk of causing significant patient harm when used in error.

Pregnancy Risk Factor D

Lactation Excretion in breast milk unknown/not recommended

Breast-Feeding Considerations It is not known if topotecan is excreted in breast milk. Due to then potential for serious adverse reactions in the nursing infant, the manufacturer recommends to discontinue breast-feeding in women who are receiving topotecan.

Use

Cervical cancer: Treatment of recurrent or resistant (stage IVB) cervical cancer (in combination with cisplatin)

Ovarian cancer: Treatment of metastatic ovarian cancer

Small cell lung cancer (SCLC): Treatment of relapsed or refractory SCLC

Unlabeled Use Treatment of acute myeloid leukemia (induction in older adults), central nervous system lesions (metastatic from lung cancer), central nervous system lymphoma (primary), Ewing's sarcoma, merkel cell cancer, osteosarcoma, rhabdomyosarcoma (pediatrics), neuroblastoma (pediatrics)

Mechanism of Action/Effect Binds to topoisomerase I and stabilizes the cleavable complex so that religation of the cleaved DNA strand cannot occur. This results in the accumulation of cleavable complexes and single-strand DNA breaks. Topotecan acts in S phase of the cell cycle.

Contraindications Hypersensitivity to topotecan or any component of the formulation; severe bone marrow depression

Canadian labeling: Additional contraindications (not in U.S. labeling): Severe renal impairment (CrCl <20 mL/minute); pregnancy; breast-feeding

Warnings/Precautions Hazardous agent - use appropriate precautions for handling and disposal (NIOSH, 2012). **[U.S. Boxed Warning]: May cause neutropenia, which may be severe or lead to infection or fatalities. Monitor blood counts frequently. Do NOT administer to patients with baseline neutrophils <1500/mm³ and platelets <100,000/mm³.** The dose-limiting toxicity is bone marrow suppression (primarily neutropenia); may also cause thrombocytopenia and anemia. Neutropenia is not cumulative overtime. In a clinical study comparing I.V. to oral topotecan, G-CSF support was administered in a higher percentage of patients receiving oral topotecan (Eckerd,

2007). Topotecan-induced neutropenia may lead to neutropenic colitis (including fatalities); should be considered in patients presenting with neutropenia, fever and abdominal pain.

Diarrhea has been reported with oral topotecan; may be severe (requiring hospitalization); incidence may be higher in the elderly; educate patients on early recognition and proper management, including diet changes, increase in fluid intake, antidiarrheals, and antibiotics. Interstitial lung disease (ILD) (with fatalities) has been reported; discontinue use in patients with confirmed ILD diagnosis; risk factors for ILD include a history of ILD, pulmonary fibrosis, lung cancer, thoracic radiation, and the use of colony-stimulating factors or medication with pulmonary toxicity; monitor pulmonary symptoms (cough, fever, dyspnea, and/or hypoxia). Use caution in renal impairment; may require dose adjustment (use in severe renal impairment is contraindicated in the Canadian labeling). Potentially significant drug-drug interactions may exist, requiring dose or frequency adjustment, additional monitoring, and/or selection of alternative therapy. Topotecan exposure is increased when oral topotecan is used concurrently with P-glycoprotein inhibitors; avoid concurrent use.

Drug Interactions

Avoid Concomitant Use

Avoid concomitant use of Topotecan with any of the following: BCG; CloZAPine; Natalizumab; P-glycoprotein/ABCB1 Inhibitors; Pimecrolimus; Tacrolimus (Topical); Tofacitinib; Vaccines (Live)

Decreased Effect

Topotecan may decrease the levels/effects of: BCG; Coccidioidin Skin Test; Sipuleucel-T; Vaccines (Inactivated); Vaccines (Live)

The levels/effects of Topotecan may be decreased by: Echinacea; Fosphenytoin-Phenytoin

Increased Effect/Toxicity

Topotecan may increase the levels/effects of: CloZAPine; Leflunomide; Natalizumab; Tofacitinib; Vaccines (Live)

The levels/effects of Topotecan may be increased by: BCRP/ABCG2 Inhibitors; Denosumab; Filgrastim; P-glycoprotein/ABCB1 Inhibitors; Pimecrolimus; Platinum Derivatives; Roflumilast; Tacrolimus (Topical); Trastuzumab

Nutritional/Ethanol Interactions Ethanol: Avoid ethanol (due to GI irritation).

Adverse Reactions

>10%:

Central nervous system: Fatigue (6% to 29%), fever (5% to 28%), pain (5% to 23%), headache (18%)

Dermatologic: Alopecia (10% to 49%), rash (16%)

◀ Gastrointestinal: Nausea (8% to 64%), vomiting (10% to 45%), diarrhea (6% to 32%; Oral: grade 3: 4%; grade 4: ≤1%; onset: 9 days), constipation (5% to 29%), abdominal pain (5% to 22%), anorexia (7% to 19%), stomatitis (18%)

Hematologic: Anemia (89% to 98%; grade 4: 7% to 37%; nadir: 15 days), neutropenia (83% to 97%; grade 4: 32% to 80%; nadir 12-15 days; duration: 7 days), leukopenia (86% to 97%; grade 4: 15% to 32%), thrombocytopenia (69% to 81%; grade 4: 6% to 27%; nadir: 15 days; duration: 3-5 days), neutropenic fever/sepsis (2% to 43%)

Neuromuscular & skeletal: Weakness (3% to 25%)

Respiratory: Dyspnea (6% to 22%), cough (15%)

Miscellaneous: Infection (≤17%)

1% to 10%:

Gastrointestinal: Obstruction (5%)

Hepatic: Liver enzymes increased (transient; 8%; grades 3/4: 4%), bilirubin increased (grades 3/4: <2%)

Neuromuscular & skeletal: Paresthesia (7%)

Respiratory: Pneumonia (8%)

Miscellaneous: Sepsis (grades 3/4: 5%)

Available Dosage Forms

Capsule, Oral:

Hycamtin: 0.25 mg, 1 mg

Solution, Intravenous:

Generic: 4 mg/4 mL (4 mL)

Solution Reconstituted, Intravenous:

Hycamtin: 4 mg (1 ea)

Generic: 4 mg (1 ea)

Solution Reconstituted, Intravenous [preservative free]:

Generic: 4 mg (1 ea)

General Dosage Range Dosage adjustment recommended in patients with renal impairment or who develop toxicities

Oral: *Adults:* 2.3 mg/m^2/day for 5 days; repeated every 21 days

I.V.: *Adults:* IVPB: 1.5 mg/m^2/day for 5 days; repeated every 21 days **or** 0.75 mg/m^2/day for 3 days; repeated every 21 days

Administration

I.V. Administer IVPB over 30 minutes. For combination chemotherapy with cisplatin, administer pretreatment hydration.

Hazardous agent; use appropriate precautions for handling and disposal (NIOSH, 2012).

Oral Administer without regard to meals. Swallow whole; do not crush, chew, or divide capsule. If vomiting occurs after dose, do not take replacement dose.

Hazardous agent; use appropriate precautions for handling and disposal (NIOSH, 2012).

Preparation for Administration Hazardous agent; use appropriate precautions for handling and disposal (NIOSH, 2012). Reconstitute

lyophilized powder with 4 mL SWFI. Further dilute in 50-100 mL D$_5$W or NS for infusion.

Storage/Stability

I.V.:

Solution for injection: Store intact vials at 2°C to 8°C (36°F to 45°F). Protect from light. Single-use vials should be discarded after initial vial entry; solutions for infusion are stable for 24 hours at room temperature after diluted.

Lyophilized powder: Store intact vials at room temperature of 20°C to 25°C (68°F to 77°F). Protect from light. Reconstituted solution is stable for up to 28 days at room temperature of 20°C to 25°C (68°F to 77°F), although the manufacturer recommends use immediately after reconstitution. Further dilute in 50-100 mL D$_5$W or NS. This solution is stable for 24 hours at room temperature (manufacturer recommendation) or up to 7 days under refrigeration (Craig, 1997).

Oral: Store at 2°C to 8°C (36°F to 46°F). Protect from light.

Nursing Actions

Physical Assessment Evaluate renal function (I & O, edema) and monitor for signs of myelosuppression, gastrointestinal disturbance (nausea, vomiting, diarrhea, pain), and dyspnea prior to each infusion and on a regular basis with oral formulation.

Patient Education

• Discuss specific use of drug and side effects with patient as it relates to treatment. (HCAHPS: During this hospital stay, were you given any medicine that you had not taken before? Before giving you any new medicine, how often did hospital staff tell you what the medicine was for? How often did hospital staff describe possible side effects in a way you could understand?)

• Patient may experience anemia, leukopenia, thrombocytopenia, fatigue, headache, nausea, dyspepsia, constipation, diarrhea, alopecia, stomatitis, or rash. Have patient report immediately to prescriber signs of infection, dyspnea, ecchymosis, discolored urine, jaundice, or inability to eat (HCAHPS).

• Educate patient about signs of a significant reaction (eg, wheezing; chest tightness; fever; itching; bad cough; blue skin color; seizures; or swelling of face, lips, tongue, or throat). **Note:** This is not a comprehensive list of all side effects. Patient should consult prescriber for additional questions.

Intended Use and Disclaimer: Should not be printed and given to patients. This information is intended to serve as a concise initial reference for healthcare professionals to use when discussing medications with a patient. You must ultimately rely on your own discretion, experience and judgment in diagnosing, treating and advising patients.

Dietary Considerations May be taken without regard to meals.

Related Information

Management of Drug Extravasations *on page 1700*

Oral Medications That Should Not Be Crushed or Altered *on page 1712*

Toremifene (tore EM i feen)

Brand Names: U.S. Fareston

Index Terms FC1157a; Toremifene Citrate

Pharmacologic Category Antineoplastic Agent, Estrogen Receptor Antagonist; Selective Estrogen Receptor Modulator (SERM)

Medication Safety Issues

Sound-alike/look-alike issues:

Toremifene may be confused with ospemifene, raloxifene

Pregnancy Risk Factor D

Lactation Excretion in breast milk unknown/not recommended

Use Treatment of metastatic breast cancer in postmenopausal women with estrogen receptor positive or estrogen receptor status unknown

Unlabeled Use Treatment of soft tissue sarcoma (desmoid tumors)

Available Dosage Forms

Tablet, Oral:

Fareston: 60 mg

General Dosage Range Oral: *Adults:* 60 mg once daily

Administration

Oral Administer orally, as a single daily dose, with or without food.

Hazardous agent; use appropriate precautions for handling and disposal (NIOSH, 2012).

Nursing Actions

Physical Assessment Monitor for thromboembolism, MI, edema, hypercalcemia, endometriosis, nausea, vomiting, and vision changes.

Patient Education

• Discuss specific use of drug and side effects with patient as it relates to treatment. (HCAHPS: During this hospital stay, were you given any medicine that you had not taken before? Before giving you any new medicine, how often did hospital staff tell you what the medicine was for? How often did hospital staff describe possible side effects in a way you could understand?)

• Patient may experience flushing, nausea, or vaginal discharge. Have patient report immediately to prescriber angina, tachycardia, syncope, dyspnea, edema or pain in leg or arm, diarrhea, paresthesia, strength differences from one side to another, or rash (HCAHPS).

• Educate patient about signs of a significant reaction (eg, wheezing; chest tightness; fever; itching; bad cough; blue skin color; seizures; or swelling of face, lips, tongue, or throat). **Note:** This is not a comprehensive list of all side effects. Patient should consult prescriber for additional questions.

Intended Use and Disclaimer: Should not be printed and given to patients. This information is intended to serve as a concise initial reference for healthcare professionals to use when discussing medications with a patient. You must ultimately rely on your own discretion, experience and judgment in diagnosing, treating and advising patients.

Related Information

Oral Medications That Should Not Be Crushed or Altered *on page 1712*

Torsemide (TORE se mide)

Brand Names: U.S. Demadex

Pharmacologic Category Antihypertensive; Diuretic, Loop

Medication Safety Issues

Sound-alike/look-alike issues:

Torsemide may be confused with furosemide

Demadex may be confused with Denorex

Pregnancy Risk Factor B

Lactation Excretion in breast milk unknown/use caution

Breast-Feeding Considerations It is not known if torsemide is excreted in breast milk. The manufacturer recommends that caution be exercised when administering torsemide to nursing women.

Use Management of edema associated with heart failure and hepatic or renal disease (including chronic renal failure); treatment of hypertension

Mechanism of Action/Effect Inhibits reabsorption of sodium and chloride in the ascending loop of Henle and distal renal tubule, interfering with the chloride-binding cotransport system, thus causing increased excretion of water, sodium, chloride, magnesium, and calcium; does not alter GFR, renal plasma flow, or acid-base balance

Contraindications Hypersensitivity to torsemide, any component of the formulation, or any sulfonylurea; anuria

Warnings/Precautions Loop diuretics are potent diuretics; excess amounts can lead to profound diuresis with fluid and electrolyte loss; close medical supervision and dose evaluation are required. Potassium supplementation and/or use of potassium-sparing diuretics may be necessary to prevent hypokalemia. Use with caution in patients with cirrhosis; avoid sudden changes in fluid and electrolyte balance and acid/base status which may lead to hepatic encephalopathy. Administration with an aldosterone antagonist or potassium-sparing diuretic may provide additional diuretic efficacy ▶

1547

and maintain normokalemia. Coadministration of antihypertensives may increase the risk of hypotension.

Monitor fluid status and renal function in an attempt to prevent oliguria, azotemia, and reversible increases in BUN and creatinine; close medical supervision of aggressive diuresis required. Ototoxicity has been demonstrated following oral administration of torsemide and following rapid I.V. administration of other loop diuretics. Other possible risk factors may include use in renal impairment, excessive doses, and concurrent use of other ototoxins (eg, aminoglycosides).

Chemical similarities are present among sulfonamides, sulfonylureas, carbonic anhydrase inhibitors, thiazides, and loop diuretics (except ethacrynic acid). Use in patients with sulfonylurea allergy is specifically contraindicated in product labeling; a risk of cross-reaction exists in patients with allergy to any of these compounds; avoid use when previous reaction has been severe. Discontinue if signs of hypersensitivity are noted.

Drug Interactions
Avoid Concomitant Use There are no known interactions where it is recommended to avoid concomitant use.

Decreased Effect
Torsemide may decrease the levels/effects of: Hypoglycemic Agents; Lithium; Neuromuscular-Blocking Agents

The levels/effects of Torsemide may be decreased by: Bile Acid Sequestrants; CYP2C9 Inducers (Strong); Dabrafenib; Fosphenytoin; Herbs (Hypertensive Properties); Methotrexate; Methylphenidate; Nonsteroidal Anti-Inflammatory Agents; Peginterferon Alfa-2b; Phenytoin; Probenecid; Salicylates; Yohimbine

Increased Effect/Toxicity
Torsemide may increase the levels/effects of: ACE Inhibitors; Allopurinol; Amifostine; Aminoglycosides; Antihypertensives; Cardiac Glycosides; CISplatin; Dofetilide; DULoxetine; Hypotensive Agents; Ivabradine; Lithium; Methotrexate; Neuromuscular-Blocking Agents; Obinutuzumab; RisperiDONE; RiTUXimab; Salicylates; Sodium Phosphates; Topiramate; Warfarin

The levels/effects of Torsemide may be increased by: Alfuzosin; Analgesics (Opioid); Beta2-Agonists; Brimonidine (Topical); Corticosteroids (Orally Inhaled); Corticosteroids (Systemic); CycloSPORINE (Systemic); CYP2C9 Inhibitors (Moderate); CYP2C9 Inhibitors (Strong); Diazoxide; Eltrombopag; Herbs (Hypotensive Properties); Licorice; MAO Inhibitors; Methotrexate; Mifepristone; Pentoxifylline; Phosphodiesterase 5 Inhibitors; Probenecid; Prostacyclin Analogues

Nutritional/Ethanol Interactions Herb/Nutraceutical: Avoid herbs with *hypertensive* properties (bayberry, blue cohosh, cayenne, ephedra, ginger,

ginseng [American], kola, licorice); may diminish the antihypertensive effect of torsemide. Avoid herbs with *hypotensive* properties (black cohosh, California poppy, coleus, golden seal, hawthorn, mistletoe, periwinkle, quinine, shepherd's purse); may enhance the hypotensive effect of torsemide.

Adverse Reactions 1% to 10%:
Cardiovascular: ECG abnormality (2%), chest pain (1%)
Central nervous system: Nervousness (1%)
Gastrointestinal: Constipation (2%), diarrhea (2%), dyspepsia (2%), nausea (2%), sore throat (2%)
Genitourinary: Excessive urination (7%)
Neuromuscular & skeletal: Arthralgia (2%), myalgia (2%), weakness (2%)
Respiratory: Rhinitis (3%), cough (2%)

Pharmacodynamics/Kinetics
Onset of Action Diuresis: Oral: Within 1 hour; Peak effect: Diuresis: Oral: 1-2 hours; Antihypertensive: Oral: 4-6 weeks (up to 12 weeks)
Duration of Action Diuresis: Oral: ~6-8 hours

Available Dosage Forms
Solution, Intravenous:
Generic: 20 mg/2 mL (2 mL); 50 mg/5 mL (5 mL)
Tablet, Oral:
Demadex: 5 mg, 10 mg, 20 mg, 100 mg
Generic: 5 mg, 10 mg, 20 mg, 100 mg

General Dosage Range
I.V.: *Adults:* 10-200 mg once daily
Oral: *Adults:* 5-200 mg once daily (maximum: 200 mg/day)

Administration
I.V. Administer over ≥2 minutes; reserve I.V. administration for situations which require rapid onset of action.

Injectable Detail pH: >8.3

Oral Administer without regard to meals; patients may be switched from the I.V. form to the oral (and vice-versa) with no change in dose.

Storage/Stability
I.V.: Store at 15°C to 30°C (59°F to 86°F). If torsemide is to be administered via continuous infusion, stability has been demonstrated through 24 hours at room temperature in plastic containers for the following fluids and concentrations:
200 mg torsemide (10 mg/mL) added to 250 mL D_5W, 250 mL NS or 500 mL 0.45% sodium chloride
50 mg torsemide (10 mg/mL) added to 500 mL D_5W, 500 mL NS, or 500 mL 0.45% sodium chloride
Tablets: Store at 15°C to 30°C (59°F to 86°F).

Nursing Actions
Physical Assessment Assess for allergy to sulfonylurea before beginning therapy. Monitor for dehydration, electrolyte imbalance, and postural hypotension on a regular basis during therapy.

Patient Education

- Discuss specific use of drug and side effects with patient as it relates to treatment. (HCAHPS: During this hospital stay, were you given any medicine that you had not taken before? Before giving you any new medicine, how often did hospital staff tell you what the medicine was for? How often did hospital staff describe possible side effects in a way you could understand?)
- Patient may experience hypokalemia, dizziness, headache, dyspepsia, nausea, xerostomia, constipation, or diarrhea. Have patient report immediately to prescriber significant weight gain, edema, hearing impairment, or rash (HCAHPS).
- Educate patient about signs of a significant reaction (eg, wheezing; chest tightness; fever; itching; bad cough; blue skin color; seizures; or swelling of face, lips, tongue, or throat). **Note:** This is not a comprehensive list of all side effects. Patient should consult prescriber for additional questions.

Intended Use and Disclaimer: Should not be printed and given to patients. This information is intended to serve as a concise initial reference for healthcare professionals to use when discussing medications with a patient. You must ultimately rely on your own discretion, experience and judgment in diagnosing, treating and advising patients.

Dietary Considerations May be taken without regard to meals; however, food slows the rate and reduces the extent of absorption and may reduce diuretic efficacy (Bard, 2004). May require increased intake of potassium-rich foods.

TraMADol (TRA ma dole)

Brand Names: U.S. ConZip; Rybix ODT [DSC]; Ultram; Ultram ER
Index Terms Tramadol Hydrochloride
Pharmacologic Category Analgesic, Opioid
Medication Safety Issues
   Sound-alike/look-alike issues:
   TraMADol may be confused with tapentadol, Toradol Trandate, traZODone, Voltaren
   Ultram may be confused with Ultane, Ultracet, Voltaren
   International issues:
   Theradol [Netherlands] may be confused with Foradil brand name for formoterol [U.S., Canada, and multiple international markets], Terazol brand name for terconazole [U.S. and Canada], and Toradol brand name for ketorolac [Canada and multiple international markets]
   Trexol [Mexico] may be confused with Trexall brand name for methotrexate [U.S.]; Truxal brand name for chlorprothixene [multiple international markets]
Pregnancy Risk Factor C
Lactation Enters breast milk/not recommended

Breast-Feeding Considerations Tramadol is excreted into breast milk. Sixteen hours following a single 100 mg I.V. dose, the amount of tramadol found in breast milk was 0.1% of the maternal dose. Use is not recommended by the manufacturer for postdelivery analgesia in nursing mothers. Some Canadian products are contraindicated for use in nursing women. Nursing infants exposed to large doses of opioids should be monitored for apnea and sedation (Montgomery, 2012).

Use Relief of moderate to moderately-severe pain Extended release formulations are indicated for patients requiring around-the-clock management of moderate to moderately-severe pain for an extended period of time

Mechanism of Action/Effect Tramadol and its active metabolite (M1) binds to μ-opiate receptors in the CNS causing inhibition of ascending pain pathways, altering the perception of and response to pain; also inhibits the reuptake of norepinephrine and serotonin, which are neurotransmitters involved in the descending inhibitory pain pathway responsible for pain relief (Grond, 2004)

Contraindications Hypersensitivity to tramadol, opioids, or any component of the formulation
Additional contraindications for Ultram®, Rybix™ ODT, and Ultram® ER: Any situation where opioids are contraindicated, including acute intoxication with alcohol, hypnotics, centrally-acting analgesics, opioids, or psychotropic drugs
Additional contraindications for ConZip: Severe/acute bronchial asthma, hypercapnia, or significant respiratory depression in the absence of appropriately monitored setting and/or resuscitative equipment

Canadian product labeling:
   Tramadol is contraindicated during or within 14 days following MAO inhibitor therapy
   Extended release formulations: Additional contraindications:
   Ralivia™, Tridural™: Severe (CrCl <30 mL/minute) renal dysfunction, severe (Child-Pugh class C) hepatic dysfunction
   Durela™ and Zytram® XL: Severe (CrCl <30 mL/minute) renal dysfunction, severe (Child-Pugh class C) hepatic dysfunction; known or suspected mechanical GI obstruction or any disease/condition that affects bowel transit; mild, intermittent or short-duration pain that can be managed with other pain medication; management of peri-operative pain; obstructive airway, acute respiratory depression, cor pulmonale, delirium tremens, seizure disorder, severe CNS depression, increased cerebrospinal or intracranial pressure, head injury, breastfeeding, pregnancy; use during labor and delivery

Warnings/Precautions Rare but serious anaphylactoid reactions (including fatalities) often following initial dosing have been reported. Pruritus, hives, bronchospasm, angioedema, toxic epidermal necrolysis (TEN) and Stevens-Johnson syndrome also have been reported with use. Previous anaphylactoid reactions to opioids may increase risks for similar reactions to tramadol. Caution patients to swallow extended release tablets whole. Rapid release and absorption of tramadol from extended release tablets that are broken, crushed, or chewed may lead to a potentially lethal overdose. May cause CNS depression, which may impair physical or mental abilities; patients must be cautioned about performing tasks which require mental alertness (eg, operating machinery or driving). May cause CNS depression and/or respiratory depression, particularly when combined with other CNS depressants. Use with caution and reduce dosage when administered to patients receiving other CNS depressants. An increased risk of seizures may occur in patients receiving serotonin reuptake inhibitors (SSRIs or anorectics), tricyclic antidepressants or other cyclic compounds (including cyclobenzaprine, promethazine), neuroleptics, drugs which may lower seizure threshold, or drugs which impair metabolism of tramadol (ie, CYP2D6 and 3A4 inhibitors). Patients with a history of seizures, or with a risk of seizures (head trauma, metabolic disorders, CNS infection, or malignancy, or during ethanol/drug withdrawal) are also at increased risk. Potentially significant drug interactions may exist, requiring dose or frequency adjustment, additional monitoring, and/or selection of alternative therapy.

Elderly (particularly >75 years of age), debilitated patients and patients with chronic respiratory disorders may be at greater risk of adverse events. Use with caution in patients with increased intracranial pressure or head injury. Avoid use in patients who are suicidal or addiction prone; use with caution in patients taking tranquilizers and/or antidepressants, or those with an emotional disturbance including depression. Healthcare provider should be alert to problems of abuse, misuse, and diversion. Use caution in heavy alcohol users. Use caution in treatment of acute abdominal conditions; may mask pain. Use tramadol with caution and reduce dosage in patients with liver disease or renal dysfunction. Avoid using extended release tablets in severe hepatic impairment. Tolerance or drug dependence may result from extended use (withdrawal symptoms have been reported); abrupt discontinuation should be avoided. Tapering of dose at the time of discontinuation limits the risk of withdrawal symptoms. Some products may contain phenylalanine.

After chronic maternal exposure to opioids, neonatal withdrawal syndrome may occur in the newborn; monitor neonate closely. Signs and symptoms include irritability, hyperactivity and abnormal sleep pattern, high pitched cry, tremor, vomiting, diarrhea and failure to gain weight.

Onset, duration and severity depend on the drug used, duration of use, maternal dose, and rate of drug elimination by the newborn. Opioid withdrawal syndrome in the neonate, unlike in adults, may be life-threatening and should be treated according to protocols developed by neonatology experts.

Drug Interactions

Avoid Concomitant Use

Avoid concomitant use of TraMADol with any of the following: Azelastine (Nasal); CarBAMazepine; Conivaptan; Fusidic Acid (Systemic); Paraldehyde; Thalidomide

Decreased Effect

TraMADol may decrease the levels/effects of: CarBAMazepine; Pegvisomant

The levels/effects of TraMADol may be decreased by: Ammonium Chloride; Antiemetics (5HT3 Antagonists); Bosentan; CarBAMazepine; CYP2D6 Inhibitors (Moderate); CYP2D6 Inhibitors (Strong); CYP3A4 Inducers (Strong); Dabrafenib; Deferasirox; Mitotane; Mixed Agonist / Antagonist Opioids; Tocilizumab

Increased Effect/Toxicity

TraMADol may increase the levels/effects of: Alcohol (Ethyl); Alvimopan; Antipsychotics; Azelastine (Nasal); CarBAMazepine; CNS Depressants; Desmopressin; Diuretics; Hydrocodone; MAO Inhibitors; Metoclopramide; Metyrosine; Paraldehyde; Pramipexole; ROPINIRole; Rotigotine; Selective Serotonin Reuptake Inhibitors; Serotonin Modulators; Thalidomide; Tricyclic Antidepressants; Vitamin K Antagonists; Zolpidem

The levels/effects of TraMADol may be increased by: Amphetamines; Anticholinergics; Antipsychotic Agents (Phenothiazines); Antipsychotics; Brimonidine (Topical); Cannabinoids; Conivaptan; Cyclobenzaprine; CYP3A4 Inhibitors (Moderate); CYP3A4 Inhibitors (Strong); Dasatinib; Doxylamine; Fusidic Acid (Systemic); HydrOXYzine; Ivacaftor; Luliconazole; Magnesium Sulfate; Mifepristone; Perampanel; Selective Serotonin Reuptake Inhibitors; Simeprevir; Sodium Oxybate; Succinylcholine; Tricyclic Antidepressants

Nutritional/Ethanol Interactions

Ethanol: May increase CNS depression; monitor for increased effects with coadministration. Caution patients about effects.

Food:

Immediate release tablet: Rate and extent of absorption were not significantly affected.

Extended release:

ConZip™: Rate and extent of absorption were unaffected.

Ultram® ER: High-fat meal reduced C_{max} and AUC, and increased T_{max} by 3 hours.

Orally disintegrating tablet: Food delays the time to peak serum concentration by 30 minutes; extent of absorption was not significantly affected.

Herb/Nutraceutical: Avoid valerian, St John's wort, kava kava, gotu kola (may increase CNS depression).

Adverse Reactions

>10%:

Cardiovascular: Flushing (8% to 16%)

Central nervous system: Dizziness (10% to 33%), headache (4% to 32%), somnolence (7% to 25%), insomnia (2% to 11%)

Dermatologic: Pruritus (3% to 12%)

Gastrointestinal: Constipation (9% to 46%), nausea (15% to 40%), vomiting (5% to 17%), dyspepsia (1% to 13%)

Neuromuscular & skeletal: Weakness (4% to 12%)

1% to 10%:

Cardiovascular: Orthostatic hypotension (2% to 5%), chest pain (1% to <5%), hypertension (1% to <5%), peripheral edema (1% to <5%), vasodilation (1% to <5%)

Central nervous system: Agitation (1% to <5%), anxiety (1% to <5%), apathy (1% to <5%), chills (1% to <5%), confusion (1% to <5%), coordination impaired (1% to <5%), depersonalization (1% to <5%), depression (1% to <5%), euphoria (1% to <5%), fever (1% to <5%), hypoesthesia (1% to <5%), lethargy (1% to <5%), nervousness (1% to <5%), pain (1% to <5%), pyrexia (1% to <5%), restlessness (1% to <5%), malaise (<1% to <5%), fatigue (2%), vertigo (2%)

Dermatologic: Dermatitis (1% to <5%), rash (1% to <5%)

Endocrine & metabolic: Hot flashes (2% to 9%), hyperglycemia (1% to <5%), menopausal symptoms (1% to <5%)

Gastrointestinal: Diarrhea (5% to 10%), xerostomia (3% to 13%), anorexia (1% to 6%), abdominal pain (1% to <5%), appetite decreased (1% to <5%), weight loss (1% to <5%), flatulence (<1% to <5%)

Genitourinary: Pelvic pain (1% to <5%), prostatic disorder (1% to <5%), urine abnormalities (1% to <5%), urinary tract infection (1% to <5%), urinary frequency (<1% to <5%), urinary retention (<1% to <5%)

Neuromuscular & skeletal: Arthralgia (1% to 5%), back pain (1% to <5%), creatine phosphokinase increased (1% to <5%), myalgia (1% to <5%), hypertonia (1% to <5%), neck pain (1% to <5%), rigors (1% to <5%), paresthesia (1% to <5%), tremor (1% to <5%)

Ocular: Blurred vision (1% to <5%), miosis (1% to <5%)

Respiratory: Bronchitis (1% to <5%), congestion (nasal/sinus) (1% to <5%), cough (1% to <5%), dyspnea (1% to <5%), nasopharyngitis (1% to <5%), pharyngitis (1% to <5%), rhinitis (1% to <5%), rhinorrhea (1% to <5%), sinusitis (1% to <5%), sneezing (1% to <5%), sore throat (1% to <5%), upper respiratory infection (1% to <5%)

Miscellaneous: Diaphoresis (2% to 9%), flu-like syndrome (1% to <5%), withdrawal syndrome (1% to <5%), shivering (<1% to <5%)

A withdrawal syndrome may include anxiety, diarrhea, hallucinations (rare), nausea, pain, piloerection, rigors, sweating, and tremor. Uncommon discontinuation symptoms may include severe anxiety, panic attacks, or paresthesia.

Pharmacodynamics/Kinetics

Onset of Action Immediate release: ~1 hour

Duration of Action 9 hours

Available Dosage Forms

Capsule, variable release, oral: 150 mg [37.5 mg (immediate release) and 112.5 mg (extended release)]

ConZip™: 100 mg [25 mg (immediate release) and 75 mg (extended release)]

ConZip™: 200 mg [50 mg (immediate release) and 150 mg (extended release)]

ConZip™: 300 mg [50 mg (immediate release) and 250 mg (extended release)]

Tablet, oral: 50 mg

Ultram®: 50 mg

Tablet, extended release, oral: 100 mg, 200 mg, 300 mg

Ultram® ER: 100 mg, 200 mg, 300 mg

General Dosage Range Dosage adjustment recommended in patients with hepatic or renal impairment

Oral:

Immediate release:

Children ≥17 years: 50-100 mg every 4-6 hours (maximum: 400 mg/day)

Adults: 50-100 mg every 4-6 hours (maximum: 400 mg/day)

Elderly >75 years: Maximum: 300 mg/day

Extended release: *Adults:* 100-300 once daily (maximum: 300 mg/day)

Administration

Oral

Immediate release: Administer without regard to meals.

Extended release: Swallow whole; do not crush, chew, or split. **Note:** Durela™, Ralivia™, and Tridural™: Canadian availability; products not available in U.S.:

ConZip™, Zytram® XL, Durela™: May administer without regard to meals.

Ultram® ER, Ralivia™, Tridural™: May administer without regard to meals, but administer in a consistent manner of either with or without meals.

Orally-disintegrating tablet: Remove from foil blister by peeling back (do not push tablet through the foil). Place tablet on tongue and allow to dissolve (may take ~1 minute); water is not needed, but may be administered with water. Do not chew, break, or split tablet.

Storage/Stability Store at 25°C (77°F); excursions permitted to 15°C to 30°C (59°F to 86°F).

◀ **Nursing Actions**

Physical Assessment Assess patient's physical and/or psychological dependence. Discontinue slowly after prolonged use.

Patient Education

• Discuss specific use of drug and side effects with patient as it relates to treatment. (HCAHPS: During this hospital stay, were you given any medicine that you had not taken before? Before giving you any new medicine, how often did hospital staff tell you what the medicine was for? How often did hospital staff describe possible side effects in a way you could understand?)

• Patient may experience constipation, fatigue, xerostomia, or insomnia. Have patient report immediately to prescriber syncope, signs of depression (ie, suicidal ideation, anxiety, emotional instability, illogical thinking), considerable asthenia, angina, difficult urination, polyuria, dyspnea, vision changes, or serotonin syndrome (ie, dizziness, severe headache, agitation, hallucinations, tachycardia, arrhythmia, flushing, tremors, hyperhidrosis, change in balance, severe nausea, significant diarrhea), (HCAHPS).

• Educate patient about signs of a significant reaction (eg, wheezing; chest tightness; fever; itching; bad cough; blue skin color; seizures; or swelling of face, lips, tongue, or throat). **Note:** This is not a comprehensive list of all side effects. Patient should consult prescriber for additional questions.

Intended Use and Disclaimer: Should not be printed and given to patients. This information is intended to serve as a concise initial reference for healthcare professionals to use when discussing medications with a patient. You must ultimately rely on your own discretion, experience and judgment in diagnosing, treating and advising patients.

Dietary Considerations Some products may contain phenylalanine.

Related Information

Oral Medications That Should Not Be Crushed or Altered *on page 1712*

Trandolapril (tran DOE la pril)

Brand Names: U.S. Mavik

Pharmacologic Category Angiotensin-Converting Enzyme (ACE) Inhibitor; Antihypertensive

Pregnancy Risk Factor D

Lactation Excretion in breast milk unknown/not recommended

Breast-Feeding Considerations It is not known if trandolapril is excreted in breast milk. Breast-feeding is not recommended by the manufacturer.

Use Treatment of hypertension alone or in combination with other antihypertensive agents; treatment of post-myocardial infarction (MI) heart failure (HF) or post-MI left ventricular (LV) dysfunction after myocardial infarction (MI)

Note: The ACCF/AHA 2013 heart failure guidelines recommend the use of ACE inhibitors, along with other guideline directed medical therapies, to prevent heart failure in patients with a reduced ejection fraction who have a history of MI (Stage B HF), to prevent heart failure in any patient with a reduced ejection fraction (Stage B HF), or to treat those with heart failure and reduced ejection fraction (Stage C HFrEF) (ACCF/AHA [Yancy, 2013]).

Unlabeled Use To delay the progression of nephropathy and reduce risks of cardiovascular events in hypertensive patients with type 1 or 2 diabetes mellitus

Mechanism of Action/Effect Competitive inhibitor of angiotensin-converting enzyme (ACE); prevents conversion of angiotensin I to angiotensin II, a potent vasoconstrictor; results in lower levels of angiotensin II which causes an increase in plasma renin activity and a reduction in aldosterone secretion

Contraindications

Hypersensitivity to trandolapril or any component of the formulation; history of angioedema related to previous treatment with an ACE inhibitor; patients with idiopathic or hereditary angioedema; concomitant use with aliskiren in patients with diabetes mellitus

Canadian labeling: Additional contraindications (not in U.S. labeling): Women who are pregnant or planning to become pregnant; breast-feeding; concomitant use with aliskiren in patients with moderate-to-severe renal impairment (GFR <60 mL/minute/1.73 m^2)

Warnings/Precautions Anaphylactic reactions may occur rarely with ACE inhibitors. At any time during treatment (especially following first dose) angioedema may occur rarely with ACE inhibitors; it may involve the head and neck (potentially compromising the airway) or the intestine (presenting with abdominal pain). African-Americans and patients with idiopathic or hereditary angioedema may be at an increased risk. Prolonged frequent monitoring may be required especially if tongue, glottis, or larynx are involved as they are associated with airway obstruction. Patients with a history of airway surgery may have a higher risk of airway obstruction. Aggressive early and appropriate management is critical. Use in patients with previous angioedema associated with ACE inhibitor therapy is contraindicated. Severe anaphylactoid reactions may be seen during hemodialysis (eg, CVVHD) with high-flux dialysis membranes (eg, AN69). Rare cases of anaphylactoid reactions have been reported in patients undergoing sensitization treatment with hymenoptera (bee, wasp) venom while receiving ACE inhibitors.

Symptomatic hypotension with or without syncope can occur with ACE inhibitors (usually with the first several doses); effects are most often observed in volume-depleted patients; correct volume depletion prior to initiation; close monitoring of patient is required especially with initial dosing and dosing increases; blood pressure must be lowered at a rate appropriate for the patient's clinical condition. Initiation of therapy in patients with ischemic heart disease or cerebrovascular disease warrants close observation due to the potential consequences posed by falling blood pressure (eg, MI, stroke). Use with caution in hypertrophic cardiomyopathy with outflow tract obstruction, severe aortic stenosis, or before, during, or immediately after major surgery. **[U.S. Boxed Warning]: Drugs that act on the renin-angiotensin system can cause injury and death to the developing fetus. Discontinue as soon as possible once pregnancy is detected.**

Hyperkalemia may occur with ACE inhibitors; risk factors include renal dysfunction, diabetes mellitus, concomitant use of potassium-sparing diuretics, potassium supplements, and/or potassium-containing salts. Use cautiously, if at all, with these agents and monitor potassium closely. Cough may occur with ACE inhibitors. Other causes of cough should be considered (eg, pulmonary congestion in patients with heart failure) and excluded prior to discontinuation.

Dosage adjustment needed in severe renal dysfunction (CrCl <30 mL/minute) or hepatic cirrhosis. May be associated with deterioration of renal function and/or increases in serum creatinine, particularly in patients with low renal blood flow (eg, renal artery stenosis, heart failure) whose glomerular filtration rate (GFR) is dependent on efferent arteriolar vasoconstriction by angiotensin II; deterioration may result in oliguria, acute renal failure, and progressive azotemia. Small increases in serum creatinine may occur following initiation; consider discontinuation only in patients with progressive and/or significant deterioration in renal function. Use with caution in patients with unstented unilateral/bilateral renal artery stenosis. When unstented bilateral renal artery stenosis is present, use is generally avoided due to the elevated risk of deterioration in renal function unless possible benefits outweigh risks. Potentially significant drug-drug interactions may exist, requiring dose or frequency adjustment, additional monitoring, and/or selection of alternative therapy.

Rare toxicities associated with ACE inhibitors include cholestatic jaundice (which may progress to fulminant hepatic necrosis), agranulocytosis, neutropenia, or leukopenia with myeloid hypoplasia. Patients with collagen vascular diseases (especially with concomitant renal impairment) or renal impairment alone may be at increased risk for hematologic toxicity; periodically monitor CBC with differential in these patients.

Drug Interactions

Avoid Concomitant Use There are no known interactions where it is recommended to avoid concomitant use.

Decreased Effect

The levels/effects of Trandolapril may be decreased by: Antacids; Aprotinin; Herbs (Hypertensive Properties); Icatibant; Lanthanum; Methylphenidate; Nonsteroidal Anti-Inflammatory Agents; Salicylates; Yohimbine

Increased Effect/Toxicity

Trandolapril may increase the levels/effects of: Allopurinol; Amifostine; Antihypertensives; AzaTHIOprine; CycloSPORINE (Systemic); DULoxetine; Ferric Gluconate; Gold Sodium Thiomalate; Hypotensive Agents; Iron Dextran Complex; Lithium; Nonsteroidal Anti-Inflammatory Agents; Obinutuzumab; RiTUXimab; Sodium Phosphates

The levels/effects of Trandolapril may be increased by: Alfuzosin; Aliskiren; Angiotensin II Receptor Blockers; Brimonidine (Topical); Canagliflozin; Diazoxide; DPP-IV Inhibitors; Eplerenone; Everolimus; Heparin; Heparin (Low Molecular Weight); Herbs (Hypotensive Properties); Loop Diuretics; MAO Inhibitors; Pentoxifylline; Phosphodiesterase 5 Inhibitors; Potassium Salts; Potassium-Sparing Diuretics; Prostacyclin Analogues; Sirolimus; Temsirolimus; Thiazide Diuretics; TiZANidine; Tolvaptan; Trimethoprim

Nutritional/Ethanol Interactions Herb/Nutraceutical: Some herbal medications may worsen hypertension (eg, licorice); others may increase the antihypertensive effects of trandolapril (eg, shepherd's purse). Management: Avoid bayberry, blue cohosh, cayenne, ephedra, ginger, ginseng (American), kola, licorice, and yohimbe. Avoid black cohosh, California poppy, coleus, golden seal, hawthorn, mistletoe, periwinkle, quinine, and shepherd's purse.

Adverse Reactions Note: Frequency ranges include data from hypertension and heart failure trials. Higher rates of adverse reactions have generally been noted in patients with CHF. However, the frequency of adverse effects associated with placebo is also increased in this population.

>1%:

Cardiovascular: Hypotension (<1% to 11%), syncope (6%), bradycardia (<1% to 5%), cardiogenic shock (4%), intermittent claudication (4%)

Central nervous system: Dizziness (1% to 23%), stroke (3%)

Endocrine & metabolic: Uric acid increased (15%), hyperkalemia (5%), hypocalcemia (5%)

Gastrointestinal: Gastritis (4%), diarrhea (1%)

Neuromuscular & skeletal: Myalgia (5%), weakness (3%)

◀ Renal: BUN increased (9%), serum creatinine increased (1% to 5%)
Respiratory: Cough (2% to 35%)

Worsening of renal function may occur in patients with bilateral renal artery stenosis or hypovolemia. In addition, a syndrome which may include fever, myalgia, arthralgia, interstitial nephritis, vasculitis, rash, eosinophilia and positive ANA, and elevated ESR has been reported with ACE inhibitors. Eosinophilic pneumonitis has also been reported with other ACE inhibitors.

Pharmacodynamics/Kinetics

Onset of Action 1-2 hours; Peak effect: Reduction in blood pressure: 6 hours

Duration of Action Prolonged; 72 hours after single dose

Available Dosage Forms

Tablet, Oral:
Mavik: 1 mg, 2 mg, 4 mg
Generic: 1 mg, 2 mg, 4 mg

General Dosage Range Dosage adjustment recommended in patients with hepatic or renal impairment

Oral: *Adults:* Initial: 1-2 mg once daily; Maintenance: 1-4 mg once daily

Storage/Stability Store at controlled room temperature of 20°C to 25°C (68°F to 77°F).

Nursing Actions

Physical Assessment Assess potential for interactions with other pharmacological agents or herbal products that may impact fluid balance or cardiac status. Monitor for hypovolemia, angioedema, and postural hypotension with first doses and on a regular basis during therapy.

Patient Education

• Discuss specific use of drug and side effects with patient as it relates to treatment. (HCAHPS: During this hospital stay, were you given any medicine that you had not taken before? Before giving you any new medicine, how often did hospital staff tell you what the medicine was for? How often did hospital staff describe possible side effects in a way you could understand?)

• Patient may experience dizziness or parageusia. Have patient report immediately to prescriber signs of infection, syncope, dyspnea, hyperhidrosis, diarrhea, significant weight gain, edema in legs or abdomen, discolored urine, jaundice, or rash (HCAHPS).

• Educate patient about signs of a significant reaction (eg, wheezing; chest tightness; fever; itching; bad cough; blue skin color; seizures; or swelling of face, lips, tongue, or throat). **Note:** This is not a comprehensive list of all side effects. Patient should consult prescriber for additional questions.

Intended Use and Disclaimer: Should not be printed and given to patients. This information is intended to serve as a concise initial reference for healthcare professionals to use when discussing medications with a patient. You must ultimately rely on your own discretion, experience and judgment in diagnosing, treating and advising patients.

Trandolapril and Verapamil
(tran DOE la pril & ver AP a mil)

Brand Names: U.S. Tarka®
Index Terms Verapamil and Trandolapril
Pharmacologic Category Angiotensin-Converting Enzyme (ACE) Inhibitor; Antihypertensive; Calcium Channel Blocker
Pregnancy Risk Factor D
Use Treatment of hypertension; however, not indicated for initial treatment of hypertension

Available Dosage Forms

Tablet, variable release: Trandolapril 2 mg [immediate release] and verapamil 180 mg [sustained release]; Trandolapril 2 mg [immediate release] and verapamil 240 mg [sustained release]; Trandolapril 4 mg [immediate release] and verapamil 240 mg [sustained release]
Tarka®:
1/240: Trandolapril 1 mg [immediate release] and verapamil 240 mg [sustained release]
2/180: Trandolapril 2 mg [immediate release] and verapamil 180 mg [sustained release]
2/240: Trandolapril 2 mg [immediate release] and verapamil 240 mg [sustained release]
4/240: Trandolapril 4 mg [immediate release] and verapamil 240 mg [sustained release]

General Dosage Range Dosage adjustment recommended in patients with hepatic or renal impairment

Oral: *Adults:* Trandolapril 1-4 mg and verapamil 180-240 mg once daily

Nursing Actions

Physical Assessment See individual agents.

Patient Education

• Discuss specific use of drug and side effects with patient as it relates to treatment. (HCAHPS: During this hospital stay, were you given any medicine that you had not taken before? Before giving you any new medicine, how often did hospital staff tell you what the medicine was for? How often did hospital staff describe possible side effects in a way you could understand?)

• Patient may experience dizziness, headache, constipation, parageusia, or edema. Have patient report immediately to prescriber hyperhidrosis, emesis, or diarrhea (HCAHPS).

• Educate patient about signs of a significant reaction (eg, wheezing; chest tightness; fever; itching; bad cough; blue skin color; seizures; or swelling of face, lips, tongue, or throat). **Note:** This is not a comprehensive list of all side effects. Patient should consult prescriber for additional questions.

Intended Use and Disclaimer: Should not be printed and given to patients. This information is intended to serve as a concise initial reference for healthcare professionals to use when discussing medications with a patient. You must ultimately rely on your own discretion, experience and judgment in diagnosing, treating and advising patients.

Related Information

Trandolapril *on page 1552*

Verapamil *on page 1597*

Tranylcypromine (tran il SIP roe meen)

Brand Names: U.S. Parnate

Index Terms Transamine Sulphate; Tranylcypromine Sulfate

Pharmacologic Category Antidepressant, Monoamine Oxidase Inhibitor

Medication Guide Available Yes

Lactation Enters breast milk

Use Treatment of major depressive episode without melancholia

Available Dosage Forms

Tablet, Oral:

Parnate: 10 mg

Generic: 10 mg

General Dosage Range Oral: *Adults:* 10-30 mg twice daily (maximum: 60 mg/day)

Nursing Actions

Physical Assessment Monitor therapeutic response (eg, mental status, mood, affect, suicide ideation) at beginning of therapy and periodically throughout. Monitor blood pressure. Observe for clinical worsening, suicidality, or unusual behavior changes, especially during the initial few months of therapy or during dosage changes.

Patient Education

• Discuss specific use of drug and side effects with patient as it relates to treatment. (HCAHPS: During this hospital stay, were you given any medicine that you had not taken before? Before giving you any new medicine, how often did hospital staff tell you what the medicine was for? How often did hospital staff describe possible side effects in a way you could understand?)

• Patient may experience presyncope, fatigue, blurred vision, illogical thinking, dizziness, headache, constipation, or insomnia. Have patient report immediately to prescriber angina, tachycardia, dyspnea, nervousness, tremors, fasciculations, behavioral problems, severe nausea, or rash (HCAHPS).

• Educate patient about signs of a significant reaction (eg, wheezing; chest tightness; fever; itching; bad cough; blue skin color; seizures; or swelling of face, lips, tongue, or throat). **Note:** This is not a comprehensive list of all side effects. Patient should consult prescriber for additional questions.

Intended Use and Disclaimer: Should not be printed and given to patients. This information is intended to serve as a concise initial reference for healthcare professionals to use when discussing medications with a patient. You must ultimately rely on your own discretion, experience and judgment in diagnosing, treating and advising patients.

Trastuzumab (tras TU zoo mab)

Brand Names: U.S. Herceptin

Index Terms anti-c-erB-2; anti-ERB-2; Conventional Trastuzumab; MOAB HER2; rhuMAb HER2; Trastuzumab (Conventional)

Pharmacologic Category Antineoplastic Agent, Anti-HER2; Antineoplastic Agent, Monoclonal Antibody

Medication Safety Issues

Sound-alike/look-alike issues:

Trastuzumab may be confused with ado-trastuzumab emtansine, pertuzumab

High alert medication:

This medication is in a class the Institute for Safe Medication Practices (ISMP) includes among its list of drug classes which have a heightened risk of causing significant patient harm when used in error.

Other safety concerns:

Conventional trastuzumab (Herceptin®) may be confused with U.S. product ado-trastuzumab emtansine (Kadcyla); products are **not** interchangeable.

Conventional trastuzumab (Herceptin®) may be confused with Canadian product trastuzumab emtansine (Kadcyla); products are **not** interchangeable.

Pregnancy Risk Factor D

Lactation Excretion in breast milk unknown/not recommended

Use Treatment (adjuvant) of HER2 overexpressing breast cancer as part of a combination regimen with doxorubicin, cyclophosphamide, and either paclitaxel or docetaxel; in combination with docetaxel and carboplatin; as a single agent following anthracycline-based combination treatment; treatment of HER2 overexpressing metastatic breast cancer in combination with paclitaxel as first-line treatment or as a single agent in patients who have received prior chemotherapy regimens for treatment of metastatic disease; treatment of HER2 overexpressing metastatic gastric or gastroesophageal junction adenocarcinoma in combination with cisplatin and either capecitabine or fluorouracil in patients who have not received prior treatment for metastatic disease

Unlabeled Use Treatment of HER2-positive metastatic breast cancer (in combination with pertuzumab and docetaxel) in patients who have not received prior anti-HER2 therapy or chemotherapy to treat metastatic disease; treatment of HER2

overexpressing metastatic breast cancer (in combination with lapatinib) which had progressed on prior trastuzumab containing therapy

Available Dosage Forms

Solution Reconstituted, Intravenous:
Herceptin: 440 mg (1 ea)

General Dosage Range Dosage adjustment recommended in patients who develop toxicities

I.V.: *Adults:* Loading dose: 4 mg/kg; Maintenance: 2 mg/kg once weekly **or** Loading dose: 8 mg/kg; Maintenance: 6 mg/kg every 3 weeks

Administration

I.V. Check label to ensure appropriate product is being administered (conventional trastuzumab and ado-trastuzumab are different products and are **NOT** interchangeable).

Administered by I.V. infusion; loading doses are infused over 90 minutes; maintenance doses may be infused over 30 minutes if tolerated. Do not administer with D_5W. **Do not administer I.V. push or by rapid bolus.**

Observe patients closely during the infusion for fever, chills, or other infusion-related symptoms. Treatment with acetaminophen, diphenhydramine, and/or meperidine is usually effective for managing infusion-related events.

Hazardous agent; use appropriate precautions for handling and disposal (meets NIOSH, 2012 criteria).

Injectable Detail pH: ~6 (reconstituted solution)

Nursing Actions

Physical Assessment Assess for signs of infusion reaction during infusion. If pregnancy inadvertently occurs during treatment, monitor amniotic fluid volume. Evaluate cardiac and respiratory function and vital signs. Monitor for arrhythmias, difficulty breathing, peripheral edema, and sudden weight gain.

Patient Education

• Discuss specific use of drug and side effects with patient as it relates to treatment. (HCAHPS: During this hospital stay, were you given any medicine that you had not taken before? Before giving you any new medicine, how often did hospital staff tell you what the medicine was for? How often did hospital staff describe possible side effects in a way you could understand?)

• Patient may experience flu-like syndrome, nausea, diarrhea, dizziness, fatigue, headache, loss of appetite, dyspepsia, rash, or rhinorrhea. Have patient report immediately to prescriber signs of infection, dyspnea, angina, tachycardia, syncope, significant weight gain, ecchymosis, or pregnancy (HCAHPS).

• Educate patient about signs of a significant reaction (eg, wheezing; chest tightness; fever; itching; bad cough; blue skin color; seizures; or swelling of face, lips, tongue, or throat). **Note:** This is not a comprehensive list of all side effects. Patient should consult prescriber for additional questions.

Intended Use and Disclaimer: Should not be printed and given to patients. This information is intended to serve as a concise initial reference for healthcare professionals to use when discussing medications with a patient. You must ultimately rely on your own discretion, experience and judgment in diagnosing, treating and advising patients.

Travelers' Diarrhea and Cholera Vaccine
(TRAV uh lerz dahy uh REE uh & KOL er uh vak SEEN)

Index Terms *Vibrio cholera* and Enterotoxigenic *Escherichia coli Vaccine*; Cholera and Traveler's Diarrhea Vaccine; Cholera Vaccine; Enterotoxigenic *Escherichia coli* and *Vibrio cholera* Vaccine; Oral Cholera Vaccine; Traveller's Diarrhea Vaccine and Cholera; WC-rBS

Pharmacologic Category Vaccine

Use Protection against travelers' diarrhea and/or cholera in adults and children ≥2 years of age who will be visiting areas where there is a risk of contracting travelers' diarrhea caused by enterotoxigenic *E. coli* (ETEC) or cholera caused by *V. cholerae* O1 (classical and El Tor biotypes; Inaba and Ogawa serotypes)

Note: The Centers for Disease Control and Prevention (CDC) *Health Information for International Travel* ("The Yellow Book") categorizes the following areas of risk (CDC, 2012):

- Low-risk countries include the United States, Canada, Australia, New Zealand, Japan, and countries in Northern and Western Europe.
- Intermediate-risk countries include those in Eastern Europe, South Africa, and some of the Caribbean islands.
- High-risk areas include most of Asia, the Middle East, Africa, Mexico, and Central and South America.

Product Availability Not available in U.S.

General Dosage Range Oral:

Children 2-6 years: Cholera: Primary immunization: 3 doses given at intervals of ≥1 week

Children ≥2 years: ETEC: Primary immunization: 2 doses given at intervals of ≥1 week

Children >6 years: Cholera: Primary immunization: 2 doses given at intervals of ≥1 week

Adults: Cholera: Primary immunization: 2 doses given at intervals of ≥1 week; ETEC: Primary immunization: 2 doses given at intervals of ≥1 week

Administration

Oral For oral use only; do not administer I.M., I.V., or SubQ. Oral administration of other medications, vaccines, and consumption of food or drink should be avoided 1 hour before and 1 hour following vaccine administration.

Administration with other vaccines (manufacturer recommendations): *Typhoid vaccine, oral:* Separate by at least 8 hours

Acetaminophen may be used when needed to provide comfort; however, routine prophylactic administration of acetaminophen to prevent fever due to vaccine use is not recommended. There is evidence of a decreased immune response to some vaccines associated with acetaminophen administration; the clinical significance of this reduction in immune response has not been established.

Nursing Actions

Physical Assessment Patient history of prior exposure to cholera vaccine should be assessed prior to treatment. Instruct patient about safe eating and drinking practices. All serious adverse reactions must be reported to the U.S. DHHS. U.S. federal law also requires entry into the patient's medical record. Instruct patient about anaphylactic treatment that should be available during use.

Patient Education

• Discuss specific use of vaccine and side effects with patient as it relates to treatment. (HCAHPS: During this hospital stay, were you given any medicine that you had not taken before? Before giving you any new medicine, how often did hospital staff tell you what the medicine was for? How often did hospital staff describe possible side effects in a way you could understand?)

• Patient may experience dyspepsia, nausea, or diarrhea. Have patient report immediately to prescriber rash (HCAHPS).

• Educate patient about signs of a significant reaction (eg, wheezing; chest tightness; fever; itching; bad cough; blue skin color; seizures; or swelling of face, lips, tongue, or throat). **Note:** This is not a comprehensive list of all side effects. Patient should consult prescriber for additional questions.

Intended Use and Disclaimer: Should not be printed and given to patients. This information is intended to serve as a concise initial reference for healthcare professionals to use when discussing medications with a patient. You must ultimately rely on your own discretion, experience and judgment in diagnosing, treating and advising patients.

Related Information

Immunization Administration Recommendations *on page 1675*

Immunization Recommendations *on page 1680*

Travoprost (TRA voe prost)

Brand Names: U.S. Travatan Z

Pharmacologic Category Ophthalmic Agent, Antiglaucoma; Prostaglandin, Ophthalmic

Medication Safety Issues

Sound-alike/look-alike issues:

Travatan® may be confused with Xalatan®

Pregnancy Risk Factor C

Lactation Excretion in breast milk unknown/use caution

Use Reduction of elevated intraocular pressure in patients with open-angle glaucoma or ocular hypertension

Available Dosage Forms

Solution, Ophthalmic:

Travatan Z: 0.004% (2.5 mL, 5 mL)

Generic: 0.004% (2.5 mL, 5 mL)

General Dosage Range Ophthalmic: *Adolescents ≥16 years and Adults:* Instill 1 drop into affected eye(s) once daily

Administration

Other May be used with other eye drops to lower intraocular pressure. If using more than one ophthalmic product, wait at least 5 minutes in between application of each medication. Remove contact lenses prior to administration and wait 15 minutes (after administration) before reinserting. Minimize contamination by not touching the eyelids or surrounding areas with the dropper tip; keep bottle tightly closed when not in use.

Nursing Actions

Patient Education

• Discuss specific use of drug and side effects with patient as it relates to treatment. (HCAHPS: During this hospital stay, were you given any medicine that you had not taken before? Before giving you any new medicine, how often did hospital staff tell you what the medicine was for? How often did hospital staff describe possible side effects in a way you could understand?)

• Patient may experience eye irritation, blurred vision, or change in eye color. Have patient report immediately to prescriber sudden vision changes, eye pain, or rash (HCAHPS).

• Educate patient about signs of a significant reaction (eg, wheezing; chest tightness; fever; itching; bad cough; blue skin color; seizures; or swelling of face, lips, tongue, or throat). **Note:** This is not a comprehensive list of all side effects. Patient should consult prescriber for additional questions.

Intended Use and Disclaimer: Should not be printed and given to patients. This information is intended to serve as a concise initial reference for healthcare professionals to use when discussing medications with a patient. You must ultimately rely on your own discretion, experience and judgment in diagnosing, treating and advising patients.

TraZODone (TRAZ oh done)

Brand Names: U.S. Oleptro [DSC]

Index Terms Desyrel; Trazodone Hydrochloride ▶

Pharmacologic Category Antidepressant, Serotonin Reuptake Inhibitor/Antagonist

Medication Safety Issues

Sound-alike/look-alike issues:

Desyrel may be confused with deferoxamine, Demerol®, Delsym®, Zestril®

TraZODone may be confused with traMADol, ziprasidone

International issues:

Desyrel [Canada, Turkey] may be confused with Deseril brand name for methysergide [Australia, Belgium, Great Britain, Netherlands]

Medication Guide Available Yes

Pregnancy Risk Factor C

Lactation Enters breast milk/use caution

Use Treatment of major depressive disorder

Unlabeled Use Potential augmenting agent for antidepressants, hypnotic

Available Dosage Forms

Tablet, Oral:

Generic: 50 mg, 100 mg, 150 mg, 300 mg

General Dosage Range Oral:

Adults: Immediate release: Initial: 150 mg/day in 3 divided doses; Maintenance: 150-600 mg/day in 3 divided doses; Extended-release: Initial: 150 mg once daily; Maximum dose: 375 mg/day

Elderly: Immediate release: Initial: 25-50 mg at bedtime; Maintenance: 25-150 mg/day at bedtime

Administration

Oral

Immediate release tablet: Dosing after meals may decrease lightheadedness and postural hypotension

Extended release tablet: Take on an empty stomach; swallow whole or as a half tablet without food. Tablet may be broken along the score line, but do not crush or chew.

Nursing Actions

Physical Assessment Monitor therapeutic response (eg, mental status, mood, affect, suicide ideation) at beginning of therapy and periodically throughout.

Patient Education

• Discuss specific use of drug and side effects with patient as it relates to treatment. (HCAHPS: During this hospital stay, were you given any medicine that you had not taken before? Before giving you any new medicine, how often did hospital staff tell you what the medicine was for? How often did hospital staff describe possible side effects in a way you could understand?)

• Patient may experience presyncope, fatigue, blurred vision, illogical thinking, dizziness, constipation, diarrhea, xerostomia, or headache. Have patient report immediately to prescriber erection lasting >4 hours, fasciculations, tremors, significant change in balance, urinary retention, severe asthenia, ecchymosis, bleeding, or rash (HCAHPS).

• Educate patient about signs of a significant reaction (eg, wheezing; chest tightness; fever; itching; bad cough; blue skin color; seizures; or swelling of face, lips, tongue, or throat). **Note:** This is not a comprehensive list of all side effects. Patient should consult prescriber for additional questions.

Intended Use and Disclaimer: Should not be printed and given to patients. This information is intended to serve as a concise initial reference for healthcare professionals to use when discussing medications with a patient. You must ultimately rely on your own discretion, experience and judgment in diagnosing, treating and advising patients.

Related Information

Oral Medications That Should Not Be Crushed or Altered *on page 1712*

Treprostinil (tre PROST in il)

Brand Names: U.S. Remodulin; Tyvaso; Tyvaso Refill; Tyvaso Starter

Index Terms Orenitram; Treprostinil Sodium

Pharmacologic Category Prostacyclin; Prostaglandin; Vasodilator

Pregnancy Risk Factor B

Lactation Excretion in breast milk unknown/use caution

Breast-Feeding Considerations It is not known if treprostinil is excreted in breast milk. The manufacturer recommends that caution be exercised when administering treprostinil to nursing women

Use

Injection: Treatment of pulmonary arterial hypertension (PAH) (WHO Group I) in patients with NYHA Class II-IV symptoms to decrease exercise-associated symptoms; to diminish clinical deterioration when transitioning from epoprostenol (I.V.)

Inhalation: Treatment of pulmonary arterial hypertension (PAH) (WHO Group I) in patients with NYHA Class III symptoms to improve exercise ability. **Note:** Nearly all controlled clinical trial experience has been with concomitant bosentan or sildenafil.

Mechanism of Action/Effect Treprostinil is a direct vasodilator of both pulmonary and systemic arterial vascular beds.

Contraindications There are no contraindications listed in the FDA-approved labeling.

Warnings/Precautions May produce symptomatic hypotension; use with caution in patients with low systemic arterial blood pressure. Abrupt withdrawal/large dosage reductions may worsen symptoms of PAH. If a SubQ or I.V. infusion is restarted within a few hours of discontinuation, the same dose rate may be used. Interruptions for longer periods may require retitration. Regardless of administration route (inhalation, I.V., or SubQ), treatment interruptions should be avoided. Immediate access to medication, back-up inhalation device, or pump and infusion sets is essential to prevent treatment interruptions. Chronic continuous I.V. infusion of treprostinil via a chronic indwelling central venous catheter has been associated with serious blood stream infections. This method of administration should be reserved for patients who are intolerant of the SubQ route or in whom the benefit outweighs the potential risks. Treprostinil should only be used by clinicians experienced in the treatment of PAH. Prior to initiation, patients should be carefully evaluated for ability to administer treprostinil, either as an I.V./SubQ infusion or inhalation, and care for the infusion system/inhalation device. Initiation of infusion must occur in a setting where adequate personnel and equipment necessary for hemodynamic monitoring and emergency treatment is available. Use with caution in patients with hepatic impairment; dose reduction is recommended for the initial dose (I.V./SubQ) in patients with mild-to-moderate hepatic insufficiency; titrate dose slowly in patients with hepatic insufficiency; has not been studied in severe hepatic impairment. Has not been studied in renal impairment; use with caution in renal impairment; titrate dose slowly in patients with renal insufficiency. Use with caution in patients ≥65 years of age. Inhalation: Safety and efficacy have not been established in patients with underlying pulmonary disease (eg, asthma, COPD). Patients with acute pulmonary infections should be monitored closely for exacerbation or reduced efficacy. Treprostinil inhibits platelet aggregation, increasing the risk of bleeding; use with caution in patients receiving concurrent anticoagulant/antiplatelet therapy.

Drug Interactions

Avoid Concomitant Use There are no known interactions where it is recommended to avoid concomitant use.

Decreased Effect

The levels/effects of Treprostinil may be decreased by: CYP2C8 Inducers (Strong)

Increased Effect/Toxicity

Treprostinil may increase the levels/effects of: Agents with Antiplatelet Properties; Anticoagulants; Antihypertensives; Highest Risk QTc-Prolonging Agents; Moderate Risk QTc-Prolonging Agents; Nonsteroidal Anti-Inflammatory Agents; Salicylates

The levels/effects of Treprostinil may be increased by: Alcohol (Ethyl); CYP2C8 Inhibitors (Strong); Mifepristone

Adverse Reactions

>10%:
Cardiovascular: Flushing (11%; inhalation: 15%)
Central nervous system: Headache (27% to 41%)
Dermatologic: Rash (14%)
Gastrointestinal: Diarrhea (25%), nausea (19% to 22%)

Local: Infusion site pain (SubQ: 85%; may improve after several months of therapy), infusion site reaction (SubQ: 83%)
Neuromuscular & skeletal: Jaw pain (13%)
Respiratory: Cough (inhalation: 54%), throat irritation/pharyngolaryngeal pain (inhalation: 25%)
1% to 10%:
Cardiovascular: Edema (9%), syncope (inhalation: 6%), hypotension (4%)
Central nervous system: Dizziness (9%)
Dermatologic: Pruritus (8%)
Respiratory: Epistaxis (inhalation), hemoptysis, pneumonia, wheezing (inhalation)

Product Availability

Orenitram extended release tablets: FDA approved December 2013; anticipated availability is June 2014.
Orenitram is indicated for the treatment of pulmonary arterial hypertension (WHO Group 1) to improve exercise capacity.

Available Dosage Forms

Solution, Inhalation:
Tyvaso: 0.6 mg/mL (2.9 mL)
Tyvaso Refill: 0.6 mg/mL (2.9 mL)
Tyvaso Starter: 0.6 mg/mL (2.9 mL)
Solution, Injection:
Remodulin: 1 mg/mL (20 mL); 2.5 mg/mL (20 mL); 5 mg/mL (20 mL); 10 mg/mL (20 mL)

General Dosage Range Dosage adjustment recommended for the I.V. infusion and SubQ routes in patients with hepatic impairment
Inhalation: *Adults:* Initial: 18 mcg (or 3 inhalations) every 4 hours 4 times/day; Maintenance: Maximum dose: 54 mcg (or 9 inhalations) 4 times/day
I.V. Infusion, SubQ: *Adults:* Initial: 0.625-1.25 ng/kg/minute; Maintenance: 1.25-40 ng/kg/minute

Administration

I.V. Avoid abrupt withdrawal (including interruptions in delivery) or rapid large dosage reductions. Immediate access to a back-up pump, infusion sets, and medication is essential to prevent treatment interruptions.
I.V. infusion: I.V. use is recommended when SubQ infusion is not tolerated or when the benefit outweighs the potential risks of an indwelling central venous catheter. Solution must be diluted in SWFI, NS, or Flolan® sterile diluent prior to use and administered by continuous infusion using a central indwelling catheter and infusion pump. The ambulatory infusion pump should be small and lightweight; have occlusion/no delivery, low battery, programming error, and motor malfunction alarms; have ± 6% accuracy of the programmed rate; and be positive pressure driven. The reservoir should be made of polyvinyl chloride, polypropylene, or glass. Peripheral infusion may be used temporarily until central line is established. Infusion sets with an in-line 0.22 or 0.2 micron filter should be used for central or peripheral administration.
Injectable Detail pH 6-7.2

◄ **Other** Avoid abrupt withdrawal (including interruptions in delivery) or rapid large dosage reductions. Immediate access to medication, a back-up inhalation device, or pump and infusion sets is essential to prevent treatment interruptions.

Inhalation: Do not mix with other medications. For inhalation only via the Tyvaso™ Inhalation System. Prior to the first treatment session of each day, transfer the entire contents of one ampule into the medicine chamber; one ampule contains sufficient volume of medication for all 4 treatment sessions in a single day. Between each session, the device should be capped and stored upright with the remaining medication inside. At the end of each day, the medicine chamber and any remaining medication must be discarded. Avoid contact of solution with eyes or skin; wash hands after handling.

SubQ infusion (preferred): Administer undiluted via continuous SubQ infusion using an appropriately-designed infusion pump. The ambulatory infusion pump should be small and lightweight; be able to adjust infusion rates in ~0.002 mL/hour increments; have occlusion/no delivery, low battery, programming error, and motor malfunction alarms; have ± 6% accuracy of the programmed rate; and be positive pressure driven. The reservoir should be made of polyvinyl chloride, polypropylene, or glass. Infusion site reactions may be helped by moving the infusion site every 3 days, local application of topical hot and cold packs, topical or oral analgesics. Injection site pain and erythema may improve after several months of treprostinil therapy.

Preparation for Administration Injection solution: For SubQ infusion, **product should not be diluted prior to use.** For I.V. infusion, dilute in SWFI, NS, or Flolan® sterile diluent to a final volume of either 50 mL or 100 mL (dependent on system reservoir and calculated dose).

Storage/Stability

Injection solution: Store vials at 25°C (77°F); excursions permitted to 15°C to 30°C (59°F to 86°F). Contents of a vial should not be used past 30 days after initial needle access into the vial. Stability for up to 48 hours at 37°C has been shown for I.V. infusion concentrations as low as 4000 ng/mL.

Solution for inhalation: Store ampules in foil packs at 25°C (77°F); excursions permitted to 15°C to 30°C (59°F to 89°F). Protect from light. Once foil pack is opened, ampules should be used within 7 days. Following transfer of solution to inhalation device, solution should remain in device for no more than 24 hours; discard unused portion.

Nursing Actions

Physical Assessment To be used only by clinicians experienced in the diagnosis and treatment of PAH. Initiation of therapy must be performed in a monitored setting. Therapy may be needed long-term; patient's ability to prepare, administer, and care for necessary equipment should be carefully assessed. Evaluate effectiveness of therapy (improved pulmonary function and quality of life). Teach patient/caregiver how to care for equipment and monitor for any malfunction. Instruct patient/caregiver to monitor vital signs on regular basis.

Patient Education

• Discuss specific use of drug and side effects with patient as it relates to treatment. (HCAHPS: During this hospital stay, were you given any medicine that you had not taken before? Before giving you any new medicine, how often did hospital staff tell you what the medicine was for? How often did hospital staff describe possible side effects in a way you could understand?)

• Patient may experience injection site pain and irritation, flushing, headache, nausea, diarrhea, jaw pain, or pharyngitis. Have patient report immediately to prescriber ecchymosis, bleeding, or rash (HCAHPS).

• Educate patient about signs of a significant reaction (eg, wheezing; chest tightness; fever; itching; bad cough; blue skin color; seizures; or swelling of face, lips, tongue, or throat). **Note:** This is not a comprehensive list of all side effects. Patient should consult prescriber for additional questions.

Intended Use and Disclaimer: Should not be printed and given to patients. This information is intended to serve as a concise initial reference for healthcare professionals to use when discussing medications with a patient. You must ultimately rely on your own discretion, experience and judgment in diagnosing, treating and advising patients.

Tretinoin (Topical) (TRET i noyn)

Brand Names: U.S. Atralin; Avita; Refissa; Renova; Renova Pump; Retin-A; Retin-A Micro; Retin-A Micro Pump; Tretin-X

Index Terms trans-Retinoic Acid; Retinoic Acid; Vitamin A Acid

Pharmacologic Category Acne Products; Retinoic Acid Derivative; Topical Skin Product, Acne

Medication Safety Issues

Sound-alike/look-alike issues:

Tretinoin may be confused with ISOtretinoin, Tenormin, triamcinolone, trientine

International issues:

Renova [U.S., Canada] may be confused with Remov brand name for nimesulide [Italy]

Pregnancy Risk Factor C

Lactation Excretion in breast milk unknown/not recommended

Use

Acne vulgaris (excluding Refissa and Renova): Treatment of acne vulgaris.

Palliation of fine wrinkles (Renova only): Adjunctive treatment for mitigation (palliation) of fine wrinkles in patients who use comprehensive skin care and sun avoidance programs.

Palliation of fine wrinkles, mottled hyperpigmentation, and facial skin roughness (Refissa only): Adjunctive treatment for mitigation (palliation) of fine wrinkles, mottled hyperpigmentation, and tactile roughness of facial skin in patients who do not achieve such palliation using comprehensive skin care and sun avoidance programs alone.

Unlabeled Use Some skin cancers

Product Availability Retin-A Micro Gel 0.08%: FDA approved January 2014; anticipated availability is currently unknown.

Available Dosage Forms

Cream, External:
Avita: 0.025% (20 g, 45 g)
Refissa: 0.05% (20 g, 40 g)
Renova: 0.02% (40 g, 60 g)
Renova Pump: 0.02% (44 g)
Retin-A: 0.025% (20 g, 45 g); 0.05% (20 g, 45 g); 0.1% (20 g, 45 g)
Tretin-X: 0.0375% (35 g); 0.075% (35 g)
Generic: 0.025% (20 g, 45 g); 0.05% (20 g, 40 g, 45 g, 60 g); 0.1% (20 g, 45 g)

Gel, External:
Atralin: 0.05% (45 g)
Avita: 0.025% (20 g, 45 g)
Retin-A: 0.01% (15 g, 45 g); 0.025% (15 g, 45 g)
Retin-A Micro: 0.04% (20 g, 45 g); 0.1% (20 g, 45 g)
Retin-A Micro Pump: 0.04% (50 g); 0.1% (50 g)
Generic: 0.01% (15 g, 45 g); 0.025% (15 g, 45 g); 0.04% (20 g, 45 g, 50 g); 0.1% (20 g, 45 g, 50 g)

Kit, External:
Tretin-X: 0.025%, 0.05%, 0.1%

General Dosage Range Topical: *Children≥10 years, Adolescents, and Adults:* Apply once daily or less frequently if necessary.

Administration

Topical Prior to application, gently wash face with a mild soap; pat dry and wait 20-30 minutes. Apply lightly to affected area before bedtime, avoiding eyes, ears, nostrils, and mouth.

Hazardous agent; use appropriate precautions for handling and disposal (NIOSH, 2012).

Nursing Actions

Patient Education
- Discuss specific use of drug and side effects with patient as it relates to treatment. (HCAHPS: During this hospital stay, were you given any medicine that you had not taken before? Before giving you any new medicine, how often did hospital staff tell you what the medicine was for? How often did hospital staff describe possible side effects in a way you could understand?)
- Patient may experience application site pain, skin irritation, or erythema (HCAHPS).
- Educate patient about signs of a significant reaction (eg, wheezing; chest tightness; fever; itching; bad cough; blue skin color; seizures; or swelling of face, lips, tongue, or throat). **Note:** This is not a comprehensive list of all side effects. Patient should consult prescriber for additional questions.

Intended Use and Disclaimer: Should not be printed and given to patients. This information is intended to serve as a concise initial reference for healthcare professionals to use when discussing medications with a patient. You must ultimately rely on your own discretion, experience and judgment in diagnosing, treating and advising patients.

Triamcinolone (Systemic)
(trye am SIN oh lone)

Brand Names: U.S. Aristospan Intra-Articular; Aristospan Intralesional; Kenalog

Index Terms Triamcinolone Acetonide, Parenteral; Triamcinolone Hexacetonide

Pharmacologic Category Corticosteroid, Systemic

Medication Safety Issues

Sound-alike/look-alike issues:
Kenalog® may be confused with Ketalar®

Other safety concerns:
TAC (occasional abbreviation for triamcinolone) is an error-prone abbreviation (mistaken as tetracaine-adrenaline-cocaine)

Pregnancy Risk Factor C

Lactation Excreted into breast milk/use caution

Breast-Feeding Considerations Corticosteroids are excreted in human milk; information specific to triamcinolone has not been located. The manufacturer notes that when used systemically, maternal use of corticosteroids have the potential to cause adverse events in a nursing infant (eg, growth suppression, interfere with endogenous corticosteroid production); therefore, caution should be used if administered to a nursing woman. A case report notes a decrease in milk production following a high-dose triamcinolone injection in a nursing mother with a previously abundant milk supply (McGuire, 2012).

Use

Intra-articular (soft tissue): Acute gouty arthritis, acute/subacute bursitis, acute tenosynovitis, epicondylitis, rheumatoid arthritis, synovitis of osteoarthritis

Intralesional: Alopecia areata, discoid lupus erythematosus, keloids, granuloma annulare lesions (localized hypertrophic, infiltrated, or inflammatory), lichen planus plaques, lichen simplex chronicus plaques, psoriatic plaques, necrobiosis lipoidica diabeticorum, cystic tumors of aponeurosis or tendon (ganglia)

Systemic: Adrenocortical insufficiency, dermatologic diseases, endocrine disorders, gastrointestinal diseases, hematologic and neoplastic disorders, nervous system disorders, nephrotic syndrome, rheumatic disorders, allergic states, respiratory diseases, systemic lupus erythematosus (SLE), and other diseases requiring antiinflammatory or immunosuppressive effects

Mechanism of Action/Effect Decreases inflammation by suppression of migration of polymorphonuclear leukocytes and reversal of increased capillary permeability; suppresses the immune system by reducing activity and volume of the lymphatic system; suppresses adrenal function at high doses

Contraindications Hypersensitivity to triamcinolone or any component of the formulation; systemic fungal infections; cerebral malaria; immune thrombocytopenia (ITP) (I.M. injection)

Warnings/Precautions May cause hypercorticism or suppression of hypothalamic-pituitary-adrenal (HPA) axis, particularly in younger children or in patients receiving high doses for prolonged periods. HPA axis suppression may lead to adrenal crisis. Withdrawal and discontinuation of a corticosteroid should be done slowly and carefully.

Acute myopathy has been reported with high-dose corticosteroids, usually in patients with neuromuscular transmission disorders; may involve ocular and/or respiratory muscles; monitor creatine kinase; recovery may be delayed. Corticosteroid use may cause psychiatric disturbances, including depression, euphoria, insomnia, mood swings, and personality changes. Pre-existing psychiatric conditions may be exacerbated by corticosteroid use. Prolonged use of corticosteroids may also increase the incidence of secondary infection, mask acute infection (including fungal infections), prolong or exacerbate viral infections, or limit response to vaccines. Exposure to chickenpox should be avoided; corticosteroids should not be used to treat ocular herpes simplex. Corticosteroids should not be used for cerebral malaria or viral hepatitis. Close observation is required in patients with latent tuberculosis and/or TB reactivity; restrict use in active TB (only in conjunction with antituberculosis treatment). Use with caution in patients with threadworm infection; may cause serious hyperinfection. Prolonged treatment with corticosteroids has been associated with the development of Kaposi's sarcoma (case reports); if noted, discontinuation of therapy should be considered. Avoid use in head injury patients.

Use with caution in patients with thyroid disease, hepatic impairment, renal impairment, cardiovascular disease, diabetes, myasthenia gravis, patients at risk for osteoporosis, patients at risk for seizures, or GI diseases (diverticulitis, peptic ulcer, ulcerative colitis) due to perforation risk. Avoid use in head injury patients. Use caution

following acute MI (corticosteroids have been associated with myocardial rupture). Because of the risk of adverse effects, systemic corticosteroids should be used cautiously in the elderly in the smallest possible effective dose for the shortest duration. Patients should not be immunized with live, viral vaccines while receiving immunosuppressive doses of corticosteroids. The ability to respond to dead viral vaccines is unknown.

Withdraw therapy with gradual tapering of dose. There have been reports of systemic corticosteroid withdrawal symptoms (eg, joint/muscle pain, lassitude, depression) when withdrawing oral inhalation therapy. Injection suspension contains benzyl alcohol; benzyl alcohol has been associated with the "gasping syndrome" in neonates and low-birth-weight infants. Administer products only via recommended route (depending on product used). Do **not** administer any triamcinolone product via the epidural or intrathecal route; serious adverse events, including fatalities, have been reported.

Drug Interactions

Avoid Concomitant Use

Avoid concomitant use of Triamcinolone (Systemic) with any of the following: Aldesleukin; BCG; Indium 111 Capromab Pendetide; Mifepristone; Natalizumab; Pimecrolimus; Tacrolimus (Topical); Tofacitinib

Decreased Effect

Triamcinolone (Systemic) may decrease the levels/effects of: Aldesleukin; Antidiabetic Agents; BCG; Calcitriol; Coccidioidin Skin Test; Corticorelin; Hyaluronidase; Indium 111 Capromab Pendetide; Isoniazid; Salicylates; Sipuleucel-T; Telaprevir; Urea Cycle Disorder Agents; Vaccines (Inactivated)

The levels/effects of Triamcinolone (Systemic) may be decreased by: Aminoglutethimide; Barbiturates; Echinacea; Mifepristone; Mitotane; Primidone; Rifamycin Derivatives

Increased Effect/Toxicity

Triamcinolone (Systemic) may increase the levels/effects of: Acetylcholinesterase Inhibitors; Amphotericin B; Deferasirox; Leflunomide; Loop Diuretics; Natalizumab; NSAID (COX-2 Inhibitor); NSAID (Nonselective); Thiazide Diuretics; Tofacitinib; Vaccines (Live); Warfarin

The levels/effects of Triamcinolone (Systemic) may be increased by: Antifungal Agents (Azole Derivatives, Systemic); Aprepitant; Calcium Channel Blockers (Nondihydropyridine); Denosumab; Estrogen Derivatives; Fluconazole; Fosaprepitant; Indacaterol; Macrolide Antibiotics; Mifepristone; Neuromuscular-Blocking Agents (Nondepolarizing); Pimecrolimus; Quinolone Antibiotics; Ritonavir; Roflumilast; Salicylates; Tacrolimus (Topical); Telaprevir; Trastuzumab

Adverse Reactions Frequency not defined; reactions reported with corticosteroid therapy in general:

Cardiovascular: Arrhythmia, bradycardia, cardiac arrest, cardiac enlargement, CHF, circulatory collapse, edema, hypertension, hypertrophic cardiomyopathy (premature infants), myocardial rupture (following recent MI), syncope, tachycardia, thromboembolism, vasculitis

Central nervous system: Arachnoiditis (I.T.), depression, emotional instability, euphoria, headache, insomnia, intracranial pressure increased, malaise, meningitis (I.T.), mood changes, neuritis, neuropathy, personality change, pseudotumor cerebri (with discontinuation), seizure, spinal cord infarction, stroke, vertigo

Dermatologic: Abscess (sterile), acne, allergic dermatitis, angioedema, atrophy (cutaneous/subcutaneous), bruising, dry skin, erythema, hair thinning, hirsutism, hyper-/hypopigmentation, hypertrichosis, impaired wound healing, lupus erythematosus-like lesions, petechiae, purpura, rash, skin test suppression, striae, thin skin

Endocrine & metabolic: Carbohydrate intolerance, Cushingoid state, diabetes mellitus, fluid retention, glucose intolerance, growth suppression (children), hypokalemia, hypokalemic alkalosis, menstrual irregularities, negative nitrogen balance, sodium retention, sperm motility altered

Gastrointestinal: Abdominal distention, appetite increased, GI hemorrhage, GI perforation, nausea, pancreatitis, peptic ulcer, ulcerative esophagitis, weight gain

Hepatic: Hepatomegaly, liver function tests increased

Local: Thrombophlebitis

Neuromuscular & skeletal: Aseptic necrosis of femoral and humeral heads, calcinosis, Charcot-like arthropathy, fractures, joint tissue damage, muscle mass loss, myopathy, osteoporosis, parasthesia, paraplegia, quadriplegia, tendon rupture, vertebral compression fractures, weakness

Ocular: Cataracts, cortical blindness, exophthalmos, glaucoma, ocular pressure increased, papilledema

Renal: Glycosuria

Respiratory: Pulmonary edema

Miscellaneous: Abnormal fat deposits, anaphylactoid reaction, anaphylaxis, diaphoresis, hiccups, infection, moon face

Available Dosage Forms

Suspension, Injection:

Aristospan Intra-Articular: 20 mg/mL (1 mL, 5 mL)

Aristospan Intralesional: 5 mg/mL (5 mL)

Kenalog: 10 mg/mL (5 mL); 40 mg/mL (1 mL, 5 mL, 10 mL)

General Dosage Range

I.M.:

Children 6-12 years: Acetonide: Initial: 40 mg; Range: 2.5-100 mg/day

Children >12 years: Acetonide: Initial: 60 mg; Range: 2.5-100 mg/day

Adults: Acetonide: Initial: 60 mg; Range: 2.5-100 mg/day, may repeat with 20-100 mg when symptoms recur; Multiple sclerosis: 160 mg/day for 1 week, then 64 mg every other day

Intra-articular: Adults: Acetonide: 2.5-80 mg; Hexacetonide: 2-20 mg

Intradermal: Adults: Acetonide: 1 mg/site

Intralesional: Adults: Acetonide: 1-30 mg (usually 1 mg/injection site); Hexacetonide: Up to 0.5 mg/sq inch

Intrasynovial: Adults: Acetonide: 5-40 mg

Tendon Sheath: Adults: Acetonide: 2.5-10 mg

Administration

I.M. Shake well before use to ensure suspension is uniform. Inspect visually to ensure no clumping; administer immediately after withdrawal so settling does not occur in the syringe. Do **not** administer any product I.V. or via the epidural or intrathecal route

Kenalog®-40 injection: For intra-articular, soft tissue or I.M. administration. When administered I.M., inject deep into the gluteal muscle using a minimum needle length of 1½ inches for adults. Obese patients may require a longer needle. Alternate sites for subsequent injections.

Other Shake well before use to ensure suspension is uniform. Inspect visually to ensure no clumping; administer immediately after withdrawal so settling does not occur in the syringe. Do **not** administer any product I.V. or via the epidural or intrathecal route.

Aristospan® (20 mg/mL concentration): For intra-articular and soft tissue administration only; a ≥23-gauge needle is preferred.

Aristospan® (5 mg/mL concentration): For intralesional or sublesional administration only; a ≥23-gauge needle is preferred.

Kenalog®-10 injection: For intra-articular or intralesional administration only. When administered intralesionally, inject directly into the lesion (ie, intradermally or subcutaneously). Tuberculin syringes with a 23- to 25-gauge needle are preferable for intralesional injections.

Kenalog®-40 injection: May administer intra-articularly or into soft tissue.

Preparation for Administration Hexacetonide injectable suspension: Avoid diluents containing parabens, phenol, or other preservatives (may cause flocculation). Suspension for intralesional use may be diluted with D_5NS, $D_{10}NS$, NS, or SWFI to a 1:1, 1:2, or 1:4 concentration. Solutions for intra-articular use, may be diluted with lidocaine 1% or 2%.

Storage/Stability Injection, suspension:

Acetonide injectable suspension: Kenalog®: Store at 20°C to 25°C (68°F to 77°F); avoid freezing. Protect from light.

Hexacetonide injectable suspension: Store at 20°C to 25°C (68°F to 77°F); avoid freezing. Protect from light. Diluted suspension stable up to 1 week.

Nursing Actions

Physical Assessment Patients with diabetes should monitor glucose levels closely (corticosteroids may alter glucose levels). When used for >10-14 days, do not discontinue abruptly; decrease dosage incrementally.

Patient Education

• Discuss specific use of drug and side effects with patient as it relates to treatment. (HCAHPS: During this hospital stay, were you given any medicine that you had not taken before? Before giving you any new medicine, how often did hospital staff tell you what the medicine was for? How often did hospital staff describe possible side effects in a way you could understand?)

• Patient may experience hyperglycemia, dyspepsia, nausea, weight gain, changes in mood, lipodystrophy, osteopenia, asthenia, skin changes, cataracts, or glaucoma. Have patient report immediately to prescriber signs of infection, tremors, tachycardia, confusion, diaphoresis, dizziness, dyspnea, first-time exposure to chickenpox, sudden vision changes, or rash (HCAHPS).

• Educate patient about signs of a significant reaction (eg, wheezing; chest tightness; fever; itching; bad cough; blue skin color; seizures; or swelling of face, lips, tongue, or throat). **Note:** This is not a comprehensive list of all side effects. Patient should consult prescriber for additional questions.

Intended Use and Disclaimer: Should not be printed and given to patients. This information is intended to serve as a concise initial reference for healthcare professionals to use when discussing medications with a patient. You must ultimately rely on your own discretion, experience and judgment in diagnosing, treating and advising patients.

Dietary Considerations Ensure adequate intake of calcium and vitamins (or consider supplementation) in patients on medium-to-high doses of systemic corticosteroids.

Triamcinolone (Nasal) (trye am SIN oh lone)

Brand Names: U.S. Nasacort Allergy 24HR [OTC]; Nasacort AQ

Index Terms Nasacort Allergy 24HR [OTC]; Triamcinolone Acetonide

Pharmacologic Category Corticosteroid, Nasal

Medication Safety Issues
Sound-alike/look-alike issues:
Nasacort may be confused with NasalCrom
Other safety concerns:
TAC (occasional abbreviation for triamcinolone) is an error-prone abbreviation (mistaken as tetracaine-adrenaline-cocaine)

Pregnancy Risk Factor C

Lactation Excretion in breast milk unknown/use caution

Use Allergic rhinitis:
Rx: Management of seasonal and perennial allergic rhinitis in adults and children 2 years and older
OTC: For the relief of hay fever and other upper respiratory allergies (eg, nasal congestion, runny nose, sneezing, itchy nose) in adults and children 2 years and older

Unlabeled Use Adjunct to antibiotics in empiric treatment of acute bacterial rhinosinusitis (ABRS) (Chow, 2012)

Dosage Forms Considerations
Nasacort AQ 16.5 g bottles contain 120 sprays.

Available Dosage Forms
Aerosol Solution, Nasal:
Nasacort Allergy 24HR [OTC]: 55 mcg/actuation
Nasacort AQ: 55 mcg/actuation (16.5 g)
Inhaler, Nasal:
Generic: 55 mcg/actuation (16.5 g)

General Dosage Range Intranasal:
Children 2 to <6 years: One spray (55 mcg) in each nostril once daily (maximum: 1 spray [55 mcg] in each nostril once daily)
Children 6 to <12 years: Initial: One spray (55 mcg) in each nostril once daily; Maintenance: 1-2 sprays (55-110 mcg) in each nostril once daily (maximum: 2 sprays [110 mcg] in each nostril once daily)
Children ≥12 years, Adolescents, and Adults: 1-2 sprays (55-110 mcg) in each nostril once daily (maximum: 2 sprays [110 mcg] in each nostril once daily)

Administration

Inhalation Shake well prior to use. Gently blow nose to clear nostrils. Avoid spraying into mouth or eyes and do **not** blow nose for 15 minutes after use. Prime prior to first use by shaking contents well and releasing 5 sprays into the air. If product is not used for more than 2 weeks, reprime with 1 spray.

Nursing Actions

Patient Education

• Discuss specific use of drug and side effects with patient as it relates to treatment. (HCAHPS: During this hospital stay, were you given any medicine that you had not taken before? Before giving you any new medicine, how often did hospital staff tell you what the medicine was for? How often did hospital staff describe possible side effects in a way you could understand?)

- Patient may experience headache. Have patient report immediately to prescriber severe rhinitis or first-time exposure to chickenpox (HCAHPS).
- Educate patient about signs of a significant reaction (eg, wheezing; chest tightness; fever; itching; bad cough; blue skin color; seizures; or swelling of face, lips, tongue, or throat). **Note:** This is not a comprehensive list of all side effects. Patient should consult prescriber for additional questions.

Intended Use and Disclaimer: Should not be printed and given to patients. This information is intended to serve as a concise initial reference for healthcare professionals to use when discussing medications with a patient. You must ultimately rely on your own discretion, experience and judgment in diagnosing, treating and advising patients.

Triamcinolone (Topical) (trye am SIN oh lone)

Brand Names: U.S. Dermasorb TA; Kenalog; Oralone; Pediaderm TA; Trianex; Triderm
Pharmacologic Category Corticosteroid, Topical
Medication Safety Issues
Sound-alike/look-alike issues:
Kenalog® may be confused with Ketalar®
Other safety concerns:
TAC (occasional abbreviation for triamcinolone) is an error-prone abbreviation (mistaken as tetra-caine-adrenaline-cocaine)
Pregnancy Risk Factor C
Lactation Excretion in breast milk unknown/use caution
Use
Oral topical: Adjunctive treatment and temporary relief of symptoms associated with oral inflammatory lesions and ulcerative lesions resulting from trauma
Topical: Inflammatory dermatoses responsive to steroids
Available Dosage Forms
Aerosol Solution, External:
Kenalog: (63 g, 100 g)
Cream, External:
Triderm: 0.1% (28.4 g, 85.2 g)
Generic: 0.025% (15 g, 80 g, 454 g); 0.1% (15 g, 30 g, 80 g, 453.6 g, 454 g); 0.5% (15 g)
Kit, External:
Dermasorb TA: 0.1%
Pediaderm TA: 0.1%
Lotion, External:
Generic: 0.025% (60 mL); 0.1% (60 mL)
Ointment, External:
Trianex: 0.05% (17 g, 85 g)
Generic: 0.025% (15 g, 80 g, 454 g); 0.1% (15 g, 80 g, 453.6 g, 454 g); 0.5% (15 g)
Paste, Mouth/Throat:
Oralone: 0.1% (5 g)
Generic: 0.1% (5 g)

General Dosage Range Topical: *Adults:* Cream, ointment: Apply thin film to affected areas 2-4 times/day; Oral: Press a small dab (about 1/4") to the lesion until a thin film develops; Spray: Apply to affected area 3-4 times/day
Administration
Topical
Oral topical: Apply small dab to lesion until a thin film develops; do not rub in. Apply at bedtime or after meals if applications are needed throughout the day.
Topical:
Ointment: Apply a thin film sparingly. Do not use on open skin or wounds. Do not occlude area unless directed; if using occluding dressing, monitor for infection.
Spray: Avoid eyes and do not inhale if spraying near face. Occlusive dressing may be used if instructed; monitor for infection.
Nursing Actions
Patient Education
- Discuss specific use of drug and side effects with patient as it relates to treatment. (HCAHPS: During this hospital stay, were you given any medicine that you had not taken before? Before giving you any new medicine, how often did hospital staff tell you what the medicine was for? How often did hospital staff describe possible side effects in a way you could understand?)
- Patient may experience xeroderma. Have patient report immediately to prescriber signs of hyperglycemia, severe stomatitis, skin changes, or significant skin irritation (HCAHPS).
- Educate patient about signs of a significant reaction (eg, wheezing; chest tightness; fever; itching; bad cough; blue skin color; seizures; or swelling of face, lips, tongue, or throat). **Note:** This is not a comprehensive list of all side effects. Patient should consult prescriber for additional questions.

Intended Use and Disclaimer: Should not be printed and given to patients. This information is intended to serve as a concise initial reference for healthcare professionals to use when discussing medications with a patient. You must ultimately rely on your own discretion, experience and judgment in diagnosing, treating and advising patients.

Triazolam (trye AY zoe lam)

Brand Names: U.S. Halcion
Pharmacologic Category Benzodiazepine

Medication Safety Issues

Sound-alike/look-alike issues:

Triazolam may be confused with alPRAZolam

Halcion® may be confused with halcinonide, Haldol®

BEERS Criteria medication:

This drug may be potentially inappropriate for use in geriatric patients (Quality of evidence - high; Strength of recommendation - strong).

Medication Guide Available Yes

Pregnancy Risk Factor X

Lactation Excretion in breast milk unknown/not recommended

Use Short-term (generally 7-10 days) treatment of insomnia

Unlabeled Use Oral sedation prior to outpatient dental procedures

Controlled Substance C-IV

Available Dosage Forms

Tablet, Oral:

Halcion: 0.25 mg

Generic: 0.125 mg, 0.25 mg

General Dosage Range Oral:

Adults: 0.125-0.25 mg at bedtime (maximum: 0.5 mg daily)

Elderly: Initial: 0.125 mg at bedtime (maximum: 0.25 mg daily)

Administration

Oral Do not take with a meal or immediately after a meal. Tablet may be crushed or swallowed whole. Onset of action is rapid; patient should take immediately before bedtime.

Nursing Actions

Physical Assessment Assess for history of addiction; long-term use can result in dependence, abuse, or tolerance. For inpatient use, institute safety measures to prevent falls.

Patient Education

• Discuss specific use of drug and side effects with patient as it relates to treatment. (HCAHPS: During this hospital stay, were you given any medicine that you had not taken before? Before giving you any new medicine, how often did hospital staff tell you what the medicine was for? How often did hospital staff describe possible side effects in a way you could understand?) • Patient may experience presyncope, fatigue, blurred vision, illogical thinking, headache, or change in balance. Have patient report immediately to prescriber depression, emotional instability, memory loss, or rash (HCAHPS).

• Educate patient about signs of a significant reaction (eg, wheezing; chest tightness; fever; itching; bad cough; blue skin color; seizures; or swelling of face, lips, tongue, or throat). **Note:** This is not a comprehensive list of all side effects. Patient should consult prescriber for additional questions.

Intended Use and Disclaimer: Should not be printed and given to patients. This information is intended to serve as a concise initial reference for healthcare professionals to use when discussing medications with a patient. You must ultimately rely on your own discretion, experience and judgment in diagnosing, treating and advising patients.

Trihexyphenidyl (trye heks ee FEN i dil)

Index Terms Artane; Benzhexol Hydrochloride; Trihexyphenidyl Hydrochloride

Pharmacologic Category Anti-Parkinson's Agent, Anticholinergic; Anticholinergic Agent

Medication Safety Issues

Sound-alike/look-alike issues:

Trihexyphenidyl may be confused with trifluoperazine

BEERS Criteria medication:

This drug may be potentially inappropriate for use in geriatric patients (Quality of evidence - moderate; Strength of recommendation - strong).

Pregnancy Risk Factor C

Lactation Excretion in breast milk unknown/use caution

Use Adjunctive treatment of Parkinson's disease; treatment of drug-induced extrapyramidal symptoms

Available Dosage Forms

Elixir, Oral:

Generic: 0.4 mg/mL (473 mL)

Tablet, Oral:

Generic: 2 mg, 5 mg

General Dosage Range Oral: *Adults:* Initial: 1 mg/day; Maintenance: 3-15 mg/day in 3-4 divided doses

Administration

Oral May be administered before or after meals; tolerated best if given in 3 daily doses and with food. High doses (>10 mg/day) may be divided into 4 doses, at meal times and at bedtime.

Nursing Actions

Physical Assessment Monitor renal function. Monitor for Parkinsonian symptoms and anticholinergic syndrome (dry mouth and mucous membranes, constipation, epigastric distress, CNS disturbances, paralytic ileus).

Patient Education

• Discuss specific use of drug and side effects with patient as it relates to treatment. (HCAHPS: During this hospital stay, were you given any medicine that you had not taken before? Before giving you any new medicine, how often did hospital staff tell you what the medicine was for? How often did hospital staff describe possible side effects in a way you could understand?) • Patient may experience dizziness, nausea, constipation, blurred vision, or xerostomia. Have patient report immediately to prescriber illogical thinking, urinary retention, or rash (HCAHPS).

• Educate patient about signs of a significant reaction (eg, wheezing; chest tightness; fever; itching; bad cough; blue skin color; seizures; or swelling of face, lips, tongue, or throat). **Note:** This is not a comprehensive list of all side effects. Patient should consult prescriber for additional questions.

Intended Use and Disclaimer: Should not be printed and given to patients. This information is intended to serve as a concise initial reference for healthcare professionals to use when discussing medications with a patient. You must ultimately rely on your own discretion, experience and judgment in diagnosing, treating and advising patients.

Trimethobenzamide (trye meth oh BEN za mide)

Brand Names: U.S. Tigan
Index Terms Trimethobenzamide HCl; Trimethobenzamide Hydrochloride
Pharmacologic Category Antiemetic
Medication Safety Issues
Sound-alike/look-alike issues:
Tigan may be confused with Tiazac, Ticlid
Trimethobenzamide may be confused with metoclopramide, trimethoprim
BEERS Criteria medication:
This drug may be potentially inappropriate for use in geriatric patients (Quality of evidence - moderate; Strength of recommendation - strong).
Lactation Excretion in breast milk unknown
Use Nausea and vomiting: Treatment of postoperative nausea and vomiting; treatment of nausea associated with gastroenteritis
Available Dosage Forms
Capsule, Oral:
Tigan: 300 mg
Generic: 300 mg
Solution, Intramuscular:
Tigan: 100 mg/mL (2 mL, 20 mL)
Generic: 100 mg/mL (2 mL, 20 mL)
General Dosage Range
I.M.: *Adults:* 200 mg 3 or 4 times daily
Oral: *Adults:* 300 mg 3 or 4 times daily
Administration
I.M. Injection: Administer I.M. only. Inject deep into upper outer quadrant of gluteal muscle. Not recommended for I.V. use.
Injectable Detail pH: ~5
Oral Capsule: Administer capsule orally.
Nursing Actions
Physical Assessment Monitor for hypovolemia, angioedema, and postural hypotension. If self-administered injection, teach patient appropriate injection technique and syringe disposal.
Patient Education
• Discuss specific use of drug and side effects with patient as it relates to treatment. (HCAHPS: During this hospital stay, were you given any

medicine that you had not taken before? Before giving you any new medicine, how often did hospital staff tell you what the medicine was for? How often did hospital staff describe possible side effects in a way you could understand?)
• Patient may experience presyncope, fatigue, blurred vision, illogical thinking, dizziness, or injection site irritation. Have patient report immediately to prescriber tremors, severe asthenia, or rash (HCAHPS).
• Educate patient about signs of a significant reaction (eg, wheezing; chest tightness; fever; itching; bad cough; blue skin color; seizures; or swelling of face, lips, tongue, or throat). **Note:** This is not a comprehensive list of all side effects. Patient should consult prescriber for additional questions.

Intended Use and Disclaimer: Should not be printed and given to patients. This information is intended to serve as a concise initial reference for healthcare professionals to use when discussing medications with a patient. You must ultimately rely on your own discretion, experience and judgment in diagnosing, treating and advising patients.

Trimethoprim (trye METH oh prim)

Brand Names: U.S. Primsol
Index Terms TMP
Pharmacologic Category Antibiotic, Miscellaneous
Pregnancy Risk Factor C
Lactation Enters breast milk/use caution
Breast-Feeding Considerations Trimethoprim is excreted in breast milk. The manufacturer recommends caution while using trimethoprim in a breast-feeding woman because trimethoprim may interfere with folic acid metabolism. Nondose-related effects could include modification of bowel flora. Also see the sulfamethoxazole/trimethoprim monograph for additional information.
Use Treatment of urinary tract infections due to susceptible strains of *E. coli, P. mirabilis, K. pneumoniae, Enterobacter* spp and coagulase-negative *Staphylococcus* including *S. saprophyticus*; acute otitis media due to susceptible strains of *S. pneumoniae* and *H. influenzae* in children
Unlabeled Use Alternative agent for *Pneumocystis jirovecii* pneumonia (in combination with dapsone)
Mechanism of Action/Effect Inhibits folic acid reduction to tetrahydrofolate, and thereby inhibits microbial growth
Contraindications Hypersensitivity to trimethoprim or any component of the formulation; megaloblastic anemia due to folate deficiency
Warnings/Precautions Use with caution in patients with impaired renal or hepatic function or with possible folate deficiency. Prolonged use may result in fungal or bacterial superinfection, ▶

including *C. difficile*-associated diarrhea (CDAD) and pseudomembranous colitis; CDAD has been observed >2 months postantibiotic treatment.

Drug Interactions

Avoid Concomitant Use

Avoid concomitant use of Trimethoprim with any of the following: BCG; Dofetilide; Leucovorin Calcium-Levoleucovorin

Decreased Effect

Trimethoprim may decrease the levels/effects of: BCG; Sodium Picosulfate; Typhoid Vaccine

The levels/effects of Trimethoprim may be decreased by: Bosentan; CYP2C9 Inducers (Strong); CYP3A4 Inducers (Strong); Dabrafenib; Deferasirox; Fosphenytoin; Herbs (CYP3A4 Inducers); Leucovorin Calcium-Levoleucovorin; Mitotane; Peginterferon Alfa-2b; Phenytoin; Tocilizumab

Increased Effect/Toxicity

Trimethoprim may increase the levels/effects of: ACE Inhibitors; Amantadine; Angiotensin II Receptor Blockers; Antidiabetic Agents (Thiazolidinedione); AzaTHIOprine; Bosentan; Carvedilol; CYP2C8 Substrates; CYP2C9 Substrates; Dapsone (Systemic); Dapsone (Topical); Digoxin; Dofetilide; Eplerenone; Fosphenytoin; Highest Risk QTc-Prolonging Agents; LamiVUDine; Memantine; Mercaptopurine; MetFORMIN; Methotrexate; Moderate Risk QTc-Prolonging Agents; Phenytoin; PRALAtrexate; Procainamide; Repaglinide; Spironolactone; Varenicline

The levels/effects of Trimethoprim may be increased by: Amantadine; CYP2C9 Inhibitors (Moderate); CYP2C9 Inhibitors (Strong); Dapsone (Systemic); Memantine; Mifepristone

Adverse Reactions Frequency not defined.

Central nervous system: Aseptic meningitis (rare), fever

Dermatologic: Maculopapular rash (3% to 7% at 200 mg/day; incidence higher with larger daily doses), erythema multiforme (rare), exfoliative dermatitis (rare), pruritus (common), phototoxic skin eruptions, Stevens-Johnson syndrome (rare), toxic epidermal necrolysis (rare)

Endocrine & metabolic: Hyperkalemia, hyponatremia

Gastrointestinal: Epigastric distress, glossitis, nausea, vomiting

Hematologic: Leukopenia, megaloblastic anemia, methemoglobinemia, neutropenia, thrombocytopenia

Hepatic: Cholestatic jaundice (rare), liver enzymes increased

Renal: BUN and creatinine increased

Miscellaneous: Anaphylaxis, hypersensitivity reactions

Available Dosage Forms

Solution, Oral:

Primsol: 50 mg/5 mL (473 mL)

Tablet, Oral:

Generic: 100 mg

General Dosage Range Dosage adjustment recommended in patients with renal impairment

Oral:

Children ≥2 months: 4-12 mg/kg/day in divided doses every 12 hours

Adults: 100 mg once daily **or** 100 mg every 12 hours **or** 200 mg every 24 hours; up to 15mg/kg/day

Administration

Oral Administer with milk or food.

Storage/Stability

Solution: Store between 15°C to 25°C (59°F to 77°F). Protect from light.

Tablets: Store at 20°C to 25°C (68°F to 77°F). Protect from light.

Nursing Actions

Physical Assessment Culture and sensitivity should be assessed prior to initiating therapy.

Patient Education

- Discuss specific use of drug and side effects with patient as it relates to treatment. (HCAHPS: During this hospital stay, were you given any medicine that you had not taken before? Before giving you any new medicine, how often did hospital staff tell you what the medicine was for? How often did hospital staff describe possible side effects in a way you could understand?)
- Patient may experience nausea, lack of appetite, or sore throat. Have patient report immediately to prescriber severe diarrhea, significant fatigue, ecchymosis, bleeding, or rash (HCAHPS).
- Educate patient about signs of a significant reaction (eg, wheezing; chest tightness; fever; itching; bad cough; blue skin color; seizures; or swelling of face, lips, tongue, or throat). **Note:** This is not a comprehensive list of all side effects. Patient should consult prescriber for additional questions.

Intended Use and Disclaimer: Should not be printed and given to patients. This information is intended to serve as a concise initial reference for healthcare professionals to use when discussing medications with a patient. You must ultimately rely on your own discretion, experience and judgment in diagnosing, treating and advising patients.

Dietary Considerations May cause folic acid deficiency, supplements may be needed. Should be taken with milk or food.

Trimipramine (trye MI pra meen)

Brand Names: U.S. Surmontil

Index Terms Trimipramine Maleate

Pharmacologic Category Antidepressant, Tricyclic (Tertiary Amine)

Medication Safety Issues

Sound-alike/look-alike issues:

Trimipramine may be confused with triamterene

BEERS Criteria medication:

This drug may be potentially inappropriate for use in geriatric patients (Quality of evidence - high [moderate for SIADH]; Strength of recommendation - strong).

Medication Guide Available Yes

Pregnancy Risk Factor C

Use Treatment of depression

Available Dosage Forms

Capsule, Oral:

Surmontil: 25 mg, 50 mg, 100 mg

General Dosage Range

Oral:

Adolescents: Initial: 50 mg/day (maximum: 100 mg/day)

Adults: 50-200 mg at bedtime (maximum: 200 mg/day [outpatient] or 300 mg/day [inpatient])

Elderly: 50-100 mg at bedtime (maximum: 100 mg/day)

Nursing Actions

Physical Assessment Monitor therapeutic response (eg, mental status, mood, affect, suicide ideation).

Patient Education

• Discuss specific use of drug and side effects with patient as it relates to treatment. (HCAHPS: During this hospital stay, were you given any medicine that you had not taken before? Before giving you any new medicine, how often did hospital staff tell you what the medicine was for? How often did hospital staff describe possible side effects in a way you could understand?)

• Patient may experience presyncope, fatigue, blurred vision, illogical thinking, dizziness, constipation, or xerostomia. Have patient report immediately to prescriber tachycardia, urinary retention, severe asthenia, nervousness and anxiety, or rash (HCAHPS).

• Educate patient about signs of a significant reaction (eg, wheezing; chest tightness; fever; itching; bad cough; blue skin color; seizures; or swelling of face, lips, tongue, or throat). **Note:** This is not a comprehensive list of all side effects. Patient should consult prescriber for additional questions.

Intended Use and Disclaimer: Should not be printed and given to patients. This information is intended to serve as a concise initial reference for healthcare professionals to use when discussing medications with a patient. You must ultimately rely on your own discretion, experience and judgment in diagnosing, treating and advising patients.

Triptorelin (trip toe REL in)

Brand Names: U.S. Trelstar Depot; Trelstar Depot Mixject; Trelstar LA; Trelstar LA Mixject; Trelstar Mixject

Index Terms AY-25650; CL-118,532; D-Trp(6)-LHRH; Detryptoreline; Triptorelin Pamoate; Tryptoreline

Pharmacologic Category Gonadotropin Releasing Hormone Agonist

Pregnancy Risk Factor X

Lactation Excretion in breast milk unknown/contraindicated

Use Palliative treatment of advanced prostate cancer

Decapeptyl® (Canadian labeling; not available in U.S.): Adjunctive therapy in women undergoing controlled ovarian hyperstimulation for assisted reproductive technologies (ART)

Unlabeled Use Treatment of endometriosis, *in vitro* fertilization, precocious puberty, uterine sarcoma; treatment of paraphilia/hypersexuality

Available Dosage Forms

Suspension Reconstituted, Intramuscular:

Trelstar Depot: 3.75 mg (1 ea)

Trelstar Depot Mixject: 3.75 mg (1 ea)

Trelstar LA: 11.25 mg (1 ea)

Trelstar LA Mixject: 11.25 mg (1 ea)

Trelstar Mixject: 22.5 mg (1 ea)

General Dosage Range I.M.: *Adults:* 3.75 mg once every 4 weeks **or** 11.25 mg once every 12 weeks **or** 22.5 mg once every 24 weeks

Administration

I.M. Administer by I.M. injection into the buttock; alternate injection sites. Administer immediately after reconstitution.

Hazardous agent; use appropriate precautions for handling and disposal (NIOSH, 2012).

Subcutaneous Decapeptyl® (Canadian availability; not available in U.S.) is administered by subcutaneous injection into the lower abdomen. If a dose is missed, it can be administered on the same day; however, do not double doses.

Hazardous agent; use appropriate precautions for handling and disposal (NIOSH, 2012).

Nursing Actions

Physical Assessment Hypersensitivity reactions, including angioedema, anaphylaxis, and anaphylactic shock, have rarely occurred; discontinue if severe reaction occurs.

Patient Education

• Discuss specific use of drug and side effects with patient as it relates to treatment. (HCAHPS: During this hospital stay, were you given any medicine that you had not taken before? Before giving you any new medicine, how often did hospital staff tell you what the medicine was for? How often did hospital staff describe possible side effects in a way you could understand?) ▶

• Patient may experience flushing, osteodynia, hematuria, urinary retention, edema, impotence, or injection site irritation. Have patient report immediately to prescriber angina, severe headache, sudden vision changes, eye pain, eye irritation, illogical thinking, polyuria, polydipsia, weight loss, or rash (HCAHPS).

• Educate patient about signs of a significant reaction (eg, wheezing; chest tightness; fever; itching; bad cough; blue skin color; seizures; or swelling of face, lips, tongue, or throat). **Note:** This is not a comprehensive list of all side effects. Patient should consult prescriber for additional questions.

Intended Use and Disclaimer: Should not be printed and given to patients. This information is intended to serve as a concise initial reference for healthcare professionals to use when discussing medications with a patient. You must ultimately rely on your own discretion, experience and judgment in diagnosing, treating and advising patients.

Ulipristal (ue li PRIS tal)

Brand Names: U.S. Ella [DSC]
Index Terms CDB-2914; Ulipristal Acetate
Pharmacologic Category Contraceptive; Progestin Receptor Modulator
Medication Safety Issues
Sound-alike/look-alike issues:
Ulipristal may be confused with ursodiol
Pregnancy Risk Factor X
Lactation Excretion in breast milk unknown/not recommended
Use Ella: Emergency contraception following unprotected intercourse or possible contraceptive failure
Fibristal [Canadian product]: Treatment of moderate-to-severe signs/symptoms of uterine fibroids in premenopausal adult women eligible for surgery. **Note:** Treatment is limited to 3 months.
General Dosage Range Oral: *Adolescents (postpubertal) and Adults:* 30 mg as a single dose
Administration
Oral
Ella: Administer with or without food at anytime during menstrual cycle. If vomiting occurs within 3 hours of administration, consider repeating dose.
Fibristal [Canadian product]: Administer orally with or without food; initiate during the first 7 days of menstrual cycle.
Hazardous agent; use appropriate precautions for handling and disposal (NIOSH, 2012).
Nursing Actions
Patient Education
• Discuss specific use of drug and side effects with patient as it relates to treatment. (HCAHPS: During this hospital stay, were you given any medicine that you had not taken before? Before

giving you any new medicine, how often did hospital staff tell you what the medicine was for? How often did hospital staff describe possible side effects in a way you could understand?)

• Patient may experience dizziness, headache, nausea, dyspepsia, menstrual pain, or menstrual irregularity. Have patient report immediately to prescriber delayed period >7 days, pregnancy, emesis, or rash (HCAHPS).

• Educate patient about signs of a significant reaction (eg, wheezing; chest tightness; fever; itching; bad cough; blue skin color; seizures; or swelling of face, lips, tongue, or throat). **Note:** This is not a comprehensive list of all side effects. Patient should consult prescriber for additional questions.

Intended Use and Disclaimer: Should not be printed and given to patients. This information is intended to serve as a concise initial reference for healthcare professionals to use when discussing medications with a patient. You must ultimately rely on your own discretion, experience and judgment in diagnosing, treating and advising patients.

Umeclidinium and Vilanterol
(ue me kli DIN ee um & VYE lan ter ol)

Brand Names: U.S. Anoro Ellipta
Index Terms Umeclidinium Bromide and Vilanterol; Vilanterol and Umeclidinium
Pharmacologic Category Anticholinergic Agent; Anticholinergic Agent, Long-Acting; Beta$_2$ Agonist; Beta$_2$-Adrenergic Agonist, Long-Acting
Medication Guide Available Yes
Pregnancy Risk Factor C
Breast-Feeding Considerations It is not known if sufficient quantities of umeclidinium or vilanterol are absorbed following inhalation to produce detectable amounts in breast milk. The manufacturer recommends that caution be exercised when administering to nursing women.
Use
Chronic obstructive pulmonary disease: Maintenance treatment of airflow obstruction in patients with chronic obstructive pulmonary disease (COPD), including chronic bronchitis and emphysema
Limitations of use: Not for the relief of acute bronchospasm or for asthma treatment
Mechanism of Action/Effect Umeclidinium, a long-acting anticholinergic, inhibits acetylcholine and causes bronchodilation. Vilanterol, a long-acting beta$_2$-agonist, relaxes bronchial smooth muscle.
Contraindications Hypersensitivity to umeclidinium, vilanterol, or any component of the formulation; severe hypersensitivity to milk proteins

Warnings/Precautions [U.S. Boxed Warning]: Long-acting beta₂-adrenergic agonists (LABAs) such as vilanterol **increase the risk of asthma-related death.** In a large, randomized, placebo-controlled U.S. clinical trial (SMART, 2006), salmeterol was associated with an increase in asthma-related deaths (when added to usual asthma therapy); risk is considered a class effect among all LABAs. A similar increase in the risk of death associated with LABAs has not been demonstrated in patients with COPD. Not indicated for treatment of asthma. Do **not** use for acute episodes of COPD. Do **not** initiate in patients with significantly worsening or acutely deteriorating COPD. Do not increase the daily dose beyond the recommended dose in this situation. Data are not available to determine if LABA use increases the risk of death in patients with COPD. Can produce paradoxical bronchospasm, which may be life threatening; discontinue use immediately.

Use with caution in patients with cardiovascular disease (arrhythmia, hypertension, or HF), diabetes mellitus, narrow-angle glaucoma, hypokalemia, seizure disorders, and thyrotoxicosis. Umeclidinium may worsen the symptoms of prostatic hyperplasia and/or bladder neck obstruction (eg, painful urination, difficulty passing urine); use with caution.

Potentially significant drug-drug interactions may exist, requiring dose or frequency adjustment, additional monitoring, and/or selection of alternative therapy. Powder for oral inhalation contains lactose; severe hypersensitivity, including anaphylaxis, may occur; use is contraindicated in patients with severe milk protein allergy.

Drug Interactions
Avoid Concomitant Use
Avoid concomitant use of Umeclidinium and Vilanterol with any of the following: Aclidinium; Anticholinergics; Beta-Blockers (Nonselective); Iobenguane I 123; Ipratropium (Oral Inhalation); Long-Acting Beta2-Agonists; Potassium Chloride; Tiotropium

Decreased Effect
Umeclidinium and Vilanterol may decrease the levels/effects of: Acetylcholinesterase Inhibitors (Central); Iobenguane I 123; Secretin

The levels/effects of Umeclidinium and Vilanterol may be decreased by: Acetylcholinesterase Inhibitors (Central); Beta-Blockers (Beta1 Selective); Beta-Blockers (Nonselective); Betahistine; Peginterferon Alfa-2b

Increased Effect/Toxicity
Umeclidinium and Vilanterol may increase the levels/effects of: AbobotulinumtoxinA; Analgesics (Opioid); Anticholinergics; Atosiban; Cannabinoids; Highest Risk QTc-Prolonging Agents; Long-Acting Beta2-Agonists; Loop Diuretics; Mirabegron; Moderate Risk QTc-Prolonging Agents; OnabotulinumtoxinA; Potassium Chloride; RimabotulinumtoxinB; Sympathomimetics; Thiazide Diuretics; Tiotropium; Topiramate

The levels/effects of Umeclidinium and Vilanterol may be increased by: Aclidinium; AtoMOXetine; Ipratropium (Oral Inhalation); MAO Inhibitors; Mifepristone; Pramlintide; Tricyclic Antidepressants

Adverse Reactions
Percentages as reported with combination product.

1% to 10%:
Cardiovascular: Chest pain (1%)
Gastrointestinal: Diarrhea (2%), constipation (1%)
Neuromuscular & skeletal: Limb pain (2%), muscle spasm (1%), neck pain (1%)
Respiratory: Pharyngitis (2%), lower respiratory tract infection (1%), sinusitis (1%)

Product Availability
Anoro Ellipta: FDA approved December 2013; anticipated availability is first quarter 2014

Available Dosage Forms
Aerosol Powder Breath Activated, Inhalation:
Anoro Ellipta: Umeclidinium 62.5 mcg and vilanterol 25 mcg per inhalation

General Dosage Range
Oral inhalation: *Adults:* Umeclidinium 62.5 mg/vilanterol 25 mcg: 1 inhalation once daily; maximum dose: 1 inhalation once daily

Administration
Inhalation Administer at the same time each day. After removing from foil tray, write the "Tray Opened" and "Discard" dates on the inhaler label. Discard device 6 weeks after it is removed from the foil tray or when the dose counter reads "0" (whichever comes first).

Storage/Stability Store at room temperature between 68°F and 77°F (20°C and 25°C); excursions are permitted between 59°F and 86°F (15°C and 30°C). Store in a dry place away from heat or sunlight. Store inside the original, unopened foil tray; remove from tray immediately prior to initial use. Discard inhaler 6 weeks after opening the foil tray or after the labeled number of inhalations have reached zero, whichever comes first.

Nursing Actions
Patient Education
- Discuss specific use of drug and side effects with patient as it relates to treatment. (HCAHPS: During this hospital stay, were you given any medicine that you had not taken before? Before giving you any new medicine, how often did hospital staff tell you what the medicine was for? How often did hospital staff describe possible side effects in a way you could understand?)
- Patient may experience pharyngitis, rhinorrhea, muscle spasm, extremity pain, constipation, diarrhea, or neck pain. Have patient report immediately to prescriber signs of hyperglycemia, signs of hypokalemia, angina, tachycardia, arrhythmia, significant nervousness and anxiety, severe headache, considerable dizziness, ▶

tremors, intolerable nausea, vision changes, ophthalmalgia, significant eye irritation, visual halos around lights, urinary retention, dysuria, or severe breathing problems (HCAHPS).
- Educate patient about signs of a significant reaction (eg, wheezing; chest tightness; fever; itching; bad cough; blue skin color; seizures; or swelling of face, lips, tongue, or throat). **Note:** This is not a comprehensive list of all side effects. Patient should consult prescriber for additional questions.

Intended Use and Disclaimer: Should not be printed and given to patients. This information is intended to serve as a concise initial reference for healthcare professionals to use when discussing medications with a patient. You must ultimately rely on your own discretion, experience and judgment in diagnosing, treating and advising patients.

Unoprostone (yoo noe PROS tone)

Brand Names: U.S. Rescula
Index Terms Unoprostone Isopropyl
Pharmacologic Category Ophthalmic Agent, Antiglaucoma; Prostaglandin, Ophthalmic
Pregnancy Risk Factor C
Lactation Excretion in breast milk unknown/use caution
Use To lower intraocular pressure (IOP) in patients with open-angle glaucoma or ocular hypertension
Available Dosage Forms
Solution, Ophthalmic:
Rescula: 0.15% (5 mL)
General Dosage Range Ophthalmic: *Adults:* Instill 1 drop into affected eye(s) twice daily
Administration
Ophthalmic May be used with other eye drops to lower intraocular pressure; if using more than one product, wait at least 5 minutes between application of each medication. Remove contact lenses prior to administration and wait 15 minutes before reinserting. Minimize contamination by not touching the eyelids or surrounding areas with the dropper tip; keep bottle tightly closed when not in use.
Nursing Actions
Patient Education
- Discuss specific use of drug and side effects with patient as it relates to treatment. (HCAHPS: During this hospital stay, were you given any medicine that you had not taken before? Before giving you any new medicine, how often did hospital staff tell you what the medicine was for? How often did hospital staff describe possible side effects in a way you could understand?)
- Patient may experience eye irritation, blurred vision, or change in eye color. Have patient report immediately to prescriber sudden vision changes, eye pain, or rash (HCAHPS).

- Educate patient about signs of a significant reaction (eg, wheezing; chest tightness; fever; itching; bad cough; blue skin color; seizures; or swelling of face, lips, tongue, or throat). **Note:** This is not a comprehensive list of all side effects. Patient should consult prescriber for additional questions.

Intended Use and Disclaimer: Should not be printed and given to patients. This information is intended to serve as a concise initial reference for healthcare professionals to use when discussing medications with a patient. You must ultimately rely on your own discretion, experience and judgment in diagnosing, treating and advising patients.

Ursodiol (ur soe DYE ol)

Brand Names: U.S. Actigall; Urso 250; Urso Forte
Index Terms Ursodeoxycholic Acid
Pharmacologic Category Gallstone Dissolution Agent
Medication Safety Issues
Sound-alike/look-alike issues:
Ursodiol may be confused with ulipristal
Pregnancy Risk Factor B
Lactation Excretion in breast milk unknown/use caution
Use
Actigall: Gallbladder stone dissolution; prevention of gallstones in obese patients experiencing rapid weight loss
Urso, Urso Forte: Primary biliary cirrhosis
Available Dosage Forms
Capsule, Oral:
Actigall: 300 mg
Generic: 300 mg
Tablet, Oral:
Urso 250: 250 mg
Urso Forte: 500 mg
Generic: 250 mg, 500 mg
General Dosage Range Oral: *Adults:* 8-15 mg/kg/day in 2-4 divided doses **or** 300 mg twice daily
Administration
Oral Do not administer with aluminum-based antacids or bile acid sequestrants. If aluminum-based antacids are needed, administer 2 hours after ursodiol; administer ursodiol 5 hours or more after bile acid sequestrants (Rust, 2000). Urso Forte can be split into halves for appropriate dosage; do not chew. Urso and Urso Forte should be taken with food.
Nursing Actions
Patient Education
- Discuss specific use of drug and side effects with patient as it relates to treatment. (HCAHPS: During this hospital stay, were you given any medicine that you had not taken before? Before giving you any new medicine, how often did

hospital staff tell you what the medicine was for? How often did hospital staff describe possible side effects in a way you could understand?)
- Patient may experience dizziness, headache, back pain, nausea, constipation, or diarrhea. Have patient report immediately to prescriber severe dyspepsia or rash (HCAHPS).
- Educate patient about signs of a significant reaction (eg, wheezing; chest tightness; fever; itching; bad cough; blue skin color; seizures; or swelling of face, lips, tongue, or throat). **Note:** This is not a comprehensive list of all side effects. Patient should consult prescriber for additional questions.

Intended Use and Disclaimer: Should not be printed and given to patients. This information is intended to serve as a concise initial reference for healthcare professionals to use when discussing medications with a patient. You must ultimately rely on your own discretion, experience and judgment in diagnosing, treating and advising patients.

ValACYclovir (val ay SYE kloe veer)

Brand Names: U.S. Valtrex
Index Terms Valacyclovir Hydrochloride
Pharmacologic Category Antiviral Agent; Antiviral Agent, Oral
Medication Safety Issues
Sound-alike/look-alike issues:
Valtrex® may be confused with Keflex®, Valcyte®, Zovirax®
ValACYclovir may be confused with acyclovir, valGANciclovir, vancomycin
Pregnancy Risk Factor B
Lactation Enters breast milk/use caution
Breast-Feeding Considerations Valacyclovir is metabolized to acyclovir; acyclovir (but not unchanged valacyclovir) can be detected in breast milk. Peak concentrations in breast milk range from 0.5-2.3 times the corresponding maternal acyclovir serum concentration. This is expected to provide a nursing infant with a dose of acyclovir equivalent to ~0.6 mg/kg/day following ingestion of valacyclovir 500 mg twice daily by the mother. The manufacturer recommends that caution be used if administered to a nursing woman. Other sources note that women with HSV infection taking valacyclovir may breast-feed as long as there are not lesions on the breast, body lesions are covered, and strict hand hygiene is practiced (ACOG, 2000; Jaiyeoba, 2012). Women with HSV who also have HIV infection should not breast-feed; complete avoidance of breast-feeding by HIV-infected women is recommended to decrease potential transmission of HIV (DHHS [perinatal], 2012).
Use Treatment of herpes zoster (shingles) in immunocompetent patients; treatment of first-episode and recurrent genital herpes; suppression of recurrent genital herpes and reduction of transmission of genital herpes in immunocompetent patients; suppression of genital herpes in HIV-infected individuals; treatment of herpes labialis (cold sores); chickenpox in immunocompetent children
Unlabeled Use Prophylaxis of cancer-related HSV, VZV, and CMV infections; treatment of cancer-related HSV, VZV infection
Mechanism of Action/Effect Valacyclovir is rapidly converted to acyclovir before it exerts its antiviral activity against HSV-1, HSV-2, or VZV. Inhibits viral DNA synthesis and replication.
Contraindications Hypersensitivity to valacyclovir, acyclovir, or any component of the formulation
Warnings/Precautions Thrombotic thrombocytopenic purpura/hemolytic uremic syndrome has occurred in immunocompromised patients (at doses of 8 g/day). Safety and efficacy have not been established for treatment/suppression of recurrent genital herpes or disseminated herpes in patients with profound immunosuppression (eg, advanced HIV with CD4 <100 cells/mm^3). CNS adverse effects (including agitation, hallucinations, confusion, delirium, seizures, and encephalopathy) have been reported. Use caution in patients with renal impairment, the elderly, and/or those receiving nephrotoxic agents. Acute renal failure has been observed in patients with renal dysfunction; dose adjustment may be required. Decreased precipitation in renal tubules may occur leading to urinary precipitation; adequately hydrate patient. For cold sores, treatment should begin at with earliest symptom (tingling, itching, burning). For genital herpes, treatment should begin as soon as possible after the first signs and symptoms (within 72 hours of onset of first diagnosis or within 24 hours of onset of recurrent episodes). For herpes zoster, treatment should begin within 72 hours of onset of rash. For chickenpox, treatment should begin with earliest sign or symptom. Use with caution in the elderly; CNS effects have been reported. Safety and efficacy have not been established in patients <2 years of age.
Drug Interactions
Avoid Concomitant Use
Avoid concomitant use of ValACYclovir with any of the following: Zoster Vaccine
Decreased Effect
ValACYclovir may decrease the levels/effects of: Zoster Vaccine
Increased Effect/Toxicity
ValACYclovir may increase the levels/effects of: Mycophenolate; Tenofovir; Zidovudine

The levels/effects of ValACYclovir may be increased by: Mycophenolate

◀ **Adverse Reactions**
>10%:
Central nervous system: Headache (13% to 38%)
Gastrointestinal: Nausea (5% to 15%), abdominal pain (1% to 11%)
Hepatic: ALT increased (≤14%), AST increased (2% to 16%)
Respiratory: Nasopharyngitis (≤16%)
1% to 10%:
Central nervous system: Fatigue (≤8%), depression (≤7%), fever (children 4%), dizziness (2% to 4%)
Dermatologic: Rash (≤8%)
Endocrine: Dysmenorrhea (≤1% to 8%), dehydration (children 2%)
Gastrointestinal: Vomiting (<1% to 6%), diarrhea (children 5%; adults <1%)
Hematologic: Thrombocytopenia (≤3%), mild leukopenia (≤1%)
Hepatic: Alkaline phosphatase increased (≤4%)
Neuromuscular & skeletal: Arthralgia (<1 to 6%)
Respiratory: Rhinorrhea (children 2%)
Miscellaneous: Herpes simplex (children 2%)

Available Dosage Forms
Tablet, Oral:
Valtrex: 500 mg, 1 g
Generic: 500 mg, 1 g
General Dosage Range Dosage adjustment recommended in patients with renal impairment
Oral:
Children 2 to <12 years: 20 mg/kg/dose 3 times daily (maximum: 1 g 3 times daily)
Children ≥12 to <18 years: 2 g every 12 hours for 1 day (cold sores) **or** 20 mg/kg/dose 3 times daily (maximum: 1 g 3 times daily) (chickenpox)
Adults: 500 mg to 1 g 1-3 times daily **or** 2 g every 12 hours for 1 day

Administration
Oral If GI upset occurs, administer with meals.
Storage/Stability Store at 15°C to 25°C (59°F to 77°F).
Nursing Actions
Physical Assessment Monitor for CNS changes (dizziness, depression), nausea, vomiting, dysmenorrhea, and arthralgia. Teach patient appropriate timing of treatment.
Patient Education
• Discuss specific use of drug and side effects with patient as it relates to treatment. (HCAHPS: During this hospital stay, were you given any medicine that you had not taken before? Before giving you any new medicine, how often did hospital staff tell you what the medicine was for? How often did hospital staff describe possible side effects in a way you could understand?)
• Patient may experience dyspepsia, leukopenia, or increased liver enzymes. Have patient report immediately to prescriber severe headache, significant nausea, considerable diarrhea, illogical thinking, difficulty speaking, sudden vision changes, ophthalmalgia, eye irritation, tremors,

difficulty with motor activity, rigidity, or petechiae (HCAHPS).
• Educate patient about signs of a significant reaction (eg, wheezing; chest tightness; fever; itching; bad cough; blue skin color; seizures; or swelling of face, lips, tongue, or throat). **Note:** This is not a comprehensive list of all side effects. Patient should consult prescriber for additional questions.

Intended Use and Disclaimer: Should not be printed and given to patients. This information is intended to serve as a concise initial reference for healthcare professionals to use when discussing medications with a patient. You must ultimately rely on your own discretion, experience and judgment in diagnosing, treating and advising patients.
Dietary Considerations May be taken with or without food.

ValGANCIclovir (val gan SYE kloh veer)

Brand Names: U.S. Valcyte
Index Terms Valganciclovir Hydrochloride
Pharmacologic Category Antiviral Agent
Medication Safety Issues
Sound-alike/look-alike issues:
Valcyte® may be confused with Valium®, Valtrex®
ValGANciclovir may be confused with valACYclovir, ganciclovir
Pregnancy Risk Factor C
Lactation Excretion in breast milk unknown/not recommended
Breast-Feeding Considerations HIV-infected mothers are discouraged from breast-feeding to decrease the potential transmission of HIV.
Use Treatment of cytomegalovirus (CMV) retinitis in patients with acquired immunodeficiency syndrome (AIDS); prevention of CMV disease in high-risk patients (donor CMV positive/recipient CMV negative) undergoing kidney, heart, or kidney/pancreas transplantation
Mechanism of Action/Effect Valganciclovir is a prodrug of ganciclovir, and is rapidly metabolized in the body to form ganciclovir. Ganciclovir inhibits the formation of viral DNA within infected cells, blocking reproduction of the virus.
Contraindications Hypersensitivity to valganciclovir, ganciclovir, or any component of the formulation
Warnings/Precautions Hazardous agent - use appropriate precautions for handling and disposal (NIOSH, 2012). **[U.S. Boxed Warning]: May cause dose- or therapy-limiting granulocytopenia, anemia, and/or thrombocytopenia;** do not use in patients with an absolute neutrophil count <500/mm^3, platelet count <25,000/mm^3, or hemoglobin <8 g/dL. Use with caution in patients with impaired renal function (dose adjustment required).

Acute renal failure (ARF) may occur; ensure adequate hydration and use with caution in patients receiving concomitant nephrotoxic agents. Elderly patients with or without pre-existing renal impairment may develop ARF; use with caution and adjust dose as needed. **[U.S. Boxed Warning]: Ganciclovir may be teratogenic, carcinogenic, and cause aspermatogenesis.** Due to its teratogenic potential, contraceptive precautions for female and male patients need to be followed during and for at least 90 days after therapy with the drug. Fertility may be temporarily or permanently impaired in males and females. Due to differences in bioavailability, valganciclovir tablets cannot be substituted for ganciclovir capsules on a one-to-one basis. The preferred dosage form for pediatric patients is the oral solution; however, valganciclovir tablets may used so long as the calculated dose is within 10% of the available tablet strength (450 mg). Not indicated for use in liver transplant patients (higher incidence of tissue-invasive CMV relative to oral ganciclovir was observed in trials). Use of valganciclovir for the treatment of congenital CMV disease has not been evaluated.

Drug Interactions

Avoid Concomitant Use

Avoid concomitant use of ValGANciclovir with any of the following: Imipenem

Decreased Effect There are no known significant interactions involving a decrease in effect.

Increased Effect/Toxicity

ValGANciclovir may increase the levels/effects of: Imipenem; Mycophenolate; Reverse Transcriptase Inhibitors (Nucleoside); Tenofovir

The levels/effects of ValGANciclovir may be increased by: Mycophenolate; Probenecid; Tenofovir

Nutritional/Ethanol Interactions Food: Coadministration with a high-fat meal increased AUC by 30%. Management: Valganciclovir should be taken with meals.

Adverse Reactions Valganciclovir is expected to share similar idiosyncratic or low incidence toxicities associated with ganciclovir.

>10%:
Cardiovascular: Hypertension (12% to 18%)
Central nervous system: Fever (9% to 31%), headache (6% to 22%), insomnia (6% to 20%)
Gastrointestinal: Diarrhea (16% to 41%), nausea (8% to 30%), vomiting (3% to 21%), abdominal pain (15%), constipation
Hematologic: Anemia (≤31%), thrombocytopenia (≤22%), neutropenia (3% to 19%)
Immunologic: Graft rejection (24%)
Neuromuscular & skeletal: Tremor (12% to 28%)
Ocular: Retinal detachment (15%)
Renal: Serum creatinine increased (S_{cr} >1.5-2.5 mg/dL: 12% to 50%; S_{cr} >2.5: 3% to 17%)

Respiratory: Cough, upper respiratory tract infection
5% to 10%:
Central nervous system: Peripheral neuropathy (9%), paresthesia (8%)
Immunologic: Organ transplant rejection (9%)
<5%:
Cardiovascular: Edema, hypotension, peripheral edema
Central nervous system: Agitation, confusion, depression, dizziness, fatigue, hallucination, pain, psychosis, seizure
Dermatologic: Acne, dermatitis, pruritus
Endocrine & metabolic: Dehydration, hyperglycemia, hyper-/hypokalemia, hypocalcemia, hypomagnesemia, hypophosphatemia
Gastrointestinal: Abdominal distention/pain, appetite (decreased), dyspepsia
Genitourinary: Urinary tract infection
Hematologic: Aplastic anemia, bleeding (potentially life-threatening due to thrombocytopenia), bone marrow depression, pancytopenia
Hepatic: Ascites, hepatic insufficiency
Local: Catheter infection (3%)
Neuromuscular & skeletal: Arthralgia, back pain, limb pain, muscle cramps, weakness
Renal: Creatinine clearance (decreased), dysuria, renal impairment
Respiratory: Dyspnea, nasopharyngitis, pharyngitis, pleural effusion, rhinorrhea
Miscellaneous: Allergic reaction, local and systemic infection (including sepsis), postoperative complication, postoperative pain, postoperative wound complication (infection, increased drainage, dehiscence)

Available Dosage Forms

Solution Reconstituted, Oral:
Valcyte: 50 mg/mL (88 mL)
Tablet, Oral:
Valcyte: 450 mg

General Dosage Range Dosage adjustment recommended in patients with renal impairment
Oral:
Children 4 months to 16 years: Dose (mg) = 7 x body surface area x creatinine clearance once daily
Children >16 years and Adults: 900 mg 1-2 times/day

Administration

Oral Valganciclovir should be taken with meals. The preferred dosage form for pediatric patients is the oral solution; however, valganciclovir tablets may used so long as the calculated dose is within 10% of the available tablet strength (450 mg).

Due to the carcinogenic and mutagenic potential, avoid direct contact with broken or crushed tablets, powder for oral solution, and oral solution. Consideration should be given to handling and disposal according to guidelines issued for ▶

antineoplastic drugs. However, there is no consensus on the need for these precautions.

Hazardous agent; use appropriate precautions for handling and disposal (NIOSH, 2012).

Preparation for Administration Hazardous agent; use appropriate precautions for handling and disposal (NIOSH, 2012).

Oral solution: Prior to dispensing, prepare the oral solution by adding 91 mL of purified water to the bottle; shake well. Discard any unused medication after 49 days. A reconstituted 100 mL bottle will only provide 88 mL of solution for administration.

Storage/Stability

Oral solution: Store dry powder at 25°C (77°F); excursions permitted to 15°C to 30°C (59°F to 86°F). Store oral solution under refrigeration at 2°C to 8°C (36°F to 46°F); do not freeze. Discard any unused medication after 49 days.

Tablet: Store at 25°C (77°F); excursions permitted to 15°C to 30°C (59°F to 86°F).

Nursing Actions

Physical Assessment Monitor for peripheral neuropathy, neutropenia, anemia, nephrotoxicity, vomiting, and bloody diarrhea on a regular basis during therapy.

Patient Education

• Discuss specific use of drug and side effects with patient as it relates to treatment. (HCAHPS: During this hospital stay, were you given any medicine that you had not taken before? Before giving you any new medicine, how often did hospital staff tell you what the medicine was for? How often did hospital staff describe possible side effects in a way you could understand?)

• Patient may experience anemia, leukopenia, thrombocytopenia, hypertension, headache, nausea, diarrhea, dyspepsia, or insomnia. Have patient report immediately to prescriber paresthesia, dyspnea, illogical thinking, fasciculations, ecchymosis, fatigue, urinary retention, or rash (HCAHPS).

• Educate patient about signs of a significant reaction (eg, wheezing; chest tightness; fever; itching; bad cough; blue skin color; seizures; or swelling of face, lips, tongue, or throat). **Note:** This is not a comprehensive list of all side effects. Patient should consult prescriber for additional questions.

Intended Use and Disclaimer: Should not be printed and given to patients. This information is intended to serve as a concise initial reference for healthcare professionals to use when discussing medications with a patient. You must ultimately rely on your own discretion, experience and judgment in diagnosing, treating and advising patients.

Dietary Considerations Should be taken with meals.

Related Information

Oral Medications That Should Not Be Crushed or Altered *on page 1712*

Valproic Acid and Derivatives
(val PROE ik AS id & dah RIV ah tives)

Brand Names: U.S. Depacon; Depakene; Depakote; Depakote ER; Depakote Sprinkles; Stavzor

Index Terms 2-Propylpentanoic Acid; 2-Propylvaleric Acid; Dipropylacetic Acid; Divalproex Sodium; DPA; Valproate Semisodium; Valproate Sodium; Valproic Acid; Valproic Acid Derivative

Pharmacologic Category Anticonvulsant, Miscellaneous; Antimanic Agent; Histone Deacetylase Inhibitor

Medication Safety Issues

Sound-alike/look-alike issues:

Depakene may be confused with Depakote

Depakote may be confused with Depakene, Depakote ER, Senokot

Depakote ER may be confused with divalproex enteric coated

Valproate sodium may be confused with vecuronium

Medication Guide Available Yes

Pregnancy Risk Factor X (migraine prophylaxis)/D (all other indications)

Lactation Enters breast milk/use caution

Breast-Feeding Considerations Valproate is excreted into breast milk. Breast milk concentrations of valproic acid have been reported as 1% to 10% of maternal concentration. The weight-adjusted dose to the infant has been calculated to be ~4% (Hagg, 2000). The manufacturer recommends that caution be used if administered to nursing women.

Use

Oral, I.V.: Monotherapy and adjunctive therapy in the treatment of patients with complex partial seizures; monotherapy and adjunctive therapy of simple and complex absence seizures; adjunctive therapy in patients with multiple seizure types that include absence seizures

Additional indications: Depakote, Depakote ER, Stavzor: Mania associated with bipolar disorder; migraine prophylaxis

Unlabeled Use Refractory status epilepticus, diabetic neuropathy

Mechanism of Action/Effect Causes increased availability of gamma-aminobutyric acid (GABA), an inhibitory neurotransmitter, to brain neurons or may enhance the action of GABA or mimic its action at postsynaptic receptor sites

Contraindications Hypersensitivity to valproic acid, divalproex, derivatives, or any component of the formulation; hepatic disease or significant impairment; urea cycle disorders; pregnant women for the prevention of migraine; known mitochondrial disorders caused by mutations in mitochondrial DNA polymerase gamma (POLG; eg, Alpers-Huttenlocher syndrome [AHS]) or children <2 years of age suspected of having a POLG-related disorder

Warnings/Precautions Hazardous agent; use appropriate precautions for handling and disposal (NIOSH, 2012). **[U.S. Boxed Warning]: Hepatic failure resulting in fatalities has occurred in patients, usually in the initial 6 months of therapy; children <2 years of age are at considerable risk. Risk is also increased in patients with hereditary neurometabolic syndromes caused by DNA mutations of the mitochondrial DNA polymerase gamma (POLG) gene (eg, Alpers-Huttenlocher syndrome [AHS]).** Other risk factors include organic brain disease, mental retardation with severe seizure disorders, congenital metabolic disorders, and patients on multiple anticonvulsants. Monitor patients closely for appearance of malaise, weakness, facial edema, anorexia, jaundice, and vomiting; discontinue immediately with signs/symptom of significant or suspected impairment. Liver function tests should be performed at baseline and at regular intervals after initiation of therapy, especially within the first 6 months. Hepatic dysfunction may progress despite discontinuing treatment. Should only be used as monotherapy and with extreme caution in children <2 years of age and/or patients at high risk for hepatotoxicity. Contraindicated with significant hepatic impairment.

[U.S. Boxed Warning]: Risk of valproate-induced acute liver failure and death is increased in patients with hereditary neurometabolic syndromes caused by DNA mutations of the mitochondrial polymerase gamma (POLG) gene (eg, Alpers-Huttenlocher syndrome [AHS]). Use is contraindicated in patients with known mitochondrial disorders caused by POLG mutations and children <2 years of age suspected of having a POLG-related disorder. Use in children ≥2 years of age suspected of having a POLG-related disorder only after other anticonvulsants have failed and with close monitoring for the development of acute liver injury. POLG mutation testing should be performed in accordance with current clinical practice.

[U.S. Boxed Warning]: Cases of life-threatening pancreatitis, occurring at the start of therapy or following years of use, have been reported in adults and children. Some cases have been hemorrhagic with rapid progression of initial symptoms to death. Promptly evaluate symptoms of abdominal pain, nausea, vomiting, and/or anorexia; should generally be discontinued if pancreatitis is diagnosed.

[U.S. Boxed Warning]: May cause teratogenic effects such as neural tube defects (eg, spina bifida) and decreased IQ scores following *in utero* exposure. Use is contraindicated in pregnant women for the prevention of migraine. **Use is not recommended in women of childbearing potential for any indication unless alternative therapies are not appropriate**, especially when used for conditions not associated with permanent injury or risk of death (eg, migraine).

May cause severe thrombocytopenia, inhibition of platelet aggregation, and bleeding. Hypersensitivity reactions affecting multiple organs have been reported in association with valproate use; may include dermatologic and/or hematologic changes (eosinophilia, neutropenia, thrombocytopenia) or symptoms of organ dysfunction.

Hyperammonemia and/or encephalopathy, sometimes fatal, have been reported following the initiation of valproate therapy and may be present with normal transaminase levels. Ammonia levels should be measured in patients who develop unexplained lethargy and vomiting, changes in mental status, or in patients who present with hypothermia (unintentional drop in core body temperature to <35°C/95°F). Discontinue therapy if ammonia levels are increased and evaluate for possible urea cycle disorder (UCD); contraindicated in patients with UCD. Evaluation of UCD should be considered for the following patients prior to the start of therapy: History of unexplained encephalopathy or coma; encephalopathy associated with protein load; pregnancy or postpartum encephalopathy; unexplained mental retardation; history of elevated plasma ammonia or glutamine; history of cyclical vomiting and lethargy; episodic extreme irritability, ataxia; low BUN or protein avoidance; family history of UCD or unexplained infant deaths (particularly male); or signs or symptoms of UCD (hyperammonemia, encephalopathy, respiratory alkalosis). Hypothermia has been reported with valproate therapy; hypothermia may or may not be associated with hyperammonemia; may also occur with concomitant topiramate therapy following topiramate initiation or dosage increase.

In vitro studies have suggested valproate stimulates the replication of HIV and CMV viruses under experimental conditions. The clinical consequence of this is unknown, but should be considered when monitoring affected patients.

Antiepileptics are associated with an increased risk of suicidal behavior/thoughts with use (regardless of indication); patients should be monitored for signs/symptoms of depression, suicidal tendencies, and other unusual behavior changes during therapy and instructed to inform their healthcare provider immediately if symptoms occur.

Intravenous valproate is not recommended for post-traumatic seizure prophylaxis in patients with acute head trauma; study results for this indication suggested increased mortality with I.V. valproate use compared to I.V. phenytoin. Anticonvulsants should not be discontinued abruptly because of the possibility of increasing seizure frequency; valproate should be withdrawn gradually to minimize the potential of increased seizure frequency, unless safety concerns require a more rapid withdrawal. Patients treated for bipolar disorder should be monitored closely for clinical worsening or suicidality; prescriptions should be written for the smallest quantity consistent with good patient care.

Reversible and irreversible cerebral and cerebellar atrophy have been reported; motor and cognitive function should be routinely monitored to assess for signs and symptoms of brain atrophy. CNS depression may occur with valproate use. Patients must be cautioned about performing tasks which require mental alertness (operating machinery or driving). Effects with other sedative drugs or ethanol may be potentiated. Use with caution in the elderly as the elderly may be more sensitive to sedating effects and dehydration; in some elderly patients with somnolence, concomitant decreases in nutritional intake and weight loss were observed. Reduce initial dosages in elderly and closely monitor fluid status, nutritional intake, somnolence, and other adverse events. Potentially significant drug-drug interactions may exist, requiring dose or frequency adjustment, additional monitoring, and/or selection of alternative therapy.

Medication residue in stool has been reported (rarely) with oral Depakote (divalproex sodium) formulations; some reports have occurred in patients with shortened GI transit times (eg, diarrhea) or anatomic GI disorders (eg, ileostomy, colostomy). In patients reporting medication residue in stool, it is recommended to monitor valproate level and clinical condition.

Drug Interactions

Avoid Concomitant Use

Avoid concomitant use of Valproic Acid and Derivatives with any of the following: Cosyntropin

Decreased Effect

Valproic Acid and Derivatives may decrease the levels/effects of: CarBAMazepine; Fosphenytoin-Phenytoin; OLANZapine; OXcarbazepine; Urea Cycle Disorder Agents

The levels/effects of Valproic Acid and Derivatives may be decreased by: Barbiturates; CarBAMazepine; Carbapenems; Ethosuximide; Fosphenytoin-Phenytoin; Methylfolate; Protease Inhibitors; Rifampin

Increased Effect/Toxicity

Valproic Acid and Derivatives may increase the levels/effects of: Barbiturates; Ethosuximide; LamoTRIgine; LORazepam; Paliperidone; Primidone; RisperiDONE; Rufinamide; Temozolomide; Tricyclic Antidepressants; Vorinostat; Zidovudine

The levels/effects of Valproic Acid and Derivatives may be increased by: ChlorproMAZINE; Cosyntropin; Felbamate; GuanFACINE; Primidone; Salicylates; Topiramate

Nutritional/Ethanol Interactions

Ethanol: Avoid ethanol (may increase CNS depression).

Food: Food may delay but does not affect the extent of absorption.

Adverse Reactions

>10%:

Central nervous system: Headache (≤31%), somnolence (≤30%), dizziness (12% to 25%), insomnia (>1% to 15%), nervousness (>1% to 11%), pain (1% to 11%)

Dermatologic: Alopecia (>1% to 24%)

Gastrointestinal: Nausea (15% to 48%), vomiting (7% to 27%), diarrhea (7% to 23%), abdominal pain (7% to 23%), dyspepsia (7% to 23%), anorexia (>1% to 12%)

Hematologic: Thrombocytopenia (1% to 24%; dose related)

Neuromuscular & skeletal: Tremor (≤57%), weakness (6% to 27%)

Ocular: Diplopia (>1% to 16%), amblyopia/blurred vision (≤12%)

Miscellaneous: Infection (≤20%), flu-like syndrome (12%)

1% to 10%:

Cardiovascular: Peripheral edema (>1% to 8%), chest pain (>1% to <5%), edema (>1% to <5%), facial edema (>1% to <5%), hypertension (>1% to <5%), hypotension (>1% to <5%), orthostatic hypotension (>1% to <5%), palpitation (>1% to <5%), tachycardia (>1% to <5%), vasodilation (>1% to <5%), arrhythmia

Central nervous system: Ataxia (>1% to 8%), amnesia (>1% to 7%), emotional lability (>1% to 6%), fever (>1% to 6%), abnormal thinking (≤6%), depression (>1% to 5%), abnormal dreams (>1% to <5%), agitation (>1% to <5%), anxiety (>1% to <5%), catatonia (>1% to <5%), chills (>1% to <5%), confusion (>1% to <5%), coordination abnormal (>1% to <5%), hallucination (>1% to <5%), malaise (>1% to <5%), personality disorder (>1% to <5%), speech disorder (>1% to <5%), tardive dyskinesia (>1% to <5%), vertigo (>1% to <5%), euphoria (1%), hypoesthesia (1%)

Dermatologic: Rash (>1% to 6%), bruising (>1% to 5%), discoid lupus erythematosus (>1% to <5%), dry skin (>1% to <5%), furunculosis (>1% to <5%), petechia (>1% to <5%), pruritus (>1% to <5%), seborrhea (>1% to <5%)

Endocrine & metabolic: Amenorrhea (>1% to <5%), dysmenorrhea (>1% to <5%), metrorrhagia (>1% to <5%), hypoproteinemia

Gastrointestinal: Weight gain (4% to 9%), weight loss (6%), appetite increased (≤6%), constipation (>1% to 5%), xerostomia (>1% to 5%), eructation (>1% to <5%), fecal incontinence (>1% to <5%), flatulence (>1% to <5%), gastroenteritis (>1% to <5%), glossitis (>1% to <5%), hematemesis (>1% to <5%), pancreatitis (>1% to <5%), periodontal abscess (>1% to <5%), stomatitis (>1% to <5%), taste perversion (>1% to <5%), dysphagia, gum hemorrhage, mouth ulceration

Genitourinary: Cystitis (>1% to 5%), dysuria (>1% to 5%), urinary frequency (>1% to <5%), urinary incontinence (>1% to <5%), vaginal hemorrhage (>1% to 5%), vaginitis (>1% to <5%)

Hepatic: ALT increased (>1% to <5%), AST increased (>1% to <5%)

Local: Injection site pain (3%), injection site reaction (2%), injection site inflammation (1%)

Neuromuscular & skeletal: Back pain (≤8%), abnormal gait (>1% to <5%), arthralgia (>1% to <5%), arthrosis (>1% to <5%), dysarthria (>1% to <5%), hypertonia (>1% to <5%), hypokinesia (>1% to <5%), leg cramps (>1% to <5%), myalgia (>1% to <5%), myasthenia (>1% to <5%), neck pain (>1% to <5%), neck rigidity (>1% to <5%), paresthesia (>1% to <5%), reflex increased (>1% to <5%), twitching (>1% to <5%)

Ocular: Nystagmus (1% to 8%), dry eyes (>1% to 5%), eye pain (>1% to 5%), abnormal vision (>1% to <5%), conjunctivitis (>1% to <5%)

Otic: Tinnitus (1% to 7%), ear pain (>1% to 5%), deafness (>1% to <5%), otitis media (>1% to <5%)

Respiratory: Pharyngitis (2% to 8%), bronchitis (5%), rhinitis (>1% to 5%), dyspnea (1% to 5%), cough (>1% to <5%), epistaxis (>1% to <5%), pneumonia (>1% to <5%), sinusitis (>1% to <5%)

Miscellaneous: Diaphoresis (1%), hiccups

Dosage Forms Considerations

Strengths of divalproex sodium and valproate sodium products are expressed in terms of valproic acid

Available Dosage Forms

Capsule, Oral:
Depakene: 250 mg
Generic: 250 mg

Capsule Delayed Release, Oral:
Stavzor: 125 mg, 250 mg, 500 mg

Capsule Sprinkle, Oral:
Depakote Sprinkles: 125 mg
Generic: 125 mg

Solution, Intravenous:
Depacon: 100 mg/mL (5 mL)
Generic: 100 mg/mL (5 mL)

Solution, Intravenous [preservative free]:
Generic: 100 mg/mL (5 mL); 500 mg/5 mL (5 mL); 100 mg/mL (5 mL)

Solution, Oral:
Generic: 250 mg/5 mL (473 mL)

Syrup, Oral:
Depakene: 250 mg/5 mL (480 mL)
Generic: 250 mg/5 mL (5 mL, 10 mL, 473 mL)

Tablet Delayed Release, Oral:
Depakote: 125 mg, 250 mg, 500 mg
Generic: 125 mg, 250 mg, 500 mg

Tablet Extended Release 24 Hour, Oral:
Depakote ER: 250 mg, 500 mg
Generic: 250 mg, 500 mg

General Dosage Range

I.V.:
Children: Initial: 15 mg/kg/day; Maximum: 60 mg/kg/day
Children ≥10 years and Adults: Initial: 10-15 mg/kg/day; Maximum: 60 mg/kg/day

Oral:
Children: Initial: 15 mg/kg/day; Maximum: 60 mg/kg/day; **Note:** Depakote ER is not recommended for use in children <10 years of age.
Children ≥10 years and Adults: Seizures: Initial: 10-15 mg/kg/day; Maximum: 60 mg/kg/day
Children ≥12 years and Adults: Migraine prophylaxis: (Stavzor) 250 mg twice daily; Maintenance: Up to 1000 mg daily
Children ≥16 years and Adults: Migraine prophylaxis (Depakote tablets): 250 mg twice daily, up to 1000 mg daily
Adults: Migraine prophylaxis (Depakote ER): 500-1000 mg once daily
Adults: Mania: Depakote tablet, Stavzor: Initial: 750 mg/day in divided doses (maximum recommended dose: 60 mg/kg/day); Depakote ER: Initial: 25 mg/kg/day given once daily (maximum recommended dose: 60 mg/kg/day)

Administration

I.V. Following dilution to final concentration, manufacturer's labeling recommends administering over 60 minutes at a rate ≤20 mg/minute. Alternatively, more rapid infusion rates of 1.5-6 mg/kg/minute have been used in clinical trials to quickly achieve therapeutic concentrations, and were generally well tolerated (Ramsay, 2003; Wheless, 2004). One study reported undiluted valproic acid administered at ≤10 mg/kg/minute (dose of ≤30 mg/kg) was well tolerated (Limdi, 2007).

Hazardous agent; use appropriate precautions for handling and disposal (NIOSH, 2012).

Oral Oral valproate products may cause GI upset; taking with food or slowly increasing the dose may decrease GI upset should it occur.

Depakote ER: Swallow whole; do not crush or chew.

Depakote Sprinkle capsules may be swallowed whole or capsule opened and sprinkled on small amount (1 teaspoonful) of soft food (eg, pudding, applesauce) to be used immediately (do not store or chew).

Depakene capsule, Stavzor: Swallow whole; do not chew.

Hazardous agent; use appropriate precautions for handling and disposal (NIOSH, 2012).

Preparation for Administration Hazardous agent; use appropriate precautions for handling and disposal (NIOSH, 2012).

I.V.: Prior to administration of the injectable solution, dilute in 50 mL of a compatible diluent.

◀ **Storage/Stability**
Oral: Store at controlled room temperature.
I.V.: Store at controlled room temperature. Stable in D₅W, NS, and LR for at least 24 hours when stored in glass or PVC.

Nursing Actions
Physical Assessment I.V.: Monitor therapeutic response (seizure activity, type, duration). Monitor for signs and symptoms of hepatic failure (malaise, weakness, facial edema, anorexia, jaundice, and vomiting), especially when used in children <2 years of age. Monitor for signs and symptoms of pancreatitis (abdominal pain, nausea, vomiting, and/or anorexia). For outpatients, monitor therapeutic effect (seizure activity, frequency, force, type, duration). Teach patient seizure safety precautions. Some adverse reactions, including hepatic failure and thrombocytopenia, can occur 3 days to 6 months after beginning therapy.

Patient Education
• Discuss specific use of drug and side effects with patient as it relates to treatment. (HCAHPS: During this hospital stay, were you given any medicine that you had not taken before? Before giving you any new medicine, how often did hospital staff tell you what the medicine was for? How often did hospital staff describe possible side effects in a way you could understand?)
• Patient may experience presyncope, fatigue, blurred vision, illogical thinking, dizziness, headache, nausea, diarrhea, dyspepsia, alopecia, asthenia, fasciculations, or insomnia. Have patient report immediately to prescriber depression, inability to eat, imbalance, ecchymosis, bleeding, discolored urine, jaundice, pregnancy, or rash (HCAHPS).
• Educate patient about signs of a significant reaction (eg, wheezing; chest tightness; fever; itching; bad cough; blue skin color; seizures; or swelling of face, lips, tongue, or throat). **Note:** This is not a comprehensive list of all side effects. Patient should consult prescriber for additional questions.

Intended Use and Disclaimer: Should not be printed and given to patients. This information is intended to serve as a concise initial reference for healthcare professionals to use when discussing medications with a patient. You must ultimately rely on your own discretion, experience and judgment in diagnosing, treating and advising patients.

Related Information
Oral Medications That Should Not Be Crushed or Altered *on page 1712*
Peak and Trough Guidelines *on page 1710*

Valrubicin (val ROO bi sin)

Brand Names: U.S. Valstar

Index Terms *N*-trifluoroacetyladriamycin-14-valerate; AD32

Pharmacologic Category Antineoplastic Agent, Anthracycline; Antineoplastic Agent, Topoisomerase II Inhibitor

Medication Safety Issues
Sound-alike/look-alike issues:
Valrubicin may be confused with DAUNOrubicin, DOXOrubicin, epirubicin, IDArubicin
Valstar® may be confused with valsartan

High alert medication:
The medication is in a class the Institute for Safe Medication Practices (ISMP) includes among its list of drug classes which have a heightened risk of causing significant patient harm when used in error.

Pregnancy Risk Factor C

Lactation Excretion in breast milk unknown/not recommended

Use Intravesical treatment of BCG-refractory bladder carcinoma *in situ*

Available Dosage Forms
Solution, Intravesical [preservative free]:
Valstar: 40 mg/mL (5 mL)

General Dosage Range Dosage adjustment recommended in patients who develop toxicities
Intravesical: *Adults:* 800 mg once weekly for 6 weeks

Administration
Other Intravesicular bladder instillation: Insert urinary catheter, empty bladder prior to instillation, slowly by gravity flow, instill 800 mg/75 mL (in 0.9% sodium chloride injection), remove catheter. Retain in the bladder for 2 hours, then void. Administer through non-PVC tubing due to the polyoxyl castor oil (Cremophor® EL) diluent. Maintain adequate hydration following treatment. Use appropriate protective gown, goggles, and gloves during administration.

Hazardous agent; use appropriate precautions for handling and disposal (NIOSH, 2012).

Nursing Actions
Physical Assessment Use caution to prevent inadvertent exposure to this medication. Monitor patient response during and following instillation (genitourinary [frequency, urgency, incontinence, dysuria, bladder spasm or pain, hematuria, urinary tract infection], rash, nausea, vomiting, myalgia, hyperglycemia).

Patient Education
• Discuss specific use of drug and side effects with patient as it relates to treatment. (HCAHPS: During this hospital stay, were you given any medicine that you had not taken before? Before giving you any new medicine, how often did hospital staff tell you what the medicine was for? How often did hospital staff describe possible side effects in a way you could understand?)
• Patient may experience bladder irritation, discolored urine, dysuria, or urinary irregularities.

Have patient report immediately to prescriber signs of infection, hematuria, urinary retention, or rash (HCAHPS).

• Educate patient about signs of a significant reaction (eg, wheezing; chest tightness; fever; itching; bad cough; blue skin color; seizures; or swelling of face, lips, tongue, or throat). **Note:** This is not a comprehensive list of all side effects. Patient should consult prescriber for additional questions.

Intended Use and Disclaimer: Should not be printed and given to patients. This information is intended to serve as a concise initial reference for healthcare professionals to use when discussing medications with a patient. You must ultimately rely on your own discretion, experience and judgment in diagnosing, treating and advising patients.

Valsartan (val SAR tan)

Brand Names: U.S. Diovan
Pharmacologic Category Angiotensin II Receptor Blocker; Antihypertensive
Medication Safety Issues
  Sound-alike/look-alike issues:
    Valsartan may be confused with losartan, Valstar, Valturna
    Diovan may be confused with Zyban
  International issues:
    Diovan [U.S., Canada, and multiple international markets] may be confused with Dianben, a brand name for metformin [Spain]
Pregnancy Risk Factor D
Lactation Excretion in breast milk unknown/not recommended
Breast-Feeding Considerations It is not known if valsartan is found in breast milk. Due to the potential for serious adverse reactions in the nursing infant, the manufacturer recommends a decision be made whether to discontinue nursing or to discontinue the drug, taking into account the importance of treatment to the mother. The Canadian labeling contraindicates use in nursing women. Breast-fed infants of mothers taking medications for hypertension should be monitored for adverse effects (Chobanian, 2003).
Use Alone or in combination with other antihypertensive agents in the treatment of primary hypertension; reduction of cardiovascular mortality in patients with left ventricular dysfunction postmyocardial infarction; treatment of heart failure (NYHA Class II-IV)

Note: The ACCF/AHA 2013 heart failure guidelines recommend the use of ARBs (ie, candesartan, losartan, and valsartan) in patients with HF with reduced ejection fraction who cannot tolerate ACE inhibitors (due to cough) to reduce morbidity and mortality. They also suggest that ARBs are reasonable first-line alternatives to ACE inhibitors

in patients already maintained on an ARB for other indications (ACCF/AHA [Yancy, 2013]).

Mechanism of Action/Effect Valsartan produces direct antagonism of the angiotensin II (AT2) receptors. Valsartan blocks the vasoconstrictor and aldosterone-secreting effects of angiotensin II. It displaces angiotensin II from the AT1 receptor and produces its blood pressure-lowering effects by antagonizing AT1-induced vasoconstriction, aldosterone release, catecholamine release, arginine vasopressin release, water intake, and hypertrophic responses. This action results in more efficient blockade of the cardiovascular effects of angiotensin II and fewer side effects than the ACE inhibitors.

Contraindications Hypersensitivity to valsartan or any component of the formulation; concomitant use with aliskiren in patients with diabetes mellitus

Canadian labeling: Additional contraindications (not in U.S. labeling): Concomitant use with aliskiren in patients with moderate-to-severe renal impairment (GFR <60 mL/minute/1.73m^2); pregnancy; breastfeeding

Warnings/Precautions [U.S. Boxed Warning]: Drugs that act on the renin-angiotensin system can cause injury and death to the developing fetus. Discontinue as soon as possible once pregnancy is detected. May cause hyperkalemia; avoid potassium supplementation unless specifically required by healthcare provider. During the initiation of therapy, hypotension may occur, particularly in patients with heart failure or post-MI patients. Use extreme caution with concurrent administration of potassium-sparing diuretics or potassium supplements, in patients with mild-to-moderate hepatic dysfunction (adjust dose), in those who may be sodium/water depleted (eg, on high-dose diuretics), and in the elderly; correct depletion first.

Use caution with unstented unilateral/bilateral renal artery stenosis. When unstented bilateral renal artery stenosis is present, use is generally avoided due to the elevated risk of deterioration in renal function unless possible benefits outweigh risks. Use with caution with preexisting renal insufficiency; significant aortic/mitral stenosis. May be associated with deterioration of renal function and/or increases in serum creatinine, particularly in patients with low renal blood flow (eg, renal artery stenosis, heart failure) whose glomerular filtration rate (GFR) is dependent on efferent arteriolar vasoconstriction by angiotensin II. Use caution in patients with severe renal impairment or significant hepatic dysfunction. Monitor renal function closely in patients with severe heart failure; changes in renal function should be anticipated and dosage adjustments of valsartan or concomitant medications may be needed. Potentially significant drug-drug interactions may exist, requiring ▶

dose or frequency adjustment, additional monitoring, and/or selection of alternative therapy.

Angioedema has been reported rarely with some angiotensin II receptor antagonists (ARBs) and may occur at any time during treatment (especially following first dose). It may involve the head and neck (potentially compromising airway) or the intestine (presenting with abdominal pain). Patients with idiopathic or hereditary angioedema or previous angioedema associated with ACE-inhibitor therapy may be at an increased risk. Prolonged frequent monitoring may be required, especially if tongue, glottis, or larynx are involved, as they are associated with airway obstruction. Patients with a history of airway surgery may have a higher risk of airway obstruction. Discontinue therapy immediately if angioedema occurs. Aggressive early management is critical. Intramuscular (I.M.) administration of epinephrine may be necessary. Do not readminister to patients who have had angioedema with ARBs.

Drug Interactions

Avoid Concomitant Use There are no known interactions where it is recommended to avoid concomitant use.

Decreased Effect
The levels/effects of Valsartan may be decreased by: Herbs (Hypertensive Properties); Methylphenidate; Nonsteroidal Anti-Inflammatory Agents; Yohimbine

Increased Effect/Toxicity
Valsartan may increase the levels/effects of: ACE Inhibitors; Amifostine; Antihypertensives; CycloSPORINE (Systemic); DULoxetine; Hydrochlorothiazide; Hypotensive Agents; Lithium; Nonsteroidal Anti-Inflammatory Agents; Obinutuzumab; Potassium-Sparing Diuretics; RiTUXimab; Sodium Phosphates

The levels/effects of Valsartan may be increased by: Alfuzosin; Aliskiren; Brimonidine (Topical); Canagliflozin; Diazoxide; Eltrombopag; Eplerenone; Heparin; Heparin (Low Molecular Weight); Herbs (Hypotensive Properties); Hydrochlorothiazide; MAO Inhibitors; Pentoxifylline; Phosphodiesterase 5 Inhibitors; Potassium Salts; Prostacyclin Analogues; Tolvaptan; Trimethoprim

Nutritional/Ethanol Interactions

Food: Decreases the peak plasma concentration and extent of absorption by 50% and 40%, respectively. Potassium supplements and/or potassium-containing salts may cause or worsen hyperkalemia. Management: Take consistently with regard to food. Consult prescriber before consuming a potassium-rich diet, potassium supplements, or salt substitutes.

Herb/Nutraceutical: Some herbal medications may worsen hypertension (eg, licorice); others may increase the antihypertensive effect of valsartan (eg, shepherd's purse). Management: Avoid bayberry, blue cohosh, cayenne, ephedra, ginger, ginseng (American), kola, licorice, and yohimbe. Avoid black cohosh, California poppy, coleus, golden seal, hawthorn, mistletoe, periwinkle, quinine, and shepherd's purse.

Adverse Reactions

>10%:

Central nervous system: Dizziness (heart failure trials 17%)

Renal: BUN increased >50% (heart failure trials 17%)

1% to 10%:

Cardiovascular: Hypotension (heart failure trials 7%; MI trial 1%), orthostatic hypotension (heart failure trials 2%), syncope (up to >1%)

Central nervous system: Dizziness (hypertension trial 2% to 8%), fatigue (heart failure trials 3%; hypertension trial 2%), postural dizziness (heart failure trials 2%), headache (heart failure trials >1%), vertigo (up to >1%)

Endocrine & metabolic: Serum potassium increased by >20% (4% to 10%), hyperkalemia (heart failure trials 2%)

Gastrointestinal: Diarrhea (heart failure trials 5%), abdominal pain (2%), nausea (heart failure trials >1%), upper abdominal pain (heart failure trials >1%)

Hematologic: Neutropenia (2%)

Neuromuscular & skeletal: Arthralgia (heart failure trials 3%), back pain (up to 3%)

Ocular: Blurred vision (heart failure trials >1%)

Renal: Creatinine doubled (MI trial 4%), creatinine increased >50% (heart failure trials 4%), renal dysfunction (up to >1%)

Respiratory: Cough (1% to 3%)

Miscellaneous: Viral infection (3%)

Pharmacodynamics/Kinetics

Onset of Action ~2 hours

Duration of Action 24 hours

Available Dosage Forms

Tablet, Oral:
Diovan: 40 mg, 80 mg, 160 mg, 320 mg

General Dosage Range Oral:
Children 6-16 years: Initial: 1.3 mg/kg once daily (maximum: 40 mg/day); Maintenance: Up to 2.7 mg/kg; 160 mg

Adults: Initial: 20-40 mg twice daily **or** 80-160 mg once daily; Maintenance: 80-160 mg twice daily (maximum: 320 mg daily)

Administration

Oral Administer with or without food.

Storage/Stability Store at 25°C (77°F); excursions permitted to 15°C to 30°C (59°F to 86°F). Protect from moisture.

Nursing Actions

Physical Assessment Assess effectiveness and interactions with other pharmacological agents and herbal products (eg, concurrent use of potassium supplements, ACE inhibitors, potassium-sparing diuretics may increase risk of hyperkalemia). Monitor for changes in renal function, dizziness, cough, headache, nausea, hypotension, and hyperkalemia.

Patient Education
- Discuss specific use of drug and side effects with patient as it relates to treatment. (HCAHPS: During this hospital stay, were you given any medicine that you had not taken before? Before giving you any new medicine, how often did hospital staff tell you what the medicine was for? How often did hospital staff describe possible side effects in a way you could understand?)
- Patient may experience hyperkalemia, dizziness, dyspepsia, back pain, diarrhea, asthenia, or worsening kidney function. Have patient report immediately to prescriber syncope, severe headache, hyperhidrosis, vomiting, weight gain, edema in legs or abdomen, rash, or pregnancy (HCAHPS).
- Educate patient about signs of a significant reaction (eg, wheezing; chest tightness; fever; itching; bad cough; blue skin color; seizures; or swelling of face, lips, tongue, or throat). **Note:** This is not a comprehensive list of all side effects. Patient should consult prescriber for additional questions.

Intended Use and Disclaimer: Should not be printed and given to patients. This information is intended to serve as a concise initial reference for healthcare professionals to use when discussing medications with a patient. You must ultimately rely on your own discretion, experience and judgment in diagnosing, treating and advising patients.

Dietary Considerations Avoid salt substitutes which contain potassium. May be taken with or without food.

Valsartan and Hydrochlorothiazide
(val SAR tan & hye droe klor oh THYE a zide)

Brand Names: U.S. Diovan HCT
Index Terms Hydrochlorothiazide and Valsartan
Pharmacologic Category Angiotensin II Receptor Blocker; Antihypertensive; Diuretic, Thiazide
Medication Safety Issues
Sound-alike/look-alike issues:
Diovan may be confused with Zyban
Pregnancy Risk Factor D
Use
U.S. labeling: Treatment of hypertension (initial, add-on, or as substitute for titrated components)
Canadian labeling: Treatment of mild-to-moderate hypertension where combination therapy is appropriate. Not indicated for initial treatment.

Available Dosage Forms
Tablet, oral: 80 mg/12.5 mg: Valsartan 80 mg and hydrochlorothiazide 12.5 mg; 160 mg/12.5 mg: Valsartan 160 mg and hydrochlorothiazide 12.5 mg; 160 mg/25 mg: Valsartan 160 mg and hydrochlorothiazide 25 mg; 320 mg/12.5 mg: Valsartan 320 mg and hydrochlorothiazide 12.5 mg;

320 mg/25 mg: Valsartan 320 mg and hydrochlorothiazide 25 mg
Diovan HCT®: 80 mg/12.5 mg: Valsartan 80 mg and hydrochlorothiazide 12.5 mg; 160 mg/12.5 mg: Valsartan 160 mg and hydrochlorothiazide 12.5 mg; 160 mg/25 mg: Valsartan 160 mg and hydrochlorothiazide 25 mg; 320 mg/12.5 mg: Valsartan 320 mg and hydrochlorothiazide 12.5 mg; 320 mg/25 mg: Valsartan 320 mg and hydrochlorothiazide 25 mg

General Dosage Range Oral: *Adults:* Valsartan 80-320 mg and hydrochlorothiazide 12.5-25 mg once daily (maximum: 25 mg daily [hydrochlorothiazide]; 320 mg daily [valsartan])

Administration
Oral Administer with or without food.

Nursing Actions
Physical Assessment See individual agents.

Patient Education
- Discuss specific use of drug and side effects with patient as it relates to treatment. (HCAHPS: During this hospital stay, were you given any medicine that you had not taken before? Before giving you any new medicine, how often did hospital staff tell you what the medicine was for? How often did hospital staff describe possible side effects in a way you could understand?)
- Patient may experience headache or dizziness. Have patient report immediately to prescriber signs of infection, signs of hyperglycemia, signs of renal or hepatic impairment, signs of pancreatitis, paresthesia, angina, sexual dysfunction, arthralgia, akathisia, dyspnea, significant weight gain, edema, ecchymosis, bleeding, or vision changes (HCAHPS).
- Educate patient about signs of a significant reaction (eg, wheezing; chest tightness; fever; itching; bad cough; blue skin color; seizures; or swelling of face, lips, tongue, or throat). **Note:** This is not a comprehensive list of all side effects. Patient should consult prescriber for additional questions.

Intended Use and Disclaimer: Should not be printed and given to patients. This information is intended to serve as a concise initial reference for healthcare professionals to use when discussing medications with a patient. You must ultimately rely on your own discretion, experience and judgment in diagnosing, treating and advising patients.

Related Information
Hydrochlorothiazide *on page 775*
Valsartan *on page 1581*

Vancomycin (van koe MYE sin)

Brand Names: U.S. First-Vancomycin 25; First-Vancomycin 50; Vancocin HCl
Index Terms Vancomycin Hydrochloride
Pharmacologic Category Glycopeptide

◀ **Medication Safety Issues**
Sound-alike/look-alike issues:
I.V. vancomycin may be confused with INVanz
Vancomycin may be confused with clindamycin, gentamicin, tobramycin, valACYclovir, vecuronium, Vibramycin

High alert medication:
The Institute for Safe Medication Practices (ISMP) includes this medication (intrathecal administration) among its list of drug classes which have a heightened risk of causing significant patient harm when used in error.

Pregnancy Risk Factor B (oral); C (injection)

Lactation Enters breast milk/not recommended

Breast-Feeding Considerations Vancomycin is excreted in human milk following I.V. administration. If given orally to the mother, the minimal systemic absorption of the dose would limit the amount available to pass into the milk. Vancomycin is recommended for the treatment of mild, moderate, or severe *Clostridium difficile* infections in breast-feeding women (Surawicz, 2013). Due to the potential for serious adverse reactions in the nursing infant, the manufacturer recommends a decision be made whether to discontinue nursing or to discontinue the drug, taking into account the importance of treatment to the mother. Nondose-related effects could include modification of bowel flora.

Use
I.V.: Treatment of patients with infections caused by staphylococcal species and streptococcal species
Oral: Treatment of *C. difficile*-associated diarrhea and treatment of enterocolitis caused by *Staphylococcus aureus* (including methicillin-resistant strains)

Unlabeled Use Bacterial endophthalmitis; treatment of infections caused by gram-positive organisms in patients who have serious allergies to beta-lactam agents; treatment of beta-lactam resistant gram-positive infections; surgical (perioperative) prophylaxis; treatment of prosthetic joint infection; group B streptococcus maternal use for neonatal prophylaxis; rectal administration for treatment of *Clostridium difficile* infection

Mechanism of Action/Effect Inhibits bacterial cell wall synthesis

Contraindications Hypersensitivity to vancomycin or any component of the formulation

Warnings/Precautions May cause nephrotoxicity although limited data suggest direct causal relationship; usual risk factors include pre-existing renal impairment, concomitant nephrotoxic medications, advanced age, and dehydration (nephrotoxicity has also been reported following treatment with oral vancomycin, typically in patients >65 years of age). If multiple sequential (≥2) serum creatinine concentrations demonstrate an increase of 0.5 mg/dL or ≥50% increase from baseline (whichever is greater) in the absence of an alternative explanation, the patient should be identified as having vancomycin-induced nephrotoxicity (Rybak, 2009). Discontinue treatment if signs of nephrotoxicity occur; renal damage is usually reversible.

May cause neurotoxicity; usual risk factors include pre-existing renal impairment, concomitant neuro-/nephrotoxic medications, advanced age, and dehydration. Ototoxicity, although rarely associated with monotherapy, is proportional to the amount of drug given and the duration of treatment. Tinnitus or vertigo may be indications of vestibular injury and impending bilateral irreversible damage. Discontinue treatment if signs of ototoxicity occur. Prolonged therapy (>1 week) or total doses exceeding 25 g may increase the risk of neutropenia; prompt reversal of neutropenia is expected after discontinuation of therapy. Prolonged use may result in fungal or bacterial superinfection, including *C. difficile*-associated diarrhea (CDAD) and pseudomembranous colitis; CDAD has been observed >2 months postantibiotic treatment. Use with caution in patients with renal impairment or those receiving other nephrotoxic or ototoxic drugs; dosage modification required in patients with impaired renal function (especially elderly). Accumulation may occur after multiple oral doses of vancomycin in patients with renal impairment; consider monitoring trough concentrations in this circumstance.

Rapid I.V. administration may result in hypotension, flushing, erythema, urticaria, and/or pruritus. Oral vancomycin is only indicated for the treatment of pseudomembranous colitis due to *C. difficile* and enterocolitis due to *S. aureus* and is not effective for systemic infections; parenteral vancomycin is not effective for the treatment of colitis due to *C. difficile* and enterocolitis due to *S. aureus*. Clinically significant serum concentrations have been reported in patients with inflammatory disorders of the intestinal mucosa who have taken oral vancomycin (multiple doses) for the treatment of *C. difficile*-associated diarrhea. Although use may be warranted, the risk for adverse reactions may be higher in this situation; consider monitoring serum trough concentrations, especially with renal insufficiency, severe colitis, concurrent rectal vancomycin administration, and/or concomitant I.V. aminoglycosides. The IDSA suggests that it is appropriate to obtain trough concentrations when a patient is receiving long courses of ≥2 g/day (Cohen, 2010). **Note:** The Infectious Disease Society of America (IDSA) and American College of Gastroenterology (ACG) recommend the use of oral metronidazole for initial treatment of mild-to-moderate *C. difficile* infection and the use of oral vancomycin for initial treatment of severe *C. difficile* infection (Cohen, 2010; Surawicz, 2013).

Drug Interactions

Avoid Concomitant Use

Avoid concomitant use of Vancomycin with any of the following: BCG; Gallium Nitrate

Decreased Effect

Vancomycin may decrease the levels/effects of: BCG; Sodium Picosulfate; Typhoid Vaccine

The levels/effects of Vancomycin may be decreased by: Bile Acid Sequestrants

Increased Effect/Toxicity

Vancomycin may increase the levels/effects of: Aminoglycosides; Colistimethate; Gallium Nitrate; Neuromuscular-Blocking Agents

The levels/effects of Vancomycin may be increased by: Nonsteroidal Anti-Inflammatory Agents

Adverse Reactions

Injection:

>10%:

Cardiovascular: Hypotension accompanied by flushing

Dermatologic: Erythematous rash on face and upper body (red neck or red man syndrome - infusion rate related)

1% to 10%:

Central nervous system: Chills, drug fever

Dermatologic: Rash

Hematologic: Eosinophilia, reversible neutropenia

Local: Phlebitis

Oral:

>10%: Gastrointestinal: Abdominal pain, bad taste (with oral solution), nausea

1% to 10%:

Cardiovascular: Peripheral edema

Central nervous system: Fatigue, fever, headache

Gastrointestinal: Diarrhea, flatulence, vomiting

Genitourinary: Urinary tract infection

Neuromuscular & skeletal: Back pain

Available Dosage Forms

Capsule, Oral:

Vancocin HCl: 125 mg, 250 mg

Generic: 125 mg, 250 mg

Solution, Intravenous:

Generic: 500 mg/100 mL (100 mL); 750 mg/150 mL (150 mL); 1 g/200 mL (200 mL)

Solution, Oral:

First-Vancomycin 25: 25 mg/mL (150 mL, 300 mL)

First-Vancomycin 50: 50 mg/mL (150 mL, 210 mL, 300 mL)

Solution Reconstituted, Intravenous:

Generic: 500 mg (1 ea); 750 mg (1 ea); 1000 mg (1 ea); 5000 mg (1 ea); 10 g (1 ea)

Solution Reconstituted, Intravenous [preservative free]:

Generic: 1000 mg (1 ea); 5000 mg (1 ea); 10 g (1 ea)

General Dosage Range

Dosage adjustment recommended in patients with renal impairment

I.V.:

Infants >1 month: 40-60 mg/kg/day in divided doses every 6 hours

Children: 40-60 mg/kg/day in divided doses every 6 hours **or** 20 mg/kg as a single dose

Adults: 30-60 mg/kg/day in divided doses every 6-12 hours **or** 500-750 mg every 6 hours **or** 1000 mg as a single dose

Intracatheter, intraventricular: *Children and Adults:* 2-5 mg/mL instilled into catheter port with a volume sufficient to fill the catheter (2-5 mL)

Intrathecal: *Children and Adults:* 5-20 mg/day

Oral:

Children: 40 mg/kg/day in 3-4 divided doses (maximum: 2000 mg/day)

Adults: 500-2000 mg/day in 3-4 divided doses (maximum: 2000 mg/day)

Administration

I.M. Do not administer I.M.

I.V. Administer vancomycin with a final concentration not to exceed 5 mg/mL by I.V. intermittent infusion over at least 60 minutes (recommended infusion period of ≥30 minutes for every 500 mg administered).

Red man syndrome may occur if the infusion is too rapid. It is not an allergic reaction, but may be characterized by hypotension and/or a maculopapular rash appearing on the face, neck, trunk, and/or upper extremities. If this should occur, slow the infusion rate to over 1$\frac{1}{2}$ to 2 hours and increase the dilution volume. Reactions are often treated with antihistamines and steroids.

Extravasation treatment: Monitor I.V. site closely; extravasation will cause serious injury with possible necrosis and tissue sloughing. Rotate infusion site frequently.

Injectable Detail pH: 3.9 (in distilled water or sodium chloride 0.9%); 2.5-4.5 (5% solution in water)

Oral Vancomycin powder for injection may be reconstituted and used for oral administration (Cohen, 2010). Reconstituted powder for injection (not premixed solution) may be administered orally by diluting the reconstituted solution in 30 mL of water; common flavoring syrups may be added to improve taste. The unflavored, diluted solution may also be administered via nasogastric tube.

Intrathecal Unlabeled route: Vancomycin is available as a powder for injection and may be diluted to 1-5 mg/mL concentration in preservative free 0.9% sodium chloride for intrathecal administration.

Intravitreal Unlabeled use: Administer vancomycin intravitreally with a final concentration of 1.0 mg/0.1 mL NS (Kelsey, 1995). **Note:** Due to retinotoxicity, some clinicians recommend using a lower dose of 0.2 mg/0.1 mL NS (Gan, 2001).

◀ **Rectal** Unlabeled route: May be administered as a retention enema per rectum (Cohen, 2010); 500 mg in 100-500 mL of NS, volume depending on length of segment being treated. If sodium chloride causes hyperchloremia could use solution with lower chloride concentration (eg, LR) (Surawicz, 2013).

Preparation for Administration Injection: Reconstitute vials with 20 mL of SWFI for each 1 g of vancomycin (10 mL/500 mg vial; 20 mL/1 g vial; 100 mL/5 g vial; 200 mL/10 g vial). The reconstituted solution must be further diluted with at least 100 mL of a compatible diluent per 500 mg of vancomycin prior to parenteral administration.

Intrathecal (unlabeled route): Vancomycin is available as a powder for injection and may be diluted to 1-5 mg/mL concentration in preservative free 0.9% sodium chloride for administration into the CSF.

Storage/Stability
Capsules: Store at controlled room temperature of 15°C to 30°C (59°F to 86°F).

Injection: Reconstituted 500 mg and 1 g vials are stable for at either room temperature or under refrigeration for 14 days. **Note:** Vials contain no bacteriostatic agent. Solutions diluted for administration in either D₅W or NS are stable under refrigeration for 14 days or at room temperature for 7 days.

Nursing Actions
Physical Assessment Culture and sensitivity tests and patient's allergy history should be evaluated prior to first dose. Use caution with renal impairment. Premedication with antihistamines may prevent or minimize "red man" reaction. Monitor infusion site closely to prevent extravasation. Monitor for hypotension, rash, neutropenia, nausea, vomiting, and auditory changes on a regular basis during therapy.

Patient Education
• Discuss specific use of drug and side effects with patient as it relates to treatment. (HCAHPS: During this hospital stay, were you given any medicine that you had not taken before? Before giving you any new medicine, how often did hospital staff tell you what the medicine was for? How often did hospital staff describe possible side effects in a way you could understand?)
• Patient may experience dyspepsia, nausea, injection site irritation, flushing, or hypotension. Have patient report immediately to prescriber severe diarrhea, significant change in balance, tinnitus, hearing impairment, urinary retention, or rash (HCAHPS).
• Educate patient about signs of a significant reaction (eg, wheezing; chest tightness; fever; itching; bad cough; blue skin color; seizures; or swelling of face, lips, tongue, or throat). **Note:** This is not a comprehensive list of all side effects. Patient should consult prescriber for additional questions.

Intended Use and Disclaimer: Should not be printed and given to patients. This information is intended to serve as a concise initial reference for healthcare professionals to use when discussing medications with a patient. You must ultimately rely on your own discretion, experience and judgment in diagnosing, treating and advising patients.

Dietary Considerations May be taken with food.
Related Information
Peak and Trough Guidelines *on page 1710*

Vandetanib (van DET a nib)

Brand Names: U.S. Caprelsa
Index Terms AZD6474; Zactima; ZD6474; Zictifa
Pharmacologic Category Antineoplastic Agent, Epidermal Growth Factor Receptor (EGFR) Inhibitor; Antineoplastic Agent, Tyrosine Kinase Inhibitor; Antineoplastic Agent, Vascular Endothelial Growth Factor (VEGF) Inhibitor
Medication Safety Issues
Sound-alike/look-alike issues:
Vandetanib may be confused with axitinib, cabozantinib, dasatinib, erlotinib, gefitinib, imatinib, lapatinib, nilotinib, PAZOPanib, SORAfenib, SUNItinib, vemurafenib, vismodegib
High alert medication:
This medication is in a class the Institute for Safe Medication Practices (ISMP) includes among its list of drug classes which have a heightened risk of causing significant patient harm when used in error.
Medication Guide Available Yes
Pregnancy Risk Factor D
Lactation Excretion in breast milk unknown/not recommended
Use Thyroid cancer: Treatment of metastatic or unresectable locally-advanced medullary thyroid cancer (symptomatic or progressive)
Available Dosage Forms
Tablet, Oral:
Caprelsa: 100 mg, 300 mg
Administration
Oral May be administered with or without food. Missed doses should be omitted if within 12 hours of the next scheduled dose. Do not crush tablet. If unable to swallow tablet whole or if nasogastric or gastrostomy tube administration is necessary, disperse one tablet in 2 ounces of water (noncarbonated only) and stir for 10 minutes to disperse (will not dissolve completely) and administer immediately. Rinse residue in glass with additional 4 ounces of water (noncarbonated only) and administer.

Hazardous agent; use appropriate precautions for handling and disposal (meets NIOSH, 2012 criteria).

Nursing Actions

Physical Assessment Instruct on proper handling; avoid direct contact with skin and mucous membranes. Check results of lab tests including thyroid levels, CBC, electrolyte levels along with ECGs, and blood pressure. Monitor bleeding, rash, breathing difficulties, shortness of breath, fever, cough, confusion, vision changes, headaches, seizures; stroke symptoms such as one-sided weakness, trouble speaking, and sun sensitivity. Inform patient they will need to sign a form prior to receiving drug. Instruct patient to avoid situations of potential injury due to bleeding possibilities.

Patient Education

- Discuss specific use of drug and side effects with patient as it relates to treatment. (HCAHPS: During this hospital stay, were you given any medicine that you had not taken before? Before giving you any new medicine, how often did hospital staff tell you what the medicine was for? How often did hospital staff describe possible side effects in a way you could understand?)
- Patient may experience hypertension, nausea, diarrhea, headache, fatigue, rash, acne, dyspepsia, or loss of appetite. Have patient report immediately to prescriber signs of infection, angina, dizziness or syncope, dyspnea, illogical thinking, strength differences from one side to another, sudden vision changes, ecchymosis, edema, significant weight gain, skin changes on hands or feet, inability to eat, or severe skin irritation (HCAHPS).
- Educate patient about signs of a significant reaction (eg, wheezing; chest tightness; fever; itching; bad cough; blue skin color; seizures; or swelling of face, lips, tongue, or throat). **Note:** This is not a comprehensive list of all side effects. Patient should consult prescriber for additional questions.

Intended Use and Disclaimer: Should not be printed and given to patients. This information is intended to serve as a concise initial reference for healthcare professionals to use when discussing medications with a patient. You must ultimately rely on your own discretion, experience and judgment in diagnosing, treating and advising patients.

Related Information

Oral Medications That Should Not Be Crushed or Altered *on page 1712*

Vardenafil (var DEN a fil)

Brand Names: U.S. Levitra; Staxyn
Index Terms Vardenafil Hydrochloride
Pharmacologic Category Phosphodiesterase-5 Enzyme Inhibitor

Medication Safety Issues

Sound-alike/look-alike issues:
Vardenafil may be confused with sildenafil, tadalafil
Levitra may be confused with Kaletra, Lexiva

Pregnancy Risk Factor B

Lactation Excretion in breast milk unknown/not indicated for use in women.

Breast-Feeding Considerations It is not known if vardenafil is excreted in breast milk. Vardenafil is not indicated for use in women.

Use Erectile dysfunction: Treatment of erectile dysfunction (ED)

Mechanism of Action/Effect Vardenafil enhances the effect of nitric oxide by inhibiting phosphodiesterase type 5 (PDE-5), resulting in smooth muscle relaxation and inflow of blood into the corpus cavernosum with sexual stimulation.

Contraindications Hypersensitivity to vardenafil or any component of the formulation; concurrent (regular or intermittent) use of organic nitrates in any form (eg, nitroglycerin, isosorbide dinitrate)

Warnings/Precautions There is a degree of cardiac risk associated with sexual activity; therefore, physicians may wish to consider the patient's cardiovascular status prior to initiating any treatment for erectile dysfunction. Use caution in patients with anatomical deformation of the penis (angulation, cavernosal fibrosis, or Peyronie's disease) and in patients who have conditions which may predispose them to priapism (sickle cell anemia, multiple myeloma, leukemia). Instruct patients to seek immediate medical attention if erection persists >4 hours.

Use is not recommended in patients with hypotension (<90/50 mm Hg); uncontrolled hypertension (>170/100 mm Hg); unstable angina or angina during intercourse; life-threatening arrhythmias, stroke, or MI within the last 6 months; cardiac failure or coronary artery disease causing unstable angina. Safety and efficacy have not been studied in these patients. Use caution in patients with left ventricular outflow obstruction (eg, aortic stenosis or hypertrophic cardiomyopathy [HCM] with outflow tract obstruction). Use caution with alpha-blockers, effective CYP3A4 inhibitors, the elderly, or those with hepatic impairment (Child-Pugh class B); dosage adjustment is needed. Concurrent use with alpha-adrenergic antagonist therapy may cause symptomatic hypotension; patients should be hemodynamically stable prior to initiating tadalafil therapy at the lowest possible dose. Avoid or limit concurrent substantial alcohol consumption as this may increase the risk of symptomatic hypotension.

Rare cases of nonarteritic ischemic optic neuropathy (NAION) have been reported; risk may be increased with history of vision loss. Other risk factors for NAION include heart disease, diabetes, hypertension, smoking, age >50 years, or history of certain eye problems. Sudden decrease or loss of ▶

hearing has been reported rarely; hearing changes may be accompanied by tinnitus and dizziness.

Safety and efficacy have not been studied in patients with the following conditions, therefore, use in these patients is not recommended at this time: Congenital QT prolongation, patients taking medications known to prolong the QT interval (avoid use in patients taking Class Ia or III antiarrhythmics); severe hepatic impairment (Child-Pugh class C); end-stage renal disease requiring dialysis; retinitis pigmentosa or other degenerative retinal disorders. The safety and efficacy of vardenafil with other treatments for erectile dysfunction have not been studied and are not recommended as combination therapy. Concomitant use with all forms of nitrates is contraindicated. If nitrate administration is medically necessary, it is not known when nitrates can be safely administered following the use of vardenafil; however, when a 20 mg (film-coated tablet) was administered 24 hours prior to a 0.4 mg sublingual dose of nitroglycerin, no changes in blood pressure or heart rate were detected. Potential underlying causes of erectile dysfunction should be evaluated prior to treatment. Some products may contain phylalanine. Some products may contain sorbitol; do not use in patients with fructose intolerance.

Drug Interactions

Avoid Concomitant Use

Avoid concomitant use of Vardenafil with any of the following: Alprostadil; Amyl Nitrite; Cobicistat; Fusidic Acid (Systemic); Phosphodiesterase 5 Inhibitors; Riociguat; Vasodilators (Organic Nitrates)

Decreased Effect

The levels/effects of Vardenafil may be decreased by: Bosentan; Etravirine

Increased Effect/Toxicity

Vardenafil may increase the levels/effects of: Alpha1-Blockers; Alprostadil; Amyl Nitrite; Antihypertensives; Bosentan; Highest Risk QTc-Prolonging Agents; Moderate Risk QTc-Prolonging Agents; Phosphodiesterase 5 Inhibitors; Riociguat; Vasodilators (Organic Nitrates)

The levels/effects of Vardenafil may be increased by: Alcohol (Ethyl); Boceprevir; Clarithromycin; Cobicistat; CYP3A4 Inhibitors (Moderate); CYP3A4 Inhibitors (Strong); Dasatinib; Erythromycin (Systemic); Fluconazole; Fusidic Acid (Systemic); Itraconazole; Ivacaftor; Ketoconazole (Systemic); Lorcaserin; Luliconazole; Mifepristone; Posaconazole; Protease Inhibitors; Sapropterin; Simeprevir; Telaprevir; Voriconazole

Nutritional/Ethanol Interactions Ethanol: Substantial consumption of ethanol may increase the risk of hypotension and orthostasis. Lower ethanol consumption has not been associated with significant changes in blood pressure or increase in orthostatic symptoms. Management: Avoid or limit ethanol consumption.

Food: High-fat meals decrease maximum serum concentration 18% to 50%. Serum concentrations/toxicity may be increased with grapefruit juice. Management: Do not take with a high-fat meal. Avoid grapefruit juice.

Adverse Reactions

>10%:
Cardiovascular: Flushing (8% to 11%)
Central nervous system: Headache (14% to 15%)
2% to 10%:
Central nervous system: Dizziness (2%)
Gastrointestinal: Dyspepsia (3% to 4%), nausea (2%)
Neuromuscular & skeletal: Back pain (2%), CPK increased (2%)
Respiratory: Rhinitis (9%), nasal congestion (3%), sinusitis (3%)
Miscellaneous: Flu-like syndrome (3%)

Pharmacodynamics/Kinetics

Onset of Action ~60 minutes

Available Dosage Forms

Tablet, Oral:
Levitra: 2.5 mg, 5 mg, 10 mg, 20 mg
Tablet Dispersible, Oral:
Staxyn: 10 mg

General Dosage Range Dosage adjustment recommended in patients with hepatic impairment or on concomitant therapy

Oral:
Adults: Film-coated tablet (Levitra): 2.5-20 mg as a single dose (maximum: 1 dose/day); Oral disintegrating tablet (Staxyn): 10 mg as a single dose (maximum: 10 mg daily)
Elderly ≥65 years: Film-coated tablet (Levitra): 2.5-5 mg as a single dose (maximum: 1 dose daily)

Administration

Oral May be administered with or without food, 60 minutes prior to sexual activity.

Oral disintegrating tablet should not be removed from blister pack until administered. Using dry hands, place immediately on tongue. Tablet will dissolve within seconds; do not take with liquid. Do not crush, split, or chew.

Storage/Stability Store at 25°C (77°F); excursions permitted to 15°C to 25°C (59°F to 86°F). Keep oral disintegrating tablets sealed in blisterpack until ready to use.

Nursing Actions

Patient Education

• Discuss specific use of drug and side effects with patient as it relates to treatment. (HCAHPS: During this hospital stay, were you given any medicine that you had not taken before? Before giving you any new medicine, how often did hospital staff tell you what the medicine was for? How often did hospital staff describe possible side effects in a way you could understand?)
• Patient may experience dizziness, flushing, headache, dyspepsia, pyrosis, rhinitis, or vision changes. Have patient report immediately to

prescriber erection lasting >4 hours, angina, tachycardia, hearing impairment, or rash (HCAHPS).

- Educate patient about signs of a significant reaction (eg, wheezing; chest tightness; fever; itching; bad cough; blue skin color; seizures; or swelling of face, lips, tongue, or throat). **Note:** This is not a comprehensive list of all side effects. Patient should consult prescriber for additional questions.

Intended Use and Disclaimer: Should not be printed and given to patients. This information is intended to serve as a concise initial reference for healthcare professionals to use when discussing medications with a patient. You must ultimately rely on your own discretion, experience and judgment in diagnosing, treating and advising patients.

Dietary Considerations Avoid grapefruit juice. Some products may contain phenylalanine. Some products may contain sorbitol; do not use in patients with fructose intolerance.

Varenicline (var e NI kleen)

Brand Names: U.S. Chantix; Chantix Continuing Month Pak; Chantix Starting Month Pak

Index Terms Varenicline Tartrate

Pharmacologic Category Partial Nicotine Agonist; Smoking Cessation Aid

Medication Guide Available Yes

Pregnancy Risk Factor C

Lactation Excretion in breast milk unknown/not recommended

Breast-Feeding Considerations It is not known if varenicline is excreted in breast milk. Due to the potential for serious adverse reactions in the nursing infant, breast-feeding is not recommended.

Use Smoking cessation: Aid to smoking cessation treatment

Mechanism of Action/Effect Decreases nicotine dependence, craving, and withdrawal

Contraindications Serious hypersensitivity or skin reactions to varenicline or any component of the formulation

Warnings/Precautions [U.S. Boxed Warning]: Serious neuropsychiatric events (including depression, suicidal thoughts, and suicide) have been reported with use; some cases may have been complicated by symptoms of nicotine withdrawal following smoking cessation. Smoking cessation (with or without treatment) is associated with nicotine withdrawal symptoms and the exacerbation of underlying psychiatric illness; however, some of the behavioral disturbances were reported in treated patients who continued to smoke. Neuropsychiatric symptoms (eg, mood disturbances, psychosis, hostility) have occurred in patients with and without pre-existing psychiatric disease; many cases resolved following therapy discontinuation

although in some cases, symptoms persisted. Ethanol consumption may increase the risk of psychiatric adverse events. Monitor all patients for behavioral changes and psychiatric symptoms (eg, agitation, depression, suicidal behavior, suicidal ideation); inform patients to discontinue treatment and contact their healthcare provider immediately if they experience any behavioral and/or mood changes. **[U.S. Boxed Warning]: Before prescribing, the risks of serious neuropsychiatric events must be weighed against the immediate and long term benefits of smoking abstinence for each patient.**

Hypersensitivity reactions (including angioedema) and rare cases of serious skin reactions (including Stevens-Johnson syndrome and erythema multiforme) have been reported. Patients should be instructed to discontinue use and contact healthcare provider if signs/symptoms occur. Treatment may increase risk of cardiovascular events. A meta-analysis of 15 clinical trials, including a placebo-controlled trial in patients with stable cardiovascular disease, showed an increased incidence of major cardiovascular events (combined outcome of cardiovascular-related death, nonfatal MI, nonfatal stroke) in patients using varenicline compared with placebo. Cardiovascular events were uncommon in both the varenicline and placebo groups. These findings did not reach statistical significance, although data was consistent. Events occurred primarily in patients with known cardiovascular disease. The meta-analysis also showed a lower incidence of all-cause and cardiovascular mortality in varenicline-treated patients, although this was not statistically significant either. Dose-dependent nausea may occur; both transient and persistent nausea has been reported. Dosage reduction may be considered for intolerable nausea. May cause CNS depression, which may impair physical or mental abilities; patients must be cautioned about performing tasks which require mental alertness (eg, operating machinery or driving). There have been postmarketing reports of traffic accidents, near-miss incidents in traffic, or other accidental injuries in patients taking varenicline.

Use caution in renal dysfunction; dosage adjustment required. Safety and efficacy of varenicline with other smoking cessation therapies have not been established; increased adverse events when used concurrently with nicotine replacement therapy.

Drug Interactions

Avoid Concomitant Use There are no known interactions where it is recommended to avoid concomitant use.

Decreased Effect There are no known significant interactions involving a decrease in effect.

◄ **Increased Effect/Toxicity**
The levels/effects of Varenicline may be increased by: Alcohol (Ethyl); H2-Antagonists; Quinolone Antibiotics; Trimethoprim

Nutritional/Ethanol Interactions Ethanol: May increase the risk of psychiatric adverse events. Caution patients about the potential effects of ethanol consumption during therapy.

Adverse Reactions
>10%:
Central nervous system: Headache (15% to 19%), insomnia (10% to 19%), abnormal dreams (9% to 13%), suicidal ideation (11%)
Gastrointestinal: Nausea (16% to 40%), vomiting (≤5% to 11%)
1% to 10%:
Cardiovascular: Angina pectoris (4%), peripheral edema (2%), myocardial infarction (1%)
Central nervous system: Malaise (≤7%), sleep disorder (≤5%), drowsiness (3%), lethargy (1% to 2%), nightmares (1% to 2%)
Dermatologic: Skin rash (≤3%)
Gastrointestinal: Flatulence (6% to 9%), constipation (5% to 8%), dysgeusia (5% to 8%), abdominal pain (≤7%), xerostomia (≤6%), dyspepsia (5%), increased appetite (3% to 4%), anorexia (≤2%), gastroesophageal reflux disease (1%)
Respiratory: Upper respiratory tract infection (5% to 7%), dyspnea (≤2%), rhinorrhea (≤1%)

Available Dosage Forms
Tablet, Oral:
Chantix: 0.5 mg, 1 mg
Chantix Continuing Month Pak: 1 mg
Chantix Starting Month Pak: 0.5 mg X 11 & 1 mg X 42

General Dosage Range Dosage adjustment recommended in patients with renal impairment or who develop toxicities
Oral: *Adults:* Days 1-3: 0.5 mg once daily; Days 4-7: 0.5 mg twice daily; Maintenance (≥ Day 8): 1 mg twice daily

Administration
Oral Administer after eating and with a full glass of water.

Storage/Stability Store at 25°C (77°F); excursions permitted to 15°C to 30°C (59°F to 86°F).

Nursing Actions
Physical Assessment Provide educational materials and counseling to support an attempt at quitting smoking. Carefully instruct patient in appropriate titration of doses. Monitor for behavioral and emotional changes, such as hostility, agitation, and suicide ideation. Monitor other medications patient is taking for potential need for dose adjustment after quitting smoking.

Patient Education
• Discuss specific use of drug and side effects with patient as it relates to treatment. (HCAHPS: During this hospital stay, were you given any medicine that you had not taken before? Before giving you any new medicine, how often did

hospital staff tell you what the medicine was for? How often did hospital staff describe possible side effects in a way you could understand?)
• Patient may experience presyncope, fatigue, blurred vision, illogical thinking, nausea, xerostomia, flatulence, dyspepsia, parageusia, insomnia, headache, or nightmares. Have patient report immediately to prescriber depression, nervousness, emotional instability, anxiety, angina, dyspnea, strength differences from one side to another, severe skin irritation, or rash (HCAHPS).
• Educate patient about signs of a significant reaction (eg, wheezing; chest tightness; fever; itching; bad cough; blue skin color; seizures; or swelling of face, lips, tongue, or throat). **Note:** This is not a comprehensive list of all side effects. Patient should consult prescriber for additional questions.

Intended Use and Disclaimer: Should not be printed and given to patients. This information is intended to serve as a concise initial reference for healthcare professionals to use when discussing medications with a patient. You must ultimately rely on your own discretion, experience and judgment in diagnosing, treating and advising patients.

Dietary Considerations Should be given with food and a full glass of water to decrease gastric upset.

Varicella Virus Vaccine
(var i SEL a VYE rus vak SEEN)

Brand Names: U.S. Varivax
Index Terms Chickenpox Vaccine; VAR; Varicella-Zoster Virus (VZV) Vaccine (Varicella); VZV Vaccine (Varicella)
Pharmacologic Category Vaccine, Live (Viral)
Medication Safety Issues
Sound-alike/look-alike issues:
Varicella virus vaccine has been given in error (instead of the indicated varicella immune globulin) to pregnant women exposed to varicella.
Other safety concerns:
Both varicella vaccine and zoster vaccine are live, attenuated strains of varicella-zoster virus. Their indications, dosing, and composition are distinct. Varicella is indicated in children to prevent chickenpox, while zoster vaccine is indicated in older individuals to prevent reactivation of the virus which causes shingles. Zoster vaccine is **not** a substitute for varicella vaccine and should not be used in children.

Lactation Excretion in breast milk unknown/use caution
Use
Varicella prevention: For the prevention of varicella in persons 12 months and older

The Advisory Committee on Immunization Practices (ACIP) recommends vaccination for all children, adolescents, and adults who do not have evidence of immunity (CDC, 2007). Vaccination is especially important for:

- Healthcare personnel
- Household contacts of immunocompromised persons
- Persons living or working in environments where transmission is likely (teachers, childcare workers, residents and staff of institutional settings)
- Persons in environments where transmission has been reported
- Nonpregnant women of childbearing age
- Adolescents and adults in households with children
- International travelers

Postexposure prophylaxis: Vaccination within 3 days (possibly 5 days) after exposure to rash is effective in preventing illness or modifying severity of disease in persons without other evidence of immunity (CDC, 2007).

Available Dosage Forms
Injectable, Subcutaneous [preservative free]:
Varivax: 1350 PFU/0.5 mL (1 ea)
General Dosage Range SubQ:
Children 12 months to 12 years: Two doses of 0.5 mL separated by ≥3 months
Adolescents ≥13 years and Adults: Two doses of 0.5 mL separated by 4 weeks
Administration
I.M. SubQ administration is recommended; however, doses inadvertently given I.M. have resulted in similar seroconversion (CDC, 2011).
I.V. Do not administer I.V.
Subcutaneous For SubQ injection only; inject in the outer aspect of upper arm or the anterolateral thigh. Administer immediately following reconstitution.

Simultaneous administration of vaccines helps ensure the patient will be fully vaccinated by the appropriate age. Simultaneous administration of vaccines is defined as administering >1 vaccine on the same day at different anatomic sites. The use of licensed combination vaccines is generally preferred over separate injections of the equivalent components. Separate vaccines should not be combined in the same syringe unless indicated by product specific labeling. Separate needles and syringes should be used for each injection. The ACIP prefers each dose of a specific vaccine in a series come from the same manufacturer when possible. Adolescents and adults should be vaccinated while seated or lying down. In general, preterm infants should be vaccinated at the same chronological age as full-term infants (CDC, 2011).

Antipyretics have not been shown to prevent febrile seizures. Antipyretics may be used to treat fever or discomfort following vaccination (CDC, 2011). One study reported that routine prophylactic administration of acetaminophen to prevent fever prior to vaccination decreased the immune response of some vaccines; the clinical significance of this reduction in immune response has not been established (Prymula, 2009).

Nursing Actions
Physical Assessment Review allergies and immunization records prior to administration. Should not be given to pregnant females. Monitor for allergic reactions after administration.
Patient Education
- Discuss specific use of vaccine and side effects with patient as it relates to treatment. (HCAHPS: During this hospital stay, were you given any medicine that you had not taken before? Before giving you any new medicine, how often did hospital staff tell you what the medicine was for? How often did hospital staff describe possible side effects in a way you could understand?)
- Patient may experience headache, nausea, diarrhea, or rhinitis. Have patient report immediately to prescriber severe asthenia or rash (HCAHPS).
- Educate patient about signs of a significant reaction (eg, wheezing; chest tightness; fever; itching; bad cough; blue skin color; seizures; or swelling of face, lips, tongue, or throat). **Note:** This is not a comprehensive list of all side effects. Patient should consult prescriber for additional questions.

Intended Use and Disclaimer: Should not be printed and given to patients. This information is intended to serve as a concise initial reference for healthcare professionals to use when discussing medications with a patient. You must ultimately rely on your own discretion, experience and judgment in diagnosing, treating and advising patients.

Related Information
Immunization Administration Recommendations *on page 1675*
Immunization Recommendations *on page 1680*

Vasopressin (vay soe PRES in)

Brand Names: U.S. Pitressin Synthetic
Index Terms 8-Arginine Vasopressin; ADH; Antidiuretic Hormone; AVP
Pharmacologic Category Antidiuretic Hormone Analog; Hormone, Posterior Pituitary

◄ **Medication Safety Issues**

High alert medication:

The Institute for Safe Medication Practices (ISMP) includes this medication (I.V. or intraosseous administration) among its list of drugs which have a heightened risk of causing significant patient harm when used in error.

Administration issues:

Use care when prescribing and/or administering vasopressin solutions. Close attention should be given to concentration of solution, route of administration, dose, and rate of administration (units/minute, units/kg/minute, units/kg/hour).

Pregnancy Risk Factor C

Lactation Enters breast milk/use caution

Use Treatment of central diabetes insipidus; differential diagnosis of diabetes insipidus

Unlabeled Use ACLS guidelines: Pulseless arrest (ventricular tachycardia [VT]/ventricular fibrillation [VF], asystole/pulseless electrical activity [PEA]); cardiac arrest secondary to anaphylaxis (unresponsive to epinephrine)

Adjunct in the treatment of GI hemorrhage and esophageal varices; adjunct in the treatment of vasodilatory shock (septic shock); donor management in brain-dead patients (hormone replacement therapy)

Available Dosage Forms

Solution, Injection:

Pitressin Synthetic: 20 units/mL (1 mL)

Generic: 20 units/mL (0.5 mL, 1 mL, 10 mL)

General Dosage Range I.M., SubQ:

Children: 2.5-10 units 2-4 times/day as needed

Adults: 5-10 units 2-4 times/day as needed

Usual Infusion Concentrations: Adult I.V. infusion: 100 units in 500 mL (concentration: 0.2 unit/mL) **or** 100 units in 100 mL (concentration: 1 unit/mL) of D$_5$W or NS

Administration

I.M. For I.M. or SubQ use (per manufacturer).

I.V. I.V. (unlabeled route): May administer as I.V. push over seconds (ACLS) or as a continuous I.V. infusion; when administered as a continuous I.V. infusion for vasodilatory shock, the use of a central venous catheter is recommended. Use extreme caution to avoid extravasation because of risk of necrosis and gangrene. In treatment of varices, infusions are often supplemented with nitroglycerin infusions to minimize cardiac effects.

Vesicant; ensure proper needle or catheter placement prior to and during infusion; avoid extravasation.

Extravasation management: If extravasation occurs, stop infusion immediately and disconnect (leave cannula/needle in place); gently aspirate extravasated solution (do **NOT** flush the line); remove needle/cannula; elevate extremity. Initiate phentolamine (or alternative antidote).

Phentolamine: Dilute 5-10 mg in 10-15 mL NS and administer into extravasation site as soon as possible after extravasation (Peberdy, 2010).

Alternatives to phentolamine (due to shortage):

Nitroglycerin topical 2% ointment (based on limited case reports in neonates/infants): Apply 4 mm/kg as a thin ribbon to the affected areas; may repeat after 8 hours if needed (Wong, 1992) **or** apply a 1-inch strip on the affected site (Denkler, 1989).

Terbutaline (based on limited case reports): Infiltrate extravasation area using a solution of terbutaline 1 mg diluted to 10 mL in NS (large extravasation site; administration volume varied from 3-10 mL) **or** 1 mg diluted in 1 mL NS (small/distal extravasation site; administration volume varied from 0.5-1 mL) (Stier, 1999).

Injectable Detail pH: 2.5-4.5 (20 units/mL solution in vial)

Topical Topical administration on nasal mucosa (unlabeled route): Administer injectable vasopressin on cotton plugs, as nasal spray, or by dropper. Should not be inhaled.

Subcutaneous For SubQ or I.M. use (per manufacturer).

Endotracheal Endotracheal (unlabeled route): If no I.V./I.O. access may give endotracheally. ACLS guidelines do not recommend a specific endotracheal dose; however, may be given endotracheally using the same I.V. dose (ACLS, 2010; Wenzel, 1997). Mix with 5-10 mL of water or normal saline, and administer down the endotracheal tube.

Nursing Actions

Physical Assessment I.V. requires use of infusion pump and close monitoring to prevent extravasation (may cause severe necrosis and gangrene). Monitor cardiac status, blood pressure, CNS status, fluid balance, and for signs or symptoms of water intoxication or intranasal irritation.

Patient Education

• Discuss specific use of drug and side effects with patient as it relates to treatment. (HCAHPS: During this hospital stay, were you given any medicine that you had not taken before? Before giving you any new medicine, how often did hospital staff tell you what the medicine was for? How often did hospital staff describe possible side effects in a way you could understand?)

• Patient may experience headache, dyspepsia, or nausea. Have patient report immediately to prescriber illogical thinking, severe asthenia, fatigue, or rash (HCAHPS).

• Educate patient about signs of a significant reaction (eg, wheezing; chest tightness; fever; itching; bad cough; blue skin color; seizures; or swelling of face, lips, tongue, or throat). **Note:** This is not a comprehensive list of all side

effects. Patient should consult prescriber for additional questions.

Intended Use and Disclaimer: Should not be printed and given to patients. This information is intended to serve as a concise initial reference for healthcare professionals to use when discussing medications with a patient. You must ultimately rely on your own discretion, experience and judgment in diagnosing, treating and advising patients.

Related Information
Management of Drug Extravasations *on page 1700*

Vecuronium (vek ue ROE nee um)

Index Terms Norcuron; ORG NC 45

Pharmacologic Category Neuromuscular Blocker Agent, Nondepolarizing

Medication Safety Issues

Sound-alike/look-alike issues:

Vecuronium may be confused with valproate sodium, vancomycin

Norcuron® may be confused with Narcan®

High alert medication:

The Institute for Safe Medication Practices (ISMP) includes this medication among its list of drugs which have a heightened risk of causing significant patient harm when used in error.

Other safety concerns:

United States Pharmacopeia (USP) 2006: The Interdisciplinary Safe Medication Use Expert Committee of the USP has recommended the following:

- Hospitals, clinics, and other practice sites should institute special safeguards in the storage, labeling, and use of these agents and should include these safeguards in staff orientation and competency training.
- Healthcare professionals should be on high alert (especially vigilant) whenever a neuromuscular-blocking agent (NMBA) is stocked, ordered, prepared, or administered.

Pregnancy Risk Factor C

Lactation Excretion in breast milk unknown/use caution

Use To facilitate endotracheal intubation and to relax skeletal muscles during surgery; to facilitate mechanical ventilation in ICU patients; does not relieve pain or produce sedation

Available Dosage Forms

Solution Reconstituted, Intravenous:

Generic: 10 mg (1 ea); 20 mg (1 ea)

Solution Reconstituted, Intravenous [preservative free]:

Generic: 10 mg (1 ea); 20 mg (1 ea)

General Dosage Range Dosage adjustment recommended in patients with hepatic impairment

I.V.: *Children ≥1 year and Adults:* Initial: 0.04-0.1 mg/kg; Maintenance: 0.01-0.015 mg/kg

every 12-15 minutes **or** 0.8-1.2 **mcg**/kg/**minute** (or 0.048-0.072 **mg**/kg/**hour**) as a continuous infusion

Usual Infusion Concentrations: Pediatric I.V. infusion: 0.1 mg/mL, 0.2 mg/mL, 1 mg/mL

Usual Infusion Concentrations: Adult I.V. infusion: 10 mg in 100 mL (concentration: 0.1 mg/mL), 20 mg in 100 mL (concentration: 0.2 mg/mL), **or** 50 mg in 50 mL (concentration: 1 mg/mL) of D_5W or NS

Administration

I.V. Concentration of 1 mg/mL may be administered by rapid I.V. injection; may also be used for I.V. infusion in fluid-restricted patients.

Injectable Detail pH: 4

Nursing Actions

Physical Assessment Ventilatory support must be instituted and maintained until adequate respiratory muscle function and/or airway protection are assured. This drug is not an anesthetic or analgesic; pain must be treated with other agents. Continuous monitoring of vital signs, cardiac status, respiratory status, and degree of neuromuscular block (objective assessment with peripheral external nerve stimulator) is mandatory during infusion and until full muscle tone has returned. It may take longer for return of muscle tone in obese or elderly patients or patients with renal or hepatic disease, dehydration, electrolyte imbalance, or severe acid/base imbalance.

Long-term use: Monitor level of neuromuscular blockade, skeletal muscle movement, and respiratory effort. Reposition patient and provide appropriate skin care, mouth care, and care of patient's eyes every 2-3 hours while sedated. Provide appropriate emotional and sensory support (auditory and environmental).

Patient Education

- Discuss specific use of drug and side effects with patient as it relates to treatment. (HCAHPS: During this hospital stay, were you given any medicine that you had not taken before? Before giving you any new medicine, how often did hospital staff tell you what the medicine was for? How often did hospital staff describe possible side effects in a way you could understand?)
- Patient may experience dizziness, flushing, or myalgia. Have patient report immediately to prescriber tachycardia or rash (HCAHPS).
- Educate patient about signs of a significant reaction (eg, wheezing; chest tightness; fever; itching; bad cough; blue skin color; seizures; or swelling of face, lips, tongue, or throat). **Note:** This is not a comprehensive list of all side effects. Patient should consult prescriber for additional questions.

Intended Use and Disclaimer: Should not be printed and given to patients. This information is intended to serve as a concise initial reference for healthcare professionals to use when discussing

medications with a patient. You must ultimately rely on your own discretion, experience and judgment in diagnosing, treating and advising patients.

Vemurafenib (vem ue RAF e nib)

Brand Names: U.S. Zelboraf
Index Terms BRAF(V600E) Kinase Inhibitor RO5185426; PLX4032; RG7204; RO5185426
Pharmacologic Category Antineoplastic Agent, BRAF Kinase Inhibitor
Medication Safety Issues
Sound-alike/look-alike issues:
Vemurafenib may be confused with axitinib, dabrafenib, regorafenib, SORAfenib, trametinib, vandetanib, vismodegib
High alert medication:
This medication is in a class the Institute for Safe Medication Practices (ISMP) includes among its list of drug classes which have a heightened risk of causing significant patient harm when used in error.

Medication Guide Available Yes
Pregnancy Risk Factor D
Lactation Excretion in breast milk unknown/not recommended
Use Melanoma:
U.S. labeling: Treatment of unresectable or metastatic melanoma in patients with a BRAFV600E mutation (as detected by an approved test); **Note:** Not recommended in patients with wild-type BRAF melanoma.
Canadian labeling: Treatment of unresectable or metastatic melanoma in patients with a BRAFV600 mutation (as identified by a validated test)
Unlabeled Use Treatment of metastatic melanoma in patients with a BRAFV600K mutation
Available Dosage Forms
Tablet, Oral:
Zelboraf: 240 mg
General Dosage Range Dosage adjustment recommended in patients who develop toxicities.
Oral: *Adults:* 960 mg twice daily
Administration
Oral Doses should be administered orally in the morning and evening, ~12 hours apart. Swallow whole with a glass of water; do not crush or chew. May be taken with or without a meal. If vomiting occurs after a dose is taken, do not take an additional dose; continue with the next scheduled dose.

Hazardous agent; use appropriate precautions for handling and disposal (meets NIOSH, 2012 criteria).

Nursing Actions
Physical Assessment Assess for signs and symptoms of arrhythmias. Check results of ECGs. Ensure serum potassium and magnesium within normal limits. Closely assess skin for any reactions or new skin lesions. This drug causes photosensitivity reactions; educate the patient on proper sun protection. Monitor for ocular toxicity: Blurred vision, pain, tearing, or irritation.
Patient Education
• Discuss specific use of drug and side effects with patient as it relates to treatment. (HCAHPS: During this hospital stay, were you given any medicine that you had not taken before? Before giving you any new medicine, how often did hospital staff tell you what the medicine was for? How often did hospital staff describe possible side effects in a way you could understand?)
• Patient may experience alopecia, arthralgia, edema in feet or hands, headache, nausea, diarrhea, fatigue, loss of appetite, rash, or xeroderma. Have patient report immediately to prescriber dizziness, syncope, tachycardia, ecchymosis, poor wound healing, severe skin irritation, mole or skin changes, inability to eat, discolored urine, jaundice, significant dyspepsia, or sudden vision changes (HCAHPS).
• Educate patient about signs of a significant reaction (eg, wheezing; chest tightness; fever; itching; bad cough; blue skin color; seizures; or swelling of face, lips, tongue, or throat). **Note:** This is not a comprehensive list of all side effects. Patient should consult prescriber for additional questions.

Intended Use and Disclaimer: Should not be printed and given to patients. This information is intended to serve as a concise initial reference for healthcare professionals to use when discussing medications with a patient. You must ultimately rely on your own discretion, experience and judgment in diagnosing, treating and advising patients.
Related Information
Oral Medications That Should Not Be Crushed or Altered *on page 1712*

Venlafaxine (ven la FAX een)

Brand Names: U.S. Effexor XR
Pharmacologic Category Antidepressant, Serotonin/Norepinephrine Reuptake Inhibitor
Medication Safety Issues
Sound-alike/look-alike issues:
Effexor may be confused with Effexor XR
BEERS Criteria medication:
This drug may be potentially inappropriate for use in geriatric patients (Quality of evidence - moderate; Strength of recommendation - strong).
Medication Guide Available Yes
Pregnancy Risk Factor C
Lactation Enters breast milk/not recommended
Breast-Feeding Considerations Venlafaxine and ODV are found in breast milk and the serum of nursing infants. Adverse events have not been

observed; however, it is recommended to monitor the infant for adverse events if the decision to breast-feed has been made. The long-term effects on neurobehavior have not been studied, thus one should prescribe venlafaxine to a mother who is breast-feeding only when the benefits outweigh the potential risks. The manufacturer does not recommend breast-feeding during therapy.

Use Treatment of major depressive disorder, generalized anxiety disorder (GAD), social anxiety disorder (social phobia), panic disorder

Unlabeled Use Obsessive-compulsive disorder (OCD); hot flashes; neuropathic pain (including diabetic neuropathy); attention-deficit/hyperactivity disorder (ADHD); post-traumatic stress disorder (PTSD); migraine prophylaxis

Mechanism of Action/Effect Venlafaxine and its active metabolite, o-desmethylvenlafaxine (ODV), inhibit the reuptake of both norepinephrine and serotonin (SNRI); improves symptoms of depression.

Contraindications Hypersensitivity to venlafaxine or any component of the formulation; use of MAO inhibitors intended to treat psychiatric disorders (concurrently or within 14 days of discontinuing the MAO inhibitor); initiation of MAO inhibitor intended to treat psychiatric disorders within 7 days of discontinuing venlafaxine; initiation of venlafaxine in a patient receiving linezolid or intravenous methylene blue

Warnings/Precautions [U.S. Boxed Warning]: Antidepressants increase the risk of suicidal thinking and behavior in children, adolescents, and young adults (18-24 years of age) with major depressive disorder (MDD) and other psychiatric disorders; consider risk prior to prescribing. Short-term studies did not show an increased risk in patients >24 years of age and showed a decreased risk in patients ≥65 years. Closely monitor for clinical worsening, suicidality, or unusual changes in behavior; the patient's family or caregiver should be instructed to closely observe the patient and communicate condition with healthcare provider. Reduced growth rate has been observed with venlafaxine therapy in children. A medication guide should be dispensed with each prescription. **Venlafaxine is not FDA approved for use in children.**

The possibility of a suicide attempt is inherent in major depression and may persist until remission occurs. Monitor for worsening of depression or suicidality, especially during initiation of therapy (generally first 1-2 months) or with dose increases or decreases. Use caution in high-risk patients. Worsening depression and severe abrupt suicidality that are not part of the presenting symptoms may require discontinuation or modification of drug therapy. The patient's family or caregiver should be alerted to monitor patients for the emergence of suicidality and associated behaviors (such as agitation, irritability, hostility, impulsivity, and hypomania) and call healthcare provider.

May worsen psychosis in some patients or precipitate a shift to mania or hypomania in patients with bipolar disorder. Patients presenting with depressive symptoms should be screened for bipolar disorder. Monotherapy in patients with bipolar disorder should be avoided. **Venlafaxine is not FDA approved for the treatment of bipolar depression.**

Potentially life-threatening serotonin syndrome (SS) has occurred with serotonergic agents (eg, SSRIs, SNRIs), particularly when used in combination with other serotonergic agents (eg, triptans, TCAs, fentanyl, lithium, tramadol, buspirone, St John's wort, tryptophan) or agents that impair metabolism of serotonin (eg, MAO inhibitors intended to treat psychiatric disorders, other MAO inhibitors [ie, linezolid and intravenous methylene blue]). Discontinue treatment (and any concomitant serotonergic agent) immediately if signs/symptoms arise.

May cause sustained increase in blood pressure or tachycardia; dose related and increases are generally modest (12-15 mm Hg diastolic). Control pre-existing hypertension prior to initiation of venlafaxine. Use caution in patients with recent history of MI, unstable heart disease, or hyperthyroidism; may cause increase in anxiety, nervousness, insomnia; may cause weight loss (use with caution in patients where weight loss is undesirable); may cause increases in serum cholesterol. Use caution with hepatic or renal impairment; dosage adjustments recommended. May cause hyponatremia/SIADH (elderly at increased risk); volume depletion (diuretics may increase risk).

Bleeding related to SSRI or SNRI use has been reported to range from relatively minor bruising and epistaxis to life-threatening hemorrhage. Interstitial lung disease and eosinophilic pneumonia have been rarely reported; may present as progressive dyspnea, cough, and/or chest pain. Prompt evaluation and possible discontinuation of therapy may be necessary. Venlafaxine may increase the risks associated with electroconvulsive therapy. Use cautiously in patients with a history of seizures. The risks of cognitive or motor impairment, as well as the potential for anticholinergic effects are very low. May cause or exacerbate sexual dysfunction. Bone fractures have been associated with antidepressant treatment. Consider the possibility of a fragility fracture if an antidepressant-treated patient presents with unexplained bone pain, point tenderness, swelling, or bruising (Rabenda, 2013; Rizzoli, 2012).

Use caution in elderly patients; may cause or exacerbate syndrome of inappropriate antidiuretic hormone secretion or hyponatremia; monitor sodium closely with initiation or dosage ▶

adjustments in older adults (Beers Criteria). Use caution in patients with increased intraocular pressure or at risk of acute narrow-angle glaucoma. Potentially significant drug-drug interactions may exist, requiring dose or frequency adjustment, additional monitoring, and/or selection of alternative therapy.

Abrupt discontinuation or interruption of antidepressant therapy has been associated with a discontinuation syndrome. Symptoms arising may vary with antidepressant however commonly include nausea, vomiting, diarrhea, headaches, lightheadedness, dizziness, diminished appetite, sweating, chills, tremors, paresthesias, fatigue, somnolence, and sleep disturbances (eg, vivid dreams, insomnia). Greater risks for developing a discontinuation syndrome have been associated with antidepressants with shorter half-lives, longer durations of treatment, and abrupt discontinuation. For antidepressants of short or intermediate half-lives, symptoms may emerge within 2-5 days after treatment discontinuation and last 7-14 days (APA, 2010; Fava, 2006; Haddad, 2001; Shelton, 2001; Warner, 2006).

Drug Interactions

Avoid Concomitant Use
Avoid concomitant use of Venlafaxine with any of the following: Conivaptan; Fusidic Acid (Systemic); Iobenguane I 123; Linezolid; MAO Inhibitors; Methylene Blue; Urokinase

Decreased Effect
Venlafaxine may decrease the levels/effects of: Alpha2-Agonists; Indinavir; Iobenguane I 123; Ioflupane I 123

The levels/effects of Venlafaxine may be decreased by: Bosentan; CYP3A4 Inducers (Strong); Dabrafenib; Deferasirox; Mitotane; Nonsteroidal Anti-Inflammatory Agents; Peginterferon Alfa-2b; Tocilizumab

Increased Effect/Toxicity
Venlafaxine may increase the levels/effects of: Agents with Antiplatelet Properties; Alpha-/Beta-Agonists; Anticoagulants; Antipsychotics; Aspirin; Collagenase (Systemic); Dabigatran Etexilate; Dofetilide; Highest Risk QTc-Prolonging Agents; Ibritumomab; Lomitapide; Methylene Blue; Moderate Risk QTc-Prolonging Agents; NSAID (Nonselective); Rivaroxaban; Salicylates; Serotonin Modulators; Thrombolytic Agents; Tositumomab and Iodine I 131 Tositumomab; TraZODone; Urokinase; Vitamin K Antagonists

The levels/effects of Venlafaxine may be increased by: Abiraterone Acetate; Alcohol (Ethyl); Antipsychotics; Conivaptan; CYP2D6 Inhibitors (Moderate); CYP2D6 Inhibitors (Strong); CYP3A4 Inhibitors (Moderate); CYP3A4 Inhibitors (Strong); Darunavir; Dasatinib; Fusidic Acid (Systemic); Glucosamine; Herbs (Anticoagulant/Antiplatelet Properties); Ibrutinib; Ivacaftor;

Linezolid; Luliconazole; MAO Inhibitors; Metoclopramide; Mifepristone; Multivitamins/Fluoride (with ADE); Multivitamins/Minerals (with ADEK, Folate, Iron); Multivitamins/Minerals (with AE, No Iron); Nonsteroidal Anti-Inflammatory Agents; Omega-3 Fatty Acids; Pentosan Polysulfate Sodium; Pentoxifylline; Propafenone; Prostacyclin Analogues; Simeprevir; Stiripentol; Tipranavir; Vitamin E; Voriconazole

Nutritional/Ethanol Interactions
Ethanol: May increase CNS depression; monitor for increased effects with coadministration. Caution patients about effects.

Herb/Nutraceutical: Avoid valerian, St John's wort, SAMe, kava kava, tryptophan (may increase risk of serotonin syndrome and/or excessive sedation).

Adverse Reactions Note: Actual frequency may be dependent upon formulation and/or indication
>10%:
Central nervous system: Headache (25% to 38%), somnolence (12% to 26%), dizziness (11% to 24%), insomnia (15% to 24%), nervousness (6% to 21%), anxiety (2% to 11%),
Gastrointestinal: Nausea (21% to 58%), xerostomia (12% to 22%), anorexia (8% to 17%), constipation (8% to 15%)
Genitourinary: Abnormal ejaculation/orgasm (2% to 19%)
Neuromuscular & skeletal: Weakness (8% to 19%)
Miscellaneous: Diaphoresis (7% to 19%)
1% to 10%:
Cardiovascular: Vasodilation (2% to 6%), hypertension (dose related; 3% in patients receiving <100 mg/day, up to 13% in patients receiving >300 mg/day), palpitation (3%), tachycardia (2%), chest pain (2%), orthostatic hypotension (1%), edema
Central nervous system: Yawning (3% to 8%), abnormal dreams (3% to 7%), chills (2% to 7%), agitation (2% to 5%), confusion (2%), abnormal thinking (2%), depersonalization (1%), depression (1% to 3%), fever, migraine, amnesia, hypoesthesia, vertigo
Dermatologic: Rash (3%), pruritus (1%), bruising
Endocrine & metabolic: Libido decreased (2% to 8%), hypercholesterolemia (5%), triglycerides increased
Gastrointestinal: Abdominal pain (8%), diarrhea (8%), vomiting (3% to 8%), dyspepsia (5% to 7%), weight loss (1% to 6%), flatulence (3% to 4%), taste perversion (2%), appetite increased, belching, weight gain
Genitourinary: Impotence (4% to 6%), urinary frequency (3%), urination impaired (2%), urinary retention (1%), metrorrhagia, prostatic disorder, vaginitis
Neuromuscular & skeletal: Tremor (1% to 10%), hypertonia (3%), paresthesia (2% to 3%), twitching (1% to 3%), arthralgia, neck pain, trismus

Ocular: Accommodation abnormal (6% to 9%), abnormal or blurred vision (4% to 6%), mydriasis (2%)

Otic: Tinnitus (2%)

Renal: Albuminuria

Respiratory: Pharyngitis (7%), sinusitis (2%), bronchitis, cough increased, dyspnea

Miscellaneous: Infection (6%), flu-like syndrome (2%), trauma (2%)

Available Dosage Forms

Capsule Extended Release 24 Hour, Oral:
Effexor XR: 37.5 mg, 75 mg, 150 mg
Generic: 37.5 mg, 75 mg, 150 mg

Tablet, Oral:
Generic: 25 mg, 37.5 mg, 50 mg, 75 mg, 100 mg

Tablet Extended Release 24 Hour, Oral:
Generic: 37.5 mg, 75 mg, 150 mg, 225 mg

General Dosage Range Dosage adjustment recommended in patients with hepatic or renal impairment

Oral:
Extended release: *Adults:* Initial: 37.5-75 mg/day once daily; Maintenance: 75-225 mg/day once daily (recommended maximum: 225 mg/day)

Immediate release: *Adults:* Initial: 75 mg/day in 2-3 divided doses; Maintenance: 75-375 mg/day in 2-3 divided doses (recommended maximum: 375 mg/day)

Administration

Oral Administer with food.

Extended-release formulations: Swallow capsule or tablet whole; do not crush or chew. Contents of capsule may be sprinkled on a spoonful of applesauce and swallowed immediately without chewing; followed with a glass of water to ensure complete swallowing of the pellets.

Storage/Stability Store at controlled room temperature of 20°C to 25°C (68°F to 77°F).

Nursing Actions

Physical Assessment Monitor blood pressure and weight/height at beginning of therapy and periodically throughout. Observe for clinical worsening, suicide ideation, or unusual behavior changes, especially during the initial few months of therapy or during dosage changes. Taper dosage when discontinuing.

Patient Education
• Discuss specific use of drug and side effects with patient as it relates to treatment. (HCAHPS: During this hospital stay, were you given any medicine that you had not taken before? Before giving you any new medicine, how often did hospital staff tell you what the medicine was for? How often did hospital staff describe possible side effects in a way you could understand?)
• Patient may experience presyncope, fatigue, blurred vision, illogical thinking, insomnia, nervousness and anxiety, headache, hyperhidrosis, nausea, constipation, xerostomia, or impotence. Have patient report immediately to prescriber dyspnea, angina, significant change in balance,

fasciculations, tremors, tachycardia, ecchymosis, bleeding, severe asthenia, or rash (HCAHPS).
• Educate patient about signs of a significant reaction (eg, wheezing; chest tightness; fever; itching; bad cough; blue skin color; seizures; or swelling of face, lips, tongue, or throat). **Note:** This is not a comprehensive list of all side effects. Patient should consult prescriber for additional questions.

Intended Use and Disclaimer: Should not be printed and given to patients. This information is intended to serve as a concise initial reference for healthcare professionals to use when discussing medications with a patient. You must ultimately rely on your own discretion, experience and judgment in diagnosing, treating and advising patients.

Dietary Considerations Should be taken with food.

Related Information
Oral Medications That Should Not Be Crushed or Altered *on page 1712*

Verapamil (ver AP a mil)

Brand Names: U.S. Calan; Calan SR; Isoptin SR; Verelan; Verelan PM

Index Terms Iproveratril Hydrochloride; Verapamil Hydrochloride

Pharmacologic Category Antianginal Agent; Antiarrhythmic Agent, Class IV; Antihypertensive; Calcium Channel Blocker; Calcium Channel Blocker, Nondihydropyridine

Medication Safety Issues

Sound-alike/look-alike issues:
Calan® may be confused with Colace®, diltiazem
Covera-HS® may be confused with Provera®
Isoptin® may be confused with Isopto® Tears
Verelan® may be confused with Voltaren®

High alert medication:
The Institute for Safe Medication Practices (ISMP) includes this medication (I.V. formulation) among its list of drug classes which have a heightened risk of causing significant patient harm when used in error.

Administration issues:
Significant differences exist between oral and I.V. dosing. Use caution when converting from one route of administration to another.

International issues:
Dilacor [Brazil] may be confused with Dilacor XR brand name for diltiazem [U.S.]

Pregnancy Risk Factor C

Lactation Enters breast milk/not recommended

Breast-Feeding Considerations Verapamil is excreted into breast milk; the estimated exposure to the nursing infant is <1% of the maternal dose. Breast-feeding is not recommended by some manufacturers. Breast-fed infants of mothers taking ▶

medications for hypertension should be monitored for adverse effects (Chobanian, 2003).

Use

Oral: Treatment of hypertension; angina pectoris (vasospastic, chronic stable, unstable) (Calan®, Covera-HS®); supraventricular tachyarrhythmia (PSVT, atrial fibrillation/flutter [rate control])

I.V.: Supraventricular tachyarrhythmia (PSVT, atrial fibrillation/flutter [rate control])

Unlabeled Use Hypertrophic cardiomyopathy; bipolar disorder (manic manifestations)

Mechanism of Action/Effect Produces relaxation of coronary vascular smooth muscle and coronary vasodilation. Increases myocardial oxygen delivery in patients with vasospastic (Prinzmetal's) angina. Slows automaticity and conduction of AV node.

Contraindications Hypersensitivity to verapamil or any component of the formulation; severe left ventricular dysfunction; hypotension (systolic pressure <90 mm Hg) or cardiogenic shock; sick sinus syndrome (except in patients with a functioning artificial ventricular pacemaker); second- or third-degree AV block (except in patients with a functioning artificial ventricular pacemaker); atrial flutter or fibrillation and an accessory bypass tract (Wolff-Parkinson-White [WPW] syndrome, Lown-Ganong-Levine syndrome)

I.V.: Additional contraindications include concurrent use of I.V. beta-blocking agents; ventricular tachycardia

Warnings/Precautions Avoid use in heart failure; can exacerbate condition; use is contraindicated in severe left ventricular dysfunction. Symptomatic hypotension with or without syncope can rarely occur; blood pressure must be lowered at a rate appropriate for the patient's clinical condition. Rare increases in hepatic enzymes can be observed. Can cause first-degree AV block or sinus bradycardia; use is contraindicated in patients with sick sinus syndrome, second- or third-degree AV block (except in patients with a functioning artificial pacemaker), or an accessory bypass tract (eg, WPW syndrome). Other conduction abnormalities are rare. Considered contraindicated in patients with wide complex tachycardias unless known to be supraventricular in origin; severe hypotension likely to occur upon administration (ACLS, 2010). Use caution when using verapamil together with a beta-blocker. Administration of I.V. verapamil and an I.V. beta-blocker within a few hours of each other may result in asystole and should be avoided; simultaneous administration is contraindicated. Use with other agents known to reduce SA node function and/or AV nodal conduction (eg, digoxin) or reduce sympathetic outflow (eg, clonidine) may increase the risk of serious bradycardia. Verapamil significantly increases digoxin serum concentrations; adjust digoxin dose. Use with caution in patients with HCM with outflow tract obstruction (especially those with high gradients, advanced heart failure, or sinus bradycardia); may be used in patients who

cannot tolerate beta-blockade. Verapamil should not be used in those with systemic hypotension or severe dyspnea at rest (Gersh, 2011; Nishimura, 2004).

Decreased neuromuscular transmission has been reported with verapamil; use with caution in patients with attenuated neuromuscular transmission (Duchenne's muscular dystrophy, myasthenia gravis); dosage reduction may be required. Use with caution in renal impairment; monitor hemodynamics and possibly ECG if severe impairment, particularly if concomitant hepatic impairment. Use with caution in patients with hepatic impairment; dosage reduction may be required; monitor hemodynamics and possibly ECG if severe impairment. May prolong recovery from nondepolarizing neuromuscular-blocking agents. Use Covera-HS® (extended-release delivery system) with caution in patients with severe GI narrowing. In patients with extremely short GI transit times (eg, <7 hours), dosage adjustment may be required; inadequate pharmacokinetic data. I.V. use for SVT for is not recommended in infants; use with caution in children as myocardial depression/hypotension may occur.

Drug Interactions

Avoid Concomitant Use

Avoid concomitant use of Verapamil with any of the following: Bosutinib; Conivaptan; Dantrolene; Disopyramide; Dofetilide; Fusidic Acid (Systemic); Ibrutinib; Ivabradine; Lomitapide; PAZOPanib; Pimozide; Pomalidomide; Simeprevir; Tolvaptan; Topotecan; Ulipristal; VinCRIStine (Liposomal)

Decreased Effect

Verapamil may decrease the levels/effects of: Clopidogrel; Ifosfamide

The levels/effects of Verapamil may be decreased by: Barbiturates; Bosentan; Calcium Salts; CarBAMazepine; CYP3A4 Inducers (Strong); Dabrafenib; Deferasirox; Herbs (CYP3A4 Inducers); Herbs (Hypertensive Properties); Methylphenidate; Mitotane; Nafcillin; P-glycoprotein/ABCB1 Inducers; Rifamycin Derivatives; Tocilizumab; Yohimbine

Increased Effect/Toxicity

Verapamil may increase the levels/effects of: Afatinib; Alcohol (Ethyl); Aliskiren; Amifostine; Amiodarone; Antihypertensives; ARIPiprazole; AtorvaSTATin; Atosiban; Avanafil; Benzodiazepines (metabolized by oxidation); Beta-Blockers; Bosentan; Bosutinib; Budesonide (Systemic, Oral Inhalation); BusPIRone; Calcium Channel Blockers (Dihydropyridine); CarBAMazepine; Cardiac Glycosides; Colchicine; Corticosteroids (Systemic); CycloSPORINE (Systemic); CYP3A4 Substrates; Dabigatran Etexilate; Disopyramide; Dofetilide; DOXOrubicin (Conventional); Dronedarone; DULoxetine; Eletriptan; Eplerenone; Everolimus; Fexofenadine; Fingolimod;

Flecainide; Fosphenytoin; Halofantrine; Hypotensive Agents; Ibrutinib; Imatinib; Ivabradine; Ivacaftor; Lithium; Lomitapide; Lovastatin; Lurasidone; Magnesium Salts; Midodrine; Neuromuscular-Blocking Agents (Nondepolarizing); Nitroprusside; Obinutuzumab; OxyCODONE; PAZOPanib; P-glycoprotein/ABCB1 Substrates; Phenytoin; Pimecrolimus; Pimozide; Pomalidomide; Propafenone; Prucalopride; QuiNIDine; Ranolazine; Red Yeast Rice; RisperiDONE; RiTUXimab; Rivaroxaban; Salicylates; Salmeterol; Saxagliptin; Simeprevir; Simvastatin; Tacrolimus (Systemic); Tacrolimus (Topical); Tolvaptan; Topotecan; Ulipristal; Vilazodone; VinCRIStine (Liposomal); Zuclopenthixol

The levels/effects of Verapamil may be increased by: Alpha1-Blockers; Anilidopiperidine Opioids; Antifungal Agents (Azole Derivatives, Systemic); AtorvaSTATin; Brimonidine (Topical); Calcium Channel Blockers (Dihydropyridine); Cimetidine; CloNIDine; Conivaptan; CycloSPORINE (Systemic); CYP3A4 Inhibitors (Moderate); CYP3A4 Inhibitors (Strong); Dantrolene; Dasatinib; Diazoxide; Dronedarone; Fluconazole; Fusidic Acid (Systemic); Grapefruit Juice; Herbs (Hypotensive Properties); Ivabradine; Ivacaftor; Luliconazole; Macrolide Antibiotics; Magnesium Salts; MAO Inhibitors; Mifepristone; Pentoxifylline; P-glycoprotein/ABCB1 Inhibitors; Phosphodiesterase 5 Inhibitors; Prostacyclin Analogues; Protease Inhibitors; QuiNIDine; Regorafenib; Simeprevir; Stiripentol; Telithromycin

Nutritional/Ethanol Interactions
Ethanol: Verapamil may increase ethanol levels. Management: Avoid or limit ethanol.

Food: Grapefruit juice may increase the serum concentration of verapamil. Management: Avoid grapefruit juice or use with caution and monitor for effects. Calan® SR and Isoptin® SR products should be taken with food or milk; other formulations may be administered without regard to meals.

Herb/Nutraceutical: St John's wort may decrease levels of verapamil. Some herbal medications have hypertensive properties (eg, licorice); others may increase or decrease the antihypertensive effect of verapamil. Management: Avoid St John's wort, bayberry, blue cohosh, cayenne, ephedra, ginger, ginseng (American), kola, licorice, and yohimbe. Avoid black cohosh, California poppy, coleus, golden seal, hawthorn, mistletoe, periwinkle, quinine, and shepherd's purse.

Adverse Reactions
>10%:
Central nervous system: Headache (1% to 12%)
Gastrointestinal: Gingival hyperplasia (≤19%), constipation (7% to 12%)
1% to 10%:
Cardiovascular: Peripheral edema (1% to 4%), hypotension (3%), CHF/pulmonary edema

(2%), AV block (1% to 2%), bradycardia (HR <50 bpm: 1%), flushing (1%)
Central nervous system: Fatigue (2% to 5%), dizziness (1% to 5%), lethargy (3%), pain (2%), sleep disturbance (1%)
Dermatologic: Rash (1% to 2%)
Gastrointestinal: Dyspepsia (3%), nausea (1% to 3%), diarrhea (2%)
Hepatic: Liver enzymes increased (1%)
Neuromuscular & skeletal: Myalgia (1%), paresthesia (1%)
Respiratory: Dyspnea (1%)
Miscellaneous: Flu-like syndrome (4%)

Pharmacodynamics/Kinetics
Onset of Action Oral (immediate release tablets): Peak effect: 1-2 hours; I.V.: Peak effect: 1-5 minutes
Duration of Action Oral: Immediate release tablets: 6-8 hours; I.V.: 10-20 minutes

Available Dosage Forms
Capsule Extended Release 24 Hour, Oral:
Verelan: 120 mg, 180 mg, 240 mg, 360 mg
Verelan PM: 100 mg, 200 mg, 300 mg
Generic: 100 mg, 120 mg, 180 mg, 200 mg, 240 mg, 300 mg, 360 mg
Solution, Intravenous:
Generic: 2.5 mg/mL (2 mL, 4 mL)
Tablet, Oral:
Calan: 80 mg, 120 mg
Generic: 40 mg, 80 mg, 120 mg
Tablet Extended Release, Oral:
Calan SR: 120 mg, 180 mg, 240 mg
Isoptin SR: 120 mg, 180 mg, 240 mg
Generic: 120 mg, 180 mg, 240 mg

General Dosage Range
I.V.:
Children 1-15 years: 0.1-0.3 mg/kg/dose (maximum: 5 mg/dose); may repeat dose (maximum for second dose: 10 mg)
Adults: Initial dose: 2.5-5 mg; Second dose: 5-10 mg (maximum: 20-30 mg total dose)
Oral:
Extended release:
Adults: 180-480 mg once daily
Elderly: Initial: 100-180 mg once daily
Immediate release: *Adults:* Initial: 80-120 mg 3 times/day; Maintenance: 80-480 mg/day in 2-4 divided doses (maximum: 480 mg/day)
Sustained release:
Adults: 120-480 mg/day in 1-2 divided doses (maximum: 480 mg/day)
Elderly: Initial: 120 mg/day once daily; Maintenance: 120-360 mg/day in 1-2 divided doses

Administration
I.V. Administer over 2 minutes (over 3 minutes in older patients [ACLS, 2010])
Injectable Detail pH: 4-6.5
Oral Do not crush or chew sustained or extended release products.
Calan® SR, Isoptin® SR: Administer with food.

Verelan®, Verelan® PM: Capsules may be opened and the contents sprinkled on 1 tablespoonful of applesauce, then swallowed immediately without chewing. Do not subdivide contents of capsules.

Storage/Stability Store at controlled room temperature of 15°C to 30°C (59°F to 86°F). Protect from light.

Nursing Actions

Physical Assessment I.V. requires use of infusion pump and continuous cardiac and hemodynamic monitoring. Monitor gums for gingival hyperplasia. Encourage good oral hygiene. Refer to dentist if indicated. Monitor cardiac status when beginning therapy, when titrating dosage, and periodically throughout.

Patient Education
- Discuss specific use of drug and side effects with patient as it relates to treatment. (HCAHPS: During this hospital stay, were you given any medicine that you had not taken before? Before giving you any new medicine, how often did hospital staff tell you what the medicine was for? How often did hospital staff describe possible side effects in a way you could understand?)
- Patient may experience dizziness, constipation, headache, or changes to gums. Have patient report immediately to prescriber angina, tachycardia, dyspnea, stomatitis, or rash (HCAHPS).
- Educate patient about signs of a significant reaction (eg, wheezing; chest tightness; fever; itching; bad cough; blue skin color; seizures; or swelling of face, lips, tongue, or throat). **Note:** This is not a comprehensive list of all side effects. Patient should consult prescriber for additional questions.

Intended Use and Disclaimer: Should not be printed and given to patients. This information is intended to serve as a concise initial reference for healthcare professionals to use when discussing medications with a patient. You must ultimately rely on your own discretion, experience and judgment in diagnosing, treating and advising patients.

Dietary Considerations Calan® SR and Isoptin® SR products may be taken with food or milk, other formulations may be administered without regard to meals; sprinkling contents of Verelan® or Verelan® PM capsule onto applesauce does not affect oral absorption.

Related Information
Oral Medications That Should Not Be Crushed or Altered *on page 1712*

Vilazodone (vil AZ oh done)

Brand Names: U.S. Viibryd
Index Terms EMD 68843; SB659746-A; Vilazodone Hydrochloride

Pharmacologic Category Antidepressant, Selective Serotonin Reuptake Inhibitor/5-HT$_{1A}$ Receptor Partial Agonist
Medication Guide Available Yes
Pregnancy Risk Factor C
Lactation Excretion in breast milk unknown/consider risk:benefit
Breast-Feeding Considerations It is not known if vilazodone is excreted in breast milk. According to the manufacturer, the decision to continue or discontinue breast-feeding during therapy should take into account the risk of exposure to the infant and the benefits of treatment to the mother. Maternal use of an SSRI during pregnancy may cause delayed milk secretion. Long-term effects on development and behavior have not been studied.
Use Treatment of major depressive disorder
Mechanism of Action/Effect Vilazodone inhibits CNS neuron serotonin uptake; minimal or no effect on reuptake of norepinephrine or dopamine. It also binds selectively with high affinity to 5-HT$_{1A}$ receptors and is a 5-HT$_{1A}$ receptor partial agonist. 5-HT$_{1A}$ receptor activity may be altered in depression and anxiety.
Contraindications Use of MAO inhibitors intended to treat psychiatric disorders (concurrently or within 14 days of discontinuing either vilazodone or the MAO inhibitor); initiation of vilazodone in a patient receiving linezolid or intravenous methylene blue
Warnings/Precautions [U.S. Boxed Warning]: Antidepressants increase the risk of suicidal thinking and behavior in children, adolescents, and young adults (18-24 years of age) with major depressive disorder (MDD) and other psychiatric disorders; consider risk prior to prescribing. Short-term studies did not show an increased risk in patients >24 years of age and showed a decreased risk in patients ≥65 years. Closely monitor patients for clinical worsening, suicidality, or unusual changes in behavior, particularly during the initial 1-2 months of therapy or during periods of dosage adjustments (increases or decreases); the patient's family or caregiver should be instructed to closely observe the patient and communicate condition with healthcare provider. A medication guide concerning the use of antidepressants should be dispensed with each prescription. **Vilazodone is not FDA approved for use in children.**

The possibility of a suicide attempt is inherent in major depression and may persist until remission occurs. Use caution in high-risk patients. Worsening depression and severe abrupt suicidality that are not part of the presenting symptoms may require discontinuation or modification of drug therapy. The patient's family or caregiver should be alerted to monitor patients for the emergence of suicidality and associated behaviors (such as agitation, irritability, hostility, impulsivity, and hypomania) and call healthcare provider.

May worsen psychosis in some patients or precipitate a shift to mania or hypomania in patients with bipolar disorder. Patients presenting with depressive symptoms should be screened for bipolar disorder. Monotherapy in patients with bipolar disorder should be avoided. **Vilazodone is not FDA approved for the treatment of bipolar depression.**

Potentially life-threatening serotonin syndrome (SS) has occurred with serotonergic agents (eg, SSRIs, SNRIs), particularly when used in combination with other serotonergic agents (eg, triptans, TCAs, fentanyl, lithium, tramadol, buspirone, St John's wort, tryptophan) or agents that impair metabolism of serotonin (eg, MAO inhibitors intended to treat psychiatric disorders, other MAO inhibitors [ie, linezolid and intravenous methylene blue]). Discontinue treatment (and any concomitant serotonergic agent) immediately if signs/symptoms arise. May increase the risks associated with electroconvulsive therapy. Bone fractures have been associated with antidepressant treatment. Consider the possibility of a fragility fracture if an antidepressant-treated patient presents with unexplained bone pain, point tenderness, swelling, or bruising (Rabenda, 2013; Rizzoli, 2012). Has a low potential to impair cognitive or motor performance; caution operating hazardous machinery or driving. Potentially significant interactions may exist, requiring dose or frequency adjustment, additional monitoring, and/or selection of alternative therapy. Consult drug interactions database for more detailed information.

Use with caution in patients with hepatic impairment, seizure disorder (or with agents that lower the seizure threshold), or in elderly patients. May cause hyponatremia/SIADH (elderly at increased risk); volume depletion and diuretics may increase risk. May cause or exacerbate sexual dysfunction.

Abrupt discontinuation or interruption of antidepressant therapy has been associated with a discontinuation syndrome. Symptoms arising may vary with antidepressant however commonly include nausea, vomiting, diarrhea, headaches, light-headedness, dizziness, diminished appetite, sweating, chills, tremors, paresthesias, fatigue, somnolence, and sleep disturbances (eg, vivid dreams, insomnia). Greater risks for developing a discontinuation syndrome have been associated with antidepressants with shorter half-lives, longer durations of treatment, and abrupt discontinuation. For antidepressants of short or intermediate half-lives, symptoms may emerge within 2-5 days after treatment discontinuation and last 7-14 days (APA, 2010; Fava, 2006; Haddad, 2001; Shelton, 2001; Warner, 2006).

Drug Interactions

Avoid Concomitant Use

Avoid concomitant use of Vilazodone with any of the following: Dosulepin; Iobenguane I 123; Linezolid; MAO Inhibitors; Methylene Blue; Pimozide; Tryptophan; Urokinase

Decreased Effect

Vilazodone may decrease the levels/effects of: Iobenguane I 123; Ioflupane I 123; Thyroid Products

The levels/effects of Vilazodone may be decreased by: Bosentan; CarBAMazepine; CYP3A4 Inducers (Strong); Cyproheptadine; Dabrafenib; Deferasirox; NSAID (COX-2 Inhibitor); NSAID (Nonselective); Peginterferon Alfa-2b; Tocilizumab

Increased Effect/Toxicity

Vilazodone may increase the levels/effects of: Agents with Antiplatelet Properties; Anticoagulants; Antidepressants (Serotonin Reuptake Inhibitor/Antagonist); Antipsychotics; Aspirin; Benzodiazepines (metabolized by oxidation); Beta-Blockers; BusPIRone; CarBAMazepine; CloZAPine; Collagenase (Systemic); Dabigatran Etexilate; Desmopressin; Dextromethorphan; Dosulepin; Galantamine; Hypoglycemic Agents; Ibritumomab; Methadone; Methylene Blue; Metoclopramide; Mexiletine; NSAID (COX-2 Inhibitor); NSAID (Nonselective); Pimozide; RisperiDONE; Rivaroxaban; Salicylates; Serotonin Modulators; Thiazide Diuretics; Thrombolytic Agents; Tositumomab and Iodine I 131 Tositumomab; TraMADol; Urokinase; Vitamin K Antagonists

The levels/effects of Vilazodone may be increased by: Alcohol (Ethyl); Analgesics (Opioid); Antipsychotics; BusPIRone; Cimetidine; CNS Depressants; Cobicistat; CYP3A4 Inhibitors (Moderate); CYP3A4 Inhibitors (Strong); Dasatinib; Glucosamine; Herbs (Anticoagulant/Antiplatelet Properties); Ibrutinib; Linezolid; Lithium; Macrolide Antibiotics; MAO Inhibitors; Metoclopramide; Metyrosine; Multivitamins/Fluoride (with ADE); Multivitamins/Minerals (with ADEK, Folate, Iron); Multivitamins/Minerals (with AE, No Iron); Omega-3 Fatty Acids; Pentosan Polysulfate Sodium; Pentoxifylline; Prostacyclin Analogues; Tipranavir; TraMADol; Tryptophan; Vitamin E

Nutritional/Ethanol Interactions

Ethanol: Ethanol may increase CNS depression. Management: Avoid or limit use and monitor for increased effects.

Food: Management: Take with food.

Herb/Nutraceutical: Avoid valerian, St John's wort, tryptophan, SAMe, kava kava, gotu kola (may increase CNS depression and/or increase the risk of serotonin syndrome).

Adverse Reactions

>10%:

Gastrointestinal: Diarrhea (28%), nausea (23%)

1% to 10%:

Cardiovascular: Palpitation (2%)

Central nervous system: Dizziness (9%), insomnia (6%), dreams abnormal (4%), fatigue (4%), ▶

◀ restlessness (3%), somnolence (3%), migraine (≥1%), sedation (≥1%)

Dermatologic: Hyperhidrosis (≥1%)

Endocrine & metabolic: Libido decreased (3% to 5%), orgasm abnormal (2% to 4%), sexual dysfunction (≤2%)

Gastrointestinal: Xerostomia (8%), vomiting (5%), dyspepsia (3%), flatulence (3%), gastroenteritis (3%), appetite increased (2%), appetite decreased (≥1%)

Genitourinary: Ejaculation delayed (2%), erectile dysfunction (2%)

Neuromuscular & skeletal: Arthralgia (3%), paresthesia (3%), jittery (2%), tremor (2%)

Ocular: Blurred vision (≥1%), dry eyes (≥1%)

Miscellaneous: Night sweats (≥1%)

Available Dosage Forms

Kit, Oral:

Viibryd: 10 & 20 & 40 mg

Tablet, Oral:

Viibryd: 10 mg, 20 mg, 40 mg

General Dosage Range Dosage adjustment recommended in patients on concomitant therapy

Oral: *Adults:* 10-40 mg once daily

Administration

Oral Administer with food.

Storage/Stability Store at 25°C (77°F); excursions permitted to 15°C to 30°C (50°F to 86°F).

Nursing Actions

Physical Assessment Assess mental status for worsening of depression, suicide ideation, anxiety, social functioning, mania, or panic attack (especially during initiation of therapy and when dosage is changed). Taper dosage slowly when discontinuing.

Patient Education

• Discuss specific use of drug and side effects with patient as it relates to treatment. (HCAHPS: During this hospital stay, were you given any medicine that you had not taken before? Before giving you any new medicine, how often did hospital staff tell you what the medicine was for? How often did hospital staff describe possible side effects in a way you could understand?)

• Patient may experience presyncope, fatigue, blurred vision, illogical thinking, dizziness, insomnia, nausea, diarrhea, xerostomia, or change in sex ability. Have patient report immediately to prescriber change in balance, fasciculations, agitation, muscle stiffness, nervousness or excitability, tachycardia, severe headache, ecchymosis, or rash (HCAHPS).

• Educate patient about signs of a significant reaction (eg, wheezing; chest tightness; fever; itching; bad cough; blue skin color; seizures; or swelling of face, lips, tongue, or throat). **Note:** This is not a comprehensive list of all side effects. Patient should consult prescriber for additional questions.

Intended Use and Disclaimer: Should not be printed and given to patients. This information is intended to serve as a concise initial reference for healthcare professionals to use when discussing medications with a patient. You must ultimately rely on your own discretion, experience and judgment in diagnosing, treating and advising patients.

Dietary Considerations Take with food.

VinBLAStine (vin BLAS teen)

Index Terms Velban; Vinblastine Sulfate; Vincaleukoblastine; VLB

Pharmacologic Category Antineoplastic Agent, Antimicrotubular; Antineoplastic Agent, Vinca Alkaloid

Medication Safety Issues

Sound-alike/look-alike issues:

VinBLAStine may be confused with vinCRIStine, vinorelbine

High alert medication:

The Institute for Safe Medication Practices (ISMP) includes this medication among its list of drug classes which have a heightened risk of causing significant patient harm when used in error.

Administration issues:

Must be dispensed in overwrap which bears the statement **"Do not remove covering until the moment of injection. Fatal if given intrathecally. For I.V. use only."** Syringes should be labeled: **"Fatal if given intrathecally. For I.V. use only."**

Pregnancy Risk Factor D

Lactation Excretion in breast milk unknown/not recommended

Breast-Feeding Considerations Due to the potential for serious adverse reactions in the nursing infant, breast-feeding is not recommended.

Use Treatment of Hodgkin's and non-Hodgkin's lymphoma; testicular cancer; breast cancer; mycosis fungoides; Kaposi's sarcoma; histiocytosis (Letterer-Siwe disease); choriocarcinoma

Unlabeled Use Treatment of bladder cancer, melanoma, nonsmall cell lung cancer (NSCLC), ovarian cancer, soft tissue sarcoma (desmoid tumors)

Mechanism of Action/Effect Vinblastine arrests cell cycle growth in metaphase. Also inhibits RNA synthesis and amino acid metabolism resulting in inhibition of metabolic pathways and cell growth.

Contraindications Significant granulocytopenia; presence of bacterial infection; I.T. administration is contraindicated (may result in death)

Warnings/Precautions Hazardous agent - use appropriate precautions for handling and disposal (NIOSH, 2012). **[U.S. Boxed Warning]: For I.V. use only. Intrathecal administration may result in death.** Must be dispensed in overwrap which bears the statement **"Do not remove covering until the moment of injection. Fatal if given**

intrathecally. For I.V. use only." [U.S. Boxed Warning]: Vinblastine is a vesicant; ensure proper needle or catheter placement prior to and during infusion. Avoid extravasation. Extravasation may cause significant irritation. Individuals administering should be experienced in vinblastine administration. If extravasation occurs, discontinue immediately and initiate appropriate extravasation management, including local injection of hyaluronidase and moderate heat application to the affected area. Use a separate vein to complete administration. Leukopenia is common; granulocytopenia may be severe with higher doses. Leukopenia may be more pronounced in cachectic patients and patients with skin ulceration. Thrombocytopenia and anemia may occur rarely.

Use with caution in patients with hepatic impairment; toxicity may be increased; may require dosage modification. Neurotoxicity is rare at clinical doses; may occur with high doses (symptoms are similar to vincristine toxicity, including peripheral neuropathy, loss of deep tendon reflexes, headache, weakness, urinary retention, and GI symptoms). May rarely cause disabling neurotoxicity (usually reversible). Itraconazole may decrease the metabolism of vinblastine via CYP3A4 inhibition and may increase the effects of vinblastine via P-glycoprotein effects; severe myelosuppression and neurotoxicity may occur. Acute shortness of breath and severe bronchospasm have been reported, most often in association with concurrent administration of mitomycin; may occur within minutes to several hours following vinblastine administration or up to 14 days following mitomycin administration; use caution in patients with pre-existing pulmonary disease. Use with caution in patients with ischemic heart disease. [U.S. Boxed Warning]: Should be administered under the supervision of an experienced cancer chemotherapy physician. Some dosage forms may contain benzyl alcohol which has been associated with "gasping syndrome" in neonates.

Drug Interactions

Avoid Concomitant Use
Avoid concomitant use of VinBLAStine with any of the following: BCG; CloZAPine; Conivaptan; Dabigatran Etexilate; Fusidic Acid (Systemic); Natalizumab; Pimecrolimus; Pimozide; Pomalidomide; Sofosbuvir; Tacrolimus (Topical); Tofacitinib; Vaccines (Live); VinCRIStine (Liposomal)

Decreased Effect
VinBLAStine may decrease the levels/effects of: Afatinib; BCG; Coccidioidin Skin Test; Dabigatran Etexilate; DOXOrubicin (Conventional); Linagliptin; P-glycoprotein/ABCB1 Substrates; Pomalidomide; Sipuleucel-T; Sofosbuvir; Vaccines (Inactivated); Vaccines (Live); VinCRIStine (Liposomal)

The levels/effects of VinBLAStine may be decreased by: Bosentan; CYP3A4 Inducers (Strong); Dabrafenib; Deferasirox; Echinacea; Herbs (CYP3A4 Inducers); Mitotane; Peginterferon Alfa-2b; P-glycoprotein/ABCB1 Inducers; Tocilizumab

Increased Effect/Toxicity
VinBLAStine may increase the levels/effects of: ARIPiprazole; CloZAPine; Dofetilide; Leflunomide; Lomitapide; MitoMYcin (Systemic); Natalizumab; Pimozide; Tofacitinib; Tolterodine; Vaccines (Live)

The levels/effects of VinBLAStine may be increased by: Conivaptan; CYP3A4 Inhibitors (Moderate); CYP3A4 Inhibitors (Strong); Dasatinib; Denosumab; Fusidic Acid (Systemic); Itraconazole; Ivacaftor; Lopinavir; Luliconazole; Macrolide Antibiotics; MAO Inhibitors; Mifepristone; P-glycoprotein/ABCB1 Inhibitors; Pimecrolimus; Posaconazole; Ritonavir; Roflumilast; Simeprevir; Stiripentol; Tacrolimus (Topical); Trastuzumab; Voriconazole

Nutritional/Ethanol Interactions Herb/Nutraceutical: Avoid St John's wort (may decrease vinblastine levels). Avoid black cohosh, dong quai in estrogen-dependent tumors.

Adverse Reactions Frequency not defined.

Common:
Cardiovascular: Hypertension
Central nervous system: Malaise
Dermatologic: Alopecia
Gastrointestinal: Constipation
Hematologic: Myelosuppression, leukopenia/granulocytopenia (nadir: 5-10 days; recovery: 7-14 days; dose-limiting toxicity)
Neuromuscular & skeletal: Bone pain, jaw pain, tumor pain

Less common:
Cardiovascular: Angina, cerebrovascular accident, coronary ischemia, ECG abnormalities, limb ischemia, MI, myocardial ischemia, Raynaud's phenomenon
Central nervous system: Depression, dizziness, headache, neurotoxicity (duration: >24 hours), seizure, vertigo
Dermatologic: Dermatitis, photosensitivity (rare), rash, skin blistering
Endocrine & metabolic: Aspermia, hyperuricemia, SIADH
Gastrointestinal: Abdominal pain, anorexia, diarrhea, gastrointestinal bleeding, hemorrhagic enterocolitis, ileus, metallic taste, nausea (mild), paralytic ileus, rectal bleeding, stomatitis, toxic megacolon, vomiting (mild)
Genitourinary: Urinary retention
Hematologic: Anemia, thrombocytopenia (recovery within a few days), thrombotic thrombocytopenic purpura
Local: Cellulitis (with extravasation), irritation, phlebitis (with extravasation), radiation recall

◀ Neuromuscular & skeletal: Deep tendon reflex loss, myalgia, paresthesia, peripheral neuritis, weakness

Ocular: Nystagmus

Otic: Auditory damage, deafness, vestibular damage

Renal: Hemolytic uremic syndrome

Respiratory: Bronchospasm, dyspnea, pharyngitis

Available Dosage Forms

Solution, Intravenous:
Generic: 1 mg/mL (10 mL)

Solution Reconstituted, Intravenous:
Generic: 10 mg (1 ea)

General Dosage Range Dosage adjustment recommended in patients with hepatic impairment

I.V.:

Children: Initial dose: 3-6.5 mg/m^2 every 7 days as needed

Adults: Initial: 3.7 mg/m^2; adjust dose every 7 days; Second dose: 5.5 mg/m^2; Third dose: 7.4 mg/m^2; Fourth dose: 9.25 mg/m^2; Fifth dose: 11.1 mg/m^2; Usual range: 5.5-7.4 mg/m^2 every 7 days; Maximum dose: 18.5 mg/m^2

Administration

I.V. For I.V. administration only. **Fatal if given intrathecally.** Administer usually as a slow (2-3 minutes) push, or a bolus (5-15 minutes) infusion; the manufacturer recommends an undiluted 1-minute infusion into a free flowing I.V. line to prevent venous irritation/extravasation. Prolonged administration times and/or increased administration volumes may increase the risk of vein irritation and extravasation.

Vesicant; ensure proper needle or catheter placement prior to and during infusion. Avoid extravasation.

Extravasation management: If extravasation occurs, stop infusion immediately and disconnect (leave cannula/needle in place); gently aspirate extravasated solution (do **NOT** flush the line); initiate hyaluronidase antidote; remove needle/cannula; apply dry warm compresses for 20 minutes 4 times a day for 1-2 days; elevate extremity (Perez Fidalgo, 2012). Remaining portion of the vinblastine dose should be infused through a separate vein.

Hyaluronidase: If needle/cannula still in place, administer 1-6 mL hyaluronidase (150 units/mL) into the existing I.V. line; the usual dose is 1 mL hyaluronidase for each 1 mL of extravasated drug (Perez Fidalgo, 2012; Schulmeister, 2011). If needle/cannula was removed, inject 1-6 mL (150 units/mL) subcutaneously in a clockwise manner using 1 mL for each 1 mL of drug extravasated (Schulmeister, 2011) **or** administer 1 mL (150 units/mL) as 5 separate 0.2 mL injections (using a 25-gauge needle) subcutaneously into the extravasation site (Polovich, 2009).

Hazardous agent; use appropriate precautions for handling and disposal (NIOSH, 2012).

Injectable Detail pH: 3.5-5

Preparation for Administration Hazardous agent; use appropriate precautions for handling and disposal (NIOSH, 2012). Reconstitute lyophilized powder to a concentration of 1 mg/mL with NS or bacteriostatic NS. For infusion, may dilute in 50 mL NS or D$_5$W; dilution in larger volumes (≥100 mL) of I.V. fluids is not recommended.

Storage/Stability Note: Must be dispensed in overwrap which bears the statement "Do not remove covering until the moment of injection. Fatal if given intrathecally. For I.V. use only." Syringes should be labeled: "Fatal if given intrathecally. For I.V. use only."

Store intact vials under refrigeration at 2°C to 8°C (36°F to 46°F). Protect from light. Solutions reconstituted in bacteriostatic NS are stable for 28 days under refrigeration.

Nursing Actions

Physical Assessment Premedication with antiemetic is advisable. Monitor infusion site closely to prevent extravasation (vesicant will cause tissue damage and necrosis). Assess renal function. Monitor for SIADH, bone marrow suppression, leukopenia, hypertension, gastrointestinal disturbance, myalgia, depression, and paresthesia throughout therapy.

Patient Education

• Discuss specific use of drug and side effects with patient as it relates to treatment. (HCAHPS: During this hospital stay, were you given any medicine that you had not taken before? Before giving you any new medicine, how often did hospital staff tell you what the medicine was for? How often did hospital staff describe possible side effects in a way you could understand?)

• Patient may experience leukopenia, hypertension, nausea, loss of appetite, constipation, stomatitis, alopecia, osteodynia, or infertility. Have patient report immediately to prescriber signs of infection, ecchymosis, angina, tachycardia, syncope, paresthesia, urinary retention, significant weight loss, severe dyspepsia, fatigue, shortness of breath, significant jaw pain, intolerable headache, or rash (HCAHPS).

• Educate patient about signs of a significant reaction (eg, wheezing; chest tightness; fever; itching; bad cough; blue skin color; seizures; or swelling of face, lips, tongue, or throat). **Note:** This is not a comprehensive list of all side effects. Patient should consult prescriber for additional questions.

Intended Use and Disclaimer: Should not be printed and given to patients. This information is intended to serve as a concise initial reference for healthcare professionals to use when discussing medications with a patient. You must ultimately rely on your own discretion, experience and

judgment in diagnosing, treating and advising patients.

Related Information

Management of Drug Extravasations *on page 1700*

VinCRIStine (vin KRIS teen)

Brand Names: U.S. Vincasar PFS

Index Terms Conventional Vincristine; Leurocristine Sulfate; Oncovin; Vincristine (Conventional); Vincristine Sulfate

Pharmacologic Category Antineoplastic Agent, Antimicrotubular; Antineoplastic Agent, Vinca Alkaloid

Medication Safety Issues

Sound-alike/look-alike issues:

VinCRIStine may be confused with vinBLAStine, vinorelbine

VinCRIStine conventional may be confused with vinCRIStine liposomal

Oncovin may be confused with Ancobon®

High alert medication:

This medication is in a class the Institute for Safe Medication Practices (ISMP) includes among its list of drug classes which have a heightened risk of causing significant patient harm when used in error.

BEERS Criteria medication:

This drug may be potentially inappropriate for use in geriatric patients (Quality of evidence - moderate; Strength of recommendation - strong).

Administration issues:

For I.V. use only. Fatal if administered by other routes. To prevent fatal inadvertent intrathecal injection, it is recommended that vincristine doses be dispensed in a small minibag. Vincristine should **NOT** be prepared during the preparation of any intrathecal medications. After preparation, keep vincristine in a location **away** from the separate storage location recommended for intrathecal medications. Vincristine should **NOT** be delivered to the patient at the same time with any medications intended for central nervous system administration.

Pregnancy Risk Factor D

Lactation Excretion in breast milk unknown/not recommended

Breast-Feeding Considerations Due to the potential for serious adverse reactions in the nursing infant, the decision to discontinue vincristine or to discontinue breast-feeding should take into account the benefits of treatment to the mother.

Use Treatment of acute lymphocytic leukemia (ALL), Hodgkin lymphoma, non-Hodgkin lymphomas, Wilms' tumor, neuroblastoma, rhabdomyosarcoma

Unlabeled Use Treatment of central nervous system tumors, chronic lymphocytic leukemia (CLL), Ewing's sarcoma, gestational trophoblastic tumors (high-risk), multiple myeloma, ovarian germ cell tumors, retinoblastoma, small cell lung cancer (SCLC); thymoma (advanced)

Mechanism of Action/Effect Binds to microtubular protein of the mitotic spindle causing metaphase arrest; cell-cycle phase specific in the M and S phases

Contraindications Patients with the demyelinating form of Charcot-Marie-Tooth syndrome

Warnings/Precautions Hazardous agent - use appropriate precautions for handling and disposal (NIOSH, 2012); avoid eye contamination.

[U.S. Boxed Warning]: For I.V. administration only; inadvertent intrathecal administration usually results in death. To prevent administration errors, the World Health Organization recommends dispensing vincristine diluted in a minibag (WHO, 2007), **if not dispensed in a minibag, affix an auxiliary label stating "For intravenous use only - fatal if given by other routes" and also place in an overwrap labeled "Do not remove covering until moment of injection."** Vincristine should **NOT** be prepared during the preparation of any intrathecal medications. After preparation, keep vincristine in a location **away** from the separate storage location recommended for intrathecal medications. Vincristine should **NOT** be delivered to the patient at the same time with any medications intended for central nervous system administration.

[U.S. Boxed Warning]: Vincristine is a vesicant; ensure proper needle or catheter placement prior to and during infusion. Avoid extravasation. Individuals administering should be experienced in vincristine administration. Extravasation may cause significant irritation. If extravasation occurs, discontinue immediately and initiate appropriate extravasation management, including local injection of hyaluronidase and moderate heat application to the affected area. Use a separate vein to complete administration.

Neurotoxicity, including alterations in mental status such as depression, confusion, or insomnia may occur; neurologic effects are dose-limiting (may require dosage reduction) and may be additive with those of other neurotoxic agents and spinal cord irradiation. Use with caution in patients with pre-existing neuromuscular disease and/or with concomitant neurotoxic agents. Constipation, paralytic ileus, intestinal necrosis and/or perforation may occur; constipation may present as upper colon impaction with an empty rectum (may require flat film of abdomen for diagnosis); generally responds to high enemas and laxatives. All patients should be on a prophylactic bowel management regimen.

Potentially significant drug-drug interactions may exist, requiring dose or frequency adjustment, additional monitoring, and/or selection of alternative therapy. Acute shortness of breath and severe bronchospasm have been reported with vinca alkaloids, usually when used in combination with mitomycin. Onset may be several minutes to hours after vincristine administration and up to 2 weeks after mitomycin. Progressive dyspnea may occur. Permanently discontinue vincristine if pulmonary dysfunction occurs.

Use with caution in patients with hepatic impairment; dosage modification required. May be associated with hepatic sinusoidal obstruction syndrome (SOS; formerly called veno-occlusive disease), increased risk in children <3 years of age; use with caution in hepatobiliary dysfunction. Monitor for signs or symptoms of hepatic SOS, including bilirubin >1.4 mg/dL, unexplained weight gain, ascites, hepatomegaly, or unexplained right upper quadrant pain (Arndt, 2004). Acute uric acid nephropathy has been reported with vincristine. Use with caution in the elderly; may cause or exacerbate syndrome of inappropriate antidiuretic hormone secretion or hyponatremia; monitor sodium closely with initiation or dosage adjustments in older adults (Beers Criteria).

Drug Interactions

Avoid Concomitant Use

Avoid concomitant use of VinCRIStine with any of the following: BCG; Conivaptan; Fusidic Acid (Systemic); Natalizumab; Pimecrolimus; Pimozide; Tacrolimus (Topical); Tofacitinib; Vaccines (Live)

Decreased Effect

VinCRIStine may decrease the levels/effects of: BCG; Cardiac Glycosides; Coccidioidin Skin Test; Fosphenytoin; Phenytoin; Sipuleucel-T; Vaccines (Inactivated); Vaccines (Live); Vitamin K Antagonists

The levels/effects of VinCRIStine may be decreased by: Bosentan; CYP3A4 Inducers (Strong); Dabrafenib; Deferasirox; Echinacea; Fosphenytoin; Herbs (CYP3A4 Inducers); Mitotane; P-glycoprotein/ABCB1 Inducers; Phenytoin; Tocilizumab

Increased Effect/Toxicity

VinCRIStine may increase the levels/effects of: ARIPiprazole; Dofetilide; Leflunomide; Lomitapide; MitoMYcin (Systemic); Natalizumab; Pimozide; Tofacitinib; Vaccines (Live); Vitamin K Antagonists

The levels/effects of VinCRIStine may be increased by: Conivaptan; CYP3A4 Inhibitors (Moderate); CYP3A4 Inhibitors (Strong); Dasatinib; Denosumab; Fusidic Acid (Systemic); Itraconazole; Ivacaftor; Lopinavir; Luliconazole; Macrolide Antibiotics; MAO Inhibitors; Mifepristone; NIFEdipine; P-glycoprotein/ABCB1 Inhibitors; Pimecrolimus; Posaconazole; Ritonavir; Roflumilast; Simeprevir; Stiripentol; Tacrolimus (Topical); Teniposide; Trastuzumab; Voriconazole

Nutritional/Ethanol Interactions Herb/Nutraceutical: St John's wort may decrease vincristine levels.

Adverse Reactions Frequency not defined.

Cardiovascular: Edema, hyper-/hypotension, MI, myocardial ischemia

Central nervous system: Ataxia, coma, cranial nerve dysfunction (auditory damage, extraocular muscle impairment, laryngeal muscle impairment, paralysis, paresis, vestibular damage, vocal cord paralysis), dizziness, fever, headache, neurotoxicity (dose-related), neuropathic pain (common), seizure, vertigo

Dermatologic toxicity: Alopecia (common), rash

Endocrine & metabolic: Hyperuricemia, parotid pain, SIADH (rare)

Gastrointestinal: Abdominal cramps, abdominal pain, anorexia, constipation (common), diarrhea, intestinal necrosis, intestinal perforation, nausea, oral ulcers, paralytic ileus, vomiting, weight loss

Genitourinary: Bladder atony, dysuria, polyuria, urinary retention

Hematologic: Anemia (mild), leukopenia (mild), thrombocytopenia (mild), thrombotic thrombocytopenic purpura

Hepatic: Hepatic sinusoidal obstruction syndrome (SOS; veno-occlusive liver disease)

Local: Phlebitis, tissue irritation/necrosis (if infiltrated)

Neuromuscular & skeletal: Back pain, bone pain, deep tendon reflex loss, difficulty walking, foot drop, gait changes, jaw pain, limb pain, motor difficulties, muscle wasting, myalgia, paralysis, paresthesia, peripheral neuropathy (common), sensorimotor dysfunction, sensory loss

Ocular: Cortical blindness (transient), nystagmus, optic atrophy with blindness

Otic: Deafness

Renal: Acute uric acid nephropathy, hemolytic uremic syndrome

Respiratory: Bronchospasm, dyspnea, pharyngeal pain

Miscellaneous: Allergic reactions (rare), anaphylaxis (rare), hypersensitivity (rare)

Available Dosage Forms

Solution, Intravenous:

Vincasar PFS: 1 mg/mL (1 mL, 2 mL)

Solution, Intravenous [preservative free]:

Generic: 1 mg/mL (1 mL, 2 mL)

General Dosage Range Dosage adjustment recommended in patients with hepatic impairment

I.V.:

Children ≤10 kg: 0.05 mg/kg once weekly (maximum: 2 mg/dose)

Children >10 kg: 1.5-2 mg/m²/dose (maximum: 2 mg/dose)

Adults: 1.4 mg/m²/dose (maximum: 2 mg/dose)

Administration

I.V. For I.V. administration only. FATAL IF GIVEN INTRATHECALLY.

Vincristine should **NOT** be delivered to the patient at the same time with any medications intended for central nervous system administration.

I.V.: Usually administered as short 5-10 minute infusion (preferred); may also be administered as a slow (1 minute) push or by a 24-hour continuous infusion (depending on the protocol).

Vesicant; ensure proper needle or catheter placement prior to and during infusion. Avoid extravasation.

Extravasation management: If extravasation occurs, stop infusion immediately and disconnect (leave cannula/needle in place); gently aspirate extravasated solution (do **NOT** flush the line); initiate hyaluronidase antidote; remove needle/cannula; apply dry warm compresses for 20 minutes 4 times a day for 1-2 days; elevate (Perez Fidalgo, 2012). Remaining portion of the vincristine dose should be infused through a separate vein.

Hyaluronidase: If needle/cannula still in place, administer 1-6 mL hyaluronidase (150 units/mL) into the existing I.V. line; the usual dose is 1 mL hyaluronidase for each 1 mL of extravasated drug (Perez Fidalgo, 2012; Schulmeister, 2011). If needle/cannula was removed, inject 1-6 mL (150 units/mL) subcutaneously in a clockwise manner using 1 mL for each 1 mL of drug extravasated (Schulmeister, 2011) **or** administer 1 mL (150 units/mL) as 5 separate 0.2 mL injections (using a 25-gauge needle) subcutaneously into the extravasation site (Polovich, 2009).

Hazardous agent; use appropriate precautions for handling and disposal (NIOSH, 2012).

Injectable Detail pH: 3.5-5.5 (solution in vial)

Preparation for Administration Hazardous agent; use appropriate precautions for handling and disposal (NIOSH, 2012).

Solutions for I.V. infusion may be mixed in NS or D_5W. **Note:** In order to prevent inadvertent intrathecal administration the World Health Organization (WHO) and the Institute for Safe Medical Practices (ISMP) recommend dispensing vincristine in a minibag (rather than a syringe). Vincristine should **NOT** be prepared during the preparation of any intrathecal medications. If dispensing vincristine in a syringe, affix an auxiliary label stating **"For intravenous use only - fatal if given by other routes"** to the syringe, and the syringe must also be packaged in the manufacturer-provided overwrap which bears the statement **"Do not remove covering until the moment of injection. For intravenous use only. Fatal if given intrathecally."**

Storage/Stability Store intact vials refrigerated at 2°C to 8°C (36°F to 46°F). Protect from light.

I.V. solution: Diluted in 25-50 mL NS or D_5W, stable for 7 days under refrigeration, or 2 days at room temperature. In ambulatory pumps, solution is stable for 7 days at room temperature. After preparation, keep vincristine in a location away from the separate storage location recommended for intrathecal medications.

Nursing Actions

Physical Assessment Premedication with antiemetic is advisable. May cause severe constipation, paralytic ileus, intestinal obstruction, necrosis, and/or perforation. Instruct patient on beginning prophylactic bowel regimen. Monitor infusion site closely to prevent extravasation. Drug is a vesicant and may cause tissue damage and necrosis. Monitor CBC with differential. Assess hepatic function, CNS status (motor difficulties, seizure, depression), and neuromuscular status (myalgia, peripheral neuropathy, jaw pain, cramping) throughout therapy.

Patient Education

- Discuss specific use of drug and side effects with patient as it relates to treatment. (HCAHPS: During this hospital stay, were you given any medicine that you had not taken before? Before giving you any new medicine, how often did hospital staff tell you what the medicine was for? How often did hospital staff describe possible side effects in a way you could understand?)
- Patient may experience constipation, fatigue, paresthesia, pain, alopecia, or infertility. Have patient report immediately to prescriber signs of infection, illogical thinking, severe dyspepsia, significant change in balance, or considerable weight gain (HCAHPS).
- Educate patient about signs of a significant reaction (eg, wheezing; chest tightness; fever; itching; bad cough; blue skin color; seizures; or swelling of face, lips, tongue, or throat). **Note:** This is not a comprehensive list of all side effects. Patient should consult prescriber for additional questions.

Intended Use and Disclaimer: Should not be printed and given to patients. This information is intended to serve as a concise initial reference for healthcare professionals to use when discussing medications with a patient. You must ultimately rely on your own discretion, experience and judgment in diagnosing, treating and advising patients.

Related Information

Management of Drug Extravasations *on page 1700*

VinCRIStine (Liposomal)

(vin KRIS teen lye po SO mal)

Brand Names: U.S. Marqibo

Index Terms Liposomal Vincristine; Liposome Vincristine; Vincristine Liposome; Vincristine Sulfate Liposome; VSLI

Pharmacologic Category Antineoplastic Agent, Antimicrotubular; Antineoplastic Agent, Vinca Alkaloid

Medication Safety Issues

Sound-alike/look-alike issues:

VinCRIStine liposomal may be confused with vinCRIStine conventional

High alert medication:

This medication is in a class the Institute for Safe Medication Practices (ISMP) includes among its list of drug classes which have a heightened risk of causing significant patient harm when used in error.

BEERS Criteria medication:

Conventional vincristine may be potentially inappropriate for use in geriatric patients (Quality of evidence - moderate; Strength of recommendation - strong).

Administration issues:

Vincristine liposomal and conventional vincristine are **NOT** interchangeable. Dosing differs between formulations; verify intended product and dose prior to preparation and administration.

For I.V. administration only. Intrathecal administration is contraindicated; inadvertent intrathecal administration has resulted in death. Liposomal vincristine should **NOT** be prepared during the preparation of any intrathecal medications. After preparation, keep liposomal vincristine in a location **away** from the separate storage location recommended for intrathecal medications. Liposomal vincristine should **NOT** be delivered to the patient at the same time with any medications intended for central nervous system administration.

Pregnancy Risk Factor D

Lactation Excretion in breast milk unknown/not recommended

Use Treatment of relapsed Philadelphia chromosome-negative (Ph-) acute lymphoblastic leukemia (ALL) in adult patients whose disease has progressed after two or more antileukemic therapies

Available Dosage Forms

Suspension, Intravenous:

Marqibo: 5 mg/31 mL (1 ea)

General Dosage Range Dosage adjustment recommended in patients with hepatic impairment or who develop toxicities.

I.V.: *Adults:* 2.25 mg/m² once every 7 days

Administration

I.V. Conventional vincristine is a vesicant. Limited information is available regarding liposomal vincristine extravasation, but may cause inflammation if extravasated; avoid extravasation. **For I.V. administration only. FATAL IF GIVEN INTRATHECALLY.** Liposomal vincristine should **NOT** be delivered to the patient at the same time as any

medications intended for central nervous system administration.

I.V.: Infuse over 1 hour. Do not administer I.V. push or bolus; do not use with in-line filters. Infusion must be completed within 12 hours of preparation.

Hazardous agent; use appropriate precautions for handling and disposal (NIOSH, 2012).

Nursing Actions

Physical Assessment Administer by I.V. route only. Check results of blood counts; hepatic and renal function tests; signs and symptoms of tumor lysis syndrome. High risk for neuropathy; monitor for jaw pain, numbness or tingling, difficulty in walking, and constipation. Encourage use of stool softener or laxative when beginning use of this medication. Monitor for pain or redness at I.V. site.

Patient Education

- Discuss specific use of drug and side effects with patient as it relates to treatment. (HCAHPS: During this hospital stay, were you given any medicine that you had not taken before? Before giving you any new medicine, how often did hospital staff tell you what the medicine was for? How often did hospital staff describe possible side effects in a way you could understand?)
- Patient may experience anemia, leukopenia, thrombocytopenia, constipation, fatigue, paresthesia, dyspepsia, emesis, diarrhea, or hair loss. Have patient report immediately to prescriber illogical thinking, significant imbalance, considerable weight gain, or rash (HCAHPS).
- Educate patient about signs of a significant reaction (eg, wheezing; chest tightness; fever; itching; bad cough; blue skin color; seizures; or swelling of face, lips, tongue, or throat). **Note:** This is not a comprehensive list of all side effects. Patient should consult prescriber for additional questions.

Intended Use and Disclaimer: Should not be printed and given to patients. This information is intended to serve as a concise initial reference for healthcare professionals to use when discussing medications with a patient. You must ultimately rely on your own discretion, experience and judgment in diagnosing, treating and advising patients.

Vinorelbine (vi NOR el been)

Brand Names: U.S. Navelbine

Index Terms Dihydroxydeoxynorvinkaleukoblastine; Vinorelbine Tartrate

Pharmacologic Category Antineoplastic Agent, Antimicrotubular; Antineoplastic Agent, Vinca Alkaloid

Medication Safety Issues

Sound-alike/look-alike issues:
Vinorelbine may be confused with vinBLAStine, vinCRIStine

High alert medication:
This medication is in a class the Institute for Safe Medication Practices (ISMP) includes among its list of drug classes which have a heightened risk of causing significant patient harm when used in error.

Administration issues:
Vinorelbine is intended **for I.V. use only**: Inadvertent intrathecal administration of other vinca alkaloids has resulted in death. Syringes containing vinorelbine should be labeled **"For I.V. use only. Fatal if given intrathecally."** Vinorelbine should **NOT** be prepared during the preparation of any intrathecal medications. After preparation, keep vinorelbine in a location **away** from the separate storage location recommended for intrathecal medications.

Pregnancy Risk Factor D

Lactation Excretion in breast milk unknown/not recommended

Breast-Feeding Considerations It is not known if vinorelbine is excreted in breast milk. Due to the potential for serious adverse reactions in the nursing infant, breast-feeding should be discontinued during treatment.

Use Treatment of nonsmall cell lung cancer (NSCLC)

Unlabeled Use Treatment of breast cancer (metastatic), cervical cancer (persistent or recurrent), Hodgkin lymphoma (relapsed or refractory), malignant pleural mesothelioma, ovarian cancer (relapsed), salivary gland cancer, small cell lung cancer, and soft tissue sarcoma (advanced)

Mechanism of Action/Effect Mitotic inhibition that causes metaphase arrest in neoplastic cells

Contraindications Pretreatment granulocyte counts <1000/mm^3

Warnings/Precautions Hazardous agent - use appropriate precautions for handling and disposal (NIOSH, 2012). **[U.S. Boxed Warning]: For I.V. use only; intrathecal administration of other vinca alkaloids has resulted in death. If dispensed in a syringe, should be labeled "for intravenous use only - fatal if given intrathecally". [U.S. Boxed Warning]: Vesicant; ensure proper needle or catheter placement prior to and during infusion. Avoid extravasation.** Extravasation may cause local tissue necrosis and/or thrombophlebitis. **[U.S. Boxed Warning]: Severe granulocytopenia may occur with treatment (may lead to infection); granulocyte counts should be ≥1000 cells/mm^3 prior to treatment initiation; dosage adjustment may be required based on blood counts (monitor blood counts prior to each dose).** Granulocytopenia is a dose-limiting toxicity; nadir is generally 7-10 days after administration and recovery occurs within the following 7-14 days. Monitor closely for infections and/or fever in patients with severe granulocytopenia. Use with extreme caution in patients with compromised marrow reserve due to prior chemotherapy or radiation therapy.

Fatal cases of interstitial pulmonary changes and ARDS have been reported (with single-agent therapy (mean onset of symptoms: 1 week); promptly evaluate changes in baseline pulmonary symptoms or any new onset pulmonary symptoms (eg, dyspnea, cough, hypoxia). Acute shortness of breath and severe bronchospasm have been reported with vinca alkaloids; usually associated with the concurrent administration of mitomycin.

Vinorelbine should **NOT** be prepared during the preparation of any intrathecal medications. After preparation, keep vinorelbine in a location **away** from the separate storage location recommended for intrathecal medications. Elimination is predominantly hepatic; while there is no evidence that toxicity is enhanced in patients with elevated transaminases, use with caution in patients with severe hepatic injury or impairment; dosage modification required for elevated total bilirubin. May cause new onset or worsening of pre-existing neuropathy; use with caution in patients with neuropathy; monitor for new or worsening sign/symptoms of neuropathy; dosage adjustment required. May cause severe constipation (grade 3-4), paralytic ileus, intestinal obstruction, necrosis, and/or perforation; some events were fatal. Potentially significant drug-drug interactions may exist, requiring dose or frequency adjustment, additional monitoring, and/or selection of alternative therapy. May have radiosensitizing effects with prior or concurrent radiation therapy; radiation recall reactions may occur in patients who have received prior radiation therapy. Avoid eye contamination (exposure may cause severe irritation). **[U.S. Boxed Warning]: Should be administered under the supervision of an experienced cancer chemotherapy physician.**

Drug Interactions

Avoid Concomitant Use

Avoid concomitant use of Vinorelbine with any of the following: BCG; CloZAPine; Conivaptan; Fusidic Acid (Systemic); Natalizumab; Pimecrolimus; Pimozide; Tacrolimus (Topical); Tofacitinib; Vaccines (Live)

Decreased Effect

Vinorelbine may decrease the levels/effects of: BCG; Coccidioidin Skin Test; Sipuleucel-T; Vaccines (Inactivated); Vaccines (Live)

The levels/effects of Vinorelbine may be decreased by: Bosentan; CYP3A4 Inducers (Strong); Dabrafenib; Deferasirox; Echinacea; Herbs (CYP3A4 Inducers); Mitotane; Peginterferon Alfa-2b; Tocilizumab

◄ **Increased Effect/Toxicity**

Vinorelbine may increase the levels/effects of: ARIPiprazole; CloZAPine; Dofetilide; Lefluno-mide; Lomitapide; MitoMYcin (Systemic); Natali-zumab; Pimozide; Tofacitinib; Vaccines (Live)

The levels/effects of Vinorelbine may be increased by: CISplatin; Conivaptan; CYP3A4 Inhibitors (Moderate); CYP3A4 Inhibitors (Strong); Dasatinib; Denosumab; Fusidic Acid (Systemic); Gefitinib; Itraconazole; Ivacaftor; Luli-conazole; Macrolide Antibiotics; Mifepristone; PACLitaxel; PACLitaxel (Protein Bound); Pime-crolimus; Posaconazole; Roflumilast; Simeprevir; Stiripentol; Tacrolimus (Topical); Trastuzumab; Voriconazole

Nutritional/Ethanol Interactions Herb/Nutra-ceutical: Avoid St John's wort (may decrease vinor-elbine levels).

Adverse Reactions Note: Reported with single-agent therapy.

>10%:

Central nervous system: Fatigue (27%)

Dermatologic: Alopecia (12% to 30%)

Gastrointestinal: Nausea (31% to 44%; grade 3: 1% to 2%), constipation (35%; grade 3: 3%), vomiting (20% to 31%; grade 3: 1% to 2%), diarrhea (12% to 17%)

Hematologic: Leukopenia (83% to 92%; grade 4: 6% to 15%), granulocytopenia (90%; grade 4: 36%; nadir: 7-10 days; recovery 14-21 days), neutropenia (85%; grade 4: 28%), anemia (83%; grades 3/4: 9%)

Hepatic: AST increased (67%; grade 3: 5%; grade 4: 1%), total bilirubin increased (5% to 13%; grade 3: 4%; grade 4: 3%)

Local: Injection site reaction (22% to 28%; includes erythema, vein discoloration), injection site pain (16%)

Neuromuscular & skeletal: Weakness (36%), peripheral neuropathy (25%; grade 3: 1%; grade 4: <1%)

Renal: Creatinine increased (13%)

1% to 10%:

Cardiovascular: Chest pain (5%)

Dermatologic: Rash (<5%)

Gastrointestinal: Paralytic ileus (1%)

Hematologic: Neutropenic fever/sepsis (8%; grade 4: 4%), thrombocytopenia (3% to 5%; grades 3/4: 1%)

Local: Phlebitis (7% to 10%)

Neuromuscular & skeletal: Loss of deep tendon reflexes (<5%), myalgia (<5%), arthralgia (<5%), jaw pain (<5%)

Otic: Ototoxicity (≤1%)

Respiratory: Dyspnea (7%)

Available Dosage Forms

Solution, Intravenous:

Navelbine: 10 mg/mL (1 mL); 50 mg/5 mL (5 mL)

Generic: 10 mg/mL (1 mL); 50 mg/5 mL (5 mL)

Solution, Intravenous [preservative free]:

Generic: 10 mg/mL (1 mL); 50 mg/5 mL (5 mL)

General Dosage Range Dosage adjustment rec-ommended in patients with hepatic or renal impair-ment or who develop toxicities

I.V.: *Adults:* 25-30 mg/m^2 every 7 days

Administration

I.V. For I.V. use only; FATAL IF GIVEN INTRA-THECALLY. Administer as a direct intravenous push or rapid bolus, over 6-10 minutes (up to 30 minutes). Longer infusions may increase the risk of pain and phlebitis. Intravenous doses should be followed by at least 75-125 mL of saline or D$_5$W to reduce the incidence of phlebitis and inflammation.

Vesicant; ensure proper needle or catheter posi-tion prior to administration. Avoid extravasation.

Extravasation management: If extravasation occurs, stop infusion immediately and disconnect (leave cannula/needle in place); gently aspirate extravasated solution (do **NOT** flush the line); initiate hyaluronidase antidote; remove needle/cannula; apply dry warm compresses for 20 minutes 4 times a day for 1-2 days; elevate extremity (Perez Fidalgo, 2012). Remaining por-tion of the vinorelbine dose should be infused through a separate vein.

Hyaluronidase: If needle/cannula still in place, administer 1-6 mL hyaluronidase (150 units/mL) into the existing I.V. line; the usual dose is 1 mL hyaluronidase for each 1 mL of extrava-sated drug (Perez Fidalgo, 2012; Schulmeister, 2011). If needle/cannula was removed, inject 1-6 mL (150 units/mL) subcutaneously in a clockwise manner using 1mL for each 1 mL of drug extravasated (Schulmeister, 2011) **or** administer 1 mL (150 units/mL) as 5 separate 0.2 mL injections (using a 25-gauge needle) subcutaneously into the extravasation site (Polovich, 2009).

Hazardous agent; use appropriate precautions for handling and disposal (NIOSH, 2012).

Injectable Detail pH: 3.5 (solution in vial)

Preparation for Administration Hazardous agent; use appropriate precautions for handling and disposal (NIOSH, 2012). Dilute in D$_5$W or NS to a final concentration of 1.5-3 mg/mL (for syringe) or D$_5$W, NS, 1/2NS, D$_5$1/2NS, LR, or Ringer's to a final concentration of 0.5-2 mg/mL (for I.V. bag). Vinorelbine should **NOT** be prepared during the preparation of any intrathecal medications.

Storage/Stability Store intact vials refrigerated at 2°C to 8°C (36°F to 46°F); do not freeze. Protect from light. Intact vials are stable at room temper-ature of 25°C (77°F) for up to 72 hours. Solutions diluted for infusion in polypropylene syringes or polyvinyl chloride bags are stable for 24 hours at 5°C to 30°C (41°F to 86°F). After preparation, keep vinorelbine in a location **away** from the separate storage location recommended for intrathecal medications.

Nursing Actions

Physical Assessment For intravenous use only; fatal if given intrathecally. Premedication with antiemetic is advisable. May cause severe constipation, paralytic ileus, intestinal obstruction, necrosis, and/or perforation. Monitor infusion site closely to prevent extravasation; may cause tissue damage and necrosis. Monitor for peripheral neuropathy. Assess pulmonary status and liver function prior to each infusion and throughout therapy.

Patient Education

• Discuss specific use of drug and side effects with patient as it relates to treatment. (HCAHPS: During this hospital stay, were you given any medicine that you had not taken before? Before giving you any new medicine, how often did hospital staff tell you what the medicine was for? How often did hospital staff describe possible side effects in a way you could understand?)

• Patient may experience anemia, leukopenia, fatigue, nausea, stomatitis, constipation, diarrhea, alopecia, or application site irritation. Have patient report immediately to prescriber signs of infection, angina, dyspnea, paresthesia, severe dyspepsia, ecchymosis, or rash (HCAHPS).

• Educate patient about signs of a significant reaction (eg, wheezing; chest tightness; fever; itching; bad cough; blue skin color; seizures; or swelling of face, lips, tongue, or throat). **Note:** This is not a comprehensive list of all side effects. Patient should consult prescriber for additional questions.

Intended Use and Disclaimer: Should not be printed and given to patients. This information is intended to serve as a concise initial reference for healthcare professionals to use when discussing medications with a patient. You must ultimately rely on your own discretion, experience and judgment in diagnosing, treating and advising patients.

Related Information

Management of Drug Extravasations *on page 1700*

Vismodegib (vis moe DEG ib)

Brand Names: U.S. Erivedge

Index Terms GDC-0449; Hedgehog Antagonist GDC-0449

Pharmacologic Category Antineoplastic Agent, Hedgehog Pathway Inhibitor

Medication Safety Issues

Sound-alike/look-alike issues:
Vismodegib may be confused with vandetanib, vemurafenib

High alert medication:
This medication is in a class the Institute for Safe Medication Practices (ISMP) includes among its list of drug classes which have a heightened risk of causing significant patient harm when used in error.

Medication Guide Available Yes

Pregnancy Risk Factor D

Lactation Excretion in breast milk unknown/not recommended

Use Basal cell carcinoma: Treatment of metastatic basal cell carcinoma, or locally-advanced basal cell carcinoma that has recurred following surgery or in patients who are not candidates for surgery, and not candidates for radiation therapy

Available Dosage Forms

Capsule, Oral:
Erivedge: 150 mg

General Dosage Range Oral: *Adults:* 150 mg once daily

Administration

Oral May be taken with or without food. Swallow capsules whole; do not open or crush. Vismodegib is associated with a moderate emetic potential; antiemetics may be needed to prevent nausea and vomiting. Hazardous agent; use appropriate precautions for handling and disposal (meets NIOSH, 2012 criteria).

Nursing Actions

Physical Assessment Educate patients of reproductive years (men and woman) about risk of pregnancy during treatment and for some time after. Patients of reproductive years may benefit from discussion about proper birth control methods. Instruct patient on inability to donate blood during treatment and for some time after therapy is completed.

Patient Education

• Discuss specific use of drug and side effects with patient as it relates to treatment. (HCAHPS: During this hospital stay, were you given any medicine that you had not taken before? Before giving you any new medicine, how often did hospital staff tell you what the medicine was for? How often did hospital staff describe possible side effects in a way you could understand?)

• Patient may experience nausea, alopecia, constipation, loss of appetite, fatigue, weight loss, diarrhea, myalgia, or arthralgia. Have patient report immediately to prescriber signs of infection, pregnancy, or rash (HCAHPS).

• Educate patient about signs of a significant reaction (eg, wheezing; chest tightness; fever; itching; bad cough; blue skin color; seizures; or swelling of face, lips, tongue, or throat). **Note:** This is not a comprehensive list of all side

effects. Patient should consult prescriber for additional questions.

Intended Use and Disclaimer: Should not be printed and given to patients. This information is intended to serve as a concise initial reference for healthcare professionals to use when discussing medications with a patient. You must ultimately rely on your own discretion, experience and judgment in diagnosing, treating and advising patients.

Related Information

Oral Medications That Should Not Be Crushed or Altered *on page 1712*

Voriconazole (vor i KOE na zole)

Brand Names: U.S. Vfend; Vfend IV
Index Terms UK109496
Pharmacologic Category Antifungal Agent, Oral; Antifungal Agent, Parenteral
Medication Safety Issues
Sound-alike/look-alike issues:
Voriconazole may be confused with fluconazole, itraconazole
Pregnancy Risk Factor D
Lactation Excretion in breast milk unknown/not recommended
Breast-Feeding Considerations It is not known if voriconazole is excreted in breast milk. Due to the potential for serious adverse reactions in the nursing infant, the manufacturer recommends a decision be made whether to discontinue nursing or to discontinue the drug, taking into account the importance of treatment to the mother.
Use Treatment of invasive aspergillosis; treatment of esophageal candidiasis; treatment of candidemia (in non-neutropenic patients); treatment of disseminated *Candida* infections of the skin and viscera; treatment of serious fungal infections caused by *Scedosporium apiospermum* and *Fusarium* spp (including *Fusarium solani*) in patients intolerant of, or refractory to, other therapy
Unlabeled Use Fungal infection prophylaxis in intermediate or high risk neutropenic cancer patients with myelodysplastic syndrome (MDS) or acute myelogenous leukemia (AML), neutropenic allogeneic hematopoietic stem cell recipients, and patients with significant graft-versus-host disease; empiric antifungal therapy (second-line) for persistent neutropenic fever; empiric treatment of fungal meningitis or osteoarticular infections; catheter-related bloodstream infections due to *Malassezia furfur*
Mechanism of Action/Effect Interferes with fungal cytochrome P450 activity (selectively inhibits 14-alpha-lanosterol demethylation), decreasing ergosterol synthesis (principal sterol in fungal cell membrane) and inhibiting fungal cell membrane formation.

Contraindications Hypersensitivity to voriconazole or any component of the formulation (cross-reaction with other azole antifungal agents may occur but has not been established, use caution); coadministration of CYP3A4 substrates which may lead to QT_c prolongation and torsade de pointes (rare); coadministration with barbiturates (long acting), carbamazepine, ergot derivatives (ergotamine and dihydroergotamine), rifampin, rifabutin, ritonavir (≥800 mg/day), sirolimus, St John's wort

Warnings/Precautions Visual changes, including blurred vision, changes in visual acuity, color perception, and photophobia, are commonly associated with treatment; postmarketing cases of optic neuritis and papilledema (lasting >1 month) have also been reported. Patients should be warned to avoid tasks which depend on vision, including operating machinery or driving. Changes are reversible on discontinuation following brief exposure/ treatment regimens (≤28 days).

Serious (and rarely fatal) hepatic reactions (eg, hepatitis, cholestasis, fulminant failure) have been observed with voriconazole. In lung transplant recipients, median time to hepatic toxicity was 14 days with the majority occurring within 30 days of therapy initiation (Luong, 2012). Use with caution in patients with serious underlying medical conditions (eg, hematologic malignancy); hepatic reactions have occurred in patients with no identifiable underlying risk factors. Liver dysfunction is usually reversible upon therapy discontinuation. Monitor liver function and bilirubin at baseline and periodically during therapy. If elevations occur, evaluate further for severe hepatic injury; discontinuation may be warranted.

Voriconazole tablets contain lactose; avoid administration in hereditary galactose intolerance, Lapp lactase deficiency, or glucose-galactose malabsorption. Suspension contains sucrose; use caution with fructose intolerance, sucrase-isomaltase deficiency, or glucose-galactose malabsorption. Avoid/limit use of intravenous formulation in patients with moderate to severe renal impairment (CrCl <50 mL/minute); injection contains excipient cyclodextrin (sulfobutyl ether beta-cyclodextrin [SBECD]), which may accumulate; consider using oral voriconazole in these patients unless benefit of injection outweighs the risk. If injection is used in patients CrCl <50 mL/minute, monitor serum creatinine closely; if increases occur, consider changing therapy to oral voriconazole.

Anaphylactoid-type reactions (eg, flushing, fever, sweating, tachycardia, chest tightness, dyspnea, nausea, pruritus, rash) may occur with I.V. infusion. Consider discontinuation of infusion if reaction is severe. Acute renal failure has been observed in severely ill patients; use with caution in patients receiving concomitant nephrotoxic medications. Evaluate renal function (particularly serum creatinine) at baseline and periodically during therapy.

Potentially significant drug-drug interactions may exist, requiring dose or frequency adjustment, additional monitoring, and/or selection of alternative therapy. Use caution in patients taking strong cytochrome P450 inducers, CYP2C9 inhibitors, and major 3A4 substrates. QT interval prolongation has been associated with voriconazole use; rare cases of arrhythmia (including torsade de pointes), cardiac arrest, and sudden death have been reported, usually in seriously ill patients with comorbidities and/or risk factors (eg, prior cardiotoxic chemotherapy, cardiomyopathy, electrolyte imbalance, or concomitant QT_c-prolonging drugs). Use with caution in these patient populations; correct electrolyte abnormalities (eg, hypokalemia, hypomagnesemia, hypocalcemia) prior to initiating therapy. Do not infuse concomitantly with blood products or short-term concentrated electrolyte solutions, even if the two infusions are running in separate intravenous lines (or cannulas).

Rare cases of malignancy (melanoma, squamous cell carcinoma [SCC]) have been reported in patients with prior onset of severe photosensitivity reactions or exposure to standard dose long-term voriconazole therapy (in lung transplant recipients, SCC increased by ~6% per 60 days with a 28% absolute risk increase at 5 years [Singer, 2012]). Other serious exfoliative cutaneous reactions, including Stevens-Johnson syndrome, have also been reported. Patient should avoid strong, direct exposure to sunlight; may cause photosensitivity, especially with long-term use. Discontinue use in patients who develop an exfoliative cutaneous reaction or a skin lesion consistent with squamous cell carcinoma or melanoma. Periodic total body skin examinations should be performed, particularly with prolonged use. Fluorosis and/or periostitis may occur during long-term therapy. If patient develops skeletal pain and radiologic findings of fluorosis or periostitis, discontinue therapy.

Voriconazole demonstrates nonlinear pharmacokinetics. Dose modifications may result in unpredictable changes in serum concentrations and contribute to toxicity. It is important to note that cutoff trough threshold values ranged widely among studies; however, an upper limit of <5.0 mg/L would be reasonable for most disease states (CDC, 2012). In patients >14 years of age or 12-14 years and weighing >50 kg, data suggest that pharmacokinetics are similar to adults (Friberg, 2012). In patients <12 years of age, the full pharmacokinetic profile for voriconazole is not completely defined, and for patients <2 years, the data are sparse. In children 2 to <12 years, current data suggests voriconazole undergoes a high degree of variability in exposure with linear elimination at lower doses and nonlinear elimination at higher doses; therefore, to achieve similar AUC as adults, increased dosage is necessary in children (Friberg, 2012; Karlsson, 2009; Walsh, 2010).

Correct electrolyte abnormalities (eg, hypokalemia, hypomagnesemia, hypocalcemia) prior to initiating therapy. Monitor pancreatic function in patients (children and adults) at risk for acute pancreatitis (eg, recent chemotherapy or hematopoietic stem cell transplantation).

Drug Interactions

Avoid Concomitant Use

Avoid concomitant use of Voriconazole with any of the following: Ado-Trastuzumab Emtansine; Alfuzosin; Apixaban; Astemizole; Atazanavir; Avanafil; Axitinib; Barbiturates; Bosutinib; Cabozantinib; CarBAMazepine; Cisapride; Conivaptan; Crizotinib; Darunavir; Dihydroergotamine; Dofetilide; Dronedarone; Eletriptan; Eplerenone; Ergoloid Mesylates; Ergonovine; Ergotamine; Everolimus; Fluconazole; Halofantrine; Highest Risk QTc-Prolonging Agents; Ibrutinib; Imatinib; Ivabradine; Lapatinib; Lomitapide; Lopinavir; Lovastatin; Lurasidone; Macitentan; Methylergonovine; Mifepristone; Nilotinib; Nisoldipine; Pimozide; Pomalidomide; QuiNIDine; Ranolazine; Red Yeast Rice; Regorafenib; Rifamycin Derivatives; Ritonavir; Rivaroxaban; Salmeterol; Silodosin; Simeprevir; Simvastatin; Sirolimus; St Johns Wort; Tamsulosin; Terfenadine; Ticagrelor; Tolvaptan; Toremifene; Ulipristal; Vemurafenib; VinCRIStine (Liposomal)

Decreased Effect

Voriconazole may decrease the levels/effects of: Amphotericin B; Atazanavir; Clopidogrel; Ifosfamide; Prasugrel; Saccharomyces boulardii; Ticagrelor

The levels/effects of Voriconazole may be decreased by: Atazanavir; Barbiturates; CarBAMazepine; CYP2C19 Inducers (Strong); CYP2C9 Inducers (Strong); Dabrafenib; Darunavir; Didanosine; Etravirine; Fosphenytoin; Lopinavir; Peginterferon Alfa-2b; Phenytoin; Reverse Transcriptase Inhibitors (Non-Nucleoside); Rifamycin Derivatives; Ritonavir; St Johns Wort; Sucralfate; Telaprevir

Increased Effect/Toxicity

Voriconazole may increase the levels/effects of: Ado-Trastuzumab Emtansine; Alfentanil; Alfuzosin; Almotriptan; Alosetron; Antineoplastic Agents (Vinca Alkaloids); Apixaban; ARIPiprazole; Astemizole; AtorvaSTATin; Avanafil; Axitinib; Bedaquiline; Benzodiazepines (metabolized by oxidation); Boceprevir; Bortezomib; Bosentan; Bosutinib; Brentuximab Vedotin; Brinzolamide; Budesonide (Nasal); Budesonide (Systemic, Oral Inhalation); BusPIRone; Busulfan; Cabozantinib; Calcium Channel Blockers; Carvedilol; Cilostazol; Cisapride; Cobicistat; Colchicine; Conivaptan; Contraceptives (Estrogens); Contraceptives (Progestins); Corticosteroids (Orally Inhaled); Corticosteroids (Systemic); CycloSPORINE (Systemic); CYP2C19 Substrates; CYP2C9 Substrates; CYP3A4 Substrates;

◀ Diclofenac (Systemic); Diclofenac (Topical); Dienogest; Dihydroergotamine; DOCEtaxel; Dofetilide; DOXOrubicin (Conventional); Dronedarone; Dutasteride; Eletriptan; Elvitegravir; Enzalutamide; Eplerenone; Ergoloid Mesylates; Ergonovine; Ergotamine; Etravirine; Everolimus; FentaNYL; Fesoterodine; Fluticasone (Nasal); Fluticasone (Oral Inhalation); Fosamprenavir; Fosphenytoin; GuanFACINE; Halofantrine; Highest Risk QTc-Prolonging Agents; Ibrutinib; Ibuprofen; Iloperidone; Imatinib; Irinotecan; Ivabradine; Ivacaftor; Ixabepilone; Lacosamide; Lapatinib; Levomilnacipran; Lomitapide; Losartan; Lovastatin; Lumefantrine; Lurasidone; Macitentan; Macrolide Antibiotics; Maraviroc; Meloxicam; Methadone; Methylergonovine; MethylPREDNISolone; Mifepristone; Moderate Risk QTc-Prolonging Agents; Nelfinavir; Nilotinib; Nisoldipine; Ospemifene; OxyCODONE; Paricalcitol; PAZOPanib; Phenytoin; Pimecrolimus; Pimozide; Pomalidomide; PONATinib; Propafenone; Proton Pump Inhibitors; QUEtiapine; QuiNIDine; Ranolazine; Red Yeast Rice; Regorafenib; Repaglinide; Reverse Transcriptase Inhibitors (Non-Nucleoside); Rifamycin Derivatives; Rilpivirine; Rivaroxaban; RomiDEPsin; Ruxolitinib; Salmeterol; Saxagliptin; Sildenafil; Silodosin; Simeprevir; Simvastatin; Sirolimus; Solifenacin; SORAfenib; Sulfonylureas; SUNItinib; Tacrolimus (Systemic); Tacrolimus (Topical); Tadalafil; Tamsulosin; Telaprevir; Terfenadine; Ticagrelor; Tofacitinib; Tolterodine; Tolvaptan; Toremifene; Ulipristal; Vardenafil; Vemurafenib; Venlafaxine; Vilazodone; VinCRIStine (Liposomal); Vitamin K Antagonists; Zolpidem; Zuclopenthixol

The levels/effects of Voriconazole may be increased by: Atazanavir; Boceprevir; Chloramphenicol; Cobicistat; Contraceptives (Estrogens); Contraceptives (Progestins); CYP2C19 Inhibitors (Moderate); CYP2C19 Inhibitors (Strong); CYP2C9 Inhibitors (Moderate); CYP2C9 Inhibitors (Strong); Etravirine; Fluconazole; Fosamprenavir; Ivabradine; Luliconazole; Macrolide Antibiotics; Mifepristone; Proton Pump Inhibitors; QTc-Prolonging Agents (Indeterminate Risk and Risk Modifying); Telaprevir

Nutritional/Ethanol Interactions

Food: Food may decrease voriconazole absorption. Management: Oral voriconazole should be taken 1 hour before or 1 hour after a meal. Maintain adequate hydration unless instructed to restrict fluid intake.

Herb/Nutraceutical: St John's wort may decrease voriconazole levels. Management: Concurrent use of St John's wort with voriconazole is contraindicated.

Adverse Reactions

>10%:
Central nervous system: Hallucination (2% to 12%; auditory and/or visual and likely serum concentration-dependent)
Ophthalmic: Visual disturbance (19%)
Renal: Increased serum creatinine (1% to 21%)
2% to 10%:
Cardiovascular: Tachycardia (≤2%)
Central nervous system: Chills (≤4%), headache (≤3%)
Dermatologic: Skin rash (≤7%)
Endocrine & metabolic: Hypokalemia (≤2%)
Gastrointestinal: Nausea (1% to 5%), vomiting (1% to 4%)
Hepatic: Increased serum alkaline phosphatase (4% to 5%), increased serum AST (2% to 4%), increased serum ALT (2% to 3%), cholestatic jaundice (1% to 2%)
Ophthalmic: Photophobia (2%)
Miscellaneous: Fever (≤6%)
<2%, postmarketing, and/or case reports (limited to important or life-threatening): Acute renal failure, adrenocortical insufficiency, agranulocytosis, alopecia, anaphylactoid reaction, anemia (aplastic, hemolytic, macrocytic, megaloblastic, or microcytic), angioedema, anorexia, anuria, arthritis, ascites, ataxia, atrial arrhythmia, atrial fibrillation, atrioventricular block, bacterial infection, bigeminy, blighted ovum, bone marrow depression, bradycardia, brain disease, bundle branch block, cardiac arrest, cardiac failure, cardiomegaly, cardiomyopathy, cellulitis, cerebral edema, cerebral hemorrhage, cerebral ischemia, cerebrovascular accident, chest pain, cholecystitis, cholelithiasis, cholestasis, chromatopsia, color blindness, coma, confusion, convulsions, corneal opacity, cyanosis, deafness, deep vein thrombophlebitis, deep vein thrombosis, delirium, dementia, dental fluorosis, depersonalization, depression, diabetes insipidus, diarrhea, discoid lupus erythematosus, disseminated intravascular coagulation, drowsiness, duodenal ulcer (active), duodenitis, dyspnea, eczema, edema, encephalitis, endocarditis, eosinophilia, erythema multiforme, esophageal ulcer, exfoliative dermatitis, extrapyramidal reaction, extrasystoles, fixed drug eruption, fungal infection, gastric ulcer, gastrointestinal hemorrhage, glucose tolerance decreased, graft versus host disease, Guillain-Barre syndrome, hematemesis, hemorrhagic cystitis, hepatic coma, hepatic failure, hepatitis, hepatomegaly, herpes simplex infection, hydronephrosis, hyperbilirubinemia, hypercholesterolemia, hyper-/hypocalcemia, hyper-/hypoglycemia, hyper-/hypomagnesemia, hyper-/hyponatremia, hyper-/hypotension, hyper-/hypothyroidism, hyperkalemia, hypersensitivity reaction, hyperuricemia, hypophosphatemia, hypoxia, impotence, increased blood urea nitrogen, increased gamma-glutamyl transferase, increased lactate dehydrogenase, increased

susceptibility to infection, intestinal perforation, intracranial hypertension, jaundice, leukopenia, lymphadenopathy, lymphangitis, maculopapular rash, malignant melanoma, melanosis, multiorgan failure, myasthenia, myocardial infarction, myopathy, nephritis, nephrosis, neuropathy, nocturnal amblyopia, nodal arrhythmia, nodule, nystagmus, oculogyric crisis, optic atrophy, optic neuritis, orthostatic hypotension, osteomalacia, osteonecrosis, osteoporosis, otitis externa, palpitations, pancreatitis, pancytopenia, papilledema, paresthesia, perforated duodenal ulcer, periosteal disease, peripheral edema, peritonitis, petechia, pleural effusion, pneumonia, prolonged bleeding time, prolonged QT interval on ECG, pruritus, pseudomembranous colitis, pseudoporphyria, psoriasis, psychosis, pulmonary edema, pulmonary embolism, purpura, rectal hemorrhage, renal insufficiency, renal tubular necrosis, respiratory distress syndrome, respiratory tract infection, retinal hemorrhage, retinitis, seizure, sepsis, skin discoloration, skin photosensitivity, splenomegaly, squamous cell carcinoma, Stevens-Johnson syndrome, subconjunctival hemorrhage, substernal pain, suicidal ideation, supraventricular extrasystole, supraventricular tachycardia, syncope, thrombocytopenia, thrombophlebitis, thrombotic thrombocytopenic purpura, tongue edema, tonic-clonic seizures, torsades de pointes, toxic epidermal necrolysis, uremia, urinary incontinence, urinary retention, urinary tract infection, urticaria, uterine hemorrhage, uveitis, vaginal hemorrhage, vasodilation, ventricular arrhythmia, ventricular fibrillation, ventricular tachycardia, visual field defect

Available Dosage Forms

Solution Reconstituted, Intravenous:
Generic: 200 mg (1 ea)
Solution Reconstituted, Intravenous [preservative free]:
Vfend IV: 200 mg (1 ea)
Suspension Reconstituted, Oral:
Vfend: 40 mg/mL (75 mL)
Generic: 40 mg/mL (75 mL)
Tablet, Oral:
Vfend: 50 mg, 200 mg
Generic: 50 mg, 200 mg

General Dosage Range Actual body weight should be used for all weight-based dosing calculations; dosage adjustment recommended in patients with hepatic impairment

I.V.: *Children ≥12 years and Adults*: Initial: 6 mg/kg every 12 hours for 2 doses; Maintenance: 3-4 mg/kg every 12 hours

Oral: *Children ≥12 years and Adults*: 100-300 mg every 12 hours

Administration

I.V. Infuse over 1-2 hours (rate not to exceed 3 mg/kg/hour). Do not administer as an I.V. bolus injection. Do not infuse **concomitantly** into same line or cannula with other drug infusions. Do not infuse **concomitantly** even in separate lines or cannulas with concentrated electrolyte solutions or blood products. May be infused simultaneously with nonconcentrated electrolytes or TPN through a separate I.V. line. If TPN is infused through a multiple lumen catheter, use a different port than used for voriconazole.

Oral Administer 1 hour before or 1 hour after a meal. Shake oral suspension for approximately 10 seconds before each use. Enteral tube feedings may decrease oral absorption; may hold tube feedings for 1 hour before and 1 hour after a voriconazole dose (Williams, 2012).

Preparation for Administration

Powder for injection: Reconstitute 200 mg vial with 19 mL of sterile water for injection (use of automated syringe is not recommended). Resultant solution (20 mL) has a concentration of 10 mg/mL. Prior to infusion, must dilute to <5 mg/mL with NS, LR, D_5WLR, D_5W$^{1/2}$NS, D_5W, D_5W with KCl 20 mEq, $^{1/2}$NS, or D_5WNS. Do not dilute with 4.2% sodium bicarbonate infusion.

Powder for oral suspension: Add 46 mL of water to the bottle to make 40 mg/mL suspension. Shake vigorously for ~1 minute. Do not refrigerate or freeze. Discard unused portion after 14 days.

Storage/Stability

Powder for injection: Store vials between 15°C to 30°C (59°F to 86°F). Reconstituted solutions are stable for up to 24 hours under refrigeration at 2°C to 8°C (36°F to 46°F).

Powder for oral suspension: Store at 2°C to 8°C (36°F to 46°F). Reconstituted oral suspension is stable for up to 14 days if stored at 15°C to 30°C (59°F to 86°F). Do not refrigerate or freeze.

Tablets: Store at 15°C to 30°C (59°F to 86°F).

Nursing Actions

Physical Assessment Allergy history should be assessed prior to beginning therapy. Monitor for vision changes (photophobia, changed visual acuity, blurred vision), hepatic toxicity (increased liver enzymes, jaundice), tachycardia, and dermatologic reactions (can be severe; periodic total body examinations should be performed).

Patient Education
• Discuss specific use of drug and side effects with patient as it relates to treatment. (HCAHPS: During this hospital stay, were you given any medicine that you had not taken before? Before giving you any new medicine, how often did hospital staff tell you what the medicine was for? How often did hospital staff describe possible side effects in a way you could understand?)
• Patient may experience headache, photophobia, blurred vision, nausea, or diarrhea. Have patient report immediately to prescriber signs of infection, dyspnea, severe edema, considerable dyspepsia, inability to eat, significant weight gain, discolored urine, jaundice, excessive osteodynia, severe asthenia, or rash (HCAHPS).

- Educate patient about signs of a significant reaction (eg, wheezing; chest tightness; fever; itching; bad cough; blue skin color; seizures; or swelling of face, lips, tongue, or throat). **Note:** This is not a comprehensive list of all side effects. Patient should consult prescriber for additional questions.

Intended Use and Disclaimer: Should not be printed and given to patients. This information is intended to serve as a concise initial reference for healthcare professionals to use when discussing medications with a patient. You must ultimately rely on your own discretion, experience and judgment in diagnosing, treating and advising patients.

Vorinostat (vor IN oh stat)

Brand Names: U.S. Zolinza
Index Terms SAHA; Suberoylanilide Hydroxamic Acid
Pharmacologic Category Antineoplastic Agent, Histone Deacetylase Inhibitor
Medication Safety Issues
Sound-alike/look-alike issues:
Vorinostat may be confused with Votrient®
High alert medication:
This medication is in a class the Institute for Safe Medication Practices (ISMP) includes among its list of drug classes which have a heightened risk of causing significant patient harm when used in error.
Pregnancy Risk Factor D
Lactation Excretion in breast milk unknown/not recommended
Breast-Feeding Considerations It is not known if vorinostat is excreted in breast milk. Due to the potential for serious adverse reactions in the nursing infant, the decision to discontinue vorinostat or to discontinue breast-feeding should take into account the benefits of treatment to the mother.
Use Cutaneous T-cell lymphoma: Treatment of cutaneous manifestations of cutaneous T-cell lymphoma (CTCL) with progressive, persistent, or recurrent disease on or following 2 systemic treatments
Mechanism of Action/Effect Histone deacetylase inhibitor; causes termination of cell growth leading to cell death
Contraindications There are no contraindications in the manufacturer's U.S. labeling.

Canadian labeling: Hypersensitivity to vorinostat or any component of the formulation; severe hepatic impairment (total bilirubin ≥3 times ULN)
Warnings/Precautions Hazardous agent - use appropriate precautions for handling and disposal (NIOSH, 2012). Pulmonary embolism and deep vein thrombosis (DVT) have been reported; monitor for signs/symptoms; use caution in patients with a history of thrombotic events. Dose-related

thrombocytopenia and/or anemia may occur; may require dosage adjustments or discontinuation; monitor blood counts (every 2 weeks for 2 months, then monthly). Gastrointestinal bleeding due to severe thrombocytopenia has been reported in patients receiving vorinostat in combination with other histone deacetylase inhibitors (eg, valproic acid); monitor platelet counts more frequently in patients receiving concomitant histone deacetylase inhibitor therapy. QT$_c$ prolongation has been observed; baseline and periodic ECGs were done in clinical trials (Duvic, 2007; Olsen, 2007). Correct electrolyte abnormalities prior to treatment and monitor and correct potassium, calcium, and magnesium levels during therapy. Use caution in patients with a history of QT$_c$ prolongation or with medications known to prolong the QT interval. May cause hyperglycemia (may be severe); monitor serum glucose and use with caution in diabetics; may require diet and/or therapy modifications. Nausea, vomiting, and diarrhea may occur; antiemetics and antidiarrheals may be required; control pre-existing nausea and vomiting prior to treatment initiation; replace fluids and electrolytes to avoid dehydration. Adverse anastomotic healing events have occurred in patients recovering from bowel surgery; use with caution in the perioperative period in patients requiring bowel surgery. May cause dizziness or fatigue; caution patients about performing tasks which require mental alertness (eg, operating machinery or driving). Use with caution in patients with hepatic impairment; dose reductions are recommended (elimination is predominantly hepatic). The Canadian labeling does not recommend use in patients with moderate hepatic impairment (total bilirubin 1.5-3 times ULN) and contraindicates use in severe hepatic impairment (bilirubin ≥3 times ULN). Potentially significant drug-drug interactions may exist, requiring dose or frequency adjustment, additional monitoring, and/or selection of alternative therapy.
Drug Interactions
Avoid Concomitant Use
Avoid concomitant use of Vorinostat with any of the following: CloZAPine
Decreased Effect There are no known significant interactions involving a decrease in effect.
Increased Effect/Toxicity
Vorinostat may increase the levels/effects of: CloZAPine; Highest Risk QTc-Prolonging Agents; Moderate Risk QTc-Prolonging Agents; Vitamin K Antagonists

The levels/effects of Vorinostat may be increased by: Mifepristone; Valproic Acid and Derivatives
Adverse Reactions
>10%:
Cardiovascular: Peripheral edema (13%)
Central nervous system: Fatigue (52%), chills (16%), dizziness (15%), headache (12%), fever (11%)

Dermatologic: Alopecia (19%), pruritus (12%)

Endocrine & metabolic: Hyperglycemia (8% to 69%; grade 3: 5%), dehydration (1% to 16%)

Gastrointestinal: Diarrhea (52%), nausea (41%), taste alteration (28%), anorexia (24%), weight loss (21%), xerostomia (16%), constipation (15%), vomiting (15%), appetite decreased (14%)

Hematologic: Thrombocytopenia (26%; grades 3/4: 6%), anemia (14%; grades 3/4: 2%)

Neuromuscular & skeletal: Muscle spasm (20%)

Renal: Proteinuria (51%), creatinine increased (16% to 47%)

Respiratory: Cough (11%), upper respiratory infection (11%)

1% to 10%:

Cardiovascular: QT_c prolongation (3% to 4%)

Dermatologic: Squamous cell carcinoma (4%)

Respiratory: Pulmonary embolism (5%)

Available Dosage Forms

Capsule, Oral:

Zolinza: 100 mg

General Dosage Range Dosage adjustment recommended in patients who develop toxicities and those with hepatic impairment

Oral: *Adults:* 400 mg once daily

Administration

Oral Administer with food. Do not open, crush, or chew capsules. Maintain adequate hydration (≥2 L/day fluids) during treatment.

Hazardous agent; use appropriate precautions for handling and disposal (NIOSH, 2012). Avoid direct skin or mucous membrane contact with crushed or broken capsules and/or capsule contents.

Storage/Stability Store at 20°C to 25°C (68°F to 77°F); excursions permitted to 15°C to 30°C (59°F to 86°F).

Nursing Actions

Physical Assessment Caution patients with diabetes to monitor serum glucose closely. Teach patient correct use and proper handling of capsules.

Patient Education

- Discuss specific use of drug and side effects with patient as it relates to treatment. (HCAHPS: During this hospital stay, were you given any medicine that you had not taken before? Before giving you any new medicine, how often did hospital staff tell you what the medicine was for? How often did hospital staff describe possible side effects in a way you could understand?)

- Patient may experience headache, presyncope, fatigue, blurred vision, illogical thinking, chills, dizziness, fasciculations, loss of appetite, hyperglycemia, nausea, diarrhea, weight loss, constipation, parageusia, alopecia, xerostomia, or edema in arms or legs. Have patient report immediately to prescriber dyspnea, angina, tachycardia, syncope, edema in abdomen, ecchymosis, or rash (HCAHPS).

- Educate patient about signs of a significant reaction (eg, wheezing; chest tightness; fever; itching; bad cough; blue skin color; seizures; or swelling of face, lips, tongue, or throat). **Note:** This is not a comprehensive list of all side effects. Patient should consult prescriber for additional questions.

Intended Use and Disclaimer: Should not be printed and given to patients. This information is intended to serve as a concise initial reference for healthcare professionals to use when discussing medications with a patient. You must ultimately rely on your own discretion, experience and judgment in diagnosing, treating and advising patients.

Dietary Considerations Take with food.

Related Information

Oral Medications That Should Not Be Crushed or Altered *on page 1712*

Vortioxetine (vor tye OX e teen)

Brand Names: U.S. Brintellix

Index Terms Lu AA21004; Vortioxetine Hydrobromide

Pharmacologic Category Antidepressant, Selective Serotonin Reuptake Inhibitor; Serotonin 5-HT$_{1A}$ Receptor Agonist; Serotonin 5-HT$_3$ Receptor Antagonist

Medication Safety Issues

Sound-alike/look-alike issues:

Vortioxetine may be confused with duloxetine, fluoxetine, paroxetine

Medication Guide Available Yes

Pregnancy Risk Factor C

Lactation Excretion unknown/not recommended

Breast-Feeding Considerations It is not known if vortioxetine is excreted into breast milk. Due to the potential for serious adverse reactions in the nursing infant, the manufacturer recommends a decision be made whether to discontinue nursing or to discontinue the drug, taking into account the importance of treatment to the mother.

Use Major depressive disorder: Treatment of major depressive disorder (MDD)

Mechanism of Action/Effect Inhibits reuptake of serotonin (5-HT); also has agonist activity at the 5-HT$_{1A}$ receptor and antagonist activity at the 5-HT$_3$ receptor.

Contraindications Hypersensitivity to vortioxetine or any component of the formulation; use of MAO inhibitors intended to treat psychiatric disorders (concurrently or within 21 days of discontinuing vortioxetine or within 14 days of discontinuing the MAO inhibitor); initiation of vortioxetine in a patient receiving linezolid or intravenous methylene blue

Warnings/Precautions [U.S. Boxed Warning]: Antidepressants increase the risk of suicidal thinking and behavior in children, adolescents, and young adults (18-24 years of age) with major depressive disorder (MDD) and other psychiatric disorders; consider risk prior to prescribing. Short-term studies did not show an increased risk in patients >24 years of age and showed a decreased risk in patients ≥65 years. Closely monitor patients for clinical worsening, suicidality, or unusual changes in behavior, particularly during the initial 1-2 months of therapy or during periods of dosage adjustments (increases or decreases); the patient's family or caregiver should be instructed to closely observe the patient and communicate condition with healthcare provider. A medication guide concerning the use of antidepressants should be dispensed with each prescription. **Vortioxetine is not approved for use in children.**

The possibility of a suicide attempt is inherent in major depression and may persist until remission occurs. Use caution in high-risk patients. Worsening depression and severe abrupt suicidality that are not part of the presenting symptoms may require discontinuation or modification of drug therapy. The patient's family or caregiver should be alerted to monitor patients for the emergence of suicidality and associated behaviors (such as agitation, irritability, hostility, aggressiveness, impulsivity, and hypomania) and call healthcare provider.

May worsen psychosis in some patients or precipitate a mixed/manic episode in patients at risk for bipolar disorder. Use with caution in patients with a family history of bipolar disorder, mania, or hypomania. Patients presenting with depressive symptoms should be screened for bipolar disorder. **Vortioxetine is not FDA approved for the treatment of bipolar depression.**

Potentially life-threatening serotonin syndrome (SS) has occurred with serotonergic antidepressants (eg, SSRIs, SNRIs), particularly when used in combination with other serotonergic agents (eg, triptans, TCAs, fentanyl, lithium, tramadol, buspirone, St John's wort, tryptophan) or agents that impair metabolism of serotonin (eg, MAO inhibitors intended to treat psychiatric disorders, other MAO inhibitors [ie, linezolid and intravenous methylene blue]). Discontinue treatment (and any concomitant serotonergic agent) immediately if signs/symptoms arise.

May impair platelet aggregation resulting in increased risk of bleeding events, particularly if used concomitantly with aspirin, NSAIDs, warfarin or other anticoagulants. Bleeding related to antidepressant use has been reported to range from relatively minor bruising and epistaxis to life-threatening hemorrhage. May cause hyponatremia/SIADH (elderly at increased risk); volume depletion (diuretics may increase risk) may occur. Use caution in elderly patients; may cause or exacerbate syndrome of inappropriate antidiuretic hormone secretion or hyponatremia; monitor sodium closely with initiation or dosage adjustments in older adults. May cause CNS depression, which may impair physical or mental abilities; patients must be cautioned about performing tasks that require mental alertness (eg, operating machinery or driving). Angioedema has been reported. Potentially significant drug-drug interactions may exist, requiring dose or frequency adjustment, additional monitoring, and/or selection of alternative therapy. Use is not recommended in severe hepatic impairment.

Abrupt discontinuation or interruption of antidepressant therapy has been associated with a discontinuation syndrome. Symptoms arising may vary with antidepressant however commonly include nausea, vomiting, diarrhea, headaches, lightheadedness, dizziness, diminished appetite, sweating, chills, tremors, paresthesias, fatigue, somnolence, and sleep disturbances (eg, vivid dreams, insomnia). Greater risks for developing a discontinuation syndrome have been associated with antidepressants with shorter half-lives, longer durations of treatment, and abrupt discontinuation. For antidepressants of short or intermediate half-lives, symptoms may emerge within 2-5 days after treatment discontinuation and last 7-14 days (APA, 2010; Fava, 2006; Haddad, 2001; Shelton, 2001; Warner, 2006).

Drug Interactions

Avoid Concomitant Use

Avoid concomitant use of Vortioxetine with any of the following: Dosulepin; Iobenguane I 123; Linezolid; MAO Inhibitors; Methylene Blue; Pimozide; Tryptophan; Urokinase

Decreased Effect

Vortioxetine may decrease the levels/effects of: Iobenguane I 123; Ioflupane I 123; Thyroid Products

The levels/effects of Vortioxetine may be decreased by: Bosentan; CarBAMazepine; CYP3A4 Inducers (Strong); Cyproheptadine; Dabrafenib; Deferasirox; NSAID (COX-2 Inhibitor); NSAID (Nonselective); Peginterferon Alfa-2b; Tocilizumab

Increased Effect/Toxicity

Vortioxetine may increase the levels/effects of: Agents with Antiplatelet Properties; Anticoagulants; Antidepressants (Serotonin Reuptake Inhibitor/Antagonist); Antipsychotics; Aspirin; Benzodiazepines (metabolized by oxidation); Beta-Blockers; BusPIRone; CarBAMazepine; CloZAPine; Collagenase (Systemic); Dabigatran Etexilate; Desmopressin; Dextromethorphan; Dosulepin; Galantamine; Hypoglycemic Agents; Ibritumomab; Methadone; Methylene Blue; Metoclopramide; Mexiletine; NSAID (COX-2 Inhibitor); NSAID (Nonselective); Pimozide; QuiNIDine;

RisperiDONE; Rivaroxaban; Salicylates; Serotonin Modulators; Thiazide Diuretics; Thrombolytic Agents; Tositumomab and Iodine I 131 Tositumomab; TraMADol; Urokinase; Vitamin K Antagonists

The levels/effects of Vortioxetine may be increased by: Abiraterone Acetate; Alcohol (Ethyl); Analgesics (Opioid); Antipsychotics; BuPROPion; BusPIRone; Cimetidine; CNS Depressants; Cobicistat; CYP2D6 Inhibitors (Moderate); CYP2D6 Inhibitors (Strong); Darunavir; Dasatinib; Glucosamine; Herbs (Anticoagulant/Antiplatelet Properties); Ibrutinib; Linezolid; Lithium; Macrolide Antibiotics; MAO Inhibitors; Metoclopramide; Metyrosine; Multivitamins/Fluoride (with ADE); Multivitamins/Minerals (with ADEK, Folate, Iron); Multivitamins/Minerals (with AE, No Iron); Omega-3 Fatty Acids; Pentosan Polysulfate Sodium; Pentoxifylline; Prostacyclin Analogues; TraMADol; Tryptophan; Vitamin E

Nutritional/Ethanol Interactions Herb/Nutraceutical: Some herbal medications may increase risk of serotonin syndrome and/or excessive sedation. Management: Avoid valerian, St John's wort, SAMe, kava kava, and tryptophan.

Adverse Reactions

>10%:

Central nervous system: Female sexual disorder (self-reporting: 1% to 2%; Arizona Sexual Experience Scale: 22% to 34%), male sexual disorder (self-reporting: 3% to 5%; Arizona Sexual Experience Scale: 10% to 29%)

Gastrointestinal: Nausea (dose-related, females >males, tolerance develops: 21% to 32%)

1% to 10%:

Central nervous system: Dizziness (8% to 9%), abnormal dreams (2% to 3%)

Dermatologic: Pruritus (2% to 3%)

Gastrointestinal: Diarrhea (7% to 10%), xerostomia (7% to 8%), constipation (5% to 6%), vomiting (3% to 6%), flatulence (2% to 3%)

Pharmacodynamics/Kinetics

Onset of Action Therapeutic: 2-4 weeks

Available Dosage Forms

Tablet, Oral:

Brintellix: 5 mg, 10 mg, 20 mg

General Dosage Range Oral: *Adults:* Initial: 10 mg once daily; Maintenance: 5-20 mg once daily.

Administration

Oral Administer without regard to meals.

Storage/Stability Store at 25°C (77°F); excursions are permitted between 15°C and 30°C (59°F and 86°F).

Nursing Actions

Physical Assessment Monitor for worsening mood, suicidal thoughts, or sudden changes in mental status.

Patient Education

- Discuss specific use of drug and side effects with patient as it relates to treatment. (HCAHPS: During this hospital stay, were you given any medicine that you had not taken before? Before giving you any new medicine, how often did hospital staff tell you what the medicine was for? How often did hospital staff describe possible side effects in a way you could understand?)
- Patient may experience nausea, xerostomia, dizziness, constipation, diarrhea, or sexual dysfunction. Have patient report immediately to prescriber signs of hyponatremia, signs of hemorrhaging, behavioral changes, insomnia, or serotonin syndrome (HCAHPS).
- Educate patient about signs of a significant reaction (eg, wheezing; chest tightness; fever; itching; bad cough; blue skin color; seizures; or swelling of face, lips, tongue, or throat). **Note:** This is not a comprehensive list of all side effects. Patient should consult prescriber for additional questions.

Intended Use and Disclaimer: Should not be printed and given to patients. This information is intended to serve as a concise initial reference for healthcare professionals to use when discussing medications with a patient. You must ultimately rely on your own discretion, experience and judgment in diagnosing, treating and advising patients.

Warfarin (WAR far in)

Brand Names: U.S. Coumadin; Jantoven

Index Terms Warfarin Sodium

Pharmacologic Category Anticoagulant; Anticoagulant, Vitamin K Antagonist

Medication Safety Issues

Sound-alike/look-alike issues:

Coumadin® may be confused with Avandia®, Cardura®, Compazine, Kemadrin

Jantoven® may be confused with Janumet®, Januvia®

High alert medication:

The Institute for Safe Medication Practices (ISMP) includes this medication among its list of drugs which have a heightened risk of causing significant patient harm when used in error.

National Patient Safety Goals:

The Joint Commission on Accreditation of Healthcare Organizations requires healthcare organizations that provide anticoagulant therapy to have a process in place to reduce the risk of anticoagulant-associated patient harm. Patients receiving anticoagulants should receive individualized care through a defined process that includes standardized ordering, dispensing, administration, monitoring and education. This does not apply to routine short-term use of anticoagulants for prevention of venous ▶

thromboembolism when the expectation is that the patient's laboratory values will remain within or close to normal values (NPSG.03.05.01).

Medication Guide Available Yes

Pregnancy Risk Factor D (women with mechanical heart valves)/X (other indications)

Lactation Does not enter breast milk/use caution

Breast-Feeding Considerations Breast-feeding women may be treated with warfarin. Based on available data, warfarin does not pass into breast milk. Women who are breast-feeding should be carefully monitored to avoid excessive anticoagulation. According to the American College of Chest Physicians (ACCP), warfarin may be used in lactating women who wish to breast-feed their infants (Bates, 2012). Monitor nursing infants for bruising or bleeding (per manufacturer).

Use Prophylaxis and treatment of thromboembolic disorders (eg, venous, pulmonary) and embolic complications arising from atrial fibrillation or cardiac valve replacement; adjunct to reduce risk of systemic embolism (eg, recurrent MI, stroke) after myocardial infarction

Unlabeled Use Prevention of recurrent transient ischemic attacks

Mechanism of Action/Effect Interferes with hepatic synthesis of vitamin K-dependent coagulation factors (II, VII, IX, X)

Contraindications Hypersensitivity to warfarin or any component of the formulation; hemorrhagic tendencies (eg, patients bleeding from the GI, respiratory, or GU tract; cerebral aneurysm; cerebrovascular hemorrhage; dissecting aortic aneurysm; spinal puncture and other diagnostic or therapeutic procedures with potential for significant bleeding; history of bleeding diathesis); recent or potential surgery of the eye or CNS; major regional lumbar block anesthesia or traumatic surgery resulting in large, open surfaces; blood dyscrasias; severe uncontrolled or malignant hypertension; pericarditis or pericardial effusion; bacterial endocarditis; unsupervised patients with conditions associated with a high potential for noncompliance; eclampsia/pre-eclampsia, threatened abortion, pregnancy (except in women with mechanical heart valves at high risk for thromboembolism)

Warnings/Precautions Hazardous agent - use appropriate precautions for handling and disposal (EPA, P-listed [>0.3%]; U-listed [<0.3%]). Use care in the selection of patients appropriate for this treatment. Ensure patient cooperation especially from the alcoholic, illicit drug user, demented, or psychotic patient; ability to comply with routine laboratory monitoring is essential. Use with caution in trauma, acute infection, moderate-severe renal insufficiency, prolonged dietary insufficiencies, moderate-severe hypertension, polycythemia vera, vasculitis, open wound, active TB, any disruption in normal GI flora, history of PUD, anaphylactic disorders, indwelling catheters, severe diabetes, and menstruating and postpartum women. Use with caution in patients with thyroid disease; warfarin responsiveness may increase (Ageno, 2012). Use with caution in protein C deficiency. Use with caution in patients with heparin-induced thrombocytopenia and DVT. Warfarin monotherapy is contraindicated in the initial treatment of active HIT. Reduced liver function, regardless of etiology, may impair synthesis of coagulation factors leading to increased warfarin sensitivity.

[U.S. Boxed Warning]: May cause major or fatal bleeding. Risk factors for bleeding include high intensity anticoagulation (INR >4), age (>65 years), variable INRs, history of GI bleeding, hypertension, cerebrovascular disease, serious heart disease, anemia, malignancy, trauma, renal insufficiency, drug-drug interactions, long duration of therapy, or known genetic deficiency in CYP2C9 activity. Patient must be instructed to report bleeding, accidents, or falls. Unrecognized bleeding sites (eg, colon cancer) may be uncovered by anticoagulation. Patient must also report any new or discontinued medications, herbal or alternative products used, or significant changes in smoking or dietary habits. Necrosis or gangrene of the skin and other tissue can occur, usually in conjunction with protein C or S deficiency. Consider alternative therapies if anticoagulation is necessary. Warfarin therapy may release atheromatous plaque emboli; symptoms depend on site of embolization, most commonly kidneys, pancreas, liver, and spleen. In some cases may lead to necrosis or death. "Purple toes syndrome," due to cholesterol microembolization, may rarely occur. The elderly may be more sensitive to anticoagulant therapy.

Presence of the CYP2C9*2 or *3 allele and/or polymorphism of the vitamin K oxidoreductase (VKORC1) gene may increase the risk of bleeding. Lower doses may be required in these patients; genetic testing may help determine appropriate dosing.

When temporary interruption is necessary before surgery, discontinue for approximately 5 days before surgery; when there is adequate hemostasis, may reinstitute warfarin therapy ~12-24 hours after surgery (evening of or next morning). Decision to safely continue warfarin therapy through the procedure and whether or not bridging of anticoagulation is necessary is dependent upon risk of perioperative bleeding and risk of thromboembolism, respectively. If risk of thromboembolism is elevated, consider bridging warfarin therapy with an alternative anticoagulant (eg, unfractionated heparin, LMWH) (Guyatt, 2012).

Drug Interactions

Avoid Concomitant Use

Avoid concomitant use of Warfarin with any of the following: Apixaban; Dabigatran Etexilate; Enzalutamide; Rivaroxaban; Streptokinase [Off Market]; Tamoxifen; Urokinase

Decreased Effect

The levels/effects of Warfarin may be decreased by: Adalimumab; Aminoglutethimide; Antineoplastic Agents; Antithyroid Agents; Aprepitant; AzaTHIOprine; Barbiturates; Bile Acid Sequestrants; Boceprevir; Bosentan; CarBAMazepine; Cloxacillin; Coenzyme Q-10; Contraceptives (Estrogens); Contraceptives (Progestins); CYP2C9 Inducers (Strong); Darunavir; Dicloxacillin; Efavirenz; Elvitegravir; Enzalutamide; Eslicarbazepine; Estrogen Derivatives; Floxacillin; Fosaprepitant; Ginseng (American); Glutethimide; Green Tea; Griseofulvin; Lopinavir; Mercaptopurine; Metreleptin; Multivitamins/Minerals (with ADEK, Folate, Iron); Nafcillin; Nelfinavir; Peginterferon Alfa-2b; Phytonadione; Progestins; Rifamycin Derivatives; Ritonavir; St Johns Wort; Sucralfate; Telaprevir; Teriflunomide; TraZODone

Increased Effect/Toxicity

Warfarin may increase the levels/effects of: Anticoagulants; Collagenase (Systemic); Deferasirox; Ethotoin; Fosphenytoin; Phenytoin; Regorafenib; Rivaroxaban; Sulfonylureas

The levels/effects of Warfarin may be increased by: Acetaminophen; Agents with Antiplatelet Properties; Allopurinol; Amiodarone; Androgens; Antineoplastic Agents; Apixaban; Atazanavir; Bicalutamide; Boceprevir; Capecitabine; Cephalosporins; Chloral Hydrate; Chloramphenicol; Cimetidine; Clopidogrel; Cloxacillin; Cobicistat; Corticosteroids (Systemic); Cranberry; CYP2C9 Inhibitors (Moderate); CYP2C9 Inhibitors (Strong); Dabigatran Etexilate; Desvenlafaxine; Dexmethylphenidate; Disulfiram; Dronedarone; Efavirenz; Erythromycin (Ophthalmic); Esomeprazole; Ethacrynic Acid; Ethotoin; Etoposide; Exenatide; Fenofibrate and Derivatives; Fenugreek; Fibric Acid Derivatives; Fluconazole; Fluorouracil (Systemic); Fluorouracil (Topical); Fosamprenavir; Fosphenytoin; Fusidic Acid (Systemic); Gefitinib; Ginkgo Biloba; Glucagon; Green Tea; Herbs (Anticoagulant/Antiplatelet Properties); HMG-CoA Reductase Inhibitors; Ibrutinib; Ifosfamide; Imatinib; Itraconazole; Ivermectin (Systemic); Ketoconazole (Systemic); Lansoprazole; Leflunomide; Levomilnacipran; Lomitapide; Macrolide Antibiotics; Methylphenidate; Metreleptin; MetroNIDAZOLE (Systemic); Miconazole (Oral); Miconazole (Topical); Mifepristone; Milnacipran; Mirtazapine; Multivitamins/Fluoride (with ADE); Multivitamins/Minerals (with ADEK, Folate, Iron); Multivitamins/Minerals (with AE, No Iron); Nelfinavir; Neomycin; NSAID (COX-2 Inhibitor); NSAID (Nonselective); Omega-3 Fatty Acids; Omeprazole; Orlistat; Penicillins; Pentosan Polysulfate Sodium; Pentoxifylline; Phenytoin; Posaconazole; Proguanil; Propafenone; Prostacyclin Analogues; QuiNIDine; QuiNINE; Quinolone Antibiotics; Ranitidine; RomiDEPsin; Salicylates; Saquinavir; Selective Serotonin Reuptake Inhibitors; Sitaxentan; SORAfenib; Streptokinase [Off Market]; Sugammadex; Sulfinpyrazone [Off Market]; Sulfonamide Derivatives; Sulfonylureas; Tamoxifen; Tegafur; Telaprevir; Tetracycline Derivatives; Thrombolytic Agents; Thyroid Products; Tibolone; Tigecycline; Tipranavir; Tolterodine; Toremifene; Torsemide; TraMADol; Tricyclic Antidepressants; Urokinase; Venlafaxine; Vitamin E; Voriconazole; Vorinostat; Zafirlukast; Zileuton

Nutritional/Ethanol Interactions

Ethanol: Acute ethanol ingestion (binge drinking) decreases the metabolism of warfarin and increases PT/INR. Chronic daily ethanol use increases the metabolism of warfarin and decreases PT/INR. Management: Avoid ethanol.

Food: The anticoagulant effects of warfarin may be decreased if taken with foods rich in vitamin K. Vitamin E may increase warfarin effect. Cranberry juice may increase warfarin effect. Management: Maintain a consistent diet; consult prescriber before making changes in diet. Take warfarin at the same time each day.

Herb/Nutraceutical: Some herbal medications (eg, St John's wort) may decrease warfarin levels and effects; many others can add additional antiplatelet activity to warfarin therapy. Management: Avoid ginseng (American), coenzyme Q_{10}, and St John's wort. Avoid cranberry, fenugreek, ginkgo biloba, glucosamine, alfalfa, anise, bilberry, bladderwrack, bromelain, cat's claw, celery, chamomile, coleus, cordyceps, dong quai, evening primrose oil, fenugreek, feverfew, garlic, ginger, ginkgo biloba, ginseng (Panax), ginseng (Siberian), grapeseed, green tea, guggul, horse chestnut seed, horseradish, licorice, omega-3-acids, prickly ash, red clover, reishi, SAMe (s-adenosylmethionine), sweet clover, turmeric, and white willow.

Adverse Reactions Bleeding is the major adverse effect of warfarin. Hemorrhage may occur at virtually any site. Risk is dependent on multiple variables, including the intensity of anticoagulation and patient susceptibility.

Cardiovascular: Vasculitis

Central nervous system: Signs/symptoms of bleeding (eg, dizziness, fatigue, fever, headache, lethargy, malaise, pain)

Dermatologic: Alopecia, bullous eruptions, dermatitis, rash, pruritus, urticaria

Gastrointestinal: Abdominal pain, diarrhea, flatulence, gastrointestinal bleeding, nausea, taste disturbance, vomiting

Genitourinary: Hematuria

Hematologic: Anemia, retroperitoneal hematoma, unrecognized bleeding sites (eg, colon cancer) may be uncovered by anticoagulation

Hepatic: Hepatitis (including cholestatic hepatitis), transaminases increased

Neuromuscular & skeletal: Osteoporosis (potential association with long-term use), paralysis, paresthesia, weakness

Respiratory: Respiratory tract bleeding, tracheobronchial calcification

Miscellaneous: Anaphylactic reaction, hypersensitivity/allergic reactions, skin necrosis, gangrene, "purple toes" syndrome

Pharmacodynamics/Kinetics

Onset of Action Anticoagulation: Oral: 24-72 hours; Peak effect: Full therapeutic effect: 5-7 days; INR may increase in 36-72 hours

Duration of Action 2-5 days

Available Dosage Forms

Solution Reconstituted, Intravenous:
Coumadin: 5 mg (1 ea)

Tablet, Oral:
Coumadin: 1 mg, 2 mg, 2.5 mg, 3 mg, 4 mg, 5 mg, 6 mg, 7.5 mg, 10 mg
Jantoven: 1 mg, 2 mg, 2.5 mg, 3 mg, 4 mg, 5 mg, 6 mg, 7.5 mg, 10 mg
Generic: 1 mg, 2 mg, 2.5 mg, 3 mg, 4 mg, 5 mg, 6 mg, 7.5 mg, 10 mg

General Dosage Range

I.V.: *Adults:* 2-5 mg once daily

Oral:
Adults: Initial: 2-5 mg daily for 2 days; Maintenance: 2-10 mg daily
Elderly: Initial: ≤5 mg/day; Maintenance: 2-5 mg/day

Administration

I.V. Administer as a slow bolus injection over 1-2 minutes. Avoid all I.M. injections.

Hazardous agent; use appropriate precautions for handling and disposal (EPA, P-listed [>0.3%]; U-listed [<0.3%]).

Injectable Detail pH: 8.1-8.3

Oral Administer with or without food. Take at the same time each day.

Hazardous agent; use appropriate precautions for handling and disposal (EPA, P-listed [>0.3%]; U-listed [<0.3%]).

Preparation for Administration Reconstitute with 2.7 mL of sterile water (yields 2 mg/mL solution).

Hazardous agent; use appropriate precautions for handling and disposal (EPA, P-listed [>0.3%]; U-listed [<0.3%]).

Storage/Stability

Injection: Prior to reconstitution, store at 15°C to 30°C (59°F to 86°F). Following reconstitution with 2.7 mL of sterile water (yields 2 mg/mL solution), stable for 4 hours at 15°C to 30°C (59°F to 86°F). Protect from light.

Tablet: Store at 15°C to 30°C (59°F to 86°F). Protect from light.

Nursing Actions

Physical Assessment Assess potential for interactions with other prescriptions, OTC medications, or herbal products patient may be taking that may affect coagulation or platelet aggregation. Monitor for bleeding from any site, rash, urticaria, gastrointestinal upset, abdominal pain, diarrhea, or hypersensitivity reaction.

Patient Education

- Discuss specific use of drug and side effects with patient as it relates to treatment. (HCAHPS: During this hospital stay, were you given any medicine that you had not taken before? Before giving you any new medicine, how often did hospital staff tell you what the medicine was for? How often did hospital staff describe possible side effects in a way you could understand?)

- Patient may experience bleeding problems, headache, or nausea. Have patient report immediately to prescriber severe dizziness, imbalance, edema, illogical thinking, excessive back pain, significant dyspepsia, melena, hematuria, hemoptysis, ecchymosis, increased menstrual bleeding, severe asthenia, considerable diarrhea, signs of infection, or rash (HCAHPS).

- Educate patient about signs of a significant reaction (eg, wheezing; chest tightness; fever; itching; bad cough; blue skin color; seizures; or swelling of face, lips, tongue, or throat). **Note:** This is not a comprehensive list of all side effects. Patient should consult prescriber for additional questions.

Intended Use and Disclaimer: Should not be printed and given to patients. This information is intended to serve as a concise initial reference for healthcare professionals to use when discussing medications with a patient. You must ultimately rely on your own discretion, experience and judgment in diagnosing, treating and advising patients.

Dietary Considerations Foods high in vitamin K (eg, beef liver, pork liver, green tea, and leafy green vegetables) inhibit anticoagulant effect. Do not change dietary habits once stabilized on warfarin therapy. A balanced diet with a consistent intake of vitamin K is essential. Avoid large amounts of alfalfa, asparagus, broccoli, Brussels sprouts, cabbage, cauliflower, green teas, kale, lettuce, spinach, turnip greens, and watercress; decreased efficacy of warfarin. It is recommended that the diet contain a CONSISTENT vitamin K content of 70-140 mcg/day. Check with healthcare provider before changing diet.

Zafirlukast (za FIR loo kast)

Brand Names: U.S. Accolate
Index Terms ICI-204,219
Pharmacologic Category Leukotriene-Receptor Antagonist

Medication Safety Issues
Sound-alike/look-alike issues:
Accolate® may be confused with Accupril®, Accutane®, Aclovate®

Pregnancy Risk Factor B

Lactation Enters breast milk/not recommended

Breast-Feeding Considerations Zafirlukast is excreted into breast milk. In women receiving zafirlukast 40 mg twice daily, maternal serum concentrations were 225 ng/mL and breast milk concentrations were 50 ng/mL. Due to the potential for adverse reactions in the nursing infant, breast-feeding is not recommended by the manufacturer.

Use Prophylaxis and chronic treatment of asthma

Mechanism of Action/Effect Leukotrienes are inflammatory mediators of asthma. Zafirlukast blocks leukotriene receptors and is able to reduce bronchoconstriction and inflammatory cell infiltration.

Contraindications Hypersensitivity to zafirlukast or any component of the formulation; hepatic impairment (including hepatic cirrhosis)

Canadian labeling: Additional contraindications (not in U.S. labeling): Patients in whom zafirlukast was discontinued due to treatment related hepatotoxicity

Warnings/Precautions Zafirlukast is not approved for use in the reversal of bronchospasm in acute asthma attacks, including status asthmaticus. Therapy with zafirlukast can be continued during acute exacerbations of asthma.

Hepatic adverse events (including hepatitis, hyperbilirubinemia, and hepatic failure) have been reported; female patients may be at greater risk. Periodic testing of liver function may be considered (early detection coupled with therapy discontinuation is generally believed to improve the likelihood of recovery). Advise patients to be alert for and to immediately report symptoms (eg, anorexia, right upper quadrant abdominal pain, nausea). If hepatic dysfunction is suspected (due to clinical signs/symptoms), discontinue use immediately and measure liver function tests (particularly ALT); resolution observed in most but not all cases upon discontinuation of therapy. Do not resume or restart if hepatic function studies indicate dysfunction. Use in patients with hepatic impairment (including hepatic cirrhosis) is contraindicated. Postmarketing reports of behavioral changes (ie, depression, insomnia) have been noted. Instruct patients to report neuropsychiatric symptoms/events during therapy.

Monitor INR closely with concomitant warfarin use. Rare cases of eosinophilic vasculitis (Churg-Strauss) have been reported in patients receiving zafirlukast (usually, but not always, associated with reduction in concurrent steroid dosage). No causal relationship established. Monitor for eosinophilic vasculitis, rash, pulmonary symptoms, cardiac symptoms, or neuropathy.

Clearance is decreased in elderly patients; C_{max} and AUC are increased approximately two- to threefold in adults ≥65 years compared to younger adults; however, no dosage adjustments are recommended in this age group. An increased proportion of zafirlukast patients >55 years of age reported infections as compared to placebo-treated patients. These infections were mostly mild or moderate in intensity and predominantly affected the respiratory tract. Infections occurred equally in both sexes, were dose-proportional to total milligrams of zafirlukast exposure, and were associated with coadministration of inhaled corticosteroids.

Drug Interactions

Avoid Concomitant Use
Avoid concomitant use of Zafirlukast with any of the following: Pimozide

Decreased Effect
The levels/effects of Zafirlukast may be decreased by: CYP2C9 Inducers (Strong); Dabrafenib; Erythromycin (Systemic); Peginterferon Alfa-2b; Theophylline Derivatives

Increased Effect/Toxicity
Zafirlukast may increase the levels/effects of: ARIPiprazole; Bosentan; Carvedilol; CYP2C9 Substrates; Dofetilide; Lomitapide; Pimozide; Theophylline Derivatives; Vitamin K Antagonists

The levels/effects of Zafirlukast may be increased by: CYP2C9 Inhibitors (Moderate); CYP2C9 Inhibitors (Strong); Mifepristone

Nutritional/Ethanol Interactions Food: Food decreases bioavailability of zafirlukast by 40%. Management: Take on an empty stomach 1 hour before or 2 hours after meals.

Adverse Reactions Incidence reported in children ≥12 years and adults unless otherwise specified.
>10%: Central nervous system: Headache (13%; children 5-11 years: 5%)
1% to 10%:
  Central nervous system: Dizziness (2%), pain (2%), fever (2%)
  Gastrointestinal: Nausea (3%), diarrhea (3%), abdominal pain (2%; children 5-11 years: 3%), vomiting (2%), dyspepsia (1%)
  Hepatic: ALT increased (2%)
  Neuromuscular & skeletal: Back pain (2%), myalgia (2%), weakness (2%)
  Miscellaneous: Infection (4%)

Available Dosage Forms
Tablet, Oral:
  Accolate: 10 mg, 20 mg
  Generic: 10 mg, 20 mg

General Dosage Range Oral:
Children 5-11 years: 10 mg twice daily
Children ≥12 years and Adults: 20 mg twice daily ▶

Administration
Oral Administer 1 hour before or 2 hours after meals.

Storage/Stability Store tablets at controlled room temperature of 20°C to 25°C (68°F to 77°F). Protect from light and moisture; dispense in original airtight container.

Nursing Actions
Physical Assessment Not for use in acute asthma attack. Monitor for liver dysfunction.

Patient Education
- Discuss specific use of drug and side effects with patient as it relates to treatment. (HCAHPS: During this hospital stay, were you given any medicine that you had not taken before? Before giving you any new medicine, how often did hospital staff tell you what the medicine was for? How often did hospital staff describe possible side effects in a way you could understand?)
- Patient may experience headache, dyspepsia, nausea, diarrhea, or hepatic impairment. Have patient report immediately to prescriber uncontrollable breathing attack, signs of infection, depression, emotional instability, nervousness and anxiety, illogical thinking, flu-like syndrome, inability to eat, discolored urine, jaundice, severe asthenia, behavioral changes, or rash (HCAHPS).
- Educate patient about signs of a significant reaction (eg, wheezing; chest tightness; fever; itching; bad cough; blue skin color; seizures; or swelling of face, lips, tongue, or throat). **Note:** This is not a comprehensive list of all side effects. Patient should consult prescriber for additional questions.

Intended Use and Disclaimer: Should not be printed and given to patients. This information is intended to serve as a concise initial reference for healthcare professionals to use when discussing medications with a patient. You must ultimately rely on your own discretion, experience and judgment in diagnosing, treating and advising patients.

Dietary Considerations Should be taken on an empty stomach (1 hour before or 2 hours after meals).

Zaleplon (ZAL e plon)

Brand Names: U.S. Sonata

Pharmacologic Category Hypnotic, Miscellaneous

Medication Safety Issues
Sound-alike/look-alike issues:
Sonata may be confused with Soriatane

Zaleplon may be confused with Zelapar, Zemplar, zolpidem, ZyPREXA Zydis

BEERS Criteria medication:
This drug may be potentially inappropriate for use in geriatric patients (Quality of evidence - moderate; Strength of recommendation - strong).

Medication Guide Available Yes

Pregnancy Risk Factor C

Lactation Enters breast milk/not recommended

Breast-Feeding Considerations Zaleplon is excreted in human milk with the highest concentration ~1 hour after administration; therefore, the manufacturer does not recommended use while breast-feeding.

Use Short-term (7-10 days) treatment of insomnia (has been demonstrated to be effective for up to 5 weeks in controlled trial)

Mechanism of Action/Effect Zaleplon is unrelated to benzodiazepines, barbiturates, or other hypnotics. However, it interacts with the benzodiazepine GABA receptor complex. Nonclinical studies have shown that it binds selectively to the brain omega-1 receptor situated on the alpha subunit of the GABA-A receptor complex.

Contraindications Hypersensitivity to zaleplon or any component of the formulation

Warnings/Precautions Symptomatic treatment of insomnia should be initiated only after careful evaluation of potential causes of sleep disturbance. Failure of sleep disturbance to resolve after 7-10 days may indicate psychiatric and/or medical illness.

Use with caution in patients with depression, particularly if suicidal risk may be present. Use with caution in patients with a history of drug dependence. Abrupt discontinuance may lead to withdrawal symptoms. Hypnotics/sedatives have been associated with abnormal thinking and behavior changes including decreased inhibition, aggression, bizarre behavior, agitation, hallucinations, and depersonalization. These changes may occur unpredictably and may indicate previously unrecognized psychiatric disorders; evaluate appropriately. May impair physical and mental capabilities. Patients must be cautioned about performing tasks which require mental alertness (operating machinery or driving). Use with caution in patients receiving other CNS depressants or psychoactive medications. Effects with other sedative drugs or ethanol may be potentiated. Postmarketing studies have indicated that the use of hypnotic/sedative agents for sleep has been associated with hypersensitivity reactions including anaphylaxis as well as angioedema. An increased risk for hazardous sleep-related activities such as sleep-driving, cooking and eating food, and making phone calls while asleep have been noted; amnesia may also occur. Evaluation is recommended in patients who report any sleep-related episodes.

Avoid chronic use (>90 days) in older adults; adverse events, including delirium, falls, fractures, has been observed with nonbenzodiazepine hypnotic use in the elderly similar to events observed with benzodiazepines. Data suggests improvements in sleep duration and latency are minimal (Beers Criteria).

Use with caution in the elderly, those with compromised respiratory function, or hepatic impairment (dosage adjustment recommended in mild-to-moderate hepatic impairment; use is not recommended in patients with severe impairment). Because of the rapid onset of action, zaleplon should be administered immediately prior to bedtime or after the patient has gone to bed and is having difficulty falling asleep. Capsules contain tartrazine (FDC yellow #5); avoid in patients with sensitivity (caution in patients with asthma).

Drug Interactions

Avoid Concomitant Use

Avoid concomitant use of Zaleplon with any of the following: Azelastine (Nasal); Paraldehyde; Sodium Oxybate; Thalidomide

Decreased Effect

The levels/effects of Zaleplon may be decreased by: Flumazenil; Rifamycin Derivatives

Increased Effect/Toxicity

Zaleplon may increase the levels/effects of: Alcohol (Ethyl); Azelastine (Nasal); Buprenorphine; CNS Depressants; Hydrocodone; Methotrimeprazine; Metyrosine; Mirtazapine; Paraldehyde; Pramipexole; ROPINIRole; Rotigotine; Selective Serotonin Reuptake Inhibitors; Sodium Oxybate; Thalidomide; Zolpidem

The levels/effects of Zaleplon may be increased by: Brimonidine (Topical); Cimetidine; Doxylamine; Droperidol; HydrOXYzine; Magnesium Sulfate; Methotrimeprazine; Perampanel; Tapentadol

Nutritional/Ethanol Interactions

Ethanol: Ethanol may increase CNS depression. Management: Avoid or limit use of ethanol and monitor for increased effects.

Food: High-fat meals prolong absorption; delay T_{max} by 2 hours, and reduce C_{max} by 35%. Management: Avoid taking after a high-fat meal.

Herb/Nutraceutical: St John's wort may decrease zaleplon levels. Some herbal medications may increase CNS depression. Management: Avoid St John's wort, valerian, kava kava, and gotu kola.

Adverse Reactions

>10%: Central nervous system: Headache (30% to 42%)

1% to 10%:

Cardiovascular: Chest pain (≥1%), peripheral edema (≤1%)

Central nervous system: Dizziness (7% to 9%), drowsiness (5% to 6%), amnesia (2% to 4%), paresthesia (3%), altered sense of smell (<1% to 2%), depersonalization (<1% to 2%),

hyperacusis (1% to 2%), hypoesthesia (<1% to 2%), malaise (<1% to 2%), abnormality in thinking (≥1%), anxiety (≥1%), depression (≥1%), migraine (≥1%), nervousness (≥1%), hypertonia (1%), confusion (≤1%), hallucination (≤1%), vertigo (≤1%)

Dermatologic: Pruritus (≥1%), skin rash (≥1%), skin photosensitivity (≤1%)

Gastrointestinal: Nausea (6% to 8%), abdominal pain (6%), anorexia (<1% to 2%), constipation (≥1%), dysgeusia (≥1%), dyspepsia (≥1%), xerostomia (≥1%), colitis (≤1%)

Genitourinary: Dysmenorrhea (3% to 4%)

Neuromuscular & skeletal: Weakness (5% to 7%), tremor (2%), arthralgia (≥1%), arthritis (≥1%), back pain (≥1%), myalgia (≥1%)

Ophthalmic: Eye pain (3% to 4%), visual disturbance (<1% to 2%), conjunctivitis (≥1%)

Otic: Otalgia (≤1%)

Respiratory: Bronchitis (≥1%), epistaxis (≤1%)

Miscellaneous: Fever (≥1%)

Pharmacodynamics/Kinetics

Onset of Action Rapid

Controlled Substance C-IV

Available Dosage Forms

Capsule, Oral:

Sonata: 5 mg, 10 mg

Generic: 5 mg, 10 mg

General Dosage Range Dosage adjustment recommended in patients with hepatic impairment

Oral:

Adults: 5-20 mg at bedtime

Elderly: 5 mg at bedtime (maximum: 10 mg/day)

Administration

Oral Administer immediately before bedtime or when the patient is in bed and cannot fall asleep.

Storage/Stability Store at controlled room temperature of 20°C to 25°C (68°F to 77°F). Protect from light.

Nursing Actions

Physical Assessment Assess for history of addiction (long-term use may result in dependence, abuse, or tolerance). For inpatient use, institute safety measures to prevent falls.

Patient Education

• Discuss specific use of drug and side effects with patient as it relates to treatment. (HCAHPS: During this hospital stay, were you given any medicine that you had not taken before? Before giving you any new medicine, how often did hospital staff tell you what the medicine was for? How often did hospital staff describe possible side effects in a way you could understand?)

• Patient may experience headache, presyncope, fatigue, blurred vision, illogical thinking, asthenia, nausea, or erythema. Have patient report immediately to prescriber depression, nervousness, emotional instability, illogical thinking, anxiety, sudden vision changes, memory loss, or rash (HCAHPS).

• Educate patient about signs of a significant reaction (eg, wheezing; chest tightness; fever; itching; bad cough; blue skin color; seizures; or swelling of face, lips, tongue, or throat). **Note:** This is not a comprehensive list of all side effects. Patient should consult prescriber for additional questions.

Intended Use and Disclaimer: Should not be printed and given to patients. This information is intended to serve as a concise initial reference for healthcare professionals to use when discussing medications with a patient. You must ultimately rely on your own discretion, experience and judgment in diagnosing, treating and advising patients.

Dietary Considerations Avoid taking with or after a heavy, high-fat meal; reduces absorption.

Zanamivir (za NA mi veer)

Brand Names: U.S. Relenza Diskhaler
Pharmacologic Category Antiviral Agent; Neuraminidase Inhibitor
Medication Safety Issues
Sound-alike/look-alike issues:
Relenza® may be confused with Albenza®, Aplenzin™
Pregnancy Risk Factor C
Lactation Excretion in breast milk unknown/use caution
Breast-Feeding Considerations It is not known if zanamivir is found in human milk and the manufacturer recommends that caution be exercised when administering zanamivir to nursing women. According to the CDC, breast-feeding while taking zanamivir can be continued. The CDC recommends that women infected with the influenza virus follow general precautions (eg, frequent hand washing) to decrease viral transmission to the child. Mothers with influenza-like illnesses at delivery should consider avoiding close contact with the infant until they have received 48 hours of antiviral medication, fever has resolved, and cough and secretions can be controlled. These measures may help decrease (but not eliminate) the risk of transmitting influenza to the newborn. During this time, breast milk can be expressed and bottle-fed to the infant by another person who is well. Protective measures, such as wearing a face mask, changing into a clean gown or clothing, and strict hand hygiene should be continued by the mother for ≥7 days after the onset of symptoms or until symptom-free for 24 hours. Infant care should be performed by a noninfected person when possible (consult current CDC guidelines). Influenza may cause serious illness in postpartum women and prompt evaluation for febrile respiratory illnesses is recommended.
Use Treatment of uncomplicated acute illness due to influenza virus A and B in patients who have

been symptomatic for no more than 2 days; prophylaxis against influenza virus A and B

The Advisory Committee on Immunization Practices (ACIP) recommends that **treatment** be considered for the following:
• Persons with severe, complicated or progressive illness
• Hospitalized persons
• Persons at higher risk for influenza complications:
  - Children <2 years of age (highest risk in children <6 months of age)
  - Adults ≥65 years of age
  - Persons with chronic disorders of the pulmonary (including asthma) or cardiovascular systems (except hypertension)
  - Persons with chronic metabolic diseases (including diabetes mellitus), hepatic disease, renal dysfunction, hematologic disorders (including sickle cell disease), or immunosuppression (including immunosuppression caused by medications or HIV)
  - Persons with neurologic/neuromuscular conditions (including conditions such as spinal cord injuries, seizure disorders, cerebral palsy, stroke, mental retardation, moderate to severe developmental delay, or muscular dystrophy) which may compromise respiratory function, the handling of respiratory secretions, or that can increase the risk of aspiration
  - Pregnant or postpartum women (≤2 weeks after delivery)
  - Persons <19 years of age on long-term aspirin therapy
  - American Indians and Alaskan Natives
  - Persons who are morbidly obese (BMI ≥40)
  - Residents of nursing homes or other chronic care facilities
• Use may also be considered for previously healthy, nonhigh-risk outpatients with confirmed or suspected influenza based on clinical judgment when treatment can be started within 48 hours of illness onset.

The ACIP recommends that **prophylaxis** be considered for the following:
• Postexposure prophylaxis may be considered for family or close contacts of suspected or confirmed cases, who are at higher risk of influenza complications, and who have not been vaccinated against the circulating strain at the time of the exposure.
• Postexposure prophylaxis may be considered for unvaccinated healthcare workers who had occupational exposure without protective equipment.
• Pre-exposure prophylaxis should only be used for persons at very high risk of influenza complications who cannot be otherwise protected at times of high risk for exposure.

- Prophylaxis should also be administered to all eligible residents of institutions that house patients at high risk when needed to control outbreaks.

Mechanism of Action/Effect Zanamivir inhibits influenza virus neuraminidase enzymes, potentially altering virus particle aggregation and release.

Contraindications Hypersensitivity to zanamivir or any component of the formulation (contains milk proteins)

Warnings/Precautions Allergic-like reactions, including anaphylaxis, oropharyngeal edema, and serious skin rashes have been reported. Rare occurrences of neuropsychiatric events (including confusion, delirium, hallucinations, and/or self-injury) have been reported from postmarketing surveillance; direct causation is difficult to establish (influenza infection may also be associated with behavioral and neurologic changes). Patients must be instructed in the use of the delivery system. Antiviral treatment should begin within 48 hours of symptom onset. However, the CDC recommends that treatment may still be beneficial and should be started in hospitalized patients with severe, complicated or progressive illness if >48 hours. Treatment should not be delayed while awaiting results of laboratory tests for influenza. Nonhospitalized persons who are not at high risk for developing severe or complicated illness and who have a mild disease are not likely to benefit if treatment is started >48 hours after symptom onset. Nonhospitalized persons who are already beginning to recover do not need treatment. Effectiveness has not been established in patients with significant underlying medical conditions or for prophylaxis of influenza in nursing home patients (per manufacturer). The CDC recommends zanamivir to be used to control institutional outbreaks of influenza when circulating strains are suspected of being resistant to oseltamivir (refer to current guidelines). Not recommended for use in patients with underlying respiratory disease, such as asthma or COPD, due to lack of efficacy and risk of serious adverse effects. Bronchospasm, decreased lung function, and other serious adverse reactions, including those with fatal outcomes, have been reported in patients with and without airway disease; discontinue with bronchospasm or signs of decreased lung function. For a patient with an underlying airway disease where a medical decision has been made to use zanamivir, a fast-acting bronchodilator should be made available, and used prior to each dose. Not a substitute for annual flu vaccination; has not been shown to reduce risk of transmission of influenza to others. Consider primary or concomitant bacterial infections. Powder for oral inhalation contains lactose; use contraindicated in patients allergic to milk proteins. The inhalation powder should only be administered via inhalation using the provided Diskhaler® delivery device. The commercially available formulation is **not** intended to be solubilized or administered via any nebulizer/mechanical ventilator; inappropriate administration has resulted in death. Safety and efficacy of repeated courses or use with hepatic impairment or severe renal impairment have not been established. Indicated for children ≥5 years of age (for influenza prophylaxis) and children ≥7 years of age (for influenza treatment); children ages 5-6 years may have inadequate inhalation (via Diskhaler®) for the treatment of influenza.

Drug Interactions

Avoid Concomitant Use There are no known interactions where it is recommended to avoid concomitant use.

Decreased Effect

Zanamivir may decrease the levels/effects of: Influenza Virus Vaccine (Live/Attenuated)

Increased Effect/Toxicity There are no known significant interactions involving an increase in effect.

Adverse Reactions Most adverse reactions occurred at a frequency which was less than or equal to the control (lactose vehicle).

>10%:

Central nervous system: Headache (prophylaxis 13% to 24%; treatment 2%)

Gastrointestinal: Throat/tonsil discomfort/pain (prophylaxis 8% to 19%)

Respiratory: Nasal signs and symptoms (prophylaxis 12% to 20%; treatment 2%), cough (prophylaxis 7% to 17%; treatment ≤2%)

Miscellaneous: Viral infection (prophylaxis 3% to 13%)

1% to 10%:

Central nervous system: Fever/chills (prophylaxis 5% to 9%; treatment <1.5%), fatigue (prophylaxis 5% to 8%; treatment <1.5%), malaise (prophylaxis 5% to 8%; treatment <1.5%), dizziness (treatment 1% to 2%)

Dermatologic: Urticaria (treatment <1.5%)

Gastrointestinal: Anorexia/appetite decreased (prophylaxis 2% to 4%), appetite increased (prophylaxis 2% to 4%), nausea (prophylaxis 1% to 2%; treatment ≤3%), diarrhea (prophylaxis 2%; treatment 2% to 3%), vomiting (prophylaxis 1% to 2%; treatment 1% to 2%), abdominal pain (treatment <1.5%)

Neuromuscular & skeletal: Muscle pain (prophylaxis 3% to 8%), musculoskeletal pain (prophylaxis 6%), arthralgia/articular rheumatism (prophylaxis 2%), arthralgia (treatment <1.5%), myalgia (treatment <1.5%)

Respiratory: Infection (ear/nose/throat; prophylaxis 2%; treatment 1% to 5%), sinusitis (treatment 3%), bronchitis (treatment 2%), nasal inflammation (prophylaxis 1%)

Available Dosage Forms

Aerosol Powder Breath Activated, Inhalation: Relenza Diskhaler: 5 mg/blister (20 ea)

General Dosage Range Oral inhalation:
Children ≥5 years: Prophylaxis: 10 mg once daily
Children ≥7 years: Treatment: 10 mg twice daily
Adolescents and Adults: Prophylaxis: 10 mg once to twice daily; Treatment: 10 mg twice daily

Administration

Inhalation Must be used with Diskhaler® delivery device. The foil blister disk containing zanamivir inhalation powder should not be manipulated, solubilized, or administered via a nebulizer. Patients who are scheduled to use an inhaled bronchodilator should use their bronchodilator prior to zanamivir. With the exception of the initial dose when used for treatment, administer at the same time each day.

Storage/Stability Store at 25°C (77°F); excursions permitted to 15°C to 30°C (59°F to 86°F). Do not puncture blister until taking a dose using the Diskhaler®.

Nursing Actions

Physical Assessment Recommendations for antiviral susceptibility and effectiveness may change. Validate with the CDC recommendations for use prior to prescribing. Therapy for treatment must be started within 48 hours of first influenza symptoms. Monitor for change in behavior.

Patient Education
- Discuss specific use of drug and side effects with patient as it relates to treatment. (HCAHPS: During this hospital stay, were you given any medicine that you had not taken before? Before giving you any new medicine, how often did hospital staff tell you what the medicine was for? How often did hospital staff describe possible side effects in a way you could understand?)
- Patient may experience headache, rhinitis, or pharyngitis. Have patient report immediately to prescriber dyspnea, behavioral problems, illogical thinking, or rash (HCAHPS).
- Educate patient about signs of a significant reaction (eg, wheezing; chest tightness; fever; itching; bad cough; blue skin color; seizures; or swelling of face, lips, tongue, or throat). **Note:** This is not a comprehensive list of all side effects. Patient should consult prescriber for additional questions.

Intended Use and Disclaimer: Should not be printed and given to patients. This information is intended to serve as a concise initial reference for healthcare professionals to use when discussing medications with a patient. You must ultimately rely on your own discretion, experience and judgment in diagnosing, treating and advising patients.

Ziconotide (zi KOE no tide)

Brand Names: U.S. Prialt
Pharmacologic Category Analgesic, Nonopioid; Calcium Channel Blocker, N-Type

Medication Safety Issues
High alert medication:
The Institute for Safe Medication Practices (ISMP) includes this medication among its list of drugs which have a heightened risk of causing significant patient harm when used in error.

Pregnancy Risk Factor C

Lactation Excretion in breast milk unknown/not recommended

Breast-Feeding Considerations It is not known if ziconotide is excreted into breast milk. Due to the potential for serious adverse reactions in the nursing infant, the manufacturer recommends a decision be made whether to discontinue nursing or to discontinue the drug, taking into account the importance of treatment to the mother.

Use Management of severe chronic pain in patients requiring intrathecal (I.T.) therapy and who are intolerant or refractory to other therapies

Mechanism of Action/Effect Ziconotide selectively binds to N-type voltage-sensitive calcium channels located on the nociceptive afferent nerves of the dorsal horn in the spinal cord. This binding is thought to block N-type calcium channels, leading to a blockade of excitatory neurotransmitter release and reducing sensitivity to painful stimuli.

Contraindications Hypersensitivity to ziconotide or any component of the formulation; history of psychosis; I.V. administration
I.T. administration is contraindicated in patients with infection at the injection site, uncontrolled bleeding, or spinal canal obstruction that impairs CSF circulation

Warnings/Precautions [U.S Boxed Warning]: Severe psychiatric symptoms and neurological impairment have been reported; interrupt or discontinue therapy if cognitive impairment, hallucinations, mood changes, or changes in consciousness occur. May cause or worsen depression and/or risk of suicide. Cognitive impairment may appear gradually during treatment and is generally reversible after discontinuation (may take up to 2 weeks for cognitive effects to reverse). Use caution in the elderly; may experience a higher incidence of confusion. Patients should be instructed to use caution in performing tasks which require alertness (eg, operating machinery or driving). May have additive effects with opioids or other CNS-depressant medications; may potentiate opioid-induced decreased GI motility; does not interact with opioid receptors or potentiate opioid-induced respiratory depression. Will not prevent or relieve symptoms associated with opioid withdrawal and opioids should not be abruptly discontinued. Unlike opioids, ziconotide therapy can be interrupted abruptly or discontinued without evidence of withdrawal.

Meningitis may occur with use of I.T. pumps; monitor for signs and symptoms of meningitis; treatment of meningitis may require removal of system and discontinuation of intrathecal therapy. Elevated serum creatine kinase can occur, particularly during the first 2 months of therapy; consider dose reduction or discontinuing if combined with new neuromuscular symptoms (myalgias, myasthenia, muscle cramps, weakness) or reduction in physical activity. Safety and efficacy have not been established with renal or hepatic dysfunction, or in pediatric patients. Should not be used in combination with intrathecal opioids.

Drug Interactions

Avoid Concomitant Use

Avoid concomitant use of Ziconotide with any of the following: Azelastine (Nasal); Paraldehyde; Thalidomide

Decreased Effect There are no known significant interactions involving a decrease in effect.

Increased Effect/Toxicity

Ziconotide may increase the levels/effects of: Alcohol (Ethyl); Azelastine (Nasal); Buprenorphine; CNS Depressants; Hydrocodone; Methotrimeprazine; Metyrosine; Mirtazapine; Paraldehyde; Pramipexole; ROPINIRole; Rotigotine; Selective Serotonin Reuptake Inhibitors; Thalidomide; Zolpidem

The levels/effects of Ziconotide may be increased by: Brimonidine (Topical); Doxylamine; Droperidol; HydrOXYzine; Magnesium Sulfate; Methotrimeprazine; Perampanel; Sodium Oxybate; Tapentadol

Nutritional/Ethanol Interactions Ethanol: May increase CNS depression; monitor for increased effects with coadministration. Caution patients about effects.

Adverse Reactions

>10%:

Central nervous system: Dizziness (46%), confusion (15% to 33%), memory impairment (7% to 22%), somnolence (17%), ataxia (14%), speech disorder (14%), headache (13%), aphasia (12%), hallucination (12%; including auditory and visual)

Gastrointestinal: Nausea (40%), diarrhea (18%), vomiting (16%)

Neuromuscular & skeletal: Creatine kinase increased (40%; ≥3 times ULN: 11%), weakness (18%), gait disturbances (14%)

Ocular: Blurred vision (12%)

2% to 10%:

Cardiovascular: Hypotension, orthostatic hypotension, peripheral edema

Central nervous system: Abnormal thinking (8%), amnesia (8%), anxiety (8%), vertigo (7%), insomnia (6%), fever (5%), paranoid reaction (3%), delirium (2%), hostility (2%), stupor (2%), agitation, attention disturbance, balance impaired, burning sensation, coordination

abnormal, depression, disorientation, fatigue, fever, hypoesthesia, irritability, lethargy, mental impairment, mood disorder, nervousness, pain, sedation

Dermatologic: Pruritus (7%)

Gastrointestinal: Anorexia (6%), taste perversion (5%), abdominal pain, appetite decreased, constipation, xerostomia

Genitourinary: Urinary retention (9%), dysuria, urinary hesitance

Neuromuscular & skeletal: Dysarthria (7%), paresthesia (7%), rigors (7%), tremor (7%), muscle spasm (6%), limb pain (5%), areflexia, muscle cramp, muscle weakness, myalgia

Ocular: Nystagmus (8%), diplopia, visual disturbance

Respiratory: Sinusitis (5%)

Miscellaneous: Diaphoresis (5%)

Available Dosage Forms

Solution, Intrathecal [preservative free]:

Prialt: 500 mcg/20 mL (20 mL); 100 mcg/mL (1 mL); 500 mcg/5 mL (5 mL)

General Dosage Range Dosage adjustment recommended in patients who develop toxicities

I.T.: *Adults:* Initial dose: ≤2.4 mcg/day (0.1 mcg/hour); Maintenance range: 2.4-19.2 mcg/day (0.1-0.8 mcg/hour) (maximum: 19.2 mcg/day [0.8 mcg/hour])

Administration

I.V. Not for I.V. administration

Other Not for I.V. administration. **For I.T. administration only** using Medtronic SynchroMed® EL, SynchroMed® II Infusion System, or CADD-Micro® ambulatory infusion pump.

Medtronic SynchroMed® EL or SynchroMed® II Infusion Systems:

Naive pump priming (first time use with ziconotide): Use 2 mL of undiluted ziconotide 25 mcg/mL solution to rinse the internal surfaces of the pump; repeat twice for a total of 3 rinses

Initial pump fill: Use only undiluted 25 mcg/mL solution and fill pump after priming. Following the initial fill only, adsorption on internal device surfaces will occur, requiring the use of the undiluted solution and refill within 14 days.

Pump refills: Contents should be emptied prior to refill. Subsequent pump refills should occur at least every 40 days if using diluted solution or at least every 84 days if using undiluted solution.

CADD-Micro® ambulatory infusion pump: Refer to manufacturer's manual for initial fill and refill instructions

pH: 4-5

Preparation for Administration Preservative free NS should be used when dilution is needed. CADD-Micro® ambulatory infusion pump: Initial fill: Dilute to final concentration of 5 mcg/mL. ▶

Medtronic SynchroMed® EL or SynchroMed® II infusion system: Prior to initial fill, rinse internal pump surfaces with 2 mL ziconotide (25 mcg/mL), repeat twice. Only the 25 mcg/mL concentration (undiluted) should be used for initial pump fill.

Storage/Stability Prior to use, store vials at 2°C to 8°C (36°F to 46°F). Once diluted, may be stored at 2°C to 8°C (36°F to 46°F) for 24 hours; refrigerate during transit. Do not freeze. Protect from light.

When using the Medtronic SynchroMed® EL or SynchroMed® II Infusion System, solutions expire as follows:

25 mcg/mL: Undiluted:
Initial fill: Use within 14 days.
Refill: Use within 84 days.
100 mcg/mL:
Undiluted: Refill: Use within 84 days.
Diluted: Refill: Use within 40 days.

Nursing Actions

Physical Assessment This medication is given intrathecally via pump. Monitor for changes in behavior, cognitive impairment, hallucinations, or changes in mood or consciousness.

Patient Education

• Discuss specific use of drug and side effects with patient as it relates to treatment. (HCAHPS: During this hospital stay, were you given any medicine that you had not taken before? Before giving you any new medicine, how often did hospital staff tell you what the medicine was for? How often did hospital staff describe possible side effects in a way you could understand?)

• Patient may experience presyncope, fatigue, blurred vision, illogical thinking, nausea, diarrhea, or asthenia. Have patient report immediately to prescriber depression, thoughts of suicide, anxiety, seizures, poor pain control, significant change in balance, severe headache, neck stiffness, considerable myalgia, or rash (HCAHPS).

• Educate patient about signs of a significant reaction (eg, wheezing; chest tightness; fever; itching; bad cough; blue skin color; seizures; or swelling of face, lips, tongue, or throat). **Note:** This is not a comprehensive list of all side effects. Patient should consult prescriber for additional questions.

Intended Use and Disclaimer: Should not be printed and given to patients. This information is intended to serve as a concise initial reference for healthcare professionals to use when discussing medications with a patient. You must ultimately rely on your own discretion, experience and judgment in diagnosing, treating and advising patients.

Zidovudine (zye DOE vyoo deen)

Brand Names: U.S. Retrovir

Index Terms Azidothymidine; AZT (error-prone abbreviation); Compound S; ZDV

Pharmacologic Category Antiretroviral, Reverse Transcriptase Inhibitor, Nucleoside (Anti-HIV)

Medication Safety Issues

Sound-alike/look-alike issues:

Azidothymidine may be confused with azaTHIOprine, aztreonam

Retrovir® may be confused with acyclovir, ritonavir

Other safety concerns:

AZT is an error-prone abbreviation (mistaken as azathioprine, aztreonam)

Pregnancy Risk Factor C

Lactation Enters breast milk/contraindicated

Breast-Feeding Considerations Concentrations of zidovudine in breast milk are similar to those in the maternal serum. Maternal or infant antiretroviral therapy does not completely eliminate the risk of postnatal HIV transmission. In addition, multiclass-resistant virus has been detected in breast-feeding infants despite maternal therapy. Therefore, in the United States, where formula is accessible, affordable, safe, and sustainable, and the risk of infant mortality due to diarrhea and respiratory infections is low, complete avoidance of breast-feeding by HIV-infected women is recommended to decrease potential transmission of HIV (DHHS [perinatal], 2012).

Use Treatment of HIV infection in combination with at least two other antiretroviral agents; prevention of maternal/fetal HIV transmission

Unlabeled Use Postexposure prophylaxis for HIV exposure as part of a multidrug regimen

Mechanism of Action/Effect Zidovudine is a thymidine analog which interferes with the HIV virus that results in inhibition of viral replication.

Contraindications Life-threatening hypersensitivity to zidovudine or any component of the formulation

Canadian labeling: Additional contraindications (not in U.S. labeling): Neutrophil count <750/mm³ or hemoglobin <7.5 g/dL (4.65 mmol/L)

Warnings/Precautions Hazardous agent - use appropriate precautions for handling and disposal (NIOSH, 2012). **[U.S. Boxed Warning]: Hematologic toxicity, including neutropenia and severe anemia have been reported with use.** Toxicity may be related to duration of use and prior bone marrow reserve. Use with caution in patients with bone marrow compromise (granulocytes <1000 cells/mm³ or hemoglobin <9.5 mg/dL); dose interruption may be required in patients who develop anemia or neutropenia. **[U.S. Boxed Warning]: Lactic acidosis and severe hepatomegaly with steatosis have been reported, including fatal cases.** Risks may be increased with liver disease, obesity, pregnancy, prolonged exposure, or in females. Suspend treatment with zidovudine in any patient who develops clinical or laboratory findings suggestive of lactic acidosis (transaminase elevation may/may not accompany hepatomegaly and steatosis). Use caution in combination with interferon alfa with or without ribavirin in HIV/HCV coinfected patients; monitor closely for hepatic decompensation, anemia, or neutropenia; dose reduction or discontinuation of interferon and/or ribavirin may be required if toxicity evident. **[U.S. Boxed Warning]: Prolonged use has been associated with symptomatic myopathy and myositis.** May cause redistribution of fat (eg, buffalo hump, peripheral wasting with increased abdominal girth, cushingoid appearance). Immune reconstitution syndrome may develop resulting in the occurrence of an inflammatory response to an indolent or residual opportunistic infection during initial HIV treatment or activation of autoimmune disorders (eg, Graves' disease, polymyositis, Guillain-Barré syndrome) later in therapy; further evaluation and treatment may be required. Hematologic toxicity may be increased due to increased serum concentrations in patients with severe hepatic impairment. Use with caution in patients with severe renal impairment; dosage adjustment recommended. Reduce dose in patients with severe renal impairment. Do not administer with combination products that contain zidovudine as one of their components (eg, COMBIVIR® [lamivudine and zidovudine] or TRIZIVIR® [abacavir sulfate, lamivudine, and zidovudine]).

Drug Interactions

Avoid Concomitant Use

Avoid concomitant use of Zidovudine with any of the following: CloZAPine; Stavudine

Decreased Effect

Zidovudine may decrease the levels/effects of: Stavudine

The levels/effects of Zidovudine may be decreased by: Clarithromycin; DOXOrubicin (Conventional); DOXOrubicin (Liposomal); Protease Inhibitors; Rifamycin Derivatives

Increased Effect/Toxicity

Zidovudine may increase the levels/effects of: CloZAPine; Ribavirin

The levels/effects of Zidovudine may be increased by: Acyclovir-Valacyclovir; Clarithromycin; DOXOrubicin (Conventional); DOXOrubicin (Liposomal); Fluconazole; Ganciclovir-Valganciclovir; Interferons; Methadone; Probenecid; Raltegravir; Valproic Acid and Derivatives

Adverse Reactions Note: Percentages noted with adults unless otherwise stated.

>10%:

Central nervous system: Headache (63%), malaise (53%), fever (children 25%)

Dermatologic: Rash (children 12%)

Gastrointestinal: Nausea (adults 51%; children 8%), anorexia (20%), vomiting (adults 17%; children 8%)

Hematologic: Macrocytosis (children >50%), anemia (neonates 22%; children 4%; adults 1%; onset 2-4 weeks)

Hepatic: Hepatomegaly (children 11%)

Respiratory: Cough (children 15%)

1% to 10%:

Cardiovascular: ECG abnormality (children <6%), edema (children <6%), heart failure (children <6%), left ventricular dilation (children <6%)

Central nervous system: Irritability (children <6%), nervousness (children <6%), chills (≥5%), fatigue (≥5%), insomnia (≥5%)

Gastrointestinal: Diarrhea (children 8%), constipation (6%), weight loss (children <6%), abdominal cramps (≥5%), abdominal pain (≥5%), dyspepsia (≥5%)

Genitourinary: Hematuria (children <6%)

Hematologic: Neutropenia (children 8%), granulocytopenia (2%; onset 6-8 weeks), thrombocytopenia (children 1%)

Hepatic: Transaminases increased (1% to 3%)

Neuromuscular & skeletal: Weakness (9%), arthralgia (≥5%), musculoskeletal pain (≥5%), myalgia (≥5%), neuropathy (≥5%)

Otic: Discharge/erythema/pain/swelling (7%)

Available Dosage Forms

Capsule, Oral:

Retrovir: 100 mg

Generic: 100 mg

Solution, Intravenous [preservative free]:

Retrovir: 10 mg/mL (20 mL)

Syrup, Oral:

Retrovir: 50 mg/5 mL (240 mL)

Generic: 50 mg/5 mL (240 mL)

Tablet, Oral:

Generic: 300 mg

General Dosage Range Dosage adjustment recommended in patients with renal impairment or who develop toxicities

I.V.:

Infants <30 weeks gestation at birth: 1.5 mg/kg/dose every 12 hours; at 4 weeks of age advance to 2.3 mg/kg/dose every 12 hours

Infants ≥30 weeks and <35 weeks gestation at birth: 1.5 mg/kg/dose every 12 hours; at 15 days of age, advance to 2.3 mg/kg/dose every 12 hours

Infants ≥35 weeks: 3 mg/kg/dose every 12 hour

Children 6 weeks to <12 years: 120 mg/m^2/dose every 6 hours **or** 20 mg/m^2/hour as a continuous infusion

Children ≥12 years and Adults: 1 mg/kg/dose every 4 hours around-the-clock **or** 2 mg/kg bolus followed by 1 mg/kg/hour continuous infusion during labor and delivery

Oral:

Infants <30 weeks gestation at birth: 2 mg/kg/dose every 12 hours; at 4 weeks of age advance to 3 mg/kg/dose every 12 hours

Infants ≥30 weeks and <35 weeks gestation at birth: 2 mg/kg/dose every 12 hours; at 15 days of age, advance to 3 mg/kg/dose every 12 hours

Infants ≥35 weeks: 4 mg/kg/dose twice daily

Children 4 weeks to <18 years: 240 mg/m² every 12 hours (maximum: 300 mg every 12 hours) **or** 160 mg/m²/dose every 8 hours (maximum: 200 mg every 8 hours)

4 to <9 kg: 12 mg/kg/dose twice daily **or** 8 mg/kg/dose 3 times/day

≥9 to <30 kg: 9 mg/kg/dose twice daily **or** 6 mg/kg/dose 3 times/day

≥30 kg and Adults: 300 mg twice daily **or** 200 mg 3 times/day

Administration

I.M. Do not give I.M.

Hazardous agent; use appropriate precautions for handling and disposal (NIOSH, 2012).

I.V. Avoid rapid infusion or bolus injection

Neonates: Infuse over 30 minutes

Adults: Infuse over 1 hour; in pregnant women, infuse loading dose over 1 hour followed by continuous infusion

Hazardous agent; use appropriate precautions for handling and disposal (NIOSH, 2012).

Injectable Detail pH: 5.5

Oral Administer around-the-clock to promote less variation in peak and trough serum levels. Oral zidovudine may be administered without regard to meals.

Hazardous agent; use appropriate precautions for handling and disposal (NIOSH, 2012).

Preparation for Administration Hazardous agent; use appropriate precautions for handling and disposal (NIOSH, 2012). Solution for injection should be diluted with D₅W to a concentration ≤4 mg/mL. Attempt to administer diluted solution within 8 hours if stored at room temperature or 24 hours if refrigerated to minimize potential for microbial-contaminated solutions (vials are single-use and do not contain preservative).

Storage/Stability

I.V.: Store undiluted vials at 15°C to 25°C (59°F to 77°F). Protect from light. When diluted, solution is physically and chemically stable for 24 hours at room temperature and 48 hours if refrigerated.

Tablets, capsules, syrup: Store at 15°C to 25°C (59°F to 77°F). Protect capsules from moisture.

Nursing Actions

Physical Assessment Allergy history should be assessed prior to beginning treatment. Monitor for lactic acidosis (elevated transaminases), anemia, neutropenia, hepatic decompensation, gastrointestinal disturbance (nausea, vomiting, diarrhea), myalgia, and peripheral neuropathy. Teach patient proper timing of multiple medications.

Patient Education
- Discuss specific use of drug and side effects with patient as it relates to treatment. (HCAHPS: During this hospital stay, were you given any medicine that you had not taken before? Before giving you any new medicine, how often did hospital staff tell you what the medicine was for? How often did hospital staff describe possible side effects in a way you could understand?)
- Patient may experience headache, nausea, loss of appetite, anemia, or leukopenia. Have patient report immediately to prescriber dyspnea, severe dyspepsia, diarrhea, discolored urine, jaundice, asthenia, or rash (HCAHPS).
- Educate patient about signs of a significant reaction (eg, wheezing; chest tightness; fever; itching; bad cough; blue skin color; seizures; or swelling of face, lips, tongue, or throat). **Note:** This is not a comprehensive list of all side effects. Patient should consult prescriber for additional questions.

Intended Use and Disclaimer: Should not be printed and given to patients. This information is intended to serve as a concise initial reference for healthcare professionals to use when discussing medications with a patient. You must ultimately rely on your own discretion, experience and judgment in diagnosing, treating and advising patients.

Dietary Considerations May be taken without regard to meals.

Related Information

Oral Medications That Should Not Be Crushed or Altered *on page 1712*

Zileuton (zye LOO ton)

Brand Names: U.S. Zyflo; Zyflo CR

Pharmacologic Category 5-Lipoxygenase Inhibitor

Pregnancy Risk Factor C

Lactation Excretion in breast milk unknown/not recommended

Breast-Feeding Considerations It is not known if zileuton is excreted into breast milk. Due to the potential tumorigenicity of zileuton in animal studies, the manufacturer does not recommend breast-feeding.

Use Prophylaxis and chronic treatment of asthma

Mechanism of Action/Effect Inhibits leukotriene formation which contributes to inflammation, edema, mucous secretion, and bronchoconstriction in the airway of the asthmatic.

Contraindications Hypersensitivity to zileuton or any component of the formulation; active liver disease or transaminase elevations ≥3 times ULN

Warnings/Precautions Not indicated for the reversal of bronchospasm in acute asthma attacks, including status asthmaticus; therapy may be continued during acute asthma exacerbations. Hepatic adverse effects have been reported (elevated transaminase levels); females >65 years and patients with pre-existing elevated transaminases may be at greater risk. Serum ALT should be monitored. Discontinue zileuton and follow transaminases until normal if patients develop clinical signs/symptoms of liver dysfunction or with transaminase levels >5 times ULN (use caution with history of liver disease and/or in those patients who consume substantial quantities of ethanol). Due to the risk of hepatotoxicity, the manufacturer does not recommend use of zileuton in children <12 years of age. Postmarketing reports of behavioral changes and sleep disorders have been noted.

Drug Interactions

Avoid Concomitant Use

Avoid concomitant use of Zileuton with any of the following: Pimozide

Decreased Effect There are no known significant interactions involving a decrease in effect.

Increased Effect/Toxicity

Zileuton may increase the levels/effects of: Pimozide; Propranolol; Theophylline; Warfarin

Nutritional/Ethanol Interactions

Ethanol: Avoid ethanol (may increase CNS depression; may increase risk of hepatic toxicity).

Food: Zyflo CR®: Improved absorption when administered with food.

Herb/Nutraceutical: St John's wort may decrease zileuton levels.

Adverse Reactions

>10%: Central nervous system: Headache (23% to 25%)

1% to 10%:

Cardiovascular: Chest pain

Central nervous system: Pain (8%), dizziness, fever, insomnia, malaise, nervousness, somnolence

Dermatologic: Pruritus, rash

Gastrointestinal: Dyspepsia (8%), diarrhea (5%), nausea (5% to 6%), abdominal pain (5%), constipation, flatulence, vomiting

Genitourinary: Urinary tract infection, vaginitis

Hematologic: Leukopenia (1% to 3%)

Hepatic: ALT increased (≥3 x ULN: 2% to 5%), hepatotoxicity

Neuromuscular & skeletal: Myalgia (7%), weakness (4%), arthralgia, hypertonia, neck pain/rigidity

Ocular: Conjunctivitis

Respiratory: Upper respiratory tract infection (9%), sinusitis (7%), pharyngolaryngeal pain (5%)

Miscellaneous: Hypersensitivity reactions, lymphadenopathy

Available Dosage Forms

Tablet, Oral:

Zyflo: 600 mg

Tablet Extended Release 12 Hour, Oral:

Zyflo CR: 600 mg

General Dosage Range Oral:

Extended release: *Children ≥12 years and Adults:* 1200 mg twice daily

Immediate release: *Children ≥12 years and Adults:* 600 mg 4 times/day

Administration

Oral

Immediate release: Administer without regard to meals.

Extended release: Do not crush, cut, or chew tablet; administer within 1 hour after morning and evening meals.

Storage/Stability Store tablets at 20°C to 25°C (68°F to 77°F). Protect from light.

Nursing Actions

Physical Assessment Not for use to relieve acute asthmatic attacks. Monitor vital signs and lung sounds prior to and periodically during therapy.

Patient Education

- Discuss specific use of drug and side effects with patient as it relates to treatment. (HCAHPS: During this hospital stay, were you given any medicine that you had not taken before? Before giving you any new medicine, how often did hospital staff tell you what the medicine was for? How often did hospital staff describe possible side effects in a way you could understand?)

- Patient may experience headache, dyspepsia, nausea, or diarrhea. Have patient report immediately to prescriber uncontrollable breathing attack, flu-like syndrome, inability to eat, discolored urine, jaundice, severe fatigue, increase inhaler usage, change in behavior, or rash (HCAHPS).

- Educate patient about signs of a significant reaction (eg, wheezing; chest tightness; fever; itching; bad cough; blue skin color; seizures; or swelling of face, lips, tongue, or throat). **Note:** This is not a comprehensive list of all side effects. Patient should consult prescriber for additional questions.

Intended Use and Disclaimer: Should not be printed and given to patients. This information is intended to serve as a concise initial reference for healthcare professionals to use when discussing medications with a patient. You must ultimately rely on your own discretion, experience and judgment in diagnosing, treating and advising patients.

Dietary Considerations
Immediate release: Take without regard to meals.
Extended release: Take with food.
Related Information
Oral Medications That Should Not Be Crushed or
Altered *on page 1712*

Ziprasidone (zi PRAS i done)

Brand Names: U.S. Geodon
Index Terms Zeldox; Ziprasidone Hydrochloride;
Ziprasidone Mesylate
Pharmacologic Category Antipsychotic Agent,
Atypical
Medication Safety Issues
Sound-alike/look-alike issues:
Ziprasidone may be confused with TraZODone
BEERS Criteria medication:
This drug may be potentially inappropriate for use
in geriatric patients (Quality of evidence - mod-
erate; Strength of recommendation - strong).
Pregnancy Risk Factor C
Lactation Excretion in breast milk unknown/not
recommended
Breast-Feeding Considerations It is not known if
ziprasidone is excreted into breast milk. Breast-
feeding is not recommended by the manufacturer.
Use Treatment of schizophrenia; treatment of acute
manic or mixed episodes associated with bipolar
disorder with or without psychosis; maintenance
treatment of bipolar disorder as an adjunct to
lithium or valproate; acute agitation in patients with
schizophrenia
Unlabeled Use Psychosis/agitation related to Alzheimer's dementia
Mechanism of Action/Effect Ziprasidone is a
benzylisothiazolylpiperazine antipsychotic which
blocks a number of CNS receptors, including dopamine, serotonin, alpha$_1$ adrenergic, and histamine
receptors. Also inhibits reuptake of serotonin and
epinephrine. Results in improvement in positive
and negative symptoms of schizophrenia.
Contraindications Hypersensitivity to ziprasidone
or any component of the formulation; history of (or
current) prolonged QT; congenital long QT syndrome; recent myocardial infarction; uncompensated heart failure; concurrent use of other QT$_c$-
prolonging agents including arsenic trioxide, chlorpromazine, class Ia antiarrhythmics (eg, disopyramide, quinidine, procainamide), class III
antiarrhythmics (eg, amiodarone, dofetilide, ibutilide, sotalol), dolasetron, droperidol, gatifloxacin,
halofantrine, levomethadyl, mefloquine, mesorida-
zine, moxifloxacin, pentamidine, pimozide, probu-
col, sparfloxacin, tacrolimus, and thioridazine
Warnings/Precautions Hazardous agent - use
appropriate precautions for handling and disposal
(NIOSH, 2012). **[U.S. Boxed Warning]: Elderly
patients with dementia-related behavioral disorders treated with antipsychotics are at an**

increased risk of death compared to placebo.
Most deaths appeared to be either cardiovascular
(eg, heart failure, sudden death) or infectious (eg,
pneumonia) in nature. Ziprasidone is not approved
for the treatment of dementia-related psychosis.

May result in QT$_c$ prolongation (dose related),
which has been associated with the development
of malignant ventricular arrhythmias (torsade de
pointes) and sudden death. Note contraindications
related to this effect. Observed prolongation was
greater than with other atypical antipsychotic
agents (risperidone, olanzapine, quetiapine), but
less than with thioridazine. Correct electrolyte disturbances, especially hypokalemia or hypomagnesemia, prior to use and throughout therapy. Use
caution in patients with bradycardia. Discontinue in
patients found to have persistent QT$_c$ intervals
>500 msec. Patients with symptoms of dizziness,
palpitations, or syncope should receive further
cardiac evaluation. May cause orthostatic hypotension. Use is contraindicated in patients with recent
acute myocardial infarction (MI), QT prolongation,
or uncompensated heart failure. Avoid use in
patients with a history of cardiac arrhythmias; use
with caution in patients with history of MI or unstable heart disease. Dyslipidemia has been reported
with atypical antipsychotics; risk profile may differ
between agents.

Leukopenia, neutropenia, and agranulocytosis
(sometimes fatal) have been reported in clinical
trials and postmarketing reports with antipsychotic
use; presence of risk factors (eg, pre-existing low
WBC or history of drug-induced leuko-/neutrope-
nia) should prompt periodic blood count assessment. Discontinue therapy at first signs of blood
dyscrasias or if absolute neutrophil count
<1000/mm^3.

May cause extrapyramidal symptoms (EPS). Risk
of dystonia (and probably other EPS) may be
greater with increased doses, use of conventional
antipsychotics, males, and younger patients.
Impaired core body temperature regulation may
occur; caution with strenuous exercise, heat exposure, dehydration, and concomitant medication
possessing anticholinergic effects; not reported in
premarketing trials of ziprasidone. Antipsychotic
use may also be associated with neuroleptic malignant syndrome (NMS). Use with caution in patients
at risk of seizures.

Atypical antipsychotics have been associated with
development of hyperglycemia. There is limited
documentation with ziprasidone and specific risk
associated with this agent is not known. Use
caution in patients with diabetes or other disorders
of glucose regulation; monitor for worsening of
glucose control. May increase prolactin levels;
clinical significance of hyperprolactinemia in
patients with breast cancer or other prolactin-
dependent tumors is unknown.

Use in elderly patients with dementia is associated with an increased risk of mortality and cerebrovascular accidents; avoid antipsychotic use for behavioral problems associated with dementia unless alternative nonpharmacologic therapies have failed and patient may harm self or others. In addition, use may cause or exacerbate syndrome of inappropriate antidiuretic hormone secretion or hyponatremia; monitor sodium closely with initiation or dosage adjustments in older adults (Beers Criteria).

Cognitive and/or motor impairment (sedation) is common with ziprasidone. Use with caution in disorders where CNS depression is a feature. Use with caution in Parkinson's disease. Antipsychotic use has been associated with esophageal dysmotility and aspiration; use with caution in patients at risk of pneumonia (ie, Alzheimer's disease). Use caution in hepatic impairment. Ziprasidone has been associated with a fairly high incidence of rash (5%). Significant weight gain has been observed with antipsychotic therapy; incidence varies with product. Monitor waist circumference and BMI. Rare cases of priapism have been reported. Use the intramuscular formulation with caution in patients with renal impairment; formulation contains cyclodextrin, an excipient which may accumulate in renal insufficiency.

The possibility of a suicide attempt is inherent in psychotic illness or bipolar disorder; use caution in high-risk patients during initiation of therapy. Prescriptions should be written for the smallest quantity consistent with good patient care.

Drug Interactions

Avoid Concomitant Use

Avoid concomitant use of Ziprasidone with any of the following: Amisulpride; Azelastine (Nasal); FLUoxetine; Highest Risk QTc-Prolonging Agents; Ivabradine; Metoclopramide; Mifepristone; Moderate Risk QTc-Prolonging Agents; Paraldehyde; Sulpiride; Thalidomide

Decreased Effect

Ziprasidone may decrease the levels/effects of: Amphetamines; Anti-Parkinson's Agents (Dopamine Agonist); Quinagolide

The levels/effects of Ziprasidone may be decreased by: CarBAMazepine; Lithium formulations

Increased Effect/Toxicity

Ziprasidone may increase the levels/effects of: Alcohol (Ethyl); Amisulpride; ARIPiprazole; Azelastine (Nasal); Buprenorphine; CNS Depressants; FLUoxetine; Highest Risk QTc-Prolonging Agents; Hydrocodone; Lomitapide; Methotrimeprazine; Methylphenidate; Paraldehyde; Serotonin Modulators; Sulpiride; Thalidomide; Zolpidem

The levels/effects of Ziprasidone may be increased by: Acetylcholinesterase Inhibitors (Central); Brimonidine (Topical); Doxylamine; FLUoxetine; HydrOXYzine; Ivabradine; Lithium formulations; Magnesium Sulfate; Methotrimeprazine; Methylphenidate; Metoclopramide; Metyrosine; Mifepristone; Moderate Risk QTc-Prolonging Agents; Perampanel; QTc-Prolonging Agents (Indeterminate Risk and Risk Modifying); Serotonin Modulators; Sodium Oxybate; Tetrabenazine

Nutritional/Ethanol Interactions

Ethanol: May increase CNS depression; monitor for increased effects with coadministration. Caution patients about effects.

Food: Administration with food increases serum levels twofold. Grapefruit juice may increase serum concentration of ziprasidone.

Herb/Nutraceutical: St John's wort may decrease serum levels of ziprasidone, due to a potential effect on CYP3A4. This has not been specifically studied. Some herbal medications may increase CNS depression. Management: Avoid kava kava, gotu kola, valerian, and St John's wort.

Adverse Reactions Note: Although minor QT_c prolongation (mean: 10 msec at 160 mg/day) may occur more frequently (incidence not specified), clinically-relevant prolongation (>500 msec) was rare (0.06%) and less than placebo (0.23%).

>10%:
Central nervous system: Extrapyramidal symptoms (2% to 31%), somnolence (8% to 31%), headache (3% to 18%), dizziness (3% to 16%)
Gastrointestinal: Nausea (4% to 12%)
1% to 10%:
Cardiovascular: Orthostatic hypotension (5%), chest pain (3%), hypertension (2% to 3%), tachycardia (2%), bradycardia (≤2%), facial edema (1%), vasodilation (≤1%)
Central nervous system: Akathisia (2% to 10%), anxiety (2% to 5%), insomnia (3%), agitation (2%), speech disorder (2%), personality disorder (2%), akinesia (≥1%), amnesia (≥1%), ataxia (≥1%), confusion (≥1%), coordination abnormal (≥1%), delirium (≥1%), dystonia (≥1%), hostility (≥1%), oculogyric crisis (≥1%), vertigo (≥1%), chills (1%), fever (1%), hypothermia (1%), psychosis (1%)
Dermatologic: Rash (4% to 5%), fungal dermatitis (2%), photosensitivity reaction (1%)
Endocrine & metabolic: Dysmenorrhea (2%)
Gastrointestinal: Weight gain (6% to 10%), constipation (2% to 9%), dyspepsia (1% to 8%), diarrhea (3% to 5%), vomiting (3% to 5%), xerostomia (1% to 5%), salivation increased (4%), tongue edema (≤3%), anorexia (2%), abdominal pain (≤2%), dysphagia (≤2%), rectal hemorrhage (≤2%), buccoglossal syndrome (≥1%)
Genitourinary: Priapism (1%)
Local: Injection site pain (7% to 9%)
Neuromuscular & skeletal: Weakness (2% to 6%), hypoesthesia (2%), myalgia (2%), paresthesia (2%), abnormal gait (≥1%), choreoathetosis ▶

(≥1%), dysarthria (≥1%), dyskinesia (≥1%), hyper-/hypokinesia (≥1%), hypotonia (≥1%), neuropathy (≥1%), tremor (≥1%), twitching (≥1%), back pain (1%), cogwheel rigidity (1%), hypertonia (1%)

Ocular: Vision abnormal (3% to 6%), diplopia (≥1%)

Respiratory: Infection (8%), rhinitis (1% to 4%), cough (3%), pharyngitis (3%), dyspnea (2%)

Miscellaneous: Diaphoresis (2%), furunculosis (2%), withdrawal syndrome (≥1%), flank pain (1%), flu-like syndrome (1%)

Available Dosage Forms

Capsule, Oral:

Geodon: 20 mg, 40 mg, 60 mg, 80 mg

Generic: 20 mg, 40 mg, 60 mg, 80 mg

Solution Reconstituted, Intramuscular:

Geodon: 20 mg (1 ea)

General Dosage Range

I.M.: *Adults:* 10 mg every 2 hours **or** 20 mg every 4 hours (maximum: 40 mg daily)

Oral: *Adults:* Initial: 20-40 mg twice daily; Maintenance: 20-80 mg twice daily (maximum: 200 mg daily)

Administration

I.M. Injection: For I.M. administration only.

Hazardous agent; use appropriate precautions for handling and disposal (NIOSH, 2012).

Oral Administer with food.

Hazardous agent; use appropriate precautions for handling and disposal (NIOSH, 2012).

Preparation for Administration Hazardous agent; use appropriate precautions for handling and disposal (NIOSH, 2012). Each vial should be reconstituted with 1.2 mL SWFI. Shake vigorously; will form a pale, pink solution containing 20 mg/mL ziprasidone.

Storage/Stability

Capsule: Store at 25°C (77°F); excursion permitted to 15°C to 30°C (59°F to 86°F).

Vials for injection: Store at 25°C (77°F); excursion permitted to 15°C to 30°C (59°F to 86°F). Protect from light. Following reconstitution, injection may be stored at room temperature up to 24 hours or under refrigeration for up to 7 days. Protect from light.

Nursing Actions

Physical Assessment Monitor weight prior to initiating therapy and at least monthly.

Patient Education

• Discuss specific use of drug and side effects with patient as it relates to treatment. (HCAHPS: During this hospital stay, were you given any medicine that you had not taken before? Before giving you any new medicine, how often did hospital staff tell you what the medicine was for? How often did hospital staff describe possible side effects in a way you could understand?)

• Patient may experience presyncope, fatigue, blurred vision, illogical thinking, dizziness,

nervousness and anxiety, nausea, constipation, weight gain, or hyperglycemia. Have patient report immediately to prescriber angina, significant change in balance, tremors, severe asthenia, polyuria, polydipsia, weight loss, significant myalgia, pregnancy, or rash (HCAHPS).

• Educate patient about signs of a significant reaction (eg, wheezing; chest tightness; fever; itching; bad cough; blue skin color; seizures; or swelling of face, lips, tongue, or throat). **Note:** This is not a comprehensive list of all side effects. Patient should consult prescriber for additional questions.

Intended Use and Disclaimer: Should not be printed and given to patients. This information is intended to serve as a concise initial reference for healthcare professionals to use when discussing medications with a patient. You must ultimately rely on your own discretion, experience and judgment in diagnosing, treating and advising patients.

Dietary Considerations Capsule: Take with food.

Related Information

Oral Medications That Should Not Be Crushed or Altered *on page 1712*

Ziv-Aflibercept (Systemic) (ziv a FLIB er sept)

Brand Names: U.S. Zaltrap

Index Terms Aflibercept I.V.; Vascular Endothelial Growth Factor Trap; VEGF Trap; VEGF Trap R1R2

Pharmacologic Category Antineoplastic Agent; Vascular Endothelial Growth Factor (VEGF) Inhibitor

Medication Safety Issues

Sound-alike/look-alike issues:

Ziv-aflibercept may be confused with aflibercept

High alert medication:

This medication is in a class the Institute for Safe Medical Practices (ISMP) includes among its list of drug classes which have a heightened risk of causing significant patient harm when used in error.

Pregnancy Risk Factor C

Lactation Excretion in breast milk unknown/not recommended

Use Colorectal cancer, metastatic: Treatment of metastatic colorectal cancer (in combination with fluorouracil, leucovorin, and irinotecan [FOLFIRI]) in patients who are resistant to or have progressed on an oxaliplatin-based regimen

Available Dosage Forms

Solution, Intravenous [preservative free]:

Zaltrap: 100 mg/4 mL (4 mL); 200 mg/8 mL (8 mL)

General Dosage Range Dosage adjustment recommended in patients who develop toxicities.

I.V.: *Adults:* 4 mg/kg every 2 weeks

Administration

I.V. Infuse over 1 hour. Do not administer I.V. push or bolus. Administer prior to any FOLFIRI component. Do not administer other medications through the same intravenous line.

Infuse via a 0.2 micron polyethersulfone filter; do not use filters made of polyvinylidene fluoride (PVDF) or nylon. Administer with one of the following types of infusion sets: Polyvinyl chloride (PVC) containing DEHP, DEHP-free PVC containing trioctyl-trimellitate (TOTM), polypropylene, polyethylene lined PVC, or polyurethane.

Injectable Detail pH: 6.2 (intact vial)

Nursing Actions

Physical Assessment Monitor blood pressure; blood counts; diarrhea in elderly patients; symptoms of GI perforation; or severe bleeding. Evaluate patients for bleeding risk; advise against surgeries or dental work while taking this drug. Monitor for mucositis. Patients at risk for DVT; evaluate for symptoms. Educate patient about discussing this drug with all doctors including dentists as drug needs to be temporarily discontinued well before surgery.

Patient Education

- Discuss specific use of drug and side effects with patient as it relates to treatment. (HCAHPS: During this hospital stay, were you given any medicine that you had not taken before? Before giving you any new medicine, how often did hospital staff tell you what the medicine was for? How often did hospital staff describe possible side effects in a way you could understand?)
- Patient may experience anemia, leukopenia, thrombocytopenia, hypertension, bleeding problems, headache, dyspepsia, weight loss, diarrhea, fatigue, loss of appetite, stomatitis, or wound that will not heal. Have patient report immediately to prescriber signs of infection, severe dizziness or syncope, edema, illogical thinking, paresthesia, or ecchymosis (HCAHPS).
- Educate patient about signs of a significant reaction (eg, wheezing; chest tightness; fever; itching; bad cough; blue skin color; seizures; or swelling of face, lips, tongue, or throat). **Note:** This is not a comprehensive list of all side effects. Patient should consult prescriber for additional questions.

Intended Use and Disclaimer: Should not be printed and given to patients. This information is intended to serve as a concise initial reference for healthcare professionals to use when discussing medications with a patient. You must ultimately rely on your own discretion, experience and judgment in diagnosing, treating and advising patients.

Zoledronic Acid (zoe le DRON ik AS id)

Brand Names: U.S. Reclast; Zometa

Index Terms CGP-42446; Zol 446; Zoledronate

Pharmacologic Category Bisphosphonate Derivative

Medication Safety Issues

Sound-alike/look-alike issues:

Zometa may be confused with Jevtana, Xgeva, Xofigo, Xtandi, Zofran, Zoladex, Zytiga

Other safety concerns:

Duplicate therapy issues: Reclast and Aclasta contain zoledronic acid, which is the same ingredient contained in Zometa; patients receiving Zometa should not be treated with Reclast or Aclasta

Medication Guide Available Yes

Pregnancy Risk Factor D

Lactation Excretion in breast milk unknown/not recommended

Breast-Feeding Considerations It is not known if zoledronic acid is excreted into breast milk. Due to the potential for serious adverse reactions in the nursing infant, the U.S. manufacturer recommends a decision be made whether to discontinue nursing or to discontinue the drug, taking into account the importance of treatment to the mother. Use in nursing women is contraindicated per the Canadian labeling.

Use

Glucocorticoid-induced osteoporosis (Reclast): Treatment and prevention of glucocorticoid-induced osteoporosis in men and women who are initiating or continuing systemic glucocorticoids in a daily dose equivalent to 7.5 mg or more of prednisone and who are expected to remain on glucocorticoids for at least 12 months.

Hypercalcemia of malignancy (Zometa): Treatment of hypercalcemia (albumin-corrected serum calcium ≥12 mg/dL) of malignancy.

Multiple myeloma and bone metastases from solid tumors (Zometa): Treatment of patients with multiple myeloma and patients with documented bone metastases from solid tumors, in conjunction with standard antineoplastic therapy.

Osteoporosis in men (Reclast): To increase bone mass in men with osteoporosis.

Paget disease of bone (Reclast): Treatment of Paget disease of bone in men and women.

Postmenopausal osteoporosis (Reclast): Treatment and prevention of osteoporosis in postmenopausal women.

Unlabeled Use Prevention of bone loss associated with aromatase inhibitor therapy in postmenopausal women with breast cancer; prevention of bone loss associated with androgen deprivation therapy in prostate cancer

Mechanism of Action/Effect A bisphosphonate which inhibits bone resorption via actions on osteoclasts or on osteoclast precursors; inhibits osteoclastic activity and skeletal calcium release induced by tumors. Decreases serum calcium and phosphorus, and increases their elimination. In osteoporosis, zoledronic acid inhibits osteoclast-mediated resorption, therefore reducing bone turnover.

Contraindications

U.S. labeling:

Hypersensitivity to zoledronic acid or any component of the product; hypocalcemia (Reclast only); CrCl <35 mL/minute and in those with evidence of acute renal impairment (Reclast only).

Documentation of allergenic cross-reactivity for bisphosphonates is limited. However, because of similarities in chemical structure and/or pharmacologic actions, the possibility of cross-sensitivity cannot be ruled out with certainty.

Canadian labeling:

All indications: Hypersensitivity to zoledronic acid or other bisphosphonates, or any component of the formulation; uncorrected hypocalcemia at the time of infusion; pregnancy, breast-feeding

Nononcology uses: Additional contraindications: Use in patients with CrCl <35 mL/minute and use in patients with evidence of acute renal impairment due to an increased risk of renal failure

Warnings/Precautions Hazardous agent - use appropriate precautions for handling and disposal (NIOSH, 2012). Osteonecrosis of the jaw (ONJ) has been reported in patients receiving bisphosphonates. Risk factors include invasive dental procedures (eg, tooth extraction, dental implants, boney surgery); a diagnosis of cancer, with concomitant chemotherapy, radiotherapy, or corticosteroids; poor oral hygiene, ill-fitting dentures; and comorbid disorders (anemia, coagulopathy, infection, pre-existing dental disease). Most reported cases occurred after I.V. bisphosphonate therapy; however, cases have been reported following oral therapy. A dental exam and preventative dentistry should be performed prior to placing patients with risk factors on chronic bisphosphonate therapy. The manufacturer's labeling states that there are no data to suggest whether discontinuing bisphosphonates in patients requiring invasive dental procedures reduces the risk of ONJ. However, other experts suggest that there is no evidence that discontinuing therapy reduces the risk of developing ONJ (Assael, 2009). The benefit/risk must be assessed by the treating physician and/or dentist/surgeon prior to any invasive dental procedure. Patients developing ONJ while on bisphosphonates should receive care by an oral surgeon.

Atypical, low-energy, or low-trauma femur fractures have been reported in patients receiving bisphosphonates. The fractures include subtrochanteric femur (bone just below the hip joint) and diaphyseal femur (long segment of the thigh bone). Some patients experience prodromal pain weeks or months before the fracture occurs. It is unclear if bisphosphonate therapy is the cause for these fractures; atypical femur fractures have also been reported in patients not taking bisphosphonates, and in patients receiving glucocorticoids. Patients receiving long-term (>3-5 years) bisphosphonate therapy may be at an increased risk. Patients presenting with thigh or groin pain with a history of receiving bisphosphonates should be evaluated for femur fracture. Consider interrupting bisphosphonate therapy in patients who develop a femoral shaft fracture; assess for fracture in the contralateral limb.

Infrequently, severe (and occasionally debilitating) musculoskeletal (bone, joint, and/or muscle) pain have been reported during bisphosphonate treatment. The onset of pain ranged from a single day to several months. Consider discontinuing therapy in patients who experience severe symptoms; symptoms usually resolve upon discontinuation. Some patients experienced recurrence when rechallenged with same drug or another bisphosphonate; avoid use in patients with a history of these symptoms in association with bisphosphonate therapy.

May cause a significant risk of hypocalcemia in patients with Paget's disease, in whom the pretreatment rate of bone turnover may be greatly elevated. Hypocalcemia, including severe and life-threatening hypocalcemia, has also been reported with oncology-related uses. Hypocalcemia must be corrected before initiation of therapy in patients with Paget's disease, osteoporosis, or oncology indications. Ensure adequate calcium and vitamin D intake during therapy. Use caution in patients with disturbances of calcium and mineral metabolism (eg, hypoparathyroidism, thyroid/parathyroid, surgery, malabsorption syndromes, excision of small intestine).

Nononcology indications: Use is contraindicated in patients with CrCl <35 mL/minute and in patients with evidence of acute renal impairment due to an increased risk of renal failure. Obtain serum creatinine and calculate creatinine clearance (using actual body weight) with the Cockcroft-Gault formula prior to each administration. In the management of osteoporosis, re-evaluate the need for continued therapy periodically; the optimal duration of treatment has not yet been determined. Consider discontinuing after 3-5 years of use in patients at low risk for fracture; following discontinuation, re-evaluate fracture risk periodically.

Oncology indications: Use caution in mild-to-moderate renal dysfunction; dosage adjustment required. In cancer patients, renal toxicity has been reported with doses >4 mg or infusions administered over 15 minutes. Risk factors for renal deterioration include pre-existing renal insufficiency and repeated doses of zoledronic acid and other bisphosphonates. Dehydration and the use of other nephrotoxic drugs which may contribute to renal deterioration should be identified and managed. Use is not recommended in patients with severe renal impairment (serum creatinine >3 mg/dL or CrCl <30 mL/minute) and bone metastases (limited data); use in patients with hypercalcemia of malignancy and severe renal impairment (serum creatinine >4.5 mg/dL for hypercalcemia of malignancy) should only be done if the benefits outweigh the risks. Diuretics should not be used before correcting hypovolemia. Renal deterioration, resulting in renal failure and dialysis has occurred in patients treated with zoledronic acid after single and multiple infusions at recommended doses of 4 mg over 15 minutes. Assess renal function prior to treatment and withhold for renal deterioration [increase in serum creatinine of 0.5 mg/dL (if baseline level normal) or increase of 1 mg/dL (if baseline level abnormal)]; treatment should be withheld until renal function returns to within 10% of baseline.

According to the American Society of Clinical Oncology (ASCO) guidelines for bisphosphonates in multiple myeloma, treatment with zoledronic acid is not recommended for asymptomatic (smoldering) or indolent myeloma or with solitary plasmacytoma (Kyle, 2007). The National Comprehensive Cancer Network (NCCN) multiple myeloma guidelines (v.2.2013) recommend bisphosphonates for all patients receiving treatment for symptomatic disease; the use of bisphosphonates in stage 1 or smoldering disease may be considered, although preferably as part of a clinical trial.

Adequate hydration is required during treatment (urine output ~2 L/day); avoid overhydration, especially in patients with heart failure. Pre-existing renal compromise, severe dehydration, and concurrent use with diuretics or other nephrotoxic drugs may increase the risk for renal impairment. Single and multiple infusions in patients with both normal and impaired renal function have been associated with renal deterioration, resulting in renal failure and dialysis or death (rare). Patients with underlying moderate-to-severe renal impairment, increased age, concurrent use of nephrotoxic or diuretic medications, or severe dehydration prior to or after zoledronic acid administration may have an increased risk of acute renal impairment or renal failure. Others with increased risk include patients with renal impairment or dehydration secondary to fever, sepsis, gastrointestinal losses, or diuretic use. If history or physical exam suggests dehydration, treatment should not be given until the patient is normovolemic. Transient increases in serum creatinine may be more pronounced in patients with impaired renal function; consider monitoring creatinine clearance in at-risk patients taking other renally-eliminated drugs.

Conjunctivitis, uveitis, episcleritis, iritis, scleritis, and orbital inflammation have been reported (infrequently) with use; further ophthalmic evaluation (and possibly therapy discontinuation) may be necessary in patients with complicated infection. Use caution in patients with aspirin-sensitive asthma (may cause bronchoconstriction) and the elderly (because decreased renal function occurs more commonly in elderly patients). Rare cases of urticaria and angioedema and very rare cases of anaphylactic reactions/shock have been reported. Do not administer Zometa and Reclast (Aclasta [Canadian brand]) to the same patient for different indications.

Drug Interactions

Avoid Concomitant Use There are no known interactions where it is recommended to avoid concomitant use.

Decreased Effect

The levels/effects of Zoledronic Acid may be decreased by: Proton Pump Inhibitors

Increased Effect/Toxicity

Zoledronic Acid may increase the levels/effects of: Deferasirox; Phosphate Supplements

The levels/effects of Zoledronic Acid may be increased by: Aminoglycosides; Nonsteroidal Anti-Inflammatory Agents; Systemic Angiogenesis Inhibitors; Thalidomide

Adverse Reactions Note: An acute reaction (eg, arthralgia, fever, flu-like symptoms, myalgia) may occur within the first 3 days following infusion in up to 44% of patients; usually resolves within 3-4 days of onset, although may take up to 14 days to resolve. The incidence may be decreased with acetaminophen (prior to infusion and for 72 hours postinfusion).

Oncology indications:
>10%:
Cardiovascular: Lower extremity edema (5% to 21%), hypotension (11%)
Central nervous system: Fatigue (39%), headache (5% to 19%), dizziness (18%), insomnia (15% to 16%), anxiety (11% to 14%), depression (14%), agitation (13%), confusion (7% to 13%), hypoesthesia (12%), rigors (11%)
Dermatologic: Alopecia (12%), dermatitis (11%)
Endocrine & metabolic: Dehydration (5% to 14%), hypophosphatemia (13%), hypokalemia (12%), hypomagnesemia (11%)
Gastrointestinal: Nausea (29% to 46%), vomiting (14% to 32%), constipation (27% to 31%), diarrhea (17% to 24%), anorexia (9% to 22%), abdominal pain (14% to 16%), weight loss (16%), decreased appetite (13%)
Genitourinary: Urinary tract infection (12% to 14%)
Hematologic & oncologic: Anemia (22% to 33%), progression of cancer (16% to 20%), neutropenia (12%)
Infection: Candidiasis (12%)

Neuromuscular & skeletal: Ostealgia (55%), weakness (5% to 24%), myalgia (23%), arthralgia (5% to 21%), back pain (15%), paresthesia (15%), limb pain (14%), skeletal pain (12%)

Renal: Renal insufficiency (8% to 17%; up to 40% in patients with abnormal baseline creatinine)

Respiratory: Dyspnea (22% to 27%), cough (12% to 22%)

Miscellaneous: Fever (32% to 44%)

1% to 10%:

Cardiovascular: Chest pain (5% to 10%)

Central nervous system: Somnolence (5% to 10%)

Endocrine & metabolic: Hypocalcemia (5% to 10%; grades 3/4: ≤1%), hypermagnesemia (grade 3: 2%)

Gastrointestinal: Dyspepsia (10%), dysphagia (5% to 10%), mucositis (5% to 10%), stomatitis (8%), sore throat (8%)

Hematologic & oncologic: Granulocytopenia (5% to 10%), pancytopenia (5% to 10%), thrombocytopenia (5% to 10%)

Infection: Infection (nonspecific; 5% to 10%)

Renal: Increased serum creatinine (grades 3/4: ≤2%)

Respiratory: Upper respiratory tract infection (10%)

Nononcology indications:

>10%:

Cardiovascular: Hypertension (5% to 13%)

Central nervous system: Pain (2% to 24%), fever (9% to 22%), headache (4% to 20%), chills (2% to 18%), fatigue (2% to 18%)

Endocrine & metabolic: Hypocalcemia (≤3%; Paget's disease 21%)

Gastrointestinal: Nausea (5% to 18%)

Immunologic: Infusion related reaction (4% to 25%)

Neuromuscular & skeletal: Arthralgia (9% to 27%), myalgia (5% to 23%), back pain (4% to 18%), limb pain (3% to 16%), musculoskeletal pain (≤12%)

Respiratory: Flu-like symptoms (1% to 11%)

1% to 10%:

Cardiovascular: Chest pain (1% to 8%), peripheral edema (3% to 6%), atrial fibrillation (1% to 3%), palpitations (≤3%)

Central nervous system: Dizziness (2% to 9%), rigors (8%), malaise (1% to 7%), hypoesthesia (≤6%), lethargy (3% to 5%), vertigo (1% to 4%), paresthesia (2%), hyperthermia (≤2%)

Dermatologic: Skin rash (2% to 3%), hyperhidrosis (≤3%)

Gastrointestinal: Abdominal pain (1% to 9%), diarrhea (5% to 8%), vomiting (2% to 8%), constipation (6% to 7%), dyspepsia (2% to 7%), abdominal discomfort (1% to 2%), anorexia (1% to 2%)

Hematologic & oncologic: Change in serum protein (C-reactive protein increased; ≤5%)

Neuromuscular & skeletal: Ostealgia (3% to 9%), arthritis (2% to 9%), shoulder pain (≤7%), neck pain (1% to 7%), weakness (2% to 6%), muscle spasm (2% to 6%), stiffness (1% to 5%), jaw pain (2% to 4%), joint swelling (≤3%)

Ophthalmic: Eye pain (≤2%)

Renal: Increased serum creatinine (2%)

Respiratory: Dyspnea (5% to 7%)

Available Dosage Forms

Concentrate, Intravenous:

Zometa: 4 mg/5 mL (5 mL)

Generic: 4 mg/5 mL (5 mL)

Concentrate, Intravenous [preservative free]:

Generic: 4 mg/5 mL (5 mL)

Solution, Intravenous:

Reclast: 5 mg/100 mL (100 mL)

Zometa: 4 mg/100 mL (100 mL)

Generic: 5 mg/100 mL (100 mL)

Solution, Intravenous [preservative free]:

Generic: 4 mg/100 mL (100 mL); 5 mg/100 mL (100 mL)

Solution Reconstituted, Intravenous:

Generic: 4 mg (1 ea)

General Dosage Range Dosage adjustment recommended in patients with renal impairment or who develop toxicities

I.V.: *Adults:*

Nononcology uses: 5 mg as a single dose, once a year or every 2 years

Oncology uses: 4 mg as a single dose or once every 3-4 weeks

Administration

I.V. If refrigerated, allow solution to reach room temperature before administration. Infuse over at least 15 minutes. Flush I.V. line with 10 mL NS flush following infusion. Infuse in a line separate from other medications. Patients must be appropriately hydrated prior to treatment. Acetaminophen after administration may reduce the incidence of acute reaction (eg, arthralgia, fever, flu-like symptoms, myalgia).

Hazardous agent; use appropriate precautions for handling and disposal (NIOSH, 2012).

Injectable Detail

Zometa: pH: ~2 (0.7% solution in water)

Reclast, Aclasta (Canadian brand): pH 6-7 (solution for infusion)

Preparation for Administration Hazardous agent; use appropriate precautions for handling and disposal (NIOSH, 2012).

Solution for injection:

Reclast, Aclasta (Canadian brand): No further preparation is necessary.

Zometa concentrate vials: Further dilute in 100 mL NS or D_5W prior to administration.

Zometa ready-to-use bottles: No further preparation is necessary. If reduced doses are required for patients with renal impairment, withdraw the appropriate volume of solution and replace with an equal amount of NS or D_5W.

Storage/Stability Solution for injection:

Aclasta (Canadian brand): Store at room temperature of 15°C to 30°C (59°F to 86°F). Keep sealed in original package until administration.

Reclast: Store at room temperature of 25°C (77°F); excursions permitted to 15°C to 30°C (59°F to 86°F). After opening, stable for 24 hours at 2°C to 8°C (36°F to 46°F). If refrigerated, allow the refrigerated solution to reach room temperature before administration.

Zometa: Store concentrate vials and ready-to-use bottles at 25°C (77°F); excursions permitted to 15°C to 30°C (59°F to 86°F). Diluted solutions for infusion which are not used immediately after preparation should be refrigerated at 2°C to 8°C (36°F to 46°F). Infusion of solution must be completed within 24 hours of preparation. The ready-to-use bottles are for single use only; if any preparation is necessary (preparing reduced dosage for patients with renal impairment), the prepared, diluted solution may be refrigerated at 2°C to 8°C (36°F to 46°F) if not used immediately. Infusion of solution must be completed within 24 hours of preparation. The previously withdrawn volume from the ready-to-use solution should be discarded; do not store or reuse.

Nursing Actions

Physical Assessment Check results of renal and calcium assessments. A thorough oral exam should be done prior to initiating any therapy. Patients need to be instructed on maintaining good oral hygiene throughout treatment. It may help to let patients know that measure is a preventative one against development of osteonecrosis of the jaw.

Patient Education

- Discuss specific use of drug and side effects with patient as it relates to treatment. (HCAHPS: During this hospital stay, were you given any medicine that you had not taken before? Before giving you any new medicine, how often did hospital staff tell you what the medicine was for? How often did hospital staff describe possible side effects in a way you could understand?)
- Patient may experience dizziness, nausea, injection site irritation, hyper-/hypotension, asthenia, dyspepsia, edema, headache, constipation, diarrhea, hypocalcemia, anemia, arthralgia, myalgia, or osteopenia. Have patient report immediately to prescriber severe jaw, groin, or thigh pain; paresthesia; fasciculations; urinary retention; or rash (HCAHPS).
- Educate patient about signs of a significant reaction (eg, wheezing; chest tightness; fever; itching; bad cough; blue skin color; seizures; or swelling of face, lips, tongue, or throat). **Note:** This is not a comprehensive list of all side effects. Patient should consult prescriber for additional questions.

Intended Use and Disclaimer: Should not be printed and given to patients. This information is intended to serve as a concise initial reference for healthcare professionals to use when discussing medications with a patient. You must ultimately rely on your own discretion, experience and judgment in diagnosing, treating and advising patients.

Dietary Considerations

Multiple myeloma or metastatic bone lesions from solid tumors: Take daily calcium supplement (500 mg) and daily multivitamin (with 400 units vitamin D).

Osteoporosis: Ensure adequate calcium and vitamin D intake; if dietary intake is inadequate, dietary supplementation is recommended. Women and men should consume:

Calcium: 1000 mg/day (men: 50-70 years) **or** 1200 mg/day (women ≥51 years and men ≥71 years) (IOM, 2011; NOF, 2013)

Vitamin D: 800-1000 IU/day (men and women ≥50 years) (NOF, 2013). Recommended Dietary Allowance (RDA): 600 IU/day (men and women ≤70 years) **or** 800 IU/day (men and women ≥71 years) (IOM, 2011).

Paget's disease: Take elemental calcium 1500 mg/day (750 mg twice daily or 500 mg 3 times/day) and vitamin D 800 units/day, particularly during the first 2 weeks after administration.

Zolmitriptan (zohl mi TRIP tan)

Brand Names: U.S. Zomig; Zomig ZMT

Index Terms 311C90

Pharmacologic Category Antimigraine Agent; Serotonin 5-HT$_{1B, 1D}$ Receptor Agonist

Medication Safety Issues

Sound-alike/look-alike issues:

ZOLMitriptan may be confused with SUMAtriptan

Pregnancy Risk Factor C

Lactation Excretion in breast milk unknown/not recommended

Breast-Feeding Considerations It is not known if zolmitriptan is excreted in breast milk. Due to the potential for serious adverse reactions in the nursing infant, the decision to continue or discontinue breast-feeding during therapy should take into account the risk of exposure to the infant and the benefits of treatment to the mother.

Use Migraines: Acute treatment of migraine with or without aura in adults

Unlabeled Use Short-term prevention of menstrual migraines

Mechanism of Action/Effect Selective agonist for serotonin receptor in cranial arteries and sensory nerves of the trigeminal system; causes vasoconstriction and relief of migraine

Contraindications Ischemic coronary artery disease (angina pectoris, history of myocardial infarction [MI], or documented silent ischemia); coronary artery vasospasm, including Prinzmetal variant angina, or other significant underlying cardiovascular disease; Wolff-Parkinson-White syndrome or arrhythmias associated with other cardiac accessory conduction pathway disorders; peripheral vascular disease; ischemic bowel disease; uncontrolled hypertension; recent use (within 24 hours) of treatment with another 5-HT$_1$ agonist, or an ergotamine-containing or ergot-type medication like dihydroergotamine or methysergide; history of stroke, transient ischemic attack, or history of hemiplegic or basilar migraine; coadministration of monoamine oxidase A (MAO A) inhibitors or use of zolmitriptan within 2 weeks of discontinuation of MAO A inhibitor therapy; hypersensitivity to zolmitriptan or any component of the formulation.

Documentation of allergenic cross-reactivity for triptans is limited. However, because of similarities in chemical structure and/or pharmacologic actions, the possibility of cross-sensitivity cannot be ruled out with certainty.

Warnings/Precautions Zolmitriptan is indicated only in patient populations with a clear diagnosis of migraine. If a patient does not respond to the first dose, the diagnosis of migraine should be reconsidered; rule out underlying neurologic disease in patients with atypical headache and in patients with no prior history of migraine. Not indicated for migraine prophylaxis (may be used off-label for menstrual migraine prophylaxis) or for the treatment of cluster headache. Acute migraine agents (eg, triptans, opioids, ergotamine, or a combination of the agents) used for 10 or more days per month may lead to worsening of headaches (medication overuse headache); withdrawal treatment may be necessary in the setting of overuse. Not for prophylactic treatment of migraine headaches. Cardiac events (coronary artery vasospasm, transient ischemia, myocardial infarction, ventricular tachycardia/fibrillation, cardiac arrest, and death) have been reported within a few hours of 5-HT$_1$ agonist administration; use in contraindicated in patients with ischemic or vasospastic coronary artery disease. Patients who experience sensations of chest pain/pressure/tightness or symptoms suggestive of angina following dosing should be evaluated for coronary artery disease or Prinzmetal's angina before receiving additional doses; if dosing is resumed and similar symptoms recur, monitor with ECG. Patients with Prinzmetal's variant angina, Wolff-Parkinson-White Syndrome or arrhythmias associated with other cardiac accessory conduction pathway disorders should not receive zolmitriptan. Should not be given to patients who have risk factors for CAD (eg, hypertension, hypercholesterolemia, smoker, obesity, diabetes, strong family history of CAD, menopause, male >40 years of age) without adequate cardiac evaluation. Patients with suspected CAD should have cardiovascular evaluation to rule out CAD before considering zolmitriptan's use; if cardiovascular evaluation negative, first dose would be safest if given in the healthcare provider's office (consider ECG monitoring). Periodic evaluation of those without cardiovascular disease, but with continued risk factors, should be done. Significant elevation in blood pressure, including hypertensive crisis, has been reported in patients with and without a history of hypertension. Use is contraindicated in patients with uncontrolled hypertension. Peripheral vascular ischemia, gastrointestinal vascular ischemia, and infarction (presenting with abdominal pain and bloody diarrhea, splenic infarction, and Raynaud's syndrome have been reported with 5-HT$_1$ agonists. In patients who experience signs or symptoms suggestive of a vasospastic reaction following use of a 5-HT$_1$ agonist, rule out a vasospastic reaction before receiving additional doses. Cerebral/subarachnoid hemorrhage and stroke have been reported with 5-HT$_1$ agonist administration and some have resulted in fatalities. Do not administer to patients with a history of stroke or TIA; discontinue use if a cerebrovascular event occurs. Rarely, partial vision loss and blindness (transient and permanent) have been reported with 5-HT$_1$ agonists. Use with caution in patients with hepatic impairment. Zomig-ZMT tablets contain phenylalanine. Symptoms of agitation, confusion, hallucinations, labile blood pressure, hyperreflexia, incoordination, myoclonus, shivering, and tachycardia (serotonin syndrome) may occur with concomitant proserotonergic drugs (eg, SSRIs, SNRIs, TCAs, MAO inhibitors, or triptans) or agents which reduce zolmitriptan's metabolism. Elderly patients are more likely to have underlying cardiovascular disease and hepatic or renal impairment; use with caution. Cardiovascular evaluation is recommended for elderly patients with other cardiovascular risk factors prior to initiation of therapy. Zomig-ZMT tablets contain phenylalanine.

Drug Interactions

Avoid Concomitant Use

Avoid concomitant use of ZOLMitriptan with any of the following: Ergot Derivatives; MAO Inhibitors

Decreased Effect There are no known significant interactions involving a decrease in effect.

Increased Effect/Toxicity

ZOLMitriptan may increase the levels/effects of: Antipsychotics; Droxidopa; Ergot Derivatives; Metoclopramide; Serotonin Modulators

The levels/effects of ZOLMitriptan may be increased by: Antipsychotics; Cimetidine; Ergot Derivatives; MAO Inhibitors; Propranolol

Adverse Reactions

>10%: Gastrointestinal: Unpleasant taste (17% to 21%)

1% to 10%:

Cardiovascular: Chest pain (1% to 4%), palpitations (≤2%), facial edema (1% to <2%)

Central nervous system: Dizziness (6% to 10%), paresthesia (5% to 10%), drowsiness (4% to 8%), local alterations in temperature sensations (5% to 7%), sensation of pressure (2% to 5%), hyperesthesia (1% to 5%), hypoesthesia (1% to 5%), flushing sensation (≤4%), pain (2% to 4%), myasthenia (≤2%), vertigo (≤2%), chills (1% to <2%), depersonalization (1% to <2%), headache (1% to <2%), insomnia (1% to <2%)

Dermatologic: Application site irritation (nasal spray 3%), diaphoresis (≤3%)

Gastrointestinal: Nausea (4% to 9%), xerostomia (2% to 5%), dyspepsia (2% to 3%), dysphagia (≤2%), abdominal pain (1% to <2%), vomiting (1% to <2%)

Hypersensitivity: Hypersensitivity reaction (≤1%)

Local: Local pain (neck/throat/jaw; 4% to 10%)

Neuromuscular & skeletal: Weakness (3% to 9%), myalgia (1% to 2%), arthralgia (1% to <2%)

Respiratory: Nasal discomfort (nasal spray 3%), constriction of the pharynx (1% to 2%), pressure on pharynx (1% to <2%)

Available Dosage Forms

Solution, Nasal:
Zomig: 2.5 mg (6 ea); 5 mg (6 ea)

Tablet, Oral:
Zomig: 2.5 mg, 5 mg
Generic: 2.5 mg, 5 mg

Tablet Dispersible, Oral:
Zomig ZMT: 2.5 mg, 5 mg
Generic: 2.5 mg, 5 mg

General Dosage Range Dosage adjustment recommended in patients with hepatic impairment

Nasal inhalation: *Adults:* 2.5 mg at the onset of migraine headache; may repeat in 2 hours if no relief (maximum: 10 mg daily)

Oral: *Adults:* 1.25-2.5 mg at the onset of migraine headache; may repeat in 2 hours if no relief (maximum: 10 mg daily)

Administration

Oral Administer as soon as migraine headache starts.

Tablet: May be broken in half to achieve a smaller initial dose.

Orally-disintegrating tablet: Must be taken whole; do not break, crush, or chew. Place on tongue and allow to dissolve. Administration with liquid is not required.

Other Nasal spray: Administer as soon as migraine headache starts. Blow nose gently prior to use. After removing protective cap, instill device into nostril. Block opposite nostril; breathe in gently through nose while pressing plunger of spray device. Breathe gently through mouth for 5-10 seconds.

Storage/Stability Store at 20°C to 25°C (68°F to 77°F). Protect tablets from light and moisture.

Nursing Actions

Physical Assessment For use only with a clear diagnosis of migraine headaches. Monitor for hypertension, cardiac events, chest pain, nausea, dizziness, paresthesia, myalgia, and pain. Teach patient proper use (treatment of acute migraine). Caution against overuse.

Patient Education

• Discuss specific use of drug and side effects with patient as it relates to treatment. (HCAHPS: During this hospital stay, were you given any medicine that you had not taken before? Before giving you any new medicine, how often did hospital staff tell you what the medicine was for? How often did hospital staff describe possible side effects in a way you could understand?)

• Patient may experience dizziness, presyncope, fatigue, blurred vision, illogical thinking, nausea, xerostomia, paresthesia, or blindness. Have patient report immediately to prescriber angina, tachycardia, syncope, change in balance, agitation, fasciculations, muscle stiffness, nervousness or excitability, strength differences from one side to another, headache, severe dyspepsia, bloody diarrhea, asthenia, or rash (HCAHPS).

• Educate patient about signs of a significant reaction (eg, wheezing; chest tightness; fever; itching; bad cough; blue skin color; seizures; or swelling of face, lips, tongue, or throat). **Note:** This is not a comprehensive list of all side effects. Patient should consult prescriber for additional questions.

Intended Use and Disclaimer: Should not be printed and given to patients. This information is intended to serve as a concise initial reference for healthcare professionals to use when discussing medications with a patient. You must ultimately rely on your own discretion, experience and judgment in diagnosing, treating and advising patients.

Dietary Considerations Some products may contain phenylalanine.

Related Information
Oral Medications That Should Not Be Crushed or Altered *on page 1712*

Zolpidem (zole PI dem)

Brand Names: U.S. Ambien; Ambien CR; Edluar; Intermezzo; Zolpimist

Index Terms Zolpidem Tartrate

Pharmacologic Category Hypnotic, Miscellaneous

◀ **Medication Safety Issues**
Sound-alike/look-alike issues:
Ambien may be confused with Abilify, Ativan, Ambi 10
Sublinox may be confused with Suboxone
Zolpidem may be confused with lorazepam, zaleplon
BEERS Criteria medication:
This drug may be potentially inappropriate for use in geriatric patients (Quality of evidence - moderate; Strength of recommendation - strong).
International issues:
Ambien [U.S., Argentina, Israel] may be confused with Amyben brand name for amiodarone [Great Britain]
Medication Guide Available Yes
Pregnancy Risk Factor C
Lactation Enters breast milk/use caution
Breast-Feeding Considerations Zolpidem is excreted in breast milk. The manufacturer recommends that caution be exercised when administering zolpidem to nursing women.
Use
Ambien, Edluar, Zolpimist: Short-term treatment of insomnia (with difficulty of sleep onset)
Ambien CR: Treatment of insomnia (with difficulty of sleep onset and/or sleep maintenance)
Intermezzo: "As needed" treatment of middle-of-the-night insomnia with ≥4 hours of sleep time remaining.
Sublinox (Canadian availability; not available in U.S.): Short-term treatment of insomnia (with difficulty of sleep onset, frequent awakenings, and/or early awakenings)
Mechanism of Action/Effect Zolpidem is structurally dissimilar to benzodiazepines but enhances the activity of γ-aminobutyric acid (GABA) resulting in increased sedation. Zolpidem exhibits minimal anxiolytic, myorelaxant, and anticonvulsant properties.
Contraindications Hypersensitivity to zolpidem or any component of the formulation

Canadian labeling: Additional contraindications (not in U.S. labeling): Significant obstructive sleep apnea syndrome and acute and/or severe impairment of respiratory function; myasthenia gravis; severe hepatic impairment; personal or family history of sleepwalking

Warnings/Precautions Should be used only after evaluation of potential causes of sleep disturbance. Failure of sleep disturbance to resolve after 7-10 days may indicate psychiatric or medical illness. Hypnotics/sedatives have been associated with abnormal thinking and behavior changes including decreased inhibition, aggression, bizarre behavior, agitation, hallucinations, and depersonalization. These changes may occur unpredictably and may indicate previously unrecognized psychiatric disorders; evaluate appropriately. Sedative/hypnotics may produce withdrawal symptoms following abrupt discontinuation. Use with caution in patients with depression; worsening of depression, including suicide or suicidal ideation has been reported with the use of hypnotics. Intentional overdose may be an issue in this population. The minimum dose that will effectively treat the individual patient should be used. Prescriptions should be written for the smallest quantity consistent with good patient care. Causes CNS depression, which may impair physical and mental capabilities. Zolpidem should only be administered when the patient is able to stay in bed a full night (7-8 hours) before being active again. Potentially significant drug-drug interactions may exist, requiring dose or frequency adjustment, additional monitoring, and/or selection of alternative therapy. Consult drug interactions database for more detailed information. Effects with other sedative drugs or ethanol may be potentiated. Canadian labeling does not recommend concomitant use with alcohol.

Use caution in patients with myasthenia gravis (contraindicated in the Canadian labeling). Avoid use in patients with sleep apnea or a history of sedative-hypnotic abuse. Postmarketing studies have indicated that the use of hypnotic/sedative agents (including zolpidem) for sleep has been associated with hypersensitivity reactions including anaphylaxis as well as angioedema. An increased risk for hazardous sleep-related activities such as sleep-driving; cooking and eating food, and making phone calls while asleep have also been noted; amnesia may also occur. Discontinue treatment in patients who report any sleep-related episodes. Canadian labeling recommends avoiding use in patients with disorders (eg, restless legs syndrome, periodic limb movement disorder, sleep apnea) that may disrupt sleep and cause frequent awakenings, potentially increasing the risk of complex sleep-related behaviors. Use with caution in patients with a history of drug dependence. Risk of abuse is increased in patients with a history or family history of alcohol or drug abuse or mental illness.

Use caution with respiratory disease (Canadian labeling contraindicates use with acute and/or severe impairment of respiratory function). Use caution with hepatic impairment (Canadian labeling contraindicates use in severe impairment); dose adjustment required. Because of the rapid onset of action, administer immediately prior to bedtime, after the patient has gone to bed and is having difficulty falling asleep, or during the middle of the night when at least 4 hours are left before waking (Intermezzo).

Use caution in the elderly; dose adjustment recommended. Closely monitor elderly or debilitated patients for impaired cognitive and/or motor performance, confusion, and potential for falling. Avoid chronic use (>90 days) in older adults; adverse events, including delirium, falls, fractures, have been observed with nonbenzodiazepine hypnotic use in the elderly similar to events observed with benzodiazepines. Data suggests improvements in sleep duration and latency are minimal (Beers Criteria).

Dosage adjustment is recommended for females; pharmacokinetic studies involving zolpidem showed a significant increase in maximum concentration and exposure in females compared to males at the same dose. When studied for the unapproved use of insomnia associated with ADHD in children, a higher incidence (~7%) of hallucinations was reported. In addition, sleep latency did not decrease compared to placebo. Zolpidem is **not** FDA- or Health Canada-approved for use in pediatric patients.

Drug Interactions

Avoid Concomitant Use

Avoid concomitant use of Zolpidem with any of the following: Azelastine (Nasal); Conivaptan; Fusidic Acid (Systemic); Paraldehyde; Sodium Oxybate; Thalidomide

Decreased Effect

The levels/effects of Zolpidem may be decreased by: Bosentan; CarBAMazepine; CYP3A4 Inducers (Strong); Dabrafenib; Deferasirox; Flumazenil; Herbs (CYP3A4 Inducers); Mitotane; Peginterferon Alfa-2b; Rifamycin Derivatives; Telaprevir; Tocilizumab

Increased Effect/Toxicity

Zolpidem may increase the levels/effects of: Alcohol (Ethyl); Azelastine (Nasal); Buprenorphine; CarBAMazepine; Hydrocodone; Methotrimeprazine; Metyrosine; Mirtazapine; Paraldehyde; Pramipexole; ROPINIRole; Rotigotine; Selective Serotonin Reuptake Inhibitors; Sodium Oxybate; Thalidomide

The levels/effects of Zolpidem may be increased by: Antifungal Agents (Azole Derivatives, Systemic); Brimonidine (Topical); CNS Depressants; Conivaptan; CYP3A4 Inhibitors (Moderate); CYP3A4 Inhibitors (Strong); Dasatinib; Doxylamine; Droperidol; Fluconazole; FluvoxaMINE; Fusidic Acid (Systemic); HydrOXYzine; Ivacaftor; Luliconazole; Magnesium Sulfate; Methotrimeprazine; Mifepristone; Perampanel; Simeprevir; Stiripentol; Tapentadol

Nutritional/Ethanol Interactions

Ethanol: May enhance the adverse/toxic effects of zolpidem. Management: Avoid use of ethanol.

Food: Maximum plasma concentration and bioavailability are decreased with food; time to peak plasma concentration is increased; half-life remains unchanged. Grapefruit juice may decrease the metabolism of zolpidem. Management: Avoid grapefruit juice.

Herb/Nutraceutical: St John's wort may decrease the levels/effects of zolpidem. Some herbal medications should be avoided due to the risk of increased CNS depression. Management: Avoid concomitant use of St John's wort. Avoid valerian, kava kava, and gotu kola.

Adverse Reactions Actual frequency may be dosage form, dose, and/or age dependent

>10%: Central nervous system: Headache (7% to 19%), drowsiness (2% to 15%), dizziness (5% to 12%)

1% to 10%:

Cardiovascular: Chest discomfort, increased blood pressure, palpitations

Central nervous system: Abnormal dreams, amnesia, anxiety, apathy, ataxia, burning sensation, confusion, depersonalization, depression, disinhibition, disorientation, drugged feeling, eating disorder (binge eating), emotional lability, equilibrium disturbance, euphoria, fatigue, hallucination, hypoesthesia, increased body temperature, insomnia, lack of concentration, lethargy, memory impairment, paresthesia, psychomotor retardation, sleep disorder, stress, vertigo

Dermatologic: Skin rash, urticaria, wrinkling of skin

Endocrine & metabolic: Hypermenorrhea

Gastrointestinal: Abdominal distress, abdominal tenderness, change in appetite, constipation, diarrhea, dyspepsia, flatulence, frequent bowel movements, gastroenteritis, gastroesophageal reflux disease, hiccups, nausea, vomiting, xerostomia

Genitourinary: Dysuria, urinary tract infection, vaginal dryness

Hypersensitivity: Hypersensitivity reaction

Neuromuscular & skeletal: Arthralgia, back pain, muscle cramps, muscle spasm, myalgia, neck pain, tremor, weakness

Ophthalmic: Accommodation disturbance, asthenopia, blurred vision, diplopia, eye redness, visual disturbance (including altered depth perception)

Otic: Labyrinthitis, tinnitus

Respiratory: Dry throat, flu-like symptoms, lower respiratory tract infection, pharyngitis, sinusitis, throat irritation, upper respiratory tract infection

Miscellaneous: Fever

Pharmacodynamics/Kinetics

Onset of Action Immediate release: 30 minutes

Duration of Action Immediate release: 6-8 hours

Controlled Substance C-IV

Available Dosage Forms

Solution, Oral:

Zolpimist: 5 mg/actuation (7.7 mL)

Tablet, Oral:

Ambien: 5 mg, 10 mg

Generic: 5 mg, 10 mg

Tablet Extended Release, Oral:

Ambien CR: 6.25 mg, 12.5 mg

Generic: 6.25 mg, 12.5 mg

Tablet Sublingual, Sublingual:

Edluar: 5 mg, 10 mg

Intermezzo: 1.75 mg, 3.5 mg

◀ **General Dosage Range** Dosage adjustment recommended in patients with hepatic impairment and concomitant medications.

Oral:

Immediate release tablet, spray:

Adults: 5 mg (females) or 5-10 mg (males) immediately before bedtime

Elderly: 5 mg immediately before bedtime

Sublingual tablet:

Adults: 5 mg (females) or 5-10 mg (males) immediately before bedtime **or** 1.75 mg (females) or 3.5 mg (males) once per night as needed

Elderly: 5 mg immediately before bedtime **or** 1.75 mg (females and males) once per night as needed

Extended release tablet:

Adults: 6.25 mg (females) or 6.25-12.5 mg (males) immediately before bedtime

Elderly: 6.25 mg immediately before bedtime

Administration

Oral Ingest immediately before bedtime due to rapid onset of action. Regardless of dosage form, do not administer with or immediately after a meal. Intermezzo should be taken in bed if patient awakes in the middle of the night (ie, if ≥4 hours left before waking) and there is difficulty in returning to sleep.

Ambien CR tablets should be swallowed whole; do not divide, crush, or chew.

Edluar, Intermezzo, or Sublinox (Canadian availability; not available in U.S.) sublingual tablets should be placed under the tongue and allowed to disintegrate; do not swallow or administer with water.

Zolpimist oral spray should be sprayed directly into the mouth over the tongue. Prior to initial use, pump should be primed by spraying 5 times. If pump is not used for at least 14 days, reprime pump with 1 spray.

Storage/Stability

Ambien, Edluar, Intermezzo: Store at 20°C to 25°C (68°F to 77°F). Protect sublingual tablets from light and moisture.

Ambien CR: Store at 15°C to 25°C (59°F to 77°F); limited excursions permitted up to 30°C (86°F).

Zolpimist: Store at 25°C (77°F); do not freeze. Avoid prolonged exposure to temperatures >30°C (86°F).

Sublinox (Canadian availability; not available in U.S.): Store at 15°C to 30°C (59°F to 86°F); protect from light and moisture.

Nursing Actions

Physical Assessment For short-term use. Assess for history of addiction; long-term use can result in dependence, abuse, or tolerance; behaviors that patient has no memory of performing after taking (driving, preparing food, or eating); periodically evaluate need for continued use. Monitor for CNS depression. For inpatient use, institute safety measures to prevent falls.

Patient Education

• Discuss specific use of drug and side effects with patient as it relates to treatment. (HCAHPS: During this hospital stay, were you given any medicine that you had not taken before? Before giving you any new medicine, how often did hospital staff tell you what the medicine was for? How often did hospital staff describe possible side effects in a way you could understand?)

• Patient may experience dizziness, presyncope, fatigue, blurred vision, illogical thinking, headache, asthenia, or nausea. Have patient report immediately to prescriber depression, nervousness, emotional instability, illogical thinking, anxiety, memory loss, or rash (HCAHPS).

• Educate patient about signs of a significant reaction (eg, wheezing; chest tightness; fever; itching; bad cough; blue skin color; seizures; or swelling of face, lips, tongue, or throat). **Note:** This is not a comprehensive list of all side effects. Patient should consult prescriber for additional questions.

Intended Use and Disclaimer: Should not be printed and given to patients. This information is intended to serve as a concise initial reference for healthcare professionals to use when discussing medications with a patient. You must ultimately rely on your own discretion, experience and judgment in diagnosing, treating and advising patients.

Dietary Considerations For faster sleep onset, do not administer with (or immediately after) a meal.

Related Information

Oral Medications That Should Not Be Crushed or Altered *on page 1712*

Zonisamide (zoe NIS a mide)

Brand Names: U.S. Zonegran

Pharmacologic Category Anticonvulsant, Miscellaneous

Medication Safety Issues

Sound-alike/look-alike issues:

Zonegran® may be confused with SINEquan®

Zonisamide may be confused with lacosamide

Medication Guide Available Yes

Pregnancy Risk Factor C

Lactation Excreted into breast milk /not recommended

Breast-Feeding Considerations Zonisamide is excreted into breast milk in concentrations similar to those in the maternal plasma and has been detected in the plasma of a nursing infant. According to the manufacturer, the decision to continue or discontinue breast-feeding during therapy should take into account the risk of exposure to the infant and the benefits of treatment to the mother.

Use Adjunct treatment of partial seizures in children >16 years of age and adults with epilepsy

Unlabeled Use Bipolar disorder

Mechanism of Action/Effect The exact mechanism of action is not known. May stabilize neuronal membranes and suppress neuronal hypersynchronization through action at sodium and calcium channels. Does not affect GABA activity.

Contraindications Hypersensitivity to zonisamide, sulfonamides, or any component of the formulation

Warnings/Precautions Hazardous agent - use appropriate precautions for handling and disposal (NIOSH, 2012). Rare, but potentially fatal sulfonamide reactions have occurred following the use of zonisamide. These reactions include Stevens-Johnson syndrome, fulminant hepatic necrosis, agranulocytosis, aplastic anemia, and toxic epidermal necrolysis, usually appearing within 2-16 weeks of drug initiation. Discontinue zonisamide if rash develops. Chemical similarities are present among sulfonamides, sulfonylureas, carbonic anhydrase inhibitors, thiazides, and loop diuretics (except ethacrynic acid). Use in patients with sulfonamide allergy is specifically contraindicated in product labeling, however, a risk of cross-reaction exists in patients with allergy to any of these compounds; avoid use when previous reaction has been severe. Use may be associated with the development of metabolic acidosis (generally dose-dependent) in certain patients; predisposing conditions/therapies include renal disease, severe respiratory disease, diarrhea, surgery, ketogenic diet, and other medications. Pediatric patients may also be at an increased risk for and may have more severe metabolic acidosis. Serum bicarbonate should be monitored in all patients prior to and during use; if metabolic acidosis occurs, consider decreasing the dose or tapering the dose to discontinue. If use continued despite acidosis, alkali treatment should be considered. Untreated metabolic acidosis may increase the risk of developing nephrolithiasis, nephrocalcinosis, osteomalacia (or rickets in children), or osteoporosis; pediatric patients may also have decreased growth rates.

Pooled analysis of trials involving various antiepileptics (regardless of indication) showed an increased risk of suicidal thoughts/behavior (incidence rate: 0.43% treated patients compared to 0.24% of patients receiving placebo); risk observed as early as 1 week after initiation and continued through duration of trials (most trials ≤24 weeks). Monitor all patients for notable changes in behavior that might indicate suicidal thoughts or depression; notify healthcare provider immediately if symptoms occur.

Discontinue zonisamide in patients who develop acute renal failure or a significant sustained increase in creatinine/BUN concentration. Kidney stones have been reported. Do not use in patients with renal impairment (GFR <50 mL/minute); use with caution in patients with hepatic impairment.

Significant CNS effects include psychiatric symptoms, psychomotor slowing, and fatigue or somnolence. Fatigue and somnolence occur within the first month of treatment, most commonly at doses of 300-500 mg/day. Effects with other sedative drugs or ethanol may be potentiated. May cause sedation, which may impair physical or mental abilities; patients must be cautioned about performing tasks which require mental alertness (eg, operating machinery or driving). Abrupt withdrawal may precipitate seizures; discontinue or reduce doses gradually.

Safety and efficacy in children <16 years of age has not been established. Decreased sweating (oligohydrosis) and hyperthermia requiring hospitalization have been reported in children. Pediatric patients may also be at an increased risk and may have more severe metabolic acidosis.

Drug Interactions
Avoid Concomitant Use
Avoid concomitant use of Zonisamide with any of the following: Azelastine (Nasal); Carbonic Anhydrase Inhibitors; Conivaptan; Fusidic Acid (Systemic); Paraldehyde; Thalidomide

Decreased Effect
Zonisamide may decrease the levels/effects of: Lithium; Methenamine; Primidone

The levels/effects of Zonisamide may be decreased by: Bosentan; CYP3A4 Inducers (Strong); Dabrafenib; Deferasirox; Fosphenytoin; Herbs (CYP3A4 Inducers); Ketorolac (Nasal); Ketorolac (Systemic); Mefloquine; Mitotane; Orlistat; PHENobarbital; Phenytoin; Tocilizumab

Increased Effect/Toxicity
Zonisamide may increase the levels/effects of: Alcohol (Ethyl); Alpha-/Beta-Agonists; Amphetamines; Anticonvulsants (Barbiturate); Anticonvulsants (Hydantoin); Azelastine (Nasal); Buprenorphine; CarBAMazepine; Carbonic Anhydrase Inhibitors; CNS Depressants; Flecainide; Hydrocodone; Memantine; MetFORMIN; Methotrimeprazine; Metyrosine; Mirtazapine; Paraldehyde; Pramipexole; Primidone; QuiNIDine; ROPINIRole; Rotigotine; Selective Serotonin Reuptake Inhibitors; Thalidomide; Zolpidem

The levels/effects of Zonisamide may be increased by: Brimonidine (Topical); Conivaptan; CYP3A4 Inhibitors (Moderate); CYP3A4 Inhibitors (Strong); Dasatinib; Doxylamine; Droperidol; Fusidic Acid (Systemic); HydrOXYzine; Ivacaftor; Luliconazole; Magnesium Sulfate; Methotrimeprazine; Mifepristone; Perampanel; Salicylates; Simeprevir; Sodium Oxybate; Stiripentol; Tapentadol

Nutritional/Ethanol Interactions
Ethanol: May increase CNS depression; monitor for increased effects with coadministration. Caution patients about effects.
Food: Food delays time to maximum concentration, but does not affect bioavailability.

Adverse Reactions Frequencies noted in patients receiving other anticonvulsants:

>10%:

Central nervous system: Somnolence (17%), dizziness (13%)

Gastrointestinal: Anorexia (13%)

1% to 10%:

Central nervous system: Headache (10%), agitation/irritability (9%), fatigue (8%), tiredness (7%), ataxia (6%), confusion (6%), concentration decreased (6%), memory impairment (6%), depression (6%), insomnia (6%), speech disorders (5%), mental slowing (4%), anxiety (3%), nervousness (2%), schizophrenic/schizophreniform behavior (2%), difficulty in verbal expression (2%), status epilepticus (1%), seizure (1%), hyperesthesia (1%), incoordination (1%)

Dermatologic: Rash (3%), bruising (2%), pruritus (1%)

Gastrointestinal: Nausea (9%), abdominal pain (6%), diarrhea (5%), dyspepsia (3%), weight loss (3%), constipation (2%), taste perversion (2%), xerostomia (2%), vomiting (1%)

Neuromuscular & skeletal: Paresthesia (4%), abnormal gait (1%), tremor (1%), weakness (1%)

Ocular: Diplopia (6%), nystagmus (4%), amblyopia (1%)

Otic: Tinnitus (1%)

Renal: Kidney stones (4%, children 3% to 8%)

Respiratory: Rhinitis (2%), pharyngitis (1%), increased cough (1%)

Miscellaneous: Flu-like syndrome (4%) accidental injury (1%)

Available Dosage Forms

Capsule, Oral:

Zonegran: 25 mg, 100 mg

Generic: 25 mg, 50 mg, 100 mg

General Dosage Range Oral: *Children >16 years and Adults:* Initial: 100 mg/day; Maintenance: 100-600 mg/day (maximum: 600 mg/day)

Administration

Oral Capsules should be swallowed whole. Dose may be administered once or twice daily. Doses of 300 mg/day and higher are associated with increased side effects. Steady-state levels are reached in 14 days.

Hazardous agent; use appropriate precautions for handling and disposal (NIOSH, 2012).

Storage/Stability Store at controlled room temperature 25°C (77°F). Protect from moisture and light.

Nursing Actions

Physical Assessment Observe and teach seizure precautions.

Patient Education

• Discuss specific use of drug and side effects with patient as it relates to treatment. (HCAHPS: During this hospital stay, were you given any medicine that you had not taken before? Before giving you any new medicine, how often did hospital staff tell you what the medicine was for? How often did hospital staff describe possible side effects in a way you could understand?)

• Patient may experience presyncope, fatigue, blurred vision, illogical thinking, dizziness, nervousness, anxiety, headache, nausea, or lack of appetite. Have patient report immediately to prescriber signs of infection, depression, dyspnea, imbalance, anhidrosis, back pain, dyspepsia, hematuria, ecchymosis, bleeding, inability to eat, severe asthenia, or rash (HCAHPS).

• Educate patient about signs of a significant reaction (eg, wheezing; chest tightness; fever; itching; bad cough; blue skin color; seizures; or swelling of face, lips, tongue, or throat). **Note:** This is not a comprehensive list of all side effects. Patient should consult prescriber for additional questions.

Intended Use and Disclaimer: Should not be printed and given to patients. This information is intended to serve as a concise initial reference for healthcare professionals to use when discussing medications with a patient. You must ultimately rely on your own discretion, experience and judgment in diagnosing, treating and advising patients.

Dietary Considerations May be taken without regard to meals.

Zoster Vaccine (ZOS ter vak SEEN)

Brand Names: U.S. Zostavax

Index Terms Herpes Zoster Vaccine; HZV; Shingles Vaccine; VZV Vaccine (Zoster)

Pharmacologic Category Vaccine, Live (Viral)

Medication Safety Issues

Administration issues:

Both varicella vaccine and zoster vaccine are live, attenuated strains of varicella-zoster virus. Their indications, dosing, and composition are distinct. Varicella vaccine is indicated for the prevention of chickenpox, while zoster vaccine is indicated in older individuals to prevent reactivation of the virus which causes shingles. Zoster vaccine is **not** a substitute for varicella vaccine and should not be used in children.

Lactation Excretion in breast milk unknown/use caution

Use

Herpes zoster prevention: Prevention of herpes zoster (shingles) in patients ≥50 years of age

The Advisory Committee on Immunization Practices (ACIP) recommends:

Routine vaccination of **all patients ≥60 years of age, including** patients who report a previous episode of zoster; patients with chronic medical conditions (eg, chronic renal failure, diabetes mellitus, rheumatoid arthritis, chronic pulmonary disease) unless those conditions are contraindications; and residents of nursing homes and other long-term care facilities ≥60 years of age without contraindications (CDC, 2008).

Although not specifically recommended for their profession, healthcare providers within the recommended age group should also receive the zoster vaccine (CDC, 2013)

Limitations of use: Not indicated for treatment of zoster or postherpetic neuralgia (PHN); not indicated for prophylaxis of primary varicella infection (chickenpox).

Available Dosage Forms

Solution Reconstituted, Subcutaneous [preservative free]:

Zostavax: 19,400 units/0.65 mL (1 ea)

General Dosage Range SubQ: *Adults ≥50 years:* 0.65 mL as a single dose

Administration

I.M. Not for I.M. administration

I.V. Not for I.V. administration

Subcutaneous Inject SubQ into the deltoid region of the upper arm. Inject immediately after reconstitution. In persons anticipating immunosuppression, give at least 14 days to 1 month prior to starting immunosuppressant (CDC, 2008).

Administration with chronic use of acyclovir, famciclovir, or valacyclovir: Discontinue ≥24 hours before administration of zoster vaccine. Do not use for ≥14 days after vaccination (CDC, 2008).

Simultaneous administration of vaccines helps ensure the patients will be fully vaccinated by the appropriate age. Simultaneous administration of vaccines is defined as administering >1 vaccine on the same day at different anatomic sites. Separate vaccines should not be combined in the same syringe unless indicated by product specific labeling. Separate needles and syringes should be used for each injection. The ACIP prefers each dose of a specific vaccine in a series come from the same manufacturer when possible. Adults should be vaccinated while seated or lying down (CDC, 2011).

Antipyretics have not been shown to prevent febrile seizures. Antipyretics may be used to treat fever or discomfort following vaccination (CDC, 2011). One study reported that routine prophylactic administration of acetaminophen to prevent fever prior to vaccination decreased the immune response of some vaccines; the clinical significance of this reduction in immune response has not been established (Prymula, 2009).

Nursing Actions

Physical Assessment Not for use in patients <50 years of age or in the treatment of active zoster outbreak. Treatment for anaphylactic/anaphylactoid reaction should be immediately available. U.S. federal law requires entry into the patient's medical record.

Patient Education

- Discuss specific use of vaccine and side effects with patient as it relates to treatment. (HCAHPS: During this hospital stay, were you given any medicine that you had not taken before? Before giving you any new medicine, how often did hospital staff tell you what the medicine was for? How often did hospital staff describe possible side effects in a way you could understand?)
- Patient may experience headache, nausea, diarrhea, or rhinitis. Have patient report immediately to prescriber severe asthenia or rash (HCAHPS).
- Educate patient about signs of a significant reaction (eg, wheezing; chest tightness; fever; itching; bad cough; blue skin color; seizures; or swelling of face, lips, tongue, or throat). **Note:** This is not a comprehensive list of all side effects. Patient should consult prescriber for additional questions.

Intended Use and Disclaimer: Should not be printed and given to patients. This information is intended to serve as a concise initial reference for healthcare professionals to use when discussing medications with a patient. You must ultimately rely on your own discretion, experience and judgment in diagnosing, treating and advising patients.

Related Information

Immunization Administration Recommendations *on page 1675*

Immunization Recommendations *on page 1680*

Zucapsaicin (zu kap SAY sin)

Pharmacologic Category Analgesic, Topical; Topical Skin Product; Transient Receptor Potential Vanilloid 1 (TRPV1) Agonist

Lactation Excretion in human breast milk is unknown/use caution

Use In conjunction with an oral NSAID or COX-2 inhibitor for short-term (≤3 months) treatment of severe pain associated with osteoarthritis of the knee that is not controlled by NSAID or COX-2 inhibitor monotherapy

Product Availability Not available in the U.S.

General Dosage Range Topical: *Adults:* Apply a pea-sized amount to each of 3 different locations around affected knee 3 times/day (minimum interval between applications: 4 hours) (maximum: 3 applications/day)

Administration

Topical For external use only on intact skin; do not apply to broken or irritated skin. Gently rub into affected knee until no residue is left on skin. Do not cover treated area with occlusive dressing. Wash hands thoroughly after application. Avoid taking a hot bath or shower immediately before or after administration (may cause burning sensation). Avoid contact with eyes, lips, and genital ▶

◄ area. Avoid concomitant application of other topical medications to treated areas.

Nursing Actions

Patient Education

- Discuss specific use of drug and side effects with patient as it relates to treatment. (HCAHPS: During this hospital stay, were you given any medicine that you had not taken before? Before giving you any new medicine, how often did hospital staff tell you what the medicine was for? How often did hospital staff describe possible side effects in a way you could understand?)
- Patient may experience skin irritation, burning, or stinging. Have patient report immediately to prescriber severe pain or rash (HCAHPS).

- Educate patient about signs of a significant reaction (eg, wheezing; chest tightness; fever; itching; bad cough; blue skin color; seizures; or swelling of face, lips, tongue, or throat). **Note:** This is not a comprehensive list of all side effects. Patient should consult prescriber for additional questions.

Intended Use and Disclaimer: Should not be printed and given to patients. This information is intended to serve as a concise initial reference for healthcare professionals to use when discussing medications with a patient. You must ultimately rely on your own discretion, experience and judgment in diagnosing, treating and advising patients.

APPENDIX TABLE OF CONTENTS

ABBREVIATIONS, ACRONYMS, AND SYMBOLS

Abbreviations Which May Be Used in This Reference

Abbreviation	Meaning
½NS	0.45% sodium chloride
5-HT	5-hydroxytryptamine
AACT	American Academy of Clinical Toxicology
AAP	American Academy of Pediatrics
AAPC	antibiotic-associated pseudomembranous colitis
ABG	arterial blood gases
ABMT	autologous bone marrow transplant
ABW	adjusted body weight
ACC	American College of Cardiology
ACE	angiotensin-converting enzyme
ACLS	advanced cardiac life support
ACOG	American College of Obstetricians and Gynecologists
ACTH	adrenocorticotrophic hormone
ADH	antidiuretic hormone
ADHD	attention-deficit/hyperactivity disorder
ADI	adequate daily intake
ADLs	activities of daily living
AED	antiepileptic drug
AHA	American Heart Association
AHCPR	Agency for Health Care Policy and Research
AIDS	acquired immunodeficiency syndrome
AIMS	Abnormal Involuntary Movement Scale
ALL	acute lymphoblastic leukemia
ALS	amyotrophic lateral sclerosis
ALT	alanine aminotransferase (formerly called SGPT)
AMA	American Medical Association
AML	acute myeloblastic leukemia
ANA	antinuclear antibodies
ANC	absolute neutrophil count
ANLL	acute nonlymphoblastic leukemia
aPTT	activated partial thromboplastin time
ARB	angiotensin receptor blocker
ARDS	acute respiratory distress syndrome
ASA-PS	American Society of Anesthesiologists – Physical Status P1: Normal, healthy patient P2: Patient having mild systemic disease P3: Patient having severe systemic disease P4: Patient having severe systemic disease which is a constant threat to life P5: Moribund patient; not expected to survive without the procedure P6: Patient declared brain-dead; organs being removed for donor purposes
AST	aspartate aminotransferase (formerly called SGOT)
ATP	adenosine triphosphate
AUC	area under the curve (area under the serum concentration-time curve)
A-V	atrial-ventricular
BDI	Beck Depression Inventory
BEC	blood ethanol concentration
BLS	basic life support
BMI	body mass index
BMT	bone marrow transplant
BP	blood pressure
BPD	bronchopulmonary disease or dysplasia
BPH	benign prostatic hyperplasia
BPRS	Brief Psychiatric Rating Scale
BSA	body surface area
BUN	blood urea nitrogen

Abbreviations Which May Be Used in This Reference *(continued)*

Abbreviation	Meaning
CABG	coronary artery bypass graft
CAD	coronary artery disease
CADD	computer ambulatory drug delivery
cAMP	cyclic adenosine monophosphate
CAN	Canadian
CAPD	continuous ambulatory peritoneal dialysis
CAS	chemical abstract service
CBC	complete blood count
CBT	cognitive behavioral therapy
CDC	Centers for Disease Control and Prevention
CF	cystic fibrosis
CFC	chlorofluorocarbons
CGI	Clinical Global Impression
CHD	coronary heart disease
CHF	congestive heart failure; chronic heart failure
CI	cardiac index
CIE	chemotherapy-induced emesis
C-II	schedule two controlled substance
C-III	schedule three controlled substance
C-IV	schedule four controlled substance
C-V	schedule five controlled substance
CIV	continuous I.V. infusion
CLL	chronic lymphocytic leukemia
C_{max}	maximum plasma concentration
C_{min}	minimum plasma concentration
CML	chronic myelogenous leukemia
CMV	cytomegalovirus
CNS	central nervous system or coagulase negative staphylococcus
COLD	chronic obstructive lung disease
COPD	chronic obstructive pulmonary disease
COX	cyclooxygenase
CPK	creatine phosphokinase
CPR	cardiopulmonary resuscitation
CrCl	creatinine clearance
CRF	chronic renal failure
CRP	C-reactive protein
CRRT	continuous renal replacement therapy
CSF	cerebrospinal fluid
CSII	continuous subcutaneous insulin infusion
CT	computed tomography
CVA	cerebrovascular accident
CVP	central venous pressure
CVVH	continuous venovenous hemofiltration
CVVHD	continuous venovenous hemodialysis
CVVHDF	continuous venovenous hemodiafiltration
CYP	cytochrome
$D_5{}^1/_4NS$	dextrose 5% in sodium chloride 0.2%
$D_5{}^1/_2NS$	dextrose 5% in sodium chloride 0.45%
D_5LR	dextrose 5% in lactated Ringer's
D_5NS	dextrose 5% in sodium chloride 0.9%
D_5W	dextrose 5% in water
$D_{10}W$	dextrose 10% in water
DBP	diastolic blood pressure
DEHP	di(3-ethylhexyl)phthalate
DIC	disseminated intravascular coagulation
DL_{co}	pulmonary diffusion capacity for carbon monoxide
DM	diabetes mellitus

Abbreviations Which May Be Used in This Reference *(continued)*

Abbreviation	Meaning
DMARD	disease modifying antirheumatic drug
DNA	deoxyribonucleic acid
DSC	discontinued
DSM-IV	Diagnostic and Statistical Manual
DVT	deep vein thrombosis
EBV	Epstein-Barr virus
ECG	electrocardiogram
ECHO	echocardiogram
ECMO	extracorporeal membrane oxygenation
ECT	electroconvulsive therapy
ED	emergency department
EEG	electroencephalogram
EF	ejection fraction
EG	ethylene glycol
EGA	estimated gestational age
EIA	enzyme immunoassay
ELBW	extremely low birth weight
ELISA	enzyme-linked immunosorbent assay
EPS	extrapyramidal side effects
ESR	erythrocyte sedimentation rate
ESRD	end stage renal disease
E.T.	endotracheal
EtOH	alcohol
FDA	Food and Drug Administration (United States)
FEV_1	forced expiratory volume exhaled after 1 second
FSH	follicle-stimulating hormone
FTT	failure to thrive
FVC	forced vital capacity
G-6-PD	glucose-6-phosphate dehydrogenase
GA	gestational age
GABA	gamma-aminobutyric acid
GAD	generalized anxiety disorder
GE	gastroesophageal
GERD	gastroesophageal reflux disease
GFR	glomerular filtration rate
GGT	gamma-glutamyltransferase
GI	gastrointestinal
GU	genitourinary
GVHD	graft versus host disease
HAM-A	Hamilton Anxiety Scale
HAM-D	Hamilton Depression Scale
HARS	HIV-associated adipose redistribution syndrome
HCAHPS	Hospital Consumer Assessment of Healthcare Providers and Systems
Hct	hematocrit
HDL-C	high density lipoprotein cholesterol
HF	heart failure
HFA	hydrofluoroalkane
HFSA	Heart Failure Society of America
Hgb	hemoglobin
HIV	human immunodeficiency virus
HMG-CoA	3-hydroxy-3-methylglutaryl-coenzyme A
HOCM	hypertrophic obstructive cardiomyopathy
HPA	hypothalamic-pituitary-adrenal
HPLC	high performance liquid chromatography
HSV	herpes simplex virus
HTN	hypertension
HUS	hemolytic uremic syndrome

Abbreviations Which May Be Used in This Reference *(continued)*

Abbreviation	Meaning
IBD	inflammatory bowel disease
IBS	irritable bowel syndrome
IBW	ideal body weight
ICD	implantable cardioverter defibrillator
ICH	intracranial hemorrhage
ICP	intracranial pressure
IDDM	insulin-dependent diabetes mellitus
IDSA	Infectious Diseases Society of America
IgG	immune globulin G
IHSS	idiopathic hypertrophic subaortic stenosis
ILCOR	International Liaison Committee on Resuscitation
I.M.	intramuscular
INR	international normalized ration
Int. unit	international unit
I.O.	intraosseous
I & O	input and output
IOP	intraocular pressure
IQ	intelligence quotient
I.T.	intrathecal
ITP	idiopathic thrombocytopenic purpura
IUGR	intrauterine growth retardation
I.V.	intravenous
IVH	intraventricular hemorrhage
IVP	intravenous push
IVPB	intravenous piggyback
JIA	juvenile idiopathic arthritis
JNC	Joint National Committee
JRA	juvenile rheumatoid arthritis
kg	kilogram
KIU	kallikrein inhibitor unit
KOH	potassium hydroxide
LAMM	L-α-acetyl methadol
LDH	lactate dehydrogenase
LDL-C	low density lipoprotein cholesterol
LE	lupus erythematosus
LFT	liver function test
LGA	large for gestational age
LH	luteinizing hormone
LP	lumbar posture
LR	lactated Ringer's
LV	left ventricular
LVEF	left ventricular ejection fraction
LVH	left ventricular hypertrophy
MAC	*Mycobacterium avium* complex
MADRS	Montgomery Asbery Depression Rating Scale
MAO	monoamine oxidase
MAOIs	monamine oxidase inhibitors
MAP	mean arterial pressure
MDD	major depressive disorder
MDRD	modification of diet in renal disease
MDRSP	multidrug resistant *streptococcus pneumoniae*
MI	myocardial infarction
MMSE	mini mental status examination
MOPP	mustargen (mechlorethamine), Oncovin® (vincristine), procarbazine, and prednisone
M/P	milk to plasma ratio
MPS I	mucopolysaccharidosis I
MRHD	maximum recommended human dose

Abbreviations Which May Be Used in This Reference *(continued)*

Abbreviation	Meaning
MRI	magnetic resonance imaging
MRSA	methicillin-resistant *Staphylococcus aureus*
MUGA	multiple gated acquisition scan
NAEPP	National Asthma Education and Prevention Program
NAS	neonatal abstinence syndrome
NCI	National Cancer Institute
ND	nasoduodenal
NF	National Formulary
NFD	Nephrogenic fibrosing dermopathy
NG	nasogastric
NIDDM	noninsulin-dependent diabetes mellitus
NIH	National Institute of Health
NIOSH	National Institute for Occupational Safety and Health
NKA	no known allergies
NKDA	No known drug allergies
NMDA	n-methyl-d-aspartate
NMS	neuroleptic malignant syndrome
NNRTI	non-nucleoside reverse transcriptase inhibitor
NRTI	nucleoside reverse transcriptase inhibitor
NS	normal saline (0.9% sodium chloride)
NSAID	nonsteroidal anti-inflammatory drug
NSF	nephrogenic systemic fibrosis
NSTEMI	Non-ST-elevation myocardial infarction
NYHA	New York Heart Association
OA	osteoarthritis
OCD	obsessive-compulsive disorder
OHSS	ovarian hyperstimulation syndrome
O.R.	operating room
OTC	over-the-counter (nonprescription)
PABA	para-aminobenzoic acid
PACTG	Pediatric AIDS Clinical Trials Group
PALS	pediatric advanced life support
PAT	paroxysmal atrial tachycardia
PCA	patient-controlled analgesia
PCP	*Pneumocystis jiroveci* pneumonia (also called *Pneumocystis carinii* pneumonia)
PCWP	pulmonary capillary wedge pressure
PD	Parkinson's disease; peritoneal dialysis
PDA	patent ductus arteriosus
PDE-5	phosphodiesterase-5
PE	pulmonary embolism
PEG tube	percutaneous endoscopic gastrostomy tube
P-gp	P-glycoprotein
PHN	post-herpetic neuralgia
PICU	Pediatric Intensive Care Unit
PID	pelvic inflammatory disease
PIP	peak inspiratory pressure
PMA	postmenstrual age
PMDD	premenstrual dysphoric disorder
PNA	postnatal age
PONV	postoperative nausea and vomiting
PPHN	persistent pulmonary hypertension of the neonate
PPN	peripheral parenteral nutrition
PROM	premature rupture of membranes
PSVT	paroxysmal supraventricular tachycardia
PT	prothrombin time
PTH	parathyroid hormone
PTSD	post-traumatic stress disorder

Abbreviations Which May Be Used in This Reference *(continued)*

Abbreviation	Meaning
PTT	partial thromboplastin time
PUD	peptic ulcer disease
PVC	premature ventricular contraction
PVD	peripheral vascular disease
PVR	peripheral vascular resistance
QT_c	corrected QT interval
QT_cF	corrected QT interval by Fredricia's formula
RA	rheumatoid arthritis
RAP	right arterial pressure
RDA	recommended daily allowance
REM	rapid eye movement
REMS	risk evaluation and mitigation strategies
RIA	radioimmunoassay
RNA	ribonucleic acid
RPLS	reversible posterior leukoencephalopathy syndrome
RSV	respiratory syncytial virus
SA	sinoatrial
SAD	seasonal affective disorder
SAH	subarachnoid hemorrhage
SBE	subacute bacterial endocarditis
SBP	systolic blood pressure
S_{cr}	serum creatinine
SERM	selective estrogen receptor modulator
SGA	small for gestational age
SGOT	serum glutamic oxaloacetic aminotransferase
SGPT	serum glutamic pyruvate transaminase
SI	International System of Units or Systeme international d'Unites
SIADH	syndrome of inappropriate antidiuretic hormone secretion
SLE	systemic lupus erythematosus
SLEDD	sustained low-efficiency daily diafiltration
SNRI	serotonin norepinephrine reuptake inhibitor
SSKI	saturated solution of potassium iodide
SSRIs	selective serotonin reuptake inhibitors
STD	sexually transmitted disease
STEM I	ST-elevation myocardial infarction
SVR	systemic vascular resistance
SVT	supraventricular tachycardia
SWFI	sterile water for injection
SWI	sterile water for injection
$T_{1/2}$	half-life
T_3	triiodothyronine
T_4	thyroxine
TB	tuberculosis
TC	total cholesterol
TCA	tricyclic antidepressant
TD	tardive dyskinesia
TG	triglyceride
TIA	transient ischemic attack
TIBC	total iron binding capacity
TMA	thrombotic microangiopathy
T_{max}	time to maximum observed concentration, plasma
TNF	tumor necrosis factor
TPN	total parenteral nutrition
TSH	thyroid stimulating hormone
TT	thrombin time
TTP	thrombotic thrombocytopenic purpura
UA	urine analysis

Abbreviations Which May Be Used in This Reference *(continued)*

Abbreviation	Meaning
UC	ulcerative colitis
ULN	upper limits of normal
URI	upper respiratory infection
USAN	United States Adopted Names
USP	United States Pharmacopeia
UTI	urinary tract infection
UV	ultraviolet
V_d	volume of distribution
V_{dss}	volume of distribution at steady-state
VEGF	vascular endothelial growth factor
VF	ventricular fibrillation
VLBW	very low birth weight
VMA	vanillylmandelic acid
VT	ventricular tachycardia
VTE	venous thromboembolism
vWD	von Willebrand disease
VZV	varicella zoster virus
WHO	World Health Organization
w/v	weight for volume
w/w	weight for weight
YBOC	Yale Brown Obsessive-Compulsive Scale
YMRS	Young Mania Rating Scale

Common Weights, Measures, or Apothecary Abbreviations

Abbreviation	Meaning
<[1]	less than
>[1]	greater than
≤	less than or equal to
≥	greater than or equal to
ac	before meals or food
ad	to, up to
ad lib	at pleasure
AM	morning
AMA	against medical advice
amp	ampul
amt	amount
aq	water
aq. dest.	distilled water
ASAP	as soon as possible
a.u.[1]	each ear
bid	twice daily
bm	bowel movement
C	Celsius, centigrade
cal	calorie
cap	capsule
cc[1]	cubic centimeter
cm	centimeter
comp	compound
cont	continue
d	day
d/c[1]	discharge
dil	dilute
disp	dispense
div	divide
dtd	give of such a dose

Common Weights, Measures, or Apothecary Abbreviations *(continued)*

Abbreviation	Meaning
Dx	diagnosis
elix, el	elixir
emp	as directed
et	and
ex aq	in water
F	Fahrenheit
f, ft	make, let be made
g	gram
gr	grain
gtt	a drop
h	hour
hs[1]	at bedtime
kcal	kilocalorie
kg	kilogram
L	liter
liq	a liquor, solution
M	molar
mcg	microgram
m. dict	as directed
mEq	milliequivalent
mg	milligram
microL	microliter
min	minute
mL	milliliter
mm	millimeter
mM	millimole
mm Hg	millimeters of mercury
mo	month
mOsm	milliosmoles
ng	nanogram
nmol	nanomole
no.	number
noc	in the night
non rep	do not repeat, no refills
NPO	nothing by mouth
NV	nausea and vomiting
O, Oct	a pint
o.d.[1]	right eye
o.l.	left eye
o.s.[1]	left eye
o.u.[1]	each eye
pc, post cib	after meals
PM	afternoon or evening
P.O.	by mouth
P.R.	rectally
prn	as needed
pulv	a powder
q	every
qad	every other day
qd[1,2]	every day, daily
qh	every hour
qid	four times a day
qod[1,2]	every other day
qs	a sufficient quantity
qs ad	a sufficient quantity to make
Rx	take, a recipe
S.L.	sublingual

Common Weights, Measures, or Apothecary Abbreviations *(continued)*

Abbreviation	Meaning
stat	at once, immediately
SubQ	subcutaneous
supp	suppository
syr	syrup
tab	tablet
tal	such
tid	three times a day
tr, tinct	tincture
trit	triturate
tsp	teaspoon
u.d.	as directed
ung	ointment
v.o.	verbal order
w.a.	while awake
x3	3 times
x4	4 times
y	year

[1]ISMP error-prone abbreviation

[2]JCAHO Do Not Use list

Additional abbreviations used and defined within a specific monograph or text piece may only apply to that text.

REFERENCES

The Institute for Safe Medication Practices (ISMP) list of Error-Prone Abbreviations, Symbols, and Dose Designations. Available at http://www.ismp.org/Tools/errorproneabbreviations.pdf

The Joint Commission Official "Do Not Use" list. Available at http://www.jointcommission.org/facts_about_the_official_/

APOTHECARY/METRIC EQUIVALENTS

Apothecary-Metric Exact Equivalents

1 gram (g)	=	15.43 grains (gr)		0.1 mg	=	1/600 gr
1 milliliter (mL)	=	16.23 minims		0.12 mg	=	1/500 gr
1 minim	=	0.06 mL		0.15 mg	=	1/400 gr
1 gr	=	64.8 milligrams (mg)		0.2 mg	=	1/300 gr
1 fluid ounce (fl oz)	=	29.57 mL		0.3 mg	=	1/200 gr
1 pint (pt)	=	473.2 mL		0.4 mg	=	1/150 gr
1 ounce (oz)	=	28.35 g		0.5 mg	=	1/120 gr
1 pound (lb)	=	453.6 g		0.6 mg	=	1/100 gr
1 killogram (kg)	=	2.2 lb		0.8 mg	=	1/80 gr
1 quart (qt)	=	946.4 mL		1 mg	=	1/65 gr

Apothecary-Metric Approximate Equivalents[1]

Liquids			Solids		
1 teaspoonful	=	5 mL	1/4 grain	=	15 mg
1 tablespoonful	=	15 mL	1/2 grain	=	30 mg
			1 grain	=	60 mg
			1 1/2 grain	=	100 mg
			5 grains	=	300 mg
			10 grains	=	600 mg

[1]Use exact equivalents for compounding and calculations requiring a high degree of accuracy.

AVERAGE WEIGHTS AND SURFACE AREAS

Average Height, Weight, and Surface Area by Age and Gender

Age	Girls			Boys		
	Height (cm)	Weight (kg)	BSA (m^2)	Height (cm)	Weight (kg)	BSA (m^2)
Birth	49.5	3.4	0.22	50	3.6	0.22
3 mo	59	5.6	0.3	61	6	0.32
6 mo	65	7.2	0.36	67	7.9	0.38
9 mo	70	8.3	0.4	72	9.3	0.43
12 mo	74.5	9.5	0.44	75.5	10.3	0.46
15 mo	77	10.3	0.47	79	11.1	0.49
18 mo	80	11	0.49	82	11.7	0.52
21 mo	83	11.6	0.52	85	12.2	0.54
2 y	86	12	0.54	87.5	12.6	0.55
2.5 y	91	13	0.57	92	13.5	0.59
3 y	94.5	13.8	0.6	96	14.3	0.62
3.5 y	97	15	0.64	98	15	0.64
4 y	101	16	0.67	102	16	0.67
4.5 y	104	17	0.7	105	17	0.7
5 y	107.5	18	0.73	109	18.5	0.75
6 y	115	20	0.80	115	21	0.82
7 y	121.5	23	0.88	122	23	0.88
8 y	127.5	25.5	0.95	127.5	26	0.96
9 y	133	29	1.04	133.5	28.5	1.03
10 y	138	33	1.12	138.5	32	1.1
11 y	144	37	1.22	143.5	36	1.2
12 y	151	41.5	1.32	149	40.5	1.29
13 y	157	46	1.42	156	45.5	1.4
14 y	160.5	49.5	1.49	163.5	51	1.52
15 y	162	52	1.53	170	56	1.63
16 y	162.5	54	1.56	173.5	61	1.71
17 y	163	55	1.58	175	64.5	1.77
Adult[1]	163.5	58	1.62	177	83.5	2.03

Data extracted from the CDC growth charts based on the 50th percentile height and weight for a given age[2]

Body surface area calculation[3]: Square root of [(Ht x Wt) / 3600]

[1]McDowell MA, Fryar CD, Hirsch R, Ogden CL. Anthropometric reference data for children and adults: U.S. population, 1999-2002. *Adv Data.* 2005;(361):1-5.

[2]Centers for Disease Control and Prevention (CDC). 2000 CDC growth charts: United States. Available at http://www.cdc.gov/growthcharts. Accessed November 16, 2007.

[3]Mosteller RD. Simplified calculation of body-surface area *N Engl J Med.* 1987;317(17):1098.

BODY SURFACE AREA OF CHILDREN AND ADULTS

Calculating Body Surface Area in Children

In a child of average size, find weight and corresponding surface area on the boxed scale to the left or use the nomogram to the right. Lay a straightedge on the correct height and weight points for the child, then read the intersecting point on the surface area scale. (**Note:** 2.2 lb = 1 kg)

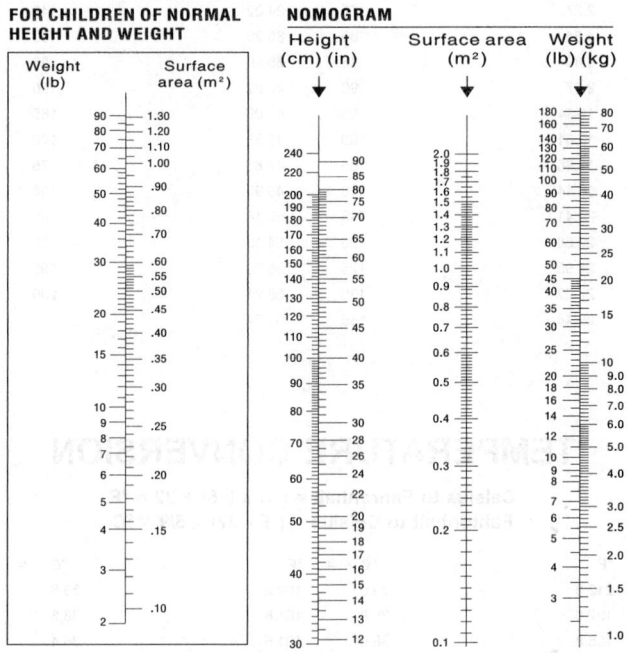

FOR CHILDREN OF NORMAL HEIGHT AND WEIGHT

NOMOGRAM

BODY SURFACE AREA FORMULA
(Adult and Pediatric)

$$BSA\ (m^2) = \sqrt{\dfrac{Ht\ (in) \times Wt\ (lb)}{3131}} \quad \text{or, in metric: } BSA\ (m^2) = \sqrt{\dfrac{Ht\ (cm) \times Wt\ (kg)}{3600}}$$

References
> Lam TK and Leung DT, "More on Simplified Calculation of Body Surface Area," *N Engl J Med*, 1988, 318(17):1130 (Letter).
> Mosteller RD, "Simplified Calculation of Body Surface Area", *N Engl J Med*, 1987, 317(17):1098 (Letter).

POUNDS/KILOGRAMS CONVERSION

1 pound = 0.45359 kilograms
1 kilogram = 2.2 pounds

lb	=	kg		lb	=	kg		lb	=	kg
1		0.45		70		31.75		140		63.50
5		2.27		75		34.02		145		65.77
10		4.54		80		36.29		150		68.04
15		6.80		85		38.56		155		70.31
20		9.07		90		40.82		160		72.58
25		11.34		95		43.09		165		74.84
30		13.61		100		45.36		170		77.11
35		15.88		105		47.63		175		79.38
40		18.14		110		49.90		180		81.65
45		20.41		115		52.16		185		83.92
50		22.68		120		54.43		190		86.18
55		24.95		125		56.70		195		88.45
60		27.22		130		58.91		200		90.72
65		29.48		135		61.24				

TEMPERATURE CONVERSION

Celsius to Fahrenheit = (°C x 9/5) + 32 = °F
Fahrenheit to Celsius = (°F - 32) x 5/9 = °C

°C	=	°F		°C	=	°F		°C	=	°F
100.0		212.0		39.0		102.2		36.8		98.2
50.0		122.0		38.8		101.8		36.6		97.9
41.0		105.8		38.6		101.5		36.4		97.5
40.8		105.4		38.4		101.1		36.2		97.2
40.6		105.1		38.2		100.8		36.0		96.8
40.4		104.7		38.0		100.4		35.8		96.4
40.2		104.4		37.8		100.1		35.6		96.1
40.0		104.0		37.6		99.7		35.4		95.7
39.8		103.6		37.4		99.3		35.2		95.4
39.6		103.3		37.2		99.0		35.0		95.0
39.4		102.9		37.0		98.6		0		32.0
39.2		102.6								

REFERENCE VALUES FOR ADULTS

CHEMISTRY

Test	Values	Remarks
Serum/Plasma		
Acetone	Negative	
Albumin	3.2-5 g/dL	
Alcohol, ethyl	Negative	
Aldolase	1.2-7.6 IU/L	
Ammonia	20-70 mcg/dL	Specimen to be placed on ice as soon as collected.
Amylase	30-110 units/L	
Bilirubin, direct	0-0.3 mg/dL	
Bilirubin, total	0.1-1.2 mg/dL	
Calcium	8.6-10.3 mg/dL	
Calcium, ionized	2.24-2.46 mEq/L	
Chloride	95-108 mEq/L	
Cholesterol, total	≤200 mg/dL	Fasted blood required – normal value affected by dietary habits. This reference range is for a general adult population.
HDL cholesterol	40-60 mg/dL	Fasted blood required – normal value affected by dietary habits.
LDL cholesterol	<160 mg/dL	If triglyceride is >400 mg/dL, LDL cannot be calculated accurately (Friedewald equation). Target LDL-C depends on patient's risk factors.
CO_2	23-30 mEq/L	
Creatine kinase (CK) isoenzymes		
CK-BB	0%	
CK-MB (cardiac)	0%-3.9%	
CK-MM (muscle)	96%-100%	
CK-MB levels must be both ≥4% and 10 IU/L to meet diagnostic criteria for CK-MB positive result consistent with myocardial injury.		
Creatine phosphokinase (CPK)	8-150 IU/L	
Creatinine	0.5-1.4 mg/dL	
Ferritin	13-300 ng/mL	
Folate	3.6-20 ng/dL	
GGT (gamma-glutamyltranspeptidase)		
male	11-63 IU/L	
female	8-35 IU/L	
GLDH	To be determined	
Glucose (preprandial)	<115 mg/dL	Goals different for diabetics.
Glucose, fasting	60-110 mg/dL	Goals different for diabetics.
Glucose, nonfasting (2-h postprandial)	<120 mg/dL	Goals different for diabetics.
Hemoglobin A_{1c}	<8	
Hemoglobin, plasma free	<2.5 mg/100 mL	
Hemoglobin, total glycosolated (Hb A_1)	4%-8%	
Iron	65-150 mcg/dL	
Iron binding capacity, total (TIBC)	250-420 mcg/dL	
Lactic acid	0.7-2.1 mEq/L	Specimen to be kept on ice and sent to lab as soon as possible.
Lactate dehydrogenase (LDH)	56-194 IU/L	

CHEMISTRY (continued)

Test	Values	Remarks
Lactate dehydrogenase (LDH) isoenzymes		
LD$_1$	20%-34%	
LD$_2$	29%-41%	
LD$_3$	15%-25%	
LD$_4$	1%-12%	
LD$_5$	1%-15%	
Flipped LD$_1$/LD$_2$ ratios (>1 may be consistent with myocardial injury) particularly when considered in combination with a recent CK-MB positive result.		
Lipase	23-208 units/L	
Magnesium	1.6-2.5 mg/dL	Increased by slight hemolysis.
Osmolality	289-308 mOsm/kg	
Phosphatase, alkaline		
adults 25-60 y	33-131 IU/L	
adults ≥61 y	51-153 IU/L	
infancy-adolescence	Values range up to 3-5 times higher than adults	
Phosphate, inorganic	2.8-4.2 mg/dL	
Potassium	3.5-5.2 mEq/L	Increased by slight hemolysis.
Prealbumin	>15 mg/dL	
Protein, total	6.5-7.9 g/dL	
AST	<35 IU/L (20-48)	
ALT (10-35)	<35 IU/L	
Sodium	134-149 mEq/L	
Thyroid stimulating hormone (TSH)		
adults ≤20 y	0.7-6.4 mIU/L	
21-54 y	0.4-4.2 mIU/L	
55-87 y	0.5-8.9 mIU/L	
Transferrin	>200 mg/dL	
Triglycerides	45-155 mg/dL	Fasted blood required.
Troponin I	<1.5 ng/mL	
Urea nitrogen (BUN)	7-20 mg/dL	
Uric acid		
male	2-8 mg/dL	
female	2-7.5 mg/dL	
Cerebrospinal Fluid		
Glucose	50-70 mg/dL	
Protein	15-45 mg/dL	CSF obtained by lumbar puncture.

Note: Bloody specimen gives erroneously high value due to contamination with blood proteins

Urine
(24-hour specimen is required for all these tests unless specified)

Test	Values	Remarks
Amylase	32-641 units/L	The value is in units/L and **not** calculated for total volume.
Amylase, fluid (random samples)		Interpretation of value left for physician, depends on the nature of fluid.
Calcium	Depends upon dietary intake	
Creatine		
male	150 mg/24 h	Higher value on children and during pregnancy.
female	250 mg/24 h	
Creatinine	1000-2000 mg/24 h	
Creatinine clearance (endogenous)		
male	85-125 mL/min	A blood sample must accompany urine specimen.
female	75-115 mL/min	

CHEMISTRY *(continued)*

Test	Values	Remarks
Glucose	1 g/24 h	
5-hydroxyindoleacetic acid	2-8 mg/24 h	
Iron	0.15 mg/24 h	Acid washed container required.
Magnesium	146-209 mg/24 h	
Osmolality	500-800 mOsm/kg	With normal fluid intake.
Oxalate	10-40 mg/24 h	
Phosphate	400-1300 mg/24 h	
Potassium	25-120 mEq/24 h	Varies with diet; the interpretation of urine electrolytes and osmolality should be left for the physician.
Sodium	40-220 mEq/24 h	
Porphobilinogen, qualitative	Negative	
Porphyrins, qualitative	Negative	
Proteins	0.05-0.1 g/24 h	
Salicylate	Negative	
Urea clearance	60-95 mL/min	A blood sample must accompany specimen.
Urea N	10-40 g/24 h	Dependent on protein intake.
Uric acid	250-750 mg/24 h	Dependent on diet and therapy.
Urobilinogen	0.5-3.5 mg/24 h	For qualitative determination on random urine, send sample to urinalysis section in Hematology Lab.
Xylose absorption test children	16%-33% of ingested xylose	

Feces

Fat, 3-day collection	<5 g/d	Value depends on fat intake of 100 g/d for 3 days preceding and during collection.

Gastric Acidity

Acidity, total, 12 h	10-60 mEq/L	Titrated at pH 7.

Blood Gases

	Arterial	Capillary	Venous
pH	7.35-7.45	7.35-7.45	7.32-7.42
pCO_2 (mm Hg)	35-45	35-45	38-52
pO_2 (mm Hg)	70-100	60-80	24-48
HCO_3 (mEq/L)	19-25	19-25	19-25
TCO_2 (mEq/L)	19-29	19-29	23-33
O_2 saturation (%)	90-95	90-95	40-70
Base excess (mEq/L)	-5 to +5	-5 to +5	-5 to +5

HEMATOLOGY

Complete Blood Count

Age	Hgb (g/dL)	Hct (%)	RBC (mill/mm³)	RDW
0-3 d	15.0-20.0	45-61	4.0-5.9	<18
1-2 wk	12.5-18.5	39-57	3.6-5.5	<17
1-6 mo	10.0-13.0	29-42	3.1-4.3	<16.5
7 mo to 2 y	10.5-13.0	33-38	3.7-4.9	<16
2-5 y	11.5-13.0	34-39	3.9-5.0	<15
5-8 y	11.5-14.5	35-42	4.0-4.9	<15
13-18 y	12.0-15.2	36-47	4.5-5.1	<14.5
Adult male	13.5-16.5	41-50	4.5-5.5	<14.5
Adult female	12.0-15.0	36-44	4.0-4.9	<14.5

Age	MCV (fL)	MCH (pg)	MCHC (%)	Plts (x 10³/mm³)
0-3 d	95-115	31-37	29-37	250-450
1-2 wk	86-110	28-36	28-38	250-450
1-6 mo	74-96	25-35	30-36	300-700
7 mo to 2 y	70-84	23-30	31-37	250-600
2-5 y	75-87	24-30	31-37	250-550
5-8 y	77-95	25-33	31-37	250-550
13-18 y	78-96	25-35	31-37	150-450
Adult male	80-100	26-34	31-37	150-450
Adult female	80-100	26-34	31-37	150-450

WBC and Differential

Age	WBC (x 10³/mm³)	Segs	Bands	Lymphs	Monos
0-3 d	9.0-35.0	32-62	<18	19-29	5-7
1-2 wk	5.0-20.0	14-34	<14	36-45	6-10
1-6 mo	6.0-17.5	13-33	<12	41-71	4-7
7 mo to 2 y	6.0-17.0	15-35	<11	45-76	3-6
2-5 y	5.5-15.5	23-45	<11	35-65	3-6
5-8 y	5.0-14.5	32-54	<11	28-48	3-6
13-18 y	4.5-13.0	34-64	<11	25-45	3-6
Adults	4.5-11.0	35-66	<11	24-44	3-6

Age	Eosinophils	Basophils	Atypical Lymphs	No. of NRBCs
0-3 d	0-2	0-1	0-8	0-2
1-2 wk	0-2	0-1	0-8	0
1-6 mo	0-3	0-1	0-8	0
7 mo to 2 y	0-3	0-1	0-8	0
2-5 y	0-3	0-1	0-8	0
5-8 y	0-3	0-1	0-8	0
13-18 y	0-3	0-1	0-8	0
Adults	0-3	0-1	0-8	0

Segs = segmented neutrophils.

Bands = band neutrophils.

Lymphs = lymphocytes.

Monos = monocytes.

Erythrocyte Sedimentation Rates and Reticulocyte Counts

Sedimentation rate, Westergren	Children	0-20 mm/h
	Adult male	0-15 mm/h
	Adult female	0-20 mm/h
Sedimentation rate, Wintrobe	Children	0-13 mm/h
	Adult male	0-10 mm/h
	Adult female	0-15 mm/h
Reticulocyte count	Newborns	2%-6%
	1-6 mo	0%-2.8%
	Adults	0.5%-1.5%

DIAGNOSTICS AND SURGICAL AIDS

Agent	Use
Aluminum chloride (Hemodent)	Hemostatic for gingival bleeding
Aminocaproic acid (Amicar)	To enhance hemostasis when fibrinolysis contributes to bleeding
Antihemophilic Factor (Recombinant) (Advate; Helixate FS; Kogenate FS; Kogenate FS Bio-Set; Recombinate; Xyntha; Xyntha Solofuse)	Prevention and treatment of hemorrhagic episodes in patients with hemophilia A (classic hemophilia or congenital factor VIII deficiency); perioperative management of hemophilia A; routine prophylaxis in patients with hemophilia A to prevent bleeding episodes (Advate; Helixate FS; Kogenate FS)
Arginine (R-Gene 10)	Pituitary function test (growth hormone)
Atopiclair (multiple ingredients)	Manage and relieve symptoms of dermatoses, including atopic dermatitis (or atopic eczema) and allergic contact dermatitis; helps to relieve dry, waxy skin by maintaining a moist skin environment; dermal donor and graft site management
Candida albicans (Monilia) (Candin)	Screen for the detection of nonresponsiveness to antigens in immunocompromised individuals
Cellulose (oxidized regenerated) (Surgicel)	Hemostatic; temporary absorbable packing for the control of capillary, venous, or small arterial hemorrhage
Collagen hemostat (eg, Actifoam; Avitene; Ultrafoam)	Adjunct to hemostasis when control of bleeding by ligature is ineffective or impractical
Corticorelin (Acthrel)	Diagnostic test used in adrenocorticotropic hormone (ACTH)-dependent Cushing's syndrome to differentiate between pituitary and ectopic production of ACTH
Cosyntropin (Cortrosyn)	Diagnostic test to differentiate primary adrenal from secondary (pituitary) adrenocortical insufficiency
Cyclopentolate (Cyclogyl)	Diagnostic procedures requiring mydriasis and cycloplegia
Cyclopentolate and phenylephrine (Cyclomydril)	Induce mydriasis greater than that produced with cyclopentolate HCl alone
Desmopressin (eg, DDAVP)	Uremic bleeding associated with acute or chronic renal failure; prevention of surgical bleeding in patients with uremia
Factor IX (recombinant) (BeneFIX; Rixubis)	Prevention and control of bleeding episodes in patients with hemophilia B; perioperative management in patients with hemophilia B
Factor VIIa (recombinant) (NovoSeven RT)	Prevention and treatment of bleeding in hemophilia A or B with inhibitors; also used to treat bleeding in patients with factor VII deficiency, acquired hemophilia, and refractory bleeding after cardiac surgery
Ferric subsulfate (Astringyn; Monsels Ferric Subsulfate)	Hemostatic in minor surgical procedures
Fibrin sealant (Artiss; Evarrest; Evicel; TachoSil; Tisseel)	Artiss: Aid in adhering autologous skin grafts in burn patients or tissue flaps during facial rhytidectomy surgery (facelift) (not indicated for hemostasis) Evarrest: Adjunct to hemostasis in open retroperitoneal, intra-abdominal, pelvic, and noncardiac thoracic surgery to control soft tissue bleeding Evicel: Adjunct to hemostasis in surgery when control of bleeding by conventional surgical techniques is ineffective or impractical TachoSil: Adjunct to hemostasis in cardiovascular surgery when control of bleeding by conventional surgical technique is ineffective or impractical Tisseel: Adjunct to hemostasis in cardiopulmonary bypass surgery (including fully heparinized patients) and splenic injury (due to blunt or penetrating trauma to the abdomen) when the control of bleeding by conventional surgical techniques is ineffective or impractical; adjunctive sealant for anastomoses following closure of colostomies
Fluorescein (AK-Fluor; Bio Glo; Fluorescite; Fluorets; Fluor-I-Strips A.T.; Ful-Glo)	Injection: Diagnostic aid in ophthalmic angiography and angioscopy Topical: To stain the anterior segment of the eye for procedures (such as fitting contact lenses), disclosing corneal injury, and in applanation tonometry
Fluorescein and benoxinate (EyeFlur; Fluress; Flurox)	For use in ophthalmic procedures when a topical disclosing agent is needed along with an anesthetic; for removal of foreign body, sutures, tonometry
Gelatin (absorbable) (Gelfilm; Gelfoam)	Adjunct to provide hemostasis in surgery; used in open prostatic surgery
Glucagon (GlucaGen)	Diagnostic aid in radiologic examinations to temporarily inhibit GI tract movement
Hydroxyamphetamine and tropicamide (Paremyd)	Short-term pupil dilation for diagnostic procedures and exams
Hydroxypropyl methylcellulose (eg, GenTeal Mild; GenTeal; Gonak; Goniosoft; Isopto Tears)	Diagnostic agent in gonioscopic examination

(continued)

Agent	Use
Indocyanine green (IC Green)	Determine hepatic function, cardiac output, and liver blood flow; ophthalmic angiography
Isosulfan blue (Lymphazurin)	Adjunct to lymphography for visualization of the lymphatic system; sentinel node identification
Mannitol (Aridol; Osmitrol; Resectisol)	Assessment of bronchial hyper-responsiveness
Methacholine (Provocholine)	Sensitive assay test for diagnosis of bronchial airway hyperactivity
Metyrapone (Metopirone)	Diagnostic test for hypothalamic-pituitary ACTH function
Perflutren lipid microspheres (Definity)	Opacification of left ventricular chamber and improvement of delineation of the left ventricular endocardial border in patients with suboptimal echocardiograms
Perflutren protein type A (Optison)	Opacification of left ventricular chamber and improvement of delineation of the left ventricular endocardial border in patients with suboptimal echocardiograms
Proparacaine (Alcaine; Parcaine)	Anesthetic for tonometry, gonioscopy; suture removal from cornea; removal of corneal foreign body; cataract extraction, glaucoma surgery; short operative procedure involving the cornea and conjunctiva
Proparacaine and fluorescein (Flucaine)	Anesthetic for tonometry, gonioscopy; suture removal from cornea; removal of corneal foreign body; cataract extraction, glaucoma surgery
Prothrombin complex concentrate (human) [(factors II, VII, IX, X), protein C, and protein S] (Kcentra)	Urgent reversal of acquired coagulation factor deficiency in patients with acute major bleeding or a need for urgent surgery/invasive procedure
Regadenoson (Lexiscan)	Radionuclide myocardial perfusion imaging (MPI) in patients unable to undergo adequate exercise stress testing
Secretin (ChiRhoStim; SecreFlo)	Secretin-stimulation testing to aid in diagnosis of pancreatic exocrine dysfunction; diagnosis of gastrinoma (Zollinger-Ellison syndrome); facilitation of endoscopic retrograde cholangiopancreatography (ERCP) visualization
Sincalide (Kinevac)	Postevacuation cholecystography; gallbladder bile sampling; stimulate pancreatic secretion for analysis; accelerate the transit of barium through the small bowel
Sodium chondroitin sulfate and sodium hyaluronate (DisCoVisc; Viscoat)	Ophthalmic surgical aid in the anterior segment during cataract extraction and intraocular lens implantation
Thrombin (topical) (Evithrom; Recothrom; Thrombi-Gel; Thrombi-Pad; Thrombin-JMI)	Hemostasis when minor bleeding from capillaries and small venules is accessible Thrombi-Gel; Thrombi-Pad: Temporary control as trauma dressing for moderate-to-severe bleeding wounds; control of surface bleeding from vascular access sites and percutaneous catheter/tubes
Thyrotropin alfa (Thyrogen)	As an adjunctive diagnostic tool for serum thyroglobulin (Tg) testing; adjunctive treatment for radioiodine ablation of thyroid tissue remnants after total or near-total thyroidectomy in patients with well-differentiated thyroid cancer without evidence of metastatic disease
Tranexamic acid (Cyklokapron; Lysteda)	Short-term use (2-8 days) in hemophilia patients to reduce or prevent hemorrhage and reduce need for replacement therapy during and following tooth extraction; used in a variety of trauma, surgical, and dental procedures where bleeding may be a problem or where bleeding is occurring
Trichophyton skin test	Assess cell-mediated immunity
Tropicamide (Mydral; Mydriacyl)	Short-acting mydriatic used in diagnostic procedures, as well as preoperatively and postoperatively; treatment of some cases of acute iritis, iridocyclitis, and keratitis
Tuberculin tests (Aplisol; Tubersol)	Skin tests in diagnosis of tuberculosis

HERBAL AND NUTRITIONAL PRODUCTS

HERBS AND COMMON NATURAL AGENTS

The authors have chosen to include this list of natural products and proposed medical claims. However, due to limited scientific investigation to support these claims, this list is not intended to imply that these claims have been scientifically proven.

Proposed Treatments

Herb	Treatment
5-HTP	Anxiety/sleep terrors, depression
Acai	Anticancer activity, antidiabetic effects, cardiovascular effects, lipid effects
African mango	Diabetes, obesity
Alfalfa	Cholesterol reduction, anti-inflammatory effects
Aloe	Burns/skin irritation, wound healing, seborrheic dermatitis/psoriasis, diabetes/hyperglycemia, anti-inflammatory effects, anticancer effects, antibacterial/anti-infective effects, gastrointestinal/inflammatory bowel disease
Alpha-lipoic acid	CNS diseases, multiple sclerosis, alzheimer disease, hearing loss, wound management, burning mouth syndrome, oxidation, diabetes, HIV and AIDS, cancer, chelation of transition and heavy metals, reduction of drug toxicity
Arginine	Diagnostic agent
Arnica	Inflammation, pain, bruising, muscle stiffness/marathon running, immune system effects
Bee pollen	Performance enhancer, prostatic conditions, premenstrual syndrome and menopausal symptoms
Beta-sitosterol	Cholesterol-lowering effects and other cardiovascular effects, immunomodulatory effects, anticancer properties, benign prostatic hyperplasia, androgenic alopecia, antimicrobial effects
Bilberry	Antioxidant effect, anti-inflammatory/allergy, cancer, cardiovascular effects, diabetes, GI effects, ophthalmic effects
Biotin	Biotin deficiency, diabetes, fingernails and hair
Bitter orange	Weight loss
Black cohosh	Menopause
Boron	Boron deficiency; bone and joint health; brain function, cognitive performance, and psychomotor function; inflammatory or immune response
Brewer's yeast	Diarrhea, immune effects, metabolic syndrome, respiratory effects
Butterbur	Allergic rhinitis, asthma, migraine
Calendula	Anti-inflammatory, dermatitis/skin conditions
Caprylidene	Alzheimer disease
Capsicum peppers	Diabetes, gastrointestinal effects, obesity, pain
Carnitine	Carnitine deficiency
Cat's claw	Anti-inflammatory, cancer
Chamomile	Anti-inflammatory, antispasmodic/antidiarrheal, skin/eczema, skin/radiation dermatitis, estrogenic activity, CNS/sensory effects, mouth (mucositis)
Chondroitin	Antiarthritic, antithrombotic
Chromium	Diabetes, hyperlipidemia, weight loss
Cinnamon	Diabetes, antioxidant effect, anti-inflammatory effect, antimicrobial activity
Clove	Anesthetic, antimicrobial, cancer
Cranberry	Cancer, urinary tract infections
Creatine	Aging, amyotrophic lateral sclerosis/motor neuron disease, other neurodegenerative disorders, exercise performance enhancement, cardiovascular disease, CNS, chronic obstructive pulmonary disease (COPD), mitochondrial disease, muscular dystrophies
Dehydroepiandrosterone (DHEA)	Assisted reproduction, cancer, cognition, metabolic effects (lipids/insulin), postmenopausal effects, schizophrenia, systemic lupus erythematosus
Devil's claw	Anti-inflammatory/analgesic effects
Dong quai	Dysmenorrhea, menstrual migraine, menopausal vasomotor symptoms
Echinacea	Cancer, immunomodulation, upper respiratory tract infection
Evening primrose oil	Atopic dermatitis/dermatologic disorders, mastalgia, menopause-associated vasomotor symptoms/premenstrual syndrome, multiple sclerosis, rheumatoid arthritis

Proposed Treatments (continued)

Herb	Treatment
Fenugreek	Cholesterol-lowering effects, glucose-lowering effects, anti-inflammatory effects, antitumor activity, antioxidant effects
Feverfew	Anti-inflammatory activity, effects on vascular smooth muscle, effects of platelets, inhibition of histamine release, chemotherapeutic activity, anticancer activity, cystic fibrosis, antioxidant effects, migraine headache and prophylactic treatment
Fish oils (docosahexaenoic acid [DHA] in LC)	Asthma/allergy, arrhythmias, coronary heart disease, CNS effects, critical illness and surgical patients, diabetes, infant development, inflammatory bowel disease, lipid-lowering effects, rheumatoid arthritis, stroke
Flax	Atherosclerosis, cancer, diabetes/metabolic syndrome
Fruit acids	Anti-aging/photoaging/actinic keratosis, dry skin and ichthyosis, melasma, acne, psoriasis, contact dermatitis, fibromyalgia
Garlic	Antimicrobial, antithrombotic effects, diabetes, dyslipidemia, hypertension, cancer
Ginger	Analgesic/anti-inflammatory effects, cancer, nausea, motion sickness, postoperative nausea, pregnancy-related nausea, inhibition of platelet aggregation
Ginkgo biloba	Alzheimer and other dementias, other CNS conditions, cancer, cardiovascular disease, diabetes, sexual dysfunction in women, stroke
Ginseng	Cancer, cardiovascular effects, CNS effects, diabetes, ergogenic effects, immunomodulatory and adaptogenic effects
Glucomannan	GI effects, antidiabetic effects, weight reduction effects, effects of lipids, effects on lung cancer, atopic disease effects
Glucosamine	Osteoarthritis
Glutathione	CNS, cancer, cardiovascular, cystic fibrosis
Goldenseal	Antimicrobial/antidiarrheal activity, cardiovascular, ophthalmic
Grape seed	Cancer, cardiovascular effects, CNS
Grapefruit	Antimicrobial effects, cardiovascular effects, cholelithiasis/nephrolithiasis
Green tea	Anogenital warts, cancer, cardiovascular effects, CNS effects, diabetes, obesity, osteoporosis, stroke (acute cerebrovascular episode), UV protection
Hawthorn	Cardiovascular disease (heart failure, blood pressure), central nervous system, hyperlipidemia
Horny goat weed	Cardiovascular, erectile dysfunction
Hyaluronic acid	Facial wrinkles and folds, lip augmentation
Inositol hexaphosphate	Skin hyperpigmentation
Kava	Anxiety, cancer, cognition
Lecithin	Hypercholesterolemia, neurologic disorders, liver disease, gallstone treatment, mania
Licorice	Antiviral, cancer, GI
L-theanine	Cancer, cardiovascular effects, CNS effects, immune system functioning
Lutein	Ophthalmic, cancer
Lycopene	Antioxidant, cancer, cardiovascular disease
Lysine	Herpes infections/cold sores, cardiovascular effects, pain management, calcium absorption and osteoporosis, glucose effects, anxiolytic effects, effects on muscle mass
Marijuana	Appetite stimulant, cancer/chemotherapy-induced nausea and vomiting, glaucoma, multiple sclerosis, pain, diabetes mellitus, inflammatory bowel disease
Maritime pine	Cardiovascular effects, erectile dysfunction, diabetes, inflammation
Melatonin	Cancer, cardiovascular effects, GI disorders, reproductive system, insomnia, jet lag/circadian misalignment, other nervous system effects
Milk thistle	Cancer, diabetes, hepatoprotective effects, dyspepsia, allergic rhinitis
Methysulfonylmethane (MSM)	Osteoarthritis, cancer, diabetes, rosacea, ichthyosis
Olive oil	Cardiovascular conditions, cancer, clinical nutrition
Pantothenic acid	Acne, hyperlipidemia, ophthalmic effects, radioprotective and adaptogen effects
Passion flower	Cardiovascular effects, CNS effects, diabetes
Pectin	Cancer, cardiovascular, chelating effects, diabetes, GI (diarrhea), gastroesophageal reflux
Peppermint	GI use (antiemetic, biliary disorders, dyspepsia, irritable bowel syndrome, smooth muscle spasm), respiratory tract, pain/sensory effects
Pineapple	Anti-inflammatory; antimicrobial; burns; ear, nose, throat/acute sinusitis; immunomodulation; malignant disease
Poison ivy	Osteoarthritis
Policosanol	Cholesterol reduction, intermittent claudication

Proposed Treatments *(continued)*

Herb	Treatment
Probiotics	Bacterial vaginosis; candidiasis, vaginal; Crohn disease, diarrhea, acute infectious; diarrhea, antibiotic-associated; diarrhea, persistent; eczema/allergic dermatitis; *Helicobacter pylori* eradication; intensive care patients, adults; irritable bowel syndrome; necrotizing enterocolitis, neonates; pancreatitis; pneumonia, ventilator-associated; respiratory tract infections/otitis media; ulcerative colitis; urinary tract infections
Progesterone	Menopause/menopausal symptoms
Quercetin	Antioxidant activity, cancer, cardiovascular disease, exercise/performance
Raspberry	Anti-inflammatory effect, cardiovascular, cancer, diabetes, pregnancy
Red yeast rice	Antibacterial activity, cancer, diabetes, hyperlipidemia
Resveratrol	Antiaging, anti-inflammatory, cancer, cardiovascular disease, diabetes, neurodegenerative conditions
Rhodiola rosea	Adaptogenic effects, cancer, depression
Rose hip	Anti-inflammatory, diabetes/metabolic syndrome
Safflower	Cardiovascular, CNS
SAMe	Depression, liver disease/hepatitis, osteoarthritis, cancer, alzheimer disease
Saw palmetto	Benign prostatic hyperplasis, cancer
Senna	Laxative
Soy	Cancer (breast, prostate, other), cardiovascular disease, diabetes, food allergy/intolerance in infants, menopausal symptoms, osteoporosis
Spirulina	Allergic rhinitis and asthma, antimicrobial activity, cancer, diabetes, dietary supplement, hyperlipidemia, immune system effects, prevention of toxicity due to metals or organic compounds, antioxidant
St John's wort	Depression, other CNS-related conditions
Sweet wormwood	Malaria, anticancer activity
Taurine	Cardiovascular effects, CNS effects, diabetes, exercise
Tea tree oil	Antibacterial, antifungal, antiviral
Turmeric	Cancer, cardiovascular effects, CNS effects, diabetes, gastrointestinal
Tyrosine	Dietary supplement
Ubiquinone	Cardiovascular disease (cardiac surgery/cardiac arrest, congestive heart failure, hypertension, Friedreich ataxia [hypertrophic cardiomyopathy], reversal of statin-induced myopathy), neurological disorders
Valerian	Anxiolytic effect, insomnia, dysmenorrhea, obsessive-compulsive disorder
Vinpocetine	Antioxidant effects, menopause, antiulcer activity, phosphodiesterase-1 inhibition, neuroprotective effects, tinnitus, antiepileptic activity, psychopharmacological effects, acute ischemic stroke, chronic cerebral vascular ischemia, pain management
Willow bark	Anticancer activity, anti-inflammatory and antioxidant activity, arthritis, lower back pain
Yohimbe	Body mass/muscle mass, erectile dysfunction, syncope/orthostatic hypotension, xerostomia (dry mouth)

IMMUNIZATION ADMINISTRATION RECOMMENDATIONS

The following tables are taken from the General Recommendations on Immunization, 2011:

- Guidelines for Spacing of Live and Inactivated Antigens
- Guidelines for Administering Antibody-Containing Products and Vaccines
- Recommended Intervals Between Administration of Antibody-Containing Products and Measles- or Varicella-Containing Vaccine, by Product and Indication for Vaccination
- Vaccination of persons with Primary and Secondary Immunodeficiencies
- Needle length and Injection Site of I.M. injections

Guidelines for Spacing of Live and Inactivated Antigens

Antigen Combination	Recommended Minimum Interval Between Doses
Two or more inactivated[1]	May be administered simultaneously or at any interval between doses
Inactivated and live	May be administered simultaneously or at any interval between doses
Two or more live injectable[2]	28 days minimum interval, if not administered simultaneously

[1]Certain experts suggest a 28-day interval between tetanus toxoid, reduced diphtheria toxoid, and reduced acellular pertussis (Tdap) vaccine and tetravalent meningococcal conjugate vaccine if they are not administered simultaneously.

[2]Live oral vaccines (eg, Ty21a typhoid vaccine and rotavirus vaccine) may be administered simultaneously or at any interval before or after inactivated or live injectable vaccines.

Adapted from American Academy of Pediatrics. Pertussis. Pickering LK, Baker CJ, Kimberlin DW, et al, eds. *Red Book*: 2009 Report of the Committee on Infectious Diseases. 28th ed. Elk Grove Village, IL: American Academy of Pediatrics; 2009;22.

Guidelines for Administering Antibody-Containing Products[1] and Vaccines

Simultaneous Administration (during the same office visit)

Products Administered	Recommended Minimum Interval Between Doses
Antibody-containing products and inactivated antigen	Can be administered simultaneously at different anatomic sites or at any time interval between doses.
Antibody-containing products and live antigen	Should **not** be administered simultaneously.[2] If simultaneous administration of measles-containing vaccine or varicella vaccine is unavoidable, administer at different sites and revaccinate or test for seroconversion after the recommended interval.

Nonsimultaneous Administration

Products Administered		Recommended Minimum Interval Between Doses
Administered first	Administered second	
Antibody-containing products	Inactivated antigen	No interval necessary
Inactivated antigen	Antibody-containing products	No interval necessary
Antibody-containing products	Live antigen	Dose-related[2,3]
Live antigen	Antibody-containing products	2 weeks[2]

[1]Blood products containing substantial amounts of immune globulin include intramuscular and intravenous immune globulin, specific hyperimmune globulin (eg, hepatitis B immune globulin, tetanus immune globulin, varicella zoster immune globulin, and rabies immune globulin), whole blood, packed red blood cells, plasma, and platelet products.

[2]Yellow fever vaccine, rotavirus vaccine, oral Ty21a typhoid vaccine, live-attenuated influenza vaccine, and zoster vaccine are exceptions to these recommendations. These live-attenuated vaccines can be administered at any time before, after, or simultaneously with an antibody-containing product.

[3]The duration of interference of antibody-containing products with the immune response to the measles component of measles-containing vaccine, and possibly varicella vaccine, is dose-related.

Recommended Intervals Between Administration of Antibody-Containing Products and Measles- or Varicella-Containing Vaccine, by Product and Indication for Vaccination

Product/Indication	Dose (mg IgG/kg) and Route[1]	Recommended Interval Before Measles- or Varicella-Containing Vaccine[2] Administration (mo)
Tetanus IG	I.M.: 250 units (10 mg IgG/kg)	3
Hepatitis A IG		
Contact prophylaxis	I.M.: 0.02 mL/kg (3.3 mg IgG/kg)	3
International travel	I.M.: 0.06 mL/kg (10 mg IgG/kg)	3
Hepatitis B IG	I.M.: 0.06 mL/kg (10 mg IgG/kg)	3
Rabies IG	I.M.: 20 int. units/kg (22 mg IgG/kg)	4
Varicella IG	I.M.: 125 units/10 kg (60-200 mg IgG/kg) (maximum: 625 units)	5
Measles prophylaxis IG		
Standard (ie, nonimmunocompromised) contact	I.M.: 0.25 mL/kg (40 mg IgG/kg)	5
Immunocompromised contact	I.M.: 0.50 mL/kg (80 mg IgG/kg)	6
Blood transfusion		
Red blood cells (RBCs), washed	I.V.: 10 mL/kg (negligible IgG/kg)	None
RBCs, adenine-saline added	I.V.: 10 mL/kg (10 mg IgG/kg)	3
Packed RBCs (hematocrit 65%)[3]	I.V.: 10 mL/kg (60 mg IgG/kg)	6
Whole blood cells (hematocrit 35% to 50%)[3]	I.V.: 10 mL/kg (80-100 mg IgG/kg)	6
Plasma/platelet products	I.V.: 10 mL/kg (160 mg IgG/kg)	7
Cytomegalovirus intravenous immune globulin (IGIV)	150 mg/kg maximum	6
IGIV		
Replacement therapy for immune deficiencies[4]	I.V.: 300-400 mg/kg[4]	8
Immune thrombocytopenic purpura treatment	I.V.: 400 mg/kg	8
Postexposure varicella prophylaxis[5]	I.V.: 400 mg/kg	8
Immune thrombocytopenic purpura treatment	I.V.: 1000 mg/kg	10
Kawasaki disease	I.V.: 2 g/kg	11
Monoclonal antibody to respiratory syncytial virus F protein (Synagis [Medimmune])[6]	I.M.: 15 mg/kg	None

HIV = human immunodeficiency virus, IG = immune globulin, IgG = immune globulin G, IGIV = intravenous immune globulin, mg IgG/kg = milligrams of immune globulin G per kilogram of body weight, I.M. = intramuscular, I.V. = intravenous, RBCs = red blood cells

[1]This table is not intended for determining the correct indications and dosages for using antibody-containing products. Unvaccinated persons might not be fully protected against measles during the entire recommended interval, and additional doses of IG or measles vaccine might be indicated after measles exposure. Concentrations of measles antibody in an IG preparation can vary by manufacturer's lot. Rates of antibody clearance after receipt of an IG preparation also might vary. Recommended intervals are extrapolated from an estimated half-life of 30 days for passively acquired antibody and an observed interference with the immune response to measles vaccine for 5 months after a dose of 80 mg IgG/kg.

[2]Does not include zoster vaccine. Zoster vaccine may be given with antibody-containing blood products.

[3]Assumes a serum IgG concentration of 16 mg/mL

[4]Measles and varicella vaccinations are recommended for children with asymptomatic or mildly symptomatic HIV infection but are contraindicated for persons with severe immunosuppression from HIV or any other immunosuppressive disorder.

[5]The investigational product VariZIG, similar to licensed varicella-zoster IG (VZIG), is a purified human IG preparation made from plasma containing high levels of anti-varicella antibodies (IgG). The interval between VariZIG and varicella vaccine (Var or MMRV) is 5 months.

[6]Contains antibody only to respiratory syncytial virus

Vaccination of Persons With Primary and Secondary Immunodeficiencies

Category	Specific Immunodeficiency	Contraindicated Vaccines[1]	Risk-Specific Recommended Vaccines[1]	Effectiveness and Comments
Primary				
B-lymphocyte (humoral)	Severe antibody deficiencies (eg, X-linked agammaglobulinemia and common variable immunodeficiency)	Oral poliovirus (OPV)[2] Smallpox Live-attenuated influenza vaccine (LAIV) BCG Ty21a (live oral typhoid) Yellow fever	Pneumococcal Consider measles and varicella vaccination	The effectiveness of any vaccine is uncertain if it depends only on the humoral response (eg, PPSV or MPSV4) IGIV interferes with the immune response to measles vaccine and possibly varicella vaccine
	Less severe antibody deficiencies (eg, selective IgA deficiency and IgG subclass deficiency)	OPV[2] BCG Yellow Fever Other live-vaccines appear to be safe	Pneumococcal	All vaccines likely effective; immune response may be attenuated
T-lymphocyte (cell-mediated and humoral)	Complete defects (eg, severe combined immunodeficiency [SCID] disease, complete DiGeorge syndrome)	All live vaccines[3,4,5]	Pneumococcal	Vaccines might be ineffective
	Partial defects (eg, most patients with DiGeorge syndrome, Wiskott-Aldrich syndrome, ataxia- telangiectasia)	All live vaccines[3,4,5]	Pneumococcal Meningococcal Hib (if not administered in infancy)	Effectiveness of any vaccine depends on degree of immune suppression
Complement	Persistent complement, properdin, or factor B deficiency	None	Pneumococcal Meningococcal	All routine vaccines likely effective
Phagocytic function	Chronic granulomatous disease, leukocyte adhesion defect, and myeloperoxidase deficiency	Live bacterial vaccines[3]	Pneumococcal[6]	All inactivated vaccines safe and likely effective; live viral vaccines likely safe and effective

Vaccination of Persons With Primary and Secondary Immunodeficiencies *continued*

Category	Specific Immunodeficiency	Contraindicated Vaccines[1]	Risk-Specific Recommended Vaccines[1]	Effectiveness and Comments
		Secondary		
	HIV/AIDS	OPV[2] Smallpox BCG LAIV Withhold MMR and varicella in severely immunocompromised persons Yellow fever vaccine might have a contraindication or a precaution depending on clinical parameters of immune function[9]	Pneumococcal Consider Hib (if not administered in infancy) and meningococcal vaccination.	MMR, varicella, rotavirus, and all inactivated vaccines, including inactivated influenza, might be effective.[7]
	Malignant neoplasm, transplantation, immunosuppressive or radiation therapy	Live viral and bacterial, depending on immune status[3,4]	Pneumococcal	Effectiveness of any vaccine depends on degree of immune suppression
	Asplenia	None	Pneumococcal Meningococcal Hib (if not administered in infancy)	All routine vaccines likely effective
	Chronic renal disease	LAIV	Pneumococcal Hepatitis B[8]	All routine vaccines likely effective

AIDS = acquired immunodeficiency syndrome; BCG = bacille Calmette-Guerin; Hib = *Haemophilus influenzae* type b; HIV = human immunodeficiency virus; IG = immunoglobulin; IGIV = immune globulin intravenous; LAIV = live, attenuated influenza vaccine; MMR = measles, mumps, and rubella; MPSV4 = quadrivalent meningococcal polysaccharide vaccine; OPV = oral poliovirus vaccine (live); PPSV = pneumococcal polysaccharide vaccine; TIV = trivalent inactivated influenza vaccine

[1]Other vaccines that are universally or routinely recommended should be administered if not contraindicated.

[2]OPV is no longer available in the United States.

[3]Live bacterial vaccines: BCG and oral Ty21a *Salmonella typhi* vaccine

[4]Live viral vaccines: MMR, MMRV, OPV, LAIV, yellow fever, zoster, rotavirus, varicella, and vaccinia (smallpox). Smallpox vaccine is not recommended for children or the general public.

[5]Regarding T-lymphocyte immunodeficiency as a contraindication for rotavirus vaccine, data exist only for severe combined immunodeficiency.

[6]Pneumococcal vaccine is not indicated for children with chronic granulomatous disease beyond age-based universal recommendations for PCV. Children with chronic granulomatous disease are not at increased risk for pneumococcal disease.

[7]HIV-infected children should receive IG after exposure to measles and may receive varicella and measles vaccine if CD4+ lymphocyte count is ≥15%.

[8]Indicated based on the risk for dialysis-based bloodborne transmission

[9]Symptomatic HIV infection or CD4+ T-lymphocyte count of <200/mm³ or <15% of total lymphocytes for children aged <6 years is a contraindication to yellow fever vaccine administration. Asymptomatic HIV infection with CD4+ T-lymphocyte count of 200-499/mm³ for persons aged ≥6 years or 15% to 24% of total lymphocytes for children aged <6 years is a precaution for yellow fever vaccine administration. Details of yellow fever vaccine recommendations are available from the CDC. (CDC. Yellow fever vaccine: recommendations of the Advisory Committee on Immunization Practices [ACIP]. *MMWR Recomm Rep.* 2010;59[No. RR-7].)

Adapted from American Academy of Pediatrics. Passive immunization. Pickering LK, Baker CJ, Kimberline DW, et al, eds. *Red Book: 2009 Report of the Committee on Infectious Diseases.* 28th ed. Elk Grove Village, IL: American Academy of Pediatrics; 2009;74-75.

Needle Length and Injection Site of I.M. for Children Aged ≤18 years (by age) and Adults Aged ≥19 years (by sex and weight)

Age Group	Needle Length	Injection Site
Children (birth to 18 y)		
Neonates[1]	5/8" (16 mm)[2]	Anterolateral thigh
Infant 1-12 mo	1" (25 mm)	Anterolateral thigh
Toddler 1-2 y	1-1¼" (25-32 mm)	Anterolateral thigh[3]
	5/8[2]-1" (16-25 mm)	Deltoid muscle of the arm
Children 3-18 y	5/8[2]-1" (16-25 mm)	Deltoid muscle of the arm[3]
	1-1¼" (25-32 mm)	Anterolateral thigh
Adults ≥19 y		
Men and women <60 kg (130 lb)	1" (25 mm)[4]	Deltoid muscle of the arm
Men and women 60-70 kg (130-152 lb)	1" (25 mm)	
Men 70-118 kg (152-260 lb)	1-1½" (25-38 mm)	
Women 70-90 kg (152-200 lb)		
Men >118 kg (260 lb)	1½" (38 mm)	
Women >90 kg (200 lb)		

I.M. = intramuscular

[1] First 28 days of life

[2] If skin is stretched tightly and subcutaneous tissues are not bunched

[3] Preferred site

[4] Some experts recommend a 5/8" needle for men and women who weigh <60 kg.

Adapted from Poland GA, Borrud A, Jacobsen RM, et al. Determination of deltoid fat pad thickness: implications for needle length in adult immunization. *JAMA*. 1997;277:1709-1711.

RECOMMENDATIONS FOR TRAVELERS

The Centers for Disease Control and Prevention (CDC) also provides guidance to assist travelers and their healthcare providers in deciding the vaccines, medications, and other measures necessary to prevent illness and injury during international travel. Available at http://wwwnc.cdc.gov/travel

REFERENCE

Centers for Disease Control and Prevention (CDC). Recommendations of the Advisory Committee on Immunization Practices (ACIP): general recommendations on immunization. *MMWR Recomm Rep*. 2011;60(2):1-61.

IMMUNIZATION RECOMMENDATIONS

Vaccine	Birth	1 mo	2 mos	4 mos	6 mos	9 mos	12 mos	15 mos	18 mos	19–23 mos	2–3 yrs	4–6 yrs	7–10 yrs	11–12 yrs	13–15 yrs	16–18 yrs
Hepatitis B[1] (HepB)	1st dose	2nd dose			3rd dose											
Rotavirus[2] (RV) RV-1 (2-dose series); RV-5 (3-dose series)			1st dose	2nd dose	see footnote 2											
Diphtheria, tetanus & acellular pertussis[3] (DTaP: <7 yrs)			1st dose	2nd dose	3rd dose		4th dose					5th dose				
Tetanus & diphtheria & acellular pertussis[4] (Tdap: ≥ 7 yrs)														(Tdap)		
Haemophilus influenzae type b[5] (Hib)			1st dose	2nd dose	see footnote 5		3rd or 4th dose, see footnote 5									
Pneumococcal conjugate[6] (PCV13)			1st dose	2nd dose	3rd dose		4th dose									
Pneumococcal polysaccharide[6] (PPSV23)																
Inactivated poliovirus[7] (IPV) (<18 years)			1st dose	2nd dose			3rd dose					4th dose				
Influenza[8] (IIV;LAIV) 2 doses for some: see footnote 8						Annual vaccination (IIV only)						Annual vaccination (IIV or LAIV)				
Measles, mumps, rubella[9] (MMR)							1st dose					2nd dose				
Varicella[10] (VAR)							1st dose					2nd dose				
Hepatitis A[11] (Hep A)							2 dose series see footnote 11									
Human papillomavirus[12] (HPV2: females only; HPV4: males and females)														(3 dose series)		
Meningococcal[13] (Hib-MenCY ≥ 6 wks; MenACWY-D ≥ 9 mos; MenACWY-CRM ≥ 2 mos.)				see footnote 13										1st dose		booster[13]

Recommended Immunization Schedule for Persons 0 to 18 Years of Age — United States, 2014[*]

- Range of recommended ages for all children.
- Range of recommended ages for catch-up immunization.
- Range of recommended ages for certain high-risk groups.
- Range of recommended ages during which catch-up is encouraged and for certain high-risk groups.
- Not routinely recommended.

NOTE: The recommendations in the tables must be read along with the following footnotes.

[*] This schedule includes recommendations in effect as of January 1, 2014. Any dose not administered at the recommended age should be administered at a subsequent visit, when indicated and feasible. The use of a combination vaccine generally is preferred over separate injections of its equivalent component vaccines. Vaccination providers should consult the relevant Advisory Committee on Immunization Practices (ACIP) statement for detailed recommendations, available online at http://www.cdc.gov/vaccines/hcp/acip-recs/index.html. Clinically significant adverse events that follow vaccination should be reported to the Vaccine Adverse Event Reporting System (VAERS) online (http://www.vaers.hhs.gov) or by telephone (800-822-7967).Suspected cases of vaccine-preventable diseases should be reported to the state or local health department. Additional information, including precautions and contraindications for vaccination, is available from CDC online (http://www.cdc.gov/vaccines/recs/vac-admin/contraindications.htm) or by telephone (800-CDC-INFO [800-232-4636]). This schedule is approved by the Advisory Committee on Immunization Practices (http://www.cdc.gov/vaccines/acip), the American Academy of Pediatrics (http://www.aap.org), the American Academy of Family Physicians (http://www.aafp.org), and the American College of Obstetricians and Gynecologists (http://www.acog.org).

This schedule includes recommendations in effect as of January 1, 2014. Any dose not administered at the recommended age should be administered at a subsequent visit, when indicated and feasible. The use of a combination vaccine generally is preferred over separate injections of its equivalent component vaccines. Vaccination providers should consult the relevant Advisory Committee on Immunization Practices (ACIP) statement for detailed recommendations, available at **http://www.cdc.gov/vaccines/hcp/acip-recs/index.-html**. Clinically significant adverse events that follow vaccination should be reported to the Vaccine Adverse Event Reporting System (VAERS), available at http://vaers.hhs.gov/index or by telephone at **(800) 822-7967**. Also see the footnotes after the following "Catch-up Immunization Schedule" for more specific information about the vaccines.

Catch-up Immunization Schedule for Persons 4 Months to 18 Years of Age Who Start Late or Who Are >1 Month Behind – United States, 2014

This table provides catch-up schedules and minimum intervals between doses for children whose vaccinations have been delayed. A vaccine series does not need to be restarted, regardless of the time that has elapsed between doses. Use the section appropriate for the child's age. Always use this table in conjunction with the previous "Recommended immunization schedule for persons aged 0 through 18 years" and the footnotes that follow.

Vaccine	Minimum Age for Dose 1	Minimum Interval Between Doses			
		Dose 1 to Dose 2	Dose 2 to Dose 3	Dose 3 to Dose 4	Dose 4 to Dose 5
Catch-up Schedule for Persons 4 Months to 6 Years of Age					
Hepatitis B[1]	Birth	4 weeks	**8 weeks** and ≥16 weeks after first dose; minimum age for final dose is 24 weeks		
Rotavirus[2]	6 weeks	**4 weeks**	**4 weeks**[2]		
Diphtheria, tetanus, and acellular pertussis[3]	6 weeks	**4 weeks**	**4 weeks**	**6 months**	**6 months**[3]
Haemophilus influenzae type b[5]	6 weeks	**4 weeks** if first dose administered at <12 months of age **8 weeks** (as final dose) if first dose administered at 12-14 months of age **No further doses needed** if first dose administered at ≥15 months of age	**4 weeks**[5] if currently <12 months of age and first dose administered at <7 months of age **8 weeks** and 12-59 months of age (as final dose)[5] if currently <12 months of age and first dose administered between 7-11 months of age (regardless of Hib vaccine [PRP-T or PRP-OMP] used for first dose); or if currently 12-59 months of age and first dose administered at <12 months of age; or if first 2 doses were PRP-OMP and administered at <12 months of age **No further doses needed** if previous dose administered at ≥15 months of age	**8 weeks** (as final dose) This dose only necessary for children 12-59 months of age who received 3 (PRP-T) doses before 12 months of age and started primary series before 7 months of age	
Pneumococcal[6]	6 weeks	**4 weeks** if first dose administered at <12 months of age **8 weeks** (as final dose for healthy children) if first dose administered at ≥12 months of age **No further doses needed** for healthy children if first dose administered at ≥24 months of age	**4 weeks** if currently <12 months of age **8 weeks** (as final dose for healthy children) if currently ≥12 months of age **No further doses needed** for healthy children if previous dose administered at ≥24 months of age	**8 weeks** (as final dose) This dose only necessary for children 12-59 months of age who received 3 doses before 12 months of age or for children at high risk who received 3 doses at any age	
Inactivated poliovirus[7]	6 weeks	**4 weeks**[7]	**4 weeks**[7]	**6 months**[7] minimum 4 years of age for final dose	
Meningococcal[13]	6 weeks	**8 weeks**[13]	See footnote 13	See footnote 13	
Measles, mumps, rubella[9]	12 months	**4 weeks**			
Varicella[10]	12 months	**3 months**			
Hepatitis A[11]	12 months	**6 months**			
Catch-up Schedule for Persons 7-18 Years of Age					
Tetanus, diphtheria; tetanus, diphtheria, and acellular pertussis[4]	7 years[4]	**4 weeks**	**4 weeks** if first dose of DTaP/DT administered at <12 months of age **6 months** if first dose of DTaP/DT administered at ≥12 months of age and then no further doses needed for catch-up	**6 months** if first dose of DTaP/DT administered at <12 months of age	
Human papillomavirus[12]	9 years	Routine dosing intervals are recommended[12]			
Hepatitis A[11]	12 months	**6 months**			
Hepatitis B[1]	Birth	**4 weeks**	**8 weeks** (and ≥16 weeks after first dose)		
Inactivated poliovirus[7]	6 weeks	**4 weeks**	**4 weeks**[7]	**6 months**[7]	
Meningococcal[13]	6 weeks	**8 weeks**[13]			
Measles, mumps, rubella[9]	12 months	**4 weeks**			
Varicella[10]	12 months	**3 months** if person is <13 years of age **4 weeks** if person is ≥13 years of age			

Footnotes to Recommended Immunization Schedule for Persons 0-18 Years of Age and the Catch-up Immunization Schedule

Note: For further guidance on the use of the vaccines mentioned below, see http://www.cdc.gov/vaccines/hcp/acip-recs/index.html. For vaccine recommendations for persons ≥19 years of age, see the adult immunization schedule.

[1]Hepatitis B vaccine (HepB) *(Minimum age: Birth)*

Routine vaccination:

At birth:

- Administer monovalent HepB vaccine to all newborns before hospital discharge.

- For infants born to hepatitis B surface antigen (HB$_s$Ag)-positive mothers, administer HepB vaccine and 0.5 mL of hepatitis B immune globulin (HBIG) within 12 hours of birth. These infants should be tested for HB$_s$Ag and antibody to HB$_s$Ag (anti-HBs) 1-2 months after completion of the HepB series at 9-18 months of age (preferably at the next well-child visit).

- If the mother's HB$_s$Ag status is unknown, within 12 hours of birth, administer HepB vaccine to all infants regardless of birth weight. For infants weighing <2000 grams, administer HBIG in addition to HepB vaccine within 12 hours of birth. Determine the mother's HB$_s$Ag status as soon as possible and, if she is HB$_s$Ag-positive, also administer HBIG for infants weighing ≥2000 grams as soon as possible but no later than 7 days of age.

Doses following the birth dose:

- The second dose should be administered at 1 or 2 months of age. Monovalent HepB vaccine should be used for doses administered before 6 weeks of age.

- Infants who did not receive a birth dose should receive 3 doses of a HepB-containing vaccine on a schedule of 0, 1-2 months, and 6 months of age starting as soon as feasible. See the previous "Catch-up Immunization Schedule".

- Administer the second dose 1-2 months after the first dose (minimum interval of 4 weeks); administer the third dose at least 8 weeks after the second dose **and** at least 16 weeks after the **first** dose. The final (third of fourth) dose in the HepB vaccine series should be administered **no earlier than 24 weeks of age**.

- Administration of a total of 4 doses of HepB vaccine is permitted when a combination vaccine containing HepB is administered after the birth dose.

Catch-up vaccination:

- Unvaccinated persons should complete a 3-dose series.

- A 2-dose series (doses separated by at least 4 months) of adult formulation Recombivax HB is licensed for use in children 11-15 years of age.

- For other catch-up guidance, see the previous "Catch-up Immunization Schedule".

[2]Rotavirus vaccine (RV) *(Minimum age: 6 weeks for both RV-1 [Rotarix] and RV-5 [RotaTeq])*

Routine vaccination:

- Administer a series of RV vaccine to all infants as follows:

  - If Rotarix is used, administer a 2-dose series at 2 and 4 months of age.

  - If RotaTeq is used, administer a 3-dose series at ages 2, 4, and 6 months of age.

  - If any dose in the series was RotaTeq or vaccine product is unknown for any dose in the series, a total of 3 doses of RV vaccine should be administered.

Catch-up vaccination:

- The maximum age for the first dose in the series is 14 weeks, 6 days; vaccination should not be initiated for infants ≥15 weeks, 0 days of age.

- The maximum age for the final dose in the series is 8 months, 0 days.

- For other catch-up guidance, see the previous "Catch-up Immunization Schedule".

[3]**Diphtheria and tetanus toxoids and acellular pertussis vaccine (DTaP)** *(Minimum age: 6 weeks; exception: DTaP-IPV [Kinrix]: 4 years)*

Routine vaccination:

- Administer a 5-dose series of DTaP vaccine at 2, 4, 6, and 15-18 months of age, and at 4-6 years of age. The fourth dose may be administered as early as 12 months of age, provided at least 6 months have elapsed since the third dose.

Catch-up vaccination:

- The fifth dose of DTaP vaccine is not necessary if the fourth dose was administered at ≥4 years of age.

- For other catch-up guidance, see the previous "Catch-up Immunization Schedule".

[4]**Tetanus and diphtheria toxoids and acellular pertussis vaccine (Tdap)** *(Minimum age: 10 years for Adacel and Boostrix)*

Routine vaccination:

- Administer 1 dose of Tdap vaccine to all adolescents 11-12 years of age.

- Tdap can be administered regardless of the interval since the last tetanus and diphtheria toxoid-containing vaccine.

- Administer 1 dose of Tdap vaccine to pregnant adolescents during each pregnancy (preferred during 27-36 weeks gestation), regardless of time since prior Td or Tdap vaccination.

Catch-up vaccination:

- Persons ≥7 years of age who are not fully immunized with DTaP vaccine series should receive Tdap vaccine as 1 (preferably the first) dose in the catch-up series; if additional doses are needed, use Td vaccine. For children 7-10 years of age who receive a dose of Tdap as part of the catch-up series, an adolescent Tdap vaccine dose at 11-12 years of age should **not** be administered. Td should be administered instead 10 years after the Tdap dose.

- Persons 11-18 years of age who have not received Tdap vaccine should receive a dose, followed by tetanus and diphtheria toxoids (Td) booster doses every 10 years thereafter.

- Inadvertent doses of DTaP vaccine:

  - If administered inadvertently to a child 7-10 years of age, may count as part of the catch-up series. This dose can count as the adolescent Tdap dose or the child can later receive a Tdap booster dose at 11-12 years of age.

  - If administered inadvertently to an adolescent 11-18 years of age, the dose should be counted as the adolescent Tdap booster.

- For other catch-up guidance, see the previous "Catch-up Immunization Schedule".

[5]***Haemophilus influenzae** **type b conjugate vaccine (Hib)** (Minimum age: 6 weeks for PRP-T [ActHIB, DTaP-IPV/Hib (Pentacel), and Hib-MenCY (MenHibrix)], PRP-OMP [PedvaxHIB or COMVAX], 12 months for PRP-T [Hiberix])*

Routine vaccination:

- Administer a 2- or 3-dose Hib vaccine primary series and a booster dose (dose 3 or 4 depending on vaccine used in primary series) at 12-15 months of age to complete a full Hib vaccine series.

- The primary series with ActHIB, MenHibrix, or Pentacel consists of 3 doses and should be administered at 2, 4, and 6 months of age. The primary series with PedvaxHIB or COMVAX consists of 2 doses and should be administered at 2 and 4 months of age; a dose at 6 months of age is not indicated.

- One booster dose (dose 3 or 4 depending on vaccine used in primary series) of any Hib vaccine should be administered at 12-15 months of age. An exception is Hiberix vaccine. Hiberix should only be used for the booster (final) dose in children 12 months to 4 years of age who have received at least 1 prior dose of Hib-containing vaccine.

- For recommendations on the use of MenHibrix in patients at increased risk for meningococcal disease, please refer to the meningococcal vaccine footnotes and also to *MMWR*, 2013, 62(RR02);1-22, available at http://www.cdc.gov/mmwr/pdf/rr/rr6202.pdf.

◀ **Catch-up vaccination:**

- If dose 1 was administered at 12-14 months of age, administer a second (final) dose at least 8 weeks after dose 1, regardless of Hib vaccine used in the primary series.

- If the first 2 doses were PRP-OMP (PedvaxHIB or COMVAX) and were administered at ≤11 months of age, the third (and final) dose should be administered at 12-15 months of age and at least 8 weeks after the second dose.

- If the first dose was administered at 7-11 months of age, administer the second dose at least 4 weeks later and a third (and final) dose at 12-15 months of age or 8 weeks after the second dose, whichever is later, regardless of Hib vaccine used for the first dose.

- If the first dose is administered at <12 months of age and the second dose is given between 12-14 months of age, a third (and final) dose should be given 8 weeks later.

- For unvaccinated children ≥15 months of age, administer only 1 dose.

- For other catch-up guidance, see the previous "Catch-up Immunization Schedule". For catch-up guidance related to MenHibrix, please see the meningococcal vaccine footnotes and also *MMWR*, 2013, 62(RR02);1-22, available at http://www.cdc.gov/mmwr/pdf/rr/rr6202.pdf.

Vaccination of persons with high-risk conditions:

- Children 12-59 months of age who are at increased risk for Hib disease, including chemotherapy recipients and whose with anatomic or functional asplenia (including sickle cell disease), human immunodeficiency virus (HIV) infection, immunoglobulin deficiency, or early component complement deficiency, who have received either no doses or only 1 dose of Hib vaccine before 12 months of age, should receive 2 additional doses of Hib vaccine 8 weeks apart; children who received ≥2 doses of Hib vaccine before 12 months of age should receive 1 additional dose.

- For patients <5 years of age undergoing chemotherapy or radiation treatment who received a Hib vaccine dose(s) within 14 days of starting therapy or during therapy, repeat the dose(s) at least 3 months following therapy completion.

- Recipients of hematopoietic stem cell transplant (HSCT) should be revaccinated with a 3-dose regimen of Hib vaccine starting 6-12 months after successful transplant, regardless of vaccination history; doses should be administered at elast 4 weeks apart.

- A single dose of any Hib-containing vaccine should be administered to unimmunized* children and adolescents ≥15 months of age undergoing an elective splenectomy; if possible, vaccine should be administered at least 14 days before the procedure.

- Hib vaccine is not routinely recommended for patients ≥5 years of age. However, 1 dose of Hib vaccine should be administered to unimmunized* persons ≥5 years of age who have anatomic or functional asplenia (including sickle cell disease) and unvaccinated persons 5-18 years of age with human immunodeficiency virus (HIV) infection.

*Patients who have not received a primary series and booster dose or at least 1 dose of Hib vaccine after 14 months of age are considered unimmunized.

⁶Pneumococcal vaccines *(Minimum age: 6 weeks for PCV13, 2 years for PPSV23)*

Routine vaccination with PCV13:

- Administer a 4-dose series of PCV13 vaccine at 2, 4, 6, and 12-15 months of age.

- For children 14-59 months of age who have received an age-appropriate series of 7-valent PCV (PCV7), administer a single supplemental dose of 13-valent PCV (PCV13).

Catch-up vaccination with PCV13:

- Administer 1 dose of PCV13 to all healthy children 24-59 months of age who are not completely vaccinated for their age.

- For other catch-up guidance, see the previous "Catch-up Immunization Schedule".

Vaccination of persons with high-risk conditions with PCV13 and PPSV23:

- All recommended PCV13 doses should be administered prior to PPSV23 vaccination if possible.

- For children 2-5 years of age with any of the following conditions: Chronic heart disease (particularly cyanotic congenital heart disease and cardiac failure); chronic lung disease (including asthma if treated with high-dose oral corticosteroid therapy); diabetes mellitus; cerebrospinal fluid leak; cochlear implant; sickle cell disease and other hemogluinopathies; anatomic or functional asplenia; HIV infection; chronic renal failure; nephrotic syndrome; diseases associated with treatment with immunosuppressive drugs or radiation therapy, including malignant neoplasms, leukemias, lymphomas, and Hodgkin disease; solid organ transplantation; or congenital immunodeficiency:

1. Administer 1 dose of PCV13 if 3 doses of PCV (PCV7 and/or PCV13) were received previously.

2. Administer 2 doses of PCV13 at least 8 weeks apart if fewer than 3 doses of PCV (PCV7 and/or PCV13) were received previously.

3. Administer 1 supplemental dose of PCV13 if 4 doses of PCV7 or other age-appropriate complete PCV7 series was received previously.

4. The minimum interval between doses of PCV (PCV7 or PCV13) is 8 weeks.

5. For children with no history of PPSV23 vaccination, administer PPSV23 at least 8 weeks after the most recent dose of PCV13.

- For children 6-18 years of age who have cerebrospinal fluid leak; cochlear implant; sickle cell disease and other hemoglobinopathies; anatomic or functional asplenia; congenital or acquired immunodeficiencies; HIV infection; chronic renal failure; nephrotic syndrome; diseases associated with treatment with immunosuppressive drugs or radiation therapy, including malignant neoplasms, leukemias, lymphomas, and Hodgkin disease; generalized malignancy; solid organ transplantation; or multiple myeloma:

  1. If neither PCV13 nor PPSV23 has been received previously, administer 1 dose of PCV13 now and 1 dose of PPSV23 at least 8 weeks later.

  2. If PCV13 has been received previously but PPSV23 has not, administer 1 dose of PPSV23 at least 8 weeks after the most recent dose of PCV13.

  3. If PPSV23 has been received but PCV13 has not, administer 1 dose of PCV13 at least 8 weeks after the most recent dose of PPSV23.

- For children 6-18 years of age with chronic heart disease (particularly cyanotic congenital heart disease and cardiac failure), chronic lung disease (including asthma if treated with high-dose oral corticosteroid therapy), diabetes mellitus, alcoholism, or chronic liver disease, who have not received PPSV23, administer 1 dose of PPSV23. If PCV13 has been received previously, then PPSV23 should be administered at least 8 weeks after any prior PCV13 dose.

- A single revaccination with PPSV23 should be administered 5 years after the first dose to children with sickle cell disease or other hemoglobinopathies; anatomic or functional asplenia; congenital or acquired immunodeficiencies; HIV infection; chronic renal failure; nephrotic syndrome; diseases associated with treatment with immunosuppressive drugs or radiation therapy, including malignant neoplasms, leukemias, lymphomas, and Hodgkin disease; generalized malignancy; solid organ transplantation; or multiple myeloma.

[7]**Inactivated poliovirus vaccine (IPV)** *(Minimum age: 6 weeks)*

Routine vaccination:

- Administer a 4-dose series of IPV at 2, 4, and 6-18 months of age and at 4-6 years of age. The final dose in the series should be administered on or after the fourth birthday and at least 6 months after the previous dose.

Catch-up vaccination:

- In the first 6 months of life, minimum age and minimum intervals are only recommended if the person is at risk for imminent exposure to circulating poliovirus (ie, travel to a polio-endemic region or during an outbreak).

- If ≥4 doses are administered before 4 years of age, an additional dose should be administered at 4-6 years of age and at least 6 months after the previous dose.

- A fourth dose is not necessary if the third dose was administered at ≥4 years of age and at least 6 months after the previous dose.

- If both OPV and IPV were administered as part of a series, a total of 4 doses should be administered, regardless of the child's current age. IPV is not routinely recommended for U.S. residents ≥18 years of age.

- For other catch-up guidance, see the previous "Catch-up Immunization Schedule".

◄ [8]**Influenza vaccines** *(Minimum age: 6 months for inactivated influenza vaccine [IIV]; 2 years for live, attenuated influenza vaccine [LAIV])*
Routine vaccination:

- Administer influenza vaccine annually to all children beginning at 6 months of age. For most healthy, nonpregnant persons 2-49 years of age, either LAIV or IIV may be used. However, LAIV should **not** be administered to some persons, including 1) those with asthma, 2) children 2-4 years of age who had wheezing in the past 12 months, or 3) those who have any other underlying medical conditions that predispose them to influenza complications. For all other contraindications to use of LAIV, see *MMWR*, 2013, 62(No. RR-7);1-43, available at http://www.cdc.gov/mmwr/pdf/rr/rr6207.pdf.

For children 6 months to 8 years of age:

- For the 2013-14 season, administer 2 doses (separated by at least 4 weeks) to children who are receiving influenza vaccine for the first time. Some children in this age group who have been vaccinated previously will also need 2 doses. For additional guidance, follow dosing guidelines in the 2013-14 ACIP influenza vaccine recommendations. See *MMWR*, 2013, 62(No. RR-7);1-43, available at http://www.cdc.gov/mmwr/pdf/rr/rr6207.pdf.

- For the 2014-15 season, follow dosing guidelines in the 2014 ACIP influenza vaccine recommendations.

For persons ≥9 years of age:

- Administer 1 dose.

[9]**Measles, mumps, and rubella vaccine (MMR)** *(Minimum age: 12 months for routine vaccination)*
Routine vaccination:

- Administer a 2-dose series of MMR vaccine at 12-15 months of age and 4-6 years of age. The second dose may be administered before 4 years of age, provided at least 4 weeks have elapsed since the first dose.

- Administer 1 dose of MMR vaccine to infants 6-11 months of age before departure from the United States for international travel. These children should be revaccinated with 2 doses of MMR vaccine, the first at 12-15 months of age (12 months if the child remains in an area where disease risk is high) and the second dose at least 4 weeks later.

- Administer 2 doses of MMR vaccine to children ≥12 months of age before departure from the United States for international travel. The first dose should be administered at ≥12 months of age and the second dose at least 4 weeks later.

Catch-up vaccination:

- Ensure that all school-aged children and adolescents have had 2 doses of MMR vaccine; the minimum interval between the 2 doses is 4 weeks.

- For other catch-up guidance, see the previous "Catch-up Immunization Schedule".

[10]**Varicella vaccine (VAR)** *(Minimum age: 12 months)*
Routine vaccination:

- Administer a 2-dose series of VAR vaccine at 12-15 months of age and 4-6 years of age. The second dose may be administered before 4 years of age, provided at least 3 months have elapsed since the first dose. If the second dose was administered at least 4 weeks after the first dose, it can be accepted as valid.

Catch-up vaccination:

- Ensure that all persons 7-18 years of age without evidence of immunity (see *MMWR*, 2007, 56[No. RR-4], available at http://www.cdc.gov/mmwr/pdf/rr/rr5604.pdf) have 2 doses of varicella vaccine. For children 7-12 years of age, the recommended minimum interval between doses is 3 months (if the second dose was administered at least 4 weeks after the first dose, it can be accepted as valid); for persons ≥13 years of age, the minimum interval between doses is 4 weeks.

- For other catch-up guidance, see the previous "Catch-up Immunization Schedule".

[11]Hepatitis A vaccine (HepA) *(Minimum age: 12 months)*
Routine vaccination:

- Initiate the 2-dose HepA vaccine series at 12-23 months of age; separate the 2 doses by 6-18 months.

- Children who have received 1 dose of HepA vaccine before 24 months of age should receive a second dose 6-18 months after the first dose.

- For any person ≥2 years of age who has not already received the HepA vaccine series, 2 doses of HepA vaccine separated by 6-18 months may be administered if immunity against hepatitis A virus infection is desired.

Catch-up vaccination:

- The minimum interval between the 2 doses is 6 months.

- For other catch-up guidance, see the previous "Catch-up Immunization Schedule".

Special populations:

- Administer 2 doses of HepA vaccine at least 6 months apart to previously unvaccinated persons who live in areas where vaccination programs target older children or who are at increased risk for infection. This includes persons traveling to or working in countries that have high or intermediate endemicity of infection; men having sex with men; users of injection and noninjection illicit drugs; persons who work with HAV-infected primates or with HAV in a research laboratory; persons with clotting-factor disorders; persons with chronic liver disease; and persons who anticipate close, personal contact (eg, household or regular babysitting) with an international adoptee during the first 60 days after arrival in the United States from a country with high or intermediate endemicity. The first dose should be administered as soon as the adoption is planned, ideally ≥2 weeks before the arrival of the adoptee.

[12]Human papillomavirus vaccines (HPV) *(Minimum age: 9 years for HPV2 [Cervarix] and HPV4 [Gardasil])*
Routine vaccination:

- Administer a 3-dose series of HPV vaccine on a schedule of 0, 1-2, and 6 months to all adolescents 11-12 years of age. Either HPV4 or HPV2 may be used for females and only HPV4 may be used for males.

- The vaccine series can be started beginning at 9 years of age.

- Administer the second dose 1-2 months after the first dose (minimum interval of 4 weeks) and administer the third dose 24 weeks after the first dose and 16 weeks after the second dose (minimum interval of 12 weeks).

Catch-up vaccination:

- Administer the vaccine series to females (either HPV2 or HPV4) and males (HPV4) at 13-18 years of age if not previously vaccinated.

- Use recommended routine dosing intervals (see above) for vaccine series catch-up.

- For other catch-up guidance, see the previous "Catch-up Immunization Schedule".

[13]Meningococcal conjugate vaccines (MCV) *(Minimum age: 6 weeks for Hib-MenCY [MenHibrix], 9 months for MenACWY-D [Menactra], 2 months for MenACWY-CRM [Menveo])*
Routine vaccination:

- Administer a single dose of Menactra or Menveo vaccine at 11-12 years of age with a booster dose at 16 years of age.

- Adolescents 11-18 years of age with human immunodeficiency virus (HIV) infection should receive a 2-dose primary series of Menactra or Menveo with at least 8 weeks between doses.

- For children 2 months to 18 years of age with high-risk conditions, see below.

Catch-up vaccination:

- Administer Menactra or Menveo vaccine at 13-18 years of age if not previously vaccinated.

- If the first dose is administered at 13-15 years of age, a booster dose should be administered at 16-18 years of age with a minimum interval of at least 8 weeks between doses.

- If the first dose is administered at ≥16 years of age, a booster dose is not needed.

- For other catch-up guidance, see the previous "Catch-up Immunization Schedule".

◀ **Vaccination of persons with high-risk conditions and other persons at increased risk of disease:**

- Children with anatomic or functional asplenia (including sickle cell disease):

  1. For children <19 months of age, administer a 4-dose infant series of MenHibrix or Menveo at 2, 4, 6, and 12-15 months of age.

  2. For children 19-23 months of age who have not completed a series of MenHibrix or Menveo, administer 2 primary doses of Menveo at least 3 months apart.

  3. For children ≥24 months of age who have not received a complete series of MenHibrix, Menveo, or Menactra, administer 2 primary doses of either Menactra or Menveo at least 2 months apart. If Menactra is administered to a child with asplenia (including sickle cell disease), do not administer Menactra until 2 years of age and at least 4 weeks after the completion of all PCV13 doses.

- Children with persistent complement component deficiency:

  1. For children <19 months of age, administer a 4-dose infant series of either MenHibrix or Menveo at 2, 4, 6, and 12-15 months of age.

  2. For children 7-23 months of age who have not initiated vaccination, two options exist depending on age and vaccine brand:

     a. For children who initiate vaccination with Menveo at 7-23 months of age, a 2-dose series should be administered with the second dose after 12 months of age and at least 3 months after the first dose.

     b. For children who initiate vaccination with Menactra at 9-23 months of age, a 2-dose series of Menactra should be administered at least 3 months apart.

     c. For children ≥24 months of age who have not received a complete series of MenHibrix, Menveo, or Menactra, administer 2 primary doses of either Menactra or Menveo at least 2 months apart.

- For children who travel to or reside in countries in which meningoccoal disease is hyperendemic or epidemic, including countries in the African meningitis belt or the Hajj, administer an age-appropriate formulation and series of Menactra or Menveo for protection against serogroups A and W meningococcal disease. Prior receipt of MenHibrix is not sufficient for children traveling to the meningitis belt or the Hajj because it does not contain serogroups A or W.

- For children at risk during a community outbreak attributable to a vaccine serogroup, administer or complete an age- and formulation-appropriate series of MenHibrix, Menactra, or Menveo.

- For booster doses among persons with high-risk conditions, refer to *MMWR*, 2013, 62(RR02);1-22, available at http://www.cdc.gov/mmwr/preview/mmwrhtml/rr6202a1.htm.

Catch-up recommendations for persons with high-risk conditions:

1. If MenHibrix is administered to achieve protection against meningococcal disease, a complete age-appropriate series of MenHibrix should be administered.

2. If the first dose of MenHibrix is given at or after 12 months of age, a total of 2 doses should be given at least 8 weeks apart to ensure protection against serogroups C and Y meningococcal disease.

3. For children who initiate vaccination with Menveo at 7-9 months of age, a 2-dose series should be administered with the second dose after 12 months of age and at least 3 months after the first dose.

4. For other catch-up recommendations for these persons, refer to *MMWR*, 2013, 62(RR02);1-22, available at http://www.cdc.gov/mmwr/preview/mmwrhtml/rr6202a1.htm.

For complete information on the use of meningococcal vaccines, including guidance related to vaccination of persons at increased risk of infection, see *MMWR*, 2013, 62(RR02);1-22, available athttp://www.cdc.gov/mmwr/preview/mmwrhtml/rr6202a1.htm

This schedule is approved by the Advisory Committee on Immunization Practices (**http://www.cdc.gov/vaccines/acip/index.html**), the American Academy of Pediatrics (**http://www.aap.org**), the American Academy of Family Physicians (**http://www.aafp.org**), and the American College of Obstetricians and Gynecologists (**http://www.acog.org**).

REFERENCE

Centers for Disease Control and Prevention (CDC). Advisory Committee on Immunization Practices (ACIP) recommended immunization schedules for persons aged 0 through 18 years and adults aged 19 years and older − United States, 2014. Available at http://www.cdc.gov/vaccines/schedules/hcp/child-adolescent.html

Recommended Adult Immunization Schedule by Vaccine and Age Group[1] — United States, 2014

Vaccine	19 to 21 years	22 to 26 years	27 to 49 years	50 to 59 years	60 to 64 years	≥ 65 years
			Age group			
Influenza[2,*]	1 dose annually					
Tetanus, diphtheria, pertussis (Td/Tdap)[3,*]	Substitute 1-time dose of Tdap for Td booster; then boost with Td every 10 y					
Varicella[4,*]	2 doses					
Human papillomavirus (HPV) female[5,*]	3 doses					
Human papillomavirus (HPV) male[5,*]	3 doses	3 doses				
Zoster[6]					1 dose	
Measles, mumps, rubella (MMR)[7,*]	1 or 2 doses					
Pneumococcal 13-valent conjugate (PCV13)[8,*]	1 dose					
Pneumococcal polysaccharide (PPSV23)[9,10]	1 or 2 doses					1 dose
Meningococcal[11,*]	1 or more doses					
Hepatitis A[12,*]	2 doses					
Hepatitis B[13,*]	3 doses					
Haemophilus influenzae type b (Hib)[14,*]	1 or 3 doses					

*Covered by the Vaccine Injury Compensation Program.

For all persons in this category who meet the age requirements and who lack documentation of vaccination or have no evidence of previous infection; zoster vaccine reccommended regardless of prior episode of zoster.

Recommended if some other risk factor is present (eg, on the basis of medical, occupational, lifestyle, or other indication).

No recommendation.

NOTE: The recommendations in the tables must be read along with the following footnotes.

Vaccines That Might Be Indicated for Adults Based on Medical and Other Indications[1]

Vaccine	Pregnancy	Immunocompromising conditions (excluding human immunodeficiency virus [HIV])[4,6,7,8,15]	HIV infection CD4+ T lymphocyte count[4,6,7,8,15] < 200 cells/µL	HIV infection CD4+ T lymphocyte count ≥ 200 cells/µL	Men who have sex with men (MSM)	Kidney failure, end-stage renal disease, receipt of hemodialysis	Heart disease, chronic lung disease, chronic alcoholism	Asplenia (including elective splenectomy and persistent complement component deficiencies)[8,14]	Chronic liver disease	Diabetes	Healthcare personnel
						Indication					
Influenza[2,*]	1 dose IIV annually				1 dose IIV or LAIV annually	1 dose IIV annually					1 dose IIV or LAIV annually
Tetanus, diphtheria, pertussis (Td/Tdap)[3,*]	1 dose Tdap each pregnancy	Substitute 1-time dose of Tdap for Td booster; then boost with Td every 10 years									
Varicella[4,*]	Contraindicated			2 doses							
Human papillomavirus (HPV) female[5,*]		3 doses through age 26 yrs				3 doses through age 26 yrs					
Human papillomavirus (HPV) male[5,*]		3 doses through age 26 yrs				3 doses through age 21 yrs					
Zoster[6]	Contraindicated			1 dose							
Measles, mumps, rubella (MMR)[7,*]	Contraindicated			1 or 2 doses							
Pneumococcal 13-valent conjugate (PCV13)[8]						1 dose	1 dose				
Pneumococcal polysaccharide (PPSV23)[9,10]							1 or 2 doses				
Meningococcal[11,*]	1 or more doses										
Hepatitis A[12,*]					2 doses						
Hepatitis B[13,*]			3 doses								
Haemophilus influenzae type b (Hib)[14,*]	post-HSCT recipients only			1 or 3 doses							

*Covered by the Vaccine Injury Compensation Program.

For all persons in this category who meet the age requirements and who lack documentation of vaccination or have no evidence of previous infection; zoster vaccine reccommended regardless of prior episode of zoster.

Recommended if some other risk factor is present (eg, on the basis of medical, occupational, lifestyle, or other indication).

No recommendation.

NOTE: The recommendations in the tables must be read along with the following footnotes.

◀ **Footnotes to Recommended Adult Immunization Schedule**
[1]**Additional information**

- Additional guidance for the use of the vaccines described in this supplement is available at http://www.cdc.gov/vaccines/hcp/acip-recs/.

- Information on vaccination recommendations when vaccination status is unknown and other general immunization information can be found in the General Recommendations on Immunization at http://www.cdc.gov/mmwr/preview/mmwrhtml/rr6002a1.htm.

- Information on travel vaccine requirements and recommendations (eg, for hepatitis A and B, meningococcal, other vaccines) is available at http://wwwnc.cdc.gov/travel/destinations/list.

- Additional information and resources regarding vaccination of pregnant women can be found at http://www.cdc.gov/vaccines/adults/rec-vac/pregnant.html.

[2]**Influenza vaccine**

- Annual vaccination against influenza is recommended for all persons ≥6 months of age.

- Persons ≥6 months of age, including pregnant women and persons with hives-only allergy to eggs, can receive the inactivated influenza vaccine (IIV). An age-appropriate IIV formulation should be used.

- Adults 18-49 years of age can receive the recombinant influenza vaccine (RIV) (FluBlok). RIV does not contain any egg protein.

- Healthy, nonpregnant persons 2-49 years of age without high-risk medical conditions can receive either intranasally administered live, attenuated influenza vaccine (LAIV) (FluMist) or IIV. Healthcare personnel who care for severely immunocompromised persons (ie, those who require care in a protected environment) should receive IIV or RIV, rather than LAIV.

- The intramuscularly or intradermally administered IIV are options for adults 18-64 years of age.

- Adults ≥65 years of age can receive the standard-dose IIV or the high-dose IIV (Fluzone High-Dose).

[3]**Tetanus, diphtheria, and acellular pertussis vaccine (Td/Tdap)**

- Administer 1 dose of Tdap vaccine to pregnant women during each pregnancy (preferred during 27-36 weeks' gestation), regardless of interval since prior Td or Tdap vaccination.

- Persons ≥11 years of age who have not received Tdap vaccine or for whom vaccine status is unknown should receive a dose of Tdap, followed by tetanus and diphtheria toxoids (Td) booster doses every 10 years thereafter. Tdap can be administered regardless of interval since the most recent tetanus or diphtheria-toxoid-containing vaccine.

- Adults with an unknown or incomplete history of completing a 3-dose primary vaccination series with Td-containing vaccines should begin or complete a primary vaccination series, including a Tdap dose.

- For unvaccinated adults, administer the first 2 doses at least 4 weeks apart and the third dose 6-12 months after the second.

- For incompletely vaccinated adults (ie, <3 doses), administer remaining doses.

- Refer to the ACIP statement for recommendations for administering Td/Tdap as prophylaxis in wound management (see footnote 1).

[4]**Varicella vaccine**

- All adults without evidence of immunity to varicella (as defined below) should receive 2 doses of single-antigen varicella vaccine or a second dose if they have received only 1 dose.

- Vaccination should be emphasized for those who have close contact with persons at high risk for severe disease (eg, healthcare personnel and family contacts of persons with immunocompromising conditions) or who are at high risk for exposure or transmission (eg, teachers; child care employees; residents and staff members of institutional settings, including correctional institutions; college students; military personnel; adolescents and adults living in households with children; nonpregnant women of childbearing age; international travelers).

- Pregnant women should be assessed for evidence of varicella immunity. Women who do not have evidence of immunity should receive the first dose of varicella vaccine upon completion or termination of pregnancy and before discharge from the healthcare facility. The second dose should be administered 4-8 weeks after the first dose.

- Evidence of immunity to varicella in adults includes any of the following:
    - Documentation of 2 doses of varicella vaccine at least 4 weeks apart
    - U.S.-born before 1980, except healthcare personnel and pregnant women
    - History of varicella based on diagnosis or verification of varicella disease by a healthcare provider
    - History of herpes zoster based on diagnosis or verification of herpes zoster disease by a healthcare provider, or
    - Laboratory evidence of immunity or laboratory confirmation of disease

[5]Human papillomavirus vaccine (HPV)

- Two vaccines are licensed for use in females, bivalent HPV vaccine (HPV2) and quadrivalent HPV vaccine (HPV4), and one HPV vaccine for use in males, HPV4.
- For females, either HPV4 or HPV2 is recommended in a 3-dose series for routine vaccination at 11 or 12 years of age, and for those 13-26 years of age, if not previously vaccinated.
- For males, HPV4 is recommended in a 3-dose series for routine vaccination at 11 or 12 years of age, and for those 13-21 years of age, if not previously vaccinated. Males 22-26 years of age may be vaccinated.
- HPV4 is recommended for men who have sex with men through 26 years of age for those who did not get any or all doses when they were younger.
- Vaccination is recommended for immunocompromised persons (including those with HIV infection) through 26 years of age for those who did not get any or all doses when they were younger.
- A complete series for either HPV4 or HPV2 consists of 3 doses. The second dose should be administered 4-8 weeks (minimum interval of 4 weeks) after the first dose; the third dose should be administered 24 weeks after the first dose and 16 weeks after the second dose (minimum interval of at least 12 weeks).
- HPV vaccines are not recommended for use in pregnant women. However, pregnancy testing is not needed before vaccination. If a woman is found to be pregnant after initiating the vaccination series, no intervention is needed; the remainder of the 3-dose series should be delayed until completion of pregnancy.

[6]Zoster vaccine

- A single dose of zoster vaccine is recommended for adults ≥60 years of age, regardless of whether they report a prior episode of herpes zoster. Although the vaccine is licensed by the U.S. Food and Drug Administration for use among and can be administered to persons ≥50 years of age, ACIP recommendes that vaccination begin at 60 years of age.
- Persons ≥60 years of age with chronic medical conditions may be vaccinated, unless their condition constitutes a contraindication, such as pregnancy or severe immunodeficiency.

[7]Measles, mumps, rubella vaccine (MMR)

- Adults born before 1957 generally are considered immune to measles and mumps. All adults born in 1957 or later should have documentation of ≥1 dose of MMR vaccine, unless they have a medical contraindication to the vaccine or laboratory evidence of immunity to each of the three diseases. Documentation of provider-diagnosed disease is not considered acceptable evidence of immunity for measles, mumps, or rubella.
- **Measles component:**
    - A routine second dose of MMR vaccine, administered a minimum of 28 days after the first dose, is recommended for adults who:
        - Are students in postsecondary educational institutions
        - Work in a healthcare facility, or
        - Plan to travel internationally
    - Persons who received inactivated (killed) measles vaccine or measles vaccine of unknown type during 1963-1967 should be revaccinated with 2 doses of MMR vaccine.

- **Mumps component:**
  - A routine second dose of MMR vaccine, administered a minimum of 28 days after the first dose, is recommended for adults who:
    - Are students in a postsecondary educational institution
    - Work in a healthcare facility, or
    - Plan to travel internationally
  - Persons vaccinated before 1979 with either killed mumps vaccine or mumps vaccine of unknown type who are at high risk for mumps infection (eg, persons who are working in a healthcare facility) should be considered for revaccination with 2 doses of MMR vaccine.
- **Rubella component:** For women of childbearing age, regardless of birth year, rubella immunity should be determined. If there is no evidence of immunity, women who are not pregnant should be vaccinated. Pregnant women who do not have evidence of immunity should receive MMR vaccine upon completion or termination of pregnancy and before discharge from the healthcare facility.
- **Healthcare personnel born before 1957:** For unvaccinated healthcare personnel born before 1957 who lack laboratory evidence of measles, mumps, and/or rubella immunity or laboratory confirmation of disease, healthcare facilities should consider vaccinating personnel with 2 doses of MMR vaccine at the appropriate interval for measles and mumps or 1 dose of MMR vaccine for rubella.

[8]Pneumococcal conjugate vaccine (PCV13)

- Adults ≥19 years of age with immunocompromising conditions (including chronic renal failure and nephrotic syndrome), functional or anatomic asplenia, cerebrospinal fluid leaks, or cochlear implants who have not previously received PCV13 or PPSV23 should receive a single dose of PCV13, followed by a dose of PPSV23 at least 8 weeks later.
- Adults ≥19 years of age with the aforementioned conditions who have previously received ≥1 dose of PPSV23 should receive a dose of PCV13 ≥1 year after the last PPSV23 dose was received. For adults who require additional doses of PPSV23, the first such dose should be given no sooner than 8 weeks after PCV13 and at least 5 years after the most recent dose of PPSV23.
- When indicated, PCV13 should be administered to patients who are uncertain of their vaccination status history and have no record of previous vaccination.
- Although PCV13 is licensed by the U.S. Food and Drug Administration for use among and can be administered to persons ≥50 years of age, ACIP recommends PCV13 for adults ≥19 years of age with the specific medical conditions noted above.

[9]Pneumococcal polysaccharide vaccine (PPSV23)

- When PCV13 is also indicated, PCV13 should be given first (see footnote 8).
- Vaccinate all persons with the following indications:
  - All adults ≥65 years of age
  - Adults <65 years of age with chronic lung disease (including chronic obstructive pulmonary disease, emphysema, and asthma), chronic cardiovascular diseases, diabetes mellitus, chronic renal failure, nephrotic syndrome, chronic liver disease (including cirrhosis), alcoholism, cochlear implants, cerebrospinal fluid leaks, immunocompromising conditions, and functional or anatomic asplenia (eg, sickle cell disease and other hemoglobinophathies, congenital or acquired asplenia, splenic dysfunction, or splenectomy [if elective splenectomy is planned, vaccinate ≥2 weeks before surgery])
  - Residents of nursing homes or long-term care facilities, and
  - Adults who smoke cigarettes
- Persons with immunocompromising conditions and other selected conditions are recommended to receive PCV13 and PPSV23 vaccines. See footnote 8 for information on timing of PCV13 and PPSV23 vaccinations.
- Persons with asymptomatic or symptomatic HIV infection should be vaccinated as soon as possible after their diagnosis.

- When cancer chemotherapy or other immunosuppressive therapy is being considered, the interval between vaccination and initiation of immunosuppresive therapy should be ≥2 weeks. Vaccination during chemotherapy or radiation therapy should be avoided.

- Routine use of PPSV23 is not recommended for American Indians/Alaska Natives or other persons <65 years of age, unless they have underlying medical conditions that are PPSV23 indications. However, public health authorities may consider recommending PPSV23 for American Indians/Alaska Natives who are living in areas where the risk for invasive pneumococcal disease is increased.

- When indicated, PPSV23 vaccine should be administered to patients who are uncertain of their vaccination status and have no record of vaccination.

[10]Revaccination with PPSV23

- One-time revaccination 5 years after the first dose of PPSV23 is recommended for persons 19-64 years of age with chronic renal failure or nephrotic syndrome, functional or anatomic asplenia (eg, sickle cell disease, splenectomy), or immunocompromising conditions.

- Persons who received 1 or 2 doses of PPSV23 before 65 years of age for any indication should receive another dose of the vaccine at ≥65 years of age if at least 5 years have passed since their previous dose.

- No further doses are needed for persons vaccinated with PPSV23 at ≥65 years of age.

[11]Meningococcal vaccine

- Administer 2 doses of quadrivalent meningococcal conjugate vaccine (MenACWY-D [Menactra]) at least 2 months apart to adults with functional asplenia or persistent complement component deficiencies. HIV infection is not an indication for routine vaccination with MenACWY-D. If an HIV-infected person of any age is vaccinated, 2 doses of MenACWY-D should be administered at least 2 months apart.

- Administer a single dose of meningococcal vaccine to microbiologists routinely exposed to isolates of Neisseria meningitidis, military recruits, persons at risk during an outbreak attributable to a vaccine serogroup, and persons who travel to or live in countries in which meningococcal disease is hyper-endemic or epidemic.

- First-year college students ≤21 years of age who are living in residence halls should be vaccinated if they have not received a dose on or after their 16th birthday.

- MenACWY-D is preferred for adults with any of the preceding indications who are ≤55 years of age, as well as for adults ≥56 years of age: a) who were vaccinated previously with MenACWY-D and are recommended for revaccination or b) for whom multiple doses are anticipated. Meningococcal poly-saccharide vaccine (MenACWY-CRM [Menveo]) is preferred for adults ≥56 years of age who have not received MenACWY-D previously and who require a single dose only (eg, travelers).

- Revaccination with MenACWY-D every 5 years is recommended for adults previously vaccinated with MenACWY-D or MenACWY-CRM who remain at increased risk for infection (eg, adults with anatomic or functional asplenia, persistent complement component deficiencies, or microbiologists).

[12]Hepatitis A vaccine

- Vaccinate any person seeking protection from hepatitis A virus (HAV) infection and persons with any of the following indications:

  – Men who have sex with men and persons who use injection or noninjection illicit drugs

  – Persons working with HAV-infected primates or with HAV in a research laboratory setting

  – Persons with chronic liver disease and persons who receive clotting factor concentrates

  – Persons traveling to or working in countries that have high or intermediate endemicity of hepatitis A, and

  – Unvaccinated persons who anticipate close personal contatct (eg, household, regular babysitting) with an international adoptee during the first 60 days after arrival in the United States from a country with high or intermediate endemicity (see footnote 1 for more information on travel recommenda-tions). The first dose of the 2-dose hepatitis A vaccine series should be administered as soon as adoption is planned, ideally ≥2 weeks before the arrival of the adoptee.

- Single-antigen vaccine formulations should be administered in a 2-dose schedule at either 0 and 6-12 months (Havrix) or 0 and 6-18 months (Vaqta). If the combined hepatitis A and hepatitis B vaccine (Twinrix) is used, administer 3 doses at 0, 1, and 6 months; alternatively, a 4-dose schedule may be used, administered on days 0, 7, and 21-30, followed by a booster dose at month 12.

◀ **[13]Hepatitis B vaccine**

- Vaccinate persons with any of the following indications and any person seeking protection from hepatitis B virus (HBV) infection:

  - Sexually active persons who are not in a long-term, mutually monogamous relationship (eg, persons with more than one sex partner during the previous 6 months), persons seeking evaluation or treatment for a sexually transmitted disease (STD), current or recent injection drug users, and men who have sex with men

  - Healthcare personnel and public safety workers who are potentially exposed to blood or other infectious body fluids

  - Persons with diabetes who are <60 years of age as soon as feasible after diagnosis and persons with diabetes who are ≥60 years of age at the discretion of the treating clinician, based on the likelihood of acquiring HBV infection, including the risk posed by an increased need for assisted blood glucose monitoring in long-term care facilities, the likelihood of experiencing chronic sequelae if infected with HBV, and the likelihood of immune response to vaccination.

  - Persons with end-stage renal disease, including patients receiving hemodialysis, persons with HIV infection, and persons with chronic liver disease

  - Household contacts and sex partners of hepatitis B surface antigen-positive persons, clients and staff members of institutions for persons with developmental disabilities, and international travelers to countries with high or intermediate prevalence of chronic HBV infection, and

  - All adults in the following settings: STD treatment facilities, HIV testing and treatment facilities, facilities providing drug-abuse treatment and prevention services, healthcare settings targeting services to injection drug users or men who have sex with men, correctional facilities, end-stage renal disease programs and facilities for chronic hemodialysis patients, and institutions and nonresidential day-care facilities for persons with developmental disabilities

- Administer missing doses to complete a 3-dose series of hepatitis B vaccine to those persons not vaccinated or not completely vaccinated. The second dose should be administered 1 month after the first dose; the third dose should be given at least 2 months after the second dose (and at least 4 months after the first dose). If the combined hepatitis A and hepatitis B vaccine (Twinrix) is used, give 3 doses at 0, 1, and 6 months; alternatively, a 4-dose Twinrix schedule, administered on days 0, 7, and 21-30, followed by a booster dose at month 12, may be used.

- Adult patients receiving hemodialysis or with other immunocompromising conditions should receive 1 dose of 40 mcg/mL (Recombivax HB) administered on a 3-dose schedule at 0, 1, and 6 months, or 2 doses of 20 mcg/mL (Engerix-B) administered simultaneously on a 4-dose schedule at 0, 1, 2, and 6 months.

[14]Haemophilus influenzae type b vaccine (Hib)

- One dose of Hib vaccine should be administered to persons who have functional or anatomic asplenia or sickle cell disease or to those who are undergoing elective splenectomy if they have not previously received Hib vaccine. Hib vaccination ≥14 days before splenectomy is suggested.

- Receipients of a hematopoietic stem cell transplant should be vaccinated with a 3-dose regimen 6-12 months after a successful transplant, regardless of vaccination history; at least 4 weeks should separate doses.

- Hib vaccine is not recommended for adults with HIV infection since their risk for Hib infection is low.

[15]Immunocompromising conditions

- Inactivated vaccines generally are acceptable (eg, pneumococcal, meningococcal, inactivated influenza vaccine) and live vaccines generally are avoided in persons with immune deficiencies or immunocompromising conditions. Information on specific conditions is available at http://www.cdc.gov/vaccines/hcp/acip-recs/index.html.

REFERENCE

Centers for Disease Control and Prevention (CDC). Advisory Committee on Immunization Practices (ACIP) recommended immunization schedules for persons aged 0 through 18 years and adults aged 19 years and older − United States, 2014. Available at http://www.cdc.gov/vaccines/schedules/hcp/adult.html

VACCINE INJURY TABLE

The Vaccine Injury Table makes it easier for some people to get compensation. The table lists and explains injuries/conditions that are presumed to be caused by vaccines. It also lists time periods in which the first symptom of these injuries/conditions must occur after receiving the vaccine. If the first symptom of these injuries/conditions occurs within the listed time period, it is presumed that the vaccine was the cause of the injury or condition, unless another cause is found. For example, if the patient received the tetanus vaccines and had a severe allergic reaction (anaphylaxis) within 4 hours after receiving the vaccine, then it is presumed that the tetanus vaccine caused the injury if no other cause is found.

If the injury/condition is not on the table or if the injury/condition did not occur within the time period on the table, it must be proven that the vaccine caused the injury/condition. Such proof must be based on medical records or opinion, which may include expert witness testimony.

Vaccine Injury Table[1]

Vaccine		Illness, Disability, Injury, or Condition Covered	Time Period for First Symptom or Manifestation of Onset or of Significant Aggravation After Vaccine Administration
Vaccines containing tetanus toxoid (eg, DTaP, DTP, DT, Td, TT)	A.	Anaphylaxis or anaphylactic shock	4 hours
	B.	Brachial neuritis	2-28 days
	C.	Any acute complication or sequela (including death) of an illness, disability, injury, or condition referred to above which illness, disability, injury, or condition arose within the time period prescribed	Not applicable
Vaccines containing whole cell pertussis bacteria, extracted or partial cell pertussis bacteria, or specific pertussis antigen(s) (eg, DTP, DTaP, P, DTP-Hib)	A.	Anaphylaxis or anaphylactic shock	4 hours
	B.	Encephalopathy (or encephalitis)	72 hours
	C.	Any acute complication or sequela (including death) of an illness, disability, injury, or condition referred to above which illness, disability, injury, or condition arose within the time period prescribed	Not applicable
Measles, mumps, and rubella vaccine or any of its components (eg, MMR, MR, M, R)	A.	Anaphylaxis or anaphylactic shock	4 hours
	B.	Encephalopathy (or encephalitis)	5-15 days
	C.	Any acute complication or sequela (including death) of an illness, disability, injury, or condition referred to above which illness, disability, injury, or condition arose within the time period prescribed	Not applicable
Vaccines containing rubella virus (eg, MMR, MR, R)	A.	Chronic arthritis	7-42 days
	B.	Any acute complication or sequela (including death) of an illness, disability, injury, or condition referred to above which illness, disability, injury, or condition arose within the time period prescribed	Not applicable
Vaccines containing measles virus (eg, MMR, MR, M)	A.	Thrombocytopenic purpura	7-30 days
	B.	Vaccine-strain measles viral infection in an immunodeficient recipient	6 months
	C.	Any acute complication or sequela (including death) of an illness, disability, injury, or condition referred to above which illness, disability, injury, or condition arose within the time period prescribed	Not applicable
Vaccines containing polio live virus (OPV)	A.	Paralytic polio	
		• In a nonimmunodeficient recipient	30 days
		• In an immunodeficient recipient	6 months
		• In a vaccine-associated community case	Not applicable
	B.	Vaccine-strain polio viral infection	
		• In a nonimmunodeficient recipient	30 days
		• In an immunodeficient recipient	6 months
		• In a vaccine-associated community case	Not applicable
	C.	Any acute complication or sequela (including death) of an illness, disability, injury, or condition referred to above which illness, disability, injury, or condition arose within the time period prescribed	Not applicable
Vaccines containing polio inactivated (eg, IPV)	A.	Anaphylaxis or anaphylactic shock	4 hours
	B.	Any acute complication or sequela (including death) of an illness, disability, injury, or condition referred to above which illness, disability, injury, or condition arose within the time period prescribed	Not applicable
Hepatitis B vaccines	A.	Anaphylaxis or anaphylactic shock	4 hours
	B.	Any acute complication or sequela (including death) of an illness, disability, injury, or condition referred to above which illness, disability, injury, or condition arose within the time period prescribed	Not applicable

Vaccine Injury Table[1] *(continued)*

Vaccine	Illness, Disability, Injury, or Condition Covered	Time Period for First Symptom or Manifestation of Onset or of Significant Aggravation After Vaccine Administration
Hemophilus influenzae type b polysaccharide conjugate vaccines	No condition specified	Not applicable
Varicella vaccine	No condition specified	Not applicable
Rotavirus vaccine	No condition specified	Not applicable
Pneumococcal conjugate vaccines	No condition specified	Not applicable
Hepatitis A vaccines	No condition specified	Not applicable
Trivalent influenza vaccines	No condition specified	Not applicable
Meningococcal vaccines	No condition specified	Not applicable
Human papillomavirus (HPV) vaccines	No condition specified	Not applicable
Any new vaccine recommended by the Centers for Disease Control and Prevention for routine administration to children, after publication by the secretary of a notice of coverage*	No condition specified	Not applicable

*Now includes all vaccines against seasonal influenza (except trivalent influenza vaccines, which are already covered), effective November 12, 2013

[1]Effective date: July 22, 2011; available at http://www.hrsa.gov/vaccinecompensation/vaccinetable.html

LATEX ALLERGY

The incidence of clinically significant latex allergy is increasing. This increase has been suggested to be due in part to the implementation of universal precautions by the CDC in 1987 secondary to the AIDS epidemic. **Because of the increased incidence of latex allergy, all patients need a complete history, including risk factor evaluation and previous evidence of clinical signs and symptoms suggesting contact dermatitis or urticaria.** For example, patients should be questioned about the presence of swelling or itching of the hands or other areas after contact with rubber gloves, condoms, diaphragms, toys, or other rubber products and about itching or swelling of the lips or mouth after dental exams, blowing up balloons, or after eating bananas, chestnuts, and avocados.

It is important today for healthcare institutions to have a comprehensive plan (including a perioperative component) in place for dealing with latex-allergic patients and healthcare personnel. In cardiovascular medicine, the high proportion of procedures and imaging modalities heightens exposure to latex allergens, usually related to rubber gloves. This is a potentially life-threatening problem, both for the patient and healthcare personnel, in situations such as the cardiac catheterization laboratory. Some institutions have avoided use of latex products throughout the hospital environment.

HYPERSENSITIVITY REACTIONS CAUSED BY LATEX

Latex-containing products can produce type I and type IV hypersensitivity reactions.

The type I (IgE-mediated) hypersensitivity reaction is the true "allergic" reaction seen with latex products. Proteins found in the latex promote the production of an antibody of the IgE class which attaches to basophils and mast cells. When the antigen (protein) is encountered again, histamine and other physiologically active mediators are released from mast cells and basophils. The clinical manifestations can include single or multiple system involvement, be mild or severe, ranging from itching to edema, and from mild hypotension to shock. It has been estimated that 10% of the true anaphylactic reactions during anesthesia are due to latex allergy. These reactions are usually seen 5-30 minutes after induction of anesthesia and start of surgery. Seventy-nine percent of type I patients previously had type IV symptoms.

In the type IV (delayed type) reaction, a contact dermatitis is seen. The preservatives, stabilizers, accelerators, and antioxidants used in the latex manufacturing process serve as the antigens for T-cell lymphocytes. The dermatitis produced can be uncomfortable, but is not life-threatening and usually occurs over a 24-hour period; limited to site of contact. Not all patients with type IV symptoms will progress to type I reactivity.

ROUTES OF EXPOSURE TO LATEX PROTEINS

It is important to consider the route of exposure of the latex protein in allergic patients as this can be a determinant of the type of reaction produced. The following table summarizes major routes of exposure.

Type of Exposure	Reaction
Direct skin contact	Localized or generalized urticaria
Mucous membrane	Rhinitis, conjunctivitis, stomatitis, angioedema; severe anaphylactic reactions and death reported
Inhalation of airborne starch-protein particles	Wheezing, bronchospasm, reduced lung compliance, episodes of desaturation and/or severe hypoxemia
Intravascular absorption of water soluble latex particles from surgical gloves	Sudden tachycardia, severe hypotension, cardiorespiratory collapse

HIGH-RISK PATIENTS

Several groups have been identified as "high-risk" for allergic reactions to latex. Special consideration should be given these individuals.

Patients having multiple surgical procedures (eg, spina bifida patients/patients with congenital urologic abnormalities). A 30% to 70% incidence of latex allergy has been reported for spina bifida patients. These patients are routinely exposed to latex-containing urinary catheters.

Healthcare providers. Latex sensitivity may be as high as 17%. Approximately 70% of adverse events reported to FDA regarding latex involve healthcare workers.

Workers with occupational exposure to natural rubber latex (eg, hairdressers, greenhouse workers, latex manufacturers).

Patients with a history of atopy, hay fever, rhinitis, asthma, or eczema. Atopy is one of the significant predisposing risk factors for latex allergy.

Patients with a history of food allergy to tropical fruits (eg, avocado, kiwi, bananas), chestnuts, stone fruits, and additional specific foods. These plants contain several proteins similar/identical to those found in latex.

Individuals with severe or anaphylactic responses to latex should consider having an Epi-Pen available at all times, and having a Medic-Alert bracelet to alert healthcare workers to the potential for life-threatening allergic reactions.

TREATMENT OF ANAPHYLACTIC REACTION

Management of an anaphylactic reaction which is thought to be due to latex allergy must be immediate. Initial therapy should consist of the following.

- Stop administration of offending agent.
- Remove all latex products (switch to nonlatex gloves and latex-free intravenous tubing). Latex-free precautions must accompany the patient throughout the perioperative and hospital stay (PACU, ICU, general floor, and discharge unit).
- Discontinue all antibiotic and blood administration.
- Maintain airway with 100% oxygen.
- Intubate the trachea (as indicated).
- Intravascular volume expansion with crystalloid or colloid.
- Epinephrine administration (see Epinephrine (Systemic, Oral Inhalation) on page 538).
- Discontinue all anesthetic agents if appropriate.
- Consider use of Military Anti-Shock Trousers (MAST).
- Display prominent signs to identify latex allergy.
- When appropriate, administer antihistamines (eg, diphenhydramine), corticosteroids (eg, hydrocortisone), catecholamine infusions (eg, norepinephrine), inhaled bronchodilators (eg, albuterol) for bronchospasm, and sodium bicarbonate (guided by arterial blood gas results). Patients should be admitted to the ICU for 24 hours following an anaphylactic reaction because of the possibility of recurrent "late-phase" reactions. To confirm a latex allergy, RAST or AlaSTAT test may be performed.
- Details of any allergic reaction should be clearly documented in the patient's chart and reported to FDA MedWatch program.
- Contact dermatitis and type IV reactions:
    - Avoid irritating skin cleansers.
    - Topical corticosteroids can be applied locally.

PERIOPERATIVE MANAGEMENT OF A LATEX ALLERGIC PATIENT

No evidence exists to demonstrate that prophylaxis before surgery prevents latex-induced anaphylactic reactions. In spite of this, prophylaxis has been used in patients with a positive history of allergy. One suggested regimen uses diphenhydramine P.O. or I.V. every 6 hours at 13, 7, and 1 hours before surgery; prednisone P.O. every 6 hours at 13, 7, and 1 hours before surgery (hydrocortisone I.V. may be substituted); and ranitidine P.O. or I.V. every 12 hours at 13 and 1 hours before surgery. This regimen is continued for 12 hours after surgery.

The key to the hospital management of the latex-allergic patient is to provide a latex-free environment. To accomplish this, the following actions should be taken.

- Substitute all items with nonlatex alternatives when possible; if there is a question concerning the latex content of a product, the manufacturer should be called.
- Gloves made of neoprene or other polymers should be used.
- Latex-based adhesives should be eliminated.
- Stopcocks should be used for drug administration instead of injection ports on I.V. tubing.
- Syringes not containing rubber tips on the plunger should be used.

- Drug products in glass ampuls should be used whenever possible; if a vial must be used, utilize a vial stopper remover so the stopper does not have to be punctured or puncture only once.

- To reduce exposure to aerosolized glove powder which is a known carrier of latex proteins, schedule the surgery as the first case of the day. Some institutions have reserved an O.R. suite for latex-allergic patients.

TESTING FOR LATEX ALLERGY

Testing for latex allergy is recommended for high-risk patients. Both *in vitro* and *in vivo* tests are available as seen in the following table.

Test	Type	Description
Skin prick (SPT)	*in vivo*	Sensitive method to confirm IgE-mediated latex hypersensitivity; correlates well with clinical presence of allergy; high sensitivity (100%), high specificity (99%)
Patch	*in vivo*	Test for type IV hypersensitivity reaction; test performed with 1 inch square of rubber glove; skin observed for contact dermatitis after 48 hours
Radioallergosorbent (RAST)	*in vitro*	Performed on the serum of patients with natural latex as the antigen; used to detect and quantify allergen specific IgE in patient's serum; positive RAST response correlates strongly with *in vivo* allergic response; sensitivity 67% to 82%
Enzymeallergosorbent (EAST)	*in vitro*	Enzyme-linked immunometric assay used to measure latex-specific IgE antibodies; can be false negatives

REFERENCES AND RECOMMENDED READING

Dakin MJ, Yentis SM. Latex allergy: a strategy for management. *Anaesthesia*. 1998; 53(8):774-781.

Hancock DL. Latex allergy. prevention and treatment. *Anesthesiol Rev*. 1994;21(5):153-163.

Katz JD, Holzman RS, Brown RH, et al. Natural rubber latex allergy: considerations for anesthesiologists. American Society of Anesthesiologists (ASA). 2005. http://ecommerce.asahq.org/publicationsAndServices/latexallergy.pdf. Accessed December 6, 2007.

Senst BL, Johnson RA. Latex allergy. *Am J Health Syst Pharm*. 1997;54(9):1071-1075.

Steelman VM. Latex allergy precautions. a research-based protocol. *Nurs Clin North Am*. 1995;30(3):475-493.

Sussman G, Gold M. Guidelines for the management of latex allergies and safe latex use in health care facilities. http://www.acaai.org/public/physicians/latex.htm

MANAGEMENT OF DRUG EXTRAVASATIONS

A potential complication of drug therapy is extravasation. A variety of symptoms, including erythema, ulceration, pain, tissue sloughing, and necrosis, are possible. A variety of drugs have been reported to cause tissue damage if extravasated.

DEFINITIONS

- **Extravasation:** Unintentional or inadvertent leakage (or instillation) of fluid out of a blood vessel into surrounding tissue

- **Irritant:** An agent that causes aching, tightness, and phlebitis with or without inflammation, but does not typically cause tissue necrosis. Irritants can cause necrosis if the extravasation is severe or left untreated.

- **Vesicant:** An agent that has the potential to cause blistering, severe tissue injury, or tissue necrosis when extravasated

- **Flare:** Local, nonpainful, possibly allergic reaction often accompanied by reddening along the vein

PREVENTING EXTRAVASATIONS

Although it is not possible to prevent all extravasations, a few precautions can minimize the risk to the patient. The vein used should be a large, intact vessel with good blood flow. Veins in the forearm (ie, basilic, cephalic, and median antebrachial) are usually good options for peripheral infusions. To minimize the risk of dislodging the catheter, avoid using veins in the hands, dorsum of the foot, and any joint space (eg, antecubital). It is important to remember to not administer chemotherapy distal to a recent venipuncture.

A frequently recommended precaution against drug extravasation is the use of a central venous catheter. Use of a central line has several advantages, including high patient satisfaction, reliable venous access, high flow rates, and rapid dilution of the drug. Many institutions encourage or require use of a vascular access device for administration of vesicant agents. Despite their benefit, central lines are not an absolute solution. Vascular access devices are subject to a number of complications. Misplacement/migration of the catheter or improper placement of the needle in accessing injection ports, and cuts, punctures, infections, or rupture of the catheter itself have all been reported.

Education of both the patient and practitioner is imperative. Educate the patient to immediately report any signs of pain, itching, tingling, burning, redness, swelling, or discomfort, all of which could be early signs of extravasation. Symptoms of extravasation which may appear later include blistering, ulceration, and necrosis. Ensure the healthcare team is informed of the risks and management strategies for both prevention and treatment of extravasations. Absence of blood return, resistance upon administration, or interruption of the I.V. flow should raise suspicion of potential extravasation.

INITIAL EXTRAVASATION MANAGEMENT

1. **Stop the infusion:** At the first suspicion of extravasation, the drug infusion and I.V. fluids should be stopped.

2. **Do NOT remove the catheter/needle:** The I.V. tubing should be disconnected, but the catheter/needle should be left in place to facilitate aspiration of fluid from the extravasation site and, if appropriate, administration of an antidote.

3. **Aspirate fluid:** To the extent possible, the extravasated drug solution should gently be removed from the subcutaneous tissues. It is important to avoid any friction or pressure to the area.

4. **Do NOT flush the line:** Flooding the infiltration site with saline or dextrose in an attempt to dilute the drug solution is not recommended.

5. **Remove the catheter/needle:** If an antidote is not going to be administered into the extravasation site, the catheter/needle should be removed. If an antidote is to be injected into the area, it should be injected through the catheter to ensure delivery of the antidote to the extravasation site. When this has been accomplished, the catheter should then be removed.

6. **Elevate:** The affected extremity should be elevated.

7. **Monitor and document:** Mark the extravasation site (using a surgical felt pen, gently draw an outline on the skin of the extravasation area) and photograph if possible. Monitor and document the event and follow-up activities according to institutional policy.

Table 1: Vesicant Agents and Extravasation Management

Extravasated Medication	Preferred Antidote	Antidote Administration	Supportive Management	Comments
Amino Acids (4.25%/parenteral nutrition)	Hyaluronidase	Hyaluronidase: Intradermal or SubQ: Inject a total of 1 mL (15 units/mL) as five separate 0.2 mL injections (using a 25-gauge needle) into area of extravasation at the leading edge in a clockwise manner (MacCara, 1983; Zenk, 1981)	Apply dry cold compresses (Hurst, 2004)	
Aminophylline	Hyaluronidase	Hyaluronidase: Intradermal or SubQ: Inject a total of 1 mL (15 units/mL) as five separate 0.2 mL injections (using a 25-gauge needle) into area of extravasation at the leading edge in a clockwise manner (MacCara, 1983; Zenk, 1981)	Apply dry cold compresses (Hurst, 2004)	
Amsacrine	No known antidote	No known antidote	Apply dry warm compresses (Schulmeister, 2011)	Not commercially available in the U.S.
Bendamustine	Sodium Thiosulfate	May be managed in the same manner as mechlorethamine extravasation (Schulmeister, 2011): Sodium thiosulfate 1/6 M solution: Inject subcutaneously into extravasation area using 2 mL for each mg of mechlorethamine suspected to have extravasated (Pérez Fidalgo, 2012; Polovich, 2009)	Apply dry cold compresses for 20 minutes 4 times/day for 1-2 days (Pérez Fidalgo, 2012)	Irritant with vesicant-like properties (reports of both irritant and vesicant reactions)
Calcium Chloride (≥10%)	Hyaluronidase	Hyaluronidase: Intradermal or SubQ: Inject a total of 1 mL (15 units/mL) as five separate 0.2 mL injections (using a 25-gauge needle) into area of extravasation at the leading edge in a clockwise manner (MacCara, 1983; Zenk, 1981)	Apply dry cold compresses (Hurst, 2004)	
Calcium Gluconate	Hyaluronidase	Hyaluronidase: Intradermal or SubQ: Inject a total of 1 mL (15 units/mL) as five separate 0.2 mL injections (using a 25-gauge needle) into area of extravasation at the leading edge in a clockwise manner (MacCara, 1983; Zenk, 1981)	Apply dry cold compresses (Hurst, 2004)	
CISplatin (>0.4 mg/mL)	Sodium Thiosulfate	Sodium thiosulfate 1/6 M solution: Inject 2 mL into existing I.V. line for each 100 mg of cisplatin extravasated; then consider also injecting 1 mL as 0.1 mL subcutaneous injections (clockwise) around the area of extravasation; may repeat subcutaneous injections several times over the next 3-4 hours (Ener, 2004) Dimethyl sulfoxide (DMSO) may also be considered an option. Apply topically to a region covering twice the affected area every 8 hours for 7 days; begin within 10 minutes of extravasation; do not cover with a dressing (Pérez Fidalgo, 2012).	Information conflicts regarding use of warm or cold compresses	
Contrast Media	Hyaluronidase	Hyaluronidase: Intradermal or SubQ: Inject a total of 1 mL (15 units/mL) as five separate 0.2 mL injections (using a 25-gauge needle) into area of extravasation at the leading edge in a clockwise manner (MacCara, 1983; Zenk, 1981) The injection of a total of 5 mL (150 units/mL) as five separate 1 mL injections around the extravasation site has been also used successfully (Rowlett, 2012)	Apply dry cold compresses (Hurst, 2004)	
DACTINomycin	No known antidote	No known antidote	Apply dry cold compress for 20 minutes 4 times/day for 1-2 days (Pérez Fidalgo, 2012)	
Dantrolene	No known antidote	No known antidote	No recommendation	
DAUNORubicin (Conventional)	Dexrazoxane or topical Dimethyl Sulfoxide (DMSO)	Adults: Dexrazoxane 1000 mg/m² (maximum dose: 2000 mg) I.V. (administer in a large vein remote from site of extravasation) over days 1 and 2, then 500 mg/m² (maximum dose: 1000 mg) I.V. over 1-2 hours day 3; begin within 6 hours after extravasation (Mouridsen, 2007; Pérez Fidalgo, 2012). Note: Reduce dexrazoxane dose by 50% in patients with moderate to severe renal impairment (CrCl <40 mL/min). Pediatrics and Adults: DMSO: Apply topically to a region covering twice the affected area every 8 hours for 7 days; begin within 10 minutes of extravasation; do not cover with a dressing (Pérez Fidalgo, 2012)	Apply dry cold compress for 20 minutes 4 times/day for 1-2 days (Pérez Fidalgo, 2012). Withhold cooling for 15 minutes before and after dexrazoxane.	If using dexrazoxane, do not use DMSO. Administer dexrazoxane through a large vein remote from area of the extravasation.

Table 1: Vesicant Agents and Extravasation Management *continued*

Extravasated Medication	Preferred Antidote	Antidote Administration	Supportive Management	Comments
Dextrose (≥10%)	Hyaluronidase	Hyaluronidase: **Dextrose 10%:** Intradermal or SubQ: Inject a total of 1 mL (15 units/mL) as five separate 0.2 mL injections (using a 25-gauge needle) into area of extravasation at the leading edge in a clockwise manner (MacCara, 1983; Zenk, 1981) **Dextrose 50%:** Injection of a total of 1 mL (150 units/mL) as five separate 0.2 mL Injections administered along the leading edge of erythema has been used successfully (Wiegand, 2010)	Apply dry cold compresses (Hurst, 2004)	
Diazepam	No known antidote	No known antidote	Apply dry cold compresses (Hurst, 2004)	
Digoxin	No known antidote	No known antidote	No recommendation	
DOCEtaxel	No known antidote	No known antidote	Information conflicts regarding use of warm or cold compresses	Irritant with vesicant-like properties (reports of both irritant and vesicant reactions)
DOPamine	Phentolamine	Phentolamine: Dilute 5-10 mg in 10-15 mL NS and administer into extravasation site as soon as possible after extravasation (Peberdy, 2010) *Alternatives to phentolamine (due to shortage):* Nitroglycerin topical 2% ointment (based on limited case reports in neonates/infants): Apply 4 mm/kg as a thin ribbon to the affected areas; may repeat after 8 hours if needed (Wong, 1992) **or** apply a 1-inch strip on the affected site (Denkler, 1989) Terbutaline (based on limited case reports): Infiltrate extravasation area using a solution of terbutaline 1 mg diluted to 10 mL in NS (large extravasation site; administration volume varied from 3-10 mL) **or** 1 mg diluted in 1 mL 0.9% NS (small/distal extravasation site; administration volume varied from 0.5-1 mL) (Stier, 1999)	Apply dry warm compresses (Hurst, 2004)	
DOXOrubicin (Conventional)	Dexrazoxane or topical DMSO	Adults: Dexrazoxane 1000 mg/m² (maximum dose: 2000 mg) I.V. (administer in a large vein remote from site of extravasation) over 1-2 hours days 1 and 2, then 500 mg/m² (maximum dose: 1000 mg) I.V. over 1-2 hours day 3; begin within 6 hours after extravasation (Mouridsen, 2007; Pérez Fidalgo, 2012). **Note:** Reduce dexrazoxane dose by 50% in patients with moderate to severe renal impairment (CrCl <40 mL/min). Pediatrics and Adults: DMSO: Apply topically to a region covering twice the affected area every 8 hours for 7 days; begin within 10 minutes of extravasation; do not cover with a dressing (Pérez Fidalgo, 2012)	Apply dry cold compress for 20 minutes 4 times/day for 1-2 days (Pérez Fidalgo, 2012). Withhold cooling for 15 minutes before and after dexrazoxane.	If using dexrazoxane, do not use DMSO. Administer dexrazoxane through a large vein remote from area of the extravasation.
EPINEPHrine	Phentolamine	Phentolamine: Dilute 5-10 mg in 10-15 mL NS and administer into extravasation site as soon as possible after extravasation (Peberdy, 2010) *Alternatives to phentolamine (due to shortage):* Nitroglycerin topical 2% ointment (based on limited case reports in neonates/infants): Apply 4 mm/kg as a thin ribbon to the affected areas; may repeat after 8 hours if needed (Wong, 1992) **or** apply a 1-inch strip on the affected site (Denkler, 1989) Terbutaline (based on limited case reports): Infiltrate extravasation area using a solution of terbutaline 1 mg diluted to 10 mL in NS (large extravasation site; administration volume varied from 3-10 mL) **or** 1 mg diluted in 1 mL NS (small/distal extravasation site; administration volume varied from 0.5-1 mL) (Stier, 1999)	Apply dry warm compresses (Hurst, 2004)	

Table 1: Vesicant Agents and Extravasation Management *continued*

Extravasated Medication	Preferred Antidote	Antidote Administration	Supportive Management	Comments
EPIrubicin	Dexrazoxane or topical DMSO	Adults: Dexrazoxane 1000 mg/m² (maximum dose: 2000 mg) I.V. (administer in a large vein remote from site of extravasation) over 1-2 hours days 1 and 2, then 500 mg/m² (maximum dose: 1000 mg) I.V. over 1-2 hours day 3; begin within 6 hours after extravasation (Mouridsen, 2007; Pérez Fidalgo, 2012). Note: Reduce dexrazoxane dose by 50% in patients with moderate to severe renal impairment (CrCl <40 mL/min). Pediatrics and Adults: DMSO: Apply topically to a region covering twice the affected area every 8 hours for 7 days; begin within 10 minutes of extravasation; do not cover with a dressing (Pérez Fidalgo, 2012)	Apply dry cold compress for 20 minutes 4 times/day for 1-2 days (Pérez Fidalgo, 2012). Withhold cooling for 15 minutes before and after dexrazoxane.	If using dexrazoxane, do not use DMSO. Administer dexrazoxane through a large vein remote from area of the extravasation.
Esmolol	No known antidote	No known antidote	No recommendation	
HydrOXYzine	No known antidote	No known antidote	No recommendation	**Note:** Labeled route of administration for parenteral hydroxyzine is by I.M. injection only; I.V. administration is contraindicated.
IDArubicin	Dexrazoxane or topical DMSO	Adults: Dexrazoxane 1000 mg/m² (maximum dose: 2000 mg) I.V. (administer in a large vein remote from site of extravasation) over 1-2 hours days 1 and 2, then 500 mg/m² (maximum dose: 1000 mg) I.V. over 1-2 hours day 3; begin within 6 hours after extravasation (Mouridsen, 2007; Pérez Fidalgo, 2012). Note: Reduce dexrazoxane dose by 50% in patients with moderate to severe renal impairment (CrCl <40 mL/min). Pediatrics and Adults: DMSO: Apply topically to a region covering twice the affected area every 8 hours for 7 days; begin within 10 minutes of extravasation; do not cover with a dressing (Pérez Fidalgo, 2012)	Apply dry cold compress for 20 minutes 4 times/day for 1-2 days (Pérez Fidalgo, 2012). Withhold cooling for 15 minutes before and after dexrazoxane.	If using dexrazoxane, do not use DMSO. Administer dexrazoxane through a large vein remote from area of the extravasation.
Mannitol (>5%)	Hyaluronidase	Hyaluronidase: SubQ: Administer multiple 0.5-1 mL injections of a 15 units/mL solution around the periphery of the extravasation (Kumar, 2003)	No recommendation	
Mechlorethamine	Sodium Thiosulfate	Sodium thiosulfate ¹⁄₆ M solution: Inject subcutaneously into extravasation area using 2 mL for each mg of mechlorethamine suspected to have extravasated (Pérez Fidalgo, 2012; Polovich, 2009)	Apply ice for 6-12 hours after sodium thiosulfate administration (Mustargen prescribing information, 2012; Polovich, 2009) **or** may apply dry cold compresses for 20 minutes 4 times/day for 1-2 days (Pérez Fidalgo, 2012)	
MitoMYcin	Topical DMSO	DMSO: Apply topically to a region covering twice the affected area every 8 hours for 7 days; begin within 10 minutes of extravasation; do not cover with a dressing (Pérez Fidalgo, 2012)	Apply dry cold compress for 20 minutes 4 times/day for 1-2 days (Pérez Fidalgo, 2012)	
MitoXANtrone	Dexrazoxane or topical DMSO	Adults: Dexrazoxane 1000 mg/m² (maximum dose: 2000 mg) I.V. (administer in a large vein remote from site of extravasation) over 1-2 hours days 1 and 2, then 500 mg/m² (maximum dose: 1000 mg) I.V. over 1-2 hours day 3; begin within 6 hours after extravasation (Mouridsen, 2007; Pérez Fidalgo, 2012). Note: Reduce dexrazoxane dose by 50% in patients with moderate to severe renal impairment (CrCl <40 mL/min). Pediatrics and Adults: DMSO: Apply topically to a region covering twice the affected area every 8 hours for 7 days; begin within 10 minutes of extravasation; do not cover with a dressing (Pérez Fidalgo, 2012)	Apply dry cold compress for 20 minutes 4 times/day for 1-2 days (Pérez Fidalgo, 2012)	Irritant with vesicant-like properties (reports of both irritant and vesicant reactions). Administer dexrazoxane through a large vein remote from area of the extravasation.
Nafcillin	Hyaluronidase	Hyaluronidase: Intradermal or SubQ: Inject a total of 1 mL (15 units/mL) as five separate 0.2 mL injections (using a 25-gauge needle) into area of extravasation at the leading edge in a clockwise manner (MacCara, 1983; Zenk, 1981)	Apply dry cold compresses (Hurst, 2004)	

Table 1: Vesicant Agents and Extravasation Management continued

Extravasated Medication	Preferred Antidote	Antidote Administration	Supportive Management	Comments
Norepinephrine	Phentolamine	Phentolamine: Dilute 5-10 mg in 10-15 mL NS and administer into extravasation site as soon as possible after extravasation (Peberdy, 2010) or dilute 5-10 mg in 10 mL NS and administer into extravasation area (within 12 hours of extravasation) (Phentolamine product information, 1999) *Alternatives to phentolamine (due to shortage):* Nitroglycerin topical 2% ointment (based on limited case reports in neonates/infants): Apply 4 mm/kg as a thin ribbon to the affected areas; may repeat after 8 hours if needed (Wong, 1992) or apply a 1-inch strip on the affected site (Denkler, 1989) Terbutaline (based on limited case reports): Infiltrate extravasation area using a solution of terbutaline 1 mg diluted to 10 mL in NS (large extravasation site; administration volume varied from 3-10 mL) or 1 mg diluted in 1 mL NS (small/distal extravasation site; administration volume varied from 0.5-1 mL) (Stier, 1999)	Apply dry warm compresses (Hurst, 2004)	
Oxaliplatin	No known antidote	No known antidote	Information conflicts regarding use of warm or cold compresses Cold compresses could potentially precipitate or exacerbate peripheral neuropathy (de Lemos, 2005)	Irritant with vesicant-like properties (reports of both irritant and vesicant reactions)
PACLitaxel	Hyaluronidase	Hyaluronidase: *If needle/cannula still in place.* Administer 1-6 mL (150 units/mL) into existing I.V. line; usual dose is 1 mL for each 1 mL of extravasated drug; if needle/cannula has been removed, inject subcutaneously in a clockwise manner around area of extravasation; may repeat several times over the next 3-4 hours (Ener, 2004)	Information conflicts regarding use of warm or cold compresses	Irritant with vesicant-like properties (reports of both irritant and vesicant reactions)
Pentamidine	No known antidote	No known antidote	Dry warm compresses (Reynolds, 2014)	Irritant with vesicant-like properties (reports of both irritant and vesicant reactions)
Phenylephrine	Phentolamine	Phentolamine: Dilute 5-10 mg in 10-15 mL NS and administer into extravasation site as soon as possible after extravasation (Peberdy, 2010) *Alternatives to phentolamine (due to shortage):* Nitroglycerin topical 2% ointment (based on limited case reports in neonates/infants): Apply 4 mm/kg as a thin ribbon to the affected areas; may repeat after 8 hours if needed (Wong, 1992) or apply a 1-inch strip on the affected site (Denkler, 1989) Terbutaline (based on limited case reports): Infiltrate extravasation area using a solution of terbutaline 1 mg diluted to 10 mL in NS (large extravasation site; administration volume varied from 3-10 mL) or 1 mg diluted in 1 mL NS (small/distal extravasation site; administration volume varied from 0.5-1 mL) (Stier, 1999)	Apply dry warm compresses (Hurst, 2004)	
Phenytoin	No antidote or Hyaluronidase	Conflicting information: Do not use antidotes (pediatrics) (Montgomery, 1999) Hyaluronidase: SubQ: Inject four separate 0.2 mL injections of 15 units/mL (using a 25-gauge needle) into area of extravasation (Sokol, 1998)	No recommendation	
Potassium Acetate (>0.1 mEq/mL)	Hyaluronidase	Hyaluronidase: Intradermal or SubQ: Inject a total of 1 mL (15 units/mL) as five separate 0.2 mL injections (using a 25-gauge needle) into area of extravasation at the leading edge in a clockwise manner (MacCara, 1983; Zenk, 1981)	Apply dry cold compresses (Hurst, 2004)	Reports of both irritant and vesicant reactions

Table 1: Vesicant Agents and Extravasation Management *continued*

Extravasated Medication	Preferred Antidote	Antidote Administration	Supportive Management	Comments
Potassium Chloride (>0.1 mEq/mL)	Hyaluronidase	Hyaluronidase: Intradermal or SubQ: Inject a total of 1 mL (15 units/mL) as five separate 0.2 mL injections (using a 25-gauge needle) into area of extravasation at the leading edge in a clockwise manner (MacCara, 1983; Zenk, 1981)	Apply dry cold compresses (Hurst, 2004)	Reports of both irritant and vesicant reactions
Promethazine	No known antidote	No known antidote	Apply dry cold compresses (Hurst, 2004)	**Note:** Preferred route of administration for promethazine is by deep intramuscular (I.M.) injection. If I.V. route is used, discontinue infusion immediately with onset of burning/pain; evaluate for inadvertent arterial injection or extravasation.
Sodium Bicarbonate (≥8.4%)	Hyaluronidase	Hyaluronidase: SubQ: Inject four to five separate 0.2 mL injections of 15 units/ mL around area of extravasation (Hurst, 2004)	Apply dry cold compresses (Hurst, 2004)	
Sodium Chloride (>1%)	No known antidote	No known antidote	Apply dry warm compresses (Hastings-Tolsma, 1993)	
Streptozocin	No known antidote	No known antidote	No recommendation	Irritant with vesicant-like properties (reports of both irritant and vesicant reactions)
Trabectedin	No known antidote	No known antidote	No recommendation	Not commercially available in the U.S.
Tromethamine	No known antidote	No known antidote	No recommendation	
Vasopressin	Phentolamine	Phentolamine: Dilute 5-10 mg in 10-15 mL NS and administer into extravasation site as soon as possible after extravasation (Peberdy, 2010) *Alternatives to phentolamine (due to shortage):* Nitroglycerin topical 2% ointment (based on limited case reports in neonates/infants): Apply 4 mm/kg as a thin ribbon to the affected areas; may repeat after 8 hours if needed (Wong, 1992) **or** apply a 1-inch strip on the affected site (Denkler, 1989) Terbutaline (based on limited case reports): Infiltrate extravasation area using a solution of terbutaline 1 mg diluted to 10 mL in NS (large extravasation site; administration volume varied from 3-10 mL) **or** 1 mg diluted in 1 mL NS (small/distal extravasation site; administration volume varied from 0.5-1 mL) (Stier, 1999)	No recommendation	
VinBLAStine	Hyaluronidase	Hyaluronidase: *If needle/cannula still in place:* Administer 1-6 mL (150 units/mL) into existing I.V. line; usual dose is 1 mL for each 1 mL of extravasated drug (Pérez Fidalgo, 2012; Schulmeister, 2011) *If needle/cannula was removed:* Inject 1-6 mL (150 units/mL) subcutaneously in a clockwise manner using 1 mL for each 1 mL of drug extravasated (Schulmeister, 2011) or administer 1 mL (150 units/mL) as five separate 0.2 mL injections (using a 25-gauge needle) into the extravasation site (Polovich, 2009)	Apply dry warm compress for 20 minutes 4 times/day for 1-2 days (Pérez Fidalgo, 2012)	

1705

Table 1: Vesicant Agents and Extravasation Management *continued*

Extravasated Medication	Preferred Antidote	Antidote Administration	Supportive Management	Comments
VinCRIStine	Hyaluronidase	Hyaluronidase: *If needle/cannula still in place:* Administer 1-6 mL (150 units/mL) into existing I.V. line; usual dose is 1 mL for each 1 mL of extravasated drug (Pérez Fidalgo, 2012; Schulmeister, 2011) *If needle/cannula was removed:* Inject 1-6 mL (150 units/mL) subcutaneously in a clockwise manner using 1 mL for each 1 mL of drug extravasated (Schulmeister, 2011) **or** administer 1 mL (150 units/mL) as five separate 0.2 mL injections (using a 25-gauge needle) into the extravasation site (Polovich, 2009)	Apply dry warm compress for 20 minutes 4 times/day for 1-2 days (Pérez Fidalgo, 2012)	
Vindesine	Hyaluronidase	Hyaluronidase: *If needle/cannula still in place:* Administer 1-6 mL (150 units/mL) into existing I.V. line; usual dose is 1 mL for each 1 mL of extravasated drug (Pérez Fidalgo, 2012; Schulmeister, 2011) *If needle/cannula was removed:* Inject 1-6 mL (150 units/mL) subcutaneously in a clockwise manner using 1 mL for each 1 mL of drug extravasated (Schulmeister, 2011) **or** administer 1 mL (150 units/mL) as five separate 0.2 mL injections (using a 25-gauge needle) into the extravasation site (Polovich, 2009)	Apply dry warm compress for 20 minutes 4 times/day for 1-2 days (Pérez Fidalgo, 2012)	Not commercially available in the U.S.
Vinorelbine	Hyaluronidase	Hyaluronidase: *If needle/cannula still in place:* Administer 1-6 mL (150 units/mL) into existing I.V. line; usual dose is 1 mL for each 1 mL of extravasated drug (Pérez Fidalgo, 2012; Schulmeister, 2011) *If needle/cannula was removed:* Inject 1-6 mL (150 units/mL) subcutaneously in a clockwise manner using 1 mL for each 1 mL of drug extravasated (Schulmeister, 2011) **or** administer 1 mL (150 units/mL) as five separate 0.2 mL injections (using a 25-gauge needle) into the extravasation site (Polovich, 2009)	Apply dry warm compress for 20 minutes 4 times/day for 1-2 days (Pérez Fidalgo, 2012)	

SUPPORTIVE MANAGEMENT

Compresses: Two issues for which there is less consensus are the application of warm or cold compresses and the use of various antidotes for extravasation management. A variety of recommendations exists for each of these concerns; however, there is no consensus concerning the proper approach.

Cold: Intermittent cooling of the area of extravasation results in vasoconstriction, potentially restricting the spread of the drug and decreasing the pain and inflammation in the area. Application of dry cold compresses for 20 minutes 4 times/day for 1-2 days is usually recommended as immediate treatment for most drug extravasations, including anthracycline, antibiotic (eg, mitomycin or dactinomycin), or alkylating agent extravasation (Pérez Fidalgo, 2012). Cold dry compresses may also be utilized in the management of nonvesicant extravasations.

Warm: Application of dry warm compresses results in a localized vasodilation and increased blood flow. Increased circulation is believed to facilitate removal of the drug from the area of extravasation. Application of dry warm compresses for 20 minutes 4 times/day for 1-2 days is generally recommended for extravasation of vinca alkaloid, taxane, and platinum derivatives (Pérez Fidalgo, 2012). Avoid moist heat. Most data are from animal studies with relatively few human case reports. Animal models indicate application of heat exacerbates the damage from anthracycline extravasations.

For some agents, such as oxaliplatin and taxanes, there are conflicting recommendations. Some reports recommend application of cold; others recommend warm.

Table 2: Antineoplastic Agents Associated With Irritation or Occasional Extravasation Reactions

Acyclovir (>7 mg/mL)	Fluorouracil
Arsenic Trioxide	Gemcitabine
Bendamustine[1]	Ibritumomab
Bleomycin	Ifosfamide
Bortezomib	Irinotecan
Busulfan	Ixabepilone
CARBOplatin	Melphalan
Carmustine	MitoXANtrone[1]
CISplatin (≤0.4 mg/mL)	Oxaliplatin[1]
Cladribine	PACLitaxel[1]
Cyclophosphamide	PACLitaxel (Protein Bound)
Dacarbazine	Pentamidine[1]
DAUNOrubicin Citrate (Liposomal)	Streptozocin[1]
DOCEtaxel[1]	Teniposide
DOXOrubicin (Liposomal)	Thiopental[1]
Etoposide	Thiotepa
Etoposide Phosphate	Topotecan

[1]Irritant with vesicant-like properties (there have been reports of both irritant and vesicant reactions)

The nurse administering the vesicant agent should monitor the patient and I.V. site frequently. Prior to drug administration, verify the patency of the I.V. line. The line should be flushed with 5-10 mL of a saline or dextrose solution (depending on compatibility) and the drug(s) infused through the side of a free-flowing I.V. line over 2-5 minutes. If an extravasation occurs, it is important to monitor the site closely at 24 hours, 1 week, 2 weeks, and as necessary for any signs and symptoms of extravasation.

EXTRAVASATION-SPECIFIC ANTIDOTES

Dexrazoxane: Dexrazoxane, a derivative of EDTA, is an intracellular chelating agent initially approved as a cardioprotective agent in patients receiving anthracycline therapy. It is believed that the cardioprotective effect of dexrazoxane is a result of chelating iron following intracellular hydrolysis. Dexrazoxane is not an effective chelator itself but is hydrolyzed intracellularly to an open-ring chelator form, which complexes with iron, other heavy metals, and doxorubicin complexes to inhibit the generation of free radicals. In the management of anthracycline-induced extravasation, dexrazoxane may act by reversibly inhibiting topoisomerase II, protecting tissue from anthracycline cytotoxicity, thereby decreasing tissue damage.

◀ Dexrazoxane is administered as 3 I.V. infusions over 1-2 hours through a different venous access location: 1000 mg/m^2 within 6 hours, 1000 mg/m^2 after 24 hours, and 500 mg/m^2 after 48 hours of the actual extravasation up to a maximum total dose of 2000 mg on days 1 and 2 and 1000 mg on day 3, respectively (Mouridsen, 2007). Localized cooling was permitted (except within 15 minutes before and after dexrazoxane infusion). Prior to administering dexrazoxane, discontinue DMSO as studies suggest the single agent is more effective than when used in combination with DMSO. **Note:** Reduce dexrazoxane dose by 50% in patients with moderate to severe renal impairment (CrCl <40 mL/minute).

Dimethyl sulfoxide (DMSO): Case reports and small studies have suggested that DMSO is an effective treatment for certain chemotherapy extravasations (anthracyclines, mitomycin, and mitoxantrone). DMSO has free-radical scavenger properties, which increases removal of vesicant drugs from tissues to minimize tissue damage in extravasation management (Pérez Fidalgo, 2012). Common dosing is to apply topically by gently painting DMSO 50% solution onto an area twice the size of the extravasation with a saturated gauze pad or cotton swab every 8 hours for 7 days (Pérez Fidalgo, 2012). Allow the site to dry. Do not cover with a dressing, as severe blistering may result. During application, DMSO may cause local erythema. Clinical reports of DMSO use are difficult to interpret due to variations in DMSO concentration (50% to 99%); the product is only commercially available in the United States at a concentration of 50% (vol/vol) solution in water.

Hyaluronidase: Hyaluronidase is an enzyme that destroys hyaluronic acid, an essential component of connective tissue. This results in increased permeability of the tissue, facilitating diffusion and absorption of fluids. It is postulated that increasing the diffusion of extravasated fluids results in more rapid absorption, thereby limiting tissue damage. In individual case reports, hyaluronidase has been reported effective in preventing tissue damage from a wide variety of agents, including vinca alkaloids, epipodophyllotoxins, and taxanes. The ESMO/EONS guidelines suggest that 150-900 units may be administered subcutaneously around the area of chemotherapy extravasation (Pérez Fidalgo, 2012). Administration as 5 separate 0.2 mL (15 units/mL) SubQ or intradermal injections into the extravasation site has been reported (MacCara, 1983). A 24-gauge or smaller needle should be used. It is recommended to use a new syringe for each injection site. If needle/cannula still in place, administration of a 1-6 mL hyaluronidase (150 units/mL) has been reported in the management of plant alkaloid extravasation (Pérez Fidalgo, 2012; Schulmeister, 2011) and paclitaxel extravasation (Ener, 2004). Refer to Table 1 for vesicant-specific management.

Phentolamine: Phentolamine minimizes tissue injury due to extravasation of norepinephrine and other sympathomimetic vasoconstrictors. Inject 5-10 mg diluted in 10-15 mL normal saline and inject/infiltrate into the extravasation area; begin as soon as possible after extravasation but within 12 hours.

Sodium thiosulfate: Sodium thiosulfate ($^1/_6$ molar) has been recommended for treatment of mechlorethamine, concentrated cisplatin, and bendamustine extravasations. Sodium thiosulfate provides a substrate for alkylation by mechlorethamine, preventing the alkylation and subsequent destruction in subcutaneous tissue.

Preparation of a $^1/_6$ molar solution of sodium thiosulfate:

- Dilute 4 mL of a sodium thiosulfate 10% solution into a syringe with 6 mL of sterile water for injection, resulting in 10 mL of $^1/_6$ molar solution

  or

- Dilute 1.6 mL of a sodium thiosulfate 25% solution with 8.4 mL of sterile water for injection, resulting in 10 mL of $^1/_6$ molar solution

Inject the $^1/_6$ molar sodium thiosulfate solution either into the existing needle/cannula or subcutaneously around the edge of the extravasation site using a tuberculin syringe, using a new syringe for each injection site. The dose of sodium thiosulfate and route of administration depend on the amount of drug extravasated. Refer to Table 1 for vesicant-specific dosing.

Topical nitroglycerin or terbutaline (alternatives to phentolamine): Terbutaline and topical nitroglycerin have been used (case reports) as alternatives to phentolamine in the event of phentolamine supply shortages. Topical nitroglycerin (2% ointment) is reported to reverse the vasoconstriction at the extravasation site caused by infiltration of sympathomimetic vasoconstrictors; case reports for use in neonates/infants suggest resolution of ischemia (Denkler, 1989; Wong, 1992).

REFERENCES

Albanell J, Baselga J. Systemic therapy emergencies. *Semin Oncol.* 2000;27(3):347-361.

Bellin MF, Jakobsen JA, Tomassin I, et al. Contrast medium extravasation injury: guidelines for prevention and management. *Eur Radiol.* 2002;12(11):2807-2812.

Bertelli G. Prevention and management of extravasation of cytotoxic drugs. *Drug Saf.* 1995;12(4):245-255.

Boyle DM, Engelking C. Vesicant extravasation: myths and realities. *Oncol Nurs Forum.* 1995;22(1):57-67.

de Lemos ML. Role of dimethylsulfoxide for mangement of chemotherapy extravasation. *J Oncol Pharm Practice.* 2004;10(4):197-200.

de Lemos ML, Walisser S. Management of extravasation of oxaliplatin. *J Oncol Pharm Pract.* 2005;11(4):159-162.

Denkler KA, Cohen BE. Reversal of dopamine extravasation injury with topical nitroglycerin ointment. *Plast Reconstr Surg.* 1989;84 (5):811-813.

Doellman D, Hadaway L, Bowe-Geddes LA, et al. Infiltration and extravasation: update on prevention and management. *J Infus Nurs.* 2009;32(4):203-211.

Dorr RT. Antidotes to vesicant chemotherapy extravasations. *Blood Rev.* 1990;4(1):41-60.

Dorr RT, Soble M, Alberts DS. Efficacy of sodium thiosulfate as a local antidote to mechlorethamine skin toxicity in the mouse. *Cancer Chemother Pharmacol.* 1988;22(4):299-302.

Ener RA, Meglathery SB, Styler M. Extravasation of systemic hemato-oncological therapies. *Ann Oncol.* 2004;15(6):858-862.

Hadaway L. Infiltration and extravasation. *Am J Nurs.* 2007;107(8):64-72.

Hastings-Tolsma MT, Yucha CB, Tompkins J, Robson L, Szeverenyi N. Effect of warm and cold applications on the resolution of I.V. infiltrations. *Res Nurs Health.* 1993;16(3):171-178.

Hurst S, McMillan M. Innovative solutions in critical care units: extravasation guidelines. *Dimens Crit Care Nurs.* 2004;23(3):125-128.

Kumar MM, Sprung J. The use of hyaluronidase to treat mannitol extravasation. *Anesth Analg.* 2003;97(4):1199-1200.

Kurul S, Saip P, Aydin T. Totally implantable venous-access ports: local problems and extravasation injury. *Lancet Oncol.* 2002;3 (11):684-692.

Larson DL. Alterations in wound healing secondary to infusion injury. *Clin Plast Surg.* 1990;17(3):509-517.

Larson DL. Treatment of tissue extravasation by antitumor agents. *Cancer.* 1982;49(9):1796-1799.

Larson DL. What is the appropriate management of tissue extravasation by antitumor agents? *Plast Reconstr Surg.* 1985;75 (3):397-405.

MacCara ME. Extravasation: a hazard of intravenous therapy. *Drug Intell Clin Pharm.* 1983;17(10):713-717.

Montgomery LA, Hanrahan K, Kottman K, Otto A, Barrett T, Hermiston B. Guideline for I.V. infiltrations in pediatric patients. *Pediatr Nurs.* 1999;25(2):167-169, 173-180.

Mouridsen HT, Langer SW, Buter J, et al. Treatment of anthracycline extravasation with savene (dexrazoxane): results from two prospective clinical multicentre studies. *Ann Oncol.* 2007;18(3):546-550.

Mustargen product information, Lundbeck, 2012

Peberdy MA, Callaway CW, Neumar RW, et al. Part 9: post-cardiac arrest care: 2010 American Heart Association guidelines for cardiopulmonary resuscitation and emergency cardiovascular care. *Circulation.* 2010;122(18 Suppl 3):S768-S786.

Pérez Fidalgo JA, García Fabregat L, Cervantes A, et al. Management of chemotherapy extravasation: ESMO-EONS clinical practice guidelines. *Ann Oncol.* 2012;23(Suppl 7):vii167-173.

Perry MC. Extravasation. *The Chemotherapy Source Book.* 4th ed. Philadelphia, PA; 2008.

Phentolamine product information, Bedford Laboratories, 1999

Polovich M, Whitford JN, Olsen M. *Chemotherapy and Biotherapy Guidelines and Recommendations for Practice.* 3rd ed. Pittsburgh, PA: Oncology Nursing Society; 2009.

Reynolds PM, Maclaren R, Mueller SW, Fish DN, Kiser TH. Management of extravasation injuries: a focused evaluation of noncytotoxic medications [published online January 13, 2014]. *Pharmacotherapy.*

Rowlett J. Extravasation of contrast media managed with recombinant human hyaluronidase. *Am J Emerg Med.* 2012;30(9):2102.

Schrijvers DL. Extravasation: a dreaded complication of chemotherapy. *Ann Oncol.* 2003;14(Suppl 3):iii26-iii30.

Schulmeister L, Camp-Sorrell D. Chemotherapy extravasation from implanted ports. *Oncol Nurs Forum.* 2000;27(3):531-538.

Schulmeister L. Extravasation management: clinical update. *Semin Oncol Nurs.* 2011;27(1):82-90.

Schulmeister L. Preventing and managing vesicant chemotherapy extravasations. *J Support Oncol.* 2010;8(5):212-215.

Sokol DK, Dahlmann A, Dunn DW. Hyaluronidase treatment for intravenous phenytoin extravasation. *J Child Neurol.* 1998;13 (5):246-247.

Stanford BL, Hardwicke F. A review of clinical experience with paclitaxel extravasations. *Support Care Cancer.* 2003;11(5):270-277.

Stier PA, Bogner MP, Webster K, Leikin JB, Burda A. Use of subcutaneous terbutaline to reverse peripheral ischemia. *Am J Emerg Med.* 1999;17(1):91-94.

Wang CL, Cohan RH, Ellis JH, Adusumilli S, Dunnick NR. Frequency, management, and outcome of extravasation of nonionic iodinated contrast medium in 69,657 intravenous injections. *Radiology.* 2007;243(1):80-87.

Wiegand R, Brown J. Hyaluronidase for the management of dextrose extravasation. *Am J Emerg Med.* 2010;28(2):257.

Wong AF, McCulloch LM, Sola A. Treatment of peripheral tissue ischemia with topical nitroglycerin ointment in neonates. *J Pediatr.* 1992;121(6):980-983.

Zenk KE. Management of intravenous extravasations. *Infusion.* 1981;5(4):77-79.

PEAK AND TROUGH GUIDELINES

Drug	When to Sample	Therapeutic Levels*	Usual Half-Life	Steady State (Ideal Sampling Time)	Potentially Toxic Levels*
Antibiotics					
Gentamicin Tobramycin	30 min after 30 min infusion Trough: <0.5 h before next dose	Peak: 3-10 mcg/mL (level dependent upon severity of infection) Trough: <2.0 mcg/mL (<1 for hospital-acquired pneumonia)	2 h (adults)	15 h	Peak: >12 mcg/mL Trough: >2 mcg/mL
Amikacin		Peak: 15-40 mcg/mL Trough: <8 mcg/mL (<4-5 for hospital-acquired pneumonia)			Peak: >40 mcg/mL Trough: >10 mcg/mL
Vancomycin	Trough: <0.5 h before next dose	Trough: ≥15-20 mcg/mL depending upon severity/type of infection	5-11 h (adults)	24-60 h	>80 mcg/mL
Anticonvulsants					
CarBAMazepine	Trough: Just before next oral dose	4-12 mcg/mL (epilepsy)	Multiple doses: 12-17 h (adults) 8-14 h (children)	Metabolism changes over the first 3-5 weeks of therapy	>15 mcg/mL
Ethosuximide	Trough: Just before next oral dose	40-100 mcg/mL	50-60 h (adults) 30 h (children)	10-13 d	
PHENobarbital	Trough: Just before next dose	20-40 mcg/mL (adults) 15-30 mcg/mL (children)	54-140 h (adults) 37-73 h (children)	~20 d	>40 mcg/mL
Phenytoin Free phenytoin	Trough: Just before next dose Draw at same time as total level	Total: 10-20 mcg/mL (children and adults) Free: l-2.5 mcg/mL	7-42 h; concentration-dependent	2-9 d	>30 mcg/mL
Primidone	Trough: Just before next dose (**Note:** Primidone is metabolized to phenobarbital; order levels separately.)	5-12 mcg/mL (adults)	Primidone: 5-15 h (variable) PEMA: 16 h (variable)	1-3 d	>15 mcg/mL
Valproic acid	Trough: Just before next dose	Seizures: 50-100 mcg/mL Mania: 50-125 mcg/mL	5-20 h	2-4 d	>150-200 mcg/mL
Bronchodilators					
Aminophylline (I.V.)	18-24 h after starting or changing a maintenance dose; given as a constant infusion	5-15 mcg/mL	Nonsmoking adult: 8 h Children: ~4 h	2 d	>20 mcg/mL
Theophylline (P.O.)	Peak levels: Not recommended Trough level: Just before next dose				

continued

Drug	When to Sample	Therapeutic Levels*	Usual Half-Life	Steady State (Ideal Sampling Time)	Potentially Toxic Levels*
		Cardiovascular Agents			
Digoxin	Trough: Just before next dose (levels drawn earlier than 6 h after a dose will be artificially elevated)	0.5-0.9 ng/mL (heart failure)	36-48 h (adults)	8-10 d	>2 ng/mL
Lidocaine	Steady-state levels are usually achieved after 6-12 h	1.5-5 mcg/mL	1.5-2 h	5-10 h	>6 mcg/mL
		Other Agents			
Amitriptyline	Trough: Just before next dose	Amitriptyline and nortriptyline (active metabolite): 80-250 ng/mL	~13-36 h	4-8 d	>300 ng/mL
CycloSPORINE		General range: 100-400 ng/mL but dependent upon organ transplanted, time after transplant, organ function, and cyclosporine toxicity		Variable	Not well-defined
Lithium		0.6-1.2 mEq/mL (acute mania) 0.8-1 mEq/mL (prevention of mania in bipolar disorder) 0.6-0.8 mEq/mL (elderly patients)	18-24 h	4-7 d	>1.5 mEq/mL

*Due to methodology differences, reference ranges may vary from laboratory to laboratory; check with the laboratory service used for their appropriate levels.

1711

ORAL MEDICATIONS THAT SHOULD NOT BE CRUSHED OR ALTERED

There are a variety of reasons for crushing tablets or capsule contents prior to administering to the patient. Patients may have nasogastric tubes which do not permit the administration of tablets or capsules, an oral solution for a particular medication may not be available from the manufacturer or readily prepared by pharmacy, patients may have difficulty swallowing capsules or tablets, or mixing of powdered medication with food or drink may make the drug more palatable.

Generally, medications which should not be crushed fall into one of the following categories:

- **Extended Release Products:** The formulation of some tablets is specialized as to allow the medication within it to be slowly released into the body. This may be accomplished by centering the drug within the core of the tablet, with a subsequent shedding of multiple layers around the core. Wax melts in the GI tract, releasing drug contained within the wax matrix (eg, OxyCONTIN). Capsules may contain beads which have multiple layers which are slowly dissolved with time.

  Common Abbreviations for Extended Release Products

CD	Controlled dose
CR	Controlled release
CRT	Controlled release tablet
LA	Long-acting
SR	Sustained release
TR	Timed release
TD	Time delay
SA	Sustained action
XL	Extended release
XR	Extended release

- **Medications Which Are Irritating to the Stomach:** Tablets which are irritating to the stomach may be enteric-coated which delays release of the drug until the time when it reaches the small intestine. Enteric-coated aspirin is an example of this.

- **Foul-Tasting Medication:** Some drugs are quite unpleasant to taste so the manufacturer coats the tablet in a sugar coating to increase its palatability. By crushing the tablet, this sugar coating is lost and the patient tastes the unpleasant tasting medication.

- **Sublingual Medication:** Medication intended for use under the tongue should not be crushed. While it appears to be obvious, it is not always easy to determine if a medication is to be used sublingually. Sublingual medications should indicate on the package that they are intended for sublingual use.

- **Effervescent Tablets:** These are tablets which, when dropped into a liquid, quickly dissolve to yield a solution. Many effervescent tablets, when crushed, lose their ability to quickly dissolve.

- **Potentially Hazardous Substances:** Certain drugs, including antineoplastic agents, hormonal agents, some antivirals, some bioengineered agents, and other miscellaneous drugs, are considered potentially hazardous when used in humans based on their characteristics. Examples of these characteristics include carcinogenicity, teratogenicity, reproductive toxicity, organ toxicity at low doses, genotoxicity, or new drugs with structural and toxicity profiles similar to existing hazardous drugs. Exposure to these substances can result in adverse effects and should be avoided. Crushing or breaking a tablet or opening a capsule of a potentially hazardous substance may increase the risk of exposure to the substance through skin contact, inhalation, or accidental ingestion. The extent of exposure, potency, and toxicity of the hazardous substance determines the health risk. Institutions have policies and procedures to follow when handling any potentially hazardous substance. **Note:** All potentially hazardous substances may not be represented in this table. Refer to institution-specific guidelines for precautions to observe when handling hazardous substances.

RECOMMENDATIONS

1. It is not advisable to crush certain medications.

2. Consult individual monographs prior to crushing capsule or tablet.

3. If crushing a tablet or capsule is contraindicated, consult with your pharmacist to determine whether an oral solution exists or can be compounded.

Drug Product	Dosage Form	Dosage Reasons/Comments
Accutane	Capsule	Mucous membrane irritant; teratogenic potential
Aciphex	Tablet	Extended release
Aciphex Sprinkle	Capsule	Slow release. Capsule may be opened and contents sprinkled on soft food (eg, applesauce, fruit- or vegetable-based baby food, yogurt) or emptied into a small amount of liquid (eg, infant formula, apple juice, pediatric electrolyte solution). Granules should not be chewed or crushed.
Actiq	Lozenge	Slow release. This lollipop delivery system requires the patient to dissolve it slowly.
Actoplus Met XR	Tablet	Variable release
Actonel	Tablet	Irritant. Chewed, crushed, or sucked tablets may cause oropharyngeal irritation.
Adalat CC	Tablet	Extended release
Adderall XR	Capsule	Extended release[1]
Adenovirus (Types 4, 7) Vaccine	Tablet	Teratogenic potential; enteric-coated; do not disrupt tablet to avoid releasing live adenovirus in upper respiratory tract
Advicor	Tablet	Variable release
Afeditab CR	Tablet	Extended release
Afinitor	Tablet	Mucous membrane irritant; teratogenic potential; hazardous substance[11]
Aggrenox	Capsule	Extended release. Capsule may be opened; contents include an aspirin tablet that may be chewed and dipyridamole pellets that may be sprinkled on applesauce.
Alavert Allergy and Sinus D-12	Tablet	Extended release
Allegra-D	Tablet	Extended release
ALPRAZolam ER	Tablet	Extended release
Altoprev	Tablet	Extended release
Ambien CR	Tablet	Extended release
Amitiza	Capsule	Manufacturer recommended
Amnesteem	Capsule	Mucous membrane irritant; teratogenic potential
Ampyra	Tablet	Extended release
Amrix	Capsule	Extended release
Aplenzin	Tablet	Extended release
Apriso	Capsule	Extended release[1]; maintain pH at ≤6
Aptivus	Capsule	Taste. Oil emulsion within spheres
Aricept 23 mg	Tablet	Film-coated; chewing or crushing may increase rate of absorption
Arava	Tablet	Teratogenic potential; hazardous substance[11]
Arthrotec	Tablet	Delayed release; enteric-coated
Asacol	Tablet	Slow release
Aspirin enteric-coated	Capsule, tablet	Delayed release; enteric-coated
Astagraf XL	Capsule	Extended release
Atelvia	Tablet	Extended release; tablet coating is an important part of the delayed release
Augmentin XR	Tablet	Extended release[2, 8]
AVINza	Capsule	Slow release[1] (not pudding)
Avodart	Capsule	Capsule should not be handled by pregnant women due to teratogenic potential[10]; hazardous substance[11]
Azulfidine EN-tabs	Tablet	Delayed release

(continued)

Drug Product	Dosage Form	Dosage Reasons/Comments
Bayer Aspirin EC	Caplet	Enteric-coated
Bayer Aspirin, Low Adult 81 mg	Tablet	Enteric-coated
Bayer Aspirin, Regular Strength 325 mg	Caplet	Enteric-coated
Biaxin XL	Tablet	Extended release
Biltricide	Tablet	Taste[8]
Bisac-Evac	Tablet	Enteric-coated[3]
Bisacodyl	Tablet	Enteric-coated[3]
Boniva	Tablet	Irritant. Chewed, crushed, or sucked tablets may cause oropharyngeal irritation.
Bosulif	Tablet	Hazardous substance[11]
Budeprion SR	Tablet	Extended release
Buproban	Tablet	Extended release
BuPROPion SR	Tablet	Extended release
Calan SR	Tablet	Extended release[8]
Campral	Tablet	Delayed release; enteric-coated
Caprelsa	Tablet	Teratogenic potential; hazardous substance[11]
Carbatrol	Capsule	Extended release[1]
Cardene SR	Capsule	Extended release
Cardizem	Tablet	Not described as slow release but releases drug over 3 hours.
Cardizem CD	Capsule	Extended release
Cardizem LA	Tablet	Extended release
Cardura XL	Tablet	Extended release
Cartia XT	Capsule	Extended release
Casodex	Tablet	Teratogenic potential; hazardous substance[11]
CeeNU	Capsule	Teratogenic potential; hazardous substance[11]
Cefaclor extended release	Tablet	Extended release
Ceftin	Tablet	Taste[2]. Use suspension for children.
Cefuroxime	Tablet	Taste[2]. Use suspension for children.
CellCept	Capsule, tablet	Teratogenic potential; hazardous substance[9,11]
Charcoal Plus DS	Tablet	Enteric-coated
Chlor-Trimeton 12-Hour	Tablet	Extended release[2]
Cipro XR	Tablet	Extended release[2]
Claravis	Capsule	Mucous membrane irritant; teratogenic potential
Claritin-D 12-Hour	Tablet	Extended release[2]
Claritin-D 24-Hour	Tablet	Extended release[2]
Colace	Capsule	Taste[5]
Colestid	Tablet	Slow release
Cometriq	Capsule	Teratogenic potential; hazardous substance[11]
Commit	Lozenge	Integrity compromised by chewing or crushing
Concerta	Tablet	Extended release
ConZip	Capsule	Variable release; tablet disruption may cause overdose
Coreg CR	Capsule	Extended release[1]; may add contents to chilled applesauce
Cotazym-S	Capsule	Enteric-coated[1]
Covera-HS	Tablet	Extended release
Creon	Capsule	Extended release[1]; enteric-coated contents
Crixivan	Capsule	Taste. Capsule may be opened and mixed with fruit puree (eg, banana).
Cymbalta	Capsule	Enteric-coated[1]; may add contents to apple juice or applesauce but not chocolate
Cytoxan	Tablet	Drug may be crushed, but manufacturer recommends using injection; hazardous substance[11]

(continued)

Drug Product	Dosage Form	Dosage Reasons/Comments
Depakene	Capsule	Slow release; mucous membrane irritant[2]; hazardous substance[11]
Depakote	Tablet	Delayed release; hazardous substance[11]
Depakote ER	Tablet	Extended release; hazardous substance[11]
Depakote Sprinkles	Capsule	Extended release[1]
Detrol LA	Capsule	Extended release
Dexedrine	Capsule	Extended release
Dexilant	Capsule	Delayed release[1]
Diamox Sequels	Capsule	Extended release
Dibenzyline	Capsule	Hazardous substance[11]
Diclegis	Tablet	Delayed release; manufacturer recommendation
Dilacor XR	Capsule	Extended release
Dilatrate-SR	Capsule	Extended release
Dilt-CD	Capsule	Extended release
Dilt-XR	Capsule	Extended release
Diltia XT	Capsule	Extended release
Ditropan XL	Tablet	Extended release
Divalproex ER	Tablet	Extended release
Donnatal Extentab	Tablet	Extended release[2]
Doxidan	Tablet	Enteric-coated[3]
Drisdol	Capsule	Liquid filled[4]
Droxia	Capsule	May be opened; wear gloves to handle; hazardous substance[11]
Duavee	Tablet	Manufacturer recommendation; hazardous substance[11]
Dulcolax	Capsule	Liquid-filled
Dulcolax	Tablet	Enteric-coated[3]
EC-Naprosyn	Tablet	Delayed release; enteric-coated
Ecotrin Adult Low Strength	Tablet	Enteric-coated
Ecotrin Maximum Strength	Tablet	Enteric-coated
Ecotrin Regular Strength	Tablet	Enteric-coated
E.E.S.	Tablet	Enteric-coated[2]
Effer-K	Tablet	Effervescent tablet[6]
Effervescent Potassium	Tablet	Effervescent tablet[6]
Effexor XR	Capsule	Extended release
Embeda	Capsule	Extended release[1]; do not give via NG tube
E-Mycin	Tablet	Enteric-coated
Enablex	Tablet	Slow release
Entocort EC	Capsule	Extended release; enteric-coated[1]
Equetro	Capsule	Extended release[1]
Ergomar	Tablet	Sublingual form[7]
Erivedge	Capsule	Teratogenic potential[11]
Eryc	Capsule	Enteric-coated
Ery-Tab	Tablet	Delayed release; enteric-coated
Erythromycin Stearate	Tablet	Enteric-coated
Erythromycin Base	Tablet	Enteric-coated
Erythromycin Delayed-Release	Capsule	Enteric-coated pellets[1]
Etoposide	Capsule	Hazardous substance[11]
Evista	Tablet	Taste; teratogenic potential[10]; hazardous substance[11]
Exalgo	Tablet	Extended release; breaking, chewing, crushing, or dissolving before ingestion or injecting increases the risk of overdose
Exjade	Tablet	Do not chew or swallow whole; do not give as tablets meant to be given as a liquid

(continued)

Drug Product	Dosage Form	Dosage Reasons/Comments
Fareston	Tablet	Teratogenic potential; hazardous substance[11]
Feldene	Capsule	Mucous membrane irritant
Fentanyl	Lozenge	Slow release; lollipop delivery system requires the patient to slowly dissolve in mouth
Fentora	Tablet	Buccal tablet; swallowing whole or crushing may reduce effectiveness
Feosol	Tablet	Enteric-coated[2]
Fergon	Tablet	Enteric-coated
Ferro-Sequels	Tablet	Slow release
Flagyl ER	Tablet	Extended release
Fleet Laxative	Tablet	Enteric-coated[3]
Flomax	Capsule	Slow release
Focalin XR	Capsule	Extended release[1]
Forfivo XL	Capsule	Extended release
Fortamet	Tablet	Extended release
Fosamax	Tablet	Mucous membrane irritant
Fosamax Plus D	Tablet	Mucous membrane irritant
Fulyzaq	Tablet	Delayed release
Gengraf	Capsule	Teratogenic potential; hazardous substance[11]
Geodon	Capsule	Hazardous substance[11]
Gleevec	Tablet	Taste[8]. May be dissolved in water or apple juice; hazardous substance[11]
GlipiZIDE XL	Tablet	Extended release
Glucophage XR	Tablet	Extended release
Glucotrol XL	Tablet	Extended release
Glumetza	Tablet	Extended release
Gralise	Tablet	Extended release
Halfprin	Tablet	Enteric-coated
Hexalen	Capsule	Teratogenic potential; hazardous substance[11]
Horizant	Tablet	Extended release
Hycamtin	Capsule	Teratogenic potential; hazardous substance[11]
Hydrea	Capsule	Can be opened and mixed with water; wear gloves to handle; hazardous substance[11]
Iclusig	Tablet	Teratogenic potential; hazardous substance[11]
Imbruvica	Capsule	Teratogenic potential; hazardous substance[11]
Imdur	Tablet	Extended release[8]
Inderal LA	Capsule	Extended release
Indomethacin SR	Capsule	Slow release[1,2]
Inlyta	Tablet	Teratogenic potential; hazardous substance[11]
InnoPran XL	Capsule	Extended release
Intelence	Tablet	Tablet should be swallowed whole and not crushed; tablet may be dispersed in water
Intermezzo	Tablet	Sublingual form[7]
Intuniv	Tablet	Extended release
Invega	Tablet	Extended release
IsoDitrate	Tablet	Extended release
Isoptin SR	Tablet	Extended release[8]
Isosorbide Dinitrate Sublingual	Tablet	Sublingual form[7]
ISOtretinoin	Capsule	Mucous membrane irritant
Jalyn	Capsule	Capsule should not be handled by pregnant women due to teratogenic potential[10]; hazardous substance[9,11]
Janumet XR	Tablet	Extended release

(continued)

Drug Product	Dosage Form	Dosage Reasons/Comments
Juxtapid	Capsule	Manufacturer recommendation
Kadian	Capsule	Extended release[1]. Do not give via NG tubes; may add contents to applesauce without crushing.
Kaletra	Tablet	Film-coated; pregnant women or women who may become pregnant should not handle crushed or broken tablets; active ingredients surrounded by wax matrix to prevent healthcare exposure
Kapidex	Capsule	Delayed release[1]
Kapvay	Tablet	Extended release
Kazano	Tablet	Not scored; manufacturer recommended
K-Dur	Tablet	Slow release
Keppra	Tablet	Taste[2]
Keppra XR	Tablet	Extended release[2]
Ketek	Tablet	Slow release
Khedezia	Tablet	Extended release
Klor-Con	Tablet	Extended release[2]
Klor-Con M	Tablet	Slow release[2]; some strengths are scored; to make liquid, place tablet in 120 mL of water; disperse 2 minutes; stir
K-Lyte/Cl	Tablet	Effervescent tablet[6]
Kombiglyze XR	Tablet	Extended release; tablet matrix may remain in stool
K-Tab	Tablet	Extended release[2]
LaMICtal XR	Tablet	Extended release
Lescol XL	Tablet	Extended release
Letairis	Tablet	Film-coated; slow release; hazardous substance[11]
Leukeran	Tablet	Teratogenic potential; hazardous substance[11]
Levbid	Tablet	Extended release[8]
Lialda	Tablet	Delayed release, enteric-coated
Lithobid	Tablet	Extended release
Lovaza	Capsule	Contents of capsule may erode walls of styrofoam or plastic materials
Luvox CR	Capsule	Extended release
Lysodren	Tablet	Hazardous substance[11]
Mag-Tab SR	Tablet	Extended release
Matulane	Capsule	Teratogenic potential; hazardous substance[11]
Maxiphen DM	Tablet	Slow release[8]
Mestinon ER	Tablet	Extended release[2]
Metadate CD	Capsule	Extended release[1]
Metadate ER	Tablet	Extended release
Metoprolol ER	Tablet	Extended release
MicroK Extencaps	Capsule	Extended release[1,2]
Minocin	Capsule	Slow release
Mirapex ER	Tablet	Extended release
Morphine sulfate extended-release	Tablet	Extended release
Motrin	Tablet	Taste[5]
Moxatag	Tablet	Extended release
MS Contin	Tablet	Extended release[2]
Mucinex	Tablet	Slow release
Mucinex DM	Tablet	Slow release[2]
Multaq	Tablet	Hazardous substance[11]
Myfortic	Tablet	Delayed release; teratogenic potential; hazardous substance[11]
Myrbetriq	Tablet	Extended release
Namenda XR	Capsule	Extended release[1]

(continued)

Drug Product	Dosage Form	Dosage Reasons/Comments
Naprelan	Tablet	Extended release
Neoral	Capsule	Teratogenic potential; hazardous substance[11]
NexIUM	Capsule	Delayed release[1]
Niaspan	Tablet	Extended release
Nicotinic Acid	Capsule, Tablet	Slow release[8]
Nifediac CC	Tablet	Extended release
Nifedical XL	Tablet	Extended release
NIFEdipine ER	Tablet	Extended release
Nitrostat	Tablet	Sublingual route[7]
Norpace CR	Capsule	Extended release; form within a special capsule
Norvir	Tablet	Crushing tablets has resulted in decreased bioavailability of drug[2]
Noxafil	Tablet	Delayed release
Nucynta ER	Tablet	Extended release; tablet disruption may cause a potentially fatal overdose
Oleptro	Tablet	Extended release[8]
Onglyza	Tablet	Film-coated
Opana ER	Tablet	Extended release; tablet disruption may cause a potentially fatal overdose
Opsumit	Tablet	Teratogenic potential; hazardous substance[11]
Oracea	Capsule	Delayed release
Oramorph SR	Tablet	Extended release[2]
Oravig	Tablet	Buccal tablet
Orphenadrine citrate ER	Tablet	Extended release
Oxtellar XR	Tablet	Extended release
OxyCONTIN	Tablet	Extended release; surrounded by wax matrix; tablet disruption may cause a potentially fatal overdose
Oxymorphone ER	Tablet	Extended release
Pancrease MT	Capsule	Enteric-coated[1]
Pancreaze	Capsule	Slow-release[1]; enteric-coated contents
Pancrelipase	Capsule	Slow-release[1]; enteric-coated contents
Paxil CR	Tablet	Extended release
Pentasa	Capsule	Slow release[1]
Pertzye	Capsule	Slow-release[1]; enteric-coated contents
Plendil	Tablet	Extended release
Pomalyst	Capsule	Teratogenic potential; hazardous substance[11]; healthcare workers should avoid contact with capsule contents/body fluids
Pradaxa	Capsule	Bioavailability increases by 75% when the pellets are taken without the capsule shell
Prevacid	Capsule	Delayed release[1]
Prevacid	Suspension	Slow release. Contains enteric-coated granules. Not for use in NG tubes; mix with water only
Prevacid SoluTab	Tablet	Orally disintegrating. Do not swallow; dissolve in water only and dispense via dosing syringe or NG tube.
PriLOSEC	Capsule	Delayed release
PriLOSEC OTC	Tablet	Delayed release
Pristiq	Tablet	Extended release
Procardia XL	Tablet	Extended release
Procysbi	Capsule	Delayed release[1]
Propecia	Tablet	Women who are, or may become, pregnant should not handle crushed or broken tablets due to teratogenic potential[10]; hazardous substance[11]
Proscar	Tablet	Women who are, or may become, pregnant should not handle crushed or broken tablets due to teratogenic potential[10]; hazardous substance[11]

(continued)

Drug Product	Dosage Form	Dosage Reasons/Comments
Protonix	Tablet	Slow release
PROzac Weekly	Capsule	Enteric-coated
Purinethol	Tablet	Teratogenic potential[10]; hazardous substance[11]
Pytest	Capsule	Hazardous substance[11]
QuiNIDine ER	Tablet	Extended release[8]; enteric-coated
Ranexa	Tablet	Slow release
Rapamune	Tablet	Hazardous substance[11]; pharmacokinetic NanoCrystal technology may be affected[2]
Rayos	Tablet	Delayed release; release is dependent upon intact coating
Razadyne ER	Capsule	Extended release
Renagel	Tablet	Expands in liquid if broken/crushed.
Renvela	Tablet	Enteric-coated[2]; expands in liquid if broken or crushed
Requip XL	Tablet	Extended release
Rescriptor	Tablet	If unable to swallow, may dissolve 100 mg tablets in water and drink; 200 mg tablets must be swallowed whole
Revlimid	Capsule	Teratogenic potential; hazardous substance[11]; healthcare workers should avoid contact with capsule contents/body fluids
RisperDAL M-Tab	Tablet	Orally disintegrating. Do not chew or break tablet; after dissolving under tongue, tablet may be swallowed
Ritalin LA	Capsule	Extended release[1]
Ritalin-SR	Tablet	Extended release
Rythmol SR	Capsule	Extended release
Ryzolt	Tablet	Extended release; tablet disruption may cause overdose
SandIMMUNE	Capsule	Teratogenic potential; hazardous substance[11]
Saphris	Tablet	Sublingual form[7]
Sensipar	Tablet	Tablets are not scored and cutting may cause inaccurate dosage
SEROquel XR	Tablet	Extended release
Sinemet CR	Tablet	Extended release[8]
Slo-Niacin	Tablet	Slow release[8]
Slow-Mag	Tablet	Delayed release
Solodyn	Tablet	Extended release
Somnote	Capsule	Liquid filled
Soriatane	Capsule	Teratogenic potential; hazardous substance[11]
Sprycel	Tablet	Film-coated. Active ingredients are surrounded by a wax matrix to prevent healthcare exposure. Women who are, or may become pregnant, should not handle crushed or broken tablets; teratogenic potential; hazardous substance[11]
Stavzor	Capsule	Delayed release; hazardous substance[11]
Stivarga	Tablet	Manufacturer recommendation; teratogenic potential; hazardous substance[11]
Strattera	Capsule	Capsule contents can cause ocular irritation.
Sudafed 12-Hour	Capsule	Extended release[2]
Sudafed 24-Hour	Capsule	Extended release[2]
Sulfazine EC	Tablet	Delayed release, enteric-coated
Sular	Tablet	Extended release
Sustiva	Tablet	Tablets should not be broken (capsules should be used if dosage adjustment needed)
Symax Duotab	Tablet	Controlled release
Symax SR	Tablet	Extended release
Syprine	Capsule	Potential risk of contact dermatitis
Tabloid	Tablet	Teratogenic potential; hazardous substance[11]
Tafinlar	Capsule	Teratogenic potential; hazardous substance[11]
Tamoxifen	Tablet	Teratogenic potential; hazardous substance[11]

(continued)

Drug Product	Dosage Form	Dosage Reasons/Comments
Targretin	Capsule	Manufacturer recommended; teratogenic potential; hazardous substance[11]
Tasigna	Capsule	Hazardous substance[11]; altering capsule may lead to high blood levels, increasing the risk of toxicity
Taztia XT	Capsule	Extended release[1]
Tecfidera	Capsule	Manufacturer recommendation; delayed release; irritant
TEGretol-XR	Tablet	Extended release[2]
Temodar	Capsule	Teratogenic potential; hazardous substance[11]. **Note:** If capsules are accidentally opened or damaged, rigorous precautions should be taken to avoid inhalation or contact of contents with the skin or mucous membranes.
Tessalon Perles	Capsule	Swallow whole; pharmacologic action may cause choking if chewed or opened and swallowed.
Tetracycline	Capsule	Hazardous substance[11]
Thalomid	Capsule	Teratogenic potential; hazardous substance[11]
Theo-24	Capsule	Extended release[1]; contains beads that dissolve through GI tract
Theochron	Tablet	Extended release
Theophylline ER	Tablet	Extended release
Tiazac	Capsule	Extended release[1]
Topamax	Capsule	Taste[1]
Topamax	Tablet	Taste
Toprol XL	Tablet	Extended release[8]
Toviaz	Tablet	Extended release
Tracleer	Tablet	Teratogenic potential; hazardous substance[10,11]; women who are or may be pregnant should not handle crushed or broken tablets
TRENtal	Tablet	Extended release
Treximet	Tablet	Unique formulation enhances rapid drug absorption
TriLipix	Capsule	Extended release
Trokendi XR	Capsule	Extended release
Tylenol Arthritis Pain	Caplet	Controlled release
Tylenol 8 Hour	Caplet	Extended release
Uceris	Tablet	Extended release; coating on tablet designed to break down at pH of ≥7
Ultram ER	Tablet	Extended release. Tablet disruption my cause a potentially fatal overdose.
Ultresa	Capsule	Delayed release; enteric-coated contents
Ultrase	Capsule	Enteric-coated[1]
Ultrase MT	Capsule	Enteric-coated[1]
Uniphyl	Tablet	Slow release
Urocit-K	Tablet	Wax-coated; prevents upper GI release
Uroxatral	Tablet	Extended release
Valcyte	Tablet	Irritant potential[2]; teratogenic potential; hazardous substance[11]
Vascepa	Capsule	Manufacturer recommendation
Verapamil SR	Tablet	Extended release[8]
Verelan	Capsule	Sustained release[1]
Verelan PM	Capsule	Extended release[1]
Vesanoid	Capsule	Teratogenic potential; hazardous substance[11]
VESIcare	Tablet	Enteric-coated
Videx EC	Capsule	Delayed release
Vimovo	Tablet	Delayed release
Viokace	Tablet	Mucous membrane irritant
Viramune XR	Tablet	Extended release[2]

(continued)

Drug Product	Dosage Form	Dosage Reasons/Comments
Voltaren-XR	Tablet	Extended release
VoSpire ER	Tablet	Extended release
Votrient	Tablet	Crushing significantly increases AUC and T_{max}; hazardous substance[11]; crushed or broken tablets may cause dangerous skin problems
Wellbutrin	Tablet	Film-coated
Wellbutrin SR	Tablet	Extended release
Wellbutrin XL	Tablet	Extended release
Xalkori	Capsule	Teratogenic potential; hazardous substance[11]
Xanax XR	Tablet	Extended release
Xeloda	Tablet	Teratogenic potential; hazardous substance[11].
Xtandi	Capsule	Teratogenic potential; hazardous substance[11]
Zegerid OTC	Capsule	Delayed release[2]
Zelboraf	Tablet	Teratogenic potential; hazardous substance[11]
Zenpep	Capsule	Delayed release[1]; enteric-coated contents
Zohydro ER	Capsule	Extended release; capsule disruption may cause a potentially fatal overdose
Zolinza	Capsule	Irritant; avoid contact with skin or mucous membranes; use gloves to handle; teratogenic potential; hazardous substance[11]
Zomig-ZMT	Tablet	Oral-disintegrating form[7]
Zortress	Tablet	Mucous membrane irritant; teratogenic potential; hazardous substance[11]
Zyban	Tablet	Slow release
Zyflo CR	Tablet	Extended release
ZyrTEC-D Allergy & Congestion	Tablet	Extended release
Zytiga	Tablet	Teratogenic potential; hazardous substance[11]; women who are or may be pregnant should wear gloves if handling tablets

[1]Capsule may be opened and the contents taken without crushing or chewing; soft food, such as applesauce or pudding, may facilitate administration; contents may generally be administered via nasogastric tube using an appropriate fluid, provided entire contents are washed down the tube.

[2]Liquid dosage forms of the product are available; however, dose, frequency of administration, and manufacturers may differ from that of the solid dosage form.

[3]Antacids and/or milk may prematurely dissolve the coating of the tablet.

[4]Capsule may be opened and the liquid contents removed for administration.

[5]The taste of this product in a liquid form would likely be unacceptable to the patient; administration via nasogastric tube should be acceptable.

[6]Effervescent tablets must be dissolved in the amount of diluent recommended by the manufacturer.

[7]Tablets are made to disintegrate under (or on) the tongue.

[8]Tablet is scored and may be broken in half without affecting release characteristics.

[9]Skin contact may enhance tumor production; avoid direct contact.

[10]Prescribing information recommends that women who are, or may become, pregnant should not handle medication, especially if crushed or broken; avoid direct contact.

[11]Potentially hazardous or hazardous substance; refer to institution-specific guidelines for precautions to observe when handling this substance.

REFERENCES

Mitchell JF. Oral dosage forms that should not be crushed. Available at http://www.ismp.org/tools/DoNotCrush.pdf. Accessed November 11, 2011.

National Institute for Occupational Safety and Health (NIOSH). NIOSH list of antineoplastic and other hazardous drugs in healthcare settings 2012. Available at http://www.cdc.gov/niosh/docs/2012-150/pdfs/2012-150.pdf. Accessed July 11, 2012.

VITAMIN K CONTENT IN SELECTED FOODS

The following list describes the relative amounts of vitamin K in foods generally considered high in vitamin K. This is a partial listing of foods with estimated portions. For more complete information, refer to the USDA National Nutrient Database for Standard Reference, Release 25, at https://www.ars.usda.gov/SP2UserFiles/Place/12354500/Data/SR25/nutrlist/sr25a430.pdf

Foods	Portion Size	Vitamin K Content (mcg)
Asparagus	1 cup	144
Asparagus	4 spears	30-48
Beet greens	1 cup	697
Broccoli	1 cup	90-220
Brussels sprouts	1 cup	219-300
Cabbage	1 cup	27-163
Collards	1 cup	773-1059
Cucumber	1 large	49
Dandelion greens	1 cup	579
Endive	1 cup	116
Kale	1 cup	1062-1147
Lettuce	1 head	130-167
Mustard greens	1 cup	830
Noodles	1 cup	162
Oil, canola	1 Tbsp	10
Oil, olive, salad, or cooking	1 Tbsp	8
Okra	1 cup	64-88
Onions	1 cup	207
Parsley	10 sprigs	164
Peas	1 cup	10-63
Spinach	1 cup	145-1027
Turnip greens	1 cup	529-851

ALPHABETICAL INDEX

Other Solutions Offered by Lexicomp

Anesthesiology & Critical Care Drug Handbook

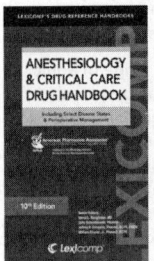

Designed for anesthesiologists, critical care practitioners, and all healthcare professionals involved in the treatment of surgical or ICU patients.

Includes: extensive drug information to support appropriate clinical management of patients; intensivist and anesthesiologist perspective; over 2000 medications most commonly used in the preoperative and critical care setting; Special Topics/Issues addressing frequently encountered patient conditions.

Drug Information Handbook

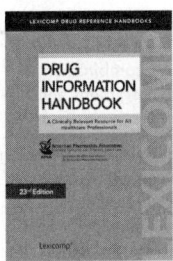

This easy-to-use drug reference is for the pharmacist, physician, or other healthcare professional requiring fast access to relevant drug information.

Over 1500 drug monographs are detailed with up to 40 fields of information per monograph. A valuable appendix offers charts and reviews of special topics such as guidelines for treatment and therapy recommendations. A pharmacologic category index is also provided.

Drug Information Handbook with International Trade Names Index

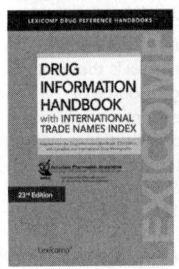

The *Drug Information Handbook with International Trade Names Index* includes the core content of our *Drug Information Handbook*, plus international drug monographs for use worldwide! This easy-to-use reference is complied especially for the pharmacist, physician, or other healthcare professional seeking quick access to extensive drug information.

Drug Information Handbook for Advanced Practice Nursing

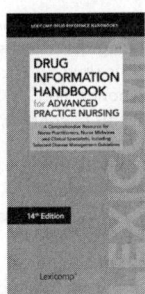

Designed to assist the advanced practice nurse with prescribing, monitoring and educating patients.

Includes: Over 4800 generic and brand names cross-referenced by page number; generic drug names and cross-references highlighted in RED; labeled and investigational indications; adult, geriatric, and pediatric dosing; and up to 75 fields of information per monograph, including Patient Education and Physical Assessment.

Other Solutions Offered by Lexicomp

Drug Information Handbook for Oncology

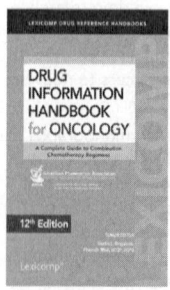

Designed for oncology professionals requiring information on combination chemotherapy regimens and dosing protocols.

Includes: monographs containing warnings, adverse reaction profiles, drug interactions, dosing for specific indications, vesicant, emetic potential, combination regimens, and more; where applicable, a special Combination Chemotherapy field links to specific oncology monographs; Special Topics such as Cancer Treatment Related Complications, Bone Marrow Transplantation, and Drug Development.

Geriatric Dosage Handbook

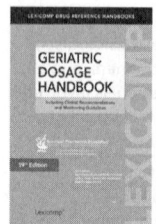

Designed for healthcare professionals managing geriatric patients.

Includes: a wide range of adult and geriatric dosing; special geriatric considerations; up to 44 key fields of information in each monograph, including Medication Safety Issues; extensive information on drug interactions, as well as dosing for patients with renal/hepatic impairment.

Pediatric & Neonatal Dosage Handbook

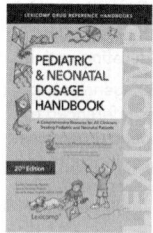

This book is designed for healthcare professionals requiring quick access to extensive pediatric drug information. Each monograph contains multiple fields of content, including usual dosage by age group, indication, and route of administration. Drug interactions, adverse reactions, extemporaneous preparations, pharmacodynamics/ pharmacokinetics data, and medication safety issues are covered.

Pediatric & Neonatal Dosage Handbook with International Trade Names Index

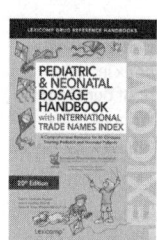

The *Pediatric & Neonatal Dosage Handbook with International Trade Names Index* is the trusted pediatric drug resource of medical professionals worldwide. The international edition contains the core content of the Lexicomp *Pediatric & Neonatal Dosage Handbook*, plus an International Trade Names Index including trade names from over 100 countries.

Other Solutions Offered by Lexicomp

Lexicomp® Online™

Lexicomp Online integrates industry-leading databases and enhanced searching technology, delivering time-sensitive clinical information at the point of care. Our easy-to-use interface and concise information eliminate the need to navigate through multiple pages or make unnecessary mouse clicks.

Lexicomp Online includes multiple databases and modules covering the following topic areas:

- Core Drug Information with Specialty Fields
- Pediatrics and Geriatrics
- Interaction Analysis
- Pharmacogenomics
- Infectious Diseases
- Laboratory Tests and Diagnostic Procedures
- Natural Products
- Patient Education
- Drug Identification
- Calculations
- I.V. Compatibility: *King® Guide to Parenteral Admixtures*™
- Toxicology

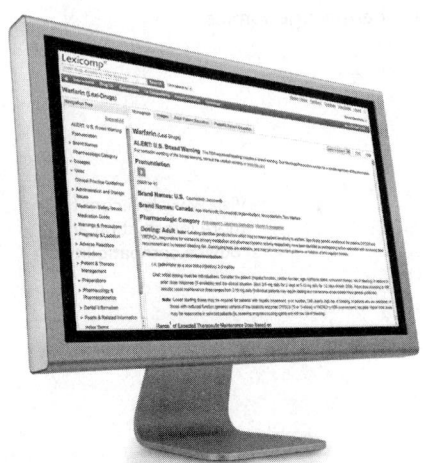

Register for a FREE 45-day trial

Visit www.lexi.com/institutions

Academic and institutional licenses available.

To order, call Customer Service at 1-866-397-3433 or visit www.lexi.com.
Outside of the U.S., call +1-330-650-6506 or visit www.lexi.com.

Other Solutions Offered by Lexicomp

Lexicomp® Mobile Apps

Apps for smartphones and tablets

At Lexicomp, we take pride in creating quality drug information for use at the point of care. Our content is not subject to third-party recommendations, but based on the contributions of our respected authors and editors, internal clinical team and thousands of professionals within the healthcare industry who continually review and validate our data.

With Lexicomp Mobile Apps, you can be confident you are accessing the most timely drug information available for mobile devices. All updates are included with your annual subscription.

Lexicomp Mobile Apps databases include:

- Adult Drug Information
- Pediatric & Neonatal Drug Information
- Pediatric Drug Information (Spanish Version)
- Drug Interactions
- Natural Products
- Toxicology
- Household Products
- Infectious Diseases
- Lab & Diagnostic Procedures
- Nursing Drug Information
- Dental Drug Information
- Oral Soft Tissue Diseases
- Pharmacogenomics

- Patient Education
- Drug ID
- Medical Calculations
- I.V. Compatibility*
- Drug Allergy & Idiosyncratic Reactions
- Pregnancy & Lactation Drug Information
- The 5-Minute Clinical Consult
- The 5-Minute Pediatric Consult
- AHFS DI® Essentials™
- Stedman's Medical Dictionary for the Health Professions and Nursing
- Stedman's Medical Abbreviations

* I.V. compatibility information © copyright King Guide Publications, Inc.

Visit www.lexi.com for more information and device compatibility!

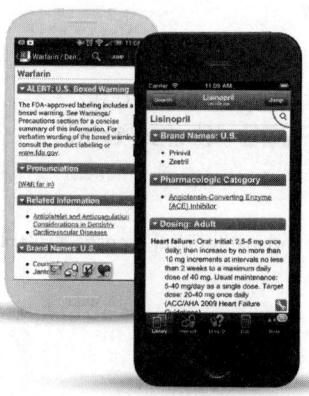

NOTES

NOTES

NOTES

NOTES

NOTES

NOTES

NOTES

NOTES